PROFESSIONAL
EDITION

2017
ICD-10-CM
FOR PHYSICIANS

INCLUDES
NETTER'S
ANATOMY
ART

Carol J. Buck
MS, CPC, CCS-P

Former Program Director
Medical Secretary Programs
Northwest Technical College
East Grand Forks, Minnesota

ELSEVIER

ELSEVIER

3251 Riverport Lane
St. Louis, Missouri 63043

2017 ICD-10-CM PHYSICIAN EDITION

ISBN: 978-0-323-43120-0

Notice

Knowledge and best practice in this field are constantly changing. As new research and experience broaden our understanding, changes in research methods, professional practices, or medical treatment may become necessary.

Practitioners and researchers must always rely on their own experience and knowledge in evaluating and using any information, methods, compounds, or experiments described herein. In using such information or methods they should be mindful of their own safety and the safety of others, including parties for whom they have a professional responsibility.

With respect to any drug or pharmaceutical products identified, readers are advised to check the most current information provided (i) on procedures featured or (ii) by the manufacturer of each product to be administered, to verify the recommended dose or formula, the method and duration of administration, and contraindications. It is the responsibility of practitioners, relying on their own experience and knowledge of their patients, to make diagnoses, to determine dosages and the best treatment for each individual patient, and to take all appropriate safety precautions.

To the fullest extent of the law, neither the Publisher nor the authors, contributors, or editors, assume any liability for any injury and/or damage to persons or property as a matter of products liability, negligence or otherwise, or from any use or operation of any methods, products, instructions, or ideas contained in the material herein.

Library of Congress Cataloging-in-Publication Data
Names: Buck, Carol J., author.
Title: 2017 ICD-10-CM for physicians / Carol J. Buck.
Other titles: ICD-10-CM for physicians
Description: Professional edition. | St. Louis, Missouri : Elsevier, [2017]
|
  Includes index. | Preceded by 2016 ICD-10-CM for physicians / Carol J.
  Buck. Professional edition. [2016].
Identifiers: LCCN 2016016068 | ISBN 9780323431200 (pbk.)
Subjects: | MESH: International statistical classification of diseases and
  related health problems. 10th revision. Clinical modification. |
  Disease--classification | International Classification of Diseases |
  Medical Records--classification | Clinical Coding--standards | Physicians
Classification: LCC RB115 | NLM WB 15 | DDC 616.001/2--dc23 LC record available at
https://lccn.loc.gov/2016016068

Director, Private Sector Education & Professional/References: Jeanne R. Olson
Content Development Manager: Luke Held
Associate Content Development Specialist: Anna Miller
Publishing Services Manager: Jeffrey Patterson
Project Manager: Lisa A. P. Bushey
Design Manager: Julia Dummitt

Printed in the United States of America

Last digit is the print number: 9 8 7 6 5 4 3 2 1

DEDICATION

To all the brave medical coders who transitioned the nation into a new coding system.
Decades of waiting finally concluded with the implementation of I-10,
and you have been the pioneers leading the way.

With greatest appreciations for your efforts!

Carol J. Buck, MS, CPC, CCS-P

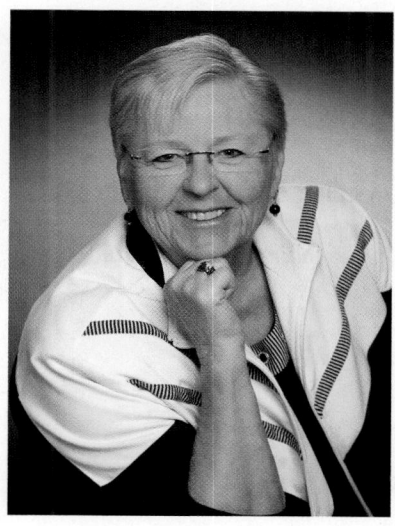

DEVELOPMENT OF THIS EDITION

Query Team

Patricia Cordy Henricksen, MS, CHCA, CPC-I, CPC, CCP-P, ASC-PM
Auditing and Coding Educator
Soterion Medical Services
Lexington, Kentucky

Jackie L. Grass, CPC
Coding and Reimbursement Specialist
Grand Forks, North Dakota

Kathleen Buchda, CPC, CPMA
Revenue Recognition
New Richmond, Wisconsin

Editorial Consultant

Jenna Price, CPC-A
President
Price Editorial Services, LLC
St. Louis, Missouri

Elsevier/MC Strategies Revenue Cycle, Coding and Compliance Staff

"Experts in providing e-learning on revenue cycle, coding and compliance."

Deborah Neville, RHIA, CCS-P
Director

Lynn-Marie D. Wozniak, MS, RHIT
Content Manager

Sandra L. Macica, MS, RHIA, CCS, ROCC
Content Manager

CONTENTS

GUIDE TO USING THE 2017 ICD-10-CM FOR PHYSICIANS

Medical coding has long been a part of the health care profession. Through the years medical coding systems have become more complex and extensive. Today, medical coding is an intricate and immense process that is present in every health care setting. The increased use of electronic submissions for health care services only increases the need for coders who understand the coding process.

2017 ICD-10-CM for Physicians, Professional Edition was developed to help meet the needs of coding professionals at all levels by offering a comprehensive coding text at a reasonable price.

All material strictly adheres to the latest government versions available at the time of printing. Updates from the *Definitions of Medicare Code Edits* (MCE) will be posted to the companion website (www. codingupdates.com) when available.

Illustrations and Items

The ICD-10-CM Tabular List contains illustrations, pictures, and items to assist you in understanding difficult terminology, diseases/conditions, or coding in a specific category. Items are always printed in ▮▮▮▮▮ ink so that the added material is not mistaken for official notations or instructions. ▮▮▮▮▮ ink is used for other annotations in the text. Your ideas on what other descriptions or illustrations should be in future editions of this text are always appreciated.

Instructional Notations

Includes Notes

Includes
The word 'Includes' appears immediately under certain categories to further define, or give examples of, the content of the category.

Excludes Notes

The ICD-10-CM has two types of excludes notes. Each note has a different definition for use, but they are both similar in that they indicate that codes excluded from each other are independent of each other.

Excludes1
A type 1 Excludes note is a pure excludes. It means "NOT CODED HERE!" An Excludes1 note indicates that the code excluded should never be used at the same time as the code above the Excludes1 note. An Excludes1 is for use when two conditions cannot occur together, such as a congenital form versus an acquired form of the same condition.

Excludes2
A type 2 Excludes note represents "NOT INCLUDED HERE." An Excludes2 note indicates that the condition excluded is not part of the condition it is excluded from but a patient may have both conditions at the same time. When an Excludes2 note appears under a code, it is acceptable to use both the code and the excluded code together.

Code First/Use Additional Code notes (etiology/manifestation paired codes)

Certain conditions have both an underlying etiology and multiple body system manifestations due to the underlying etiology. For such conditions the ICD-10-CM has a coding convention that requires the underlying condition be sequenced first, followed by the manifestation. Wherever such a combination exists, there is a "use additional code" note at the etiology code, and a "code first" note at the manifestation code. These instructional notes indicate the proper sequencing order of the codes, etiology followed by manifestation.

In most cases the manifestation codes will have in the code title, "in diseases classified elsewhere." Codes with this title are a component of the etiology/manifestation convention. The code title indicates that it is a manifestation code. "In diseases classified elsewhere" codes are never permitted to be used as first-listed or principal diagnosis codes. They must be used in conjunction with an underlying condition code, and they must be listed following the underlying condition.

Use additional
The words indicate an instructional note that another code may be needed.

Code first
The words indicate an instructional note that directs the coder to sequence the underlying condition before the manifestation.

Code also
A "code also" note instructs that two codes may be required to fully describe a condition, but the sequencing of the two codes is discretionary, depending on the severity of the conditions and the reason for the encounter.

Unspecified
The highlight indicates that although the code is valid as a principal (first-listed) diagnosis, it is not as specific as other codes without the highlight.

7th characters and placeholder X

For codes less than 6 characters that require a 7th character a placeholder X should be assigned for all characters less than 6. The 7th character must always be the 7th character of a code.

Annotated

Throughout the manual, revisions, additions, and deleted codes or words are indicated by the following symbols:

◀|||| **Revised:** Revisions within the line or code from the previous edition are indicated by the arrow.

◀   **New:** Additions to the previous edition are indicated by the triangle.

deleted   **Deleted:** Deletions from the previous edition are struck through.

ICD-10-CM Tabular List Symbols

●   **Use Additional Character(s):** The red stop sign cautions that the code requires additional character(s) to ensure the greatest specificity.

X   For codes less than 6 characters that require a 7th character, a placeholder X should be assigned for all characters less than 6. The 7th character must always be the 7th character of a code.

OGCR   The *Official Guidelines for Coding and Reporting* symbol includes the placement of a portion of a guideline as that guideline pertains to the code by which it is located. The complete OGCR are located in Part I.

▶   **Manifestation Code:** Describes the manifestation of an underlying disease, not the disease itself, and therefore should not be assigned as a principal diagnosis, according to the *Definitions of Medicare Code Edits* (MCE).

Age conflict: The *Definitions of Medicare Code Edits* (MCE) detects inconsistencies between a patient's age and diagnosis. For example, a 5-year-old patient with benign prostatic hypertrophy or a 78-year-old pregnant female.

The diagnosis is clinically and virtually impossible in a patient of the stated age. Therefore, either the diagnosis or the age is presumed to be incorrect. There are four age categories for diagnoses in the *Definitions of Medicare Code Edits* (MCE):

N   • Newborn. Age of Ø years; a subset of diagnoses intended only for newborns and neonates (e.g., fetal distress, perinatal jaundice).

P   • Pediatric. Age range is Ø-17 years inclusive (e.g., Reye's syndrome, routine child health exam).

M   • Maternity. Age range is 12-55 years inclusive (e.g., diabetes in pregnancy, antepartum pulmonary complication).

A   • Adult. Age range is 15-124 years inclusive (e.g., senile delirium, mature cataract).

♀♂   **Sex conflict:** *Definitions of Medicare Code Edits* (MCE) detects inconsistencies between a patient's sex and any diagnosis or procedure on the patient's record. For example, a male patient with cervical cancer (diagnosis) or a female patient with a prostatectomy (procedure). In both instances, the indicated diagnosis or the procedure conflicts with the stated sex of the patient. Therefore, either the patient's diagnosis, procedure, or sex is presumed to be incorrect.

Coding Clinic Identifies the year, quarter, and page number that presents information about an ICD-10-CM code in the American Hospital Association's *Coding Clinic*® for ICD-10-CM.

Visit codingupdates.com for the full list of 2017 Present on Admission codes.

SYMBOLS AND CONVENTIONS

ICD-10-CM Tabular

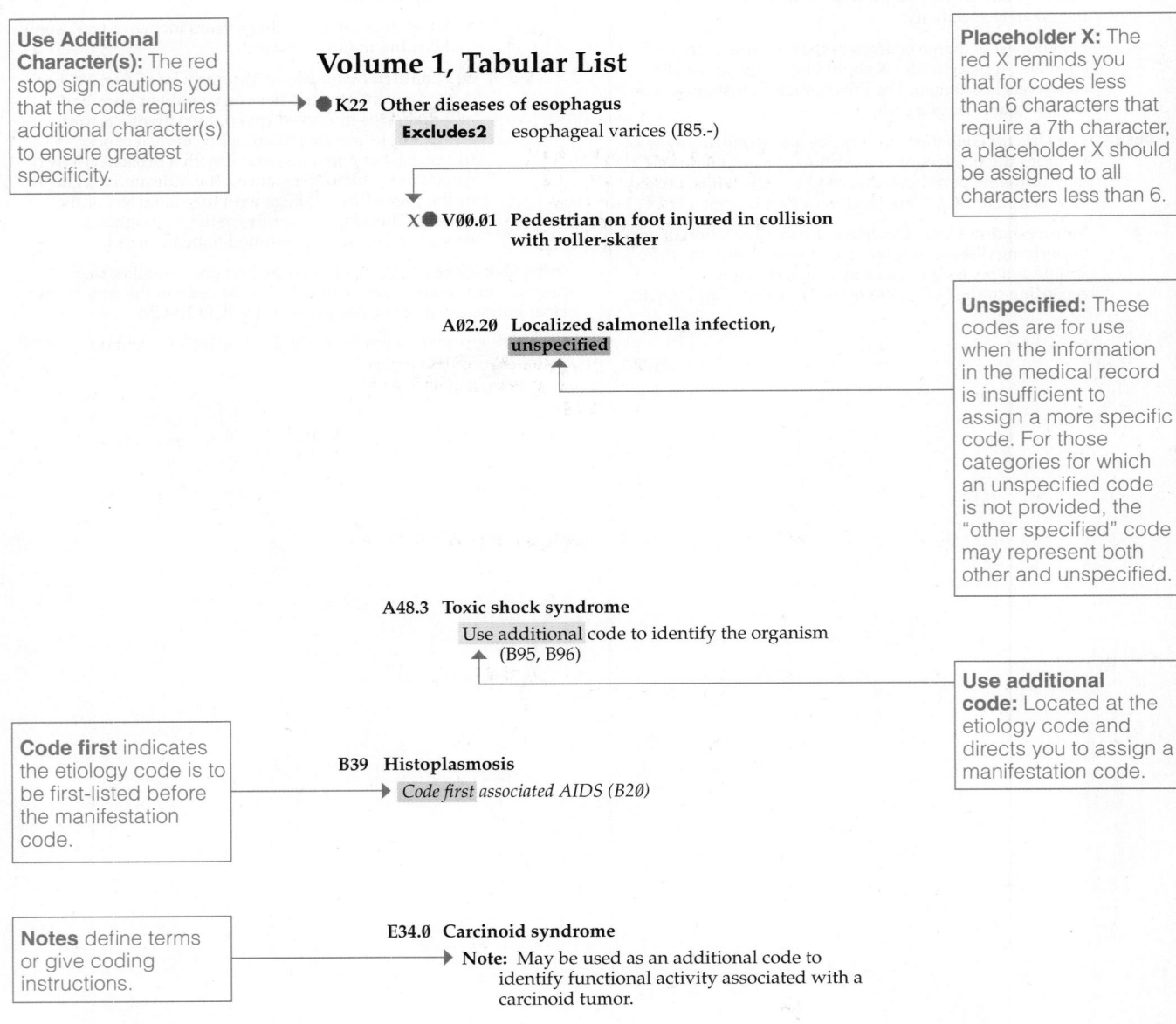

Use Additional Character(s): The red stop sign cautions you that the code requires additional character(s) to ensure greatest specificity.

Volume 1, Tabular List

● **K22** Other diseases of esophagus

Excludes2 esophageal varices (I85.-)

X ● **V00.01** Pedestrian on foot injured in collision with roller-skater

A02.20 Localized salmonella infection, **unspecified**

A48.3 Toxic shock syndrome
Use additional code to identify the organism (B95, B96)

B39 Histoplasmosis
Code first associated AIDS (B20)

E34.0 Carcinoid syndrome
Note: May be used as an additional code to identify functional activity associated with a carcinoid tumor.

Placeholder X: The red X reminds you that for codes less than 6 characters that require a 7th character, a placeholder X should be assigned to all characters less than 6.

Unspecified: These codes are for use when the information in the medical record is insufficient to assign a more specific code. For those categories for which an unspecified code is not provided, the "other specified" code may represent both other and unspecified.

Use additional code: Located at the etiology code and directs you to assign a manifestation code.

Code first indicates the etiology code is to be first-listed before the manifestation code.

Notes define terms or give coding instructions.

Codes or index entries are for purposes of illustration only and may not be current.

OGCR Section I.C.6.B.5.

Neoplasm Related Pain Code G89.3 is assigned to pain documented as being related, associated or due to cancer, primary or secondary malignancy, or tumor. This code is assigned regardless of whether the pain is acute or chronic.

OGCR: The *Official Guidelines for Coding and Reporting* are placed near the codes to which they refer and are highlighted.

I70.2   **Atherosclerosis of native arteries of the extremities**
Mönckeberg's (medial) sclerosis

Use additional code, if applicable, to identify chronic total occlusion of artery of extremity (I70.92)

code, if applicable, directs the coder to other conditions that may be appropriate to report.

I74   **Arterial embolism and thrombosis**
Includes   embolic infarction
embolic occlusion
thrombotic infarction
thrombotic occlusion

The word "and" should be interpreted to mean either "and" or "or" when it appears in a statement.

Bold typeface is used on all codes and titles.

I83.001   **Varicose veins of unspecified lower extremity with ulcer of thigh**

"with" should be interpreted to mean "associated with" or "due to."

K73.2   Chronic active hepatitis, not elsewhere classified

"not elsewhere classified" or **NEC** identifies a code that is assigned only when the information at hand specifies a condition for which no more specific code is available.

"not otherwise specified" or **NOS** is equivalent to unspecified.

W13.9   Fall from, out of or through building, not otherwise specified

Codes or index entries are for purposes of illustration only and may not be current.

Excludes1 means "NOT CODED HERE!" An Excludes1 note indicates that the code excluded should never be assigned at the same time as the code above the Excludes1 note.

Includes: This note appears immediately under a three-character code title to further define, or give examples of, the content.

Codes titled "other" or "other specified" are for use when the information in the medical record provides detail for which a specific code does not exist.

Pediatric Age, 0-17, according to the *Definitions of Medicare Code Edits* (MCE).

Females Only according to the *Definitions of Medicare Code Edits* (MCE).

M19 **Other and unspecified osteoarthritis**
　　　Excludes1　polyarthritis (M15.-)
　　　Excludes2　arthrosis of spine (M47.-)
　　　　　　　　　hallux rigidus (M20.2)
　　　　　　　　　osteoarthritis of spine (M47.-)

A06 **Amebiasis**
　　　Includes　　infection due to Entamoeba histolytica

E26.01 **Conn's syndrome**
　　　　　Code also adrenal adenoma (D35.0)

E25.8 **Other adrenogenital disorders**

O00.2 **Ovarian pregnancy**　　　　　　　　M

P02.20 **Newborn (suspected to be) affected by unspecified morphological and functional abnormalities of placenta**　　N

L21.0 **Seborrhea capitis**　　　　　　　　P
　　　　　Cradle cap

G30.1 **Alzheimer's disease with late onset**　　A

B37.3 **Candidiasis of vulva and vagina** ♀

C60.1 **Malignant neoplasm of glans penis** ♂

Excludes2 represents "NOT INCLUDED HERE." An Excludes2 note indicates that the condition excluded is not part of the condition represented by the code, but a patient may have both conditions at the same time and it is acceptable to use both the code and the excluded code together, when appropriate.

Code also instructs that two codes may be required to fully describe a condition, but this note does not provide sequencing direction.

Maternity DX (Diagnosis) for ages 12-55 according to the *Definitions of Medicare Code Edits* (MCE).

Newborn, Age 0, according to the *Definitions of Medicare Code Edits* (MCE).

Adult Age, 15-124, according to the *Definitions of Medicare Code Edits* (MCE).

Males Only according to the *Definitions of Medicare Code Edits* (MCE).

Codes or index entries are for purposes of illustration only and may not be current.

▷ **H22** *Disorders of iris and ciliary body in diseases classified elsewhere*

Code first *underlying disease, such as:*
gout (M1A-, M10.-)

Manifestation according to the *Definitions of Medicare Code Edits* (MCE).

G14 **Postpolio syndrome**

Includes   Postpolio myelitic syndrome

Excludes 1   sequelae of poliomyelitis (B91)

B96.5 **Pseudomonas (aeruginosa) (mallei) (pseudomallei) as the cause of diseases classified elsewhere**
▶ Coding Clinic: 2015, Q1, P18

Coding Clinic identifies the year, quarter, and page number that presents information about an ICD-10-PCS code in the American Hospital Association's *Coding Clinic®*.

Codes or index entries are for purposes of illustration only and may not be current.

Alphabetic Index

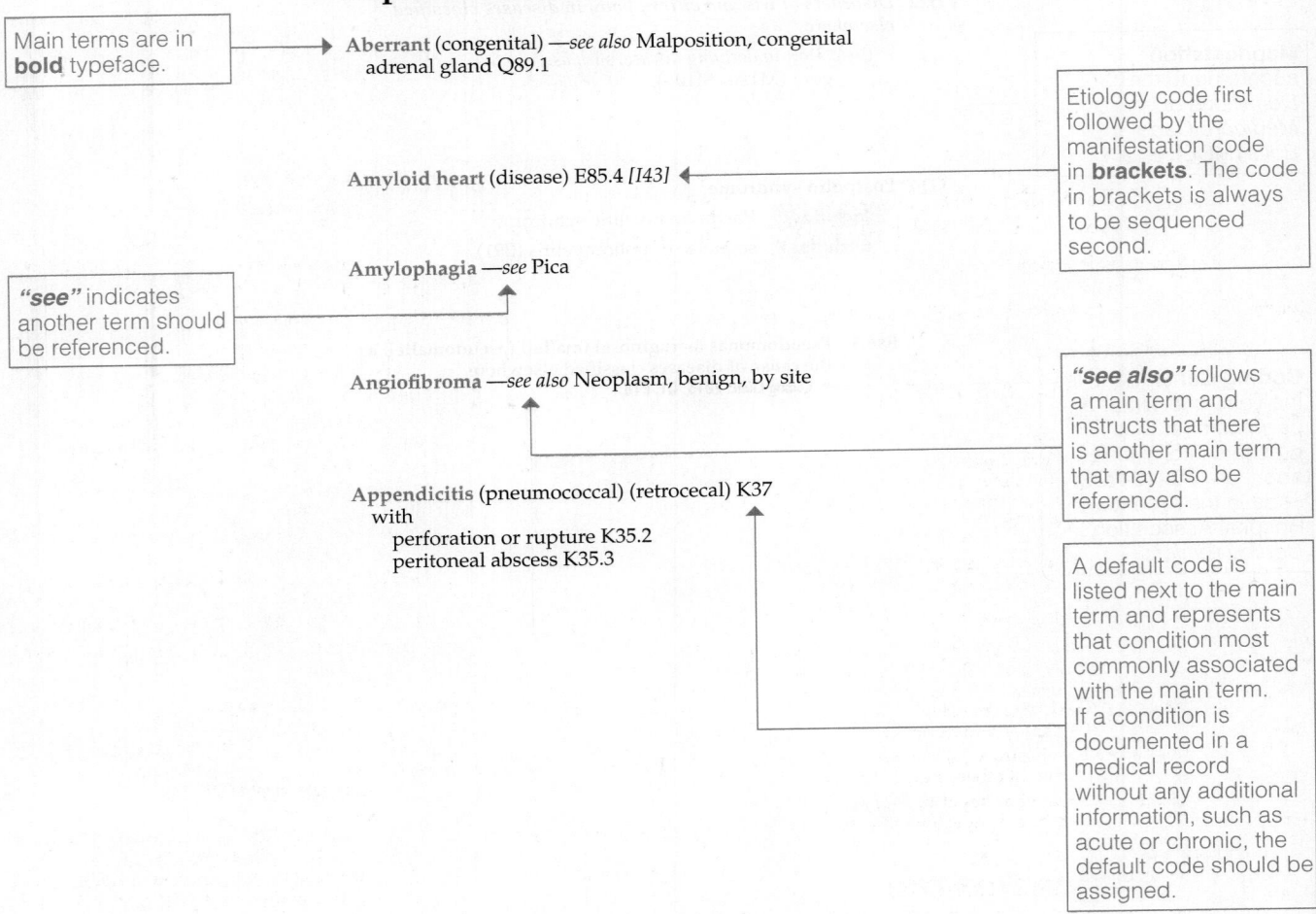

Main terms are in **bold** typeface.

Aberrant (congenital) —*see also* Malposition, congenital
    adrenal gland Q89.1

Etiology code first followed by the manifestation code in **brackets**. The code in brackets is always to be sequenced second.

Amyloid heart (disease) E85.4 *[I43]*

Amylophagia —*see* Pica

"**see**" indicates another term should be referenced.

Angiofibroma —*see also* Neoplasm, benign, by site

"**see also**" follows a main term and instructs that there is another main term that may also be referenced.

Appendicitis (pneumococcal) (retrocecal) K37
    with
        perforation or rupture K35.2
        peritoneal abscess K35.3

A default code is listed next to the main term and represents that condition most commonly associated with the main term. If a condition is documented in a medical record without any additional information, such as acute or chronic, the default code should be assigned.

Codes or index entries are for purposes of illustration only and may not be current.

GUIDE TO THE 2017 ICD-10-CM UPDATES

CHAPTER 1

CERTAIN INFECTIOUS AND PARASITIC DISEASES (A00-B99)

A40 **Streptococcal sepsis**
Code first
Revised   postprocedural streptococcal sepsis (T81.4-)

A41 **Other sepsis**
Code first
Revised   postprocedural sepsis (T81.4-)
Deleted   **Excludes1**   sepsis NOS (A41.9)

New   **A92.5** **Zika virus disease**
New   Zika virus fever
New   Zika virus infection
New   Zika NOS

     B17.9 **Acute viral hepatitis, unspecified**
New   Acute infectious hepatitis NOS

B18 **Chronic viral hepatitis**
New   **Includes**   Carrier of viral hepatitis
     B18.1 **Chronic viral hepatitis B without delta-agent**
New   Carrier of viral hepatitis B
     B18.2 **Chronic viral hepatitis C**
New   Carrier of viral hepatitis C
     B18.8 **Other chronic viral hepatitis**
New   Carrier of other viral hepatitis
     B18.9 **Chronic viral hepatitis, unspecified**
New   Carrier of unspecified viral hepatitis

CHAPTER 2

NEOPLASMS (C00-D49)

C00 Malignant neoplasm of lip
C01 Malignant neoplasm of base of tongue
C02 Malignant neoplasm of other and unspecified parts of tongue
C03 Malignant neoplasm of gum
C04 Malignant neoplasm of floor of mouth
C05 Malignant neoplasm of palate
C06 Malignant neoplasm of other and unspecified parts of mouth
C07 Malignant neoplasm of parotid gland
C08 Malignant neoplasm of other and unspecified major salivary glands
C09 Malignant neoplasm of tonsil
C10 Malignant neoplasm of oropharynx
C11 Malignant neoplasm of nasopharynx
C12 Malignant neoplasm of pyriform sinus
C13 Malignant neoplasm of hypopharynx
C14 Malignant neoplasm of other and ill-defined sites in the lip, oral cavity and pharynx
     Use additional code to identify:
Revised   history of tobacco dependence (Z87.891)

MALIGNANT NEOPLASM OF DIGESTIVE ORGANS (C15-C26)

New   **Excludes2**   gastrointestinal stromal tumors (C49.A-)

C25 **Malignant neoplasm of pancreas**
New   Code also exocrine pancreatic insufficiency (K86.81)

C32 Malignant neoplasm of larynx
C33 Malignant neoplasm of trachea
C34 Malignant neoplasm of bronchus and lung
C39 Malignant neoplasm of other and ill-defined sites in the respiratory system and intrathoracic organs
     Use additional code to identify:
Revised   history of tobacco dependence (Z87.891)

New   **C49.A** **Gastrointestinal stromal tumor**
New   **C49.A0** **Gastrointestinal stromal tumor, unspecified site**
New   **C49.A1** **Gastrointestinal stromal tumor of esophagus**
New   **C49.A2** **Gastrointestinal stromal tumor of stomach**
New   **C49.A3** **Gastrointestinal stromal tumor of small intestine**
New   **C49.A4** **Gastrointestinal stromal tumor of large intestine**
New   **C49.A5** **Gastrointestinal stromal tumor of rectum**
New   **C49.A9** **Gastrointestinal stromal tumor of other sites**

C61 **Malignant neoplasm of prostate**
New   Use additional code to identify:
New   hormone sensitivity status (Z19.1-Z19.2)
New   rising PSA following treatment for malignant neoplasm of prostate (R97.21)

Revised   **C7A.094** **Malignant carcinoid tumor of the foregut unspecified**
Revised   **C7A.095** **Malignant carcinoid tumor of the midgut unspecified**
Revised   **C7A.096** **Malignant carcinoid tumor of the hindgut unspecified**

C78 **Secondary malignant neoplasm of respiratory and digestive organs**
Deleted   **Excludes1**   lymph node metastases (C77.0)
New   **Excludes2**   lymph node metastases (C77.0)
     C78.89 **Secondary malignant neoplasm of other digestive organs**
New   Code also exocrine pancreatic insufficiency (K86.81)

C79 **Secondary malignant neoplasm of other and unspecified sites**
Deleted   **Excludes1**   lymph node metastases (C77.0)
New   **Excludes2**   lymph node metastases (C77.0)

Revised   **C81.1** **Nodular sclerosis Hodgkin lymphoma**
New   Nodular sclerosis classical Hodgkin lymphoma
Revised   **C81.10** **Nodular sclerosis Hodgkin lymphoma, unspecified site**
Revised   **C81.11** **Nodular sclerosis Hodgkin lymphoma, lymph nodes of head, face, and neck**
Revised   **C81.12** **Nodular sclerosis Hodgkin lymphoma, intrathoracic lymph nodes**
Revised   **C81.13** **Nodular sclerosis Hodgkin lymphoma, intra-abdominal lymph nodes**
Revised   **C81.14** **Nodular sclerosis Hodgkin lymphoma, lymph nodes of axilla and upper limb**
Revised   **C81.15** **Nodular sclerosis Hodgkin lymphoma, lymph nodes of inguinal region and lower limb**

Revised	C81.16	Nodular sclerosis Hodgkin lymphoma, intrapelvic lymph nodes
Revised	C81.17	Nodular sclerosis Hodgkin lymphoma, spleen
Revised	C81.18	Nodular sclerosis Hodgkin lymphoma, lymph nodes of multiple sites
Revised	C81.19	Nodular sclerosis Hodgkin lymphoma, extranodal and solid organ sites

Revised C81.2 **Mixed cellularity Hodgkin lymphoma**
New   Mixed cellularity classical Hodgkin lymphoma

Revised	C81.20	Mixed cellularity Hodgkin lymphoma, unspecified site
Revised	C81.21	Mixed cellularity Hodgkin lymphoma, lymph nodes of head, face, and neck
Revised	C81.22	Mixed cellularity Hodgkin lymphoma, intrathoracic lymph nodes
Revised	C81.23	Mixed cellularity Hodgkin lymphoma, intra-abdominal lymph nodes
Revised	C81.24	Mixed cellularity Hodgkin lymphoma, lymph nodes of axilla and upper limb
Revised	C81.25	Mixed cellularity Hodgkin lymphoma, lymph nodes of inguinal region and lower limb
Revised	C81.26	Mixed cellularity Hodgkin lymphoma, intrapelvic lymph nodes
Revised	C81.27	Mixed cellularity Hodgkin lymphoma, spleen
Revised	C81.28	Mixed cellularity Hodgkin lymphoma, lymph nodes of multiple sites
Revised	C81.29	Mixed cellularity Hodgkin lymphoma, extranodal and solid organ sites

Revised C81.3 **Lymphocyte depleted Hodgkin lymphoma**
New   Lymphocyte depleted classical Hodgkin lymphoma

Revised	C81.30	Lymphocyte depleted Hodgkin lymphoma, unspecified site
Revised	C81.31	Lymphocyte depleted Hodgkin lymphoma, lymph nodes of head, face, and neck
Revised	C81.32	Lymphocyte depleted Hodgkin lymphoma, intrathoracic lymph nodes
Revised	C81.33	Lymphocyte depleted Hodgkin lymphoma, intra-abdominal lymph nodes
Revised	C81.34	Lymphocyte depleted Hodgkin lymphoma, lymph nodes of axilla and upper limb
Revised	C81.35	Lymphocyte depleted Hodgkin lymphoma, lymph nodes of inguinal region and lower limb
Revised	C81.36	Lymphocyte depleted Hodgkin lymphoma, intrapelvic lymph nodes
Revised	C81.37	Lymphocyte depleted Hodgkin lymphoma, spleen
Revised	C81.38	Lymphocyte depleted Hodgkin lymphoma, lymph nodes of multiple sites
Revised	C81.39	Lymphocyte depleted Hodgkin lymphoma, extranodal and solid organ sites

Revised C81.4 **Lymphocyte-rich Hodgkin lymphoma**
New   Lymphocyte-rich classical Hodgkin lymphoma

Revised	C81.40	Lymphocyte-rich Hodgkin lymphoma, unspecified site
Revised	C81.41	Lymphocyte-rich Hodgkin lymphoma, lymph nodes of head, face, and neck
Revised	C81.42	Lymphocyte-rich Hodgkin lymphoma, intrathoracic lymph nodes
Revised	C81.43	Lymphocyte-rich Hodgkin lymphoma, intra-abdominal lymph nodes
Revised	C81.44	Lymphocyte-rich Hodgkin lymphoma, lymph nodes of axilla and upper limb
Revised	C81.45	Lymphocyte-rich Hodgkin lymphoma, lymph nodes of inguinal region and lower limb
Revised	C81.46	Lymphocyte-rich Hodgkin lymphoma, intrapelvic lymph nodes
Revised	C81.47	Lymphocyte-rich Hodgkin lymphoma, spleen
Revised	C81.48	Lymphocyte-rich Hodgkin lymphoma, lymph nodes of multiple sites
Revised	C81.49	Lymphocyte-rich Hodgkin lymphoma, extranodal and solid organ sites

Revised C81.7 **Other Hodgkin lymphoma**
New   Other classical Hodgkin lymphoma

Revised	C81.70	Other Hodgkin lymphoma, unspecified site
Revised	C81.71	Other Hodgkin lymphoma, lymph nodes of head, face, and neck
Revised	C81.72	Other Hodgkin lymphoma, intrathoracic lymph nodes
Revised	C81.73	Other Hodgkin lymphoma, intra-abdominal lymph nodes
Revised	C81.74	Other Hodgkin lymphoma, lymph nodes of axilla and upper limb
Revised	C81.75	Other Hodgkin lymphoma, lymph nodes of inguinal region and lower limb
Revised	C81.76	Other Hodgkin lymphoma, intrapelvic lymph nodes
Revised	C81.77	Other Hodgkin lymphoma, spleen
Revised	C81.78	Other Hodgkin lymphoma, lymph nodes of multiple sites
Revised	C81.79	Other Hodgkin lymphoma, extranodal and solid organ sites

C94.20 **Acute megakaryoblastic leukemia not having achieved remission**
Revised   Acute megakaryoblastic leukemia with failed remission

D00.0 **Carcinoma in situ of lip, oral cavity and pharynx**
Use additional code to identify:
Revised   history of tobacco dependence (Z87.891)

D01.3 **Carcinoma in situ of anus and anal canal**
New   Anal intraepithelial neoplasia III [AIN III]
New   Severe dysplasia of anus
New   **Excludes1** anal intraepithelial neoplasia I and II [AIN I and AIN II] (K62.82)

D02 **Carcinoma in situ of middle ear and respiratory system**
Use additional code to identify:
Revised   history of tobacco dependence (Z87.891)

D07.5 **Carcinoma in situ of prostate**
Revised   **Excludes1** dysplasia (mild) (moderate) of prostate (N42.3-)
New   prostatic intraepithelial neoplasia II [PIN II] (N42.3-)

Revised D10.3 **Benign neoplasm of other and unspecified parts of mouth**

D16.4 **Benign neoplasm of bones of skull and face**
Deleted   **Excludes1** benign neoplasm of lower jaw bone (D16.5)
New   **Excludes2** benign neoplasm of lower jaw bone (D16.5)

D27 **Benign neoplasm of ovary**
Revised **Excludes2** corpus albicans cyst (N83.2-)
Revised   corpus luteum cyst (N83.1-)
Revised   follicular (atretic) cyst (N83.0-)
Revised   graafian follicle cyst (N83.0-)
Revised   ovarian cyst NEC (N83.2-)
Revised   ovarian retention cyst (N83.2-)

Revised D3A.094 **Benign carcinoid tumor of the foregut, unspecified**
Revised D3A.095 **Benign carcinoid tumor of the midgut, unspecified**
Revised D3A.096 **Benign carcinoid tumor of the hindgut, unspecified**
Revised D46.2 **Refractory anemia with excess of blasts [RAEB]**

New	**D47.Z2**	**Castleman disease**
New		Code also if applicable human herpesvirus 8 infection (B10.89)
New		**Excludes2** Kaposi's sarcoma (C46-)
	D49.2	**Neoplasm of unspecified behavior of bone, soft tissue, and skin**
Revised		**Excludes1** neoplasm of unspecified behavior of skin of genital organs (D49.59)
New	**D49.51**	**Neoplasm of unspecified behavior of kidney**
New	**D49.511**	**Neoplasm of unspecified behavior of right kidney**
New	**D49.512**	**Neoplasm of unspecified behavior of left kidney**
New	**D49.519**	**Neoplasm of unspecified behavior of unspecified kidney**
New	**D49.59**	**Neoplasm of unspecified behavior of other genitourinary organ**

CHAPTER 3

DISEASES OF THE BLOOD AND BLOOD-FORMING ORGANS AND CERTAIN DISORDERS INVOLVING THE IMMUNE MECHANISM (D50-D89)

	D61.81	**Pancytopenia**
Deleted		**Excludes1** pancytopenia (due to) (with) myelodysplastic syndromes (D46.-)
New		**Excludes2** pancytopenia (due to) (with) myelodysplastic syndromes (D46.-)
	D64.81	**Anemia due to antineoplastic chemotherapy**
Deleted		**Excludes1** anemia in neoplastic disease (D63.0)
New		**Excludes2** anemia in neoplastic disease (D63.0)
	D68.62	**Lupus anticoagulant syndrome**
Revised		**Excludes1** lupus anticoagulant (LAC) finding without diagnosis (R76.0)
	D76	**Other specified diseases with participation of lymphoreticular and reticulohistiocytic tissue**
New		**Excludes1** histiocytic medullary reticulosis (C96.9)
New		leukemic reticuloendotheliosis (C91.4-)
New		lipomelanotic reticulosis (I89.8)
Deleted		leukemic reticuloendotheliosis or reticulosis (C91.4-)
Deleted		lipomelanotic reticuloendotheliosis or reticulosis (I89.8)
New		malignant reticulosis (C86.0)
New		nonlipid reticuloendotheliosis (C96.0)
Revised	**D78.2**	**Postprocedural hemorrhage of the spleen following a procedure**
Revised	**D78.21**	**Postprocedural hemorrhage of the spleen following a procedure on the spleen**
Revised	**D78.22**	**Postprocedural hemorrhage of the spleen following other procedure**
New	**D78.3**	**Postprocedural hematoma and seroma of the spleen following a procedure**
New	**D78.31**	**Postprocedural hematoma of the spleen following a procedure on the spleen**
New	**D78.32**	**Postprocedural hematoma of the spleen following other procedure**
New	**D78.33**	**Postprocedural seroma of the spleen following a procedure on the spleen**
New	**D78.34**	**Postprocedural seroma of the spleen following other procedure**

New	**D89.4**	**Mast cell activation syndrome and related disorders**
New		**Excludes1** aggressive systemic mastocytosis (C96.2)
New		cutaneous mastocytosis (Q82.2)
New		indolent systemic mastocytosis (D47.0)
New		malignant mastocytoma (C96.2)
New		mast cell leukemia (C94.3-)
New		mastocytoma (D47.0)
New		systemic mastocytosis associated with a clonal hematologic non-mast cell lineage disease (SM-AHNMD) (D47.0)
New	**D89.40**	**Mast cell activation, unspecified**
New		Mast cell activation disorder, unspecified
New		Mast cell activation syndrome, NOS
New	**D89.41**	**Monoclonal mast cell activation syndrome**
New	**D89.42**	**Idiopathic mast cell activation syndrome**
New	**D89.43**	**Secondary mast cell activation**
New		Secondary mast cell activation syndrome
New		Code also underlying etiology, if known
New	**D89.49**	**Other mast cell activation disorder**
New		Other mast cell activation syndrome

CHAPTER 4

ENDOCRINE, NUTRITIONAL AND METABOLIC DISEASES (E00-E89)

	E08	**Diabetes mellitus due to underlying condition**
Revised		Use additional code to identify control using:
New		insulin (Z79.4)
New		oral antidiabetic drugs (Z79.84)
New		oral hypoglycemic drugs (Z79.84)
	E08.32	**Diabetes mellitus due to underlying condition with mild nonproliferative diabetic retinopathy**
New		One of the following 7th characters is to be assigned to codes in subcategory E08.32 to designate laterality of the disease:

New	1 right eye
New	2 left eye
New	3 bilateral
New	9 unspecified eye

	E08.33	**Diabetes mellitus due to underlying condition with moderate nonproliferative diabetic retinopathy**
New		One of the following 7th characters is to be assigned to codes in subcategory E08.33 to designate laterality of the disease:

New	1 right eye
New	2 left eye
New	3 bilateral
New	9 unspecified eye

	E08.34	**Diabetes mellitus due to underlying condition with severe nonproliferative diabetic retinopathy**
New		One of the following 7th characters is to be assigned to codes in subcategory E08.34 to designate laterality of the disease:

New	1 right eye
New	2 left eye
New	3 bilateral
New	9 unspecified eye

E08.35 Diabetes mellitus due to underlying condition with proliferative diabetic retinopathy

New   One of the following 7th characters is to be assigned to codes in subcategory E08.35 to designate laterality of the disease:

New
New
New
New

1	right eye
2	left eye
3	bilateral
9	unspecified eye

New   E08.352 Diabetes mellitus due to underlying condition with proliferative diabetic retinopathy with traction retinal detachment involving the macula

New   E08.353 Diabetes mellitus due to underlying condition with proliferative diabetic retinopathy with traction retinal detachment not involving the macula

New   E08.354 Diabetes mellitus due to underlying condition with proliferative diabetic retinopathy with combined traction retinal detachment and rhegmatogenous retinal detachment

New   E08.355 Diabetes mellitus due to underlying condition with stable proliferative diabetic retinopathy

New E08.37 Diabetes mellitus due to underlying condition with diabetic macular edema, resolved following treatment

New   One of the following 7th characters is to be assigned to code E08.37 to designate laterality of the disease:

New
New
New
New

1	right eye
2	left eye
3	bilateral
9	unspecified eye

E09 Drug or chemical induced diabetes mellitus
Revised   Use additional code to identify control using:
New   insulin (Z79.4)
New   oral antidiabetic drugs (Z79.84)
New   oral hypoglycemic drugs (Z79.84)

E09.32 Drug or chemical induced diabetes mellitus with mild nonproliferative diabetic retinopathy

New   One of the following 7th characters is to be assigned to codes in subcategory E09.32 to designate laterality of the disease:

New
New
New
New

1	right eye
2	left eye
3	bilateral
9	unspecified eye

E09.33 Drug or chemical induced diabetes mellitus with moderate nonproliferative diabetic retinopathy

New   One of the following 7th characters is to be assigned to codes in subcategory E09.33 to designate laterality of the disease:

New
New
New
New

1	right eye
2	left eye
3	bilateral
9	unspecified eye

E09.34 Drug or chemical induced diabetes mellitus with severe nonproliferative diabetic retinopathy

New   One of the following 7th characters is to be assigned to codes in subcategory E09.34 to designate laterality of the disease:

New
New
New
New

1	right eye
2	left eye
3	bilateral
9	unspecified eye

E09.35 Drug or chemical induced diabetes mellitus with proliferative diabetic retinopathy

New   One of the following 7th characters is to be assigned to codes in subcategory E09.35 to designate laterality of the disease:

New
New
New
New

1	right eye
2	left eye
3	bilateral
9	unspecified eye

New   E09.352 Drug or chemical induced diabetes mellitus with proliferative diabetic retinopathy with traction retinal detachment involving the macula

New   E09.353 Drug or chemical induced diabetes mellitus with proliferative diabetic retinopathy with traction retinal detachment not involving the macula

New   E09.354 Drug or chemical induced diabetes mellitus with proliferative diabetic retinopathy with combined traction retinal detachment and rhegmatogenous retinal detachment

New   E09.355 Drug or chemical induced diabetes mellitus with stable proliferative diabetic retinopathy

E09.37 Drug or chemical induced diabetes mellitus with diabetic macular edema, resolved following treatment

New   One of the following 7th characters is to be assigned to code E09.37 to designate laterality of the disease:

New
New
New
New

1	right eye
2	left eye
3	bilateral
9	unspecified eye

E10.32 Type 1 diabetes mellitus with mild nonproliferative diabetic retinopathy

New   One of the following 7th characters is to be assigned to codes in subcategory E10.32 to designate laterality of the disease:

New
New
New
New

1	right eye
2	left eye
3	bilateral
9	unspecified eye

E10.33 Type 1 diabetes mellitus with moderate nonproliferative diabetic retinopathy

New   One of the following 7th characters is to be assigned to codes in subcategory E10.33 to designate laterality of the disease:

New
New
New
New

1	right eye
2	left eye
3	bilateral
9	unspecified eye

E10.34   Type 1 diabetes mellitus with severe nonproliferative diabetic retinopathy

New

One of the following 7th characters is to be assigned to codes in subcategory E10.34 to designate laterality of the disease:

New   1   right eye
New   2   left eye
New   3   bilateral
New   9   unspecified eye

E10.35   Type 1 diabetes mellitus with proliferative diabetic retinopathy

New

One of the following 7th characters is to be assigned to codes in subcategory E10.35 to designate laterality of the disease:

New   1   right eye
New   2   left eye
New   3   bilateral
New   9   unspecified eye

New   **E10.352   Type 1 diabetes mellitus with proliferative diabetic retinopathy with traction retinal detachment involving the macula**

New   **E10.353   Type 1 diabetes mellitus with proliferative diabetic retinopathy with traction retinal detachment not involving the macula**

New   **E10.354   Type 1 diabetes mellitus with proliferative diabetic retinopathy with combined traction retinal detachment and rhegmatogenous retinal detachment**

New   **E10.355   Type 1 diabetes mellitus with stable proliferative diabetic retinopathy**

New   **E10.37   Type 1 diabetes mellitus with diabetic macular edema, resolved following treatment**

One of the following 7th characters is to be assigned to code E10.37 to designate laterality of the disease:

New   1   right eye
New   2   left eye
New   3   bilateral
New   9   unspecified eye

E11   Type 2 diabetes mellitus

Revised   Use additional code to identify control using:
New   insulin (Z79.4)
New   oral antidiabetic drugs (Z79.84)
New   oral hypoglycemic drugs (Z79.84)

   E11.32   Type 2 diabetes mellitus with mild nonproliferative diabetic retinopathy

New

One of the following 7th characters is to be assigned to codes in subcategory E11.32 to designate laterality of the disease:

New   1   right eye
New   2   left eye
New   3   bilateral
New   9   unspecified eye

   E11.33   Type 2 diabetes mellitus with moderate nonproliferative diabetic retinopathy

New

One of the following 7th characters is to be assigned to codes in subcategory E11.33 to designate laterality of the disease:

New   1   right eye
New   2   left eye
New   3   bilateral
New   9   unspecified eye

E11.34   Type 2 diabetes mellitus with severe nonproliferative diabetic retinopathy

New

One of the following 7th characters is to be assigned to codes in subcategory E11.34 to designate laterality of the disease:

New   1   right eye
New   2   left eye
New   3   bilateral
New   9   unspecified eye

E11.35   Type 2 diabetes mellitus with proliferative diabetic retinopathy

New

One of the following 7th characters is to be assigned to codes in subcategory E11.35 to designate laterality of the disease:

New   1   right eye
New   2   left eye
New   3   bilateral
New   9   unspecified eye

New   **E11.352   Type 2 diabetes mellitus with proliferative diabetic retinopathy with traction retinal detachment involving the macula**

New   **E11.353   Type 2 diabetes mellitus with proliferative diabetic retinopathy with traction retinal detachment not involving the macula**

New   **E11.354   Type 2 diabetes mellitus with proliferative diabetic retinopathy with combined traction retinal detachment and rhegmatogenous retinal detachment**

New   **E11.355   Type 2 diabetes mellitus with stable proliferative diabetic retinopathy**

New   **E11.37   Type 2 diabetes mellitus with diabetic macular edema, resolved following treatment**

New

One of the following 7th characters is to be assigned to code E11.37 to designate laterality of the disease:

New   1   right eye
New   2   left eye
New   3   bilateral
New   9   unspecified eye

E13   Other specified diabetes mellitus

Revised   Use additional code to identify control using:
New   insulin (Z79.4)
New   oral antidiabetic drugs (Z79.84)
New   oral hypoglycemic drugs (Z79.84)

New   **Excludes1**   type 1 diabetes mellitus (E10.-)

   E13.32   Other specified diabetes mellitus with mild nonproliferative diabetic retinopathy

New

One of the following 7th characters is to be assigned to codes in subcategory E13.32 to designate laterality of the disease:

New   1   right eye
New   2   left eye
New   3   bilateral
New   9   unspecified eye

E13.33   Other specified diabetes mellitus with moderate nonproliferative diabetic retinopathy

New
One of the following 7th characters is to be assigned to codes in subcategory E13.33 to designate laterality of the disease:

New	1 right eye
New	2 left eye
New	3 bilateral
New	9 unspecified eye

E13.34   Other specified diabetes mellitus with severe nonproliferative diabetic retinopathy

New
One of the following 7th characters is to be assigned to codes in subcategory E13.34 to designate laterality of the disease:

New	1 right eye
New	2 left eye
New	3 bilateral
New	9 unspecified eye

E13.35   Other specified diabetes mellitus with proliferative diabetic retinopathy

New
One of the following 7th characters is to be assigned to codes in subcategory E13.35 to designate laterality of the disease:

New	1 right eye
New	2 left eye
New	3 bilateral
New	9 unspecified eye

New   **E13.352   Other specified diabetes mellitus with proliferative diabetic retinopathy with traction retinal detachment involving the macula**

New   **E13.353   Other specified diabetes mellitus with proliferative diabetic retinopathy with traction retinal detachment not involving the macula**

New   **E13.354   Other specified diabetes mellitus with proliferative diabetic retinopathy with combined traction retinal detachment and rhegmatogenous retinal detachment**

New   **E13.355   Other specified diabetes mellitus with stable proliferative diabetic retinopathy**

E13.37   Other specified diabetes mellitus with diabetic macular edema, resolved following treatment

New
One of the following 7th characters is to be assigned to code E13.37 to designate laterality of the disease:

New	1 right eye
New	2 left eye
New	3 bilateral
New	9 unspecified eye

E16.0   Drug-induced hypoglycemia without coma

New   **Excludes1**   diabetes with hypoglycemia without coma (E09.692)

E16.1   Other hypoglycemia

New   **Excludes1**   diabetes with hypoglycemia (E08.649, E10.649, E11.649, E13.649)

E16.2   Hypoglycemia, unspecified

New   **Excludes1**   diabetes with hypoglycemia (E08.649, E10.649, E11.649, E13.649)

E29   Testicular dysfunction

Revised   **Excludes1**   Klinefelter's syndrome (Q98.0-Q98.1, Q98.4)

E66.2   Morbid (severe) obesity with alveolar hypoventilation

New   Obesity hypoventilation syndrome (OHS)

E78.0   Pure hypercholesterolemia

Deleted   Familial hypercholesterolemia
Deleted   Fredrickson's hyperlipoproteinemia, type IIa
Deleted   Hyperbetalipoproteinemia
Deleted   Hyperlipidemia, Group A
Deleted   Low-density-lipoprotein-type [LDL] hyperlipoproteinemia

New   **E78.00   Pure hypercholesterolemia, unspecified**

New   Fredrickson's hyperlipoproteinemia, type IIa
New   Hyperbetalipoproteinemia
New   Low-density-lipoprotein-type [LDL] hyperlipoproteinemia

New   **E78.01   Familial hypercholesterolemia**

E84   Cystic fibrosis

New   Code also exocrine pancreatic insufficiency (K86.81)

E85.0   Non-neuropathic heredofamilial amyloidosis

Deleted   Familial Mediterranean fever

E86   Volume depletion

New   Use additional code(s) for any associated disorders of electrolyte and acid-base balance (E87.-)

E88.42   MERRF syndrome

Revised   Code also progressive myoclonic epilepsy (G40.3-)

Revised   **E89.81   Postprocedural hemorrhage of an endocrine system organ or structure following a procedure**

Revised   **E89.810   Postprocedural hemorrhage of an endocrine system organ or structure following an endocrine system procedure**

Revised   **E89.811   Postprocedural hemorrhage of an endocrine system organ or structure following other procedure**

New   **E89.82   Postprocedural hematoma and seroma of an endocrine system organ or structure**

New   **E89.820   Postprocedural hematoma of an endocrine system organ or structure following an endocrine system procedure**

New   **E89.821   Postprocedural hematoma of an endocrine system organ or structure following other procedure**

New   **E89.822   Postprocedural seroma of an endocrine system organ or structure following an endocrine system procedure**

New   **E89.823   Postprocedural seroma of an endocrine system organ or structure following other procedure**

CHAPTER 5

MENTAL, BEHAVIORAL AND NEURODEVELOPMENTAL DISORDERS (F01-F99)

F01.50   Vascular dementia without behavioral disturbance

New   Major neurocognitive disorder without behavioral disturbance

	F01.51	**Vascular dementia with behavioral disturbance**
New		Major neurocognitive disorder due to vascular disease, with behavioral disturbance
New		Major neurocognitive disorder with aggressive behavior
New		Major neurocognitive disorder with combative behavior
New		Major neurocognitive disorder with violent behavior

F02   Dementia in other diseases classified elsewhere

Code first the underlying physiological condition, such as:

New		dementia with Parkinsonism (G31.83)
New		Huntington's disease (G10)
New		prion disease (A81.9)
New		traumatic brain injury (S06.-)
New	**Includes**	Major neurocognitive disorder in other diseases classified elsewhere
Deleted	**Excludes1**	dementia with Parkinsonism (G31.83)

	F02.80	**Dementia in other diseases classified elsewhere without behavioral disturbance**
New		Major neurocognitive disorder in other diseases classified elsewhere
	F02.81	**Dementia in other diseases classified elsewhere with behavioral disturbance**
New		Major neurocognitive disorder in other diseases classified elsewhere with aggressive behavior
New		Major neurocognitive disorder in other diseases classified elsewhere with combative behavior
New		Major neurocognitive disorder in other diseases classified elsewhere with violent behavior

	F06.1	**Catatonic disorder due to known physiological condition**
New		Catatonia associated with another mental disorder
New		Catatonia NOS
	F10.10	**Alcohol abuse, uncomplicated**
New		Alcohol use disorder, mild
	F10.14	**Alcohol abuse with alcohol-induced mood disorder**
New		Alcohol use disorder, mild, with alcohol-induced bipolar or related disorder
New		Alcohol use disorder, mild, with alcohol-induced depressive disorder
	F10.20	**Alcohol dependence, uncomplicated**
New		Alcohol use disorder, moderate
New		Alcohol use disorder, severe
	F10.22	**Alcohol dependence with intoxication**
		Acute drunkenness (in alcoholism)
Deleted	**Excludes1**	alcohol dependence with withdrawal (F10.23-)
New	**Excludes2**	alcohol dependence with withdrawal (F10.23-)
	F10.23	**Alcohol dependence with withdrawal**
Deleted	**Excludes1**	alcohol dependence with intoxication (F10.22-)
New	**Excludes2**	alcohol dependence with intoxication (F10.22-)
	F10.24	**Alcohol dependence with alcohol-induced mood disorder**
New		Alcohol use disorder, moderate, with alcohol-induced bipolar or related disorder
New		Alcohol use disorder, moderate, with alcohol-induced depressive disorder
New		Alcohol use disorder, severe, with alcohol-induced bipolar or related disorder
New		Alcohol use disorder, severe, with alcohol-induced depressive disorder

	F10.26	**Alcohol dependence with alcohol-induced persisting amnestic disorder**
New		Alcohol use disorder, moderate, with alcohol-induced major neurocognitive disorder, amnestic-confabulatory type
New		Alcohol use disorder, severe, with alcohol-induced major neurocognitive disorder, amnestic-confabulatory type
	F10.27	**Alcohol dependence with alcohol-induced persisting dementia**
New		Alcohol use disorder, moderate, with alcohol-induced major neurocognitive disorder, nonamnestic-confabulatory type
New		Alcohol use disorder, severe, with alcohol-induced major neurocognitive disorder, nonamnestic-confabulatory type
	F10.288	**Alcohol dependence with other alcohol-induced disorder**
New		Alcohol use disorder, moderate, with alcohol-induced mild neurocognitive disorder
New		Alcohol use disorder, severe, with alcohol-induced mild neurocognitive disorder
	F10.94	**Alcohol use, unspecified with alcohol-induced mood disorder**
New		Alcohol-induced bipolar or related disorder, without use disorder
New		Alcohol-induced depressive disorder, without use disorder
	F10.959	**Alcohol use, unspecified with alcohol-induced psychotic disorder, unspecified**
New		Alcohol-induced psychotic disorder without use disorder
	F10.96	**Alcohol use, unspecified with alcohol-induced persisting amnestic disorder**
New		Alcohol-induced major neurocognitive disorder, amnestic-confabulatory type, without use disorder
	F10.97	**Alcohol use, unspecified with alcohol-induced persisting dementia**
New		Alcohol-induced major neurocognitive disorder, nonamnestic-confabulatory type, without use disorder
	F10.980	**Alcohol use, unspecified with alcohol-induced anxiety disorder**
New		Alcohol-induced anxiety disorder, without use disorder
	F10.981	**Alcohol use, unspecified with alcohol-induced sexual dysfunction**
New		Alcohol-induced sexual dysfunction, without use disorder
	F10.982	**Alcohol use, unspecified with alcohol-induced sleep disorder**
New		Alcohol-induced sleep disorder, without use disorder
	F10.988	**Alcohol use, unspecified with other alcohol-induced disorder**
New		Alcohol-induced mild neurocognitive disorder, without use disorder
	F11.10	**Opioid abuse, uncomplicated**
New		Opioid use disorder, mild
	F11.14	**Opioid abuse with opioid-induced mood disorder**
New		Opioid use disorder, mild, with opioid-induced depressive disorder

	F11.20	**Opioid dependence, uncomplicated**
New		Opioid use disorder, moderate
New		Opioid use disorder, severe
	F11.24	**Opioid dependence with opioid-induced mood disorder**
New		Opioid use disorder, moderate, with opioid-induced depressive disorder
	F11.921	**Opioid use, unspecified with intoxication delirium**
New		Opioid-induced delirium
	F11.94	**Opioid use, unspecified with opioid-induced mood disorder**
New		Opioid-induced depressive disorder, without use disorder
	F11.981	**Opioid use, unspecified with opioid-induced sexual dysfunction**
New		Opioid-induced sexual dysfunction, without use disorder
	F11.982	**Opioid use, unspecified with opioid-induced sleep disorder**
New		Opioid-induced sleep disorder, without use disorder
	F11.988	**Opioid use, unspecified with other opioid-induced disorder**
New		Opioid-induced anxiety disorder, without use disorder
	F12.10	**Cannabis abuse, uncomplicated**
New		Cannabis use disorder, mild
	F12.188	**Cannabis abuse with other cannabis-induced disorder**
New		Cannabis use disorder, mild, with cannabis-induced sleep disorder
	F12.2	**Cannabis dependence**
	F12.20	**Cannabis dependence, uncomplicated**
New		Cannabis use disorder, moderate
New		Cannabis use disorder, severe
	F12.288	**Cannabis dependence with other cannabis-induced disorder**
New		Cannabis use disorder, moderate, with cannabis-induced sleep disorder
New		Cannabis use disorder, severe, with cannabis-induced sleep disorder
New		Cannabis withdrawal
	F12.959	**Cannabis use, unspecified with psychotic disorder, unspecified**
New		Cannabis-induced psychotic disorder, without use disorder
	F12.980	**Cannabis use, unspecified with anxiety disorder**
New		Cannabis-induced anxiety disorder, without use disorder
	F12.988	**Cannabis use, unspecified with other cannabis-induced disorder**
New		Cannabis-induced sleep disorder, without use disorder
	F13.10	**Sedative, hypnotic or anxiolytic abuse, uncomplicated**
New		Sedative, hypnotic, or anxiolytic use disorder, mild

	F13.14	**Sedative, hypnotic or anxiolytic abuse with sedative, hypnotic or anxiolytic-induced mood disorder**
New		Sedative, hypnotic, or anxiolytic use disorder, mild, with sedative, hypnotic, or anxiolytic-induced bipolar or related disorder
New		Sedative, hypnotic, or anxiolytic use disorder, mild, with sedative, hypnotic, or anxiolytic-induced depressive disorder
	F13.23	**Sedative, hypnotic or anxiolytic dependence with withdrawal**
New		Sedative, hypnotic, or anxiolytic use disorder, moderate
New		Sedative, hypnotic, or anxiolytic use disorder, severe
	F13.232	**Sedative, hypnotic or anxiolytic dependence with withdrawal with perceptual disturbance**
New		Sedative, hypnotic, or anxiolytic withdrawal with perceptual disturbances
	F13.239	**Sedative, hypnotic or anxiolytic dependence with withdrawal, unspecified**
New		Sedative, hypnotic, or anxiolytic withdrawal without perceptual disturbances
	F13.24	**Sedative, hypnotic or anxiolytic dependence with sedative, hypnotic or anxiolytic-induced mood disorder**
New		Sedative, hypnotic, or anxiolytic use disorder, moderate, with sedative, hypnotic, or anxiolytic-induced bipolar or related disorder
New		Sedative, hypnotic, or anxiolytic use disorder, moderate, with sedative, hypnotic, or anxiolytic-induced depressive disorder
New		Sedative, hypnotic, or anxiolytic use disorder, severe, with sedative, hypnotic, or anxiolytic-induced bipolar or related disorder
New		Sedative, hypnotic, or anxiolytic use disorder, severe, with sedative, hypnotic, or anxiolytic-induced depressive disorder
	F13.27	**Sedative, hypnotic or anxiolytic dependence with sedative, hypnotic or anxiolytic-induced persisting dementia**
New		Sedative, hypnotic, or anxiolytic use disorder, moderate, with sedative, hypnotic, or anxiolytic-induced major neurocognitive disorder
New		Sedative, hypnotic, or anxiolytic use disorder, severe, with sedative, hypnotic, or anxiolytic-induced major neurocognitive disorder
	F13.288	**Sedative, hypnotic or anxiolytic dependence with other sedative, hypnotic or anxiolytic-induced disorder**
New		Sedative, hypnotic, or anxiolytic use disorder, moderate, with sedative, hypnotic, or anxiolytic-induced mild neurocognitive disorder
New		Sedative, hypnotic, or anxiolytic use disorder, severe, with sedative, hypnotic, or anxiolytic-induced mild neurocognitive disorder

F13.921 Sedative, hypnotic or anxiolytic use, unspecified with intoxication delirium

New   Sedative, hypnotic, or anxiolytic-induced delirium

F13.94 Sedative, hypnotic or anxiolytic use, unspecified with sedative, hypnotic or anxiolytic-induced mood disorder

New   Sedative, hypnotic, or anxiolytic-induced bipolar or related disorder, without use disorder

New   Sedative, hypnotic, or anxiolytic-induced depressive disorder, without use disorder

F13.959 Sedative, hypnotic or anxiolytic use, unspecified with sedative, hypnotic or anxiolytic-induced psychotic disorder, unspecified

New   Sedative, hypnotic, or anxiolytic-induced psychotic disorder, without use disorder

F13.97 Sedative, hypnotic or anxiolytic use, unspecified with sedative, hypnotic or anxiolytic-induced persisting dementia

New   Sedative, hypnotic, or anxiolytic-induced major neurocognitive disorder, without use disorder

F13.980 Sedative, hypnotic or anxiolytic use, unspecified with sedative, hypnotic or anxiolytic-induced anxiety disorder

New   Sedative, hypnotic, or anxiolytic-induced anxiety disorder, without use disorder

F13.981 Sedative, hypnotic or anxiolytic use, unspecified with sedative, hypnotic or anxiolytic-induced sexual dysfunction

New   Sedative, hypnotic, or anxiolytic-induced sexual dysfunction disorder, without use disorder

F13.982 Sedative, hypnotic or anxiolytic use, unspecified with sedative, hypnotic or anxiolytic-induced sleep disorder

New   Sedative, hypnotic, or anxiolytic-induced sleep disorder, without use disorder

F13.988 Sedative, hypnotic or anxiolytic use, unspecified with other sedative, hypnotic or anxiolytic-induced disorder

New   Sedative, hypnotic, or anxiolytic-induced mild neurocognitive disorder

F14.10 Cocaine abuse, uncomplicated

New   Cocaine use disorder, mild

F14.14 Cocaine abuse with cocaine-induced mood disorder

New   Cocaine use disorder, mild, with cocaine-induced bipolar or related disorder

New   Cocaine use disorder, mild, with cocaine-induced depressive disorder

F14.188 Cocaine abuse with other cocaine-induced disorder

New   Cocaine use disorder, mild, with cocaine-induced obsessive-compulsive or related disorder

F14.20 Cocaine dependence, uncomplicated

New   Cocaine use disorder, moderate

New   Cocaine use disorder, severe

F14.24 Cocaine dependence with cocaine-induced mood disorder

New   Cocaine use disorder, moderate, with cocaine-induced bipolar or related disorder

New   Cocaine use disorder, moderate, with cocaine-induced depressive disorder

New   Cocaine use disorder, severe, with cocaine-induced bipolar or related disorder

New   Cocaine use disorder, severe, with cocaine-induced depressive disorder

F14.288 Cocaine dependence with other cocaine-induced disorder

New   Cocaine use disorder, moderate, with cocaine-induced obsessive-compulsive or related disorder

      Cocaine use disorder, severe, with cocaine-induced obsessive-compulsive or related disorder

F14.94 Cocaine use, unspecified with cocaine-induced mood disorder

New   Cocaine-induced bipolar or related disorder, without use disorder

New   Cocaine-induced depressive disorder, without use disorder

F14.959 Cocaine use, unspecified with cocaine-induced psychotic disorder, unspecified

New   Cocaine-induced psychotic disorder, without use disorder

F14.980 Cocaine use, unspecified with cocaine-induced anxiety disorder

New   Cocaine-induced anxiety disorder, without use disorder

F14.981 Cocaine use, unspecified with cocaine-induced sexual dysfunction

New   Cocaine-induced sexual dysfunction, without use disorder

F14.982 Cocaine use, unspecified with cocaine-induced sleep disorder

New   Cocaine-induced sleep disorder, without use disorder

F14.988 Cocaine use, unspecified with other cocaine-induced disorder

New   Cocaine-induced obsessive-compulsive or related disorder

F15.10 Other stimulant abuse, uncomplicated

New   Amphetamine type substance use disorder, mild

New   Other or unspecified stimulant use disorder, mild

F15.122 Other stimulant abuse with intoxication with perceptual disturbance

New   Amphetamine or other stimulant use disorder, mild, with amphetamine or other stimulant intoxication, with perceptual disturbances

F15.129   **Other stimulant abuse with intoxication, unspecified**

New   Amphetamine or other stimulant use disorder, mild, with amphetamine or other stimulant intoxication, without perceptual disturbances

F15.14   **Other stimulant abuse with stimulant-induced mood disorder**

New   Amphetamine or other stimulant use disorder, mild, with amphetamine or other stimulant-induced bipolar or related disorder

New   Amphetamine or other stimulant use disorder, mild, with amphetamine or other stimulant-induced depressive disorder

F15.188   **Other stimulant abuse with other stimulant-induced disorder**

New   Amphetamine or other stimulant use disorder, mild, with amphetamine or other stimulant-induced obsessive-compulsive or related disorder

F15.20   **Other stimulant dependence, uncomplicated**

New   Amphetamine type substance use disorder, moderate

New   Amphetamine type substance use disorder, severe

New   Other or unspecified stimulant use disorder, moderate

New   Other or unspecified stimulant use disorder, severe

F15.222   **Other stimulant dependence with intoxication with perceptual disturbance**

New   Amphetamine or other stimulant use disorder, moderate, with amphetamine or other stimulant intoxication, with perceptual disturbances

New   Amphetamine or other stimulant use disorder, severe, with amphetamine or other stimulant intoxication, with perceptual disturbances

F15.229   **Other stimulant dependence with intoxication, unspecified**

New   Amphetamine or other stimulant use disorder, moderate, with amphetamine or other stimulant intoxication, without perceptual disturbances

New   Amphetamine or other stimulant use disorder, severe, with amphetamine or other stimulant intoxication, without perceptual disturbances

F15.23   **Other stimulant dependence with withdrawal**

New   Amphetamine or other stimulant withdrawal

F15.24   **Other stimulant dependence with stimulant-induced mood disorder**

New   Amphetamine or other stimulant use disorder, moderate, with amphetamine or other stimulant-induced bipolar or related disorder

New   Amphetamine or other stimulant use disorder, moderate, with amphetamine or other stimulant-induced depressive disorder

New   Amphetamine or other stimulant use disorder, severe, with amphetamine or other stimulant-induced bipolar or related disorder

New   Amphetamine or other stimulant use disorder, severe, with amphetamine or other stimulant-induced depressive disorder

F15.288   **Other stimulant dependence with other stimulant-induced disorder**

New   Amphetamine or other stimulant use disorder, moderate, with amphetamine or other stimulant-induced obsessive-compulsive or related disorder

New   Amphetamine or other stimulant use disorder, severe, with amphetamine or other stimulant-induced obsessive-compulsive or related disorder

F15.921   **Other stimulant use, unspecified with intoxication delirium**

New   Amphetamine or other stimulant-induced delirium

F15.929   **Other stimulant use, unspecified with intoxication, unspecified**

New   Caffeine intoxication

F15.93   **Other stimulant use, unspecified with withdrawal**

New   Caffeine withdrawal

F15.94   **Other stimulant use, unspecified with stimulant-induced mood disorder**

New   Amphetamine or other stimulant-induced bipolar or related disorder, without use disorder

New   Amphetamine or other stimulant-induced depressive disorder, without use disorder

F15.959   **Other stimulant use, unspecified with stimulant-induced psychotic disorder, unspecified**

New   Amphetamine or other stimulant-induced psychotic disorder, without use disorder

F15.980   **Other stimulant use, unspecified with stimulant-induced anxiety disorder**

New   Amphetamine or other stimulant-induced anxiety disorder, without use disorder

New   Caffeine-induced anxiety disorder, without use disorder

F15.981 Other stimulant use, unspecified with stimulant-induced sexual dysfunction

New
  Amphetamine or other stimulant-induced sexual dysfunction, without use disorder

F15.982 Other stimulant use, unspecified with stimulant-induced sleep disorder

New
  Amphetamine or other stimulant-induced sleep disorder, without use disorder

New
  Caffeine-induced sleep disorder, without use disorder

F15.988 Other stimulant use, unspecified with other stimulant-induced disorder

New
  Amphetamine or other stimulant-induced obsessive-compulsive or related disorder, without use disorder

F16.10 Hallucinogen abuse, uncomplicated

New Other hallucinogen use disorder, mild
New Phencyclidine use disorder, mild

F16.14 Hallucinogen abuse with hallucinogen-induced mood disorder

New
  Other hallucinogen use disorder, mild, with other hallucinogen-induced bipolar or related disorder

New
  Other hallucinogen use disorder, mild, with other hallucinogen-induced depressive disorder

New
  Phencyclidine use disorder, mild, with phencyclidine-induced bipolar or related disorder

New
  Phencyclidine use disorder, mild, with phencyclidine-induced depressive disorder

F16.20 Hallucinogen dependence, uncomplicated

New Other hallucinogen use disorder, moderate
New Other hallucinogen use disorder, severe
New Phencyclidine use disorder, moderate
New Phencyclidine use disorder, severe

F16.24 Hallucinogen dependence with hallucinogen-induced mood disorder

New
  Other hallucinogen use disorder, moderate, with other hallucinogen-induced bipolar or related disorder

New
  Other hallucinogen use disorder, moderate, with other hallucinogen-induced depressive disorder

New
  Other hallucinogen use disorder, severe, with other hallucinogen-induced bipolar or related disorder

New
  Other hallucinogen use disorder, severe, with other hallucinogen-induced depressive disorder

New
  Phencyclidine use disorder, moderate, with phencyclidine-induced bipolar or related disorder

New
  Phencyclidine use disorder, moderate, with phencyclidine-induced depressive disorder

New
  Phencyclidine use disorder, severe, with phencyclidine-induced bipolar or related disorder

New
  Phencyclidine use disorder, severe, with phencyclidine-induced depressive disorder

F16.921 Hallucinogen use, unspecified with intoxication with delirium

New
  Other hallucinogen intoxication delirium

F16.94 Hallucinogen use, unspecified with hallucinogen-induced mood disorder

New
  Other hallucinogen-induced bipolar or related disorder, without use disorder

New
  Other hallucinogen-induced depressive disorder, without use disorder

New
  Phencyclidine-induced bipolar or related disorder, without use disorder

New
  Phencyclidine-induced depressive disorder, without use disorder

F16.959 Hallucinogen use, unspecified with hallucinogen-induced psychotic disorder, unspecified

New
  Other hallucinogen-induced psychotic disorder, without use disorder

New
  Phencyclidine-induced psychotic disorder, without use disorder

F16.980 Hallucinogen use, unspecified with hallucinogen-induced anxiety disorder

New
  Other hallucinogen-induced anxiety disorder, without use disorder

New
  Phencyclidine-induced anxiety disorder, without use disorder

F17.200 Nicotine dependence, unspecified, uncomplicated

New Tobacco use disorder, mild
New Tobacco use disorder, moderate
New Tobacco use disorder, severe

F17.203 Nicotine dependence unspecified, with withdrawal

New Tobacco withdrawal

F18.10 Inhalant abuse, uncomplicated

New Inhalant use disorder, mild

F18.14 Inhalant abuse with inhalant-induced mood disorder

New
  Inhalant use disorder, mild, with inhalant-induced depressive disorder

F18.17 Inhalant abuse with inhalant-induced dementia

New
  Inhalant use disorder, mild, with inhalant-induced major neurocognitive disorder

F18.188 Inhalant abuse with other inhalant-induced disorder

New
  Inhalant use disorder, mild, with inhalant-induced mild neurocognitive disorder

F18.20 Inhalant dependence, uncomplicated

New Inhalant use disorder, moderate
New Inhalant use disorder, severe

F18.24 Inhalant dependence with inhalant-induced mood disorder

New
  Inhalant use disorder, moderate, with inhalant-induced depressive disorder

New
  Inhalant use disorder, severe, with inhalant-induced depressive disorder

F18.27 Inhalant dependence with inhalant-induced dementia

New
  Inhalant use disorder, moderate, with inhalant-induced major neurocognitive disorder

New
  Inhalant use disorder, severe, with inhalant-induced major neurocognitive disorder

F18.288   Inhalant dependence with other inhalant-induced disorder

New   Inhalant use disorder, moderate, with inhalant-induced mild neurocognitive disorder

New   Inhalant use disorder, severe, with inhalant-induced mild neurocognitive disorder

F18.94   Inhalant use, unspecified with inhalant-induced mood disorder

New   Inhalant-induced depressive disorder

F18.97   Inhalant use, unspecified with inhalant-induced persisting dementia

New   Inhalant-induced major neurocognitive disorder

F18.988   Inhalant use, unspecified with other inhalant-induced disorder

New   Inhalant-induced mild neurocognitive disorder

F19.10   Other psychoactive substance abuse, uncomplicated

New   Other (or unknown) substance use disorder, mild

F19.14   Other psychoactive substance abuse with psychoactive substance-induced mood disorder

New   Other (or unknown) substance use disorder, mild, with other (or unknown) substance-induced bipolar or related disorder

New   Other (or unknown) substance use disorder, mild, with other (or unknown) substance-induced depressive disorder

F19.17   Other psychoactive substance abuse with psychoactive substance-induced persisting dementia

New   Other (or unknown) substance use disorder, mild, with other (or unknown) substance-induced major neurocognitive disorder

F19.188   Other psychoactive substance abuse with other psychoactive substance-induced disorder

New   Other (or unknown) substance use disorder, mild, with other (or unknown) substance-induced mild neurocognitive disorder

New   Other (or unknown) substance use disorder, mild, with other (or unknown) substance-induced obsessive-compulsive or related disorder

F19.20   Other psychoactive substance dependence, uncomplicated

New   Other (or unknown) substance use disorder, moderate

New   Other (or unknown) substance use disorder, severe

F19.24   Other psychoactive substance dependence with psychoactive substance-induced mood disorder

New.   Other (or unknown) substance use disorder, moderate, with other (or unknown) substance-induced bipolar or related disorder

New   Other (or unknown) substance use disorder, moderate, with other (or unknown) substance-induced depressive disorder

New   Other (or unknown) substance use disorder, severe, with other (or unknown) substance-induced bipolar or related disorder

New   Other (or unknown) substance use disorder, severe, with other (or unknown) substance-induced depressive disorder

F19.27   Other psychoactive substance dependence with psychoactive substance-induced persisting dementia

New   Other (or unknown) substance use disorder, moderate, with other (or unknown) substance-induced major neurocognitive disorder

New   Other (or unknown) substance use disorder, severe, with other (or unknown) substance-induced major neurocognitive disorder

F19.288   Other psychoactive substance dependence with other psychoactive substance-induced disorder

New   Other (or unknown) substance use disorder, moderate, with other (or unknown) substance-induced mild neurocognitive disorder

New   Other (or unknown) substance use disorder, severe, with other (or unknown) substance-induced mild neurocognitive disorder

New   Other (or unknown) substance use disorder, moderate, with other (or unknown) substance-induced obsessive-compulsive or related disorder

New   Other (or unknown) substance use disorder, severe, with other (or unknown) substance-induced obsessive-compulsive or related disorder

F19.921   Other psychoactive substance use, unspecified with intoxication with delirium

New   Other (or unknown) substance-induced delirium

F19.94   Other psychoactive substance use, unspecified with psychoactive substance-induced mood disorder

New   Other (or unknown) substance-induced bipolar or related disorder, without use disorder

New   Other (or unknown) substance-induced depressive disorder, without use disorder

F19.959   Other psychoactive substance use, unspecified with psychoactive substance-induced psychotic disorder, unspecified

New   Other or unknown substance-induced psychotic disorder, without use disorder

F19.97   Other psychoactive substance use, unspecified with psychoactive substance-induced persisting dementia

New   Other (or unknown) substance-induced major neurocognitive disorder, without use disorder

F19.980   Other psychoactive substance use, unspecified with psychoactive substance-induced anxiety disorder

New   Other (or unknown) substance-induced anxiety disorder, without use disorder

F19.981   Other psychoactive substance use, unspecified with psychoactive substance-induced sexual dysfunction

New   Other (or unknown) substance-induced sexual dysfunction, without use disorder

	F19.982	**Other psychoactive substance use, unspecified with psychoactive substance-induced sleep disorder**
New		Other (or unknown) substance-induced sleep disorder, without use disorder
	F19.988	**Other psychoactive substance use, unspecified with other psychoactive substance-induced disorder**
New		Other (or unknown) substance-induced mild neurocognitive disorder, without use disorder
New		Other (or unknown) substance-induced obsessive-compulsive or related disorder, without use disorder

	F20.3	**Undifferentiated schizophrenia**
Revised		**Excludes2** post-schizophrenic depression (F32.89)

	F32.8	**Other depressive episodes**
Deleted		Atypical depression
Deleted		Post-schizophrenic depression
Deleted		Single episode of 'masked' depression NOS
New	**F32.81**	**Premenstrual dysphoric disorder**
New		**Excludes1** premenstrual tension syndrome (N94.3)
New	**F32.89**	**Other specified depressive episodes**
New		Atypical depression
New		Post-schizophrenic depression
New		Single episode of 'masked' depression NOS

	F34.1	**Dysthymic disorder**
New		Persistent depressive disorder
	F34.8	**Other persistent mood [affective] disorders**
New	**F34.81**	**Disruptive mood dysregulation disorder**
New	**F34.89**	**Other specified persistent mood disorders**

F42		**Obsessive-compulsive disorder**
Deleted		Anancastic neurosis
Deleted		Obsessive-compulsive neurosis
New	**F42.2**	**Mixed obsessional thoughts and acts**
New	**F42.3**	**Hoarding disorder**
New	**F42.4**	**Excoriation (skin-picking) disorder**
New		**Excludes1** factitial dermatitis (L98.1)
New		other specified behavioral and emotional disorders with onset usually occurring in early childhood and adolescence (F98.8)
New	**F42.8**	**Other obsessive-compulsive disorder**
New		Anancastic neurosis
New		Obsessive-compulsive neurosis
New	**F42.9**	**Obsessive-compulsive disorder, unspecified**

	F43.8	**Other reactions to severe stress**
New		Other specified trauma and stressor-related disorder
	F43.9	**Reaction to severe stress, unspecified**
New		Trauma and stressor-related disorder, NOS

	F44.0	**Dissociative amnesia**
New		**Excludes1** dissociative amnesia with dissociative fugue (F44.1)
	F44.1	**Dissociative fugue**
		Dissociative amnesia with dissociative fugue

	F45.1	**Undifferentiated somatoform disorder**
New		Somatic symptom disorder
	F45.21	**Hypochondriasis**
New		Illness anxiety disorder

	F50.0	**Anorexia nervosa**
Revised		**Excludes1** psychogenic loss of appetite (F50.89)
	F50.8	**Other eating disorders**
Deleted		Pica in adults
Deleted		Psychogenic loss of appetite
New	**F50.81**	**Binge eating disorder**
New	**F50.89**	**Other specified eating disorder**
New		Pica in adults
New		Psychogenic loss of appetite

	F52.0	**Hypoactive sexual desire disorder**
Deleted		Anhedonia (sexual)
New		Sexual anhedonia
	F52.22	**Female sexual arousal disorder**
Deleted		Frigidity
	F52.32	**Male orgasmic disorder**
New		Delayed ejaculation

	F52.6	**Dyspareunia not due to a substance or known physiological condition**
New		Genito-pelvic pain penetration disorder
Revised		**Excludes2** dyspareunia (due to a known physiological condition) (N94.1-)

	F60.5	**Obsessive-compulsive personality disorder**
Revised		**Excludes2** obsessive-compulsive disorder (F42-)

	F64.0	**Transsexualism**
New		Gender identity disorder in adolescence and adulthood
New		Gender dysphoria in adolescents and adults
Revised	**F64.1**	**Dual role transvestism**
Deleted		Dual role transvestism
Deleted		Transvestism
	F64.2	**Gender identity disorder of childhood**
New		Gender dysphoria in children
Revised		**Excludes1** gender identity disorder in adolescence and adulthood (F64.0)

	F80.0	**Phonological disorder**
New		Speech-sound disorder
	F80.8	**Other developmental disorders of speech or language**
New	**F80.82**	**Social pragmatic communication disorder**
New		**Excludes1** Asperger's syndrome (F84.5)
New		autistic disorder (F84.0)

	F84.0	**Autistic disorder**
New		Autism spectrum disorder

F88		**Other disorders of psychological development**
New		Global developmental delay
New		Other specified neurodevelopmental disorder

F89		**Unspecified disorder of psychological development**
New		Neurodevelopmental disorder NOS

	F91.8	**Other conduct disorders**
New		Other specified conduct disorder
New		Other specified disruptive disorder
	F91.9	**Conduct disorder, unspecified**
New		Disruptive disorder NOS

	F95.0	**Transient tic disorder**
New		Provisional tic disorder

F98		**Other behavioral and emotional disorders with onset usually occurring in childhood and adolescence**
Revised		**Excludes2** obsessive-compulsive disorder (F42-)
	F98.4	**Stereotyped movement disorders**
Revised		**Excludes2** compulsions in obsessive-compulsive disorder (F42-)

CHAPTER 6
DISEASES OF THE NERVOUS SYSTEM
(G00-G99)

G00.1 Pneumococcal meningitis
New   Meningitis due to Streptococcal pneumoniae

     G31.84 Mild cognitive impairment, so stated
Revised   Excludes1 cognitive deficits following (sequelae of) cerebral hemorrhage or infarction (I69.01-, I69.11-, I69.21-, I69.31-, I69.81-, I69.91-)

G40 Epilepsy and recurrent seizures
Deleted   Excludes1 hippocampal sclerosis (G93.81)
Deleted   mesial temporal sclerosis (G93.81)
Deleted   temporal sclerosis (G93.81)
Deleted   Todd's paralysis (G83.8)
New   Excludes2 hippocampal sclerosis (G93.81)
New   mesial temporal sclerosis (G93.81)
New   temporal sclerosis (G93.81)
New   Todd's paralysis (G83.84)

G56.0 Carpal tunnel syndrome
New   G56.03 Carpal tunnel syndrome, bilateral upper limbs
G56.1 Other lesions of median nerve
New   G56.13 Other lesions of median nerve, bilateral upper limbs
G56.2 Lesion of ulnar nerve
New   G56.23 Lesion of ulnar nerve, bilateral upper limbs
G56.3 Lesion of radial nerve
New   G56.33 Lesion of radial nerve, bilateral upper limbs
G56.4 Causalgia of upper limb
New   G56.43 Causalgia of bilateral upper limbs
G56.8 Other specified mononeuropathies of upper limb
New   G56.83 Other specified mononeuropathies of bilateral upper limbs
G56.9 Unspecified mononeuropathy of upper limb
New   G56.93 Unspecified mononeuropathy of bilateral upper limbs

G57.0 Lesion of sciatic nerve
New   G57.03 Lesion of sciatic nerve, bilateral lower limbs
G57.1 Meralgia paresthetica
New   G57.13 Meralgia paresthetica, bilateral lower limbs
G57.2 Lesion of femoral nerve
New   G57.23 Lesion of femoral nerve, bilateral lower limbs
G57.3 Lesion of lateral popliteal nerve
New   G57.33 Lesion of lateral popliteal nerve, bilateral lower limbs
G57.4 Lesion of medial popliteal nerve
New   G57.43 Lesion of medial popliteal nerve, bilateral lower limbs
G57.5 Tarsal tunnel syndrome
New   G57.53 Tarsal tunnel syndrome, bilateral lower limbs
G57.6 Lesion of plantar nerve
New   G57.63 Lesion of plantar nerve, bilateral lower limbs
G57.7 Causalgia of lower limb
New   G57.73 Causalgia of bilateral lower limbs
G57.8 Other specified mononeuropathies of lower limb
New   G57.83 Other specified mononeuropathies of bilateral lower limbs
G57.9 Unspecified mononeuropathy of lower limb
New   G57.93 Unspecified mononeuropathy of bilateral lower limbs

    G61.8 Other inflammatory polyneuropathies
New   G61.82 Multifocal motor neuropathy
New   MMN

G89 Pain, not elsewhere classified
Revised   Excludes2 pain from prosthetic devices, implants, and grafts (T82.84, T83.84, T84.84, T85.84-)

G97 Intraoperative and postprocedural complications and disorders of nervous system, not elsewhere classified
Revised **G97.5 Postprocedural hemorrhage of a nervous system organ or structure following a procedure**
Revised   G97.51 Postprocedural hemorrhage of a nervous system organ or structure following a nervous system procedure
Revised   G97.52 Postprocedural hemorrhage of a nervous system organ or structure following other procedure
New **G97.6 Postprocedural hematoma and seroma of a nervous system organ or structure following a procedure**
New   G97.61 Postprocedural hematoma of a nervous system organ or structure following a nervous system procedure
New   G97.62 Postprocedural hematoma of a nervous system organ or structure following other procedure
New   G97.63 Postprocedural seroma of a nervous system organ or structure following a nervous system procedure
New   G97.64 Postprocedural seroma of a nervous system organ or structure following other procedure

CHAPTER 7
DISEASES OF THE EYE AND ADNEXA
(H00-H59)

H34.81 Central retinal vein occlusion
New   One of the following 7th characters is to be assigned to codes in subcategory H34.81 to designate the severity of the occlusion:
New   0 with macular edema
New   1 with retinal neovascularization
New   2 stable
New   Old central retinal vein occlusion

H34.83 Tributary (branch) retinal vein occlusion
New   One of the following 7th characters is to be assigned to codes in subcategory H34.83 to designate the severity of the occlusion:
New   0 with macular edema
New   1 with retinal neovascularization
New   2 stable
New   Old tributary (branch) retinal vein occlusion

H35.31 Nonexudative age-related macular degeneration
New   Dry age-related macular degeneration
New   One of the following 7th characters is to be assigned to codes in subcategory H35.31 to designate the stage of the disease:
New   0 stage unspecified
New   1 early dry stage
New   2 intermediate dry stage
New   3 advanced atrophic without subfoveal involvement
New   advanced dry stage
New   4 advanced atrophic with subfoveal involvement

New	H35.311	Nonexudative age-related macular degeneration, right eye
New	H35.312	Nonexudative age-related macular degeneration, left eye
New	H35.313	Nonexudative age-related macular degeneration, bilateral
New	H35.319	Nonexudative age-related macular degeneration, unspecified eye
	H35.32	Exudative age-related macular degeneration
New		Wet age-related macular degeneration
New		One of the following 7th characters is to be assigned to codes in subcategory H35.32 to designate the stage of the disease:

New	0	stage unspecified
New	1	with active choroidal neovascularization
New	2	with inactive choroidal neovascularization
New		with involuted or regressed neovascularization
New	3	with inactive scar

New	H35.321	Exudative age-related macular degeneration, right eye
New	H35.322	Exudative age-related macular degeneration, left eye
New	H35.323	Exudative age-related macular degeneration, bilateral
New	H35.329	Exudative age-related macular degeneration, unspecified eye
	H40.11	Primary open-angle glaucoma
New	H40.111	Primary open-angle glaucoma, right eye
New	H40.112	Primary open-angle glaucoma, left eye
New	H40.113	Primary open-angle glaucoma, bilateral
New	H40.119	Primary open-angle glaucoma, unspecified eye

	H42	Glaucoma in diseases classified elsewhere
Revised	**Excludes1**	glaucoma (in) onchocerciasis (B73.02)
Deleted		diabetes mellitus (E08.39, E09.39, E10.39, E11.39, E13.39)
Deleted		onchocerciasis (B73.02)
Revised		glaucoma (in) syphilis (A52.71)
Revised		glaucoma (in) tuberculous (A18.59)
New	**Excludes2**	glaucoma (in) diabetes mellitus (E08.39, E09.39, E10.39, E11.39, E13.39)

	H53.0	Amblyopia ex anopsia
New	H53.04	Amblyopia suspect
New	H53.041	Amblyopia suspect, right eye
New	H53.042	Amblyopia suspect, left eye
New	H53.043	Amblyopia suspect, bilateral
	H53.049	Amblyopia suspect, unspecified eye

	H59	Intraoperative and postprocedural complications and disorders of eye and adnexa, not elsewhere classified
Revised	H59.3	Postprocedural hemorrhage, hematoma, and seroma of eye and adnexa following other procedure
Revised	H59.31	Postprocedural hemorrhage of eye and adnexa following an ophthalmic procedure
Revised	H59.311	Postprocedural hemorrhage of right eye and avdnexa following an ophthalmic procedure
Revised	H59.312	Postprocedural hemorrhage of left eye and adnexa following an ophthalmic procedure
Revised	H59.313	Postprocedural hemorrhage of eye and adnexa following an ophthalmic procedure, bilateral

Revised	H59.319	Postprocedural hemorrhage of unspecified eye and adnexa following an ophthalmic procedure
Revised	H59.32	Postprocedural hemorrhage of eye and adnexa following other procedure
Revised	H59.321	Postprocedural hemorrhage of right eye and adnexa following other procedure
Revised	H59.322	Postprocedural hemorrhage of left eye and adnexa following other procedure
Revised	H59.323	Postprocedural hemorrhage of eye and adnexa following other procedure, bilateral
Revised	H59.329	Postprocedural hemorrhage of unspecified eye and adnexa following other procedure
New	H59.33	Postprocedural hematoma of eye and adnexa following an ophthalmic procedure
New	H59.331	Postprocedural hematoma of right eye and adnexa following an ophthalmic procedure
New	H59.332	Postprocedural hematoma of left eye and adnexa following an ophthalmic procedure
New	H59.333	Postprocedural hematoma of eye and adnexa following an ophthalmic procedure, bilateral
New	H59.339	Postprocedural hematoma of unspecified eye and adnexa following an ophthalmic procedure
New	H59.34	Postprocedural hematoma of eye and adnexa following other procedure
New	H59.341	Postprocedural hematoma of right eye and adnexa following other procedure
New	H59.342	Postprocedural hematoma of left eye and adnexa following other procedure
New	H59.343	Postprocedural hematoma of eye and adnexa following other procedure, bilateral
New	H59.349	Postprocedural hematoma of unspecified eye and adnexa following other procedure
New	H59.35	Postprocedural seroma of eye and adnexa following an ophthalmic procedure
New	H59.351	Postprocedural seroma of right eye and adnexa following an ophthalmic procedure
New	H59.352	Postprocedural seroma of left eye and adnexa following an ophthalmic procedure
New	H59.353	Postprocedural seroma of eye and adnexa following an ophthalmic procedure, bilateral
New	H59.359	Postprocedural seroma of unspecified eye and adnexa following an ophthalmic procedure
New	H59.36	Postprocedural seroma of eye and adnexa following other procedure
New	H59.361	Postprocedural seroma of right eye and adnexa following other procedure
New	H59.362	Postprocedural seroma of left eye and adnexa following other procedure
New	H59.363	Postprocedural seroma of eye and adnexa following other procedure, bilateral
New	H59.369	Postprocedural seroma of unspecified eye and adnexa following other procedure

CHAPTER 8

DISEASES OF THE EAR AND MASTOID PROCESS (H60-H95)

	H65	Nonsuppurative otitis media
	H66	Suppurative and unspecified otitis media
		Use additional code to identify:
New		history of tobacco dependence (Z87.891)

	H90	Conductive and sensorineural hearing loss	
New		H90.A	Conductive and sensorineural hearing loss with restricted hearing on the contralateral side
New		H90.A1	Conductive hearing loss, unilateral, with restricted hearing on the contralateral side
New			H90.A11 Conductive hearing loss, unilateral, right ear with restricted hearing on the contralateral side
New			H90.A12 Conductive hearing loss, unilateral, left ear with restricted hearing on the contralateral side
New		H90.A2	Sensorineural hearing loss, unilateral, with restricted hearing on the contralateral side
New			H90.A21 Sensorineural hearing loss, unilateral, right ear, with restricted hearing on the contralateral side
New			H90.A22 Sensorineural hearing loss, unilateral, left ear, with restricted hearing on the contralateral side
New		H90.A3	Mixed conductive and sensorineural hearing loss, unilateral with restricted hearing on the contralateral side
New			H90.A31 Mixed conductive and sensorineural hearing loss, unilateral, right ear with restricted hearing on the contralateral side
New			H90.A32 Mixed conductive and sensorineural hearing loss, unilateral, left ear with restricted hearing on the contralateral side
	H93	Other disorders of ear, not elsewhere classified	
New		H93.A	Pulsatile tinnitus
New			H93.A1 Pulsatile tinnitus, right ear
New			H93.A2 Pulsatile tinnitus, left ear
New			H93.A3 Pulsatile tinnitus, bilateral
New			H93.A9 Pulsatile tinnitus, unspecified ear
	H95	Intraoperative and postprocedural complications and disorders of ear and mastoid process, not elsewhere classified	
Revised		H95.4	Postprocedural hemorrhage of ear and mastoid process following a procedure
Revised			H95.41 Postprocedural hemorrhage of ear and mastoid process following a procedure on the ear and mastoid process
Revised			H95.42 Postprocedural hemorrhage of ear and mastoid process following other procedure
New		H95.5	Postprocedural hematoma and seroma of ear and mastoid process following a procedure
New			H95.51 Postprocedural hematoma of ear and mastoid process following a procedure on the ear and mastoid process
New			H95.52 Postprocedural hematoma of ear and mastoid process following other procedure
New			H95.53 Postprocedural seroma of ear and mastoid process following a procedure on the ear and mastoid process
New			H95.54 Postprocedural seroma of ear and mastoid process following other procedure

CHAPTER 9   DISEASES OF THE CIRCULATORY SYSTEM (I00-I99)

This chapter contains the following blocks:

Revised	I10-I16	Hypertensive diseases

HYPERTENSIVE DISEASES (I10-I16)

		Use additional code to identify:
Revised		history of tobacco dependence (Z87.891)
New	**Excludes2**	hypertensive disease complicating pregnancy, childbirth and the puerperium (O10-O11, O13-O16)

New	I16	Hypertensive crisis	
New		Code also any identified hypertensive disease (I10-I15)	
New		I16.0	Hypertensive urgency
New		I16.1	Hypertensive emergency
New		I16.9	Hypertensive crisis, unspecified

ISCHEMIC HEART DISEASES (I20-I25)

Revised		Use additional code to identify presence of hypertension (I10-I16)

	I20	Angina pectoris	
		Use additional code to identify:	
Revised		history of tobacco dependence (Z87.891)	
		I20.8	Other forms of angina pectoris
New			Stable angina

	I21	ST elevation (STEMI) and non-ST elevation (NSTEMI) myocardial infarction
	I22	Subsequent ST elevation (STEMI) and non-ST elevation (NSTEMI) myocardial infarction
	I25	Chronic ischemic heart disease
		Use additional code to identify:
Revised		history of tobacco dependence (Z87.891)

	I42	Cardiomyopathy	
Deleted		**Excludes1**	ischemic cardiomyopathy (I25.5)
Deleted			peripartum cardiomyopathy (O90.3)
New		**Excludes2**	ischemic cardiomyopathy (I25.5)
New			peripartum cardiomyopathy (O90.3)
	I50	Heart failure	
Deleted		**Excludes1**	cardiac arrest (I46.-)
New		**Excludes2**	cardiac arrest (I46.-)
		I50.9	Heart failure, unspecified
Deleted			**Excludes1** fluid overload (E87.70)
New			**Excludes2** fluid overload (E87.70)

CEREBROVASCULAR DISEASES (I60-I69)

		Use additional code to identify presence of:
Revised		history of tobacco dependence (Z87.891)

	I60	Nontraumatic subarachnoid hemorrhage	
Deleted		**Excludes1**	sequelae of subarachnoid hemorrhage (I69.0-)
New		**Excludes2**	sequelae of subarachnoid hemorrhage (I69.0-)
		I60.2	Nontraumatic subarachnoid hemorrhage from anterior communicating artery
Deleted			I60.20 Nontraumatic subarachnoid hemorrhage from unspecified anterior communicating artery
Deleted			I60.21 Nontraumatic subarachnoid hemorrhage from right anterior communicating artery
Deleted			I60.22 Nontraumatic subarachnoid hemorrhage from left anterior communicating artery
	I61	Nontraumatic intracerebral hemorrhage	
Deleted		**Excludes1**	sequelae of intracerebral hemorrhage (I69.1-)
New		**Excludes2**	sequelae of intracerebral hemorrhage (I69.1-)

	I62	**Other and unspecified nontraumatic intracranial hemorrhage**
Deleted		**Excludes1** sequelae of intracerebral hemorrhage (I69.2)
New		**Excludes2** sequelae of intracranial hemorrhage (I69.2)

	I63	**Cerebral infarction**
New		Use additional code, if known, to indicate National Institutes of Health Stroke Scale (NIHSS) score (R29.7-)
Deleted		**Excludes1** sequelae of cerebral infarction (I69.3-)
New		**Excludes2** sequelae of cerebral infarction (I69.3-)

New	I63.013	Cerebral infarction due to thrombosis of bilateral vertebral arteries
	I63.03	Cerebral infarction due to thrombosis of carotid artery
New	I63.033	Cerebral infarction due to thrombosis of bilateral carotid arteries
New	I63.113	Cerebral infarction due to embolism of bilateral vertebral arteries
New	I63.133	Cerebral infarction due to embolism of bilateral carotid arteries
New	I63.213	Cerebral infarction due to unspecified occlusion or stenosis of bilateral vertebral arteries
New	I63.233	Cerebral infarction due to unspecified occlusion or stenosis of bilateral carotid arteries
New	I63.313	Cerebral infarction due to thrombosis of bilateral middle cerebral arteries
New	I63.323	Cerebral infarction due to thrombosis of bilateral anterior arteries
New	I63.333	Cerebral infarction to thrombosis of bilateral posterior arteries
New	I63.343	Cerebral infarction to thrombosis of bilateral cerebellar arteries
New	I63.413	Cerebral infarction due to embolism of bilateral middle cerebral arteries
New	I63.423	Cerebral infarction due to embolism of bilateral anterior cerebral arteries
New	I63.433	Cerebral infarction due to embolism of bilateral posterior cerebral arteries
New	I63.443	Cerebral infarction due to embolism of bilateral cerebellar arteries
New	I63.513	Cerebral infarction due to unspecified occlusion or stenosis of bilateral middle arteries
New	I63.523	Cerebral infarction due to unspecified occlusion or stenosis of bilateral anterior arteries
New	I63.533	Cerebral infarction due to unspecified occlusion or stenosis of bilateral posterior arteries
New	I63.543	Cerebral infarction due to unspecified occlusion or stenosis of bilateral cerebellar arteries

	I67	**Other cerebrovascular diseases**
Deleted		**Excludes1** sequelae of the listed conditions (I69.8)
New		**Excludes2** sequelae of the listed conditions (I69.8)

New	I69.010	Attention and concentration deficit following nontraumatic subarachnoid hemorrhage
New	I69.011	Memory deficit following nontraumatic subarachnoid hemorrhage
New	I69.012	Visuospatial deficit and spatial neglect following nontraumatic subarachnoid hemorrhage
New	I69.013	Psychomotor deficit following nontraumatic subarachnoid hemorrhage
New	I69.014	Frontal lobe and executive function deficit following nontraumatic subarachnoid hemorrhage
New	I69.015	Cognitive social or emotional deficit following nontraumatic subarachnoid hemorrhage
New	I69.018	Other symptoms and signs involving cognitive functions following nontraumatic subarachnoid hemorrhage
New	I69.019	Unspecified symptoms and signs involving cognitive functions following nontraumatic subarachnoid hemorrhage
New	I69.110	Attention and concentration deficit following nontraumatic intracerebral hemorrhage
New	I69.111	Memory deficit following nontraumatic intracerebral hemorrhage
New	I69.112	Visuospatial deficit and spatial neglect following nontraumatic intracerebral hemorrhage
New	I69.113	Psychomotor deficit following nontraumatic intracerebral hemorrhage
New	I69.114	Frontal lobe and executive function deficit following nontraumatic intracerebral hemorrhage
New	I69.115	Cognitive social or emotional deficit following nontraumatic intracerebral hemorrhage
New	I69.118	Other symptoms and signs involving cognitive functions following nontraumatic intracerebral hemorrhage
New	I69.119	Unspecified symptoms and signs involving cognitive functions following nontraumatic intracerebral hemorrhage
	I69.123	Fluency disorder following nontraumatic intracerebral hemorrhage
Revised		Stuttering following nontraumatic intracerebral hemorrhage

I69.21 Cognitive deficits following other nontraumatic intracranial hemorrhage

New   I69.210 Attention and concentration deficit following other nontraumatic intracranial hemorrhage

New   I69.211 Memory deficit following other nontraumatic intracranial hemorrhage

New   I69.212 Visuospatial deficit and spatial neglect following other nontraumatic intracranial hemorrhage

New   I69.213 Psychomotor deficit following other nontraumatic intracranial hemorrhage

New   I69.214 Frontal lobe and executive function deficit following other nontraumatic intracranial hemorrhage

New   I69.215 Cognitive social or emotional deficit following other nontraumatic intracranial hemorrhage

New   I69.218 Other symptoms and signs involving cognitive functions following other nontraumatic intracranial hemorrhage

New   I69.219 Unspecified symptoms and signs involving cognitive functions following other nontraumatic intracranial hemorrhage

I69.223 Fluency disorder following other nontraumatic intracranial hemorrhage

Revised   Stuttering following other nontraumatic intracranial hemorrhage

New   I69.310 Attention and concentration deficit following cerebral infarction

New   I69.311 Memory deficit following cerebral infarction

New   I69.312 Visuospatial deficit and spatial neglect following cerebral infarction

New   I69.313 Psychomotor deficit following cerebral infarction

New   I69.314 Frontal lobe and executive function deficit following cerebral infarction

New   I69.315 Cognitive social or emotional deficit following cerebral infarction

New   I69.318 Other symptoms and signs involving cognitive functions following cerebral infarction

New   I69.319 Unspecified symptoms and signs involving cognitive functions following cerebral infarction

I69.323 Fluency disorder following cerebral infarction

Revised   Stuttering following cerebral infarction

New   I69.810 Attention and concentration deficit following other cerebrovascular disease

New   I69.811 Memory deficit following other cerebrovascular disease

New   I69.812 Visuospatial deficit and spatial neglect following other cerebrovascular disease

New   I69.813 Psychomotor deficit following other cerebrovascular disease

New   I69.814 Frontal lobe and executive function deficit following other cerebrovascular disease

New   I69.815 Cognitive social or emotional deficit following other cerebrovascular disease

New   I69.818 Other symptoms and signs involving cognitive functions following other cerebrovascular disease

New   I69.819 Unspecified symptoms and signs involving cognitive functions following other cerebrovascular disease

I69.823 Fluency disorder following other cerebrovascular disease

Revised   Stuttering following other cerebrovascular disease

New   I69.910 Attention and concentration deficit following unspecified cerebrovascular disease

New   I69.911 Memory deficit following unspecified cerebrovascular disease

New   I69.912 Visuospatial deficit and spatial neglect following unspecified cerebrovascular disease

New   I69.913 Psychomotor deficit following unspecified cerebrovascular disease

New   I69.914 Frontal lobe and executive function deficit following unspecified cerebrovascular disease

New   I69.915 Cognitive social or emotional deficit following unspecified cerebrovascular disease

New   I69.918 Other symptoms and signs involving cognitive functions following unspecified cerebrovascular disease

New   I69.919 Unspecified symptoms and signs involving cognitive functions following unspecified cerebrovascular disease

I69.923 Fluency disorder following unspecified cerebrovascular disease

Revised   Stuttering following unspecified cerebrovascular disease

I70   Atherosclerosis

   Use additional code to identify:

Revised   history of tobacco dependence (Z87.891)

I72   Other aneurysm

New   **Excludes2** dissection of precerebral artery, congenital (nonruptured) (Q28.1)

New   I72.5   Aneurysm of other precerebral arteries
New   Aneurysm of basilar artery (trunk)
New   **Excludes2** aneurysm of carotid artery (I72.Ø)
New   aneurysm of vertebral artery (I72.6)
New   dissection of carotid artery (I77.71)
New   dissection of other precerebral arteries (I77.75)
New   dissection of vertebral artery (I77.74)

New   I72.6   Aneurysm of vertebral artery
New   **Excludes2** dissection of vertebral artery (I77.74)

I74   Arterial embolism and thrombosis

Revised   **Excludes2** mesenteric embolism and thrombosis (K55.Ø-)

New		I77.70	Dissection of unspecified artery
		I77.74	Dissection of vertebral artery
New			**Excludes2** aneurysm of vertebral artery (I72.6)
New		I77.75	Dissection of other precerebral arteries
New			Dissection of basilar artery (trunk)
New			**Excludes2** aneurysm of carotid artery (I72.0)
New			aneurysm of other precerebral arteries (I72.5)
New			aneurysm of vertebral artery (I72.6)
New			dissection of carotid artery (I77.71)
New			dissection of vertebral artery (I77.74)
New		I77.76	Dissection of artery of upper extremity
New		I77.77	Dissection of artery of lower extremity
Revised		I77.79	Dissection of other specified artery
	I82	**Other venous embolism and thrombosis**	
Revised		**Excludes2** mesenteric (K55.0-)	
Deleted	**I83.1**	**Varicose veins of lower extremities with inflammation**	
		Stasis dermatitis	
New	**I87.2**	**Venous insufficiency (chronic) (peripheral)**	
		Stasis dermatitis	
New		**Excludes1** stasis dermatitis with varicose veins of lower extremities (I83.1-, I83.2-)	
	I89	**Other noninfective disorders of lymphatic vessels and lymph nodes**	
Revised		**Excludes1** chylocele, tunica vaginalis (nonfilarial) NOS (N50.89)	
	I96	**Gangrene, not elsewhere classified**	
Revised		**Excludes1** gangrene in diabetes mellitus (E08-E13 with .52)	
Revised	**I97.6**	**Postprocedural hemorrhage, hematoma and seroma of a circulatory system organ or structure following a procedure**	
Revised		I97.61	Postprocedural hemorrhage of a circulatory system organ or structure following a circulatory system procedure
Revised			I97.610 Postprocedural hemorrhage of a circulatory system organ or structure following a cardiac catheterization
Revised			I97.611 Postprocedural hemorrhage of a circulatory system organ or structure following cardiac bypass
Revised			I97.618 Postprocedural hemorrhage of a circulatory system organ or structure following other circulatory system procedure
Revised		I97.62	Postprocedural hemorrhage, hematoma and seroma of a circulatory system organ or structure following other procedure
New			I97.620 Postprocedural hemorrhage of a circulatory system organ or structure following other procedure
New			I97.621 Postprocedural hematoma of a circulatory system organ or structure following other procedure
New			I97.622 Postprocedural seroma of a circulatory system organ or structure following other procedure

New		I97.63	Postprocedural hematoma of a circulatory system organ or structure following a circulatory system procedure
New			I97.630 Postprocedural hematoma of a circulatory system organ or structure following a cardiac catheterization
New			I97.631 Postprocedural hematoma of a circulatory system organ or structure following cardiac bypass
New			I97.638 Postprocedural hematoma of a circulatory system organ or structure following other circulatory system procedure
New		I97.64	Postprocedural seroma of a circulatory system organ or structure following a circulatory system procedure
New			I97.640 Postprocedural seroma of a circulatory system organ or structure following a cardiac catheterization
New			I97.641 Postprocedural seroma of a circulatory system organ or structure following cardiac bypass
New			I97.648 Postprocedural seroma of a circulatory system organ or structure following other circulatory system procedure
Revised		I97.820	Postprocedural cerebrovascular infarction following cardiac surgery
Revised		I97.821	Postprocedural cerebrovascular infarction following other surgery

CHAPTER 10

DISEASES OF THE RESPIRATORY SYSTEM (J00-J99)

J31	Chronic rhinitis, nasopharyngitis and pharyngitis
J32	Chronic sinusitis
J33	Nasal polyp
J35	Chronic diseases of tonsils and adenoids
J37	Chronic laryngitis and laryngotracheitis
J38	Diseases of vocal cords and larynx, not elsewhere classified
J40	Bronchitis, not specified as acute or chronic
J41	Simple and mucopurulent chronic bronchitis
J42	Unspecified chronic bronchitis
J43	Emphysema
J44	Other chronic obstructive pulmonary disease

Revised	Use additional code to identify: history of tobacco dependence (Z87.891)
Deleted	**Excludes1** lung diseases due to external agents (J60-J70)
New	**Excludes2** lung diseases due to external agents (J60-J70)

	J45	Asthma
	J47	Bronchiectasis
Revised		Use additional code to identify: history of tobacco dependence (Z87.891)
		J47.0 Bronchiectasis with acute lower respiratory infection
New		Use additional code to identify the infection
	J81	Pulmonary edema
Revised		Use additional code to identify: history of tobacco dependence (Z87.891)

		J84.89	Other specified interstitial pulmonary diseases
Deleted			Organizing pneumonia due to known underlying cause
Revised		J95.83	Postprocedural hemorrhage of a respiratory system organ or structure following a procedure
Revised		J95.830	Postprocedural hemorrhage of a respiratory system organ or structure following a respiratory system procedure
Revised		J95.831	Postprocedural hemorrhage of a respiratory system organ or structure following other procedure
New		J95.86	Postprocedural hematoma and seroma of a respiratory system organ or structure following a procedure
New		J95.860	Postprocedural hematoma of a respiratory system organ or structure following a respiratory system procedure
New		J95.861	Postprocedural hematoma of a respiratory system organ or structure following other procedure
New		J95.862	Postprocedural seroma of a respiratory system organ or structure following a respiratory system procedure
New		J95.863	Postprocedural seroma of a respiratory system organ or structure following other procedure

J98   **Other respiratory disorders**

Use additional code to identify:

Revised   history of tobacco dependence (Z87.891)

J98.5   **Diseases of mediastinum, not elsewhere classified**

Deleted	Fibrosis of mediastinum
Deleted	Hernia of mediastinum
Deleted	Retraction of mediastinum
Deleted	Mediastinitis

New	J98.51	**Mediastinitis**
New		Code first underlying condition, if applicable, such as postoperative mediastinitis (T81.-)
New	J98.59	**Other diseases of mediastinum, not elsewhere classified**
New		Fibrosis of mediastinum
New		Hernia of mediastinum
New		Retraction of mediastinum

CHAPTER 11

DISEASES OF THE DIGESTIVE SYSTEM (K00-K95)

K02   **Dental caries**

New	**Includes**	caries of dentine
New		dental cavities
New		early childhood caries
New		pre-eruptive caries
New		recurrent caries (dentino enamel junction) (enamel) (to the pulp)

	K02.52	**Dental caries on pit and fissure surface penetrating into dentin**
New		Primary dental caries, cervical origin

K04.0   **Pulpitis**

Deleted	Reversible pulpitis
Deleted	Irreversible pulpitis
New	K04.01	**Reversible pulpitis**
New	K04.02	**Irreversible pulpitis**

K05   **Gingivitis and periodontal diseases**

Use additional code to identify:

Revised   history of tobacco dependence (Z87.891)

	K05.00	**Acute gingivitis, plaque induced**
New		Plaque induced gingival disease

K05.1   **Chronic gingivitis**

New		Pregnancy associated gingivitis
New		Code first, if applicable, diseases of the digestive system complicating pregnancy (O99.61-)
New	K05.211	Aggressive periodontitis, localized, slight
New	K05.212	Aggressive periodontitis, localized, moderate
New	K05.213	Aggressive periodontitis, localized, severe
New	K05.219	Aggressive periodontitis, localized, unspecified severity
New	K05.221	Aggressive periodontitis, generalized, slight
New	K05.222	Aggressive periodontitis, generalized, moderate
New	K05.223	Aggressive periodontitis, generalized, severe
New	K05.229	Aggressive periodontitis, generalized, unspecified severity
New	K05.311	Chronic periodontitis, localized, slight
New	K05.312	Chronic periodontitis, localized, moderate
New	K05.313	Chronic periodontitis, localized, severe
New	K05.319	Chronic periodontitis, localized, unspecified severity
New	K05.321	Chronic periodontitis, generalized, slight
New	K05.322	Chronic periodontitis, generalized, moderate
New	K05.323	Chronic periodontitis, generalized, severe
New	K05.329	Chronic periodontitis, generalized, unspecified severity

K05.5   **Other periodontal diseases**

New	Combined periodontic-endodontic lesion
New	Narrow gingival width (of periodontal soft tissue)

New	K06.3	**Horizontal alveolar bone loss**

K06.8   **Other specified disorders of gingiva and edentulous alveolar ridge**

New	Vertical ridge deficiency

K08.8   **Other specified disorders of teeth and supporting structures**

Deleted	Enlargement of alveolar ridge NOS
Deleted	Irregular alveolar process
Deleted	Toothache NOS

New	K08.81	**Primary occlusal trauma**
New	K08.82	**Secondary occlusal trauma**
New	K08.89	**Other specified disorders of teeth and supporting structures**
New		Enlargement of alveolar ridge NOS
New		Insufficient anatomic crown height
New		Insufficient clinical crown length
New		Irregular alveolar process
New		Toothache NOS

K11	**Diseases of salivary glands**
K12	**Stomatitis and related lesions**
K13	**Other diseases of lip and oral mucosa**
K14	**Diseases of tongue**

Use additional code to identify:

Revised   history of tobacco dependence (Z87.891)

	K35.3	**Acute appendicitis with localized peritonitis**
Revised		Acute appendicitis with or without perforation or rupture with peritonitis NOS

NONINFECTIVE ENTERITIS AND COLITIS (K50–K52)

Revised   **Excludes1** megacolon (K59.3-)

K52.2 Allergic and dietetic gastroenteritis and colitis

New   **Excludes2** allergic eosinophilic colitis (K52.82)
New   allergic eosinophilic esophagitis (K20.0)
New   allergic eosinophilic gastritis (K52.81)
New   allergic eosinophilic gastroenteritis (K52.81)
New   food protein-induced proctocolitis (K52.82)

New   **K52.21 Food protein-induced enterocolitis syndrome**
New   Use additional code for hypovolemic shock, if present (R57.1)

New   **K52.22 Food protein-induced enteropathy**

K52.29 Other allergic and dietetic gastroenteritis and colitis
New   Food hypersensitivity gastroenteritis or colitis
New   Immediate gastrointestinal hypersensitivity

New   **K52.3 Indeterminate colitis**
New   Colonic inflammatory bowel disease unclassified (IBDU)
New   **Excludes1** unspecified colitis (K52.9)

K52.81 Eosinophilic gastritis or gastroenteritis
            Eosinophilic enteritis
Deleted   **Excludes1** eosinophilic esophagitis (K20.0)
New   **Excludes2** eosinophilic esophagitis (K20.0)

K52.82 Eosinophilic colitis
New   Allergic proctocolitis
New   Food-induced eosinophilic proctocolitis
New   Food protein-induced proctocolitis
New   Milk protein-induced proctocolitis

New   **K52.83 Microscopic colitis**
New   **K52.831 Collagenous colitis**
New   **K52.832 Lymphocytic colitis**
New   **K52.838 Other microscopic colitis**
New   **K52.839 Microscopic colitis, unspecified**

K52.89 Other specified noninfective gastroenteritis and colitis
Deleted   Collagenous colitis
Deleted   Lymphocytic colitis
Deleted   Microscopic colitis (collagenous or lymphocytic)

K55.0 Acute vascular disorders of intestine
Deleted   Acute fulminant ischemic colitis
Deleted   Acute intestinal infarction
Deleted   Acute small intestine ischemia
Deleted   Necrosis of intestine
Deleted   Subacute ischemic colitis

New   **K55.01 Acute (reversible) ischemia of small intestine**
New   **K55.011 Focal (segmental) acute (reversible) ischemia of small intestine**
New   **K55.012 Diffuse acute (reversible) ischemia of small intestine**
New   **K55.019 Acute (reversible) ischemia of small intestine, extent unspecified**

New   **K55.02 Acute infarction of small intestine**
New   Gangrene of small intestine
New   Necrosis of small intestine
New   **K55.021 Focal (segmental) acute infarction of small intestine**
New   **K55.022 Diffuse acute infarction of small intestine**
New   **K55.029 Acute infarction of small intestine, extent unspecified**

New   **K55.03 Acute (reversible) ischemia of large intestine**
New   Acute fulminant ischemic colitis
New   Subacute ischemic colitis
New   **K55.031 Focal (segmental) acute (reversible) ischemia of large intestine**
New   **K55.032 Diffuse acute (reversible) ischemia of large intestine**
New   **K55.039 Acute (reversible) ischemia of large intestine, extent unspecified**

New   **K55.04 Acute infarction of large intestine**
New   Gangrene of large intestine
New   Necrosis of large intestine
New   **K55.041 Focal (segmental) acute infarction of large intestine**
New   **K55.042 Diffuse acute infarction of large intestine**
New   **K55.049 Acute infarction of large intestine, extent unspecified**

New   **K55.05 Acute (reversible) ischemia of intestine, part unspecified**
New   **K55.051 Focal (segmental) acute (reversible) ischemia of intestine, part unspecified**
New   **K55.052 Diffuse acute (reversible) ischemia of intestine, part unspecified**
New   **K55.059 Acute (reversible) ischemia of intestine, part and extent unspecified**

New   **K55.06 Acute infarction of intestine, part unspecified**
New   Acute intestinal infarction
New   Gangrene of intestine
New   Necrosis of intestine
New   **K55.061 Focal (segmental) acute infarction of intestine, part unspecified**
New   **K55.062 Diffuse acute infarction of intestine, part unspecified**
New   **K55.069 Acute infarction of intestine, part and extent unspecified**

New   **K55.3 Necrotizing enterocolitis**
New   **Excludes1** necrotizing enterocolitis of newborn (P77.-)
New   **Excludes2** necrotizing enterocolitis due to Clostridium difficile (A04.7)
New   **K55.30 Necrotizing enterocolitis, unspecified**
New   Necrotizing enterocolitis, NOS
New   **K55.31 Stage 1 necrotizing enterocolitis**
New   Necrotizing enterocolitis without pneumatosis, without perforation
New   **K55.32 Stage 2 necrotizing enterocolitis**
New   Necrotizing enterocolitis with pneumatosis, without perforation
New   **K55.33 Stage 3 necrotizing enterocolitis**
New   Necrotizing enterocolitis with perforation
New   Necrotizing enterocolitis with pneumatosis and perforation

New   **K58.1 Irritable bowel syndrome with constipation**
New   **K58.2 Mixed irritable bowel syndrome**
New   **K58.8 Other irritable bowel syndrome**

K59.0 Constipation
New   Use additional code for adverse effect, if applicable, to identify drug (T36-T50 with fifth or sixth character 5)

New   **K59.03 Drug induced constipation**
New   Use additional code for adverse effect, if applicable, to identify drug (T36-T50 with fifth or sixth character 5)

New   **K59.04 Chronic idiopathic constipation**
New   Functional constipation

New   **K59.09 Other constipation**
New   Chronic constipation

	K59.3	**Megacolon, not elsewhere classified**
Deleted		Toxic colon
New	**K59.31**	**Toxic megacolon**
New	**K59.39**	**Other megacolon**
New		Megacolon NOS

K72 Hepatic failure, not elsewhere classified

Deleted **Includes** acute hepatitis NEC, with hepatic failure
Deleted **Excludes1** viral hepatitis with hepatic coma (B15-B19)
New **Excludes2** viral hepatitis with hepatic coma (B15-B19)

K72.0 Acute and subacute hepatic failure
New Acute non-viral hepatitis NOS

K75.0 Abscess of liver
New **Excludes2** acute or subacute hepatitis NOS (B17.9)
New acute or subacute non-viral hepatitis (K72.0)
New chronic hepatitis NEC (K73.8)

K76.7 Hepatorenal syndrome
Revised **Excludes1** postprocedural hepatorenal syndrome (K91.83)

K85 Acute pancreatitis
Deleted **Includes** abscess of pancreas
Deleted acute necrosis of pancreas
Deleted gangrene of (gangrenous) pancreas
Deleted hemorrhagic pancreatitis
Deleted infective necrosis of pancreas
Deleted suppurative pancreatitis

New **K85.00 Idiopathic acute pancreatitis without necrosis or infection**
New **K85.01 Idiopathic acute pancreatitis with uninfected necrosis**
New **K85.02 Idiopathic acute pancreatitis with infected necrosis**
New **K85.10 Biliary acute pancreatitis without necrosis or infection**
New **K85.11 Biliary acute pancreatitis with uninfected necrosis**
New **K85.12 Biliary acute pancreatitis with infected necrosis**
New **K85.20 Alcohol induced acute pancreatitis without necrosis or infection**
New **K85.21 Alcohol induced acute pancreatitis with uninfected necrosis**
New **K85.22 Alcohol induced acute pancreatitis with infected necrosis**
New **K85.30 Drug induced acute pancreatitis without necrosis or infection**
New **K85.31 Drug induced acute pancreatitis with uninfected necrosis**
New **K85.32 Drug induced acute pancreatitis with infected necrosis**
New **K85.80 Other acute pancreatitis without necrosis or infection**
New **K85.81 Other acute pancreatitis with uninfected necrosis**
New **K85.82 Other acute pancreatitis with infected necrosis**
New **K85.90 Acute pancreatitis without necrosis or infection, unspecified**
New **K85.91 Acute pancreatitis with uninfected necrosis, unspecified**
New **K85.92 Acute pancreatitis with infected necrosis, unspecified**

K86.0 Alcohol-induced chronic pancreatitis
New Code also exocrine pancreatic insufficiency (K86.81)
Revised **Excludes2** alcohol induced acute pancreatitis (K85.2-)

K86.1 Other chronic pancreatitis
New Code also exocrine pancreatic insufficiency (K86.81)

K86.8 Other specified diseases of pancreas
Deleted Aseptic pancreatic necrosis
Deleted Atrophy of pancreas
Deleted Calculus of pancreas
Deleted Cirrhosis of pancreas
Deleted Fibrosis of pancreas
Deleted Pancreatic fat necrosis
Deleted Pancreatic infantilism
Deleted Pancreatic necrosis NOS

New **K86.81 Exocrine pancreatic insufficiency**
New **K86.89 Other specified diseases of pancreas**
New Aseptic pancreatic necrosis, unrelated to acute pancreatitis
New Atrophy of pancreas
New Calculus of pancreas
New Cirrhosis of pancreas
New Fibrosis of pancreas
New Pancreatic fat necrosis, unrelated to acute pancreatitis
New Pancreatic infantilism
New Pancreatic necrosis NOS, unrelated to acute pancreatitis

K90.0 Celiac disease
New Celiac disease with steatorrhea
Deleted Idiopathic steatorrhea
New Code also exocrine pancreatic insufficiency (K86.81)

K90.4 Other malabsorption due to intolerance
Deleted Malabsorption due to intolerance to carbohydrate
Deleted Malabsorption due to intolerance to fat
Deleted Malabsorption due to intolerance to protein
Deleted Malabsorption due to intolerance to starch
New **K90.41 Non-celiac gluten sensitivity**
New Gluten sensitivity NOS
New Non-celiac gluten sensitive enteropathy
New **K90.49 Malabsorption due to intolerance, not elsewhere classified**
New Malabsorption due to intolerance to carbohydrate
New Malabsorption due to intolerance to fat
New Malabsorption due to intolerance to protein
New Malabsorption due to intolerance to starch

Revised **K91.61 Intraoperative hemorrhage and hematoma of a digestive system organ or structure complicating a digestive system procedure**

Revised **K91.84 Postprocedural hemorrhage of a digestive system organ or structure following a procedure**
Revised **K91.840 Postprocedural hemorrhage of a digestive system organ or structure following a digestive system procedure**
Revised **K91.841 Postprocedural hemorrhage of a digestive system organ or structure following other procedure**

New **K91.87 Postprocedural hematoma and seroma of a digestive system organ or structure following a procedure**
New **K91.870 Postprocedural hematoma of a digestive system organ or structure following a digestive system procedure**
New **K91.871 Postprocedural hematoma of a digestive system organ or structure following other procedure**

New | K91.872 | Postprocedural seroma of a digestive system organ or structure following a digestive system procedure

New | K91.873 | Postprocedural seroma of a digestive system organ or structure following other procedure

CHAPTER 12

DISEASES OF THE SKIN AND SUBCUTANEOUS TISSUE (L00-L99)

L02.2 Cutaneous abscess, furuncle and carbuncle of trunk

Revised | Excludes2 | abscess of breast (N61.1)

L03.211 Cellulitis of face

New | Excludes2 | abscess of orbit (H05.01-)
Revised | | cellulitis of orbit (H05.01-)

L03.213 Periorbital cellulitis
New | Preseptal cellulitis

L03.31 Cellulitis of trunk

Revised | Excludes2 | cellulitis of breast NOS (N61.0)

L05.01 Pilonidal cyst with abscess

Deleted | Parasacral dimple with abscess
New | Excludes2 | congenital sacral dimple (Q82.6)
New | | parasacral dimple (Q82.6)

L05.91 Pilonidal cyst without abscess

Deleted | Parasacral dimple
New | Excludes2 | congenital sacral dimple (Q82.6)
New | | parasacral dimple (Q82.6)

DERMATITIS AND ECZEMA (L20-L30)

Revised | Excludes2 | stasis dermatitis (I87.2)

L30 Other and unspecified dermatitis

Revised | Excludes2 | stasis dermatitis (I87.2)

L50.2 Urticaria due to cold and heat

New | Excludes2 | familial cold urticaria (M04.2)

L70 Acne

Revised | **L70.5 Acné excoriée**
New | Acné excoriée des jeunes filles

Revised | **L76.2 Postprocedural hemorrhage of skin and subcutaneous tissue following a procedure**

Revised | **L76.21 Postprocedural hemorrhage of skin and subcutaneous tissue following a dermatologic procedure**

Revised | **L76.22 Postprocedural hemorrhage of skin and subcutaneous tissue following other procedure**

New | **L76.3 Postprocedural hematoma and seroma of skin and subcutaneous tissue following a procedure**

New | **L76.31 Postprocedural hematoma of skin and subcutaneous tissue following a dermatologic procedure**

New | **L76.32 Postprocedural hematoma of skin and subcutaneous tissue following other procedure**

New | **L76.33 Postprocedural seroma of skin and subcutaneous tissue following a dermatologic procedure**

New | **L76.34 Postprocedural seroma of skin and subcutaneous tissue following other procedure**

L82 Seborrheic keratosis
New | Includes | basal cell papilloma

L89.521 Pressure ulcer of left ankle, stage 1
Revised | Pressure pre-ulcer skin changes limited to persistent focal edema, left ankle

L98.1 Factitial dermatitis
New | Excludes1 | Excoriation (skin-picking) disorder (F42.4)

L98.7 Excessive and redundant skin and subcutaneous tissue
New | Loose or sagging skin following bariatric surgery weight loss
New | Loose or sagging skin following dietary weight loss
New | Loose or sagging skin, NOS
New | Excludes2 | acquired excess or redundant skin of eyelid (H02.3-)
New | | congenital excess or redundant skin of eyelid (Q10.3)
New | | skin changes due to chronic exposure to nonionizing radiation (L57.-)

CHAPTER 13

DISEASES OF THE MUSCULOSKELETAL SYSTEM AND CONNECTIVE TISSUE (M00-M99)

This chapter contains the following blocks:

New | M04 | Autoinflammatory syndromes
New | M97 | Periprosthetic fracture around internal prosthetic joint

AUTOINFLAMMATORY SYNDROMES (M04)

New | **M04 Autoinflammatory syndromes**
New | Excludes2 | Crohn's disease (K50.-)
New | **M04.1 Periodic fever syndromes**
New | Familial Mediterranean fever
New | Hyperimmunoglobin D syndrome
New | Mevalonate kinase deficiency
New | Tumor necrosis factor receptor associated periodic syndrome [TRAPS]
New | **M04.2 Cryopyrin-associated periodic syndromes**
New | Chronic infantile neurological, cutaneous and articular syndrome [CINCA]
New | Familial cold autoinflammatory syndrome
New | Familial cold urticaria
New | Muckle-Wells syndrome
New | Neonatal onset multisystemic inflammatory disorder [NOMID]
New | **M04.8 Other autoinflammatory syndromes**
New | Blau syndrome
New | Deficiency of interleukin 1 receptor antagonist [DIRA]
New | Majeed syndrome
New | Periodic fever, aphthous stomatitis, pharyngitis, and adenopathy syndrome [PFAPA]
New | Pyogenic arthritis, pyoderma gangrenosum, and acne syndrome [PAPA]
New | **M04.9 Autoinflammatory syndrome, unspecified**

M1A Chronic gout
Deleted | Excludes1 | acute gout (M10.-)
New | Excludes2 | acute gout (M10.-)

M10 Gout
Deleted | Gout NOS
Deleted | Excludes1 | chronic gout (M1A.-)
New | Excludes2 | chronic gout (M1A.-)

M20.1 Hallux valgus (acquired)
Deleted | Bunion
New | Excludes2 | bunion (M21.6-)

M21.1 Varus deformity, not elsewhere classified
Revised | Excludes1 | metatarsus varus (Q66.22)

	M21.6	Other acquired deformities of foot		
Revised		**Excludes2**	deformities of toe (acquired) (M20.1-M20.6-)	
New		M21.61	Bunion	
New			M21.611	Bunion of right foot
New			M21.612	Bunion of left foot
New			M21.619	Bunion of unspecified foot
New		M21.62	Bunionette	
New			M21.621	Bunionette of right foot
New			M21.622	Bunionette of left foot
New			M21.629	Bunionette of unspecified foot

New	M25.5	Pain in joint		
New		M25.54	Pain in joints of hand	
New			M25.541	Pain in joints of right hand
New			M25.542	Pain in joints of left hand
New			M25.549	Pain in joints of unspecified hand
New				Pain in joints of hand NOS
New			M26.601	Right temporomandibular joint disorder, unspecified
New			M26.602	Left temporomandibular joint disorder, unspecified
New			M26.603	Bilateral temporomandibular joint disorder, unspecified
New			M26.609	Unspecified temporomandibular joint disorder, unspecified side
New				Temporomandibular joint disorder NOS
New			M26.611	Adhesions and ankylosis of right temporomandibular joint
New			M26.612	Adhesions and ankylosis of left temporomandibular joint
New			M26.613	Adhesions and ankylosis of bilateral temporomandibular joint
New			M26.619	Adhesions and ankylosis of temporomandibular joint, unspecified side
New			M26.621	Arthralgia of right temporomandibular joint
New			M26.622	Arthralgia of left temporomandibular joint
New			M26.623	Arthralgia of bilateral temporomandibular joint
New			M26.629	Arthralgia of temporomandibular joint, unspecified side
New			M26.631	Articular disc disorder of right temporomandibular joint
New			M26.632	Articular disc disorder of left temporomandibular joint
New			M26.633	Articular disc disorder of bilateral temporomandibular joint
New			M26.639	Articular disc disorder of temporomandibular joint, unspecified side

	M48.5	Collapsed vertebra, not elsewhere classified		
New				Compression fracture of vertebra NOS
		M50.02	Cervical disc disorder with myelopathy, mid-cervical region	
Deleted				C4-C5 disc disorder with myelopathy
Deleted				C5-C6 disc disorder with myelopathy
Deleted				C6-C7 disc disorder with myelopathy
			M50.020	Cervical disc disorder with myelopathy, mid-cervical region, unspecified level

			M50.021	Cervical disc disorder at C4-C5 level with myelopathy
				C4-C5 disc disorder with myelopathy
			M50.022	Cervical disc disorder at C5-C6 level with myelopathy
				C5-C6 disc disorder with myelopathy
			M50.023	Cervical disc disorder at C6-C7 level with myelopathy
				C6-C7 disc disorder with myelopathy
		M50.12	Cervical disc disorder with radiculopathy, mid-cervical region	
Deleted				C4-C5 disc disorder with radiculopathy
Deleted				C5 radiculopathy due to disc disorder
Deleted				C5-C6 disc disorder with radiculopathy
Deleted				C6 radiculopathy due to disc disorder
Deleted				C6-C7 disc disorder with radiculopathy
Deleted				C7 radiculopathy due to disc disorder
New			M50.120	Mid-cervical disc disorder, unspecified
New			M50.121	Cervical disc disorder at C4-C5 level with radiculopathy
New				C4-C5 disc disorder with radiculopathy
New				C5 radiculopathy due to disc disorder
New			M50.122	Cervical disc disorder at C5-C6 level with radiculopathy
New				C5-C6 disc disorder with radiculopathy
New				C6 radiculopathy due to disc disorder
New			M50.123	Cervical disc disorder at C6-C7 level with radiculopathy
New				C6-C7 disc disorder with radiculopathy
New				C7 radiculopathy due to disc disorder
		M50.22	Other cervical disc displacement, mid-cervical region	
Deleted				Other C4-C5 cervical disc displacement
Deleted				Other C5-C6 cervical disc displacement
Deleted				Other C6-C7 cervical disc displacement
New			M50.220	Other cervical disc displacement, mid-cervical region, unspecified level
New			M50.221	Other cervical disc displacement at C4-C5 level
New				Other C4-C5 cervical disc displacement
New			M50.222	Other cervical disc displacement at C5-C6 level
New				Other C5-C6 cervical disc displacement
New			M50.223	Other cervical disc displacement at C6-C7 level
New				Other C6-C7 cervical disc displacement
		M50.32	Other cervical disc degeneration, mid-cervical region	
Deleted				Other C4-C5 cervical disc displacement
Deleted				Other C5-C6 cervical disc displacement
Deleted				Other C6-C7 cervical disc displacement
New			M50.320	Other cervical disc degeneration, mid-cervical region, unspecified level
New			M50.321	Other cervical disc degeneration at C4-C5 level
New				Other C4-C5 cervical disc degeneration
New			M50.322	Other cervical disc degeneration at C5-C6 level
New				Other C5-C6 cervical disc degeneration
New			M50.323	Other cervical disc degeneration at C6-C7 level
New				Other C6-C7 cervical disc degeneration

	M50.82 **Other cervical disc disorders, mid-cervical region**
Deleted	Other C4-C5 cervical disc disorders
Deleted	Other C5-C6 cervical disc disorders
Deleted	Other C6-C7 cervical disc disorders
New	**M50.820** **Other cervical disc disorders, mid-cervical region, unspecified level**
New	**M50.821** **Other cervical disc disorders at C4-C5 level**
New	Other C4-C5 cervical disc disorders
New	**M50.822** **Other cervical disc disorders at C5-C6 level**
New	Other C5-C6 cervical disc disorders
New	**M50.823** **Other cervical disc disorders at C6-C7 level**
New	Other C6-C7 cervical disc disorders
	M50.92 **Cervical disc disorder, unspecified, mid-cervical region**
Deleted	C4-C5 cervical disc disorder, unspecified
Deleted	C5-C6 cervical disc disorder, unspecified
Deleted	C6-C7 cervical disc disorder, unspecified
New	**M50.920** **Unspecified cervical disc disorder, mid-cervical region, unspecified level**
New	**M50.921** **Unspecified cervical disc disorder at C4-C5 level**
New	Unspecified C4-C5 cervical disc disorder
New	**M50.922** **Unspecified cervical disc disorder at C5-C6 level**
New	Unspecified C5-C6 cervical disc disorder
New	**M50.923** **Unspecified cervical disc disorder at C6-C7 level**
New	Unspecified C6-C7 cervical disc disorder
	M62.5 **Muscle wasting and atrophy, not elsewhere classified**
New	**Excludes1** sarcopenia (M62.84)
	M62.81 **Muscle weakness (generalized)**
New	**Excludes1** muscle weakness in sarcopenia (M62.84)
New	**M62.84** **Sarcopenia**
New	Age-related sarcopenia
New	*Code first underlying disease, if applicable, such as:*
New	disorders of myoneural junction and muscle disease in diseases classified elsewhere (G73.-)
New	other and unspecified myopathies (G72.-)
New	primary disorders of muscles (G71.-)
	M71.5 **Other bursitis, not elsewhere classified**
Revised	**Excludes2** bursitis of shoulder (M75.5) bursitis of tibial collateral [Pellegrini-Stieda] (M76.4-)
New	**M84.7** **Nontraumatic fracture, not elsewhere classified**
New	**M84.75** **Atypical femoral fracture**
New	The appropriate 7th character is to be added to each code from M84.75:

A	initial encounter for fracture
D	subsequent encounter for fracture with routine healing
G	subsequent encounter for fracture with delayed healing
K	subsequent encounter for fracture with nonunion
P	subsequent encounter for fracture with malunion
S	sequela

New	**M84.750** Atypical femoral fracture, **unspecified**
New	**M84.751** Incomplete atypical femoral fracture, right leg
New	**M84.752** Incomplete atypical femoral fracture, left leg
New	**M84.753** Incomplete atypical femoral fracture, **unspecified** leg
New	**M84.754** Complete transverse atypical femoral fracture, right leg
New	**M84.755** Complete transverse atypical femoral fracture, left leg
New	**M84.756** Complete transverse atypical femoral fracture, **unspecified** leg
New	**M84.757** Complete oblique atypical femoral fracture, right leg
New	**M84.758** Complete oblique atypical femoral fracture, left leg
New	**M84.759** Complete oblique atypical femoral fracture, **unspecified** leg
	M90 **Osteopathies in diseases classified elsewhere**
Revised	**Excludes1** diabetes mellitus (E08-E13 with .69-)
	M96 **Intraoperative and postprocedural complications and disorders of musculoskeletal system, not elsewhere classified**
New	**Excludes2** periprosthetic fracture around internal prosthetic joint (M97.-)
Revised	**M96.83** **Postprocedural hemorrhage of a musculoskeletal structure following a procedure**
Revised	**M96.830** **Postprocedural hemorrhage of a musculoskeletal structure following a musculoskeletal system procedure**
Revised	**M96.831** **Postprocedural hemorrhage of a musculoskeletal structure following other procedure**
New	**M96.84** **Postprocedural hematoma and seroma of a musculoskeletal structure following a procedure**
New	**M96.840** **Postprocedural hematoma of a musculoskeletal structure following a musculoskeletal system procedure**
New	**M96.841** **Postprocedural hematoma of a musculoskeletal structure following other procedure**
New	**M96.842** **Postprocedural seroma of a musculoskeletal structure following a musculoskeletal system procedure**
New	**M96.843** **Postprocedural seroma of a musculoskeletal structure following other procedure**

New	**PERIPROSTHETIC FRACTURE AROUND INTERNAL PROSTHETIC JOINT (M97)**
New	**M97** **Periprosthetic fracture around internal prosthetic joint**
New	**Excludes2** fracture of bone following insertion of orthopedic implant, joint prosthesis or bone plate (M96.6-)
New	breakage (fracture) of prosthetic joint (T84.01-)
New	The appropriate 7th character is to be added to each code from category M97:

A	initial encounter
D	subsequent encounter
S	sequela

(rows marked *New* for A, D, S)

New	**M97.0** **Periprosthetic fracture around internal prosthetic hip joint**
New	**M97.01** **Periprosthetic fracture around internal prosthetic right hip joint**
New	**M97.02** **Periprosthetic fracture around internal prosthetic left hip joint**

New	**M97.1**	**Periprosthetic fracture around internal prosthetic knee joint**
New		**M97.11 Periprosthetic fracture around internal prosthetic right knee joint**
New		**M97.12 Periprosthetic fracture around internal prosthetic left knee joint**
New	**M97.2**	**Periprosthetic fracture around internal prosthetic ankle joint**
New		**M97.21 Periprosthetic fracture around internal prosthetic right ankle joint**
New		**M97.22 Periprosthetic fracture around internal prosthetic left ankle joint**
New	**M97.3**	**Periprosthetic fracture around internal prosthetic shoulder joint**
New		**M97.31 Periprosthetic fracture around internal prosthetic right shoulder joint**
New		**M97.32 Periprosthetic fracture around internal prosthetic left shoulder joint**
New	**M97.4**	**Periprosthetic fracture around internal prosthetic elbow joint**
New		**M97.41 Periprosthetic fracture around internal prosthetic right elbow joint**
New		**M97.42 Periprosthetic fracture around internal prosthetic left elbow joint**
New	**M97.8**	**Periprosthetic fracture around other internal prosthetic joint**
New		Periprosthetic fracture around internal prosthetic finger joint
New		Periprosthetic fracture around internal prosthetic spinal joint
New		Periprosthetic fracture around internal prosthetic toe joint
New		Periprosthetic fracture around internal prosthetic wrist joint
New		Use additional code to identify the joint (Z96.6-)
New	**M97.9**	**Periprosthetic fracture around unspecified internal prosthetic joint**

CHAPTER 14

DISEASES OF THE GENITOURINARY SYSTEM (N00-N99)

Revised	**N10**	**Acute pyelonephritis**
Revised		Acute tubulo-interstitial nephritis
New	**N13.0**	**Hydronephrosis with ureteropelvic junction obstruction**
New		Hydronephrosis due to acquired occlusion of ureteropelvic junction
New		**Excludes2** Hydronephrosis with ureteropelvic junction obstruction due to calculus (N13.2)
Revised	**N13.6**	**Pyonephrosis**
		Conditions in N13.0-N13.5 with infection
	N36.0	**Urethral fistula**
New		**Excludes1** urethroscrotal fistula (N50.89)
	N36.8	**Other specified disorders of urethra**
New		**Excludes1** congenital urethrocele (Q64.7)
New		female urethrocele (N81.0)
	N39.42	**Incontinence without sensory awareness**
		Insensible (urinary) incontinence
	N39.49	**Other specified urinary incontinence**
New		**N39.491 Coital incontinence**
New		**N39.492 Postural (urinary) incontinence**
	N40	**Benign prostatic hyperplasia**
Deleted		**Includes** benign prostatic hyperplasia
New		enlarged prostate
Revised	**N40.0**	**Benign prostatic hyperplasia without lower urinary tract symptoms**
Revised	**N40.1**	**Benign prostatic hyperplasia with lower urinary tract symptoms**

	N42.3	**Dysplasia of prostate**
Deleted		Prostatic intraepithelial neoplasia I (PIN I)
Deleted		Prostatic intraepithelial neoplasia II (PIN II)
Deleted		**Excludes1** prostatic intraepithelial neoplasia III (PIN III) (D07.5)
New		**N42.30 Unspecified dysplasia of prostate**
New		**N42.31 Prostatic intraepithelial neoplasia**
New		PIN
New		Prostatic intraepithelial neoplasia I (PIN I)
New		Prostatic intraepithelial neoplasia II (PIN II)
New		**Excludes1** prostatic intraepithelial neoplasia III (PIN III) (D07.5)
New		**N42.32 Atypical small acinar proliferation of prostate**
New		**N42.39 Other dysplasia of prostate**
	N50.8	**Other specified disorders of male genital organs**
Deleted		Atrophy of scrotum, seminal vesicle, spermatic cord, tunica vaginalis and vas deferens
Deleted		Edema of scrotum, seminal vesicle, spermatic cord, testis, tunica vaginalis and vas deferens
Deleted		Hypertrophy of scrotum, seminal vesicle, spermatic cord, testis, tunica vaginalis and vas deferens
Deleted		Ulcer of scrotum, seminal vesicle, spermatic cord, testis, tunica vaginalis and vas deferens
Deleted		Chylocele, tunica vaginalis (nonfilarial) NOS
Deleted		Urethroscrotal fistula
Deleted		Stricture of spermatic cord, tunica vaginalis, and vas deferens
New		**N50.81 Testicular pain**
New		**N50.811 Right testicular pain**
New		**N50.812 Left testicular pain**
New		**N50.819 Testicular pain, unspecified**
New		**N50.82 Scrotal pain**
New		**N50.89 Other specified disorders of the male genital organs**
New		Atrophy of scrotum, seminal vesicle, spermatic cord, tunica vaginalis and vas deferens
New		Chylocele, tunica vaginalis (nonfilarial) NOS
New		Edema of scrotum, seminal vesicle, spermatic cord, tunica vaginalis and vas deferens
New		Hypertrophy of scrotum, seminal vesicle, spermatic cord, tunica vaginalis and vas deferens
New		Stricture of spermatic cord, tunica vaginalis, and vas deferens
New		Ulcer of scrotum, seminal vesicle, spermatic cord, testis, tunica vaginalis and vas deferens
New		Urethroscrotal fistula
Revised	**N52.3**	**Postprocedural erectile dysfunction**
New		**N52.35 Erectile dysfunction following radiation therapy**
New		**N52.36 Erectile dysfunction following interstitial seed therapy**
New		**N52.37 Erectile dysfunction following prostate ablative therapy**
New		Erectile dysfunction following cryotherapy
New		Erectile dysfunction following other prostate ablative therapies
New		Erectile dysfunction following ultrasound ablative therapies
Revised		**N52.39 Other and unspecified postprocedural erectile dysfunction**
	N61	**Inflammatory disorders of breast**
Deleted		Abscess (acute) (chronic) (nonpuerperal) of areola
Deleted		Abscess (acute) (chronic) (nonpuerperal) of breast
Deleted		Carbuncle of breast
Deleted		Infective mastitis (acute) (subacute) (nonpuerperal)
Deleted		Mastitis (acute) (subacute) (nonpuerperal) NOS
New		**N61.0 Mastitis without abscess**
New		Infective mastitis (acute) (nonpuerperal) (subacute)
New		Mastitis (acute) (nonpuerperal) (subacute) NOS
New		Cellulitis (acute) (nonpuerperal) (subacute) of breast NOS
New		Cellulitis (acute) (nonpuerperal) (subacute) of nipple NOS

New	**N61.1**		**Abscess of the breast and nipple**
New			Abscess (acute) (chronic) (nonpuerperal) of areola
New			Abscess (acute) (chronic) (nonpuerperal) of breast
New			Carbuncle of breast
New			Mastitis with abscess

	N64.1	**Fat necrosis of breast**
Revised		*Code first breast necrosis due to breast graft (T85.898)*

	N81	**Female genital prolapse**	
Revised		**Excludes1**	prolapse and hernia of ovary and fallopian tube (N83.4-)

New		**N83.00**	**Follicular cyst of ovary, unspecified side**
New		**N83.01**	**Follicular cyst of right ovary**
New		**N83.02**	**Follicular cyst of left ovary**
New		**N83.10**	**Corpus luteum cyst of ovary, unspecified side**
New		**N83.11**	**Corpus luteum cyst of right ovary**
New		**N83.12**	**Corpus luteum cyst of left ovary**
		N83.20	**Unspecified ovarian cysts**
New		**N83.201**	**Unspecified ovarian cyst, right side**
New		**N83.202**	**Unspecified ovarian cyst, left side**
New		**N83.209**	**Unspecified ovarian cyst, unspecified side**
New			Ovarian cyst, NOS
New		**N83.291**	**Other ovarian cyst, right side**
New		**N83.292**	**Other ovarian cyst, left side**
New		**N83.299**	**Other ovarian cyst, unspecified side**
New		**N83.311**	**Acquired atrophy of right ovary**
New		**N83.312**	**Acquired atrophy of left ovary**
New		**N83.319**	**Acquired atrophy of ovary, unspecified side**
New			Acquired atrophy of ovary, NOS
New		**N83.321**	**Acquired atrophy of right fallopian tube**
New		**N83.322**	**Acquired atrophy of left fallopian tube**
New		**N83.329**	**Acquired atrophy of fallopian tube, unspecified side**
New			Acquired atrophy of fallopian tube, NOS
New		**N83.331**	**Acquired atrophy of right ovary and fallopian tube**
New		**N83.332**	**Acquired atrophy of left ovary and fallopian tube**
New		**N83.339**	**Acquired atrophy of ovary and fallopian tube, unspecified side**
New			Acquired atrophy of ovary and fallopian tube, NOS
New		**N83.40**	**Prolapse and hernia of ovary and fallopian tube, unspecified side**
New			Prolapse and hernia of ovary and fallopian tube, NOS
New		**N83.41**	**Prolapse and hernia of right ovary and fallopian tube**
New		**N83.42**	**Prolapse and hernia of left ovary and fallopian tube**
New		**N83.511**	**Torsion of right ovary and ovarian pedicle**
New		**N83.512**	**Torsion of left ovary and ovarian pedicle**

New		**N83.519**	**Torsion of ovary and ovarian pedicle, unspecified side**
New			Torsion of ovary and ovarian pedicle, NOS
New		**N83.521**	**Torsion of right fallopian tube**
New		**N83.522**	**Torsion of left fallopian tube**
New		**N83.529**	**Torsion of fallopian tube, unspecified side**
New			Torsion of fallopian tube, NOS

New	**N83.6**	**Hematosalpinx**	
Revised		**Excludes1**	tubal pregnancy (O00.1-)

	N90.6	**Hypertrophy of vulva**	
Deleted			Hypertrophy of labia
New		**N90.60**	**Unspecified hypertrophy of vulva**
New			Unspecified hypertrophy of labia
New		**N90.61**	**Childhood asymmetric labium majus enlargement**
New			CALME
New		**N90.69**	**Other specified hypertrophy of vulva**
New			Other specified hypertrophy of labia

New	**N93.1**	**Pre-pubertal vaginal bleeding**	
New		**N94.10**	**Unspecified dyspareunia**
New		**N94.11**	**Superficial (introital) dyspareunia**
New		**N94.12**	**Deep dyspareunia**
New		**N94.19**	**Other specified dyspareunia**
	N94.3	**Premenstrual tension syndrome**	
New		**Excludes1**	Premenstrual dysphoric disorder (F32.81)
Revised		**N99.113**	**Postprocedural anterior bulbous urethral stricture**
New		**N99.115**	**Postprocedural fossa navicularis urethral stricture**

	N99.5	**Complications of stoma of urinary tract**	
Revised		**Excludes2**	mechanical complication of urinary catheter (T83.0-)
Revised		**N99.52**	**Complication of incontinent external stoma of urinary tract**
Revised		**N99.520**	**Hemorrhage of incontinent external stoma of urinary tract**
Revised		**N99.521**	**Infection of incontinent external stoma of urinary tract**
Revised		**N99.522**	**Malfunction of incontinent external stoma of urinary tract**
New		**N99.523**	**Herniation of incontinent stoma of urinary tract**
New		**N99.524**	**Stenosis of incontinent stoma of urinary tract**
Revised		**N99.528**	**Other complication of incontinent external stoma of urinary tract**
Revised		**N99.53**	**Complication of continent stoma of urinary tract**
Revised		**N99.530**	**Hemorrhage of continent stoma of urinary tract**
Revised		**N99.531**	**Infection of continent stoma of urinary tract**
Revised		**N99.532**	**Malfunction of continent stoma of urinary tract**
New		**N99.533**	**Herniation of continent stoma of urinary tract**
New		**N99.534**	**Stenosis of continent stoma of urinary tract**
Revised		**N99.538**	**Other complication of continent stoma of urinary tract**
Revised		**N99.82**	**Postprocedural hemorrhage of a genitourinary system organ or structure following a procedure**
Revised		**N99.820**	**Postprocedural hemorrhage of a genitourinary system organ or structure following a genitourinary system procedure**

Revised		N99.821	Postprocedural hemorrhage of a genitourinary system organ or structure following other procedure
New	N99.84		Postprocedural hematoma and seroma of a genitourinary system organ or structure following a procedure
New		N99.840	Postprocedural hematoma of a genitourinary system organ or structure following a genitourinary system procedure
New		N99.841	Postprocedural hematoma of a genitourinary system organ or structure following other procedure
New		N99.842	Postprocedural seroma of a genitourinary system organ or structure following a genitourinary system procedure
New		N99.843	Postprocedural seroma of a genitourinary system organ or structure following other procedure

CHAPTER 15

PREGNANCY, CHILDBIRTH AND THE PUERPERIUM (O00-O9A)

Revised			Use additional code from category Z3A, Weeks of gestation, to identify the specific week of the pregnancy, if known.
	O00.0		Abdominal pregnancy
New		O00.00	Abdominal pregnancy without intrauterine pregnancy
New			Abdominal pregnancy NOS
New		O00.01	Abdominal pregnancy with intrauterine pregnancy
	O00.1		Tubal pregnancy
New		O00.10	Tubal pregnancy without intrauterine pregnancy
New			Tubal pregnancy NOS
New		O00.11	Tubal pregnancy with intrauterine pregnancy
	O00.2		Ovarian pregnancy
New		O00.20	Ovarian pregnancy without intrauterine pregnancy
New			Ovarian pregnancy NOS
New		O00.21	Ovarian pregnancy with intrauterine pregnancy
New	O00.8		Other ectopic pregnancy
New		O00.80	Other ectopic pregnancy without intrauterine pregnancy
New			Other ectopic pregnancy NOS
New		O00.81	Other ectopic pregnancy with intrauterine pregnancy
New	O00.9		Ectopic pregnancy, unspecified
New		O00.90	Unspecified ectopic pregnancy without intrauterine pregnancy
New			Ectopic pregnancy NOS
New		O00.91	Unspecified ectopic pregnancy with intrauterine pregnancy
Revised	O09.1		Supervision of pregnancy with history of ectopic pregnancy
Revised		O09.10	Supervision of pregnancy with history of ectopic pregnancy, unspecified trimester
Revised		O09.11	Supervision of pregnancy with history of ectopic pregnancy, first trimester
Revised		O09.12	Supervision of pregnancy with history of ectopic pregnancy, second trimester
Revised		O09.13	Supervision of pregnancy with history of ectopic pregnancy, third trimester

New	O09.A		Supervision of pregnancy with history of molar pregnancy
New		O09.A0	Supervision of pregnancy with history of molar pregnancy, unspecified trimester
New		O09.A1	Supervision of pregnancy with history of molar pregnancy, first trimester
New		O09.A2	Supervision of pregnancy with history of molar pregnancy, second trimester
New		O09.A3	Supervision of pregnancy with history of molar pregnancy, third trimester
		O09.81	Supervision of pregnancy resulting from assisted reproductive technology
New			**Excludes2** gestational carrier status (Z33.3)
New	O11.4		Pre-existing hypertension with pre-eclampsia, complicating childbirth
New	O11.5		Pre-existing hypertension with pre-eclampsia, complicating the puerperium
New		O12.04	Gestational edema, complicating childbirth
New		O12.05	Gestational edema, complicating the puerperium
New		O12.14	Gestational proteinuria, complicating childbirth
New		O12.15	Gestational proteinuria, complicating the puerperium
New		O12.24	Gestational edema with proteinuria, complicating childbirth
New		O12.25	Gestational edema with proteinuria, complicating the puerperium
	O13		Gestational [pregnancy-induced] hypertension without significant proteinuria
New			**Includes** transient hypertension of pregnancy
New	O13.4		Gestational [pregnancy-induced] hypertension without significant proteinuria, complicating childbirth
New	O13.5		Gestational [pregnancy-induced] hypertension without significant proteinuria, complicating the puerperium
New		O14.04	Mild to moderate pre-eclampsia, complicating childbirth
New		O14.05	Mild to moderate pre-eclampsia, complicating the puerperium
New		O14.14	Severe pre-eclampsia complicating childbirth
New		O14.15	Severe pre-eclampsia, complicating the puerperium
New		O14.24	HELLP syndrome, complicating childbirth
New		O14.25	HELLP syndrome, complicating the puerperium
New		O14.94	Unspecified pre-eclampsia, complicating childbirth
New		O14.95	Unspecified pre-eclampsia, complicating the puerperium
Revised	O15.0		Eclampsia complicating pregnancy
Revised		O15.00	Eclampsia complicating pregnancy, unspecified trimester
Revised		O15.02	Eclampsia complicating pregnancy, second trimester
Revised		O15.03	Eclampsia complicating pregnancy, third trimester
Revised	O15.1		Eclampsia complicating labor
Revised	O15.2		Eclampsia complicating the puerperium
New	O16.4		Unspecified maternal hypertension, complicating childbirth
New	O16.5		Unspecified maternal hypertension, complicating the puerperium

Revised	**O24.0**		**Pre-existing type 1 diabetes mellitus, in pregnancy, childbirth and the puerperium**	
Revised		**O24.01**	**Pre-existing type 1 diabetes mellitus, in pregnancy**	
Revised			**O24.011**	**Pre-existing type 1 diabetes mellitus, in pregnancy, first trimester**
Revised			**O24.012**	**Pre-existing type 1 diabetes mellitus, in pregnancy, second trimester**
Revised			**O24.013**	**Pre-existing type 1 diabetes mellitus, in pregnancy, third trimester**
Revised			**O24.019**	**Pre-existing type 1 diabetes mellitus, in pregnancy, unspecified trimester**
Revised		**O24.02**	**Pre-existing type 1 diabetes mellitus, in childbirth**	
Revised		**O24.03**	**Pre-existing type 1 diabetes mellitus, in the puerperium**	
Revised	**O24.1**		**Pre-existing type 2 diabetes mellitus, in pregnancy, childbirth and the puerperium**	
Revised		**O24.11**	**Pre-existing type 2 diabetes mellitus, in pregnancy**	
Revised			**O24.111**	**Pre-existing type 2 diabetes mellitus, in pregnancy, first trimester**
Revised			**O24.112**	**Pre-existing type 2 diabetes mellitus, in pregnancy, second trimester**
Revised			**O24.113**	**Pre-existing type 2 diabetes mellitus, in pregnancy, third trimester**
Revised			**O24.119**	**Pre-existing type 2 diabetes mellitus, in pregnancy, unspecified trimester**
Revised		**O24.12**	**Pre-existing type 2 diabetes mellitus, in childbirth**	
Revised		**O24.13**	**Pre-existing type 2 diabetes mellitus, in the puerperium**	
New			**O24.415**	**Gestational diabetes mellitus in pregnancy, controlled by oral hypoglycemic drugs**
New				Gestational diabetes mellitus in pregnancy, controlled by oral antidiabetic drugs
New			**O24.425**	**Gestational diabetes mellitus in childbirth, controlled by oral hypoglycemic drugs**
New				Gestational diabetes mellitus in childbirth, controlled by oral antidiabetic drugs
New			**O24.435**	**Gestational diabetes mellitus in puerperium, controlled by oral hypoglycemic drugs**
New				Gestational diabetes mellitus in puerperium, controlled by oral antidiabetic drugs
	O33.7		**Maternal care for disproportion due to other fetal deformities**	
New			One of the following 7th characters is to be assigned to code O33.7. 7th character 0 is for single gestations and multiple gestations where the fetus is unspecified. 7th characters 1 through 9 are for cases of multiple gestations to identify the fetus for which the code applies. The appropriate code from category O30, Multiple gestation, must also be assigned when assigning code O33.7 with a 7th character of 1 through 9.	

New	0	not applicable or unspecified
New	1	fetus 1
New	2	fetus 2
New	3	fetus 3
New	4	fetus 4
New	5	fetus 5
New	9	other fetus

	O34.0		**Maternal care for congenital malformation of uterus**	
New			Maternal care for double uterus	
New			Maternal care for uterus bicornis	
New			**O34.211**	**Maternal care for low transverse scar from previous cesarean delivery**
New			**O34.212**	**Maternal care for vertical scar from previous cesarean delivery**
New				Maternal care for classical scar from previous cesarean delivery
New			**O34.219**	**Maternal care for unspecified type scar from previous cesarean delivery**
New		**O34.29**	**Maternal care due to uterine scar from other previous surgery**	
New			Maternal care due to uterine scar from other transmural uterine incision	
		O42.02	**Full-term premature rupture of membranes, onset of labor within 24 hours of rupture**	
Revised			Premature rupture of membranes at or after 37 completed weeks of gestation, onset of labor within 24 hours of rupture	
		O42.12	**Full-term premature rupture of membranes, onset of labor more than 24 hours following rupture**	
Revised			Premature rupture of membranes at or after 37 completed weeks of gestation, onset of labor more than 24 hours following rupture	
		O42.92	**Full-term premature rupture of membranes, unspecified as to length of time between rupture and onset of labor**	
Revised			Premature rupture of membranes at or after 37 completed weeks of gestation, unspecified as to length of time between rupture and onset of labor	
Revised	**O44.0**		**Complete placenta previa NOS or without hemorrhage**	
Deleted			Low implantation of placenta specified as without hemorrhage	
New			Placenta previa NOS	
Revised		**O44.00**	**Complete placenta previa NOS or without hemorrhage, unspecified trimester**	
Revised		**O44.01**	**Complete placenta previa NOS or without hemorrhage, first trimester**	
Revised		**O44.02**	**Complete placenta previa NOS or without hemorrhage, second trimester**	
Revised		**O44.03**	**Complete placenta previa NOS or without hemorrhage, third trimester**	
Revised	**O44.1**		**Complete placenta previa with hemorrhage**	
Deleted			Complete placenta previa with hemorrhage	
Deleted			Low implantation of placenta, NOS or with hemorrhage	
Deleted			Marginal placenta previa, NOS or with hemorrhage	
Deleted			Partial placenta previa, NOS or with hemorrhage	
Deleted			Total placenta previa, NOS or with hemorrhage	
Revised		**O44.10**	**Complete placenta previa with hemorrhage, unspecified trimester**	
Revised		**O44.11**	**Complete placenta previa with hemorrhage, first trimester**	
Revised		**O44.12**	**Complete placenta previa with hemorrhage, second trimester**	
Revised		**O44.13**	**Complete placenta previa with hemorrhage, third trimester**	
New	**O44.2**		**Partial placenta previa without hemorrhage**	
			Marginal placenta previa, NOS or without hemorrhage	
New		**O44.20**	**Partial placenta previa NOS or without hemorrhage, unspecified trimester**	
New		**O44.21**	**Partial placenta previa NOS or without hemorrhage, first trimester**	

New		O44.22 Partial placenta previa NOS or without hemorrhage, second trimester
New		O44.23 Partial placenta previa NOS or without hemorrhage, third trimester
New	O44.3	Partial placenta previa with hemorrhage
New		Marginal placenta previa with hemorrhage
New		O44.30 Partial placenta previa with hemorrhage, unspecified trimester
New		O44.31 Partial placenta previa with hemorrhage, first trimester
New		O44.32 Partial placenta previa with hemorrhage, second trimester
New		O44.33 Partial placenta previa with hemorrhage, third trimester
New	O44.4	Low lying placenta NOS or without hemorrhage
New		Low implantation of placenta NOS or without hemorrhage
New		O44.40 Low lying placenta NOS or without hemorrhage, unspecified trimester
New		O44.41 Low lying placenta NOS or without hemorrhage, first trimester
New		O44.42 Low lying placenta NOS or without hemorrhage, second trimester
New		O44.43 Low lying placenta NOS or without hemorrhage, third trimester
New	O44.5	Low lying placenta with hemorrhage
New		Low implantation of placenta with hemorrhage
New		O44.50 Low lying placenta with hemorrhage, unspecified trimester
New		O44.51 Low lying placenta with hemorrhage, first trimester
New		O44.52 Low lying placenta with hemorrhage, second trimester
New		O44.53 Low lying placenta with hemorrhage, third trimester
New		O70.20 Third degree perineal laceration during delivery, unspecified
New		O70.21 Third degree perineal laceration during delivery, IIIa
New		Third degree perineal laceration during delivery with less than 50% of external anal sphincter (EAS) thickness torn
New		O70.22 Third degree perineal laceration during delivery, IIIb
New		Third degree perineal laceration during delivery with more than 50% external anal sphincter (EAS) thickness torn
New		O70.23 Third degree perineal laceration during delivery, IIIc
New		Third degree perineal laceration during delivery with both external anal sphincter (EAS) and internal anal sphincter (IAS) torn
Revised		O99.33 Tobacco use disorder complicating pregnancy, childbirth, and the puerperium
New		Smoking complicating pregnancy, childbirth, and the puerperium
New		Use additional code from category F17 to identify type of tobacco nicotine dependence
	O99.6	Diseases of the digestive system complicating pregnancy, childbirth and the puerperium
New		Excludes2 hemorrhoids in pregnancy (O22.4-)
		O99.82 Streptococcus B carrier state complicating pregnancy, childbirth and the puerperium
New		Excludes1 Carrier of streptococcus group B (GBS) in a nonpregnant woman (Z22.330)

CHAPTER 16

CERTAIN CONDITIONS ORIGINATING IN THE PERINATAL PERIOD (P00-P96)

NEWBORN AFFECTED BY MATERNAL FACTORS AND BY COMPLICATIONS OF PREGNANCY, LABOR, AND DELIVERY (P00-P04)

Revised		Note: These codes are for use when the listed maternal conditions are specified as the cause of confirmed morbidity or potential morbidity which have their origin in the perinatal period (before birth through the first 28 days after birth).
Revised	P00	Newborn affected by maternal conditions that may be unrelated to present pregnancy
New		Excludes2 encounter for observation of newborn for suspected diseases and conditions ruled out (Z05.-)
New		newborn affected by maternal complications of pregnancy (P01.-)
Revised	P00.0	Newborn affected by maternal hypertensive disorders
Revised		Newborn affected by maternal conditions classifiable to O10-O11, O13-O16
Revised	P00.1	Newborn affected by maternal renal and urinary tract diseases
Revised		Newborn affected by maternal conditions classifiable to N00-N39
Revised	P00.2	Newborn affected by maternal infectious and parasitic diseases
Revised		Newborn affected by maternal infectious disease classifiable to A00-B99, J09 and J10
Revised	P00.3	Newborn affected by other maternal circulatory and respiratory diseases
Revised		Newborn affected by maternal conditions classifiable to I00-I99, J00-J99, Q20-Q34 and not included in P00.0, P00.2
Revised	P00.4	Newborn affected by maternal nutritional disorders
Revised		Newborn affected by maternal disorders classifiable to E40-E64
Revised	P00.5	Newborn affected by maternal injury
Revised		Newborn affected by maternal conditions classifiable to O9A.2-
Revised	P00.6	Newborn affected by surgical procedure on mother
Revised		Newborn affected by amniocentesis
Revised	P00.7	Newborn affected by other medical procedures on mother, not elsewhere classified
Revised		Newborn affected by radiation to mother
Revised	P00.8	Newborn affected by other maternal conditions
Revised		P00.81 Newborn affected by periodontal disease in mother
Revised		P00.89 Newborn affected by other maternal conditions
Revised		Newborn affected by conditions classifiable to T80-T88
Revised		Newborn affected by maternal genital tract or other localized infections
Revised		Newborn affected by maternal systemic lupus erythematosus
Revised	P00.9	Newborn affected by unspecified maternal condition
Revised	P01	Newborn affected by maternal complications of pregnancy
New		Excludes2 encounter for observation of newborn for suspected diseases and conditions ruled out (Z05.-)
Revised	P01.0	Newborn affected by incompetent cervix
Revised	P01.1	Newborn affected by premature rupture of membranes
Revised	P01.2	Newborn affected by oligohydramnios
Revised	P01.3	Newborn affected by polyhydramnios
Revised		Newborn affected by hydramnios
Revised	P01.4	Newborn affected by ectopic pregnancy
Revised		Newborn affected by abdominal pregnancy
Revised	P01.5	Newborn affected by multiple pregnancy
Revised		Newborn affected by triplet (pregnancy)
Revised		Newborn affected by twin (pregnancy)

Revised	P01.6	**Newborn affected by maternal death**	

Revised   P01.6   **Newborn affected by maternal death**

Revised   P01.7   **Newborn affected by malpresentation before labor**

Revised   Newborn affected by breech presentation before labor

Revised   Newborn affected by external version before labor

Revised   Newborn affected by face presentation before labor

Revised   Newborn affected by transverse lie before labor

Revised   Newborn affected by unstable lie before labor

Revised   P01.8   **Newborn affected by other maternal complications of pregnancy**

Revised   P01.9   **Newborn affected by maternal complication of pregnancy, unspecified**

Revised   P02   **Newborn affected by complications of placenta, cord and membranes**

New   **Excludes2**   encounter for observation of newborn for suspected diseases and conditions ruled out (Z05.-)

Revised   P02.0   **Newborn affected by placenta previa**

Revised   P02.1   **Newborn affected by other forms of placental separation and hemorrhage**

Revised   Newborn affected by abruptio placenta

Revised   Newborn affected by accidental hemorrhage

Revised   Newborn affected by antepartum hemorrhage

Revised   Newborn affected by damage to placenta from amniocentesis, cesarean delivery or surgical induction

Revised   Newborn affected by maternal blood loss

Revised   Newborn affected by premature separation of placenta

Revised   P02.2   **Newborn affected by other and unspecified morphological and functional abnormalities of placenta**

Revised   P02.20   **Newborn affected by unspecified morphological and functional abnormalities of placenta**

Revised   P02.29   **Newborn affected by other morphological and functional abnormalities of placenta**

Revised   Newborn affected by placental dysfunction

Revised   Newborn affected by placental infarction

Revised   Newborn affected by placental insufficiency

Revised   P02.3   **Newborn affected by placental transfusion syndromes**

Revised   Newborn affected by placental and cord abnormalities resulting in twin-to-twin or other transplacental transfusion

Revised   P02.4   **Newborn affected by prolapsed cord**

Revised   P02.5   **Newborn affected by other compression of umbilical cord**

Revised   Newborn affected by umbilical cord (tightly) around neck

Revised   Newborn affected by entanglement of umbilical cord

Revised   Newborn affected by knot in umbilical cord

Revised   P02.6   **Newborn affected by other and unspecified conditions of umbilical cord**

Revised   P02.60   **Newborn affected by unspecified conditions of umbilical cord**

Revised   P02.69   **Newborn affected by other conditions of umbilical cord**

Revised   Newborn affected by short umbilical cord

Revised   Newborn affected by vasa previa

Revised   P02.7   **Newborn affected by chorioamnionitis**

Revised   Newborn affected by amnionitis

Revised   Newborn affected by membranitis

Revised   Newborn affected by placentitis

Revised   P02.8   **Newborn affected by other abnormalities of membranes**

Revised   P02.9   **Newborn affected by abnormality of membranes, unspecified**

Revised   P03   **Newborn affected by other complications of labor and delivery**

New   **Excludes2**   encounter for observation of newborn for suspected diseases and conditions ruled out (Z05.-)

Revised   P03.0   **Newborn affected by breech delivery and extraction**

Revised   P03.1   **Newborn affected by other malpresentation, malposition and disproportion during labor and delivery**

Revised   Newborn affected by contracted pelvis

Revised   Newborn affected by conditions classifiable to O64-O66

Revised   Newborn affected by persistent occipitoposterior

Revised   Newborn affected by transverse lie

Revised   P03.2   **Newborn affected by forceps delivery**

Revised   P03.3   **Newborn affected by delivery by vacuum extractor [ventouse]**

Revised   P03.4   **Newborn affected by Cesarean delivery**

Revised   P03.5   **Newborn affected by precipitate delivery**

Revised   Newborn affected by rapid second stage

Revised   P03.6   **Newborn affected by abnormal uterine contractions**

Revised   Newborn affected by conditions classifiable to O62.-, except O62.3

Revised   Newborn affected by hypertonic labor

Revised   Newborn affected by uterine inertia

Revised   P03.8   **Newborn affected by other specified complications of labor and delivery**

Revised   P03.81   **Newborn affected by abnormality in fetal (intrauterine) heart rate or rhythm**

Revised   P03.810   **Newborn affected by abnormality in fetal (intrauterine) heart rate or rhythm before the onset of labor**

Revised   P03.811   **Newborn affected by abnormality in fetal (intrauterine) heart rate or rhythm during labor**

Revised   P03.819   **Newborn affected by abnormality in fetal (intrauterine) heart rate or rhythm, unspecified as to time of onset**

Revised   P03.89   **Newborn affected by other specified complications of labor and delivery**

Revised   Newborn affected by abnormality of maternal soft tissues

Revised   Newborn affected by conditions classifiable to O60-O75 and by procedures used in labor and delivery not included in P02.- and P03.0-P03.6

Revised   Newborn affected by induction of labor

Revised   P03.9   **Newborn affected by complication of labor and delivery, unspecified**

Revised   P04   **Newborn affected by noxious substances transmitted via placenta or breast milk**

New   **Excludes2**   congenital malformations (Q00-Q99)
encounter for observation of newborn for suspected diseases and conditions ruled out (Z05.-)

Revised   P04.0   **Newborn affected by maternal anesthesia and analgesia in pregnancy, labor and delivery**

        Newborn affected by reactions and intoxications from maternal opiates and tranquilizers administered during labor and delivery

Revised   P04.1   **Newborn affected by other maternal medication**

Revised   Newborn affected by cancer chemotherapy

Revised   Newborn affected by cytotoxic drugs

Revised   P04.2   **Newborn affected by maternal use of tobacco**

        Newborn affected by exposure in utero to tobacco smoke

Revised   P04.3   **Newborn affected by maternal use of alcohol**

        P04.4   **Newborn affected by maternal use of drugs of addiction**

Revised   P04.41   **Newborn affected by maternal use of cocaine**

Revised   P04.49   **Newborn affected by maternal use of other drugs of addiction**

Revised   **Excludes2**   newborn affected by maternal anesthesia and analgesia (P04.0)

Revised	P04.5	Newborn affected by maternal use of nutritional chemical substances
Revised	P04.6	Newborn affected by maternal exposure to environmental chemical substances
Revised	P04.8	Newborn affected by other maternal noxious substances
Revised	P04.9	Newborn affected by maternal noxious substance, unspecified
	P05.0	Newborn light for gestational age
New		Weight below but length above 10th percentile for gestational age
New	P05.09	Newborn light for gestational age, 2500 grams and over
New		Newborn light for gestational age, other
	P05.1	Newborn small for gestational age
		Weight and length below 10th percentile for gestational age
New	P05.19	Newborn small for gestational age, other
New		Newborn small for gestational age, 2500 grams and over

P07   Disorders of newborn related to short gestation and low birth weight, not elsewhere classified

Deleted	**Excludes1**	low birth weight due to slow fetal growth and fetal malnutrition (P05.-)
	P07.0	Extremely low birth weight newborn
New	**Excludes1**	low birth weight due to slow fetal growth and fetal malnutrition (P05.-)
	P07.1	Other low birth weight newborn
New	**Excludes1**	low birth weight due to slow fetal growth and fetal malnutrition (P05.-)
	P96.5	Complication to newborn due to (fetal) intrauterine procedure
Revised	**Excludes2**	newborn affected by amniocentesis (P00.6)

CHAPTER 17
CONGENITAL MALFORMATIONS, DEFORMATIONS AND CHROMOSOMAL ABNORMALITIES (Q00-Q99)

	Q25.1	Coarctation of aorta
New		Stenosis of aorta
	Q25.2	Atresia of aorta
New	Q25.21	Interruption of aortic arch
New		Atresia of aortic arch
New	Q25.29	Other atresia of aorta
New		Atresia of aorta
	Q25.4	Other congenital malformations of aorta
Deleted		Absence of aorta
Deleted		Aneurysm of sinus of Valsalva (ruptured)
Deleted		Aplasia of aorta
Deleted		Congenital aneurysm of aorta
Deleted		Congenital malformations of aorta
Deleted		Congenital dilatation of aorta
Deleted		Double aortic arch [vascular ring of aorta]
Deleted		Hypoplasia of aorta
Deleted		Persistent convolutions of aortic arch
Deleted		Persistent right aortic arch
New	Q25.40	Congenital malformation of aorta unspecified
New	Q25.41	Absence and aplasia of aorta
New	Q25.42	Hypoplasia of aorta
New	Q25.43	Congenital aneurysm of aorta
		Congenital aneurysm of aortic root
		Congenital aneurysm of aortic sinus
New	Q25.44	Congenital dilation of aorta
New	Q25.45	Double aortic arch
		Vascular ring of aorta
New	Q25.46	Tortuous aortic arch
		Persistent convolutions of aortic arch

New	Q25.47	Right aortic arch
		Persistent right aortic arch
New	Q25.48	Anomalous origin of subclavian artery
New	Q25.49	Other congenital malformations of aorta
	Q52.12	Longitudinal vaginal septum
Deleted		Longitudinal vaginal septum with or without obstruction
New	Q52.120	Longitudinal vaginal septum, nonobstructing
New	Q52.121	Longitudinal vaginal septum, obstructing, right side
New	Q52.122	Longitudinal vaginal septum, obstructing, left side
New	Q52.123	Longitudinal vaginal septum, microperforate, right side
New	Q52.124	Longitudinal vaginal septum, microperforate, left side
New	Q52.129	Other and unspecified longitudinal vaginal septum
New	Q66.21	Congenital metatarsus primus varus
New	Q66.22	Congenital metatarsus adductus
		Congenital metatarsus varus
New	Q82.6	Congenital sacral dimple
New		Parasacral dimple
New	**Excludes2**	pilonidal cyst with abscess (L05.01)
New		pilonidal cyst without abscess (L05.91)
New	Q87.82	Arterial tortuosity syndrome

CHAPTER 18
SYMPTOMS, SIGNS AND ABNORMAL CLINICAL AND LABORATORY FINDINGS, NOT ELSEWHERE CLASSIFIED (R00-R99)

	R00	Abnormalities of heart beat
Deleted	**Excludes1**	specified arrhythmias (I47-I49)
New	**Excludes2**	specified arrhythmias (I47-I49)
	R01.1	Cardiac murmur, unspecified
New		Systolic murmur NOS

SYMPTOMS AND SIGNS INVOLVING THE DIGESTIVE SYSTEM AND ABDOMEN (R10-R19)

Deleted	**Excludes1**	congenital or infantile pylorospasm (Q40.0)
Deleted		gastrointestinal hemorrhage (K92.0-K92.2)
Deleted		intestinal obstruction (K56.-)
Deleted		newborn gastrointestinal hemorrhage (P54.0-P54.3)
Deleted		newborn intestinal obstruction (P76.-)
Deleted		pylorospasm (K31.3)
Deleted		signs and symptoms involving the urinary system (R30-R39)
Deleted		symptoms referable to female genital organs (N94.-)
Deleted		symptoms referable to male genital organs (N48-N50)
New	**Excludes2**	congenital or infantile pylorospasm (Q40.0)
New		gastrointestinal hemorrhage (K92.0-K92.2)
New		intestinal obstruction (K56.-)
New		newborn gastrointestinal hemorrhage (P54.0-P54.3)
New		newborn intestinal obstruction (P76.-)
New		pylorospasm (K31.3)
New		signs and symptoms involving the urinary system (R30-R39)
New		symptoms referable to female genital organs (N94.-)
New		symptoms referable to male genital organs (N48-N50)

	R11		Nausea and vomiting	
Revised		**Excludes1**	psychogenic vomiting (F50.89)	
New	R29.7		National Institutes of Health Stroke Scale (NIHSS) score	
New			*Code first the type of cerebral infarction (I63-)*	
New		R29.70	NIHSS score 0-9	
New			R29.700	NIHSS score 0
New			R29.701	NIHSS score 1
New			R29.702	NIHSS score 2
New			R29.703	NIHSS score 3
New			R29.704	NIHSS score 4
New			R29.705	NIHSS score 5
New			R29.706	NIHSS score 6
New			R29.707	NIHSS score 7
New			R29.708	NIHSS score 8
New			R29.709	NIHSS score 9
New		R29.71	NIHSS score 10-19	
New			R29.710	NIHSS score 10
New			R29.711	NIHSS score 11
New			R29.712	NIHSS score 12
New			R29.713	NIHSS score 13
New			R29.714	NIHSS score 14
New			R29.715	NIHSS score 15
New			R29.716	NIHSS score 16
New			R29.717	NIHSS score 17
New			R29.718	NIHSS score 18
New			R29.719	NIHSS score 19
New		R29.72	NIHSS score 20-29	
New			R29.720	NIHSS score 20
New			R29.721	NIHSS score 21
New			R29.722	NIHSS score 22
New			R29.723	NIHSS score 23
New			R29.724	NIHSS score 24
New			R29.725	NIHSS score 25
New			R29.726	NIHSS score 26
New			R29.727	NIHSS score 27
New			R29.728	NIHSS score 28
New			R29.729	NIHSS score 29
New		R29.73	NIHSS score 30-39	
New			R29.730	NIHSS score 30
New			R29.731	NIHSS score 31
New			R29.732	NIHSS score 32
New			R29.733	NIHSS score 33
New			R29.734	NIHSS score 34
New			R29.735	NIHSS score 35
New			R29.736	NIHSS score 36
New			R29.737	NIHSS score 37
New			R29.738	NIHSS score 38
New			R29.739	NIHSS score 39
New		R29.74	NIHSS score 40-42	
New			R29.740	NIHSS score 40
New			R29.741	NIHSS score 41
New			R29.742	NIHSS score 42
New		R31.21	Asymptomatic microscopic hematuria	
New			AMH	
New		R31.29	Other microscopic hematuria	
New		R39.19	Other difficulties with micturition	
New			R39.191	Need to immediately re-void
New			R39.192	Position dependent micturition
New			R39.198	Other difficulties with micturition
New		R39.82	Chronic bladder pain	

SYMPTOMS AND SIGNS INVOLVING COGNITION, PERCEPTION, EMOTIONAL STATE AND BEHAVIOR (R40-R46)

Deleted		**Excludes1**	symptoms and signs constituting part of a pattern of mental disorder (F01-F99)
New		**Excludes2**	symptoms and signs constituting part of a pattern of mental disorder (F01-F99)
	R40.2	Coma	
Revised		**Note:**	One code from each subcategory R40.21-R40-23 is required to complete the coma scale
		R40.24	Glasgow coma scale, total score
Deleted			Use codes R40.21- through R40.23- only when the individual score(s) are documented
New			Note: Assign a code from subcategory R40.24, when only the total coma score is documented
New			The following appropriate 7th character is to be added to subcategory R40.24-:

New	0	unspecified time
New	1	in the field [EMT or ambulance]
New	2	at arrival to emergency department
New	3	at hospital admission
New	4	24 hours or more after hospital admission

		R41.84	Other specified cognitive deficit
New		**Excludes1**	cognitive deficits as sequelae of cerebrovascular disease (I69.01-, I69.11-, I69.21-, I69.31-, I69.81-, I69.91-)
		R46.81	Obsessive-compulsive behavior
Revised		**Excludes1**	obsessive-compulsive disorder (F42-)
		R50.82	Postprocedural fever
Revised		**Excludes1**	postprocedural infection (T81.4-)
	R53.1	Weakness	
New		**Excludes1**	sarcopenia (M62.84)
	R54	Age-related physical debility	
New		**Excludes1**	sarcopenia (M62.84)
	R63.0	Anorexia	
Revised		**Excludes1**	loss of appetite of nonorganic origin (F50.89)
	R65.2	Severe sepsis	
		Code first underlying infection, such as:	
Revised			infection following a procedure (T81.4-)
		R68.84	Jaw pain
Revised		**Excludes1**	temporomandibular joint arthralgia (M26.62-)

ABNORMAL FINDINGS ON EXAMINATION OF BLOOD, WITHOUT DIAGNOSIS (R70-R79)

Deleted	**Excludes1**	abnormalities (of)(on):
Deleted		abnormal findings on antenatal screening of mother (O28.-)
Deleted		coagulation hemorrhagic disorders (D65-D68)
Deleted		lipids (E78.-)
Deleted		platelets and thrombocytes (D69.-)
Deleted		white blood cells classified elsewhere (D70-D72)
Deleted		diagnostic abnormal findings classified elsewhere - see Alphabetical Index
Deleted		hemorrhagic and hematological disorders of newborn (P50-P61)
New	**Excludes2**	abnormal findings on antenatal screening of mother (O28.-)
New		abnormalities of lipids (E78.-)
New		abnormalities of platelets and thrombocytes (D69.-)
New		abnormalities of white blood cells classified elsewhere (D70-D72)
New		coagulation hemorrhagic disorders (D65-D68)
New		diagnostic abnormal findings classified elsewhere —*see* Alphabetical Index
New		hemorrhagic and hematological disorders of newborn (P50-P61)

New	**R73.03**	**Prediabetes**
New		Latent diabetes
	R73.09	**Other abnormal glucose**
Deleted		Latent diabetes
Deleted		Prediabetes
	R78.81	**Bacteremia**
Revised	**Excludes1**	sepsis-code to specified infection
	R82.7	**Abnormal findings on microbiological examination of urine**
Deleted		Positive culture findings of urine
New	**R82.71**	**Bacteriuria**
New	**R82.79**	**Other abnormal findings on microbiological examination of urine**
New		Positive culture findings of urine
	R93.4	**Abnormal findings on diagnostic imaging of urinary organs**
Deleted		Filling defect of bladder found on diagnostic imaging
Deleted		Filling defect of kidney found on diagnostic imaging
Deleted		Filling defect of ureter found on diagnostic imaging
Deleted	**Excludes1**	hypertrophy of kidney (N28.81)
New	**Excludes2**	hypertrophy of kidney (N28.81)
New	**R93.41**	**Abnormal radiologic findings on diagnostic imaging of renal pelvis, ureter, or bladder**
New		Filling defect of bladder found on diagnostic imaging
New		Filling defect of renal pelvis found on diagnostic imaging
New		Filling defect of ureter found on diagnostic imaging
New	**R93.42**	**Abnormal radiologic findings on diagnostic imaging of kidney**
New	**R93.421**	**Abnormal radiologic findings on diagnostic imaging of right kidney**
New	**R93.422**	**Abnormal radiologic findings on diagnostic imaging of left kidney**
New	**R93.429**	**Abnormal radiologic findings on diagnostic imaging of unspecified kidney**
New	**R93.49**	**Abnormal radiologic findings on diagnostic imaging of other urinary organs**

New	R97.20	Elevated prostate specific antigen [PSA]
New	R97.21	Rising PSA following treatment for malignant neoplasm of prostate

CHAPTER 19

INJURY, POISONING AND CERTAIN OTHER CONSEQUENCES OF EXTERNAL CAUSES (S00-T88)

	S00.8		**Superficial injury of other parts of head**
New			Superficial injuries of face [any part]
New		S02.101	Fracture of base of skull, right side
New		S02.102	Fracture of base of skull, left side
New		S02.109	Fracture of base of skull, unspecified side
Revised		S02.110	Type I occipital condyle fracture, unspecified side
Revised		S02.111	Type II occipital condyle fracture, unspecified side
Revised		S02.112	Type III occipital condyle fracture, unspecified side
Revised		S02.118	Other fracture of occiput, unspecified side
New		S02.11A	Type I occipital condyle fracture, right side
New		S02.11B	Type I occipital condyle fracture, left side
New		S02.11C	Type II occipital condyle fracture, right side
New		S02.11D	Type II occipital condyle fracture, left side
New		S02.11E	Type III occipital condyle fracture, right side
New		S02.11F	Type III occipital condyle fracture, left side
New		S02.11G	Other fracture of occiput, right side
New		S02.11H	Other fracture of occiput, left side
New	S02.30		Fracture of orbital floor, unspecified side
New	S02.31		Fracture of orbital floor, right side
New	S02.32		Fracture of orbital floor, left side
Revised		S02.400	Malar fracture, unspecified side
Revised		S02.401	Maxillary fracture, unspecified side
Revised		S02.402	Zygomatic fracture, unspecified side
New		S02.40A	Malar fracture, right side
New		S02.40B	Malar fracture, left side
New		S02.40C	Maxillary fracture, right side
New		S02.40D	Maxillary fracture, left side
New		S02.40E	Zygomatic fracture, right side
New		S02.40F	Zygomatic fracture, left side
Revised		S02.600	Fracture of unspecified part of body of mandible, unspecified side
New		S02.601	Fracture of unspecified part of body of right mandible
New		S02.602	Fracture of unspecified part of body of left mandible
New		S02.610	Fracture of condylar process of mandible, unspecified side
New		S02.611	Fracture of condylar process of right mandible
New		S02.612	Fracture of condylar process of left mandible

New		S02.620	Fracture of subcondylar process of mandible, unspecified side
New		S02.621	Fracture of subcondylar process of right mandible
New		S02.622	Fracture of subcondylar process of left mandible
New		S02.630	Fracture of coronoid process of mandible, unspecified side
New		S02.631	Fracture of coronoid process of right mandible
New		S02.632	Fracture of coronoid process of left mandible
New		S02.640	Fracture of ramus of mandible, unspecified side
New		S02.641	Fracture of ramus of right mandible
New		S02.642	Fracture of ramus of left mandible
New		S02.650	Fracture of angle of mandible, unspecified side
New		S02.651	Fracture of angle of right mandible
New		S02.652	Fracture of angle of left mandible
New		S02.670	Fracture of alveolus of mandible, unspecified side
New		S02.671	Fracture of alveolus of right mandible
New		S02.672	Fracture of alveolus of left mandible
New	S02.80		Fracture of other specified skull and facial bones, unspecified side
New	S02.81		Fracture of other specified skull and facial bones, right side
New	S02.82		Fracture of other specified skull and facial bones, left side
New	S03.00		Dislocation of jaw, unspecified side
New	S03.01		Dislocation of jaw, right side
New	S03.02		Dislocation of jaw, left side
New	S03.03		Dislocation of jaw, bilateral side
New	S03.40		Sprain of jaw, unspecified side
New	S03.41		Sprain of jaw, right side
New	S03.42		Sprain of jaw, left side
New	S03.43		Sprain of jaw, bilateral side
	S06.0		Concussion
Revised		Excludes1	concussion with other intracranial injuries classified in subcategories S06.1- to S06.6- , S06.81- and S06.82- code to specified intracranial injury
Deleted		~~S06.0X2~~	~~Concussion with loss of consciousness of 31 minutes to 59 minutes~~
Deleted		~~S06.0X3~~	~~Concussion with loss of consciousness of 1 hour to 5 hours 59 minutes~~
Deleted		~~S06.0X4~~	~~Concussion with loss of consciousness of 6 hours to 24 hours~~
Deleted		~~S06.0X5~~	~~Concussion with loss of consciousness greater than 24 hours with return to pre-existing conscious level~~
Deleted		~~S06.0X6~~	~~Concussion with loss of consciousness greater than 24 hours without return to pre-existing conscious level with patient surviving~~

Deleted		~~S06.0X7~~	~~Concussion with loss of consciousness of any duration with death due to brain injury prior to regaining consciousness~~
Deleted		~~S06.0X8~~	~~Concussion with loss of consciousness of any duration with death due to other cause prior to regaining consciousness~~
	S06.89		Other specified intracranial injury
New		Excludes1	concussion (S06.0X-)
	S06.9		Unspecified intracranial injury
New			Traumatic brain injury NOS
New		Excludes1	conditions classifiable to S06.0- to S06.8-code to specified intracranial injury
		S34.101	Unspecified injury to L$_1$ level of lumbar spinal cord
New			Unspecified injury to lumbar spinal cord level 1
		S34.102	Unspecified injury to L$_2$ level of lumbar spinal cord
New			Unspecified injury to lumbar spinal cord level 2
		S34.103	Unspecified injury to L$_3$ level of lumbar spinal cord
New			Unspecified injury to lumbar spinal cord level 3
		S34.104	Unspecified injury to L$_4$ level of lumbar spinal cord
New			Unspecified injury to lumbar spinal cord level 4
		S34.105	Unspecified injury to L$_5$ level of lumbar spinal cord
New			Unspecified injury to lumbar spinal cord level 5
		S34.111	Complete lesion of L$_1$ level of lumbar spinal cord
New			Complete lesion of lumbar spinal cord level 1
		S34.112	Complete lesion of L$_2$ level of lumbar spinal cord
New			Complete lesion of lumbar spinal cord level 2
		S34.113	Complete lesion of L$_3$ level of lumbar spinal cord
New			Complete lesion of lumbar spinal cord level 3
		S34.114	Complete lesion of L$_4$ level of lumbar spinal cord
New			Complete lesion of lumbar spinal cord level 4
		S34.115	Complete lesion of L$_5$ level of lumbar spinal cord
New			Complete lesion of lumbar spinal cord level 5
		S34.121	Incomplete lesion of L$_1$ level of lumbar spinal cord
New			Incomplete lesion of lumbar spinal cord level 1
		S34.122	Incomplete lesion of L$_2$ level of lumbar spinal cord
New			Incomplete lesion of lumbar spinal cord level 2
		S34.123	Incomplete lesion of L$_3$ level of lumbar spinal cord
New			Incomplete lesion of lumbar spinal cord level 3
		S34.124	Incomplete lesion of L$_4$ level of lumbar spinal cord
New			Incomplete lesion of lumbar spinal cord level 4
		S34.125	Incomplete lesion of L$_5$ level of lumbar spinal cord
New			Incomplete lesion of lumbar spinal cord level 5

Revised		S49.031	Salter-Harris Type III physeal fracture of upper end of humerus, right arm
Revised		S49.032	Salter-Harris Type III physeal fracture of upper end of humerus, left arm
Revised		S49.039	Salter-Harris Type III physeal fracture of upper end of humerus, unspecified arm
Revised	S49.13		Salter-Harris Type III physeal fracture of lower end of humerus
Revised		S49.131	Salter-Harris Type III physeal fracture of lower end of humerus, right arm
Revised		S49.132	Salter-Harris Type III physeal fracture of lower end of humerus, left arm
Revised		S49.139	Salter-Harris Type III physeal fracture of lower end of humerus, unspecified arm
Revised	S54.8X		Injury of other nerves at forearm level
Revised		S54.8X1	Injury of other nerves at forearm level, right arm
Revised		S54.8X2	Injury of other nerves at forearm level, left arm
Revised		S54.8X9	Injury of other nerves at forearm level, unspecified arm

S92.0   Fracture of calcaneus

New   **Excludes2** Physeal fracture of calcaneus (S99.0-)

S92.3   Fracture of metatarsal bone(s)

New   **Excludes2** Physeal fracture of metatarsal (S99.1-)

S92.4   Fracture of great toe

New   **Excludes2** Physeal fracture of phalanx of toe (S99.2-)

S92.5   Fracture of lesser toe(s)

New   **Excludes2** Physeal fracture of phalanx of toe (S99.2-)

New	S92.8		Other fracture of foot, except ankle
New	S92.81		Other fracture of foot
			Sesamoid fracture of foot
New		S92.811	Other fracture of right foot
New		S92.812	Other fracture of left foot
New		S92.819	Other fracture of unspecified foot

S99   Other and unspecified injuries of ankle and foot

Deleted   The appropriate 7th character is to be added to each code from subcategories S99

Deleted	A	initial encounter
Deleted	D	subsequent encounter
Deleted	S	sequela

New   S99.0   Physeal fracture of calcaneus

New   The appropriate 7th character is to be added to each code from subcategories S99.0

New	A	initial encounter for closed fracture
New	B	initial encounter for open fracture
New	D	subsequent encounter for fracture with routine healing
New	G	subsequent encounter for fracture with delayed healing
New	K	subsequent encounter for fracture with nonunion
New	P	subsequent encounter for fracture with malunion
New	S	sequela

New	S99.00		Unspecified physeal fracture of calcaneus
New		S99.001	Unspecified physeal fracture of right calcaneus

New		S99.002	Unspecified physeal fracture of left calcaneus
New		S99.009	Unspecified physeal fracture of unspecified calcaneus
New	S99.01		Salter-Harris Type I physeal fracture of calcaneus
New		S99.011	Salter-Harris Type I physeal fracture of right calcaneus
New		S99.012	Salter-Harris Type I physeal fracture of left calcaneus
New		S99.019	Salter-Harris Type I physeal fracture of unspecified calcaneus
New	S99.02		Salter-Harris Type II physeal fracture of calcaneus
New		S99.021	Salter-Harris Type II physeal fracture of right calcaneus
New		S99.022	Salter-Harris Type II physeal fracture of left calcaneus
New		S99.029	Salter-Harris Type II physeal fracture of unspecified calcaneus
New	S99.03		Salter-Harris Type III physeal fracture of calcaneus
New		S99.031	Salter-Harris Type III physeal fracture of right calcaneus
New		S99.032	Salter-Harris Type III physeal fracture of left calcaneus
New		S99.039	Salter-Harris Type III physeal fracture of unspecified calcaneus
New	S99.04		Salter-Harris Type IV physeal fracture of calcaneus
New		S99.041	Salter-Harris Type IV physeal fracture of right calcaneus
New		S99.042	Salter-Harris Type IV physeal fracture of left calcaneus
New		S99.049	Salter-Harris Type IV physeal fracture of unspecified calcaneus
New	S99.09		Other physeal fracture of calcaneus
New		S99.091	Other physeal fracture of right calcaneus
New		S99.092	Other physeal fracture of left calcaneus
New		S99.099	Other physeal fracture of unspecified calcaneus

New   S99.1   Physeal fracture of metatarsal

New   The appropriate 7th character is to be added to each code from subcategories S99.1

New	A	initial encounter for closed fracture
New	B	initial encounter for open fracture
New	D	subsequent encounter for fracture with routine healing
New	G	subsequent encounter for fracture with delayed healing
New	K	subsequent encounter for fracture with nonunion
New	P	subsequent encounter for fracture with malunion
New	S	sequela

New	S99.10		Unspecified physeal fracture of metatarsal
New		S99.101	Unspecified physeal fracture of right metatarsal
New		S99.102	Unspecified physeal fracture of left metatarsal
New		S99.109	Unspecified physeal fracture of unspecified metatarsal
New	S99.11		Salter-Harris Type I physeal fracture of metatarsal
New		S99.111	Salter-Harris Type I physeal fracture of right metatarsal
New		S99.112	Salter-Harris Type I physeal fracture of left metatarsal

New		S99.119	Salter-Harris Type I physeal fracture of unspecified metatarsal
New	S99.12		Salter-Harris Type II physeal fracture of metatarsal
New		S99.121	Salter-Harris Type II physeal fracture of right metatarsal
New		S99.122	Salter-Harris Type II physeal fracture of left metatarsal
New		S99.129	Salter-Harris Type II physeal fracture of unspecified metatarsal
New	S99.13		Salter-Harris Type III physeal fracture of metatarsal
New		S99.131	Salter-Harris Type III physeal fracture of right metatarsal
New		S99.132	Salter-Harris Type III physeal fracture of left metatarsal
New		S99.139	Salter-Harris Type III physeal fracture of unspecified metatarsal
New	S99.14		Salter-Harris Type IV physeal fracture of metatarsal
New		S99.141	Salter-Harris Type IV physeal fracture of right metatarsal
New		S99.142	Salter-Harris Type IV physeal fracture of left metatarsal
New		S99.149	Salter-Harris Type IV physeal fracture of unspecified metatarsal
New	S99.19		Other physeal fracture of metatarsal
New		S99.191	Other physeal fracture of right metatarsal
New		S99.192	Other physeal fracture of left metatarsal
New		S99.199	Other physeal fracture of unspecified metatarsal
New	S99.2		Physeal fracture of phalanx of toe
New			The appropriate 7th character is to be added to each code from subcategories S99.2

New	A initial encounter for closed fracture
New	B initial encounter for open fracture
New	D subsequent encounter for fracture with routine healing
New	G subsequent encounter for fracture with delayed healing
New	K subsequent encounter for fracture with nonunion
New	P subsequent encounter for fracture with malunion
	S sequela

New	S99.20		Unspecified physeal fracture of phalanx of toe
New		S99.201	Unspecified physeal fracture of phalanx of right toe
New		S99.202	Unspecified physeal fracture of phalanx of right toe
New		S99.209	Unspecified physeal fracture of phalanx of unspecified toe
New	S99.21		Salter-Harris Type I physeal fracture of phalanx of toe
New		S99.211	Salter-Harris Type I physeal fracture of phalanx of right toe
New		S99.212	Salter-Harris Type I physeal fracture of phalanx of left toe
New		S99.219	Salter-Harris Type I physeal fracture of phalanx of unspecified toe
New	S99.22		Salter-Harris Type II physeal fracture of phalanx of toe
New		S99.221	Salter-Harris Type II physeal fracture of phalanx of right toe
New		S99.222	Salter-Harris Type II physeal fracture of phalanx of left toe
New		S99.229	Salter-Harris Type II physeal fracture of phalanx of unspecified toe

New	S99.23		Salter-Harris Type III physeal fracture of phalanx of toe
New		S99.231	Salter-Harris Type III physeal fracture of phalanx of right toe
New		S99.232	Salter-Harris Type III physeal fracture of phalanx of left toe
New		S99.239	Salter-Harris Type III physeal fracture of phalanx of unspecified toe
New	S99.24		Salter-Harris Type IV physeal fracture of phalanx of toe
New		S99.241	Salter-Harris Type IV physeal fracture of phalanx of right toe
New		S99.242	Salter-Harris Type IV physeal fracture of phalanx of left toe
New		S99.249	Salter-Harris Type IV physeal fracture of phalanx of unspecified toe
New	S99.29		Other physeal fracture of phalanx of toe
New		S99.291	Other physeal fracture of phalanx of right toe
New		S99.292	Other physeal fracture of phalanx of left toe
New		S99.299	Other physeal fracture of phalanx of unspecified toe
	S99.8		Other specified injuries of ankle and foot
New			The appropriate 7th character is to be added to each code from subcategory S99.8

New	A initial encounter
New	D subsequent encounter
New	S sequela

	S99.9	Unspecified injury of ankle and foot
New		The appropriate 7th character is to be added to each code from subcategory S99.9

New	A initial encounter
New	D subsequent encounter
New	S sequela

	T17.32	Food in larynx
Revised		Bones in larynx
	T61	Toxic effect of noxious substances eaten as seafood
		Excludes1 allergic reaction to food, such as:
Deleted		gastroenteritis (noninfective) (K52.2)
New		food protein-induced enterocolitis syndrome (K52.21)
New		food protein-induced enteropathy (K52.22)
New		gastroenteritis (noninfective) (K52.29)
	T62	Toxic effect of other noxious substances eaten as food
		Excludes1 allergic reaction to food, such as:
Deleted		gastroenteritis (noninfective) (K52.2)
New		food protein-induced enterocolitis syndrome (K52.21)
New		food protein-induced enteropathy (K52.22)
New		gastroenteritis (noninfective) (K52.29)
	T78.05	Anaphylactic reaction due to tree nuts and seeds
Deleted		**Excludes1** anaphylactic reaction due to peanuts (T78.01)
New		**Excludes2** anaphylactic reaction due to peanuts (T78.01)
	T78.1	Other adverse food reactions, not elsewhere classified
Revised		Use additional code to identify the type of reaction, if applicable
Revised		**Excludes2** allergic and dietetic gastroenteritis and colitis (K52.29)
New		food protein-induced enterocolitis syndrome (K52.21)
New		food protein-induced enteropathy (K52.22)

T78.4   **Other and unspecified allergy**

Excludes1   specified types of allergic reaction such as:

Revised   allergic diarrhea (K52.29)

Revised   allergic gastroenteritis and colitis (K52.29)

New   food protein-induced enterocolitis syndrome (K52.21)

New   food protein-induced enteropathy (K52.22)

T80.1   **Vascular complications following infusion, transfusion and therapeutic injection**

Revised   **Excludes2**   vascular complications specified as due to prosthetic devices, implants and grafts (T82.8-, T83.8-, T84.8-, T85.8-)

T80.2   **Infections following infusion, transfusion and therapeutic injection**

Revised   **Excludes2**   postprocedural infections (T81.4-)

T80.21   **Infection due to central venous catheter**

New   Infection due to pulmonary artery catheter (Swan-Ganz catheter)

T80.211   **Bloodstream infection due to central venous catheter**

New   Bloodstream infection due to pulmonary artery catheter

T80.212   **Local infection due to central venous catheter**

New   Local infection due to pulmonary artery catheter

T80.218   **Other infection due to central venous catheter**

New   Other infection due to pulmonary artery catheter

T80.219   **Unspecified infection due to central venous catheter**

New   Unspecified infection due to pulmonary artery catheter

T80.6   **Other serum reactions**

Revised   **Excludes2**   serum hepatitis (B16-B19)

T81.12   **Postprocedural septic shock**

Revised   Postprocedural endotoxic shock resulting from a procedure, not elsewhere classified

Revised   Postprocedural gram-negative shock resulting from a procedure, not elsewhere classified

T81.7   **Vascular complications following a procedure, not elsewhere classified**

Revised   **Excludes2**   embolism due to prosthetic devices, implants and grafts (T82.8-, T83.81, T84.8-, T85.1-)

Revised   T82.81   **Embolism due to cardiac and vascular prosthetic devices, implants and grafts**

Revised   T82.817   **Embolism due to cardiac prosthetic devices, implants and grafts**

Revised   T82.818   **Embolism due to vascular prosthetic devices, implants and grafts**

Revised   T82.82   **Fibrosis due to cardiac and vascular prosthetic devices, implants and grafts**

Revised   T82.827   **Fibrosis due to cardiac prosthetic devices, implants and grafts**

Revised   T82.828   **Fibrosis due to vascular prosthetic devices, implants and grafts**

Revised   T82.83   **Hemorrhage due to cardiac and vascular prosthetic devices, implants and grafts**

Revised   T82.837   **Hemorrhage due to cardiac prosthetic devices, implants and grafts**

Revised   T82.838   **Hemorrhage due to vascular prosthetic devices, implants and grafts**

Revised   T82.84   **Pain due to cardiac and vascular prosthetic devices, implants and grafts**

Revised   T82.847   **Pain due to cardiac prosthetic devices, implants and grafts**

Revised   T82.848   **Pain due to vascular prosthetic devices, implants and grafts**

Revised   T82.85   **Stenosis due to cardiac and vascular prosthetic devices, implants and grafts**

New   T82.855   **Stenosis of coronary artery stent**

New   In-stent stenosis (restenosis) of coronary artery stent

New   Restenosis of coronary artery stent

New   T82.856   **Stenosis of peripheral vascular stent**

New   In-stent stenosis (restenosis) of peripheral vascular stent

New   Restenosis of peripheral vascular stent

Revised   T82.857   **Stenosis of other cardiac prosthetic devices, implants and grafts**

Revised   T82.858   **Stenosis of other vascular prosthetic devices, implants and grafts**

Revised   T82.86   **Thrombosis of cardiac and vascular prosthetic devices, implants and grafts**

Revised   T82.867   **Thrombosis due to cardiac prosthetic devices, implants and grafts**

Revised   T82.868   **Thrombosis due to vascular prosthetic devices, implants and grafts**

Revised   T83.0   **Mechanical complication of urinary catheter**

Revised   T83.01   **Breakdown (mechanical) of urinary catheter**

New   T83.011   **Breakdown (mechanical) of indwelling urethral catheter**

New   T83.012   **Breakdown (mechanical) of nephrostomy catheter**

Revised   T83.018   **Breakdown (mechanical) of other urinary catheter**

New   Breakdown (mechanical) of Hopkins catheter

New   Breakdown (mechanical) of ileostomy catheter

New   Breakdown (mechanical) urostomy catheter

Revised   T83.02   **Displacement of urinary catheter**

Revised   Malposition of urinary catheter

New   T83.021   **Displacement of indwelling urethral catheter**

New   T83.022   **Displacement of nephrostomy catheter**

Revised   T83.028   **Displacement of other urinary catheter**

New   Displacement of Hopkins catheter

New   Displacement of ileostomy catheter

New   Displacement of urostomy catheter

Revised   T83.03   **Leakage of urinary catheter**

New   T83.031   **Leakage of indwelling urethral catheter**

New   T83.032   **Leakage of nephrostomy catheter**

Revised	T83.038	**Leakage of other urinary catheter**
New		Leakage of Hopkins catheter
New		Leakage of ileostomy catheter
New		Leakage of urostomy catheter
Revised	T83.09	**Other mechanical complication of urinary catheter**
Revised		Obstruction (mechanical) of urinary catheter
Revised		Perforation of urinary catheter
Revised		Protrusion of urinary catheter
New	T83.091	**Other mechanical complication of indwelling urethral catheter**
New	T83.092	**Other mechanical complication of nephrostomy catheter**
Revised	T83.098	**Other mechanical complication of other urinary catheter**
New		Other mechanical complication of Hopkins catheter
New		Other mechanical complication of ileostomy catheter
New		Other mechanical complication of urostomy catheter
	T83.110	**Breakdown (mechanical) of urinary electronic stimulator device**
New		**Excludes2** Breakdown (mechanical) of electrode (lead) for sacral nerve neuro-stimulator (T85.111)
New		Breakdown (mechanical) of implanted electronic sacral neuro-stimulator, pulse generator or receiver (T85.113)
Revised	T83.111	**Breakdown (mechanical) of implanted urinary sphincter**
Revised	T83.112	**Breakdown (mechanical) of indwelling ureteral stent**
New	T83.113	**Breakdown (mechanical) of other urinary stents**
New		Breakdown (mechanical) of ileal conduit stent
New		Breakdown (mechanical) of nephroureteral stent
	T83.120	**Displacement of urinary electronic stimulator device**
New		**Excludes2** Displacement of electrode (lead) for sacral nerve neuro-stimulator (T85.121)
New		Displacement of implanted electronic sacral neuro-stimulator, pulse generator or receiver (T85.123)
Revised	T83.121	**Displacement of implanted urinary sphincter**
Revised	T83.122	**Displacement of indwelling ureteral stent**
New	T83.123	**Displacement of other urinary stents**
New		Displacement of ileal conduit stent
New		Displacement of nephroureteral stent
Revised	T83.190	**Other mechanical complication of urinary electronic stimulator device**
New		**Excludes2** Other mechanical complication of electrode (lead) for sacral nerve neuro-stimulator (T85.191)
New		Other mechanical complication of implanted electronic sacral neuro-stimulator, pulse generator or receiver (T85.193)
Revised	T83.191	**Other mechanical complication of implanted urinary sphincter**
Revised	T83.192	**Other mechanical complication of indwelling ureteral stent**
New	T83.193	**Other mechanical complication of other urinary stent**
New		Other mechanical complication of ileal conduit stent
New		Other mechanical complication of nephroureteral stent
New	T83.24	**Erosion of graft of urinary organ**
New	T83.25	**Exposure of graft of urinary organ**
	T83.32	**Displacement of intrauterine contraceptive device**
New		Missing string of intrauterine contraceptive device
Revised	T83.410	**Breakdown (mechanical) of implanted penile prosthesis**
New		Breakdown (mechanical) of penile prosthesis cylinder
New		Breakdown (mechanical) of penile prosthesis pump
New		Breakdown (mechanical) of penile prosthesis reservoir
New	T83.411	**Breakdown (mechanical) of implanted testicular prosthesis**
Revised	T83.420	**Displacement of implanted penile prosthesis**
New		Displacement of penile prosthesis cylinder
New		Displacement of penile prosthesis pump
New		Displacement of penile prosthesis reservoir
New	T83.421	**Displacement of implanted testicular prosthesis**

Revised		T83.490	**Other mechanical complication of implanted penile prosthesis**
New			Other mechanical complication of penile prosthesis cylinder
New			Other mechanical complication of penile prosthesis pump
New			Other mechanical complication of penile prosthesis reservoir
New		T83.491	**Other mechanical complication of implanted testicular prosthesis**
Revised	T83.51		**Infection and inflammatory reaction due to urinary catheter**
New		T83.510	**Infection and inflammatory reaction due to cystostomy catheter**
New		T83.511	**Infection and inflammatory reaction due to indwelling urethral catheter**
New		T83.512	**Infection and inflammatory reaction due to nephrostomy catheter**
New		T83.518	**Infection and inflammatory reaction due to other urinary catheter**
New			Infection and inflammatory reaction due to Hopkins catheter
New			Infection and inflammatory reaction due to ileostomy catheter
New			Infection and inflammatory reaction due to urostomy catheter
New		T83.590	**Infection and inflammatory reaction due to implanted urinary neurostimulation device**
New			**Excludes2** Infection and inflammatory reaction due to electrode lead of sacral nerve neurostimulator (T85.732)
New			Infection and inflammatory reaction due to pulse generator or receiver of sacral nerve neurostimulator (T85.734)
New		T83.591	**Infection and inflammatory reaction due to implanted urinary sphincter**
New		T83.592	**Infection and inflammatory reaction due to indwelling ureteral stent**
New		T83.593	**Infection and inflammatory reaction due to other urinary stents**
New			Infection and inflammatory reaction due to ileal conduit stents
New			Infection and inflammatory reaction due to nephroureteral stent
New		T83.598	**Infection and inflammatory reaction due to other prosthetic device, implant and graft in urinary system**

New		T83.61	**Infection and inflammatory reaction due to implanted penile prosthesis**
New			Infection and inflammatory reaction due to penile prosthesis cylinder
New			Infection and inflammatory reaction due to penile prosthesis pump
New			Infection and inflammatory reaction due to penile prosthesis reservoir
New		T83.62	**Infection and inflammatory reaction due to implanted testicular prosthesis**
New		T83.69	**Infection and inflammatory reaction due to other prosthetic device, implant and graft in genital tract**
Revised		T83.711	**Erosion of implanted vaginal mesh to surrounding organ or tissue**
Revised			Erosion of implanted vaginal mesh into pelvic floor muscles
New		T83.712	**Erosion of implanted urethral mesh to surrounding organ or tissue**
New			Erosion of implanted female urethral sling
New			Erosion of implanted male urethral sling
New			Erosion of implanted urethral mesh into pelvic floor muscles
New		T83.713	**Erosion of implanted urethral bulking agent to surrounding organ or tissue**
New		T83.714	**Erosion of implanted ureteral bulking agent to surrounding organ or tissue**
Revised		T83.718	**Erosion of other implanted mesh to organ or tissue**
New		T83.719	**Erosion of other prosthetic materials to surrounding organ or tissue**
	T83.72		**Exposure of implanted mesh and other prosthetic materials into surrounding organ or tissue**
New			Extrusion of implanted mesh
Revised		T83.721	**Exposure of implanted vaginal mesh into vagina**
Revised			Exposure of implanted vaginal mesh through vaginal wall
New		T83.722	**Exposure of implanted urethral mesh into urethra**
New			Exposure of implanted female urethral sling
New			Exposure of implanted male urethral sling
New			Exposure of implanted urethral mesh through urethral wall
New		T83.723	**Exposure of implanted urethral bulking agent into urethra**
New		T83.724	**Exposure of implanted ureteral bulking agent into ureter**
Revised		T83.728	**Exposure of other implanted mesh into organ or tissue**
New		T83.729	**Exposure of other prosthetic materials into organ or tissue**
New		T83.79	**Other specified complications due to other genitourinary prosthetic materials**
	T83.8		**Other specified complications of genitourinary prosthetic devices, implants and grafts**
Revised		T83.81	**Embolism due to genitourinary prosthetic devices, implants and grafts**
Revised		T83.82	**Fibrosis due to genitourinary prosthetic devices, implants and grafts**

Revised	T83.83	**Hemorrhage due to genitourinary prosthetic devices, implants and grafts**
Revised	T83.84	**Pain due to genitourinary prosthetic devices, implants and grafts**
Revised	T83.85	**Stenosis due to genitourinary prosthetic devices, implants and grafts**
Revised	T83.86	**Thrombosis due to genitourinary prosthetic devices, implants and grafts**
Deleted	~~T84.04~~	~~Periprosthetic fracture around internal prosthetic joint~~
Deleted		**Excludes2** breakage (fracture) of prosthetic joint (T84.01)
Deleted	~~T84.040~~	~~Periprosthetic fracture around internal prosthetic right hip joint~~
Deleted	~~T84.041~~	~~Periprosthetic fracture around internal prosthetic left hip joint~~
Deleted	~~T84.042~~	~~Periprosthetic fracture around internal prosthetic right knee joint~~
Deleted	~~T84.043~~	~~Periprosthetic fracture around internal prosthetic left knee joint~~
Deleted	~~T84.048~~	~~Periprosthetic fracture around other internal prosthetic joint~~
Deleted		Use additional code to identify the joint (Z96.6-)
Deleted	~~T84.049~~	~~Periprosthetic fracture around unspecified internal prosthetic joint~~
Revised	T85.110	**Breakdown (mechanical) of implanted electronic neurostimulator of brain electrode (lead)**
Revised	T85.111	**Breakdown (mechanical) of implanted electronic neurostimulator of peripheral nerve electrode (lead)**
New		Breakdown of electrode (lead) for cranial nerve neurostimulators
New		Breakdown of electrode (lead) for gastric neurostimulator
New		Breakdown of electrode (lead) for sacral nerve neurostimulator
New		Breakdown of electrode (lead) for vagal nerve neurostimulators
Revised	T85.112	**Breakdown (mechanical) of implanted electronic neurostimulator of spinal cord electrode (lead)**
New	T85.113	**Breakdown (mechanical) of implanted electronic neurostimulator, generator**
New		Breakdown (mechanical) of implanted electronic neurostimuator generator, brain, peripheral, gastric, spinal
New		Breakdown (mechanical) of implanted electronic sacral neurostimulator, pulse generator or receiver
Revised	T85.120	**Displacement of implanted electronic neurostimulator of brain electrode (lead)**
Revised	T85.121	**Displacement of implanted electronic neurostimulator of peripheral nerve electrode (lead)**
New		Displacement of electrode (lead) for cranial nerve neurostimulators
New		Displacement of electrode (lead) for gastric neurostimulator
New		Displacement of electrode (lead) for sacral nerve neurostimulator
New		Displacement of electrode (lead) for vagal nerve neurostimulators
Revised	T85.122	**Displacement of implanted electronic neurostimulator of spinal cord electrode (lead)**
New	T85.123	**Displacement of implanted electronic neurostimulator, generator**
New		Displacement of implanted electronic neurostimulator generator, brain, peripheral, gastric, spinal
New		Displacement of implanted electronic sacral neurostimulator, pulse generator or receiver
Revised	T85.190	**Other mechanical complication of implanted electronic neurostimulator of brain electrode (lead)**
Revised	T85.191	**Other mechanical complication of implanted electronic neurostimulator of peripheral nerve electrode (lead)**
New		Other mechanical complication of electrode (lead) for cranial nerve neurostimulators
New		Other mechanical complication of electrode (lead) for gastric neurostimulator
New		Other mechanical complication of electrode (lead) for sacral nerve neurostimulator
New		Other mechanical complication of electrode (lead) for vagal nerve neurostimulators
Revised	T85.192	**Other mechanical complication of implanted electronic neurostimulator of spinal cord electrode (lead)**
New	T85.193	**Other mechanical complication of implanted electronic neurostimulator, generator**
New		Other mechanical complication of implanted electronic neurostimulator generator, brain, peripheral, gastric, spinal
New		Other mechanical complication of implanted electronic sacral neurostimulator, pulse generator or receiver

Revised	T85.610	**Breakdown (mechanical) of cranial or spinal infusion catheter**
New		Breakdown (mechanical) of epidural infusion catheter
New		Breakdown (mechanical) of intrathecal infusion catheter
New		Breakdown (mechanical) of subarachnoid infusion catheter
New		Breakdown (mechanical) of subdural infusion catheter
New	T85.615	**Breakdown (mechanical) of other nervous system device, implant or graft**
New		Breakdown (mechanical) of intrathecal infusion pump
Revised	T85.620	**Displacement of cranial or spinal infusion catheter**
New		Displacement of epidural infusion catheter
New		Displacement of intrathecal infusion catheter
New		Displacement of subarachnoid infusion catheter
New		Displacement of subdural infusion catheter
New	T85.625	**Displacement of other nervous system device, implant or graft**
New		Displacement of intrathecal infusion pump
Revised	T85.630	**Leakage of cranial or spinal infusion catheter**
New		Leakage of epidural infusion catheter
New		Leakage of intrathecal infusion catheter
New		Leakage of subdural infusion catheter
New		Leakage of subarachnoid infusion catheter
New	T85.635	**Leakage of other nervous system device, implant or graft**
New		Leakage of intrathecal infusion pump
Revised	T85.690	**Other mechanical complication of cranial or spinal infusion catheter**
New		Other mechanical complication of epidural infusion catheter
New		Other mechanical complication of intrathecal infusion catheter
New		Other mechanical complication of subarachnoid infusion catheter
New		Other mechanical complication of subdural infusion catheter
New	T85.695	**Other mechanical complication of other nervous system device, implant or graft**
New		Other mechanical complication of intrathecal infusion pump

New	T85.73	**Infection and inflammatory reaction due to nervous system devices, implants and graft**
New	T85.730	**Infection and inflammatory reaction due to ventricular intracranial (communicating) shunt**
New	T85.731	**Infection and inflammatory reaction due to implanted electronic neurostimulator of brain, electrode (lead)**
New	T85.732	**Infection and inflammatory reaction due to implanted electronic neurostimulator of peripheral nerve, electrode (lead)**
New		Infection and inflammatory reaction due to electrode (lead) for cranial nerve neurostimulators
New		Infection and inflammatory reaction due to electrode (lead) for gastric neurostimulator
New		Infection and inflammatory reaction due to electrode (lead) for sacral nerve neurostimulator
New		Infection and inflammatory reaction due to electrode (lead) for vagal nerve neurostimulators
New	T85.733	**Infection and inflammatory reaction due to implanted electronic neurostimulator of spinal cord, electrode (lead)**
New	T85.734	**Infection and inflammatory reaction due to implanted electronic neurostimulator, generator**
New		Generator pocket infection
New	T85.735	**Infection and inflammatory reaction due to cranial or spinal infusion catheter**
New		Infection and inflammatory reaction due to epidural catheter
New		Infection and inflammatory reaction due to intrathecal infusion catheter
New		Infection and inflammatory reaction due to subarachnoid catheter
New		Infection and inflammatory reaction due to subdural catheter
New	T85.738	**Infection and inflammatory reaction due to other nervous system device, implant or graft**
New		Infection and inflammatory reaction due to intrathecal infusion pump
New	T85.810	**Embolism due to nervous system prosthetic devices, implants and grafts**
New	T85.818	**Embolism due to other internal prosthetic devices, implants and grafts**
New	T85.820	**Fibrosis due to nervous system prosthetic devices, implants and grafts**
New	T85.828	**Fibrosis due to other internal prosthetic devices, implants and grafts**
New	T85.830	**Hemorrhage due to nervous system prosthetic devices, implants and grafts**

New		T85.838	**Hemorrhage due to other internal prosthetic devices, implants and grafts**
New		T85.840	**Pain due to nervous system prosthetic devices, implants and grafts**
New		T85.848	**Pain due to other internal prosthetic devices, implants and grafts**
New		T85.850	**Stenosis due to nervous system prosthetic devices, implants and grafts**
New		T85.858	**Stenosis due to other internal prosthetic devices, implants and grafts**
New		T85.860	**Thrombosis due to nervous system prosthetic devices, implants and grafts**
New		T85.868	**Thrombosis due to other internal prosthetic devices, implants and grafts**
	T85.89		**Other specified complication of internal prosthetic devices, implants and grafts, not elsewhere classified**
New			Erosion or breakdown of subcutaneous device pocket
New		T85.890	**Other specified complication of nervous system prosthetic devices, implants and grafts**
New		T85.898	**Other specified complication of other internal prosthetic devices, implants and grafts**
New	T88.53		**Unintended awareness under general anesthesia during procedure**
New		**Excludes2**	personal history of unintended awareness under general anesthesia (Z92.84)

CHAPTER 20
EXTERNAL CAUSES OF MORBIDITY (V00-Y99)

This chapter contains the following blocks:

New	X50	Overexertion and strenuous or repetitive movements
Revised	X92-Y09	Assault

TRANSPORT ACCIDENTS (V00-V99)

Deleted **Note:** This section is structured in 12 groups. Those relating to land transport accidents (V01-V89) reflect the victim's mode of transport and are subdivided to identify the victim's 'counterpart' or the type of event. The vehicle of which the injured person is an occupant is identified in the first two characters since it is seen as the most important factor to identify for prevention purposes. A transport accident is one in which the vehicle involved must be moving or running or in use for transport purposes at the time of the accident.

New **Note:** This section is structured in 12 groups. Those relating to land transport accidents (V00-V89) reflect the victim's mode of transport and are subdivided to identify the victim's 'counterpart' or the type of event. The vehicle of which the injured person is an occupant is identified in the first two characters since it is seen as the most important factor to identify for prevention purposes. A transport accident is one in which the vehicle involved must be moving or running or in use for transport purposes at the time of the accident.

Revised **Note:** Definitions related to transport accidents:

Revised (a) A transport accident (V00-V99) is any accident involving a device designed primarily for, or used at the time primarily for, conveying persons or good from one place to another.

Revised (e) A pedestrian is any person involved in an accident who was not at the time of the accident riding in or on a motor vehicle, railway train, streetcar or animal-drawn or other vehicle, or on a pedal cycle or animal. This includes, a person changing a tire, working on a parked car, or a person on foot. It also includes the user of a pedestrian conveyance such as a baby-stroller, ice-skates, skis, sled, roller skates, a skateboard, nonmotorized or motorized wheelchair, motorized mobility scooter, or nonmotorized scooter.

Revised (h) A person on the outside of a vehicle is any person being transported by a vehicle but not occupying the space normally reserved for the driver or passengers, or the space intended for the transport of property. This includes a person travelling on the bodywork, bumper, fender, roof, running board or step of a vehicle, as well as, hanging on the outside of the vehicle.

Revised (k) A motorcycle is a two-wheeled motor vehicle with one or two riding saddles and sometimes with a third wheel for the support of a sidecar. The sidecar is considered part of the motorcycle. This includes a moped, motor scooter, or motorized bicycle.

Revised (n) A car [automobile] is a four-wheeled motor vehicle designed primarily for carrying up to 7 persons. A trailer being towed by the car is considered part of the car. It does not include a van or minivan—see definition (o)

Revised (t) A special vehicle mainly used on industrial premises is a motor vehicle designed primarily for use within the buildings and premises of industrial or commercial establishments. This includes battery-powered airport passenger vehicles or baggage/mail trucks, forklifts, coal-cars in a coal mine, logging cars and trucks used in mines or quarries.

Revised (w) A special all-terrain vehicle is a motor vehicle of special design to enable it to negotiate over rough or soft terrain, snow or sand. Examples of special design are high construction, special wheels and tires, tracks, and support on a cushion of air. This includes snow mobiles, all-terrain vehicles (ATV), and dune buggies. It does not include passenger vehicle designated as sport utility vehicles (SUV).

Deleted ~~V47.01 Driver of sport utility vehicle injured in collision with fixed or stationary object in nontraffic accident~~

Deleted ~~V47.02 Driver of other type car injured in collision with fixed or stationary object in nontraffic accident~~

Deleted ~~V47.11 Passenger of sport utility vehicle injured in collision with fixed or stationary object in nontraffic accident~~

Deleted ~~V47.12 Passenger of other type car injured in collision with fixed or stationary object in nontraffic accident~~

Deleted ~~V47.31 Unspecified occupant of sport utility vehicle injured in collision with fixed or stationary object in nontraffic accident~~

Deleted ~~V47.32 Unspecified occupant of other type car injured in collision with fixed or stationary object in nontraffic accident~~

Deleted ~~V47.51 Driver of sport utility vehicle injured in collision with fixed or stationary object in traffic accident~~

Deleted ~~V47.52 Driver of other type car injured in collision with fixed or stationary object in traffic accident~~

Deleted ~~V47.61 Passenger of sport utility vehicle injured in collision with fixed or stationary object in traffic accident~~

Deleted ~~V47.62 Passenger of other type car injured in collision with fixed or stationary object in traffic accident~~

Deleted		~~V47.91 Unspecified occupant of sport utility vehicle injured in collision with fixed or stationary object in traffic accident~~
Deleted		~~V47.92 Unspecified occupant of other type car injured in collision with fixed or stationary object in traffic accident~~

EXPOSURE TO INANIMATE MECHANICAL FORCES (W20-W49)

Revised	**Excludes1**	assault (X92-Y09)
	W25	**Contact with sharp glass**
		Excludes2 glass embedded in skin (W45)
Revised	W26	**Contact with other sharp objects**
New		**Excludes2** sharp object(s) embedded in skin (W45)
New		W26.2 **Contact with edge of stiff paper**
New		Paper cut
New		W26.8 **Contact with other sharp object(s), not elsewhere classified**
New		Contact with tin can lid
New		W26.9 **Contact with unspecified sharp object(s)**
	W45	**Foreign body or object entering through skin**
New		**Includes** foreign body or object embedded in skin nail embedded in skin
Revised		**Excludes2** contact with other sharp object(s) (W26.-)
Deleted		~~W45.1 Paper entering through skin~~
Deleted		~~Paper cut~~
Deleted		~~W45.2 Lid of can entering through skin~~
	W89	**Exposure to man-made visible and ultraviolet light**
Deleted		**Excludes2** exposure to sunlight (X32)
New		**Excludes1** exposure to sunlight (X32)
	X32	**Exposure to sunlight**
Deleted		**Excludes1** radiation-related disorders of the skin and subcutaneous tissue (L55-L59)
	X39.0	**Exposure to natural radiation**
Revised		**Excludes1** contact with and (suspected) exposure to radon and other naturally occuring radiation (Z77.123)

OVEREXERTION AND STRENUOUS OR REPETITIVE MOVEMENTS (X50)

New	X50	**Overexertion and strenuous or repetitive movements**
New		The appropriate 7th character is to be added to each code from category X50

New	A	initial encounter
New	D	subsequent encounter
New	S	sequela

New	X50.0	**Overexertion from strenuous movement or load**
New		Lifting heavy objects
New		Lifting weights
New	X50.1	**Overexertion from prolonged static or awkward postures**
New		Prolonged bending
New		Prolonged kneeling
New		Prolonged reaching
New		Prolonged sitting
New		Prolonged standing
New		Prolonged twisting
New		Static bending
New		Static kneeling
New		Static reaching
New		Static sitting
New		Static standing
New		Static twisting
New	X50.3	**Overexertion from repetitive movements**
New		Use of hand as hammer
New		**Excludes2** Overuse from prolonged static or awkward postures (X50.1)
New	X50.9	**Other and unspecified overexertion or strenuous movements or postures**
New		Contact pressure
New		Contact stress

Deleted		**ASSAULT (X92-Y08)**
New		**ASSAULT (X92-Y09)**

MISADVENTURES TO PATIENTS DURING SURGICAL AND MEDICAL CARE (Y62-Y69)

New	**Excludes1**	surgical and medical procedures as the cause of abnormal reaction of the patient, without mention of misadventure at the time of the procedure (Y83-Y84)
Deleted	**Excludes2**	surgical and medical procedures as the cause of abnormal reaction of the patient, without mention of misadventure at the time of the procedure (Y83-Y84)

MEDICAL DEVICES ASSOCIATED WITH ADVERSE INCIDENTS IN DIAGNOSTIC AND THERAPEUTIC USE (Y70-Y82)

Deleted	**Excludes1**	misadventure to patients during surgical and medical care, classifiable to (Y62-Y69)
Deleted		later complications following use of medical devices without breakdown or malfunctioning of device (Y83-Y84)
New	**Excludes2**	breakdown or malfunctioning of medical device (after implantation) (during procedure) (ongoing use) (Y70-Y82)
New		later complications following use of medical devices without breakdown or malfunctioning of device (Y83-Y84)
New		misadventure to patients during surgical and medical care, classifiable to (Y62-Y69)
New		surgical and other medical procedures as the cause of abnormal reaction of the patient, or of later complication, without mention of misadventure at the time of the procedure (Y83-Y84)

SURGICAL AND OTHER MEDICAL PROCEDURES AS THE CAUSE OF ABNORMAL REACTION OF THE PATIENT, OR OF LATER COMPLICATION, WITHOUT MENTION OF MISADVENTURE AT THE TIME OF THE PROCEDURE (Y83-Y84)

New	**Excludes2**	breakdown or malfunctioning of medical device (after implantation) (during procedure) (ongoing use) (Y70-Y82)
Revised	Y92.4	**Street, highway and other paved roadways as the place of occurrence of the external cause**
New	Y93.85	**Activity, choking game**
New		Activity, blackout game
New		Activity, fainting game
New		Activity, pass out game

CHAPTER 21
FACTORS INFLUENCING HEALTH STATUS AND CONTACT WITH HEALTH SERVICES (Z00-Z99)

This chapter contains the following blocks:

Deleted	Z20-Z28	Persons with potential health hazards related to communicable diseases
New	Z19	Hormone sensitivity malignancy status
New	Z20-Z29	Persons with potential health hazards related to communicable diseases

	Z01.411	**Encounter for gynecological examination (general) (routine) with abnormal findings**
New		Use additional code to identify any abnormal findings
	Z01.419	**Encounter for gynecological examination (general) (routine) without abnormal findings**
Deleted		Use additional code to identify any abnormal findings

New	**Z05**	**Encounter for observation and evaluation of newborn for suspected diseases and conditions ruled out**
New		This category is to be used for newborns, within the neonatal period (the first 28 days of life), who are suspected of having an abnormal condition unrelated to exposure from the mother or the birth process, but without signs or symptoms, and which, after examination and observation, is ruled out.
New		**Excludes2** newborn observation for suspected condition, related to exposure from the mother or birth process (P00-P04)
New	**Z05.0**	**Observation and evaluation of newborn for suspected cardiac condition ruled out**
New	**Z05.1**	**Observation and evaluation of newborn for suspected infectious condition ruled out**
New	**Z05.2**	**Observation and evaluation of newborn for suspected neurological condition ruled out**
New	**Z05.3**	**Observation and evaluation of newborn for suspected respiratory condition ruled out**
New	**Z05.4**	**Observation and evaluation of newborn for suspected genetic, metabolic or immunologic condition ruled out**
New	**Z05.41**	**Observation and evaluation of newborn for suspected genetic condition ruled out**
New	**Z05.42**	**Observation and evaluation of newborn for suspected metabolic condition ruled out**
New	**Z05.43**	**Observation and evaluation of newborn for suspected immunologic condition ruled out**
New	**Z05.5**	**Observation and evaluation of newborn for suspected gastrointestinal condition ruled out**
New	**Z05.6**	**Observation and evaluation of newborn for suspected genitourinary condition ruled out**
New	**Z05.7**	**Observation and evaluation of newborn for suspected skin, subcutaneous, musculoskeletal and connective tissue condition ruled out**
New	**Z05.71**	**Observation and evaluation of newborn for suspected skin and subcutaneous tissue condition ruled out**
New	**Z05.72**	**Observation and evaluation of newborn for suspected musculoskeletal condition ruled out**
New	**Z05.73**	**Observation and evaluation of newborn for suspected connective tissue condition ruled out**
New	**Z05.8**	**Observation and evaluation of newborn for other specified suspected condition ruled out**
New	**Z05.9**	**Observation and evaluation of newborn for unspecified suspected condition ruled out**
	Z12.4	**Encounter for screening for malignant neoplasm of cervix**
Deleted		**Excludes1** encounter for screening for human papillomavirus (Z11.51)
New		**Excludes2** encounter for screening for human papillomavirus (Z11.51)

New **HORMONE SENSITIVITY MALIGNANCY STATUS (Z19)**

New	**Z19**	**Hormone sensitivity malignancy status**
New		*Code first* malignant neoplasm —*see* Table of Neoplasms, by site, malignant
New	**Z19.1**	**Hormone sensitive malignancy status**
New	**Z19.2**	**Hormone resistant malignancy status**
New		Castrate resistant prostate malignancy status

Deleted **PERSONS WITH POTENTIAL HEALTH HAZARDS RELATED TO COMMUNICABLE DISEASES (Z20-Z28)**

New **PERSONS WITH POTENTIAL HEALTH HAZARDS RELATED TO COMMUNICABLE DISEASES (Z20-Z29)**

	Z22	**Carrier of infectious disease**
New		**Excludes2** carrier of viral hepatitis (B18.-)
	Z22.330	**Carrier of Group B streptococcus**
New		**Excludes1** Carrier of streptococcus group B (GBS) complicating pregnancy, childbirth and the puerperium (O99.82-)
Deleted		~~Z22.5 Carrier of viral hepatitis~~
Deleted		~~Z22.50 Carrier of unspecified viral hepatitis~~
Deleted		~~Z22.51 Carrier of viral hepatitis B~~
Deleted		~~Hepatitis B surface antigen [HBsAg] carrier~~
Deleted		~~Z22.52 Carrier of viral hepatitis C~~
Deleted		~~Z22.59 Carrier of other viral hepatitis~~
New	**Z29**	**Encounter for other prophylactic measures**
New		**Excludes1** desensitization to allergens (Z51.6)
New		prophylactic surgery (Z40.-)
New	**Z29.1**	**Encounter for prophylactic immunotherapy**
New		Encounter for administration of immunoglobulin
New	**Z29.11**	**Encounter for prophylactic immunotherapy for respiratory syncytial virus (RSV)**
New	**Z29.12**	**Encounter for prophylactic antivenin**
New	**Z29.13**	**Encounter for prophylactic Rho(D) immune globulin**
New	**Z29.14**	**Encounter for prophylactic rabies immune globin**
New	**Z29.3**	**Encounter for prophylactic fluoride administration**
New	**Z29.8**	**Encounter for other specified prophylactic measures**
New	**Z29.9**	**Encounter for prophylactic measures, unspecified**
New	**Z30.015**	**Encounter for initial prescription of vaginal ring hormonal contraceptive**
New	**Z30.016**	**Encounter for initial prescription of transdermal patch hormonal contraceptive device**
New	**Z30.017**	**Encounter for initial prescription of implantable subdermal contraceptive**
New	**Z30.018**	**Encounter for initial prescription of other contraceptives**
New		Encounter for initial prescription of barrier contraception
New		Encounter for initial prescription of diaphragm
New	**Z30.44**	**Encounter for surveillance of vaginal ring hormonal contraceptive device**
New	**Z30.45**	**Encounter for surveillance of transdermal patch hormonal contraceptive device**
New	**Z30.46**	**Encounter for surveillance of implantable subdermal contraceptive**
New		Encounter for checking, reinsertion or removal of implantable subdermal contraceptive
New	**Z30.49**	**Encounter for surveillance of other contraceptives**
New		Encounter for surveillance of barrier contraception
New		Encounter for surveillance of diaphragm

New   **Z31.7** **Encounter for procreative management and counseling for gestational carrier**
New   **Excludes1** pregnant state, gestational carrier (Z33.3)

New   **Z33.1** **Pregnant state, incidental**
New   **Excludes1** pregnant state, gestational carrier (Z33.3)

New   **Z33.3** **Pregnant state, gestational carrier**
New   **Excludes1** encounter for procreative management and counseling for gestational carrier (Z31.7)

        Z3A **Weeks of gestation**
Revised   **Note:** Codes from category Z3A are for use, only on the maternal record, to indicate the weeks of gestation of the pregnancy, if known.

        Z45.01 **Encounter for adjustment and management of cardiac pacemaker**
New   Encounter for adjustment and management of cardiac resynchronization therapy pacemaker (CRT-P)
        Z45.02 **Encounter for adjustment and management of automatic implantable cardiac defibrillator**
New   Encounter for adjustment and management of cardiac resynchronization therapy defibrillator (CRT-D)

Revised **Z51** **Encounter for other aftercare and medical care**
New   **Z51.6** **Encounter for desensitization to allergens**

New   **Z53.3** **Procedure converted to open procedure**
New   **Z53.31** **Laparoscopic surgical procedure converted to open procedure**
New   **Z53.32** **Thoracoscopic surgical procedure converted to open procedure**
New   **Z53.33** **Arthroscopic surgical procedure converted to open procedure**
New   **Z53.39** **Other specified procedure converted to open procedure**

        Z77 **Other contact with and (suspected) exposures hazardous to health**
Revised   **Excludes2** newborn affected by noxious substances transmitted via placenta or breast milk (P04.-)

        Z79 **Long term (current) drug therapy**
New   **Excludes2** long term (current) use of oral antidiabetic drugs (Z79.84)
New   long term (current) use of oral hypoglycemic drugs (Z79.84)
New   **Z79.84** **Long term (current) use of oral hypoglycemic drugs**
New   Long term (current) use of oral antidiabetic drugs
New   **Excludes2** long term (current) use of insulin (Z79.4)

        Z79.891 **Long term (current) use of opiate analgesic**
Revised   **Excludes1** methadone use NOS (F11.9-)

New   **Z83.42** **Family history of familial hypercholesterolemia**

New   **Z84.82** **Family history of sudden infant death syndrome**
New   Family history of SIDS

        Z85 **Personal history of malignant neoplasm**
            Use additional code to identify:
Revised   history of tobacco dependence (Z87.891)
        Z85.8 **Personal history of malignant neoplasms of other organs and systems**
Revised   Conditions classifiable to C00-C14, C40-C49, C69-C75, C7A.098, C76-C79

New   **Z86.00** **Personal history of in-situ neoplasm**
            Conditions classifiable to D00-D09
New   **Z86.001** **Personal history of in-situ neoplasm of cervix uteri**
                Personal history of cervical intraepithelial neoplasia III [CIN III]
        Z86.008 **Personal history of in-situ neoplasm of other site**
New   Personal history of vaginal intraepithelial neoplasia III [VAIN III]
New   Personal history of vulvar intraepithelial neoplasia III [VIN III]
        Z87.41 **Personal history of dysplasia of the female genital tract**
New   **Excludes1** personal history of intraepithelial neoplasia III of female genital tract (Z87.001, Z87.008)

        Z90.41 **Acquired absence of pancreas**
New   Code also exocrine pancreatic insufficiency (K86.81)

        Z92.84 **Personal history of unintended awareness under general anesthesia**
New   **Excludes2** unintended awareness under general anesthesia during procedure (T88.53)

        Z95.0 **Presence of cardiac pacemaker**
New   Presence of cardiac resynchronization therapy (CRT-P) pacemaker
New   **Excludes1** adjustment or management of cardiac device (Z45.0-)
        Z95.1 **Presence of aortocoronary bypass graft**
New   Presence of coronary artery bypass graft
        Z95.810 **Presence of automatic (implantable) cardiac defibrillator**
New   Presence of cardiac resynchronization therapy defibrillator (CRT-D)
New   Presence of cardioverter-defribrillator (ICD)

        Z97.5 **Presence of (intrauterine) contraceptive device**
Revised   **Excludes1** checking, reinsertion or removal of implantable subdermal contraceptive (Z30.46)
New   checking, reinsertion or removal of intrauterine contraceptive device (Z30.43-)

        Z98.89 **Other specified postprocedural states**
Deleted   Personal history of surgery, not elsewhere classified
New   **Z98.890** **Other specified postprocedural states**
New   Personal history of surgery, not elsewhere classified
New   **Z98.891** **History of uterine scar from previous surgery**
New   **Excludes1** Maternal care due to uterine scar from previous surgery (O34.2-)

        Z99.2 **Dependence on renal dialysis**
Deleted   **Excludes1** noncompliance with renal dialysis (Z91.15)
New   **Excludes2** noncompliance with renal dialysis (Z91.15)

Introduction

ICD-10-CM Official Guidelines for Coding and Reporting 2017
Narrative changes appear in **bold** text
Items <u>underlined</u> have been moved within the guidelines since the 2016 version
Italics are used to indicate revisions to heading changes

The Centers for Medicare and Medicaid Services (CMS) and the National Center for Health Statistics (NCHS), two departments within the U.S. Federal Government's Department of Health and Human Services (DHHS) provide the following guidelines for coding and reporting using the International Classification of Diseases, 10th Revision, Clinical Modification (ICD-10-CM). These guidelines should be used as a companion document to the official version of the ICD-10-CM as published on the NCHS website. The ICD-10-CM is a morbidity classification published by the United States for classifying diagnoses and reason for visits in all health care settings. The ICD-10-CM is based on the ICD-10, the statistical classification of disease published by the World Health Organization (WHO).

These guidelines have been approved by the four organizations that make up the Cooperating Parties for the ICD-10-CM: the American Hospital Association (AHA), the American Health Information Management Association (AHIMA), CMS, and NCHS.

These guidelines are a set of rules that have been developed to accompany and complement the official conventions and instructions provided within the ICD-10-CM itself. The instructions and conventions of the classification take precedence over guidelines. These guidelines are based on the coding and sequencing instructions in the Tabular List and Alphabetic Index of ICD-10-CM, but provide additional instruction. Adherence to these guidelines when assigning ICD-10-CM diagnosis codes is required under the Health Insurance Portability and Accountability Act (HIPAA). The diagnosis codes (Tabular List and Alphabetic Index) have been adopted under HIPAA for all healthcare settings. A joint effort between the healthcare provider and the coder is essential to achieve complete and accurate documentation, code assignment, and reporting of diagnoses and procedures. These guidelines have been developed to assist both the healthcare provider and the coder in identifying those diagnoses that are to be reported. The importance of consistent, complete documentation in the medical record cannot be overemphasized. Without such documentation accurate coding cannot be achieved. The entire record should be reviewed to determine the specific reason for the encounter and the conditions treated.

The term encounter is used for all settings, including hospital admissions. In the context of these guidelines, the term provider is used throughout the guidelines to mean physician or any qualified health care practitioner who is legally accountable for establishing the patient's diagnosis. Only this set of guidelines, approved by the Cooperating Parties, is official.

The guidelines are organized into sections. Section I includes the structure and conventions of the classification and general guidelines that apply to the entire classification, and chapter-specific guidelines that correspond to the chapters as they are arranged in the classification. Section II includes guidelines for selection of principal diagnosis for non-outpatient settings. Section III includes guidelines for reporting additional diagnoses in non-outpatient settings. Section IV is for outpatient coding and reporting. It is necessary to review all sections of the guidelines to fully understand all of the rules and instructions needed to code properly.

ICD-10-CM Official Guidelines for Coding and Reporting

Section I. Conventions, general coding guidelines and chapter specific guidelines

A. Conventions for the ICD-10-CM
  1. The Alphabetic Index and Tabular List
  2. Format and Structure:
  3. Use of codes for reporting purposes
  4. Placeholder character
  5. 7th Characters
  6. Abbreviations
     a. Alphabetic Index abbreviations
     b. Tabular List abbreviations
  7. Punctuation
  8. Use of "and"
  9. Other and Unspecified codes
     a. "Other" codes
     b. "Unspecified" codes
  10. Includes Notes
  11. Inclusion terms
  12. Excludes Notes
     a. Excludes1
     b. Excludes2
  13. Etiology/manifestation convention ("code first", "use additional code" and "in diseases classified elsewhere" notes)
  14. "And"
  15. "With"
  16. "See" and "See Also"
  17. "Code also note"
  18. Default codes
  19. Code assignment and Clinical Criteria
B. General Coding Guidelines
  1. Locating a code in the ICD-10-CM
  2. Level of Detail in Coding
  3. Code or codes from A00.0 through T88.9, Z00-Z99.8
  4. Signs and symptoms
  5. Conditions that are an integral part of a disease process
  6. Conditions that are not an integral part of a disease process
  7. Multiple coding for a single condition
  8. Acute and Chronic Conditions
  9. Combination Code
  10. Sequela (Late Effects)
  11. Impending or Threatened Condition
  12. Reporting Same Diagnosis Code More than Once
  13. Laterality
  14. Documentation for BMI, *Depth of* Non-pressure ulcers, Pressure Ulcer Stages, Coma Scale, and *NIH Stroke Scale*
  15. Syndromes
  16. Documentation of Complications of Care
  17. Borderline Diagnosis
  18. Use of Sign/Symptom/Unspecified Codes
C. Chapter-Specific Coding Guidelines
  1. Chapter 1: Certain Infectious and Parasitic Diseases (A00-B99)
     a. Human Immunodeficiency Virus (HIV) Infections
     b. Infectious agents as the cause of diseases classified to other chapters
     c. Infections resistant to antibiotics
     d. Sepsis, Severe Sepsis, and Septic Shock
     e. Methicillin Resistant *Staphylococcus aureus* (MRSA) Conditions
     f. Zika virus infection
  2. Chapter 2: Neoplasms (C00-D49)
     a. Treatment directed at the malignancy
     b. Treatment of secondary site
     c. Coding and sequencing of complications
     d. Primary malignancy previously excised
     e. Admissions/Encounters involving chemotherapy, immunotherapy and radiation therapy
     f. Admission/encounter to determine extent of malignancy
     g. Symptoms, signs, and abnormal findings listed in Chapter 18 associated with neoplasms
     h. Admission/encounter for pain control/ management
     i. Malignancy in two or more noncontiguous sites
     j. Disseminated malignant neoplasm, unspecified
     k. Malignant neoplasm without specification of site
     l. Sequencing of neoplasm codes
     m. Current malignancy versus personal history of malignancy
     n. Leukemia, Multiple Myeloma, and Malignant Plasma Cell Neoplasms in remission versus personal history
     o. Aftercare following surgery for neoplasm
     p. Follow-up care for completed treatment of a malignancy
     q. Prophylactic organ removal for prevention of malignancy
     r. Malignant neoplasm associated with transplanted organ
  3. Chapter 3: Disease of the blood and blood-forming organs and certain disorders involving the immune mechanism (D50-D89)
  4. Chapter 4: Endocrine, Nutritional, and Metabolic Diseases (E00-E89)
     a. Diabetes mellitus
  5. Chapter 5: Mental, Behavioral and Neurodevelopmental disorders (F01 – F99)
     a. Pain disorders related to psychological factors
     b. Mental and behavioral disorders due to psychoactive substance use
  6. Chapter 6: Diseases of the Nervous System (G00-G99)
     a. Dominant/nondominant side
     b. Pain - Category G89
  7. Chapter 7: Diseases of the Eye and Adnexa (H00-H59)
     a. Glaucoma
  8. Chapter 8: Diseases of the Ear and Mastoid Process (H60-H95)
  9. Chapter 9: Diseases of the Circulatory System (I00-I99)
     a. Hypertension
     b. Atherosclerotic Coronary Artery Disease and Angina
     c. Intraoperative and Postprocedural Cerebrovascular Accident
     d. Sequelae of Cerebrovascular Disease
     e. Acute myocardial infarction (AMI)

Section II. Selection of Principal Diagnosis

A. Codes for symptoms, signs, and ill-defined conditions
B. Two or more interrelated conditions, each potentially meeting the definition for principal diagnosis
C. Two or more diagnoses that equally meet the definition for principal diagnosis
D. Two or more comparative or contrasting conditions
E. A symptom(s) followed by contrasting/comparative diagnoses
F. Original treatment plan not carried out
G. Complications of surgery and other medical care
H. Uncertain Diagnosis

I. Admission from Observation Unit
  1. Admission Following Medical Observation
  2. Admission Following Post-Operative Observation
J. Admission from Outpatient Surgery
K. Admissions/Encounters for Rehabilitation

Section III. Reporting Additional Diagnoses

A. Previous conditions
B. Abnormal findings
C. Uncertain Diagnosis

Section IV. Diagnostic Coding and Reporting Guidelines for Outpatient Services

A. Selection of first-listed condition
  1. Outpatient Surgery
  2. Observation Stay
B. Codes from A00.0 through T88.9, Z00-Z99
C. Accurate reporting of ICD-10-CM diagnosis codes
D. Codes that describe symptoms and signs
E. Encounters for circumstances other than a disease or injury
F. Level of Detail in Coding
  1. ICD-10-CM codes with 3, 4, 5, 6, or 7 characters
  2. Use of full number of characters required for a code
G. ICD-10-CM code for the diagnosis, condition, problem, or other reason for encounter/visit
H. Uncertain diagnosis
I. Chronic diseases
J. Code all documented conditions that coexist
K. Patients receiving diagnostic services only
L. Patients receiving therapeutic services only
M. Patients receiving preoperative evaluations only
N. Ambulatory surgery
O. Routine outpatient prenatal visits
P. Encounters for general medical examinations with abnormal findings
Q. Encounters for routine health screenings

Appendix I: Present on Admission Reporting Guidelines

Section I. Conventions, general coding guidelines and chapter specific guidelines

The conventions, general guidelines and chapter-specific guidelines are applicable to all health care settings unless otherwise indicated. The conventions and instructions of the classification take precedence over guidelines.

A. Conventions for the ICD-10-CM

The conventions for the ICD-10-CM are the general rules for use of the classification independent of the guidelines. These conventions are incorporated within the Alphabetic Index and Tabular List of the ICD-10-CM as instructional notes.

1. The Alphabetic Index and Tabular List

The ICD-10-CM is divided into the Alphabetic Index, an alphabetical list of terms and their corresponding code, and the Tabular List, a structured list of codes divided into chapters based on body system or condition. The Alphabetic Index consists of the following parts: the Index of Diseases and Injury, the Index of External Causes of Injury, the Table of Neoplasms and the Table of Drugs and Chemicals.

See Section I.C2. General guidelines
See Section I.C.19. Adverse effects, poisoning, underdosing and toxic effects

2. Format and Structure:

The ICD-10-CM Tabular List contains categories, subcategories and codes. Characters for categories, subcategories and codes may be either a letter or a number. All categories are 3 characters. A three-character category that has no further subdivision is equivalent to a code. Subcategories are either 4 or 5 characters. Codes may be 3, 4, 5, 6 or 7 characters. That is, each level of subdivision after a category is a subcategory. The final level of subdivision is a code. Codes that have applicable 7th characters are still referred to as codes, not subcategories. A code that has an applicable 7th character is considered invalid without the 7th character.

The ICD-10-CM uses an indented format for ease in reference

3. Use of codes for reporting purposes

For reporting purposes only codes are permissible, not categories or subcategories, and any applicable 7th character is required.

4. Placeholder character

The ICD-10-CM utilizes a placeholder character "X". The "X" is used as a placeholder at certain codes to allow for future expansion. An example of this is at the poisoning, adverse effect and underdosing codes, categories T36-T50. Where a placeholder exists, the X must be used in order for the code to be considered a valid code.

5. 7th Characters

Certain ICD-10-CM categories have applicable 7th characters. The applicable 7th character is required for all codes within the category, or as the notes in the Tabular List instruct. The 7th character must always be the 7th character in the data field. If a code that requires a 7th character is not 6 characters, a placeholder X must be used to fill in the empty characters.

6. Abbreviations

a. Alphabetic Index abbreviations

NEC "Not elsewhere classifiable"
This abbreviation in the Alphabetic Index represents "other specified". When a specific code is not available for a condition the Alphabetic Index directs the coder to the "other specified" code in the Tabular List.

NOS "Not otherwise specified"
This abbreviation is the equivalent of unspecified.

b. Tabular List abbreviations

NEC "Not elsewhere classifiable"
This abbreviation in the Tabular List represents "other specified". When a specific code is not available for a condition, the Tabular List includes an NEC entry under a code to identify the code as the "other specified" code.

NOS "Not otherwise specified"
This abbreviation is the equivalent of unspecified.

7. Punctuation

[ ] Brackets are used in the Tabular List to enclose synonyms, alternative wording or explanatory phrases. Brackets are used in the Alphabetic Index to identify manifestation codes.

( ) Parentheses are used in both the Alphabetic Index and Tabular List to enclose supplementary words that may be present or absent in the statement of a disease or procedure without affecting the code number to which it is assigned. The terms within the parentheses are referred to as nonessential modifiers. The nonessential modifiers in the Alphabetic Index to Diseases apply to subterms following a main term except when a nonessential modifier and a subentry are mutually exclusive, the subentry takes precedence. For example, in the ICD-10-CM Alphabetic Index under the main term Enteritis, "acute" is a nonessential modifier and "chronic" is a subentry. In this case, the nonessential modifier "acute" does not apply to the subentry "chronic".

: Colons are used in the Tabular List after an incomplete term which needs one or more of the modifiers following the colon to make it assignable to a given category.

8. Use of "and".

See Section I.A.14. Use of the term "And"

9. Other and Unspecified codes

a. "Other" codes

Codes titled "other" or "other specified" are for use when the information in the medical record provides detail for which a specific code does not exist. Alphabetic Index entries with NEC in the line designate "other" codes in the Tabular List. These Alphabetic Index entries represent specific disease entities for which no specific code exists so the term is included within an "other" code.

b. "Unspecified" codes

Codes titled "unspecified" are for use when the information in the medical record is insufficient to assign a more specific code. For those categories for which an unspecified code is not provided, the "other specified" code may represent both other and unspecified.

See Section I.B.18 Use of Signs/Symptom/Unspecified Codes

10. Includes Notes

This note appears immediately under a three-character code title to further define, or give examples of, the content of the category.

11. Inclusion terms

List of terms is included under some codes. These terms are the conditions for which that code is to be used. The terms may be synonyms of the code title, or, in the case of "other specified" codes, the terms are a list of the various conditions assigned to that code. The inclusion terms are not necessarily exhaustive. Additional terms found only in the Alphabetic Index may also be assigned to a code.

12. Excludes Notes

The ICD-10-CM has two types of excludes notes. Each type of note has a different definition for use but they are all similar in that they indicate that codes excluded from each other are independent of each other.

a. Excludes1

A type 1 Excludes note is a pure excludes note. It means "NOT CODED HERE!" An Excludes1 note indicates that the code excluded should never be used at the same time as the code above the Excludes1 note. An Excludes1 is used when two conditions cannot occur together, such as a congenital form versus an acquired form of the same condition.

An exception to the Excludes1 definition is the circumstance when the two conditions are unrelated to each other. If it is not clear whether the two conditions involving an Excludes1 note are related or not, query the provider. For example, code F45.8, Other somatoform disorders, has an Excludes1 note for "sleep related teeth grinding (G47.63)," because "teeth grinding" is an inclusion term under F45.8. Only one of these two codes should be assigned for teeth grinding. However psychogenic dysmenorrhea is also an inclusion term under F45.8, and a patient could have both this condition and sleep related teeth grinding. In this case, the two conditions are clearly unrelated to each other, and so it would be appropriate to report F45.8 and G47.63 together.

b. Excludes2

A Type 2 Excludes note represents "Not included here." An excludes2 note indicates that the condition excluded is not part of the condition represented by the code, but a patient may have both conditions at the same time. When an Excludes2 note appears under a code, it is acceptable to use both the code and the excluded code together, when appropriate.

13. Etiology/manifestation convention ("code first", "use additional code" and "in diseases classified elsewhere" notes)

Certain conditions have both an underlying etiology and multiple body system manifestations

GUIDELINES (ICD-10-CM)

due to the underlying etiology. For such conditions, the ICD-10-CM has a coding convention that requires the underlying condition be sequenced first, **if applicable,** followed by the manifestation. Wherever such a combination exists, there is a "use additional code" note at the etiology code, and a "code first" note at the manifestation code. These instructional notes indicate the proper sequencing order of the codes, etiology followed by manifestation.

In most cases the manifestation codes will have in the code title, "in diseases classified elsewhere." Codes with this title are a component of the etiology/ manifestation convention. The code title indicates that it is a manifestation code. "In diseases classified elsewhere" codes are never permitted to be used as first-listed or principal diagnosis codes. They must be used in conjunction with an underlying condition code and they must be listed following the underlying condition. See category F02, Dementia in other diseases classified elsewhere, for an example of this convention.

There are manifestation codes that do not have "in diseases classified elsewhere" in the title. For such codes, there is a "use additional code" note at the etiology code and a "code first" note at the manifestation code and the rules for sequencing apply.

In addition to the notes in the Tabular List, these conditions also have a specific Alphabetic Index entry structure. In the Alphabetic Index both conditions are listed together with the etiology code first followed by the manifestation codes in brackets. The code in brackets is always to be sequenced second.

An example of the etiology/manifestation convention is dementia in Parkinson's disease. In the Alphabetic Index, code G20 is listed first, followed by code F02.80 or F02.81 in brackets. Code G20 represents the underlying etiology, Parkinson's disease, and must be sequenced first, whereas codes F02.80 and F02.81 represent the manifestation of dementia in diseases classified elsewhere, with or without behavioral disturbance.

"Code first" and "Use additional code" notes are also used as sequencing rules in the classification for certain codes that are not part of an etiology/manifestation combination.

See Section I.B.7. Multiple coding for a single condition.

14. "And"

The word "and" should be interpreted to mean either "and" or "or" when it appears in a title.

For example, cases of "tuberculosis of bones", "tuberculosis of joints" and "tuberculosis of bones and joints" are classified to subcategory A18.0, Tuberculosis of bones and joints.

15. "With"

The word "with" should be interpreted to mean "associated with" or "due to" when it appears in a code title, the Alphabetic Index, or an instructional note in the Tabular List. **The classification presumes a causal relationship between the two conditions linked by these terms in the Alphabetic Index or Tabular List. These conditions should be coded as related even in the absence of provider documentation explicitly linking them, unless the documentation clearly states the conditions are unrelated. For conditions not specifically linked by these relational terms in the classification, provider documentation must link the conditions in order to code them as related.**

The word "with" in the Alphabetic Index is sequenced immediately following the main term, not in alphabetical order.

16. "See" and "See Also"

The "see" instruction following a main term in the Alphabetic Index indicates that another term should be referenced. It is necessary to go to the main term referenced with the "see" note to locate the correct code.

A "see also" instruction following a main term in the Alphabetic Index instructs that there is another main term that may also be referenced that may provide additional Alphabetic Index entries that may be useful. It is not necessary to follow the "see also" note when the original main term provides the necessary code.

17. "Code also" note

A "code also" note instructs that two codes may be required to fully describe a condition, but this note does not provide sequencing direction.

18. Default codes

A code listed next to a main term in the ICD-10-CM Alphabetic Index is referred to as a default code. The default code represents that condition that is most commonly associated with the main term, or is the unspecified code for the condition. If a condition is documented in a medical record (for example, appendicitis) without any additional information, such as acute or chronic, the default code should be assigned.

19. Code assignment and Clinical Criteria

The assignment of a diagnosis code is based on the provider's diagnostic statement that the condition exists. The provider's statement that the patient has a particular condition is sufficient. Code assignment is not based on clinical criteria used by the provider to establish the diagnosis.

B. General Coding Guidelines

1. Locating a code in the ICD-10-CM

To select a code in the classification that corresponds to a diagnosis or reason for visit documented in a medical record, first locate the term in the Alphabetic Index, and then verify the code in the Tabular List. Read and be guided by instructional notations that appear in both the Alphabetic Index and the Tabular List.

It is essential to use both the Alphabetic Index and Tabular List when locating and assigning a code. The Alphabetic Index does not always provide the full code. Selection of the full code, including laterality and any applicable 7th character can only be done in the Tabular List. A dash (-) at the end of an Alphabetic Index entry indicates that additional characters are required. Even if a dash is not included at the Alphabetic Index entry, it is necessary to refer to the Tabular List to verify that no 7th character is required.

2. **Level of Detail in Coding**
   Diagnosis codes are to be used and reported at their highest number of characters available.

   ICD-10-CM diagnosis codes are composed of codes with 3, 4, 5, 6 or 7 characters. Codes with three characters are included in ICD-10-CM as the heading of a category of codes that may be further subdivided by the use of fourth and/or fifth characters and/or sixth characters, which provide greater detail.

   A three-character code is to be used only if it is not further subdivided. A code is invalid if it has not been coded to the full number of characters required for that code, including the 7th character, if applicable.

3. **Code or codes from A00.0 through T88.9, Z00-Z99.8**
   The appropriate code or codes from A00.0 through T88.9, Z00-Z99.8 must be used to identify diagnoses, symptoms, conditions, problems, complaints or other reason(s) for the encounter/visit.

4. **Signs and symptoms**
   Codes that describe symptoms and signs, as opposed to diagnoses, are acceptable for reporting purposes when a related definitive diagnosis has not been established (confirmed) by the provider. Chapter 18 of ICD-10-CM, Symptoms, Signs, and Abnormal Clinical and Laboratory Findings, Not Elsewhere Classified (codes R00.0 - R99) contains many, but not all codes for symptoms.
   See Section I.B.18 Use of Signs/Symptom/ Unspecified Codes

5. **Conditions that are an integral part of a disease process**
   Signs and symptoms that are associated routinely with a disease process should not be assigned as additional codes, unless otherwise instructed by the classification.

6. **Conditions that are not an integral part of a disease process**
   Additional signs and symptoms that may not be associated routinely with a disease process should be coded when present.

7. **Multiple coding for a single condition**
   In addition to the etiology/manifestation convention that requires two codes to fully describe a single condition that affects multiple body systems, there are other single conditions that also require more than one code. "Use additional code" notes are found in the Tabular List at codes that are not part of an etiology/manifestation pair where a secondary code is useful to fully describe

a condition. The sequencing rule is the same as the etiology/manifestation pair, "use additional code" indicates that a secondary code should be added.

For example, for bacterial infections that are not included in chapter 1, a secondary code from category B95, Streptococcus, Staphylococcus, and Enterococcus, as the cause of diseases classified elsewhere, or B96, Other bacterial agents as the cause of diseases classified elsewhere, may be required to identify the bacterial organism causing the infection. A "use additional code" note will normally be found at the infectious disease code, indicating a need for the organism code to be added as a secondary code.

"Code first" notes are also under certain codes that are not specifically manifestation codes but may be due to an underlying cause. When there is a "code first" note and an underlying condition is present, the underlying condition should be sequenced first.

"Code, if applicable, any causal condition first," notes indicate that this code may be assigned as a principal diagnosis when the causal condition is unknown or not applicable. If a causal condition is known, then the code for that condition should be sequenced as the principal or first-listed diagnosis.

Multiple codes may be needed for sequela, complication codes and obstetric codes to more fully describe a condition. See the specific guidelines for these conditions for further instruction.

8. **Acute and Chronic Conditions**
   If the same condition is described as both acute (subacute) and chronic, and separate subentries exist in the Alphabetic Index at the same indentation level, code both and sequence the acute (subacute) code first.

9. **Combination Code**
   A combination code is a single code used to classify:
   Two diagnoses, or
   A diagnosis with an associated secondary process (manifestation)
   A diagnosis with an associated complication
   Combination codes are identified by referring to subterm entries in the Alphabetic Index and by reading the inclusion and exclusion notes in the Tabular List.

   Assign only the combination code when that code fully identifies the diagnostic conditions involved or when the Alphabetic Index so directs. Multiple coding should not be used when the classification provides a combination code that clearly identifies all of the elements documented in the diagnosis. When the combination code lacks necessary specificity in describing the manifestation or complication, an additional code should be used as a secondary code.

10. **Sequela (Late Effects)**
    A sequela is the residual effect (condition produced) after the acute phase of an illness or injury has terminated. There is no time limit on when a sequela code can be used. The residual may

be apparent early, such as in cerebral infarction, or it may occur months or years later, such as that due to a previous injury. Examples of sequela include: scar formation resulting from a burn, deviated septum due to a nasal fracture, and infertility due to tubal occlusion from old tuberculosis. Coding of sequela generally requires two codes sequenced in the following order: the condition or nature of the sequela is sequenced first. The sequela code is sequenced second.

An exception to the above guidelines are those instances where the code for the sequela is followed by a manifestation code identified in the Tabular List and title, or the sequela code has been expanded (at the fourth, fifth or sixth character levels) to include the manifestation(s). The code for the acute phase of an illness or injury that led to the sequela is never used with a code for the late effect.

> See Section I.C.9. Sequelae of cerebrovascular disease
> See Section I.C.15. Sequelae of complication of pregnancy, childbirth and the puerperium
> See Section I.C.19. Application of 7th characters for Chapter 19

11. **Impending or Threatened Condition**
Code any condition described at the time of discharge as "impending" or "threatened" as follows:

If it did occur, code as confirmed diagnosis.

If it did not occur, reference the Alphabetic Index to determine if the condition has a subentry term for "impending" or "threatened" and also reference main term entries for "Impending" and for "Threatened."

If the subterms are listed, assign the given code.

If the subterms are not listed, code the existing underlying condition(s) and not the condition described as impending or threatened.

12. **Reporting Same Diagnosis Code More than Once**
Each unique ICD-10-CM diagnosis code may be reported only once for an encounter. This applies to bilateral conditions when there are no distinct codes identifying laterality or two different conditions classified to the same ICD-10-CM diagnosis code.

13. **Laterality**
Some ICD-10-CM codes indicate laterality, specifying whether the condition occurs on the left, right or is bilateral. If no bilateral code is provided and the condition is bilateral, assign separate codes for both the left and right side. If the side is not identified in the medical record, assign the code for the unspecified side.

When a patient has a bilateral condition and each side is treated during separate encounters, assign the "bilateral" code (as the condition still exists on both sides), including for the encounter to treat the first side. For the second encounter for treatment after one side has previously been treated and the condition no longer exists on that side, assign the appropriate unilateral code for the side where the condition still exists (e.g., cataract surgery performed on each eye in separate encounters). The bilateral code would not be assigned for the subsequent encounter, as the patient no longer has the condition in the previously-treated site. If the treatment on the first side did not completely resolve the condition, then the bilateral code would still be appropriate.

14. **Documentation for BMI, *Depth of* Non-pressure ulcers, Pressure Ulcer Stages, Coma Scale, *and* NIH Stroke Scale**
For the Body Mass Index (BMI), depth of non-pressure chronic ulcers, pressure ulcer stage, **coma scale, and NIH stroke scale (NIHSS) codes,** code assignment may be based on medical record documentation from clinicians who are not the patient's provider (i.e., physician or other qualified healthcare practitioner legally accountable for establishing the patient's diagnosis), since this information is typically documented by other clinicians involved in the care of the patient (e.g., a dietitian often documents the BMI, a nurse often documents the pressure ulcer stages, **and an emergency medical technician often documents the coma scale**). However, the associated diagnosis (such as overweight, obesity, **acute stroke,** or pressure ulcer) must be documented by the patient's provider. If there is conflicting medical record documentation, either from the same clinician or different clinicians, the patient's attending provider should be queried for clarification.

The BMI, **coma scale, and NIHSS** codes should only be reported as secondary diagnoses.

15. **Syndromes**
Follow the Alphabetic Index guidance when coding syndromes. In the absence of Alphabetic Index guidance, assign codes for the documented manifestations of the syndrome. Additional codes for manifestations that are not an integral part of the disease process may also be assigned when the condition does not have a unique code.

16. **Documentation of Complications of Care**
Code assignment is based on the provider's documentation of the relationship between the condition and the care or procedure, **unless otherwise instructed by the classification.** The guideline extends to any complications of care, regardless of the chapter the code is located in. It is important to note that not all conditions that occur during or following medical care or surgery are classified as complications. There must be a cause-and-effect relationship between the care provided and the condition, and an indication in the documentation that it is a complication. Query the provider for clarification, if the complication is not clearly documented.

17. **Borderline Diagnosis**
If the provider documents a "borderline" diagnosis at the time of discharge, the diagnosis is coded as confirmed, unless the classification provides a specific entry (e.g., borderline diabetes). If a borderline condition has a specific index entry in ICD-10-CM, it should be coded as such. Since

borderline conditions are not uncertain diagnoses, no distinction is made between the care setting (inpatient versus outpatient). Whenever the documentation is unclear regarding a borderline condition, coders are encouraged to query for clarification.

18. Use of Sign/Symptom/Unspecified Codes

Sign/symptom and "unspecified" codes have acceptable, even necessary, uses. While specific diagnosis codes should be reported when they are supported by the available medical record documentation and clinical knowledge of the patient's health condition, there are instances when signs/symptoms or unspecified codes are the best choices for accurately reflecting the healthcare encounter. Each healthcare encounter should be coded to the level of certainty known for that encounter.

If a definitive diagnosis has not been established by the end of the encounter, it is appropriate to report codes for sign(s) and/or symptom(s) in lieu of a definitive diagnosis. When sufficient clinical information isn't known or available about a particular health condition to assign a more specific code, it is acceptable to report the appropriate "unspecified" code (e.g., a diagnosis of pneumonia has been determined, but not the specific type). Unspecified codes should be reported when they are the codes that most accurately reflect what is known about the patient's condition at the time of that particular encounter. It would be inappropriate to select a specific code that is not supported by the medical record documentation or conduct medically unnecessary diagnostic testing in order to determine a more specific code.

C. Chapter-Specific Coding Guidelines

In addition to general coding guidelines, there are guidelines for specific diagnoses and/or conditions in the classification. Unless otherwise indicated, these guidelines apply to all health care settings. Please refer to Section II for guidelines on the selection of principal diagnosis.

1. Chapter 1: Certain Infectious and Parasitic Diseases (A00-B99)

a. Human Immunodeficiency Virus (HIV) Infections

1) Code only confirmed cases

Code only confirmed cases of HIV infection/illness. This is an exception to the hospital inpatient guideline Section II, H.

In this context, "confirmation" does not require documentation of positive serology or culture for HIV; the provider's diagnostic statement that the patient is HIV positive, or has an HIV-related illness is sufficient.

2) Selection and sequencing of HIV codes

(a) Patient admitted for HIV-related condition

If a patient is admitted for an HIV-related condition, the principal diagnosis should be B20,

Human immunodeficiency virus [HIV] disease followed by additional diagnosis codes for all reported HIV-related conditions.

(b) Patient with HIV disease admitted for unrelated condition

If a patient with HIV disease is admitted for an unrelated condition (such as a traumatic injury), the code for the unrelated condition (e.g., the nature of injury code) should be the principal diagnosis. Other diagnoses would be B20 followed by additional diagnosis codes for all reported HIV-related conditions.

(c) Whether the patient is newly diagnosed

Whether the patient is newly diagnosed or has had previous admissions/encounters for HIV conditions is irrelevant to the sequencing decision.

(d) Asymptomatic human immunodeficiency virus

Z21, Asymptomatic human immunodeficiency virus [HIV] infection status, is to be applied when the patient without any documentation of symptoms is listed as being "HIV positive," "known HIV," "HIV test positive," or similar terminology. Do not use this code if the term "AIDS" is used or if the patient is treated for any HIV-related illness or is described as having any condition(s) resulting from his/her HIV positive status; use B20 in these cases.

(e) Patients with inconclusive HIV serology

Patients with inconclusive HIV serology, but no definitive diagnosis or manifestations of the illness, may be assigned code R75, Inconclusive laboratory evidence of human immunodeficiency virus [HIV].

(f) Previously diagnosed HIV-related illness

Patients with any known prior diagnosis of an HIV-related illness should be coded to B20. Once a patient has developed an HIV-related illness, the patient should always be assigned code B20 on every subsequent admission/encounter. Patients previously diagnosed with any HIV illness (B20) should never be assigned to R75 or Z21, Asymptomatic human immunodeficiency virus [HIV] infection status.

(g) HIV Infection in Pregnancy, Childbirth and the Puerperium

During pregnancy, childbirth or the puerperium, a patient admitted (or presenting for a health care encounter) because of an HIV-related illness should receive a principal diagnosis code of O98.7-, Human immunodeficiency [HIV] disease complicating pregnancy, childbirth and the puerperium, followed by B20 and the code(s) for the HIV-related illness(es). Codes from Chapter 15 always take sequencing priority.

Patients with asymptomatic HIV infection status admitted (or presenting for a health care encounter) during pregnancy, childbirth, or the puerperium should receive codes of O98.7- and Z21.

GUIDELINES (ICD-10-CM)

(h) Encounters for testing for HIV

If a patient is being seen to determine his/her HIV status, use code Z11.4, Encounter for screening for human immunodeficiency virus [HIV]. Use additional codes for any associated high risk behavior.

If a patient with signs or symptoms is being seen for HIV testing, code the signs and symptoms. An additional counseling code Z71.7, Human immunodeficiency virus [HIV] counseling, may be used if counseling is provided during the encounter for the test.

When a patient returns to be informed of his/her HIV test results and the test result is negative, use code Z71.7, Human immunodeficiency virus [HIV] counseling.

If the results are positive, see previous guidelines and assign codes as appropriate.

b. Infectious agents as the cause of diseases classified to other chapters

Certain infections are classified in chapters other than Chapter 1 and no organism is identified as part of the infection code. In these instances, it is necessary to use an additional code from Chapter 1 to identify the organism. A code from category B95, Streptococcus, Staphylococcus, and Enterococcus as the cause of diseases classified to other chapters, B96, Other bacterial agents as the cause of diseases classified to other chapters, or B97, Viral agents as the cause of diseases classified to other chapters, is to be used as an additional code to identify the organism. An instructional note will be found at the infection code advising that an additional organism code is required.

c. Infections resistant to antibiotics

Many bacterial infections are resistant to current antibiotics. It is necessary to identify all infections documented as antibiotic resistant. Assign a code from category Z16, Resistance to antimicrobial drugs, following the infection code only if the infection code does not identify drug resistance.

d. Sepsis, Severe Sepsis, and Septic Shock

1) Coding of Sepsis and Severe Sepsis

(a) Sepsis

For a diagnosis of sepsis, assign the appropriate code for the underlying systemic infection. If the type of infection or causal organism is not further specified, assign code A41.9, Sepsis, unspecified organism.

A code from subcategory R65.2, Severe sepsis, should not be assigned unless severe sepsis or an associated acute organ dysfunction is documented.

(i) Negative or inconclusive blood cultures and sepsis
Negative or inconclusive blood cultures do not preclude a diagnosis of sepsis in patients with clinical evidence of the condition, however, the provider should be queried.

(ii) Urosepsis
The term urosepsis is a nonspecific term. It is not to be considered synonymous with sepsis. It has no default code in the Alphabetic Index. Should a provider use this term, he/she must be queried for clarification.

(iii) Sepsis with organ dysfunction
If a patient has sepsis and associated acute organ dysfunction or multiple organ dysfunction (MOD), follow the instructions for coding severe sepsis.

(iv) Acute organ dysfunction that is not clearly associated with the sepsis
If a patient has sepsis and an acute organ dysfunction, but the medical record documentation indicates that the acute organ dysfunction is related to a medical condition other than the sepsis, do not assign a code from subcategory R65.2, Severe sepsis. An acute organ dysfunction must be associated with the sepsis in order to assign the severe sepsis code. If the documentation is not clear as to whether an acute organ dysfunction is related to the sepsis or another medical condition, query the provider.

(b) Severe sepsis

The coding of severe sepsis requires a minimum of 2 codes: first a code for the underlying systemic infection, followed by a code from subcategory R65.2, Severe sepsis. If the causal organism is not documented, assign code A41.9, Sepsis, unspecified organism, for the infection. Additional code(s) for the associated acute organ dysfunction are also required.

Due to the complex nature of severe sepsis, some cases may require querying the provider prior to assignment of the codes.

2) Septic shock

(a) Septic shock generally refers to circulatory failure associated with severe sepsis, and therefore, it represents a type of acute organ dysfunction.

For all cases of septic shock, the code for the systemic infection should be sequenced first, followed by code R65.21, Severe sepsis with septic shock or code T81.12, Postprocedural septic shock. Any additional codes for the other acute organ dysfunctions should also be assigned. As noted in the sequencing instructions in the Tabular List, the code for septic shock cannot be assigned as a principal diagnosis.

3) Sequencing of severe sepsis

If severe sepsis is present on admission, and meets the definition of principal diagnosis, the underlying systemic infection should be assigned as principal diagnosis followed by the appropriate code from subcategory R65.2 as required by the sequencing rules in the Tabular List. A code from subcategory R65.2 can never be assigned as a principal diagnosis.

When severe sepsis develops during an encounter (it was not present on admission) the underlying systemic infection and the appropriate code from subcategory R65.2 should be assigned as secondary diagnoses.

Severe sepsis may be present on admission but the diagnosis may not be confirmed until sometime after admission. If the documentation is not clear whether severe sepsis was present on admission, the provider should be queried.

4) Sepsis and severe sepsis with a localized infection

If the reason for admission is both sepsis or severe sepsis and a localized infection, such as pneumonia or cellulitis, a code(s) for the underlying systemic infection should be assigned first and the code for the localized infection should be assigned as a secondary diagnosis. If the patient has severe sepsis, a code from subcategory R65.2 should also be assigned as a secondary diagnosis. If the patient is admitted with a localized infection, such as pneumonia, and sepsis/severe sepsis doesn't develop until after admission, the localized infection should be assigned first, followed by the appropriate sepsis/severe sepsis codes.

5) Sepsis due to a postprocedural infection

(a) Documentation of causal relationship

As with all postprocedural complications, code assignment is based on the provider's documentation of the relationship between the infection and the procedure.

(b) Sepsis due to a postprocedural infection

For such cases, the postprocedural infection code, such as, T80.2, Infections following infusion, transfusion, and therapeutic injection, T81.4, Infection following a procedure, T88.0, Infection following immunization, or O86.0, Infection of obstetric surgical wound, should be coded first, followed by the code for the specific infection. If the patient has severe sepsis the appropriate code from subcategory R65.2 should also be assigned with the additional code(s) for any acute organ dysfunction.

(c) Postprocedural infection and postprocedural septic shock

In cases where a postprocedural infection has occurred and has resulted in severe sepsis the code for the precipitating complication such as code T81.4, Infection following a procedure, or O86.0, Infection of obstetrical surgical wound should be coded first followed by code R65.20, Severe sepsis without septic shock. A Code for the systemic infection should also be assigned.

If a postprocedural infection has resulted in postprocedural septic shock, the code for the precipitating complication such as code T81.4, Infection following a procedure, or O86.0, Infection of obstetrical surgical wound should be coded first followed by code T81.12-, Postprocedural septic shock. A code for the systemic infection should also be assigned.

6) Sepsis and severe sepsis associated with a noninfectious process (condition)

In some cases a noninfectious process (condition), such as trauma, may lead to an infection which can result in sepsis or severe sepsis. If sepsis or severe sepsis is documented as associated with a noninfectious condition, such as a burn or serious injury, and this condition meets the definition for principal diagnosis, the code for the noninfectious condition should be sequenced first, followed by the code for the resulting infection. If severe sepsis is present, a code from subcategory R65.2 should also be assigned with any associated organ dysfunction(s) codes. It is not necessary to assign a code from subcategory R65.1, Systemic inflammatory response syndrome (SIRS) of non-infectious origin, for these cases.

If the infection meets the definition of principal diagnosis it should be sequenced before the non-infectious condition. When both the associated non-infectious condition and the infection meet the definition of principal diagnosis either may be assigned as principal diagnosis.

Only one code from category R65, Symptoms and signs specifically associated with systemic inflammation and infection, should be assigned. Therefore, when a non-infectious condition leads to an infection resulting in severe sepsis, assign the appropriate code from subcategory R65.2, Severe sepsis. Do not additionally assign a code from subcategory R65.1, Systemic inflammatory response syndrome (SIRS) of non-infectious origin.

See Section I.C.18. SIRS due to non-infectious process

7) Sepsis and septic shock complicating abortion, pregnancy, childbirth, and the puerperium

See Section I.C.15. Sepsis and septic shock complicating abortion, pregnancy, childbirth and the puerperium

8) Newborn sepsis

See Section I.C.16. f. Bacterial sepsis of Newborn

e. Methicillin Resistant Staphylococcus aureus (MRSA) Conditions

1) Selection and sequencing of MRSA codes

(a) Combination codes for MRSA infection

When a patient is diagnosed with an infection that is due to methicillin resistant *Staphylococcus aureus* (MRSA), and that infection has a combination code that includes the causal organism (e.g., sepsis, pneumonia) assign the appropriate combination code for the condition (e.g., code A41.02, Sepsis

GUIDELINES (ICD-10-CM)

due to Methicillin resistant Staphylococcus aureus or code J15.212, Pneumonia due to Methicillin resistant Staphylococcus aureus). Do not assign code B95.62, Methicillin resistant Staphylococcus aureus infection as the cause of diseases classified elsewhere, as an additional code because the combination code includes the type of infection and the MRSA organism. Do not assign a code from subcategory Z16.11, Resistance to penicillins, as an additional diagnosis.

See Section C.1. for instructions on coding and sequencing of sepsis and severe sepsis.

(b) Other codes for MRSA infection

When there is documentation of a current infection (e.g., wound infection, stitch abscess, urinary tract infection) due to MRSA, and that infection does not have a combination code that includes the causal organism, assign the appropriate code to identify the condition along with code B95.62, Methicillin resistant Staphylococcus aureus infection as the cause of diseases classified elsewhere for the MRSA infection. Do not assign a code from subcategory Z16.11, Resistance to penicillins.

(c) Methicillin susceptible Staphylococcus aureus (MSSA) and MRSA colonization

The condition or state of being colonized or carrying MSSA or MRSA is called colonization or carriage, while an individual person is described as being colonized or being a carrier. Colonization means that MSSA or MSRA is present on or in the body without necessarily causing illness. A positive MRSA colonization test might be documented by the provider as "MRSA screen positive" or "MRSA nasal swab positive".

Assign code Z22.322, Carrier or suspected carrier of Methicillin resistant Staphylococcus aureus, for patients documented as having MRSA colonization. Assign code Z22.321, Carrier or suspected carrier of Methicillin susceptible Staphylococcus aureus, for patient documented as having MSSA colonization. Colonization is not necessarily indicative of a disease process or as the cause of a specific condition the patient may have unless documented as such by the provider.

(d) MRSA colonization and infection

If a patient is documented as having both MRSA colonization and infection during a hospital admission, code Z22.322, Carrier or suspected carrier of Methicillin resistant Staphylococcus aureus, and a code for the MRSA infection may both be assigned.

f. Zika virus infections

1) Code only confirmed cases

Code only a confirmed diagnosis of Zika virus (A92.5, Zika virus disease) as documented by the provider. This is an exception to the hospital inpatient guideline Section II, H.

In this context, "confirmation" does not require documentation of the type of test performed; the physician's diagnostic statement that the condition is confirmed is sufficient. This code should be assigned regardless of the stated mode of transmission.

If the provider documents "suspected", "possible" or "probable" Zika, do not assign code A92.5. Assign a code(s) explaining the reason for encounter (such as fever, rash, or joint pain) or Z20.828, Contact with and (suspected) exposure to other viral communicable diseases.

2. **Chapter 2: Neoplasms (C00-D49)**
General guidelines

Chapter 2 of the ICD-10-CM contains the codes for most benign and all malignant neoplasms. Certain benign neoplasms, such as prostatic adenomas, may be found in the specific body system chapters. To properly code a neoplasm it is necessary to determine from the record if the neoplasm is benign, in-situ, malignant, or of uncertain histologic behavior. If malignant, any secondary (metastatic) sites should also be determined.

Primary malignant neoplasms overlapping site boundaries

A primary malignant neoplasm that overlaps two or more contiguous (next to each other) sites should be classified to the subcategory/ code .8 ('overlapping lesion'), unless the combination is specifically indexed elsewhere. For multiple neoplasms of the same site that are not contiguous such as tumors in different quadrants of the same breast, codes for each site should be assigned.

Malignant neoplasm of ectopic tissue

Malignant neoplasms of ectopic tissue are to be coded to the site of origin mentioned, e.g., ectopic pancreatic malignant neoplasms involving the stomach are coded to pancreas, unspecified (C25.9).

The neoplasm table in the Alphabetic Index should be referenced first. However, if the histological term is documented, that term should be referenced first, rather than going immediately to the Neoplasm Table, in order to determine which column in the Neoplasm Table is appropriate. For example, if the documentation indicates "adenoma," refer to the term in the Alphabetic Index to review the entries under this term and the instructional note to "see also neoplasm, by site, benign." The table provides the proper code based on the type of neoplasm and the site. It is important to select the proper column in the table that corresponds to the type of neoplasm. The Tabular List should then be referenced to verify that the correct code has been selected from the table and that a more specific site code does not exist.

See Section I.C.21. Factors influencing health status and contact with health services, Status, for information regarding Z15.0, codes for genetic susceptibility to cancer.

a. **Treatment directed at the malignancy**

If the treatment is directed at the malignancy, designate the malignancy as the principal diagnosis.

The only exception to this guideline is if a patient admission/encounter is solely for the administration of chemotherapy, immunotherapy or radiation therapy, assign the appropriate Z51.— code as the first-listed or principal diagnosis, and the diagnosis or problem for which the service is being performed as a secondary diagnosis.

b. **Treatment of secondary site**

When a patient is admitted because of a primary neoplasm with metastasis and treatment is directed toward the secondary site only, the secondary neoplasm is designated as the principal diagnosis even though the primary malignancy is still present.

c. **Coding and sequencing of complications**

Coding and sequencing of complications associated with the malignancies or with the therapy thereof are subject to the following guidelines:

1) **Anemia associated with malignancy**

When admission/encounter is for management of an anemia associated with the malignancy, and the treatment is only for anemia, the appropriate code for the malignancy is sequenced as the principal or first-listed diagnosis followed by the appropriate code for the anemia (such as code D63.0, Anemia in neoplastic disease).

2) **Anemia associated with chemotherapy, immunotherapy and radiation therapy**

When the admission/encounter is for management of an anemia associated with an adverse effect of the administration of chemotherapy or immunotherapy and the only treatment is for the anemia, the anemia code is sequenced first followed by the appropriate codes for the neoplasm and the adverse effect (T45.1X5, Adverse effect of antineoplastic and immunosuppressive drugs).

When the admission/encounter is for management of an anemia associated with an adverse effect of radiotherapy, the anemia code should be sequenced first, followed by the appropriate neoplasm code and code Y84.2, Radiological procedure and radiotherapy as the cause of abnormal reaction of the patient, or of later complication, without mention of misadventure at the time of the procedure.

3) **Management of dehydration due to the malignancy**

When the admission/encounter is for management of dehydration due to the malignancy and only the dehydration is being treated (intravenous rehydration), the dehydration is sequenced first, followed by the code(s) for the malignancy.

4) **Treatment of a complication resulting from a surgical procedure**

When the admission/encounter is for treatment of a complication resulting from a surgical procedure, designate the complication as the principal or first-listed diagnosis if treatment is directed at resolving the complication.

d. **Primary malignancy previously excised**

When a primary malignancy has been previously excised or eradicated from its site and there is no further treatment directed to that site and there is no evidence of any existing primary malignancy, a code from category Z85, Personal history of malignant neoplasm, should be used to indicate the former site of the malignancy. Any mention of extension, invasion, or metastasis to another site is coded as a secondary malignant neoplasm to that site. The secondary site may be the principal or first-listed with the Z85 code used as a secondary code.

e. **Admissions/Encounters involving chemotherapy, immunotherapy and radiation therapy**

1) **Episode of care involves surgical removal of neoplasm**

When an episode of care involves the surgical removal of a neoplasm, primary or secondary site, followed by adjunct chemotherapy or radiation treatment during the same episode of care, the code for the neoplasm should be assigned as principal or first-listed diagnosis.

2) **Patient admission/encounter solely for administration of chemotherapy, immunotherapy and radiation therapy**

If a patient admission/encounter is solely for the administration of chemotherapy, immunotherapy or radiation therapy assign code Z51.0, Encounter for antineoplastic radiation therapy, or Z51.11, Encounter for antineoplastic chemotherapy, or Z51.12, Encounter for antineoplastic immunotherapy as the first-listed or principal diagnosis. If a patient receives more than one of these therapies during the same admission more than one of these codes may be assigned, in any sequence.

The malignancy for which the therapy is being administered should be assigned as a secondary diagnosis.

3) **Patient admitted for radiation therapy, chemotherapy or immunotherapy and develops complications**

When a patient is admitted for the purpose of radiotherapy, immunotherapy or chemotherapy and develops complications such as uncontrolled nausea and vomiting or dehydration, the principal or first-listed diagnosis is Z51.0, Encounter for antineoplastic radiation therapy, or Z51.11, Encounter for antineoplastic chemotherapy, or Z51.12, Encounter for antineoplastic immunotherapy followed by any codes for the complications.

f. **Admission/encounter to determine extent of malignancy**

When the reason for admission/encounter is to determine the extent of the malignancy, or for a procedure such as paracentesis or thoracentesis, the primary malignancy or appropriate metastatic site is designated as the principal or first-listed diagnosis, even though chemotherapy or radiotherapy is administered.

g. Symptoms, signs, and abnormal findings listed in Chapter 18 associated with neoplasms

Symptoms, signs, and ill-defined conditions listed in Chapter 18 characteristic of, or associated with, an existing primary or secondary site malignancy cannot be used to replace the malignancy as principal or first-listed diagnosis, regardless of the number of admissions or encounters for treatment and care of the neoplasm.

See section I.C.21. Factors influencing health status and contact with health services, Encounter for prophylactic organ removal.

h. Admission/encounter for pain control/ management

See Section I.C.6. for information on coding admission/ encounter for pain control/management.

i. Malignancy in two or more noncontiguous sites

A patient may have more than one malignant tumor in the same organ. These tumors may represent different primaries or metastatic disease, depending on the site. Should the documentation be unclear, the provider should be queried as to the status of each tumor so that the correct codes can be assigned.

j. Disseminated malignant neoplasm, unspecified

Code C80.0, Disseminated malignant neoplasm, unspecified, is for use only in those cases where the patient has advanced metastatic disease and no known primary or secondary sites are specified. It should not be used in place of assigning codes for the primary site and all known secondary sites.

k. Malignant neoplasm without specification of site

Code C80.1, Malignant (primary) neoplasm, unspecified, equates to Cancer, unspecified. This code should only be used when no determination can be made as to the primary site of a malignancy. This code should rarely be used in the inpatient setting.

l. Sequencing of neoplasm codes

1) Encounter for treatment of primary malignancy

If the reason for the encounter is for treatment of a primary malignancy, assign the malignancy as the principal/first-listed diagnosis. The primary site is to be sequenced first, followed by any metastatic sites.

2) Encounter for treatment of secondary malignancy

When an encounter is for a primary malignancy with metastasis and treatment is directed toward the metastatic (secondary) site(s) only, the metastatic site(s) is designated as the principal/ first-listed diagnosis. The primary malignancy is coded as an additional code.

3) Malignant neoplasm in a pregnant patient

When a pregnant woman has a malignant neoplasm, a code from subcategory O9A.1-, Malignant neoplasm complicating pregnancy, childbirth, and the puerperium, should be sequenced first, followed by the appropriate code from Chapter 2 to indicate the type of neoplasm.

4) Encounter for complication associated with a neoplasm

When an encounter is for management of a complication associated with a neoplasm, such as dehydration, and the treatment is only for the complication, the complication is coded first, followed by the appropriate code(s) for the neoplasm.

The exception to this guideline is anemia. When the admission/encounter is for management of an anemia associated with the malignancy, and the treatment is only for anemia, the appropriate code for the malignancy is sequenced as the principal or first-listed diagnosis followed by code D63.0, Anemia in neoplastic disease.

5) Complication from surgical procedure for treatment of a neoplasm

When an encounter is for treatment of a complication resulting from a surgical procedure performed for the treatment of the neoplasm, designate the complication as the principal/ first-listed diagnosis. See guideline regarding the coding of a current malignancy versus personal history to determine if the code for the neoplasm should also be assigned.

6) Pathologic fracture due to a neoplasm

When an encounter is for a pathological fracture due to a neoplasm, and the focus of treatment is the fracture, a code from subcategory M84.5, Pathological fracture in neoplastic disease, should be sequenced first, followed by the code for the neoplasm.

If the focus of treatment is the neoplasm with an associated pathological fracture, the neoplasm code should be sequenced first, followed by a code from M84.5 for the pathological fracture.

m. Current malignancy versus personal history of malignancy

When a primary malignancy has been excised but further treatment, such as an additional surgery for the malignancy, radiation therapy or chemotherapy is directed to that site, the primary malignancy code should be used until treatment is completed.

When a primary malignancy has been previously excised or eradicated from its site, there is no further treatment (of the malignancy) directed to that site, and there is no evidence of any existing primary malignancy, a code from category Z85, Personal history of malignant neoplasm, should be used to indicate the former site of the malignancy.

See Section I.C.21. Factors influencing health status and contact with health services, History (of)

n. Leukemia, Multiple Myeloma, and Malignant Plasma Cell Neoplasms in remission versus personal history

The categories for leukemia, and category C90, Multiple myeloma and malignant plasma cell neoplasms, have codes indicating whether or not the leukemia has achieved remission. There are also codes Z85.6, Personal history of leukemia, and Z85.79, Personal history of other malignant neoplasms of lymphoid, hematopoietic and related tissues. If the documentation is unclear, as to whether the leukemia has achieved remission, the provider should be queried.

See Section I.C.21. Factors influencing health status and contact with health services, History (of)

o. Aftercare following surgery for neoplasm
See Section I.C.21. Factors influencing health status and contact with health services, Aftercare

p. Follow-up care for completed treatment of a malignancy
See Section I.C.21. Factors influencing health status and contact with health services, Follow-up

q. Prophylactic organ removal for prevention of malignancy
See Section I.C. 21, Factors influencing health status and contact with health services, Prophylactic organ removal

r. Malignant neoplasm associated with transplanted organ
A malignant neoplasm of a transplanted organ should be coded as a transplant complication. Assign first the appropriate code from category T86.-, Complications of transplanted organs and tissue, followed by code C80.2, Malignant neoplasm associated with transplanted organ. Use an additional code for the specific malignancy.

3. Chapter 3: Disease of the blood and blood-forming organs and certain disorders involving the immune mechanism (D50-D89)
Reserved for future guideline expansion

4. Chapter 4: Endocrine, Nutritional, and Metabolic Diseases (E00-E89)

a. Diabetes mellitus
The diabetes mellitus codes are combination codes that include the type of diabetes mellitus, the body system affected, and the complications affecting that body system. As many codes within a particular category as are necessary to describe all of the complications of the disease may be used. They should be sequenced based on the reason for a particular encounter. Assign as many codes from categories E08 – E13 as needed to identify all of the associated conditions that the patient has.

1) Type of diabetes
The age of a patient is not the sole determining factor, though most type 1 diabetics develop the condition before reaching puberty. For this reason type 1 diabetes mellitus is also referred to as juvenile diabetes.

2) Type of diabetes mellitus not documented
If the type of diabetes mellitus is not documented in the medical record the default is E11.-, Type 2 diabetes mellitus.

3) Diabetes mellitus and the use of insulin oral hypoglycemics
If the documentation in a medical record does not indicate the type of diabetes but does indicate that the patient uses insulin, code E11, Type 2 diabetes mellitus, should be assigned. Code Z79.4, Long-term (current) use of insulin, **or Z79.84, Long term (current) use of oral hypoglycemic drugs,** should also be assigned to indicate that the patient uses insulin **or hypoglycemic drugs**. Code Z79.4 should not be assigned if insulin is given temporarily to bring a type 2 patient's blood sugar under control during an encounter.

4) Diabetes mellitus in pregnancy and gestational diabetes
See Section I.C.15. Diabetes mellitus in pregnancy.
See Section I.C.15. Gestational (pregnancy induced) diabetes

5) Complications due to insulin pump malfunction

(a) Underdose of insulin due to insulin pump failure
An underdose of insulin due to an insulin pump failure should be assigned to a code from subcategory T85.6, Mechanical complication of other specified internal and external prosthetic devices, implants and grafts, that specifies the type of pump malfunction, as the principal or first-listed code, followed by code T38.3X6-, Underdosing of insulin and oral hypoglycemic [antidiabetic] drugs. Additional codes for the type of diabetes mellitus and any associated complications due to the underdosing should also be assigned.

(b) Overdose of insulin due to insulin pump failure
The principal or first-listed code for an encounter due to an insulin pump malfunction resulting in an overdose of insulin, should also be T85.6-, Mechanical complication of other specified internal and external prosthetic devices, implants and grafts, followed by code T38.3X1-, Poisoning by insulin and oral hypoglycemic [antidiabetic] drugs, accidental (unintentional).

6) Secondary diabetes mellitus
Codes under categories E08, Diabetes mellitus due to underlying condition, E09, Drug or chemical induced diabetes mellitus and E13, Other specified diabetes mellitus, identify complications/manifestations associated with secondary diabetes mellitus. Secondary diabetes is always caused by another condition or event (e.g., cystic fibrosis, malignant neoplasm of pancreas, pancreatectomy, adverse effect of drug, or poisoning).

(a) Secondary diabetes mellitus and the use of insulin or hypoglycemic drugs
For patients who routinely use insulin **or hypoglycemic drugs,** code Z79.4, Long-term (current) use of insulin, **or Z79.84, Long term (current) use of oral hypoglycemic drugs** should also be assigned. Code Z79.4 should not be assigned if insulin is given temporarily to bring a patient's blood sugar under control during an encounter.

(b) Assigning and sequencing secondary diabetes codes and its causes
The sequencing of the secondary diabetes codes in relationship to codes for the cause of the diabetes is based on the Tabular List instructions for categories E08, E09 and E13.

(i) **Secondary diabetes mellitus due to pancreatectomy** For postpancreatectomy diabetes mellitus (lack of insulin due to the surgical removal of all or part of the pancreas), assign code E89.1, Postprocedural hypoinsulinemia. Assign a code from category E13 and a code from subcategory Z90.41-, Acquired absence of pancreas, as additional codes.

(ii) **Secondary diabetes due to drugs** Secondary diabetes may be caused by an adverse effect of correctly administered medications, poisoning or sequela of poisoning.

See section I.C.19.e for coding of adverse effects and poisoning, and section I.C.20 for external cause code reporting.

5. **Chapter 5: Mental, Behavioral and Neurodevelopmental disorders (F01 – F99)**

a. Pain disorders related to psychological factors

Assign code F45.41, for pain that is exclusively related to psychological disorders. As indicated by the Excludes 1 note under category G89, a code from category G89 should not be assigned with code F45.41

Code F45.42, Pain disorders with related psychological factors, should be used with a code from category G89, Pain, not elsewhere classified, if there is documentation of a psychological component for a patient with acute or chronic pain.

See Section I.C.6. Pain

c. Mental and behavioral disorders due to psychoactive substance use

1) In Remission

Selection of codes for "in remission" for categories F10-F19, Mental and behavioral disorders due to psychoactive substance use (categories F10-F19 with -.21) requires the provider's clinical judgment. The appropriate codes for "in remission" are assigned only on the basis of provider documentation (as defined in the Official Guidelines for Coding and Reporting).

2) Psychoactive Substance Use, Abuse And Dependence

When the provider documentation refers to use, abuse and dependence of the same substance (e.g. alcohol, opioid, cannabis, etc.), only one code should be assigned to identify the pattern of use based on the following hierarchy:

- If both use and abuse are documented, assign only the code for abuse
- If both abuse and dependence are documented, assign only the code for dependence
- If use, abuse and dependence are all documented, assign only the code for dependence
- If both use and dependence are documented, assign only the code for dependence.

3) Psychoactive Substance Use

As with all other diagnoses, the codes for psychoactive substance use (F10.9-, F11.9-, F12.9-, F13.9-, F14.9-, F15.9-, F16.9-) should only be assigned based on provider documentation and when they meet the definition of a reportable diagnosis (see Section III, Reporting Additional Diagnoses). The codes are to be used only when the psychoactive substance use is associated with a mental or behavioral disorder, and such a relationship is documented by the provider.

6. **Chapter 6: Diseases of the Nervous System (G00-G99)**

a. Dominant/nondominant side

Codes from category G81, Hemiplegia and hemiparesis, and subcategories, G83.1, Monoplegia of lower limb, G83.2, Monoplegia of upper limb, and G83.3, Monoplegia, unspecified, identify whether the dominant or nondominant side is affected. Should the affected side be documented, but not specified as dominant or nondominant, and the classification system does not indicate a default, code selection is as follows:

- For ambidextrous patients, the default should be dominant.
- If the left side is affected, the default is non-dominant.
- If the right side is affected, the default is dominant.

b. Pain - Category G89

1) General coding information

Codes in category G89, Pain, not elsewhere classified, may be used in conjunction with codes from other categories and chapters to provide more detail about acute or chronic pain and neoplasm-related pain, unless otherwise indicated below.

If the pain is not specified as acute or chronic, post-thoracotomy, postprocedural, or neoplasm-related, do not assign codes from category G89.

A code from category G89 should not be assigned if the underlying (definitive) diagnosis is known, unless the reason for the encounter is pain control/management and not management of the underlying condition.

When an admission or encounter is for a procedure aimed at treating the underlying condition (e.g., spinal fusion, kyphoplasty), a code for the underlying condition (e.g., vertebral fracture, spinal stenosis) should be assigned as the principal diagnosis. No code from category G89 should be assigned.

(a) Category G89 Codes as Principal or First-Listed Diagnosis

Category G89 codes are acceptable as principal diagnosis or the first-listed code:

- When pain control or pain management is the reason for the admission/encounter (e.g., a patient with displaced intervertebral disc, nerve impingement and severe back pain presents for injection of steroid into the spinal canal). The underlying cause of the pain should be reported as an additional diagnosis, if known.

- When a patient is admitted for the insertion of a neurostimulator for pain control, assign the appropriate pain code as the principal or first-listed diagnosis. When an admission or encounter is for a procedure aimed at treating the underlying condition and a neurostimulator is inserted for pain control during the same admission/encounter, a code for the underlying condition should be assigned as the principal diagnosis and the appropriate pain code should be assigned as a secondary diagnosis.

(b) Use of Category G89 Codes in Conjunction with Site Specific Pain Codes

(i) Assigning Category G89 and Site-Specific Pain Codes

Codes from category G89 may be used in conjunction with codes that identify the site of pain (including codes from chapter 18) if the category G89 code provides additional information. For example, if the code describes the site of the pain, but does not fully describe whether the pain is acute or chronic, then both codes should be assigned.

(ii) Sequencing of Category G89 Codes with Site-Specific Pain Codes

The sequencing of category G89 codes with site-specific pain codes (including chapter 18 codes), is dependent on the circumstances of the encounter/admission as follows:

- If the encounter is for pain control or pain management, assign the code from category G89 followed by the code identifying the specific site of pain (e.g., encounter for pain management for acute neck pain from trauma is assigned code G89.11, Acute pain due to trauma, followed by code M54.2, Cervicalgia, to identify the site of pain).
- If the encounter is for any other reason except pain control or pain management, and a related definitive diagnosis has not been established (confirmed) by the provider, assign the code for the specific site of pain first, followed by the appropriate code from category G89.

2) Pain due to devices, implants and grafts
See Section I.C.19. Pain due to medical devices

3) Postoperative Pain
The provider's documentation should be used to guide the coding of postoperative pain, as well as *Section III. Reporting Additional Diagnoses* and *Section IV. Diagnostic Coding and Reporting in the Outpatient Setting*.

The default for post-thoracotomy and other postoperative pain not specified as acute or chronic is the code for the acute form.

Routine or expected postoperative pain immediately after surgery should not be coded.

(a) Postoperative pain not associated with specific postoperative complication
Postoperative pain not associated with a specific postoperative complication is assigned to the appropriate postoperative pain code in category G89.

(b) Postoperative pain associated with specific postoperative complication
Postoperative pain associated with a specific postoperative complication (such as painful wire sutures) is assigned to the appropriate code(s) found in Chapter 19, Injury, poisoning, and certain other consequences of external causes. If appropriate, use additional code(s) from category G89 to identify acute or chronic pain (G89.18 or G89.28).

4) Chronic pain
Chronic pain is classified to subcategory G89.2. There is no time frame defining when pain becomes chronic pain. The provider's documentation should be used to guide use of these codes.

5) Neoplasm Related Pain
Code G89.3 is assigned to pain documented as being related, associated or due to cancer, primary or secondary malignancy, or tumor. This code is assigned regardless of whether the pain is acute or chronic.

This code may be assigned as the principal or first-listed code when the stated reason for the admission/encounter is documented as pain control/pain management. The underlying neoplasm should be reported as an additional diagnosis.

When the reason for the admission/encounter is management of the neoplasm and the pain associated with the neoplasm is also documented, code G89.3 may be assigned as an additional diagnosis. It is not necessary to assign an additional code for the site of the pain.

See Section I.C.2 for instructions on the sequencing of neoplasms for all other stated reasons for the admission/encounter (except for pain control/pain management).

6) Chronic pain syndrome
Central pain syndrome (G89.0) and chronic pain syndrome (G89.4) are different than the term "chronic pain," and therefore codes should only be used when the provider has specifically documented this condition.

See Section I.C.5. Pain disorders related to psychological factors

7. Chapter 7: Diseases of the Eye and Adnexa (H00-H59)
a. Glaucoma
1) Assigning Glaucoma Codes
Assign as many codes from category H40, Glaucoma, as needed to identify the type of glaucoma, the affected eye, and the glaucoma stage.

2) Bilateral glaucoma with same type and stage

When a patient has bilateral glaucoma and both eyes are documented as being the same type and stage, and there is a code for bilateral glaucoma, report only the code for the type of glaucoma, bilateral, with the seventh character for the stage.

When a patient has bilateral glaucoma and both eyes are documented as being the same type and stage, and the classification does not provide a code for bilateral glaucoma (i.e. subcategories H40.10, H40.11 and H40.20) report only one code for the type of glaucoma with the appropriate seventh character for the stage.

3) Bilateral glaucoma stage with different types or stages

When a patient has bilateral glaucoma and each eye is documented as having a different type or stage, and the classification distinguishes laterality, assign the appropriate code for each eye rather than the code for bilateral glaucoma.

When a patient has bilateral glaucoma and each eye is documented as having a different type, and the classification does not distinguish laterality (i.e. subcategories H40.10, H40.11 and H40.20), assign one code for each type of glaucoma with the appropriate seventh character for the stage.

When a patient has bilateral glaucoma and each eye is documented as having the same type, but different stage, and the classification does not distinguish laterality (i.e. subcategories H40.10, H40.11 and H40.20), assign a code for the type of glaucoma for each eye with the seventh character for the specific glaucoma stage documented for each eye.

4) Patient admitted with glaucoma and stage evolves during the admission

If a patient is admitted with glaucoma and the stage progresses during the admission, assign the code for highest stage documented.

5) Indeterminate stage glaucoma

Assignment of the seventh character "4" for "indeterminate stage" should be based on the clinical documentation. The seventh character "4" is used for glaucomas whose stage cannot be clinically determined. This seventh character should not be confused with the seventh character "0", unspecified, which should be assigned when there is no documentation regarding the stage of the glaucoma.

8. **Chapter 8: Diseases of the Ear and Mastoid Process (H60-H95)**
Reserved for future guideline expansion

9. **Chapter 9: Diseases of the Circulatory System (I00-I99)**

a. Hypertension
The classification presumes a causal relationship between hypertension and heart involvement and between hypertension and kidney involvement, as the two conditions are linked by the term "with" in the Alphabetic Index. These conditions should be coded as related even in the absence of provider documentation explicitly linking them, unless the documentation clearly states the conditions are unrelated.

For hypertension and conditions not specifically linked by relational terms such as "with," "associated with" or "due to" in the classification, provider documentation must link the conditions in order to code them as related.

1) Hypertension with Heart Disease
Hypertension with heart conditions classified to I50.- or I51.4-I51.9, are assigned to, a code from category I11, Hypertensive heart disease. Use an additional code from category I50, Heart failure, to identify the type of heart failure in those patients with heart failure.

The same heart conditions (I50.-, I51.4-I51.9) with hypertension are coded separately **if the provider has specifically documented a different cause.** Sequence according to the circumstances of the admission/encounter.

2) Hypertensive Chronic Kidney Disease
Assign codes from category I12, Hypertensive chronic kidney disease, when both hypertension and a condition classifiable to category N18, Chronic kidney disease (CKD), are present. **CKD should not be coded as hypertensive if the physician has specifically documented a different cause.**

The appropriate code from category N18 should be used as a secondary code with a code from category I12 to identify the stage of chronic kidney disease.
See Section I.C.14. Chronic kidney disease.

If a patient has hypertensive chronic kidney disease and acute renal failure, an additional code for the acute renal failure is required.

3) Hypertensive Heart and Chronic Kidney Disease
Assign codes from combination category I13, Hypertensive heart and chronic kidney disease, when **there is hypertension with both heart and kidney involvement.** If heart failure is present, assign an additional code from category I50 to identify the type of heart failure.

The appropriate code from category N18, Chronic kidney disease, should be used as a secondary code with a code from category I13 to identify the stage of chronic kidney disease.
See Section I.C.14. Chronic kidney disease.

The codes in category I13, Hypertensive heart and chronic kidney disease, are combination codes that include hypertension, heart disease and chronic kidney disease. The Includes note at I13 specifies that the conditions included at I11 and I12 are included together in I13. If a patient has hypertension, heart disease and chronic kidney disease then a code from I13 should be used, not individual codes for hypertension, heart disease and chronic kidney disease, or codes from I11 or I12.

For patients with both acute renal failure and chronic kidney disease an additional code for acute renal failure is required.

4) Hypertensive Cerebrovascular Disease
For hypertensive cerebrovascular disease, first assign the appropriate code from categories I60-I69, followed by the appropriate hypertension code.

5) Hypertensive Retinopathy
Subcategory H35.0, Background retinopathy and retinal vascular changes, should be used with a code from category I10 – I15, Hypertensive disease to include the systemic hypertension. The sequencing is based on the reason for the encounter.

6) Hypertension, Secondary
Secondary hypertension is due to an underlying condition. Two codes are required: one to identify the underlying etiology and one from category I15 to identify the hypertension. Sequencing of codes is determined by the reason for admission/encounter.

7) Hypertension, Transient
Assign code R03.0, Elevated blood pressure reading without diagnosis of hypertension, unless patient has an established diagnosis of hypertension. Assign code O13.-, Gestational [pregnancy-induced] hypertension without significant proteinuria, or O14.-, Pre-eclampsia, for transient hypertension of pregnancy.

8) Hypertension, Controlled
This diagnostic statement usually refers to an existing state of hypertension under control by therapy. Assign the appropriate code from categories I10-I15, Hypertensive diseases.

9) Hypertension, Uncontrolled
Uncontrolled hypertension may refer to untreated hypertension or hypertension not responding to current therapeutic regimen. In either case, assign the appropriate code from categories I10-I15, Hypertensive diseases.

10) Hypertensive Crisis
Assign a code from category I16, Hypertensive crisis, for documented hypertensive urgency, hypertensive emergency or unspecified hypertensive crisis. Code also any identified hypertensive disease (I10-I15). The sequencing is based on the reason for the encounter.

b. Atherosclerotic Coronary Artery Disease and Angina
ICD-10-CM has combination codes for atherosclerotic heart disease with angina pectoris. The subcategories for these codes are I25.11, Atherosclerotic heart disease of native coronary artery with angina pectoris and I25.7, Atherosclerosis of coronary artery bypass graft(s) and coronary artery of transplanted heart with angina pectoris.

When using one of these combination codes it is not necessary to use an additional code for angina pectoris. A causal relationship can be assumed in a patient with both atherosclerosis and angina pectoris, unless the documentation indicates the angina is due to something other than the atherosclerosis.

If a patient with coronary artery disease is admitted due to an acute myocardial infarction (AMI), the AMI should be sequenced before the coronary artery disease.

See Section I.C.9. Acute myocardial infarction (AMI)

c. Intraoperative and Postprocedural Cerebrovascular Accident
Medical record documentation should clearly specify the cause-and-effect relationship between the medical intervention and the cerebrovascular accident in order to assign a code for intraoperative or postprocedural cerebrovascular accident.

Proper code assignment depends on whether it was an infarction or hemorrhage and whether it occurred intraoperatively or postoperatively. If it was a cerebral hemorrhage, code assignment depends on the type of procedure performed.

d. Sequelae of Cerebrovascular Disease

1) Category I69, Sequelae of Cerebrovascular disease
Category I69 is used to indicate conditions classifiable to categories I60-I67 as the causes of sequela (neurologic deficits), themselves classified elsewhere. These "late effects" include neurologic deficits that persist after initial onset of conditions classifiable to categories I60-I67. The neurologic deficits caused by cerebrovascular disease may be present from the onset or may arise at any time after the onset of the condition classifiable to categories I60-I67.

Codes from category I69, Sequelae of cerebrovascular disease, that specify hemiplegia, hemiparesis and monoplegia identify whether the dominant or nondominant side is affected. Should the affected side be documented, but not specified as dominant or nondominant, and the classification system does not indicate a default, code selection is as follows:

- For ambidextrous patients, the default should be dominant.
- If the left side is affected, the default is non-dominant.
- If the right side is affected, the default is dominant.

2) Codes from category I69 with codes from I60-I67
Codes from category I69 may be assigned on a health care record with codes from I60-I67, if the patient has a current cerebrovascular disease and deficits from an old cerebrovascular disease.

3) Codes from category I69 and Personal history of transient ischemic attack (TIA) and cerebral infarction (Z86.73)
Codes from category I69 should not be assigned if the patient does not have neurologic deficits.

See Section I.C.21. 4. History (of) for use of personal history codes

e. Acute myocardial infarction (AMI)

1) ST elevation myocardial infarction (STEMI) and non ST elevation myocardial infarction (NSTEMI)

The ICD-10-CM codes for acute myocardial infarction (AMI) identify the site, such as anterolateral wall or true posterior wall. Subcategories I21.0-I21.2 and code I21.3 are used for ST elevation myocardial infarction (STEMI). Code I21.4, Non-ST elevation (NSTEMI) myocardial infarction, is used for non ST elevation myocardial infarction (NSTEMI) and nontransmural MIs.

If NSTEMI evolves to STEMI, assign the STEMI code. If STEMI converts to NSTEMI due to thrombolytic therapy, it is still coded as STEMI.

For encounters occurring while the myocardial infarction is equal to, or less than, four weeks old, including transfers to another acute setting or a postacute setting, and the myocardial infarction **meets the definition for "other diagnoses" (see Section III, Reporting Additional Diagnoses)**, codes from category I21 may continue to be reported. For encounters after the 4 week time frame and the patient is still receiving care related to the myocardial infarction, the appropriate aftercare code should be assigned, rather than a code from category I21. For old or healed myocardial infarctions not requiring further care, code I25.2, Old myocardial infarction, may be assigned.

2) Acute myocardial infarction, unspecified

Code I21.3, ST elevation (STEMI) myocardial infarction of unspecified site, is the default for unspecified acute myocardial infarction. If only STEMI or transmural MI without the site is documented, assign code I21.3.

3) AMI documented as nontransmural or subendocardial but site provided

If an AMI is documented as nontransmural or subendocardial, but the site is provided, it is still coded as a subendocardial AMI.

See Section I.C.21.3 for information on coding status post administration of tPA in a different facility within the last 24 hours.

4) Subsequent acute myocardial infarction

A code from category I22, Subsequent ST elevation (STEMI) and non ST elevation (NSTEMI) myocardial infarction, is to be used when a patient who has suffered an AMI has a new AMI within the 4 week time frame of the initial AMI. A code from category I22 must be used in conjunction with a code from category I21. The sequencing of the I22 and I21 codes depends on the circumstances of the encounter.

10. Chapter 10: Diseases of the Respiratory System (J00-J99)

a. Chronic Obstructive Pulmonary Disease [COPD] and Asthma

1) Acute exacerbation of chronic obstructive bronchitis and asthma

The codes in categories J44 and J45 distinguish between uncomplicated cases and those in acute exacerbation. An acute exacerbation is a worsening or a decompensation of a chronic condition. An acute exacerbation is not equivalent to an infection superimposed on a chronic condition, though an exacerbation may be triggered by an infection.

b. Acute Respiratory Failure

1) Acute respiratory failure as principal diagnosis

A code from subcategory J96.0, Acute respiratory failure, or subcategory J96.2, Acute and chronic respiratory failure, may be assigned as a principal diagnosis when it is the condition established after study to be chiefly responsible for occasioning the admission to the hospital, and the selection is supported by the Alphabetic Index and Tabular List. However, chapter-specific coding guidelines (such as obstetrics, poisoning, HIV, newborn) that provide sequencing direction take precedence.

2) Acute respiratory failure as secondary diagnosis

Respiratory failure may be listed as a secondary diagnosis if it occurs after admission, or if it is present on admission, but does not meet the definition of principal diagnosis.

3) Sequencing of acute respiratory failure and another acute condition

When a patient is admitted with respiratory failure and another acute condition, (e.g., myocardial infarction, cerebrovascular accident, aspiration pneumonia), the principal diagnosis will not be the same in every situation. This applies whether the other acute condition is a respiratory or nonrespiratory condition. Selection of the principal diagnosis will be dependent on the circumstances of admission. If both the respiratory failure and the other acute condition are equally responsible for occasioning the admission to the hospital, and there are no chapter-specific sequencing rules, the guideline regarding two or more diagnoses that equally meet the definition for principal diagnosis *(Section II, C.)* may be applied in these situations.

If the documentation is not clear as to whether acute respiratory failure and another condition are equally responsible for occasioning the admission, query the provider for clarification.

c. Influenza due to certain identified influenza viruses

Code only confirmed cases of influenza due to certain identified influenza viruses (category J09), and due to other identified influenza virus (category J10). This is an exception to the hospital inpatient guideline Section II, H. (Uncertain Diagnosis).

In this context, "confirmation" does not require documentation of positive laboratory testing specific for avian or other novel influenza A or other identified influenza virus. However, coding should be based on the provider's diagnostic statement that the patient has avian influenza, or other novel influenza A, for category J09, or has another particular identified strain of influenza, such as H1N1 or H3N2, but not identified as novel or variant, for category J10.

If the provider records "suspected" or "possible" or "probable" avian influenza, or novel influenza, or other identified influenza, then the appropriate influenza code from category J11, Influenza due to unidentified influenza virus, should be assigned. A code from category J09, Influenza due to certain identified influenza viruses, should not be assigned nor should a code from category J10, Influenza due to other identified influenza virus.

d. Ventilator associated Pneumonia

1) Documentation of Ventilator associated Pneumonia

As with all procedural or postprocedural complications, code assignment is based on the provider's documentation of the relationship between the condition and the procedure.

Code J95.851, Ventilator associated pneumonia, should be assigned only when the provider has documented ventilator associated pneumonia (VAP). An additional code to identify the organism (e.g., Pseudomonas aeruginosa, code B96.5) should also be assigned. Do not assign an additional code from categories J12-J18 to identify the type of pneumonia.

Code J95.851 should not be assigned for cases where the patient has pneumonia and is on a mechanical ventilator and the provider has not specifically stated that the pneumonia is ventilator-associated pneumonia. If the documentation is unclear as to whether the patient has a pneumonia that is a complication attributable to the mechanical ventilator, query the provider.

2) Ventilator associated Pneumonia Develops after Admission

A patient may be admitted with one type of pneumonia (e.g., code J13, Pneumonia due to Streptococcus pneumonia) and subsequently develop VAP. In this instance, the principal diagnosis would be the appropriate code from categories J12-J18 for the pneumonia diagnosed at the time of admission. Code J95.851, Ventilator associated pneumonia, would be assigned as an additional diagnosis when the provider has also documented the presence of ventilator associated pneumonia.

11. Chapter 11: Diseases of the Digestive System (K00-K95)

Reserved for future guideline expansion

12. Chapter 12: Diseases of the Skin and Subcutaneous Tissue (L00-L99)

a. Pressure ulcer stage codes

1) Pressure ulcer stages

Codes from category L89, Pressure ulcer, identify the site of the pressure ulcer as well as the stage of the ulcer.

The ICD-10-CM classifies pressure ulcer stages based on severity, which is designated by stages 1-4, unspecified stage and unstageable.

Assign as many codes from category L89 as needed to identify all the pressure ulcers the patient has, if applicable.

2) Unstageable pressure ulcers

Assignment of the code for unstageable pressure ulcer (L89.--0) should be based on the clinical documentation. These codes are used for pressure ulcers whose stage cannot be clinically determined (e.g., the ulcer is covered by eschar or has been treated with a skin or muscle graft) and pressure ulcers that are documented as deep tissue injury but not documented as due to trauma. This code should not be confused with the codes for unspecified stage (L89.--9). When there is no documentation regarding the stage of the pressure ulcer, assign the appropriate code for unspecified stage (L89.--9).

3) Documented pressure ulcer stage

Assignment of the pressure ulcer stage code should be guided by clinical documentation of the stage or documentation of the terms found in the Alphabetic Index. For clinical terms describing the stage that are not found in the Alphabetic Index, and there is no documentation of the stage, the provider should be queried.

4) Patients admitted with pressure ulcers documented as healed

No code is assigned if the documentation states that the pressure ulcer is completely healed.

5) Patients admitted with pressure ulcers documented as healing

Pressure ulcers described as healing should be assigned the appropriate pressure ulcer stage code based on the documentation in the medical record. If the documentation does not provide information about the stage of the healing pressure ulcer, assign the appropriate code for unspecified stage.

If the documentation is unclear as to whether the patient has a current (new) pressure ulcer or if the patient is being treated for a healing pressure ulcer, query the provider.

For ulcers that were present on admission but healed at the time of discharge, assign the code for the site and stage of the pressure ulcer at the time of admission.

6) Patient admitted with pressure ulcer evolving into another stage during the admission

If a patient is admitted with a pressure ulcer at one stage and it progresses to a higher stage, **two separate codes should be assigned: one code for the site and stage of the ulcer on admission and a second code for the same ulcer site and the highest stage reported during the stay.**

13. Chapter 13: Diseases of the Musculoskeletal System and Connective Tissue (M00-M99)

a. Site and laterality

Most of the codes within Chapter 13 have site and laterality designations. The site represents the bone, joint or the muscle involved. For some conditions where more than one bone, joint or muscle is usually involved, such as osteoarthritis, there is a "multiple sites" code available. For categories where no multiple site code is provided and more than one bone, joint or muscle is involved, multiple codes should be used to indicate the different sites involved.

1) Bone versus joint
For certain conditions, the bone may be affected at the upper or lower end, (e.g., avascular necrosis of bone, M87, Osteoporosis, M80, M81). Though the portion of the bone affected may be at the joint, the site designation will be the bone, not the joint.

b. Acute traumatic versus chronic or recurrent musculoskeletal conditions
Many musculoskeletal conditions are a result of previous injury or trauma to a site, or are recurrent conditions. Bone, joint or muscle conditions that are the result of a healed injury are usually found in chapter 13. Recurrent bone, joint or muscle conditions are also usually found in chapter 13. Any current, acute injury should be coded to the appropriate injury code from chapter 19. Chronic or recurrent conditions should generally be coded with a code from chapter 13. If it is difficult to determine from the documentation in the record which code is best to describe a condition, query the provider.

c. Coding of Pathologic Fractures
7th character A is for use as long as the patient is receiving active treatment for the fracture. While the patient may be seen by a new or different provider over the course of treatment for a pathological fracture, assignment of the 7th character is based on whether the patient is undergoing active treatment and not whether the provider is seeing the patient for the first time.

7th character, D is to be used for encounters after the patient has completed active treatment. The other 7th characters, listed under each subcategory in the Tabular List, are to be used for subsequent encounters for **routine care of fractures during the healing and recovery phase as well as** treatment of problems associated with the healing, such as malunions, nonunions, and sequelae.

Care for complications of surgical treatment for fracture repairs during the healing or recovery phase should be coded with the appropriate complication codes.

See Section I.C.19. Coding of traumatic fractures.

d. Osteoporosis
Osteoporosis is a systemic condition, meaning that all bones of the musculoskeletal system are affected. Therefore, site is not a component of the codes under category M81, Osteoporosis without current pathological fracture. The site codes under category M80, Osteoporosis with current pathological fracture, identify the site of the fracture, not the osteoporosis.

1) Osteoporosis without pathological fracture
Category M81, Osteoporosis without current pathological fracture, is for use for patients

with osteoporosis who do not currently have a pathologic fracture due to the osteoporosis, even if they have had a fracture in the past. For patients with a history of osteoporosis fractures, status code Z87.310, Personal history of (healed) osteoporosis fracture, should follow the code from M81.

2) Osteoporosis with current pathological fracture
Category M80, Osteoporosis with current pathological fracture, is for patients who have a current pathologic fracture at the time of an encounter. The codes under M80 identify the site of the fracture. A code from category M80, not a traumatic fracture code, should be used for any patient with known osteoporosis who suffers a fracture, even if the patient had a minor fall or trauma, if that fall or trauma would not usually break a normal, healthy bone.

14. Chapter 14: Diseases of Genitourinary System (N00-N99)

a. Chronic kidney disease

1) Stages of chronic kidney disease (CKD)
The ICD-10-CM classifies CKD based on severity. The severity of CKD is designated by stages 1-5. Stage 2, code N18.2, equates to mild CKD; stage 3, code N18.3, equates to moderate CKD; and stage 4, code N18.4, equates to severe CKD. Code N18.6, End stage renal disease (ESRD), is assigned when the provider has documented end-stage-renal disease (ESRD).

If both a stage of CKD and ESRD are documented, assign code N18.6 only.

2) Chronic kidney disease and kidney transplant status
Patients who have undergone kidney transplant may still have some form of chronic kidney disease CKD because the kidney transplant may not fully restore kidney function. Therefore, the presence of CKD alone does not constitute a transplant complication. Assign the appropriate N18 code for the patient's stage of CKD and code Z94.0, Kidney transplant status. If a transplant complication such as failure or rejection or other transplant complication is documented, see section I.C.19.g for information on coding complications of a kidney transplant. If the documentation is unclear as to whether the patient has a complication of the transplant, query the provider.

3) Chronic kidney disease with other conditions
Patients with CKD may also suffer from other serious conditions, most commonly diabetes mellitus and hypertension. The sequencing of the CKD code in relationship to codes for other contributing conditions is based on the conventions in the Tabular List.

See I.C.9. Hypertensive chronic kidney disease.
See I.C.19. Chronic kidney disease and kidney transplant complications.

15. **Chapter 15: Pregnancy, Childbirth, and the Puerperium (O00-O9A)**

    a. **General Rules for Obstetric Cases**

       1) **Codes from chapter 15 and sequencing priority**

    Obstetric cases require codes from chapter 15, codes in the range O00-O9A, Pregnancy, Childbirth, and the Puerperium. Chapter 15 codes have sequencing priority over codes from other chapters. Additional codes from other chapters may be used in conjunction with chapter 15 codes to further specify conditions. Should the provider document that the pregnancy is incidental to the encounter, then code Z33.1, Pregnant state, incidental, should be used in place of any chapter 15 codes. It is the provider's responsibility to state that the condition being treated is not affecting the pregnancy.

       2) **Chapter 15 codes used only on the maternal record**

    Chapter 15 codes are to be used only on the maternal record, never on the record of the newborn.

       3) **Final character for trimester**

    The majority of codes in Chapter 15 have a final character indicating the trimester of pregnancy. The timeframes for the trimesters are indicated at the beginning of the chapter. If trimester is not a component of a code it is because the condition always occurs in a specific trimester, or the concept of trimester of pregnancy is not applicable. Certain codes have characters for only certain trimesters because the condition does not occur in all trimesters, but it may occur in more than just one.

    Assignment of the final character for trimester should be based on the provider's documentation of the trimester (or number of weeks) for the current admission/encounter. This applies to the assignment of trimester for pre-existing conditions as well as those that develop during or are due to the pregnancy. The provider's documentation of the number of weeks may be used to assign the appropriate code identifying the trimester.

    Whenever delivery occurs during the current admission, and there is an "in childbirth" option for the obstetric complication being coded, the "in childbirth" code should be assigned.

       4) **Selection of trimester for inpatient admissions that encompass more than one trimester**

    In instances when a patient is admitted to a hospital for complications of pregnancy during one trimester and remains in the hospital into a subsequent trimester, the trimester character for the antepartum complication code should be assigned on the basis of the trimester when the complication developed, not the trimester of the discharge. If the condition developed prior to the current admission/encounter or represents a pre-existing condition, the trimester character for the trimester at the time of the admission/encounter should be assigned.

       5) **Unspecified trimester**

    Each category that includes codes for trimester has a code for "unspecified trimester." The "unspecified trimester" code should rarely be used, such as when the documentation in the record is insufficient to determine the trimester and it is not possible to obtain clarification.

       6) **7th character for Fetus Identification**

    Where applicable, a 7th character is to be assigned for certain categories (O31, O32, O33.3 - O33.6, O35, O36, O40, O41, O60.1, O60.2, O64, and O69) to identify the fetus for which the complication code applies.

    Assign 7th character "0":
    - For single gestations
    - When the documentation in the record is insufficient to determine the fetus affected and it is not possible to obtain clarification.
    - When it is not possible to clinically determine which fetus is affected.

    b. **Selection of OB Principal or First-listed Diagnosis**

       1) **Routine outpatient prenatal visits**

    For routine outpatient prenatal visits when no complications are present, a code from category Z34, Encounter for supervision of normal pregnancy, should be used as the first-listed diagnosis. These codes should not be used in conjunction with chapter 15 codes.

       2) *Supervision of High-Risk Pregnancy*

    Codes from category O09, Supervision of high-risk pregnancy, are intended for use only during the prenatal period. For complications during the labor or delivery episode as a result of a high-risk pregnancy, assign the applicable complication codes from Chapter 15. If there are no complications during the labor or delivery episode, assign code O80, Encounter for full-term uncomplicated delivery.

    For routine prenatal outpatient visits for patients with high-risk pregnancies, a code from category O09, Supervision of high-risk pregnancy, should be used as the first-listed diagnosis. Secondary chapter 15 codes may be used in conjunction with these codes if appropriate.

       3) **Episodes when no delivery occurs**

    In episodes when no delivery occurs, the principal diagnosis should correspond to the principal complication of the pregnancy which necessitated the encounter. Should more than one complication exist, all of which are treated or monitored, any of the complications codes may be sequenced first.

       4) **When a delivery occurs**

    When an obstetric patient is admitted and delivers during that admission, the condition that prompted the admission should be sequenced as the principal diagnosis. If multiple conditions prompted the admission, sequence the one most related to the delivery as the principal

diagnosis. **A code for any complication of the delivery should be assigned as an additional diagnosis.** In cases of cesarean delivery, if the patient was admitted with a condition that resulted in the performance of a cesarean procedure, that condition should be selected as the principal diagnosis. If the reason for the admission was unrelated to the condition resulting in the cesarean delivery, the condition related to the reason for the admission should be selected as the principal diagnosis.

5) Outcome of delivery

A code from category Z37, Outcome of delivery, should be included on every maternal record when a delivery has occurred. These codes are not to be used on subsequent records or on the newborn record.

c. Pre-existing conditions versus conditions due to the pregnancy

Certain categories in Chapter 15 distinguish between conditions of the mother that existed prior to pregnancy (pre-existing) and those that are a direct result of pregnancy. When assigning codes from Chapter 15, it is important to assess if a condition was pre-existing prior to pregnancy or developed during or due to the pregnancy in order to assign the correct code.

Categories that do not distinguish between pre-existing and pregnancy-related conditions may be used for either. It is acceptable to use codes specifically for the puerperium with codes complicating pregnancy and childbirth if a condition arises postpartum during the delivery encounter.

d. Pre-existing hypertension in pregnancy

Category O10, Pre-existing hypertension complicating pregnancy, childbirth and the puerperium, includes codes for hypertensive heart and hypertensive chronic kidney disease. When assigning one of the O10 codes that includes hypertensive heart disease or hypertensive chronic kidney disease, it is necessary to add a secondary code from the appropriate hypertension category to specify the type of heart failure or chronic kidney disease.

See Section I.C.9. Hypertension.

e. Fetal Conditions Affecting the Management of the Mother

1) Codes from categories O35 and O36

Codes from categories O35, Maternal care for known or suspected fetal abnormality and damage, and O36, Maternal care for other fetal problems, are assigned only when the fetal condition is actually responsible for modifying the management of the mother, i.e., by requiring diagnostic studies, additional observation, special care, or termination of pregnancy. The fact that the fetal condition exists does not justify assigning a code from this series to the mother's record.

2) In utero surgery

In cases when surgery is performed on the fetus, a diagnosis code from category O35, Maternal care for known or suspected fetal abnormality and damage, should be assigned identifying the fetal condition. Assign the appropriate procedure code for the procedure performed.

No code from Chapter 16, the perinatal codes, should be used on the mother's record to identify fetal conditions. Surgery performed in utero on a fetus is still to be coded as an obstetric encounter.

f. HIV Infection in Pregnancy, Childbirth and the Puerperium

During pregnancy, childbirth or the puerperium, a patient admitted because of an HIV-related illness should receive a principal diagnosis from subcategory O98.7-, Human immunodeficiency [HIV] disease complicating pregnancy, childbirth and the puerperium, followed by the code(s) for the HIV-related illness(es).

Patients with asymptomatic HIV infection status admitted during pregnancy, childbirth, or the puerperium should receive codes of O98.7- and Z21, Asymptomatic human immunodeficiency virus [HIV] infection status.

g. Diabetes mellitus in pregnancy

Diabetes mellitus is a significant complicating factor in pregnancy. Pregnant women who are diabetic should be assigned a code from category O24, Diabetes mellitus in pregnancy, childbirth, and the puerperium, first, followed by the appropriate diabetes code(s) (E08-E13) from Chapter 4.

h. Long term use of insulin and oral hypoglycemics

Code Z79.4, Long-term (current) use of insulin, or **code Z79.84, Long-term (current) use of oral hypoglycemic drugs,** should also be assigned if the diabetes mellitus is being treated with insulin **or oral medications. If the patient is treated with both oral medications and insulin, only the code for insulin-controlled should be assigned.**

i. Gestational (pregnancy induced) diabetes

Gestational (pregnancy induced) diabetes can occur during the second and third trimester of pregnancy in women who were not diabetic prior to pregnancy. Gestational diabetes can cause complications in the pregnancy similar to those of pre-existing diabetes mellitus. It also puts the woman at greater risk of developing diabetes after the pregnancy. Codes for gestational diabetes are in subcategory O24.4, Gestational diabetes mellitus. No other code from category O24, Diabetes mellitus in pregnancy, childbirth, and the puerperium, should be used with a code from O24.4.

The codes under subcategory O24.4 include diet controlled, insulin controlled, **and controlled by oral hypoglycemic drugs.** If a patient with gestational diabetes is treated with both diet and insulin, only the code for insulin-controlled is required. **If a patient with gestational diabetes is treated with both diet and oral hypoglycemic medications, only the code for "controlled by oral hypoglycemic drugs" is required.** Code Z79.4, Long-term (current) use of insulin **or code Z79.84, Long-term (current) use of oral hypoglycemic drugs,** should not be assigned with codes from subcategory O24.4.

An abnormal glucose tolerance in pregnancy is assigned a code from subcategory O99.81, Abnormal glucose complicating pregnancy, childbirth, and the puerperium.

j. Sepsis and septic shock complicating abortion, pregnancy, childbirth and the puerperium

When assigning a chapter 15 code for sepsis complicating abortion, pregnancy, childbirth, and the puerperium, a code for the specific type of infection should be assigned as an additional diagnosis. If severe sepsis is present, a code from subcategory R65.2, Severe sepsis, and code(s) for associated organ dysfunction(s) should also be assigned as additional diagnoses.

k. Puerperal sepsis

Code O85, Puerperal sepsis, should be assigned with a secondary code to identify the causal organism (e.g., for a bacterial infection, assign a code from category B95-B96, Bacterial infections in conditions classified elsewhere). A code from category A40, Streptococcal sepsis, or A41, Other sepsis, should not be used for puerperal sepsis. If applicable, use additional codes to identify severe sepsis (R65.2-) and any associated acute organ dysfunction.

l. Alcohol and tobacco use during pregnancy, childbirth and the puerperium

1) Alcohol use during pregnancy, childbirth and the puerperium

Codes under subcategory O99.31, Alcohol use complicating pregnancy, childbirth, and the puerperium, should be assigned for any pregnancy case when a mother uses alcohol during the pregnancy or postpartum. A secondary code from category F10, Alcohol related disorders, should also be assigned to identify manifestations of the alcohol use.

2) Tobacco use during pregnancy, childbirth and the puerperium

Codes under subcategory O99.33, Smoking (tobacco) complicating pregnancy, childbirth, and the puerperium, should be assigned for any pregnancy case when a mother uses any type of tobacco product during the pregnancy or postpartum. A secondary code from category F17, Nicotine dependence, should also be assigned to identify the type of nicotine dependence.

m. Poisoning, toxic effects, adverse effects and underdosing in a pregnant patient

A code from subcategory O9A.2, Injury, poisoning and certain other consequences of external causes complicating pregnancy, childbirth, and the puerperium, should be sequenced first, followed by the appropriate injury, poisoning, toxic effect, adverse effect or underdosing code, and then the additional code(s) that specifies the condition caused by the poisoning, toxic effect, adverse effect or underdosing.

See Section I.C.19. Adverse effects, poisoning, underdosing and toxic effects.

n. Normal Delivery, Code O80

1) Encounter for full term uncomplicated delivery

Code O80 should be assigned when a woman is admitted for a full-term normal delivery and delivers a single, healthy infant without any complications antepartum, during the delivery, or postpartum during the delivery episode. Code O80 is always a principal diagnosis. It is not to be used if any other code from chapter 15 is needed to describe a current complication of the antenatal, delivery, or perinatal period. Additional codes from other chapters may be used with code O80 if they are not related to or are in any way complicating the pregnancy.

2) Uncomplicated delivery with resolved antepartum complication

Code O80 may be used if the patient had a complication at some point during the pregnancy, but the complication is not present at the time of the admission for delivery.

3) Outcome of delivery for O80

Z37.0, Single live birth, is the only outcome of delivery code appropriate for use with O80.

o. The Peripartum and Postpartum Periods

1) Peripartum and Postpartum periods

The postpartum period begins immediately after delivery and continues for six weeks following delivery. The peripartum period is defined as the last month of pregnancy to five months postpartum.

2) Peripartum and postpartum complication

A postpartum complication is any complication occurring within the six-week period.

3) Pregnancy-related complications after 6 week period

Chapter 15 codes may also be used to describe pregnancy-related complications after the peripartum or postpartum period if the provider documents that a condition is pregnancy related.

4) Admission for routine postpartum care following delivery outside hospital

When the mother delivers outside the hospital prior to admission and is admitted for routine postpartum care and no complications are noted, code Z39.0, Encounter for care and examination of mother immediately after delivery, should be assigned as the principal diagnosis.

5) Pregnancy associated cardiomyopathy

Pregnancy associated cardiomyopathy, code O90.3, is unique in that it may be diagnosed in the third trimester of pregnancy but may continue to progress months after delivery. For this reason, it is referred to as peripartum cardiomyopathy. Code O90.3 is only for use when the cardiomyopathy develops as a result of pregnancy in a woman who did not have pre-existing heart disease.

p. Code O94, Sequelae of complication of pregnancy, childbirth, and the puerperium

1) Code O94

Code O94, Sequelae of complication of pregnancy, childbirth, and the puerperium, is for use in those cases when an initial complication of a pregnancy develops a sequelae requiring care or treatment at a future date.

2) After the initial postpartum period

This code may be used at any time after the initial postpartum period.

3) Sequencing of Code O94

This code, like all sequela codes, is to be sequenced following the code describing the sequelae of the complication.

q. *Termination of Pregnancy and Spontaneous abortions*

1) Abortion with Liveborn Fetus

When an attempted termination of pregnancy results in a liveborn fetus assign code Z33.2, Encounter for elective termination of pregnancy and a code from category Z37, Outcome of Delivery.

2) Retained Products of Conception following an abortion

Subsequent encounters for retained products of conception following a spontaneous abortion or elective termination of pregnancy are assigned the appropriate code from category O03, Spontaneous abortion, or codes O07.4, Failed attempted termination of pregnancy without complication and Z33.2, Encounter for elective termination of pregnancy. This advice is appropriate even when the patient was discharged previously with a discharge diagnosis of complete abortion.

3) Complications leading to abortion

Codes from Chapter 15 may be used as additional codes to identify any documented complications of the pregnancy in conjunction with codes in categories in O07 and O08.

r. Abuse in a pregnant patient

For suspected or confirmed cases of abuse of a pregnant patient, a code(s) from subcategories O9A.3, Physical abuse complicating pregnancy, childbirth, and the puerperium, O9A.4, Sexual abuse complicating pregnancy, childbirth, and the puerperium, and O9A.5, Psychological abuse complicating pregnancy, childbirth, and the puerperium, should be sequenced first, followed by the appropriate codes (if applicable) to identify any associated current injury due to physical abuse, sexual abuse, and the perpetrator of abuse.

See Section I.C.19. Adult and child abuse, neglect and other maltreatment.

16. Chapter 16: Certain Conditions Originating in the Perinatal Period (P00-P96)

For coding and reporting purposes the perinatal period is defined as before birth through the 28th day following birth. The following guidelines are provided for reporting purposes

a. General Perinatal Rules

1) Use of Chapter 16 Codes

Codes in this chapter are <u>never</u> for use on the maternal record. Codes from Chapter 15, the obstetric chapter, are never permitted on the newborn record. Chapter 16 codes may be used throughout the life of the patient if the condition is still present.

2) Principal Diagnosis for Birth Record

When coding the birth episode in a newborn record, assign a code from category Z38, Liveborn infants according to place of birth and type of delivery, as the principal diagnosis. A code from category Z38 is assigned only once, to a newborn at the time of birth. If a newborn is transferred to another institution, a code from category Z38 should not be used at the receiving hospital.

A code from category Z38 is used only on the newborn record, not on the mother's record.

3) Use of Codes from other Chapters with Codes from Chapter 16

Codes from other chapters may be used with codes from chapter 16 if the codes from the other chapters provide more specific detail. Codes for signs and symptoms may be assigned when a definitive diagnosis has not been established. If the reason for the encounter is a perinatal condition, the code from chapter 16 should be sequenced first.

4) Use of Chapter 16 Codes after the Perinatal Period

Should a condition originate in the perinatal period, and continue throughout the life of the patient, the perinatal code should continue to be used regardless of the patient's age.

5) Birth process or community acquired conditions

If a newborn has a condition that may be either due to the birth process or community acquired and the documentation does not indicate which it is, the default is due to the birth process and the code from Chapter 16 should be used. If the condition is community-acquired, a code from Chapter 16 should not be assigned.

6) Code all clinically significant conditions

All clinically significant conditions noted on routine newborn examination should be coded. A condition is clinically significant if it requires:

- clinical evaluation; or
- therapeutic treatment; or
- diagnostic procedures; or

- extended length of hospital stay; or
- increased nursing care and/or monitoring; or
- has implications for future health care needs

Note: The perinatal guidelines listed above are the same as the general coding guidelines for "additional diagnoses", except for the final point regarding implications for future health care needs. Codes should be assigned for conditions that have been specified by the provider as having implications for future health care needs.

b. Observation and Evaluation of Newborns for Suspected Conditions not Found

1) Assign a code from category Z05, Observation and evaluation of newborns and infants for suspected conditions ruled out, to identify those instances when a healthy newborn is evaluated for a suspected condition that is determined after study not to be present. Do not use a code from category Z05 when the patient has identified signs or symptoms of a suspected problem; in such cases code the sign or symptom.

2) A code from category Z05 may also be assigned as a principal or first-listed code for readmissions or encounters when the code from category Z38 code no longer applies. Codes from category Z05 are for use only for healthy newborns and infants for which no condition after study is found to be present.

3) Z05 on a birth record

A code from category Z05 is to be used as a secondary code after the code from category Z38, Liveborn infants according to place of birth and type of delivery.

c. Coding Additional Perinatal Diagnoses

1) **Assigning codes for conditions that require treatment**

Assign codes for conditions that require treatment or further investigation, prolong the length of stay, or require resource utilization.

2) **Codes for conditions specified as having implications for future health care needs**

Assign codes for conditions that have been specified by the provider as having implications for future health care needs.

Note: This guideline should not be used for adult patients.

d. Prematurity and Fetal Growth Retardation

Providers utilize different criteria in determining prematurity. A code for prematurity should not be assigned unless it is documented. Assignment of codes in categories P05, Disorders of newborn related to slow fetal growth and fetal malnutrition, and P07, Disorders of newborn related to short gestation and low birth weight, not elsewhere classified, should be based on the recorded birth weight and estimated gestational age. Codes from category P05 should not be assigned with codes from category P07.

When both birth weight and gestational age are available, two codes from category P07 should be assigned, with the code for birth weight sequenced before the code for gestational age.

e. Low birth weight and immaturity status

Codes from category P07, Disorders of newborn related to short gestation and low birth weight, not elsewhere classified, are for use for a child or adult who was premature or had a low birth weight as a newborn and this is affecting the patient's current health status.

See Section I.C.21. Factors influencing health status and contact with health services, Status.

f. Bacterial Sepsis of Newborn

Category P36, Bacterial sepsis of newborn, includes congenital sepsis. If a perinate is documented as having sepsis without documentation of congenital or community acquired, the default is congenital and a code from category P36 should be assigned. If the P36 code includes the causal organism, an additional code from category B95, Streptococcus, Staphylococcus, and Enterococcus as the cause of diseases classified elsewhere, or B96, Other bacterial agents as the cause of diseases classified elsewhere, should not be assigned. If the P36 code does not include the causal organism, assign an additional code from category B96. If applicable, use additional codes to identify severe sepsis (R65.2-) and any associated acute organ dysfunction.

g. Stillbirth

Code P95, Stillbirth, is only for use in institutions that maintain separate records for stillbirths. No other code should be used with P95. Code P95 should not be used on the mother's record.

17. **Chapter 17: Congenital malformations, deformations, and chromosomal abnormalities (Q00-Q99)**

Assign an appropriate code(s) from categories Q00-Q99, Congenital malformations, deformations, and chromosomal abnormalities when a malformation/deformation or chromosomal abnormality is documented. A malformation/deformation/or chromosomal abnormality may be the principal/first-listed diagnosis on a record or a secondary diagnosis.

When a malformation/deformation/or chromosomal abnormality does not have a unique code assignment, assign additional code(s) for any manifestations that may be present.

When the code assignment specifically identifies the malformation/deformation/or chromosomal abnormality, manifestations that are an inherent component of the anomaly should not be coded separately. Additional codes should be assigned for manifestations that are not an inherent component.

Codes from Chapter 17 may be used throughout the life of the patient. If a congenital malformation or deformity has been corrected, a personal history code should be used to identify the history of the malformation or deformity. Although present at birth, malformation/deformation/or chromosomal

27

abnormality may not be identified until later in life. Whenever the condition is diagnosed by the physician, it is appropriate to assign a code from codes Q00-Q99.

For the birth admission, the appropriate code from category Z38, Liveborn infants, according to place of birth and type of delivery, should be sequenced as the principal diagnosis, followed by any congenital anomaly codes, Q00-Q99.

18. **Chapter 18: Symptoms, signs, and abnormal clinical and laboratory findings, not elsewhere classified (R00-R99)**
Chapter 18 includes symptoms, signs, abnormal results of clinical or other investigative procedures, and ill-defined conditions regarding which no diagnosis classifiable elsewhere is recorded. Signs and symptoms that point to a specific diagnosis have been assigned to a category in other chapters of the classification.

 a. **Use of symptom codes**
Codes that describe symptoms and signs are acceptable for reporting purposes when a related definitive diagnosis has not been established (confirmed) by the provider.

 b. **Use of a symptom code with a definitive diagnosis code**
Codes for signs and symptoms may be reported in addition to a related definitive diagnosis when the sign or symptom is not routinely associated with that diagnosis, such as the various signs and symptoms associated with complex syndromes. The definitive diagnosis code should be sequenced before the symptom code.

Signs or symptoms that are associated routinely with a disease process should not be assigned as additional codes, unless otherwise instructed by the classification.

 c. **Combination codes that include symptoms**
ICD-10-CM contains a number of combination codes that identify both the definitive diagnosis and common symptoms of that diagnosis. When using one of these combination codes, an additional code should not be assigned for the symptom.

 d. **Repeated falls**
Code R29.6, Repeated falls, is for use for encounters when a patient has recently fallen and the reason for the fall is being investigated.

Code Z91.81, History of falling, is for use when a patient has fallen in the past and is at risk for future falls. When appropriate, both codes R29.6 and Z91.81 may be assigned together.

 e. **Coma scale**
The coma scale codes (R40.2-) can be used in conjunction with traumatic brain injury codes, acute cerebrovascular disease or sequelae of cerebrovascular disease codes. These codes are primarily for use by trauma registries, but they may be used in any setting where this information is collected. **The coma scale may also be used to assess the status of the central nervous system for other non-trauma conditions, such as monitoring patients in the intensive care unit regardless of medical condition.** The coma scale codes should be sequenced after the diagnosis code(s).

These codes, one from each subcategory, are needed to complete the scale. The 7th character indicates when the scale was recorded. The 7th character should match for all three codes.

At a minimum, report the initial score documented on presentation at your facility. This may be a score from the emergency medicine technician (EMT) or in the emergency department. If desired, a facility may choose to capture multiple coma scale scores.

Assign code R40.24, Glasgow coma scale, total score, when only the total score is documented in the medical record and not the individual score(s).

 f. **Functional quadriplegia**
Functional quadriplegia (code R53.2) is the lack of ability to use one's limbs or to ambulate due to extreme debility. It is not associated with neurologic deficit or injury, and code R53.2 should not be used for cases of neurologic quadriplegia. It should only be assigned if functional quadriplegia is specifically documented in the medical record.

 g. **SIRS due to Non-Infectious Process**
The systemic inflammatory response syndrome (SIRS) can develop as a result of certain non-infectious disease processes, such as trauma, malignant neoplasm, or pancreatitis. When SIRS is documented with a noninfectious condition, and no subsequent infection is documented, the code for the underlying condition, such as an injury, should be assigned, followed by code R65.10, Systemic inflammatory response syndrome (SIRS) of non-infectious origin without acute organ dysfunction, or code R65.11, Systemic inflammatory response syndrome (SIRS) of non-infectious origin with acute organ dysfunction. If an associated acute organ dysfunction is documented, the appropriate code(s) for the specific type of organ dysfunction(s) should be assigned in addition to code R65.11. If acute organ dysfunction is documented, but it cannot be determined if the acute organ dysfunction is associated with SIRS or due to another condition (e.g., directly due to the trauma), the provider should be queried.

 h. **Death NOS**
Code R99, Ill-defined and unknown cause of mortality, is only for use in the very limited circumstance when a patient who has already died is brought into an emergency department or other healthcare facility and is pronounced dead upon arrival. It does not represent the discharge disposition of death.

 i. **NIHSS Stroke Scale**
The NIH stroke scale (NIHSS) codes (R29.7- -) can be used in conjunction with acute stroke codes (I63) to identify the patient's neurological status and the severity of the stroke. The stroke scale codes should be sequenced after the acute stroke diagnosis code(s).

At a minimum, report the initial score documented. If desired, a facility may choose to capture multiple stroke scale scores.

See Section I.B.14. for information concerning the medical record documentation that may be used for assignment of the NIHSS codes.

19. **Chapter 19: Injury, poisoning, and certain other consequences of external causes (S00-T88)**

   a. **Application of 7th Characters in Chapter 19**
   Most categories in chapter 19 have a 7th character requirement for each applicable code. Most categories in this chapter have three 7th character values (with the exception of fractures): A, initial encounter, D, subsequent encounter and S, sequela. Categories for traumatic fractures have additional 7th character values. While the patient may be seen by a new or different provider over the course of treatment for an injury, assignment of the 7th character is based on whether the patient is undergoing active treatment and not whether the provider is seeing the patient for the first time.

   For complication codes, active treatment refers to treatment for the condition described by the code, even though it may be related to an earlier precipitating problem. For example, code T84.50XA, Infection and inflammatory reaction due to unspecified internal joint prosthesis, initial encounter, is used when active treatment is provided for the infection, even though the condition relates to the prosthetic device, implant or graft that was placed at a previous encounter.

   7th character "A", initial encounter is used **for each encounter where** the patient is receiving active treatment for the condition.

   7th character "D" subsequent encounter is used for encounters after the patient has **completed** active treatment of the condition and is receiving routine care for the condition during the healing or recovery phase.

   The aftercare Z codes should not be used for aftercare for conditions such as injuries or poisonings, where 7th characters are provided to identify subsequent care. For example, for aftercare of an injury, assign the acute injury code with the 7th character "D" (subsequent encounter).

   7th character "S", sequela, is for use for complications or conditions that arise as a direct result of a condition, such as scar formation after a burn. The scars are sequelae of the burn. When using 7th character "S", it is necessary to use both the injury code that precipitated the sequela and the code for the sequela itself. The "S" is added only to the injury code, not the sequela code. The 7th character "S" identifies the injury responsible for the sequela. The specific type of sequela (e.g. scar) is sequenced first, followed by the injury code.

   See Section I.B.10. Sequelae, (Late Effects)

   b. **Coding of Injuries**
   When coding injuries, assign separate codes for each injury unless a combination code is provided, in which case the combination code is assigned. Code T07, Unspecified multiple injuries should not be assigned in the inpatient setting unless information for a more specific code is not available. Traumatic injury codes (S00-T14.9) are not to be used for normal, healing surgical wounds or to identify complications of surgical wounds.

   The code for the most serious injury, as determined by the provider and the focus of treatment, is sequenced first.

   1) **Superficial injuries**
   Superficial injuries such as abrasions or contusions are not coded when associated with more severe injuries of the same site.

   2) **Primary injury with damage to nerves/ blood vessels**
   When a primary injury results in minor damage to peripheral nerves or blood vessels, the primary injury is sequenced first with additional code(s) for injuries to nerves and spinal cord (such as category S04), and/or injury to blood vessels (such as category S15). When the primary injury is to the blood vessels or nerves, that injury should be sequenced first.

   c. **Coding of Traumatic Fractures**
   The principles of multiple coding of injuries should be followed in coding fractures. Fractures of specified sites are coded individually by site in accordance with both the provisions within categories S02, S12, S22, S32, S42, S49, S52, S59, S62, S72, S79, S82, S89, S92 and the level of detail furnished by medical record content.

   A fracture not indicated as open or closed should be coded to closed. A fracture not indicated whether displaced or not displaced should be coded to displaced.

   More specific guidelines are as follows:

   1) **Initial vs. Subsequent Encounter for Fractures**
   Traumatic fractures are coded using the appropriate 7th character for initial encounter (A, B, C) **for each encounter where** the patient is receiving active treatment for the fracture. The appropriate 7th character for initial encounter should also be assigned for a patient who delayed seeking treatment for the fracture or nonunion.

   Fractures are coded using the appropriate 7th character for subsequent care for encounters after the patient has completed active treatment of the fracture and is receiving routine care for the fracture during the healing or recovery phase.

   Care for complications of surgical treatment for fracture repairs during the healing or recovery phase should be coded with the appropriate complication codes.

   Care of complications of fractures, such as malunion and nonunion, should be reported with the appropriate 7th character for subsequent care with nonunion (K, M, N,) or subsequent care with malunion (P, Q, R).

   Malunion/nonunion: The appropriate 7th character for initial encounter should also be assigned for a patient who delayed seeking treatment for the fracture or nonunion.

The open fracture designations in the assignment of the 7th character for fractures of the forearm, femur and lower leg, including ankle are based on the Gustilo open fracture classification. When the Gustilo classification type is not specified for an open fracture, the 7th character for open fracture type I or II should be assigned (B, E, H, M, Q).

A code from category M80, not a traumatic fracture code, should be used for any patient with known osteoporosis who suffers a fracture, even if the patient had a minor fall or trauma, if that fall or trauma would not usually break a normal, healthy bone.

See Section I.C.13. Osteoporosis.

The aftercare Z codes should not be used for aftercare for traumatic fractures. For aftercare of a traumatic fracture, assign the acute fracture code with the appropriate 7th character.

2) Multiple fractures sequencing

Multiple fractures are sequenced in accordance with the severity of the fracture.

d. Coding of Burns and Corrosions

The ICD-10-CM makes a distinction between burns and corrosions. The burn codes are for thermal burns, except sunburns, that come from a heat source, such as a fire or hot appliance. The burn codes are also for burns resulting from electricity and radiation. Corrosions are burns due to chemicals. The guidelines are the same for burns and corrosions.

Current burns (T20-T25) are classified by depth, extent and by agent (X code). Burns are classified by depth as first degree (erythema), second degree (blistering), and third degree (full-thickness involvement). Burns of the eye and internal organs (T26-T28) are classified by site, but not by degree.

1) Sequencing of burn and related condition codes

Sequence first the code that reflects the highest degree of burn when more than one burn is present.

    a. When the reason for the admission or encounter is for treatment of external multiple burns, sequence first the code that reflects the burn of the highest degree.

    b. When a patient has both internal and external burns, the circumstances of admission govern the selection of the principal diagnosis or first-listed diagnosis.

    c. When a patient is admitted for burn injuries and other related conditions such as smoke inhalation and/or respiratory failure, the circumstances of admission govern the selection of the principal or first-listed diagnosis.

2) Burns of the same local site

Classify burns of the same local site (three-character category level, T20-T28) but of different degrees to the subcategory identifying the highest degree recorded in the diagnosis.

3) Non-healing burns

Non-healing burns are coded as acute burns.

Necrosis of burned skin should be coded as a non-healed burn.

4) Infected Burn

For any documented infected burn site, use an additional code for the infection.

5) Assign separate codes for each burn site

When coding burns, assign separate codes for each burn site. Category T30, Burn and corrosion, body region unspecified is extremely vague and should rarely be used.

6) Burns and Corrosions Classified According to Extent of Body Surface Involved

Assign codes from category T31, Burns classified according to extent of body surface involved, or T32, Corrosions classified according to extent of body surface involved, when the site of the burn is not specified or when there is a need for additional data. It is advisable to use category T31 as additional coding when needed to provide data for evaluating burn mortality, such as that needed by burn units. It is also advisable to use category T31 as an additional code for reporting purposes when there is mention of a third-degree burn involving 20 percent or more of the body surface.

Categories T31 and T32 are based on the classic "rule of nines" in estimating body surface involved: head and neck are assigned nine percent, each arm nine percent, each leg 18 percent, the anterior trunk 18 percent, posterior trunk 18 percent, and genitalia one percent. Providers may change these percentage assignments where necessary to accommodate infants and children who have proportionately larger heads than adults, and patients who have large buttocks, thighs, or abdomen that involve burns.

7) Encounters for treatment of sequela of burns

Encounters for the treatment of the late effects of burns or corrosions (i.e., scars or joint contractures) should be coded with a burn or corrosion code with the 7th character "S" for sequela.

8) Sequelae with a late effect code and current burn

When appropriate, both a code for a current burn or corrosion with 7th character "A" or "D" and a burn or corrosion code with 7th character "S" may be assigned on the same record (when both a current burn and sequelae of an old burn exist). Burns and corrosions do not heal at the same rate and a current healing wound may still exist with sequela of a healed burn or corrosion.

See Section I.B.10. Sequela, (Late Effects)

9) Use of an external cause code with burns and corrosions

An external cause code should be used with burns and corrosions to identify the source and intent of the burn, as well as the place where it occurred.

GUIDELINES (ICD-10-CM)

e. **Adverse Effects, Poisoning , Underdosing and Toxic Effects**

Codes in categories T36-T65 are combination codes that include the substance that was taken as well as the intent. No additional external cause code is required for poisonings, toxic effects, adverse effects and underdosing codes.

1) **Do not code directly from the Table of Drugs**

Do not code directly from the Table of Drugs and Chemicals. Always refer back to the Tabular List.

2) **Use as many codes as necessary to describe**

Use as many codes as necessary to describe completely all drugs, medicinal or biological substances.

3) **If the same code would describe the causative agent**

If the same code would describe the causative agent for more than one adverse reaction, poisoning, toxic effect or underdosing, assign the code only once.

4) **If two or more drugs, medicinal or biological substances**

If two or more drugs, medicinal or biological substances are reported, code each individually unless a combination code is listed in the Table of Drugs and Chemicals.

5) **The occurrence of drug toxicity is classified in ICD-10-CM as follows:**

(a) Adverse Effect

When coding an adverse effect of a drug that has been correctly prescribed and properly administered, assign the appropriate code for the nature of the adverse effect followed by the appropriate code for the adverse effect of the drug (T36-T50). The code for the drug should have a 5th or 6th character "5" (for example T36.0X5-) Examples of the nature of an adverse effect are tachycardia, delirium, gastrointestinal hemorrhaging, vomiting, hypokalemia, hepatitis, renal failure, or respiratory failure.

(b) Poisoning

When coding a poisoning or reaction to the improper use of a medication (e.g., overdose, wrong substance given or taken in error, wrong route of administration), first assign the appropriate code from categories T36-T50. The poisoning codes have an associated intent as their 5th or 6th character (accidental, intentional self-harm, assault and undetermined). **If the intent of the poisoning is unknown or unspecified, code the intent as accidental intent. The undetermined intent is only for use if the documentation in the record specifies that the intent cannot be determined.** Use additional code(s) for all manifestations of poisonings.

If there is also a diagnosis of abuse or dependence of the substance, the abuse or dependence is assigned as an additional code.

Examples of poisoning include:

(i) Error was made in drug prescription Errors made in drug prescription or in the administration of the drug by provider, nurse, patient, or other person.

(ii) Overdose of a drug intentionally taken If an overdose of a drug was intentionally taken or administered and resulted in drug toxicity, it would be coded as a poisoning.

(iii) Nonprescribed drug taken with correctly prescribed and properly administered drug. If a nonprescribed drug or medicinal agent was taken in combination with a correctly prescribed and properly administered drug, any drug toxicity or other reaction resulting from the interaction of the two drugs would be classified as a poisoning.

(iv) Interaction of drug(s) and alcohol. When a reaction results from the interaction of a drug(s) and alcohol, this would be classified as poisoning.

See Section I.C.4. if poisoning is the result of insulin pump malfunctions.

(c) Underdosing

Underdosing refers to taking less of a medication than is prescribed by a provider or a manufacturer's instruction. For underdosing, assign the code from categories T36-T50 (fifth or sixth character "6").

Codes for underdosing should never be assigned as principal or first-listed codes. If a patient has a relapse or exacerbation of the medical condition for which the drug is prescribed because of the reduction in dose, then the medical condition itself should be coded.

Noncompliance (Z91.12-, Z91.13-) or complication of care (Y63.6-Y63.9) codes are to be used with an underdosing code to indicate intent, if known.

(d) Toxic Effects

When a harmful substance is ingested or comes in contact with a person, this is classified as a toxic effect. The toxic effect codes are in categories T51-T65.

Toxic effect codes have an associated intent: accidental, intentional self-harm, assault and undetermined.

f. **Adult and child abuse, neglect and other maltreatment**

Sequence first the appropriate code from categories T74.- (Adult and child abuse, neglect and other maltreatment, confirmed) or T76.- (Adult and child abuse, neglect and other maltreatment, suspected) for abuse, neglect and other maltreatment, followed by any accompanying mental health or injury code(s).

If the documentation in the medical record states abuse or neglect it is coded as confirmed (T74.-). It is coded as suspected if it is documented as suspected (T76.-).

For cases of confirmed abuse or neglect an external cause code from the assault section (X92-**Y09**) should be added to identify the cause of any physical injuries. A perpetrator code (Y07) should be added when the perpetrator of the abuse is known. For suspected cases of abuse or neglect, do not report external cause or perpetrator code.

If a suspected case of abuse, neglect or mistreatment is ruled out during an encounter code Z04.71, Encounter for examination and observation following alleged physical adult abuse, ruled out, or code Z04.72, Encounter for examination and observation following alleged child physical abuse, ruled out, should be used, not a code from T76.

If a suspected case of alleged rape or sexual abuse is ruled out during an encounter code Z04.41, Encounter for examination and observation following alleged **adult rape** or code Z04.42, Encounter for examination and observation following alleged **child** rape, should be used, not a code from T76.

See Section I.C.15. Abuse in a pregnant patient.

g. **Complications of care**

1) **General guidelines for complications of care**

(a) **Documentation of complications of care**

See Section I.B.16. for information on documentation of complications of care.

2) **Pain due to medical devices**

Pain associated with devices, implants or grafts left in a surgical site (for example painful hip prosthesis) is assigned to the appropriate code(s) found in Chapter 19, Injury, poisoning, and certain other consequences of external causes. Specific codes for pain due to medical devices are found in the T code section of the ICD-10-CM. Use additional code(s) from category G89 to identify acute or chronic pain due to presence of the device, implant or graft (G89.18 or G89.28).

3) **Transplant complications**

(a) **Transplant complications other than kidney**

Codes under category T86, Complications of transplanted organs and tissues, are for use for both complications and rejection of transplanted organs. A transplant complication code is only assigned if the complication affects the function of the transplanted organ. Two codes are required to fully describe a transplant complication: the appropriate code from category T86 and a secondary code that identifies the complication.

Pre-existing conditions or conditions that develop after the transplant are not coded as complications unless they affect the function of the transplanted organs.

See I.C.21. for transplant organ removal status
See I.C.2. for malignant neoplasm associated with transplanted organ.

(b) **Kidney transplant complications**

Patients who have undergone kidney transplant may still have some form of chronic kidney disease (CKD) because the kidney transplant may not fully restore kidney function. Code T86.1- should be assigned for documented complications of a kidney transplant, such as transplant failure or rejection or other transplant complication. Code T86.1- should not be assigned for post kidney transplant patients who have chronic kidney (CKD) unless a transplant complication such as transplant failure or rejection is documented. If the documentation is unclear as to whether the patient has a complication of the transplant, query the provider.

Conditions that affect the function of the transplanted kidney, other than CKD, should be assigned a code from subcategory T86.1, Complications of transplanted organ, Kidney, and a secondary code that identifies the complication.

For patients with CKD following a kidney transplant, but who do not have a complication such as failure or rejection, *see section I.C.14. Chronic kidney disease and kidney transplant status.*

4) **Complication codes that include the external cause**

As with certain other T codes, some of the complications of care codes have the external cause included in the code. The code includes the nature of the complication as well as the type of procedure that caused the complication. No external cause code indicating the type of procedure is necessary for these codes.

5) **Complications of care codes within the body system chapters**

Intraoperative and postprocedural complication codes are found within the body system chapters with codes specific to the organs and structures of that body system. These codes should be sequenced first, followed by a code(s) for the specific complication, if applicable.

20. **Chapter 20: External Causes of Morbidity (V00-Y99)**

The external causes of morbidity codes should never be sequenced as the first-listed or principal diagnosis.

External cause codes are intended to provide data for injury research and evaluation of injury prevention strategies. These codes capture how the injury or health condition happened (cause), the intent (unintentional or accidental; or intentional, such as suicide or assault), the place where the event occurred the activity of the patient at the time of the event, and the person's status (e.g., civilian, military).

There is no national requirement for mandatory ICD-10-CM external cause code reporting. Unless a provider is subject to a state-based external cause code reporting mandate or these codes are required by a particular payer, reporting of ICD-10-CM codes in Chapter 20, External Causes of Morbidity, is not required. In the absence of a mandatory reporting requirement, providers are encouraged to voluntarily report external cause codes, as they provide valuable data for injury research and evaluation of injury prevention strategies.

a. **General External Cause Coding Guidelines**

1) **Used with any code in the range of A00.0-T88.9, Z00-Z99**

An external cause code may be used with any code in the range of A00.0-T88.9, Z00-Z99, classification that is a health condition due to an external cause. Though they are most applicable to injuries, they are also valid for use with such things as infections or diseases due to an external source, and other health conditions, such as a heart attack that occurs during strenuous physical activity.

2) **External cause code used for length of treatment**

Assign the external cause code, with the appropriate 7th character (initial encounter, subsequent encounter or sequela) for each encounter for which the injury or condition is being treated.

Most categories in chapter 20 have a 7th character requirement for each applicable code. Most categories in this chapter have three 7th character values: A, initial encounter, D, subsequent encounter and S, sequela. While the patient may be seen by a new or different provider over the course of treatment for an injury or condition, assignment of the 7th character for external cause should match the 7th character of the code assigned for the associated injury or condition for the encounter.

3) **Use the full range of external cause codes**

Use the full range of external cause codes to completely describe the cause, the intent, the place of occurrence and if applicable, the activity of the patient at the time of the event, and the patient's status, for all injuries, and other health conditions due to an external cause.

4) **Assign as many external cause codes as necessary**

Assign as many external cause codes as necessary to fully explain each cause. If only one external code can be recorded, assign the code most related to the principal diagnosis.

5) **The selection of the appropriate external cause code**

The selection of the appropriate external cause code is guided by the Alphabetic Index of External Causes and by Inclusion and Exclusion notes in the Tabular List.

6) **External cause code can never be a principal diagnosis**

An external cause code can never be a principal (first-listed) diagnosis.

7) **Combination external cause codes**

Certain of the external cause codes are combination codes that identify sequential events that result in an injury, such as a fall which results in striking against an object. The injury may be due to either event or both. The combination external cause code used should correspond to the sequence of events regardless of which caused the most serious injury.

8) **No external cause code needed in certain circumstances**

No external cause code from Chapter 20 is needed if the external cause and intent are included in a code from another chapter (e.g. T36.0X1- Poisoning by penicillins, accidental (unintentional)).

b. **Place of Occurrence Guideline**

Codes from category Y92, Place of occurrence of the external cause, are secondary codes for use after other external cause codes to identify the location of the patient at the time of injury or other condition.

Generally, a place of occurrence code is assigned only once, at the initial encounter for treatment. However, in the rare instance that a new injury occurs during hospitalization, an additional place of occurrence code may be assigned. No 7th characters are used for Y92. Only one code from Y92 should be recorded on a medical record.

Do not use place of occurrence code Y92.9 if the place is not stated or is not applicable.

c. **Activity Code**

Assign a code from category Y93, Activity code, to describe the activity of the patient at the time the injury or other health condition occurred.

An activity code is used only once, at the initial encounter for treatment. Only one code from Y93 should be recorded on a medical record.

The activity codes are not applicable to poisonings, adverse effects, misadventures or sequela.

Do not assign Y93.9, Unspecified activity, if the activity is not stated.

A code from category Y93 is appropriate for use with external cause and intent codes if identifying the activity provides additional information about the event.

d. **Place of Occurrence, Activity, and Status Codes Used with other External Cause Code**

When applicable, place of occurrence, activity, and external cause status codes are sequenced after the main external cause code(s). Regardless of the number of external cause codes assigned, there should be only one place of occurrence code, one activity code, and one external cause status code assigned to an encounter.

e. If the Reporting Format Limits the Number of External Cause Codes

If the reporting format limits the number of external cause codes that can be used in reporting clinical data, report the code for the cause/intent most related to the principal diagnosis. If the format permits capture of additional external cause codes, the cause/intent, including medical misadventures, of the additional events should be reported rather than the codes for place, activity, or external status.

f. Multiple External Cause Coding Guidelines

More than one external cause code is required to fully describe the external cause of an illness or injury. The assignment of external cause codes should be sequenced in the following priority:

If two or more events cause separate injuries, an external cause code should be assigned for each cause. The first-listed external cause code will be selected in the following order:

External codes for child and adult abuse take priority over all other external cause codes.

See Section I.C.19., Child and Adult abuse guidelines.

External codes for terrorism events take priority over all other external cause codes except child and adult abuse.

External cause codes for cataclysmic events take priority over all other external cause codes except child and adult abuse and terrorism.

External cause codes for transport accidents take priority over all other external cause codes except cataclysmic events, child and adult abuse and terrorism.

Activity and external cause status codes are assigned following all causal (intent) external cause codes.

The first-listed external cause code should correspond to the cause of the most serious diagnosis due to an assault, accident, or self-harm, following the order of hierarchy listed above.

g. Child and Adult Abuse Guideline

Adult and child abuse, neglect and maltreatment are classified as assault. Any of the assault codes may be used to indicate the external cause of any injury resulting from the confirmed abuse.

For confirmed cases of abuse, neglect and maltreatment, when the perpetrator is known, a code from Y07, Perpetrator of maltreatment and neglect, should accompany any other assault codes.

See Section I.C.19. Adult and child abuse, neglect and other maltreatment

h. Unknown or Undetermined Intent Guideline

If the intent (accident, self-harm, assault) of the cause of an injury or other condition is unknown or unspecified, code the intent as accidental intent. All transport accident categories assume accidental intent.

1) Use of undetermined intent

External cause codes for events of undetermined intent are only for use if the documentation in the record specifies that the intent cannot be determined.

i. Sequelae (Late Effects) of External Cause Guidelines

1) Sequelae external cause codes

Sequela are reported using the external cause code with the 7th character "S" for sequela. These codes should be used with any report of a late effect or sequela resulting from a previous injury.

See Section I.B.10. Sequela, (Late Effects)

2) Sequela external cause code with a related current injury

A sequela external cause code should never be used with a related current nature of injury code.

3) Use of sequela external cause codes for subsequent visits

Use a late effect external cause code for subsequent visits when a late effect of the initial injury is being treated. Do not use a late effect external cause code for subsequent visits for follow-up care (e.g., to assess healing, to receive rehabilitative therapy) of the injury when no late effect of the injury has been documented.

j. Terrorism Guidelines

1) Cause of injury identified by the Federal Government (FBI) as terrorism

When the cause of an injury is identified by the Federal Government (FBI) as terrorism, the first-listed external cause code should be a code from category Y38, Terrorism. The definition of terrorism employed by the FBI is found at the inclusion note at the beginning of category Y38. Use additional code for place of occurrence (Y92.-). More than one Y38 code may be assigned if the injury is the result of more than one mechanism of terrorism.

2) Cause of an injury is suspected to be the result of terrorism

When the cause of an injury is suspected to be the result of terrorism a code from category Y38 should not be assigned. Suspected cases should be classified as assault.

3) Code Y38.9, Terrorism, secondary effects

Assign code Y38.9, Terrorism, secondary effects, for conditions occurring subsequent to the terrorist event. This code should not be assigned for conditions that are due to the initial terrorist act.

It is acceptable to assign code Y38.9 with another code from Y38 if there is an injury due to the initial terrorist event and an injury that is a subsequent result of the terrorist event.

k. External cause status

A code from category Y99, External cause status, should be assigned whenever any other external cause code is assigned for an encounter, including an Activity code, except for the events noted below. Assign a code from category Y99, External cause status, to indicate the work status of the person at the time the event occurred. The status code indicates whether the event occurred during military activity, whether a non-military person was at work, whether an individual including a student or volunteer was involved in a non-work activity at the time of the causal event.

A code from Y99, External cause status, should be assigned, when applicable, with other external cause codes, such as transport accidents and falls. The external cause status codes are not applicable to poisonings, adverse effects, misadventures or late effects.

Do not assign a code from category Y99 if no other external cause codes (cause, activity) are applicable for the encounter.

An external cause status code is used only once, at the initial encounter for treatment. Only one code from Y99 should be recorded on a medical record.

Do not assign code Y99.9, Unspecified external cause status, if the status is not stated.

21. **Chapter 21: Factors influencing health status and contact with health services (Z00-Z99)**
    Note: The chapter specific guidelines provide additional information about the use of Z codes for specified encounters.

    a. Use of Z codes in any healthcare setting
    Z codes are for use in any healthcare setting. Z codes may be used as either a first-listed (principal diagnosis code in the inpatient setting) or secondary code, depending on the circumstances of the encounter. Certain Z codes may only be used as first-listed or principal diagnosis.

    b. Z Codes indicate a reason for an encounter
    Z codes are not procedure codes. A corresponding procedure code must accompany a Z code to describe any procedure performed.

    c. Categories of Z Codes
    1) Contact/Exposure
    Category Z20 indicates contact with, and suspected exposure to, communicable diseases. These codes are for patients who do not show any sign or symptom of a disease but are suspected to have been exposed to it by close personal contact with an infected individual or are in an area where a disease is epidemic.

    Category Z77, Other contact with and (suspected) exposures hazardous to health, indicates contact with and suspected exposures hazardous to health.

    Contact/exposure codes may be used as a first-listed code to explain an encounter for testing, or, more commonly, as a secondary code to identify a potential risk.

    2) Inoculations and vaccinations
    Code Z23 is for encounters for inoculations and vaccinations. It indicates that a patient is being seen to receive a prophylactic inoculation against a disease. Procedure codes are required to identify the actual administration of the injection and the type(s) of immunizations given. Code Z23 may be used as a secondary code if the inoculation is given as a routine part of preventive health care, such as a well-baby visit.

    3) Status
    Status codes indicate that a patient is either a carrier of a disease or has the sequelae or residual of a past disease or condition. This includes such things as the presence of prosthetic or mechanical devices resulting from past treatment. A status code is informative, because the status may affect the course of treatment and its outcome. A status code is distinct from a history code. The history code indicates that the patient no longer has the condition.

    A status code should not be used with a diagnosis code from one of the body system chapters, if the diagnosis code includes the information provided by the status code. For example, code Z94.1, Heart transplant status, should not be used with a code from subcategory T86.2, Complications of heart transplant. The status code does not provide additional information. The complication code indicates that the patient is a heart transplant patient.

    For encounters for weaning from a mechanical ventilator, assign a code from subcategory J96.1, Chronic respiratory failure, followed by code Z99.11, Dependence on respirator [ventilator] status.

    The status Z codes/categories are:
    Z14   Genetic carrier
           Genetic carrier status indicates that a person carries a gene, associated with a particular disease, which may be passed to offspring who may develop that disease. The person does not have the disease and is not at risk of developing the disease.
    Z15   Genetic susceptibility to disease Genetic susceptibility indicates that a person has a gene that increases the risk of that person developing the disease.
    Codes from category Z15 should not be used as principal or first-listed codes. If the patient has the condition to which he/she is susceptible, and that condition is the reason for the encounter, the code for the current condition should be sequenced first. If the patient is being seen for follow-up after completed treatment for this condition, and the condition no longer exists, a follow-up code should be sequenced first, followed by the appropriate personal history and genetic susceptibility codes. If the purpose of the encounter is genetic counseling associated with procreative management, code Z31.5, Encounter for genetic counseling, should be assigned as the first-listed code, followed by a code from category Z15. Additional codes should be assigned for any applicable family or personal history.
    Z16   Resistance to antimicrobial drugs
           This code indicates that a patient has a condition that is resistant to antimicrobial drug treatment. Sequence the infection code first.

Z17 Estrogen receptor status

Z18 Retained foreign body fragments

Z19 Hormone sensitivity malignancy status

Z21 Asymptomatic HIV infection status This code indicates that a patient has tested positive for HIV but has manifested no signs or symptoms of the disease.

Z22 Carrier of infectious disease Carrier status indicates that a person harbors the specific organisms of a disease without manifest symptoms and is capable of transmitting the infection.

Z28.3 Underimmunization status

Z33.1 Pregnant state, incidental This code is a secondary code only for use when the pregnancy is in no way complicating the reason for visit. Otherwise, a code from the obstetric chapter is required.

Z66 Do not resuscitate

This code may be used when it is documented by the provider that a patient is on do not resuscitate status at any time during the stay.

Z67 Blood type

Z68 Body mass index (BMI)
As with all other secondary diagnosis codes, the BMI codes should only be assigned when they meet the definition of a reportable diagnosis (see Section III, Reporting Additional Diagnoses).

Z74.01 Bed confinement status

Z76.82 Awaiting organ transplant status

Z78 Other specified health status

Code Z78.1, Physical restraint status, may be used when it is documented by the provider that a patient has been put in restraints during the current encounter. Please note that this code should not be reported when it is documented by the provider that a patient is temporarily restrained during a procedure.

Z79 Long-term (current) drug therapy

Codes from this category indicate a patient's continuous use of a prescribed drug (including such things as aspirin therapy) for the long-term treatment of a condition or for prophylactic use. It is not for use for patients who have addictions to drugs. This subcategory is not for use of medications for detoxification or maintenance programs to prevent withdrawal symptoms in patients with drug dependence (e.g., methadone maintenance for opiate dependence). Assign the appropriate code for the drug dependence instead.

Assign a code from Z79 if the patient is receiving a medication for an extended period as a prophylactic measure (such as for the prevention of deep vein thrombosis) or as treatment of a chronic condition (such as arthritis) or a disease requiring a lengthy course of treatment (such as cancer). Do not assign a code from category Z79 for medication being administered for a brief period of time to treat an acute illness or injury (such as a course of antibiotics to treat acute bronchitis).

Z88 Allergy status to drugs, medicaments and biological substances Except: Z88.9, Allergy status to unspecified drugs, medicaments and biological substances status

Z89 Acquired absence of limb

Z90 Acquired absence of organs, not elsewhere classified

Z91.0- Allergy status, other than to drugs and biological substances

Z92.82 Status post administration of tPA (rtPA) in a different facility within the last 24 hours prior to admission to a current facility Assign code Z92.82, Status post administration of tPA (rtPA) in a different facility within the last 24 hours prior to admission to current facility, as a secondary diagnosis when a patient is received by transfer into a facility and documentation indicates they were administered tissue plasminogen activator (tPA) within the last 24 hours prior to admission to the current facility. This guideline applies even if the patient is still receiving the tPA at the time they are received into the current facility. The appropriate code for the condition for which the tPA was administered (such as cerebrovascular disease or myocardial infarction) should be assigned first. Code Z92.82 is only applicable to the receiving facility record and not to the transferring facility record.

Z93 Artificial opening status

Z94 Transplanted organ and tissue status

Z95 Presence of cardiac and vascular implants and grafts

Z96 Presence of other functional implants

Z97 Presence of other devices

Z98 Other postprocedural states

Assign code Z98.85, Transplanted organ removal status, to indicate that a transplanted organ has been previously removed. This code should not be assigned for the encounter in which the transplanted organ is removed. The complication necessitating removal of the transplant organ should be assigned for that encounter.

See section I.C.19. for information on the coding of organ transplant complications.

Z99 Dependence on enabling machines and devices, not elsewhere classified

Note: Categories Z89-Z90 and Z93-Z99 are for use only if there are no complications or malfunctions of the organ or tissue replaced, the amputation site or the equipment on which the patient is dependent.

4) History (of)

There are two types of history Z codes, personal and family. Personal history codes explain a patient's past medical condition that no longer exists and is not receiving any treatment, but that has the potential for recurrence, and therefore may require continued monitoring.

Family history codes are for use when a patient has a family member(s) who has had a particular disease that causes the patient to be at higher risk of also contracting the disease.

Personal history codes may be used in conjunction with follow-up codes and family history codes may be used in conjunction with screening codes to explain the need for a test or procedure. History codes are also acceptable on any medical record regardless of the reason for visit. A history of an illness, even if no longer present, is important information that may alter the type of treatment ordered.

The history Z code categories are:

Z8Ø	Family history of primary malignant neoplasm
Z81	Family history of mental and behavioral disorders
Z82	Family history of certain disabilities and chronic diseases (leading to disablement)
Z83	Family history of other specific disorders
Z84	Family history of other conditions
Z85	Personal history of malignant neoplasm
Z86	Personal history of certain other diseases
Z87	Personal history of other diseases and conditions
Z91.4-	Personal history of psychological trauma, not elsewhere classified
Z91.5	Personal history of self-harm
Z91.8-	Other specified personal risk factors, not elsewhere classified Exception: Z91.83, Wandering in diseases classified elsewhere
Z92	Personal history of medical treatment Except: Z92.Ø, Personal history of contraception Except: Z92.82, Status post administration of tPA (rtPA) in a different facility within the last 24 hours prior to admission to a current facility

5) Screening

Screening is the testing for disease or disease precursors in seemingly well individuals so that early detection and treatment can be provided for those who test positive for the disease (e.g., screening mammogram).

The testing of a person to rule out or confirm a suspected diagnosis because the patient has some sign or symptom is a diagnostic examination, not a screening. In these cases, the sign or symptom is used to explain the reason for the test.

A screening code may be a first-listed code if the reason for the visit is specifically the screening exam. It may also be used as an additional code if the screening is done during an office visit for other health problems. A screening code is not necessary if the screening is inherent to a routine examination, such as a pap smear done during a routine pelvic examination.

Should a condition be discovered during the screening then the code for the condition may be assigned as an additional diagnosis.

The Z code indicates that a screening exam is planned. A procedure code is required to confirm that the screening was performed.

The screening Z codes/categories:

Z11	Encounter for screening for infectious and parasitic diseases
Z12	Encounter for screening for malignant neoplasms
Z13	Encounter for screening for other diseases and disorders Except: Z13.9, Encounter for screening, unspecified
Z36	Encounter for antenatal screening for mother

6) Observation

There are **three** observation Z code categories. They are for use in very limited circumstances when a person is being observed for a suspected condition that is ruled out. The observation codes are not for use if an injury or illness or any signs or symptoms related to the suspected condition are present. In such cases the diagnosis/symptom code is used with the corresponding external cause code.

The observation codes are to be used as principal diagnosis only. **The only exception to this is when the principal diagnosis is required to be a code from category Z38, Liveborn infants according to place of birth and type of delivery. Then a code from category ZØ5, Encounter for observation and evaluation of newborn for suspected diseases and conditions ruled out, is sequenced after the Z38 code.** Additional codes may be used in addition to the observation code, but only if they are unrelated to the suspected condition being observed.

Codes from subcategory ZØ3.7 Encounter for suspected maternal and fetal conditions ruled out, may either be used as a first-listed or as an additional code assignment depending on the case. They are for use in very limited circumstances on a maternal record when an encounter is for a suspected maternal or fetal condition that is ruled out during that encounter (for example, a maternal or fetal condition may be suspected due to an abnormal test result). These codes should not be used when the condition is confirmed. In those cases, the confirmed condition should be coded. In addition, these codes are not for use if an illness or any signs or symptoms related to the suspected condition or problem are present. In such cases the diagnosis/symptom code is used.

GUIDELINES (ICD-10-CM)

Additional codes may be used in addition to the code from subcategory Z03.7, but only if they are unrelated to the suspected condition being evaluated.

Codes from subcategory Z03.7 may not be used for encounters for antenatal screening of mother. *See Section I.C.21. Screening.*

For encounters for suspected fetal condition that are inconclusive following testing and evaluation, assign the appropriate code from category O35, O36, O40 or O41.

The observation Z code categories:

Z03 Encounter for medical observation for suspected diseases and conditions ruled out

Z04 Encounter for examination and observation for other reasons Except: Z04.9, Encounter for examination and observation for unspecified reason

Z05 Encounter for observation and evaluation of newborn for suspected diseases and conditions ruled out

7) Aftercare

Aftercare visit codes cover situations when the initial treatment of a disease has been performed and the patient requires continued care during the healing or recovery phase, or for the long-term consequences of the disease. The aftercare Z code should not be used if treatment is directed at a current, acute disease. The diagnosis code is to be used in these cases.

Exceptions to this rule are codes Z51.0, Encounter for antineoplastic radiation therapy, and codes from subcategory Z51.1, Encounter for antineoplastic chemotherapy and immunotherapy. These codes are to be first-listed, followed by the diagnosis code when a patient's encounter is solely to receive radiation therapy, chemotherapy, or immunotherapy for the treatment of a neoplasm. If the reason for the encounter is more than one type of antineoplastic therapy, code Z51.0 and a code from subcategory Z51.1 may be assigned together, in which case one of these codes would be reported as a secondary diagnosis.

The aftercare Z codes should also not be used for aftercare for injuries. For aftercare of an injury, assign the acute injury code with the appropriate 7th character (for subsequent encounter).

The aftercare codes are generally first-listed to explain the specific reason for the encounter. An aftercare code may be used as an additional code when some type of aftercare is provided in addition to the reason for admission and no diagnosis code is applicable. An example of this would be the closure of a colostomy during an encounter for treatment of another condition.

Aftercare codes should be used in conjunction with other aftercare codes or diagnosis codes to provide better detail on the specifics of an aftercare encounter visit, unless otherwise directed by the classification. Should a patient receive multiple types of antineoplastic therapy during the same encounter, code Z51.0, Encounter for antineoplastic radiation therapy, and codes from subcategory Z51.1, Encounter for antineoplastic chemotherapy and immunotherapy, may be used together on a record. The sequencing of multiple aftercare codes depends on the circumstances of the encounter.

Certain aftercare Z code categories need a secondary diagnosis code to describe the resolving condition or sequelae. For others, the condition is included in the code title.

Additional Z code aftercare category terms include fitting and adjustment, and attention to artificial openings.

Status Z codes may be used with aftercare Z codes to indicate the nature of the aftercare. For example code Z95.1, Presence of aortocoronary bypass graft, may be used with code Z48.812, Encounter for surgical aftercare following surgery on the circulatory system, to indicate the surgery for which the aftercare is being performed. A status code should not be used when the aftercare code indicates the type of status, such as using Z43.0, Encounter for attention to tracheostomy, with Z93.0, Tracheostomy status.

The aftercare Z category/codes:

Z42 Encounter for plastic and reconstructive surgery following medical procedure or healed injury

Z43 Encounter for attention to artificial openings

Z44 Encounter for fitting and adjustment of external prosthetic device

Z45 Encounter for adjustment and management of implanted device

Z46 Encounter for fitting and adjustment of other devices

Z47 Orthopedic aftercare

Z48 Encounter for other postprocedural aftercare

Z49 Encounter for care involving renal dialysis

Z51 Encounter for other aftercare **and medical care**

8) Follow-up

The follow-up codes are used to explain continuing surveillance following completed treatment of a disease, condition, or injury. They imply that the condition has been fully treated and no longer exists. They should not be confused with aftercare codes, or injury codes with a 7th character for subsequent encounter, that explain ongoing care of a healing condition or its sequelae. Follow-up codes may be used in conjunction with history codes to provide the full picture of the healed condition and its treatment. The follow-up code is sequenced first, followed by the history code.

A follow-up code may be used to explain multiple visits. Should a condition be found to have recurred on the follow-up visit, then the diagnosis code for the condition should be assigned in place of the follow-up code.

The follow-up Z code categories:

Z08   Encounter for follow-up examination after completed treatment for malignant neoplasm

Z09   Encounter for follow-up examination after completed treatment for conditions other than malignant neoplasm

Z39   Encounter for maternal postpartum care and examination

9) Donor

Codes in category Z52, Donors of organs and tissues, are used for living individuals who are donating blood or other body tissue. These codes are only for individuals donating for others, not for self-donations. They are not used to identify cadaveric donations.

10) Counseling

Counseling Z codes are used when a patient or family member receives assistance in the aftermath of an illness or injury, or when support is required in coping with family or social problems. They are not used in conjunction with a diagnosis code when the counseling component of care is considered integral to standard treatment.

The counseling Z codes/categories:

Z30.0-   Encounter for general counseling and advice on contraception

Z31.5   Encounter for genetic counseling

Z31.6-   Encounter for general counseling and advice on procreation

Z32.2   Encounter for childbirth instruction

Z32.3   Encounter for childcare instruction

Z69   Encounter for mental health services for victim and perpetrator of abuse

Z70   Counseling related to sexual attitude, behavior and orientation

Z71   Persons encountering health services for other counseling and medical advice, not elsewhere classified

Z76.81   Expectant mother prebirth pediatrician visit

11) Encounters for Obstetrical and Reproductive Services

See Section I.C.15. Pregnancy, Childbirth, and the Puerperium, for further instruction on the use of these codes.

Z codes for pregnancy are for use in those circumstances when none of the problems or complications included in the codes from the Obstetrics chapter exist (a routine prenatal visit or postpartum care). Codes in category Z34, Encounter for supervision of normal pregnancy, are always first listed and are not to be used with any other code from the OB chapter.

Codes in category Z3A, Weeks of gestation, may be assigned to provide additional information about the pregnancy. **Category Z3A codes should not be assigned for pregnancies with abortive outcomes (categories O00-O08), elective termination of pregnancy (code Z33.32), nor for postpartum conditions, as category Z3A is not applicable to**

these conditions. The date of the admission should be used to determine weeks of gestation for inpatient admissions that encompass more than one gestational week.

The outcome of delivery, category Z37, should be included on all maternal delivery records. It is always a secondary code. Codes in category Z37 should not be used on the newborn record.

Z codes for family planning (contraceptive) or procreative management and counseling should be included on an obstetric record either during the pregnancy or the postpartum stage, if applicable.

Z codes/categories for obstetrical and reproductive services:

Z30   Encounter for contraceptive management

Z31   Encounter for procreative management

Z32.2   Encounter for childbirth instruction

Z32.3   Encounter for childcare instruction

Z33   Pregnant state

Z34   Encounter for supervision of normal pregnancy

Z36   Encounter for antenatal screening of mother

Z3A   Weeks of gestation

Z37   Outcome of delivery

Z39   Encounter for maternal postpartum care and examination

Z76.81   Expectant mother prebirth pediatrician visit

12) Newborns and Infants

See Section I.C.16. Newborn (Perinatal) Guidelines, for further instruction on the use of these codes.

Newborn Z codes/categories:

Z76.1   Encounter for health supervision and care of foundling

Z00.1-   Encounter for routine child health examination

Z38   Liveborn infants according to place of birth and type of delivery

13) Routine and administrative examinations

The Z codes allow for the description of encounters for routine examinations, such as, a general check-up, or, examinations for administrative purposes, such as, a pre-employment physical. The codes are not to be used if the examination is for diagnosis of a suspected condition or for treatment purposes. In such cases the diagnosis code is used. During a routine exam, should a diagnosis or condition be discovered, it should be coded as an additional code. Pre-existing and chronic conditions and history codes may also be included as additional codes as long as the examination is for administrative purposes and not focused on any particular condition.

Some of the codes for routine health examinations distinguish between "with" and "without" abnormal findings. Code assignment depends on the information that is known at the time the encounter is being coded. For example, if no abnormal findings were found during the examination, but the encounter is being coded before test results are back, it is acceptable to assign the code for "without abnormal findings." When assigning a code for "with abnormal findings," additional code(s) should be assigned to identify the specific abnormal finding(s).

Pre-operative examination and pre-procedural laboratory examination Z codes are for use only in those situations when a patient is being cleared for a procedure or surgery and no treatment is given.

The Z codes/categories for routine and administrative examinations:

Z00 Encounter for general examination without complaint, suspected or reported diagnosis

Z01 Encounter for other special examination without complaint, suspected or reported diagnosis

Z02 Encounter for administrative examination
Except: Z02.9, Encounter for administrative examinations, unspecified

Z32.0- Encounter for pregnancy test

14) Miscellaneous Z codes

The miscellaneous Z codes capture a number of other health care encounters that do not fall into one of the other categories. Certain of these codes identify the reason for the encounter; others are for use as additional codes that provide useful information on circumstances that may affect a patient's care and treatment.

Prophylactic Organ Removal

For encounters specifically for prophylactic removal of an organ (such as prophylactic removal of breasts due to a genetic susceptibility to cancer or a family history of cancer), the principal or first-listed code should be a code from category Z40, Encounter for prophylactic surgery, followed by the appropriate codes to identify the associated risk factor (such as genetic susceptibility or family history).

If the patient has a malignancy of one site and is having prophylactic removal at another site to prevent either a new primary malignancy or metastatic disease, a code for the malignancy should also be assigned in addition to a code from subcategory Z40.0, Encounter for prophylactic surgery for risk factors related to malignant neoplasms. A Z40.0 code should not be assigned if the patient is having organ removal for treatment of a malignancy, such as the removal of the testes for the treatment of prostate cancer.

Miscellaneous Z codes/categories:

Z28 Immunization not carried out
Except: Z28.3, Underimmunization status

Z29 Encounter for other prophylactic measures

Z40 Encounter for prophylactic surgery

Z41 Encounter for procedures for purposes other than remedying health state
Except: Z41.9, Encounter for procedure for purposes other than remedying health state, unspecified

Z53 Persons encountering health services for specific procedures and treatment, not carried out

Z55 Problems related to education and literacy

Z56 Problems related to employment and unemployment

Z57 Occupational exposure to risk factors

Z58 Problems related to physical environment

Z59 Problems related to housing and economic circumstances

Z60 Problems related to social environment

Z62 Problems related to upbringing

Z63 Other problems related to primary support group, including family circumstances

Z64 Problems related to certain psychosocial circumstances

Z65 Problems related to other psychosocial circumstances

Z72 Problems related to lifestyle
Note: These codes should be assigned only when the documentation specifies that the patient has an associated problem

Z73 Problems related to life management difficulty

Z74 Problems related to care provider dependency Except: Z74.01, Bed confinement status

Z75 Problems related to medical facilities and other health care

Z76.0 Encounter for issue of repeat prescription

Z76.3 Healthy person accompanying sick person

Z76.4 Other boarder to healthcare facility

Z76.5 Malingerer [conscious simulation]

Z91.1- Patient's noncompliance with medical treatment and regimen

Z91.83 Wandering in diseases classified elsewhere

Z91.89 Other specified personal risk factors, not elsewhere classified

15) Nonspecific Z codes

Certain Z codes are so non-specific, or potentially redundant with other codes in the classification, that there can be little justification for their use in the inpatient setting. Their use in the outpatient setting should be limited to those instances when there is no further documentation to permit more precise coding. Otherwise, any sign or symptom or any other reason for visit that is captured in another code should be used.

Nonspecific Z codes/categories:

Z02.9 Encounter for administrative examinations, unspecified

Z04.9 Encounter for examination and observation for unspecified reason

Z13.9 Encounter for screening, unspecified

Z41.9   Encounter for procedure for purposes other than remedying health state, unspecified

Z52.9   Donor of unspecified organ or tissue

Z86.59   Personal history of other mental and behavioral disorders

Z88.9   Allergy status to unspecified drugs, medicaments and biological substances status

Z92.0   Personal history of contraception

16) Z Codes That May Only be Principal/First-Listed Diagnosis

The following Z codes/categories may only be reported as the principal/first-listed diagnosis, except when there are multiple encounters on the same day and the medical records for the encounters are combined:

Z00   Encounter for general examination without complaint, suspected or reported diagnosis
Except: Z00.6

Z01   Encounter for other special examination without complaint, suspected or reported diagnosis

Z02   Encounter for administrative examination

Z03   Encounter for medical observation for suspected diseases and conditions ruled out

Z04   Encounter for examination and observation for other reasons

Z33.2   Encounter for elective termination of pregnancy

Z31.81   Encounter for male factor infertility in female patient

Z31.83   Encounter for assisted reproductive fertility procedure cycle

Z31.84   Encounter for fertility preservation procedure

Z34   Encounter for supervision of normal pregnancy

Z39   Encounter for maternal postpartum care and examination

Z38   Liveborn infants according to place of birth and type of delivery

Z42   Encounter for plastic and reconstructive surgery following medical procedure or healed injury

Z51.0   Encounter for antineoplastic radiation therapy

Z51.1-   Encounter for antineoplastic chemotherapy and immunotherapy

Z52   Donors of organs and tissues Except: Z52.9, Donor of unspecified organ or tissue

Z76.1   Encounter for health supervision and care of foundling

Z76.2   Encounter for health supervision and care of other healthy infant and child

Z99.12   Encounter for respirator [ventilator] dependence during power failure

Section II. Selection of Principal Diagnosis

The circumstances of inpatient admission always govern the selection of principal diagnosis. The principal diagnosis is defined in the Uniform Hospital Discharge Data Set (UHDDS) as "that condition established after study to be chiefly responsible for occasioning the admission of the patient to the hospital for care."

The UHDDS definitions are used by hospitals to report inpatient data elements in a standardized manner. These data elements and their definitions can be found in the July 31, 1985, Federal Register (Vol. 50, No, 147), pp. 31038-40.

Since that time the application of the UHDDS definitions has been expanded to include all nonoutpatient settings (acute care, short term, long term care and psychiatric hospitals; home health agencies; rehab facilities; nursing homes, etc). **The UHDDS definitions also apply to hospice services (all levels of care).**

In determining principal diagnosis, coding conventions in the ICD-10-CM, the Tabular List and Alphabetic Index take precedence over these official coding guidelines.

(See Section I.A., Conventions for the ICD-10-CM)

The importance of consistent, complete documentation in the medical record cannot be overemphasized. Without such documentation the application of all coding guidelines is a difficult, if not impossible, task.

A. Codes for symptoms, signs, and ill-defined conditions

Codes for symptoms, signs, and ill-defined conditions from Chapter 18 are not to be used as principal diagnosis when a related definitive diagnosis has been established.

B. Two or more interrelated conditions, each potentially meeting the definition for principal diagnosis.

When there are two or more interrelated conditions (such as diseases in the same ICD-10-CM chapter or manifestations characteristically associated with a certain disease) potentially meeting the definition of principal diagnosis, either condition may be sequenced first, unless the circumstances of the admission, the therapy provided, the Tabular List, or the Alphabetic Index indicate otherwise.

C. Two or more diagnoses that equally meet the definition for principal diagnosis

In the unusual instance when two or more diagnoses equally meet the criteria for principal diagnosis as determined by the circumstances of admission, diagnostic workup and/or therapy provided, and the Alphabetic Index, Tabular List, or another coding guidelines does not provide sequencing direction, any one of the diagnoses may be sequenced first.

D. Two or more comparative or contrasting conditions.

In those rare instances when two or more contrasting or comparative diagnoses are documented as "either/or" (or similar terminology), they are coded as if the diagnoses

GUIDELINES (ICD-10-CM)

were confirmed and the diagnoses are sequenced according to the circumstances of the admission. If no further determination can be made as to which diagnosis should be principal, either diagnosis may be sequenced first.

E. A symptom(s) followed by contrasting/ comparative diagnoses
GUIDELINE HAS BEEN DELETED EFFECTIVE OCTOBER 1, 2014

F. Original treatment plan not carried out
Sequence as the principal diagnosis the condition, which after study occasioned the admission to the hospital, even though treatment may not have been carried out due to unforeseen circumstances.

G. Complications of surgery and other medical care
When the admission is for treatment of a complication resulting from surgery or other medical care, the complication code is sequenced as the principal diagnosis. If the complication is classified to the T80-T88 series and the code lacks the necessary specificity in describing the complication, an additional code for the specific complication should be assigned.

H. Uncertain Diagnosis
If the diagnosis documented at the time of discharge is qualified as "probable", "suspected", "likely", "questionable", "possible", or "still to be ruled out", or other similar terms indicating uncertainty, code the condition as if it existed or was established. The bases for these guidelines are the diagnostic workup, arrangements for further workup or observation, and initial therapeutic approach that correspond most closely with the established diagnosis.

Note: This guideline is applicable only to inpatient admissions to short-term, acute, long-term care and psychiatric hospitals.

I. Admission from Observation Unit

1. Admission Following Medical Observation
When a patient is admitted to an observation unit for a medical condition, which either worsens or does not improve, and is subsequently admitted as an inpatient of the same hospital for this same medical condition, the principal diagnosis would be the medical condition which led to the hospital admission.

2. Admission Following Post-Operative Observation
When a patient is admitted to an observation unit to monitor a condition (or complication) that develops following outpatient surgery, and then is subsequently admitted as an inpatient of the same hospital, hospitals should apply the Uniform Hospital Discharge Data Set (UHDDS) definition of principal diagnosis as "that condition established after study to be chiefly responsible for occasioning the admission of the patient to the hospital for care."

J. Admission from Outpatient Surgery
When a patient receives surgery in the hospital's outpatient surgery department and is subsequently admitted for continuing inpatient care at the same hospital, the following guidelines should be followed in selecting the principal diagnosis for the inpatient admission:
- If the reason for the inpatient admission is a complication, assign the complication as the principal diagnosis.
- If no complication, or other condition, is documented as the reason for the inpatient admission, assign the reason for the outpatient surgery as the principal diagnosis.
- If the reason for the inpatient admission is another condition unrelated to the surgery, assign the unrelated condition as the principal diagnosis.

K. Admissions/Encounters for Rehabilitation
When the purpose for the admission/encounter is rehabilitation, sequence first the code for the condition for which the service is being performed. For example, for an admission/encounter for rehabilitation for right-sided dominant hemiplegia following a cerebrovascular infarction, report code I69.351, Hemiplegia and hemiparesis following cerebral infarction affecting right dominant side, as the first-listed or principal diagnosis.

If the condition for which the rehabilitation service is no longer present, report the appropriate aftercare code as the first-listed or principal diagnosis. For example, if a patient with severe degenerative osteoarthritis of the hip, underwent hip replacement and the current encounter/ admission is for rehabilitation, report code Z47.1, Aftercare following joint replacement surgery, as the first-listed or principal diagnosis.

See Section I.C.21.c.7, Factors influencing health states and contact with health services, Aftercare.

Section III. Reporting Additional Diagnoses

GENERAL RULES FOR OTHER (ADDITIONAL) DIAGNOSES
For reporting purposes the definition for "other diagnoses" is interpreted as additional conditions that affect patient care in terms of requiring:
clinical evaluation; or
therapeutic treatment; or
diagnostic procedures; or
extended length of hospital stay; or
increased nursing care and/or monitoring.

The UHDDS item #11-b defines Other Diagnoses as "all conditions that coexist at the time of admission, that develop subsequently, or that affect the treatment received and/or the length of stay. Diagnoses that relate to an earlier episode which have no bearing on the current hospital stay are to be excluded." UHDDS definitions apply to inpatients in acute care, short-term, long term care and psychiatric hospital setting. The UHDDS definitions are used by acute care short-term hospitals to report inpatient data elements in a standardized manner. These data elements and their definitions can be found in the July 31, 1985, Federal Register (Vol. 50, No, 147), pp. 31038-40.

Since that time the application of the UHDDS definitions has been expanded to include all nonoutpatient settings (acute care, short term, long term care and psychiatric hospitals; home health agencies; rehab facilities; nursing homes, etc). **The UHDDS definitions also apply to hospice services (all levels of care).**

The following guidelines are to be applied in designating "other diagnoses" when neither the Alphabetic Index nor the Tabular List in ICD-10-CM provide direction. The listing of the diagnoses in the patient record is the responsibility of the attending provider.

A. Previous conditions

If the provider has included a diagnosis in the final diagnostic statement, such as the discharge summary or the face sheet, it should ordinarily be coded. Some providers include in the diagnostic statement resolved conditions or diagnoses and status-post procedures from previous admission that have no bearing on the current stay. Such conditions are not to be reported and are coded only if required by hospital policy.

However, history codes (categories Z80-Z87) may be used as secondary codes if the historical condition or family history has an impact on current care or influences treatment.

B. Abnormal findings

Abnormal findings (laboratory, x-ray, pathologic, and other diagnostic results) are not coded and reported unless the provider indicates their clinical significance. If the findings are outside the normal range and the attending provider has ordered other tests to evaluate the condition or prescribed treatment, it is appropriate to ask the provider whether the abnormal finding should be added.

Please note: This differs from the coding practices in the outpatient setting for coding encounters for diagnostic tests that have been interpreted by a provider.

C. Uncertain Diagnosis

If the diagnosis documented at the time of discharge is qualified as "probable", "suspected", "likely", "questionable", "possible", or "still to be ruled out" or other similar terms indicating uncertainty, code the condition as if it existed or was established. The bases for these guidelines are the diagnostic workup, arrangements for further workup or observation, and initial therapeutic approach that correspond most closely with the established diagnosis.

Note: This guideline is applicable only to inpatient admissions to short-term, acute, long-term care and psychiatric hospitals.

Section IV. Diagnostic Coding and Reporting Guidelines for Outpatient Services

These coding guidelines for outpatient diagnoses have been approved for use by hospitals/ providers in coding and reporting hospital-based outpatient services and provider-based office visits. **Guidelines in Section I, Conventions, general coding guidelines and chapter-specific guidelines, should also be applied for outpatient services and office visits.**

Information about the use of certain abbreviations, punctuation, symbols, and other conventions used in the ICD-10-CM Tabular List (code numbers and titles), can be found in Section IA of these guidelines, under "Conventions Used in the Tabular List." Section I.B. contains general guidelines that apply to the entire classification. Section I.C. contains chapter-specific guidelines that correspond to the chapters as they are arranged in the classification. Information about the correct sequence to use in finding a code is also described in Section I.

The terms encounter and visit are often used interchangeably in describing outpatient service contacts and, therefore, appear together in these guidelines without distinguishing one from the other.

Though the conventions and general guidelines apply to all settings, coding guidelines for outpatient and provider reporting of diagnoses will vary in a number of instances from those for inpatient diagnoses, recognizing that:

The Uniform Hospital Discharge Data Set (UHDDS) definition of principal diagnosis **does not apply to hospital-based outpatient services and provider-based office visits.**

Coding guidelines for inconclusive diagnoses (probable, suspected, rule out, etc.) were developed for inpatient reporting and do not apply to outpatients.

A. Selection of first-listed condition

In the outpatient setting, the term first-listed diagnosis is used in lieu of principal diagnosis.

In determining the first-listed diagnosis the coding conventions of ICD-10-CM, as well as the general and disease specific guidelines take precedence over the outpatient guidelines.

Diagnoses often are not established at the time of the initial encounter/visit. It may take two or more visits before the diagnosis is confirmed.

The most critical rule involves beginning the search for the correct code assignment through the Alphabetic Index. Never begin searching initially in the Tabular List as this will lead to coding errors.

1. Outpatient Surgery

When a patient presents for outpatient surgery (same day surgery), code the reason for the surgery as the first-listed diagnosis (reason for the encounter), even if the surgery is not performed due to a contraindication.

2. Observation Stay

When a patient is admitted for observation for a medical condition, assign a code for the medical condition as the first-listed diagnosis.

GUIDELINES (ICD-10-CM)

When a patient presents for outpatient surgery and develops complications requiring admission to observation, code the reason for the surgery as the first reported diagnosis (reason for the encounter), followed by codes for the complications as secondary diagnoses.

B. Codes from A00.0 through T88.9, Z00-Z99
The appropriate code(s) from A00.0 through T88.9, Z00-Z99 must be used to identify diagnoses, symptoms, conditions, problems, complaints, or other reason(s) for the encounter/visit.

C. Accurate reporting of ICD-10-CM diagnosis codes
For accurate reporting of ICD-10-CM diagnosis codes, the documentation should describe the patient's condition, using terminology which includes specific diagnoses as well as symptoms, problems, or reasons for the encounter. There are ICD-10-CM codes to describe all of these.

D. Codes that describe symptoms and signs
Codes that describe symptoms and signs, as opposed to diagnoses, are acceptable for reporting purposes when a diagnosis has not been established (confirmed) by the provider. Chapter 18 of ICD-10-CM, Symptoms, Signs, and Abnormal Clinical and Laboratory Findings Not Elsewhere Classified (codes R00-R99) contain many, but not all codes for symptoms.

E. Encounters for circumstances other than a disease or injury
ICD-10-CM provides codes to deal with encounters for circumstances other than a disease or injury. The Factors Influencing Health Status and Contact with Health Services codes (Z00-Z99) are provided to deal with occasions when circumstances other than a disease or injury are recorded as diagnosis or problems.
See Section I.C.21. Factors influencing health status and contact with health services.

F. Level of Detail in Coding
1. ICD-10-CM codes with 3, 4, 5, 6 or 7 characters
ICD-10-CM is composed of codes with 3, 4, 5, 6 or 7 characters. Codes with three characters are included in ICD-10-CM as the heading of a category of codes that may be further subdivided by the use of fourth, fifth, sixth or seventh characters to provide greater specificity.
2. Use of full number of characters required for a code
A three-character code is to be used only if it is not further subdivided. A code is invalid if it has not been coded to the full number of characters required for that code, including the 7th character, if applicable.

G. ICD-10-CM code for the diagnosis, condition, problem, or other reason for encounter/visit
List first the ICD-10-CM code for the diagnosis, condition, problem, or other reason for encounter/visit shown in the medical record to be chiefly responsible for the services provided. List additional codes that describe any coexisting conditions. In some cases the first-listed diagnosis may be a symptom when a diagnosis has not been established (confirmed) by the physician.

H. Uncertain diagnosis
Do not code diagnoses documented as "probable", "suspected," "questionable," "rule out," or "working diagnosis" or other similar terms indicating uncertainty. Rather, code the condition(s) to the highest degree of certainty for that encounter/visit, such as symptoms, signs, abnormal test results, or other reason for the visit.
Please note: This differs from the coding practices used by short-term, acute care, long-term care and psychiatric hospitals.

I. Chronic diseases
Chronic diseases treated on an ongoing basis may be coded and reported as many times as the patient receives treatment and care for the condition(s)

J. Code all documented conditions that coexist
Code all documented conditions that coexist at the time of the encounter/visit, and require or affect patient care treatment or management. Do not code conditions that were previously treated and no longer exist. However, history codes (categories Z80-Z87) may be used as secondary codes if the historical condition or family history has an impact on current care or influences treatment.

K. Patients receiving diagnostic services only
For patients receiving diagnostic services only during an encounter/visit, sequence first the diagnosis, condition, problem, or other reason for encounter/visit shown in the medical record to be chiefly responsible for the outpatient services provided during the encounter/visit. Codes for other diagnoses (e.g., chronic conditions) may be sequenced as additional diagnoses.
For encounters for routine laboratory/radiology testing in the absence of any signs, symptoms, or associated diagnosis, assign Z01.89, Encounter for other specified special examinations. If routine testing is performed during the same encounter as a test to evaluate a sign, symptom, or diagnosis, it is appropriate to assign both the Z code and the code describing the reason for the non-routine test.
For outpatient encounters for diagnostic tests that have been interpreted by a physician, and the final report is available at the time of coding, code any confirmed or definitive diagnosis(es) documented in the interpretation. Do not code related signs and symptoms as additional diagnoses.
Please note: This differs from the coding practice in the hospital inpatient setting regarding abnormal findings on test results.

L. Patients receiving therapeutic services only
For patients receiving therapeutic services only during an encounter/visit, sequence first the diagnosis, condition, problem, or other reason for encounter/visit shown in the medical record to be chiefly responsible for the outpatient services provided during the encounter/visit. Codes for other diagnoses (e.g., chronic conditions) may be sequenced as additional diagnoses.

The only exception to this rule is that when the primary reason for the admission/encounter is chemotherapy or radiation therapy, the appropriate Z code for the service is listed first, and the diagnosis or problem for which the service is being performed listed second.

M. Patients receiving preoperative evaluations only
For patients receiving preoperative evaluations only, sequence first a code from subcategory Z01.81, Encounter for pre-procedural examinations, to describe the pre-op consultations. Assign a code for the condition to describe the reason for the surgery as an additional diagnosis. Code also any findings related to the pre-op evaluation.

N. Ambulatory surgery
For ambulatory surgery, code the diagnosis for which the surgery was performed. If the postoperative diagnosis is known to be different from the preoperative diagnosis at the time the diagnosis is confirmed, select the postoperative diagnosis for coding, since it is the most definitive.

O. Routine outpatient prenatal visits
See Section I.C.15. Routine outpatient prenatal visits.

P. Encounters for general medical examinations with abnormal findings
The subcategories for encounters for general medical examinations, Z00.0-, provide codes for with and without abnormal findings. Should a general medical examination result in an abnormal finding, the code for general medical examination with abnormal finding should be assigned as the first-listed diagnosis. **An examination with abnormal findings refers to a condition/diagnosis that is newly identified or a change in severity of a chronic condition (such as uncontrolled hypertension, or an acute exacerbation of chronic obstructive pulmonary disease) during a routine physical examination.** A secondary code for the abnormal finding should also be coded.

Q. Encounters for routine health screenings
See Section I.C.21. Factors influencing health status and contact with health services, Screening

Appendix I
Present on Admission Reporting Guidelines

Introduction

These guidelines are to be used as a supplement to the *ICD-10-CM Official Guidelines for Coding and Reporting* to facilitate the assignment of the Present on Admission (POA) indicator for each diagnosis and external cause of injury code reported on claim forms (UB-04 and 837 Institutional).

These guidelines are not intended to replace any guidelines in the main body of the *ICD-10-CM Official Guidelines for Coding and Reporting*. The POA guidelines are not intended to provide guidance on when a condition should be coded, but rather, how to apply the POA indicator to the final set of diagnosis codes that have been assigned in accordance with Sections I, II, and III of the official coding guidelines. Subsequent to the assignment of the ICD-10-CM codes, the POA indicator should then be assigned to those conditions that have been coded.

As stated in the Introduction to the ICD-10-CM Official Guidelines for Coding and Reporting, a joint effort between the healthcare provider and the coder is essential to achieve complete and accurate documentation, code assignment, and reporting of diagnoses and procedures. The importance of consistent, complete documentation in the medical record cannot be overemphasized. Medical record documentation from any provider involved in the care and treatment of the patient may be used to support the determination of whether a condition was present on admission or not. In the context of the official coding guidelines, the term "provider" means a physician or any qualified healthcare practitioner who is legally accountable for establishing the patient's diagnosis.

These guidelines are not a substitute for the provider's clinical judgment as to the determination of whether a condition was/was not present on admission. The provider should be queried regarding issues related to the linking of signs/symptoms, timing of test results, and the timing of findings.

Please see the CDC website for the detailed list of ICD-10-CM codes that do not require the use of a POA indicator (ftp://ftp.cdc.gov/pub/Health_Statistics/NCHS/Publications/ICD10CM/2017/). The conditions on this exempt list represent categories and/or codes for circumstances regarding the healthcare encounter or factors influencing health status that do not represent a current disease or injury or are always present on admission.

General Reporting Requirements

All claims involving inpatient admissions to general acute care hospitals or other facilities that are subject to a law or regulation mandating collection of present on admission information.

Present on admission is defined as present at the time the order for inpatient admission occurs—conditions that develop during an outpatient encounter, including emergency department, observation, or outpatient surgery, are considered as present on admission.

POA indicator is assigned to principal and secondary diagnoses (as defined in Section II of the Official Guidelines for Coding and Reporting) and the external cause of injury codes.

Issues related to inconsistent, missing, conflicting or unclear documentation must still be resolved by the provider.

If a condition would not be coded and reported based on UHDDS definitions and current official coding guidelines, then the POA indicator would not be reported.

Reporting Options

Y - Yes

N - No

U - Unknown

W - Clinically undetermined

Unreported/Not used - (Exempt from POA reporting)

Reporting Definitions

Y = present at the time of inpatient admission

N = not present at the time of inpatient admission

U = documentation is insufficient to determine if condition is present on admission

W = provider is unable to clinically determine whether condition was present on admission or not

Timeframe for POA Identification and Documentation

There is no required timeframe as to when a provider (per the definition of "provider" used in these guidelines) must identify or document a condition to be present on admission. In some clinical situations, it may not be possible for a provider to make a definitive diagnosis (or a condition may not be recognized or reported by the patient) for a period of time after admission. In some cases it may be several days before the provider arrives at a definitive diagnosis. This does not mean that the condition was not present on admission. Determination of whether the condition was present on admission or not will be based on the applicable POA guideline as identified in this document, or on the provider's best clinical judgment.

If at the time of code assignment the documentation is unclear as to whether a condition was present on admission or not, it is appropriate to query the provider for clarification.

Assigning the POA Indicator

Condition is on the "Exempt from Reporting" list

Leave the "present on admission" field blank if the condition is on the list of ICD-10-CM codes for which this field is not applicable. This is the only circumstance in which the field may be left blank.

POA Explicitly Documented

Assign Y for any condition the provider explicitly documents as being present on admission.

Assign N for any condition the provider explicitly documents as not present at the time of admission.

Conditions diagnosed prior to inpatient admission

Assign "Y" for conditions that were diagnosed prior to admission (example: hypertension, diabetes mellitus, asthma)

Conditions diagnosed during the admission but clearly present before admission

Assign "Y" for conditions diagnosed during the admission that were clearly present but not diagnosed until after admission occurred.

Diagnoses subsequently confirmed after admission are considered present on admission if at the time of admission they are documented as suspected, possible, rule out, differential diagnosis, or constitute an underlying cause of a symptom that is present at the time of admission.

Condition develops during outpatient encounter prior to inpatient admission

Assign Y for any condition that develops during an outpatient encounter prior to a written order for inpatient admission.

Documentation does not indicate whether condition was present on admission

Assign "U" when the medical record documentation is unclear as to whether the condition was present on admission. "U" should not be routinely assigned and used only in very limited circumstances. Coders are encouraged to query the providers when the documentation is unclear.

Documentation states that it cannot be determined whether the condition was or was not present on admission

Assign "W" when the medical record documentation indicates that it cannot be clinically determined whether or not the condition was present on admission.

Chronic condition with acute exacerbation during the admission

If a single code identifies both the chronic condition and the acute exacerbation, see POA guidelines pertaining to **codes that contain multiple clinical concepts**.

If a single code only identifies the chronic condition and not the acute exacerbation (e.g., acute exacerbation of chronic leukemia), assign "Y."

Conditions documented as possible, probable, suspected, or rule out at the time of discharge

If the final diagnosis contains a possible, probable, suspected, or rule out diagnosis, and this diagnosis was based on signs, symptoms or clinical findings suspected at the time of inpatient admission, assign "Y."

If the final diagnosis contains a possible, probable, suspected, or rule out diagnosis, and this diagnosis was based on signs, symptoms or clinical findings that were not present on admission, assign "N".

Conditions documented as impending or threatened at the time of discharge

If the final diagnosis contains an impending or threatened diagnosis, and this diagnosis is based on symptoms or clinical findings that were present on admission, assign "Y".

If the final diagnosis contains an impending or threatened diagnosis, and this diagnosis is based on symptoms or clinical findings that were not present on admission, assign "N".

Acute and Chronic Conditions

Assign "Y" for acute conditions that are present at time of admission and N for acute conditions that are not present at time of admission.

Assign "Y" for chronic conditions, even though the condition may not be diagnosed until after admission.

If a single code identifies both an acute and chronic condition, see the POA guidelines for codes **that contain multiple clinical concepts.**

Codes **That Contain Multiple Clinical Concepts**

Assign "N" if at least one of the clinical concepts included in the code was not present on admission (e.g., COPD with acute exacerbation and the exacerbation was not present on admission; gastric ulcer that does not start bleeding until after admission; asthma patient develops status asthmaticus after admission).

Assign "Y" if all of the **clinical concepts included in the code** were present on admission (e.g., **duodenal ulcer that perforates prior to admission**).

For infection codes that include the causal organism, assign "Y" if the infection (or signs of the infection) **were** present on admission, even though the culture results may not be known until after admission (e.g., patient is admitted with pneumonia and the provider documents Pseudomonas as the causal organism a few days later).

Same Diagnosis Code for Two or More Conditions

When the same ICD-10-CM diagnosis code applies to two or more conditions during the same encounter (e.g. two separate conditions classified to the same ICD-10-CM diagnosis code):

Assign "Y" if all conditions represented by the single ICD-10-CM code were present on admission (e.g. bilateral unspecified age-related cataracts).

Assign "N" if any of the conditions represented by the single ICD-10-CM code was not present on admission (e.g. traumatic secondary and recurrent hemorrhage and seroma is assigned to a single code T79.2, but only one of the conditions was present on admission).

Obstetrical conditions

Whether or not the patient delivers during the current hospitalization does not affect assignment of the POA indicator. The determining factor for POA assignment is whether the pregnancy complication or obstetrical condition described by the code was present at the time of admission or not.

If the pregnancy complication or obstetrical condition was present on admission (e.g., patient admitted in preterm labor), assign "Y".

If the pregnancy complication or obstetrical condition was not present on admission (e.g., 2nd degree laceration during delivery, postpartum hemorrhage that occurred during current hospitalization, fetal distress develops after admission), assign "N".

If the obstetrical code includes more than one diagnosis and any of the diagnoses identified by the code were not present on admission assign "N".

(e.g., Category O11, Pre-existing hypertension with pre-eclampsia)

Perinatal conditions

Newborns are not considered to be admitted until after birth. Therefore, any condition present at birth or that developed in utero is considered present at admission and should be assigned "Y". This includes conditions that occur during delivery (e.g., injury during delivery, meconium aspiration, exposure to streptococcus B in the vaginal canal).

Congenital conditions and anomalies

Assign "Y" for congenital conditions and anomalies except for categories Q00-Q99, Congenital anomalies, which are on the exempt list. Congenital conditions are always considered present on admission.

External cause of injury codes

Assign "Y" for any external cause code representing an external cause of morbidity that occurred prior to inpatient admission (e.g., patient fell out of bed at home, patient fell out of bed in emergency room prior to admission).

Assign "N" for any external cause code representing an external cause of morbidity that occurred during inpatient hospitalization (e.g., patient fell out of hospital bed during hospital stay, patient experienced an adverse reaction to a medication administered after inpatient admission).

Anterior view

Left gastric nodes

Hepatic nodes

Pyloric nodes

Splenic nodes

Superior pancreatic nodes

Celiac nodes

Superior mesenteric nodes (central superior group)

Pancreaticoduodenal nodes

Cystic node (of Calot)

Hepatic portal vein

Celiac nodes

Posterior view

Superior pancreatic nodes

Splenic vein

Inferior mesenteric vein

Superior mesenteric artery and vein

Hepatic nodes around bile ducts and proper hepatic artery

Pancreaticoduodenal nodes

Superior mesenteric nodes (central superior group)

Plate 315 Lymph Vessels and Nodes of Pancreas. (Netter: Atlas of Human Anatomy, 4 ed, 2006, Saunders.)

Dermatome pattern

Levels of principal dermatomes

C5	Clavicles
C5, 6, 7	Lateral parts of upper limbs
C8; T1	Medial sides of upper limbs
C6	Thumb
C6, 7, 8	Hand
C8	Ring and little fingers
T4	Level of nipples
T10	Level of umbilicus
T12	Inguinal or groin regions
L1, 2, 3, 4	Anterior and inner surfaces of lower limbs
L4, 5; S1	Foot
L4	Medial side of great toe
L5; S1, 2	Outer and posterior sides of lower limbs
S1	Lateral margin of foot and little toe
S2, 3, 4	Perineum

Plate 164 Dermatomes. (Netter: Atlas of Human Anatomy, 4 ed, 2006, Saunders.)

Female: frontal section

Peritoneum
Body of bladder
Fundus of bladder
Interureteric crest
Left ureteric orifice
Trigone of bladder
Neck of bladder
Paravesical endopelvic fascia and vesical venous plexus
Vesical fascia
Tendinous arch of levator ani muscle
Obturator internus muscle
Levator ani muscle
Tendinous arch of pelvic fascia
Urethra
Sphincter urethrae muscle
Perineal membrane
Inferior pubic ramus
Crus of clitoris and ischiocavernosus muscle
Bulb of vestibule and bulbospongiosus muscle
Deep perineal (investing or Gallaudet's) fascia
Superficial perineal (Colles') fascia

Round ligament of uterus

Vagina

Male: frontal section

Body of bladder
Fundus of bladder
Ductus (vas) deferens
Interureteric crest
Right ureteric orifice
Trigone of bladder
Neck of bladder
Paravesical endopelvic fascia and vesical venous plexus
Tendinous arch of levator ani muscle
Uvula of bladder
Obturator internus muscle
Levator ani muscle
Capsule of prostate
Prostate and prostatic urethra
Seminal colliculus
Bulbourethral (Cowper's) gland
Perineal membrane and sphincter urethrae muscle
Bulbous portion of spongy urethra
Corpus spongiosum and bulbospongiosus muscle
Deep perineal (investing or Gallaudet's) fascia

Peritoneum

Internal urethral sphincter

Tendinous arch of pelvic fascia

Anterior recess of ischio-anal fossa

Inferior pubic ramus

Crus of penis and ischiocavernosus muscle

Superficial perineal (Colles') fascia

Plate 366   Urinary Bladder: Female and Male. (Netter: Atlas of Human Anatomy, 4 ed, 2006, Saunders.)

51

Sites of ectopic implantation

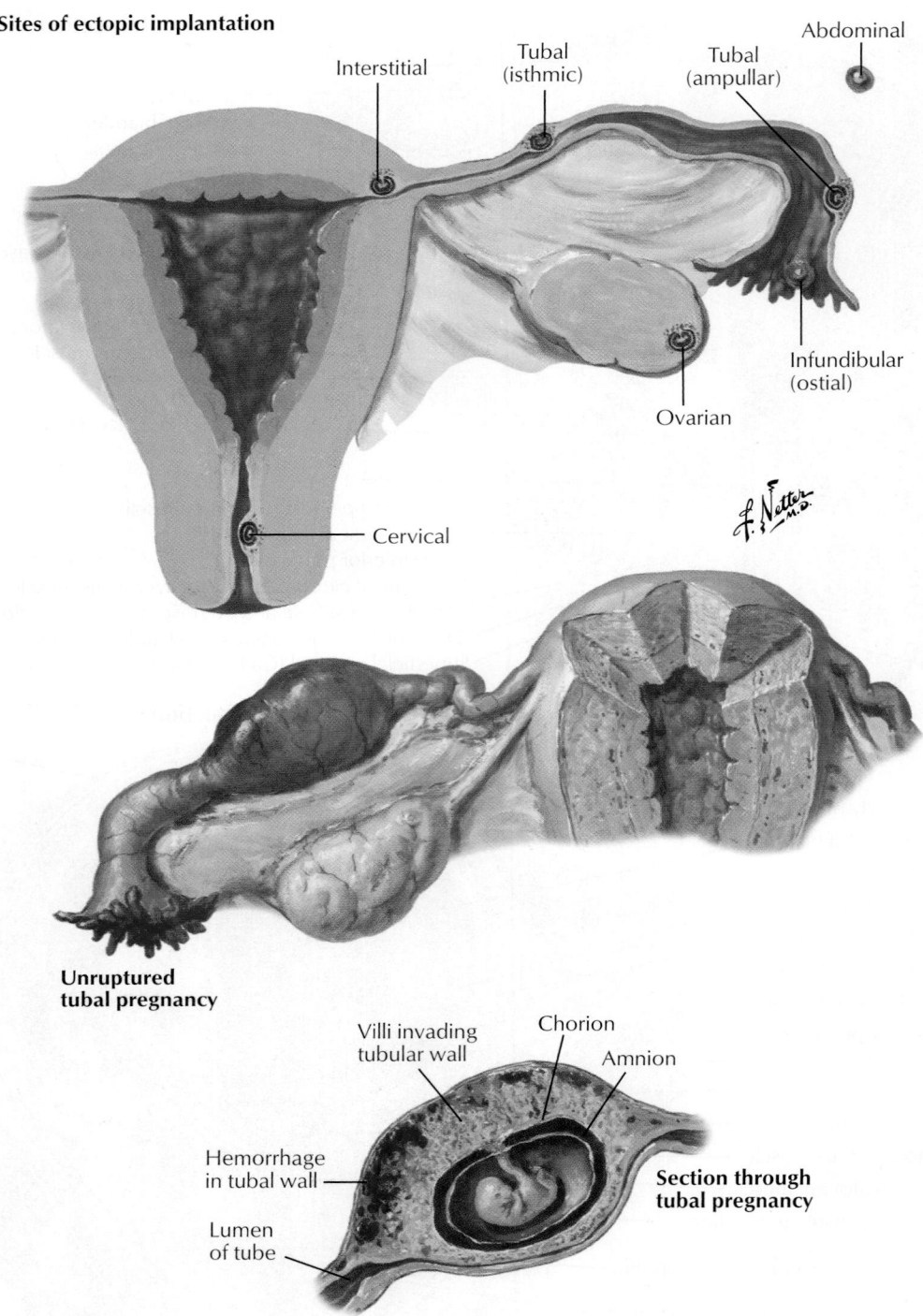

Interstitial

Tubal (isthmic)

Tubal (ampullar)

Abdominal

Infundibular (ostial)

Ovarian

Cervical

Unruptured tubal pregnancy

Villi invading tubular wall

Chorion

Amnion

Hemorrhage in tubal wall

Section through tubal pregnancy

Lumen of tube

Plate 375   Ectopic Pregnancy. (Netter: Atlas of Human Anatomy, 4 ed, 2006, Saunders.)

Skin of penis

Superficial fascia of penis (Colles' fascia)

Deep (Buck's) fascia of penis

Testicular artery

Ductus deferens

Artery to ductus deferens

Genital branch of genitofemoral nerve

Pampiniform (venous) plexus

Epididymis

Appendix of epididymis

Appendix of testis

Testis (covered by visceral layer of tunica vaginalis)

Parietal layer of tunica vaginalis

Superficial inguinal ring

External spermatic fascia

Cremaster muscle and fascia

Septum of scrotum (formed by dartos fascia)

Superficial (dartos) fascia of scrotum

Skin of scrotum

Superficial (dartos) fascia of scrotum

External spermatic fascia

Cremaster muscle and fascia

Internal spermatic fascia

Parietal layer of tunica vaginalis

Epididymis

Testis (covered by visceral layer of tunica vaginalis)

Skin of scrotum

Plate 387   Scrotum and Contents. (Netter: Atlas of Human Anatomy, 4 ed, 2006, Saunders.)

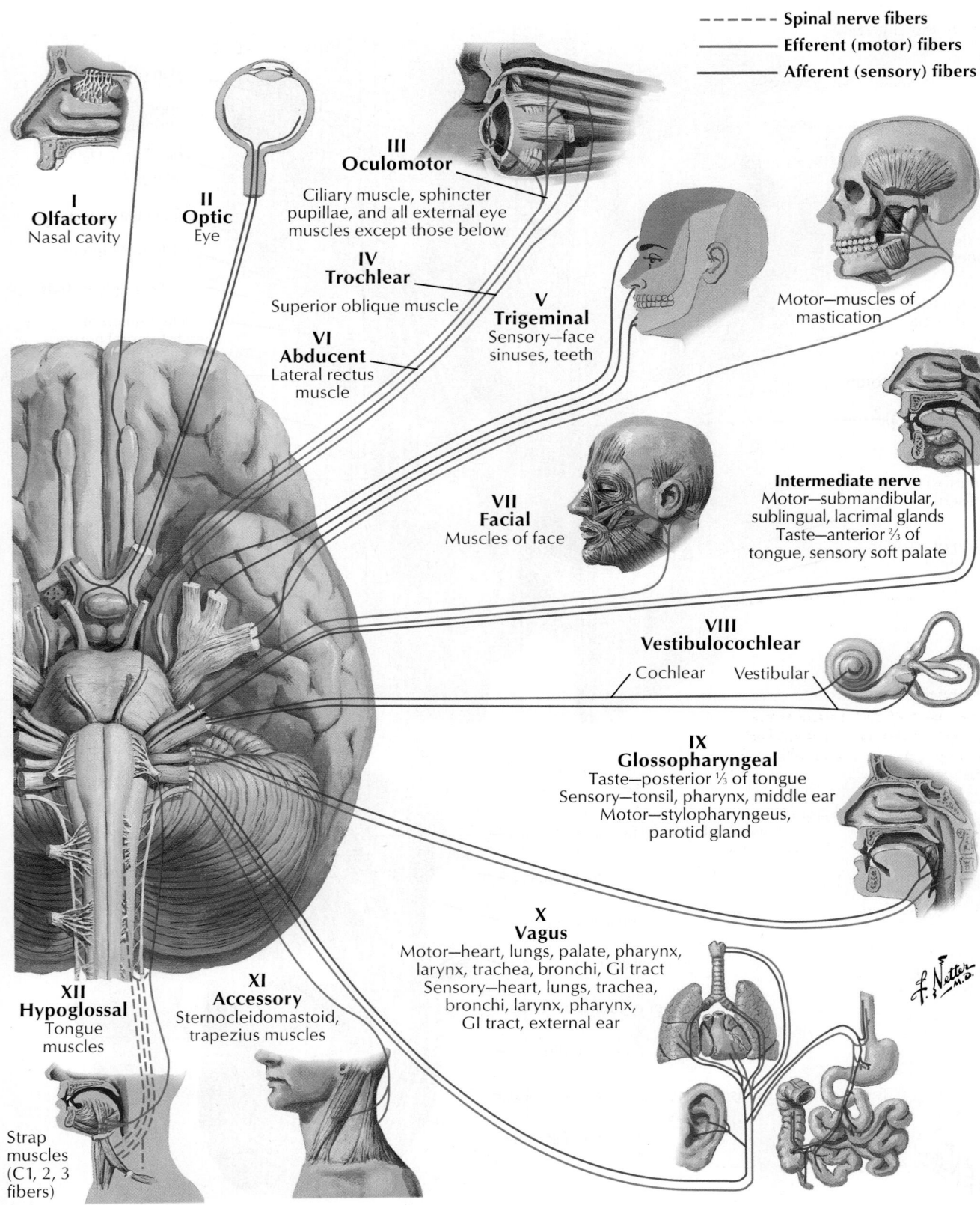

- - - - Spinal nerve fibers
———— Efferent (motor) fibers
———— Afferent (sensory) fibers

I Olfactory
Nasal cavity

II Optic
Eye

III Oculomotor
Ciliary muscle, sphincter pupillae, and all external eye muscles except those below

IV Trochlear
Superior oblique muscle

VI Abducent
Lateral rectus muscle

V Trigeminal
Sensory—face sinuses, teeth
Motor—muscles of mastication

VII Facial
Muscles of face

Intermediate nerve
Motor—submandibular, sublingual, lacrimal glands
Taste—anterior ⅔ of tongue, sensory soft palate

VIII Vestibulocochlear
Cochlear   Vestibular

IX Glossopharyngeal
Taste—posterior ⅓ of tongue
Sensory—tonsil, pharynx, middle ear
Motor—stylopharyngeus, parotid gland

X Vagus
Motor—heart, lungs, palate, pharynx, larynx, trachea, bronchi, GI tract
Sensory—heart, lungs, trachea, bronchi, larynx, pharynx, GI tract, external ear

XII Hypoglossal
Tongue muscles

Strap muscles (C1, 2, 3 fibers)

XI Accessory
Sternocleidomastoid, trapezius muscles

Plate 118   Cranial Nerves (Motor and Sensory Distribution): Schema. (Netter: Atlas of Human Anatomy, 4 ed, 2006, Saunders.)

Superior view

Supratrochlear nerve

Medial rectus muscle

Superior oblique muscle

Infratrochlear nerve

Nasociliary nerve

Trochlear nerve (IV)

Common tendinous ring

Ophthalmic nerve (V₁)

Optic nerve (II)

Internal carotid artery and nerve plexus

Oculomotor nerve (III)

Trochlear nerve (IV)

Abducent nerve (VI)

Tentorium cerebelli

Medial branch
Lateral branch } Supraorbital nerve

Levator palpebrae superioris muscle

Superior rectus muscle

Lacrimal gland

Lacrimal nerve

Lateral rectus muscle

Frontal nerve

Maxillary nerve (V₂)

Meningeal branch of maxillary nerve

Mandibular nerve (V₃)

Lesser petrosal nerve

Meningeal branch of mandibular nerve

Greater petrosal nerve

Trigeminal (semilunar) ganglion

Tentorial (meningeal) branch of ophthalmic nerve

Superior view:
levator palpebrae superioris, superior rectus, and superior oblique muscles partially cut away

Supratrochlear nerve (cut)

Supraorbital nerve branches (cut)

Infratrochlear nerve

Anterior ethmoidal nerve

Optic nerve (II)

Posterior ethmoidal nerve

Superior branch of oculomotor nerve (III) (cut)

Nasociliary nerve

Internal carotid plexus

Trochlear nerve (IV) (cut)

Oculomotor nerve (III)

Abducent nerve (VI)

Long ciliary nerves

Short ciliary nerves

Lacrimal nerve

Ciliary ganglion

Parasympathetic root of ciliary ganglion (from inferior branch of oculomotor nerve)

Sympathetic root of ciliary ganglion (from internal carotid plexus)

Sensory root of ciliary ganglion (from nasociliary nerve)

Branches to inferior and medial rectus muscles

Abducent nerve (VI)

Inferior branch of oculomotor nerve (III)

Lacrimal nerve

Frontal nerve (cut)

Ophthalmic nerve (V₁)

f. Netter M.D.

NETTER'S ANATOMY ILLUSTRATIONS

Plate 86 Nerves of Orbit. (Netter: Atlas of Human Anatomy, 4 ed, 2006, Saunders.)

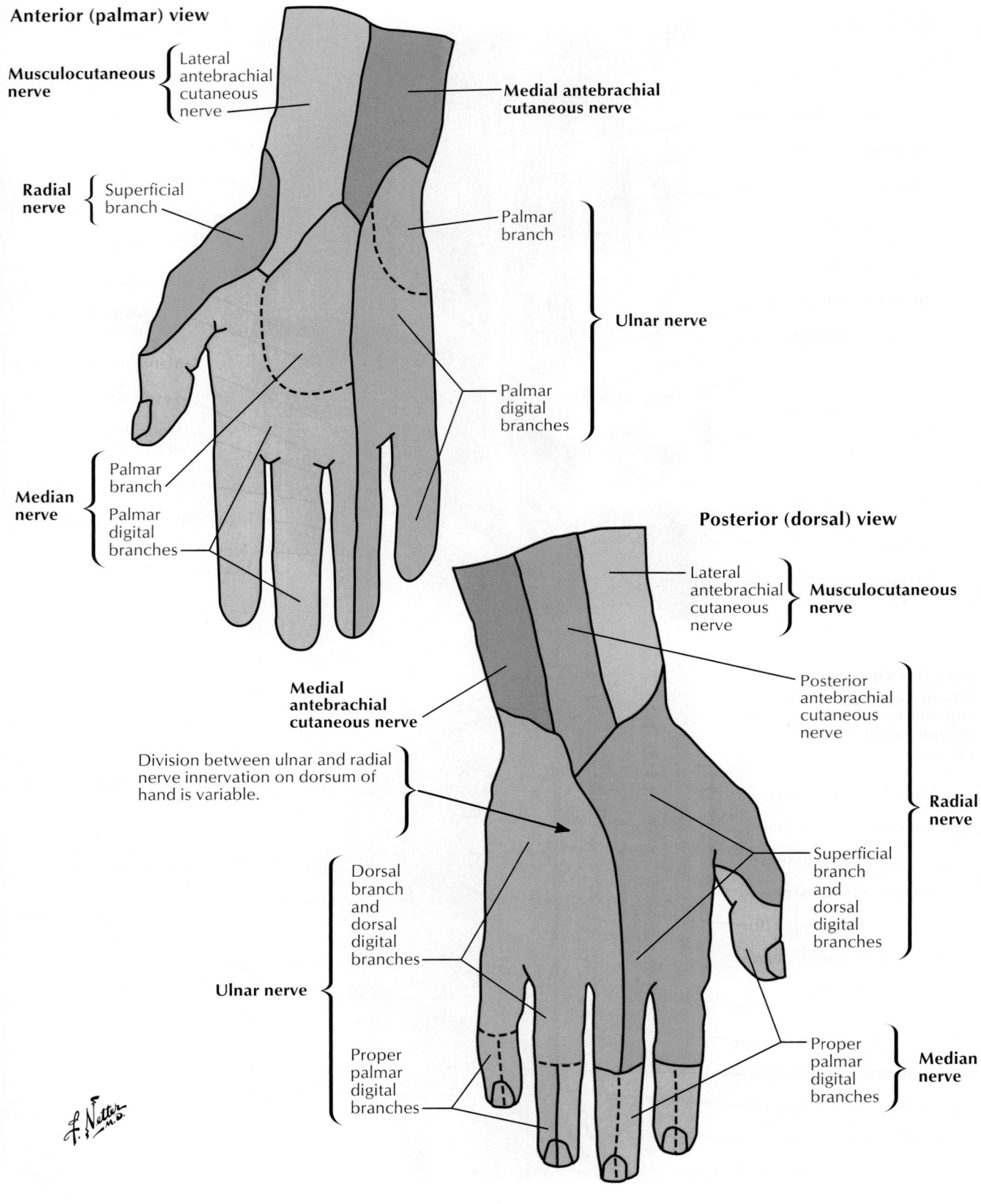

Anterior (palmar) view

Musculocutaneous nerve

Lateral antebrachial cutaneous nerve

Medial antebrachial cutaneous nerve

Radial nerve
Superficial branch

Palmar branch

Ulnar nerve

Palmar digital branches

Median nerve
Palmar branch
Palmar digital branches

Posterior (dorsal) view

Lateral antebrachial cutaneous nerve

Musculocutaneous nerve

Posterior antebrachial cutaneous nerve

Medial antebrachial cutaneous nerve

Division between ulnar and radial nerve innervation on dorsum of hand is variable.

Radial nerve

Superficial branch and dorsal digital branches

Dorsal branch and dorsal digital branches

Ulnar nerve

Proper palmar digital branches

Proper palmar digital branches

Median nerve

Plate 472 Cutaneous Innervation of Wrist and Hand. (Netter: Atlas of Human Anatomy, 4 ed, 2006, Saunders.)

Anterior view

Deltoid muscle

Coracobrachialis muscle

Biceps brachii muscle { Short head (*cut*)
Long head (*cut*)

Musculocutaneous nerve

Brachialis muscle

Biceps brachii muscle (*cut*) and tendon

Lateral antebrachial cutaneous nerve
(from musculocutaneous nerve)

Radial nerve { Deep branch
Superficial branch

Supinator muscle

Brachioradialis muscle

Radial artery

Pronator teres muscle (*partially cut*)

Median nerve

Flexor pollicis longus muscle

Flexor carpi radialis
tendon (*cut*)

Flexor retinaculum
(transverse carpal
ligament)

Superficial branch
of radial nerve

Recurrent (motor)
branch of
median nerve to
thenar muscles

Common palmar
digital branches
of median nerve

Proper palmar
digital branches
of median nerve

Intercostobrachial nerve

Medial brachial
cutaneous nerve

Radial nerve

Ulnar nerve

Medial antebrachial
cutaneous nerve

Median nerve

Brachial artery

Bicipital aponeurosis

Humeral head (*cut*)
Ulnar head } Pronator teres muscle

Flexor carpi radialis muscle (*cut*)

Humeroulnar head
Radial head } Flexor digitorum superficialis muscle (*cut*)

Flexor digitorum profundus muscle

Flexor carpi ulnaris muscle

Ulnar artery and nerve

Dorsal branch of ulnar nerve

Flexor digitorum superficialis tendons (*cut*)

Deep palmar branch of ulnar artery and deep branch of ulnar nerve

Superficial branch of ulnar nerve

Superficial palmar arch (*cut*)

Common palmar digital branch of ulnar nerve

Communicating branch of median nerve with ulnar nerve

Proper palmar digital branches of ulnar nerve

Plate 473 Arteries and Nerves of Upper Limb. (Netter: Atlas of Human Anatomy, 4 ed, 2006, Saunders.)

57

NETTER'S ANATOMY ILLUSTRATIONS

Lateral cutaneous branch of subcostal nerve

Inguinal ligament (Poupart's)

Superficial circumflex iliac vein

Femoral branches of genitofemoral nerve

Lateral femoral cutaneous nerve

Saphenous opening (fossa ovalis)

Fascia lata

Anterior cutaneous branches of femoral nerve

Patellar nerve plexus

Branches of lateral sural cutaneous nerve (from common fibular [peroneal] nerve)

Deep fascia of leg (crural fascia)

Superficial fibular (peroneal) nerve
Medial dorsal cutaneous branch

Intermediate dorsal cutaneous branch

Small saphenous vein and lateral dorsal cutaneous nerve (from sural nerve)

Lateral dorsal digital nerve and vein of 5th toe

Dorsal metatarsal veins

Dorsal digital nerves and veins

Superficial epigastric vein

Ilioinguinal nerve (scrotal branch) (usually passes through superficial inguinal ring)

Genital branch of genitofemoral nerve

Femoral vein

Superficial external pudendal vein

Accessory saphenous vein

Great saphenous vein

Cutaneous branches of obturator nerve

Infrapatellar branch of saphenous nerve

Saphenous nerve (terminal branch of femoral nerve)

Great saphenous vein

Dorsal digital nerves

Dorsal venous arch

Dorsal digital nerve and vein of medial side of great toe

Dorsal digital branch of deep fibular (peroneal) nerve

Plate 544   Superficial Nerves and Veins of Lower Limb: Anterior View. (Netter: Atlas of Human Anatomy, 4 ed, 2006, Saunders.)

Lateral cutaneous branch of iliohypogastric nerve

Iliac crest

Medial clunial nerves (from dorsal rami of S1, 2, 3)

Superior clunial nerves (from dorsal rami of L1, 2, 3)

Inferior clunial nerves (from posterior femoral cutaneous nerve)

Perforating cutaneous nerve (from dorsal rami of S1, 2, 3)

Branches of posterior femoral cutaneous nerve

Branches of lateral femoral cutaneous nerve

Accessory saphenous vein

Branch of femoral cutaneous nerve

Branch of cutaneous branch of femoral nerve

Terminal branches of posterior femoral cutaneous nerve

Great saphenous vein

Lateral sural cutaneous nerve (from common fibular [peroneal] nerve)

Small saphenous vein

Sural communicating nerve

Branches of saphenous nerve

Medial sural cutaneous nerve (from tibial nerve)

Sural nerve

Lateral calcaneal branches of sural nerve

Medial calcaneal branches of tibial nerve

Lateral dorsal cutaneous nerve (continuation of sural nerve)

Plantar cutaneous branches of medial plantar nerve

Plantar cutaneous branches of lateral plantar nerve

Plate 545   Superficial Nerves and Veins of Lower Limb: Posterior View. (Netter: Atlas of Human Anatomy, 4 ed, 2006, Saunders.)

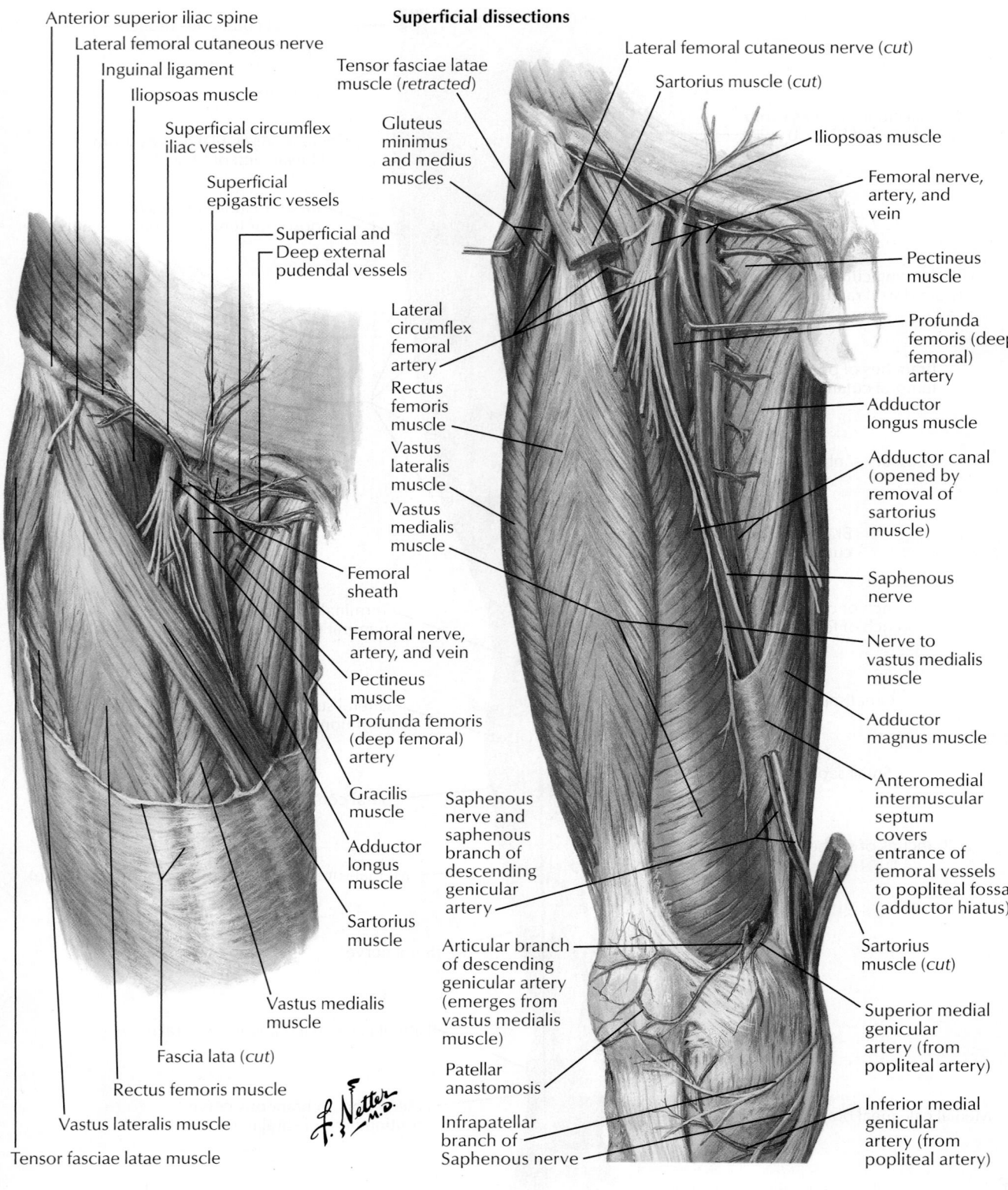

Anterior superior iliac spine
Lateral femoral cutaneous nerve
Inguinal ligament
Iliopsoas muscle
Superficial circumflex iliac vessels
Superficial epigastric vessels
Superficial and Deep external pudendal vessels

Superficial dissections

Tensor fasciae latae muscle (*retracted*)
Gluteus minimus and medius muscles
Lateral circumflex femoral artery
Rectus femoris muscle
Vastus lateralis muscle
Vastus medialis muscle

Lateral femoral cutaneous nerve (*cut*)
Sartorius muscle (*cut*)
Iliopsoas muscle
Femoral nerve, artery, and vein
Pectineus muscle
Profunda femoris (deep femoral) artery
Adductor longus muscle
Adductor canal (opened by removal of sartorius muscle)
Saphenous nerve
Nerve to vastus medialis muscle
Adductor magnus muscle
Anteromedial intermuscular septum covers entrance of femoral vessels to popliteal fossa (adductor hiatus)
Sartorius muscle (*cut*)
Superior medial genicular artery (from popliteal artery)
Inferior medial genicular artery (from popliteal artery)

Femoral sheath
Femoral nerve, artery, and vein
Pectineus muscle
Profunda femoris (deep femoral) artery
Gracilis muscle
Adductor longus muscle
Sartorius muscle
Vastus medialis muscle
Fascia lata (*cut*)
Rectus femoris muscle
Vastus lateralis muscle
Tensor fasciae latae muscle

Saphenous nerve and saphenous branch of descending genicular artery
Articular branch of descending genicular artery (emerges from vastus medialis muscle)
Patellar anastomosis
Infrapatellar branch of Saphenous nerve

Plate 500   Arteries and Nerves of Thigh: Anterior Views. (Netter: Atlas of Human Anatomy, 4 ed, 2006, Saunders.)

NETTER'S ANATOMY ILLUSTRATIONS

Deep dissection

Deep circumflex iliac artery

Lateral femoral cutaneous nerve

Sartorius muscle (*cut*)

Iliopsoas muscle

Tensor fasciae latae muscle (*retracted*)

Gluteus medius and minimus muscles

Femoral nerve

Rectus femoris muscle (*cut*)

Ascending, transverse and descending branches of Lateral circumflex femoral artery

Medial circumflex femoral artery

Pectineus muscle (*cut*)

Profunda femoris (deep femoral) artery

Perforating branches

Adductor longus muscle (*cut*)

Vastus lateralis muscle

Vastus intermedius muscle

Rectus femoris muscle (*cut*)

Saphenous nerve

Anteromedial intermuscular septum (*opened*)

Vastus medialis muscle

Quadriceps femoris tendon

Patella and patellar anastomosis

Medial patellar retinaculum

Patellar ligament

External iliac artery and vein

Inguinal ligament (Poupart's)

Femoral artery and vein (*cut*)

Pectineus muscle (*cut*)

Obturator canal

Obturator externus muscle

Adductor longus muscle (*cut*)

Anterior branch and Posterior branch of obturator nerve

Quadratus femoris muscle

Adductor brevis muscle

Branches of posterior branch of obturator nerve

Adductor magnus muscle

Gracilis muscle

Cutaneous branch of obturator nerve

Femoral artery and vein (*cut*)

Descending genicular artery
Articular branch
Saphenous branch

Adductor hiatus

Sartorius muscle (*cut*)

Adductor magnus tendon

Adductor tubercle on medial epicondyle of femur

Superior medial genicular artery (from popliteal artery)

Infrapatellar branch of Saphenous nerve

Inferior medial genicular artery (from popliteal artery)

Plate 501 Arteries and Nerves of Thigh: Posterior View. (Netter: Atlas of Human Anatomy, 4 ed, 2006, Saunders.)

Deep dissection

Superior clunial nerves

Gluteus maximus muscle (*cut*)

Medial clunial nerves

Inferior gluteal artery and nerve

Pudendal nerve

Nerve to obturator internus
(and superior gemellus)

Posterior femoral
cutaneous nerve

Sacrotuberous ligament

Ischial tuberosity

Inferior clunial nerves (*cut*)

Adductor magnus muscle

Gracilis muscle

Sciatic nerve

Muscular branches of sciatic nerve

Semitendinosus muscle (*retracted*)

Semimembranosus muscle

Sciatic nerve

Articular branch

Adductor hiatus

Popliteal vein and artery

Superior medial genicular artery

Medial epicondyle of femur

Tibial nerve

Gastrocnemius muscle (medial head)

Medial sural cutaneous nerve

Small saphenous vein

Iliac crest

Gluteal aponeurosis and
gluteus medius muscle (*cut*)

Superior gluteal artery and nerve

Gluteus minimus muscle

Tensor fasciae latae muscle

Piriformis muscle

Gluteus medius muscle (*cut*)

Superior gemellus muscle

Greater trochanter of femur

Obturator internus muscle

Inferior gemellus muscle

Gluteus maximus muscle (*cut*)

Quadratus femoris muscle

Medial circumflex femoral
artery

Vastus lateralis muscle
and iliotibial tract

Adductor minimus part of
adductor magnus muscle

1st perforating artery (from
profunda femoris artery)

Adductor magnus muscle

2nd and 3rd perforating arteries
(from profunda femoris artery)

4th perforating artery (from
profunda femoris artery)

Long head (*retracted*) ⎫ Biceps femoris
Short head ⎭ muscle

Superior lateral genicular artery

Common fibular (peroneal) nerve

Plantaris muscle

Gastrocnemius muscle (lateral head)

Lateral sural cutaneous nerve

Plate 502 Arteries and Nerves of Thigh: Posterior View. (Netter: Atlas of Human Anatomy, 4 ed, 2006, Saunders.)

Horizontal section

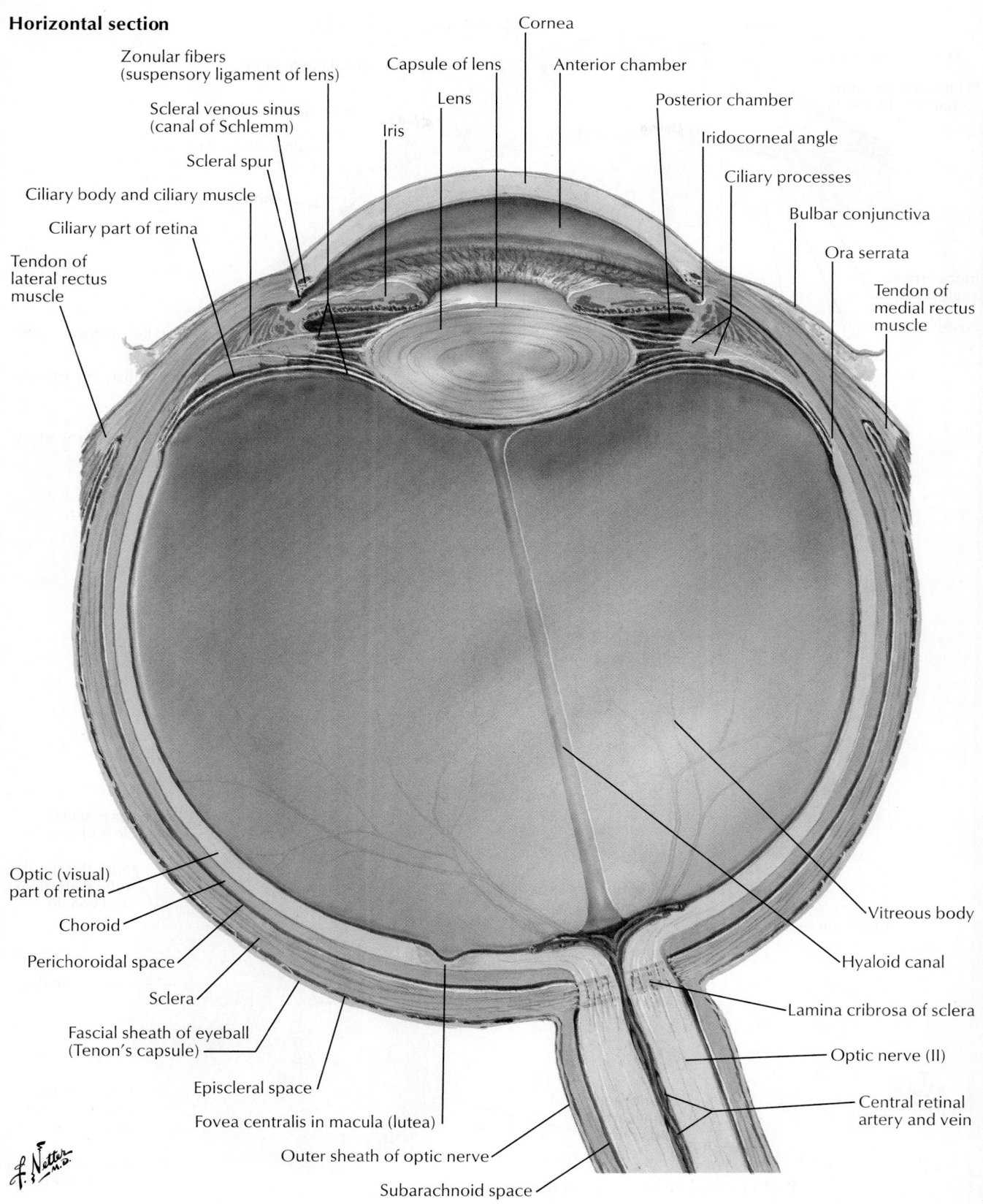

Zonular fibers (suspensory ligament of lens)

Scleral venous sinus (canal of Schlemm)

Scleral spur

Ciliary body and ciliary muscle

Ciliary part of retina

Tendon of lateral rectus muscle

Capsule of lens

Lens

Iris

Cornea

Anterior chamber

Posterior chamber

Iridocorneal angle

Ciliary processes

Bulbar conjunctiva

Ora serrata

Tendon of medial rectus muscle

Optic (visual) part of retina

Choroid

Perichoroidal space

Sclera

Fascial sheath of eyeball (Tenon's capsule)

Episcleral space

Fovea centralis in macula (lutea)

Outer sheath of optic nerve

Subarachnoid space

Vitreous body

Hyaloid canal

Lamina cribrosa of sclera

Optic nerve (II)

Central retinal artery and vein

NETTER'S ANATOMY ILLUSTRATIONS

Plate 87 Eyeball. (Netter: Atlas of Human Anatomy, 4 ed, 2006, Saunders.)

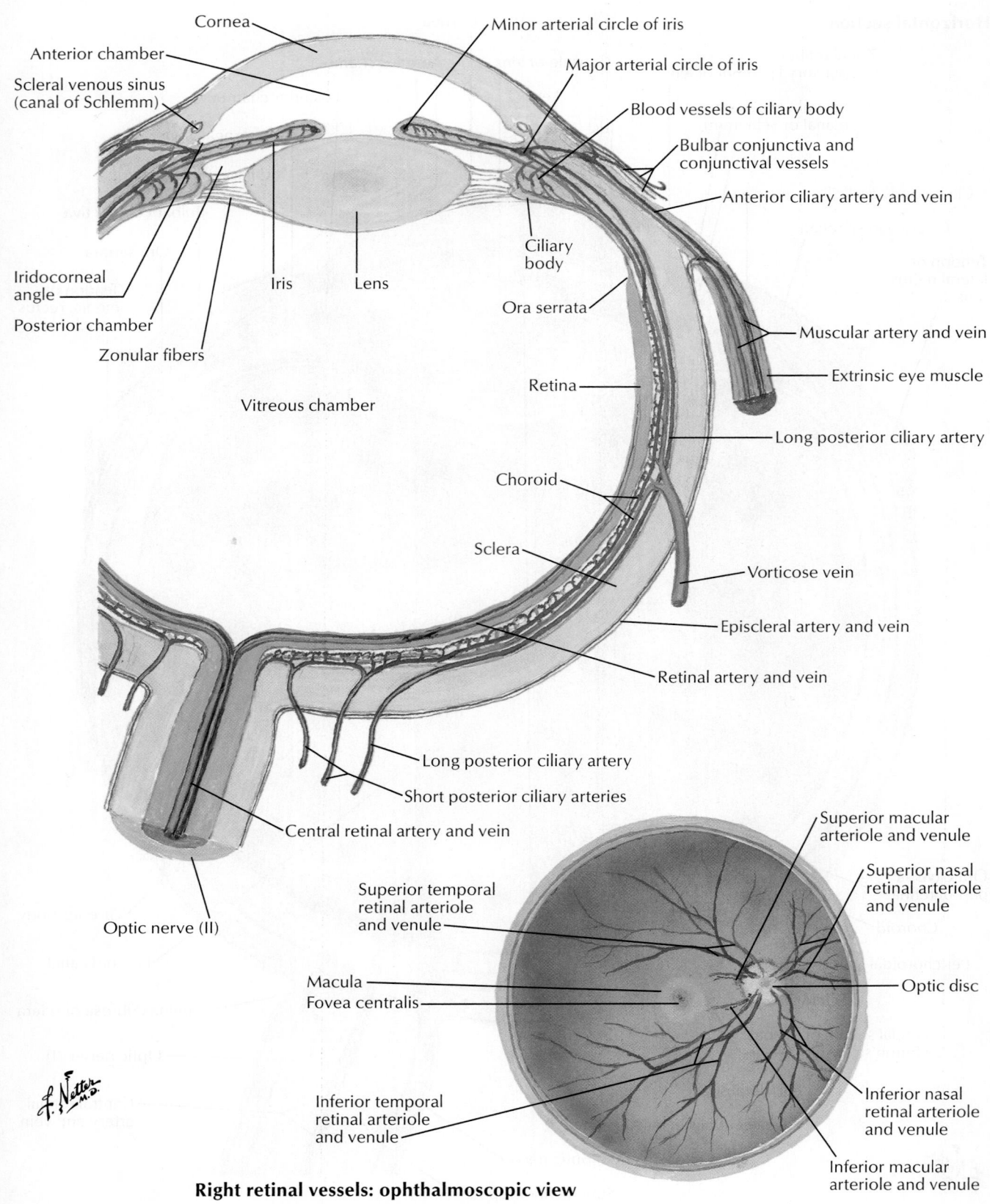

Cornea

Anterior chamber

Scleral venous sinus (canal of Schlemm)

Minor arterial circle of iris

Major arterial circle of iris

Blood vessels of ciliary body

Bulbar conjunctiva and conjunctival vessels

Anterior ciliary artery and vein

Ciliary body

Ora serrata

Iridocorneal angle

Iris

Lens

Posterior chamber

Zonular fibers

Vitreous chamber

Retina

Choroid

Sclera

Muscular artery and vein

Extrinsic eye muscle

Long posterior ciliary artery

Vorticose vein

Episcleral artery and vein

Retinal artery and vein

Long posterior ciliary artery

Short posterior ciliary arteries

Central retinal artery and vein

Optic nerve (II)

Superior temporal retinal arteriole and venule

Macula

Fovea centralis

Inferior temporal retinal arteriole and venule

Superior macular arteriole and venule

Superior nasal retinal arteriole and venule

Optic disc

Inferior nasal retinal arteriole and venule

Inferior macular arteriole and venule

Right retinal vessels: ophthalmoscopic view

Plate 90 Intrinsic Arteries and Veins of Eye. (Netter: Atlas of Human Anatomy, 4 ed, 2006, Saunders.)

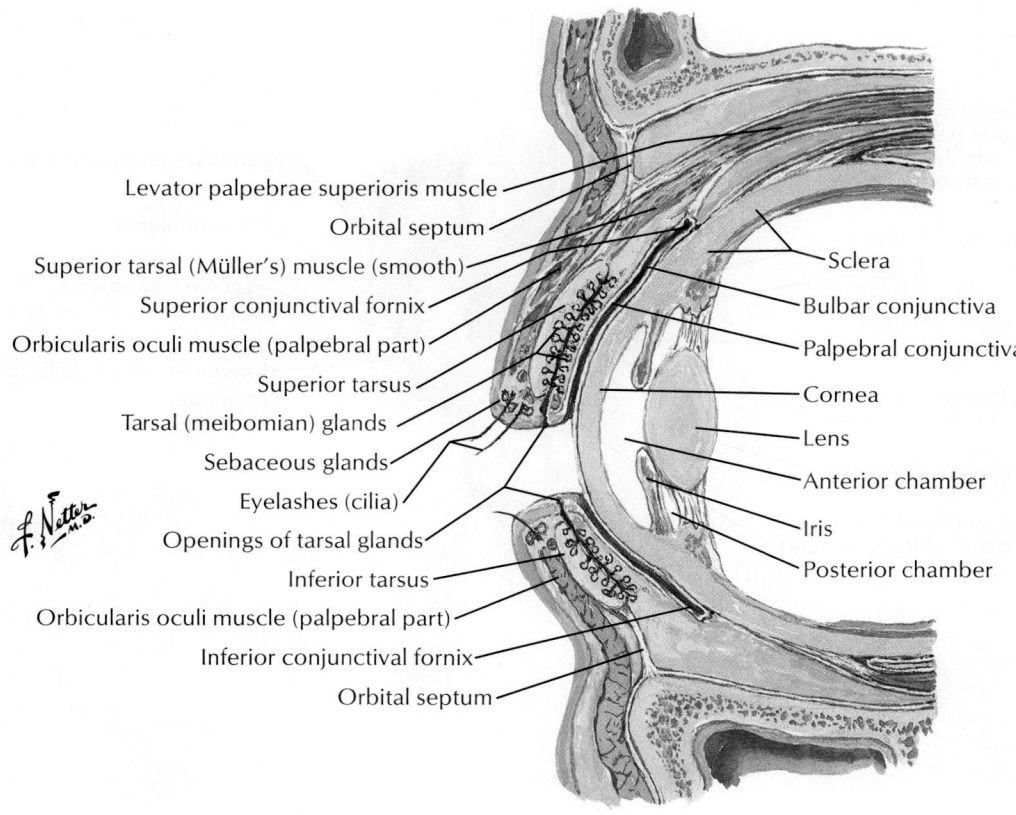

Levator palpebrae superioris muscle
Orbital septum
Superior tarsal (Müller's) muscle (smooth)
Superior conjunctival fornix
Orbicularis oculi muscle (palpebral part)
Superior tarsus
Tarsal (meibomian) glands
Sebaceous glands
Eyelashes (cilia)
Openings of tarsal glands
Inferior tarsus
Orbicularis oculi muscle (palpebral part)
Inferior conjunctival fornix
Orbital septum

Sclera
Bulbar conjunctiva
Palpebral conjunctiva
Cornea
Lens
Anterior chamber
Iris
Posterior chamber

Plate 81, Middle   Eyelids. (Netter: Atlas of Human Anatomy, 4 ed, 2006, Saunders.)

Superior palpebral conjunctiva:
tarsal (meibomian) glands
shining through

Seen through { Pupil
cornea { Iris

Corneoscleral junction
(corneal limbus)

Bulbar conjunctiva
over sclera

Inferior conjunctival fornix

Inferior palpebral conjunctiva:
tarsal glands shining through

Superior lacrimal papilla and
punctum

Plica semilunaris

Lacrimal caruncle in
lacrimal lake (lacus lacrimalis)

Inferior lacrimal papilla and
punctum

Plate 81, Upper Eyelid. (Netter: Atlas of Human Anatomy, 4 ed, 2006, Saunders.)

Orbital part of lacrimal gland

Palpebral part of lacrimal gland

Excretory ducts of lacrimal gland

Plica semilunaris

Lacrimal caruncle

Inferior lacrimal papilla and punctum

Superior lacrimal papilla and punctum

Lacrimal canaliculi

Lacrimal sac

Nasolacrimal duct

Opening of nasolacrimal duct

Frontal bone (cut away)

Orbital part of lacrimal gland

Palpebral part of lacrimal gland

Excretory ducts of lacrimal gland

Plica semilunaris and lacrimal lake

Lacrimal caruncle

Inferior lacrimal papilla and punctum

Opening of nasolacrimal duct

Superior lacrimal papilla and punctum

Lacrimal canaliculi

Lacrimal sac

Nasolacrimal duct

Middle nasal concha

Nasal cavity

Inferior nasal concha (cut)

Inferior nasal meatus

Plate 82 Lacrimal Apparatus. (Netter: Atlas of Human Anatomy, 4 ed, 2006, Saunders.)

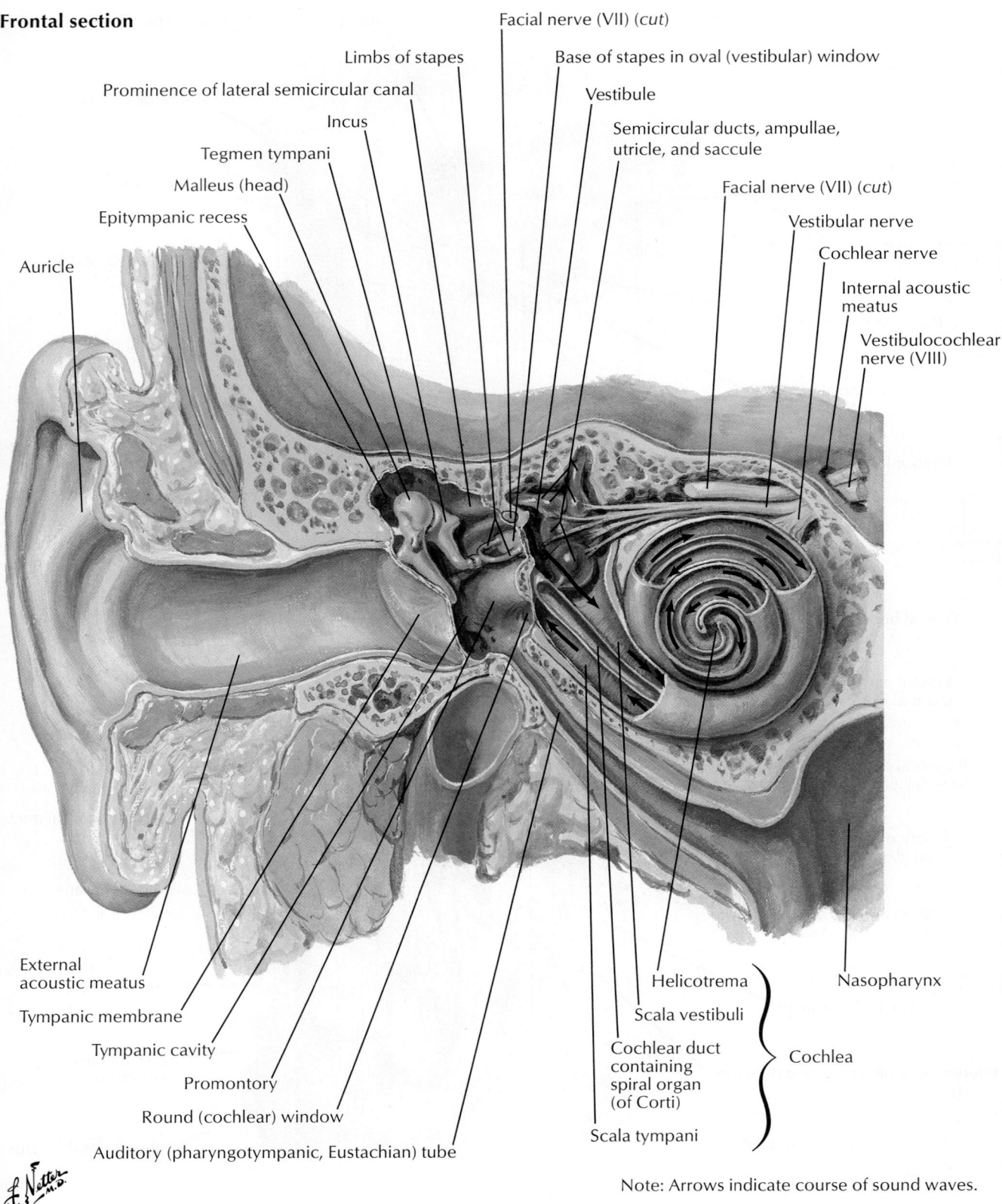

Facial nerve (VII) (*cut*)

Limbs of stapes

Base of stapes in oval (vestibular) window

Prominence of lateral semicircular canal

Vestibule

Incus

Semicircular ducts, ampullae, utricle, and saccule

Tegmen tympani

Malleus (head)

Facial nerve (VII) (*cut*)

Epitympanic recess

Vestibular nerve

Cochlear nerve

Auricle

Internal acoustic meatus

Vestibulocochlear nerve (VIII)

External acoustic meatus

Tympanic membrane

Tympanic cavity

Promontory

Round (cochlear) window

Auditory (pharyngotympanic, Eustachian) tube

Helicotrema

Scala vestibuli

Cochlear duct containing spiral organ (of Corti)

Scala tympani

Nasopharynx

Cochlea

Note: Arrows indicate course of sound waves.

Plate 92 Pathway of Sound Reception. (Netter: Atlas of Human Anatomy, 4 ed, 2006, Saunders.)

Medial wall of tympanic cavity: lateral view

Mastoid antrum

Prominence of lateral semicircular canal

Prominence of facial canal

Geniculum (geniculate ganglion) of facial nerve

Greater petrosal nerve

Base of stapes in fossa of oval (vestibular) window

Limbs of stapes

Pyramidal eminence

Chorda tympani nerve (*cut*)

Mastoid cells

Tendon of stapedius muscle

Fossa of round (cochlear) window

Facial nerve (VII) in stylomastoid foramen

Jugular fossa

Tympanic cells

Tensor tympani muscle (*tendon cut*)

Auditory (pharyngotympanic, Eustachian) tube

Levator veli palatini muscle

Promontory with tympanic nerve (of Jacobson) and plexus under mucosa

Internal carotid artery

Plate 94 Tympanic Cavity. (Netter: Atlas of Human Anatomy, 4 ed, 2006, Saunders.)

Otoscopic view of right tympanic membrane

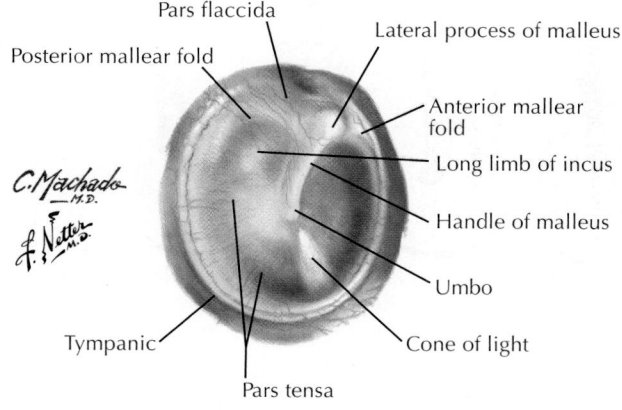

Pars flaccida

Posterior mallear fold

Lateral process of malleus

Anterior mallear fold

Long limb of incus

Handle of malleus

Umbo

Cone of light

Tympanic

Pars tensa

Plate 93 Tympanic Cavity. (Netter: Atlas of Human Anatomy, 4 ed, 2006, Saunders.)

Dissected right bony labyrinth (otic capsule): membranous labyrinth removed

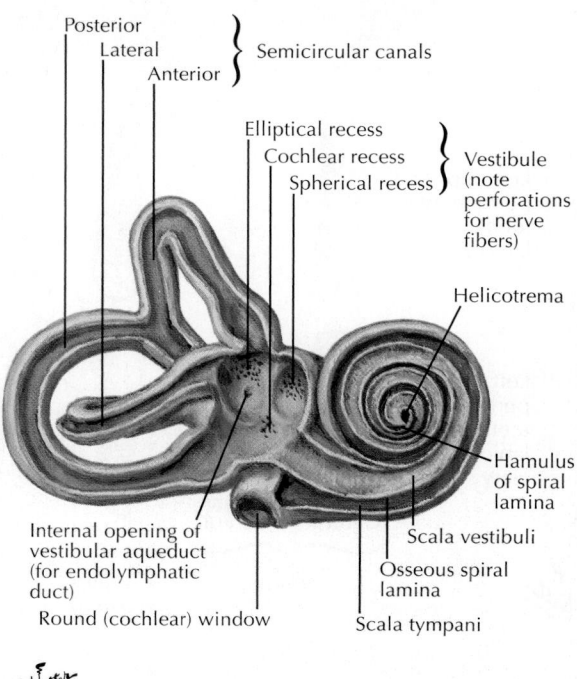

Posterior

Lateral

Anterior

Semicircular canals

Elliptical recess

Cochlear recess

Spherical recess

Vestibule (note perforations for nerve fibers)

Helicotrema

Hamulus of spiral lamina

Scala vestibuli

Osseous spiral lamina

Scala tympani

Internal opening of vestibular aqueduct (for endolymphatic duct)

Round (cochlear) window

Plate 95 Bony Membranous Labyrinth. (Netter: Atlas of Human Anatomy, 4 ed, 2006, Saunders.)

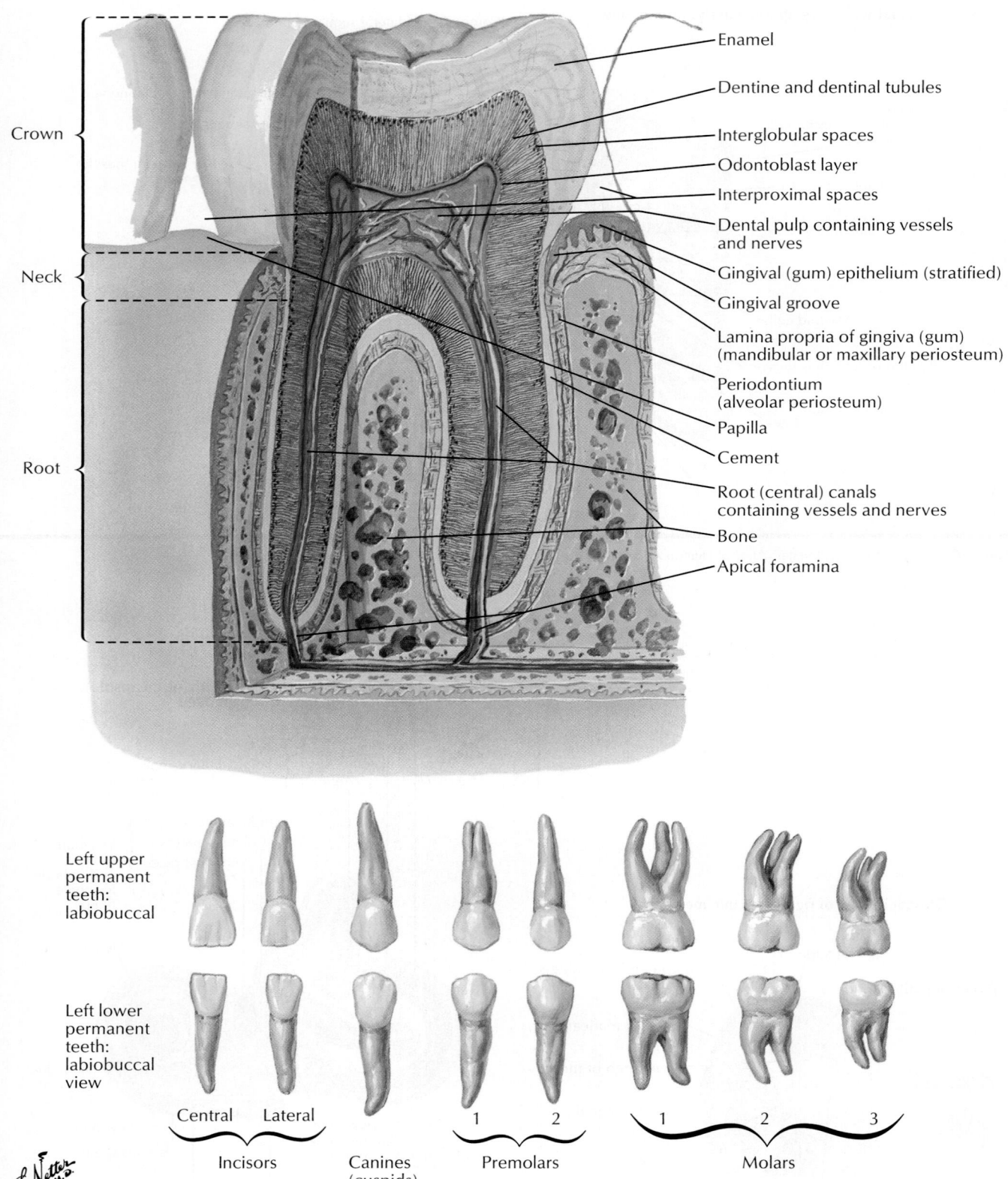

Crown

Neck

Root

Enamel

Dentine and dentinal tubules

Interglobular spaces

Odontoblast layer

Interproximal spaces

Dental pulp containing vessels and nerves

Gingival (gum) epithelium (stratified)

Gingival groove

Lamina propria of gingiva (gum) (mandibular or maxillary periosteum)

Periodontium (alveolar periosteum)

Papilla

Cement

Root (central) canals containing vessels and nerves

Bone

Apical foramina

Left upper permanent teeth: labiobuccal

Left lower permanent teeth: labiobuccal view

Central   Lateral

1   2

1   2   3

Incisors

Canines (cuspids)

Premolars

Molars

Plate 57   Teeth. (Netter: Atlas of Human Anatomy, 4 ed, 2006, Saunders.)

Tongue

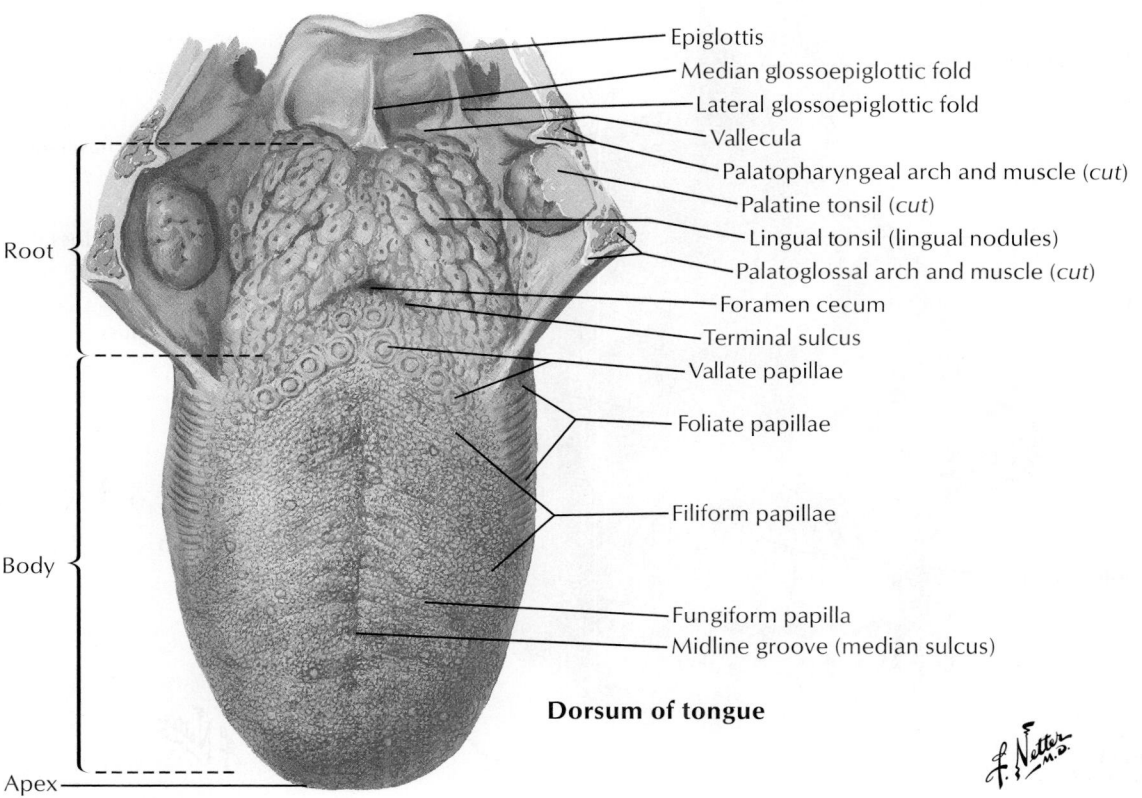

Epiglottis

Median glossoepiglottic fold

Lateral glossoepiglottic fold

Vallecula

Palatopharyngeal arch and muscle (*cut*)

Palatine tonsil (*cut*)

Lingual tonsil (lingual nodules)

Palatoglossal arch and muscle (*cut*)

Foramen cecum

Terminal sulcus

Vallate papillae

Foliate papillae

Filiform papillae

Fungiform papilla

Midline groove (median sulcus)

Root

Body

Apex

Dorsum of tongue

Plate 58   Tongue. (Netter: Atlas of Human Anatomy, 4 ed, 2006, Saunders.)

71

NETTER'S ANATOMY ILLUSTRATIONS

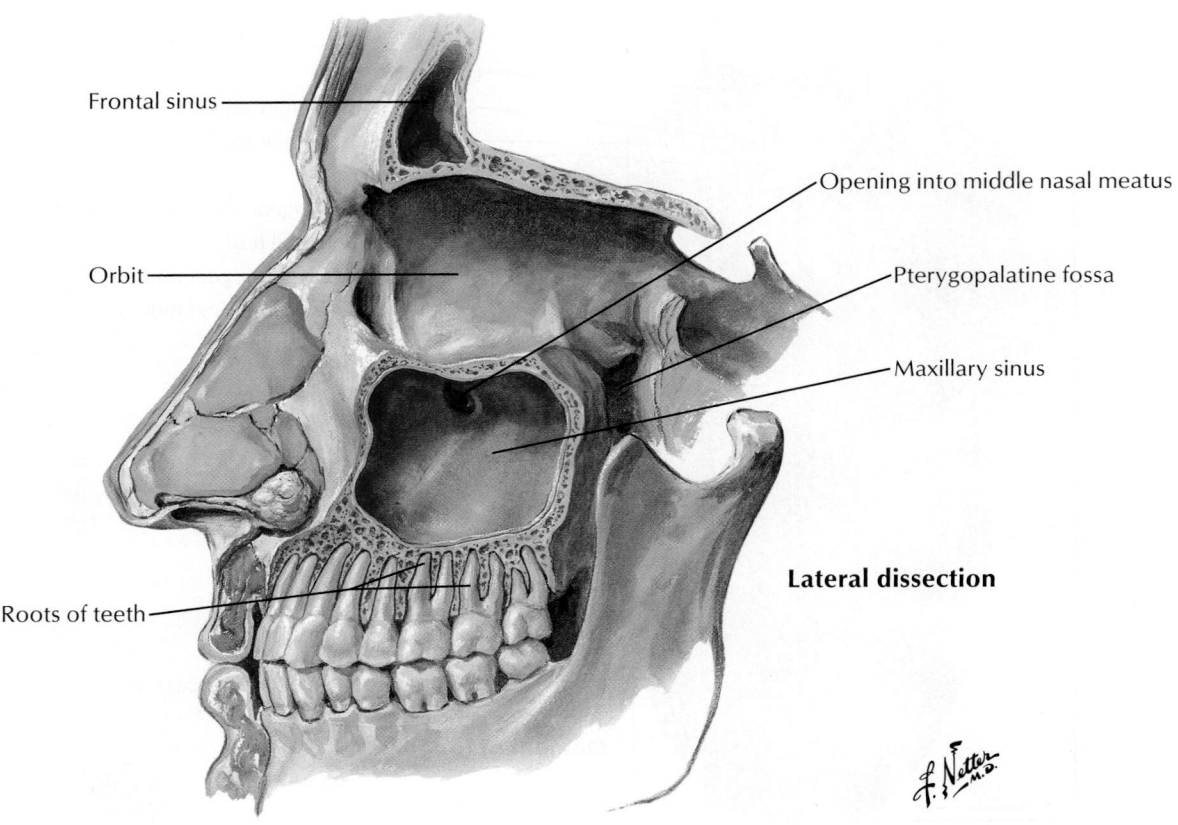

Frontal sinus

Opening into middle nasal meatus

Orbit

Pterygopalatine fossa

Maxillary sinus

Roots of teeth

Lateral dissection

Plate 49 Paranasal Sinuses. (Netter: Atlas of Human Anatomy, 4 ed, 2006, Saunders.)

72

Superficial temporal artery and vein and auriculotemporal nerve

Branches of facial nerve

Transverse facial artery

Accessory parotid gland

Parotid duct

Buccinator muscle (*cut*)

Masseter muscle

Lingual nerve

Submandibular ganglion

Tongue

Frenulum of tongue

Sublingual fold with openings of sublingual ducts

Sublingual caruncle with opening of submandibular duct

Sublingual gland

Submandibular duct

Sublingual artery and vein

Mylohyoid muscle (*cut*)

Digastric muscle (anterior belly)

Submandibular gland

Facial artery and vein

Hyoid bone

Parotid gland

Retromandibular vein (anterior and posterior branches)

Digastric muscle (posterior belly)

Stylohyoid muscle

External jugular vein

Sternocleidomastoid muscle

Common trunk receiving facial, anterior branch of retromandibular, and lingual veins (common facial vein)

Internal jugular vein

External carotid artery

Parotid gland: totally serous

Submandibular gland: mostly serous, partially mucous

Sublingual gland: almost completely mucous

Plate 61   Salivary Glands. (Netter: Atlas of Human Anatomy, 4 ed, 2006, Saunders.)

73

Coronary Arteries: Arteriographic Views

Right coronary artery: left anterior oblique view

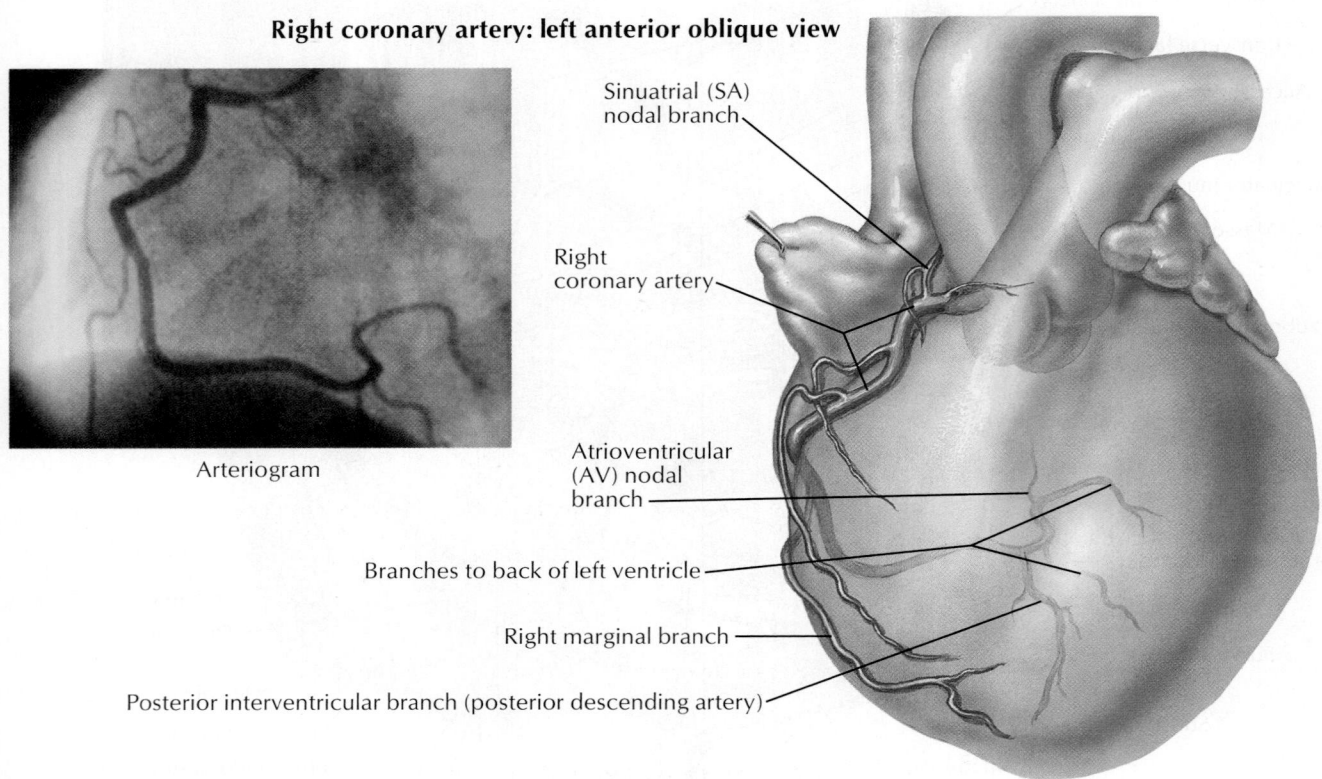

Arteriogram

Sinuatrial (SA) nodal branch

Right coronary artery

Atrioventricular (AV) nodal branch

Branches to back of left ventricle

Right marginal branch

Posterior interventricular branch (posterior descending artery)

Right coronary artery: right anterior oblique view

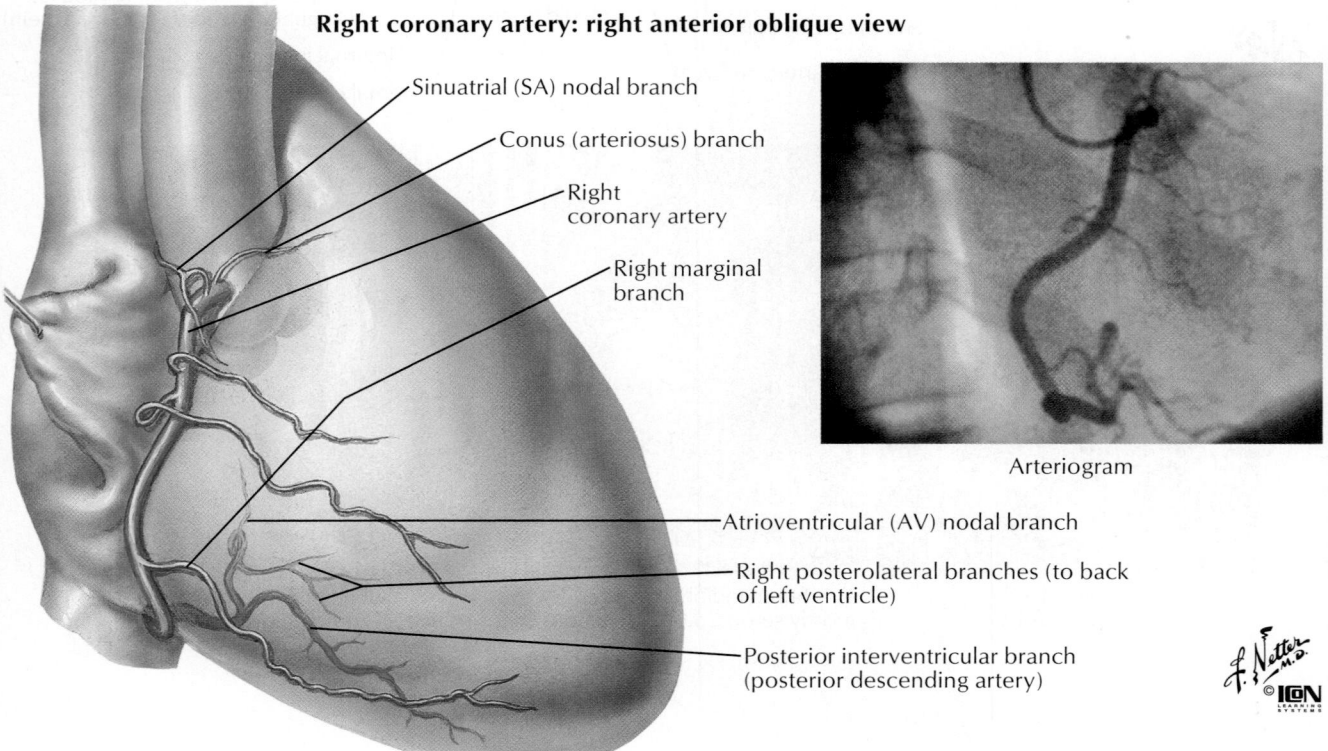

Sinuatrial (SA) nodal branch

Conus (arteriosus) branch

Right coronary artery

Right marginal branch

Arteriogram

Atrioventricular (AV) nodal branch

Right posterolateral branches (to back of left ventricle)

Posterior interventricular branch (posterior descending artery)

Plate 218 Coronary Arteries: Arteriographic Views. (Netter: Atlas of Human Anatomy, 4 ed, 2006, Saunders.)

74

Left coronary artery: left anterior oblique view

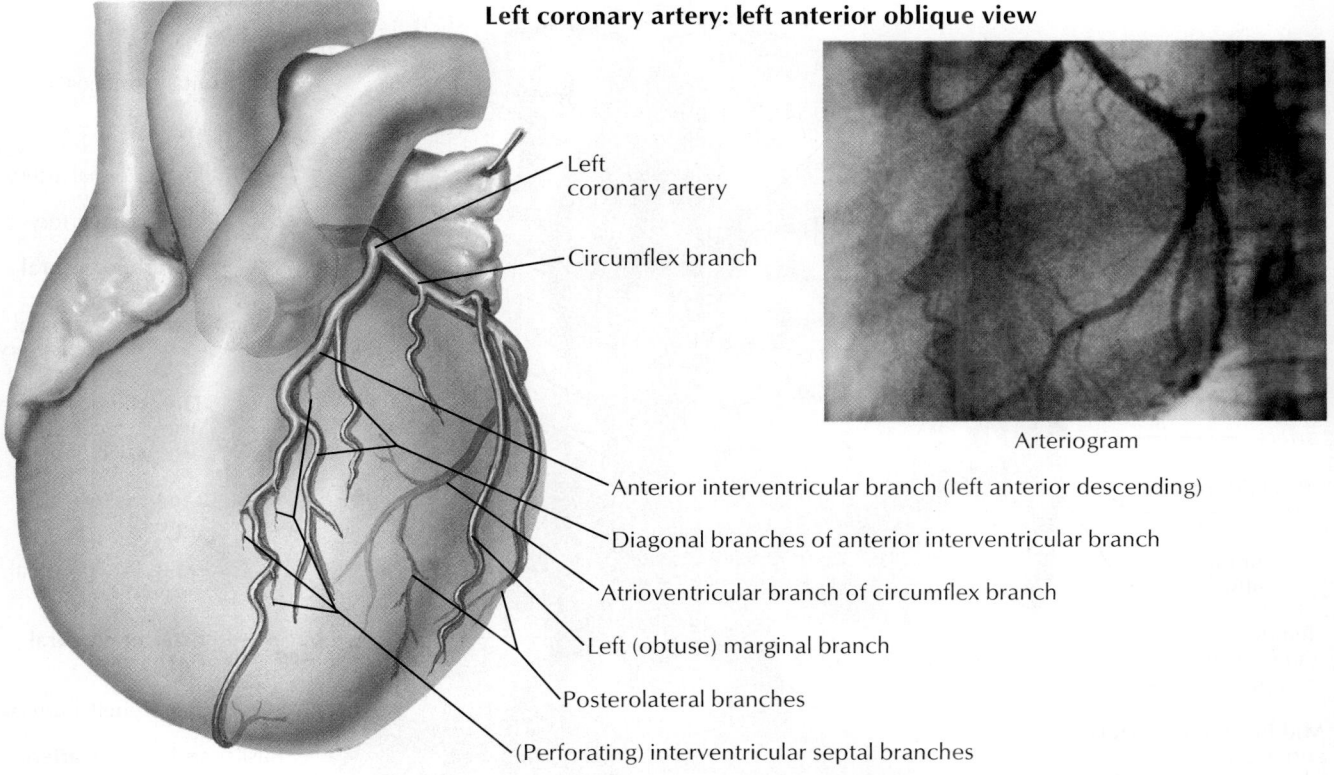

Left coronary artery

Circumflex branch

Arteriogram

Anterior interventricular branch (left anterior descending)

Diagonal branches of anterior interventricular branch

Atrioventricular branch of circumflex branch

Left (obtuse) marginal branch

Posterolateral branches

(Perforating) interventricular septal branches

Left coronary artery: right anterior oblique view

Left coronary artery

Anterior interventricular branch (left anterior descending)

Circumflex branch

(Perforating) interventricular septal branches

Arteriogram

Left (obtuse) marginal branch

Posterolateral branches

Diagonal branch of Anterior interventricular branch

Atrioventricular branch of circumflex branch

Plate 219   Coronary Arteries: Arteriographic Views. (Netter: Atlas of Human Anatomy, 4 ed, 2006, Saunders.)

75

NETTER'S ANATOMY ILLUSTRATIONS

Corpus callosum

Anterolateral central (lenticulostriate) arteries

Lateral frontobasal (orbitofrontal) artery

Prefrontal artery

Precentral (pre-Rolandic) and central (Rolandic) sulcal arteries

Anterior parietal (postcentral sulcal) artery

Posterior parietal artery

Branch to angular gyrus

Temporal branches (anterior, middle, and posterior)

Middle cerebral artery and branches (deep in lateral cerebral [Sylvian] sulcus)

Anterior communicating artery

Posterior communicating artery

Anterior inferior cerebellar artery (AICA)

Posterior spinal artery

Paracentral artery

Medial frontal branches

Pericallosal artery

Callosomarginal artery

Polar frontal artery

Anterior cerebral arteries

Medial frontobasal (orbitofrontal) artery

Distal medial striate artery (recurrent artery of Heubner)

Internal carotid artery

Anterior choroidal artery

Posterior cerebral artery

Superior cerebellar artery

Basilar and pontine arteries

Labyrinthine (internal acoustic) artery

Vertebral artery

Posterior inferior cerebellar artery (PICA)

Anterior spinal artery

Corpus striatum (caudate and lentiform nuclei)

Anterolateral central (lenticulostriate) arteries

Insula (island of Reil)

Limen of insula

Precentral (pre-Rolandic), central (Rolandic) sulcal, and parietal arteries

Lateral cerebral (Sylvian) sulcus

Temporal branches of middle cerebral artery

Temporal lobe

Middle cerebral artery

Internal carotid artery

Falx cerebri

Callosomarginal arteries and Pericallosal arteries (branches of anterior cerebral arteries)

Trunk of corpus callosum

Internal capsule

Septum pellucidum

Rostrum of corpus callosum

Anterior cerebral arteries

Distal medial striate artery (recurrent artery of Heubner)

Anterior communicating artery

Optic chiasm

Plate 141 Arteries of Brain: Frontal View and Section. (Netter: Atlas of Human Anatomy, 4 ed, 2006, Saunders.)

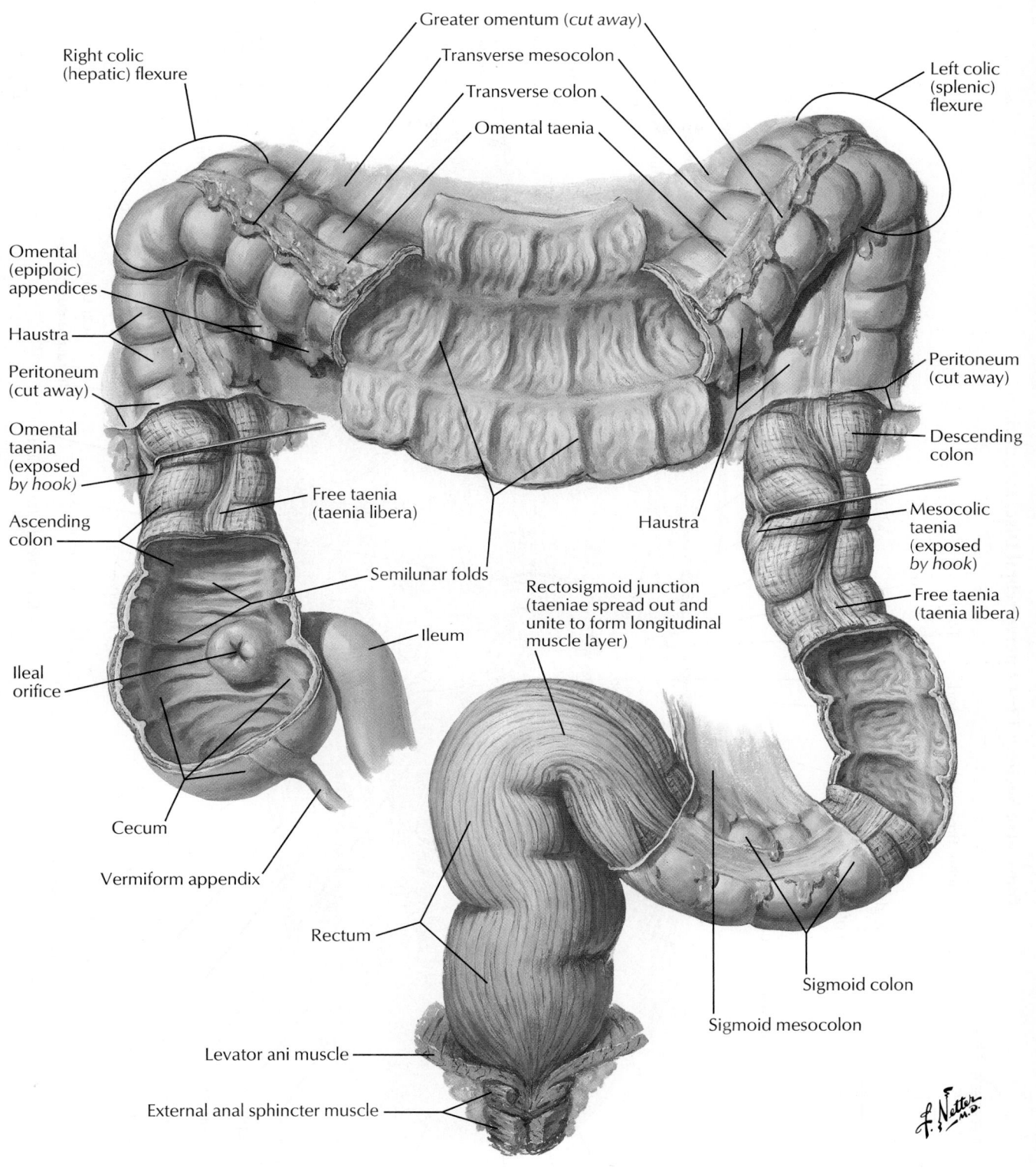

Right colic (hepatic) flexure

Greater omentum (*cut away*)

Transverse mesocolon

Transverse colon

Omental taenia

Left colic (splenic) flexure

Omental (epiploic) appendices

Haustra

Peritoneum (cut away)

Omental taenia (exposed *by hook*)

Ascending colon

Ileal orifice

Cecum

Vermiform appendix

Free taenia (taenia libera)

Semilunar folds

Ileum

Rectosigmoid junction (taeniae spread out and unite to form longitudinal muscle layer)

Haustra

Peritoneum (cut away)

Descending colon

Mesocolic taenia (exposed *by hook*)

Free taenia (taenia libera)

Rectum

Levator ani muscle

External anal sphincter muscle

Sigmoid colon

Sigmoid mesocolon

Plate 284 Mucosa and Musculature of Large Intestine. (Netter: Atlas of Human Anatomy, 4 ed, 2006, Saunders.)

Transverse Section: T3–4 Intervertebral Disc, Manubrium

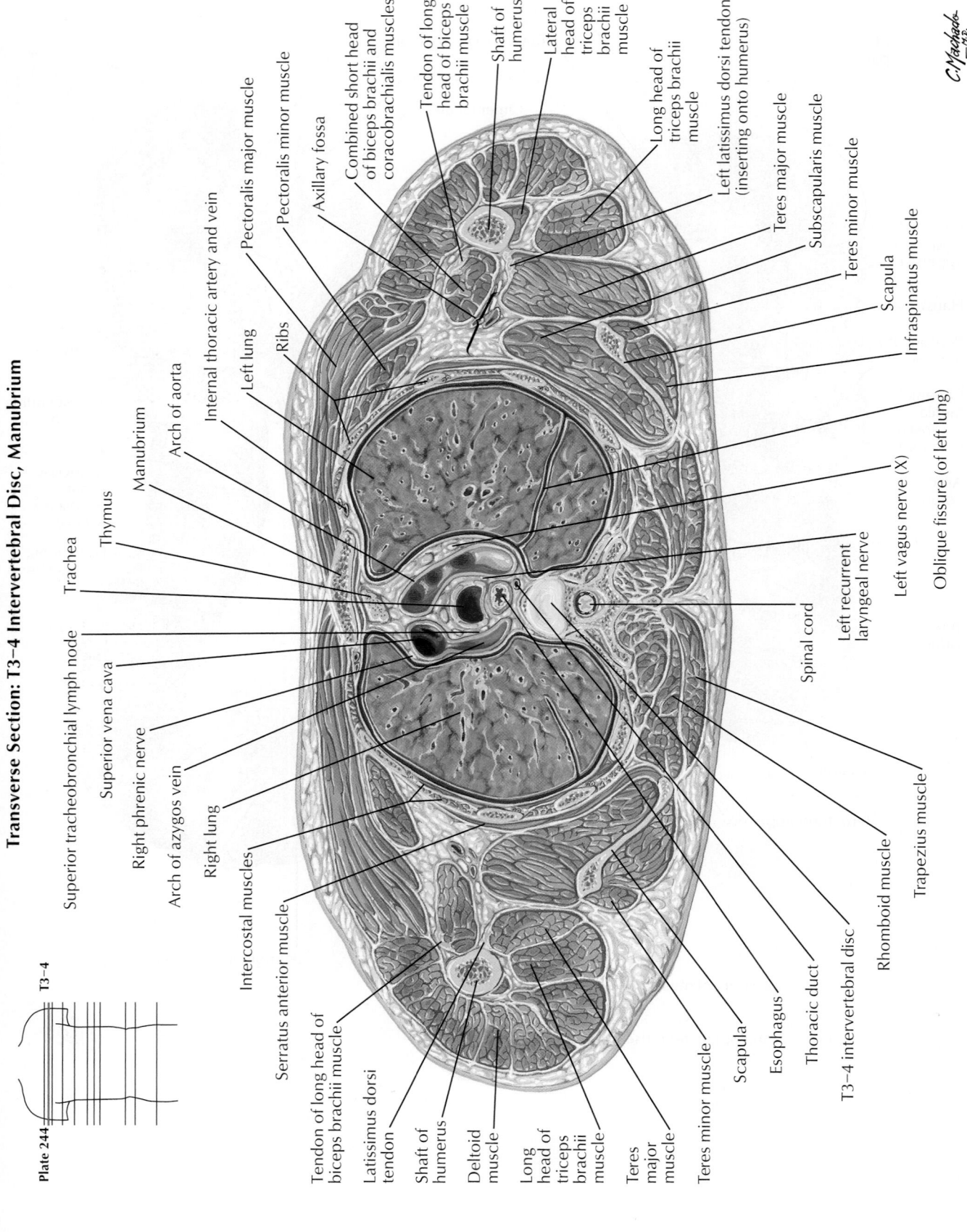

C. Machado —M.D.

Plate 244

T3–4

Superior tracheobronchial lymph node

Trachea

Thymus

Manubrium

Arch of aorta

Internal thoracic artery and vein

Left lung

Ribs

Axillary fossa

Pectoralis minor muscle

Pectoralis major muscle

Combined short head of biceps brachii and coracobrachialis muscles

Tendon of long head of biceps brachii muscle

Shaft of humerus

Lateral head of triceps brachii muscle

Long head of triceps brachii muscle

Left latissimus dorsi tendon (inserting onto humerus)

Teres major muscle

Subscapularis muscle

Teres minor muscle

Scapula

Infraspinatus muscle

Oblique fissure (of left lung)

Left vagus nerve (X)

Left recurrent laryngeal nerve

Spinal cord

Trapezius muscle

Rhomboid muscle

T3–4 intervertebral disc

Thoracic duct

Esophagus

Scapula

Teres minor muscle

Teres major muscle

Long head of triceps brachii muscle

Deltoid muscle

Shaft of humerus

Latissimus dorsi tendon

Tendon of long head of biceps brachii muscle

Serratus anterior muscle

Intercostal muscles

Right lung

Arch of azygos vein

Right phrenic nerve

Superior vena cava

Plate 244 Cross Section of Thorax at T3-4 Disc Level. (Netter: Atlas of Human Anatomy, 4 ed, 2006, Saunders.)

Right knee in extension: posterior view

Posterior cruciate ligament

Anterior cruciate ligament

Posterior meniscofemoral ligament

Lateral condyle of femur (articular surface)

Popliteus tendon

Fibular collateral ligament

Lateral meniscus

Head of fibula

Adductor tubercle on medial epicondyle of femur

Medial condyle of femur (articular surface)

Medial meniscus

Tibial collateral ligament

Medial condyle of tibia

Plate 509   Knee: Cruciate and Collateral Ligaments. (Netter: Atlas of Human Anatomy, 4 ed, 2006, Saunders.)

79

Paramedian (sagittal) dissection

Ureter

Uterine (fallopian) tube

Ovary

Ligament of ovary

Round ligament of uterus

Broad ligament (*cut*)

Superior pubic ramus (*cut*)

Inferior pubic ramus (*cut*)

Ischiocavernosus muscle

Body of clitoris

Labia minora

Labium majus

Rectouterine pouch (of Douglas)

Peritoneum (*cut edge*)

Vesicouterine pouch

Rectum

Ureter

Urinary bladder

Vagina

Pelvic diaphragm (levator ani muscle)

Deep transverse perineal muscle (*cut*)

External anal sphincter muscle

Median (sagittal) section

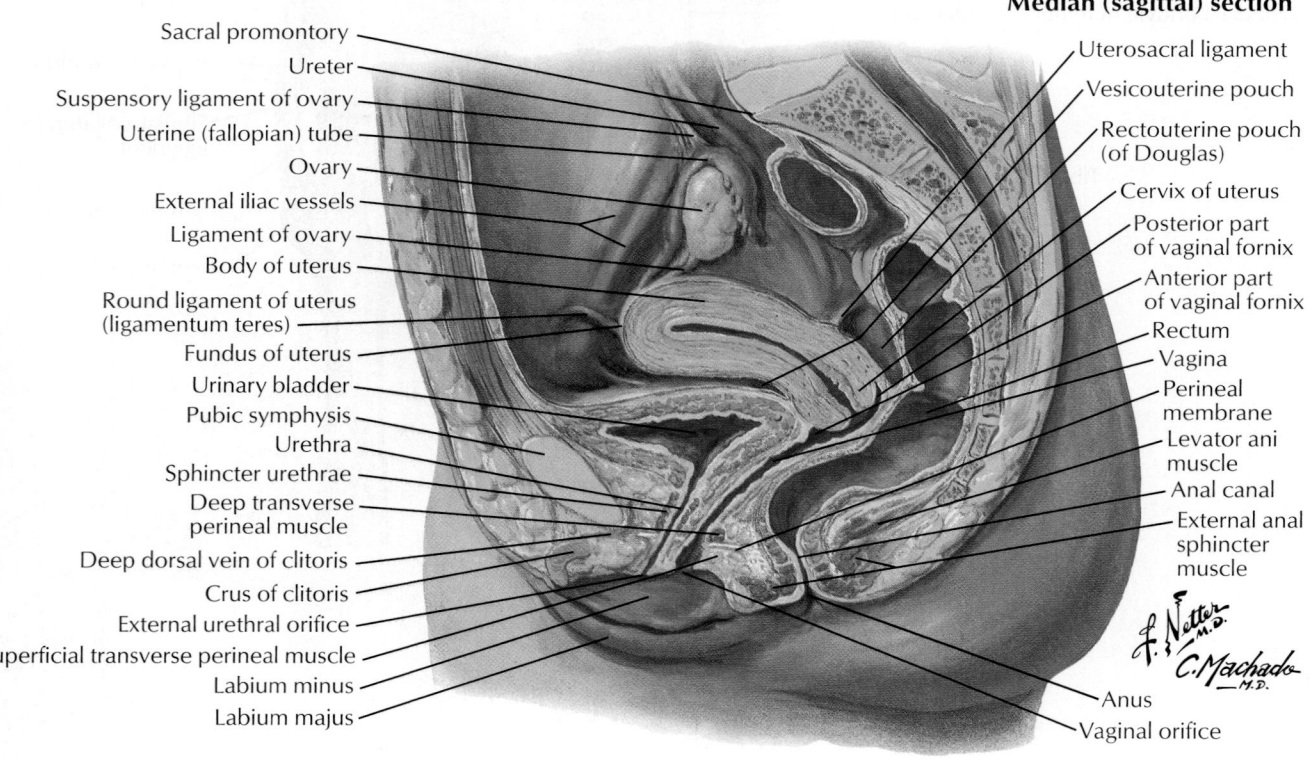

Sacral promontory

Ureter

Suspensory ligament of ovary

Uterine (fallopian) tube

Ovary

External iliac vessels

Ligament of ovary

Body of uterus

Round ligament of uterus (ligamentum teres)

Fundus of uterus

Urinary bladder

Pubic symphysis

Urethra

Sphincter urethrae

Deep transverse perineal muscle

Deep dorsal vein of clitoris

Crus of clitoris

External urethral orifice

Superficial transverse perineal muscle

Labium minus

Labium majus

Uterosacral ligament

Vesicouterine pouch

Rectouterine pouch (of Douglas)

Cervix of uterus

Posterior part of vaginal fornix

Anterior part of vaginal fornix

Rectum

Vagina

Perineal membrane

Levator ani muscle

Anal canal

External anal sphincter muscle

Anus

Vaginal orifice

F. Netter M.D.

C. Machado M.D.

Plate 360   Pelvic Viscera and Perineum: Female. (Netter: Atlas of Human Anatomy, 4 ed, 2006, Saunders.)

Alphabetic Index

A

Aarskog's syndrome Q87.1
Abandonment —*see* Maltreatment
Abasia (-astasia) (hysterical) F44.4
Abderhalden-Kaufmann-Lignac syndrome
   (cystinosis) E72.04
Abdomen, abdominal —*see also* condition
   acute R10.0
   angina K55.1
   muscle deficiency syndrome Q79.4
Abdominalgia —*see* Pain, abdominal
Abduction contracture, hip or other joint —*see*
   Contraction, joint
Aberrant (congenital) —*see also* Malposition,
   congenital
   adrenal gland Q89.1
   artery (peripheral) Q27.8
     basilar NEC Q28.1
     cerebral Q28.3
     coronary Q24.5
     digestive system Q27.8
     eye Q15.8
     lower limb Q27.8
     precerebral Q28.1
     pulmonary Q25.79
     renal Q27.2
     retina Q14.1
     specified site NEC Q27.8
     subclavian Q27.8
     upper limb Q27.8
     vertebral Q28.1
   breast Q83.8
   endocrine gland NEC Q89.2
   hepatic duct Q44.5
   pancreas Q45.3
   parathyroid gland Q89.2
   pituitary gland Q89.2
   sebaceous glands, mucous membrane,
     mouth, congenital Q38.6
   spleen Q89.09
   subclavian artery Q27.8
   thymus (gland) Q89.2
   thyroid gland Q89.2
   vein (peripheral) NEC Q27.8
     cerebral Q28.3
     digestive system Q27.8
     lower limb Q27.8
     precerebral Q28.1
     specified site NEC Q27.8
     upper limb Q27.8
Aberration
   distantial —*see* Disturbance, visual
   mental F99
Abetalipoproteinemia E78.6
Abiotrophy R68.89
Ablatio, ablation
   retinae —*see* Detachment, retina
Ablepharia, ablepharon Q10.3
Abnormal, abnormality, abnormalities —*see*
   also Anomaly
   acid-base balance (mixed) E87.4
   albumin R77.0
   alphafetoprotein R77.2
   alveolar ridge K08.9
   anatomical relationship Q89.9
   apertures, congenital, diaphragm
     Q79.1
   auditory perception H93.29-
     diplacusis —*see* Diplacusis
     hyperacusis —*see* Hyperacusis
     recruitment —*see* Recruitment, auditory
     threshold shift —*see* Shift, auditory
       threshold
   autosomes Q99.9
     fragile site Q95.5
   basal metabolic rate R94.8
   biosynthesis, testicular androgen
     E29.1
   bleeding time R79.1

Abnormal, abnormality, abnormalities —
(Continued)
   blood level (of)
     cobalt R79.0
     copper R79.0
     iron R79.0
     lithium R78.89
     magnesium R79.0
     mineral NEC R79.0
     zinc R79.0
   blood pressure
     elevated R03.0
     low reading (nonspecific) R03.1
   blood sugar R73.09
   blood-gas level R79.81
   bowel sounds R19.15
     absent R19.11
     hyperactive R19.12
   brain scan R94.02
   breathing R06.9
   caloric test R94.138
   cerebrospinal fluid R83.9
     cytology R83.6
     drug level R83.2
     enzyme level R83.0
     hormones R83.1
     immunology R83.4
     microbiology R83.5
     nonmedicinal level R83.3
     specified type NEC R83.8
   chemistry, blood R79.9
     C-reactive protein R79.82
     drugs —*see* Findings, abnormal, in blood
     gas level R79.81
     minerals R79.0
     pancytopenia D61.818
     PTT R79.1
     specified NEC R79.89
     toxins —*see* Findings, abnormal, in
       blood
   chest sounds (friction) (rales) R09.89
   chromosome, chromosomal Q99.9
     with more than three X chromosomes,
       female Q97.1
     analysis result R89.8
      bronchial washings R84.8
      cerebrospinal fluid R83.8
      cervix uteri NEC R87.89
      nasal secretions R84.8
      nipple discharge R89.8
      peritoneal fluid R85.89
      pleural fluid R84.8
      prostatic secretions R86.8
      saliva R85.89
      seminal fluid R86.8
      sputum R84.8
      synovial fluid R89.8
      throat scrapings R84.8
      vagina R87.89
      vulva R87.89
      wound secretions R89.8
     dicentric replacement Q93.2
     ring replacement Q93.2
     sex Q99.8
      female phenotype Q97.9
        specified NEC Q97.8
      male phenotype Q98.9
        specified NEC Q98.8
      structural male Q98.6
     specified NEC Q99.8
   clinical findings NEC R68.89
   coagulation D68.9
     newborn, transient P61.6
     profile R79.1
     time R79.1
   communication —*see* Fistula
   conjunctiva, vascular H11.41-
   coronary artery Q24.5
   cortisol-binding globulin E27.8
   course, eustachian tube Q17.8

Abnormal, abnormality, abnormalities —
(Continued)
   creatinine clearance R94.4
   cytology
     anus R85.619
      atypical squamous cells cannot
        exclude high grade squamous
        intraepithelial lesion (ASC-H)
        R85.611
      atypical squamous cells of undetermined
        significance (ASC-US) R85.610
      cytologic evidence of malignancy
        R85.614
      high grade squamous intraepithelial
        lesion (HGSIL) R85.613
      human papillomavirus (HPV) DNA test
        high risk positive R85.81
        low risk postive R85.82
      inadequate smear R85.615
      low grade squamous intraepithelial
        lesion (LGSIL) R85.612
      satisfactory anal smear but lacking
        transformation zone R85.616
      specified NEC R85.618
      unsatisfactory smear R85.615
     female genital organs —*see* Abnormal,
       Papanicolaou (smear)
   dark adaptation curve H53.61
   dentofacial NEC —*see* Anomaly, dentofacial
   development, developmental Q89.9
     central nervous system Q07.9
   diagnostic imaging
     abdomen, abdominal region NEC R93.5
     biliary tract R93.2
     bladder R93.41 ◀
     breast R92.8
     central nervous system NEC R90.89
     cerebrovascular NEC R90.89
     coronary circulation R93.1
     digestive tract NEC R93.3
     gastrointestinal (tract) R93.3
     genitourinary organs R93.8
     head R93.0
     heart R93.1
     intrathoracic organ NEC R93.8
     kidney R93.42- ◀
     limbs R93.6
     liver R93.2
     lung (field) R91.8
     musculoskeletal system NEC R93.7
     renal pelvis R93.41 ◀
     retroperitoneum R93.5
     site specified NEC R93.8
     skin and subcutaneous tissue R93.8
     skull R93.0
     ~~urinary organs R93.4~~
     urinary organs specified NEC R93.49 ◀
     ureter R93.41 ◀
   direction, teeth, fully erupted M26.30
   ear ossicles, acquired NEC H74.39-
     ankylosis —*see* Ankylosis, ear ossicles
     discontinuity —*see* Discontinuity, ossicles,
       ear
     partial loss —*see* Loss, ossicles, ear (partial)
   Ebstein Q22.5
   echocardiogram R93.1
   echoencephalogram R90.81
   echogram —*see* Abnormal, diagnostic
     imaging
   electrocardiogram [ECG] [EKG] R94.31
   electroencephalogram [EEG] R94.01
   electrolyte —*see* Imbalance, electrolyte
   electromyogram [EMG] R94.131
   electro-oculogram [EOG] R94.110
   electrophysiological intracardiac studies
     R94.39
   electroretinogram [ERG] R94.111
   erythrocytes
     congenital, with perinatal jaundice D58.9
   feces (color) (contents) (mucus) R19.5

Abnormal, abnormality, abnormalities —
(Continued)
finding —see Findings, abnormal, without
diagnosis
fluid
amniotic —see Abnormal, specimen,
specified
cerebrospinal —see Abnormal,
cerebrospinal fluid
peritoneal —see Abnormal, specimen,
digestive organs
pleural —see Abnormal, specimen,
respiratory organs
synovial —see Abnormal, specimen,
specified
thorax (bronchial washings) (pleural
fluid) —see Abnormal, specimen,
respiratory organs
vaginal —see Abnormal, specimen, female
genital organs
form
teeth K00.2
uterus —see Anomaly, uterus
function studies
auditory R94.120
bladder R94.8
brain R94.09
cardiovascular R94.30
ear R94.128
endocrine NEC R94.7
eye NEC R94.118
kidney R94.4
liver R94.5
nervous system
central NEC R94.09
peripheral NEC R94.138
pancreas R94.8
placenta R94.8
pulmonary R94.2
special senses NEC R94.128
spleen R94.8
thyroid R94.6
vestibular R94.121
gait —see Gait
hysterical F44.4
gastrin secretion E16.4
globulin R77.1
cortisol-binding E27.8
thyroid-binding E07.89
glomerular, minor —see also N00-N07 with
fourth character .0 N05.0
glucagon secretion E16.3
glucose tolerance (test) (non-fasting)
R73.09
gravitational (G) forces or states (effect of)
T75.81
hair (color) (shaft) L67.9
specified NEC L67.8
hard tissue formation in pulp (dental)
K04.3
head movement R25.0
heart
rate R00.9
specified NEC R00.8
shadow R93.1
sounds NEC R01.2
hemoglobin (disease) —see also Disease,
hemoglobin D58.2
trait —see Trait, hemoglobin, abnormal
histology NEC R89.7
immunological findings R89.4
in serum R76.9
specified NEC R76.8
increase in appetite R63.2
involuntary movement —see Abnormal,
movement, involuntary
jaw closure M26.51
karyotype R89.8
kidney function test R94.4
knee jerk R29.2
leukocyte (cell) (differential) NEC D72.9

Abnormal, abnormality, abnormalities —
(Continued)
liver
loss of
height R29.890
weight R63.4
mammogram NEC R92.8
calcification (calculus) R92.1
microcalcification R92.0
Mantoux test R76.11
movement (disorder) —see also Disorder,
movement
head R25.0
involuntary R25.9
fasciculation R25.3
of head R25.0
spasm R25.2
specified type NEC R25.8
tremor R25.1
myoglobin (Aberdeen) (Annapolis) R89.7
neonatal screening P09
oculomotor study R94.113
palmar creases Q82.8
Papanicolaou (smear)
anus R85.619
atypical squamous cells cannot
exclude high grade squamous
intraepithelial lesion (ASC-H)
R85.611
atypical squamous cells of undetermined
significance (ASC-US) R85.610
cytologic evidence of malignancy
R85.614
high grade squamous intraepithelial
lesion (HGSIL) R85.613
human papillomavirus (HPV)
DNA test
high risk positive R85.81
low risk postive R85.82
inadequate smear R85.615
low grade squamous intraepithelial
lesion (LGSIL) R85.612
satisfactory anal smear but lacking
transformation zone R85.616
specified NEC R85.618
unsatisfactory smear R85.615
bronchial washings R84.6
cerebrospinal fluid R83.6
cervix R87.619
atypical squamous cells cannot
exclude high grade squamous
intraepithelial lesion (ASC-H)
R87.611
atypical squamous cells of undetermined
significance (ASC-US) R87.610
cytologic evidence of malignancy
R87.614
high grade squamous intraepithelial
lesion (HGSIL) R87.613
inadequate smear R87.615
low grade squamous intraepithelial
lesion (LGSIL) R87.612
non-atypical endometrial cells
R87.618
satisfactory cervical smear but
lacking transformation zone
R87.616
specified NEC R87.618
thin preparaton R87.619
unsatisfactory smear R87.615
nasal secretions R84.6
nipple discharge R89.6
peritoneal fluid R85.69
pleural fluid R84.6
prostatic secretions R86.6
saliva R85.69
seminal fluid R86.6
sites NEC R89.6
sputum R84.6
synovial fluid R89.6
throat scrapings R84.6

Abnormal, abnormality, abnormalities —
(Continued)
Papanicolaou (smear) (Continued)
vagina R87.629
atypical squamous cells cannot
exclude high grade squamous
intraepithelial lesion (ASC-H)
R87.621
atypical squamous cells of
undetermined significance
(ASC-US) R87.620
cytologic evidence of malignancy
R87.624
high grade squamous intraepithelial
lesion (HGSIL) R87.623
inadequate smear R87.625
low grade squamous intraepithelial
lesion (LGSIL) R87.622
specified NEC R87.628
thin preparation R87.629
unsatisfactory smear R87.625
vulva R87.69
wound secretions R89.6
partial thromboplastin time (PTT) R79.1
pelvis (bony) —see Deformity, pelvis
percussion, chest (tympany) R09.89
periods (grossly) —see Menstruation
phonocardiogram R94.39
plantar reflex R29.2
plasma
protein R77.9
specified NEC R77.8
viscosity R70.1
pleural (folds) Q34.0
posture R29.3
product of conception O02.9
specified type NEC O02.89
prothrombin time (PT) R79.1
pulmonary
artery, congenital Q25.79
function, newborn P28.89
test results R94.2
pulsations in neck R00.2
pupillary H21.56-
function (reaction) (reflex) —see Anomaly,
pupil, function
radiological examination —see Abnormal,
diagnostic imaging
red blood cell (s) (morphology) (volume)
R71.8
reflex —see Reflex
renal function test R94.4
response to nerve stimulation R94.130
retinal correspondence H53.31
retinal function study R94.111
rhythm, heart —see also Arrhythmia
saliva —see Abnormal, specimen, digestive
organs
scan
kidney R94.4
liver R93.2
thyroid R94.6
secretion
gastrin E16.4
glucagon E16.3
semen, seminal fluid —see Abnormal,
specimen, male genital organs
serum level (of)
acid phosphatase R74.8
alkaline phosphatase R74.8
amylase R74.8
enzymes R74.9
specified NEC R74.8
lipase R74.8
triacylglycerol lipase R74.8
shape
gravid uterus —see Anomaly, uterus
sinus venosus Q21.1
size, tooth, teeth K00.2
spacing, tooth, teeth, fully erupted
M26.30

Abnormal, abnormality, abnormalities —
(Continued)
specimen
digestive organs (peritoneal fluid) (saliva)
R85.9
cytology R85.69
drug level R85.2
enzyme level R85.0
histology R85.7
hormones R85.1
immunology R85.4
microbiology R85.5
nonmedicinal level R85.3
specified type NEC R85.89
female genital organs (secretions) (smears)
R87.9
cytology R87.69
cervix R87.619
human papillomavirus (HPV) DNA
test
high risk positive R87.810
low risk positive R87.820
inadequate (unsatisfactory) smear
R87.615
non-atypical endometrial cells
R87.618
specified NEC R87.618
vagina R87.629
human papillomavirus (HPV) DNA
test
high risk positive R87.811
low risk positive R87.821
inadequate (unsatisfactory) smear
R87.625
vulva R87.69
drug level R87.2
enzyme level R87.0
histological R87.7
hormones R87.1
immunology R87.4
microbiology R87.5
nonmedicinal level R87.3
specified type NEC R87.89
male genital organs (prostatic secretions)
(semen) R86.9
cytology R86.6
drug level R86.2
enzyme level R86.0
histological R86.7
hormones R86.1
immunology R86.4
microbiology R86.5
nonmedicinal level R86.3
specified type NEC R86.8
nipple discharge —see Abnormal,
specimen, specified
respiratory organs (bronchial washings)
(nasal secretions) (pleural fluid)
(sputum) R84.9
cytology R84.6
drug level R84.2
enzyme level R84.0
histology R84.7
hormones R84.1
immunology R84.4
microbiology R84.5
nonmedicinal level R84.3
specified type NEC R84.8
specified organ, system and tissue NOS
R89.9
cytology R89.6
drug level R89.2
enzyme level R89.0
histology R89.7
hormones R89.1
immunology R89.4
microbiology R89.5
nonmedicinal level R89.3
specified type NEC R89.8
synovial fluid —see Abnormal, specimen,
specified

Abnormal, abnormality, abnormalities —
(Continued)
specimen (Continued)
thorax (bronchial washings) (pleural
fluids) —see Abnormal, specimen,
respiratory organs
vagina (secretion) (smear) R87.629
vulva (secretion) (smear) R87.69
wound secretion —see Abnormal,
specimen, specified
spermatozoa —see Abnormal, specimen, male
genital organs
sputum (amount) (color) (odor) R09.3
stool (color) (contents) (mucus) R19.5
bloody K92.1
guaiac positive R19.5
synchondrosis Q78.8
thermography —see also Abnormal,
diagnostic imaging R93.8
thyroid-binding globulin E07.89
tooth, teeth (form) (size) K00.2
toxicology (findings) R78.9
transport protein E88.09
tumor marker NEC R97.8
ultrasound results —see Abnormal, diagnostic
imaging
umbilical cord complicating delivery O69.9
urination NEC R39.198 ◀▥
urine (constituents) R82.90
bile R82.2
cytological examination R82.8
drugs R82.5
fat R82.0
glucose R81
heavy metals R82.6
hemoglobin R82.3
histological examination R82.8
ketones R82.4
microbiological examination (culture)
R82.79 ◀▥
myoglobin R82.1
positive culture R82.79 ◀▥
protein —see Proteinuria
specified substance NEC R82.99
chromoabnormality NEC R82.91
substances nonmedical R82.6
uterine hemorrhage —see Hemorrhage,
uterus
vectorcardiogram R94.39
visually evoked potential (VEP) R94.112
white blood cells D72.9
specified NEC D72.89
X-ray examination —see Abnormal,
diagnostic imaging
Abnormity (any organ or part) —see Anomaly
Abocclusion M26.29
hemolytic disease (newborn) P55.1
incompatibility reaction ABO —see
Complication (s), transfusion,
incompatibility reaction, ABO
Abolition, language R48.8
Aborter, habitual or recurrent —see Loss (of),
pregnancy, recurrent
Abortion (complete) (spontaneous) O03.9
with
retained products of conception - see
Abortion, incomplete
attempted (elective) (failed) O07.4
complicated by O07.30
afibrinogenemia O07.1
cardiac arrest O07.36
chemical damage of pelvic organ (s)
O07.34
circulatory collapse O07.31
cystitis O07.38
defibrination syndrome O07.1
electrolyte imbalance O07.33
embolism (air) (amniotic fluid) (blood
clot) (fat) (pulmonary) (septic)
(soap) O07.2
endometritis O07.0

Abortion (Continued)
attempted (Continued)
complicated by (Continued)
genital tract and pelvic infection O07.0
hemolysis O07.1
hemorrhage (delayed) (excessive) O07.1
infection
genital tract or pelvic O07.0
urinary tract tract O07.38
intravascular coagulation O07.1
laceration of pelvic organ(s) O07.34
metabolic disorder O07.33
oliguria O07.32
oophoritis O07.0
parametritis O07.0
pelvic peritonitis O07.0
perforation of pelvic organ(s) O07.34
renal failure or shutdown O07.32
salpingitis or salpingo-oophoritis O07.0
sepsis O07.37
shock O07.31
specified condition NEC O07.39
tubular necrosis (renal) O07.32
uremia O07.32
urinary tract infection O07.38
venous complication NEC O07.35
embolism (air) (amniotic fluid) (blood
clot) (fat) (pulmonary) (septic)
(soap) O07.2
complicated (by) (following) O03.80
afibrinogenemia O03.6
cardiac arrest O03.86
chemical damage of pelvic organ (s) O03.84
circulatory collapse O03.81
cystitis O03.88
defibrination syndrome O03.6
electrolyte imbalance O03.83
embolism (air) (amniotic fluid) (blood
clot) (fat) (pulmonary) (septic) (soap)
O03.7
endometritis O03.5
genital tract and pelvic infection O03.5
hemolysis O03.6
hemorrhage (delayed) (excessive) O03.6
infection
genital tract or pelvic O03.5
urinary tract O03.88
intravascular coagulation O03.6
laceration of pelvic organ (s) O03.84
metabolic disorder O03.83
oliguria O03.82
oophoritis O03.5
parametritis O03.5
pelvic peritonitis O03.5
perforation of pelvic organ (s) O03.84
renal failure or shutdown O03.82
salpingitis or salpingo-oophoritis O03.5
sepsis O03.87
shock O03.81
specified condition NEC O03.89
tubular necrosis (renal) O03.82
uremia O03.82
urinary tract infection O03.88
venous complication NEC O03.85
embolism (air) (amniotic fluid) (blood
clot) (fat) (pulmonary) (septic)
(soap) O03.7
failed —see Abortion, attempted
habitual or recurrent N96
with current abortion —see categories
O03-O06
without current pregnancy N96
care in current pregnancy O26.2-
incomplete (spontaneous) O03.4
complicated (by) (following) O03.30
afibrinogenemia O03.1
cardiac arrest O03.36
chemical damage of pelvic organ (s)
O03.34
circulatory collapse O03.31
cystitis O03.38

◀ New   ◀▥ Revised   ~~deleted~~ Deleted

Abortion *(Continued)*
  incomplete *(Continued)*
    complicated *(Continued)*
      defibrination syndrome O03.1
      electrolyte imbalance O03.33
      embolism (air) (amniotic fluid) (blood
          clot) (fat) (pulmonary) (septic)
          (soap) O03.2
      endometritis O03.0
      genital tract and pelvic infection O03.0
      hemolysis O03.1
      hemorrhage (delayed) (excessive)
          O03.1
      infection
        genital tract or pelvic O03.0
        urinary tract O03.38
      intravascular coagulation O03.1
      laceration of pelvic organ (s) O03.34
      metabolic disorder O03.33
      oliguria O03.32
      oophoritis O03.0
      parametritis O03.0
      pelvic peritonitis O03.0
      perforation of pelvic organ (s) O03.34
      renal failure or shutdown O03.32
      salpingitis or salpingo-oophoritis O03.0
      sepsis O03.37
      shock O03.31
      specified condition NEC O03.39
      tubular necrosis (renal) O03.32
      uremia O03.32
      urinary infection O03.38
      venous complication NEC O03.35
        embolism (air) (amniotic fluid) (blood
            clot) (fat) (pulmonary) (septic)
            (soap) O03.2
  induced (encounter for) Z33.2
    complicated by O04.80
      afibrinogenemia O04.6
      cardiac arrest O04.86
      chemical damage of pelvic organ (s)
          O04.84
      circulatory collapse O04.81
      cystitis O04.88
      defibrination syndrome O04.6
      electrolyte imbalance O04.83
      embolism (air) (amniotic fluid) (blood
          clot) (fat) (pulmonary) (septic)
          (soap) O04.7
      endometritis O04.5
      genital tract and pelvic infection O04.5
      hemolysis O04.6
      hemorrhage (delayed) (excessive) O04.6
      infection
        genital tract or pelvic O04.5
        urinary tract O04.88
      intravascular coagulation O04.6
      laceration of pelvic organ (s) O04.84
      metabolic disorder O04.83
      oliguria O04.82
      oophoritis O04.5
      parametritis O04.5
      pelvic peritonitis O04.5
      perforation of pelvic organ (s) O04.84
      renal failure or shutdown O04.82
      salpingitis or salpingo-oophoritis O04.5
      sepsis O04.87
      shock O04.81
      specified condition NEC O04.89
      tubular necrosis (renal) O04.82
      uremia O04.82
      urinary tract infection O04.88
      venous complication NEC O04.85
        embolism (air) (amniotic fluid) (blood
            clot) (fat) (pulmonary) (septic)
            (soap) O04.7
  missed O02.1
  spontaneous —*see* Abortion (complete)
      (spontaneous)
    threatened O20.0
  threatened (spontaneous) O20.0

Abortion *(Continued)*
  tubal O00.10 ◄▥▥▥
    with intrauterine pregnancy O00.11 ◄
Abortus fever A23.1
Aboulomania F60.7
Abrami's disease D59.8
Abramov-Fiedler myocarditis (acute isolated
    myocarditis) I40.1
Abrasion T14.8
  abdomen, abdominal (wall) S30.811
  alveolar process S00.512
  ankle S90.51-
  antecubital space —*see* Abrasion, elbow
  anus S30.817
  arm (upper) S40.81-
  auditory canal —*see* Abrasion, ear
  auricle —*see* Abrasion, ear
  axilla —*see* Abrasion, arm
  back, lower S30.810
  breast S20.11-
  brow S00.81
  buttock S30.810
  calf —*see* Abrasion, leg
  canthus —*see* Abrasion, eyelid
  cheek S00.81
    internal S00.512
  chest wall —*see* Abrasion, thorax
  chin S00.81
  clitoris S30.814
  cornea S05.0-
  costal region —*see* Abrasion, thorax
  dental K03.1
  digit (s)
    foot —*see* Abrasion, toe
    hand —*see* Abrasion, finger
  ear S00.41-
  elbow S50.31-
  epididymis S30.813
  epigastric region S30.811
  epiglottis S10.11
  esophagus (thoracic) S27.818
    cervical S10.11
  eyebrow —*see* Abrasion, eyelid
  eyelid S00.21-
  face S00.81
  finger (s) S60.41-
    index S60.41-
    little S60.41-
    middle S60.41-
    ring S60.41-
  flank S30.811
  foot (except toe (s) alone) S90.81-
    toe —*see* Abrasion, toe
  forearm S50.81-
    elbow only —*see* Abrasion, elbow
  forehead S00.81
  genital organs, external
    female S30.816
    male S30.815
  groin S30.811
  gum S00.512
  hand S60.51-
  head S00.91
    ear —*see* Abrasion, ear
    eyelid —*see* Abrasion, eyelid
    lip S00.511
    nose S00.31
    oral cavity S00.512
    scalp S00.01
    specified site NEC S00.81
  heel —*see* Abrasion, foot
  hip S70.21-
  inguinal region S30.811
  interscapular region S20.419
  jaw S00.81
  knee S80.21-
  labium (majus) (minus) S30.814
  larynx S10.11
  leg (lower) S80.81-
    knee —*see* Abrasion, knee
    upper —*see* Abrasion, thigh

Abrasion *(Continued)*
  lip S00.511
  lower back S30.810
  lumbar region S30.810
  malar region S00.81
  mammary —*see* Abrasion, breast
  mastoid region S00.81
  mouth S00.512
  nail
    finger —*see* Abrasion, finger
    toe —*see* Abrasion, toe
  nape S10.81
  nasal S00.31
  neck S10.91
    specified site NEC S10.81
    throat S10.11
  nose S00.31
  occipital region S00.01
  oral cavity S00.512
  orbital region —*see* Abrasion, eyelid
  palate S00.512
  palm —*see* Abrasion, hand
  parietal region S00.01
  pelvis S30.810
  penis S30.812
  perineum
    female S30.814
    male S30.810
  periocular area —*see* Abrasion, eyelid
  phalanges
    finger —*see* Abrasion, finger
    toe —*see* Abrasion, toe
  pharynx S10.11
  pinna —*see* Abrasion, ear
  popliteal space —*see* Abrasion, knee
  prepuce S30.812
  pubic region S30.810
  pudendum
    female S30.816
    male S30.815
  sacral region S30.810
  scalp S00.01
  scapular region —*see* Abrasion, shoulder
  scrotum S30.813
  shin —*see* Abrasion, leg
  shoulder S40.21-
  skin NEC T14.8
  sternal region S20.319
  submaxillary region S00.81
  submental region S00.81
  subungual
    finger (s) —*see* Abrasion, finger
    toe (s) —*see* Abrasion, toe
  supraclavicular fossa S10.81
  supraorbital S00.81
  temple S00.81
  temporal region S00.81
  testis S30.813
  thigh S70.31-
  thorax, thoracic (wall) S20.91
    back S20.41-
    front S20.31-
  throat S10.11
  thumb S60.31-
  toe (s) (lesser) S90.416
    great S90.41-
  tongue S00.512
  tooth, teeth (dentifrice) (habitual) (hard
      tissues) (occupational) (ritual)
      (traditional) K03.1
  trachea S10.11
  tunica vaginalis S30.813
  tympanum, tympanic membrane —*see*
      Abrasion, ear
  uvula S00.512
  vagina S30.814
  vocal cords S10.11
  vulva S30.814
  wrist S60.81-
Abrism —*see* Poisoning, food, noxious,
    plant

Abruptio placentae O45.9-
  with
    afibrinogenemia O45.01-
    coagulation defect O45.00-
      specified NEC O45.09-
    disseminated intravascular coagulation O45.02-
    hypofibrinogenemia O45.01-
  specified NEC O45.8-
Abruption, placenta —see Abruptio placentae
Abscess (connective tissue) (embolic) (fistulous) (infective) (metastatic) (multiple) (pernicious) (pyogenic) (septic) L02.91
  with
    diverticular disease (intestine) K57.80
      with bleeding K57.81
      large intestine K57.20
        with
          bleeding K57.21
          small intestine K57.40
            with bleeding K57.41
        small intestine K57.00
          with
            bleeding K57.01
            large intestine K57.40
              with bleeding K57.41
    lymphangitis - code by site under Abscess
  abdomen, abdominal
    cavity K65.1
    wall L02.211
  abdominopelvic K65.1
  accessory sinus —see Sinusitis
  adrenal (capsule) (gland) E27.8
  alveolar K04.7
    with sinus K04.6
  amebic A06.4
    brain (and liver or lung abscess) A06.6
    genitourinary tract A06.82
    liver (without mention of brain or lung abscess) A06.4
    lung (and liver) (without mention of brain abscess) A06.5
    specified site NEC A06.89
    spleen A06.89
  anerobic A48.0
  ankle —see Abscess, lower limb
  anorectal K61.2
  antecubital space —see Abscess, upper limb
  antrum (chronic) (Highmore) —see Sinusitis, maxillary
  anus K61.0
  apical (tooth) K04.7
    with sinus (alveolar) K04.6
  appendix K35.3
  areola (acute) (chronic) (nonpuerperal) N61.1 ◀
    puerperal, postpartum or gestational —see Infection, nipple
  arm (any part) —see Abscess, upper limb
  artery (wall) I77.89
  atheromatous I77.2
  auricle, ear —see Abscess, ear, external
  axilla (region) L02.41-
    lymph gland or node L04.2
  back (any part, except buttock) L02.212
  Bartholin's gland N75.1
    with
      abortion —see Abortion, by type complicated by, sepsis
      ectopic or molar pregnancy O08.0
    following ectopic or molar pregnancy O08.0
  Bezold's —see Mastoiditis, acute
  bilharziasis B65.1
  bladder (wall) —see Cystitis, specified type NEC
  bone (subperiosteal) —see also Osteomyelitis, specified type NEC
    accessory sinus (chronic) —see Sinusitis
    chronic or old —see Osteomyelitis, chronic
    jaw (lower) (upper) M27.2

Abscess (Continued)
  bone (Continued)
    mastoid —see Mastoiditis, acute, subperiosteal
    petrous —see Petrositis
    spinal (tuberculous) A18.01
      nontuberculous —see Osteomyelitis, vertebra
  bowel K63.0
  brain (any part) (cystic) (otogenic) G06.0
    amebic (with abscess of any other site) A06.6
    gonococcal A54.82
    pheomycotic (chromomycotic) B43.1
    tuberculous A17.81
  breast (acute) (chronic) (nonpuerperal) N61.1 ◀
    newborn P39.0
    puerperal, postpartum, gestational —see Mastitis, obstetric, purulent
  broad ligament N73.2
    acute N73.0
    chronic N73.1
  Brodie's (localized) (chronic) M86.8X-
  bronchi J98.09
  buccal cavity K12.2
  bulbourethral gland N34.0
  bursa M71.00
    ankle M71.07-
    elbow M71.02-
    foot M71.07-
    hand M71.04-
    hip M71.05-
    knee M71.06-
    multiple sites M71.09
    pharyngeal J39.1
    shoulder M71.01-
    specified site NEC M71.08
    wrist M71.03-
  buttock L02.31
  canthus —see Blepharoconjunctivitis
  cartilage —see Disorder, cartilage, specified type NEC
  cecum K35.3
  cerebellum, cerebellar G06.0
    sequelae G09
  cerebral (embolic) G06.0
    sequelae G09
  cervical (meaning neck) L02.11
    lymph gland or node L04.0
  cervix (stump) (uteri) —see Cervicitis
  cheek (external) L02.01
    inner K12.2
  chest J86.9
    with fistula J86.0
    wall L02.213
  chin L02.01
  choroid —see Inflammation, chorioretinal
  circumtonsillar J36
  cold (lung) (tuberculous) —see also Tuberculosis, abscess, lung
    articular —see Tuberculosis, joint
  colon K63.0
  colostomy K94.02
  conjunctiva —see Conjunctivitis, acute
  cornea H16.31-
  corpus
    cavernosum N48.21
    luteum —see Oophoritis
  Cowper's gland N34.0
  cranium G06.0
  cul-de-sac (Douglas') (posterior) —see Peritonitis, pelvic, female
  cutaneous —see Abscess, by site
  dental K04.7
    with sinus (alveolar) K04.6
  dentoalveolar K04.7
    with sinus K04.6
  diaphragm, diaphragmatic K65.1
  Douglas' cul-de-sac or pouch —see Peritonitis, pelvic, female
  Dubois A50.59

Abscess (Continued)
  ear (middle) —see also Otitis, media, suppurative
    acute —see Otitis, media, suppurative, acute
    external H60.0-
  entamebic —see Abscess, amebic
  enterostomy K94.12
  epididymis N45.4
  epidural G06.2
    brain G06.0
    spinal cord G06.1
  epiglottis J38.7
  epiploon, epiploic K65.1
  erysipelatous —see Erysipelas
  esophagus K20.8
  ethmoid (bone) (chronic) (sinus) J32.2
  external auditory canal —see Abscess, ear, external
  extradural G06.2
    brain G06.0
      sequelae G09
    spinal cord G06.1
  extraperitoneal K68.19
  eye —see Endophthalmitis, purulent
  eyelid H00.03-
  face (any part, except ear, eye and nose) L02.01
  fallopian tube —see Salpingitis
  fascia M72.8
  fauces J39.1
  fecal K63.0
  femoral (region) —see Abscess, lower limb
  filaria, filarial —see Infestation, filarial
  finger (any) —see also Abscess, hand
    nail —see Cellulitis, finger
  foot L02.61-
  forehead L02.01
  frontal sinus (chronic) J32.1
  gallbladder K81.0
  genital organ or tract
    female (external) N76.4
    male N49.9
      multiple sites N49.8
      specified NEC N49.8
  gestational mammary O91.11-
  gestational subareolar O91.11-
  gingival —see Peridontitis, aggressive, localized ◀
  gland, glandular (lymph) (acute) —see Lymphadenitis, acute
  gluteal (region) L02.31
  gonorrheal —see Gonococcus
  groin L02.214
  gum —see Peridontitis, aggressive, localized ◀
  hand L02.51-
  head NEC L02.811
    face (any part, except ear, eye and nose) L02.01
  heart —see Carditis
  heel —see Abscess, foot
  helminthic —see Infestation, helminth
  hepatic (cholangitic) (hematogenic) (lymphogenic) (pylephlebitic) K75.0
    amebic A06.4
  hip (region) —see Abscess, lower limb
  ileocecal K35.3
  ileostomy (bud) K94.12
  iliac (region) L02.214
    fossa K35.3
  infraclavicular (fossa) —see Abscess, upper limb
  inguinal (region) L02.214
    lymph gland or node L04.1
  intestine, intestinal NEC K63.0
    rectal K61.1
  intra-abdominal —see also Abscess, peritoneum K65.1
    postoperative T81.4
      retroperitoneal K68.11
    postprocedural T81.43 ◀
      retroperitoneal K68.11 ◀
  intra-muscular, postprocedural T81.42 ◀

◀ New   ◀▐ Revised   ~~deleted~~ Deleted

Abscess *(Continued)*
  intracranial G06.0
  intramammary —*see* Abscess, breast
  intraorbital —*see* Abscess, orbit
  intraperitoneal K65.1
  intrasphincteric (anus) K61.4
  intraspinal G06.1
  intratonsillar J36
  ischiorectal (fossa) K61.3
  jaw (bone) (lower) (upper) M27.2
  joint —*see* Arthritis, pyogenic or pyemic
    spine (tuberculous) A18.01
      nontuberculous —*see* Spondylopathy,
        infective
  kidney N15.1
    with calculus N20.0
      with hydronephrosis N13.6
    puerperal (postpartum) O86.21
  knee —*see also* Abscess, lower limb
    joint M00.9
  labium (majus) (minus) N76.4
  lacrimal
    caruncle —*see* Inflammation, lacrimal,
      passages, acute
    gland —*see* Dacryoadenitis
    passages (duct) (sac) —*see* Inflammation,
      lacrimal, passages, acute
  lacunar N34.0
  larynx J38.7
  lateral (alveolar) K04.7
    with sinus K04.6
  leg (any part) —*see* Abscess, lower limb
  lens H27.8
  lingual K14.0
    tonsil J36
  lip K13.0
  Littre's gland N34.0
  liver (cholangitic) (hematogenic)
      (lymphogenic) (pylephlebitic)
      (pyogenic) K75.0
    amebic (due to Entamoeba histolytica)
        (dysenteric) (tropical) A06.4
      with
        brain abscess (and liver or lung
          abscess) A06.6
        lung abscess A06.5
  loin (region) L02.211
  lower limb L02.41-
  lumbar (tuberculous) A18.01
    nontuberculous L02.212
  lung (miliary) (putrid) J85.2
    with pneumonia J85.1
      due to specified organism (*see*
        Pneumonia, in (due to))
    amebic (with liver abscess) A06.5
      with
        brain abscess A06.6
        pneumonia A06.5
  lymph, lymphatic, gland or node (acute) —*see
    also* Lymphadenitis, acute
    mesentery I88.0
  malar M27.2
  mammary gland —*see* Abscess, breast
  marginal, anus K61.0
  mastoid —*see* Mastoiditis, acute
  maxilla, maxillary M27.2
    molar (tooth) K04.7
      with sinus K04.6
    premolar K04.7
    sinus (chronic) J32.0
  mediastinum J85.3
  meibomian gland —*see* Hordeolum
  meninges G06.2
  mesentery, mesenteric K65.1
  mesosalpinx —*see* Salpingitis
  mons pubis L02.215
  mouth (floor) K12.2
  muscle —*see* Myositis, infective
  myocardium I40.0
  nabothian (follicle) —*see* Cervicitis
  nasal J32.9
  nasopharyngeal J39.1

Abscess *(Continued)*
  navel L02.216
    newborn P38.9
      with mild hemorrhage P38.1
      without hemorrhage P38.9
  neck (region) L02.11
    lymph gland or node L04.0
  nephritic —*see* Abscess, kidney
  nipple N61.1 ◀▥
    associated with
      lactation —*see* Pregnancy, complicated
        by ◀▥
      pregnancy —*see* Pregnancy, complicated
        by
  nose (external) (fossa) (septum) J34.0
    sinus (chronic) —*see* Sinusitis
  omentum K65.1
  operative wound T81.40 ◀▥
  orbit, orbital —*see* Cellulitis, orbit
  otogenic G06.0
  ovary, ovarian (corpus luteum) —*see*
      Oophoritis
  oviduct —*see* Oophoritis
  palate (soft) K12.2
    hard M27.2
  palmar (space) —*see* Abscess, hand
  pancreas (duct) —*see* Pancreatitis, acute
  parafrenal N48.21
  parametric, parametrium N73.2
    acute N73.0
    chronic N73.1
  paranephric N15.1
  parapancreatic —*see* Pancreatitis, acute
  parapharyngeal J39.0
  pararectal K61.1
  parasinus —*see* Sinusitis
  parauterine (*see also* Disease, pelvis,
      inflammatory) N73.2
  paravaginal —*see* Vaginitis
  parietal region (scalp) L02.811
  parodontal —*see* Peridontitis, aggressive,
      localized ◀▥
  parotid (duct) (gland) K11.3
    region K12.2
  pectoral (region) L02.213
  pelvis, pelvic
    female —*see* Disease, pelvis, inflammatory
    male, peritoneal K65.1
  penis N48.21
    gonococcal (accessory gland) (periurethral)
      A54.1
  perianal K61.0
  periapical K04.7
    with sinus (alveolar) K04.6
  periappendicular K35.3
  pericardial I30.1
  pericecal K35.3
  pericemental —*see* Peridontitis, aggressive,
      localized ◀▥
  pericholecystic —*see* Cholecystitis, acute
  pericoronal —*see* Peridontitis, aggressive,
      localized ◀▥
  peridental —*see* Peridontitis, aggressive,
      localized ◀▥
  perimetric —*see also* Disease, pelvis,
      inflammatory N73.2
  perinephric, perinephritic —*see* Abscess,
      kidney
  perineum, perineal (superficial) L02.215
    urethra N34.0
  periodontal (parietal) —*see* Peridontitis,
      aggressive, localized ◀▥
    apical K04.7
  periosteum, periosteal —*see also*
      Osteomyelitis, specified type NEC
    with osteomyelitis —*see also* Osteomyelitis,
      specified type NEC
    acute —*see* Osteomyelitis, acute
    chronic —*see* Osteomyelitis, chronic
  peripharyngeal J39.0
  peripleuritic J86.9
    with fistula J86.0

Abscess *(Continued)*
  periprostatic N41.2
  perirectal K61.1
  perirenal (tissue) —*see* Abscess, kidney
  perisinuous (nose) —*see* Sinusitis
  peritoneum, peritoneal (perforated)
      (ruptured) K65.1
    with appendicitis K35.3
    pelvic
      female —*see* Peritonitis, pelvic, female
        K65.1
      male K65.1
    postoperative T81.43 ◀▥
    puerperal, postpartum, childbirth O85
    tuberculous A18.31
  peritonsillar J36
  perityphlic K35.3
  periureteral N28.89
  periurethral N34.0
    gonococcal (accessory gland) (periurethral)
      A54.1
  periuterine —*see also* Disease, pelvis,
      inflammatory N73.2
  perivesical —*see* Cystitis, specified type NEC
  petrous bone —*see* Petrositis
  phagedenic NOS L02.91
    chancroid A57
  pharynx, pharyngeal (lateral) J39.1
  pilonidal L05.01
  pituitary (gland) E23.6
  pleura J86.9
    with fistula J86.0
  popliteal —*see* Abscess, lower limb
  postcecal K35.3
  postlaryngeal J38.7
  postnasal J34.0
  postoperative (any site) T81.40 ◀▥
    retroperitoneal K68.11
  postpharyngeal J39.0
  posttonsillar J36
  post-typhoid A01.09
  pouch of Douglas —*see* Peritonitis, pelvic,
      female
  premammary —*see* Abscess, breast
  prepatellar —*see* Abscess, lower limb
  prostate N41.2
    gonococcal (acute) (chronic) A54.22
  psoas muscle K68.12
  puerperal - code by site under Puerperal,
      abscess
  pulmonary —*see* Abscess, lung
  pulp, pulpal (dental) K04.01 ◀▥
    irreversible K04.02 ◀
    reversible K04.01 ◀
  rectovaginal septum K63.0
  rectovesical —*see* Cystitis, specified type NEC
  rectum K61.1
  renal —*see* Abscess, kidney
  retina —*see* Inflammation, chorioretinal
  retrobulbar —*see* Abscess, orbit
  retrocecal K65.1
  retrolaryngeal J38.7
  retromammary —*see* Abscess, breast
  retroperitoneal NEC K68.19
    postprocedural K68.11
  retropharyngeal J39.0
  retrouterine —*see* Peritonitis, pelvic, female
  retrovesical —*see* Cystitis, specified type NEC
  root, tooth K04.7
    with sinus (alveolar) K04.6
  round ligament —*see also* Disease, pelvis,
      inflammatory N73.2
  rupture (spontaneous) NOS L02.91
  sacrum (tuberculous) A18.01
    nontuberculous M46.28
  salivary (duct) (gland) K11.3
  scalp (any part) L02.811
  scapular —*see* Osteomyelitis, specified type
      NEC
  sclera —*see* Scleritis
  scrofulous (tuberculous) A18.2
  scrotum N49.2

Abscess (Continued)
seminal vesicle N49.0
septal, dental K04.7
  with sinus (alveolar) K04.6
serous —see Periostitis
shoulder (region) —see Abscess, upper limb
sigmoid K63.0
sinus (accessory) (chronic) (nasal) —see also
  Sinusitis
  intracranial venous (any) G06.0
Skene's duct or gland N34.0
skin —see Abscess, by site
specified site NEC L02.818
spermatic cord N49.1
sphenoidal (sinus) (chronic) J32.3
spinal cord (any part) (staphylococcal) G06.1
  tuberculous A17.81
spine (column) (tuberculous) A18.01
  epidural G06.1
  nontuberculous —see Osteomyelitis,
    vertebra
spleen D73.3
  amebic A06.89
stitch T81.48 ◀▥
subarachnoid G06.2
  brain G06.0
  spinal cord G06.1
subareolar —see Abscess, breast
subcecal K35.3
subcutaneous —see also Abscess, by site
  pheomycotic (chromomycotic) B43.2
  postprocedural T81.41 ◀
subdiaphragmatic K65.1
subdural G06.2
  brain G06.0
    sequelae G09
  spinal cord G06.1
subgaleal L02.811
subhepatic K65.1
sublingual K12.2
  gland K11.3
submammary —see Abscess, breast
submandibular (region) (space) (triangle) K12.2
  gland K11.3
submaxillary (region) L02.01
  gland K11.3
submental L02.01
  gland K11.3
subperiosteal —see Osteomyelitis, specified
  type NEC
subphrenic K65.1
  postoperative T81.43 ◀▥
suburethral N34.0
sudoriparous L75.8
supraclavicular (fossa) —see Abscess, upper
  limb
suprapelvic, acute N73.0
suprarenal (capsule) (gland) E27.8
sweat gland L74.8
tear duct —see Inflammation, lacrimal,
  passages, acute
temple L02.01
temporal region L02.01
temporosphenoidal G06.0
tendon (sheath) M65.00
  ankle M65.07-
  foot M65.07-
  forearm M65.03-
  hand M65.04-
  lower leg M65.06-
  pelvic region M65.05-
  shoulder region M65.01-
  specified site NEC M65.08
  thigh M65.05-
  upper arm M65.02-
testis N45.4
thigh —see Abscess, lower limb
thorax J86.9
  with fistula J86.0
throat J39.1
thumb —see also Abscess, hand
  nail —see Cellulitis, finger

Abscess (Continued)
thymus (gland) E32.1
thyroid (gland) E06.0
toe (any) —see also Abscess, foot
  nail —see Cellulitis, toe
tongue (staphylococcal) K14.0
tonsil (s) (lingual) J36
tonsillopharyngeal J36
tooth, teeth (root) K04.7
  with sinus (alveolar) K04.6
  supporting structures NEC —see
    Peridontitis, aggressive, localized ◀▥
trachea J39.8
trunk L02.219
  abdominal wall L02.211
  back L02.212
  chest wall L02.213
  groin L02.214
  perineum L02.215
  umbilicus L02.216
tubal —see Salpingitis
tuberculous —see Tuberculosis, abscess
tubo-ovarian —see Salpingo-oophoritis
tunica vaginalis N49.1
umbilicus L02.216
upper
  limb L02.41-
  respiratory J39.8
urethral (gland) N34.0
urinary N34.0
uterus, uterine (wall) —see also Endometritis
  ligament —see also Disease, pelvis,
    inflammatory N73.2
  neck —see Cervicitis
uvula K12.2
vagina (wall) —see Vaginitis
vaginorectal —see Vaginitis
vas deferens N49.1
vermiform appendix K35.3
vertebra (column) (tuberculous) A18.01
  nontuberculous —see Osteomyelitis,
    vertebra
vesical —see Cystitis, specified type NEC
vesico-uterine pouch —see Peritonitis, pelvic,
  female
vitreous (humor) —see Endophthalmitis,
  purulent
vocal cord J38.3
von Bezold's —see Mastoiditis, acute
vulva N76.4
vulvovaginal gland N75.1
web space —see Abscess, hand
wound T81.40 ◀▥
wrist —see Abscess, upper limb
Absence (of) (organ or part) (complete or
  partial)
adrenal (gland) (congenital) Q89.1
  acquired E89.6
albumin in blood E88.09
alimentary tract (congenital) Q45.8
  upper Q40.8
alveolar process (acquired) —see Anomaly,
  alveolar
ankle (acquired) Z89.44-
anus (congenital) Q42.3
  with fistula Q42.2
aorta (congenital) Q25.41 ◀▥
appendix, congenital Q42.8
arm (acquired) Z89.20-
  above elbow Z89.22-
    congenital (with hand present) —see
      Agenesis, arm, with hand present
    and hand —see Agenesis, forearm,
      and hand
  below elbow Z89.21-
    congenital (with hand present) —see
      Agenesis, arm, with hand present
    and hand —see Agenesis, forearm,
      and hand
  congenital —see Defect, reduction, upper
    limb

Absence (Continued)
arm (Continued)
  shoulder (following explantation of
    shoulder joint prosthesis) (joint) (with
    or without presence of antibiotic-
    impregnated cement spacer) Z89.23-
  congenital (with hand present) —see
    Agenesis, arm, with hand present
artery (congenital) (peripheral) Q27.8
  brain Q28.3
  coronary Q24.5
  pulmonary Q25.79
  specified NEC Q27.8
  umbilical Q27.0
atrial septum (congenital) Q21.1
auditory canal (congenital) (external) Q16.1
auricle (ear), congenital Q16.0
bile, biliary duct, congenital Q44.5
bladder (acquired) Z90.6
  congenital Q64.5
bowel sounds R19.11
brain Q00.0
  part of Q04.3
breast (s) (and nipple (s)) (acquired) Z90.1-
  congenital Q83.8
broad ligament Q50.6
bronchus (congenital) Q32.4
canaliculus lacrimalis, congenital Q10.4
cerebellum (vermis) Q04.3
cervix (acquired) (with uterus) Z90.710
  with remaining uterus Z90.712
  congenital Q51.5
chin, congenital Q18.8
cilia (congenital) Q10.3
  acquired —see Madarosis
clitoris (congenital) Q52.6
coccyx, congenital Q76.49
cold sense R20.8
congenital
  lumen —see Atresia
  organ or site NEC —see Agenesis
  septum —see Imperfect, closure
corpus callosum Q04.0
cricoid cartilage, congenital Q31.8
diaphragm (with hernia), congenital Q79.1
digestive organ (s) or tract, congenital Q45.8
  acquired NEC Z90.49
  upper Q40.8
ductus arteriosus Q28.8
duodenum (acquired) Z90.49
  congenital Q41.0
ear, congenital Q16.9
  acquired H93.8-
  auricle Q16.0
  external Q16.0
  inner Q16.5
  lobe, lobule Q17.8
  middle, except ossicles Q16.4
    ossicles Q16.3
  ossicles Q16.3
ejaculatory duct (congenital) Q55.4
endocrine gland (congenital) NEC Q89.2
  acquired E89.89
epididymis (congenital) Q55.4
  acquired Z90.79
epiglottis, congenital Q31.8
esophagus (congenital) Q39.8
  acquired (partial) Z90.49
eustachian tube (congenital) Q16.2
extremity (acquired) Z89.9
  congenital Q73.0
  knee (following explantation of knee joint
    prosthesis) (joint) (with or without
    presence of antibiotic-impregnated
    cement spacer) Z89.52-
  lower (above knee) Z89.619
    below knee Z89.51-
  upper —see Absence, arm
eye (acquired) Z90.01
  congenital Q11.1
  muscle (congenital) Q10.3

◀ New   ◀▥ Revised   ~~deleted~~ Deleted

Absence (Continued)
  eyeball (acquired) Z90.01
  eyelid (fold) (congenital) Q10.3
    acquired Z90.01
  face, specified part NEC Q18.8
  fallopian tube (s) (acquired) Z90.79
    congenital Q50.6
  family member (causing problem in home)
      NEC —see also Disruption, family Z63.32
  femur, congenital —see Defect, reduction,
      lower limb, longitudinal, femur
  fibrinogen (congenital) D68.2
    acquired D65
  finger (s) (acquired) Z89.02-
    congenital —see Agenesis, hand
  foot (acquired) Z89.43-
    congenital —see Agenesis, foot
  forearm (acquired) —see Absence, arm, below
      elbow
  gallbladder (acquired) Z90.49
    congenital Q44.0
  gamma globulin in blood D80.1
    hereditary D80.0
  genital organs
    acquired (female) (male) Z90.79
    female, congenital Q52.8
      external Q52.71
      internal NEC Q52.8
    male, congenital Q55.8
  genitourinary organs, congenital NEC
    female Q52.8
    male Q55.8
  globe (acquired) Z90.01
    congenital Q11.1
  glottis, congenital Q31.8
  hand and wrist (acquired) Z89.11-
    congenital —see Agenesis, hand
  head, part (acquired) NEC Z90.09
  heat sense R20.8
  hip (following explantation of hip joint
      prosthesis) (joint) (with or without
      presence of antibiotic-impregnated
      cement spacer) Z89.62-
  hymen (congenital) Q52.4
  ileum (acquired) Z90.49
    congenital Q41.2
  immunoglobulin, isolated NEC D80.3
    IgA D80.2
    IgG D80.3
    IgM D80.4
  incus (acquired) —see Loss, ossicles, ear
    congenital Q16.3
  inner ear, congenital Q16.5
  intestine (acquired) (small) Z90.49
    congenital Q41.9
      specified NEC Q41.8
    large Z90.49
      congenital Q42.9
        specified NEC Q42.8
  iris, congenital Q13.1
  jejunum (acquired) Z90.49
    congenital Q41.1
  joint
    acquired
      hip (following explantation of hip
          joint prosthesis) (with or without
          presence of antibiotic-impregnated
          cement spacer) Z89.62-
      knee (following explantation of knee
          joint prosthesis) (with or without
          presence of antibiotic-impregnated
          cement spacer) Z89.52-
      shoulder (following explantation of
          shoulder joint prosthesis) (with
          or without presence of antibiotic-
          impregnated cement spacer)
          Z89.23-
    congenital NEC Q74.8
  kidney (s) (acquired) Z90.5
    congenital Q60.2
      bilateral Q60.1
      unilateral Q60.0

Absence (Continued)
  knee (following explantation of knee joint
      prosthesis) (joint) (with or without
      presence of antibiotic-impregnated
      cement spacer) Z89.52-
  labyrinth, membranous Q16.5
  larynx (congenital) Q31.8
    acquired Z90.02
  leg (acquired) (above knee) Z89.61-
    below knee (acquired) Z89.51-
    congenital —see Defect, reduction, lower
        limb
  lens (acquired) —see also Aphakia
    congenital Q12.3
    post cataract extraction Z98.4-
  limb (acquired) —see Absence, extremity
  lip Q38.6
  liver (congenital) Q44.7
  lung (fissure) (lobe) (bilateral) (unilateral)
      (congenital) Q33.3
    acquired (any part) Z90.2
  menstruation —see Amenorrhea
  muscle (congenital) (pectoral) Q79.8
    ocular Q10.3
  neck, part Q18.8
  neutrophil —see Agranulocytosis
  nipple (s) (with breast (s)) (acquired) Z90.1-
    congenital Q83.2
  nose (congenital) Q30.1
    acquired Z90.09
  organ
    of Corti, congenital Q16.5
    or site, congenital NEC Q89.8
      acquired NEC Z90.89
  osseous meatus (ear) Q16.4
  ovary (acquired)
    bilateral Z90.722
    congenital
      bilateral Q50.02
      unilateral Q50.01
    unilateral Z90.721
  oviduct (acquired)
    bilateral Z90.722
    congenital Q50.6
    unilateral Z90.721
  pancreas (congenital) Q45.0
    acquired Z90.410
      complete Z90.410
      partial Z90.411
      total Z90.410
  parathyroid gland (acquired) E89.2
    congenital Q89.2
  patella, congenital Q74.1
  penis (congenital) Q55.5
    acquired Z90.79
  pericardium (congenital) Q24.8
  pituitary gland (congenital) Q89.2
    acquired E89.3
  prostate (acquired) Z90.79
    congenital Q55.4
  pulmonary valve Q22.0
  punctum lacrimale (congenital) Q10.4
  radius, congenital —see Defect, reduction,
      upper limb, longitudinal, radius
  rectum (congenital) Q42.1
    with fistula Q42.0
    acquired Z90.49
  respiratory organ NOS Q34.9
  rib (acquired) Z90.89
    congenital Q76.6
  sacrum, congenital Q76.49
  salivary gland (s), congenital Q38.4
  scrotum, congenital Q55.29
  seminal vesicles (congenital) Q55.4
    acquired Z90.79
  septum
    atrial (congenital) Q21.1
    between aorta and pulmonary artery Q21.4
    ventricular (congenital) Q20.4
  sex chromosome
    female phenotype Q97.8
    male phenotype Q98.8

Absence (Continued)
  skull bone (congenital) Q75.8
    with
      anencephaly Q00.0
      encephalocele —see Encephalocele
      hydrocephalus Q03.9
        with spina bifida —see Spina
            bifida, by site, with
            hydrocephalus
      microcephaly Q02
  spermatic cord, congenital Q55.4
  spine, congenital Q76.49
  spleen (congenital) Q89.01
    acquired Z90.81
  sternum, congenital Q76.7
  stomach (acquired) (partial) Z90.3
    congenital Q40.2
  superior vena cava, congenital
      Q26.8
  teeth, tooth (congenital) K00.0
    acquired (complete) K08.109
      class I K08.101
      class II K08.102
      class III K08.103
      class IV K08.104
      due to
        caries K08.139
          class I K08.131
          class II K08.132
          class III K08.133
          class IV K08.134
        periodontal disease K08.129
          class I K08.121
          class II K08.122
          class III K08.123
          class IV K08.124
        specified NEC K08.199
          class I K08.191
          class II K08.192
          class III K08.193
          class IV K08.194
        trauma K08.119
          class I K08.111
          class II K08.112
          class III K08.113
          class IV K08.114
    partial K08.409
      class I K08.401
      class II K08.402
      class III K08.403
      class IV K08.404
      due to
        caries K08.439
          class I K08.431
          class II K08.432
          class III K08.433
          class IV K08.434
        periodontal disease K08.429
          class I K08.421
          class II K08.422
          class III K08.423
          class IV K08.424
        specified NEC K08.499
          class I K08.491
          class II K08.492
          class III K08.493
          class IV K08.494
        trauma K08.419
          class I K08.411
          class II K08.412
          class III K08.413
          class IV K08.414
  tendon (congenital) Q79.8
  testis (congenital) Q55.0
    acquired Z90.79
  thumb (acquired) Z89.01-
    congenital —see Agenesis, hand
  thymus gland Q89.2
  thyroid (gland) (acquired) E89.0
    cartilage, congenital Q31.8
    congenital E03.1

Absence *(Continued)*
  toe (s) (acquired) Z89.42-
    with foot —*see* Absence, foot and
      ankle
    congenital —*see* Agenesis, foot
    great Z89.41-
  tongue, congenital Q38.3
  trachea (cartilage), congenital Q32.1
  transverse aortic arch, congenital
    Q25.49 ◄▥
  tricuspid valve Q22.4
  umbilical artery, congenital Q27.0
  upper arm and forearm with hand present,
    congenital —*see* Agenesis, arm, with
    hand present
  ureter (congenital) Q62.4
    acquired Z90.6
  urethra, congenital Q64.5
  uterus (acquired) Z90.710
    with cervix Z90.710
      with remaining cervical stump
        Z90.711
    congenital Q51.0
  uvula, congenital Q38.5
  vagina, congenital Q52.0
  vas deferens (congenital) Q55.4
    acquired Z90.79
  vein (peripheral) congenital NEC
    Q27.8
    cerebral Q28.3
    digestive system Q27.8
    great Q26.8
    lower limb Q27.8
    portal Q26.5
    precerebral Q28.1
    specified site NEC Q27.8
    upper limb Q27.8
  vena cava (inferior) (superior), congenital
    Q26.8
  ventricular septum Q20.4
  vertebra, congenital Q76.49
  vulva, congenital Q52.71
  wrist (acquired) Z89.12-
Absorbent system disease I87.8
Absorption
  carbohydrate, disturbance K90.49 ◄▥
  chemical —*see* Table of Drugs and
    Chemicals
    through placenta (newborn) P04.9
      environmental substance P04.6
      nutritional substance P04.5
      obstetric anesthetic or analgesic drug
        P04.0
  drug NEC —*see* Table of Drugs and
    Chemicals
    addictive
      through placenta (newborn) P04.49
        cocaine P04.41
    medicinal
      through placenta (newborn) P04.1
    through placenta (newborn) P04.1
      obstetric anesthetic or analgesic drug
        P04.0
  fat, disturbance K90.49 ◄▥
    pancreatic K90.3
  noxious substance —*see* Table of Drugs and
    Chemicals
  protein, disturbance K90.49 ◄▥
  starch, disturbance K90.49 ◄▥
  toxic substance —*see* Table of Drugs and
    Chemicals
  uremic —*see* Uremia
Abstinence symptoms, syndrome
  alcohol F10.239
    with delirium F10.231
  cocaine F14.23
  neonatal P96.1
  nicotine —*see* Dependence, drug, nicotine,
    with, withdrawal
  opioid F11.93
    with dependence F11.23

Abstinence symptoms, syndrome *(Continued)*
  psychoactive NEC F19.939
    with
      delirium F19.931
      dependence F19.239
        with
          delirium F19.231
          perceptual disturbance F19.232
        uncomplicated F19.230
      perceptual disturbance F19.932
    uncomplicated F19.930
  sedative F13.939
    with
      delirium F13.931
      dependence F13.239
        with
          delirium F13.231
          perceptual disturbance F13.232
        uncomplicated F13.230
      perceptual disturbance F13.932
    uncomplicated F13.930
  stimulant NEC F15.93
    with dependence F15.23
Abulia R68.89
Abulomania F60.7
Abuse
  adult —*see* Maltreatment, adult
    as reason for
      couple seeking advice (including
        offender) Z63.0
  alcohol (non-dependent) F10.10
    with
      anxiety disorder F10.180
      intoxication F10.129
        with delirium F10.121
        uncomplicated F10.120
      mood disorder F10.14
      other specified disorder F10.188
      psychosis F10.159
        delusions F10.150
        hallucinations F10.151
      sexual dysfunction F10.181
      sleep disorder F10.182
      unspecified disorder F10.19
    counseling and surveillance Z71.41
  amphetamine (or related substance) —*see*
    Abuse, drug, stimulant NEC
  analgesics (non-prescribed) (over the counter)
    F55.8
  antacids F55.0
  antidepressants —*see* Abuse, drug,
    psychoactive NEC
  anxiolytic —*see* Abuse, drug, sedative
  barbiturates —*see* Abuse, drug, sedative
  caffeine —*see* Abuse, drug, stimulant NEC
  cannabis, cannabinoids —*see* Abuse, drug,
    cannabis
  child —*see* Maltreatment, child
  cocaine —*see* Abuse, drug, cocaine
  drug NEC (non-dependent) F19.10
    with sleep disorder F19.182
    amphetamine type —*see* Abuse, drug,
      stimulant NEC
    analgesics (non-prescribed) (over the
      counter) F55.8
    antacids F55.0
    antidepressants —*see* Abuse, drug,
      psychoactive NEC
    anxiolytics —*see* Abuse, drug, sedative
    barbiturates —*see* Abuse, drug, sedative
    caffeine —*see* Abuse, drug, stimulant NEC
    cannabis F12.10
      with
        anxiety disorder F12.180
        intoxication F12.129
          with
            delirium F12.121
            perceptual disturbance
              F12.122
          uncomplicated F12.120
        other specified disorder F12.188

Abuse *(Continued)*
  drug NEC *(Continued)*
    cannabis *(Continued)*
      with *(Continued)*
        psychosis F12.159
          delusions F12.150
          hallucinations F12.151
        unspecified disorder F12.19
    cocaine F14.10
      with
        anxiety disorder F14.180
        intoxication F14.129
          with
            delirium F14.121
            perceptual disturbance F14.122
          uncomplicated F14.120
        mood disorder F14.14
        other specified disorder F14.188
        psychosis F14.159
          delusions F14.150
          hallucinations F14.151
        sexual dysfunction F14.181
        sleep disorder F14.182
        unspecified disorder F14.19
    counseling and surveillance Z71.51
    hallucinogen F16.10
      with
        anxiety disorder F16.180
        flashbacks F16.183
        intoxication F16.129
          with
            delirium F16.121
            perceptual disturbance F16.122
          uncomplicated F16.120
        mood disorder F16.14
        other specified disorder F16.188
        perception disorder, persisting F16.183
        psychosis F16.159
          delusions F16.150
          hallucinations F16.151
        unspecified disorder F16.19
    hashish —*see* Abuse, drug, cannabis
    herbal or folk remedies F55.1
    hormones F55.3
    hypnotics —*see* Abuse, drug, sedative
    inhalant F18.10
      with
        anxiety disorder F18.180
        dementia, persisting F18.17
        intoxication F18.129
          with delirium F18.121
          uncomplicated F18.120
        mood disorder F18.14
        other specified disorder F18.188
        psychosis F18.159
          delusions F18.150
          hallucinations F18.151
        unspecified disorder F18.19
    laxatives F55.2
    LSD —*see* Abuse, drug, hallucinogen
    marihuana —*see* Abuse, drug, cannabis
    morphine type (opioids) —*see* Abuse, drug,
      opioid
    opioid F11.10
      with
        intoxication F11.129
          with
            delirium F11.121
            perceptual disturbance F11.122
          uncomplicated F11.120
        mood disorder F11.14
        other specified disorder F11.188
        psychosis F11.159
          delusions F11.150
          hallucinations F11.151
        sexual dysfunction F11.181
        sleep disorder F11.182
        unspecified disorder F11.19
    PCP (phencyclidine) (or related
      substance) —*see* Abuse, drug,
      hallucinogen

Abuse (Continued)
  drug NEC (Continued)
    psychoactive NEC F19.10
      with
        amnestic disorder F19.16
        anxiety disorder F19.180
        dementia F19.17
        intoxication F19.129
          with
            delirium F19.121
            perceptual disturbance
              F19.122
          uncomplicated F19.120
        mood disorder F19.14
        other specified disorder F19.188
        psychosis F19.159
          delusions F19.150
          hallucinations F19.151
        sexual dysfunction F19.181
        sleep disorder F19.182
        unspecified disorder F19.19
    sedative, hypnotic or anxiolytic F13.10
      with
        anxiety disorder F13.180
        intoxication F13.129
          with delirium F13.121
          uncomplicated F13.120
        mood disorder F13.14
        other specified disorder F13.188
        psychosis F13.159
          delusions F13.150
          hallucinations F13.151
        sexual dysfunction F13.181
        sleep disorder F13.182
        unspecified disorder F13.19
    solvent —see Abuse, drug, inhalant
    steroids F55.3
    stimulant NEC F15.10
      with
        anxiety disorder F15.180
        intoxication F15.129
          with
            delirium F15.121
            perceptual disturbance F15.122
          uncomplicated F15.120
        mood disorder F15.14
        other specified disorder F15.188
        psychosis F15.159
          delusions F15.150
          hallucinations F15.151
        sexual dysfunction F15.181
        sleep disorder F15.182
        unspecified disorder F15.19
    tranquilizers —see Abuse, drug, sedative
    vitamins F55.4
  hallucinogens —see Abuse, drug,
      hallucinogen
  hashish —see Abuse, drug, cannabis
  herbal or folk remedies F55.1
  hormones F55.3
  hypnotic —see Abuse, drug, sedative
  inhalant —see Abuse, drug, inhalant
  laxatives F55.2
  LSD —see Abuse, drug, hallucinogen
  marihuana —see Abuse, drug, cannabis
  morphine type (opioids) —see Abuse, drug,
      opioid
  non-psychoactive substance NEC F55.8
    antacids F55.0
    folk remedies F55.1
    herbal remedies F55.1
    hormones F55.3
    laxatives F55.2
    steroids F55.3
    vitamins F55.4
  opioids —see Abuse, drug, opioid
  PCP (phencyclidine) (or related substance) —
      see Abuse, drug, hallucinogen
  physical (adult) (child) —see Maltreatment
  psychoactive substance —see Abuse, drug,
      psychoactive NEC

Abuse (Continued)
  psychological (adult) (child) —see
      Maltreatment
  sedative —see Abuse, drug, sedative
  sexual —see Maltreatment
  solvent —see Abuse, drug, inhalant
  steroids F55.3
  vitamins F55.4
Acalculia R48.8
  developmental F81.2
Acanthamebiasis (with) B60.10
  conjunctiva B60.12
  keratoconjunctivitis B60.13
  meningoencephalitis B60.11
  other specified B60.19
Acanthocephaliasis B83.8
Acanthocheilonemiasis B74.4
Acanthocytosis E78.6
Acantholysis L11.9
Acanthosis (acquired) (nigricans) L83
  benign Q82.8
  congenital Q82.8
  seborrheic L82.1
    inflamed L82.0
  tongue K14.3
Acapnia E87.3
Acarbia E87.2
Acardia, acardius Q89.8
Acardiacus amorphus Q89.8
Acardiotrophia I51.4
Acariasis B88.0
  scabies B86
Acarodermatitis (urticarioides) B88.0
Acarophobia F40.218
Acatalasemia, acatalasia E80.3
Acathisia (drug induced) G25.71
Accelerated atrioventricular conduction
    I45.6
Accentuation of personality traits (type A)
    Z73.1
Accessory (congenital)
  adrenal gland Q89.1
  anus Q43.4
  appendix Q43.4
  atrioventricular conduction I45.6
  auditory ossicles Q16.3
  auricle (ear) Q17.0
  biliary duct or passage Q44.5
  bladder Q64.79
  blood vessels NEC Q27.9
    coronary Q24.5
  bone NEC Q79.8
  breast tissue, axilla Q83.1
  carpal bones Q74.0
  cecum Q43.4
  chromosome (s) NEC (nonsex) Q92.9
    with complex rearrangements NEC
        Q92.5
    seen only at prometaphase
        Q92.8
    13 —see Trisomy, 13
    18 —see Trisomy, 18
    21 —see Trisomy, 21
    partial Q92.9
    sex
      female phenotype Q97.8
  coronary artery Q24.5
  cusp (s), heart valve NEC Q24.8
    pulmonary Q22.3
  cystic duct Q44.5
  digit (s) Q69.9
  ear (auricle) (lobe) Q17.0
  endocrine gland NEC Q89.2
  eye muscle Q10.3
  eyelid Q10.3
  face bone (s) Q75.8
  fallopian tube (fimbria) (ostium)
      Q50.6
  finger (s) Q69.0
  foreskin N47.8
  frontonasal process Q75.8

Accessory (Continued)
  gallbladder Q44.1
  genital organ (s)
    female Q52.8
      external Q52.79
      internal NEC Q52.8
    male Q55.8
  genitourinary organs NEC Q89.8
    female Q52.8
    male Q55.8
  hallux Q69.2
  heart Q24.8
    valve NEC Q24.8
      pulmonary Q22.3
  hepatic ducts Q44.5
  hymen Q52.4
  intestine (large) (small) Q43.4
  kidney Q63.0
  lacrimal canal Q10.6
  leaflet, heart valve NEC Q24.8
  ligament, broad Q50.6
  liver Q44.7
    duct Q44.5
  lobule (ear) Q17.0
  lung (lobe) Q33.1
  muscle Q79.8
  navicular of carpus Q74.0
  nervous system, part NEC Q07.8
  nipple Q83.3
  nose Q30.8
  organ or site not listed —see Anomaly,
      by site
  ovary Q50.31
  oviduct Q50.6
  pancreas Q45.3
  parathyroid gland Q89.2
  parotid gland (and duct) Q38.4
  pituitary gland Q89.2
  preauricular appendage Q17.0
  prepuce N47.8
  renal arteries (multiple) Q27.2
  rib Q76.6
    cervical Q76.5
  roots (teeth) K00.2
  salivary gland Q38.4
  sesamoid bones Q74.8
    foot Q74.2
    hand Q74.0
  skin tags Q82.8
  spleen Q89.09
  sternum Q76.7
  submaxillary gland Q38.4
  tarsal bones Q74.2
  teeth, tooth K00.1
  tendon Q79.8
  thumb Q69.1
  thymus gland Q89.2
  thyroid gland Q89.2
  toes Q69.2
  tongue Q38.3
  tooth, teeth K00.1
  tragus Q17.0
  ureter Q62.5
  urethra Q64.79
  urinary organ or tract NEC Q64.8
  uterus Q51.2
  vagina Q52.10
  valve, heart NEC Q24.8
    pulmonary Q22.3
  vertebra Q76.49
  vocal cords Q31.8
  vulva Q52.79
Accident
  birth —see Birth, injury
  cardiac —see Infarct, myocardium
  cerebral I63.9
  cerebrovascular (embolic) (ischemic)
      (thrombotic) I63.9
    aborted I63.9
    hemorrhagic —see Hemorrhage,
        intracranial, intracerebral

Accident (*Continued*)
  cerebrovascular (*Continued*)
    old (without sequelae) Z86.73
      with sequelae (of) —*see* Sequelae,
        infarction, cerebral
  coronary —*see* Infarct, myocardium
  craniovascular I63.9
  vascular, brain I63.9
Accidental —*see* condition
Accommodation (disorder) —*see also* condition
  hysterical paralysis of F44.89
  insufficiency of H52.4
  paresis —*see* Paresis, of accommodation
  spasm —*see* Spasm, of accommodation
Accouchement —*see* Delivery
Accreta placenta O43.21-
Accretio cordis (nonrheumatic) I31.0
Accretions, tooth, teeth K03.6
Acculturation difficulty Z60.3
Accumulation secretion, prostate N42.89
Acephalia, acephalism, acephalus, acephaly
  Q00.0
Acephalobrachia monster Q89.8
Acephalochirus monster Q89.8
Acephalogaster Q89.8
Acephalostomus monster Q89.8
Acephalothorax Q89.8
Acerophobia F40.298
Acetonemia R79.89
  in Type 1 diabetes E10.10
    with coma E10.11
Acetonuria R82.4
Achalasia (cardia) (esophagus) K22.0
  congenital Q39.5
  pylorus Q40.0
  sphincteral NEC K59.8
Ache (s) —*see* Pain
Acheilia Q38.6
Achillobursitis —*see* Tendinitis, Achilles
Achillodynia —*see* Tendinitis, Achilles
Achlorhydria, achlorhydric (neurogenic)
  K31.83
  anemia D50.8
  diarrhea K31.83
  psychogenic F45.8
  secondary to vagotomy K91.1
Achluophobia F40.228
Acholia K82.8
Acholuric jaundice (familial)
  (splenomegalic) —*see also* Spherocytosis
  acquired D59.8
Achondrogenesis Q77.0
Achondroplasia (osteosclerosis congenita)
  Q77.4
Achroma, cutis L80
Achromat (ism), achromatopsia (acquired)
  (congenital) H53.51
Achromia, congenital —*see* Albinism
Achromia parasitica B36.0
Achylia gastrica K31.89
  psychogenic F45.8
Acid
  burn —*see* Corrosion
  deficiency
    amide nicotinic E52
    ascorbic E54
    folic E53.8
    nicotinic E52
    pantothenic E53.8
  intoxication E87.2
  peptic disease K30
  phosphatase deficiency E83.39
  stomach K30
    psychogenic F45.8
Acidemia E87.2
  argininosuccinic E72.22
  isovaleric E71.110
  metabolic (newborn) P19.9
    first noted before onset of labor P19.0
    first noted during labor P19.1
    noted at birth P19.2

Acidemia (*Continued*)
  methylmalonic E71.120
  pipecolic E72.3
  propionic E71.121
Acidity, gastric (high) K30
  psychogenic F45.8
Acidocytopenia —*see* Agranulocytosis
Acidocytosis D72.1
Acidopenia —*see* Agranulocytosis
Acidosis (lactic) (respiratory) E87.2
  in Type 1 diabetes E10.10
    with coma E10.11
  kidney, tubular N25.89
  lactic E87.2
  metabolic NEC E87.2
    with respiratory acidosis E87.4
    late, of newborn P74.0
  mixed metabolic and respiratory,
    newborn P84
  newborn P84
  renal (hyperchloremic) (tubular)
    N25.89
  respiratory E87.2
    complicated by
      metabolic
        acidosis E87.4
        alkalosis E87.4
Aciduria
  argininosuccinic E72.22
  glutaric (type I) E72.3
    type II E71.313
    type III E71.5-
  orotic (congenital) (hereditary) (pyrimidine
    deficiency) E79.8
    anemia D53.0
Acladiosis (skin) B36.0
Aclasis, diaphyseal Q78.6
Acleistocardia Q21.1
Aclusion —*see* Anomaly, dentofacial,
  malocclusion
Acne L70.9
  artificialis L70.8
  atrophica L70.2
  cachecticorum (Hebra) L70.8
  conglobata L70.1
  cystic L70.0
  decalvans L66.2
  ~~excoriée des jeunes filles L70.5~~
  excoriée (des jeunes filles) L70.5 ◀
  frontalis L70.2
  indurata L70.0
  infantile L70.4
  keloid L73.0
  lupoid L70.2
  necrotic, necrotica (miliaris) L70.2
  neonatal L70.4
  nodular L70.0
  occupational L70.8
  picker's L70.5
  pustular L70.0
  rodens L70.2
  rosacea L71.9
  specified NEC L70.8
  tropica L70.3
  varioliformis L70.2
  vulgaris L70.0
Acnitis (primary) A18.4
Acosta's disease T70.29
Acoustic —*see* condition
Acousticophobia F40.298
Acquired —*see also* condition
  immunodeficiency syndrome (AIDS) B20
Acrania Q00.0
Acroangiodermatitis I78.9
Acroasphyxia, chronic I73.89
Acrobystitis N47.7
Acrocephalopolysyndactyly Q87.0
Acrocephalosyndactyly Q87.0
Acrocephaly Q75.0
Acrochondrohyperplasia —*see* Syndrome,
  Marfan's

Acrocyanosis I73.8
  newborn P28.2
    meaning transient blue hands and feet -
      omit code
Acrodermatitis L30.8
  atrophicans (chronica) L90.4
  continua (Hallopeau) L40.2
  enteropathica (hereditary) E83.2
  Hallopeau's L40.2
  infantile papular L44.4
  perstans L40.2
  pustulosa continua L40.2
  recalcitrant pustular L40.2
Acrodynia —*see* Poisoning, mercury
Acromegaly, acromegalia E22.0
Acromelalgia I73.81
Acromicria, acromikria Q79.8
Acronyx L60.0
Acropachy, thyroid —*see* Thyrotoxicosis
Acroparesthesia (simple) (vasomotor) I73.89
Acropathy, thyroid —*see* Thyrotoxicosis
Acrophobia F40.241
Acroposthitis N47.7
Acroscleriasis, acroscleroderma,
  acrosclerosis —*see* Sclerosis, systemic
Acrosphacelus I96
Acrospiroma, eccrine —*see* Neoplasm, skin,
  benign
Acrostealgia —*see* Osteochondropathy
Acrotrophodynia —*see* Immersion
ACTH ectopic syndrome E24.3
Actinic —*see* condition
Actinobacillosis, actinobacillus A28.8
  mallei A24.0
  muris A25.1
Actinomyces israelii (infection) —*see*
  Actinomycosis
Actinomycetoma (foot) B47.1
Actinomycosis, actinomycotic A42.9
  with pneumonia A42.0
  abdominal A42.1
  cervicofacial A42.2
  cutaneous A42.89
  gastrointestinal A42.1
  pulmonary A42.0
  sepsis A42.7
  specified site NEC A42.89
Actinoneuritis G62.82
Action, heart
  disorder I49.9
  irregular I49.9
    psychogenic F45.8
Activated protein C resistance D68.51
Activation ◀
  mast cell (disorder) (syndrome) D89.40 ◀
    idiopathic D89.42 ◀
    monoclonal D89.41 ◀
    secondary D89.43 ◀
    specified type NEC D89.49 ◀
Active —*see* condition
Acute —*see also* condition
  abdomen R10.0
  gallbladder —*see* Cholecystitis, acute
Acyanotic heart disease (congenital) Q24.9
Acystia Q64.5
Adair-Dighton syndrome (brittle bones and
  blue sclera, deafness) Q78.0
Adamantinoblastoma —*see* Ameloblastoma
Adamantinoma —*see also* Cyst, calcifying
  odontogenic
  long bones C40.90
    lower limb C40.2-
    upper limb C40.0-
  malignant C41.1
    jaw (bone) (lower) C41.1
      upper C41.0
  tibial C40.2-
Adamantoblastoma —*see* Ameloblastoma
Adams-Stokes (-Morgagni) **disease or**
  syndrome I45.9
Adaption reaction —*see* Disorder, adjustment

◀ New   ◀III Revised   ~~deleted~~ Deleted

Addiction —*see also* Dependence F19.20
  alcohol, alcoholic (ethyl) (methyl) (wood)
      (without remission) F10.20
    with remission F10.21
  drug —*see* Dependence, drug
  ethyl alcohol (without remission) F10.20
    with remission F10.21
  heroin —*see* Dependence, drug, opioid
  methyl alcohol (without remission) F10.20
    with remission F10.21
  methylated spirit (without remission) F10.20
    with remission F10.21
  morphine(-like substances) —*see*
      Dependence, drug, opioid
  nicotine —*see* Dependence, drug, nicotine
  opium and opioids —*see* Dependence, drug,
      opioid
  tobacco —*see* Dependence, drug, nicotine
Addisonian crisis E27.2
Addison's
  anemia (pernicious) D51.0
  disease (bronze) or syndrome E27.1
    tuberculous A18.7
  keloid L94.0
Addison-Biermer anemia (pernicious) D51.0
Addison-Schilder complex E71.528
Additional —*see also* Accessory
  chromosome (s) Q99.8
    21 —*see* Trisomy, 21
    sex —*see* Abnormal, chromosome, sex
Adduction contracture, hip or other joint —*see*
      Contraction, joint
Adenitis —*see also* Lymphadenitis
  acute, unspecified site L04.9
  axillary I88.9
    acute L04.2
    chronic or subacute I88.1
  Bartholin's gland N75.8
  bulbourethral gland —*see* Urethritis
  cervical I88.9
    acute L04.0
    chronic or subacute I88.1
  chancroid (Hemophilus ducreyi) A57
  chronic, unspecified site I88.1
  Cowper's gland —*see* Urethritis
  due to Pasteurella multocida (p. septica) A28.0
  epidemic, acute B27.09
  gangrenous L04.9
  gonorrheal NEC A54.89
  groin I88.9
    acute L04.1
    chronic or subacute I88.1
  infectious (acute) (epidemic) B27.09
  inguinal I88.9
    acute L04.1
    chronic or subacute I88.1
  lymph gland or node, except mesenteric I88.9
    acute —*see* Lymphadenitis, acute
    chronic or subacute I88.1
  mesenteric (acute) (chronic) (nonspecific)
      (subacute) I88.0
  parotid gland (suppurative) —*see*
      Sialoadenitis
  salivary gland (any) (suppurative) —*see*
      Sialoadenitis
  scrofulous (tuberculous) A18.2
  Skene's duct or gland —*see* Urethritis
  strumous, tuberculous A18.2
  subacute, unspecified site I88.1
  sublingual gland (suppurative) —*see*
      Sialoadenitis
  submandibular gland (suppurative) —*see*
      Sialoadenitis
  submaxillary gland (suppurative) —*see*
      Sialoadenitis
  tuberculous —*see* Tuberculosis, lymph gland
  urethral gland —*see* Urethritis
  Wharton's duct (suppurative) —*see*
      Sialoadenitis
Adenoacanthoma —*see* Neoplasm, malignant,
      by site

Adenoameloblastoma —*see* Cyst, calcifying
      odontogenic
Adenocarcinoid (tumor) —*see* Neoplasm,
      malignant, by site
Adenocarcinoma —*see also* Neoplasm,
      malignant, by site
  acidophil
    specified site —*see* Neoplasm, malignant,
        by site
    unspecified site C75.1
  adrenal cortical C74.0-
  alveolar —*see* Neoplasm, lung, malignant
  apocrine
    breast —*see* Neoplasm, breast, malignant
    in situ
      breast D05.8-
      specified site NEC —*see* Neoplasm, skin,
          in situ
      unspecified site D04.9
    specified site NEC —*see* Neoplasm, skin,
        malignant
    unspecified site C44.99
  basal cell
    specified site —*see* Neoplasm, skin,
        malignant
    unspecified site C08.9
  basophil
    specified site —*see* Neoplasm, malignant,
        by site
    unspecified site C75.1
  bile duct type C22.1
    liver C22.1
    specified site NEC —*see* Neoplasm,
        malignant, by site
    unspecified site C22.1
  bronchiolar —*see* Neoplasm, lung, malignant
  bronchioloalveolar —*see* Neoplasm, lung,
      malignant
  ceruminous C44.29-
  cervix, in situ (*see also* Carcinoma, cervix
      uteri, in situ) D06.9
  chromophobe
    specified site —*see* Neoplasm, malignant,
        by site
    unspecified site C75.1
  diffuse type
    specified site —*see* Neoplasm, malignant,
        by site
    unspecified site C16.9
  duct
    infiltrating
      with Paget's disease —*see* Neoplasm,
          breast, malignant
      specified site —*see* Neoplasm,
          malignant, by site
      unspecified site (female) C50.91-
        male C50.92-
    specified site —*see* Neoplasm, malignant,
        by site
    unspecified site
      female C56.9
      male C61
  eosinophil
    specified site —*see* Neoplasm, malignant,
        by site
    unspecified site C75.1
  follicular
    with papillary C73
    moderately differentiated C73
    specified site —*see* Neoplasm, malignant,
        by site
    trabecular C73
    unspecified site C73
    well differentiated C73
  Hurthle cell C73
  in
    adenomatous
      polyposis coli C18.9
  infiltrating duct
    with Paget's disease —*see* Neoplasm,
        breast, malignant

Adenocarcinoma (*Continued*)
  infiltrating duct (*Continued*)
    specified site —*see* Neoplasm, malignant,
        by site
    unspecified site (female) C50.91-
      male C50.92-
  inflammatory
    specified site —*see* Neoplasm, malignant,
        by site
    unspecified site (female) C50.91-
      male C50.92-
  intestinal type
    specified site —*see* Neoplasm, malignant,
        by site
    unspecified site C16.9
  intracystic papillary
  intraductal
    breast D05.1-
    noninfiltrating
      breast D05.1-
    papillary
      with invasion
        specified site —*see* Neoplasm,
            malignant, by site
        unspecified site (female) C50.91-
          male C50.92-
      breast D05.1-
      specified site NEC —*see* Neoplasm, in
          situ, by site
      unspecified site D05.1-
    specified site NEC —*see* Neoplasm, in
        situ, by site
    unspecified site D05.1-
  papillary
    with invasion
      specified site —*see* Neoplasm,
          malignant, by site
      unspecified site (female) C50.91-
        male C50.92-
    breast D05.1-
    specified site —*see* Neoplasm, in situ,
        by site
    unspecified site D05.1-
  specified site NEC —*see* Neoplasm, in situ,
      by site
  unspecified site D05.1-
  islet cell
    with exocrine, mixed
      specified site —*see* Neoplasm,
          malignant, by site
      unspecified site C25.9
    pancreas C25.4
    specified site NEC —*see* Neoplasm,
        malignant, by site
    unspecified site C25.4
  lobular
    in situ
      breast D05.0-
      specified site NEC —*see* Neoplasm, in
          situ, by site
      unspecified site D05.0-
    specified site —*see* Neoplasm, malignant,
        by site
    unspecified site (female) C50.91-
      male C50.92-
  mucoid —*see also* Neoplasm, malignant, by site
    cell
      specified site —*see* Neoplasm,
          malignant, by site
      unspecified site C75.1
  nonencapsulated sclerosing C73
  papillary
    with follicular C73
    follicular variant C73
    intraductal (noninfiltrating)
      with invasion
        specified site —*see* Neoplasm,
            malignant, by site
        unspecified site (female) C50.91-
          male C50.92-
      breast D05.1-

Adenocarcinoma *(Continued)*
  papillary *(Continued)*
    intraductal *(Continued)*
      specified site NEC —*see* Neoplasm, in situ, by site
      unspecified site D05.1-
    serous
      specified site —*see* Neoplasm, malignant, by site
      unspecified site C56.9
  papillocystic
    specified site —*see* Neoplasm, malignant, by site
    unspecified site C56.9
  pseudomucinous
    specified site —*see* Neoplasm, malignant, by site
    unspecified site C56.9
  renal cell C64-
  sebaceous —*see* Neoplasm, skin, malignant, by site
  serous —*see also* Neoplasm, malignant, by site
    papillary
      specified site —*see* Neoplasm, malignant, by site
      unspecified site C56.9
  sweat gland —*see* Neoplasm, skin, malignant
  water-clear cell C75.0
Adenocarcinoma-in-situ —*see also* Neoplasm, in situ, by site
  breast D05.9-
Adenofibroma
  clear cell —*see* Neoplasm, benign, by site
  endometrioid D27.9
    borderline malignancy D39.10
    malignant C56-
  mucinous
    specified site —*see* Neoplasm, benign, by site
    unspecified site D27.9
  papillary
    specified site —*see* Neoplasm, benign, by site
    unspecified site D27.9
  prostate —*see* Enlargement, enlarged, prostate
  serous
    specified site —*see* Neoplasm, benign, by site
    unspecified site D27.9
  specified site —*see* Neoplasm, benign, by site
  unspecified site D27.9
Adenofibrosis
  breast —*see* Fibroadenosis, breast
  endometrioid N80.0
Adenoiditis (chronic) J35.02
  with tonsillitis J35.03
  acute J03.90
    recurrent J03.91
    specified organism NEC J03.80
      recurrent J03.81
    staphylococcal J03.80
      recurrent J03.81
    streptococcal J03.00
      recurrent J03.01
Adenoids —*see* condition
Adenolipoma —*see* Neoplasm, benign, by site
Adenolipomatosis, Launois-Bensaude E88.89
Adenolymphoma
  specified site —*see* Neoplasm, benign, by site
  unspecified site D11.9
Adenoma —*see also* Neoplasm, benign, by site
  acidophil
    specified site —*see* Neoplasm, benign, by site
    unspecified site D35.2
  acidophil-basophil, mixed
    specified site —*see* Neoplasm, benign, by site
    unspecified site D35.2

Adenoma *(Continued)*
  adrenal (cortical) D35.00
    clear cell D35.00
    compact cell D35.00
    glomerulosa cell D35.00
    heavily pigmented variant D35.00
    mixed cell D35.00
  alpha-cell
    pancreas D13.7
    specified site NEC —*see* Neoplasm, benign, by site
    unspecified site D13.7
  alveolar D14.30
  apocrine
    breast D24-
    specified site NEC —*see* Neoplasm, skin, benign, by site
    unspecified site D23.9
  basal cell D11.9
  basophil
    specified site —*see* Neoplasm, benign, by site
    unspecified site D35.2
  basophil-acidophil, mixed
    specified site —*see* Neoplasm, benign, by site
    unspecified site D35.2
  beta-cell
    pancreas D13.7
    specified site NEC —*see* Neoplasm, benign, by site
    unspecified site D13.7
  bile duct D13.4
    common D13.5
    extrahepatic D13.5
    intrahepatic D13.4
    specified site NEC —*see* Neoplasm, benign, by site
    unspecified site D13.4
  black D35.00
  bronchial D38.1
    cylindroid type —*see* Neoplasm, lung, malignant
  ceruminous D23.2-
  chief cell D35.1
  chromophobe
    specified site —*see* Neoplasm, benign, by site
    unspecified site D35.2
  colloid
    specified site —*see* Neoplasm, benign, by site
    unspecified site D34
  duct
  eccrine, papillary —*see* Neoplasm, skin, benign
  endocrine, multiple
    single specified site —*see* Neoplasm, uncertain behavior, by site
    two or more specified sites D44-
    unspecified site D44.9
  endometrioid —*see also* Neoplasm, benign
    borderline malignancy —*see* Neoplasm, uncertain behavior, by site
  eosinophil
    specified site —*see* Neoplasm, malignant, by site
    unspecified site D35.2
  fetal
    specified site —*see* Neoplasm, benign, by site
    unspecified site D34
  follicular
    specified site —*see* Neoplasm, benign, by site
    unspecified site D34
  hepatocellular D13.4
  Hurthle cell D34
  islet cell
    pancreas D13.7
    specified site NEC —*see* Neoplasm, benign, by site
    unspecified site D13.7

Adenoma *(Continued)*
  liver cell D13.4
  macrofollicular
    specified site —*see* Neoplasm, benign, by site
    unspecified site D34
  malignant, malignum —*see* Neoplasm, malignant, by site
  microcystic
    pancreas D13.6 ◀▥
    specified site NEC —*see* Neoplasm, benign, by site
    unspecified site D13.6 ◀▥
  microfollicular
    specified site —*see* Neoplasm, benign, by site
    unspecified site D34
  mucoid cell
    specified site —*see* Neoplasm, benign, by site
    unspecified site D35.2
  multiple endocrine
    single specified site —*see* Neoplasm, uncertain behavior, by site
    two or more specified sites D44-
    unspecified site D44.9
  nipple D24-
  papillary —*see also* Neoplasm, benign, by site
    eccrine —*see* Neoplasm, skin, benign, by site
  Pick's tubular
    specified site —*see* Neoplasm, benign, by site
    unspecified site
      female D27.9
      male D29.20
  pleomorphic
    carcinoma in —*see* Neoplasm, salivary gland, malignant
      specified site —*see* Neoplasm, malignant, by site
    unspecified site C08.9
  polypoid —*see also* Neoplasm, benign
    adenocarcinoma in —*see* Neoplasm, malignant, by site
    adenocarcinoma in situ —*see* Neoplasm, in situ, by site
  prostate —*see* Neoplasm, benign, prostate
  rete cell D29.20
  sebaceous —*see* Neoplasm, skin, benign
  Sertoli cell
    specified site —*see* Neoplasm, benign, by site
    unspecified site
      female D27.9
      male D29.20
  skin appendage —*see* Neoplasm, skin, benign
  sudoriferous gland —*see* Neoplasm, skin, benign
  sweat gland —*see* Neoplasm, skin, benign
  testicular
    specified site —*see* Neoplasm, benign, by site
    unspecified site
      female D27.9
      male D29.20
  tubular —*see also* Neoplasm, benign, by site
    adenocarcinoma in —*see* Neoplasm, malignant, by site
    adenocarcinoma in situ —*see* Neoplasm, in situ, by site
    Pick's
      specified site —*see* Neoplasm, benign
      unspecified site
        female D27.9
        male D29.20
  tubulovillous —*see also* Neoplasm, benign, by site
    adenocarcinoma in —*see* Neoplasm, malignant, by site
    adenocarcinoma in situ —*see* Neoplasm, in situ, by site

Adenoma (Continued)
  villous —see Neoplasm, uncertain behavior,
    by site
      adenocarcinoma in —see Neoplasm,
        malignant, by site
      adenocarcinoma in situ —see Neoplasm, in
        situ, by site
  water-clear cell D35.1
Adenomatosis
  endocrine (multiple) E31.20
    single specified site —see Neoplasm,
      uncertain behavior, by site
  erosive of nipple D24-
  pluriendocrine —see Adenomatosis,
    endocrine
  pulmonary D38.1
    malignant —see Neoplasm, lung,
      malignant
  specified site —see Neoplasm, benign, by site
  unspecified site D12.6
Adenomatous
  goiter (nontoxic) E04.9
    with hyperthyroidism —see Hyper-
      thyroidism, with, goiter, nodular
    toxic —see Hyperthyroidism, with, goiter,
      nodular
Adenomyoma —see also Neoplasm, benign, by
  site
  prostate —see Enlarged, prostate
Adenomyometritis N80.0
Adenomyosis N80.0
Adenopathy (lymph gland) R59.9
  generalized R59.1
  inguinal R59.0
  localized R59.0
  mediastinal R59.0
  mesentery R59.0
  syphilitic (secondary) A51.49
  tracheobronchial R59.0
    tuberculous A15.4
      primary (progressive) A15.7
  tuberculous —see also Tuberculosis, lymph
    gland
    tracheobronchial A15.4
      primary (progressive) A15.7
Adenosalpingitis —see Salpingitis
Adenosarcoma —see Neoplasm, malignant, by
  site
Adenosclerosis I88.8
Adenosis (sclerosing) breast —see
  Fibroadenosis, breast
Adenovirus, as cause of disease classified
  elsewhere B97.0
Adentia (complete) (partial) —see Absence,
  teeth
Adherent —see also Adhesions
  labia (minora) N90.89
  pericardium (nonrheumatic) I31.0
    rheumatic I09.2
  placenta (with hemorrhage) O72.0
    without hemorrhage O73.0
  prepuce, newborn N47.0
  scar (skin) L90.5
  tendon in scar L90.5
Adhesions, adhesive (postinfective) K66.0
  with intestinal obstruction K56.5
  abdominal (wall) —see Adhesions,
    peritoneum
  appendix K38.8
  bile duct (common) (hepatic) K83.8
  bladder (sphincter) N32.89
  bowel —see Adhesions, peritoneum
  cardiac I31.0
    rheumatic I09.2
  cecum —see Adhesions, peritoneum
  cervicovaginal N88.1
    congenital Q52.8
    postpartal O90.89
      old N88.1
  cervix N88.1
  ciliary body NEC —see Adhesions, iris

Adhesions, adhesive (Continued)
  clitoris N90.89
  colon —see Adhesions, peritoneum
  common duct K83.8
  congenital —see also Anomaly, by site
    fingers —see Syndactylism, complex,
      fingers
    omental, anomalous Q43.3
    peritoneal Q43.3
    tongue (to gum or roof of mouth)
      Q38.3
  conjunctiva (acquired) H11.21-
    congenital Q15.8
  cystic duct K82.8
  diaphragm —see Adhesions, peritoneum
  due to foreign body —see Foreign body
  duodenum —see Adhesions, peritoneum
  ear
    middle H74.1-
  epididymis N50.89 ◀▦
  epidural —see Adhesions, meninges
  epiglottis J38.7
  eyelid H02.59
  female pelvis N73.6
  gallbladder K82.8
  globe H44.89
  heart I31.0
    rheumatic I09.2
  ileocecal (coil) —see Adhesions, peritoneum
  ileum —see Adhesions, peritoneum
  intestine —see also Adhesions, peritoneum
    with obstruction K56.5
  intra-abdominal —see Adhesions, peritoneum
  iris H21.50-
    anterior H21.51-
    goniosynechiae H21.52-
    posterior H21.54-
    to corneal graft T85.898 ◀▦
  joint —see Ankylosis
    knee M23.8X
    temporomandibular M26.61- ◀▦
  labium (majus) (minus), congenital Q52.5
  liver —see Adhesions, peritoneum
  lung J98.4
  mediastinum J98.59 ◀▦
  meninges (cerebral) (spinal) G96.12
    congenital Q07.8
    tuberculous (cerebral) (spinal) A17.0
  mesenteric —see Adhesions, peritoneum
  nasal (septum) (to turbinates) J34.89
  ocular muscle —see Strabismus, mechanical
  omentum —see Adhesions, peritoneum
  ovary N73.6
    congenital (to cecum, kidney or omentum)
      Q50.39
  paraovarian N73.6
  pelvic (peritoneal)
    female N73.6
      postprocedural N99.4
    male —see Adhesions, peritoneum
    postpartal (old) N73.6
    tuberculous A18.17
  penis to scrotum (congenital) Q55.8
  periappendiceal —see also Adhesions,
    peritoneum
  pericardium (nonrheumatic) I31.0
    focal I31.8
    rheumatic I09.2
    tuberculous A18.84
  pericholecystic K82.8
  perigastric —see Adhesions, peritoneum
  periovarian N73.6
  periprostatic N42.89
  perirectal —see Adhesions, peritoneum
  perirenal N28.89
  peritoneum, peritoneal (postinfective)
    (postprocedural) K66.0
    with obstruction (intestinal) K56.5
    congenital Q43.3
    pelvic, female N73.6
      postprocedural N99.4

Adhesions, adhesive (Continued)
  peritoneum, peritoneal (Continued)
    postpartal, pelvic N73.6
      to uterus N73.6
    peritubal N73.6
    periureteral N28.89
    periuterine N73.6
    perivesical N32.89
    perivesicular (seminal vesicle) N50.89 ◀▦
    pleura, pleuritic J94.8
      tuberculous NEC A15.6
    pleuropericardial J94.8
    postoperative (gastrointestinal tract)
      K66.0
      with obstruction K91.3
      due to foreign body accidentally left
        in wound —see Foreign body,
        accidentally left during a procedure
    pelvic peritoneal N99.4
    urethra —see Stricture, urethra,
      postprocedural
    vagina N99.2
  postpartal, old (vulva or perineum) N90.89
  preputial, prepuce N47.5
  pulmonary J98.4
  pylorus —see Adhesions, peritoneum
  sciatic nerve —see Lesion, nerve, sciatic
  seminal vesicle N50.89 ◀▦
  shoulder (joint) —see Capsulitis, adhesive
  sigmoid flexure —see Adhesions, peritoneum
  spermatic cord (acquired) N50.89 ◀▦
    congenital Q55.4
  spinal canal G96.12
  stomach —see Adhesions, peritoneum
  subscapular —see Capsulitis, adhesive
  temporomandibular M26.61- ◀▦
  tendinitis —see also Tenosynovitis, specified
    type NEC
    shoulder —see Capsulitis, adhesive
  testis N44.8
  tongue, congenital (to gum or roof of mouth)
    Q38.3
    acquired K14.8
  trachea J39.8
  tubo-ovarian N73.6
  tunica vaginalis N44.8
  uterus N73.6
    internal N85.6
    to abdominal wall N73.6
  vagina (chronic) N89.5
    postoperative N99.2
  vitreomacular H43.82-
  vitreous H43.89
  vulva N90.89
Adiaspiromycosis B48.8
Adie (-Holmes) pupil or syndrome —see
  Anomaly, pupil, function, tonic pupil
Adiponecrosis neonatorum P83.8
Adiposis —see also Obesity
  cerebralis E23.6
  dolorosa E88.2
Adiposity —see also Obesity
  heart —see Degeneration, myocardial
  localized E65
Adiposogenital dystrophy E23.6
Adjustment
  disorder —see Disorder, adjustment
  implanted device —see Encounter (for),
    adjustment (of)
  prosthesis, external —see Fitting
  reaction —see Disorder, adjustment
Administration of tPA (rtPA) in a different
  facility within the last 24 hours prior to
  admission to current facility Z92.82
Admission (for) —see also Encounter (for)
  adjustment (of)
    artificial
      arm Z44.00-
        complete Z44.01-
        partial Z44.02-
      eye Z44.2

Admission *(Continued)*
 adjustment *(Continued)*
  artificial *(Continued)*
   leg Z44.10-
    complete Z44.11-
    partial Z44.12-
   brain neuropacemaker Z46.2
    implanted Z45.42
   breast
    implant Z45.81
    prosthesis (external) Z44.3
   colostomy belt Z46.89
   contact lenses Z46.0
   cystostomy device Z46.6
   dental prosthesis Z46.3
   device NEC
    abdominal Z46.89
    implanted Z45.89
     cardiac Z45.09
      defibrillator (with synchronous
       cardiace pacemaker) Z45.02
      pacemaker (cardiac
       resynchronization therapy
       (CRT-P)) Z45.018 ◀▥▥
       pulse generator Z45.010
      resynchronization therapy
       defibrillator (CRT-D) Z45.02 ◀
    hearing device Z45.328
     bone conduction Z45.320
     cochlear Z45.321
    infusion pump Z45.1
    nervous system Z45.49
     CSF drainage Z45.41
     hearing device —*see* Admission,
      adjustment, device, implanted,
      hearing device
     neuropacemaker Z45.42
     visual substitution Z45.31
    specified NEC Z45.89
    vascular access Z45.2
    visual substitution Z45.31
   nervous system Z46.2
    implanted —*see* Admission,
     adjustment, device, implanted,
     nervous system
   orthodontic Z46.4
   prosthetic Z44.9
    arm —*see* Admission, adjustment,
     artificial, arm
    breast Z44.3
    dental Z46.3
    eye Z44.2
    leg —*see* Admission, adjustment,
     artificial, leg
    specified type NEC Z44.8
   substitution
    auditory Z46.2
     implanted —*see* Admission,
      adjustment, device, implanted,
      hearing device
    nervous system Z46.2
     implanted —*see* Admission,
      adjustment, device, implanted,
      nervous system
    visual Z46.2
     implanted Z45.31
    urinary Z46.6
   hearing aid Z46.1
    implanted —*see* Admission, adjustment,
     device, implanted, hearing device
   ileostomy device Z46.89
   intestinal appliance or device NEC Z46.89
   neuropacemaker (brain) (peripheral nerve)
    (spinal cord) Z46.2
    implanted Z45.42
   orthodontic device Z46.4
   orthopedic (brace) (cast) (device) (shoes)
    Z46.89
   pacemaker (cardiac resynchronization
    therapy (CRT-P)) ◀▥▥
    cardiac Z45.018
     pulse generator Z45.010

Admission *(Continued)*
 adjustment *(Continued)*
  pacemaker *(Continued)*
   nervous system Z46.2
    implanted Z45.42
   portacath (port-a-cath) Z45.2
   prosthesis Z44.9
    arm —*see* Admission, adjustment,
     artificial, arm
    breast Z44.3
    dental Z46.3
    eye Z44.2
    leg —*see* Admission, adjustment,
     artificial, leg
    specified NEC Z44.8
   spectacles Z46.0
 aftercare *(see also* Aftercare) Z51.89
  postpartum
   immediately after delivery Z39.0
   routine follow-up Z39.2
  radiation therapy (antineoplastic) Z51.0
 attention to artificial opening (of) Z43.9
  artificial vagina Z43.7
  colostomy Z43.3
  cystostomy Z43.5
  enterostomy Z43.4
  gastrostomy Z43.1
  ileostomy Z43.2
  jejunostomy Z43.4
  nephrostomy Z43.6
  specified site NEC Z43.8
   intestinal tract Z43.4
   urinary tract Z43.6
  tracheostomy Z43.0
  ureterostomy Z43.6
  urethrostomy Z43.6
 breast augmentation or reduction Z41.1
 breast reconstruction following mastectomy
  Z42.1
 change of
  dressing (nonsurgical) Z48.00
  neuropacemaker device (brain) (peripheral
   nerve) (spinal cord) Z46.2
   implanted Z45.42
  surgical dressing Z48.01
 circumcision, ritual or routine (in absence of
  diagnosis) Z41.2
 clinical research investigation (control)
  (normal comparison) (participant) Z00.6
 contraceptive management Z30.9
 cosmetic surgery NEC Z41.1
 counseling *(see also* Counseling)
  dietary Z71.3
  gestational carrier Z31.7 ◀
  HIV Z71.7
  human immunodeficiency virus Z71.7
  nonattending third party Z71.0
  procreative management NEC Z31.69
 delivery, full-term, uncomplicated O80
  cesarean, without indication O82
 desensitization to allergens Z51.6 ◀
 dietary surveillance and counseling Z71.3
 ear piercing Z41.3
 examination at health care facility (adult) —
  see also Examination Z00.00
  with abnormal findings Z00.01
  clinical research investigation (control)
   (normal comparison) (participant)
   Z00.6
  dental Z01.20
   with abnormal findings Z01.21
  donor (potential) Z00.5
  ear Z01.10
   with abnormal findings NEC Z01.118
  eye Z01.00
   with abnormal findings Z01.01
  general, specified reason NEC Z00.8
  hearing Z01.10
   with abnormal findings NEC Z01.118
  postpartum checkup Z39.2
  psychiatric (general) Z00.8
   requested by authority Z04.6

Admission *(Continued)*
 examination at health care facility *(Continued)*
  vision Z01.00
   with abnormal findings Z01.01
 fitting (of)
  artificial
   arm —*see* Admission, adjustment,
    artificial, arm
   eye Z44.2
   leg —*see* Admission, adjustment,
    artificial, leg
  brain neuropacemaker Z46.2
   implanted Z45.42
  breast prosthesis (external) Z44.3
  colostomy belt Z46.89
  contact lenses Z46.0
  cystostomy device Z46.6
  dental prosthesis Z46.3
  dentures Z46.3
  device NEC
   abdominal Z46.89
   nervous system Z46.2
    implanted —*see* Admission,
     adjustment, device, implanted,
     nervous system
   orthodontic Z46.4
   prosthetic Z44.9
    breast Z44.3
    dental Z46.3
    eye Z44.2
   substitution
    auditory Z46.2
     implanted —*see* Admission,
      adjustment, device, implanted,
      hearing device
    nervous system Z46.2
     implanted —*see* Admission,
      adjustment, device, implanted,
      nervous system
    visual Z46.2
     implanted Z45.31
  hearing aid Z46.1
  ileostomy device Z46.89
  intestinal appliance or device NEC Z46.89
  neuropacemaker (brain) (peripheral nerve)
   (spinal cord) Z46.2
   implanted Z45.42
  orthodontic device Z46.4
  orthopedic device (brace) (cast) (shoes)
   Z46.89
  prosthesis Z44.9
   arm —*see* Admission, adjustment,
    artificial, arm
   breast Z44.3
   dental Z46.3
   eye Z44.2
   leg —*see* Admission, adjustment,
    artificial, leg
   specified type NEC Z44.8
  spectacles Z46.0
 follow-up examination Z09
 intrauterine device management Z30.431
  initial prescription Z30.014
 mental health evaluation Z00.8
  requested by authority Z04.6
 observation —*see* Observation
 Papanicolaou smear, cervix Z12.4
  for suspected malignant neoplasm Z12.4
 plastic and reconstructive surgery following
  medical procedure or healed injury
  NEC Z42.8
 plastic surgery, cosmetic NEC Z41.1
 postpartum observation
  immediately after delivery Z39.0
  routine follow-up Z39.2
 poststerilization (for restoration) Z31.0
  aftercare Z31.42
 procreative management Z31.9
 prophylactic (measure) —*see also* Encounter,
  prophylactic measures ◀▥▥
  organ removal Z40.00
   breast Z40.01
   ovary Z40.02

◀ New   ▥▥ Revised   ~~deleted~~ Deleted

Admission *(Continued)*
  prophylactic *(Continued)*
    organ removal *(Continued)*
      specified organ NEC Z40.09
      testes Z40.09
    vaccination Z23
  psychiatric examination (general) Z00.8
    requested by authority Z04.6
  radiation therapy (antineoplastic) Z51.0
  reconstructive surgery following medical
      procedure or healed injury NEC Z42.8
  removal of
    cystostomy catheter Z43.5
    drains Z48.03
    dressing (nonsurgical) Z48.00
    implantable subdermal contraceptive
        Z30.46 ◀
    intrauterine contraceptive device Z30.432
    neuropacemaker (brain) (peripheral nerve)
        (spinal cord) Z46.2
      implanted Z45.42
    staples Z48.02
    surgical dressing Z48.01
    sutures Z48.02
    ureteral stent Z46.6
  respirator [ventilator] use during power
      failure Z99.12
  restoration of organ continuity
      (poststerilization) Z31.0
    aftercare Z31.42
  sensitivity test —*see also* Test, skin
    allergy NEC Z01.82
    Mantoux Z11.1
  tuboplasty following previous sterilization
      Z31.0
    aftercare Z31.42
  vasoplasty following previous sterilization
      Z31.0
    aftercare Z31.42
  vision examination Z01.00
    with abnormal findings Z01.01
  waiting period for admission to other facility
      Z75.1
Adnexitis (suppurative) —*see*
    Salpingo-oophoritis
Adolescent X-linked adrenoleukodystrophy
    E71.521
Adrenal (gland) —*see* condition
Adrenalism, tuberculous A18.7
Adrenalitis, adrenitis E27.8
  autoimmune E27.1
  meningococcal, hemorrhagic A39.1
Adrenarche, premature E27.0
Adrenocortical syndrome —*see* Cushing's,
    syndrome
Adrenogenital syndrome E25.9
  acquired E25.8
  congenital E25.0
  salt loss E25.0
Adrenogenitalism, congenital E25.0
Adrenoleukodystrophy E71.529
  neonatal E71.511
  X-linked E71.529
    Addison only phenotype E71.528
    Addison-Schilder E71.528
    adolescent E71.521
    adrenomyeloneuropathy E71.522
    childhood cerebral E71.520
    other specified E71.528
Adrenomyeloneuropathy E71.522
Adventitious bursa —*see* Bursopathy, specified
    type NEC
Adverse effect —*see* Table of Drugs and
    Chemicals, categories T36-T50, with 6th
    character 5
Advice —*see* Counseling
Adynamia (episodica) (hereditary) (periodic)
    G72.3
Aeration lung imperfect, newborn —*see*
    Atelectasis
Aerobullosis T70.3
Aerocele —*see* Embolism, air

Aerodermectasia
  subcutaneous (traumatic) T79.7
Aerodontalgia T70.29
Aeroembolism T70.3
Aerogenes capsulatus infection A48.0
Aero-otitis media T70.0
Aerophagy, aerophagia (psychogenic) F45.8
Aerophobia F40.228
Aerosinusitis T70.1
Aerotitis T70.0
Affection —*see* Disease
Afibrinogenemia —*see also* Defect, coagulation
    D68.8
  acquired D65
  congenital D68.2
  following ectopic or molar pregnancy O08.1
  in abortion —*see* Abortion, by type,
      complicated by, afibrinogenemia
  puerperal O72.3
African
  sleeping sickness B56.9
  tick fever A68.1
  trypanosomiasis B56.9
    gambian B56.0
    rhodesian B56.1
Aftercare —*see also* Care Z51.89
  following surgery (for) (on)
    amputation Z47.81
    attention to
      drains Z48.03
      dressings (nonsurgical) Z48.00
        surgical Z48.01
      sutures Z48.02
    circulatory system Z48.812
    delayed (planned) wound closure Z48.1
    digestive system Z48.815
    explantation of joint prosthesis (staged
        procedure)
      hip Z47.32
      knee Z47.33
      shoulder Z47.31
    genitourinary system Z48.816
    joint replacement Z47.1
    neoplasm Z48.3
    nervous system Z48.811
    oral cavity Z48.814
    organ transplant
      bone marrow Z48.290
      heart Z48.21
      heart-lung Z48.280
      kidney Z48.22
      liver Z48.23
      lung Z48.24
      multiple organs NEC Z48.288
      specified NEC Z48.298
    orthopedic NEC Z47.89
    planned wound closure Z48.1
    removal of internal fixation device Z47.2
    respiratory system Z48.813
    scoliosis Z47.82
    sense organs Z48.810
    skin and subcutaneous tissue Z48.817
    specified body system
      circulatory Z48.812
      digestive Z48.815
      genitourinary Z48.816
      nervous Z48.811
      oral cavity Z48.814
      respiratory Z48.813
      sense organs Z48.810
      skin and subcutaneous tissue Z48.817
      teeth Z48.814
    specified NEC Z48.89
    spinal Z48.89
    teeth Z48.814
  fracture — code to fracture with seventh
      character D
  involving
    removal of
      drains Z48.03
      dressings (nonsurgical) Z48.00

Aftercare *(Continued)*
  involving *(Continued)*
    removal of *(Continued)*
      staples Z48.02
      surgical dressings Z48.01
      sutures Z48.02
    neuropacemaker (brain) (peripheral nerve)
        (spinal cord) Z46.2
      implanted Z45.42
    orthopedic NEC Z47.89
    postprocedural —*see* Aftercare, following
        surgery
After-cataract —*see* Cataract, secondary
Agalactia (primary) O92.3
  elective, secondary or therapeutic O92.5
Agammaglobulinemia (acquired (secondary))
    (nonfamilial) D80.1
  with
    immunoglobulin-bearing B-lymphocytes
        D80.1
    lymphopenia D81.9
  autosomal recessive (Swiss type) D80.0
  Bruton's X-linked D80.0
  common variable (CVAgamma) D80.1
  congenital sex-linked D80.0
  hereditary D80.0
  lymphopenic D81.9
  Swiss type (autosomal recessive) D80.0
  X-linked (with growth hormone deficiency)
      (Bruton) D80.0 ◀▥
Aganglionosis (bowel) (colon) Q43.1
Age (old) —*see* Senility
Agenesis
  adrenal (gland) Q89.1
  alimentary tract (complete) (partial) NEC
      Q45.8
    upper Q40.8
  anus, anal (canal) Q42.3
    with fistula Q42.2
  aorta Q25.41 ◀▥
  appendix Q42.8
  arm (complete) Q71.0-
    with hand present Q71.1-
  artery (peripheral) Q27.9
    brain Q28.3
    coronary Q24.5
    pulmonary Q25.79
    specified NEC Q27.8
    umbilical Q27.0
  auditory (canal) (external) Q16.1
  auricle (ear) Q16.0
  bile duct or passage Q44.5
  bladder Q64.5
  bone Q79.9
  brain Q00.0
    part of Q04.3
  breast (with nipple present) Q83.8
    with absent nipple Q83.0
  bronchus Q32.4
  canaliculus lacrimalis Q10.4
  carpus —*see* Agenesis, hand
  cartilage Q79.9
  cecum Q42.8
  cerebellum Q04.3
  cervix Q51.5
  chin Q18.8
  cilia Q10.3
  circulatory system, part NOS Q28.9
  clavicle Q74.0
  clitoris Q52.6
  coccyx Q76.49
  colon Q42.9
    specified NEC Q42.8
  corpus callosum Q04.0
  cricoid cartilage Q31.8
  diaphragm (with hernia) Q79.1
  digestive organ (s) or tract (complete)
      (partial) NEC Q45.8
    upper Q40.8
  ductus arteriosus Q28.8
  duodenum Q41.0

Agenesis (Continued)
  ear Q16.9
    auricle Q16.0
    lobe Q17.8
  ejaculatory duct Q55.4
  endocrine (gland) NEC Q89.2
  epiglottis Q31.8
  esophagus Q39.8
  eustachian tube Q16.2
  eye Q11.1
    adnexa Q15.8
  eyelid (fold) Q10.3
  face
    bones NEC Q75.8
    specified part NEC Q18.8
  fallopian tube Q50.6
  femur —see Defect, reduction, lower limb,
      longitudinal, femur
  fibula —see Defect, reduction, lower limb,
      longitudinal, fibula
  finger (complete) (partial) —see Agenesis,
      hand
  foot (and toes) (complete) (partial) Q72.3-
  forearm (with hand present) —see Agenesis,
      arm, with hand present
    and hand Q71.2-
  gallbladder Q44.0
  gastric Q40.2
  genitalia, genital (organ (s))
    female Q52.8
      external Q52.71
      internal NEC Q52.8
    male Q55.8
  glottis Q31.8
  hair Q84.0
  hand (and fingers) (complete) (partial) Q71.3-
  heart Q24.8
    valve NEC Q24.8
      pulmonary Q22.0
  hepatic Q44.7
  humerus —see Defect, reduction, upper limb
  hymen Q52.4
  ileum Q41.2
  incus Q16.3
  intestine (small) Q41.9
    large Q42.9
      specified NEC Q42.8
  iris (dilator fibers) Q13.1
  jaw M26.09
  jejunum Q41.1
  kidney (s) (partial) Q60.2
    bilateral Q60.1
    unilateral Q60.0
  labium (majus) (minus) Q52.71
  labyrinth, membranous Q16.5
  lacrimal apparatus Q10.4
  larynx Q31.8
  leg (complete) Q72.0-
    with foot present Q72.1-
    lower leg (with foot present) —see
        Agenesis, leg, with foot present
      and foot Q72.2-
  lens Q12.3
  limb (complete) Q73.0
    lower —see Agenesis, leg
    upper —see Agenesis, arm
  lip Q38.0
  liver Q44.7
  lung (fissure) (lobe) (bilateral) (unilateral)
      Q33.3
  mandible, maxilla M26.09
  metacarpus —see Agenesis, hand
  metatarsus —see Agenesis, foot
  muscle Q79.8
    eyelid Q10.3
    ocular Q15.8
  musculoskeletal system NEC Q79.8
  nail (s) Q84.3
  neck, part Q18.8
  nerve Q07.8
  nervous system, part NEC Q07.8

Agenesis (Continued)
  nipple Q83.2
  nose Q30.1
  nuclear Q07.8
  organ
    of Corti Q16.5
    or site not listed —see Anomaly, by site
  osseous meatus (ear) Q16.1
  ovary
    bilateral Q50.02
    unilateral Q50.01
  oviduct Q50.6
  pancreas Q45.0
  parathyroid (gland) Q89.2
  parotid gland (s) Q38.4
  patella Q74.1
  pelvic girdle (complete) (partial) Q74.2
  penis Q55.5
  pericardium Q24.8
  pituitary (gland) Q89.2
  prostate Q55.4
  punctum lacrimale Q10.4
  radioulnar —see Defect, reduction, upper
      limb
  radius —see Defect, reduction, upper limb,
      longitudinal, radius
  rectum Q42.1
    with fistula Q42.0
  renal Q60.2
    bilateral Q60.1
    unilateral Q60.0
  respiratory organ NEC Q34.8
  rib Q76.6
  roof of orbit Q75.8
  round ligament Q52.8
  sacrum Q76.49
  salivary gland Q38.4
  scapula Q74.0
  scrotum Q55.29
  seminal vesicles Q55.4
  septum
    atrial Q21.1
    between aorta and pulmonary artery
        Q21.4
    ventricular Q20.4
  shoulder girdle (complete) (partial) Q74.0
  skull (bone) Q75.8
    with
      anencephaly Q00.0
      encephalocele —see Encephalocele
      hydrocephalus Q03.9
        with spina bifida —see Spina bifida, by
            site, with hydrocephalus
      microcephaly Q02
  spermatic cord Q55.4
  spinal cord Q06.0
  spine Q76.49
  spleen Q89.01
  sternum Q76.7
  stomach Q40.2
  submaxillary gland (s) (congenital) Q38.4
  tarsus —see Agenesis, foot
  tendon Q79.8
  testicle Q55.0
  thymus (gland) Q89.2
  thyroid (gland) E03.1
    cartilage Q31.8
  tibia —see Defect, reduction, lower limb,
      longitudinal, tibia
  tibiofibular —see Defect, reduction, lower
      limb, specified type NEC
  toe (and foot) (complete) (partial) —see
      Agenesis, foot
  tongue Q38.3
  trachea (cartilage) Q32.1
  ulna —see Defect, reduction, upper limb,
      longitudinal, ulna
  upper limb —see Agenesis, arm
  ureter Q62.4
  urethra Q64.5
  urinary tract NEC Q64.8

Agenesis (Continued)
  uterus Q51.0
  uvula Q38.5
  vagina Q52.0
  vas deferens Q55.4
  vein (s) (peripheral) Q27.9
    brain Q28.3
    great NEC Q26.8
    portal Q26.5
  vena cava (inferior) (superior) Q26.8
  vermis of cerebellum Q04.3
  vertebra Q76.49
  vulva Q52.71
Ageusia R43.2
Agitated —see condition
Agitation R45.1
Aglossia (congenital) Q38.3
Aglossia-adactylia syndrome Q87.0
Aglycogenosis E74.00
Agnosia (body image) (other senses) (tactile)
    R48.1
  developmental F88
  verbal R48.1
    auditory R48.1
      developmental F80.2
    developmental F80.2
  visual (object) R48.3
Agoraphobia F40.00
  with panic disorder F40.01
  without panic disorder F40.02
Agrammatism R48.8
Agranulocytopenia —see Agranulocytosis
Agranulocytosis (chronic) (cyclical) (genetic)
    (infantile) (periodic) (pernicious) (see also
    Neutropenia) D70.9
  congenital D70.0
  cytoreductive cancer chemotherapy sequela
      D70.1
  drug-induced D70.2
    due to cytoreductive cancer chemotherapy
        D70.1
  due to infection D70.3
  secondary D70.4
    drug-induced D70.2
      due to cytoreductive cancer
          chemotherapy D70.1
Agraphia (absolute) R48.8
  with alexia R48.0
  developmental F81.81
Ague (dumb) —see Malaria
Agyria Q04.3
Ahumada-del Castillo syndrome E23.0
Aichomophobia F40.298
AIDS (related complex) B20
Ailment heart —see Disease, heart
Ailurophobia F40.218
Ainhum (disease) L94.6
AIN —see Neoplasia, intraepithelial, anal ◀
AIPHI (acute idiopathic pulmonary hemorrhage
    in infants (over 28 days old)) R04.81
Air
  anterior mediastinum J98.2
  compressed, disease T70.3
  conditioner lung or pneumonitis J67.7
  embolism (artery) (cerebral) (any site) T79.0
    with ectopic or molar pregnancy O08.2
    due to implanted device NEC —see
        Complications, by site and type,
        specified NEC
    following
      abortion —see Abortion by type,
          complicated by, embolism
      ectopic or molar pregnancy O08.2
    infusion, therapeutic injection or
        transfusion T80.0
    in pregnancy, childbirth or puerperium —
        see Embolism, obstetric
    traumatic T79.0
  hunger, psychogenic F45.8
  rarefied, effects of —see Effect, adverse, high
      altitude
  sickness T75.3

Airplane sickness T75.3
Akathisia (drug-induced) (treatment- induced) G25.71
   neuroleptic induced (acute) G25.71
Akinesia R29.898
Akinetic mutism R41.89
Akureyri's disease G93.3
Alactasia, congenital E73.0
Alagille's syndrome Q44.7
Alastrim B03
Albers-Schönberg syndrome Q78.2
Albert's syndrome —see Tendinitis, Achilles
Albinism, albino E70.30
   with hematologic abnormality E70.339
      Chédiak-Higashi syndrome E70.330
      Hermansky-Pudlak syndrome E70.331
      other specified E70.338
   I E70.320
   II E70.321
   ocular E70.319
      autosomal recessive E70.311
      other specified E70.318
      X-linked E70.310
   oculocutaneous E70.329
      other specified E70.328
      tyrosinase (ty) negative E70.320
      tyrosinase (ty) positive E70.321
   other specified E70.39
Albinismus E70.30
Albright (-McCune)(-Sternberg) syndrome Q78.1
Albuminous —see condition
Albuminuria, albuminuric (acute) (chronic) (subacute) —see also Proteinuria R80.9
   complicating pregnancy —see Proteinuria, gestational
      with
         gestational hypertension —see Pre-eclampsia
         pre-existing hypertension —see Hypertension, complicating pregnancy, pre-existing, with, pre-eclampsia
   gestational —see Proteinuria, gestational
      with
         gestational hypertension —see Pre-eclampsia
         pre-existing hypertension —see Hypertension, complicating pregnancy, pre-existing, with, pre-eclampsia
   orthostatic R80.2
   postural R80.2
   pre-eclamptic —see Pre-eclampsia
   scarlatinal A38.8
Albuminurophobia F40.298
Alcaptonuria E70.29
Alcohol, alcoholic, alcohol-induced
   addiction (without remission) F10.20
      with remission F10.21
   amnestic disorder, persisting F10.96
      with dependence F10.26
   anxiety disorder F10.980 ◄
   bipolar and related disorder F10.94 ◄
   brain syndrome, chronic F10.97
      with dependence F10.27
   cardiopathy I42.6
   counseling and surveillance Z71.41
      family member Z71.42
   delirium (acute) (tremens) (withdrawal) F10.231
      with intoxication F10.921
         in
            abuse F10.121
            dependence F10.221
   dementia F10.97
      with dependence F10.27
   depressive disorder F10.94 ◄
   deterioration F10.97
      with dependence F10.27

Alcohol, alcoholic, alcohol-induced (Continued)
   hallucinosis (acute) F10.951
      in
         abuse F10.151
         dependence F10.251
   insanity F10.959
   intoxication (acute) (without dependence) F10.129
      with
         delirium F10.121
         dependence F10.229
            with delirium F10.221
            uncomplicated F10.220
         uncomplicated F10.120
   jealousy F10.988
   Korsakoff's, Korsakov's, Korsakow's F10.26
   liver K70.9
      acute —see Disease, liver, alcoholic, hepatitis
   major neurocognitive disorder, amnestic-confabulatory type F10.96 ◄
   major neurocognitive disorder, nonamnestic-confabulatory type F10.97 ◄
   mania (acute) (chronic) F10.959
   mild neurocognitive disorder F10.988 ◄
   paranoia, paranoid (type) psychosis F10.950
   pellagra E52
   poisoning, accidental (acute) NEC —see Table of Drugs and Chemicals, alcohol, poisoning
   psychosis —see Psychosis, alcoholic
   psychotic disorder F10.959 ◄
   sexual dysfunction F10.981 ◄
   sleep disorder F10.982 ◄
   withdrawal (without convulsions) F10.239
      with delirium F10.231
Alcoholism (chronic) (without remission) F10.20
   with
      psychosis —see Psychosis, alcoholic remission F10.21
   Korsakov's F10.96
      with dependence F10.26
Alder (-Reilly) anomaly or syndrome (leukocyte granulation) D72.0
Aldosteronism E26.9
   familial (type I) E26.02
   glucocorticoid-remediable E26.02
   primary (due to (bilateral) adrenal hyperplasia) E26.09
   primary NEC E26.09
   secondary E26.1
   specified NEC E26.89
Aldosteronoma D44.10
Aldrich(-Wiskott) syndrome (eczema-thrombocytopenia) D82.0
Alektorophobia F40.218
Aleppo boil B55.1
Aleukemic —see condition Aleukia
   congenital D70.0
   hemorrhagica D61.9
      congenital D61.09
   splenica D73.1
Alexia R48.0
   developmental F81.0
   secondary to organic lesion R48.0
Algoneurodystrophy M89.00
   ankle M89.07-
   foot M89.07-
   forearm M89.03-
   hand M89.04-
   lower leg M89.06-
   multiple sites M89.0-
   shoulder M89.01-
   specified site NEC M89.08
   thigh M89.05-
   upper arm M89.02-
Algophobia F40.298
Alienation, mental —see Psychosis
Alkalemia E87.3

Alkalosis E87.3
   metabolic E87.3
      with respiratory acidosis E87.4
   respiratory E87.3
Alkaptonuria E70.29
Allen-Masters syndrome N83.8
Allergy, allergic (reaction) (to) T78.40
   air-borne substance NEC (rhinitis) J30.89
   alveolitis (extrinsic) J67.9
      due to
         Aspergillus clavatus J67.4
         Cryptostroma corticale J67.6
         organisms (fungal, thermophilic actinomycete) growing in ventilation (air conditioning) systems J67.7
      specified type NEC J67.8
   anaphylactic reaction or shock T78.2
   angioneurotic edema T78.3
   animal (dander) (epidermal) (hair) (rhinitis) J30.81
   bee sting (anaphylactic shock) —see Toxicity, venom, arthropod, bee
   biological —see Allergy, drug
   colitis —see also Colitis, allergic K52.29 ◄▥
   dander (animal) (rhinitis) J30.81
   dandruff (rhinitis) J30.81
   dental restorative material (existing) K08.55
   dermatitis —see Dermatitis, contact, allergic
   diathesis —see History, allergy
   drug, medicament & biological (any) (external) (internal) T78.40
      correct substance properly administered —see Table of Drugs and Chemicals, by drug, adverse effect
      wrong substance given or taken NEC (by accident) —see Table of Drugs and Chemicals, by drug, poisoning
   due to pollen J30.1
   dust (house) (stock) (rhinitis) J30.89
      with asthma —see Asthma, allergic extrinsic
   eczema —see Dermatitis, contact, allergic
   epidermal (animal) (rhinitis) J30.81
   feathers (rhinitis) J30.89
   food (any) (ingested) NEC T78.1
      anaphylactic shock —see Shock, anaphylactic, due to food
      dermatitis —see Dermatitis, due to, food
      dietary counseling and surveillance Z71.3
      in contact with skin L23.6
      rhinitis J30.5
      status (without reaction) Z91.018
         eggs Z91.012
         milk products Z91.011
         peanuts Z91.010
         seafood Z91.013
         specified NEC Z91.018
   gastrointestinal —see also specific type of allergic reaction ◄▥
      meaning colitis —see also Colitis, allergic) K52.29 ◄
      meaning gastroenteritis —see also Gastroenteritis, allergic) K52.29 ◄
      meaning other adverse food reaction not elsewhere classified T78.1 ◄
   grain J30.1
   grass (hay fever) (pollen) J30.1
      asthma —see Asthma, allergic extrinsic
   hair (animal) (rhinitis) J30.81
   history (of) —see History, allergy
   horse serum —see Allergy, serum
   inhalant (rhinitis) J30.89
      pollen J30.1
   kapok (rhinitis) J30.89
   medicine —see Allergy, drug
   milk protein —see also Allergy, food Z91.011 ◄▥
      anaphylactic reaction T78.07 ◄
      dermatitis L27.2 ◄
      enterocolitis syndrome K52.21 ◄
      enteropathy K52.22 ◄
      gastroenteritis K52.29 ◄

Allergy, allergic *(Continued)*
  milk protein *(Continued)*
    gastroesophageal reflux —*see also* Reaction, adverse, food) K21.9 ◄
      with esophagitis K21.0 ◄
    proctocolitis K52.82 ◄]
  nasal, seasonal due to pollen J30.1
  pneumonia J82
  pollen (any) (hay fever) J30.1
    asthma —*see* Asthma, allergic extrinsic
  primrose J30.1
  primula J30.1
  proctocolitis K52.82 ◄
  purpura D69.0
  ragweed (hay fever) (pollen) J30.1
    asthma —*see* Asthma, allergic extrinsic
  rose (pollen) J30.1
  seasonal NEC J30.2
  Senecio jacobae (pollen) J30.1
  serum —*see also* Reaction, serum T80.69
    anaphylactic shock T80.59
  shock (anaphylactic) T78.2
    due to
      administration of blood and blood
        products T80.51
      adverse effect of correct medicinal
        substance properly administered
        T88.6
      immunization T80.52
      serum NEC T80.59
      vaccination T80.52
  specific NEC T78.49
  tree (any) (hay fever) (pollen) J30.1
    asthma —*see* Asthma, allergic extrinsic
  upper respiratory J30.9
  urticaria L50.0
  vaccine —*see* Allergy, serum
  wheat —*see* Allergy, food
Allescheriasis B48.2
Alligator skin disease Q80.9
Allocheiria, allochiria R20.8
Almeida's disease —*see*
  Paracoccidioidomycosis
Alopecia (hereditaria) (seborrheica) L65.9
  androgenic L64.9
    drug-induced L64.0
    specified NEC L64.8
  areata L63.9
    ophiasis L63.2
    specified NEC L63.8
    totalis L63.0
    universalis L63.1
  cicatricial L66.9
    specified NEC L66.8
  circumscripta L63.9
  congenital, congenitalis Q84.0
  due to cytotoxic drugs NEC L65.8
  mucinosa L65.2
  postinfective NEC L65.8
  postpartum L65.0
  premature L64.8
  specific (syphilitic) A51.32
  specified NEC L65.8
  syphilitic (secondary) A51.32
  totalis (capitis) L63.0
  universalis (entire body) L63.1
  X-ray L58.1
Alpers' disease G31.81
Alpine sickness T70.29
Alport syndrome Q87.81
ALTE (apparent life threatening event) in
  newborn and infant R68.13
Alteration (of), Altered
  ~~awareness, transient R40.4~~
  awareness ◄
    transient R40.4 ◄
    unintended under general anesthesia,
      during procedure T88.53 ◄
  mental status R41.82
  pattern of family relationships affecting child
    Z62.898

Alteration (of), Altered *(Continued)*
  sensation
    following
      cerebrovascular disease I69.998
        cerebral infarction I69.398
        intracerebral hemorrhage I69.198
        nontraumatic intracranial hemorrhage
          NEC I69.298
        specified disease NEC I69.898
        subarachnoid hemorrhage I69.098
Alternating —*see* condition
Altitude, high (effects) —*see* Effect, adverse,
  high altitude
Aluminosis (of lung) J63.0
Alveolitis
  allergic (extrinsic) —*see* Pneumonitis,
    hypersensitivity
  due to
    Aspergillus clavatus J67.4
    Cryptostroma corticale J67.6
  fibrosing (cryptogenic) (idiopathic) J84.112
  jaw M27.3
  sicca dolorosa M27.3
Alveolus, alveolar —*see* condition
Alymphocytosis D72.810
  thymic (with immunodeficiency) D82.1
Alymphoplasia, thymic D82.1
Alzheimer's disease or sclerosis —*see* Disease,
  Alzheimer's
Amastia (with nipple present) Q83.8
  with absent nipple Q83.0
Amathophobia F40.228
Amaurosis (acquired) (congenital) —*see also*
  Blindness
  fugax G45.3
  hysterical F44.6
  Leber's congenital H35.50
  uremic —*see* Uremia
Amaurotic idiocy (infantile) (juvenile) (late) E75.4
Amaxophobia F40.248
Ambiguous genitalia Q56.4
Amblyopia (congenital) (ex anopsia) (partial)
  (suppression) H53.00-
  anisometropic —*see* Amblyopia, refractive
  deprivation H53.01-
  hysterical F44.6
  nocturnal —*see also* Blindness, night
    vitamin A deficiency E50.5
  refractive H53.02-
  strabismic H53.03-
  suspect H53.04- ◄
  tobacco H53.8
  toxic NEC H53.8
  uremic —*see* Uremia
Ameba, amebic (histolytica) —*see also* Amebiasis
  abscess (liver) A06.4
Amebiasis A06.9
  with abscess —*see* Abscess, amebic
  acute A06.0
  chronic (intestine) A06.1
    with abscess —*see* Abscess, amebic
  cutaneous A06.7
  cutis A06.7
  cystitis A06.81
  genitourinary tract NEC A06.82
  hepatic —*see* Abscess, liver, amebic
  intestine A06.0
  nondysenteric colitis A06.2
  skin A06.7
  specified site NEC A06.89
Ameboma (of intestine) A06.3
Amelia Q73.0
  lower limb —*see* Agenesis, leg
  upper limb —*see* Agenesis, arm
Ameloblastoma —*see also* Cyst, calcifying
  odontogenic
  long bones C40.9-
    lower limb C40.2-
    upper limb C40.0-
  malignant C41.1
    jaw (bone) (lower) C41.1
      upper C41.0
  tibial C40.2-

Amelogenesis imperfecta K00.5
  nonhereditaria (segmentalis) K00.4
Amenorrhea N91.2
  hyperhormonal E28.8
  primary N91.0
  secondary N91.1
Amentia —*see* Disability, intellectual
  Meynert's (nonalcoholic) F04
American
  leishmaniasis B55.2
  mountain tick fever A93.2
Ametropia —*see* Disorder, refraction
AMH (asymptomatic microscopic hematuria)
  R31.21 ◄
Amianthosis J61
Amimia R48.8
Amino-acid disorder E72.9
  anemia D53.0
Aminoacidopathy E72.9
Aminoaciduria E72.9
Amnes (t)ic syndrome (post-traumatic) F04
  induced by
    alcohol F10.96
      with dependence F10.26
    psychoactive NEC F19.96
      with
        abuse F19.16
        dependence F19.26
    sedative F13.96
      with dependence F13.26
Amnesia R41.3
  anterograde R41.1
  auditory R48.8
  dissociative F44.0
    with dissociative fugue F44.1 ◄
  hysterical F44.0
  postictal in epilepsy —*see* Epilepsy
  psychogenic F44.0
  retrograde R41.2
  transient global G45.4
Amnion, amniotic —*see* condition
Amnionitis —*see* Pregnancy, complicated by
Amok F68.8
Amoral traits F60.89
Amphetamine (or other stimulant) —
  induced ◄
  anxiety disorder F15.980 ◄
  bipolar and related disorder F15.94 ◄
  delirium F15.921 ◄
  depressive disorder F15.94 ◄
  obsessive-compulsive and related disorder
    F15.988 ◄
  psychotic disorder F15.959 ◄
  sexual dysfunction F15.981 ◄
  sleep disorder F15.982 ◄
  stimulant withdrawal F15.23 ◄
Ampulla
  lower esophagus K22.8
  phrenic K22.8
Amputation —*see also* Absence, by site,
  acquired
  neuroma (postoperative) (traumatic) —*see*
    Complications, amputation stump,
    neuroma
  stump (surgical)
    abnormal, painful, or with complication
      (late) —*see* Complications,
      amputation stump
    healed or old NOS Z89.9
  traumatic (complete) (partial)
    arm (upper) (complete) S48.91-
      at
        elbow S58.01-
          partial S58.02-
        shoulder joint (complete) S48.01-
          partial S48.02-
      between
        elbow and wrist (complete) S58.11-
          partial S58.12-
        shoulder and elbow (complete) S48.11-
          partial S48.12-
      partial S48.92-

Amputation *(Continued)*
 traumatic *(Continued)*
  breast (complete) S28.21-
   partial S28.22-
  clitoris (complete) S38.211
   partial S38.212
  ear (complete) S08.11-
   partial S08.12-
  finger (complete) (metacarpophalangeal)
    S68.11-
   index S68.11-
   little S68.11-
   middle S68.11-
   partial S68.12-
    index S68.12-
    little S68.12-
    middle S68.12-
    ring S68.12-
   ring S68.11-
   thumb —*see* Amputation, traumatic,
     thumb
   transphalangeal (complete) S68.61-
    index S68.61-
    little S68.61-
    middle S68.61-
    partial S68.62-
     index S68.62-
     little S68.62-
     middle S68.62-
     ring S68.62-
    ring S68.61-
  foot (complete) S98.91-
   at ankle level S98.01-
    partial S98.02-
   midfoot S98.31-
    partial S98.32-
   partial S98.92-
  forearm (complete) S58.91-
   at elbow level (complete) S58.01-
    partial S58.02-
   between elbow and wrist (complete)
     S58.11-
    partial S58.12-
   partial S58.92-
  genital organ (s) (external)
   female (complete) S38.211
    partial S38.212
   male
    penis (complete) S38.221
     partial S38.222
    scrotum (complete) S38.231
     partial S38.232
    testes (complete) S38.231
     partial S38.232
  hand (complete) (wrist level) S68.41-
   finger (s) alone —*see* Amputation,
     traumatic, finger
   partial S68.42-
   thumb alone —*see* Amputation,
     traumatic, thumb
   transmetacarpal (complete) S68.71-
    partial S68.72-
  head
   ear —*see* Amputation, traumatic, ear
   nose (partial) S08.812
    complete S08.811
   part S08.89
    scalp S08.0
  hip (and thigh) (complete) S78.91-
   at hip joint (complete) S78.01-
    partial S78.02-
   between hip and knee (complete) S78.11-
    partial S78.12-
   partial S78.92-
  labium (majus) (minus) (complete) S38.21-
   partial S38.21-
  leg (lower) S88.91-
   at knee level S88.01-
    partial S88.02-
   between knee and ankle S88.11-
    partial S88.12-
   partial S88.92-

Amputation *(Continued)*
 traumatic *(Continued)*
  nose (partial) S08.812
   complete S08.811
  penis (complete) S38.221
   partial S38.222
  scrotum (complete) S38.231
   partial S38.232
  shoulder —*see* Amputation, traumatic, arm
   at shoulder joint —*see* Amputation,
     traumatic, arm, at shoulder joint
  testes (complete) S38.231
   partial S38.232
  thigh —*see* Amputation, traumatic, hip
  thorax, part of S28.1
   breast —*see* Amputation, traumatic,
     breast
  thumb (complete) (metacarpophalangeal)
    S68.01-
   partial S68.02-
   transphalangeal (complete) S68.51-
    partial S68.52-
  toe (lesser) S98.13-
   great S98.11-
    partial S98.12-
   more than one S98.21-
    partial S98.22-
   partial S98.14-
  vulva (complete) S38.211
   partial S38.212
Amputee (bilateral) (old) Z89.9
Amsterdam dwarfism Q87.1
Amusia R48.8
 developmental F80.89
Amyelencephalus, amyelencephaly Q00.0
Amyelia Q06.0
Amygdalitis —*see* Tonsillitis
Amygdalolith J35.8
Amyloid heart (disease) E85.4 *[I43]*
Amyloidosis (generalized) (primary) E85.9
 with lung involvement E85.4 *[J99]*
 familial E85.2
 genetic E85.2
 heart E85.4 *[I43]*
 hemodialysis-associated E85.3
 liver E85.4 *[K77]*
 localized E85.4
 neuropathic heredofamilial E85.1
 non-neuropathic heredofamilial E85.0
 organ limited E85.4
 Portuguese E85.1
 pulmonary E85.4 *[J99]*
 secondary systemic E85.3
 skin (lichen) (macular) E85.4 *[L99]*
 specified NEC E85.8
 subglottic E85.4 *[J99]*
Amylopectinosis (brancher enzyme deficiency)
   E74.03
Amylophagia —*see* Pica
Amyoplasia congenita Q79.8
Amyotonia M62.89
 congenita G70.2
Amyotrophia, amyotrophy, amyotrophic G71.8
 congenita Q79.8
 diabetic —*see* Diabetes, amyotrophy
 lateral sclerosis G12.21
 neuralgic G54.5
 spinal progressive G12.21
Anacidity, gastric K31.83
 psychogenic F45.8
Anaerosis of newborn P28.89
Analbuminemia E88.09
Analgesia —*see* Anesthesia
Analphalipoproteinemia E78.6
Anaphylactic
 purpura D69.0
 shock or reaction —*see* Shock, anaphylactic
Anaphylactoid shock or reaction —*see* Shock,
   anaphylactic
Anaphylactoid syndrome of pregnancy
   O88.01-

Anaphylaxis —*see* Shock, anaphylactic
Anaplasia cervix —*see also* Dysplasia, cervix
   N87.9
Anaplasmosis, human A77.49
Anarthria R47.1
Anasarca R60.1
 cardiac —*see* Failure, heart, congestive
 lung J18.2
 newborn P83.2
 nutritional E43
 pulmonary J18.2
 renal N04.9
Anastomosis
 aneurysmal —*see* Aneurysm
 arteriovenous ruptured brain I60.8
 intestinal K63.89
  complicated NEC K91.89
   involving urinary tract N99.89
 retinal and choroidal vessels (congenital)
   Q14.8
Anatomical narrow angle H40.03-
Ancylostoma, ancylostomiasis (braziliense)
   (caninum) (ceylanicum) (duodenale) B76.0
 Necator americanus B76.1
Andersen's disease (glycogen storage) E74.09
Anderson-Fabry disease E75.21
Andes disease T70.29
Andrews' disease (bacterid) L08.89
Androblastoma
 benign
  specified site —*see* Neoplasm, benign, by
    site
  unspecified site
   female D27.9
   male D29.20
 malignant
  specified site —*see* Neoplasm, malignant,
    by site
  unspecified site
   female C56.9
   male C62.90
 specified site —*see* Neoplasm, uncertain
   behavior, by site
 tubular
  with lipid storage
   specified site —*see* Neoplasm, benign,
     by site
   unspecified site
    female D27.9
    male D29.20
  specified site —*see* Neoplasm, benign, by site
  unspecified site
   female D27.9
   male D29.20
 unspecified site
  female D39.10
  male D40.10
Androgen insensitivity syndrome —*see also*
   Syndrome, androgen insensitivity E34.50
Androgen resistance syndrome —*see also*
   Syndrome, androgen insensitivity
   E34.50
Android pelvis Q74.2
 with disproportion (fetopelvic) O33.3
  causing obstructed labor O65.3
Androphobia F40.290
Anectasis, pulmonary (newborn) —*see*
   Atelectasis
Anemia (essential) (general) (hemoglobin
   deficiency) (infantile) (primary)
   (profound) D64.9
 with (due to) (in)
  disorder of
   anaerobic glycolysis D55.2
    pentose phosphate pathway D55.1
   koilonychia D50.9
 achlorhydric D50.8
 achrestic D53.1
 Addison (-Biermer) (pernicious) D51.0
 agranulocytic —*see* Agranulocytosis
 amino-acid-deficiency D53.0

Anemia (Continued)
  aplastic D61.9
    congenital D61.09
    drug-induced D61.1
    due to
      drugs D61.1
      external agents NEC D61.2
      infection D61.2
      radiation D61.2
    idiopathic D61.3
    red cell (pure) D60.9
      chronic D60.0
      congenital D61.01
      specified type NEC D60.8
      transient D60.1
    specified type NEC D61.89
    toxic D61.2
  aregenerative
    congenital D61.09
  asiderotic D50.9
  atypical (primary) D64.9
  Baghdad spring D55.0
  Balantidium coli A07.0
  Biermer's (pernicious) D51.0
  blood loss (chronic) D50.0
    acute D62
  bothriocephalus B70.0 [D63.8]
  brickmaker's B76.9 [D63.8]
  cerebral I67.89
  childhood D58.9
  chlorotic D50.8
  chronic
    blood loss D50.0
    hemolytic D58.9
      idiopathic D59.9
    simple D53.9
  chronica congenita aregenerativa D61.09
  combined system disease NEC D51.0 [G32.0]
    due to dietary vitamin B12 deficiency
      D51.3 [G32.0]
  complicating pregnancy, childbirth
    or puerperium —see Pregnancy,
    complicated by (management affected
    by), anemia
  congenital P61.4
    aplastic D61.09
    due to isoimmunization NOS P55.9
    dyserythropoietic, dyshematopoietic D64.4
    following fetal blood loss P61.3
    Heinz body D58.2
    hereditary hemolytic NOS D58.9
    pernicious D51.0
    spherocytic D58.0
  Cooley's (erythroblastic) D56.1
  cytogenic D51.0
  deficiency D53.9
    2, 3 diphosphoglycurate mutase D55.2
    2, 3 PG D55.2
    6 phosphogluconate dehydrogenase D55.1
    6-PGD D55.1
    amino-acid D53.0
    combined B12 and folate D53.1
    enzyme D55.9
      drug-induced (hemolytic) D59.2
      glucose-6-phosphate dehydrogenase
        (G6PD) D55.0
      glycolytic D55.2
      nucleotide metabolism D55.3
      related to hexose monophosphate
        (HMP) shunt pathway NEC D55.1
      specified type NEC D55.8
    erythrocytic glutathione D55.1
    folate D52.9
      dietary D52.0
      drug-induced D52.1
    folic acid D52.9
      dietary D52.0
      drug-induced D52.1
    G SH D55.1
    G6PD D55.0
    GGS-R D55.1

Anemia (Continued)
  deficiency (Continued)
    glucose-6-phosphate dehydrogenase D55.0
    glutathione reductase D55.1
    glyceraldehyde phosphate dehydrogenase
      D55.2
    hexokinase D55.2
    iron D50.9
      secondary to blood loss (chronic) D50.0
    nutritional D53.9
      with
        poor iron absorption D50.8
        specified deficiency NEC D53.8
    phosphofructo-aldolase D55.2
    phosphoglycerate kinase D55.2
    PK D55.2
    protein D53.0
    pyruvate kinase D55.2
    transcobalamin II D51.2
    triose-phosphate isomerase D55.2
    vitamin B12 NOS D51.9
      dietary D51.3
      due to
        intrinsic factor deficiency D51.0
        selective vitamin B12 malabsorption
          with proteinuria D51.1
      pernicious D51.0
      specified type NEC D51.8
  Diamond-Blackfan (congenital hypoplastic)
    D61.01
  dibothriocephalus B70.0 [D63.8]
  dimorphic D53.1
  diphasic D53.1
  Diphyllobothrium (Dibothriocephalus) B70.0
    [D63.8]
  due to (in) (with)
    antineoplastic chemotherapy D64.81
    blood loss (chronic) D50.0
      acute D62
    chemotherapy, antineoplastic D64.81
    chronic disease classified elsewhere NEC
      D63.8
    chronic kidney disease D63.1
    deficiency
      amino-acid D53.0
      copper D53.8
      folate (folic acid) D52.9
        dietary D52.0
        drug-induced D52.1
      molybdenum D53.8
      protein D53.0
      zinc D53.8
    dietary vitamin B12 deficiency D51.3
    disorder of
      glutathione metabolism D55.1
      nucleotide metabolism D55.3
    drug —see Anemia, by type —see also Table
      of Drugs and Chemicals
    end stage renal disease D63.1
    enzyme disorder D55.9
    fetal blood loss P61.3
    fish tapeworm (D latum) infestation B70.0
      [D63.8]
    hemorrhage (chronic) D50.0
      acute D62
    impaired absorption D50.9
    loss of blood (chronic) D50.0
      acute D62
    myxedema E03.9 [D63.8]
    Necator americanus B76.1 [D63.8]
    prematurity P61.2
    selective vitamin B12 malabsorption with
      proteinuria D51.1
    transcobalamin II deficiency D51.2
  Dyke-Young type (secondary) (symptomatic)
    D59.1
  dyserythropoietic (congenital) D64.4
  dyshematopoietic (congenital) D64.4
  Egyptian B76.9 [D63.8]
  elliptocytosis —see Elliptocytosis
  enzyme-deficiency, drug-induced D59.2

Anemia (Continued)
  epidemic —see also Ancylostomiasis B76.9
    [D63.8]
  erythroblastic
    familial D56.1
    newborn —see also Disease, hemolytic P55.9
    of childhood D56.1
  erythrocytic glutathione deficiency D55.1
  erythropoietin-resistant anemia (EPO
    resistant anemia) D63.1
  Faber's (achlorhydric anemia) D50.9
  factitious (self-induced blood letting) D50.0
  familial erythroblastic D56.1
  Fanconi's (congenital pancytopenia) D61.09
  favism D55.0
  fish tapeworm (D. latum) infestation B70.0
    [D63.8]
  folate (folic acid) deficiency D52.9
  glucose-6-phosphate dehydrogenase (G6PD)
    deficiency D55.0
  glutathione-reductase deficiency D55.1
  goat's milk D52.0
  granulocytic —see Agranulocytosis
  Heinz body, congenital D58.2
  hemolytic D58.9
    acquired D59.9
      with hemoglobinuria NEC D59.6
      autoimmune NEC D59.1
      infectious D59.4
      specified type NEC D59.8
      toxic D59.4
    acute D59.9
      due to enzyme deficiency specified type
        NEC D55.8
      Lederer's D59.1
    autoimmune D59.1
      drug-induced D59.0
    chronic D58.9
      idiopathic D59.9
    cold type (secondary) (symptomatic) D59.1
    congenital (spherocytic) —see
      Spherocytosis
    due to
      cardiac conditions D59.4
      drugs (nonautoimmune) D59.2
        autoimmune D59.0
      enzyme disorder D55.9
        drug-induced D59.2
      presence of shunt or other internal
        prosthetic device D59.4
    familial D58.9
    hereditary D58.9
      due to enzyme disorder D55.9
        specified type NEC D55.8
      specified type NEC D58.8
    idiopathic (chronic) D59.9
    mechanical D59.4
    microangiopathic D59.4
    nonautoimmune D59.4
      drug-induced D59.2
    nonspherocytic
      congenital or hereditary NEC D55.8
        glucose-6-phosphate dehydrogenase
          deficiency D55.0
        pyruvate kinase deficiency D55.2
      type
        I D55.1
        II D55.2
      type
        I D55.1
        II D55.2
    secondary D59.4
      autoimmune D59.1
    specified (hereditary) type NEC D58.8
    Stransky-Regala type —see also
      Hemoglobinopathy D58.8
    symptomatic D59.4
      autoimmune D59.1
    toxic D59.4
    warm type (secondary) (symptomatic)
      D59.1

◀ New   ◀▥ Revised   ~~deleted~~ Deleted

Anemia *(Continued)*
  hemorrhagic (chronic) D50.0
    acute D62
  Herrick's D57.1
  hexokinase deficiency D55.2
  hookworm B76.9 *[D63.8]*
  hypochromic (idiopathic) (microcytic)
      (normoblastic) D50.9
    due to blood loss (chronic) D50.0
      acute D62
    familial sex-linked D64.0
    pyridoxine-responsive D64.3
    sideroblastic, sex-linked D64.0
  hypoplasia, red blood cells D61.9
    congenital or familial D61.01
  hypoplastic (idiopathic) D61.9
    congenital or familial (of childhood)
        D61.01
  hypoproliferative (refractive) D61.9
  idiopathic D64.9
    aplastic D61.3
    hemolytic, chronic D59.9
  in (due to) (with)
    chronic kidney disease D63.1
    end stage renal disease D63.1
    failure, kidney (renal) D63.1
    neoplastic disease —*see also* Neoplasm
        D63.0
  intertropical —*see also* Ancylostomiasis D63.8
  iron deficiency D50.9
    secondary to blood loss (chronic) D50.0
      acute D62
    specified type NEC D50.8
  Joseph-Diamond-Blackfan (congenital
      hypoplastic) D61.01
  Lederer's (hemolytic) D59.1
  leukoerythroblastic D61.82
  macrocytic D53.9
    nutritional D52.0
    tropical D52.8
  malarial (*see also* Malaria) B54 *[D63.8]*
  malignant (progressive) D51.0
  malnutrition D53.9
  marsh (*see also* Malaria) B54 *[D63.8]*
  Mediterranean (with other
      hemoglobinopathy) D56.9
  megaloblastic D53.1
    combined B12 and folate deficiency
        D53.1
    hereditary D51.1
    nutritional D52.0
    orotic aciduria D53.0
    refractory D53.1
    specified type NEC D53.1
  megalocytic D53.1
  microcytic (hypochromic) D50.9
    due to blood loss (chronic) D50.0
      acute D62
    familial D56.8
  microdrepanocytosis D57.40
  microelliptopoikilocytic (Rietti-Greppi-
      Micheli) D56.9
  miner's B76.9 *[D63.8]*
  myelodysplastic D46.9
  myelofibrosis D75.81
  myelogenous D64.89
  myelopathic D64.89
  myelophthisic D61.82
  myeloproliferative D47.Z9
  newborn P61.4
    due to
      ABO (antibodies, isoimmunization,
          maternal/fetal incompatibility)
          P55.1
      Rh (antibodies, isoimmunization,
          maternal/fetal incompatibility)
          P55.0
    following fetal blood loss P61.3
    posthemorrhagic (fetal) P61.3
  nonspherocytic hemolytic —*see* Anemia,
      hemolytic, nonspherocytic

Anemia *(Continued)*
  normocytic (infectional) D64.9
    due to blood loss (chronic) D50.0
      acute D62
    myelophthisic D61.82
  nutritional (deficiency) D53.9
    with
      poor iron absorption D50.8
      specified deficiency NEC D53.8
    megaloblastic D52.0
  of prematurity P61.2
  orotaciduric (congenital) (hereditary) D53.0
  osteosclerotic D64.89
  ovalocytosis (hereditary) —*see* Elliptocytosis
  paludal —*see also* Malaria B54 *[D63.8]*
  pernicious (congenital) (malignant)
      (progressive) D51.0
  pleochromic D64.89
    of sprue D52.8
  posthemorrhagic (chronic) D50.0
    acute D62
    newborn P61.3
  postoperative (postprocedural)
    due to (acute) blood loss D62
      chronic blood loss D50.0
    specified NEC D64.9
  postpartum O90.81
  pressure D64.89
  progressive D64.9
    malignant D51.0
    pernicious D51.0
  protein-deficiency D53.0
  pseudoleukemica infantum D64.89
  pure red cell D60.9
    congenital D61.01
  pyridoxine-responsive D64.3
  pyruvate kinase deficiency D55.2
  refractory D46.4
    with
      excess of blasts D46.20
        1 (RAEB 1) D46.21
        2 (RAEB 2) D46.22
        in transformation (RAEB T) —*see*
            Leukemia, acute myeloblastic
      hemochromatosis D46.1
      sideroblasts (ring) (RARS) D46.1
    without ring sideroblasts, so stated D46.0
    without sideroblasts without excess of
        blasts D46.0
    megaloblastic D53.1
    sideroblastic D46.1
    sideropenic D50.9
  Rietti-Greppi-Micheli D56.9
  scorbutic D53.2
  secondary to
    blood loss (chronic) D50.0
      acute D62
    hemorrhage (chronic) D50.0
      acute D62
  semiplastic D61.89
  sickle-cell —*see* Disease, sickle-cell
  sideroblastic D64.3
    hereditary D64.0
    hypochromic, sex-linked D64.0
    pyridoxine-responsive NEC D64.3
    refractory D46.1
    secondary (due to)
      disease D64.1
      drugs and toxins D64.2
    specified type NEC D64.3
  sideropenic (refractory) D50.9
    due to blood loss (chronic) D50.0
      acute D62
  simple chronic D53.9
  specified type NEC D64.89
  spherocytic (hereditary) —*see* Spherocytosis
  splenic D64.89
  splenomegalic D64.89
  stomatocytosis D58.8
  syphilitic (acquired) (late) A52.79 *[D63.8]*
  target cell D64.89

Anemia *(Continued)*
  thalassemia D56.9
  thrombocytopenic —*see* Thrombocytopenia
  toxic D61.2
  tropical B76.9 *[D63.8]*
    macrocytic D52.8
  tuberculous A18.89 *[D63.8]*
  vegan D51.3
  vitamin
    B6-responsive D64.3
    B12 deficiency (dietary) pernicious D51.0
  von Jaksch's D64.89
  Witts' (achlorhydric anemia) D50.8
Anemophobia F40.228
Anencephalus, anencephaly Q00.0
Anergasia —*see* Psychosis, organic
Anesthesia, anesthetic R20.0
  complication or reaction NEC —*see also*
      Complications, anesthesia T88.59
    due to
      correct substance properly
          administered —*see* Table of Drugs
          and Chemicals, by drug, adverse
          effect
      overdose or wrong substance given —*see*
          Table of Drugs and Chemicals, by
          drug, poisoning
      unintended awareness under general
          anesthesia during procedure
          T88.53 ◀
        personal history of Z92.84 ◀
  cornea H18.81-
  dissociative F44.6
  functional (hysterical) F44.6
  hyperesthetic, thalamic G89.0
  hysterical F44.6
  local skin lesion R20.0
  sexual (psychogenic) F52.1
  shock (due to) T88.2
  skin R20.0
  testicular N50.9
Anetoderma (maculosum) (of) L90.8
  Jadassohn-Pellizzari L90.2
  Schweninger-Buzzi L90.1
Aneurin deficiency E51.9
Aneurysm (anastomotic) (artery) (cirsoid)
    (diffuse) (false) (fusiform) (multiple)
    (saccular) I72.9
  abdominal (aorta) I71.4
    ruptured I71.3
    syphilitic A52.01
  aorta, aortic (nonsyphilitic) I71.9
    abdominal I71.4
      ruptured I71.3
    arch I71.2
      ruptured I71.1
    arteriosclerotic I71.9
      ruptured I71.8
    ascending I71.2
      ruptured I71.1
    congenital Q25.43 ◀▥
    descending I71.9
      abdominal I71.4
        ruptured I71.3
      ruptured I71.8
      thoracic I71.2
        ruptured I71.1
    root Q25.43 ◀
    ruptured I71.8
    sinus, congenital Q25.43 ◀▥
    syphilitic A52.01
    thoracic I71.2
      ruptured I71.1
    thoracoabdominal I71.6
      ruptured I71.5
    thorax, thoracic (arch) I71.2
      ruptured I71.1
    transverse I71.2
      ruptured I71.1
    valve (heart) —*see also* Endocarditis, aortic
        I35.8

Angina *(Continued)*
  spasm-induced —*see* Angina, with
      documented spasm
  specified NEC I20.8
  stable I20.8 ◀▥
  stenocardia —*see* Angina, specified NEC
  stridulous, diphtheritic A36.2
  tonsil J36
  trachealis J05.0
  unstable I20.0
  variant —*see* Angina, with documented
      spasm
  Vincent's A69.1
  worsening effort —*see* Angina, unstable
Angioblastoma —*see* Neoplasm, connective
  tissue, uncertain behavior
Angiocholecystitis —*see* Cholecystitis, acute
Angiocholitis —*see also* Cholecystitis, acute K83.0
Angiodysgenesis spinalis G95.19
Angiodysplasia (cecum) (colon) K55.20
  with bleeding K55.21
  duodenum (and stomach) K31.819
    with bleeding K31.811
  stomach (and duodenum) K31.819
    with bleeding K31.811
Angioedema (allergic) (any site) (with urticaria)
  T78.3
  hereditary D84.1
Angioendothelioma —*see* Neoplasm, uncertain
  behavior, by site
  benign D18.00
    intra-abdominal D18.03
    intracranial D18.02
    skin D18.01
    specified site NEC D18.09
  bone —*see* Neoplasm, bone, malignant
  Ewing's —*see* Neoplasm, bone, malignant
Angioendotheliomatosis C85.8-
Angiofibroma —*see also* Neoplasm, benign, by
  site
  juvenile
    specified site —*see* Neoplasm, benign, by
      site
    unspecified site D10.6
Angiohemophilia (A) (B) D68.0
Angioid streaks (choroid) (macula) (retina)
  H35.33
Angiokeratoma —*see* Neoplasm, skin, benign
  corporis diffusum E75.21
Angioleiomyoma —*see* Neoplasm, connective
  tissue, benign
Angiolipoma —*see also* Lipoma
  infiltrating —*see* Lipoma
Angioma —*see also* Hemangioma, by site
  capillary I78.1
  hemorrhagicum hereditaria I78.0
  intra-abdominal D18.03
  intracranial D18.02
  malignant —*see* Neoplasm, connective tissue,
    malignant
  plexiform D18.00
    intra-abdominal D18.03
    intracranial D18.02
    skin D18.01
    specified site NEC D18.09
  senile I78.1
  serpiginosum L81.7
  skin D18.01
  specified site NEC D18.09
  spider I78.1
  stellate I78.1
  venous Q28.3
Angiomatosis Q82.8
  bacillary A79.89
  encephalotrigeminal Q85.8
  hemorrhagic familial I78.0
  hereditary familial I78.0
  liver K76.4
Angiomyolipoma —*see* Lipoma
Angiomyoliposarcoma —*see* Neoplasm,
  connective tissue, malignant

Angiomyoma —*see* Neoplasm, connective
  tissue, benign
Angiomyosarcoma —*see* Neoplasm, connective
  tissue, malignant
Angiomyxoma —*see* Neoplasm, connective
  tissue, uncertain behavior
Angioneurosis F45.8
Angioneurotic edema (allergic) (any site) (with
  urticaria) T78.3
  hereditary D84.1
Angiopathia, angiopathy I99.9
  cerebral I67.9
    amyloid E85.4 [I68.0]
  diabetic (peripheral) —*see* Diabetes,
    angiopathy
  peripheral I73.9
    diabetic —*see* Diabetes, angiopathy
    specified type NEC I73.89
  retinae syphilitica A52.05
  retinalis (juvenilis)
    diabetic —*see* Diabetes, retinopathy
    proliferative —*see* Retinopathy,
      proliferative
Angiosarcoma —*see also* Neoplasm, connective
  tissue, malignant
  liver C22.3
Angiosclerosis —*see* Arteriosclerosis
Angiospasm (peripheral) (traumatic) (vessel)
  I73.9
  brachial plexus G54.0
  cerebral G45.9
  cervical plexus G54.2
  nerve
    arm —*see* Mononeuropathy, upper limb
      axillary G54.0
      median —*see* Lesion, nerve, median
      ulnar —*see* Lesion, nerve, ulnar
    axillary G54.0
    leg —*see* Mononeuropathy, lower limb
    median —*see* Lesion, nerve, median
    plantar —*see* Lesion, nerve, plantar
    ulnar —*see* Lesion, nerve, ulnar
Angiospastic disease or edema I73.9
Angiostrongyliasis
  due to
    Parastrongylus
      cantonensis B83.2
      costaricensis B81.3
  intestinal B81.3
Anguillulosis —*see* Strongyloidiasis
Angulation
  cecum —*see* Obstruction, intestine
  coccyx (acquired) —*see also* subcategory
    M43.8
    congenital NEC Q76.49
  femur (acquired) —*see also* Deformity, limb,
    specified type NEC, thigh
    congenital Q74.2
  intestine (large) (small) —*see* Obstruction,
    intestine
  sacrum (acquired) —*see also* subcategory M43.8
    congenital NEC Q76.49
  sigmoid (flexure) —*see* Obstruction, intestine
  spine —*see* Dorsopathy, deforming, specified
    NEC
  tibia (acquired) —*see also* Deformity, limb,
    specified type NEC, lower leg
    congenital Q74.2
  ureter N13.5
    with infection N13.6
  wrist (acquired) —*see also* Deformity, limb,
    specified type NEC, forearm
    congenital Q74.0
Angulus infectiosus (lips) K13.0
Anhedonia R45.84
  sexual F52.0 ◀
Anhidrosis L74.4
~~Anhydration, anhydremia E86.0~~
  ~~with~~
    ~~hypernatremia E87.0~~
    ~~hyponatremia E87.1~~

Anhydration E86.0 ◀
Anhydremia E86.0
  ~~with~~
    ~~hypernatremia E87.0~~
    ~~hyponatremia E87.1~~
Anidrosis L74.4
Aniridia (congenital) Q13.1
Anisakiasis (infection) (infestation) B81.0
Anisakis larvae infestation B81.0
Aniseikonia H52.32
Anisocoria (pupil) H57.02
  congenital Q13.2
Anisocytosis R71.8
Anisometropia (congenital) H52.31
Ankle —*see* condition
Ankyloblepharon (eyelid) (acquired) —*see also*
  Blepharophimosis
  filiforme (adnatum) (congenital) Q10.3
  total Q10.3
Ankyloglossia Q38.1
Ankylosis (fibrous) (osseous) (joint) M24.60
  ankle M24.67-
  arthrodesis status Z98.1
  cricoarytenoid (cartilage) (joint) (larynx) J38.7
  dental K03.5
  ear ossicles H74.31-
  elbow M24.62-
  foot M24.67-
  hand M24.64-
  hip M24.65-
  incostapedial joint (infectional) —*see*
    Ankylosis, ear ossicles
  jaw (temporomandibular) M26.61- ◀▥
  knee M24.66-
  lumbosacral (joint) M43.27
  postoperative (status) Z98.1
  produced by surgical fusion, status Z98.1
  sacro-iliac (joint) M43.28
  shoulder M24.61-
  spine (joint) —*see also* Fusion, spine
    spondylitic —*see* Spondylitis, ankylosing
  surgical Z98.1
  temporomandibular M26.61- ◀▥
  tooth, teeth (hard tissues) K03.5
  wrist M24.63-
Ankylostoma —*see* Ancylostoma
Ankylostomiasis —*see* Ancylostomiasis
Ankylurethria —*see* Stricture, urethra
Annular —*see also* condition
  detachment, cervix N88.8
  organ or site, congenital NEC —*see* Distortion
  pancreas (congenital) Q45.1
Anodontia (complete) (partial) (vera) K00.0
  acquired K08.10
Anomaly, anomalous (congenital) (unspecified
  type) Q89.9
  abdominal wall NEC Q79.59
  acoustic nerve Q07.8
  adrenal (gland) Q89.1
  Alder (-Reilly) (leukocyte granulation) D72.0
  alimentary tract Q45.9
    upper Q40.9
  alveolar M26.70
    hyperplasia M26.79
      mandibular M26.72
      maxillary M26.71
    hypoplasia M26.79
      mandibular M26.74
      maxillary M26.73
    ridge (process) M26.79
    specified NEC M26.79
  ankle (joint) Q74.2
  anus Q43.9
  aorta (arch) NEC Q25.40 ◀▥
    coarctation (preductal) (postductal) Q25.1
  aortic cusp or valve Q23.9
  appendix Q43.8
  apple peel syndrome Q41.1
  aqueduct of Sylvius Q03.0
    with spina bifida —*see* Spina bifida, with
      hydrocephalus

Anomaly, anomalous *(Continued)*
  arm Q74.0
  arteriovenous NEC
    coronary Q24.5
    gastrointestinal Q27.33
      acquired —*see* Angiodysplasia
  artery (peripheral) Q27.9
    basilar NEC Q28.1
    cerebral Q28.3
    coronary Q24.5
    digestive system Q27.8
    eye Q15.8
    great Q25.9
      specified NEC Q25.8
    lower limb Q27.8
    peripheral Q27.9
      specified NEC Q27.8
    pulmonary NEC Q25.79
    renal Q27.2
    retina Q14.1
    specified site NEC Q27.8
    subclavian Q27.8
      origin Q25.48 ◀
    umbilical Q27.0
    upper limb Q27.8
    vertebral NEC Q28.1
  aryteno-epiglottic folds Q31.8
  atrial
    bands or folds Q20.8
    septa Q21.1
  atrioventricular
    excitation I45.6
    septum Q21.0
  auditory canal Q17.8
  auricle
    ear Q17.8
      causing impairment of hearing
        Q16.9
    heart Q20.8
  Axenfeld's Q15.0
  back Q89.9
  band
    atrial Q20.8
    heart Q24.8
    ventricular Q24.8
  Bartholin's duct Q38.4
  biliary duct or passage Q44.5
  bladder Q64.70
    absence Q64.5
    diverticulum Q64.6
    exstrophy Q64.10
      cloacal Q64.12
      extroversion Q64.19
      specified type NEC Q64.19
      supravesical fissure Q64.11
    neck obstruction Q64.31
    specified type NEC Q64.79
  bone Q79.9
    arm Q74.0
    face Q75.9
    leg Q74.2
    pelvic girdle Q74.2
    shoulder girdle Q74.0
    skull Q75.9
      with
        anencephaly Q00.0
        encephalocele —*see* Encephalocele
        hydrocephalus Q03.9
          with spina bifida —*see* Spina bifida,
            by site, with hydrocephalus
        microcephaly Q02
  brain (multiple) Q04.9
    vessel Q28.3
  breast Q83.9
  broad ligament Q50.6
  bronchus Q32.4
  bulbus cordis Q21.9
  bursa Q79.9
  canal of Nuck Q52.4
  canthus Q10.3
  capillary Q27.9

Anomaly, anomalous *(Continued)*
  cardiac Q24.9
    chambers Q20.9
      specified NEC Q20.8
    septal closure Q21.9
      specified NEC Q21.8
    valve NEC Q24.8
      pulmonary Q22.3
  cardiovascular system Q28.8
  carpus Q74.0
  caruncle, lacrimal Q10.6
  cascade stomach Q40.2
  cauda equina Q06.3
  cecum Q43.9
  cerebral Q04.9
    vessels Q28.3
  cervix Q51.9
  Chédiak-Higashi(-Steinbrinck) (congenital
    gigantism of peroxidase granules)
    E70.330
  cheek Q18.9
  chest wall Q67.8
    bones Q76.9
  chin Q18.9
  chordae tendineae Q24.8
  choroid Q14.3
    plexus Q07.8
  chromosomes, chromosomal Q99.9
    D (1) —*see* condition, chromosome 13
    E (3) —*see* condition, chromosome 18
    G —*see* condition, chromosome 21
    sex
      female phenotype Q97.8
      gonadal dysgenesis (pure) Q99.1
      Klinefelter's Q98.4
      male phenotype Q98.9
      Turner's Q96.9
    specified NEC Q99.8
  cilia Q10.3
  circulatory system Q28.9
  clavicle Q74.0
  clitoris Q52.6
  coccyx Q76.49
  colon Q43.9
  common duct Q44.5
  communication
    coronary artery Q24.5
    left ventricle with right atrium Q21.0
  concha (ear) Q17.3
  connection
    portal vein Q26.5
    pulmonary venous Q26.4
      partial Q26.3
      total Q26.2
    renal artery with kidney Q27.2
  cornea (shape) Q13.4
  coronary artery or vein Q24.5
  cranium —*see* Anomaly, skull
  cricoid cartilage Q31.8
  cystic duct Q44.5
  dental
    alveolar —*see* Anomaly, alveolar
    arch relationship M26.20
      specified NEC M26.29
  dentofacial M26.9
    alveolar —*see* Anomaly, alveolar
    dental arch relationship M26.20
      specified NEC M26.29
    functional M26.50
      specified NEC M26.59
    jaw-cranial base relationship M26.10
      asymmetry M26.12
        maxillary M26.11
      specified type NEC M26.19
    jaw size M26.00
      macrogenia M26.05
      mandibular
        hyperplasia M26.03
        hypoplasia M26.04
      maxillary
        hyperplasia M26.01
        hypoplasia M26.02

Anomaly, anomalous *(Continued)*
  dentofacial *(Continued)*
    jaw size *(Continued)*
      microgenia M26.06
      specified type NEC M26.09
    malocclusion M26.4
      dental arch relationship NEC M26.29
      jaw-cranial base relationship —*see*
        Anomaly, dentofacial, jaw-cranial
        base relationship
      jaw size —*see* Anomaly, dentofacial, jaw
        size
    specified type NEC M26.89
    temporomandibular joint M26.60- ◀▥
      adhesions M26.61- ◀▥
      ankylosis M26.61- ◀▥
      arthralgia M26.62- ◀▥
      articular disc M26.63- ◀▥
      specified type NEC M26.69
    tooth position, fully erupted M26.30
      specified NEC M26.39
  dermatoglyphic Q82.8
  diaphragm (apertures) NEC Q79.1
  digestive organ (s) or tract Q45.9
    lower Q43.9
    upper Q40.9
  distance, interarch (excessive) (inadequate)
    M26.25
  distribution, coronary artery Q24.5
  ductus
    arteriosus Q25.0
    botalli Q25.0
  duodenum Q43.9
  dura (brain) Q04.9
    spinal cord Q06.9
  ear (external) Q17.9
    causing impairment of hearing Q16.9
    inner Q16.5
    middle (causing impairment of hearing)
      Q16.4
    ossicles Q16.3
  Ebstein's (heart) (tricuspid valve) Q22.5
  ectodermal Q82.9
  Eisenmenger's (ventricular septal defect)
    Q21.8
  ejaculatory duct Q55.4
  elbow Q74.0
  endocrine gland NEC Q89.2
  epididymis Q55.4
  epiglottis Q31.8
  esophagus Q39.9
  eustachian tube Q17.8
  eye Q15.9
    anterior segment Q13.9
      specified NEC Q13.89
    posterior segment Q14.9
      specified NEC Q14.8
    ptosis (eyelid) Q10.0
    specified NEC Q15.8
  eyebrow Q18.8
  eyelid Q10.3
    ptosis Q10.0
  face Q18.9
    bone(s) Q75.9
  fallopian tube Q50.6
  fascia Q79.9
  femur NEC Q74.2
  fibula NEC Q74.2
  finger Q74.0
  fixation, intestine Q43.3
  flexion (joint) NOS Q74.9
    hip or thigh Q65.89
  foot NEC Q74.2
    varus (congenital) Q66.3
  foramen
    Botalli Q21.1
    ovale Q21.1
  forearm Q74.0
  forehead Q75.8
  form, teeth K00.2
  fovea centralis Q14.1

◀ New   ◀▥ Revised   ~~deleted~~ Deleted

Anomaly, anomalous *(Continued)*
  frontal bone —*see* Anomaly, skull
  gallbladder (position) (shape) (size) Q44.1
  Gartner's duct Q52.4
  gastrointestinal tract Q45.9
  genitalia, genital organ (s) or system
    female Q52.9
      external Q52.70
      internal NOS Q52.9
    male Q55.9
      hydrocele P83.5
      specified NEC Q55.8
  genitourinary NEC
    female Q52.9
    male Q55.9
  Gerbode Q21.0
  glottis Q31.8
  granulation or granulocyte, genetic
      (constitutional) (leukocyte) D72.0
  gum Q38.6
  gyri Q07.9
  hair Q84.2
  hand Q74.0
  hard tissue formation in pulp K04.3
  head —*see* Anomaly, skull
  heart Q24.9
    auricle Q20.8
    bands or folds Q24.8
    fibroelastosis cordis I42.4
    obstructive NEC Q22.6
    patent ductus arteriosus (Botalli) Q25.0
    septum Q21.9
      auricular Q21.1
      interatrial Q21.1
      interventricular Q21.0
        with pulmonary stenosis or atresia,
          dextraposition of aorta and
          hypertrophy of right ventricle
          Q21.3
      specified NEC Q21.8
      ventricular Q21.0
        with pulmonary stenosis or atresia,
          dextraposition of aorta and
          hypertrophy of right ventricle
          Q21.3
    tetralogy of Fallot Q21.3
    valve NEC Q24.8
      aortic
        bicuspid valve Q23.1
        insufficiency Q23.1
        stenosis Q23.0
          subaortic Q24.4
      mitral
        insufficiency Q23.3
        stenosis Q23.2
      pulmonary Q22.3
        atresia Q22.0
        insufficiency Q22.2
        stenosis Q22.1
          infundibular Q24.3
          subvalvular Q24.3
      tricuspid
        atresia Q22.4
        stenosis Q22.4
    ventricle Q20.8
  heel NEC Q74.2
  Hegglin's D72.0
  hemianencephaly Q00.0
  hemicephaly Q00.0
  hemicrania Q00.0
  hepatic duct Q44.5
  hip NEC Q74.2
  hourglass stomach Q40.2
  humerus Q74.0
  hydatid of Morgagni
    female Q50.5
    male (epididymal) Q55.4
      testicular Q55.29
  hymen Q52.4
  hypersegmentation of neutrophils, hereditary
      D72.0

Anomaly, anomalous *(Continued)*
  hypophyseal Q89.2
  ileocecal (coil) (valve) Q43.9
  ileum Q43.9
  ilium NEC Q74.2
  integument Q84.9
    specified NEC Q84.8
  interarch distance (excessive) (inadequate)
      M26.25
  intervertebral cartilage or disc Q76.49
  intestine (large) (small) Q43.9
    with anomalous adhesions, fixation or
      malrotation Q43.3
  iris Q13.2
  ischium NEC Q74.2
  jaw —*see* Anomaly, dentofacial
    alveolar —*see* Anomaly, alveolar
  jaw-cranial base relationship —*see*
      Anomaly, dentofacial, jaw-cranial
      base relationship
  jejunum Q43.8
  joint Q74.9
    specified NEC Q74.8
  Jordan's D72.0
  kidney(s) (calyx) (pelvis) Q63.9
    artery Q27.2
    specified NEC Q63.8
  Klippel-Feil (brevicollis) Q76.1
  knee Q74.1
  labium (majus) (minus) Q52.70
  labyrinth, membranous Q16.5
  lacrimal apparatus or duct Q10.6
  larynx, laryngeal (muscle) Q31.9
    web (bed) Q31.0
  lens Q12.9
  leukocytes, genetic D72.0
    granulation (constitutional) D72.0
  lid (fold) Q10.3
  ligament Q79.9
    broad Q50.6
    round Q52.8
  limb Q74.9
    lower NEC Q74.2
      reduction deformity —*see* Defect,
        reduction, lower limb
    upper Q74.0
  lip Q38.0
  liver Q44.7
    duct Q44.5
  lower limb NEC Q74.2
  lumbosacral (joint) (region) Q76.49
    kyphosis —*see* Kyphosis, congenital
    lordosis —*see* Lordosis, congenital
  lung (fissure) (lobe) Q33.9
  mandible —*see* Anomaly, dentofacial
  maxilla —*see* Anomaly, dentofacial
  May (-Hegglin) D72.0
  meatus urinarius NEC Q64.79
  meningeal bands or folds Q07.9
    constriction of Q07.8
    spinal Q06.9
  meninges Q07.9
    cerebral Q04.8
    spinal Q06.9
  meningocele Q05.9
  mesentery Q45.9
  metacarpus Q74.0
  metatarsus NEC Q74.2
  middle ear Q16.4
    ossicles Q16.3
  mitral (leaflets) (valve) Q23.9
    insufficiency Q23.3
    specified NEC Q23.8
    stenosis Q23.2
  mouth Q38.6
  Müllerian —*see also* Anomaly, by site
    uterus NEC Q51.818
  multiple NEC Q89.7
  muscle Q79.9
    eyelid Q10.3
  musculoskeletal system, except limbs Q79.9

Anomaly, anomalous *(Continued)*
  myocardium Q24.8
  nail Q84.6
  narrowness, eyelid Q10.3
  nasal sinus (wall) Q30.8
  neck (any part) Q18.9
  nerve Q07.9
    acoustic Q07.8
    optic Q07.8
  nervous system (central) Q07.9
  nipple Q83.9
  nose, nasal (bones) (cartilage) (septum)
      (sinus) Q30.9
    specified NEC Q30.8
  ocular muscle Q15.8
  omphalomesenteric duct Q43.0
  opening, pulmonary veins Q26.4
  optic
    disc Q14.2
    nerve Q07.8
  opticociliary vessels Q13.2
  orbit (eye) Q10.7
  organ Q89.9
    of Corti Q16.5
  origin
    artery
      innominate Q25.8
      pulmonary Q25.79
      renal Q27.2
      subclavian Q25.48 ◀▦
  osseous meatus (ear) Q16.1
  ovary Q50.39
  oviduct Q50.6
  palate (hard) (soft) NEC Q38.5
  pancreas or pancreatic duct Q45.3
  papillary muscles Q24.8
  parathyroid gland Q89.2
  paraurethral ducts Q64.79
  parotid (gland) Q38.4
  patella Q74.1
  Pelger-Huët (hereditary hyposegmentation)
      D72.0
  pelvic girdle NEC Q74.2
  pelvis (bony) NEC Q74.2
    rachitic E64.3
  penis (glans) Q55.69
  pericardium Q24.8
  peripheral vascular system Q27.9
  Peter's Q13.4
  pharynx Q38.8
  pigmentation L81.9
    congenital Q82.8
  pituitary (gland) Q89.2
  pleural (folds) Q34.0
  portal vein Q26.5
    connection Q26.5
  position, tooth, teeth, fully erupted M26.30
    specified NEC M26.39
  precerebral vessel Q28.1
  prepuce Q55.69
  prostate Q55.4
  pulmonary Q33.9
    artery NEC Q25.79
    valve Q22.3
      atresia Q22.0
      insufficiency Q22.2
      specified type NEC Q22.3
      stenosis Q22.1
        infundibular Q24.3
        subvalvular Q24.3
    venous connection Q26.4
      partial Q26.3
      total Q26.2
  pupil Q13.2
    function H57.00
      anisocoria H57.02
      Argyll Robertson pupil H57.01
      miosis H57.03
      mydriasis H57.04
      specified type NEC H57.09
      tonic pupil H57.05-

Anomaly, anomalous *(Continued)*
 pylorus Q40.3
 radius Q74.0
 rectum Q43.9
 reduction (extremity) (limb)
  femur (longitudinal) —*see* Defect,
   reduction, lower limb, longitudinal,
   femur
  fibula (longitudinal) —*see* Defect,
   reduction, lower limb, longitudinal,
   fibula
  lower limb —*see* Defect, reduction, lower
   limb
  radius (longitudinal) —*see* Defect,
   reduction, upper limb, longitudinal,
   radius
  tibia (longitudinal) —*see* Defect, reduction,
   lower limb, longitudinal, tibia
  ulna (longitudinal) —*see* Defect, reduction,
   upper limb, longitudinal, ulna
  upper limb —*see* Defect, reduction, upper
   limb
 refraction —*see* Disorder, refraction
 renal Q63.9
  artery Q27.2
  pelvis Q63.9
   specified NEC Q63.8
 respiratory system Q34.9
  specified NEC Q34.8
 retina Q14.1
 rib Q76.6
  cervical Q76.5
 Rieger's Q13.81
 rotation —*see* Malrotation
  hip or thigh Q65.89
 round ligament Q52.8
 sacroiliac (joint) NEC Q74.2
 sacrum NEC Q76.49
  kyphosis —*see* Kyphosis, congenital
  lordosis —*see* Lordosis, congenital
 saddle nose, syphilitic A50.57
 salivary duct or gland Q38.4
 scapula Q74.0
 scrotum —*see* Malformation, testis and
  scrotum
 sebaceous gland Q82.9
 seminal vesicles Q55.4
 sense organs NEC Q07.8
 sex chromosomes NEC —*see also* Anomaly,
  chromosomes
  female phenotype Q97.8
  male phenotype Q98.9
 shoulder (girdle) (joint) Q74.0
 sigmoid (flexure) Q43.9
 simian crease Q82.8
 sinus of Valsalva Q25.49 ◀▦
 skeleton generalized Q78.9
 skin (appendage) Q82.9
 skull Q75.9
  with
   anencephaly Q00.0
   encephalocele —*see* Encephalocele
   hydrocephalus Q03.9
    with spina bifida —*see* Spina bifida, by
     site, with hydrocephalus
   microcephaly Q02
 specified organ or site NEC Q89.8
 spermatic cord Q55.4
 spine, spinal NEC Q76.49
  column NEC Q76.49
   kyphosis —*see* Kyphosis, congenital
   lordosis —*see* Lordosis, congenital
  cord Q06.9
  nerve root Q07.8
 spleen Q89.09
  agenesis Q89.01
 stenonian duct Q38.4
 sternum NEC Q76.7
 stomach Q40.3
 submaxillary gland Q38.4
 tarsus NEC Q74.2

Anomaly, anomalous *(Continued)*
 tendon Q79.9
 testis —*see* Malformation, testis and
  scrotum
 thigh NEC Q74.2
 thorax (wall) Q67.8
  bony Q76.9
 throat Q38.8
 thumb Q74.0
 thymus gland Q89.2
 thyroid (gland) Q89.2
  cartilage Q31.8
 tibia NEC Q74.2
  saber A50.56
 toe Q74.2
 tongue Q38.3
 tooth, teeth K00.9
  eruption K00.6
  position, fully erupted M26.30
  spacing, fully erupted M26.30
 trachea (cartilage) Q32.1
 tragus Q17.9
 tricuspid (leaflet) (valve) Q22.9
  atresia or stenosis Q22.4
  Ebstein's Q22.5
 Uhl's (hypoplasia of myocardium, right
  ventricle) Q24.8
 ulna Q74.0
 umbilical artery Q27.0
 union
  cricoid cartilage and thyroid cartilage
   Q31.8
  thyroid cartilage and hyoid bone
   Q31.8
  trachea with larynx Q31.8
 upper limb Q74.0
 urachus Q64.4
 ureter Q62.8
  obstructive NEC Q62.39
   cecoureterocele Q62.32
   orthotopic ureterocele Q62.31
 urethra Q64.70
  absence Q64.5
  double Q64.74
  fistula to rectum Q64.73
  obstructive Q64.39
   stricture Q64.32
  prolapse Q64.71
  specified type NEC Q64.79
 urinary tract Q64.9
 uterus Q51.9
  with only one functioning horn Q51.4
 uvula Q38.5
 vagina Q52.4
 valleculae Q31.8
 valve (heart) NEC Q24.8
  coronary sinus Q24.5
  inferior vena cava Q24.8
  pulmonary Q22.3
  sinus coronario Q24.5
  venae cavae inferioris Q24.8
 vas deferens Q55.4
 vascular Q27.9
  brain Q28.3
  ring Q25.45 ◀▦
 vein (s) (peripheral) Q27.9
  brain Q28.3
  cerebral Q28.3
  coronary Q24.5
  developmental Q28.3
  great Q26.9
   specified NEC Q26.8
 vena cava (inferior) (superior) Q26.9
 venous —*see* Anomaly, vein (s)
 venous return Q26.8
 ventricular
  bands or folds Q24.8
  septa Q21.0
 vertebra Q76.49
  kyphosis —*see* Kyphosis, congenital
  lordosis —*see* Lordosis, congenital

Anomaly, anomalous *(Continued)*
 vesicourethral orifice Q64.79
 vessel (s) Q27.9
  optic papilla Q14.2
  precerebral Q28.1
 vitelline duct Q43.0
 vitreous body or humor Q14.0
 vulva Q52.70
 wrist (joint) Q74.0
Anomia R48.8
Anonychia (congenital) Q84.3
 acquired L60.8
Anophthalmos, anophthalmus (congenital)
  (globe) Q11.1
 acquired Z90.01
Anopia, anopsia H53.46-
 quadrant H53.46-
Anorchia, anorchism, anorchidism Q55.0
Anorexia R63.0
 hysterical F44.89
 nervosa F50.00
  atypical F50.9
  binge-eating type F50.2
   with purging F50.02
  restricting type F50.01
Anorgasmy, psychogenic (female)
  F52.31
 male F52.32
Anosmia R43.0
 hysterical F44.6
 postinfectional J39.8
Anosognosia R41.89
Anosteoplasia Q78.9
Anovulatory cycle N97.0
Anoxemia R09.02
 newborn P84
Anoxia (pathological) R09.02
 altitude T70.29
 cerebral G93.1
  complicating
   anesthesia (general) (local) or other
    sedation T88.59
   in labor and delivery O74.3
   in pregnancy O29.21-
    postpartum, puerperal O89.2
  delivery (cesarean) (instrumental)
   O75.4
  during a procedure G97.81
  newborn P84
  resulting from a procedure G97.82
 due to
  drowning T75.1
  high altitude T70.29
 heart —*see* Insufficiency, coronary
 intrauterine P84
 myocardial —*see* Insufficiency, coronary
 newborn P84
 spinal cord G95.11
 systemic (by suffocation) (low content in
  atmosphere) —*see* Asphyxia,
  traumatic
Anteflexion —*see* Anteversion
Antenatal
 care (normal pregnancy) Z34.90
 screening (encounter for) of mother
  Z36
Antepartum —*see* condition
Anterior —*see* condition
Antero-occlusion M26.220
Anteversion
 cervix —*see* Anteversion, uterus
 femur (neck), congenital Q65.89
 uterus, uterine (cervix) (postinfectional)
  (postpartal, old) N85.4
  congenital Q51.818
  in pregnancy or childbirth —*see* Pregnancy,
   complicated by
Anthophobia F40.228
Anthracosilicosis J60
Anthracosis (lung) (occupational) J60
 lingua K14.3

◀ New   ◀▦ Revised   ~~deleted~~ Deleted

Anthrax A22.9
  with pneumonia A22.1
  cerebral A22.8
  colitis A22.2
  cutaneous A22.0
  gastrointestinal A22.2
  inhalation A22.1
  intestinal A22.2
  meningitis A22.8
  pulmonary A22.1
  respiratory A22.1
  sepsis A22.7
  specified manifestation NEC A22.8
Anthropoid pelvis Q74.2
  with disproportion (fetopelvic) O33.0
Anthropophobia F40.10
  generalized F40.11
Antibodies, maternal (blood group) —see
    Isoimmunization, affecting management
    of pregnancy
  anti-D —see Isoimmunization, affecting
    management of pregnancy, Rh
    newborn P55.0
Antibody
  anticardiolipin R76.0
    with
      hemorrhagic disorder D68.312
      hypercoagulable state D68.61
  antiphosphatidylglycerol R76.0
    with
      hemorrhagic disorder D68.312
      hypercoagulable state D68.61
  antiphosphatidylinositol R76.0
    with
      hemorrhagic disorder D68.312
      hypercoagulable state D68.61
  antiphosphatidylserine R76.0
    with
      hemorrhagic disorder D68.312
      hypercoagulable state D68.61
  antiphospholipid R76.0
    with
      hemorrhagic disorder D68.312
      hypercoagulable state D68.61
Anticardiolipin syndrome D68.61
Anticoagulant, circulating (intrinsic) —see also -
    Disorder, hemorrhagic D68.318
  drug-induced (extrinsic) —see also - Disorder,
    hemorrhagic D68.32
  iatrogenic D68.32 ◀
Antidiuretic hormone syndrome E22.2
Antimonial cholera —see Poisoning,
    antimony
Antiphospholipid
  antibody
    with hemorrhagic disorder D68.312
  syndrome D68.61
Antisocial personality F60.2
Antithrombinemia —see Circulating
    anticoagulants
Antithromboplastinemia D68.318
Antithromboplastinogenemia D68.318
Antitoxin complication or reaction —see
    Complications, vaccination
Antlophobia F40.228
Antritis J32.0
  maxilla J32.0
    acute J01.00
      recurrent J01.01
  stomach K29.60
    with bleeding K29.61
Antrum, antral —see condition
Anuria R34
  calculous (impacted) (recurrent) —see also
      Calculus, urinary N20.9
  following
    abortion —see Abortion by type
        complicated by, renal failure
    ectopic or molar pregnancy O08.4
  newborn P96.0
  postprocedural N99.0

Anuria (Continued)
  postrenal N13.8
  traumatic (following crushing) T79.5
Anus, anal —see condition
Anusitis K62.89
Anxiety F41.9
  depression F41.8
  episodic paroxysmal F41.0
  generalized F41.1
  hysteria F41.8
  neurosis F41.1
  panic type F41.0
  reaction F41.1
  separation, abnormal (of childhood) F93.0
  specified NEC F41.8
  state F41.1
Aorta, aortic —see condition
Aortectasia —see Ectasia, aorta
  with aneurysm —see Aneurysm, aorta
Aortitis (nonsyphilitic) (calcific) I77.6
  arteriosclerotic I70.0
  Doehle-Heller A52.02
  luetic A52.02
  rheumatic —see Endocarditis, acute,
      rheumatic
  specific (syphilitic) A52.02
  syphilitic A52.02
    congenital A50.54 [I79.1]
Apathetic thyroid storm —see Thyrotoxicosis
Apathy R45.3
Apeirophobia F40.228
Apepsia K30
  psychogenic F45.8
Aperistalsis, esophagus K22.0
Apertognathia M26.29
Apert's syndrome Q87.0
Aphagia R13.0
  psychogenic F50.9
Aphakia (acquired) (postoperative) H27.0-
  congenital Q12.3
Aphasia (amnestic) (global) (nominal)
    (semantic) (syntactic) R47.01
  acquired, with epilepsy (Landau-Kleffner
      syndrome) —see Epilepsy, specified
      NEC
  auditory (developmental) F80.2
  developmental (receptive type) F80.2
    expressive type F80.1
    Wernicke's F80.2
  following
    cerebrovascular disease I69.920
      cerebral infarction I69.320
      intracerebral hemorrhage I69.120
      nontraumatic intracranial hemorrhage
          NEC I69.220
      specified disease NEC I69.820
      subarachnoid hemorrhage I69.020
    primary progressive G31.01 [F02.80]
      with behavioral disturbance G31.01
          [F02.81]
    progressive isolated G31.01 [F02.80]
      with behavioral disturbance G31.01
          [F02.81]
  sensory F80.2
  syphilis, tertiary A52.19
  Wernicke's (developmental) F80.2
Aphonia (organic) R49.1
  hysterical F44.4
  psychogenic F44.4
Aphthae, aphthous —see also condition
  Bednar's K12.0
  cachectic K14.0
  epizootic B08.8
  fever B08.8
  oral (recurrent) K12.0
  stomatitis (major) (minor) K12.0
  thrush B37.0
  ulcer (oral) (recurrent) K12.0
    genital organ (s) NEC
      female N76.6
      male N50.89 ◀║
  larynx J38.7

Apical —see condition
Apiphobia F40.218
Aplasia —see also Agenesis
  abdominal muscle syndrome Q79.4
  alveolar process (acquired) —see Anomaly,
      alveolar
    congenital Q38.6
  aorta (congenital) Q25.41 ◀║
  axialis extracorticalis (congenita) E75.29
  bone marrow (myeloid) D61.9
    congenital D61.01
  brain Q00.0
    part of Q04.3
  bronchus Q32.4
  cementum K00.4
  cerebellum Q04.3
  cervix (congenital) Q51.5
  congenital pure red cell D61.01
  corpus callosum Q04.0
  cutis congenita Q84.8
  erythrocyte congenital D61.01
  extracortical axial E75.29
  eye Q11.1
  fovea centralis (congenital) Q14.1
  gallbladder, congenital Q44.0
  iris Q13.1
  labyrinth, membranous Q16.5
  limb (congenital) Q73.8
    lower —see Defect, reduction, lower limb
    upper —see Agenesis, arm
  lung, congenital (bilateral) (unilateral) Q33.3
  pancreas Q45.0
  parathyroid-thymic D82.1
  Pelizaeus-Merzbacher E75.29
  penis Q55.5
  prostate Q55.4
  red cell (with thymoma) D60.9
    acquired D60.9
      due to drugs D60.9
    adult D60.9
    chronic D60.0
    congenital D61.01
    constitutional D61.01
    due to drugs D60.9
    hereditary D61.01
    of infants D61.01
    primary D61.01
    pure D61.01
      due to drugs D60.9
    specified type NEC D60.8
    transient D60.1
  round ligament Q52.8
  skin Q84.8
  spermatic cord Q55.4
  spleen Q89.01
  testicle Q55.0
  thymic, with immunodeficiency D82.1
  thyroid (congenital) (with myxedema)
      E03.1
  uterus Q51.0
  ventral horn cell Q06.1
Apnea, apneic (of) (spells) R06.81
  newborn NEC P28.4
    obstructive P28.4
    sleep (central) (obstructive) (primary)
        P28.3
  prematurity P28.4
  sleep G47.30
    central (primary) G47.31
      in conditions classified elsewhere
          G47.37
    obstructive (adult) (pediatric) G47.33
    primary central G47.31
    specified NEC G47.39
Apneumatosis, newborn P28.0
Apocrine metaplasia (breast) —see Dysplasia,
    mammary, specified type NEC
Apophysitis (bone) —see also
    Osteochondropathy
  calcaneus M92.8
  juvenile M92.9

Apoplectiform convulsions (cerebral ischemia) I67.82

Apoplexia, apoplexy, apoplectic
  adrenal A39.1
  heart (auricle) (ventricle) —see Infarct, myocardium
  heat T67.0
  hemorrhagic (stroke) —see Hemorrhage, intracranial
  meninges, hemorrhagic —see Hemorrhage, intracranial, subarachnoid
  uremic N18.9 [I68.8]

Appearance
  bizarre R46.1
  specified NEC R46.89
  very low level of personal hygiene R46.0

Appendage
  epididymal (organ of Morgagni) Q55.4
  intestine (epiploic) Q43.8
  preauricular Q17.0
  testicular (organ of Morgagni) Q55.29

Appendicitis (pneumococcal) (retrocecal) K37
  with
    perforation or rupture K35.2
    peritoneal abscess K35.3
    peritonitis NEC K35.3
      generalized (with perforation or rupture) K35.2
      localized (with perforation or rupture) K35.3
  acute (catarrhal) (fulminating) (gangrenous) (obstructive) (retrocecal) (suppurative) K35.80
    with
      peritoneal abscess K35.3
      peritonitis NEC K35.3
        generalized (with perforation or rupture) K35.2
        localized (with perforation or rupture) K35.3
    specified NEC K35.89
  amebic A06.89
  chronic (recurrent) K36
  exacerbation —see Appendicitis, acute
  gangrenous —see Appendicitis, acute
  healed (obliterative) K36
  interval K36
  neurogenic K36
  obstructive K36
  recurrent K36
  relapsing K36
  subacute (adhesive) K36
  subsiding K36
  suppurative —see Appendicitis, acute
  tuberculous A18.32

Appendicopathia oxyurica B80

Appendix, appendicular —see also condition
  epididymis Q55.4
  Morgagni
    female Q50.5
    male (epididymal) Q55.4
      testicular Q55.29
  testis Q55.29

Appetite
  depraved —see Pica
  excessive R63.2
  lack or loss —see also Anorexia R63.0
    nonorganic origin F50.89 ◀▥
    psychogenic F50.89 ◀▥
  perverted (hysterical) —see Pica

Apple peel syndrome Q41.1

Apprehension state F41.1

Apprehensiveness, abnormal F41.9

Approximal wear K03.0

Apraxia (classic) (ideational) (ideokinetic) (ideomotor) (motor) (verbal) R48.2
  following
    cerebrovascular disease I69.990
      cerebral infarction I69.390
        intracerebral hemorrhage I69.190

Apraxia (Continued)
  following (Continued)
    cerebrovascular disease (Continued)
      nontraumatic intracranial hemorrhage NEC I69.290
      specified disease NEC I69.890
      subarachnoid hemorrhage I69.090
  oculomotor, congenital H51.8

Aptyalism K11.7

Apudoma —see Neoplasm, uncertain behavior, by site

Aqueous misdirection H40.83-

Arabicum elephantiasis —see Infestation, filarial

Arachnitis —see Meningitis

Arachnodactyly —see Syndrome, Marfan's

Arachnoiditis (acute) (adhesive) (basal) (brain) (cerebrospinal) —see Meningitis

Arachnophobia F40.210

Arboencephalitis, Australian A83.4

Arborization block (heart) I45.5

ARC (AIDS-related complex) B20

Arches —see condition

Arcuate uterus Q51.810

Arcuatus uterus Q51.810

Arcus (cornea) senilis —see Degeneration, cornea, senile

Arc-welder's lung J63.4

Areflexia R29.2

Areola —see condition

Argentaffinoma —see also Neoplasm, uncertain behavior, by site
  malignant —see Neoplasm, malignant, by site
  syndrome E34.0

Argininemia E72.21

Arginosuccinic aciduria E72.22

Argyll Robertson phenomenon, pupil or syndrome (syphilitic) A52.19
  atypical H57.09
  nonsyphilitic H57.09

Argyria, argyriasis
  conjunctival H11.13-
  from drug or medicament —see Table of Drugs and Chemicals, by substance

Argyrosis, conjunctival H11.13-

Arhinencephaly Q04.1

Ariboflavinosis E53.0

Arm —see condition

Arnold-Chiari disease, obstruction or syndrome (type II) Q07.00
  with
    hydrocephalus Q07.02
      with spina bifida Q07.03
    spina bifida Q07.01
      with hydrocephalus Q07.03
  type III —see Encephalocele
  type IV Q04.8

Aromatic amino-acid metabolism disorder E70.9
  specified NEC E70.8

Arousals, confusional G47.51

Arrest, arrested
  cardiac I46.9
    complicating
      abortion —see Abortion, by type, complicated by, cardiac arrest
      anesthesia (general) (local) or other sedation —see Table of Drugs and Chemicals, by drug
        in labor and delivery O74.2
        in pregnancy O29.11-
          postpartum, puerperal O89.1
      delivery (cesarean) (instrumental) O75.4
    due to
      cardiac condition I46.2
      specified condition NEC I46.8
    intraoperative I97.71-
    newborn P29.81
    postprocedural I97.12-
      obstetric procedure O75.4

Arrest, arrested (Continued)
  cardiorespiratory —see Arrest, cardiac
  circulatory —see Arrest, cardiac
  deep transverse O64.0
  development or growth
    bone —see Disorder, bone, development or growth
    child R62.50
    tracheal rings Q32.1
    epiphyseal
      complete
        femur M89.15-
        humerus M89.12-
        tibia M89.16-
        ulna M89.13-
      forearm M89.13-
        specified NEC M89.13-
        ulna —see Arrest, epiphyseal, by type, ulna
      lower leg M89.16-
        specified NEC M89.168
        tibia —see Arrest, epiphyseal, by type, tibia
      partial
        femur M89.15-
        humerus M89.12-
        tibia M89.16-
        ulna M89.13-
      specified NEC M89.18
  granulopoiesis —see Agranulocytosis
  growth plate —see Arrest, epiphyseal
  heart —see Arrest, cardiac
  legal, anxiety concerning Z65.3
  physeal —see Arrest, epiphyseal
  respiratory R09.2
    newborn P28.81
  sinus I45.5
  spermatogenesis (complete) —see Azoospermia
    incomplete —see Oligospermia
  transverse (deep) O64.0

Arrhenoblastoma
  benign
    specified site —see Neoplasm, benign, by site
    unspecified site
      female D27.9
      male D29.20
  malignant
    specified site —see Neoplasm, malignant, by site
    unspecified site
      female C56.9
      male C62.90
  specified site —see Neoplasm, uncertain behavior, by site
  unspecified site
    female D39.10
    male D40.10

Arrhythmia (auricle)(cardiac) (juvenile) (nodal) (reflex)(sinus)(supraventricular) (transitory)(ventricle) I49.9
  block I45.9
  extrasystolic I49.49
  newborn
    bradycardia P29.12
      occurring before birth P03.819
        before onset of labor P03.810
        during labor P03.811
    tachycardia P29.11
  psychogenic F45.8
  specified NEC I49.8
  vagal R55
  ventricular re-entry I47.0

Arrillaga-Ayerza syndrome (pulmonary sclerosis with pulmonary hypertension) I27.0

Arsenical pigmentation L81.8
  from drug or medicament —see Table of Drugs and Chemicals

Arsenism —see Poisoning, arsenic

Arterial —*see* condition
Arteriofibrosis —*see* Arteriosclerosis
Arteriolar sclerosis —*see* Arteriosclerosis
Arteriolith —*see* Arteriosclerosis
Arteriolitis I77.6
  necrotizing, kidney I77.5
  renal —*see* Hypertension, kidney
Arteriolosclerosis —*see* Arteriosclerosis
Arterionephrosclerosis —*see* Hypertension,
  kidney
Arteriopathy I77.9
Arteriosclerosis, arteriosclerotic (diffuse)
  (obliterans) (of) (senile) (with calcification)
  I70.90
  aorta I70.0
  arteries of extremities —*see* Arteriosclerosis,
    extremities
  brain I67.2
  bypass graft
    coronary —*see* Arteriosclerosis, coronary,
      bypass graft
    extremities —*see* Arteriosclerosis,
      extremities, bypass graft
  cardiac —*see* Disease, heart, ischemic,
    atherosclerotic
  cardiopathy —*see* Disease, heart, ischemic,
    atherosclerotic
  cardiorenal —*see* Hypertension, cardiorenal
  cardiovascular —*see* Disease, heart, ischemic,
    atherosclerotic
  carotid —*see also* Occlusion, artery, carotid
    I65.2-
  central nervous system I67.2
  cerebral I67.2
  cerebrovascular I67.2
  coronary (artery) I25.10
    bypass graft I25.810
      with
        angina pectoris I25.709
          with documented spasm I25.701
          specified type NEC I25.708
          unstable I25.700
        ischemic chest pain I25.709
      autologous artery I25.810
        with
          angina pectoris I25.729
            with documented spasm I25.721
            specified type I25.728
            unstable I25.720
          ischemic chest pain I25.729
      autologous vein I25.810
        with
          angina pectoris I25.719
            with documented spasm I25.711
            specified type I25.718
            unstable I25.710
          ischemic chest pain I25.719
      nonautologous biological I25.810
        with
          angina pectoris I25.739
            with documented spasm I25.731
            specified type I25.738
            unstable I25.730
          ischemic chest pain I25.739
      specified type NEC I25.810
        with
          angina pectoris I25.799
            with documented spasm I25.791
            specified type I25.798
            unstable I25.790
          ischemic chest pain I25.799
    due to
      calcified coronary lesion (severely) I25.84
      lipid rich plaque I25.83
    native vessel
      with
        angina pectoris I25.119
          with documented spasm I25.111
          specified type NEC I25.118
          unstable I25.110
        ischemic chest pain I25.119

Arteriosclerosis, arteriosclerotic *(Continued)*
  coronary *(Continued)*
    transplanted heart I25.811
      bypass graft I25.812
        with
          angina pectoris I25.769
            with documented spasm
              I25.761
            specified type I25.768
            unstable I25.760
          ischemic chest pain I25.769
      native coronary artery I25.811
        with
          angina pectoris I25.759
            with documented spasm I25.751
            specified type I25.758
            unstable I25.750
          ischemic chest pain I25.759
  extremities (native arteries) I70.209
    bypass graft I70.309
      autologous vein graft I70.409
        leg I70.409
          with
            gangrene (and intermittent
              claudication, rest pain and
              ulcer) I70.469
            intermittent claudication
              I70.419
            rest pain (and intermittent
              claudication) I70.429
        bilateral I70.403
          with
            gangrene (and intermittent
              claudication, rest pain
              and ulcer) I70.463
            intermittent claudication
              I70.413
            rest pain (and intermittent
              claudication) I70.423
          specified type NEC I70.493
        left I70.402
          with
            gangrene (and intermittent
              claudication, rest pain
              and ulcer) I70.462
            intermittent claudication
              I70.412
            rest pain (and intermittent
              claudication) I70.422
            ulceration (and intermittent
              claudication and rest
              pain) I70.449
              ankle I70.443
              calf I70.442
              foot site NEC I70.445
              heel I70.444
              lower leg NEC I70.448
              midfoot I70.444
              thigh I70.441
          specified type NEC I70.492
        right I70.401
          with
            gangrene (and intermittent
              claudication, rest pain
              and ulcer) I70.461
            intermittent claudication
              I70.411
            rest pain (and intermittent
              claudication) I70.421
            ulceration (and intermittent
              claudication and rest
              pain) I70.439
              ankle I70.433
              calf I70.432
              foot site NEC I70.435
              heel I70.434
              lower leg NEC I70.438
              midfoot I70.434
              thigh I70.431
          specified type NEC I70.491
        specified type NEC I70.499

Arteriosclerosis, arteriosclerotic *(Continued)*
  extremities *(Continued)*
    bypass graft *(Continued)*
      autologous vein graft *(Continued)*
        specified NEC I70.408
          with
            gangrene (and intermittent
              claudication, rest pain and
              ulcer) I70.468
            intermittent claudication I70.418
            rest pain (and intermittent
              claudication) I70.428
            ulceration (and intermittent
              claudication and rest pain)
              I70.45
          specified type NEC I70.498
        leg I70.309
          with
            gangrene (and intermittent
              claudication, rest pain and
              ulcer) I70.369
            intermittent claudication I70.319
            rest pain (and intermittent
              claudication) I70.329
        bilateral I70.303
          with
            gangrene (and intermittent
              claudication, rest pain and
              ulcer) I70.363
            intermittent claudication I70.313
            rest pain (and intermittent
              claudication) I70.323
          specified type NEC I70.393
        left I70.302
          with
            gangrene (and intermittent
              claudication, rest pain and
              ulcer) I70.362
            intermittent claudication I70.312
            rest pain (and intermittent
              claudication) I70.322
            ulceration (and intermittent
              claudication and rest pain)
              I70.349
              ankle I70.343
              calf I70.342
              foot site NEC I70.345
              heel I70.344
              lower leg NEC I70.348
              midfoot I70.344
              thigh I70.341
          specified type NEC I70.392
        right I70.301
          with
            gangrene (and intermittent
              claudication, rest pain and
              ulcer) I70.361
            intermittent claudication I70.311
            rest pain (and intermittent
              claudication) I70.321
            ulceration (and intermittent
              claudication and rest pain)
              I70.339
              ankle I70.333
              calf I70.332
              foot site NEC I70.335
              heel I70.334
              lower leg NEC I70.338
              midfoot I70.334
              thigh I70.331
          specified type NEC I70.391
        specified type NEC I70.399
      nonautologous biological graft I70.509
        leg I70.509
          with
            gangrene (and intermittent
              claudication, rest pain and
              ulcer) I70.569
            intermittent claudication I70.519
            rest pain (and intermittent
              claudication) I70.529

Arteriosclerosis, arteriosclerotic (Continued)
extremities (Continued)
bypass graft (Continued)
nonautologous biological graft
(Continued)
leg (Continued)
bilateral I70.503
with
gangrene (and intermittent
claudication, rest pain
and ulcer) I70.563
intermittent claudication
I70.513
rest pain (and intermittent
claudication) I70.523
specified type NEC I70.593
left I70.502
with
gangrene (and intermittent
claudication, rest pain
and ulcer) I70.562
intermittent claudication
I70.512
rest pain (and intermittent
claudication)
I70.522
ulceration (and intermittent
claudication and rest
pain) I70.549
ankle I70.543
calf I70.542
foot site NEC I70.545
heel I70.544
lower leg NEC I70.548
midfoot I70.544
thigh I70.541
specified type NEC I70.592
right I70.501
with
gangrene (and intermittent
claudication, rest pain
and ulcer) I70.561
intermittent claudication
I70.511
rest pain (and intermittent
claudication) I70.521
ulceration (and intermittent
claudication and rest
pain) I70.539
ankle I70.533
calf I70.532
foot site NEC I70.535
heel I70.534
lower leg NEC I70.538
midfoot I70.534
thigh I70.531
specified type NEC I70.591
specified type NEC I70.599
specified NEC I70.508
with
gangrene (and intermittent
claudication, rest pain and
ulcer) I70.568
intermittent claudication
I70.518
rest pain (and intermittent
claudication) I70.528
ulceration (and intermittent
claudication and rest pain)
I70.55
specified type NEC I70.598
nonbiological graft I70.609
leg I70.609
with
gangrene (and intermittent
claudication, rest pain and
ulcer) I70.669
intermittent claudication
I70.619
rest pain (and intermittent
claudication) I70.629

Arteriosclerosis, arteriosclerotic (Continued)
extremities (Continued)
bypass graft (Continued)
nonbiological graft (Continued)
leg (Continued)
bilateral I70.603
with
gangrene (and intermittent
claudication, rest
pain and ulcer)
I70.663
intermittent claudication
I70.613
rest pain (and intermittent
claudication) I70.623
specified type NEC I70.693
left I70.602
with
gangrene (and intermittent
claudication, rest
pain and ulcer)
I70.662
intermittent claudication
I70.612
rest pain (and intermittent
claudication) I70.622
ulceration (and intermittent
claudication and rest
pain) I70.649
ankle I70.643
calf I70.642
foot site NEC I70.645
heel I70.644
lower leg NEC I70.648
midfoot I70.644
thigh I70.641
specified type NEC I70.692
right I70.601
with
gangrene (and intermittent
claudication, rest pain
and ulcer) I70.661
intermittent claudication
I70.611
rest pain (and intermittent
claudication) I70.621
ulceration (and intermittent
claudication and rest
pain) I70.639
ankle I70.633
calf I70.632
foot site NEC I70.635
heel I70.634
lower leg NEC I70.638
midfoot I70.634
thigh I70.631
specified type NEC I70.691
specified type NEC I70.699
specified NEC I70.608
with
gangrene (and intermittent
claudication, rest pain and
ulcer) I70.668
intermittent claudication
I70.618
rest pain (and intermittent
claudication) I70.628
ulceration (and intermittent
claudication and rest pain)
I70.65
specified type NEC I70.698
specified graft NEC I70.709
leg I70.709
with
gangrene (and intermittent
claudication, rest pain and
ulcer) I70.769
intermittent claudication
I70.719
rest pain (and intermittent
claudication) I70.729

Arteriosclerosis, arteriosclerotic (Continued)
extremities (Continued)
bypass graft (Continued)
specified graft NEC (Continued)
leg (Continued)
bilateral I70.703
with
gangrene (and intermittent
claudication, rest pain
and ulcer) I70.763
intermittent claudication
I70.713
rest pain (and intermittent
claudication) I70.723
specified type NEC I70.793
left I70.702
with
gangrene (and intermittent
claudication, rest pain
and ulcer) I70.762
intermittent claudication
I70.712
rest pain (and intermittent
claudication) I70.722
ulceration (and intermittent
claudication and rest
pain) I70.749
ankle I70.743
calf I70.742
foot site NEC I70.745
heel I70.744
lower leg NEC I70.748
midfoot I70.744
thigh I70.741
specified type NEC I70.792
right I70.701
with
gangrene (and intermittent
claudication, rest pain
and ulcer) I70.761
intermittent claudication
I70.711
rest pain (and intermittent
claudication) I70.721
ulceration (and intermittent
claudication and rest
pain) I70.739
ankle I70.733
calf I70.732
foot site NEC I70.735
heel I70.734
lower leg NEC I70.738
midfoot I70.734
thigh I70.731
specified type NEC I70.791
specified type NEC I70.799
specified NEC I70.708
with
gangrene (and intermittent
claudication, rest pain and
ulcer) I70.768
intermittent claudication
I70.718
rest pain (and intermittent
claudication) I70.728
ulceration (and intermittent
claudication and rest pain)
I70.75
specified type NEC I70.798
specified NEC I70.308
with
gangrene (and intermittent
claudication, rest pain and
ulcer) I70.368
intermittent claudication I70.318
rest pain (and intermittent
claudication) I70.328
ulceration (and intermittent
claudication and rest pain)
I70.35
specified type NEC I70.398

◀ New ◀╟╟ Revised ~~deleted~~ Deleted

Arteriosclerosis, arteriosclerotic (Continued)
extremities (Continued)
  leg I70.209
    with
      gangrene (and intermittent
        claudication, rest pain and ulcer)
        I70.269
      intermittent claudication I70.219
      rest pain (and intermittent
        claudication) I70.229
  bilateral I70.203
    with
      gangrene (and intermittent
        claudication, rest pain and
        ulcer) I70.263
      intermittent claudication I70.213
      rest pain (and intermittent
        claudication) I70.223
      specified type NEC I70.293
  left I70.202
    with
      gangrene (and intermittent
        claudication, rest pain and
        ulcer) I70.262
      intermittent claudication I70.212
      rest pain (and intermittent
        claudication) I70.222
      ulceration (and intermittent
        claudication and rest pain)
        I70.249
        ankle I70.243
        calf I70.242
        foot site NEC I70.245
        heel I70.244
        lower leg NEC I70.248
        midfoot I70.244
        thigh I70.241
      specified type NEC I70.292
  right I70.201
    with
      gangrene (and intermittent
        claudication, rest pain and
        ulcer) I70.261
      intermittent claudication I70.211
      rest pain (and intermittent
        claudication) I70.221
      ulceration (and intermittent
        claudication and rest pain)
        I70.239
        ankle I70.233
        calf I70.232
        foot site NEC I70.235
        heel I70.234
        lower leg NEC I70.238
        midfoot I70.234
        thigh I70.231
      specified type NEC I70.291
  specified type NEC I70.299
  specified site NEC I70.208
    with
      gangrene (and intermittent
        claudication, rest pain and ulcer)
        I70.268
      intermittent claudication I70.218
      rest pain (and intermittent
        claudication) I70.228
      ulceration (and intermittent
        claudication and rest pain) I70.25
      specified type NEC I70.298
generalized I70.91
heart (disease) —see Arteriosclerosis,
  coronary (artery)
kidney —see Hypertension, kidney
medial —see Arteriosclerosis, extremities
mesenteric (artery) K55.1
Mönckeberg's —see Arteriosclerosis,
  extremities
myocarditis I51.4
peripheral (of extremities) —see
  Arteriosclerosis, extremities
pulmonary (idiopathic) I27.0

Arteriosclerosis, arteriosclerotic (Continued)
renal (arterioles) —see also Hypertension,
  kidney
  artery I70.1
retina (vascular) I70.8 [H35.0-]
specified artery NEC I70.8
spinal (cord) G95.19
vertebral (artery) I67.2
Arteriospasm I73.9
Arteriovenous —see condition
Arteritis I77.6
allergic M31.0
aorta (nonsyphilitic) I77.6
  syphilitic A52.02
aortic arch M31.4
brachiocephalic M31.4
brain I67.7
  syphilitic A52.04
cerebral I67.7
  in
    diseases classified elsewhere I68.2
    systemic lupus erythematosus M32.19
  listerial A32.89
  syphilitic A52.04
  tuberculous A18.89
coronary (artery) I25.89
  rheumatic I01.8
    chronic I09.89
  syphilitic A52.06
cranial (left) (right), giant cell M31.6
deformans —see Arteriosclerosis
giant cell NEC M31.6
  with polymyalgia rheumatica M31.5
necrosing or necrotizing M31.9
  specified NEC M31.8
nodosa M30.0
obliterans —see Arteriosclerosis
pulmonary I28.8
rheumatic —see Fever, rheumatic
senile —see Arteriosclerosis
suppurative I77.2
syphilitic (general) A52.09
  brain A52.04
  coronary A52.06
  spinal A52.09
temporal, giant cell M31.6
young female aortic arch syndrome M31.4
Artery, arterial —see also condition
abscess I77.89
single umbilical Q27.0
Arthralgia (allergic) —see also Pain, joint
in caisson disease T70.3
temporomandibular M26.62
Arthritis, arthritic (acute) (chronic)
  (nonpyogenic) (subacute) M19.90
allergic —see Arthritis, specified form NEC
ankylosing (crippling) (spine) —see also
  Spondylitis, ankylosing
  sites other than spine —see Arthritis,
    specified form NEC
atrophic —see Osteoarthritis
  spine —see Spondylitis, ankylosing
back —see Spondylopathy, inflammatory
blennorrhagic (gonococcal) A54.42
Charcot's —see Arthropathy, neuropathic
diabetic —see Diabetes, arthropathy,
  neuropathic
syringomyelic G95.0
chylous (filarial) —see also category M01
  B74.9
climacteric (any site) NEC —see Arthritis,
  specified form NEC
crystal (-induced) —see Arthritis, in, crystals
deformans —see Osteoarthritis
degenerative —see Osteoarthritis
due to or associated with
  acromegaly E22.0
  brucellosis —see Brucellosis
  caisson disease T70.3
  diabetes —see Diabetes, arthropathy
  dracontiasis —see also category M01 B72

Arthritis, arthritic (Continued)
due to or associated with (Continued)
  enteritis NEC
    regional —see Enteritis, regional
  erysipelas —see also category M01 A46
  erythema
    epidemic A25.1
    nodosum L52
  filariasis NOS B74.9
  glanders A24.0
  helminthiasis —see also category M01 B83.9
  hemophilia D66 [M36.2]
  Henoch-(Schönlein) purpura D69.0 [M36.4]
  human parvovirus —see also category M01
    B97.6
  infectious disease NEC —see category M01
  leprosy (see also category M01) —see also
    Leprosy A30.9
  Lyme disease A69.23
  mycobacteria —see also category M01
    A31.8
  parasitic disease NEC —see also category
    M01 B89
  paratyphoid fever (see also category M01)
    —see also Fever, paratyphoid A01.4
  rat bite fever —see also category M01
    A25.1
  regional enteritis —see Enteritis, regional
  respiratory disorder NOS J98.9
  serum sickness —see also Reaction, serum
    T80.69
  syringomyelia G95.0
  typhoid fever A01.04
epidemic erythema A25.1
febrile —see Fever, rheumatic
gonococcal A54.42
gouty (acute) —see Gout ◀⣿
in (due to)
  acromegaly —see also subcategory
    M14.8- E22.0
  amyloidosis —see also subcategory
    M14.8- E85.4
  bacterial disease —see also subcategory
    M01 A49.9
  Behçet's syndrome M35.2
  caisson disease —see also subcategory
    M14.8- T70.3
  coliform bacilli (Escherichia coli) —see
    Arthritis, in, pyogenic organism NEC
  crystals M11.9
    dicalcium phosphate —see Arthritis, in,
      crystals, specified type NEC
    hydroxyapatite M11.0-
    pyrophosphate —see Arthritis, in,
      crystals, specified type NEC
    specified type NEC M11.80
      ankle M11.87-
      elbow M11.82-
      foot joint M11.87-
      hand joint M11.84-
      hip M11.85-
      knee M11.86-
      multiple sites M11.8-
      shoulder M11.81-
      vertebrae M11.88
      wrist M11.83-
  dermatoarthritis, lipoid E78.81
  dracontiasis (dracunculiasis) —see also
    category M01 B72
  endocrine disorder NEC —see also
    subcategory M14.8- E34.9
  enteritis, infectious NEC —see also category
    M01 A09
    specified organism NEC —see also
      category M01 A08.8
  erythema
    multiforme —see also subcategory
      M14.8- L51.9
    nodosum —see also subcategory
      M14.8- L52
  gout —see Gout ◀⣿

Arthritis, arthritic *(Continued)*
  in *(Continued)*
    helminthiasis NEC —*see also* category M01
      B83.9
    hemochromatosis —*see also* subcategory
      M14.8- E83.118
    hemoglobinopathy NEC D58.2 *[M36.3]*
    hemophilia NEC D66 *[M36.2]*
    Hemophilus influenzae M00.8- *[B96.3]*
    Henoch(-Schönlein) purpura D69.0 *[M36.4]*
    hyperparathyroidism NEC —*see also*
      subcategory M14.8- E21.3
    hypersensitivity reaction NEC T78.49
      [M36.4]
    hypogammaglobulinemia —*see also*
      subcategory M14.8- D80.1
    hypothyroidism NEC —*see also*
      subcategory M14.8- E03.9
    infection —*see* Arthritis, pyogenic or
      pyemic
      spine —*see* Spondylopathy, infective
    infectious disease NEC —*see* category M01
    leprosy —*see also* category M01 A30.9
    leukemia NEC C95.9- *[M36.1]*
    lipoid dermatoarthritis E78.81
    Lyme disease A69.23
    Mediterranean fever, familial —*see also*
      subcategory M14.8- M04.1 ◀▦
    Meningococcus A39.83
    metabolic disorder NEC —*see also*
      subcategory M14.8- E88.9
    multiple myelomatosis C90.0- *[M36.1]*
    mumps B26.85
    mycosis NEC —*see also* category M01 B49
    myelomatosis (multiple) C90.0- *[M36.1]*
    neurological disorder NEC G98.0
    ochronosis —*see also* subcategory
      M14.8- E70.29
    O'nyong-nyong —*see also* category M01
      A92.1
    parasitic disease NEC —*see also* category
      M01 B89
    paratyphoid fever —*see also* category M01
      A01.4
    Pseudomonas —*see* Arthritis, pyogenic,
      bacterial NEC
    psoriasis L40.50
    pyogenic organism NEC —*see* Arthritis,
      pyogenic, bacterial NEC
    Reiter's disease —*see* Reiter's disease
    respiratory disorder NEC —*see also*
      subcategory M14.8- J98.9
    reticulosis, malignant —*see also*
      subcategory M14.8- C86.0
    rubella B06.82
    Salmonella (arizonae) (cholerae-suis)
      (enteritidis) (typhimurium)
      A02.23
    sarcoidosis D86.86
    specified bacteria NEC —*see* Arthritis,
      pyogenic, bacterial NEC
    sporotrichosis B42.82
    syringomyelia G95.0
    thalassemia NEC D56.9 *[M36.3]*
    tuberculosis —*see* Tuberculosis, arthritis
    typhoid fever A01.04
    urethritis, Reiter's —*see* Reiter's disease
    viral disease NEC —*see also* category M01
      B34.9
  infectious or infective —*see also* Arthritis,
    pyogenic or pyemic
    spine —*see* Spondylopathy, infective
  juvenile M08.90
    with systemic onset —*see* Still's disease
    ankle M08.97-
    elbow M08.92-
    foot joint M08.97-
    hand joint M08.94-
    hip M08.95-
    knee M08.96-
    multiple site M08.99

Arthritis, arthritic *(Continued)*
  juvenile *(Continued)*
    pauciarticular M08.40
      ankle M08.47-
      elbow M08.42-
      foot joint M08.47-
      hand joint M08.44-
      hip M08.45-
      knee M08.46-
      shoulder M08.41-
      vertebrae M08.48
      wrist M08.43-
    psoriatic L40.54
    rheumatoid —*see* Arthritis, rheumatoid,
      juvenile
    shoulder M08.91-
    specified type NEC M08.80
      ankle M08.87-
      elbow M08.82-
      foot joint M08.87-
      hand joint M08.84-
      hip M08.85-
      knee M08.86-
      multiple site M08.89
      shoulder M08.81-
      specified joint NEC M08.88
      vertebrae M08.88
      wrist M08.83-
    vertebra M08.98
    wrist M08.93-
  meaning osteoarthritis —*see* Osteoarthritis
  meningococcal A39.83
  menopausal (any site) NEC —*see* Arthritis,
    specified form NEC
  mutilans (psoriatic) L40.52
  mycotic NEC —*see also* category M01 B49
  neuropathic (Charcot) —*see* Arthropathy,
    neuropathic
    diabetic —*see* Diabetes, arthropathy,
      neuropathic
    nonsyphilitic NEC G98.0
    syringomyelic G95.0
  ochronotic —*see also* subcategory
    M14.8- E70.29
  palindromic (any site) —*see* Rheumatism,
    palindromic
  pneumococcal M00.10
    ankle M00.17-
    elbow M00.12-
    foot joint —*see* Arthritis, pneumococcal,
      ankle
    hand joint M00.14-
    hip M00.15-
    knee M00.16-
    multiple site M00.19
    shoulder M00.11-
    vertebra M00.18
    wrist M00.13-
  postdysenteric —*see* Arthropathy,
    postdysenteric
  postmeningococcal A39.84
  postrheumatic, chronic —*see* Arthropathy,
    postrheumatic, chronic
  primary progressive —*see also* Arthritis,
    specified form NEC
    spine —*see* Spondylitis, ankylosing
  psoriatic L40.50
  purulent (any site except spine) —*see*
    Arthritis, pyogenic or pyemic
    spine —*see* Spondylopathy, infective
  pyogenic or pyemic (any site except spine)
    M00.9
    bacterial NEC M00.80
      ankle M00.87-
      elbow M00.82-
      foot joint —*see* Arthritis, pyogenic,
        bacterial NEC, ankle
      hand joint M00.84-
      hip M00.85-
      knee M00.86-
      multiple site M00.89

Arthritis, arthritic *(Continued)*
  pyogenic or pyemic *(Continued)*
    bacterial NEC *(Continued)*
      shoulder M00.81-
      vertebra M00.88
      wrist M00.83-
    pneumococcal —*see* Arthritis,
      pneumococcal
    spine —*see* Spondylopathy, infective
    staphylococcal —*see* Arthritis,
      staphylococcal
    streptococcal —*see* Arthritis, streptococcal
      NEC
    pneumococcal —*see* Arthritis,
      pneumococcal
  reactive —*see* Reiter's disease
  rheumatic —*see also* Arthritis, rheumatoid
    acute or subacute —*see* Fever, rheumatic
  rheumatoid M06.9
    with
      carditis —*see* Rheumatoid, carditis
      endocarditis —*see* Rheumatoid, carditis
      heart involvement NEC —*see*
        Rheumatoid, carditis
      lung involvement —*see* Rheumatoid,
        lung
      myocarditis —*see* Rheumatoid, carditis
      myopathy —*see* Rheumatoid, myopathy
      pericarditis —*see* Rheumatoid, carditis
      polyneuropathy —*see* Rheumatoid,
        polyneuropathy
      rheumatoid factor —*see* Arthritis,
        rheumatoid, seropositive
      splenoadenomegaly and leukopenia —
        see Felty's syndrome
      vasculitis —*see* Rheumatoid, vasculitis
      visceral involvement NEC —*see*
        Rheumatoid, arthritis, with
        involvement of organs NEC
    juvenile (with or without rheumatoid
      factor) M08.00
    ankle M08.07-
    elbow M08.02-
    foot joint M08.07-
    hand joint M08.04-
    hip M08.05-
    knee M08.06-
    multiple site M08.09
    shoulder M08.01-
    vertebra M08.08
    wrist M08.03-
    seronegative M06.00
    ankle M06.07-
    elbow M06.02-
    foot joint M06.07-
    hand joint M06.04-
    hip M06.05-
    knee M06.06-
    multiple sites M06.09
    shoulder M06.01-
    vertebra M06.08
    wrist M06.03-
    seropositive M05.9
      without organ involvement M05.70
        ankle M05.77-
        elbow M05.72-
        foot joint M05.77-
        hand joint M05.74-
        hip M05.75-
        knee M05.76-
        multiple sites M05.79
        shoulder M05.71-
        vertebra —*see* Spondylitis, ankylosing
        wrist M05.73-
    specified NEC M05.80
      ankle M05.87-
      elbow M05.82-
      foot joint M05.87-
      hand joint M05.84-
      hip M05.85-
      knee M05.86-

Arthritis, arthritic (Continued)
  rheumatoid (Continued)
    specified NEC (Continued)
      multiple sites M05.89
      shoulder M05.81-
      vertebra —see Spondylitis, ankylosing
      wrist M05.83-
    specified type NEC M06.80
      ankle M06.87-
      elbow M06.82-
      foot joint M06.87-
      hand joint M06.84-
      hip M06.85-
      knee M06.86-
      multiple site M06.89
      shoulder M06.81-
      vertebra M06.88
      wrist M06.83-
    spine —see Spondylitis, ankylosing
  rubella B06.82
  scorbutic —see also subcategory M14.8- E54
  senile or senescent —see Osteoarthritis
  septic (any site except spine) —see Arthritis,
      pyogenic or pyemic
    spine —see Spondylopathy, infective
  serum (nontherapeutic) (therapeutic) —see
      Arthropathy, postimmunization
  specified form NEC M13.80
    ankle M13.87-
    elbow M13.82-
    foot joint M13.87-
    hand joint M13.84-
    hip M13.85-
    knee M13.86-
    multiple site M13.89
    shoulder M13.81-
    specified joint NEC M13.88
    wrist M13.83-
  spine —see also Spondylopathy,
      inflammatory
    infectious or infective NEC —see
        Spondylopathy, infective
    Marie-Strümpell —see Spondylitis,
        ankylosing
    pyogenic —see Spondylopathy, infective
    rheumatoid —see Spondylitis, ankylosing
    traumatic (old) —see Spondylopathy,
        traumatic
    tuberculous A18.01
  staphylococcal M00.00
    ankle M00.07-
    elbow M00.02-
    foot joint —see Arthritis, staphylococcal,
        ankle
    hand joint M00.04-
    hip M00.05-
    knee M00.06-
    multiple site M00.09
    shoulder M00.01-
    vertebra M00.08
    wrist M00.03-
  streptococcal NEC M00.20
    ankle M00.27-
    elbow M00.22-
    foot joint —see Arthritis, streptococcal,
        ankle
    hand joint M00.24-
    hip M00.25-
    knee M00.26-
    multiple site M00.29
    shoulder M00.21-
    vertebra M00.28
    wrist M00.23-
  suppurative —see Arthritis, pyogenic or
      pyemic
  syphilitic (late) A52.16
    congenital A50.55 [M12.80]
  syphilitica deformans (Charcot) A52.16
  temporomandibular M26.69
  toxic of menopause (any site) —see Arthritis,
      specified form NEC

Arthritis, arthritic (Continued)
  transient —see Arthropathy, specified form
      NEC
  traumatic (chronic) —see Arthropathy,
      traumatic
  tuberculous A18.02
    spine A18.01
  uratic —see Gout ◀▥
  urethritica (Reiter's) —see Reiter's disease
  vertebral —see Spondylopathy, inflammatory
  villous (any site) —see Arthropathy, specified
      form NEC
Arthrocele —see Effusion, joint
Arthrodesis status Z98.1
Arthrodynia —see also Pain, joint
Arthrodysplasia Q74.9
Arthrofibrosis, joint —see Ankylosis
Arthrogryposis (congenital) Q68.8
  multiplex congenita Q74.3
Arthrokatadysis M24.7
Arthropathy (see also Arthritis) M12.9
  Charcot's —see Arthropathy, neuropathic
    diabetic —see Diabetes, arthropathy,
        neuropathic
    syringomyelic G95.0
  cricoarytenoid J38.7
  crystal(-induced) —see Arthritis, in, crystals
  diabetic NEC —see Diabetes, arthropathy
  distal interphalangeal, psoriatic L40.51
  enteropathic M07.60
    ankle M07.67-
    elbow M07.62-
    foot joint M07.67-
    hand joint M07.64-
    hip M07.65-
    knee M07.66-
    multiple site M07.69
    shoulder M07.61-
    vertebra M07.68
    wrist M07.63-
  following intestinal bypass M02.00
    ankle M02.07-
    elbow M02.02-
    foot joint M02.07-
    hand joint M02.04-
    hip M02.05-
    knee M02.06-
    multiple site M02.09
    shoulder M02.01-
    vertebra M02.08
    wrist M02.03-
  gouty —see also Gout ◀▥
    in (due to)
      Lesch-Nyhan syndrome E79.1 [M14.8-]
      sickle-cell disorders D57- [M14.8-]
  hemophilic NEC D66 [M36.2]
    in (due to)
      hyperparathyroidism NEC E21.3 [M14.8-]
      metabolic disease NOS E88.9 [M14.8-]
  in (due to)
    acromegaly E22.0 [M14.8-]
    amyloidosis E85.4 [M14.8-]
    blood disorder NOS D75.9 [M36.3]
    diabetes —see Diabetes, arthropathy
    endocrine disease NOS E34.9 [M14.8-]
    erythema
      multiforme L51.9 [M14.8-]
      nodosum L52 [M14.8-]
    hemochromatosis E83.118 [M14.8-]
    hemoglobinopathy NEC D58.2 [M36.3]
    hemophilia NEC D66 [M36.2]
    Henoch-Schönlein purpura D69.0 [M36.4]
    hyperthyroidism E05.90 [M14.8-]
    hypothyroidism E03.9 [M14.8-]
    infective endocarditis I33.0 [M12.80]
    leukemia NEC C95.9- [M36.1]
    malignant histiocytosis C96.A [M36.1]
    metabolic disease NOS E88.9 [M14.8-]
    multiple myeloma C90.0- [M36.1]
    neoplastic disease NOS (see also Neoplasm)
        D49.9 [M36.1]

Arthropathy (Continued)
  hemochromatosis (Continued)
    nutritional deficiency —see also
        subcategory M14.8- E63.9
    psoriasis NOS L40.50
    sarcoidosis D86.86
    syphilis (late) A52.77
      congenital A50.55 [M12.80]
    thyrotoxicosis —see also subcategory
        M14.8- E05.90
    ulcerative colitis K51.90 [M07.60]
    viral hepatitis (postinfectious) NEC B19.9
        [M12.80]
    Whipple's disease —see also subcategory
        M14.8- K90.81
  Jaccoud —see Arthropathy, postrheumatic,
      chronic
  juvenile —see Arthritis, juvenile
    psoriatic L40.54
  mutilans (psoriatic) L40.52
  neuropathic (Charcot) M14.60
    ankle M14.67-
    diabetic —see Diabetes, arthropathy,
        neuropathic
    elbow M14.62-
    foot joint M14.67-
    hand joint M14.64-
    hip M14.65-
    knee M14.66-
    multiple site M14.69
    nonsyphilitic NEC G98.0
    shoulder M14.61-
    syringomyelic G95.0
    vertebra M14.68
    wrist M14.63-
  osteopulmonary —see Osteoarthropathy,
      hypertrophic, specified NEC
  postdysenteric M02.10
    ankle M02.17-
    elbow M02.12-
    foot joint M02.17-
    hand joint M02.14-
    hip M02.15-
    knee M02.16-
    multiple site M02.19
    shoulder M02.11-
    vertebra M02.18
    wrist M02.13-
  postimmunization M02.20
    ankle M02.27-
    elbow M02.22-
    foot joint M02.27-
    hand joint M02.24-
    hip M02.25-
    knee M02.26-
    multiple site M02.29
    shoulder M02.21-
    vertebra M02.28
    wrist M02.23-
  postinfectious NEC B99 [M12.80]
    in (due to)
      enteritis due to Yersinia enterocolitica
          A04.6 [M12.80]
      syphilis A52.77
      viral hepatitis NEC B19.9
          [M12.80]
  postrheumatic, chronic (Jaccoud)
      M12.00
    ankle M12.07-
    elbow M12.02-
    foot joint M12.07-
    hand joint M12.04-
    hip M12.05-
    knee M12.06-
    multiple site M12.09
    shoulder M12.01-
    specified joint NEC M12.08
    vertebrae M12.08
    wrist M12.03-
  psoriatic NEC L40.59
    interphalangeal, distal L40.51

Arthropathy *(Continued)*
  reactive M02.9
    in (due to)
      infective endocarditis I33.0 [M02.9]
      specified type NEC M02.80
        ankle M02.87-
        elbow M02.82-
        foot joint M02.87-
        hand joint M02.84-
        hip M02.85-
        knee M02.86-
        multiple site M02.89
        shoulder M02.81-
        vertebra M02.88
        wrist M02.83-
  specified form NEC M12.80
    ankle M12.87-
    elbow M12.82-
    foot joint M12.87-
    hand joint M12.84-
    hip M12.85-
    knee M12.86-
    multiple site M12.89
    shoulder M12.81-
    specified joint NEC M12.88
    vertebrae M12.88
    wrist M12.83-
  syringomyelic G95.0
  tabes dorsalis A52.16
  tabetic A52.16
  transient —*see* Arthropathy, specified form
      NEC
  traumatic M12.50
    ankle M12.57-
    elbow M12.52-
    foot joint M12.57-
    hand joint M12.54-
    hip M12.55-
    knee M12.56-
    multiple site M12.59
    shoulder M12.51-
    specified joint NEC M12.58
    vertebrae M12.58
    wrist M12.53-
Arthropyosis —*see* Arthritis, pyogenic or pyemic
Arthrosis (deformans) (degenerative)
      (localized) —*see also* Osteoarthritis
      M19.90
  spine —*see* Spondylosis
Arthus' phenomenon or reaction T78.41
  due to
    drug —*see* Table of Drugs and Chemicals,
        by drug
Articular —*see* condition
Articulation, reverse (teeth) M26.24
Artificial
  insemination complication —*see*
      Complications, artificial, fertilization
  opening status (functioning) (without
      complication) Z93.9
    anus (colostomy) Z93.3
    colostomy Z93.3
    cystostomy Z93.50
      appendico-vesicostomy Z93.52
      cutaneous Z93.51
      specified NEC Z93.59
    enterostomy Z93.4
    gastrostomy Z93.1
    ileostomy Z93.2
    intestinal tract NEC Z93.4
    jejunostomy Z93.4
    nephrostomy Z93.6
    specified site NEC Z93.8
    tracheostomy Z93.0
    ureterostomy Z93.6
    urethrostomy Z93.6
    urinary tract NEC Z93.6
    vagina Z93.8
  vagina status Z93.8
Arytenoid —*see* condition
Asbestosis (occupational) J61

ASC-H (atypical squamous cells cannot exclude
      high grade squamous intraepithelial lesion
      on cytologic smear)
  anus R85.611
  cervix R87.611
  vagina R87.621
ASC-US (atypical squamous cells of
      undetermined significance on cytologic
      smear)
  anus R85.610
  cervix R87.610
  vagina R87.620
Ascariasis B77.9
  with
    complications NEC B77.89
    intestinal complications B77.0
    pneumonia, pneumonitis B77.81
Ascaridosis, ascaridiasis —*see* Ascariasis
Ascaris (infection) (infestation)
      (lumbricoides) —*see* Ascariasis
Ascending —*see* condition
Aschoff's bodies —*see* Myocarditis,
      rheumatic
Ascites (abdominal) R18.8
  cardiac I50.9
  chylous (nonfilarial) I89.8
    filarial —*see* Infestation, filarial
  due to
    cirrhosis, alcoholic K70.31
    hepatitis
      alcoholic K70.11
      chronic active K71.51
    S. japonicum B65.2
  heart I50.9
  malignant R18.0
  pseudochylous R18.8
  syphilitic A52.74
  tuberculous A18.31
Aseptic —*see* condition
Asherman's syndrome N85.6
Asialia K11.7
Asiatic cholera —*see* Cholera
Asimultagnosia (simultanagnosia)
      R48.3
Askin's tumor —*see* Neoplasm, connective
      tissue, malignant
Asocial personality F60.2
Asomatognosia R41.4
Aspartylglucosaminuria E77.1
Asperger's disease or syndrome F84.5
Aspergilloma —*see* Aspergillosis
Aspergillosis (with pneumonia) B44.9
  bronchopulmonary, allergic B44.81
  disseminated B44.7
  generalized B44.7
  pulmonary NEC B44.1
    allergic B44.81
    invasive B44.0
  specified NEC B44.89
  tonsillar B44.2
Aspergillus (flavus) (fumigatus) (infection)
      (terreus) —*see* Aspergillosis
Aspermatogenesis —*see* Azoospermia
Aspermia (testis) —*see* Azoospermia
Asphyxia, asphyxiation (by) R09.01
  antenatal P84
  birth P84
  bunny bag —*see* Asphyxia, due to,
      mechanical threat to breathing, trapped
      in bed clothes
  crushing S28.0
  drowning T75.1
  gas, fumes, or vapor —*see* Table of Drugs and
      Chemicals
  inhalation —*see* Inhalation
  intrauterine P84
  local I73.00
    with gangrene I73.01
  mucus —*see also* Foreign body, respiratory
      tract, causing asphyxia
  newborn P84

Asphyxia, asphyxiation *(Continued)*
  pathological R09.01
  postnatal P84
    mechanical —*see* Asphyxia, due to,
        mechanical threat to breathing
  prenatal P84
  reticularis R23.1
  strangulation —*see* Asphyxia, due to,
      mechanical threat to breathing
  submersion T75.1
  traumatic T71.9
    due to
      crushed chest S28.0
      foreign body (in) —*see* Foreign body,
          respiratory tract, causing asphyxia
      low oxygen content of ambient air T71.20
        due to
          being trapped in
            low oxygen environment T71.29
              in car trunk T71.221
                circumstances undetermined
                    T71.224
                done with intent to harm by
                    another person T71.223
                    self T71.222
              in refrigerator T71.231
                circumstances undetermined
                    T71.234
                done with intent to harm by
                    another person T71.233
                    self T71.232
            cave-in T71.21
      mechanical threat to breathing
          (accidental) T71.191
        circumstances undetermined T71.194
        done with intent to harm by
            another person T71.193
            self T71.192
        hanging T71.161
          circumstances undetermined
              T71.164
          done with intent to harm by
              another person T71.163
              self T71.162
        plastic bag T71.121
          circumstances undetermined
              T71.124
          done with intent to harm by
              another person T71.123
              self T71.122
        smothering
          in furniture T71.151
            circumstances undetermined
                T71.154
            done with intent to harm by
                another person T71.153
                self T71.152
          under
            another person's body T71.141
              circumstances undetermined
                  T71.144
              done with intent to harm
                  T71.143
            pillow T71.111
              circumstances undetermined
                  T71.114
              done with intent to harm by
                  another person T71.113
                  self T71.112
        trapped in bed clothes T71.131
          circumstances undetermined
              T71.134
          done with intent to harm by
              another person T71.133
              self T71.132
  vomiting, vomitus —*see* Foreign body,
      respiratory tract, causing asphyxia
Aspiration
  amniotic (clear) fluid (newborn) P24.10
    with
      pneumonia (pneumonitis) P24.11
      respiratory symptoms P24.11

◀ New   ◀◀ Revised   ~~deleted~~ Deleted

Aspiration *(Continued)*
blood
  newborn (without respiratory symptoms)
    P24.20
    with
      pneumonia (pneumonitis) P24.21
      respiratory symptoms P24.21
    specified age NEC —*see* Foreign body,
      respiratory tract
  bronchitis J69.0
  food or foreign body (with asphyxiation) —
    see Asphyxia, food
  liquor (amnii) (newborn) P24.10
    with
      pneumonia (pneumonitis) P24.11
      respiratory symptoms P24.11
  meconium (newborn) (without respiratory
    symptoms) P24.00
    with
      pneumonitis (pneumonitis) P24.01
      respiratory symptoms P24.01
  milk (newborn) (without respiratory
    symptoms) P24.30
    with
      pneumonia (pneumonitis) P24.31
      respiratory symptoms P24.31
    specified age NEC —*see* Foreign body,
      respiratory tract
  mucus —*see also* Foreign body, by site,
    causing asphyxia
    newborn P24.10
      with
        pneumonia (pneumonitis) P24.11
        respiratory symptoms P24.11
  neonatal P24.9
    specific NEC (without respiratory
      symptoms) P24.80
      with
        pneumonia (pneumonitis) P24.81
        respiratory symptoms P24.81
  newborn P24.9
    specific NEC (without respiratory
      symptoms) P24.80
      with
        pneumonia (pneumonitis) P24.81
        respiratory symptoms P24.81
  pneumonia J69.0
  pneumonitis J69.0
  syndrome of newborn —*see* Aspiration, by
    substance, with pneumonia
  vernix caseosa (newborn) P24.80
    with
      pneumonia (pneumonitis) P24.81
      respiratory symptoms P24.81
  vomitus —*see also* Foreign body, respiratory
    tract
    newborn (without respiratory symptoms)
      P24.30
      with
        pneumonia (pneumonitis)
          P24.31
        respiratory symptoms P24.31
Asplenia (congenital) Q89.01
  postsurgical Z90.81
Assam fever B55.0
Assault, sexual —*see* Maltreatment
Assmann's focus NEC A15.0
Astasia (-abasia) (hysterical) F44.4
Asteatosis cutis L85.3
Astereognosia, astereognosis R48.1
Asterixis R27.8
  in liver disease K71.3
Asteroid hyalitis —*see* Deposit, crystalline
Asthenia, asthenic R53.1
  cardiac —*see also* Failure, heart I50.9
    psychogenic F45.8
  cardiovascular —*see also* Failure, heart
    I50.9
    psychogenic F45.8
  heart —*see also* Failure, heart I50.9
    psychogenic F45.8

Asthenia, asthenic *(Continued)*
  hysterical F44.4
  myocardial —*see also* Failure, heart
    I50.9
    psychogenic F45.8
  nervous F48.8
  neurocirculatory F45.8
  neurotic F48.8
  psychogenic F48.8
  psychoneurotic F48.8
  psychophysiologic F48.8
  reaction (psychophysiologic) F48.8
  senile R54
Asthenopia —*see also* Discomfort, visual
  hysterical F44.6
  psychogenic F44.6
Asthenospermia —*see* Abnormal, specimen,
  male genital organs
Asthma, asthmatic (bronchial) (catarrh)
  (spasmodic) J45.909
  with
    chronic obstructive bronchitis
      J44.9
      with
        acute lower respiratory infection J44.0
        exacerbation (acute) J44.1
    chronic obstructive pulmonary disease
      J44.9
      with
        acute lower respiratory infection
          J44.0
        exacerbation (acute) J44.1
    exacerbation (acute) J45.901
    hay fever —*see* Asthma, allergic extrinsic
    rhinitis, allergic —*see* Asthma, allergic
      extrinsic
    status asthmaticus J45.902
  allergic extrinsic J45.909
    with
      exacerbation (acute) J45.901
      status asthmaticus J45.902
  atopic —*see* Asthma, allergic extrinsic
  cardiac —*see* Failure, ventricular, left
  cardiobronchial I50.1
  childhood J45.909
    with
      exacerbation (acute) J45.901
      status asthmaticus J45.902
  chronic obstructive J44.9
    with
      acute lower respiratory infection
        J44.0
      exacerbation (acute) J44.1
  collier's J60
  cough variant J45.991
  detergent J69.8
  due to
    detergent J69.8
    inhalation of fumes J68.3
  eosinophilic J82
  extrinsic, allergic —*see* Asthma, allergic
    extrinsic
  grinder's J62.8
  hay —*see* Asthma, allergic extrinsic
  heart I50.1
  idiosyncratic —*see* Asthma, nonallergic
  intermittent (mild) J45.20
    with
      exacerbation (acute) J45.21
      status asthmaticus J45.22
  intrinsic, nonallergic —*see* Asthma,
    nonallergic
  Kopp's E32.8
  late-onset J45.909
    with
      exacerbation (acute) J45.901
      status asthmaticus J45.902
  mild intermittent J45.20
    with
      exacerbation (acute) J45.21
      status asthmaticus J45.22

Asthma, asthmatic *(Continued)*
  mild persistent J45.30
    with
      exacerbation (acute) J45.31
      status asthmaticus J45.32
  Millar's (laryngismus stridulus) J38.5
  miner's J60
  mixed J45.909
    with
      exacerbation (acute) J45.901
      status asthmaticus J45.902
  moderate persistent J45.40
    with
      exacerbation (acute) J45.41
      status asthmaticus J45.42
  nervous —*see* Asthma, nonallergic
  nonallergic (intrinsic) J45.909
    with
      exacerbation (acute) J45.901
      status asthmaticus J45.902
  persistent
    mild J45.30
      with
        exacerbation (acute) J45.31
        status asthmaticus J45.32
    moderate J45.40
      with
        exacerbation (acute) J45.41
        status asthmaticus J45.42
    severe J45.50
      with
        exacerbation (acute) J45.51
        status asthmaticus J45.52
  platinum J45.998
  pneumoconiotic NEC J64
  potter's J62.8
  predominantly allergic J45.909
  psychogenic F54
  pulmonary eosinophilic J82
  red cedar J67.8
  Rostan's I50.1
  sandblaster's J62.8
  sequoiosis J67.8
  severe persistent J45.50
    with
      exacerbation (acute) J45.51
      status asthmaticus J45.52
  specified NEC J45.998
  stonemason's J62.8
  thymic E32.8
  tuberculous —*see* Tuberculosis, pulmonary
  Wichmann's (laryngismus stridulus) J38.5
  wood J67.8
Astigmatism (compound) (congenital) H52.20-
  irregular H52.21-
  regular H52.22-
Astraphobia F40.220
Astroblastoma
  specified site —*see* Neoplasm, malignant, by
    site
  unspecified site C71.9
Astrocytoma (cystic)
  anaplastic
    specified site —*see* Neoplasm, malignant,
      by site
    unspecified site C71.9
  fibrillary
    specified site —*see* Neoplasm, malignant,
      by site
    unspecified site C71.9
  fibrous
    specified site —*see* Neoplasm, malignant,
      by site
    unspecified site C71.9
  gemistocytic
    specified site —*see* Neoplasm, malignant,
      by site
    unspecified site C71.9
  juvenile
    specified site —*see* Neoplasm, malignant,
      by site
    unspecified site C71.9

Astrocytoma *(Continued)*
  pilocytic
    specified site —*see* Neoplasm, malignant,
      by site
    unspecified site C71.9
  piloid
    specified site —*see* Neoplasm, malignant,
      by site
    unspecified site C71.9
  protoplasmic
    specified site —*see* Neoplasm, malignant,
      by site
    unspecified site C71.9
  specified site NEC —*see* Neoplasm,
    malignant, by site
  subependymal D43.2
    giant cell
      specified site —*see* Neoplasm, uncertain
        behavior, by site
      unspecified site D43.2
    specified site —*see* Neoplasm, uncertain
      behavior, by site
    unspecified site D43.2
  unspecified site C71.9
Astroglioma
  specified site —*see* Neoplasm, malignant, by
    site
  unspecified site C71.9
Asymbolia R48.8
Asymmetry —*see also* Distortion
  between native and reconstructed breast
    N65.1
  face Q67.0
  jaw (lower) —*see* Anomaly, dentofacial, jaw-
    cranial base relationship, asymmetry
Asynergia, asynergy R27.8
  ventricular I51.89
Asystole (heart) —*see* Arrest, cardiac
At risk
  for falling Z91.81
Ataxia, ataxy, ataxic R27.0
  acute R27.8
  brain (hereditary) G11.9
  cerebellar (hereditary) G11.9
    with defective DNA repair G11.3
    alcoholic G31.2
    early-onset G11.1
    in
      alcoholism G31.2
      myxedema E03.9 *[G13.2]*
      neoplastic disease —*see also* Neoplasm
        D49.9 *[G32.81]* ◀▥
        specified disease NEC G32.81
    late-onset (Marie's) G11.2
  cerebral (hereditary) G11.9
  congenital nonprogressive G11.0
  family, familial —*see* Ataxia, hereditary
  following
    cerebrovascular disease I69.993
      cerebral infarction I69.393
      intracerebral hemorrhage I69.193
      nontraumatic intracranial hemorrhage
        NEC I69.293
      specified disease NEC I69.893
      subarachnoid hemorrhage I69.093
  Friedreich's (heredofamilial) (cerebellar)
    (spinal) G11.1
  gait R26.0
    hysterical F44.4
  general R27.8
  gluten M35.9 *[G32.81]*
    with celiac disease K90.0 *[G32.81]*
  hereditary G11.9
    with neuropathy G60.2
    cerebellar —*see* Ataxia, cerebellar
    spastic G11.4
    specified NEC G11.8
    spinal (Friedreich's) G11.1
  heredofamilial —*see* Ataxia, hereditary
  Hunt's G11.1
  hysterical F44.4

Ataxia, ataxy, ataxic *(Continued)*
  locomotor (progressive) (syphilitic) (partial)
    (spastic) A52.11
    diabetic —*see* Diabetes, ataxia
  Marie's (cerebellar) (heredofamilial) (late-
    onset) G11.2
  nonorganic origin F44.4
  nonprogressive, congenital G11.0
  psychogenic F44.4
  Roussy-Lévy G60.0
  Sanger-Brown's (hereditary) G11.2
  spastic hereditary G11.4
  spinal
    hereditary (Friedreich's) G11.1
    progressive (syphilitic) A52.11
  spinocerebellar, X-linked recessive G11.1
  telangiectasia (Louis-Bar) G11.3
Ataxia-telangiectasia (Louis-Bar) G11.3
Atelectasis (massive) (partial) (pressure)
  (pulmonary) J98.11
  newborn P28.10
    due to resorption P28.11
    partial P28.19
    primary P28.0
    secondary P28.19
  primary (newborn) P28.0
  tuberculous —*see* Tuberculosis, pulmonary
Atelocardia Q24.9
Atelomyelia Q06.1
Atheroembolism
  of
    extremities
      lower I75.02-
      upper I75.01-
    kidney I75.81
    specified NEC I75.89
Atheroma, atheromatous —*see also*
    Arteriosclerosis I70.90
  aorta, aortic I70.0
    valve —*see also* Endocarditis, aortic I35.8
  aorto-iliac I70.0
  artery —*see* Arteriosclerosis
  basilar (artery) I67.2
  carotid (artery) (common) (internal) I67.2
  cerebral (arteries) I67.2
  coronary (artery) I25.10
    with angina pectoris —*see* Arteriosclerosis,
      coronary (artery)
  degeneration —*see* Arteriosclerosis
  heart, cardiac —*see* Disease, heart, ischemic,
    atherosclerotic
  mitral (valve) I34.8
  myocardium, myocardial —*see* Disease, heart,
    ischemic, atherosclerotic
  pulmonary valve (heart) —*see also*
    Endocarditis, pulmonary I37.8
  tricuspid (heart) (valve) I36.8
  valve, valvular —*see* Endocarditis
  vertebral (artery) I67.2
Atheromatosis —*see* Arteriosclerosis
Atherosclerosis —*see also* Arteriosclerosis
  coronary
    artery I25.10
      with angina pectoris —*see*
        Arteriosclerosis, coronary (artery),
      due to
        calcified coronary lesion (severely)
          I25.84
        lipid rich plaque I25.83
    transplanted heart I25.811
      bypass graft I25.812
        with angina pectoris —*see*
          Arteriosclerosis, coronary (artery)
      native coronary artery I25.811
        with angina pectoris —*see*
          Arteriosclerosis, coronary (artery)
Athetosis (acquired) R25.8
  bilateral (congenital) G80.3
  congenital (bilateral) (double) G80.3
  double (congenital) G80.3
  unilateral R25.8

Athlete's
  foot B35.3
  heart I51.7
Athrepsia E41
Athyrea (acquired) —*see also* Hypothyroidism
  congenital E03.1
Atonia, atony, atonic
  bladder (sphincter) (neurogenic) N31.2
  capillary I78.8
  cecum K59.8
    psychogenic F45.8
  colon —*see* Atony, intestine
  congenital P94.2
  esophagus K22.8
  intestine K59.8
    psychogenic F45.8
  stomach K31.89
    neurotic or psychogenic F45.8
  uterus (during labor) O62.2
    with hemorrhage (postpartum) O72.1
    postpartum (with hemorrhage) O72.1
      without hemorrhage O75.89
Atopy —*see* History, allergy
Atransferrinemia, congenital E88.09
Atresia, atretic
  alimentary organ or tract NEC Q45.8
    upper Q40.8
  ani, anus, anal (canal) Q42.3
    with fistula Q42.2
  aorta (ring) Q25.29 ◀▥
  aortic (orifice) (valve) Q23.0
    arch Q25.21 ◀▥
    congenital with hypoplasia of ascending
      aorta and defective development of
      left ventricle (with mitral stenosis)
      Q23.4
    in hypoplastic left heart syndrome Q23.4
  aqueduct of Sylvius Q03.0
    with spina bifida —*see* Spina bifida, with
      hydrocephalus
  artery NEC Q27.8
    cerebral Q28.3
    coronary Q24.5
    digestive system Q27.8
    eye Q15.8
    lower limb Q27.8
    pulmonary Q25.5
    specified site NEC Q27.8
    umbilical Q27.0
    upper limb Q27.8
  auditory canal (external) Q16.1
  bile duct (common) (congenital) (hepatic)
    Q44.2
    acquired —*see* Obstruction, bile duct
  bladder (neck) Q64.39
    obstruction Q64.31
  bronchus Q32.4
  cecum Q42.8
  cervix (acquired) N88.2
    congenital Q51.828
    in pregnancy or childbirth —*see* Anomaly,
      cervix, in pregnancy or childbirth
      causing obstructed labor O65.5
  choana Q30.0
  colon Q42.9
    specified NEC Q42.8
  common duct Q44.2
  cricoid cartilage Q31.8
  cystic duct Q44.2
    acquired K82.8
      with obstruction K82.0
  digestive organs NEC Q45.8
  duodenum Q41.0
  ear canal Q16.1
  ejaculatory duct Q55.4
  epiglottis Q31.8
  esophagus Q39.0
    with tracheoesophageal fistula Q39.1
  eustachian tube Q17.8
  fallopian tube (congenital) Q50.6
    acquired N97.1

◀ New   ◀▥ Revised   ~~deleted~~ Deleted

Atresia, atretic (Continued)
follicular cyst N83.0- ◀▥
foramen of
Luschka Q03.1
with spina bifida —see Spina bifida, with
hydrocephalus
Magendie Q03.1
with spina bifida —see Spina bifida, with
hydrocephalus
gallbladder Q44.1
genital organ
external
female Q52.79
male Q55.8
internal
female Q52.8
male Q55.8
glottis Q31.8
gullet Q39.0
with tracheoesophageal fistula Q39.1
heart valve NEC Q24.8
pulmonary Q22.0
tricuspid Q22.4
hymen Q52.3
acquired (postinfective) N89.6
ileum Q41.2
intestine (small) Q41.9
large Q42.9
specified NEC Q42.8
iris, filtration angle Q15.0
jejunum Q41.1
lacrimal apparatus Q10.4
larynx Q31.8
meatus urinarius Q64.33
mitral valve Q23.2
in hypoplastic left heart syndrome
Q23.4
nares (anterior) (posterior) Q30.0
nasopharynx Q34.8
nose, nostril Q30.0
acquired J34.89
organ or site NEC Q89.8
osseous meatus (ear) Q16.1
oviduct (congenital) Q50.6
acquired N97.1
parotid duct Q38.4
acquired K11.8
pulmonary (artery) Q25.5
valve Q22.0
pulmonic Q22.0
pupil Q13.2
rectum Q42.1
with fistula Q42.0
salivary duct Q38.4
acquired K11.8
sublingual duct Q38.4
acquired K11.8
submandibular duct Q38.4
acquired K11.8
submaxillary duct Q38.4
acquired K11.8
thyroid cartilage Q31.8
trachea Q32.1
tricuspid valve Q22.4
ureter Q62.10
pelvic junction Q62.11
vesical orifice Q62.12
ureteropelvic junction Q62.11
ureterovesical orifice Q62.12
urethra (valvular) Q64.39
stricture Q64.32
urinary tract NEC Q64.8
uterus Q51.818
acquired N85.8
vagina (congenital) Q52.4
acquired (postinfectional) (senile)
N89.5
vas deferens Q55.3
vascular NEC Q27.8
cerebral Q28.3
digestive system Q27.8

Atresia, atretic (Continued)
vascular NEC (Continued)
lower limb Q27.8
specified site NEC Q27.8
upper limb Q27.8
vein NEC Q27.8
digestive system Q27.8
great Q26.8
lower limb Q27.8
portal Q26.5
pulmonary Q26.3
specified site NEC Q27.8
upper limb Q27.8
vena cava (inferior) (superior) Q26.8
vesicourethral orifice Q64.31
vulva Q52.79
acquired N90.5
Atrichia, atrichosis —see Alopecia
Atrophia —see also Atrophy
cutis senilis L90.8
due to radiation L57.8
gyrata of choroid and retina H31.23
senilis R54
dermatological L90.8
due to radiation (nonionizing) (solar)
L57.8
unguium L60.3
congenita Q84.6
Atrophie blanche (en plaque) (de Milian) L95.0
Atrophoderma, atrophodermia (of) L90.9
diffusum (idiopathic) L90.4
maculatum L90.8
et striatum L90.8
due to syphilis A52.79
syphilitic A51.39
neuriticum L90.8
Pasini and Pierini L90.3
pigmentosum Q82.1
reticulatum symmetricum faciei L66.4
senile L90.8
due to radiation (nonionizing) (solar) L57.8
vermiculata (cheeks) L66.4
Atrophy, atrophic (of)
adrenal (capsule) (gland) E27.49
primary (autoimmune) E27.1
alveolar process or ridge (edentulous) K08.20
anal sphincter (disuse) N81.84
appendix K38.8
arteriosclerotic —see Arteriosclerosis
bile duct (common) (hepatic) K83.8
bladder N32.89
neurogenic N31.8
blanche (en plaque) (of Milian) L95.0
bone (senile) NEC —see also Disorder, bone,
specified type NEC
due to
tabes dorsalis (neurogenic) A52.11
brain (cortex) (progressive) G31.9
frontotemporal circumscribed G31.01
[F02.80]
with behavioral disturbance G31.01
[F02.81]
senile NEC G31.1
breast N64.2
obstetric —see Disorder, breast, specified
type NEC
buccal cavity K13.79
cardiac —see Degeneration, myocardial
cartilage (infectional) (joint) —see Disorder,
cartilage, specified NEC
cerebellar —see Atrophy, brain
cerebral —see Atrophy, brain
cervix (mucosa) (senile) (uteri) N88.8
menopausal N95.8
Charcot-Marie-Tooth G60.0
choroid (central) (macular) (myopic) (retina)
H31.10-
diffuse secondary H31.12-
gyrate H31.23
senile H31.11-
ciliary body —see Atrophy, iris

Atrophy, atrophic (Continued)
conjunctiva (senile) H11.89
corpus cavernosum N48.89
cortical —see Atrophy, brain
cystic duct K82.8
Déjérine-Thomas G23.8
disuse NEC —see Atrophy, muscle
Duchenne-Aran G12.21
ear H93.8-
edentulous alveolar ridge K08.20
endometrium (senile) N85.8
cervix N88.8
enteric K63.89
epididymis N50.89 ◀▥
eyeball —see Disorder, globe, degenerated
condition, atrophy
eyelid (senile) —see Disorder, eyelid,
degenerative
facial (skin) L90.9
fallopian tube (senile) N83.32- ◀▥
with ovary N83.33- ◀▥
fascioscapulohumeral (Landouzy- Déjérine)
G71.0
fatty, thymus (gland) E32.8
gallbladder K82.8
gastric K29.40
with bleeding K29.41
gastrointestinal K63.89
glandular I89.8
globe H44.52-
gum —see also Recession, gingival K06.0 ◀▥
hair L67.8
heart (brown) —see Degeneration, myocardial
hemifacial Q67.4
Romberg G51.8
infantile E41
paralysis, acute —see Poliomyelitis,
paralytic
intestine K63.89
iris (essential) (progressive) H21.26-
specified NEC H21.29
kidney (senile) (terminal) —see also Sclerosis,
renal N26.1
congenital or infantile Q60.5
bilateral Q60.4
unilateral Q60.3
hydronephrotic —see Hydronephrosis
lacrimal gland (primary) H04.14-
secondary H04.15-
Landouzy-Déjérine G71.0
laryngitis, infective J37.0
larynx J38.7
Leber's optic (hereditary) H47.22
lip K13.0
liver (yellow) K72.90
with coma K72.91
acute, subacute K72.00
with coma K72.01
chronic K72.10
with coma K72.11
lung (senile) J98.4
macular (dermatological) L90.8
syphilitic, skin A51.39
striated A52.79
mandible (edentulous) K08.20
minimal K08.21
moderate K08.22
severe K08.23
maxilla K08.20
minimal K08.24
moderate K08.25
severe K08.26
muscle, muscular (diffuse) (general)
(idiopathic) (primary) M62.50
ankle M62.57-
Duchenne-Aran G12.21
foot M62.57-
forearm M62.53-
hand M62.54-
infantile spinal G12.0
lower leg M62.56-

Atrophy, atrophic *(Continued)*
  muscle, muscular *(Continued)*
    multiple sites M62.59
    myelopathic —*see* Atrophy, muscle, spinal
    myotonic G71.11
    neuritic G58.9
    neuropathic (peroneal) (progressive) G60.0
    pelvic (disuse) N81.84
    peroneal G60.0
    progressive (bulbar) G12.21
      adult G12.1
      infantile (spinal) G12.0
      spinal G12.9
        adult G12.1
        infantile G12.0
    pseudohypertrophic G71.0
    shoulder region M62.51-
    specified site NEC M62.58
    spinal G12.9
      adult form G12.1
      Aran-Duchenne G12.21
      childhood form, type II G12.1
      distal G12.1
      hereditary NEC G12.1
      infantile, type I (Werdnig- Hoffmann) G12.0
      juvenile form, type III (Kugelberg- Welander) G12.1
      progressive G12.21
      scapuloperoneal form G12.1
      specified NEC G12.8
    syphilitic A52.78
    thigh M62.55-
    upper arm M62.52-
  myocardium —*see* Degeneration, myocardial
  myometrium (senile) N85.8
    cervix N88.8
  myopathic NEC —*see* Atrophy, muscle
  myotonia G71.11
  nail L60.3
  nasopharynx J31.1
  nerve —*see also* Disorder, nerve
    abducens —*see* Strabismus, paralytic, sixth nerve
    accessory G52.8
    acoustic or auditory —*see* subcategory H93.3
    cranial G52.9
      eighth (auditory) —*see* subcategory H93.3
      eleventh (accessory) G52.8
      fifth (trigeminal) G50.8
      first (olfactory) G52.0
      fourth (trochlear) —*see* Strabismus, paralytic, fourth nerve
      second (optic) H47.20
      sixth (abducens) —*see* Strabismus, paralytic, sixth nerve
      tenth (pneumogastric) (vagus) G52.2
      third (oculomotor) —*see* Strabismus, paralytic, third nerve
      twelfth (hypoglossal) G52.3
    hypoglossal G52.3
    oculomotor —*see* Strabismus, paralytic, third nerve
    olfactory G52.0
    optic (papillomacular bundle)
      syphilitic (late) A52.15
        congenital A50.44
    pneumogastric G52.2
    trigeminal G50.8
    trochlear —*see* Strabismus, paralytic, fourth nerve
    vagus (pneumogastric) G52.2
  neurogenic, bone, tabetic A52.11
  nutritional E41
  old age R54
  olivopontocerebellar G23.8

Atrophy, atrophic *(Continued)*
  optic (nerve) H47.20
    glaucomatous H47.23-
    hereditary H47.22
    primary H47.21-
    specified type NEC H47.29-
    syphilitic (late) A52.15
      congenital A50.44
  orbit H05.31-
  ovary (senile) N83.31- ◀▥
    with fallopian tube N83.33- ◀▥
  oviduct (senile) —*see* Atrophy, fallopian tube
  palsy, diffuse (progressive) G12.22
  pancreas (duct) (senile) K86.89 ◀▥
  parotid gland K11.0
  pelvic muscle N81.84
  penis N48.89
  pharynx J39.2
  pluriglandular E31.8
    autoimmune E31.0
  polyarthritis M15.9
  prostate N42.89
  pseudohypertrophic (muscle) G71.0
  renal —*see also* Sclerosis, renal N26.1
  retina, retinal (postinfectional) H35.89
  rhinitis J31.0
  salivary gland K11.0
  scar L90.5
  sclerosis, lobar (of brain) G31.09 *[F02.80]*
    with behavioral disturbance G31.09 *[F02.81]*
  scrotum N50.89 ◀▥
  seminal vesicle N50.89 ◀▥
  senile R54
    due to radiation (nonionizing) (solar) L57.8
  skin (patches) (spots) L90.9
    degenerative (senile) L90.8
    due to radiation (nonionizing) (solar) L57.8
    senile L90.8
  spermatic cord N50.89 ◀▥
  spinal (acute) (cord) G95.89
    muscular —*see* Atrophy, muscle, spinal
    paralysis G12.20
      acute —*see* Poliomyelitis, paralytic
      meaning progressive muscular atrophy G12.21
  spine (column) —*see* Spondylopathy, specified NEC
  spleen (senile) D73.0
  stomach K29.40
    with bleeding K29.41
  striate (skin) L90.6
    syphilitic A52.79
  subcutaneous L90.9
  sublingual gland K11.0
  submandibular gland K11.0
  submaxillary gland K11.0
  Sudeck's —*see* Algoneurodystrophy
  suprarenal (capsule) (gland) E27.49
    primary E27.1
  systemic affecting central nervous system in
    myxedema E03.9 *[G13.2]*
    neoplastic disease —*see also* Neoplasm D49.9 *[G13.1]*
    specified disease NEC G13.8
  tarso-orbital fascia, congenital Q10.3
  testis N50.0
  thenar, partial —*see* Syndrome, carpal tunnel
  thymus (fatty) E32.8
  thyroid (gland) (acquired) E03.4
    with cretinism E03.1
    congenital (with myxedema) E03.1
  tongue (senile) K14.8
    papillae K14.4
  trachea J39.8
  tunica vaginalis N50.89 ◀▥
  turbinate J34.89
  tympanic membrane (nonflaccid) H73.82-
    flaccid H73.81-
  upper respiratory tract J39.8

Atrophy, atrophic *(Continued)*
  uterus, uterine (senile) N85.8
    cervix N88.8
    due to radiation (intended effect) N85.8
      adverse effect or misadventure N99.89
  vagina (senile) N95.2
  vas deferens N50.89 ◀▥
  vascular I99.8
  vertebra (senile) —*see* Spondylopathy, specified NEC
  vulva (senile) N90.5
  Werdnig-Hoffmann G12.0
  yellow —*see* Failure, hepatic
Attack, attacks
  with alteration of consciousness (with automatisms) —*see* Epilepsy, localization-related, symptomatic, with complex partial seizures
  without alteration of consciousness —*see* Epilepsy, localization-related, symptomatic, with simple partial seizures
  Adams-Stokes I45.9
  akinetic —*see* Epilepsy, generalized, specified NEC
  angina —*see* Angina
  atonic —*see* Epilepsy, generalized, specified NEC
  benign shuddering G25.83
  cataleptic —*see* Catalepsy
  coronary —*see* Infarct, myocardium
  cyanotic, newborn P28.2
  drop NEC R55
  epileptic —*see* Epilepsy
  heart —*see* infarct, myocardium
  hysterical F44.9
  jacksonian —*see* Epilepsy, localization-related, symptomatic, with simple partial seizures
  myocardium, myocardial —*see* Infarct, myocardium
  myoclonic —*see* Epilepsy, generalized, specified NEC
  panic F41.0
  psychomotor —*see* Epilepsy, localization-related, symptomatic, with complex partial seizures
  salaam —*see* Epilepsy, spasms
  schizophreniform, brief F23
  shuddering, benign G25.83
  Stokes-Adams I45.9
  syncope R55
  transient ischemic (TIA) G45.9
    specified NEC G45.8
  unconsciousness R55
    hysterical F44.89
  vasomotor R55
  vasovagal (paroxysmal) (idiopathic) R55
Attention (to)
  artificial
    opening (of) Z43.9
      digestive tract NEC Z43.4
        colon Z43.3
        ilium Z43.2
        stomach Z43.1
      specified NEC Z43.8
      trachea Z43.0
      urinary tract NEC Z43.6
        cystostomy Z43.5
        nephrostomy Z43.6
        ureterostomy Z43.6
        urethrostomy Z43.6
      vagina Z43.7
  colostomy Z43.3
  cystostomy Z43.5
  deficit disorder or syndrome F98.8
    with hyperactivity —*see* Disorder, attention-deficit hyperactivity
  gastrostomy Z43.1
  ileostomy Z43.2

◀ New   ◀▥ Revised   ~~deleted~~ Deleted

Attention (*Continued*)
jejunostomy Z43.4
nephrostomy Z43.6
surgical dressings Z48.01
sutures Z48.02
tracheostomy Z43.0
ureterostomy Z43.6
urethrostomy Z43.6
Attrition
gum —*see also* Recession, gingival K06.0 ◀▥
tooth, teeth (excessive) (hard tissues) K03.0
Atypical, atypism —*see also* condition
cells (on cytolgocial smear) (endocervical)
(endometrial) (glandular)
cervix R87.619
vagina R87.629
cervical N87.9
endometrium N85.9
hyperplasia N85.00
parenting situation Z62.9
Auditory —*see* condition
Aujeszky's disease B33.8
Aurantiasis, cutis E67.1
Auricle, auricular —*see also* condition
cervical Q18.2
Auriculotemporal syndrome G50.8
Austin Flint murmur (aortic insufficiency)
I35.1
Australian
Q fever A78
X disease A83.4
Autism, autistic (childhood) (infantile) F84.0
atypical F84.9
spectrum disorder F84.0 ◀
Autodigestion R68.89
Autoerythrocyte sensitization (syndrome)
D69.2
Autographism L50.3
Autoimmune
disease (systemic) M35.9
inhibitors to clotting factors D68.311
lymphoproliferative syndrome [ALPS]
D89.82
thyroiditis E06.3
Autointoxication R68.89
Automatism G93.89
with temporal sclerosis G93.81
epileptic —*see* Epilepsy, localization- related,
symptomatic, with complex partial
seizures

Automatism (*Continued*)
paroxysmal, idiopathic —*see* Epilepsy,
localization-related, symptomatic, with
complex partial seizures
Autonomic, autonomous
bladder (neurogenic) N31.2
hysteria seizure F44.5
Autosensitivity, erythrocyte D69.2
Autosensitization, cutaneous L30.2
Autosome —*see* condition by chromosome
involved
Autotopagnosia R48.1
Autotoxemia R68.89
Autumn —*see* condition
Avellis' syndrome G46.8
Aversion
oral R63.3
newborn P92.-
nonorganic origin F98.2
sexual F52.1
Aviator's
disease or sickness —*see* Effect, adverse, high
altitude
ear T70.0
Avitaminosis (multiple) —*see also* Deficiency,
vitamin E56.9
B E53.9
with
beriberi E51.11
pellagra E52
B2 E53.0
B6 E53.1
B12 E53.8
D E55.9
with rickets E55.0
G E53.0
K E56.1
nicotinic acid E52
AVNRT (atrioventricular nodal re-entrant
tachycardia) I47.1
AVRT (atrioventricular nodal re-entrant
tachycardia) I47.1
Avulsion (traumatic)
blood vessel —*see* Injury, blood vessel
bone —*see* Fracture, by site
cartilage —*see also* Dislocation, by site
symphyseal (inner), complicating delivery
O71.6
external site other than limb —*see* Wound,
open, by site

Avulsion (*Continued*)
eye S05.7-
head (intracranial)
external site NEC S08.89
scalp S08.0
internal organ or site —*see* Injury, by site
joint —*see also* Dislocation, by site
capsule —*see* Sprain, by site
kidney S37.06-
ligament —*see* Sprain, by site
limb —*see also* Amputation, traumatic,
by site
skin and subcutaneous tissue —*see* Wound,
open, by site
muscle —*see* Injury, muscle
nerve (root) —*see* Injury, nerve
scalp S08.0
skin and subcutaneous tissue —*see* Wound,
open, by site
spleen S36.032
symphyseal cartilage (inner), complicating
delivery O71.6
tendon —*see* Injury, muscle
tooth S03.2
Awareness of heart beat R00.2
Axenfeld's
anomaly or syndrome Q15.0
degeneration (calcareous) Q13.4
Axilla, axillary —*see also* condition
breast Q83.1
Axonotmesis —*see* Injury, nerve
Ayerza's disease or syndrome (pulmonary
artery sclerosis with pulmonary
hypertension) I27.0
Azoospermia (organic) N46.01
due to
drug therapy N46.021
efferent duct obstruction N46.023
infection N46.022
radiation N46.024
specified cause NEC N46.029
systemic disease N46.025
Azotemia R79.89
meaning uremia N19
Aztec ear Q17.3
Azygos
continuation inferior vena cava Q26.8
lobe (lung) Q33.1

B

Baastrup's disease —see Kissing spine
Babesiosis B60.0
Babington's disease (familial hemorrhagic telangiectasia) I78.0
Babinski's syndrome A52.79
Baby
  crying constantly R68.11
  floppy (syndrome) P94.2
Bacillary —see condition
Bacilluria R82.71 ◀
Bacillus —see also Infection, bacillus
  abortus infection A23.1
  anthracis infection A22.9
  coli infection —see also Escherichia coli B96.20
  Flexner's A03.1
  mallei infection A24.0
  Shiga's A03.0
  suipestifer infection —see Infection, salmonella
Back —see condition
Backache (postural) M54.9
  sacroiliac M53.3
  specified NEC M54.89
Backflow —see Reflux
Backward reading (dyslexia) F81.0
Bacteremia R78.81
  with sepsis —see Sepsis
Bactericholia —see Cholecystitis, acute
Bacterid, bacteride (pustular) L40.3
Bacterium, bacteria, bacterial
  agent NEC, as cause of disease classified elsewhere B96.89
  in blood —see Bacteremia
  in urine —see Bacteriuria
Bacteriuria, bacteruria R82.71 ◀
  asymptomatic R82.71 ◀
Bacteroides
  fragilis, as cause of disease classified elsewhere B96.6
Bad
  heart —see Disease, heart
  trip
    due to drug abuse —see Abuse, drug, hallucinogen
    due to drug dependence —see Dependence, drug, hallucinogen
Baelz's disease (cheilitis glandularis apostematosa) K13.0
Baerensprung's disease (eczema marginatum) B35.6
Bagasse disease or pneumonitis J67.1
Bagassosis J67.1
Baker's cyst —see Cyst, Baker's
Bakwin-Krida syndrome (metaphyseal dysplasia) Q78.5 ◀
Balancing side interference M26.56
Balanitis (circinata) (erosiva) (gangrenosa) (phagedenic) (vulgaris) N48.1
  amebic A06.82
  candidal B37.42
  due to Haemophilus ducreyi A57
  gonococcal (acute) (chronic) A54.09
  xerotica obliterans N48.0
Balanoposthitis N47.6
  gonococcal (acute) (chronic) A54.09
  ulcerative (specific) A63.8
Balanorrhagia —see Balanitis
Balantidiasis, balantidiosis A07.0
Bald tongue K14.4
Baldness —see also Alopecia
  male-pattern —see Alopecia, androgenic
Balkan grippe A78
Balloon disease —see Effect, adverse, high altitude
Balo's disease (concentric sclerosis) G37.5
Bamberger-Marie disease —see Osteoarthropathy, hypertrophic, specified type NEC
Bancroft's filariasis B74.0

Band (s)
  adhesive —see Adhesions, peritoneum
  anomalous or congenital —see also Anomaly, by site
    heart (atrial) (ventricular) Q24.8
    intestine Q43.3
    omentum Q43.3
  cervix N88.1
  constricting, congenital Q79.8
  gallbladder (congenital) Q44.1
  intestinal (adhesive) —see Adhesions, peritoneum
  obstructive
    intestine K56.5
    peritoneum K56.5
  periappendiceal, congenital Q43.3
  peritoneal (adhesive) —see Adhesions, peritoneum
  uterus N73.6
    internal N85.6
  vagina N89.5
Bandemia D72.825
Bandl's ring (contraction), complicating delivery O62.4
Bangkok hemorrhagic fever A91
Bang's disease (brucella abortus) A23.1
Bankruptcy, anxiety concerning Z59.8
Bannister's disease T78.3
  hereditary D84.1
Banti's disease or syndrome (with cirrhosis) (with portal hypertension) K76.6
Bar, median, prostate —see Enlargement, enlarged, prostate
Barcoo disease or rot —see Ulcer, skin
Barlow's disease E54
Barodontalgia T70.29
Baron Münchausen syndrome —see Disorder, factitious
Barosinusitis T70.1
Barotitis T70.0
Barotrauma T70.29
  odontalgia T70.29
  otitic T70.0
  sinus T70.1
Barraquer (-Simons) disease or syndrome (progressive lipodystrophy) E88.1
Barré-Guillain disease or syndrome G61.0
Barré-Liéou syndrome (posterior cervical sympathetic) M53.0
Barrel chest M95.4
Barrett's
  disease —see Barrett's, esophagus
  esophagus K22.70
    with dysplasia K22.719
      high grade K22.711
      low grade K22.710
    without dysplasia K22.70
  syndrome —see Barrett's, esophagus
  ulcer K22.10
    with bleeding K22.11
    without bleeding K22.10
Barth syndrome E78.71
Bársony (-Polgár) (-Teschendorf) syndrome (corkscrew esophagus) K22.4
Bartholinitis (suppurating) N75.8
  gonococcal (acute) (chronic) (with abscess) A54.1
Bartonellosis A44.9
  cutaneous A44.1
  mucocutaneous A44.1
  specified NEC A44.8
  systemic A44.0
Barton's fracture S52.56-
Bartter's syndrome E26.81
Basal —see condition
Basan's (hidrotic) ectodermal dysplasia Q82.4
Baseball finger —see Dislocation, finger
Basedow's disease (exophthalmic goiter) —see Hyperthyroidism, with, goiter
Basic —see condition
Basilar —see condition

Bason's (hidrotic) ectodermal dysplasia Q82.4
Basopenia —see Agranulocytosis
Basophilia D72.824
Basophilism (cortico-adrenal) (Cushing's) (pituitary) E24.0
Bassen-Kornzweig disease or syndrome E78.6
Bat ear Q17.5
Bateman's
  disease B08.1
  purpura (senile) D69.2
Bathing cramp T75.1
Bathophobia F40.248
Batten (-Mayou) disease E75.4
  retina E75.4 [H36]
Batten-Steinert syndrome G71.11
Battered —see Maltreatment
Battey Mycobacterium infection A31.0
Battle exhaustion F43.0
Battledore placenta O43.19-
Baumgarten-Cruveilhier cirrhosis, disease or syndrome K74.69
Bauxite fibrosis (of lung) J63.1
Bayle's disease (general paresis) A52.17
Bazin's disease (primary) (tuberculous) A18.4
Beach ear —see Swimmer's, ear
Beaded hair (congenital) Q84.1
Béal conjunctivitis or syndrome B30.2
Beard's disease (neurasthenia) F48.8
Beat (s)
  atrial, premature I49.1
  ectopic I49.49
  elbow —see Bursitis, elbow
  escaped, heart I49.49
  hand —see Bursitis, hand
  knee —see Bursitis, knee
  premature I49.40
    atrial I49.1
    auricular I49.1
    supraventricular I49.1
Beau's
  disease or syndrome —see Degeneration, myocardial
  lines (transverse furrows on fingernails) L60.4
Bechterev's syndrome —see Spondylitis, ankylosing
Beck's syndrome (anterior spinal artery occlusion) I65.8
Becker's
  cardiomyopathy I42.8
  disease
    idiopathic mural endomyocardial disease I42.3
    myotonia congenita, recessive form G71.12
  dystrophy G71.0
  pigmented hairy nevus D22.5
Beckwith-Wiedemann syndrome Q87.3
Bed confinement status Z74.01
Bed sore —see Ulcer, pressure, by site
Bedbug bite (s) —see Bite (s), by site, superficial, insect
Bedclothes, asphyxiation or suffocation by —see Asphyxia, traumatic, due to, mechanical, trapped
Bednar's
  aphthae K12.0
  tumor —see Neoplasm, malignant, by site
Bedridden Z74.01
Bedsore —see Ulcer, pressure, by site
Bedwetting —see Enuresis
Bee sting (with allergic or anaphylactic shock) —see Toxicity, venom, arthropod, bee
Beer drinker's heart (disease) I42.6
Begbie's disease (exophthalmic goiter) —see Hyperthyroidism, with, goiter
Behavior
  antisocial
    adult Z72.811
    child or adolescent Z72.810
  disorder, disturbance —see Disorder, conduct
  disruptive —see Disorder, conduct

◀ New   ◀◀ Revised   ~~deleted~~ Deleted

Behavior *(Continued)*
  drug seeking Z76.5 ◀▦
  inexplicable R46.2
  marked evasiveness R46.5
  obsessive-compulsive R46.81
  overactivity R46.3
  poor responsiveness R46.4
  self-damaging (life-style) Z72.89
  sleep-incompatible Z72.821
  slowness R46.4
  specified NEC R46.89
  strange (and inexplicable) R46.2
  suspiciousness R46.5
  type A pattern Z73.1
  undue concern or preoccupation with
    stressful events R46.6
  verbosity and circumstantial detail obscuring
    reason for contact R46.7
Behcet's disease or syndrome M35.2
Behr's disease —*see* Degeneration, macula
Beigel's disease or morbus (white piedra)
  B36.2
Bejel A65
Bekhterev's syndrome —*see* Spondylitis,
  ankylosing
Belching —*see* Eructation
Bell's
  mania F30.8
  palsy, paralysis G51.0
    infant or newborn P11.3
  spasm G51.3
Bence Jones albuminuria or proteinuria NEC
  R80.3
Bends T70.3
Benedikt's paralysis or syndrome G46.3
Benign (*see also* condition)
  prostatic hyperplasia —*see* Hyperplasia,
    prostate
Bennett's fracture (displaced) S62.21-
Benson's disease —*see* Deposit, crystalline
Bent
  back (hysterical) F44.4
  nose M95.0
    congenital Q67.4
Bereavement (uncomplicated) Z63.4
Bergeron's disease (hysterical chorea) F44.4
Berger's disease —*see* Nephropathy, IgA
Beriberi (dry) E51.11
  heart (disease) E51.12
  polyneuropathy E51.11
  wet E51.12
    involving circulatory system E51.11
Berlin's disease or edema (traumatic) S05.8X-
Berlock (berloque) dermatitis L56.2
Bernard-Horner syndrome G90.2
Bernard-Soulier disease or thrombopathia
  D69.1
Bernhardt (-Roth) disease —*see*
  Mononeuropathy, lower limb, meralgia
  paresthetica
Bernheim's syndrome —*see* Failure, heart,
  congestive
Bertielliasis B71.8
Berylliosis (lung) J63.2
Besnier-Boeck (-Schaumann) disease —*see*
  Sarcoidosis
Besnier's
  lupus pernio D86.3
  prurigo L20.0
Bestiality F65.89
Best's disease H35.50
Beta-mercaptolactate-cysteine disulfiduria
  E72.09
Betalipoproteinemia, broad or floating E78.2
Betting and gambling Z72.6
  pathological (compulsive) F63.0
Bezoar T18.9
  intestine T18.3
  stomach T18.2
Bezold's abscess —*see* Mastoiditis, acute
Bianchi's syndrome R48.8

Bicornate or bicornis uterus Q51.3
  in pregnancy or childbirth O34.0- ◀▦
    causing obstructed labor O65.5
Bicuspid aortic valve Q23.1
Biedl-Bardet syndrome Q87.89
Bielschowsky (-Jansky) disease E75.4
Biermer's (pernicious) anemia or disease D51.0
Biett's disease L93.0
Bifid (congenital)
  apex, heart Q24.8
  clitoris Q52.6
  kidney Q63.8
  nose Q30.2
  patella Q74.1
  scrotum Q55.29
  toe NEC Q74.2
  tongue Q38.3
  ureter Q62.8
  uterus Q51.3
  uvula Q35.7
Biforis uterus (suprasimplex) Q51.3
Bifurcation (congenital)
  gallbladder Q44.1
  kidney pelvis Q63.8
  renal pelvis Q63.8
  rib Q76.6
  tongue, congenital Q38.3
  trachea Q32.1
  ureter Q62.8
  urethra Q64.74
  vertebra Q76.49
Big spleen syndrome D73.1
Bigeminal pulse R00.8
Bilateral —*see* condition
Bile
  duct —*see* condition
  pigments in urine R82.2
Bilharziasis —*see also* Schistosomiasis
  chyluria B65.0
  cutaneous B65.3
  galacturia B65.0
  hematochyluria B65.0
  intestinal B65.1
  lipemia B65.9
  lipuria B65.0
  oriental B65.2
  piarhemia B65.9
  pulmonary NOS B65.9 *[J99]*
    pneumonia B65.9 *[J17]*
  tropical hematuria B65.0
  vesical B65.0
Biliary —*see* condition
Bilirubin metabolism disorder E80.7
  specified NEC E80.6
Bilirubinemia, familial nonhemolytic E80.4
Bilirubinuria R82.2
Biliuria R82.2
Bilocular stomach K31.2
Binswanger's disease I67.3
Biparta, bipartite
  carpal scaphoid Q74.0
  patella Q74.1
  vagina Q52.10
Bird
  face Q75.8
  fancier's disease or lung J67.2
Birt-Hogg-Dube syndrome Q87.89
Birth
  complications in mother —*see* Delivery,
    complicated
  compression during NOS P15.9
  defect —*see* Anomaly
  immature (less than 37 completed weeks) —
    see Preterm, newborn
    extremely (less than 28 completed
      weeks) —*see* Immaturity, extreme
  inattention, at or after —*see* Maltreatment,
    child, neglect
  injury NOS P15.9
    basal ganglia P11.1
    brachial plexus NEC P14.3

Birth *(Continued)*
  injury NOS *(Continued)*
    brain (compression) (pressure)
      P11.2
    central nervous system NOS P11.9
    cerebellum P11.1
    cerebral hemorrhage P10.1
    external genitalia P15.5
    eye P15.3
    face P15.4
    fracture
      bone P13.9
        specified NEC P13.8
      clavicle P13.4
      femur P13.2
      humerus P13.3
      long bone, except femur P13.3
      radius and ulna P13.3
      skull P13.0
      spine P11.5
      tibia and fibula P13.3
    intracranial P11.2
      laceration or hemorrhage P10.9
        specified NEC P10.8
    intraventricular hemorrhage P10.2
    laceration
      brain P10.1
      by scalpel P15.8
      peripheral nerve P14.9
    liver P15.0
    meninges
      brain P11.1
      spinal cord P11.5
    nerve
      brachial plexus P14.3
      cranial NEC (except facial) P11.4
      facial P11.3
      peripheral P14.9
      phrenic (paralysis) P14.2
    paralysis
      facial nerve P11.3
      spinal P11.5
    penis P15.5
    rupture
      spinal cord P11.5
    scalp P12.9
    scalpel wound P15.8
    scrotum P15.5
    skull NEC P13.1
      fracture P13.0
    specified type NEC P15.8
    spinal cord P11.5
    spine P11.5
    spleen P15.1
    sternomastoid (hematoma) P15.2
    subarachnoid hemorrhage P10.3
    subcutaneous fat necrosis P15.6
    subdural hemorrhage P10.0
    tentorial tear P10.4
    testes P15.5
    vulva P15.5
  lack of care, at or after —*see* Maltreatment,
    child, neglect
  neglect, at or after —*see* Maltreatment, child,
    neglect
  palsy or paralysis, newborn, NOS (birth
    injury) P14.9
  premature (infant) —*see* Preterm,
    newborn
  shock, newborn P96.89
  trauma —*see* Birth, injury
  weight
    4000 grams to 4499 grams P08.1
    4500 grams or more P08.0
    low (2499 grams or less) —*see* Low,
      birthweight
      extremely (999 grams or less) —*see* Low,
        birthweight, extreme
Birthmark Q82.5
Bisalbuminemia E88.09
Biskra's button B55.1

Bite (s) (animal) (human)
  abdomen, abdominal
    wall S31.159
      with penetration into peritoneal cavity
        S31.659
      epigastric region S31.152
        with penetration into peritoneal cavity
          S31.652
      left
        lower quadrant S31.154
          with penetration into peritoneal
            cavity S31.654
        upper quadrant S31.151
          with penetration into peritoneal
            cavity S31.651
      periumbilic region S31.155
        with penetration into peritoneal cavity
          S31.655
      right
        lower quadrant S31.153
          with penetration into peritoneal
            cavity S31.653
        upper quadrant S31.150
          with penetration into peritoneal
            cavity S31.650
      superficial NEC S30.871
        insect S30.861
  alveolar (process) —*see* Bite, oral cavity
  amphibian (venomous) —*see* Venom, bite,
    amphibian
  animal —*see also* Bite, by site
    venomous —*see* Venom
  ankle S91.05-
    superficial NEC S90.57-
      insect S90.56-
  antecubital space —*see* Bite, elbow
  anus S31.835
    superficial NEC S30.877
      insect S30.867
  arm (upper) S41.15-
    lower —*see* Bite, forearm
    superficial NEC S40.87-
      insect S40.86-
  arthropod NEC —*see* Venom, bite,
    arthropod
  auditory canal (external) (meatus) —
    see Bite, ear
  auricle, ear —*see* Bite, ear
  axilla —*see* Bite, arm
  back —*see also* Bite, thorax, back
    lower S31.050
      with penetration into retroperitoneal
        space S31.051
      superficial NEC S30.870
        insect S30.860
  bedbug —*see* Bite (s), by site, superficial,
    insect
  breast S21.05-
    superficial NEC S20.17-
      insect S20.16-
  brow —*see* Bite, head, specified site NEC
  buttock S31.805
    left S31.825
    right S31.815
    superficial NEC S30.870
      insect S30.860
  calf —*see* Bite, leg
  canaliculus lacrimalis —*see* Bite, eyelid
  canthus, eye —*see* Bite, eyelid
  centipede —*see* Toxicity, venom, arthropod,
    centipede
  cheek (external) S01.45-
    internal —*see* Bite, oral cavity
    superficial NEC S00.87
      insect S00.86
  chest wall —*see* Bite, thorax
  chigger B88.0
  chin —*see* Bite, head, specified site
    NEC
  clitoris —*see* Bite, vulva
  costal region —*see* Bite, thorax

Bite *(Continued)*
  digit (s)
    hand —*see* Bite, finger
    toe —*see* Bite, toe
  ear (canal) (external) S01.35-
    superficial NEC S00.47-
      insect S00.46-
  elbow S51.05-
    superficial NEC S50.37-
      insect S50.36-
  epididymis —*see* Bite, testis
  epigastric region —*see* Bite, abdomen
  epiglottis —*see* Bite, neck, specified site
    NEC
  esophagus, cervical S11.25
    superficial NEC S10.17
      insect S10.16
  eyebrow —*see* Bite, eyelid
  eyelid S01.15-
    superficial NEC S00.27-
      insect S00.26-
  face NEC —*see* Bite, head, specified site
    NEC
  finger (s) S61.259
    with
      damage to nail S61.359
    index S61.258
      with
        damage to nail S61.358
      left S61.251
        with
          damage to nail S61.351
      right S61.250
        with
          damage to nail S61.350
      superficial NEC S60.478
        insect S60.46-
    little S61.25-
      with
        damage to nail S61.35-
      superficial NEC S60.47-
        insect S60.46-
    middle S61.25-
      with
        damage to nail S61.35-
      superficial NEC S60.47-
        insect S60.46-
    ring S61.25-
      with
        damage to nail S61.35-
      superficial NEC S60.47-
        insect S60.46-
    superficial NEC S60.479
      insect S60.469
    thumb —*see* Bite, thumb
  flank —*see* Bite, abdomen, wall
  flea —*see* Bite, by site, superficial,
    insect
  foot (except toe (s) alone) S91.35-
    superficial NEC S90.87-
      insect S90.86-
    toe —*see* Bite, toe
  forearm S51.85-
    elbow only —*see* Bite, elbow
    superficial NEC S50.87-
      insect S50.86-
  forehead —*see* Bite, head, specified site
    NEC
  genital organs, external
    female S31.552
      superficial NEC S30.876
        insect S30.866
      vagina and vulva —*see* Bite, vulva
    male S31.551
      penis —*see* Bite, penis
      scrotum —*see* Bite, scrotum
      superficial NEC S30.875
        insect S30.865
      testes —*see* Bite, testis
  groin —*see* Bite, abdomen, wall
  gum —*see* Bite, oral cavity

Bite *(Continued)*
  hand S61.45-
    finger —*see* Bite, finger
    superficial NEC S60.57-
      insect S60.56-
    thumb —*see* Bite, thumb
  head S01.95
    cheek —*see* Bite, cheek
    ear —*see* Bite, ear
    eyelid —*see* Bite, eyelid
    lip —*see* Bite, lip
    nose —*see* Bite, nose
    oral cavity —*see* Bite, oral cavity
    scalp —*see* Bite, scalp
    specified site NEC S01.85
      superficial NEC S00.87
        insect S00.86
    superficial NEC S00.97
      insect S00.96
    temporomandibular area —*see* Bite, cheek
  heel —*see* Bite, foot
  hip S71.05-
    superficial NEC S70.27-
      insect S70.26-
  hymen S31.45
  hypochondrium —*see* Bite, abdomen, wall
  hypogastric region —*see* Bite, abdomen, wall
  inguinal region —*see* Bite, abdomen, wall
  insect —*see* Bite, by site, superficial, insect
  instep —*see* Bite, foot
  interscapular region —*see* Bite, thorax, back
  jaw —*see* Bite, head, specified site NEC
  knee S81.05-
    superficial NEC S80.27-
      insect S80.26-
  labium (majus) (minus) —*see* Bite, vulva
  lacrimal duct —*see* Bite, eyelid
  larynx S11.015
    superficial NEC S10.17
      insect S10.16
  leg (lower) S81.85-
    ankle —*see* Bite, ankle
    foot —*see* Bite, foot
    knee —*see* Bite, knee
    superficial NEC S80.87-
      insect S80.86-
    toe —*see* Bite, toe
    upper —*see* Bite, thigh
  lip S01.551
    superficial NEC S00.571
      insect S00.561
  lizard (venomous) —*see* Venom, bite, reptile
  loin —*see* Bite, abdomen, wall
  lower back —*see* Bite, back, lower
  lumbar region —*see* Bite, back, lower
  malar region —*see* Bite, head, specified site
    NEC
  mammary —*see* Bite, breast
  marine animals (venomous) —*see* Toxicity,
    venom, marine animal
  mastoid region —*see* Bite, head, specified site
    NEC
  mouth —*see* Bite, oral cavity
  nail
    finger —*see* Bite, finger
    toe —*see* Bite, toe
  nape —*see* Bite, neck, specified site NEC
  nasal (septum) (sinus) —*see* Bite, nose
  nasopharynx —*see* Bite, head, specified site
    NEC
  neck S11.95
    involving
      cervical esophagus —*see* Bite,
        esophagus, cervical
      larynx —*see* Bite, larynx
      pharynx —*see* Bite, pharynx
      thyroid gland S11.15
      trachea —*see* Bite, trachea
    specified site NEC S11.85
      superficial NEC S10.87
        insect S10.86

◀ New   ◀▥ Revised   ~~deleted~~ Deleted

Bite (Continued)
  neck (Continued)
    superficial NEC S10.97
      insect S10.96
    throat S11.85
      superficial NEC S10.17
        insect S10.16
  nose (septum) (sinus) S01.25
    superficial NEC S00.37
      insect S00.36
  occipital region —see Bite, scalp
  oral cavity S01.552
    superficial NEC S00.572
      insect S00.562
  orbital region —see Bite, eyelid
  palate —see Bite, oral cavity
  palm —see Bite, hand
  parietal region —see Bite, scalp
  pelvis S31.050
    with penetration into retroperitoneal space
      S31.051
    superficial NEC S30.870
      insect S30.860
  penis S31.25
    superficial NEC S30.872
      insect S30.862
  perineum
    female —see Bite, vulva
    male —see Bite, pelvis
  periocular area (with or without lacrimal
      passages) —see Bite, eyelid
  phalanges
    finger —see Bite, finger
    toe —see Bite, toe
  pharynx S11.25
    superficial NEC S10.17
      insect S10.16
  pinna —see Bite, ear
  poisonous —see Venom
  popliteal space —see Bite, knee
  prepuce —see Bite, penis
  pubic region —see Bite, abdomen, wall
  rectovaginal septum —see Bite, vulva
  red bug B88.0
  reptile NEC —see also Venom, bite,
      reptile
    nonvenomous —see Bite, by site
    snake —see Venom, bite, snake
  sacral region —see Bite, back, lower
  sacroiliac region —see Bite, back, lower
  salivary gland —see Bite, oral cavity
  scalp S01.05
    superficial NEC S00.07
      insect S00.06
  scapular region —see Bite, shoulder
  scrotum S31.35
    superficial NEC S30.873
      insect S30.863
  sea-snake (venomous) —see Toxicity, venom,
      snake, sea snake
  shin —see Bite, leg
  shoulder S41.05-
    superficial NEC S40.27-
      insect S40.26-
  snake —see also Venom, bite, snake
    nonvenomous —see Bite, by site
  spermatic cord —see Bite, testis
  spider (venomous) —see Toxicity, venom,
      spider
    nonvenomous —see Bite, by site,
        superficial, insect
  sternal region —see Bite, thorax, front
  submaxillary region —see Bite, head,
      specified site NEC
  submental region —see Bite, head, specified
      site NEC
  subungual
    finger (s) —see Bite, finger
    toe —see Bite, toe
  superficial —see Bite, by site, superficial
  supraclavicular fossa S11.85

Bite (Continued)
  supraorbital —see Bite, head, specified site
      NEC
  temple, temporal region —see Bite, head,
      specified site NEC
  temporomandibular area —see Bite, cheek
  testis S31.35
    superficial NEC S30.873
      insect S30.863
  thigh S71.15-
    superficial NEC S70.37-
      insect S70.36-
  thorax, thoracic (wall) S21.95
    back S21.25-
      with penetration into thoracic cavity
        S21.45-
    breast —see Bite, breast
    front S21.15-
      with penetration into thoracic cavity
        S21.35-
    superficial NEC S20.97
      back S20.47-
      front S20.37-
      insect S20.96
        back S20.46-
        front S20.36-
  throat —see Bite, neck, throat
  thumb S61.05-
    with
      damage to nail S61.15-
    superficial NEC S60.37-
      insect S60.36-
  thyroid S11.15
    superficial NEC S10.87
      insect S10.86
  toe (s) S91.15-
    with
      damage to nail S91.25-
    great S91.15-
      with
        damage to nail S91.25-
    lesser S91.15-
      with
        damage to nail S91.25-
    superficial NEC S90.47-
      great S90.47-
      insect S90.46-
        great S90.46-
  tongue S01.552
  trachea S11.025
    superficial NEC S10.17
      insect S10.16
  tunica vaginalis —see Bite, testis
  tympanum, tympanic membrane —see Bite,
      ear
  umbilical region S31.155
  uvula —see Bite, oral cavity
  vagina —see Bite, vulva
  venomous —see Venom
  vocal cords S11.035
    superficial NEC S10.17
      insect S10.16
  vulva S31.45
    superficial NEC S30.874
      insect S30.864
  wrist S61.55-
    superficial NEC S60.87-
      insect S60.86-
Biting, cheek or lip K13.1
Biventricular failure (heart) I50.9
Björck (-Thorson) syndrome (malignant
    carcinoid) E34.0
Black
  death A20.9
  eye S00.1-
  hairy tongue K14.3
  heel (foot) S90.3-
  lung (disease) J60
  palm (hand) S60.22-
Blackfan-Diamond anemia or syndrome
    (congenital hypoplastic anemia) D61.01

Blackhead L70.0
Blackout R55
Bladder —see condition
Blast (air) (hydraulic) (immersion) (underwater)
  blindness S05.8X-
  injury
    abdomen or thorax —see Injury, by site
    ear (acoustic nerve trauma) —see Injury,
        nerve, acoustic, specified type NEC
  syndrome NEC T70.8
Blastoma —see Neoplasm, malignant, by site
  pulmonary —see Neoplasm, lung, malignant
Blastomycosis, blastomycotic B40.9
  Brazilian —see Paracoccidioidomycosis
  cutaneous B40.3
  disseminated B40.7
  European —see Cryptococcosis
  generalized B40.7
  keloidal B48.0
  North American B40.9
  primary pulmonary B40.0
  pulmonary B40.2
    acute B40.0
    chronic B40.1
  skin B40.3
  South American —see Paracoccidioidomycosis
  specified NEC B40.89
Bleb (s) R23.8
  emphysematous (lung) (solitary) J43.9
  endophthalmitis H59.43
  filtering (vitreous), after glaucoma surgery
      Z98.83
  inflamed (infected), postprocedural H59.40
    stage 1 H59.41
    stage 2 H59.42
    stage 3 H59.43
  lung (ruptured) J43.9
    congenital —see Atelectasis
    newborn P25.8
  subpleural (emphysematous) J43.9
Blebitis, postprocedural H59.40
  stage 1 H59.41
  stage 2 H59.42
  stage 3 H59.43
Bleeder (familial) (hereditary) —see Hemophilia
Bleeding —see also Hemorrhage
  anal K62.5
  anovulatory N97.0
  atonic, following delivery O72.1
  capillary I78.8
    puerperal O72.2
  contact (postcoital) N93.0
  due to uterine subinvolution N85.3
  ear —see Otorrhagia
  excessive, associated with menopausal onset
      N92.4
  familial —see Defect, coagulation
  following intercourse N93.0
  gastrointestinal K92.2
  hemorrhoids —see Hemorrhoids
  intermenstrual (regular) N92.3
    irregular N92.1
  intraoperative —see Complication,
      intraoperative, hemorrhage
  irregular N92.6
  menopausal N92.4
  newborn, intraventricular —see
      Newborn, affected by, hemorrhage,
      intraventricular
  nipple N64.59
  nose R04.0
  ovulation N92.3
  postclimacteric N95.0
  postcoital N93.0
  postmenopausal N95.0
  postoperative —see Complication,
      postprocedural, hemorrhage
  preclimacteric N92.4
  pre-pubertal vaginal N93.1 ◄
  puberty (excessive, with onset of menstrual
      periods) N92.2

Bleeding *(Continued)*
  rectum, rectal K62.5
    newborn P54.2
  tendencies —*see* Defect, coagulation
  throat R04.1
  tooth socket (post-extraction) K91.840
  umbilical stump P51.9
  uterus, uterine NEC N93.9
    climacteric N92.4
    dysfunctional of functional N93.8
    menopausal N92.4
    preclimacteric or premenopausal N92.4
    unrelated to menstrual cycle N93.9
  vagina, vaginal (abnormal) N93.9
    dysfunctional or functional N93.8
    newborn P54.6
    pre-pubertal N93.1 ◄
  vicarious N94.89
Blennorrhagia, blennorrhagic —*see* Gonorrhea
Blennorrhea (acute) (chronic) —*see also*
    Gonorrhea
  inclusion (neonatal) (newborn) P39.1
  lower genitourinary tract (gonococcal)
    A54.00
  neonatorum (gonococcal ophthalmia)
    A54.31
Blepharelosis —*see* Entropion
Blepharitis (angularis) (ciliaris) (eyelid)
    (marginal) (nonulcerative) H01.009
  herpes zoster B02.39
  left H01.006
    lower H01.005
    upper H01.004
  right H01.003
    lower H01.002
    upper H01.001
  squamous H01.029
    left H01.026
      lower H01.025
      upper H01.024
    right H01.023
      lower H01.022
      upper H01.021
  ulcerative H01.019
    left H01.016
      lower H01.015
      upper H01.014
    right H01.013
      lower H01.012
      upper H01.011
Blepharochalasis H02.30
  congenital Q10.0
  left H02.36
    lower H02.35
    upper H02.34
  right H02.33
    lower H02.32
    upper H02.31
Blepharoclonus H02.59
Blepharoconjunctivitis H10.50-
  angular H10.52-
  contact H10.53-
  ligneous H10.51-
Blepharophimosis (eyelid) H02.529
  congenital Q10.3
  left H02.526
    lower H02.525
    upper H02.524
  right H02.523
    lower H02.522
    upper H02.521
Blepharoptosis H02.40-
  congenital Q10.0
  mechanical H02.41-
  myogenic H02.42-
  neurogenic H02.43-
  paralytic H02.43-
Blepharopyorrhea, gonococcal A54.39
Blepharospasm G24.5
  drug induced G24.01
Blighted ovum O02.0

Blind —*see also* Blindness
  bronchus (congenital) Q32.4
  loop syndrome K90.2
    congenital Q43.8
  sac, fallopian tube (congenital) Q50.6
  spot, enlarged —*see* Defect, visual field,
    localized, scotoma, blind spot area
  tract or tube, congenital NEC —*see* Atresia,
    by site
Blindness (acquired) (congenital) (both eyes)
    H54.0
  blast S05.8X-
  color —*see* Deficiency, color vision
  concussion S05.8X-
  cortical H47.619
    left brain H47.612
    right brain H47.611
  day H53.11
  due to injury (current episode) S05.9-
    sequelae — code to injury with seventh
      character S
  eclipse (total) —*see* Retinopathy, solar
  emotional (hysterical) F44.6
  face H53.16
  hysterical F44.6
  legal (both eyes) (USA definition) H54.8
  mind R48.8
  night H53.60
    abnormal dark adaptation curve H53.61
    acquired H53.62
    congenital H53.63
    specified type NEC H53.69
    vitamin A deficiency E50.5
  one eye (other eye normal) H54.40
    left (normal vision on right) H54.42
      low vision on right H54.12
    low vision, other eye H54.10
    right (normal vision on left) H54.41
      low vision on left H54.11
  psychic R48.8
  river B73.01
  snow —*see* Photokeratitis
  sun, solar —*see* Retinopathy, solar
  transient —*see* Disturbance, vision, subjective,
    loss, transient
  traumatic (current episode) S05.9-
  word (developmental) F81.0
    acquired R48.0
    secondary to organic lesion R48.0
Blister (nonthermal)
  abdominal wall S30.821
  alveolar process S00.522
  ankle S90.52-
  antecubital space —*see* Blister, elbow
  anus S30.827
  arm (upper) S40.82-
  auditory canal —*see* Blister, ear
  auricle —*see* Blister, ear
  axilla —*see* Blister, arm
  back, lower S30.820
  beetle dermatitis L24.89
  breast S20.12-
  brow S00.82
  calf —*see* Blister, leg
  canthus —*see* Blister, eyelid
  cheek S00.82
    internal S00.522
  chest wall —*see* Blister, thorax
  chin S00.82
  costal region —*see* Blister, thorax
  digit (s)
    foot —*see* Blister, toe
    hand —*see* Blister, finger
  due to burn —*see* Burn, by site, second degree
  ear S00.42-
  elbow S50.32-
  epiglottis S10.12
  esophagus, cervical S10.12
  eyebrow —*see* Blister, eyelid
  eyelid S00.22-
  face S00.82

Blister *(Continued)*
  fever B00.1
  finger (s) S60.429
    index S60.42-
    little S60.42-
    middle S60.42-
    ring S60.42-
  foot (except toe (s) alone) S90.82-
    toe —*see* Blister, toe
  forearm S50.82-
    elbow only —*see* Blister, elbow
  forehead S00.82
  fracture - omit code
  genital organ
    female S30.826
    male S30.825
  gum S00.522
  hand S60.52-
  head S00.92
    ear —*see* Blister, ear
    eyelid —*see* Blister, eyelid
    lip S00.521
    nose S00.32
    oral cavity S00.522
    scalp S00.02
    specified site NEC S00.82
  heel —*see* Blister, foot
  hip S70.22-
  interscapular region S20.429
  jaw S00.82
  knee S80.22-
  larynx S10.12
  leg (lower) S80.82-
    knee —*see* Blister, knee
    upper —*see* Blister, thigh
  lip S00.521
  malar region S00.82
  mammary —*see* Blister, breast
  mastoid region S00.82
  mouth S00.522
  multiple, skin, nontraumatic R23.8
  nail
    finger —*see* Blister, finger
    toe —*see* Blister, toe
  nasal S00.32
  neck S10.92
    specified site NEC S10.82
    throat S10.12
  nose S00.32
  occipital region S00.02
  oral cavity S00.522
  orbital region —*see* Blister, eyelid
  palate S00.522
  palm —*see* Blister, hand
  parietal region S00.02
  pelvis S30.820
  penis S30.822
  periocular area —*see* Blister, eyelid
  phalanges
    finger —*see* Blister, finger
    toe —*see* Blister, toe
  pharynx S10.12
  pinna —*see* Blister, ear
  popliteal space —*see* Blister, knee
  scalp S00.02
  scapular region —*see* Blister, shoulder
  scrotum S30.823
  shin —*see* Blister, leg
  shoulder S40.22-
  sternal region S20.329
  submaxillary region S00.82
  submental region S00.82
  subungual
    finger (s) —*see* Blister, finger
    toe (s) —*see* Blister, toe
  supraclavicular fossa S10.82
  supraorbital S00.82
  temple S00.82
  temporal region S00.82
  testis S30.823
  thermal —*see* Burn, second degree, by site

◄ New   ◄|||| Revised   ~~deleted~~ Deleted

Blister (Continued)
thigh S70.32-
thorax, thoracic (wall) S20.92
back S20.42-
front S20.32-
throat S10.12
thumb S60.32-
toe (s) S90.42-
great S90.42-
tongue S00.522
trachea S10.12
tympanum, tympanic membrane —see Blister,
ear
upper arm —see Blister, arm (upper)
uvula S00.522
vagina S30.824
vocal cords S10.12
vulva S30.824
wrist S60.82-
Bloating R14.0
Bloch-Sulzberger disease or syndrome Q82.3
Block, blocked
alveolocapillary J84.10
arborization (heart) I45.5
arrhythmic I45.9
atrioventricular (incomplete) (partial) I44.30
with atrioventricular dissociation I44.2
complete I44.2
congenital Q24.6
congenital Q24.6
first degree I44.0
second degree (types I and II) I44.1
specified NEC I44.39
third degree I44.2
types I and II I44.1
auriculoventricular —see Block,
atrioventricular
bifascicular (cardiac) I45.2
bundle-branch (complete) (false) (incomplete)
I45.4
bilateral I45.2
left I44.7
with right bundle branch block I45.2
hemiblock I44.60
anterior I44.4
posterior I44.5
incomplete I44.7
with right bundle branch block I45.2
right I45.10
with
left bundle branch block I45.2
left fascicular block I45.2
specified NEC I45.19
Wilson's type I45.19
cardiac I45.9
conduction I45.9
complete I44.2
fascicular (left) I44.60
anterior I44.4
posterior I44.5
right I45.0
specified NEC I44.69
foramen Magendie (acquired) G91.1
congenital Q03.1
with spina bifida —see Spina bifida, by
site, with hydrocephalus
heart I45.9
bundle branch I45.4
bilateral I45.2
complete (atrioventricular) I44.2
congenital Q24.6
first degree (atrioventricular) I44.0
second degree (atrioventricular) I44.1
specified type NEC I45.5
third degree (atrioventricular) I44.2
hepatic vein I82.0
intraventricular (nonspecific) I45.4
bundle branch
bilateral I45.2
kidney N28.9
postcystoscopic or postprocedural N99.0

Block, blocked (Continued)
Mobitz (types I and II) I44.1
myocardial —see Block, heart
nodal I45.5
organ or site, congenital NEC —see Atresia,
by site
portal (vein) I81
second degree (types I and II) I44.1
sinoatrial I45.5
sinoauricular I45.5
third degree I44.2
trifascicular I45.3
tubal N97.1
vein NOS I82.90
Wenckebach (types I and II) I44.1
Blockage —see Obstruction
Blocq's disease F44.4
Blood
constituents, abnormal R78.9
disease D75.9
donor —see Donor, blood
dyscrasia D75.9
with
abortion —see Abortion, by type,
complicated by, hemorrhage
ectopic pregnancy O08.1
molar pregnancy O08.1
following ectopic or molar pregnancy
O08.1
newborn P61.9
puerperal, postpartum O72.3
flukes NEC —see Schistosomiasis
in
feces K92.1
occult R19.5
urine —see Hematuria
mole O02.0
occult in feces R19.5
pressure
decreased, due to shock following injury
T79.4
examination only Z01.30
fluctuating I99.8
high —see Hypertension
borderline R03.0
incidental reading, without diagnosis of
hypertension R03.0
low —see also Hypotension
incidental reading, without diagnosis of
hypotension R03.1
spitting —see Hemoptysis
staining cornea —see Pigmentation, cornea,
stromal
transfusion
reaction or complication —see
Complications, transfusion
type
A (Rh positive) Z67.10
Rh negative Z67.11
AB (Rh positive) Z67.30
Rh negative Z67.31
B (Rh positive) Z67.20
Rh negative Z67.21
O (Rh positive) Z67.40
Rh negative Z67.41
Rh (positive) Z67.90
negative Z67.91
vessel rupture —see Hemorrhage
vomiting —see Hematemesis
Blood-forming organs, disease D75.9
Bloodgood's disease —see Mastopathy,
cystic
Bloom (-Machacek)(-Torre) **syndrome**
Q82.8
Blount's disease or osteochondrosis —see
Osteochondrosis, juvenile, tibia
Blue
baby Q24.9
diaper syndrome E72.09
dome cyst (breast) —see Cyst, breast
dot cataract Q12.0

Blue (Continued)
nevus D22.9
sclera Q13.5
with fragility of bone and deafness Q78.0
toe syndrome I75.02-
Blueness —see Cyanosis
Blues, postpartal O90.6
baby O90.6
Blurring, visual H53.8
Blushing (abnormal) (excessive) R23.2
BMI —see Body, mass index
Boarder, hospital NEC Z76.4
accompanying sick person Z76.3
healthy infant or child Z76.2
foundling Z76.1
Bockhart's impetigo L01.02
Bodechtel-Guttman disease (subacute
sclerosing panencephalitis) A81.1
Boder-Sedgwick syndrome (ataxia-
telangiectasia) G11.3
Body, bodies
Aschoff's —see Myocarditis, rheumatic
asteroid, vitreous —see Deposit, crystalline
cytoid (retina) —see Occlusion, artery, retina
drusen (degenerative) (macula) (retinal) —see
also Degeneration, macula, drusen
optic disc —see Drusen, optic disc
foreign —see Foreign body
loose
joint, except knee —see Loose, body, joint
knee M23.4-
sheath, tendon —see Disorder, tendon,
specified type NEC
mass index (BMI)
adult
19 or less Z68.1
20.0-20.9 Z68.20
21.0-21.9 Z68.21
22.0-22.9 Z68.22
23.0-23.9 Z68.23
24.0-24.9 Z68.24
25.0-25.9 Z68.25
26.0-26.9 Z68.26
27.0-27.9 Z68.27
28.0-28.9 Z68.28
29.0-29.9 Z68.29
30.0-30.9 Z68.30
31.0-31.9 Z68.31
32.0-32.9 Z68.32
33.0-33.9 Z68.33
34.0-34.9 Z68.34
35.0-35.9 Z68.35
36.0-36.9 Z68.36
37.0-37.9 Z68.37
38.0-38.9 Z68.38
39.0-39.9 Z68.39
40.0-44.9 Z68.41
45.0-49.9 Z68.42
50.0-59.9 Z68.43
60.0-69.9 Z68.44
70 and over Z68.45
pediatric
5th percentile to less than 85th percentile
for age Z68.52
85th percentile to less than 95th
percentile for age Z68.53
greater than or equal to ninety-fifth
percentile for age Z68.54
less than fifth percentile for age Z68.51
Mooser's A75.2
rice —see also Loose, body, joint
knee M23.4-
rocking F98.4
Boeck's
disease or sarcoid —see Sarcoidosis
lupoid (miliary) D86.3
Boerhaave's syndrome (spontaneous
esophageal rupture) K22.3
Boggy
cervix N88.8
uterus N85.8

Boil —see also Furuncle, by site
  Aleppo B55.1
  Baghdad B55.1
  Delhi B55.1
  lacrimal
    gland —see Dacryoadenitis
    passages (duct) (sac) —see Inflammation,
      lacrimal, passages, acute
  Natal B55.1
  orbit, orbital —see Abscess, orbit
  tropical B55.1
Bold hives —see Urticaria
Bombé, iris —see Membrane, pupillary
Bone —see condition
Bonnevie-Ullrich syndrome —see also Turner's
  syndrome Q87.1
Bonnier's syndrome —see subcategory H81.8
Bonvale dam fever T73.3
Bony block of joint —see Ankylosis
BOOP (bronchiolitis obliterans organized
  pneumonia) J84.89
Borderline
  diabetes mellitus R73.03
  hypertension R03.0
  osteopenia M85.8-
  pelvis, with obstruction during labor O65.1
  personality F60.3
Borna disease A83.9
Bornholm disease B33.0
Boston exanthem A88.0
Botalli, ductus (patent) (persistent) Q25.0
Bothriocephalus latus infestation B70.0
Botulism (foodborne intoxication) A05.1
  infant A48.51
  non-foodborne A48.52
  wound A48.52
Bouba —see Yaws
Bouchard's nodes (with arthropathy) M15.2
Bouffée délirante F23
Bouillaud's disease or syndrome (rheumatic
  heart disease) I01.9
Bourneville's disease Q85.1
Boutonniere deformity (finger) —see
  Deformity, finger, boutonniere
Bouveret (-Hoffmann) syndrome (paroxysmal
  tachycardia) I47.9
Bovine heart —see Hypertrophy, cardiac
Bowel —see condition
Bowen's
  dermatosis (precancerous) —see Neoplasm,
    skin, in situ
  disease —see Neoplasm, skin, in situ
  epithelioma —see Neoplasm, skin, in situ
  type
    epidermoid carcinoma-in-situ —see
      Neoplasm, skin, in situ
    intraepidermal squamous cell carcinoma —
      see Neoplasm, skin, in situ
Bowing
  femur —see also Deformity, limb, specified
    type NEC, thigh
    congenital Q68.3
  fibula —see also Deformity, limb, specified
    type NEC, lower leg
    congenital Q68.4
  forearm —see Deformity, limb, specified type
    NEC, forearm
  leg (s), long bones, congenital Q68.5
  radius —see Deformity, limb, specified type
    NEC, forearm
  tibia —see also Deformity, limb, specified type
    NEC, lower leg
    congenital Q68.4
Bowleg (s) (acquired) M21.16-
  congenital Q68.5
  rachitic E64.3
Boyd's dysentery A03.2
Brachial —see condition
Brachycardia R00.1
Brachycephaly Q75.0
Bradley's disease A08.19

Bradyarrhythmia, cardiac I49.8
Bradycardia (sinoatrial) (sinus) (vagal) R00.1
  neonatal P29.12
  reflex G90.09
  tachycardia syndrome I49.5
Bradykinesia R25.8
Bradypnea R06.89
Bradytachycardia I49.5
Brailsford's disease or osteochondrosis —see
  Osteochondrosis, juvenile, radius
Brain —see also condition
  death G93.82
  syndrome —see Syndrome, brain
Branched-chain amino-acid disorder E71.2
Branchial —see condition
  cartilage, congenital Q18.2
Branchiogenic remnant (in neck) Q18.0
Brandt's syndrome (acrodermatitis
  enteropathica) E83.2
Brash (water) R12
Bravais-jacksonian epilepsy —see Epilepsy,
  localization-related, symptomatic, with
  simple partial seizures
Braxton Hicks contractions —see False, labor
Brazilian leishmaniasis B55.2
BRBPR K62.5
Break, retina (without detachment) H33.30-
  with retinal detachment —see Detachment,
    retina
  horseshoe tear H33.31-
  multiple H33.33-
  round hole H33.32-
Breakdown
  device, graft or implant —see also
    Complications, by site and type,
    mechanical T85.618
    arterial graft NEC —see Complication,
      cardiovascular device, mechanical,
      vascular
    breast (implant) T85.41
    catheter NEC T85.618
      cystostomy T83.010
      dialysis (renal) T82.41
        intraperitoneal T85.611
      Hopkins T83.018
      ileostomy T83.018
      infusion NEC T82.514
        cranial T85.610
        epidural T85.610
        intrathecal T85.610
        spinal T85.610
        subarachnoid T85.610
        subdural T85.610
      urinary (indwelling) T83.018
      nephrostomy T83.012
      urethral indwelling T83.011
      urinary NEC T83.018
      urostomy T83.018
    electronic (electrode) (pulse generator)
      (stimulator)
      bone T84.310
      cardiac T82.119
        electrode T82.110
        pulse generator T82.111
        specified type NEC T82.118
      nervous system —see Complication,
        prosthetic device, mechanical,
        electronic nervous system stimulator
      urinary —see Complication,
        genitourinary, device, urinary,
        mechanical
    fixation, internal (orthopedic) NEC —see
      Complication, fixation device,
      mechanical
    gastrointestinal —see Complications,
      prosthetic device, mechanical,
      gastrointestinal device
    genital NEC T83.418
      intrauterine contraceptive device T83.31
      penile prosthesis (cylinder) (implanted)
        (pump) (resevoir) T83.410
      testicular prosthesis T83.411

Breakdown (Continued)
  device, graft or implant (Continued)
    heart NEC —see Complication,
      cardiovascular device, mechanical
    intrathecal infusion pump T85.615
    joint prosthesis —see Complications...,
      joint prosthesis,internal, mechanical,
      by site
    nervous system, specified device NEC
      T85.615
    ocular NEC —see Complications, prosthetic
      device, mechanical, ocular device
    orthopedic NEC —see Complication,
      orthopedic, device, mechanical
    specified NEC T85.618
    subcutaneous device pocket
      nervous system prosthetic device,
        implant, or graft T85.890
      other internal prosthetic device, implant,
        or graft T85.898
    sutures, permanent T85.612
      used in bone repair —see Complications,
        fixation device, internal
        (orthopedic), mechanical
    urinary NEC T83.118
      graft T83.21
      sphincter, implanted T83.111
      stent (ileal conduit) (nephroureteral)
        T83.113
      ureteral indwelling T83.112
    vascular NEC —see Complication,
      cardiovascular device, mechanical
    ventricular intracranial shunt T85.01
  nervous F48.8
  perineum O90.1
  respirator J95.850
    specified NEC J95.859
  ventilator J95.850
    specified NEC J95.859
Breast —see also condition
  buds E30.1
    in newborn P96.89
  dense R92.2
  nodule N63
Breath
  foul R19.6
  holder, child R06.89
  holding spell R06.89
  shortness R06.02
Breathing
  labored —see Hyperventilation
  mouth R06.5
    causing malocclusion M26.5
  periodic R06.3
    high altitude G47.32
Breathlessness R06.81
Breda's disease —see Yaws
Breech presentation (mother) O32.1
  causing obstructed labor O64.1
  footling O32.8
    causing obstructed labor O64.8
  incomplete O32.8
    causing obstructed labor O64.8
Breisky's disease N90.4
Brennemann's syndrome I88.0
Brenner
  tumor (benign) D27.9
    borderline malignancy D39.1-
    malignant C56
    proliferating D39.1
Bretonneau's disease or angina A36.0
Breus' mole O02.0
Brevicollis Q76.49
Brickmakers' anemia B76.9 [D63.8]
Bridge, myocardial Q24.5
Bright red blood per rectum (BRBPR) K62.5
Bright's disease —see also Nephritis
  arteriosclerotic —see Hypertension, kidney
Brill (-Zinsser) disease (recrudescent typhus)
  A75.1
  flea-borne A75.2
  louse-borne A75.1

◀ New   ◀⫶⫶ Revised   ~~deleted~~ Deleted

Brill-Symmers' disease C82.90
Brion-Kayser disease —*see* Fever, parathyroid
Briquet's disorder or syndrome F45.0
Brissaud's
    infantilism or dwarfism E23.0
    motor-verbal tic F95.2
Brittle
    bones disease Q78.0
    nails L60.3
        congenital Q84.6
Broad —*see also* condition
    beta disease E78.2
    ligament laceration syndrome N83.8
Broad- or floating-betalipoproteinemia E78.2
Brock's syndrome (atelectasis due to enlarged
    lymph nodes) J98.19
Brocq-Duhring disease (dermatitis
    herpetiformis) L13.0
Brodie's abscess or disease M86.8X-
Broken
    arches —*see also* Deformity, limb, flat foot
    arm (meaning upper limb) —*see* Fracture, arm
    back —*see* Fracture, vertebra
    bone —*see* Fracture
    implant or internal device —*see*
        Complications, by site and type,
        mechanical
    leg (meaning lower limb) —*see* Fracture, leg
    nose S02.2
    tooth, teeth —*see* Fracture, tooth
Bromhidrosis, bromidrosis L75.0
Bromidism, bromism G92
    chronic (dependence) F13.20
    due to
        correct substance properly administered —
            see Table of Drugs and Chemicals, by
            drug, adverse effect
        overdose or wrong substance given or
            taken —*see* Table of Drugs and
            Chemicals, by drug, poisoning
Bromidrosiphobia F40.298
Bronchi, bronchial —*see* condition
Bronchiectasis (cylindrical) (diffuse) (fusiform)
    (localized) (saccular) J47.9
    with
        acute
            bronchitis J47.0
            lower respiratory infection J47.0
        exacerbation (acute) J47.1
    congenital Q33.4
    tuberculous NEC —*see* Tuberculosis,
        pulmonary
Bronchiolectasis —*see* Bronchiectasis
Bronchiolitis (acute) (infective) (subacute) J21.9
    with
        bronchospasm or obstruction J21.9
        influenza, flu or grippe —*see* Influenza,
            with, respiratory manifestations NEC
    chemical (chronic) J68.4
        acute J68.0
    chronic (fibrosing) (obliterative) J44.9
    due to
        external agent —*see* Bronchitis, acute, due to
        human metapneumovirus J21.1
        respiratory syncytial virus J21.0
        specified organism NEC J21.8
    fibrosa obliterans J44.9
    influenzal —*see* Influenza, with, respiratory
        manifestations NEC
    obliterans J42
        with organizing pneumonia (BOOP) J84.89
    obliterative (chronic) (subacute) J44.9
        due to chemicals, gases, fumes or vapors
            (inhalation) J68.4
        due to fumes or vapors J68.4
    respiratory, interstitial lung disease J84.115
Bronchitis (diffuse) (fibrinous) (hypostatic)
    (infective) (membranous) J40
    with
        influenza, flu or grippe —*see* Influenza,
            with, respiratory manifestations NEC

Bronchitis (*Continued*)
    with (*Continued*)
        obstruction (airway) (lung) J44.9
        tracheitis (15 years of age and above) J40
            acute or subacute J20.9
            chronic J42
            under 15 years of age J20.9
    acute or subacute (with bronchospasm or
        obstruction) J20.9
        with
            bronchiectasis J47.0
            chronic obstructive pulmonary disease
                J44.0
        chemical (due to gases, fumes or vapors)
            J68.0
        due to
            fumes or vapors J68.0
            Haemophilus influenzae J20.1
            Mycoplasma pneumoniae J20.0
            radiation J70.0
            specified organism NEC J20.8
            Streptococcus J20.2
            virus
                coxsackie J20.3
                echovirus J20.7
                parainfluenzae J20.4
                respiratory syncytial J20.5
                rhinovirus J20.6
        viral NEC J20.8
    allergic (acute) J45.909
        with
            exacerbation (acute) J45.901
            status asthmaticus J45.902
    arachidic T17.528
    aspiration (due to fumes or vapors) J68.0
    asthmatic J45.9
        chronic J44.9
            with
                acute lower respiratory infection J44.0
                exacerbation (acute) J44.1
    capillary —*see* Pneumonia, broncho
    caseous (tuberculous) A15.5
    Castellani's A69.8
    catarrhal (15 years of age and above) J40
        acute —*see* Bronchitis, acute
        chronic J41.0
        under 15 years of age J20.9
    chemical (acute) (subacute) J68.0
        chronic J68.4
        due to fumes or vapors J68.0
            chronic J68.4
    chronic J42
        with
            airways obstruction J44.9
            tracheitis (chronic) J42
        asthmatic (obstructive) J44.9
        catarrhal J41.0
        chemical (due to fumes or vapors) J68.4
        due to
            chemicals, gases, fumes or vapors
                (inhalation) J68.4
            radiation J70.1
            tobacco smoking J41.0
        emphysematous J44.9
        mucopurulent J41.1
        non-obstructive J41.0
        obliterans J44.9
        obstructive J44.9
        purulent J41.1
        simple J41.0
    croupous —*see* Bronchitis, acute
    due to gases, fumes or vapors (chemical)
        J68.0
    emphysematous (obstructive) J44.9
    exudative —*see* Bronchitis, acute
    fetid J41.1
    grippal —*see* Influenza, with, respiratory
        manifestations NEC
    in those under 15 years age —*see* Bronchitis,
        acute
    chronic —*see* Bronchitis, chronic

Bronchitis (*Continued*)
    influenzal —*see* Influenza, with, respiratory
        manifestations NEC
    mixed simple and mucopurulent J41.8
    moulder's J62.8
    mucopurulent (chronic) (recurrent) J41.1
        acute or subacute J20.9
        simple (mixed) J41.8
    obliterans (chronic) J44.9
    obstructive (chronic) (diffuse) J44.9
    pituitous J41.1
    pneumococcal, acute or subacute J20.2
    pseudomembranous, acute or subacute —*see*
        Bronchitis, acute
    purulent (chronic) (recurrent) J41.1
        acute or subacute —*see* Bronchitis, acute
    putrid J41.1
    senile (chronic) J42
    simple and mucopurulent (mixed) J41.8
    smokers' J41.0
    spirochetal NEC A69.8
    subacute —*see* Bronchitis, acute
    suppurative (chronic) J41.1
        acute or subacute —*see* Bronchitis, acute
    tuberculous A15.5
    under 15 years of age —*see* Bronchitis, acute
        chronic —*see* Bronchitis, chronic
    viral NEC, acute or subacute —*see also*
        Bronchitis, acute J20.8
Bronchoalveolitis J18.0
Bronchoaspergillosis B44.1
Bronchocele meaning goiter E04.0
Broncholithiasis J98.09
    tuberculous NEC A15.5
Bronchomalacia J98.09
    congenital Q32.2
Bronchomycosis NOS B49 [*J99*]
    candidal B37.1
Bronchopleuropneumonia —*see* Pneumonia,
    broncho
Bronchopneumonia —*see* Pneumonia, broncho
Bronchopneumonitis —*see* Pneumonia,
    broncho
Bronchopulmonary —*see* condition
Bronchopulmonitis —*see* Pneumonia, broncho
Bronchorrhagia (*see* Hemoptysis)
Bronchorrhea J98.09
    acute J20.9
    chronic (infective) (purulent) J42
Bronchospasm (acute) J98.01
    with
        bronchiolitis, acute J21.9
        bronchitis, acute (conditions in J20) —*see*
            Bronchitis, acute
    due to external agent —*see* condition,
        respiratory, acute, due to
    exercise induced J45.990
Bronchospirochetosis A69.8
    Castellani A69.8
Bronchostenosis J98.09
Bronchus —*see* condition
Brontophobia F40.220
Bronze baby syndrome P83.8
Brooke's tumor —*see* Neoplasm, skin, benign
Brown enamel of teeth (hereditary) K00.5
Brown's sheath syndrome H50.61-
Brown-Séquard disease, paralysis or
    syndrome G83.81
Bruce sepsis A23.0
Brucellosis (infection) A23.9
    abortus A23.1
    canis A23.3
    dermatitis A23.9
    melitensis A23.0
    mixed A23.8
    sepsis A23.9
        melitensis A23.0
        specified NEC A23.8
    suis A23.2
Bruck-de Lange disease Q87.1
Bruck's disease —*see* Deformity, limb

Brugsch's syndrome Q82.8
Bruise (skin surface intact) —see also Contusion
with
    open wound —see Wound, open
  internal organ —see Injury, by site
  newborn P54.5
  scalp, due to birth injury, newborn P12.3
  umbilical cord O69.5
Bruit (arterial) R09.89
  cardiac R01.1
Brush burn —see Abrasion, by site
Bruton's X-linked agammaglobulinemia D80.0
Bruxism
  psychogenic F45.8
  sleep related G47.63
Bubbly lung syndrome P27.0
Bubo I88.8
  blennorrhagic (gonococcal) A54.89
  chancroidal A57
  climatic A55
  due to Haemophilus ducreyi A57
  gonococcal A54.89
  indolent (nonspecific) I88.8
  inguinal (nonspecific) I88.8
    chancroidal A57
    climatic A55
    due to H. ducreyi A57
    infective I88.8
  scrofulous (tuberculous) A18.2
  soft chancre A57
  suppurating —see Lymphadenitis, acute
  syphilitic (primary) A51.0
    congenital A50.07
  tropical A55
  virulent (chancroidal) A57
Bubonic plague A20.0
Bubonocele —see Hernia, inguinal
Buccal —see condition
Buchanan's disease or osteochondrosis M91.0
Buchem's syndrome (hyperostosis corticalis)
  M85.2
Bucket-handle fracture or tear (semilunar
  cartilage) —see Tear, meniscus
Budd-Chiari syndrome (hepatic vein
  thrombosis) I82.0
Budgerigar fancier's disease or lung
  J67.2
Buds
  breast E30.1
    in newborn P96.89
Buerger's disease (thromboangiitis obliterans)
  I73.1
Bulbar —see condition
Bulbus cordis (left ventricle) (persistent)
  Q21.8
Bulimia (nervosa) F50.2
  atypical F50.9
  normal weight F50.9
Bulky
  stools R19.5
  uterus N85.2
Bulla (e) R23.8
  lung (emphysematous) (solitary) J43.9
    newborn P25.8
Bullet wound —see also Wound, open
  fracture - code as Fracture, by site
  internal organ —see Injury, by site
Bundle
  branch block (complete) (false)
    (incomplete) —see Block, bundle-branch
  of His —see condition
Bunion M21.61- ◀▥
  tailor's M21.62- ◀
Bunionette M21.62- ◀
Buphthalmia, buphthalmos (congenital) Q15.0
Burdwan fever B55.0
Bürger-Grütz disease or syndrome E78.3
Buried
  penis (congenital) Q55.64
    acquired N48.83
  roots K08.3

Burke's syndrome K86.89 ◀▥
Burkitt
  cell leukemia C91.0-
  lymphoma (malignant) C83.7-
    small noncleaved, diffuse C83.7-
    spleen C83.77
    undifferentiated C83.7-
  tumor C83.7-
  type
    acute lymphoblastic leukemia C91.0-
    undifferentiated C83.7-
Burn (electricity) (flame) (hot gas, liquid or hot
  object) (radiation) (steam) (thermal) T30.0
  abdomen, abdominal (muscle) (wall)
    T21.02
    first degree T21.12
    second degree T21.22
    third degree T21.32
  above elbow T22.039
    first degree T22.139
    left T22.032
      first degree T22.132
      second degree T22.232
      third degree T22.332
    right T22.031
      first degree T22.131
      second degree T22.231
      third degree T22.331
    second degree T22.239
    third degree T22.339
  acid (caustic) (external) (internal) —see
    Corrosion, by site
  alimentary tract NEC T28.2
    esophagus T28.1
    mouth T28.0
    pharynx T28.0
  alkaline (caustic) (external) (internal) —see
    Corrosion, by site
  ankle T25.019
    first degree T25.119
    left T25.012
      first degree T25.112
      second degree T25.212
      third degree T25.312
    multiple with foot —see Burn, lower, limb,
      multiple, ankle and foot
    right T25.011
      first degree T25.111
      second degree T25.211
      third degree T25.311
    second degree T25.219
    third degree T25.319
  anus —see Burn, buttock
  arm (lower) (upper) —see Burn, upper,
    limb
  axilla T22.049
    first degree T22.149
    left T22.042
      first degree T22.142
      second degree T22.242
      third degree T22.342
    right T22.041
      first degree T22.141
      second degree T22.241
      third degree T22.341
    second degree T22.249
    third degree T22.349
  back (lower) T21.04
    first degree T21.14
    second degree T21.24
    third degree T21.34
    upper T21.03
      first degree T21.13
      second degree T21.23
      third degree T21.33
  blisters - code as Burn, second degree, by site
  breast (s) —see Burn, chest wall
  buttock (s) T21.05
    first degree T21.15
    second degree T21.25
    third degree T21.35

Burn (Continued)
  calf T24.039
    first degree T24.139
    left T24.032
      first degree T24.132
      second degree T24.232
      third degree T24.332
    right T24.031
      first degree T24.131
      second degree T24.231
      third degree T24.331
    second degree T24.239
    third degree T24.339
  canthus (eye) —see Burn, eyelid
  caustic acid or alkaline —see Corrosion, by
    site
  cervix T28.3
  cheek T20.06
    first degree T20.16
    second degree T20.26
    third degree T20.36
  chemical (acids) (alkalines) (caustics) (external)
    (internal) —see Corrosion, by site
  chest wall T21.01
    first degree T21.11
    second degree T21.21
    third degree T21.31
  chin T20.03
    first degree T20.13
    second degree T20.23
    third degree T20.33
  colon T28.2
  conjunctiva (and cornea) —see Burn, cornea
  cornea (and conjunctiva) T26.1-
    chemical —see Corrosion, cornea
  corrosion (external) (internal) —see
    Corrosion, by site
  deep necrosis of underlying tissue - code as
    Burn, third degree, by site
  dorsum of hand T23.069
    first degree T23.169
    left T23.062
      first degree T23.162
      second degree T23.262
      third degree T23.362
    right T23.061
      first degree T23.161
      second degree T23.261
      third degree T23.361
    second degree T23.269
    third degree T23.369
  due to ingested chemical agent —see
    Corrosion, by site
  ear (auricle) (external) (canal) T20.01
    first degree T20.11
    second degree T20.21
    third degree T20.31
  elbow T22.029
    first degree T22.129
    left T22.022
      first degree T22.122
      second degree T22.222
      third degree T22.322
    right T22.021
      first degree T22.121
      second degree T22.221
      third degree T22.321
    second degree T22.229
    third degree T22.329
  epidermal loss - code as Burn, second degree,
    by site
  erythema, erythematous - code as Burn, first
    degree, by site
  esophagus T28.1
  extent (percentage of body surface)
    less than 10 percent T31.0
    10-19 percent T31.10
      with 0-9 percent third degree burns
        T31.10
      with 10-19 percent third degree burns
        T31.11

Burn *(Continued)*
  extent *(Continued)*
    20-29 percent T31.20
      with 0-9 percent third degree burns
        T31.20
      with 10-19 percent third degree burns
        T31.21
      with 20-29 percent third degree burns
        T31.22
    30-39 percent T31.30
      with 0-9 percent third degree burns
        T31.30
      with 10-19 percent third degree burns
        T31.31
      with 20-29 percent third degree burns
        T31.32
      with 30-39 percent third degree burns
        T31.33
    40-49 percent T31.40
      with 0-9 percent third degree burns
        T31.40
      with 10-19 percent third degree burns
        T31.41
      with 20-29 percent third degree burns
        T31.42
      with 30-39 percent third degree burns
        T31.43
      with 40-49 percent third degree burns
        T31.44
    50-59 percent T31.50
      with 0-9 percent third degree burns T31.50
      with 10-19 percent third degree burns
        T31.51
      with 20-29 percent third degree burns
        T31.52
      with 30-39 percent third degree burns
        T31.53
      with 40-49 percent third degree burns
        T31.54
      with 50-59 percent third degree burns
        T31.55
    60-69 percent T31.60
      with 0-9 percent third degree burns T31.60
      with 10-19 percent third degree burns
        T31.61
      with 20-29 percent third degree burns
        T31.62
      with 30-39 percent third degree burns
        T31.63
      with 40-49 percent third degree burns
        T31.64
      with 50-59 percent third degree burns
        T31.65
      with 60-69 percent third degree burns
        T31.66
    70-79 percent T31.70
      with 0-9 percent third degree burns T31.70
      with 10-19 percent third degree burns
        T31.71
      with 20-29 percent third degree burns
        T31.72
      with 30-39 percent third degree burns
        T31.73
      with 40-49 percent third degree burns
        T31.74
      with 50-59 percent third degree burns
        T31.75
      with 60-69 percent third degree burns
        T31.76
      with 70-79 percent third degree burns
        T31.77
    80-89 percent T31.80
      with 0-9 percent third degree burns T31.80
      with 10-19 percent third degree burns
        T31.81
      with 20-29 percent third degree burns
        T31.82
      with 30-39 percent third degree burns
        T31.83
      with 40-49 percent third degree burns
        T31.84

Burn *(Continued)*
  extent *(Continued)*
    80-89 percent T31.80 *(Continued)*
      with 50-59 percent third degree burns
        T31.85
      with 60-69 percent third degree burns
        T31.86
      with 70-79 percent third degree burns
        T31.87
      with 80-89 percent third degree burns
        T31.88
    90 percent or more T31.90
      with 0-9 percent third degree burns T31.90
      with 10-19 percent third degree burns
        T31.91
      with 20-29 percent third degree burns
        T31.92
      with 30-39 percent third degree burns
        T31.93
      with 40-49 percent third degree burns
        T31.94
      with 50-59 percent third degree burns
        T31.95
      with 60-69 percent third degree burns
        T31.96
      with 70-79 percent third degree burns
        T31.97
      with 80-89 percent third degree burns
        T31.98
      with 90 percent or more third degree
        burns T31.99
  extremity —*see* Burn, limb
  eye (s) and adnexa T26.4-
    with resulting rupture and destruction of
      eyeball T26.2-
    conjunctival sac —*see* Burn, cornea
    cornea —*see* Burn, cornea
    lid —*see* Burn, eyelid
    periocular area —*see* Burn, eyelid
    specified site NEC T26.3-
  eyeball —*see* Burn, eye
  eyelid (s) T26.0-
    chemical —*see* Corrosion, eyelid
  face —*see* Burn, head
  finger T23.029
    first degree T23.129
    left T23.022
      first degree T23.122
      second degree T23.222
      third degree T23.322
    multiple sites (without thumb) T23.039
      with thumb T23.049
        first degree T23.149
        left T23.042
          first degree T23.142
          second degree T23.242
          third degree T23.342
        right T23.041
          first degree T23.141
          second degree T23.241
          third degree T23.341
        second degree T23.249
        third degree T23.349
      first degree T23.139
      left T23.032
        first degree T23.132
        second degree T23.232
        third degree T23.332
      right T23.031
        first degree T23.131
        second degree T23.231
        third degree T23.331
      second degree T23.239
      third degree T23.339
    right T23.021
      first degree T23.121
      second degree T23.221
      third degree T23.321
    second degree T23.229
    third degree T23.329
  flank —*see* Burn, abdominal wall

Burn *(Continued)*
  foot T25.029
    first degree T25.129
    left T25.022
      first degree T25.122
      second degree T25.222
      third degree T25.322
    multiple with ankle —*see* Burn, lower,
      limb, multiple, ankle and foot
    right T25.021
      first degree T25.121
      second degree T25.221
      third degree T25.321
    second degree T25.229
    third degree T25.329
  forearm T22.019
    first degree T22.119
    left T22.012
      first degree T22.112
      second degree T22.212
      third degree T22.312
    right T22.011
      first degree T22.111
      second degree T22.211
      third degree T22.311
    second degree T22.219
    third degree T22.319
  forehead T20.06
    first degree T20.16
    second degree T20.26
    third degree T20.36
  fourth degree - code as Burn, third degree,
    by site
  friction —*see* Burn, by site
  from swallowing caustic or corrosive
    substance NEC —*see* Corrosion,
    by site
  full thickness skin loss - code as Burn, third
    degree, by site
  gastrointestinal tract NEC T28.2
    from swallowing caustic or corrosive
      substance T28.7
  genital organs
    external
      female T21.07
        first degree T21.17
        second degree T21.27
        third degree T21.37
      male T21.06
        first degree T21.16
        second degree T21.26
        third degree T21.36
    internal T28.3
      from caustic or corrosive substance
        T28.8
  groin —*see* Burn, abdominal wall
  hand (s) T23.009
    back —*see* Burn, dorsum of hand
    finger —*see* Burn, finger
    first degree T23.109
    left T23.002
      first degree T23.102
      second degree T23.202
      third degree T23.302
    multiple sites with wrist T23.099
      first degree T23.199
      left T23.092
        first degree T23.192
        second degree T23.292
        third degree T23.392
      right T23.091
        first degree T23.191
        second degree T23.291
        third degree T23.391
      second degree T23.299
      third degree T23.399
    palm —*see* Burn, palm
    right T23.001
      first degree T23.101
      second degree T23.201
      third degree T23.301

Burn *(Continued)*
  hand *(Continued)*
    second degree T23.209
    third degree T23.309
    thumb —*see* Burn, thumb
  head (and face) (and neck) T20.00
    cheek —*see* Burn, cheek
    chin —*see* Burn, chin
    ear —*see* Burn, ear
    eye (s) only —*see* Burn, eye
    first degree T20.10
    forehead —*see* Burn, forehead
    lip —*see* Burn, lip
    multiple sites T20.09
      first degree T20.19
      second degree T20.29
      third degree T20.39
    neck —*see* Burn, neck
    nose —*see* Burn, nose
    scalp —*see* Burn, scalp
    second degree T20.20
    third degree T20.30
  hip (s) —*see* Burn, thigh ◄▦
  inhalation —*see* Burn, respiratory tract
    caustic or corrosive substance (fumes) —*see* Corrosion, respiratory tract
  internal organ (s) T28.40
    alimentary tract T28.2
      esophagus T28.1
    eardrum T28.41
    esophagus T28.1
    from caustic or corrosive substance (swallowing) NEC —*see* Corrosion, by site
    genitourinary T28.3
    mouth T28.0
    pharynx T28.0
    respiratory tract —*see* Burn, respiratory tract
    specified organ NEC T28.49
  interscapular region —*see* Burn, back, upper
  intestine (large) (small) T28.2
  knee T24.029
    first degree T24.129
    left T24.022
      first degree T24.122
      second degree T24.222
      third degree T24.322
    right T24.021
      first degree T24.121
      second degree T24.221
      third degree T24.321
    second degree T24.229
    third degree T24.329
  labium (majus) (minus) —*see* Burn, genital organs, external, female
  lacrimal apparatus, duct, gland or sac —*see* Burn, eye, specified site NEC
  larynx T27.0
    with lung T27.1
  leg (s) (lower) (upper) —*see* Burn, lower, limb
  lightning —*see* Burn, by site
  limb (s)
    lower (except ankle or foot alone) —*see* Burn, lower, limb
    upper —*see* Burn, upper limb
  lip (s) T20.02
    first degree T20.12
    second degree T20.22
    third degree T20.32
  lower
    back —*see* Burn, back
    limb T24.009
      ankle —*see* Burn, ankle
      calf —*see* Burn, calf
      first degree T24.109
      foot —*see* Burn, foot
      hip —*see* Burn, thigh
      knee —*see* Burn, knee

Burn *(Continued)*
  lower *(Continued)*
    limb *(Continued)*
      left T24.002
        first degree T24.102
        second degree T24.202
        third degree T24.302
      multiple sites, except ankle and foot T24.099
        ankle and foot T25.099
          first degree T25.199
          left T25.092
            first degree T25.192
            second degree T25.292
            third degree T25.392
          right T25.091
            first degree T25.191
            second degree T25.291
            third degree T25.391
          second degree T25.299
          third degree T25.399
        first degree T24.199
        left T24.092
          first degree T24.192
          second degree T24.292
          third degree T24.392
        right T24.091
          first degree T24.191
          second degree T24.291
          third degree T24.391
        second degree T24.299
        third degree T24.399
      right T24.001
        first degree T24.101
        second degree T24.201
        third degree T24.301
      second degree T24.209
      thigh —*see* Burn, thigh
      third degree T24.309
      toe —*see* Burn, toe
  lung (with larynx and trachea) T27.1
  mouth T28.0
  neck T20.07
    first degree T20.17
    second degree T20.27
    third degree T20.37
  nose (septum) T20.04
    first degree T20.14
    second degree T20.24
    third degree T20.34
  ocular adnexa —*see* Burn, eye
  orbit region —*see* Burn, eyelid
  palm T23.059
    first degree T23.159
    left T23.052
      first degree T23.152
      second degree T23.252
      third degree T23.352
    right T23.051
      first degree T23.151
      second degree T23.251
      third degree T23.351
    second degree T23.259
    third degree T23.359
  partial thickness - code as Burn, unspecified degree, by site
  pelvis —*see* Burn, trunk
  penis —*see* Burn, genital organs, external, male
  perineum
    female —*see* Burn, genital organs, external, female
    male —*see* Burn, genital organs, external, male
  periocular area —*see* Burn, eyelid
  pharynx T28.0
  rectum T28.2
  respiratory tract T27.3
    larynx —*see* Burn, larynx
    specified part NEC T27.2
    trachea —*see* Burn, trachea

Burn *(Continued)*
  sac, lacrimal —*see* Burn, eye, specified site NEC
  scalp T20.05
    first degree T20.15
    second degree T20.25
    third degree T20.35
  scapular region T22.069
    first degree T22.169
    left T22.062
      first degree T22.162
      second degree T22.262
      third degree T22.362
    right T22.061
      first degree T22.161
      second degree T22.261
      third degree T22.361
    second degree T22.269
    third degree T22.369
  sclera —*see* Burn, eye, specified site NEC
  scrotum —*see* Burn, genital organs, external, male
  shoulder T22.059
    first degree T22.159
    left T22.052
      first degree T22.152
      second degree T22.252
      third degree T22.352
    right T22.051
      first degree T22.151
      second degree T22.251
      third degree T22.351
    second degree T22.259
    third degree T22.359
  stomach T28.2
  temple —*see* Burn, head
  testis —*see* Burn, genital organs, external, male
  thigh T24.019
    first degree T24.119
    left T24.012
      first degree T24.112
      second degree T24.212
      third degree T24.312
    right T24.011
      first degree T24.111
      second degree T24.211
      third degree T24.311
    second degree T24.219
    third degree T24.319
  thorax (external) —*see* Burn, trunk
  throat (meaning pharynx) T28.0
  thumb (s) T23.019
    first degree T23.119
    left T23.012
      first degree T23.112
      second degree T23.212
      third degree T23.312
    multiple sites with fingers T23.049
      first degree T23.149
      left T23.042
        first degree T23.142
        second degree T23.242
        third degree T23.342
      right T23.041
        first degree T23.141
        second degree T23.241
        third degree T23.341
      second degree T23.249
      third degree T23.349
    right T23.011
      first degree T23.111
      second degree T23.211
      third degree T23.311
    second degree T23.219
    third degree T23.319
  toe T25.039
    first degree T25.139
    left T25.032
      first degree T25.132
      second degree T25.232
      third degree T25.332

◄ New   ◄▦ Revised   ~~deleted~~ Deleted

Burn *(Continued)*
  toe *(Continued)*
    right T25.031
      first degree T25.131
      second degree T25.231
      third degree T25.331
    second degree T25.239
    third degree T25.339
  tongue T28.0
  tonsil (s) T28.0
  trachea T27.0
    with lung T27.1
  trunk T21.00
    abdominal wall —*see* Burn, abdominal wall
    anus —*see* Burn, buttock
    axilla —*see* Burn, upper limb
    back —*see* Burn, back
    breast —*see* Burn, chest wall
    buttock —*see* Burn, buttock
    chest wall —*see* Burn, chest wall
    first degree T21.10
    flank —*see* Burn, abdominal wall
    genital
      female —*see* Burn, genital organs, external, female
      male —*see* Burn, genital organs, external, male
    groin —*see* Burn, abdominal wall
    interscapular region —*see* Burn, back, upper
    labia —*see* Burn, genital organs, external, female
    lower back —*see* Burn, back
    penis —*see* Burn, genital organs, external, male
    perineum
      female —*see* Burn, genital organs, external, female
      male —*see* Burn, genital organs, external, male
    scapula region —*see* Burn, scapular region
    scrotum —*see* Burn, genital organs, external, male
    second degree T21.20
    specified site NEC T21.09
      first degree T21.19
      second degree T21.29
      third degree T21.39
    testes —*see* Burn, genital organs, external, male
    third degree T21.30
    upper back —*see* Burn, back, upper
    vulva —*see* Burn, genital organs, external, female
  unspecified site with extent of body surface involved specified
    less than 10 percent T31.0
    10-19 percent (0-9 percent third degree) T31.10
      with 10-19 percent third degree T31.11
    20-29 percent (0-9 percent third degree) T31.20
      with
        10-19 percent third degree T31.21
        20-29 percent third degree T31.22
    30-39 percent (0-9 percent third degree) T31.30
      with
        10-19 percent third degree T31.31
        20-29 percent third degree T31.32
        30-39 percent third degree T31.33
    40-49 percent (0-9 percent third degree) T31.40
      with
        10-19 percent third degree T31.41
        20-29 percent third degree T31.42
        30-39 percent third degree T31.43
        40-49 percent third degree T31.44

Burn *(Continued)*
  unspecified site with extent of body surface involved specified *(Continued)*
    50-59 percent (0-9 percent third degree) T31.50
      with
        10-19 percent third degree T31.51
        20-29 percent third degree T31.52
        30-39 percent third degree T31.53
        40-49 percent third degree T31.54
        50-59 percent third degree T31.55
    60-69 percent (0-9 percent third degree) T31.60
      with
        10-19 percent third degree T31.61
        20-29 percent third degree T31.62
        30-39 percent third degree T31.63
        40-49 percent third degree T31.64
        50-59 percent third degree T31.65
        60-69 percent third degree T31.66
    70-79 percent (0-9 percent third degree) T31.70
      with
        10-19 percent third degree T31.71
        20-29 percent third degree T31.72
        30-39 percent third degree T31.73
        40-49 percent third degree T31.74
        50-59 percent third degree T31.75
        60-69 percent third degree T31.76
        70-79 percent third degree T31.77
    80-89 percent (0-9 percent third degree) T31.80
      with
        10-19 percent third degree T31.81
        20-29 percent third degree T31.82
        30-39 percent third degree T31.83
        40-49 percent third degree T31.84
        50-59 percent third degree T31.85
        60-69 percent third degree T31.86
        70-79 percent third degree T31.87
        80-89 percent third degree T31.88
    90 percent or more (0-9 percent third degree) T31.90
      with
        10-19 percent third degree T31.91
        20-29 percent third degree T31.92
        30-39 percent third degree T31.93
        40-49 percent third degree T31.94
        50-59 percent third degree T31.95
        60-69 percent third degree T31.96
        70-79 percent third degree T31.97
        80-89 percent third degree T31.98
        90-99 percent third degree T31.99
  upper limb T22.00
    above elbow —*see* Burn, above elbow
    axilla —*see* Burn, axilla
    elbow —*see* Burn, elbow
    first degree T22.10
    forearm —*see* Burn, forearm
    hand —*see* Burn, hand
    interscapular region —*see* Burn, back, upper
    multiple sites T22.099
      first degree T22.199
      left T22.092
        first degree T22.192
        second degree T22.292
        third degree T22.392
      right T22.091
        first degree T22.191
        second degree T22.291
        third degree T22.391
      second degree T22.299
      third degree T22.399
    scapular region —*see* Burn, scapular region
    second degree T22.20
    shoulder —*see* Burn, shoulder
    third degree T22.30
    wrist —*see* Burn, wrist
  uterus T28.3
  vagina T28.3

Burn *(Continued)*
  vulva —*see* Burn, genital organs, external, female
  wrist T23.079
    first degree T23.179
    left T23.072
      first degree T23.172
      second degree T23.272
      third degree T23.372
    multiple sites with hand T23.099
      first degree T23.199
      left T23.092
        first degree T23.192
        second degree T23.292
        third degree T23.392
      right T23.091
        first degree T23.191
        second degree T23.291
        third degree T23.391
      second degree T23.299
      third degree T23.399
    right T23.071
      first degree T23.171
      second degree T23.271
      third degree T23.371
    second degree T23.279
    third degree T23.379
Burnett's syndrome E83.52
Burning
  feet syndrome E53.9
  sensation R20.8
  tongue K14.6
Burn-out (state) Z73.0
Burns' disease or osteochondrosis —*see* Osteochondrosis, juvenile, ulna
Bursa —*see* condition
Bursitis M71.9
  Achilles —*see* Tendinitis, Achilles
  adhesive —*see* Bursitis, specified NEC
  ankle —*see* Enthesopathy, lower limb, ankle, specified type NEC
  calcaneal —*see* Enthesopathy, foot, specified type NEC
  collateral ligament, tibial —*see* Bursitis, tibial collateral
  due to use, overuse, pressure —*see also* Disorder, soft tissue, due to use, specified type NEC
    specified NEC —*see* Disorder, soft tissue, due to use, specified NEC
  Duplay's M75.0
  elbow NEC M70.3-
    olecranon M70.2-
  finger —*see* Disorder, soft tissue, due to use, specified type NEC, hand
  foot —*see* Enthesopathy, foot, specified type NEC
  gonococcal A54.49
  gouty —*see* Gout ◄||||
  hand M70.1-
  hip NEC M70.7-
    trochanteric M70.6-
  infective NEC M71.10
    abscess —*see* Abscess, bursa
    ankle M71.17-
    elbow M71.12-
    foot M71.17-
    hand M71.14-
    hip M71.15-
    knee M71.16-
    multiple sites M71.19
    shoulder M71.11-
    specified site NEC M71.18
    wrist M71.13-
  ischial —*see* Bursitis, hip
  knee NEC M70.5-
    prepatellar M70.4-
  occupational NEC —*see also* Disorder, soft tissue, due to use
  olecranon —*see* Bursitis, elbow, olecranon
  pharyngeal J39.1

Bursitis *(Continued)*
  popliteal —*see* Bursitis, knee
  prepatellar M70.4-
  radiohumeral M77.8
  rheumatoid M06.20
    ankle M06.27-
    elbow M06.22-
    foot joint M06.27-
    hand joint M06.24-
    hip M06.25-
    knee M06.26-
    multiple site M06.29
    shoulder M06.21-
    vertebra M06.28
    wrist M06.23-
  scapulohumeral —*see* Bursitis, shoulder
  semimembranous muscle (knee) —*see*
    Bursitis, knee
  shoulder M75.5-
    adhesive —*see* Capsulitis, adhesive
  specified NEC M71.50
    ankle M71.57-
    due to use, overuse or pressure —*see*
      Disorder, soft tissue, due to, use
    elbow M71.52-
    foot M71.57-
    hand M71.54-

Bursitis *(Continued)*
  specified NEC *(Continued)*
    hip M71.55-
    knee M71.56-
    shoulder —*see* Bursitis, shoulder
    specified site NEC M71.58
    tibial collateral M76.4-
    wrist M71.53-
  subacromial —*see* Bursitis, shoulder
  subcoracoid —*see* Bursitis, shoulder
  subdeltoid —*see* Bursitis, shoulder
  syphilitic A52.78
  Thornwaldt, Tornwaldt J39.2
  tibial collateral M76.4- ◄▥
  toe —*see* Enthesopathy, foot, specified type
    NEC
  trochanteric (area) —*see* Bursitis, hip,
    trochanteric
  wrist —*see* Bursitis, hand
Bursopathy M71.9
  specified type NEC M71.80
    ankle M71.87-
    elbow M71.82-
    foot M71.87-
    hand M71.84-
    hip M71.85-
    knee M71.86-

Bursopathy *(Continued)*
  specified type NEC *(Continued)*
    multiple sites M71.89
    shoulder M71.81-
    specified site NEC M71.88
    wrist M71.83-
Burst stitches or sutures (complication of
  surgery) T81.31
  external operation wound T81.31
  internal operation wound T81.32
Buruli ulcer A31.1
Bury's disease L95.1
Buschke's
  disease B45.3
  scleredema —*see* Sclerosis, systemic
Busse-Buschke disease B45.3
Buttock —*see* condition
Button
  Biskra B55.1
  Delhi B55.1
  oriental B55.1
Buttonhole deformity (finger) —*see* Deformity,
  finger, boutonniere
Bwamba fever A92.8
Byssinosis J66.0
Bywaters' syndrome T79.5

C

Cachexia R64
 cancerous R64
 cardiac —see Disease, heart
 dehydration E86.0
  ~~with~~
   ~~hypernatremia E87.0~~
   ~~hyponatremia E87.1~~
 due to malnutrition R64
 exophthalmic —see Hyperthyroidism
 heart —see Disease, heart
 hypophyseal E23.0
 hypopituitary E23.0
 lead —see Poisoning, lead
 malignant R64
 marsh —see Malaria
 nervous F48.8
 old age R54
 paludal —see Malaria
 pituitary E23.0
 renal N28.9
 saturnine —see Poisoning, lead
 senile R54
 Simmonds' E23.0
 splenica D73.0
 strumipriva E03.4
 tuberculous NEC —see Tuberculosis
Café au lait spots L81.3
Caffeine-induced ◀
 anxiety disorder F15.980 ◀
 sleep disorder F15.982 ◀
Caffey's syndrome Q78.8
Caisson disease T70.3
Cake kidney Q63.1
Caked breast (puerperal, postpartum) O92.79
Calabar swelling B74.3
Calcaneal spur —see Spur, bone, calcaneal
Calcaneo-apophysitis M92.8
Calcareous —see condition
Calcicosis J62.8
Calciferol (vitamin D) deficiency E55.9
 with rickets E55.0
Calcification
 adrenal (capsule) (gland) E27.49
  tuberculous E35 [B90.8]
 aorta I70.0
 artery (annular) —see Arteriosclerosis
 auricle (ear) —see Disorder, pinna, specified
   type NEC
 basal ganglia G23.8
 bladder N32.89
  due to Schistosoma hematobium
    B65.0
 brain (cortex) —see Calcification, cerebral
 bronchus J98.09
 bursa M71.40
  ankle M71.47-
  elbow M71.42-
  foot M71.47-
  hand M71.44-
  hip M71.45-
  knee M71.46-
  multiple sites M71.49
  shoulder M75.3-
  specified site NEC M71.48
  wrist M71.43-
 cardiac —see Degeneration, myocardial
 cerebral (cortex) G93.89
  artery I67.2
 cervix (uteri) N88.8
 choroid plexus G93.89
 conjunctiva —see Concretion, conjunctiva
 corpora cavernosa (penis) N48.89
 cortex (brain) —see Calcification, cerebral
 dental pulp (nodular) K04.2
 dentinal papilla K00.4
 fallopian tube N83.8
 falx cerebri G96.19
 gallbladder K82.8
 general E83.59

Calcification (Continued)
 heart —see also Degeneration, myocardial
  valve —see Endocarditis
 idiopathic infantile arterial (IIAC) Q28.8
 intervertebral cartilage or disc
    (postinfective) —see Disorder, disc,
    specified NEC
 intracranial —see Calcification, cerebral
 joint —see Disorder, joint, specified type NEC
 kidney N28.89
  tuberculous N29 [B90.1]
 larynx (senile) J38.7
 lens —see Cataract, specified NEC
 lung (active) (postinfectional) J98.4
  tuberculous B90.9
 lymph gland or node (postinfectional) I89.8
  tuberculous —see also Tuberculosis, lymph
    gland B90.8
 mammographic R92.1
 massive (paraplegic) —see Myositis,
    ossificans, in, quadriplegia
 medial —see Arteriosclerosis, extremities
 meninges (cerebral) (spinal) G96.19
 metastatic E83.59
 Mönckeberg's —see Arteriosclerosis,
    extremities
 muscle M61.9
  due to burns —see Myositis, ossificans, in,
    burns
  paralytic —see Myositis, ossificans, in,
    quadriplegia
  specified type NEC M61.40
   ankle M61.47-
   foot M61.47-
   forearm M61.43-
   hand M61.44-
   lower leg M61.46-
   multiple sites M61.49
   pelvic region M61.45-
   shoulder region M61.41-
   specified site NEC M61.48
   thigh M61.45-
   upper arm M61.42-
 myocardium, myocardial —see Degeneration,
    myocardial
 ovary N83.8
 pancreas K86.89 ◀▥
 penis N48.89
 periarticular —see Disorder, joint, specified
    type NEC
 pericardium —see also Pericarditis I31.1
 pineal gland E34.8
 pleura J94.8
  postinfectional J94.8
  tuberculous NEC B90.9
 pulpal (dental) (nodular) K04.2
 sclera H15.89
 spleen D73.89
 subcutaneous L94.2
 suprarenal (capsule) (gland) E27.49
 tendon (sheath) —see also Tenosynovitis,
    specified type NEC
  with bursitis, synovitis or tenosynovitis —
    see Tendinitis, calcific
 trachea J39.8
 ureter N28.89
 vitreous —see Deposit, crystalline
Calcified —see Calcification
Calcinosis (interstitial) (tumoral) (universalis)
    E83.59
 with Raynaud's phenomenon, esophageal
    dysfunction, sclerodactyly,
    telangiectasia (CREST syndrome) M34.1
 circumscripta (skin) L94.2
 cutis L94.2
Calciphylaxis —see also Calcification, by site
    E83.59
Calcium
 deposits —see Calcification, by site
 metabolism disorder E83.50
 salts or soaps in vitreous —see Deposit,
    crystalline

Calciuria R82.99
Calculi —see Calculus
Calculosis, intrahepatic —see Calculus, bile
    duct
Calculus, calculi, calculous
 ampulla of Vater —see Calculus, bile duct
 anuria (impacted) (recurrent) —see also
    Calculus, urinary N20.9
 appendix K38.1
 bile duct (common) (hepatic) K80.50
  with
   calculus of gallbladder —see Calculus,
     gallbladder and bile duct
   cholangitis K80.30
    with
     cholecystitis —see Calculus, bile
       duct, with cholecystitis
     obstruction K80.31
    acute K80.32
     with
      chronic cholangitis K80.36
       with obstruction K80.37
      obstruction K80.33
    chronic K80.34
     with
      acute cholangitis K80.36
       with obstruction K80.37
      obstruction K80.35
   cholecystitis (with cholangitis) K80.40
    with obstruction K80.41
    acute K80.42
     with
      chronic cholecystitis K80.46
       with obstruction K80.47
      obstruction K80.43
    chronic K80.44
     with
      acute cholecystitis K80.46
       with obstruction K80.47
      obstruction K80.45
   obstruction K80.51
  biliary —see also Calculus, gallbladder
   specified NEC K80.80
    with obstruction K80.81
  bilirubin, multiple —see Calculus,
    gallbladder
  bladder (encysted) (impacted) (urinary)
    (diverticulum) N21.0
  bronchus J98.09
  calyx (kidney) (renal) —see Calculus, kidney
  cholesterol (pure) (solitary) —see Calculus,
    gallbladder
  common duct (bile) —see Calculus, bile duct
  conjunctiva —see Concretion, conjunctiva
  cystic N21.0
   duct —see Calculus, gallbladder
  dental (subgingival) (supragingival)
    K03.6
  diverticulum
   bladder N21.0
   kidney N20.0
  epididymis N50.89 ◀▥
  gallbladder K80.20
   with
    bile duct calculus —see Calculus,
      gallbladder and bile duct
    cholecystitis K80.10
     with obstruction K80.11
     acute K80.00
      with
       chronic cholecystitis K80.12
        with obstruction K80.13
       obstruction K80.01
     chronic K80.10
      with
       acute cholecystitis K80.12
        with obstruction K80.13
       obstruction K80.11
    specified NEC K80.18
     with obstruction K80.19
    obstruction K80.21

Calculus, calculi, calculous *(Continued)*
 gallbladder and bile duct K80.70
  with
    cholecystitis K80.60
     with obstruction K80.61
     acute K80.62
      with
       chronic cholecystitis K80.66
        with obstruction K80.67
        obstruction K80.63
      chronic K80.64
       with
        acute cholecystitis K80.66
         with obstruction K80.67
         obstruction K80.65
     obstruction K80.71
  hepatic (duct) —*see* Calculus, bile duct
  hepatobiliary K80.80
   with obstruction K80.81
  ileal conduit N21.8
  intestinal (impaction) (obstruction) K56.49
  kidney (impacted) (multiple) (pelvis)
     (recurrent) (staghorn) N20.0
   with calculus, ureter N20.2
   congenital Q63.8
  lacrimal passages —*see* Dacryolith
  liver (impacted) —*see* Calculus, bile duct
  lung J98.4
  mammographic R92.1
  nephritic (impacted) (recurrent) —*see*
     Calculus, kidney
  nose J34.89
  pancreas (duct) K86.89 ◀▥
  parotid duct or gland K11.5
  pelvis, encysted —*see* Calculus, kidney
  prostate N42.0
  pulmonary J98.4
  pyelitis (impacted) (recurrent) N20.0
   with hydronephrosis N13.2
  pyelonephritis (impacted) (recurrent) —*see*
     category N20
   with hydronephrosis N13.2
  renal (impacted) (recurrent) —*see* Calculus,
     kidney
  salivary (duct) (gland) K11.5
  seminal vesicle N50.89 ◀▥
  staghorn —*see* Calculus, kidney
  Stensen's duct K11.5
  stomach K31.89
  sublingual duct or gland K11.5
   congenital Q38.4
  submandibular duct, gland or region K11.5
  submaxillary duct, gland or region K11.5
  suburethral N21.8
  tonsil J35.8
  tooth, teeth (subgingival) (supragingival)
     K03.6
  tunica vaginalis N50.89 ◀▥
  ureter (impacted) (recurrent) N20.1
   with calculus, kidney N20.2
    with hydronephrosis N13.2
     with infection N13.6
  urethra (impacted) N21.1
  urinary (duct) (impacted) (passage) (tract)
     N20.9
   with hydronephrosis N13.2
    with infection N13.6
   in (due to)
   lower N21.9
    specified NEC N21.8
  vagina N89.8
  vesical (impacted) N21.0
  Wharton's duct K11.5
  xanthine E79.8 *[N22]*
Calicectasis N28.89
Caliectasis N28.89
California
 disease B38.9
 encephalitis A83.5
Caligo cornea —*see* Opacity, cornea, central
Callositas, callosity (infected) L84

Callus (infected) L84
 bone —*see* Osteophyte
   excessive, following fracture - code as
     Sequelae of fracture
CALME (childhood asymmetric labium majus
   enlargement) N90.61 ◀
Calorie deficiency or malnutrition —*see also*
   Malnutrition E46
Calvé-Perthes disease —*see* Legg-Calve-Perthes
   disease
Calvé's disease —*see* Osteochondrosis, juvenile,
   spine
Calvities —*see* Alopecia, androgenic
Cameroon fever —*see* Malaria
Camptocormia (hysterical) F44.4
Camurati-Engelmann syndrome Q78.3
Canal —*see also* condition
 atrioventricular common Q21.2
Canaliculitis (lacrimal) (acute) (subacute) H04.33-
 Actinomyces A42.89
 chronic H04.42-
Canavan's disease E75.29
Canceled procedure (surgical) Z53.9
 because of
   contraindication Z53.09
     smoking Z53.01
   left against medical advice (AMA) Z53.21
   patient's decision Z53.20
     for reasons of belief or group pressure
       Z53.1
     specified reason NEC Z53.29
   specified reason NEC Z53.8
Cancer —*see also* Neoplasm, by site, malignant
 bile duct type, liver C22.1
 blood —*see* Leukemia
 breast —*see also* Neoplasm, breast, malignant
   C50.91-
 hepatocellular C22.0
 lung —*see also* Neoplasm, lung, malignant
   C34.90-
 ovarian —*see also* Neoplasm, ovary,
   malignant C56.9-
 unspecified site (primary) C80.1
Cancer (o)phobia F45.29
Cancerous —*see* Neoplasm, malignant, by site
Cancrum oris A69.0
Candidiasis, candidal B37.9
 balanitis B37.42
 bronchitis B37.1
 cheilitis B37.83
 congenital P37.5
 cystitis B37.41
 disseminated B37.7
 endocarditis B37.6
 enteritis B37.82
 esophagitis B37.81
 intertrigo B37.2
 lung B37.1
 meningitis B37.5
 mouth B37.0
 nails B37.2
 neonatal P37.5
 onychia B37.2
 oral B37.0
 osteomyelitis B37.89
 otitis externa B37.84
 paronychia B37.2
 perionyxis B37.2
 pneumonia B37.1
 proctitis B37.82
 pulmonary B37.1
 pyelonephritis B37.49
 sepsis B37.7
 skin B37.2
 specified site NEC B37.89
 stomatitis B37.0
 systemic B37.7
 urethritis B37.41
 urogenital site NEC B37.49
 vagina B37.3
 vulva B37.3
 vulvovaginitis B37.3

Candidid L30.2
Candidosis —*see* Candidiasis
Candiru infection or infestation B88.8
Canities (premature) L67.1
 congenital Q84.2
Canker (mouth) (sore) K12.0
 rash A38.9
Cannabinosis J66.2
Cannabis induced ◀
 anxiety disorder F12.980 ◀
 psychotic disorder F12.959 ◀
 sleep disorder F12.988 ◀
Canton fever A75.9
Cantrell's syndrome Q87.89
Capillariasis (intestinal) B81.1
 hepatic B83.8
Capillary —*see* condition
Caplan's syndrome —*see* Rheumatoid, lung
Capsule —*see* condition
Capsulitis (joint) —*see also* Enthesopathy
 adhesive (shoulder) M75.0-
 hepatic K65.8
 labyrinthine —*see* Otosclerosis, specified NEC
 thyroid E06.9
Caput
 crepitus Q75.8
 medusae I86.8
 succedaneum P12.81
Car sickness T75.3
Carapata (disease) A68.0
Carate —*see* Pinta
Carbon lung J60
Carbuncle L02.93
 abdominal wall L02.231
 anus K61.0
 auditory canal, external —*see* Abscess, ear,
   external
 auricle ear —*see* Abscess, ear, external
 axilla L02.43-
 back (any part) L02.232
 breast N61.1 ◀▥
 buttock L02.33
 cheek (external) L02.03
 chest wall L02.233
 chin L02.03
 corpus cavernosum N48.21
 ear (any part) (external) (middle) —*see*
   Abscess, ear, external
 external auditory canal —*see* Abscess, ear,
   external
 eyelid —*see* Abscess, eyelid
 face NEC L02.03
 femoral (region) —*see* Carbuncle, lower limb
 finger —*see* Carbuncle, hand
 flank L02.231
 foot L02.63-
 forehead L02.03
 genital —*see* Abscess, genital
 gluteal (region) L02.33
 groin L02.234
 hand L02.53-
 head NEC L02.831
 heel —*see* Carbuncle, foot
 hip —*see* Carbuncle, lower limb
 kidney —*see* Abscess, kidney
 knee —*see* Carbuncle, lower limb
 labium (majus) (minus) N76.4
 lacrimal
   gland —*see* Dacryoadenitis
   passages (duct) (sac) —*see* Inflammation,
     lacrimal, passages, acute
 leg —*see* Carbuncle, lower limb
 lower limb L02.43-
 malignant A22.0
 navel L02.236
 neck L02.13
 nose (external) (septum) J34.0
 orbit, orbital —*see* Abscess, orbit
 palmar (space) —*see* Carbuncle, hand
 partes posteriores L02.33
 pectoral region L02.233
 penis N48.21

◀ New   ◀▥ Revised   ~~deleted~~ Deleted

Carbuncle *(Continued)*
    perineum L02.235
    pinna —*see* Abscess, ear, external
    popliteal —*see* Carbuncle, lower limb
    scalp L02.831
    seminal vesicle N49.0
    shoulder —*see* Carbuncle, upper limb
    specified site NEC L02.838
    temple (region) L02.03
    thumb —*see* Carbuncle, hand
    toe —*see* Carbuncle, foot
    trunk L02.239
        abdominal wall L02.231
        back L02.232
        chest wall L02.233
        groin L02.234
        perineum L02.235
        umbilicus L02.236
    umbilicus L02.236
    upper limb L02.43-
    urethra N34.0
    vulva N76.4
Carbunculus —*see* Carbuncle
Carcinoid (tumor) —*see* Tumor, carcinoid
Carcinoidosis E34.0
Carcinoma (malignant) —*see also* Neoplasm, by
        site, malignant
    acidophil
        specified site —*see* Neoplasm, malignant,
            by site
        unspecified site C75.1
    acidophil-basophil, mixed
        specified site —*see* Neoplasm, malignant,
            by site
        unspecified site C75.1
    adnexal (skin) —*see* Neoplasm, skin,
        malignant
    adrenal cortical C74.0-
    alveolar —*see* Neoplasm, lung, malignant
        cell —*see* Neoplasm, lung, malignant
    ameloblastic C41.1
        upper jaw (bone) C41.0
    apocrine
        breast —*see* Neoplasm, breast, malignant
        specified site NEC —*see* Neoplasm, skin,
            malignant
        unspecified site C44.99
    basal cell (pigmented) (*see also* Neoplasm,
        skin, malignant) C44.91
        fibro-epithelial —*see* Neoplasm, skin,
            malignant
        morphea —*see* Neoplasm, skin, malignant
        multicentric —*see* Neoplasm, skin, malignant
    basaloid
    basal-squamous cell, mixed —*see* Neoplasm,
        skin, malignant
    basophil
        specified site —*see* Neoplasm, malignant,
            by site
        unspecified site C75.1
    basophil-acidophil, mixed
        specified site —*see* Neoplasm, malignant,
            by site
        unspecified site C75.1
    basosquamous —*see* Neoplasm, skin, malignant
    bile duct
        with hepatocellular, mixed C22.0
        liver C22.1
        specified site NEC —*see* Neoplasm,
            malignant, by site
        unspecified site C22.1
    branchial or branchiogenic C10.4
    bronchial or bronchogenic —*see* Neoplasm,
        lung, malignant
    bronchiolar —*see* Neoplasm, lung, malignant
    bronchioloalveolar —*see* Neoplasm, lung,
        malignant
    C cell
        specified site —*see* Neoplasm, malignant,
            by site
        unspecified site C73
    ceruminous C44.29-

Carcinoma *(Continued)*
    cervix uteri
        in situ D06.9
            endocervix D06.0
            exocervix D06.1
            specified site NEC D06.7
    chorionic
        specified site —*see* Neoplasm, malignant,
            by site
        unspecified site
            female C58
            male C62.90
    chromophobe
        specified site —*see* Neoplasm, malignant,
            by site
        unspecified site C75.1
    cloacogenic
        specified site —*see* Neoplasm, malignant,
            by site
        unspecified site C21.2
    diffuse type
        specified site —*see* Neoplasm, malignant,
            by site
        unspecified site C16.9
    duct (cell)
        with Paget's disease —*see* Neoplasm,
            breast, malignant
        infiltrating
            with lobular carcinoma (in situ)
                specified site —*see* Neoplasm,
                    malignant, by site
                unspecified site (female) C50.91-
                    male C50.92-
            specified site —*see* Neoplasm,
                malignant, by site
            unspecified site (female) C50.91-
                male C50.92-
    ductal
        with lobular
            specified site —*see* Neoplasm,
                malignant, by site
            unspecified site (female) C50.91-
                male C50.92-
    ductular, infiltrating
        specified site —*see* Neoplasm, malignant,
            by site
        unspecified site (female) C50.91-
            male C50.92-
    embryonal
        liver C22.7
    endometrioid
        specified site —*see* Neoplasm, malignant,
            by site
        unspecified site
            female C56.9
            male C61
    eosinophil
        specified site —*see* Neoplasm, malignant,
            by site
        unspecified site C75.1
    epidermoid —*see also* Neoplasm, skin
        malignant
        in situ, Bowen's type —*see* Neoplasm, skin,
            in situ
    fibroepithelial, basal cell —*see* Neoplasm,
        skin, malignant
    follicular
        with papillary (mixed) C73
        moderately differentiated C73
        pure follicle C73
        specified site —*see* Neoplasm, malignant,
            by site
        trabecular C73
        unspecified site C73
        well differentiated C73
    generalized, with unspecified primary site
        C80.0
    glycogen-rich —*see* Neoplasm, breast,
        malignant
    granulosa cell C56-
    hepatic cell C22.0

Carcinoma *(Continued)*
    hepatocellular C22.0
        with bile duct, mixed C22.0
        fibrolamellar C22.0
    hepatocholangiolitic C22.0
    Hurthle cell C73
    in
        adenomatous
            polyposis coli C18.9
        pleomorphic adenoma —*see* Neoplasm,
            salivary glands, malignant
        situ —*see* Carcinoma-in-situ
    infiltrating
        duct
            with lobular
                specified site —*see* Neoplasm,
                    malignant, by site
                unspecified site (female) C50.91-
                    male C50.92
            with Paget's disease —*see* Neoplasm,
                breast, malignant
            specified site —*see* Neoplasm,
                malignant
            unspecified site (female) C50.91-
                male C50.92-
        ductular
            specified site —*see* Neoplasm,
                malignant
            unspecified site (female) C50.91-
                male C50.92-
        lobular
            specified site —*see* Neoplasm,
                malignant
            unspecified site (female) C50.91-
                male C50.92-
    inflammatory
        specified site —*see* Neoplasm, malignant
        unspecified site (female) C50.91-
            male C50.92-
    intestinal type
        specified site —*see* Neoplasm, malignant,
            by site
        unspecified site C16.9
    intracystic
        noninfiltrating —*see* Neoplasm, in situ,
            by site
    intraductal (noninfiltrating)
        with Paget's disease —*see* Neoplasm,
            breast, malignant
        breast D05.1-
        papillary
            with invasion
                specified site —*see* Neoplasm,
                    malignant, by site
                unspecified site (female) C50.91-
                    male C50.92-
            breast D05.1-
            specified site NEC —*see* Neoplasm,
                in situ, by site
            unspecified site (female) D05.1-
        specified site NEC —*see* Neoplasm,
            in situ, by site
        unspecified site (female) D05.1-
    intraepidermal —*see* Neoplasm, in situ
        squamous cell, Bowen's type —*see*
            Neoplasm, skin, in situ
    intraepithelial —*see* Neoplasm, in situ,
        by site
        squamous cell —*see* Neoplasm, in situ,
            by site
    intraosseous C41.1
        upper jaw (bone) C41.0
    islet cell
        with exocrine, mixed
            specified site —*see* Neoplasm,
                malignant, by site
            unspecified site C25.9
        pancreas C25.4
        specified site NEC —*see* Neoplasm,
            malignant, by site
        unspecified site C25.4

Carcinoma *(Continued)*
 juvenile, breast —*see* Neoplasm, breast,
  malignant
 large cell
  small cell
   specified site —*see* Neoplasm,
    malignant, by site
   unspecified site C34.90
 Leydig cell (testis)
  specified site —*see* Neoplasm, malignant,
   by site
  unspecified site
   female C56.9
   male C62.90
 lipid-rich (female) C50.91-
  male C50.92-
 liver cell C22.0
 liver NEC C22.7
 lobular (infiltrating)
  with intraductal
   specified site —*see* Neoplasm,
    malignant, by site
   unspecified site (female) C50.91-
    male C50.92-
  noninfiltrating
   breast D05.0-
   specified site NEC —*see* Neoplasm, in
    situ, by site
   unspecified site D05.0-
  specified site —*see* Neoplasm, malignant,
   by site
  unspecified site (female) C50.91-
   male C50.92-
 medullary
  with
   amyloid stroma
    specified site —*see* Neoplasm,
     malignant, by site
    unspecified site C73
   lymphoid stroma
    specified site —*see* Neoplasm,
     malignant, by site
    unspecified site (female) C50.91-
     male C50.92-
 Merkel cell C4A.9
  anal margin C4A.51
  anal skin C4A.51
  canthus C4A.1-
  ear and external auricular canal C4A.2-
  external auricular canal C4A.2-
  eyelid, including canthus C4A.1-
  face C4A.30
   specified NEC C4A.39
  hip C4A.7-
  lip C4A.0
  lower limb, including hip C4A.7-
  neck C4A.4
  nodal presentation C7B.1
  nose C4A.31
  overlapping sites C4A.8
  perianal skin C4A.51
  scalp C4A.4
  secondary C7B.1
  shoulder C4A.6-
  skin of breast C4A.52
  trunk NEC C4A.59
  upper limb, including shoulder C4A.6-
  visceral metastatic C7B.1
 metastatic —*see* Neoplasm, secondary
 metatypical —*see* Neoplasm, skin, malignant
 morphea, basal cell —*see* Neoplasm, skin,
  malignant
 mucoid
  cell
   specified site —*see* Neoplasm,
    malignant, by site
   unspecified site C75.1
 neuroendocrine —*see also* Tumor,
  neuroendocrine
  high grade, any site C7A.1
  poorly differentiated, any site C7A.1

Carcinoma *(Continued)*
 nonencapsulated sclerosing C73
 noninfiltrating
  intracystic —*see* Neoplasm, in situ, by site
  intraductal
   breast D05.1-
   papillary
    breast D05.1-
    specified site NEC —*see* Neoplasm, in
     situ, by site
    unspecified site D05.1-
   specified site —*see* Neoplasm, in situ,
    by site
   unspecified site D05.1-
  lobular
   breast D05.0-
   specified site NEC —*see* Neoplasm, in
    situ, by site
   unspecified site (female) D05.0-
 oat cell
  specified site —*see* Neoplasm, malignant,
   by site
  unspecified site C34.90
 odontogenic C41.1
  upper jaw (bone) C41.0
 papillary
  with follicular (mixed) C73
  follicular variant C73
  intraductal (noninfiltrating)
   with invasion
    specified site —*see* Neoplasm,
     malignant, by site
    unspecified site (female) C50.91-
     male C50.92-
   breast D05.1-
   specified site NEC —*see* Neoplasm, in
    situ, by site
   unspecified site D05.1-
  serous
   specified site —*see* Neoplasm,
    malignant, by site
   surface
    specified site —*see* Neoplasm,
     malignant, by site
    unspecified site C56.9
   unspecified site C56.9
 papillocystic
  specified site —*see* Neoplasm, malignant,
   by site
  unspecified site C56.9
 parafollicular cell
  specified site —*see* Neoplasm, malignant,
   by site
  unspecified site C73
 pilomatrix —*see* Neoplasm, skin, malignant
 pseudomucinous
  specified site —*see* Neoplasm, malignant,
   by site
  unspecified site C56.9
 renal cell C64-
 Schmincke —*see* Neoplasm, nasopharynx,
  malignant
 Schneiderian
  specified site —*see* Neoplasm, malignant,
   by site
  unspecified site C30.0
 sebaceous —*see* Neoplasm, skin, malignant
 secondary —*see also* Neoplasm, secondary,
  by site
  Merkel cell C7B.1
 secretory, breast —*see* Neoplasm, breast,
  malignant
 serous
  papillary
   specified site —*see* Neoplasm,
    malignant, by site
   unspecified site C56.9
  surface, papillary
   specified site —*see* Neoplasm,
    malignant, by site
   unspecified site C56.9

Carcinoma *(Continued)*
 Sertoli cell
  specified site —*see* Neoplasm, malignant,
   by site
  unspecified site C62.90
   female C56.9
   male C62.90
 skin appendage —*see* Neoplasm, skin,
  malignant
 small cell
  fusiform cell
   specified site —*see* Neoplasm,
    malignant, by site
   unspecified site C34.90
  intermediate cell
   specified site —*see* Neoplasm,
    malignant, by site
   unspecified site C34.90
  large cell
   specified site —*see* Neoplasm,
    malignant, by site
   unspecified site C34.90
 solid
  with amyloid stroma
   specified site —*see* Neoplasm,
    malignant, by site
   unspecified site C73
  microinvasive
   specified site —*see* Neoplasm,
    malignant, by site
   unspecified site C53.9
 sweat gland —*see* Neoplasm, skin,
  malignant
 theca cell C56.-
 thymic C37
 unspecified site (primary) C80.1
 water-clear cell C75.0
Carcinoma-in-situ —*see also* Neoplasm, in situ,
 by site
 breast NOS D05.9-
  specified type NEC D05.8-
 epidermoid —*see also* Neoplasm, in situ, by
  site
  with questionable stromal invasion
   cervix D06.9
   specified site NEC —*see* Neoplasm, in
    situ, by site
   unspecified site D06.9
  Bowen's type —*see* Neoplasm, skin,
   in situ
 intraductal
  breast D05.1-
  specified site NEC —*see* Neoplasm, in situ,
   by site
  unspecified site D05.1-
 lobular
  with
   infiltrating duct
    breast (female) C50.91-
     male C50.92-
    specified site NEC —*see* Neoplasm,
     malignant
    unspecified site (female) C50.91-
     male C50.92-
   intraductal
    breast D05.8-
    specified site NEC —*see* Neoplasm, in
     situ, by site
    unspecified site (female) D05.8-
  breast D05.0-
  specified site NEC —*see* Neoplasm, in situ,
   by site
  unspecified site D05.0-
 squamous cell —*see also* Neoplasm, in situ,
  by site
  with questionable stromal invasion
   cervix D06.9
   specified site NEC —*see* Neoplasm, in
    situ, by site
   unspecified site D06.9
Carcinomaphobia F45.29

◀ New   ◀▦ Revised   ~~deleted~~ Deleted

Carcinomatosis C80.0
　peritonei C78.6
　unspecified site (primary) (secondary) C80.0
Carcinosarcoma —see Neoplasm, malignant, by site
　embryonal —see Neoplasm, malignant, by site
Cardia, cardial —see condition
Cardiac —see also condition
　death, sudden —see Arrest, cardiac
　pacemaker
　　in situ Z95.0
　　management or adjustment Z45.018
　tamponade I31.4
Cardialgia —see Pain, precordial
Cardiectasis —see Hypertrophy, cardiac
Cardiochalasia K21.9
Cardiomalacia I51.5
Cardiomegalia glycogenica diffusa E74.02 [I43]
Cardiomegaly —see also Hypertrophy, cardiac
　congenital Q24.8
　glycogen E74.02 [I43]
　idiopathic I51.7
Cardiomyoliposis I51.5
Cardiomyopathy (familial) (idiopathic) I42.9
　alcoholic I42.6
　amyloid E85.4 [I43]
　arteriosclerotic —see Disease, heart, ischemic, atherosclerotic
　beriberi E51.12
　cobalt-beer I42.6
　congenital I42.4
　congestive I42.0
　constrictive NOS I42.5
　dilated I42.0
　due to
　　alcohol I42.6
　　beriberi E51.12
　　cardiac glycogenosis E74.02 [I43]
　　drugs I42.7
　　external agents NEC I42.7
　　Friedreich's ataxia G11.1
　　myotonia atrophica G71.11 [I43]
　　progressive muscular dystrophy G71.0
　glycogen storage E74.02 [I43]
　hypertensive —see Hypertension, heart
　hypertrophic (nonobstructive) I42.2
　　obstructive I42.1
　　　congenital Q24.8
　in
　　Chagas' disease (chronic) B57.2
　　　acute B57.0
　　sarcoidosis D86.85
　ischemic I25.5
　metabolic E88.9 [I43]
　　thyrotoxic E05.90 [I43]
　　　with thyroid storm E05.91 [I43]
　newborn I42.8
　　congenital I42.4
　nutritional E63.9 [I43]
　　beriberi E51.12
　obscure of Africa I42.8
　peripartum O90.3
　postpartum O90.3
　restrictive NEC I42.5
　rheumatic I09.0
　secondary I42.9
　stress induced I51.81
　takotsubo I51.81
　thyrotoxic E05.90 [I43]
　　with thyroid storm E05.91 [I43]
　toxic NEC I42.7
　tuberculous A18.84
　viral B33.24
Cardionephritis —see Hypertension, cardiorenal
Cardionephropathy —see Hypertension, cardiorenal
Cardionephrosis —see Hypertension, cardiorenal
Cardiopathia nigra I27.0

Cardiopathy —see also Disease, heart I51.9
　idiopathic I42.9
　mucopolysaccharidosis E76.3 [I52]
Cardiopericarditis —see Pericarditis
Cardiophobia F45.29
Cardiorenal —see condition
Cardiorrhexis —see Infarct, myocardium
Cardiosclerosis —see Disease, heart, ischemic, atherosclerotic
Cardiosis —see Disease, heart
Cardiospasm (esophagus) (reflex) (stomach) K22.0
　congenital Q39.5
　　with megaesophagus Q39.5
Cardiostenosis —see Disease, heart
Cardiosymphysis I31.0
Cardiovascular —see condition
Carditis (acute) (bacterial) (chronic) (subacute) I51.89
　meningococcal A39.50
　rheumatic —see Disease, heart, rheumatic
　rheumatoid —see Rheumatoid, carditis
　viral B33.20
Care (of) (for) (following)
　child (routine) Z76.2
　family member (handicapped) (sick)
　　creating problem for family Z63.6
　　provided away from home for holiday relief Z75.5
　　unavailable, due to
　　　absence (person rendering care) (sufferer) Z74.2
　　　inability (any reason) of person rendering care Z74.2
　foundling Z76.1
　holiday relief Z75.5
　improper —see Maltreatment
　lack of (at or after birth) (infant) —see Maltreatment, child, neglect
　lactating mother Z39.1
　palliative Z51.5
　postpartum
　　immediately after delivery Z39.0
　　routine follow-up Z39.2
　respite Z75.5
　unavailable, due to
　　absence of person rendering care Z74.2
　　inability (any reason) of person rendering care Z74.2
　well-baby Z76.2
Caries
　bone NEC A18.03
　dental (dentino enamel junction) (early childhood) (of dentine) (pre-eruptive) (recurrent) (to the pulp) K02.9 ◀
　　arrested (coronal) (root) K02.3
　　chewing surface
　　　limited to enamel K02.51
　　　penetrating into dentin K02.52
　　　penetrating into pulp K02.53
　　coronal surface
　　　chewing surface
　　　　limited to enamel K02.51
　　　　penetrating into dentin K02.52
　　　　penetrating into pulp K02.53
　　　pit and fissure surface
　　　　limited to enamel K02.51
　　　　penetrating into dentin K02.52
　　　　penetrating into pulp K02.53
　　　smooth surface
　　　　limited to enamel K02.61
　　　　penetrating into dentin K02.62
　　　　penetrating into pulp K02.63
　　pit and fissure surface
　　　limited to enamel K02.51
　　　penetrating into dentin K02.52
　　　penetrating into pulp K02.53
　　primary, cervical origin K02.52 ◀
　　root K02.7

Caries (Continued)
　dental (Continued)
　　smooth surface
　　　limited to enamel K02.61
　　　penetrating into dentin K02.62
　　　penetrating into pulp K02.63
　　external meatus —see Disorder, ear, external, specified type NEC
　　hip (tuberculous) A18.02
　　initial (tooth)
　　　chewing surface K02.51
　　　pit and fissure surface K02.51
　　　smooth surface K02.61
　　knee (tuberculous) A18.02
　　labyrinth —see subcategory H83.8
　　limb NEC (tuberculous) A18.03
　　mastoid process (chronic) —see Mastoiditis, chronic
　　　tuberculous A18.03
　　middle ear —see subcategory H74.8
　　nose (tuberculous) A18.03
　　orbit (tuberculous) A18.03
　　ossicles, ear —see Abnormal, ear ossicles
　　petrous bone —see Petrositis
　　root (dental) (tooth) K02.7
　　sacrum (tuberculous) A18.01
　　spine, spinal (column) (tuberculous) A18.01
　　syphilitic A52.77
　　　congenital (early) A50.02 [M90.80]
　　tooth, teeth —see Caries, dental
　　tuberculous A18.03
　　vertebra (column) (tuberculous) A18.01
Carious teeth —see Caries, dental
Carneous mole O02.0
Carnitine insufficiency E71.40
Carotid body or sinus syndrome G90.01
Carotidynia G90.01
Carotinemia (dietary) E67.1
Carotinosis (cutis) (skin) E67.1
Carpal tunnel syndrome —see Syndrome, carpal tunnel
Carpenter's syndrome Q87.0
Carpopedal spasm —see Tetany
Carr-Barr-Plunkett syndrome Q97.1
Carrier (suspected) of
　amebiasis Z22.1
　bacterial disease NEC Z22.39
　　diphtheria Z22.2
　　intestinal infectious NEC Z22.1
　　　typhoid Z22.0
　　meningococcal Z22.31
　　sexually transmitted Z22.4
　　specified NEC Z22.39
　　staphylococcal (Methicillin susceptible) Z22.321
　　　Methicillin resistant Z22.322
　　streptococcal Z22.338
　　　group B Z22.330
　　　　complicating pregnancy or delivery O99.82- ◀
　　typhoid Z22.0
　cholera Z22.1
　diphtheria Z22.2
　gastrointestinal pathogens NEC Z22.1
　genetic Z14.8
　　cystic fibrosis Z14.1
　　hemophilia A (asymptomatic) Z14.01
　　　symptomatic Z14.02
　gestational, pregnant Z33.1 ◀
　gonorrhea Z22.4
　HAA (hepatitis Australian-antigen) B18.8 ◀║
　HB (c)(s)-AG B18.1 ◀║
　hepatitis (viral) B18.9 ◀║
　　Australia-antigen (HAA) B18.8 ◀║
　　B surface antigen (HBsAg) B18.1 ◀║
　　　with acute delta- (super)infection B17.0
　　C B18.2 ◀║
　　specified NEC B18.8 ◀║
　human T-cell lymphotropic virus type-1 (HTLV-1) infection Z22.6

C

Carrier of *(Continued)*
  infectious organism Z22.9
    specified NEC Z22.8
  meningococci Z22.31
  Salmonella typhosa Z22.0
  serum hepatitis —*see* Carrier, hepatitis
  staphylococci (Methicillin susceptible) Z22.321
    Methicillin resistant Z22.322
  streptococci Z22.338
    group B Z22.330
      complicating pregnancy or delivery
        O99.82- ◀
  syphilis Z22.4
  typhoid Z22.0
  venereal disease NEC Z22.4
Carrion's disease A44.0
Carter's relapsing fever (Asiatic) A68.1
Cartilage —*see* condition
Caruncle (inflamed)
  conjunctiva (acute) —*see* Conjunctivitis, acute
  labium (majus) (minus) N90.89
  lacrimal —*see* Inflammation, lacrimal,
    passages
  myrtiform N89.8
  urethral (benign) N36.2
Cascade stomach K31.2
Caseation lymphatic gland (tuberculous) A18.2
Cassidy (-Scholte) syndrome (malignant
    carcinoid) E34.0
Castellani's disease A69.8
Castration, traumatic, male S38.231
Casts in urine R82.99
Cat
  cry syndrome Q93.4
  ear Q17.3
  eye syndrome Q92.8
Catabolism, senile R54
Catalepsy (hysterical) F44.2
  schizophrenic F20.2
Cataplexy (idiopathic) —*see* - Narcolepsy
Cataract (cortical) (immature) (incipient) H26.9
  with
    neovascularization —*see* Cataract,
      complicated
  age-related —*see* Cataract, senile
  anterior
    and posterior axial embryonal Q12.0
    pyramidal Q12.0
  associated with
    galactosemia E74.21 *[H28]*
    myotonic disorders G71.19 *[H28]*
  blue Q12.0
  central Q12.0
  cerulean Q12.0
  complicated H26.20
    with
      neovascularization H26.21-
      ocular disorder H26.22-
    glaucomatous flecks H26.23-
  congenital Q12.0
  coraliform Q12.0
  coronary Q12.0
  crystalline Q12.0
  diabetic —*see* Diabetes, cataract
  drug-induced H26.3-
  due to
    ocular disorder —*see* Cataract, complicated
    radiation H26.8
  electric H26.8
  extraction status Z98.4-
  glass-blower's H26.8
  heat ray H26.8
  heterochromic —*see* Cataract, complicated
  hypermature —*see* Cataract, senile,
    morgagnian type
  in (due to)
    chronic iridocyclitis —*see* Cataract,
      complicated
    diabetes —*see* Diabetes, cataract
    endocrine disease E34.9 *[H28]*
    eye disease —*see* Cataract, complicated

Cataract *(Continued)*
  in (due to) *(Continued)*
    hypoparathyroidism E20.9 *[H28]*
    malnutrition-dehydration E46 *[H28]*
    metabolic disease E88.9 *[H28]*
    myotonic disorders G71.19 *[H28]*
    nutritional disease E63.9 *[H28]*
  infantile —*see* Cataract, presenile
  irradiational —*see* Cataract, specified NEC
  juvenile —*see* Cataract, presenile
  malnutrition-dehydration E46 *[H28]*
  morgagnian —*see* Cataract, senile,
    morgagnian type
  myotonic G71.19 *[H28]*
  myxedema E03.9 *[H28]*
  nuclear
    embryonal Q12.0
    sclerosis —*see* Cataract, senile, nuclear
  presenile H26.00-
    combined forms H26.06-
    cortical H26.01-
    lamellar —*see* Cataract, presenile, cortical
    nuclear H26.03-
    specified NEC H26.09
    subcapsular polar (anterior) H26.04-
      posterior H26.05-
    zonular —*see* Cataract, presenile, cortical
  secondary H26.40
    Soemmering's ring H26.41-
    specified NEC H26.49-
    to eye disease —*see* Cataract, complicated
  senile H25.9
    brunescens —*see* Cataract, senile, nuclear
    combined forms H25.81-
    coronary —*see* Cataract, senile, incipient
    cortical H25.01-
    hypermature —*see* Cataract, senile,
      morgagnian type
    incipient (mature) (total) H25.09-
      cortical —*see* Cataract, senile, cortical
      subcapsular —*see* Cataract, senile,
        subcapsular
    morgagnian type (hypermature) H25.2-
    nuclear (sclerosis) H25.1-
    polar subcapsular (anterior) (posterior) —
      see Cataract, senile, incipient
    punctate —*see* Cataract, senile, incipient
    specified NEC H25.89
    subcapsular polar (anterior) H25.03-
      posterior H25.04-
  snowflake —*see* Diabetes, cataract
  specified NEC H26.8
  toxic —*see* Cataract, drug-induced
  traumatic H26.10-
    localized H26.11-
    partially resolved H26.12-
    total H26.13-
  zonular (perinuclear) Q12.0
Cataracta —*see also* Cataract
  brunescens —*see* Cataract, senile, nuclear
  centralis pulverulenta Q12.0
  cerulea Q12.0
  complicata —*see* Cataract, complicated
  congenita Q12.0
  coralliformis Q12.0
  coronaria Q12.0
  diabetic —*see* Diabetes, cataract
  membranacea
    accreta —*see* Cataract, secondary
    congenita Q12.0
  nigra —*see* Cataract, senile, nuclear
  sunflower —*see* Cataract, complicated
Catarrh, catarrhal (acute) (febrile) (infectious)
    (inflammation) *(see also* condition) J00
  bronchial —*see* Bronchitis
  chest —*see* Bronchitis
  chronic J31.0
  due to congenital syphilis A50.03
  enteric —*see* Enteritis
  eustachian H68.009
  fauces —*see* Pharyngitis

Catarrh, catarrhal *(Continued)*
  gastrointestinal —*see* Enteritis
  gingivitis K05.00
    nonplaque induced K05.01
    plaque induced K05.00
  hay —*see* Fever, hay
  intestinal —*see* Enteritis
  larynx, chronic J37.0
  liver B15.9
    with hepatic coma B15.0
  lung —*see* Bronchitis
  middle ear, chronic —*see* Otitis, media,
    nonsuppurative, chronic, serous
  mouth K12.1
  nasal (chronic) —*see* Rhinitis
  nasobronchial J31.1
  nasopharyngeal (chronic) J31.1
    acute J00
  pulmonary —*see* Bronchitis
  spring (eye) (vernal) —*see* Conjunctivitis,
    acute, atopic
  summer (hay) —*see* Fever, hay
  throat J31.2
  tubotympanal —*see also* Otitis, media,
    nonsuppurative
    chronic —*see* Otitis, media,
      nonsuppurative, chronic, serous
Catatonia (schizophrenic) F20.2
Catatonic
  disorder due to known physiologic condition
    F06.1
  schizophrenia F20.2
  stupor R40.1
Cat-scratch —*see also* Abrasion
  disease or fever A28.1
Cauda equina —*see* condition
Cauliflower ear M95.1-
Causalgia (upper limb) G56.4-
  lower limb G57.7-
Cause
  external, general effects T75.89
Caustic burn —*see* Corrosion, by site
Cavare's disease (familial periodic paralysis)
    G72.3
Cave-in, injury
  crushing (severe) —*see* Crush
  suffocation —*see* Asphyxia, traumatic, due to
    low oxygen, due to cave-in
Cavernitis (penis) N48.29
Cavernositis N48.29
Cavernous —*see* condition
Cavitation of lung —*see also* Tuberculosis,
    pulmonary
  nontuberculous J98.4
Cavities, dental —*see* Caries, dental
Cavity
  lung —*see* Cavitation of lung
  optic papilla Q14.2
  pulmonary —*see* Cavitation of lung
Cavovarus foot, congenital Q66.1
Cavus foot (congenital) Q66.7
  acquired —*see* Deformity, limb, foot, specified
    NEC
Cazenave's disease L10.2
Cecitis K52.9
  with perforation, peritonitis, or rupture K65.8
Cecum —*see* condition
Celiac
  artery compression syndrome I77.4
  disease (with steatorrhea) K90.0 ◀▥
  infantilism K90.0
Cell (s), cellular —*see also* condition
  in urine R82.99
Cellulitis (diffuse) (phlegmonous) (septic)
    (suppurative) L03.90
  abdominal wall L03.311
  anaerobic A48.0
  ankle —*see* Cellulitis, lower limb
  anus K61.0
  arm —*see* Cellulitis, upper limb
  auricle (ear) —*see* Cellulitis, ear

Cellulitis (Continued)
 axilla L03.11-
 back (any part) L03.312
 breast (acute) (nonpuerperal) (subacute)
  N61.0 ◀
  nipple N61.0 ◀
 broad ligament
  acute N73.0
 buttock L03.317
 cervical (meaning neck) L03.221
 cervix (uteri) —see Cervicitis
 cheek (external) L03.211
  internal K12.2
 chest wall L03.313
 chronic L03.90
 clostridial A48.0
 corpus cavernosum N48.22
 digit
  finger —see Cellulitis, finger
  toe —see Cellulitis, toe
 Douglas' cul-de-sac or pouch
  acute N73.0
 drainage site (following operation) T81.48 ◀⃕
 ear (external) H60.1-
 eosinophilic (granulomatous) L98.3
 erysipelatous —see Erysipelas
 external auditory canal —see Cellulitis, ear
 eyelid —see Abscess, eyelid
 face NEC L03.211
 finger (intrathecal) (periosteal)
  (subcutaneous) (subcuticular) L03.01-
 foot —see Cellulitis, lower limb
 gangrenous —see Gangrene
 genital organ NEC
  female (external) N76.4
  male N49.9
   multiple sites N49.8
   specified NEC N49.8
 gluteal (region) L03.317
 gonococcal A54.89
 groin L03.314
 hand —see Cellulitis, upper limb
 head NEC L03.811
  face (any part, except ear, eye and nose)
   L03.211
 heel —see Cellulitis, lower limb
 hip —see Cellulitis, lower limb
 jaw (region) L03.211
 knee —see Cellulitis, lower limb
 labium (majus) (minus) —see Vulvitis
 lacrimal passages —see Inflammation,
  lacrimal, passages
 larynx J38.7
 leg —see Cellulitis, lower limb
 lip K13.0
 lower limb L03.11-
  toe —see Cellulitis, toe
 mouth (floor) K12.2
 multiple sites, so stated L03.90
 nasopharynx J39.1
 navel L03.316
  newborn P38.9
   with mild hemorrhage P38.1
   without hemorrhage P38.9
 neck (region) L03.221
 nipple (acute) (nonpuerperal) (subacute)
  N61.0 ◀
 nose (septum) (external) J34.0
 orbit, orbital H05.01-
 palate (soft) K12.2
 pectoral (region) L03.313
 pelvis, pelvic (chronic)
  female —see also Disease, pelvis,
   inflammatory N73.2
   acute N73.0
  following ectopic or molar pregnancy
   O08.0
  male K65.0
 penis N48.22
 perineal, perineum L03.315
 periorbital L03.213 ◀

Cellulitis (Continued)
 perirectal K61.1
 peritonsillar J36
 periurethral N34.0
 periuterine —see also Disease, pelvis,
  inflammatory N73.2
  acute N73.0
 pharynx J39.1
 preseptal L03.213 ◀
 rectum K61.1
 retroperitoneal K68.9
 round ligament
  acute N73.0
 scalp (any part) L03.811
 scrotum N49.2
 seminal vesicle N49.0
 shoulder —see Cellulitis, upper limb
 specified site NEC L03.818
 submandibular (region) (space) (triangle)
  K12.2
  gland K11.3
 submaxillary (region) K12.2
  gland K11.3
 thigh —see Cellulitis, lower limb
 thumb (intrathecal) (periosteal)
  (subcutaneous) (subcuticular) —see
  Cellulitis, finger
 toe (intrathecal) (periosteal) (subcutaneous)
  (subcuticular) L03.03-
 tonsil J36
 trunk L03.319
  abdominal wall L03.311
  back (any part) L03.312
  buttock L03.317
  chest wall L03.313
  groin L03.314
  perineal, perineum L03.315
  umbilicus L03.316
 tuberculous (primary) A18.4
 umbilicus L03.316
 upper limb L03.11-
  axilla —see Cellulitis, axilla
  finger —see Cellulitis, finger
  thumb —see Cellulitis, finger
 vaccinal T88.0
 vocal cord J38.3
 vulva —see Vulvitis
 wrist —see Cellulitis, upper limb
Cementoblastoma, benign —see Cyst,
 calcifying odontogenic
Cementoma —see Cyst, calcifying odontogenic
Cementoperiostitis —see Periodontitis
Cementosis K03.4
Central auditory processing disorder H93.25
Central pain syndrome G89.0
Cephalematocele, cephal (o)hematocele
 newborn P52.8
  birth injury P10.8
 traumatic —see Hematoma, brain
Cephalematoma, cephalhematoma (calcified)
 newborn (birth injury) P12.0
 traumatic —see Hematoma, brain
Cephalgia, cephalalgia —see also Headache
 histamine G44.009
  intractable G44.001
  not intractable G44.009
 trigeminal autonomic (TAC) NEC G44.099
  intractable G44.091
  not intractable G44.099
Cephalic —see condition
Cephalitis —see Encephalitis
Cephalocele —see Encephalocele
Cephalomenia N94.89
Cephalopelvic —see condition
Cerclage (with cervical incompetence) in
 pregnancy —see Incompetence, cervix, in
 pregnancy
Cerebellitis —see Encephalitis
Cerebellum, cerebellar —see condition
Cerebral —see condition
Cerebritis —see Encephalitis

Cerebro-hepato-renal syndrome Q87.89
Cerebromalacia —see Softening, brain
 sequelae of cerebrovascular disease I69.398
Cerebroside lipidosis E75.22
Cerebrospasticity (congenital) G80.1
Cerebrospinal —see condition
Cerebrum —see condition
Ceroid-lipofuscinosis, neuronal E75.4
Cerumen (accumulation) (impacted) H61.2-
Cervical —see also condition
 auricle Q18.2
 dysplasia in pregnancy —see Abnormal,
  cervix, in pregnancy or childbirth
 erosion in pregnancy —see Abnormal, cervix,
  in pregnancy or childbirth
 fibrosis in pregnancy —see Abnormal, cervix,
  in pregnancy or childbirth
 fusion syndrome Q76.1
 rib Q76.5
 shortening (complicating pregnancy)
  O26.87-
Cervicalgia M54.2
Cervicitis (acute) (chronic) (nonvenereal)
 (senile (atrophic)) (subacute) (with
 ulceration) N72
 with
  abortion —see Abortion, by type
   complicated by genital tract and
   pelvic infection
  ectopic pregnancy O08.0
  molar pregnancy O08.0
 chlamydial A56.09
 gonococcal A54.03
 herpesviral A60.03
 puerperal (postpartum) O86.11
 syphilitic A52.76
 trichomonal A59.09
 tuberculous A18.16
Cervicocolpitis (emphysematosa) (see also
 Cervicitis) N72
Cervix —see condition
Cesarean delivery, previous, affecting
 management of pregnancy O34.219 ◀⃕
 classical (vertical) scar O34.212 ◀
 low transverse scar O34.211 ◀
Céstan (-Chenais) paralysis or syndrome G46.3
Céstan-Raymond syndrome I65.8
Cestode infestation B71.9
 specified type NEC B71.8
Cestodiasis B71.9
Chabert's disease A22.9
Chacaleh E53.8
Chafing L30.4
Chagas' (-Mazza) disease (chronic) B57.2
 with
  cardiovascular involvement NEC B57.2
  digestive system involvement B57.30
   megacolon B57.32
   megaesophagus B57.31
   other specified B57.39
  megacolon B57.32
  megaesophagus B57.31
  myocarditis B57.2
  nervous system involvement B57.40
   meningitis B57.41
   meningoencephalitis B57.42
   other specified B57.49
  specified organ involvement NEC B57.5
 acute (with) B57.1
  cardiovascular NEC B57.0
  myocarditis B57.0
Chagres fever B50.9
Chairridden Z74.09
Chalasia (cardiac sphincter) K21.9
Chalazion H00.19
 left H00.16
  lower H00.15
  upper H00.14
 right H00.13
  lower H00.12
  upper H00.11

Chalcosis —see also Disorder, globe, degenerative, chalcosis
- cornea —see Deposit, cornea
- crystalline lens —see Cataract, complicated
- retina H35.89

Chalicosis (pulmonum) J62.8

Chancre (any genital site) (hard) (hunterian) (mixed) (primary) (seronegative) (seropositive) (syphilitic) A51.0
- congenital A50.07
- conjunctiva NEC A51.2
- Ducrey's A57
- extragenital A51.2
- eyelid A51.2
- lip A51.2
- nipple A51.2
- Nisbet's A57
- of
  - carate A67.0
  - pinta A67.0
  - yaws A66.0
- palate, soft A51.2
- phagedenic A57
- simple A57
- soft A57
  - bubo A57
  - palate A51.2
- urethra A51.0
- yaws A66.0

Chancroid (anus) (genital) (penis) (perineum) (rectum) (urethra) (vulva) A57

Chandler's disease (osteochondritis dissecans, hip) —see Osteochondritis, dissecans, hip

Change (s) (in) (of) —see also Removal
- arteriosclerotic —see Arteriosclerosis
- bone —see also Disorder, bone
  - diabetic —see Diabetes, bone change
- bowel habit R19.4
- cardiorenal (vascular) —see Hypertension, cardiorenal
- cardiovascular —see Disease, cardiovascular
- circulatory I99.9
- cognitive (mild) (organic) R41.89
- color, tooth, teeth
  - during formation K00.8
  - posteruptive K03.7
- contraceptive device Z30.433
- corneal membrane H18.30
  - Bowman's membrane fold or rupture H18.31-
  - Descemet's membrane
    - fold H18.32-
    - rupture H18.33-
- coronary —see Disease, heart, ischemic
- degenerative, spine or vertebra —see Spondylosis
- dental pulp, regressive K04.2
- dressing (nonsurgical) Z48.00
  - surgical Z48.01
- heart —see Disease, heart
- hip joint —see Derangement, joint, hip
- hyperplastic larynx J38.7
- hypertrophic
  - nasal sinus J34.89
  - turbinate, nasal J34.3
  - upper respiratory tract J39.8
- indwelling catheter Z46.6
- inflammatory —see also Inflammation
  - sacroiliac M46.1
- job, anxiety concerning Z56.1
- joint —see Derangement, joint
- life —see Menopause
- mental status R41.82
- minimal (glomerular) —see also N00-N07
  - with fourth character .0 N05.0
- myocardium, myocardial —see Degeneration, myocardial - of life —see Menopause
- pacemaker Z45.018
  - pulse generator Z45.010

Change (Continued)
- personality (enduring) F68.8
  - due to (secondary to)
    - general medical condition F07.0
  - secondary (nonspecific) F60.89
- regressive, dental pulp K04.2
- renal —see Disease, renal
- retina H35.9
  - myopic H44.2-
- sacroiliac joint M53.3
- senile —see also condition R54
- sensory R20.8
- skin R23.9
  - acute, due to ultraviolet radiation L56.9
    - specified NEC L56.8
  - chronic, due to nonionizing radiation L57.9
    - specified NEC L57.8
  - cyanosis R23.0
  - flushing R23.2
  - pallor R23.1
  - petechiae R23.3
  - specified change NEC R23.8
  - swelling —see Mass, localized
  - texture R23.4
- trophic
  - arm —see Mononeuropathy, upper limb
  - leg —see Mononeuropathy, lower limb
- vascular I99.9
- vasomotor I73.9
- voice R49.9
  - psychogenic F44.4
  - specified NEC R49.8

Changing sleep-work schedule, affecting sleep G47.26

Changuinola fever A93.1

Chapping skin T69.8

Charcot-Marie-Tooth disease, paralysis or syndrome G60.0

Charcot's
- arthropathy —see Arthropathy, neuropathic
- cirrhosis K74.3
- disease (tabetic arthropathy) A52.16
- joint (disease) (tabetic) A52.16
  - diabetic —see Diabetes, with, arthropathy
  - syringomyelic G95.0
- syndrome (intermittent claudication) I73.9

CHARGE association Q89.8

Charley-horse (quadriceps) M62.831
- traumatic (quadriceps) S76.11-

Charlouis' disease —see Yaws

Cheadle's disease E54

Checking (of)
- cardiac pacemaker (battery) (electrode (s)) Z45.018
  - pulse generator Z45.010
- implantable subdermal contraceptive Z30.46 ◀
- intrauterine contraceptive device Z30.431

Check-up —see Examination

Chédiak-Higashi (-Steinbrinck) syndrome (congenital gigantism of peroxidase granules) E70.330

Cheek —see condition

Cheese itch B88.0

Cheese-washer's lung J67.8

Cheese-worker's lung J67.8

Cheilitis (acute) (angular) (catarrhal) (chronic) (exfoliative) (gangrenous) (glandular) (infectional) (suppurative) (ulcerative) (vesicular) K13.0
- actinic (due to sun) L56.8
  - other than from sun L59.8
- candidal B37.83

Cheilodynia K13.0

Cheiloschisis —see Cleft, lip

Cheilosis (angular) K13.0
- with pellagra E52
- due to
  - vitamin B2 (riboflavin) deficiency E53.0

Cheiromegaly M79.89

Cheiropompholyx L30.1

Cheloid —see Keloid

Chemical burn —see Corrosion, by site

Chemodectoma —see Paraganglioma, nonchromaffin

Chemosis, conjunctiva —see Edema, conjunctiva

Chemotherapy (session) (for)
- cancer Z51.11
- neoplasm Z51.11

Cherubism M27.8

Chest —see condition

Cheyne-Stokes breathing (respiration) R06.3

Chiari's
- disease or syndrome (hepatic vein thrombosis) I82.0
- malformation
  - type I G93.5
  - type II —see Spina bifida
- net Q24.8

Chicago disease B40.9

Chickenpox —see Varicella

Chiclero ulcer or sore B55.1

Chigger (infestation) B88.0

Chignon (disease) B36.8
- newborn (from vacuum extraction) (birth injury) P12.1

Chilaiditi's syndrome (subphrenic displacement, colon) Q43.3

Chilblain (s) (lupus) T69.1

Child
- custody dispute Z65.3

Childbirth —see Delivery

Childhood
- cerebral X-linked adrenoleukodystrophy E71.520
- period of rapid growth Z00.2

Chill (s) R68.83
- with fever R50.9
- without fever R68.83
- congestive in malarial regions B54

Chilomastigiasis A07.8

Chimera 46,XX/46,XY Q99.0

Chin —see condition

Chinese dysentery A03.9

Chionophobia F40.228

Chitral fever A93.1

Chlamydia, chlamydial A74.9
- cervicitis A56.09
- conjunctivitis A74.0
- cystitis A56.01
- endometritis A56.11
- epididymitis A56.19
- female
  - pelvic inflammatory disease A56.11
  - pelviperitonitis A56.11
- orchitis A56.19
- peritonitis A74.81
- pharyngitis A56.4
- proctitis A56.3
- psittaci (infection) A70
- salpingitis A56.11
- sexually-transmitted infection NEC A56.8
- specified NEC A74.89
- urethritis A56.01
- vulvovaginitis A56.02

Chlamydiosis —see Chlamydia

Chloasma (skin) (idiopathic) (symptomatic) L81.1
- eyelid H02.719
  - hyperthyroid E05.90 [H02.719]
    - with thyroid storm E05.91 [H02.719]
  - left H02.716
    - lower H02.715
    - upper H02.714
  - right H02.713
    - lower H02.712
    - upper H02.711

Chloroma C92.3-

Chlorosis D50.9
- Egyptian B76.9 [D63.8]
- miner's B76.9 [D63.8]

Chlorotic anemia D50.8

Chocolate cyst (ovary) N80.1
Choked
  disc or disk —*see* Papilledema
  on food, phlegm, or vomitus NOS —*see*
    Foreign body, by site
  while vomiting NOS —*see* Foreign body, by
    site
Chokes (resulting from bends) T70.3
Choking sensation R09.89
Cholangiectasis K83.8
Cholangiocarcinoma
  with hepatocellular carcinoma, combined
    C22.0
  liver C22.1
  specified site NEC —*see* Neoplasm,
    malignant, by site
  unspecified site C22.1
Cholangiohepatitis K83.8
  due to fluke infestation B66.1
Cholangiohepatoma C22.0
Cholangiolitis (acute) (chronic) (extrahepatic)
    (gangrenous) (intrahepatic) K83.0
  paratyphoidal —*see* Fever, paratyphoid
  typhoidal A01.09
Cholangioma D13.4
  malignant —*see* Cholangiocarcinoma
Cholangitis (ascending) (primary) (recurrent)
    (sclerosing) (secondary) (stenosing)
    (suppurative) K83.0
  with calculus, bile duct —*see* Calculus, bile
    duct, with cholangitis
  chronic nonsuppurative destructive K74.3
Cholecystectasia K82.8
Cholecystitis K81.9
  with
    calculus, stones in
      bile duct (common) (hepatic) —
        see Calculus, bile duct, with
          cholecystitis
      cystic duct —*see* Calculus, gallbladder,
        with cholecystitis
      gallbladder —*see* Calculus, gallbladder,
        with cholecystitis
    choledocholithiasis —*see* Calculus, bile
      duct, with cholecystitis
    cholelithiasis —*see* Calculus, gallbladder,
      with cholecystitis
  acute (emphysematous) (gangrenous)
    (suppurative) K81.0
    with
      calculus, stones in
        cystic duct —*see* Calculus,
          gallbladder, with cholecystitis,
          acute
        gallbladder —*see* Calculus,
          gallbladder, with cholecystitis,
          acute
      choledocholithiasis —*see* Calculus, bile
        duct, with cholecystitis, acute
      cholelithiasis —*see* Calculus,
        gallbladder, with cholecystitis,
        acute
    chronic cholecystitis K81.2
      with gallbladder calculus K80.12
        with obstruction K80.13
  chronic K81.1
    with acute cholecystitis K81.2
      with gallbladder calculus K80.12
        with obstruction K80.13
  emphysematous (acute) —*see* Cholecystitis,
    acute
  gangrenous —*see* Cholecystitis, acute
  paratyphoidal, current A01.4
  suppurative —*see* Cholecystitis, acute
  typhoidal A01.09
Cholecystolithiasis —*see* Calculus, gallbladder
Choledochitis (suppurative) K83.0
Choledocholith —*see* Calculus, bile duct
Choledocholithiasis (common duct) (hepatic
    duct) —*see* Calculus, bile duct
  cystic —*see* Calculus, gallbladder
  typhoidal A01.09

Cholelithiasis (cystic duct) (gallbladder)
    (impacted) (multiple) —*see* Calculus,
    gallbladder
  bile duct (common) (hepatic) —*see* Calculus,
    bile duct
  hepatic duct —*see* Calculus, bile duct
  specified NEC K80.80
    with obstruction K80.81
Cholemia —*see also* Jaundice
  familial (simple) (congenital) E80.4
  Gilbert's E80.4
Choleperitoneum, choleperitonitis K65.3
Cholera (Asiatic) (epidemic) (malignant) A00.9
  antimonial —*see* Poisoning, antimony
  classical A00.0
  due to Vibrio cholerae 01 A00.9
    biovar cholerae A00.0
    biovar eltor A00.1
    el tor A00.1
  el tor A00.1
Cholerine —*see* Cholera
Cholestasis NEC K83.1
  with hepatocyte injury K71.0
  due to total parenteral nutrition (TPN) K76.89
  pure K71.0
Cholesteatoma (ear) (middle) (with reaction)
    H71.9-
  attic H71.0-
  external ear (canal) H60.4-
  mastoid H71.2-
  postmastoidectomy cavity (recurrent) —*see*
    Complications, postmastoidectomy,
    recurrent cholesteatoma
  recurrent (postmastoidectomy) —*see*
    Complications, postmastoidectomy,
    recurrent cholesteatoma
  tympanum H71.1-
Cholesteatosis, diffuse H71.3-
Cholesteremia E78.00 ◀▥
Cholesterin in vitreous —*see* Deposit, crystalline
Cholesterol
  deposit
    retina H35.89
    vitreous —*see* Deposit, crystalline
  elevated (high) E78.00 ◀▥
    with elevated (high) triglycerides E78.2
    screening for Z13.220
  imbibition of gallbladder K82.4
Cholesterolemia (essential) (pure) E78.00 ◀▥
  familial E78.01 ◀
  hereditary E78.01 ◀
Cholesterolosis, cholesterosis (gallbladder)
    K82.4
  cerebrotendinous E75.5
Cholocolic fistula K82.3
Choluria R82.2
Chondritis M94.8X9
  aurical H61.03-
  costal (Tietze's) M94.0
  external ear H61.03-
  patella, posttraumatic —*see* Chondromalacia,
    patella
  pinna H61.03-
  purulent M94.8X-
  tuberculous NEC A18.02
    intervertebral A18.01
Chondroblastoma —*see also* Neoplasm, bone,
    benign
  malignant —*see* Neoplasm, bone, malignant
Chondrocalcinosis M11.20
  ankle M11.27-
  elbow M11.22-
  familial M11.10
    ankle M11.17-
    elbow M11.12-
    foot joint M11.17-
    hand joint M11.14-
    hip M11.15-
    knee M11.16-
    multiple site M11.19
    shoulder M11.11-

Chondrocalcinosis (*Continued*)
  familial (*Continued*)
    vertebrae M11.18
    wrist M11.13-
  foot joint M11.27-
  hand joint M11.24-
  hip M11.25-
  knee M11.26-
  multiple site M11.29
  shoulder M11.21-
  specified type NEC M11.20
    ankle M11.27-
    elbow M11.22-
    foot joint M11.27-
    hand joint M11.24-
    hip M11.25-
    knee M11.26-
    multiple site M11.29
    shoulder M11.21-
    vertebrae M11.28
    wrist M11.23-
  vertebrae M11.28
  wrist M11.23-
Chondrodermatitis nodularis helicis or
    anthelicis —*see* Perichondritis, ear
Chondrodysplasia Q78.9
  with hemangioma Q78.4
  calcificans congenita Q77.3
  fetalis Q77.4
  metaphyseal (Jansen's) (McKusick's)
    (Schmid's) Q78.8 ◀▥
  punctata Q77.3
Chondrodystrophy, chondrodystrophia
    (familial) (fetalis) (hypoplastic) Q78.9
  calcificans congenita Q77.3
  myotonic (congenital) G71.13
  punctata Q77.3
Chondroectodermal dysplasia Q77.6
Chondrogenesis imperfecta Q77.4
Chondrolysis M94.35-
Chondroma —*see also* Neoplasm, cartilage,
    benign
  juxtacortical —*see* Neoplasm, bone, benign
  periosteal —*see* Neoplasm, bone, benign
Chondromalacia (systemic) M94.20
  acromioclavicular joint M94.21-
  ankle M94.27-
  elbow M94.22-
  foot joint M94.27-
  glenohumeral joint M94.21-
  hand joint M94.24-
  hip M94.25-
  knee M94.26-
    patella M22.4-
  multiple sites M94.29
  patella M22.4-
  rib M94.28
  sacroiliac joint M94.259
  shoulder M94.21-
  sternoclavicular joint M94.21-
  vertebral joint M94.28
  wrist M94.23-
Chondromatosis —*see also* Neoplasm, cartilage,
    uncertain behavior
  internal Q78.4
Chondromyxosarcoma —*see* Neoplasm,
    cartilage, malignant
Chondro-osteodysplasia (Morquio-Brailsford
    type) E76.219
Chondro-osteodystrophy E76.29
Chondro-osteoma —*see* Neoplasm, bone, benign
Chondropathia tuberosa M94.0
Chondrosarcoma —*see* Neoplasm, cartilage,
    malignant
  juxtacortical —*see* Neoplasm, bone, malignant
  mesenchymal —*see* Neoplasm, connective
    tissue, malignant
  myxoid —*see* Neoplasm, cartilage, malignant
Chordee (nonvenereal) N48.89
  congenital Q54.4
  gonococcal A54.09

Chorditis (fibrinous) (nodosa) (tuberosa) J38.2
Chordoma —see Neoplasm, vertebral (column),
   malignant
Chorea (chronic) (gravis) (posthemiplegic)
   (senile) (spasmodic) G25.5
   with
      heart involvement I02.0
         active or acute (conditions in I01-) I02.0
         rheumatic I02.9
            with valvular disorder I02.0
         rheumatic heart disease (chronic) (inactive)
            (quiescent) — code to rheumatic heart
            condition involved
   drug-induced G25.4
   habit F95.8
   hereditary G10
   Huntington's G10
   hysterical F44.4
   minor I02.9
      with heart involvement I02.0
   progressive G25.5
      hereditary G10
   rheumatic (chronic) I02.9
      with heart involvement I02.0
   Sydenham's I02.9
      with heart involvement —see Chorea, with
         rheumatic heart disease
      nonrheumatic G25.5
Choreoathetosis (paroxysmal) G25.5
Chorioadenoma (destruens) D39.2
Chorioamnionitis O41.12-
Chorioangioma D26.7
Choriocarcinoma —see Neoplasm, malignant,
   by site
   combined with
      embryonal carcinoma —see Neoplasm,
         malignant, by site
      other germ cell elements —see Neoplasm,
         malignant, by site
      teratoma —see Neoplasm, malignant, by
         site
   specified site —see Neoplasm, malignant, by
      site
   unspecified site
      female C58
      male C62.90
Chorioencephalitis (acute) (lymphocytic)
   (serous) A87.2
Chorioepithelioma —see Choriocarcinoma
Choriomeningitis (acute) (lymphocytic)
   (serous) A87.2
Chorionepithelioma —see Choriocarcinoma
Chorioretinitis —see also Inflammation,
   chorioretinal
   disseminated —see also Inflammation,
      chorioretinal, disseminated
      in neurosyphilis A52.19
   Egyptian B76.9 [D63.8]
   focal —see also Inflammation, chorioretinal,
      focal
   histoplasmic B39.9 [H32]
   in (due to)
      histoplasmosis B39.9 [H32]
      syphilis (secondary) A51.43
         late A52.71
      toxoplasmosis (acquired) B58.01
         congenital (active) P37.1 [H32]
      tuberculosis A18.53
   juxtapapillary, juxtapapillaris —see
      Inflammation, chorioretinal, focal,
      juxtapapillary
   leprous A30.9 [H32]
   miner's B76.9 [D63.8]
   progressive myopia (degeneration) H44.2-
   syphilitic (secondary) A51.43
      congenital (early) A50.01 [H32]
         late A50.32
      late A52.71
   tuberculous A18.53
Chorioretinopathy, central serous H35.71-
Choroid —see condition

Choroideremia H31.21
Choroiditis —see Chorioretinitis
Choroidopathy —see Disorder, choroid
Choroidoretinitis —see Chorioretinitis
Choroidoretinopathy, central serous —see
   Chorioretinopathy, central serous
Christian-Weber disease M35.6
Christmas disease D67
Chromaffinoma —see also Neoplasm, benign,
   by site
   malignant —see Neoplasm, malignant, by site
Chromatopsia —see Deficiency, color vision
Chromhidrosis, chromidrosis L75.1
Chromoblastomycosis —see Chromomycosis
Chromoconversion R82.91
Chromomycosis B43.9
   brain abscess B43.1
   cerebral B43.1
   cutaneous B43.0
   skin B43.0
   specified NEC B43.8
   subcutaneous abscess or cyst B43.2
Chromophytosis B36.0
Chromosome —see condition by chromosome
   involved
   D (1) —see condition, chromosome 13
   E (3) —see condition, chromosome 18
   G —see condition, chromosome 21
Chromotrichomycosis B36.8
Chronic —see condition
   fracture —see Fracture, pathological
Churg-Strauss syndrome M30.1
Chyle cyst, mesentery I89.8
Chylocele (nonfilarial) I89.8
   filarial —see also Infestation, filarial B74.9
      [N51]
   tunica vaginalis N50.89 ◀═
      filarial —see also Infestation, filarial B74.9
         [N51]
Chylomicronemia (fasting) (with
   hyperprebetalipoproteinemia) E78.3
Chylopericardium I31.3
   acute I30.9
Chylothorax (nonfilarial) I89.8
   filarial —see also Infestation, filarial B74.9
      [J91.8]
Chylous —see condition
Chyluria (nonfilarial) R82.0
   due to
      bilharziasis B65.0
      Brugia (malayi) B74.1
         timori B74.2
      schistosomiasis (bilharziasis) B65.0
      Wuchereria (bancrofti) B74.0
   filarial —see Infestation, filarial
Cicatricial (deformity) —see Cicatrix
Cicatrix (adherent) (contracted) (painful)
   (vicious) —see also Scar L90.5
   adenoid (and tonsil) J35.8
   alveolar process M26.79
   anus K62.89
   auricle —see Disorder, pinna, specified type
      NEC
   bile duct (common) (hepatic) K83.8
   bladder N32.89
   bone —see Disorder, bone, specified type
      NEC
   brain G93.89
   cervix (postoperative) (postpartal) N88.1
   common duct K83.8
   cornea H17.9
      tuberculous A18.59
   duodenum (bulb), obstructive K31.5
   esophagus K22.2
   eyelid —see Disorder, eyelid function
   hypopharynx J39.2
   lacrimal passages —see Obstruction, lacrimal
   larynx J38.7
   lung J98.4
   middle ear —see subcategory H74.8
   mouth K13.79

Cicatrix (Continued)
   muscle M62.89
      with contracture —see Contraction, muscle
         NEC
   nasopharynx J39.2
   palate (soft) K13.79
   penis N48.89
   pharynx J39.2
   prostate N42.89
   rectum K62.89
   retina —see Scar, chorioretinal
   semilunar cartilage —see Derangement,
      meniscus
   seminal vesicle N50.89 ◀═
   skin L90.5
      infected L08.89
      postinfective L90.5
      tuberculous B90.8
   specified site NEC L90.5
   throat J39.2
   tongue K14.8
   tonsil (and adenoid) J35.8
   trachea J39.8
   tuberculous NEC B90.9
   urethra N36.8
   uterus N85.8
   vagina N89.8
      postoperative N99.2
   vocal cord J38.3
   wrist, constricting (annular) L90.5
CIDP (chronic inflammatory demyelinating
   polyneuropathy) G61.81
CIN —see Neoplasia, intraepithelial, cervix
CINCA (chronic infantile neurological, cutaneous
   and articular syndrome) M04.2 ◀
Cinchonism —see Deafness, ototoxic
   correct substance properly administered —see
      Table of Drugs and Chemicals, by drug,
      adverse effect
   overdose or wrong substance given or
      taken —see Table of Drugs and
      Chemicals, by drug, poisoning
Circle of Willis —see condition
Circular —see condition
Circulating anticoagulants —see also - Disorder,
   hemorrhagic D68.318
   due to drugs —see also - Disorder,
      hemorrhagic D68.32
   following childbirth O72.3
Circulation
   collateral, any site I99.8
   defective (lower extremity) I99.8
      congenital Q28.9
   embryonic Q28.9
   failure (peripheral) R57.9
      newborn P29.89
   fetal, persistent P29.3
   heart, incomplete Q28.9
Circulatory system —see condition
Circulus senilis (cornea) —see Degeneration,
   cornea, senile
Circumcision (in absence of medical indication)
   (ritual) (routine) Z41.2
Circumscribed —see condition
Circumvallate placenta O43.11-
Cirrhosis, cirrhotic (hepatic) (liver)
   K74.60
   alcoholic K70.30
      with ascites K70.31
   atrophic —see Cirrhosis, liver
   Baumgarten-Cruveilhier K74.69
   biliary (cholangiolitic) (cholangitic)
      (hypertrophic) (obstructive)
      (pericholangiolitic) K74.5
      due to
         Clonorchiasis B66.1
         flukes B66.3
      primary K74.3
      secondary K74.4
   cardiac (of liver) K76.1
   Charcot's K74.3

Coats' disease (exudative retinopathy) —see
    Retinopathy, exudative
Cocaine-induced ◄
    anxiety disorder F14.980 ◄
    bipolar and related disorder F14.94 ◄
    depressive disorder F14.94 ◄
    obsessive-compulsive and related disorder
        F14.988 ◄
    psychotic disorder F14.959 ◄
    sleep disorder F14.982 ◄
    sexual dysfunction F14.981 ◄
Cocainism —see Disorder, cocaine use ◄▥
Coccidioidomycosis B38.9
    cutaneous B38.3
    disseminated B38.7
    generalized B38.7
    meninges B38.4
    prostate B38.81
    pulmonary B38.2
        acute B38.0
        chronic B38.1
    skin B38.3
    specified NEC B38.89
Coccidioidosis —see Coccidioidomycosis
Coccidiosis (intestinal) A07.3
Coccydynia, coccygodynia M53.3
Coccyx —see condition
Cochin-China diarrhea K90.1
Cockayne's syndrome Q87.1
Cocked up toe —see Deformity, toe, specified
    NEC
Cock's peculiar tumor L72.3
Codman's tumor —see Neoplasm, bone,
    benign
Coenurosis B71.8
Coffee-worker's lung J67.8
Cogan's syndrome H16.32-
    oculomotor apraxia H51.8
Coitus, painful (female) N94.10 ◄▥
    male N53.12
    psychogenic F52.6
Cold J00
    with influenza, flu, or grippe —see Influenza,
        with, respiratory manifestations NEC
    agglutinin disease or hemoglobinuria
        (chronic) D59.1
    bronchial —see Bronchitis
    chest —see Bronchitis
    common (head) J00
    effects of T69.9
        specified effect NEC T69.8
    excessive, effects of T69.9
        specified effect NEC T69.8
    exhaustion from T69.8
    exposure to T69.9
        specified effect NEC T69.8
    head J00
    injury syndrome (newborn) P80.0
    on lung —see Bronchitis
    rose J30.1
    sensitivity, auto-immune D59.1
    virus J00
Coldsore B00.1
Colibacillosis A49.8
    as the cause of other disease (see also
        Escherichia coli) B96.20
    generalized A41.50
Colic (bilious) (infantile) (intestinal) (recurrent)
    (spasmodic) R10.83
    abdomen R10.83
        psychogenic F45.8
    appendix, appendicular K38.8
    bile duct —see Calculus, bile duct
    biliary —see Calculus, bile duct
    common duct —see Calculus, bile duct
    cystic duct —see Calculus, gallbladder
    Devonshire NEC —see Poisoning, lead
    gallbladder —see Calculus, gallbladder
    gallstone —see Calculus, gallbladder
        gallbladder or cystic duct —see Calculus,
            gallbladder

Colic (Continued)
    hepatic (duct) —see Calculus, bile duct
    hysterical F45.8
    kidney N23
    lead NEC —see Poisoning, lead
    mucous K58.9
        with diarrhea K58.0
        psychogenic F54
    nephritic N23
    painter's NEC —see Poisoning, lead
    pancreas K86.89 ◄▥
    psychogenic F45.8
    renal N23
    saturnine NEC —see Poisoning, lead
    ureter N23
    urethral N36.8
        due to calculus N21.1
    uterus NEC N94.89
        menstrual —see Dysmenorrhea
    worm NOS B83.9
Colicystitis —see Cystitis
Colitis (acute) (catarrhal) (chronic)
    (noninfective) (hemorrhagic) (see also
    Enteritis) K52.9
    allergic K52.29 ◄▥
        with ◄
            food protein-induced enterocolitis
                syndrome K52.21 ◄
            proctocolitis K52.82 ◄
    amebic (acute) —see also Amebiasis A06.0
        nondysenteric A06.2
    anthrax A22.2
    bacillary —see Infection, Shigella
    balantidial A07.0
    Clostridium difficile A04.7
    coccidial A07.3
    collagenous K52.831 ◄▥
    cystica superficialis K52.89
    dietary counseling and surveillance (for)
        Z71.3
    dietetic —see also Colitis, allergic K52.29 ◄▥
    drug-induced K52.1
    due to radiation K52.0
    eosinophilic K52.82
    food hypersensitivity —see also Colitis,
        allergic K52.29 ◄▥
    giardial A07.1
    granulomatous —see Enteritis, regional, large
        intestine
    infectious —see Enteritis, infectious
    indeterminate, so stated K52.3 ◄
    ischemic K55.9
        acute (subacute) —see also Ischemia,
            intestine, acute K55.039 ◄▥
        chronic K55.1
        due to mesenteric artery insufficiency
            K55.1
        fulminant (acute) —see also Ischemia,
            intestine, acute K55.039 ◄▥
    left sided K51.50
        with
            abscess K51.514
            complication K51.519
                specified NEC K51.518
            fistula K51.513
            obstruction K51.512
            rectal bleeding K51.511
    lymphocytic K52.832 ◄▥
    membranous
        psychogenic F54
    microscopic K52.839 ◄▥
        specified NEC K52.838 ◄
    mucous —see Syndrome, irritable, bowel
        psychogenic F54
    noninfective K52.9
        specified NEC K52.89
    polyposa —see Polyp, colon, inflammatory
    protozoal A07.9
    pseudomembranous A04.7
    pseudomucinous —see Syndrome, irritable,
        bowel

Colitis (Continued)
    regional —see Enteritis, regional, large
        intestine
    segmental —see Enteritis, regional, large
        intestine
    septic —see Enteritis, infectious
    spastic K58.9
        with diarrhea K58.0
        psychogenic F54
    staphylococcal A04.8
        foodborne A05.0
    subacute ischemic —see also Ischemia,
        intestine, acute K55.039 ◄▥
    thromboulcerative —see also Ischemia,
        intestine, acute K55.039 ◄▥
    toxic NEC K52.1
        due to Clostridium difficile A04.7
    transmural —see Enteritis, regional, large
        intestine
    trichomonal A07.8
    tuberculous (ulcerative) A18.32
    ulcerative (chronic) K51.90
        with
            complication K51.919
                abscess K51.914
                fistula K51.913
                obstruction K51.912
                rectal bleeding K51.911
                specified complication NEC K51.918
        enterocolitis —see Enterocolitis, ulcerative
        ileocolitis —see Ileocolitis, ulcerative
        mucosal proctocolitis —see Proctocolitis,
            mucosal
        proctitis —see Proctitis, ulcerative
        pseudopolyposis —see Polyp, colon,
            inflammatory
        psychogenic F54
        rectosigmoiditis —see Rectosigmoiditis,
            ulcerative
        specified type NEC K51.80
            with
                complication K51.819
                    abscess K51.814
                    fistula K51.813
                    obstruction K51.812
                    rectal bleeding K51.811
                    specified complication NEC
                        K51.818
Collagenosis, collagen disease (nonvascular)
    (vascular) M35.9
    cardiovascular I42.8
    reactive perforating L87.1
    specified NEC M35.8
Collapse R55
    adrenal E27.2
    cardiorespiratory R57.0
    cardiovascular R57.0
        newborn P29.89
    circulatory (peripheral) R57.9
        during or after labor and delivery O75.1
        following ectopic or molar pregnancy
            O08.3
        newborn P29.89
    during or
        after labor and delivery O75.1
        resulting from a procedure, not elsewhere
            classified T81.10
    external ear canal —see Stenosis, external ear
        canal
    general R55
    heart —see Disease, heart
    heat T67.1
    hysterical F44.89
    labyrinth, membranous (congenital) Q16.5
    lung (massive) —see also Atelectasis J98.19
        pressure due to anesthesia (general) (local)
            or other sedation T88.2
            during labor and delivery O74.1
            in pregnancy O29.02-
            postpartum, puerperal O89.09
    myocardial —see Disease, heart

Collapse (Continued)
  nervous F48.8
  neurocirculatory F45.8
  nose M95.0
  postoperative T81.10
  pulmonary —see also Atelectasis J98.19
    newborn —see Atelectasis
  trachea J39.8
  tracheobronchial J98.09
  valvular —see Endocarditis
  vascular (peripheral) R57.9
    during or after labor and delivery O75.1
    following ectopic or molar pregnancy
      O08.3
    newborn P29.89
  vertebra M48.50-
    cervical region M48.52-
    cervicothoracic region M48.53-
    in (due to)
      metastasis —see Collapse, vertebra, in,
        specified disease NEC
      osteoporosis —see also Osteoporosis
        M80.88
        cervical region M80.88
        cervicothoracic region M80.88
        lumbar region M80.88
        lumbosacral region M80.88
        multiple sites M80.88
        occipito-atlanto-axial region M80.88
        sacrococcygeal region M80.88
        thoracic region M80.88
        thoracolumbar region M80.88
      specified disease NEC M48.50-
        cervical region M48.52-
        cervicothoracic region M48.53-
        lumbar region M48.56-
        lumbosacral region M48.57-
        occipito-atlanto-axial region M48.51-
        sacrococcygeal region M48.58-
        thoracic region M48.54-
        thoracolumbar region M48.55-
    lumbar region M48.56-
    lumbosacral region M48.57-
    occipito-atlanto-axial region M48.51-
    sacrococcygeal region M48.58-
    thoracic region M48.54-
    thoracolumbar region M48.55-
Collateral —see also condition
  circulation (venous) I87.8
  dilation, veins I87.8
Colles' fracture S52.53-
Collet (-Sicard) syndrome G52.7
Collier's asthma or lung J60
Collodion baby Q80.2
Colloid nodule (of thyroid) (cystic) E04.1
Coloboma (iris) Q13.0
  eyelid Q10.3
  fundus Q14.8
  lens Q12.2
  optic disc (congenital) Q14.2
    acquired H47.31-
Coloenteritis —see Enteritis
Colon —see condition
Colonization
  MRSA (Methicillin resistant Staphylococcus
    aureus) Z22.322
  MSSA (Methicillin susceptible
    Staphylococcus aureus) Z22.321
  status —see Carrier (suspected) of
Coloptosis K63.4
Color blindness —see Deficiency, color vision
Colostomy
  attention to Z43.3
  fitting or adjustment Z46.89
  malfunctioning K94.03
  status Z93.3
Colpitis (acute) —see Vaginitis
Colpocele N81.5
Colpocystitis —see Vaginitis
Colpospasm N94.2
Column, spinal, vertebral —see condition

Coma R40.20
  with
    motor response (none) R40.231
      abnormal R40.233
      extension R40.232
      flexion withdrawal R40.234
    motor response (none) (Continued)
      localizes pain R40.235
      obeys commands R40.236
    opening of eyes (never) R40.211
      in response to
        pain R40.212
        sound R40.213
      spontaneous R40.214
    verbal response (none) R40.221
      confused conversation R40.224
      inappropriate words R40.223
      incomprehensible words R40.222
      oriented R40.225
  eclamptic —see Eclampsia
  epileptic —see Epilepsy
  Glasgow, scale score —see Glasgow coma
    scale
  hepatic —see Failure, hepatic, by type, with
    coma
  hyperglycemic (diabetic) —see Diabetes,
    by type, with hyperosmolarity, with
    coma ◀▦
  hyperosmolar (diabetic) —see Diabetes,
    by type, with hyperosmolarity, with
    coma ◀▦
  hypoglycemic (diabetic) —see Diabetes, by
    type, with hypoglycemia, with coma ◀▦
    nondiabetic E15
  in diabetes —see Diabetes, coma
  insulin-induced —see Coma, hypoglycemic
  myxedematous E03.5
  newborn P91.5
  persistent vegetative state R40.3
  specified NEC, without documented
    Glasgow coma scale score, or with
    partial Glasgow coma scale score
    reported R40.244
Comatose —see Coma
Combat fatigue F43.0
Combined —see condition
Comedo, comedones (giant) L70.0
Comedocarcinoma —see also Neoplasm, breast,
    malignant
  noninfiltrating
    breast D05.8-
    specified site —see Neoplasm, in situ,
      by site
    unspecified site D05.8-
Comedomastitis —see Ectasia, mammary duct
Comminuted fracture - code as Fracture, closed
Common
  arterial trunk Q20.0
  atrioventricular canal Q21.2
  atrium Q21.1
  cold (head) J00
  truncus (arteriosus) Q20.0
  variable immunodeficiency —see
    Immunodeficiency, common variable
  ventricle Q20.4
Commotio, commotion (current)
  brain —see Injury, intracranial, concussion
  cerebri —see Injury, intracranial, concussion
  retinae S05.8X-
  spinal cord —see Injury, spinal cord,
    by region
  spinalis —see Injury, spinal cord, by region
Communication
  between
    base of aorta and pulmonary artery
      Q21.4
    left ventricle and right atrium Q20.5
    pericardial sac and pleural sac Q34.8
    pulmonary artery and pulmonary vein,
      congenital Q25.72
  congenital between uterus and digestive or
    urinary tract Q51.7

Compartment syndrome (deep) (posterior)
    (traumatic) T79.A0
  abdomen T79.A3
  lower extremity (hip, buttock, thigh, leg, foot,
    toes) T79.A2
  nontraumatic
    abdomen M79.A3
    lower extremity (hip, buttock, thigh, leg,
      foot, toes) M79.A2-
    specified site NEC M79.A9
    upper extremity (shoulder, arm, forearm,
      wrist, hand, fingers) M79.A1-
  specified site NEC T79.A9
  upper extremity (shoulder, arm, forearm,
    wrist, hand, fingers) T79.A1
Compensation
  failure —see Disease, heart
  neurosis, psychoneurosis —see Disorder,
    factitious
Complaint —see also Disease
  bowel, functional K59.9
    psychogenic F45.8
  intestine, functional K59.9
    psychogenic F45.8
  kidney —see Disease, renal
  miners' J60
Complete —see condition
Complex
  Addison-Schilder E71.528
  cardiorenal —see Hypertension, cardiorenal
  Costen's M26.69
  disseminated mycobacterium avium-
    intracellulare (DMAC) A31.2
  Eisenmenger's (ventricular septal defect)
    I27.89
  hypersexual F52.8
  jumped process, spine —see Dislocation,
    vertebra
  primary, tuberculous A15.7
  Schilder-Addison E71.528
  subluxation (vertebral) M99.19
    abdomen M99.19
    acromioclavicular M99.17
    cervical region M99.11
    cervicothoracic M99.11
    costochondral M99.18
    costovertebral M99.18
    head region M99.10
    hip M99.15
    lower extremity M99.16
    lumbar region M99.13
    lumbosacral M99.13
    occipitocervical M99.10
    pelvic region M99.15
    pubic M99.15
    rib cage M99.18
    sacral region M99.14
    sacrococcygeal M99.14
    sacroiliac M99.14
    specified NEC M99.19
    sternochondral M99.18
    sternoclavicular M99.17
    thoracic region M99.12
    thoracolumbar M99.12
    upper extremity M99.17
  Taussig-Bing (transposition, aorta and
    overriding pulmonary artery) Q20.1
Complication (s) (from) (of)
  accidental puncture or laceration during a
    procedure (of) —see Complications,
    intraoperative (intraprocedural),
    puncture or laceration
  amputation stump (surgical) (late) NEC
    T87.9
    dehiscence T87.81
    infection or inflammation T87.40
      lower limb T87.4-
      upper limb T87.4-
    necrosis T87.50
      lower limb T87.5-
      upper limb T87.5-

Complication *(Continued)*
  amputation stump (surgical) (late) (NEC)
      (Continued)
    neuroma T87.3Ø
      lower limb T87.3-
      upper limb T87.3-
    specified type NEC T87.89
  anastomosis (and bypass) —*see also*
      Complications, prosthetic device or
      implant
    intestinal (internal) NEC K91.89
      involving urinary tract N99.89
    urinary tract (involving intestinal tract)
        N99.89
    vascular —*see* Complications,
        cardiovascular device or implant
  anesthesia, anesthetic —*see also* Anesthesia,
      complication T88.59
    brain, postpartum, puerperal O89.2
    cardiac
      in
        labor and delivery O74.2
        pregnancy O29.19-
      postpartum, puerperal O89.1
    central nervous system
      in
        labor and delivery O74.3
        pregnancy O29.29-
      postpartum, puerperal O89.2
    difficult or failed intubation T88.4
      in pregnancy O29.6-
    failed sedation (conscious) (moderate)
        during procedure T88.52
    general, unintended awareness during
        procedure T88.53 ◀
    hyperthermia, malignant T88.3
    hypothermia T88.51
    intubation failure T88.4
    malignant hyperthermia T88.3
    pulmonary
      in
        labor and delivery O74.1
        pregnancy NEC O29.Ø9-
      postpartum, puerperal O89.Ø9
    shock T88.2
    spinal and epidural
      in
        labor and delivery NEC O74.6
          headache O74.5
        pregnancy NEC O29.5X-
      postpartum, puerperal NEC O89.5
          headache O89.4
    unintended awareness under general
        anesthesia during procedure T88.53 ◀
  anti-reflux device —*see* Complications,
      esophageal anti-reflux device
  aortic (bifurcation) graft —*see* Complications,
      graft, vascular
  aortocoronary (bypass) graft —*see*
      Complications, coronary artery (bypass)
      graft
  aortofemoral (bypass) graft —*see*
      Complications, extremity artery
      (bypass) graft
  arteriovenous
    fistula, surgically created T82.9
      embolism T82.818
      fibrosis T82.828
      hemorrhage T82.838
      infection or inflammation T82.7
      mechanical
        breakdown T82.51Ø
        displacement T82.52Ø
        leakage T82.53Ø
        malposition T82.52Ø
        obstruction T82.59Ø
        perforation T82.59Ø
        protrusion T82.59Ø
      pain T82.848
      specified type NEC T82.898
      stenosis T82.858
      thrombosis T82.868

Complication *(Continued)*
  arteriovenous *(Continued)*
    shunt, surgically created T82.9
      embolism T82.818
      fibrosis T82.828
      hemorrhage T82.838
      infection or inflammation T82.7
      mechanical
        breakdown T82.511
        displacement T82.521
        leakage T82.531
        malposition T82.521
        obstruction T82.591
        perforation T82.591
        protrusion T82.591
      pain T82.848
      specified type NEC T82.898
      stenosis T82.858
      thrombosis T82.868
  arthroplasty —*see* Complications, joint
      prosthesis
  artificial
    fertilization or insemination N98.9
      attempted introduction (of)
        embryo in embryo transfer
            N98.3
        ovum following in vitro fertilization
            N98.2
      hyperstimulation of ovaries
          N98.1
      infection N98.Ø
      specified NEC N98.8
    heart T82.9
      embolism T82.817
      fibrosis T82.827
      hemorrhage T82.837
      infection or inflammation T82.7
      mechanical
        breakdown T82.512
        displacement T82.522
        leakage T82.532
        malposition T82.522
        obstruction T82.592
        perforation T82.592
        protrusion T82.592
      pain T82.847
      specified type NEC T82.897
      stenosis T82.857
      thrombosis T82.867
    opening
      cecostomy —*see* Complications,
          colostomy
      colostomy —*see* Complications,
          colostomy
      cystostomy —*see* Complications,
          cystostomy
      enterostomy —*see* Complications,
          enterostomy
      gastrostomy —*see* Complications,
          gastrostomy
      ileostomy —*see* Complications,
          enterostomy
      jejunostomy —*see* Complications,
          enterostomy
      nephrostomy —*see* Complications,
          stoma, urinary tract
      tracheostomy —*see* Complications,
          tracheostomy
      ureterostomy —*see* Complications,
          stoma, urinary tract
      urethrostomy —*see* Complications,
          stoma, urinary tract
  balloon implant or device
    gastrointestinal T85.9
      embolism T85.818 ◀▥
      fibrosis T85.828 ◀▥
      hemorrhage T85.838 ◀▥
      infection and inflammation T85.79
      pain T85.848 ◀▥
      specified type NEC T85.898 ◀▥
      stenosis T85.858 ◀▥
      thrombosis T85.868 ◀▥

Complication *(Continued)*
  balloon implant or device *(Continued)*
    vascular (counterpulsation) T82.9
      embolism T82.818
      fibrosis T82.828
      hemorrhage T82.838
      infection or inflammation T82.7
      mechanical
        breakdown T82.513
        displacement T82.523
        leakage T82.533
        malposition T82.523
        obstruction T82.593
        perforation T82.593
        protrusion T82.593
      pain T82.848
      specified type NEC T82.898
      stenosis T82.858
      thrombosis T82.868
  bariatric procedure
    gastric band procedure K95.Ø9
      infection K95.Ø1
    specified procedure NEC K95.89
      infection K95.81
  bile duct implant (prosthetic) T85.9
    embolism T85.818 ◀▥
    fibrosis T85.828 ◀▥
    hemorrhage T85.838 ◀▥
    infection and inflammation T85.79
    mechanical
      breakdown T85.51Ø
      displacement T85.52Ø
      malfunction T85.51Ø
      malposition T85.52Ø
      obstruction T85.59Ø
      perforation T85.59Ø
      protrusion T85.59Ø
      specified NEC T85.59Ø
    pain T85.848 ◀▥
    specified type NEC T85.898 ◀▥
    stenosis T85.858 ◀▥
    thrombosis T85.868 ◀▥
  bladder device (auxiliary) —*see*
      Complications, genitourinary, device or
      implant, urinary system
  bleeding (postoperative) —*see* Complication,
      postoperative, hemorrhage
    intraoperative —*see* Complication,
        intraoperative, hemorrhage
  blood vessel graft —*see* Complications, graft,
      vascular
  bone
    device NEC T84.9
      embolism T84.81
      fibrosis T84.82
      hemorrhage T84.83
      infection or inflammation T84.7
      mechanical
        breakdown T84.318
        displacement T84.328
        malposition T84.328
        obstruction T84.398
        perforation T84.398
        protrusion T84.398
      pain T84.84
      specified type NEC T84.89
      stenosis T84.85
      thrombosis T84.86
    graft —*see* Complications, graft, bone
    growth stimulator (electrode) —*see*
        Complications, electronic stimulator
        device, bone
    marrow transplant —*see* Complications,
        transplant, bone, marrow
  brain neurostimulator (electrode) —*see*
      Complications, electronic stimulator
      device, brain
  breast implant (prosthetic) T85.9
    capsular contracture T85.44
    embolism T85.818 ◀▥
    fibrosis T85.828 ◀▥

◀ New   ◀▥ Revised   ~~deleted~~ Deleted

Complication (Continued)
  breast implant (prosthetic) (Continued)
    hemorrhage T85.838 ◀llll
    infection and inflammation T85.79
    mechanical
      breakdown T85.41
      displacement T85.42
      leakage T85.43
      malposition T85.42
      obstruction T85.49
      perforation T85.49
      protrusion T85.49
      specified NEC T85.49
    pain T85.848 ◀llll
    specified type NEC T85.898 ◀llll
    stenosis T85.858 ◀llll
    thrombosis T85.868 ◀llll
  bypass —see also Complications, prosthetic device or implant
    aortocoronary —see Complications, coronary artery (bypass) graft
    arterial —see also Complications, graft, vascular
      extremity —see Complications, extremity artery (bypass) graft
  cardiac —see also Disease, heart
    device, implant or graft T82.9
      embolism T82.817
      fibrosis T82.827
      hemorrhage T82.837
      infection or inflammation T82.7
        valve prosthesis T82.6
      mechanical
        breakdown T82.519
          specified device NEC T82.518
        displacement T82.529
          specified device NEC T82.528
        leakage T82.539
          specified device NEC T82.538
        malposition T82.529
          specified device NEC T82.528
        obstruction T82.599
          specified device NEC T82.598
        perforation T82.599
          specified device NEC T82.598
        protrusion T82.599
          specified device NEC T82.598
      pain T82.847
      specified type NEC T82.897
      stenosis T82.857
      thrombosis T82.867
  cardiovascular device, graft or implant T82.9
    aortic graft —see Complications, graft, vascular
    arteriovenous
      fistula, artificial —see Complication, arteriovenous, fistula, surgically created
      shunt —see Complication, arteriovenous, shunt, surgically created
    artificial heart —see Complication, artificial, heart
    balloon (counterpulsation) device —see Complication, balloon implant, vascular
    carotid artery graft —see Complications, graft, vascular
    coronary bypass graft —see Complication, coronary artery (bypass) graft
    dialysis catheter (vascular) —see Complication, catheter, dialysis
    electronic T82.9
      electrode T82.9
        embolism T82.817
        fibrosis T82.827
        hemorrhage T82.837
        infection T82.7
        mechanical
          breakdown T82.110
          displacement T82.120

Complication (Continued)
  cardiovascular device, graft or implant (Continued)
    electronic (Continued)
      electrode (Continued)
        mechanical (Continued)
          leakage T82.190
          obstruction T82.190
          perforation T82.190
          protrusion T82.190
          specified type NEC T82.190
        pain T82.847
        specified NEC T82.897
        stenosis T82.857
        thrombosis T82.867
      embolism T82.817
      fibrosis T82.827
      hemorrhage T82.837
      infection T82.7
      mechanical
        breakdown T82.119
        displacement T82.129
        leakage T82.199
        obstruction T82.199
        perforation T82.199
        protrusion T82.199
        specified type NEC T82.199
      pain T82.847
      pulse generator T82.9
        embolism T82.817
        fibrosis T82.827
        hemorrhage T82.837
        infection T82.7
        mechanical
          breakdown T82.111
          displacement T82.121
          leakage T82.191
          obstruction T82.191
          perforation T82.191
          protrusion T82.191
          specified type NEC T82.191
        pain T82.847
        specified NEC T82.897
        stenosis T82.857
        thrombosis T82.867
      specified condition NEC T82.897
      specified device NEC T82.9
        embolism T82.817
        fibrosis T82.827
        hemorrhage T82.837
        infection T82.7
        mechanical
          breakdown T82.118
          displacement T82.128
          leakage T82.198
          obstruction T82.198
          perforation T82.198
          protrusion T82.198
          specified type NEC T82.198
        pain T82.847
        specified NEC T82.897
        stenosis T82.857
        thrombosis T82.867
      stenosis T82.857
      thrombosis T82.867
    extremity artery graft —see Complication, extremity artery (bypass) graft
    femoral artery graft —see Complication, extremity artery (bypass) graft
    heart
      transplant —see Complication, transplant, heart
      valve —see Complication, prosthetic device, heart valve
        graft —see Complication, heart, valve, graft
    heart-lung transplant —see Complication, transplant, heart, with lung
    infection or inflammation T82.7
    umbrella device —see Complication, umbrella device, vascular

Complication (Continued)
  cardiovascular device, graft or implant (Continued)
    vascular graft (or anastomosis) —see Complication, graft, vascular
  carotid artery (bypass) graft —see Complications, graft, vascular
  catheter (device) NEC —see also Complications, prosthetic device or implant
    cranial infusion ◀
      infection and inflammation T85.735 ◀
      mechanical ◀
        breakdown T85.610 ◀
        displacement T85.620 ◀
        leakage T85.630 ◀
        malfunction T85.690 ◀
        malposition T85.620 ◀
        obstruction T85.690 ◀
        perforation T85.690 ◀
        protrusion T85.690 ◀
        specified NEC T85.690 ◀
    cystostomy T83.9
      embolism T83.81
      fibrosis T83.82
      hemorrhage T83.83
      infection and inflammation T83.510 ◀llll
      mechanical
        breakdown T83.010
        displacement T83.020
        leakage T83.030
        malposition T83.020
        obstruction T83.090
        perforation T83.090
        protrusion T83.090
        specified NEC T83.090
      pain T83.84
      specified type NEC T83.89
      stenosis T83.85
      thrombosis T83.86
    dialysis (vascular) T82.9
      embolism T82.818
      fibrosis T82.828
      hemorrhage T82.838
      infection and inflammation T82.7
      intraperitoneal —see Complications, catheter, intraperitoneal
      mechanical
        breakdown T82.41
        displacement T82.42
        leakage T82.43
        malposition T82.42
        obstruction T82.49
        perforation T82.49
        protrusion T82.49
      pain T82.848
      specified type NEC T82.898
      stenosis T82.858
      thrombosis T82.868
    epidural infusion T85.9
      embolism T85.810 ◀llll
      fibrosis T85.820 ◀llll
      hemorrhage T85.830 ◀llll
      infection and inflammation T85.735 ◀llll
      mechanical
        breakdown T85.610
        displacement T85.620
        leakage T85.630
        malfunction T85.610
        malposition T85.620
        obstruction T85.690
        perforation T85.690
        protrusion T85.690
        specified NEC T85.690
      pain T85.840 ◀llll
      specified type NEC T85.890 ◀llll
      stenosis T85.850 ◀llll
      thrombosis T85.860 ◀llll
    intraperitoneal dialysis T85.9
      embolism T85.818 ◀llll
      fibrosis T85.828 ◀llll

Complication *(Continued)*
  catheter NEC *(Continued)*
    intraperitoneal dialysis *(Continued)*
      hemorrhage T85.838 ◄▥
      infection and inflammation T85.71
      mechanical
        breakdown T85.611
        displacement T85.621
        leakage T85.631
        malfunction T85.611
        malposition T85.621
        obstruction T85.691
        perforation T85.691
        protrusion T85.691
        specified NEC T85.691
      pain T85.848 ◄▥
      specified type NEC T85.898 ◄▥
      stenosis T85.858 ◄▥
      thrombosis T85.868 ◄▥
    intrathecal infusion ◄
      infection and inflammation T85.735 ◄
      mechanical ◄
        breakdown T85.610 ◄
        displacement T85.620 ◄
        leakage T85.630 ◄
        malfunction T85.690 ◄
        malposition T85.620 ◄
        obstruction T85.690 ◄
        perforation T85.690 ◄
        protrusion T85.690 ◄
        specified NEC T85.690 ◄
    intravenous infusion T82.9
      embolism T82.818
      fibrosis T82.828
      hemorrhage T82.838
      infection or inflammation T82.7
      mechanical
        breakdown T82.514
        displacement T82.524
        leakage T82.534
        malposition T82.524
        obstruction T82.594
        perforation T82.594
        protrusion T82.594
      pain T82.848
      specified type NEC T82.898
      stenosis T82.858
      thrombosis T82.868
    spinal infusion ◄
      infection and inflammation T85.735 ◄
      mechanical ◄
        breakdown T85.610 ◄
        displacement T85.620 ◄
        leakage T85.630 ◄
        malfunction T85.690 ◄
        malposition T85.620 ◄
        obstruction T85.690 ◄
        perforation T85.690 ◄
        protrusion T85.690 ◄
        specified NEC T85.690 ◄
    subarachnoid infusion ◄
      infection and inflammation T85.735 ◄
      mechanical ◄
        breakdown T85.610 ◄
        displacement T85.620 ◄
        leakage T85.630 ◄
        malfunction T85.690 ◄
        malposition T85.620 ◄
        obstruction T85.690 ◄
        perforation T85.690 ◄
        protrusion T85.690 ◄
        specified NEC T85.690 ◄
    subdural infusion T85.9
      embolism T85.810 ◄▥
      fibrosis T85.820 ◄▥
      hemorrhage T85.830 ◄▥
      infection and inflammation T85.735 ◄▥
      mechanical
        breakdown T85.610
        displacement T85.620
        leakage T85.630

Complication *(Continued)*
  catheter NEC *(Continued)*
    subdural infusion *(Continued)*
      mechanical *(Continued)*
        malfunction T85.610
        malposition T85.620
        obstruction T85.690
        perforation T85.690
        protrusion T85.690
        specified NEC T85.690
      pain T85.840 ◄▥
      specified type NEC T85.890 ◄▥
      stenosis T85.850 ◄▥
      thrombosis T85.860 ◄▥
    ~~urethral, indwelling T83.9~~
      ~~displacement T83.028~~
      ~~embolism T83.81~~
      ~~fibrosis T83.82~~
      ~~hemorrhage T83.83~~
      ~~infection and inflammation T83.51~~
      ~~leakage T83.038~~
      ~~malposition T83.028~~
      ~~mechanical~~
        ~~breakdown T83.018~~
      ~~obstruction (mechanical) T83.098~~
      ~~pain T83.84~~
      ~~perforation T83.098~~
      ~~protrusion T83.098~~
      ~~specified type NEC T83.098~~
      ~~stenosis T83.85~~
      ~~thrombosis T83.86~~
    ~~urinary (indwelling) —see Complications,~~
      ~~catheter, urethral, indwelling~~
    urethral T83.9 ◄
      displacement T83.028 ◄
      embolism T83.81 ◄
      fibrosis T83.82 ◄
      hemorrhage T83.83 ◄
      indwelling ◄
        breakdown T83.011 ◄
        displacement T83.021 ◄
        infection and inflammation T83.511 ◄
        leakage T83.031 ◄
        specified complication NEC T83.091 ◄
      infection and inflammation T83.511 ◄
      leakage T83.038 ◄
      malposition T83.028 ◄
      mechanical ◄
        breakdown T83.011 ◄
      obstruction (mechanical) T83.091 ◄
      pain T83.84 ◄
      perforation T83.091 ◄
      protrusion T83.091 ◄
      specified type NEC T83.091 ◄
      stenosis T83.85 ◄
      thrombosis T83.86 ◄
    urinary NEC ◄
      breakdown T83.018 ◄
      displacement T83.028 ◄
      infection and inflammation T83.518 ◄
      leakage T83.038 ◄
      specified complication NEC T83.098 ◄
  cecostomy (stoma) —see Complications,
    colostomy
  cesarean delivery wound NEC O90.89
    disruption O90.0
    hematoma O90.2
    infection (following delivery) O86.0
  chemotherapy (antineoplastic) NEC T88.7
  chin implant (prosthetic) —see Complication,
    prosthetic device or implant, specified
    NEC
  circulatory system I99.8
    intraoperative I97.88
    postprocedural I97.89
      following cardiac surgery I97.19-
        postcardiotomy syndrome I97.0
      hypertension I97.3
      lymphedema after mastectomy I97.2
      postcardiotomy syndrome I97.0
      specified NEC I97.89

Complication *(Continued)*
  colostomy (stoma) K94.00
    hemorrhage K94.01
    infection K94.02
    malfunction K94.03
    mechanical K94.03
    specified complication NEC
      K94.09
  contraceptive device, intrauterine —
    see Complications, intrauterine,
    contraceptive device
  cord (umbilical) —*see* Complications,
    umbilical cord
  corneal graft —*see* Complications, graft,
    cornea
  coronary artery (bypass) graft T82.9
    atherosclerosis —*see* Arteriosclerosis,
      coronary (artery)
    embolism T82.818
    fibrosis T82.828
    hemorrhage T82.838
    infection and inflammation T82.7
    mechanical
      breakdown T82.211
      displacement T82.212
      leakage T82.213
      malposition T82.212
      obstruction T82.218
      perforation T82.218
      protrusion T82.218
      specified NEC T82.218
    pain T82.848
    specified type NEC T82.898 ◄▥
    stenosis T82.858
    thrombosis T82.868
  counterpulsation device (balloon), intra-
    aortic —*see* Complications, balloon
    implant, vascular
  cystostomy (stoma) N99.518
    catheter —*see* Complications, catheter,
      cystostomy
    hemorrhage N99.510
    infection N99.511
    malfunction N99.512
    specified type NEC N99.518
  delivery —*see also* Complications, obstetric
    O75.9
    procedure (instrumental) (manual)
      (surgical) O75.4
    specified NEC O75.89
  dialysis (peritoneal) (renal) —*see also*
    Complications, infusion
    catheter (vascular) —*see* Complication,
      catheter, dialysis
      peritoneal, intraperitoneal —*see*
        Complications, catheter,
        intraperitoneal
  dorsal column (spinal) neurostimulator —*see*
    Complications, electronic stimulator
    device, spinal cord
  drug NEC T88.7
  ear procedure —*see also* Disorder, ear
    intraoperative H95.88-
      hematoma —*see* Complications,
        intraoperative, hematoma (of),
        ear ◄▥
      hemorrhage —*see* Complications,
        intraoperative, hemorrhage (of),
        ear ◄▥
      laceration —*see* Complications,
        intraoperative, puncture or
        laceration..., ear
      seroma —*see* Complications,
        postprocedural, seroma (of),
        mastoid process ◄
      specified NEC H95.88-
    postoperative H95.89-
      external ear canal stenosis H95.81-
      hematoma —*see* Complications,
        postprocedural, hemorrhage
        (hematoma) (of), ear

◄ New   ◄▥ Revised   ~~deleted~~ Deleted

Complication (Continued)
  ear procedure (Continued)
    postoperative (Continued)
      hemorrhage —see Complications,
        postprocedural, hemorrhage
        (hematoma) (of), ear
      postmastoidectomy —see Complications,
        postmastoidectomy
      specified NEC H95.89-
  ectopic pregnancy O08.9
    damage to pelvic organs O08.6
    embolism O08.2
    genital infection O08.0
    hemorrhage (delayed) (excessive) O08.1
    metabolic disorder O08.5
    renal failure O08.4
    shock O08.3
    specified type NEC O08.0
    venous complication NEC O08.7
  electronic stimulator device
    bladder (urinary) —see Complications,
      electronic stimulator device, urinary
    bone T84.9
      breakdown T84.310
      displacement T84.320
      embolism T84.81
      fibrosis T84.82
      hemorrhage T84.83
      infection or inflammation T84.7
      malfunction T84.310
      malposition T84.320
      mechanical NEC T84.390
      obstruction T84.390
      pain T84.84
      perforation T84.390
      protrusion T84.390
      specified type NEC T84.89
      stenosis T84.85
      thrombosis T84.86
    brain T85.9
      embolism T85.810 ◀▥
      fibrosis T85.820 ◀▥
      hemorrhage T85.830 ◀▥
      infection and inflammation T85.731 ◀▥
      mechanical
        breakdown T85.110
        displacement T85.120
        leakage T85.190
        malposition T85.120
        obstruction T85.190
        perforation T85.190
        protrusion T85.190
        specified NEC T85.190
      pain T85.840 ◀▥
      specified type NEC T85.890 ◀▥
      stenosis T85.850 ◀▥
      thrombosis T85.860 ◀▥
    cardiac (defibrillator) (pacemaker) —see
      Complications, cardiovascular device
      or implant, electronic
    generator (brain) (gastric) (peripheral)
      (sacral) (spinal) ◀
      breakdown T85.113 ◀
      displacement T85.123 ◀
      leakage T85.193 ◀
      malposition T85.123 ◀
      obstruction T85.193 ◀
      perforation T85.193 ◀
      protrusion T85.193 ◀
      specified type NEC T85.193 ◀
    muscle T84.9
      breakdown T84.418
      displacement T84.428
      embolism T84.81
      fibrosis T84.82
      hemorrhage T84.83
      infection or inflammation T84.7
      mechanical NEC T84.498
      pain T84.84
      specified type NEC T84.89
      stenosis T84.85
      thrombosis T84.86

Complication (Continued)
  electronic stimulator device (Continued)
    nervous system T85.9
      brain —see Complications, electronic
        stimulator device, brain
      cranial nerve —see Complications,
        electronic stimulator device,
        peripheral nerve ◀
      embolism T85.810 ◀▥
      fibrosis T85.820 ◀▥
      gastric nerve —see Complications,
        electronic stimulator device,
        peripheral nerve ◀
      hemorrhage T85.830 ◀▥
      infection and inflammation T85.738 ◀▥
      mechanical
        breakdown T85.118
        displacement T85.128
        leakage T85.199
        malposition T85.128
        obstruction T85.199
        perforation T85.199
        protrusion T85.199
        specified NEC T85.199
      pain T85.840 ◀▥
      peripheral nerve —see Complications,
        electronic stimulator device,
        peripheral nerve
      sacral nerve —see Complications,
        electronic stimulator device,
        peripheral nerve ◀
      specified type NEC T85.890 ◀▥
      spinal cord —see Complications,
        electronic stimulator device, spinal
        cord
      stenosis T85.850 ◀▥
      thrombosis T85.860 ◀▥
      vagal nerve —see Complications,
        electronic stimulator device,
        peripheral nerve ◀
    peripheral nerve T85.9
      embolism T85.810 ◀▥
      fibrosis T85.820 ◀▥
      hemorrhage T85.830 ◀▥
      infection and inflammation T85.732 ◀▥
      mechanical
        breakdown T85.111
        displacement T85.121
        leakage T85.191
        malposition T85.121
        obstruction T85.191
        perforation T85.191
        protrusion T85.191
        specified NEC T85.191
      pain T85.840 ◀▥
      specified type NEC T85.890 ◀▥
      stenosis T85.850 ◀▥
      thrombosis T85.860 ◀▥
    spinal cord T85.9
      embolism T85.810 ◀▥
      fibrosis T85.820 ◀▥
      hemorrhage T85.830 ◀▥
      infection and inflammation T85.733 ◀▥
      mechanical
        breakdown T85.112
        displacement T85.122
        leakage T85.192
        malposition T85.122
        obstruction T85.192
        perforation T85.192
        protrusion T85.192
        specified NEC T85.192
      pain T85.840 ◀▥
      specified type NEC T85.890 ◀▥
      stenosis T85.850 ◀▥
      thrombosis T85.860 ◀▥
    urinary T83.9
      embolism T83.81
      fibrosis T83.82
      hemorrhage T83.83
      infection and inflammation T83.598 ◀▥

Complication (Continued)
  electronic stimulator device (Continued)
    urinary (Continued)
      mechanical
        breakdown T83.110
        displacement T83.120
        malposition T83.120
        perforation T83.190
        protrusion T83.190
        specified NEC T83.190
      pain T83.84
      specified type NEC T83.89
      stenosis T83.85
      thrombosis T83.86
  electroshock therapy T88.9
    specified NEC T88.8
  endocrine E34.9
    postprocedural
      adrenal hypofunction E89.6
      hypoinsulinemia E89.1
      hypoparathyroidism E89.2
      hypopituitarism E89.3
      hypothyroidism E89.0
      ovarian failure E89.40
        asymptomatic E89.40
        symptomatic E89.41
      specified NEC E89.89
      testicular hypofunction E89.5
  endodontic treatment NEC M27.59
  enterostomy (stoma) K94.10
    hemorrhage K94.11
    infection K94.12
    malfunction K94.13
    mechanical K94.13
    specified complication NEC K94.19
  episiotomy, disruption O90.1
  esophageal anti-reflux device T85.9
    embolism T85.818 ◀▥
    fibrosis T85.828 ◀▥
    hemorrhage T85.838 ◀▥
    infection and inflammation T85.79
    mechanical
      breakdown T85.511
      displacement T85.521
      malfunction T85.511
      malposition T85.521
      obstruction T85.591
      perforation T85.591
      protrusion T85.591
      specified NEC T85.591
    pain T85.848 ◀▥
    specified type NEC T85.898 ◀▥
    stenosis T85.858 ◀▥
    thrombosis T85.868 ◀▥
  esophagostomy K94.30
    hemorrhage K94.31
    infection K94.32
    malfunction K94.33
    mechanical K94.33
    specified complication NEC K94.39
  extracorporeal circulation T80.90
  extremity artery (bypass) graft T82.9
    arteriosclerosis —see Arteriosclerosis,
      extremities, bypass graft
    embolism T82.818
    fibrosis T82.828
    hemorrhage T82.838
    infection and inflammation T82.7
    mechanical
      breakdown T82.318
        femoral artery T82.312
      displacement T82.328
        femoral artery T82.322
      leakage T82.338
        femoral artery T82.332
      malposition T82.328
        femoral artery T82.322
      obstruction T82.398
        femoral artery T82.392
      perforation T82.398
        femoral artery T82.392

Complication *(Continued)*
  extremity artery (bypass) graft *(Continued)*
    mechanical *(Continued)*
      protrusion T82.398
        femoral artery T82.392
      pain T82.848
      specified type NEC T82.898
      stenosis T82.858
      thrombosis T82.868
  eye H57.9
    corneal graft —*see* Complications, graft,
      cornea
    implant (prosthetic) T85.9
      embolism T85.818 ◄‖‖
      fibrosis T85.828 ◄‖‖
      hemorrhage T85.838 ◄‖‖
      infection and inflammation T85.79
      mechanical
        breakdown T85.318
        displacement T85.328
        leakage T85.398
        malposition T85.328
        obstruction T85.398
        perforation T85.398
        protrusion T85.398
        specified NEC T85.398
      pain T85.848 ◄‖‖
      specified type NEC T85.898 ◄‖‖
      stenosis T85.858 ◄‖‖
      thrombosis T85.868 ◄‖‖
    intraocular lens —*see* Complications,
      intraocular lens
    orbital prosthesis —*see* Complications,
      orbital prosthesis
  female genital N94.9
    device, implant or graft NEC —*see*
      Complications, genitourinary, device
      or implant, genital tract
  femoral artery (bypass) graft —*see*
    Complication, extremity artery (bypass)
    graft
  fixation device, internal (orthopedic) T84.9
    infection and inflammation T84.60
      arm T84.61-
        humerus T84.61-
        radius T84.61-
        ulna T84.61-
      leg T84.629
        femur T84.62-
        fibula T84.62-
        tibia T84.62-
      specified site NEC T84.69
      spine T84.63
    mechanical
      breakdown
        limb T84.119
          carpal T84.210
          femur T84.11-
          fibula T84.11-
          humerus T84.11-
          metacarpal T84.210
          metatarsal T84.213
          phalanx
            foot T84.213
            hand T84.210
          radius T84.11-
          tarsal T84.213
          tibia T84.11-
          ulna T84.11-
        specified bone NEC T84.218
        spine T84.216
      displacement
        limb T84.129
          carpal T84.220
          femur T84.12-
          fibula T84.12-
          humerus T84.12-
          metacarpal T84.220
          metatarsal T84.223
          phalanx
            foot T84.223
            hand T84.220

Complication *(Continued)*
  fixation device, internal *(Continued)*
    mechanical *(Continued)*
      displacement *(Continued)*
        limb *(Continued)*
          radius T84.12-
          tarsal T84.223
          tibia T84.12-
          ulna T84.12-
        specified bone NEC T84.228
        spine T84.226
      malposition —*see* Complications,
        fixation device, internal,
        mechanical, displacement
      obstruction —*see* Complications, fixation
        device, internal, mechanical,
        specified type NEC
      perforation —*see* Complications, fixation
        device, internal, mechanical,
        specified type NEC
      protrusion —*see* Complications, fixation
        device, internal, mechanical,
        specified type NEC
      specified type NEC
        limb T84.199
          carpal T84.290
          femur T84.19-
          fibula T84.19-
          humerus T84.19-
          metacarpal T84.290
          metatarsal T84.293
          phalanx
            foot T84.293
            hand T84.290
          radius T84.19-
          tarsal T84.293
          tibia T84.19-
          ulna T84.19-
        specified bone NEC T84.298
        vertebra T84.296
    specified type NEC T84.89
      embolism T84.81
      fibrosis T84.82
      hemorrhage T84.83
      pain T84.84
      specified complication NEC T84.89
      stenosis T84.85
      thrombosis T84.86
  following
    acute myocardial infarction NEC I23.8
      aneurysm (false) (of cardiac wall) (of
        heart wall) (ruptured) I23.3
      angina I23.7
      atrial
        septal defect I23.1
        thrombosis I23.6
      cardiac wall rupture I23.3
      chordae tendinae rupture I23.4
      defect
        septal
          atrial (heart) I23.1
          ventricular (heart) I23.2
      hemopericardium I23.0
      papillary muscle rupture I23.5
      rupture
        cardiac wall I23.3
          with hemopericardium I23.0
        chordae tendineae I23.4
        papillary muscle I23.5
      specified NEC I23.8
      thrombosis
        atrium I23.6
        auricular appendage I23.6
        ventricle (heart) I23.6
      ventricular
        septal defect I23.2
        thrombosis I23.6
    ectopic or molar pregnancy
      O08.9
      cardiac arrest O08.81
      sepsis O08.82

Complication *(Continued)*
  following *(Continued)*
    ectopic or molar pregnancy *(Continued)*
      specified type NEC O08.89
      urinary tract infection O08.83
    termination of pregnancy —*see* Abortion
  gastrointestinal K92.9
    bile duct prosthesis —*see* Complications,
      bile duct implant
    esophageal anti-reflux device —*see*
      Complications, esophageal
      anti-reflux device
    postoperative
      colostomy —*see* Complications,
        colostomy
      dumping syndrome K91.1
      enterostomy —*see* Complications,
        enterostomy
      gastrostomy —*see* Complications,
        gastrostomy
      malabsorption NEC K91.2
      obstruction K91.3
      postcholecystectomy syndrome K91.5
      specified NEC K91.89
      vomiting after GI surgery K91.0
    prosthetic device or implant
      bile duct prosthesis —*see* Complications,
        bile duct implant
      esophageal anti-reflux device —*see*
        Complications, esophageal anti-
        reflux device
      specified type NEC
        embolism T85.818 ◄‖‖
        fibrosis T85.828 ◄‖‖
        hemorrhage T85.838 ◄‖‖
        mechanical
          breakdown T85.518
          displacement T85.528
          malfunction T85.518
          malposition T85.528
          obstruction T85.598
          perforation T85.598
          protrusion T85.598
          specified NEC T85.598
        pain T85.848 ◄‖‖
        specified complication NEC
          T85.898 ◄‖‖
        stenosis T85.858 ◄‖‖
        thrombosis T85.868 ◄‖‖
  gastrostomy (stoma) K94.20
    hemorrhage K94.21
    infection K94.22
    malfunction K94.23
    mechanical K94.23
    specified complication NEC K94.29
  genitourinary
    device or implant T83.9
      genital tract T83.9
        infection or inflammation T83.69 ◄‖‖
        intrauterine contraceptive device —*see*
          Complications, intrauterine,
          contraceptive device
        mechanical —*see* Complications, by
          device, mechanical
        mesh —*see* Complications, mesh
        penile prosthesis —*see* Complications,
          prosthetic device, penile
        specified type NEC T83.89
          embolism T83.81
          fibrosis T83.82
          hemorrhage T83.83
          pain T83.84
          specified complication NEC T83.89
          stenosis T83.85
          thrombosis T83.86
        vaginal mesh —*see* Complications,
          mesh
      urinary system T83.9
        cystostomy catheter —*see*
          Complication, catheter,
          cystostomy

◄ New   ◄‖‖ Revised   ~~deleted~~ Deleted

Complication *(Continued)*
  genitourinary *(Continued)*
    device or implant *(Continued)*
      urinary system *(Continued)*
        electronic stimulator —*see*
            Complications, electronic
            stimulator device, urinary
        indwelling urethral catheter —*see*
            Complications, catheter, urethral,
            indwelling
        infection or inflammation T83.598 ◀⫿⫿
          ~~indwelling urinary catheter T83.51~~
          indwelling urethral catheter
              T83.511 ◀
        kidney transplant —*see* Complication,
            transplant, kidney
        organ graft —*see* Complication, graft,
            urinary organ
        specified type NEC T83.89
          embolism T83.81
          fibrosis T83.82
          hemorrhage T83.83
          mechanical T83.198
            breakdown T83.118
            displacement T83.128
            malfunction T83.118
            malposition T83.128
            obstruction T83.198
            perforation T83.198
            protrusion T83.198
            specified NEC T83.198
          sphincter, implanted T83.191 ◀
          stent (ileal conduit) (nephroureteral)
              T83.193 ◀
          ureteral indwelling T83.192 ◀
          pain T83.84
          specified complication NEC T83.89
          stenosis T83.85
          thrombosis T83.86
        sphincter implant —*see*
            Complications, implant, urinary
            sphincter
    postprocedural
      pelvic peritoneal adhesions N99.4
      renal failure N99.0
      specified NEC N99.89
      stoma —*see* Complications, stoma,
          urinary tract
      urethral stricture —*see* Stricture, urethra,
          postprocedural
      vaginal
        adhesions N99.2
        vault prolapse N99.3
  graft (bypass) (patch) —*see also*
        Complications, prosthetic device or
        implant
    aorta —*see* Complications, graft, vascular
    arterial —*see* Complication, graft, vascular
    bone T86.839
      failure T86.831
      infection T86.832
      mechanical T84.318
        breakdown T84.318
        displacement T84.328
        protrusion T84.398
        specified type NEC T84.398
      rejection T86.830
      specified type NEC T86.838
    carotid artery —*see* Complications, graft,
        vascular
    cornea T86.849
      failure T86.841
      infection T86.842
      mechanical T85.398
        breakdown T85.318
        displacement T85.328
        protrusion T85.398
        specified type NEC T85.398
      rejection T86.840
      retroprosthetic membrane T85.398
      specified type NEC T86.848

Complication *(Continued)*
  graft *(Continued)*
    femoral artery (bypass) —*see* Complication,
        extremity artery (bypass) graft
    genital organ or tract —*see* Complications,
        genitourinary, device or implant,
        genital tract
    muscle T84.9
      breakdown T84.410
      displacement T84.420
      embolism T84.81
      fibrosis T84.82
      hemorrhage T84.83
      infection and inflammation T84.7
      mechanical NEC T84.490
      pain T84.84
      specified type NEC T84.89
      stenosis T84.85
      thrombosis T84.86
    nerve —*see* Complication, prosthetic device
        or implant, specified NEC
    skin —*see* Complications, prosthetic device
        or implant, skin graft
    tendon T84.9
      breakdown T84.410
      displacement T84.420
      embolism T84.81
      fibrosis T84.82
      hemorrhage T84.83
      infection and inflammation T84.7
      mechanical NEC T84.490
      pain T84.84
      specified type NEC T84.89
      stenosis T84.85
      thrombosis T84.86
    urinary organ T83.9
      embolism T83.81
      fibrosis T83.82
      hemorrhage T83.83
      infection and inflammation
          T83.598 ◀⫿⫿
        indwelling urethral catheter
            T83.511 ◀⫿⫿
      mechanical
        breakdown T83.21
        displacement T83.22
        erosion T83.24 ◀
        exposure T83.25 ◀
        leakage T83.23
        malposition T83.22
        obstruction T83.29
        perforation T83.29
        protrusion T83.29
        specified NEC T83.29
      pain T83.84
      specified type NEC T83.89
      stenosis T83.85
      thrombosis T83.86
    vascular T82.9
      embolism T82.818
      femoral artery —*see* Complication,
          extremity artery (bypass) graft
      fibrosis T82.828
      hemorrhage T82.838
      mechanical
        breakdown T82.319
          aorta (bifurcation) T82.310
          carotid artery T82.311
          specified vessel NEC T82.318
        displacement T82.329
          aorta (bifurcation) T82.320
          carotid artery T82.321
          specified vessel NEC T82.328
        leakage T82.339
          aorta (bifurcation) T82.330
          carotid artery T82.331
          specified vessel NEC T82.338
        malposition T82.329
          aorta (bifurcation) T82.320
          carotid artery T82.321
          specified vessel NEC T82.328

Complication *(Continued)*
  graft *(Continued)*
    vascular *(Continued)*
      mechanical *(Continued)*
        obstruction T82.399
          aorta (bifurcation) T82.390
          carotid artery T82.391
          specified vessel NEC T82.398
        perforation T82.399
          aorta (bifurcation) T82.390
          carotid artery T82.391
          specified vessel NEC T82.398
        protrusion T82.399
          aorta (bifurcation) T82.390
          carotid artery T82.391
          specified vessel NEC T82.398
      pain T82.848
      specified complication NEC
          T82.898
      stenosis T82.858
      thrombosis T82.868
  heart I51.9
    assist device
      infection and inflammation T82.7
    following acute myocardial infarction —
        see Complications, following, acute
        myocardial infarction
    postoperative —*see* Complications,
        circulatory system
    transplant —*see* Complication, transplant,
        heart
      and lung (s) —*see* Complications,
          transplant, heart, with lung
    valve
      graft (biological) T82.9
        embolism T82.817
        fibrosis T82.827
        hemorrhage T82.837
        infection and inflammation
            T82.7
        mechanical T82.228
          breakdown T82.221
          displacement T82.222
          leakage T82.223
          malposition T82.222
          obstruction T82.228
          perforation T82.228
          protrusion T82.228
        pain T82.847
        specified type NEC T82.897
        stenosis T82.857
        thrombosis T82.867
      prosthesis T82.9
        embolism T82.817
        fibrosis T82.827
        hemorrhage T82.837
        infection or inflammation T82.6
        mechanical T82.09
          breakdown T82.01
          displacement T82.02
          leakage T82.03
          malposition T82.02
          obstruction T82.09
          perforation T82.09
          protrusion T82.09
        pain T82.847
        specified type NEC T82.897
          mechanical T82.09
        stenosis T82.857
        thrombosis T82.867
  hematoma
    intraoperative —*see* Complication,
        intraoperative, hemorrhage
    postprocedural —*see* Complication,
        postprocedural, hematoma ◀⫿⫿
  hemodialysis —*see* Complications, dialysis
  hemorrhage
    intraoperative —*see* Complication,
        intraoperative, hemorrhage
    postprocedural —*see* Complication,
        postprocedural, hemorrhage

Complication *(Continued)*
  ileostomy (stoma) —*see* Complications,
      enterostomy
  immunization (procedure) —*see*
      Complications, vaccination
  implant —*see also* Complications, by site and
      type
    urinary sphincter T83.9
      embolism T83.81
      fibrosis T83.82
      hemorrhage T83.83
      infection and inflammation
          T83.591 ⬅
      mechanical
        breakdown T83.111
        displacement T83.121
        leakage T83.191
        malposition T83.121
        obstruction T83.191
        perforation T83.191
        protrusion T83.191
        specified NEC T83.191
      pain T83.84
      specified type NEC T83.89
      stenosis T83.85
      thrombosis T83.86
  infusion (procedure) T80.90
    air embolism T80.0
    blood —*see* Complications, transfusion
    catheter —*see* Complications, catheter
    infection T80.29
    pump —*see* Complications, cardiovascular,
        device or implant
    sepsis T80.29
    serum reaction —*see also* Reaction, serum
        T80.69
      anaphylactic shock —*see also* Shock,
          anaphylactic T80.59
    specified type NEC T80.89
  inhalation therapy NEC T81.81
  injection (procedure) T80.90
    drug reaction —*see* Reaction, drug
    infection T80.29
    sepsis T80.29
    serum (prophylactic) (therapeutic) —*see*
        Complications, vaccination
    specified type NEC T80.89
    vaccine (any) —*see* Complications,
        vaccination
  inoculation (any) —*see* Complications,
      vaccination
  insulin pump
    infection and inflammation T85.72
    mechanical
      breakdown T85.614
      displacement T85.624
      leakage T85.633
      malposition T85.624
      obstruction T85.694
      perforation T85.694
      protrusion T85.694
      specified NEC T85.694
  intestinal pouch NEC K91.858
  intraocular lens (prosthetic) T85.9
    embolism T85.818 ⬅
    fibrosis T85.828 ⬅
    hemorrhage T85.838 ⬅
    infection and inflammation
        T85.79
    mechanical
      breakdown T85.21
      displacement T85.22
      malposition T85.22
      obstruction T85.29
      perforation T85.29
      protrusion T85.29
      specified NEC T85.29
    pain T85.848 ⬅
    specified type NEC T85.898 ⬅
    stenosis T85.858 ⬅
    thrombosis T85.868 ⬅

Complication *(Continued)*
  intraoperative (intraprocedural)
    cardiac arrest
      during cardiac surgery I97.710
      during other surgery I97.711
    cardiac functional disturbance NEC
      during cardiac surgery I97.790
      during other surgery I97.791
    hemorrhage (hematoma) (of)
      circulatory system organ or structure
        during cardiac bypass I97.411
        during cardiac catheterization I97.410
        during other circulatory system
            procedure I97.418
        during other procedure I97.42
      digestive system organ
        during procedure on digestive system
            K91.61
        during procedure on other organ
            K91.62
      ear
        during procedure on ear and mastoid
            process H95.21
        during procedure on other organ
            H95.22
      endocrine system organ or structure
        during procedure on endocrine
            system organ or structure E36.01
        during procedure on other organ
            E36.02
      eye and adnexa
        during ophthalmic procedure H59.11-
        during other procedure H59.12-
      genitourinary organ or structure
        during procedure on genitourinary
            organ or structure N99.61
        during procedure on other organ
            N99.62
      mastoid process
        during procedure on ear and mastoid
            process H95.21
        during procedure on other organ
            H95.22
      musculoskeletal structure
        during musculoskeletal surgery
            M96.810
        during non-orthopedic surgery
            M96.811
        during orthopedic surgery M96.810
      nervous system
        during a nervous system procedure
            G97.31
        during other procedure G97.32
      respiratory system
        during other procedure J95.62
        during procedure on respiratory
            system organ or structure J95.61
      skin and subcutaneous tissue
        during a dermatologic procedure
            L76.01
        during a procedure on other organ
            L76.02
      spleen
        during a procedure on other organ
            D78.02
        during a procedure on the spleen
            D78.01
    puncture or laceration (accidental)
        (unintentional) (of)
      brain
        during a nervous system procedure
            G97.48
        during other procedure G97.49
      circulatory system organ or structure
        during circulatory system procedure
            I97.51
        during other procedure I97.52
      digestive system
        during procedure on digestive system
            K91.71
        during procedure on other organ
            K91.72

Complication *(Continued)*
  intraoperative *(Continued)*
    puncture or laceration *(Continued)*
      ear
        during procedure on ear and mastoid
            process H95.31
        during procedure on other organ
            H95.32
      endocrine system organ or structure
        during procedure on endocrine
            system organ or structure E36.11
        during procedure on other organ
            E36.12
      eye and adnexa
        during ophthalmic procedure H59.21-
        during other procedure H59.22-
      genitourinary organ or structure
        during procedure on genitourinary
            organ or structure N99.71
        during procedure on other organ
            N99.72
      mastoid process
        during procedure on ear and mastoid
            process H95.31
        during procedure on other organ
            H95.32
      musculoskeletal structure
        during musculoskeletal surgery
            M96.820
        during non-orthopedic surgery
            M96.821
        during orthopedic surgery M96.820
      nervous system
        during a nervous system procedure
            G97.48
        during other procedure G97.49
      respiratory system
        during other procedure J95.72
        during procedure on respiratory
            system organ or structure J95.71
      skin and subcutaneous tissue
        during a dermatologic procedure
            L76.11
        during a procedure on other organ
            L76.12
      spleen
        during a procedure on other organ
            D78.12
        during a procedure on the spleen
            D78.11
    specified NEC
      circulatory system I97.88
      digestive system K91.81
      ear H95.88
      endocrine system E36.8
      eye and adnexa H59.88
      genitourinary system N99.81
      mastoid process H95.88
      musculoskeletal structure M96.89
      nervous system G97.81
      respiratory system J95.88
      skin and subcutaneous tissue L76.81
      spleen D78.81
  intraperitoneal catheter (dialysis)
      (infusion) —*see* Complications, catheter,
      intraperitoneal
  intrathecal infusion pump ◄
    infection and inflammation T85.738 ◄
    mechanical ◄
      breakdown T85.615 ◄
      displacement T85.625 ◄
      leakage T85.635 ◄
      malfunction T85.695 ◄
      malposition T85.625 ◄
      obstruction T85.695 ◄
      perforation T85.695 ◄
      protrusion T85.695 ◄
      specified NEC T85.695 ◄
  intrauterine
    contraceptive device
      embolism T83.81
      fibrosis T83.82

◄ New   ⬅ Revised   ~~deleted~~ Deleted

Complication (Continued)
  intrauterine (Continued)
    contraceptive device (Continued)
      hemorrhage T83.83
      infection and inflammation T83.69 ◄▥
      mechanical
        breakdown T83.31
        displacement T83.32
        malposition T83.32
        obstruction T83.39
        perforation T83.39
        protrusion T83.39
        specified NEC T83.39
      pain T83.84
      specified type NEC T83.89
      stenosis T83.85
      thrombosis T83.86
    procedure (fetal), to newborn P96.5
  jejunostomy (stoma) —see Complications,
      enterostomy
  joint prosthesis, internal T84.9
    breakage (fracture) T84.01-
    dislocation T84.02-
    fracture T84.01-
    infection or inflammation T84.50
      hip T84.5-
      knee T84.5-
      specified joint NEC T84.59
    instability T84.02-
    malposition —see Complications, joint
        prosthesis, mechanical, displacement
    mechanical
      breakage, broken T84.01-
      dislocation T84.02-
      fracture T84.01-
      instability T84.02-
      leakage —see Complications, joint
          prosthesis, mechanical, specified
          NEC
      loosening T84.039
        hip T84.03-
        knee T84.03-
        specified joint NEC T84.038
      obstruction —see Complications, joint
          prosthesis, mechanical, specified
          NEC
      perforation —see Complications, joint
          prosthesis, mechanical, specified
          NEC
      periprosthetic
        fracture T84.049
          hip T84.04-
          knee T84.04-
          other specified joint T84.048
      osteolysis T84.059 ◄
        hip T84.05- ◄
        knee T84.05- ◄
        other specified joint T84.058 ◄
      protrusion —see Complications, joint
          prosthesis, mechanical, specified
          NEC
      specified complication NEC T84.099
        hip T84.09-
        knee T84.09-
        other specified joint T84.098
      subluxation T84.02-
      wear of articular bearing surface T84.069
        hip T84.06-
        knee T84.06-
        other specified joint T84.068
    specified joint NEC T84.89
      embolism T84.81
      fibrosis T84.82
      hemorrhage T84.83
      pain T84.84
      specified complication NEC T84.89
      stenosis T84.85
      thrombosis T84.86
    subluxation T84.02-
  kidney transplant —see Complications,
      transplant, kidney

Complication (Continued)
  labor O75.9
    specified NEC O75.89
  liver transplant (immune or nonimmune) —
      see Complications, transplant, liver
  lumbar puncture G97.1
    cerebrospinal fluid leak G97.0
    headache or reaction G97.1
  lung transplant —see Complications,
      transplant, lung
    and heart —see Complications, transplant,
        lung, with heart
  male genital N50.9
    device, implant or graft —see
        Complications, genitourinary, device
        or implant, genital tract
    postprocedural or postoperative —see
        Complications, genitourinary,
        postprocedural
    specified NEC N99.89
  mastoid (process) procedure
    intraoperative H95.88-
      hematoma —see Complications,
          intraoperative, hemorrhage
          (hematoma) (of), mastoid
          process
      hemorrhage —see Complications,
          intraoperative, hemorrhage
          (hematoma) (of), mastoid
          process
      laceration —see Complications,
          intraoperative, puncture or
          laceration..., mastoid
          process
      specified NEC H95.88-
    postmastoidectomy —see Complications,
        postmastoidectomy
    postoperative H95.89-
      external ear canal stenosis H95.81-
      hematoma —see Complications...,
          postprocedural, hematoma (of),
          mastoid process ◄▥
      hemorrhage —see Complications...,
          postprocedural, hemorrhage (of),
          mastoid process ◄▥
      postmastoidectomy —see Complications,
          postmastoidectomy
      seroma —see Complications,
          postprocedural, seroma (of),
          mastoid process ◄
      specified NEC H95.89-
    mastoidectomy cavity —see Complications,
        postmastoidectomy
  mechanical —see Complications, by site and
      type, mechanical
  medical procedures (see also Complication(s),
      intraoperative) T88.9
  metabolic E88.9
    postoperative E89.89
    specified NEC E89.89
  molar pregnancy NOS O08.9
    damage to pelvic organs O08.6
    embolism O08.2
    genital infection O08.0
    hemorrhage (delayed) (excessive) O08.1
    metabolic disorder O08.5
    renal failure O08.4
    shock O08.3
    specified type NEC O08.0
    venous complication NEC O08.7
  musculoskeletal system —see also
      Complication, intraoperative
      (intraprocedural), by site
    device, implant or graft NEC —see
        Complications, orthopedic, device or
        implant
    internal fixation (nail) (plate) (rod) —see
        Complications, fixation device,
        internal
    joint prosthesis —see Complications, joint
        prosthesis

Complication (Continued)
  musculoskeletal system (Continued)
    postoperative (postprocedural) M96.89
      with osteoporosis —see Osteoporosis
      fracture following insertion of device —
          see Fracture, following insertion of
          orthopedic implant, joint prosthesis
          or bone plate
      joint instability after prosthesis removal
          M96.89
      lordosis M96.4
      postlaminectomy syndrome NEC M96.1
        kyphosis M96.2 ◄▥
      pseudarthrosis M96.0
      specified complication NEC M96.89
    post radiation M96.89
      kyphosis M96.3
      scoliosis M96.5
      specified complication NEC M96.89
  nephrostomy (stoma) —see Complications,
      stoma, urinary tract, external NEC
  nervous system G98.8
    central G96.9
    device, implant or graft —see also
        Complication, prosthetic device or
        implant, specified NEC
      electronic stimulator (electrode (s)) —
          see Complications, electronic
          stimulator device
      specified NEC ◄
        infection and inflammation T85.738 ◄
        mechanical T85.695 ◄
          breakdown T85.615 ◄
          displacement T85.625 ◄
          leakage T85.635 ◄
          malfunction T85.695 ◄
          malposition T85.625 ◄
          obstruction T85.695 ◄
          perforation T85.695 ◄
          protrusion T85.695 ◄
          specified NEC T85.695 ◄
      ventricular shunt —see Complications,
          ventricular shunt
    electronic stimulator (electrode (s)) —see
        Complications, electronic stimulator
        device
    postprocedural G97.82
      intracranial hypotension G97.2
      specified NEC G97.82
      spinal fluid leak G97.0
  newborn, due to intrauterine (fetal)
      procedure P96.5
  nonabsorbable (permanent) sutures —see
      Complication, sutures, permanent
  obstetric O75.9
    procedure (instrumental) (manual)
        (surgical) specified NEC O75.4
    specified NEC O75.89
    surgical wound NEC O90.89
      hematoma O90.2
      infection O86.0
  ocular lens implant —see Complications,
      intraocular lens
  ophthalmologic
    postprocedural bleb —see Blebitis
  orbital prosthesis T85.9
    embolism T85.818 ◄▥
    fibrosis T85.828 ◄▥
    hemorrhage T85.838 ◄▥
    infection and inflammation T85.79
    mechanical
      breakdown T85.31-
      displacement T85.32-
      malposition T85.32-
      obstruction T85.39-
      perforation T85.39-
      protrusion T85.39-
      specified NEC T85.39-
    pain T85.848 ◄▥
    specified type NEC T85.898 ◄▥
    stenosis T85.858 ◄▥
    thrombosis T85.868 ◄▥

Complication *(Continued)*
  organ or tissue transplant (partial) (total) —
    see Complications, transplant
  orthopedic —*see also* Disorder, soft tissue
    device or implant T84.9
      bone
        device or implant —*see* Complication,
          bone, device NEC
        graft —*see* Complication, graft, bone
      breakdown T84.418
      displacement T84.428
      electronic bone stimulator —*see*
        Complications, electronic
        stimulator device, bone
      embolism T84.81
      fibrosis T84.82
      fixation device —*see* Complication,
        fixation device, internal
      hemorrhage T84.83
      infection or inflammation T84.7
      joint prosthesis —*see* Complication, joint
        prosthesis, internal
      malfunction T84.418
      malposition T84.428
      mechanical NEC T84.498
      muscle graft —*see* Complications, graft,
        muscle
      obstruction T84.498
      pain T84.84
      perforation T84.498
      protrusion T84.498
      specified complication NEC T84.89
      stenosis T84.85
      tendon graft —*see* Complications, graft,
        tendon
      thrombosis T84.86
    fracture (following insertion of device) —
      see Fracture, following insertion of
      orthopedic implant, joint prosthesis
      or bone plate
    postprocedural M96.89
      fracture —*see* Fracture, following
        insertion of orthopedic implant,
        joint prosthesis or bone plate
      postlaminectomy syndrome NEC M96.1
        kyphosis M96.3
        lordosis M96.4
      postradiation
        kyphosis M96.2
        scoliosis M96.5
      pseudarthrosis post-fusion M96.0
      specified type NEC M96.89
  pacemaker (cardiac) —*see* Complications,
    cardiovascular device or implant,
    electronic
  pancreas transplant —*see* Complications,
    transplant, pancreas
  penile prosthesis (implant) —*see*
    Complications, prosthetic device, penile
  perfusion NEC T80.90
  perineal repair (obstetrical) NEC O90.89
    disruption O90.1
    hematoma O90.2
    infection (following delivery) O86.0
  phototherapy T88.9
    specified NEC T88.8
  postmastoidectomy NEC H95.19-
    cyst, mucosal H95.13-
    granulation H95.12-
    inflammation, chronic H95.11-
    recurrent cholesteatoma H95.0-
  postoperative —*see* Complications,
    postprocedural
    circulatory —*see* Complications, circulatory
      system
    ear —*see* Complications, ear
    endocrine —*see* Complications,
      endocrine
    eye —*see* Complications, eye
    lumbar puncture G97.1
      cerebrospinal fluid leak G97.0

Complication *(Continued)*
  postoperative *(Continued)*
    nervous system (central) (peripheral) —*see*
      Complications, nervous system
    respiratory system —*see* Complications,
      respiratory system
  postprocedural —*see also* Complications,
    surgical procedure
    cardiac arrest
      following cardiac surgery I97.120
      following other surgery I97.121
    cardiac functional disturbance NEC
      following cardiac surgery I97.190
      following other surgery I97.191
    cardiac insufficiency
      following cardiac surgery I97.110
      following other surgery I97.111
    chorioretinal scars following retinal
      surgery H59.81-
    following cataract surgery
      cataract (lens) fragments H59.02-
      cystoid macular edema H59.03-
      specified NEC H59.09-
      vitreous (touch) syndrome H59.01-
    heart failure
      following cardiac surgery I97.130
      following other surgery I97.131
    hematoma (of) ◀
      circulatory system organ or structure ◀
        following cardiac bypass I97.631 ◀
        following cardiac catheterization
          I97.630 ◀
        following other circulatory system
          procedure I97.638 ◀
        following other procedure I97.621 ◀
      digestive system ◀
        following procedure on digestive
          system K91.870 ◀
        following procedure on other organ
          K91.871 ◀
      ear ◀
        following other procedure H95.52 ◀
        following procedure on ear and
          mastoid process H95.51 ◀
      endocrine system ◀
        following endocrine system procedure
          E89.820 ◀
        following other procedure E89.821 ◀
      eye and adnexa ◀
        following ophthalmic procedure
          H59.33- ◀
        following other procedure H59.34- ◀
      genitourinary organ or structure ◀
        following procedure on genitourinary
          organ or structure N99.840 ◀
        following procedure on other organ
          N99.841 ◀
      mastoid process ◀
        following other procedure H95.52 ◀
        following procedure on ear and
          mastoid process H95.51 ◀
      musculoskeletal structure ◀
        following musculoskeletal surgery
          M96.840 ◀
        following non-orthopedic surgery
          M96.841 ◀
        following orthopedic surgery
          M96.840 ◀
      nervous system ◀
        following nervous system procedure
          G97.61 ◀
        following other procedure G97.62 ◀
      respiratory system ◀
        following other procedure J95.861 ◀
        following procedure on respiratory
          system organ or structure
          J95.860 ◀
      skin and subcutaneous tissue ◀
        following dermatologic procedure
          L76.31 ◀
        following procedure on other organ
          L76.32 ◀

Complication *(Continued)*
  postprocedural *(Continued)*
    hematoma *(Continued)*
      spleen ◀
        following procedure on other organ
          D78.32 ◀
        following procedure on the spleen
          D78.31 ◀
    hemorrhage (of) ◀▥
      circulatory system organ or structure
        ~~following a cardiac bypass I97.611~~
        ~~following a cardiac catheterization~~
          ~~I97.610~~
        following cardiac bypass I97.611 ◀
        following cardiac catheterization
          I97.610 ◀
        following other circulatory system
          procedure I97.618
        following other procedure I97.620 ◀▥
      digestive system
        following procedure on digestive
          system K91.840
        following procedure on other organ
          K91.841
      ear
        following other procedure H95.42
        following procedure on ear and
          mastoid process H95.41
      endocrine system
        following endocrine system procedure
          E89.810
        following other procedure E89.811
      eye and adnexa
        following ophthalmic procedure
          H59.31-
        following other procedure H59.32-
      genitourinary organ or structure
        following procedure on
          genitourinary organ or
          structure N99.820
        following procedure on other organ
          N99.821
      mastoid process
        following other procedure H95.42
        following procedure on ear and
          mastoid process H95.41
      musculoskeletal structure
        following musculoskeletal surgery
          M96.830
        following non-orthopedic surgery
          M96.831
        following orthopedic surgery M96.830
      nervous system
        ~~following a nervous system procedure~~
          ~~G97.51~~
        following nervous system procedure
          G97.51 ◀
        following other procedure G97.52
      respiratory system
        following other procedure J95.831
        following procedure on respiratory
          system organ or structure J95.830
      skin and subcutaneous tissue
        ~~following a dermatologic procedure~~
          ~~L76.21~~
        following dermatologic procedure
          L76.21 ◀
        following a procedure on other organ
          L76.22
      spleen
        following procedure on other organ
          D78.22
        following procedure on the spleen
          D78.21
    seroma (of) ◀
      circulatory system organ or structure ◀
        following cardiac bypass I97.641 ◀
        following cardiac catheterization
          I97.640 ◀
        following other circulatory system
          procedure I97.648 ◀
        following other procedure I97.622 ◀

◀ New   ◀▥ Revised   ~~deleted~~ Deleted

C

Complication *(Continued)*
  postprocedural *(Continued)*
    seroma *(Continued)*
      digestive system ◄
        following procedure on digestive system K91.872 ◄
        following procedure on other organ K91.873 ◄
      ear ◄
        following other procedure H95.54 ◄
        following procedure on ear and mastoid process H95.53 ◄
      endocrine system ◄
        following endocrine system procedure E89.822 ◄
        following other procedure E89.823 ◄
      eye and adnexa ◄
        following ophthalmic procedure H59.35-
        following other procedure H59.36- ◄
      genitourinary organ or structure ◄
        following procedure on genitourinary organ or structure N99.842 ◄
        following procedure on other organ N99.843 ◄
      mastoid process ◄
        following other procedure H95.54 ◄
        following procedure on ear and mastoid process H95.53 ◄
      musculoskeletal structure ◄
        following musculoskeletal surgery M96.842 ◄
        following non-orthopedic surgery M96.843 ◄
        following orthopedic surgery M96.842 ◄
      nervous system ◄
        following nervous system procedure G97.63 ◄
        following other procedure G97.64 ◄
      respiratory system ◄
        following other procedure J95.863 ◄
        following procedure on respiratory system organ or structure J95.862 ◄
      skin and subcutaneous tissue ◄
        following dermatologic procedure L76.33 ◄
        following procedure on other organ L76.34 ◄
      spleen ◄
        following procedure on other organ D78.34 ◄
        following procedure on the spleen D78.33 ◄
    specified NEC
      circulatory system I97.89
      digestive K91.89
      ear H95.89
      endocrine E89.89
      eye and adnexa H59.89
      genitourinary N99.89
      mastoid process H95.89
      metabolic E89.89
      musculoskeletal structure M96.89
      nervous system G97.82
      respiratory system J95.89
      skin and subcutaneous tissue L76.82
      spleen D78.89
  pregnancy NEC —see Pregnancy, complicated by
  prosthetic device or implant T85.9
    bile duct —see Complications, bile duct implant
    breast —see Complications, breast implant
    bulking agent ◄
      ureteral ◄
        erosion T83.714 ◄
        exposure T83.724 ◄
      urethral ◄
        erosion T83.713 ◄
        exposure T83.723 ◄

Complication *(Continued)*
  prosthetic device or implant *(Continued)*
    cardiac and vascular NEC —see Complications, cardiovascular device or implant
    corneal transplant —see Complications, graft, cornea
    electronic nervous system stimulator —see Complications, electronic stimulator device
    epidural infusion catheter —see Complications, catheter, epidural
    esophageal anti-reflux device —see Complications, esophageal anti-reflux device
    genital organ or tract —see Complications, genitourinary, device or implant, genital tract
      specified NEC T83.79 ◄
    heart valve —see Complications, heart, valve, prosthesis
    infection or inflammation T85.79
      intestine transplant T86.892
      liver transplant T86.43
      lung transplant T86.812
      pancreas transplant T86.892
      skin graft T86.822
    intraocular lens —see Complications, intraocular lens
    intraperitoneal (dialysis) catheter — see Complications, catheter, intraperitoneal
    joint —see Complications, joint prosthesis, internal
    mechanical NEC T85.698
      dialysis catheter (vascular) —see also Complication, catheter, dialysis, mechanical
        peritoneal —see Complication, catheter, intraperitoneal, mechanical
      gastrointestinal device T85.598
      ocular device T85.398
      subdural (infusion) catheter T85.690
      suture, permanent T85.692
        that for bone repair —see Complications, fixation device, internal (orthopedic), mechanical
      ventricular shunt
        breakdown T85.01
        displacement T85.02
        leakage T85.03
        malposition T85.02
        obstruction T85.09
        perforation T85.09
        protrusion T85.09
        specified NEC T85.09
    mesh
      erosion (to surrounding organ or tissue) T83.717 ◄▥
        urethral (into pelvic floor muscles) T83.712 ◄
        vaginal (into pelvic floor muscles) T83.711
      exposure (into surrounding organ or tissue) T83.727 ◄▥
        urethral (through urethral wall) T83.722 ◄
        vaginal (into vagina) (through vaginal wall) T83.721
    orbital —see Complications, orbital prosthesis
    penile T83.9
      embolism T83.81
      fibrosis T83.82
      hemorrhage T83.83
      infection and inflammation T83.61 ◄▥
      mechanical
        breakdown T83.410
        displacement T83.420
        leakage T83.490
        malposition T83.420

Complication *(Continued)*
  prosthetic device or implant *(Continued)*
    penile *(Continued)*
      mechanical *(Continued)*
        obstruction T83.490
        perforation T83.490
        protrusion T83.490
        specified NEC T83.490
      pain T83.84
      specified type NEC T83.89
      stenosis T83.85
      thrombosis T83.86
    prosthetic materials NEC
      erosion (to surrounding organ or tissue) T83.718
        ~~vaginal (into pelvic floor muscles) T83.711~~
      exposure (into surrounding organ or tissue) T83.728
        ~~vaginal (into vagina) (through vaginal wall) T83.721~~
    skin graft T86.829
      artificial skin or decellularized allodermis
        embolism T85.818 ◄▥
        fibrosis T85.828 ◄▥
        hemorrhage T85.838 ◄▥
        infection and inflammation T85.79
        mechanical
          breakdown T85.613
          displacement T85.623
          malfunction T85.613
          malposition T85.623
          obstruction T85.693
          perforation T85.693
          protrusion T85.693
          specified NEC T85.693
        pain T85.848 ◄▥
        specified type NEC T85.898 ◄▥
        stenosis T85.858 ◄▥
        thrombosis T85.868 ◄▥
      failure T86.821
      infection T86.822
      rejection T86.820
      specified NEC T86.828
    sling ◄
      urethral (female) (male) ◄
        erosion T83.712 ◄
        exposure T83.722 ◄
    specified NEC T85.9
      embolism T85.818 ◄▥
      fibrosis T85.828 ◄▥
      hemorrhage T85.838 ◄▥
      infection and inflammation T85.79
      mechanical
        breakdown T85.618
        displacement T85.628
        leakage T85.638
        malfunction T85.618
        malposition T85.628
        obstruction T85.698
        perforation T85.698
        protrusion T85.698
        specified NEC T85.698
      pain T85.848 ◄▥
      specified type NEC T85.898 ◄▥
      stenosis T85.858 ◄▥
      thrombosis T85.868 ◄▥
    subdural infusion catheter —see Complications, catheter, subdural
    sutures —see Complications, sutures
    urinary organ or tract NEC —see Complications, genitourinary, device or implant, urinary system
    vascular —see Complications, cardiovascular device or implant
    ventricular shunt —see Complications, ventricular shunt (device)
  puerperium —see Puerperal
  puncture, spinal G97.1
    cerebrospinal fluid leak G97.0
    headache or reaction G97.1

Complication (Continued)
  pyelogram N99.89
  radiation
    kyphosis M96.2
    scoliosis M96.5
  reattached
    extremity (infection) (rejection)
      lower T87.1X-
      upper T87.0X-
    specified body part NEC T87.2
  reconstructed breast
    asymmetry between native and
      reconstructed breast N65.1
    deformity N65.0
    disproportion between native and
      reconstructed breast N65.1
    excess tissue N65.1
    misshappen N65.0
  reimplant NEC —see also Complications,
    prosthetic device or implant
    limb (infection) (rejection) —see
      Complications, reattached,
      extremity
    organ (partial) (total) —see Complications,
      transplant
    prosthetic device NEC —see Complications,
      prosthetic device
  renal N28.9
    allograft —see Complications, transplant,
      kidney
    dialysis —see Complications, dialysis
  respirator
    mechanical J95.850
      specified NEC J95.859
  respiratory system J98.9
    device, implant or graft —see
      Complication, prosthetic device or
      implant, specified NEC
    lung transplant —see Complications,
      prosthetic device or implant, lung
      transplant
    postoperative J95.89
      air leak J95.812
      Mendelson's syndrome (chemical
        pneumonitis) J95.4
      pneumothorax J95.811
      pulmonary insufficiency (acute) (after
        nonthoracic surgery) J95.2
        chronic J95.3
        following thoracic surgery J95.1
      respiratory failure (acute) J95.821
        acute and chronic J95.822
      specified NEC J95.89
      subglottic stenosis J95.5
      tracheostomy complication —see
        Complications, tracheostomy
    therapy T81.89
  sedation during labor and delivery O74.9
    cardiac O74.2
    central nervous system O74.3
    pulmonary NEC O74.1
  shunt —see also Complications, prosthetic
    device or implant
    arteriovenous —see Complications,
      arteriovenous, shunt
    ventricular (communicating) —see
      Complications, ventricular shunt
  skin
    graft T86.829
      failure T86.821
      infection T86.822
      rejection T86.820
      specified type NEC T86.828
  spinal
    anesthesia —see Complications, anesthesia,
      spinal
    catheter (epidural) (subdural) —see
      Complications, catheter
    puncture or tap G97.1
      cerebrospinal fluid leak G97.0
      headache or reaction G97.1

Complication (Continued)
  stent
    bile duct —see Complications, bile duct
      prosthesis
    ureteral indwelling ◀
      breakdown T83.112 ◀
      displacement T83.122 ◀
      leakage T83.192 ◀
      malposition T83.122 ◀
      obstruction T83.192 ◀
      perforation T83.192 ◀
      protrusion T83.192 ◀
      specified NEC T83.192 ◀
    urinary (ileal conduit) (nephroureteral)
      T83.193 ◀
      embolism T83.81 ◀
      fibrosis T83.82 ◀
      hemorrhage T83.83 ◀
      infection and inflammation T83.593 ◀
      mechanical ◀
        breakdown T83.113 ◀
        displacement T83.123 ◀
        leakage T83.193 ◀
        malposition T83.123 ◀
        obstruction T83.193 ◀
        perforation T83.193 ◀
        protrusion T83.193 ◀
        specified NEC T83.193 ◀
      pain T83.84 ◀
      specified type NEC T83.89 ◀
      stenosis T83.85 ◀
      thrombosis T83.86 ◀
    vascular ◀
      end stent stenosis —see Restenosis,
        stent ◀
      in stent stenosis —see Restenosis,
        stent ◀
  stoma
    digestive tract
      colostomy —see Complications,
        colostomy
      enterostomy —see Complications,
        enterostomy
      esophagostomy —see Complications,
        esophagostomy
      gastrostomy —see Complications,
        gastrostomy
    urinary tract N99.528 ◀▥
      continent N99.538 ◀
        hemorrhage N99.530 ◀
        herniation N99.533 ◀
        infection N99.531 ◀
        malfunction N99.532 ◀
        specified type NEC N99.538 ◀
        stenosis N99.534 ◀
      cystostomy —see Complications,
        cystostomy
      external NOS N99.528 ◀
        hemorrhage N99.520
        infection N99.521
        malfunction N99.522
        specified type NEC N99.528
      hemorrhage N99.520 ◀▥
      herniation N99.523 ◀
      incontinent N99.528 ◀
        hemorrhage N99.520 ◀
        herniation N99.523 ◀
        infection N99.521 ◀
        malfunction N99.522 ◀
        specified type NEC N99.528 ◀
        stenosis N99.524 ◀
      infection N99.521 ◀
      malfunction N99.522 ◀▥
      specified type NEC N99.528 ◀▥
      stenosis N99.524 ◀
  stomach banding —see Complication (s),
    bariatric procedure
  stomach stapling —see Complication (s),
    bariatric procedure
  surgical material, nonabsorbable —see
    Complication, suture, permanent

Complication (Continued)
  surgical procedure (on) T81.9
    amputation stump (late) —see
      Complications, amputation stump
    cardiac —see Complications, circulatory
      system
    cholesteatoma, recurrent —see
      Complications, postmastoidectomy,
      recurrent cholesteatoma
    circulatory (early) —see Complications,
      circulatory system
    digestive system —see Complications,
      gastrointestinal
    dumping syndrome (postgastrectomy)
      K91.1
    ear —see Complications, ear
    elephantiasis or lymphedema I97.89
      postmastectomy I97.2
    emphysema (surgical) T81.82
    endocrine —see Complications, endocrine
    eye —see Complications, eye
    fistula (persistent postoperative) T81.83
    foreign body inadvertently left in wound
      (sponge) (suture) (swab) —see
      Foreign body, accidentally left during
      a procedure
    gastrointestinal —see Complications,
      gastrointestinal
    genitourinary NEC N99.89
    hematoma
      intraoperative —see Complication,
        intraoperative, hemorrhage
      postprocedural —see Complication,
        postprocedural, hematoma ◀▥
    hemorrhage
      intraoperative —see Complication,
        intraoperative, hemorrhage
      postprocedural —see Complication,
        postprocedural, hemorrhage
    hepatic failure K91.82
    hyperglycemia (postpancreatectomy) E89.1
    hypoinsulinemia (postpancreatectomy)
      E89.1
    hypoparathyroidism
      (postparathyroidectomy) E89.2
    hypopituitarism (posthypophysectomy)
      E89.3
    hypothyroidism (post-thyroidectomy)
      E89.0
    intestinal obstruction K91.3
    intracranial hypotension following
      ventricular shunting
      (ventriculostomy) G97.2
    lymphedema I97.89
      postmastectomy I97.2
    malabsorption (postsurgical) NEC K91.2
      osteoporosis —see Osteoporosis,
        postsurgical malabsorption
    mastoidectomy cavity NEC —see
      Complications, postmastoidectomy
    metabolic E89.89
      specified NEC E89.89
    musculoskeletal —see Complications,
      musculoskeletal system
    nervous system (central) (peripheral) —see
      Complications, nervous system
    ovarian failure E89.40
      asymptomatic E89.40
      symptomatic E89.41
    peripheral vascular —see Complications,
      surgical procedure, vascular
    postcardiotomy syndrome I97.0
    postcholecystectomy syndrome K91.5
    postcommissurotomy syndrome I97.0
    postgastrectomy dumping syndrome K91.1
    postlaminectomy syndrome NEC M96.1
      kyphosis M96.3
    postmastectomy lymphedema syndrome
      I97.2
    postmastoidectomy cholesteatoma —see
      Complications, postmastoidectomy,
      recurrent cholesteatoma

◀ New   ◀▥ Revised   deleted Deleted

Complication *(Continued)*
  surgical procedure *(Continued)*
    postvagotomy syndrome K91.1
    postvalvulotomy syndrome I97.0
    pulmonary insufficiency (acute) J95.2
      chronic J95.3
      following thoracic surgery J95.1
    reattached body part —*see* Complications, reattached
    respiratory —*see* Complications, respiratory system
    shock (hypovolemic) T81.19
    spleen (postoperative) D78.89
      intraoperative D78.81
    stitch abscess T81.48
    subglottic stenosis (postsurgical) J95.5
    testicular hypofunction E89.5
    transplant —*see* Complications, organ or tissue transplant
    urinary NEC N99.89
    vaginal vault prolapse (posthysterectomy) N99.3
    vascular (peripheral)
      artery T81.719
        mesenteric T81.710
        renal T81.711
        specified NEC T81.718
      vein T81.72
    wound infection T81.40
  suture, permanent (wire) NEC T85.9
    with repair of bone —*see* Complications, fixation device, internal
    embolism T85.818
    fibrosis T85.828
    hemorrhage T85.838
    infection and inflammation T85.79
    mechanical
      breakdown T85.612
      displacement T85.622
      malfunction T85.612
      malposition T85.622
      obstruction T85.692
      perforation T85.692
      protrusion T85.692
      specified NEC T85.692
    pain T85.848
    specified type NEC T85.898
    stenosis T85.858
    thrombosis T85.868
  tracheostomy J95.00
    granuloma J95.09
    hemorrhage J95.01
    infection J95.02
    malfunction J95.03
    mechanical J95.03
    obstruction J95.03
    specified type NEC J95.09
    tracheo-esophageal fistula J95.04
  transfusion (blood) (lymphocytes) (plasma) T80.92
    air embolism T80.0
    circulatory overload E87.71
    febrile nonhemolytic transfusion reaction R50.84
    hemochromatosis E83.111
    hemolysis T80.89
    hemolytic reaction (antigen unspecified) T80.919
    incompatibility reaction (antigen unspecified) T80.919
      ABO T80.30
        delayed serologic (DSTR) T80.39
        hemolytic transfusion reaction (HTR) (unspecified time after transfusion) T80.319
        acute (AHTR) (less than 24 hours after transfusion) T80.310
        delayed (DHTR) (24 hours or more after transfusion) T80.311
        specified NEC T80.39

Complication *(Continued)*
  transfusion *(Continued)*
    incompatibility reaction *(Continued)*
      acute (antigen unspecified) T80.910
      delayed (antigen unspecified) T80.911
      delayed serologic (DSTR) T80.89
      Non-ABO (minor antigens (Duffy) (Kell) (Kidd) (Lewis) (M) (N) (P) (S)) T80.A0
        delayed serologic (DSTR) T80.A9
        hemolytic transfusion reaction (HTR) (unspecified time after transfusion) T80.A19
        acute (AHTR) (less than 24 hours after transfusion) T80.A10
        delayed (DHTR) (24 hours or more after transfusion) T80.A11
        specified NEC T80.A9
      Rh (antigens (C) (c) (D) (E) (e)) (factor) T80.40
        delayed serologic (DSTR) T80.49
        hemolytic transfusion reaction (HTR) (unspecified time after transfusion) T80.419
        acute (AHTR) (less than 24 hours after transfusion) T80.410
        delayed (DHTR) (24 hours or more after transfusion) T80.411
        specified NEC T80.49
    infection T80.29
      acute T80.22
    reaction NEC T80.89
    sepsis T80.29
    shock T80.89
  transplant T86.90
    bone T86.839
      failure T86.831
      infection T86.832
      rejection T86.830
      specified type NEC T86.838
    bone marrow T86.00
      failure T86.02
      infection T86.03
      rejection T86.01
      specified type NEC T86.09
    cornea T86.849
      failure T86.841
      infection T86.842
      rejection T86.840
      specified type NEC T86.848
    failure T86.92
    heart T86.20
      with lung T86.30
      cardiac allograft vasculopathy T86.290
        failure T86.32
        infection T86.33
        rejection T86.31
        specified type NEC T86.39
      failure T86.22
      infection T86.23
      rejection T86.21
      specified type NEC T86.298
    infection T86.93
    intestine T86.859
      failure T86.851
      infection T86.852
      rejection T86.850
      specified type NEC T86.858
    kidney T86.10
      failure T86.12
      infection T86.13
      rejection T86.11
      specified type NEC T86.19
    liver T86.40
      failure T86.42
      infection T86.43
      rejection T86.41
      specified type NEC T86.49
    lung T86.819
      with heart T86.30
        failure T86.32
        infection T86.33

Complication *(Continued)*
  transplant *(Continued)*
    lung *(Continued)*
      with heart *(Continued)*
        rejection T86.31
        specified type NEC T86.39
      failure T86.811
      infection T86.812
      rejection T86.810
      specified type NEC T86.818
    malignant neoplasm C80.2
    pancreas T86.899
      failure T86.891
      infection T86.892
      rejection T86.890
      specified type NEC T86.898
    peripheral blood stem cells T86.5
    post-transplant lymphoproliferative disorder (PTLD) D47.Z1
    rejection T86.91
    skin T86.829
      failure T86.821
      infection T86.822
      rejection T86.820
      specified type NEC T86.828
    specified
      tissue T86.899
        failure T86.891
        infection T86.892
        rejection T86.890
        specified type NEC T86.898
      type NEC T86.99
    stem cell (from peripheral blood) (from umbilical cord) T86.5
    umbilical cord stem cells T86.5
  trauma (early) T79.9
    specified NEC T79.8
  ultrasound therapy NEC T88.9
  umbilical cord NEC
    complicating delivery O69.9
      specified NEC O69.89
  umbrella device, vascular T82.9
    embolism T82.818
    fibrosis T82.828
    hemorrhage T82.838
    infection or inflammation T82.7
    mechanical
      breakdown T82.515
      displacement T82.525
      leakage T82.535
      malposition T82.525
      obstruction T82.595
      perforation T82.595
      protrusion T82.595
    pain T82.848
    specified type NEC T82.898
    stenosis T82.858
    thrombosis T82.868
  urethral catheter —*see* Complications, catheter, urethral, indwelling
  vaccination T88.1
    anaphylaxis NEC T80.52
    arthropathy —*see* Arthropathy, postimmunization
    cellulitis T88.0
    encephalitis or encephalomyelitis G04.02
    infection (general) (local) NEC T88.0
    meningitis G03.8
    myelitis G04.02
    protein sickness T80.62
    rash T88.1
    reaction (allergic) T88.1
      serum T80.62
    sepsis T88.0
    serum intoxication, sickness, rash, or other serum reaction NEC T80.62
      anaphylactic shock T80.52
    shock (allergic) (anaphylactic) T80.52
    vaccinia (generalized) (localized) T88.1
  vas deferens device or implant —*see* Complications, genitourinary, device or implant, genital tract

Complication *(Continued)*
  vascular I99.9
    device or implant T82.9
      embolism T82.818
      fibrosis T82.828
      hemorrhage T82.838
      infection or inflammation T82.7
      mechanical
        breakdown T82.519
          specified device NEC T82.518
        displacement T82.529
          specified device NEC T82.528
        leakage T82.539
          specified device NEC T82.538
        malposition T82.529
          specified device NEC T82.528
        obstruction T82.599
          specified device NEC T82.598
        perforation T82.599
          specified device NEC T82.598
        protrusion T82.599
          specified device NEC T82.598
      pain T82.848
      specified type NEC T82.898
      stenosis T82.858
      thrombosis T82.868
    dialysis catheter —*see* Complication,
        catheter, dialysis
    following infusion, therapeutic injection or
        transfusion T80.1
    graft T82.9
      embolism T82.818
      fibrosis T82.828
      hemorrhage T82.838
      mechanical
        breakdown T82.319
          aorta (bifurcation) T82.310
          carotid artery T82.311
          specified vessel NEC T82.318
        displacement T82.329
          aorta (bifurcation) T82.320
          carotid artery T82.321
          specified vessel NEC T82.328
        leakage T82.339
          aorta (bifurcation) T82.330
          carotid artery T82.331
          specified vessel NEC T82.338
        malposition T82.329
          aorta (bifurcation) T82.320
          carotid artery T82.321
          specified vessel NEC T82.328
        obstruction T82.399
          aorta (bifurcation) T82.390
          carotid artery T82.391
          specified vessel NEC T82.398
        perforation T82.399
          aorta (bifurcation) T82.390
          carotid artery T82.391
          specified vessel NEC T82.398
        protrusion T82.399
          aorta (bifurcation) T82.390
          carotid artery T82.391
          specified vessel NEC T82.398
      pain T82.848
      specified complication NEC T82.898
      stenosis T82.858
      thrombosis T82.868
    postoperative —*see* Complications,
        postoperative, circulatory
    vena cava device (filter) (sieve) (umbrella) —
        see Complications, umbrella device,
        vascular
    ventilation therapy NEC T81.81
    ventilator
      mechanical J95.850
        specified NEC J95.859
    ventricular (communicating) shunt (device)
        T85.9
      embolism T85.810 ◀▥
      fibrosis T85.820 ◀▥
      hemorrhage T85.830 ◀▥

Complication *(Continued)*
  ventricular shunt *(Continued)*
    infection and inflammation T85.730 ◀▥
    mechanical
      breakdown T85.01
      displacement T85.02
      leakage T85.03
      malposition T85.02
      obstruction T85.09
      perforation T85.09
      protrusion T85.09
      specified NEC T85.09
    pain T85.840 ◀▥
    specified type NEC T85.890 ◀▥
    stenosis T85.850 ◀▥
    thrombosis T85.860 ◀▥
  wire suture, permanent (implanted) —*see*
      Complications, suture, permanent
Compressed air disease T70.3
Compression
  with injury - code by Nature of injury
  artery I77.1
    celiac, syndrome I77.4
  brachial plexus G54.0
  brain (stem) G93.5
    due to
      contusion (diffuse) —*see* Injury,
          intracranial, diffuse
        focal —*see* Injury, intracranial, focal
      injury NEC —*see* Injury, intracranial,
          diffuse
      traumatic —*see* Injury, intracranial, diffuse
  bronchus J98.09
  cauda equina G83.4
  celiac (artery) (axis) I77.4
  cerebral —*see* Compression, brain
  cervical plexus G54.2
  cord
    spinal —*see* Compression, spinal
    umbilical —*see* Compression, umbilical
        cord
  cranial nerve G52.9
    eighth —*see* subcategory H93.3
    eleventh G52.8
    fifth G50.8
    first G52.0
    fourth —*see* Strabismus, paralytic, fourth
        nerve
    ninth G52.1
    second —*see* Disorder, nerve, optic
    seventh G52.8
    sixth —*see* Strabismus, paralytic, sixth
        nerve
    tenth G52.2
    third —*see* Strabismus, paralytic, third
        nerve
    twelfth G52.3
  diver's squeeze T70.3
  during birth (newborn) P15.9
  esophagus K22.2
  eustachian tube —*see* Obstruction, eustachian
      tube, cartilaginous
  facies Q67.1
  fracture
    nontraumatic NOS —*see* Collapse,
        vertebra ◀
    pathological —*see* Fracture, pathological ◀
    traumatic —*see* Fracture, traumatic ◀
  heart —*see* Disease, heart
  intestine —*see* Obstruction, intestine
  laryngeal nerve, recurrent G52.2
    with paralysis of vocal cords and larynx
        J38.00
      bilateral J38.02
      unilateral J38.01
  lumbosacral plexus G54.1
  lung J98.4
  lymphatic vessel I89.0
  medulla —*see* Compression, brain
  nerve —*see also* Disorder, nerve G58.9
    arm NEC —*see* Mononeuropathy, upper
        limb

Compression *(Continued)*
  nerve *(Continued)*
    axillary G54.0
    cranial —*see* Compression, cranial nerve
    leg NEC —*see* Mononeuropathy, lower
        limb
    median (in carpal tunnel) —*see* Syndrome,
        carpal tunnel
    optic —*see* Disorder, nerve, optic
    plantar —*see* Lesion, nerve, plantar
    posterior tibial (in tarsal tunnel) —*see*
        Syndrome, tarsal tunnel
    root or plexus NOS (in) G54.9
      intervertebral disc disorder NEC —
          see Disorder, disc, with,
          radiculopathy
        with myelopathy —*see* Disorder, disc,
            with, myelopathy
      neoplastic disease —*see also* Neoplasm
          D49.9 *[G55]*
      spondylosis —*see* Spondylosis, with
          radiculopathy
    sciatic (acute) —*see* Lesion, nerve, sciatic
    sympathetic G90.8
    traumatic —*see* Injury, nerve
    ulnar —*see* Lesion, nerve, ulnar
    upper extremity NEC —*see*
        Mononeuropathy, upper limb
  spinal (cord) G95.20
    by displacement of intervertebral disc
        NEC —*see also* Disorder, disc, with,
        myelopathy
    nerve root NOS G54.9
      due to displacement of intervertebral
          disc NEC —*see* Disorder, disc, with,
          radiculopathy
        with myelopathy —*see* Disorder, disc,
            with, myelopathy
    specified NEC G95.29
    spondylogenic (cervical) (lumbar,
        lumbosacral) (thoracic) —*see*
        Spondylosis, with myelopathy NEC
    anterior —*see* Syndrome, anterior, spinal
        artery, compression
    traumatic —*see* Injury, spinal cord, by
        region
  subcostal nerve (syndrome) —*see*
      Mononeuropathy, upper limb, specified
      NEC
  sympathetic nerve NEC G90.8
  syndrome T79.5
  trachea J39.8
  ulnar nerve (by scar tissue) —*see* Lesion,
      nerve, ulnar
  umbilical cord
    complicating delivery O69.2
      cord around neck O69.1
      prolapse O69.0
      specified NEC O69.2
  ureter N13.5
  vein I87.1
  vena cava (inferior) (superior) I87.1
Compulsion, compulsive
  gambling F63.0
  neurosis F42.8 ◀▥
  personality F60.5
  states F42.8 ◀▥
  swearing F42.8 ◀▥
    in Gilles de la Tourette's syndrome F95.2
  tics and spasms F95.9
Concato's disease (pericardial polyserositis)
    A19.9
  nontubercular I31.1
  pleural —*see* Pleurisy, with effusion
Concavity chest wall M95.4
Concealed penis Q55.69
Concern (normal) about sick person in family
    Z63.6
Concrescence (teeth) K00.2
Concretio cordis I31.1
  rheumatic I09.2

◀ New   ◀▥ Revised   ~~deleted~~ Deleted

Concretion —see also Calculus
  appendicular K38.1
  canaliculus —see Dacryolith
  clitoris N90.89
  conjunctiva H11.12-
  eyelid —see Disorder, eyelid, specified type NEC
  lacrimal passages —see Dacryolith
  prepuce (male) N47.8
  salivary gland (any) K11.5
  seminal vesicle N50.89 ◄▥
  tonsil J35.8
Concussion (brain) (cerebral) (current) S06.0X9 ◄▥
  with ◄
    loss of consciousness of 30 minutes or less S06.0X1 ◄
    loss of consciousness of unspecified duration S06.0X9 ◄
  blast (air) (hydraulic) (immersion) (underwater)
    abdomen or thorax —see Injury, blast, by site
    ear with acoustic nerve injury —see Injury, nerve, acoustic, specified type NEC
  cauda equina S34.3
  conus medullaris S34.02
  ocular S05.8X-
  spinal (cord)
    cervical S14.0
    lumbar S34.01
    sacral S34.02
    thoracic S24.0
  syndrome F07.81
  Without loss of consciousness S06.0X0 ◄
Condition —see Disease
Conditions arising in the perinatal period — see Newborn, affected by
Conduct disorder —see Disorder, conduct
Condyloma A63.0
  acuminatum A63.0
  gonorrheal A54.09
  latum A51.31
  syphilitic A51.31
    congenital A50.07
  venereal, syphilitic A51.31
Conflagration —see also Burn
  asphyxia (by inhalation of gases, fumes or vapors) —see also Table of Drugs and Chemicals T59.9-
Conflict (with) —see also Discord
  family Z73.9
  marital Z63.0
    involving divorce or estrangement Z63.5
  parent-child Z62.820
    parent-adopted child Z62.821
    parent-biological child Z62.820
    parent-foster child Z62.822
  social role NEC Z73.5
Confluent —see condition
Confusion, confused R41.0
  epileptic F05
  mental state (psychogenic) F44.89
  psychogenic F44.89
  reactive (from emotional stress, psychological trauma) F44.89
Confusional arousals G47.51
Congelation T69.9
Congenital —see also condition
  aortic septum Q25.49 ◄▥
  intrinsic factor deficiency D51.0
  malformation —see Anomaly
Congestion, congestive
  bladder N32.89
  bowel K63.89
  brain G93.89
  breast N64.59
  bronchial J98.09
  catarrhal J31.0
  chest R09.89
  chill, malarial —see Malaria

Congestion, congestive (Continued)
  circulatory NEC I99.8
  duodenum K31.89
  eye —see Hyperemia, conjunctiva
  facial, due to birth injury P15.4
  general R68.89
  glottis J37.0
  heart —see Failure, heart, congestive
  hepatic K76.1
  hypostatic (lung) —see Edema, lung
  intestine K63.89
  kidney N28.89
  labyrinth —see subcategory H83.8
  larynx J37.0
  liver K76.1
  lung R09.89
    active or acute —see Pneumonia
  malaria, malarial —see Malaria
  nasal R09.81
  nose R09.81
  orbit, orbital —see also Exophthalmos
    inflammatory (chronic) —see Inflammation, orbit
  ovary N83.8
  pancreas K86.89 ◄▥
  pelvic, female N94.89
  pleural J94.8
  prostate (active) N42.1
  pulmonary —see Congestion, lung
  renal N28.89
  retina H35.81
  seminal vesicle N50.1
  spinal cord G95.19
  spleen (chronic) D73.2
  stomach K31.89
  trachea —see Tracheitis
  urethra N36.8
  uterus N85.8
    with subinvolution N85.3
  venous (passive) I87.8
  viscera R68.89
Congestive —see Congestion
Conical
  cervix (hypertrophic elongation) N88.4
  cornea —see Keratoconus
  teeth K00.2
Conjoined twins Q89.4
Conjugal maladjustment Z63.0
  involving divorce or estrangement Z63.5
Conjunctiva —see condition
Conjunctivitis (staphylococcal) (streptococcal) NOS H10.9
  Acanthamoeba B60.12
  acute H10.3-
    atopic H10.1-
    chemical —see also Corrosion, cornea H10.21-
    mucopurulent H10.02-
      follicular H10.01-
    pseudomembranous H10.22-
    serous except viral H10.23-
      viral —see Conjunctivitis, viral
    toxic H10.21-
  adenoviral (acute) (follicular) B30.1
  allergic (acute) —see Conjunctivitis, acute, atopic
    chronic H10.45
      vernal H10.44
  anaphylactic —see Conjunctivitis, acute, atopic
  Apollo B30.3
  atopic (acute) —see Conjunctivitis, acute, atopic
  Béal's B30.2
  blennorrhagic (gonococcal) (neonatorum) A54.31
  chemical (acute) —see also Corrosion, cornea H10.21-
  chlamydial A74.0
    due to trachoma A71.1
  neonatal P39.1

Conjunctivitis (Continued)
  chronic (nodosa) (petrificans) (phlyctenular) H10.40-
    allergic H10.45
      vernal H10.44
    follicular H10.43-
    giant papillary H10.41-
    simple H10.42-
    vernal H10.44
  coxsackievirus 24 B30.3
  diphtheritic A36.86
  due to
    dust —see Conjunctivitis, acute, atopic
    filariasis B74.9
    mucocutaneous leishmaniasis B55.2
  enterovirus type 70 (hemorrhagic) B30.3
  epidemic (viral) B30.9
    hemorrhagic B30.3
  gonococcal (neonatorum) A54.31
  granular (trachomatous) A71.1
    sequelae (late effect) B94.0
  hemorrhagic (acute) (epidemic) B30.3
  herpes zoster B02.31
  in (due to)
    Acanthamoeba B60.12
    adenovirus (acute) (follicular) B30.1
    Chlamydia A74.0
    coxsackievirus 24 B30.3
    diphtheria A36.86
    enterovirus type 70 (hemorrhagic) B30.3
    filariasis B74.9
    gonococci A54.31
    herpes (simplex) virus B00.53
      zoster B02.31
    infectious disease NEC B99
    meningococci A39.89
    mucocutaneous leishmaniasis B55.2
    rosacea L71.9
    syphilis (late) A52.71
    zoster B02.31
  inclusion A74.0
  infantile P39.1
    gonococcal A54.31
  Koch-Weeks' —see Conjunctivitis, acute, mucopurulent
  light —see Conjunctivitis, acute, atopic
  ligneous —see Blepharoconjunctivitis, ligneous
  meningococcal A39.89
  mucopurulent —see Conjunctivitis, acute, mucopurulent
  neonatal P39.1
    gonococcal A54.31
  Newcastle B30.8
  of Béal B30.2
  parasitic
    filariasis B74.9
    mucocutaneous leishmaniasis B55.2
  Parinaud's H10.89
  petrificans H10.89
  rosacea L71.9
  specified NEC H10.89
  swimming-pool B30.1
  trachomatous A71.1
    acute A71.0
    sequelae (late effect) B94.0
  traumatic NEC H10.89
  tuberculous A18.59
  tularemic A21.1
  tularensis A21.1
  viral B30.9
    due to
      adenovirus B30.1
      enterovirus B30.3
    specified NEC B30.8
Conjunctivochalasis H11.82-
Connective tissue —see condition
Conn's syndrome E26.01
Conradi (-Hunermann) disease Q77.3
Consanguinity Z84.3
  counseling Z71.89

Conscious simulation (of illness) Z76.5
Consecutive —*see* condition
Consolidation lung (base) —*see* Pneumonia, lobar
Constipation (atonic) (neurogenic) (simple) (spastic) K59.00
  chronic K59.09 ◀
    idiopathic K59.04 ◀
  drug-induced K59.03 ◀▥
  functional K59.04 ◀
  outlet dysfunction K59.02
  psychogenic F45.8
  slow transit K59.01
  specified NEC K59.09
Constitutional —*see also* condition
  substandard F60.7
Constitutionally substandard F60.7
Constriction —*see also* Stricture
  auditory canal —*see* Stenosis, external ear canal
  bronchial J98.09
  duodenum K31.5
  esophagus K22.2
  external
    abdomen, abdominal (wall) S30.841
    alveolar process S00.542
    ankle S90.54-
    antecubital space —*see* Constriction, external, forearm
    arm (upper) S40.84-
    auricle —*see* Constriction, external, ear
    axilla —*see* Constriction, external, arm
    back, lower S30.840
    breast S20.14-
    brow S00.84
    buttock S30.840
    calf —*see* Constriction, external, leg
    canthus —*see* Constriction, external, eyelid
    cheek S00.84
      internal S00.542
    chest wall —*see* Constriction, external, thorax
    chin S00.84
    clitoris S30.844
    costal region —*see* Constriction, external, thorax
    digit (s)
      foot —*see* Constriction, external, toe
      hand —*see* Constriction, external, finger
    ear S00.44-
    elbow S50.34-
    epididymis S30.843
    epigastric region S30.841
    esophagus, cervical S10.14
    eyebrow —*see* Constriction, external, eyelid
    eyelid S00.24-
    face S00.84
    finger (s) S60.44-
      index S60.44-
      little S60.44-
      middle S60.44-
      ring S60.44-
    flank S30.841
    foot (except toe (s) alone) S90.84-
      toe —*see* Constriction, external, toe
    forearm S50.84-
      elbow only —*see* Constriction, external, elbow
    forehead S00.84
    genital organs, external
      female S30.846
      male S30.845
    groin S30.841
    gum S00.542
    hand S60.54-
    head S00.94
      ear —*see* Constriction, external, ear
      eyelid —*see* Constriction, external, eyelid
      lip S00.541
      nose S00.34
      oral cavity S00.542

Constriction *(Continued)*
  external *(Continued)*
    head *(Continued)*
      scalp S00.04
      specified site NEC S00.84
    heel —*see* Constriction, external, foot
    hip S70.24-
    inguinal region S30.841
    interscapular region S20.449
    jaw S00.84
    knee S80.24-
    labium (majus) (minus) S30.844
    larynx S10.14
    leg (lower) S80.84-
      knee —*see* Constriction, external, knee
      upper —*see* Constriction, external, thigh
    lip S00.541
    lower back S30.840
    lumbar region S30.840
    malar region S00.84
    mammary —*see* Constriction, external, breast
    mastoid region S00.84
    mouth S00.542
    nail
      finger —*see* Constriction, external, finger
      toe —*see* Constriction, external, toe
    nasal S00.34
    neck S10.94
      specified site NEC S10.84
      throat S10.14
    nose S00.34
    occipital region S00.04
    oral cavity S00.542
    orbital region —*see* Constriction, external, eyelid
    palate S00.542
    palm —*see* Constriction, external, hand
    parietal region S00.04
    pelvis S30.840
    penis S30.842
    perineum
      female S30.844
      male S30.840
    periocular area —*see* Constriction, external, eyelid
    phalanges
      finger —*see* Constriction, external, finger
      toe —*see* Constriction, external, toe
    pharynx S10.14
    pinna —*see* Constriction, external, ear
    popliteal space —*see* Constriction, external, knee
    prepuce S30.842
    pubic region S30.840
    pudendum
      female S30.846
      male S30.845
    sacral region S30.840
    scalp S00.04
    scapular region —*see* Constriction, external, shoulder
    scrotum S30.843
    shin —*see* Constriction, external, leg
    shoulder S40.24-
    sternal region S20.349
    submaxillary region S00.84
    submental region S00.84
    subungual
      finger (s) —*see* Constriction, external, finger
      toe (s) —*see* Constriction, external, toe
    supraclavicular fossa S10.84
    supraorbital S00.84
    temple S00.84
    temporal region S00.84
    testis S30.843
    thigh S70.34-
    thorax, thoracic (wall) S20.94
      back S20.44-
      front S20.34-

Constriction *(Continued)*
  external *(Continued)*
    throat S10.14
    thumb S60.34-
    toe (s) (lesser) S90.44-
      great S90.44-
    tongue S00.542
    trachea S10.14
    tunica vaginalis S30.843
    uvula S00.542
    vagina S30.844
    vulva S30.844
    wrist S60.84-
  gallbladder —*see* Obstruction, gallbladder
  intestine —*see* Obstruction, intestine
  larynx J38.6
    congenital Q31.8
      specified NEC Q31.8
      subglottic Q31.1
  organ or site, congenital NEC —*see* Atresia, by site
  prepuce (acquired) (congenital) N47.1
  pylorus (adult hypertrophic) K31.1
    congenital or infantile Q40.0
    newborn Q40.0
  ring dystocia (uterus) O62.4
  spastic —*see also* Spasm
    ureter N13.5
  ureter N13.5
    with infection N13.6
  urethra —*see* Stricture, urethra
  visual field (peripheral) (functional) —*see* Defect, visual field
Constrictive —*see* condition
Consultation
  without complaint or sickness Z71.9
    feared complaint unfounded Z71.1
    specified reason NEC Z71.89
  medical —*see* Counseling, medical
  religious Z71.81
  specified reason NEC Z71.89
  spiritual Z71.81
Consumption —*see* Tuberculosis
Contact (with) —*see also* Exposure (to)
  acariasis Z20.7
  AIDS virus Z20.6
  air pollution Z77.110
  algae and algae toxins Z77.121
  algae bloom Z77.121
  anthrax Z20.810
  aromatic (hazardous) compounds NEC Z77.028
  aromatic amines Z77.020
  aromatic dyes NOS Z77.028
  arsenic Z77.010
  asbestos Z77.090
  bacterial disease NEC Z20.818
  benzene Z77.021
  blue-green algae bloom Z77.121
  body fluids (potentially hazardous) Z77.21
  brown tide Z77.121
  chemicals (chiefly nonmedicinal) (hazardous) NEC Z77.098
  cholera Z20.09
  chromium compounds Z77.018
  communicable disease Z20.9
    bacterial NEC Z20.818
    specified NEC Z20.89
    viral NEC Z20.828
  cyanobacteria bloom Z77.121
  dyes Z77.098
  Escherichia coli (E. coli) Z20.01
  fiberglass —*see* Table of Drugs and Chemicals, fiberglass
  German measles Z20.4
  gonorrhea Z20.2
  hazardous metals NEC Z77.018
  hazardous substances NEC Z77.29
  hazards in the physical environment NEC Z77.128
  hazards to health NEC Z77.9

Contact (Continued)
  HIV Z20.6
  HTLV-III/LAV Z20.6
  human immunodeficiency virus (HIV) Z20.6
  infection Z20.9
    specified NEC Z20.89
  infestation (parasitic) NEC Z20.7
  intestinal infectious disease NEC Z20.09
    Escherichia coli (E. coli) Z20.01
  lead Z77.011
  meningococcus Z20.811
  mold (toxic) Z77.120
  nickel dust Z77.018
  noise Z77.122
  parasitic disease Z20.7
  pediculosis Z20.7
  pfiesteria piscicida Z77.121
  poliomyelitis Z20.89
  pollution
    air Z77.110
    environmental NEC Z77.118
    soil Z77.112
    water Z77.111
  polycyclic aromatic hydrocarbons Z77.028
  rabies Z20.3
  radiation, naturally occurring NEC Z77.123
  radon Z77.123
  red tide (Florida) Z77.121
  rubella Z20.4
  sexually-transmitted disease Z20.2
  smallpox (laboratory) Z20.89
  syphilis Z20.2
  tuberculosis Z20.1
  uranium Z77.012
  varicella Z20.820
  venereal disease Z20.2
  viral disease NEC Z20.828
  viral hepatitis Z20.5
  water pollution Z77.111
Contamination, food —see Intoxication,
    foodborne
Contraception, contraceptive
  advice Z30.09
  counseling Z30.09
  device (intrauterine) (in situ) Z97.5
    causing menorrhagia T83.83
    checking Z30.431
    complications —see Complications,
        intrauterine, contraceptive device
    in place Z97.5
    initial prescription Z30.014
    reinsertion Z30.433
    removal Z30.432
    replacement Z30.433
  emergency (postcoital) Z30.012
  initial prescription Z30.019
    barrier Z30.018 ◄
    diaphragm Z30.018 ◄
    injectable Z30.013
    intrauterine device Z30.014
    pills Z30.011
    postcoital (emergency) Z30.012
    specified type NEC Z30.018
    subdermal implantable Z30.017 ◄▥
    transdermal patch hormonal Z30.016 ◄
    vaginal ring hormonal Z30.015 ◄
  maintenance Z30.40
    barrier Z30.49 ◄
    diaphragm Z30.49 ◄
    examination Z30.8
    injectable Z30.42
    intrauterine device Z30.431
    pills Z30.41
    specified type NEC Z30.49
    subdermal implantable Z30.46 ◄▥
    transdermal patch hormonal Z30.45 ◄
    vaginal ring hormonal Z30.44 ◄
  management Z30.9
    specified NEC Z30.8
  postcoital (emergency) Z30.012
  prescription Z30.019
    repeat Z30.40

Contraception, contraceptive (Continued)
  sterilization Z30.2
  surveillance (drug) —see Contraception,
    maintenance
Contraction (s), contracture, contracted
  Achilles tendon —see also Short, tendon,
      Achilles
    congenital Q66.89
  amputation stump (surgical) (flexion) (late)
      next proximal joint T87.89
  anus K59.8
  bile duct (common) (hepatic) K83.8
  bladder N32.89
    neck or sphincter N32.0
  bowel, cecum, colon or intestine, any part —
      see Obstruction, intestine
  Braxton Hicks —see False, labor
  breast implant, capsular T85.44
  bronchial J98.09
  burn (old) —see Cicatrix
  cervix —see Stricture, cervix
  cicatricial —see Cicatrix
  conjunctiva, trachomatous, active A71.1
    sequelae (late effect) B94.0
  Dupuytren's M72.0
  eyelid —see Disorder, eyelid function
  fascia (lata) (postural) M72.8
    Dupuytren's M72.0
    palmar M72.0
    plantar M72.2
  finger NEC —see also Deformity, finger
    congenital Q68.1
    joint —see Contraction, joint, hand
  flaccid —see Contraction, paralytic
  gallbladder K82.0
  heart valve —see Endocarditis
  hip —see Contraction, joint, hip
  hourglass
    bladder N32.89
      congenital Q64.79
    gallbladder K82.0
      congenital Q44.1
    stomach K31.89
      congenital Q40.2
      psychogenic F45.8
    uterus (complicating delivery) O62.4
  hysterical F44.4
  internal os —see Stricture, cervix
  joint (abduction) (acquired) (adduction)
      (flexion) (rotation) M24.50
    ankle M24.57-
    congenital NEC Q68.8
      hip Q65.89
    elbow M24.52-
    foot joint M24.57-
    hand joint M24.54-
    hip M24.55-
      congenital Q65.89
    hysterical F44.4
    knee M24.56-
    shoulder M24.51-
    wrist M24.53-
  kidney (granular) (secondary) N26.9
    congenital Q63.8
    hydronephritic —see Hydronephrosis
        Page N26.2
    pyelonephritic —see Pyelitis, chronic
    tuberculous A18.11
  ligament —see also Disorder, ligament
    congenital Q79.8
  muscle (postinfective) (postural) NEC M62.40
    with contracture of joint —see Contraction,
        joint
    ankle M62.47-
    congenital Q79.8
      sternocleidomastoid Q68.0
    extraocular —see Strabismus
    eye (extrinsic) —see Strabismus
    foot M62.47-
    forearm M62.43-
    hand M62.44-

Contraction, contracture, contracted
    (Continued)
  muscle (Continued)
    hysterical F44.4
    ischemic (Volkmann's) T79.6
    lower leg M62.46-
    multiple sites M62.49
    pelvic region M62.45-
    posttraumatic —see Strabismus, paralytic
    psychogenic F45.8
      conversion reaction F44.4
    shoulder region M62.41-
    specified site NEC M62.48
    thigh M62.45-
    upper arm M62.42-
  neck —see Torticollis
  ocular muscle —see Strabismus
  organ or site, congenital NEC —see Atresia,
      by site
  outlet (pelvis) —see Contraction, pelvis
  palmar fascia M72.0
  paralytic
    joint —see Contraction, joint
    muscle —see also Contraction, muscle NEC
      ocular —see Strabismus, paralytic
  pelvis (acquired) (general) M95.5
    with disproportion (fetopelvic) O33.1
      causing obstructed labor O65.1
      inlet O33.2
      mid-cavity O33.3
      outlet O33.3
  plantar fascia M72.2
  premature
    atrium I49.1
    auriculoventricular I49.49
    heart I49.49
    junctional I49.2
    supraventricular I49.1
    ventricular I49.3
  prostate N42.89
  pylorus NEC —see also Pylorospasm
    psychogenic F45.8
  rectum, rectal (sphincter) K59.8
  ring (Bandl's) (complicating delivery) O62.4
  scar —see Cicatrix
  spine —see Dorsopathy, deforming
  sternocleidomastoid (muscle), congenital
      Q68.0
  stomach K31.89
    hourglass K31.89
      congenital Q40.2
      psychogenic F45.8
    psychogenic F45.8
  tendon (sheath) M62.40
    with contracture of joint —see Contraction,
        joint
    Achilles —see Short, tendon, Achilles
    ankle M62.47-
      Achilles —see Short, tendon, Achilles
    foot M62.47-
    forearm M62.43-
    hand M62.44-
    lower leg M62.46-
    multiple sites M62.49
    neck M62.48
    pelvic region M62.45-
    shoulder region M62.41-
    specified site NEC M62.48
    thigh M62.45-
    thorax M62.48
    trunk M62.48
    upper arm M62.42-
  toe —see Deformity, toe, specified NEC
  ureterovesical orifice (postinfectional) N13.5
    with infection N13.6
  urethra —see also Stricture, urethra
    orifice N32.0
  uterus N85.8
    abnormal NEC O62.9
    clonic (complicating delivery) O62.4
    dyscoordinate (complicating delivery) O62.4

Contraction, contracture, contracted
    (Continued)
  uterus (Continued)
    hourglass (complicating delivery) O62.4
    hypertonic O62.4
    hypotonic NEC O62.2
    inadequate
      primary O62.0
      secondary O62.1
    incoordinate (complicating delivery) O62.4
    poor O62.2
    tetanic (complicating delivery) O62.4
  vagina (outlet) N89.5
  vesical N32.89
    neck or urethral orifice N32.0
  visual field —see Defect, visual field,
      generalized
  Volkmann's (ischemic) T79.6
Contusion (skin surface intact) T14.8
  abdomen, abdominal (muscle) (wall) S30.1
  adnexa, eye NEC S05.8X-
  adrenal gland S37.812
  alveolar process S00.532
  ankle S90.0-
  antecubital space —see Contusion, forearm
  anus S30.3
  arm (upper) S40.02-
    lower (with elbow) —see Contusion,
        forearm
  auditory canal —see Contusion, ear
  auricle —see Contusion, ear
  axilla —see Contusion, arm, upper
  back —see also Contusion, thorax, back
    lower S30.0
  bile duct S36.13
  bladder S37.22
  bone NEC T14.8
  brain (diffuse) —see Injury, intracranial, diffuse
    focal —see Injury, intracranial, focal
  brainstem S06.38-
  breast S20.0-
  broad ligament S37.892
  brow S00.83
  buttock S30.0
  canthus, eye S00.1-
  cauda equina S34.3
  cerebellar, traumatic S06.37-
  cerebral S06.33-
    left side S06.32-
    right side S06.31-
  cheek S00.83
    internal S00.532
  chest (wall) —see Contusion, thorax
  chin S00.83
  clitoris S30.23
  colon —see Injury, intestine, large, contusion
  common bile duct S36.13
  conjunctiva S05.1-
    with foreign body (in conjunctival sac) —
        see Foreign body, conjunctival sac
  conus medullaris (spine) S34.139
  cornea —see Contusion, eyeball
    with foreign body —see Foreign body,
        cornea
  corpus cavernosum S30.21
  cortex (brain) (cerebral) —see Injury,
      intracranial, diffuse
    focal —see Injury, intracranial, focal
  costal region —see Contusion, thorax
  cystic duct S36.13
  diaphragm S27.802
  duodenum S36.420
  ear S00.43-
  elbow S50.0-
    with forearm —see Contusion, forearm
  epididymis S30.22
  epigastric region S30.1
  epiglottis S10.0
  esophagus (thoracic) S27.812
    cervical S10.0
  eyeball S05.1-

Contusion (Continued)
  eyebrow S00.1-
  eyelid (and periocular area) S00.1-
  face NEC S00.83
  fallopian tube S37.529
    bilateral S37.522
    unilateral S37.521
  femoral triangle S30.1
  finger (s) S60.00
    with damage to nail (matrix) S60.10
    index S60.02-
      with damage to nail S60.12-
    little S60.05-
      with damage to nail S60.15-
    middle S60.03-
      with damage to nail S60.13-
    ring S60.04-
      with damage to nail S60.14-
    thumb —see Contusion, thumb
  flank S30.1
  foot (except toe (s) alone) S90.3-
    toe —see Contusion, toe
  forearm S50.1-
    elbow only —see Contusion, elbow
  forehead S00.83
  gallbladder S36.122
  genital organs, external
    female S30.202
    male S30.201
  globe (eye) —see Contusion, eyeball
  groin S30.1
  gum S00.532
  hand S60.22-
    finger (s) —see Contusion, finger
    wrist —see Contusion, wrist
  head S00.93
    ear —see Contusion, ear
    eyelid —see Contusion, eyelid
    lip S00.531
    nose S00.33
    oral cavity S00.532
    scalp S00.03
    specified part NEC S00.83
  heart —see also Injury, heart S26.91 ◀
  heel —see Contusion, foot
  hepatic duct S36.13
  hip S70.0-
  ileum S36.428
  iliac region S30.1
  inguinal region S30.1
  interscapular region S20.229
  intra-abdominal organ S36.92
    colon —see Injury, intestine, large, contusion
    liver S36.112
    pancreas —see Contusion, pancreas
    rectum S36.62
    small intestine —see Injury, intestine, small,
        contusion
    specified organ NEC S36.892
    spleen —see Contusion, spleen
    stomach S36.32
  iris (eye) —see Contusion, eyeball
  jaw S00.83
  jejunum S36.428
  kidney S37.01-
    major (greater than 2 cm) S37.02-
    minor (less than 2 cm) S37.01-
  knee S80.0-
  labium (majus) (minus) S30.23
  lacrimal apparatus, gland or sac S05.8X-
  larynx S10.0
  leg (lower) S80.1-
    knee —see Contusion, knee
  lens —see Contusion, eyeball
  lip S00.531
  liver S36.112
  lower back S30.0
  lumbar region S30.0
  lung S27.329
    bilateral S27.322
    unilateral S27.321

Contusion (Continued)
  malar region S00.83
  mastoid region S00.83
  membrane, brain —see Injury, intracranial,
      diffuse
    focal —see Injury, intracranial, focal
  mesentery S36.892
  mesosalpinx S37.892
  mouth S00.532
  muscle —see Contusion, by site
  nail
    finger —see Contusion, finger, with
        damage to nail
    toe —see Contusion, toe, with damage to
        nail
  nasal S00.33
  neck S10.93
    specified site NEC S10.83
    throat S10.0
  nerve —see Injury, nerve
  newborn P54.5
  nose S00.33
  occipital
    lobe (brain) —see Injury, intracranial,
        diffuse
    focal —see Injury, intracranial,
        focal
    region (scalp) S00.03
  orbit (region) (tissues) S05.1-
  ovary S37.429
    bilateral S37.422
    unilateral S37.421
  palate S00.532
  pancreas S36.229
    body S36.221
    head S36.220
    tail S36.222
  parietal
    lobe (brain) —see Injury, intracranial,
        diffuse
    focal —see Injury, intracranial, focal
    region (scalp) S00.03
  pelvic organ S37.92
    adrenal gland S37.812
    bladder S37.22
    fallopian tube —see Contusion, fallopian
        tube
    kidney —see Contusion, kidney
    ovary —see Contusion, ovary
    prostate S37.822
    specified organ NEC S37.892
    ureter S37.12
    urethra S37.32
    uterus S37.62
  pelvis S30.0
  penis S30.21
  perineum
    female S30.23
    male S30.0
  periocular area S00.1-
  peritoneum S36.81
  periurethral tissue —see Contusion,
      urethra
  pharynx S10.0
  pinna —see Contusion, ear
  popliteal space —see Contusion, knee
  prepuce S30.21
  prostate S37.822
  pubic region S30.1
  pudendum
    female S30.202
    male S30.201
  quadriceps femoris —see Contusion, thigh
  rectum S36.62
  retroperitoneum S36.892
  round ligament S37.892
  sacral region S30.0
  scalp S00.03
    due to birth injury P12.3
  scapular region —see Contusion, shoulder
  sclera —see Contusion, eyeball

◀ New   ◀▥ Revised   ~~deleted~~ Deleted

Contusion *(Continued)*
 scrotum S30.22
 seminal vesicle S37.892
 shoulder S40.01-
 skin NEC T14.8
 small intestine —*see* Injury, intestine, small,
  contusion
 spermatic cord S30.22
 spinal cord —*see* Injury, spinal cord, by region
  cauda equina S34.3
  conus medullaris S34.139
 spleen S36.029
  major S36.021
  minor S36.020
 sternal region S20.219
 stomach S36.32
 subconjunctival S05.1-
 subcutaneous NEC T14.8
 submaxillary region S00.83
 submental region S00.83
 subperiosteal NEC T14.8
 subungual
  finger —*see* Contusion, finger, with
   damage to nail
  toe —*see* Contusion, toe, with damage to
   nail
 supraclavicular fossa S10.83
 supraorbital S00.83
 suprarenal gland S37.812
 temple (region) S00.83
 temporal
  lobe (brain) —*see* Injury, intracranial,
   diffuse
  focal —*see* Injury, intracranial, focal
  region S00.83
 testis S30.22
 thigh S70.1-
 thorax (wall) S20.20
  back S20.22-
  front S20.21-
 throat S10.0
 thumb S60.01-
  with damage to nail S60.11-
 toe (s) (lesser) S90.12-
  with damage to nail S90.22-
  great S90.11-
   with damage to nail S90.21-
   specified type NEC S90.221
 tongue S00.532
 trachea (cervical) S10.0
  thoracic S27.52
 tunica vaginalis S30.22
 tympanum, tympanic membrane —*see*
  Contusion, ear
 ureter S37.12
 urethra S37.32
 urinary organ NEC S37.892
 uterus S37.62
 uvula S00.532
 vagina S30.23
 vas deferens S37.892
 vesical S37.22
 vocal cord (s) S10.0
 vulva S30.23
 wrist S60.21-
Conus (congenital) (any type) Q14.8
 cornea —*see* Keratoconus
 medullaris syndrome G95.81
Conversion hysteria, neurosis or reaction F44.9
Converter, tuberculosis (test reaction) R76.11
Conviction (legal), anxiety concerning Z65.0
 with imprisonment Z65.1
Convulsions (idiopathic) —*see also* Seizure(s)
 R56.9
 apoplectiform (cerebral ischemia) I67.82
 benign neonatal (familial) —see Epilepsy,
  generalized, idiopathic
 dissociative F44.5
 epileptic —*see* Epilepsy
 epileptiform, epileptoid —*see* Seizure,
  epileptiform

Convulsions *(Continued)*
 ether (anesthetic) —*see* Table of Drugs and
  Chemicals, by drug
 febrile R56.00
  with status epilepticus G40.901
  complex R56.01
   with status epilepticus G40.901
  simple R56.00
 hysterical F44.5
 infantile P90
  epilepsy —*see* Epilepsy
 jacksonian —*see* Epilepsy, localization-
  related, symptomatic, with simple
  partial seizures
 myoclonic G25.3
 neonatal, benign (familial) —see Epilepsy,
  generalized, idiopathic
 newborn P90
 obstetrical (nephritic) (uremic) —*see*
  Eclampsia
 paretic A52.17
 post traumatic R56.1
 psychomotor —*see* Epilepsy, localization-
  related, symptomatic, with complex
  partial seizures
 recurrent R56.9
 reflex R25.8
 scarlatinal A38.8
 tetanus, tetanic —*see* Tetanus
 thymic E32.8
Convulsive —*see also* Convulsions
Cooley's anemia D56.1
Coolie itch B76.9
Cooper's
 disease —*see* Mastopathy, cystic
 hernia —*see* Hernia, abdomen, specified site
  NEC
Copra itch B88.0
Coprophagy F50.89 ◀▥
Coprophobia F40.298
Coproporphyria, hereditary E80.29
Cor
 biloculare Q20.8
 bovis, bovinum —*see* Hypertrophy, cardiac
 pulmonale (chronic) I27.81
  acute I26.09
 triatriatum, triatrium Q24.2
 triloculare Q20.8
  biatrium Q20.4
  biventriculare Q21.1
Corbus' disease (gangrenous balanitis) N48.1
Cord —*see also* condition
 around neck (tightly) (with compression)
  complicating delivery O69.1
 bladder G95.89
  tabetic A52.19
Cordis ectopia Q24.8
Corditis (spermatic) N49.1
Corectopia Q13.2
Cori's disease (glycogen storage) E74.03
Corkhandler's disease or lung J67.3
Corkscrew esophagus K22.4
Corkworker's disease or lung J67.3
Corn (infected) L84
Cornea —*see also* condition
 donor Z52.5
 plana Q13.4
Cornelia de Lange syndrome Q87.1
Cornu cutaneum L85.8
Cornual gestation or pregnancy O00.80 ◀▥
 with intrauterine pregnancy O00.81 ◀
Coronary (artery) —*see* condition
Coronavirus, as cause of disease classified
 elsewhere B97.29
 SARS-associated B97.21
Corpora —*see also* condition
 amylacea, prostate N42.89
 cavernosa —*see* condition
Corpulence —*see* Obesity
Corpus —*see* condition
Corrected transposition Q20.5

Corrosion (injury) (acid) (caustic) (chemical)
 (lime) (external) (internal) T30.4
 abdomen, abdominal (muscle) (wall) T21.42
  first degree T21.52
  second degree T21.62
  third degree T21.72
 above elbow T22.439
  first degree T22.539
  left T22.432
   first degree T22.532
   second degree T22.632
   third degree T22.732
  right T22.431
   first degree T22.531
   second degree T22.631
   third degree T22.731
  second degree T22.639
  third degree T22.739
 alimentary tract NEC T28.7
 ankle T25.419
  first degree T25.519
  left T25.412
   first degree T25.512
   second degree T25.612
   third degree T25.712
  multiple with foot —*see* Corrosion, lower,
   limb, multiple, ankle and foot
  right T25.411
   first degree T25.511
   second degree T25.611
   third degree T25.711
  second degree T25.619
  third degree T25.719
 anus —*see* Corrosion, buttock
 arm (s) (meaning upper limb (s)) —*see*
  Corrosion, upper limb
 axilla T22.449
  first degree T22.549
  left T22.442
   first degree T22.542
   second degree T22.642
   third degree T22.742
  right T22.441
   first degree T22.541
   second degree T22.641
   third degree T22.741
  second degree T22.649
  third degree T22.749
 back (lower) T21.44
  first degree T21.54
  second degree T21.64
  third degree T21.74
  upper T21.43
   first degree T21.53
   second degree T21.63
   third degree T21.73
 blisters - code as Corrosion, second degree,
  by site
 breast (s) —*see* Corrosion, chest wall
 buttock (s) T21.45
  first degree T21.55
  second degree T21.65
  third degree T21.75
 calf T24.439
  first degree T24.539
  left T24.432
   first degree T24.532
   second degree T24.632
   third degree T24.732
  right T24.431
   first degree T24.531
   second degree T24.631
   third degree T24.731
  second degree T24.639
  third degree T24.739
 canthus (eye) —*see* Corrosion, eyelid
 cervix T28.8
 cheek T20.46
  first degree T20.56
  second degree T20.66
  third degree T20.76

Corrosion (Continued)
  chest wall T21.41
    first degree T21.51
    second degree T21.61
    third degree T21.71
  chin T20.43
    first degree T20.53
    second degree T20.63
    third degree T20.73
  colon T28.7
  conjunctiva (and cornea) —*see* Corrosion, cornea
  cornea (and conjunctiva) T26.6-
  deep necrosis of underlying tissue - code as Corrosion, third degree, by site
  dorsum of hand T23.469
    first degree T23.569
    left T23.462
      first degree T23.562
      second degree T23.662
      third degree T23.762
    right T23.461
      first degree T23.561
      second degree T23.661
      third degree T23.761
    second degree T23.669
    third degree T23.769
  ear (auricle) (external) (canal) T20.41
    drum T28.91
    first degree T20.51
    second degree T20.61
    third degree T20.71
  elbow T22.429
    first degree T22.529
    left T22.422
      first degree T22.522
      second degree T22.622
      third degree T22.722
    right T22.421
      first degree T22.521
      second degree T22.621
      third degree T22.721
    second degree T22.629
    third degree T22.729
  entire body —*see* Corrosion, multiple body regions
  epidermal loss - code as Corrosion, second degree, by site
  epiglottis T27.4
  erythema, erythematous - code as Corrosion, first degree, by site
  esophagus T28.6
  extent (percentage of body surface)
    less than 10 percent T32.0
    10-19 percent (0-9 percent third degree) T32.10
      with 10-19 percent third degree T32.11
    20-29 percent (0-9 percent third degree) T32.20
      with
        10-19 percent third degree T32.21
        20-29 percent third degree T32.22
    30-39 percent (0-9 percent third degree) T32.30
      with
        10-19 percent third degree T32.31
        20-29 percent third degree T32.32
        30-39 percent third degree T32.33
    40-49 percent (0-9 percent third degree) T32.40
      with
        10-19 percent third degree T32.41
        20-29 percent third degree T32.42
        30-39 percent third degree T32.43
        40-49 percent third degree T32.44
    50-59 percent (0-9 percent third degree) T32.50
      with
        10-19 percent third degree T32.51
        20-29 percent third degree T32.52

Corrosion (Continued)
  extent (Continued)
    50-59 percent (Continued)
      with (Continued)
        30-39 percent third degree T32.53
        40-49 percent third degree T32.54
        50-59 percent third degree T32.55
    60-69 percent (0-9 percent third degree) T32.60
      with
        10-19 percent third degree T32.61
        20-29 percent third degree T32.62
        30-39 percent third degree T32.63
        40-49 percent third degree T32.64
        50-59 percent third degree T32.65
        60-69 percent third degree T32.66
    70-79 percent (0-9 percent third degree) T32.70
      with
        10-19 percent third degree T32.71
        20-29 percent third degree T32.72
        30-39 percent third degree T32.73
        40-49 percent third degree T32.74
        50-59 percent third degree T32.75
        60-69 percent third degree T32.76
        70-79 percent third degree T32.77
    80-89 percent (0-9 percent third degree) T32.80
      with
        10-19 percent third degree T32.81
        20-29 percent third degree T32.82
        30-39 percent third degree T32.83
        40-49 percent third degree T32.84
        50-59 percent third degree T32.85
        60-69 percent third degree T32.86
        70-79 percent third degree T32.87
        80-89 percent third degree T32.88
    90 percent or more (0-9 percent third degree) T32.90
      with
        10-19 percent third degree T32.91
        20-29 percent third degree T32.92
        30-39 percent third degree T32.93
        40-49 percent third degree T32.94
        50-59 percent third degree T32.95
        60-69 percent third degree T32.96
        70-79 percent third degree T32.97
        80-89 percent third degree T32.98
        90-99 percent third degree T32.99
  extremity —*see* Corrosion, limb
  eye (s) and adnexa T26.9-
    with resulting rupture and destruction of eyeball T26.7-
    conjunctival sac —*see* Corrosion, cornea
    cornea —*see* Corrosion, cornea
    lid —*see* Corrosion, eyelid
    periocular area —*see* Corrosion eyelid
    specified site NEC T26.8-
  eyeball —*see* Corrosion, eye
  eyelid (s) T26.5-
  face —*see* Corrosion, head
  finger T23.429
    first degree T23.529
    left T23.422
      first degree T23.522
      second degree T23.622
      third degree T23.722
    multiple sites (without thumb) T23.439
      with thumb T23.449
        first degree T23.549
        left T23.442
          first degree T23.542
          second degree T23.642
          third degree T23.742
        right T23.441
          first degree T23.541
          second degree T23.641
          third degree T23.741
      second degree T23.649
      third degree T23.749

Corrosion (Continued)
  finger (Continued)
    multiple sites (Continued)
      first degree T23.539
      left T23.432
        first degree T23.532
        second degree T23.632
        third degree T23.732
      right T23.431
        first degree T23.531
        second degree T23.631
        third degree T23.731
      second degree T23.639
      third degree T23.739
    right T23.421
      first degree T23.521
      second degree T23.621
      third degree T23.721
    second degree T23.629
    third degree T23.729
  flank —*see* Corrosion, abdomen
  foot T25.429
    first degree T25.529
    left T25.422
      first degree T25.522
      second degree T25.622
      third degree T25.722
    multiple with ankle —*see* Corrosion, lower, limb, multiple, ankle and foot
    right T25.421
      first degree T25.521
      second degree T25.621
      third degree T25.721
    second degree T25.629
    third degree T25.729
  forearm T22.419
    first degree T22.519
    left T22.412
      first degree T22.512
      second degree T22.612
      third degree T22.712
    right T22.411
      first degree T22.511
      second degree T22.611
      third degree T22.711
    second degree T22.619
    third degree T22.719
  forehead T20.46
    first degree T20.56
    second degree T20.66
    third degree T20.76
  fourth degree - code as Corrosion, third degree, by site
  full thickness skin loss - code as Corrosion, third degree, by site
  gastrointestinal tract NEC T28.7
  genital organs
    external
      female T21.47
        first degree T21.57
        second degree T21.67
        third degree T21.77
      male T21.46
        first degree T21.56
        second degree T21.66
        third degree T21.76
    internal T28.8
  groin —*see* Corrosion, abdominal wall
  hand (s) T23.409
    back —*see* Corrosion, dorsum of hand
    finger —*see* Corrosion, finger
    first degree T23.509
    left T23.402
      first degree T23.502
      second degree T23.602
      third degree T23.702
    multiple sites with wrist T23.499
      first degree T23.599
      left T23.492
        first degree T23.592
        second degree T23.692
        third degree T23.792

Corrosion *(Continued)*
    hand (s) *(Continued)*
        multiple sites *(Continued)*
            right T23.491
                first degree T23.591
                second degree T23.691
                third degree T23.791
            second degree T23.699
            third degree T23.799
        palm —*see* Corrosion, palm
        right T23.401
            first degree T23.501
            second degree T23.601
            third degree T23.701
        second degree T23.609
        third degree T23.709
        thumb —*see* Corrosion, thumb
    head (and face) (and neck) T20.40
        cheek —*see* Corrosion, cheek
        chin —*see* Corrosion, chin
        ear —*see* Corrosion, ear
        eye (s) only —*see* Corrosion, eye
        first degree T20.50
        forehead —*see* Corrosion, forehead
        lip —*see* Corrosion, lip
        multiple sites T20.49
            first degree T20.59
            second degree T20.69
            third degree T20.79
        neck —*see* Corrosion, neck
        nose —*see* Corrosion, nose
        scalp —*see* Corrosion, scalp
        second degree T20.60
        third degree T20.70
    hip (s) —*see* Corrosion, lower, limb
    inhalation —*see* Corrosion, respiratory
        tract
    internal organ (s) *(see also* Corrosion, by site)
        T28.90
        alimentary tract T28.7
            esophagus T28.6
        esophagus T28.6
        genitourinary T28.8
        mouth T28.5
        pharynx T28.5
        specified organ NEC T28.99
    interscapular region —*see* Corrosion, back,
        upper
    intestine (large) (small) T28.7
    knee T24.429
        first degree T24.529
        left T24.422
            first degree T24.522
            second degree T24.622
            third degree T24.722
        right T24.421
            first degree T24.521
            second degree T24.621
            third degree T24.721
        second degree T24.629
        third degree T24.729
    labium (majus) (minus) —*see* Corrosion,
        genital organs, external, female
    lacrimal apparatus, duct, gland or sac —*see*
        Corrosion, eye, specified site NEC
    larynx T27.4
        with lung T27.5
    leg (s) (meaning lower limb (s)) —*see*
        Corrosion, lower limb
    limb (s)
        lower —*see* Corrosion, lower, limb
        upper —*see* Corrosion, upper limb
    lip (s) T20.42
        first degree T20.52
        second degree T20.62
        third degree T20.72
    lower
        back —*see* Corrosion, back
        limb T24.409
            ankle —*see* Corrosion, ankle
            calf —*see* Corrosion, calf

Corrosion *(Continued)*
    lower *(Continued)*
        limb *(Continued)*
            first degree T24.509
            foot —*see* Corrosion, foot
            hip —*see* Corrosion, thigh
            knee —*see* Corrosion, knee
            left T24.402
                first degree T24.502
                second degree T24.602
                third degree T24.702
            multiple sites, except ankle and foot
                T24.499
                ankle and foot T25.499
                    first degree T25.599
                    left T25.492
                        first degree T25.592
                        second degree T25.692
                        third degree T25.792
                    right T25.491
                        first degree T25.591
                        second degree T25.691
                        third degree T25.791
                    second degree T25.699
                    third degree T25.799
                first degree T24.599
                left T24.492
                    first degree T24.592
                    second degree T24.692
                    third degree T24.792
                right T24.491
                    first degree T24.591
                    second degree T24.691
                    third degree T24.791
                second degree T24.699
                third degree T24.799
            right T24.401
                first degree T24.501
                second degree T24.601
                third degree T24.701
            second degree T24.609
            thigh —*see* Corrosion, thigh
            third degree T24.709
    lung (with larynx and trachea)
        T27.5
    mouth T28.5
    neck T20.47
        first degree T20.57
        second degree T20.67
        third degree T20.77
    nose (septum) T20.44
        first degree T20.54
        second degree T20.64
        third degree T20.74
    ocular adnexa —*see* Corrosion, eye
    orbit region —*see* Corrosion, eyelid
    palm T23.459
        first degree T23.559
        left T23.452
            first degree T23.552
            second degree T23.652
            third degree T23.752
        right T23.451
            first degree T23.551
            second degree T23.651
            third degree T23.751
        second degree T23.659
        third degree T23.759
    partial thickness - code as Corrosion,
        unspecified degree, by site
    pelvis —*see* Corrosion, trunk
    penis —*see* Corrosion, genital organs,
        external, male
    perineum
        female —*see* Corrosion, genital organs,
            external, female
        male —*see* Corrosion, genital organs,
            external, male
    periocular area —*see* Corrosion, eyelid
    pharynx T28.5
    rectum T28.7

Corrosion *(Continued)*
    respiratory tract T27.7
        larynx —*see* Corrosion, larynx
        specified part NEC T27.6
        trachea —*see* Corrosion, larynx
    sac, lacrimal —*see* Corrosion, eye,
        specified site NEC
    scalp T20.45
        first degree T20.55
        second degree T20.65
        third degree T20.75
    scapular region T22.469
        first degree T22.569
        left T22.462
            first degree T22.562
            second degree T22.662
            third degree T22.762
        right T22.461
            first degree T22.561
            second degree T22.661
            third degree T22.761
        second degree T22.669
        third degree T22.769
    sclera —*see* Corrosion, eye, specified site
        NEC
    scrotum —*see* Corrosion, genital organs,
        external, male
    shoulder T22.459
        first degree T22.559
        left T22.452
            first degree T22.552
            second degree T22.652
            third degree T22.752
        right T22.451
            first degree T22.551
            second degree T22.651
            third degree T22.751
        second degree T22.659
        third degree T22.759
    stomach T28.7
    temple —*see* Corrosion, head
    testis —*see* Corrosion, genital organs,
        external, male
    thigh T24.419
        first degree T24.519
        left T24.412
            first degree T24.512
            second degree T24.612
            third degree T24.712
        right T24.411
            first degree T24.511
            second degree T24.611
            third degree T24.711
        second degree T24.619
        third degree T24.719
    thorax (external) —*see* Corrosion, trunk
    throat (meaning pharynx) T28.5
    thumb (s) T23.419
        first degree T23.519
        left T23.412
            first degree T23.512
            second degree T23.612
            third degree T23.712
        multiple sites with fingers T23.449
            first degree T23.549
            left T23.442
                first degree T23.542
                second degree T23.642
                third degree T23.742
            right T23.441
                first degree T23.541
                second degree T23.641
                third degree T23.741
            second degree T23.649
            third degree T23.749
        right T23.411
            first degree T23.511
            second degree T23.611
            third degree T23.711
        second degree T23.619
        third degree T23.719

Corrosion (Continued)
  toe T25.439
    first degree T25.539
    left T25.432
      first degree T25.532
      second degree T25.632
      third degree T25.732
    right T25.431
      first degree T25.531
      second degree T25.631
      third degree T25.731
    second degree T25.639
    third degree T25.739
  tongue T28.5
  tonsil (s) T28.5
  total body —see Corrosion, multiple body
      regions
  trachea T27.4
    with lung T27.5
  trunk T21.40
    abdominal wall —see Corrosion,
        abdominal wall
    anus —see Corrosion, buttock
    axilla —see Corrosion, upper limb
    back —see Corrosion, back
    breast —see Corrosion, chest wall
    buttock —see Corrosion, buttock
    chest wall —see Corrosion, chest wall
    first degree T21.50
    flank —see Corrosion, abdominal wall
    genital
      female —see Corrosion, genital organs,
          external, female
      male —see Corrosion, genital organs,
          external, male
    groin —see Corrosion, abdominal wall
    interscapular region —see Corrosion, back,
        upper
    labia —see Corrosion, genital organs,
        external, female
    lower back —see Corrosion, back
    penis —see Corrosion, genital organs,
        external, male
    perineum
      female —see Corrosion, genital organs,
          external, female
      male —see Corrosion, genital organs,
          external, male
    scapular region —see Corrosion, upper
        limb
    scrotum —see Corrosion, genital organs,
        external, male
    second degree T21.60
    shoulder —see Corrosion, upper limb
    specified site NEC T21.49
      first degree T21.59
      second degree T21.69
      third degree T21.79
    testes —see Corrosion, genital organs,
        external, male
    third degree T21.70
    upper back —see Corrosion, back, upper
    vagina T28.8
    vulva —see Corrosion, genital organs,
        external, female
  unspecified site with extent of body surface
      involved specified
    less than 10 percent T32.0
    10-19 percent (0-9 percent third degree)
        T32.10
      with 10-19 percent third degree T32.11
    20-29 percent (0-9 percent third degree)
        T32.20
      with
        10-19 percent third degree T32.21
        20-29 percent third degree T32.22
    30-39 percent (0-9 percent third degree)
        T32.30
      with
        10-19 percent third degree T32.31
        20-29 percent third degree T32.32
        30-39 percent third degree T32.33

Corrosion (Continued)
  unspecified site with extent of body surface
      involved specified (Continued)
    40-49 percent (0-9 percent third degree)
        T32.40
      with
        10-19 percent third degree T32.41
        20-29 percent third degree T32.42
        30-39 percent third degree T32.43
        40-49 percent third degree T32.44
    50-59 percent (0-9 percent third degree)
        T32.50
      with
        10-19 percent third degree T32.51
        20-29 percent third degree T32.52
        30-39 percent third degree T32.53
        40-49 percent third degree T32.54
        50-59 percent third degree T32.55
    60-69 percent (0-9 percent third degree)
        T32.60
      with
        10-19 percent third degree T32.61
        20-29 percent third degree T32.62
        30-39 percent third degree T32.63
        40-49 percent third degree T32.64
        50-59 percent third degree T32.65
        60-69 percent third degree T32.66
    70-79 percent (0-9 percent third degree)
        T32.70
      with
        10-19 percent third degree T32.71
        20-29 percent third degree T32.72
        30-39 percent third degree T32.73
        40-49 percent third degree T32.74
        50-59 percent third degree T32.75
        60-69 percent third degree T32.76
        70-79 percent third degree T32.77
    80-89 percent (0-9 percent third degree)
        T32.80
      with
        10-19 percent third degree T32.81
        20-29 percent third degree T32.82
        30-39 percent third degree T32.83
        40-49 percent third degree T32.84
        50-59 percent third degree T32.85
        60-69 percent third degree T32.86
        70-79 percent third degree T32.87
        80-89 percent third degree T32.88
    90 percent or more (0-9 percent third
        degree) T32.90
      with
        10-19 percent third degree T32.91
        20-29 percent third degree T32.92
        30-39 percent third degree T32.93
        40-49 percent third degree T32.94
        50-59 percent third degree T32.95
        60-69 percent third degree T32.96
        70-79 percent third degree T32.97
        80-89 percent third degree T32.98
        90-99 percent third degree T32.99
  upper limb (axilla) (scapular region) T22.40
    above elbow —see Corrosion, above elbow
    axilla —see Corrosion, axilla
    elbow —see Corrosion, elbow
    first degree T22.50
    forearm —see Corrosion, forearm
    hand —see Corrosion, hand
    interscapular region —see Corrosion, back,
        upper
    multiple sites T22.499
      first degree T22.599
      left T22.492
        first degree T22.592
        second degree T22.692
        third degree T22.792
      right T22.491
        first degree T22.591
        second degree T22.691
        third degree T22.791
      second degree T22.699
      third degree T22.799

Corrosion (Continued)
  upper limb (axilla) (scapular region)
      (Continued)
    scapular region —see Corrosion, scapular
        region
    second degree T22.60
    shoulder —see Corrosion, shoulder
    third degree T22.70
    wrist —see Corrosion, hand
  uterus T28.8
  vagina T28.8
  vulva —see Corrosion, genital organs,
      external, female
  wrist T23.479
    first degree T23.579
    left T23.472
      first degree T23.572
      second degree T23.672
      third degree T23.772
    multiple sites with hand T23.499
      first degree T23.599
      left T23.492
        first degree T23.592
        second degree T23.692
        third degree T23.792
      right T23.491
        first degree T23.591
        second degree T23.691
        third degree T23.791
      second degree T23.699
      third degree T23.799
    right T23.471
      first degree T23.571
      second degree T23.671
      third degree T23.771
    second degree T23.679
    third degree T23.779
Corrosive burn —see Corrosion
Corsican fever —see Malaria
Cortical —see condition
Cortico-adrenal —see condition
Coryza (acute) J00
  with grippe or influenza —see Influenza,
      with, respiratory manifestations
      NEC
  syphilitic
    congenital (chronic) A50.05
Costen's syndrome or complex M26.69
Costiveness —see Constipation
Costochondritis M94.0
Cot death R99
Cotard's syndrome F22
Cotia virus B08.8
Cotton wool spots (retinal) H35.81
Cotungo's disease —see Sciatica
Cough (affected) (chronic) (epidemic) (nervous)
    R05
  with hemorrhage —see Hemoptysis
  bronchial R05
    with grippe or influenza —see Influenza,
        with, respiratory manifestations
        NEC
  functional F45.8
  hysterical F45.8
  laryngeal, spasmodic R05
  psychogenic F45.8
  smokers' J41.0
  tea taster's B49
Counseling (for) Z71.9
  abuse NEC
    perpetrator Z69.82
    victim Z69.81
  alcohol abuser Z71.41
    family Z71.42
  child abuse
    nonparental
      perpetrator Z69.021
      victim Z69.020
    parental
      perpetrator Z69.011
      victim Z69.010

◀ New   ◀▥ Revised   ~~deleted~~ Deleted

Counseling (Continued)
 consanguinity Z71.89
 contraceptive Z30.09
 dietary Z71.3
 drug abuser Z71.51
  family member Z71.52
 family Z71.89
 fertility preservation (prior to cancer therapy) (prior to removal of gonads) Z31.62
 for non-attending third party Z71.0
  related to sexual behavior or orientation Z70.2
 genetic NEC Z31.5
 gestational carrier Z31.7 ◀
 health (advice) (education) (instruction) —see Counseling, medical
 human immunodeficiency virus (HIV) Z71.7
 impotence Z70.1
 insulin pump use Z46.81
 medical (for) Z71.9
  boarding school resident Z59.3
  consanguinity Z71.89
  feared complaint and no disease found Z71.1
  human immunodeficiency virus (HIV) Z71.7
  institutional resident Z59.3
  on behalf of another Z71.0
   related to sexual behavior or orientation Z70.2
  person living alone Z60.2
  specified reason NEC Z71.89
 natural family planning
  procreative Z31.61
  to avoid pregnancy Z30.02
 perpetrator (of)
  abuse NEC Z69.82
  child abuse
   non-parental Z69.021
   parental Z69.011
  rape NEC Z69.82
  spousal abuse Z69.12
 procreative NEC Z31.69
  fertility preservation (prior to cancer therapy) (prior to removal of gonads) Z31.62
  using natural family planning Z31.61
 promiscuity Z70.1
 rape victim Z69.81
 religious Z71.81
 sex, sexual (related to) Z70.9
  attitude (s) Z70.0
  behavior or orientation Z70.1
  combined concerns Z70.3
  non-responsiveness Z70.1
  on behalf of third party Z70.2
  specified reason NEC Z70.8
 specified reason NEC Z71.89
 spiritual Z71.81
 spousal abuse (perpetrator) Z69.12
  victim Z69.11
 substance abuse Z71.89
  alcohol Z71.41
  drug Z71.51
  tobacco Z71.6
 tobacco use Z71.6
 use (of)
  insulin pump Z46.81
 victim (of)
  abuse Z69.81
  child abuse
   by parent Z69.010
   non-parental Z69.020
  rape NEC Z69.81
Coupled rhythm R00.8
Couvelaire syndrome or uterus (complicating delivery) O45.8X-
Cowperitis —see Urethritis
Cowper's gland —see condition

Cowpox B08.010
 due to vaccination T88.1
Coxa
 magna M91.4-
 plana M91.2-
 valga (acquired) —see also Deformity, limb, specified type NEC, thigh
  congenital Q65.81
  sequelae (late effect) of rickets E64.3
 vara (acquired) —see also Deformity, limb, specified type NEC, thigh
  congenital Q65.82
  sequelae (late effect) of rickets E64.3
Coxalgia, coxalgic (nontuberculous) —see also Pain, joint, hip
 tuberculous A18.02
Coxitis —see Monoarthritis, hip
Coxsackie (virus) (infection) B34.1
 as cause of disease classified elsewhere B97.11
 carditis B33.20
 central nervous system NEC A88.8
 endocarditis B33.21
 enteritis A08.39
 meningitis (aseptic) A87.0
 myocarditis B33.22
 pericarditis B33.23
 pharyngitis B08.5
 pleurodynia B33.0
 specific disease NEC B33.8
Crabs, meaning pubic lice B85.3
Crack baby P04.41
Cracked nipple N64.0
 associated with
  lactation O92.13
  pregnancy O92.11-
  puerperium O92.12
Cracked tooth K03.81
Cradle cap L21.0
Craft neurosis F48.8
Cramp (s) R25.2
 abdominal —see Pain, abdominal
 bathing T75.1
 colic R10.83
  psychogenic F45.8
 due to immersion T75.1
 fireman T67.2
 heat T67.2
 immersion T75.1
 intestinal —see Pain, abdominal
  psychogenic F45.8
 leg, sleep related G47.62
 limb (lower) (upper) NEC R25.2
  sleep related G47.62
 linotypist's F48.8
  organic G25.89
 muscle (limb) (general) R25.2
  due to immersion T75.1
  psychogenic F45.8
 occupational (hand) F48.8
  organic G25.89
 salt-depletion E87.1
 sleep related, leg G47.62
 stoker's T67.2
 swimmer's T75.1
 telegrapher's F48.8
  organic G25.89
 typist's F48.8
  organic G25.89
 uterus N94.89
  menstrual —see Dysmenorrhea
 writer's F48.8
  organic G25.89
Cranial —see condition
Craniocleidodysostosis Q74.0
Craniofenestria (skull) Q75.8
Craniolacunia (skull) Q75.8
Craniopagus Q89.4
Craniopathy, metabolic M85.2
Craniopharyngeal —see condition
Craniopharyngioma D44.4
Craniorachischisis (totalis) Q00.1

Cranioschisis Q75.8
Craniostenosis Q75.0
Craniosynostosis Q75.0
Craniotabes (cause unknown) M83.8
 neonatal P96.3
 rachitic E64.3
 syphilitic A50.56
Cranium —see condition
Craw-craw —see Onchocerciasis
Creaking joint —see Derangement, joint, specified type NEC
Creeping
 eruption B76.9
 palsy or paralysis G12.22
Crenated tongue K14.8
Creotoxism A05.9
Crepitus
 caput Q75.8
 joint —see Derangement, joint, specified type NEC
Crescent or conus choroid, congenital Q14.3
CREST syndrome M34.1
Cretin, cretinism (congenital) (endemic) (nongoitrous) (sporadic) E00.9
 pelvis
  with disproportion (fetopelvic) O33.0
   causing obstructed labor O65.0
 type
  hypothyroid E00.1
  mixed E00.2
  myxedematous E00.1
  neurological E00.0
Creutzfeldt-Jakob disease or syndrome (with dementia) A81.00
 familial A81.09
 iatrogenic A81.09
 specified NEC A81.09
 sporadic A81.09
 variant (vCJD) A81.01
Crib death R99
Cribriform hymen Q52.3
Cri-du-chat syndrome Q93.4
Crigler-Najjar disease or syndrome E80.5
Crime, victim of Z65.4
Crimean hemorrhagic fever A98.0
Criminalism F60.2
Crisis
 abdomen R10.0
 acute reaction F43.0
 addisonian E27.2
 adrenal (cortical) E27.2
 celiac K90.0
 Dietl's N13.8
 emotional —see also Disorder, adjustment
  acute reaction to stress F43.0
  specific to childhood and adolescence F93.8
 glaucomatocyclitic —see Glaucoma, secondary, inflammation
 heart —see Failure, heart
 nitritoid I95.2
  correct substance properly administered — see Table of Drugs and Chemicals, by drug, adverse effect
  overdose or wrong substance given or taken —see Table of Drugs and Chemicals, by drug, poisoning
 oculogyric H51.8
  psychogenic F45.8
 Pel's (tabetic) A52.11
 psychosexual identity F64.2
 renal N28.0
 sickle-cell D57.00
  with
   acute chest syndrome D57.01
   splenic sequestration D57.02
 state (acute reaction) F43.0
 tabetic A52.11
 thyroid —see Thyrotoxicosis with thyroid storm
 thyrotoxic —see Thyrotoxicosis with thyroid storm

Crocq's disease (acrocyanosis) I73.89
Crohn's disease —see Enteritis, regional
Crooked septum, nasal J34.2
Cross syndrome E70.328
Crossbite (anterior) (posterior) M26.24
Cross-eye —see Strabismus, convergent
     concomitant
Croup, croupous (catarrhal) (infectious)
     (inflammatory) (nondiphtheritic) J05.0
   bronchial J20.9
   diphtheritic A36.2
   false J38.5
   spasmodic J38.5
     diphtheritic A36.2
   stridulous J38.5
     diphtheritic A36.2
Crouzon's disease Q75.1
Crowding, tooth, teeth, fully erupted M26.31
CRST syndrome M34.1
Cruchet's disease A85.8
Cruelty in children —see also Disorder, conduct
Crural ulcer —see Ulcer, lower limb
Crush, crushed, crushing T14.8
   abdomen S38.1
   ankle S97.0-
   arm (upper) (and shoulder) S47.-
   axilla —see Crush, arm
   back, lower S38.1
   buttock S38.1
   cheek S07.0
   chest S28.0
   cranium S07.1
   ear S07.0
   elbow S57.0-
   extremity
     lower
       ankle —see Crush, ankle
       below knee —see Crush, leg
       foot —see Crush, foot
       hip —see Crush, hip
       knee —see Crush, knee
       thigh —see Crush, thigh
       toe —see Crush, toe
     upper
       below elbow S67.9-
       elbow —see Crush, elbow
       finger —see Crush, finger
       forearm —see Crush, forearm
       hand —see Crush, hand
       thumb —see Crush, thumb
       upper arm —see Crush, arm
       wrist —see Crush, wrist
   face S07.0
   finger (s) S67.1-
     with hand (and wrist) —see Crush, hand,
          specified site NEC
     index S67.19-
     little S67.19-
     middle S67.19-
     ring S67.19-
     thumb —see Crush, thumb
   foot S97.8-
     toe —see Crush, toe
   forearm S57.8-
   genitalia, external
     female S38.002
       vagina S38.03
       vulva S38.03
     male S38.001
       penis S38.01
       scrotum S38.02
       testis S38.02
   hand (except fingers alone) S67.2-
     with wrist S67.4-
   head S07.9
     specified NEC S07.8
   heel —see Crush, foot
   hip S77.0-
     with thigh S77.2-
   internal organ (abdomen, chest, or pelvis)
       NEC T14.8

Crush, crushed, crushing (Continued)
   knee S87.0-
   labium (majus) (minus) S38.03
   larynx S17.0
   leg (lower) S87.8-
     knee —see Crush, knee
   lip S07.0
   lower
     back S38.1
     leg —see Crush, leg
   neck S17.9
   nerve —see Injury, nerve
   nose S07.0
   pelvis S38.1
   penis S38.01
   scalp S07.8
   scapular region —see Crush, arm
   scrotum S38.02
   severe, unspecified site T14.8
   shoulder (and upper arm) —see Crush, arm
   skull S07.1
   syndrome (complication of trauma) T79.5
   testis S38.02
   thigh S77.1-
     with hip S77.2-
   throat S17.8
   thumb S67.0-
     with hand (and wrist) —see Crush, hand,
          specified site NEC
   toe (s) S97.10-
     great S97.11-
     lesser S97.12-
   trachea S17.0
   vagina S38.03
   vulva S38.03
   wrist S67.3-
     with hand S67.4-
Crusta lactea L21.0
Crusts R23.4
Crutch paralysis —see Injury, brachial plexus
Cruveilhier-Baumgarten cirrhosis, disease or
     syndrome K74.69
Cruveilhier's atrophy or disease G12.8
Crying (constant) (continuous) (excessive)
   child, adolescent, or adult R45.83
   infant (baby) (newborn) R68.11
Cryofibrinogenemia D89.2
Cryoglobulinemia (essential) (idiopathic)
     (mixed) (primary) (purpura) (secondary)
     (vasculitis) D89.1
   with lung involvement D89.1 [J99]
Cryptitis (anal) (rectal) K62.89
Cryptococcosis, cryptococcus (infection)
     (neoformans) B45.9
   bone B45.3
   cerebral B45.1
   cutaneous B45.2
   disseminated B45.7
   generalized B45.7
   meningitis B45.1
   meningocerebralis B45.1
   osseous B45.3
   pulmonary B45.0
   skin B45.2
   specified NEC B45.8
Cryptopapillitis (anus) K62.89
Cryptophthalmos Q11.2
   syndrome Q87.0
Cryptorchid, cryptorchism, cryptorchidism
     Q53.9
   bilateral Q53.20
     abdominal Q53.21
     perineal Q53.22
   unilateral Q53.10
     abdominal Q53.11
     perineal Q53.12
Cryptosporidiosis A07.2
   hepatobiliary B88.8
   respiratory B88.8
Cryptostromosis J67.6
Crystalluria R82.99

Cubitus
   congenital Q68.8
   valgus (acquired) M21.0-
     congenital Q68.8
     sequelae (late effect) of rickets E64.3
   varus (acquired) M21.1-
     congenital Q68.8
     sequelae (late effect) of rickets E64.3
Cultural deprivation or shock Z60.3
Curling esophagus K22.4
Curling's ulcer —see Ulcer, peptic, acute
Curschmann (-Batten) (-Steinert) disease or
     syndrome G71.11
Curse, Ondine's —see Apnea, sleep
Curvature
   organ or site, congenital NEC —see Distortion
   penis (lateral) Q55.61
   Pott's (spinal) A18.01
   radius, idiopathic, progressive (congenital)
     Q74.0
   spine (acquired) (angular) (idiopathic)
     (incorrect) (postural) —see Dorsopathy,
     deforming
     congenital Q67.5
     due to or associated with
       Charcot-Marie-Tooth disease —see also
          subcategory M49.8 G60.0
       osteitis
          deformans M88.88
          fibrosa cystica —see also subcategory
            M49.8 E21.0
     tuberculosis (Pott's curvature) A18.01
     sequelae (late effect) of rickets E64.3
     tuberculous A18.01
Cushingoid due to steroid therapy E24.2
   correct substance properly administered —see
     Table of Drugs and Chemicals, by drug,
     adverse effect
   overdose or wrong substance given or
     taken —see Table of Drugs and
     Chemicals, by drug, poisoning
Cushing's
   syndrome or disease E24.9
     drug-induced E24.2
     iatrogenic E24.2
     pituitary-dependent E24.0
     specified NEC E24.8
   ulcer —see Ulcer, peptic, acute
Cusp, Carabelli - omit code
Cut (external) —see also Laceration
   muscle —see Injury, muscle
Cutaneous —see also condition
   hemorrhage R23.3
   larva migrans B76.9
Cutis —see also condition
   hyperelastica Q82.8
     acquired L57.4
   laxa (hyperelastica) —see Dermatolysis
   marmorata R23.8
   osteosis L94.2
   pendula —see Dermatolysis
   rhomboidalis nuchae L57.2
   verticis gyrata Q82.8
     acquired L91.8
Cyanosis R23.0
   due to
     patent foramen botalli Q21.1
     persistent foramen ovale Q21.1
   enterogenous D74.8
   paroxysmal digital —see Raynaud's disease
     with gangrene I73.01
   retina, retinal H35.89
Cyanotic heart disease I24.9
   congenital Q24.9
Cycle
   anovulatory N97.0
   menstrual, irregular N92.6
Cyclencephaly Q04.9
Cyclical vomiting (see also Vomiting, cyclical)
     G43.A0
   psychogenic F50.89

◀ New   ◀ Revised   deleted Deleted

Cyclitis —see also Iridocyclitis H20.9
  chronic —see Iridocyclitis, chronic
  Fuchs' heterochromic H20.81-
  granulomatous —see Iridocyclitis, chronic
  lens-induced —see Iridocyclitis,
    lens-induced
  posterior H30.2-
Cycloid personality F34.0
Cyclophoria H50.54
Cyclopia, cyclops Q87.0
Cyclopism Q87.0
Cyclosporiasis A07.4
Cyclothymia F34.0
Cyclothymic personality F34.0
Cyclotropia H50.41-
Cylindroma —see also Neoplasm, malignant,
  by site
  eccrine dermal —see Neoplasm, skin,
    benign
  skin —see Neoplasm, skin, benign
Cylindruria R82.99
Cynanche
  diphtheritic A36.2
  tonsillaris J36
Cynophobia F40.218
Cynorexia R63.2
Cyphosis —see Kyphosis
Cyprus fever —see Brucellosis
Cyst (colloid) (mucous) (simple) (retention)
  adenoid (infected) J35.8
  adrenal gland E27.8
    congenital Q89.1
  air, lung J98.4
  allantoic Q64.4
  alveolar process (jaw bone) M27.40
  amnion, amniotic O41.8X-
  aneurysmal M27.49 ◄
  anterior
    chamber (eye) —see Cyst, iris
    nasopalatine K09.1
  antrum J34.1
  anus K62.89
  apical (tooth) (periodontal) K04.8
  appendix K38.8
  arachnoid, brain (acquired) G93.0
    congenital Q04.6
  arytenoid J38.7
  Baker's M71.2-
    ruptured M66.0
    tuberculous A18.02
  Bartholin's gland N75.0
  bile duct (common) (hepatic) K83.5
  bladder (multiple) (trigone) N32.89
  blue dome (breast) —see Cyst, breast
  bone (local) NEC M85.60
    aneurysmal M85.50
      ankle M85.57-
      foot M85.57-
      forearm M85.53-
      hand M85.54-
      jaw M27.49
      lower leg M85.56-
      multiple site M85.59
      neck M85.58
      rib M85.58
      shoulder M85.51-
      skull M85.58
      specified site NEC M85.58
      thigh M85.55-
      toe M85.57-
      upper arm M85.52-
      vertebra M85.58
    solitary M85.40
      ankle M85.47-
      fibula M85.46-
      foot M85.47-
      hand M85.44-
      humerus M85.42-
      jaw M27.49
      neck M85.48
      pelvis M85.45-

Cyst (Continued)
  bone NEC (Continued)
    solitary (Continued)
      radius M85.43-
      rib M85.48
      shoulder M85.41-
      skull M85.48
      specified site NEC M85.48
      tibia M85.46-
      toe M85.47-
      ulna M85.43-
      vertebra M85.48
    specified type NEC M85.60
      ankle M85.67-
      foot M85.67-
      forearm M85.63-
      hand M85.64-
      jaw M27.40
        developmental (nonodontogenic) K09.1
          odontogenic K09.0
        latent M27.0
      lower leg M85.66-
      multiple site M85.69
      neck M85.68
      rib M85.68
      shoulder M85.61-
      skull M85.68
      specified site NEC M85.68
      thigh M85.65-
      toe M85.67-
      upper arm M85.62-
      vertebra M85.68
  brain (acquired) G93.0
    congenital Q04.6
    hydatid B67.99 [G94]
    third ventricle (colloid), congenital
      Q04.6
  branchial (cleft) Q18.0
  branchiogenic Q18.0
  breast (benign) (blue dome) (pedunculated)
    (solitary) N60.0-
    involution —see Dysplasia, mammary,
      specified type NEC
    sebaceous —see Dysplasia, mammary,
      specified type NEC
  broad ligament (benign) N83.8
  bronchogenic (mediastinal) (sequestration)
    J98.4
    congenital Q33.0
  buccal K09.8
  bulbourethral gland N36.8
  bursa, bursal NEC M71.30
    with rupture —see Rupture, synovium
    ankle M71.37-
    elbow M71.32-
    foot M71.37-
    hand M71.34-
    hip M71.35-
    multiple sites M71.39
    pharyngeal J39.2
    popliteal space —see Cyst, Baker's
    shoulder M71.31-
    specified site NEC M71.38
    wrist M71.33-
  calcifying odontogenic D16.5
    upper jaw (bone) (maxilla) D16.4
  canal of Nuck (female) N94.89
    congenital Q52.4
  canthus —see Cyst, conjunctiva
  carcinomatous —see Neoplasm, malignant,
    by site
  cauda equina G95.89
  cavum septi pellucidi —see Cyst, brain
  celomic (pericardium) Q24.8
  cerebellopontine (angle) —see Cyst, brain
  cerebellum —see Cyst, brain
  cerebral —see Cyst, brain
  cervical lateral Q18.0 ◄
  cervix NEC N88.8
    embryonic Q51.6
    nabothian N88.8

Cyst (Continued)
  chiasmal optic NEC —see Disorder, optic,
    chiasm
  chocolate (ovary) N80.1
  choledochus, congenital Q44.4
  chorion O41.8X-
  choroid plexus G93.0
  ciliary body —see Cyst, iris
  clitoris N90.7
  colon K63.89
  common (bile) duct K83.5
  congenital NEC Q89.8
    adrenal gland Q89.1
    epiglottis Q31.8
    esophagus Q39.8
    fallopian tube Q50.4
    kidney Q61.00
      more than one (multiple) Q61.02
        specified as polycystic Q61.3
          adult type Q61.2
          infantile type NEC Q61.19
            collecting duct dilation Q61.11
      solitary Q61.01
    larynx Q31.8
    liver Q44.6
    lung Q33.0
    mediastinum Q34.1
    ovary Q50.1
    oviduct Q50.4
    periurethral (tissue) Q64.79
    prepuce Q55.69
    salivary gland (any) Q38.4
    sublingual Q38.6
    submaxillary gland Q38.6
    thymus (gland) Q89.2
    tongue Q38.3
    ureterovesical orifice Q62.8
    vulva Q52.79
  conjunctiva H11.44-
  cornea H18.89-
  corpora quadrigemina G93.0
  corpus
    albicans N83.29- ◄
    luteum (hemorrhagic) (ruptured)
      N83.1- ◄
  Cowper's gland (benign) (infected) N36.8
  cranial meninges G93.0
  craniobuccal pouch E23.6
  craniopharyngeal pouch E23.6
  cystic duct K82.8
  Cysticercus —see Cysticercosis
  Dandy-Walker Q03.1
    with spina bifida —see Spina bifida
  dental (root) K04.8
    developmental K09.0
    eruption K09.0
    primordial K09.0
  dentigerous (mandible) (maxilla) K09.0
  dermoid —see Neoplasm, benign, by site
    with malignant transformation C56.-
    implantation
      external area or site (skin) NEC
        L72.0
      iris —see Cyst, iris, implantation
      vagina N89.8
      vulva N90.7
    mouth K09.8
    oral soft tissue K09.8
    sacrococcygeal —see Cyst, pilonidal
  developmental K09.1
    odontogenic K09.0
    oral region (nonodontogenic) K09.1
    ovary, ovarian Q50.1
  dura (cerebral) G93.0
    spinal G96.19
  ear (external) Q18.1
  echinococcal —see Echinococcus
  embryonic
    cervix uteri Q51.6
    fallopian tube Q50.4
    vagina Q51.6

Cyst *(Continued)*
  endometrium, endometrial (uterus) N85.8
    ectopic —*see* Endometriosis
  enterogenous Q43.8
  epidermal, epidermoid (inclusion) *(see also*
    Cyst, skin)* L72.0
    mouth K09.8
    oral soft tissue K09.8
  epididymis N50.3
  epiglottis J38.7
  epiphysis cerebri E34.8
  epithelial (inclusion) L72.0
  epoophoron Q50.5
  eruption K09.0
  esophagus K22.8
  ethmoid sinus J34.1
  external female genital organs NEC N90.7
  eye NEC H57.8
    congenital Q15.8
  eyelid (sebaceous) H02.829
    infected —*see* Hordeolum
    left H02.826
      lower H02.825
      upper H02.824
    right H02.823
      lower H02.822
      upper H02.821
  fallopian tube N83.8
    congenital Q50.4
  fimbrial (twisted) Q50.4
  fissural (oral region) K09.1
  follicle (graafian) (hemorrhagic) N83.0- ◀▦
    nabothian N88.8
  follicular (atretic) (hemorrhagic) (ovarian)
    N83.0- ◀▦
    dentigerous K09.0
    odontogenic K09.0
    skin L72.9
    specified NEC L72.8
  frontal sinus J34.1
  gallbladder K82.8
  ganglion —*see* Ganglion
  Gartner's duct Q52.4
  gingiva K09.0
  gland of Moll —*see* Cyst, eyelid
  globulomaxillary K09.1
  graafian follicle (hemorrhagic) N83.0- ◀▦
  granulosal lutein (hemorrhagic) N83.1- ◀▦
  hemangiomatous D18.00
    intra-abdominal D18.03
    intracranial D18.02
    skin D18.01
    specified site NEC D18.09
  hemorrhagic M27.49 ◀
  hydatid —*see also* Echinococcus B67.90
    brain B67.99 *[G94]*
    liver —*see also* Cyst, liver, hydatid B67.8
    lung NEC B67.99 *[J99]*
    Morgagni
      female Q50.5
      male (epididymal) Q55.4
        testicular Q55.29
    specified site NEC B67.99
  hymen N89.8
    embryonic Q52.4
  hypopharynx J39.2
  hypophysis, hypophyseal (duct) (recurrent)
    E23.6
    cerebri E23.6
  implantation (dermoid)
    external area or site (skin) NEC L72.0
    iris —*see* Cyst, iris, implantation
    vagina N89.8
    vulva N90.7
  incisive canal K09.1
  inclusion (epidermal) (epithelial)
    (epidermoid) (squamous) L72.0
    not of skin - code under Cyst, by site
  intestine (large) (small) K63.89
  intracranial —*see* Cyst, brain
  intraligamentous —*see also* Disorder, ligament
    knee —*see* Derangement, knee

Cyst *(Continued)*
  intrasellar E23.6
  iris H21.309
    exudative H21.31-
    idiopathic H21.30-
    implantation H21.32-
    parasitic H21.33-
    pars plana (primary) H21.34-
      exudative H21.35-
  jaw (bone) M27.40
    aneurysmal M27.49
    developmental (odontogenic) K09.0
    fissural K09.1
    hemorrhagic M27.49
    traumatic M27.49
  joint NEC —*see* Disorder, joint, specified type
    NEC
  kidney (acquired) N28.1
    calyceal —*see* Hydronephrosis
    congenital Q61.00
    more than one (multiple) Q61.02
      specified as polycystic Q61.3
        adult type (autosomal dominant)
          Q61.2
        infantile type (autosomal recessive)
          NEC Q61.19
            collecting duct dilation Q61.11
    pyelogenic —*see* Hydronephrosis
    simple N28.1
    solitary (single) Q61.01
      acquired N28.1
  labium (majus) (minus) N90.7
    sebaceous N90.7
  lacrimal —*see also* Disorder, lacrimal system,
    specified NEC
    gland H04.13-
    passages or sac —*see* Disorder, lacrimal
      system, specified NEC
  larynx J38.7
  lateral periodontal K09.0
  lens H27.8
    congenital Q12.8
  lip (gland) K13.0
  liver (idiopathic) (simple) K76.89
    congenital Q44.6
    hydatid B67.8
      granulosus B67.0
      multilocularis B67.5
  lung J98.4
    congenital Q33.0
    giant bullous J43.9
  lutein N83.1- ◀▦
  lymphangiomatous D18.1
  lymphoepithelial, oral soft tissue K09.8
  macula —*see* Degeneration, macula, hole
  malignant —*see* Neoplasm, malignant, by site
  mammary gland —*see* Cyst, breast
  mandible M27.40
    dentigerous K09.0
    radicular K04.8
  maxilla M27.40
    dentigerous K09.0
    radicular K04.8
  medial, face and neck Q18.8
  median
    anterior maxillary K09.1
    palatal K09.1
  mediastinum, congenital Q34.1
  meibomian (gland) —*see* Chalazion
    infected —*see* Hordeolum
  membrane, brain G93.0
  meninges (cerebral) G93.0
    spinal G96.19
  meniscus, knee —*see* Derangement, knee,
    meniscus, cystic
  mesentery, mesenteric K66.8
    chyle I89.8
  mesonephric duct
    female Q50.5
    male Q55.4
  milk N64.89

Cyst *(Continued)*
  Morgagni (hydatid)
    female Q50.5
    male (epididymal) Q55.4
      testicular Q55.29
  mouth K09.8
  Müllerian duct Q50.4
    appendix testis Q55.29
    cervix Q51.6
    fallopian tube Q50.4
    female Q50.4
    male Q55.29
    prostatic utricle Q55.4
    vagina (embryonal) Q52.4
  multilocular (ovary) D39.10
    benign —*see* Neoplasm, benign, by site
  myometrium N85.8
  nabothian (follicle) (ruptured) N88.8
  nasoalveolar K09.1
  nasolabial K09.1
  nasopalatine (anterior) (duct) K09.1
  nasopharynx J39.2
  neoplastic —*see* Neoplasm, uncertain
    behavior, by site
    benign —*see* Neoplasm, benign, by site
  nervous system NEC G96.8
  neuroenteric (congenital) Q06.8
  nipple —*see* Cyst, breast
  nose (turbinates) J34.1
    sinus J34.1
  odontogenic, developmental K09.0
  omentum (lesser) K66.8
    congenital Q45.8
  ora serrata —*see* Cyst, retina, ora serrata
  oral
    region K09.9
      developmental (nonodontogenic) K09.1
      specified NEC K09.8
    soft tissue K09.9
      specified NEC K09.8
  orbit H05.81-
  ovary, ovarian (twisted) N83.20- ◀▦
    adherent N83.20- ◀▦
    chocolate N80.1
    corpus
      albicans N83.29- ◀▦
      luteum (hemorrhagic) N83.1- ◀▦
    dermoid D27.9
    developmental Q50.1
    due to failure of involution NEC N83.20- ◀▦
    endometrial N80.1
    follicular (graafian) (hemorrhagic) N83.0- ◀▦
    hemorrhagic N83.20- ◀▦
    in pregnancy or childbirth O34.8-
      with obstructed labor O65.5
    multilocular D39.10
    pseudomucinous D27.9
    retention N83.29- ◀▦
    serous N83.20- ◀▦
    specified NEC N83.29- ◀▦
    theca lutein (hemorrhagic) N83.1- ◀▦
    tuberculous A18.18
  oviduct N83.8
  palate (median) (fissural) K09.1
  palatine papilla (jaw) K09.1
  pancreas, pancreatic (hemorrhagic) (true) K86.2
    congenital Q45.2
    false K86.3
  paralabral
    hip M24.85-
    shoulder S43.43-
  paramesonephric duct Q50.4
    female Q50.4
    male Q55.29
  paranephric N28.1
  paraphysis, cerebri, congenital Q04.6
  parasitic B89
  parathyroid (gland) E21.4
  paratubal N83.8
  paraurethral duct N36.8
  paroophoron Q50.5

Cyst (Continued)
  parotid gland K11.6
  parovarian Q50.5
  pelvis, female N94.89
    in pregnancy or childbirth O34.8-
      causing obstructed labor O65.5
  penis (sebaceous) N48.89
  periapical K04.8
  pericardial (congenital) Q24.8
    acquired (secondary) I31.8
  pericoronal K09.0
  periodontal K04.8
    lateral K09.0
  peripelvic (lymphatic) N28.1
  peritoneum K66.8
    chylous I89.8
  periventricular, acquired, newborn P91.1
  pharynx (wall) J39.2
  pilar L72.11
  pilonidal (infected) (rectum) L05.91
    with abscess L05.01
    malignant C44.59-
  pituitary (duct) (gland) E23.6
  placenta O43.19-
  pleura J94.8
  popliteal —see Cyst, Baker's
  porencephalic Q04.6
    acquired G93.0
  postanal (infected) —see Cyst, pilonidal
  postmastoidectomy cavity (mucosal) —see
      Complications, postmastoidectomy, cyst
  preauricular Q18.1
  prepuce N47.4
    congenital Q55.69
  primordial (jaw) K09.0
  prostate N42.83
  pseudomucinous (ovary) D27.9
  pupillary, miotic H21.27-
  radicular (residual) K04.8
  radiculodental K04.8
  ranular K11.8
  Rathke's pouch E23.6
  rectum (epithelium) (mucous) K62.89
  renal —see Cyst, kidney
  residual (radicular) K04.8
  retention (ovary) N83.29- ◀▦
    salivary gland K11.6
  retina H33.19-
    ora serrata H33.11-
    parasitic H33.12-
  retroperitoneal K68.9
  sacrococcygeal (dermoid) —see Cyst,
      pilonidal
  salivary gland or duct (mucous extravasation
      or retention) K11.6
  Sampson's N80.1
  sclera H15.89
  scrotum L72.9
    sebaceous L72.3
  sebaceous (duct) (gland) L72.3
    breast —see Dysplasia, mammary, specified
        type NEC
    eyelid —see Cyst, eyelid
    genital organ NEC
      female N94.89
      male N50.89 ◀▦
    scrotum L72.3
  semilunar cartilage (knee) (multiple) —see
      Derangement, knee, meniscus, cystic
  seminal vesicle N50.89 ◀▦
  serous (ovary) N83.20- ◀▦
  sinus (accessory) (nasal) J34.1
  Skene's gland N36.8
  skin L72.9
    breast —see Dysplasia, mammary, specified
        type NEC
    epidermal, epidermoid L72.0
    epithelial L72.0
    eyelid —see Cyst, eyelid
    genital organ NEC
      female N90.7
      male N50.89 ◀▦

Cyst (Continued)
  skin (Continued)
    inclusion L72.0
    scrotum L72.9
    sebaceous L72.3
    sweat gland or duct L74.8
  solitary
    bone —see Cyst, bone, solitary
    jaw M27.40
    kidney N28.1
  spermatic cord N50.89 ◀▦
  sphenoid sinus J34.1
  spinal meninges G96.19
  spleen NEC D73.4
    congenital Q89.09
    hydatid —see also Echinococcus B67.99 [D77]
  Stafne's M27.0
  subarachnoid intrasellar R93.0
  subcutaneous, pheomycotic (chromomycotic)
      B43.2
  subdural (cerebral) G93.0
    spinal cord G96.19
  sublingual gland K11.6
  submandibular gland K11.6
  submaxillary gland K11.6
  suburethral N36.8
  suprarenal gland E27.8
  suprasellar —see Cyst, brain
  sweat gland or duct L74.8
  synovial —see also Cyst, bursa
    ruptured —see Rupture, synovium
  tarsal —see Chalazion
  tendon (sheath) —see Disorder, tendon,
      specified type NEC
  testis N44.2
    tunica albuginea N44.1
  theca lutein (ovary) N83.1- ◀▦
  Thornwaldt's J39.2
  thymus (gland) E32.8
  thyroglossal duct (infected) (persistent)
      Q89.2
  thyroid (gland) E04.1
  thyrolingual duct (infected) (persistent)
      Q89.2
  tongue K14.8
  tonsil J35.8
  tooth —see Cyst, dental
  Tornwaldt's J39.2
  trichilemmal (proliferating) L72.12
  trichodermal L72.12
  tubal (fallopian) N83.8
    inflammatory —see Salpingitis, chronic
  tubo-ovarian N83.8
    inflammatory N70.13
  tunica
    albuginea testis N44.1
    vaginalis N50.89 ◀▦
  turbinate (nose) J34.1
  Tyson's gland N48.89
  urachus, congenital Q64.4
  ureter N28.89
  ureterovesical orifice N28.89
  urethra, urethral (gland) N36.8
  uterine ligament N83.8
  uterus (body) (corpus) (recurrent)
      N85.8
    embryonic Q51.818
      cervix Q51.6
  vagina, vaginal (implantation) (inclusion)
      (squamous cell) (wall) N89.8
    embryonic Q52.4
  vallecula, vallecular (epiglottis) J38.7
  vesical (orifice) N32.89
  vitreous body H43.89
  vulva (implantation) (inclusion) N90.7
    congenital Q52.79
    sebaceous gland N90.7
  vulvovaginal gland N90.7
  wolffian
    female Q50.5
    male Q55.4

Cystadenocarcinoma —see Neoplasm,
    malignant, by site
  bile duct C22.1
  endometrioid —see Neoplasm, malignant,
      by site
    specified site —see Neoplasm, malignant,
        by site
    unspecified site
      female C56.9
      male C61
  mucinous
    papillary
      specified site —see Neoplasm,
          malignant, by site
      unspecified site C56.9
    specified site —see Neoplasm, malignant,
        by site
    unspecified site C56.9
  papillary
    mucinous
      specified site —see Neoplasm,
          malignant, by site
      unspecified site C56.9
    pseudomucinous
      specified site —see Neoplasm,
          malignant, by site
      unspecified site C56.9
    serous
      specified site —see Neoplasm,
          malignant, by site
      unspecified site C56.9
    specified site —see Neoplasm, malignant,
        by site
    unspecified site C56.9
  pseudomucinous
    papillary
      specified site —see Neoplasm,
          malignant, by site
      unspecified site C56.9
    specified site —see Neoplasm, malignant,
        by site
    unspecified site C56.9
  serous
    papillary
      specified site —see Neoplasm,
          malignant, by site
      unspecified site C56.9
    specified site —see Neoplasm, malignant,
        by site
    unspecified site C56.9
Cystadenofibroma
  clear cell —see Neoplasm, benign, by site
  endometrioid D27.9
    borderline malignancy D39.1-
    malignant C56.-
  mucinous
    specified site —see Neoplasm, benign, by site
    unspecified site D27.9
  serous
    specified site —see Neoplasm, benign, by site
    unspecified site D27.9
  specified site —see Neoplasm, benign, by site
  unspecified site D27.9
Cystadenoma —see also Neoplasm, benign, by
    site
  bile duct D13.4
  endometrioid —see Neoplasm, benign, by site
    borderline malignancy —see Neoplasm,
        uncertain behavior, by site
    malignant —see Neoplasm, malignant, by site
  mucinous
    borderline malignancy
      ovary C56.-
      specified site NEC —see Neoplasm,
          uncertain behavior, by site
      unspecified site C56.9
    papillary
      borderline malignancy
        ovary C56.-
        specified site NEC —see Neoplasm,
            uncertain behavior, by site
        unspecified site C56.9

Cystadenoma *(Continued)*
  mucinous *(Continued)*
    papillary *(Continued)*
      specified site —*see* Neoplasm, benign,
        by site
      unspecified site D27.9
    specified site —*see* Neoplasm, benign, by site
    unspecified site D27.9
  papillary
    borderline malignancy
      ovary C56-
      specified site NEC —*see* Neoplasm,
        uncertain behavior, by site
      unspecified site C56.9
    lymphomatosum
      specified site —*see* Neoplasm, benign,
        by site
      unspecified site D11.9
    mucinous
      borderline malignancy
        ovary C56.-
        specified site NEC —*see* Neoplasm,
          uncertain behavior, by site
        unspecified site C56.9
      specified site —*see* Neoplasm, benign,
        by site
      unspecified site D27.9
    pseudomucinous
      borderline malignancy
        ovary C56.-
        specified site NEC —*see* Neoplasm,
          uncertain behavior, by site
        unspecified site C56.9
      specified site —*see* Neoplasm, benign,
        by site
      unspecified site D27.9
    serous
      borderline malignancy
        ovary C56.-
        specified site NEC —*see* Neoplasm,
          uncertain behavior, by site
        unspecified site C56.9
      specified site —*see* Neoplasm, benign,
        by site
      unspecified site D27.9
    specified site —*see* Neoplasm, benign, by site
    unspecified site D27.9
  pseudomucinous
    borderline malignancy
      ovary C56.-
      specified site NEC —*see* Neoplasm,
        uncertain behavior, by site
      unspecified site C56.9
    papillary
      borderline malignancy
        ovary C56.-
        specified site NEC —*see* Neoplasm,
          uncertain behavior, by site
        unspecified site C56.9
      specified site —*see* Neoplasm, benign,
        by site
      unspecified site D27.9
    specified site —*see* Neoplasm, benign, by site
    unspecified site D27.9
  serous
    borderline malignancy
      ovary C56.-
      specified site NEC —*see* Neoplasm,
        uncertain behavior, by site
      unspecified site C56.9
    papillary
      borderline malignancy
        ovary C56.-
        specified site NEC —*see* Neoplasm,
          uncertain behavior, by site
        unspecified site C56.9
      specified site —*see* Neoplasm, benign,
        by site
      unspecified site D27.9
    specified site —*see* Neoplasm, benign, by site
    unspecified site D27.9

Cystathionine synthase deficiency E72.11
Cystathioninemia E72.19
Cystathioninuria E72.19
Cystic —*see also* condition
  breast (chronic) —*see* Mastopathy, cystic
  corpora lutea (hemorrhagic) N83.1- ◀━
  duct —*see* condition
  eyeball (congenital) Q11.0
  fibrosis —*see* Fibrosis, cystic
  kidney (congenital) Q61.9
    adult type Q61.2
    infantile type Q61.19
      collecting duct dilatation Q61.11
    medullary Q61.5
  liver, congenital Q44.6
  lung disease J98.4
    congenital Q33.0
  mastitis, chronic —*see* Mastopathy, cystic
  medullary, kidney Q61.5
  meniscus —*see* Derangement, knee,
    meniscus, cystic
  ovary N83.20- ◀━
Cysticercosis, cysticerciasis B69.9
  with
    epileptiform fits B69.0
    myositis B69.81
  brain B69.0
  central nervous system B69.0
  cerebral B69.0
  ocular B69.1
  specified NEC B69.89
Cysticercus cellulose infestation —*see*
    Cysticercosis
Cystinosis (malignant) E72.04
Cystinuria E72.01
Cystitis (exudative) (hemorrhagic) (septic)
    (suppurative) N30.90
  with
    fibrosis —*see* Cystitis, chronic, interstitial
    hematuria N30.91
    leukoplakia —*see* Cystitis, chronic,
      interstitial
    malakoplakia —*see* Cystitis, chronic,
      interstitial
    metaplasia —*see* Cystitis, chronic, interstitial
    prostatitis N41.3
  acute N30.00
    with hematuria N30.01
    of trigone N30.30
      with hematuria N30.31
  allergic —*see* Cystitis, specified type NEC
  amebic A06.81
  bilharzial B65.9 *[N33]*
  blennorrhagic (gonococcal) A54.01
  bullous —*see* Cystitis, specified type NEC
  calculous N21.0
  chlamydial A56.01
  chronic N30.20
    with hematuria N30.21
    interstitial N30.10
      with hematuria N30.11
    of trigone N30.30
      with hematuria N30.31
    specified NEC N30.20
      with hematuria N30.21
  cystic (a) —*see* Cystitis, specified type NEC
  diphtheritic A36.85
  echinococcal
    granulosus B67.39
    multilocularis B67.69
  emphysematous —*see* Cystitis, specified type
    NEC
  encysted —*see* Cystitis, specified type NEC
  eosinophilic —*see* Cystitis, specified type
    NEC
  follicular —*see* Cystitis, of trigone
  gangrenous —*see* Cystitis, specified type
    NEC
  glandularis —*see* Cystitis, specified type
    NEC

Cystitis *(Continued)*
  gonococcal A54.01
  incrusted —*see* Cystitis, specified type
    NEC
  interstitial (chronic) —*see* Cystitis, chronic,
    interstitial
  irradiation N30.40
    with hematuria N30.41
  irritation —*see* Cystitis, specified type
    NEC
  malignant —*see* Cystitis, specified type
    NEC
  of trigone N30.30
    with hematuria N30.31
  panmural —*see* Cystitis, chronic, interstitial
  polyposa —*see* Cystitis, specified type NEC
  prostatic N41.3
  puerperal (postpartum) O86.22
  radiation —*see* Cystitis, irradiation
  specified type NEC N30.80
    with hematuria N30.81
  subacute —*see* Cystitis, chronic
  submucous —*see* Cystitis, chronic, interstitial
  syphilitic (late) A52.76
  trichomonal A59.03
  tuberculous A18.12
  ulcerative —*see* Cystitis, chronic, interstitial
Cystocele (-urethrocele)
  female N81.10
    with prolapse of uterus —*see* Prolapse,
      uterus
    lateral N81.12
    midline N81.11
    paravaginal N81.12
  in pregnancy or childbirth O34.8-
    causing obstructed labor O65.5
  male N32.89
Cystolithiasis N21.0
Cystoma —*see also* Neoplasm, benign, by site
  endometrial, ovary N80.1
  mucinous
    specified site —*see* Neoplasm, benign, by site
    unspecified site D27.9
  serous
    specified site —*see* Neoplasm, benign, by site
    unspecified site D27.9
  simple (ovary) N83.29- ◀━
Cystoplegia N31.2
Cystoptosis N32.89
Cystopyelitis —*see* Pyelonephritis
Cystorrhagia N32.89
Cystosarcoma phyllodes D48.6-
  benign D24-
  malignant —*see* Neoplasm, breast, malignant
Cystostomy
  attention to Z43.5
  complication —*see* Complications, cystostomy
  status Z93.50
    appendico-vesicostomy Z93.52
    cutaneous Z93.51
    specified NEC Z93.59
Cystourethritis —*see* Urethritis
Cystourethrocele —*see also* Cystocele
  female N81.10
    with uterine prolapse —*see* Prolapse,
      uterus
    lateral N81.12
    midline N81.11
    paravaginal N81.12
  male N32.89
Cytomegalic inclusion disease
  congenital P35.1
Cytomegalovirus infection B25.9
Cytomycosis (reticuloendothelial) B39.4
Cytopenia D75.9
  refractory
    with multilineage dysplasia D46.A
      and ring sideroblasts (RCMD RS) D46.B
Czerny's disease (periodic hydrarthrosis of the
    knee) —*see* Effusion, joint, knee

◀ New   ◀━ Revised   ~~deleted~~ Deleted

D

Daae (-Finsen) disease (epidemic pleurodynia) B33.0
Dabney's grip B33.0
Da Costa's syndrome F45.8
Dacryoadenitis, dacryadenitis H04.00-
 acute H04.01-
 chronic H04.02-
Dacryocystitis H04.30-
 acute H04.32-
 chronic H04.41-
 neonatal P39.1
 phlegmonous H04.31-
 syphilitic A52.71
  congenital (early) A50.01
 trachomatous, active A71.1
  sequelae (late effect) B94.0
Dacryocystoblenorrhea —see Inflammation, lacrimal, passages, chronic
Dacryocystocele —see Disorder, lacrimal system, changes
Dacryolith, dacryolithiasis H04.51-
Dacryoma —see Disorder, lacrimal system, changes
Dacryopericystitis —see Dacryocystitis
Dacryops H04.11-
Dacryostenosis —see also Stenosis, lacrimal
 congenital Q10.5
Dactylitis
 bone —see Osteomyelitis
 sickle-cell D57.00
  Hb C D57.219
  Hb SS D57.00
  specified NEC D57.819
 skin L08.9
 syphilitic A52.77
 tuberculous A18.03
Dactylolysis spontanea (ainhum) L94.6
Dactylosymphysis Q70.9
 fingers —see Syndactylism, complex, fingers
 toes —see Syndactylism, complex, toes
Damage
 arteriosclerotic —see Arteriosclerosis
 brain (nontraumatic) G93.9
  anoxic, hypoxic G93.1
   resulting from a procedure G97.82
  child NEC G80.9
  due to birth injury P11.2
 cardiorenal (vascular) —see Hypertension, cardiorenal
 cerebral NEC —see Damage, brain
 coccyx, complicating delivery O71.6
 coronary —see Disease, heart, ischemic
 eye, birth injury P15.3
 liver (nontraumatic) K76.9
  alcoholic K70.9
  due to drugs —see Disease, liver, toxic
  toxic —see Disease, liver, toxic
 medication T88.7
 pelvic
  joint or ligament, during delivery O71.6
  organ NEC
   during delivery O71.5
   following ectopic or molar pregnancy O08.6
 renal —see Disease, renal
 subendocardium, subendocardial —see Degeneration, myocardial
 vascular I99.9
Dana-Putnam syndrome (subacute combined sclerosis with pernicious anemia) —see Degeneration, combined
Danbolt (-Cross) syndrome (acrodermatitis enteropathica) E83.2
Dandruff L21.0
Dandy-Walker syndrome Q03.1
 with spina bifida —see Spina bifida
Danlos' syndrome Q79.6
Darier (-White) disease (congenital) Q82.8
 meaning erythema annulare centrifugum L53.1

Darier-Roussy sarcoid D86.3
Darling's disease or histoplasmosis B39.4
Darwin's tubercle Q17.8
Dawson's (inclusion body) encephalitis A81.1
De Beurmann (-Gougerot) disease B42.1
De la Tourette's syndrome F95.2
De Lange's syndrome Q87.1
De Morgan's spots (senile angiomas) I78.1
De Quervain's
 disease (tendon sheath) M65.4
 syndrome E34.51
 thyroiditis (subacute granulomatous thyroiditis) E06.1
De Toni-Fanconi (-Debré) syndrome E72.09
 with cystinosis E72.04
Dead
 fetus, retained (mother) O36.4
  early pregnancy O02.1
 labyrinth —see subcategory H83.2
 ovum, retained O02.0
Deaf nonspeaking NEC H91.3
Deafmutism (acquired) (congenital) NEC H91.3
 hysterical F44.6
 syphilitic, congenital —see also subcategory H94.8 A50.09
Deafness (acquired) (complete) (hereditary) (partial) H91.9-
 with blue sclera and fragility of bone Q78.0
 auditory fatigue —see Deafness, specified type NEC
 aviation T70.0
  nerve injury —see Injury, nerve, acoustic, specified type NEC
 boilermaker's —see subcategory H83.3
 central —see Deafness, sensorineural
 conductive H90.2
  and sensorineural, mixed H90.8
  bilateral H90.6
  and sensorineural ◄
   mixed H90.8 ◄
    bilateral H90.6 ◄
  bilateral H90.0
  unilateral H90.1-
   with restricted hearing on the contralateral side H90.A- ◄
 congenital H90.5
  with blue sclera and fragility of bone Q78.0
 due to toxic agents —see Deafness, ototoxic
 emotional (hysterical) F44.6
 functional (hysterical) F44.6
 high frequency H91.9-
 hysterical F44.6
 low frequency H91.9-
 mental R48.8
 mixed conductive and sensorineural H90.8
  bilateral H90.6
  unilateral H90.7-
 nerve —see Deafness, sensorineural
 neural —see Deafness, sensorineural
 noise-induced —see also subcategory H83.3
  nerve injury —see Injury, nerve, acoustic, specified type NEC
 nonspeaking H91.3
 ototoxic —see subcategory H91.0
 perceptive —see Deafness, sensorineural
 psychogenic (hysterical) F44.6
 sensorineural H90.5
  and conductive, mixed H90.8
  bilateral H90.6
  and conductive ◄
   mixed H90.8 ◄
    bilateral H90.6 ◄
  bilateral H90.3
  unilateral H90.4-
   with restricted hearing on the contralateral side H90.A- ◄
 sensory —see Deafness, sensorineural
 specified type NEC —see subcategory H91.8
 sudden (idiopathic) H91.2-

Deafness (Continued)
 syphilitic A52.15
 transient ischemic H93.01-
 traumatic —see Injury, nerve, acoustic, specified type NEC
 word (developmental) H93.25
Death (cause unknown) (of) (unexplained) (unspecified cause) R99
 brain G93.82
 cardiac (sudden) (with successful resuscitation) — code to underlying disease
  family history of Z82.41
  personal history of Z86.74
 family member (assumed) Z63.4
Debility (chronic) (general) (nervous) R53.81
 congenital or neonatal NOS P96.9
 nervous R53.81
 old age R54
 senile R54
Débove's disease (splenomegaly) R16.1
Decalcification
 bone —see Osteoporosis
 teeth K03.89
Decapsulation, kidney N28.89
Decay
 dental —see Caries, dental
 senile R54
 tooth, teeth —see Caries, dental
Deciduitis (acute)
 following ectopic or molar pregnancy O08.0
Decline (general) —see Debility
 cognitive, age-associated R41.81
Decompensation
 cardiac (acute) (chronic) —see Disease, heart
 cardiovascular —see Disease, cardiovascular
 heart —see Disease, heart
 hepatic —see Failure, hepatic
 myocardial (acute) (chronic) —see Disease, heart
 respiratory J98.8
Decompression sickness T70.3
Decrease (d)
 absolute neutrophile count —see Neutropenia
 blood
  platelets —see Thrombocytopenia
  pressure R03.1
   due to shock following
    injury T79.4
    operation T81.19
 estrogen E28.39
  postablative E89.40
   asymptomatic E89.40
   symptomatic E89.41
 fragility of erythrocytes D58.8
 function
  lipase (pancreatic) K90.3
  ovary in hypopituitarism E23.0
  parenchyma of pancreas K86.89 ◄
  pituitary (gland) (anterior) (lobe) E23.0
   posterior (lobe) E23.0
 functional activity R68.89
 glucose R73.09
 hematocrit R71.0
 hemoglobin R71.0
 leukocytes D72.819
  specified NEC D72.818
 libido R68.82
 lymphocytes D72.810
 platelets D69.6
 respiration, due to shock following injury T79.4
 sexual desire R68.82
 tear secretion NEC —see Syndrome, dry eye
 tolerance
  fat K90.49 ◄
  glucose R73.09
  pancreatic K90.3
  salt and water E87.8
 vision NEC H54.7
 white blood cell count D72.819
  specified NEC D72.818

Decubitus (ulcer) —see Ulcer, pressure, by site
   cervix N86
Deepening acetabulum —see Derangement,
      joint, specified type NEC, hip
Defect, defective Q89.9
   3-beta-hydroxysteroid dehydrogenase E25.0
   11-hydroxylase E25.0
   21-hydroxylase E25.0
   abdominal wall, congenital Q79.59
   antibody immunodeficiency D80.9
   aorticopulmonary septum Q21.4
   atrial septal (ostium secundum type) Q21.1
      following acute myocardial infarction
         (current complication) I23.1
      ostium primum type Q21.2
   atrioventricular
      canal Q21.2
      septum Q21.2
   auricular septal Q21.1
   bilirubin excretion NEC E80.6
   biosynthesis, androgen (testicular) E29.1
   bulbar septum Q21.0
   catalase E80.3
   cell membrane receptor complex (CR3) D71
   circulation I99.9
      congenital Q28.9
      newborn Q28.9
   coagulation (factor) —see also Deficiency,
         factor D68.9
      with
         ectopic pregnancy O08.1
         molar pregnancy O08.1
      acquired D68.4
      antepartum with hemorrhage —see
            Hemorrhage, antepartum, with
            coagulation defect
      due to
         liver disease D68.4
         vitamin K deficiency D68.4
      hereditary NEC D68.2
      intrapartum O67.0
      newborn, transient P61.6
      postpartum O72.3
      specified type NEC D68.8
   complement system D84.1
   conduction (heart) I45.9
      bone —see Deafness, conductive
   congenital, organ or site not listed —see
         Anomaly, by site
   coronary sinus Q21.1
   cushion, endocardial Q21.2
   degradation, glycoprotein E77.1
   dental bridge, crown, fillings —see Defect,
         dental restoration
   dental restoration K08.50
      specified NEC K08.59
   dentin (hereditary) K00.5
   Descemet's membrane, congenital Q13.89
   developmental —see also Anomaly
      cauda equina Q06.3
   diaphragm
      with elevation, eventration or hernia —see
            Hernia, diaphragm
      congenital Q79.1
         with hernia Q79.0
         gross (with hernia) Q79.0
   ectodermal, congenital Q82.9
   Eisenmenger's Q21.8
   enzyme
      catalase E80.3
      peroxidase E80.3
   esophagus, congenital Q39.9
   extensor retinaculum M62.89
   fibrin polymerization D68.2
   filling
      bladder R93.41 ◀▥▥
      kidney R93.42- ◀▥▥
      renal pelvis R93.41 ◀
      stomach R93.3
      ureter R93.41 ◀▥▥
      urinary organs, specified NEC R93.49 ◀

Defect, defective (Continued)
   Gerbode Q21.0
   glycoprotein degradation E77.1
   Hageman (factor) D68.2
   hearing —see Deafness
   high grade F70
   interatrial septal Q21.1
   interauricular septal Q21.1
   interventricular septal Q21.0
      with dextroposition of aorta, pulmonary
            stenosis and hypertrophy of right
            ventricle Q21.3
      in tetralogy of Fallot Q21.3
   learning (specific) —see Disorder, learning
   lymphocyte function antigen-1 (LFA-1) D84.0
   lysosomal enzyme, post-translational
         modification E77.0
   major osseous M89.70
      ankle M89.77-
      carpus M89.74-
      clavicle M89.71-
      femur M89.75-
      fibula M89.76-
      fingers M89.74-
      foot M89.77-
      forearm M89.73-
      hand M89.74-
      humerus M89.72-
      lower leg M89.76-
      metacarpus M89.74-
      metatarsus M89.77-
      multiple sites M89.79
      pelvic region M89.75-
      pelvis M89.75-
      radius M89.73-
      scapula M89.71-
      shoulder region M89.71-
      specified NEC M89.78
      tarsus M89.77-
      thigh M89.75-
      tibia M89.76-
      toes M89.77-
      ulna M89.73-
   mental —see Disability, intellectual
   modification, lysosomal enzymes, post-
         translational E77.0
   obstructive, congenital
      renal pelvis Q62.39
      ureter Q62.39
         atresia —see Atresia, ureter
         cecoureterocele Q62.32
         megaureter Q62.2
         orthotopic ureterocele Q62.31
   osseous, major M89.70
      ankle M89.77-
      carpus M89.74-
      clavicle M89.71-
      femur M89.75-
      fibula M89.76-
      fingers M89.74-
      foot M89.77-
      forearm M89.73-
      hand M89.74-
      humerus M89.72-
      lower leg M89.76-
      metacarpus M89.74-
      metatarsus M89.77-
      multiple sites M89.9
      pelvic region M89.75-
      pelvis M89.75-
      radius M89.73-
      scapula M89.71-
      shoulder region M89.71-
      specified NEC M89.78
      tarsus M89.77-
      thigh M89.75-
      tibia M89.76-
      toes M89.77-
      ulna M89.73-
   osteochondral NEC —see also Deformity
         M95.8-

Defect, defective (Continued)
   ostium
      primum Q21.2
      secundum Q21.1
   peroxidase E80.3
   placental blood supply —see Insufficiency,
         placental
   platelets, qualitative D69.1
      constitutional D68.0
   postural NEC, spine —see Dorsopathy,
         deforming
   reduction
      limb Q73.8
         lower Q72.9-
            absence —see Agenesis, leg
            foot —see Agenesis, foot
            longitudinal
               femur Q72.4-
               fibula Q72.6-
               tibia Q72.5-
            specified type NEC Q72.89-
            split foot Q72.7-
         specified type NEC Q73.8
         upper Q71.9-
            absence —see Agenesis, arm
            forearm —see Agenesis, forearm
            hand —see Agenesis, hand
            lobster-claw hand Q71.6-
            longitudinal
               radius Q71.4-
               ulna Q71.5-
            specified type NEC Q71.89-
   renal pelvis Q63.8
      obstructive Q62.39
   respiratory system, congenital Q34.9
   restoration, dental K08.50
      specified NEC K08.59
   retinal nerve bundle fibers H35.89
   septal (heart) NOS Q21.9
      acquired (atrial) (auricular) (ventricular)
            (old) I51.0
      atrial Q21.1
         concurrent with acute myocardial
               infarction —see Infarct,
               myocardium
         following acute myocardial infarction
               (current complication) I23.1
      ventricular —see also Defect, ventricular
            septal Q21.0
   sinus venosus Q21.1
   speech R47.9
      developmental F80.9
      specified NEC R47.89
   Taussig-Bing (aortic transposition and
         overriding pulmonary artery) Q20.1
   teeth, wedge K03.1
   vascular (local) I99.9
      congenital Q27.9
   ventricular septal Q21.0
      concurrent with acute myocardial
            infarction —see Infarct, myocardium
      following acute myocardial infarction
            (current complication) I23.2
      in tetralogy of Fallot Q21.3
   vision NEC H54.7
   visual field H53.40
      bilateral
         heteronymous H53.47
         homonymous H53.46-
      generalized contraction H53.48-
      localized
         arcuate H53.43-
         scotoma (central area) H53.41-
            blind spot area H53.42-
         sector H53.43-
      specified type NEC H53.45-
   voice R49.9
      specified NEC R49.8
   wedge, tooth, teeth (abrasion) K03.1
Deferentitis N49.1
   gonorrheal (acute) (chronic) A54.23

Defibrination (syndrome) D65
  antepartum —*see* Hemorrhage, antepartum,
        with coagulation defect, disseminated
        intravascular coagulation
  following ectopic or molar pregnancy O08.1
  intrapartum O67.0
  newborn P60
  postpartum O72.3
Deficiency, deficient
  3-beta hydroxysteroid dehydrogenase E25.0
  11-hydroxylase E25.0
  21-hydroxylase E25.0
  5-alpha reductase (with male
        pseudohermaphroditism) E29.1
  abdominal muscle syndrome Q79.4
  AC globulin (congenital) (hereditary) D68.2
    acquired D68.4
  accelerator globulin (Ac G) (blood) D68.2
  acid phosphatase E83.39
  activating factor (blood) D68.2
  adenosine deaminase (ADA) D81.3
  aldolase (hereditary) E74.19
  alpha-1-antitrypsin E88.01
  amino-acids E72.9
  anemia —*see* Anemia
  aneurin E51.9
  antibody with
    hyperimmunoglobulinemia D80.6
    near-normal immunoglobins D80.6
  antidiuretic hormone E23.2
  anti-hemophilic
    factor (A) D66
      B D67
      C D68.1
    globulin (AHG) NEC D66
  antithrombin (antithrombin III) D68.59
  ascorbic acid E54
  attention (disorder) (syndrome) F98.8
    with hyperactivity —*see* Disorder,
        attention-deficit hyperactivity
  autoprothrombin
    I D68.2
    II D67
    C D68.2
  beta-glucuronidase E76.29
  biotin E53.8
  biotin-dependent carboxylase D81.819
  biotinidase D81.810
  brancher enzyme (amylopectinosis) E74.03
  C1 esterase inhibitor (C1-INH) D84.1
  calciferol E55.9
    with
      adult osteomalacia M83.8
      rickets —*see* Rickets
  calcium (dietary) E58
  calorie, severe E43
    with marasmus E41
      and kwashiorkor E42
  cardiac —*see* Insufficiency, myocardial
  carnitine E71.40
    due to
      hemodialysis E71.43
      inborn errors of metabolism E71.42
      Valproic acid therapy E71.43
    iatrogenic E71.43
    muscle palmityltransferase E71.314
    primary E71.41
    secondary E71.448
  carotene E50.9
  central nervous system G96.8
  ceruloplasmin (Wilson) E83.01
  choline E53.8
  Christmas factor D67
  chromium E61.4
  clotting (blood) —*see also* Deficiency,
        coagulation factor D68.9
  clotting factor NEC (hereditary) —*see also*
        Deficiency, factor D68.2
  coagulation NOS D68.9
    with
      ectopic pregnancy O08.1
      molar pregnancy O08.1

Deficiency, deficient *(Continued)*
  coagulation NOS *(Continued)*
    acquired (any) D68.4
    antepartum hemorrhage —*see*
        Hemorrhage, antepartum, with
        coagulation defect
    clotting factor NEC —*see also* Deficiency,
        factor D68.2
    due to
      hyperprothrombinemia D68.4
      liver disease D68.4
      vitamin K deficiency D68.4
    newborn, transient P61.6
    postpartum O72.3
    specified NEC D68.8
  cognitive F09
  color vision H53.50
    achromatopsia H53.51
    acquired H53.52
    deuteranomaly H53.53
    protanomaly H53.54
    specified type NEC H53.59
    tritanomaly H53.55
  combined glucocorticoid and
        mineralocorticoid E27.49
  contact factor D68.2
  copper (nutritional) E61.0
  corticoadrenal E27.40
    primary E27.1
  craniofacial axis Q75.0
  cyanocobalamin E53.8
  debrancher enzyme (limit dextrinosis) E74.03
  dehydrogenase
    long chain/very long chain acyl CoA
        E71.310
    medium chain acyl CoA E71.311
    short chain acyl CoA E71.312
  diet E63.9
  dihydropyrimidine dehydrogenase (DPD)
        E88.89
  disaccharidase E73.9
  edema —*see* Malnutrition, severe
  endocrine E34.9
  energy-supply —*see* Malnutrition
  enzymes, circulating NEC E88.09
  ergosterol E55.9
    with
      adult osteomalacia M83.8
      rickets —*see* Rickets
  essential fatty acid (EFA) E63.0
  factor —*see also* Deficiency, coagulation
    Hageman D68.2
    I (congenital) (hereditary) D68.2
    II (congenital) (hereditary) D68.2
    IX (congenital) (functional) (hereditary)
        (with functional defect) D67
    multiple (congenital) D68.8
      acquired D68.4
    V (congenital) (hereditary) D68.2
    VII (congenital) (hereditary) D68.2
    VIII (congenital) (functional) (hereditary)
        (with functional defect) D66
      with vascular defect D68.0
    X (congenital) (hereditary) D68.2
    XI (congenital) (hereditary) D68.1
    XII (congenital) (hereditary) D68.2
    XIII (congenital) (hereditary) D68.2
  femoral, proximal focal (congenital) —
        see Defect, reduction, lower limb,
        longitudinal, femur
  fibrin-stabilizing factor (congenital)
        (hereditary) D68.2
    acquired D68.4
  fibrinase D68.2
  fibrinogen (congenital) (hereditary) D68.2
    acquired D65
  folate E53.8
  folic acid E53.8
  foreskin N47.3
  fructokinase E74.11
  fructose 1,6-diphosphatase E74.19

Deficiency, deficient *(Continued)*
  fructose-1-phosphate aldolase E74.19
  galactokinase E74.29
  galactose-1-phosphate uridyl transferase
        E74.29
  gammaglobulin in blood D80.1
    hereditary D80.0
  glass factor D68.2
  glucocorticoid E27.49
    mineralocorticoid E27.49
  glucose-6-phosphatase E74.01
  glucose-6-phosphate dehydrogenase anemia
        D55.0
  glucuronyl transferase E80.5
  glycogen synthetase E74.09
  gonadotropin (isolated) E23.0
  growth hormone (idiopathic) (isolated) E23.0
  Hageman factor D68.2
  hemoglobin D64.9
  hepatophosphorylase E74.09
  homogentisate 1,2-dioxygenase E70.29
  hormone
    anterior pituitary (partial) NEC E23.0
      growth E23.0
    growth (isolated) E23.0
    pituitary E23.0
    testicular E29.1
  hypoxanthine-(guanine)-
        phosphoribosyltransferase (HG-PRT)
        (total HG-PRT) E79.1
  immunity D84.9
    cell-mediated D84.8
      with thrombocytopenia and eczema
        D82.0
    combined D81.9
    humoral D80.9
    IgA (secretory) D80.2
    IgG D80.3
    IgM D80.4
  immuno —*see* Immunodeficiency
  immunoglobulin, selective
    A (IgA) D80.2
    G (IgG) (subclasses) D80.3
    M (IgM) D80.4
  inositol (B complex) E53.8
  intrinsic
    factor (congenital) D51.0
    sphincter N36.42
      with urethral hypermobility N36.43
  iodine E61.8
    congenital syndrome —*see* Syndrome,
        iodine-deficiency, congenital
  iron E61.1
    anemia D50.9
  kalium E87.6
  kappa-light chain D80.8
  labile factor (congenital) (hereditary) D68.2
    acquired D68.4
  lacrimal fluid (acquired) —*see also* Syndrome,
        dry eye
    congenital Q10.6
  lactase
    congenital E73.0
    secondary E73.1
  Laki-Lorand factor D68.2
  lecithin cholesterol acyltransferase E78.6
  lipocaic K86.89 ◀▥
  lipoprotein (familial) (high density) E78.6
  liver phosphorylase E74.09
  lysosomal alpha-1, 4 glucosidase E74.02
  magnesium E61.2
  major histocompatibility complex
    class I D81.6
    class II D81.7
  manganese E61.3
  menadione (vitamin K) E56.1
    newborn P53
  mental (familial) (hereditary) —*see* Disability,
        intellectual
  methylenetetrahydrofolate reductase
        (MTHFR) E72.12

Deficiency, deficient (Continued)
  mevalonate kinase M04.1 ◀
  mineral NEC E61.8
  mineralocorticoid E27.49
    with glucocorticoid E27.49
  molybdenum (nutritional) E61.5
  moral F60.2
  multiple nutrient elements E61.7
  muscle
    carnitine (palmityltransferase) E71.314
    phosphofructokinase E74.09
  myoadenylate deaminase E79.2
  myocardial —see Insufficiency, myocardial
  myophosphorylase E74.04
  NADH diaphorase or reductase (congenital) D74.0
  NADH-methemoglobin reductase (congenital) D74.0
  natrium E87.1
  niacin (amide) (-tryptophan) E52
  nicotinamide E52
  nicotinic acid E52
  number of teeth —see Anodontia
  nutrient element E61.9
    multiple E61.7
    specified NEC E61.8
  nutrition, nutritional E63.9
    sequelae —see Sequelae, nutritional deficiency
    specified NEC E63.8
  of interleukin 1 receptor antagonist [DIRA] M04.8 ◀
  ornithine transcarbamylase E72.4
  ovarian E28.39
  oxygen —see Anoxia
  pantothenic acid E53.8
  parathyroid (gland) E20.9
  perineum (female) N81.89
  phenylalanine hydroxylase E70.1
  phosphoenolpyruvate carboxykinase E74.4
  phosphofructokinase E74.19
  phosphomannomutase E74.8
  phosphomannose isomerase E74.8
  phosphomannosyl mutase E74.8
  phosphorylase kinase, liver E74.09
  pituitary hormone (isolated) E23.0
  plasma thromboplastin
    antecedent (PTA) D68.1
    component (PTC) D67
  platelet NEC D69.1
    constitutional D68.0
  polyglandular E31.8
    autoimmune E31.0
  potassium (K) E87.6
  prepuce N47.3
  proaccelerin (congenital) (hereditary) D68.2
    acquired D68.4
  proconvertin factor (congenital) (hereditary) D68.2
    acquired D68.4
  protein —see also Malnutrition E46
    anemia D53.0
    C D68.59
    S D68.59
  prothrombin (congenital) (hereditary) D68.2
    acquired D68.4
  Prower factor D68.2
  pseudocholinesterase E88.09
  PTA (plasma thromboplastin antecedent) D68.1
  PTC (plasma thromboplastin component) D67
  purine nucleoside phosphorylase (PNP) D81.5
  pyracin (alpha) (beta) E53.1
  pyridoxal E53.1
  pyridoxamine E53.1
  pyridoxine (derivatives) E53.1
  pyruvate
    carboxylase E74.4
    dehydrogenase E74.4
  riboflavin (vitamin B2) E53.0

Deficiency, deficient (Continued)
  salt E87.1
  secretion
    ovary E28.39
    salivary gland (any) K11.7
    urine R34
  selenium (dietary) E59
  serum antitrypsin, familial E88.01
  short stature homeobox gene (SHOX)
    with
      dyschondrosteosis Q78.8
      short stature (idiopathic) E34.3
      Turner's syndrome Q96.9
  sodium (Na) E87.1
  SPCA (factor VII) D68.2
  sphincter, intrinsic N36.42
    with urethral hypermobility N36.43
  stable factor (congenital) (hereditary) D68.2
    acquired D68.4
  Stuart-Prower (factor X) D68.2
  sucrase E74.39
  sulfatase E75.29
  sulfite oxidase E72.19
  thiamin, thiaminic (chloride) E51.9
    beriberi (dry) E51.11
    wet E51.12
  thrombokinase D68.2
    newborn P53
  thyroid (gland) —see Hypothyroidism
  tocopherol E56.0
  tooth bud K00.0
  transcobalamine II (anemia) D51.2
  vanadium E61.6
  vascular I99.9
  vasopressin E23.2
  vertical ridge K06.8 ◀
  viosterol —see Deficiency, calciferol
  vitamin (multiple) NOS E56.9
    A E50.9
      with
        Bitot's spot (corneal) E50.1
        follicular keratosis E50.8
        keratomalacia E50.4
        manifestations NEC E50.8
        night blindness E50.5
        scar of cornea, xerophthalmic E50.6
        xeroderma E50.8
        xerophthalmia E50.7
        xerosis
          conjunctival E50.0
          and Bitot's spot E50.1
          cornea E50.2
          and ulceration E50.3
      sequelae E64.1
    B (complex) NOS E53.9
      with
        beriberi (dry) E51.11
        wet E51.12
        pellagra E52
    B1 NOS E51.9
      beriberi (dry) E51.11
        with circulatory system manifestations E51.11
        wet E51.12
    B12 E53.8
    B2 (riboflavin) E53.0
    B6 E53.1
    C E54
      sequelae E64.2
    D E55.9
      with
        adult osteomalacia M83.8
        rickets —see Rickets
      25-hydroxylase E83.32
    E E56.0
    folic acid E53.8
    G E53.0
    group B E53.9
      specified NEC E53.8

Deficiency, deficient (Continued)
  vitamin (Continued)
    H (biotin) E53.8
    K E56.1
      of newborn P53
    nicotinic E52
    P E56.8
    PP (pellagra-preventing) E52
    specified NEC E56.8
    thiamin E51.9
      beriberi —see Beriberi
  zinc, dietary E60
Deficit —see also Deficiency
  attention and concentration R41.840
    following ◀
      cerebral infarction I69.310 ◀
      cerebrovascular disease I69.910 ◀
        specified disease NEC I69.810 ◀
      nontraumatic ◀
        intracerebral hemorrhage I69.110 ◀
        specified intracranial hemorrhage NEC I69.210 ◀
        subarachnoid hemorrhage I69.010 ◀
  disorder —see Attention, deficit
  ~~cognitive communication R41.841~~
  cognitive ◀
    communication R41.841 ◀
    emotional ◀
      following ◀
        cerebral infarction I69.315 ◀
        cerebrovascular disease I69.915 ◀
          specified disease NEC I69.815 ◀
        nontraumatic ◀
          intracerebral hemorrhage I69.115 ◀
          specified intracranial hemorrhage NEC I69.215 ◀
          subarachnoid hemorrhage I69.015 ◀
    following ◀
      cerebral infarction I69.319 ◀
      cerebrovascular disease I69.919 ◀
        specified disease NEC I69.819 ◀
      nontraumatic ◀
        intracerebral hemorrhage I69.119 ◀
        specified intracranial hemorrhage NEC I69.219 ◀
        subarachnoid hemorrhage I69.019 ◀
    social ◀
      following ◀
        cerebral infarction I69.315 ◀
        cerebrovascular disease I69.915 ◀
          specified disease NEC I69.815 ◀
        nontraumatic ◀
          intracerebral hemorrhage I69.115 ◀
          specified intracranial hemorrhage NEC I69.215 ◀
          subarachnoid hemorrhage I69.015 ◀
  cognitive NEC R41.89
    following
      cerebral infarction I69.318 ◀▥
      cerebrovascular disease I69.918 ◀▥
        specified disease NEC I69.818 ◀▥
      ~~intracerebral hemorrhage I69.11~~
      ~~nontraumatic intracranial hemorrhage NEC I69.21~~
      nontraumatic ◀
        intracerebral hemorrhage I69.118 ◀
        specified intracranial hemorrhage NEC I69.218 ◀
        subarachnoid hemorrhage I69.018 ◀
      ~~subarachnoid hemorrhage I69.01~~
  concentration R41.840
  executive function R41.844
    following ◀
      cerebral infarction I69.314 ◀
      cerebrovascular disease I69.914 ◀
        specified disease NEC I69.814 ◀
      nontraumatic ◀
        intracerebral hemorrhage I69.114 ◀
        specified intracranial hemorrhage NEC I69.214 ◀
        subarachnoid hemorrhage I69.014 ◀

◀ New   ◀▥ Revised   ~~deleted~~ Deleted

Deficit *(Continued)*
frontal lobe R41.844
following ◀
cerebral infarction I69.314 ◀
cerebrovascular disease I69.914 ◀
specified disease NEC I69.814 ◀
nontraumatic ◀
intracerebral hemorrhage I69.114 ◀
specified intracranial hemorrhage
NEC I69.214 ◀
subarachnoid hemorrhage I69.014 ◀
memory ◀
following ◀
cerebral infarction I69.311 ◀
cerebrovascular disease I69.911 ◀
specified disease NEC I69.811 ◀
nontraumatic ◀
intracerebral hemorrhage I69.111 ◀
specified intracranial hemorrhage
NEC I69.211 ◀
subarachnoid hemorrhage
I69.011 ◀
neurologic NEC R29.818
ischemic
reversible (RIND) I63.9
prolonged (PRIND) I63.9
oxygen R09.02
prolonged reversible ischemic neurologic
(PRIND) I63.9
psychomotor R41.843
following ◀
cerebral infarction I69.313 ◀
cerebrovascular disease I69.913 ◀
specified disease NEC I69.813 ◀
nontraumatic ◀
intracerebral hemorrhage I69.113 ◀
specified intracranial hemorrhage
NEC I69.213 ◀
subarachnoid hemorrhage
I69.013 ◀
visuospatial R41.842
following ◀
cerebral infarction I69.312 ◀
cerebrovascular disease I69.912 ◀
specified disease NEC I69.812 ◀
nontraumatic ◀
intracerebral hemorrhage I69.112 ◀
specified intracranial hemorrhage
NEC I69.212 ◀
subarachnoid hemorrhage I69.012 ◀
Deflection
radius —*see* Deformity, limb, specified type
NEC, forearm
septum (acquired) (nasal) (nose) J34.2
spine —*see* Curvature, spine
turbinate (nose) J34.2
Defluvium
capillorum —*see* Alopecia
ciliorum —*see* Madarosis
unguium L60.8
Deformity Q89.9
abdomen, congenital Q89.9
abdominal wall
acquired M95.8
congenital Q79.59
acquired (unspecified site) M95.9
adrenal gland Q89.1
alimentary tract, congenital Q45.9
upper Q40.9
ankle (joint) (acquired) —*see also* Deformity,
limb, lower leg
abduction —*see* Contraction, joint, ankle
congenital Q68.8
contraction —*see* Contraction, joint,
ankle
specified type NEC —*see* Deformity, limb,
foot, specified NEC
anus (acquired) K62.89
congenital Q43.9
aorta (arch) (congenital) Q25.40 ◀▥
acquired I77.89

Deformity *(Continued)*
aortic
arch, acquired I77.89
cusp or valve (congenital) Q23.8
acquired —*see also* Endocarditis, aortic
I35.8
arm (acquired) (upper) —*see also* Deformity,
limb, upper arm
congenital Q68.8
forearm —*see* Deformity, limb, forearm
artery (congenital) (peripheral) NOS Q27.9
acquired I77.89
coronary (acquired) I25.9
congenital Q24.5
umbilical Q27.0
atrial septal Q21.1
auditory canal (external) (congenital) —*see
also* Malformation, ear, external
acquired —*see* Disorder, ear, external,
specified type NEC
auricle
ear (congenital) —*see also* Malformation,
ear, external
acquired —*see* Disorder, pinna,
deformity
back —*see* Dorsopathy, deforming
bile duct (common) (congenital) (hepatic)
Q44.5
acquired K83.8
biliary duct or passage (congenital) Q44.5
acquired K83.8
bladder (neck) (trigone) (sphincter)
(acquired) N32.89
congenital Q64.79
bone (acquired) NOS M95.9
congenital Q79.9
turbinate M95.0
brain (congenital) Q04.9
acquired G93.89
reduction Q04.3
breast (acquired) N64.89
congenital Q83.9
reconstructed N65.0
bronchus (congenital) Q32.4
acquired NEC J98.09
bursa, congenital Q79.9
canaliculi (lacrimalis) (acquired) —*see also*
Disorder, lacrimal system, changes
congenital Q10.6
canthus, acquired —*see* Disorder, eyelid,
specified type NEC
capillary (acquired) I78.8
cardiovascular system, congenital Q28.9
caruncle, lacrimal (acquired) —*see also*
Disorder, lacrimal system, changes
congenital Q10.6
cascade, stomach K31.2
cecum (congenital) Q43.9
acquired K63.89
cerebral, acquired G93.89
congenital Q04.9
cervix (uterus) (acquired) NEC N88.8
congenital Q51.9
cheek (acquired) M95.2
congenital Q18.9
chest (acquired) (wall) M95.4
congenital Q67.8
sequelae (late effect) of rickets E64.3
chin (acquired) M95.2
congenital Q18.9
choroid (congenital) Q14.3
acquired H31.8
plexus Q07.8
acquired G96.19
cicatricial —*see* Cicatrix
cilia, acquired —*see* Disorder, eyelid,
specified type NEC
clavicle (acquired) M95.8
congenital Q68.8
clitoris (congenital) Q52.6
acquired N90.89
clubfoot —*see* Clubfoot

Deformity *(Continued)*
coccyx (acquired) —*see* subcategory M43.8
colon (congenital) Q43.9
acquired K63.89
concha (ear), congenital —*see also*
Malformation, ear, external
acquired —*see* Disorder, pinna, deformity
cornea (acquired) H18.70
congenital Q13.4
descemetocele —*see* Descemetocele
ectasia —*see* Ectasia, cornea
specified NEC H18.79-
staphyloma —*see* Staphyloma, cornea
coronary artery (acquired) I25.9
congenital Q24.5
cranium (acquired) —*see* Deformity, skull
cricoid cartilage (congenital) Q31.8
acquired J38.7
cystic duct (congenital) Q44.5
acquired K82.8
Dandy-Walker Q03.1
with spina bifida —*see* Spina bifida
diaphragm (congenital) Q79.1
acquired J98.6
digestive organ NOS Q45.9
ductus arteriosus Q25.0
duodenal bulb K31.89
duodenum (congenital) Q43.9
acquired K31.89
dura —*see* Deformity, meninges
ear (acquired) —*see also* Disorder, pinna,
deformity
congenital (external) Q17.9
internal Q16.5
middle Q16.4
ossicles Q16.3
ossicles Q16.3
ectodermal (congenital) NEC Q84.9
ejaculatory duct (congenital) Q55.4
acquired N50.89 ◀▥
elbow (joint) (acquired) —*see also* Deformity,
limb, upper arm
congenital Q68.8
contraction —*see* Contraction, joint, elbow
endocrine gland NEC Q89.2
epididymis (congenital) Q55.4
acquired N50.89 ◀▥
epiglottis (congenital) Q31.8
acquired J38.7
esophagus (congenital) Q39.9
acquired K22.8
eustachian tube (congenital) NEC Q17.8
eye, congenital Q15.9
eyebrow (congenital) Q18.8
eyelid (acquired) —*see also* Disorder, eyelid,
specified type NEC
congenital Q10.3
face (acquired) M95.2
congenital Q18.9
fallopian tube, acquired N83.8
femur (acquired) —*see* Deformity, limb,
specified type NEC, thigh
fetal
with fetopelvic disproportion O33.7
causing obstructed labor O66.3
finger (acquired) M20.00-
boutonniere M20.02-
congenital Q68.1
flexion contracture —*see* Contraction, joint,
hand
mallet finger M20.01-
specified NEC M20.09-
swan-neck M20.03-
flexion (joint) (acquired) —*see also* Deformity,
limb, flexion M21.20
congenital NOS Q74.9
hip Q65.89
foot (acquired) —*see also* Deformity, limb,
lower leg
cavovarus (congenital) Q66.1
congenital NOS Q66.9
specified type NEC Q66.89

Deformity *(Continued)*
  foot *(Continued)*
    specified type NEC —*see* Deformity, limb,
      foot, specified NEC
    valgus (congenital) Q66.6
      acquired —*see* Deformity, valgus, ankle
    varus (congenital) NEC Q66.3
      acquired —*see* Deformity, varus, ankle
  forearm (acquired) —*see also* Deformity, limb,
    forearm
    congenital Q68.8
  forehead (acquired) M95.2
    congenital Q75.8
  frontal bone (acquired) M95.2
    congenital Q75.8
  gallbladder (congenital) Q44.1
    acquired K82.8
  gastrointestinal tract (congenital) NOS
    Q45.9
    acquired K63.89
  genitalia, genital organ (s) or system NEC
    female (congenital) Q52.9
      acquired N94.89
      external Q52.70
    male (congenital) Q55.9
      acquired N50.89 ◀▥
  globe (eye) (congenital) Q15.8
    acquired H44.89
  gum, acquired NEC K06.8
  hand (acquired) —*see* Deformity, limb,
    hand
    congenital Q68.1
  head (acquired) M95.2
    congenital Q75.8
  heart (congenital) Q24.9
    septum Q21.9
      auricular Q21.1
      ventricular Q21.0
    valve (congenital) NEC Q24.8
      acquired —*see* Endocarditis
  heel (acquired) —*see* Deformity, foot
  hepatic duct (congenital) Q44.5
    acquired K83.8
  hip (joint) (acquired) —*see also* Deformity,
    limb, thigh
    congenital Q65.9
    due to (previous) juvenile
      osteochondrosis —*see* Coxa, plana
    flexion —*see* Contraction, joint, hip
  hourglass —*see* Contraction, hourglass
  humerus (acquired) M21.82-
    congenital Q74.0
  hypophyseal (congenital) Q89.2
  ileocecal (coil) (valve) (acquired) K63.89
    congenital Q43.9
  ileum (congenital) Q43.9
    acquired K63.89
  ilium (acquired) M95.5
    congenital Q74.2
  integument (congenital) Q84.9
  intervertebral cartilage or disc (acquired) —
    see Disorder, disc, specified NEC
  intestine (large) (small) (congenital) NOS
    Q43.9
    acquired K63.89
  intrinsic minus or plus (hand) —*see*
    Deformity, limb, specified type NEC,
    forearm
  iris (acquired) H21.89
    congenital Q13.2
  ischium (acquired) M95.5
    congenital Q74.2
  jaw (acquired) (congenital) M26.9
  joint (acquired) NEC M21.90
    congenital Q68.8
    elbow M21.92-
    hand M21.94-
    hip M21.95-
    knee M21.96-
    shoulder M21.92-
    wrist M21.93-

Deformity *(Continued)*
  kidney (s) (calyx) (pelvis) (congenital) Q63.9
    acquired N28.89
    artery (congenital) Q27.2
      acquired I77.89
  Klippel-Feil (brevicollis) Q76.1
  knee (acquired) NEC —*see also* Deformity,
    limb, lower leg
    congenital Q68.2
  labium (majus) (minus) (congenital) Q52.79
    acquired N90.89
  lacrimal passages or duct (congenital) NEC
    Q10.6
    acquired —*see* Disorder, lacrimal system,
      changes
  larynx (muscle) (congenital) Q31.8
    acquired J38.7
    web (glottic) Q31.0
  leg (upper) (acquired) NEC —*see also*
    Deformity, limb, thigh
    congenital Q68.8
    lower leg —*see* Deformity, limb, lower leg
  lens (acquired) H27.8
    congenital Q12.9
  lid (fold) (acquired) —*see also* Disorder,
    eyelid, specified type NEC
    congenital Q10.3
  ligament (acquired) —*see* Disorder, ligament
    congenital Q79.9
  limb (acquired) M21.90
    clawfoot M21.53-
    clawhand M21.51-
    clubfoot M21.54-
    clubhand M21.52-
    congenital, except reduction deformity
      Q74.9
    flat foot M21.4-
    flexion M21.20
      ankle M21.27-
      elbow M21.22-
      finger M21.24-
      hip M21.25-
      knee M21.26-
      shoulder M21.21-
      toe M21.27-
      wrist M21.23-
    foot
      claw —*see* Deformity, limb, clawfoot
      club —*see* Deformity, limb, clubfoot
      drop M21.37-
      flat —*see* Deformity, limb, flat foot
      specified NEC M21.6X-
    forearm M21.93-
    hand M21.94-
    lower leg M21.96-
    specified type NEC M21.80
      forearm M21.83-
      lower leg M21.86-
      thigh M21.85-
      upper arm M21.82-
    thigh M21.95-
    unequal length M21.70
      short site is
        femur M21.75-
        fibula M21.76-
        humerus M21.72-
        radius M21.73-
        tibia M21.76-
        ulna M21.73-
    upper arm M21.92-
    valgus —*see* Deformity, valgus
    varus —*see* Deformity, varus
    wrist drop M21.33-
  lip (acquired) NEC K13.0
    congenital Q38.0
  liver (congenital) Q44.7
    acquired K76.89
  lumbosacral (congenital) (joint) (region) Q76.49
    acquired —*see* subcategory M43.8
    kyphosis —*see* Kyphosis, congenital
    lordosis —*see* Lordosis, congenital

Deformity *(Continued)*
  lung (congenital) Q33.9
    acquired J98.4
  lymphatic system, congenital Q89.9
  Madelung's (radius) Q74.0
  mandible (acquired) (congenital) M26.9
  maxilla (acquired) (congenital) M26.9
  meninges or membrane (congenital) Q07.9
    cerebral Q04.8
      acquired G96.19
    spinal cord (congenital) G96.19
      acquired G96.19
  metacarpus (acquired) —*see* Deformity, limb,
    forearm
    congenital Q74.0
  metatarsus (acquired) —*see* Deformity,
    foot
    congenital Q66.9
  middle ear (congenital) Q16.4
    ossicles Q16.3
  mitral (leaflets) (valve) I05.8
    parachute Q23.2
    stenosis, congenital Q23.2
  mouth (acquired) K13.79
    congenital Q38.6
  multiple, congenital NEC Q89.7
  muscle (acquired) M62.89
    congenital Q79.9
      sternocleidomastoid Q68.0
  musculoskeletal system (acquired) M95.9
    congenital Q79.9
    specified NEC M95.8
  nail (acquired) L60.8
    congenital Q84.6
  nasal —*see* Deformity, nose
  neck (acquired) M95.3
    congenital Q18.9
      sternocleidomastoid Q68.0
  nervous system (congenital) Q07.9
  nipple (congenital) Q83.9
    acquired N64.89
  nose (acquired) (cartilage) M95.0
    bone (turbinate) M95.0
    congenital Q30.9
      bent or squashed Q67.4
    saddle M95.0
      syphilitic A50.57
    septum (acquired) J34.2
      congenital Q30.8
    sinus (wall) (congenital) Q30.8
      acquired M95.0
    syphilitic (congenital) A50.57
      late A52.73
  ocular muscle (congenital) Q10.3
    acquired —*see* Strabismus, mechanical
  opticociliary vessels (congenital) Q13.2
  orbit (eye) (acquired) H05.30
    atrophy —*see* Atrophy, orbit
    congenital Q10.7
    due to
      bone disease NEC H05.32-
      trauma or surgery H05.33-
    enlargement —*see* Enlargement, orbit
    exostosis —*see* Exostosis, orbit
  organ of Corti (congenital) Q16.5
  ovary (congenital) Q50.39
    acquired N83.8
  oviduct, acquired N83.8
  palate (congenital) Q38.5
    acquired M27.8
    cleft (congenital) —*see* Cleft, palate
  pancreas (congenital) Q45.3
    acquired K86.89 ◀▥
  parathyroid (gland) Q89.2
  parotid (gland) (congenital) Q38.4
    acquired K11.8
  patella (acquired) —*see* Disorder, patella,
    specified NEC
  pelvis, pelvic (acquired) (bony) M95.5
    with disproportion (fetopelvic) O33.0
      causing obstructed labor O65.0

Deformity *(Continued)*
  pelvis, pelvic *(Continued)*
    congenital Q74.2
    rachitic sequelae (late effect) E64.3
  penis (glans) (congenital) Q55.69
    acquired N48.89
  pericardium (congenital) Q24.8
    acquired —*see* Pericarditis
  pharynx (congenital) Q38.8
    acquired J39.2
  pinna, acquired —*see also* Disorder, pinna,
      deformity
    congenital Q17.9
  pituitary (congenital) Q89.2
  posture —*see* Dorsopathy, deforming
  prepuce (congenital) Q55.69
    acquired N47.8
  prostate (congenital) Q55.4
    acquired N42.89
  pupil (congenital) Q13.2
    acquired —*see* Abnormality, pupillary
  pylorus (congenital) Q40.3
    acquired K31.89
  rachitic (acquired), old or healed E64.3
  radius (acquired) —*see also* Deformity, limb,
      forearm
    congenital Q68.8
  rectum (congenital) Q43.9
    acquired K62.89
  reduction (extremity) (limb), congenital *(see
      also* condition and site) Q73.8
    brain Q04.3
    lower —*see* Defect, reduction, lower limb
    upper —*see* Defect, reduction, upper
        limb
  renal —*see* Deformity, kidney
  respiratory system (congenital) Q34.9
  rib (acquired) M95.4
    congenital Q76.6
      cervical Q76.5
  rotation (joint) (acquired) —*see* Deformity,
      limb, specified site NEC
    congenital Q74.9
    hip —*see* Deformity, limb, specified type
        NEC, thigh
      congenital Q65.89
  sacroiliac joint (congenital) Q74.2
    acquired —*see* subcategory M43.8
  sacrum (acquired) —*see* subcategory
      M43.8
  saddle
    back —*see* Lordosis
    nose M95.0
      syphilitic A50.57
  salivary gland or duct (congenital) Q38.4
    acquired K11.8
  scapula (acquired) M95.8
    congenital Q68.8
  scrotum (congenital) —*see also* Malformation,
      testis and scrotum
    acquired N50.89 ◀▥
  seminal vesicles (congenital) Q55.4
    acquired N50.89 ◀▥
  septum, nasal (acquired) J34.2
  shoulder (joint) (acquired) —*see* Deformity,
      limb, upper arm
    congenital Q74.0
    contraction —*see* Contraction, joint,
        shoulder
  sigmoid (flexure) (congenital) Q43.9
    acquired K63.89
  skin (congenital) Q82.9
  skull (acquired) M95.2
    congenital Q75.8
      with
        anencephaly Q00.0
        encephalocele —*see* Encephalocele
        hydrocephalus Q03.9
          with spina bifida —*see* Spina bifida,
              by site, with hydrocephalus
        microcephaly Q02

Deformity *(Continued)*
  soft parts, organs or tissues (of pelvis)
    in pregnancy or childbirth NEC O34.8-
      causing obstructed labor O65.5
  spermatic cord (congenital) Q55.4
    acquired N50.89 ◀▥
    torsion —*see* Torsion, spermatic cord
  spinal —*see* Dorsopathy, deforming
    column (acquired) —*see* Dorsopathy,
        deforming
    congenital Q67.5
    cord (congenital) Q06.9
      acquired G95.89
    nerve root (congenital) Q07.9
  spine (acquired) —*see also* Dorsopathy,
      deforming
    congenital Q67.5
    rachitic E64.3
    specified NEC —*see* Dorsopathy,
        deforming, specified NEC
  spleen
    acquired D73.89
    congenital Q89.09
  Sprengel's (congenital) Q74.0
  sternocleidomastoid (muscle), congenital
      Q68.0
  sternum (acquired) M95.4
    congenital NEC Q76.7
  stomach (congenital) Q40.3
    acquired K31.89
  submandibular gland (congenital) Q38.4
  submaxillary gland (congenital) Q38.4
    acquired K11.8
  talipes —*see* Talipes
  testis (congenital) —*see also* Malformation,
      testis and scrotum
    acquired N44.8
    torsion —*see* Torsion, testis
  thigh (acquired) —*see also* Deformity, limb,
      thigh
    congenital NEC Q68.8
  thorax (acquired) (wall) M95.4
    congenital Q67.8
    sequelae of rickets E64.3
  thumb (acquired) —*see also* Deformity, finger
    congenital NEC Q68.1
  thymus (tissue) (congenital) Q89.2
  thyroid (gland) (congenital) Q89.2
    cartilage Q31.8
      acquired J38.7
  tibia (acquired) —*see also* Deformity, limb,
      specified type NEC, lower leg
    congenital NEC Q68.8
    saber (syphilitic) A50.56
  toe (acquired) M20.6-
    congenital Q66.9
    hallux rigidus M20.2-
    hallux valgus M20.1-
    hallux varus M20.3-
    hammer toe M20.4-
    specified NEC M20.5X-
  tongue (congenital) Q38.3
    acquired K14.8
  tooth, teeth K00.2
  trachea (rings) (congenital) Q32.1
    acquired J39.8
  transverse aortic arch (congenital)
      Q25.49 ◀▥
  tricuspid (leaflets) (valve) I07.8
    atresia or stenosis Q22.4
    Ebstein's Q22.5
  trunk (acquired) M95.8
    congenital Q89.9
  ulna (acquired) —*see also* Deformity, limb,
      forearm
    congenital NEC Q68.8
  urachus, congenital Q64.4
  ureter (opening) (congenital) Q62.8
    acquired N28.89
  urethra (congenital) Q64.79
    acquired N36.8

Deformity *(Continued)*
  urinary tract (congenital) Q64.9
    urachus Q64.4
  uterus (congenital) Q51.9
    acquired N85.8
  uvula (congenital) Q38.5
  vagina (acquired) N89.8
    congenital Q52.4
  valgus NEC M21.00
    ankle M21.07-
    elbow M21.02-
    hip M21.05-
    knee M21.06-
  valve, valvular (congenital) (heart) Q24.8
    acquired —*see* Endocarditis
  varus NEC M21.10
    ankle M21.17-
    elbow M21.12-
    hip M21.15
    knee M21.16-
    tibia —*see* Osteochondrosis, juvenile, tibia
  vas deferens (congenital) Q55.4
    acquired N50.89 ◀▥
  vein (congenital) Q27.9
    great Q26.9
  vertebra —*see* Dorsopathy, deforming
  vertical talus (congenital) Q66.80
    left foot Q66.82
    right foot Q66.81
  vesicourethral orifice (acquired) N32.89
    congenital NEC Q64.79
  vessels of optic papilla (congenital) Q14.2
  visual field (contraction) —*see* Defect, visual
      field
  vitreous body, acquired H43.89
  vulva (congenital) Q52.79
    acquired N90.89
  wrist (joint) (acquired) —*see also* Deformity,
      limb, forearm
    congenital Q68.8
    contraction —*see* Contraction, joint, wrist
Degeneration, degenerative
  adrenal (capsule) (fatty) (gland) (hyaline)
      (infectional) E27.8
  amyloid —*see also* Amyloidosis E85.9
  anterior cornua, spinal cord G12.29
  anterior labral S43.49-
  aorta, aortic I70.0
    fatty I77.89
  aortic valve (heart) —*see* Endocarditis,
      aortic
  arteriovascular —*see* Arteriosclerosis
  artery, arterial (atheromatous) (calcareous) —
      see also Arteriosclerosis
    cerebral, amyloid E85.4 *[I68.0]*
    medial —*see* Arteriosclerosis, extremities
  articular cartilage NEC —*see* Derangement,
      joint, articular cartilage, by site
  atheromatous —*see* Arteriosclerosis
  basal nuclei or ganglia G23.9
    specified NEC G23.8
  bone NEC —*see* Disorder, bone, specified
      type NEC
  brachial plexus G54.0
  brain (cortical) (progressive) G31.9
    alcoholic G31.2
    arteriosclerotic I67.2
    childhood G31.9
      specified NEC G31.89
    cystic G31.89
      congenital Q04.6
    in
      alcoholism G31.2
      beriberi E51.2
      cerebrovascular disease I67.9
      congenital hydrocephalus Q03.9
        with spina bifida —*see also* Spina
            bifida
      Fabry-Anderson disease E75.21
      Gaucher's disease E75.22
      Hunter's syndrome E76.1

Degeneration, degenerative (Continued)
  brain (Continued)
    in (Continued)
      lipidosis
        cerebral E75.4
        generalized E75.6
      mucopolysaccharidosis —see
        Mucopolysaccharidosis
      myxedema E03.9 [G32.89]
      neoplastic disease —see also Neoplasm
        D49.6 [G32.89]
      Niemann-Pick disease E75.249 [G32.89]
      sphingolipidosis E75.3 [G32.89]
      vitamin B12 deficiency E53.8 [G32.89]
    senile NEC G31.1
  breast N64.89
  Bruch's membrane —see Degeneration,
    choroid
  capillaries (fatty) I78.8
    amyloid E85.8 [I79.8]
  cardiac —see also Degeneration, myocardial
    valve, valvular —see Endocarditis
  cardiorenal —see Hypertension, cardiorenal
  cardiovascular —see also Disease,
    cardiovascular
    renal —see Hypertension, cardiorenal
  cerebellar NOS G31.9
    alcoholic G31.2
    primary (hereditary) (sporadic) G11.9
  cerebral —see Degeneration, brain
  cerebrovascular I67.9
    due to hypertension I67.4
  cervical plexus G54.2
  cervix N88.8
    due to radiation (intended effect) N88.8
      adverse effect or misadventure N99.89
  chamber angle H21.21-
  changes, spine or vertebra —see Spondylosis
  chorioretinal —see also Degeneration, choroid
    hereditary H31.20
  choroid (colloid) (drusen) H31.10-
    atrophy —see Atrophy, choroidal
    hereditary —see Dystrophy, choroidal,
      hereditary
  ciliary body H21.22-
  cochlear —see subcategory H83.8
  combined (spinal cord) (subacute) E53.8
    [G32.0]
    with anemia (pernicious) D51.0 [G32.0]
      due to dietary vitamin B12 deficiency
        D51.3 [G32.0]
    in (due to)
      vitamin B12 deficiency E53.8 [G32.0]
        anemia D51.9 [G32.0]
  conjunctiva H11.10
    concretions —see Concretion, conjunctiva
    deposits —see Deposit, conjunctiva
    pigmentations —see Pigmentation,
      conjunctiva
    pinguecula —see Pinguecula
    xerosis —see Xerosis, conjunctiva
  cornea H18.40
    calcerous H18.43
      band keratopathy H18.42-
    familial, hereditary —see Dystrophy, cornea
    hyaline (of old scars) H18.49
    keratomalacia —see Keratomalacia
    nodular H18.45-
    peripheral H18.46-
    senile H18.41-
    specified type NEC H18.49
  cortical (cerebellar) (parenchymatous)
    G31.89
    alcoholic G31.2
    diffuse, due to arteriopathy I67.2
  corticobasal G31.85
  cutis L98.8
    amyloid E85.4 [L99]
  dental pulp K04.2
  disc disease —see Degeneration,
    intervertebral disc NEC

Degeneration, degenerative (Continued)
  dorsolateral (spinal cord) —see Degeneration,
    combined
  extrapyramidal G25.9
  eye, macular —see also Degeneration, macula
    congenital or hereditary —see Dystrophy,
      retina
  facet joints —see Spondylosis
  fatty
    liver NEC K76.0
      alcoholic K70.0
  grey matter (brain) (Alpers') G31.81
  heart —see also Degeneration, myocardial
    amyloid E85.4 [I43]
    atheromatous —see Disease, heart,
      ischemic, atherosclerotic
    ischemic —see Disease, heart, ischemic
  hepatolenticular (Wilson's) E83.01
  hepatorenal K76.7
  hyaline (diffuse) (generalized)
    localized —see Degeneration, by site
  infrapatellar fat pad M79.4
  intervertebral disc NOS
    with
      myelopathy —see Disorder, disc, with,
        myelopathy
      radiculitis or radiculopathy —see
        Disorder, disc, with, radiculopathy
    cervical, cervicothoracic —see Disorder,
      disc, cervical, degeneration
      with
        myelopathy —see Disorder, disc,
          cervical, with myelopathy
        neuritis, radiculitis or
          radiculopathy —see Disorder,
          disc, cervical, with neuritis
    lumbar region M51.36
      with
        myelopathy M51.06
        neuritis, radiculitis, radiculopathy or
          sciatica M51.16
    lumbosacral region M51.37
      with
        neuritis, radiculitis, radiculopathy or
          sciatica M51.17
    sacrococcygeal region M53.3
    thoracic region M51.34
      with
        myelopathy M51.04
        neuritis, radiculitis, radiculopathy
          M51.14
    thoracolumbar region M51.35
      with
        myelopathy M51.05
        neuritis, radiculitis, radiculopathy
          M51.15
  intestine, amyloid E85.4
  iris (pigmentary) H21.23-
  ischemic —see Ischemia
  joint disease —see Osteoarthritis
  kidney N28.89
    amyloid E85.4 [N29]
    cystic, congenital Q61.9
    fatty N28.89
    polycystic Q61.3
      adult type (autosomal dominant)
        Q61.2
      infantile type (autosomal recessive) NEC
        Q61.19
        collecting duct dilatation Q61.11
  Kuhnt-Junius —see also Degeneration, macula
    H35.32-
  lens —see Cataract
  lenticular (familial) (progressive) (Wilson's)
    (with cirrhosis of liver) E83.01
  liver (diffuse) NEC K76.89
    amyloid E85.4 [K77]
    cystic K76.89
      congenital Q44.6
    fatty NEC K76.0
      alcoholic K70.0

Degeneration, degenerative (Continued)
  liver (Continued)
    hypertrophic K76.89
    parenchymatous, acute or subacute
      K72.00
      with coma K72.01
    pigmentary K76.89
    toxic (acute) K71.9
  lung J98.4
  lymph gland I89.8
    hyaline I89.8
  macula, macular (acquired) (age-related)
    (senile) H35.30
    angioid streaks H35.33
    atrophic age-related H35.31-
    congenital or hereditary —see Dystrophy,
      retina
    cystoid H35.35-
    drusen H35.36-
    dry age-related H35.31-
    exudative H35.32-
    hole H35.34-
    nonexudative H35.31-
    puckering H35.37-
    toxic H35.38-
    wet age-related H35.32-
  membranous labyrinth, congenital (causing
    impairment of hearing) Q16.5
  meniscus —see Derangement, meniscus
  mitral —see Insufficiency, mitral
  Mönckeberg's —see Arteriosclerosis,
    extremities
  motor centers, senile G31.1
  multi-system G90.3
  mural —see Degeneration, myocardial
  muscle (fatty) (fibrous) (hyaline)
    (progressive) M62.89
    heart —see Degeneration, myocardial
  myelin, central nervous system G37.9
  myocardial, myocardium (fatty) (hyaline)
    (senile) I51.5
    with rheumatic fever (conditions in I00)
      I09.0
      active, acute or subacute I01.2
        with chorea I02.0
      inactive or quiescent (with chorea) I09.0
    hypertensive —see Hypertension, heart
    rheumatic —see Degeneration, myocardial,
      with rheumatic fever
    syphilitic A52.06
  nasal sinus (mucosa) J32.9
    frontal J32.1
    maxillary J32.0
  nerve —see Disorder, nerve
  nervous system G31.9
    alcoholic G31.2
    amyloid E85.4 [G99.8]
    autonomic G90.9
    fatty G31.89
    specified NEC G31.89
  nipple N64.89
  olivopontocerebellar (hereditary) (familial)
    G23.8
  osseous labyrinth —see subcategory H83.8
  ovary N83.8
    cystic N83.20-
    microcystic N83.20-
  pallidal pigmentary (progressive) G23.0
  pancreas K86.89
    tuberculous A18.83
  penis N48.89
  pigmentary (diffuse) (general)
    localized —see Degeneration, by site
    pallidal (progressive) G23.0
  pineal gland E34.8
  pituitary (gland) E23.6
  popliteal fat pad M79.4
  posterolateral (spinal cord) —see
    Degeneration, combined
  pulmonary valve (heart) I37.8
  pulp (tooth) K04.2

◀ New   ◀║ Revised   deleted Deleted

Degeneration, degenerative (Continued)
pupillary margin H21.24-
renal —see Degeneration, kidney
retina H35.9
hereditary (cerebroretinal) (congenital) (juvenile) (macula) (peripheral) (pigmentary) —see Dystrophy, retina
Kuhnt-Junius —see also Degeneration, macula H35.32- ◀▥▥
macula (cystic) (exudative) (hole) (nonexudative) (pseudohole) (senile) (toxic) —see Degeneration, macula
peripheral H35.40
lattice H35.41-
microcystoid H35.42-
paving stone H35.43-
secondary
pigmentary H35.45-
vitreoretinal H35.46-
senile reticular H35.44-
pigmentary (primary) —see also Dystrophy, retina
secondary —see Degeneration, retina, peripheral, secondary
posterior pole —see Degeneration, macula
saccule, congenital (causing impairment of hearing) Q16.5
senile R54
brain G31.1
cardiac, heart or myocardium —see Degeneration, myocardial
motor centers G31.1
vascular —see Arteriosclerosis
sinus (cystic) —see also Sinusitis
polypoid J33.1
skin L98.8
amyloid E85.4 [L99]
colloid L98.8
spinal (cord) G31.89
amyloid E85.4 [G32.89]
combined (subacute) —see Degeneration, combined
dorsolateral —see Degeneration, combined
familial NEC G31.89
fatty G31.89
funicular —see Degeneration, combined
posterolateral —see Degeneration, combined
subacute combined —see Degeneration, combined
tuberculous A17.81
spleen D73.0
amyloid E85.4 [D77]
stomach K31.89
striatonigral G23.2
suprarenal (capsule) (gland) E27.8
synovial membrane (pulpy) —see Disorder, synovium, specified type NEC
tapetoretinal —see Dystrophy, retina
thymus (gland) E32.8
fatty E32.8
thyroid (gland) E07.89
tricuspid (heart) (valve) I07.9
tuberculous NEC —see Tuberculosis
turbinate J34.89
uterus (cystic) N85.8
vascular (senile) —see Arteriosclerosis
hypertensive —see Hypertension
vitreoretinal, secondary —see Degeneration, retina, peripheral, secondary, vitreoretinal
vitreous (body) H43.81-
Wallerian —see Disorder, nerve
Wilson's hepatolenticular E83.01
Deglutition
paralysis R13.0
hysterical F44.4
pneumonia J69.0
Degos' disease I77.89
Dehiscence (of)
amputation stump T87.81
cesarean wound O90.0

Dehiscence (Continued)
closure of
cornea T81.31
craniotomy T81.32
fascia (muscular) (superficial) T81.32
internal organ or tissue T81.32
laceration (external) (internal) T81.33
ligament T81.32
mucosa T81.31
muscle or muscle flap T81.32
ribs or rib cage T81.32
skin and subcutaneous tissue (full-thickness) (superficial) T81.31
skull T81.32
sternum (sternotomy) T81.32
tendon T81.32
traumatic laceration (external) (internal) T81.33
episiotomy O90.1
operation wound NEC T81.31
external operation wound (superficial) T81.31
internal operation wound (deep) T81.32
perineal wound (postpartum) O90.1
traumatic injury wound repair T81.33
wound T81.30
traumatic repair T81.33
Dehydration E86.0
~~hypertonic E87.0~~
~~hypotonic E87.1~~
newborn P74.1
Déjérine-Roussy syndrome G93.89
Déjérine-Sottas disease or neuropathy (hypertrophic) G60.0
Déjérine-Thomas atrophy G23.8
Delay, delayed
any plane in pelvis
complicating delivery O66.9
birth or delivery NOS O63.9
closure, ductus arteriosus (Botalli) P29.3
coagulation —see Defect, coagulation
conduction (cardiac) (ventricular) I45.9
delivery, second twin, triplet, etc O63.2
development R62.50
global F88
intellectual (specific) F81.9
language F80.9
due to hearing loss F80.4
learning F81.9
pervasive F84.9
physiological R62.50
specified stage NEC R62.0
reading F81.0
sexual E30.0
speech F80.9
due to hearing loss F80.4
spelling F81.81
ejaculation F52.32 ◀
gastric emptying K30
menarche E30.0
menstruation (cause unknown) N91.0
milestone R62.0
passage of meconium (newborn) P76.0
primary respiration P28.9
puberty (constitutional) E30.0
separation of umbilical cord P96.82
sexual maturation, female E30.0
sleep phase syndrome G47.21
union, fracture —see Fracture, by site
vaccination Z28.9
Deletion (s)
autosome Q93.9
identified by fluorescence in situ hybridization (FISH) Q93.89
identified by in situ hybridization (ISH) Q93.89
chromosome
with complex rearrangements NEC Q93.7
part of NEC Q93.5
seen only at prometaphase Q93.89

Deletion (Continued)
chromosome (Continued)
short arm
4 Q93.3
5p Q93.4
22q11.2 Q93.81
specified NEC Q93.89
long arm chromosome 18 or 21 Q93.89
with complex rearrangements NEC Q93.7
microdeletions NEC Q93.88
Delhi boil or button B55.1
Delinquency (juvenile) (neurotic) F91.8
group Z72.810
Delinquent immunization status Z28.3
Delirium, delirious (acute or subacute) (not alcohol or drug-induced) (with dementia) R41.0
alcoholic (acute) (tremens) (withdrawal) F10.921
with intoxication F10.921
in
abuse F10.121
dependence F10.221
due to (secondary to)
alcohol
intoxication F10.921
in
abuse F10.121
dependence F10.221
withdrawal F10.231
amphetamine intoxication F15.921
in
abuse F15.121
dependence F15.221
anxiolytic
intoxication F13.921
in
abuse F13.121
dependence F13.221
withdrawal F13.231
cannabis intoxication (acute) F12.921
in
abuse F12.121
dependence F12.221
cocaine intoxication (acute) F14.921
in
abuse F14.121
dependence F14.221
general medical condition F05
hallucinogen intoxication F16.921
in
abuse F16.121
dependence F16.221
hypnotic
intoxication F13.921
in
abuse F13.121
dependence F13.221
withdrawal F13.231
inhalant intoxication (acute) F18.921
in
abuse F18.121
dependence F18.221
multiple etiologies F05
opioid intoxication (acute) F11.921
in
abuse F11.121
dependence F11.221
other (or unknown) substance F19.921 ◀
phencyclidine intoxication (acute) F16.921
in
abuse F16.121
dependence F16.221
psychoactive substance NEC intoxication (acute) F19.921
in
abuse F19.121
dependence F19.221

Delirium, delirious *(Continued)*
  due to *(Continued)*
    sedative
      intoxication F13.921
        in
          abuse F13.121
          dependence F13.221
      withdrawal F13.231
    unknown etiology F05
  exhaustion F43.0
  hysterical F44.89
  postprocedural (postoperative) F05
  puerperal F05
  thyroid —*see* Thyrotoxicosis with thyroid
      storm
  traumatic —*see* Injury, intracranial
  tremens (alcohol-induced) F10.231
    sedative-induced F13.231
Delivery (childbirth) (labor)
  arrested active phase O62.1
  cesarean (for)
    without indication O82
    abnormal
      pelvis (bony) (deformity) (major) NEC
          with disproportion (fetopelvic)
          O33.0
        with obstructed labor O65.0
      presentation or position O32.9
    abruptio placentae —*see also* Abruptio
        placentae O45.9-
    acromion presentation O32.2
    atony, uterus O62.2
    breech presentation O32.1
      incomplete O32.8
    brow presentation O32.3
    cephalopelvic disproportion O33.9
    cerclage O34.3-
    chin presentation O32.3
    cicatrix of cervix O34.4-
    contracted pelvis (general)
      inlet O33.2
      outlet O33.3
    cord presentation or prolapse O69.0
    cystocele O34.8-
    deformity (acquired) (congenital)
      pelvic organs or tissues NEC O34.8-
      pelvis (bony) NEC O33.0
    disproportion NOS O33.9
    eclampsia —*see* Eclampsia
    face presentation O32.3
    failed
      forceps O66.5
      induction of labor O61.9
        instrumental O61.1
        mechanical O61.1
        medical O61.0
        specified NEC O61.8
        surgical O61.1
      trial of labor NOS O66.40
        following previous cesarean delivery
          O66.41
      vacuum extraction O66.5
      ventouse O66.5
    fetal-maternal hemorrhage O43.01-
    hemorrhage (intrapartum) O67.9
      with coagulation defect O67.0
      specified cause NEC O67.8
    high head at term O32.4
    hydrocephalic fetus O33.6
    incarceration of uterus O34.51-
    incoordinate uterine action O62.4
    increased size, fetus O33.5
    inertia, uterus O62.2
      primary O62.0
      secondary O62.1
    lateroversion, uterus O34.59-
    mal lie O32.9
    malposition
      fetus O32.9
      pelvic organs or tissues NEC O34.8-
      uterus NEC O34.59-

Delivery *(Continued)*
  cesarean *(Continued)*
    malpresentation NOS O32.9
    oblique presentation O32.2
    occurring after 37 completed weeks of
        gestation but before 39 completed
        weeks gestation due to (spontaneous)
        onset of labor O75.82
    oversize fetus O33.5
    pelvic tumor NEC O34.8-
    placenta previa O44.0- ◀
      complete O44.0- ◀
      with hemorrhage O44.1- ◀
      without hemorrhage O44.0-
    placental insufficiency O36.51-
    planned, occurring after 37 completed
        weeks of gestation but before 39
        completed weeks gestation due to
        (spontaneous) onset of labor O75.82
    polyp, cervix O34.4-
      causing obstructed labor O65.5
    poor dilatation, cervix O62.0
    pre-eclampsia O14.94 ◀
      mild O14.04 ◀
      moderate O14.04 ◀
      severe O14.14 ◀
        with hemolysis, elevated liver
            enzymes and low platelet count
            (HELLP) O14.24 ◀
    previous
      cesarean delivery O34.219 ◀
        classical (vertical) scar O34.212 ◀
        low transverse scar O34.211 ◀
      surgery (to)
        cervix O34.4-
        gynecological NEC O34.8-
        rectum O34.7-
        uterus O34.29
        vagina O34.6-
    prolapse
      arm or hand O32.2
      uterus O34.52-
    prolonged labor NOS O63.9
    rectocele O34.8-
    retroversion
      uterus O34.53-
    rigid
      cervix O34.4-
      pelvic floor O34.8-
      perineum O34.7-
      vagina O34.6-
      vulva O34.7-
    sacculation, pregnant uterus O34.59-
    scar (s)
      cervix O34.4-
      cesarean delivery O34.219 ◀
        classical (vertical) O34.212 ◀
        low transverse O34.211 ◀
      transmural uterine O34.29 ◀
      uterus O34.29
    Shirodkar suture in situ O34.3-
    shoulder presentation O32.2
    stenosis or stricture, cervix O34.4-
    streptococcus B carrier state O99.824
    streptococcus group B (GBS) carrier state
        O99.824 ◀
    transmural uterine scar O34.29 ◀
    transverse presentation or lie O32.2
    tumor, pelvic organs or tissues NEC O34.8-
      cervix O34.4-
    umbilical cord presentation or prolapse
        O69.0
  completely normal case O80
  complicated O75.9
    by
      abnormal, abnormality (of)
        forces of labor O62.9
          specified type NEC O62.8
        glucose O99.814
        uterine contractions NOS O62.9
      abruptio placentae —*see also* Abruptio
          placentae O45.9-

Delivery *(Continued)*
  complicated *(Continued)*
    by *(Continued)*
      abuse
        physical O9A.32
        psychological O9A.52
        sexual O9A.42
      adherent placenta O72.0
        without hemorrhage O73.0
      alcohol use O99.314
      anemia (pre-existing) O99.02
      anesthetic death O74.8
      annular detachment of cervix O71.3
      atony, uterus O62.2
      attempted vacuum extraction and
          forceps O66.5
      Bandl's ring O62.4
      bariatric surgery status O99.844
      biliary tract disorder O26.62
      bleeding —*see* Delivery, complicated by,
          hemorrhage
      blood disorder NEC O99.12
      cervical dystocia (hypotonic) O62.2
        primary O62.0
        secondary O62.1
      circulatory system disorder O99.42
      compression of cord (umbilical) NEC
          O69.2
      condition NEC O99.89
      contraction, contracted ring O62.4
      cord (umbilical)
        around neck
          with compression O69.1
          without compression O69.81
        bruising O69.5
        complication O69.9
          specified NEC O69.89
        compression NEC O69.2
        entanglement O69.2
          without compression O69.82
        hematoma O69.5
        presentation O69.0
        prolapse O69.0
        short O69.3
        thrombosis (vessels) O69.5
        vascular lesion O69.5
      Couvelaire uterus O45.8X-
      damage to (injury to) NEC
        perineum O71.82
        periurethral tissue O71.82
        vulva O71.82
      delay following rupture of membranes
          (spontaneous) —*see* Pregnancy,
          complicated by, premature rupture
          of membranes
      depressed fetal heart tones O76
      diabetes O24.92
        gestational O24.429
          diet controlled O24.420
          insulin controlled O24.424
          oral drug controlled (antidiabetic)
              (hypoglycemic) O24.425 ◀
        pre-existing O24.32
          specified NEC O24.82
          type 1 O24.02
          type 2 O24.12
      diastasis recti (abdominis) O71.89
      dilatation
        bladder O66.8
        cervix incomplete, poor or slow O62.0
      disease NEC O99.89
      disruptio uteri —*see* Delivery,
          complicated by, rupture, uterus
      drug use O99.324
      dysfunction, uterus NOS O62.9
        hypertonic O62.4
        hypotonic O62.2
          primary O62.0
          secondary O62.1
        incoordinate O62.4
      eclampsia O15.1
      embolism (pulmonary) —*see* Embolism,
          obstetric

◀ New   ◀▥ Revised   ~~deleted~~ Deleted

Delivery *(Continued)*
  complicated *(Continued)*
    by *(Continued)*
      endocrine, nutritional or metabolic disease NEC O99.284
      failed
        attempted vaginal birth after previous cesarean delivery O66.41
        induction of labor O61.9
          instrumental O61.1
          mechanical O61.1
          medical O61.0
          specified NEC O61.8
          surgical O61.1
        trial of labor O66.40
      female genital mutilation O65.5
      fetal
        abnormal acid-base balance O68
        acidemia O68
        acidosis O68
        alkalosis O68
        death, early O02.1
        deformity O66.3
        heart rate or rhythm (abnormal) (non-reassuring) O76
        hypoxia O77.8
        stress O77.9
          due to drug administration O77.1
          electrocardiographic evidence of O77.8
          specified NEC O77.8
          ultrasound evidence of O77.8
      fever during labor O75.2
      gastric banding status O99.844
      gastric bypass status O99.844
      gastrointestinal disease NEC O99.62
      ~~gestational diabetes O24.429~~
        ~~diet controlled O24.420~~
        ~~insulin (and diet) controlled O24.424~~
      gestational ◀
        diabetes O24.429 ◀
          diet controlled O24.420 ◀
          insulin (and diet) controlled O24.424 ◀
          oral drug controlled (antidiabetic) (hypoglycemic) O24.425 ◀
        edema O12.04 ◀
          with proteinuria O12.24 ◀
        proteinuria O12.14 ◀
      gonorrhea O98.22
      hematoma O71.7
        ischial spine O71.7
        pelvic O71.7
        vagina O71.7
        vulva or perineum O71.7
      hemorrhage (uterine) O67.9
        associated with
          afibrinogenemia O67.0
          coagulation defect O67.0
          hyperfibrinolysis O67.0
          hypofibrinogenemia O67.0
        due to
          low implantation of placenta O44.5- ◀
          low-lying placenta O44.5- ◀◀
          placenta previa O44.1-
            marginal O44.3- ◀
            partial O44.3- ◀
          premature separation of placenta (normally implanted) (*see also* Abruptio placentae) O45.9-
          retained placenta O72.0
          uterine leiomyoma O67.8
        placenta NEC O67.8
        postpartum NEC (atonic) (immediate) O72.1
          with retained or trapped placenta O72.0
          delayed O72.2
          secondary O72.2
          third stage O72.0

Delivery *(Continued)*
  complicated *(Continued)*
    by *(Continued)*
      hourglass contraction, uterus O62.4
      hypertension, hypertensive (pre-existing) —*see* Hypertension, complicated by, childbirth (labor)
      hypotension O26.5-
      incomplete dilatation (cervix) O62.0
      incoordinate uterus contractions O62.4
      inertia, uterus O62.2
        during latent phase of labor O62.0
        primary O62.0
        secondary O62.1
      infection (maternal) O98.92
        carrier state NEC O99.834
        gonorrhea O98.22
        human immunodeficiency virus (HIV) O98.72
        sexually transmitted NEC O98.32
        specified NEC O98.82
        syphilis O98.12
        tuberculosis O98.02
        viral hepatitis O98.42
        viral NEC O98.52
      injury (to mother) (*see also* Delivery, complicated, by, damage to) O71.9
        nonobstetric O9A.22
          caused by abuse —*see* Delivery, complicated by, abuse
      intrauterine fetal death, early O02.1
      inversion, uterus O71.2
      laceration (perineal) O70.9
        anus (sphincter) O70.4
          with third degree laceration —*see also* Delivery, complicated, by, laceration, perineum, third degree O70.20
            with mucosa O70.3
          without third degree laceration O70.4
        bladder (urinary) O71.5
        bowel O71.5
        cervix (uteri) O71.3
        fourchette O70.0
        hymen O70.0
        labia O70.0
        pelvic
          floor O70.1
          organ NEC O71.5
        perineum, perineal O70.9
          first degree O70.0
          fourth degree O70.3
          muscles O70.1
          second degree O70.1
          skin O70.0
          slight O70.0
          third degree O70.20 ◀◀
            with ◀
              both external anal sphincter (EAS) and internal anal sphincter (IAS) torn (IIIc) O70.23 ◀
              less than 50% of external anal sphincter (EAS) thickness torn (IIIa) O70.21 ◀
              more than 50% external anal sphincter (EAS) thickness torn (IIIb) O70.22 ◀
            IIIa O70.21 ◀
            IIIb O70.22 ◀
            IIIc O70.23 ◀
        peritoneum (pelvic) O71.5
        rectovaginal (septum) (without perineal laceration) O71.4
          with perineum —*see also* Delivery, complicated, by, laceration, perineum, third degree O70.20 ◀◀
          with anal or rectal mucosa O70.3

Delivery *(Continued)*
  complicated *(Continued)*
    by *(Continued)*
      laceration *(Continued)*
        specified NEC O71.89
        sphincter ani —*see* Delivery, complicated, by, laceration, anus (sphincter)
        urethra O71.5
        uterus O71.81
          before labor O71.81
        vagina, vaginal (deep) (high) (without perineal laceration) O71.4
          with perineum O70.0
          muscles, with perineum O70.1
        vulva O70.0
      liver disorder O26.62
      malignancy O9A.12
      malnutrition O25.2
      malposition, malpresentation O32.9 —*see also* Delivery, complicated by, obstruction
        without obstruction O32.9 —*see also* Delivery, complicated by, obstruction
        breech O32.1
        compound O32.6
        face (brow) (chin) O32.3
        footling O38.8
        high head O32.4
        oblique O32.2
        specified NEC O32.8
        transverse O32.2
        unstable lie O32.0
        placenta O44.0- ◀◀
          ~~without hemorrhage O44.0-~~
          with hemorrhage O44.1- ◀
        uterus or cervix O65.5
      meconium in amniotic fluid O77.0
      mental disorder NEC O99.344
      metrorrhexis —*see* Delivery, complicated by, rupture, uterus
      nervous system disorder O99.354
      obesity (pre-existing) O99.214
      obesity surgery status O99.844
      obstetric trauma O71.9
        specified NEC O71.89
      obstructed labor
        due to
          breech (complete) (frank) presentation O64.1
            incomplete O64.8
          brow presenation O64.3
          buttock presentation O64.1
          chin presentation O64.2
          compound presentation O64.5
          contracted pelvis O65.1
          deep transverse arrest O64.0
          deformed pelvis O65.0
          dystocia (fetal) O66.9
            due to
              conjoined twins O66.3
              fetal
                abnormality NEC O66.3
                ascites O66.3
                hydrops O66.3
                meningomyelocele O66.3
                sacral teratoma O66.3
                tumor O66.3
             hydrocephalic fetus O66.3
          shoulder O66.0
          face presentation O64.2
          fetopelvic disproportion O65.4
          footling presentation O64.8
          impacted shoulders O66.0
          incomplete rotation of fetal head O64.0
          large fetus O66.2
          locked twins O66.1
          malposition O64.9
            specified NEC O64.8
          malpresentation O64.9
            specified NEC O64.8

◀ New ◀▥ Revised ~~deleted~~ Deleted

Dementia (Continued)
in (Continued)
psychoactive drug F19.97
with dependence F19.27
inhalants F18.97
with dependence F18.27
sedatives, hypnotics or anxiolytics
F13.97
with dependence F13.27
sedatives, hypnotics or anxiolytics F13.97
with dependence F13.27
systemic lupus erythematosus
M32.- [F02.80]
with behavioral disturbance
M32.- [F02.81]
trypanosomiasis
African B56.9 [F02.80]
with behavioral disturbance B56.9
[F02.81]
unknown etiology F03
vitamin B12 deficiency E53.8 [F02.80]
with behavioral disturbance E53.8
[F02.81]
volatile solvents F18.97
with dependence F18.27
infantile, infantilis F84.3
Lewy body G31.83 [F02.80]
with behavioral disturbance G31.83
[F02.81]
multi-infarct —see Dementia, vascular
paralytica, paralytic (syphilitic) A52.17
[F02.80]
with behavioral disturbance A52.17
[F02.81]
juvenilis A50.45
paretic A52.17
praecox —see Schizophrenia
presenile F03
Alzheimer's type —see Disease,
Alzheimer's, early onset
primary degenerative F03
progressive, syphilitic A52.17
senile F03
with acute confusional state F05
Alzheimer's type —see Disease,
Alzheimer's, late onset
depressed or paranoid type F03
vascular (acute onset) (mixed) (multi-infarct)
(subcortical) F01.50
with behavioral disturbance F01.51
Demineralization, bone —see Osteoporosis
Demodex folliculorum (infestation) B88.0
Demophobia F40.248
Demoralization R45.3
Demyelination, demyelinization
central nervous system G37.9
specified NEC G37.8
corpus callosum (central) G37.1
disseminated, acute G36.9
specified NEC G36.8
global G35
in optic neuritis G36.0
Dengue (classical) (fever) A90
hemorrhagic A91
sandfly A93.1
Dennie-Marfan syphilitic syndrome
A50.45
Dens evaginatus, in dente or invaginatus
K00.2
Dense breasts R92.2
Density
increased, bone (disseminated) (generalized)
(spotted) —see Disorder, bone, density
and structure, specified type NEC
lung (nodular) J98.4
Dental —see also condition
examination Z01.20
with abnormal findings Z01.21
restoration
aesthetically inadequate or displeasing
K08.56

Dental (Continued)
restoration (Continued)
defective K08.50
specified NEC K08.59
failure of marginal integrity K08.51
failure of periodontal anatomical integrity
K08.54
Dentia praecox K00.6
Denticles (pulp) K04.2
Dentigerous cyst K09.0
Dentin
irregular (in pulp) K04.3
opalescent K00.5
secondary (in pulp) K04.3
sensitive K03.89
Dentinogenesis imperfecta K00.5
Dentinoma —see Cyst, calcifying odontogenic
Dentition (syndrome) K00.7
delayed K00.6
difficult K00.7
precocious K00.6
premature K00.6
retarded K00.6
Dependence (on) (syndrome) F19.20
with remission F19.21
alcohol (ethyl) (methyl) (without remission)
F10.20
with
amnestic disorder, persisting F10.26
anxiety disorder F10.280
dementia, persisting F10.27
intoxication F10.229
with delirium F10.221
uncomplicated F10.220
mood disorder F10.24
psychotic disorder F10.259
with
delusions F10.250
hallucinations F10.251
remission F10.21
sexual dysfunction F10.281
sleep disorder F10.282
specified disorder NEC F10.288
withdrawal F10.239
with
delirium F10.231
perceptual disturbance F10.232
uncomplicated F10.230
counseling and surveillance Z71.41
amobarbital —see Dependence, drug,
sedative
amphetamine (s) (type) —see Dependence,
drug, stimulant NEC
amytal (sodium) —see Dependence, drug,
sedative
analgesic NEC F55.8
anesthetic (agent) (gas) (general) (local)
NEC —see Dependence, drug,
psychoactive NEC
anxiolytic NEC —see Dependence, drug,
sedative
barbital (s) —see Dependence, drug, sedative
barbiturate (s) (compounds) (drugs
classifiable to T42) —see Dependence,
drug, sedative
benzedrine —see Dependence, drug,
stimulant NEC
bhang —see Dependence, drug, cannabis
bromide (s) NEC —see Dependence, drug,
sedative
caffeine —see Dependence, drug, stimulant
NEC
cannabis (sativa) (indica) (resin) (derivatives)
(type) —see Dependence, drug, cannabis
chloral (betaine) (hydrate) —see Dependence,
drug, sedative
chlordiazepoxide —see Dependence, drug,
sedative
coca (leaf) (derivatives) —see Dependence,
drug, cocaine
cocaine —see Dependence, drug, cocaine

Dependence (Continued)
codeine —see Dependence, drug, opioid
combinations of drugs F19.20
dagga —see Dependence, drug, cannabis
demerol —see Dependence, drug, opioid
dexamphetamine —see Dependence, drug,
stimulant NEC
dexedrine —see Dependence, drug, stimulant
NEC
dextromethorphan —see Dependence, drug,
opioid
dextromoramide —see Dependence, drug,
opioid
dextro-nor-pseudo-ephedrine —see
Dependence, drug, stimulant NEC
dextrorphan —see Dependence, drug, opioid
diazepam —see Dependence, drug, sedative
dilaudid —see Dependence, drug, opioid
D-lysergic acid diethylamide —see
Dependence, drug, hallucinogen
drug NEC F19.20
with sleep disorder F19.282
cannabis F12.20
with
anxiety disorder F12.280
intoxication F12.229
with
delirium F12.221
perceptual disturbance F12.222
uncomplicated F12.220
other specified disorder F12.288
psychosis F12.259
delusions F12.250
hallucinations F12.251
unspecified disorder F12.29
in remission F12.21
cocaine F14.20
with
anxiety disorder F14.280
intoxication F14.229
with
delirium F14.221
perceptual disturbance F14.222
uncomplicated F14.220
mood disorder F14.24
other specified disorder F14.288
psychosis F14.259
delusions F14.250
hallucinations F14.251
sexual dysfunction F14.281
sleep disorder F14.282
unspecified disorder F14.29
withdrawal F14.23
in remission F14.21
withdrawal symptoms in newborn P96.1
counseling and surveillance Z71.51
hallucinogen F16.20
with
anxiety disorder F16.280
flashbacks F16.283
intoxication F16.229
with delirium F16.221
uncomplicated F16.220
mood disorder F16.24
other specified disorder F16.288
perception disorder, persisting F16.283
psychosis F16.259
delusions F16.250
hallucinations F16.251
unspecified disorder F16.29
in remission F16.21
in remission F19.21
inhalant F18.20
with
anxiety disorder F18.280
dementia, persisting F18.27
intoxication F18.229
with delirium F18.221
uncomplicated F18.220
mood disorder F18.24
other specified disorder F18.288

Dependence *(Continued)*
  drug NEC *(Continued)*
    inhalant *(Continued)*
      with *(Continued)*
        psychosis F18.259
          delusions F18.250
          hallucinations F18.251
        unspecified disorder F18.29
      in remission F18.21
    nicotine F17.200
      with disorder F17.209
        remission F17.201
        specified disorder NEC F17.208
        withdrawal F17.203
      chewing tobacco F17.220
        with disorder F17.229
          remission F17.221
          specified disorder NEC F17.228
          withdrawal F17.223
      cigarettes F17.210
        with disorder F17.219
          remission F17.211
          specified disorder NEC F17.218
          withdrawal F17.213
      specified product NEC F17.290
        with disorder F17.299
          remission F17.291
          specified disorder NEC F17.298
          withdrawal F17.293
    opioid F11.20
      with
        intoxication F11.229
          with
            delirium F11.221
            perceptual disturbance F11.222
          uncomplicated F11.220
        mood disorder F11.24
        other specified disorder F11.288
        psychosis F11.259
          delusions F11.250
          hallucinations F11.251
        sexual dysfunction F11.281
        sleep disorder F11.282
        unspecified disorder F11.29
        withdrawal F11.23
      in remission F11.21
    psychoactive NEC F19.20
      with
        amnestic disorder F19.26
        anxiety disorder F19.280
        dementia F19.27
        intoxication F19.229
          with
            delirium F19.221
            perceptual disturbance
              F19.222
          uncomplicated F19.220
        mood disorder F19.24
        other specified disorder F19.288
        psychosis F19.259
          delusions F19.250
          hallucinations F19.251
        sexual dysfunction F19.281
        sleep disorder F19.282
        unspecified disorder F19.29
        withdrawal F19.239
          with
            delirium F19.231
            perceptual disturbance
              F19.232
          uncomplicated F19.230
    sedative, hypnotic or anxiolytic F13.20
      with
        amnestic disorder F13.26
        anxiety disorder F13.280
        dementia, persisting F13.27
        intoxication F13.229
          with delirium F13.221
          uncomplicated F13.220
        mood disorder F13.24
        other specified disorder F13.288

Dependence *(Continued)*
  drug NEC *(Continued)*
    sedative, hypnotic or anxiolytic *(Continued)*
      with *(Continued)*
        psychosis F13.259
          delusions F13.250
          hallucinations F13.251
        sexual dysfunction F13.281
        sleep disorder F13.282
        unspecified disorder F13.29
        withdrawal F13.239
          with
            delirium F13.231
            perceptual disturbance F13.232
          uncomplicated F13.230
      in remission F13.21
    stimulant NEC F15.20
      with
        anxiety disorder F15.280
        intoxication F15.229
          with
            delirium F15.221
            perceptual disturbance F15.222
          uncomplicated F15.220
        mood disorder F15.24
        other specified disorder F15.288
        psychosis F15.259
          delusions F15.250
          hallucinations F15.251
        sexual dysfunction F15.281
        sleep disorder F15.282
        unspecified disorder F15.29
        withdrawal F15.23
      in remission F15.21
    ethyl
      alcohol (without remission) F10.20
        with remission F10.21
      bromide —*see* Dependence, drug,
        sedative
      carbamate F19.20
      chloride F19.20
      morphine —*see* Dependence, drug, opioid
    ganja —*see* Dependence, drug, cannabis
    glue (airplane) (sniffing) —*see* Dependence,
      drug, inhalant
    glutethimide —*see* Dependence, drug,
      sedative
    hallucinogenics —*see* Dependence, drug,
      hallucinogen
    hashish —*see* Dependence, drug, cannabis
    hemp —*see* Dependence, drug, cannabis
    heroin (salt) (any) —*see* Dependence, drug,
      opioid
    hypnotic NEC —*see* Dependence, drug,
      sedative
    Indian hemp —*see* Dependence, drug,
      cannabis
    inhalants —*see* Dependence, drug, inhalant
    khat —*see* Dependence, drug, stimulant NEC
    laudanum —*see* Dependence, drug, opioid
    LSD (-25) (derivatives) —*see* Dependence,
      drug, hallucinogen
    luminal —*see* Dependence, drug, sedative
    lysergic acid —*see* Dependence, drug,
      hallucinogen
    maconha —*see* Dependence, drug, cannabis
    marihuana —*see* Dependence, drug, cannabis
    meprobamate —*see* Dependence, drug,
      sedative
    mescaline —*see* Dependence, drug,
      hallucinogen
    methadone —*see* Dependence, drug, opioid
    methamphetamine (s) —*see* Dependence,
      drug, stimulant NEC
    methaqualone —*see* Dependence, drug,
      sedative
    methyl
      alcohol (without remission) F10.20
        with remission F10.21
      bromide —*see* Dependence, drug, sedative
      morphine —*see* Dependence, drug, opioid

Dependence *(Continued)*
  methyl *(Continued)*
    phenidate —*see* Dependence, drug,
      stimulant NEC
    sulfonal —*see* Dependence, drug, sedative
  morphine (sulfate) (sulfite) (type) —*see*
    Dependence, drug, opioid
  narcotic (drug) NEC —*see* Dependence, drug,
    opioid
  nembutal —*see* Dependence, drug, sedative
  neraval —*see* Dependence, drug, sedative
  neravan —*see* Dependence, drug, sedative
  neurobarb —*see* Dependence, drug, sedative
  nicotine —*see* Dependence, drug, nicotine
  nitrous oxide F19.20
  nonbarbiturate sedatives and tranquilizers
    with similar effect —*see* Dependence,
    drug, sedative
  on
    artificial heart (fully implantable)
      (mechanical) Z95.812
    aspirator Z99.0
    care provider (because of) Z74.9
      impaired mobility Z74.09
      need for
        assistance with personal care Z74.1
        continuous supervision Z74.3
      no other household member able to
        render care Z74.2
      specified reason NEC Z74.8
    machine Z99.89
      enabling NEC Z99.89
      specified type NEC Z99.89
    renal dialysis (hemodialysis) (peritoneal)
      Z99.2
    respirator Z99.11
    ventilator Z99.11
    wheelchair Z99.3
  opiate —*see* Dependence, drug, opioid
  opioids —*see* Dependence, drug, opioid
  opium (alkaloids) (derivatives) (tincture) —
    see Dependence, drug, opioid
  oxygen (long-term) (supplemental) Z99.81
  paraldehyde —*see* Dependence, drug,
    sedative
  paregoric —*see* Dependence, drug, opioid
  PCP (phencyclidine) (or related substance) —
    see Dependence, drug, hallucinogen ◀▥▥
  pentobarbital —*see* Dependence, drug,
    sedative
  pentobarbitone (sodium) —*see* Dependence,
    drug, sedative
  pentothal —*see* Dependence, drug, sedative
  peyote —*see* Dependence, drug, hallucinogen
  phencyclidine (PCP) (or related substance) —
    see Dependence, drug, hallucinogen ◀▥▥
  phenmetrazine —*see* Dependence, drug,
    stimulant NEC
  phenobarbital —*see* Dependence, drug,
    sedative
  polysubstance F19.20
  psilocibin, psilocin, psilocyn, psilocyline —*see*
    Dependence, drug, hallucinogen
  psychostimulant NEC —*see* Dependence,
    drug, stimulant NEC
  secobarbital —*see* Dependence, drug, sedative
  seconal —*see* Dependence, drug, sedative
  sedative NEC —*see* Dependence, drug,
    sedative
  specified drug NEC —*see* Dependence, drug
  stimulant NEC —*see* Dependence, drug,
    stimulant NEC
  substance NEC —*see* Dependence, drug
  supplemental oxygen Z99.81
  tobacco —*see* Dependence, drug, nicotine
    counseling and surveillance Z71.6
  tranquilizer NEC —*see* Dependence, drug,
    sedative
  vitamin B6 E53.1
  volatile solvents —*see* Dependence, drug,
    inhalant

◀ New   ◀▥▥ Revised   ~~deleted~~ Deleted

Dependency
  care-provider Z74.9
  passive F60.7
  reactions (persistent) F60.7
Depersonalization (in neurotic state) (neurotic)
    (syndrome) F48.1
Depletion
  extracellular fluid E86.9
  plasma E86.1
  potassium E87.6
    nephropathy N25.89
  salt or sodium E87.1
    causing heat exhaustion or prostration T67.4
    nephropathy N28.9
  volume NOS E86.9
Deployment (current) (military) status Z56.82
  in theater or in support of military war,
      peacekeeping and humanitarian
      operations Z56.82
  personal history of Z91.82
    military war, peacekeeping and
        humanitarian deployment (current or
        past conflict) Z91.82
  returned from Z91.82
Depolarization, premature I49.40
  atrial I49.1
  junctional I49.2
  specified NEC I49.49
  ventricular I49.3
Deposit
  bone in Boeck's sarcoid D86.89
  calcareous, calcium —see Calcification
  cholesterol
    retina H35.89
    vitreous (body) (humor) —see Deposit,
        crystalline
  conjunctiva H11.11-
  cornea H18.00-
    argentous H18.02-
    due to metabolic disorder H18.03-
    Kayser-Fleischer ring H18.04-
    pigmentation —see Pigmentation, cornea
  crystalline, vitreous (body) (humor) H43.2-
  hemosiderin in old scars of cornea —see
      Pigmentation, cornea, stromal
  metallic in lens —see Cataract, specified NEC
  skin R23.8
  tooth, teeth (betel) (black) (green) (materia
      alba) (orange) (tobacco) K03.6
  urate, kidney —see Calculus, kidney
Depraved appetite —see Pica
Depressed
  HDL cholesterol E78.6
Depression (acute) (mental) F32.9
  agitated (single episode) F32.2
  anaclitic —see Disorder, adjustment
  anxiety F41.8
    persistent F34.1
  arches —see also Deformity, limb, flat foot
  atypical (single episode) F32.89 ◀▥
    recurrent episode F33.8 ◀
  basal metabolic rate R94.8
  bone marrow D75.89
  central nervous system R09.2
  cerebral R29.818
    newborn P91.4
  cerebrovascular I67.9
  chest wall M95.4
  climacteric (single episode) F32.89 ◀▥
    recurrent episode F33.8 ◀
  endogenous (without psychotic symptoms)
      F33.2
    with psychotic symptoms F33.3
  functional activity R68.89
  hysterical F44.89
  involutional (single episode) F32.89 ◀▥
    recurrent episode F33.8 ◀
  major F32.9
    with psychotic symptoms F32.3
    recurrent —see Disorder, depressive,
        recurrent

Depression (Continued)
  manic-depressive —see Disorder, depressive,
      recurrent
  masked (single episode) F32.89 ◀▥
  medullary G93.89
  menopausal (single episode) F32.89 ◀▥
    recurrent episode F33.8 ◀
  metatarsus —see Depression, arches
  monopolar F33.9
  nervous F34.1
  neurotic F34.1
  nose M95.0
  postnatal F53
  postpartum F53
  post-psychotic of schizophrenia F32.89 ◀▥
  post-schizophrenic F32.89 ◀▥
  psychogenic (reactive) (single episode) F32.9
  psychoneurotic F34.1
  psychotic (single episode) F32.3
    recurrent F33.3
  reactive (psychogenic) (single episode) F32.9
    psychotic (single episode) F32.3
  recurrent —see Disorder, depressive,
      recurrent
  respiratory center G93.89
  seasonal —see Disorder, depressive, recurrent
  senile F03
  severe, single episode F32.2
  situational F43.21
  skull Q67.4
  specified NEC (single episode) F32.89 ◀▥
  sternum M95.4
  visual field —see Defect, visual field
  vital (recurrent) (without psychotic
      symptoms) F33.2
    with psychotic symptoms F33.3
    single episode F32.2
Deprivation
  cultural Z60.3
  effects NOS T73.9
    specified NEC T73.8
  emotional NEC Z65.8
    affecting infant or child —see
        Maltreatment, child, psychological
  food T73.0
  protein —see Malnutrition
  sleep Z72.820
  social Z60.4
    affecting infant or child —see
        Maltreatment, child, psychological
  specified NEC T73.8
  vitamins —see Deficiency, vitamin
  water T73.1
Derangement
  ankle (internal) —see Derangement, joint,
      ankle
  cartilage (articular) NEC —see Derangement,
      joint, articular cartilage, by site
    recurrent —see Dislocation, recurrent
  cruciate ligament, anterior, current injury —
      see Sprain, knee, cruciate, anterior
  elbow (internal) —see Derangement, joint,
      elbow
  hip (joint) (internal) (old) —see Derangement,
      joint, hip
  joint (internal) M24.9
    ankylosis —see Ankylosis
    articular cartilage M24.10
      ankle M24.17-
      elbow M24.12-
      foot M24.17-
      hand M24.14-
      hip M24.15-
      knee NEC M23.9-
      loose body —see Loose, body
      shoulder M24.11-
      wrist M24.13-
    contracture —see Contraction, joint
    current injury —see also Dislocation
      knee, meniscus or cartilage —see Tear,
          meniscus

Derangement (Continued)
  joint (Continued)
    dislocation
      pathological —see Dislocation,
          pathological
      recurrent —see Dislocation, recurrent
    knee —see Derangement, knee
    ligament —see Disorder, ligament
    loose body —see Loose, body
    recurrent —see Dislocation, recurrent
    specified type NEC M24.80
      ankle M24.87-
      elbow M24.82-
      foot joint M24.87-
      hand joint M24.84-
      hip M24.85-
      shoulder M24.81-
      wrist M24.83-
    temporomandibular M26.69
  knee (recurrent) M23.9-
    ligament disruption, spontaneous
        M23.60-
      anterior cruciate M23.61-
      capsular M23.67-
      instability, chronic M23.5-
      lateral collateral M23.64-
      medial collateral M23.63-
      posterior cruciate M23.62-
    loose body M23.4-
    meniscus M23.30-
      cystic M23.00-
        lateral M23.002
          anterior horn M23.04-
          posterior horn M23.05-
          specified NEC M23.06-
        medial M23.005
          anterior horn M23.01-
          posterior horn M23.02-
          specified NEC M23.03-
      degenerate —see Derangement, knee,
          meniscus, specified NEC
      detached —see Derangement, knee,
          meniscus, specified NEC
      due to old tear or injury M23.20-
        lateral M23.20-
          anterior horn M23.24-
          posterior horn M23.25-
          specified NEC M23.26-
        medial M23.20-
          anterior horn M23.21-
          posterior horn M23.22-
          specified NEC M23.23-
      retained —see Derangement, knee,
          meniscus, specified NEC
      specified NEC M23.30-
        lateral M23.30-
          anterior horn M23.34-
          posterior horn M23.35-
          specified NEC M23.36-
        medial M23.30-
          anterior horn M23.31-
          posterior horn M23.32-
          specified NEC M23.33-
    old M23.8X-
    specified NEC —see subcategory M23.8
  low back NEC —see Dorsopathy, specified
      NEC
  meniscus —see Derangement, knee,
      meniscus
  mental —see Psychosis
  patella, specified NEC —see Disorder,
      patella, derangement NEC
  semilunar cartilage (knee) —see
      Derangement, knee, meniscus,
      specified NEC
  shoulder (internal) —see Derangement,
      joint, shoulder
Dercum's disease E88.2
Derealization (neurotic) F48.1
Dermal —see condition
Dermaphytid —see Dermatophytosis

Dermatitis (eczematous) L30.9
  ab igne L59.0
  acarine B88.0
  actinic (due to sun) L57.8
    other than from sun L59.8
  allergic —see Dermatitis, contact, allergic
  ambustionis, due to burn or scald —see Burn
  amebic A06.7
  ammonia L22
  arsenical (ingested) L27.8
  artefacta L98.1
    psychogenic F54
  atopic L20.9
    psychogenic F54
    specified NEC L20.89
  autoimmune progesterone L30.8
  berlock, berloque L56.2
  blastomycotic B40.3
  blister beetle L24.89
  bullous, bullosa L13.9
    mucosynechial, atrophic L12.1
    seasonal L30.8
    specified NEC L13.8
  calorica L59.0
    due to burn or scald —see Burn
  caterpillar L24.89
  cercarial B65.3
  combustionis L59.0
    due to burn or scald —see Burn
  congelationis T69.1
  contact (occupational) L25.9
    allergic L23.9
      due to
        adhesives L23.1
        cement L23.5
        chemical products NEC L23.5
        chromium L23.0
        cosmetics L23.2
        dander (cat) (dog) L23.81
        drugs in contact with skin L23.3
        dyes L23.4
        food in contact with skin L23.6
        hair (cat) (dog) L23.81
        insecticide L23.5
        metals L23.0
        nickel L23.0
        plants, non-food L23.7
        plastic L23.5
        rubber L23.5
        specified agent NEC L23.89
      due to
        cement L25.3
        chemical products NEC L25.3
        cosmetics L25.0
        dander (cat) (dog) L23.81
        drugs in contact with skin L25.1
        dyes L25.2
        food in contact with skin L25.4
        hair (cat) (dog) L23.81
        plants, non-food L25.5
        specified agent NEC L25.8
      irritant L24.9
        due to
          cement L24.5 ◀▦
          chemical products NEC L24.5
          cosmetics L24.3
          detergents L24.0
          drugs in contact with skin L24.4
          food in contact with skin L24.6
          oils and greases L24.1
          plants, non-food L24.7
          solvents L24.2
          specified agent NEC L24.89
  contusiformis L52
  diabetic —see E08-E13 with .620
  diaper L22
  diphtheritica A36.3
  dry skin L85.3
  due to
    acetone (contact) (irritant) L24.2
    acids (contact) (irritant) L24.5

Dermatitis (Continued)
  due to (Continued)
    adhesive (s) (allergic) (contact) (plaster)
        L23.1
      irritant L24.5
    alcohol (irritant) (skin contact) (substances in
        category T51) L24.2
      taken internally L27.8
    alkalis (contact) (irritant) L24.5
    arsenic (ingested) L27.8
    carbon disulfide (contact) (irritant) L24.2
    caustics (contact) (irritant) L24.5
    cement (contact) L25.3
    cereal (ingested) L27.2
    chemical (s) NEC L25.3
      taken internally L27.8
    chlorocompounds L24.2
    chromium (contact) (irritant) L24.81
    coffee (ingested) L27.2
    cold weather L30.8
    cosmetics (contact) L25.0
      allergic L23.2
      irritant L24.3
    cyclohexanes L24.2
    dander (cat) (dog) L23.81
    Demodex species B88.0
    Dermanyssus gallinae B88.0
    detergents (contact) (irritant) L24.0
    dichromate L24.81
    drugs and medicaments (generalized)
        (internal use) L27.0
      external —see Dermatitis, due to, drugs,
          in contact with skin
      in contact with skin L25.1
        allergic L23.3
        irritant L24.4
      localized skin eruption L27.1
      specified substance —see Table of Drugs
          and Chemicals
    dyes (contact) L25.2
      allergic L23.4
      irritant L24.89
    epidermophytosis —see Dermatophytosis
    esters L24.2
    external irritant NEC L24.9
    fish (ingested) L27.2
    flour (ingested) L27.2
    food (ingested) L27.2
      in contact with skin L25.4
    fruit (ingested) L27.2
    furs (allergic) (contact) L23.81
    glues —see Dermatitis, due to, adhesives
    glycols L24.2
    greases NEC (contact) (irritant) L24.1
    hair (cat) (dog) L23.81
    hot
      objects and materials —see Burn
      weather or places L59.0
    hydrocarbons L24.2
    infrared rays L59.8
    ingestion, ingested substance L27.9
      chemical NEC L27.8
      drugs and medicaments —see
          Dermatitis, due to, drugs
      food L27.2
      specified NEC L27.8
    insecticide in contact with skin L24.5
    internal agent L27.9
      drugs and medicaments (generalized) —
          see Dermatitis, due to, drugs
      food L27.2
    irradiation —see Dermatitis, due to,
        radioactive substance
    ketones L24.2
    lacquer tree (allergic) (contact) L23.7
    light (sun) NEC L57.8
      acute L56.8
      other L59.8
    Liponyssoides sanguineus B88.0
    low temperature L30.8
    meat (ingested) L27.2

Dermatitis (Continued)
  due to (Continued)
    metals, metal salts (contact) (irritant)
        L24.81
    milk (ingested) L27.2
    nickel (contact) (irritant) L24.81
    nylon (contact) (irritant) L24.5
    oils NEC (contact) (irritant) L24.1
    paint solvent (contact) (irritant) L24.2
    petroleum products (contact) (irritant)
        (substances in T52) L24.2
    plants NEC (contact) L25.5
      allergic L23.7
      irritant L24.7
    plasters (adhesive) (any) (allergic) (contact)
        L23.1
      irritant L24.5
    plastic (contact) L25.3
    preservatives (contact) —see Dermatitis,
        due to, chemical, in contact with
        skin
    primrose (allergic) (contact) L23.7
    primula (allergic) (contact) L23.7
    radiation L59.8
      nonionizing (chronic exposure) L57.8
      sun NEC L57.8
        acute L56.8
    radioactive substance L58.9
      acute L58.0
      chronic L58.1
    radium L58.9
      acute L58.0
      chronic L58.1
    ragweed (allergic) (contact) L23.7
    Rhus (allergic) (contact) (diversiloba)
        (radicans) (toxicodendron) (venenata)
        (verniciflua) L23.7
    rubber (contact) L24.5
    Senecio jacobaea (allergic) (contact)
        L23.7
    solvents (contact) (irritant) (substances in
        categories T52) L24.2
    specified agent NEC (contact) L25.8
      allergic L23.89
      irritant L24.89
    sunshine NEC L57.8
      acute L56.8
    tetrachlorethylene (contact) (irritant)
        L24.2
    toluene (contact) (irritant) L24.2
    turpentine (contact) L24.2
    ultraviolet rays (sun NEC) (chronic
        exposure) L57.8
      acute L56.8
    vaccine or vaccination L27.0
      specified substance —see Table of Drugs
          and Chemicals
    varicose veins —see Varix, leg, with,
        inflammation
    X-rays L58.9
      acute L58.0
      chronic L58.1
  dyshydrotic L30.1
  dysmenorrheica N94.6
  escharotica —see Burn
  exfoliative, exfoliativa (generalized) L26
    neonatorum L00
  eyelid —see also Dermatosis, eyelid
    allergic H01.119
      left H01.116
        lower H01.115
        upper H01.114
      right H01.113
        lower H01.112
        upper H01.111
    contact —see Dermatitis, eyelid,
        allergic
    due to
      Demodex species B88.0
      herpes (zoster) B02.39
        simplex B00.59

Dermatitis (Continued)
eyelid (Continued)
eczematous H01.139
left H01.136
lower H01.135
upper H01.134
right H01.133
lower H01.132
upper H01.131
facta, factitia, factitial L98.1
psychogenic F54
flexural NEC L20.82
friction L30.4
fungus B36.9
specified type NEC B36.8
gangrenosa, gangrenous infantum L08.0
harvest mite B88.0
heat L59.0
herpesviral, vesicular (ear) (lip) B00.1
herpetiformis (bullous) (erythematous)
(pustular) (vesicular) L13.0
juvenile L12.2
senile L12.0
hiemalis L30.8
hypostatic, hypostatica —see Varix, leg, with,
inflammation
infectious eczematoid L30.3
infective L30.3
irritant —see Dermatitis, contact, irritant
Jacquet's (diaper dermatitis) L22
Leptus B88.0
lichenified NEC L28.0
medicamentosa (generalized) (internal
use) —see Dermatitis, due to drugs
mite B88.0
multiformis L13.0
juvenile L12.2
napkin L22
neurotica L13.0
nummular L30.0
papillaris capillitii L73.0
pellagrous E52
perioral L71.0
photocontact L56.2
polymorpha dolorosa L13.0
pruriginosa L13.0
pruritic NEC L30.8
psychogenic F54
purulent L08.0
pustular
contagious B08.02
subcorneal L13.1
pyococcal L08.0
pyogenica L08.0
repens L40.2
Ritter's (exfoliativa) L00
Schamberg's L81.7
schistosome B65.3
seasonal bullous L30.8
seborrheic L21.9
infantile L21.1
specified NEC L21.8
sensitization NOS L23.9
septic L08.0
solare L57.8
specified NEC L30.8
stasis I87.2
~~with varicose ulcer —see Varix, leg, with~~
~~ulcer, with inflammation~~
with ◄
varicose ulcer —see Varix, leg, with ulcer,
with inflammation ◄
varicose veins —see Varix, leg, with,
inflammation ◄
due to postthrombotic syndrome —see
Syndrome, postthrombotic
suppurative L08.0
traumatic NEC L30.4
trophoneurotica L13.0
ultraviolet (sun) (chronic exposure) L57.8
acute L56.8

Dermatitis (Continued)
varicose —see Varix, leg, with, inflammation
vegetans L10.1
verrucosa B43.0
vesicular, herpesviral B00.1
Dermatoarthritis, lipoid E78.81
Dermatochalasis, eyelid H02.839
left H02.836
lower H02.835
upper H02.834
right H02.833
lower H02.832
upper H02.831
Dermatofibroma (lenticulare) —see Neoplasm,
skin, benign
protuberans —see Neoplasm, skin, uncertain
behavior
Dermatofibrosarcoma (pigmented)
(protuberans) —see Neoplasm, skin,
malignant
Dermatographia L50.3
Dermatolysis (exfoliativa) (congenital)
Q82.8
acquired L57.4
eyelids —see Blepharochalasis
palpebrarum —see Blepharochalasis
senile L57.4
Dermatomegaly NEC Q82.8
Dermatomucosomyositis M33.10
with
myopathy M33.12
respiratory involvement M33.11
specified organ involvement NEC
M33.19
Dermatomycosis B36.9
furfuracea B36.0
specified type NEC B36.8
Dermatomyositis (acute) (chronic) —see also
Dermatopolymyositis
in (due to) neoplastic disease —see also
Neoplasm D49.9 [M36.0]
Dermatoneuritis of children —see Poisoning,
mercury
Dermatophilosis A48.8
Dermatophytid L30.2
Dermatophytide —see Dermatophytosis
Dermatophytosis (epidermophyton) (infection)
(Microsporum) (tinea) (Trichophyton)
B35.9
beard B35.0
body B35.4
capitis B35.0
corporis B35.4
deep-seated B35.8
disseminated B35.8
foot B35.3
granulomatous B35.8
groin B35.6
hand B35.2
nail B35.1
perianal (area) B35.6
scalp B35.0
specified NEC B35.8
Dermatopolymyositis M33.90
with
myopathy M33.92
respiratory involvement M33.91
specified organ involvement NEC
M33.99
in neoplastic disease (see also Neoplasm)
D49.9 [M36.0]
juvenile M33.00
with
myopathy M33.02
respiratory involvement M33.01
specified organ involvement NEC
M33.09
specified NEC M33.10
myopathy M33.12
respiratory involvement M33.11
specified organ involvement NEC M33.19

Dermatopolyneuritis —see Poisoning, mercury
Dermatorrhexis Q79.6
acquired L57.4
Dermatosclerosis —see also Scleroderma
localized L94.0
Dermatosis L98.9
Andrews' L08.89
Bowen's —see Neoplasm, skin, in situ
bullous L13.9
specified NEC L13.8
exfoliativa L26
eyelid (noninfectious)
dermatitis —see Dermatitis, eyelid
discoid lupus erythematosus —see Lupus,
erythematosus, eyelid
xeroderma —see Xeroderma, acquired,
eyelid
factitial L98.1
febrile neutrophilic L98.2
gonococcal A54.89
herpetiformis L13.0
juvenile L12.2
linear IgA L13.8
menstrual NEC L98.8
neutrophilic, febrile L98.2
occupational —see Dermatitis, contact
papulosa nigra L82.1
pigmentary L81.9
progressive L81.7
Schamberg's L81.7
psychogenic F54
purpuric, pigmented L81.7
pustular, subcorneal L13.1
transient acantholytic L11.1
Dermographia, dermographism L50.3
Dermoid (cyst) —see also Neoplasm, benign,
by site
with malignant transformation C56-
due to radiation (nonionizing) L57.8
Dermopathy
infiltrative with thyrotoxicosis —see
Thyrotoxicosis
nephrogenic fibrosing L90.8
Dermophytosis —see Dermatophytosis
Descemetocele H18.73-
Descemet's membrane —see condition
Descending —see condition
Descensus uteri —see Prolapse, uterus
Desert
rheumatism B38.0
sore —see Ulcer, skin
Desertion (newborn) —see Maltreatment
Desmoid (extra-abdominal) (tumor) —see
Neoplasm, connective tissue, uncertain
behavior
abdominal D48.1
Despondency F32.9
Desquamation, skin R23.4
Destruction, destructive —see also Damage
articular facet —see also Derangement, joint,
specified type NEC
knee M23.8X-
vertebra —see Spondylosis
bone —see also Disorder, bone, specified type
NEC
syphilitic A52.77
joint —see also Derangement, joint, specified
type NEC
sacroiliac M53.3
rectal sphincter K62.89
septum (nasal) J34.89
tuberculous NEC —see Tuberculosis
tympanum, tympanic membrane
(nontraumatic) —see Disorder,
tympanic membrane, specified
NEC
vertebral disc —see Degeneration,
intervertebral disc
Destructiveness —see also Disorder, conduct
adjustment reaction —see Disorder,
adjustment

Desultory labor O62.2
Detachment
    cartilage —*see* Sprain
    cervix, annular N88.8
        complicating delivery O71.3
    choroid (old) (postinfectional) (simple)
            (spontaneous) H31.40-
        hemorrhagic H31.41-
        serous H31.42-
    ligament —*see* Sprain
    meniscus (knee) —*see also* Derangement,
            knee, meniscus, specified NEC
        current injury —*see* Tear, meniscus
        due to old tear or injury —*see*
                Derangement, knee, meniscus, due
                to old tear
    retina (without retinal break) (serous) H33.2-
        with retinal:
            break H33.00-
                giant H33.03-
                multiple H33.02-
                single H33.01-
            dialysis H33.04-
        pigment epithelium —*see* Degeneration,
                retina, separation of layers, pigment
                epithelium detachment
        rhegmatogenous —*see* Detachment, retina,
                with retinal, break
        specified NEC H33.8
        total H33.05-
        traction H33.4-
    vitreous (body) H43.81
Detergent asthma J69.8
Deterioration
    epileptic F06.8
    general physical R53.81
    heart, cardiac —*see* Degeneration, myocardial
    mental —*see* Psychosis
    myocardial, myocardium —*see* Degeneration,
            myocardial
    senile (simple) R54
Deuteranomaly (anomalous trichromat) H53.53
Deuteranopia (complete) (incomplete) H53.53
Development
    abnormal, bone Q79.9
    arrested R62.50
        bone —*see* Arrest, development or growth,
                bone
        child R62.50
        due to malnutrition E45
    defective, congenital —*see also* Anomaly, by
            site
        cauda equina Q06.3
        left ventricle Q24.8
            in hypoplastic left heart syndrome
                    Q23.4
        valve Q24.8
            pulmonary Q22.3
    delayed (*see also* Delay, development) R62.50
        arithmetical skills F81.2
        language (skills) (expressive) F80.1
        learning skill F81.9
        mixed skills F88
        motor coordination F82
        reading F81.0
        specified learning skill NEC F81.89
        speech F80.9
        spelling F81.81
        written expression F81.81
    imperfect, congenital —*see also* Anomaly, by
            site
        heart Q24.9
        lungs Q33.6
    incomplete
        bronchial tree Q32.4
        organ or site not listed —*see* Hypoplasia,
                by site
        respiratory system Q34.9
    sexual, precocious NEC E30.1
    tardy, mental (*see also* Disability, intellectual)
            F79

Developmental —*see* condition
    ~~testing, child —see Examination, child~~
    testing, infant or child —*see* Examination,
            child ◀
Devergie's disease (pityriasis rubra pilaris)
        L44.0
Deviation (in)
    conjugate palsy (eye) (spastic) H51.0
    esophagus (acquired) K22.8
    eye, skew H51.8
    midline (jaw) (teeth) (dental arch) M26.29
        specified site NEC —*see* Malposition
    nasal septum J34.2
        congenital Q67.4
    opening and closing of the mandible M26.53
    organ or site, congenital NEC —*see*
            Malposition, congenital
    septum (nasal) (acquired) J34.2
        congenital Q67.4
    sexual F65.9
        bestiality F65.89
        erotomania F52.8
        exhibitionism F65.2
        fetishism, fetishistic F65.0
            transvestism F65.1
        frotteurism F65.81
        masochism F65.51
        multiple F65.89
        necrophilia F65.89
        nymphomania F52.8
        pederosis F65.4
        pedophilia F65.4
        sadism, sadomasochism F65.52
        satyriasis F52.8
        specified type NEC F65.89
        transvestism F64.1
        voyeurism F65.3
    teeth, midline M26.29
    trachea J39.8
    ureter, congenital Q62.61
Device
    cerebral ventricle (communicating) in situ
            Z98.2
    contraceptive —*see* Contraceptive, device
    drainage, cerebrospinal fluid, in situ Z98.2
Devic's disease G36.0
Devil's
    grip B33.0
    pinches (purpura simplex) D69.2
Devitalized tooth K04.99
Devonshire colic —*see* Poisoning, lead
Dextraposition, aorta Q20.3
    in tetralogy of Fallot Q21.3
Dextrinosis, limit (debrancher enzyme
        deficiency) E74.03
Dextrocardia (true) Q24.0
    with
        complete transposition of viscera Q89.3
        situs inversus Q89.3
Dextrotransposition, aorta Q20.3
d-glycericacidemia E72.59
Dhat syndrome F48.8
Dhobi itch B35.6
Di George's syndrome D82.1
Di Guglielmo's disease C94.0-
Diabetes, diabetic (mellitus) (sugar) E11.9
    with
        amyotrophy E11.44
        arthropathy NEC E11.618
        autonomic (poly)neuropathy E11.43
        cataract E11.36
        Charcot's joints E11.610
        chronic kidney disease E11.22
        circulatory complication NEC E11.59
        complication E11.8
            specified NEC E11.69
        dermatitis E11.620
        foot ulcer E11.621
        gangrene E11.52
        gastroparalysis E11.43 ◀
        gastroparesis E11.43

Diabetes, diabetic (Continued)
    with (Continued)
        glomerulonephrosis, intracapillary E11.21
        glomerulosclerosis, intercapillary E11.21
        hyperglycemia E11.65
        hyperosmolarity E11.00
            with coma E11.01
        hypoglycemia E11.649
            with coma E11.641
        kidney complications NEC E11.29
        Kimmelsteil-Wilson disease E11.21
        loss of protective sensation (LOPS) —*see*
                Diabetes, by type, with neuropathy
        mononeuropathy E11.41
        myasthenia E11.44
        necrobiosis lipoidica E11.620
        nephropathy E11.21
        neuralgia E11.42
        neurologic complication NEC E11.49
        neuropathic arthropathy E11.610
        neuropathy E11.40
        ophthalmic complication NEC E11.39
        oral complication NEC E11.638
        osteomyelitis E11.69 ◀
        periodontal disease E11.630
        peripheral angiopathy E11.51
            with gangrene E11.52
        polyneuropathy E11.42
        renal complication NEC E11.29
        renal tubular degeneration E11.29
        retinopathy E11.319
            with macular edema E11.311
                resolved following treatment
                        E11.37 ◀
            nonproliferative E11.329
                with macular edema E11.321
                mild E11.329
                    with macular edema E11.321
                moderate E11.339
                    with macular edema E11.331
                severe E11.349
                    with macular edema E11.341
            proliferative E11.359
                ~~with macular edema E11.351~~
                with ◀
                    combined traction retinal
                            detachment and
                            rhegmatogenous retinal
                            detachment E11.354 ◀
                    macular edema E11.351 ◀
                    stable proliferative diabetic
                            retinopathy E11.355 ◀
                    traction retinal detachment
                            involving the macula
                            E11.352 ◀
                    traction retinal detachment not
                            involving the macula
                            E11.353 ◀
        skin complication NEC E11.628
        skin ulcer NEC E11.622
    brittle —*see* Diabetes, type 1 ◀
    bronzed E83.110
    complicating pregnancy —*see* Pregnancy,
            complicated by, diabetes
    dietary counseling and surveillance Z71.3
    due to ◀
        autoimmune process —*see* Diabetes,
                type 1 ◀
        immune mediated pancreatic islet beta-cell
                destruction —*see* Diabetes, type 1 ◀
    due to drug or chemical E09.9
        with
            amyotrophy E09.44
            arthropathy NEC E09.618
            autonomic (poly)neuropathy E09.43
            cataract E09.36
            Charcot's joints E09.610
            chronic kidney disease E09.22
            circulatory complication NEC E09.59
            complication E09.8
                specified NEC E09.69

◀ New   ◀|||| Revised   ~~deleted~~ Deleted

Diabetes, diabetic (Continued)
 due to drug or chemical (Continued)
  with (Continued)
   dermatitis E09.620
   foot ulcer E09.621
   gangrene E09.52
   gastroparalysis E09.43 ◄
   gastroparesis E09.43
   glomerulonephrosis, intracapillary E09.21
   glomerulosclerosis, intercapillary E09.21
   hyperglycemia E09.65
   hyperosmolarity E09.00
    with coma E09.01
   hypoglycemia E09.649
    with coma E09.641
   ketoacidosis E09.10
    with coma E09.11
   kidney complications NEC E09.29
   Kimmelsteil-Wilson disease E09.21
   mononeuropathy E09.41
   myasthenia E09.44
   necrobiosis lipoidica E09.620
   nephropathy E09.21
   neuralgia E09.42
   neurologic complication NEC E09.49
   neuropathic arthropathy E09.610
   neuropathy E09.40
   ophthalmic complication NEC E09.39
   oral complication NEC E09.638
   periodontal disease E09.630
   peripheral angiopathy E09.51
    with gangrene E09.52
   polyneuropathy E09.42
   renal complication NEC E09.29
   renal tubular degeneration E09.29
   retinopathy E09.319
    with macular edema E09.311
     resolved following treatment E09.37 ◄
    nonproliferative E09.329
     with macular edema E09.321
     mild E09.329
      with macular edema E09.321
     moderate E09.339
      with macular edema E09.331
     severe E09.349
      with macular edema E09.341
    proliferative E09.359
     with macular edema E09.351
     with ◄
      combined traction retinal detachment and rhegmatogenous retinal detachment E09.354 ◄
      macular edema E09.351 ◄
      stable proliferative diabetic retinopathy E09.355 ◄
      traction retinal detachment involving the macula E09.352 ◄
      traction retinal detachment not involving the macula E09.353 ◄
   skin complication NEC E09.628
   skin ulcer NEC E09.622
 due to underlying condition E08.9
  with
   amyotrophy E08.44
   arthropathy NEC E08.618
   autonomic (poly)neuropathy E08.43
   cataract E08.36
   Charcot's joints E08.610
   chronic kidney disease E08.22
   circulatory complication NEC E08.59
   complication E08.8
    specified NEC E08.69
   dermatitis E08.620
   foot ulcer E08.621
   gangrene E08.52
   gastroparalysis E08.43 ◄

Diabetes, diabetic (Continued)
 due to underlying condition (Continued)
  with (Continued)
   gastroparesis E08.43
   glomerulonephrosis, intracapillary E08.21
   glomerulosclerosis, intercapillary E08.21
   hyperglycemia E08.69
   hyperosmolarity E08.00
    with coma E08.01
   hypoglycemia E08.649
    with coma E08.641
   ketoacidosis E08.10
    with coma E08.11
   kidney complications NEC E08.29
   Kimmelsteil-WIlson disease E08.21
   mononeuropathy E08.41
   myasthenia E08.44
   necrobiosis lipoidica E08.620
   nephropathy E08.21
   neuralgia E08.42
   neurologic complication NEC E08.49
   neuropathic arthropathy E08.610
   neuropathy E08.40
   ophthalmic complication NEC E08.39
   oral complication NEC E08.638
   periodontal disease E08.630
   peripheral angiopathy E08.51
    with gangrene E08.52
   polyneuropathy E08.42
   renal complication NEC E08.29
   renal tubular degeneration E08.29
   retinopathy E08.319
    with macular edema E08.311
     resolved following treatment E08.37 ◄
    nonproliferative E08.329
     with macular edema E08.321
     mild E08.329
      with macular edema E08.321
     moderate E08.339
      with macular edema E08.331
     severe E08.349
      with macular edema E08.341
    proliferative E08.359
     with macular edema E08.351
     with ◄
      combined traction retinal detachment and rhegmatogenous retinal detachment E08.354 ◄
      macular edema E08.351 ◄
      stable proliferative diabetic retinopathy E08.355 ◄
      traction retinal detachment involving the macula E08.352 ◄
      traction retinal detachment not involving the macula E08.353 ◄
   skin complication NEC E08.628
   skin ulcer NEC E08.622
 gestational (in pregnancy) O24.419
  affecting newborn P70.0
  diet-controlled O24.410
  in childbirth O24.429
   diet-controlled O24.420
   insulin (and diet) controlled O24.424
   oral drug controlled (antidiabetic) (hypoglycemic) O24.425 ◄
  insulin (and diet) controlled O24.414
  oral drug controlled (antidiabetic) (hypoglycemic) O24.415 ◄
  puerperal O24.439
   diet-controlled O24.430
   insulin (and diet) controlled O24.434
   oral drug controlled (antidiabetic) (hypoglycemic) O24.435 ◄
 hepatogenous E13.9
 idiopathic —see Diabetes, type 1 ◄

Diabetes, diabetic (Continued)
 inadequately controlled — code to Diabetes, by type, with hyperglycemia
 insipidus E23.2
  nephrogenic N25.1
  pituitary E23.2
  vasopressin resistant N25.1
 insulin dependent — code to type of diabetes
 juvenile-onset —see Diabetes, type 1
 ketosis-prone —see Diabetes, type 1
 latent R73.03 ◄
 neonatal (transient) P70.2
 non-insulin dependent — code to type of diabetes
 out of control — code to Diabetes, by type, with hyperglycemia
 phosphate E83.39
 poorly controlled — code to Diabetes, by type, with hyperglycemia
 postpancreatectomy —see Diabetes, specified type NEC
 postprocedural —see Diabetes, specified type NEC
 secondary diabetes mellitus NEC —see Diabetes, specified type NEC
 specified type NEC E13.9
  with
   amyotrophy E13.44
   arthropathy NEC E13.618
   autonomic (poly)neuropathy E13.43
   cataract E13.36
   Charcot's joints E13.610
   chronic kidney disease E13.22
   circulatory complication NEC E13.59
   complication E13.8
    specified NEC E13.69
   dermatitis E13.620
   foot ulcer E13.621
   gangrene E13.52
   gastroparalysis E13.43 ◄
   gastroparesis E13.43
   glomerulonephrosis, intracapillary E13.21
   glomerulosclerosis, intercapillary E13.21
   hyperglycemia E13.65
   hyperosmolarity E13.00
    with coma E13.01
   hypoglycemia E13.649
    with coma E13.641
   ketoacidosis E13.10
    with coma E13.11
   kidney complications NEC E13.29
   Kimmelsteil-Wilson disease E13.21
   mononeuropathy E13.41
   myasthenia E13.44
   necrobiosis lipoidica E13.620
   nephropathy E13.21
   neuralgia E13.42
   neurologic complication NEC E13.49
   neuropathic arthropathy E13.610
   neuropathy E13.40
   ophthalmic complication NEC E13.39
   oral complication NEC E13.638
   periodontal disease E13.630
   peripheral angiopathy E13.51
    with gangrene E13.52
   polyneuropathy E13.42
   renal complication NEC E13.29
   renal tubular degeneration E13.29
   retinopathy E13.319
    with macular edema E13.311
     resolved following treatment E13.37 ◄
    nonproliferative E13.329
     with macular edema E13.321
     mild E13.329
      with macular edema E13.321
     moderate E13.339
      with macular edema E13.331
     severe E13.349
      with macular edema E13.341

Diabetes, diabetic *(Continued)*
  specified type NEC *(Continued)*
    with *(Continued)*
      retinopathy *(Continued)*
        proliferative E13.359
          ~~with macular edema E13.351~~ ◄
          with ◄
            combined traction retinal detachment and rhegmatogenous retinal detachment E13.354 ◄
            macular edema E13.351 ◄
            stable proliferative diabetic retinopathy E13.355 ◄
            traction retinal detachment involving the macula E13.352 ◄
            traction retinal detachment not involving the macula E13.353 ◄
      skin complication NEC E13.628
      skin ulcer NEC E13.622
  steroid-induced —*see* Diabetes, due to, drug or chemical
  type 1 E10.9
    with
      amyotrophy E10.44
      arthropathy NEC E10.618
      autonomic (poly)neuropathy E10.43
      cataract E10.36
      Charcot's joints E10.610
      chronic kidney disease E10.22
      circulatory complication NEC E10.59
      complication E10.8
        specified NEC E10.69
      dermatitis E10.620
      foot ulcer E10.621
      gangrene E10.52
      gastroparalysis E10.43 ◄
      gastroparesis E10.43
      glomerulonephrosis, intracapillary E10.21
      glomerulosclerosis, intercapillary E10.21
      hyperglycemia E10.65
      hypoglycemia E10.649
        with coma E10.641
      ketoacidosis E10.10
        with coma E10.11
      kidney complications NEC E10.29
      Kimmelsteil-Wilson disease E10.21
      mononeuropathy E10.41
      myasthenia E10.44
      necrobiosis lipoidica E10.620
      nephropathy E10.21
      neuralgia E10.42
      neurologic complication NEC E10.49
      neuropathic arthropathy E10.610
      neuropathy E10.40
      ophthalmic complication NEC E10.39
      oral complication NEC E10.638
      periodontal disease E10.630
      peripheral angiopathy E10.51
        with gangrene E10.52
      polyneuropathy E10.42
      renal complication NEC E10.29
      renal tubular degeneration E10.29
      retinopathy E10.319
        with macular edema E10.311
          resolved following treatment E10.37 ◄
        nonproliferative E10.329
          with macular edema E10.321
          mild E10.329
            with macular edema E10.321
          moderate E10.339
            with macular edema E10.331
          severe E10.349
            with macular edema E10.341

Diabetes, diabetic *(Continued)*
  type 1 *(Continued)*
    with *(Continued)*
      retinopathy *(Continued)*
        proliferative E10.359
          ~~with macular edema E10.351~~ ◄
          with ◄
            combined traction retinal detachment and rhegmatogenous retinal detachment E13.354 ◄
            macular edema E13.351 ◄
            stable proliferative diabetic retinopathy E13.355 ◄
            traction retinal detachment involving the macula E13.352 ◄
            traction retinal detachment not involving the macula E13.353 ◄
      skin complication NEC E10.628
      skin ulcer NEC E10.622
  type 2 E11.9
    with
      amyotrophy E11.44
      arthropathy NEC E11.618
      autonomic (poly)neuropathy E11.43
      cataract E11.36
      Charcot's joints E11.610
      chronic kidney disease E11.22
      circulatory complication NEC E11.59
      complication E11.8
        specified NEC E11.69
      dermatitis E11.620
      foot ulcer E11.621
      gangrene E11.52
      gastroparalysis E11.43 ◄
      gastroparesis E11.43
      glomerulonephrosis, intracapillary E11.21
      glomerulosclerosis, intercapillary E11.21
      hyperglycemia E11.65
      hyperosmolarity E11.00
        with coma E11.01
      hypoglycemia E11.649
        with coma E11.641
      kidney complications NEC E11.29
      Kimmelsteil-Wilson disease E11.21
      mononeuropathy E11.41
      myasthenia E11.44
      necrobiosis lipoidica E11.620
      nephropathy E11.21
      neuralgia E11.42
      neurologic complication NEC E11.49
      neuropathic arthropathy E11.610
      neuropathy E11.40
      ophthalmic complication NEC E11.39
      oral complication NEC E11.638
      periodontal disease E11.630
      peripheral angiopathy E11.51
        with gangrene E11.52
      polyneuropathy E11.42
      renal complication NEC E11.29
      renal tubular degeneration E11.29
      retinopathy E11.319
        with macular edema E11.311
          resolved following treatment E11.37 ◄
        nonproliferative E11.329
          with macular edema E11.321
          mild E11.329
            with macular edema E11.321
          moderate E11.339
            with macular edema E11.331
          severe E11.349
            with macular edema E11.341
        proliferative E11.359
          ~~with macular edema E11.351~~
          with ◄
            combined traction retinal detachment and rhegmatogenous retinal detachment E11.354 ◄

Diabetes, diabetic *(Continued)*
  type 2 *(Continued)*
    with *(Continued)*
      retinopathy *(Continued)*
        proliferative *(Continued)*
          with *(Continued)*
            macular edema E11.351 ◄
            stable proliferative diabetic retinopathy E11.355 ◄
            traction retinal detachment involving the macula E11.352 ◄
            traction retinal detachment not involving the macula E11.353 ◄
      skin complication NEC E11.628
      skin ulcer NEC E11.622
  uncontrolled
    meaning ◄
      hyperglycemia —*see* Diabetes, by type, with, hyperglycemia ◄
      hypoglycemia —*see* Diabetes, by type, with, hypoglycemia ◄
Diacyclothrombopathia D69.1
Diagnosis deferred R69
Dialysis (intermittent) (treatment)
  noncompliance (with) Z91.15
  renal (hemodialysis) (peritoneal), status Z99.2
  retina, retinal —*see* Detachment, retina, with retinal, dialysis
Diamond-Blackfan anemia (congenital hypoplastic) D61.01
Diamond-Gardener syndrome (autoerythrocyte sensitization) D69.2
Diaper rash L22
Diaphoresis (excessive) R61
Diaphragm —*see* condition
Diaphragmalgia R07.1
Diaphragmatitis, diaphragmitis J98.6
Diaphysial aclasis Q78.6
Diaphysitis —*see* Osteomyelitis, specified type NEC
Diarrhea, diarrheal (disease) (infantile) (inflammatory) R19.7
  achlorhydric K31.83
  allergic K52.29 ◄
    due to ◄
      colitis —*see* Colitis, allergic ◄
      enteritis —*see* Enteritis, allergic ◄
  amebic —*see also* Amebiasis A06.0
    with abscess —*see* Abscess, amebic
    acute A06.0
    chronic A06.1
    nondysenteric A06.2
  bacillary —*see* Dysentery, bacillary
  balantidial A07.0
  cachectic NEC K52.89
  Chilomastix A07.8
  choleriformis A00.1
  chronic (noninfectious) K52.9
  coccidial A07.3
  Cochin-China K90.1
    strongyloidiasis B78.0
  Dientamoeba A07.8
  dietetic —*see also* Diarrhea, allergic K52.29 ◄
  drug-induced K52.1
  due to
    bacteria A04.9
      specified NEC A04.8
    Campylobacter A04.5
    Capillaria philippinensis B81.1
    Clostridium difficile A04.7
    Clostridium perfringens (C) (F) A04.8
    Cryptosporidium A07.2
    drugs K52.1
    Escherichia coli A04.4
      enteroaggregative A04.4
      enterohemorrhagic A04.3
      enteroinvasive A04.2
      enteropathogenic A04.0

◄ New   ◄▥ Revised   ~~deleted~~ Deleted

Diarrhea, diarrheal *(Continued)*
  due to *(Continued)*
    Escherichia coli *(Continued)*
      enterotoxigenic A04.1
      specified NEC A04.4
    food hypersensitivity —*see also* Diarrhea,
        allergic K52.29 ◀▥
    Necator americanus B76.1
    S. japonicum B65.2
    specified organism NEC A08.8
      bacterial A04.8
      viral A08.39
    Staphylococcus A04.8
    Trichuris trichiuria B79
    virus —*see* Enteritis, viral
    Yersinia enterocolitica A04.6
  dysenteric A09
  endemic A09
  epidemic A09
  flagellate A07.9
  Flexner's (ulcerative) A03.1
  functional K59.1
    following gastrointestinal surgery K91.89
    psychogenic F45.8
  Giardia lamblia A07.1
  giardial A07.1
  hill K90.1
  infectious A09
  malarial —*see* Malaria
  mite B88.0
  mycotic NEC B49
  neonatal (noninfectious) P78.3
  nervous F45.8
  neurogenic K59.1
  noninfectious K52.9
  postgastrectomy K91.1
  postvagotomy K91.1
  protozoal A07.9
    specified NEC A07.8
  psychogenic F45.8
  specified
    bacterium NEC A04.8
    virus NEC A08.39
  strongyloidiasis B78.0
  toxic K52.1
  trichomonal A07.8
  tropical K90.1
  tuberculous A18.32
  viral —*see* Enteritis, viral
Diastasis
  cranial bones M84.88
    congenital NEC Q75.8
  joint (traumatic) —*see* Dislocation
  muscle M62.00
    ankle M62.07-
    congenital Q79.8
    foot M62.07-
    forearm M62.03-
    hand M62.04-
    lower leg M62.06-
    pelvic region M62.05-
    shoulder region M62.01-
    specified site NEC M62.08
    thigh M62.05-
    upper arm M62.02-
  recti (abdomen)
    complicating delivery O71.89
    congenital Q79.59
Diastema, tooth, teeth, fully erupted M26.32
Diastematomyelia Q06.2
Diataxia, cerebral G80.4
Diathesis
  allergic —*see* History, allergy
  bleeding (familial) D69.9
  cystine (familial) E72.00
  gouty —*see* Gout
  hemorrhagic (familial) D69.9
    newborn NEC P53
  spasmophilic R29.0
Diaz's disease or osteochondrosis (juvenile)
    (talus) —*see* Osteochondrosis, juvenile,
    tarsus

Dibothriocephalus, dibothriocephaliasis
    (latus) (infection) (infestation) B70.0
  larval B70.1
Dicephalus, dicephaly Q89.4
Dichotomy, teeth K00.2
Dichromat, dichromatopsia (congenital) —*see*
    Deficiency, color vision
Dichuchwa A65
Dicroceliasis B66.2
Didelphia, didelphys —*see* Double uterus
Didymytis N45.1
  with orchitis N45.3
Dietary
  inadequacy or deficiency E63.9
  surveillance and counseling Z71.3
Dietl's crisis N13.8
Dieulafoy lesion (hemorrhagic)
  duodenum K31.82
  esophagus K22.8
  intestine (colon) K63.81
  stomach K31.82
Difficult, difficulty (in)
  acculturation Z60.3
  feeding R63.3
    newborn P92.9
      breast P92.5
      specified NEC P92.8
    nonorganic (infant or child) F98.29
  intubation, in anesthesia T88.4
  mechanical, gastroduodenal stoma K91.89
    causing obstruction K91.3
  micturition ◀
    need to immediately re-void R39.191 ◀
    position dependent R39.192 ◀
    specified NEC R39.198 ◀
  reading (developmental) F81.0
    secondary to emotional disorders F93.9
  spelling (specific) F81.81
    with reading disorder F81.89
    due to inadequate teaching Z55.8
  swallowing —*see* Dysphagia
  walking R26.2
  work
    conditions NEC Z56.5
    schedule Z56.3
Diffuse —*see* condition
DiGeorge's syndrome (thymic hypoplasia)
    D82.1
Digestive —*see* condition
Dihydropyrimidine dehydrogenase disease
    (DPD) E88.89
Diktyoma —*see* Neoplasm, malignant, by site
Dilaceration, tooth K00.4
Dilatation
  anus K59.8
    venule —*see* Hemorrhoids
  aorta (focal) (general) —*see* Ectasia, aorta
    with aneurysm —*see* Aneurysm, aorta
    congenital Q25.44 ◀
  artery —*see* Aneurysm
  bladder (sphincter) N32.89
    congenital Q64.79
  blood vessel I99.8
  bronchial J47.9
    with
      exacerbation (acute) J47.1
      lower respiratory infection J47.0
  calyx (due to obstruction) —*see*
      Hydronephrosis
  capillaries I78.8
  cardiac (acute) (chronic) —*see also*
      Hypertrophy, cardiac
    congenital Q24.8
      valve NEC Q24.8
        pulmonary Q22.3
    valve —*see* Endocarditis
  cavum septi pellucidi Q06.8
  cervix (uteri) —*see also* Incompetency,
      cervix
    incomplete, poor, slow complicating
        delivery O62.0

Dilatation *(Continued)*
  colon K59.39 ◀▥
    congenital Q43.1
    psychogenic F45.8
    toxic K59.31 ◀
  common duct (acquired) K83.8
    congenital Q44.5
  cystic duct (acquired) K82.8
    congenital Q44.5
  duct, mammary —*see* Ectasia, mammary duct
  duodenum K59.8
  esophagus K22.8
    congenital Q39.5
    due to achalasia K22.0
  eustachian tube, congenital Q17.8
  gallbladder K82.8
  gastric —*see* Dilatation, stomach
  heart (acute) (chronic) —*see also* Hypertrophy,
      cardiac
    congenital Q24.8
    valve —*see* Endocarditis
  ileum K59.8
    psychogenic F45.8
  jejunum K59.8
    psychogenic F45.8
  kidney (calyx) (collecting structures) (cystic)
      (parenchyma) (pelvis) (idiopathic)
      N28.89
  lacrimal passages or duct —*see* Disorder,
      lacrimal system, changes
  lymphatic vessel I89.0
  mammary duct —*see* Ectasia, mammary duct
  Meckel's diverticulum (congenital) Q43.0
    malignant —*see* Table of Neoplasms, small
        intestine, malignant
  myocardium (acute) (chronic) —*see*
      Hypertrophy, cardiac organ or site,
      congenital NEC —*see* Distortion
  pancreatic duct K86.89 ◀▥
  pericardium —*see* Pericarditis
  pharynx J39.2
  prostate N42.89
  pulmonary
    artery (idiopathic) I28.8
    valve, congenital Q22.3
  pupil H57.04
  rectum K59.39 ◀▥
  saccule, congenital Q16.5
  salivary gland (duct) K11.8
  sphincter ani K62.89
  stomach K31.89
    acute K31.0
    psychogenic F45.8
  submaxillary duct K11.8
  trachea, congenital Q32.1
  ureter (idiopathic) N28.82
    congenital Q62.2
    due to obstruction N13.4
  urethra (acquired) N36.8
  vasomotor I73.9
  vein I86.8
  ventricular, ventricle (acute) (chronic) —*see
      also* Hypertrophy, cardiac
    cerebral, congenital Q04.8
  venule NEC I86.8
  vesical orifice N32.89
Dilated, dilation —*see* Dilatation
Diminished, diminution
  hearing (acuity) —*see* Deafness
  sense or sensation (cold) (heat) (tactile)
      (vibratory) R20.8
  vision NEC H54.7
  vital capacity R94.2
Diminuta taenia B71.0
Dimitri-Sturge-Weber disease Q85.8
Dimple
  ~~parasacral, pilonidal or postanal —*see* Cyst,~~
      ~~pilonidal~~
  congenital sacral Q82.6 ◀
  parasacral Q82.6 ◀
  pilonidal or postanal —*see* Cyst, pilonidal ◀

Dioctophyme renalis (infection) (infestation) B83.8
Dipetalonemiasis B74.4
Diphallus Q55.69
Diphtheria, diphtheritic (gangrenous) (hemorrhagic) A36.9
  carrier (suspected) Z22.2
  cutaneous A36.3
  faucial A36.0
  infection of wound A36.3
  laryngeal A36.2
  myocarditis A36.81
  nasal, anterior A36.89
  nasopharyngeal A36.1
  neurological complication A36.89
  pharyngeal A36.0
  specified site NEC A36.89
  tonsillar A36.0
Diphyllobothriasis (intestine) B70.0
  larval B70.1
Diplacusis H93.22-
Diplegia (upper limbs) G83.0
  congenital (cerebral) G80.8
  facial G51.0
  lower limbs G82.20
  spastic G80.1
Diplococcus, diplococcal —see condition
Diplopia H53.2
Dipsomania F10.20
  with
    psychosis —see Psychosis, alcoholic
    remission F10.21
Dipylidiasis B71.1
DIRA (deficiency of interleukin 1 receptor antagonist) M04.8 ◀
Direction, teeth, abnormal, fully erupted M26.30
Dirofilariasis B74.8
Dirt-eating child F98.3
Disability, disabilities
  heart —see Disease, heart
  intellectual F79
    with
      autistic features F84.9
    mild (I.Q. 50-69) F70
    moderate (I.Q. 35-49) F71
    profound (I.Q. under 20) F73
    severe (I.Q. 20-34) F72
    specified level NEC F78
  knowledge acquisition F81.9
  learning F81.9
  limiting activities Z73.6
  spelling, specific F81.81
Disappearance of family member Z63.4
Disarticulation —see Amputation
  meaning traumatic amputation —see Amputation, traumatic
Discharge (from)
  abnormal finding in —see Abnormal, specimen
  breast (female) (male) N64.52
  diencephalic autonomic idiopathic —see Epilepsy, specified NEC
  ear —see also Otorrhea
    blood —see Otorrhagia
  excessive urine R35.8
  nipple N64.52
  penile R36.9
  postnasal R09.82
  prison, anxiety concerning Z65.2
  urethral R36.9
    without blood R36.0
    hematospermia R36.1
  vaginal N89.8
Discitis, diskitis M46.40
  cervical region M46.42
  cervicothoracic region M46.43
  lumbar region M46.46
  lumbosacral region M46.47
  multiple sites M46.49
  occipito-atlanto-axial region M46.41

Discitis, diskitis (Continued)
  pyogenic —see Infection, intervertebral disc, pyogenic
  sacrococcygeal region M46.48
  thoracic region M46.44
  thoracolumbar region M46.45
Discoid
  meniscus (congenital) Q68.6
  semilunar cartilage (congenital) —see Derangement, knee, meniscus, specified NEC
Discoloration
  nails L60.8
  teeth (posteruptive) K03.7
    during formation K00.8
Discomfort
  chest R07.89
  visual H53.14-
Discontinuity, ossicles, ear H74.2-
Discord (with)
  boss Z56.4
  classmates Z55.4
  counselor Z64.4
  employer Z56.4
  family Z63.8
  fellow employees Z56.4
  in-laws Z63.1
  landlord Z59.2
  lodgers Z59.2
  neighbors Z59.2
  probation officer Z64.4
  social worker Z64.4
  teachers Z55.4
  workmates Z56.4
Discordant connection
  atrioventricular (congenital) Q20.5
  ventriculoarterial Q20.3
Discrepancy
  centric occlusion maximum intercuspation M26.55
  leg length (acquired) —see Deformity, limb, unequal length
    congenital —see Defect, reduction, lower limb
  uterine size date O26.84-
Discrimination
  ethnic Z60.5
  political Z60.5
  racial Z60.5
  religious Z60.5
  sex Z60.5
Disease, diseased —see also Syndrome
  absorbent system I87.8
  acid-peptic K30
  Acosta's T70.29
  Adams-Stokes (-Morgagni) (syncope with heart block) I45.9
  Addison's anemia (pernicious) D51.0
  adenoids (and tonsils) J35.9
  adrenal (capsule) (cortex) (gland) (medullary) E27.9
    hyperfunction E27.0
    specified NEC E27.8
  ainhum L94.6
  airway
    obstructive, chronic J44.9
      due to
        cotton dust J66.0
        specific organic dusts NEC J66.8
    reactive —see Asthma
  akamushi (scrub typhus) A75.3
  Albers-Schönberg (marble bones) Q78.2
  Albert's —see Tendinitis, Achilles
  alimentary canal K63.9
  alligator-skin Q80.9
    acquired L85.0
  alpha heavy chain C88.3
  alpine T70.29
  altitude T70.20

Disease, diseased (Continued)
  alveolar ridge
    edentulous K06.9
      specified NEC K06.8
  alveoli, teeth K08.9
  Alzheimer's G30.9 [F02.80]
    with behavioral disturbance G30.9 [F02.81]
    early onset G30.0 [F02.80]
      with behavioral disturbance G30.0 [F02.81]
    late onset G30.1 [F02.80]
      with behavioral disturbance G30.1 [F02.81]
    specified NEC G30.8 [F02.80]
      with behavioral disturbance G30.8 [F02.81]
  amyloid —see Amyloidosis
  Andersen's (glycogenosis IV) E74.09
  Andes T70.29
  Andrews' (bacterid) L08.89
  angiospastic I73.9
    cerebral G45.9
    vein I87.8
  anterior
    chamber H21.9
    horn cell G12.29
  antiglomerular basement membrane (anti-GBM) antibody M31.0
    tubulo-interstitial nephritis N12
  antral —see Sinusitis, maxillary
  anus K62.9
    specified NEC K62.89
  aorta (nonsyphilitic) I77.9
    syphilitic NEC A52.02
  aortic (heart) (valve) I35.9
    rheumatic I06.9
  Apollo B30.3
  aponeuroses —see Enthesopathy
  appendix K38.9
    specified NEC K38.8
  aqueous (chamber) H21.9
  Arnold-Chiari —see Arnold-Chiari disease
  arterial I77.9
    occlusive —see Occlusion, by site
      due to stricture or stenosis I77.1
  arteriocardiorenal —see Hypertension, cardiorenal
  arteriolar (generalized) (obliterative) I77.9
  arteriorenal —see Hypertension, kidney
  arteriosclerotic —see also Arteriosclerosis
    cardiovascular —see Disease, heart, ischemic, atherosclerotic
    coronary (artery) —see Disease, heart, ischemic, atherosclerotic
    heart —see Disease, heart, ischemic, atherosclerotic
  artery I77.9
    cerebral I67.9
    coronary I25.10
      with angina pectoris —see Arteriosclerosis, coronary (artery),
  arthropod-borne NOS (viral) A94
    specified type NEC A93.8
  atticoantral, chronic H66.20
    left H66.22
      with right H66.23
    right H66.21
      with left H66.23
  auditory canal —see Disorder, ear, external
  auricle, ear NEC —see Disorder, pinna
  Australian X A83.4
  autoimmune (systemic) NOS M35.9
    hemolytic (cold type) (warm type) D59.1
      drug-induced D59.0
    thyroid E06.3
  aviator's —see Effect, adverse, high altitude
  Ayala's Q78.5
  Ayerza's (pulmonary artery sclerosis with pulmonary hypertension) I27.0

◀ New   ◀▥ Revised   ~~deleted~~ Deleted

Disease, diseased *(Continued)*
 Babington's (familial hemorrhagic
  telangiectasia) I78.Ø
 bacterial A49.9
  specified NEC A48.8
  zoonotic A28.9
   specified type NEC A28.8
 Baelz's (cheilitis glandularis apostematosa)
  K13.Ø
 bagasse J67.1
 balloon —*see* Effect, adverse, high altitude
 Bang's (brucella abortus) A23.1
 Bannister's T78.3
 barometer makers' —*see* Poisoning, mercury
 Barraquer (-Simons') (progressive
  lipodystrophy) E88.1
 Barrett's —*see* Barrett's, esophagus
 Bartholin's gland N75.9
 basal ganglia G25.9
  degenerative G23.9
   specified NEC G23.8
  specified NEC G25.89
 Basedow's (exophthalmic goiter) —*see*
  Hyperthyroidism, with, goiter (diffuse)
 Bateman's BØ8.1
 Batten-Steinert G71.11
 Battey A31.Ø
 Beard's (neurasthenia) F48.8
 Becker
  idiopathic mural endomyocardial I42.3
  myotonia congenita G71.12
 Begbie's (exophthalmic goiter) —*see*
  Hyperthyroidism, with, goiter (diffuse)
 behavioral, organic FØ7.9
 Beigel's (white piedra) B36.2
 Benson's —*see* Deposit, crystalline
 Bernard-Soulier (thrombopathy) D69.1
 Bernhardt (-Roth) —*see* Mononeuropathy,
  lower limb, meralgia paresthetica
 Biermer's (pernicious anemia) D51.Ø
 bile duct (common) (hepatic) K83.9
  with calculus, stones —*see* Calculus, bile
   duct
  specified NEC K83.8
 biliary (tract) K83.9
  specified NEC K83.8
 Billroth's —*see* Spina bifida
 bird fancier's J67.2
 black lung J6Ø
 bladder N32.9
  in (due to)
   schistosomiasis (bilharziasis) B65.Ø [N33]
  specified NEC N32.89
 bleeder's D66
 blood D75.9
  forming organs D75.9
  vessel I99.9
 Bloodgood's —*see* Mastopathy, cystic
 Bodechtel-Guttmann (subacute sclerosing
  panencephalitis) A81.1
 bone —*see also* Disorder, bone
  aluminum M83.4
  fibrocystic NEC
   jaw M27.49
 bone-marrow D75.9
 Borna A83.9
 Bornholm (epidemic pleurodynia) B33.Ø
 Bouchard's (myopathic dilatation of the
  stomach) K31.Ø
 Bouillaud's (rheumatic heart disease) IØ1.9
 Bourneville (-Brissaud) (tuberous sclerosis)
  Q85.1
 Bouveret (-Hoffmann) (paroxysmal
  tachycardia) I47.9
 bowel K63.9
  functional K59.9
   psychogenic F45.8
 brain G93.9
  arterial, artery I67.9
  arteriosclerotic I67.2
  congenital QØ4.9

Disease, diseased *(Continued)*
 brain *(Continued)*
  degenerative —*see* Degeneration, brain
  inflammatory —*see* Encephalitis
  organic G93.9
   arteriosclerotic I67.2
  parasitic NEC B71.9 *[G94]*
  senile NEC G31.1
  specified NEC G93.89
 breast *(see also* Disorder, breast) N64.9
  cystic (chronic) —*see* Mastopathy, cystic
  fibrocystic —*see* Mastopathy, cystic
  Paget's
   female, unspecified side C5Ø.91-
   male, unspecified side C5Ø.92-
  specified NEC N64.89
 Breda's —*see* Yaws
 Bretonneau's (diphtheritic malignant angina)
  A36.Ø
 Bright's —*see* Nephritis
  arteriosclerotic —*see* Hypertension, kidney
 Brill's (recrudescent typhus) A75.1
 Brill-Zinsser (recrudescent typhus) A75.1
 Brion-Kayser —*see* Fever, paratyphoid
 broad
  beta E78.2
  ligament (noninflammatory) N83.9
   inflammatory —*see* Disease, pelvis,
    inflammatory
   specified NEC N83.8
 Brocq-Duhring (dermatitis herpetiformis)
  L13.Ø
 Brocq's
  meaning
   dermatitis herpetiformis L13.Ø
   prurigo L28.2
 bronchopulmonary J98.4
 bronchus NEC J98.Ø9
 bronze Addison's E27.1
  tuberculous A18.7
 budgerigar fancier's J67.2
 Buerger's (thromboangiitis obliterans)
  I73.1
 bullous L13.9
  chronic of childhood L12.2
  specified NEC L13.8
 Bürger-Grütz (essential familial
  hyperlipemia) E78.3
 bursa —*see* Bursopathy
 caisson T70.3
 California —*see* Coccidioidomycosis
 capillaries I78.9
  specified NEC I78.8
 Carapata A68.Ø
 cardiac —*see* Disease, heart
 cardiopulmonary, chronic I27.9
 cardiorenal (hepatic) (hypertensive)
  (vascular) —*see* Hypertension,
  cardiorenal
 cardiovascular (atherosclerotic) I25.1Ø
  with angina pectoris —*see* Arteriosclerosis,
   coronary (artery),
  congenital Q28.9
  hypertensive —*see* Hypertension, heart
  newborn P29.9
   specified NEC P29.89
  renal (hypertensive) —*see* Hypertension,
   cardiorenal
  syphilitic (asymptomatic) A52.ØØ
 cartilage —*see* Disorder, cartilage
 Castellani's A69.8
 Castleman (unicentric) (multicentric)
  D47.Z2 ◀
  HHV-8-associated —*see also* Herpesvirus,
   human, 8 D47.Z2 ◀
 cat-scratch A28.1
 Cavare's (familial periodic paralysis) G72.3
 cecum K63.9
 celiac (adult) (infantile) (with steatorrhea)
  K9Ø.Ø ◀▥
 cellular tissue L98.9

Disease, diseased *(Continued)*
 central core G71.2
 cerebellar, cerebellum —*see* Disease, brain
 cerebral —*see also* Disease, brain
  degenerative —*see* Degeneration, brain
 cerebrospinal G96.9
 cerebrovascular I67.9
  acute I67.89
   embolic I63.4-
   thrombotic I63.3-
  arteriosclerotic I67.2
  specified NEC I67.89
 cervix (uteri) (noninflammatory) N88.9
  inflammatory —*see* Cervicitis
  specified NEC N88.8
 Chabert's A22.9
 Chandler's (osteochondritis dissecans, hip) —
  see Osteochondritis, dissecans, hip
 Charlouis —*see* Yaws
 Chédiak-Steinbrinck (-Higashi) (congenital
  gigantism of peroxidase granules)
  E70.33Ø
 chest J98.9
 Chiari's (hepatic vein thrombosis) I82.Ø
 Chicago B4Ø.9
 Chignon B36.8
 chigo, chigoe B88.1
 childhood granulomatous D71
 Chinese liver fluke B66.1
 chlamydial A74.9
  specified NEC A74.89
 cholecystic K82.9
 choroid H31.9
  specified NEC H31.8
 Christmas D67
 chronic bullous of childhood L12.2
 chylomicron retention E78.3
 ciliary body H21.9
  specified NEC H21.89
 circulatory (system) NEC I99.8
  newborn P29.9
  syphilitic A52.ØØ
   congenital A5Ø.54
 coagulation factor deficiency (congenital) —
  see Defect, coagulation
 coccidioidal —*see* Coccidioidomycosis
 cold
  agglutinin or hemoglobinuria D59.1
   paroxysmal D59.6
  hemagglutinin (chronic) D59.1
 collagen NOS (nonvascular) (vascular) M35.9
  specified NEC M35.8
 colon K63.9
  functional K59.9
   congenital Q43.2
  ischemic —*see also* Ischemia, intestine,
   acute K55.Ø39 ◀▥
 colonic inflammatory bowel, unclassified
  (IBDU) K52.3 ◀
 combined system —*see* Degeneration,
  combined
 compressed air T70.3
 Concato's (pericardial polyserositis) A19.9
  nontubercular I31.1
  pleural —*see* Pleurisy, with effusion
 conjunctiva H11.9
  chlamydial A74.Ø
  specified NEC H11.89
  viral B3Ø.9
   specified NEC B3Ø.8
 connective tissue, systemic (diffuse) M35.9
  in (due to)
   hypogammaglobulinemia D8Ø.1 *[M36.8]*
   ochronosis E70.29 *[M36.8]*
  specified NEC M35.8
 Conor and Bruch's (boutonneuse fever) A77.1
 Cooper's —*see* Mastopathy, cystic
 Cori's (glycogenosis III) E74.Ø3
 corkhandler's or corkworker's J67.3
 cornea H18.9
  specified NEC H18.89-

Disease, diseased *(Continued)*
  coronary (artery) —*see* Disease, heart,
    ischemic, atherosclerotic
    congenital Q24.5
    ostial, syphilitic (aortic) (mitral)
      (pulmonary) A52.03
  corpus cavernosum N48.9
    specified NEC N48.89
  Cotugno's —*see* Sciatica
  coxsackie (virus) NEC B34.1
  cranial nerve NOS G52.9
  Creutzfeldt-Jakob —*see* Creutzfeldt- Jakob
    disease or syndrome
  Crocq's (acrocyanosis) I73.89
  Crohn's —*see* Enteritis, regional
  Curschmann G71.11
  cystic
    breast (chronic) —*see* Mastopathy, cystic
    kidney, congenital Q61.9
    liver, congenital Q44.6
    lung J98.4
      congenital Q33.0
  cytomegalic inclusion (generalized) B25.9
    with pneumonia B25.0
    congenital P35.1
  cytomegaloviral B25.9
    specified NEC B25.8
  Czerny's (periodic hydrarthrosis of the
    knee) —*see* Effusion, joint, knee
  Daae (-Finsen) (epidemic pleurodynia) B33.0
  Darling's —*see* Histoplasmosis capsulati
  Débove's (splenomegaly) R16.1
  deer fly —*see* Tularemia
  Degos' I77.8
  demyelinating, demyelinizating (nervous
    system) G37.9
    multiple sclerosis G35
    specified NEC G37.8
  dense deposit —*see also* N00-N07 with fourth
    character .6 N05.6
  deposition, hydroxyapatite —*see* Disease,
    hydroxyapatite deposition
  de Quervain's (tendon sheath) M65.4
    thyroid (subacute granulomatous
      thyroiditis) E06.1
  Devergie's (pityriasis rubra pilaris) L44.0
  Devic's G36.0
  diaphorase deficiency D74.0
  diaphragm J98.6
  diarrheal, infectious NEC A09
  digestive system K92.9
    specified NEC K92.89
  disc, degenerative —*see* Degeneration,
    intervertebral disc
  discogenic —*see also* Displacement,
    intervertebral disc NEC
    with myelopathy —*see* Disorder, disc, with,
      myelopathy
  diverticular —*see* Diverticula
  Dubois (thymus) A50.59 *[E35]*
  Duchenne-Griesinger G71.0
  Duchenne's
    muscular dystrophy G71.0
    pseudohypertrophy, muscles G71.0
  ductless glands E34.9
  Duhring's (dermatitis herpetiformis) L13.0
  duodenum K31.9
    specified NEC K31.89
  Dupré's (meningism) R29.1
  Dupuytren's (muscle contracture) M72.0
  Durand-Nicholas-Favre (climatic bubo) A55
  Duroziez's (congenital mitral stenosis) Q23.2
  ear —*see* Disorder, ear
  Eberth's —*see* Fever, typhoid
  Ebola (virus) A98.4
  Ebstein's heart Q22.5
  Echinococcus —*see* Echinococcus
  echovirus NEC B34.1
  Eddowes' (brittle bones and blue sclera) Q78.0
  edentulous (alveolar) ridge K06.9
    specified NEC K06.8

Disease, diseased *(Continued)*
  Edsall's T67.2
  Eichstedt's (pityriasis versicolor) B36.0
  Ellis-van Creveld (chondroectodermal
    dysplasia) Q77.6
  end stage renal (ESRD) N18.6
    due to hypertension I12.0
  endocrine glands or system NEC E34.9
  endomyocardial (eosinophilic) I42.3
  English (rickets) E55.0
  enteroviral, enterovirus NEC B34.1
    central nervous system NEC A88.8
  epidemic B99.9
    specified NEC B99.8
  epididymis N50.9
  Erb (-Landouzy) G71.0
  Erdheim-Chester (ECD) E88.89
  esophagus K22.9
    functional K22.4
    psychogenic F45.8
    specified NEC K22.8
  Eulenburg's (congenital paramyotonia)
    G71.19
  eustachian tube —*see* Disorder, eustachian tube
  external
    auditory canal —*see* Disorder, ear, external
    ear —*see* Disorder, ear, external
  extrapyramidal G25.9
    specified NEC G25.89
  eye H57.9
    anterior chamber H21.9
    inflammatory NEC H57.8
    muscle (external) —*see* Strabismus
    specified NEC H57.8
    syphilitic —*see* Oculopathy, syphilitic
  eyeball H44.9
    specified NEC H44.89
  eyelid —*see* Disorder, eyelid
    specified NEC —*see* Disorder, eyelid,
      specified type NEC
  eyeworm of Africa B74.3
  facial nerve (seventh) G51.9
    newborn (birth injury) P11.3
  Fahr (of brain) G23.8
  Fahr Volhard (of kidney) I12.-
  fallopian tube (noninflammatory) N83.9
    inflammatory —*see* Salpingo-oophoritis
    specified NEC N83.8
  familial periodic paralysis G72.3
  Fanconi's (congenital pancytopenia) D61.09
  fascia NEC —*see also* Disorder, muscle
    inflammatory —*see* Myositis
    specified NEC M62.89
  Fauchard's (periodontitis) —*see* Periodontitis
  Favre-Durand-Nicolas (climatic bubo) A55
  Fede's K14.0
  Feer's —*see* Poisoning, mercury
  female pelvic inflammatory —*see also* Disease,
    pelvis, inflammatory N73.9
    syphilitic (secondary) A51.42
    tuberculous A18.17
  Fernels' (aortic aneurysm) I71.9
  fibrocaseous of lung —*see* Tuberculosis,
    pulmonary
  fibrocystic —*see* Fibrocystic disease
  Fiedler's (leptospiral jaundice) A27.0
  fifth B08.3
  file-cutter's —*see* Poisoning, lead
  fish-skin Q80.9
    acquired L85.0
  Flajani (-Basedow) (exophthalmic goiter) —
    see Hyperthyroidism, with, goiter
    (diffuse)
  flax-dresser's J66.1
  fluke —*see* Infestation, fluke
  foot and mouth B08.8
  foot process N04.9
  Forbes' (glycogenosis III) E74.03
  Fordyce-Fox (apocrine miliaria) L75.2
  Fordyce's (ectopic sebaceous glands) (mouth)
    Q38.6

Disease, diseased *(Continued)*
  Forestier's (rhizomelic pseudopolyarthritis)
    M35.3
    meaning ankylosing hyperostosis —*see*
      Hyperostosis, ankylosing
  Fothergill's
    neuralgia —*see* Neuralgia, trigeminal
    scarlatina anginosa A38.9
  Fournier (gangrene) N49.3
    female N76.89
  fourth B08.8
  Fox (-Fordyce) (apocrine miliaria) L75.2
  Francis' —*see* Tularemia
  Franklin C88.2
  Frei's (climatic bubo) A55
  Friedreich's
    combined systemic or ataxia G11.1
    myoclonia G25.3
  frontal sinus —*see* Sinusitis, frontal
  fungus NEC B49
  Gaisböck's (polycythemia hypertonica) D75.1
  gallbladder K82.9
    calculus —*see* Calculus, gallbladder
    cholecystitis —*see* Cholecystitis
    cholesterolosis K82.4
    fistula —*see* Fistula, gallbladder
    hydrops K82.1
    obstruction —*see* Obstruction, gallbladder
    perforation K82.2
    specified NEC K82.8
  gamma heavy chain C88.2
  Gamna's (siderotic splenomegaly) D73.2
  Gamstorp's (adynamia episodica hereditaria)
    G72.3
  Gandy-Nanta (siderotic splenomegaly) D73.2
  ganister J62.8
  gastric —*see* Disease, stomach
  gastroesophageal reflux (GERD) K21.9
    with esophagitis K21.0
  gastrointestinal (tract) K92.9
    amyloid E85.4
    functional K59.9
      psychogenic F45.8
    specified NEC K92.89
  Gee (-Herter) (-Heubner) (-Thaysen)
    (nontropical sprue) K90.0
  genital organs
    female N94.9
    male N50.9
  Gerhardt's (erythromelalgia) I73.81
  Gibert's (pityriasis rosea) L42
  Gierke's (glycogenosis I) E74.01
  Gilles de la Tourette's (motor-verbal tic) F95.2
  gingiva K06.9
    plaque induced K05.00 ◀
    specified NEC K06.8
  gland (lymph) I89.9
  Glanzmann's (hereditary hemorrhagic
    thrombasthenia) D69.1
  glass-blower's (cataract) —*see* Cataract,
    specified NEC
    salivary gland hypertrophy K11.1
  Glisson's —*see* Rickets
  globe H44.9
    specified NEC H44.89
  glomerular —*see also* Glomerulonephritis
    with edema —*see* Nephrosis
    acute —*see* Nephritis, acute
    chronic —*see* Nephritis, chronic
    minimal change N05.0
    rapidly progressive N01.9
  glycogen storage E74.00
    Andersen's E74.09
    Cori's E74.03
    Forbes' E74.03
    generalized E74.00
    glucose-6-phosphatase deficiency E74.01
    heart E74.02 *[I43]*
    hepatorenal E74.09
    Hers' E74.09
    liver and kidney E74.09

◀ New   ◀▦ Revised   ~~deleted~~ Deleted

Disease, diseased *(Continued)*
  glycogen storage *(Continued)*
    McArdle's E74.04
    muscle phosphofructokinase E74.09
    myocardium E74.02 *[143]*
    Pompe's E74.02
    Tauri's E74.09
    type Ø E74.09
    type I E74.01
    type II E74.02
    type III E74.03
    type IV E74.09
    type V E74.04
    type VI-XI E74.09
    Von Gierke's E74.01
  Goldstein's (familial hemorrhagic
      telangiectasia) I78.0
  gonococcal NOS A54.9
  graft-versus-host (GVH) D89.813
    acute D89.810
    acute on chronic D89.812
    chronic D89.811
  grainhandler's J67.8
  granulomatous (childhood) (chronic) D71
  Graves' (exophthalmic goiter) —*see*
      Hyperthyroidism, with, goiter
      (diffuse)
  Griesinger's —*see* Ancylostomiasis
  Grisel's M43.6
  Gruby's (tinea tonsurans) B35.0
  Guillain-Barré G61.0
  Guinon's (motor-verbal tic) F95.2
  gum K06.9
  gynecological N94.9
  H (Hartnup's) E72.02
  Haff —*see* Poisoning, mercury
  Hageman (congenital factor XII deficiency)
      D68.2
  hair (color) (shaft) L67.9
    follicles L73.9
      specified NEC L73.8
  Hamman's (spontaneous mediastinal
      emphysema) J98.2
  hand, foot and mouth B08.4
  Hansen's —*see* Leprosy
  Hantavirus, with pulmonary manifestations
      B33.4
    with renal manifestations A98.5
  Harada's H30.81-
  Hartnup (pellagra-cerebellar ataxia-renal
      aminoaciduria) E72.02
  Hart's (pellagra-cerebellar ataxia-renal
      aminoaciduria) E72.02
  Hashimoto's (struma lymphomatosa) E06.3
  Hb —*see* Disease, hemoglobin
  heart (organic) I51.9
    with
      pulmonary edema (acute) —*see also*
          Failure, ventricular, left I50.1
      rheumatic fever (conditions in I00)
          active I01.9
            with chorea I02.0
            specified NEC I01.8
          inactive or quiescent (with chorea)
              I09.9
            specified NEC I09.89
    amyloid E85.4 *[143]*
    aortic (valve) I35.9
    arteriosclerotic or sclerotic (senile) —
        see Disease, heart, ischemic,
        atherosclerotic
    artery, arterial —*see* Disease, heart,
        ischemic, atherosclerotic
    beer drinkers' I42.6
    beriberi (wet) E51.12
    black I27.0
    congenital Q24.9
      cyanotic Q24.9
      specified NEC Q24.8
    coronary —*see* Disease, heart, ischemic
    cryptogenic I51.9

Disease, diseased *(Continued)*
  heart *(Continued)*
    fibroid —*see* Myocarditis
    functional I51.89
      psychogenic F45.8
    glycogen storage E74.02 *[143]*
    gonococcal A54.83
    hypertensive —*see* Hypertension, heart
    hyperthyroid —*see also* Hyperthyroidism
        E05.90 *[143]*
      with thyroid storm E05.91 *[143]*
    ischemic (chronic or with a stated duration
        of over 4 weeks) I25.9
      atherosclerotic (of) I25.10
        with angina pectoris —*see*
            Arteriosclerosis, coronary
            (artery)
        coronary artery bypass graft —*see*
            Arteriosclerosis, coronary
            (artery),
      cardiomyopathy I25.5
      diagnosed on ECG or other special
          investigation, but currently
          presenting no symptoms I25.6
      silent I25.6
      specified form NEC I25.89
    kyphoscoliotic I27.1
    meningococcal A39.50
      endocarditis A39.51
      myocarditis A39.52
      pericarditis A39.53
    mitral I05.9
      specified NEC I05.8
    muscular —*see* Degeneration, myocardial
    psychogenic (functional) F45.8
    pulmonary (chronic) I27.9
      in schistosomiasis B65.9 *[152]*
      specified NEC I27.89
    rheumatic (chronic) (inactive) (old)
        (quiescent) (with chorea) I09.9
      active or acute I01.9
        with chorea (acute) (rheumatic)
            (Sydenham's) I02.0
      specified NEC I09.89
    senile —*see* Myocarditis
    syphilitic A52.06
      aortic A52.03
        aneurysm A52.01
      congenital A50.54 *[152]*
    thyrotoxic —*see also* Thyrotoxicosis E05.90
        [143]
      with thyroid storm E05.91 *[143]*
    valve, valvular (obstructive)
        (regurgitant) —*see also* Endocarditis
      congenital NEC Q24.8
        pulmonary Q22.3
    vascular —*see* Disease, cardiovascular
  heavy chain NEC C88.2
    alpha C88.3
    gamma C88.2
    mu C88.2
  Hebra's
    pityriasis
      maculata et circinata L42
      rubra pilaris L44.0
    prurigo L28.2
  hematopoietic organs D75.9
  hemoglobin or Hb
    abnormal (mixed) NEC D58.2
      with thalassemia D56.9
    AS genotype D57.3
    Bart's D56.0
    C (Hb-C) D58.2
      with other abnormal hemoglobin NEC
          D58.2
      elliptocytosis D58.1
      Hb-S D57.2-
      sickle-cell D57.2-
      thalassemia D56.8
    Constant Spring D58.2
    D (Hb-D) D58.2

Disease, diseased *(Continued)*
  hemoglobin or Hb *(Continued)*
    E (Hb-E) D58.2
    E-beta thalassemia D56.5
    elliptocytosis D58.1
    H (Hb-H) (thalassemia) D56.0
      with other abnormal hemoglobin NEC
          D56.9
      Constant Spring D56.0
    I thalassemia D56.9
    M D74.0
    S or SS D57.1
    SC D57.2-
    SD D57.8-
    SE D57.8-
    spherocytosis D58.0
    unstable, hemolytic D58.2
  hemolytic (newborn) P55.9
    autoimmune (cold type) (warm type) D59.1
    drug-induced D59.0
    due to or with
      incompatibility
        ABO (blood group) P55.1
        blood (group) (Duffy) (K(ell)) (Kidd)
            (Lewis) (M) (S) NEC P55.8
        Rh (blood group) (factor) P55.0
        Rh negative mother P55.0
    specified type NEC P55.8
    unstable hemoglobin D58.2
  hemorrhagic D69.9
    newborn P53
  Henoch (-Schönlein) (purpura nervosa) D69.0
  hepatic —*see* Disease, liver
  hepatobiliary K83.9
    toxic K71.9
  hepatolenticular E83.01
  heredodegenerative NEC
    spinal cord G95.89
  herpesviral, disseminated B00.7
  Hers' (glycogenosis VI) E74.09
  Herter (-Gee) (-Heubner) (nontropical sprue)
      K90.0
  Heubner-Herter (nontropical sprue) K90.0
  high fetal gene or hemoglobin thalassemia
      D56.9
  Hildenbrand's —*see* Typhus
  hip (joint) M25.9
    congenital Q65.89
    suppurative M00.9
    tuberculous A18.02
  His (-Werner) (trench fever) A79.0
  Hodgson's I71.2
    ruptured I71.1
  Holla —*see* Spherocytosis
  hookworm B76.9
    specified NEC B76.8
  host-versus-graft D89.813
    acute D89.810
    acute on chronic D89.812
    chronic D89.811
  human immunodeficiency virus (HIV) B20
  Huntington's G10
  Hutchinson's (cheiropompholyx) —*see*
      Hutchinson's disease
  hyaline (diffuse) (generalized)
      membrane (lung) (newborn) P22.0
      adult J80
  hydatid —*see* Echinococcus
  hydroxyapatite deposition M11.00
    ankle M11.07-
    elbow M11.02-
    foot joint M11.07-
    hand joint M11.04-
    hip M11.05-
    knee M11.06-
    multiple site M11.09
    shoulder M11.01-
    vertebra M11.08
    wrist M11.03-
  hyperkinetic —*see* Hyperkinesia
  hypertensive —*see* Hypertension

◄ New   ◄▥ Revised   ~~deleted~~ Deleted

Disease, diseased *(Continued)*
  hypophysis E23.7
  Iceland G93.3
  I-cell E77.0
  immune D89.9
  immunoproliferative (malignant) C88.9
    small intestinal C88.3
    specified NEC C88.8
  inclusion B25.9
    salivary gland B25.9
  infectious, infective B99.9
    congenital P37.9
      specified NEC P37.8
      viral P35.9
        specified type NEC P35.8
    specified NEC B99.8
  inflammatory
    penis N48.29
      abscess N48.21
      cellulitis N48.22
    prepuce N47.7
      balanoposthitis N47.6
    tubo-ovarian —*see* Salpingo-oophoritis
  intervertebral disc —*see also* Disorder, disc
    with myelopathy —*see* Disorder, disc, with,
      myelopathy
    cervical, cervicothoracic —*see* Disorder,
      disc, cervical
      with
        myelopathy —*see* Disorder, disc,
          cervical, with myelopathy
        neuritis, radiculitis or
          radiculopathy —*see* Disorder,
          disc, cervical, with neuritis
      specified NEC —*see* Disorder, disc,
        cervical, specified type NEC
    lumbar (with)
      myelopathy M51.06
      neuritis, radiculitis, radiculopathy or
        sciatica M51.16
      specified NEC M51.86
    lumbosacral (with)
      neuritis, radiculitis, radiculopathy or
        sciatica M51.17
      specified NEC M51.87
    specified NEC —*see* Disorder, disc,
      specified NEC
    thoracic (with)
      myelopathy M51.04
      neuritis, radiculitis or radiculopathy
        M51.14
      specified NEC M51.84
    thoracolumbar (with)
      myelopathy M51.05
      neuritis, radiculitis or radiculopathy
        M51.15
      specified NEC M51.85
  intestine K63.9
    functional K59.9
      psychogenic F45.8
      specified NEC K59.8
    organic K63.9
    protozoal A07.9
    specified NEC K63.89
  iris H21.9
    specified NEC H21.89
  iron metabolism or storage E83.10
  island (scrub typhus) A75.3
  itai-itai —*see* Poisoning, cadmium
  Jakob-Creutzfeldt —*see* Creutzfeldt- Jakob
    disease or syndrome
  jaw M27.9
    fibrocystic M27.49
    specified NEC M27.8
  jigger B88.1
  joint —*see also* Disorder, joint
    Charcot's —*see* Arthropathy, neuropathic
      (Charcot)
    degenerative —*see* Osteoarthritis
      multiple M15.9
      spine —*see* Spondylosis

Disease, diseased *(Continued)*
  joint *(Continued)*
    hypertrophic —*see* Osteoarthritis
    sacroiliac M53.3
    specified NEC —*see* Disorder, joint,
      specified type NEC
    spine NEC —*see* Dorsopathy
    suppurative —*see* Arthritis, pyogenic or
      pyemic
  Jourdain's (acute gingivitis) K05.00
    nonplaque induced K05.01
    plaque induced K05.00
  Kaschin-Beck (endemic polyarthritis)
    M12.10
    ankle M12.17-
    elbow M12.12-
    foot joint M12.17-
    hand joint M12.14-
    hip M12.15-
    knee M12.16-
    multiple site M12.19
    shoulder M12.11-
    vertebra M12.18
    wrist M12.13-
  Katayama B65.2
  Kedani (scrub typhus) A75.3
  Keshan E59
  kidney (functional) (pelvis) N28.9
    chronic N18.9
      hypertensive —*see* Hypertension, kidney
      stage 1 N18.1
      stage 2 (mild) N18.2
      stage 3 (moderate) N18.3
      stage 4 (severe) N18.4
      stage 5 N18.5
    complicating pregnancy —*see* Pregnancy,
      complicated by, renal disease
    cystic (congenital) Q61.9
    diabetic - see E08-E13 with .22
    fibrocystic (congenital) Q61.8
    hypertensive —*see* Hypertension, kidney
    in (due to)
      schistosomiasis (bilharziasis) B65.9 *[N29]*
    multicystic Q61.4
    polycystic Q61.3
      adult type Q61.2
      childhood type NEC Q61.19
        collecting duct dilatation Q61.11
  Kimmelstiel (-Wilson) (intercapillary polycystic
    (congenital) glomerulosclerosis) —*see*
    E08-E13 with .21
  Kimura D21.9
    specified site (see Neoplasm, connective
      tissue benign)
  Kinnier Wilson's (hepatolenticular
    degeneration) E83.01
  kissing —*see* Mononucleosis, infectious
  Klebs' —*see also* Glomerulonephritis N05.-
  Klippel-Feil (brevicollis) Q76.1
  Köhler-Pellegrini-Stieda (calcification, knee
    joint) —*see* Bursitis, tibial collateral
  Kok Q89.8
  König's (osteochondritis dissecans) —*see*
    Osteochondritis, dissecans
  Korsakoff's (nonalcoholic) F04
    alcoholic F10.96
      with dependence F10.26
  Kostmann's (infantile genetic
    agranulocytosis) D70.0
  kuru A81.81
  Kyasanur Forest A98.2
  labyrinth, ear —*see* Disorder, ear, inner
  lacrimal system —*see* Disorder, lacrimal
    system
  Lafora's —*see* Epilepsy, generalized,
    idiopathic
  Lancereaux-Mathieu (leptospiral jaundice)
    A27.0
  Landry's G61.0
  Larrey-Weil (leptospiral jaundice) A27.0
  larynx J38.7

Disease, diseased *(Continued)*
  legionnaires' A48.1
    nonpneumonic A48.2
  Lenegre's I44.2
  lens H27.9
    specified NEC H27.8
  Lev's (acquired complete heart block) I44.2
  Lewy body (dementia) G31.83 *[F02.80]*
    with behavioral disturbance G31.83 *[F02.81]*
  Lichtheim's (subacute combined sclerosis
    with pernicious anemia) D51.0
  Lightwood's (renal tubular acidosis) N25.89
  Lignac's (cystinosis) E72.04
  lip K13.0
  lipid-storage E75.6
    specified NEC E75.5
  Lipschütz's N76.6
  liver (chronic) (organic) K76.9
    alcoholic (chronic) K70.9
      acute —*see* Disease, liver, alcoholic,
        hepatitis
      cirrhosis K70.30
        with ascites K70.31
      failure K70.40
        with coma K70.41
      fatty liver K70.0
      fibrosis K70.2
      hepatitis K70.10
        with ascites K70.11
      sclerosis K70.2
    cystic, congenital Q44.6
    drug-induced (idiosyncratic) (toxic)
      (predictable) (unpredictable) —*see*
      Disease, liver, toxic
    end stage K72.90
      due to hepatitis —*see* Hepatitis
    fatty, nonalcoholic (NAFLD) K76.0
      alcoholic K70.0
    fibrocystic (congenital) Q44.6
    fluke
      Chinese B66.1
      oriental B66.1
      sheep B66.3
    glycogen storage E74.09 *[K77]*
    in (due to)
      schistosomiasis (bilharziasis) B65.9 *[K77]*
    inflammatory K75.9
      alcoholic K70.1
      specified NEC K75.89
    polycystic (congenital) Q44.6
    toxic K71.9
      with
        cholestasis K71.0
        cirrhosis (liver) K71.7
        fibrosis (liver) K71.7
        focal nodular hyperplasia K71.8
        hepatic granuloma K71.8
        hepatic necrosis K71.10
          with coma K71.11
        hepatitis NEC K71.6
          acute K71.2
          chronic
            active K71.50
              with ascites K71.51
            lobular K71.4
            persistent K71.3
          lupoid K71.50
            with ascites K71.51
        peliosis hepatis K71.8
        veno-occlusive disease (VOD) of liver
          K71.8
      veno-occlusive K76.5
  Lobo's (keloid blastomycosis) B48.0
  Lobstein's (brittle bones and blue sclera) Q78.0
  Ludwig's (submaxillary cellulitis) K12.2
  lumbosacral region M53.87
  lung J98.4
    black J60
    congenital Q33.9
    cystic J98.4
      congenital Q33.0

◄ New   ◄▬ Revised   ~~deleted~~ Deleted

Disease, diseased *(Continued)*
 lung *(Continued)*
  fibroid (chronic) —*see* Fibrosis, lung
  fluke B66.4
   oriental B66.4
  in
   amyloidosis E85.4 *[J99]*
   sarcoidosis D86.0
   Sjögren's syndrome M35.02
   systemic
    lupus erythematosus M32.13
    sclerosis M34.81
  interstitial J84.9
   of childhood, specified NEC J84.848
   respiratory bronchiolitis J84.115
   specified NEC J84.89
  obstructive (chronic) J44.9
   with
    acute
     bronchitis J44.0
      exacerbation NEC J44.1
      lower respiratory infection J44.0
    alveolitis, allergic J67.9
    asthma J44.9
    bronchiectasis J47.9
     with
      exacerbation (acute) J47.1
      lower respiratory infection J47.0
    bronchitis J44.9
     with
      exacerbation (acute) J44.1
      lower respiratory infection J44.0
    emphysema J44.9
    hypersensitivity pneumonitis J67.9
   decompensated J44.1
    with
     exacerbation (acute) J44.1
  polycystic J98.4
   congenital Q33.0
  rheumatoid (diffuse) (interstitial) —*see*
    Rheumatoid, lung
 Lutembacher's (atrial septal defect with
   mitral stenosis) Q21.1
 Lyme A69.20
 lymphatic (gland) (system) (channel) (vessel)
   I89.9
 lymphoproliferative D47.9
  specified NEC D47.Z9
  T-gamma D47.Z9
  X-linked D82.3
 Magitot's M27.2
 malarial —*see* Malaria
 malignant —*see also* Neoplasm, malignant,
   by site
 Manson's B65.1
 maple bark J67.6
 maple-syrup-urine E71.0
 Marburg (virus) A98.3
 Marion's (bladder neck obstruction) N32.0
 Marsh's (exophthalmic goiter) —*see*
   Hyperthyroidism, with, goiter (diffuse)
 mastoid (process) —*see* Disorder, ear, middle
 Mathieu's (leptospiral jaundice) A27.0
 Maxcy's A75.2
 McArdle (-Schmid-Pearson) (glycogenosis
   V) E74.04
 mediastinum J98.59 ◄▥
 medullary center (idiopathic) (respiratory)
   G93.89
 Meige's (chronic hereditary edema) Q82.0
 meningococcal —*see* Infection, meningococcal
 mental F99
  organic F09
 mesenchymal M35.9
 mesenteric embolic —*see also* Ischemia,
   intestine, acute K55.039 ◄▥
 metabolic, metabolism E88.9
  bilirubin E80.7
 metal-polisher's J62.8
 metastatic —*see also* Neoplasm, secondary, by
   site C79.9

Disease, diseased *(Continued)*
 microvascular — code to condition
 microvillus
  atrophy Q43.8
  inclusion (MVD) Q43.8
 middle ear —*see* Disorder, ear, middle
 Mikulicz' (dryness of mouth, absent or
   decreased lacrimation) K11.8
 Milroy's (chronic hereditary edema) Q82.0
 Minamata —*see* Poisoning, mercury
 minicore G71.2
 Minor's G95.19
 Minot's (hemorrhagic disease, newborn) P53
 Minot-von Willebrand-Jürgens
   (angiohemophilia) D68.0
 Mitchell's (erythromelalgia) I73.81
 mitral (valve) I05.9
  nonrheumatic I34.9
 mixed connective tissue M35.1
 moldy hay J67.0
 Monge's T70.29
 Morgagni-Adams-Stokes (syncope with heart
   block) I45.9
 Morgagni's (syndrome) (hyperostosis
   frontalis interna) M85.2
 Morton's (with metatarsalgia) —*see* Lesion,
   nerve, plantar
 Morvan's G60.8
 motor neuron (bulbar) (familial) (mixed type)
   (spinal) G12.20
  amyotrophic lateral sclerosis G12.21
  progressive bulbar palsy G12.22
  specified NEC G12.29
 moyamoya I67.5
 mu heavy chain disease C88.2
 multicore G71.2
 muscle —*see also* Disorder, muscle
  inflammatory —*see* Myositis
  ocular (external) —*see* Strabismus
 musculoskeletal system, soft tissue —*see also*
   Disorder, soft tissue
  specified NEC —*see* Disorder, soft tissue,
    specified type NEC
 mushroom workers' J67.5
 mycotic B49
 myelodysplastic, not classified C94.6
 myeloproliferative, not classified C94.6
  chronic D47.1
 myocardium, myocardial —*see also*
   Degeneration, myocardial I51.5
  primary (idiopathic) I42.9
 myoneural G70.9
 Naegeli's D69.1
 nails L60.9
  specified NEC L60.8
 Nairobi (sheep virus) A93.8
 nasal J34.9
 nemaline body G71.2
 nerve —*see* Disorder, nerve
 nervous system G98.8
  autonomic G90.9
  central G96.9
   specified NEC G96.8
  congenital Q07.9
  parasympathetic G90.9
  specified NEC G98.8
  sympathetic G90.9
  vegetative G90.9
 neuromuscular system G70.9
 Newcastle B30.8
 Nicolas (-Durand)-Favre (climatic bubo)
   A55
 nipple N64.9
  Paget's C50.01-
   female C50.01-
   male C50.02-
 Nishimoto (-Takeuchi) I67.5
 nonarthropod-borne NOS (viral) B34.9
  enterovirus NEC B34.1
 nonautoimmune hemolytic D59.4
  drug-induced D59.2

Disease, diseased *(Continued)*
 Nonne-Milroy-Meige (chronic hereditary
   edema) Q82.0
 nose J34.9
 nucleus pulposus —*see* Disorder, disc
 nutritional E63.9
 oast-house-urine E72.19
 ocular
  herpesviral B00.50
  zoster B02.30
 obliterative vascular I77.1
 Ohara's —*see* Tularemia
 Opitz's (congestive splenomegaly)
   D73.2
 Oppenheim-Urbach (necrobiosis lipoidica
   diabeticorum) —*see* E08-E13 with .620
 optic nerve NEC —*see* Disorder, nerve, optic
   orbit —*see* Disorder, orbit
 Oriental liver fluke B66.1
 Oriental lung fluke B66.4
 Ormond's N13.5
 Oropouche virus A93.0
 Osler-Rendu (familial hemorrhagic
   telangiectasia) I78.0
 osteofibrocystic E21.0
 Otto's M24.7
 outer ear —*see* Disorder, ear, external
 ovary (noninflammatory) N83.9
  cystic N83.20- ◄▥
  inflammatory —*see* Salpingo-oophoritis
  polycystic E28.2
  specified NEC N83.8
 Owren's (congenital) —*see* Defect,
   coagulation
 pancreas K86.9
  cystic K86.2
  fibrocystic E84.9
  specified NEC K86.89 ◄▥
 panvalvular I08.9
  specified NEC I08.8
 parametrium (noninflammatory) N83.9
 parasitic B89
  cerebral NEC B71.9 *[G94]*
  intestinal NOS B82.9
  mouth B37.0
  skin NOS B88.9
  specified type —*see* Infestation
  tongue B37.0
 parathyroid (gland) E21.5
  specified NEC E21.4
 Parkinson's G20
 parodontal K05.6
 Parrot's (syphilitic osteochondritis) A50.02
 Parry's (exophthalmic goiter) —*see*
   Hyperthyroidism, with, goiter (diffuse)
 Parson's (exophthalmic goiter) —*see*
   Hyperthyroidism, with, goiter (diffuse)
 Paxton's (white piedra) B36.2
 pearl-worker's —*see* Osteomyelitis, specified
   type NEC
 Pellegrini-Stieda (calcification, knee joint) —
   see Bursitis, tibial collateral
 pelvis, pelvic
  female NOS N94.9
   specified NEC N94.89
  gonococcal (acute) (chronic) A54.24
  inflammatory (female) N73.9
   acute N73.0
   chlamydial A56.11 ◄
   chronic N73.1
   specified NEC N73.8
   syphilitic (secondary) A51.42
    late A52.76
   tuberculous A18.17
  organ, female N94.9
  peritoneum, female NEC N94.89
 penis N48.9
  inflammatory N48.29
   abscess N48.21
   cellulitis N48.22
  specified NEC N48.89

Disease, diseased *(Continued)*
  periapical tissues NOS K04.90
  periodontal K05.6
    specified NEC K05.5
  periosteum —*see* Disorder, bone, specified
        type NEC
  peripheral
    arterial I73.9
    autonomic nervous system G90.9
    nerves —*see* Polyneuropathy
    vascular NOS I73.9
  peritoneum K66.9
    pelvic, female NEC N94.89
    specified NEC K66.8
  persistent mucosal (middle ear) H66.20
    left H66.22
      with right H66.23
    right H66.21
      with left H66.23
  Petit's —*see* Hernia, abdomen, specified site
        NEC
  pharynx J39.2
    specified NEC J39.2
  Phocas' —*see* Mastopathy, cystic
  photochromogenic (acid-fast bacilli)
        (pulmonary) A31.0
    nonpulmonary A31.9
  Pick's G31.01 *[F02.80]*
    with behavioral disturbance G31.01
        [F02.81]
    brain G31.01 *[F02.80]* ◀
      with behavioral disturbance G31.01
        [F02.81] ◀
    of pericardium (pericardial pseudocirrhosis
        of liver) I31.1 ◀
  pigeon fancier's J67.2
  pineal gland E34.8
  pink —*see* Poisoning, mercury
  Pinkus' (lichen nitidus) L44.1
  pinworm B80
  Piry virus A93.8
  pituitary (gland) E23.7
  pituitary-snuff-taker's J67.8
  pleura (cavity) J94.9
    specified NEC J94.8
  pneumatic drill (hammer) T75.21
  Pollitzer's (hidradenitis suppurativa)
        L73.2
  polycystic
    kidney or renal Q61.3
      adult type Q61.2
      childhood type NEC Q61.19
        collecting duct dilatation Q61.11
    liver or hepatic Q44.6
    lung or pulmonary J98.4
      congenital Q33.0
    ovary, ovaries E28.2
    spleen Q89.09
  polyethylene T84.05-
  Pompe's (glycogenosis II) E74.02
  Posadas-Wernicke B38.9
  Potain's (pulmonary edema) —*see* Edema,
        lung
  prepuce N47.8
    inflammatory N47.7
      balanoposthitis N47.6
  Pringle's (tuberous sclerosis) Q85.1
  prion, central nervous system A81.9
    specified NEC A81.89
  prostate N42.9
    specified NEC N42.89
  protozoal B64
    acanthamebiasis —*see* Acanthamebiasis
    African trypanosomiasis —*see* African
        trypanosomiasis
    babesiosis B60.0
    Chagas disease —*see* Chagas disease
    intestine, intestinal A07.9
    leishmaniasis —*see* Leishmaniasis
    malaria —*see* Malaria
    naegleriasis B60.2

Disease, diseased *(Continued)*
  protozoal *(Continued)*
    pneumocystosis B59
    specified organism NEC B60.8
    toxoplasmosis —*see* Toxoplasmosis
  pseudo-Hurler's E77.0
  psychiatric F99
  psychotic —*see* Psychosis
  Puente's (simple glandular cheilitis) K13.0
  puerperal —*see also* Puerperal O90.89
  pulmonary —*see also* Disease, lung
    artery I28.9
    chronic obstructive J44.9
      with
        acute bronchitis J44.0
        exacerbation (acute) J44.1
        lower respiratory infection (acute)
          J44.0
      decompensated J44.1
        with
          exacerbation (acute) J44.1
    heart I27.9
      specified NEC I27.89
    hypertensive (vascular) I27.0
    valve I37.9
      rheumatic I09.89
  pulp (dental) NOS K04.90
  pulseless M31.4
  Putnam's (subacute combined sclerosis with
        pernicious anemia) D51.0
  Pyle (-Cohn) (metaphyseal dysplasia)
        Q78.5 ◀▥
  ragpicker's or ragsorter's A22.1
  Raynaud's —*see* Raynaud's disease
  reactive airway —*see* Asthma
  Reclus' (cystic) —*see* Mastopathy,
        cystic
  rectum K62.9
    specified NEC K62.89
  Refsum's (heredopathia atactica
        polyneuritiformis) G60.1
  renal (functional) (pelvis) —*see also* Disease,
        kidney N28.9
    with
      edema —*see* Nephrosis
      glomerular lesion —*see*
          Glomerulonephritis
        with edema —*see* Nephrosis
      interstitial nephritis N12
    acute N28.9
    chronic —*see also* Disease, kidney, chronic
        N18.9
    cystic, congenital Q61.9
    diabetic —*see* E08-E13 with .22
    end-stage (failure) N18.6
      due to hypertension I12.0
    fibrocystic (congenital) Q61.8
    hypertensive —*see* Hypertension,
        kidney
    lupus M32.14
    phosphate-losing (tubular) N25.0
    polycystic (congenital) Q61.3
      adult type Q61.2
      childhood type NEC Q61.19
        collecting duct dilatation Q61.11
    rapidly progressive N01.9
    subacute N01.9
  Rendu-Osler-Weber (familial hemorrhagic
        telangiectasia) I78.0
  renovascular (arteriosclerotic) —*see*
        Hypertension, kidney
  respiratory (tract) J98.9
    acute or subacute NOS J06.9
      due to
        chemicals, gases, fumes or vapors
          (inhalation) J68.3
        external agent J70.9
          specified NEC J70.8
        radiation J70.0
        smoke inhalation J70.5
    noninfectious J39.8

Disease, diseased *(Continued)*
  respiratory *(Continued)*
    chronic NOS J98.9
      due to
        chemicals, gases, fumes or vapors
          J68.4
        external agent J70.9
          specified NEC J70.8
        radiation J70.1
      newborn P27.9
        specified NEC P27.8
    due to
      chemicals, gases, fumes or vapors J68.9
        acute or subacute NEC J68.3
        chronic J68.4
      external agent J70.9
        specified NEC J70.8
    newborn P28.9
      specified type NEC P28.89
    upper J39.9
      acute or subacute J06.9
      noninfectious NEC J39.8
      specified NEC J39.8
      streptococcal J06.9
  retina, retinal H35.9
    Batten's or Batten-Mayou E75.4 *[H36]*
    specified NEC H35.89
  rheumatoid —*see* Arthritis, rheumatoid
  rickettsial NOS A79.9
    specified type NEC A79.89
  Riga (-Fede) (cachectic aphthae) K14.0
  Riggs' (compound periodontitis) —*see*
        Periodontitis
  Ritter's L00
  Rivalta's (cervicofacial actinomycosis)
        A42.2
  Robles' (onchocerciasis) B73.01
  Roger's (congenital interventricular septal
        defect) Q21.0
  Rosenthal's (factor XI deficiency) D68.1
  Ross River B33.1
  Rossbach's (hyperchlorhydria) K30
  Rotes Quérol —*see* Hyperostosis, ankylosing
  Roth (-Bernhardt) —*see* Mononeuropathy,
        lower limb, meralgia paresthetica
  Runeberg's (progressive pernicious anemia)
        D51.0
  sacroiliac NEC M53.3
  salivary gland or duct K11.9
    inclusion B25.9
    specified NEC K11.8
    virus B25.9
  sandworm B76.9
  Schimmelbusch's —*see* Mastopathy, cystic
  Schmorl's —*see* Schmorl's disease or nodes
  Schönlein (-Henoch) (purpura rheumatica)
        D69.0
  Schottmüller's —*see* Fever, paratyphoid
  Schultz's (agranulocytosis) —*see*
        Agranulocytosis
  Schwalbe-Ziehen-Oppenheim G24.1
  Schwartz-Jampel G71.13
  sclera H15.9
    specified NEC H15.89
  scrofulous (tuberculous) A18.2
  scrotum N50.9
  sebaceous glands L73.9
  semilunar cartilage, cystic —*see also*
        Derangement, knee, meniscus, cystic
  seminal vesicle N50.9
  serum NEC —*see also* Reaction, serum T80.69
  sexually transmitted A64
    anogenital
      herpesviral infection —*see* Herpes,
          anogenital
      warts A63.0
    chancroid A57
    chlamydial infection —*see* Chlamydia
    gonorrhea —*see* Gonorrhea
    granuloma inguinale A58
    specified organism NEC A63.8

◀ New   ◀▥ Revised   ~~deleted~~ Deleted

Disease, diseased (Continued)
  sexually transmitted (Continued)
    syphilis —see Syphilis
    trichomoniasis —see Trichomoniasis
  Sézary C84.1-
  shimamushi (scrub typhus) A75.3
  shipyard B30.0
  sickle-cell D57.1
    with crisis (vasoocclusive pain) D57.00
      with
        acute chest syndrome D57.01
        splenic sequestration D57.02
    elliptocytosis D57.8-
    Hb-C D57.20
      with crisis (vasoocclusive pain) D57.219
        with
          acute chest syndrome D57.211
          splenic sequestration D57.212
      without crisis D57.20
    Hb-SD D57.80
      with crisis D57.819
        with
          acute chest syndrome D57.811
          splenic sequestration D57.812
    Hb-SE D57.80
      with crisis D57.819
        with
          acute chest syndrome D57.811
          splenic sequestration D57.812
    specified NEC D57.80
      with crisis D57.819
        with
          acute chest syndrome D57.811
          splenic sequestration D57.812
    spherocytosis D57.80
      with crisis D57.819
        with
          acute chest syndrome D57.811
          splenic sequestration D57.812
    thalassemia D57.40
      with crisis (vasoocclusive pain) D57.419
        with
          acute chest syndrome D57.411
          splenic sequestration D57.412
      without crisis D57.40
  silo-filler's J68.8
    bronchitis J68.0
    pneumonitis J68.0
    pulmonary edema J68.1
  simian B B00.4
  Simons' (progressive lipodystrophy) E88.1
  sin nombre virus B33.4
  sinus —see Sinusitis
  Sirkari's B55.0
  sixth B08.20
    due to human herpesvirus 6 B08.21
    due to human herpesvirus 7 B08.22
  skin L98.9
    due to metabolic disorder NEC E88.9
      [L99]
    specified NEC L98.8
  slim (HIV) B20
  small vessel I73.9
  Sneddon-Wilkinson (subcorneal pustular
    dermatosis) L13.1
  South African creeping B88.0
  spinal (cord) G95.9
    congenital Q06.9
    specified NEC G95.89
  spine —see also Spondylopathy
    joint —see Dorsopathy
    tuberculous A18.01
  spinocerebellar (hereditary) G11.9
    specified NEC G11.8
  spleen D73.9
    amyloid E85.4 [D77]
    organic D73.9
    polycystic Q89.09
    postinfectional D73.89
  sponge-diver's —see Toxicity, venom, marine
    animal, sea anemone

Disease, diseased (Continued)
  Startle Q89.8
  Steinert's G71.11
  Sticker's (erythema infectiosum) B08.3
  Stieda's (calcification, knee joint) —see
    Bursitis, tibial collateral
  Stokes' (exophthalmic goiter) —see
    Hyperthyroidism, with, goiter (diffuse)
  Stokes-Adams (syncope with heart block)
    I45.9
  stomach K31.9
    functional, psychogenic F45.8
    specified NEC K31.89
  stonemason's J62.8
  storage
    glycogen —see Disease, glycogen storage
    mucopolysaccharide —see
      Mucopolysaccharidosis
  striatopallidal system NEC G25.89
  Stuart-Prower (congenital factor X deficiency)
    D68.2
  Stuart's (congenital factor X deficiency) D68.2
  subcutaneous tissue —see Disease, skin
  supporting structures of teeth K08.9
    specified NEC K08.89 ◄▥
  suprarenal (capsule) (gland) E27.9
    hyperfunction E27.0
    specified NEC E27.8
  sweat glands L74.9
    specified NEC L74.8
  Sweeley-Klionsky E75.21
  Swift (-Feer) —see Poisoning, mercury
  swimming-pool granuloma A31.1
  Sylvest's (epidemic pleurodynia) B33.0
  sympathetic nervous system G90.9
  synovium —see Disorder, synovium
  syphilitic —see Syphilis
  systemic tissue mast cell C96.2
  tanapox (virus) B08.71
  Tangier E78.6
  Tarral-Besnier (pityriasis rubra pilaris) L44.0
  Tauri's E74.09
  tear duct —see Disorder, lacrimal system
  tendon, tendinous —see also Disorder, tendon
    nodular —see Trigger finger
  terminal vessel I73.9
  testis N50.9
  thalassemia Hb-S —see Disease, sickle-cell,
    thalassemia
  Thaysen-Gee (nontropical sprue) K90.0
  Thomsen G71.12
  throat J39.2
    septic J02.0
  thromboembolic —see Embolism
  thymus (gland) E32.9
    specified NEC E32.8
  thyroid (gland) E07.9
    heart —see also Hyperthyroidism E05.90
      [I43]
      with thyroid storm E05.91 [I43]
    specified NEC E07.8
  Tietze's M94.0
  tongue K14.9
    specified NEC K14.89
  tonsils, tonsillar (and adenoids) J35.9
  tooth, teeth K08.9
    hard tissues K03.9
      specified NEC K03.89
    pulp NEC K04.99
    specified NEC K08.89 ◄▥
  Tourette's F95.2
  trachea NEC J39.8
  tricuspid I07.9
    nonrheumatic I36.9
  triglyceride-storage E75.5
  trophoblastic —see Mole, hydatidiform
  tsutsugamushi A75.3
  tube (fallopian) (noninflammatory) N83.9
    inflammatory —see Salpingitis
    specified NEC N83.8
  tuberculous NEC —see Tuberculosis

Disease, diseased (Continued)
  tubo-ovarian (noninflammatory) N83.9
    inflammatory —see Salpingo-oophoritis
    specified NEC N83.8
  tubotympanic, chronic —see Otitis, media,
    suppurative, chronic, tubotympanic
  tubulo-interstitial N15.9
    specified NEC N15.8
  tympanum —see Disorder, tympanic
    membrane
  Uhl's Q24.8
  Underwood's (sclerema neonatorum) P83.0
  Unverricht (-Lundborg) —see Epilepsy,
    generalized, idiopathic
  Urbach-Oppenheim (necrobiosis lipoidica
    diabeticorum) —see E08-E13 with .620
  ureter N28.9
    in (due to)
      schistosomiasis (bilharziasis) B65.0 [N29]
  urethra N36.9
    specified NEC N36.8
  urinary (tract) N39.9
    bladder N32.9
      specified NEC N32.89
    specified NEC N39.8
  uterus (noninflammatory) N85.9
    infective —see Endometritis
    inflammatory —see Endometritis
    specified NEC N85.8
  uveal tract (anterior) H21.9
    posterior H31.9
  vagabond's B85.1
  vagina, vaginal (noninflammatory) N89.9
    inflammatory NEC N76.89
    specified NEC N89.8
  valve, valvular I38
    multiple I08.9
      specified NEC I08.8
  van Creveld-von Gierke (glycogenosis I)
    E74.01
  vas deferens N50.9
  vascular I99.9
    arteriosclerotic —see Arteriosclerosis
    ciliary body NEC —see Disorder, iris,
      vascular
    hypertensive —see Hypertension
    iris NEC —see Disorder, iris, vascular
    obliterative I77.1
      peripheral I73.9
    occlusive I99.8
    peripheral (occlusive) I73.9
      in diabetes mellitus —see E08-E13 with .51
    vasomotor I73.9
  vasospastic I73.9
  vein I87.9
  venereal —see also Disease, sexually
    transmitted A64
    chlamydial NEC A56.8
      anus A56.3
      genitourinary NOS A56.2
      pharynx A56.4
      rectum A56.3
    fifth A55
    sixth A55
    specified nature or type NEC A63.8
  vertebra, vertebral —see also Spondylopathy
    disc —see Disorder, disc
  vibration —see Vibration, adverse effects
  viral, virus —see also Disease, by type of virus
    B34.9
    arbovirus NOS A94
    arthropod-borne NOS A94
    congenital P35.9
      specified NEC P35.8
    Hanta (with renal manifestations)
      (Dobrava) (Puumala) (Seoul) A98.5
      with pulmonary manifestations (Andes)
        (Bayou) (Bermejo) (Black Creek
        Canal) (Choclo) (Juquitiba) (Laguna
        negra) (Lechiguanas) (New York)
        (Oran) (Sin nombre) B33.4

Disease, diseased *(Continued)*
  viral, virus *(Continued)*
    Hantaan (Korean hemorrhagic fever) A98.5
    human immunodeficiency (HIV) B20
    Kunjin A83.4
    nonarthropod-borne NOS B34.9
    Powassan A84.8
    Rocio (encephalitis) A83.6
    Sin nombre (Hantavirus) (cardio)-
      pulmonary syndrome B33.4
    Tahyna B33.8
    vesicular stomatitis A93.8
  vitreous H43.9
    specified NEC H43.89
  vocal cord J38.3
  Volkmann's, acquired T79.6
  von Eulenburg's (congenital paramyotonia)
    G71.19
  von Gierke's (glycogenosis I) E74.01
  von Graefe's —*see* Strabismus, paralytic,
    ophthalmoplegia, progressive
  von Willebrand (-Jürgens) (angiohemophilia)
    D68.0
  Vrolik's (osteogenesis imperfecta) Q78.0
  vulva (noninflammatory) N90.9
    inflammatory NEC N76.89
    specified NEC N90.89
  Wallgren's (obstruction of splenic vein with
    collateral circulation) I87.8
  Wassilieff's (leptospiral jaundice) A27.0
  wasting NEC R64
    due to malnutrition E41
  Waterhouse-Friderichsen A39.1
  Wegner's (syphilitic osteochondritis) A50.02
  Weil's (leptospiral jaundice of lung) A27.0
  Weir Mitchell's (erythromelalgia) I73.81
  Werdnig-Hoffmann G12.0
  Wermer's E31.21
  Werner-His (trench fever) A79.0
  Werner-Schultz (neutropenic splenomegaly)
    D73.81
  Wernicke-Posadas B38.9
  whipworm B79
  white blood cells D72.9
    specified NEC D72.89
  white matter R90.82
  white-spot, meaning lichen sclerosus et
    atrophicus L90.0
    penis N48.0
    vulva N90.4
  Wilkie's K55.1
  Wilkinson-Sneddon (subcorneal pustular
    dermatosis) L13.1
  Willis' —*see* Diabetes
  Wilson's (hepatolenticular degeneration)
    E83.01
  woolsorter's A22.1
  yaba monkey tumor B08.72
  yaba pox (virus) B08.72
  Zika virus A92.5 ◀
  zoonotic, bacterial A28.9
    specified type NEC A28.8
Disfigurement (due to scar) L90.5
Disgerminoma —*see* Dysgerminoma
DISH (diffuse idiopathic skeletal
  hyperostosis) —*see* Hyperostosis,
  ankylosing
Disinsertion, retina —*see* Detachment, retina
Dislocatable hip, congenital Q65.6
Dislocation (articular)
  with fracture —*see* Fracture
  acromioclavicular (joint) S43.10-
    with displacement
      100%-200% S43.12-
      more than 200% S43.13-
    inferior S43.14-
    posterior S43.15-
  ankle S93.0-
  astragalus —*see* Dislocation, ankle
  atlantoaxial S13.121
  atlantooccipital S13.111

Dislocation *(Continued)*
  atloidooccipital S13.111
  breast bone S23.29
  capsule, joint code by site under Dislocation
  carpal (bone) —*see* Dislocation, wrist
  carpometacarpal (joint) NEC S63.05-
    thumb S63.04-
  cartilage (joint) - code by site under
    Dislocation
  cervical spine (vertebra) —*see* Dislocation,
    vertebra, cervical
  chronic —*see* Dislocation, recurrent
  clavicle —*see* Dislocation, acromioclavicular
    joint
  coccyx S33.2
  congenital NEC Q68.8
  coracoid —*see* Dislocation, shoulder
  costal cartilage S23.29
  costochondral S23.29
  cricoarytenoid articulation S13.29
  cricothyroid articulation S13.29
  dorsal vertebra —*see* Dislocation, vertebra,
    thoracic
  ear ossicle —*see* Discontinuity, ossicles, ear
  elbow S53.10-
    congenital Q68.8
    pathological —*see* Dislocation, pathological
      NEC, elbow
    radial head alone —*see* Dislocation, radial
      head
    recurrent —*see* Dislocation, recurrent,
      elbow
    traumatic S53.10-
      anterior S53.11-
      lateral S53.14-
      medial S53.13-
      posterior S53.12-
      specified type NEC S53.19-
  eye, nontraumatic —*see* Luxation, globe
  eyeball, nontraumatic —*see* Luxation, globe
  femur
    distal end —*see* Dislocation, knee
    proximal end —*see* Dislocation, hip
  fibula
    distal end —*see* Dislocation, ankle
    proximal end —*see* Dislocation, knee
  finger S63.25-
    index S63.25-
    interphalangeal S63.27-
      distal S63.29-
        index S63.29-
        little S63.29-
        middle S63.29-
        ring S63.29-
      index S63.27-
      little S63.27-
      middle S63.27-
      proximal S63.28-
        index S63.28-
        little S63.28-
        middle S63.28-
        ring S63.28-
      ring S63.27-
    little S63.25-
    metacarpophalangeal S63.26-
      index S63.26-
      little S63.26-
      middle S63.26-
      ring S63.26-
    middle S63.25-
    recurrent —*see* Dislocation, recurrent,
      finger
    ring S63.25-
    thumb —*see* Dislocation, thumb
  foot S93.30-
    recurrent —*see* Dislocation, recurrent,
      foot
    specified site NEC S93.33-
    tarsal joint S93.31-
    tarsometatarsal joint S93.32-
    toe —*see* Dislocation, toe

Dislocation *(Continued)*
  fracture —*see* Fracture
  glenohumeral (joint) —*see* Dislocation,
    shoulder
  glenoid —*see* Dislocation, shoulder
  habitual —*see* Dislocation, recurrent
  hip S73.00-
    anterior S73.03-
      obturator S73.02-
    central S73.04-
    congenital (total) Q65.2
      bilateral Q65.1
      partial Q65.5
        bilateral Q65.4
        unilateral Q65.3-
      unilateral Q65.0-
    developmental M24.85-
    pathological —*see* Dislocation, pathological
      NEC, hip
    posterior S73.01-
    recurrent —*see* Dislocation, recurrent,
      hip
  humerus, proximal end —*see* Dislocation,
    shoulder
  incomplete —*see* Subluxation, by site
  incus —*see* Discontinuity, ossicles, ear
  infracoracoid —*see* Dislocation, shoulder
  innominate (pubic junction) (sacral junction)
    S33.39
    acetabulum —*see* Dislocation, hip
  interphalangeal (joint (s))
    finger S63.279
      distal S63.29-
        index S63.29-
        little S63.29-
        middle S63.29-
        ring S63.29-
      index S63.27-
      little S63.27-
      middle S63.27-
      proximal S63.28-
        index S63.28-
        little S63.28-
        middle S63.28-
        ring S63.28-
      ring S63.27-
    foot or toe —*see* Dislocation, toe
    thumb S63.12-
      distal joint S63.14-
      proximal joint S63.13-
  jaw (cartilage) (meniscus) S03.0- ◀▥
  joint prosthesis —*see* Complications, joint
    prosthesis, mechanical, displacement,
    by site
  knee S83.106
    cap —*see* Dislocation, patella
    congenital Q68.2
    old M23.8X-
    patella —*see* Dislocation, patella
    pathological —*see* Dislocation, pathological
      NEC, knee
    proximal tibia
      anteriorly S83.11-
      laterally S83.14-
      medially S83.13-
      posteriorly S83.12-
    recurrent —*see also* Derangement, knee,
      specified NEC
    specified type NEC S83.19-
  lacrimal gland H04.16-
  lens (complete) H27.10-
    anterior H27.12-
    congenital Q12.1
    ocular implant —*see* Complications,
      intraocular lens
    partial H27.11-
    posterior H27.13-
    traumatic S05.8X-
  ligament code by site under Dislocation
  lumbar (vertebra) —*see* Dislocation, vertebra,
    lumbar

Dislocation *(Continued)*
  lumbosacral (vertebra) —*see also* Dislocation,
    vertebra, lumbar
    congenital Q76.49
  mandible S03.0- ◀▥
  meniscus (knee) —*see* Tear, meniscus
    other sites code by site under Dislocation
  metacarpal (bone)
    distal end —*see* Dislocation, finger
    proximal end S63.06-
  metacarpophalangeal (joint)
    finger S63.26-
      index S63.26-
      little S63.26-
      middle S63.26-
      ring S63.26-
      thumb S63.11-
  metatarsal (bone) —*see* Dislocation, foot
  metatarsophalangeal (joint (s)) —*see*
    Dislocation, toe
  midcarpal (joint) S63.03-
  midtarsal (joint) —*see* Dislocation, foot
  neck S13.20
    specified site NEC S13.29
    vertebra —*see* Dislocation, vertebra,
      cervical
  nose (septal cartilage) S03.1
  occipitoatloid S13.111
  old —*see* Derangement, joint, specified type
    NEC
  ossicles, ear —*see* Discontinuity, ossicles, ear
  partial —*see* Subluxation, by site
  patella S83.006
    congenital Q74.1
    lateral S83.01-
    recurrent (nontraumatic) M22.0-
      incomplete M22.1-
    specified type NEC S83.09-
  pathological NEC M24.30
    ankle M24.37-
    elbow M24.32-
    foot joint M24.37-
    hand joint M24.34-
    hip M24.35-
    knee M24.36-
    lumbosacral joint —*see* subcategory M53.2
    pelvic region —*see* Dislocation,
      pathological, hip
    sacroiliac —*see* subcategory M53.2
    shoulder M24.31-
    wrist M24.33-
  pelvis NEC S33.30
    specified NEC S33.39
  phalanx
    finger or hand —*see* Dislocation, finger
    foot or toe —*see* Dislocation, toe
  prosthesis, internal —*see* Complications,
    prosthetic device, by site, mechanical
  radial head S53.006
    anterior S53.01-
    posterior S53.02-
    specified type NEC S53.09-
  radiocarpal (joint) S63.02-
  radiohumeral (joint) —*see* Dislocation, radial
    head
  radioulnar (joint)
    distal S63.01-
    proximal —*see* Dislocation, elbow
  radius
    distal end —*see* Dislocation, wrist
    proximal end —*see* Dislocation, radial head
  recurrent M24.40
    ankle M24.47-
    elbow M24.42-
    finger M24.44-
    foot joint M24.47-
    hand joint M24.44-
    hip M24.45-
    knee M24.46-
      patella —*see* Dislocation, patella,
        recurrent

Dislocation *(Continued)*
  recurrent *(Continued)*
    patella —*see* Dislocation, patella, recurrent
    sacroiliac —*see* subcategory M53.2
    shoulder M24.41-
    toe M24.47-
    vertebra —*see also* subcategory M43.5
      atlantoaxial M43.4
        with myelopathy M43.3
    wrist M24.43-
  rib (cartilage) S23.29
  sacrococcygeal S33.2
  sacroiliac (joint) (ligament) S33.2
    congenital Q74.2
    recurrent —*see* subcategory M53.2
  sacrum S33.2
  scaphoid (bone) (hand) (wrist) —*see*
    Dislocation, wrist
    foot —*see* Dislocation, foot
  scapula —*see* Dislocation, shoulder, girdle,
    scapula
  semilunar cartilage, knee —*see* Tear, meniscus
  septal cartilage (nose) S03.1
  septum (nasal) (old) J34.2
  sesamoid bone code by site under Dislocation
  shoulder (blade) (ligament) (joint) (traumatic)
    S43.006
    acromioclavicular —*see* Dislocation,
      acromioclavicular
    chronic —*see* Dislocation, recurrent,
      shoulder
    congenital Q68.8
    girdle S43.30-
      scapula S43.31-
      specified site NEC S43.39-
    humerus S43.00-
      anterior S43.01-
      inferior S43.03-
      posterior S43.02-
    pathological —*see* Dislocation, pathological
      NEC, shoulder
    recurrent —*see* Dislocation, recurrent,
      shoulder
    specified type NEC S43.08-
  spine
    cervical —*see* Dislocation, vertebra, cervical
    congenital Q76.49
    due to birth trauma P11.5
    lumbar —*see* Dislocation, vertebra, lumbar
    thoracic —*see* Dislocation, vertebra,
      thoracic
  spontaneous —*see* Dislocation, pathological
  sternoclavicular (joint) S43.206
    anterior S43.21-
    posterior S43.22-
  sternum S23.29
  subglenoid —*see* Dislocation, shoulder
  symphysis pubis S33.4
  talus —*see* Dislocation, ankle
  tarsal (bone (s)) (joint (s)) —*see* Dislocation,
    foot
  tarsometatarsal (joint (s)) —*see* Dislocation,
    foot
  temporomandibular (joint) S03.0- ◀▥
  thigh, proximal end —*see* Dislocation, hip
  thorax S23.20
    specified site NEC S23.29
    vertebra —*see* Dislocation, vertebra
  thumb S63.10-
    interphalangeal joint —*see* Dislocation,
      interphalangeal (joint), thumb
    metacarpophalangeal joint —*see*
      Dislocation, metacarpophalangeal
      (joint), thumb
  thyroid cartilage S13.29
  tibia
    distal end —*see* Dislocation, ankle
    proximal end —*see* Dislocation, knee
  tibiofibular (joint)
    distal —*see* Dislocation, ankle
    superior —*see* Dislocation, knee

Dislocation *(Continued)*
  toe (s) S93.106
    great S93.10-
      interphalangeal joint S93.11-
      metatarsophalangeal joint S93.12-
    interphalangeal joint S93.119
    lesser S93.106
      interphalangeal joint S93.11-
      metatarsophalangeal joint S93.12-
    metatarsophalangeal joint S93.12-
  tooth S03.2
  trachea S23.29
  ulna
    distal end S63.07-
    proximal end —*see* Dislocation, elbow
  ulnohumeral (joint) —*see* Dislocation, elbow
  vertebra (articular process) (body)
    (traumatic)
    cervical S13.101
      atlantoaxial joint S13.121
      atlantooccipital joint S13.111
      atloidooccipital joint S13.111
      joint between
        C0 and C1 S13.111
        C1 and C2 S13.121
        C2 and C3 S13.131
        C3 and C4 S13.141
        C4 and C5 S13.151
        C5 and C6 S13.161
        C6 and C7 S13.171
        C7 and T1 S13.181
      occipitoatloid joint S13.111
    congenital Q76.49
    lumbar S33.101
      joint between
        L1 and L2 S33.111
        L2 and L3 S33.121
        L3 and L4 S33.131
        L4 and L5 S33.141
    nontraumatic —*see* Displacement,
      intervertebral disc
    partial —*see* Subluxation, by site
    recurrent NEC —*see* subcategory
      M43.5
    thoracic S23.101
      joint between
        T1 and T2 S23.111
        T2 and T3 S23.121
        T3 and T4 S23.123
        T4 and T5 S23.131
        T5 and T6 S23.133
        T6 and T7 S23.141
        T7 and T8 S23.143
        T8 and T9 S23.151
        T9 and T10 S23.153
        T10 and T11 S23.161
        T11 and T12 S23.163
        T12 and L1 S23.171
  wrist (carpal bone) S63.006
    carpometacarpal joint —*see* Dislocation,
      carpometacarpal (joint)
    distal radioulnar joint —*see* Dislocation,
      radioulnar (joint), distal
    metacarpal bone, proximal —*see*
      Dislocation, metacarpal (bone),
      proximal end
    midcarpal —*see* Dislocation, midcarpal
      (joint)
    radiocarpal joint —*see* Dislocation,
      radiocarpal (joint)
    recurrent —*see* Dislocation, recurrent,
      wrist
    specified site NEC S63.09-
    ulna —*see* Dislocation, ulna, distal end
  xiphoid cartilage S23.29
Disorder (of) —*see also* Disease
  acantholytic L11.9
    specified NEC L11.8
  acute
    psychotic —*see* Psychosis, acute
    stress F43.0

Disorder (Continued)
  adjustment (grief) F43.20
    with
      anxiety F43.22
        with depressed mood F43.23
      conduct disturbance F43.24
        with emotional disturbance F43.25
      depressed mood F43.21
        with anxiety F43.23
      other specified symptom F43.29
  adrenal (capsule) (gland) (medullary) E27.9
    specified NEC E27.8
  adrenogenital E25.9
    drug-induced E25.8
    iatrogenic E25.8
    idiopathic E25.8
  adult personality (and behavior) F69
    specified NEC F68.8
  affective (mood) —see Disorder, mood
  aggressive, unsocialized F91.1
  alcohol-related F10.99
    with
      amnestic disorder, persisting F10.96
      anxiety disorder F10.980
      dementia, persisting F10.97
      intoxication F10.929
        with delirium F10.921
        uncomplicated F10.920
      mood disorder F10.94
      other specified F10.988
      psychotic disorder F10.959
        with
          delusions F10.950
          hallucinations F10.951
      sexual dysfunction F10.981
      sleep disorder F10.982
  alcohol use ◄
    mild F10.10 ◄
      with ◄
        alcohol-induced ◄
          anxiety disorder F10.180 ◄
          bipolar and related disorder
            F10.14 ◄
          depressive disorder F10.14 ◄
          psychotic disorder F10.159 ◄
          sexual dysfunction F10.181 ◄
          sleep disorder F10.182 ◄
        alcohol intoxication F10.129 ◄
          delirium F10.121 ◄
    moderate or severe F10.20 ◄
      with ◄
        alcohol-induced ◄
          anxiety disorder F10.280 ◄
          bipolar and related disorder
            F10.24 ◄
          depressive disorder F10.24 ◄
          major neurocognitive disorder,
            amnestic-confabulatory type
            F10.26 ◄
          major neurocognitive disorder,
            nonamnestic-confabulatory
            type F10.27 ◄
          mild neurocognitive disorder
            F10.288 ◄
          psychotic disorder F10.259 ◄
          sexual dysfunction F10.281 ◄
          sleep disorder F10.282 ◄
        alcohol intoxication F10.229 ◄
          delirium F10.221 ◄
  allergic —see Allergy
  alveolar NEC J84.09
  amino-acid
    cystathioninuria E72.19
    cystinosis E72.04
    cystinuria E72.01
    glycinuria E72.09
    homocystinuria E72.11
    metabolism —see Disturbance,
      metabolism, amino-acid
    specified NEC E72.8
    neonatal, transitory P74.8

Disorder (Continued)
  amino-acid (Continued)
    renal transport NEC E72.09
    transport NEC E72.09
  amnesic, amnestic
    alcohol-induced F10.96
      with dependence F10.26
    due to (secondary to) general medical
      condition F04
    psychoactive NEC-induced F19.96
      with
        abuse F19.16
        dependence F19.26
    sedative, hypnotic or anxiolytic-
      induced F13.96
      with dependence F13.26
  amphetamine-type substance use ◄
    mild F15.10 ◄
    moderate F15.20 ◄
    severe F15.20 ◄
  amphetamine (or other stimulant)
    use ◄
    mild ◄
      with ◄
        amphetamine (or other stimulant)
          -induced ◄
          anxiety disorder F15.180 ◄
          bipolar and related disorder
            F15.14 ◄
          depressive disorder F15.14 ◄
          obsessive-compulsive and related
            disorder F15.188 ◄
          psychotic disorder F15.159 ◄
          sexual dysfunction F15.181 ◄
        amphetamine, cocaine, or other
          stimulant intoxication ◄
          with perceptual disturbances
            F15.122 ◄
          without perceptual disturbances
            F15.129 ◄
          intoxication delirium F15.121 ◄
    moderate or severe ◄
      with ◄
        amphetamine (or other stimulant)
          -induced ◄
          anxiety disorder F15.280 ◄
          obsessive-compulsive and related
            disorder F15.288 ◄
          sexual dysfunction F15.281 ◄
          bipolar and related disorder
            F15.24 ◄
          depressive disorder F15.24 ◄
          psychotic disorder F15.259 ◄
        amphetamine, cocaine, or other
          stimulant intoxication ◄
          with perceptual disturbances
            F15.222 ◄
          without perceptual disturbances
            F15.229 ◄
          intoxication delirium F15.221 ◄
  anaerobic glycolysis with anemia
    D55.2
  anxiety F41.9
    due to (secondary to)
      alcohol F10.980
      amphetamine F15.980
        in
          abuse F15.180
          dependence F15.280
      anxiolytic F13.980
        in
          abuse F13.180
          dependence F13.280
      caffeine F15.980
        in
          abuse F15.180
          dependence F15.280
      cannabis F12.980
        in
          abuse F12.180
          dependence F12.280

Disorder (Continued)
  anxiety (Continued)
    due to (Continued)
      cocaine F14.980
        in
          abuse F14.180
          dependence F14.180
      general medical condition F06.4
      hallucinogen F16.980
        in
          abuse F16.180
          dependence F16.280
      hypnotic F13.980
        in
          abuse F13.180
          dependence F13.280
      inhalant F18.980
        in
          abuse F18.180
          dependence F18.280
      phencyclidine F16.980
        in
          abuse F16.180
          dependence F16.280
      psychoactive substance NEC F19.980
        in
          abuse F19.180
          dependence F19.280
      sedative F13.980
        in
          abuse F13.180
          dependence F13.280
      volatile solvents F18.980
        in
          abuse F18.180
          dependence F18.280
    generalized F41.1
    illness F45.21 ◄
    mixed
      with depression (mild) F41.8
      specified NEC F41.3
    organic F06.4
    phobic F40.9
      of childhood F40.8
    specified NEC F41.8
  aortic valve —see Endocarditis, aortic
  aromatic amino-acid metabolism E70.9
    specified NEC E70.8
  arteriole NEC I77.89
  artery NEC I77.89
  articulation —see Disorder, joint
  attachment (childhood)
    disinhibited F94.2
    reactive F94.1
  attention-deficit hyperactivity (adolescent)
    (adult) (child) F98.8 ◄▥
    combined type F90.2
    hyperactive type F90.1
    inattentive type F90.0
    specified type NEC F90.8
  attention-deficit without hyperactivity
    (adolescent) (adult) (child) F90.0
  auditory processing (central) H93.25
  autism spectrum F84.0 ◄
  autistic F84.0
  autonomic nervous system G90.9
    specified NEC G90.8
  avoidant, child or adolescent F40.10
  avoidant ◄
    child or adolescent F40.10 ◄
    restrictive food intake F50.89 ◄
  balance
    acid-base E87.8
      mixed E87.4
    electrolyte E87.8
    fluid NEC E87.8
  behavioral (disruptive) —see Disorder, conduct
  beta-amino-acid metabolism E72.8
  bile acid and cholesterol metabolism E78.70
    Barth syndrome E78.71
    other specified E78.79
    Smith-Lemli-Opitz syndrome E78.72

◄ New   ◄▥ Revised   ~~deleted~~ Deleted

Disorder *(Continued)*
  bilirubin excretion E80.6
  binge eating F50.81 ◀
  binocular
    movement H51.9
      convergence
        excess H51.12
        insufficiency H51.11
      internuclear ophthalmoplegia —*see*
          Ophthalmoplegia, internuclear
      palsy of conjugate gaze H51.0
      specified type NEC H51.8
    vision NEC —*see* Disorder, vision,
        binocular
  bipolar (I) F31.9
    current episode
      depressed F31.9
        with psychotic features F31.5
        without psychotic features
            F31.30
          mild F31.31
          moderate F31.32
          severe (without psychotic features)
              F31.4
            with psychotic features
                F31.5
      hypomanic F31.0
      manic F31.9
        with psychotic features F31.2
        without psychotic features F31.10
          mild F31.11
          moderate F31.12
          severe (without psychotic features)
              F31.13
            with psychotic features F31.2
      mixed F31.60
        mild F31.61
        moderate F31.62
        severe (without psychotic features)
            F31.63
          with psychotic features F31.64
        severe depression (without psychotic
            features) F31.4
          with psychotic features F31.5
    II F31.81
    in remission (currently) F31.70
      in full remission
        most recent episode
          depressed F31.76
          hypomanic F31.72
          manic F31.74
          mixed F31.78
      in partial remission
        most recent episode
          depressed F31.75
          hypomanic F31.71
          manic F31.73
          mixed F31.77
    organic F06.30
    single manic episode F30.9
      mild F30.11
      moderate F30.12
      hhsevere (without psychotic symptoms)
          F30.13
        with psychotic symptoms F30.2
    specified NEC F31.89
  bladder N32.9
    functional NEC N31.9
    in schistosomiasis B65.0 *[N33]*
    specified NEC N32.89
  bleeding D68.9
  blood D75.9
    in congenital early syphilis A50.09 *[D77]*
  body dysmorphic F45.22
  bone M89.9
    continuity M84.9
      specified type NEC M84.80
        ankle M84.87-
        fibula M84.86-
        foot M84.87-
        hand M84.84-

Disorder *(Continued)*
  bone *(Continued)*
    continuity *(Continued)*
      specified type *(Continued)*
        humerus M84.82-
        neck M84.88
        pelvis M84.859
        radius M84.83-
        rib M84.88
        shoulder M84.81-
        skull M84.88
        thigh M84.85-
        tibia M84.86-
        ulna M84.83-
        vertebra M84.88
    density and structure M85.9
      cyst —*see also* Cyst, bone, specified type
          NEC
        aneurysmal —*see* Cyst, bone,
            aneurysmal
        solitary —*see* Cyst, bone, solitary
      diffuse idiopathic skeletal
          hyperostosis —*see* Hyperostosis,
          ankylosing
      fibrous dysplasia (monostotic) —*see*
          Dysplasia, fibrous, bone
      fluorosis —*see* Fluorosis, skeletal
      hyperostosis of skull M85.2
      osteitis condensans —*see* Osteitis,
          condensans
      specified type NEC M85.8-
        ankle M85.87-
        foot M85.87-
        forearm M85.83-
        hand M85.84-
        lower leg M85.86-
        multiple sites M85.89
        neck M85.88
        rib M85.88
        shoulder M85.81-
        skull M85.88
        thigh M85.85-
        upper arm M85.82-
        vertebra M85.88
    development and growth NEC
        M89.20
      carpus M89.24-
      clavicle M89.21-
      femur M89.25-
      fibula M89.26-
      finger M89.24-
      humerus M89.22-
      ilium M89.259
      ischium M89.259
      metacarpus M89.24-
      metatarsus M89.27-
      multiple sites M89.29
      neck M89.28
      radius M89.23-
      rib M89.28
      scapula M89.21-
      skull M89.28
      tarsus M89.27-
      tibia M89.26-
      toe M89.27-
      ulna M89.23-
      vertebra M89.28
    specified type NEC M89.8X-
  brachial plexus G54.0
  branched-chain amino-acid metabolism
      E71.2
    specified NEC E71.19
  breast N64.9
    agalactia —*see* Agalactia
    associated with
      lactation O92.70
        specified NEC O92.79
      pregnancy O92.20
        specified NEC O92.29
      puerperium O92.20
        specified NEC O92.29

Disorder *(Continued)*
  breast *(Continued)*
    cracked nipple —*see* Cracked nipple
    galactorrhea —*see* Galactorrhea
    hypogalactia O92.4
    lactation disorder NEC O92.79
    mastitis —*see* Mastitis
    nipple infection —*see* Infection, nipple
    retracted nipple —*see* Retraction, nipple
    specified type NEC N64.89
  Briquet's F45.0
  bullous, in diseases classified elsewhere
      L14
  caffeine use ◀
    mild ◀
      with ◀
        caffeine-induced ◀
          anxiety disorder F15.180 ◀
          sleep disorder F15.182 ◀
    moderate or severe ◀
      with ◀
        caffeine-induced ◀
          anxiety disorder F15.280 ◀
          sleep disorder F15.282 ◀
  cannabis use
    ~~due to drug abuse —see Abuse, drug,~~
        ~~cannabis~~
    ~~due to drug dependence —see~~
        ~~Dependence, drug, cannabis~~
    mild F12.10 ◀
      with ◀
        cannabis-induced ◀
          anxiety disorder F12.180 ◀
          psychotic disorder F12.159 ◀
          sleep disorder F12.188 ◀
        cannabis intoxication delirium
            F12.121 ◀
          with perceptual disturbances
              F12.122 ◀
          without perceptual disturbances
              F12.129 ◀
    moderate or severe F12.20 ◀
      with ◀
        cannabis-induced ◀
          anxiety disorder F12.280 ◀
          psychotic disorder F12.259 ◀
          sleep disorder F12.288 ◀
        cannabis intoxication
          with perceptual disturbances
              F12.222 ◀
          without perceptual disturbances
              F12.229 ◀
        delirium F12.221 ◀
  carbohydrate
    absorption, intestinal NEC E74.39
    metabolism (congenital) E74.9
      specified NEC E74.8
  cardiac, functional I51.89
  carnitine metabolism E71.40
  cartilage M94.9
    articular NEC —*see* Derangement, joint,
        articular cartilage
    chondrocalcinosis —*see*
        Chondrocalcinosis
    specified type NEC M94.8X-
      articular —*see* Derangement, joint,
          articular cartilage
      multiple sites M94.8X0
  catatonia (due to known physiological
      condition) (with another mental
      disorder) F06.1 ◀
  catatonic
    due to (secondary to) known physiological
        condition F06.1
    organic F06.1
  central auditory processing H93.25
  cervical
    region NEC M53.82
    root (nerve) NEC G54.2
  character NOS F60.9
  childhood disintegrative NEC F84.3

Disorder *(Continued)*
  cholesterol and bile acid metabolism E78.70
    Barth syndrome E78.71
    other specified E78.79
    Smith-Lemli-Opitz syndrome E78.72
  choroid H31.9
    atrophy —*see* Atrophy, choroid
    degeneration —*see* Degeneration, choroid
    detachment —*see* Detachment, choroid
    dystrophy —*see* Dystrophy, choroid
    hemorrhage —*see* Hemorrhage, choroid
    rupture —*see* Rupture, choroid
    scar —*see* Scar, chorioretinal
    solar retinopathy —*see* Retinopathy, solar
    specified type NEC H31.8
  ciliary body —*see* Disorder, iris
    degeneration —*see* Degeneration, ciliary body
  coagulation (factor) (*see also* Defect, coagulation) D68.9
    newborn, transient P61.6
  cocaine use ◄
    mild F14.10 ◄
      with ◄
        amphetamine, cocaine, or other stimulant intoxication ◄
          with perceptual disturbances F14.122 ◄
          without perceptual disturbances F14.129 ◄
        cocaine-induced ◄
          anxiety disorder F14.180 ◄
          bipolar and related disorder F14.14 ◄
          depressive disorder F14.14 ◄
          obsessive-compulsive and related disorder F14.188 ◄
          psychotic disorder F14.159 ◄
          sexual dysfunction F14.181 ◄
          sleep disorder F14.182 ◄
        cocaine intoxication delirium F14.121 ◄
    moderate or severe F14.20 ◄
      with ◄
        amphetamine, cocaine, or other stimulant intoxication ◄
          with perceptual disturbances F14.222 ◄
          without perceptual disturbances F14.229 ◄
        cocaine-induced ◄
          anxiety disorder F14.280 ◄
          bipolar and related disorder F14.24 ◄
          depressive disorder F14.24 ◄
          obsessive-compulsive and related disorder F14.288 ◄
          psychotic disorder F14.259 ◄
          sexual dysfunction F14.281 ◄
          sleep disorder F14.282 ◄
        cocaine intoxication delirium F14.221 ◄
  coccyx NEC M53.3
  cognitive F09
    due to (secondary to) general medical condition F09
    persisting R41.89
      due to
        alcohol F10.97
          with dependence F10.27
        anxiolytics F13.97
          with dependence F13.27
        hypnotics F13.97
          with dependence F13.27
        sedatives F13.97
          with dependence F13.27
        specified substance NEC F19.97
          with
            abuse F19.17
            dependence F19.27

Disorder *(Continued)*
  communication F80.9
    social pragmatic F80.82 ◄
  conduct (childhood) F91.9
    adjustment reaction —*see* Disorder, adjustment
    adolescent onset type F91.2
    childhood onset type F91.1
    compulsive F63.9
    confined to family context F91.0
    depressive F91.8
    group type F91.2
    hyperkinetic —*see* Disorder, attention-deficit hyperactivity
    oppositional defiance F91.3
    socialized F91.2
    solitary aggressive type F91.1
    specified NEC F91.8
    unsocialized (aggressive) F91.1
  conduction, heart I45.9
  congenital glycosylation (CDG) E74.8
  conjunctiva H11.9
    infection —*see* Conjunctivitis
  connective tissue, localized L94.9
    specified NEC L94.8
  conversion (functional neurological symptom disorder) ◄▭
    with ◄
      abnormal movement F44.4 ◄
      anesthesia or sensory loss F44.6 ◄
      attacks or seizures F44.5 ◄
      mixed symptoms F44.7 ◄
      special sensory symptoms F44.6 ◄
      speech symptoms F44.4 ◄
      swallowing symptoms F44.4 ◄
      weakness or paralysis F44.4 ◄
  convulsive (secondary) —*see* Convulsions
  cornea H18.9
    deformity —*see* Deformity, cornea
    degeneration —*see* Degeneration, cornea
    deposits —*see* Deposit, cornea
    due to contact lens H18.82-
      specified as edema —*see* Edema, cornea
    edema —*see* Edema, cornea
    keratitis —*see* Keratitis
    keratoconjunctivitis —*see* Keratoconjunctivitis
    membrane change —*see* Change, corneal membrane
    neovascularization —*see* Neovascularization, cornea
    scar —*see* Opacity, cornea
    specified type NEC H18.89-
    ulcer —*see* Ulcer, cornea
  corpus cavernosum N48.9
  cranial nerve —*see* Disorder, nerve, cranial
  cyclothymic F34.0
  defiant oppositional F91.3
  delusional (persistent) (systematized) F22
    induced F24
  depersonalization F48.1
  depressive F32.9
    major F32.9
      with psychotic symptoms F32.3
      in remission (full) F32.5
        partial F32.4
      recurrent F33.9
      single episode F32.9
        mild F32.0
        moderate F32.1
        severe (without psychotic symptoms) F32.2
          with psychotic symptoms F32.3
    organic F06.31
    persistent F34.1 ◄
    recurrent F33.9
      current episode
        mild F33.0
        moderate F33.1

Disorder *(Continued)*
  depressive *(Continued)*
    recurrent *(Continued)*
      current episode *(Continued)*
        severe (without psychotic symptoms) F33.2
          with psychotic symptoms F33.3
      in remission F33.40
        full F33.42
        partial F33.41
      specified NEC F33.8
    single episode —*see* Episode, depressive
    specified NEC F32.89 ◄
  developmental F89
    arithmetical skills F81.2
    coordination (motor) F82
    expressive writing F81.81
    language F80.9
      expressive F80.1
      mixed receptive and expressive F80.2
      receptive type F80.2
      specified NEC F80.89
    learning F81.9
      arithmetical F81.2
      reading F81.0
    mixed F88
    motor coordination or function F82
    pervasive F84.9
      specified NEC F84.8
    phonological F80.0
    reading F81.0
    scholastic skills —*see also* Disorder, learning
      mixed F81.89
    specified NEC F88
    speech F80.9
      articulation F80.0
      specified NEC F80.89
    written expression F81.81
  diaphragm J98.6
  digestive (system) K92.9
    newborn P78.9
      specified NEC P78.89
    postprocedural —*see* Complication, gastrointestinal
    psychogenic F45.8
  disc (intervertebral) M51.9
    with
      myelopathy
        cervical region M50.00
        cervicothoracic region M50.03
        high cervical region M50.01
        lumbar region M51.06
        mid-cervical region M50.020 ◄▭
        sacrococcygeal region M53.3
        thoracic region M51.04
        thoracolumbar region M51.05
      radiculopathy
        cervical region M50.10
        cervicothoracic region M50.13
        high cervical region M50.11
        lumbar region M51.16
        lumbosacral region M51.17
        mid-cervical region M50.120 ◄▭
        sacrococcygeal region M53.3
        thoracic region M51.14
        thoracolumbar region M51.15
    cervical M50.90
      with
        myelopathy M50.00
          C2-C3 M50.01
          C3-C4 M50.01
          C4-C5 M50.021 ◄▭
          C5-C6 M50.022 ◄▭
          C6-C7 M50.023 ◄▭
          C7-T1 M50.03
          cervicothoracic region M50.03
          high cervical region M50.01
          mid-cervical region M50.020 ◄▭

◄ New   ◄▭ Revised   ~~deleted~~ Deleted

Disorder (Continued)
disc (Continued)
cervical (Continued)
with (Continued)
neuritis, radiculitis or radiculopathy
M50.10
C2-C3 M50.11
C3-C4 M50.11
C4-C5 M50.121 ◀▥
C5-C6 M50.122 ◀▥
C6-C7 M50.123 ◀▥
C7-T1 M50.13
cervicothoracic region M50.13
high cervical region M50.11
mid-cervical region M50.120 ◀▥
C2-C3 M50.91
C3-C4 M50.91
C4-C5 M50.921 ◀▥
C5-C6 M50.922 ◀▥
C6-C7 M50.923 ◀▥
C7-T1 M50.93
cervicothoracic region M50.93
degeneration M50.30
C2-C3 M50.31
C3-C4 M50.31
C4-C5 M50.321 ◀▥
C5-C6 M50.322 ◀▥
C6-C7 M50.323 ◀▥
C7-T1 M50.33
cervicothoracic region M50.33
high cervical region M50.31
mid-cervical region M50.320 ◀▥
displacement M50.20
C2-C3 M50.21
C3-C4 M50.21
C4-C5 M50.221 ◀▥
C5-C6 M50.222 ◀▥
C6-C7 M50.223 ◀▥
C7-T1 M50.23
cervicothoracic region M50.23
high cervical region M50.21
mid-cervical region M50.220 ◀▥
high cervical region M50.91
mid-cervical region M50.920 ◀▥
specified type NEC M50.80
C2-C3 M50.81
C3-C4 M50.81
C4-C5 M50.821 ◀▥
C5-C6 M50.822 ◀▥
C6-C7 M50.823 ◀▥
C7-T1 M50.83
cervicothoracic region M50.83
high cervical region M50.81
mid-cervical region M50.820 ◀▥
specified NEC
lumbar region M51.86
lumbosacral region M51.87
sacrococcygeal region M53.3
thoracic region M51.84
thoracolumbar region M51.85
disinhibited attachment (childhood) F94.2
disintegrative, childhood NEC F84.3
disruptive F91.9 ◀
mood dysregulation F34.81 ◀
specified NEC F91.8 ◀
disruptive behavior F91.9 ◀▥
dissocial personality F60.2
dissociative F44.9
affecting
motor function F44.4
and sensation F44.7
sensation F44.6
and motor function F44.7
brief reactive F43.0
due to (secondary to) general medical
condition F06.8
mixed F44.7
organic F06.8
other specified NEC F44.89
double heterozygous sickling —see Disease,
sickle-cell

dream anxiety F51.5
drug induced hemorrhagic D68.32
drug related F19.99
abuse —see Abuse, drug
dependence —see Dependence, drug
dysmorphic body F45.22 ◀▥
dysthymic F34.1
ear H93.9-
bleeding —see Otorrhagia
deafness —see Deafness
degenerative H93.09-
discharge —see Otorrhea
external H61.9-
auditory canal stenosis —see Stenosis,
external ear canal
exostosis —see Exostosis, external ear
canal
impacted cerumen —see Impaction,
cerumen
otitis —see Otitis, externa
perichondritis —see Perichondritis, ear
pinna —see Disorder, pinna
specified type NEC H61.89-
in diseases classified elsewhere
H62.8X-
inner H83.9-
vestibular dysfunction —see Disorder,
vestibular function
middle H74.9-
adhesive H74.1-
ossicle —see Abnormal, ear ossicles
polyp —see Polyp, ear (middle)
specified NEC, in diseases classified
elsewhere H75.8-
postprocedural —see Complications, ear,
procedure
specified NEC, in diseases classified
elsewhere H94.8-
eating (adult) (psychogenic) F50.9
anorexia —see Anorexia
binge F50.81 ◀
bulimia F50.2
child F98.29
pica F98.3
rumination disorder F98.21
pica F50.89 ◀▥
childhood F98.3
electrolyte (balance) NEC E87.8
with
abortion —see Abortion by type
complicated by specified condition
NEC
ectopic pregnancy O08.5
molar pregnancy O08.5
acidosis (metabolic) (respiratory)
E87.2
alkalosis (metabolic) (respiratory)
E87.3
elimination, transepidermal L87.9
specified NEC L87.8
emotional (persistent) F34.9
of childhood F93.9
specified NEC F93.8
endocrine E34.9
postprocedural E89.89
specified NEC E89.89
erectile (male) (organic) —see also
Dysfunction, sexual, male, erectile
N52.9
nonorganic F52.21
erythematous —see Erythema
esophagus K22.9
functional K22.4
psychogenic F45.8
eustachian tube H69.9-
infection —see Salpingitis, eustachian
obstruction —see Obstruction, eustachian
tube
patulous —see Patulous, eustachian tube
specified NEC H69.8-

Disorder (Continued)
extrapyramidal G25.9
in diseases classified elsewhere —see
category G26
specified type NEC G25.89
eye H57.9
postprocedural —see Complication,
postprocedural, eye
eyelid H02.9
cyst —see Cyst, eyelid
degenerative H02.70
chloasma —see Chloasma, eyelid
madarosis —see Madarosis
specified type NEC H02.79
vitiligo —see Vitiligo, eyelid
xanthelasma —see Xanthelasma
dermatochalasis —see Dermato-chalasis
edema —see Edema, eyelid
elephantiasis —see Elephantiasis, eyelid
foreign body, retained —see Foreign body,
retained, eyelid
function H02.59
abnormal innervation syndrome —see
Syndrome, abnormal innervation
blepharochalasis —see Blepharochalasis
blepharoclonus —see Blepharoclonus
blepharophimosis —see
Blepharophimosis
blepharoptosis —see Blepharoptosis
lagophthalmos —see Lagophthalmos
lid retraction —see Retraction, lid
hypertrichosis —see Hypertrichosis, eyelid
specified type NEC H02.89
vascular H02.879
left H02.876
lower H02.875
upper H02.874
right H02.873
lower H02.872
upper H02.871
factitious F68.10
with predominantly
physical symptoms F68.12
with psychological symptoms F68.13
psychological symptoms F68.11
with physical symptoms F68.13
factor, coagulation —see Defect, coagulation
fatty acid
metabolism E71.30
specified NEC E71.39
oxidation
LCAD E71.310
MCAD E71.311
SCAD E71.312
specified deficiency NEC E71.318
feeding (infant or child) —see also Disorder,
eating R63.3-
feigned (with obvious motivation) Z76.5
without obvious motivation —see Disorder,
factitious
female
hypoactive sexual desire F52.0
orgasmic F52.31
sexual arousal F52.22
fibroblastic M72.9
specified NEC M72.8
fluency
adult onset F98.5
childhood onset F80.81
following
cerebral infarction I69.323
cerebrovascular disease I69.923
specified disease NEC I69.823
intracerebral hemorrhage I69.123
nontraumatic intracranial hemorrhage
NEC I69.223
subarachnoid hemorrhage I69.023
in conditions classified elsewhere R47.82
fluid balance E87.8
follicular (skin) L73.9
specified NEC L73.8

Disorder (Continued)
  fructose metabolism E74.10
    essential fructosuria E74.11
    fructokinase deficiency E74.11
    fructose-1, 6-diphosphatase deficiency
        E74.19
    hereditary fructose intolerance E74.12
    other specified E74.19
  functional polymorphonuclear neutrophils
      D71
  gallbladder, biliary tract and pancreas in
      diseases classified elsewhere K87
  gamma-glutamyl cycle E72.8
  gastric (functional) K31.9
    motility K30
    psychogenic F45.8
    secretion K30
  gastrointestinal (functional) NOS K92.9
    newborn P78.9
    psychogenic F45.8
  gender-identity or -role F64.9
    childhood F64.2
    effect on relationship F66
    of adolescence or adulthood F64.0 ◀▥
      nontranssexual F64.8 ◀
    specified NEC F64.8
    uncertainty F66
  genito-pelvic pain penetration F52.6 ◀
  genitourinary system
    female N94.9
    male N50.9
    psychogenic F45.8
  globe H44.9
    degenerated condition H44.50
      absolute glaucoma H44.51-
      atrophy H44.52-
      leucocoria H44.53-
    degenerative H44.30
      chalcosis H44.31-
      myopia H44.2-
      siderosis H44.32-
      specified type NEC H44.39-
    endophthalmitis —see Endophthalmitis
    foreign body, retained —see Foreign body,
        intraocular, old, retained
    hemophthalmos —see Hemophthalmos
    hypotony H44.40
      due to
        ocular fistula H44.42-
        specified disorder NEC H44.43-
      flat anterior chamber H44.41-
      primary H44.44-
    luxation —see Luxation, globe
    specified type NEC H44.89
  glomerular (in) N05.9
    amyloidosis E85.4 [N08]
    cryoglobulinemia D89.1 [N08]
    disseminated intravascular coagulation
        D65 [N08]
    Fabry's disease E75.21 [N08]
    familial lecithin cholesterol acyltransferase
        deficiency E78.6 [N08]
    Goodpasture's syndrome M31.0
    hemolytic-uremic syndrome D59.3
    Henoch (-Schönlein) purpura D69.0 [N08]
    malariae malaria B52.0
    microscopic polyangiitis M31.7 [N08]
    multiple myeloma C90.0- [N08]
    mumps B26.83
    schistosomiasis B65.9 [N08]
    sepsis NEC A41.- [N08]
      streptococcal A40.- [N08]
    sickle-cell disorders D57.- [N08]
    strongyloidiasis B78.9 [N08]
    subacute bacterial endocarditis I33.0 [N08]
    syphilis A52.75
    systemic lupus erythematosus M32.14
    thrombotic thrombocytopenic purpura
        M31.1 [N08]
    Waldenström macroglobulinemia C88.0
        [N08]
    Wegener's granulomatosis M31.31

Disorder (Continued)
  gluconeogenesis E74.4
  glucosaminoglycan metabolism —
      see Disorder, metabolism,
      glucosaminoglycan
  glycine metabolism E72.50
    d-glycericacidemia E72.59
    hyperhydroxyprolinemia E72.59
    hyperoxaluria E72.53
    hyperprolinemia E72.59
    non-ketotic hyperglycinemia E72.51
    oxalosis E72.53
    oxaluria E72.53
    sarcosinemia E72.59
    trimethylaminuria E72.52
  glycoprotein metabolism E77.9
    specified NEC E77.8
  habit (and impulse) F63.9
    involving sexual behavior NEC F65.9
    specified NEC F63.89
  hallucinogen use ◀
    mild F16.10 ◀
      with ◀
        hallucinogen-induced ◀
          anxiety disorder F16.180 ◀
          bipolar and related disorder
              F16.14 ◀
          depressive disorder F16.14 ◀
          psychotic disorder F16.159 ◀
        hallucinogen intoxication delirium
            F16.121 ◀
        other hallucinogen intoxication
            F16.129 ◀
    moderate or severe F16.20 ◀
      with ◀
        hallucinogen-induced ◀
          anxiety disorder F16.280 ◀
          bipolar and related disorder
              F16.24 ◀
          depressive disorder F16.24 ◀
          psychotic disorder F16.259 ◀
        hallucinogen intoxication delirium
            F16.221 ◀
        other hallucinogen intoxication
            F16.229 ◀
  heart action I49.9
  hematological D75.9
    newborn (transient) P61.9
      specified NEC P61.8
  hematopoietic organs D75.9
  hemorrhagic NEC D69.9
    drug-induced D68.32
    due to
      extrinsic circulating anticoagulants
          D68.32
      increase in
        anti-IIa D68.32
        anti-Xa D68.32
      intrinsic
        circulating anticoagulants
            D68.318
        increase in
          antithrombin D68.318
          anti-VIIIa D68.318
          anti-IXa D68.318
          anti-XIa D68.318
    following childbirth O72.3
  hemostasis —see Defect, coagulation
  histidine metabolism E70.40
    histidinemia E70.41
    other specified E70.49
  hoarding F42.3 ◀
  hyperkinetic —see Disorder, attention-deficit
      hyperactivity
  hyperleucine-isoleucinemia E71.19
  hypervalinemia E71.19
  hypoactive sexual desire F52.0
  hypochondriacal F45.20
    body dysmorphic F45.22
    neurosis F45.21
    other specified F45.29

Disorder (Continued)
  identity
    dissociative F44.81
    illness anxiety F45.21 ◀
    of childhood F93.8
  immune mechanism (immunity) D89.9
    specified type NEC D89.89
  impaired renal tubular function
      N25.9
    specified NEC N25.89
  impulse (control) F63.9
  inflammatory
    pelvic, in diseases classified elsewhere —
        see category N74
    penis N48.29
      abscess N48.21
      cellulitis N48.22
  inhalant use ◀
    mild F18.10 ◀
      with ◀
        inhalant-induced ◀
          anxiety disorder F18.180 ◀
          depressive disorder F18.14 ◀
          major neurocognitive disorder
              F18.17 ◀
          mild neurocognitive disorder
              F18.188 ◀
          psychotic disorder F18.159 ◀
        inhalant intoxication F18.129 ◀
        inhalant intoxication delirium
            F18.121 ◀
    moderate or severe F18.20 ◀
      with ◀
        inhalant-induced ◀
          anxiety disorder F18.280 ◀
          depressive disorder F18.24 ◀
          major neurocognitive disorder
              F18.27 ◀
          mild neurocognitive disorder
              F18.288 ◀
          psychotic disorder F18.259 ◀
        inhalant intoxication F18.229 ◀
        inhalant intoxication delirium
            F18.221 ◀
  integument, newborn P83.9
    specified NEC P83.8
  intermittent explosive F63.81
  internal secretion pancreas —see Increased,
      secretion, pancreas, endocrine
  intestine, intestinal
    carbohydrate absorption NEC E74.39
      postoperative K91.2
    functional NEC K59.9
      postoperative K91.89
    psychogenic F45.8
    vascular K55.9
      chronic K55.1
      specified NEC K55.8
  intraoperative (intraprocedural) —see
      Complications, intraoperative
  involuntary emotional expression (IEED)
      F48.2
  iris H21.9
    adhesions —see Adhesions, iris
    atrophy —see Atrophy, iris
    chamber angle recession —see Recession,
        chamber angle
    cyst —see Cyst, iris
    degeneration —see Degeneration, iris
    in diseases classified elsewhere H22
    iridodialysis —see Iridodialysis
    iridoschisis —see Iridoschisis
    miotic pupillary cyst —see Cyst, pupillary
    pupillary
      abnormality —see Abnormality,
          pupillary
      membrane —see Membrane, pupillary
    specified type NEC H21.89
    vascular NEC H21.1X-
  iron metabolism E83.10
    specified NEC E83.19

◀ New   ◀▥ Revised   deleted Deleted

Disorder *(Continued)*
  isovaleric acidemia E71.110
  jaw, developmental M27.0
    temporomandibular —*see also* Anomaly,
      dentofacial, temporomandibular joint
      M26.60- ◀▥
  joint M25.9
    derangement —*see* Derangement, joint
    effusion —*see* Effusion, joint
    fistula —*see* Fistula, joint
    hemarthrosis —*see* Hemarthrosis
    instability —*see* Instability, joint
    osteophyte —*see* Osteophyte
    pain —*see* Pain, joint
    psychogenic F45.8
    specified type NEC M25.80
      ankle M25.87-
      elbow M25.82-
      foot joint M25.87-
      hand joint M25.84-
      hip M25.85-
      knee M25.86-
      shoulder M25.81-
      wrist M25.83-
    stiffness —*see* Stiffness, joint
  ketone metabolism E71.32
  kidney N28.9
    functional (tubular) N25.9
    in
      schistosomiasis B65.9 [N29]
    tubular function N25.9
    specified NEC N25.89
  lacrimal system H04.9
    changes H04.69
    fistula —*see* Fistula, lacrimal
    gland H04.19
      atrophy —*see* Atrophy, lacrimal
        gland
      cyst —*see* Cyst, lacrimal, gland
      dacryops —*see* Dacryops
      dislocation —*see* Dislocation, lacrimal
        gland
      dry eye syndrome —*see* Syndrome, dry
        eye
      infection —*see* Dacryoadenitis
      granuloma —*see* Granuloma, lacrimal
      inflammation —*see* Inflammation, lacrimal
      obstruction —*see* Obstruction, lacrimal
      specified NEC H04.89
  lactation NEC O92.79
  language (developmental) F80.9
    expressive F80.1
    mixed receptive and expressive F80.2
    receptive F80.2
  late luteal phase dysphoric N94.89
  learning (specific) F81.9
    acalculia R48.8
    alexia R48.0
    mathematics F81.2
    reading F81.0
    specified NEC F81.89
    spelling F81.81
    written expression F81.81
  lens H27.9
    aphakia —*see* Aphakia
    cataract —*see* Cataract
    dislocation —*see* Dislocation, lens
    specified type NEC H27.8
  ligament M24.20
    ankle M24.27-
    attachment, spine —*see* Enthesopathy,
      spinal
    elbow M24.22-
    foot joint M24.27-
    hand joint M24.24-
    hip M24.25-
    knee —*see* Derangement, knee, specified
      NEC
    shoulder M24.21-
    vertebra M24.28
    wrist M24.23-

Disorder *(Continued)*
  ligamentous attachments —*see also*
    Enthesopathy
    spine —*see* Enthesopathy, spinal
  lipid
    metabolism, congenital E78.9
    storage E75.6
      specified NEC E75.5
  lipoprotein
    deficiency (familial) E78.6
    metabolism E78.9
      specified NEC E78.89
  liver K76.9
    malarial B54 [K77]
  low back —*see also* Dorsopathy, specified
    NEC
  lumbosacral
    plexus G54.1
    root (nerve) NEC G54.4
  lung, interstitial, drug-induced J70.4
    acute J70.2
    chronic J70.3
  lymphoproliferative, post-transplant (PTLD)
    D47.Z1
  lysine and hydroxylysine metabolism E72.3
  major neurocognitive —*see* Dementia, in (due
    to) ◀
  male
    erectile (organic) —*see also* Dysfunction,
      sexual, male, erectile N52.9
      nonorganic F52.21
    hypoactive sexual desire F52.0
    orgasmic F52.32
  manic F30.9
    organic F06.33
  mast cell activation —*see* Activation, mast
    cell ◀
  mastoid —*see also* Disorder, ear, middle
    postprocedural —*see* Complications, ear,
      procedure
  meniscus —*see* Derangement, knee, meniscus
  menopausal N95.9
    specified NEC N95.8
  menstrual N92.6
    psychogenic F45.8
    specified NEC N92.5
  mental (or behavioral) (nonpsychotic) F99
    due to (secondary to)
      amphetamine
        due to drug abuse —*see* Abuse, drug,
          stimulant
        due to drug dependence —*see*
          Dependence, drug, stimulant
      brain disease, damage and dysfunction
        F09
      caffeine use
        due to drug abuse —*see* Abuse, drug,
          stimulant
        due to drug dependence —*see*
          Dependence, drug, stimulant
      cannabis use
        due to drug abuse —*see* Abuse, drug,
          cannabis
        due to drug dependence —*see*
          Dependence, drug, cannabis
      general medical condition F09
      sedative or hypnotic use
        due to drug abuse —*see* Abuse, drug,
          sedative
        due to drug dependence —*see*
          Dependence, drug, sedative
      tobacco (nicotine) use —*see* Dependence,
        drug, nicotine
    following organic brain damage F07.9
      frontal lobe syndrome F07.0
      personality change F07.0
      postconcussional syndrome F07.81
      specified NEC F07.89
    infancy, childhood or adolescence F98.9
    neurotic —*see* Neurosis
    organic or symptomatic F09

Disorder *(Continued)*
  mental *(Continued)*
    presenile, psychotic F03
    problem NEC
    psychoneurotic —*see* Neurosis
    psychotic —*see* Psychosis
    puerperal F53
    senile, psychotic NEC F03
  metabolic, amino acid, transitory, newborn
    P74.8
  metabolism NOS E88.9
    amino-acid E72.9
      aromatic E70.9
        albinism —*see* Albinism
        histidine E70.40
          histidinemia E70.41
          other specified E70.49
        hyperphenylalaninemia E70.1
          classical phenylketonuria E70.0
        other specified E70.8
        tryptophan E70.5
        tyrosine E70.20
          hypertyrosinemia E70.21
          other specified E70.29
      branched chain E71.2
        3-methylglutaconic aciduria E71.111
        hyperleucine-isoleucinemia E71.19
        hypervalinemia E71.19
        isovaleric acidemia E71.110
        maple syrup urine disease E71.0
        methylmalonic acidemia E71.120
        organic aciduria NEC E71.118
        other specified E71.19
        proprionate NEC E71.128
        proprionic acidemia E71.121
      glycine E72.50
        d-glycericacidemia E72.59
        hyperhydroxyprolinemia E72.59
        hyperoxaluria E72.53
        hyperprolinemia E72.59
        non-ketotic hyperglycinemia E72.51
        other specified E72.59
        sarcosinemia E72.59
        trimethylaminuria E72.52
      hydroxylysine E72.3
      lysine E72.3
      ornithine E72.4
      other specified E72.8
        beta-amino acid E72.8
        gamma-glutamyl cycle E72.8
      straight-chain E72.8
      sulfur-bearing E72.10
        homocystinuria E72.11
        methylenetetrahydrofolate reductase
          deficiency E72.12
        other specified E72.19
    bile acid and cholesterol metabolism
      E78.70
    bilirubin E80.7
      specified NEC E80.6
    calcium E83.50
      hypercalcemia E83.52
      hypocalcemia E83.51
      other specified E83.59
    carbohydrate E74.9
      specified NEC E74.8
    cholesterol and bile acid metabolism
      E78.70
    congenital E88.9
    copper E83.00
      specified type NEC E83.09
      Wilson's disease E83.01
    cystinuria E72.01
    fructose E74.10
    galactose E74.20
    glucosaminoglycan E76.9
      mucopolysaccharidosis —*see*
        Mucopolysaccharidosis
      specified NEC E76.8
    glutamine E72.8
    glycine E72.50

Disorder *(Continued)*
  metabolism *(Continued)*
    glycogen storage (hepatorenal) E74.09
    glycoprotein E77.9
      specified NEC E77.8
    glycosaminoglycan E76.9
      specified NEC E76.8
    in labor and delivery O75.89
    iron E83.10
    isoleucine E71.19
    leucine E71.19
    lipoid E78.9
    lipoprotein E78.9
      specified NEC E78.89
    magnesium E83.40
      hypermagnesemia E83.41
      hypomagnesemia E83.42
      other specified E83.49
    mineral E83.9
      specified NEC E83.89
    mitochondrial E88.40
      MELAS syndrome E88.41
      MERRF syndrome (myoclonic epilepsy
        associated with ragged-red fibers)
        E88.42
      other specified E88.49
    ornithine E72.4
    phosphatases E83.30
    phosphorus E83.30
      acid phosphatase deficiency E83.39
      hypophosphatasia E83.39
      hypophosphatemia E83.39
        familial E83.31
      other specified E83.39
      pseudovitamin D deficiency E83.32
    plasma protein NEC E88.09
    porphyrin —*see* Porphyria
    postprocedural E89.89
      specified NEC E89.89
    purine E79.9
      specified NEC E79.8
    pyrimidine E79.9
      specified NEC E79.8
    pyruvate E74.4
    serine E72.8
    sodium E87.8
    specified NEC E88.89
    threonine E72.8
    valine E71.19
    zinc E83.2
  methylmalonic acidemia E71.120
  micturition NEC —*see also* Difficulty,
      micturition R39.198 ◀▥
    feeling of incomplete emptying R39.14
    hesitancy R39.11
    poor stream R39.12
    psychogenic F45.8
    split stream R39.13
    straining R39.16
    urgency R39.15
  mild neurocognitive G31.84 ◀
  mitochondrial metabolism E88.40
  mitral (valve) —*see* Endocarditis, mitral
  mixed
    anxiety and depressive F41.8
    of scholastic skills (developmental)
      F81.89
    receptive expressive language F80.2
  mood F39
    bipolar —*see* Disorder, bipolar
    depressive —*see* Disorder, depressive
    due to (secondary to)
      alcohol F10.94
      amphetamine F15.94
        in
          abuse F15.14
          dependence F15.24
      anxiolytic F13.94
        in
          abuse F13.14
          dependence F13.24

Disorder *(Continued)*
  mood *(Continued)*
    due to *(Continued)*
      cocaine F14.94
        in
          abuse F14.14
          dependence F14.24
      general medical condition F06.30
      hallucinogen F16.94
        in
          abuse F16.14
          dependence F16.24
      hypnotic F13.94
        in
          abuse F13.14
          dependence F13.24
      inhalant F18.94
        in
          abuse F18.14
          dependence F18.24
      opioid F11.94
        in
          abuse F11.14
          dependence F11.24
      phencyclidine (PCP) F16.94
        in
          abuse F16.14
          dependence F16.24
      physiological condition F06.30
        with
          depressive features F06.31
          major depressive-like episode
            F06.32
          manic features F06.33
          mixed features F06.34
      psychoactive substance NEC F19.94
        in
          abuse F19.14
          dependence F19.24
      sedative F13.94
        in
          abuse F13.14
          dependence F13.24
      volatile solvents F18.94
        in
          abuse F18.14
          dependence F18.24
    manic episode F30.9
      with psychotic symptoms F30.2
      without psychotic symptoms F30.10
        mild F30.11
        moderate F30.12
        severe F30.13
      in remission (full) F30.4
        partial F30.3
      specified type NEC F30.8
    organic F06.30
      right hemisphere F07.89
    persistent F34.9
      cyclothymia F34.0
      dysthymia F34.1
      specified type NEC F34.89 ◀▥
    recurrent F39
    right hemisphere organic F07.89
  movement G25.9
    drug-induced G25.70
      akathisia G25.71
      specified NEC G25.79
    hysterical F44.4
    in diseases classified elsewhere —*see*
      category G26
    periodic limb G47.61
      sleep related G47.61
    sleep related NEC G47.69
    specified NEC G25.89
    stereotyped F98.4
    treatment-induced G25.9
  multiple personality F44.81
  muscle M62.9
    attachment, spine —*see* Enthesopathy,
      spinal

Disorder *(Continued)*
  muscle *(Continued)*
    in trichinellosis —*see* Trichinellosis, with
      muscle disorder
    psychogenic F45.8
    specified type NEC M62.89
    tone, newborn P94.9
      specified NEC P94.8
  muscular
    attachments —*see also* Enthesopathy
      spine —*see* Enthesopathy, spinal
    urethra N36.44
  musculoskeletal system, soft tissue —*see*
      Disorder, soft tissue
    postprocedural M96.89
    psychogenic F45.8
  myoneural G70.9
    due to lead G70.1
    specified NEC G70.89
    toxic G70.1
  myotonic NEC G71.19
  nail, in diseases classified elsewhere L62
  neck region NEC —*see* Dorsopathy, specified
      NEC
  neonatal onset multisystemic inflammatory
      (NOMID) M04.2 ◀
  nerve G58.9
    abducent NEC —*see* Strabismus, paralytic,
      sixth nerve
    accessory G52.8
    acoustic —*see* subcategory H93.3
    auditory —*see* subcategory H93.3
    auriculotemporal G50.8
    axillary G54.0
    cerebral —*see* Disorder, nerve, cranial
    cranial G52.9
      eighth —*see* subcategory H93.3
      eleventh G52.8
      fifth G50.9
      first G52.0
      fourth NEC —*see* Strabismus, paralytic,
        fourth nerve
      multiple G52.7
      ninth G52.1
      second NEC —*see* Disorder, nerve, optic
      seventh NEC G51.8
      sixth NEC —*see* Strabismus, paralytic,
        sixth nerve
      specified NEC G52.8
      tenth G52.2
      third NEC —*see* Strabismus, paralytic,
        third nerve
      twelfth G52.3
    entrapment —*see* Neuropathy, entrapment
    facial G51.9
      specified NEC G51.8
    femoral —*see* Lesion, nerve, femoral
    glossopharyngeal NEC G52.1
    hypoglossal G52.3
    intercostal G58.0
    lateral
      cutaneous of thigh —*see*
        Mononeuropathy, lower limb,
        meralgia paresthetica
      popliteal —*see* Lesion, nerve, popliteal
    lower limb —*see* Mononeuropathy, lower
      limb
    medial popliteal —*see* Lesion, nerve,
      popliteal, medial
    median NEC —*see* Lesion, nerve, median
    multiple G58.7
    oculomotor NEC —*see* Strabismus,
      paralytic, third nerve
    olfactory G52.0
    optic NEC H47.09-
      hemorrhage into sheath —*see*
        Hemorrhage, optic nerve
      ischemic H47.01-
    peroneal —*see* Lesion, nerve, popliteal
    phrenic G58.8
    plantar —*see* Lesion, nerve, plantar

◀ New   ◀▥ Revised   ~~deleted~~ Deleted

Disorder *(Continued)*
  nerve *(Continued)*
    pneumogastric G52.2
    posterior tibial —*see* Syndrome, tarsal
      tunnel
    radial —*see* Lesion, nerve, radial
    recurrent laryngeal G52.2
    root G54.9
      cervical G54.2
      lumbosacral G54.1
      specified NEC G54.8
      thoracic G54.3
    sciatic NEC —*see* Lesion, nerve, sciatic
    specified NEC G58.8
      lower limb —*see* Mononeuropathy,
        lower limb, specified NEC
      upper limb —*see* Mononeuropathy,
        upper limb, specified NEC
    sympathetic G90.9
    tibial —*see* Lesion, nerve, popliteal,
      medial
    trigeminal G50.9
      specified NEC G50.8
    trochlear NEC —*see* Strabismus, paralytic,
      fourth nerve
    ulnar —*see* Lesion, nerve, ulnar
    upper limb —*see* Mononeuropathy, upper
      limb
    vagus G52.2
  nervous system G98.8
    autonomic (peripheral) G90.9
      specified NEC G90.8
    central G96.9
      specified NEC G96.8
    parasympathetic G90.9
    specified NEC G98.8
    sympathetic G90.9
    vegetative G90.9
  neurocognitive ◄
    major ◄
      with ◄
        aggressive behavior F01.51 ◄
        combative behavior F01.51 ◄
        violent behavior F01.51 ◄
      due to vascular disease, with behavioral
        disturbance F01.51 ◄
      in (due to) (other diseases classified
        elsewhere) —*see also* Dementia, in
        (due to) F02.80 ◄
        with ◄
          aggressive behavior F02.81 ◄
          combative behavior F02.81 ◄
          violent behavior F02.81 ◄
        without behavioral disturbance
          F01.50 ◄
    mild G31.84 ◄
  neurodevelopmental F89 ◄
    specified NEC F88 ◄
  neurohypophysis NEC E23.3
  neurological NEC R29.818
  neuromuscular G70.9
    hereditary NEC G71.9
    specified NEC G70.89
    toxic G70.1
  neurotic F48.9
    specified NEC F48.8
  neutrophil, polymorphonuclear D71
  nicotine use —*see* Dependence, drug,
    nicotine
  nightmare F51.5
  nose J34.9
    specified NEC J34.89
  obsessive-compulsive F42.9 ◄▥
  odontogenesis NOS K00.9
  opioid use
    with
      opioid-induced psychotic disorder
        F11.959
        with
          delusions F11.950
          hallucinations F11.951

Disorder *(Continued)*
  opioid use *(Continued)*
    due to drug abuse —*see* Abuse, drug,
      opioid
    due to drug dependence —*see* Dependence,
      drug, opioid
    mild F11.10 ◄
      with ◄
        opioid-induced ◄
          anxiety disorder F11.188 ◄
          depressive disorder F11.14 ◄
          sexual dysfunction F11.181 ◄
        opioid intoxication ◄
          with perceptual disturbances
            F11.122 ◄
          delirium F11.121 ◄
          without perceptual disturbances
            F11.129 ◄
    moderate or severe F11.20 ◄
      with ◄
        opioid-induced ◄
          anxiety disorder F11.288 ◄
          anxiety disorder F11.988 ◄
          depressive disorder F11.24 ◄
          depressive disorder F11.94 ◄
          sexual dysfunction F11.281 ◄
          sexual dysfunction F11.981 ◄
        opioid intoxication ◄
          with perceptual disturbances
            F11.222 ◄
          delirium F11.221 ◄
          without perceptual disturbances
            F11.229 ◄
  oppositional defiant F91.3
  optic
    chiasm H47.49
      due to
        inflammatory disorder H47.41
        neoplasm H47.42
        vascular disorder H47.43
    disc H47.39-
      coloboma —*see* Coloboma, optic disc
      drusen —*see* Drusen, optic disc
      pseudopapilledema —*see*
        Pseudopapilledema
    radiations —*see* Disorder, visual, pathway
    tracts —*see* Disorder, visual, pathway
  orbit H05.9
    cyst —*see* Cyst, orbit
    deformity —*see* Deformity, orbit
    edema —*see* Edema, orbit
    enophthalmos —*see* Enophthalmos
    exophthalmos —*see* Exophthalmos
    hemorrhage —*see* Hemorrhage, orbit
    inflammation —*see* Inflammation, orbit
    myopathy —*see* Myopathy, extraocular
      muscles
    retained foreign body —*see* Foreign body,
      orbit, old
    specified type NEC H05.89
  organic
    anxiety F06.4
    catatonic F06.1
    delusional F06.2
    dissociative F06.8
    emotionally labile (asthenic) F06.8
    mood (affective) F06.30
    schizophrenia-like F06.2
  orgasmic (female) F52.31
    male F52.32
  ornithine metabolism E72.4
  overanxious F41.1
    of childhood F93.8
  pain
    with related psychological factors F45.42
    exclusively related to psychological factors
      F45.41
    genito-pelvic penetration disorder
      F52.6 ◄
  pancreatic internal secretion E16.9
    specified NEC E16.8

Disorder *(Continued)*
  panic F41.0
    with agoraphobia F40.01
  papulosquamous L44.9
    in diseases classified elsewhere L45
    specified NEC L44.8
  paranoid F22
    induced F24
    shared F24
  parathyroid (gland) E21.5
    specified NEC E21.4
  parietoalveolar NEC J84.09
  paroxysmal, mixed R56.9
  patella M22.9-
    chondromalacia —*see* Chondromalacia,
      patella
    derangement NEC M22.3X-
    recurrent
      dislocation —*see* Dislocation, patella,
        recurrent
      subluxation —*see* Dislocation, patella,
        recurrent, incomplete
    specified NEC M22.8X-
  patellofemoral M22.2X-
  pentose phosphate pathway with anemia
    D55.1
  perception, due to hallucinogens F16.983
    in
      abuse F16.183
      dependence F16.283
  peripheral nervous system NEC G64
  peroxisomal E71.50
    biogenesis
      neonatal adrenoleukodystrophy E71.511
      specified disorder NEC E71.518
      Zellweger syndrome E71.510
    rhizomelic chondrodysplasia punctata
      E71.540
    specified form NEC E71.548
      group 1 E71.518
      group 2 E71.53
      group 3 E71.542
    X-linked adrenoleukodystrophy
      E71.529
      adolescent E71.521
      adrenomyeloneuropathy E71.522
      childhood E71.520
      specified form NEC E71.528
    Zellweger-like syndrome E71.541
  persistent
    (somatoform) pain F45.41
    affective (mood) F34.9
  personality —*see also* Personality F60.9
    affective F34.0
    aggressive F60.3
    amoral F60.2
    anankastic F60.5
    antisocial F60.2
    anxious F60.6
    asocial F60.2
    asthenic F60.7
    avoidant F60.6
    borderline F60.3
    change (secondary) due to general medical
      condition F07.0
    compulsive F60.5
    cyclothymic F34.0
    dependent (passive) F60.7
    depressive F34.1
    dissocial F60.2
    emotional instability F60.3
    expansive paranoid F60.0
    explosive F60.3
    following organic brain damage
      F07.9
    histrionic F60.4
    hyperthymic F34.0
    hypothymic F34.1
    hysterical F60.4
    immature F60.89
    inadequate F60.7

Disorder *(Continued)*
  personality *(Continued)*
    labile F60.3
    mixed (nonspecific) F60.89
    moral deficiency F60.2
    narcissistic F60.81
    negativistic F60.89
    obsessional F60.5
    obsessive (-compulsive) F60.5
    organic F07.9
    overconscientious F60.5
    paranoid F60.0
    passive (-dependent) F60.7
    passive-aggressive F60.89
    pathological NEC F60.9
    pseudosocial F60.2
    psychopathic F60.2
    schizoid F60.1
    schizotypal F21
    self-defeating F60.7
    specified NEC F60.89
    type A F60.5
    unstable (emotional) F60.3
  pervasive, developmental F84.9
  phencyclidine use ◄
    mild F16.10 ◄
      with ◄
        phencyclidine-induced ◄
          anxiety disorder F16.180 ◄
          bipolar and related disorder
            F16.14 ◄
          depressive disorder F16.14 ◄
          psychotic disorder F16.159 ◄
        phencyclidine intoxication
          F16.129 ◄
        phencyclidine intoxication delirium
          F16.121 ◄
    moderate or severe F16.20 ◄
      with ◄
        phencyclidine-induced ◄
          anxiety disorder F16.280 ◄
          bipolar and related disorder
            F16.24 ◄
          depressive disorder F16.24 ◄
          psychotic disorder F16.259 ◄
        phencyclidine intoxication F16.229 ◄
        phencyclidine intoxication delirium
          F16.221 ◄
  phobic anxiety, childhood F40.8
  phosphate-losing tubular N25.0
  pigmentation L81.9
    choroid, congenital Q14.3
    diminished melanin formation L81.6
    iron L81.8
    specified NEC L81.8
  pinna (noninfective) H61.10-
    deformity, acquired H61.11-
    hematoma H61.12-
    perichondritis —see Perichondritis, ear
    specified type NEC H61.19-
  pituitary gland E23.7
    iatrogenic (postprocedural) E89.3
    specified NEC E23.6
  platelets D69.1
  plexus G54.9
    specified NEC G54.8
  polymorphonuclear neutrophils D71
  porphyrin metabolism —see Porphyria
  postconcussional F07.81
  posthallucinogen perception F16.983
    in
      abuse F16.183
      dependence F16.283
  postmenopausal N95.9
    specified NEC N95.8
  postprocedural (postoperative) —see
    Complications, postprocedural
  post-transplant lymphoproliferative D47.z1
  post-traumatic stress (PTSD) F43.10
    acute F43.11
    chronic F43.12

Disorder *(Continued)*
  premenstrual dysphoric (PMDD) F32.81 ◄⊪
  prepuce N47.8
  propionic acidemia E71.121
  prostate N42.9
    specified NEC N42.89
  psychogenic NOS —see also condition F45.9
    anxiety F41.8
    appetite F50.9
    asthenic F48.8
    cardiovascular (system) F45.8
    compulsive F42.8 ◄⊪
    cutaneous F54
    depressive F32.9
    digestive (system) F45.8
    dysmenorrheic F45.8
    dyspneic F45.8
    endocrine (system) F54
    eye NEC F45.8
    feeding —see Disorder, eating
    functional NEC F45.8
    gastric F45.8
    gastrointestinal (system) F45.8
    genitourinary (system) F45.8
    heart (function) (rhythm) F45.8
    hyperventilatory F45.8
    hypochondriacal —see Disorder,
      hypochondriacal
    intestinal F45.8
    joint F45.8
    learning F81.9
    limb F45.8
    lymphatic (system) F45.8
    menstrual F45.8
    micturition F45.8
    monoplegic NEC F44.4
    motor F44.4
    muscle F45.8
    musculoskeletal F45.8
    neurocirculatory F45.8
    obsessive F42.8 ◄⊪
    occupational F48.8
    organ or part of body NEC F45.8
    paralytic NEC F44.4
    phobic F40.9
    physical NEC F45.8
    rectal F45.8
    respiratory (system) F45.8
    rheumatic F45.8
    sexual (function) F52.9
    skin (allergic) (eczematous) F54
    sleep F51.9
    specified part of body NEC F45.8
    stomach F45.8
  psychological F99
    associated with
      disease classified elsewhere F54
      sexual
        development F66
        relationship F66
        uncertainty about gender identity
          F64.9 ◄⊪
  psychomotor NEC F44.4
    hysterical F44.4
  psychoneurotic —see also Neurosis
    mixed NEC F48.8
  psychophysiologic —see Disorder,
    somatoform
  psychosexual F65.9
    development F66
    identity of childhood F64.2
  psychosomatic NOS —see Disorder,
    somatoform
    multiple F45.0
    undifferentiated F45.1
  psychotic —see Psychosis
    transient (acute) F23
  puberty E30.9
    specified NEC E30.8
  pulmonary (valve) —see Endocarditis,
    pulmonary

Disorder *(Continued)*
  purine metabolism E79.9
  pyrimidine metabolism E79.9
  pyruvate metabolism E74.4
  reactive attachment (childhood) F94.1
  reading R48.0
    developmental (specific) F81.0
  receptive language F80.2
  receptor, hormonal, peripheral —see also
      Syndrome, androgen insensitivity
      E34.50
  recurrent brief depressive F33.8
  reflex R29.2
  refraction H52.7
    aniseikonia H52.32
    anisometropia H52.31
    astigmatism —see Astigmatism
    hypermetropia —see Hypermetropia
    myopia —see Myopia
    presbyopia H52.4
    specified NEC H52.6
  relationship F68.8
    due to sexual orientation F66
  REM sleep behavior G47.52
  renal function, impaired (tubular) N25.9
  resonance R49.9
    specified NEC R49.8
  respiratory function, impaired —see also
      Failure, respiration
    postprocedural —see Complication,
      postoperative, respiratory system
    psychogenic F45.8
  retina H35.9
    angioid streaks H35.33
    changes in vascular appearance H35.01-
    degeneration —see Degeneration, retina
    dystrophy (hereditary) —see Dystrophy,
      retina
    edema H35.81
    hemorrhage —see Hemorrhage, retina
    ischemia H35.82
    macular degeneration —see Degeneration,
      macula
    microaneurysms H35.04-
    microvascular abnormality NEC
      H35.09
    neovascularization —see
      Neovascularization, retina
    retinopathy —see Retinopathy
    separation of layers H35.70
      central serous chorioretinopathy
        H35.71-
      pigment epithelium detachment (serous)
        H35.72-
      hemorrhagic H35.73-
    specified type NEC H35.89
    telangiectasis —see Telangiectasis, retina
    vasculitis —see Vasculitis, retina
  retroperitoneal K68.9
  right hemisphere organic affective F07.89
  rumination (infant or child) F98.21
  sacrum, sacrococcygeal NEC M53.3
  schizoaffective F25.9
    bipolar type F25.0
    depressive type F25.1
    manic type F25.0
    mixed type F25.0
    specified NEC F25.8
  schizoid of childhood F84.5
  schizophreniform F20.81
    brief F23
  schizotypal (personality) F21
  secretion, thyrocalcitonin E07.0
  sedative, hypnotic, or anxiolytic use ◄
    mild F13.10 ◄
      with ◄
        sedative, hypnotic, or anxiolytic-
          induced ◄
          anxiety disorder F13.180 ◄
          bipolar and related disorder
            F13.14 ◄

◄ New   ◄⊪ Revised   ~~deleted~~ Deleted

Disorder *(Continued)*
  sedative, hypnotic, or anxiolytic use
    (Continued)
    mild *(Continued)*
      with *(Continued)*
        sedative, hypnotic, or anxiolytic-
          induced *(Continued)*
          depressive disorder F13.14 ◄
          psychotic disorder F13.159 ◄
          sexual dysfunction F13.181 ◄
        sedative, hypnotic, or anxiolytic
          intoxication F13.129 ◄
        sedative, hypnotic, or anxiolytic
          intoxication delirium F13.121 ◄
    moderate or severe F13.20 ◄
      with ◄
        sedative, hypnotic, or anxiolytic-
          induced ◄
          anxiety disorder F13.280 ◄
          bipolar and related disorder
            F13.24 ◄
          depressive disorder F13.24 ◄
          major neurocognitive disorder
            F13.27 ◄
          mild neurocognitive disorder
            F13.288 ◄
          psychotic disorder F13.259 ◄
          sexual dysfunction F13.281 ◄
        sedative, hypnotic, or anxiolytic
          intoxication F13.229 ◄
        sedative, hypnotic, or anxiolytic
          intoxication delirium F13.221 ◄
  seizure —*see also* Epilepsy G40.909
    intractable G40.919
      with status epilepticus G40.911
  semantic pragmatic F80.89
    with autism F84.0
  sense of smell R43.1
    psychogenic F45.8
  separation anxiety, of childhood F93.0
  sexual
    arousal, female F52.22
    aversion F52.1
    function, psychogenic F52.9
    maturation F66
    nonorganic F52.9
    preference —*see also* Deviation, sexual
      F65.9
      fetishistic transvestism F65.1
    relationship F66
  shyness, of childhood and adolescence F40.10
  sibling rivalry F93.8
  sickle-cell (sickling) (homozygous) —*see*
    Disease, sickle-cell
    heterozygous D57.3
    specified type NEC D57.8-
    trait D57.3
  sinus (nasal) J34.9
    specified NEC J34.89
  skin L98.9
    atrophic L90.9
      specified NEC L90.8
    granulomatous L92.9
      specified NEC L92.8
    hypertrophic L91.9
      specified NEC L91.8
    infiltrative NEC L98.6
    newborn P83.9
      specified NEC P83.8
    picking F42.4 ◄
    psychogenic (allergic) (eczematous) F54
  sleep G47.9
    breathing-related —*see* Apnea, sleep
    circadian rhythm G47.20
      advance sleep phase type G47.22
      delayed sleep phase type G47.21
      due to
        alcohol
          abuse F10.182
          dependence F10.282
          use F10.982

Disorder *(Continued)*
  sleep *(Continued)*
    circadian rhythm *(Continued)*
      due to *(Continued)*
        amphetamines
          abuse F15.182
          dependence F15.282
          use F15.982
        caffeine
          abuse F15.182
          dependence F15.282
          use F15.982
        cocaine
          abuse F14.182
          dependence F14.282
          use F14.982
        drug NEC
          abuse F19.182
          dependence F19.282
          use F19.982
        opioid
          abuse F11.182
          dependence F11.282
          use F11.982
        psychoactive substance NEC
          abuse F19.182
          dependence F19.282
          use F19.982
        sedative, hypnotic, or anxiolytic
          abuse F13.182
          dependence F13.282
          use F13.982
        stimulant NEC
          abuse F15.182
          dependence F15.282
          use F15.982
      free running type G47.24
      in conditions classified elsewhere
        G47.27
      irregular sleep wake type
        G47.23
      jet lag type G47.25
      shift work type G47.26
      specified NEC G47.29
    due to
      alcohol
        abuse F10.182
        dependence F10.282
        use F10.982
      amphetamine
        abuse F15.182
        dependence F15.282
        use F15.982
      anxiolytic
        abuse F13.182
        dependence F13.282
        use F13.982
      caffeine
        abuse F15.182
        dependence F15.282
        use F15.982
      cocaine
        abuse F14.182
        dependence F14.282
        use F14.982
      drug NEC
        abuse F19.182
        dependence F19.282
        use F19.982
      hypnotic
        abuse F13.182
        dependence F13.282
        use F13.982
      opioid
        abuse F11.182
        dependence F11.282
        use F11.982
      psychoactive substance NEC
        abuse F19.182
        dependence F19.282
        use F19.982

Disorder *(Continued)*
  sleep *(Continued)*
    due to *(Continued)*
      sedative
        abuse F13.182
        dependence F13.282
        use F13.982
      stimulant NEC
        abuse F15.182
        dependence F15.282
        use F15.982
    emotional F51.9
    excessive somnolence —*see* Hypersomnia
    hypersomnia type —*see* Hypersomnia
    initiating or maintaining —*see* Insomnia
    nightmares F51.5
    nonorganic F51.9
      specified NEC F51.8
    parasomnia type G47.50
    specified NEC G47.8
    terrors F51.4
    walking F51.3
  sleep-wake pattern or schedule —*see*
    Disorder, sleep, circadian rhythm
  social
    anxiety of childhood F40.10
    functioning in childhood F94.9
      specified NEC F94.8
    pragmatic F80.82 ◄
  soft tissue M79.9
    ankle M79.9
    due to use, overuse and pressure
      M70.90
      ankle M70.97-
      bursitis —*see* Bursitis
      foot M70.97-
      forearm M70.93-
      hand M70.94-
      lower leg M70.96-
      multiple sites M70.99
      pelvic region M70.95-
      shoulder region M70.91-
      specified site NEC M70.98
      specified type NEC M70.80
        ankle M70.87-
        foot M70.87-
        forearm M70.83-
        hand M70.84-
        lower leg M70.86-
        multiple sites M70.89
        pelvic region M70.85-
        shoulder region M70.81-
        specified site NEC M70.88
        thigh M70.85-
        upper arm M70.82-
      thigh M70.95-
      upper arm M70.92-
    foot M79.9
    forearm M79.9
    hand M79.9
    lower leg M79.9
    multiple sites M79.9
    occupational —*see* Disorder, soft tissue,
      due to use, overuse and pressure
    pelvic region M79.9
    shoulder region M79.9
    specified type NEC M79.89
    thigh M79.9
    upper arm M79.9
  somatic symptom F45.1 ◄
  somatization F45.0
  somatoform F45.9
    pain (persistent) F45.41
    somatization (multiple) (long-lasting) F45.0
    specified NEC F45.8
    undifferentiated F45.1
  somnolence, excessive —*see* Hypersomnia
  specific
    arithmetical F81.2
    developmental, of motor F82
    reading F81.0

◀ New   ▥ Revised   ~~deleted~~ Deleted

Disorder (*Continued*)
  white blood cells D72.9
    specified NEC D72.89
  withdrawing, child or adolescent
    F40.10
Disorientation R41.0
Displacement, displaced
  acquired traumatic of bone, cartilage, joint,
    tendon NEC —*see* Dislocation
  adrenal gland (congenital) Q89.1
  appendix, retrocecal (congenital) Q43.8
  auricle (congenital) Q17.4
  bladder (acquired) N32.89
    congenital Q64.19
  brachial plexus (congenital) Q07.8
  brain stem, caudal (congenital) Q04.8
  canaliculus (lacrimalis), congenital Q10.6
  cardia through esophageal hiatus (congenital)
    Q40.1
  cerebellum, caudal (congenital) Q04.8
  cervix —*see* Malposition, uterus
  colon (congenital) Q43.3
  device, implant or graft —*see also*
    Complications, by site and type,
    mechanical T85.628
    arterial graft NEC —*see* Complication,
      cardiovascular device, mechanical,
      vascular
    breast (implant) T85.42
    catheter NEC T85.628
      dialysis (renal) T82.42
        intraperitoneal T85.621
      infusion NEC T82.524
        spinal (epidural) (subdural)
          T85.620
      urinary ◀▥
        cystostomy T83.020
        Hopkins T83.028 ◀
        ileostomy T83.028 ◀
        indwelling T83.021 ◀
        nephrostomy T83.022 ◀
        specified NEC T83.028 ◀
        urostomy T83.028 ◀
    electronic (electrode) (pulse generator)
      (stimulator) —*see* Complication,
      electronic stimulator
    fixation, internal (orthopedic) NEC —*see*
      Complication, fixation device,
      mechanical
    gastrointestinal —*see* Complications,
      prosthetic device, mechanical,
      gastrointestinal device
    genital NEC T83.428
      intrauterine contraceptive device (string)
        T83.32 ◀▥
      penile prosthesis (cylinder) (implanted)
        (pump) (resevoir) T83.420 ◀▥
      testicular prosthesis T83.421 ◀
    heart NEC —*see* Complication,
      cardiovascular device, mechanical
    joint prosthesis —*see* Complications, joint
      prosthesis, mechanical
    ocular —*see* Complications, prosthetic
      device, mechanical, ocular device
    orthopedic NEC —*see* Complication,
      orthopedic, device or graft,
      mechanical
    specified NEC T85.628
    urinary NEC T83.128 ◀▥
      graft T83.22
      sphincter, implanted T83.121 ◀
      stent (ileal conduit) (nephroureteral)
        T83.123 ◀
        ureteral indwelling T83.122 ◀
    vascular NEC —*see* Complication,
      cardiovascular device, mechanical
    ventricular intracranial shunt T85.02
  electronic stimulator
    bone T84.320
    cardiac —*see* Complications, cardiac
      device, electronic

Displacement, displaced (*Continued*)
  electronic stimulator (*Continued*)
    nervous system —*see* Complication,
      prosthetic device, mechanical,
      electronic nervous system
      stimulator
    urinary —*see* Complications, electronic
      stimulator, urinary
  esophageal mucosa into cardia of stomach,
    congenital Q39.8
  esophagus (acquired) K22.8
    congenital Q39.8
  eyeball (acquired) (lateral) (old) —*see*
    Displacement, globe
    congenital Q15.8
    current —*see* Avulsion, eye
  fallopian tube (acquired) N83.4- ◀▥
    congenital Q50.6
    opening (congenital) Q50.6
  gallbladder (congenital) Q44.1
  gastric mucosa (congenital) Q40.2
  globe (acquired) (old) (lateral) H05.21-
    current —*see* Avulsion, eye
  heart (congenital) Q24.8
    acquired I51.89
  hymen (upward) (congenital) Q52.4
  intervertebral disc NEC
    with myelopathy —*see* Disorder, disc, with,
      myelopathy
    cervical, cervicothoracic (with)
      M50.20
      myelopathy —*see* Disorder, disc,
        cervical, with myelopathy
      neuritis, radiculitis or radiculopathy —
        see Disorder, disc, cervical, with
        neuritis
    due to trauma —*see* Dislocation, vertebra
    lumbar region M51.26
      with
        neuritis, radiculitis, radiculopathy or
          sciatica M51.16
    lumbosacral region M51.27
      with
        myelopathy M51.07
        neuritis, radiculitis, radiculopathy or
          sciatica M51.17
    sacrococcygeal region M53.3
    thoracic region M51.24
      with
        myelopathy M51.04
        neuritis, radiculitis, radiculopathy
          M51.14
    thoracolumbar region M51.25
      with
        myelopathy M51.05
        neuritis, radiculitis, radiculopathy
          M51.15
  intrauterine device (string) T83.32 ◀▥
  kidney (acquired) N28.83
    congenital Q63.2
  lachrymal, lacrimal apparatus or duct
    (congenital) Q10.6
  lens, congenital Q12.1
  macula (congenital) Q14.1
  Meckel's diverticulum Q43.0
    malignant —*see* Table of Neoplasms, small
      intestine, malignant
  nail (congenital) Q84.6
    acquired L60.8
  opening of Wharton's duct in mouth Q38.4
  organ or site, congenital NEC —*see*
    Malposition, congenital
  ovary (acquired) N83.4- ◀▥
    congenital Q50.39
    free in peritoneal cavity (congenital)
      Q50.39
    into hernial sac N83.4- ◀▥
  oviduct (acquired) N83.4- ◀▥
    congenital Q50.6
  parathyroid (gland) E21.4
  parotid gland (congenital) Q38.4

Displacement, displaced (*Continued*)
  punctum lacrimale (congenital) Q10.6
  sacro-iliac (joint) (congenital) Q74.2
    current injury S33.2
    old —*see* subcategory M53.2
  salivary gland (any) (congenital) Q38.4
  spleen (congenital) Q89.09
  stomach, congenital Q40.2
  sublingual duct Q38.4
  tongue (downward) (congenital) Q38.3
  tooth, teeth, fully erupted M26.30
    horizontal M26.33
    vertical M26.34
  trachea (congenital) Q32.1
  ureter or ureteric opening or orifice
    (congenital) Q62.62
  uterine opening of oviducts or fallopian tubes
    Q50.6
  uterus, uterine —*see* Malposition, uterus
  ventricular septum Q21.0
    with rudimentary ventricle Q20.4
Disproportion
  between native and reconstructed breast N65.1
  fiber-type G71.2
Disruptio uteri —*see* Rupture, uterus
Disruption (of)
  ciliary body NEC H21.89
  closure of
    cornea T81.31
    craniotomy T81.32
    fascia (muscular) (superficial) T81.32
    internal organ or tissue T81.32
    laceration (external) (internal) T81.33
    ligament T81.32
    mucosa T81.31
    muscle or muscle flap T81.32
    ribs or rib cage T81.32
    skin and subcutaneous tissue (full-
      thickness) (superficial) T81.31
    skull T81.32
    sternum (sternotomy) T81.32
    tendon T81.32
    traumatic laceration (external) (internal)
      T81.33
  family Z63.8
    due to
      absence of family member due to
        military deployment Z63.31
      absence of family member NEC Z63.32
      alcoholism and drug addiction in family
        Z63.72
      bereavement Z63.4
      death (assumed) or disappearance of
        family member Z63.4
      divorce or separation Z63.5
      drug addiction in family Z63.72
      return of family member from military
        deployment (current or past
        conflict) Z63.71
      stressful life events NEC Z63.79
  iris NEC H21.89
  ligament (s) —*see also* Sprain
    knee
      current injury —*see* Dislocation, knee
      old (chronic) —*see* Derangement, knee,
        ligament, instability, chronic
      spontaneous NEC —*see* Derangement,
        knee, disruption ligament
  ossicular chain —*see* Discontinuity, ossicles, ear
  pelvic ring (stable) S32.810
    unstable S32.811
  traumatic injury wound repair T81.33
  wound T81.30
    episiotomy O90.1
    operation T81.31
      cesarean O90.0
      external operation wound (superficial)
        T81.31
      internal operation wound (deep) T81.32
    perineal (obstetric) O90.1
  traumatic injury repair T81.33

Dissatisfaction with
  employment Z56.9
  school environment Z55.4
Dissecting —see condition
Dissection
  aorta I71.00
    abdominal I71.02
    thoracic I71.01
    thoracoabdominal I71.03
  artery I77.70 ◄▥
    basilar (trunk) I77.75 ◄
    carotid I77.71
    cerebral (nonruptured) I67.0
      ruptured —see Hemorrhage, intracranial,
        subarachnoid
    coronary I25.42
    extremity ◄
      lower I77.77 ◄
      upper I77.76 ◄
    iliac I77.72 ◄
    precerebral ◄
      congenital (nonruptured) Q28.1 ◄
      specified site NEC I77.75 ◄
    renal I77.73
    specified NEC I77.79
    vertebral I77.74
  traumatic —see Wound, open, by site
  vascular I99.8
  wound —see Wound, open
Disseminated —see condition
Dissociation
  auriculoventricular or atrioventricular (AV)
    (any degree) (isorhythmic) I45.89
    with heart block I44.2
  interference I45.89
Dissociative reaction, state F44.9
Dissolution, vertebra —see Osteoporosis
Distension, distention
  abdomen R14.0
  bladder N32.89
  cecum K63.89
  colon K63.89
  gallbladder K82.8
  intestine K63.89
  kidney N28.89
  liver K76.89
  seminal vesicle N50.89 ◄▥
  stomach K31.89
    acute K31.0
    psychogenic F45.8
  ureter —see Dilatation, ureter
  uterus N85.8
Distoma hepaticum infestation B66.3
Distomiasis B66.9
  bile passages B66.3
  hemic B65.9
  hepatic B66.3
    due to Clonorchis sinensis B66.1
  intestinal B66.5
  liver B66.3
    due to Clonorchis sinensis B66.1
  lung B66.4
  pulmonary B66.4
Distomolar (fourth molar) K00.1
Disto-occlusion (Division I) (Division II)
  M26.212
Distortion (s) (congenital)
  adrenal (gland) Q89.1
  arm NEC Q68.8
  bile duct or passage Q44.5
  bladder Q64.79
  brain Q04.9
  cervix (uteri) Q51.9
  chest (wall) Q67.8
    bones Q76.8
  clavicle Q74.0
  clitoris Q52.6
  coccyx Q76.49
  common duct Q44.5
  coronary Q24.5
  cystic duct Q44.5

Distortion (Continued)
  ear (auricle) (external) Q17.3
    inner Q16.5
    middle Q16.4
      ossicles Q16.3
  endocrine NEC Q89.2
  eustachian tube Q17.8
  eye (adnexa) Q15.8
  face bone (s) NEC Q75.8
  fallopian tube Q50.6
  femur NEC Q68.8
  fibula NEC Q68.8
  finger (s) Q68.1
  foot Q66.9
  genitalia, genital organ (s)
    female Q52.8
      external Q52.79
      internal NEC Q52.8
  gyri Q04.8
  hand bone (s) Q68.1
  heart (auricle) (ventricle) Q24.8
    valve (cusp) Q24.8
  hepatic duct Q44.5
  humerus NEC Q68.8
  hymen Q52.4
  intrafamilial communications
    Z63.8
  jaw NEC M26.89
  labium (majus) (minus) Q52.79
  leg NEC Q68.8
  lens Q12.8
  liver Q44.7
  lumbar spine Q76.49
    with disproportion O33.8
      causing obstructed labor O65.0
  lumbosacral (joint) (region) Q76.49
    kyphosis —see Kyphosis, congenital
    lordosis —see Lordosis, congenital
  nerve Q07.8
  nose Q30.8
  organ
    of Corti Q16.5
    or site not listed —see Anomaly, by site
      ossicles, ear Q16.3
  oviduct Q50.6
  pancreas Q45.3
  parathyroid (gland) Q89.2
  pituitary (gland) Q89.2
  radius NEC Q68.8
  sacroiliac joint Q74.2
  sacrum Q76.49
  scapula Q74.0
  shoulder girdle Q74.0
  skull bone (s) NEC Q75.8
    with
      anencephalus Q00.0
      encephalocele —see Encephalocele
      hydrocephalus Q03.9
        with spina bifida —see Spina bifida,
          with hydrocephalus
      microcephaly Q02
  spinal cord Q06.8
  spine Q76.49
    kyphosis —see Kyphosis, congenital
    lordosis —see Lordosis, congenital
  spleen Q89.09
  sternum NEC Q76.7
  thorax (wall) Q67.8
    bony Q76.8
  thymus (gland) Q89.2
  thyroid (gland) Q89.2
  tibia NEC Q68.8
  toe (s) Q66.9
  tongue Q38.3
  trachea (cartilage) Q32.1
  ulna NEC Q68.8
  ureter Q62.8
  urethra Q64.79
    causing obstruction Q64.39
  uterus Q51.9
  vagina Q52.4

Distortion (Continued)
  vertebra Q76.49
    kyphosis —see Kyphosis, congenital
    lordosis —see Lordosis, congenital
  visual —see also Disturbance, vision
    shape and size H53.15
  vulva Q52.79
  wrist (bones) (joint) Q68.8
Distress
  abdomen —see Pain, abdominal
  acute respiratory R06.00 ◄▥
    syndrome (adult) (child) J80 ◄
  epigastric R10.13
  fetal P84
    complicating pregnancy —see Stress, fetal
  gastrointestinal (functional) K30
    psychogenic F45.8
  intestinal (functional) NOS K59.9
    psychogenic F45.8
  maternal, during labor and delivery O75.0
  respiratory (adult) (child) R06.00 ◄▥
    ~~adult J80~~
    ~~child J80~~
    newborn P22.9
      specified NEC P22.8
    orthopnea R06.01
    psychogenic F45.8
    shortness of breath R06.02
    specified type NEC R06.09
Distribution vessel, atypical Q27.9
  coronary artery Q24.5
  precerebral Q28.1
Districhiasis L68.8
Disturbance (s) —see also Disease
  absorption K90.9
    calcium E58
    carbohydrate K90.49 ◄▥
    fat K90.49 ◄▥
      pancreatic K90.3
    protein K90.49 ◄▥
    starch K90.49 ◄▥
    vitamin —see Deficiency, vitamin
  acid-base equilibrium E87.8
    mixed E87.4
  activity and attention (with hyperkinesis) —
    see Disorder, attention-deficit
    hyperactivity
  amino acid transport E72.00
  assimilation, food K90.9
  auditory nerve, except deafness —see
    subcategory H93.3
  behavior —see Disorder, conduct
  blood clotting (mechanism) —see also Defect,
    coagulation D68.9
  cerebral
    nerve —see Disorder, nerve, cranial
    status, newborn P91.9
      specified NEC P91.8
  circulatory I99.9
  conduct —see also Disorder, conduct F91.9
    adjustment reaction —see Disorder,
      adjustment
    compulsive F63.9
    disruptive F91.9
    hyperkinetic —see Disorder, attention-
      deficit hyperactivity
    socialized F91.2
    specified NEC F91.8
    unsocialized F91.1
  coordination R27.8
  cranial nerve —see Disorder, nerve, cranial
  deep sensibility —see Disturbance,
    sensation
  digestive K30
    psychogenic F45.8
  electrolyte —see also Imbalance, electrolyte
    newborn, transitory P74.4
      hyperammonemia P74.6
      potassium balance P74.3
      sodium balance P74.2
      specified type NEC P74.4

◄ New   ◄▥ Revised   ~~deleted~~ Deleted

Disturbance *(Continued)*
 emotions specific to childhood and
   adolescence F93.9
  with
   anxiety and fearfulness NEC F93.8
   elective mutism F94.0
   oppositional disorder F91.3
   sensitivity (withdrawal) F40.10
   shyness F40.10
   social withdrawal F40.10
  involving relationship problems
    F93.8
  mixed F93.8
  specified NEC F93.8
 endocrine (gland) E34.9
  neonatal, transitory P72.9
   specified NEC P72.8
 equilibrium R42
 fructose metabolism E74.10
 gait —*see* Gait
  hysterical F44.4
  psychogenic F44.4
 gastrointestinal (functional) K30
  psychogenic F45.8
 habit, child F98.9
 hearing, except deafness and tinnitus —*see*
   Abnormal, auditory perception
 heart, functional (conditions in I44-I50)
  due to presence of (cardiac) prosthesis
    I97.19-
  postoperative I97.89
   cardiac surgery I97.19-
 hormones E34.9
 innervation uterus (parasympathetic)
   (sympathetic) N85.8
 keratinization NEC
  gingiva K05.10
   nonplaque induced K05.11
   plaque induced K05.10
  lip K13.0
  oral (mucosa) (soft tissue) K13.29
  tongue K13.29
 learning (specific) —*see* Disorder,
   learning
 memory —*see* Amnesia
  mild, following organic brain damage
    F06.8
 mental F99
  associated with diseases classified
    elsewhere F54
 metabolism E88.9
  with
   abortion —*see* Abortion, by type with
     other specified complication
   ectopic pregnancy O08.5
   molar pregnancy O08.5
  amino-acid E72.9
   aromatic E70.9
   branched-chain E71.2
   straight-chain E72.8
   sulfur-bearing E72.10
  ammonia E72.20
  arginine E72.21
  arginosuccinic acid E72.22
  carbohydrate E74.9
  cholesterol E78.9
  citrulline E72.23
  cystathionine E72.19
  general E88.9
  glutamine E72.8
  histidine E70.40
  homocystine E72.19
  hydroxylysine E72.3
  in labor or delivery O75.89
  iron E83.10
  lipoid E78.9
  lysine E72.3
  methionine E72.19
  neonatal, transitory P74.9
   calcium and magnesium P71.9
    specified type NEC P71.8

Disturbance *(Continued)*
 metabolism *(Continued)*
  neonatal, transitory *(Continued)*
   carbohydrate metabolism P70.9
    specified type NEC P70.8
   specified NEC P74.8
  ornithine E72.4
  phosphate E83.39
  sodium NEC E87.8
  threonine E72.8
  tryptophan E70.5
  tyrosine E70.20
  urea cycle E72.20
 motor R29.2
 nervous, functional R45.0
 neuromuscular mechanism (eye), due to
   syphilis A52.15
 nutritional E63.9
  nail L60.3
 ocular motion H51.9
  psychogenic F45.8
 oculogyric H51.8
  psychogenic F45.8
 oculomotor H51.9
  psychogenic F45.8
 olfactory nerve R43.1
 optic nerve NEC —*see* Disorder, nerve, optic
 oral epithelium, including tongue NEC
   K13.29
 perceptual due to
  alcohol withdrawal F10.232
  amphetamine intoxication F15.922
   in
    abuse F15.122
    dependence F15.222
  anxiolytic withdrawal F13.232
  cannabis intoxication (acute) F12.922
   in
    abuse F12.122
    dependence F12.222
  cocaine intoxication (acute) F14.922
   in
    abuse F14.122
    dependence F14.222
  hypnotic withdrawal F13.232
  opioid intoxication (acute) F11.922
   in
    abuse F11.122
    dependence F11.222
  phencyclidine intoxication (acute)
    F16.122 ◀▥
   ~~in~~
    ~~abuse F19.122~~
    ~~dependence F19.222~~
  sedative withdrawal F13.232
 personality (pattern) (trait) —*see also*
   Disorder, personality F60.9
  following organic brain damage F07.9
 polyglandular E31.9
  specified NEC E31.8
 potassium balance, newborn P74.3
 psychogenic F45.9
 psychomotor F44.4
 psychophysical visual H53.16
 pupillary —*see* Anomaly, pupil, function
 reflex R29.2
 rhythm, heart I49.9
 salivary secretion K11.7
 sensation (cold) (heat) (localization) (tactile
   discrimination) (texture) (vibratory)
   NEC R20.9
  hysterical F44.6
  skin R20.9
   anesthesia R20.0
   hyperesthesia R20.3
   hypoesthesia R20.1
   paresthesia R20.2
   specified type NEC R20.8
  smell R43.9
   and taste (mixed) R43.8
   anosmia R43.0

Disturbance *(Continued)*
 sensation *(Continued)*
  smell *(Continued)*
   parosmia R43.1
   specified NEC R43.8
  taste R43.9
   and smell (mixed) R43.8
   parageusia R43.2
   specified NEC R43.8
 sensory —*see* Disturbance, sensation
 situational (transient) —*see also* Disorder,
   adjustment
  acute F43.0
 sleep G47.9
  nonorganic origin F51.9
 smell —*see* Disturbance, sensation,
   smell
 sociopathic F60.2
 sodium balance, newborn P74.2
 speech R47.9
  developmental F80.9
  specified NEC R47.89
 stomach (functional) K31.9
 sympathetic (nerve) G90.9
 taste —*see* Disturbance, sensation,
   taste
 temperature
  regulation, newborn P81.9
   specified NEC P81.8
  sense R20.8
   hysterical F44.6
 tooth
  eruption K00.6
  formation K00.4
  structure, hereditary NEC K00.5
 touch —*see* Disturbance, sensation
 vascular I99.9
  arteriosclerotic —*see* Arteriosclerosis
 vasomotor I73.9
 vasospastic I73.9
 vision, visual H53.9
  following
   cerebral infarction I69.398
   cerebrovascular disease I69.998
    specified NEC I69.898
   intracerebral hemorrhage I69.198
   nontraumatic intracranial hemorrhage
     NEC I69.298
   specified disease NEC I69.898
   subarachnoid hemorrhage I69.098
  psychophysical H53.16
  specified NEC H53.8
  subjective H53.10
   day blindness H53.11
   discomfort H53.14-
   distortions of shape and size
     H53.15
   loss
    sudden H53.13-
    transient H53.12-
   specified type NEC H53.19
 voice R49.9
  psychogenic F44.4
  specified NEC R49.8
Diuresis R35.8
Diver's palsy, paralysis or squeeze T70.3
Diverticulitis (acute) K57.92
 bladder —*see* Cystitis
 ileum —*see* Diverticulitis, intestine, small
 intestine K57.92
  with
   abscess, perforation or peritonitis
     K57.80
    with bleeding K57.81
   bleeding K57.93
  congenital Q43.8
  large K57.32
   with
    abscess, perforation or peritonitis
      K57.20
     with bleeding K57.21

Diverticulitis *(Continued)*
  intestine *(Continued)*
    large *(Continued)*
      with *(Continued)*
        bleeding K57.33
        small intestine K57.52
          with
            abscess, perforation or peritonitis
              K57.40
              with bleeding K57.41
            bleeding K57.53
      small K57.12
        with
          abscess, perforation or peritonitis
            K57.00
            with bleeding K57.01
          bleeding K57.13
          large intestine K57.52
            with
              abscess, perforation or peritonitis
                K57.40
                with bleeding K57.41
              bleeding K57.53
Diverticulosis K57.90
  with bleeding K57.91
  large intestine K57.30
    with
      bleeding K57.31
      small intestine K57.50
        with bleeding K57.51
  small intestine K57.10
    with
      bleeding K57.11
      large intestine K57.50
        with bleeding K57.51
Diverticulum, diverticula (multiple) K57.90
  appendix (noninflammatory) K38.2
  bladder (sphincter) N32.3
    congenital Q64.6
  bronchus (congenital) Q32.4
    acquired J98.09
  calyx, calyceal (kidney) N28.89
  cardia (stomach) K31.4
  cecum —*see* Diverticulosis, intestine, large
    congenital Q43.8
  colon —*see* Diverticulosis, intestine, large
    congenital Q43.8
  duodenum —*see* Diverticulosis, intestine,
    small
    congenital Q43.8
  epiphrenic (esophagus) K22.5
  esophagus (congenital) Q39.6
    acquired (epiphrenic) (pulsion) (traction)
      K22.5
  eustachian tube —*see* Disorder, eustachian
    tube, specified NEC
  fallopian tube N83.8
  gastric K31.4
  heart (congenital) Q24.8
  ileum —*see* Diverticulosis, intestine, small
  jejunum —*see* Diverticulosis, intestine, small
  kidney (pelvis) (calyces) N28.89
    with calculus —*see* Calculus, kidney
  Meckel's (displaced) (hypertrophic) Q43.0
    malignant —*see* Table of Neoplasms, small
      intestine, malignant
  midthoracic K22.5
  organ or site, congenital NEC —*see* Distortion
  pericardium (congenital) (cyst) Q24.8
    acquired I31.8
  pharyngoesophageal (congenital) Q39.6
    acquired K22.5
  pharynx (congenital) Q38.7
  rectosigmoid —*see* Diverticulosis, intestine,
    large
    congenital Q43.8
  rectum —*see* Diverticulosis, intestine, large
  Rokitansky's K22.5
  seminal vesicle N50.89 ◀▥
  sigmoid —*see* Diverticulosis, intestine, large
    congenital Q43.8

Diverticulum, diverticula *(Continued)*
  stomach (acquired) K31.4
    congenital Q40.2
  trachea (acquired) J39.8
  ureter (acquired) N28.89
    congenital Q62.8
  ureterovesical orifice N28.89
  urethra (acquired) N36.1
    congenital Q64.79
  ventricle, left (congenital) Q24.8
  vesical N32.3
    congenital Q64.6
  Zenker's (esophagus) K22.5
Division
  cervix uteri (acquired) N88.8
  glans penis Q55.69
  labia minora (congenital) Q52.79
  ligament (partial or complete) (current) —*see
    also* Sprain
    with open wound —*see* Wound, open
  muscle (partial or complete) (current) —*see
    also* Injury, muscle
    with open wound —*see* Wound, open
  nerve (traumatic) —*see* Injury, nerve
  spinal cord —*see* Injury, spinal cord,
    by region
  vein I87.8
Divorce, causing family disruption Z63.5
Dix-Hallpike neurolabyrinthitis —*see*
  Neuronitis, vestibular
Dizziness R42
  hysterical F44.89
  psychogenic F45.8
DMAC (disseminated mycobacterium avium-
  intracellulare complex) A31.2
DNR (do not resuscitate) Z66
Doan-Wiseman syndrome (primary splenic
  neutropenia) —*see* Agranulocytosis
Doehle-Heller aortitis A52.02
Dog bite —*see* Bite
Dohle body panmyelopathic syndrome
  D72.0
Dolichocephaly Q67.2
Dolichocolon Q43.8
Dolichostenomelia —*see* Syndrome, Marfan's
Donohue's syndrome E34.8
Donor (organ or tissue) Z52.9
  blood (whole) Z52.000
    autologous Z52.010
    specified component (lymphocytes)
      (platelets) NEC Z52.008
      autologous Z52.018
      specified donor NEC Z52.098
    specified donor NEC Z52.090
    stem cells Z52.001
      autologous Z52.011
      specified donor NEC Z52.091
  bone Z52.20
    autologous Z52.21
    marrow Z52.3
    specified type NEC Z52.29
  cornea Z52.5
  egg (Oocyte) Z52.819
    age 35 and over Z52.812
      anonymous recipient Z52.812
      designated recipient Z52.813
    under age 35 Z52.810
      anonymous recipient Z52.810
      designated recipient Z52.811
  kidney Z52.4
  liver Z52.6
  lung Z52.89
  lymphocyte —*see* Donor, blood, specified
    components NEC
  Oocyte —*see* Donor, egg
  platelets Z52.008
  potential, examination of Z00.5
  semen Z52.89
  skin Z52.10
    autologous Z52.11
    specified type NEC Z52.19

Donor *(Continued)*
  specified organ or tissue NEC Z52.89
  sperm Z52.89
Donovanosis A58
Dorsalgia M54.9
  psychogenic F45.41
  specified NEC M54.89
Dorsopathy M53.9
  deforming M43.9
    specified NEC —*see* subcategory M43.8
  specified NEC M53.80
    cervical region M53.82
    cervicothoracic region M53.83
    lumbar region M53.86
    lumbosacral region M53.87
    occipito-atlanto-axial region M53.81
    sacrococcygeal region M53.88
    thoracic region M53.84
    thoracolumbar region M53.85
Double
  albumin E88.09
  aortic arch Q25.45 ◀▥
  auditory canal Q17.8
  auricle (heart) Q20.8
  bladder Q64.79
  cervix Q51.820
    with doubling of uterus (and vagina) Q51.10
      with obstruction Q51.11
  inlet ventricle Q20.4
  kidney with double pelvis (renal) Q63.0
  meatus urinarius Q64.75
  monster Q89.4
  outlet
    left ventricle Q20.2
    right ventricle Q20.1
  pelvis (renal) with double ureter Q62.5
  tongue Q38.3
  ureter (one or both sides) Q62.5
    with double pelvis (renal) Q62.5
  urethra Q64.74
  urinary meatus Q64.75
  uterus Q51.2
    with
      doubling of cervix (and vagina)
        Q51.10
        with obstruction Q51.11
    in pregnancy or childbirth O34.59-
      causing obstructed labor O65.5
  vagina Q52.10
    with doubling of uterus (and cervix)
      Q51.10
      with obstruction Q51.11
  vision H53.2
  vulva Q52.79
Douglas' pouch, cul-de-sac —*see* condition
Down syndrome Q90.9
  meiotic nondisjunction Q90.0
  mitotic nondisjunction Q90.1
  mosaicism Q90.1
  translocation Q90.2
DPD (dihydropyrimidine dehydrogenase
  deficiency) E88.89
Dracontiasis B72
Dracunculiasis, dracunculosis B72
Dream state, hysterical F44.89
Drepanocytic anemia —*see* Disease, sickle-cell
Dresbach's syndrome (elliptocytosis) D58.1
Dreschlera (hawaiiensis) (infection) B43.8
Dressler's syndrome I24.1
Drift, ulnar —*see* Deformity, limb, specified
  type NEC, forearm
Drinking (alcohol)
  excessive, to excess NEC (without
    dependence) F10.10
    habitual (continual) (without remission)
      F10.20
      with remission F10.21
Drip, postnasal (chronic) R09.82
  due to
    allergic rhinitis —*see* Rhinitis, allergic
    common cold J00

Drip, postnasal (*Continued*)
  due to (*Continued*)
    gastroesophageal reflux —*see* Reflux,
      gastroesophageal
    nasopharyngitis —*see* Nasopharyngitis
    other known condition — code to
      condition
    sinusitis —*see* Sinusitis
Droop
  facial R29.810
    cerebrovascular disease I69.992
      cerebral infarction I69.392
      intracerebral hemorrhage I69.192
      nontraumatic intracranial hemorrhage
        NEC I69.292
      specified disease NEC I69.892
      subarachnoid hemorrhage I69.092
Drop (in)
  attack NEC R55
  finger —*see* Deformity, finger
  foot —*see* Deformity, limb, foot, drop
  hematocrit (precipitous) R71.0
  hemoglobin R71.0
  toe —*see* Deformity, toe, specified NEC
  wrist —*see* Deformity, limb, wrist drop
Dropped heart beats I45.9
Dropsy, dropsical —*see also* Hydrops
  abdomen R18.8
  brain —*see* Hydrocephalus
  cardiac, heart —*see* Failure, heart, congestive
  gangrenous —*see* Gangrene
  heart —*see* Failure, heart, congestive
  kidney —*see* Nephrosis
  lung —*see* Edema, lung
  newborn due to isoimmunization P56.0
  pericardium —*see* Pericarditis
Drowned, drowning (near) T75.1
Drowsiness R40.0
Drug
  abuse counseling and surveillance Z71.51
  addiction —*see* Dependence
  dependence —*see* Dependence
  habit —*see* Dependence
  harmful use —*see* Abuse, drug
  induced fever R50.2
  overdose —*see* Table of Drugs and Chemicals,
    by drug, poisoning
  poisoning —*see* Table of Drugs and
    Chemicals, by drug, poisoning
  resistant organism infection —*see also*
    Resistant, organism, to, drug Z16.30
  therapy
    long term (current) (prophylactic) —*see*
      Therapy, drug long-term (current)
      (prophylactic)
    short term - omit code
  wrong substance given or taken in error —*see*
    Table of Drugs and Chemicals, by drug,
    poisoning
Drunkenness (without dependence) F10.129
  acute in alcoholism F10.229
  chronic (without remission) F10.20
    with remission F10.21
  pathological (without dependence) F10.129
    with dependence F10.229
  sleep F51.9
Drusen
  macula (degenerative) (retina) —*see*
    Degeneration, macula, drusen
  optic disc H47.32-
Dry, dryness —*see also* condition
  larynx J38.7
  mouth R68.2
    due to dehydration E86.0
  nose J34.89
  socket (teeth) M27.3
  throat J39.2
DSAP L56.5
Duane's syndrome H50.81-
Dubin-Johnson disease or syndrome E80.6
Dubois' disease (thymus gland) A50.59 [E35]

Dubowitz' syndrome Q87.1
Duchenne-Aran muscular atrophy G12.21
Duchenne-Griesinger disease G71.0
Duchenne's
  disease or syndrome
    motor neuron disease G12.22
    muscular dystrophy G71.0
  locomotor ataxia (syphilitic) A52.11
  paralysis
    birth injury P14.0
    due to or associated with
      motor neuron disease G12.22
      muscular dystrophy G71.0
Ducrey's chancre A57
Duct, ductus —*see* condition
Duhring's disease (dermatitis herpetiformis)
  L13.0
Dullness, cardiac (decreased) (increased) R01.2
Dumb ague —*see* Malaria
Dumbness —*see* Aphasia
Dumdum fever B55.0
Dumping syndrome (postgastrectomy) K91.1
Duodenitis (nonspecific) (peptic) K29.80
  with bleeding K29.81
Duodenocholangitis —*see* Cholangitis
Duodenum, duodenal —*see* condition
Duplay's bursitis or periarthritis —*see*
  Tendinitis, calcific, shoulder
Duplication, duplex —*see also* Accessory
  alimentary tract Q45.8
  anus Q43.4
  appendix (and cecum) Q43.4
  biliary duct (any) Q44.5
  bladder Q64.79
  cecum (and appendix) Q43.4
  cervix Q51.820
  chromosome NEC
    with complex rearrangements NEC
      Q92.5
    seen only at prometaphase Q92.8
  cystic duct Q44.5
  digestive organs Q45.8
  esophagus Q39.8
  frontonasal process Q75.8
  intestine (large) (small) Q43.4
  kidney Q63.0
  liver Q44.7
  pancreas Q45.3
  penis Q55.69
  respiratory organs NEC Q34.8
  salivary duct Q38.4
  spinal cord (incomplete) Q06.2
  stomach Q40.2
Dupré's disease (meningism) R29.1
Dupuytren's contraction or disease M72.0
Durand-Nicolas-Favre disease A55
Durotomy (inadvertent) (incidental) G97.41
Duroziez's disease (congenital mitral stenosis)
  Q23.2
Dutton's relapsing fever (West African) A68.1
Dwarfism E34.3
  achondroplastic Q77.4
  congenital E34.3
  constitutional E34.3
  hypochondroplastic Q77.4
  hypophyseal E23.0
  infantile E34.3
  Laron-type E34.3
  Lorain (-Levi) type E23.0
  metatropic Q77.8
  nephrotic-glycosuric (with
    hypophosphatemic rickets) E72.09
  nutritional E45
  pancreatic K86.89 ◄▥
  pituitary E23.0
  renal N25.0
  thanatophoric Q77.1
Dyke-Young anemia (secondary)
  (symptomatic) D59.1
Dysacusis —*see* Abnormal, auditory
  perception

Dysadrenocortism E27.9
  hyperfunction E27.0
Dysarthria R47.1
  following
    cerebral infarction I69.322
    cerebrovascular disease I69.922
      specified disease NEC I69.822
    intracerebral hemorrhage I69.122
    nontraumatic intracranial hemorrhage
      NEC I69.222
    subarachnoid hemorrhage I69.022
Dysautonomia (familial) G90.1
Dysbarism T70.3
Dysbasia R26.2
  angiosclerotica intermittens I73.9
  hysterical F44.4
  lordotica (progressiva) G24.1
  nonorganic origin F44.4
  psychogenic F44.4
Dysbetalipoproteinemia (familial) E78.2
Dyscalculia R48.8
  developmental F81.2
Dyschezia K59.00
Dyschondroplasia (with hemangiomata)
  Q78.4
Dyschromia (skin) L81.9
Dyscollagenosis M35.9
Dyscranio-pygo-phalangy Q87.0
Dyscrasia
  blood (with) D75.9
    antepartum hemorrhage —*see*
      Hemorrhage, antepartum, with
      coagulation defect
    intrapartum hemorrhage O67.0
    newborn P61.9
      specified type NEC P61.8
    puerperal, postpartum O72.3
    polyglandular, pluriglandular E31.9
Dysendocrinism E34.9
Dysentery, dysenteric (catarrhal) (diarrhea)
  (epidemic) (hemorrhagic) (infectious)
  (sporadic) (tropical) A09
  abscess, liver A06.4
  amebic —*see also* Amebiasis A06.0
    with abscess —*see* Abscess, amebic
    acute A06.0
    chronic A06.1
  arthritis —*see also* category M01 A09
    bacillary —*see also* category M01 A03.9
  bacillary A03.9
    arthritis —*see also* category M01
      A03.9
    Boyd A03.2
    Flexner A03.1
    Schmitz (-Stutzer) A03.0
    Shiga (-Kruse) A03.0
    Shigella A03.9
      boydii A03.2
      dysenteriae A03.0
      flexneri A03.1
      group A A03.0
      group B A03.1
      group C A03.2
      group D A03.3
      sonnei A03.3
      specified type NEC A03.8
    Sonne A03.3
    specified type NEC A03.8
  balantidial A07.0
  Balantidium coli A07.0
  Boyd's A03.2
  candidal B37.82
  Chilomastix A07.8
  Chinese A03.9
  coccidial A07.3
  Dientamoeba (fragilis) A07.8
  Embadomonas A07.8
  Entamoeba, entambic —*see* Dysentery,
    amebic
  Flexner-Boyd A03.2
  Flexner's A03.1

Dysentery, dysenteric *(Continued)*
  Giardia lamblia A07.1
  Hiss-Russell A03.1
  Lamblia A07.1
  leishmanial B55.0
  malarial —*see* Malaria
  metazoal B82.0
  monilial B37.82
  protozoal A07.9
  Salmonella A02.0
  schistosomal B65.1
  Schmitz (-Stutzer) A03.0
  Shiga (-Kruse) A03.0
  Shigella NOS —*see* Dysentery, bacillary
  Sonne A03.3
  strongyloidiasis B78.0
  trichomonal A07.8
  viral —*see also* Enteritis, viral A08.4
Dysequilibrium R42
Dysesthesia R20.8
  hysterical F44.6
Dysfibrinogenemia (congenital) D68.2
Dysfunction
  adrenal E27.9
    hyperfunction E27.0
  autonomic
    due to alcohol G31.2
    somatoform F45.8
  bladder N31.9
    neurogenic NOS —*see* Dysfunction,
      bladder, neuromuscular
    neuromuscular NOS N31.9
      atonic (motor) (sensory) N31.2
      autonomous N31.2
      flaccid N31.2
      nonreflex N31.2
      reflex N31.1
      specified NEC N31.8
      uninhibited N31.0
  bleeding, uterus N93.8
  cerebral G93.89
  colon K59.9
    psychogenic F45.8
  colostomy K94.03
  cystic duct K82.8
  cystostomy (stoma) —*see* Complications,
    cystostomy
  ejaculatory N53.19
    anejaculatory orgasm N53.13
    painful N53.12
    premature F52.4
    retarded N53.11
  endocrine NOS E34.9
  endometrium N85.8
  enterostomy K94.13
  erectile —*see* Dysfunction, sexual, male,
    erectile ◄
  gallbladder K82.8
  gastrostomy (stoma) K94.23
  gland, glandular NOS E34.9
  heart I51.89
  hemoglobin D75.89
  hepatic K76.89
  hypophysis E23.7
  hypothalamic NEC E23.3
  ileostomy (stoma) K94.13
  jejunostomy (stoma) K94.13
  kidney —*see* Disease, renal
  labyrinthine —*see* subcategory H83.2
  left ventricular, following sudden emotional
    stress I51.81
  liver K76.89
  male —*see* Dysfunction, sexual, male
  orgasmic (female) F52.31
    male F52.32
  ovary E28.9
    specified NEC E28.8
  papillary muscle I51.89
  parathyroid E21.4
  physiological NEC R68.89
    psychogenic F59

Dysfunction *(Continued)*
  pineal gland E34.8
  pituitary (gland) E23.3
  platelets D69.1
  polyglandular E31.9
    specified NEC E31.8
  psychophysiologic F59
  psychosexual F52.9
    with
      dyspareunia F52.6
      premature ejaculation F52.4
      vaginismus F52.5
  pylorus K31.9
  rectum K59.9
    psychogenic F45.8
  reflex (sympathetic) —*see* Syndrome, pain,
    complex regional I
  segmental —*see* Dysfunction, somatic
  senile R54
  sexual (due to) R37
    alcohol F10.981
    amphetamine F15.981
      in
        abuse F15.181
        dependence F15.281
    anxiolytic F13.981
      in
        abuse F13.181
        dependence F13.281
    cocaine F14.981
      in
        abuse F14.181
        dependence F14.281
    excessive sexual drive F52.8
    failure of genital response (male) F52.21
      female F52.22
    female N94.9
      aversion F52.1
      dyspareunia N94.10 ◀▥
        psychogenic F52.6
      frigidity F52.22
      nymphomania F52.8
      orgasmic F52.31
      psychogenic F52.9
        aversion F52.1
        dyspareunia F52.6
        frigidity F52.22
        nymphomania F52.8
        orgasmic F52.31
        vaginismus F52.5
      vaginismus N94.2
        psychogenic F52.5
    hypnotic F13.981
      in
        abuse F13.181
        dependence F13.281
    inhibited orgasm (female) F52.31
      male F52.32
    lack
      of sexual enjoyment F52.1
      or loss of sexual desire F52.0
    male N53.9
      anejaculatory orgasm N53.13
      ejaculatory N53.19
        painful N53.12
        premature F52.4
        retarded N53.11
      erectile N52.9
        drug induced N52.2
        due to
          disease classified elsewhere N52.1
          drug N52.2
        postoperative (postprocedural) N52.39
          following
            cryotherapy N52.37 ◀
            interstitial seed therapy
              N52.36 ◀
            prostate ablative therapy
              N52.37 ◀
            prostatectomy N52.34
              radical N52.31

Dysfunction *(Continued)*
  sexual *(Continued)*
    male *(Continued)*
      erectile *(Continued)*
        postoperative *(Continued)*
          following *(Continued)*
            radiation therapy N52.35 ◀
            radical cystectomy N52.32
            ultrasound ablative therapy
              N52.37 ◀
            urethral surgery N52.33
          psychogenic F52.21
          specified cause NEC N52.8
          vasculogenic
            arterial insufficiency N52.01
              with corporo-venous occlusive
                N52.03
            corporo-venous occlusive N52.02
              with arterial insufficiency N52.03
        impotence —*see* Dysfunction, sexual,
          male, erectile
        psychogenic F52.9
          aversion F52.1
          erectile F52.21
          orgasmic F52.32
          premature ejaculation F52.4
          satyriasis F52.8
          specified type NEC F52.8
        specified type NEC N53.8
      nonorganic F52.9
        specified NEC F52.8
      opioid F11.981
        in
          abuse F11.181
          dependence F11.281
      orgasmic dysfunction (female) F52.31
        male F52.32
      premature ejaculation F52.4
      psychoactive substances NEC F19.981
        in
          abuse F19.181
          dependence F19.281
      psychogenic F52.9
      sedative F13.981
        in
          abuse F13.181
          dependence F13.281
      sexual aversion F52.1
      vaginismus (nonorganic) (psychogenic)
        F52.5
  sinoatrial node I49.5
  somatic M99.09
    abdomen M99.09
    acromioclavicular M99.07
    cervical region M99.01
    cervicothoracic M99.01
    costochondral M99.08
    costovertebral M99.08
    head region M99.00
    hip M99.05
    lower extremity M99.06
    lumbar region M99.03
    lumbosacral M99.03
    occipitocervical M99.00
    pelvic region M99.05
    pubic M99.05
    rib cage M99.08
    sacral region M99.04
    sacrococcygeal M99.04
    sacroiliac M99.04
    specified NEC M99.09
    sternochondral M99.08
    sternoclavicular M99.07
    thoracic region M99.02
    thoracolumbar M99.02
    upper extremity M99.07
  somatoform autonomic F45.8
  stomach K31.89
    psychogenic F45.8
  suprarenal E27.9
    hyperfunction E27.0

◀ New   ◀▥ Revised   ~~deleted~~ Deleted

Dysfunction *(Continued)*
  symbolic R48.9
    specified type NEC R48.8
  temporomandibular (joint) M26.69
    joint-pain syndrome M26.62- ◀▥
  testicular (endocrine) E29.9
    specified NEC E29.8
  thymus E32.9
  thyroid E07.9
  ureterostomy (stoma) —*see* Complications,
    stoma, urinary tract
  urethrostomy (stoma) —*see* Complications,
    stoma, urinary tract
  uterus, complicating delivery O62.9
    hypertonic O62.4
    hypotonic O62.2
      primary O62.0
      secondary O62.1
  ventricular I51.9
    with congestive heart failure I50.9-
      left, reversible, following sudden
        emotional stress I51.81
Dysgenesis
  gonadal (due to chromosomal anomaly)
    Q96.9
    pure Q99.1
  renal Q60.5
    bilateral Q60.4
    unilateral Q60.3
  reticular D72.0
  tidal platelet D69.3
Dysgerminoma
  specified site —*see* Neoplasm, malignant,
    by site
  unspecified site
    female C56.9
    male C62.90
Dysgeusia R43.2
Dysgraphia R27.8
Dyshidrosis, dysidrosis L30.1
Dyskaryotic cervical smear R87.619
Dyskeratosis L85.8
  cervix —*see* Dysplasia, cervix
  congenital Q82.8
  uterus NEC N85.8
Dyskinesia G24.9
  biliary (cystic duct or gallbladder) K82.8
  drug induced
    orofacial G24.01
  esophagus K22.4
  hysterical F44.4
  intestinal K59.8
  nonorganic origin F44.4
  orofacial (idiopathic) G24.4
    drug induced G24.01
  psychogenic F44.4
  subacute, drug induced G24.01
  tardive G24.01
    neuroleptic induced G24.01
  trachea J39.8
  tracheobronchial J98.09
Dyslalia (developmental) F80.0
Dyslexia R48.0
  developmental F81.0
Dyslipidemia E78.5
  depressed HDL cholesterol E78.6
  elevated fasting triglycerides E78.1
Dysmaturity —*see also* Light for dates
  pulmonary (newborn) (Wilson-Mikity) P27.0
Dysmenorrhea (essential) (exfoliative) N94.6
  congestive (syndrome) N94.6
  primary N94.4
  psychogenic F45.8
  secondary N94.5
Dysmetabolic syndrome X E88.81
Dysmetria R27.8
Dysmorphism (due to)
  alcohol Q86.0
  exogenous cause NEC Q86.8
  hydantoin Q86.1
  warfarin Q86.2

Dysmorphophobia (nondelusional)
    F45.22
  delusional F22
Dysnomia R47.01
Dysorexia R63.0
  psychogenic F50.89 ◀▥
Dysostosis
  cleidocranial, cleidocranialis Q74.0
  craniofacial Q75.1
  Fairbank's (idiopathic familial generalized
    osteophytosis) Q78.9
  mandibulofacial (incomplete)
    Q75.4
  multiplex E76.01
  oculomandibular Q75.5
Dyspareunia (female) N94.10 ◀▥
  deep N94.12 ◀
  male N53.12
  nonorganic F52.6
  psychogenic F52.6
  secondary N94.19 ◀▥
  specified NEC N94.19 ◀
  superficial (introital) N94.11 ◀
Dyspepsia R10.13
  atonic K30
  functional (allergic) (congenital)
    (gastrointestinal) (occupational) (reflex)
    K30
  intestinal K59.8
  nervous F45.8
  neurotic F45.8
  psychogenic F45.8
Dysphagia R13.10
  cervical R13.19
  following
    cerebral infarction I69.391
    cerebrovascular disease I69.991
      specified NEC I69.891
    intracerebral hemorrhage I69.191
    nontraumatic intracranial hemorrhage
      NEC I69.291
    specified disease NEC I69.891
    subarachnoid hemorrhage I69.091
  functional (hysterical) F45.8
  hysterical F45.8
  nervous (hysterical) F45.8
  neurogenic R13.19
  oral phase R13.11
  oropharyngeal phase R13.12
  pharyneal phase R13.13
  pharyngoesophageal phase R13.14
  psychogenic F45.8
  sideropenic D50.1
  spastica K22.4
  specified NEC R13.19
Dysphagocytosis, congenital D71
Dysphasia R47.02
  developmental
    expressive type F80.1
    receptive type F80.2
  following
    cerebrovascular disease I69.921
      cerebral infarction I69.321
      intracerebral hemorrhage I69.121
    nontraumatic intracranial hemorrhage NEC
      I69.221
      specified disease NEC I69.821
      subarachnoid hemorrhage I69.021
Dysphonia R49.0
  functional F44.4
  hysterical F44.4
  psychogenic F44.4
  spastica J38.3
  ~~Dysphoria, postpartal O90.6~~
Dysphoria ◀
  gender ◀
    in ◀
      adolescence and adulthood F64.0 ◀
      children F64.2 ◀
      postpartal O90.6 ◀
Dyspituitarism E23.3

Dysplasia —*see also* Anomaly
  acetabular, congenital Q65.89
  alveolar capillary, with vein misalignment
    J84.843
  anus (histologically confirmed) (mild)
    (moderate) K62.82
    severe D01.3
  arrhythmogenic right ventricular I42.8
  arterial, fibromuscular I77.3
  asphyxiating thoracic (congenital) Q77.2
  brain Q07.9
  bronchopulmonary, perinatal P27.1
  cervix (uteri) N87.9
    mild N87.0
    moderate N87.1
    severe D06.9
  chondroectodermal Q77.6
  colon D12.6
  craniometaphyseal Q78.58 ◀▥
  dentinal K00.5
  diaphyseal, progressive Q78.3
  dystrophic Q77.5
  ectodermal (anhidrotic) (congenital)
    (hereditary) Q82.4
    hydrotic Q82.8
  epithelial, uterine cervix —*see* Dysplasia,
    cervix
  eye (congenital) Q11.2
  fibrous
    bone NEC (monostotic) M85.00
      ankle M85.07-
      foot M85.07-
      forearm M85.03-
      hand M85.04-
      lower leg M85.06-
      multiple site M85.09
      neck M85.08
      rib M85.08
      shoulder M85.01-
      skull M85.08
      specified site NEC M85.08
      thigh M85.05-
      toe M85.07-
      upper arm M85.02-
      vertebra M85.08
    diaphyseal, progressive Q78.3
    jaw M27.8
    polyostotic Q78.1
  florid osseous —*see also* Cyst, calcifying
    odontogenic
  high grade, focal D12.6
  hip, congenital Q65.89
  joint, congenital Q74.8
  kidney Q61.4
    multicystic Q61.4
  leg Q74.2
  lung, congenital (not associated with short
    gestation) Q33.6
  mammary (gland) (benign) N60.9-
    cyst (solitary) —*see* Cyst, breast
    cystic —*see* Mastopathy, cystic
    duct ectasia —*see* Ectasia, mammary
      duct
    fibroadenosis —*see* Fibroadenosis, breast
    fibrosclerosis —*see* Fibrosclerosis, breast
    specified type NEC N60.8-
  metaphyseal Q78.5 ◀▥
  muscle Q79.8
  oculodentodigital Q87.0
  periapical (cemental) (cemento-osseous) —*see*
    Cyst, calcifying odontogenic
  periosteum —*see* Disorder, bone, specified
    type NEC
  polyostotic fibrous Q78.1
  prostate —*see also* Neoplasia, intraepithelial,
    prostate N42.30 ◀▥
    severe D07.5
    specified NEC N42.39 ◀
  renal Q61.4
    multicystic Q61.4
  retinal, congenital Q14.1

Dysplasia (Continued)
  right ventricular, arrhythmogenic I42.8
  septo-optic Q04.4
  skin L98.8
  spinal cord Q06.1
  spondyloepiphyseal Q77.7
  thymic, with immunodeficiency D82.1
  vagina N89.3
    mild N89.0
    moderate N89.1
    severe NEC D07.2
  vulva N90.3
    mild N90.0
    moderate N90.1
    severe NEC D07.1
Dyspnea (nocturnal) (paroxysmal)
    R06.00
  asthmatic (bronchial) J45.909
    with
      bronchitis J45.909
        with
          exacerbation (acute) J45.901
          status asthmaticus J45.902
        chronic J44.9
      exacerbation (acute) J45.901
      status asthmaticus J45.902
    cardiac —see Failure, ventricular, left
  cardiac —see Failure, ventricular, left
  functional F45.8
  hyperventilation R06.4
  hysterical F45.8
  newborn P28.89
  psychogenic F45.8
  shortness of breath R06.02
  specified type NEC R06.09
Dyspraxia R27.8
  developmental (syndrome) F82
Dysproteinemia E88.09
Dysreflexia, autonomic G90.4
Dysrhythmia
  cardiac I49.9
    newborn
      bradycardia P29.12
        occurring before birth P03.819
          before onset of labor P03.810
          during labor P03.811
      tachycardia P29.11
    postoperative I97.89
  cerebral or cortical —see Epilepsy
Dyssomnia —see Disorder, sleep
Dyssynergia
  biliary K83.8
  bladder sphincter N36.44
  cerebellaris myoclonica (Hunt's ataxia)
    G11.1
Dysthymia F34.1
Dysthyroidism E07.9
Dystocia O66.9
  affecting newborn P03.1
  cervical (hypotonic) O62.2
    affecting newborn P03.6
    primary O62.0
    secondary O62.1
  contraction ring O62.4

Dystocia (Continued)
  fetal O66.9
    abnormality NEC O66.3
    conjoined twins O66.3
    oversize O66.2
  maternal O66.9
  positional O64.9
  shoulder (girdle) O66.0
    causing obstructed labor O66.0
  uterine NEC O62.4
Dystonia G24.9
  deformans progressiva G24.1
  drug induced NEC G24.09
    acute G24.02
    specified NEC G24.09
  familial G24.1
  idiopathic G24.1
    familial G24.1
    nonfamilial G24.2
    orofacial G24.4
  lenticularis G24.8
  musculorum deformans G24.1
  neuroleptic induced (acute) G24.02
  orofacial (idiopathic) G24.4
  oromandibular G24.4
    due to drug G24.01
  specified NEC G24.8
  torsion (familial) (idiopathic) G24.1
    acquired G24.8
    genetic G24.1
  symptomatic (nonfamilial) G24.2
Dystonic movements R25.8
Dystrophy, dystrophia
  adiposogenital E23.6
  Becker's type G71.0
  cervical sympathetic G90.2
  choroid (hereditary) H31.20
    central areolar H31.22
    choroideremia H31.21
    gyrate atrophy H31.23
    specified type NEC H31.29
  cornea (hereditary) H18.50
    endothelial H18.51
    epithelial H18.52
    granular H18.53
    lattice H18.54
    macular H18.55
    specified type NEC H18.59
  Duchenne's type G71.0
  due to malnutrition E45
  Erb's G71.0
  Fuchs' H18.51
  Gower's muscular G71.0
  hair L67.8
  infantile neuraxonal G31.89
  Landouzy-Déjérine G71.0
  Leyden-Möbius G71.0
  muscular G71.0
    benign (Becker type) G71.0
    congenital (hereditary) (progressive)
      (with specific morphological
      abnormalities of the muscle fiber)
      G71.0
      myotonic G71.11

Dystrophy, dystrophia (Continued)
  muscular (Continued)
    distal G71.0
    Duchenne type G71.0
    Emery-Dreifuss G71.0
    Erb type G71.0
    facioscapulohumeral G71.0
    Gower's G71.0
    hereditary (progressive) G71.0
    Landouzy-Déjérine type G71.0
    limb-girdle G71.0
    myotonic G71.11
    progressive (hereditary) G71.0
      Charcot-Marie (-Tooth) type
        G60.0
      pseudohypertrophic (infantile)
        G71.0
      severe (Duchenne type) G71.0
  myocardium, myocardial —see
      Degeneration, myocardial
  nail L60.3
    congenital Q84.6
  nutritional E45
  ocular G71.0
  oculocerebrorenal E72.03
  oculopharyngeal G71.0
  ovarian N83.8
  polyglandular E31.8
  reflex (neuromuscular) (sympathetic) —
      see Syndrome, pain, complex
      regional I
  retinal (hereditary) H35.50
    in
      lipid storage disorders E75.6
        [H36]
      systemic lipidoses E75.6 [H36]
    involving
      pigment epithelium H35.54
      sensory area H35.53
    pigmentary H35.52
    vitreoretinal H35.51
  Salzmann's nodular —see Degeneration,
      cornea, nodular
  scapuloperoneal G71.0
  skin NEC L98.8
  sympathetic (reflex) —see Syndrome, pain,
      complex regional I
    cervical G90.2
  tapetoretinal H35.54
  thoracic, asphyxiating Q77.2
  unguium L60.3
    congenital Q84.6
  vitreoretinal H35.51
  vulva N90.4
  yellow (liver) —see Failure, hepatic
Dysuria R30.0
  psychogenic F45.8

◀ New   ◀▥ Revised   ~~deleted~~ Deleted

E

Eales' disease H35.06-
Ear —*see also* condition
 piercing Z41.3
 ~~tropical B36.8~~
 tropical NEC B36.9 [H62.40] ◀
  in ◀
   aspergillosis B44.89 ◀
   candidiasis B37.84 ◀
   moniliasis B37.84 ◀
  wax (impacted) H61.20
   left H61.22
    with right H61.23
   right H61.21
    with left H61.23
Earache —*see* subcategory H92.0
Early satiety R68.81
Eaton-Lambert syndrome—*see* Syndrome,
  Lambert-Eaton
Eberth's disease (typhoid fever) A01.00
Ebola virus disease A98.4
Ebstein's anomaly or syndrome (heart) Q22.5
Eccentro-osteochondrodysplasia E76.29
Ecchondroma —*see* Neoplasm, bone, benign
Ecchondrosis D48.0
Ecchymosis R58
 conjunctiva —*see* Hemorrhage, conjunctiva
 eye (traumatic) —*see* Contusion, eyeball
 eyelid (traumatic) —*see* Contusion, eyelid
 newborn P54.5
 spontaneous R23.3
 traumatic —*see* Contusion
Echinococciasis —*see* Echinococcus
Echinococcosis —*see* Echinococcus
Echinococcus (infection) B67.90
 granulosus B67.4
  bone B67.2
  liver B67.0
  lung B67.1
  multiple sites B67.32
  specified site NEC B67.39
  thyroid B67.31 ◀▥
 liver NOS B67.8
  granulosus B67.0
  multilocularis B67.5
 lung NEC B67.99
  granulosus B67.1
  multilocularis B67.69
 multilocularis B67.7
  liver B67.5
  multiple sites B67.61
  specified site NEC B67.69
 specified site NEC B67.99
  granulosus B67.39
  multilocularis B67.69
 thyroid NEC B67.99
  granulosus B67.31 ◀▥
  multilocularis B67.69 [E35]
Echinorhynchiasis B83.8
Echinostomiasis B66.8
Echolalia R48.8
Echovirus, as cause of disease classified
  elsewhere B97.12
Eclampsia, eclamptic (coma) (convulsions)
  (delirium) (with hypertension) NEC O15.9
 complicating ◀
  labor and delivery O15.1 ◀
  postpartum O15.2 ◀
  pregnancy O15.0- ◀
  puerperium O15.2 ◀
 ~~during labor and delivery O15.1~~
 ~~postpartum O15.2~~
 ~~pregnancy O15.0-~~
 ~~puerperal O15.2~~
Economic circumstances affecting care Z59.9
Economo's disease A85.8
Ectasia, ectasis
 annuloaortic I35.8
 aorta I77.819
  with aneurysm —*see* Aneurysm, aorta
  abdominal I77.811

Ectasia, ectasis (*Continued*)
 aorta (*Continued*)
  thoracic I77.810
  thoracoabdominal I77.812
 breast —*see* Ectasia, mammary duct
 capillary I78.8
 cornea H18.71-
 gastric antral vascular (GAVE) K31.819
  with hemorrhage K31.811
  without hemorrhage K31.819
 mammary duct N60.4-
 salivary gland (duct) K11.8
 sclera —*see* Sclerectasia
Ecthyma L08.0
 contagiosum B08.02
 gangrenosum L08.0
 infectiosum B08.02
Ectocardia Q24.8
Ectodermal dysplasia (anhidrotic) Q82.4
Ectodermosis erosiva pluriorificialis
  L51.1
Ectopic, ectopia (congenital)
 abdominal viscera Q45.8
  due to defect in anterior abdominal wall
    Q79.59
 ACTH syndrome E24.3
 adrenal gland Q89.1
 anus Q43.5
 atrial beats I49.1
 beats I49.49
  atrial I49.1
  ventricular I49.3
 bladder Q64.10
 bone and cartilage in lung Q33.5
 brain Q04.8
 breast tissue Q83.8
 cardiac Q24.8
 cerebral Q04.8
 cordis Q24.8
 endometrium —*see* Endometriosis
 gastric mucosa Q40.2
 gestation —*see* Pregnancy, by site
 heart Q24.8
 hormone secretion NEC E34.2
 kidney (crossed) (pelvis) Q63.2
 lens, lentis Q12.1
 mole —*see* Pregnancy, by site
 organ or site NEC —*see* Malposition,
   congenital
 pancreas Q45.3
 pregnancy —*see* Pregnancy, ectopic
 pupil —*see* Abnormality, pupillary
 renal Q63.2
 sebaceous glands of mouth Q38.6
 spleen Q89.09
 testis Q53.00
  bilateral Q53.02
  unilateral Q53.01
 thyroid Q89.2
 tissue in lung Q33.5
 ureter Q62.63
 ventricular beats I49.3
 vesicae Q64.10
Ectromelia Q73.8
 lower limb —*see* Defect, reduction, limb,
   lower, specified type NEC
 upper limb —*see* Defect, reduction, limb,
   upper, specified type NEC
Ectropion H02.109
 cervix N86
  with cervicitis N72
 congenital Q10.1
 eyelid (paralytic) H02.109
  cicatricial H02.119
   left H02.116
    lower H02.115
    upper H02.114
   right H02.113
    lower H02.112
    upper H02.111
  congenital Q10.1

Ectropion (*Continued*)
 eyelid (*Continued*)
  left H02.106
   lower H02.105
   upper H02.104
  mechanical H02.129
   left H02.126
    lower H02.125
    upper H02.124
   right H02.123
    lower H02.122
    upper H02.121
  right H02.103
   lower H02.102
   upper H02.101
  senile H02.139
   left H02.136
    lower H02.135
    upper H02.134
   right H02.133
    lower H02.132
    upper H02.131
  spastic H02.149
   left H02.146
    lower H02.145
    upper H02.144
   right H02.143
    lower H02.142
    upper H02.141
 iris H21.89
 lip (acquired) K13.0
  congenital Q38.0
 urethra N36.8
 uvea H21.89
Eczema (acute) (chronic) (erythematous)
   (fissum) (rubrum) (squamous) (*see also*
   Dermatitis) L30.9
 contact —*see* Dermatitis, contact
 dyshydrotic L30.1
 external ear —*see* Otitis, externa, acute,
   eczematoid
 flexural L20.82
 herpeticum B00.0
 hypertrophicum L28.0
 hypostatic —*see* Varix, leg, with,
   inflammation
 impetiginous L01.1
 infantile (due to any substance) L20.83
  intertriginous L21.1
  seborrheic L21.1
 intertriginous NEC L30.4
  infantile L21.1
 intrinsic (allergic) L20.84
 lichenified NEC L28.0
 marginatum (hebrae) B35.6
 pustular L30.3
 stasis I87.2 ◀▥
  with varicose veins —*see* Varix, leg, with,
    inflammation ◀
 vaccination, vaccinatum T88.1
 varicose —*see* Varix, leg, with, inflammation
Eczematid L30.2
Eddowes (-Spurway) syndrome Q78.0
Edema, edematous (infectious) (pitting)
   (toxic) R60.9
 with nephritis —*see* Nephrosis
 allergic T78.3
 amputation stump (surgical) (sequelae
   (late effect)) T87.89
 angioneurotic (allergic) (any site) (with
   urticaria) T78.3
  hereditary D84.1
 angiospastic I73.9
 Berlin's (traumatic) S05.8X-
 brain (cytotoxic) (vasogenic) G93.6
  due to birth injury P11.0
   newborn (anoxia or hypoxia) P52.4
    birth injury P11.0
  traumatic —*see* Injury, intracranial,
    cerebral edema
 cardiac —*see* Failure, heart, congestive

Edema, edematous (Continued)
  cardiovascular —see Failure, heart, congestive
  cerebral —see Edema, brain
  cerebrospinal —see Edema, brain
  cervix (uteri) (acute) N88.8
    puerperal, postpartum O90.89
  chronic hereditary Q82.0
  circumscribed, acute T78.3
    hereditary D84.1
  conjunctiva H11.42-
  cornea H18.2-
    idiopathic H18.22-
    secondary H18.23-
      due to contact lens H18.21-
  due to
    lymphatic obstruction I89.0
    salt retention E87.0
  epiglottis —see Edema, glottis
  essential, acute T78.3
    hereditary D84.1
  extremities, lower —see Edema, legs
  eyelid NEC H02.849
    left H02.846
      lower H02.845
      upper H02.844
    right H02.843
      lower H02.842
      upper H02.841
  familial, hereditary Q82.0
  famine —see Malnutrition, severe
  generalized R60.1
  glottis, glottic, glottidis (obstructive) (passive)
      J38.4
    allergic T78.3
      hereditary D84.1
  heart —see Failure, heart, congestive
  heat T67.7
  hereditary Q82.0
  inanition —see Malnutrition, severe
  intracranial G93.6
  iris H21.89
  joint —see Effusion, joint
  larynx —see Edema, glottis
  legs R60.0
    due to venous obstruction I87.1
    hereditary Q82.0
  localized R60.0
    due to venous obstruction I87.1
  lower limbs —see Edema, legs
  lung J81.1
    with heart condition or failure —see
        Failure, ventricular, left
    acute J81.0
    chemical (acute) J68.1
      chronic J68.1
    chronic J81.1
      due to
        chemicals, gases, fumes or vapors
            (inhalation) J68.1
        external agent J70.9
          specified NEC J70.8
        radiation J70.1
    due to
      chemicals, fumes or vapors (inhalation)
          J68.1
      external agent J70.9
        specified NEC J70.8
      high altitude T70.29
      near drowning T75.1
      radiation J70.0
    meaning failure, left ventricle I50.1
  lymphatic I89.0
    due to mastectomy I97.2
  macula H35.81
    cystoid, following cataract surgery —see
        Complications, postprocedural,
        following cataract surgery
    diabetic —see Diabetes, by type, with,
        retinopathy, with macular edema
  malignant —see Gangrene, gas
  Milroy's Q82.0

Edema, edematous (Continued)
  nasopharynx J39.2
  newborn P83.30
    hydrops fetalis —see Hydrops, fetalis
    specified NEC P83.39
  nutritional —see also Malnutrition, severe
      with dyspigmentation, skin and hair E40
  optic disc or nerve —see Papilledema
  orbit H05.22-
  pancreas K86.89 ◀▥
  papilla, optic —see Papilledema
  penis N48.89
  periodic T78.3
    hereditary D84.1
  pharynx J39.2
  pulmonary —see Edema, lung
  Quincke's T78.3
    hereditary D84.1
  renal —see Nephrosis
  retina H35.81
    diabetic —see Diabetes, by type, with,
        retinopathy, with macular edema
  salt E87.0
  scrotum N50.89 ◀▥
  seminal vesicle N50.89 ◀▥
  spermatic cord N50.89 ◀▥
  spinal (cord) (vascular) (nontraumatic) G95.19
  starvation —see Malnutrition, severe
  stasis —see Hypertension, venous, (chronic)
  subglottic —see Edema, glottis
  supraglottic —see Edema, glottis
  testis N44.8
  tunica vaginalis N50.89 ◀▥
  vas deferens N50.89 ◀▥
  vulva (acute) N90.89
Edentulism —see Absence, teeth, acquired
Edsall's disease T67.2
Educational handicap Z55.9
  specified NEC Z55.8
Edward's syndrome —see Trisomy, 18
Effect, adverse
  abnormal gravitational (G) forces or states
      T75.81
  abuse —see Maltreatment
  air pressure T70.9
    specified NEC T70.8
  altitude (high) —see Effect, adverse, high
      altitude
  anesthesia —see also Anesthesia T88.59
    in labor and delivery O74.9
    in pregnancy NEC O29.3-
    local, toxic
      in labor and delivery O74.4-
      in pregnancy NEC O29.3- ◀
      postpartum, puerperal O89.3
    postpartum, puerperal O89.9
    specified NEC T88.59
      in labor and delivery O74.8
      postpartum, puerperal O89.8
    spinal and epidural T88.59
      headache T88.59
        in labor and delivery O74.5
        postpartum, puerperal O89.4
      specified NEC
        in labor and delivery O74.6
        postpartum, puerperal O89.5
  antitoxin —see Complications, vaccination
  atmospheric pressure T70.9
    due to explosion T70.8
    high T70.3
    low —see Effect, adverse, high altitude
    specified effect NEC T70.8
  biological, correct substance properly
      administered —see Effect, adverse, drug
  blood (derivatives) (serum) (transfusion) —
      see Complications, transfusion
  chemical substance —see Table of Drugs and
      Chemicals
  cold (temperature) (weather) T69.9
    chilblains T69.1
    frostbite —see Frostbite
    specified effect NEC T69.8

Effect, adverse (Continued)
  drugs and medicaments T88.7
    specified drug —see Table of Drugs and
        Chemicals, by drug, adverse effect
    specified effect — code to condition
  electric current, electricity (shock) T75.4
    burn —see Burn
  exertion (excessive) T73.3
  exposure —see Exposure
  external cause NEC T75.89
  foodstuffs T78.1
    allergic reaction —see Allergy, food
      causing anaphylaxis —see Shock,
          anaphylactic, due to food
    noxious —see Poisoning, food, noxious
  gases, fumes, or vapors T59.9-
    specified agent —see Table of Drugs and
        Chemicals
  glue (airplane) sniffing
    due to drug abuse —see Abuse, drug,
        inhalant
    due to drug dependence —see Dependence,
        drug, inhalant
  heat —see Heat
  high altitude NEC T70.29
    anoxia T70.29
    on
      ears T70.0
      sinuses T70.1
    polycythemia D75.1
  high pressure fluids T70.4
  hot weather —see Heat
  hunger T73.0
  immersion, foot —see Immersion
  immunization —see Complications,
      vaccination
  immunological agents —see Complications,
      vaccination
  infrared (radiation) (rays) NOS T66
    dermatitis or eczema L59.8
  infusion —see Complications, infusion
  lack of care of infants —see Maltreatment,
      child
  lightning —see Lightning
  medical care T88.9
    specified NEC T88.8
  medicinal substance, correct, properly
      administered —see Effect, adverse, drug
  motion T75.3
  noise, on inner ear —see subcategory H83.3
  overheated places —see Heat
  psychosocial, of work environment Z56.5
  radiation (diagnostic) (infrared) (natural
      source) (therapeutic) (ultraviolet)
      (X-ray) NOS T66
    dermatitis or eczema —see Dermatitis, due
        to, radiation
    fibrosis of lung J70.1
    pneumonitis J70.0
    pulmonary manifestations
      acute J70.0
      chronic J70.1
    skin L59.9
  radioactive substance NOS
    dermatitis or eczema —see Radiodermatitis
  reduced temperature T69.9
    immersion foot or hand —see Immersion
    specified effect NEC T69.8
  serum NEC (see also Reaction, serum) T80.69
  specified NEC T78.8
    external cause NEC T75.89
  strangulation —see Asphyxia, traumatic
  submersion T75.1
  thirst T73.1
  toxic —see Toxicity
  transfusion —see Complications, transfusion
  ultraviolet (radiation) (rays) NOS T66
    burn —see Burn
    dermatitis or eczema —see Dermatitis, due
        to, ultraviolet rays
      acute L56.8

◀ New   ◀▥ Revised   ~~deleted~~ Deleted

Effect, adverse *(Continued)*
vaccine (any) —*see* Complications, vaccination
vibration —*see* Vibration, adverse effects
water pressure NEC T70.9
specified NEC T70.8
weightlessness T75.82
whole blood —*see* Complications, transfusion
work environment Z56.5
Effect (s) (of) (from) —*see* Effect, adverse NEC
Effects, late —*see* Sequelae
Effluvium
anagen L65.1
telogen L65.0
Effort syndrome (psychogenic) F45.8
Effusion
amniotic fluid —*see* Pregnancy, complicated by, prematue rupture of membranes
brain (serous) G93.6
bronchial —*see* Bronchitis
cerebral G93.6
cerebrospinal —*see also* Meningitis
vessel G93.6
chest —*see* Effusion, pleura
chylous, chyliform (pleura) J94.0
intracranial G93.6
joint M25.40
ankle M25.47-
elbow M25.42-
foot joint M25.47-
hand joint M25.44-
hip M25.45-
knee M25.46-
shoulder M25.41-
specified joint NEC M25.48
wrist M25.43-
malignant pleural J91.0
meninges —*see* Meningitis
pericardium, pericardial (noninflammatory) I31.3
acute —*see* Pericarditis, acute
peritoneal (chronic) R18.8
pleura, pleurisy, pleuritic, pleuropericardial J90
chylous, chyliform J94.0
due to systemic lupus erythematosis M32.13
influenzal —*see* Influenza, with, respiratory manifestations NEC
malignant J91.0
newborn P28.89
tuberculous NEC A15.6
primary (progressive) A15.7
spinal —*see* Meningitis
thorax, thoracic —*see* Effusion, pleura
Egg shell nails L60.3
congenital Q84.6
Egyptian splenomegaly B65.1
Ehlers-Danlos syndrome Q79.6
Ehrlichiosis A77.40
due to
E. chafeensis A77.41
E. sennetsu A79.81
specified organism NEC A77.49
Eichstedt's disease B36.0
Eisenmenger's
complex or syndrome I27.89
defect Q21.8
Ejaculation
delayed F52.32 ◄
painful N53.12
premature F52.4
retarded N53.11
retrograde N53.14
semen, painful N53.12
psychogenic F52.6
Ekbom's syndrome (restless legs) G25.81
Ekman's syndrome (brittle bones and blue sclera) Q78.0
Elastic skin Q82.8
acquired L57.4

Elastofibroma —*see* Neoplasm, connective tissue, benign
Elastoma (juvenile) Q82.8
Miescher's L87.2
Elastomyofibrosis I42.4
Elastosis
actinic, solar L57.8
atrophicans (senile) L57.4
perforans serpiginosa L87.2
senilis L57.4
Elbow —*see* condition
Electric current, electricity, effects (concussion) (fatal) (nonfatal) (shock) T75.4
burn —*see* Burn
Electric feet syndrome E53.8
Electrocution T75.4
from electroshock gun (taser) T75.4
Electrolyte imbalance E87.8
with
abortion —*see* Abortion by type, complicated by, electrolyte imbalance
ectopic pregnancy O08.5
molar pregnancy O08.5
Elephantiasis (nonfilarial) I89.0
arabicum —*see* Infestation, filarial
bancroftian B74.0
congenital (any site) (hereditary) Q82.0
due to
Brugia (malayi) B74.1
timori B74.2
mastectomy I97.2
Wuchereria (bancrofti) B74.0
eyelid H02.859
left H02.856
lower H02.855
upper H02.854
right H02.853
lower H02.852
upper H02.851
filarial, filariensis —*see* Infestation, filarial
glandular I89.0
graecorum A30.9
lymphangiectatic I89.0
lymphatic vessel I89.0
due to mastectomy I97.2
scrotum (nonfilarial) I89.0
streptococcal I89.0
surgical I97.89
postmastectomy I97.2
telangiectodes I89.0
vulva (nonfilarial) N90.89
Elevated, elevation
antibody titer R76.0
basal metabolic rate R94.8
blood pressure —*see also* Hypertension
reading (incidental) (isolated) (nonspecific), no diagnosis of hypertension R03.0
blood sugar R73.9
body temperature (of unknown origin) R50.9
C-reactive protein (CRP) R79.82
cancer antigen 125 [CA 125] R97.1
carcinoembryonic antigen [CEA] R97.0
cholesterol E78.00 ◄
with high triglycerides E78.2
conjugate, eye H51.0
diaphragm, congenital Q79.1
erythrocyte sedimentation rate R70.0
fasting glucose R73.01
fasting triglycerides E78.1
finding on laboratory examination —*see* Findings, abnormal, inconclusive, without diagnosis, by type of exam
GFR (glomerular filtration rate) —*see* Findings, abnormal, inconclusive, without diagnosis, by type of exam
glucose tolerance (oral) R73.02
immunoglobulin level R76.8
indoleacetic acid R82.5
lactic acid dehydrogenase (LDH) level R74.0
leukocytes D72.829
lipoprotein a level E78.8

Elevated, elevation *(Continued)*
liver function
study R94.5
test R79.89
alkaline phosphatase R74.8
aminotransferase R74.0
bilirubin R17
hepatic enzyme R74.8
lactate dehydrogenase R74.0
lymphocytes D72.820
prostate specific antigen [PSA] R97.20 ◄
Rh titer —*see* Complication (s), transfusion, incompatibility reaction, Rh (factor)
scapula, congenital Q74.0
sedimentation rate R70.0
SGOT R74.0
SGPT R74.0
transaminase level R74.0
triglycerides E78.1
with high cholesterol E78.2
tumor associated antigens [TAA] NEC R97.8
tumor specific antigens [TSA] NEC R97.8
urine level of
17-ketosteroids R82.5
catecholamine R82.5
indoleacetic acid R82.5
steroids R82.5
vanillylmandelic acid (VMA) R82.5
venous pressure I87.8
white blood cell count D72.829
specified NEC D72.828
Elliptocytosis (congenital) (hereditary) D58.1
Hb C (disease) D58.1
hemoglobin disease D58.1
sickle-cell (disease) D57.8-
trait D57.3
Ellison-Zollinger syndrome E16.4
Ellis-van Creveld syndrome (chondroectodermal dysplasia) Q77.6
Elongated, elongation (congenital) —*see also* Distortion
bone Q79.9
cervix (uteri) Q51.828
acquired N88.4
hypertrophic N88.4
colon Q43.8
common bile duct Q44.5
cystic duct Q44.5
frenulum, penis Q55.69
labia minora (acquired) N90.69 ◄
ligamentum patellae Q74.1
petiolus (epiglottidis) Q31.8
tooth, teeth K00.2
uvula Q38.6
Eltor cholera A00.1
Emaciation (due to malnutrition) E41
Embadomoniasis A07.8
Embedded tooth, teeth K01.0
root only K08.3
Embolic —*see* condition
Embolism (multiple) (paradoxical) I74.9
air (any site) (traumatic) T79.0
following
abortion —*see* Abortion by type complicated by embolism
ectopic pregnancy O08.2
infusion, therapeutic injection or transfusion T80.0
molar pregnancy O08.2
procedure NEC
artery T81.719
mesenteric T81.710
renal T81.711
specified NEC T81.718
vein T81.72
in pregnancy, childbirth or puerperium —*see* Embolism, obstetric
amniotic fluid (pulmonary) —*see also* Embolism, obstetric
following
abortion —*see* Abortion by type complicated by embolism

Embolism *(Continued)*
  amniotic fluid *(Continued)*
    following *(Continued)*
      ectopic pregnancy O08.2
      molar pregnancy O08.2
  aorta, aortic I74.10
    abdominal I74.09
      saddle I74.01
    bifurcation I74.09
    saddle I74.01
    thoracic I74.11
  artery I74.9
    auditory, internal I65.8
    basilar —*see* Occlusion, artery, basilar
    carotid (common) (internal) —*see*
        Occlusion, artery, carotid
    cerebellar (anterior inferior) (posterior
        inferior) (superior) I66.3
    cerebral —*see* Occlusion, artery, cerebral
    choroidal (anterior) I66.8
    communicating posterior I66.8
    coronary —*see also* Infarct, myocardium
      not resulting in infarction I24.0
    extremity I74.4
      lower I74.3
      upper I74.2
    hypophyseal I66.8
    iliac I74.5
    limb I74.4
      lower I74.3
      upper I74.2
    mesenteric (with gangrene) —*see also*
        Ischemia, intestine, acute K55.09 ◀▥
    ophthalmic —*see* Occlusion, artery, retina
    peripheral I74.4
    pontine I66.8
    precerebral —*see* Occlusion, artery,
        precerebral
    pulmonary —*see* Embolism, pulmonary
    renal N28.0
    retinal —*see* Occlusion, artery, retina
    septic I76
    specified NEC I74.8
    vertebral —*see* Occlusion, artery, vertebral
  basilar (artery) I65.1
  blood clot
    following
      abortion —*see* Abortion by type
          complicated by embolism
      ectopic or molar pregnancy O08.2
    in pregnancy, childbirth or puerperium —
        see Embolism, obstetric
  brain —*see also* Occlusion, artery, cerebral
    following
      abortion —*see* Abortion by type
          complicated by embolism
      ectopic or molar pregnancy O08.2
    puerperal, postpartum, childbirth —*see*
        Embolism, obstetric
  capillary I78.8
  cardiac —*see also* Infarct, myocardium
    not resulting in infarction I51.3 ◀▥
  carotid (artery) (common) (internal) —*see*
      Occlusion, artery, carotid
  cavernous sinus (venous) —*see* Embolism,
      intracranial venous sinus
  cerebral —*see* Occlusion, artery, cerebral
  cholesterol —*see* Atheroembolism
  coronary (artery or vein) (systemic) —*see*
      Occlusion, coronary
  due to device, implant or graft —*see also*
      Complications, by site and type,
      specified NEC
    arterial graft NEC T82.818
    breast (implant) T85.818 ◀▥
    catheter NEC T85.818 ◀▥
      dialysis (renal) T82.818
        intraperitoneal T85.818 ◀▥
      infusion NEC T82.818
        spinal (epidural) (subdural) T85.810 ◀▥
      urinary (indwelling) T83.81

Embolism *(Continued)*
  due to device, implant or graft *(Continued)*
    electronic (electrode) (pulse generator)
        (stimulator)
      bone T84.81
      cardiac T82.817
      nervous system (brain) (peripheral
          nerve) (spinal) T85.810 ◀▥
      urinary T83.81
    fixation, internal (orthopedic) NEC T84.81
    gastrointestinal (bile duct) (esophagus)
        T85.818 ◀▥
    genital NEC T83.81
    heart (graft) (valve) T82.817
    joint prosthesis T84.81
    ocular (corneal graft) (orbital implant)
        T85.818 ◀▥
    orthopedic (bone graft) NEC T86.838
    specified NEC T85.818 ◀▥
    urinary (graft) NEC T83.81
    vascular NEC T82.818
    ventricular intracranial shunt T85.810 ◀▥
  extremities
    lower —*see* Embolism, vein, lower
        extremity
      arterial I74.3
    upper I74.2
  eye H34.9
  fat (cerebral) (pulmonary) (systemic) T79.1
    complicating delivery —*see* Embolism,
        obstetric
    following
      abortion —*see* Abortion by type
          complicated by embolism
      ectopic or molar pregnancy O08.2
  following
    abortion —*see* Abortion by type
        complicated by embolism
    ectopic or molar pregnancy O08.2
    infusion, therapeutic injection or
        transfusion
      air T80.0
  heart (fatty) —*see also* Infarct, myocardium
    not resulting in infarction I51.3 ◀▥
  hepatic (vein) I82.0
  in pregnancy, childbirth or puerperium —*see*
      Embolism, obstetric
  intestine (artery) (vein) (with gangrene) —*see*
      also Ischemia, intestine, acute K55.039 ◀▥
  intracranial —*see also* Occlusion, artery,
      cerebral
    venous sinus (any) G08
      nonpyogenic I67.6
  intraspinal venous sinuses or veins G08
    nonpyogenic G95.19
  kidney (artery) N28.0
  lateral sinus (venous) —*see* Embolism,
      intracranial, venous sinus
  leg —*see* Embolism, vein, lower extremity
    arterial I74.3
  longitudinal sinus (venous) —*see* Embolism,
      intracranial, venous sinus
  lung (massive) —*see* Embolism, pulmonary
  meninges I66.8
  mesenteric (artery) (vein) (with gangrene) —
      see also Ischemia, intestine, acute
      K55.059 ◀▥
  obstetric (in) (pulmonary)
    childbirth O88.22 ◀▥
      air O88.02
      amniotic fluid O88.12
      blood clot O88.22
      fat O88.82
      pyemic O88.32
      septic O88.32
      specified type NEC O88.82
    pregnancy O88.21- ◀▥
      air O88.01-
      amniotic fluid O88.11-
      blood clot O88.21-
      fat O88.81-

Embolism *(Continued)*
  obstetric *(Continued)*
    pregnancy *(Continued)*
      pyemic O88.31-
      septic O88.31-
      specified type NEC O88.81-
    puerperal O88.23 ◀▥
      air O88.03
      amniotic fluid O88.13
      blood clot O88.23
      fat O88.83
      pyemic O88.33
      septic O88.33
      specified type NEC O88.83
  ophthalmic —*see* Occlusion, artery, retina
  penis N48.81
  peripheral artery NOS I74.4
  pituitary E23.6
  popliteal (artery) I74.3
  portal (vein) I81
  postoperative, postprocedural
    artery T81.719
      mesenteric T81.710
      renal T81.711
      specified NEC T81.718
    vein T81.72
  precerebral artery —*see* Occlusion, artery,
      precerebral
  puerperal —*see* Embolism, obstetric
  pulmonary (acute) (artery) (vein) I26.99
    with acute cor pulmonale I26.09
    chronic I27.82
    following
      abortion —*see* Abortion by type
          complicated by embolism
      ectopic or molar pregnancy O08.2
    healed or old Z86.711
    in pregnancy, childbirth or puerperium —
        see Embolism, obstetric
    personal history of Z86.711
    saddle I26.92
      with acute cor pulmonale I26.02
    septic I26.90
      with acute cor pulmonale I26.01
  pyemic (multiple) I76
    following
      abortion —*see* Abortion by type
          complicated by embolism
      ectopic or molar pregnancy O08.2
    Hemophilus influenzae A41.3
    pneumococcal A40.3
      with pneumonia J13
    puerperal, postpartum, childbirth (any
        organism) —*see* Embolism, obstetric
    specified organism NEC A41.89
    staphylococcal A41.2
    streptococcal A40.9
  renal (artery) N28.0
    vein I82.3
  retina, retinal —*see* Occlusion, artery,
      retina
  saddle
    abdominal aorta I74.01
    pulmonary artery I26.92
      with acute cor pulmonale I26.02
  septic (arterial) I76
    complicating abortion —*see* Abortion, by
        type, complicated by, embolism
  sinus —*see* Embolism, intracranial, venous
      sinus
  soap complicating abortion —*see* Abortion,
      by type, complicated by, embolism
  spinal cord G95.19
    pyogenic origin G06.1
  spleen, splenic (artery) I74.8
  upper extremity I74.2
  vein (acute) I82.90
    antecubital I82.61-
      chronic I82.71-
    axillary I82.A1-
      chronic I82.A2-

◀ New   ◀▥ Revised   ~~deleted~~ Deleted

Embolism (Continued)
vein (Continued)
basilic I82.61-
chronic I82.71-
brachial I82.62-
chronic I82.72-
brachiocephalic (innominate) I82.290
chronic I82.291
cephalic I82.61-
chronic I82.71-
chronic I82.91
deep (DVT) I82.40-
calf I82.4Z-
chronic I82.5Z-
lower leg I82.4Z-
chronic I82.5Z-
thigh I82.4Y-
chronic I82.5Y-
upper leg I82.4Y
chronic I82.5y--
femoral I82.41-
chronic I82.51-
iliac (iliofemoral) I82.42-
chronic I82.52-
innominate I82.290
chronic I82.291
internal jugular I82.C1-
chronic I82.C2-
lower extremity
deep I82.40-
chronic I82.50-
specified NEC I82.49-
chronic NEC I82.59-
distal
deep I82.4Z-
proximal
deep I82.4Y-
chronic I82.5Y-
superficial I82.81-
popliteal I82.43-
chronic I82.53-
radial I82.62-
chronic I82.72-
renal I82.3
saphenous (greater) (lesser) I82.81-
specified NEC I82.890
chronic NEC I82.891
subclavian I82.B1-
chronic I82.B2-
thoracic NEC I82.290
chronic I82.291
tibial I82.44-
chronic I82.54-
ulnar I82.62-
chronic I82.72-
upper extremity I82.60-
chronic I82.70-
deep I82.62-
chronic I82.72-
superficial I82.61-
chronic I82.71-
vena cava
inferior (acute) I82.220
chronic I82.221
superior (acute) I82.210
chronic I82.211
venous sinus G08
vessels of brain —see Occlusion, artery,
cerebral
Embolus —see Embolism
Embryoma —see also Neoplasm, uncertain
behavior, by site
benign —see Neoplasm, benign, by site
kidney C64.-
liver C22.0
malignant —see also Neoplasm, malignant,
by site
kidney C64.-
liver C22.0
testis C62.9-
descended (scrotal) C62.1-
undescended C62.0-

Embryoma (Continued)
testis C62.9-
descended (scrotal) C62.1-
undescended C62.0-
Embryonic
circulation Q28.9
heart Q28.9
vas deferens Q55.4
Embryopathia NOS Q89.9
Embryotoxon Q13.4
Emesis —see Vomiting
Emotional lability R45.86
Emotionality, pathological F60.3
Emotogenic disease —see Disorder,
psychogenic
Emphysema (atrophic) (bullous) (chronic)
(interlobular) (lung) (obstructive)
(pulmonary) (senile) (vesicular)
J43.9
cellular tissue (traumatic) T79.7
surgical T81.82
centrilobular J43.2
compensatory J98.3
congenital (interstitial) P25.0
conjunctiva H11.89
connective tissue (traumatic) T79.7
surgical T81.82
due to chemicals, gases, fumes or vapors
J68.4
eyelid (s) —see Disorder, eyelid, specified
type NEC
surgical T81.82
traumatic T79.7
interstitial J98.2
congenital P25.0
perinatal period P25.0
laminated tissue T79.7
surgical T81.82
mediastinal J98.2
newborn P25.2
orbit, orbital —see Disorder, orbit, specified
type NEC
panacinar J43.1
panlobular J43.1
specified NEC J43.8
subcutaneous (traumatic) T79.7
nontraumatic J98.2
postprocedural T81.82
surgical T81.82
surgical T81.82
thymus (gland) (congenital) E32.8
traumatic (subcutaneous) T79.7
unilateral J43.0
Empty nest syndrome Z60.0
Empyema (acute) (chest) (double) (pleura)
(supradiaphragmatic) (thorax) J86.9
with fistula J86.0
accessory sinus (chronic) —see Sinusitis
antrum (chronic) —see Sinusitis, maxillary
brain (any part) —see Abscess, brain
ethmoidal (chronic) (sinus) —see Sinusitis,
ethmoidal
extradural —see Abscess, extradural
frontal (chronic) (sinus) —see Sinusitis,
frontal
gallbladder K81.0
mastoid (process) (acute) —see Mastoiditis,
acute
maxilla, maxillary M27.2
sinus (chronic) —see Sinusitis,
maxillary
nasal sinus (chronic) —see Sinusitis
sinus (accessory) (chronic) (nasal) —see
Sinusitis
sphenoidal (sinus) (chronic) —see Sinusitis,
sphenoidal
subarachnoid —see Abscess, extradural
subdural —see Abscess, subdural
tuberculous A15.6
ureter —see Ureteritis
ventricular —see Abscess, brain

En coup de sabre lesion L94.1
Enamel pearls K00.2
Enameloma K00.2
Enanthema, viral B09
Encephalitis (chronic) (hemorrhagic)
(idiopathic) (nonepidemic) (spurious)
(subacute) G04.90
acute —see also Encephalitis, viral A86
disseminated G04.00
infectious G04.01
noninfectious G04.81
postimmunization (postvaccination)
G04.02
postinfectious G04.01
inclusion body A85.8
necrotizing hemorrhagic G04.30
postimmunization G04.32
postinfectious G04.31
specified NEC G04.39
arboviral, arbovirus NEC A85.2
arthropod-borne NEC (viral) A85.2
Australian A83.4
California (virus) A83.5
Central European (tick-borne) A84.1
Czechoslovakian A84.1
Dawson's (inclusion body) A81.1
diffuse sclerosing A81.1
disseminated, acute G04.00
due to
cat scratch disease A28.1
human immunodeficiency virus (HIV)
disease B20 [G05.3]
malaria —see Malaria
rickettsiosis —see Rickettsiosis
smallpox inoculation G04.02
typhus —see Typhus
Eastern equine A83.2
endemic (viral) A86
epidemic NEC (viral) A86
equine (acute) (infectious) (viral) A83.9
Eastern A83.2
Venezuelan A92.2
Western A83.1
Far Eastern (tick-borne) A84.0
following vaccination or other immunization
procedure G04.02
herpes zoster B02.0
herpesviral B00.4
due to herpesvirus 6 B10.01
due to herpesvirus 7 B10.09
specified NEC B10.09
Ilheus (virus) A83.8
in (due to)
actinomycosis A42.82
adenovirus A85.1
African trypanosomiasis B56.9 [G05.3]
Chagas' disease (chronic) B57.42
cytomegalovirus B25.8
enterovirus A85.0
herpes (simplex) virus B00.4
due to herpesvirus 6 B10.01
due to herpesvirus 7 B10.09
specified NEC B10.09
infectious disease NEC B99 [G05.3]
influenza —see Influenza, with,
encephalopathy
listeriosis A32.12
measles B05.0
mumps B26.2
naegleriasis B60.2
parasitic disease NEC B89 [G05.3]
poliovirus A80.9 [G05.3]
rubella B06.01
syphilis
congenital A50.42
late A52.14
systemic lupus erythematosus M32.19
toxoplasmosis (acquired) B58.2
congenital P37.1
tuberculosis A17.82
zoster B02.0

Encephalitis (Continued)
inclusion body A81.1
infectious (acute) (virus) NEC A86
Japanese (B type) A83.0
La Crosse A83.5
lead —see Poisoning, lead
lethargica (acute) (infectious) A85.8
louping ill A84.8
lupus erythematosus, systemic M32.19
lymphatica A87.2
Mengo A85.8
meningococcal A39.81
Murray Valley A83.4
otitic NEC H66.40 [G05.3]
parasitic NOS B71.9
periaxial G37.0
periaxialis (concentrica) (diffuse) G37.5
postchickenpox B01.11
postexanthematous NEC B09
postimmunization G04.02
postinfectious NEC G04.01
postmeasles B05.0
postvaccinal G04.02
postvaricella B01.11
postviral NEC A86
Powassan A84.8
Rasmussen G04.81
Rio Bravo A85.8
Russian
autumnal A83.0
spring-summer (taiga) A84.0
saturnine —see Poisoning, lead
specified NEC G04.81
St. Louis A83.3
subacute sclerosing A81.1
summer A83.0
suppurative G04.81
tick-borne A84.9
Torula, torular (cryptococcal) B45.1
toxic NEC G92
trichinosis B75 [G05.3]
type
B A83.0
C A83.3
van Bogaert's A81.1
Venezuelan equine A92.2
Vienna A85.8
viral, virus A86
arthropod-borne NEC A85.2
mosquito-borne A83.9
Australian X disease A83.4
California virus A83.5
Eastern equine A83.2
Japanese (B type) A83.0
Murray Valley A83.4
specified NEC A83.8
St. Louis A83.3
type B A83.0
type C A83.3
Western equine A83.1
tick-borne A84.9
biundulant A84.1
central European A84.1
Czechoslovakian A84.1
diphasic meningoencephalitis A84.1
Far Eastern A84.0
Russian spring-summer (taiga)
A84.0
specified NEC A84.8
specified type NEC A85.8
Western equine A83.1
Encephalocele Q01.9
frontal Q01.0
nasofrontal Q01.1
occipital Q01.2
specified NEC Q01.8
Encephalocystocele —see Encephalocele
Encephaloduroarteriomyosynangiosis
(EDAMS) I67.5
Encephalomalacia (brain) (cerebellar)
(cerebral) —see Softening, brain

Encephalomeningitis —see
Meningoencephalitis
Encephalomeningocele —see Encephalocele
Encephalomeningomyelitis —see
Meningoencephalitis
Encephalomyelitis —see also Encephalitis
G04.90
acute disseminated G04.00
infectious G04.01
noninfectious G04.81
postimmunization G04.02
postinfectious G04.01
acute necrotizing hemorrhagic G04.30
postimmunization G04.32
postinfectious G04.31
specified NEC G04.39
benign myalgic G93.3
equine A83.9
Eastern A83.2
Venezuelan A92.2
Western A83.1
in diseases classified elsewhere G05.3
myalgic, benign G93.3
postchickenpox B01.11
postinfectious NEC G04.01
postmeasles B05.0
postvaccinal G04.02
postvaricella B01.11
rubella B06.01
specified NEC G04.81
Venezuelan equine A92.2
Encephalomyelocele —see Encephalocele
Encephalomyelomeningitis —see
Meningoencephalitis
Encephalomyelopathy G96.9
Encephalomyeloradiculitis (acute) G61.0
Encephalomyeloradiculoneuritis (acute)
(Guillain-Barré) G61.0
Encephalomyeloradiculopathy G96.9
Encephalopathia hyperbilirubinemica,
newborn P57.9
due to isoimmunization (conditions in P55)
P57.0
Encephalopathy (acute) G93.40
acute necrotizing hemorrhagic G04.30
postimmunization G04.32
postinfectious G04.31
specified NEC G04.39
alcoholic G31.2
anoxic —see Damage, brain, anoxic
arteriosclerotic I67.2
centrolobar progressive (Schilder) G37.0
congenital Q07.9
degenerative, in specified disease NEC
G32.89
due to
drugs (see also Table of Drugs and
Chemicals) G92
demyelinating callosal G37.1
hepatic —see Failure, hepatic
hyperbilirubinemic, newborn P57.9
due to isoimmunization (conditions in P55)
P57.0
hypertensive I67.4
hypoglycemic E16.2
hypoxic —see Damage, brain, anoxic
hypoxic ischemic P91.60
mild P91.61
moderate P91.62
severe P91.63
in (due to) (with)
birth injury P11.1
hyperinsulinism E16.1 [G94]
influenza —see Influenza, with,
encephalopathy
lack of vitamin (see also Deficiency, vitamin)
E56.9 [G32.89]
neoplastic disease (see also Neoplasm)
D49.9 [G13.1]
serum (see also Reaction, serum) T80.69
syphilis A52.17

Encephalopathy (Continued)
in (Continued)
trauma (postconcussional) F07.81
current injury —see Injury, intracranial
vaccination G04.02
lead —see Poisoning, lead
metabolic G93.41
drug induced G92
toxic G92
myoclonic, early, symptomatic —see Epilepsy,
generalized, specified NEC
necrotizing, subacute (Leigh) G31.82
pellagrous E52 [G32.89]
portosystemic —see Failure, hepatic
postcontusional F07.81
current injury —see Injury, intracranial,
diffuse
posthypoglycemic (coma) E16.1 [G94]
postradiation G93.89
saturnine —see Poisoning, lead
septic G93.41
specified NEC G93.49
spongioform, subacute (viral) A81.09
toxic G92
metabolic G92
traumatic (postconcussional) F07.81
current injury —see Injury, intracranial
vitamin B deficiency NEC E53.9 [G32.89]
vitamin B1 E51.2
Wernicke's E51.2
Encephalorrhagia —see Hemorrhage,
intracranial, intracerebral
Encephalosis, posttraumatic F07.81
Enchondroma —see also Neoplasm, bone,
benign
Enchondromatosis (cartilaginous) (multiple)
Q78.4
Encopresis R15.9
functional F98.1
nonorganic origin F98.1
psychogenic F98.1
Encounter (with health service) (for) Z76.89
adjustment and management (of)
breast implant Z45.81
implanted device NEC Z45.89
myringotomy device (stent) (tube)
Z45.82
administrative purpose only Z02.9
examination for
adoption Z02.82
armed forces Z02.3
disability determination Z02.71
driving license Z02.4
employment Z02.1
insurance Z02.6
medical certificate NEC Z02.79
paternity testing Z02.81
residential institution admission Z02.2
school admission Z02.0
sports Z02.5
specified reason NEC Z02.89
aftercare —see Aftercare
antenatal screening Z36
assisted reproductive fertility procedure cycle
Z31.83
blood typing Z01.83
Rh typing Z01.83
breast augmentation or reduction Z41.1
breast implant exchange (different material)
(different size) Z45.81
breast reconstruction following mastectomy
Z42.1
check-up —see Examination
chemotherapy for neoplasm Z51.11
colonoscopy, screening Z12.11
counseling —see Counseling
delivery, full-term, uncomplicated O80
cesarean, without indication O82
desensitization to allergens Z51.6 ◀
ear piercing Z41.3
examination —see Examination

◀ New   ◀▥ Revised   ~~deleted~~ Deleted

Encounter (Continued)
    expectant parent (s) (adoptive) pre-birth
            pediatrician visit Z76.81
    fertility preservation procedure (prior to
            cancer therapy) (prior to removal of
            gonads) Z31.84
    fitting (of) —see Fitting (and adjustment) (of)
    genetic
        counseling Z31.5
        testing —see Test, genetic
    hearing conservation and treatment
            Z01.12
    immunotherapy for neoplasm Z51.12
    in vitro fertilization cycle Z31.83
    instruction (in)
        child care (postpartal) (prenatal) Z32.3
        childbirth Z32.2
        natural family planning
            procreative Z31.61
            to avoid pregnancy Z30.02
    insulin pump titration Z46.81
    joint prosthesis insertion following prior
            explantation of joint prosthesis (staged
            procedure)
        hip Z47.32
        knee Z47.33
        shoulder Z47.31
    laboratory (as part of a general medical
            examination) Z00.00
        with abnormal findings Z00.01
    mental health services (for)
        abuse NEC
            perpetrator Z69.82
            victim Z69.81
        child abuse
            nonparental
                perpetrator Z69.021
                victim Z69.020
            parental
                perpetrator Z69.011
                victim Z69.010
        spousal or partner abuse
            perpetrator Z69.12
            victim Z69.11
    observation (for) (ruled out)
        exposure to (suspected)
            anthrax Z03.810
            biological agent NEC Z03.818
    pediatrician visit, by expectant parent (s)
            (adoptive) Z76.81
    plastic and reconstructive surgery following
            medical procedure or healed injury
            NEC Z42.8
    pregnancy
        supervision of —see Pregnancy,
            supervision of
        test Z32.00
            result negative Z32.02
            result positive Z32.01
    procreative management and counseling for
            gestational carrier Z31.7 ◄
    prophylactic measures Z29.9 ◄
        antivenin Z29.12 ◄
        fluoride administration Z29.3 ◄
        immunotherapy for respiratory syncytial
            virus (RSV) Z29.11 ◄
        rabies immune globin Z29.14 ◄
        Rho (D) immune globulin Z29.13 ◄
        specified NEC Z29.8 ◄
    radiation therapy (antineoplastic) Z51.0
    radiological (as part of a general medical
            examination) Z00.00
        with abnormal findings Z00.01
    reconstructive surgery following medical
            procedure or healed injury NEC
            Z42.8
    removal (of) —see also Removal
        artificial
            arm Z44.00-
                complete Z44.01-
                partial Z44.02-

Encounter (Continued)
    removal (Continued)
        artificial (Continued)
            eye Z44.2-
            leg Z44.10-
                complete Z44.11-
                partial Z44.12-
        breast implant Z45.81
            tissue expander (without synchronous
                insertion of permanent implant)
                Z45.81
        device Z46.9
            specified NEC Z46.89
        external
            fixation device — code to fracture with
                seventh character D
            prosthesis, prosthetic device Z44.9
                breast Z44.3-
                specified NEC Z44.8
        implanted device NEC Z45.89
        insulin pump Z46.81
        internal fixation device Z47.2
        myringotomy device (stent) (tube) Z45.82
        nervous system device NEC Z46.2
            brain neuropacemaker Z46.2
            visual substitution device Z46.2
                implanted Z45.31
        non-vascular catheter Z46.82
        orthodontic device Z46.4
        stent
            ureteral Z46.6
        urinary device Z46.6
    repeat cervical smear to confirm findings of
            recent normal smear following initial
            abnormal smear Z01.42
    respirator [ventilator] use during power
            failure (Z99.12)
    Rh typing Z01.83
    screening —see Screening
    specified NEC Z76.89
    sterilization Z30.2
    suspected condition, ruled out
        amniotic cavity and membrane Z03.71
        cervical shortening Z03.75
        fetal anomaly Z03.73
        fetal growth Z03.74
        maternal and fetal conditions NEC Z03.79
        oligohydramnios Z03.71
        placental problem Z03.72
        polyhydramnios Z03.71
    suspected exposure (to), ruled out
        anthrax Z03.810
        biological agents NEC Z03.818
    termination of pregnancy, elective Z33.2
    testing —see Test
    therapeutic drug level monitoring Z51.81
    titration, insulin pump Z46.81
    to determine fetal viability of pregnancy
            O36.80
    training
        insulin pump Z46.81
    X-ray of chest (as part of a general medical
            examination Z00.00)
        with abnormal findings Z00.01
Encystment —see Cyst
Endarteritis (bacterial, subacute) (infective)
        I77.6
    brain I67.7
    cerebral or cerebrospinal I67.7
    deformans —see Arteriosclerosis
    embolic —see Embolism
    obliterans —see also Arteriosclerosis
        pulmonary I28.8
    pulmonary I28.8
    retina —see Vasculitis, retina
    senile —see Arteriosclerosis
    syphilitic A52.09
        brain or cerebral A52.04
        congenital A50.54 [I79.8]
    tuberculous A18.89
Endemic —see condition

Endocarditis (chronic) (marantic) (nonbacterial)
        (thrombotic) (valvular) I38
    with rheumatic fever (conditions in I00)
        active —see Endocarditis, acute, rheumatic
        inactive or quiescent (with chorea) I09.1
    acute or subacute I33.9
        infective I33.0
        rheumatic (aortic) (mitral) (pulmonary)
            (tricuspid) I01.1
            with chorea (acute) (rheumatic)
                (Sydenham's) I02.0
    aortic (heart) (nonrheumatic) (valve) I35.8
        with
            mitral disease I08.0
                with tricuspid (valve) disease I08.3
                active or acute I01.1
                    with chorea (acute) (rheumatic)
                        (Sydenham's) I02.0
            rheumatic fever (conditions in I00)
                active —see Endocarditis, acute,
                    rheumatic
                inactive or quiescent (with chorea)
                    I06.9
            tricuspid (valve) disease I08.2
                with mitral (valve) disease I08.3
        acute or subacute I33.9
        arteriosclerotic I35.8
        rheumatic I06.9
            with mitral disease I08.0
                with tricuspid (valve) disease I08.3
                active or acute I01.1
                    with chorea (acute) (rheumatic)
                        (Sydenham's) I02.0
            active or acute I01.1
                with chorea (acute) (rheumatic)
                    (Sydenham's) I02.0
            specified NEC I06.8
        specified cause NEC I35.8
        syphilitic A52.03
    arteriosclerotic I38
    atypical verrucous (Libman-Sacks) M32.11
    bacterial (acute) (any valve) (subacute)
        I33.0
    candidal B37.6
    congenital Q24.8
    constrictive I33.0
    Coxiella burnetii A78 [I39]
    Coxsackie B33.21
    due to
        prosthetic cardiac valve T82.6
        Q fever A78 [I39]
        Serratia marcescens I33.0
        typhoid (fever) A01.02
    gonococcal A54.83
    infectious or infective (acute) (any valve)
        (subacute) I33.0
    lenta (acute) (any valve) (subacute) I33.0
    Libman-Sacks M32.11
    listerial A32.82
    Löffler's I42.3
    malignant (acute) (any valve) (subacute) I33.0
    meningococcal A39.51
    mitral (chronic) (double) (fibroid) (heart)
        (inactive) (valve) (with chorea) I05.9
        with
            aortic (valve) disease I08.0
                with tricuspid (valve) disease I08.3
                active or acute I01.1
                    with chorea (acute) (rheumatic)
                        (Sydenham's) I02.0
            rheumatic fever (conditions in I00)
                active —see Endocarditis, acute,
                    rheumatic
                inactive or quiescent (with chorea)
                    I05.9
            tricuspid (valve) disease I08.1
                with aortic (valve) disease I08.3
        active or acute I01.1
            with chorea (acute) (rheumatic)
                (Sydenham's) I02.0
        bacterial I33.0

Endocarditis (Continued)
  mitral (Continued)
    arteriosclerotic I34.8
    nonrheumatic I34.8
      acute or subacute I33.9
    specified NEC I05.8
  monilial B37.6
  multiple valves I08.9
    specified disorders I08.8
  mycotic (acute) (any valve) (subacute) I33.0
  pneumococcal (acute) (any valve) (subacute)
      I33.0
  pulmonary (chronic) (heart) (valve) I37.8
    with rheumatic fever (conditions in I00)
      active —see Endocarditis, acute,
          rheumatic
      inactive or quiescent (with chorea)
          I09.89
        with aortic, mitral or tricuspid disease
            I08.8
    acute or subacute I33.9
      rheumatic I01.1
        with chorea (acute) (rheumatic)
            (Sydenham's) I02.0
    arteriosclerotic I37.8
    congenital Q22.2
    rheumatic (chronic) (inactive) (with chorea)
        I09.89
      active or acute I01.1
        with chorea (acute) (rheumatic)
            (Sydenham's) I02.0
    syphilitic A52.03
  purulent (acute) (any valve) (subacute) I33.0
  Q fever A78 [I39]
  rheumatic (chronic) (inactive) (with chorea)
      I09.1
    active or acute (aortic) (mitral)
        (pulmonary) (tricuspid) I01.1
      with chorea (acute) (rheumatic)
          (Sydenham's) I02.0
  rheumatoid —see Rheumatoid, carditis
  septic (acute) (any valve) (subacute) I33.0
  streptococcal (acute) (any valve) (subacute)
      I33.0
  subacute —see Endocarditis, acute
  suppurative (acute) (any valve) (subacute)
      I33.0
  syphilitic A52.03
  toxic I33.9
  tricuspid (chronic) (heart) (inactive)
      (rheumatic) (valve) (with chorea) I07.9
    with
      aortic (valve) disease I08.2
        mitral (valve) disease I08.3
      mitral (valve) disease I08.1
        aortic (valve) disease I08.3
      rheumatic fever (conditions in I00)
        active —see Endocarditis, acute,
            rheumatic
        inactive or quiescent (with chorea)
            I07.8
    active or acute I01.1
      with chorea (acute) (rheumatic)
          (Sydenham's) I02.0
    arteriosclerotic I36.8
    nonrheumatic I36.8
      acute or subacute I33.9
    specified cause, except rheumatic I36.8
  tuberculous —see Tuberculosis, endocarditis
  typhoid A01.02
  ulcerative (acute) (any valve) (subacute) I33.0
  vegetative (acute) (any valve) (subacute) I33.0
  verrucous (atypical) (nonbacterial)
      (nonrheumatic) M32.11
Endocardium, endocardial —see also condition
  cushion defect Q21.2
Endocervicitis —see also Cervicitis
  due to intrauterine (contraceptive) device
      T83.69 ◀▥
  hyperplastic N72
Endocrine —see condition

Endocrinopathy, pluriglandular E31.9
Endodontic
  overfill M27.52
  underfill M27.53
Endodontitis K04.01 ◀▥
  irreversible K04.02 ◀
  reversible K04.01 ◀
Endomastoiditis —see Mastoiditis
Endometrioma N80.9
Endometriosis N80.9
  appendix N80.5
  bladder N80.8
  bowel N80.5
  broad ligament N80.3
  cervix N80.0
  colon N80.5
  cul-de-sac (Douglas') N80.3
  exocervix N80.0
  fallopian tube N80.2
  female genital organ NEC N80.8
  gallbladder N80.8
  in scar of skin N80.6
  internal N80.0
  intestine N80.5
  lung N80.8
  myometrium N80.0
  ovary N80.1
  parametrium N80.3
  pelvic peritoneum N80.3
  peritoneal (pelvic) N80.3
  rectovaginal septum N80.4
  rectum N80.5
  round ligament N80.3
  skin (scar) N80.6
  specified site NEC N80.8
  stromal D39.0
  umbilicus N80.8
  uterus (internal) N80.0
  vagina N80.4
  vulva N80.8
Endometritis (decidual) (nonspecific) (purulent)
    (senile (atrophic) (suppurative) N71.9
  with ectopic pregnancy O08.0
  acute N71.0
  blenorrhagic (gonococcal) (acute) (chronic)
      A54.24
  cervix, cervical (with erosion or ectropion) —
      see also Cervicitis
    hyperplastic N72
  chlamydial A56.11
  chronic N71.1
  following
    abortion —see Abortion by type
        complicated by genital infection
    ectopic or molar pregnancy O08.0
  gonococcal, gonorrheal (acute) (chronic) A54.24
  hyperplastic —see also Hyperplasia,
        endometrial N85.00-
    cervix N72
  puerperal, postpartum, childbirth O86.12
  subacute N71.0
  tuberculous A18.17
Endometrium —see condition
Endomyocardiopathy, South African I42.3
Endomyocarditis —see Endocarditis
Endomyofibrosis I42.3
Endomyometritis —see Endometritis
Endopericarditis —see Endocarditis
Endoperineuritis —see Disorder, nerve
Endophlebitis —see Phlebitis
Endophthalmia —see Endophthalmitis,
    purulent
Endophthalmitis (acute) (infective) (metastatic)
    (subacute) H44.009
  bleb associated H59.4 —see also Bleb,
      inflamed (infected), postprocedural
  gonorrheal A54.39
  in (due to)
    cysticercosis B69.1
    onchocerciasis B73.01
    toxocariasis B83.0

Endophthalmitis (Continued)
  panuveitis —see Panuveitis
  parasitic H44.12-
  purulent H44.00-
    panophthalmitis —see Panophthalmitis
    vitreous abscess H44.02-
  specified NEC H44.19
  sympathetic —see Uveitis, sympathetic
Endosalpingioma D28.2
Endosalpingiosis N94.89
Endosteitis —see Osteomyelitis
Endothelioma, bone —see Neoplasm, bone,
    malignant
Endotheliosis (hemorrhagic infectional) D69.8
Endotoxemia — code to condition
Endotrachelitis —see Cervicitis
Engelmann (-Camurati) syndrome Q78.3
English disease —see Rickets
Engman's disease L30.3
Engorgement
  breast N64.59
    newborn P83.4
    puerperal, postpartum O92.79
  lung (passive) —see Edema, lung
  pulmonary (passive) —see Edema, lung
  stomach K31.89
  venous, retina —see Occlusion, retina, vein,
      engorgement
Enlargement, enlarged —see also Hypertrophy
  adenoids J35.2
    with tonsils J35.3
  alveolar ridge K08.89 ◀▥
    congenital —see Anomaly, alveolar
  apertures of diaphragm (congenital)
      Q79.1
  gingival K06.1
  heart, cardiac —see Hypertrophy, cardiac
  labium majus, childhood asymmetric
      (CALME) N90.61 ◀
  lacrimal gland, chronic H04.03-
  liver —see Hypertrophy, liver
  lymph gland or node R59.9
    generalized R59.1
    localized R59.0
  orbit H05.34-
  organ or site, congenital NEC —see Anomaly,
      by site
  parathyroid (gland) E21.0
  pituitary fossa R93.0
  prostate N40.0
    with lower urinary tract symptoms (LUTS)
        N40.1
    without lower urinary tract symptoms
        (LUTS) N40.0
  sella turcica R93.0
  spleen —see Splenomegaly
  thymus (gland) (congenital) E32.0
  thyroid (gland) —see Goiter
  tongue K14.8
  tonsils J35.1
    with adenoids J35.3
  uterus N85.2
Enophthalmos H05.40-
  due to
    orbital tissue atrophy H05.41-
    trauma or surgery H05.42-
Enostosis M27.8
Entamebic, entamebiasis —see Amebiasis
Entanglement
  umbilical cord (s) O69.2
    with compression O69.2
      without compression O69.82
    around neck (with compression) O69.1
      without compression O69.81
    of twins in monoamniotic sac O69.2
Enteralgia —see Pain, abdominal
Enteric —see condition
Enteritis (acute) (diarrheal) (hemorrhagic)
    (noninfective) K52.9 ◀▥
  adenovirus A08.2
  aertrycke infection A02.0

◀ New   ◀▥ Revised   ~~deleted~~ Deleted

Enteritis *(Continued)*
  allergic K52.29 ◀▥
    with ◀
      eosinophilic gastritis or gastroenteritis
        K52.81 ◀
      food protein-induced enterocolitis
        syndrome K52.21 ◀
      food protein-induced enteropathy
        K52.22 ◀
    amebic (acute) A06.0
      with abscess —*see* Abscess, amebic
      chronic A06.1
        with abscess —*see* Abscess, amebic
        nondysenteric A06.2
      nondysenteric A06.2
    astrovirus A08.32
    bacillary NOS A03.9
    bacterial A04.9
      specified NEC A04.8
    calicivirus A08.31
    candidal B37.82
    Chilomastix A07.8
    choleriformis A00.1
    chronic (noninfectious) K52.9
      ulcerative —*see* Colitis, ulcerative
    cicatrizing (chronic) —*see* Enteritis, regional,
      small intestine
    Clostridium
      botulinum (food poisoning) A05.1
      difficile A04.7
    coccidial A07.3
    coxsackie virus A08.39
    dietetic —*see also* Enteritis, allergic
      K52.29 ◀▥
    drug-induced K52.1
    due to
      astrovirus A08.32
      calicivirus A08.31
      coxsackie virus A08.39
      drugs K52.1
      echovirus A08.39
      enterovirus NEC A08.39
      food hypersensitivity —*see also* Enteritis,
        allergic K52.29 ◀▥
      infectious organism (bacterial) (viral) —*see*
        Enteritis, infectious
      torovirus A08.39
      Yersinia enterocolitica A04.6
    echovirus A08.39
    eltor A00.1
    enterovirus NEC A08.39
    eosinophilic K52.81
    epidemic (infectious) A09
    fulminant —*see also* Ischemia, intestine, acute
      K55.019 ◀▥
    gangrenous —*see* Enteritis, infectious
    giardial A07.1
    infectious NOS A09
      due to
        adenovirus A08.2
        Aerobacter aerogenes A04.8
        Arizona (bacillus) A02.0
        bacteria NOS A04.9
          specified NEC A04.8
        Campylobacter A04.5
        Clostridium difficile A04.7
        Clostridium perfringens A04.8
        Enterobacter aerogenes A04.8
        enterovirus A08.39
        Escherichia coli A04.4
          enteroaggregative A04.4
          enterohemorrhagic A04.3
          enteroinvasive A04.2
          enteropathogenic A04.0
          enterotoxigenic A04.1
          specified NEC A04.4
        specified
          bacteria NEC A04.8
          virus NEC A08.39
        Staphylococcus A04.8

Enteritis *(Continued)*
  infectious NOS *(Continued)*
    due to *(Continued)*
      virus NEC A08.4
        specified type NEC A08.39
      Yersinia enterocolitica A04.6
      specified organism NEC A08.8
    influenzal —*see* Influenza, with, digestive
      manifestations
    ischemic K55.9
      acute —*see also* Ischemia, intestine, acute
        K55.019 ◀▥
      chronic K55.1
    microsporidial A07.8
    mucomembranous, myxomembranous —*see*
      Syndrome, irritable bowel
    mucous —*see* Syndrome, irritable bowel
    necroticans A05.2
    necrotizing of newborn —*see* Enterocolitis,
      necrotizing, in newborn
    neurogenic —*see* Syndrome, irritable
      bowel
    newborn necrotizing —*see* Enterocolitis,
      necrotizing, in newborn
    noninfectious K52.9
    norovirus A08.11
    parasitic NEC B82.9
    paratyphoid (fever) —*see* Fever,
      paratyphoid
    protozoal A07.9
      specified NEC A07.8
    radiation K52.0
    regional (of) K50.90
      with
        complication K50.919
          abscess K50.914
          fistula K50.913
          intestinal obstruction K50.912
          rectal bleeding K50.911
          specified complication NEC
            K50.918
      colon —*see* Enteritis, regional, large
        intestine
      duodenum —*see* Enteritis, regional, small
        intestine
      ileum —*see* Enteritis, regional, small
        intestine
      jejunum —*see* Enteritis, regional, small
        intestine
      large bowel —*see* Enteritis, regional, large
        intestine
      large intestine (colon) (rectum) K50.10
        with
          complication K50.119
            abscess K50.114
            fistula K50.113
            intestinal obstruction K50.112
            rectal bleeding K50.111
            small intestine (duodenum) (ileum)
              (jejunum) involvement
              K50.80
              with
                complication K50.819
                  abscess K50.814
                  fistula K50.813
                  intestinal obstruction
                    K50.812
                  rectal bleeding K50.811
                  specified complication NEC
                    K50.818
            specified complication NEC
              K50.118
      rectum —*see* Enteritis, regional, large
        intestine
      small intestine (duodenum) (ileum)
        (jejunum) K50.00
        with
          complication K50.019
            abscess K50.014
            fistula K50.013
            intestinal obstruction K50.012

Enteritis *(Continued)*
  regional *(Continued)*
    small intestine *(Continued)*
      with *(Continued)*
        complication *(Continued)*
          large intestine (colon) (rectum)
            involvement K50.80
            with
              complication K50.819
                abscess K50.814
                fistula K50.813
                intestinal obstruction K50.812
                rectal bleeding K50.811
                specified complication NEC
                  K50.818
          rectal bleeding K50.011
          specified complication NEC K50.018
    rotaviral A08.0
    Salmonella, salmonellosis (arizonae)
      (cholerae-suis) (enteritidis)
      (typhimurium) A02.0
    segmental —*see* Enteritis, regional
    septic A09
    Shigella —*see* Infection, Shigella
    small round structured NEC A08.19
    spasmodic, spastic —*see* Syndrome, irritable
      bowel
    staphylococcal A04.8
      due to food A05.0
    torovirus A08.39
    toxic NEC K52.1
      due to Clostridium difficile A04.7
    trichomonal A07.8
    tuberculous A18.32
    typhosa A01.00
    ulcerative (chronic) —*see* Colitis, ulcerative
    viral A08.4
      adenovirus A08.2
      enterovirus A08.39
      Rotavirus A08.0
      small round structured NEC A08.19
      specified NEC A08.39
      virus specified NEC A08.39
Enterobiasis B80
Enterobius vermicularis (infection) (infestation)
  B80
Enterocele —*see also* Hernia, abdomen
  pelvic, pelvis (acquired) (congenital) N81.5
  vagina, vaginal (acquired) (congenital)
    NEC N81.5
Enterocolitis —*see also* Enteritis K52.9
  due to Clostridium difficile A04.7
  fulminant ischemic —*see also* Ischemia,
    intestine, acute K55.059 ◀▥
  granulomatous —*see* Enteritis, regional
  hemorrhagic (acute) —*see also* Ischemia,
    intestine, acute K55.059 ◀▥
    chronic K55.1
  infectious NEC A09
  ischemic K55.9
  necrotizing K55.30 ◀▥
    with ◀
      perforation K55.33 ◀
      pneumatosis K55.32 ◀
      and perforation K55.33 ◀
    due to Clostridium difficile A04.7
    in non-newborn K55.30 ◀
      stage 1 (without pneumatosis, without
        perforation) K55.31 ◀
      stage 2 (with pneumatosis, without
        perforation) K55.32 ◀
      stage 3 (with pneumatosis, with
        perforation) K55.33 ◀
    in newborn P77.9
      stage 1 (without pneumatosis, without
        perforation) P77.1
      stage 2 (with pneumatosis, without
        perforation) P77.2
      stage 3 (with pneumatosis, with
        perforation) P77.3
    without pneumatosis or perforation
      K55.31 ◀

◀ New   ◀▥ Revised   ~~deleted~~ Deleted

233

Enterocolitis (Continued)
  noninfectious K52.9
    newborn —see Enterocolitis, necrotizing, in
      newborn
  pseudomembranous (newborn) A04.7
  radiation K52.0
    newborn —see Enterocolitis, necrotizing, in
      newborn
  ulcerative (chronic) —see Pancolitis,
    ulcerative (chronic)
Enterogastritis —see Enteritis
Enteropathy K63.9
  food protein-induced enterocolitis K52.22 ◀
  gluten-sensitive K90.0
    non-celiac K90.41 ◀
  hemorrhagic, terminal —see also Ischemia,
    intestine, acute K55.059 ◀▥
  protein-losing K90.49 ◀▥
Enteroperitonitis —see Peritonitis
Enteroptosis K63.4
Enterorrhagia K92.2
Enterospasm —see also Syndrome, irritable,
  bowel
  psychogenic F45.8
Enterostenosis —see also Obstruction, intestine
  K56.69
Enterostomy
  complication —see Complication,
    enterostomy
  status Z93.4
Enterovirus, as cause of disease classified
    elsewhere B97.10
  coxsackievirus B97.11
  echovirus B97.12
  other specified B97.19
Enthesopathy (peripheral) M77.9
  Achilles tendinitis —see Tendinitis,
    Achilles
  ankle and tarsus M77.9
    specified type NEC —see Enthesopathy,
      foot, specified type NEC
  anterior tibial syndrome M76.81-
  calcaneal spur —see Spur, bone, calcaneal
  elbow region M77.8
    lateral epicondylitis —see Epicondylitis,
      lateral
    medial epicondylitis —see Epicondylitis,
      medial
  foot NEC M77.9
    metatarsalgia —see Metatarsalgia
    specified type NEC M77.5-
  forearm M77.9
  gluteal tendinitis —see Tendinitis, gluteal
  hand M77.9
  hip —see Enthesopathy, lower limb, specified
    type NEC
  iliac crest spur —see Spur, bone, iliac crest
  iliotibial band syndrome —see Syndrome,
    iliotibial band
  knee —see Enthesopathy, lower limb, lower
    leg, specified type NEC
  lateral epicondylitis —see Epicondylitis,
    lateral
  lower limb (excluding foot) M76.9
    Achilles tendinitis —see Tendinitis, Achilles
    anterior tibial syndrome M76.81-
    gluteal tendinitis —see Tendinitis, gluteal
    iliac crest spur —see Spur, bone, iliac crest
    iliotibial band syndrome —see Syndrome,
      iliotibial band
    patellar tendinitis —see Tendinitis, patellar
    pelvic region —see Enthesopathy, lower
      limb, specified type NEC
    peroneal tendinitis —see Tendinitis,
      peroneal
    posterior tibial syndrome M76.82-
    psoas tendinitis —see Tendinitis, psoas
    shoulder M77.9
    specified type NEC M76.89-
    tibial collateral bursitis —see Bursitis, tibial
      collateral

Enthesopathy (Continued)
  medial epicondylitis —see Epicondylitis,
    medial
  multiple sites M77.9
  patellar tendinitis —see Tendinitis, patellar
  pelvis M77.9
  periarthritis of wrist —see Periarthritis,
    wrist
  peroneal tendinitis —see Tendinitis, peroneal
  posterior tibial syndrome M76.82-
  psoas tendinitis —see Tendinitis, psoas
  shoulder region —see Lesion, shoulder
  specified site NEC M77.9
  specified type NEC M77.8
  spinal M46.00
    cervical region M46.02
    cervicothoracic region M46.03
    lumbar region M46.06
    lumbosacral region M46.07
    multiple sites M46.09
    occipito-atlanto-axial region M46.01
    sacrococcygeal region M46.08
    thoracic region M46.04
    thoracolumbar region M46.05
  tibial collateral bursitis —see Bursitis, tibial
    collateral
  upper arm M77.9
  wrist and carpus NEC M77.8
    calcaneal spur —see Spur, bone, calcaneal
    periarthritis of wrist —see Periarthritis,
      wrist
Entomophobia F40.218
Entomophthoromycosis B46.8
Entrance, air into vein —see Embolism, air
Entrapment, nerve —see Neuropathy,
    entrapment
Entropion (eyelid) (paralytic) H02.009
  cicatricial H02.019
    left H02.016
      lower H02.015
      upper H02.014
    right H02.013
      lower H02.012
      upper H02.011
  congenital Q10.2
  left H02.006
    lower H02.005
    upper H02.004
  mechanical H02.029
    left H02.026
      lower H02.025
      upper H02.024
    right H02.023
      lower H02.022
      upper H02.021
  right H02.003
    lower H02.002
    upper H02.001
  senile H02.039
    left H02.036
      lower H02.035
      upper H02.034
    right H02.033
      lower H02.032
      upper H02.031
  spastic H02.049
    left H02.046
      lower H02.045
      upper H02.044
    right H02.043
      lower H02.042
      upper H02.041
Enucleated eye (traumatic, current) S05.7-
Enuresis R32
  functional F98.0
  habit disturbance F98.0
  nocturnal N39.44
    psychogenic F98.0
  nonorganic origin F98.0
  psychogenic F98.0
Eosinopenia —see Agranulocytosis

Eosinophilia (allergic) (hereditary) (idiopathic)
    (secondary) D72.1
  with
    angiolymphoid hyperplasia (ALHE)
      D18.01
  infiltrative J82
  Löffler's J82
  peritoneal —see Peritonitis, eosinophilic
  pulmonary NEC J82
  tropical (pulmonary) J82
Eosinophilia-myalgia syndrome M35.8
Ependymitis (acute) (cerebral) (chronic)
    (granular) —see Encephalomyelitis
Ependymoblastoma
  specified site —see Neoplasm, malignant, by
    site
  unspecified site C71.9
Ependymoma (epithelial) (malignant)
  anaplastic
    specified site —see Neoplasm, malignant,
      by site
    unspecified site C71.9
  benign
    specified site —see Neoplasm, benign, by
      site
    unspecified site D33.2
  myxopapillary D43.2
    specified site —see Neoplasm, uncertain
      behavior, by site
    unspecified site D43.2
  papillary D43.2
    specified site —see Neoplasm, uncertain
      behavior, by site
    unspecified site D43.2
  specified site —see Neoplasm, malignant, by
    site
  unspecified site C71.9
Ependymopathy G93.89
Ephelis, ephelides L81.2
Epiblepharon (congenital) Q10.3
Epicanthus, epicanthic fold (eyelid)
    (congenital) Q10.3
Epicondylitis (elbow)
  lateral M77.1-
  medial M77.0-
Epicystitis —see Cystitis
Epidemic —see condition
Epidermidalization, cervix —see Dysplasia,
    cervix
Epidermis, epidermal —see condition
Epidermodysplasia verruciformis B07.8
Epidermolysis
  bullosa (congenital) Q81.9
    acquired L12.30
      drug-induced L12.31
      specified cause NEC L12.35
    dystrophica Q81.2
    letalis Q81.1
    simplex Q81.0
    specified NEC Q81.8
  necroticans combustiformis L51.2
    due to drug —see Table of Drugs and
      Chemicals, by drug
Epidermophytid —see Dermatophytosis
Epidermophytosis (infected) —see
    Dermatophytosis
Epididymis —see condition
Epididymitis (acute) (nonvenereal) (recurrent)
    (residual) N45.1
  with orchitis N45.3
  blennorrhagic (gonococcal) A54.23
  caseous (tuberculous) A18.15
  chlamydial A56.19
  filarial —see also Infestation, filarial B74.9
    [N51]
  gonococcal A54.23
  syphilitic A52.76
  tuberculous A18.15
Epididymo-orchitis —see also Epididymitis
  N45.3
Epidural —see condition

◀ New   ◀▥ Revised   ~~deleted~~ Deleted

Epigastrium, epigastric —*see* condition
Epigastrocele —*see* Hernia, ventral
Epiglottis —*see* condition
Epiglottitis, epiglottiditis (acute) J05.10
  with obstruction J05.11
  chronic J37.0
Epignathus Q89.4
Epilepsia partialis continua —*see also*
  Kozhevnikof's epilepsy G40.1-
Epilepsy, epileptic, epilepsia (attack)
  (cerebral) (convulsion) (fit) (seizure)
  G40.909

> Note: the following terms are to be
> considered equivalent to intractable:
> pharmacoresistant (pharmacologically
> resistant), treatment resistant, refractory
> (medically) and poorly controlled

  with
    complex partial seizures —*see* Epilepsy,
      localization-related, symptomatic,
      with complex partial seizures
    grand mal seizures on awakening —
      see Epilepsy, generalized, specified
      NEC
    myoclonic absences —*see* Epilepsy,
      generalized, specified NEC
    myoclonic-astatic seizures —*see* Epilepsy,
      generalized, specified NEC
    simple partial seizures —*see* Epilepsy,
      localization-related, symptomatic,
      with simple partial seizures
  akinetic —*see* Epilepsy, generalized, specified
    NEC
  benign childhood with centrotemporal EEG
    spikes —*see* Epilepsy, localization-
    related, idiopathic
  benign myoclonic in infancy G40.80-
  Bravais-jacksonian —*see* Epilepsy,
    localization-related, symptomatic,
    with simple partial seizures
  childhood
    with occipital EEG paroxysms —*see*
      Epilepsy, localization-related,
      idiopathic
    absence G40.A09
      intractable G40.A19
        with status epilepticus G40.A11
        without status epilepticus G40.A19
      not intractable G40.A09
        with status epilepticus G40.A01
        without status epilepticus
          G40.A09
  climacteric —*see* Epilepsy, specified NEC
  cysticercosis B69.0
  deterioration (mental) F06.8
  due to syphilis A52.19
  focal —*see* Epilepsy, localization-related,
    symptomatic, with simple partial
    seizures
  generalized
    idiopathic G40.309
      intractable G40.319
        with status epilepticus G40.311
        without status epilepticus G40.319
      not intractable G40.309
        with status epilepticus G40.301
        without status epilepticus G40.309
    specified NEC G40.409
      intractable G40.419
        with status epilepticus G40.411
        without status epilepticus G40.419
      not intractable G40.409
        with status epilepticus G40.401
        without status epilepticus G40.409
  impulsive petit mal —*see* Epilepsy, juvenile
    myoclonic
  intractable G40.919
    with status epilepticus G40.911
    without status epilepticus G40.919

Epilepsy, epileptic, epilepsia *(Continued)*
  juvenile absence G40.A09
    intractable G40.A19
      with status epilepticus G40.A11
      without status epilepticus G40.A19
    not intractable G40.A09
      with status epilepticus G40.A01
      without status epilepticus G40.A09
  juvenile myoclonic G40.B11
    intractable G40.B19
      with status epilepticus G40.B11
      without status epilepticus G40.B19
    not intractable G40.B09
      with status epilepticus G40.B01
      without status epilepticus G40.B09
  localization-related (focal) (partial)
    idiopathic G40.009
      with seizures of localized onset G40.009
        intractable G40.019
          with status epilepticus G40.011
          without status epilepticus G40.019
        not intractable G40.009
          with status epilepticus G40.001
          without status epilepticus G40.009
    symptomatic
      with complex partial seizures G40.209
        intractable G40.219
          with status epilepticus G40.211
          without status epilepticus G40.219
        not intractable G40.209
          with status epilepticus G40.201
          without status epilepticus
            G40.209
      with simple partial seizures G40.109
        intractable G40.119
          with status epilepticus G40.111
          without status epilepticus
            G40.119
        not intractable G40.109
          with status epilepticus G40.101
          without status epilepticus G40.109
  myoclonus, myoclonic —*see* Epilepsy,
    generalized, specified NEC ◀
  progressive —*see* Epilepsy, generalized,
    idiopathic ◀
  not intractable G40.909
    with status epilepticus G40.901
    without status epilepticus G40.909
  on awakening —*see* Epilepsy, generalized,
    specified NEC
  parasitic NOS B71.9 *[G94]*
  partialis continua —*see also* Kozhevnikof's
    epilepsy G40.1-
  peripheral —*see* Epilepsy, specified NEC
  procursiva —*see* Epilepsy, localization-
    related, symptomatic, with simple
    partial seizures
  progressive (familial) myoclonic —*see*
    Epilepsy, generalized, idiopathic
  reflex —*see* Epilepsy, specified NEC
  related to
    alcohol G40.509
      not intractable G40.509
        with status epilepticus G40.501
        without status epliepticus G40.509
    drugs G40.509
      not intractable G40.509
        with status epilepticus G40.501
        without status epliepticus G40.509
    external causes G40.509
      not intractable G40.509
        with status epilepticus G40.501
        without status epilepticus G40.509
    hormonal changes G40.509
      not intractable G40.509
        with status epilepticus G40.501
        without status epilepticus G40.509
    sleep deprivation G40.509
      not intractable G40.509
        with status epilepticus G40.501
        without status epliepticus G40.509

Epilepsy, epileptic, epilepsia *(Continued)*
  related to *(Continued)*
    stress G40.509
      not intractable G40.509
        with status epilepticus G40.501
        without status epliepticus G40.509
    somatomotor —*see* Epilepsy, localization-
      related, symptomatic, with simple
      partial seizures
    somatosensory —*see* Epilepsy, localization-
      related, symptomatic, with simple
      partial seizures
  spasms G40.822
    intractable G40.824
      with status epilepticus G40.823
      without status epilepticus G40.824
    not intractable G40.822
      with status epilepticus G40.821
      without status epilepticus G40.822
  specified NEC G40.802
    intractable G40.804
      with status epilepticus G40.803
      without status epilepticus G40.804
    not intractable G40.802
      with status epilepticus G40.801
      without status epilepticus G40.802
  syndromes
    generalized
      idiopathic G40.309
        intractable G40.319
          with status epilepticus G40.311
          without status epilepticus G40.319
        not intractable G40.309
          with status epilepticus G40.301
          without status epilepticus G40.309
      specified NEC G40.409
        intractable G40.419
          with status epilepticus G40.411
          without status epilepticus G40.419
        not intractable G40.409
          with status epilepticus G40.401
          without status epilepticus G40.409
    localization-related (focal) (partial)
      idiopathic G40.009
        with seizures of localized onset
          G40.009
        intractable G40.019
          with status epilepticus G40.011
          without status epilepticus
            G40.019
        not intractable G40.009
          with status epilepticus G40.001
          without status epilepticus
            G40.009
    symptomatic
      with complex partial seizures
        G40.209
      intractable G40.219
        with status epilepticus G40.211
        without status epilepticus
          G40.219
      not intractable G40.209
        with status epilepticus G40.201
        without status epilepticus G40.209
      with simple partial seizures G40.109
        intractable G40.119
          with status epilepticus G40.111
          without status epilepticus G40.119
        not intractable G40.109
          with status epilepticus G40.101
          without status epilepticus G40.109
    specified NEC G40.802
      intractable G40.804
        with status epilepticus G40.803
        without status epilepticus G40.804
      not intractable G40.802
        with status epilepticus G40.801
        without status epilepticus G40.802
  tonic (-clonic) —*see* Epilepsy, generalized,
    specified NEC
  twilight F05

Epilepsy, epileptic, epilepsia *(Continued)*
 uncinate (gyrus) —*see* Epilepsy, localization-related, symptomatic, with complex partial seizures
 Unverricht (-Lundborg) (familial myoclonic) — *see* Epilepsy, generalized, idiopathic
 visceral —*see* Epilepsy, specified NEC
 visual —*see* Epilepsy, specified NEC
Epiloia Q85.1
Epimenorrhea N92.0
Epipharyngitis —*see* Nasopharyngitis
Epiphora H04.20-
 due to
  excess lacrimation H04.21-
  insufficient drainage H04.22-
Epiphyseal arrest —*see* Arrest, epiphyseal
Epiphyseolysis, epiphysiolysis —*see* Osteochondropathy
Epiphysitis —*see also* Osteochondropathy
 juvenile M92.9
 syphilitic (congenital) A50.02
Epiplocele —*see* Hernia, abdomen
Epiploitis —*see* Peritonitis
Epiplosarcomphalocele —*see* Hernia, umbilicus
Episcleritis (suppurative) H15.10-
 in (due to)
  syphilis A52.71
  tuberculosis A18.51
 nodular H15.12-
 periodica fugax H15.11-
  angioneurotic —*see* Edema, angioneurotic
 syphilitic (late) A52.71
 tuberculous A18.51
Episode
 affective, mixed F39
 depersonalization (in neurotic state) F48.1
 depressive F32.9
  major F32.9
   mild F32.0
   moderate F32.1
   severe (without psychotic symptoms) F32.2
    with psychotic symptoms F32.3
  recurrent F33.9
   brief F33.8
  specified NEC F32.89 ◀
 hypomanic F30.8
 manic F30.9
  with
   psychotic symptoms F30.2
   remission (full) F30.4
    partial F30.3
  without psychotic symptoms F30.10
   mild F30.11
   moderate F30.12
   severe (without psychotic symptoms) F30.13
    with psychotic symptoms F30.2
  other specified F30.8
  recurrent F31.89
 psychotic F23
  organic F06.8
 schizophrenic (acute) NEC, brief F23
Epispadias (female) (male) Q64.0
Episplenitis D73.89
Epistaxis (multiple) R04.0
 hereditary I78.0
 vicarious menstruation N94.89
Epithelioma (malignant) —*see also* Neoplasm, malignant, by site
 adenoides cysticum —*see* Neoplasm, skin, benign
 basal cell —*see* Neoplasm, skin, malignant
 benign —*see* Neoplasm, benign, by site
 Bowen's —*see* Neoplasm, skin, in situ
 calcifying, of Malherbe —*see* Neoplasm, skin, benign
 external site —*see* Neoplasm, skin, malignant
 intraepidermal, Jadassohn —*see* Neoplasm, skin, benign
 squamous cell —*see* Neoplasm, malignant, by site

Epitheliomatosis pigmented Q82.1
Epitheliopathy, multifocal placoid pigment H30.14-
Epithelium, epithelial —*see* condition
Epituberculosis (with atelectasis) (allergic) A15.7
Eponychia Q84.6
Epstein's
 nephrosis or syndrome —*see* Nephrosis
 pearl K09.8
Epulis (gingiva) (fibrous) (giant cell) K06.8
Equinia A24.0
Equinovarus (congenital) (talipes) Q66.0
 acquired —*see* Deformity, limb, clubfoot
Equivalent
 convulsive (abdominal) —*see* Epilepsy, specified NEC
 epileptic (psychic) —*see* Epilepsy, localization-related, symptomatic, with complex partial seizures
Erb (-Duchenne) paralysis (birth injury) (newborn) P14.0
Erb's
 disease G71.0
 palsy, paralysis (brachial) (birth) (newborn) P14.0
 spinal (spastic) syphilitic A52.17
 pseudohypertrophic muscular dystrophy G71.0
Erb-Goldflam disease or syndrome G70.00
 with exacerbation (acute) G70.01
 in crisis G70.01
Erdheim's syndrome (acromegalic macrospondylitis) E22.0
Erection, painful (persistent) —*see* Priapism
Ergosterol deficiency (vitamin D) E55.9
 with
  adult osteomalacia M83.8
  rickets —*see* Rickets
Ergotism —*see also* Poisoning, food, noxious, plant
 from ergot used as drug (migraine therapy) —*see* Table of Drugs and Chemicals
Erosio interdigitalis blastomycetica B37.2
Erosion
 artery I77.2
  without rupture I77.89
 bone —*see* Disorder, bone, density and structure, specified NEC
 bronchus J98.09
 cartilage (joint) —*see* Disorder, cartilage, specified type NEC
 cervix (uteri) (acquired) (chronic) (congenital) N86
  with cervicitis N72
 cornea (nontraumatic) —*see* Ulcer, cornea
  recurrent H18.83-
  traumatic —*see* Abrasion, cornea
 dental (idiopathic) (occupational) (due to diet, drugs or vomiting) K03.2
 duodenum, postpyloric —*see* Ulcer, duodenum
 esophagus K22.10
  with bleeding K22.11
 gastric —*see* Ulcer, stomach
 gastrojejunal —*see* Ulcer, gastrojejunal
 implanted mesh —*see* Complications, mesh
 intestine K63.3
 lymphatic vessel I89.8
 pylorus, pyloric (ulcer) —*see* Ulcer, stomach
 spine, aneurysmal A52.09
 stomach —*see* Ulcer, stomach
 subcutaneous device pocket ◀
  nervous system prosthetic device, implant, or graft T85.890 ◀
  other internal prosthetic device, implant, or graft T85.898 ◀
 teeth (idiopathic) (occupational) (due to diet, drugs or vomiting) K03.2
 urethra N36.8
 uterus N85.8

Erotomania F52.8
Error
 metabolism, inborn —*see* Disorder, metabolism
 refractive —*see* Disorder, refraction
Eructation R14.2
 nervous or psychogenic F45.8
Eruption
 creeping B76.9
 drug (generalized) (taken internally) L27.0
  fixed L27.1
  in contact with skin —*see* Dermatitis, due to drugs
  localized L27.1
 Hutchinson, summer L56.4
 Kaposi's varicelliform B00.0
 napkin L22
 polymorphous light (sun) L56.4
 recalcitrant pustular L13.8
 ringed R23.8
 skin (nonspecific) R21
  creeping (meaning hookworm) B76.9
  due to inoculation/vaccination (generalized) —*see also* Dermatitis, due to, vaccine L27.0
   localized L27.1
  erysipeloid A26.0
  feigned L98.1
  Kaposi's varicelliform B00.0
  lichenoid L28.0
  meaning dermatitis —*see* Dermatitis
  toxic NEC L53.0
 tooth, teeth, abnormal (incomplete) (late) (premature) (sequence) K00.6
 vesicular R23.8
Erysipelas (gangrenous) (infantile) (newborn) (phlegmonous) (suppurative) A46
 external ear A46 [H62.40]
 puerperal, postpartum O86.89
Erysipeloid A26.9
 cutaneous (Rosenbach's) A26.0
 disseminated A26.8
 sepsis A26.7
 specified NEC A26.8
Erythema, erythematous (infectional) (inflammation) L53.9
 ab igne L59.0
 annulare (centrifugum) (rheumaticum) L53.1
 arthriticum epidemicum A25.1
 brucellum —*see* Brucellosis
 chronic figurate NEC L53.3
 chronicum migrans (Borrelia burgdorferi) A69.20
 diaper L22
 due to
  chemical NEC L53.0
   in contact with skin L24.5
  drug (internal use) —*see* Dermatitis, due to, drugs
 elevatum diutinum L95.1
 endemic E52
 epidemic, arthritic A25.1
 figuratum perstans L53.3
 gluteal L22
 heat - code by site under Burn, first degree
 ichthyosiforme congenitum bullous Q80.3
 in diseases classified elsewhere L54
 induratum (nontuberculous) L52
  tuberculous A18.4
 infectiosum B08.3
 intertrigo L30.4
 iris L51.9
 marginatum L53.2
  in (due to) acute rheumatic fever I00
 medicamentosum —*see* Dermatitis, due to, drugs
 migrans A26.0
  chronicum A69.20
  tongue K14.1

◀ New ◀▥ Revised ~~deleted~~ Deleted

Erythema, erythematous (Continued)
  multiforme (major) (minor) L51.9
    bullous, bullosum L51.1
    conjunctiva L51.1
    nonbullous L51.0
    pemphigoides L12.0
    specified NEC L51.8
  napkin L22
  neonatorum P83.8
    toxic P83.1
  nodosum L52
    tuberculous A18.4
  palmar L53.8
  pernio T69.1
  rash, newborn P83.8
  scarlatiniform (recurrent) (exfoliative)
    L53.8
  solare L55.0
  specified NEC L53.8
  toxic, toxicum NEC L53.0
    newborn P83.1
  tuberculous (primary) A18.4
Erythematous, erythematosus —see condition
Erythermalgia (primary) I73.81
Erythralgia I73.81
Erythrasma L08.1
Erythredema (polyneuropathy) —see Poisoning,
    mercury
Erythremia (acute) C94.0-
  chronic D45
  secondary D75.1
Erythroblastopenia —see also Aplasia, red cell
    D60.9
  congenital D61.01
Erythroblastophthisis D61.09
Erythroblastosis (fetalis) (newborn) P55.9
  due to
    ABO (antibodies) (incompatibility)
      (isoimmunization) P55.1
    Rh (antibodies) (incompatibility)
      (isoimmunization) P55.0
Erythrocyanosis (crurum) I73.89
Erythrocythemia —see Erythremia
Erythrocytosis (megalosplenic) (secondary)
    D75.1
  familial D75.0
  oval, hereditary —see Elliptocytosis
  secondary D75.1
  stress D75.1
Erythroderma (secondary) —see also Erythema
    L53.9
  bullous ichthyosiform, congenital Q80.3
  desquamativum L21.1
  ichthyosiform, congenital (bullous) Q80.3
  neonatorum P83.8
  psoriaticum L40.8
Erythrodysesthesia, palmar plantar (PPE) L27.1
Erythrogenesis imperfecta D61.09
Erythroleukemia C94.0-
Erythromelalgia I73.81
Erythrophagocytosis D75.89
Erythrophobia F40.298
Erythroplakia, oral epithelium, and tongue
    K13.29
Erythroplasia (Queyrat) D07.4
  specified site —see Neoplasm, skin, in situ
  unspecified site D07.4
Escherichia coli (E. coli), as cause of disease
    classified elsewhere B96.20
  non-O157 Shiga toxin-producing (with
    known O group) B96.22
  non-Shiga toxin-producing B96.29
  O157 with confirmation of Shiga toxin when
    H antigen is unknown, or is not H7
    B96.21
  O157:H- (nonmotile) with confirmation of
    Shiga toxin B96.21
  O157:H7 with or without confirmation of
    Shiga toxin-production B96.21
  Shiga toxin-producing (with unspecified O
    group) (STEC) B96.23

Escherichia coli (Continued)
  O157 B96.21
  O157:H7 with or without confirmation of
    Shiga toxin-production B96.21
    specified NEC B96.22
  specified NEC B96.29
Esophagismus K22.4
Esophagitis (acute) (alkaline) (chemical)
    (chronic) (infectional) (necrotic) (peptic)
    (postoperative) K20.9
  candidal B37.81
  due to gastrointestinal reflux disease K21.0
  eosinophilic K20.0
  reflux K21.0
  specified NEC K20.8
  tuberculous A18.83
  ulcerative K22.10
    with bleeding K22.11
Esophagocele K22.5
Esophagomalacia K22.8
Esophagospasm K22.4
Esophagostenosis K22.2
Esophagostomiasis B81.8
Esophagotracheal —see condition
Esophagus —see condition
Esophoria H50.51
  convergence, excess H51.12
  divergence, insufficiency H51.8
Esotropia —see Strabismus, convergent
    concomitant
Espundia B55.2
Essential —see condition
Esthesioneuroblastoma C30.0
Esthesioneurocytoma C30.0
Esthesioneuroepithelioma C30.0
Esthiomene A55
Estivo-autumnal malaria (fever) B50.9
Estrangement (marital) Z63.5
  parent-child NEC Z62.890
Estriasis —see Myiasis
Ethanolism —see Alcoholism
Etherism —see Dependence, drug, inhalant
Ethmoid, ethmoidal —see condition
Ethmoiditis (chronic) (nonpurulent)
    (purulent) —see also Sinusitis, ethmoidal
  influenzal —see Influenza, with, respiratory
    manifestations NEC
  Woakes' J33.1
Ethylism —see Alcoholism
Eulenburg's disease (congenital paramyotonia)
    G71.19
Eumycetoma B47.0
Eunuchoidism E29.1
  hypogonadotropic E23.0
European blastomycosis —see Cryptococcosis
Eustachian —see condition
Evaluation (for) (of)
  development state
    adolescent Z00.3
    period of
      delayed growth in childhood Z00.70
        with abnormal findings Z00.71
      rapid growth in childhood Z00.2
    puberty Z00.3
  growth and developmental state (period of
    rapid growth) Z00.2
    delayed growth Z00.70
      with abnormal findings Z00.71
  mental health (status) Z00.8
    requested by authority Z04.6
  period of
    delayed growth in childhood Z00.70
      with abnormal findings Z00.71
    rapid growth in childhood Z00.2
  suspected condition —see Observation
Evans syndrome D69.41
Event, apparent life threatening in newborn
    and infant (ALTE) R68.13
Eventration —see also Hernia, ventral
  colon into chest —see Hernia, diaphragm
  diaphragm (congenital) Q79.1

Eversion
  bladder N32.89
  cervix (uteri) N86
    with cervicitis N72
  foot NEC —see also Deformity, valgus, ankle
    congenital Q66.6
  punctum lacrimale (postinfectional) (senile)
    H04.52-
  ureter (meatus) N28.89
  urethra (meatus) N36.8
  uterus N81.4
Evidence
  cytologic
    of malignancy on anal smear R85.614
    of malignancy on cervical smear R87.614
    of malignancy on vaginal smear R87.624
Evisceration
  birth injury P15.8
  traumatic NEC
    eye —see Enucleated eye
Evulsion —see Avulsion
Ewing's sarcoma or tumor —see Neoplasm,
    bone, malignant
Examination (for) (following) (general) (of)
    (routine) Z00.00
  with abnormal findings Z00.01
  abuse, physical (alleged), ruled out
    adult Z04.71
    child Z04.72
  adolescent (development state) Z00.3
  alleged rape or sexual assault (victim), ruled
    out
    adult Z04.41
    child Z04.42
  allergy Z01.82
  annual (adult) (periodic) (physical) Z00.00
    with abnormal findings Z00.01
    gynecological Z01.419
      with abnormal findings Z01.411
  antibody response Z01.84
  blood —see Examination, laboratory
  blood pressure Z01.30
    with abnormal findings Z01.31
  cancer staging —see Neoplasm, malignant,
    by site
  cervical Papanicolaou smear Z12.4
    as part of routine gynecological
      examination Z01.419
      with abnormal findings Z01.411
  child (over 28 days old) Z00.129
    with abnormal findings Z00.121
    under 28 days old —see Newborn,
      examination
  clinical research control or normal
    comparison (control) (participant) Z00.6
  contraceptive (drug) maintenance (routine)
    Z30.8
    device (intrauterine) Z30.431
  dental Z01.20
    with abnormal findings Z01.21
  developmental —see Examination, child
  donor (potential) Z00.5
  ear Z01.10
    with abnormal findings NEC Z01.118
  eye Z01.00
    with abnormal findings Z01.01
  following
    accident NEC Z04.3
      transport Z04.1
      work Z04.2
    assault, alleged, ruled out
      adult Z04.71
      child Z04.72
    motor vehicle accident Z04.1
    treatment (for) Z09
      combined NEC Z09
        fracture Z09
        malignant neoplasm Z08
      malignant neoplasm Z08
      mental disorder Z09
      specified condition NEC Z09

◀ New   ◀||| Revised   deleted Deleted

Examination (Continued)
  follow-up (routine) (following) Z09
    chemotherapy NEC Z09
      malignant neoplasm Z08
    fracture Z09
    malignant neoplasm Z08
    postpartum Z39.2
    psychotherapy Z09
    radiotherapy NEC Z09
      malignant neoplasm Z08
    surgery NEC Z09
      malignant neoplasm Z08
  gynecological Z01.419
    with abnormal findings Z01.411
    for contraceptive maintenance Z30.8
  health —see Examination, medical
  hearing Z01.10
    with abnormal findings NEC Z01.118
    following failed hearing screening Z01.110
  immunity status testing Z01.84
  laboratory (as part of a general medical
        examination) Z00.00
    with abnormal findings Z00.01
    preprocedural Z01.812
  lactating mother Z39.1
  medical (adult) (for) (of) Z00.00
    with abnormal findings Z00.01
    administrative purpose only Z02.9
      specified NEC Z02.89
    admission to
      armed forces Z02.3
      old age home Z02.2
      prison Z02.89
      residential institution Z02.2
      school Z02.0
        following illness or medical treatment
            Z02.0
      summer camp Z02.89
    adoption Z02.82
    blood alcohol or drug level Z02.83
    camp (summer) Z02.89
    clinical research, normal subject (control)
        (participant) Z00.6
    control subject in clinical research (normal
        comparison) (participant) Z00.6
    donor (potential) Z00.5
    driving license Z02.4
    general (adult) Z00.00
      with abnormal findings Z00.01
    immigration Z02.89
    insurance purposes Z02.6
    marriage Z02.89
    medicolegal reasons NEC Z04.8
    naturalization Z02.89
    participation in sport Z02.5
    paternity testing Z02.81
    population survey Z00.8
    pre-employment Z02.1
    pre-operative —see Examination,
        pre-procedural
    pre-procedural
      cardiovascular Z01.810
      respiratory Z01.811
      specified NEC Z01.818
    preschool children
      for admission to school Z02.0
    prisoners
      for entrance into prison Z02.89
    recruitment for armed forces Z02.3
    specified NEC Z00.8
    sport competition Z02.5
  medicolegal reason NEC Z04.8
  newborn —see Newborn, examination
  pelvic (annual) (periodic) Z01.419
    with abnormal findings Z01.411
  period of rapid growth in childhood Z00.2
  periodic (adult) (annual) (routine) Z00.00
    with abnormal findings Z00.01
  physical (adult) —see also Examination,
      medical Z00.00
    sports Z02.5

Examination (Continued)
  postpartum
    immediately after delivery Z39.0
    routine follow-up Z39.2
  pre-chemotherapy (antineoplastic) Z01.818
  prenatal (normal pregnancy) —see also
      Pregnancy, normal Z34.9-
  pre-procedural (pre-operative)
    cardiovascular Z01.810
    laboratory Z01.812
    respiratory Z01.811
    specified NEC Z01.818
  prior to chemotherapy (antineoplastic)
      Z01.818
  psychiatric NEC Z00.8
    follow-up not needing further care Z09
    requested by authority Z04.6
  radiological (as part of a general medical
      examination) Z00.00
    with abnormal findings Z00.01
  repeat cervical smear to confirm findings of
      recent normal smear following initial
      abnormal smear Z01.42
  skin (hypersensitivity) Z01.82
  special —see also Examination, by type Z01.89
    specified type NEC Z01.89
  specified type or reason NEC Z04.8
  teeth Z01.20
    with abnormal findings Z01.21
  urine —see Examination, laboratory
  vision Z01.00
    with abnormal findings Z01.01
Exanthem, exanthema —see also Rash
  with enteroviral vesicular stomatitis B08.4
  Boston A88.0
  epidemic with meningitis A88.0 [G02]
  subitum B08.20
    due to human herpesvirus 6 B08.21
    due to human herpesvirus 7 B08.22
  viral, virus B09
    specified type NEC B08.8
Excess, excessive, excessively
  alcohol level in blood R78.0
  androgen (ovarian) E28.1
  attrition, tooth, teeth K03.0
  carotene, carotin (dietary) E67.1
  cold, effects of T69.9
    specified effect NEC T69.8
  convergence H51.12
  crying
    in child, adolescent, or adult R45.83
    in infant R68.11
  development, breast N62
  divergence H51.8
  drinking (alcohol) NEC (without
      dependence) F10.10
    habitual (continual) (without remission)
        F10.20
  eating R63.2
  estrogen E28.0
  fat —see also Obesity
    in heart —see Degeneration, myocardial
    localized E65
  foreskin N47.8
  gas R14.0
  glucagon E16.3
  heat —see Heat
  intermaxillary vertical dimension of fully
      erupted teeth M26.37
  interocclusal distance of fully erupted teeth
      M26.37
  kalium E87.5
  large
    colon K59.39
      congenital Q43.8
    infant P08.0
    organ or site, congenital NEC —see
        Anomaly, by site
  long
    organ or site, congenital NEC —see
        Anomaly, by site

Excess, excessive, excessively (Continued)
  menstruation (with regular cycle) N92.0
    with irregular cycle N92.1
  napping Z72.821
  natrium E87.0
  number of teeth K00.1
  nutrient (dietary) NEC R63.2
  potassium (K) E87.5
  salivation K11.7
  secretion —see also Hypersecretion
    milk O92.6
    sputum R09.3
    sweat R61
  sexual drive F52.8
  short
    organ or site, congenital NEC —see
        Anomaly, by site
    umbilical cord in labor or delivery O69.3
  skin, eyelid (acquired) —see Blepharochalasis
    congenital Q10.3
  skin L98.7 ◀
    and subcutaneous tissue L98.7 ◀
    eyelid (acquired) —see Blepharochalasis ◀
      congenital Q10.3 ◀
  sodium (Na) E87.0
  spacing of fully erupted teeth M26.32
  sputum R09.3
  sweating R61
  thirst R63.1
    due to deprivation of water T73.1
  tuberosity of jaw M26.07
  vitamin
    A (dietary) E67.0
      administered as drug (prolonged
          intake) —see Table of Drugs and
          Chemicals, vitamins, adverse
          effect
      overdose or wrong substance given or
          taken —see Table of Drugs and
          Chemicals, vitamins, poisoning
    D (dietary) E67.3
      administered as drug (prolonged
          intake) —see Table of Drugs and
          Chemicals, vitamins, adverse effect
      overdose or wrong substance given or
          taken —see Table of Drugs and
          Chemicals, vitamins, poisoning
  weight
    gain R63.5
    loss R63.4
Excitability, abnormal, under minor stress
    (personality disorder) F60.3
Excitation
  anomalous atrioventricular I45.6
  psychogenic F30.8
  reactive (from emotional stress, psychological
      trauma) F30.8
Excitement
  hypomanic F30.8
  manic F30.9
  mental, reactive (from emotional stress,
      psychological trauma) F30.8
  state, reactive (from emotional stress,
      psychological trauma) F30.8
Excoriation (traumatic) —see also Abrasion
  neurotic L98.1
  skin picking disorder F42.4 ◀
Exfoliation
  due to erythematous conditions according to
      extent of body surface involved L49.0
    10-19 percent of body surface L49.1
    20-29 percent of body surface L49.2
    30-39 percent of body surface L49.3
    40-49 percent of body surface L49.4
    50-59 percent of body surface L49.5
    60-69 percent of body surface L49.6
    70-79 percent of body surface L49.7
    80-89 percent of body surface L49.8
    90-99 percent of body surface L49.9
    less than 10 percent of body surface L49.0
  teeth, due to systemic causes K08.0

◀ New   ◀▥ Revised   ~~deleted~~ Deleted

Exfoliative —*see* condition
Exhaustion, exhaustive (physical NEC) R53.83
  battle F43.0
  cardiac—*see* Failure, heart
  delirium F43.0
  due to
    cold T69.8
    excessive exertion T73.3
    exposure T73.2
    neurasthenia F48.8
  heart —*see* Failure, heart
  heat —*see also* Heat, exhaustion T67.5
    due to
      salt depletion T67.4
      water depletion T67.3
  maternal, complicating delivery O75.81
  mental F48.8
  myocardium, myocardial —*see* Failure, heart
  nervous F48.8
  old age R54
  psychogenic F48.8
  psychosis F43.0
  senile R54
  vital NEC Z73.0
Exhibitionism F65.2
Exocervicitis —*see* Cervicitis
Exomphalos Q79.2
  meaning hernia —*see* Hernia, umbilicus
Exophoria H50.52
  convergence, insufficiency H51.11
  divergence, excess H51.8
Exophthalmos H05.2-
  congenital Q15.8
  constant NEC H05.24-
  displacement, globe —*see* Displacement,
    globe
  due to thyrotoxicosis (hyperthyroidism) —*see*
    Hyperthyroidism, with, goiter (diffuse)
  dysthyroid —*see* Hyperthyroidism, with,
    goiter (diffuse)
  goiter —*see* Hyperthyroidism, with, goiter
    (diffuse)
  intermittent NEC H05.25-
  malignant —*see* Hyperthyroidism, with,
    goiter (diffuse)
  orbital
    edema —*see* Edema, orbit
    hemorrhage —*see* Hemorrhage, orbit
  pulsating NEC H05.26-
  thyrotoxic, thyrotropic —*see*
    Hyperthyroidism, with, goiter (diffuse)
Exostosis —*see also* Disorder, bone
  cartilaginous —*see* Neoplasm, bone, benign
  congenital (multiple) Q78.6
  external ear canal H61.81-
  gonococcal A54.49
  jaw (bone) M27.8
  multiple, congenital Q78.6
  orbit H05.35-
  osteocartilaginous —*see* Neoplasm, bone,
    benign
  syphilitic A52.77
Exotropia —*see* Strabismus, divergent
    concomitant
Explanation of
  investigation finding Z71.2
  medication Z71.89
Exposure (to) —*see also* Contact, with T75.89
  acariasis Z20.7
  AIDS virus Z20.6
  air pollution Z77.110
  algae and algae toxins Z77.121
  algae bloom Z77.121
  anthrax Z20.810
  aromatic amines Z77.020
  aromatic (hazardous) compounds NEC
    Z77.028
  aromatic dyes NOS Z77.028

Exposure (*Continued*)
  arsenic Z77.010
  asbestos Z77.090
  bacterial disease NEC Z20.818
  benzene Z77.021
  blue-green algae bloom Z77.121
  body fluids (potentially hazardous) Z77.21
  brown tide Z77.121
  chemicals (chiefly nonmedicinal) (hazardous)
    NEC Z77.098
  cholera Z20.09
  chromium compounds Z77.018
  cold, effects of T69.9
    specified effect NEC T69.8
  communicable disease Z20.9
    bacterial NEC Z20.818
    specified NEC Z20.89
    viral NEC Z20.828
  cyanobacteria bloom Z77.121
  disaster Z65.5
  discrimination Z60.5
  dyes Z77.098
  effects of T73.9
  environmental tobacco smoke (acute)
    (chronic) Z77.22
  Escherichia coli (E. coli) Z20.01
  exhaustion due to T73.2
  fiberglass —*see* Table of Drugs and
    Chemicals, fiberglass
  German measles Z20.4
  gonorrhea Z20.2
  hazardous metals NEC Z77.018
  hazardous substances NEC Z77.29
  hazards in the physical environment NEC
    Z77.128
  hazards to health NEC Z77.9
  human immunodeficiency virus (HIV) Z20.6
  human T-lymphotropic virus type-1 (HTLV-1)
    Z20.89
  implanted
    mesh —*see* Complications, mesh
    prosthetic materials NEC —*see*
      Complications, prosthetic materials
      NEC
  infestation (parasitic) NEC Z20.7
  intestinal infectious disease NEC Z20.09
    Escherichia coli (E. coli) Z20.01
  lead Z77.011
  meningococcus Z20.811
  mold (toxic) Z77.120
  nickel dust Z77.018
  noise Z77.122
  occupational
    air contaminants NEC Z57.39
    dust Z57.2
    environmental tobacco smoke Z57.31
    extreme temperature Z57.6
    noise Z57.0
    radiation Z57.1
    risk factors Z57.9
      specified NEC Z57.8
    toxic agents (gases) (liquids) (solids)
      (vapors) in agriculture Z57.4
    toxic agents (gases) (liquids) (solids)
      (vapors) in industry NEC Z57.5
    vibration Z57.7
  parasitic disease NEC Z20.7
  pediculosis Z20.7
  persecution Z60.5
  pfiesteria piscicida Z77.121
  poliomyelitis Z20.89
  pollution
    air Z77.110
    environmental NEC Z77.118
    soil Z77.112
    water Z77.111
  polycyclic aromatic hydrocarbons
    Z77.028

Exposure (*Continued*)
  prenatal (drugs) (toxic chemicals) —*see*
    Newborn, affected by, noxious
    substances transmitted via placenta or
    breast milk ⬅
  rabies Z20.3
  radiation, naturally occurring NEC Z77.123
  radon Z77.123
  red tide (Florida) Z77.121
  rubella Z20.4
  second hand tobacco smoke (acute) (chronic)
    Z77.22
    in the perinatal period P96.81
  sexually-transmitted disease Z20.2
  smallpox (laboratory) Z20.89
  syphilis Z20.2
  terrorism Z65.4
  torture Z65.4
  tuberculosis Z20.1
  uranium Z77.012
  varicella Z20.820
  venereal disease Z20.2
  viral disease NEC Z20.828
  war Z65.5
  water pollution Z77.111
Exsanguination —*see* Hemorrhage
Exstrophy
  abdominal contents Q45.8
  bladder Q64.10
    cloacal Q64.12
    specified type NEC Q64.19
    supravesical fissure Q64.11
Extensive —*see* condition
Extra —*see also* Accessory
  marker chromosomes (normal individual)
    Q92.61
    in abnormal individual Q92.62
  rib Q76.6
    cervical Q76.5
Extrasystoles (supraventricular) I49.49
  atrial I49.1
  auricular I49.1
  junctional I49.2
  ventricular I49.3
Extrauterine gestation or pregnancy —*see*
    Pregnancy, by site
Extravasation
  blood R58
  chyle into mesentery I89.8
  pelvicalyceal N13.8
  pyelosinus N13.8
  urine (from ureter) R39.0
  vesicant agent
    antineoplastic chemotherapy T80.810
    other agent NEC T80.818
Extremity —*see* condition, limb
Extrophy —*see* Exstrophy
Extroversion
  bladder Q64.19
  uterus N81.4
    complicating delivery O71.2
    postpartal (old) N81.4
Extruded tooth (teeth) M26.34
Extrusion
  breast implant (prosthetic) T85.42
  eye implant (globe) (ball) T85.328
  intervertebral disc —*see* Displacement,
    intervertebral disc
  ocular lens implant (prosthetic) —*see*
    Complications, intraocular lens
  vitreous —*see* Prolapse, vitreous
Exudate
  pleural —*see* Effusion, pleura
  retina H35.89
Exudative —*see* condition
Eye, eyeball, eyelid —*see* condition
Eyestrain —*see* Disturbance, vision, subjective
Eyeworm disease of Africa B74.3

F

Faber's syndrome (achlorhydric anemia) D50.9
Fabry (-Anderson) disease E75.21
Faciocephalalgia, autonomic —*see also*
    Neuropathy, peripheral, autonomic G90.09
Factor (s)
  psychic, associated with diseases classified
      elsewhere F54
  psychological
    affecting physical conditions F54
    or behavioral
      affecting general medical condition F54
      associated with disorders or diseases
        classified elsewhere F54
Fahr disease (of brain) G23.8
Fahr Volhard disease (of kidney) I12.-
Failure, failed
  abortion —*see* Abortion, attempted
  aortic (valve) I35.8
    rheumatic I06.8
  attempted abortion —*see* Abortion, attempted
  biventricular I50.9
  bone marrow —*see* Anemia, aplastic
  cardiac —*see* Failure, heart
  cardiorenal (chronic) I50.9
    hypertensive I13.2
  cardiorespiratory (*see also* Failure, heart)
    R09.2
  cardiovascular (chronic) —*see* Failure, heart
  cerebrovascular I67.9
  cervical dilatation in labor O62.0
  circulation, circulatory (peripheral) R57.9
    newborn P29.89
  compensation —*see* Disease, heart
  compliance with medical treatment or
    regimen —*see* Noncompliance
  congestive —*see* Failure, heart, congestive
  dental implant (endosseous) M27.69
    due to
      failure of dental prosthesis M27.63
      lack of attached gingiva M27.62
      occlusal trauma (poor prosthetic design)
        M27.62
      parafunctional habits M27.62
      periodontal infection (peri-implantitis)
        M27.62
      poor oral hygiene M27.62
    osseointegration M27.61
      due to
        complications of systemic disease
          M27.61
        poor bone quality M27.61
      iatrogenic M27.61
    post-osseointegration
      biological M27.62
      due to complications of systemic disease
        M27.62
      iatrogenic M27.62
      mechanical M27.63
    pre-integration M27.61
    pre-osseointegration M27.61
    specified NEC M27.69
  descent of head (at term) of pregnancy
    (mother) O32.4
  endosseous dental implant —*see* Failure,
    dental implant
  engagement of head (term of pregnancy)
    (mother) O32.4
  erection (penile) —*see also* Dysfunction,
    sexual, male, erectile N52.9
    ~~nonorgqanic F52.21~~
    nonorganic F52.21 ◀
  examination (s), anxiety concerning Z55.2
  expansion terminal respiratory units
    (newborn) (primary) P28.0
  forceps NOS (with subsequent cesarean
    delivery) O66.5
  gain weight (child over 28 days old) R62.51
    adult R62.7
    newborn P92.6

Failure, failed (*Continued*)
  genital response (male) F52.21
    female F52.22
  heart (acute) (senile) (sudden) I50.9
    with
      acute pulmonary edema —*see* Failure,
        ventricular, left
      decompensation —*see* Failure, heart,
        congestive
      dilatation —*see* Disease, heart
    arteriosclerotic I70.90
    biventricular I50.9
    combined left-right sided I50.9
    compensated I50.9
    complicating
      anesthesia (general) (local) or other
        sedation
        in labor and delivery O74.2
        in pregnancy O29.12-
        postpartum, puerperal O89.1
      delivery (cesarean) (instrumental) O75.4
    congestive (compensated)
      (decompensated) I50.9
      with rheumatic fever (conditions in I00)
        active I01.8
        inactive or quiescent (with chorea)
          I09.81
      newborn P29.0
      rheumatic (chronic) (inactive) (with
        chorea) I09.81
        active or acute I01.8
        with chorea I02.0
    decompensated I50.9
    degenerative —*see* Degeneration,
      myocardial
    diastolic (congestive) I50.30
      acute (congestive) I50.31
        and (on) chronic (congestive) I50.33
      chronic (congestive) I50.32
        and (on) acute (congestive) I50.33
      combined with systolic (congestive)
        I50.40
        acute (congestive) I50.41
          and (on) chronic (congestive)
            I50.43
        chronic (congestive) I50.42
          and (on) acute (congestive) I50.43
    due to presence of cardiac prosthesis
      I97.13-
    following cardiac surgery I97.13-
    high output NOS I50.9
    hypertensive —*see* Hypertension, heart
    left (ventricular) —*see* Failure, ventricular,
      left
    low output (syndrome) NOS I50.9
    newborn P29.0
    organic —*see* Disease, heart
    peripartum O90.3
    postprocedural I97.13-
    rheumatic (chronic) (inactive) I09.9
    right (ventricular) (secondary to left
      heart failure) —*see* Failure, heart,
      congestive
    systolic (congestive) I50.20
      acute (congestive) I50.21
        and (on) chronic (congestive)
          I50.23
      chronic (congestive) I50.22
        and (on) acute (congestive) I50.23
      combined with diastolic (congestive)
        I50.40
        acute (congestive) I50.41
          and (on) chronic (congestive)
            I50.43
        chronic (congestive) I50.42
          and (on) acute (congestive)
            I50.43
    thyrotoxic —*see also* Thyrotoxicosis
      E05.90 [*I43*]
      with thyroid storm E05.91 [*I43*]
    valvular —*see* Endocarditis

Failure, failed (*Continued*)
  hepatic K72.90
    with coma K72.91
    acute or subacute K72.00
      with coma K72.01
      due to drugs K71.10
        with coma K71.11
      alcoholic (acute) (chronic) (subacute)
        K70.40
      with coma K70.41
    chronic K72.10
      with coma K72.11
      due to drugs (acute) (subacute) (chronic)
        K71.10
        with coma K71.11
    due to drugs (acute) (subacute) (chronic)
      K71.10
      with coma K71.11
    postprocedural K91.82
  hepatorenal K76.7
  induction (of labor) O61.9
    abortion —*see* Abortion, attempted
    by
      oxytocic drugs O61.0
      prostaglandins O61.0
    instrumental O61.1
    mechanical O61.1
    medical O61.0
    specified NEC O61.8
    surgical O61.1
  intubation during anesthesia T88.4
    in pregnancy O29.6-
    labor and delivery O74.7
    postpartum, puerperal O89.6
  involution, thymus (gland) E32.0
  kidney —*see also* Disease, kidney, chronic N19
    acute —*see* Failure, renal, acute N17.9-
    diabetic —*see* E08-E13 with .22
  lactation (complete) O92.3
    partial O92.4
  Leydig's cell, adult E29.1
  liver —*see* Failure, hepatic
  menstruation at puberty N91.0
  mitral I05.8
  myocardial, myocardium —*see also* Failure,
    heart I50.9
    chronic —*see also* Failure, heart, congestive
      I50.9
    congestive —*see also* Failure, heart,
      congestive I50.9
  orgasm (female) (psychogenic) F52.31
    male F52.32
  ovarian (primary) E28.39
    iatrogenic E89.40
      asymptomatic E89.40
      symptomatic E89.41
    postprocedural (postablative)
      (postirradiation) (postsurgical)
      E89.40
      asymptomatic E89.40
      symptomatic E89.41
  ovulation causing infertility N97.0
  polyglandular, autoimmune E31.0
  prosthetic joint implant —*see* Complications,
    joint prosthesis, mechanical,
    breakdown, by site
  renal N19
    with
      tubular necrosis (acute) N17.0
    acute N17.9
      with
        cortical necrosis N17.1
        medullary necrosis N17.2
        tubular necrosis N17.0
      specified NEC N17.8
    chronic N18.9
      hypertensive —*see* Hypertension,
        kidney
    congenital P96.0
    end stage (chronic) N18.6
      due to hypertension I12.0

Failure, failed (Continued)
  renal (Continued)
    following
      abortion —see Abortion by type
        complicated by specified
        condition NEC
      crushing T79.5
      ectopic or molar pregnancy O08.4
      labor and delivery (acute) O90.4
    hypertensive —see Hypertension,
      kidney
    postprocedural N99.0
    respiration, respiratory J96.9
      with
        hypercapnia J96.92
        hypoxia J96.91
      acute J96.00
        with
          hypercapnia J96.02
          hypoxia J96.01
      acute and (on) chronic J96.20
        with
          hypercapnia J96.22
          hypoxia J96.21
      center G93.89
      chronic J96.10
        with
          hypercapnia J96.12
          hypoxia J96.11
      newborn P28.5
      postprocedural (acute) J95.821
        acute and chronic J95.822
    rotation
      cecum Q43.3
      colon Q43.3
      intestine Q43.3
      kidney Q63.2
    sedation (conscious) (moderate) during
      procedure T88.52
      history of Z92.83
    segmentation —see also Fusion
      fingers —see Syndactylism, complex,
        fingers
      vertebra Q76.49
        with scoliosis Q76.3
    seminiferous tubule, adult E29.1
    senile (general) R54
    sexual arousal (male) F52.21
      female F52.22
    testicular endocrine function E29.1
    to thrive (child over 28 days old)
      R62.51
      adult R62.7
      newborn P92.6
    transplant T86.92
      bone T86.831
        marrow T86.02
      cornea T86.841
      heart T86.22
        with lung (s) T86.32
      intestine T86.851
      kidney T86.12
      liver T86.42
      lung (s) T86.811
        with heart T86.32
      pancreas T86.891
      skin (allograft) (autograft) T86.821
      specified organ or tissue NEC T86.891
      stem cell (peripheral blood) (umbilical
        cord) T86.5
    trial of labor (with subsequent cesarean
      delivery) O66.40
      following previous cesarean delivery
        O66.41
    tubal ligation N99.89
    urinary —see Disease, kidney, chronic
    vacuum extraction NOS (with subsequent
      cesarean delivery) O66.5
    vasectomy N99.89
    ventouse NOS (with subsequent cesarean
      delivery) O66.5

Failure, failed (Continued)
  ventricular —see also Failure, heart I50.9
    left I50.1
      with rheumatic fever (conditions in I00)
        active I01.8
          with chorea I02.0
        inactive or quiescent (with chorea)
          I09.81
      rheumatic (chronic) (inactive) (with
        chorea) I09.81
        active or acute I01.8
          with chorea I02.0
    right —see also Failure, heart, congestive
      I50.9
  vital centers, newborn P91.8
Fainting (fit) R55
Fallen arches —see Deformity, limb, flat foot
Falling, falls (repeated) R29.6
  any organ or part —see Prolapse
Fallopian
  insufflation Z31.41
  tube —see condition
Fallot's
  pentalogy Q21.8
  tetrad or tetralogy Q21.3
  triad or trilogy Q22.3
False —see also condition
  croup J38.5
  joint —see Nonunion, fracture
  labor (pains) O47.9
    at or after 37 completed weeks of gestation
      O47.1
    before 37 completed weeks of gestation
      O47.0-
  passage, urethra (prostatic) N36.5
  pregnancy F45.8
Family, familial —see also condition
  disruption Z63.8
    involving divorce or separation Z63.5
  Li-Fraumeni (syndrome) Z15.01
  planning advice Z30.09
  problem Z63.9
    specified NEC Z63.8
  retinoblastoma C69.2-
Famine (effects of) T73.0
  edema —see Malnutrition, severe
Fanconi (-de Toni)(-Debré) **syndrome** E72.09
  with cystinosis E72.04
Fanconi's anemia (congenital pancytopenia)
  D61.09
Farber's disease or syndrome E75.29
Farcy A24.0
Farmer's
  lung J67.0
  skin L57.8
Farsightedness —see Hypermetropia
Fascia —see condition
Fasciculation R25.3
Fasciitis M72.9
  diffuse (eosinophilic) M35.4
  infective M72.8
    necrotizing M72.6
  necrotizing M72.6
  nodular M72.4
  perirenal (with ureteral obstruction)
    N13.5
    with infection N13.6
  plantar M72.2
  specified NEC M72.8
  traumatic (old) M72.8
    current - code by site under Sprain
Fascioliasis B66.3
Fasciolopsis, fasciolopsiasis (intestinal)
  B66.5
Fascioscapulohumeral myopathy G71.0
Fast pulse R00.0
Fat
  embolism —see Embolism, fat
  excessive —see also Obesity
    in heart —see Degeneration, myocardial
  in stool R19.5

Fat (Continued)
  localized (pad) E65
    heart —see Degeneration, myocardial
    knee M79.4
    retropatellar M79.4
  necrosis
    breast N64.1
    mesentery K65.4
    omentum K65.4
  pad E65
    knee M79.4
Fatigue R53.83
  auditory deafness —see Deafness
  chronic R53.82
  combat F43.0
  general R53.83
    psychogenic F48.8
  heat (transient) T67.6
  muscle M62.89
  myocardium —see Failure, heart
  neoplasm-related R53.0
  nervous, neurosis F48.8
  operational F48.8
  psychogenic (general) F48.8
  senile R54
  voice R49.8
Fatness —see Obesity
Fatty —see also condition
  apron E65
  degeneration —see Degeneration, fatty
  heart (enlarged) —see Degeneration,
    myocardial
  liver NEC K76.0
    alcoholic K70.0
    nonalcoholic K76.0
  necrosis —see Degeneration, fatty
Fauces —see condition
Fauchard's disease (periodontitis) —see
  Periodontitis
Faucitis J02.9
Favism (anemia) D55.0
Favus —see Dermatophytosis
Fazio-Londe disease or syndrome
  G12.1
Fear complex or reaction F40.9
Fear of —see Phobia
Feared complaint unfounded Z71.1
Febris, febrile —see also Fever
  flava —see also Fever, yellow A95.9
  melitensis A23.0
  pestis —see Plague
  recurrens —see Fever, relapsing
  rubra A38.9
Fecal
  incontinence R15.9
  smearing R15.1
  soiling R15.1
  urgency R15.2
Fecalith (impaction) K56.41
  appendix K38.1
  congenital P76.8
Fede's disease K14.0
**Feeble rapid pulse due to shock following
  injury** T79.4
Feeble-minded F70
Feeding
  difficulties R63.3
  problem R63.3
    newborn P92.9
      specified NEC P92.8
    nonorganic (adult) —see Disorder,
      eating
Feeling (of)
  foreign body in throat R09.89
Feer's disease —see Poisoning, mercury
Feet —see condition
Feigned illness Z76.5
Feil-Klippel syndrome (brevicollis) Q76.1
Feinmesser's (hidrotic) **ectodermal dysplasia**
  Q82.4
Felinophobia F40.218

Felon —*see also* Cellulitis, digit
  with lymphangitis —*see* Lymphangitis, acute,
    digit
Felty's syndrome M05.00
  ankle M05.07-
  elbow M05.02-
  foot joint M05.07-
  hand joint M05.04-
  hip M05.05-
  knee M05.06-
  multiple site M05.09
  shoulder M05.01-
  vertebra —*see* Spondylitis, ankylosing
  wrist M05.03-
Female genital cutting status —*see* Female
    genital mutilation status (FGM)
Female genital mutilation status (FGM) N90.810
  specified NEC N90.818
  type I (clitorectomy status) N90.811
  type II (clitorectomy with excision of labia
    minora status) N90.812
  type III (infibulation status) N90.813
  type IV N90.818
Femur, femoral —*see* condition
Fenestration, fenestrated —*see also* Imperfect,
    closure
  aortico-pulmonary Q21.4
  cusps, heart valve NEC Q24.8
    pulmonary Q22.3
  pulmonic cusps Q22.3
Fernell's disease (aortic aneurysm) I71.9
Fertile eunuch syndrome E23.0
Fetid
  breath R19.6
  sweat L75.0
Fetishism F65.0
  transvestic F65.1
Fetus, fetal —*see also* condition
  alcohol syndrome (dysmorphic) Q86.0
  compressus O31.0-
  hydantoin syndrome Q86.1
  lung tissue P28.0
  papyraceous O31.0-
Fever (inanition) (of unknown origin)
    (persistent) (with chills) (with rigor) R50.9
  abortus A23.1
  Aden (dengue) A90
  African tick-borne A68.1
  American
    mountain (tick) A93.2
    spotted A77.0
  aphthous B08.8
  arbovirus, arboviral A94
    hemorrhagic A94
    specified NEC A93.8
  Argentinian hemorrhagic A96.0
  Assam B55.0
  Australian Q A78
  Bangkok hemorrhagic A91
  Barmah forest A92.8
  Bartonella A44.0
  bilious, hemoglobinuric B50.8
  blackwater B50.8
  blister B00.1
  Bolivian hemorrhagic A96.1
  Bonvale dam T73.3
  boutonneuse A77.1
  brain —*see* Encephalitis
  Brazilian purpuric A48.4
  breakbone A90
  Bullis A77.0
  Bunyamwera A92.8
  Burdwan B55.0
  Bwamba A92.8
  Cameroon —*see* Malaria
  Canton A75.9
  catarrhal (acute) J00
    chronic J31.0
  cat-scratch A28.1
  Central Asian hemorrhagic A98.0
  cerebral —*see* Encephalitis

Fever *(Continued)*
  cerebrospinal meningococcal A39.0
  Chagres B50.9
  Chandipura A92.8
  Changuinola A93.1
  Charcot's (biliary) (hepatic) (intermittent) —
    see Calculus, bile duct
  Chikungunya (viral) (hemorrhagic)
    A92.0
  Chitral A93.1
  Colombo —*see* Fever, paratyphoid
  Colorado tick (virus) A93.2
  congestive (remittent) —*see* Malaria
  Congo virus A98.0
  continued malarial B50.9
  Corsican —*see* Malaria
  Crimean-Congo hemorrhagic A98.0
  Cyprus —*see* Brucellosis
  dandy A90
  deer fly —*see* Tularemia
  dengue (virus) A90
    hemorrhagic A91
    sandfly A93.1
  desert B38.0
  drug induced R50.2
  due to
    conditions classified elsewhere
      R50.81
    heat T67.0
  enteric A01.00
  enteroviral exanthematous (Boston
    exanthem) A88.0
  ephemeral (of unknown origin) R50.9
  epidemic hemorrhagic A98.5
  erysipelatous —*see* Erysipelas
  estivo-autumnal (malarial) B50.9
  famine A75.0
  five day A79.0
  following delivery O86.4
  Fort Bragg A27.89
  gastroenteric A01.00
  gastromalarial —*see* Malaria
  Gibraltar —*see* Brucellosis
  glandular —*see* Mononucleosis, infectious
  Guama (viral) A92.8
  Haverhill A25.1
  hay (allergic) J30.1
    with asthma (bronchial) J45.909
      with
        exacerbation (acute) J45.901
        status asthmaticus J45.902
    due to
      allergen other than pollen J30.89
      pollen, any plant or tree J30.1
  heat (effects) T67.0
  hematuric, bilious B50.8
  hemoglobinuric (malarial) (bilious) B50.8
  hemorrhagic (arthropod-borne) NOS A94
    with renal syndrome A98.5
    arenaviral A96.9
      specified NEC A96.8
    Argentinian A96.0
    Bangkok A91
    Bolivian A96.1
    Central Asian A98.0
    Chikungunya A92.0
    Crimean-Congo A98.0
    dengue (virus) A91
    epidemic A98.5
    Junin (virus) A96.0
    Korean A98.5
    Kyasanur forest A98.2
    Machupo (virus) A96.1
    mite-borne A93.8
    mosquito-borne A92.8
    Omsk A98.1
    Philippine A91
    Russian A98.5
    Singapore A91
    Southeast Asia A91
    Thailand A91

Fever *(Continued)*
  hemorrhagic NOS *(Continued)*
    tick-borne NEC A93.8
    viral A99
      specified NEC A98.8
  hepatic —*see* Cholecystitis
  herpetic —*see* Herpes
  icterohemorrhagic A27.0
  Indiana A93.8
  infective B99.9
    specified NEC B99.8
  intermittent (bilious) —*see also* Malaria
    of unknown origin R50.9
    pernicious B50.9
  iodide R50.2
  Japanese river A75.3
  jungle —*see also* Malaria
    yellow A95.0
  Junin (virus) hemorrhagic A96.0
  Katayama B65.2
  kedani A75.3
  Kenya (tick) A77.1
  Kew Garden A79.1
  Korean hemorrhagic A98.5
  Lassa A96.2
  Lone Star A77.0
  Machupo (virus) hemorrhagic A96.1
  malaria, malarial —*see* Malaria
  Malta A23.9
  Marseilles A77.1
  marsh —*see* Malaria
  Mayaro (viral) A92.8
  Mediterranean —*see also* Brucellosis A23.9
    familial M04.1 ◀||||
    tick A77.1
  meningeal —*see* Meningitis
  Meuse A79.0
  Mexican A75.2
  mianeh A68.1
  miasmatic —*see* Malaria
  mosquito-borne (viral) A92.9
    hemorrhagic A92.8
  mountain —*see also* Brucellosis
    meaning Rocky Mountain spotted fever
      A77.0
    tick (American) (Colorado) (viral) A93.2
  Mucambo (viral) A92.8
  mud A27.9
  Neapolitan —*see* Brucellosis
  neutropenic D70.9
  newborn P81.9
    environmental P81.0
  Nine-Mile A78
  non-exanthematous tick A93.2
  North Asian tick-borne A77.2
  Omsk hemorrhagic A98.1
  O'nyong-nyong (viral) A92.1
  Oropouche (viral) A93.0
  Oroya A44.0
  paludal —*see* Malaria
  Panama (malarial) B50.9
  Pappataci A93.1
  paratyphoid A01.4
    A A01.1
    B A01.2
    C A01.3
  parrot A70
  periodic (Mediterranean) M04.1 ◀||||
  persistent (of unknown origin) R50.9
  petechial A39.0
  pharyngoconjunctival B30.2
  Philippine hemorrhagic A91
  phlebotomus A93.1
  Piry (virus) A93.8
  Pixuna (viral) A92.8
  Plasmodium ovale B53.0
  polioviral (nonparalytic) A80.4
  Pontiac A48.2
  postimmunization R50.83
  postoperative R50.82
    due to infection T81.40 ◀||||

◀ New   ◀|||| Revised   ~~deleted~~ Deleted

Fever *(Continued)*
  posttransfusion R50.84
  postvaccination R50.83
  presenting with conditions classified
      elsewhere R50.81
  pretibial A27.89
  puerperal O86.4
  Q A78
  quadrilateral A78
  quartan (malaria) B52.9
  Queensland (coastal) (tick) A77.3
  quintan A79.0
  rabbit —*see* Tularemia
  rat-bite A25.9
      due to
          Spirillum A25.0
          Streptobacillus moniliformis A25.1
  recurrent —*see* Fever, relapsing
  relapsing (Borrelia) A68.9
      Carter's (Asiatic) A68.1
      Dutton's (West African) A68.1
      Koch's A68.9
      louse-borne A68.0
      Novy's
          louse-borne A68.0
          tick-borne A68.1
      Obermeyer's (European) A68.0
      tick-borne A68.1
  remittent (bilious) (congestive) (gastric) —*see*
      Malaria
  rheumatic (active) (acute) (chronic) (subacute)
      I00
      with central nervous system involvement
          I02.9
      active with heart involvement —*see*
          category I01
      inactive or quiescent with
          cardiac hypertrophy I09.89
          carditis I09.9
          endocarditis I09.1
              aortic (valve) I06.9
                  with mitral (valve) disease I08.0
              mitral (valve) I05.9
                  with aortic (valve) disease I08.0
              pulmonary (valve) I09.89
              tricuspid (valve) I07.8
          heart disease NEC I09.89
          heart failure (congestive) (conditions in
              I50.9) I09.81
          left ventricular failure (conditions in
              I50.1) I09.81
          myocarditis, myocardial degeneration
              (conditions in I51.4) I09.0
          pancarditis I09.9
          pericarditis I09.2
  Rift Valley (viral) A92.4
  Rocky Mountain spotted A77.0
  rose J30.1
  Ross River B33.1
  Russian hemorrhagic A98.5
  San Joaquin (Valley) B38.0
  sandfly A93.1
  Sao Paulo A77.0
  scarlet A38.9
  seven day (leptospirosis) (autumnal)
      (Japanese) A27.89
      dengue A90
  shin-bone A79.0
  Singapore hemorrhagic A91
  solar A90
  Songo A98.5
  sore B00.1
  South African tick-bite A68.1
  Southeast Asia hemorrhagic A91
  spinal —*see* Meningitis
  spirillary A25.0
  splenic —*see* Anthrax
  spotted A77.9
      American A77.0
      Brazilian A77.0
      cerebrospinal meningitis A39.0

Fever *(Continued)*
  spotted *(Continued)*
      Colombian A77.0
      due to Rickettsia
          australis A77.3
          conorii A77.1
          rickettsii A77.0
          sibirica A77.2
          specified type NEC A77.8
      Ehrlichiosis A77.40
          due to
              E. chafeensis A77.41
              specified organism NEC A77.49
      Rocky Mountain A77.0
  steroid R50.2
  streptobacillary A25.1
  subtertian B50.9
  Sumatran mite A75.3
  sun A90
  swamp A27.9
  swine A02.8
  sylvatic, yellow A95.0
  Tahyna B33.8
  tertian —*see* Malaria, tertian
  Thailand hemorrhagic A91
  thermic T67.0
  three-day A93.1
  tick
      American mountain A93.2
      Colorado A93.2
      Kemerovo A93.8
      Mediterranean A77.1
      mountain A93.2
      nonexanthematous A93.2
      Quaranfil A93.8
  tick-bite NEC A93.8
  tick-borne (hemorrhagic) NEC A93.8
  trench A79.0
  tsutsugamushi A75.3
  typhogastric A01.00
  typhoid (abortive) (hemorrhagic)
      (intermittent) (malignant) A01.00
      complicated by
          arthritis A01.04
          heart involvement A01.02
          meningitis A01.01
          osteomyelitis A01.05
          pneumonia A01.03
          specified NEC A01.09
  typhomalarial —*see* Malaria
  typhus —*see* Typhus (fever)
  undulant —*see* Brucellosis
  unknown origin R50.9
  uveoparotid D86.89
  valley B38.0
  Venezuelan equine A92.2
  vesicular stomatitis A93.8
  viral hemorrhagic —*see* Fever, hemorrhagic,
      by type of virus
  Volhynian A79.0
  Wesselsbron (viral) A92.8
  West
      African B50.8
      Nile (viral) A92.30
          with
              complications NEC A92.39
              cranial nerve disorders A92.32
              encephalitis A92.31
              encephalomyelitis A92.31
              neurologic manifestation NEC
                  A92.32
              optic neuritis A92.32
              polyradiculitis A92.32
  Whitmore's —*see* Melioidosis
  Wolhynian A79.0
  worm B83.9
  yellow A95.9
      jungle A95.0
      sylvatic A95.0
      urban A95.1
  Zika virus A92.5 ◀

Fibrillation
  atrial or auricular (established) I48.91
      chronic I48.2
      paroxysmal I48.0
      permanent I48.2
      persistent I48.1
  cardiac I49.8
  heart I49.8
  muscular M62.89
  ventricular I49.01
Fibrin
  ball or bodies, pleural (sac) J94.1
  chamber, anterior (eye) (gelatinous
      exudate) —*see* Iridocyclitis, acute
Fibrinogenolysis —*see* Fibrinolysis
Fibrinogenopenia D68.8
  acquired D65
  congenital D68.2
Fibrinolysis (hemorrhagic) (acquired) D65
  antepartum hemorrhage —*see* Hemorrhage,
      antepartum, with coagulation defect
  following
      abortion —*see* Abortion by type
          complicated by hemorrhage
      ectopic or molar pregnancy O08.1
  intrapartum O67.0
  newborn, transient P60
  postpartum O72.3
Fibrinopenia (hereditary) D68.2
  acquired D68.4
Fibrinopurulent —*see* condition
Fibrinous —*see* condition
Fibroadenoma
  cellular intracanalicular D24-
  giant D24-
  intracanalicular
      cellular D24-
      giant D24-
      specified site —*see* Neoplasm, benign, by
          site
      unspecified site D24-
  juvenile D24-
  pericanalicular
      specified site —*see* Neoplasm, benign, by
          site
      unspecified site D24-
  phyllodes D24-
  prostate D29.1
  specified site NEC —*see* Neoplasm, benign,
      by site
  unspecified site D24-
Fibroadenosis, breast (chronic) (cystic) (diffuse)
      (periodic) (segmental) N60.2-
Fibroangioma —*see also* Neoplasm, benign, by
      site
  juvenile
      specified site —*see* Neoplasm, benign, by
          site
      unspecified site D10.6
Fibrochondrosarcoma —*see* Neoplasm,
      cartilage, malignant
Fibrocystic
  disease —*see also* Fibrosis, cystic
      breast —*see* Mastopathy, cystic
      jaw M27.49
      kidney (congenital) Q61.8
      liver Q44.6
      pancreas E84.9
  kidney (congenital) Q61.8
Fibrodysplasia ossificans progressiva —*see*
      Myositis, ossificans, progressiva
Fibroelastosis (cordis) (endocardial)
      (endomyocardial) I42.4
Fibroid (tumor) —*see also* Neoplasm, connective
      tissue, benign
  disease, lung (chronic) —*see* Fibrosis, lung
  heart (disease) —*see* Myocarditis
  in pregnancy or childbirth O34.1-
      causing obstructed labor O65.5
  induration, lung (chronic) —*see* Fibrosis, lung
  lung —*see* Fibrosis, lung

Fibroid (*Continued*)
pneumonia (chronic) —*see* Fibrosis, lung
uterus D25.9
Fibrolipoma —*see* Lipoma
Fibroliposarcoma —*see* Neoplasm, connective tissue, malignant
Fibroma —*see also* Neoplasm, connective tissue, benign
  ameloblastic —*see* Cyst, calcifying odontogenic
  bone (nonossifying) —*see* Disorder, bone, specified type NEC
    ossifying —*see* Neoplasm, bone, benign
  cementifying —*see* Neoplasm, bone, benign
  chondromyxoid —*see* Neoplasm, bone, benign
  desmoplastic —*see* Neoplasm, connective tissue, uncertain behavior
  durum —*see* Neoplasm, connective tissue, benign
  fascial —*see* Neoplasm, connective tissue, benign
  invasive —*see* Neoplasm, connective tissue, uncertain behavior
  molle —*see* Lipoma
  myxoid —*see* Neoplasm, connective tissue, benign
  nasopharynx, nasopharyngeal (juvenile) D10.6
  nonosteogenic (nonossifying) —*see* Dysplasia, fibrous
  odontogenic (central) —*see* Cyst, calcifying odontogenic
  ossifying —*see* Neoplasm, bone, benign
  periosteal —*see* Neoplasm, bone, benign
  soft —*see* Lipoma
Fibromatosis M72.9
  abdominal —*see* Neoplasm, connective tissue, uncertain behavior
  aggressive —*see* Neoplasm, connective tissue, uncertain behavior
  congenital generalized —*see* Neoplasm, connective tissue, uncertain behavior
  Dupuytren's M72.0
  gingival K06.1
  palmar (fascial) M72.0
  plantar (fascial) M72.2
  pseudosarcomatous (proliferative) (subcutaneous) M72.4
  retroperitoneal D48.3
  specified NEC M72.8
Fibromyalgia M79.7
Fibromyoma —*see also* Neoplasm, connective tissue, benign
  uterus (corpus) —*see also* Leiomyoma, uterus
    in pregnancy or childbirth —*see* Fibroid, in pregnancy or childbirth
    causing obstructed labor O65.5
Fibromyositis M79.7
Fibromyxolipoma D17.9
Fibromyxoma —*see* Neoplasm, connective tissue, benign
Fibromyxosarcoma —*see* Neoplasm, connective tissue, malignant
Fibro-odontoma, ameloblastic —*see* Cyst, calcifying odontogenic
Fibro-osteoma —*see* Neoplasm, bone, benign
Fibroplasia, retrolental H35.17
Fibropurulent —*see* condition
Fibrosarcoma —*see also* Neoplasm, connective tissue, malignant
  ameloblastic C41.1
    upper jaw (bone) C41.0
  congenital —*see* Neoplasm, connective tissue, malignant
  fascial —*see* Neoplasm, connective tissue, malignant
  infantile —*see* Neoplasm, connective tissue, malignant

Fibrosarcoma (*Continued*)
  odontogenic C41.1
    upper jaw (bone) C41.0
  periosteal —*see* Neoplasm, bone, malignant
Fibrosclerosis
  breast N60.3-
  multifocal M35.5
  penis (corpora cavernosa) N48.6
Fibrosis, fibrotic
  adrenal (gland) E27.8
  amnion O41.8X-
  anal papillae K62.89
  arteriocapillary —*see* Arteriosclerosis
  bladder N32.89
    interstitial —*see* Cystitis, chronic, interstitial
    localized submucosal —*see* Cystitis, chronic, interstitial
    panmural —*see* Cystitis, chronic, interstitial
  breast —*see* Fibrosclerosis, breast
  capillary —*see also* Arteriosclerosis I70.90
    lung (chronic) —*see* Fibrosis, lung
  cardiac —*see* Myocarditis
  cervix N88.8
  chorion O41.8X-
  corpus cavernosum (sclerosing) N48.6
  cystic (of pancreas) E84.9
    with
      distal intestinal obstruction syndrome E84.19
      fecal impaction E84.19
      intestinal manifestations NEC E84.19
      pulmonary manifestations E84.0
      specified manifestations NEC E84.8
  due to device, implant or graft —*see also* Complications, by site and type, specified NEC T85.828 ◀▥
    arterial graft NEC T82.828
    breast (implant) T85.828 ◀▥
    catheter NEC T85.828 ◀▥
      dialysis (renal) T82.828
        intraperitoneal T85.828 ◀▥
      infusion NEC T82.828
        spinal (epidural) (subdural) T85.820 ◀▥
      urinary (indwelling) T83.82
    electronic (electrode) (pulse generator) (stimulator)
      bone T84.82
      cardiac T82.827
      nervous system (brain) (peripheral nerve) (spinal) T85.820 ◀▥
      urinary T83.82
    fixation, internal (orthopedic) NEC T84.82
    gastrointestinal (bile duct) (esophagus) T85.828 ◀▥
    genital NEC T83.82
    heart NEC T82.827
    joint prosthesis T84.82
    ocular (corneal graft) (orbital implant) NEC T85.828 ◀▥
    orthopedic NEC T84.82
    specified NEC T85.828 ◀▥
    urinary NEC T83.82
    vascular NEC T82.828
    ventricular intracranial shunt T85.820 ◀▥
  ejaculatory duct N50.89 ◀▥
  endocardium —*see* Endocarditis
  endomyocardial (tropical) I42.3
  epididymis N50.89 ◀▥
  eye muscle —*see* Strabismus, mechanical
  heart —*see* Myocarditis
  hepatic —*see* Fibrosis, liver
  hepatolienal (portal hypertension) K76.6
  hepatosplenic (portal hypertension) K76.6
  infrapatellar fat pad M79.4
  intrascrotal N50.89 ◀▥
  kidney N26.9
  liver K74.0
    with sclerosis K74.2
    alcoholic K70.2

Fibrosis, fibrotic (*Continued*)
  lung (atrophic) (chronic) (confluent) (massive) (perialveolar) (peribronchial) J84.10
    with
      anthracosilicosis J60
      anthracosis J60
      asbestosis J61
      bagassosis J67.1
      bauxite J63.1
      berylliosis J63.2
      byssinosis J66.0
      calcicosis J62.8
      chalicosis J62.8
      dust reticulation J64
      farmer's lung J67.0
      ganister disease J62.8
      graphite J63.3
      pneumoconiosis NOS J64
      siderosis J63.4
      silicosis J62.8
    capillary J84.10
    congenital P27.8
    diffuse (idiopathic) J84.10
      chemicals, gases, fumes or vapors (inhalation) J68.4
      interstitial J84.10
        acute J84.114
      talc J62.0
    following radiation J70.1
    idiopathic J84.112
    postinflammatory J84.10
    silicotic J62.8
    tuberculous —*see* Tuberculosis, pulmonary
  lymphatic gland I89.8
  median bar —*see* Hyperplasia, prostate
  mediastinum (idiopathic) J98.59 ◀▥
  meninges G96.19
  myocardium, myocardial —*see* Myocarditis
  ovary N83.8
  oviduct N83.8
  pancreas K86.89 ◀▥
  penis NEC N48.6
  pericardium I31.0
  perineum, in pregnancy or childbirth O34.7-
    causing obstructed labor O65.5
  pleura J94.1
  popliteal fat pad M79.4
  prostate (chronic) —*see* Hyperplasia, prostate
  pulmonary —*see also* Fibrosis, lung J84.10
    congenital P27.8
    idiopathic J84.112
  rectal sphincter K62.89
  retroperitoneal, idiopathic (with ureteral obstruction) N13.5
    with infection N13.6
  sclerosing mesenteric (idiopathic) K65.4
  scrotum N50.89 ◀▥
  seminal vesicle N50.89 ◀▥
  senile R54
  skin L90.5
  spermatic cord N50.89 ◀▥
  spleen D73.89
    in schistosomiasis (bilharziasis) B65.9 [D77]
  subepidermal nodular —*see* Neoplasm, skin, benign
  submucous (oral) (tongue) K13.5
  testis N44.8
    chronic, due to syphilis A52.76
  thymus (gland) E32.8
  tongue, submucous K13.5
  tunica vaginalis N50.89 ◀▥
  uterus (non-neoplastic) N85.8
  vagina N89.8
  valve, heart —*see* Endocarditis
  vas deferens N50.89 ◀▥
  vein I87.8
Fibrositis (periarticular) M79.7
  nodular, chronic (Jaccoud's) (rheumatoid) —*see* Arthropathy, postrheumatic, chronic

◀ New   ◀▥ Revised   ~~deleted~~ Deleted

Fibrothorax J94.1

Fibrotic —see Fibrosis

Fibrous —see condition

Fibroxanthoma —see also Neoplasm, connective tissue, benign
  atypical —see Neoplasm, connective tissue, uncertain behavior
  malignant —see Neoplasm, connective tissue, malignant

Fibroxanthosarcoma —see Neoplasm, connective tissue, malignant

Fiedler's
  disease (icterohemorrhagic leptospirosis) A27.0
  myocarditis (acute) I40.1

Fifth disease B08.3
  venereal A55

Filaria, filarial, filariasis —see Infestation, filarial

Filatov's disease —see Mononucleosis, infectious

File-cutter's disease —see Poisoning, lead

Filling defect
  biliary tract R93.2
  bladder R93.41 ◄▥
  duodenum R93.3
  gallbladder R93.2
  gastrointestinal tract R93.3
  intestine R93.3
  kidney R93.42- ◄▥
  stomach R93.3
  ureter R93.41 ◄▥
  urinary organs, specified NEC R93.49 ◄

Fimbrial cyst Q50.4

Financial problem affecting care NOS Z59.9
  bankruptcy Z59.8
  foreclosure on loan Z59.8

Findings, abnormal, inconclusive, without diagnosis —see also Abnormal
  17-ketosteroids, elevated R82.5
  acetonuria R82.4
  alcohol in blood R78.0
  anisocytosis R71.8
  antenatal screening of mother O28.9
    biochemical O28.1
    chromosomal O28.5
    cytological O28.2
    genetic O28.5
    hematological O28.0
    radiological O28.4
    specified NEC O28.8
    ultrasonic O28.3
  antibody titer, elevated R76.0
  anticardiolipin antibody R76.0
  antiphosphatidylglycerol antibody R76.0
  antiphosphatidylinositol antibody R76.0
  antiphosphatidylserine antibody R76.0
  antiphospholipid antibody R76.0
  bacteriuria R82.71 ◄▥
  bicarbonate E87.8
  bile in urine R82.2
  blood sugar R73.09
    high R73.9
    low (transient) E16.2
  body fluid or substance, specified NEC R88.8
  casts, urine R82.99
  catecholamines R82.5
  cells, urine R82.99
  chloride E87.8
  cholesterol E78.9
    high E78.00 ◄▥
      with high triglycerides E78.2
  chyluria R82.0
  cloudy
    dialysis effluent R88.0
    urine R82.90
  creatinine clearance R94.4
  crystals, urine R82.99
  culture
    blood R78.81
    positive —see Positive, culture
  echocardiogram R93.1

Findings, abnormal, inconclusive, without diagnosis (Continued)
  electrolyte level, urinary R82.99
  function study NEC R94.8
    bladder R94.8
    endocrine NEC R94.7
      thyroid R94.6
    kidney R94.4
    liver R94.5
    pancreas R94.8
    placenta R94.8
    pulmonary R94.2
    spleen R94.8
  gallbladder, nonvisualization R93.2
  glucose (tolerance test) (non-fasting) R73.09
  glycosuria R81
  heart
    shadow R93.1
    sounds R01.2
  hematinuria R82.3
  hematocrit drop (precipitous) R71.0
  hemoglobinuria R82.3
  human papillomavirus (HPV) DNA test positive
    cervix
      high risk R87.810
      low risk R87.820
    vagina
      high risk R87.811
      low risk R87.821
  in blood (of substance not normally found in blood) R78.9
    addictive drug NEC R78.4
    alcohol (excessive level) R78.0
    cocaine R78.2
    hallucinogen R78.3
    heavy metals (abnormal level) R78.79
    lead R78.71
    lithium (abnormal level) R78.89
    opiate drug R78.1
    psychotropic drug R78.5
    specified substance NEC R78.89
    steroid agent R78.6
  indoleacetic acid, elevated R82.5
  ketonuria R82.4
  lactic acid dehydrogenase (LDH) R74.0
  liver function test R79.89
  mammogram NEC R92.8
    calcification (calculus) R92.1
    inconclusive result (due to dense breasts) R92.2
    microcalcification R92.0
  mediastinal shift R93.8
  melanin, urine R82.99
  myoglobinuria R82.1
  neonatal screening P09
  nonvisualization of gallbladder R93.2
  odor of urine NOS R82.90
  Papanicolaou cervix R87.619
    non-atypical endometrial cells R87.618
  pneumoencephalogram R93.0
  poikilocytosis R71.8
  potassium (deficiency) E87.6
    excess E87.5
  PPD R76.11
  radiologic (X-ray) R93.8
    abdomen R93.5
    biliary tract R93.2
    breast R92.8
    gastrointestinal tract R93.3
    genitourinary organs R93.8
    head R93.0
    inconclusive due to excess body fat of patient R93.9
    intrathoracic organs NEC R93.1
    placenta R93.8
    retroperitoneum R93.5
    skin R93.8
    skull R93.0
    subcutaneous tissue R93.8

Findings, abnormal, inconclusive, without diagnosis (Continued)
  red blood cell (count) (morphology) (sickling) (volume) R71.8
  scan NEC R94.8
    bladder R94.8
    bone R94.8
    kidney R94.4
    liver R93.2
    lung R94.2
    pancreas R94.8
    placental R94.8
    spleen R94.8
    thyroid R94.6
  sedimentation rate, elevated R70.0
  SGOT R74.0
  SGPT R74.0
  sodium (deficiency) E87.1
    excess E87.0
  specified body fluid NEC R88.8
  stress test R94.39
  thyroid (function) (metabolic rate) (scan) (uptake) R94.6
  transaminase (level) R74.0
  triglycerides E78.9
    high E78.1
      with high cholesterol E78.2
  tuberculin skin test (without active tuberculosis) R76.11
  urine R82.90
    acetone R82.4
    bacteria R82.71 ◄▥
    bile R82.2
    casts or cells R82.99
    chyle R82.0
    culture positive R82.79 ◄▥
    glucose R81
    hemoglobin R82.3
    ketone R82.4
    sugar R81
  vanillylmandelic acid (VMA), elevated R82.5
  vectorcardiogram (VCG) R94.39
  ventriculogram R93.0
  white blood cell (count) (differential) (morphology) D72.9
  xerography R92.8

Finger —see condition

Fire, Saint Anthony's —see Erysipelas

Fire-setting
  pathological (compulsive) F63.1

Fish hook stomach K31.89

Fishmeal-worker's lung J67.8

Fissure, fissured
  anus, anal K60.2
    acute K60.0
    chronic K60.1
    congenital Q43.8
  ear, lobule, congenital Q17.8
  epiglottis (congenital) Q31.8
  larynx J38.7
    congenital Q31.8
  lip K13.0
    congenital —see Cleft, lip
  nipple N64.0
    associated with
      lactation O92.13
      pregnancy O92.11-
      puerperium O92.12
  nose Q30.2
  palate (congenital) —see Cleft, palate
  skin R23.4
  spine (congenital) —see also Spina bifida
    with hydrocephalus —see Spina bifida, by site, with hydrocephalus
  tongue (acquired) K14.5
    congenital Q38.3

Fistula (cutaneous) L98.8
  abdomen (wall) K63.2
    bladder N32.2
    intestine NEC K63.2

Fistula *(Continued)*
  abdomen *(Continued)*
    ureter N28.89
    uterus N82.5
  abdominorectal K63.2
  abdominosigmoidal K63.2
  abdominothoracic J86.0
  abdominouterine N82.5
    congenital Q51.7
  abdominovesical N32.2
  accessory sinuses —*see* Sinusitis
  actinomycotic —*see* Actinomycosis
  alveolar antrum —*see* Sinusitis, maxillary
  alveolar process K04.6
  anorectal K60.5
  antrobuccal —*see* Sinusitis, maxillary
  antrum —*see* Sinusitis, maxillary
  anus, anal (recurrent) (infectional) K60.3
    congenital Q43.6
      with absence, atresia and stenosis Q42.2
    tuberculous A18.32
  aorta-duodenal I77.2
  appendix, appendicular K38.3
  arteriovenous (acquired) (nonruptured) I77.0
    brain I67.1
      congenital Q28.2
        ruptured I60.8
      ruptured I60.8
    cerebral —*see* Fistula, arteriovenous, brain
    congenital (peripheral) —*see also*
        Malformation, arteriovenous
      brain Q28.2
        ruptured I60.8
      coronary Q24.5
      pulmonary Q25.72
    coronary I25.41
      congenital Q24.5
    pulmonary I28.0
      congenital Q25.72
    surgically created (for dialysis) Z99.2
      complication —*see* Complication,
          arteriovenous, fistula, surgically
          created
    traumatic —*see* Injury, blood vessel
  artery I77.2
  aural (mastoid) —*see* Mastoiditis, chronic
  auricle —*see also* Disorder, pinna, specified
      type NEC
    congenital Q18.1
  Bartholin's gland N82.8
  bile duct (common) (hepatic) K83.3
    with calculus, stones —*see* Calculus, bile
        duct
  biliary (tract) —*see* Fistula, bile duct
  bladder (sphincter) NEC —*see also* Fistula,
      vesico- N32.2
    into seminal vesicle N32.2
  bone —*see also* Disorder, bone, specified type
      NEC
    with osteomyelitis, chronic —*see*
        Osteomyelitis, chronic, with draining
        sinus
  brain G93.89
    arteriovenous (acquired) I67.1
      congenital Q28.2
  branchial (cleft) Q18.0
  branchiogenous Q18.0
  breast N61.0 ◀▥
    puerperal, postpartum or gestational, due
        to mastitis (purulent) —*see* Mastitis,
        obstetric, purulent
  bronchial J86.0
  bronchocutaneous, bronchomediastinal,
      bronchopleural,
      bronchopleuromediastinal (infective)
      J86.0
    tuberculous NEC A15.5
  bronchoesophageal J86.0
    congenital Q39.2
      with atresia of esophagus Q39.1
  bronchovisceral J86.0

Fistula *(Continued)*
  buccal cavity (infective) K12.2
  cecosigmoidal K63.2
  cecum K63.2
  cerebrospinal (fluid) G96.0
  cervical, lateral Q18.1
  cervicoaural Q18.1
  cervicosigmoidal N82.4
  cervicovesical N82.1
  cervix N82.8
  chest (wall) J86.0
  cholecystenteric —*see* Fistula, gallbladder
  cholecystocolic —*see* Fistula, gallbladder
  cholecystocolonic —*see* Fistula, gallbladder
  cholecystoduodenal —*see* Fistula,
      gallbladder
  cholecystogastric —*see* Fistula, gallbladder
  cholecystointestinal —*see* Fistula,
      gallbladder
  choledochoduodenal —*see* Fistula,
      bile duct
  cholocolic K82.3
  coccyx —*see* Sinus, pilonidal
  colon K63.2
  colostomy K94.09
  common duct —*see* Fistula, bile duct
  congenital, site not listed —*see* Anomaly, by
      site
  coronary, arteriovenous I25.41
    congenital Q24.5
  costal region J86.0
  cul-de-sac, Douglas' N82.8
  cystic duct —*see also* Fistula, gallbladder
    congenital Q44.5
  dental K04.6
  diaphragm J86.0
  duodenum K31.6
  ear (external) (canal) —*see* Disorder, ear,
      external, specified type NEC
  enterocolic K63.2
  enterocutaneous K63.2
  enterouterine N82.4
    congenital Q51.7
  enterovaginal N82.4
    congenital Q52.2
    large intestine N82.3
    small intestine N82.2
  enterovesical N32.1
  epididymis N50.89 ◀▥
    tuberculous A18.15
  esophagobronchial J86.0
    congenital Q39.2
      with atresia of esophagus Q39.1
  esophagocutaneous K22.8
  esophagopleural-cutaneous J86.0
  esophagotracheal J86.0
    congenital Q39.2
      with atresia of esophagus Q39.1
  esophagus K22.8
    congenital Q39.2
      with atresia of esophagus Q39.1
  ethmoid —*see* Sinusitis, ethmoidal
  eyeball (cornea) (sclera) —*see* Disorder, globe,
      hypotony
  eyelid H01.8
  fallopian tube, external N82.5
  fecal K63.2
    congenital Q43.6
  from periapical abscess K04.6
  frontal sinus —*see* Sinusitis, frontal
  gallbladder K82.3
    with calculus, cholelithiasis, stones —*see*
        Calculus, gallbladder
  gastric K31.6
  gastrocolic K31.6
    congenital Q40.2
    tuberculous A18.32
  gastroenterocolic K31.6
  gastroesophageal K31.6
  gastrojejunal K31.6
  gastrojejunocolic K31.6

Fistula *(Continued)*
  genital tract (female) N82.9
    specified NEC N82.8
    to intestine NEC N82.4
    to skin N82.5
  hepatic artery-portal vein, congenital Q26.6
  hepatopleural J86.0
  hepatopulmonary J86.0
  ileorectal or ileosigmoidal K63.2
  ileovaginal N82.2
  ileovesical N32.1
  ileum K63.2
  in ano K60.3
    tuberculous A18.32
  inner ear (labyrinth) —*see* subcategory H83.1
  intestine NEC K63.2
  intestinocolonic (abdominal) K632
  intestinoureteral N28.89
  intestinouterine N82.4
  intestinovaginal N82.4
    large intestine N82.3
    small intestine N82.2
  intestinovesical N32.1
  ischiorectal (fossa) K61.3
  jejunum K63.2
  joint M25.10
    ankle M25.17-
    elbow M25.12-
    foot joint M25.17-
    hand joint M25.14-
    hip M25.15-
    knee M25.16-
    shoulder M25.11-
    specified joint NEC M25.18
    tuberculous —*see* Tuberculosis, joint
    vertebrae M25.18
    wrist M25.13-
  kidney N28.89
  labium (majus) (minus) N82.8
  labyrinth —*see* subcategory H83.1
  lacrimal (gland) (sac) H04.61-
  lacrimonasal duct —*see* Fistula, lacrimal
  laryngotracheal, congenital Q34.8
  larynx J38.7
  lip K13.0
    congenital Q38.0
  lumbar, tuberculous A18.01
  lung J86.0
  lymphatic I89.8
  mammary (gland) N61.0 ◀▥
  mastoid (process) (region) —*see* Mastoiditis,
      chronic
  maxillary J32.0
  medial, face and neck Q18.8
  mediastinal J86.0
  mediastinobronchial J86.0
  mediastinocutaneous J86.0
  middle ear —*see* subcategory H74.8
  mouth K12.2
  nasal J34.89
    sinus —*see* Sinusitis
  nasopharynx J39.2
  nipple N64.0
  nose J34.89
  oral (cutaneous) K12.2
    maxillary J32.0
    nasal (with cleft palate) —*see* Cleft, palate
  orbit, orbital —*see* Disorder, orbit, specified
      type NEC
  oroantral J32.0
  oviduct, external N82.5
  palate (hard) M27.8
  pancreatic K86.89 ◀▥
  pancreaticoduodenal K86.89 ◀▥
  parotid (gland) K11.4
    region K12.2
  penis N48.89
  perianal K60.3
  pericardium (pleura) (sac) —*see* Pericarditis
  pericecal K63.2
  perineorectal K60.4
  perineosigmoidal K63.2

Fistula *(Continued)*
perineum, perineal (with urethral
  involvement) NEC N36.0
    tuberculous A18.13
    ureter N28.89
perirectal K60.4
  tuberculous A18.32
peritoneum K65.9
pharyngoesophageal J39.2
pharynx J39.2
  branchial cleft (congenital) Q18.0
pilonidal (infected) (rectum) —*see* Sinus,
  pilonidal
pleura, pleural, pleurocutaneous,
  pleuroperitoneal J86.0
    tuberculous NEC A15.6
pleuropericardial I31.8
portal vein-hepatic artery, congenital Q26.6
postauricular H70.81-
postoperative, persistent T81.83
  specified site —*see* Fistula, by site
preauricular (congenital) Q18.1
prostate N42.89
pulmonary J86.0
  arteriovenous I28.0
    congenital Q25.72
  tuberculous —*see* Tuberculosis, pulmonary
pulmonoperitoneal J86.0
rectolabial N82.4
rectosigmoid (intercommunicating) K63.2
rectoureteral N28.89
rectourethral N36.0
  congenital Q64.73
rectouterine N82.4
  congenital Q51.7
rectovaginal N82.3
  congenital Q52.2
  tuberculous A18.18
rectovesical N32.1
  congenital Q64.79
rectovesicovaginal N82.3
rectovulval N82.4
  congenital Q52.79
rectum (to skin) K60.4
  congenital Q43.6
    with absence, atresia and stenosis Q42.0
  tuberculous A18.32
renal N28.89
retroauricular —*see* Fistula, postauricular
salivary duct or gland (any) K11.4
  congenital Q38.4
scrotum (urinary) N50.89 ◀▦
  tuberculous A18.15
semicircular canals —*see* subcategory H83.1
sigmoid K63.2
  to bladder N32.1
sinus —*see* Sinusitis
skin L98.8
  to genital tract (female) N82.5
splenocolic D73.89
stercoral K63.2
stomach K31.6
sublingual gland K11.4
submandibular gland K11.4
submaxillary (gland) K11.4
  region K12.2
thoracic J86.0
  duct I89.8
thoracoabdominal J86.0
thoracogastric J86.0
thoracointestinal J86.0
thorax J86.0
thyroglossal duct Q89.2
thyroid E07.89
trachea, congenital (external) (internal) Q32.1
tracheoesophageal J86.0
  congenital Q39.2
    with atresia of esophagus Q39.1
  following tracheostomy J95.04
traumatic arteriovenous —*see* Injury, blood
  vessel, by site

Fistula *(Continued)*
tuberculous - code by site under
  Tuberculosis
typhoid A01.09
umbilicourinary Q64.8
urachus, congenital Q64.4
ureter (persistent) N28.89
ureteroabdominal N28.89
ureterorectal N28.89
ureterosigmoido-abdominal N28.89
ureterovaginal N82.1
ureterovesical N32.2
urethra N36.0
  congenital Q64.79
  tuberculous A18.13
urethroperineal N36.0
urethroperineovesical N32.2
urethrorectal N36.0
  congenital Q64.73
urethroscrotal N50.89 ◀▦
urethrovaginal N82.1
urethrovesical N32.2
urinary (tract) (persistent) (recurrent)
  N36.0
uteroabdominal N82.5
  congenital Q51.7
uteroenteric, uterointestinal N82.4
  congenital Q51.7
uterorectal N82.4
  congenital Q51.7
uteroureteric N82.1
uterourethral Q51.7
uterovaginal N82.8
uterovesical N82.1
  congenital Q51.7
uterus N82.8
vagina (postpartal) (wall) N82.8
vaginocutaneous (postpartal) N82.5
vaginointestinal NEC N82.4
  large intestine N82.3
  small intestine N82.2
vaginoperineal N82.5
vasocutaneous, congenital Q55.7
vesical NEC N32.2
vesicoabdominal N32.2
vesicocervicovaginal N82.1
vesicocolic N32.1
vesicocutaneous N32.2
vesicoenteric N32.1
vesicointestinal N32.1
vesicometrorectal N82.4
vesicoperineal N32.2
vesicorectal N32.1
  congenital Q64.79
vesicosigmoidal N32.1
vesicosigmoidovaginal N82.3
vesicoureteral N32.2
vesicoureterovaginal N82.1
vesicourethral N32.2
vesicourethrorectal N32.1
vesicouterine N82.1
  congenital Q51.7
vesicovaginal N82.0
vulvorectal N82.4
  congenital Q52.79
Fit R56.9
epileptic —*see* Epilepsy
fainting R55
hysterical F44.5
newborn P90
Fitting (and adjustment) (of)
artificial
  arm —*see* Admission, adjustment, artificial,
    arm
  breast Z44.3
  eye Z44.2
  leg —*see* Admission, adjustment, artificial,
    leg
automatic implantable cardiac defibrillator
  (with synchronous cardiac pacemaker)
  Z45.02

Fitting *(Continued)*
brain neuropacemaker Z46.2
  implanted Z45.42
cardiac defibrillator —*see* Fitting (and
  adjustment) (of), automatic implantable
  cardiac defibrillator
catheter, non-vascular Z46.82
colostomy belt Z46.89
contact lenses Z46.0
CRT-D (resynchronization therapy
  defibrillator) Z45.02 ◀
CRT-P (cardiac resynchronization therapy
  pacemaker) Z45.018 ◀
  pulse generator Z45.010 ◀
cystostomy device Z46.6
defibrillator, cardiac —*see* Fitting (and
  adjustment) (of), automatic implantable
  cardiac defibrillator
dentures Z46.3
device NOS Z46.9
  abdominal Z46.89
  gastrointestinal NEC Z46.59
  implanted NEC Z45.89
  nervous system Z46.2
    implanted —*see* Admission, adjustment,
      device, implanted, nervous
      system
  orthodontic Z46.4
  orthoptic Z46.0
  orthotic Z46.89
  prosthetic (external) Z44.9
    breast Z44.3
    dental Z46.3
    eye Z44.2
    specified NEC Z44.8
  specified NEC Z46.89
  substitution
    auditory Z46.2
      implanted —*see* Admission,
        adjustment, device, implanted,
        hearing device
    nervous system Z46.2
      implanted —*see* Admission,
        adjustment, device, implanted,
        nervous system
    visual Z46.2
      implanted Z45.31
  urinary Z46.6
gastric lap band Z46.51
gastrointestinal appliance NEC Z46.59
glasses (reading) Z46.0
hearing aid Z46.1
ileostomy device Z46.89
insulin pump Z46.81
intestinal appliance NEC Z46.89
myringotomy device (stent) (tube) Z45.82
neuropacemaker Z46.2
  implanted Z45.42
non-vascular catheter Z46.82
orthodontic device Z46.4
orthopedic device (brace) (cast) (corset)
  (shoes) Z46.89
pacemaker (cardiac) (cardiac
  resynchronization therapy (CRT-P))
  Z45.018 ◀▦
  nervous system (brain) (peripheral nerve)
    (spinal cord) Z46.2
    implanted Z45.42
  pulse generator Z45.010
portacath (port-a-cath) Z45.2
prosthesis (external) Z44.9
  arm —*see* Admission, adjustment, artificial,
    arm
  breast Z44.3
  dental Z46.3
  eye Z44.2
  leg —*see* Admission, adjustment, artificial,
    leg
  specified NEC Z44.8
spectacles Z46.0
wheelchair Z46.89

Fitzhugh-Curtis syndrome
  due to
    Chlamydia trachomatis A74.81
    Neisseria gonorrhorea (gonococcal
      peritonitis) A54.85
Fitz's syndrome (acute hemorrhagic
  pancreatitis) —see also Pancreatitis, acute
  K85.80 ◄▥
Fixation
  joint —see Ankylosis
  larynx J38.7
  stapes —see Ankylosis, ear ossicles
    deafness —see Deafness, conductive
  uterus (acquired) —see Malposition, uterus
  vocal cord J38.3
Flabby ridge K06.8
Flaccid —see also condition
  palate, congenital Q38.5
Flail
  chest S22.5-
    newborn (birth injury) P13.8
  joint (paralytic) M25.20
    ankle M25.27-
    elbow M25.22-
    foot joint M25.27-
    hand joint M25.24-
    hip M25.25-
    knee M25.26-
    shoulder M25.21-
    specified joint NEC M25.28
    wrist M25.23-
Flajani's disease —see Hyperthyroidism, with,
  goiter (diffuse)
Flap, liver K71.3
Flashbacks (residual to hallucinogen use) F16.283
Flat
  chamber (eye) —see Disorder, globe,
    hypotony, flat anterior chamber
  chest, congenital Q67.8
  foot (acquired) (fixed type) (painful)
    (postural) —see also Deformity, limb,
    flat foot
    congenital (rigid) (spastic) (everted) Q66.5-
    rachitic sequelae (late effect) E64.3
  organ or site, congenital NEC —see Anomaly,
    by site
  pelvis M95.5
    with disproportion (fetopelvic) O33.0
      causing obstructed labor O65.0
    congenital Q74.2
Flatau-Schilder disease G37.0
Flatback syndrome M40.30
  lumbar region M40.36
  lumbosacral region M40.37
  thoracolumbar region M40.35
Flattening
  head, femur M89.8X5
  hip —see Coxa, plana
  lip (congenital) Q18.8
  nose (congenital) Q67.4
    acquired M95.0
Flatulence R14.3
  psychogenic F45.8
Flatus R14.3
  vaginalis N89.8
Flax-dresser's disease J66.1
Flea bite —see Injury, bite, by site, superficial,
  insect
Flecks, glaucomatous (subcapsular) —see
  Cataract, complicated
Fleischer (-Kayser) ring (cornea) H18.04-
Fleshy mole O02.0
Flexibilitas cerea —see Catalepsy
Flexion
  amputation stump (surgical) T87.89
  cervix —see Malposition, uterus
  contracture, joint —see Contraction, joint
  deformity, joint —see also Deformity, limb,
    flexion M21.20
    hip, congenital Q65.89
  uterus —see also Malposition, uterus
    lateral —see Lateroversion, uterus

Flexner-Boyd dysentery A03.2
Flexner's dysentery A03.1
Flexure —see Flexion
Flint murmur (aortic insufficiency) I35.1
Floater, vitreous —see Opacity, vitreous
Floating
  cartilage (joint) —see also Loose, body, joint
    knee —see Derangement, knee, loose body
  gallbladder, congenital Q44.1
  kidney N28.89
    congenital Q63.8
  spleen D73.89
Flooding N92.0
Floor —see condition
Floppy
  baby syndrome (nonspecific) P94.2
  iris syndrome (intraoperative) (IFIS) H21.81
  nonrheumatic mitral valve syndrome I34.1
Flu —see also Influenza
  avian —see also Influenza, due to, identified
    novel influenza A virus J09.X2
  bird —see also Influenza, due to, identified
    novel influenza A virus J09.X2
  intestinal NEC A08.4
  swine (viruses that normally cause infections
    in pigs) —see also Influenza, due to,
    identified novel influenza A virus
    J09.X2
Fluctuating blood pressure I99.8
Fluid
  abdomen R18.8
  chest J94.8
  heart —see Failure, heart, congestive
  joint —see Effusion, joint
  loss (acute) E86.9
    ~~with~~
      ~~hypernatremia E87.0~~
      ~~hyponatremia E87.1~~
  lung —see Edema, lung
  overload E87.70
    specified NEC E87.79
  peritoneal cavity R18.8
  pleural cavity J94.8
  retention R60.9
Flukes NEC —see also Infestation, fluke
  blood NEC —see Schistosomiasis
  liver B66.3
Fluor (vaginalis) N89.8
  trichomonal or due to Trichomonas
    (vaginalis) A59.00
Fluorosis
  dental K00.3
  skeletal M85.10
    ankle M85.17-
    foot M85.17-
    forearm M85.13-
    hand M85.14-
    lower leg M85.16-
    multiple site M85.19
    neck M85.18
    rib M85.18
    shoulder M85.11-
    skull M85.18
    specified site NEC M85.18
    thigh M85.15-
    toe M85.17-
    upper arm M85.12-
    vertebra M85.18
Flush syndrome E34.0
Flushing R23.2
  menopausal N95.1
Flutter
  atrial or auricular I48.92
    atypical I48.4
    type I I48.3
    type II I48.4
    typical I48.3
  heart I49.8
    atrial or auricular I48.92
      atypical I48.4
      type I I48.3

Fistula (Continued)
  heart (Continued)
    atrial or auricular (Continued)
      type II I48.4
      typical I48.3
      ventricular I49.02
    ventricular I49.02
FNHTR (febrile nonhemolytic transfusion
  reaction) R50.84
Fochier's abscess - code by site under Abscess
Focus, Assmann's —see Tuberculosis,
  pulmonary
Fogo selvagem L10.3
Foix-Alajouanine syndrome G95.19
Fold, folds (anomalous) —see also Anomaly,
  by site
  Descemet's membrane —see Change, corneal
    membrane, Descemet's, fold
  epicanthic Q10.3
  heart Q24.8
Folie à deux F24
Follicle
  cervix (nabothian) (ruptured) N88.8
  graafian, ruptured, with hemorrhage
    N83.0- ◄▥
  nabothian N88.8
Follicular —see condition
Folliculitis (superficial) L73.9
  abscedens et suffodiens L66.3
  cyst N83.0- ◄▥
  decalvans L66.2
  deep —see Furuncle, by site
  gonococcal (acute) (chronic) A54.01
  keloid, keloidalis L73.0
  pustular L01.02
  ulerythematosa reticulata L66.4
Folliculome lipidique
  specified site —see Neoplasm, benign,
    by site
  unspecified site
    female D27.9
    male D29.20
Følling's disease E70.0
Follow-up —see Examination, follow-up
Fong's syndrome (hereditary osteo-
  onychodysplasia) Q87.2 ◄▥
Food
  allergy L27.2
  asphyxia (from aspiration or inhalation) —see
    Foreign body, by site
  choked on —see Foreign body, by site
  deprivation T73.0
    specified kind of food NEC E63.8
  intoxication —see Poisoning, food
  lack of T73.0
  poisoning —see Poisoning, food
  rejection NEC —see Disorder, eating
  strangulation or suffocation —see Foreign
    body, by site
  toxemia —see Poisoning, food
Foot —see condition
Foramen ovale (nonclosure) (patent)
  (persistent) Q21.1
Forbes' glycogen storage disease E74.03
Fordyce-Fox disease L75.2
Fordyce's disease (mouth) Q38.6
Forearm —see condition
Foreign body
  with
    laceration —see Laceration, by site, with
      foreign body
    puncture wound —see Puncture, by site,
      with foreign body
  accidentally left following a procedure
    T81.509
    aspiration T81.506
      resulting in
        adhesions T81.516
        obstruction T81.526
        perforation T81.536
        specified complication NEC T81.596

◄ New   ◄▥ Revised   ~~deleted~~ Deleted

Foreign body *(Continued)*
  accidentally left following a procedure
    (Continued)
    cardiac catheterization T81.505
      resulting in
        acute reaction T81.60
          aseptic peritonitis T81.61
          specified NEC T81.69
        adhesions T81.515
        obstruction T81.525
        perforation T81.535
        specified complication NEC T81.595
      causing
        acute reaction T81.60
          aseptic peritonitis T81.61
          specified complication NEC T81.69
        adhesions T81.519
        aseptic peritonitis T81.61
        obstruction T81.529
        perforation T81.539
        specified complication NEC T81.599
    endoscopy T81.504
      resulting in
        adhesions T81.514
        obstruction T81.524
        perforation T81.534
        specified complication NEC T81.594
    immunization T81.503
      resulting in
        adhesions T81.513
        obstruction T81.523
        perforation T81.533
        specified complication NEC T81.593
    infusion T81.501
      resulting in
        adhesions T81.511
        obstruction T81.521
        perforation T81.531
        specified complication NEC T81.591
    injection T81.503
      resulting in
        adhesions T81.513
        obstruction T81.523
        perforation T81.533
        specified complication NEC T81.593
    kidney dialysis T81.502
      resulting in
        adhesions T81.512
        obstruction T81.522
        perforation T81.532
        specified complication NEC T81.592
    packing removal T81.507
      resulting in
        acute reaction T81.60
          aseptic peritonitis T81.61
          specified NEC T81.69
        adhesions T81.517
        obstruction T81.527
        perforation T81.537
        specified complication NEC T81.597
    puncture T81.506
      resulting in
        adhesions T81.516
        obstruction T81.526
        perforation T81.536
        specified complication NEC T81.596
    specified procedure NEC T81.508
      resulting in
        acute reaction T81.60
          aseptic peritonitis T81.61
          specified NEC T81.69
        adhesions T81.518
        obstruction T81.528
        perforation T81.538
        specified complication NEC
          T81.598
    surgical operation T81.500
      resulting in
        acute reaction T81.60
          aseptic peritonitis T81.61
          specified NEC T81.69

Foreign body *(Continued)*
  accidentally left following a procedure
    (Continued)
    surgical operation *(Continued)*
      resulting in *(Continued)*
        adhesions T81.510
        obstruction T81.520
        perforation T81.530
        specified complication NEC T81.590
    transfusion T81.501
      resulting in
        adhesions T81.511
        obstruction T81.521
        perforation T81.531
        specified complication NEC T81.591
  alimentary tract T18.9
    anus T18.5
    colon T18.4
    esophagus —*see* Foreign body, esophagus
    mouth T18.0
    multiple sites T18.8
    rectosigmoid (junction) T18.5
    rectum T18.5
    small intestine T18.3
    specified site NEC T18.8
    stomach T18.2
  anterior chamber (eye) S05.5-
  auditory canal —*see* Foreign body, entering
    through orifice, ear
  bronchus T17.508
    causing
      asphyxiation T17.500
        food (bone) (seed) T17.520
        gastric contents (vomitus) T17.510
        specified type NEC T17.590
      injury NEC T17.508
        food (bone) (seed) T17.528
        gastric contents (vomitus) T17.518
        specified type NEC T17.598
  canthus —*see* Foreign body, conjunctival sac
  ciliary body (eye) S05.5-
  conjunctival sac T15.1-
  cornea T15.0-
  entering through orifice
    accessory sinus T17.0
    alimentary canal T18.9
      multiple parts T18.8
      specified part NEC T18.8
    alveolar process T18.0
    antrum (Highmore's) T17.0
    anus T18.5
    appendix T18.4
    auditory canal —*see* Foreign body, entering
      through orifice, ear
    auricle —*see* Foreign body, entering
      through orifice, ear
    bladder T19.1
    bronchioles —*see* Foreign body, respiratory
      tract, specified site NEC
    bronchus (main) —*see* Foreign body,
      bronchus
    buccal cavity T18.0
    canthus (inner) —*see* Foreign body,
      conjunctival sac
    cecum T18.4
    cervix (canal) (uteri) T19.3
    colon T18.4
    conjunctival sac —*see* Foreign body,
      conjunctival sac
    cornea —*see* Foreign body, cornea
    digestive organ or tract NOS T18.9
      multiple parts T18.8
      specified part NEC T18.8
    duodenum T18.3
    ear (external) T16.-
    esophagus —*see* Foreign body, esophagus
    eye (external) NOS T15.9-
      conjunctival sac —*see* Foreign body,
        conjunctival sac
      cornea —*see* Foreign body, cornea
      specified part NEC T15.8-

Foreign body *(Continued)*
  entering through orifice *(Continued)*
    eyeball —*see also* Foreign body, entering
      through orifice, eye, specified part
      NEC
      with penetrating wound —*see* Puncture,
        eyeball
    eyelid —*see also* Foreign body, conjunctival
      sac
      with
        laceration —*see* Laceration, eyelid,
          with foreign body
        puncture —*see* Puncture, eyelid, with
          foreign body
        superficial injury —*see* Foreign body,
          superficial, eyelid
    gastrointestinal tract T18.9
      multiple parts T18.8
      specified part NEC T18.8
    genitourinary tract T19.9
      multiple parts T19.8
      specified part NEC T19.8
    globe —*see* Foreign body, entering through
      orifice, eyeball
    gum T18.0
    Highmore's antrum T17.0
    hypopharynx —*see* Foreign body, pharynx
    ileum T18.3
    intestine (small) T18.3
      large T18.4
    lacrimal apparatus (punctum) —*see*
      Foreign body, entering through
      orifice, eye, specified part NEC
    large intestine T18.4
    larynx —*see* Foreign body, larynx
    lung —*see* Foreign body, respiratory tract,
      specified site NEC
    maxillary sinus T17.0
    mouth T18.0
    nasal sinus T17.0
    nasopharynx —*see* Foreign body, pharynx
    nose (passage) T17.1
    nostril T17.1
    oral cavity T18.0
    palate T18.0
    penis T19.4
    pharynx —*see* Foreign body, pharynx
    piriform sinus —*see* Foreign body, pharynx
    rectosigmoid (junction) T18.5
    rectum T18.5
    respiratory tract —*see* Foreign body,
      respiratory tract
    sinus (accessory) (frontal) (maxillary)
      (nasal) T17.0
      piriform —*see* Foreign body, pharynx
    small intestine T18.3
    stomach T18.2
    suffocation by —*see* Foreign body, by site
    tear ducts or glands —*see* Foreign body,
      entering through orifice, eye,
      specified part NEC
    throat —*see* Foreign body, pharynx
    tongue T18.0
    tonsil, tonsillar (fossa) —*see* Foreign body,
      pharynx
    trachea —*see* Foreign body, trachea
    ureter T19.8
    urethra T19.0
    uterus (any part) T19.3
    vagina T19.2
    vulva T19.2
  esophagus T18.108
    causing
      injury NEC T18.108
        food (bone) (seed) T18.128
        gastric contents (vomitus) T18.118
        specified type NEC T18.198
      tracheal compression T18.100
        food (bone) (seed) T18.120
        gastric contents (vomitus) T18.110
        specified type NEC T18.190

Foreign body (Continued)
  felling of, in throat R09.89
  fragment —see Retained, foreign body
      fragments (type of)
  genitourinary tract T19.9
    bladder T19.1
    multiple parts T19.8
    penis T19.4
    specified site NEC T19.8
    urethra T19.0
    uterus T19.3
      IUD Z97.5
    vagina T19.2
      contraceptive device Z97.5
    vulva T19.2
  granuloma (old) (soft tissue) —see also
      Granuloma, foreign body
    skin L92.3
  in
    laceration —see Laceration, by site, with
        foreign body
    puncture wound —see Puncture, by site,
        with foreign body
    soft tissue (residual) M79.5
  inadvertently left in operation wound —see
      Foreign body, accidentally left during a
      procedure
  ingestion, ingested NOS T18.9
  inhalation or inspiration —see Foreign body,
      by site
  internal organ, not entering through a natural
      orifice - code as specific injury with
      foreign body
  intraocular S05.5-
    old, retained (nonmagnetic) H44.70-
      anterior chamber H44.71-
      ciliary body H44.72-
      iris H44.72-
      lens H44.73-
      magnetic H44.60-
        anterior chamber H44.61-
        ciliary body H44.62-
        iris H44.62-
        lens H44.63-
        posterior wall H44.64-
        specified site NEC H44.69-
        vitreous body H44.65-
      posterior wall H44.74-
      specified site NEC H44.79-
      vitreous body H44.75-
    iris —see Foreign body, intraocular
  lacrimal punctum —see Foreign body,
      entering through orifice, eye, specified
      part NEC
  larynx T17.308
    causing
      asphyxiation T17.300
        food (bone) (seed) T17.320
        gastric contents (vomitus) T17.310
        specified type NEC T17.390
      injury NEC T17.308
        food (bone) (seed) T17.328
        gastric contents (vomitus) T17.318
        specified type NEC T17.398
  lens —see Foreign body, intraocular
  ocular muscle S05.4-
    old, retained —see Foreign body, orbit, old
  old or residual
    soft tissue (residual) M79.5
  operation wound, left accidentally —see
      Foreign body, accidentally left during a
      procedure
  orbit S05.4-
    old, retained H05.5-
  pharynx T17.208
    causing
      asphyxiation T17.200
        food (bone) (seed) T17.220
        gastric contents (vomitus)
            T17.210
        specified type NEC T17.290

Foreign body (Continued)
  pharynx (Continued)
    causing (Continued)
      injury NEC T17.208
        food (bone) (seed) T17.228
        gastric contents (vomitus) T17.218
        specified type NEC T17.298
  respiratory tract T17.908
    bronchioles —see Foreign body, respiratory
        tract, specified site NEC
    bronchus —see Foreign body, bronchus
    causing
      asphyxiation T17.900
        food (bone) (seed) T17.920
        gastric contents (vomitus) T17.910
        specified type NEC T17.990
      injury NEC T17.908
        food (bone) (seed) T17.928
        gastric contents (vomitus) T17.918
        specified type NEC T17.998
    larynx —see Foreign body, larynx
    lung —see Foreign body, respiratory tract,
        specified site NEC
    multiple parts —see Foreign body,
        respiratory tract, specified site NEC
    nasal sinus T17.0
    nasopharynx —see Foreign body, pharynx
    nose T17.1
    nostril T17.1
    pharynx —see Foreign body, pharynx
    specified site NEC T17.808
      causing
        asphyxiation T17.800
          food (bone) (seed) T17.820
          gastric contents (vomitus) T17.810
          specified type NEC T17.890
        injury NEC T17.808
          food (bone) (seed) T17.828
          gastric contents (vomitus) T17.818
          specified type NEC T17.898
    throat —see Foreign body, pharynx
    trachea —see Foreign body, trachea
  retained (old) (nonmagnetic) (in)
    anterior chamber (eye) —see Foreign body,
        intraocular, old, retained, anterior
        chamber
      magnetic —see Foreign body, intraocular,
          old, retained, magnetic, anterior
          chamber
    ciliary body —see Foreign body,
        intraocular, old, retained, ciliary body
      magnetic —see Foreign body, intraocular,
          old, retained, magnetic, ciliary
          body
    eyelid H02.819
      left H02.816
        lower H02.815
        upper H02.814
      right H02.813
        lower H02.812
        upper H02.811
    fragments —see Retained, foreign body
        fragments (type of)
    globe —see Foreign body, intraocular, old,
        retained
      magnetic —see Foreign body, intraocular,
          old, retained, magnetic
    intraocular —see Foreign body, intraocular,
        old, retained
      magnetic —see Foreign body, intraocular,
          old, retained, magnetic
    iris —see Foreign body, intraocular, old,
        retained, iris
      magnetic —see Foreign body, intraocular,
          old, retained, magnetic, iris
    lens —see Foreign body, intraocular, old,
        retained, lens
      magnetic —see Foreign body, intraocular,
          old, retained, magnetic, lens
    muscle —see Foreign body, retained, soft
        tissue

Foreign body (Continued)
  retained (Continued)
    orbit —see Foreign body, orbit, old
    posterior wall of globe —see Foreign body,
        intraocular, old, retained, posterior
        wall
      magnetic —see Foreign body, intraocular,
          old, retained, magnetic, posterior
          wall
    retrobulbar —see Foreign body, orbit, old,
        retrobulbar
    soft tissue M79.5
    vitreous —see Foreign body, intraocular,
        old, retained, vitreous body
      magnetic —see Foreign body, intraocular,
          old, retained, magnetic, vitreous
          body
  retina S05.5-
  superficial, without open wound
    abdomen, abdominal (wall) S30.851
    alveolar process S00.552
    ankle S90.55-
    antecubital space —see Foreign body,
        superficial, forearm
    anus S30.857
    arm (upper) S40.85-
    auditory canal —see Foreign body,
        superficial, ear
    auricle —see Foreign body, superficial, ear
    axilla —see Foreign body, superficial, arm
    back, lower S30.850
    breast S20.15-
    brow S00.85
    buttock S30.850
    calf —see Foreign body, superficial, leg
    canthus —see Foreign body, superficial,
        eyelid
    cheek S00.85
      internal S00.552
    chest wall —see Foreign body, superficial,
        thorax
    chin S00.85
    clitoris S30.854
    costal region —see Foreign body,
        superficial, thorax
    digit (s)
      foot —see Foreign body, superficial, toe
      hand —see Foreign body, superficial,
          finger
    ear S00.45-
    elbow S50.35-
    epididymis S30.853
    epigastric region S30.851
    epiglottis S10.15
    esophagus, cervical S10.15
    eyebrow —see Foreign body, superficial,
        eyelid
    eyelid S00.25-
    face S00.85
    finger (s) S60.459
      index S60.45-
      little S60.45-
      middle S60.45-
      ring S60.45-
    flank S30.851
    foot (except toe (s) alone) S90.85-
      toe —see Foreign body, superficial, toe
    forearm S50.85-
      elbow only —see Foreign body,
          superficial, elbow
    forehead S00.85
    genital organs, external
      female S30.856
      male S30.855
    groin S30.851
    gum S00.552
    hand S60.55-
    head S00.95
      ear —see Foreign body, superficial, ear
      eyelid —see Foreign body, superficial,
          eyelid

◀ New   ◀═ Revised   ~~deleted~~ Deleted

Foreign body *(Continued)*
  superficial, without open wound *(Continued)*
    head *(Continued)*
      lip S00.551
      nose S00.35
      oral cavity S00.552
      scalp S00.05
      specified site NEC S00.85
    heel —*see* Foreign body, superficial, foot
    hip S70.25-
    inguinal region S30.851
    interscapular region S20.459
    jaw S00.85
    knee S80.25-
    labium (majus) (minus) S30.854
    larynx S10.15
    leg (lower) S80.85-
      knee —*see* Foreign body, superficial, knee
      upper —*see* Foreign body, superficial, thigh
    lip S00.551
    lower back S30.850
    lumbar region S30.850
    malar region S00.85
    mammary —*see* Foreign body, superficial, breast
    mastoid region S00.85
    mouth S00.552
    nail
      finger —*see* Foreign body, superficial, finger
      toe —*see* Foreign body, superficial, toe
    nape S10.85
    nasal S00.35
    neck S10.95
      specified site NEC S10.85
      throat S10.15
    nose S00.35
    occipital region S00.05
    oral cavity S00.552
    orbital region —*see* Foreign body, superficial, eyelid
    palate S00.552
    palm —*see* Foreign body, superficial, hand
    parietal region S00.05
    pelvis S30.850
    penis S30.852
    perineum
      female S30.854
      male S30.850
    periocular area —*see* Foreign body, superficial, eyelid
    phalanges
      finger —*see* Foreign body, superficial, finger
      toe —*see* Foreign body, superficial, toe
    pharynx S10.15
    pinna —*see* Foreign body, superficial, ear
    popliteal space —*see* Foreign body, superficial, knee
    prepuce S30.852
    pubic region S30.850
    pudendum
      female S30.856
      male S30.855
    sacral region S30.850
    scalp S00.05
    scapular region —*see* Foreign body, superficial, shoulder
    scrotum S30.853
    shin —*see* Foreign body, superficial, leg
    shoulder S40.25-
    sternal region S20.359
    submaxillary region S00.85
    submental region S00.85
    subungual
      finger (s) —*see* Foreign body, superficial, finger
      toe (s) —*see* Foreign body, superficial, toe

Foreign body *(Continued)*
  superficial, without open wound *(Continued)*
    supraclavicular fossa S10.85
    supraorbital S00.85
    temple S00.85
    temporal region S00.85
    testis S30.853
    thigh S70.35-
    thorax, thoracic (wall) S20.95
      back S20.45-
      front S20.35-
    throat S10.15
    thumb S60.35-
    toe (s) (lesser) S90.456
      great S90.45-
    tongue S00.552
    trachea S10.15
    tunica vaginalis S30.853
    tympanum, tympanic membrane —*see* Foreign body, superficial, ear
    uvula S00.552
    vagina S30.854
    vocal cords S10.15
    vulva S30.854
    wrist S60.85-
  swallowed T18.9
  trachea T17.408
    causing
      asphyxiation T17.400
        food (bone) (seed) T17.420
        gastric contents (vomitus) T17.410
        specified type NEC T17.490
      injury NEC T17.408
        food (bone) (seed) T17.428
        gastric contents (vomitus) T17.418
        specified type NEC T17.498
  type of fragment —*see* Retained, foreign body fragments (type of)
  vitreous (humor) S05.5-
Forestier's disease (rhizomelic pseudopolyarthritis) M35.3-
  meaning ankylosing hyperostosis —*see* Hyperostosis, ankylosing
Formation
  hyalin in cornea —*see* Degeneration, cornea
  sequestrum in bone (due to infection) —*see* Osteomyelitis, chronic
  valve
    colon, congenital Q43.8
    ureter (congenital) Q62.39
Formication R20.2
Fort Bragg fever A27.89
Fossa —*see also* condition
  pyriform —*see* condition
Foster-Kennedy syndrome H47.14-
Fothergill's
  disease (trigeminal neuralgia) —*see also* Neuralgia, trigeminal
  scarlatina anginosa A38.9
Foul breath R19.6
Foundling Z76.1
Fournier disease or gangrene N49.3
  female N76.89
Fourth
  cranial nerve —*see* condition
  molar K00.1
Foville's (peduncular) disease or syndrome G46.3
Fox (-Fordyce) disease (apocrine miliaria) L75.2
Fracture, burst —*see* Fracture, traumatic, by site
Fracture, chronic —*see* Fracture, pathological
Fracture, insufficiency —*see* Fracture, pathologic, by site
Fracture, nontraumatic, NEC ◄
  atypical ◄
    femur M84.750- ◄
      complete ◄
        oblique M84.759 ◄
          left side M84.758 ◄
          right side M84.757 ◄

Fracture, nontraumatic *(Continued)*
  atypical *(Continued)*
    femur *(Continued)*
      complete *(Continued)*
        transverse M84.756 ◄
          left side M84.755 ◄
          right side M84.754 ◄
      incomplete M84.753 ◄
        left side M84.752 ◄
        right side M84.751 ◄
Fracture, pathological (pathologic) —*see also* Fracture, traumatic M84.40
  ankle M84.47-
  carpus M84.44-
  clavicle M84.41-
  compression (not due to trauma) —*see also* Collapse, vertebra M48.50- ◄
  dental implant M27.63
  dental restorative material K08.539
    with loss of material K08.531
    without loss of material K08.530
  due to
    neoplastic disease NEC —*see also* Neoplasm M84.50
      ankle M84.57-
      carpus M84.54-
      clavicle M84.51-
      femur M84.55-
      fibula M84.56-
      finger M84.54-
      hip M84.559
      humerus M84.52-
      ilium M84.550
      ischium M84.550
      metacarpus M84.54-
      metatarsus M84.57-
      neck M84.58
      pelvis M84.550
      radius M84.53-
      rib M84.58
      scapula M84.51-
      skull M84.58
      specified site NEC M84.58
      tarsus M84.57-
      tibia M84.56-
      toe M84.57-
      ulna M84.53-
      vertebra M84.58
    osteoporosis M80.00 ◄▦
      disuse —*see* Osteoporosis, specified type NEC, with pathological fracture
      drug-induced —*see* Osteoporosis, drug induced, with pathological fracture
      idiopathic —*see* Osteoporosis, specified type NEC, with pathological fracture
      postmenopausal —*see* Osteoporosis, postmenopausal, with pathological fracture
      postoophorectomy —*see* Osteoporosis, postoophorectomy, with pathological fracture
      postsurgical malabsorption —*see* Osteoporosis, specified type NEC, with pathological fracture
      specified cause NEC —*see* Osteoporosis, specified type NEC, with pathological fracture
    specified disease NEC M84.60
      ankle M84.67-
      carpus M84.64-
      clavicle M84.61-
      femur M84.65-
      fibula M84.66-
      finger M84.64-
      hip M84.65-
      humerus M84.62-
      ilium M84.650
      ischium M84.650
      metacarpus M84.64-
      metatarsus M84.67-

Fracture, pathological *(Continued)*
  due to *(Continued)*
    specified disease NEC *(Continued)*
      neck M84.68
      radius M84.63-
      rib M84.68
      scapula M84.61-
      skull M84.68
      tarsus M84.67-
      tibia M84.66-
      toe M84.67-
      ulna M84.63-
      vertebra M84.68
  femur M84.45-
  fibula M84.46-
  finger M84.44-
  hip M84.459
  humerus M84.42-
  ilium M84.454
  ischium M84.454
  joint prosthesis —*see* Complications, joint
    prosthesis, mechanical, breakdown, by
    site
    periprosthetic —*see* Fracture, pathological,
      periprosthetic ◀▥
  metacarpus M84.44-
  metatarsus M84.47-
  neck M84.48
  pelvis M84.454
  periprosthetic M97.9 ◀
    ankle M97.2- ◀
    elbow M97.4- ◀
    finger M97.8 ◀
    hip M97.0- ◀
    knee M97.1- ◀
    other specified joint M97.8 ◀
    shoulder M97.3- ◀
    spinal joint M97.8 ◀
    toe joint M97.8 ◀
    wrist joint M97.8 ◀
  radius M84.43-
  restorative material (dental) K08.539
    with loss of material K08.531
    without loss of material K08.530
  rib M84.48
  scapula M84.41-
  skull M84.48
  tarsus M84.47-
  tibia M84.46-
  toe M84.47-
  ulna M84.43-
  vertebra M84.48
Fracture, traumatic (abduction) (adduction)
  (separation) —*see also* Fracture,
  pathological T14.8
  acetabulum S32.40-
    column
      anterior (displaced) (iliopubic)
        S32.43-
        nondisplaced S32.436
      posterior (displaced) (ilioischial)
        S32.443
        nondisplaced S32.44-
    dome (displaced) S32.48-
      nondisplaced S32.48
    specified NEC S32.49-
    transverse (displaced) S32.45-
      with associated posterior wall fracture
        (displaced) S32.46-
        nondisplaced S32.46-
      nondisplaced S32.45-
    wall
      anterior (displaced) S32.41-
        nondisplaced S32.41-
      medial (displaced) S32.47-
        nondisplaced S32.47-
      posterior (displaced) S32.42-
        with associated transverse fracture
          (displaced) S32.46-
          nondisplaced S32.46-
        nondisplaced S32.42-

Fracture, traumatic *(Continued)*
  acromion —*see* Fracture, scapula, acromial
    process
  ankle S82.899
    bimalleolar (displaced) S82.84-
      nondisplaced S82.84-
    lateral malleolus only (displaced) S82.6-
      nondisplaced S82.6-
    medial malleolus (displaced) S82.5-
      associated with Maisonneuve's
        fracture —*see* Fracture,
        Maisonneuve's
      nondisplaced S82.5-
    talus —*see* Fracture, tarsal, talus
    trimalleolar (displaced) S82.85-
      nondisplaced S82.85-
  arm (upper) —*see also* Fracture, humerus,
    shaft
    humerus —*see* Fracture, humerus
    radius —*see* Fracture, radius
    ulna —*see* Fracture, ulna
  astragalus —*see* Fracture, tarsal, talus
  atlas —*see* Fracture, neck, cervical vertebra,
    first
  axis —*see* Fracture, neck, cervical vertebra,
    second
  back —*see* Fracture, vertebra
  Barton's —*see* Barton's fracture
  base of skull —*see* Fracture, skull, base
  basicervical (basal) (femoral) S72.0
  Bennett's —*see* Bennett's fracture
  bimalleolar —*see* Fracture, ankle,
    bimalleolar
  blow-out S02.3- ◀▥
  bone NEC T14.8
    birth injury P13.9
    following insertion of orthopedic implant,
      joint prosthesis or bone plate —*see*
      Fracture, following insertion of
      orthopedic implant, joint prosthesis
      or bone plate
    in (due to) neoplastic disease NEC —*see*
      Fracture, pathological, due to,
      neoplastic disease
    pathological (cause unknown) —*see*
      Fracture, pathological
  breast bone —*see* Fracture, sternum
  bucket handle (semilunar cartilage) —*see*
    Tear, meniscus
  burst —*see* Fracture, traumatic, by site
  calcaneus —*see* Fracture, tarsal, calcaneus
  carpal bone (s) S62.10-
    capitate (displaced) S62.13-
      nondisplaced S62.13-
    cuneiform —*see* Fracture, carpal bone,
      triquetrum
    hamate (body) (displaced) S62.143
      hook process (displaced) S62.15-
        nondisplaced S62.15-
      nondisplaced S62.14-
    larger multangular —*see* Fracture, carpal
      bones, trapezium
    lunate (displaced) S62.12-
      nondisplaced S62.12-
    navicular S62.00-
      distal pole (displaced) S62.01-
        nondisplaced S62.01-
      middle third (displaced) S62.02-
        nondisplaced S62.02-
      proximal third (displaced) S62.03-
        nondisplaced S62.03-
      volar tuberosity —*see* Fracture, carpal
        bones, navicular, distal pole
    os magnum —*see* Fracture, carpal bones,
      capitate
    pisiform (displaced) S62.16-
      nondisplaced S62.16-
    semilunar —*see* Fracture, carpal bones,
      lunate
    smaller multangular —*see* Fracture, carpal
      bones, trapezoid

Fracture, traumatic *(Continued)*
  carpal bone (s) *(Continued)*
    trapezium (displaced) S62.17-
      nondisplaced S62.17-
    trapezoid (displaced) S62.18-
      nondisplaced S62.18-
    triquetrum (displaced) S62.11-
      nondisplaced S62.11-
    unciform —*see* Fracture, carpal bones,
      hamate
  cervical —*see* Fracture, vertebra, cervical
  clavicle S42.00-
    acromial end (displaced) S42.03-
      nondisplaced S42.03-
    birth injury P13.4
    lateral end —*see* Fracture, clavicle, acromial
      end
    shaft (displaced) S42.02-
      nondisplaced S42.02-
    sternal end (anterior) (displaced) S42.01-
      nondisplaced S42.01-
      posterior S42.01-
  coccyx S32.2
  collapsed —*see* Collapse, vertebra
  collar bone —*see* Fracture, clavicle
  Colles' —*see* Colles' fracture
  ~~compression, not due to trauma —see~~
    ~~Collapse, vertebra~~
  coronoid process —*see* Fracture, ulna, upper
    end, coronoid process
  corpus cavernosum penis S39.840
  costochondral cartilage S23.41
  costochondral, costosternal junction —*see*
    Fracture, rib
  cranium —*see* Fracture, skull
  cricoid cartilage S12.8
  cuboid (ankle) —*see* Fracture, tarsal, cuboid
  cuneiform
    foot —*see* Fracture, tarsal, cuneiform
    wrist —*see* Fracture, carpal, triquetrum
  delayed union —*see* Delay, union, fracture
  dental restorative material K08.539
    with loss of material K08.531
    without loss of material K08.530
  due to
    birth injury —*see* Birth, injury, fracture
    osteoporosis —*see* Osteoporosis, with
      fracture
  Dupuytren's —*see* Fracture, ankle, lateral
    malleolus
  elbow S42.40-
  ethmoid (bone) (sinus) —*see* Fracture, skull,
    base
  face bone S02.92
  fatigue —*see also* Fracture, stress
    vertebra M48.40
      cervical region M48.42
      cervicothoracic region M48.43
      lumbar region M48.46
      lumbosacral region M48.47
      occipito-atlanto-axial region M48.41
      sacrococcygeal region M48.48
      thoracic region M48.44
      thoracolumbar region M48.45
  femur, femoral S72.9-
    basicervical (basal) S72.0
    birth injury P13.2
    capital epiphyseal S79.01-
    condyles, epicondyles —*see* Fracture,
      femur, lower end
    distal end —*see* Fracture, femur,
      lower end
    epiphysis
      head —*see* Fracture, femur, upper end,
        epiphysis
      lower —*see* Fracture, femur, lower end,
        epiphysis
      upper —*see* Fracture, femur, upper end,
        epiphysis
    following insertion of implant, prosthesis
      or plate M96.66-

◀ New   ▥ Revised   ~~deleted~~ Deleted

Fracture, traumatic *(Continued)*
  femur, femoral *(Continued)*
    head —*see* Fracture, femur, upper end,
        head
    intertrochanteric —*see* Fracture, femur,
        trochanteric
    intratrochanteric —*see* Fracture, femur,
        trochanteric
    lower end S72.40-
        condyle (displaced) S72.41-
            lateral (displaced) S72.42-
                nondisplaced S72.42-
            medial (displaced) S72.43-
                nondisplaced S72.43-
            nondisplaced S72.41-
        epiphysis (displaced) S72.44-
            nondisplaced S72.44-
        physeal S79.10-
            Salter-Harris
                Type I S79.11-
                Type II S79.12-
                Type III S79.13-
                Type IV S79.14-
            specified NEC S79.19-
        specified NEC S72.49-
        supracondylar (displaced) S72.45-
            with intracondylar extension
                (displaced) S72.46-
                nondisplaced S72.46-
            nondisplaced S72.45-
        torus S72.47-
    neck —*see* Fracture, femur, upper end, neck
    pertrochanteric —*see* Fracture, femur,
        trochanteric
    shaft (lower third) (middle third) (upper
        third) S72.30-
        comminuted (displaced) S72.35-
            nondisplaced S72.35-
        oblique (displaced) S72.33-
            nondisplaced S72.33-
        segmental (displaced) S72.36-
            nondisplaced S72.36-
        specified NEC S72.39-
        spiral (displaced) S72.34-
            nondisplaced S72.34-
        transverse (displaced) S72.32-
            nondisplaced S72.32-
    specified site NEC —*see* subcategory S72.8
    subcapital (displaced) S72.01-
    subtrochanteric (region) (section)
        (displaced) S72.2-
        nondisplaced S72.2-
    transcervical —*see* Fracture, femur, upper
        end, neck
    transtrochanteric —*see* Fracture, femur,
        trochanteric
    trochanteric S72.10-
        apophyseal (displaced) S72.13-
            nondisplaced S72.13-
        greater trochanter (displaced) S72.11-
            nondisplaced S72.11-
        intertrochanteric (displaced) S72.14-
            nondisplaced S72.14-
        lesser trochanter (displaced) S72.12-
            nondisplaced S72.12-
    upper end S72.00-
        apophyseal (displaced) S72.13-
            nondisplaced S72.13-
        cervicotrochanteric —*see* Fracture,
            femur, upper end, neck, base
        epiphysis (displaced) S72.02-
            nondisplaced S72.02-
        head S72.05-
            articular (displaced) S72.06-
                nondisplaced S72.06-
            specified NEC S72.09-
        intertrochanteric (displaced) S72.14-
            nondisplaced S72.14-
        intracapsular S72.01-
        midcervical (displaced) S72.03-
            nondisplaced S72.03-

Fracture, traumatic *(Continued)*
  femur, femoral *(Continued)*
    upper end *(Continued)*
        neck S72.00-
            base (displaced) S72.04-
                nondisplaced S72.04-
            specified NEC S72.09-
        pertrochanteric —*see* Fracture, femur,
            upper end, trochanteric
        physeal S79.00-
            Salter-Harris type I S79.01-
            specified NEC S79.09-
        subcapital (displaced) S72.01-
        subtrochanteric (displaced) S72.2-
            nondisplaced S72.2-
        transcervical —*see* Fracture, femur,
            upper end, midcervical
        trochanteric S72.10-
            greater (displaced) S72.11-
                nondisplaced S72.11-
            lesser (displaced) S72.12-
                nondisplaced S72.12-
  fibula (shaft) (styloid) S82.40-
    comminuted (displaced) S82.45-
        nondisplaced S82.45-
    following insertion of implant, prosthesis
        or plate M96.67-
    involving ankle or malleolus —*see*
        Fracture, fibula, lateral malleolus
    lateral malleolus (displaced)
        S82.6-
        nondisplaced S82.6-
    lower end
        physeal S89.30-
            Salter-Harris
                Type I S89.31-
                Type II S89.32-
                specified NEC S89.39-
            specified NEC S82.83-
            torus S82.82-
    oblique (displaced) S82.43-
        nondisplaced S82.43-
    segmental (displaced) S82.46-
        nondisplaced S82.46-
    specified NEC S82.49-
    spiral (displaced) S82.44-
        nondisplaced S82.44-
    transverse (displaced) S82.42-
        nondisplaced S82.42-
    upper end
        physeal S89.20-
            Salter-Harris
                Type I S89.21-
                Type II S89.22-
                specified NEC S89.29-
            specified NEC S82.83-
            torus S82.81-
  finger (except thumb) S62.60-
    distal phalanx (displaced) S62.63-
        nondisplaced S62.66-
    index S62.60-
        distal phalanx (displaced) S62.63-
            nondisplaced S62.66-
        medial phalanx (displaced) S62.62-
            nondisplaced S62.65-
        proximal phalanx (displaced) S62.61-
            nondisplaced S62.64-
    little S62.60-
        distal phalanx (displaced) S62.63-
            nondisplaced S62.66-
        medial phalanx (displaced) S62.62-
            nondisplaced S62.65-
        proximal phalanx (displaced) S62.61-
            nondisplaced S62.64-
    medial phalanx (displaced) S62.62-
        nondisplaced S62.65-
    middle S62.60-
        distal phalanx (displaced) S62.63-
            nondisplaced S62.66-
        medial phalanx (displaced) S62.62-
            nondisplaced S62.65-

Fracture, traumatic *(Continued)*
  finger *(Continued)*
    middle *(Continued)*
        proximal phalanx (displaced) S62.61-
            nondisplaced S62.64-
    proximal phalanx (displaced) S62.61-
        nondisplaced S62.64-
    ring S62.60-
        distal phalanx (displaced) S62.63-
            nondisplaced S62.66-
        medial phalanx (displaced) S62.62-
            nondisplaced S62.65-
        proximal phalanx (displaced) S62.61-
            nondisplaced S62.64-
    thumb —*see* Fracture, thumb
  following insertion (intraoperative)
        (postoperative) of orthopedic implant,
        joint prosthesis or bone plate M96.69
    femur M96.66-
    fibula M96.67-
    humerus M96.62-
    pelvis M96.65
    radius M96.63-
    specified bone NEC M96.69
    tibia M96.67-
    ulna M96.63-
  foot S92.90-
    astragalus —*see* Fracture, tarsal, talus
    calcaneus —*see* Fracture, tarsal, calcaneus
    cuboid —*see* Fracture, tarsal, cuboid
    cuneiform —*see* Fracture, tarsal, cuneiform
    metatarsal —*see* Fracture, metatarsal
    navicular —*see* Fracture, tarsal, navicular
    sesamoid S92.81- ◀
    specified NEC S92.81- ◀
    talus —*see* Fracture, tarsal, talus
    tarsal —*see* Fracture, tarsal
    toe —*see* Fracture, toe
  forearm S52.9-
    radius —*see* Fracture, radius
    ulna —*see* Fracture, ulna
  fossa (anterior) (middle) (posterior) S02.19
  frontal (bone) (skull) S02.0
    sinus S02.19
  glenoid (cavity) (scapula) —*see* Fracture,
        scapula, glenoid cavity
  greenstick —*see* Fracture, by site
  hallux —*see* Fracture, toe, great
  hand S62.9-
    carpal —*see* Fracture, carpal bone
    finger (except thumb) —*see* Fracture, finger
    metacarpal —*see* Fracture, metacarpal
    navicular (scaphoid) (hand) —*see* Fracture,
        carpal bone, navicular
    thumb —*see* Fracture, thumb
  healed or old
    with complications - code by Nature of the
        complication
  heel bone —*see* Fracture, tarsal, calcaneus
  Hill-Sachs S42.29-
  hip —*see* Fracture, femur, neck
  humerus S42.30-
    anatomical neck —*see* Fracture, humerus,
        upper end
    articular process —*see* Fracture, humerus,
        lower end
    capitellum —*see* Fracture, humerus, lower
        end, condyle, lateral
    distal end —*see* Fracture, humerus, lower
        end
    epiphysis
        lower —*see* Fracture, humerus, lower
            end, physeal
        upper —*see* Fracture, humerus, upper
            end, physeal
    external condyle —*see* Fracture, humerus,
        lower end, condyle, lateral
    following insertion of implant, prosthesis
        or plate M96.62-
    great tuberosity —*see* Fracture, humerus,
        upper end, greater tuberosity

Fracture, traumatic (Continued)
  humerus (Continued)
    intercondylar —see Fracture, humerus,
        lower end
    internal epicondyle —see Fracture,
        humerus, lower end, epicondyle,
        medial
    lesser tuberosity —see Fracture, humerus,
        upper end, lesser tuberosity
    lower end S42.40-
      condyle
        lateral (displaced) S42.45-
          nondisplaced S42.45-
        medial (displaced) S42.46-
          nondisplaced S42.46-
      epicondyle
        lateral (displaced) S42.43-
          nondisplaced S42.43-
        medial (displaced) S42.44-
          incarcerated S42.44-
          nondisplaced S42.44-
      physeal S49.10-
        Salter-Harris
          Type I S49.11-
          Type II S49.12-
          Type III S49.13-
          Type IV S49.14-
          specified NEC S49.19-
      specified NEC (displaced) S42.49-
        nondisplaced S42.49-
      supracondylar (simple) (displaced)
          S42.41-
        with intercondylar fracture —see
            Fracture, humerus, lower end ◄
        comminuted (displaced) S42.42-
          nondisplaced S42.42-
        nondisplaced S42.41-
      torus S42.48-
      transcondylar (displaced) S42.47-
        nondisplaced S42.47-
    proximal end —see Fracture, humerus,
        upper end
    shaft S42.30-
      comminuted (displaced) S42.35-
        nondisplaced S42.35-
      greenstick S42.31-
      oblique (displaced) S42.33-
        nondisplaced S42.33-
      segmental (displaced) S42.36-
        nondisplaced S42.36-
      specified NEC S42.39-
      spiral (displaced) S42.34-
        nondisplaced S42.34-
      transverse (displaced) S42.32-
        nondisplaced S42.32-
    supracondylar —see Fracture, humerus,
        lower end
    surgical neck —see Fracture, humerus,
        upper end, surgical neck
    trochlea —see Fracture, humerus, lower
        end, condyle, medial
    tuberosity —see Fracture, humerus, upper
        end
    upper end S42.20-
      anatomical neck —see Fracture, humerus,
          upper end, specified NEC
      articular head —see Fracture, humerus,
          upper end, specified NEC
      epiphysis —see Fracture, humerus,
          upper end, physeal
      greater tuberosity (displaced) S42.25-
        nondisplaced S42.25-
      lesser tuberosity (displaced) S42.26-
        nondisplaced S42.26-
      physeal S49.00-
        Salter-Harris
          Type I S49.01-
          Type II S49.02-
          Type III S49.03-
          Type IV S49.04-
          specified NEC S49.09-

Fracture, traumatic (Continued)
  humerus (Continued)
    upper end (Continued)
      specified NEC (displaced) S42.29-
        nondisplaced S42.29-
      surgical neck (displaced) S42.21-
        four-part S42.24-
        nondisplaced S42.21-
        three-part S42.23-
        two-part (displaced) S42.22-
          nondisplaced S42.22-
      torus S42.27-
      transepiphyseal —see Fracture, humerus,
          upper end, physeal
  hyoid bone S12.8
  ilium S32.30-
    with disruption of pelvic ring —see
        Disruption, pelvic ring
    avulsion (displaced) S32.31-
      nondisplaced S32.31-
    specified NEC S32.39-
  impaction, impacted - code as Fracture, by
      site
  innominate bone —see Fracture, ilium
  instep —see Fracture, foot
  ischium S32.60-
    with disruption of pelvic ring —see
        Disruption, pelvic ring
    avulsion (displaced) S32.61-
      nondisplaced S32.61-
    specified NEC S32.69-
  jaw (bone) (lower) —see Fracture, mandible
    upper —see Fracture, maxilla
  joint prosthesis —see Complications, joint
      prosthesis, mechanical, breakdown, by
      site
    periprosthetic —see Fracture, traumatic,
        periprosthetic ◄▥
  knee cap —see Fracture, patella
  larynx S12.8
  late effects —see Sequelae, fracture
  leg (lower) S82.9-
    ankle —see Fracture, ankle
    femur —see Fracture, femur
    fibula —see Fracture, fibula
    malleolus —see Fracture, ankle
    patella —see Fracture, patella
    specified site NEC S82.89-
    tibia —see Fracture, tibia
  lumbar spine —see Fracture, vertebra, lumbar
  lumbosacral spine S32.9
  Maisonneuve's (displaced) S82.86-
    nondisplaced S82.86-
  malar bone —see also Fracture, maxilla
      S02.400
    left side S02.40B ◄
    right side S02.40A ◄
  malleolus —see Fracture, ankle
  malunion —see Fracture, by site
  mandible (lower jawbone) S02.609
    alveolus S02.67- ◄▥
    angle (of jaw) S02.65- ◄▥
    body, unspecified S02.600-
      left side S02.602 ◄
      right side S02.601 ◄
    condylar process S02.61- ◄▥
    coronoid process S02.63- ◄▥
    ramus, unspecified S02.64- ◄▥
    specified site NEC S02.69
    subcondylar process S02.62- ◄▥
    symphysis S02.66
  manubrium (sterni) S22.21
    dissociation from sternum S22.23
  march —see Fracture, traumatic, stress, by site
  maxilla, maxillary (bone) (sinus) (superior)
      (upper jaw) S02.401
    alveolus S02.42
    inferior —see Fracture, mandible
    LeFort I S02.411
    LeFort II S02.412
    LeFort III S02.413

Fracture, traumatic (Continued)
  maxilla, maxillary (Continued)
    left side S02.40D ◄
    right side S02.40C ◄
  metacarpal S62.309
    base (displaced) S62.319
      nondisplaced S62.349
    fifth S62.30-
      base (displaced) S62.31-
        nondisplaced S62.34-
      neck (displaced) S62.33-
        nondisplaced S62.36-
      shaft (displaced) S62.32-
        nondisplaced S62.35-
      specified NEC S62.398
    first S62.20-
      base NEC (displaced) S62.23-
        nondisplaced S62.23-
      Bennett's —see Bennett's fracture
      neck (displaced) S62.25-
        nondisplaced S62.25-
      shaft (displaced) S62.24-
        nondisplaced S62.24-
      specified NEC S62.29-
    fourth S62.30-
      base (displaced) S62.31-
        nondisplaced S62.34-
      neck (displaced) S62.33-
        nondisplaced S62.36-
      shaft (displaced) S62.32-
        nondisplaced S62.35-
      specified NEC S62.39-
    neck (displaced) S62.33-
      nondisplaced S62.36-
    Rolando's —see Rolando's fracture
    second S62.30-
      base (displaced) S62.31-
        nondisplaced S62.34-
      neck (displaced) S62.33-
        nondisplaced S62.36-
      shaft (displaced) S62.32-
        nondisplaced S62.35-
      specified NEC S62.39-
    shaft (displaced) S62.32-
      nondisplaced S62.35-
    specified NEC S62.399
    third S62.30-
      base (displaced) S62.31-
        nondisplaced S62.34-
      neck (displaced) S62.33-
        nondisplaced S62.36-
      shaft (displaced) S62.32-
        nondisplaced S62.35-
      specified NEC S62.39-
  metastatic —see Fracture, pathological,
      due to, neoplastic disease —see also
      Neoplasm
  metatarsal bone S92.30-
    fifth (displaced) S92.35-
      nondisplaced S92.35-
    first (displaced) S92.31-
      nondisplaced S92.31-
    fourth (displaced) S92.34-
      nondisplaced S92.34-
    physeal S99.10- ◄
      Salter-Harris ◄
        Type I S99.11- ◄
        Type II S99.12- ◄
        Type III S99.13- ◄
        Type IV S99.14- ◄
        specified NEC S99.19- ◄
    second (displaced) S92.32-
      nondisplaced S92.32-
    third (displaced) S92.33-
      nondisplaced S92.33-
  Monteggia's —see Monteggia's
      fracture
  multiple
    hand (and wrist) NEC —see Fracture, by
        site
    ribs —see Fracture, rib, multiple

◄ New   ◄▥ Revised   ~~deleted~~ Deleted

Fracture, traumatic *(Continued)*
  nasal (bone (s)) S02.2
  navicular (scaphoid) (foot) —*see also* Fracture, tarsal, navicular
    hand —*see* Fracture, carpal, navicular
  neck S12.9
    cervical vertebra S12.9
      fifth (displaced) S12.400
        nondisplaced S12.401
        specified type NEC (displaced) S12.490
          nondisplaced S12.491
      first (displaced) S12.000
        burst (stable) S12.01
          unstable S12.02
        lateral mass (displaced) S12.040
          nondisplaced S12.041
        nondisplaced S12.001
        posterior arch (displaced) S12.030
          nondisplaced S12.031
        specified type NEC (displaced) S12.090
          nondisplaced S12.091
      fourth (displaced) S12.300
        nondisplaced S12.301
        specified type NEC (displaced) S12.390
          nondisplaced S12.391
      second (displaced) S12.100
        dens (anterior) (displaced) (type II) S12.110
          nondisplaced S12.112
          posterior S12.111
          specified type NEC (displaced) S12.120
            nondisplaced S12.121
        nondisplaced S12.101
        specified type NEC (displaced) S12.190
          nondisplaced S12.191
      seventh (displaced) S12.600
        nondisplaced S12.601
        specified type NEC (displaced) S12.690
          displaced S12.691
          nondisplaced S12.691 ◀
      sixth (displaced) S12.500
        nondisplaced S12.501
        specified type NEC (displaced) S12.590
          displaced S12.591
          nondisplaced S12.591 ◀
      third (displaced) S12.200
        nondisplaced S12.201
        specified type NEC (displaced) S12.290
          displaced S12.291
          nondisplaced S12.291 ◀
    hyoid bone S12.8
    larynx S12.8
    specified site NEC S12.8
    thyroid cartilage S12.8
    trachea S12.8
  neoplastic NEC —*see* Fracture, pathological, due to, neoplastic disease
  neural arch —*see* Fracture, vertebra
  newborn —*see* Birth, injury, fracture
  nontraumatic —*see* Fracture, pathological
  nonunion —*see* Nonunion, fracture
  nose, nasal (bone) (septum) S02.2
  occiput —*see* Fracture, skull, base, occiput
  odontoid process —*see* Fracture, neck, cervical vertebra, second
  olecranon (process) (ulna) —*see* Fracture, ulna, upper end, olecranon process
  orbit, orbital (bone) (region) S02.8- ◀▥
    floor (blow-out) S02.3- ◀▥
    roof S02.19
  os
    calcis —*see* Fracture, tarsal, calcaneus
    magnum —*see* Fracture, carpal, capitate
    pubis —*see* Fracture, pubis
  palate S02.8- ◀▥
  parietal bone (skull) S02.0

Fracture, traumatic *(Continued)*
  patella S82.00-
    comminuted (displaced) S82.04-
      nondisplaced S82.04-
    longitudinal (displaced) S82.02-
      nondisplaced S82.02-
    osteochondral (displaced) S82.01-
      nondisplaced S82.01-
    specified NEC S82.09-
    transverse (displaced) S82.03-
      nondisplaced S82.03-
  pedicle (of vertebral arch) —*see* Fracture, vertebra
  pelvis, pelvic (bone) S32.9
    acetabulum —*see* Fracture, acetabulum
    circle —*see* Disruption, pelvic ring
    following insertion of implant, prosthesis or plate M96.65
    ilium —*see* Fracture, ilium
    ischium —*see* Fracture, ischium
    multiple
      with disruption of pelvic ring (circle) — *see* Disruption, pelvic ring
      without disruption of pelvic ring (circle) S32.82
    pubis —*see* Fracture, pubis
    sacrum —*see* Fracture, sacrum
    specified site NEC S32.89
  periprosthetic, around internal prosthetic joint M97.9 ◀
    ankle M97.2- ◀
    elbow M97.4- ◀
    finger M97.8- ◀
    hip M97.0- ◀
    knee M97.1-- ◀
    shoulder M97.3- ◀
    specified joint NEC M97.8 ◀
    spine M97.8 ◀
    toe M97.8 ◀
    wrist M97.8 ◀
  phalanx
    foot —*see* Fracture, toe
    hand —*see* Fracture, finger
  pisiform —*see* Fracture, carpal, pisiform
  pond —*see* Fracture, skull
  prosthetic device, internal —*see* Complications, prosthetic device, by site, mechanical
  pubis S32.50-
    with disruption of pelvic ring —*see* Disruption, pelvic ring
    specified site NEC S32.59-
    superior rim S32.59-
  radius S52.9-
    distal end —*see* Fracture, radius, lower end
    following insertion of implant, prosthesis or plate M96.63-
    head —*see* Fracture, radius, upper end, head
    lower end S52.50-
      Barton's —*see* Barton's fracture
      Colles' —*see* Colles' fracture
      extraarticular NEC S52.55-
      intraarticular NEC S52.57-
      physeal S59.20-
        Salter-Harris
          Type I S59.21-
          Type II S59.22-
          Type III S59.23-
          Type IV S59.24-
        specified NEC S59.29-
      Smith's —*see* Smith's fracture
      specified NEC S52.59-
      styloid process (displaced) S52.51-
        nondisplaced S52.51-
      torus S52.52-
    neck —*see* Fracture, radius, upper end
    proximal end —*see* Fracture, radius, upper end

Fracture, traumatic *(Continued)*
  radius *(Continued)*
    shaft S52.30-
      bent bone S52.38-
      comminuted (displaced) S52.35-
        nondisplaced S52.35-
      Galeazzi's —*see* Galeazzi's fracture
      greenstick S52.31-
      oblique (displaced) S52.33-
        nondisplaced S52.33-
      segmental (displaced) S52.36-
        nondisplaced S52.36-
      specified NEC S52.39-
      spiral (displaced) S52.34-
        nondisplaced S52.34-
      transverse (displaced) S52.32-
        nondisplaced S52.32-
    upper end S52.10-
      head (displaced) S52.12-
        nondisplaced S52.12-
      neck (displaced) S52.13-
        nondisplaced S52.13-
      physeal S59.10-
        Salter-Harris
          Type I S59.11-
          Type II S59.12-
          Type III S59.13-
          Type IV S59.14-
        specified NEC S59.19-
      specified NEC S52.18-
      torus S52.11-
  ramus
    inferior or superior, pubis —*see* Fracture, pubis
    mandible —*see* Fracture, mandible
  restorative material (dental) K08.539
    with loss of material K08.531
    without loss of material K08.530
  rib S22.3-
    with flail chest —*see* Flail, chest
    multiple S22.4-
      with flail chest —*see* Flail, chest
  root, tooth —*see* Fracture, tooth
  sacrum S32.10-
    specified NEC S32.19
    Type
      1 S32.14
      2 S32.15
      3 S32.16
      4 S32.17
    Zone
      I S32.119
        displaced (minimally) S32.111
          severely S32.112
        nondisplaced S32.110
      II S32.129
        displaced (minimally) S32.121
          severely S32.122
        nondisplaced S32.120
      III S32.139
        displaced (minimally) S32.131
          severely S32.132
        nondisplaced S32.130
  scaphoid (hand) —*see also* Fracture, carpal, navicular
    foot —*see* Fracture, tarsal, navicular
  scapula S42.10-
    acromial process (displaced) S42.12-
      nondisplaced S42.12-
    body (displaced) S42.11-
      nondisplaced S42.11-
    coracoid process (displaced) S42.13-
      nondisplaced S42.13-
    glenoid cavity (displaced) S42.14-
      nondisplaced S42.14-
    neck (displaced) S42.15-
      nondisplaced S42.15-
    specified NEC S42.19-
  semilunar bone, wrist —*see* Fracture, carpal, lunate
  sequelae —*see* Sequelae, fracture

◀ New   ◀▥ Revised   ~~deleted~~ Deleted

255

Fracture, traumatic *(Continued)*
  sesamoid bone
    foot S92.81- ◀
    hand —*see* Fracture, carpal
    other —*see* Fracture, traumatic, by site ◀
    ~~other - code by site under Fracture~~
  shepherd's —*see* Fracture, tarsal, talus
  shoulder (girdle) S42.9-
    blade —*see* Fracture, scapula
  sinus (ethmoid) (frontal) S02.19
  skull S02.91
    base S02.10- ◀▥
      occiput S02.119
        condyle S02.113
          type I S02.110
            left side S02.11B ◀
            right side S02.11A ◀
          type II S02.111
            left side S02.11D ◀
            right side S02.11C ◀
          type III S02.112
            left side S02.11F ◀
            right side S02.11E ◀
          specified NEC S02.118 ◀
            left side S02.11H ◀
            right side S02.11G ◀
          ~~specified NEC S02.118~~
      specified NEC S02.19- ◀▥
    birth injury P13.0
    frontal bone S02.0
    parietal bone S02.0
    specified site NEC S02.8
    temporal bone S02.19
    vault S02.0
  Smith's —*see* Smith's fracture
  sphenoid (bone) (sinus) S02.19
  spine —*see* Fracture, vertebra
  spinous process —*see* Fracture, vertebra
  spontaneous (cause unknown) —*see* Fracture,
      pathological
  stave (of thumb) —*see* Fracture, metacarpal,
      first
  sternum S22.20
    with flail chest —*see* Flail, chest
    body S22.22
    manubrium S22.21
    xiphoid (process) S22.24
  stress M84.30
    ankle M84.37-
    carpus M84.34-
    clavicle M84.31-
    femoral neck M84.359
    femur M84.35-
    fibula M84.36-
    finger M84.34-
    hip M84.359
    humerus M84.32-
    ilium M84.350
    ischium M84.350
    metacarpus M84.34-
    metatarsus M84.37-
    neck —*see* Fracture, fatigue, vertebra
    pelvis M84.350
    radius M84.33-
    rib M84.38
    scapula M84.31-
    skull M84.38
    tarsus M84.37-
    tibia M84.36-
    toe M84.37-
    ulna M84.33-
    vertebra —*see* Fracture, fatigue, vertebra
  supracondylar, elbow —*see* Fracture,
      humerus, lower end, supracondylar
  symphysis pubis —*see* Fracture, pubis
  talus (ankle bone) —*see* Fracture, tarsal, talus
  tarsal bone (s) S92.20-
    astragalus —*see* Fracture, tarsal, talus
    calcaneus S92.00-
      anterior process (displaced) S92.02-
        nondisplaced S92.02-

Fracture, traumatic *(Continued)*
  tarsal bone *(Continued)*
    calcaneus *(Continued)*
      body (displaced) S92.01-
        nondisplaced S92.01-
      extraarticular NEC (displaced) S92.05-
        nondisplaced S92.05-
      intraarticular (displaced) S92.06-
        nondisplaced S92.06-
      physeal S99.00- ◀
        Salter-Harris ◀
          Type I S99.01- ◀
          Type II S99.02- ◀
          Type III S99.03- ◀
          Type IV S99.04- ◀
          specified NEC S99.09- ◀
      tuberosity (displaced) S92.04-
        avulsion (displaced) S92.03-
          nondisplaced S92.03-
        nondisplaced S92.04-
    cuboid (displaced) S92.21-
      nondisplaced S92.21-
    cuneiform
      intermediate (displaced) S92.23-
        nondisplaced S92.23-
      lateral (displaced) S92.22-
        nondisplaced S92.22-
      medial (displaced) S92.24-
        nondisplaced S92.24-
    navicular (displaced) S92.25-
      nondisplaced S92.25-
    scaphoid —*see* Fracture, tarsal, navicular
    talus S92.10-
      avulsion (displaced) S92.15-
        nondisplaced S92.15-
      body (displaced) S92.12-
        nondisplaced S92.12-
      dome (displaced) S92.14-
        nondisplaced S92.14-
      head (displaced) S92.12-
        nondisplaced S92.12-
      lateral process (displaced) S92.14-
        nondisplaced S92.14-
      neck (displaced) S92.11-
        nondisplaced S92.11-
      posterior process (displaced) S92.13-
        nondisplaced S92.13-
      specified NEC S92.19-
  temporal bone (styloid) S02.19
  thorax (bony) S22.9
    with flail chest —*see* Flail, chest
    rib S22.3-
      multiple S22.4-
        with flail chest —*see* Flail, chest
    sternum S22.20
      body S22.22
      manubrium S22.21
      xiphoid process S22.24
    vertebra (displaced) S22.009
      burst (stable) S22.001
        unstable S22.002
      eighth S22.069
        burst (stable) S22.061
          unstable S22.062
        specified type NEC S22.068
        wedge compression S22.060
      eleventh S22.089
        burst (stable) S22.081
          unstable S22.082
        specified type NEC S22.088
        wedge compression S22.080
      fifth S22.059
        burst (stable) S22.051
          unstable S22.052
        specified type NEC S22.058
        wedge compression S22.050
      first S22.019
        burst (stable) S22.011
          unstable S22.012
        specified type NEC S22.018
        wedge compression S22.010

Fracture, traumatic *(Continued)*
  thorax *(Continued)*
    vertebra *(Continued)*
      fourth S22.049
        burst (stable) S22.041
          unstable S22.042
        specified type NEC S22.048
        wedge compression S22.040
      ninth S22.079
        burst (stable) S22.071
          unstable S22.072
        specified type NEC S22.078
        wedge compression S22.070
      nondisplaced S22.001
      second S22.029
        burst (stable) S22.021
          unstable S22.022
        specified type NEC S22.028
        wedge compression S22.020
      seventh S22.069
        burst (stable) S22.061
          unstable S22.062
        specified type NEC S22.068
        wedge compression S22.060
      sixth S22.059
        burst (stable) S22.051
          unstable S22.052
        specified type NEC S22.058
        wedge compression S22.050
      specified type NEC S22.008
      tenth S22.079
        burst (stable) S22.071
          unstable S22.072
        specified type NEC S22.078
        wedge compression S22.070
      third S22.039
        burst (stable) S22.031
          unstable S22.032
        specified type NEC S22.038
        wedge compression S22.030
      twelfth S22.089
        burst (stable) S22.081
          unstable S22.082
        specified type NEC S22.088
        wedge compression S22.080
      wedge compression S22.000
  thumb S62.50-
    distal phalanx (displaced) S62.52-
      nondisplaced S62.52-
    proximal phalanx (displaced)
        S62.51-
      nondisplaced S62.51-
  thyroid cartilage S12.8
  tibia (shaft) S82.20-
    comminuted (displaced) S82.25-
      nondisplaced S82.25-
    condyles —*see* Fracture, tibia, upper end
    distal end —*see* Fracture, tibia, lower end
    epiphysis
      lower —*see* Fracture, tibia, lower end
      upper —*see* Fracture, tibia, upper end
    following insertion of implant, prosthesis
        or plate M96.67-
    head (involving knee joint) —*see* Fracture,
        tibia, upper end
    intercondyloid eminence —*see* Fracture,
        tibia, upper end
    involving ankle or malleolus —*see*
        Fracture, ankle, medial malleolus
    lower end S82.30-
      physeal S89.10-
        Salter-Harris
          Type I S89.11-
          Type II S89.12-
          Type III S89.13-
          Type IV S89.14-
          specified NEC S89.19-
      pilon (displaced) S82.87-
        nondisplaced S82.87-
      specified NEC S82.39-
      torus S82.31-

◀ New   ◀▥ Revised   ~~deleted~~ Deleted

Fracture, traumatic *(Continued)*
  tibia *(Continued)*
    malleolus —*see* Fracture, ankle, medial malleolus
    oblique (displaced) S82.23-
      nondisplaced S82.23-
    pilon —*see* Fracture, tibia, lower end, pilon
    proximal end —*see* Fracture, tibia, upper end
    segmental (displaced) S82.26-
      nondisplaced S82.26-
    specified NEC S82.29-
    spine —*see* Fracture, upper end, spine
    spiral (displaced) S82.24-
      nondisplaced S82.24-
    transverse (displaced) S82.22-
      nondisplaced S82.22-
    tuberosity —*see* Fracture, tibia, upper end, tuberosity
    upper end S82.10-
      bicondylar (displaced) S82.14-
        nondisplaced S82.14-
      lateral condyle (displaced) S82.12-
        nondisplaced S82.12-
      medial condyle (displaced) S82.13-
        nondisplaced S82.13-
      physeal S89.00-
        Salter-Harris
          Type I S89.01-
          Type II S89.02-
          Type III S89.03-
          Type IV S89.04-
        specified NEC S89.09-
      plateau —*see* Fracture, tibia, upper end, bicondylar
      specified NEC S82.19-
      spine (displaced) S82.11-
        nondisplaced S82.11-
      torus S82.16-
      tuberosity (displaced) S82.15-
        nondisplaced S82.15-
  toe S92.91-
    great (displaced) S92.40-
      distal phalanx (displaced) S92.42-
        nondisplaced S92.42-
      nondisplaced S92.40-
      proximal phalanx (displaced) S92.41-
        nondisplaced S92.41-
      specified NEC S92.49-
    lesser (displaced) S92.50-
      distal phalanx (displaced) S92.53-
        nondisplaced S92.53-
      medial phalanx (displaced) S92.52-
        nondisplaced S92.52-
      nondisplaced S92.50-
      proximal phalanx (displaced) S92.51-
        nondisplaced S92.51-
      specified NEC S92.59-
    physeal ◀
      phalanx S99.20- ◀
        Salter-Harris ◀
          Type I S99.21- ◀
          Type II S99.22- ◀
          Type III S99.23- ◀
          Type IV S99.24- ◀
        specified NEC S99.29- ◀
  tooth (root) S02.5
  trachea (cartilage) S12.8
  transverse process —*see* Fracture, vertebra
  trapezium or trapezoid bone —*see* Fracture, carpal
  trimalleolar —*see* Fracture, ankle, trimalleolar
  triquetrum (cuneiform of carpus) —*see* Fracture, carpal, triquetrum
  trochanter —*see* Fracture, femur, trochanteric
  tuberosity (external) —*see* Fracture, traumatic, by site ◀||||

Fracture, traumatic *(Continued)*
  ulna (shaft) S52.20-
    bent bone S52.28-
    coronoid process —*see* Fracture, ulna, upper end, coronoid process
    distal end —*see* Fracture, ulna, lower end
    following insertion of implant, prosthesis or plate M96.63-
    head S52.00-
    lower end S52.60-
      physeal S59.00-
        Salter-Harris
          Type I S59.01-
          Type II S59.02-
          Type III S59.03-
          Type IV S59.04-
        specified NEC S59.09-
      specified NEC S52.69-
      styloid process (displaced) S52.61-
        nondisplaced S52.61-
      torus S52.62-
    proximal end —*see* Fracture, ulna, upper end
    shaft S52.20-
      comminuted (displaced) S52.25-
        nondisplaced S52.25-
      greenstick S52.21-
      Monteggia's —*see* Monteggia's fracture
      oblique (displaced) S52.23-
        nondisplaced S52.23-
      segmental (displaced) S52.26-
        nondisplaced S52.26-
      specified NEC S52.29-
      spiral (displaced) S52.24-
        nondisplaced S52.24-
      transverse (displaced) S52.22-
        nondisplaced S52.22-
    upper end S52.00-
      coronoid process (displaced) S52.04-
        nondisplaced S52.04-
      olecranon process (displaced) S52.02-
        with intraarticular extension S52.03-
        nondisplaced S52.02-
          with intraarticular extension S52.03-
      specified NEC S52.09-
      torus S52.01-
  unciform —*see* Fracture, carpal, hamate
  vault of skull S02.0
  vertebra, vertebral (arch) (body) (column) (neural arch) (pedicle) (spinous process) (transverse process)
    atlas —*see* Fracture, neck, cervical vertebra, first
    axis —*see* Fracture, neck, cervical vertebra, second
    cervical (teardrop) S12.9
      axis —*see* Fracture, neck, cervical vertebra, second
      first (atlas) —*see* Fracture, neck, cervical vertebra, first
      second (axis) —*see* Fracture, neck, cervical vertebra, second
    chronic M84.48
    coccyx S32.2
    dorsal —*see* Fracture, thorax, vertebra
    lumbar S32.009
      burst (stable) S32.001
        unstable S32.002
      fifth S32.059
        burst (stable) S32.051
          unstable S32.052
        specified type NEC S32.058
        wedge compression S32.050
      first S32.019
        burst (stable) S32.011
          unstable S32.012
        specified type NEC S32.018
        wedge compression S32.010

Fracture, traumatic *(Continued)*
  vertebra, vertebral *(Continued)*
    lumbar *(Continued)*
      fourth S32.049
        burst (stable) S32.041
          unstable S32.042
        specified type NEC S32.048
        wedge compression S32.040
      second S32.029
        burst (stable) S32.021
          unstable S32.022
        specified type NEC S32.028
        wedge compression S32.020
      specified type NEC S32.008
      third S32.039
        burst (stable) S32.031
          unstable S32.032
        specified type NEC S32.038
        wedge compression S32.030
      wedge compression S32.000
    metastatic —*see* Collapse, vertebra, in, specified disease NEC —*see also* Neoplasm
    newborn (birth injury) P11.5
    sacrum S32.10
      specified NEC S32.19
      Type
        1 S32.14
        2 S32.15
        3 S32.16
        4 S32.17
      Zone
        I S32.119
          displaced (minimally) S32.111
            severely S32.112
          nondisplaced S32.110
        II S32.129
          displaced (minimally) S32.121
            severely S32.122
          nondisplaced S32.120
        III S32.139
          displaced (minimally) S32.131
            severely S32.132
          nondisplaced S32.130
    thoracic —*see* Fracture, thorax, vertebra
    vertex S02.0
    vomer (bone) S02.2
    wrist S62.10-
      carpal —*see* Fracture, carpal bone
      navicular (scaphoid) (hand) —*see* Fracture, carpal, navicular
    xiphisternum, xiphoid (process) S22.24
    zygoma S02.442
      left side S02.40F ◀
      right side S02.40E ◀
Fragile, fragility
  autosomal site Q95.5
  bone, congenital (with blue sclera) Q78.0
  capillary (hereditary) D69.8
  hair L67.8
  nails L60.3
  non-sex chromosome site Q95.5
  X chromosome Q99.2
Fragilitas
  crinium L67.8
  ossium (with blue sclerae) (hereditary) Q78.0
  unguium L60.3
    congenital Q84.6
Fragments, cataract (lens), following cataract surgery H59.02-
  retained foreign body —*see* Retained, foreign body fragments (type of)
Frailty (frail) R54
  mental R41.81
Frambesia, frambesial (tropica) —*see also* Yaws
  initial lesion or ulcer A66.0
  primary A66.0
Frambeside
  gummatous A66.4
  of early yaws A66.2

Frambesioma A66.1
Franceschetti-Klein (-Wildervanck) disease or
    syndrome Q75.4
Francis' disease —see Tularemia
Franklin disease C88.2
Frank's essential thrombocytopenia D69.3
Fraser's syndrome Q87.0
Freckle (s) L81.2
    malignant melanoma in —see Melanoma
    melanotic (Hutchinson's) —see Melanoma,
        in situ
    retinal D49.81
Frederickson's hyperlipoproteinemia, type
    I and V E78.3
    IIA E78.00 ◀▥
    IIB and III E78.2
    IV E78.1
Freeman Sheldon syndrome Q87.0
Freezing —see also Effect, adverse, cold T69.9
Freiberg's disease (infraction of metatarsal
    head or osteochondrosis) —see
        Osteochondrosis, juvenile, metatarsus
Frei's disease A55
Fremitus, friction, cardiac R01.2
Frenum, frenulum
    external os Q51.828
    tongue (shortening) (congenital) Q38.1
Frequency micturition (nocturnal) R35.0
    psychogenic F45.8
Frey's syndrome
    auriculotemporal G50.8
    hyperhidrosis L74.52
Friction
    burn —see Burn, by site
    fremitus, cardiac R01.2
    precordial R01.2
    sounds, chest R09.89
Friderichsen-Waterhouse syndrome or disease
    A39.1
Friedländer's B (bacillus) NEC —see also
    condition A49.8
Friedreich's
    ataxia G11.1
    combined systemic disease G11.1
    facial hemihypertrophy Q67.4
    sclerosis (cerebellum) (spinal cord)
        G11.1
Frigidity F52.22
Fröhlich's syndrome E23.6
Frontal —see also condition
    lobe syndrome F07.0
Frostbite (superficial) T33.90
    with
        partial thickness skin loss —see Frostbite
            (superficial), by site
        tissue necrosis T34.90
    abdominal wall T33.3
        with tissue necrosis T34.3
    ankle T33.81-
        with tissue necrosis T34.81-
    arm T33.4-
    with tissue necrosis T34.4-
        finger (s) —see Frostbite, finger
        hand —see Frostbite, hand
        wrist —see Frostbite, wrist
    ear T33.01-
        with tissue necrosis T34.01-
    face T33.09
        with tissue necrosis T34.09
    finger T33.53-
        with tissue necrosis T34.53-
    foot T33.82-
        with tissue necrosis T34.82-
    hand T33.52-
        with tissue necrosis T34.52-
    head T33.09
        with tissue necrosis T34.09
        ear —see Frostbite, ear
        nose —see Frostbite, nose
    hip (and thigh) T33.6-
        with tissue necrosis T34.6-

Frostbite (Continued)
    knee T33.7-
        with tissue necrosis T34.7-
    leg T33.9-
        with tissue necrosis T34.9-
        ankle —see Frostbite, ankle
        foot —see Frostbite, foot
        knee —see Frostbite, knee
        lower T33.7-
            with tissue necrosis T34.7-
        thigh —see Frostbite, hip
        toe —see Frostbite, toe
    limb
        lower T33.99
            with tissue necrosis T34.99
        upper —see Frostbite, arm
    neck T33.1
        with tissue necrosis T34.1
    nose T33.02
        with tissue necrosis T34.02
    pelvis T33.3
        with tissue necrosis T34.3
    specified site NEC T33.99
        with tissue necrosis T34.99
    thigh —see Frostbite, hip
    thorax T33.2
        with tissue necrosis T34.2
    toes T33.83-
        with tissue necrosis T34.83-
    trunk T33.99
        with tissue necrosis T34.99
    wrist T33.51-
        with tissue necrosis T34.51-
Frotteurism F65.81
Frozen —see also Effect, adverse, cold T69.9
    pelvis (female) N94.89
        male K66.8
    shoulder —see Capsulitis, adhesive
Fructokinase deficiency E74.11
Fructose 1,6 diphosphatase deficiency E74.19
Fructosemia (benign) (essential) E74.12
Fructosuria (benign) (essential) E74.11
Fuchs'
    black spot (myopic) H44.2-
    dystrophy (corneal endothelium) H18.51
    heterochromic cyclitis —see Cyclitis, Fuchs'
        heterochromic
Fucosidosis E77.1
Fugue R68.89
    dissociative F44.1
    hysterical (dissociative) F44.1
    postictal in epilepsy —see Epilepsy
    reaction to exceptional stress (transient)
        F43.0
Fulminant, fulminating —see condition
Functional —see also condition
    bleeding (uterus) N93.8
Functioning, intellectual, borderline R41.83
Fundus —see condition
Fungemia NOS B49
Fungus, fungous
    cerebral G93.89
    disease NOS B49
    infection —see Infection, fungus
Funiculitis (acute) (chronic) (endemic) N49.1
    gonococcal (acute) (chronic) A54.23
    tuberculous A18.15
Funnel
    breast (acquired) M95.4
        congenital Q67.6
        sequelae (late effect) of rickets E64.3
    chest (acquired) M95.4
        congenital Q67.6
        sequelae (late effect) of rickets E64.3
    pelvis (acquired) M95.5
        with disproportion (fetopelvic) O33.3
            causing obstructed labor O65.3
        congenital Q74.2
FUO (fever of unknown origin) R50.9
Furfur L21.0
    microsporon B36.0

Furrier's lung J67.8
Furrowed K14.5
    nail (s) (transverse) L60.4
        congenital Q84.6
    tongue K14.5
        congenital Q38.3
Furuncle L02.92
    abdominal wall L02.221
    ankle —see Furuncle, lower limb
    antecubital space —see Furuncle, upper limb
    anus K61.0
    arm —see Furuncle, upper limb
    auditory canal, external —see Abscess, ear,
        external
    auricle (ear) —see Abscess, ear, external
    axilla (region) L02.42-
    back (any part) L02.222
    breast N61.1 ◀▥
    buttock L02.32
    cheek (external) L02.02
    chest wall L02.223
    chin L02.02
    corpus cavernosum N48.21
    ear, external —see Abscess, ear, external
    external auditory canal —see Abscess, ear,
        external
    eyelid —see Abscess, eyelid
    face L02.02
    femoral (region) —see Furuncle, lower
        limb
    finger —see Furuncle, hand
    flank L02.221
    foot L02.62-
    forehead L02.02
    gluteal (region) L02.32
    groin L02.224
    hand L02.52-
    head L02.821
        face L02.02
    hip —see Furuncle, lower limb
    kidney —see Abscess, kidney
    knee —see Furuncle, lower limb
    labium (majus) (minus) N76.4
    lacrimal
        gland —see Dacryoadenitis
        passages (duct) (sac) —see Inflammation,
            lacrimal, passages, acute
    leg (any part) —see Furuncle, lower limb
    lower limb L02.42-
    malignant A22.0
    mouth K12.2
    navel L02.226
    neck L02.12
    nose J34.0
    orbit, orbital —see Abscess, orbit
    palmar (space) —see Furuncle, hand
    partes posteriores L02.32
    pectoral region L02.223
    penis N48.21
    perineum L02.225
    pinna —see Abscess, ear, external
    popliteal —see Furuncle, lower limb
    prepatellar —see Furuncle, lower limb
    scalp L02.821
    seminal vesicle N49.0
    shoulder —see Furuncle, upper limb
    specified site NEC L02.828
    submandibular K12.2
    temple (region) L02.02
    thumb —see Furuncle, hand
    toe —see Furuncle, foot
    trunk L02.229
        abdominal wall L02.221
        back L02.222
        chest wall L02.223
        groin L02.224
        perineum L02.225
        umbilicus L02.226
    umbilicus L02.226
    upper limb L02.42-
    vulva N76.4

◀ New   ▥ Revised   ~~deleted~~ Deleted

Furunculosis —*see* Furuncle
Fused —*see* Fusion, fused
Fusion, fused (congenital)
  astragaloscaphoid Q74.2
  atria Q21.1
  auditory canal Q16.1
  auricles, heart Q21.1
  binocular with defective stereopsis H53.32
  bone Q79.8
  cervical spine M43.22
  choanal Q30.0
  commissure, mitral valve Q23.2
  cusps, heart valve NEC Q24.8
    mitral Q23.2
    pulmonary Q22.1
    tricuspid Q22.4
  ear ossicles Q16.3
  fingers Q70.0-
  hymen Q52.3
  joint (acquired) —*see also* Ankylosis
    congenital Q74.8
  kidneys (incomplete) Q63.1
  labium (majus) (minus) Q52.5
  larynx and trachea Q34.8

Fusion, fused (*Continued*)
  limb, congenital Q74.8
    lower Q74.2
    upper Q74.0
  lobes, lung Q33.8
  lumbosacral (acquired) M43.27
    arthrodesis status Z98.1
    congenital Q76.49
    postprocedural status Z98.1
  nares, nose, nasal, nostril (s) Q30.0
  organ or site not listed —*see* Anomaly, by site
  ossicles Q79.9
    auditory Q16.3
  pulmonic cusps Q22.1
  ribs Q76.6
  sacroiliac (joint) (acquired) M43.28
    arthrodesis status Z98.1
    congenital Q74.2
    postprocedural status Z98.1
  spine (acquired) NEC M43.20
    arthrodesis status Z98.1
    cervical region M43.22
    cervicothoracic region M43.23
    congenital Q76.49

Fusion, fused (*Continued*)
  spine (*Continued*)
    lumbar M43.26
    lumbosacral region M43.27
    occipito-atlanto-axial region M43.21
    postoperative status Z98.1
    sacrococcygeal region M43.28
    thoracic region M43.24
    thoracolumbar region M43.25
  sublingual duct with submaxillary duct at
    opening in mouth Q38.4
  testes Q55.1
  toes Q70.2
  tooth, teeth K00.2
  trachea and esophagus Q39.8
  twins Q89.4
  vagina Q52.4
  ventricles, heart Q21.0
  vertebra (arch) —*see* Fusion, spine
  vulva Q52.5
Fusospirillosis (mouth) (tongue) (tonsil)
  A69.1
Fussy baby R68.12

G

Gain in weight (abnormal) (excessive) —*see also* Weight, gain
Gaisböck's disease (polycythemia hypertonica) D75.1
Gait abnormality R26.9
    ataxic R26.0
    falling R29.6
    hysterical (ataxic) (staggering) F44.4
    paralytic R26.1
    spastic R26.1
    specified type NEC R26.89
    staggering R26.0
    unsteadiness R26.81
    walking difficulty NEC R26.2
Galactocele (breast) N64.89
    puerperal, postpartum O92.79
Galactokinase deficiency E74.29
Galactophoritis N61.0 ◀▥▥
    gestational, puerperal, postpartum O91.2-
Galactorrhea O92.6
    not associated with childbirth N64.3
Galactosemia (classic) (congenital) E74.21
Galactosuria E74.29
Galacturia R82.0
    schistosomiasis (bilharziasis) B65.0
Galeazzi's fracture S52.37-
Galen's vein —*see* condition
Galeophobia F40.218
Gall duct —*see* condition
Gallbladder —*see also* condition
    acute K81.0
Gallop rhythm R00.8
Gallstone (colic) (cystic duct) (gallbladder) (impacted) (multiple) —*see also* Calculus, gallbladder
    with
        cholecystitis —*see* Calculus, gallbladder, with cholecystitis
        bile duct (common) (hepatic) —*see* Calculus, bile duct
    causing intestinal obstruction K56.3
    specified NEC K80.80
        with obstruction K80.81
Gambling Z72.6
    pathological (compulsive) F63.0
Gammopathy (of undetermined significance [MGUS]) D47.2
    associated with lymphoplasmacytic dyscrasia D47.2
    monoclonal D47.2
    polyclonal D89.0
Gamna's disease (siderotic splenomegaly) D73.1
Gamophobia F40.298
Gampsodactylia (congenital) Q66.7
Gamstorp's disease (adynamia episodica hereditaria) G72.3
Gandy-Nanta disease (siderotic splenomegaly) D73.1
Gang
    membership offenses Z72.810
Gangliocytoma D36.10
Ganglioglioma —*see* Neoplasm, uncertain behavior, by site
Ganglion (compound) (diffuse) (joint) (tendon (sheath)) M67.40
    ankle M67.47-
    foot M67.47-
    forearm M67.43-
    hand M67.44-
    lower leg M67.46-
    multiple sites M67.49
    of yaws (early) (late) A66.6
    pelvic region M67.45-
    periosteal —*see* Periostitis
    shoulder region M67.41-
    specified site NEC M67.48
    thigh region M67.45-
    tuberculous A18.09
    upper arm M67.42-
    wrist M67.43-

Ganglioneuroblastoma —*see* Neoplasm, nerve, malignant
Ganglioneuroma D36.10
    malignant —*see* Neoplasm, nerve, malignant
Ganglioneuromatosis D36.10
Ganglionitis
    fifth nerve —*see* Neuralgia, trigeminal
    gasserian (postherpetic) (postzoster) B02.21
    geniculate G51.1
        newborn (birth injury) P11.3
        postherpetic, postzoster B02.21
    herpes zoster B02.21
    postherpetic geniculate B02.21
Gangliosidosis E75.10
    GM1 E75.19
    GM2 E75.00
        other specified E75.09
        Sandhoff disease E75.01
        Tay-Sachs disease E75.02
    GM3 E75.19
    mucolipidosis IV E75.11
Gangosa A66.5
Gangrene, gangrenous (connective tissue) (dropsical) (dry) (moist) (skin) (ulcer) —*see also* Necrosis I96
    with diabetes (mellitus) —*see* Diabetes, gangrene
    abdomen (wall) I96
    alveolar M27.3
    appendix K35.80
        with
            perforation or rupture K35.2
            peritoneal abscess K35.3
            peritonitis NEC K35.3
                generalized (with perforation or rupture) K35.2
                localized (with perforation or rupture) K35.3
    arteriosclerotic (general) (senile) —*see* Arteriosclerosis, extremities, with, gangrene
    auricle I96
    Bacillus welchii A48.0
    bladder (infectious) —*see* Cystitis, specified type NEC
    bowel, cecum, or colon —*see* Gangrene, intestine
    Clostridium perfringens or welchii A48.0
    cornea H18.89-
    corpora cavernosa N48.29
        noninfective N48.89
    cutaneous, spreading I96
    decubital —*see* Ulcer, pressure, by site
    diabetic (any site) —*see* Diabetes, gangrene
    emphysematous —*see* Gangrene, gas
    epidemic —*see* Poisoning, food, noxious, plant
    epididymis (infectional) N45.1
    erysipelas —*see* Erysipelas
    extremity (lower) (upper) I96
    Fournier N49.3
        female N76.89
    fusospirochetal A69.0
    gallbladder —*see* Cholecystitis, acute
    gas (bacillus) A48.0
        following
            abortion —*see* Abortion by type complicated by infection
            ectopic or molar pregnancy O08.0
    glossitis K14.0
    hernia —*see* Hernia, by site, with gangrene
    intestine, intestinal (hemorrhagic) (massive) —*see also* Infarct, intestine K55.069 ◀▥▥
        with
            mesenteric embolism —*see also* Infarct, intestine K55.069 ◀▥▥
            obstruction —*see* Obstruction, intestine
    laryngitis J04.0
    limb (lower) (upper) I96

Gangrene, gangrenous (Continued)
    lung J85.0
        spirochetal A69.8
    lymphangitis I89.1
    Meleney's (synergistic) —*see* Ulcer, skin
    mesentery —*see also* Infarct, intestine K55.069 ◀▥▥
        with
            embolism —*see also* Infarct, intestine K55.069 ◀▥▥
            intestinal obstruction —*see* Obstruction, intestine
    mouth A69.0
    ovary —*see* Oophoritis
    pancreas —*see* Pancreatitis, acute ◀▥▥
    penis N48.29
        noninfective N48.89
    perineum I96
    pharynx —*see also* Pharyngitis
        Vincent's A69.1
    presenile I73.1
    progressive synergistic —*see* Ulcer, skin
    pulmonary J85.0
    pulpal (dental) K04.1
    quinsy J36
    Raynaud's (symmetric gangrene) I73.01
    retropharyngeal J39.2
    scrotum N49.3
        noninfective N50.89 ◀▥▥
    senile (atherosclerotic) —*see* Arteriosclerosis, extremities, with, gangrene
    spermatic cord N49.1
        noninfective N50.89 ◀▥▥
    spine I96
    spirochetal NEC A69.8
    spreading cutaneous I96
    stomatitis A69.0
    symmetrical I73.01
    testis (infectional) N45.2
        noninfective N44.8
    throat —*see also* Pharyngitis
        diphtheritic A36.0
        Vincent's A69.1
    thyroid (gland) E07.89
    tooth (pulp) K04.1
    tuberculous NEC —*see* Tuberculosis
    tunica vaginalis N49.1
        noninfective N50.89 ◀▥▥
    umbilicus I96
    uterus —*see* Endometritis
    uvulitis K12.2
    vas deferens N49.1
        noninfective N50.89 ◀▥▥
    vulva N76.89
Ganister disease J62.8
Ganser's syndrome (hysterical) F44.89
Gardner-Diamond syndrome (autoerythrocyte sensitization) D69.2
Gargoylism E76.01
Garré's disease, osteitis (sclerosing), osteomyelitis —*see* Osteomyelitis, specified type NEC
Garrod's pad, knuckle M72.1
Gartner's duct
    cyst Q52.4
    persistent Q50.6
Gas R14.3
    asphyxiation, inhalation, poisoning, suffocation NEC —*see* Table of Drugs and Chemicals
    excessive R14.0
    gangrene A48.0
        following
            abortion —*see* Abortion by type complicated by infection
            ectopic or molar pregnancy O08.0
    on stomach R14.0
    pains R14.1
Gastralgia —*see also* Pain, abdominal
Gastrectasis K31.0
    psychogenic F45.8
Gastric —*see* condition

◀ New   ◀▥▥ Revised   ~~deleted~~ Deleted

Gastrinoma
  malignant
    pancreas C25.4
    specified site NEC —*see* Neoplasm,
      malignant, by site
    unspecified site C25.4
  specified site —*see* Neoplasm, uncertain
    behavior
  unspecified site D37.9
Gastritis (simple) K29.70
  with bleeding K29.71
  acute (erosive) K29.00
    with bleeding K29.01
  alcoholic K29.20
    with bleeding K29.21
  allergic K29.60
    with bleeding K29.61
  atrophic (chronic) K29.40
    with bleeding K29.41
  chronic (antral) (fundal) K29.50
    with bleeding K29.51
    atrophic K29.40
      with bleeding K29.41
    superficial K29.30
      with bleeding K29.31
  dietary counseling and surveillance Z71.3
  due to diet deficiency E63.9
  eosinophilic K52.81
  giant hypertrophic K29.60
    with bleeding K29.61
  granulomatous K29.60
    with bleeding K29.61
  hypertrophic (mucosa) K29.60
    with bleeding K29.61
  nervous F54
  spastic K29.60
    with bleeding K29.61
  specified NEC K29.60
    with bleeding K29.61
  superficial chronic K29.30
    with bleeding K29.31
  tuberculous A18.83
  viral NEC A08.4
Gastrocarcinoma —*see* Neoplasm, malignant,
  stomach
Gastrocolic —*see* condition
Gastrodisciasis, gastrodiscoidiasis B66.8
Gastroduodenitis K29.90
  with bleeding K29.91
  virus, viral A08.4
    specified type NEC A08.39
Gastrodynia —*see* Pain, abdominal
Gastroenteritis (acute) (chronic) (noninfectious)
    (*see also* Enteritis) K52.9
  allergic K52.29 ◀▥
  with ◀
    eosinophilic gastritis or gastroenteritis
      K52.81 ◀
    food protein-induced enterocolitis
      syndrome K52.21 ◀
    food protein-induced enteropathy
      K52.22 ◀
  dietetic —*see also* Gastroenteritis, allergic
    K52.29 ◀▥
  drug-induced K52.1
  due to
    Cryptosporidium A07.2
    drugs K52.1
    food poisoning —*see* Intoxication,
      foodborne
    radiation K52.0
  eosinophilic K52.81
  epidemic (infectious) A09
  food hypersensitivity —*see also*
    Gastroenteritis, allergic K52.29 ◀▥
  infectious —*see* Enteritis, infectious
  influenzal —*see* Influenza, with
    gastroenteritis
  noninfectious K52.9
    specified NEC K52.89
  rotaviral A08.0

Gastroenteritis *(Continued)*
  Salmonella A02.0
  toxic K52.1
  viral NEC A08.4
    acute infectious A08.39
      type Norwalk A08.11
    infantile (acute) A08.39
    Norwalk agent A08.11
    rotaviral A08.0
    severe of infants A08.39
    specified type NEC A08.39
Gastroenteropathy —*see also* Gastroenteritis
    K52.9
  acute, due to Norovirus A08.11
  acute, due to Norwalk agent A08.11
  infectious A09
Gastroenteroptosis K63.4
Gastroesophageal laceration-hemorrhage
    syndrome K22.6
Gastrointestinal —*see* condition
Gastrojejunal —*see* condition
Gastrojejunitis —*see also* Enteritis K52.9
Gastrojejunocolic —*see* condition
Gastroliths K31.89
Gastromalacia K31.89
Gastroparalysis K31.84
  diabetic —*see* Diabetes, gastroparalysis
Gastroparesis K31.84
  diabetic —*see* Diabetes, by type, with
    gastroparesis
Gastropathy K31.9
  congestive portal K31.89
  erythematous K29.70
  exudative K90.89
  portal hypertensive K31.89
Gastroptosis K31.89
Gastrorrhagia K92.2
  psychogenic F45.8
Gastroschisis (congenital) Q79.3
Gastrospasm (neurogenic) (reflex) K31.89
  neurotic F45.8
  psychogenic F45.8
Gastrostaxis —*see* Gastritis, with bleeding
Gastrostenosis K31.89
Gastrostomy
  attention to Z43.1
  status Z93.1
Gastrosuccorrhea (continuous) (intermittent)
    K31.89
  neurotic F45.8
  psychogenic F45.8
Gatophobia F40.218
Gaucher's disease or splenomegaly (adult)
    (infantile) E75.22
Gee (-Herter)(-Thaysen) disease (nontropical
    sprue) K90.0
Gélineau's syndrome G47.419
  with cataplexy G47.411
Gemination, tooth, teeth K00.2
Gemistocytoma
  specified site —*see* Neoplasm, malignant, by
    site
  unspecified site C71.9
General, generalized —*see* condition
Genetic
  carrier (status)
    cystic fibrosis Z14.1
    hemophilia A (asymptomatic) Z14.01
      symptomatic Z14.02
    specified NEC Z14.8
  susceptibility to disease NEC Z15.89
    malignant neoplasm Z15.09
      breast Z15.01
      endometrium Z15.04
      ovary Z15.02
      prostate Z15.03
      specified NEC Z15.09
    multiple endocrine neoplasia Z15.81
Genital —*see* condition
Genito-anorectal syndrome A55
Genitourinary system —*see* condition

Genu
  congenital Q74.1
  extrorsum (acquired) —*see also* Deformity,
    varus, knee
    congenital Q74.1
    sequelae (late effect) of rickets E64.3
  introrsum (acquired) —*see also* Deformity,
    valgus, knee
    congenital Q74.1
    sequelae (late effect) of rickets E64.3
  rachitic (old) E64.3
  recurvatum (acquired) —*see also* Deformity,
    limb, specified type NEC, lower leg
    congenital Q68.2
    sequelae (late effect) of rickets E64.3
  valgum (acquired) (knock-knee) M21.06-
    congenital Q74.1
    sequelae (late effect) of rickets E64.3
  varum (acquired) (bowleg) M21.16-
    congenital Q74.1
    sequelae (late effect) of rickets E64.3
Geographic tongue K14.1
Geophagia —*see* Pica
Geotrichosis B48.3
  stomatitis B48.3
Gephyrophobia F40.242
Gerbode defect Q21.0
GERD (gastroesophageal reflux disease) K21.9
Gerhardt's
  disease (erythromelalgia) I73.81
  syndrome (vocal cord paralysis)
    J38.00
    bilateral J38.02
    unilateral J38.01
German measles —*see also* Rubella
  exposure to Z20.4
Germinoblastoma (diffuse) C85.9-
  follicular C82.9-
Germinoma —*see* Neoplasm, malignant, by site
Gerontoxon —*see* Degeneration, cornea, senile
Gerstmann-Sträussler-Scheinker syndrome
    (GSS) A81.82
Gerstmann's syndrome R48.8
  developmental F81.2
Gestation (period) —*see also* Pregnancy
  ectopic —*see* Pregnancy, by site
  multiple O30.9-
    greater than quadruplets —*see* Pregnancy,
      multiple (gestation), specified NEC
    specified NEC —*see* Pregnancy, multiple
      (gestation), specified NEC
Gestational
  mammary abscess O91.11-
  purulent mastitis O91.11-
  subareolar abscess O91.11-
Ghon tubercle, primary infection A15.7
Ghost
  teeth K00.4
  vessels (cornea) H16.41-
Ghoul hand A66.3
Gianotti-Crosti disease L44.4
Giant
  cell
    epulis K06.8
    peripheral granuloma K06.8
  esophagus, congenital Q39.5
  kidney, congenital Q63.3
  urticaria T78.3
    hereditary D84.1
Giardiasis A07.1
Gibert's disease or pityriasis L42
Giddiness R42
  hysterical F44.89
  psychogenic F45.8
Gierke's disease (glycogenosis I) E74.01
Gigantism (cerebral) (hypophyseal) (pituitary)
    E22.0
  constitutional E34.4
Gilbert's disease or syndrome E80.4
Gilchrist's disease B40.9
Gilford-Hutchinson disease E34.8

Gilles de la Tourette's disease or syndrome
(motor-verbal tic) F95.2
Gingivitis K05.10
acute (catarrhal) K05.00
necrotizing A69.1
nonplaque induced K05.01
plaque induced K05.00
chronic (desquamative) (hyperplastic)
(simple marginal) (pregnancy
associated) (ulcerative) K05.10 ◀▥
nonplaque induced K05.11
plaque induced K05.10
expulsiva —see Periodontitis
necrotizing ulcerative (acute) A69.1
pellagrous E52
acute necrotizing A69.1
Vincent's A69.1
Gingivoglossitis K14.0
Gingivopericementitis —see Periodontitis
Gingivosis —see Gingivitis, chronic
Gingivostomatitis K05.10
herpesviral B00.2
necrotizing ulcerative (acute) A69.1
Gland, glandular —see condition
Glanders A24.0
Glanzmann (-Naegeli) disease or
thrombasthenia D69.1
Glasgow coma scale
total score
3-8 R40.243
9-12 R40.242
13-15 R40.241
Glass-blower's disease (cataract) —see
Cataract, specified NEC
Glaucoma H40.9
with
increased episcleral venous pressure
H40.81-
pseudoexfoliation of lens —see Glaucoma,
open angle, primary, capsular
absolute H44.51-
angle-closure (primary) H40.20-
acute (attack) (crisis) H40.21-
chronic H40.22-
intermittent H40.23-
residual stage H40.24-
borderline H40.00-
capsular (with pseudoexfoliation of lens) —
see Glaucoma, open angle, primary,
capsular
childhood Q15.0
closed angle —see Glaucoma, angle-closure
congenital Q15.0
corticosteroid-induced —see Glaucoma,
secondary, drugs
hypersecretion H40.82-
in (due to)
amyloidosis E85.4 [H42]
aniridia Q13.1 [H42]
concussion of globe —see Glaucoma,
secondary, trauma
dislocation of lens —see Glaucoma,
secondary
disorder of lens NEC —see Glaucoma,
secondary
drugs —see Glaucoma, secondary, drugs
endocrine disease NOS E34.9 [H42]
eye
inflammation —see Glaucoma,
secondary, inflammation
trauma —see Glaucoma, secondary,
trauma
hypermature cataract —see Glaucoma,
secondary
iridocyclitis —see Glaucoma, secondary,
inflammation
lens disorder —see Glaucoma, secondary,
Lowe's syndrome E72.03 [H42]
metabolic disease NOS E88.9 [H42]
ocular disorders NEC —see Glaucoma,
secondary

Glaucoma (Continued)
in (due to) (Continued)
onchocerciasis B73.02
pupillary block —see Glaucoma, secondary
retinal vein occlusion —see Glaucoma,
secondary
Rieger's anomaly Q13.81 [H42]
rubeosis of iris —see Glaucoma, secondary
tumor of globe —see Glaucoma, secondary
infantile Q15.0
low tension —see Glaucoma, open angle,
primary, low-tension
malignant H40.83-
narrow angle —see Glaucoma, angle-closure
newborn Q15.0
noncongestive (chronic) —see Glaucoma,
open angle
nonobstructive —see Glaucoma, open angle
obstructive —see also Glaucoma,
angle-closure
due to lens changes —see Glaucoma,
secondary
open angle H40.10-
primary H40.11-
capsular (with pseudoexfoliation of lens)
H40.14-
low-tension H40.12-
pigmentary H40.13-
residual stage H40.15-
phacolytic —see Glaucoma, secondary
pigmentary —see Glaucoma, open angle,
primary, pigmentary
postinfectious —see Glaucoma, secondary,
inflammation
secondary (to) H40.5-
drugs H40.6-
inflammation H40.4-
trauma H40.3-
simple (chronic) H40.11- ◀▥
simplex H40.11- ◀▥
specified type NEC H40.89
suspect H40.00-
syphilitic A52.71
traumatic —see also Glaucoma, secondary,
trauma
newborn (birth injury) P15.3
tuberculous A18.59
Glaucomatous flecks (subcapsular) —see
Cataract, complicated
Glazed tongue K14.4
Gleet (gonococcal) A54.01
Glénard's disease K63.4
Glioblastoma (multiforme)
with sarcomatous component
specified site —see Neoplasm, malignant,
by site
unspecified site C71.9
giant cell
specified site —see Neoplasm, malignant,
by site
unspecified site C71.9
specified site —see Neoplasm, malignant, by
site
unspecified site C71.9
Glioma (malignant)
astrocytic
specified site —see Neoplasm, malignant,
by site
unspecified site C71.9
mixed
specified site —see Neoplasm, malignant,
by site
unspecified site C71.9
nose Q30.8
specified site NEC —see Neoplasm,
malignant, by site
subependymal D43.2
specified site —see Neoplasm, uncertain
behavior, by site
unspecified site D43.2
unspecified site C71.9

Gliomatosis cerebri C71.0
Glioneuroma —see Neoplasm, uncertain
behavior, by site
Gliosarcoma
specified site —see Neoplasm, malignant, by
site
unspecified site C71.9
Gliosis (cerebral) G93.89
spinal G95.89
Glisson's disease —see Rickets
Globinuria R82.3
Globus (hystericus) F45.8
Glomangioma D18.00
intra-abdominal D18.03
intracranial D18.02
skin D18.01
specified site NEC D18.09
Glomangiomyoma D18.00
intra-abdominal D18.03
intracranial D18.02
skin D18.01
specified site NEC D18.09
Glomangiosarcoma —see Neoplasm, connective
tissue, malignant
Glomerular
disease in syphilis A52.75
nephritis —see Glomerulonephritis
Glomerulitis —see Glomerulonephritis
Glomerulonephritis —see also Nephritis N05.9
with
edema —see Nephrosis
minimal change N05.0
minor glomerular abnormality N05.0
acute N00.9
chronic N03.9
crescentic (diffuse) NEC —see also N00-N07
with fourth character .7 N05.7
dense deposit —see also N00-N07 with fourth
character .6 N05.6
diffuse
crescentic —see also N00-N07 with fourth
character .7 N05.7
endocapillary proliferative —see also
N00N07 with fourth character .4
N05.4
membranous —see also N00-N07 with
fourth character .2 N05.2
mesangial proliferative —see also N00-N07
with fourth character .3 N05.3
mesangiocapillary —see also N00-N07 with
fourth character .5 N05.5
sclerosing N05.8
endocapillary proliferative (diffuse) NEC —
see also N00-N07 with fourth character
.4 N05.4
extracapillary NEC —see also N00-N07 with
fourth character .7 N05.7
focal (and segmental) —see also N00-N07 with
fourth character .1 N05.1
hypocomplementemic —see
Glomerulonephritis,
membranoproliferative
IgA —see Nephropathy, IgA
immune complex (circulating) NEC
N05.8
in (due to)
amyloidosis E85.4 [N08]
bilharziasis B65.9 [N08]
cryoglobulinemia D89.1 [N08]
defibrination syndrome D65 [N08]
diabetes mellitus —see Diabetes,
glomerulosclerosis
disseminated intravascular coagulation
D65 [N08]
Fabry (-Anderson) disease E75.21 [N08]
Goodpasture's syndrome M31.0
hemolytic-uremic syndrome D59.3
Henoch (-Schönlein) purpura D69.0
[N08]
lecithin cholesterol acyltransferase
deficiency E78.6 [N08]

◀ New   ◀▥ Revised   ~~deleted~~ Deleted

Glomerulonephritis (Continued)
in (Continued)
microscopic polyangiitis M31.7 [N08]
multiple myeloma C90.0- [N08]
Plasmodium malariae B52.0
schistosomiasis B65.9 [N08]
sepsis A41.9- [N08]
streptococcal A40- [N08]
sickle-cell disorders D57.- [N08]
strongyloidiasis B78.9 [N08]
subacute bacterial endocarditis I33.0
[N08]
syphilis (late) congenital A50.59 [N08]
systemic lupus erythematosus M32.14
thrombotic thrombocytopenic purpura
M31.1 [N08]
typhoid fever A01.09
Waldenström macroglobulinemia C88.0
[N08]
Wegener's granulomatosis M31.31
latent or quiescent N03.9
lobular, lobulonodular —see
Glomerulonephritis,
membranoproliferative
membranoproliferative (diffuse) (type 1
or 3) —see also N00-N07 with fourth
character .5 N05.5
dense deposit (type 2) NEC —see also
N00-N07 with fourth character .6
N05.6
membranous (diffuse) NEC —see also
N00-N07 with fourth character .2 N05.2
mesangial
IgA/IgG —see Nephropathy, IgA
proliferative (diffuse) NEC —see also
N00-N07 with fourth character .3
N05.3
mesangiocapillary (diffuse) NEC —see also
N00-N07 with fourth character .5 N05.5
necrotic, necrotizing NEC —see also N00-N07
with fourth character .8 N05.8
nodular —see Glomerulonephritis,
membranoproliferative
poststreptococcal NEC N05.9
acute N00.9
chronic N03.9
rapidly progressive N01.9
proliferative NEC —see also N00-N07 with
fourth character .8 N05.8
diffuse (lupus) M32.14
rapidly progressive N01.9
sclerosing, diffuse N05.8
specified pathology NEC —see also N00-N07
with fourth character .8 N05.8
subacute N01.9
Glomerulopathy —see Glomerulonephritis
Glomerulosclerosis —see also Sclerosis, renal
intercapillary (nodular) (with diabetes) —see
Diabetes, glomerulosclerosis
intracapillary —see Diabetes,
glomerulosclerosis
Glossagra K14.6
Glossalgia K14.6
Glossitis (chronic superficial) (gangrenous)
(Moeller's) K14.0
areata exfoliativa K14.1
atrophic K14.4
benign migratory K14.1
cortical superficial, sclerotic K14.0
Hunter's D51.0
interstitial, sclerous K14.0
median rhomboid K14.2
pellagrous E52
superficial, chronic K14.0
Glossocele K14.8
Glossodynia K14.6
exfoliativa K14.4
Glossoncus K14.8
Glossopathy K14.9
Glossophytia K14.3
Glossoplegia K14.8

Glossoptosis K14.8
Glossopyrosis K14.6
Glossotrichia K14.3
Glossy skin L90.8
Glottis —see condition
Glottitis —see also Laryngitis J04.0
Glucagonoma
pancreas
benign D13.7
malignant C25.4
uncertain behavior D37.8
specified site NEC
benign —see Neoplasm, benign, by site
malignant —see Neoplasm, malignant, by
site
uncertain behavior —see Neoplasm,
uncertain behavior, by site
unspecified site
benign D13.7
malignant C25.4
uncertain behavior D37.8
Glucoglycinuria E72.51
Glucose-galactose malabsorption E74.39
Glue
ear —see Otitis, media, nonsuppurative,
chronic, mucoid
sniffing (airplane) —see Abuse, drug,
inhalant
dependence —see Dependence, drug,
inhalant
Glutaric aciduria E72.3
Glycinemia E72.51
Glycinuria (renal) (with ketosis) E72.09
Glycogen
infiltration —see Disease, glycogen storage
storage disease —see Disease, glycogen
storage
Glycogenosis (diffuse) (generalized) —see also
Disease, glycogen storage
cardiac E74.02 [I43]
diabetic, secondary —see Diabetes,
glycogenosis, secondary
pulmonary interstitial J84.842
Glycopenia E16.2
Glycosuria R81
renal E74.8
Gnathostoma spinigerum (infection)
(infestation), **gnathostomiasis** (wandering
swelling) B83.1
Goiter (plunging) (substernal) E04.9
with
hyperthyroidism (recurrent) —see
Hyperthyroidism, with, goiter
thyrotoxicosis —see Hyperthyroidism,
with, goiter
adenomatous —see Goiter, nodular
cancerous C73
congenital (nontoxic) E03.0
diffuse E03.0
parenchymatous E03.0
transitory, with normal functioning
P72.0
cystic E04.2
due to iodine-deficiency E01.1
due to
enzyme defect in synthesis of thyroid
hormone E07.1
iodine-deficiency (endemic) E01.2
dyshormonogenetic (familial) E07.1
endemic (iodine-deficiency) E01.2
diffuse E01.0
multinodular E01.1
exophthalmic —see Hyperthyroidism, with,
goiter
iodine-deficiency (endemic) E01.2
diffuse E01.0
multinodular E01.1
nodular E01.1
lingual Q89.2
lymphadenoid E06.3
malignant C73

Goiter (Continued)
multinodular (cystic) (nontoxic) E04.2
toxic or with hyperthyroidism E05.20
with thyroid storm E05.21
neonatal NEC P72.0
nodular (nontoxic) (due to) E04.9
with
hyperthyroidism E05.20
with thyroid storm E05.21
thyrotoxicosis E05.20
with thyroid storm E05.21
endemic E01.1
iodine-deficiency E01.1
sporadic E04.9
toxic E05.20
with thyroid storm E05.21
nontoxic E04.9
diffuse (colloid) E04.0
multinodular E04.2
simple E04.0
specified NEC E04.8
uninodular E04.1
simple E04.0
toxic —see Hyperthyroidism, with, goiter
uninodular (nontoxic) E04.1
toxic or with hyperthyroidism E05.10
with thyroid storm E05.11
Goiter-deafness syndrome E07.1
Goldberg syndrome Q89.8
Goldberg-Maxwell syndrome E34.51
Goldblatt's hypertension or kidney I70.1
Goldenhar (-Gorlin) syndrome Q87.0
Goldflam-Erb disease or syndrome G70.00
with exacerbation (acute) G70.01
in crisis G70.01
Goldscheider's disease Q81.8
Goldstein's disease (familial hemorrhagic
telangiectasia) I78.0
Golfer's elbow —see Epicondylitis, medial
Gonadoblastoma
specified site —see Neoplasm, uncertain
behavior, by site
unspecified site
female D39.10
male D40.10
Gonecystitis —see Vesiculitis
Gongylonemiasis B83.8
Goniosynechiae —see Adhesions, iris,
goniosynechiae
Gonococcemia A54.86
Gonococcus, gonococcal (disease) (infection)
—see also condition A54.9
anus A54.6
bursa, bursitis A54.49
conjunctiva, conjunctivitis (neonatorum)
A54.31
endocardium A54.83
eye A54.30
conjunctivitis A54.31
iridocyclitis A54.32
keratitis A54.33
newborn A54.31
other specified A54.39
fallopian tubes (acute) (chronic) A54.24
genitourinary (organ) (system) (tract) (acute)
A54.00
lower A54.00
with abscess (accessory gland)
(periurethral) A54.1
upper —see also condition A54.29
heart A54.83
iridocyclitis A54.32
joint A54.42
lymphatic (gland) (node) A54.89
meninges, meningitis A54.81
musculoskeletal A54.40
arthritis A54.42
osteomyelitis A54.43
other specified A54.49
spondylopathy A54.41
pelviperitonitis A54.24
pelvis (acute) (chronic) A54.24

Gonococcus, gonococcal *(Continued)*
pharynx A54.5
proctitis A54.6
pyosalpinx (acute) (chronic) A54.24
rectum A54.6
skin A54.89
specified site NEC A54.89
tendon sheath A54.49
throat A54.5
urethra (acute) (chronic) A54.01
with abscess (accessory gland)
(periurethral) A54.1
vulva (acute) (chronic) A54.02
Gonocytoma
specified site —*see* Neoplasm, uncertain
behavior, by site
unspecified site
female D39.10
male D40.10
Gonorrhea (acute) (chronic) A54.9
Bartholin's gland (acute) (chronic) (purulent)
A54.02
with abscess (accessory gland)
(periurethral) A54.1
bladder A54.01
cervix A54.03
conjunctiva, conjunctivitis (neonatorum)
A54.31
contact Z20.2
Cowper's gland (with abscess) A54.1
exposure to Z20.2
fallopian tube (acute) (chronic) A54.24
kidney (acute) (chronic) A54.21
lower genitourinary tract A54.00
with abscess (accessory gland)
(periurethral) A54.1
ovary (acute) (chronic) A54.24
pelvis (acute) (chronic) A54.24
female pelvic inflammatory disease A54.24
penis A54.09
prostate (acute) (chronic) A54.22
seminal vesicle (acute) (chronic) A54.23
specified site not listed —*see also* Gonococcus
A54.89
spermatic cord (acute) (chronic) A54.23
urethra A54.01
with abscess (accessory gland)
(periurethral) A54.1
vagina A54.02
vas deferens (acute) (chronic) A54.23
vulva A54.02
Goodall's disease A08.19
Goodpasture's syndrome M31.0
Gopalan's syndrome (burning feet) E53.0
Gorlin-Chaudry-Moss syndrome Q87.0
Gottron's papules L94.4
Gougerot's syndrome (trisymptomatic) L81.7
Gougerot-Blum syndrome (pigmented
purpuric lichenoid dermatitis) L81.7
Gougerot-Carteaud disease or syndrome
(confluent reticulate papillomatosis) L83
Gouley's syndrome (constrictive pericarditis)
I31.1
Goundou A66.6
Gout, chronic (*see also* Gout, gouty) M1A.9-
drug-induced M1A.20
ankle M1A.27-
elbow M1A.22-
foot joint M1A.27-
hand joint M1A.24-
hip M1A.25-
knee M1A.26-
multiple site M1A.29-
shoulder M1A.21-
vertebrae M1A.28
wrist M1A.23-
idiopathic M1A.00
ankle M1A.07-
elbow M1A.02-
foot joint M1A.07-
hand joint M1A.04-

Gout, chronic *(Continued)*
idiopathic *(Continued)*
hip M1A.05-
knee M1A.06-
multiple site M1A.09
shoulder M1A.01-
vertebrae M1A.08
wrist M1A.03-
in (due to) renal impairment M1A.30
ankle M1A.37-
elbow M1A.32-
foot joint M1A.37-
hand joint M1A.34-
hip M1A.35-
knee M1A.36-
multiple site M1A.39
shoulder M1A.31-
vertebrae M1A.38
wrist M1A.33-
lead-induced M1A.10
ankle M1A.17-
elbow M1A.12-
foot joint M1A.17-
hand joint M1A.14-
hip M1A.15-
knee M1A.16-
multiple site M1A.19
shoulder M1A.11-
vertebrae M1A.18
wrist M1A.13-
primary —*see* Gout, chronic, idiopathic
saturnine —*see* Gout, chronic, lead-induced
secondary NEC M1A.40
ankle M1A.47-
elbow M1A.42-
foot joint M1A.47-
hand joint M1A.44-
hip M1A.45-
knee M1A.46-
multiple site M1A.49
shoulder M1A.41-
vertebrae M1A.48
wrist M1A.43-
syphilitic —*see also* subcategory M14.8-
A52.77
tophi M1A.9
Gout, gouty (acute) (attack) (flare) —*see also*
Gout, chronic M10.9-
drug-induced M10.20
ankle M10.27-
elbow M10.22-
foot joint M10.27-
hand joint M10.24-
hip M10.25-
knee M10.26-
multiple site M10.29
shoulder M10.21-
vertebrae M10.28
wrist M10.23-
idiopathic M10.00
ankle M10.07-
elbow M10.02-
foot joint M10.07-
hand joint M10.04-
hip M10.05-
knee M10.06-
multiple site M10.09
shoulder M10.01-
vertebrae M10.08
wrist M10.03-
in (due to) renal impairment M10.30
ankle M10.37-
elbow M10.32-
foot joint M10.37-
hand joint M10.34-
hip M10.35-
knee M10.36-
multiple site M10.39
shoulder M10.31-
vertebrae M10.38
wrist M10.33-

Gout, gouty *(Continued)*
lead-induced M10.10
ankle M10.17-
elbow M10.12-
foot joint M10.17-
hand joint M10.14-
hip M10.15-
knee M10.16-
multiple site M10.19
shoulder M10.11-
vertebrae M10.18
wrist M10.13-
primary —*see* Gout, idiopathic
saturnine —*see* Gout, lead-induced
secondary NEC M10.40
ankle M10.47-
elbow M10.42-
foot joint M10.47-
hand joint M10.44-
hip M10.45-
knee M10.46-
multiple site M10.49
shoulder M10.41-
vertebrae M10.48
wrist M10.43-
syphilitic —*see also* subcategory M14.8-
A52.77
tophi NEC —*see* Gout, chronic
Gower's
muscular dystrophy G71.0
syndrome (vasovagal attack) R55
Gradenigo's syndrome —*see* Otitis, media,
suppurative, acute
Graefe's disease —*see* Strabismus, paralytic,
ophthalmoplegia, progressive
Graft-versus-host disease D89.813
acute D89.810
acute on chronic D89.812
chronic D89.811
Grain mite (itch) B88.0
Grainhandler's disease or lung J67.8
Grand mal —*see* Epilepsy, generalized,
specified NEC
Grand multipara status only (not pregnant)
Z64.1
pregnant —*see* Pregnancy, complicated by,
grand multiparity
Granite worker's lung J62.8
Granular —*see also* condition
inflammation, pharynx J31.2
kidney (contracting) —*see* Sclerosis, renal
liver K74.69
Granulation tissue (abnormal) (excessive) L92.9
postmastoidectomy cavity —*see*
Complications, postmastoidectomy,
granulation
Granulocytopenia (primary) (malignant) —*see*
Agranulocytosis
Granuloma L92.9
abdomen K66.8
from residual foreign body L92.3
pyogenicum L98.0
actinic L57.5
annulare (perforating) L92.0
apical K04.5
aural —*see* Otitis, externa, specified NEC
beryllium (skin) L92.3
bone
eosinophilic C96.6
from residual foreign body —*see*
Osteomyelitis, specified type NEC
lung C96.6
brain (any site) G06.0
schistosomiasis B65.9 [G07]
canaliculus lacrimalis —*see* Granuloma,
lacrimal
candidal (cutaneous) B37.2
cerebral (any site) G06.0
coccidioidal (primary) (progressive) B38.7
lung B38.1
meninges B38.4

Granuloma (Continued)
　colon K63.89
　conjunctiva H11.22-
　dental K04.5
　ear, middle —see Cholesteatoma
　eosinophilic C96.6
　　bone C96.6
　　lung C96.6
　　oral mucosa K13.4
　　skin L92.2
　eyelid H01.8
　facial (e) L92.2
　foreign body (in soft tissue) NEC M60.20
　　ankle M60.27-
　　foot M60.27-
　　forearm M60.23-
　　hand M60.24-
　　in operation wound —see Foreign body,
　　　accidentally left during a procedure
　　lower leg M60.26-
　　pelvic region M60.25-
　　shoulder region M60.21-
　　skin L92.3
　　specified site NEC M60.28
　　subcutaneous tissue L92.3
　　thigh M60.25-
　　upper arm M60.22-
　gangraenescens M31.2
　genito-inguinale A58
　giant cell (central) (reparative) (jaw) M27.1
　　gingiva (peripheral) K06.8
　gland (lymph) I88.8
　hepatic NEC K75.3
　　in (due to)
　　　berylliosis J63.2 [K77]
　　　sarcoidosis D86.89
　Hodgkin C81.9
　ileum K63.89
　infectious B99.9
　　specified NEC B99.8
　inguinale (Donovan) (venereal) A58
　intestine NEC K63.89
　intracranial (any site) G06.0
　intraspinal (any part) G06.1
　iridocyclitis —see Iridocyclitis, chronic
　jaw (bone) (central) M27.1
　　reparative giant cell M27.1
　kidney —see also Infection, kidney N15.8
　lacrimal H04.81-
　larynx J38.7
　lethal midline (faciale (e)) M31.2
　liver NEC —see Granuloma, hepatic
　lung (infectious) —see also Fibrosis, lung
　　coccidioidal B38.1
　　eosinophilic C96.6
　Majocchi's B35.8
　malignant (facial (e)) M31.2
　mandible (central) M27.1
　midline (lethal) M31.2
　monilial (cutaneous) B37.2
　nasal sinus —see Sinusitis
　operation wound T81.89
　　foreign body —see Foreign body,
　　　accidentally left during a procedure
　　stitch T81.89
　　talc —see Foreign body, accidentally left
　　　during a procedure
　oral mucosa K13.4
　orbit, orbital H05.11-
　paracoccidioidal B41.8
　penis, venereal A58
　periapical K04.5
　peritoneum K66.8
　　due to ova of helminths NOS —see also
　　　Helminthiasis B83.9 [K67]
　postmastoidectomy cavity —see
　　　Complications, postmastoidectomy,
　　　recurrent cholesteatoma
　prostate N42.89
　pudendi (ulcerating) A58
　pulp, internal (tooth) K03.3

Granuloma (Continued)
　pyogenic, pyogenicum (of) (skin) L98.0
　　gingiva K06.8
　　maxillary alveolar ridge K04.5
　　oral mucosa K13.4
　rectum K62.89
　reticulohistiocytic D76.3
　rubrum nasi L74.8
　Schistosoma —see Schistosomiasis
　septic (skin) L98.0
　silica (skin) L92.3
　sinus (accessory) (infective) (nasal) —see
　　　Sinusitis
　skin L92.9
　　from residual foreign body L92.3
　　pyogenicum L98.0
　spine
　　syphilitic (epidural) A52.19
　　tuberculous A18.01
　stitch (postoperative) T81.89
　suppurative (skin) L98.0
　swimming pool A31.1
　talc —see also Granuloma, foreign body
　　in operation wound —see Foreign body,
　　　accidentally left during a procedure
　telangiectaticum (skin) L98.0
　tracheostomy J95.09
　trichophyticum B35.8
　tropicum A66.4
　umbilicus L92.9
　urethra N36.8
　uveitis —see Iridocyclitis, chronic
　vagina A58
　venereum A58
　vocal cord J38.3
Granulomatosis L92.9
　lymphoid C83.8-
　miliary (listerial) A32.89
　necrotizing, respiratory M31.30
　progressive septic D71
　specified NEC L92.8
　Wegener's M31.30
　　with renal involvement M31.31
Granulomatous tissue (abnormal) (excessive)
　　L92.9
Granulosis rubra nasi L74.8
Graphite fibrosis (of lung) J63.3
Graphospasm F48.8
　organic G25.89
Grating scapula M89.8X1
Gravel (urinary) —see Calculus, urinary
Graves' disease —see Hyperthyroidism, with,
　　goiter
Gravis —see condition
Grawitz tumor C64.-
Gray syndrome (newborn) P93.0
Grayness, hair (premature) L67.1
　congenital Q84.2
Green sickness D50.8
Greenfield's disease
　meaning
　　concentric sclerosis (encephalitis periaxialis
　　　concentrica) G37.5
　　metachromatic leukodystrophy E75.25
Greenstick fracture - code as Fracture, by site
Grey syndrome (newborn) P93.0
Grief F43.21
　prolonged F43.29
　reaction —see also Disorder, adjustment F43.20
Griesinger's disease B76.9
Grinder's lung or pneumoconiosis J62.8
Grinding, teeth
　psychogenic F45.8
　sleep related G47.63
Grip
　Dabney's B33.0
　devil's B33.0
Grippe, grippal —see also Influenza
　Balkan A78
　summer, of Italy A93.1
Grisel's disease M43.6
Groin —see condition

Grooved tongue K14.5
Ground itch B76.9
Grover's disease or syndrome L11.1
Growing pains, children R29.898
Growth (fungoid) (neoplastic) (new) —see also
　　Neoplasm
　adenoid (vegetative) J35.8
　benign —see Neoplasm, benign, by site
　malignant —see Neoplasm, malignant, by site
　rapid, childhood Z00.2
　secondary —see Neoplasm, secondary, by site
Gruby's disease B35.0
Gubler-Millard paralysis or syndrome G46.3
Guerin-Stern syndrome Q74.3
Guidance, insufficient anterior (occlusal) M26.54
Guillain-Barré disease or syndrome G61.0
　sequelae G65.0
Guinea worms (infection) (infestation) B72
Guinon's disease (motor-verbal tic) F95.2
Gull's disease E03.4
Gum —see condition
Gumboil K04.7
　with sinus K04.6
Gumma (syphilitic) A52.79
　artery A52.09
　　cerebral A52.04
　bone A52.77
　　of yaws (late) A66.6
　brain A52.19
　cauda equina A52.19
　central nervous system A52.3
　ciliary body A52.71
　congenital A50.59
　eyelid A52.71
　heart A52.06
　intracranial A52.19
　iris A52.71
　kidney A52.75
　larynx A52.73
　leptomeninges A52.19
　liver A52.74
　meninges A52.19
　myocardium A52.06
　nasopharynx A52.73
　neurosyphilitic A52.3
　nose A52.73
　orbit A52.71
　palate (soft) A52.79
　penis A52.76
　pericardium A52.06
　pharynx A52.73
　pituitary A52.79
　scrofulous (tuberculous) A18.4
　skin A52.79
　specified site NEC A52.79
　spinal cord A52.19
　tongue A52.79
　tonsil A52.73
　trachea A52.73
　tuberculous A18.4
　ulcerative due to yaws A66.4
　ureter A52.75
　yaws A66.4
　　bone A66.6
Gunn's syndrome Q07.8
Gunshot wound —see also Wound, open
　fracture - code as Fracture, by site
　internal organs —see Injury, by site
Gynandrism Q56.0
Gynandroblastoma
　specified site —see Neoplasm, uncertain
　　behavior, by site
　unspecified site
　　female D39.10
　　male D40.10
Gynecological examination (periodic) (routine)
　　Z01.419
　with abnormal findings Z01.411
Gynecomastia N62
Gynephobia F40.291
Gyrate scalp Q82.8

H

H (Hartnup's) disease E72.02
Haas' disease or osteochondrosis (juvenile)
   (head of humerus) —see Osteochondrosis,
   juvenile, humerus
Habit, habituation
   bad sleep Z72.821
   chorea F95.8
   disturbance, child F98.9
   drug —see Dependence, drug
   irregular sleep Z72.821
   laxative F55.2
   spasm —see Tic
   tic —see Tic
Haemophilus (H.) influenzae, as cause of
   disease classified elsewhere B96.3
Haff disease —see Poisoning, mercury
Hageman's factor defect, deficiency or disease
   D68.2
Haglund's disease or osteochondrosis
   (juvenile) (os tibiale externum) —see
   Osteochondrosis, juvenile, tarsus
Hailey-Hailey disease Q82.8
Hair —see also condition
   plucking F63.3
      in stereotyped movement disorder F98.4
   tourniquet syndrome —see also Constriction,
      external, by site
      finger S60.44-
      penis S30.842
      thumb S60.34-
      toe S90.44-
Hairball in stomach T18.2
Hair-pulling, pathological (compulsive) F63.3
Hairy black tongue K14.3
Half vertebra Q76.49
Halitosis R19.6
Hallerman-Streiff syndrome Q87.0
Hallervorden-Spatz disease G23.0
Hallopeau's acrodermatitis or disease L40.2
Hallucination R44.3
   auditory R44.0
   gustatory R44.2
   olfactory R44.2
   specified NEC R44.2
   tactile R44.2
   visual R44.1
Hallucinosis (chronic) F28
   alcoholic (acute) F10.951
      in
         abuse F10.151
         dependence F10.251
   drug-induced F19.951
      cannabis F12.951
      cocaine F14.951
      hallucinogen F16.151
      in
         abuse F19.151
            cannabis F12.151
            cocaine F14.151
            hallucinogen F16.151
            inhalant F18.151
            opioid F11.151
            sedative, anxiolytic or hypnotic
               F13.151
            stimulant NEC F15.151
         dependence F19.251
            cannabis F12.251
            cocaine F14.251
            hallucinogen F16.251
            inhalant F18.251
            opioid F11.251
            sedative, anxiolytic or hypnotic
               F13.251
            stimulant NEC F15.251
      inhalant F18.951
      opioid F11.951
      sedative, anxiolytic or hypnotic F13.951
      stimulant NEC F15.951
   organic F06.0

Hallux
   deformity (acquired) NEC M20.5X-
   limitus M20.5X-
   malleus (acquired) NEC M20.3-
   rigidus (acquired) M20.2-
      congenital Q74.2
      sequelae (late effect) of rickets E64.3
   valgus (acquired) M20.1-
      congenital Q66.6
   varus (acquired) M20.3-
      congenital Q66.3
Halo, visual H53.19
Hamartoma, hamartoblastoma Q85.9
   epithelial (gingival), odontogenic, central
      or peripheral —see Cyst, calcifying
      odontogenic
Hamartosis Q85.9
Hamman-Rich syndrome J84.114
Hammer toe (acquired) NEC —see also
   Deformity, toe, hammer toe
   congenital Q66.89
   sequelae (late effect) of rickets E64.3
Hand —see condition
Hand-foot syndrome L27.1
Handicap, handicapped
   educational Z55.9
      specified NEC Z55.8
Hand-Schüller-Christian disease or syndrome
   C96.5
Hanging (asphyxia) (strangulation)
   (suffocation) —see Asphyxia, traumatic,
   due to mechanical threat
Hangnail —see also Cellulitis, digit
   with lymphangitis —see Lymphangitis, acute,
      digit
Hangover (alcohol) F10.129
Hanhart's syndrome Q87.0
Hanot-Chauffard (-Troisier) syndrome E83.19
Hanot's cirrhosis or disease K74.3
Hansen's disease —see Leprosy
Hantaan virus disease (Korean hemorrhagic
   fever) A98.5
Hantavirus disease (with renal manifestations)
   (Dobrava) (Puumala) (Seoul) A98.5
   with pulmonary manifestations (Andes)
      (Bayou) (Bermejo) (Black Creek Canal)
      (Choclo) (Juquitiba) (Laguna negra)
      (Lechiguanas) (New York) (Oran) (Sin
      nombre) B33.4
Happy puppet syndrome Q93.5
Harada's disease or syndrome H30.81-
Hardening
   artery —see Arteriosclerosis
   brain G93.89
Harelip (complete) (incomplete) —see Cleft, lip
Harlequin (newborn) Q80.4
Harley's disease D59.6
Harmful use (of)
   alcohol F10.10
   anxiolytics —see Abuse, drug, sedative
   cannabinoids —see Abuse, drug, cannabis
   cocaine —see Abuse, drug, cocaine
   drug —see Abuse, drug
   hallucinogens —see Abuse, drug,
      hallucinogen
   hypnotics —see Abuse, drug, sedative -
      opioids —see Abuse, drug, opioid
   PCP (phencyclidine) —see Abuse, drug,
      hallucinogen
   sedatives —see Abuse, drug, sedative
   stimulants NEC —see Abuse, drug, stimulant
Harris' lines —see Arrest, epiphyseal
Hartnup's disease E72.02
Harvester's lung J67.0
Harvesting ovum for in vitro fertilization
   Z31.83
Hashimoto's disease or thyroiditis E06.3
Hashitoxicosis (transient) E06.3
Hassal-Henle bodies or warts (cornea) H18.49
Haut mal —see Epilepsy, generalized, specified
   NEC

Haverhill fever A25.1
Hay fever —see also Fever, hay J30.1
Hayem-Widal syndrome D59.8
Haygarth's nodes M15.8
Haymaker's lung J67.0
Hb (abnormal)
   Bart's disease D56.0
   disease —see Disease, hemoglobin
   trait —see Trait
Head —see condition
Headache R51
   allergic NEC G44.89
   associated with sexual activity
      G44.82
   chronic daily R51
   cluster G44.009
      chronic G44.029
         intractable G44.021
         not intractable G44.029
      episodic G44.019
         intractable G44.011
         not intractable G44.019
      intractable G44.001
      not intractable G44.009
   cough (primary) G44.83
   daily chronic R51
   drug-induced NEC G44.40
      intractable G44.41
      not intractable G44.40
   exertional (primary) G44.84
   histamine G44.009
      intractable G44.001
      not intractable G44.009
   hypnic G44.81
   lumbar puncture G97.1
   medication overuse G44.40
      intractable G44.41
      not intractable G44.40
   menstrual —see Migraine, menstrual
   migraine (type) —see also Migraine
      G43.909
   nasal septum R51
   neuralgiform, short lasting unilateral, with
      conjunctival injection and tearing
      (SUNCT) G44.059
      intractable G44.051
      not intractable G44.059
   new daily persistent (NDPH) G44.52
   orgasmic G44.82
   periodic syndromes in adults and children
      G43.C0
      with refractory migraine G43.C1
      intractable G43.C1
      not intractable G43.C0
      without refractory migraine G43.C0
   postspinal puncture G97.1
   post-traumatic G44.309
      acute G44.319
         intractable G44.311
         not intractable G44.319
      chronic G44.329
         intractable G44.321
         not intractable G44.329
      intractable G44.301
      not intractable G44.309
   pre-menstrual —see Migraine, menstrual
   preorgasmic G44.82
   primary
      cough G44.83
      exertional G44.84
      stabbing G44.85
      thunderclap G44.53
   rebound G44.40
      intractable G44.41
      not intractable G44.40
   short lasting unilateral neuralgiform, with
      conjunctival injection and tearing
      (SUNCT) G44.059
      intractable G44.051
      not intractable G44.059
   specified syndrome NEC G44.89

◀ New   ◀▥ Revised   ~~deleted~~ Deleted

Headache *(Continued)*
  spinal and epidural anesthesia - induced
      T88.59
    in labor and delivery O74.5
    in pregnancy O29.4-
    postpartum, puerperal O89.4
  spinal fluid loss (from puncture) G97.1
  stabbing (primary) G44.85
  tension (-type) G44.209
    chronic G44.229
      intractable G44.221
      not intractable G44.229
    episodic G44.219
      intractable G44.211
      not intractable G44.219
    intractable G44.201
    not intractable G44.209
  thunderclap (primary) G44.53
  vascular NEC G44.1
Healthy
  infant
    accompanying sick mother Z76.3
    receiving care Z76.2
  person accompanying sick person Z76.3
Hearing examination Z01.10
  with abnormal findings NEC Z01.118
  following failed hearing screening Z01.110
  for hearing conservation and treatment
      Z01.12
Heart —*see* condition
Heart beat
  abnormality R00.9
    specified NEC R00.8
  awareness R00.2
  rapid R00.0
  slow R00.1
Heartburn R12
  psychogenic F45.8
Heat (effects) T67.9
  apoplexy T67.0
  burn —*see also* Burn L55.9
  collapse T67.1
  cramps T67.2
  dermatitis or eczema L59.0
  edema T67.7
  erythema - code by site under Burn, first
      degree
  excessive T67.9
    specified effect NEC T67.8
  exhaustion T67.5
    anhydrotic T67.3
    due to
      salt (and water) depletion T67.4
      water depletion T67.3
        with salt depletion T67.4
  fatigue (transient) T67.6
  fever T67.0
  hyperpyrexia T67.0
  prickly L74.0
  prostration —*see* Heat, exhaustion
  pyrexia T67.0
  rash L74.0
  specified effect NEC T67.8
  stroke T67.0
  sunburn —*see* Sunburn
  syncope T67.1
Heavy-for-dates NEC (infant) (4000g to 4499g)
      P08.1
  exceptionally (4500g or more) P08.0
Hebephrenia, hebephrenic (schizophrenia)
      F20.1
Heberden's disease or nodes (with
      arthropathy) M15.1
Hebra's
  pityriasis L26
  prurigo L28.2
Heel —*see* condition
Heerfordt's disease D86.89
Hegglin's anomaly or syndrome D72.0
Heilmeyer-Schoner disease D45
Heine-Medin disease A80.9

Heinz body anemia, congenital D58.2
Heliophobia F40.228
Heller's disease or syndrome F84.3
HELLP syndrome (hemolysis, elevated liver
      enzymes and low platelet count) O14.2-
  complicating ◄
    childbirth O14.24 ◄
    puerperium O14.25 ◄
Helminthiasis —*see also* Infestation, helminth
  Ancylostoma B76.0
  intestinal B82.0
    mixed types (types classifiable to more
        than one of the titles B65.0-B81.3 and
        B81.8) B81.4
    specified type NEC B81.8
  mixed types (intestinal) (types classifiable to
      more than one of the titles B65.0-B81.3
      and B81.8) B81.4
  Necator (americanus) B76.1
  specified type NEC B83.8
Heloma L84
Hemangioblastoma —*see* Neoplasm,
      connective tissue, uncertain behavior
  malignant —*see* Neoplasm, connective tissue,
      malignant
Hemangioendothelioma —*see also* Neoplasm,
      uncertain behavior, by site
  benign D18.00
    intra-abdominal D18.03
    intracranial D18.02
    skin D18.01
    specified site NEC D18.09
  bone (diffuse) —*see* Neoplasm, bone,
      malignant
  epithelioid —*see also* Neoplasm, uncertain
      behavior, by site
    malignant —*see* Neoplasm, malignant, by
        site
  malignant —*see* Neoplasm, connective tissue,
      malignant
Hemangiofibroma —*see* Neoplasm, benign,
      by site
Hemangiolipoma —*see* Lipoma
Hemangioma D18.00
  arteriovenous D18.00
    intra-abdominal D18.03
    intracranial D18.02
    skin D18.01
    specified site NEC D18.09
  capillary D18.00
    intra-abdominal D18.03
    intracranial D18.02
    skin D18.01
    specified site NEC D18.09
  cavernous D18.00
    intra-abdominal D18.03
    intracranial D18.02
    skin D18.01
    specified site NEC D18.09
  epithelioid D18.00
    intra-abdominal D18.03
    intracranial D18.02
    skin D18.01
    specified site NEC D18.09
  histiocytoid D18.00
    intra-abdominal D18.03
    intracranial D18.02
    skin D18.01
    specified site NEC D18.09
  infantile D18.00
    intra-abdominal D18.03
    intracranial D18.02
    skin D18.01
    specified site NEC D18.09
  intra-abdominal D18.03
  intracranial D18.02
  intramuscular D18.00
    intra-abdominal D18.03
    intracranial D18.02
    skin D18.01
    specified site NEC D18.09

Hemangioma *(Continued)*
  intrathoracic structures D18.09 ◄
  juvenile D18.00
  malignant —*see* Neoplasm, connective tissue,
      malignant
  plexiform D18.00
    intra-abdominal D18.03
    intracranial D18.02
    skin D18.01
    specified site NEC D18.09
  racemose D18.00
    intra-abdominal D18.03
    intracranial D18.02
    skin D18.01
    specified site NEC D18.09
  sclerosing —*see* Neoplasm, skin, benign
  simplex D18.00
    intra-abdominal D18.03
    intracranial D18.02
    skin D18.01
    specified site NEC D18.09
  skin D18.01
  specified site NEC D18.09
  venous D18.00
    intra-abdominal D18.03
    intracranial D18.02
    skin D18.01
    specified site NEC D18.09
  verrucous keratotic D18.00
    intra-abdominal D18.03
    intracranial D18.02
    skin D18.01
    specified site NEC D18.09
Hemangiomatosis (systemic) I78.8
  involving single site —*see* Hemangioma
Hemangiopericytoma —*see also* Neoplasm,
      connective tissue, uncertain behavior
  benign —*see* Neoplasm, connective tissue,
      benign
  malignant —*see* Neoplasm, connective tissue,
      malignant
Hemangiosarcoma —*see* Neoplasm, connective
      tissue, malignant
Hemarthrosis (nontraumatic) M25.00
  ankle M25.07-
  elbow M25.02-
  foot joint M25.07-
  hand joint M25.04-
  hip M25.05-
  in hemophilic arthropathy —*see* Arthropathy,
      hemophilic
  knee M25.06-
  shoulder M25.01-
  specified joint NEC M25.08
  traumatic —*see* Sprain, by site
  vertebrae M25.08
  wrist M25.03-
Hematemesis K92.0
  with ulcer - code by site under Ulcer, with
      hemorrhage K27.4
  newborn, neonatal P54.0
    due to swallowed maternal blood
        P78.2
Hematidrosis L74.8
Hematinuria —*see also* Hemoglobinuria
  malarial B50.8
Hematobilia K83.8
Hematocele
  female NEC N94.89
    with ectopic pregnancy O00.90 ◄▥
      with intrauterine pregnancy O00.91 ◄
    ovary N83.8
  male N50.1
Hematochezia —*see also* Melena K92.1
Hematochyluria —*see also* Infestation, filarial
  schistosomiasis (bilharziasis) B65.0
Hematocolpos (with hematometra or
      hematosalpinx) N89.7
Hematocornea —*see* Pigmentation, cornea,
      stromal
Hematogenous —*see* condition

Hematoma (traumatic) (skin surface intact) —
see also Contusion
with
injury of internal organs —see Injury, by site
open wound —see Wound, open
amputation stump (surgical) (late) T87.89
aorta, dissecting I71.00
abdominal I71.02
thoracic I71.01
thoracoabdominal I71.03
aortic intramural —see Dissection, aorta
arterial (complicating trauma) —see Injury,
blood vessel, by site
auricle —see Contusion, ear
nontraumatic —see Disorder, pinna,
hematoma
birth injury NEC P15.8
brain (traumatic)
with
cerebral laceration or contusion
(diffuse) —see Injury, intracranial,
diffuse
focal —see Injury, intracranial, focal
cerebellar, traumatic S06.37-
intracerebral, traumatic —see Injury,
intracranial, intracerebral
hemorrhage
newborn NEC P52.4
birth injury P10.1
nontraumatic —see Hemorrhage,
intracranial
subarachnoid, arachnoid, traumatic —see
Injury, intracranial, subarachnoid
hemorrhage
subdural, traumatic —see Injury,
intracranial, subdural hemorrhage
breast (nontraumatic) N64.89
broad ligament (nontraumatic) N83.7
traumatic S37.892
cerebellar, traumatic S06.37-
cerebral —see Hematoma, brain
cerebrum S06.36-
left S06.35-
right S06.34-
cesarean delivery wound O90.2
complicating delivery (perineal) (pelvic)
(vagina) (vulva) O71.7
corpus cavernosum (nontraumatic) N48.89
epididymis (nontraumatic) N50.1
epidural (traumatic) —see Injury, intracranial,
epidural hemorrhage
spinal —see Injury, spinal cord, by region
episiotomy O90.2
face, birth injury P15.4
genital organ NEC (nontraumatic)
female (nonobstetric) N94.89
traumatic S30.202
male N50.1
traumatic S30.201
internal organs —see Injury, by site
intracerebral, traumatic —see Injury,
intracranial, intracerebral hemorrhage
intraoperative —see Complications,
intraoperative, hemorrhage
labia (nontraumatic) (nonobstetric) N90.8
liver (subcapsular) (nontraumatic) K76.89
birth injury P15.0
mediastinum —see Injury, intrathoracic
mesosalpinx (nontraumatic) N83.7
traumatic S37.898
muscle - code by site under Contusion
nontraumatic
muscle M79.81
soft tissue M79.81
obstetrical surgical wound O90.2
orbit, orbital (nontraumatic) —see also
Hemorrhage, orbit
traumatic —see Contusion, orbit
pelvis (female) (nontraumatic) (nonobstetric)
N94.89
obstetric O71.7
traumatic —see Injury, by site

Hematoma (Continued)
penis (nontraumatic) N48.89
birth injury P15.5
perianal (nontraumatic) K64.5
perineal S30.23
complicating delivery O71.7
perirenal —see Injury, kidney
pinna —see Contusion, ear
nontraumatic —see Disorder, pinna,
hematoma
placenta O43.89-
postoperative (postprocedural) —see
Complication, postprocedural,
hematoma ◄▦
retroperitoneal (nontraumatic) K66.1
traumatic S36.892
scrotum, superficial S30.22
birth injury P15.5
seminal vesicle (nontraumatic) N50.1
traumatic S37.892
spermatic cord (traumatic) S37.892
nontraumatic N50.1
spinal (cord) (meninges) —see also Injury,
spinal cord, by region
newborn (birth injury) P11.5
spleen D73.5
intraoperative —see Complications,
intraoperative, hemorrhage, spleen
postprocedural (postoperative) —see
Complications, postprocedural,
hemorrhage, spleen
sternocleidomastoid, birth injury P15.2
sternomastoid, birth injury P15.2
subarachnoid (traumatic) —see Injury,
intracranial, subarachnoid hemorrhage
newborn (nontraumatic) P52.5
due to birth injury P10.3
nontraumatic —see Hemorrhage,
intracranial, subarachnoid
subdural (traumatic) —see Injury, intracranial,
subdural hemorrhage
newborn (localized) P52.8
birth injury P10.0
nontraumatic —see Hemorrhage,
intracranial, subdural
superficial, newborn P54.5
testis (nontraumatic) N50.1
birth injury P15.5
tunica vaginalis (nontraumatic) N50.1
umbilical cord, complicating delivery
O69.5
uterine ligament (broad) (nontraumatic)
N83.7
traumatic S37.892
vagina (ruptured) (nontraumatic) N89.8
complicating delivery O71.7
vas deferens (nontraumatic) N50.1
traumatic S37.892
vitreous —see Hemorrhage, vitreous
vulva (nontraumatic) (nonobstetric) N90.89
complicating delivery O71.7
newborn (birth injury) P15.5
Hematometra N85.7
with hematocolpos N89.7
Hematomyelia (central) G95.19
newborn (birth injury) P11.5
traumatic T14.8
Hematomyelitis G04.90
Hematoperitoneum —see Hemoperitoneum
Hematophobia F40.230
Hematopneumothorax (see Hemothorax)
Hematopoiesis, cyclic D70.4
Hematoporphyria —see Porphyria
Hematorachis, hematorrhachis G95.19
newborn (birth injury) P11.5
Hematosalpinx N83.6
with
hematocolpos N89.7
hematometra N85.7
with hematocolpos N89.7
infectional —see Salpingitis

Hematospermia R36.1
Hematothorax (see Hemothorax)
Hematuria R31.9
benign (familial) (of childhood) —see also
Hematuria, idiopathic
essential microscopic R31.1
due to sulphonamide, sulfonamide —see Table
of Drugs and Chemicals, by drug
endemic —see also Schistosomiasis B65.0
gross R31.0
idiopathic N02.9
with glomerular lesion
crescentic (diffuse) glomerulonephritis
N02.7
dense deposit disease N02.6
endocapillary proliferative
glomerulonephritis N02.4
focal and segmental hyalinosis or
sclerosis N02.1
membranoproliferative (diffuse) N02.5
membranous (diffuse) N02.2
mesangial proliferative (diffuse) N02.3
mesangiocapillary (diffuse) N02.5
minor abnormality N02.0
proliferative NEC N02.8
specified pathology NEC N02.8
intermittent —see Hematuria, idiopathic
malarial B50.8
microscopic NEC (with symptoms) R31.29 ◄▦
asymptomatic R31.21 ◄
benign essential R31.1
paroxysmal —see also Hematuria, idiopathic
nocturnal D59.5
persistent —see Hematuria, idiopathic
recurrent —see Hematuria, idiopathic
tropical —see also Schistosomiasis B65.0
tuberculous A18.13
Hemeralopia (day blindness) H53.11
vitamin A deficiency E50.5
Hemi-akinesia R41.4
Hemianalgesia R20.0
Hemianencephaly Q00.0
Hemianesthesia R20.0
Hemianopia, hemianopsia (heteronymous)
H53.47
homonymous H53.46-
syphilitic A52.71
Hemiathetosis R25.8
Hemiatrophy R68.89
cerebellar G31.9
face, facial, progressive (Romberg) G51.8
tongue K14.8
Hemiballism (us) G25.5
Hemicardia Q24.8
Hemicephalus, hemicephaly Q00.0
Hemichorea G25.5
Hemicolitis, left —see Colitis, left sided
Hemicrania
congenital malformation Q00.0
continua G44.51
meaning migraine —see also Migraine G43.909
paroxysmal G44.039
chronic G44.049
intractable G44.041
not intractable G44.049
episodic G44.039
intractable G44.031
not intractable G44.039
intractable G44.031
not intractable G44.039
Hemidystrophy —see Hemiatrophy
Hemiectromelia Q73.8
Hemihypalgesia R20.8
Hemihypesthesia R20.1
Hemi-inattention R41.4
Hemimelia Q73.8
lower limb —see Defect, reduction, lower
limb, specified type NEC
upper limb —see Defect, reduction, upper
limb, specified type NEC
Hemiparalysis —see Hemiplegia
Hemiparesis —see Hemiplegia

◄ New   ◄▦ Revised   ~~deleted~~ Deleted

Hemiparesthesia R20.2
Hemiparkinsonism G20
Hemiplegia G81.9-
  alternans facialis G83.89
  ascending NEC G81.90
    spinal G95.89
  congenital (cerebral) G80.8
    spastic G80.2
  embolic (current episode) I63.4-
  flaccid G81.0-
  following
    cerebrovascular disease I69.959
      cerebral infarction I69.35-
      intracerebral hemorrhage I69.15-
      nontraumatic intracranial hemorrhage
        NEC I69.25-
      specified disease NEC I69.85-
      stroke NOS I69.35-
      subarachnoid hemorrhage I69.05-
  hysterical F44.4
  newborn NEC P91.8
    birth injury P11.9
  spastic G81.1-
    congenital G80.2
  thrombotic (current episode) I63.3- ◀▥
Hemisection, spinal cord —see Injury, spinal
    cord, by region
Hemispasm (facial) R25.2
Hemisporosis B48.8
Hemitremor R25.1
Hemivertebra Q76.49
  failure of segmentation with scoliosis Q76.3
  fusion with scoliosis Q76.3
Hemochromatosis E83.119
  with refractory anemia D46.1
  due to repeated red blood cell transfusion
    E83.111
  hereditary (primary) E83.110
  primary E83.110
  specified NEC E83.118
Hemoglobin —see also condition
  abnormal (disease) —see Disease, hemoglobin
  AS genotype D57.3
  Constant Spring D58.2
  E-beta thalassemia D56.5
  fetal, hereditary persistence (HPFH) D56.4
  H Constant Spring D56.0
  low NOS D64.9
  S (Hb S), heterozygous D57.3
Hemoglobinemia D59.9
  due to blood transfusion T80.89
  paroxysmal D59.6
    nocturnal D59.5
Hemoglobinopathy (mixed) D58.2
  with thalassemia D56.8
  sickle-cell D57.1
    with thalassemia D57.40
      with crisis (vasoocclusive pain) D57.419
        with
          acute chest syndrome D57.411
          splenic sequestration D57.412
      without crisis D57.40
Hemoglobinuria R82.3
  with anemia, hemolytic, acquired (chronic)
    NEC D59.6
  cold (agglutinin) (paroxysmal) (with
    Raynaud's syndrome) D59.6
  due to exertion or hemolysis NEC D59.6
  intermittent D59.6
  malarial B50.8
  march D59.6
  nocturnal (paroxysmal) D59.5
  paroxysmal (cold) D59.6
    nocturnal D59.5
Hemolymphangioma D18.1
Hemolysis
  intravascular
    with
      abortion —see Abortion, by type,
        complicated by, hemorrhage
      ectopic or molar pregnancy O08.1

Hemolysis (Continued)
  intravascular (Continued)
    with (Continued)
      hemorrhage
        antepartum —see Hemorrhage,
          antepartum, with coagulation
          defect
        intrapartum —see also Hemorrhage,
          complicating, delivery O67.0
    postpartum O72.3
  neonatal (excessive) P58.9
    specified NEC P58.8
Hemolytic —see condition
Hemopericardium I31.2
  following acute myocardial infarction
    (current complication) I23.0
  newborn P54.8
  traumatic —see Injury, heart, with
    hemopericardium
Hemoperitoneum K66.1
  infectional K65.9
  traumatic S36.899
    with open wound —see Wound, open, with
      penetration into peritoneal cavity
Hemophilia (classical) (familial) (hereditary)
    D66
  A D66
  B D67
  C D68.1
  acquired D68.311
  autoimmune D68.311
  calcipriva —see also Defect, coagulation D68.4
  nonfamilial —see also Defect, coagulation
    D68.4
  secondary D68.311
  vascular D68.0
Hemophthalmos H44.81-
Hemopneumothorax —see also Hemothorax
  traumatic S27.2
Hemoptysis R04.2
  newborn P26.9
  tuberculous —see Tuberculosis, pulmonary
Hemorrhage, hemorrhagic (concealed) R58
  abdomen R58
  accidental antepartum —see Hemorrhage,
    antepartum
  acute idiopathic pulmonary, in infants
    R04.81
  adenoid J35.8
  adrenal (capsule) (gland) E27.49
    medulla E27.8
    newborn P54.4
  after delivery —see Hemorrhage, postpartum
  alveolar
    lung, newborn P26.8
    process K08.89 ◀▥
  alveolus K08.89 ◀▥
  amputation stump (surgical) T87.89
  anemia (chronic) D50.0
    acute D62
  antepartum (with) O46.90
    with coagulation defect O46.00-
      afibrinogenemia O46.01-
      disseminated intravascular coagulation
        O46.02-
      hypofibrinogenemia O46.01-
      specified defect NEC O46.09-
    before 20 weeks gestation O20.9
      specified type NEC O20.8
      threatened abortion O20.0
    due to
      abruptio placenta —see also Abruptio
        placentae O45.9-
      leiomyoma, uterus —see Hemorrhage,
        antepartum, specified cause NEC
      placenta previa O44.1-
    specified cause NEC —see subcategory
      O46.8X-
  anus (sphincter) K62.5
  apoplexy (stroke) —see Hemorrhage,
    intracranial, intracerebral

Hemorrhage, hemorrhagic (Continued)
  arachnoid —see Hemorrhage, intracranial,
    subarachnoid
  artery R58
    brain —see Hemorrhage, intracranial,
      intracerebral
  basilar (ganglion) I61.0
  bladder N32.89
  bowel K92.2
    newborn P54.3
  brain (miliary) (nontraumatic) —see
      Hemorrhage, intracranial, intracerebral
    due to
      birth injury P10.1
      syphilis A52.05
    epidural or extradural (traumatic) —
        see Injury, intracranial, epidural
        hemorrhage
    newborn P52.4
      birth injury P10.1
    subarachnoid —see Hemorrhage,
      intracranial, subarachnoid
    subdural —see Hemorrhage, intracranial,
      subdural
  brainstem (nontraumatic) I61.3
    traumatic S06.38-
  breast N64.59
  bronchial tube —see Hemorrhage, lung
  bronchopulmonary —see Hemorrhage, lung
  bronchus —see Hemorrhage, lung
  bulbar I61.5
  capillary I78.8
    primary D69.8
  cecum K92.2
  cerebellar, cerebellum (nontraumatic) I61.4
    newborn P52.6
    traumatic S06.37-
  cerebral, cerebrum —see also Hemorrhage,
      intracranial, intracerebral
    lobe I61.1
    newborn (anoxic) P52.4
      birth injury P10.1
  cerebromeningeal I61.8
  cerebrospinal —see Hemorrhage, intracranial,
    intracerebral
  cervix (uteri) (stump) NEC N88.8
  chamber, anterior (eye) —see Hyphema
  childbirth —see Hemorrhage, complicating,
    delivery
  choroid H31.30-
    expulsive H31.31-
  ciliary body —see Hyphema
  cochlea —see subcategory H83.8
  colon K92.2
  complicating
    abortion —see Abortion, by type,
      complicated by, hemorrhage
    delivery O67.9
      associated with coagulation defect
        (afibrinogenemia) (DIC)
        (hyperfibrinolysis) O67.0
      specified cause NEC O67.8
    surgical procedure —see Hemorrhage,
      intraoperative
  conjunctiva H11.3-
    newborn P54.8
  cord, newborn (stump) P51.9
  corpus luteum (ruptured) cyst N83.1- ◀▥
  cortical (brain) I61.1
  cranial —see Hemorrhage, intracranial
  cutaneous R23.3
    due to autosensitivity, erythrocyte D69.2
    newborn P54.5
  delayed
    following ectopic or molar pregnancy
      O08.1
    postpartum O72.2
  diathesis (familial) D69.9
  disease D69.9
    newborn P53
    specified type NEC D69.8

Hemorrhage, hemorrhagic (Continued)
  due to or associated with
    afibrinogenemia or other coagulation defect
        (conditions in categories D65-D69)
      antepartum —see Hemorrhage,
          antepartum, with coagulation
          defect
      intrapartum O67.0
    dental implant M27.61
    device, implant or graft —see also
        Complications, by site and type,
        specified NEC T85.838 ◄▬
      arterial graft NEC T82.838
      breast T85.838 ◄▬
      catheter NEC T85.838 ◄▬
        dialysis (renal) T82.838
          intraperitoneal T85.838 ◄▬
        infusion NEC T82.838
          spinal (epidural) (subdural)
              T85.830 ◄▬
        urinary (indwelling) T83.83
      electronic (electrode) (pulse generator)
          (stimulator)
        bone T84.83
        cardiac T82.837
        nervous system (brain) (peripheral
            nerve) (spinal) T85.830 ◄▬
        urinary T83.83
      fixation, internal (orthopedic) NEC T84.83
      gastrointestinal (bile duct) (esophagus)
          T85.838 ◄▬
      genital NEC T83.83
      heart NEC T82.837
      joint prosthesis T84.83
      ocular (corneal graft) (orbital implant)
          NEC T85.838 ◄▬
      orthopedic NEC T84.83
        bone graft T86.838
      specified NEC T85.838 ◄▬
      urinary NEC T83.83
      vascular NEC T82.838
      ventricular intracranial shunt T85.838 ◄▬
  duodenum, duodenal K92.2
    ulcer —see Ulcer, duodenum, with
        hemorrhage
  dura mater —see Hemorrhage, intracranial,
      subdural
  endotracheal —see Hemorrhage, lung
  epicranial subaponeurotic (massive), birth
      injury P12.2
  epidural (traumatic) —see also Injury,
      intracranial, epidural hemorrhage
    nontraumatic I62.1
  esophagus K22.8
    varix I85.01
      secondary I85.11
  excessive, following ectopic gestation
      (subsequent episode) O08.1
  extradural (traumatic) —see Injury,
      intracranial, epidural hemorrhage
    birth injury P10.8
    newborn (anoxic) (nontraumatic) P52.8
    nontraumatic I62.1
  eye NEC H57.8
    fundus —see Hemorrhage, retina
    lid —see Disorder, eyelid, specified type
        NEC
  fallopian tube N83.6
  fibrinogenolysis —see Fibrinolysis
  fibrinolytic (acquired) —see Fibrinolysis
  from
    ear (nontraumatic) —see Otorrhagia
    tracheostomy stoma J95.01
  fundus, eye —see Hemorrhage, retina
  funis —see Hemorrhage, umbilicus, cord
  gastric —see Hemorrhage, stomach
  gastroenteric K92.2
    newborn P54.3
  gastrointestinal (tract) K92.2
    newborn P54.3
  genital organ, male N50.1

Hemorrhage, hemorrhagic (Continued)
  genitourinary (tract) NOS R31.9
  gingiva K06.8
  globe (eye) —see Hemophthalmos
  graafian follicle cyst (ruptured) N83.0- ◄▬
  gum K06.8
  heart I51.89
  hypopharyngeal (throat) R04.1
  intermenstrual (regular) N92.3
    irregular N92.1
  internal (organs) NEC R58
    capsule I61.0
    ear —see subcategory H83.8
    newborn P54.8
  intestine K92.2
    newborn P54.3
  intra-abdominal R58
  intra-alveolar (lung), newborn P26.8
  intracerebral (nontraumatic) —see
      Hemorrhage, intracranial,
      intracerebral
  intracranial (nontraumatic) I62.9
    birth injury P10.9
    epidural, nontraumatic I62.1
    extradural, nontraumatic I62.1
    intracerebral (nontraumatic) (in) I61.9
      brain stem I61.3
      cerebellum I61.4
      hemisphere I61.2
        cortical (superficial) I61.1
        subcortical (deep) I61.0
      intraoperative
        during a nervous system procedure
            G97.31
        during other procedure G97.32
      intraventricular I61.5
      multiple localized I61.6
      newborn P52.4
        birth injury P10.1
      postprocedural
        following a nervous system procedure
            G97.51
        following other procedure
            G97.52
      specified NEC I61.8
      superficial I61.1
      traumatic (diffuse) —see Injury,
          intracranial, diffuse
      focal —see Injury, intracranial, focal
    newborn P52.9
      specified NEC P52.8
    subarachnoid (nontraumatic) (from)
        I60.9
      intracranial (cerebral) artery I60.7
        anterior communicating I60.2 ◄▬
        basilar I60.4
        carotid siphon and bifurcation
            I60.0-
        communicating I60.7
          anterior I60.2 ◄▬
          posterior I60.3-
        middle cerebral I60.1-
        posterior communicating I60.3-
        specified artery NEC I60.6
        vertebral I60.5-
      newborn P52.5
        birth injury P10.3
      specified NEC I60.8
      traumatic S06.6X-
    subdural (nontraumatic) I62.00
      acute I62.01
      birth injury P10.0
      chronic I62.03
      newborn (anoxic) (hypoxic) P52.8
        birth injury P10.0
      spinal G95.19
      subacute I62.02
      traumatic —see Injury, intracranial,
          subdural hemorrhage
    traumatic —see Injury, intracranial, focal
        brain injury

Hemorrhage, hemorrhagic (Continued)
  intramedullary NEC G95.19
  intraocular —see Hemophthalmos
  intraoperative, intraprocedural —see
      Complication, hemorrhage (hematoma),
      intraoperative (intraprocedural), by site
  intrapartum —see Hemorrhage, complicating,
      delivery
  intrapelvic
    female N94.89
    male K66.1
  intraperitoneal K66.1
  intrapontine I61.3
  intraprocedural —see Complication,
      hemorrhage (hematoma), intraoperative
      (intraprocedural), by site
  intrauterine N85.7
    complicating delivery —see also Hemorrhage,
        complicating, delivery O67.9
    postpartum —see Hemorrhage, postpartum
  intraventricular I61.5
    newborn (nontraumatic) —see also Newborn,
        affected by, hemorrhage P52.3
      due to birth injury P10.2
      grade
        1 P52.0
        2 P52.1
        3 P52.21
        4 P52.22
  intravesical N32.89
  iris (postinfectional) (postinflammatory)
      (toxic) —see Hyphema
  joint (nontraumatic) —see Hemarthrosis
  kidney N28.89
  knee (joint) (nontraumatic) —see
      Hemarthrosis, knee
  labyrinth —see subcategory H83.8
  lenticular striate artery I61.0
  ligature, vessel —see Hemorrhage,
      postoperative
  liver K76.89
  lung R04.89
    newborn P26.9
      massive P26.1
      specified NEC P26.8
    tuberculous —see Tuberculosis, pulmonary
  massive umbilical, newborn P51.0
  mediastinum —see Hemorrhage, lung
  medulla I61.3
  membrane (brain) I60.8
    spinal cord —see Hemorrhage, spinal cord
  meninges, meningeal (brain) (middle) I60.8
    spinal cord —see Hemorrhage, spinal cord
  mesentery K66.1
  metritis —see Endometritis
  mouth K13.79
  mucous membrane NEC R58
    newborn P54.8
  muscle M62.89
  nail (subungual) L60.8
  nasal turbinate R04.0
    newborn P54.8
  navel, newborn P51.9
  newborn P54.9
    specified NEC P54.8
  nipple N64.59
  nose R04.0
    newborn P54.8
  omentum K66.1
  optic nerve (sheath) H47.02-
  orbit, orbital H05.23-
  ovary NEC N83.8
  oviduct N83.6
  pancreas K86.89 ◄▬
  parathyroid (gland) (spontaneous) E21.4
  parturition —see Hemorrhage, complicating,
      delivery
  penis N48.89
  pericardium, pericarditis I31.2
  peritoneum, peritoneal K66.1
  peritonsillar tissue J35.8
    due to infection J36

◄ New   ◄▬ Revised   ~~deleted~~ Deleted

Hemorrhage, hemorrhagic *(Continued)*
petechial R23.3
due to autosensitivity, erythrocyte D69.2
pituitary (gland) E23.6
pleura —*see* Hemorrhage, lung
polioencephalitis, superior E51.2
polymyositis —*see* Polymyositis
pons, pontine I61.3
posterior fossa (nontraumatic) I61.8
newborn P52.6
postmenopausal N95.0
postnasal R04.0
postoperative —*see* Complications,
postprocedural, hemorrhage, by site
postpartum NEC (following delivery of
placenta) O72.1
delayed or secondary O72.2
retained placenta O72.0
third stage O72.0
pregnancy —*see* Hemorrhage, antepartum
preretinal —*see* Hemorrhage, retina
prostate N42.1
puerperal —*see* Hemorrhage, postpartum
delayed or secondary O72.2
pulmonary R04.89
newborn P26.9
massive P26.1
specified NEC P26.8
tuberculous —*see* Tuberculosis, pulmonary
purpura (primary) D69.3
rectum (sphincter) K62.5
newborn P54.2
recurring, following initial hemorrhage at
time of injury T79.2
renal N28.89
respiratory passage or tract R04.9
specified NEC R04.89
retina, retinal (vessels) H35.6-
diabetic —*see* Diabetes, retinal, hemorrhage
retroperitoneal R58
scalp R58
scrotum N50.1
secondary (nontraumatic) R58
following initial hemorrhage at time of
injury T79.2
seminal vesicle N50.1
skin R23.3
newborn P54.5
slipped umbilical ligature P51.8
spermatic cord N50.1
spinal (cord) G95.19
newborn (birth injury) P11.5
spleen D73.5
intraoperative —*see* Complications,
intraoperative, hemorrhage, spleen
postprocedural —*see* Complications,
postprocedural, hemorrhage, spleen
stomach K92.2
newborn P54.3
ulcer —*see* Ulcer, stomach, with
hemorrhage
subarachnoid (nontraumatic) —*see*
Hemorrhage, intracranial, subarachnoid
subconjunctival —*see also* Hemorrhage,
conjunctiva
birth injury P15.3
subcortical (brain) I61.0
subcutaneous R23.3
subdiaphragmatic R58
subdural (acute) (nontraumatic) —*see*
Hemorrhage, intracranial, subdural
subependymal
newborn P52.0
with intraventricular extension P52.1
and intracerebral extension P52.22
subgaleal P12.2 ◀|||
subhyaloid —*see* Hemorrhage, retina
subperiosteal —*see* Disorder, bone, specified
type NEC
subretinal —*see* Hemorrhage, retina
subtentorial —*see* Hemorrhage, intracranial,
subdural

Hemorrhage, hemorrhagic *(Continued)*
subungual L60.8
suprarenal (capsule) (gland) E27.49
newborn P54.4
tentorium (traumatic) NEC —*see*
Hemorrhage, brain
newborn (birth injury) P10.4
testis N50.1
third stage (postpartum) O72.0
thorax —*see* Hemorrhage, lung
throat R04.1
thymus (gland) E32.8
thyroid (cyst) (gland) E07.89
tongue K14.8
tonsil J35.8
trachea —*see* Hemorrhage, lung
tracheobronchial R04.89
newborn P26.0
traumatic — code to specific injury
cerebellar —*see* Hemorrhage, brain
intracranial —*see* Hemorrhage, brain
recurring or secondary (following initial
hemorrhage at time of injury)
T79.2
tuberculous NEC —*see also* Tuberculosis,
pulmonary A15.0
tunica vaginalis N50.1
ulcer - code by site under Ulcer, with
hemorrhage K27.4
umbilicus, umbilical
cord
after birth, newborn P51.9
complicating delivery O69.5
newborn P51.9
massive P51.0
slipped ligature P51.8
stump P51.9
urethra (idiopathic) N36.8
uterus, uterine (abnormal) N93.9
climacteric N92.4
complicating delivery —*see* Hemorrhage,
complicating, delivery
dysfunctional or functional N93.8
intermenstrual (regular) N92.3
irregular N92.1
postmenopausal N95.0
postpartum —*see* Hemorrhage,
postpartum
preclimacteric or premenopausal N92.4
prepubertal N93.8
pubertal N92.2
vagina (abnormal) N93.9
newborn P54.6
vas deferens N50.1
vasa previa O69.4
ventricular I61.5
vesical N32.89
viscera NEC R58
newborn P54.8
vitreous (humor) (intraocular) H43.1-
vulva N90.89
Hemorrhoids (bleeding) (without mention of
degree) K64.9
1st degree (grade/stage I) (without prolapse
outside of anal canal) K64.0
2nd degree (grade/stage II) (that
prolapse with straining but retract
spontaneously) K64.1
3rd degree (grade/stage III) (that prolapse
with straining and require manual
replacement back inside anal canal)
K64.2
4th degree (grade/stage IV) (with prolapsed
tissue that cannot be manually replaced)
K64.3
complicating
pregnancy O22.4
puerperium O87.2
external K64.4
with
thrombosis K64.5

Hemorrhoids *(Continued)*
internal (without mention of degree) K64.8
prolapsed K64.8
skin tags
anus K64.4
residual K64.4
specified NEC K64.8
strangulated —*see also* Hemorrhoids, by
degree K64.8
thrombosed —*see also* Hemorrhoids, by
degree K64.5
ulcerated —*see also* Hemorrhoids, by degree
K64.8
Hemosalpinx N83.6
with
hematocolpos N89.7
hematometra N85.7
with hematocolpos N89.7
Hemosiderosis (dietary) E83.19
pulmonary, idiopathic E83.1 *[J84.03]*
transfusion T80.89
Hemothorax (bacterial) (nontuberculous) J94.2
newborn P54.8
traumatic S27.1
with pneumothorax S27.2
tuberculous NEC A15.6
Henoch (-Schönlein) disease or syndrome
(purpura) D69.0
Henpue, henpuye A66.6
Hepar lobatum (syphilitic) A52.74
Hepatalgia K76.89
Hepatitis K75.9
acute B17.9
with coma K72.01
with hepatic failure —*see* Failure, hepatic
alcoholic —*see* Hepatitis, alcoholic
infectious B15.9 ◀|||
~~with hepatic coma B15.0~~
non-viral K72.0 ◀
viral B17.9
alcoholic (acute) (chronic) K70.10
with ascites K70.11
amebic —*see* Abscess, liver, amebic
anicteric (viral) —*see* Hepatitis, viral
antigen-associated (HAA) —*see* Hepatitis, B
Australia-antigen (positive) —*see* Hepatitis, B
autoimmune K75.4
B B19.10
with hepatic coma B19.11
acute B16.9
with
delta-agent (coinfection) (without
hepatic coma) B16.1
with hepatic coma B16.0
hepatic coma (without delta-agent
coinfection) B16.2
chronic B18.1
with delta-agent B18.0
bacterial NEC K75.89
C (viral) B19.20
with hepatic coma B19.21
acute B17.10
with hepatic coma B17.11
chronic B18.2
catarrhal (acute) B15.9
with hepatic coma B15.0
cholangiolitic K75.89
cholestatic K75.89
chronic K73.9
active NEC K73.2
lobular NEC K73.1
persistent NEC K73.0
specified NEC K73.8
cytomegaloviral B25.1
due to ethanol (acute) (chronic) —*see*
Hepatitis, alcoholic
epidemic B15.9
with hepatic coma B15.0
fulminant NEC (viral) —*see* Hepatitis, viral
granulomatous NEC K75.3
herpesviral B00.81

Hepatitis *(Continued)*
history of
B Z86.19
C Z86.19
homologous serum —*see* Hepatitis, viral,
type B
in (due to)
mumps B26.81
toxoplasmosis (acquired) B58.1
congenital (active) P37.1 *[K77]*
infectious, infective B15.9 ◄▬
with hepatic coma B15.0
acute (subacute) B17.9 ◄
chronic B18.9 ◄
inoculation —*see* Hepatitis, viral, type B
interstitial (chronic) K74.69
lupoid NEC K75.2
malignant NEC (with hepatic failure)
K72.90
with coma K72.91
neonatal giant cell P59.29
neonatal (idiopathic) (toxic) P59.29
newborn P59.29
postimmunization —*see* Hepatitis, viral,
type B
post-transfusion —*see* Hepatitis, viral, type B
reactive, nonspecific K75.2
serum —*see* Hepatitis, viral, type B
specified type NEC
with hepatic failure —*see* Failure, hepatic
syphilitic (late) A52.74
congenital (early) A50.08 *[K77]*
late A50.59 *[K77]*
secondary A51.45
toxic —*see also* Disease, liver, toxic K71.6
tuberculous A18.83
viral, virus B19.9
with hepatic coma B19.0
acute B17.9
chronic B18.9
specified NEC B18.8
type
B B18.1
with delta-agent B18.0
C B18.2
congenital P35.3
coxsackie B33.8 *[K77]*
cytomegalic inclusion B25.1
in remission, any type — code to Hepatitis,
chronic, by type
non-A, non-B B17.8
specified type NEC (with or without coma)
B17.8
type
A B15.9
with hepatic coma B15.0
B B19.10
with hepatic coma B19.11
acute B16.9
with
delta-agent (coinfection) (without
hepatic coma) B16.1
with hepatic coma B16.0
hepatic coma (without delta-
agent coinfection) B16.2
chronic B18.1
with delta-agent B18.0
C B19.20
with hepatic coma B19.21
acute B17.10
with hepatic coma B17.11
chronic B18.2
E B17.2
non-A, non-B B17.8
Hepatization lung (acute) —*see* Pneumonia,
lobar
Hepatoblastoma C22.2
Hepatocarcinoma C22.0
Hepatocholangiocarcinoma C22.0
Hepatocholangioma, benign D13.4
Hepatocholangitis K75.89

Hepatolenticular degeneration E83.01
Hepatoma (malignant) C22.0
benign D13.4
embryonal C22.0
Hepatomegaly —*see also* Hypertrophy, liver
with splenomegaly R16.2
congenital Q44.7
in mononucleosis
gammaherpesviral B27.09
infectious specified NEC B27.89
Hepatoptosis K76.89
Hepatorenal syndrome following labor and
delivery O90.4
Hepatosis K76.89
Hepatosplenomegaly R16.2
hyperlipemic (Bürger-Grütz type) E78.3 *[K77]*
Hereditary —*see* condition
Heredodegeneration, macular —*see* Dystrophy,
retina
Heredopathia atactica polyneuritiformis G60.1
Heredosyphilis —*see* Syphilis, congenital
Herlitz' syndrome Q81.1
Hermansky-Pudlak syndrome E70.331
Hermaphrodite, hermaphroditism (true) Q56.0
46,XX with streak gonads Q99.1
46,XX/46,XY Q99.0
46,XY with streak gonads Q99.1
chimera 46,XX/46,XY Q99.0
Hernia, hernial (acquired) (recurrent) K46.9
with
gangrene —*see* Hernia, by site, with,
gangrene
incarceration —*see* Hernia, by site, with,
obstruction
irreducible —*see* Hernia, by site, with,
obstruction
obstruction —*see* Hernia, by site, with,
obstruction
strangulation —*see* Hernia, by site, with,
obstruction
abdomen, abdominal K46.9
with
gangrene (and obstruction) K46.1
obstruction K46.0
femoral —*see* Hernia, femoral
incisional —*see* Hernia, incisional
inguinal —*see* Hernia, inguinal
specified site NEC K45.8
with
gangrene (and obstruction) K45.1
obstruction K45.0
umbilical —*see* Hernia, umbilical
wall —*see* Hernia, ventral
appendix —*see* Hernia, abdomen
bladder (mucosa) (sphincter)
congenital (female) (male) Q79.51
female —*see* Cystocele
male N32.89
brain, congenital —*see* Encephalocele
cartilage, vertebra —*see* Displacement,
intervertebral disc
cerebral, congenital —*see also* Encephalocele
endaural Q01.8
ciliary body (traumatic) S05.2-
colon —*see* Hernia, abdomen
Cooper's —*see* Hernia, abdomen, specified
site NEC
crural —*see* Hernia, femoral
diaphragm, diaphragmatic K44.9
with
gangrene (and obstruction) K44.1
obstruction K44.0
congenital Q79.0
direct (inguinal) —*see* Hernia, inguinal
diverticulum, intestine —*see* Hernia,
abdomen
double (inguinal) —*see* Hernia, inguinal,
bilateral
due to adhesions (with obstruction) K56.5
epigastric —*see also* Hernia, ventral K43.9
esophageal hiatus —*see* Hernia, hiatal

Hernia, hernial *(Continued)*
external (inguinal) —*see* Hernia, inguinal
fallopian tube N83.4- ◄▬
fascia M62.89
femoral K41.90
with
gangrene (and obstruction) K41.40
not specified as recurrent K41.40
recurrent K41.41
obstruction K41.30
not specified as recurrent K41.30
recurrent K41.31
bilateral K41.20
with
gangrene (and obstruction) K41.10
not specified as recurrent K41.10
recurrent K41.11
obstruction K41.00
not specified as recurrent K41.00
recurrent K41.01
not specified as recurrent K41.20
recurrent K41.21
not specified as recurrent K41.90
recurrent K41.91
unilateral K41.90
with
gangrene (and obstruction) K41.40
not specified as recurrent K41.40
recurrent K41.41
obstruction K41.30
not specified as recurrent K41.30
recurrent K41.31
not specified as recurrent K41.90
recurrent K41.91
foramen magnum G93.5
congenital Q01.8
funicular (umbilical) —*see also* Hernia,
umbilicus
spermatic (cord) —*see* Hernia, inguinal
gastrointestinal tract —*see* Hernia, abdomen
Hesselbach's —*see* Hernia, femoral, specified
site NEC
hiatal (esophageal) (sliding) K44.9
with
gangrene (and obstruction) K44.1
obstruction K44.0
congenital Q40.1
hypogastric —*see* Hernia, ventral
incarcerated —*see also* Hernia, by site, with
obstruction
with gangrene —*see* Hernia, by site, with
gangrene
incisional K43.92
with
gangrene (and obstruction) K43.1
obstruction K43.0
indirect (inguinal) —*see* Hernia, inguinal
inguinal (direct) (external) (funicular)
(indirect) (internal) (oblique) (scrotal)
(sliding) K40.90
with
gangrene (and obstruction) K40.40
not specified as recurrent K40.40
recurrent K40.41
obstruction K40.30
not specified as recurrent K40.30
recurrent K40.31
bilateral K40.20
with
gangrene (and obstruction)
K40.10
not specified as recurrent
K40.10
recurrent K40.11
obstruction K40.00
not specified as recurrent K40.00
recurrent K40.01
not specified as recurrent K40.20
recurrent K40.21
not specified as recurrent K40.90
recurrent K40.91

◄ New ◄▬ Revised ~~deleted~~ Deleted

Hernia, hernial (Continued)
  inguinal (Continued)
    unilateral K40.90
      with
        gangrene (and obstruction) K40.40
          not specified as recurrent K40.40
          recurrent K40.41
        obstruction K40.30
          not specified as recurrent K40.30
          recurrent K40.31
      not specified as recurrent K40.90
      recurrent K40.91
  internal —see also Hernia, abdomen
    inguinal —see Hernia, inguinal
  interstitial —see Hernia, abdomen
  intervertebral cartilage or disc —see
      Displacement, intervertebral disc
  intestine, intestinal —see Hernia, by site
  intra-abdominal —see Hernia, abdomen
  iris (traumatic) S05.2-
  irreducible —see also Hernia, by site, with
      obstruction
    with gangrene —see Hernia, by site, with
        gangrene
  ischiatic —see Hernia, abdomen, specified
      site NEC
  ischiorectal —see Hernia, abdomen, specified
      site NEC
  lens (traumatic) S05.2-
  linea (alba) (semilunaris) —see Hernia,
      ventral
  Littre's —see Hernia, abdomen
  lumbar —see Hernia, abdomen, specified site
      NEC
  lung (subcutaneous) J98.4
  mediastinum J98.59 ◄⫶⫶
  mesenteric (internal) —see Hernia, abdomen
  midline —see Hernia, ventral
  muscle (sheath) M62.89
  nucleus pulposus —see Displacement,
      intervertebral disc
  oblique (inguinal) —see Hernia, inguinal
  obstructive —see also Hernia, by site, with
      obstruction
    with gangrene —see Hernia, by site, with
        gangrene
  obturator —see Hernia, abdomen, specified
      site NEC
  omental —see Hernia, abdomen
  ovary N83.4- ◄⫶⫶
  oviduct N83.4- ◄⫶⫶
  paraesophageal —see also Hernia, diaphragm
    congenital Q40.1
  parastomal K43.5
    with
      gangrene (and obstruction) K43.4
      obstruction K43.3
  paraumbilical —see Hernia, umbilicus
  perineal —see Hernia, abdomen, specified
      site NEC
  Petit's —see Hernia, abdomen, specified site
      NEC
  postoperative —see Hernia, incisional
  pregnant uterus —see Abnormal, uterus in
      pregnancy or childbirth
  prevesical N32.89
  properitoneal —see Hernia, abdomen,
      specified site NEC
  pudendal —see Hernia, abdomen, specified
      site NEC
  rectovaginal N81.6
  retroperitoneal —see Hernia, abdomen,
      specified site NEC
  Richter's —see Hernia, abdomen, with
      obstruction
  Rieux's, Riex's —see Hernia, abdomen,
      specified site NEC
  sac condition (adhesion) (dropsy)
      (inflammation) (laceration)
      (suppuration) - code by site under
      Hernia

Hernia, hernial (Continued)
  sciatic —see Hernia, abdomen, specified site
      NEC
  scrotum, scrotal —see Hernia, inguinal
  sliding (inguinal) —see also Hernia,
      inguinal
    hiatus —see Hernia, hiatal
  spigelian —see Hernia, ventral
  spinal —see Spina bifida
  strangulated —see also Hernia, by site, with
      obstruction
    with gangrene —see Hernia, by site, with
        gangrene
  subxiphoid —see Hernia, ventral
  supra-umbilicus —see Hernia, ventral
  tendon —see Disorder, tendon, specified type
      NEC
  Treitz's (fossa) —see Hernia, abdomen,
      specified site NEC
  tunica vaginalis Q55.29
  umbilicus, umbilical K42.9
    with
      gangrene (and obstruction) K42.1
      obstruction K42.0
  ureter N28.89
  urethra, congenital Q64.79
  urinary meatus, congenital Q64.79
  uterus N81.4
    pregnant —see Abnormal, uterus in
        pregnancy or childbirth
  vaginal (anterior) (wall) —see Cystocele
  Velpeau's —see Hernia, femoral
  ventral K43.9
    with
      gangrene (and obstruction) K43.7
      obstruction K43.6
    incisional K43.2
      with
        gangrene (and obstruction) K43.1
        obstruction K43.0
      recurrent —see Hernia, incisional
    specified NEC K43.9
      with
        gangrene (and obstruction) K43.7
        obstruction K43.6
  vesical
    congenital (female) (male) Q79.51
    female —see Cystocele
    male N32.89
  vitreous (into wound) S05.2-
    into anterior chamber —see Prolapse,
        vitreous
Herniation —see also Hernia
  brain (stem) G93.5
  cerebral G93.5
  mediastinum J98.59 ◄⫶⫶
  nucleus pulposus —see Displacement,
      intervertebral disc
Herpangina B08.5
Herpes, herpesvirus, herpetic B00.9
  anogenital A60.9
    perianal skin A60.1
    rectum A60.1
    urogenital tract A60.00
      cervix A60.03
      male genital organ NEC A60.02
      penis A60.01
      specified site NEC A60.09
      vagina A60.04
      vulva A60.04
  blepharitis (zoster) B02.39
    simplex B00.59
  circinatus B35.4
    bullosus L12.0
  conjunctivitis (simplex) B00.53
    zoster B02.31
  cornea B02.33
  encephalitis B00.4
    due to herpesvirus 6 B10.01
    due to herpesvirus 7 B10.09
    specified NEC B10.09

Herpes, herpesvirus, herpetic (Continued)
  eye (zoster) B02.30
    simplex B00.50
  eyelid (zoster) B02.39
    simplex B00.59
  facialis B00.1
  febrilis B00.1
  geniculate ganglionitis B02.21
  genital, genitalis A60.00
    female A60.09
    male A60.02
  gestational, gestationis O26.4-
  gingivostomatitis B00.2
  human B00.9
    1 —see Herpes, simplex
    2 —see Herpes, simplex
    3 —see Varicella
    4 —see Mononucleosis, Epstein-Barr (virus)
    5 —see Disease, cytomegalic inclusion
        (generalized)
    6
      encephalitis B10.01
      specified NEC B10.81
    7
      encephalitis B10.09
      specified NEC B10.82
    8 B10.89
  infection NEC B10.89
    Kaposi's sarcoma associated B10.89
  iridocyclitis (simplex) B00.51
    zoster B02.32
  iris (vesicular erythema multiforme) L51.9
  iritis (simplex) B00.51
  Kaposi's sarcoma associated B10.89
  keratitis (simplex) (dendritic) (disciform)
      (interstitial) B00.52
    zoster (interstitial) B02.33
  keratoconjunctivitis (simplex) B00.52
    zoster B02.33
  labialis B00.1
  lip B00.1
  meningitis (simplex) B00.3
    zoster B02.1
  ophthalmicus (zoster) NEC B02.30
    simplex B00.50
  penis A60.01
  perianal skin A60.1
  pharyngitis, pharyngotonsillitis B00.2
  rectum A60.1
  scrotum A60.02
  sepsis B00.7
  simplex B00.9
    complicated NEC B00.89
    congenital P35.2
    conjunctivitis B00.53
    external ear B00.1
    eyelid B00.59
    hepatitis B00.81
    keratitis (interstitial) B00.52
    myelitis B00.82
    specified complication NEC B00.89
    visceral B00.89
  stomatitis B00.2
  tonsurans B35.0
  visceral B00.89
  vulva A60.04
  whitlow B00.89
  zoster —see also condition B02.9
    auricularis B02.21
    complicated NEC B02.8
    conjunctivitis B02.31
    disseminated B02.7
    encephalitis B02.0
    eye(lid) B02.39
    geniculate ganglionitis B02.21
    keratitis (interstitial) B02.33
    meningitis B02.1
    myelitis B02.24
    neuritis, neuralgia B02.29
    ophthalmicus NEC B02.30
    oticus B02.21

Herpes, herpesvirus, herpetic (Continued)
  zoster (Continued)
    polyneuropathy B02.23
    specified complication NEC B02.8
    trigeminal neuralgia B02.22
Herpesvirus (human) —see Herpes
Herpetophobia F40.218
Herrick's anemia —see Disease, sickle-cell
Hers' disease E74.09
Herter-Gee syndrome K90.0
Herxheimer's reaction R68.89
Hesitancy
  of micturition R39.11
  urinary R39.11
Hesselbach's hernia —see Hernia, femoral,
    specified site NEC
Heterochromia (congenital) Q13.2
  cataract —see Cataract, complicated
  cyclitis (Fuchs) —see Cyclitis, Fuchs'
    heterochromic
  hair L67.1
  iritis —see Cyclitis, Fuchs' heterochromic
  retained metallic foreign body
    (nonmagnetic) —see Foreign body,
    intraocular, old, retained
    magnetic —see Foreign body, intraocular,
    old, retained, magnetic
  uveitis —see Cyclitis, Fuchs' heterochromic
Heterophoria —see Strabismus, heterophoria
Heterophyes, heterophyiasis (small intestine)
    B66.8
Heterotopia, heterotopic —see also Malposition,
    congenital
  cerebralis Q04.8
Heterotropia —see Strabismus
Heubner-Herter disease K90.0
Hexadactylism Q69.9
HGSIL (cytology finding) (high grade
    squamous intraepithelial lesion on
    cytologic smear) (Pap smear finding)
  anus R85.613
  cervix R87.613
    biopsy (histology) finding — see Neoplasia,
      intraepithelial, cervix, grade II or
      grade III
  vagina R87.623
    biopsy (histology) finding — see Neoplasia,
      intraepithelial, vagina, grade II or
      grade III
Hibernoma —see Lipoma
Hiccup, hiccough R06.6
  epidemic B33.0
  psychogenic F45.8
Hidden penis (congenital) Q55.64
  acquired N48.83
Hidradenitis (axillaris) (suppurative) L73.2
Hidradenoma (nodular) —see also Neoplasm,
    skin, benign
  clear cell —see Neoplasm, skin, benign
  papillary —see Neoplasm, skin, benign
Hidrocystoma —see Neoplasm, skin, benign
High
  altitude effects T70.20
    anoxia T70.29
    on
      ears T70.0
      sinuses T70.1
    polycythemia D75.1
  arch
    foot Q66.7
    palate, congenital Q38.5
  arterial tension —see Hypertension
  basal metabolic rate R94.8
  blood pressure —see also Hypertension
    borderline R03.0
    reading (incidental) (isolated)
      (nonspecific), without diagnosis of
      hypertension R03.0
  cholesterol E78.00
    with high triglycerides E78.2
  diaphragm (congenital) Q79.1

High (Continued)
  expressed emotional level within family
    Z63.8
  head at term O32.4
  palate, congenital Q38.5
  risk
    infant NEC Z76.2
    sexual behavior (heterosexual) Z72.51
      bisexual Z72.53
      homosexual Z72.52
  temperature (of unknown origin) R50.9
  thoracic rib Q76.6
  triglycerides E78.1
    with high cholesterol E78.2
Hildenbrand's disease A75.0
Hilum —see condition
Hip —see condition
Hippel's disease Q85.8
Hippophobia F40.218
Hippus H57.09
Hirschsprung's disease or megacolon Q43.1
Hirsutism, hirsuties L68.0
Hirudiniasis
  external B88.3
  internal B83.4
Hiss-Russell dysentery A03.1
Histidinemia, histidinuria E70.41
Histiocytoma —see also Neoplasm, skin, benign
  fibrous —see also Neoplasm, skin, benign
    atypical —see Neoplasm, connective tissue,
      uncertain behavior
    malignant —see Neoplasm, connective
      tissue, malignant
Histiocytosis D76.3
  acute differentiated progressive C96.0
  Langerhans' cell NEC C96.6
    multifocal X
      multisystemic (disseminated) C96.0
      unisystemic C96.5
    pulmonary, adult (adult PLCH) J84.82
    unifocal (X) C96.6
  lipid, lipoid D76.3
    essential E75.29
  malignant C96.A
  mononuclear phagocytes NEC D76.1
    Langerhans' cells C96.6
  non-Langerhans cell D76.3
  polyostotic sclerosing D76.3
  sinus, with massive lymphadenopathy
    D76.3
  syndrome NEC D76.3
  X NEC C96.6
    acute (progressive) C96.0
    chronic C96.6
    multifocal C96.5
    multisystemic C96.0
    unifocal C96.6
Histoplasmosis B39.9
  with pneumonia NEC B39.2
  African B39.5
  American —see Histoplasmosis, capsulati
  capsulati B39.4
    disseminated B39.3
    generalized B39.3
    pulmonary B39.2
      acute B39.0
      chronic B39.1
  Darling's B39.4
  duboisii B39.5
  lung NEC B39.2
History
  family (of) —see also History, personal (of)
    alcohol abuse Z81.1
    allergy NEC Z84.89
    anemia Z83.2
    arthritis Z82.61
    asthma Z82.5
    blindness Z82.1
    cardiac death (sudden) Z82.41
    carrier of genetic disease Z84.81
    chromosomal anomaly Z82.79

History (Continued)
  family (Continued)
    chronic
      disabling disease NEC Z82.8
      lower respiratory disease Z82.5
    colonic polyps Z83.71
    congenital malformations and
      deformations Z82.79
      polycystic kidney Z82.71
    consanguinity Z84.3
    deafness Z82.2
    diabetes mellitus Z83.3
    disability NEC Z82.8
    disease or disorder (of)
      allergic NEC Z84.89
      behavioral NEC Z81.8
      blood and blood-forming organs Z83.2
      cardiovascular NEC Z82.49
      chronic disabling NEC Z82.8
      digestive Z83.79
      ear NEC Z83.52
      endocrine NEC Z83.49
      eye NEC Z83.518
        glaucoma Z83.511
      familial hypercholesterolemia Z83.42 ◀
      genitourinary NEC Z84.2
      glaucoma Z83.511
      hematological Z83.2
      immune mechanism Z83.2
      infectious NEC Z83.1
      ischemic heart Z82.49
      kidney Z84.1
      mental NEC Z81.8
      metabolic Z83.49
      musculoskeletal NEC Z82.69
      neurological NEC Z82.0
      nutritional Z83.49
      parasitic NEC Z83.1
      psychiatric NEC Z81.8
      respiratory NEC Z83.6
      skin and subcutaneous tissue NEC Z84.0
      specified NEC Z84.89
    drug abuse NEC Z81.3
    epilepsy Z82.0
    familial hypercholesterolemia Z83.42 ◀
    genetic disease carrier Z84.81
    glaucoma Z83.511
    hearing loss Z82.2
    human immunodeficiency virus (HIV)
      infection Z83.0
    Huntington's chorea Z82.0
    intellectual disability Z81.0
    leukemia Z80.6
    malignant neoplasm (of) NOS Z80.9
      bladder Z80.52
      breast Z80.3
      bronchus Z80.1
      digestive organ Z80.0
      gastrointestinal tract Z80.0
      genital organ Z80.49
        ovary Z80.41
        prostate Z80.42
        specified organ NEC Z80.49
        testis Z80.43
      hematopoietic NEC Z80.7
      intrathoracic organ NEC Z80.2
      kidney Z80.51
      lung Z80.1
      lymphatic NEC Z80.7
      ovary Z80.41
      prostate Z80.42
      respiratory organ NEC Z80.2
      specified site NEC Z80.8
      testis Z80.43
      trachea Z80.1
      urinary organ or tract Z80.59
        bladder Z80.52
        kidney Z80.51
    mental
      disorder NEC Z81.8
    multiple endocrine neoplasia (MEN)
      syndrome Z83.41

◀ New   ◀▥ Revised   ~~deleted~~ Deleted

History *(Continued)*
  family *(Continued)*
    osteoporosis Z82.62
    polycystic kidney Z82.71
    polyps (colon) Z83.71
    psychiatric disorder Z81.8
    psychoactive substance abuse NEC Z81.3
    respiratory condition NEC Z83.6
      asthma and other lower respiratory
        conditions Z82.5
    self-harmful behavior Z81.8
    SIDS (sudden infant death syndrome)
      Z84.82 ◀
    skin condition Z84.0
    specified condition NEC Z84.89
    stroke (cerebrovascular) Z82.3
    substance abuse NEC Z81.4
      alcohol Z81.1
      drug NEC Z81.3
      psychoactive NEC Z81.3
      tobacco Z81.2
    sudden cardiac death Z82.41
    sudden ◀
      cardiac death Z82.41 ◀
      infant death syndrome (SIDS) Z84.82 ◀
    tobacco abuse Z81.2
    violence, violent behavior Z81.8
    visual loss Z82.1
  personal (of) —*see also* History, family (of)
    abuse
      adult Z91.419
        physical and sexual Z91.410
        psychological Z91.411
      childhood Z62.819
        physical Z62.810
        psychological Z62.811
        sexual Z62.810
    alcohol dependence F10.21
    allergy (to) Z88.9
      analgesic agent NEC Z88.6
      anesthetic Z88.4
      antibiotic agent NEC Z88.1
      anti-infective agent NEC Z88.3
      contrast media Z91.041
      drugs, medicaments and biological
        substances Z88.9
        specified NEC Z88.8
      food Z91.018
        additives Z91.02
        eggs Z91.012
        milk products Z91.011
        peanuts Z91.010
        seafood Z91.013
        specified food NEC Z91.018
      insect Z91.038
        bee Z91.030
      latex Z91.040
      medicinal agents Z88.9
        specified NEC Z88.8
      narcotic agent NEC Z88.5
      nonmedicinal agents Z91.048
      penicillin Z88.0
      serum Z88.7
      specified NEC Z91.09
      sulfonamides Z88.2
      vaccine Z88.7
    anaphylactic shock Z87.892
    anaphylaxis Z87.892
    behavioral disorders Z86.59
    benign carcinoid tumor Z86.012
    benign neoplasm Z86.018
      brain Z86.011
      carcinoid Z86.012
      colonic polyps Z86.010
    brain injury (traumatic) Z87.820
    breast implant removal Z98.86
    calculi, renal Z87.442
    cancer —*see* History, personal (of),
      malignant neoplasm (of)
    cardiac arrest (death), successfully
      resuscitated Z86.74

History *(Continued)*
  personal *(Continued)*
    cerebral infarction without residual deficit
      Z86.73
    cervical dysplasia Z87.410
    chemotherapy for neoplastic condition
      Z92.21
    childhood abuse —*see* History, personal
      (of), abuse
    cleft lip (corrected) Z87.730
    cleft palate (corrected) Z87.730
    collapsed vertebra (healed) Z87.311
      due to osteoporosis Z87.310
    combat and operational stress reaction
      Z86.51
    congenital malformation (corrected)
      Z87.798
      circulatory system (corrected) Z87.74
      digestive system (corrected) NEC
        Z87.738
      ear (corrected) Z87.720
      eye (corrected) Z87.721
      face and neck (corrected) Z87.790
      genitourinary system (corrected) NEC
        Z87.718
      heart (corrected) Z87.74
      integument (corrected) Z87.76
      limb (s) (corrected) Z87.76
      musculoskeletal system (corrected)
        Z87.76
      neck (corrected) Z87.790
      nervous system (corrected) NEC
        Z87.728
      respiratory system (corrected) Z87.75
      sense organs (corrected) NEC Z87.728
      specified NEC Z87.798
    contraception Z92.0
    deployment (military) Z91.82
    diabetic foot ulcer Z86.31
    disease or disorder (of) Z87.898
      blood and blood-forming organs Z86.2
      circulatory system Z86.79
        specified condition NEC Z86.79
      connective tissue NEC Z87.39
      digestive system Z87.19
        colonic polyp Z86.010
        peptic ulcer disease Z87.11
        specified condition NEC Z87.19
      ear Z86.69
      endocrine Z86.39
        diabetic foot ulcer Z86.31
        gestational diabetes Z86.32
        specified type NEC Z86.39
      eye Z86.69
      genital (track) system NEC
        female Z87.42
        male Z87.438
      hematological Z86.2
      Hodgkin Z85.71
      immune mechanism Z86.2
      infectious Z86.19
        malaria Z86.13
        Methicillin resistant Staphylococcus
          aureus (MRSA) Z86.14
        poliomyelitis Z86.12
        specified NEC Z86.19
        tuberculosis Z86.11
      mental NEC Z86.59
      metabolic Z86.39
        diabetic foot ulcer Z86.31
        gestational diabetes Z86.32
        specified type NEC Z86.39
      musculoskeletal NEC Z87.39
      nervous system Z86.69
      nutritional Z86.39
      parasitic Z86.19
      respiratory system NEC Z87.09
      sense organs Z86.69
      skin Z87.2
      specified site or type NEC Z87.898
      subcutaneous tissue Z87.2

History *(Continued)*
  personal *(Continued)*
    disease or disorder (of) *(Continued)*
      trophoblastic Z87.59
      urinary system NEC Z87.448
    drug dependence —*see* Dependence, drug,
      by type, in remission
    drug therapy
      antineoplastic chemotherapy Z92.21
      estrogen Z92.23
      immunosupression Z92.25
      inhaled steroids Z92.240
      monoclonal drug Z92.22
      specified NEC Z92.29
      steroid Z92.241
      systemic steroids Z92.241
    dysplasia
      cervical (mild) (moderate) Z87.410 ◀
        severe (grade III) Z86.001 ◀
      prostatic Z87.430
      vaginal Z87.411
      vulvar (mild) (moderate) Z87.412 ◀
        severe (grade III) Z86.008 ◀
    embolism (venous) Z86.718
      pulmonary Z86.711
    encephalitis Z86.61
    estrogen therapy Z92.23
    extracorporeal membrane oxygenation
      (ECMO) Z92.81
    failed conscious sedation Z92.83
    failed moderate sedation Z92.83
    fall, falling Z91.81
    fracture (healed)
      fatigue Z87.312
      fragility Z87.310
      osteoporosis Z87.310
      pathological NEC Z87.311
      stress Z87.312
      traumatic Z87.81
    gestational diabetes Z86.32
    hepatitis
      B Z86.19
      C Z86.19
    Hodgkin disease Z85.71
    hyperthermia, malignant Z88.4
    hypospadias (corrected) Z87.710
    hysterectomy Z90.710
    immunosupression therapy Z92.25
    in situ neoplasm
      breast Z86.000
      cervix uteri Z86.001
      specified NEC Z86.008
    infection NEC Z86.19
      central nervous system Z86.61
      Methicillin resistant Staphylococcus
        aureus (MRSA) Z86.14
      urinary (tract) Z87.41
    injury NEC Z87.828
    in utero procedure during pregnancy
      Z98.870
    in utero procedure while a fetus Z98.871
    irradiation Z92.3
    kidney stones Z87.442
    leukemia Z85.6
    lymphoma (non-Hodgkin) Z85.72
    malignant melanoma (skin) Z85.820
    malignant neoplasm (of) Z85.9
      accessory sinuses Z85.22
      anus NEC Z85.048
        carcinoid Z85.040
      bladder Z85.51
      bone Z85.830
      brain Z85.841
      breast Z85.3
      bronchus NEC Z85.118
        carcinoid Z85.110
      carcinoid —*see* History, personal (of),
        malignant neoplasm, by site,
        carcinioid
      cervix Z85.41
      colon NEC Z85.038
        carcinoid Z85.030

History *(Continued)*
  personal *(Continued)*
    malignant neoplasm *(Continued)*
      digestive organ Z85.00
        specified NEC Z85.09
      endocrine gland NEC Z85.858
      epididymis Z85.48
      esophagus Z85.01
      eye Z85.840
      gastrointestinal tract —*see* History, malignant neoplasm, digestive organ
      genital organ
        female Z85.40
          specified NEC Z85.44
        male Z85.45
          specified NEC Z85.49
      hematopoietic NEC Z85.79
      intrathoracic organ Z85.20-
      kidney NEC Z85.528
        carcinoid Z85.520
      large intestine NEC Z85.038
        carcinoid Z85.030
      larynx Z85.21
      liver Z85.05
      lung NEC Z85.118
        carcinoid Z85.110
      mediastinum Z85.29
      Merkel cell Z85.821
      middle ear Z85.22
      nasal cavities Z85.22
      nervous system NEC Z85.848
      oral cavity Z85.819
        specified site NEC Z85.818
      ovary Z85.43
      pancreas Z85.07
      pelvis Z85.53
      pharynx Z85.819
        specified site NEC Z85.818
      pleura Z85.29
      prostate Z85.46
      rectosigmoid junction NEC Z85.048
        carcinoid Z85.040
      rectum NEC Z85.048
        carcinoid Z85.040
      respiratory organ Z85.20
      sinuses, accessory Z85.22
      skin NEC Z85.828
        melanoma Z85.820
        Merkel cell Z85.821
      small intestine NEC Z85.068
        carcinoid Z85.060
      soft tissue Z85.831
      specified site NEC Z85.89
      stomach NEC Z85.028
        carcinoid Z85.020
      testis Z85.47
      thymus NEC Z85.238
        carcinoid Z85.230
      thyroid Z85.850
      tongue Z85.810
      trachea Z85.12
      ureter Z85.54
      urinary organ or tract Z85.50
        specified NEC Z85.59
      uterus Z85.42
    maltreatment Z91.89
    medical treatment NEC Z92.89
    melanoma (malignant) (skin) Z85.820
    meningitis Z86.61
    mental disorder Z86.59
    Merkel cell carcinoma (skin) Z85.821
    Methicillin resistant Staphylococcus aureus (MRSA) Z86.14
    military deployment Z91.82
    military war, peacekeeping and humanitarian deployment (current or past conflict) Z91.82
    myocardial infarction (old) I25.2
    neglect (in)
      adult Z91.412
      childhood Z62.812

History *(Continued)*
  personal *(Continued)*
    neoplasm
      benign Z86.018
        brain Z86.011
        colon polyp Z86.010
      in situ
        breast Z86.000
        cervix uteri Z86.001
        specified NEC Z86.008
      malignant —*see* History of, malignant neoplasm
      uncertain behavior Z86.03
    nephrotic syndrome Z87.441
    nicotine dependence Z87.891
    noncompliance with medical treatment or regimen —*see* Noncompliance
    nutritional deficiency Z86.39
    obstetric complications Z87.59
      childbirth Z87.59
      pregnancy Z87.59
      pre-term labor Z87.51
      puerperium Z87.59
    osteoporosis fractures Z87.31
    parasuicide (attempt) Z91.5
    physical trauma NEC Z87.828
      self-harm or suicide attempt Z91.5
    pneumonia (recurrent) Z87.01
    poisoning NEC Z91.89
      self-harm or suicide attempt Z91.5
    poor personal hygiene Z91.89
    preterm labor Z87.51
    procedure during pregnancy Z98.870
    procedure while a fetus Z98.871
    prolonged reversible ischemic neurologic deficit (PRINO) Z86.73
    prostatic dysplasia Z87.430
    psychiatric disorder NEC Z87.89
    psychological
      abuse
        adult Z91.411
        child Z62.811
      trauma, specified NEC Z91.49
    radiation therapy Z92.3
    removal
      implant
        breast Z98.86
    renal calculi Z87.442
    respiratory condition NEC Z87.09
    retained foreign body fully removed Z87.821
    risk factors NEC Z91.89
    self-harm Z91.5
    self-poisoning attempt Z91.5
    sex reassignment Z87.890
    sleep-wake cycle problem Z72.821
    specified NEC Z87.898
    steroid therapy (systemic) Z92.241
      inhaled Z92.240
    stroke without residual deficits Z86.73
    substance abuse NEC F10-F19 with fifth character 1
    sudden cardiac arrest Z86.74
    sudden cardiac death successfully resuscitated Z86.74
    suicide attempt Z91.5
    surgery NEC Z98.890 ◀▥
      with uterine scar Z98.891 ◀
      sex reassignment Z87.890
      transplant —*see* Transplant
    thrombophlebitis Z86.72
    thrombosis (venous) Z86.718
      pulmonary Z86.711
    tobacco dependence Z87.891
    transient ischemic attack (TIA) without residual deficits Z86.73
    trauma (physical) NEC Z87.828
      psychological NEC Z91.49
      self-harm Z91.5
    traumatic brain injury Z87.820
    unhealthy sleep-wake cycle Z72.821

History *(Continued)*
  personal *(Continued)*
    unintended awareness under general anesthesia Z92.84 ◀
    urinary (recurrent) (tract) infection (s) Z87.440
    urinary calculi Z87.42
    uterine scar from previous surgery Z98.891 ◀
    vaginal dysplasia Z87.411
    venous thrombosis or embolism Z86.718
      pulmonary Z86.711
    vulvar dysplasia Z87.412
His-Werner disease A79.0
HIV —*see also* Human, immunodeficiency virus B20
  laboratory evidence (nonconclusive) R75
  nonconclusive test (in infants) R75
  positive, seropositive Z21
Hives (bold) —*see* Urticaria
Hoarseness R49.0
Hobo Z59.0
Hodgkin disease —*see* Lymphoma, Hodgkin
Hodgson's disease I71.2
  ruptured I71.1
Hoffa-Kastert disease E88.89
Hoffa's disease E88.89
Hoffmann-Bouveret syndrome I47.9
Hoffmann's syndrome E03.9 *[G73.7]*
Hole (round)
  macula H35.34-
  retina (without detachment) —*see* Break, retina, round hole
    with detachment —*see* Detachment, retina, with retinal, break
Holiday relief care Z75.5
Hollenhorst's plaque —*see* Occlusion, artery, retina
Hollow foot (congenital) Q66.7
  acquired —*see* Deformity, limb, foot, specified NEC
Holoprosencephaly Q04.2
Holt-Oram syndrome Q87.2
Homelessness Z59.0
Homesickness —*see* Disorder, adjustment
Homocystinemia, homocystinuria E72.11
Homogentisate 1,2-dioxygenase deficiency E70.29
Homologous serum hepatitis (prophylactic) (therapeutic) —*see* Hepatitis, viral, type B
Honeycomb lung J98.4
  congenital Q33.0
Hooded
  clitoris Q52.6
  penis Q55.69
Hookworm (anemia) (disease) (infection) (infestation) B76.9
  specified NEC B76.8
Hordeolum (eyelid) (externum) (recurrent) H00.019
  internum H00.029
    left H00.026
      lower H00.025
      upper H00.024
    right H00.023
      lower H00.022
      upper H00.021
  left H00.016
    lower H00.015
    upper H00.014
  right H00.013
    lower H00.012
    upper H00.011
Horn
  cutaneous L85.8
  nail L60.2
    congenital Q84.6
Horner (-Claude Bernard) syndrome G90.2
  traumatic —*see* Injury, nerve, cervical sympathetic

Horseshoe kidney (congenital) Q63.1
Horton's headache or neuralgia G44.099
  intractable G44.091
  not intractable G44.099
Hospital hopper syndrome —see Disorder,
    factitious
Hospitalism in children —see Disorder,
    adjustment
Hostility R45.5
  towards child Z62.3
Hot flashes
  menopausal N95.1
Hourglass (contracture) —see also Contraction,
    hourglass
  stomach K31.89
    congenital Q40.2
    stricture K31.2
Household, housing circumstance affecting
    care Z59.9
  specified NEC Z59.8
Housemaid's knee —see Bursitis, prepatellar
Hudson (-Stähli) line (cornea) —see
    Pigmentation, cornea, anterior
Human
  bite (open wound) —see also Bite
    intact skin surface —see Bite, superficial
  herpesvirus —see Herpes
  immunodeficiency virus (HIV) disease
      (infection) B20
    asymptomatic status Z21
    contact Z20.6
    counseling Z71.7
    dementia B20 [F02.80]
      with behavioral disturbance B20 [F02.81]
    exposure to Z20.6
    laboratory evidence R75
    type-2 (HIV 2) as cause of disease classified
        elsewhere B97.35
  papillomavirus (HPV)
    DNA test positive
      high risk
        cervix R87.810
        vagina R87.811
      low risk
        cervix R87.820
        vagina R87.821
    screening for Z11.51
  T-cell lymphotropic virus
    type-1 (HTLV-I) infection B33.3
      as cause of disease classified elsewhere
          B97.33
      carrier Z22.6
    type-2 (HTLV-II) as cause of disease
        classified elsewhere B97.34
Humidifier lung or pneumonitis J67.7
Humiliation (experience) in childhood Z62.898
Humpback (acquired) —see Kyphosis
Hunchback (acquired) —see Kyphosis
Hunger T73.0
  air, psychogenic F45.8
Hungry bone syndrome E83.81
Hunner's ulcer —see Cystitis, chronic,
    interstitial
Hunter's
  glossitis D51.0
  syndrome E76.1
Huntington's disease or chorea G10
  with dementia G10 [F02.80]
    with behavioral disturbance G10 [F02.81]
Hunt's
  disease or syndrome (herpetic geniculate
      ganglionitis) B02.21
  dyssynergia cerebellaris myoclonica G11.1
  neuralgia B02.21
Hurler (-Scheie) disease or syndrome E76.02
Hurst's disease G36.1
Hurthle cell
  adenocarcinoma C73
  adenoma D34
  carcinoma C73
  tumor D34

Hutchinson-Boeck disease or syndrome —see
    Sarcoidosis
Hutchinson-Gilford disease or syndrome E34.8
Hutchinson's
  disease, meaning
    angioma serpiginosum L81.7
    pompholyx (cheiropompholyx) L30.1
    prurigo estivalis L56.4
    summer eruption or summer prurigo L56.4
  melanotic freckle —see Melanoma, in situ
    malignant melanoma in —see Melanoma
  teeth or incisors (congenital syphilis) A50.52
  triad (congenital syphilis) A50.53
Hyalin plaque, sclera, senile H15.89
Hyaline membrane (disease) (lung)
    (pulmonary) (newborn) P22.0
Hyalinosis
  cutis (et mucosae) E78.89
  focal and segmental (glomerular) —see also
      N00-N07 with fourth character .1 N05.1
Hyalitis, hyalosis, asteroid —see also Deposit,
    crystalline
  syphilitic (late) A52.71
Hydatid
  cyst or tumor —see Echinococcus
  mole —see Hydatidiform mole
  Morgagni
    female Q50.5
    male (epididymal) Q55.4
      testicular Q55.29
Hydatidiform mole (benign) (complicating
    pregnancy) (delivered) (undelivered)
    O01.9
  classical O01.0
  complete O01.0
  incomplete O01.1
  invasive D39.2
  malignant D39.2
  partial O01.1
Hydatidosis —see Echinococcus
Hydradenitis (axillaris) (suppurative) L73.2
Hydradenoma —see Hidradenoma
Hydramnios O40.-
Hydrancephaly, hydranencephaly Q04.3
  with spina bifida —see Spina bifida, with
      hydrocephalus
Hydrargyrism NEC —see Poisoning, mercury
Hydrarthrosis —see also Effusion, joint
  gonococcal A54.42
  intermittent M12.40
    ankle M12.47-
    elbow M12.42-
    foot joint M12.47-
    hand joint M12.44-
    hip M12.45-
    knee M12.46-
    multiple site M12.49
    shoulder M12.41-
    specified joint NEC M12.48
    wrist M12.43-
  of yaws (early) (late) —see also subcategory
      M14.8- A66.6
  syphilitic (late) A52.77
    congenital A50.55 [M12.80]
Hydremia D64.89
Hydrencephalocele (congenital) —see
    Encephalocele
Hydrencephalomeningocele (congenital) —see
    Encephalocele
Hydroa R23.8
  aestivale L56.4
  vacciniforme L56.4
Hydroadenitis (axillaris) (suppurative) L73.2
Hydrocalycosis —see Hydronephrosis
Hydrocele (spermatic cord) (testis) (tunica
    vaginalis) N43.3
  canal of Nuck N94.89
  communicating N43.2
    congenital P83.5
  congenital P83.5
  encysted N43.0

Hydrocele (Continued)
  female NEC N94.89
  infected N43.1
  newborn P83.5
  round ligament N94.89
  specified NEC N43.2
  spinalis —see Spina bifida
  vulva N90.89
Hydrocephalus (acquired) (external) (internal)
    (malignant) (recurrent) G91.9
  aqueduct Sylvius stricture Q03.0
  causing disproportion O33.6
    with obstructed labor O66.3
  communicating G91.0
  congenital (external) (internal) Q03.9
    with spina bifida Q05.4
      cervical Q05.0
      dorsal Q05.1
      lumbar Q05.2
      lumbosacral Q05.2
      sacral Q05.3
      thoracic Q05.1
      thoracolumbar Q05.1
    specified NEC Q03.8
  due to toxoplasmosis (congenital) P37.1
  foramen Magendie block (acquired) G91.1
    congenital —see also Hydrocephalus,
        congenital Q03.1
  in (due to)
    infectious disease NEC B89 [G91.4]
    neoplastic disease NEC (see also Neoplasm)
        G91.4
    parasitic disease B89 [G91.4]
  newborn Q03.9
    with spina bifida —see Spina bifida, with
        hydrocephalus
  noncommunicating G91.1
  normal pressure G91.2
    secondary G91.0
  obstructive G91.1
  otitic G93.2
  post-traumatic NEC G91.3
  secondary G91.4
    post-traumatic G91.3
  specified NEC G91.8
  syphilitic, congenital A50.49
Hydrocolpos (congenital) N89.8
Hydrocystoma —see Neoplasm, skin, benign
Hydroencephalocele (congenital) —see
    Encephalocele
Hydroencephalomeningocele (congenital) —
    see Encephalocele
Hydrohematopneumothorax —see Hemothorax
Hydromeningitis —see Meningitis
Hydromeningocele (spinal) —see also Spina
    bifida
  cranial —see Encephalocele
Hydrometra N85.8
Hydrometrocolpos N89.8
Hydromicrocephaly Q02
Hydromphalos (since birth) Q45.8
Hydromyelia Q06.4
Hydromyelocele —see Spina bifida
Hydronephrosis (atrophic) (early)
    (functionless) (intermittent) (primary)
    (secondary) NEC N13.30
  with
    infection N13.6
    obstruction (by) (of)
      renal calculus N13.2
        with infection N13.6
      ureteral NEC N13.1
        with infection N13.6
        calculus N13.2
          with infection N13.6
      ureteropelvic junction (congenital) Q62.0
        with infection N13.6
        acquired N13.0 ◄
          with infection N13.6 ◄
      ureteral stricture NEC N13.1
        with infection N13.6

Hydronephrosis NEC (Continued)
  congenital Q62.0
    due to acquired occlusion of ureteropelvic
      junction N13.0 ◀
    specified type NEC N13.39
    tuberculous A18.11
Hydropericarditis —see Pericarditis
Hydropericardium —see Pericarditis
Hydroperitoneum R18.8
Hydrophobia —see Rabies
Hydrophthalmos Q15.0
Hydropneumohemothorax —see Hemothorax
Hydropneumopericarditis —see Pericarditis
Hydropneumopericardium —see Pericarditis
Hydropneumothorax J94.8
  traumatic —see Injury, intrathoracic, lung
  tuberculous NEC A15.6
Hydrops R60.9
  abdominis R18.8
  articulorum intermittens —see Hydrarthrosis,
    intermittent
  cardiac —see Failure, heart, congestive
  causing obstructed labor (mother) O66.3
  endolymphatic H81.0-
  fetal —see Pregnancy, complicated by,
    hydrops, fetalis
  fetalis P83.2
    due to
      ABO isoimmunization P56.0
      alpha thalassemia D56.0
      hemolytic disease P56.90
        specified NEC P56.99
      isoimmunization (ABO) (Rh) P56.0
      other specified nonhemolytic disease
        NEC P83.2
      Rh incompatibility P56.0
    during pregnancy —see Pregnancy,
      complicated by, hydrops, fetalis
  gallbladder K82.1
  joint —see Effusion, joint
  labyrinth H81.0
  newborn (idiopathic) P83.2
    due to
      ABO isoimmunization P56.0
      alpha thalassemia D56.0
      hemolytic disease P56.90
        specified NEC P56.99
      isoimmunization (ABO) (Rh) P56.0
      Rh incompatibility P56.0
  nutritional —see Malnutrition, severe
  pericardium —see Pericarditis
  pleura —see Hydrothorax
  spermatic cord —see Hydrocele
Hydropyonephrosis N13.6
Hydrorachis Q06.4
Hydrorrhea (nasal) J34.89
  pregnancy —see Rupture, membranes,
    premature
Hydrosadenitis (axillaris) (suppurative) L73.2
Hydrosalpinx (fallopian tube) (follicularis)
  N70.11
Hydrothorax (double) (pleura) J94.8
  chylous (nonfilarial) I89.8
    filarial —see also Infestation, filarial B74.9
      [J91.8]
  traumatic —see Injury, intrathoracic
  tuberculous NEC (non primary) A15.6
Hydroureter —see also Hydronephrosis N13.4
  with infection N13.6
  congenital Q62.39
Hydroureteronephrosis —see Hydronephrosis
Hydrourethra N36.8
Hydroxykynureninuria E70.8
Hydroxylysinemia E72.3
Hydroxyprolinemia E72.59
Hygiene, sleep
  abuse Z72.821
  inadequate Z72.821
  poor Z72.821
Hygroma (congenital) (cystic) D18.1
  praepatellare, prepatellar —see Bursitis,
    prepatellar

Hymen —see condition
Hymenolepis, hymenolepiasis (diminuta)
  (infection) (infestation) (nana) B71.0
Hypalgesia R20.8
Hyperacidity (gastric) K31.89
  psychogenic F45.8
Hyperactive, hyperactivity F90.9
  basal cell, uterine cervix —see Dysplasia,
    cervix
  bowel sounds R19.12
  cervix epithelial (basal) —see Dysplasia,
    cervix
  child F90.9
    attention deficit —see Disorder, attention-
      deficit hyperactivity
  detrusor muscle N32.81
  gastrointestinal K31.89
    psychogenic F45.8
  nasal mucous membrane J34.3
  stomach K31.89
  thyroid (gland) —see Hyperthyroidism
Hyperacusis H93.23-
Hyperadrenalism E27.5
Hyperadrenocorticism E24.9
  congenital E25.0
  iatrogenic E24.2
    correct substance properly administered —
      see Table of Drugs and Chemicals, by
      drug, adverse effect
    overdose or wrong substance given or
      taken —see Table of Drugs and
      Chemicals, by drug, poisoning
  not associated with Cushing's syndrome E27.0
  pituitary-dependent E24.0
Hyperaldosteronism E26.9
  familial (type I) E26.02
  glucocorticoid-remediable E26.02
  primary (due to (bilateral) adrenal
    hyperplasia) E26.09
  primary NEC E26.09
  secondary E26.1
  specified NEC E26.89
Hyperalgesia R20.8
Hyperalimentation R63.2
  carotene, carotin E67.1
  specified NEC E67.8
  vitamin
    A E67.0
    D E67.3
Hyperaminoaciduria
  arginine E72.21
  cystine E72.01
  lysine E72.3
  ornithine E72.4
Hyperammonemia (congenital) E72.20
Hyperazotemia —see Uremia
Hyperbetalipoproteinemia (familial) E78.00 ◀╍╍
  with prebetalipoproteinemia E78.2
Hyperbilirubinemia
  constitutional E80.6
  familial conjugated E80.6
  neonatal (transient) —see Jaundice, newborn
Hypercalcemia, hypocalciuric, familial E83.52
Hypercalciuria, idiopathic E83.52
Hypercapnia R06.89
  newborn P84
Hypercarotenemia, hypercarotinemia (dietary)
  E67.1
Hypercementosis K03.4
Hyperchloremia E87.8
Hyperchlorhydria K31.89
  neurotic F45.8
  psychogenic F45.8
Hypercholesterinemia —see
  Hypercholesterolemia
Hypercholesterolemia (essential) (primary)
  (pure) E78.00 ◀╍╍
  with hyperglyceridemia, endogenous E78.2
  dietary counseling and surveillance Z71.3
  familial E78.01 ◀
  hereditary E78.01 ◀

Hyperchylia gastrica, psychogenic F45.8
Hyperchylomicronemia (familial) (primary)
  E78.3
  with hyperbetalipoproteinemia E78.3
Hypercoagulable (state) D68.59
  activated protein C resistance D68.51
  antithrombin (III) deficiency D68.59
  factor V Leiden mutation D68.51
  primary NEC D68.59
  protein C deficiency D68.59
  protein S deficiency D68.59
  prothrombin gene mutation D68.52
  secondary D68.69
  specified NEC D68.69
Hypercoagulation (state) D68.59
Hypercorticalism, pituitary-dependent E24.0
Hypercorticosolism —see Cushing's, syndrome
Hypercorticosteronism E24.2
  correct substance properly administered —see
    Table of Drugs and Chemicals, by drug,
    adverse effect
  overdose or wrong substance given or
    taken —see Table of Drugs and
    Chemicals, by drug, poisoning
Hypercortisonism E24.2
  correct substance properly administered —see
    Table of Drugs and Chemicals, by drug,
    adverse effect
  overdose or wrong substance given or
    taken —see Table of Drugs and
    Chemicals, by drug, poisoning
Hyperekplexia Q89.8
Hyperelectrolytemia E87.8
Hyperemesis R11.10
  with nausea R11.2
  gravidarum (mild) O21.0
    with
      carbohydrate depletion O21.1
      dehydration O21.1
      electrolyte imbalance O21.1
      metabolic disturbance O21.1
      severe (with metabolic disturbance) O21.1
  projectile R11.12
  psychogenic F45.8
Hyperemia (acute) (passive) R68.89
  anal mucosa K62.89
  bladder N32.89
  cerebral I67.89
  conjunctiva H11.43-
  ear internal, acute —see subcategory H83.0
  enteric K59.8
  eye —see Hyperemia, conjunctiva
  eyelid (active) (passive) —see Disorder,
    eyelid, specified type NEC
  intestine K59.8
  iris —see Disorder, iris, vascular
  kidney N28.89
  labyrinth —see subcategory H83.0
  liver (active) K76.89
  lung (passive) —see Edema, lung
  pulmonary (passive) —see Edema, lung
  renal N28.89
  retina H35.89
  stomach K31.89
Hyperesthesia (body surface) R20.3
  larynx (reflex) J38.7
    hysterical F44.89
  pharynx (reflex) J39.2
    hysterical F44.89
Hyperestrogenism (drug-induced) (iatrogenic)
  E28.0
Hyperexplexia Q89.8
Hyperfibrinolysis —see Fibrinolysis
Hyperfructosemia E74.19
Hyperfunction
  adrenal cortex, not associated with Cushing's
    syndrome E27.0
  medulla E27.5
    adrenomedullary E27.5
  virilism E25.9
    congenital E25.0

◀ New   ╍╍ Revised   ~~deleted~~ Deleted

Hyperfunction (Continued)
  ovarian E28.8
  pancreas K86.89 ◀▥
  parathyroid (gland) E21.3
  pituitary (gland) (anterior) E22.9
    specified NEC E22.8
  polyglandular E31.1
  testicular E29.0
Hypergammaglobulinemia D89.2
  polyclonal D89.0
  Waldenström D89.0
Hypergastrinemia E16.4
Hyperglobulinemia R77.1
Hyperglycemia, hyperglycemic (transient) R73.9
  coma —see Diabetes, by type, with coma
  postpancreatectomy E89.1
Hyperglyceridemia (endogenous) (essential)
    (familial) (hereditary) (pure) E78.1
  mixed E78.3
Hyperglycinemia (non-ketotic) E72.51
Hypergonadism
  ovarian E28.8
  testicular (primary) (infantile) E29.0
Hyperheparinemia D68.32
Hyperhidrosis, hyperidrosis R61
  focal
    primary L74.519
      axilla L74.510
      face L74.511
      palms L74.512
      soles L74.513
    secondary L74.52
  generalized R61
  localized
    primary L74.519
      axilla L74.510
      face L74.511
      palms L74.512
      soles L74.513
    secondary L74.52
  psychogenic F45.8
  secondary R61
    focal L74.52
Hyperhistidinemia E70.41
Hyperhomocysteinemia E72.11
Hyperhydroxyprolinemia E72.59
Hyperinsulinism (functional) E16.1
  with
    coma (hypoglycemic) E15
    encephalopathy E16.1 [G94]
  ectopic E16.1
  therapeutic misadventure (from
      administration of insulin) —see
      subcategory T38.3
Hyperkalemia E87.5
Hyperkeratosis —see also Keratosis L85.9
  cervix N88.0
  due to yaws (early) (late) (palmar or plantar)
      A66.3
  follicularis Q82.8
    penetrans (in cutem) L87.0
  palmoplantaris climacterica L85.1
  pinta A67.1
  senile (with pruritus) L57.0
  universalis congenita Q80.8
  vocal cord J38.3
  vulva N90.4
Hyperkinesia, hyperkinetic (disease) (reaction)
    (syndrome) (childhood) (adolescence) —see
    also Disorder, attention-deficit hyperactivity
  heart I51.89
Hyperleucine-isoleucinemia E71.19
Hyperlipemia, hyperlipidemia E78.5
  combined E78.2
    familial E78.4
  group
    A E78.00 ◀▥
    B E78.1
    C E78.2
    D E78.3
  mixed E78.2
  specified NEC E78.4

Hyperlipidosis E75.6
  hereditary NEC E75.5
Hyperlipoproteinemia E78.5
  Fredrickson's type
    I E78.3
    IIa E78.00 ◀▥
    IIb E78.2
    III E78.2
    IV E78.1
    V E78.3
  low-density-lipoprotein-type (LDL) E78.00 ◀▥
  very-low-density-lipoprotein-type (VLDL)
      E78.1
Hyperlucent lung, unilateral J43.0
Hyperlysinemia E72.3
Hypermagnesemia E83.41
  neonatal P71.8
Hypermenorrhea N92.0
Hypermethioninemia E72.19
Hypermetropia (congenital) H52.0-
Hypermobility, hypermotility
  cecum —see Syndrome, irritable bowel
  coccyx —see subcategory M53.2
  colon —see Syndrome, irritable bowel
    psychogenic F45.8
  ileum K58.9
  intestine —see also Syndrome, irritable bowel
      K58.9
    psychogenic F45.8
  meniscus (knee) —see Derangement, knee,
      meniscus
  scapula —see Instability, joint, shoulder
  stomach K31.89
    psychogenic F45.8
  syndrome M35.7
  urethra N36.41
    with intrinsic sphincter deficiency N36.43
Hypernasality R49.21
Hypernatremia E87.0
Hypernephroma C64.-
Hyperopia —see Hypermetropia
Hyperorexia nervosa F50.2
Hyperornithinemia E72.4
Hyperosmia R43.1
Hyperosmolality E87.0
Hyperostosis (monomelic) —see also Disorder,
    bone, density and structure, specified NEC
  ankylosing (spine) M48.10
    cervical region M48.12
    cervicothoracic region M48.13
    lumbar region M48.16
    lumbosacral region M48.17
    multiple sites M48.19
    occipito-atlanto-axial region M48.11
    sacrococcygeal region M48.18
    thoracic region M48.14
    thoracolumbar region M48.15
  cortical (skull) M85.2
    infantile M89.8X-
  frontal, internal of skull M85.2
  interna frontalis M85.2
  skeletal, diffuse idiopathic —see
      Hyperostosis, ankylosing
  skull M85.2
    congenital Q75.8
  vertebral, ankylosing —see Hyperostosis,
      ankylosing
Hyperovarism E28.8
Hyperoxaluria (primary) E72.53
Hyperparathyroidism E21.3
  primary E21.0
  secondary (renal) N25.81
    non-renal E21.1
  specified NEC E21.2
  tertiary E21.2
Hyperpathia R20.8
Hyperperistalsis R19.2
  psychogenic F45.8
Hyperpermeability, capillary I78.8
Hyperphagia R63.2
Hyperphenylalaninemia NEC E70.1

Hyperphoria (alternating) H50.53
Hyperphosphatemia E83.39
Hyperpiesis, hyperpiesia —see Hypertension
Hyperpigmentation —see also Pigmentation
  melanin NEC L81.4
  postinflammatory L81.0
Hyperpinealism E34.8
Hyperpituitarism E22.9
Hyperplasia, hyperplastic
  adenoids J35.2
  adrenal (capsule) (cortex) (gland) E27.8
    with
      sexual precocity (male) E25.9
        congenital E25.0
      virilism, adrenal E25.9
        congenital E25.0
      virilization (female) E25.9
        congenital E25.0
    congenital E25.0
    salt-losing E25.0
  adrenomedullary E27.5
  angiolymphoid, eosinophilia (ALHE) D18.01
  appendix (lymphoid) K38.0
  artery, fibromuscular I77.3
  bone —see also Hypertrophy, bone
    marrow D75.89
  breast —see also Hypertrophy, breast
    ductal (atypical) N60.9-
  C-cell, thyroid E07.0
  cementation (tooth) (teeth) K03.4
  cervical gland R59.0
  cervix (uteri) (basal cell) (endometrium)
      (polypoid) —see also Dysplasia, cervix
    congenital Q51.828
  clitoris, congenital Q52.6
  denture K06.2
  endocervicitis N72
  endometrium, endometrial (adenomatous)
      (benign) (cystic) (glandular) (glandular-
      cystic) (polypoid) N85.00
    with atypia N85.02
    cervix —see Dysplasia, cervix
    complex (without atypia) N85.01
    simple (without atypia) N85.01
  epithelial L85.9
    focal, oral, including tongue K13.29
    nipple N62
    skin L85.9
    tongue K13.29
    vaginal wall N89.3
  erythroid D75.89
  fibromuscular of artery (carotid) (renal)
      I77.3
  genital
    female NEC N94.89
    male N50.89 ◀▥
  gingiva K06.1
  glandularis cystica uteri (interstitialis) —see
      also Hyperplasia, endometrial N85.00-
  gum K06.1
  hymen, congenital Q52.4
  irritative, edentulous (alveolar) K06.2
  jaw M26.09
    alveolar M26.79
      lower M26.03
        alveolar M26.72
      upper M26.01
        alveolar M26.71
  kidney (congenital) Q63.3
  labia N90.69 ◀▥
    epithelial N90.3
  liver (congenital) Q44.7
    nodular, focal K76.89
  lymph gland or node R59.9
  mandible, mandibular M26.03
    alveolar M26.72
    unilateral condylar M27.8
  maxilla, maxillary M26.01
    alveolar M26.71
  myometrium, myometrial N85.2
  neuroendocrine cell, of infancy J84.841

Hyperplasia, hyperplastic *(Continued)*
  nose
    lymphoid J34.89
    polypoid J33.9
  oral mucosa (irritative) K13.6
  organ or site, congenital NEC —*see* Anomaly,
    by site
  ovary N83.8
  palate, papillary (irritative) K13.6
  pancreatic islet cells E16.9
    alpha E16.8
      with excess
        gastrin E16.4
        glucagon E16.3
    beta E16.1
  parathyroid (gland) E21.0
  pharynx (lymphoid) J39.2
  prostate (adenofibromatous) (nodular)
    N40.0
    with lower urinary tract symptoms (LUTS)
      N40.1
    without lower urinary tract symptoms
      (LUTS) N40.0
  renal artery I77.89
  reticulo-endothelial (cell) D75.89
  salivary gland (any) K11.1
  Schimmelbusch's —*see* Mastopathy,
    cystic
  suprarenal capsule (gland) E27.8
  thymus (gland) (persistent) E32.0
  thyroid (gland) —*see* Goiter
  tonsils (faucial) (infective) (lingual)
    (lymphoid) J35.1
    with adenoids J35.3
  unilateral condylar M27.8
  uterus, uterine N85.2
    endometrium (glandular) —*see also*
      Hyperplasia, endometrial
      N85.00-
  vulva N90.69 ◀▥
    epithelial N90.3
Hyperpnea —*see* Hyperventilation
Hyperpotassemia E87.5
Hyperprebetalipoproteinemia (familial)
  E78.1
Hyperprolactinemia E22.1
Hyperprolinemia (type I) (type II) E72.59
Hyperproteinemia E88.09
Hyperprothrombinemia, causing coagulation
  factor deficiency D68.4
Hyperpyrexia R50.9
  heat (effects) T67.0
  malignant, due to anesthetic T88.3
  rheumatic —*see* Fever, rheumatic
  unknown origin R50.9
Hyper-reflexia R29.2
Hypersalivation K11.7
Hypersecretion
  ACTH (not associated with Cushing's
    syndrome) E27.0
    pituitary E24.0
  adrenaline E27.5
  adrenomedullary E27.5
  androgen (testicular) E29.0
    ovarian (drug-induced) (iatrogenic) E28.1
  calcitonin E07.0
  catecholamine E27.5
  corticoadrenal E24.9
  cortisol E24.9
  epinephrine E27.5
  estrogen E28.0
  gastric K31.89
    psychogenic F45.8
  gastrin E16.4
  glucagon E16.3
  hormone (s)
    ACTH (not associated with Cushing's
      syndrome) E27.0
      pituitary E24.0
    antidiuretic E22.2
    growth E22.0

Hypersecretion *(Continued)*
  hormone *(Continued)*
    intestinal NEC E34.1
    ovarian androgen E28.1
    pituitary E22.9
    testicular E29.0
    thyroid stimulating E05.80
      with thyroid storm E05.81
  insulin —*see* Hyperinsulinism
  lacrimal glands —*see* Epiphora
  medulloadrenal E27.5
  milk O92.6
  ovarian androgens E28.1
  salivary gland (any) K11.7
  thyrocalcitonin E07.0
  upper respiratory J39.8
Hypersegmentation, leukocytic, hereditary
  D72.0
Hypersensitive, hypersensitiveness,
  hypersensitivity —*see also* Allergy
  carotid sinus G90.01
  colon —*see* Irritable, colon
  drug T88.7
  gastrointestinal K52.29 ◀▥
    immediate K52.29 ◀
    psychogenic F45.8
  labyrinth —*see* subcategory H83.2
  pain R20.8
  pneumonitis —*see* Pneumonitis,
    allergic
  reaction T78.40
    upper respiratory tract NEC J39.3
Hypersomnia (organic) G47.10
  due to
    alcohol
      abuse F10.182
      dependence F10.282
      use F10.982
    amphetamines
      abuse F15.182
      dependence F15.282
      use F15.982
    caffeine
      abuse F15.182
      dependence F15.282
      use F15.982
    cocaine
      abuse F14.182
      dependence F14.282
      use F14.982
    drug NEC
      abuse F19.182
      dependence F19.282
      use F19.982
    medical condition G47.14
    mental disorder F51.13
    opioid
      abuse F11.182
      dependence F11.282
      use F11.982
    psychoactive substance NEC
      abuse F19.182
      dependence F19.282
      use F19.982
    sedative, hypnotic, or anxiolytic
      abuse F13.182
      dependence F13.282
      use F13.982
    stimulant NEC
      abuse F15.182
      dependence F15.282
      use F15.982
  idiopathic G47.11
    with long sleep time G47.11
    without long sleep time G47.12
  menstrual related G47.13
  nonorganic origin F51.11
    specified NEC F51.19
  not due to a substance or known
    physiological condition F51.11
    specified NEC F51.19

Hypersomnia *(Continued)*
  primary F51.11
  recurrent G47.13
  specified NEC G47.19
Hypersplenia, hypersplenism D73.1
Hyperstimulation, ovaries (associated with
  induced ovulation) N98.1
Hypersusceptibility —*see* Allergy
Hypertelorism (ocular) (orbital) Q75.2
Hypertension, hypertensive (accelerated)
  (benign) (essential) (idiopathic)
  (malignant) (systemic) I10
  with
    heart involvement (conditions in
      I51.4-I51.9 due to hypertension) —*see*
      Hypertension, heart
    kidney involvement —*see* Hypertension,
      kidney
  benign, intracranial G93.2
  borderline R03.0
  cardiorenal (disease) I13.10
    with heart failure I13.0
      with stage 1 through stage 4 chronic
        kidney disease I13.0
      with stage 5 or end stage renal disease
        I13.2
    without heart failure I13.10
      with stage 1 through stage 4 chronic
        kidney disease I13.10
      with stage 5 or end stage renal disease
        I13.11
  cardiovascular
    disease (arteriosclerotic) (sclerotic) —*see*
      Hypertension, heart
    renal (disease) —*see* Hypertension,
      cardiorenal
  chronic venous —*see* Hypertension, venous
    (chronic)
  complicating
    childbirth (labor) O16.4 ◀▥
      ~~with~~
        ~~heart disease O10.12~~
          ~~with renal disease O10.32~~
        ~~renal disease O10.22~~
          ~~with heart disease O10.32~~
      ~~essential O10.02~~
      pre-existing O10.92 ◀
        with ◀
          heart disease O10.12 ◀
            with renal disease
              O10.32 ◀
          pre-eclampsia O11.4 ◀
          renal disease O10.22 ◀
            with heart disease
              O10.32 ◀
      essential O10.02 ◀
      secondary O10.42
    pregnancy O16.-
      with edema —*see also* Pre-eclampsia
        O14.9-
      gestational (pregnancy induced)
        (without proteinuria) O13.- ◀▥
        with proteinuria O14.9-
          mild pre-eclampsia O14.0-
          moderate pre-eclampsia
            O14.0-
          severe pre-eclampsia O14.1-
            with hemolysis, elevated liver
              enzymes and low platelet
              count (HELLP) O14.2-
      pre-existing O10.91-
        with
          heart disease O10.11-
            with renal disease O10.31-
          pre-eclampsia —*see* category
            O11 ◀▥
          renal disease O10.21-
            with heart disease O10.31-
        essential O10.01-
        secondary O10.41-
      transient O13.- ◀

◀ New   ◀▥ Revised   ~~deleted~~ Deleted

Hypertension, hypertensive *(Continued)*
  complicating *(Continued)*
    puerperium pre-existing O16.5 ◄▯
      ~~with~~
        ~~heart disease O10.13~~
          ~~with renal disease O10.33~~
        ~~renal disease O10.23~~
          ~~with heart disease O10.33~~
      ~~essential O10.03~~
      pre-existing ◄
        with ◄
          heart disease O10.13 ◄
            with renal disease O10.33 ◄
          pre-eclampsia O11.5 ◄
          renal disease O10.23 ◄
            with heart disease O10.33 ◄
        essential O10.03 ◄
      pregnancy-induced O13.9
      secondary O10.43
  crisis I16.9 ◄
  due to
    endocrine disorders I15.2
    pheochromocytoma I15.2
    renal disorders NEC I15.1
      arterial I15.0
    renovascular disorders I15.0
    specified disease NEC I15.8
  emergency I16.2 ◄
  encephalopathy I67.4
  gestational (without significant proteinuria)
    (pregnancy-induced) (transient)
    O13.-
    with significant proteinuria —*see*
      Pre-eclampsia
    complicating ◄
      delivery O13.4 ◄
      puerperium O13.5 ◄
  Goldblatt's I70.1
  heart (disease) (conditions in I51.4-I51.9 due
    to hypertension) I11.9
    with
      heart failure (congestive) I11.0
      kidney disease (chronic) —*see*
        Hypertension, cardiorenal
  intracranial (benign) G93.2
  kidney I12.9
    with
      heart disease —*see* Hypertension,
        cardiorenal
      stage 1 through stage 4 chronic kidney
        disease I12.9
      stage 5 chronic kidney disease (CKD)
        or end stage renal disease (ESRD)
        I12.0
  lesser circulation I27.0
  maternal O16.- ◄
  newborn P29.2
    pulmonary (persistent) P29.3
  ocular H40.05-
  pancreatic duct — code to underlying
    condition
    with chronic pancreatitis K86.1
  portal (due to chronic liver disease)
    (idiopathic) K76.6
    gastropathy K31.89
    in (due to) schistosomiasis (bilharziasis)
      B65.9 *[K77]*
  postoperative I97.3
  psychogenic F45.8
  pulmonary (artery) (secondary) NEC
    I27.2
    with
      cor pulmonale (chronic) I27.2
        acute I26.09
      right heart ventricular strain/failure
        I27.2
        acute I26.09
    of newborn (persistent) P29.3
    primary (idiopathic) I27.0
  renal —*see* Hypertension, kidney
  renovascular I15.0

Hypertension, hypertensive *(Continued)*
  secondary NEC I15.9
    due to
      endocrine disorders I15.2
      pheochromocytoma I15.2
      renal disorders NEC I15.1
        arterial I15.0
      renovascular disorders I15.0
    specified NEC I15.8
  transient, of pregnancy O13.- ◄
  urgency I16.0 ◄
  venous (chronic)
    due to
      deep vein thrombosis —*see* Syndrome,
        postthrombotic
    idiopathic I87.309
      with
        inflammation I87.32-
          with ulcer I87.33-
        specified complication NEC I87.39-
        ulcer I87.31-
          with inflammation I87.33-
      asymptomatic I87.30-
Hypertensive urgency —*see* Hypertension
Hyperthecosis ovary E28.8
Hyperthermia (of unknown origin) —*see also*
  Hyperpyrexia
  malignant, due to anesthesia T88.3
  newborn P81.9
    environmental P81.0
Hyperthyroid (recurrent) —*see*
  Hyperthyroidism
Hyperthyroidism (latent) (pre-adult)
  (recurrent) E05.90
  with
    goiter (diffuse) E05.00
      with thyroid storm E05.01
      nodular (multinodular) E05.20
        with thyroid storm E05.21
        uninodular E05.10
          with thyroid storm E05.11
    storm E05.91
  due to ectopic thyroid tissue E05.30
    with thyroid storm E05.31
  neonatal, transitory P72.1
  specified NEC E05.80
    with thyroid storm E05.81
Hypertony, hypertonia, hypertonicity
  bladder N31.8
  congenital P94.1
  stomach K31.89
    psychogenic F45.8
  uterus, uterine (contractions) (complicating
    delivery) O62.4
Hypertrichosis L68.9
  congenital Q84.2
  eyelid H02.869
    left H02.866
      lower H02.865
      upper H02.864
    right H02.863
      lower H02.862
      upper H02.861
  lanuginosa Q84.2
    acquired L68.1
  localized L68.2
  specified NEC L68.8
Hypertriglyceridemia, essential E78.1
Hypertrophy, hypertrophic
  adenofibromatous, prostate —*see*
    Enlargement, enlarged, prostate
  adenoids (infective) J35.2
    with tonsils J35.3
  adrenal cortex E27.8
  alveolar process or ridge —*see* Anomaly,
    alveolar
  anal papillae K62.89
  artery I77.89
    congenital NEC Q27.8
      digestive system Q27.8
      lower limb Q27.8

Hypertrophy, hypertrophic *(Continued)*
  artery *(Continued)*
    congenital NEC *(Continued)*
      specified site NEC Q27.8
      upper limb Q27.8
  auricular —*see* Hypertrophy, cardiac
  Bartholin's gland N75.8
  bile duct (common) (hepatic) K83.8
  bladder (sphincter) (trigone) N32.89
  bone M89.30
    carpus M89.34-
    clavicle M89.31-
    femur M89.35-
    fibula M89.36-
    finger M89.34-
    humerus M89.32-
    ilium M89.359
    ischium M89.359
    metacarpus M89.34-
    metatarsus M89.37-
    multiple sites M89.39
    neck M89.38
    radius M89.33-
    rib M89.38
    scapula M89.31-
    skull M89.38
    tarsus M89.37-
    tibia M89.36-
    toe M89.37-
    ulna M89.33-
    vertebra M89.38
  brain G93.89
  breast N62
    cystic —*see* Mastopathy, cystic
    newborn P83.4
    pubertal, massive N62
    puerperal, postpartum —*see* Disorder,
      breast, specified type NEC
    senile (parenchymatous) N62
  cardiac (chronic) (idiopathic) I51.7
    with rheumatic fever (conditions in I00)
      active I01.8
      inactive or quiescent (with chorea) I09.89
    congenital NEC Q24.8
    fatty —*see* Degeneration, myocardial
    hypertensive —*see* Hypertension, heart
    rheumatic (with chorea) I09.89
      active or acute I01.8
        with chorea I02.0
    valve —*see* Endocarditis
  cartilage —*see* Disorder, cartilage, specified
    type NEC
  cecum —*see* Megacolon
  cervix (uteri) N88.8
    congenital Q51.828
    elongation N88.4
  clitoris (cirrhotic) N90.89
    congenital Q52.6
  colon —*see also* Megacolon
    congenital Q43.2
  conjunctiva, lymphoid H11.89
  corpora cavernosa N48.89
  cystic duct K82.8
  duodenum K31.89
  endometrium (glandular) —*see also*
    Hyperplasia, endometrial N85.00-
    cervix N88.8
  epididymis N50.89 ◄▯
  esophageal hiatus (congenital) Q79.1
    with hernia —*see* Hernia, hiatal
  eyelid —*see* Disorder, eyelid, specified type
    NEC
  fat pad E65
    knee (infrapatellar) (popliteal) (prepatellar)
      (retropatellar) M79.4
  foot (congenital) Q74.2
  frenulum, frenum (tongue) K14.8
    lip K13.0
  gallbladder K82.8
  gastric mucosa K29.60
    with bleeding K29.61

Hypertrophy, hypertrophic *(Continued)*
gland, glandular R59.9
  generalized R59.1
  localized R59.0
gum (mucous membrane) K06.1
heart (idiopathic) —*see also* Hypertrophy,
    cardiac
  valve —*see also* Endocarditis I38
hemifacial Q67.4
hepatic —*see* Hypertrophy, liver
hiatus (esophageal) Q79.1
hilus gland R59.0
hymen, congenital Q52.4
ileum K63.89
intestine NEC K63.89
jejunum K63.89
kidney (compensatory) N28.81
  congenital Q63.3
labium (majus) (minus) N90.60 ◀⃜
ligament —*see* Disorder, ligament
lingual tonsil (infective) J35.1
  with adenoids J35.3
lip K13.0
  congenital Q18.6
liver R16.0
  acute K76.89
  cirrhotic —*see* Cirrhosis, liver
  congenital Q44.7
  fatty —*see* Fatty, liver
lymph, lymphatic gland R59.9
  generalized R59.1
  localized R59.0
  tuberculous —*see* Tuberculosis, lymph
    gland
mammary gland —*see* Hypertrophy, breast
Meckel's diverticulum (congenital) Q43.0
  malignant —*see* Table of Neoplasms, small
    intestine, malignant
median bar —*see* Hyperplasia, prostate
meibomian gland —*see* Chalazion
meniscus, knee, congenital Q74.1
metatarsal head —*see* Hypertrophy, bone,
    metatarsus
metatarsus —*see* Hypertrophy, bone,
    metatarsus
mucous membrane
  alveolar ridge K06.2
  gum K06.1
  nose (turbinate) J34.3
muscle M62.89
muscular coat, artery I77.89
myocardium —*see also* Hypertrophy, cardiac
  idiopathic I42.2
myometrium N85.2
nail L60.2
  congenital Q84.5
nasal J34.89
  alae J34.89
  bone J34.89
  cartilage J34.89
  mucous membrane (septum) J34.3
  sinus J34.89
  turbinate J34.3
nasopharynx, lymphoid (infectional) (tissue)
    (wall) J35.2
nipple N62
organ or site, congenital NEC —*see* Anomaly,
    by site - ovary N83.8
palate (hard) M27.8
  soft K13.79
pancreas, congenital Q45.3
parathyroid (gland) E21.0
parotid gland K11.1
penis N48.89
pharyngeal tonsil J35.2
pharynx J39.2
  lymphoid (infectional) (tissue) (wall)
    J35.2
pituitary (anterior) (fossa) (gland) E23.6
prepuce (congenital) N47.8
  female N90.89

Hypertrophy, hypertrophic *(Continued)*
prostate —*see* Enlargement, enlarged,
    prostate
  congenital Q55.4
pseudomuscular G71.0
pylorus (adult) (muscle) (sphincter)
    K31.1
  congenital or infantile Q40.0
rectal, rectum (sphincter) K62.89
rhinitis (turbinate) J31.0
salivary gland (any) K11.1
  congenital Q38.4
scaphoid (tarsal) —*see* Hypertrophy, bone,
    tarsus
scar L91.0
scrotum N50.89 ◀⃜
seminal vesicle N50.89 ◀⃜
sigmoid —*see* Megacolon
skin L91.9
  specified NEC L91.8
spermatic cord N50.89 ◀⃜
spleen —*see* Splenomegaly
spondylitis —*see* Spondylosis
stomach K31.89
sublingual gland K11.1
submandibular gland K11.1
suprarenal cortex (gland) E27.8
synovial NEC M67.20
  acromioclavicular M67.21-
  ankle M67.27-
  elbow M67.22-
  foot M67.27-
  hand M67.24-
  hip M67.25-
  knee M67.26-
  multiple sites M67.29
  specified site NEC M67.28
  wrist M67.23-
tendon —*see* Disorder, tendon, specified type
    NEC
testis N44.8
  congenital Q55.29
thymic, thymus (gland) (congenital)
    E32.0
thyroid (gland) —*see* Goiter
toe (congenital) Q74.2
  acquired —*see also* Deformity, toe, specified
    NEC
tongue K14.8
  congenital Q38.2
  papillae (foliate) K14.3
tonsils (faucial) (infective) (lingual)
    (lymphoid) J35.1
  with adenoids J35.3
tunica vaginalis N50.89 ◀⃜
ureter N28.89
urethra N36.8
uterus N85.2
  neck (with elongation) N88.4
  puerperal O90.89
uvula K13.79
vagina N89.8
vas deferens N50.89 ◀⃜
vein I87.8
ventricle, ventricular (heart) —*see also*
    Hypertrophy, cardiac
  congenital Q24.8
  in tetralogy of Fallot Q21.3
verumontanum N36.8
vocal cord J38.3
vulva N90.60 ◀⃜
  stasis (nonfilarial) N90.69 ◀⃜
Hypertropia H50.2-
Hypertyrosinemia E70.21
Hyperuricemia (asymptomatic)
    E79.0
Hypervalinemia E71.19
Hyperventilation (tetany) R06.4
  hysterical F45.8
  psychogenic F45.8
  syndrome F45.8

Hypervitaminosis (dietary) NEC E67.8
  A E67.0
    administered as drug (prolonged intake) —
      see Table of Drugs and Chemicals,
      vitamins, adverse effect
    overdose or wrong substance given or
      taken —*see* Table of Drugs and
      Chemicals, vitamins, poisoning
  B6 E67.2
  D E67.3
    administered as drug (prolonged intake) —
      see Table of Drugs and Chemicals,
      vitamins, adverse effect
    overdose or wrong substance given or
      taken —*see* Table of Drugs and
      Chemicals, vitamins, poisoning
  K E67.8
    administered as drug (prolonged intake) —
      see Table of Drugs and Chemicals,
      vitamins, adverse effect
    overdose or wrong substance given or
      taken —*see* Table of Drugs and
      Chemicals, vitamins, poisoning
Hypervolemia E87.70
  specified NEC E87.79
Hypesthesia R20.1
  cornea —*see* Anesthesia, cornea
Hyphema H21.0-
  traumatic S05.1-
Hypoacidity, gastric K31.89
  psychogenic F45.8
Hypoadrenalism, hypoadrenia E27.40
  primary E27.1
  tuberculous A18.7
Hypoadrenocorticism E27.40
  pituitary E23.0
  primary E27.1
Hypoalbuminemia E88.09
Hypoaldosteronism E27.40
Hypoalphalipoproteinemia E78.6
Hypobarism T70.29
Hypobaropathy T70.29
Hypobetalipoproteinemia (familial)
    E78.6
Hypocalcemia E83.51
  dietary E58
  neonatal P71.1
    due to cow's milk P71.0
  phosphate-loading (newborn) P71.1
Hypochloremia E87.8
Hypochlorhydria K31.89
  neurotic F45.8
  psychogenic F45.8
Hypochondria, hypochondriac,
    hypochondriasis (reaction) F45.21
  sleep F51.03
Hypochondrogenesis Q77.0
Hypochondroplasia Q77.4
Hypochromasia, blood cells D50.8
Hypodontia —*see* Anodontia
Hypoeosinophilia D72.89
Hypoesthesia R20.1
Hypofibrinogenemia D68.8
  acquired D65
  congenital (hereditary) D68.2
Hypofunction
  adrenocortical E27.40
    drug-induced E27.3
    postprocedural E89.6
    primary E27.1
  adrenomedullary, postprocedural E89.6
  cerebral R29.818
  corticoadrenal NEC E27.40
  intestinal K59.8
  labyrinth —*see* subcategory H83.2
  ovary E28.39
  pituitary (gland) (anterior) E23.0
  testicular E29.1
    postprocedural (postsurgical)
      (postirradiation) (iatrogenic) E89.5
Hypogalactia O92.4

◀ New   ◀⃜ Revised   ~~deleted~~ Deleted

Hypogammaglobulinemia —*see also*
  Agammaglobulinemia D80.1
  hereditary D80.0
  nonfamilial D80.1
  transient, of infancy D80.7
Hypogenitalism (congenital) —*see*
  Hypogonadism
Hypoglossia Q38.3
Hypoglycemia (spontaneous) E16.2
  coma E15
    diabetic —*see* Diabetes, coma
  diabetic —*see* Diabetes, hypoglycemia
  dietary counseling and surveillance Z71.3
  drug-induced E16.0
    with coma (nondiabetic) E15
  due to insulin E16.0
    with coma (nondiabetic) E15
    therapeutic misadventure —*see*
      subcategory T38.3
  functional, nonhyperinsulinemic E16.1
  iatrogenic E16.0
    with coma (nondiabetic) E15
  in infant of diabetic mother P70.1
    gestational diabetes P70.0
  infantile E16.1
  leucine-induced E71.19
  neonatal (transitory) P70.4
    iatrogenic P70.3
  reactive (not drug-induced) E16.1
  transitory neonatal P70.4
Hypogonadism
  female E28.39
  hypogonadotropic E23.0
  male E29.1
  ovarian (primary) E28.39
  pituitary E23.0
  testicular (primary) E29.1
Hypohidrosis, hypoidrosis L74.4
Hypoinsulinemia, postprocedural E89.1
Hypokalemia E87.6
Hypoleukocytosis —*see* Agranulocytosis
Hypolipoproteinemia (alpha) (beta) E78.6
Hypomagnesemia E83.42
  neonatal P71.2
Hypomania, hypomanic reaction F30.8
Hypomenorrhea —*see* Oligomenorrhea
Hypometabolism R63.8
Hypomotility
  gastrointestinal (tract) K31.89
    psychogenic F45.8
  intestine K59.8
    psychogenic F45.8
  stomach K31.89
    psychogenic F45.8
Hyponasality R49.22
Hyponatremia E87.1
Hypo-osmolality E87.1
Hypo-ovarianism, hypo-ovarism E28.39
Hypoparathyroidism E20.9
  familial E20.8
  idiopathic E20.0
  neonatal, transitory P71.4
  postprocedural E89.2
  specified NEC E20.8
Hypoperfusion (in)
  newborn P96.89
Hypopharyngitis —*see* Laryngopharyngitis
Hypophoria H50.53
Hypophosphatemia, hypophosphatasia
  (acquired) (congenital) (renal) E83.39
  familial E83.31
Hypophyseal, hypophysis —*see also* condition
  dwarfism E23.0
  gigantism E22.0
Hypopiesis —*see* Hypotension
Hypopinealism E34.8
Hypopituitarism (juvenile) E23.0
  drug-induced E23.1
  due to
    hypophysectomy E89.3
    radiotherapy E89.3

Hypopituitarism (*Continued*)
  iatrogenic NEC E23.1
  postirradiation E89.3
  postpartum O99.285 ◄▪▪▪▪
  postprocedural E89.3
Hypoplasia, hypoplastic
  adrenal (gland), congenital Q89.1
  alimentary tract, congenital Q45.8
    upper Q40.8
  anus, anal (canal) Q42.3
    with fistula Q42.2
  aorta, aortic Q25.42 ◄▪▪▪▪
    ascending, in hypoplastic left heart
      syndrome Q23.4
    valve Q23.1
      in hypoplastic left heart syndrome
        Q23.4
  areola, congenital Q83.8
  arm (congenital) —*see* Defect, reduction,
    upper limb
  artery (peripheral) Q27.8
    brain (congenital) Q28.3
    coronary Q24.5
    digestive system Q27.8
    lower limb Q27.8
    pulmonary Q25.79
      functional, unilateral J43.0
    retinal (congenital) Q14.1
    specified site NEC Q27.8
    umbilical Q27.0
    upper limb Q27.8
  auditory canal Q17.8
    causing impairment of hearing Q16.9
  biliary duct or passage Q44.5
  bone NOS Q79.9
    face Q75.8
    marrow D61.9
      megakaryocytic D69.49
    skull —*see* Hypoplasia, skull
  brain Q02
    gyri Q04.3
    part of Q04.3
  breast (areola) N64.82
  bronchus Q32.4
  cardiac Q24.8
  carpus —*see* Defect, reduction, upper limb,
    specified type NEC
  cartilage hair Q78.8 ◄▪▪▪▪
  cecum Q42.8
  cementum K00.4
  cephalic Q02
  cerebellum Q04.3
  cervix (uteri), congenital Q51.821
  clavicle (congenital) Q74.0
  coccyx Q76.49
  colon Q42.9
    specified NEC Q42.8
  corpus callosum Q04.0
  cricoid cartilage Q31.2
  digestive organ (s) or tract NEC Q45.8
    upper (congenital) Q40.8
  ear (auricle) (lobe) Q17.2
    middle Q16.4
  enamel of teeth (neonatal) (postnatal)
    (prenatal) K00.4
  endocrine (gland) NEC Q89.2
  endometrium N85.8
  epididymis (congenital) Q55.4
  epiglottis Q31.2
  erythroid, congenital D61.01
  esophagus (congenital) Q39.8
  eustachian tube Q17.8
  eye Q11.2
  eyelid (congenital) Q10.3
  face Q18.8
    bone (s) Q75.8
  femur (congenital) —*see* Defect,
    reduction, lower limb, specified
    type NEC
  fibula (congenital) —*see* Defect, reduction,
    lower limb, specified type NEC

Hypoplasia, hypoplastic (*Continued*)
  finger (congenital) —*see* Defect, reduction,
    upper limb, specified type NEC
  focal dermal Q82.8
  foot —*see* Defect, reduction, lower limb,
    specified type NEC
  gallbladder Q44.0
  genitalia, genital organ (s)
    female, congenital Q52.8
      external Q52.79
      internal NEC Q52.8
    in adiposogenital dystrophy E23.6
  glottis Q31.2
  hair Q84.2
  hand (congenital) —*see* Defect, reduction,
    upper limb, specified type NEC
  heart Q24.8
  humerus (congenital) —*see* Defect, reduction,
    upper limb, specified type NEC
  intestine (small) Q41.9
    large Q42.9
      specified NEC Q42.8
  jaw M26.09
    alveolar M26.79
    lower M26.04
      alveolar M26.74
    upper M26.02
      alveolar M26.73
  kidney (s) Q60.5
    bilateral Q60.4
    unilateral Q60.3
  labium (majus) (minus), congenital Q52.79
  larynx Q31.2
  left heart syndrome Q23.4
  leg (congenital) —*see* Defect, reduction, lower
    limb
  limb Q73.8
    lower (congenital) —*see* Defect, reduction,
      lower limb
    upper (congenital) —*see* Defect, reduction,
      upper limb
  liver Q44.7
  lung (lobe) (not associated with short
    gestation) Q33.6
    associated with immaturity, low birth
      weight, prematurity, or short
      gestation P28.0
  mammary (areola), congenital Q83.8
  mandible, mandibular M26.04
    alveolar M26.74
    unilateral condylar M27.8
  maxillary M26.02
    alveolar M26.73
  medullary D61.9
  megakaryocytic D69.49
  metacarpus —*see* Defect, reduction, upper
    limb, specified type NEC
  metatarsus —*see* Defect, reduction, lower
    limb, specified type NEC
  muscle Q79.8
  nail (s) Q84.6
  nose, nasal Q30.1
  optic nerve H47.03-
  osseous meatus (ear) Q17.8
  ovary, congenital Q50.39
  pancreas Q45.0
  parathyroid (gland) Q89.2
  parotid gland Q38.4
  patella Q74.1
  pelvis, pelvic girdle Q74.2
  penis (congenital) Q55.62
  peripheral vascular system Q27.8
    digestive system Q27.8
    lower limb Q27.8
    specified site NEC Q27.8
    upper limb Q27.8
  pituitary (gland) (congenital) Q89.2
  pulmonary (not associated with short
    gestation) Q33.6
    artery, functional J43.0
    associated with short gestation P28.0

Hypoplasia, hypoplastic (Continued)
  radioulnar —see Defect, reduction, upper
      limb, specified type NEC
  radius —see Defect, reduction, upper limb
  rectum Q42.1
      with fistula Q42.0
  respiratory system NEC Q34.8
  rib Q76.6
  right heart syndrome Q22.6
  sacrum Q76.49
  scapula Q74.0
  scrotum Q55.1
  shoulder girdle Q74.0
  skin Q82.8
  skull (bone) Q75.8
      with
          anencephaly Q00.0
          encephalocele —see Encephalocele
          hydrocephalus Q03.9
              with spina bifida —see Spina bifida, by
                  site, with hydrocephalus
          microcephaly Q02
  spinal (cord) (ventral horn cell)
      Q06.1
  spine Q76.49
  sternum Q76.7
  tarsus —see Defect, reduction, lower limb,
      specified type NEC
  testis Q55.1
  thymic, with immunodeficiency D82.1
  thymus (gland) Q89.2
      with immunodeficiency D82.1
  thyroid (gland) E03.1
      cartilage Q31.2
  tibiofibular (congenital) —see Defect,
      reduction, lower limb, specified type
      NEC
  toe —see Defect, reduction, lower limb,
      specified type NEC
  tongue Q38.3
  Turner's K00.4
  ulna (congenital) —see Defect, reduction,
      upper limb
  umbilical artery Q27.0
  unilateral condylar M27.8
  ureter Q62.8
  uterus, congenital Q51.811
  vagina Q52.4
  vascular NEC peripheral Q27.8
      brain Q28.3
      digestive system Q27.8
      lower limb Q27.8
      specified site NEC Q27.8
      upper limb Q27.8
  vein (s) (peripheral) Q27.8
      brain Q28.3
      digestive system Q27.8
      great Q26.8
      lower limb Q27.8
      specified site NEC Q27.8
      upper limb Q27.8
  vena cava (inferior) (superior) Q26.8
  vertebra Q76.49
  vulva, congenital Q52.79
  zonule (ciliary) Q12.8

Hypopotassemia E87.6
Hypoproconvertinemia, congenital
    (hereditary) D68.2
Hypoproteinemia E77.8
Hypoprothrombinemia (congenital)
    (hereditary) (idiopathic) D68.2
    acquired D68.4
    newborn, transient P61.6
Hypoptyalism K11.7
Hypopyon (eye) (anterior chamber) —see
    Iridocyclitis, acute, hypopyon
Hypopyrexia R68.0
Hyporeflexia R29.2
Hyposecretion
    ACTH E23.0
    antidiuretic hormone E23.2
    ovary E28.39
    salivary gland (any) K11.7
    vasopressin E23.2
Hyposegmentation, leukocytic, hereditary
    D72.0
Hyposiderinemia D50.9
Hypospadias Q54.9
    balanic Q54.0
    coronal Q54.0
    glandular Q54.0
    penile Q54.1
    penoscrotal Q54.2
    perineal Q54.3
    specified NEC Q54.8
Hypospermatogenesis —see Oligospermia
Hyposplenism D73.0
Hypostasis pulmonary, passive —see Edema,
    lung
Hypostatic —see condition
Hyposthenuria N28.89
Hypotension (arterial) (constitutional) I95.9
    chronic I95.89
    drug-induced I95.2
    due to (of) hemodialysis I95.3
    iatrogenic I95.89
    idiopathic (permanent) I95.0
    intracranial, following ventricular shunting
        (ventriculostomy) G97.2
    intra-dialytic I95.3
    maternal, syndrome (following labor and
        delivery) O26.5-
    neurogenic, orthostatic G90.3
    orthostatic (chronic) I95.1
        due to drugs I95.2
        neurogenic G90.3
    postoperative I95.81
    postural I95.1
    specified NEC I95.89
Hypothermia (accidental) T68
    due to anesthesia, anesthetic T88.51
    low environmental temperature T68
    neonatal P80.9
        environmental (mild) NEC P80.8
        mild P80.8
        severe (chronic) (cold injury syndrome)
            P80.0
        specified NEC P80.8
    not associated with low environmental
        temperature R68.0

Hypothyroidism (acquired) E03.9
    congenital (without goiter) E03.1
        with goiter (diffuse) E03.0
    due to
        exogenous substance NEC E03.2
        iodine-deficiency, acquired E01.8
            subclinical E02
        irradiation therapy E89.0
        medicament NEC E03.2
        P-aminosalicylic acid (PAS) E03.2
        phenylbutazone E03.2
        resorcinol E03.2
        sulfonamide E03.2
        surgery E89.0
        thiourea group drugs E03.2
    iatrogenic NEC E03.2
    iodine-deficiency (acquired) E01.8
        congenital —see Syndrome, iodine-
            deficiency, congenital
        subclinical E02
    neonatal, transitory P72.2
    postinfectious E03.3
    postirradiation E89.0
    postprocedural E89.0
    postsurgical E89.0
    specified NEC E03.8
    subclinical, iodine-deficiency related
        E02
Hypotonia, hypotonicity, hypotony
    bladder N31.2
    congenital (benign) P94.2
    eye —see Disorder, globe, hypotony
Hypotrichosis —see Alopecia
Hypotropia H50.2-
Hypoventilation R06.89
    congenital central alveolar G47.35
    sleep related
        idiopathic nonobstructive alveolar
            G47.34
        in conditions classified elsewhere
            G47.36
Hypovitaminosis —see Deficiency, vitamin
Hypovolemia E86.1
    surgical shock T81.19
    traumatic (shock) T79.4
Hypoxemia R09.02
    newborn P84
    sleep related, in conditions classified
        elsewhere G47.36
Hypoxia —see also Anoxia R09.02
    cerebral, during a procedure NEC G97.81
        postprocedural NEC G97.82
    intrauterine P84
    myocardial —see Insufficiency, coronary
    newborn P84
    sleep-related G47.34
Hypsarrhythmia —see Epilepsy, generalized,
    specified NEC
Hysteralgia, pregnant uterus O26.89-
Hysteria, hysterical (conversion) (dissociative
    state) F44.9
    anxiety F41.8
    convulsions F44.5
    psychosis, acute F44.9
Hysteroepilepsy F44.5

◄ New   ◄⁗ Revised   ~~deleted~~ Deleted

I

IBDU (colonic inflammatory bowel dissease unclassified) K52.3 ◄
Ichthyoparasitism due to Vandellia cirrhosa B88.8
Ichthyosis (congenital) Q80.9
  acquired L85.0
  fetalis Q80.4
  hystrix Q80.8
  lamellar Q80.2
  lingual K13.29
  palmaris and plantaris Q82.8
  simplex Q80.0
  vera Q80.8
  vulgaris Q80.0
  X-linked Q80.1
Ichthyotoxism —see Poisoning, fish
  bacterial —see Intoxication, foodborne
Icteroanemia, hemolytic (acquired) D59.9
  congenital —see Spherocytosis
Icterus —see also Jaundice
  conjunctiva R17
  gravis, newborn P55.0
  hematogenous (acquired) D59.9
  hemolytic (acquired) D59.9
    congenital —see Spherocytosis
  hemorrhagic (acute) (leptospiral) (spirochetal) A27.0
    newborn P53
  infectious B15.9
    with hepatic coma B15.0
    leptospiral A27.0
    spirochetal A27.0
  neonatorum —see Jaundice, newborn
  newborn P59.9
  spirochetal A27.0
Ictus solaris, solis T67.0
Ideation
  homicidal R45.850
  suicidal R45.851
Identity disorder (child) F64.9
  gender role F64.2
  psychosexual F64.2
Idioglossia F80.0
Idiopathic —see condition
Idiot, idiocy (congenital) F73
  amaurotic (Bielschowsky(-Jansky)) (family) (infantile (late)) (juvenile (late)) (Vogt-Spielmeyer) E75.4
  microcephalic Q02
Id reaction (due to bacteria) L30.2
IgE asthma J45.909
IIAC (idiopathic infantile arterial calcification) Q28.8
Ileitis (chronic) (noninfectious) —see also Enteritis K52.9
  backwash —see Pancolitis, ulcerative (chronic)
  infectious A09
  regional (ulcerative) —see Enteritis, regional, small intestine
  segmental —see Enteritis, regional
  terminal (ulcerative) —see Enteritis, regional, small intestine
Ileocolitis —see also Enteritis K52.9
  infectious A09
  regional —see Enteritis, regional
Ileostomy
  attention to Z43.2
  malfunctioning K94.13
  status Z93.2
    with complication —see Complications, enterostomy
Ileotyphus —see Typhoid
Ileum —see condition
Ileus (bowel) (colon) (inhibitory) (intestine) K56.7
  adynamic K56.0
  due to gallstone (in intestine) K56.3
  duodenal (chronic) K31.5

Ileus (Continued)
  gallstone K56.3
  mechanical NEC K56.69
  meconium P76.0
    in cystic fibrosis E84.11
    meaning meconium plug (without cystic fibrosis) P76.0
  myxedema K59.8
  neurogenic K56.0
    Hirschsprung's disease or megacolon Q43.1
  newborn
    due to meconium P76.0
      in cystic fibrosis E84.11
      meaning meconium plug (without cystic fibrosis) P76.0
    transitory P76.1
  obstructive K56.69
  paralytic K56.0
Iliac —see condition
Iliotibial band syndrome M76.3-
Illiteracy Z55.0
Illness —see also Disease R69
  manic-depressive —see Disorder, bipolar
Imbalance R26.89
  autonomic G90.8
  constituents of food intake E63.1
  electrolyte E87.8
    with
      abortion —see Abortion by type, complicated by, electrolyte imbalance
      molar pregnancy O08.5
    due to hyperemesis gravidarum O21.1
    following ectopic or molar pregnancy O08.5
    neonatal, transitory NEC P74.4
      potassium P74.3
      sodium P74.2
  endocrine E34.9
  eye muscle NOS H50.9
  hormone E34.9
  hysterical F44.4
  labyrinth —see subcategory H83.2
  posture R29.3
  protein-energy —see Malnutrition
  sympathetic G90.8
Imbecile, imbecility (I.Q. 35-49) F71
Imbedding, intrauterine device T83.39
Imbibition, cholesterol (gallbladder) K82.4
Imbrication, teeth, fully erupted M26.30
Imerslund (-Gräsbeck) syndrome D51.1
Immature —see also Immaturity
  birth (less than 37 completed weeks) —see Preterm, newborn
  extremely (less than 28 completed weeks) —see Immaturity, extreme
  personality F60.89
Immaturity (less than 37 completed weeks) —see also Preterm, newborn
  extreme of newborn (less than 28 completed weeks of gestation) (less than 196 completed days of gestation) (unspecified weeks of gestation) P07.20
    gestational age
      23 completed weeks (23 weeks, 0 days through 23 weeks, 6 days) P07.22
      24 completed weeks (24 weeks, 0 days through 24 weeks, 6 days) P07.23
      25 completed weeks (25 weeks, 0 days through 25 weeks, 6 days) P07.24
      26 completed weeks (26 weeks, 0 days through 26 weeks, 6 days) P07.25
      27 completed weeks (27 weeks, 0 days through 27 weeks, 6 days) P07.26
      less than 23 completed weeks P07.21
  fetus or infant light-for-dates —see Light-for-dates
  lung, newborn P28.0
  organ or site NEC —see Hypoplasia
  pulmonary, newborn P28.0
  reaction F60.89
  sexual (female) (male), after puberty E30.0

Immersion T75.1
  foot T69.02-
  hand T69.01-
Immobile, immobility
  complete, due to severe physical disability or frailty R53.2
  intestine K59.8
  syndrome (paraplegic) M62.3
Immune reconstitution (inflammatory) syndrome [IRIS] D89.3
Immunization —see also Vaccination
  ABO —see Incompatibility, ABO
    in newborn P55.1
  complication —see Complications, vaccination
  encounter for Z23
  not done (not carried out) Z28.9
    because (of)
      acute illness of patient Z28.01
      allergy to vaccine (or component) Z28.04
      caregiver refusal Z28.82
      chronic illness of patient Z28.02
      contraindication NEC Z28.09
      group pressure Z28.1
      guardian refusal Z28.82
      immune compromised state of patient Z28.03
      parent refusal Z28.82
      patient's belief Z28.1
      patient had disease being vaccinated against Z28.81
      patient refusal Z28.21
      religious beliefs of patient Z28.1
      specified reason NEC Z28.89
        of patient Z28.29
      unspecified patient reason Z28.20
  Rh factor
    affecting management of pregnancy NEC O36.09-
    anti-D antibody O36.01-
    from transfusion —see Complication (s), transfusion, incompatibility reaction, Rh (factor)
Immunocytoma C83.0-
Immunodeficiency D84.9
  with
    adenosine-deaminase deficiency D81.3
    antibody defects D80.9
      specified type NEC D80.8
    hyperimmunoglobulinemia D80.6
    increased immunoglobulin M (IgM) D80.5
    major defect D82.9
      specified type NEC D82.8
    partial albinism D82.8
    short-limbed stature D82.2
    thrombocytopenia and eczema D82.0
  antibody with
    hyperimmunoglobulinemia D80.6
    near-normal immunoglobulins D80.6
  autosomal recessive, Swiss type D80.0
  combined D81.9
    biotin-dependent carboxylase D81.819
    biotinidase D81.810
    holocarboxylase synthetase D81.818
    specified type NEC D81.818
    severe (SCID) D81.9
      with
        low or normal B-cell numbers D81.2
        low T- and B-cell numbers D81.1
        reticular dysgenesis D81.0
    specified type NEC D81.89
  common variable D83.9
    with
      abnormalities of B-cell numbers and function D83.0
      autoantibodies to B- or T-cells D83.2
      immunoregulatory T-cell disorders D83.1
    specified type NEC D83.8
  following hereditary defective response to Epstein-Barr virus (EBV) D82.3

Immunodeficiency (Continued)
  selective, immunoglobulin
    A (IgA) D80.2
    G (IgG) (subclasses) D80.3
    M (IgM) D80.4
  severe combined (SCID) D81.9
  specified type NEC D84.8
  X-linked, with increased IgM D80.5
Immunotherapy (encounter for)
  antineoplastic Z51.12
Impaction, impacted
  bowel, colon, rectum —see also Impaction,
    fecal K56.49
    by gallstone K56.3
  calculus —see Calculus
  cerumen (ear) (external) H61.2-
  cuspid —see Impaction, tooth
  dental (same or adjacent tooth) K01.1
  fecal, feces K56.41
  fracture —see Fracture, by site
  gallbladder —see Calculus, gallbladder
  gallstone (s) —see Calculus, gallbladder
    bile duct (common) (hepatic) —see
      Calculus, bile duct
    cystic duct —see Calculus, gallbladder
    in intestine, with obstruction (any part)
      K56.3
  intestine (calculous) NEC —see also
    Impaction, fecal K56.49
    gallstone, with ileus K56.3
  intrauterine device (IUD) T83.39
  molar —see Impaction, tooth
  shoulder, causing obstructed labor O66.0
  tooth, teeth K01.1
  turbinate J34.89
Impaired, impairment (function)
  auditory discrimination —see Abnormal,
    auditory perception
  cognitive, mild, so stated G31.84
  dual sensory Z73.82
  fasting glucose R73.01
  glucose tolerance (oral) R73.02
  hearing —see Deafness
  heart —see Disease, heart
  kidney N28.9
    disorder resulting from N25.9
      specified NEC N25.89
  liver K72.90
    with coma K72.91
  mastication K08.89
  mild cognitive, so stated G31.84
  mobility
    ear ossicles —see Ankylosis, ear ossicles
    requiring care provider Z74.09
  myocardium, myocardial —see Insufficiency,
    myocardial
  rectal sphincter R19.8
  renal (acute) (chronic) N28.9
    disorder resulting from N25.9
      specified NEC N25.89
  vision NEC H54.7
    both eyes H54.3
Impediment, speech R47.9
  psychogenic (childhood) F98.8
  slurring R47.81
  specified NEC R47.89
Impending
  coronary syndrome I20.0
  delirium tremens F10.239
  myocardial infarction I20.0
Imperception auditory (acquired) —see also
    Deafness
  congenital H93.25
Imperfect
  aeration, lung (newborn) NEC —see
    Atelectasis
  closure (congenital)
    alimentary tract NEC Q45.8
      lower Q43.8
      upper Q40.8
    atrioventricular ostium Q21.2

Imperfect (Continued)
  closure (Continued)
    atrium (secundum) Q21.1
    branchial cleft or sinus Q18.0
    choroid Q14.3
    cricoid cartilage Q31.8
    cusps, heart valve NEC Q24.8
      pulmonary Q22.3
    ductus
      arteriosus Q25.0
      Botalli Q25.0
    ear drum (causing impairment of hearing)
      Q16.4
    esophagus with communication to
      bronchus or trachea Q39.1
    eyelid Q10.3
    foramen
      botalli Q21.1
      ovale Q21.1
    genitalia, genital organ (s) or system
      female Q52.8
        external Q52.79
        internal NEC Q52.8
      male Q55.8
    glottis Q31.8
    interatrial ostium or septum Q21.1
    interauricular ostium or septum Q21.1
    interventricular ostium or septum Q21.0
    larynx Q31.8
    lip —see Cleft, lip
    nasal septum Q30.3
    nose Q30.2
    omphalomesenteric duct Q43.0
    optic nerve entry Q14.2
    organ or site not listed —see Anomaly, by
      site
    ostium
      interatrial Q21.1
      interauricular Q21.1
      interventricular Q21.0
    palate —see Cleft, palate
    preauricular sinus Q18.1
    retina Q14.1
    roof of orbit Q75.8
    sclera Q13.5
    septum
      aorticopulmonary Q21.4
      atrial (secundum) Q21.1
      between aorta and pulmonary artery
        Q21.4
      heart Q21.9
      interatrial (secundum) Q21.1
      interauricular (secundum) Q21.1
      interventricular Q21.0
        in tetralogy of Fallot Q21.3
      nasal Q30.3
      ventricular Q21.0
        with pulmonary stenosis or atresia,
          dextraposition of aorta, and
          hypertrophy of right ventricle
          Q21.3
        in tetralogy of Fallot Q21.3
    skull Q75.0
      with
        anencephaly Q00.0
        encephalocele —see Encephalocele
        hydrocephalus Q03.9
          with spina bifida —see Spina bifida,
            by site, with hydrocephalus
        microcephaly Q02
    spine (with meningocele) —see Spina
      bifida
    trachea Q32.1
    tympanic membrane (causing impairment
      of hearing) Q16.4
    uterus Q51.818
    vitelline duct Q43.0
  erection —see Dysfunction, sexual, male,
    erectile
  fusion —see Imperfect, closure
  inflation, lung (newborn) —see Atelectasis

Imperfect (Continued)
  posture R29.3
  rotation, intestine Q43.3
  septum, ventricular Q21.0
Imperfectly descended testis —see Cryptorchid
Imperforate (congenital) —see also Atresia
  anus Q42.3
    with fistula Q42.2
  cervix (uteri) Q51.828
  esophagus Q39.0
    with tracheoesophageal fistula Q39.1
  hymen Q52.3
  jejunum Q41.1
  pharynx Q38.8
  rectum Q42.1
    with fistula Q42.0
  urethra Q64.39
  vagina Q52.4
Impervious (congenital) —see also Atresia
  anus Q42.3
    with fistula Q42.2
  bile duct Q44.2
  esophagus Q39.0
    with tracheoesophageal fistula Q39.1
  intestine (small) Q41.9
    large Q42.9
      specified NEC Q42.8
  rectum Q42.1
    with fistula Q42.0
  ureter —see Atresia, ureter
  urethra Q64.39
Impetiginization of dermatoses L01.1
Impetigo (any organism) (any site) (circinate)
    (contagiosa) (simplex) (vulgaris)
    L01.00
  Bockhart's L01.02
  bullous, bullosa L01.03
  external ear L01.00 [H62.40]
  follicularis L01.02
  furfuracea L30.5
  herpetiformis L40.1
    nonobstetrical L40.1
  neonatorum L01.03
  nonbullous L01.01
  specified type NEC L01.09
  ulcerative L01.09
Impingement (on teeth)
  soft tissue
    anterior M26.81
    posterior M26.82
Implant, endometrial N80.9
Implantation
  anomalous —see Anomaly, by site
    ureter Q62.63
  cyst
    external area or site (skin) NEC L72.0
    iris —see Cyst, iris, implantation
    vagina N89.8
    vulva N90.7
  dermoid (cyst) —see Implantation, cyst
Impotence (sexual) N52.9
  counseling Z70.1
  organic origin —see also Dysfunction, sexual,
    male, erectile N52.9
  psychogenic F52.21
Impression, basilar Q75.8
Imprisonment, anxiety concerning Z65.1
Improper care (child) (newborn) —see
    Maltreatment
Improperly tied umbilical cord (causing
    hemorrhage) P51.8
Impulsiveness (impulsive) R45.87
Inability to swallow —see Aphagia
Inaccessible, inaccessibility
  health care NEC Z75.3
    due to
      waiting period Z75.2
        for admission to facility elsewhere
          Z75.1
    other helping agencies Z75.4
Inactive —see condition

◀ New   ◀▥ Revised   ~~deleted~~ Deleted

Inadequate, inadequacy
  aesthetics of dental restoration K08.56
  biologic, constitutional, functional, or social
    F60.7
  development
    child R62.50
    genitalia
      after puberty NEC E30.0
      congenital
        female Q52.8
          external Q52.79
          internal Q52.8
        male Q55.8
    lungs Q33.6
      associated with short gestation P28.0
    organ or site not listed —see Anomaly, by
      site
  diet (causing nutritional deficiency) E63.9
  eating habits Z72.4
  environment, household Z59.1
  family support Z63.8
  food (supply) NEC Z59.4
    hunger effects T73.0
  functional F60.7
  household care, due to
    family member
      handicapped or ill Z74.2
      on vacation Z75.5
      temporarily away from home Z74.2
    technical defects in home Z59.1
    temporary absence from home of person
      rendering care Z74.2
  housing (heating) (space) Z59.1
  income (financial) Z59.6
  intrafamilial communication Z63.8
  material resources Z59.9
  mental —see Disability, intellectual
  parental supervision or control of child Z62.0
  personality F60.7
  pulmonary
    function R06.89
      newborn P28.5
    ventilation, newborn P28.5
  sample of cytologic smear
    anus R85.615
    cervix R87.615
    vagina R87.625
  social F60.7
    insurance Z59.7
    skills NEC Z73.4
  supervision of child by parent Z62.0
  teaching affecting education Z55.8
  welfare support Z59.7
Inanition R64
  with edema —see Malnutrition, severe
  due to
    deprivation of food T73.0
    malnutrition —see Malnutrition
  fever R50.9
Inappropriate
  change in quantitative human chorionic
    gonadotropin (hCG) in early pregnancy
    O02.81
  diet or eating habits Z72.4
  level of quantitative human chorionic
    gonadotropin (hCG) for gestational age
    in early pregnancy O02.81
  secretion
    antidiuretic hormone (ADH) (excessive)
      E22.2
    deficiency E23.2
    pituitary (posterior) E22.2
Inattention at or after birth —see Neglect
Incarceration, incarcerated
  enterocele K46.0
    gangrenous K46.1
  epiplocele K46.0
    gangrenous K46.1
  exomphalos K42.0 ◄
    gangrenous K42.1 ◄
  ~~exophthalmos K42.0~~
    ~~gangrenous K42.1~~

Incarceration, incarcerated (Continued)
  hernia —see also Hernia, by site, with
    obstruction
    with gangrene —see Hernia, by site, with
      gangrene
  iris, in wound —see Injury, eye, laceration,
    with prolapse
  lens, in wound —see Injury, eye, laceration,
    with prolapse
  omphalocele K42.0
  prison, anxiety concerning Z65.1
  rupture —see Hernia, by site
  sarcoepiplocele K46.0
    gangrenous K46.1
  sarcoepiplomphalocele K42.0
    with gangrene K42.1
  uterus N85.8
    gravid O34.51-
      causing obstructed labor O65.5
Incised wound
  external —see Laceration
  internal organs —see Injury, by site
Incision, incisional
  hernia K43.2
    with
      gangrene (and obstruction) K43.1
      obstruction K43.0
  surgical, complication —see Complications,
    surgical procedure
  traumatic
    external —see Laceration
    internal organs —see Injury, by site
Inclusion
  azurophilic leukocytic D72.0
  blennorrhea (neonatal) (newborn) P39.1
  gallbladder in liver (congenital) Q44.1
Incompatibility
  ABO
    affecting management of pregnancy
      O36.11-
      anti-A sensitization O36.11-
      anti-B sensitization O36.19-
      specified NEC O36.19-
    infusion or transfusion reaction —see
      Complication (s), transfusion,
      incompatibility reaction, ABO
    newborn P55.1
  blood (group) (Duffy) (K(ell)) (Kidd) (Lewis)
    (M) (S) NEC
    affecting management of pregnancy
      O36.11-
      anti-A sensitization O36.11-
      anti-B sensitization O36.19-
    infusion or transfusion reaction T80.89
    newborn P55.8
  divorce or estrangement Z63.5
  Rh (blood group) (factor) Z31.82
    affecting management of pregnancy NEC
      O36.09-
      anti-D antibody O36.01-
    infusion or transfusion reaction —see
      Complication (s), transfusion,
      incompatibility reaction, Rh (factor)
    newborn P55.0
  rhesus —see Incompatibility, Rh
Incompetency, incompetent, incompetence
  annular
    aortic (valve) —see Insufficiency, aortic
    mitral (valve) I34.0
    pulmonary valve (heart) I37.1
  aortic (valve) —see Insufficiency, aortic
  cardiac valve —see Endocarditis
  cervix, cervical (os) N88.3
    in pregnancy O34.3-
  chronotropic I45.89
    with
      autonomic dysfunction G90.8
      ischemic heart disease I25.89
      left ventricular dysfunction I51.89
      sinus node dysfunction I49.8
  esophagogastric (junction) (sphincter) K22.0

Incompetency, incompetent, incompetence
    (Continued)
  mitral (valve) —see Insufficiency, mitral
  pelvic fundus N81.89
  pubocervical tissue N81.82
  pulmonary valve (heart) I37.1
    congenital Q22.3
  rectovaginal tissue N81.83
  tricuspid (annular) (valve) —see Insufficiency,
    tricuspid
  valvular —see Endocarditis
    congenital Q24.8
  vein, venous (saphenous) (varicose) —see
    Varix, leg
Incomplete —see also condition
  bladder, emptying R33.9
  defecation R15.0
  expansion lungs (newborn) NEC —see
    Atelectasis
  rotation, intestine Q43.3
Inconclusive
  diagnostic imaging due to excess body fat of
    patient R93.9
  findings on diagnostic imaging of breast NEC
    R92.8
  mammogram (due to dense breasts) R92.2
Incontinence R32
  anal sphincter R15.9
  coital N39.491 ◄
  feces R15.9
    nonorganic origin F98.1
  insensible (urinary) N39.42 ◄
  overflow N39.490
  postural (urinary) N39.492 ◄
  psychogenic F45.8
  rectal R15.9
  reflex N39.498
  stress (female) (male) N39.3
    and urge N39.46
  urethral sphincter R32
  urge N39.41
    and stress (female) (male) N39.46
  urine (urinary) R32
    continuous N39.45
    due to cognitive impairment, or severe
      physical disability or immobility
      R39.81
    functional R39.81
    insensible N39.42 ◄
    mixed (stress and urge) N39.46
    nocturnal N39.44
    nonorganic origin F98.0
    overflow N39.490
    post dribbling N39.43
    postural N39.492 ◄
    reflex N39.498
    specified NEC N39.498
    stress (female) (male) N39.3
      and urge N39.46
    total N39.498
    unaware N39.42
    urge N39.41
      and stress (female) (male) N39.46
Incontinentia pigmenti Q82.3
Incoordinate, incoordination
  esophageal-pharyngeal (newborn) —see
    Dysphagia
  muscular R27.8
  uterus (action) (contractions) (complicating
    delivery) O62.4
Increase, increased
  abnormal, in development R63.8
  androgens (ovarian) E28.1
  anticoagulants (antithrombin) (anti-VIIIa)
    (anti-IXa) (anti-Xa) (anti-XIa) —see
    Circulating anticoagulants
  cold sense R20.8
  estrogen E28.0
  function
    adrenal
      cortex —see Cushing's, syndrome
      medulla E27.5

Increase, increased (Continued)
  function (Continued)
    pituitary (gland) (anterior) (lobe) E22.9
      posterior E22.2
    heat sense R20.8
    intracranial pressure (benign) G93.2
    permeability, capillaries I78.8
    pressure, intracranial G93.2
    secretion
      gastrin E16.4
      glucagon E16.3
      pancreas, endocrine E16.9
        growth hormone-releasing hormone E16.8
        pancreatic polypeptide E16.8
        somatostatin E16.8
        vasoactive-intestinal polypeptide E16.8
    sphericity, lens Q12.4
    splenic activity D73.1
    venous pressure I87.8
      portal K76.6
Increta placenta O43.22-
Incrustation, cornea, foreign body (lead)
  (zinc) —see Foreign body, cornea
Incyclophoria H50.54
Incyclotropia —see Cyclotropia
Indeterminate sex Q56.4
India rubber skin Q82.8
Indigestion (acid) (bilious) (functional) K30
  catarrhal K31.89
  due to decomposed food NOS A05.9
  nervous F45.8
  psychogenic F45.8
Indirect —see condition
Induratio penis plastica N48.6
Induration, indurated
  brain G93.89
  breast (fibrous) N64.51
    puerperal, postpartum O92.29
  broad ligament N83.8
  chancre
    anus A51.1
    congenital A50.07
    extragenital NEC A51.2
  corpora cavernosa (penis) (plastic) N48.6
  liver (chronic) K76.89
  lung (black) (chronic) (fibroid) —see also
    Fibrosis, lung J84.10
    essential brown J84.03
  penile (plastic) N48.6
  phlebitic —see Phlebitis
  skin R23.4
Inebriety (without dependence) —see Alcohol,
  intoxication
Inefficiency, kidney N28.9
Inelasticity, skin R23.4
Inequality, leg (length) (acquired) —see also
  Deformity, limb, unequal length
  congenital —see Defect, reduction, lower
    limb
  lower leg —see Deformity, limb, unequal
    length
Inertia
  bladder (neurogenic) N31.2
  stomach K31.89
    psychogenic F45.8
  uterus, uterine during labor O62.2
    during latent phase of labor O62.0
    primary O62.0
    secondary O62.1
  vesical (neurogenic) N31.2
Infancy, infantile, infantilism —see also
  condition
  celiac K90.0
  genitalia, genitals (after puberty) E30.0
  Herter's (nontropical sprue) K90.0
  intestinal K90.0
  Lorain E23.0
  pancreatic K86.89 ◄▪▪▪
  pelvis M95.5
    with disproportion (fetopelvic) O33.1
      causing obstructed labor O65.1

Infancy, infantile, infantilism (Continued)
  pituitary E23.0
  renal N25.0
  uterus —see Infantile, genitalia
Infant (s) —see also Infancy
  excessive crying R68.11
  irritable child R68.12
  lack of care —see Neglect
  liveborn (singleton) Z38.2
    born in hospital Z38.00
      by cesarean Z38.01
    born outside hospital Z38.1
    multiple NEC Z38.8
      born in hospital Z38.68
        by cesarean Z38.69
      born outside hospital Z38.7
    quadruplet Z38.8
      born in hospital Z38.63
        by cesarean Z38.64
      born outside hospital Z38.7
    quintuplet Z38.8
      born in hospital Z38.65
        by cesarean Z38.66
      born outside hospital Z38.7
    triplet Z38.8
      born in hospital Z38.61
        by cesarean Z38.62
      born outside hospital Z38.7
    twin Z38.5
      born in hospital Z38.30
        by cesarean Z38.31
      born outside hospital Z38.4
  of diabetic mother (syndrome of) P70.1
    gestational diabetes P70.0
Infantile —see also condition
  genitalia, genitals E30.0
  os, uterine E30.0
  penis E30.0
  testis E29.1
  uterus E30.0
Infantilism —see Infancy
Infarct, infarction
  adrenal (capsule) (gland) E27.49
  appendices epiploicae —see also Infarct,
    intestine K55.069 ◄▪▪▪
  bowel —see also Infarct, intestine K55.069 ◄▪▪▪
  brain (stem) —see Infarct, cerebral
  breast N64.89
  brewer's (kidney) N28.0
  cardiac —see Infarct, myocardium
  cerebellar —see Infarct, cerebral
  cerebral —see also Occlusion, artery cerebral
    or precerebral, with infarction I63.9-
    aborted I63.9
    cortical I63.9
    due to
      cerebral venous thrombosis,
        nonpyogenic I63.6
      embolism
        cerebral arteries I63.4-
        precerebral arteries I63.1-
      occlusion NEC
        cerebral arteries I63.5-
        precerebral arteries I63.2-
      stenosis NEC
        cerebral arteries I63.5-
        precerebral arteries I63.2-
      thrombosis
        cerebral artery I63.3-
        precerebral artery I63.0-
    intraoperative
      during cardiac surgery I97.810
      during other surgery I97.811
    postprocedural
      following cardiac surgery I97.820
      following other surgery I97.821
    specified NEC I63.8
  colon (acute) (agnogenic) (embolic)
    (hemorrhagic) (nonocclusive)
    (nonthrombotic) (occlusive) (segmental)
    (thrombotic) (with gangrene) —see also
    Infarct, intestine K55.049 ◄▪▪▪

Infarct, infarction (Continued)
  coronary artery —see Infarct, myocardium
  embolic —see Embolism
  fallopian tube N83.8
  gallbladder K82.8
  heart —see Infarct, myocardium
  hepatic K76.3
  hypophysis (anterior lobe) E23.6
  impending (myocardium) I20.0
  intestine (acute) (agnogenic) (embolic)
    (hemorrhagic) (nonocclusive)
    (nonthrombotic) (occlusive) (thrombotic)
    (with gangrene) K55.069 ◄▪▪▪
    diffuse K55.062 ◄
    focal K55.061 ◄
    large K55.049 ◄
      diffuse K55.042 ◄
      focal K55.041 ◄
    small K55.029 ◄
      diffuse K55.022 ◄
      focal K55.021 ◄
  kidney N28.0
  liver K76.3
  lung (embolic) (thrombotic) —see Embolism,
    pulmonary
  lymph node I89.8
  mesentery, mesenteric (embolic) (thrombotic)
    (with gangrene) —see also Infarct,
    intestine K55.069 ◄▪▪▪
  muscle (ischemic) M62.20
    ankle M62.27-
    foot M62.27-
    forearm M62.23-
    hand M62.24-
    lower leg M62.26-
    pelvic region M62.25-
    shoulder region M62.21-
    specified site NEC M62.28
    thigh M62.25-
    upper arm M62.22-
  myocardium, myocardial (acute) (with stated
    duration of 4 weeks or less) I21.3
    diagnosed on ECG, but presenting no
      symptoms I25.2
    healed or old I25.2
    intraoperative
      during cardiac surgery I97.790
      during other surgery I97.791
    non-Q wave I21.4
    non-ST elevation (NSTEMI) I21.4
      subsequent I22.2
    nontransmural I21.4
    past (diagnosed on ECG or other
      investigation, but currently
      presenting no symptoms) I25.2
    postprocedural
      following cardiac surgery I97.190
      following other surgery I97.191
    Q wave (see also, Infarct, myocardium, by
      site) I21.3
    ST elevation (STEMI) I21.3
      anterior (anteroapical) (anterolateral)
        (anteroseptal) (Q wave) (wall)
        I21.09
        subsequent I22.0
      inferior (diaphragmatic) (inferolateral)
        (inferoposterior) (wall) NEC I21.19
        subsequent I22.1
      inferoposterior transmural (Q wave)
        I21.11
      involving
        coronary artery of anterior wall NEC
          I21.09
        coronary artery of inferior wall NEC
          I21.19
        diagonal coronary artery I21.02
        left anterior descending coronary
          artery I21.02
        left circumflex coronary artery
          I21.21
        left main coronary artery I21.01

◄ New   ◄▪▪▪ Revised   ~~deleted~~ Deleted

Infarct, infarction *(Continued)*
  myocardium, myocardial *(Continued)*
    ST elevation (STEMI) *(Continued)*
      involving *(Continued)*
        oblique marginal coronary artery I21.21
        right coronary artery I21.11
        lateral (apical-lateral) (basal-lateral)
            (high) I21.29
          subsequent I22.8
        posterior (posterobasal) (posterolateral)
            (posteroseptal) (true) I21.29
          subsequent I22.8
        septal I21.29
          subsequent I22.8
        specified NEC I21.29
          subsequent I22.8
      subsequent I22.9
    subsequent (recurrent) (reinfarction) I22.9
      anterior (anteroapical) (anterolateral)
          (anteroseptal) (wall) I22.0
      diaphragmatic (wall) I22.1
      inferior (diaphragmatic) (inferolateral)
          (inferoposterior) (wall) I22.1
      lateral (apical-lateral) (basal-lateral)
          (high) I22.8
      non-ST elevation (NSTEMI) I22.2
      posterior (posterobasal) (posterolateral)
          (posteroseptal) (true) I22.8
      septal I22.8
      specified NEC I22.8
      ST elevation I22.9
        anterior (anteroapical) (anterolateral)
            (anteroseptal) (wall) I22.0
        inferior (diaphragmatic) (inferolateral)
            (inferoposterior) (wall) I22.1
        specified NEC I22.8
    subendocardial I22.2
    transmural I22.9
      anterior (anteroapical) (anterolateral)
          (anteroseptal) (wall) I22.0
      diaphragmatic (wall) I22.1
      inferior (diaphragmatic) (inferolateral)
          (inferoposterior) (wall) I22.1
      lateral (apical-lateral) (basal-lateral)
          (high) I22.8
      posterior (posterobasal)
          (posterolateral) (posteroseptal)
          (true) I22.8
      specified NEC I22.8
  syphilitic A52.06
  transmural I21.3
    anterior (anteroapical) (anterolateral)
        (anteroseptal) (Q wave) (wall) NEC
        I21.09
    inferior (diaphragmatic) (inferolateral)
        (inferoposterior) (Q wave) (wall)
        NEC I21.19
    inferoposterior (Q wave) I21.11
    lateral (apical-lateral) (basal-lateral)
        (high) NEC I21.29
    posterior (posterobasal) (posterolateral)
        (posteroseptal) (true) NEC I21.29
    septal NEC I21.29
    specified NEC I21.29
  nontransmural I21.4
  omentum —*see also* Infarct, intestine
      K55.069 ◄▥
  ovary N83.8
  pancreas K86.89 ◄▥
  papillary muscle —*see* Infarct, myocardium
  parathyroid gland E21.4
  pituitary (gland) E23.6
  placenta O43.81-
  prostate N42.89
  pulmonary (artery) (vein) (hemorrhagic) —
      see Embolism, pulmonary
  renal (embolic) (thrombotic) N28.0
  retina, retinal (artery) —*see* Occlusion, artery,
      retina
  spinal (cord) (acute) (embolic) (nonembolic)
      G95.11

Infarct, infarction *(Continued)*
  spleen D73.5
    embolic or thrombotic I74.8
  subendocardial (acute) (nontransmural)
      I21.4
  suprarenal (capsule) (gland) E27.49
  testis N50.1
  thrombotic —*see also* Thrombosis
    artery, arterial —*see* Embolism
  thyroid (gland) E07.89
  ventricle (heart) —*see* Infarct, myocardium
Infecting —*see* condition
Infection, infected, infective (opportunistic)
    B99.9
  with
    drug resistant organism —*see* Resistance
        (to), drug —*see also* specific organism
    lymphangitis —*see* Lymphangitis
    organ dysfunction (acute) R65.20
      with septic shock R65.21
  abscess (skin) - code by site under Abscess
  Absidia —*see* Mucormycosis
  Acanthamoeba —*see* Acanthamebiasis
  Acanthocheilonema (perstans) (streptocerca)
      B74.4
  accessory sinus (chronic) —*see* Sinusitis
  achorion —*see* Dermatophytosis
  Acremonium falciforme B47.0
  acromioclavicular M00.9
  Actinobacillus (actinomycetem-comitans)
      A28.8
    mallei A24.0
    muris A25.1
  Actinomadura B47.1
  Actinomyces (israelii) —*see also*
      Actinomycosis A42.9
  Actinomycetales —*see* Actinomycosis
  actinomycotic NOS —*see* Actinomycosis
  adenoid (and tonsil) J03.90
    chronic J35.02
  adenovirus NEC
    as cause of disease classified elsewhere
        B97.0
    unspecified nature or site B34.0
  aerogenes capsulatus A48.0
  aertrycke —*see* Infection, salmonella
  alimentary canal NOS —*see* Enteritis,
      infectious
  Allescheria boydii B48.2
  Alternaria B48.8
  alveolus, alveolar (process) K04.7
  Ameba, amebic (histolytica) —*see* Amebiasis
  amniotic fluid, sac or cavity O41.10-
    chorioamnionitis O41.12-
    placentitis O41.14-
  amputation stump (surgical) —*see*
      Complication, amputation stump,
      infection
  Ancylostoma (duodenalis) B76.0
  Anisakiasis, Anisakis larvae B81.0
  anthrax —*see* Anthrax
  antrum (chronic) —*see* Sinusitis, maxillary
  anus, anal (papillae) (sphincter) K62.89
  arbovirus (arbor virus) A94
    specified type NEC A93.8
  artificial insemination N98.0
  Ascaris lumbricoides —*see* Ascariasis
  Ascomycetes B47.0
  Aspergillus (flavus) (fumigatus) (terreus) —
      see Aspergillosis
  atypical
    acid-fast (bacilli) —*see* Mycobacterium,
        atypical
    mycobacteria —*see* Mycobacterium,
        atypical
    virus A81.9
      specified type NEC A81.89
  auditory meatus (external) —*see* Otitis,
      externa, infective
  auricle (ear) —*see* Otitis, externa, infective
  axillary gland (lymph) L04.2

Infection, infected, infective *(Continued)*
  Bacillus A49.9
    abortus A23.1
    anthracis —*see* Anthrax
    Ducrey's (any location) A57
    Flexner's A03.1
    Friedländer's NEC A49.8
    gas (gangrene) A48.0
    mallei A24.0
    melitensis A23.0
    paratyphoid, paratyphosus A01.4
      A A01.1
      B A01.2
      C A01.3
    Shiga (-Kruse) A03.0
    suipestifer —*see* Infection, salmonella
    swimming pool A31.1
    typhosa A01.00
    welchii —*see* Gangrene, gas
  bacterial NOS A49.9
    as cause of disease classified elsewhere
        B96.89
      Bacteroides fragilis [B. fragilis] B96.6
      Clostridium perfringens [C. perfringens]
          B96.7
      Enterobacter sakazakii B96.89
      Enterococcus B95.2
      Escherichia coli [E. coli] (*see also*
          Escherichia coli) B96.20
      Helicobacter pylori [H.pylori]
          B96.81
      Hemophilus influenzae [H. influenzae]
          B96.3
      Klebsiella pneumoniae [K. pneumoniae]
          B96.1
      Mycoplasma pneumoniae [M.
          pneumoniae] B96.0
      Proteus (mirabilis) (morganii) B96.4
      Pseudomonas (aeruginosa) (mallei)
          (pseudomallei) B96.5
      Staphylococcus B95.8
        aureus (methicillin susceptible)
            (MSSA) B95.61
          methicillin resistant (MRSA)
              B95.62
        specified NEC B95.7
      Streptococcus B95.5
        group A B95.0
        group B B95.1
        pneumoniae B95.3
        specified NEC B95.4
      Vibrio vulnificus B96.82
    specified NEC A48.8
  Bacterium
    paratyphosum A01.4
      A A01.1
      B A01.2
      C A01.3
    typhosum A01.00
  Bacteroides NEC A49.8
    fragilis, as cause of disease classified
        elsewhere B96.6
  Balantidium coli A07.0
  Bartholin's gland N75.8
  Basidiobolus B46.8
  bile duct (common) (hepatic) —*see*
      Cholangitis
  bladder —*see* Cystitis
  Blastomyces, blastomycotic —*see also*
      Blastomycosis
    brasiliensis —*see* Paracoccidioidomycosis
    dermatitidis —*see* Blastomycosis
    European —*see* Cryptococcosis
    Loboi B48.0
    North American B40.9
    South American —*see*
        Paracoccidioidomycosis
  bleb, postprocedure —*see* Blebitis
  bone —*see* Osteomyelitis
  Bordetella —*see* Whooping cough
  Borrelia bergdorfi A69.20

Infection, infected, infective (Continued)
  brain —see also Encephalitis G04.90
    membranes —see Meningitis
    septic G06.0
      meninges —see Meningitis, bacterial
  branchial cyst Q18.0
  breast —see Mastitis
  bronchus —see Bronchitis
  Brucella A23.9
    abortus A23.1
    canis A23.3
    melitensis A23.0
    mixed A23.8
    specified NEC A23.8
    suis A23.2
  Brugia (malayi) B74.1
    timori B74.2
  bursa —see Bursitis, infective
  buttocks (skin) L08.9
  Campylobacter, intestinal A04.5
    as cause of disease classified elsewhere
      B96.81
  Candida (albicans) (tropicalis) —see
      Candidiasis
  candiru B88.8
  Capillaria (intestinal) B81.1
    hepatica B83.8
    philippinensis B81.1
  cartilage —see Disorder, cartilage, specified
      type NEC
  catheter-related bloodstream (CRBSI) T80.211
  cat liver fluke B66.0
  cellulitis - code by site under Cellulitis
  central line-associated T80.219
    bloodstream (CLABSI) T80.211
    specified NEC T80.218
  Cephalosporium falciforme B47.0
  cerebrospinal —see Meningitis
  cervical gland (lymph) L04.0
  cervix —see Cervicitis
  cesarean delivery wound (puerperal) O86.0
  cestodes —see Infestation, cestodes
  chest J22
  Chilomastix (intestinal) A07.8
  Chlamydia, chlamydial A74.9
    anus A56.3
    genitourinary tract A56.2
      lower A56.00
      specified NEC A56.19
    lymphogranuloma A55
    pharynx A56.4
    psittaci A70
    rectum A56.3
    sexually transmitted NEC A56.8
  cholera —see Cholera
  Cladosporium
    bantianum (brain abscess) B43.1
    carrionii B43.0
    castellanii B36.1
    trichoides (brain abscess) B43.1
    werneckii B36.1
  Clonorchis (sinensis) (liver) B66.1
  Clostridium NEC
    bifermentans A48.0
    botulinum (food poisoning) A05.1
      infant A48.51
      wound A48.52
    difficile
      as cause of disease classified elsewhere
        B96.89
      foodborne (disease) A04.7
      gas gangrene A48.0
      necrotizing enterocolitis A04.7
      sepsis A41.4
    gas-forming NEC A48.0
    histolyticum A48.0
    novyi, causing gas gangrene A48.0
    oedematiens A48.0
    perfringens
      as cause of disease classified elsewhere
        B96.7
      due to food A05.2

Infection, infected, infective (Continued)
  Clostridium (Continued)
    perfringens (Continued)
      foodborne (disease) A05.2
      gas gangrene A48.0
      sepsis A41.4
    septicum, causing gas gangrene A48.0
    sordellii, causing gas gangrene A48.0
    welchii
      as cause of disease classified elsewhere
        B96.7
      foodborne (disease) A05.2
      gas gangrene A48.0
      necrotizing enteritis A05.2
      sepsis A41.4
  Coccidioides (immitis) —see
      Coccidioidomycosis
  colon —see Enteritis, infectious
  colostomy K94.02
  common duct —see Cholangitis
  congenital P39.9
    Candida (albicans) P37.5
    cytomegalovirus P35.1
    hepatitis, viral P35.3
    herpes simplex P35.2
    infectious or parasitic disease P37.9
      specified NEC P37.8
    listeriosis (disseminated) P37.2
    malaria NEC P37.4
      falciparum P37.3
    Plasmodium falciparum P37.3
    poliomyelitis P35.8
    rubella P35.0
    skin P39.4
    toxoplasmosis (acute) (subacute) (chronic)
        P37.1
    tuberculosis P37.0
    urinary (tract) P39.3
    vaccinia P35.8
    virus P35.9
      specified type NEC P35.8
  Conidiobolus B46.8
  coronavirus NEC B34.2
    as cause of disease classified elsewhere
        B97.29
    severe acute respiratory syndrome (SARS
        associated) B97.21
  corpus luteum —see Salpingo-oophoritis
  Corynebacterium diphtheriae —see
      Diphtheria
  cotia virus B08.8
  Coxiella burnetii A78
  coxsackie —see Coxsackie
  Cryptococcus neoformans —see
      Cryptococcosis
  Cryptosporidium A07.2
  Cunninghamella —see Mucormycosis
  cyst —see Cyst
  cystic duct —see also Cholecystitis K81.9
  Cysticercus cellulosae —see Cysticercosis
  cytomegalovirus, cytomegaloviral B25.9
    congenital P35.1
    maternal, maternal care for (suspected)
        damage to fetus O35.3
    mononucleosis B27.10
      with
        complication NEC B27.19
        meningitis B27.12
        polyneuropathy B27.11
  delta-agent (acute), in hepatitis B carrier
      B17.0
  dental (pulpal origin) K04.7
  Deuteromycetes B47.0
  Dicrocoelium dendriticum B66.2
  Dipetalonema (perstans) (streptocerca) B74.4
  diphtherial —see Diphtheria
  Diphyllobothrium (adult) (latum) (pacificum)
      B70.0
    larval B70.1
  Diplogonoporus (grandis) B71.8
  Dipylidium caninum B67.4

Infection, infected, infective (Continued)
  Dirofilaria B74.8
  Dracunculus medinensis B72
  Drechslera (hawaiiensis) B43.8
  Ducrey Haemophilus (any location) A57
  due to or resulting from
    artificial insemination N98.0
    central venous catheter T80.219
      bloodstream T80.211
      exit or insertion site T80.212
      localized T80.212
      port or reservoir T80.212
      specified NEC T80.218
      tunnel T80.212
    device, implant or graft —see also
        Complications, by site and type,
        infection or inflammation
        T85.79
      arterial graft NEC T82.7
      breast (implant) T85.79
      catheter NEC T85.79
        dialysis (renal) T82.7
          intraperitoneal T85.71
        infusion NEC T82.7
          cranial T85.735 ◄
          intrathecal T85.735 ◄
          spinal (epidural) (subdural)
            T85.735 ◄▥
          subarachnoid T85.735 ◄
        urinary T83.518 ◄▥
          cystostomy T83.510 ◄
          Hopkins T83.518 ◄
          ileostomy T83.518 ◄
          nephrostomy T83.512 ◄
          specified NEC T83.518 ◄
          urethral indwelling T83.511 ◄
          urostomy T83.518 ◄
      electronic (electrode) (pulse generator)
          (stimulator)
        bone T84.7
        cardiac T82.7
        nervous system T85.738 ◄▥
          brain T85.731 ◄
          cranial nerve T85.732 ◄
          gastric nerve T85.732 ◄
          generator pocket T85.734 ◄
          neurostimulator generator
            T85.734 ◄
          peripheral nerve T85.732 ◄
          sacral nerve T85.732 ◄
          spinal cord T85.733 ◄
          vagal nerve T85.732 ◄
        urinary T83.590 ◄▥
      fixation, internal (orthopedic) NEC —see
          Complication, fixation device,
          infection
      gastrointestinal (bile duct) (esophagus)
          T85.79
        neurostimulator electrode (lead)
            T85.732 ◄
      genital NEC T83.69 ◄▥
      heart NEC T82.7
        valve (prosthesis) T82.6
          graft T82.7
      joint prosthesis —see Complication, joint
          prosthesis, infection
      ocular (corneal graft) (orbital implant)
          NEC T85.79
      orthopedic NEC T84.7
      penile (cylinder) (pump) (resevoir)
          T83.61 ◄
      specified NEC T85.79
      testicular T83.62 ◄
      urinary NEC T83.598 ◄▥
        ileal conduit stent T83.593 ◄
        implanted neurostimulation
            T83.590 ◄
        implanted sphincter T83.591 ◄
        indwelling ureteral stent T83.592 ◄
        nephroureteral stent T83.593 ◄
        specified stent NEC T83.593 ◄

◄ New   ◄▥ Revised   ~~deleted~~ Deleted

Infection, infected, infective *(Continued)*
  due to or resulting from *(Continued)*
    device, implant or graft *(Continued)*
      vascular NEC T82.7
      ~~ventricular intracranial shunt T85.79~~
      ventricular intracranial (communicating) shunt T85.730 ◀
    Hickman catheter T80.219
      bloodstream T80.211
      localized T80.212
      specified NEC T80.218
    immunization or vaccination T88.0
    infusion, injection or transfusion NEC T80.29
      acute T80.22
    injury NEC - code by site under Wound, open
    peripherally inserted central catheter (PICC) T80.219
      bloodstream T80.211
      localized T80.212
      specified NEC T80.218
    portacath (port-a-cath) T80.219
      bloodstream T80.211
      localized T80.212
      specified NEC T80.218
    pulmonary artery catheter —*see* Infection, due to or resulting from, central venous catheter ◀
    surgery T81.40 ◀▥
    Swan Ganz catheter —*see* Infection, due to or resulting from, central venous catheter ◀
    triple lumen catheter T80.219
      bloodstream T80.211
      localized T80.212
      specified NEC T80.218
    umbilical venous catheter T80.219
      bloodstream T80.211
      localized T80.212
      specified NEC T80.218
  during labor NEC O75.3
  ear (middle) —*see also* Otitis media
    external —*see* Otitis, externa, infective
    inner —*see* subcategory H83.0
  Eberthella typhosa A01.00
  Echinococcus —*see* Echinococcus
  echovirus
    as cause of disease classified elsewhere B97.12
    unspecified nature or site B34.1
  endocardium I33.0
  endocervix —*see* Cervicitis
  Entamoeba —*see* Amebiasis
  enteric —*see* Enteritis, infectious
  Enterobacter sakazakii B96.89
  Enterobius vermicularis B80
  enterostomy K94.12
  enterovirus B34.1
    as cause of disease classified elsewhere B97.10
      coxsackievirus B97.11
      echovirus B97.12
      specified NEC B97.19
  Entomophthora B46.8
  Epidermophyton —*see* Dermatophytosis
  epididymis —*see* Epididymitis
  episiotomy (puerperal) O86.0
  Erysipelothrix (insidiosa) (rhusiopathiae) —*see* Erysipeloid
  erythema infectiosum B08.3
  Escherichia (E.) coli NEC A49.8
    as cause of disease classified elsewhere — *see also* Escherichia coli B96.20
    congenital P39.8
      sepsis P36.4
    generalized A41.51
    intestinal —*see* Enteritis, infectious, due to, Escherichia coli
  ethmoidal (chronic) (sinus) —*see* Sinusitis, ethmoidal

Infection, infected, infective *(Continued)*
  eustachian tube (ear) —*see* Salpingitis, eustachian
  external auditory canal (meatus) NEC —*see* Otitis, externa, infective
  eye (purulent) —*see* Endophthalmitis, purulent
  eyelid —*see* Inflammation, eyelid
  fallopian tube —*see* Salpingo-oophoritis
  Fasciola (gigantica) (hepatica) (indica) B66.3
  Fasciolopsis (buski) B66.5
  filarial —*see* Infestation, filarial
  finger (skin) L08.9
    nail L03.01-
      fungus B35.1
  fish tapeworm B70.0
    larval B70.1
  flagellate, intestinal A07.9
  fluke —*see* Infestation, fluke
  focal
    teeth (pulpal origin) K04.7
    tonsils J35.01
  Fonsecaea (compactum) (pedrosoi) B43.0
  food —*see* Intoxication, foodborne
  foot (skin) L08.9
    dermatophytic fungus B35.3
  Francisella tularensis —*see* Tularemia
  frontal (sinus) (chronic) —*see* Sinusitis, frontal
  fungus NOS B49
    beard B35.0
    dermatophytic —*see* Dermatophytosis
    foot B35.3
    groin B35.6
    hand B35.2
    nail B35.1
    pathogenic to compromised host only B48.8
    perianal (area) B35.6
    scalp B35.0
    skin B36.9
      foot B35.3
      hand B35.2
      toenails B35.1
  Fusarium B48.8
  gallbladder —*see* Cholecystitis
  gas bacillus —*see* Gangrene, gas
  gastrointestinal —*see* Enteritis, infectious
  generalized NEC —*see* Sepsis
  generator pocket, implanted electronic neurostimulator T85.734 ◀
  genital organ or tract
    female —*see* Disease, pelvis, inflammatory
    male N49.9
      multiple sites N49.8
      specified NEC N49.8
  Ghon tubercle, primary A15.7
  Giardia lamblia A07.1
  gingiva (chronic) K05.10
    acute K05.00
      nonplaque induced K05.01
      plaque induced K05.00
    nonplaque induced K05.11
    plaque induced K05.10
  glanders A24.0
  glenosporopsis B48.0
  Gnathostoma (spinigerum) B83.1
  Gongylonema B83.8
  gonococcal —*see* Gonococcus
  gram-negative bacilli NOS A49.9
  guinea worm B72
  gum (chronic) K05.10
    acute K05.00
      nonplaque induced K05.01
      plaque induced K05.00
    nonplaque induced K05.11
    plaque induced K05.10
  Haemophilus —*see* Infection, Hemophilus
  heart —*see* Carditis

Infection, infected, infective *(Continued)*
  Helicobacter pylori A04.8
    as cause of disease classified elsewhere B96.81
  helminths B83.9
    intestinal B82.0
      mixed (types classifiable to more than one of the titles B65.0-B81.3 and B81.8) B81.4
      specified type NEC B81.8
    specified type NEC B83.8
  Hemophilus
    aegyptius, systemic A48.4
    ducrey (any location) A57
    generalized A41.3
    influenzae NEC A49.2
      as cause of disease classified elsewhere B96.3
  herpes (simplex) —*see also* Herpes
    congenital P35.2
    disseminated B00.7
    zoster B02.9
  herpesvirus, herpesviral —*see* Herpes
  Heterophyes (heterophyes) B66.8
  hip (joint) NEC M00.9
    due to internal joint prosthesis
      left T84.52
      right T84.51
    skin NEC L08.9
  Histoplasma —*see* Histoplasmosis
    American B39.4
    capsulatum B39.4
  hookworm B76.9
  human
    papilloma virus A63.0
    T-cell lymphotropic virus type-1 (HTLV-1) B33.3
  hydrocele N43.0
  Hymenolepis B71.0
  hypopharynx —*see* Pharyngitis
  inguinal (lymph) glands L04.1
    due to soft chancre A57
  intervertebral disc, pyogenic M46.30
    cervical region M46.32
    cervicothoracic region M46.33
    lumbar region M46.36
    lumbosacral region M46.37
    multiple sites M46.39
    occipito-atlanto-axial region M46.31
    sacrococcygeal region M46.38
    thoracic region M46.34
    thoracolumbar region M46.35
  intestine, intestinal —*see* Enteritis, infectious
    specified NEC A08.8
  intra-amniotic affecting newborn NEC P39.2
  Isospora belli or hominis A07.3
  Japanese B encephalitis A83.0
  jaw (bone) (lower) (upper) M27.2
  joint NEC M00.9
    due to internal joint prosthesis T84.50
  kidney (cortex) (hematogenous) N15.9
    with calculus N20.0
      with hydronephrosis N13.6
    following ectopic gestation O08.83
    pelvis and ureter (cystic) N28.85
    puerperal (postpartum) O86.21
    specified NEC N15.8
  Klebsiella (K.) pneumoniae NEC A49.8
    as cause of disease classified elsewhere B96.1
  knee (joint) NEC M00.9
    due to internal joint prosthesis
      left T84.54
      right T84.53
    joint M00.9
    skin L08.9
  Koch's —*see* Tuberculosis
  labia (majora) (minora) (acute) —*see* Vulvitis
  lacrimal
    gland —*see* Dacryoadenitis
    passages (duct) (sac) —*see* Inflammation, lacrimal, passages

Infection, infected, infective (*Continued*)
lancet fluke B66.2
larynx NEC J38.7
leg (skin) NOS L08.9
Legionella pneumophila A48.1
   nonpneumonic A48.2
Leishmania —*see also* Leishmaniasis
   aethiopica B55.1
   braziliensis B55.2
   chagasi B55.0
   donovani B55.0
   infantum B55.0
   major B55.1
   mexicana B55.1
   tropica B55.1
lentivirus, as cause of disease classified
   elsewhere B97.31
Leptosphaeria senegalensis B47.0
Leptospira interrogans A27.9
   autumnalis A27.89
   canicola A27.89
   hebdomadis A27.89
   icterohaemorrhagiae A27.0
   pomona A27.89
   specified type NEC A27.89
leptospirochetal NEC —*see* Leptospirosis
Listeria monocytogenes —*see also* Listeriosis
   congenital P37.2
Loa loa B74.3
   with conjunctival infestation B74.3
   eyelid B74.3
Loboa loboi B48.0
local, skin (staphylococcal) (streptococcal)
   L08.9
   abscess - code by site under Abscess
   cellulitis - code by site under Cellulitis
   specified NEC L08.89
   ulcer —*see* Ulcer, skin
Loefflerella mallei A24.0
lung —*see also* Pneumonia J18.9
   atypical Mycobacterium A31.0
   spirochetal A69.8
   tuberculous —*see* Tuberculosis,
     pulmonary
   virus —*see* Pneumonia, viral
lymph gland —*see also* Lymphadenitis,
   acute
   mesenteric I88.0
lymphoid tissue, base of tongue or posterior
   pharynx, NEC (chronic) J35.03
Madurella (grisea) (mycetomii) B47.0
major
   following ectopic or molar pregnancy
     O08.0
   puerperal, postpartum, childbirth O85
Malassezia furfur B36.0
Malleomyces
   mallei A24.0
   pseudomallei (whitmori) —*see* Melioidosis
mammary gland N61.0 ◀▥
Mansonella (ozzardi) (perstans) (streptocerca)
   B74.4
mastoid —*see* Mastoiditis
maxilla, maxillary M27.2
   sinus (chronic) —*see* Sinusitis,
     maxillary
mediastinum J98.51 ◀▥
Medina (worm) B72
meibomian cyst or gland —*see* Hordeolum
meninges —*see* Meningitis, bacterial
meningococcal —*see also* condition
   A39.9
   adrenals A39.1
   brain A39.81
   cerebrospinal A39.0
   conjunctiva A39.89
   endocardium A39.51
   heart A39.50
     endocardium A39.51
     myocardium A39.52
     pericardium A39.53

Infection, infected, infective (*Continued*)
meningococcal (*Continued*)
   joint A39.83
   meninges A39.0
   meningococcemia A39.4
     acute A39.2
     chronic A39.3
   myocardium A39.52
   pericardium A39.53
   retrobulbar neuritis A39.82
   specified site NEC A39.89
mesenteric lymph nodes or glands NEC
   I88.0
Metagonimus B66.8
metatarsophalangeal M00.9
methicillin
   resistant Staphylococcus aureus (MRSA)
     A49.02
   susceptible Staphylococcus aureus (MSSA)
     A49.01
Microsporum, microsporic —*see*
   Dermatophytosis
mixed flora (bacterial) NEC A49.8
Monilia —*see* Candidiasis
Monosporium apiospermum B48.2
mouth, parasitic B37.0
Mucor —*see* Mucormycosis
muscle NEC —*see* Myositis, infective
mycelium NOS B49
mycetoma B47.9
   actinomycotic NEC B47.1
   mycotic NEC B47.0
Mycobacterium, mycobacterial —*see*
   Mycobacterium
Mycoplasma NEC A49.3
   pneumoniae, as cause of disease classified
     elsewhere B96.0
mycotic NOS B49
   pathogenic to compromised host only
     B48.8
   skin NOS B36.9
myocardium NEC I40.0
nail (chronic)
   with lymphangitis —*see* Lymphangitis,
     acute, digit
   finger L03.01-
     fungus B35.1
   ingrowing L60.0
   toe L03.03-
     fungus B35.1
nasal sinus (chronic) —*see* Sinusitis
nasopharynx —*see* Nasopharyngitis
navel L08.82
Necator americanus B76.1
Neisseria —*see* Gonococcus
Neotestudina rosatii B47.0
newborn P39.9
   intra-amniotic NEC P39.2
   skin P39.4
   specified type NEC P39.8
nipple N61.0 ◀▥
   associated with
     lactation O91.03
     pregnancy O91.01-
     puerperium O91.02
Nocardia —*see* Nocardiosis
obstetrical surgical wound (puerperal)
   O86.0
Oesophagostomum (apiostomum)
   B81.8
Oestrus ovis —*see* Myiasis
Oidium albicans B37.9
Onchocerca (volvulus) —*see* Onchocerciasis -
   oncovirus, as cause of disease classified
     elsewhere B97.32
operation wound T81.40 ◀▥
Opisthorchis (felineus) (viverrini) B66.0
orbit, orbital —*see* Inflammation, orbit
orthopoxvirus NEC B08.09
ovary —*see* Salpingo-oophoritis
Oxyuris vermicularis B80

Infection, infected, infective (*Continued*)
pancreas (acute) —*see* Pancreatitis, acute ◀▥
   abscess —*see* Pancreatitis, acute
   specified NEC —*see also* Pancreatitis, acute
     K85.80 ◀▥
papillomavirus, as cause of disease classified
   elsewhere B97.7
papovavirus NEC B34.4
Paracoccidioides brasiliensis —*see*
   Paracoccidioidomycosis
Paragonimus (westermani) B66.4
parainfluenza virus B34.8
parameningococcus NOS A39.9
parapoxvirus B08.60
   specified NEC B08.69
parasitic B89
Parastrongylus
   cantonensis B83.2
   costaricensis B81.3
   paratyphoid A01.4
     Type A A01.1
     Type B A01.2
     Type C A01.3
paraurethral ducts N34.2
parotid gland —*see* Sialoadenitis
parvovirus NEC B34.3
   as cause of disease classified elsewhere
     B97.6
Pasteurella NEC A28.0
   multocida A28.0
   pestis —*see* Plague
   pseudotuberculosis A28.0
   septica (cat bite) (dog bite) A28.0
   tularensis —*see* Tularemia
pelvic, female —*see* Disease, pelvis,
   inflammatory
Penicillium (marneffei) B48.4
penis (glans) (retention) NEC N48.29
periapical K04.5
peridental, periodontal K05.20
   generalized —*see* Peridontitis, aggressive,
     generalized ◀▥
   localized —*see* Peridontitis, aggressive,
     localized ◀▥
perinatal period P39.9
   specified type NEC P39.8
perineal repair (puerperal) O86.0
periorbital —*see* Inflammation, orbit
perirectal K62.89
perirenal —*see* Infection, kidney
peritoneal —*see* Peritonitis
periureteral N28.89
Petriellidium boydii B48.2
pharynx —*see also* Pharyngitis
   coxsackievirus B08.5
   posterior, lymphoid (chronic) J35.03
Phialophora
   gougerotii (subcutaneous abscess or cyst)
     B43.2
   jeanselmei (subcutaneous abscess or cyst)
     B43.2
   verrucosa (skin) B43.0
Piedraia hortae B36.3
pinta A67.9
   intermediate A67.1
   late A67.2
   mixed A67.3
   primary A67.0
pinworm B80
pityrosporum furfur B36.0
pleuro-pneumonia-like organism (PPLO)
   NEC A49.3
   as cause of disease classified elsewhere
     B96.0
pneumococcus, pneumococcal NEC A49.1
   as cause of disease classified elsewhere
     B95.3
   generalized (purulent) A40.3
   with pneumonia J13
Pneumocystis carinii (pneumonia) B59
Pneumocystis jiroveci (pneumonia) B59

◀ New   ◀▥ Revised   ~~deleted~~ Deleted

Infection, infected, infective *(Continued)*
  port or reservoir T80.212
  postoperative T81.40 ◀▥
  postoperative wound T81.40 ◀▥
  postprocedural T81.40 ◀▥
    deep incisional surgical site T81.42 ◀
    organ and space surgical site T81.43 ◀
    sepsis T81.49 ◀
    specified surgical site NEC T81.48 ◀
    superficial incisional surgical site T81.41 ◀
  postvaccinal T88.0
  prepuce NEC N47.7
    with penile inflammation N47.6
  prion —*see* Disease, prion, central nervous system
  prostate (capsule) —*see* Prostatitis
  Proteus (mirabilis) (morganii) (vulgaris) NEC A49.8
    as cause of disease classified elsewhere B96.4
  protozoal NEC B64
    intestinal A07.9
      specified NEC A07.8
    specified NEC B60.8
  Pseudoallescheria boydii B48.2
  Pseudomonas NEC A49.8
    as cause of disease classified elsewhere B96.5
    mallei A24.0
    pneumonia J15.1
    pseudomallei —*see* Melioidosis
  puerperal O86.4
    genitourinary tract NEC O86.89
    major or generalized O85
    minor O86.4
    specified NEC O86.89
  pulmonary —*see* Infection, lung
  purulent —*see* Abscess
  Pyrenochaeta romeroi B47.0
  Q fever A78
  rectum (sphincter) K62.89
  renal —*see also* Infection, kidney
    pelvis and ureter (cystic) N28.85
  reovirus, as cause of disease classified elsewhere B97.5
  respiratory (tract) NEC J98.8
    acute J22
    chronic J98.8
    influenzal (upper) (acute) —*see* Influenza, with, respiratory manifestations NEC
    lower (acute) J22
      chronic —*see* Bronchitis, chronic
    rhinovirus J00
    syncytial virus, as cause of disease classified elsewhere B97.4
    upper (acute) NOS J06.9
      chronic J39.8
      streptococcal J06.9
      viral NOS J06.9
  resulting from
    presence of internal prosthesis, implant, graft —*see* Complications, by site and type, infection
  retortamoniasis A07.8
  retroperitoneal NEC K68.9
  retrovirus B33.3
    as cause of disease classified elsewhere B97.30
      human
        immunodeficiency, type 2 (HIV 2) B97.35
        T-cell lymphotropic
          type I (HTLV-I) B97.33
          type II (HTLV-II) B97.34
      lentivirus B97.31
      oncovirus B97.32
      specified NEC B97.39
  Rhinosporidium (seeberi) B48.1
  rhinovirus
    as cause of disease classified elsewhere B97.89
    unspecified nature or site B34.8

Infection, infected, infective *(Continued)*
  Rhizopus —*see* Mucormycosis
  rickettsial NOS A79.9
  roundworm (large) NEC B82.0
    Ascariasis —*see also* Ascariasis B77.9
  rubella —*see* Rubella
  Saccharomyces —*see* Candidiasis
  salivary duct or gland (any) —*see* Sialoadenitis
  Salmonella (aertrycke) (arizonae) (callinarum) (cholerae-suis) (enteritidis) (suipestifer) (typhimurium) A02.9
    with
      (gastro) enteritis A02.0
      sepsis A02.1
      specified manifestation NEC A02.8
    due to food (poisoning) A02.9
    hirschfeldii A01.3
    localized A02.20
      arthritis A02.23
      meningitis A02.21
      osteomyelitis A02.24
      pneumonia A02.22
      pyelonephritis A02.25
      specified NEC A02.29
    paratyphi A01.4
      A A01.1
      B A01.2
      C A01.3
    schottmuelleri A01.2
    typhi, typhosa —*see* Typhoid
  Sarcocystis A07.8
  scabies B86
  Schistosoma —*see* Infestation, Schistosoma
  scrotum (acute) NEC N49.2
  seminal vesicle —*see* Vesiculitis
  septic
    localized, skin —*see* Abscess
  sheep liver fluke B66.3
  Shigella A03.9
    boydii A03.2
    dysenteriae A03.0
    flexneri A03.1
    group
      A A03.0
      B A03.1
      C A03.2
      D A03.3
    Schmitz (-Stutzer) A03.0
    schmitzii A03.0
    shigae A03.0
    sonnei A03.3
    specified NEC A03.8
  shoulder (joint) NEC M00.9
    due to internal joint prosthesis T84.59
    skin NEC L08.9
  sinus (accessory) (chronic) (nasal) —*see also* Sinusitis
    pilonidal —*see* Sinus, pilonidal
    skin NEC L08.89
  Skene's duct or gland —*see* Urethritis
  skin (local) (staphylococcal) (streptococcal) L08.9
    abscess - code by site under Abscess
    cellulitis - code by site under Cellulitis
    due to fungus B36.9
      specified type NEC B36.8
    mycotic B36.9
      specified type NEC B36.8
    newborn P39.4
    ulcer —*see* Ulcer, skin
  slow virus A81.9
    specified NEC A81.89
  Sparganum (mansoni) (proliferum) (baxteri) B70.1
  specific —*see also* Syphilis
    to perinatal period —*see* Infection, congenital
  specified NEC B99.8
  spermatic cord NEC N49.1

Infection, infected, infective *(Continued)*
  sphenoidal (sinus) —*see* Sinusitis, sphenoidal
  spinal cord NOS —*see also* Myelitis G04.91
    abscess G06.1
    meninges —*see* Meningitis
    streptococcal G04.89
  Spirillum A25.0
  spirochetal NOS A69.9
    lung A69.8
    specified NEC A69.8
  Spirometra larvae B70.1
  spleen D73.89
  Sporotrichum, Sporothrix (schenckii) —*see* Sporotrichosis
  staphylococcal, unspecified site
    aureus (methicillin susceptible) (MSSA) A49.01
      methicillin resistant (MRSA) A49.02
    as cause of disease classified elsewhere B95.8
      aureus (methicillin susceptible) (MSSA) B95.61
      methicillin resistant (MRSA) B95.62
      specified NEC B95.7
    food poisoning A05.0
    generalized (purulent) A41.2
    pneumonia —*see* Pneumonia, staphylococcal
  Stellantchasmus falcatus B66.8
  streptobacillus moniliformis A25.1
  streptococcal NEC A49.1
    as cause of disease classified elsewhere B95.5
    B genitourinary complicating
      childbirth O98.82
      pregnancy O98.81-
      puerperium O98.83
    congenital
      sepsis P36.10
        group B P36.0
        specified NEC P36.19
    generalized (purulent) A40.9
  Streptomyces B47.1
  Strongyloides (stercoralis) —*see* Strongyloidiasis
  stump (amputation) (surgical) —*see* Complication, amputation stump, infection
  subcutaneous tissue, local L08.9
  suipestifer —*see* Infection, salmonella
  swimming pool bacillus A31.1
  Taenia —*see* Infestation, Taenia
  Taeniarhynchus saginatus B68.1
  tapeworm —*see* Infestation, tapeworm
  tendon (sheath) —*see* Tenosynovitis, infective NEC
  Ternidens diminutus B81.8
  testis —*see* Orchitis
  threadworm B80
  throat —*see* Pharyngitis
  thyroglossal duct K14.8
  toe (skin) L08.9
    cellulitis L03.03-
      fungus B35.1
    nail L03.03-
      fungus B35.1
  tongue NEC K14.0
    parasitic B37.0
  tonsil (and adenoid) (faucial) (lingual) (pharyngeal) —*see* Tonsillitis
  tooth, teeth K04.7
    irreversible K04.02 ◀
    periapical K04.7
    peridental, periodontal K05.20
      generalized —*see* Peridontitis, aggressive, generalized ◀▥
      localized —*see* Peridontitis, aggressive, localized ◀▥

Infection, infected, infective (Continued)
  tooth, teeth (Continued)
    pulp K04.01 ⬅
    reversible K04.01 ◀
    socket M27.3
  TORCH —see Infection, congenital
    without active infection P00.2
  Torula histolytica —see Cryptococcosis
  Toxocara (canis) (cati) (felis) B83.0
  Toxoplasma gondii —see Toxoplasma
  trachea, chronic J42
  trematode NEC —see Infestation, fluke
  trench fever A79.0
  Treponema pallidum —see Syphilis
  Trichinella (spiralis) B75
  Trichomonas A59.9
    cervix A59.09
    intestine A07.8
    prostate A59.02
    specified site NEC A59.8
    urethra A59.03
    urogenitalis A59.00
    vagina A59.01
    vulva A59.01
  Trichophyton, trichophytic —see
    Dermatophytosis
  Trichosporon (beigelii) cutaneum B36.2
  Trichostrongylus B81.2
  Trichuris (trichiura) B79
  Trombicula (irritans) B88.0
  Trypanosoma
    brucei
      gambiense B56.0
      rhodesiense B56.1
    cruzi —see Chagas' disease
  tubal —see Salpingo-oophoritis
  tuberculous NEC —see Tuberculosis
  tubo-ovarian —see Salpingo-oophoritis
  tunica vaginalis N49.1
  tunnel T80.212
  tympanic membrane NEC —see Myringitis
  typhoid (abortive) (ambulant) (bacillus) —see
    Typhoid
  typhus A75.9
    flea-borne A75.2
    mite-borne A75.3
    recrudescent A75.1
    tick-borne A77.9
      African A77.1
      North Asian A77.2
  umbilicus L08.82
  ureter N28.86
  urethra —see Urethritis
  urinary (tract) N39.0
    bladder —see Cystitis
    complicating
      pregnancy O23.4-
        specified type NEC O23.3-
    kidney —see Infection, kidney
    newborn P39.3
    puerperal (postpartum) O86.20
    tuberculous A18.13
    urethra —see Urethritis
  uterus, uterine —see Endometritis
  vaccination T88.0
  vaccinia not from vaccination B08.011
  vagina (acute) —see Vaginitis
  varicella B01.9
  varicose veins —see Varix
  vas deferens NEC N49.1
  vesical —see Cystitis
  Vibrio
    cholerae A00.0
      El Tor A00.1
    parahaemolyticus (food poisoning)
      A05.3
    vulnificus
      as cause of disease classified elsewhere
        B96.82
      foodborne intoxication A05.5
  Vincent's (gum) (mouth) (tonsil) A69.1

Infection, infected, infective (Continued)
  virus, viral NOS B34.9
    adenovirus
      as cause of disease classified elsewhere
        B97.0
      unspecified nature or site B34.0
    arborvirus, arbovirus arthropod-borne A94
    as cause of disease classified elsewhere
      B97.89
      adenovirus B97.0
      coronavirus B97.29
        SARS-associated B97.21
      coxsackievirus B97.11
      echovirus B97.12
      enterovirus B97.10
        coxsackievirus B97.11
        echovirus B97.12
        specified NEC B97.19
      human
        immunodeficiency, type 2 (HIV 2)
          B97.35
        metapneumovirus B97.81
        T-cell lymphotropic,
          type I (HTLV-I) B97.33
          type II (HTLV-II) B97.34
      papillomavirus B97.7
      parvovirus B97.6
      reovirus B97.5
      respiratory syncytial B97.4
      retrovirus B97.30
        human
          immunodeficiency, type 2 (HIV 2)
            B97.35
          T-cell lymphotropic,
            type I (HTLV-I) B97.33
            type II (HTLV-II) B97.34
        lentivirus B97.31
        oncovirus B97.32
        specified NEC B97.39
      specified NEC B97.89
    central nervous system A89
      atypical A81.9
        specified NEC A81.89
      enterovirus NEC A88.8
        meningitis A87.0
      slow virus A81.9
        specified NEC A81.89
      specified NEC A88.8
    chest J98.8
    cotia B08.8
    coxsackie —see also Infection, coxsackie B34.1
      as cause of disease classified elsewhere
        B97.11
    ECHO
      as cause of disease classified elsewhere
        B97.12
      unspecified nature or site B34.1
    encephalitis, tick-borne A84.9
    enterovirus, as cause of disease classified
      elsewhere B97.10
      coxsackievirus B97.11
      echovirus B97.12
      specified NEC B97.19
    exanthem NOS B09
    human metapneumovirus as cause of
      disease classified elsewhere B97.81
    human papilloma as cause of disease
      classified elsewhere B97.7
    intestine —see Enteritis, viral
    respiratory syncytial
      as cause of disease classified elsewhere
        B97.4
      bronchopneumonia J12.1
      common cold syndrome J00
      nasopharyngitis (acute) J00
    rhinovirus
      as cause of disease classified elsewhere
        B97.89
      unspecified nature or site B34.8
    slow A81.9
      specified NEC A81.89

Infection, infected, infective (Continued)
  virus, viral NOS (Continued)
    specified type NEC B33.8
      as cause of disease classified elsewhere
        B97.89
      unspecified nature or site B34.8
    unspecified nature or site B34.9
    West Nile —see Virus, West Nile
  vulva (acute) —see Vulvitis
  West Nile —see Virus, West Nile
  whipworm B79
  worms B83.9
    specified type NEC B83.8
  Wuchereria (bancrofti) B74.0
    malayi B74.1
    yatapoxvirus B08.70
      specified NEC B08.79
  yeast (see also Candidiasis) B37.9
  yellow fever —see Fever, yellow
  Yersinia
    enterocolitica (intestinal) A04.6
    pestis —see Plague
    pseudotuberculosis A28.2
  Zeis' gland —see Hordeolum
  Zika virus A92.5 ◀
  zoonotic bacterial NOS A28.9
  Zopfia senegalensis B47.0
Infective, infectious —see condition
Infertility
  female N97.9
    age-related N97.8
    associated with
      anovulation N97.0
      cervical (mucus) disease or anomaly
        N88.3
      congenital anomaly
        cervix N88.3
        fallopian tube N97.1
        uterus N97.2
        vagina N97.8
      dysmucorrhea N88.3
      fallopian tube disease or anomaly N97.1
      pituitary-hypothalamic origin E23.0
      specified origin NEC N97.8
      Stein-Leventhal syndrome E28.2
      uterine disease or anomaly N97.2
      vaginal disease or anomaly N97.8
    due to
      cervical anomaly N88.3
      fallopian tube anomaly N97.1
      ovarian failure E28.39
      Stein-Leventhal syndrome E28.2
      uterine anomaly N97.2
      vaginal anomaly N97.8
    nonimplantation N97.2
    origin
      cervical N88.3
      tubal (block) (occlusion) (stenosis) N97.1
      uterine N97.2
      vaginal N97.8
  male N46.9
    azoospermia N46.01
      extratesticular cause N46.029
        drug therapy N46.021
        efferent duct obstruction N46.023
        infection N46.022
        radiation N46.024
        specified cause NEC N46.029
        systemic disease N46.025
    oligospermia N46.11
      extratesticular cause N46.129
        drug therapy N46.121
        efferent duct obstruction N46.123
        infection N46.122
        radiation N46.124
        specified cause NEC N46.129
        systemic disease N46.125
    specified type NEC N46.8
Infestation B88.9
  Acanthocheilonema (perstans) (streptocerca)
    B74.4

◀ New   ⬅ Revised   ~~deleted~~ Deleted

Infestation (Continued)
  Acariasis B88.Ø
    demodex folliculorum B88.Ø
    sarcoptes scabiei B86
    trombiculae B88.Ø
  Agamofilaria streptocerca B74.4
  Ancylostoma, ankylostoma (braziliense)
      (caninum) (ceylanicum) (duodenale)
      B76.Ø
    americanum B76.1
    new world B76.1
  Anisakis larvae, anisakiasis B81.Ø
  arthropod NEC B88.2
  Ascaris lumbricoides —see Ascariasis
  Balantidium coli AØ7.Ø
  beef tapeworm B68.1
  Bothriocephalus (latus) B7Ø.Ø
    larval B7Ø.1
  broad tapeworm B7Ø.Ø
    larval B7Ø.1
  Brugia (malayi) B74.1
    timori B74.2
  candiru B88.8
  Capillaria
    hepatica B83.8
    philippinensis B81.1
  cat liver fluke B66.Ø
  cestodes B71.9
    diphyllobothrium —see Infestation,
        diphyllobothrium
    dipylidiasis B71.1
    hymenolepiasis B71.Ø
    specified type NEC B71.8
  chigger B88.Ø
  chigo, chigoe B88.1
  Clonorchis (sinensis) (liver) B66.1
  coccidial AØ7.3
  crab-lice B85.3
  Cysticercus cellulosae —see Cysticercosis
  Demodex (folliculorum) B88.Ø
  Dermanyssus gallinae B88.Ø
  Dermatobia (hominis) —see Myiasis
  Dibothriocephalus (latus) B7Ø.Ø
    larval B7Ø.1
  Dicrocoelium dendriticum B66.2
  Diphyllobothrium (adult) (latum) (intestinal)
      (pacificum) B7Ø.Ø
    larval B7Ø.1
  Diplogonoporus (grandis) B71.8
  Dipylidium caninum B67.4
  Distoma hepaticum B66.3
  dog tapeworm B67.4
  Dracunculus medinensis B72
  dragon worm B72
  dwarf tapeworm B71.Ø
  Echinococcus —see Echinococcus
  Echinostomum ilocanum B66.8
  Entamoeba (histolytica) —see Infection,
      Ameba
  Enterobius vermicularis B8Ø
  eyelid
    in (due to)
      leishmaniasis B55.1
      loiasis B74.3
      onchocerciasis B73.Ø9
      phthiriasis B85.3
      parasitic NOS B89
  eyeworm B74.3
  Fasciola (gigantica) (hepatica) (indica) B66.3
  Fasciolopsis (buski) (intestine) B66.5
  filarial B74.9
    bancroftian B74.Ø
    conjunctiva B74.9
    due to
      Acanthocheilonema (perstans)
          (streptocerca) B74.4
      Brugia (malayi) B74.1
        timori B74.2
      Dracunculus medinensis B72
      guinea worm B72
      loa loa B74.3

Infestation (Continued)
  filarial (Continued)
    due to (Continued)
      Mansonella (ozzardi) (perstans)
          (streptocerca) B74.4
      Onchocerca volvulus B73.ØØ
        eye B73.ØØ
        eyelid B73.Ø9
      Wuchereria (bancrofti) B74.Ø
      Malayan B74.1
      ozzardi B74.4
      specified type NEC B74.8
  fish tapeworm B7Ø.Ø
    larval B7Ø.1
  fluke B66.9
    blood NOS —see Schistosomiasis
    cat liver B66.Ø
    intestinal B66.5
    lancet B66.2
    liver (sheep) B66.3
      cat B66.Ø
      Chinese B66.1
      due to clonorchiasis B66.1
      oriental B66.1
    lung (oriental) B66.4
    sheep liver B66.3
    specified type NEC B66.8
  fly larvae —see Myiasis
  Gasterophilus (intestinalis) —see Myiasis
  Gastrodiscoides hominis B66.8
  Giardia lamblia AØ7.1
  Gnathostoma (spinigerum) B83.1
  Gongylonema B83.8
  guinea worm B72
  helminth B83.9
    angiostrongyliasis B83.2
      intestinal B81.3
    gnathostomiasis B83.1
    hirudiniasis, internal B83.4
    intestinal B82.Ø
      angiostrongyliasis B81.3
      anisakiasis B81.Ø
      ascariasis —see Ascariasis
      capillariasis B81.1
      cysticercosis —see Cysticercosis
      diphyllobothriasis —see Infestation,
          diphyllobothriasis
      dracunculiasis B72
      echinococcus —see Echinococcosis
      enterobiasis B8Ø
      filariasis —see Infestation, filarial
      fluke —see Infestation, fluke
      hookworm —see Infestation, hookworm
      mixed (types classifiable to more than
          one of the titles B65.Ø-B81.3 and
          B81.8) B81.4
      onchocerciasis —see Onchocerciasis
      schistosomiasis —see Infestation,
          schistosoma
      specified
        cestode NEC —see Infestation, cestode
        type NEC B81.8
      strongyloidiasis —see Strongyloidiasis
      taenia —see Infestation, taenia
      trichinellosis B75
      trichostrongyliasis B81.2
      trichuriasis B79
    specified type NEC B83.8
    syngamiasis B83.3
    visceral larva migrans B83.Ø
  Heterophyes (heterophyes) B66.8
  hookworm B76.9
    ancylostomiasis B76.Ø
    necatoriasis B76.1
    specified type NEC B76.8
  Hymenolepis (diminuta) (nana) B71.Ø
  intestinal NEC B82.9
  leeches (aquatic) (land) —see Hirudiniasis
  Leishmania —see Leishmaniasis
  lice, louse —see Infestation, Pediculus
  Linguatula B88.8

Infestation (Continued)
  Liponyssoides sanguineus B88.Ø
  Loa loa B74.3
    conjunctival B74.3
    eyelid B74.3
  louse —see Infestation, Pediculus
  maggots —see Myiasis
  Mansonella (ozzardi) (perstans) (streptocerca)
      B74.4
  Medina (worm) B72
  Metagonimus (yokogawai) B66.8
  microfilaria streptocerca —see Onchocerciasis
    eye B73.ØØ
    eyelid B73.Ø9
  mites B88.9
    scabic B86
  Monilia (albicans) —see Candidiasis
  mouth B37.Ø
  Necator americanus B76.1
  nematode NEC (intestinal) B82.Ø
    Ancylostoma B76.Ø
    conjunctiva NEC B83.9
    Enterobius vermicularis B8Ø
    Gnathostoma spinigerum B83.1
    physaloptera B8Ø
    specified NEC B81.8
    trichostrongylus B81.2
    trichuris (trichuria) B79
  Oesophagostomum (apiostomum) B81.8
  Oestrus ovis —see also Myiasis B87.9
  Onchocerca (volvulus) —see Onchocerciasis
  Opisthorchis (felineus) (viverrini) B66.Ø
  orbit, parasitic NOS B89
  Oxyuris vermicularis B8Ø
  Paragonimus (westermani) B66.4
  parasite, parasitic B89
    eyelid B89
    intestinal NOS B82.9
    mouth B37.Ø
    skin B88.9
    tongue B37.Ø
  Parastrongylus
    cantonensis B83.2
    costaricensis B81.3
  Pediculus B85.2
    body B85.1
    capitis (humanus) (any site) B85.Ø
    corporis (humanus) (any site) B85.1
    head B85.Ø
    mixed (classifiable to more than one of the
        titles B85.Ø-B85.3) B85.4
    pubis (any site) B85.3
  Pentastoma B88.8
  Phthirus (pubis) (any site) B85.3
    with any infestation classifiable to
        B85.Ø-B85.2 B85.4
  pinworm B8Ø
  pork tapeworm (adult) B68.Ø
  protozoal NEC B64
    intestinal AØ7.9
      specified NEC AØ7.8
    specified NEC B6Ø.8
  pubic, louse B85.3
  rat tapeworm B71.Ø
  red bug B88.Ø
  roundworm (large) NEC B82.Ø
    Ascariasis —see also Ascariasis B77.9
  sandflea B88.1
  Sarcoptes scabiei B86
  scabies B86
  Schistosoma B65.9
    bovis B65.8
    cercariae B65.3
    haematobium B65.Ø
    intercalatum B65.8
    japonicum B65.2
    mansoni B65.1
    mattheei B65.8
    mekongi B65.8
    specified type NEC B65.8
    spindale B65.8

Infestation (Continued)
  screw worms —see Myiasis
  skin NOS B88.9
  Sparganum (mansoni) (proliferum) (baxteri)
    B70.1
    larval B70.1
  specified type NEC B88.8
  Spirometra larvae B70.1
  Stellantchasmus falcatus B66.8
  Strongyloides stercoralis —see
    Strongyloidiasis
  Taenia B68.9
    diminuta B71.0
    echinococcus —see Echinococcus
    mediocanellata B68.1
    nana B71.0
    saginata B68.1
    solium (intestinal form) B68.0
      larval form —see Cysticercosis
  Taeniarhynchus saginatus B68.1
  tapeworm B71.9
    beef B68.1
    broad B70.0
      larval B70.1
    dog B67.4
    dwarf B71.0
    fish B70.0
      larval B70.1
    pork B68.0
    rat B71.0
  Ternidens diminutus B81.8
  Tetranychus molestissimus B88.0
  threadworm B80
  tongue B37.0
  Toxocara (canis) (cati) (felis) B83.0
  trematode (s) NEC —see Infestation, fluke
  Trichinella (spiralis) B75
  Trichocephalus B79
  Trichomonas —see Trichomoniasis
  Trichostrongylus B81.2
  Trichuris (trichiura) B79
  Trombicula (irritans) B88.0
  Tunga penetrans B88.1
  Uncinaria americana B76.1
  Vandellia cirrhosa B88.8
  whipworm B79
  worms B83.9
    intestinal B82.0
  Wuchereria (bancrofti) B74.0
Infiltrate, infiltration
  amyloid (generalized) (localized) —see
    Amyloidosis
  calcareous NEC R89.7
    localized —see Degeneration, by site
  calcium salt R89.7
  cardiac
    fatty —see Degeneration, myocardial
    glycogenic E74.02 [I43]
  corneal —see Edema, cornea
  eyelid —see Inflammation, eyelid
  glycogen, glycogenic —see Disease, glycogen
    storage
  heart, cardiac
    fatty —see Degeneration, myocardial
    glycogenic E74.02 [I43]
  inflammatory in vitreous H43.89
  kidney N28.89
  leukemic —see Leukemia
  liver K76.89
    fatty —see Fatty, liver NEC
    glycogen —see also Disease, glycogen
      storage E74.03 [K77]
  lung R91.8
    eosinophilic J82
  lymphatic —see also Leukemia, lymphatic
    C91.9-
    gland I88.9
  muscle, fatty M62.89
  myocardium, myocardial
    fatty —see Degeneration, myocardial
    glycogenic E74.02 [I43]

Infiltrate, infiltration (Continued)
  on chest x-ray R91.8
  pulmonary R91.8
    with eosinophilia J82
  skin (lymphocytic) L98.6
  thymus (gland) (fatty) E32.8
  urine R39.0
  vesicant agent
    antineoplastic chemotherapy T80.810
    other agent NEC T80.818
  vitreous body H43.89
Infirmity R68.89
  senile R54
Inflammation, inflamed, inflammatory (with
  exudation)
  abducent (nerve) —see Strabismus, paralytic,
    sixth nerve
  accessory sinus (chronic) —see Sinusitis
  adrenal (gland) E27.8
  alveoli, teeth M27.3
    scorbutic E54
  anal canal, anus K62.89
  antrum (chronic) —see Sinusitis, maxillary
  appendix —see Appendicitis
  arachnoid —see Meningitis
  areola N61.0 ◀▥
    puerperal, postpartum or gestational —see
      Infection, nipple
  areolar tissue NOS L08.9
  artery —see Arteritis
  auditory meatus (external) —see Otitis,
    externa
  Bartholin's gland N75.8
  bile duct (common) (hepatic) or passage —see
    Cholangitis
  bladder —see Cystitis
  bone —see Osteomyelitis
  brain —see also Encephalitis
    membrane —see Meningitis
  breast N61.0 ◀▥
    puerperal, postpartum, gestational —see
      Mastitis, obstetric
  broad ligament —see Disease, pelvis,
    inflammatory
  bronchi —see Bronchitis
  catarrhal J00
  cecum —see Appendicitis
  cerebral —see also Encephalitis
    membrane —see Meningitis
  cerebrospinal
    meningococcal A39.0
  cervix (uteri) —see Cervicitis
  chest J98.8
  chorioretinal H30.9-
    cyclitis —see Cyclitis
    disseminated H30.10-
      generalized H30.13-
      peripheral H30.12-
      posterior pole H30.11-
    epitheliopathy —see Epitheliopathy
    focal H30.00-
      juxtapapillary H30.01-
      macular H30.04-
      paramacular —see Inflammation,
        chorioretinal, focal, macular
      peripheral H30.03-
      posterior pole H30.02-
    specified type NEC H30.89-
  choroid —see Inflammation, chorioretinal
  chronic, postmastoidectomy cavity —see
    Complications, postmastoidectomy,
    inflammation
  colon —see Enteritis
  connective tissue (diffuse) NEC —see
    Disorder, soft tissue, specified type
    NEC
  cornea —see Keratitis
  corpora cavernosa N48.29
  cranial nerve —see Disorder, nerve, cranial
  Douglas' cul-de-sac or pouch (chronic)
    N73.0

Inflammation, inflamed, inflammatory
  (Continued)
  due to device, implant or graft —see also
    Complications, by site and type,
    infection or inflammation
    arterial graft T82.7
    breast (implant) T85.79
    catheter T85.79
      dialysis (renal) T82.7
        intraperitoneal T85.71
      infusion T82.7
        cranial T85.735 ◀
        intrathecal T85.735 ◀
        spinal (epidural) (subdural)
          T85.735 ◀▥
        subarachnoid T85.735 ◀
      urinary T83.518 ◀▥
        cystostomy T83.510 ◀
        Hopkins T83.518 ◀
        ileostomy T83.518 ◀
        nephrostomy T83.512 ◀
        specified NEC T83.518 ◀
        urethral indwelling T83.511 ◀
        urostomy T83.518 ◀
    electronic (electrode) (pulse generator)
      (stimulator)
      bone T84.7
      cardiac T82.7
      nervous system T85.738 ◀▥
        brain T85.731 ◀
        cranial nerve T85.732 ◀
        gastric nerve T85.732 ◀
        neurostimulator generator T85.734 ◀
        peripheral nerve T85.732 ◀
        sacral nerve T85.732 ◀
        spinal cord T85.733 ◀
        vagal nerve T85.732 ◀
      urinary T83.590 ◀▥
    fixation, internal (orthopedic) NEC —see
      Complication, fixation device,
      infection
    gastrointestinal (bile duct) (esophagus)
      T85.79
    neurostimulator electrode (lead)
      T85.732 ◀
    genital NEC T83.69 ◀▥
    heart NEC T82.7
      valve (prosthesis) T82.6
        graft T82.7
    joint prosthesis —see Complication, joint
      prosthesis, infection
    ocular (corneal graft) (orbital implant)
      NEC T85.79
    orthopedic NEC T84.7
    penile (cylinder) (pump) (resevoir)
      T83.61 ◀
    specified NEC T85.79
    testicular T83.62 ◀
    urinary NEC T83.598 ◀▥
      ileal conduit stent T83.593 ◀
      implanted neurostimulation T83.590 ◀
      implanted sphincter T83.591 ◀
      indwelling ureteral stent T83.592 ◀
      nephroureteral stent T83.593 ◀
      specified stent NEC T83.593 ◀
    vascular NEC T82.7
    ~~ventricular intracranial shunt T85.79~~
    ventricular intracranial (communicating)
      shunt T85.730 ◀
  duodenum K29.80
    with bleeding K29.81
  dura mater —see Meningitis
  ear (middle) —see also Otitis, media
    external —see Otitis, externa
    inner —see subcategory H83.0
  epididymis —see Epididymitis
  esophagus K20.9
  ethmoidal (sinus) (chronic) —see Sinusitis,
    ethmoidal
  eustachian tube (catarrhal) —see Salpingitis,
    eustachian

◀ New   ◀▥ Revised   ~~deleted~~ Deleted

Inflammation, inflamed, inflammatory
(Continued)
eyelid H01.9
abscess —see Abscess, eyelid
blepharitis —see Blepharitis
chalazion —see Chalazion
dermatosis (noninfectious) —see
Dermatosis, eyelid
hordeolum —see Hordeolum
specified NEC H01.8
fallopian tube —see Salpingo-oophoritis
fascia —see Myositis
follicular, pharynx J31.2
frontal (sinus) (chronic) —see Sinusitis, frontal
gallbladder —see Cholecystitis
gastric —see Gastritis
gastrointestinal —see Enteritis
genital organ (internal) (diffuse)
female —see Disease, pelvis, inflammatory
male N49.9
multiple sites N49.8
specified NEC N49.8
gland (lymph) —see Lymphadenitis
glottis —see Laryngitis
granular, pharynx J31.2
gum K05.10
nonplaque induced K05.11
plaque induced K05.10
heart —see Carditis
hepatic duct —see Cholangitis
ileoanal (internal) pouch K91.850
ileum —see also Enteritis
regional or terminal —see Enteritis, regional
intestinal pouch K91.850
intestine (any part) —see Enteritis
jaw (acute) (bone) (chronic) (lower)
(suppurative) (upper) M27.2
joint NEC —see Arthritis
sacroiliac M46.1
kidney —see Nephritis
knee (joint) M13.169
tuberculous A18.02
labium (majus) (minus) —see Vulvitis
lacrimal
gland —see Dacryoadenitis
passages (duct) (sac) —see also
Dacryocystitis
canaliculitis —see Canaliculitis, lacrimal
larynx —see Laryngitis
leg NOS L08.9
lip K13.0
liver (capsule) —see also Hepatitis
chronic K73.9
suppurative K75.0
lung (acute) —see also Pneumonia
chronic J98.4
lymphatic vessel —see Lymphangitis
lymph gland or node —see Lymphadenitis
maxilla, maxillary M27.2
sinus (chronic) —see Sinusitis, maxillary
membranes of brain or spinal cord —see
Meningitis
meninges —see Meningitis
mouth K12.1
muscle —see Myositis
myocardium —see Myocarditis
nasal sinus (chronic) —see Sinusitis
nasopharynx —see Nasopharyngitis
navel L08.82
nerve NEC —see Neuralgia
nipple N61.0 ◀▥
puerperal, postpartum or gestational —see
Infection, nipple
nose —see Rhinitis
oculomotor (nerve) —see Strabismus,
paralytic, third nerve
optic nerve —see Neuritis, optic
orbit (chronic) H05.10
acute H05.00
abscess —see Abscess, orbit
cellulitis —see Cellulitis, orbit

Inflammation, inflamed, inflammatory
(Continued)
orbit (chronic) (Continued)
acute (Continued)
osteomyelitis —see Osteomyelitis,
orbit
periostitis —see Periostitis, orbital
tenonitis —see Tenonitis, eye
granuloma —see Granuloma, orbit
myositis —see Myositis, orbital
ovary —see Salpingo-oophoritis
oviduct —see Salpingo-oophoritis
pancreas (acute) —see Pancreatitis
parametrium N73.0
parotid region L08.9
pelvis, female —see Disease, pelvis,
inflammatory
penis (corpora cavernosa) N48.29
perianal K62.89
pericardium —see Pericarditis
perineum (female) (male) L08.9
perirectal K62.89
peritoneum —see Peritonitis
periuterine —see Disease, pelvis,
inflammatory
perivesical —see Cystitis
petrous bone (acute) (chronic) —see Petrositis
pharynx (acute) —see Pharyngitis
pia mater —see Meningitis
pleura —see Pleurisy
polyp, colon —see also Polyp, colon,
inflammatory K51.40
prostate —see also Prostatitis
specified type NEC N41.8
rectosigmoid —see Rectosigmoiditis
rectum —see also Proctitis K62.89
respiratory, upper —see also Infection,
respiratory, upper J06.9
acute, due to radiation J70.0
chronic, due to external agent —see
condition, respiratory, chronic, due to
due to
chemicals, gases, fumes or vapors
(inhalation) J68.2
radiation J70.1
retina —see Chorioretinitis
retrocecal —see Appendicitis
retroperitoneal —see Peritonitis
salivary duct or gland (any) (suppurative) —
see Sialoadenitis
scorbutic, alveoli, teeth E54
scrotum N49.2
seminal vesicle —see Vesiculitis
sigmoid —see Enteritis
sinus —see Sinusitis
Skene's duct or gland —see Urethritis
skin L08.9
spermatic cord N49.1
sphenoidal (sinus) —see Sinusitis, sphenoidal
spinal
cord —see Encephalitis
membrane —see Meningitis
nerve —see Disorder, nerve
spine —see Spondylopathy, inflammatory
spleen (capsule) D73.89
stomach —see Gastritis
subcutaneous tissue L08.9
suprarenal (gland) E27.8
synovial —see Tenosynovitis
tendon (sheath) NEC —see Tenosynovitis
testis —see Orchitis
throat (acute) —see Pharyngitis
thymus (gland) E32.8
thyroid (gland) —see Thyroiditis
tongue K14.0
tonsil —see Tonsillitis
trachea —see Tracheitis
trochlear (nerve) —see Strabismus, paralytic,
fourth nerve
tubal —see Salpingo-oophoritis
tuberculous NEC —see Tuberculosis

Inflammation, inflamed, inflammatory
(Continued)
tubo-ovarian —see Salpingo-oophoritis
tunica vaginalis N49.1
tympanic membrane —see Tympanitis
umbilicus, umbilical L08.82
uterine ligament —see Disease, pelvis,
inflammatory
uterus (catarrhal) —see Endometritis
uveal tract (anterior) NOS —see also
Iridocyclitis
posterior —see Chorioretinitis
vagina —see Vaginitis
vas deferens N49.1
vein —see also Phlebitis
intracranial or intraspinal (septic) G08
thrombotic I80.9
leg —see Phlebitis, leg
lower extremity —see Phlebitis, leg
vocal cord J38.3
vulva —see Vulvitis
Wharton's duct (suppurative) —see
Sialoadenitis
Inflation, lung, imperfect (newborn) —see
Atelectasis
Influenza (bronchial) (epidemic) (respiratory
(upper)) (unidentified influenza virus)
J11.1
with
digestive manifestations J11.2
encephalopathy J11.81
enteritis J11.2
gastroenteritis J11.2
gastrointestinal manifestations J11.2
laryngitis J11.1
myocarditis J11.82
otitis media J11.83
pharyngitis J11.1
pneumonia J11.00
specified type J11.08
respiratory manifestations NEC J11.1
specified manifestation NEC J11.89
A/H5N1 —see also Influenza, due to,
identified novel influenza A virus J09.X2
avian —see also Influenza, due to, identified
novel influenza A virus J09.X2
bird —see also Influenza, due to, identified
novel influenza A virus J09.X2
novel (2009) H1N1 influenza —see also
Influenza, due to, identified influenza
virus NEC J10.1
novel influenza A/H1N1 —see also Influenza,
due to, identified influenza virus NEC
J10.1
due to
avian (see also Influenza, due to, identified
novel influenza A virus) J09.X2
identified influenza virus NEC J10.1
with
digestive manifestations J10.2
encephalopathy J10.81
enteritis J10.2
gastroenteritis J10.2
gastrointestinal manifestations J10.2
laryngitis J10.1
myocarditis J10.82
otitis media J10.83
pharyngitis J10.1
pneumonia (unspecified type) J10.00
with same identified influenza virus
J10.01
specified type NEC J10.08
respiratory manifestations NEC J10.1
specified manifestation NEC J10.89
identified novel influenza A virus J09.X2
with
digestive manifestations J09.X3
encephalopathy J09.X9
enteritis J09.X3
gastroenteritis J09.X3
gastrointestinal manifestations J09.X3

Influenza *(Continued)*
  due to *(Continued)*
    identified novel influenza A virus
      (Continued)
      with *(Continued)*
        laryngitis J09.X2
        myocarditis J09.X9
        otitis media J09.X9
        pharyngitis J09.X2
        pneumonia J09.X1
        respiratory manifestations NEC J09.X2
        specified manifestation NEC J09.X9
        upper respiratory symptoms J09.X2
    of other animal origin, not bird or swine *(see also* Influenza, due to, identified novel influenza A virus) J09.X2
    swine (viruses that normally cause infections in pigs) —*see also* Influenza, due to, identified novel influenza A virus J09.X2
Influenza-like disease —*see* Influenza
Influenzal —*see* Influenza
Infraction, Freiberg's (metatarsal head) —*see* Osteochondrosis, juvenile, metatarsus
Infraeruption of tooth (teeth) M26.34
Infusion complication, misadventure, or reaction —*see* Complications, infusion
Ingestion
  chemical —*see* Table of Drugs and Chemicals, by substance, poisoning
  drug or medicament
    correct substance properly administered —*see* Table of Drugs and Chemicals, by drug, adverse effect
    overdose or wrong substance given or taken —*see* Table of Drugs and Chemicals, by drug, poisoning
  foreign body —*see* Foreign body, alimentary tract
  tularemia A21.3
Ingrowing
  hair (beard) L73.1
  nail (finger) (toe) L60.0
Inguinal —*see also* condition
  testicle Q53.9
    bilateral Q53.21
    unilateral Q53.11
Inhalant-induced ◄
  anxiety disorder F18.980 ◄
  depressive disorder F18.94 ◄
  major neurocognitive disorder F18.97 ◄
  mild neurocognitive disorder F18.988 ◄
  psychotic disorder F18.959 ◄
Inhalation
  anthrax A22.1
  flame T27.3
  food or foreign body —*see* Foreign body, by site
  gases, fumes, or vapors NEC T59.9-
    specified agent —*see* Table of Drugs and Chemicals, by substance
  liquid or vomitus —*see* Asphyxia
  meconium (newborn) P24.00
    with
      with respiratory symptoms P24.01
      pneumonia (pneumonitis) P24.01
  mucus —*see* Asphyxia, mucus
  oil or gasoline (causing suffocation) —*see* Foreign body, by site
  smoke J70.5
    due to chemicals, gases, fumes and vapors J68.9
  steam —*see* Toxicity, vapors
  stomach contents or secretions —*see* Foreign body, by site
    due to anesthesia (general) (local) or other sedation T88.59
    in labor and delivery O74.0
    in pregnancy O29.01-
    postpartum, puerperal O89.01

Inhibition, orgasm
  female F52.31
  male F52.32
Inhibitor, systemic lupus erythematosus (presence of) D68.62
Iniencephalus, iniencephaly Q00.2
Injection, traumatic jet (air) (industrial) (water) (paint or dye) T70.4
Injury —*see also* specified injury type T14.90
  abdomen, abdominal S39.91
    blood vessel —*see* Injury, blood vessel, abdomen
    cavity —*see* Injury, intra-abdominal
    contusion S30.1
    internal —*see* Injury, intra-abdominal
    intra-abdominal organ —*see* Injury, intra-abdominal
    nerve —*see* Injury, nerve, abdomen
    open —*see* Wound, open, abdomen
    specified NEC S39.81
    superficial —*see* Injury, superficial, abdomen
  Achilles tendon S86.00-
    laceration S86.02-
    specified type NEC S86.09-
    strain S86.01-
  acoustic, resulting in deafness —*see* Injury, nerve, acoustic
  adrenal (gland) S37.819
    contusion S37.812
    laceration S37.813
    specified type NEC S37.818
  alveolar (process) S09.93
  ankle S99.91-
    contusion —*see* Contusion, ankle
    dislocation —*see* Dislocation, ankle
    fracture —*see* Fracture, ankle
    nerve —*see* Injury, nerve, ankle
    open —*see* Wound, open, ankle
    specified type NEC S99.81-
    sprain —*see* Sprain, ankle
    superficial —*see* Injury, superficial, ankle
  anterior chamber, eye —*see* Injury, eye, specified site NEC
  anus —*see* Injury, abdomen
  aorta (thoracic) S25.00
    abdominal S35.00
      laceration (minor) (superficial) S35.01
        major S35.02
      specified type NEC S35.09
    laceration (minor) (superficial) S25.01
      major S25.02
    specified type NEC S25.09
  arm (upper) S49.9-
    blood vessel —*see* Injury, blood vessel, arm
    contusion —*see* Contusion, arm, upper
    fracture —*see* Fracture, humerus
    lower —*see* Injury, forearm
    muscle —*see* Injury, muscle, shoulder
    nerve —*see* Injury, nerve, arm
    open —*see* Wound, open, arm
    specified type NEC S49.8-
    superficial —*see* Injury, superficial, arm
  artery (complicating trauma) —*see also* Injury, blood vessel, by site
    cerebral or meningeal —*see* Injury, intracranial
  auditory canal (external) (meatus) S09.91
  auricle, auris, ear S09.91
  axilla —*see* Injury, shoulder
  back —*see* Injury, back, lower
  bile duct S36.13
  birth —*see also* Birth, injury P15.9
  bladder (sphincter) S37.20
    at delivery O71.5
    contusion S37.22
    laceration S37.23
    obstetrical trauma O71.5
    specified type NEC S37.29

Injury *(Continued)*
  blast (air) (hydraulic) (immersion) (underwater) NEC T14.8
    acoustic nerve trauma —*see* Injury, nerve, acoustic
    bladder —*see* Injury, bladder
    brain —*see* Concussion
    colon —*see* Injury, intestine, large, blast injury
    ear (primary) S09.31-
      secondary S09.39-
    generalized T70.8
    lung —*see* Injury, intrathoracic, lung, blast injury
    multiple body organs T70.8
    peritoneum S36.81
    rectum S36.61
    retroperitoneum S36.898
    small intestine S36.419
      duodenum S36.410
      specified site NEC S36.418
    specified
      intra-abdominal organ NEC S36.898
      pelvic organ NEC S37.899
  blood vessel NEC T14.8
    abdomen S35.9-
      aorta —*see* Injury, aorta, abdominal
      celiac artery —*see* Injury, blood vessel, celiac artery
      iliac vessel —*see* Injury, blood vessel, iliac
      laceration S35.91
      mesenteric vessel —*see* Injury, mesenteric
      portal vein —*see* Injury, blood vessel, portal vein
      renal vessel —*see* Injury, blood vessel, renal
      specified vessel NEC S35.8X-
      splenic vessel —*see* Injury, blood vessel, splenic
      vena cava —*see* Injury, vena cava, inferior
    ankle —*see* Injury, blood vessel, foot
    aorta (abdominal) (thoracic) —*see* Injury, aorta
    arm (upper) NEC S45.90-
      forearm —*see* Injury, blood vessel, forearm
      laceration S45.91-
      specified
        site NEC S45.80-
          laceration S45.81-
          specified type NEC S45.89-
        type NEC S45.99-
      superficial vein S45.30-
        laceration S45.31-
        specified type NEC S45.39-
    axillary
      artery S45.00-
        laceration S45.01-
        specified type NEC S45.09-
      vein S45.20-
        laceration S45.21-
        specified type NEC S45.29-
    azygos vein —*see* Injury, blood vessel, thoracic, specified site NEC
    brachial
      artery S45.10-
        laceration S45.11-
        specified type NEC S45.19-
      vein S45.20-
        laceration S45.219
        specified type NEC S45.29-
    carotid artery (common) (external) (internal, extracranial) S15.00-
      internal, intracranial S06.8-
      laceration (minor) (superficial) S15.01-
        major S15.02-
      specified type NEC S15.09-

Injury (Continued)
　blood vessel NEC (Continued)
　　celiac artery S35.219
　　　branch S35.299
　　　　laceration (minor) (superficial) S35.291
　　　　　major S35.292
　　　　specified NEC S35.298
　　　　laceration (minor) (superficial) S35.211
　　　　　major S35.212
　　　　specified type NEC S35.218
　　cerebral —see Injury, intracranial
　　deep plantar —see Injury, blood vessel,
　　　　plantar artery
　　digital (hand) —see Injury, blood vessel,
　　　　finger
　　dorsal
　　　artery (foot) S95.00-
　　　　laceration S95.01-
　　　　specified type NEC S95.09-
　　　vein (foot) S95.20-
　　　　laceration S95.21-
　　　　specified type NEC S95.29-
　　due to accidental laceration during
　　　　procedure —see Laceration, accidental
　　　　complicating surgery
　　extremity —see Injury, blood vessel, limb
　　femoral
　　　artery (common) (superficial) S75.00-
　　　　laceration (minor) (superficial)
　　　　　S75.01-
　　　　　major S75.02-
　　　　specified type NEC S75.09-
　　　vein (hip level) (thigh level) S75.10-
　　　　laceration (minor) (superficial) S75.11-
　　　　　major S75.12-
　　　　specified type NEC S75.19-
　　finger S65.50-
　　　index S65.50-
　　　　laceration S65.51-
　　　　specified type NEC S65.59-
　　　laceration S65.51-
　　　little S65.50-
　　　　laceration S65.51-
　　　　specified type NEC S65.59-
　　　middle S65.50-
　　　　laceration S65.51-
　　　　specified type NEC S65.59-
　　　specified type NEC S65.59-
　　　thumb —see Injury, blood vessel, thumb
　　foot S95.90-
　　　dorsal
　　　　artery —see Injury, blood vessel,
　　　　　dorsal, artery
　　　　vein —see Injury, blood vessel, dorsal,
　　　　　vein
　　　laceration S95.91-
　　　plantar artery —see Injury, blood vessel,
　　　　plantar artery
　　　specified
　　　　site NEC S95.80-
　　　　　laceration S95.81-
　　　　　specified type NEC S95.89-
　　　　specified type NEC S95.99-
　　forearm S55.90-
　　　laceration S55.91-
　　　radial artery —see Injury, blood vessel,
　　　　radial artery
　　　specified
　　　　site NEC S55.80-
　　　　　laceration S55.81-
　　　　　specified type NEC S55.89-
　　　　type NEC S55.99-
　　　ulnar artery —see Injury, blood vessel,
　　　　ulnar artery
　　　vein S55.20-
　　　　laceration S55.21-
　　　　specified type NEC S55.29-
　　gastric
　　　artery —see Injury, mesenteric, artery,
　　　　branch
　　　vein —see Injury, blood vessel, abdomen

Injury (Continued)
　blood vessel NEC (Continued)
　　gastroduodenal artery —see Injury,
　　　mesenteric, artery, branch
　　greater saphenous vein (lower leg level)
　　　S85.30-
　　　hip (and thigh) level S75.20-
　　　　laceration (minor) (superficial) S75.21-
　　　　　major S75.22-
　　　　specified type NEC S75.29-
　　　laceration S85.31-
　　　specified type NEC S85.39-
　　hand (level) S65.90-
　　　finger —see Injury, blood vessel, finger
　　　laceration S65.91-
　　　palmar arch —see Injury, blood vessel,
　　　　palmar arch
　　　radial artery —see Injury, blood vessel,
　　　　radial artery, hand
　　　specified
　　　　site NEC S65.80-
　　　　　laceration S65.81-
　　　　　specified type NEC S65.89-
　　　　type NEC S65.99-
　　　thumb —see Injury, blood vessel,
　　　　thumb
　　　ulnar artery —see Injury, blood vessel,
　　　　ulnar artery, hand
　　head S09.0
　　　intracranial —see Injury, intracranial
　　　multiple S09.0
　　hepatic
　　　artery —see Injury, mesenteric, artery
　　　vein —see Injury, vena cava, inferior
　　hip S75.90-
　　　femoral artery —see Injury, blood vessel,
　　　　femoral, artery
　　　femoral vein —see Injury, blood vessel,
　　　　femoral, vein
　　　greater saphenous vein —see Injury,
　　　　blood vessel, greater saphenous,
　　　　hip level
　　　laceration S75.91-
　　　specified
　　　　site NEC S75.80-
　　　　　laceration S75.81-
　　　　　specified type NEC S75.89-
　　　　type NEC S75.99-
　　hypogastric (artery) (vein) —see Injury,
　　　blood vessel, iliac
　　iliac S35.5-
　　　artery S35.51-
　　　specified vessel NEC S35.5-
　　　uterine vessel —see Injury, blood vessel,
　　　　uterine
　　　vein S35.51-
　　innominate —see Injury, blood vessel,
　　　thoracic, innominate
　　intercostal (artery) (vein) —see Injury,
　　　blood vessel, thoracic, intercostal
　　jugular vein (external) S15.20-
　　　internal S15.30-
　　　　laceration (minor) (superficial) S15.31-
　　　　　major S15.32-
　　　　specified type NEC S15.39-
　　　laceration (minor) (superficial) S15.21-
　　　　major S15.22-
　　　specified type NEC S15.29-
　　leg (level) (lower) S85.90-
　　　greater saphenous —see Injury, blood
　　　　vessel, greater saphenous
　　　laceration S85.91-
　　　lesser saphenous —see Injury, blood
　　　　vessel, lesser saphenous
　　　peroneal artery —see Injury, blood
　　　　vessel, peroneal artery
　　　popliteal
　　　　artery —see Injury, blood vessel,
　　　　　popliteal, artery
　　　　vein —see Injury, blood vessel,
　　　　　popliteal, vein

Injury (Continued)
　blood vessel NEC (Continued)
　　leg (level) (lower) (Continued)
　　　specified
　　　　site NEC S85.80-
　　　　　laceration S85.81-
　　　　　specified type NEC S85.89-
　　　　type NEC S85.99-
　　　thigh —see Injury, blood vessel, hip
　　　tibial artery —see Injury, blood vessel,
　　　　tibial artery
　　lesser saphenous vein (lower leg level)
　　　S85.40-
　　　laceration S85.41-
　　　specified type NEC S85.49-
　　limb
　　　lower —see Injury, blood vessel, leg
　　　upper —see Injury, blood vessel, arm
　　lower back —see Injury, blood vessel,
　　　abdomen
　　　specified NEC —see Injury, blood
　　　　vessel, abdomen, specified, site
　　　　NEC
　　mammary (artery) (vein) —see Injury,
　　　blood vessel, thoracic, specified site
　　　NEC
　　mesenteric (inferior) (superior)
　　　artery —see Injury, mesenteric, artery
　　　vein —see Injury, mesenteric, vein
　　neck S15.9
　　　specified site NEC S15.8
　　ovarian (artery) (vein) —see subcategory
　　　S35.8
　　palmar arch (superficial) S65.20-
　　　deep S65.30-
　　　　laceration S65.31-
　　　　specified type NEC S65.39-
　　　laceration S65.21-
　　　specified type NEC S65.29-
　　pelvis —see Injury, blood vessel, abdomen
　　　specified NEC —see Injury, blood vessel,
　　　　abdomen, specified, site NEC
　　peroneal artery S85.20-
　　　laceration S85.21-
　　　specified type NEC S85.29-
　　plantar artery (deep) (foot) S95.10-
　　　laceration S95.11-
　　　specified type NEC S95.19-
　　popliteal
　　　artery S85.00-
　　　　laceration S85.01-
　　　　specified type NEC S85.09-
　　　vein S85.50-
　　　　laceration S85.51-
　　　　specified type NEC S85.59-
　　portal vein S35.319
　　　laceration S35.311
　　　specified type NEC S35.318
　　precerebral —see Injury, blood vessel, neck
　　pulmonary (artery) (vein) —see Injury,
　　　blood vessel, thoracic, pulmonary
　　radial artery (forearm level) S55.10-
　　　hand and wrist (level) S65.10-
　　　　laceration S65.11-
　　　　specified type NEC S65.19-
　　　laceration S55.11-
　　　specified type NEC S55.19-
　　renal
　　　artery S35.40-
　　　　laceration S35.41-
　　　　specified NEC S35.49-
　　　vein S35.40-
　　　　laceration S35.41-
　　　　specified NEC S35.49-
　　saphenous vein (greater) (lower leg
　　　level) —see Injury, blood vessel,
　　　greater saphenous
　　　hip and thigh level —see Injury, blood
　　　　vessel, greater saphenous, hip level
　　　lesser —see Injury, blood vessel, lesser
　　　　saphenous

Injury (Continued)
  blood vessel NEC (Continued)
    shoulder
      specified NEC —see Injury, blood vessel,
        arm, specified site NEC
      superficial vein —see Injury, blood
        vessel, arm, superficial vein
    specified NEC T14.8
    splenic
      artery —see Injury, blood vessel, celiac
        artery, branch
      vein S35.329
        laceration S35.321
        specified NEC S35.328
    subclavian —see Injury, blood vessel,
      thoracic, innominate
    thigh —see Injury, blood vessel, hip
    thoracic S25.90
      aorta S25.00
        laceration (minor) (superficial) S25.01
          major S25.02
        specified type NEC S25.09
      azygos vein —see Injury, blood vessel,
        thoracic, specified, site NEC
      innominate
        artery S25.10-
          laceration (minor) (superficial)
            S25.11-
            major S25.12-
          specified type NEC S25.19-
        vein S25.30-
          laceration (minor) (superficial)
            S25.31-
            major S25.32-
          specified type NEC S25.39-
      intercostal S25.50-
        laceration S25.51-
        specified type NEC S25.59-
      laceration S25.91
      mammary vessel —see Injury, blood
        vessel, thoracic, specified, site NEC
      pulmonary S25.40-
        laceration (minor) (superficial) S25.41-
          major S25.42-
        specified type NEC S25.49-
      specified
        site NEC S25.80-
          laceration S25.81-
          specified type NEC S25.89-
        type NEC S25.99
      subclavian —see Injury, blood vessel,
        thoracic, innominate
      vena cava (superior) S25.20
        laceration (minor) (superficial) S25.21
          major S25.22
        specified type NEC S25.29
    thumb S65.40-
      laceration S65.41-
      specified type NEC S65.49-
    tibial artery S85.10-
      anterior S85.13-
        laceration S85.14-
        specified injury NEC S85.15-
      laceration S85.11-
      posterior S85.16-
        laceration S85.17-
        specified injury NEC S85.18-
      specified injury NEC S85.12-
    ulnar artery (forearm level) S55.00-
      hand and wrist (level) S65.00-
        laceration S65.01-
        specified type NEC S65.09-
      laceration S55.01-
      specified type NEC S55.09-
    upper arm (level) —see Injury, blood vessel,
      arm
    superficial vein —see Injury, blood
      vessel, arm, superficial vein
    uterine S35.5-
      artery S35.53-
      vein S35.53-

Injury (Continued)
  blood vessel NEC (Continued)
    vena cava —see Injury, vena cava
    vertebral artery S15.10-
      laceration (minor) (superficial) S15.11-
        major S15.12-
      specified type NEC S15.19-
    wrist (level) —see Injury, blood vessel,
      hand
  brachial plexus S14.3
    newborn P14.3
  brain (traumatic) S06.9-
    diffuse (axonal) S06.2X-
    focal S06.30-
    ~~traumatic — see category S06~~
  brainstem S06.38-
  breast NOS S29.9
  broad ligament —see Injury, pelvic organ,
    specified site NEC
  bronchus, bronchi —see Injury, intrathoracic,
    bronchus
  brow S09.90
  buttock S39.92
  canthus, eye S05.90
  cardiac plexus —see Injury, nerve, thorax,
    sympathetic
  cauda equina S34.3
  cavernous sinus —see Injury, intracranial
  cecum —see Injury, colon
  celiac ganglion or plexus —see Injury, nerve,
    lumbosacral, sympathetic
  cerebellum —see Injury, intracranial
  cerebral —see Injury, intracranial
  cervix (uteri) —see Injury, uterus
  cheek (wall) S09.93
  chest —see Injury, thorax
  childbirth (newborn) —see also Birth, injury
    maternal NEC O71.9
  chin S09.93
  choroid (eye) —see Injury, eye, specified site
    NEC
  clitoris S39.94
  coccyx —see also Injury, back, lower
    complicating delivery O71.6
  colon —see Injury, intestine, large
  common bile duct —see Injury, liver
  conjunctiva (superficial) —see Injury, eye,
    conjunctiva
  conus medullaris —see Injury, spinal, sacral
    cord
    spermatic (pelvic region) S37.898
      scrotal region S39.848
    spinal —see Injury, spinal cord, by region
  cornea —see Injury, eye, specified site NEC
    abrasion —see Injury, eye, cornea, abrasion
  cortex (cerebral) —see also Injury, intracranial
    visual —see Injury, nerve, optic
  costal region NEC S29.9
  costochondral NEC S29.9
  cranial
    cavity —see Injury, intracranial
    nerve —see Injury, nerve, cranial
  crushing —see Crush
  cutaneous sensory nerve
  cystic duct —see Injury, liver
  deep tissue —see Contusion, by site
    meaning pressure ulcer —see Ulcer,
      pressure, unstageable, by site
  delivery (newborn) P15.9
    maternal NEC O71.9
  Descemet's membrane —see Injury, eyeball,
    penetrating
  diaphragm —see Injury, intrathoracic,
    diaphragm
  duodenum —see Injury, intestine, small,
    duodenum
  ear (auricle) (external) (canal) S09.91
    abrasion —see Abrasion, ear
    bite —see Bite, ear
    blister —see Blister, ear
    bruise —see Contusion, ear

Injury (Continued)
  ear (Continued)
    contusion —see Contusion, ear
    external constriction —see Constriction,
      external, ear
    hematoma —see Hematoma, ear
    inner —see Injury, ear, middle
    laceration —see Laceration, ear
    middle S09.30-
      blast —see Injury, blast, ear
      specified NEC S09.39-
    puncture —see Puncture, ear
    superficial —see Injury, superficial, ear
  eighth cranial nerve (acoustic or auditory) —
    see Injury, nerve, acoustic
  elbow S59.90-
    contusion —see Contusion, elbow
    dislocation —see Dislocation, elbow
    fracture —see Fracture, ulna, upper end
    open —see Wound, open, elbow
    specified NEC S59.80-
    sprain —see Sprain, elbow
    superficial —see Injury, superficial, elbow
  eleventh cranial nerve (accessory) —see
    Injury, nerve, accessory
  epididymis S39.94
  epigastric region S39.91
  epiglottis NEC S19.89
  esophageal plexus —see Injury, nerve, thorax,
    sympathetic
  esophagus (thoracic part) —see also Injury,
    intrathoracic, esophagus
    cervical NEC S19.85
  eustachian tube S09.30-
  eye S05.9-
    avulsion S05.7-
    ball —see Injury, eyeball
    conjunctiva S05.0-
    cornea
      abrasion S05.0-
      laceration S05.3-
        with prolapse S05.2-
    lacrimal apparatus S05.8X-
    orbit penetration S05.4-
    specified site NEC S05.8X-
  eyeball S05.8X-
    contusion S05.1-
    penetrating S05.6-
      with
        foreign body S05.5-
        prolapse or loss of intraocular tissue
          S05.2-
      without prolapse or loss of intraocular
        tissue S05.3-
    specified type NEC S05.8-
  eyebrow S09.93
  eyelid S09.93
    abrasion —see Abrasion, eyelid
    contusion —see Contusion, eyelid
    open —see Wound, open, eyelid
  face S09.93
  fallopian tube S37.509
    bilateral S37.502
      blast injury S37.512
      contusion S37.522
      laceration S37.532
      specified type NEC S37.592
    blast injury (primary) S37.519
      bilateral S37.512
      secondary —see Injury, fallopian tube,
        specified type NEC
      unilateral S37.511
    contusion S37.529
      bilateral S37.522
      unilateral S37.521
    laceration S37.539
      bilateral S37.532
      unilateral S37.531
    specified type NEC S37.599
      bilateral S37.592
      unilateral S37.591

◀ New   ◀▥ Revised   ~~deleted~~ Deleted

Injury (Continued)
fallopian tube (Continued)
  unilateral S37.501
    blast injury S37.511
    contusion S37.521
    laceration S37.531
    specified type NEC S37.591
fascia —see Injury, muscle
fifth cranial nerve (trigeminal) —see Injury,
  nerve, trigeminal
finger (nail) S69.9-
  blood vessel —see Injury, blood vessel,
    finger
  contusion —see Contusion, finger
  dislocation —see Dislocation, finger
  fracture —see Fracture, finger
  muscle —see Injury, muscle, finger
  nerve —see Injury, nerve, digital, finger
  open —see Wound, open, finger
  specified NEC S69.8-
  sprain —see Sprain, finger
  superficial —see Injury, superficial, finger
first cranial nerve (olfactory) —see Injury,
  nerve, olfactory
flank —see Injury, abdomen
foot S99.92-
  blood vessel —see Injury, blood vessel, foot
  contusion —see Contusion, foot
  dislocation —see Dislocation, foot
  fracture —see Fracture, foot
  muscle —see Injury, muscle, foot
  open —see Wound, open, foot
  specified type NEC S99.82-
  sprain —see Sprain, foot
  superficial —see Injury, superficial, foot
forceps NOS P15.9
forearm S59.91-
  blood vessel —see Injury, blood vessel,
    forearm
  contusion —see Contusion, forearm
  fracture —see Fracture, forearm
  muscle —see Injury, muscle, forearm
  nerve —see Injury, nerve, forearm
  open —see Wound, open, forearm
  specified NEC S59.81-
  superficial —see Injury, superficial,
    forearm
forehead S09.90
fourth cranial nerve (trochlear) —see Injury,
  nerve, trochlear
gallbladder S36.129
  contusion S36.122
  laceration S36.123
  specified NEC S36.128
ganglion
  celiac, coeliac —see Injury, nerve,
    lumbosacral, sympathetic
  gasserian —see Injury, nerve, trigeminal
  stellate —see Injury, nerve, thorax,
    sympathetic
  thoracic sympathetic —see Injury, nerve,
    thorax, sympathetic
gasserian ganglion —see Injury, nerve,
  trigeminal
gastric artery —see Injury, blood vessel, celiac
  artery, branch
gastroduodenal artery —see Injury, blood
  vessel, celiac artery, branch
gastrointestinal tract —see Injury,
  intra-abdominal
  with open wound into abdominal cavity —
    see Wound, open, with penetration
    into peritoneal cavity
  colon —see Injury, intestine, large
  rectum —see Injury, intestine, large, rectum
    with open wound into abdominal cavity
      S36.61
  small intestine —see Injury, intestine, small
  specified site NEC —see Injury, intra-
    abdominal, specified, site NEC
  stomach —see Injury, stomach

Injury (Continued)
genital organ (s)
  external S39.94
    specified NEC S39.848
  internal S37.90
    fallopian tube —see Injury, fallopian tube
    ovary —see Injury, ovary
    prostate —see Injury, prostate
    seminal vesicle —see Injury, pelvis,
      organ, specified site NEC
    uterus —see Injury, uterus
    vas deferens —see Injury, pelvis, organ,
      specified site NEC
  obstetrical trauma O71.9
gland
  lacrimal laceration —see Injury, eye,
    specified site NEC
  salivary S09.93 ◄▥
  thyroid NEC S19.84
globe (eye) S05.90
  specified NEC S05.8X-
groin —see Injury, abdomen
gum S09.90
hand S69.9-
  blood vessel —see Injury, blood vessel,
    hand
  contusion —see Contusion, hand
  fracture —see Fracture, hand
  muscle —see Injury, muscle, hand
  nerve —see Injury, nerve, hand
  open —see Wound, open, hand
  specified NEC S69.8-
  sprain —see Sprain, hand
  superficial —see Injury, superficial, hand
head S09.90
  with loss of consciousness S06.9-
  specified NEC S09.8-
heart S26.90
  with hemopericardium S26.00
    contusion S26.01
    laceration (mild) S26.020
      major S26.022
      moderate S26.021
    specified type NEC S26.09
  without hemopericardium S26.10
    contusion S26.11
    laceration S26.12
    specified type NEC S26.19
  contusion S26.91
  laceration S26.92
  specified type NEC S26.99
heel —see Injury, foot
hepatic
  artery —see Injury, blood vessel, celiac
    artery, branch
  duct —see Injury, liver
  vein —see Injury, vena cava, inferior
hip S79.91-
  blood vessel —see Injury, blood vessel,
    hip
  contusion —see Contusion, hip
  dislocation —see Dislocation, hip
  fracture —see Fracture, femur, neck
  muscle —see Injury, muscle, hip
  nerve —see Injury, nerve, hip
  open —see Wound, open, hip
  specified NEC S79.81-
  sprain —see Sprain, hip
  superficial —see Injury, superficial, hip
hymen S39.94
hypogastric
  blood vessel —see Injury, blood vessel, iliac
  plexus —see Injury, nerve, lumbosacral,
    sympathetic
ileum —see Injury, intestine, small
iliac region S39.91
instrumental (during surgery) —see
  Laceration, accidental complicating
  surgery
  birth injury —see Birth, injury
  nonsurgical —see Injury, by site

Injury (Continued)
instrumental (Continued)
  obstetrical O71.9
    bladder O71.5
    cervix O71.3
    high vaginal O71.4
    perineal NOS O70.9
    urethra O71.5
    uterus O71.5
      with rupture or perforation O71.1
internal T14.8
  aorta —see Injury, aorta
  bladder (sphincter) —see Injury, bladder
    with
      ectopic or molar pregnancy O08.6
      following ectopic or molar pregnancy
        O08.6
      obstetrical trauma O71.5
  bronchus, bronchi —see Injury,
    intrathoracic, bronchus
  cecum —see Injury, intestine, large
  cervix (uteri) —see also Injury, uterus
    with ectopic or molar pregnancy O08.6
    following ectopic or molar pregnancy
      O08.6
    obstetrical trauma O71.3
  chest —see Injury, intrathoracic
  gastrointestinal tract —see Injury,
    intra-abdominal
  heart —see Injury, heart
  intestine NEC —see Injury, intestine
  intrauterine —see Injury, uterus
  mesentery —see Injury, intra-abdominal,
    specified, site NEC
  pelvis, pelvic (organ) S37.90
    following ectopic or molar pregnancy
      (subsequent episode) O08.6
    obstetrical trauma NEC O71.5
    rupture or perforation O71.1
    specified NEC S39.83
  rectum —see Injury, intestine, large,
    rectum
  stomach —see Injury, stomach
  ureter —see Injury, ureter
  urethra (sphincter) following ectopic or
    molar pregnancy O08.6
  uterus —see Injury, uterus
interscapular area —see Injury, thorax
intestine
  large S36.509
    ascending (right) S36.500
      blast injury (primary) S36.510
        secondary S36.590
      contusion S36.520
      laceration S36.530
      specified type NEC S36.590
    blast injury (primary) S36.519
      ascending (right) S36.510
      descending (left) S36.512
      rectum S36.61
      sigmoid S36.513
      specified site NEC S36.518
      transverse S36.511
    contusion S36.529
      ascending (right) S36.520
      descending (left) S36.522
      rectum S36.62
      sigmoid S36.523
      specified site NEC S36.528
      transverse S36.521
    descending (left) S36.502
      blast injury (primary) S36.512
        secondary S36.592
      contusion S36.522
      laceration S36.532
      specified type NEC S36.592
    laceration S36.539
      ascending (right) S36.530
      descending (left) S36.532
      rectum S36.63
      sigmoid S36.533

Injury *(Continued)*
  intestine *(Continued)*
    large *(Continued)*
      laceration *(Continued)*
        specified site NEC S36.538
        transverse S36.531
      rectum S36.60
        blast injury (primary) S36.61
          secondary S36.69
        contusion S36.62
        laceration S36.63
        specified type NEC S36.69
      sigmoid S36.503
        blast injury (primary) S36.513
          secondary S36.593
        contusion S36.523
        laceration S36.533
        specified type NEC S36.593
      specified
        site NEC S36.508
          blast injury (primary) S36.518
            secondary S36.598
          contusion S36.528
          laceration S36.538
          specified type NEC S36.598
        type NEC S36.599
          ascending (right) S36.590
          descending (left) S36.592
          rectum S36.69
          sigmoid S36.593
          specified site NEC S36.598
          transverse S36.591
      transverse S36.501
        blast injury (primary) S36.511
          secondary S36.591
        contusion S36.521
        laceration S36.531
        specified type NEC S36.591
    small S36.409
      blast injury (primary) S36.419
        duodenum S36.410
        secondary S36.499
          duodenum S36.490
          specified site NEC S36.498
        specified site NEC S36.418
      contusion S36.429
        duodenum S36.420
        specified site NEC S36.428
      duodenum S36.400
        blast injury (primary) S36.410
          secondary S36.490
        contusion S36.420
        laceration S36.430
        specified NEC S36.490
      laceration S36.439
        duodenum S36.430
        specified site NEC S36.438
      specified
        site NEC S36.408
        type NEC S36.499
          duodenum S36.490
          specified site NEC S36.498
  intra-abdominal S36.90
    adrenal gland —*see* Injury, adrenal gland
    bladder —*see* Injury, bladder
    colon —*see* Injury, intestine, large
    contusion S36.92
    fallopian tube —*see* Injury, fallopian tube
    gallbladder —*see* Injury, gallbladder
    intestine —*see* Injury, intestine
    kidney —*see* Injury, kidney
    laceration S36.93
    liver —*see* Injury, liver
    ovary —*see* Injury, ovary
    pancreas —*see* Injury, pancreas
    pelvic NOS S37.90
    peritoneum —*see* Injury, intra-abdominal, specified, site NEC
    prostate —*see* Injury, prostate
    rectum —*see* Injury, intestine, large, rectum

Injury *(Continued)*
  intra-abdominal *(Continued)*
    retroperitoneum —*see* Injury, intra-abdominal, specified, site NEC
    seminal vesicle —*see* Injury, pelvis, organ, specified site NEC
    small intestine —*see* Injury, intestine, small
    specified
      pelvic S37.90
        specified
          site NEC S37.899
            specified type NEC S37.898
          type NEC S37.99
      site NEC S36.899
        contusion S36.892
        laceration S36.893
        specified type NEC S36.898
      type NEC S36.99
    spleen —*see* Injury, spleen
    stomach —*see* Injury, stomach
    ureter —*see* Injury, ureter
    urethra —*see* Injury, urethra
    uterus —*see* Injury, uterus
    vas deferens —*see* Injury, pelvis, organ, specified site NEC
  intracranial (traumatic) S06.9-
    cerebellar hemorrhage, traumatic —*see* Injury, intracranial, focal
    cerebral edema, traumatic S06.1X-
      diffuse S06.1X-
      focal S06.1X-
    diffuse (axonal) S06.2X-
    epidural hemorrhage (traumatic) S06.4X-
    focal brain injury S06.30-
      contusion —*see* Contusion, cerebral
      laceration —*see* Laceration, cerebral
    intracerebral hemorrhage, traumatic S06.36-
      left side S06.35-
      right side S06.34-
    subarachnoid hemorrhage, traumatic S06.6X-
    subdural hemorrhage, traumatic S06.5X-
  intraocular —*see* Injury, eyeball, penetrating
  intrathoracic S27.9
    bronchus S27.409
      bilateral S27.402
      blast injury (primary) S27.419
        bilateral S27.412
        secondary —*see* Injury, intrathoracic, bronchus, specified type NEC
        unilateral S27.411
      contusion S27.429
        bilateral S27.422
        unilateral S27.421
      laceration S27.439
        bilateral S27.432
        unilateral S27.431
      specified type NEC S27.499
        bilateral S27.492
        unilateral S27.491
      unilateral S27.401
    diaphragm S27.809
      contusion S27.802
      laceration S27.803
      specified type NEC S27.808
    esophagus (thoracic) S27.819
      contusion S27.812
      laceration S27.813
      specified type NEC S27.818
    heart —*see* Injury, heart
    hemopneumothorax S27.2
    hemothorax S27.1
    lung S27.309
      aspiration J69.0
      bilateral S27.302
      blast injury (primary) S27.319
        bilateral S27.312
        secondary —*see* Injury, intrathoracic, lung, specified type NEC
        unilateral S27.311

Injury *(Continued)*
  intrathoracic *(Continued)*
    bronchus *(Continued)*
      contusion S27.329
        bilateral S27.322
        unilateral S27.321
      laceration S27.339
        bilateral S27.332
        unilateral S27.331
      specified type NEC S27.399
        bilateral S27.392
        unilateral S27.391
      unilateral S27.301
    pleura S27.60
      laceration S27.63
      specified type NEC S27.69
    pneumothorax S27.0
    specified organ NEC S27.899
      contusion S27.892
      laceration S27.893
      specified type NEC S27.898
    thoracic duct —*see* Injury, intrathoracic, specified organ NEC
    thymus gland —*see* Injury, intrathoracic, specified organ NEC
    trachea, thoracic S27.50
      blast (primary) S27.51
      contusion S27.52
      laceration S27.53
      specified type NEC S27.59
  iris —*see* Injury, eye, specified site NEC
    penetrating —*see* Injury, eyeball, penetrating
  jaw S09.93
  jejunum —*see* Injury, intestine, small
  joint NOS T14.8
    old or residual —*see* Disorder, joint, specified type NEC
  kidney S37.00-
    acute (nontraumatic) N17.9
    contusion —*see* Contusion, kidney
    laceration —*see* Laceration, kidney
    specified NEC S37.09-
  knee S89.9-
    contusion —*see* Contusion, knee
    dislocation —*see* Dislocation, knee
    meniscus (lateral) (medial) —*see* Sprain, knee, specified site NEC
      old injury or tear —*see* Derangement, knee, meniscus, due to old injury
    open —*see* Wound, open, knee
    specified NEC S89.8-
    sprain —*see* Sprain, knee
    superficial —*see* Injury, superficial, knee
  labium (majus) (minus) S39.94
  labyrinth, ear S09.30-
  lacrimal apparatus, duct, gland, or sac —*see* Injury, eye, specified site NEC
  larynx NEC S19.81
  leg (lower) S89.9-
    blood vessel —*see* Injury, blood vessel, leg
    contusion —*see* Contusion, leg
    fracture —*see* Fracture, leg
    muscle —*see* Injury, muscle, leg
    nerve —*see* Injury, nerve, leg
    open —*see* Wound, open, leg
    specified NEC S89.8-
    superficial —*see* Injury, superficial, leg
  lens, eye —*see* Injury, eye, specified site NEC
    penetrating —*see* Injury, eyeball, penetrating
  limb NEC T14.8
  lip S09.93
  liver S36.119
    contusion S36.112
    laceration S36.113
      major (stellate) S36.116
      minor S36.114
      moderate S36.115
    specified NEC S36.118
  lower back S39.92
    specified NEC S39.82

Injury (Continued)
  lumbar, lumbosacral (region) S39.92
    plexus —see Injury, lumbosacral plexus
  lumbosacral plexus S34.4
  lung —see also Injury, intrathoracic, lung
    aspiration J69.0
    transfusion-related (TRALI) J95.84
  lymphatic thoracic duct —see Injury,
    intrathoracic, specified organ NEC
  malar region S09.93
  mastoid region S09.90
  maxilla S09.93
  mediastinum —see Injury, intrathoracic,
    specified organ NEC
  membrane, brain —see Injury, intracranial
  meningeal artery —see Injury, intracranial,
    subdural hemorrhage
  meninges (cerebral) —see Injury, intracranial
  mesenteric
    artery
      branch S35.299
        laceration (minor) (superficial) S35.291
          major S35.292
          specified NEC S35.298
      inferior S35.239
        laceration (minor) (superficial) S35.231
          major S35.232
          specified NEC S35.238
      superior S35.229
        laceration (minor) (superficial) S35.221
          major S35.222
          specified NEC S35.228
    plexus (inferior) (superior) —see Injury,
      nerve, lumbosacral, sympathetic
    vein
      inferior S35.349
        laceration S35.341
        specified NEC S35.348
      superior S35.339
        laceration S35.331
        specified NEC S35.338
  mesentery —see Injury, intra-abdominal,
    specified site NEC
  mesosalpinx —see Injury, pelvic organ,
    specified site NEC
  middle ear S09.30-
  midthoracic region NOS S29.9
  mouth S09.93
  multiple NOS T07
  muscle (and fascia) (and tendon)
    abdomen S39.001
      laceration S39.021
      specified type NEC S39.091
      strain S39.011
    abductor
      thumb, forearm level —see Injury,
        muscle, thumb, abductor
    adductor
      thigh S76.20-
        laceration S76.22-
        specified type NEC S76.29-
        strain S76.21-
    ankle —see Injury, muscle, foot
    anterior muscle group, at leg level (lower)
      S86.20-
      laceration S86.22-
      specified type NEC S86.29-
      strain S86.21-
    arm (upper) —see Injury, muscle,
      shoulder
    biceps (parts NEC) S46.20-
      laceration S46.22-
      long head S46.10-
        laceration S46.12-
        specified type NEC S46.19-
        strain S46.11-
      specified type NEC S46.29-
      strain S46.21-
    extensor
      finger (s) (other than thumb) —see Injury,
        muscle, finger by site, extensor

Injury (Continued)
  muscle (Continued)
    extensor (Continued)
      forearm level, specified NEC —see
        Injury, muscle, forearm, extensor
      thumb —see Injury, muscle, thumb,
        extensor
      toe (large) (ankle level) (foot level) —see
        Injury, muscle, toe, extensor
    finger
      extensor (forearm level) S56.40-
        hand level S66.309
          laceration S66.329
          specified type NEC S66.399
          strain S66.319
        laceration S56.429
        specified type NEC S56.499
        strain S56.419
      flexor (forearm level) S56.10-
        hand level S66.109
          laceration S66.129
          specified type NEC S66.199
          strain S66.119
        laceration S56.129
        specified type NEC S56.199
        strain S56.119
      index
        extensor (forearm level)
          hand level S66.308
            laceration S66.32-
            specified type NEC S66.39-
            strain S66.31-
          specified type NEC S56.492-
        flexor (forearm level)
          hand level S66.108
            laceration S66.12-
            specified type NEC
              S66.19-
            strain S66.11-
          specified type NEC S56.19-
          strain S56.11-
        intrinsic S66.50-
          laceration S66.52-
          specified type NEC S66.59-
          strain S66.51-
      intrinsic S66.509
        laceration S66.529
        specified type NEC S66.599
        strain S66.519
      little
        extensor (forearm level)
          hand level S66.30-
            laceration S66.32-
            specified type NEC S66.39-
            strain S66.31-
          laceration S56.42-
          specified type NEC S56.49-
          strain S56.41-
        flexor (forearm level)
          hand level S66.10-
            laceration S66.12-
            specified type NEC S66.19-
            strain S66.11-
          laceration S56.12-
          specified type NEC S56.19-
          strain S56.11-
        intrinsic S66.50-
          laceration S66.52-
          specified type NEC S66.59-
          strain S66.51-
      middle
        extensor (forearm level)
          hand level S66.30-
            laceration S66.32-
            specified type NEC
              S66.39-
            strain S66.31-
          laceration S56.42-
          specified type NEC
            S56.49-
          strain S56.41-

Injury (Continued)
  muscle (Continued)
    finger (Continued)
      middle (Continued)
        flexor (forearm level)
          hand level S66.10-
            laceration S66.12-
            specified type NEC
              S66.19-
            strain S66.11-
          laceration S56.12-
          specified type NEC S56.19-
          strain S56.11-
        intrinsic S66.50-
          laceration S66.52-
          specified type NEC S66.59-
          strain S66.51-
      ring
        extensor (forearm level)
          hand level S66.30-
            laceration S66.32-
            specified type NEC S66.39-
            strain S66.31-
          laceration S56.42-
          specified type NEC S56.49-
          strain S56.41-
        flexor (forearm level)
          hand level S66.10-
            laceration S66.12-
            specified type NEC S66.19-
            strain S66.11-
          laceration S56.12-
          specified type NEC S56.19-
          strain S56.11-
        intrinsic S66.50-
          laceration S66.52-
          specified type NEC S66.59-
          strain S66.51-
    flexor
      finger(s) (other than thumb) — see Injury,
        muscle, finger
      forearm level, specified NEC — see
        Injury, muscle, forearm, flexor
      thumb —see Injury, muscle, thumb,
        flexor
      toe (long) (ankle level) (foot level) —see
        Injury, muscle, toe, flexor
    foot S96.90-
      intrinsic S96.20-
        laceration S96.22-
        specified type NEC S96.29-
        strain S96.21-
      laceration S96.92-
      long extensor, toe —see Injury, muscle,
        toe, extensor
      long flexor, toe —see Injury, muscle, toe,
        flexor
      specified
        site NEC S96.80-
          laceration S96.82-
          specified type NEC
            S96.89-
          strain S96.81-
        type NEC S96.99-
      strain S96.91-
    forearm (level) S56.90-
      extensor S56.50-
        laceration S56.52-
        specified type NEC S56.59-
        strain S56.51-
      flexor S56.20-
        laceration S56.22-
        specified type NEC S56.29-
        strain S56.21-
      laceration S56.92-
      specified S56.99-
        site NEC S56.80-
          laceration S56.82-
          strain S56.81-
        type NEC S56.89-
      strain S56.91-

Injury (Continued)
  muscle (Continued)
    hand (level) S66.90-
      laceration S66.92-
      specified
        site NEC S66.80-
          laceration S66.82-
          specified type NEC S66.89-
          strain S66.81-
        type NEC S66.99-
      strain S66.91-
    head S09.10
      laceration S09.12
      specified type NEC S09.19
      strain S09.11
    hip NEC S76.00-
      laceration S76.02-
      specified type NEC S76.09-
      strain S76.01-
    intrinsic
      ankle and foot level —see Injury, muscle,
        foot, intrinsic
      finger (other than thumb) —see Injury,
        muscle, finger by site, intrinsic
      foot (level) —see Injury, muscle, foot,
        intrinsic
      thumb —see Injury, muscle, thumb,
        intrinsic
    leg (level) (lower) S86.90-
      Achilles tendon —see Injury, Achilles
        tendon
      anterior muscle group —see Injury,
        muscle, anterior muscle
        group
      laceration S86.92-
      peroneal muscle group —see Injury,
        muscle, peroneal muscle group
      posterior muscle group —see Injury,
        muscle, posterior muscle group,
        leg level
      specified
        site NEC S86.80-
          laceration S86.82-
          specified type NEC
            S86.89-
          strain S86.81-
        type NEC S86.99-
      strain S86.91-
    long
      extensor toe, at ankle and foot level —see
        Injury, muscle, toe, extensor
      flexor, toe, at ankle and foot level —see
        Injury, muscle, toe, flexor
      head, biceps —see Injury, muscle, biceps,
        long head
    lower back S39.002
      laceration S39.022
      specified type NEC S39.092
      strain S39.012
    neck (level) S16.9
      laceration S16.2
      specified type NEC S16.8
      strain S16.1
    pelvis S39.003
      laceration S39.023
      specified type NEC S39.093
      strain S39.013
    peroneal muscle group, at leg level (lower)
      S86.30-
      laceration S86.32-
      specified type NEC S86.39-
      strain S86.31-
    posterior muscle (group)
      leg level (lower) S86.10-
        laceration S86.12-
        specified type NEC S86.19-
        strain S86.11-
      thigh level S76.30-
        laceration S76.32-
        specified type NEC S76.39-
        strain S76.31-

Injury (Continued)
  muscle (Continued)
    quadriceps (thigh) S76.10-
      laceration S76.12-
      specified type NEC S76.19-
      strain S76.11-
    shoulder S46.90-
      laceration S46.92-
      rotator cuff —see Injury, rotator cuff
      specified site NEC S46.80-
        laceration S46.82-
        specified type NEC S46.89-
        strain S46.81-
      specified type NEC S46.99-
      strain S46.91-
    thigh NEC (level) S76.90-
      adductor —see Injury, muscle, adductor,
        thigh
      laceration S76.92-
      posterior muscle (group) —see Injury,
        muscle, posterior muscle, thigh
        level
      quadriceps —see Injury, muscle,
        quadriceps
      specified
        site NEC S76.80-
          laceration S76.82-
          specified type NEC S76.89-
          strain S76.81-
        type NEC S76.99-
      strain S76.91-
    thorax (level) S29.009
      back wall S29.002
      front wall S29.001
      laceration S29.029
        back wall S29.022
        front wall S29.021
      specified type NEC S29.099
        back wall S29.092
        front wall S29.091
      strain S29.019
        back wall S29.012
        front wall S29.011
    thumb
      abductor (forearm level) S56.30-
        laceration S56.32-
        specified type NEC S56.39-
        strain S56.31-
      extensor (forearm level) S56.30-
        hand level S66.20-
          laceration S66.22-
          specified type NEC S66.29-
          strain S66.21-
        laceration S56.32-
        specified type NEC S56.39-
        strain S56.31-
      flexor (forearm level) S56.00-
        hand level S66.00-
          laceration S66.02-
          specified type NEC S66.09-
          strain S66.01-
        laceration S56.02-
        specified type NEC S56.09-
        strain S56.01-
        wrist level —see Injury, muscle,
          thumb, flexor, hand level
      intrinsic S66.40-
        laceration S66.42-
        specified type NEC S66.49-
        strain S66.41-
    toe —see also Injury, muscle, foot
      extensor, long S96.10-
        laceration S96.12-
        specified type NEC
          S96.19-
        strain S96.11-
      flexor, long S96.00-
        laceration S96.02-
        specified type NEC
          S96.09-
        strain S96.01-

Injury (Continued)
  muscle (Continued)
    triceps S46.30-
      laceration S46.32-
      specified type NEC S46.39-
      strain S46.31-
    wrist (and hand) level —see Injury, muscle,
      hand
  musculocutaneous nerve —see Injury, nerve,
    musculocutaneous
  myocardium —see Injury, heart
  nape —see Injury, neck
  nasal (septum) (sinus) S09.92
  nasopharynx S09.92
  neck S19.9
    specified NEC S19.80
      specified site NEC S19.89
  nerve NEC T14.8
    abdomen S34.9
      peripheral S34.6
      specified site NEC S34.8
    abducens S04.4-
      contusion S04.4-
      laceration S04.4-
      specified type NEC S04.4-
    abducent —see Injury, nerve,
      abducens
    accessory S04.7-
      contusion S04.7-
      laceration S04.7-
      specified type NEC S04.7-
    acoustic S04.6-
      contusion S04.6-
      laceration S04.6-
      specified type NEC S04.6-
    ankle S94.9-
      cutaneous sensory S94.3-
      specified site NEC —see subcategory S94.8
    anterior crural, femoral —see Injury, nerve,
      femoral
    arm (upper) S44.9-
      axillary —see Injury, nerve, axillary
      cutaneous —see Injury, nerve, cutaneous,
        arm
      median —see Injury, nerve, median,
        upper arm
      musculocutaneous —see Injury, nerve,
        musculocutaneous
      radial —see Injury, nerve, radial, upper
        arm
      specified site NEC —see subcategory
        S44.8
      ulnar —see Injury, nerve, ulnar, arm
    auditory —see Injury, nerve, acoustic
    axillary S44.3-
    brachial plexus —see Injury, brachial plexus
    cervical sympathetic S14.5
    cranial S04.9
      contusion S04.9
      eighth (acoustic or auditory) —see Injury,
        nerve, acoustic
      eleventh (accessory) —see Injury, nerve,
        accessory
      fifth (trigeminal) —see Injury, nerve,
        trigeminal
      first (olfactory) —see Injury, nerve,
        olfactory
      fourth (trochlear) —see Injury, nerve,
        trochlear
      laceration S04.9
      ninth (glossopharyngeal) —see Injury,
        nerve, glossopharyngeal
      second (optic) —see Injury, nerve, optic
      seventh (facial) —see Injury, nerve, facial
      sixth (abducent) —see Injury, nerve,
        abducens
      specified
        nerve NEC S04.89-
          contusion S04.89-
          laceration S04.89-
          specified type NEC S04.89-
        type NEC S04.9

◄ New   ◄═ Revised   ~~deleted~~ Deleted

Injury *(Continued)*
nerve NEC *(Continued)*
cranial *(Continued)*
tenth (pneumogastric or vagus) —*see* Injury, nerve, vagus
third (oculomotor) —*see* Injury, nerve, oculomotor
twelfth (hypoglossal) —*see* Injury, nerve, hypoglossal
cutaneous sensory
ankle (level) S94.3-
arm (upper) (level) S44.5-
foot (level) —*see* Injury, nerve, cutaneous sensory, ankle
forearm (level) S54.3-
hip (level) S74.2-
leg (lower level) S84.2-
shoulder (level) —*see* Injury, nerve, cutaneous sensory, arm
thigh (level) —*see* Injury, nerve, cutaneous sensory, hip
deep peroneal —*see* Injury, nerve, peroneal, foot
digital
finger S64.4-
index S64.49-
little S64.49-
middle S64.49-
ring S64.49-
thumb S64.3-
toe —*see* Injury, nerve, ankle, specified site NEC
eighth cranial (acoustic or auditory) —*see* Injury, nerve, acoustic
eleventh cranial (accessory) —*see* Injury, nerve, accessory
facial S04.5-
contusion S04.5-
laceration S04.5-
newborn P11.3
specified type NEC S04.5-
femoral (hip level) (thigh level) S74.1-
fifth cranial (trigeminal) —*see* Injury, nerve, trigeminal
finger (digital) —*see* Injury, nerve, digital, finger
first cranial (olfactory) —*see* Injury, nerve, olfactory
foot S94.9-
cutaneous sensory S94.3-
deep peroneal S94.2-
lateral plantar S94.0-
medial plantar S94.1-
specified site NEC —*see* subcategory S94.8
forearm (level) S54.9-
cutaneous sensory —*see* Injury, nerve, cutaneous sensory, forearm
median —*see* Injury, nerve, median
radial —*see* Injury, nerve, radial
specified site NEC —*see* subcategory S54.8
ulnar —*see* Injury, nerve, ulnar
fourth cranial (trochlear) —*see* Injury, nerve, trochlear
glossopharyngeal S04.89-
specified type NEC S04.89-
hand S64.9-
median —*see* Injury, nerve, median, hand
radial —*see* Injury, nerve, radial, hand
specified NEC —*see* subcategory S64.8
ulnar —*see* Injury, nerve, ulnar, hand
hip (level) S74.9-
cutaneous sensory —*see* Injury, nerve, cutaneous sensory, hip
femoral —*see* Injury, nerve, femoral
sciatic —*see* Injury, nerve, sciatic
specified site NEC —*see* subcategory S74.8

Injury *(Continued)*
nerve NEC *(Continued)*
hypoglossal S04.89-
specified type NEC S04.89-
lateral plantar S94.0-
leg (lower) S84.9-
cutaneous sensory —*see* Injury, nerve, cutaneous sensory, leg
peroneal —*see* Injury, nerve, peroneal
specified site NEC —*see* subcategory S84.8
tibial —*see* Injury, nerve, tibial
upper —*see* Injury, nerve, thigh
lower
back —*see* Injury, nerve, abdomen, specified site NEC
peripheral —*see* Injury, nerve, abdomen, peripheral
limb —*see* Injury, nerve, leg
lumbar plexus —*see* Injury, nerve, lumbosacral, sympathetic
lumbar spinal —*see* Injury, nerve, spinal, lumbar
lumbosacral
plexus —*see* Injury, nerve, lumbosacral, sympathetic
sympathetic S34.5
medial plantar S94.1-
median (forearm level) S54.1-
hand (level) S64.1-
upper arm (level) S44.1-
wrist (level) —*see* Injury, nerve, median, hand
musculocutaneous S44.4-
musculospiral (upper arm level) —*see* Injury, nerve, radial, upper arm
neck S14.9
peripheral S14.4
specified site NEC S14.8
sympathetic S14.5
ninth cranial (glossopharyngeal) —*see* Injury, nerve, glossopharyngeal
oculomotor S04.1-
contusion S04.1-
laceration S04.1-
specified type NEC S04.1-
olfactory S04.81-
specified type NEC S04.81-
optic S04.01-
contusion S04.01-
laceration S04.01-
specified type NEC S04.01-
pelvic girdle —*see* Injury, nerve, hip
pelvis —*see* Injury, nerve, abdomen, specified site NEC
peripheral —*see* Injury, nerve, abdomen, peripheral
peripheral NEC T14.8
abdomen —*see* Injury, nerve, abdomen, peripheral
lower back —*see* Injury, nerve, abdomen, peripheral
neck —*see* Injury, nerve, neck, peripheral
pelvis —*see* Injury, nerve, abdomen, peripheral
specified NEC T14.8
peroneal (lower leg level) S84.1-
foot S94.2-
plexus
brachial —*see* Injury, brachial plexus
celiac, coeliac —*see* Injury, nerve, lumbosacral, sympathetic
mesenteric, inferior —*see* Injury, nerve, lumbosacral, sympathetic
sacral —*see* Injury, lumbosacral plexus
spinal
brachial —*see* Injury, brachial plexus
lumbosacral —*see* Injury, lumbosacral plexus

Injury *(Continued)*
nerve NEC *(Continued)*
pneumogastric —*see* Injury, nerve, vagus
radial (forearm level) S54.2-
hand (level) S64.2-
upper arm (level) S44.2-
wrist (level) —*see* Injury, nerve, radial, hand
root —*see* Injury, nerve, spinal, root
sacral plexus —*see* Injury, lumbosacral plexus
sacral spinal —*see* Injury, nerve, spinal, sacral
sciatic (hip level) (thigh level) S74.0-
second cranial (optic) —*see* Injury, nerve, optic
seventh cranial (facial) —*see* Injury, nerve, facial
shoulder —*see* Injury, nerve, arm
sixth cranial (abducent) —*see* Injury, nerve, abducens
spinal
plexus —*see* Injury, nerve, plexus, spinal
root
cervical S14.2
dorsal S24.2
lumbar S34.21
sacral S34.22
thoracic —*see* Injury, nerve, spinal, root, dorsal
splanchnic —*see* Injury, nerve, lumbosacral, sympathetic
sympathetic NEC —*see* Injury, nerve, lumbosacral, sympathetic
cervical —*see* Injury, nerve, cervical sympathetic
tenth cranial (pneumogastric or vagus) —*see* Injury, nerve, vagus
thigh (level) —*see* Injury, nerve, hip
cutaneous sensory —*see* Injury, nerve, cutaneous sensory, hip
femoral —*see* Injury, nerve, femoral
sciatic —*see* Injury, nerve, sciatic
specified NEC —*see* Injury, nerve, hip
third cranial (oculomotor) —*see* Injury, nerve, oculomotor
thorax S24.9
peripheral S24.3
specified site NEC S24.8
sympathetic S24.4
thumb, digital —*see* Injury, nerve, digital, thumb
tibial (lower leg level) (posterior) S84.0-
toe —*see* Injury, nerve, ankle
trigeminal S04.3-
contusion S04.3-
laceration S04.3-
specified type NEC S04.3-
trochlear S04.2-
contusion S04.2-
laceration S04.2-
specified type NEC S04.2-
twelfth cranial (hypoglossal) —*see* Injury, nerve, hypoglossal
ulnar (forearm level) S54.0-
arm (upper) (level) S44.0-
hand (level) S64.0-
wrist (level) —*see* Injury, nerve, ulnar, hand
vagus S04.89-
specified type NEC S04.89-
wrist (level) —*see* Injury, nerve, hand
ninth cranial nerve (glossopharyngeal) —*see* Injury, nerve, glossopharyngeal
nose (septum) S09.92
obstetrical O71.9
specified NEC O71.89
occipital (region) (scalp) S09.90
lobe —*see* Injury, intracranial
optic chiasm S04.02
optic radiation S04.03-

Injury *(Continued)*
  optic tract and pathways S04.03-
  orbit, orbital (region) —*see* Injury, eye
    penetrating (with foreign body) —*see*
      Injury, eye, orbit, penetrating
    specified NEC —*see* Injury, eye, specified
      site NEC
  ovary, ovarian S37.409
    bilateral S37.402
      contusion S37.422
      laceration S37.432
      specified type NEC S37.492
    blood vessel —*see* Injury, blood vessel,
      ovarian
    contusion S37.429
      bilateral S37.422
      unilateral S37.421
    laceration S37.439
      bilateral S37.432
      unilateral S37.431
    specified type NEC S37.499
      bilateral S37.492
      unilateral S37.491
    unilateral S37.401
      contusion S37.421
      laceration S37.431
      specified type NEC S37.491
  palate (hard) (soft) S09.93
  pancreas S36.209
    body S36.201
      contusion S36.221
      laceration S36.231
        major S36.261
        minor S36.241
        moderate S36.251
      specified type NEC S36.291
    contusion S36.229
    head S36.200
      contusion S36.220
      laceration S36.230
        major S36.260
        minor S36.240
        moderate S36.250
      specified type NEC S36.290
    laceration S36.239
      major S36.269
      minor S36.249
      moderate S36.259
    specified type NEC S36.299
    tail S36.202
      contusion S36.222
      laceration S36.232
        major S36.262
        minor S36.242
        moderate S36.252
      specified type NEC S36.292
  parietal (region) (scalp) S09.90
    lobe —*see* Injury, intracranial
  patellar ligament (tendon) S76.10-
    laceration S76.12-
    specified NEC S76.19-
    strain S76.11-
  pelvis, pelvic (floor) S39.93
    complicating delivery O70.1
    joint or ligament, complicating delivery
      O71.6
    organ S37.90
      with ectopic or molar pregnancy O08.6
      complication of abortion —*see* Abortion
      contusion S37.92
      following ectopic or molar pregnancy
        O08.6
      laceration S37.93
      obstetrical trauma NEC O71.5
      specified
        site NEC S37.899
          contusion S37.892
          laceration S37.893
          specified type NEC S37.898
        type NEC S37.99
    specified NEC S39.83

Injury *(Continued)*
  penis S39.94
  perineum S39.94
  peritoneum S36.81
    laceration S36.893
  periurethral tissue —*see* Injury, urethra
    complicating delivery O71.82
  phalanges
    foot —*see* Injury, foot
    hand —*see* Injury, hand
  pharynx NEC S19.85
  pleura —*see* Injury, intrathoracic, pleura
  plexus
    brachial —*see* Injury, brachial plexus
    cardiac —*see* Injury, nerve, thorax,
      sympathetic
    celiac, coeliac —*see* Injury, nerve,
      lumbosacral, sympathetic
    esophageal —*see* Injury, nerve, thorax,
      sympathetic
    hypogastric —*see* Injury, nerve,
      lumbosacral, sympathetic
    lumbar, lumbosacral —*see* Injury,
      lumbosacral plexus
    mesenteric —*see* Injury, nerve, lumbosacral,
      sympathetic
    pulmonary —*see* Injury, nerve, thorax,
      sympathetic
  postcardiac surgery (syndrome) I97.0
  prepuce S39.94
  prostate S37.829
    contusion S37.822
    laceration S37.823
    specified type NEC S37.828
  pubic region S39.94
  pudendum S39.94
  pulmonary plexus —*see* Injury, nerve, thorax,
    sympathetic
  rectovaginal septum NEC S39.83
  rectum —*see* Injury, intestine, large, rectum
  retina —*see* Injury, eye, specified site NEC
    penetrating —*see* Injury, eyeball,
      penetrating
  retroperitoneal —*see* Injury, intra-abdominal,
    specified site NEC
  rotator cuff (muscle (s)) (tendon (s)) S46.00-
    laceration S46.02-
    specified type NEC S46.09-
    strain S46.01-
  round ligament —*see* Injury, pelvic organ,
    specified site NEC
  sacral plexus —*see* Injury, lumbosacral
    plexus
  salivary duct or gland S09.93
  scalp S09.90
    newborn (birth injury) P12.9
      due to monitoring (electrode) (sampling
        incision) P12.4
      specified NEC P12.89
        caput succedaneum P12.81
  scapular region —*see* Injury, shoulder
  sclera —*see* Injury, eye, specified site NEC
    penetrating —*see* Injury, eyeball,
      penetrating
  scrotum S39.94
  second cranial nerve (optic) —*see* Injury,
    nerve, optic
  seminal vesicle —*see* Injury, pelvic organ,
    specified site NEC
  seventh cranial nerve (facial) —*see* Injury,
    nerve, facial
  shoulder S49.9-
    blood vessel —*see* Injury, blood vessel,
      arm
    contusion —*see* Contusion, shoulder
    dislocation —*see* Dislocation, shoulder
    fracture —*see* Fracture, shoulder
    muscle —*see* Injury, muscle, shoulder
    nerve —*see* Injury, nerve, shoulder
    open —*see* Wound, open, shoulder
    specified type NEC S49.8-

Injury *(Continued)*
  shoulder *(Continued)*
    sprain —*see* Sprain, shoulder girdle
    superficial —*see* Injury, superficial,
      shoulder
  sinus
    cavernous —*see* Injury, intracranial
    nasal S09.92
  sixth cranial nerve (abducent) —*see* Injury,
    nerve, abducens
  skeleton, birth injury P13.9
    specified part NEC P13.8
  skin NEC T14.8
    surface intact —*see* Injury, superficial
  skull NEC S09.90
  specified NEC T14.8
  spermatic cord (pelvic region) S37.898
    scrotal region S39.848
  spinal (cord)
    cervical (neck) S14.109
      anterior cord syndrome S14.139
        C1 level S14.131
        C2 level S14.132
        C3 level S14.133
        C4 level S14.134
        C5 level S14.135
        C6 level S14.136
        C7 level S14.137
        C8 level S14.138
      Brown-Séquard syndrome S14.149
        C1 level S14.141
        C2 level S14.142
        C3 level S14.143
        C4 level S14.144
        C5 level S14.145
        C6 level S14.146
        C7 level S14.147
        C8 level S14.148
      C1 level S14.101
      C2 level S14.102
      C3 level S14.103
      C4 level S14.104
      C5 level S14.105
      C6 level S14.106
      C7 level S14.107
      C8 level S14.108
      central cord syndrome S14.129
        C1 level S14.121
        C2 level S14.122
        C3 level S14.123
        C4 level S14.124
        C5 level S14.125
        C6 level S14.126
        C7 level S14.127
        C8 level S14.128
      complete lesion S14.119
        C1 level S14.111
        C2 level S14.112
        C3 level S14.113
        C4 level S14.114
        C5 level S14.115
        C6 level S14.116
        C7 level S14.117
        C8 level S14.118
      concussion S14.0
      edema S14.0
      incomplete lesion specified NEC S14.159
        C1 level S14.151
        C2 level S14.152
        C3 level S14.153
        C4 level S14.154
        C5 level S14.155
        C6 level S14.156
        C7 level S14.157
        C8 level S14.158
      posterior cord syndrome S14.159
        C1 level S14.151
        C2 level S14.152
        C3 level S14.153
        C4 level S14.154
        C5 level S14.155

◀ New   ⬷ Revised   ~~deleted~~ Deleted

Injury (Continued)
  spinal (Continued)
    cervical (Continued)
      posterior cord syndrome (Continued)
        C6 level S14.156
        C7 level S14.157
        C8 level S14.158
      dorsal —see Injury, spinal, thoracic
      lumbar S34.109
        complete lesion S34.119
          L1 level S34.111
          L2 level S34.112
          L3 level S34.113
          L4 level S34.114
          L5 level S34.115
        concussion S34.01
        edema S34.01
        incomplete lesion S34.129
          L1 level S34.121
          L2 level S34.122
          L3 level S34.123
          L4 level S34.124
          L5 level S34.125
        L1 level S34.101
        L2 level S34.102
        L3 level S34.103
        L4 level S34.104
        L5 level S34.105
      nerve root NEC
        cervical —see Injury, nerve, spinal, root,
          cervical
        dorsal —see Injury, nerve, spinal, root,
          dorsal
        lumbar S34.21
        sacral S34.22
        thoracic —see Injury, nerve, spinal, root,
          dorsal
      plexus
        brachial —see Injury, brachial plexus
        lumbosacral —see Injury, lumbosacral
          plexus
      sacral S34.139
        complete lesion S34.131
        incomplete lesion S34.132
      thoracic S24.109
        anterior cord syndrome S24.139
          T1 level S24.131
          T2-T6 level S24.132
          T7-T10 level S24.133
          T11-T12 level S24.134
        Brown-Séquard syndrome
          S24.149
          T1 level S24.141
          T2-T6 level S24.142
          T7-T10 level S24.143
          T11-T12 level S24.144
        complete lesion S24.119
          T1 level S24.111
          T2-T6 level S24.112
          T7-T10 level S24.113
          T11-T12 level S24.114
        concussion S24.0
        edema S24.0
        incomplete lesion specified NEC
          S24.159
          T1 level S24.151
          T2-T6 level S24.152
          T7-T10 level S24.153
          T11-T12 level S24.154
        posterior cord syndrome
          S24.159
          T1 level S24.151
          T2-T6 level S24.152
          T7-T10 level S24.153
          T11-T12 level S24.154
        T1 level S24.101
        T2-T6 level S24.102
        T7-T10 level S24.103
        T11-T12 level S24.104
  splanchnic nerve —see Injury, nerve,
    lumbosacral, sympathetic

Injury (Continued)
  spleen S36.00
    contusion S36.029
      major S36.021
      minor S36.020
    laceration S36.039
      major (massive) (stellate) S36.032
      moderate S36.031
      superficial (capsular) (minor) S36.030
    specified type NEC S36.09
  splenic artery —see Injury, blood vessel, celiac
    artery, branch
  stellate ganglion —see Injury, nerve, thorax,
    sympathetic
  sternal region S29.9
  stomach S36.30
    contusion S36.32
    laceration S36.33
    specified type NEC S36.39
  subconjunctival —see Injury, eye, conjunctiva
  subcutaneous NEC T14.8
  submaxillary region S09.93
  submental region S09.93
  subungual
    fingers —see Injury, hand
    toes —see Injury, foot
  superficial NEC T14.8
    abdomen, abdominal (wall) S30.92
      abrasion S30.811
      bite S30.871
        insect S30.861
      contusion S30.1
      external constriction S30.841
      foreign body S30.851
    abrasion —see Abrasion, by site
    adnexa, eye NEC —see Injury, eye,
      specified site NEC
    alveolar process —see Injury, superficial,
      oral cavity
    ankle S90.91-
      abrasion —see Abrasion, ankle
      bite —see Bite, ankle
      blister —see Blister, ankle
      contusion —see Contusion, ankle
      external constriction —see Constriction,
        external, ankle
      foreign body —see Foreign body,
        superficial, ankle
    anus S30.98
    arm (upper) S40.92-
      abrasion —see Abrasion, arm
      bite —see Bite, superficial, arm
      blister —see Blister, arm (upper)
      contusion —see Contusion, arm
      external constriction —see Constriction,
        external, arm
      foreign body —see Foreign body,
        superficial, arm
    auditory canal (external) (meatus) —see
      Injury, superficial, ear
    auricle —see Injury, superficial, ear
    axilla —see Injury, superficial, arm
    back —see also Injury, superficial, thorax,
      back
      lower S30.91
        abrasion S30.810
        contusion S30.0
        external constriction S30.840
        superficial
          bite NEC S30.870
            insect S30.860
          foreign body S30.850
    bite NEC —see Bite, superficial NEC, by site
    blister —see Blister, by site
    breast S20.10-
      abrasion —see Abrasion, breast
      bite —see Bite, superficial, breast
      contusion —see Contusion, breast
      external constriction —see Constriction,
        external, breast
      foreign body —see Foreign body,
        superficial, breast

Injury (Continued)
  superficial NEC (Continued)
    brow —see Injury, superficial, head,
      specified NEC
    buttock S30.91
    calf —see Injury, superficial, leg
    canthus, eye —see Injury, superficial,
      periocular area
    cheek (external) —see Injury, superficial,
      head, specified NEC
      internal —see Injury, superficial, oral
        cavity
    chest wall —see Injury, superficial, thorax
    chin —see Injury, superficial, head NEC
    clitoris S30.95
    conjunctiva —see Injury, eye, conjunctiva
      with foreign body (in conjunctival
        sac) —see Foreign body,
        conjunctival sac
    contusion —see Contusion, by site
    costal region —see Injury, superficial, thorax
    digit (s)
      hand —see Injury, superficial, finger
    ear (auricle) (canal) (external) S00.40-
      abrasion —see Abrasion, ear
      bite —see Bite, superficial, ear
      contusion —see Contusion, ear
      external constriction —see Constriction,
        external, ear
      foreign body —see Foreign body,
        superficial, ear
    elbow S50.90-
      abrasion —see Abrasion, elbow
      bite —see Bite, superficial, elbow
      blister —see Blister, elbow
      contusion —see Contusion, elbow
      external constriction —see Constriction,
        external, elbow
      foreign body —see Foreign body,
        superficial, elbow
    epididymis S30.94
    epigastric region S30.92
    epiglottis —see Injury, superficial, throat
    esophagus
      cervical —see Injury, superficial, throat
    external constriction —see Constriction,
      external, by site
    extremity NEC T14.8
    eyeball NEC —see Injury, eye, specified
      site NEC
    eyebrow —see Injury, superficial,
      periocular area
    eyelid S00.20-
      abrasion —see Abrasion, eyelid
      bite —see Bite, superficial, eyelid
      contusion —see Contusion, eyelid
      external constriction —see Constriction,
        external, eyelid
      foreign body —see Foreign body,
        superficial, eyelid
    face NEC —see Injury, superficial, head,
      specified NEC
    finger (s) S60.949
      abrasion —see Abrasion, finger
      bite —see Bite, superficial, finger
      blister —see Blister, finger
      contusion —see Contusion, finger
      external constriction —see Constriction,
        external, finger
      foreign body —see Foreign body,
        superficial, finger
      index S60.94-
      insect bite —see Bite, by site, superficial,
        insect
      little S60.94-
      middle S60.94-
      ring S60.94-
    flank S30.92
    foot S90.92-
      abrasion —see Abrasion, foot
      bite —see Bite, foot

Injury *(Continued)*
  superficial NEC *(Continued)*
    foot *(Continued)*
      blister —*see* Blister, foot
      contusion —*see* Contusion, foot
      external constriction —*see* Constriction, external, foot
      foreign body —*see* Foreign body, superficial, foot
    forearm S50.91-
      abrasion —*see* Abrasion, forearm
      bite —*see* Bite, forearm, superficial
      blister —*see* Blister, forearm
      contusion —*see* Contusion, forearm
      elbow only —*see* Injury, superficial, elbow
      external constriction —*see* Constriction, external, forearm
      foreign body —*see* Foreign body, superficial, forearm
    forehead —*see* Injury, superficial, head NEC
    foreign body —*see* Foreign body, superficial
    genital organs, external
      female S30.97
      male S30.96
    globe (eye) —*see* Injury, eye, specified site NEC
    groin S30.92
    gum —*see* Injury, superficial, oral cavity
    hand S60.92-
      abrasion —*see* Abrasion, hand
      bite —*see* Bite, superficial, hand
      contusion —*see* Contusion, hand
      external constriction —*see* Constriction, external, hand
      foreign body —*see* Foreign body, superficial, hand
    head S00.90
      ear —*see* Injury, superficial, ear
      eyelid —*see* Injury, superficial, eyelid
      nose S00.30
      oral cavity S00.502
      scalp S00.00
      specified site NEC S00.80
    heel —*see* Injury, superficial, foot
    hip S70.91-
      abrasion —*see* Abrasion, hip
      bite —*see* Bite, superficial, hip
      blister —*see* Blister, hip
      contusion —*see* Contusion, hip
      external constriction —*see* Constriction, external, hip
      foreign body —*see* Foreign body, superficial, hip
    iliac region —*see* Injury, superficial, abdomen
    inguinal region —*see* Injury, superficial, abdomen
    insect bite —*see* Bite, by site, superficial, insect
    interscapular region —*see* Injury, superficial, thorax, back
    jaw —*see* Injury, superficial, head, specified NEC
    knee S80.91-
      abrasion —*see* Abrasion, knee
      bite —*see* Bite, superficial, knee
      blister —*see* Blister, knee
      contusion —*see* Contusion, knee
      external constriction —*see* Constriction, external, knee
      foreign body —*see* Foreign body, superficial, knee
    labium (majus) (minus) S30.95
    lacrimal (apparatus) (gland) (sac) —*see* Injury, eye, specified site NEC
    larynx —*see* Injury, superficial, throat
    leg (lower) S80.92-
      abrasion —*see* Abrasion, leg
      bite —*see* Bite, superficial, leg

Injury *(Continued)*
  superficial NEC *(Continued)*
    leg *(Continued)*
      contusion —*see* Contusion, leg
      external constriction —*see* Constriction, external, leg
      foreign body —*see* Foreign body, superficial, leg
      knee —*see* Injury, superficial, knee
    limb NEC T14.8
    lip S00.501
    lower back S30.91
    lumbar region S30.91
    malar region —*see* Injury, superficial, head, specified NEC
    mammary —*see* Injury, superficial, breast
    mastoid region —*see* Injury, superficial, head, specified NEC
    mouth —*see* Injury, superficial, oral cavity
    muscle NEC T14.8
    nail NEC T14.8
      finger —*see* Injury, superficial, finger
      toe —*see* Injury, superficial, toe
    nasal (septum) —*see* Injury, superficial, nose
    neck S10.90
      specified site NEC S10.80
    nose (septum) S00.30
    occipital region —*see* Injury, superficial, scalp
    oral cavity S00.502
    orbital region —*see* Injury, superficial, periocular area
    palate —*see* Injury, superficial, oral cavity
    palm —*see* Injury, superficial, hand
    parietal region —*see* Injury, superficial, scalp
    pelvis S30.91
      girdle —*see* Injury, superficial, hip
    penis S30.93
    perineum
      female S30.95
      male S30.91
    periocular area S00.20-
      abrasion —*see* Abrasion, eyelid
      bite —*see* Bite, superficial, eyelid
      contusion —*see* Contusion, eyelid
      external constriction —*see* Constriction, external, eyelid
      foreign body —*see* Foreign body, superficial, eyelid
    phalanges
      finger —*see* Injury, superficial, finger
      toe —*see* Injury, superficial, toe
    pharynx —*see* Injury, superficial, throat
    pinna —*see* Injury, superficial, ear
    popliteal space —*see* Injury, superficial, knee
    prepuce S30.93
    pubic region S30.91
    pudendum
      female S30.97
      male S30.96
    sacral region S30.91
    scalp S00.00
    scapular region —*see* Injury, superficial, shoulder
    sclera —*see* Injury, eye, specified site NEC
    scrotum S30.94
    shin —*see* Injury, superficial, leg
    shoulder S40.91-
      abrasion —*see* Abrasion, shoulder
      bite —*see* Bite, superficial, shoulder
      blister —*see* Blister, shoulder
      contusion —*see* Contusion, shoulder
      external constriction —*see* Constriction, external, shoulder
      foreign body —*see* Foreign body, superficial, shoulder

Injury *(Continued)*
  superficial NEC *(Continued)*
    skin NEC T14.8
    sternal region —*see* Injury, superficial, thorax, front
    subconjunctival —*see* Injury, eye, specified site NEC
    subcutaneous NEC T14.8
    submaxillary region —*see* Injury, superficial, head, specified NEC
    submental region —*see* Injury, superficial, head, specified NEC
    subungual
      finger (s) —*see* Injury, superficial, finger
      toe (s) —*see* Injury, superficial, toe
    supraclavicular fossa —*see* Injury, superficial, neck
    supraorbital —*see* Injury, superficial, head, specified NEC
    temple —*see* Injury, superficial, head, specified NEC
    temporal region —*see* Injury, superficial, head, specified NEC
    testis S30.94
    thigh S70.92-
      abrasion —*see* Abrasion, thigh
      bite —*see* Bite, superficial, thigh
      blister —*see* Blister, thigh
      contusion —*see* Contusion, thigh
      external constriction —*see* Constriction, external, thigh
      foreign body —*see* Foreign body, superficial, thigh
    thorax, thoracic (wall) S20.90
      abrasion —*see* Abrasion, thorax
      back S20.40-
      bite —*see* Bite, thorax, superficial
      blister —*see* Blister, thorax
      contusion —*see* Contusion, thorax
      external constriction —*see* Constriction, external, thorax
      foreign body —*see* Foreign body, superficial, thorax
      front S20.30-
    throat S10.10
      abrasion S10.11
      bite S10.17
        insect S10.16
      blister S10.12
      contusion S10.0
      external constriction S10.14
      foreign body S10.15
    thumb S60.93-
      abrasion —*see* Abrasion, thumb
      bite —*see* Bite, superficial, thumb
      blister —*see* Blister, thumb
      contusion —*see* Contusion, thumb
      external constriction —*see* Constriction, external, thumb
      foreign body —*see* Foreign body, superficial, thumb
      insect bite —*see* Bite, by site, superficial, insect
      specified type NEC S60.39-
    toe (s) S90.93-
      abrasion —*see* Abrasion, toe
      bite —*see* Bite, toe
      blister —*see* Blister, toe
      contusion —*see* Contusion, toe
      external constriction —*see* Constriction, external, toe
      foreign body —*see* Foreign body, superficial, toe
      great S90.93-
    tongue —*see* Injury, superficial, oral cavity
    tooth, teeth —*see* Injury, superficial, oral cavity
    trachea S10.10
    tunica vaginalis S30.94
    tympanum, tympanic membrane —*see* Injury, superficial, ear

◀ New   ◀▥ Revised   ~~deleted~~ Deleted

Injury (Continued)
  superficial NEC (Continued)
    uvula —see Injury, superficial, oral cavity
    vagina S30.95
    vocal cords —see Injury, superficial, throat
    vulva S30.95
    wrist S60.91-
  supraclavicular region —see Injury, neck
  supraorbital S09.93
  suprarenal gland (multiple) —see Injury,
      adrenal
  surgical complication (external or internal
      site) —see Laceration, accidental
      complicating surgery
  temple S09.90
  temporal region S09.90
  tendon —see also Injury, muscle, by site
    abdomen —see Injury, muscle, abdomen
    Achilles —see Injury, Achilles tendon
    lower back —see Injury, muscle, lower back
    pelvic organs —see Injury, muscle, pelvis
  tenth cranial nerve (pneumogastric or
      vagus) —see Injury, nerve, vagus
  testis S39.94
  thigh S79.92-
    blood vessel —see Injury, blood vessel, hip
    contusion —see Contusion, thigh
    fracture —see Fracture, femur
    muscle —see Injury, muscle, thigh
    nerve —see Injury, nerve, thigh
    open —see Wound, open, thigh
    specified NEC S79.82-
    superficial —see Injury, superficial, thigh
  third cranial nerve (oculomotor) —see Injury,
      nerve, oculomotor
  thorax, thoracic S29.9
    blood vessel —see Injury, blood vessel,
        thorax
    cavity —see Injury, intrathoracic
    dislocation —see Dislocation, thorax
    external (wall) S29.9
      contusion —see Contusion, thorax
      nerve —see Injury, nerve, thorax
      open —see Wound, open, thorax
      specified NEC S29.8
      sprain —see Sprain, thorax
      superficial —see Injury, superficial,
          thorax
    fracture —see Fracture, thorax
    internal —see Injury, intrathoracic
    intrathoracic organ —see Injury,
        intrathoracic
    sympathetic ganglion —see Injury, nerve,
        thorax, sympathetic
  throat —see also Injury, neck S19.9
  thumb S69.9-
    blood vessel —see Injury, blood vessel,
        thumb
    contusion —see Contusion, thumb
    dislocation —see Dislocation, thumb
    fracture —see Fracture, thumb
    muscle —see Injury, muscle, thumb
    nerve —see Injury, nerve, digital, thumb
    open —see Wound, open, thumb
    specified NEC S69.8-
    sprain —see Sprain, thumb
    superficial —see Injury, superficial, thumb
  thymus (gland) —see Injury, intrathoracic,
      specified organ NEC
  thyroid (gland) NEC S19.84
  toe S99.92-
    contusion —see Contusion, toe
    dislocation —see Dislocation, toe
    fracture —see Fracture, toe
    muscle —see Injury, muscle, toe
    open —see Wound, open, toe
    specified type NEC S99.82-
    sprain —see Sprain, toe
    superficial —see Injury, superficial, toe
  tongue S09.93
  tonsil S09.93

Injury (Continued)
  tooth S09.93
  trachea (cervical) NEC S19.82
    thoracic —see Injury, intrathoracic, trachea,
        thoracic
  transfusion-related acute lung (TRALI) J95.84
  tunica vaginalis S39.94
  twelfth cranial nerve (hypoglossal) —see
      Injury, nerve, hypoglossal
  ureter S37.10
    contusion S37.12
    laceration S37.13
    specified type NEC S37.19
  urethra (sphincter) S37.30
    at delivery O71.5
    contusion S37.32
    laceration S37.33
    specified type NEC S37.38
  urinary organ S37.899
    contusion S37.92
    laceration S37.93
    specified
      site NEC S37.899
        contusion S37.892
        laceration S37.893
        specified type NEC S37.898
      type NEC S37.99
  uterus, uterine S37.60
    with ectopic or molar pregnancy O08.6
    blood vessel —see Injury, blood vessel, iliac
    contusion S37.62
    laceration S37.63
      cervix at delivery O71.3
    rupture associated with obstetrics —see
        Rupture, uterus
    specified type NEC S37.69
  uvula S09.93
  vagina S39.93
    abrasion S30.814
    bite S31.45
      insect S30.864
      superficial NEC S30.874
    contusion S30.23
    crush S38.03
    during delivery —see Laceration, vagina,
        during delivery
    external constriction S30.844
    insect bite S30.864
    laceration S31.41
      with foreign body S31.42
    open wound S31.40
    puncture S31.43
      with foreign body S31.44
    superficial S30.95
      foreign body S30.854
  vas deferens —see Injury, pelvic organ,
      specified site NEC
  vascular NEC T14.8
  vein —see Injury, blood vessel
  vena cava (superior) S25.20
    inferior S35.10
      laceration (minor) (superficial) S35.11
        major S35.12
      specified type NEC S35.19
    laceration (minor) (superficial) S25.21
      major S25.22
    specified type NEC S25.29
  vesical (sphincter) —see Injury, bladder
  visual cortex S04.04-
  vitreous (humor) S05.90
    specified NEC S05.8X-
  vocal cord NEC S19.83
  vulva S39.94
    abrasion S30.814
    bite S31.45
      insect S30.864
      superficial NEC S30.874
    contusion S30.23
    crush S38.03
    during delivery —see Laceration,
        perineum, female, during delivery

Injury (Continued)
  vulva (Continued)
    external constriction S30.844
    insect bite S30.864
    laceration S31.41
      with foreign body S31.42
    open wound S31.40
    puncture S31.43
      with foreign body S31.44
    superficial S30.95
      foreign body S30.854
  whiplash (cervical spine) S13.4
  wrist S69.9-
    blood vessel —see Injury, blood vessel,
        hand
    contusion —see Contusion, wrist
    dislocation —see Dislocation, wrist
    fracture —see Fracture, wrist
    muscle —see Injury, muscle, hand
    nerve —see Injury, nerve, hand
    open —see Wound, open, wrist
    specified NEC S69.8-
    sprain —see Sprain, wrist
    superficial —see Injury, superficial, wrist
Inoculation —see also Vaccination
  complication or reaction —see Complications,
      vaccination
Insanity, insane —see also Psychosis
  adolescent —see Schizophrenia
  confusional F28
    acute or subacute F05
  delusional F22
  senile F03
Insect
  bite —see Bite, by site, superficial, insect
  venomous, poisoning NEC (by) —see Venom,
      arthropod
Insensitivity
  adrenocorticotropin hormone (ACTH)
      E27.49
  androgen E34.50
    complete E34.51
    partial E34.52
Insertion
  cord (umbilical) lateral or velamentous
      O43.12-
  intrauterine contraceptive device (encounter
      for) —see Intrauterine contraceptive
      device
Insolation (sunstroke) T67.0
Insomnia (organic) G47.00
  without objective findings F51.02
  adjustment F51.02
  adjustment disorder F51.02
  behavioral, of childhood Z73.819
    combined type Z73.812
    limit setting type Z73.811
    sleep-onset association type Z73.810
  childhood Z73.819
  chronic F51.04
    somatized tension F51.04
  conditioned F51.04
  due to
    alcohol
      abuse F10.182
      dependence F10.282
      use F10.982
    amphetamines
      abuse F15.182
      dependence F15.282
      use F15.982
    anxiety disorder F51.05
    caffeine
      abuse F15.182
      dependence F15.282
      use F15.982
    cocaine
      abuse F14.182
      dependence F14.282
      use F14.982
    depression F51.05

Insomnia *(Continued)*
  due to *(Continued)*
    drug NEC
      abuse F19.182
      dependence F19.282
      use F19.982
    medical condition G47.01
    mental disorder NEC F51.05
    opioid
      abuse F11.182
      dependence F11.282
      use F11.982
    psychoactive substance NEC
      abuse F19.182
      dependence F19.282
      use F19.982
    sedative, hypnotic, or anxiolytic
      abuse F13.182
      dependence F13.282
      use F13.982
    stimulant NEC
      abuse F15.182
      dependence F15.282
      use F15.982
  fatal familial (FFI) A81.83
  idiopathic F51.01
  learned F51.3
  nonorganic origin F51.01
  not due to a substance or known
      physiological condition F51.01
    specified NEC F51.09
  paradoxical F51.03
  primary F51.01
  psychiatric F51.05
  psychophysiologic F51.04
  related to psychopathology F51.05
  short-term F51.02
  specified NEC G47.09
  stress-related F51.02
  transient F51.02
Inspiration
  food or foreign body —*see* Foreign body, by
    site
  mucus —*see* Asphyxia, mucus
Inspissated bile syndrome (newborn)
    P59.1
Instability
  emotional (excessive) F60.3
  joint (post-traumatic) M25.30
    ankle M25.37-
    due to old ligament injury —*see* Disorder,
      ligament
    elbow M25.32-
    flail —*see* Flail, joint
    foot M25.37-
    hand M25.34-
    hip M25.35-
    knee M25.36-
    lumbosacral —*see* subcategory M53.2
    prosthesis —*see* Complications, joint
      prosthesis, mechanical, displacement,
      by site
    sacroiliac —*see* subcategory M53.2
    secondary to
      old ligament injury —*see* Disorder,
        ligament
      removal of joint prosthesis M96.89
    shoulder (region) M25.31-
    spine —*see* subcategory M53.2
    wrist M25.33-
  knee (chronic) M23.5-
  lumbosacral —*see* subcategory M53.2
  nervous F48.8
  personality (emotional) F60.3
  spine —*see* Instability, joint, spine
  vasomotor R55
Institutional syndrome (childhood)
    F94.2
Institutionalization, affecting child
    Z62.22
  disinhibited attachment F94.2

Insufficiency, insufficient
  accommodation, old age H52.4
  adrenal (gland) E27.40
    primary E27.1
  adrenocortical E27.40
    drug-induced E27.3
    iatrogenic E27.3
    primary E27.1
  anatomic crown height K08.89 ◀
  anterior (occlusal) guidance M26.54
  anus K62.89
  aortic (valve) I35.1
    with
      mitral (valve) disease I08.0
        with tricuspid (valve) disease I08.3
      stenosis I35.2
      tricuspid (valve) disease I08.2
        with mitral (valve) disease I08.3
    congenital Q23.1
    rheumatic I06.1
      with
        mitral (valve) disease I08.0
          with tricuspid (valve) disease
            I08.3
        stenosis I06.2
          with mitral (valve) disease I08.0
            with tricuspid (valve) disease
              I08.3
        tricuspid (valve) disease I08.2
          with mitral (valve) disease I08.3
    specified cause NEC I35.1
    syphilitic A52.03
  arterial I77.1
    basilar G45.0
    carotid (hemispheric) G45.1
    cerebral I67.81
    coronary (acute or subacute) I24.8
    mesenteric K55.1
    peripheral I73.9
    precerebral (multiple) (bilateral) G45.2
    vertebral G45.0
  arteriovenous I99.8
  biliary K83.8
  cardiac —*see also* Insufficiency, myocardial
    due to presence of (cardiac) prosthesis
      I97.11-
    postprocedural I97.11-
  cardiorenal, hypertensive I13.2
  cardiovascular —*see* Disease, cardiovascular
  cerebrovascular (acute) I67.81
    with transient focal neurological signs and
      symptoms G45.8
  circulatory NEC I99.8
    newborn P29.89
  clinical crown length K08.89 ◀
  convergence H51.11
  coronary (acute or subacute) I24.8
    chronic or with a stated duration of over 4
      weeks I25.89
  corticoadrenal E27.40
    primary E27.1
  dietary E63.9
  divergence H51.8
  food T73.0
  gastroesophageal K22.8
  gonadal
    ovary E28.39
    testis E29.1
  heart —*see also* Insufficiency, myocardial
    newborn P29.0
    valve —*see* Endocarditis
  hepatic —*see* Failure, hepatic
  idiopathic autonomic G90.09
  interocclusal distance of fully erupted teeth
    (ridge) M26.36
  kidney N28.9
    acute N28.9
    chronic N18.9
  lacrimal (secretion) H04.12-
    passages —*see* Stenosis, lacrimal
  liver —*see* Failure, hepatic

Insufficiency, insufficient *(Continued)*
  lung —*see* Insufficiency, pulmonary
  mental (congenital) —*see* Disability,
    intellectual
  mesenteric K55.1
  mitral (valve) I34.0
    with
      aortic valve disease I08.0
        with tricuspid (valve) disease
          I08.3
      obstruction or stenosis I05.2
        with aortic valve disease I08.0
      tricuspid (valve) disease I08.1
        with aortic (valve) disease I08.3
    congenital Q23.3
    rheumatic I05.1
      with
        aortic valve disease I08.0
          with tricuspid (valve) disease I08.3
        obstruction or stenosis I05.2
          with aortic valve disease I08.0
            with tricuspid (valve) disease
              I08.3
        tricuspid (valve) disease I08.1
          with aortic (valve) disease I08.3
      active or acute I01.1
        with chorea, rheumatic (Sydenham's)
          I02.0
    specified cause, except rheumatic
      I34.0
  muscle —*see also* Disease, muscle
    heart —*see* Insufficiency, myocardial
    ocular NEC H50.9
  myocardial, myocardium (with
    arteriosclerosis) I50.9
    with
      rheumatic fever (conditions in I00)
        I09.0
        active, acute or subacute I01.2
          with chorea I02.0
        inactive or quiescent (with chorea)
          I09.0
    congenital Q24.8
    hypertensive —*see* Hypertension, heart
    newborn P29.0
    rheumatic I09.0
      active, acute, or subacute I01.2
    syphilitic A52.06
  nourishment T73.0
  pancreatic K86.89 ◀IIII
    exocrine K86.81 ◀
  parathyroid (gland) E20.9
  peripheral vascular (arterial) I73.9
  pituitary E23.0
  placental (mother) O36.51-
  platelets D69.6
  prenatal care affecting management of
    pregnancy O09.3-
  progressive pluriglandular E31.0
  pulmonary J98.4
    acute, following surgery (nonthoracic)
      J95.2
      thoracic J95.1
    chronic, following surgery J95.3
    following
      shock J98.4
      trauma J98.4
    newborn P28.5
    valve I37.1
      with stenosis I37.2
      congenital Q22.2
      rheumatic I09.89
        with aortic, mitral or tricuspid (valve)
          disease I08.8
  pyloric K31.89
  renal (acute) N28.9
    chronic N18.9
  respiratory R06.89
    newborn P28.5
  rotation —*see* Malrotation
  sleep syndrome F51.12

◀ New   ◀IIII Revised   ~~deleted~~ Deleted

Insufficiency, insufficient *(Continued)*
  social insurance Z59.7
  suprarenal E27.40
    primary E27.1
  tarso-orbital fascia, congenital Q10.3
  testis E29.1
  thyroid (gland) (acquired) E03.9
    congenital E03.1
  tricuspid (valve) (rheumatic) I07.1
    with
      aortic (valve) disease I08.2
        with mitral (valve) disease I08.3
      mitral (valve) disease I08.1
        with aortic (valve) disease I08.3
      obstruction or stenosis I07.2
        with aortic (valve) disease I08.2
          with mitral (valve) disease
          I08.3
    congenital Q22.8
    nonrheumatic I36.1
      with stenosis I36.2
  urethral sphincter R32
  valve, valvular (heart) —*see* Endocarditis
    congenital Q24.8
  vascular I99.8
    intestine K55.9
      acute —*see also* Ischemia, intestine, acute
        K55.059 ◀▥
    mesenteric K55.1
    peripheral I73.9
    renal —*see* Hypertension, kidney
  velopharyngeal
    acquired K13.79
    congenital Q38.8
  venous (chronic) (peripheral) I87.2
  ventricular —*see* Insufficiency, myocardial
  welfare support Z59.7
Insufflation, fallopian Z31.41
Insular —*see* condition
Insulinoma
  pancreas
    benign D13.7
    malignant C25.4
    uncertain behavior D37.8
  specified site
    benign —*see* Neoplasm, by site, benign
    malignant —*see* Neoplasm, by site,
      malignant
    uncertain behavior —*see* Neoplasm, by site,
      uncertain behavior
  unspecified site
    benign D13.7
    malignant C25.4
    uncertain behavior D37.8
Insuloma —*see* Insulinoma
Interference
  balancing side M26.56
  non-working side M26.56
Intermenstrual —*see* condition
Intermittent —*see* condition
Internal —*see* condition
Interrogation
  cardiac defibrillator (automatic) (implantable)
    Z45.02
  cardiac pacemaker Z45.018
  cardiac (event) (loop) recorder Z45.09
  infusion pump (implanted) (intrathecal)
    Z45.1
  neurostimulator Z46.2
Interruption
  aortic arch Q25.21 ◀
  phase-shift, sleep cycle —*see* Disorder, sleep,
    circadian rhythm
  sleep phase-shift, or 24 hour sleep-wake
    cycle —*see* Disorder, sleep, circadian
    rhythm
Interstitial —*see* condition
Intertrigo L30.4
  labialis K13.0
Intervertebral disc —*see* condition
Intestine, intestinal —*see* condition

Intolerance
  carbohydrate K90.49 ◀▥
  disaccharide, hereditary E73.0
  fat NEC K90.49 ◀▥
    pancreatic K90.3
  food K90.49 ◀▥
    dietary counseling and surveillance Z71.3
  fructose E74.10
    hereditary E74.12
  glucose(-galactose) E74.39
  gluten K90.01 ◀▥
  lactose E73.9
    specified NEC E73.8
  lysine E72.3
  milk NEC K90.49 ◀▥
    lactose E73.9
  protein K90.49 ◀▥
  starch NEC K90.49 ◀▥
  sucrose (-isomaltose) E74.31
Intoxicated NEC (without dependence) —*see*
  Alcohol, intoxication
Intoxication
  acid E87.2
  alcoholic (acute) (without dependence) —*see*
    Alcohol, intoxication
  alimentary canal K52.1
  amphetamine (without dependence) —
    see Abuse, drug, stimulant, with
    intoxication
    with dependence —*see* Dependence, drug,
      stimulant, with intoxication
  anxiolytic (acute) (without dependence) —*see*
    Abuse, drug, sedative, with intoxication
    with dependence —*see* Dependence, drug,
      sedative, with intoxication
  caffeine F15.929 ◀▥
    with dependence —*see* Dependence, drug,
      stimulant, with intoxication
  cannabinoids (acute) (without dependence) —
    see Use, cannabis, with intoxication ◀▥
    ~~with dependence —see Dependence, drug,~~
    ~~cannabis, with intoxication~~
    with ◀
      abuse —*see* Abuse, drug, cannabis, with
        intoxication ◀
      dependence —*see* Dependence, drug,
        cannabis, with intoxication ◀
  chemical —*see* Table of Drugs and Chemicals
    via placenta or breast milk —*see* -
      Absorption, chemical, through
      placenta
  cocaine (acute) (without dependence) —*see*
    Abuse, drug, cocaine, with intoxication
    with dependence —*see* Dependence, drug,
      cocaine, with intoxication
  drug
    acute (without dependence) —*see* Abuse,
      drug, by type with intoxication
      with dependence —*see* Dependence,
        drug, by type with intoxication
    addictive
      via placenta or breast milk —*see*
        Absorption, drug, addictive,
        through placenta
    newborn P93.8
      gray baby syndrome P93.0
    overdose or wrong substance given or
      taken —*see* Table of Drugs and
      Chemicals, by drug, poisoning
  enteric K52.1
  foodborne A05.9
    bacterial A05.9
    classical (Clostridium botulinum) A05.1
    due to
      Bacillus cereus A05.4
      bacterium A05.9
        specified NEC A05.8
      Clostridium
        botulinum A05.1
        perfringens A05.2
        welchii A05.2

Intoxication *(Continued)*
  foodborne *(Continued)*
    due to *(Continued)*
      Salmonella A02.9
        with
          (gastro) enteritis A02.0
          localized infection (s) A02.20
            arthritis A02.23
            meningitis A02.21
            osteomyelitis A02.24
            pneumonia A02.22
            pyelonephritis A02.25
            specified NEC A02.29
          sepsis A02.1
          specified manifestation NEC
            A02.8
      Staphylococcus A05.0
      Vibrio
        parahaemolyticus A05.3
        vulnificus A05.5
    enterotoxin, staphylococcal A05.0
    noxious —*see* Poisoning, food, noxious
  gastrointestinal K52.1
  hallucinogenic (without dependence) —*see*
    Abuse, drug, hallucinogen, with
    intoxication
    with dependence —*see* Dependence, drug,
      hallucinogen, with intoxication
  hypnotic (acute) (without dependence) —*see*
    Abuse, drug, sedative, with intoxication
    with dependence —*see* Dependence, drug,
      sedative, with intoxication
  inhalant (acute) (without dependence) —*see*
    Abuse, drug, inhalant, with intoxication
    with dependence —*see* Dependence, drug,
      inhalant, with intoxication
  meaning
    inebriation —*see* category F10
    poisoning —*see* Table of Drugs and
      Chemicals
  methyl alcohol (acute) (without
    dependence) —*see* Alcohol, intoxication
  opioid (acute) (without dependence) —*see*
    Abuse, drug, opioid, with intoxication
    with dependence —*see* Dependence, drug,
      opioid, with intoxication
  pathologic NEC (without dependence) —*see*
    Alcohol, intoxication
  phencyclidine (without dependence) —*see*
    Abuse, drug, hallucinogen, with
    intoxication ◀▥
    with dependence —*see* Dependence, drug,
      hallucinogen, with intoxication ◀▥
  potassium (K) E87.5
  psychoactive substance NEC (without
    dependence) —*see* Abuse, drug,
    psychoactive NEC, with intoxication
    with dependence —*see* Dependence, drug,
      psychoactive NEC, with intoxication
  sedative (acute) (without dependence) —*see*
    Abuse, drug, sedative, with intoxication
    with dependence —*see* Dependence, drug,
      sedative, with intoxication
  serum —*see also* Reaction, serum T80.69
  uremic —*see* Uremia
  volatile solvents (acute) (without
    dependence) —*see* Abuse, drug, inhalant,
    with intoxication
    with dependence —*see* Dependence, drug,
      inhalant, with intoxication
  water E87.79
Intracranial —*see* condition
Intrahepatic gallbladder Q44.1
Intraligamentous —*see* condition
Intrathoracic —*see also* condition
  kidney Q63.2
Intrauterine contraceptive device
  checking Z30.431
  in situ Z97.5
  insertion Z30.430
    immediately following removal Z30.433

Intrauterine contraceptive device *(Continued)*
  management Z30.431
  reinsertion Z30.433
  removal Z30.432
  replacement Z30.433
  retention in pregnancy O26.3-
Intraventricular —*see* condition
Intrinsic deformity —*see* Deformity
Intubation, difficult or failed T88.4
Intumescence, lens (eye) (cataract) —*see* Cataract
Intussusception (bowel) (colon) (enteric) (ileocecal)
    (ileocolic) (intestine) (rectum) K56.1
  appendix K38.8
  congenital Q43.8
  ureter (with obstruction) N13.5
Invagination (bowel, colon, intestine or rectum)
    K56.1
Inversion
  albumin-globulin (A-G) ratio E88.09
  bladder N32.89
  cecum —*see* Intussusception
  cervix N88.8
  chromosome in normal individual Q95.1
  circadian rhythm —*see* Disorder, sleep,
    circadian rhythm
  nipple N64.59
    congenital Q83.8
    gestational —*see* Retraction, nipple
    puerperal, postpartum —*see* Retraction,
      nipple
  nyctohemeral rhythm —*see* Disorder, sleep,
    circadian rhythm
  optic papilla Q14.2
  organ or site, congenital NEC —*see* Anomaly,
    by site
  sleep rhythm —*see* Disorder, sleep, circadian
    rhythm
  testis (congenital) Q55.29
  uterus (chronic) (postinfectional) (postpartal,
    old) N85.5
    postpartum O71.2
  vagina (posthysterectomy) N99.3
  ventricular Q20.5
Investigation —*see also* Examination Z04.9
  clinical research subject (control) (normal
    comparison) (participant) Z00.6
Involuntary movement, abnormal R25.9
Involution, involutional —*see also* condition
  breast, cystic —*see* Dysplasia, mammary,
    specified type NEC
  depression (single episode) F32.89 ◀▥
    recurrent episode F33.9
  melancholia (single episode) F32.89 ◀▥
    recurrent episode F33.8 ◀
  ovary, senile —*see* Atrophy, ovary
  thymus failure E32.8
I.Q.
  under 20 F73
  20-34 F72
  35-49 F71
  50-69 F70
IRDS (type I) P22.0
  type II P22.1
Irideremia Q13.1
Iridis rubeosis —*see* Disorder, iris, vascular
Iridochoroiditis (panuveitis) —*see* Panuveitis
Iridocyclitis H20.9-
  acute H20.0-
    hypopyon H20.05-
    primary H20.01-
    recurrent H20.02-
    secondary (noninfectious) H20.04-
      infectious H20.03-
  chronic H20.1-
  due to allergy —*see* Iridocyclitis, acute,
    secondary
  endogenous —*see* Iridocyclitis, acute, primary
  Fuchs' —*see* Cyclitis, Fuchs' heterochromic
  gonococcal A54.32
  granulomatous —*see* Iridocyclitis, chronic
  herpes, herpetic (simplex) B00.51
    zoster B02.32

Iridocyclitis *(Continued)*
  hypopyon —*see* Iridocyclitis, acute, hypopyon
  in (due to)
    ankylosing spondylitis M45.9
    gonococcal infection A54.32
    herpes (simplex) virus B00.51
      zoster B02.32
    infectious disease NOS B99
    parasitic disease NOS B89 *[H22]*
    sarcoidosis D86.83
    syphilis A51.43
    tuberculosis A18.54
    zoster B02.32
  lens-induced H20.2-
  nongranulomatous —*see* Iridocyclitis, acute
  recurrent —*see* Iridocyclitis, acute, recurrent
  rheumatic —*see* Iridocyclitis, chronic
  subacute —*see* Iridocyclitis, acute
  sympathetic —*see* Uveitis, sympathetic
  syphilitic (secondary) A51.43
  tuberculous (chronic) A18.54
  Vogt-Koyanagi H20.82-
Iridocyclochoroiditis (panuveitis) —*see*
    Panuveitis
Iridodialysis H21.53-
Iridodonesis H21.89
Iridoplegia (complete) (partial) (reflex) H57.09
Iridoschisis H21.25-
Iris —*see also* condition
  bombé —*see* Membrane, pupillary
Iritis —*see also* Iridocyclitis
  chronic —*see* Iridocyclitis, chronic
  diabetic —*see* E08-E13 with .39
  due to
    herpes simplex B00.51
    leprosy A30.9 *[H22]*
  gonococcal A54.32
  gouty —*see also* Gout, by type M10.9 *[H22]* ◀▥
  granulomatous —*see* Iridocyclitis, chronic
  lens induced —*see* Iridocyclitis, lens-induced
  papulosa (syphilitic) A52.71
  rheumatic —*see* Iridocyclitis, chronic
  syphilitic (secondary) A51.43
    congenital (early) A50.01
    late A52.71
  tuberculous A18.54
Iron —*see* condition
Iron-miner's lung J63.4
Irradiated enamel (tooth, teeth) K03.89
Irradiation effects, adverse T66
Irreducible, irreducibility —*see* condition
Irregular, irregularity
  action, heart I49.9
  alveolar process K08.89 ◀▥
  bleeding N92.6
  breathing R06.89
  contour of cornea (acquired) —*see* Deformity,
    cornea
    congenital Q13.4
  contour, reconstructed breast N65.0
  dentin (in pulp) K04.3
  eye movements H55.89
    nystagmus —*see* Nystagmus
    saccadic H55.81
  labor O62.2
  menstruation (cause unknown) N92.6
  periods N92.6
  prostate N42.9
  pupil —*see* Abnormality, pupillary
  reconstructed breast N65.0
  respiratory R06.89
  septum (nasal) J34.2
  shape, organ or site, congenital NEC —*see*
    Distortion
  sleep-wake pattern (rhythm) G47.23
Irritable, irritability R45.4
  bladder N32.89
  bowel (syndrome) K58.9
    with diarrhea K58.0
    with ◀
      constipation K58.1 ◀
      diarrhea K58.0 ◀

Irritable, irritability *(Continued)*
  bowel (syndrome) *(Continued)*
    mixed K58.2 ◀
    psychogenic F45.8
    specified NEC K58.8 ◀
  bronchial —*see* Bronchitis
  cerebral, in newborn P91.3
  colon —*see also* Irritable, bowel K58.9 ◀▥
    with diarrhea K58.0
    psychogenic F45.8
  duodenum K59.8
  heart (psychogenic) F45.8
  hip —*see* Derangement, joint, specified type
    NEC, hip
  ileum K59.8
  infant R68.12
  jejunum K59.8
  rectum K59.8
  stomach K31.89
    psychogenic F45.8
  sympathetic G90.8
  urethra N36.8
Irritation
  anus K62.89
  axillary nerve G54.0
  bladder N32.89
  brachial plexus G54.0
  bronchial —*see* Bronchitis
  cervical plexus G54.2
  cervix —*see* Cervicitis
  choroid, sympathetic —*see* Endophthalmitis
  cranial nerve —*see* Disorder, nerve, cranial
  gastric K31.89
    psychogenic F45.8
  globe, sympathetic —*see* Uveitis, sympathetic
  labyrinth —*see* subcategory H83.2
  lumbosacral plexus G54.1
  meninges (traumatic) —*see* Injury, intracranial
    nontraumatic —*see* Meningismus
  nerve —*see* Disorder, nerve
  nervous R45.0
  penis N48.89
  perineum NEC L29.3
  peripheral autonomic nervous system
    G90.8
  peritoneum —*see* Peritonitis
  pharynx J39.2
  plantar nerve —*see* Lesion, nerve, plantar
  spinal (cord) (traumatic) —*see also* Injury, spinal
    cord, by region
    nerve G58.9
      root NEC —*see* Radiculopathy
      nontraumatic —*see* Myelopathy
  stomach K31.89
    psychogenic F45.8
  sympathetic nerve NEC G90.8
  ulnar nerve —*see* Lesion, nerve, ulnar
  vagina N89.8
Ischemia, ischemic I99.8
  bowel (transient)
    acute —*see also* Ischemia, intestine, acute
      K55.059 ◀▥
    chronic K55.1
    due to mesenteric artery insufficiency K55.1
  brain —*see* Ischemia, cerebral
  cardiac (*see* Disease, heart, ischemic)
  cardiomyopathy I25.5
  cerebral (chronic) (generalized) I67.82
    arteriosclerotic I67.2
    intermittent G45.9
    newborn P91.0
    recurrent focal G45.8
    transient G45.9
  colon chronic (due to mesenteric artery
    insufficiency) K55.1
  coronary —*see* Disease, heart, ischemic
  demand (coronary) —*see also* Angina I24.8
  heart (chronic or with a stated duration of over
    4 weeks) I25.9
    acute or with a stated duration of 4 weeks or
      less I24.9
    subacute I24.9

◀ New   ◀▥ Revised   ~~deleted~~ Deleted

Ischemia, ischemic (Continued)
  infarction, muscle —see Infarct, muscle
  intestine (large) (small) (transient) K55.9
    acute K55.059 ◀▥
      diffuse K55.052 ◀
      focal K55.051 ◀
      large K55.039 ◀
        diffuse K55.032 ◀
        focal K55.031 ◀
      small K55.019 ◀
        diffuse K55.012 ◀
        focal K55.011 ◀
    chronic K55.1
    due to mesenteric artery insufficiency
        K55.1
  kidney N28.0
  mesenteric, acute —see also Ischemia, intestine,
      acute K55.059 ◀▥
  muscle, traumatic T79.6
  myocardium, myocardial (chronic or with a
      stated duration of over 4 weeks) I25.9
    acute, without myocardial infarction
        I51.3 ◀▥
    silent (asymptomatic) I25.6
    transient of newborn P29.4
  renal N28.0
  retina, retinal —see Occlusion, artery, retina
  small bowel
    acute K55.019 ◀▥
      diffuse K55.012 ◀
      focal K55.011 ◀
    chronic K55.1
    due to mesenteric artery insufficiency K55.1
  spinal cord G95.11
  subendocardial —see Insufficiency, coronary
  supply (coronary) —see also Angina I25.9
    due to vasospasm I20.1
Ischial spine —see condition
Ischialgia —see Sciatica
Ischiopagus Q89.4
Ischium, ischial —see condition
Ischuria R34

Iselin's disease or osteochondrosis —see
    Osteochondrosis, juvenile, metatarsus
Islands of
  parotid tissue in
    lymph nodes Q38.6
    neck structures Q38.6
  submaxillary glands in
    fascia Q38.6
    lymph nodes Q38.6
    neck muscles Q38.6
Islet cell tumor, pancreas D13.7
Isoimmunization NEC —see also Incompatibility
  affecting management of pregnancy (ABO)
      (with hydrops fetalis) O36.11-
    anti-A sensitization O36.11-
    anti-B sensitization O36.19-
    anti-c sensitization O36.09-
    anti-C sensitization O36.09-
    anti-e sensitization O36.09-
    anti-E sensitization O36.09-
    Rh NEC O36.09-
      anti-D antibody O36.01-
    specified NEC O36.19-
  newborn P55.9
    with
      hydrops fetalis P56.0
      kernicterus P57.0
    ABO (blood groups) P55.1
    Rhesus (Rh) factor P55.0
    specified type NEC P55.8
Isolation, isolated
  dwelling Z59.8
  family Z63.79
  social Z60.4
Isoleucinosis E71.19
Isomerism atrial appendages (with asplenia or
    polysplenia) Q20.6
Isosporiasis, isosporosis A07.3
Isovaleric acidemia E71.110
Issue of
  medical certificate Z02.79
    for disability determination Z02.71

Issue of (Continued)
  repeat prescription (appliance) (glasses)
      (medicinal substance, medicament,
      medicine) Z76.0
    contraception —see Contraception
Itch, itching —see also Pruritus
  baker's L23.6
  barber's B35.0
  bricklayer's L24.5
  cheese B88.0
  clam digger's B65.3
  coolie B76.9
  copra B88.0
  dew B76.9
  dhobi B35.6
  filarial —see Infestation, filarial
  grain B88.0
  grocer's B88.0
  ground B76.9
  harvest B88.0
  jock B35.6
  Malabar B35.5
    beard B35.0
    foot B35.3
    scalp B35.0
  meaning scabies B86
  Norwegian B86
  perianal L29.0
  poultrymen's B88.0
  sarcoptic B86
  scabies B86
  scrub B88.0
  straw B88.0
  swimmer's B65.3
  water B76.9
  winter L29.8
Ivemark's syndrome (asplenia with congenital
    heart disease) Q89.01
Ivory bones Q78.2
Ixodiasis NEC B88.8

J

Jaccoud's syndrome —*see* Arthropathy, postrheumatic, chronic
Jackson's
  membrane Q43.3
  paralysis or syndrome G83.89
  veil Q43.3
Jacquet's dermatitis (diaper dermatitis) L22
Jadassohn-Pellizari's disease or anetoderma L90.2
Jadassohn's
  blue nevus —*see* Nevus
  intraepidermal epithelioma —*see* Neoplasm, skin, benign
Jaffe-Lichtenstein (-Uehlinger) syndrome —*see* Dysplasia, fibrous, bone NEC
Jakob-Creutzfeldt disease or syndrome —*see* Creutzfeldt-Jakob disease or syndrome
Jaksch-Luzet disease D64.89
Jamaican
  neuropathy G92
  paraplegic tropical ataxic-spastic syndrome G92
Janet's disease F48.8
Janiceps Q89.4
Jansky-Bielschowsky amaurotic idiocy E75.4
Japanese
  B-type encephalitis A83.0
  river fever A75.3
Jaundice (yellow) R17
  acholuric (familial) (splenomegalic) —*see also* Spherocytosis
    acquired D59.8
  breast-milk (inhibitor) P59.3
  catarrhal (acute) B15.9
    with hepatic coma B15.0
  cholestatic (benign) R17
  due to or associated with
    delayed conjugation P59.8
      associated with (due to) preterm delivery P59.0
    preterm delivery P59.0
  epidemic (catarrhal) B15.9
    with hepatic coma B15.0
    leptospiral A27.0
    spirochetal A27.0
  familial nonhemolytic (congenital) (Gilbert) E80.4
    Crigler-Najjar E80.5
  febrile (acute) B15.9
    with hepatic coma B15.0
    leptospiral A27.0
    spirochetal A27.0
  hematogenous D59.9
  hemolytic (acquired) D59.9
    congenital —*see* Spherocytosis

Jaundice (*Continued*)
  hemorrhagic (acute) (leptospiral) (spirochetal) A27.0
  infectious (acute) (subacute) B15.9
    with hepatic coma B15.0
    leptospiral A27.0
    spirochetal A27.0
  leptospiral (hemorrhagic) A27.0
  malignant (without coma) K72.90
    with coma K72.91
  neonatal —*see* Jaundice, newborn
  newborn P59.9
    due to or associated with
      ABO
        antibodies P55.1
        incompatibility, maternal/fetal P55.1
        isoimmunization P55.1
      absence or deficiency of enzyme system for bilirubin conjugation (congenital) P59.8
      bleeding P58.1
      breast milk inhibitors to conjugation P59.3
        associated with preterm delivery P59.0
      bruising P58.0
      Crigler-Najjar syndrome E80.5
      delayed conjugation P59.8
        associated with preterm delivery P59.0
      drugs or toxins
        given to newborn P58.42
        transmitted from mother P58.41
      excessive hemolysis P58.9
        due to
          bleeding P58.1
          bruising P58.0
          drugs or toxins
            given to newborn P58.42
            transmitted from mother P58.41
          infection P58.2
          polycythemia P58.3
          swallowed maternal blood P58.5
        specified type NEC P58.8
      galactosemia E74.21
      Gilbert syndrome E80.4
      hemolytic disease P55.9
        ABO isoimmunization P55.1
        Rh isoimmunization P55.0
        specified NEC P55.8
      hepatocellular damage P59.20
        specified NEC P59.29
      hereditary hemolytic anemia P58.8
      hypothyroidism, congenital E03.1
      incompatibility, maternal/fetal NOS P55.9
      infection P58.2

Jaundice (*Continued*)
  newborn (*Continued*)
    due to or associated with (*Continued*)
      inspissated bile syndrome P59.1
      isoimmunization NOS P55.9
      mucoviscidosis E84.9
      polycythemia P58.3
      preterm delivery P59.0
      Rh
        antibodies P55.0
        incompatibility, maternal/fetal P55.0
        isoimmunization P55.0
      specified cause NEC P59.8
      swallowed maternal blood P58.5
      spherocytosis (congenital) D58.0
    nonhemolytic congenital familial (Gilbert) E80.4
    nuclear, newborn —*see also* Kernicterus of newborn P57.9
    obstructive —*see also* Obstruction, bile duct K83.1
    post-immunization —*see* Hepatitis, viral, type, B
    post-transfusion —*see* Hepatitis, viral, type, B
    regurgitation —*see also* Obstruction, bile duct K83.1
    serum (homologous) (prophylactic) (therapeutic) —*see* Hepatitis, viral, type, B
    spirochetal (hemorrhagic) A27.0
    symptomatic R17
      newborn P59.9
Jaw —*see* condition
Jaw-winking phenomenon or syndrome Q07.8
Jealousy
  alcoholic F10.988
  childhood F93.8
  sibling F93.8
Jejunitis —*see* Enteritis
Jejunostomy status Z93.4
Jejunum, jejunal —*see* condition
Jensen's disease —*see* Inflammation, chorioretinal, focal, juxtapapillary
Jerks, myoclonic G25.3
Jervell-Lange-Nielsen syndrome I45.81
Jeune's disease Q77.2
Jigger disease B88.1
Job's syndrome (chronic granulomatous disease) D71
Joint —*see also* condition
  mice —*see* Loose, body, joint
    knee M23.4-
Jordan's anomaly or syndrome D72.0
Joseph-Diamond-Blackfan anemia (congenital hypoplastic) D61.01
Jungle yellow fever A95.0
Jüngling's disease —*see* Sarcoidosis
Juvenile —*see* condition

◀ New   ◀▦ Revised   ~~deleted~~ Deleted

K

Kahler's disease C90.0-
Kakke E51.11
Kala-azar B55.0
Kallmann's syndrome E23.0
Kanner's syndrome (autism) —*see* Psychosis, childhood
Kaposi's
  dermatosis (xeroderma pigmentosum) Q82.1
  lichen ruber L44.0
    acuminatus L44.0
  sarcoma
    colon C46.4
    connective tissue C46.1
    gastrointestinal organ C46.4
    lung C46.5-
    lymph node (multiple) C46.3
    palate (hard) (soft) C46.2
    rectum C46.4
    skin (multiple sites) C46.0
    specified site NEC C46.7
    stomach C46.4
    unspecified site C46.9
  varicelliform eruption B00.0
  vaccinia T88.1
Kartagener's syndrome or triad (sinusitis, bronchiectasis, situs inversus) Q89.3
Karyotype
  with abnormality except iso (Xq) Q96.2
  45,X Q96.0
  46,X
    iso (Xq) Q96.1
  46,XX Q98.3
    with streak gonads Q50.32
    hermaphrodite (true) Q99.1
    male Q98.3
  46,XY
    with streak gonads Q56.1
    female Q97.3
    hermaphrodite (true) Q99.1
  47,XXX Q97.0
  47,XXY Q98.0
  47,XYY Q98.5
Kaschin-Beck disease —*see* Disease, Kaschin-Beck
Katayama's disease or fever B65.2
Kawasaki's syndrome M30.3
Kayser-Fleischer ring (cornea) (pseudosclerosis) H18.04-
Kaznelson's syndrome (congenital hypoplastic anemia) D61.01
Kearns-Sayre syndrome H49.81-
Kedani fever A75.3
Kelis L91.0
Kelly (-Patterson) syndrome (sideropenic dysphagia) D50.1
Keloid, cheloid L91.0
  acne L73.0
  Addison's L94.0
  cornea —*see* Opacity, cornea
  Hawkin's L91.0
  scar L91.0
Keloma L91.0
Kenya fever A77.1
Keratectasia —*see also* Ectasia, cornea
  congenital Q13.4
Keratinization of alveolar ridge mucosa
  excessive K13.23
  minimal K13.22
Keratinized residual ridge mucosa
  excessive K13.23
  minimal K13.22
Keratitis (nodular) (nonulcerative) (simple) (zonular) H16.9
  with ulceration (central) (marginal) (perforated) (ring) —*see* Ulcer, cornea
  actinic —*see* Photokeratitis
  arborescens (herpes simplex) B00.52
  areolar H16.11-
  bullosa H16.8

Keratitis (Continued)
  deep H16.309
    specified type NEC H16.399
  dendritic (a) (herpes simplex) B00.52
  disciform (is) (herpes simplex) B00.52
    varicella B01.81
  filamentary H16.12-
  gonococcal (congenital or prenatal) A54.33
  herpes, herpetic (simplex) B00.52
    zoster B02.33
  in (due to)
    acanthamebiasis B60.13
    adenovirus B30.0
    exanthema —*see also* Exanthem B09
    herpes (simplex) virus B00.52
    measles B05.81
    syphilis A50.31
    tuberculosis A18.52
    zoster B02.33
  interstitial (nonsyphilitic) H16.30-
    diffuse H16.32-
    herpes, herpetic (simplex) B00.52
      zoster B02.33
    sclerosing H16.33-
    specified type NEC H16.39-
    syphilitic (congenital) (late) A50.31
    tuberculous A18.52
  macular H16.11-
  nummular H16.11-
  oyster shuckers' H16.8
  parenchymatous —*see* Keratitis, interstitial
  petrificans H16.8
  postmeasles B05.81
  punctata
    leprosa A30.9 [H16.14-]
    syphilitic (profunda) A50.31
  punctate H16.14-
  purulent H16.8
  rosacea L71.8
  sclerosing H16.33-
  specified type NEC H16.8
  stellate H16.11-
  striate H16.11-
  superficial H16.10-
    with conjunctivitis —*see* Keratoconjunctivitis
    due to light —*see* Photokeratitis
  suppurative H16.8
  syphilitic (congenital) (prenatal) A50.31
  trachomatous A71.1
    sequelae B94.0
  tuberculous A18.52
  vesicular H16.8
  xerotic —*see also* Keratomalacia H16.8
    vitamin A deficiency E50.4
Keratoacanthoma L85.8
Keratocele —*see* Descemetocele
Keratoconjunctivitis H16.20-
  Acanthamoeba B60.13
  adenoviral B30.0
  epidemic B30.0
  exposure H16.21-
  herpes, herpetic (simplex) B00.52
    zoster B02.33
  in exanthema —*see also* Exanthem B09
  infectious B30.0
  lagophthalmic —*see* Keratoconjunctivitis, specified type NEC
  neurotrophic H16.23-
  phlyctenular H16.25-
  postmeasles B05.81
  shipyard B30.0
  sicca (Sjogren's) M35.0-
    not Sjogren's H16.22-
  specified type NEC H16.29-
  tuberculous (phlyctenular) A18.52
  vernal H16.26-
Keratoconus H18.60-
  congenital Q13.4
  stable H18.61-
  unstable H18.62-

Keratocyst (dental) (odontogenic) —*see* Cyst, calcifying odontogenic
Keratoderma, keratodermia (congenital) (palmaris et plantaris) (symmetrical) Q82.8
  acquired L85.1
    in diseases classified elsewhere L86
  climactericum L85.1
  gonococcal A54.89
  gonorrheal A54.89
  punctata L85.2
  Reiter's —*see* Reiter's disease
Keratodermatocele —*see* Descemetocele
Keratoglobus H18.79
  congenital Q15.8
    with glaucoma Q15.0
Keratohemia —*see* Pigmentation, cornea, stromal
Keratoiritis —*see also* Iridocyclitis
  syphilitic A50.39
  tuberculous A18.54
Keratoma L57.0
  palmaris and plantaris hereditarium Q82.8
  senile L57.0
Keratomalacia H18.44-
  vitamin A deficiency E50.4
Keratomegaly Q13.4
Keratomycosis B49
  nigrans, nigricans (palmaris) B36.1
Keratopathy H18.9
  band H18.42-
  bullous H18.1-
  bullous (aphakic), following cataract surgery H59.01-
Keratoscleritis, tuberculous A18.52
Keratosis L57.0
  actinic L57.0
  arsenical L85.8
  congenital, specified NEC Q80.8
  female genital NEC N94.89
  follicularis Q82.8
    acquired L11.0
    congenita Q82.8
    et parafollicularis in cutem penetrans L87.0
    spinulosa (decalvans) Q82.8
    vitamin A deficiency E50.8
  gonococcal A54.89
  male genital (external) N50.89
  nigricans L83
  obturans, external ear (canal) —*see* Cholesteatoma, external ear
  palmaris et plantaris (inherited) (symmetrical) Q82.8
    acquired L85.1
  penile N48.89
  pharynx J39.2
  pilaris, acquired L85.8
  punctata (palmaris et plantaris) L85.2
  scrotal N50.89
  seborrheic L82.1
    inflamed L82.0
  senile L57.0
  solar L57.0
  tonsillaris J35.8
  vagina N89.4
  vegetans Q82.8
  vitamin A deficiency E50.8
  vocal cord J38.3
Kerato-uveitis —*see* Iridocyclitis
Kerion (celsi) B35.0
Kernicterus of newborn (not due to isoimmunization) P57.9
  due to isoimmunization (conditions in P55.0-P55.9) P57.0
  specified type NEC P57.8
Kerunoparalysis T75.09
Keshan disease E59
Ketoacidosis E87.2
  diabetic —*see* Diabetes, by type, with ketoacidosis
Ketonuria R82.4

Ketosis NEC E88.89
   diabetic —*see* Diabetes, by type, with
      ketoacidosis
Kew Garden fever A79.1
Kidney —*see* condition
Kienböck's disease —*see also* Osteochondrosis,
   juvenile, hand, carpal lunate
   adult M93.1
Kimmelstiel (-Wilson) disease —*see* Diabetes,
   Kimmelstiel (-Wilson) disease
Kimura disease D21.9
   specified site (see Neoplasm, connective
      tissue benign)
Kink, kinking
   artery I77.1
   hair (acquired) L67.8
   ileum or intestine —*see* Obstruction,
      intestine
   Lane's —*see* Obstruction, intestine
   organ or site, congenital NEC —*see* Anomaly,
      by site
   ureter (pelvic junction) N13.5
      with
         hydronephrosis N13.1
            with infection N13.6
         pyelonephritis (chronic) N11.1
      congenital Q62.39
   vein (s) I87.8
      caval I87.1
      peripheral I87.1
Kinnier Wilson's disease (hepatolenticular
   degeneration) E83.01
Kissing spine M48.20
   cervical region M48.22
   cervicothoracic region M48.23
   lumbar region M48.26
   lumbosacral region M48.27
   occipito-atlanto-axial region M48.21
   thoracic region M48.24
   thoracolumbar region M48.25
Klatskin's tumor C24.0
Klauder's disease A26.8
Klebs' disease —*see also* Glomerulonephritis
   N05.-
Klebsiella (K.) pneumoniae, as cause of
   disease classified elsewhere B96.1
Klein (e)-Levin syndrome G47.13
Kleptomania F63.2
Klinefelter's syndrome Q98.4
   karyotype 47,XXY Q98.0
   male with more than two X chromosomes
      Q98.1
Klippel-Feil deficiency, disease, or syndrome
   (brevicollis) Q76.1
Klippel's disease I67.2
Klippel-Trenaunay (-Weber) syndrome
   Q87.2
Klumpke (-Déjerine) palsy, paralysis (birth)
   (newborn) P14.1
Knee —*see* condition
Knock knee (acquired) M21.06-
   congenital Q74.1

Knot (s)
   intestinal, syndrome (volvulus) K56.2
   surfer S89.8-
   umbilical cord (true) O69.2
Knotting (of)
   hair L67.8
   intestine K56.2
Knuckle pad (Garrod's) M72.1
Koch's
   infection —*see* Tuberculosis
   relapsing fever A68.9
Koch-Weeks' conjunctivitis —*see*
   Conjunctivitis, acute, mucopurulent
Köebner's syndrome Q81.8
Köenig's disease (osteochondritis dissecans) —
   see Osteochondritis, dissecans
Köhler-Pellegrini-Steida disease or syndrome
   (calcification, knee joint) —*see* Bursitis,
   tibial collateral
Köhler's disease
   patellar —*see* Osteochondrosis, juvenile,
      patella
   tarsal navicular —*see* Osteochondrosis,
      juvenile, tarsus
Koilonychia L60.3
   congenital Q84.6
Kojevnikov's, epilepsy —*see* Kozhevnikof's
   epilepsy
Koplik's spots B05.9
Kopp's asthma E32.8
Korsakoff's (Wernicke) disease, psychosis or
   syndrome (alcoholic) F10.96
   with dependence F10.26
   drug-induced
      due to drug abuse —*see* Abuse, drug, by
         type, with amnestic disorder
      due to drug dependence —*see* Dependence,
         drug, by type, with amnestic disorder
   nonalcoholic F04
Korsakov's disease, psychosis or syndrome —
   see Korsakoff's disease
Korsakow's disease, psychosis or syndrome —
   see Korsakoff's disease
Kostmann's disease or syndrome (infantile
   genetic agranulocytosis) —*see*
   Agranulocytosis
Kozhevnikof's epilepsy G40.109
   intractable G40.119
      with status epilepticus G40.111
      without status epilepticus G40.119
   not intractable G40.109
      with status epilepticus G40.101
      without status epilepticus G40.109
Krabbe's
   disease E75.23
   syndrome, congenital muscle hypoplasia
      Q79.8
Kraepelin-Morel disease —*see* Schizophrenia
Kraft-Weber-Dimitri disease Q85.8
Kraurosis
   ani K62.89
   penis N48.0

Kraurosis (*Continued*)
   vagina N89.8
   vulva N90.4
Kreotoxism A05.9
Krukenberg's
   spindle —*see* Pigmentation, cornea, posterior
   tumor C79.6-
Kufs' disease E75.4
Kugelberg-Welander disease G12.1
Kuhnt-Junius degeneration —*see also*
   Degeneration, macula H35.32- ◄▥
Kümmell's disease or spondylitis —*see*
   Spondylopathy, traumatic
Kupffer cell sarcoma C22.3
Kuru A81.81
Kussmaul's
   disease M30.0
   respiration E87.2
      in diabetic acidosis —*see* Diabetes, by type,
         with ketoacidosis
Kwashiorkor E40
   marasmic, marasmus type E42
Kyasanur Forest disease A98.2
Kyphoscoliosis, kyphoscoliotic (acquired) —
   see also Scoliosis M41.9
   congenital Q67.5
   heart (disease) I27.1
   sequelae of rickets E64.3
   tuberculous A18.01
Kyphosis, kyphotic (acquired) M40.209
   cervical region M40.202
   cervicothoracic region M40.203
   congenital Q76.419
      cervical region Q76.412
      cervicothoracic region Q76.413
      occipito-atlanto-axial region Q76.411
      thoracic region Q76.414
      thoracolumbar region Q76.415
   Morquio-Brailsford type (spinal) —*see also*
      subcategory M49.8 E76.219
   postlaminectomy M96.3
   postradiation therapy M96.2
   postural (adolescent) M40.00
      cervicothoracic region M40.03
      thoracic region M40.04
      thoracolumbar region M40.05
   secondary NEC M40.10
      cervical region M40.12
      cervicothoracic region M40.13
      thoracic region M40.14
      thoracolumbar region M40.15
   sequelae of rickets E64.3
   specified type NEC M40.299
      cervical region M40.292
      cervicothoracic region M40.293
      thoracic region M40.294
      thoracolumbar region M40.295
   syphilitic, congenital A50.56
   thoracic region M40.204
   thoracolumbar region M40.205
   tuberculous A18.01
Kyrle disease L87.0

◄ New   ◄▥ Revised   ~~deleted~~ Deleted

L

Labia, labium —*see* condition
Labile
　blood pressure R09.89
　vasomotor system I73.9
Labioglossal paralysis G12.29
Labium leporinum —*see* Cleft, lip
Labor —*see* Delivery
Labored breathing —*see* Hyperventilation
Labyrinthitis (circumscribed) (destructive)
　　(diffuse) (inner ear) (latent) (purulent)
　　(suppurative) (*see also* subcategory)
　　H83.0
　syphilitic A52.79
Laceration
　with abortion —*see* Abortion, by type,
　　　complicated by laceration of pelvic
　　　organs
　abdomen, abdominal
　　wall S31.119
　　　with
　　　　foreign body S31.129
　　　　penetration into peritoneal cavity
　　　　　S31.619
　　　　　with foreign body S31.629
　　　epigastric region S31.112
　　　　with
　　　　　foreign body S31.122
　　　　　penetration into peritoneal cavity
　　　　　　S31.612
　　　　　　with foreign body S31.622
　　　left
　　　　lower quadrant S31.114
　　　　　with
　　　　　　foreign body S31.124
　　　　　　penetration into peritoneal cavity
　　　　　　　S31.614
　　　　　　　with foreign body S31.624
　　　　upper quadrant S31.111
　　　　　with
　　　　　　foreign body S31.121
　　　　　　penetration into peritoneal cavity
　　　　　　　S31.611
　　　　　　　with foreign body S31.621
　　　periumbilic region S31.115
　　　　with
　　　　　foreign body S31.125
　　　　　penetration into peritoneal cavity
　　　　　　S31.615
　　　　　　with foreign body S31.625
　　　right
　　　　lower quadrant S31.113
　　　　　with
　　　　　　foreign body S31.123
　　　　　　penetration into peritoneal cavity
　　　　　　　S31.613
　　　　　　　with foreign body S31.623
　　　　upper quadrant S31.110
　　　　　with
　　　　　　foreign body S31.120
　　　　　　penetration into peritoneal cavity
　　　　　　　S31.610
　　　　　　　with foreign body S31.620
　accidental, complicating surgery —*see*
　　　Complications, surgical, accidental
　　　puncture or laceration
　Achilles tendon S86.02-
　adrenal gland S37.813
　alveolar (process) —*see* Laceration, oral cavity
　ankle S91.01-
　　with
　　　foreign body S91.02-
　antecubital space —*see* Laceration, elbow
　anus (sphincter) S31.831
　　with
　　　ectopic or molar pregnancy O08.6
　　　foreign body S31.832
　　complicating delivery —*see* Delivery,
　　　complicated, by, laceration, anus
　　　(sphincter)

Laceration *(Continued)*
　anus *(Continued)*
　　following ectopic or molar pregnancy
　　　O08.6
　　nontraumatic, nonpuerperal —*see* Fissure,
　　　anus
　arm (upper) S41.11-
　　with foreign body S41.12-
　　lower —*see* Laceration, forearm
　auditory canal (external) (meatus) —*see*
　　　Laceration, ear
　auricle, ear —*see* Laceration, ear
　axilla —*see* Laceration, arm
　back —*see also* Laceration, thorax, back
　　lower S31.010
　　　with
　　　　foreign body S31.020
　　　　　with penetration into
　　　　　　retroperitoneal space S31.021
　　　　penetration into retroperitoneal space
　　　　　S31.011
　bile duct S36.13
　bladder S37.23
　　with ectopic or molar pregnancy O08.6
　　following ectopic or molar pregnancy
　　　O08.6
　　obstetrical trauma O71.5
　blood vessel —*see* Injury, blood vessel
　bowel —*see also* Laceration, intestine
　　with ectopic or molar pregnancy O08.6
　　complicating abortion —*see* Abortion,
　　　by type, complicated by, specified
　　　condition NEC
　　following ectopic or molar pregnancy
　　　O08.6
　　obstetrical trauma O71.5
　brain (any part) (cortex) (diffuse)
　　　(membrane) —*see also* Injury,
　　　intracranial, diffuse
　　during birth P10.8
　　　with hemorrhage P10.1
　　focal —*see* Injury, intracranial, focal brain
　　　injury
　brainstem S06.38-
　breast S21.01-
　　with foreign body S21.02-
　broad ligament S37.893
　　with ectopic or molar pregnancy O08.6
　　following ectopic or molar pregnancy
　　　O08.6
　　laceration syndrome N83.8
　　obstetrical trauma O71.6
　　syndrome (laceration) N83.8
　buttock S31.801
　　with foreign body S31.802
　　left S31.821
　　　with foreign body S31.822
　　right S31.811
　　　with foreign body S31.812
　calf —*see* Laceration, leg
　canaliculus lacrimalis —*see* Laceration,
　　　eyelid
　canthus, eye —*see* Laceration, eyelid
　capsule, joint —*see* Sprain
　causing eversion of cervix uteri (old) N86
　central (perineal), complicating delivery
　　　O70.9
　cerebellum, traumatic S06.37-
　cerebral S06.33-
　　during birth P10.8
　　　with hemorrhage P10.1
　　left side S06.32-
　　right side S06.31-
　cervix (uteri)
　　with ectopic or molar pregnancy O08.6
　　following ectopic or molar pregnancy
　　　O08.6
　　nonpuerperal, nontraumatic N88.1
　　obstetrical trauma (current) O71.3
　　old (postpartal) N88.1
　　traumatic S37.63

Laceration *(Continued)*
　cheek (external) S01.41-
　　with foreign body S01.42-
　　internal —*see* Laceration, oral cavity
　chest wall —*see* Laceration, thorax
　chin —*see* Laceration, head, specified site
　　　NEC
　chordae tendinae NEC I51.1
　　concurrent with acute myocardial
　　　infarction —*see* Infarct, myocardium
　　following acute myocardial infarction
　　　(current complication) I23.4
　clitoris —*see* Laceration, vulva
　colon —*see* Laceration, intestine, large,
　　　colon
　common bile duct S36.13
　cortex (cerebral) —*see* Injury, intracranial,
　　　diffuse
　costal region —*see* Laceration, thorax
　cystic duct S36.13
　diaphragm S27.803
　digit (s)
　　foot —*see* Laceration, toe
　　hand —*see* Laceration, finger
　duodenum S36.430
　ear (canal) (external) S01.31-
　　with foreign body S01.32-
　　drum S09.2-
　elbow S51.01-
　　with
　　　foreign body S51.02-
　epididymis —*see* Laceration, testis
　epigastric region —*see* Laceration, abdomen,
　　　wall, epigastric region
　esophagus K22.8
　　traumatic
　　　cervical S11.21
　　　　with foreign body S11.22
　　　thoracic S27.813
　eye (ball) S05.3-
　　with prolapse or loss of intraocular tissue
　　　S05.2-
　　penetrating S05.6-
　eyebrow —*see* Laceration, eyelid
　eyelid S01.11-
　　with foreign body S01.12-
　face NEC —*see* Laceration, head, specified
　　　site NEC
　fallopian tube S37.539
　　bilateral S37.532
　　unilateral S37.531
　finger (s) S61.219
　　with
　　　damage to nail S61.319
　　　　with
　　　　　foreign body S61.329
　　　foreign body S61.229
　　index S61.218
　　　with
　　　　damage to nail S61.318
　　　　　with
　　　　　　foreign body S61.328
　　　　foreign body S61.228
　　　left S61.211
　　　　with
　　　　　damage to nail S61.311
　　　　　　with
　　　　　　　foreign body S61.321
　　　　　foreign body S61.221
　　　right S61.210
　　　　with
　　　　　damage to nail S61.310
　　　　　　with
　　　　　　　foreign body S61.320
　　　　　foreign body S61.220
　　little S61.218
　　　with
　　　　damage to nail S61.318
　　　　　with
　　　　　　foreign body S61.328
　　　　foreign body S61.228

Laceration *(Continued)*
  finger *(Continued)*
    little *(Continued)*
      left S61.217
        with
          damage to nail S61.317
            with
              foreign body S61.327
          foreign body S61.227
      right S61.216
        with
          damage to nail S61.316
            with
              foreign body S61.326
          foreign body S61.226
    middle S61.218
      with
        damage to nail S61.318
          with
            foreign body S61.328
        foreign body S61.228
      left S61.213
        with
          damage to nail S61.313
            with
              foreign body S61.323
          foreign body S61.223
      right S61.212
        with
          damage to nail S61.312
            with
              foreign body S61.322
          foreign body S61.222
    ring S61.218
      with
        damage to nail S61.318
          with
            foreign body S61.328
        foreign body S61.228
      left S61.215
        with
          damage to nail S61.315
            with
              foreign body S61.325
          foreign body S61.225
      right S61.214
        with
          damage to nail S61.314
            with
              foreign body S61.324
          foreign body S61.224
  flank S31.119
    with foreign body S31.129
  foot (except toe (s) alone) S91.319
    with foreign body S91.329
    left S91.312
      with foreign body S91.322
    right S91.311
      with foreign body S91.321
    toe —*see* Laceration, toe
  forearm S51.819
    with
      foreign body S51.829
    elbow only —*see* Laceration, elbow
    left S51.812
      with
        foreign body S51.822
    right S51.811
      with
        foreign body S51.821
  forehead S01.81
    with foreign body S01.82
  fourchette O70.0
    with ectopic or molar pregnancy O08.6
    complicating delivery O70.0
    following ectopic or molar pregnancy O08.6
  gallbladder S36.123

Laceration *(Continued)*
  genital organs, external
    female S31.512
      with foreign body S31.522
      vagina —*see* Laceration, vagina
      vulva —*see* Laceration, vulva
    male S31.511
      with foreign body S31.521
      penis —*see* Laceration, penis
      scrotum —*see* Laceration, scrotum
      testis —*see* Laceration, testis
  groin —*see* Laceration, abdomen, wall
  gum —*see* Laceration, oral cavity
  hand S61.419
    with
      foreign body S61.429
    finger —*see* Laceration, finger
    left S61.412
      with
        foreign body S61.422
    right S61.411
      with
        foreign body S61.421
    thumb —*see* Laceration, thumb
  head S01.91
    with foreign body S01.92
    cheek —*see* Laceration, cheek
    ear —*see* Laceration, ear
    eyelid —*see* Laceration, eyelid
    lip —*see* Laceration, lip
    nose —*see* Laceration, nose
    oral cavity —*see* Laceration, oral cavity
    scalp S01.01
      with foreign body S01.02
    specified site NEC S01.81
      with foreign body S01.82
    temporomandibular area —*see* Laceration, cheek
  heart —*see* Injury, heart, laceration
  heel —*see* Laceration, foot
  hepatic duct S36.13
  hip S71.019
    with foreign body S71.029
    left S71.012
      with foreign body S71.022
    right S71.011
      with foreign body S71.021
  hymen —*see* Laceration, vagina
  hypochondrium —*see* Laceration, abdomen, wall
  hypogastric region —*see* Laceration, abdomen, wall
  ileum S36.438
  inguinal region —*see* Laceration, abdomen, wall
  instep —*see* Laceration, foot
  internal organ —*see* Injury, by site
  interscapular region —*see* Laceration, thorax, back
  intestine
    large
      colon S36.539
        ascending S36.530
        descending S36.532
        sigmoid S36.533
        specified site NEC S36.538
      rectum S36.63
        transverse S36.531
    small S36.439
      duodenum S36.430
      specified site NEC S36.438
  intra-abdominal organ S36.93
    intestine —*see* Laceration, intestine
    liver —*see* Laceration, liver
    pancreas —*see* Laceration, pancreas
    peritoneum S36.81
    specified site NEC S36.893
    spleen —*see* Laceration, spleen
    stomach —*see* Laceration, stomach

Laceration *(Continued)*
  intracranial NEC —*see also* Injury, intracranial, diffuse
    birth injury P10.9
  jaw —*see* Laceration, head, specified site NEC
  jejunum S36.438
  joint capsule —*see* Sprain, by site
  kidney S37.03-
    major (greater than 3 cm) (massive) (stellate) S37.06-
    minor (less than 1 cm) S37.04-
    moderate (1 to 3 cm) S37.05-
    multiple S37.06-
  knee S81.01-
    with foreign body S81.02-
  labium (majus) (minus) —*see* Laceration, vulva
  lacrimal duct —*see* Laceration, eyelid
  large intestine —*see* Laceration, intestine, large
  larynx S11.011
    with foreign body S11.012
  leg (lower) S81.819
    with foreign body S81.829
    foot —*see* Laceration, foot
    knee —*see* Laceration, knee
    left S81.812
      with foreign body S81.822
    right S81.811
      with foreign body S81.821
    upper —*see* Laceration, thigh
  ligament —*see* Sprain
  lip S01.511
    with foreign body S01.521
  liver S36.113
    major (stellate) S36.116
    minor S36.114
    moderate S36.115
  loin —*see* Laceration, abdomen, wall
  lower back —*see* Laceration, back, lower
  lumbar region —*see* Laceration, back, lower
  lung S27.339
    bilateral S27.332
    unilateral S27.331
  malar region —*see* Laceration, head, specified site NEC
  mammary —*see* Laceration, breast
  mastoid region —*see* Laceration, head, specified site NEC
  meninges —*see* Injury, intracranial, diffuse
  meniscus —*see* Tear, meniscus
  mesentery S36.893
  mesosalpinx S37.893
  mouth —*see* Laceration, oral cavity
  muscle —*see* Injury, muscle, by site, laceration
  nail
    finger —*see* Laceration, finger, with damage to nail
    toe —*see* Laceration, toe, with damage to nail
  nasal (septum) (sinus) —*see* Laceration, nose
  nasopharynx —*see* Laceration, head, specified site NEC
  neck S11.91
    with foreign body S11.92
    involving
      cervical esophagus S11.21
        with foreign body S11.22
      larynx —*see* Laceration, larynx
      pharynx —*see* Laceration, pharynx
      thyroid gland —*see* Laceration, thyroid gland
      trachea —*see* Laceration, trachea
    specified site NEC S11.81
      with foreign body S11.82
  nerve —*see* Injury, nerve
  nose (septum) (sinus) S01.21
    with foreign body S01.22
  ocular NOS S05.3-
    adnexa NOS S01.11-

◀ New   ◀|||| Revised   ~~deleted~~ Deleted

Laceration *(Continued)*
 oral cavity S01.512
  with foreign body S01.522
 orbit (eye) —*see* Wound, open, ocular, orbit
 ovary S37.439
  bilateral S37.432
  unilateral S37.431
 palate —*see* Laceration, oral cavity
 palm —*see* Laceration, hand
 pancreas S36.239
  body S36.231
   major S36.261
   minor S36.241
   moderate S36.251
  head S36.230
   major S36.260
   minor S36.240
   moderate S36.250
  major S36.269
  minor S36.249
  moderate S36.259
  tail S36.232
   major S36.262
   minor S36.242
   moderate S36.252
 pelvic S31.010
  with
   foreign body S31.020
    penetration into retroperitoneal cavity S31.021
   penetration into retroperitoneal cavity S31.011
  floor —*see also* Laceration, back, lower
   with ectopic or molar pregnancy O08.6
   complicating delivery O70.1
   following ectopic or molar pregnancy O08.6
   old (postpartal) N81.89
  organ S37.93
   with ectopic or molar pregnancy O08.6
   adrenal gland S37.813
   bladder S37.23
   fallopian tube —*see* Laceration, fallopian tube
   following ectopic or molar pregnancy O08.6
   kidney —*see* Laceration, kidney
   obstetrical trauma O71.5
   ovary —*see* Laceration, ovary
   prostate S37.823
   specified site NEC S37.893
   ureter S37.13
   urethra S37.33
   uterus S37.63
 penis S31.21
  with foreign body S31.22
 perineum
  female S31.41
   with
    ectopic or molar pregnancy O08.6
    foreign body S31.42
   during delivery O70.9
    first degree O70.0
    fourth degree O70.3
    second degree O70.1
    third degree —*see also* Delivery, complicated, by, laceration, perineum, third degree O70.20 ◄⫶⫶⫶
   old (postpartal) N81.89
   postpartal N81.89
   secondary (postpartal) O90.1
  male S31.119
   with foreign body S31.129
 periocular area (with or without lacrimal passages) —*see* Laceration, eyelid
 peritoneum S36.893
 periumbilic region —*see* Laceration, abdomen, wall, periumbilic

Laceration *(Continued)*
 periurethral tissue —*see* Laceration, urethra
 phalanges
  finger —*see* Laceration, finger
  toe —*see* Laceration, toe
 pharynx S11.21
  with foreign body S11.22
 pinna —*see* Laceration, ear
 popliteal space —*see* Laceration, knee
 prepuce —*see* Laceration, penis
 prostate S37.823
 pubic region S31.119
  with foreign body S31.129
 pudendum —*see* Laceration, genital organs, external
 rectovaginal septum —*see* Laceration, vagina
 rectum S36.63
 retroperitoneum S36.893
 round ligament S37.893
 sacral region —*see* Laceration, back, lower
 sacroiliac region —*see* Laceration, back, lower
 salivary gland —*see* Laceration, oral cavity
 scalp S01.01
  with foreign body S01.02
 scapular region —*see* Laceration, shoulder
 scrotum S31.31
  with foreign body S31.32
 seminal vesicle S37.893
 shin —*see* Laceration, leg
 shoulder S41.019
  with foreign body S41.029
  left S41.012
   with foreign body S41.022
  right S41.011
   with foreign body S41.021
 small intestine —*see* Laceration, intestine, small
 spermatic cord —*see* Laceration, testis
 spinal cord (meninges) —*see also* Injury, spinal cord, by region
  due to injury at birth P11.5
  newborn (birth injury) P11.5
 spleen S36.039
  major (massive) (stellate) S36.032
  moderate S36.031
  superficial (minor) S36.030
 sternal region —*see* Laceration, thorax, front
 stomach S36.33
 submaxillary region —*see* Laceration, head, specified site NEC
 submental region —*see* Laceration, head, specified site NEC
 subungual
  finger (s) —*see* Laceration, finger, with damage to nail
  toe (s) —*see* Laceration, toe, with damage to nail
 suprarenal gland —*see* Laceration, adrenal gland
 temple, temporal region —*see* Laceration, head, specified site NEC
 temporomandibular area —*see* Laceration, cheek
 tendon —*see* Injury, muscle, by site, laceration
  Achilles S86.02-
 tentorium cerebelli —*see* Injury, intracranial, diffuse
 testis S31.31
  with foreign body S31.32
 thigh S71.11-
  with foreign body S71.12-
 thorax, thoracic (wall) S21.91
  with foreign body S21.92
   back S21.22-
    with penetration into thoracic cavity S21.42-
   front S21.12-
    with penetration into thoracic cavity S21.32-

Laceration *(Continued)*
 thorax, thoracic *(Continued)*
  back S21.21-
   with
    foreign body S21.22-
     with penetration into thoracic cavity S21.42-
    penetration into thoracic cavity S21.41-
  breast —*see* Laceration, breast
  front S21.11-
   with
    foreign body S21.12-
     with penetration into thoracic cavity S21.32-
    penetration into thoracic cavity S21.31-
 thumb S61.019
  with
   damage to nail S61.119
    with foreign body S61.129
   foreign body S61.029
  left S61.012
   with
    damage to nail S61.112
     with foreign body S61.122
    foreign body S61.022
  right S61.011
   with
    damage to nail S61.111
     with foreign body S61.121
    foreign body S61.021
 thyroid gland S11.11
  with foreign body S11.12
 toe (s) S91.119
  with
   damage to nail S91.219
    with foreign body S91.229
   foreign body S91.129
  great S91.113
   with
    damage to nail S91.213
     with foreign body S91.223
    foreign body S91.123
   left S91.112
    with
     damage to nail S91.212
      with foreign body S91.222
     foreign body S91.122
   right S91.111
    with
     damage to nail S91.211
      with foreign body S91.221
     foreign body S91.121
  lesser S91.116
   with
    damage to nail S91.216
     with foreign body S91.226
    foreign body S91.126
   left S91.115
    with
     damage to nail S91.215
      with foreign body S91.225
     foreign body S91.125
   right S91.114
    with
     damage to nail S91.214
      with foreign body S91.224
     foreign body S91.124
 tongue —*see* Laceration, oral cavity

Laceration *(Continued)*
trachea S11.021
  with foreign body S11.022
tunica vaginalis —*see* Laceration, testis
tympanum, tympanic membrane —*see*
    Laceration, ear, drum
umbilical region S31.115
  with foreign body S31.125
ureter S37.13
urethra S37.33
  with or following ectopic or molar
     pregnancy O08.6
  obstetrical trauma O71.5
urinary organ NEC S37.893
uterus S37.63
  with ectopic or molar pregnancy O08.6
  following ectopic or molar pregnancy
    O08.6
  nonpuerperal, nontraumatic N85.8
  obstetrical trauma NEC O71.81
  old (postpartal) N85.8
uvula —*see* Laceration, oral cavity
vagina S31.41
  with
    ectopic or molar pregnancy O08.6
    foreign body S31.42
  during delivery O71.4
    with perineal laceration —*see* Laceration,
     perineum, female, during delivery
  following ectopic or molar pregnancy
    O08.6
  nonpuerperal, nontraumatic N89.8
  old (postpartal) N89.8
vas deferens S37.893
vesical —*see* Laceration, bladder
vocal cords S11.031
  with foreign body S11.032
vulva S31.41
  with
    ectopic or molar pregnancy O08.6
    foreign body S31.42
  complicating delivery O70.0
  following ectopic or molar pregnancy
    O08.6
  nonpuerperal, nontraumatic N90.89
  old (postpartal) N90.89
wrist S61.519
  with
    foreign body S61.529
  left S61.512
    with
     foreign body S61.522
  right S61.511
    with
     foreign body S61.521
Lack of
achievement in school Z55.3
adequate
  food Z59.4
  intermaxillary vertical dimension of fully
    erupted teeth M26.36
  sleep Z72.820
appetite (*see* Anorexia) R63.0
awareness R41.9
care
  in home Z74.2
  of infant (at or after birth) T76.02
    confirmed T74.02
cognitive functions R41.9
coordination R27.9
  ataxia R27.0
  specified type NEC R27.8
development (physiological) R62.50
  failure to thrive (child over 28 days old)
    R62.51
    adult R62.7
    newborn P92.6
  short stature R62.52
  specified type NEC R62.59
energy R53.83
financial resources Z59.6

Lack of *(Continued)*
food T73.0
growth R62.52
heating Z59.1
housing (permanent) (temporary) Z59.0
  adequate Z59.1
learning experiences in childhood Z62.898
leisure time (affecting life-style) Z73.2
material resources Z59.9
memory —*see also* Amnesia
  mild, following organic brain damage F06.8
ovulation N97.0
parental supervision or control of child Z62.0
person able to render necessary care Z74.2
physical exercise Z72.3
play experience in childhood Z62.898
posterior occlusal support M26.57
relaxation (affecting life-style) Z73.2
sexual
  desire F52.0
  enjoyment F52.1
shelter Z59.0
sleep (adequate) Z72.820
supervision of child by parent Z62.0
support, posterior occlusal M26.57
water T73.1
Lacrimal —*see* condition
Lacrimation, abnormal —*see* Epiphora
Lacrimonasal duct —*see* condition
Lactation, lactating (breast) (puerperal,
    postpartum)
associated
  cracked nipple O92.13
  retracted nipple O92.03
defective O92.4
disorder NEC O92.79
excessive O92.6
failed (complete) O92.3
  partial O92.4
mastitis NEC —*see* Mastitis, obstetric
mother (care and/or examination) Z39.1
nonpuerperal N64.3
Lacticemia, excessive E87.2
Lacunar skull Q75.8
Laennec's cirrhosis K70.30 ◀▥
~~alcoholic K70.30~~
  ~~with ascites K70.31~~
  with ascites K70.31 ◀
  nonalcoholic K74.69 ◀
Lafora's disease —*see* Epilepsy, generalized,
    idiopathic
Lag, lid (nervous) —*see* Retraction, lid
Lagophthalmos (eyelid) (nervous) H02.209
cicatricial H02.219
  left H02.216
    lower H02.215
    upper H02.214
  right H02.213
    lower H02.212
    upper H02.211
keratoconjunctivitis —*see* Keratoconjunctivitis
left H02.206
  lower H02.205
  upper H02.204
mechanical H02.229
  left H02.226
    lower H02.225
    upper H02.224
  right H02.223
    lower H02.222
    upper H02.221
paralytic H02.239
  left H02.236
    lower H02.235
    upper H02.234
  right H02.233
    lower H02.232
    upper H02.231
right H02.203
  lower H02.202
  upper H02.201

Laki-Lorand factor deficiency —*see* Defect,
    coagulation, specified type NEC
Lalling F80.0
Lambert-Eaton syndrome —*see* Syndrome,
    Lambert-Eaton
Lambliasis, lambliosis A07.1
Landau-Kleffner syndrome —*see* Epilepsy,
    specified NEC
**Landouzy-Déjérine dystrophy or
    facioscapulohumeral atrophy** G71.0
Landouzy's disease (icterohemorrhagic
    leptospirosis) A27.0
Landry-Guillain-Barré, syndrome or paralysis
    G61.0
Landry's disease or paralysis G61.0
Lane's
band Q43.3
kink —*see* Obstruction, intestine
syndrome K90.2
Langdon Down's syndrome —*see* Trisomy, 21
Lapsed immunization schedule status Z28.3
Large
baby (regardless of gestational age) (4000g to
    4499g) P08.1
ear, congenital Q17.1
physiological cup Q14.2
stature R68.89
Large-for-dates NEC (infant) (4000g to 4499g)
    P08.1
affecting management of pregnancy O36.6-
exceptionally (4500g or more) P08.0
**Larsen-Johansson disease
    orosteochondrosis** —*see* Osteochondrosis,
    juvenile, patella
Larsen's syndrome (flattened facies and
    multiple congenital dislocations) Q74.8
Larva migrans
cutaneous B76.9
  Ancylostoma B76.0
visceral B83.0
Laryngeal —*see* condition
Laryngismus (stridulus) J38.5
congenital P28.89
diphtheritic A36.2
Laryngitis (acute) (edematous) (fibrinous)
    (infective) (infiltrative) (malignant)
    (membranous) (phlegmonous)
    (pneumococcal) (pseudomembranous)
    (septic) (subglottic) (suppurative)
    (ulcerative) J04.0
with
  influenza, flu, or grippe —*see* Influenza,
    with, laryngitis
  tracheitis (acute) —*see* Laryngotracheitis
atrophic J37.0
catarrhal J37.0
chronic J37.0
  with tracheitis (chronic) J37.1
diphtheritic A36.2
due to external agent —*see* Inflammation,
    respiratory, upper, due to
Hemophilus influenzae J04.0
H. influenzae J04.0
hypertrophic J37.0
influenzal —*see* Influenza, with, respiratory
    manifestations NEC
obstructive J05.0
sicca J37.0
spasmodic J05.0
  acute J04.0
streptococcal J04.0
stridulous J05.0
syphilitic (late) A52.73
  congenital A50.59 *[J99]*
    early A50.03 *[J99]*
tuberculous A15.5
Vincent's A69.1
Laryngocele (congenital) (ventricular) Q31.3
Laryngofissure J38.7
congenital Q31.8
Laryngomalacia (congenital) Q31.5

Laryngopharyngitis (acute) J06.0
  chronic J37.0
  due to external agent —*see* Inflammation,
    respiratory, upper, due to
Laryngoplegia J38.00
  bilateral J38.02
  unilateral J38.01
Laryngoptosis J38.7
Laryngospasm J38.5
Laryngostenosis J38.6
Laryngotracheitis (acute) (Infectional)
    (infective) (viral) J04.2
  atrophic J37.1
  catarrhal J37.1
  chronic J37.1
  diphtheritic A36.2
  due to external agent —*see* Inflammation,
    respiratory, upper, due to
  Hemophilus influenzae J04.2
  hypertrophic J37.1
  influenzal —*see* Influenza, with, respiratory
    manifestations NEC
  pachydermic J38.7
  sicca J37.1
  spasmodic J38.5
    acute J05.0
  streptococcal J04.2
  stridulous J38.5
  syphilitic (late) A52.73
    congenital A50.59 *[J99]*
      early A50.03 *[J99]*
  tuberculous A15.5
  Vincent's A69.1
Laryngotracheobronchitis —*see* Bronchitis
Larynx, laryngeal —*see* condition
Lassa fever A96.2
Lassitude —*see* Weakness
Late
  talker R62.0
  walker R62.0
Late effect (s) —*see* Sequelae
Latent —*see* condition
Laterocession —*see* Lateroversion
Lateroflexion —*see* Lateroversion
Lateroversion
  cervix —*see* Lateroversion, uterus
  uterus, uterine (cervix) (postinfectional)
    (postpartal, old) N85.4
    congenital Q51.818
    in pregnancy or childbirth O34.59-
Lathyrism —*see* Poisoning, food, noxious, plant
Launois' syndrome (pituitary gigantism) E22.0
Launois-Bensaude adenolipomatosis E88.89
Laurence-Moon (-Bardet)-Biedl syndrome
    Q87.89
Lax, laxity —*see also* Relaxation
  ligament (ous) —*see also* Disorder, ligament
    familial M35.7
    knee —*see* Derangement, knee
  skin (acquired) L57.4
    congenital Q82.8
Laxative habit F55.2
Lazy leukocyte syndrome D70.8
Lead miner's lung J63.6
Leak, leakage
  air NEC J93.82
    postprocedural J95.812
  amniotic fluid —*see* Rupture, membranes,
    premature
  blood (microscopic), fetal, into maternal
    circulation affecting management of
    pregnancy —*see* Pregnancy, complicated
    by
  cerebrospinal fluid G96.0
    from spinal (lumbar) puncture G97.0
  device, implant or graft —*see also*
    Complications, by site and type,
    mechanical
    arterial graft NEC —*see* Complication,
      cardiovascular device, mechanical,
      vascular

Leak, leakage (Continued)
  device, implant or graft (Continued)
    breast (implant) T85.43
    catheter NEC T85.638
      dialysis (renal) T82.43
        intraperitoneal T85.631
      infusion NEC T82.534
        spinal (epidural) (subdural) T85.630
        urinary, indwelling T83.038
        cystostomy T83.030
      urinary T83.038 ◄
        cystostomy T83.030 ◄
        Hopkins T83.038 ◄
        ileostomy T83.038 ◄
        indwelling T83.031 ◄
        nephrostomy T83.032 ◄
        specified NEC T83.038 ◄
        urostomy T83.038 ◄
    gastrointestinal —*see* Complications,
      prosthetic device, mechanical,
      gastrointestinal device
    genital NEC T83.498
      penile prosthesis (cylinder) (implanted)
        (pump) (resevoir) T83.490 ◄▥
      testicular prosthesis T83.491 ◄
    heart NEC —*see* Complication,
      cardiovascular device, mechanical
    joint prosthesis —*see* Complications, joint
      prosthesis, mechanical, specified
      NEC, by site
    ocular NEC —*see* Complications, prosthetic
      device, mechanical, ocular device
    orthopedic NEC —*see* Complication,
      orthopedic, device, mechanical
    persistent air J93.82
    specified NEC T85.638
    urinary NEC —*see also* Complication,
      genitourinary, device, urinary,
      mechanical
      graft T83.23
    vascular NEC —*see* Complication,
      cardiovascular device, mechanical
    ventricular intracranial shunt T85.03
  urine —*see* Incontinence
Leaky heart —*see* Endocarditis
Learning defect (specific) F81.9
Leather bottle stomach C16.9
Leber's
  congenital amaurosis H35.50
  optic atrophy (hereditary) H47.22
Lederer's anemia D59.1
Leeches (external) —*see* Hirudiniasis
Leg —*see* condition
Legg (-Calvé)-Perthes disease, syndrome or
    osteochondrosis M91.1-
Legionellosis A48.1
  nonpneumonic A48.2
Legionnaires'
  disease A48.1
    nonpneumonic A48.2
  pneumonia A48.1
Leigh's disease G31.82
Leiner's disease L21.1
Leiofibromyoma —*see* Leiomyoma
Leiomyoblastoma —*see* Neoplasm, connective
    tissue, benign
Leiomyofibroma —*see also* Neoplasm,
    connective tissue, benign
  uterus (cervix) (corpus) D25.9
Leiomyoma —*see also* Neoplasm, connective
    tissue, benign
  bizarre —*see* Neoplasm, connective tissue,
    benign
  cellular —*see* Neoplasm, connective tissue,
    benign
  epithelioid —*see* Neoplasm, connective
    tissue, benign
  uterus (cervix) (corpus) D25.9
    intramural D25.1
    submucous D25.0
    subserosal D25.2

Leiomyoma (Continued)
  vascular —*see* Neoplasm, connective tissue,
    benign
Leiomyoma, leiomyomatosis (intravascular) —
    see Neoplasm, connective tissue, uncertain
    behavior
Leiomyosarcoma —*see also* Neoplasm,
    connective tissue, malignant
  epithelioid —*see* Neoplasm, connective
    tissue, malignant
  myxoid —*see* Neoplasm, connective tissue,
    malignant
Leishmaniasis B55.9
  American (mucocutaneous) B55.2
    cutaneous B55.1
  Asian Desert B55.1
  Brazilian B55.2
  cutaneous (any type) B55.1
    dermal —*see also* Leishmaniasis, cutaneous
      post-kala-azar B55.0
    eyelid B55.1
  infantile B55.0
  Mediterranean B55.0
  mucocutaneous (American) (New World)
    B55.2
  naso-oral B55.2
  nasopharyngeal B55.2
  old world B55.1
  tegumentaria diffusa B55.1
  visceral B55.0
Leishmanoid, dermal —*see also* Leishmaniasis,
    cutaneous
  post-kala-azar B55.0
Lenegre's disease I44.2
Lengthening, leg —*see* Deformity, limb,
    unequal length
Lennert's lymphoma —*see* Lymphoma,
    Lennert's
Lennox-Gastaut syndrome G40.812
  intractable G40.814
    with status epilepticus G40.813
    without status epilepticus G40.814
  not intractable G40.812
    with status epilepticus G40.811
    without status epilepticus G40.812
Lens —*see* condition
Lenticonus (anterior) (posterior) (congenital)
    Q12.8
Lenticular degeneration, progressive E83.01
Lentiglobus (posterior) (congenital) Q12.8
Lentigo (congenital) L81.4
  maligna —*see also* Melanoma, in situ
    melanoma —*see* Melanoma
Lentivirus, as cause of disease classified
    elsewhere B97.31
Leontiasis
  ossium M85.2
  syphilitic (late) A52.78
    congenital A50.59
Lepothrix A48.8
Lepra —*see* Leprosy
Leprechaunism E34.8
Leprosy A30.-
  with muscle disorder A30.9 *[M63.80]*
    ankle A30.9 *[M63.87-]*
    foot A30.9 *[M63.87-]*
    forearm A30.9 *[M63.83-]*
    hand A30.9 *[M63.84-]*
    lower leg A30.9 *[M63.86-]*
    multiple sites A30.9 *[M63.89]*
    pelvic region A30.9 *[M63.85-]*
    shoulder region A30.9 *[M63.81-]*
    specified site NEC A30.9 *[M63.88]*
    thigh A30.9 *[M63.85-]*
    upper arm A30.9 *[M63.82-]*
  anesthetic A30.9
  BB A30.3
  BL A30.4
  borderline (infiltrated) (neuritic) A30.3
    lepromatous A30.4
    tuberculoid A30.2

◄ New   ◄▥ Revised   ~~deleted~~ Deleted   **321**

Leprosy (Continued)
- BT A30.2
- dimorphous (infiltrated) (neuritic) A30.3
- I A30.0
- indeterminate (macular) (neuritic) A30.0
- lepromatous (diffuse) (infiltrated) (macular) (neuritic) (nodular) A30.5
- LL A30.5
- macular (early) (neuritic) (simple) A30.9
- maculoanesthetic A30.9
- mixed A30.3
- neural A30.9
- nodular A30.5
- primary neuritic A30.3
- specified type NEC A30.8
- TT A30.1
- tuberculoid (major) (minor) A30.1

Leptocytosis, hereditary D56.9
Leptomeningitis (chronic) (circumscribed) (hemorrhagic) (nonsuppurative) —see Meningitis
Leptomeningopathy G96.19
Leptospiral —see condition
Leptospirochetal —see condition
Leptospirosis A27.9
- canicola A27.89
- due to Leptospira interrogans serovar icterohaemorrhagiae A27.0
- icterohemorrhagica A27.0
- pomona A27.89
- Weil's disease A27.0

Leptus dermatitis B88.0
Leriche's syndrome (aortic bifurcation occlusion) I74.09
Leri's pleonosteosis Q78.8
Leri-Weill syndrome Q77.8
Lermoyez' syndrome —see Vertigo, peripheral NEC
Lesch-Nyhan syndrome E79.1
Leser-Trélat disease L82.1
- inflamed L82.0

Lesion (s) (nontraumatic)
- abducens nerve —see Strabismus, paralytic, sixth nerve
- alveolar process K08.9
- angiocentric immunoproliferative D47.Z9
- anorectal K62.9
- aortic (valve) I35.9
- auditory nerve —see subcategory H93.3
- basal ganglion G25.9
- bile duct —see Disease, bile duct
- biomechanical M99.9
  - specified type NEC M99.89
    - abdomen M99.89
    - acromioclavicular M99.87
    - cervical region M99.81
    - cervicothoracic M99.81
    - costochondral M99.88
    - costovertebral M99.88
    - head region M99.80
    - hip M99.85
    - lower extremity M99.86
    - lumbar region M99.83
    - lumbosacral M99.83
    - occipitocervical M99.80
    - pelvic region M99.85
    - pubic M99.85
    - rib cage M99.88
    - sacral region M99.84
    - sacrococcygeal M99.84
    - sacroiliac M99.84
    - specified NEC M99.89
    - sternochondral M99.88
    - sternoclavicular M99.87
    - thoracic region M99.82
    - thoracolumbar M99.82
    - upper extremity M99.87
- bladder N32.9
- bone —see Disorder, bone
- brachial plexus G54.0

Lesion (Continued)
- brain G93.9
  - congenital Q04.9
  - vascular I67.9
    - degenerative I67.9
    - hypertensive I67.4
- buccal cavity K13.79
- calcified —see Calcification
- canthus —see Disorder, eyelid
- carate —see Pinta, lesions
- cardia K31.9 ◀▥
- cardiac —see also Disease, heart I51.9
  - congenital Q24.9
  - valvular —see Endocarditis
- cauda equina G83.4
- cecum K63.9
- cerebral —see Lesion, brain
- cerebrovascular I67.9
  - degenerative I67.9
  - hypertensive I67.4
- cervical (nerve) root NEC G54.2
- chiasmal —see Disorder, optic, chiasm
- chorda tympani G51.8
- coin, lung R91.1
- colon K63.9
- combined periodontic - endodontic K05.5 ◀
- congenital —see Anomaly, by site
- conjunctiva H11.9
- conus medullaris —see Injury, conus medullaris
- coronary artery —see Ischemia, heart
- cranial nerve G52.9
  - eighth —see Disorder, ear
  - eleventh G52.9
  - fifth G50.9
  - first G52.0
  - fourth —see Strabismus, paralytic, fourth nerve
  - seventh G51.9
  - sixth —see Strabismus, paralytic, sixth nerve
  - tenth G52.2
  - twelfth G52.3
- cystic —see Cyst
- degenerative —see Degeneration
- duodenum K31.9
- edentulous (alveolar) ridge, associated with trauma, due to traumatic occlusion K06.2
- en coup de sabre L94.1
- eyelid —see Disorder, eyelid
- gasserian ganglion G50.8
- gastric K31.9
- gastroduodenal K31.9
- gastrointestinal K63.9
- gingiva, associated with trauma K06.2
- glomerular
  - focal and segmental —see also N00-N07 with fourth character .1 N05.1
  - minimal change —see also N00-N07 with fourth character .0 N05.0
- heart (organic) —see Disease, heart
- hyperchromic, due to pinta (carate) A67.1
- hyperkeratotic —see Hyperkeratosis
- hypothalamic E23.7
- ileocecal K63.9
- ileum K63.9
- iliohypogastric nerve G57.8-
- inflammatory —see Inflammation
- intestine K63.9
- intracerebral —see Lesion, brain
- intrachiasmal (optic) —see Disorder, optic, chiasm
- intracranial, space-occupying R90.0
- joint —see Disorder, joint
  - sacroiliac (old) M53.3
- keratotic —see Keratosis
- kidney —see Disease, renal
- laryngeal nerve (recurrent) G52.2
- lip K13.0

Lesion (Continued)
- liver K76.9
- lumbosacral
  - plexus G54.1
  - root (nerve) NEC G54.4
- lung (coin) R91.1
- maxillary sinus J32.0
- mitral I05.9
- Morel-Lavallée —see Hematoma, by site
- motor cortex NEC G93.89
- mouth K13.79
- nerve G58.9
  - femoral G57.2-
  - median G56.1-
    - carpal tunnel syndrome —see Syndrome, carpal tunnel
  - plantar G57.6-
  - popliteal (lateral) G57.3-
    - medial G57.4-
  - radial G56.3-
  - sciatic G57.0-
  - spinal —see Injury, nerve, spinal
  - ulnar G56.2-
- nervous system, congenital Q07.9
- nonallopathic —see Lesion, biomechanical
- nose (internal) J34.89
- obstructive —see Obstruction
- obturator nerve G57.8-
- oral mucosa K13.70
- organ or site NEC —see Disease, by site
- osteolytic —see Osteolysis
- peptic K27.9
- periodontal, due to traumatic occlusion K05.5
- pharynx J39.2
- pigment, pigmented (skin) L81.9
- pinta —see Pinta, lesions
- polypoid —see Polyp
- prechiasmal (optic) —see Disorder, optic, chiasm
- primary —see also Syphilis, primary A51.0
  - carate A67.0
  - pinta A67.0
  - yaws A66.0
- pulmonary J98.4
  - valve I37.9
- pylorus K31.9
- rectosigmoid K63.9
- retina, retinal H35.9
- sacroiliac (joint) (old) M53.3
- salivary gland K11.9
  - benign lymphoepithelial K11.8
- saphenous nerve G57.8-
- sciatic nerve G57.0-
- secondary —see Syphilis, secondary
- shoulder (region) M75.9-
  - specified NEC M75.8-
- sigmoid K63.9
- sinus (accessory) (nasal) J34.89
- skin L98.9
  - suppurative L08.0
- SLAP S43.43-
- spinal cord G95.9
  - congenital Q06.9
- spleen D73.89
- stomach K31.9
- superior glenoid labrum S43.43-
- syphilitic —see Syphilis
- tertiary —see Syphilis, tertiary
- thoracic root (nerve) NEC G54.3
- tonsillar fossa J35.9
- tooth, teeth K08.9
  - white spot
    - chewing surface K02.51
    - pit and fissure surface K02.51
    - smooth surface K02.61
- traumatic —see specific type of injury by site
- tricuspid (valve) I07.9
  - nonrheumatic I36.9
- trigeminal nerve G50.9

◀ New   ◀▥ Revised   ~~deleted~~ Deleted

Lesion (Continued)
  ulcerated or ulcerative —see Ulcer, skin
  uterus N85.9
  vagus nerve G52.2
  valvular —see Endocarditis
  vascular I99.9
    affecting central nervous system I67.9
    following trauma NEC T14.8
    umbilical cord, complicating delivery
        O69.5
  warty —see Verruca
  white spot (tooth)
    chewing surface K02.51
    pit and fissure surface K02.51
    smooth surface K02.61
Lethargic —see condition
Lethargy R53.83
Letterer-Siwe's disease C96.0
Leukemia, leukemic C95.9-
  acute basophilic C94.8-
  acute bilineal C95.0-
  acute erythroid C94.0-
  acute lymphoblastic C91.0-
  acute megakaryoblastic C94.2-
  acute megakaryocytic C94.2-
  acute mixed lineage C95.0-
  acute monoblastic (monoblastic/monocytic)
      C93.0-
  acute monocytic (monoblastic/monocytic)
      C93.0-
  acute myeloblastic (minimal differentiation)
      (with maturation) C92.0-
  acute myeloid
    with
      11q23-abnormality C92.6-
      dysplasia of remaining hematopoesis
          and/or myelodysplastic disease in
          its history C92.A-
      multilineage dysplasia C92.A-
      variation of MLL-gene C92.6-
    M6 (a)(b) C94.0-
    M7 C94.2-
  acute myelomonocytic C92.5-
  acute promyelocytic C92.4-
  adult T-cell (HTLV-1-associated)
      (acute variant) (chronic variant)
      (lymphomatoid variant) (smouldering
      variant) C91.5-
  aggressive NK-cell C94.8-
  AML (1/ETO) (M0) (M1) (M2) (without a
      FAB classification) C92.0-
  AML M3 C92.4-
  AML M4 (Eo with inv(16) or t(16;16))
      C92.5-
  AML M5 C93.0-
  AML M5a C93.0-
  AML M5b C93.0-
  AML Me with t (15;17) and variants C92.4-
  atypical chronic myeloid, BCR/ABL-negative
      C92.2-
  biphenotypic acute C95.0-
  blast cell C95.0-
  Burkitt-type, mature B-cell C91.A-
  chronic lymphocytic, of B-cell type C91.1-
  chronic monocytic C93.1-
  chronic myelogenous (Philadelphia
      chromosome (Ph1) positive) (t(9;22))
      (q34;q11) (with crisis of blast cells)
      C92.1-
  chronic myeloid, BCR/ABL-positive C92.1-
    atypical, BCR/ABL-negative C92.2-
  chronic myelomonocytic C93.1-
  chronic neutrophilic D47.1
  CMML (-1) (-2) (with eosinophilia) C93.1-
  granulocytic —see also Category C92 C92.9-
  hairy-cell C91.4-
  juvenile myelomonocytic C93.3-
  lymphoid C91.9-
    specified NEC C91.Z-
  mast cell C94.3-
  mature B-cell, Burkitt-type C91.A-

Leukemia, leukemic (Continued)
  monocytic (subacute) C93.9-
    specified NEC C93.Z-
  myelogenous —see also Category C92 C92.9-
  myeloid C92.9-
    specified NEC C92.Z-
  plasma cell C90.1-
  plasmacytic C90.1-
  prolymphocytic
    of B-cell type C91.3-
    of T-cell type C91.6-
  specified NEC C94.8-
  stem cell, of unclear lineage C95.0-
  subacute lymphocytic C91.9-
  T-cell large granular lymphocytic C91.Z-
  unspecified cell type C95.9-
    acute C95.0-
    chronic C95.1-
Leukemoid reaction —see also Reaction,
    leukemoid D72.823-
Leukoaraiosis (hypertensive) I67.81
Leukoariosis —see Leukoaraiosis
Leukocoria —see Disorder, globe, degenerated
    condition, leucocoria
Leukocytopenia D72.819
Leukocytosis D72.829
  eosinophilic D72.1
Leukoderma, leukodermia NEC L81.5
  syphilitic A51.39
    late A52.79
Leukodystrophy E75.29
Leukoedema, oral epithelium K13.29
Leukoencephalitis G04.81
  acute (subacute) hemorrhagic G36.1
    postimmunization or postvaccinal G04.02
  postinfectious G04.01
  subacute sclerosing A81.1
  van Bogaert's (sclerosing) A81.1
Leukoencephalopathy —see also
    Encephalopathy G93.49
  Binswanger's I67.3
  heroin vapor G92
  metachromatic E75.25
  multifocal (progressive) A81.2
  postimmunization and postvaccinal G04.02
  progressive multifocal A81.2
  reversible, posterior G93.6
  van Bogaert's (sclerosing) A81.1
  vascular, progressive I67.3
Leukoerythroblastosis D75.9
Leukokeratosis —see also Leukoplakia
  mouth K13.21
  nicotina palati K13.24
  oral mucosa K13.21
  tongue K13.21
  vocal cord J38.3
Leukokraurosis vulva (e) N90.4
Leukoma (cornea) —see also Opacity, cornea
  adherent H17.0-
  interfering with central vision —see Opacity,
      cornea, central
Leukomalacia, cerebral, newborn P91.2
  periventricular P91.2
Leukomelanopathy, hereditary D72.0
Leukonychia (punctata) (striata) L60.8
  congenital Q84.4
Leukopathia unguium L60.8
  congenital Q84.4
Leukopenia D72.819
  basophilic D72.818
  chemotherapy (cancer) induced D70.1
  congenital D70.0
  cyclic D70.0
  drug induced NEC D70.2
    due to cytoreductive cancer chemotherapy
        D70.1
  eosinophilic D72.818
  familial D70.0
  infantile genetic D70.0
  malignant D70.9
  periodic D70.0
  transitory neonatal P61.5

Leukopenic —see condition
Leukoplakia
  anus K62.89
  bladder (postinfectional) N32.89
  buccal K13.21
  cervix (uteri) N88.0
  esophagus K22.8
  gingiva K13.21
  hairy (oral mucosa) (tongue) K13.3
  kidney (pelvis) N28.89
  larynx J38.7
  lip K13.21
  mouth K13.21
  oral epithelium, including tongue (mucosa)
      K13.21
  palate K13.21
  pelvis (kidney) N28.89
  penis (infectional) N48.0
  rectum K62.89
  syphilitic (late) A52.79
  tongue K13.21
  ureter (postinfectional) N28.89
  urethra (postinfectional) N36.8
  uterus N85.8
  vagina N89.4
  vocal cord J38.3
  vulva N90.4
Leukorrhea N89.8
  due to Trichomonas (vaginalis)
      A59.00
  trichomonal A59.00
Leukosarcoma C85.9
Levocardia (isolated) Q24.1
  with situs inversus Q89.3
Levotransposition Q20.5
Lev's disease or syndrome (acquired complete
    heart block) I44.2
Levulosuria —see Fructosuria
Levurid L30.2
Lewy body (ies) (dementia) (disease)
    G31.83
Leyden-Moebius dystrophy G71.0
Leydig cell
  carcinoma
    specified site —see Neoplasm, malignant,
        by site
    unspecified site
      female C56.9-
      male C62.9-
  tumor
    benign
      specified site —see Neoplasm, benign,
          by site
      unspecified site
        female D27.-
        male D29.2-
    malignant
      specified site —see Neoplasm,
          malignant, by site
      unspecified site
        female C56.-
        male C62.9-
    specified site —see Neoplasm, uncertain
        behavior, by site
    unspecified site
      female D39.1-
      male D40.1-
Leydig-Sertoli cell tumor
  specified site —see Neoplasm, benign,
      by site
  unspecified site
    female D27.-
    male D29.2-
LGSIL (Low grade squamous intraepithelial
    lesion on cytologic smear of)
  anus R85.612
  cervix R87.612
  vagina R87.622
Liar, pathologic F60.2
Libido
  decreased R68.82

Libman-Sacks disease M32.11
Lice (infestation) B85.2
  body (Pediculus corporis) B85.1
  crab B85.3
  head (Pediculus capitis) B85.0
  mixed (classifiable to more than one of the
      titles B85.0-B85.3) B85.4
  pubic (Phthirus pubis) B85.3
Lichen L28.0
  albus L90.0
    penis N48.0
    vulva N90.4
  amyloidosis E85.4 *[L99]*
  atrophicus L90.0
    penis N48.0
    vulva N90.4
  congenital Q82.8
  myxedematosus L98.5
  nitidus L44.1
  pilaris Q82.8
    acquired L85.8
  planopilaris L66.1
  planus (chronicus) L43.9
    annularis L43.8
    bullous L43.1
    follicular L66.1
    hypertrophic L43.0
    moniliformis L44.3
    of Wilson L43.9
    specified NEC L43.8
    subacute (active) L43.3
    tropicus L43.3
  ruber
    acuminatus L44.0
    moniliformis L44.3
    planus L43.9
  sclerosus (et atrophicus) L90.0
    penis N48.0
    vulva N90.4
  scrofulosus (primary) (tuberculous) A18.4
  simplex (chronicus) (circumscriptus) L28.0
  striatus L44.2
  urticatus L28.2
Lichenification L28.0
Lichenoides tuberculosis (primary) A18.4
Lichtheim's disease or syndrome —see
      Degeneration, combined
Lien migrans D73.89
Ligament —see condition
Light
  for gestational age —see Light for dates
  headedness R42
Light-for-dates (infant) P05.00
  with weight of
    499 grams or less P05.01
    500-749 grams P05.02
    750-999 grams P05.03
    1000-1249 grams P05.04
    1250-1499 grams P05.05
    1500-1749 grams P05.06
    1750-1999 grams P05.07
    2000-2499 grams P05.08
    2500 grams and over P05.09 ◄
  affecting management of pregnancy O36.59-
  and small-for-dates —see Small for dates
  specified NEC P05.09 ◄
Lightning (effects) (stroke) (struck by) T75.00
  burn —see Burn
  foot E53.8
  shock T75.01
  specified effect NEC T75.09
Lightwood-Albright syndrome N25.89
Lightwood's disease or syndrome (renal
      tubular acidosis) N25.89
Lignac (-de Toni) (-Fanconi) (-Debré) disease or
      syndrome E72.09
  with cystinosis E72.04
Ligneous thyroiditis E06.5
Likoff's syndrome I20.8
Limb —see condition
Limbic epilepsy personality syndrome F07.0

Limitation, limited
  activities due to disability Z73.6
  cardiac reserve —see Disease, heart
  eye muscle duction, traumatic —see
      Strabismus, mechanical
  mandibular range of motion M26.52
Lindau (-von Hippel) disease Q85.8
Line (s)
  Beau's L60.4
  Harris' —see Arrest, epiphyseal
  Hudson's (cornea) —see Pigmentation,
      cornea, anterior
  Stähli's (cornea) —see Pigmentation, cornea,
      anterior
Linea corneae senilis —see Change, cornea,
      senile
Lingua
  geographica K14.1
  nigra (villosa) K14.3
  plicata K14.5
  tylosis K13.29
Lingual —see condition
Linguatulosis B88.8
Linitis (gastric) plastica C16.9
Lip —see condition
Lipedema —see Edema
Lipemia —see also Hyperlipidemia
  retina, retinalis E78.3
Lipidosis E75.6
  cerebral (infantile) (juvenile) (late) E75.4
  cerebroretinal E75.4
  cerebroside E75.22
  cholesterol (cerebral) E75.5
  glycolipid E75.21
  hepatosplenomegalic E78.3
  sphingomyelin —see Niemann-Pick disease
      or syndrome
  sulfatide E75.29
Lipoadenoma —see Neoplasm, benign, by site
Lipoblastoma —see Lipoma
Lipoblastomatosis —see Lipoma
Lipochondrodystrophy E76.01
Lipochrome histiocytosis (familial) D71
Lipodermatosclerosis —see Varix, leg, with,
      inflammation
  ulcerated —see Varix, leg, with, ulcer, with
      inflammation by site
Lipodystrophia progressiva E88.1
Lipodystrophy (progressive) E88.1
  insulin E88.1
  intestinal K90.81
  mesenteric K65.4
Lipofibroma —see Lipoma
Lipofuscinosis, neuronal (with ceroidosis)
      E75.4
Lipogranuloma, sclerosing L92.8
Lipogranulomatosis E78.89
Lipoid —see also condition
  histiocytosis D76.3
    essential E75.29
  nephrosis N04.9
  proteinosis of Urbach E78.89
Lipoidemia —see Hyperlipidemia
Lipoidosis —see Lipidosis
Lipoma D17.9
  fetal D17.9
    fat cell D17.9
  infiltrating D17.9
  intramuscular D17.9
  pleomorphic D17.9
  site classification
    arms (skin) (subcutaneous) D17.2-
    connective tissue D17.30
      intra-abdominal D17.5
      intrathoracic D17.4
      peritoneum D17.79
      retroperitoneum D17.79
      specified site NEC D17.39
      spermatic cord D17.6
    face (skin) (subcutaneous) D17.0
    genitourinary organ NEC D17.72

Lipoma (Continued)
  site classification (Continued)
    head (skin) (subcutaneous) D17.0
    intra-abdominal D17.5
    intrathoracic D17.4
    kidney D17.71
    legs (skin) (subcutaneous) D17.2-
    neck (skin) (subcutaneous) D17.0
    peritoneum D17.79
    retroperitoneum D17.79
    skin D17.30
      specified site NEC D17.39
    specified site NEC D17.79
    spermatic cord D17.6
    subcutaneous D17.30
      specified site NEC D17.39
    trunk (skin) (subcutaneous) D17.1
    unspecified D17.9
  spindle cell D17.9
Lipomatosis E88.2
  dolorosa (Dercum) E88.2
  fetal —see Lipoma
  Launois-Bensaude E88.89
Lipomyoma —see Lipoma
Lipomyxoma —see Lipoma
Lipomyxosarcoma —see Neoplasm, connective
      tissue, malignant
Lipoprotein metabolism disorder E78.9
Lipoproteinemia E78.5
  broad-beta E78.2
  floating-beta E78.2
  hyper-pre-beta E78.1
Liposarcoma —see also Neoplasm, connective
      tissue, malignant
  dedifferentiated —see Neoplasm, connective
      tissue, malignant
  differentiated type —see Neoplasm,
      connective tissue, malignant
  embryonal —see Neoplasm, connective tissue,
      malignant
  mixed type —see Neoplasm, connective
      tissue, malignant
  myxoid —see Neoplasm, connective tissue,
      malignant
  pleomorphic —see Neoplasm, connective
      tissue, malignant
  round cell —see Neoplasm, connective tissue,
      malignant
  well differentiated type —see Neoplasm,
      connective tissue, malignant
Liposynovitis prepatellaris E88.89
Lipping, cervix N86
Lipschütz disease or ulcer N76.6
Lipuria R82.0
  schistosomiasis (bilharziasis) B65.0
Lisping F80.0
Lissauer's paralysis A52.17
Lissencephalia, lissencephaly Q04.3
Listeriosis, listerellosis A32.9
  congenital (disseminated) P37.2
  cutaneous A32.0
  neonatal, newborn (disseminated) P37.2
  oculoglandular A32.81
  specified NEC A32.89
Lithemia E79.0
Lithiasis —see Calculus
Lithosis J62.8
Lithuria R82.99
Litigation, anxiety concerning Z65.3
Little leaguer's elbow —see Epicondylitis,
      medial
Little's disease G80.9
Littre's
  gland —see condition
  hernia —see Hernia, abdomen
Littritis —see Urethritis
Livedo (annularis) (racemosa) (reticularis)
      R23.1
Liver —see condition
Living alone (problems with) Z60.2
  with handicapped person Z74.2

◄ New   ◄IIII Revised   ~~deleted~~ Deleted

Lloyd's syndrome —*see* Adenomatosis, endocrine
Loa loa, loaiasis, loasis B74.3
Lobar —*see* condition
Lobomycosis B48.0
Lobo's disease B48.0
Lobotomy syndrome F07.0
Lobstein (-Ekman) disease or syndrome Q78.0
Lobster-claw hand Q71.6-
Lobulation (congenital) —*see also* Anomaly, by site
  kidney, Q63.1
  liver, abnormal Q44.7
  spleen Q89.09
Lobule, lobular —*see* condition
Local, localized —*see* condition
Locked twins causing obstructed labor O66.1
Locked-in state G83.5
Locking
  joint —*see* Derangement, joint, specified type NEC
    knee —*see* Derangement, knee
Lockjaw —*see* Tetanus
Löffler's
  endocarditis I42.3
  eosinophilia J82
  pneumonia J82
  syndrome (eosinophilic pneumonitis) J82
Loiasis (with conjunctival infestation) (eyelid) B74.3
Lone Star fever A77.0
Long
  labor O63.9
    first stage O63.0
    second stage O63.1
  QT syndrome I45.81
Long-term (current) (prophylactic) drug therapy (use of)
  agents affecting estrogen receptors and estrogen levels NEC Z79.818
  anastrozole (Arimidex) Z79.811
  antibiotics Z79.2
    short-term use - omit code
  anticoagulants Z79.01
  anti-inflammatory, non-steroidal (NSAID) Z79.1
  antiplatelet Z79.02
  antithrombotics Z79.02
  aromatase inhibitors Z79.811
  aspirin Z79.82
  birth control pill or patch Z79.3
  bisphosphonates Z79.83
  contraceptive, oral Z79.3
  drug, specified NEC Z79.899
  estrogen receptor downregulators Z79.818
  Evista Z79.810
  exemestane (Aromasin) Z79.811
  Fareston Z79.810
  fulvestrant (Faslodex) Z79.818
  gonadotropin-releasing hormone (GnRH) agonist Z79.818
  goserelin acetate (Zoladex) Z79.818
  hormone replacement (postmenopausal) Z79.890
  insulin Z79.4
  letrozole (Femara) Z79.811
  leuprolide acetate (leuprorelin) (Lupron) Z79.818
  megestrol acetate (Megace) Z79.818
  methadone for pain management Z79.891
  Nolvadex Z79.810
  non-steroidal anti-inflammatories (NSAID) Z79.1
  opiate analgesic Z79.891
  oral contraceptive Z79.3
  oral ◄
    antidiabetic Z79.84 ◄
    contraceptive Z79.3 ◄
    hypoglycemic Z79.84 ◄
  raloxifene (Evista) Z79.810

Long-term (*Continued*)
  selective estrogen receptor modulators (SERMs) Z79.810
  steroids
    inhaled Z79.51
    systemic Z79.52
  tamoxifen (Nolvadex) Z79.810
  toremifene (Fareston) Z79.810
Longitudinal stripes or grooves, nails L60.8
  congenital Q84.6
Loop
  intestine —*see* Volvulus
  vascular on papilla (optic) Q14.2
Loose —*see also* condition
  body
    joint M24.00
      ankle M24.07-
      elbow M24.02-
      hand M24.04-
      hip M24.05-
      knee M23.4-
      shoulder (region) M24.01-
      specified site NEC M24.08
      toe M24.07-
      vertebra M24.08
      wrist M24.03-
    knee M23.4-
    sheath, tendon —*see* Disorder, tendon, specified type NEC
  cartilage —*see* Loose, body, joint
  skin and subcutaneous tissue (following bariatric surgery weight loss) (following dietary weight loss) L98.7 ◄
  tooth, teeth K08.89 ◄▥
Loosening
  aseptic
    joint prosthesis —*see* Complications, joint prosthesis, mechanical, loosening, by site
    epiphysis —*see* Osteochondropathy
  mechanical
    joint prosthesis —*see* Complications, joint prosthesis, mechanical, loosening, by site
Looser-Milkman (-Debray) syndrome M83.8
Lop ear (deformity) Q17.3
Lorain (-Levi) short stature syndrome E23.0
Lordosis M40.50
  acquired —*see* Lordosis, specified type NEC
  congenital Q76.429
    lumbar region Q76.426
    lumbosacral region Q76.427
    sacral region Q76.428
    sacrococcygeal region Q76.428
    thoracolumbar region Q76.425
  lumbar region M40.56
  lumbosacral region M40.57
  postsurgical M96.4
  postural —*see* Lordosis, specified type NEC
  rachitic (late effect) (sequelae) E64.3
  sequelae of rickets E64.3
  specified type NEC M40.40
    lumbar region M40.46
    lumbosacral region M40.47
    thoracolumbar region M40.45
  thoracolumbar region M40.55
  tuberculous A18.01
Loss (of)
  appetite (*see* Anorexia) R63.0
    hysterical F50.89 ◄▥
    nonorganic origin F50.89 ◄▥
    psychogenic F50.89 ◄▥
  blood —*see* Hemorrhage
  bone —*see* Loss, substance of, bone ◄
  consciousness, transient R55
    traumatic —*see* Injury, intracranial
  control, sphincter, rectum R15.9
    nonorganic origin F98.1
  elasticity, skin R23.4

Loss (*Continued*)
  family (member) in childhood Z62.898
  fluid (acute) E86.9
    with
      hypernatremia E87.0
      hyponatremia E87.1
  function of labyrinth —*see* subcategory H83.2
  hair, nonscarring —*see* Alopecia
  hearing —*see also* Deafness
    central NOS H90.5
    conductive H90.2 ◄
      bilateral H90.0 ◄
      unilateral ◄
        with ◄
          restricted hearing on the contralateral side H90.A1- ◄
          unrestricted hearing on the contralateral side H90.1- ◄
    mixed conductive and sensorineural hearing loss H90.8 ◄
      bilateral H90.6 ◄
      unilateral ◄
        with ◄
          restricted hearing on the contralateral side H90.A3- ◄
          unrestricted hearing on the contralateral side H90.7- ◄
    neural NOS H90.5
    perceptive NOS H90.5
    sensorineural NOS H90.5
      bilateral H90.3 ◄
      unilateral ◄
        with ◄
          restricted hearing on the contralateral side H90.A2- ◄
          unrestricted hearing on the contralateral side H90.4- ◄
    sensory NOS H90.5
  height R29.890
  limb or member, traumatic, current —*see* Amputation, traumatic
  love relationship in childhood Z62.898
  memory —*see also* Amnesia
    mild, following organic brain damage F06.8
  mind —*see* Psychosis
  occlusal vertical dimension of fully erupted teeth M26.37
  organ or part —*see* Absence, by site, acquired
  ossicles, ear (partial) H74.32-
  parent in childhood Z63.4
  pregnancy, recurrent N96
    without current pregnancy N96
    care in current pregnancy O26.2-
  recurrent pregnancy —*see* Loss, pregnancy, recurrent
  self-esteem, in childhood Z62.898
  sense of
    smell —*see* Disturbance, sensation, smell
    taste —*see* Disturbance, sensation, taste
    touch R20.8
  sensory R44.9
    dissociative F44.6
  sexual desire F52.0
  sight (acquired) (complete) (congenital) —*see* Blindness
  substance of
    bone —*see* Disorder, bone, density and structure, specified NEC
      horizontal alveolar K06.3 ◄
    cartilage —*see* Disorder, cartilage, specified type NEC
      auricle (ear) —*see* Disorder, pinna, specified type NEC
    vitreous (humor) H15.89
  tooth, teeth —*see* Absence, teeth, acquired
  vision, visual H54.7
    both eyes H54.3
    one eye H54.60
      left (normal vision on right) H54.62
      right (normal vision on left) H54.61

Loss *(Continued)*
  vision, visual *(Continued)*
    specified as blindness —*see* Blindness
    subjective
      sudden H53.13-
      transient H53.12-
    vitreous —*see* Prolapse, vitreous
    voice —*see* Aphonia
    weight (abnormal) (cause unknown) R63.4
Louis-Bar syndrome (ataxia-telangiectasia)
    G11.3
Louping ill (encephalitis) A84.8
Louse, lousiness —*see* Lice
Low
  achiever, school Z55.3
  back syndrome M54.5
  basal metabolic rate R94.8
  birthweight (2499 grams or less) P07.10
    with weight of
      1000-1249 grams P07.14
      1250-1499 grams P07.15
      1500-1749 grams P07.16
      1750-1999 grams P07.17
      2000-2499 grams P07.18
    extreme (999 grams or less) P07.00
      with weight of
        499 grams or less P07.01
        500-749 grams P07.02
        750-999 grams P07.03
    for gestational age —*see* Light for dates
  blood pressure —*see also* Hypotension
    reading (incidental) (isolated) (nonspecific)
      R03.1
  cardiac reserve —*see* Disease, heart
  function —*see also* Hypofunction
    kidney N28.9
  hematocrit D64.9
  hemoglobin D64.9
  income Z59.6
  level of literacy Z55.0
  lying
    kidney N28.89
    organ or site, congenital —*see* Malposition,
      congenital
  output syndrome (cardiac) —*see* Failure,
    heart
  platelets (blood) —*see* Thrombocytopenia
  reserve, kidney N28.89
  salt syndrome E87.1
  self esteem R45.81
  set ears Q17.4
  vision H54.2
    one eye (other eye normal) H54.50
      left (normal vision on right) H54.52
      other eye blind —*see* Blindness
      right (normal vision on left) H54.51
Low-density-lipoprotein-type (LDL)
    hyperlipoproteinemia E78.00 ◄▥
Lowe's syndrome E72.03
Lown-Ganong-Levine syndrome I45.6
LSD reaction (acute) (without dependence)
    F16.90
  with dependence F16.20
L-shaped kidney Q63.8
Ludwig's angina or disease K12.2
Lues (venerea), luetic —*see* Syphilis
Luetscher's syndrome (dehydration) E86.0
Lumbago, lumbalgia M54.5
  with sciatica M54.4-
    due to intervertebral disc disorder
      M51.17
  due to displacement, intervertebral disc
    M51.27
    with sciatica M51.17
Lumbar —*see* condition
Lumbarization, vertebra, congenital Q76.49
Lumbermen's itch B88.0
Lump —*see* Mass
Lunacy —*see* Psychosis
Lung —*see* condition
Lupoid (miliary) of Boeck D86.3

Lupus
  anticoagulant D68.62
    with
      hemorrhagic disorder D68.312
      hypercoagulable state D68.62
    finding without diagnosis R76.0
  discoid (local) L93.0
  erythematosus (discoid) (local) L93.0
    disseminated —*see* Lupus, erythematosus,
      systemic
    eyelid H01.129
      left H01.126
        lower H01.125
        upper H01.124
      right H01.123
        lower H01.122
        upper H01.121
    profundus L93.2
    specified NEC L93.2
    subacute cutaneous L93.1
    systemic M32.9
      with organ or system involvement
        M32.10
        endocarditis M32.11
        lung M32.13
        pericarditis M32.12
        renal (glomerular) M32.14
          tubulo-interstitial M32.15
        specified organ or system NEC
          M32.19
      drug-induced M32.0
      inhibitor (presence of) D68.62
        with
          hemorrhagic disorder D68.312
          hypercoagulable state D68.62
        finding without diagnosis R76.0
      specified NEC M32.8
  exedens A18.4
  hydralazine M32.0
    correct substance properly administered —
      see Table of Drugs and Chemicals, by
      drug, adverse effect
    overdose or wrong substance given or
      taken —*see* Table of Drugs and
      Chemicals, by drug, poisoning
  nephritis (chronic) M32.14
  nontuberculous, not disseminated L93.0
  panniculitis L93.2
  pernio (Besnier) D86.3
  systemic —*see* Lupus, erythematosus,
    systemic
  tuberculous A18.4
    eyelid A18.4
  vulgaris A18.4
    eyelid A18.4
Luteinoma D27.-
Lutembacher's disease or syndrome (atrial
    septal defect with mitral stenosis)
    Q21.1
Luteoma D27.-
Lutz (-Splendore-de Almeida) disease —*see*
    Paracoccidioidomycosis
Luxation —*see also* Dislocation
  eyeball (nontraumatic) —*see* Luxation, globe
    birth injury P15.3
  globe, nontraumatic H44.82-
  lacrimal gland —*see* Dislocation, lacrimal
    gland
  lens (old) (partial) (spontaneous)
    congenital Q12.1
    syphilitic A50.39
Lycanthropy F22
Lyell's syndrome L51.2
  due to drug L51.2
    correct substance properly administered —
      see Table of Drugs and Chemicals, by
      drug, adverse effect
    overdose or wrong substance given or
      taken —*see* Table of Drugs and
      Chemicals, by drug, poisoning
Lyme disease A69.20

Lymph
  gland or node —*see* condition
  scrotum —*see* Infestation, filarial
Lymphadenitis I88.9
  with ectopic or molar pregnancy O08.0
  acute L04.9
    axilla L04.2
    face L04.0
    head L04.0
    hip L04.3
    limb
      lower L04.3
      upper L04.2
    neck L04.0
    shoulder L04.2
    specified site NEC L04.8
    trunk L04.1
  anthracosis (occupational) J60
  any site, except mesenteric I88.9
    chronic I88.1
    subacute I88.1
  breast
    gestational —*see* Mastitis, obstetric
    puerperal, postpartum (nonpurulent)
      O91.22
  chancroidal (congenital) A57
  chronic I88.1
    mesenteric I88.0
  due to
    Brugia (malayi) B74.1
      timori B74.2
    chlamydial lymphogranuloma A55
    diphtheria (toxin) A36.89
    lymphogranuloma venereum A55
    Wuchereria bancrofti B74.0
  following ectopic or molar pregnancy O08.0
  gonorrheal A54.89
  infective —*see* Lymphadenitis, acute
  mesenteric (acute) (chronic) (nonspecific)
      (subacute) I88.0
    due to Salmonella typhi A01.09
    tuberculous A18.39
  mycobacterial A31.8
  purulent —*see* Lymphadenitis, acute
  pyogenic —*see* Lymphadenitis, acute
  regional, nonbacterial I88.8
  septic —*see* Lymphadenitis, acute
  subacute, unspecified site I88.1
  suppurative —*see* Lymphadenitis, acute
  syphilitic (early) (secondary) A51.49
    late A52.79
  tuberculous —*see* Tuberculosis, lymph gland
  venereal (chlamydial) A55
Lymphadenoid goiter E06.3
Lymphadenopathy (generalized) R59.1
  angioimmunoblastic, with dysproteinemia
      (AILD) C86.5
  due to toxoplasmosis (acquired) B58.89
    congenital (acute) (subacute) (chronic)
      P37.1
  localized R59.0
  syphilitic (early) (secondary) A51.49
Lymphadenosis R59.1
Lymphangiectasis I89.0
  conjunctiva H11.89
  postinfectional I89.0
  scrotum I89.0
Lymphangiectatic elephantiasis, nonfilarial
    I89.0
Lymphangioendothelioma D18.1
  malignant —*see* Neoplasm, connective tissue,
    malignant
Lymphangioleiomyomatosis J84.81
Lymphangioma D18.1
  capillary D18.1
  cavernous D18.1
  cystic D18.1
  malignant —*see* Neoplasm, connective tissue,
    malignant
Lymphangiomyoma D18.1
Lymphangiomyomatosis J84.81

◄ New   ◄▥ Revised   ~~deleted~~ Deleted

Lymphangiosarcoma —see Neoplasm, connective tissue, malignant

Lymphangitis I89.1
  with
    abscess - code by site under Abscess
    cellulitis - code by site under Cellulitis
    ectopic or molar pregnancy O08.0
  acute L03.91
    abdominal wall L03.321
    ankle —see Lymphangitis, acute, lower limb
    arm —see Lymphangitis, acute, upper limb
    auricle (ear) —see Lymphangitis, acute, ear
    axilla L03.12-
    back (any part) L03.322
    buttock L03.327
    cervical (meaning neck) L03.222
    cheek (external) L03.212
    chest wall L03.323
    digit
      finger —see Lymphangitis, acute, finger
      toe —see Lymphangitis, acute, toe
    ear (external) H60.1-
    external auditory canal —see Lymphangitis, acute, ear
    eyelid —see Abscess, eyelid
    face NEC L03.212
    finger (intrathecal) (periosteal) (subcutaneous) (subcuticular) L03.02-
    foot —see Lymphangitis, acute, lower limb
    gluteal (region) L03.327
    groin L03.324
    hand —see Lymphangitis, acute, upper limb
    head NEC L03.891
      face (any part, except ear, eye and nose) L03.212
    heel —see Lymphangitis, acute, lower limb
    hip —see Lymphangitis, acute, lower limb
    jaw (region) L03.212
    knee —see Lymphangitis, acute, lower limb
    leg —see Lymphangitis, acute, lower limb
    lower limb L03.12-
      toe —see Lymphangitis, acute, toe
    navel L03.326
    neck (region) L03.222
    orbit, orbital —see Cellulitis, orbit
    pectoral (region) L03.323
    perineal, perineum L03.325
    scalp (any part) L03.891
    shoulder —see Lymphangitis, acute, upper limb
    specified site NEC L03.898
    thigh —see Lymphangitis, acute, lower limb
    thumb (intrathecal) (periosteal) (subcutaneous) (subcuticular) —see Lymphangitis, acute, finger
    toe (intrathecal) (periosteal) (subcutaneous) (subcuticular) L03.04-
    trunk L03.329
      abdominal wall L03.321
      back (any part) L03.322
      buttock L03.327
      chest wall L03.323
      groin L03.324
      perineal, perineum L03.325
      umbilicus L03.326
    umbilicus L03.326
    upper limb L03.12-
      axilla —see Lymphangitis, acute, axilla
      finger —see Lymphangitis, acute, finger
      thumb —see Lymphangitis, acute, finger
    wrist —see Lymphangitis, acute, upper limb
  breast
    gestational —see Mastitis, obstetric
  chancroidal A57
  chronic (any site) I89.1

Lymphangitis (Continued)
  due to
    Brugia (malayi) B74.1
      timori B74.2
    Wuchereria bancrofti B74.0
  following ectopic or molar pregnancy O08.89
  penis
    acute N48.29
    gonococcal (acute) (chronic) A54.09
  puerperal, postpartum, childbirth O86.89
  strumous, tuberculous A18.2
  subacute (any site) I89.1
  tuberculous —see Tuberculosis, lymph gland

Lymphatic (vessel) —see condition

Lymphatism E32.8

Lymphectasia I89.0

Lymphedema (acquired) —see also Elephantiasis
  congenital Q82.0
  hereditary (chronic) (idiopathic) Q82.0
  postmastectomy I97.2
  praecox I89.0
  secondary I89.0
  surgical NEC I97.89
    postmastectomy (syndrome) I97.2

Lymphoblastic —see condition

Lymphoblastoma (diffuse) —see Lymphoma, lymphoblastic (diffuse)
  giant follicular —see Lymphoma, lymphoblastic (diffuse)
  macrofollicular —see Lymphoma, lymphoblastic (diffuse)

Lymphocele I89.8

Lymphocytic
  chorioencephalitis (acute) (serous) A87.2
  choriomeningitis (acute) (serous) A87.2
  meningoencephalitis A87.2

Lymphocytoma, benign cutis L98.8

Lymphocytopenia D72.810

Lymphocytosis (symptomatic) D72.820
  infectious (acute) B33.8

Lymphoepithelioma —see Neoplasm, malignant, by site

Lymphogranuloma (malignant) —see also Lymphoma, Hodgkin
  chlamydial A55
  inguinale A55
  venereum (any site) (chlamydial) (with stricture of rectum) A55

Lymphogranulomatosis (malignant) —see also Lymphoma, Hodgkin
  benign (Boeck's sarcoid) (Schaumann's) D86.1

Lymphohistiocytosis, hemophagocytic (familial) D76.1

Lymphoid —see condition

Lymphoma (of) (malignant) C85.90
  adult T-cell (HTLV-1-associated) (acute variant) (chronic variant) (lymphomatoid variant) (smouldering variant) C91.5-
  anaplastic large cell
    ALK-negative C84.7-
    ALK-positive C84.6-
    CD30-positive C84.6-
    primary cutaneous C86.6
  angioimmunoblastic T-cell C86.5
  BALT C88.4
  B-cell C85.1-
  B-precursor C83.5-
  blastic NK-cell C86.4
  bronchial-associated lymphoid tissue [BALT-lymphoma] C88.4
  Burkitt (atypical) C83.7-
  Burkitt-like C83.7-
  centrocytic C83.1-
  cutaneous follicle center C82.6-
  cutaneous T-cell C84.A-
  diffuse follicle center C82.5-
  diffuse large cell C83.3-
    anaplastic C83.3-
    B-cell C83.3-

Lymphoma (Continued)
  diffuse large cell (Continued)
    CD30-positive C83.3-
    centroblastic C83.3-
    immunoblastic C83.3-
    plasmablastic C83.3-
    subtype not specified C83.3-
    T-cell rich C83.3-
  enteropathy-type (associated) (intestinal) T-cell C86.2
  extranodal marginal zone B-cell lymphoma of mucosa-associated lymphoid tissue [MALT-lymphoma] C88.4
  extranodal NK/T-cell, nasal type C86.0
  follicular C82.9-
    grade
      I C82.0-
      II C82.1-
      III C82.2-
      IIIa C82.3-
      IIIb C82.4-
    specified NEC C82.8-
  hepatosplenic T-cell (alpha-beta) (gamma-delta) C86.1
  histiocytic C85.9-
    true C96.A
  Hodgkin C81.9
    classical C81.7-
      lymphocyte-rich C81.4-
      lymphocytic depletion C81.3-
      mixed cellularity C81.2-
      nodular sclerosis C81.1-
      specified NEC C81.7-
    lymphocyte-rich (classical) C81.4- ◄
    lymphocyte depleted (classical) C81.3- ◄
    mixed cellularity (classical) C81.2- ◄
    nodular sclerosis (classical) C81.1- ◄
    specified NEC (classical) C81.7- ◄
    lymphocyte-rich classical C81.4-
    lymphocyte depleted classical C81.3-
    mixed cellularity classical C81.2-
    nodular
      lymphocyte predominant C81.0-
      sclerosis classical C81.1-
      sclerosis (classical) C81.1- ◄
  intravascular large B-cell C83.8-
  Lennert's C84.4-
  lymphoblastic (diffuse) C83.5-
  lymphoblastic B-cell C83.5-
  lymphoblastic T-cell C83.5-
  lymphoepithelioid C84.4-
  lymphoplasmacytic C83.0-
    with IgM-production C88.0
  MALT C88.4
  mantle cell C83.1-
  mature T-cell NEC C84.4-
  mature T/NK-cell C84.9-
    specified NEC C84.Z-
  mediastinal (thymic) large B-cell C85.2-
  Mediterranean C88.3
  mucosa-associated lymphoid tissue [MALT-lymphoma] C88.4
  NK/T cell C84.9-
  nodal marginal zone C83.0-
  non-follicular (diffuse) C83.9-
    specified NEC C83.8-
  non-Hodgkin —see also Lymphoma, by type C85.9-
    specified NEC C85.8-
  non-leukemic variant of B-CLL C83.0-
  peripheral T-cell, not classified C84.4-
  primary cutaneous
    anaplastic large cell C86.6
    CD30-positive large T-cell C86.6
  primary effusion B-cell C83.8-
  SALT C88.4
  skin-associated lymphoid tissue [SALT-lymphoma] C88.4

Lymphoma *(Continued)*
  small cell B-cell C83.0-
  splenic marginal zone C83.0-
  subcutaneous panniculitis-like T-cell
      C86.3
  T-precursor C83.5-
  true histiocytic C96.A
Lymphomatosis —*see* Lymphoma

Lymphopathia venereum, veneris A55
Lymphopenia D72.810
Lymphoplasmacytic leukemia —*see* Leukemia,
    chronic lymphocytic, B-cell type
Lymphoproliferation, X-linked disease
    D82.3
Lymphoreticulosis, benign (of inoculation)
    A28.1

Lymphorrhea I89.8
Lymphosarcoma (diffuse) —*see also* Lymphoma
    C85.9-
Lymphostasis I89.8
Lypemania —*see* Melancholia
Lysine and hydroxylysine metabolism
    disorder E72.3
Lyssa —*see* Rabies

◀ New ◀▥ Revised ~~deleted~~ Deleted

M

Macacus ear Q17.3
Maceration, wet feet, tropical (syndrome)
    T69.02-
MacLeod's syndrome J43.0
Macrocephalia, macrocephaly Q75.3
Macrocheilia, macrochilia (congenital)Q18.6
Macrocolon —see also Megacolon Q43.1
Macrocornea Q15.8
    with glaucoma Q15.0
Macrocytic —see condition
Macrocytosis D75.89
Macrodactylia, macrodactylism (fingers)
        (thumbs) Q74.0
    toes Q74.2
Macrodontia K00.2
Macrogenia M26.05
Macrogenitosomia (adrenal) (male) (praecox)
        E25.9
    congenital E25.0
Macroglobulinemia (idiopathic) (primary)
        C88.0
    monoclonal (essential) D47.2
    Waldenström C88.0
Macroglossia (congenital) Q38.2
    acquired K14.8
Macrognathia, macrognathism (congenital)
        (mandibular) (maxillary) M26.09
Macrogyria (congenital) Q04.8
Macrohydrocephalus —see Hydrocephalus
Macromastia —see Hypertrophy, breast
Macrophthalmos Q11.3
    in congenital glaucoma Q15.0
Macropsia H53.15
Macrosigmoid K59.39 ◄▥
    congenital Q43.2
Macrospondylitis, acromegalic E22.0
Macrostomia (congenital) Q18.4
Macrotia (external ear) (congenital) Q17.1
Macula
    cornea, corneal —see Opacity, cornea
    degeneration (atrophic) (exudative)
            (senile) —see also Degeneration, macula
        hereditary —see Dystrophy, retina
Maculae ceruleae — B85.1
Maculopathy, toxic —see Degeneration, macula,
        toxic
Madarosis (eyelid) H02.729
    left H02.726
        lower H02.725
        upper H02.724
    right H02.723
        lower H02.722
        upper H02.721
Madelung's
    deformity (radius) Q74.0
    disease
        radial deformity Q74.0
        symmetrical lipomas, neck E88.89
Madness —see Psychosis
Madura
    foot B47.9
        actinomycotic B47.1
        mycotic B47.0
Maduromycosis B47.0
Maffucci's syndrome Q78.4
Magnesium metabolism disorder —see
        Disorder, metabolism, magnesium
Main en griffe (acquired) —see also Deformity,
        limb, clawhand
    congenital Q74.0
Maintenance (encounter for)
    antineoplastic chemotherapy Z51.11
    antineoplastic radiation therapy Z51.0
    methadone F11.20
Majocchi's
    disease L81.7
    granuloma B35.8
Major —see condition
Malabar itch (any site) B35.5

Malabsorption K90.9
    calcium K90.89
    carbohydrate K90.49 ◄▥
    disaccharide E73.9
    fat K90.49 ◄▥
    galactose E74.20
    glucose(-galactose) E74.39
    intestinal K90.9
        specified NEC K90.89
    isomaltose E74.31
    lactose E73.9
    methionine E72.19
    monosaccharide E74.39
    postgastrectomy K91.2
    postsurgical K91.2
    protein K90.49 ◄▥
    starch K90.49 ◄▥
    sucrose E74.39
    syndrome K90.9
        postsurgical K91.2
Malacia, bone (adult) M83.9
    juvenile —see Rickets
Malacoplakia
    bladder N32.89
    pelvis (kidney) N28.89
    ureter N28.89
    urethra N36.8
Malacosteon, juvenile —see Rickets
Maladaptation —see Maladjustment
Maladie de Roger Q21.0
Maladjustment
    conjugal Z63.0
        involving divorce or estrangement Z63.5
    educational Z55.4
    family Z63.9
    marital Z63.0
        involving divorce or estrangement Z63.5
    occupational NEC Z56.89
    simple, adult —see Disorder, adjustment
    situational —see Disorder, adjustment
    social Z60.9
        due to
            acculturation difficulty Z60.3
            discrimination and persecution
                (perceived) Z60.5
            exclusion and isolation Z60.4
            life-cycle (phase of life) transition Z60.0
            rejection Z60.4
            specified reason NEC Z60.8
Malaise R53.81
Malakoplakia —see Malacoplakia
Malaria, malarial (fever) B54
    with
        blackwater fever B50.8
            hemoglobinuric (bilious) B50.8
            hemoglobinuria B50.8
    accidentally induced (therapeutically) - code
            by type under Malaria
    algid B50.9
    cerebral B50.0 [G94]
    clinically diagnosed (without parasitological
            confirmation) B54
    congenital NEC P37.4
        falciparum P37.3
    congestion, congestive B54
    continued (fever) B50.9
    estivo-autumnal B50.9
    falciparum B50.9
        with complications NEC B50.8
            cerebral B50.0 [G94]
            severe B50.8
        hemorrhagic B54
        malariae B52.9
            with
                complications NEC B52.8
                glomerular disorder B52.0
    malignant (tertian) —see Malaria, falciparum
    mixed infections — code to first listed type
            in B50-B53
    ovale B53.0
    parasitologically confirmed NEC B53.8

Malaria, malarial (Continued)
    pernicious, acute —see Malaria, falciparum
    Plasmodium (P.)
        falciparum NEC —see Malaria, falciparum
        malariae NEC B52.9
            with Plasmodium
                falciparum (and or vivax) —see
                    Malaria, falciparum
                vivax —see also Malaria, vivax
                    and falciparum —see Malaria,
                        falciparum
        ovale B53.0
            with Plasmodium malariae —see also
                Malaria, malariae
                and vivax —see also Malaria, vivax
                    and falciparum —see Malaria,
                        falciparum
        simian B53.1
            with Plasmodium malariae —see also
                Malaria, malariae
                and vivax —see also Malaria, vivax
                    and falciparum —see Malaria,
                        falciparum
        vivax NEC B51.9
            with Plasmodium falciparum —see
                Malaria, falciparum
    quartan —see Malaria, malariae
    quotidian —see Malaria, falciparum
    recurrent B54
    remittent B54
    specified type NEC (parasitologically
            confirmed) B53.8
    spleen B54
    subtertian (fever) —see Malaria, falciparum
    tertian (benign) —see also Malaria, vivax
        malignant B50.9
    tropical B50.9
    typhoid B54
    vivax B51.9
        with
            complications NEC B51.8
            ruptured spleen B51.0
Malassez's disease (cystic) N50.89 ◄▥
Malassimilation K90.9
Mal de los pintos —see Pinta
Mal de mer T75.3
Maldescent, testis Q53.9
    bilateral Q53.20
        abdominal Q53.21
        perineal Q53.22
    unilateral Q53.10
        abdominal Q53.11
        perineal Q53.12
Maldevelopment —see also Anomaly
    brain Q07.9
    colon Q43.9
    hip Q74.2
        congenital dislocation Q65.2
            bilateral Q65.1
            unilateral Q65.0-
    mastoid process Q75.8
    middle ear Q16.4
        except ossicles Q16.4
        ossicles Q16.3
    ossicles Q16.3
    spine Q76.49
    toe Q74.2
Male type pelvis Q74.2
    with disproportion (fetopelvic) O33.3
        causing obstructed labor O65.3
Malformation (congenital) —see also Anomaly
    adrenal gland Q89.1
    affecting multiple systems with skeletal
            changes NEC Q87.5
    alimentary tract Q45.9
        specified type NEC Q45.8
        upper Q40.9
            specified type NEC Q40.8
    aorta Q25.40 ◄▥
        absence Q25.41 ◄
        aneurysm, congenital Q25.43 ◄

Malformation *(Continued)*
 aorta *(Continued)*
  aplasia Q25.41 ◀
  atresia Q25.29 ◀▥
   aortic arch Q25.21 ◀
  coarctation (preductal) (postductal) Q25.1
  dilatation, congenital Q25.44 ◀
  hypoplasia Q25.42 ◀
  patent ductus arteriosus Q25.0
  specified type NEC Q25.49 ◀▥
  stenosis Q25.1 ◀▥
   supravalvular Q25.3 ◀
 aortic valve Q23.9
  specified NEC Q23.8
 arteriovenous, aneurysmatic (congenital)
   Q27.30
  brain Q28.2
  cerebral Q28.2
  peripheral Q27.30
   digestive system Q27.33
   lower limb Q27.32
   other specified site Q27.39
   renal vessel Q27.34
   upper limb Q27.31
  precerebral vessels (nonruptured)
    Q28.0
 auricle
  ear (congenital) Q17.3
   acquired H61.119
    left H61.112
     with right H61.113
    right H61.111
     with left H61.113
 bile duct Q44.5
 bladder Q64.79
  aplasia Q64.5
  diverticulum Q64.6
  exstrophy —*see* Exstrophy, bladder
  neck obstruction Q64.31
 bone Q79.9
  face Q75.9
   specified type NEC Q75.8
  skull Q75.9
   specified type NEC Q75.8
 brain (multiple) Q04.9
  arteriovenous Q28.2
  specified type NEC Q04.8
 branchial cleft Q18.2
 breast Q83.9
  specified type NEC Q83.8
 broad ligament Q50.6
 bronchus Q32.4
 bursa Q79.9
 cardiac
  chambers Q20.9
   specified type NEC Q20.8
  septum Q21.9
   specified type NEC Q21.8
 cerebral Q04.9
  vessels Q28.3
 cervix uteri Q51.9
  specified type NEC Q51.828
 Chiari
  Type I G93.5
  Type II Q07.01
 choroid (congenital) Q14.3
  plexus Q07.8
 circulatory system Q28.9
 cochlea Q16.5
 cornea Q13.4
 coronary vessels Q24.5
 corpus callosum (congenital) Q04.0
 diaphragm Q79.1
 digestive system NEC, specified type NEC
   Q45.8
 dura Q07.9
  brain Q04.9
  spinal Q06.9
 ear Q17.9
  causing impairment of hearing
    Q16.9

Malformation *(Continued)*
 ear *(Continued)*
  external Q17.9
   accessory auricle Q17.0
   causing impairment of hearing Q16.9
    absence of
     auditory canal Q16.1
     auricle Q16.0
   macrotia Q17.1
   microtia Q17.2
   misplacement Q17.4
   misshapen NEC Q17.3
   prominence Q17.5
   specified type NEC Q17.8
  inner Q16.5
  middle Q16.4
   absence of eustachian tube Q16.2
   ossicles (fusion) Q16.3
  ossicles Q16.3
  specified type NEC Q17.8
 epididymis Q55.4
 esophagus Q39.9
  specified type NEC Q39.8
 eye Q15.9
  lid Q10.3
  specified NEC Q15.8
 fallopian tube Q50.6
 genital organ —*see* Anomaly, genitalia
 great
  artery Q25.9
   aorta —*see* Malformation, aorta
   pulmonary artery —*see* Malformation,
     pulmonary, artery
   specified type NEC Q25.8
  vein Q26.9
   anomalous
    portal venous connection Q26.5
    pulmonary venous connection Q26.4
     partial Q26.3
     total Q26.2
   persistent left superior vena cava Q26.1
   portal vein-hepatic artery fistula Q26.6
   specified type NEC Q26.8
   vena cava stenosis, congenital Q26.0
 gum Q38.6
 hair Q84.2
 heart Q24.9
  specified type NEC Q24.8
 integument Q84.9
  specified type NEC Q84.8
 internal ear Q16.5
 intestine Q43.9
  specified type NEC Q43.8
 iris Q13.2
 joint Q74.9
  ankle Q74.2
  lumbosacral Q76.49
  sacroiliac Q74.2
  specified type NEC Q74.8
 kidney Q63.9
  accessory Q63.0
  giant Q63.3
  horseshoe Q63.1
  hydronephrosis Q62.0
  malposition Q63.2
  specified type NEC Q63.8
 lacrimal apparatus Q10.6
 lingual Q38.3
 lip Q38.0
 liver Q44.7
 lung Q33.9
 meninges or membrane (congenital)
   Q07.9
  cerebral Q04.8
  spinal (cord) Q06.9
 middle ear Q16.4
  ossicles Q16.3
 mitral valve Q23.9
  specified NEC Q23.8
 Mondini's (congenital) (malformation,
   cochlea) Q16.5

Malformation *(Continued)*
 mouth (congenital) Q38.6
 multiple types NEC Q89.7
 musculoskeletal system Q79.9
 myocardium Q24.8
 nail Q84.6
 nervous system (central) Q07.9
 nose Q30.9
  specified type NEC Q30.8
 optic disc Q14.2
 orbit Q10.7
 ovary Q50.39
 palate Q38.5
 parathyroid gland Q89.2
 pelvic organs or tissues NEC
  in pregnancy or childbirth O34.8-
   causing obstructed labor O65.5
 penis Q55.69
  aplasia Q55.5
  curvature (lateral) Q55.61
  hypoplasia Q55.62
 pericardium Q24.8
 peripheral vascular system Q27.9
  specified type NEC Q27.8
 pharynx Q38.8
 precerebral vessels Q28.1
 prostate Q55.4
 pulmonary
  arteriovenous Q25.72
  artery Q25.9
   atresia Q25.5
   specified type NEC Q25.79
   stenosis Q25.6
  valve Q22.3
 renal artery Q27.2
 respiratory system Q34.9
 retina Q14.1
 scrotum —*see* Malformation, testis and
   scrotum
 seminal vesicles Q55.4
 sense organs NEC Q07.9
 skin Q82.9
 specified NEC Q89.8
 spinal
  cord Q06.9
  nerve root Q07.8
 spine Q76.49
  kyphosis —*see* Kyphosis, congenital
  lordosis —*see* Lordosis, congenital
 spleen Q89.09
 stomach Q40.3
  specified type NEC Q40.2
 teeth, tooth K00.9
 tendon Q79.9
 testis and scrotum Q55.20
  aplasia Q55.0
  hypoplasia Q55.1
  polyorchism Q55.21
  retractile testis Q55.22
  scrotal transposition Q55.23
  specified NEC Q55.29
 thorax, bony Q76.9
 throat Q38.8
 thyroid gland Q89.2
 tongue (congenital) Q38.3
  hypertrophy Q38.2
  tie Q38.1
 trachea Q32.1
 tricuspid valve Q22.9
  specified type NEC Q22.8
 umbilical cord NEC (complicating delivery)
   O69.89
 umbilicus Q89.9
 ureter Q62.8
  agenesis Q62.4
  duplication Q62.5
  malposition —*see* Malposition, congenital,
    ureter
  obstructive defect —*see* Defect, obstructive,
    ureter
  vesico-uretero-renal reflux Q62.7

◀ New   ◀▥ Revised   ~~deleted~~ Deleted

Malformation (Continued)
  urethra Q64.79
    aplasia Q64.5
    duplication Q64.74
    posterior valves Q64.2
    prolapse Q64.71
    stricture Q64.32
  urinary system Q64.9
  uterus Q51.9
    specified type NEC Q51.818
  vagina Q52.4
  vascular system, peripheral Q27.9
  vas deferens Q55.4
    atresia Q55.3
  venous —see Anomaly, vein (s)
  vulva Q52.70
Malfunction —see also Dysfunction
  cardiac electronic device T82.119
    electrode T82.110
    pulse generator T82.111
    specified type NEC T82.118
  catheter device NEC T85.618
    cystostomy T83.010
    dialysis (renal) (vascular) T82.41
      intraperitoneal T85.611
    infusion NEC T82.514
      cranial T85.610 ◀
      epidural T85.610 ◀
      intrathecal T85.610 ◀
      spinal T85.610 ◀ⅢⅢ
      subarachnoid T85.610 ◀
      subdural T85.610 ◀
      urinary, indwelling T83.018
    urinary —see also Breakdown, device,
      catheter T83.018 ◀
  colostomy K94.03
    valve K94.03
  cystostomy (stoma) N99.512
    catheter T83.010
  enteric stoma K94.13
  enterostomy K94.13
  esophagostomy K94.33
  gastroenteric K31.89
  gastrostomy K94.23
  ileostomy K94.13
    valve K94.13
  intrathecal infusion pump T85.615 ◀
  jejunostomy K94.13
  nervous system device, implant or graft,
    specified NEC T85.615 ◀
  pacemaker —see Malfunction, cardiac
    electronic device
  prosthetic device, internal —see
    Complications, prosthetic device, by
    site, mechanical
  tracheostomy J95.03
  urinary device NEC —see Complication,
    genitourinary, device, urinary,
    mechanical
  valve
    colostomy K94.03
    heart T82.09
    ileostomy K94.13
  vascular graft or shunt NEC —see
    Complication, cardiovascular device,
    mechanical, vascular
  ventricular (communicating shunt) T85.01
Malherbe's tumor —see Neoplasm, skin, benign
Malibu disease L98.8-
Malignancy —see also Neoplasm, malignant,
  by site
  unspecified site (primary) C80.1
Malignant —see condition
Malingerer, malingering Z76.5
Mallet finger (acquired) —see Deformity, finger,
  mallet finger
  congenital Q74.0
  sequelae of rickets E64.3
Malleus A24.0
Mallory's bodies R89.7
Mallory-Weiss syndrome K22.6

Malnutrition E46
  degree
    first E44.1
    mild (protein) E44.1
    moderate (protein) E44.0
    second E44.0
    severe (protein-energy) E43
      intermediate form E42
        with
          kwashiorkor (and marasmus) E42
          marasmus E41
    third E43
  following gastrointestinal surgery K91.2
  intrauterine
    light-for-dates —see Light for dates
    small-for-dates —see Small for dates
  lack of care, or neglect (child) (infant) T76.02
    confirmed T74.02
  malignant E40
  protein E46
    calorie E46
      mild E44.1
      moderate E44.0
      severe E43
        intermediate form E42
          with
            kwashiorkor (and marasmus)
              E42
            marasmus E41
    energy E46
      mild E44.1
      moderate E44.0
      severe E43
        intermediate form E42
          with
            kwashiorkor (and marasmus)
              E42
            marasmus E41
  severe (protein-energy) E43
    with
      kwashiorkor (and marasmus) E42
      marasmus E41
Malocclusion (teeth) M26.4
  Angle's M26.219
    class I M26.211
    class II M26.212
    class III M26.213
  due to
    abnormal swallowing M26.59
    mouth breathing M26.59
    tongue, lip or finger habits M26.59
  temporomandibular (joint) M26.69
Malposition
  cervix —see Malposition, uterus
  congenital
    adrenal (gland) Q89.1
    alimentary tract Q45.8
      lower Q43.8
      upper Q40.8
    aorta Q25.49 ◀ⅢⅢ
    appendix Q43.8
    arterial trunk Q20.0
    artery (peripheral) Q27.8
      coronary Q24.5
      digestive system Q27.8
      lower limb Q27.8
      pulmonary Q25.79
      specified site NEC Q27.8
      upper limb Q27.8
    auditory canal Q17.8
      causing impairment of hearing Q16.9
    auricle (ear) Q17.4
      causing impairment of hearing Q16.9
    cervical Q18.2
    biliary duct or passage Q44.5
    bladder (mucosa) —see Exstrophy,
      bladder
    brachial plexus Q07.8
    brain tissue Q04.8
    breast Q83.8
    bronchus Q32.4

Malposition (Continued)
  congenital (Continued)
    cecum Q43.8
    clavicle Q74.0
    colon Q43.8
    digestive organ or tract NEC Q45.8
      lower Q43.8
      upper Q40.8
    ear (auricle) (external) Q17.4
      ossicles Q16.3
    endocrine (gland) NEC Q89.2
    epiglottis Q31.8
    eustachian tube Q17.8
    eye Q15.8
    facial features Q18.8
    fallopian tube Q50.6
    finger (s) Q68.1
      supernumerary Q69.0
    foot Q66.9
    gallbladder Q44.1
    gastrointestinal tract Q45.8
    genitalia, genital organ (s) or tract
      female Q52.8
        external Q52.79
        internal NEC Q52.8
      male Q55.8
    glottis Q31.8
    hand Q68.1
    heart Q24.8
      dextrocardia Q24.0
        with complete transposition of viscera
          Q89.3
    hepatic duct Q44.5
    hip (joint) Q65.89
    intestine (large) (small) Q43.8
      with anomalous adhesions, fixation or
        malrotation Q43.3
    joint NEC Q68.8
    kidney Q63.2
    larynx Q31.8
    limb Q68.8
      lower Q68.8
      upper Q68.8
    liver Q44.7
    lung (lobe) Q33.8
    nail (s) Q84.6
    nerve Q07.8
    nervous system NEC Q07.8
    nose, nasal (septum) Q30.8
    organ or site not listed —see Anomaly,
      by site
    ovary Q50.39
    pancreas Q45.3
    parathyroid (gland) Q89.2
    patella Q74.1
    peripheral vascular system Q27.8
    pituitary (gland) Q89.2
    respiratory organ or system NEC
      Q34.8
    rib (cage) Q76.6
      supernumerary in cervical region
        Q76.5
    scapula Q74.0
    shoulder Q74.0
    spinal cord Q06.8
    spleen Q89.09
    sternum NEC Q76.7
    stomach Q40.2
    symphysis pubis Q74.2
    thymus (gland) Q89.2
    thyroid (gland) (tissue) Q89.2
      cartilage Q31.8
    toe (s) Q66.9
      supernumerary Q69.2
    tongue Q38.3
    trachea Q32.1
    ureter Q62.60
      deviation Q62.61
      displacement Q62.62
      ectopia Q62.63
      specified type NEC Q62.69

M

Malposition *(Continued)*
  congenital *(Continued)*
    uterus Q51.818
    vein (s) (peripheral) Q27.8
      great Q26.8
    vena cava (inferior) (superior) Q26.8
  device, implant or graft —*see also*
    Complications, by site and type,
    mechanical T85.628
    arterial graft NEC —*see* Complication,
      cardiovascular device, mechanical,
      vascular
    breast (implant) T85.42
    catheter NEC T85.628
      cystostomy T83.020
      dialysis (renal) T82.42
        intraperitoneal T85.621
      infusion NEC T82.524
        spinal (epidural) (subdural) T85.620
      urinary, indwelling T83.028
      urinary —*see also* Displacement, device,
        catheter, urinary T83.028 ◀
    electronic (electrode) (pulse generator)
      (stimulator)
      bone T84.320
      cardiac T82.129
        electrode T82.120
        pulse generator T82.121
        specified type NEC T82.128
      nervous system —*see* Complication,
        prosthetic device, mechanical,
        electronic nervous system
        stimulator
      urinary —*see* Complication,
        genitourinary, device, urinary,
        mechanical
    fixation, internal (orthopedic) NEC —*see*
      Complication, fixation device,
      mechanical
    gastrointestinal —*see* Complications,
      prosthetic device, mechanical,
      gastrointestinal device
    genital NEC T83.428
      intrauterine contraceptive device (string)
        T83.32 ◀▥
      penile prosthesis (cylinder) (implanted)
        (pump) (resevoir) T83.420 ◀▥
      testicular prosthesis T83.421 ◀
    heart NEC —*see* Complication,
      cardiovascular device, mechanical
    joint prosthesis —*see* Complication, joint
      prosthesis, mechanical
    ocular NEC —*see* Complications, prosthetic
      device, mechanical, ocular device
    orthopedic NEC —*see* Complication,
      orthopedic, device, mechanical
    specified NEC T85.628
    urinary NEC —*see also* Complication,
      genitourinary, device, urinary,
      mechanical
      graft T83.22
    vascular NEC —*see* Complication,
      cardiovascular device, mechanical
    ventricular intracranial shunt T85.02
  fetus —*see* Pregnancy, complicated by
    (management affected by), presentation,
    fetal
  gallbladder K82.8
  gastrointestinal tract, congenital Q45.8
  heart, congenital NEC Q24.8
  joint prosthesis —*see* Complications, joint
    prosthesis, mechanical, displacement,
    by site
  stomach K31.89
    congenital Q40.2
  tooth, teeth, fully erupted M26.30
  uterus (acute) (acquired) (adherent)
    (asymptomatic) (postinfectional)
    (postpartal, old) N85.4
    anteflexion or anteversion N85.4
      congenital Q51.818

Malposition *(Continued)*
  uterus *(Continued)*
    flexion N85.4
      lateral —*see* Lateroversion, uterus
    inversion N85.5
    lateral (flexion) (version) —*see*
      Lateroversion, uterus
    in pregnancy or childbirth —*see*
      subcategory O34.5
    retroflexion or retroversion —*see*
      Retroversion, uterus
Malposture R29.3
Malrotation
  cecum Q43.3
  colon Q43.3
  intestine Q43.3
  kidney Q63.2
Malta fever —*see* Brucellosis
Maltreatment
  adult
    abandonment
      confirmed T74.01
      suspected T76.01
    confirmed T74.91
    history of Z91.419
    neglect
      confirmed T74.01
      suspected T76.01
    physical abuse
      confirmed T74.11
      suspected T76.11
    psychological abuse
      confirmed T74.31
      history of Z91.411
      suspected T76.31
    sexual abuse
      confirmed T74.21
      suspected T76.21
    suspected T76.91
  child
    abandonment
      confirmed T74.02
      suspected T76.02
    confirmed T74.92
    history of —*see* History, personal (of),
      abuse
    neglect
      confirmed T74.02
      history of —*see* History, personal (of),
        abuse
      suspected T76.02
    physical abuse
      confirmed T74.12
      history of —*see* History, personal (of),
        abuse
      suspected T76.12
    psychological abuse
      confirmed T74.32
      history of —*see* History, personal (of),
        abuse
      suspected T76.32
    sexual abuse
      confirmed T74.22
      history of —*see* History, personal (of),
        abuse
      suspected T76.22
    suspected T76.92
    personal history of Z91.89
Maltworker's lung J67.4
Malunion, fracture —*see* Fracture, by site
Mammillitis N61.0 ◀▥
  puerperal, postpartum O91.02
Mammitis —*see* Mastitis
Mammogram (examination) Z12.39
  routine Z12.31
Mammoplasia N62
Management (of)
  bone conduction hearing device (implanted)
    Z45.320
  cardiac pacemaker NEC Z45.018
  cerebrospinal fluid drainage device Z45.41

Management *(Continued)*
  cochlear device (implanted) Z45.321
  contraceptive Z30.9
    specified NEC Z30.8
  implanted device Z45.9
    specified NEC Z45.89
  infusion pump Z45.1
  procreative Z31.9
    male factor infertility in female Z31.81
    specified NEC Z31.89
  prosthesis (external) —*see also* Fitting Z44.9
    implanted Z45.9
      specified NEC Z45.89
  renal dialysis catheter Z49.01
  vascular access device Z45.2
Mangled —*see* specified injury by site
Mania (monopolar) —*see also* Disorder, mood,
  manic episode
  with psychotic symptoms F30.2
  without psychotic symptoms F30.10
    mild F30.11
    moderate F30.12
    severe F30.13
  Bell's F30.8
  chronic (recurrent) F31.89
  hysterical F44.89
  puerperal F30.8
  recurrent F31.89
Manic-depressive insanity, psychosis, or
  syndrome —*see* Disorder, bipolar
Mannosidosis E77.1
Mansonelliasis, mansonellosis B74.4
Manson's
  disease B65.1
  schistosomiasis B65.1
Manual —*see* condition
Maple-bark-stripper's lung (disease) J67.6
Maple-syrup-urine disease E71.0
Marable's syndrome (celiac artery
  compression) I77.4
Marasmus E41
  due to malnutrition E41
  intestinal E41
  nutritional E41
  senile R54
  tuberculous NEC —*see* Tuberculosis
Marble
  bones Q78.2
  skin R23.8
Marburg virus disease A98.3
March
  fracture —*see* Fracture, traumatic, stress, by
    site
  hemoglobinuria D59.6
Marchesani (-Weill) syndrome Q87.0
Marchiafava (-Bignami) syndrome or disease
  G37.1
Marchiafava-Micheli syndrome D59.5
Marcus Gunn's syndrome Q07.8
Marfan's syndrome —*see* Syndrome, Marfan's
Marie-Bamberger disease —*see*
  Osteoarthropathy, hypertrophic, specified
  NEC
Marie-Charcot-Tooth neuropathic muscular
  atrophy G60.0
Marie's
  cerebellar ataxia (late-onset) G11.2
  disease or syndrome (acromegaly) E22.0
Marie-Strümpell arthritis, disease or
  spondylitis —*see* Spondylitis, ankylosing
Marion's disease (bladder neck obstruction)
  N32.0
Marital conflict Z63.0
Mark
  port wine Q82.5
  raspberry Q82.5
  strawberry Q82.5
  stretch L90.6
  tattoo L81.8
Marker heterochromatin —*see* Extra, marker
  chromosomes

Maroteaux-Lamy syndrome (mild) (severe) E76.29
Marrow (bone)
  arrest D61.9
  poor function D75.89
Marseilles fever A77.1
Marsh fever —see Malaria
Marshall's (hidrotic) ectodermal dysplasia Q82.4
Marsh's disease (exophthalmic goiter) E05.00
  with storm E05.01
Masculinization (female) with adrenal hyperplasia E25.9
  congenital E25.0
Masculinovoblastoma D27.-
Masochism (sexual) F65.51
Mason's lung J62.8
Mass
  abdominal R19.00
    epigastric R19.06
    generalized R19.07
    left lower quadrant R19.04
    left upper quadrant R19.02
    periumbilic R19.05
    right lower quadrant R19.03
    right upper quadrant R19.01
    specified site NEC R19.09
  breast N63
  chest R22.2
  cystic —see Cyst
  ear H93.8-
  head R22.0
  intra-abdominal (diffuse) (generalized) —see Mass, abdominal
  kidney N28.89
  liver R16.0
  localized (skin) R22.9
    chest R22.2
    head R22.0
    limb
      lower R22.4-
      upper R22.3-
    neck R22.1
    trunk R22.2
  lung R91.8
  malignant —see Neoplasm, malignant, by site
  neck R22.1
  pelvic (diffuse) (generalized) —see Mass, abdominal
  specified organ NEC —see Disease, by site
  splenic R16.1
  substernal thyroid —see Goiter
  superficial (localized) R22.9
  umbilical (diffuse) (generalized) R19.09
Massive —see condition
Mast cell
  disease, systemic tissue D47.0
  leukemia C94.3-
  sarcoma C96.2
  tumor D47.0
    malignant C96.2
Mastalgia N64.4
Masters-Allen syndrome N83.8
Mastitis (acute) (diffuse) (nonpuerperal) (subacute) N61.0 ◀▦
  with abscess N61.1 ◀
  chronic (cystic) —see Mastopathy, cystic
  cystic (Schimmelbusch's type) —see Mastopathy, cystic
  fibrocystic —see Mastopathy, cystic
  infective N61.0 ◀▦
    newborn P39.0
  interstitial, gestational or puerperal —see Mastitis, obstetric
  neonatal (noninfective) P83.4
    infective P39.0
  obstetric (interstitial) (nonpurulent)
    associated with
      lactation O91.23
      pregnancy O91.21-
      puerperium O91.22

Mastitis (Continued)
  obstetric (Continued)
    purulent
      associated with
        lactation O91.13
        pregnancy O91.11-
        puerperium O91.12
    periductal —see Ectasia, mammary duct
    phlegmonous —see Mastopathy, cystic
    plasma cell —see Ectasia, mammary duct
    without abscess N61.0 ◀
Mastocytoma D47.0
  malignant C96.2
Mastocytosis Q82.2
  aggressive systemic C96.2
  indolent systemic D47.0
  malignant C96.2
  systemic, associated with clonal hematopoetic non-mast-cell disease (SM-AHNMD) D47.0
Mastodynia N64.4
Mastoid —see condition
Mastoidalgia —see subcategory H92.0
Mastoiditis (coalescent) (hemorrhagic) (suppurative) H70.9-
  acute, subacute H70.00-
    complicated NEC H70.09-
    subperiosteal H70.01-
  chronic (necrotic) (recurrent) H70.1-
  in (due to)
    infectious disease NEC B99 [H75.0-]
    parasitic disease NEC B89 [H75.0-]
    tuberculosis A18.03
  petrositis —see Petrositis
  postauricular fistula —see Fistula, postauricular
  specified NEC H70.89-
  tuberculous A18.03
Mastopathy, mastopathia N64.9
  chronica cystica —see Mastopathy, cystic
  cystic (chronic) (diffuse) N60.1
    with epithelial proliferation N60.3-
  diffuse cystic —see Mastopathy, cystic
  estrogenic, oestrogenica N64.89
  ovarian origin N64.89
Mastoplasia, mastoplastia N62
Masturbation (excessive) F98.8
Maternal care (for) —see Pregnancy (complicated by) (management affected by)
Matheiu's disease (leptospiral jaundice) A27.0
Mauclaire's disease or osteochondrosis —see Osteochondrosis, juvenile, hand, metacarpal
Maxcy's disease A75.2
Maxilla, maxillary —see condition
May (-Hegglin) anomaly or syndrome D72.0
McArdle (-Schmid)(-Pearson) disease (glycogen storage) E74.04
McCune-Albright syndrome Q78.1
McQuarrie's syndrome (idiopathic familial hypoglycemia) E16.2
Meadow's syndrome Q86.1
Measles (black) (hemorrhagic) (suppressed) B05.9
  with
    complications NEC B05.89
    encephalitis B05.0
    intestinal complications B05.4
    keratitis (keratoconjunctivitis) B05.81
    meningitis B05.1
    otitis media B05.3
    pneumonia B05.2
  French —see Rubella
  German —see Rubella
  Liberty —see Rubella
Meatitis, urethral —see Urethritis
Meatus, meatal —see condition
Meat-wrappers' asthma J68.9

Meckel-Gruber syndrome Q61.9
Meckel's diverticulitis, diverticulum (displaced) (hypertrophic) Q43.0
Meconium
  ileus, newborn P76.0
    in cystic fibrosis E84.11
    meaning meconium plug (without cystic fibrosis) P76.0
  obstruction, newborn P76.0
    due to fecaliths P76.0
    in mucoviscidosis E84.11
  peritonitis P78.0
  plug syndrome (newborn) NEC P76.0
Median —see also condition
  arcuate ligament syndrome I77.4
  bar (prostate) (vesical orifice) —see Hyperplasia, prostate
  rhomboid glossitis K14.2
Mediastinal shift R93.8
Mediastinitis (acute) (chronic) J98.51 ◀▦
  syphilitic A52.73
  tuberculous A15.8
Mediastinopericarditis —see also Pericarditis
  acute I30.9
  adhesive I31.0
  chronic I31.8
  rheumatic I09.2
Mediastinum, mediastinal —see condition
Medicine poisoning —see Table of Drugs and Chemicals, by drug, poisoning
Mediterranean
  fever —see Brucellosis
    familial M04.1 ◀▦
    tick A77.1
  kala-azar B55.0
  leishmaniasis B55.0
  tick fever A77.1
Medulla —see condition
Medullary cystic kidney Q61.5
Medullated fibers
  optic (nerve) Q14.8
  retina Q14.1
Medulloblastoma
  desmoplastic C71.6
  specified site —see Neoplasm, malignant, by site
  unspecified site C71.6
Medulloepithelioma —see also Neoplasm, malignant, by site
  teratoid —see Neoplasm, malignant, by site
Medullomyoblastoma
  specified site —see Neoplasm, malignant, by site
  unspecified site C71.6
Meekeren-Ehlers-Danlos syndrome Q79.6
Megacolon (acquired) (functional) (not Hirschsprung's disease) (in) K59.39 ◀▦
  Chagas' disease B57.32
  congenital, congenitum (aganglionic) Q43.1
  Hirschsprung's (disease) Q43.1
  toxic NEC K59.31 ◀▦
    due to Clostridium difficile A04.7
Megaesophagus (functional) K22.0
  congenital Q39.5
  in (due to) Chagas' disease B57.31
Megalencephaly Q04.5
Megalerythema (epidemic) B08.3
Megaloappendix Q43.8
Megalocephalus, megalocephaly NEC Q75.3
Megalocornea Q15.8
  with glaucoma Q15.0
Megalocytic anemia D53.1
Megalodactylia (fingers) (thumbs) (congenital) Q74.0
  toes Q74.2
Megaloduodenum Q43.8
Megaloesophagus (functional) K22.0
  congenital Q39.5

M

Megalogastria (acquired) K31.89
  congenital Q40.2
Megalophthalmos Q11.3
Megalopsia H53.15
Megalosplenia —*see* Splenomegaly
Megaloureter N28.82
  congenital Q62.2
Megarectum K62.89
Megasigmoid K59.39 ◀▥▥
  congenital Q43.2
Megaureter N28.82
  congenital Q62.2
Megavitamin-B6 syndrome E67.2
Megrim —*see* Migraine
Meibomian
  cyst, infected —*see* Hordeolum
  gland —*see* condition
  sty, stye —*see* Hordeolum
Meibomitis —*see* Hordeolum
Meige-Milroy disease (chronic hereditary
      edema) Q82.0
Meige's syndrome Q82.0
Melalgia, nutritional E53.8
Melancholia F32.9
  climacteric (single episode) F32.89 ◀▥▥
    recurrent episode F33.8 ◀▥▥
  hypochondriac F45.29
  intermittent (single episode) F32.89 ◀▥▥
    recurrent episode F33.8 ◀▥▥
  involutional (single episode) F32.89 ◀▥▥
    recurrent episode F33.8 ◀▥▥
  menopausal (single episode) F32.89 ◀▥▥
    recurrent episode F33.8 ◀▥▥
  puerperal F32.89 ◀▥▥
  reactive (emotional stress or trauma) F32.3
  recurrent F33.9
  senile F03
  stuporous (single episode) F32.89 ◀▥▥
    recurrent episode F33.8 ◀▥▥
Melanemia R79.89
Melanoameloblastoma —*see* Neoplasm, bone,
      benign
Melanoblastoma —*see* Melanoma
Melanocarcinoma —*see* Melanoma
Melanocytoma, eyeball D31.9- ◀▥▥
Melanocytosis, neurocutaneous Q82.8
Melanoderma, melanodermia L81.4
Melanodontia, infantile K03.89
Melanodontoclasia K03.89
Melanoepithelioma —*see* Melanoma
Melanoma (malignant) C43.9
  acral lentiginous, malignant —*see* Melanoma,
      skin, by site
  amelanotic —*see* Melanoma, skin, by site
  balloon cell —*see* Melanoma, skin, by site
  benign —*see* Nevus
  desmoplastic, malignant —*see* Melanoma,
      skin, by site
  epithelioid cell —*see* Melanoma, skin, by site
    with spindle cell, mixed —*see* Melanoma,
        skin, by site
  in
    giant pigmented nevus —*see* Melanoma,
        skin, by site
    Hutchinson's melanotic freckle —*see*
        Melanoma, skin, by site
    junctional nevus —*see* Melanoma, skin,
        by site
    precancerous melanosis —*see* Melanoma,
        skin, by site
  in situ D03.9
    abdominal wall D03.59
    ala nasi D03.39
    ankle D03.7-
    anus, anal (margin) (skin) D03.51
    arm D03.6-
    auditory canal D03.2-
    auricle (ear) D03.2-
    auricular canal (external) D03.2-
    axilla, axillary fold D03.59
    back D03.59

Melanoma *(Continued)*
  in situ *(Continued)*
    breast D03.52
    brow D03.39
    buttock D03.59
    canthus (eye) D03.1-
    cheek (external) D03.39
    chest wall D03.59
    chin D03.39
    choroid D03.8
    conjunctiva D03.8
    ear (external) D03.2-
    external meatus (ear) D03.2-
    eye D03.8
    eyebrow D03.39
    eyelid (lower) (upper) D03.1-
    face D03.30
      specified NEC D03.39
    female genital organ (external) NEC D03.8
    finger D03.6-
    flank D03.59
    foot D03.7-
    forearm D03.6-
    forehead D03.39
    foreskin D03.8
    gluteal region D03.59
    groin D03.59
    hand D03.6-
    heel D03.7-
    helix D03.2-
    hip D03.7-
    interscapular region D03.59
    iris D03.8
    jaw D03.39
    knee D03.7-
    labium (majus) (minus) D03.8
    lacrimal gland D03.8
    leg D03.7-
    lip (lower) (upper) D03.0
    lower limb NEC D03.7-
    male genital organ (external) NEC
        D03.8
    nail D03.9
      finger D03.6-
      toe D03.7-
    neck D03.4
    nose (external) D03.39
    orbit D03.8
    penis D03.8
    perianal skin D03.51
    perineum D03.51
    pinna D03.2-
    popliteal fossa or space D03.7-
    prepuce D03.8
    pudendum D03.8
    retina D03.8
    retrobulbar D03.8
    scalp D03.4
    scrotum D03.8
    shoulder D03.6-
    specified site NEC D03.8
    submammary fold D03.52
    temple D03.39
    thigh D03.7-
    toe D03.7-
    trunk NEC D03.59
    umbilicus D03.59
    upper limb NEC D03.6-
    vulva D03.8
  juvenile —*see* Nevus
  malignant, of soft parts except skin —*see*
      Neoplasm, connective tissue, malignant
  metastatic
    breast C79.81
    genital organ C79.82
    specified site NEC C79.89
  neurotropic, malignant —*see* Melanoma, skin,
      by site
  nodular —*see* Melanoma, skin, by site
  regressing, malignant —*see* Melanoma, skin,
      by site

Melanoma *(Continued)*
  skin C43.9
    abdominal wall C43.59
    ala nasi C43.31
    ankle C43.7-
    anus, anal (skin) C43.51
    arm C43.6-
    auditory canal (external) C43.2-
    auricle (ear) C43.2-
    auricular canal (external) C43.2-
    axilla, axillary fold C43.59
    back C43.59
    breast (female) (male) C43.52
    brow C43.39
    buttock C43.59
    canthus (eye) C43.1-
    cheek (external) C43.39
    chest wall C43.59
    chin C43.39
    ear (external) C43.2-
    elbow C43.6-
    external meatus (ear) C43.2-
    eyebrow C43.39
    eyelid (lower) (upper) C43.1-
    face C43.30
      specified NEC C43.39
    female genital organ (external) NEC
        C51.9
    finger C43.6-
    flank C43.59
    foot C43.7-
    forearm C43.6-
    forehead C43.39
    foreskin C60.0
    glabella C43.39
    gluteal region C43.59
    groin C43.59
    hand C43.6-
    heel C43.7-
    helix C43.2-
    hip C43.7-
    interscapular region C43.59
    jaw (external) C43.39
    knee C43.7-
    labium C51.9
      majus C51.0
      minus C51.1
    leg C43.7-
    lip (lower) (upper) C43.0
    lower limb NEC C43.7-
    male genital organ (external) NEC
        C63.9
    nail
      finger C43.6-
      toe C43.7-
    nasolabial groove C43.39
    nates C43.59
    neck C43.4
    nose (external) C43.31
    overlapping site C43.8
    palpebra C43.1-
    penis C60.9
    perianal skin C43.51
    perineum C43.51
    pinna C43.2-
    popliteal fossa or space C43.7-
    prepuce C60.0
    pudendum C51.9
    scalp C43.4
    scrotum C63.2
    shoulder C43.6-
    skin NEC C43.9
    submammary fold C43.52
    temple C43.39
    thigh C43.7-
    toe C43.7-
    trunk NEC C43.59
    umbilicus C43.59
    upper limb NEC C43.6-
    vulva C51.9
      overlapping sites C51.8

◀ New   ◀▥▥ Revised   ~~deleted~~ Deleted

Melanoma (Continued)
  spindle cell
    with epithelioid, mixed —see Melanoma,
        skin, by site
      type A C69.4-
      type B C69.4-
    superficial spreading —see Melanoma, skin,
        by site
Melanosarcoma —see also Melanoma
  epithelioid cell —see Melanoma
Melanosis L81.4
  addisonian E27.1
    tuberculous A18.7
  adrenal E27.1
  colon K63.89
  conjunctiva —see Pigmentation, conjunctiva
    congenital Q13.89
  cornea (presenile) (senile) —see also
        Pigmentation, cornea
    congenital Q13.4
  eye NEC H57.8
    congenital Q15.8
  lenticularis progressiva Q82.1
  liver K76.89
  precancerous —see also Melanoma, in situ
    malignant melanoma in —see Melanoma
  Riehl's L81.4
  sclera H15.89
    congenital Q13.89
  suprarenal E27.1
  tar L81.4
  toxic L81.4
Melanuria R82.99
MELAS syndrome E88.41
Melasma L81.1
  adrenal (gland) E27.1
  suprarenal (gland) E27.1
Melena K92.1
  with ulcer - code by site under Ulcer, with
      hemorrhage K27.4
  due to swallowed maternal blood P78.2
  newborn, neonatal P54.1
    due to swallowed maternal blood P78.2
Meleney's
  gangrene (cutaneous) —see Ulcer, skin
  ulcer (chronic undermining) —see Ulcer, skin
Melioidosis A24.9
  acute A24.1
  chronic A24.2
  fulminating A24.1
  pneumonia A24.1
  pulmonary (chronic) A24.2
    acute A24.1
    subacute A24.2
  sepsis A24.1
  specified NEC A24.3
  subacute A24.2
Melitensis, febris A23.0
Melkersson (-Rosenthal) syndrome G51.2
Mellitus, diabetes —see Diabetes
Melorheostosis (bone) —see Disorder, bone,
    density and structure, specified NEC
Meloschisis Q18.4
Melotia Q17.4
Membrana
  capsularis lentis posterior Q13.89
  epipapillaris Q14.2
Membranacea placenta O43.19-
Membranaceous uterus N85.8
Membrane (s), membranous —see also condition
  cyclitic —see Membrane, pupillary
  folds, congenital —see Web
  Jackson's Q43.3
  over face of newborn P28.9
  premature rupture —see Rupture,
      membranes, premature
  pupillary H21.4-
    persistent Q13.89
  retained (with hemorrhage) (complicating
      delivery) O72.2
    without hemorrhage O73.1

Membrane (s), membranous (Continued)
  secondary cataract —see Cataract, secondary
  unruptured (causing asphyxia) —see
      Asphyxia, newborn
  vitreous —see Opacity, vitreous, membranes
      and strands
Membranitis —see Chorioamnionitis
Memory disturbance, lack or loss —see also
      Amnesia
  mild, following organic brain damage F06.8
Menadione deficiency E56.1
Menarche
  delayed E30.0
  precocious E30.1
Mendacity, pathologic F60.2
Mendelson's syndrome (due to anesthesia)
      J95.4
  in labor and delivery O74.0
  in pregnancy O29.01-
  obstetric O74.0
  postpartum, puerperal O89.01
Ménétrier's disease or syndrome K29.60
  with bleeding K29.61
Ménière's disease, syndrome or vertigo H81.0-
Meninges, meningeal —see condition
Meningioma —see also Neoplasm, meninges,
      benign
  angioblastic —see Neoplasm, meninges,
      benign
  angiomatous —see Neoplasm, meninges,
      benign
  endotheliomatous —see Neoplasm, meninges,
      benign
  fibroblastic —see Neoplasm, meninges,
      benign
  fibrous —see Neoplasm, meninges, benign
  hemangioblastic —see Neoplasm, meninges,
      benign
  hemangiopericytic —see Neoplasm,
      meninges, benign
  malignant —see Neoplasm, meninges,
      malignant
  meningiothelial —see Neoplasm, meninges,
      benign
  meningotheliomatous —see Neoplasm,
      meninges, benign
  mixed —see Neoplasm, meninges, benign
  multiple —see Neoplasm, meninges,
      uncertain behavior
  papillary —see Neoplasm, meninges,
      uncertain behavior
  psammomatous —see Neoplasm, meninges,
      benign
  syncytial —see Neoplasm, meninges, benign
  transitional —see Neoplasm, meninges,
      benign
Meningiomatosis (diffuse) —see Neoplasm,
      meninges, uncertain behavior
Meningism —see Meningismus
Meningismus (infectional) (pneumococcal)
      R29.1
  due to serum or vaccine R29.1
  influenzal —see Influenza, with,
      manifestations NEC
Meningitis (basal) (basic) (brain) (cerebral)
      (cervical) (congestive) (diffuse)
      (hemorrhagic) infantile) (membranous)
      (metastatic) (nonspecific) (pontine)
      (progressive) (simple) (spinal) (subacute)
      (sympathetic) (toxic) G03.9
  abacterial G03.0
  actinomycotic A42.81
  adenoviral A87.1
  arbovirus A87.8
  aseptic (acute) G03.0
  bacterial G00.9
    Escherichia coli (E. coli) G00.8
    Friedländer (bacillus) G00.8
    gram-negative G00.9
    H. influenzae G00.0
    Klebsiella G00.8

Meningitis (Continued)
  bacterial (Continued)
    pneumococcal G00.1
    specified organism NEC G00.8
    staphylococcal G00.3
    streptococcal (acute) G00.2
  benign recurrent (Mollaret) G03.2
  candidal B37.5
  caseous (tuberculous) A17.0
  cerebrospinal A39.0
  chronic NEC G03.1
  clear cerebrospinal fluid NEC G03.0
  coxsackievirus A87.0
  cryptococcal B45.1
  diplococcal (gram positive) A39.0
  echovirus A87.0
  enteroviral A87.0
  eosinophilic B83.2
  epidemic NEC A39.0
  Escherichia coli (E. coli) G00.8
  fibrinopurulent G00.9
    specified organism NEC G00.8
  Friedländer (bacillus) G00.8
  gonococcal A54.81
  gram-negative cocci G00.9
  gram-positive cocci G00.9
  Haemophilus (influenzae) G00.0
  H. influenzae G00.0
  in (due to)
    adenovirus A87.1
    African trypanosomiasis B56.9 [G02]
    anthrax A22.8
    bacterial disease NEC A48.8 [G01]
    Chagas' disease (chronic) B57.41
    chickenpox B01.0
    coccidioidomycosis B38.4
    Diplococcus pneumoniae G00.1
    enterovirus A87.0
    herpes (simplex) virus B00.3
      zoster B02.1
    infectious mononucleosis B27.92
    leptospirosis A27.81
    Listeria monocytogenes A32.11
    Lyme disease A69.21
    measles B05.1
    mumps (virus) B26.1
    neurosyphilis (late) A52.13
    parasitic disease NEC B89 [G02]
    poliovirus A80.9 [G02]
    preventive immunization, inoculation or
        vaccination G03.8
    rubella B06.02
    Salmonella infection A02.21
    specified cause NEC G03.8
    Streptococcal pneumoniae G00.1 ◄
    typhoid fever A01.01
    varicella B01.0
    viral disease NEC A87.8
    whooping cough A37.90
    zoster B02.1
  infectious G00.9
  influenzal (H. influenzae) G00.0
  Klebsiella G00.8
  leptospiral (aseptic) A27.81
  lymphocytic (acute) (benign) (serous) A87.2
  meningococcal A39.0
  Mima polymorpha G00.8
  Mollaret (benign recurrent) G03.2
  monilial B37.5
  mycotic NEC B49 [G02]
  Neisseria A39.0
  nonbacterial G03.0
  nonpyogenic NEC G03.0
  ossificans G96.19
  pneumococcal G00.1
  pneumococcal streptococcus pneumoniae
      G00.1 ◄
  poliovirus A80.9 [G02]
  postmeasles B05.1
  purulent G00.9
    specified organism NEC G00.8

Meningitis (Continued)
  pyogenic G00.9
    specified organism NEC G00.8
    Salmonella (arizonae) (Cholerae-Suis)
      (enteritidis) (typhimurium) A02.21
  septic G00.9
    specified organism NEC G00.8
  serosa circumscripta NEC G03.0
  serous NEC G93.2
  specified organism NEC G00.8
  sporotrichosis B42.81
  staphylococcal G00.3
  sterile G03.0
  Streptococcal (acute) G00.2 ◄▥
    pneumoniae G00.1 ◄
  suppurative G00.9
    specified organism NEC G00.8
  syphilitic (late) (tertiary) A52.13
    acute A51.41
    congenital A50.41
    secondary A51.41
  Torula histolytica (cryptococcal) B45.1
  traumatic (complication of injury)
    T79.8
  tuberculous A17.0
  typhoid A01.01
  viral NEC A87.9
  Yersinia pestis A20.3
Meningocele (spinal) —see also Spina bifida
  with hydrocephalus —see Spina bifida, by
    site, with hydrocephalus
  acquired (traumatic) G96.19
  cerebral —see Encephalocele
Meningocerebritis —see Meningoencephalitis
Meningococcemia A39.4
  acute A39.2
  chronic A39.3
Meningococcus, meningococcal —see also
    condition A39.9
  adrenalitis, hemorrhagic A39.1
  carrier (suspected) of Z22.31
  meningitis (cerebrospinal) A39.0
Meningoencephalitis —see also Encephalitis
    G04.90
  acute NEC —see also Encephalitis, viral A86
  bacterial NEC G04.2
  California A83.5
  diphasic A84.1
  eosinophilic B83.2
  epidemic A39.81
  herpesviral, herpetic B00.4
    due to herpesvirus 6 B10.01
    due to herpesvirus 7 B10.09
    specified NEC B10.09
  in (due to)
    blastomycosis NEC B40.81
    diseases classified elsewhere G05.3
    free-living amebae B60.2
    Hemophilus influenzae (H. influenzae)
      G00.0 ◄▥
    herpes B00.4
      due to herpesvirus 6 B10.01
      due to herpesvirus 7 B10.09
      specified NEC B10.09
    H. influenzae G00.0
    Lyme disease A69.22
    mercury —see subcategory T56.1
    mumps B26.2
    Naegleria (amebae) (organisms) (fowleri)
      B60.2
    Parastrongylus cantonensis B83.2
    toxoplasmosis (acquired) B58.2
      congenital P37.1
  infectious (acute) (viral) A86
  influenzal (H. influenzae) G00.0 ◄▥
  Listeria monocytogenes A32.12
  lymphocytic (serous) A87.2
  mumps B26.2
  parasitic NEC B89 [G05.3]
  pneumococcal G04.2 ◄▥
  primary amebic B60.2

Meningoencephalitis (Continued)
  specific (syphilitic) A52.14
  specified organism NEC G04.81
  staphylococcal G04.2
  streptococcal G04.2
  syphilitic A52.14
  toxic NEC G92
    due to mercury —see subcategory T56.1
  tuberculous A17.82
  virus NEC A86
Meningoencephalocele —see also
    Encephalocele
  syphilitic A52.19
  congenital A50.49
Meningoencephalomyelitis —see also
    Meningoencephalitis
  acute NEC (viral) A86
    disseminated G04.00
      postimmunization or postvaccination
        G04.02
      postinfectious G04.01
  due to
    actinomycosis A42.82
    Torula B45.1
    Toxoplasma or toxoplasmosis (acquired)
      B58.2
    congenital P37.1
  postimmunization or postvaccination G04.02
Meningoencephalomyelopathy G96.9
Meningoencephalopathy G96.9
Meningomyelitis —see also
    Meningoencephalitis
  bacterial NEC G04.2
  blastomycotic NEC B40.81
  cryptococcal B45.1
  in diseases classified elsewhere G05.4
  meningococcal A39.81
  syphilitic A52.14
  tuberculous A17.82
Meningomyelocele —see also Spina bifida
  syphilitic A52.19
Meningomyeloneuritis —see
    Meningoencephalitis
Meningoradiculitis —see Meningitis
Meningovascular —see condition
Menkes' disease or syndrome E83.09
  meaning maple-syrup-urine disease E71.0
Menometrorrhagia N92.1
Menopause, menopausal (asymptomatic)
    (state) Z78.0
  arthritis (any site) NEC —see Arthritis,
    specified form NEC
  bleeding N92.4
  depression (single episode) F32.89 ◄▥
    agitated (single episode) F32.2
      recurrent episode F33.9
    psychotic (single episode) F32.89 ◄▥
      recurrent episode F33.8 ◄▥
    recurrent episode F33.9
  melancholia (single episode) F32.89 ◄▥
    recurrent episode F33.8 ◄▥
  paranoid state F22
  premature E28.319
    asymptomatic E28.319
      postirradiation E89.40
      postsurgical E89.40
    symptomatic E28.310
      postirradiation E89.41
      postsurgical E89.41
  psychosis NEC F28
  symptomatic N95.1
  toxic polyarthritis NEC —see Arthritis,
    specified form NEC
Menorrhagia (primary) N92.0
  climacteric N92.4
    menopausal N92.4
  menopausal N92.4
  postclimacteric N95.0
  postmenopausal N95.0
  preclimacteric or premenopausal N92.4
  pubertal (menses retained) N92.2

Menostaxis N92.0
Menses, retention N94.89
Menstrual —see Menstruation
Menstruation
  absent —see Amenorrhea
  anovulatory N97.0
  cycle, irregular N92.6
  delayed N91.0
  disorder N93.9
    psychogenic F45.8
  during pregnancy O20.8
  excessive (with regular cycle) N92.0
    with irregular cycle N92.1
    at puberty N92.2
  frequent N92.0
  infrequent —see Oligomenorrhea
  irregular N92.6
    specified NEC N92.5
  latent N92.5
  membranous N92.5
  painful —see also Dysmenorrhea N94.6
    primary N94.4
    psychogenic F45.8
    secondary N94.5
  passage of clots N92.0
  precocious E30.1
  protracted N92.5
  rare —see Oligomenorrhea
  retained N94.89
  retrograde N92.5
  scanty —see Oligomenorrhea
  suppression N94.89
  vicarious (nasal) N94.89
Mental —see also condition
  deficiency —see Disability, intellectual
  deterioration —see Psychosis
  disorder —see Disorder, mental
  exhaustion F48.8
  insufficiency (congenital) —see Disability,
    intellectual
  observation without need for further medical
    care Z03.89
  retardation —see Disability, intellectual
  subnormality —see Disability, intellectual
  upset —see Disorder, mental
Meralgia paresthetica G57.1-
Mercurial —see condition
Mercurialism —see subcategory T56.1
MERRF syndrome (myoclonic epilepsy
    associated with ragged-red fiber)
    E88.42
Merkel cell tumor —see Carcinoma,
    Merkel cell
Merocele —see Hernia, femoral
Meromelia
  lower limb —see Defect, reduction, lower
    limb
    intercalary
      femur —see Defect, reduction, lower
        limb, specified type NEC
        tibiofibular (complete) (incomplete) —
          see Defect, reduction, lower
          limb
  upper limb —see Defect, reduction, upper
    limb
    intercalary, humeral, radioulnar —see
      Agenesis, arm, with hand present
Merzbacher-Pelizaeus disease E75.29
Mesaortitis —see Aortitis
Mesarteritis —see Arteritis
Mesencephalitis —see Encephalitis
Mesenchymoma —see also Neoplasm,
    connective tissue, uncertain behavior
  benign —see Neoplasm, connective tissue,
    benign
  malignant —see Neoplasm, connective tissue,
    malignant
Mesenteritis
  retractile K65.4
  sclerosing K65.4
Mesentery, mesenteric —see condition

Mesiodens, mesiodentes K00.1
Mesio-occlusion M26.213
Mesocolon —*see* condition
Mesonephroma (malignant) —*see* Neoplasm,
malignant, by site
benign —*see* Neoplasm, benign, by site
Mesophlebitis —*see* Phlebitis
Mesostromal dysgenesia Q13.89
Mesothelioma (malignant) C45.9
benign
mesentery D19.1
mesocolon D19.1
omentum D19.1
peritoneum D19.1
pleura D19.0
specified site NEC D19.7
unspecified site D19.9
biphasic C45.9
benign
mesentery D19.1
mesocolon D19.1
omentum D19.1
peritoneum D19.1
pleura D19.0
specified site NEC D19.7
unspecified site D19.9
cystic D48.4
epithelioid C45.9
benign
mesentery D19.1
mesocolon D19.1
omentum D19.1
peritoneum D19.1
pleura D19.0
specified site NEC D19.7
unspecified site D19.9
fibrous C45.9
benign
mesentery D19.1
mesocolon D19.1
omentum D19.1
peritoneum D19.1
pleura D19.0
specified site NEC D19.7
unspecified site D19.9
site classification
liver C45.7
lung C45.7
mediastinum C45.7
mesentery C45.1
mesocolon C45.1
omentum C45.1
pericardium C45.2
peritoneum C45.1
pleura C45.0
parietal C45.0
retroperitoneum C45.7
specified site NEC C45.7
unspecified C45.9
Metabolic syndrome E88.81
Metagonimiasis B66.8
Metagonimus infestation (intestine) B66.8
Metal
pigmentation L81.8
polisher's disease J62.8
Metamorphopsia H53.15
Metaplasia
apocrine (breast) —*see* Dysplasia, mammary,
specified type NEC
cervix (squamous) —*see* Dysplasia, cervix
endometrium (squamous) (uterus) N85.8
esophagus K22.7- ◀▥
kidney (pelvis) (squamous) N28.89
myelogenous D73.1
myeloid (agnogenic) (megakaryocytic)
D73.1
spleen D73.1
squamous cell, bladder N32.89
Metastasis, metastatic
abscess —*see* Abscess
calcification E83.59

Metastasis, metastatic *(Continued)*
cancer
from specified site —*see* Neoplasm,
malignant, by site
to specified site —*see* Neoplasm, secondary,
by site
deposits (in) —*see* Neoplasm, secondary, by
site
disease *(see also* Neoplasm, secondary, by site)
C79.9
spread (to) —*see* Neoplasm, secondary, by site
Metastrongyliasis B83.8
Metatarsalgia M77.4-
anterior G57.6-
Morton's G57.6-
Metatarsus, metatarsal —*see also* condition
adductus, congenital Q66.22 ◀
valgus (abductus), congenital Q66.6
varus (congenital) Q66.22 ◀▥
primus Q66.21 ◀
Methadone use —*see* Use, opioid ◀▥
Methemoglobinemia D74.9
acquired (with sulfhemoglobinemia) D74.8
congenital D74.0
enzymatic (congenital) D74.0
Hb M disease D74.0
hereditary D74.0
toxic D74.8
Methemoglobinuria —*see* Hemoglobinuria
Methioninemia E72.19
Methylmalonic acidemia E71.120
Metritis (catarrhal) (hemorrhagic) (septic)
(suppurative) —*see also* Endometritis
cervical —*see* Cervicitis
Metropathia hemorrhagica N93.8
Metroperitonitis —*see* Peritonitis, pelvic, female
Metrorrhagia N92.1
climacteric N92.4
menopausal N92.4
postpartum NEC (atonic) (following delivery
of placenta) O72.1
delayed or secondary O72.2
preclimacteric or premenopausal N92.4
psychogenic F45.8
Metrorrhexis —*see* Rupture, uterus
Metrosalpingitis N70.91
Metrostaxis N93.8
Metrovaginitis —*see* Endometritis
Meyer-Schwickerath and Weyers syndrome
Q87.0
Meynert's amentia (nonalcoholic) F04
alcoholic F10.96
with dependence F10.26
Mibelli's disease (porokeratosis) Q82.8
Mice, joint —*see* Loose, body, joint
knee M23.4
Micrencephalon, micrencephaly Q02
Microalbuminuria R80.9
Microaneurysm, retinal —*see also* Disorder,
retina, microaneurysms
diabetic —*see* E08-E13 with .31
Microangiopathy (peripheral) I73.9
thrombotic M31.1
Microcalcifications, breast R92.0
Microcephalus, microcephalic, microcephaly
Q02
due to toxoplasmosis (congenital) P37.1
Microcheilia Q18.7
Microcolon (congenital) Q43.8
Microcornea (congenital) Q13.4
Microcytic —*see* condition D57.40
Microdeletions NEC Q93.88
Microdontia K00.2
Microdrepanocytosis D57.40
with crisis (vasoocclusive pain) D57.419
with
acute chest syndrome D57.411
splenic sequestration D57.412
Microembolism
atherothrombotic —*see* Atheroembolism
retinal —*see* Occlusion, artery, retina

Microencephalon Q02
Microfilaria streptocerca infestation —*see*
Onchocerciasis
Microgastria (congenital) Q40.2
Microgenia M26.06
Microgenitalia, congenital
female Q52.8
male Q55.8
Microglioma —*see* Lymphoma, non-Hodgkin,
specified NEC
Microglossia (congenital) Q38.3
Micrognathia, micrognathism (congenital)
(mandibular) (maxillary) M26.09
Microgyria (congenital) Q04.3
Microinfarct of heart —*see* Insufficiency,
coronary
Microlentia (congenital) Q12.8
Microlithiasis, alveolar, pulmonary J84.02
Micromastia N64.82
Micromyelia (congenital) Q06.8
Micropenis Q55.62
Microphakia (congenital) Q12.8
Microphthalmos, microphthalmia (congenital)
Q11.2
due to toxoplasmosis P37.1
Micropsia H53.15
Microscopic polyangiitis (polyarteritis) M31.7
Microsporidiosis B60.8
intestinal A07.8
Microsporon furfur infestation B36.0
Microsporosis —*see also* Dermatophytosis
nigra B36.1
Microstomia (congenital) Q18.5
Microtia (congenital) (external ear) Q17.2
Microtropia H50.40
Microvillus inclusion disease (MVD) (MVID)
Q43.8
Micturition
disorder NEC —*see also* Difficulty, micturition
R39.198 ◀▥
psychogenic F45.8
frequency R35.0
psychogenic F45.8
hesitancy R39.11
incomplete emptying R39.14
nocturnal R35.1
painful R30.9
dysuria R30.0
psychogenic F45.8
tenesmus R30.1
poor stream R39.12
position dependent R39.192 ◀
split stream R39.13
straining R39.16
urgency R39.15
Mid plane —*see* condition
Middle
ear —*see* condition
lobe (right) syndrome J98.19
Miescher's elastoma L87.2
Mietens' syndrome Q87.2
Migraine (idiopathic) G43.909
with refractory migraine G43.919
with status migrainosus G43.911
without status migrainosus G43.919
with aura (acute-onset) (prolonged) (typical)
(without headache) G43.109
with refractory migraine G43.119
with status migrainosus G43.111
without status migrainosus G43.119
intractable G43.119
with status migrainosus G43.111
without status migrainosus G43.119
not intractable G43.109
with status migrainosus G43.101
without status migrainosus G43.109
persistent G43.509
with cerebral infarction G43.609
with refractory migraine G43.619
with status migrainosus G43.611
without status migrainosus G43.619

M

Migraine (Continued)
  with aura (Continued)
    persistent (Continued)
      with cerebral infarction (Continued)
        intractable G43.619
          with status migrainosus G43.611
          without status migrainosus G43.619
        not intractable G43.609
          with status migrainosus G43.601
          without status migrainosus G43.609
        without refractory migraine G43.609
          with status migrainosus G43.601
          without status migrainosus G43.609
      without cerebral infarction G43.509
        with refractory migraine G43.519
          with status migrainosus G43.511
          without status migrainosus G43.519
        intractable G43.519
          with status migrainosus G43.511
          without status migrainosus G43.519
        not intractable G43.509
          with status migrainosus G43.501
          without status migrainosus G43.509
        without refractory migraine G43.509
          with status migrainosus G43.501
          without status migrainosus G43.509
    without mention of refractory migraine G43.109
      with status migrainosus G43.101
      without status migrainosus G43.109
  abdominal G43.D0
    with refractory migraine G43.D1
    intractable G43.D1
    not intractable G43.D0
    without refractory migraine G43.D0
  basilar —see Migraine, with aura
  classical —see Migraine, with aura
  common —see Migraine, without aura
  complicated G43.109
  equivalents —see Migraine, with aura
  familiar —see Migraine, hemiplegic
  hemiplegic G43.409
    with refractory migraine G43.419
      with status migrainosus G43.411
      without status migrainosus G43.419
    intractable G43.419
      with status migrainosus G43.411
      without status migrainosus G43.419
    not intractable G43.409
      with status migrainosus G43.401
      without status migrainosus G43.409
    without refractory migraine G43.409
      with status migrainosus G43.401
      without status migrainosus G43.409
  intractable G43.919
    with status migrainosus G43.911
    without status migrainosus G43.919
  menstrual G43.829
    with refractory migraine G43.839
      with status migrainosus G43.831
      without status migrainosus G43.839
    intractable G43.839
      with status migrainosus G43.831
      without status migrainosus G43.839
    not intractable G43.829
      with status migrainosus G43.821
      without status migrainosus G43.829
    without refractory migraine G43.829
      with status migrainosus G43.821
      without status migrainosus G43.829
  menstrually related —see Migraine, menstrual
  not intractable G43.909
    with status migrainosus G43.901
    without status migrainosus G43.919
  ophthalmoplegic G43.B0
    with refractory migraine G43.B1
    intractable G43.B1
    not intractable G43.B0
      without refractory migraine G43.B0

Migraine (Continued)
  persistent aura (with, without) cerebral infarction —see Migraine, with aura, persistent
  preceded or accompanied by transient focal neurological phenomena —see Migraine, with aura
  pre-menstrual —see Migraine, menstrual
  pure menstrual —see Migraine, menstrual
  retinal —see Migraine, with aura
  specified NEC G43.809
    intractable G43.819
      with status migrainosus G43.811
      without status migrainosus G43.819
    not intractable G43.809
      with status migrainosus G43.801
      without status migrainosus G43.809
  sporadic —see Migraine, hemiplegic
  transformed —see Migraine, without aura, chronic
  triggered seizures —see Migraine, with aura
  without aura G43.009
    with refractory migraine G43.019
      with status migrainosus G43.011
      without status migrainosus G43.019
    chronic G43.709
      with refractory migraine G43.719
        with status migrainosus G43.711
        without status migrainosus G43.719
      intractable
        with status migrainosus G43.711
        without status migrainosus G43.719
      not intractable
        with status migrainosus G43.701
        without status migrainosus G43.709
      without refractory migraine G43.709
        with status migrainosus G43.701
        without status migrainosus G43.709
    intractable
      with status migrainosus G43.011
      without status migrainosus G43.019
    not intractable
      with status migrainosus G43.001
      without status migrainosus G43.009
    without mention of refractory migraine G43.009
      with status migrainosus G43.001
      without status migrainosus G43.009
    without refractory migraine G43.909
      with status migrainosus G43.901
      without status migrainosus G43.919
Migrant, social Z59.0
Migration, anxiety concerning Z60.3
Migratory, migrating —see also condition
  person Z59.0
  testis Q55.29
Mikity-Wilson disease or syndrome P27.0
Mikulicz' disease or syndrome K11.8
Miliaria L74.3
  alba L74.1
  apocrine L75.2
  crystallina L74.1
  profunda L74.2
  rubra L74.0
  tropicalis L74.2
Miliary —see condition
Milium L72.0
  colloid L57.8
Milk
  crust L21.0
  excessive secretion O92.6
  poisoning —see Poisoning, food, noxious
  retention O92.79
  sickness —see Poisoning, food, noxious
  spots I31.0
Milk-alkali disease or syndrome E83.52
Milk-leg (deep vessels) (nonpuerperal) —see Embolism, vein, lower extremity
  complicating pregnancy O22.3-
  puerperal, postpartum, childbirth O87.1

Milkman's disease or syndrome M83.8
Milky urine —see Chyluria
Millard-Gubler (-Foville) paralysis or syndrome G46.3
Millar's asthma J38.5
Miller-Fisher syndrome G61.0
Mills' disease —see Hemiplegia
Millstone maker's pneumoconiosis J62.8
Milroy's disease (chronic hereditary edema) Q82.0
Minamata disease T56.1- ◀▥
Miners' asthma or lung J60
Minkowski-Chauffard syndrome —see Spherocytosis
Minor —see condition
Minor's disease (hematomyelia) G95.19
Minot's disease (hemorrhagic disease), newborn P53
Minot-von Willebrand-Jurgens disease or syndrome (angiohemophilia) D68.0
Minus (and plus) hand (intrinsic) —see Deformity, limb, specified type NEC, forearm
Miosis (pupil) H57.03
Mirizzi's syndrome (hepatic duct stenosis) K83.1
Mirror writing F81.0
Misadventure (of) (prophylactic) (therapeutic) — see also Complications T88.9
  administration of insulin (by accident) —see subcategory T38.3
  infusion —see Complications, infusion
  local applications (of fomentations, plasters, etc.) T88.9
    burn or scald —see Burn
    specified NEC T88.8
  medical care (early) (late) T88.9
    adverse effect of drugs or chemicals —see Table of Drugs and Chemicals
  medical care (early) (late)
    burn or scald —see Burn
    specified NEC T88.8
  specified NEC T88.8
  surgical procedure (early) (late) —see Complications, surgical procedure
  transfusion —see Complications, transfusion
  vaccination or other immunological procedure —see Complications, vaccination
Miscarriage O03.9
Misdirection, aqueous H40.83-
Misperception, sleep state F51.02
Misplaced, misplacement
  ear Q17.4
  kidney (acquired) N28.89
    congenital Q63.2
  organ or site, congenital NEC —see Malposition, congenital
Missed
  abortion O02.1
  delivery O36.4
Missing —see also Absence ◀▥
  string of intrauterine contraceptive device T83.32 ◀
Misuse of drugs F19.99
Misuse of drugs F19.99
Mitchell's disease (erythromelalgia) I73.81
Mite (s) (infestation) B88.9
  diarrhea B88.0
  grain (itch) B88.0
  hair follicle (itch) B88.0
  in sputum B88.0
Mitral —see condition
Mittelschmerz N94.0
Mixed —see condition
MMN (multifocal motor neuropathy) G61.82 ◀
MNGIE (Mitochondrial Neurogastrointestinal Encephalopathy) syndrome E88.49
Mobile, mobility
  cecum Q43.3
  excessive —see Hypermobility
  gallbladder, congenital Q44.1

Mobile, mobility *(Continued)*
  kidney N28.89
  organ or site, congenital NEC —*see*
    Malposition, congenital
Mobitz heart block (atrioventricular) I44.1
Moebius, Möbius
  disease (ophthalmoplegic migraine) —*see*
    Migraine, ophthalmoplegic
  syndrome Q87.0
    congenital oculofacial paralysis (with other
      anomalies) Q87.0
    ophthalmoplegic migraine —*see* Migraine,
      ophthalmoplegic
Moeller's glossitis K14.0
Mohr's syndrome (Types I and II) Q87.0
Mola destruens D39.2
Molar pregnancy O02.0
Molarization of premolars K00.2
Molding, head (during birth) - omit code
Mole (pigmented) —*see also* Nevus
  blood O02.0
  Breus' O02.0
  cancerous —*see* Melanoma
  carneous O02.0
  destructive D39.2
  fleshy O02.0
  hydatid, hydatidiform (benign) (complicating
    pregnancy) (delivered) (undelivered)
    O01.9
    classical O01.0
    complete O01.0
    incomplete O01.1
    invasive D39.2
    malignant D39.2
    partial O01.1
  intrauterine O02.0
  invasive (hydatidiform) D39.2
  malignant
    meaning
      malignant hydatidiform mole D39.2
      melanoma —*see* Melanoma
  nonhydatidiform O02.0
  nonpigmented —*see* Nevus
  pregnancy NEC O02.0
  skin —*see* Nevus
  tubal O00.10 ◄▥
    with intrauterine pregnancy O00.11 ◄
  vesicular —*see* Mole, hydatidiform
Molimen, molimina (menstrual) N94.3
Molluscum contagiosum (epitheliale) B08.1
**Mönckeberg's arteriosclerosis, disease, or
  sclerosis** —*see* Arteriosclerosis, extremities
Mondini's malformation (cochlea) Q16.5
Mondor's disease I80.8
Monge's disease T70.29
Monilethrix (congenital) Q84.1
Moniliasis —*see also* Candidiasis B37.9
  neonatal P37.5
Monitoring (encounter for)
  therapeutic drug level Z51.81
Monkey malaria B53.1
Monkeypox B04
Monoarthritis M13.10
  ankle M13.17-
  elbow M13.12-
  foot joint M13.17-
  hand joint M13.14-
  hip M13.15-
  knee M13.16-
  shoulder M13.11-
  wrist M13.13-
Monoblastic —*see* condition
Monochromat (ism), **monochromatopsia**
  (acquired) (congenital) H53.51
Monocytic —*see* condition
Monocytopenia D72.818
Monocytosis (symptomatic) D72.821
Monomania —*see* Psychosis
Mononeuritis G58.9
  cranial nerve —*see* Disorder, nerve,
    cranial

Mononeuritis *(Continued)*
  femoral nerve G57.2-
  lateral
    cutaneous nerve of thigh G57.1-
    popliteal nerve G57.3-
  lower limb G57.9-
    specified nerve NEC G57.8-
  medial popliteal nerve G57.4-
  median nerve G56.1-
  multiplex G58.7
  plantar nerve G57.6-
  posterior tibial nerve G57.5-
  radial nerve G56.3-
  sciatic nerve G57.0-
  specified NEC G58.8
  tibial nerve G57.4-
  ulnar nerve G56.2-
  upper limb G56.9-
    specified nerve NEC G56.8-
  vestibular —*see* subcategory H93.3
Mononeuropathy G58.9
  carpal tunnel syndrome —*see* Syndrome,
    carpal tunnel
  diabetic NEC —*see* E08-E13 with .41
  femoral nerve —*see* Lesion, nerve, femoral
  ilioinguinal nerve G57.8-
  in diseases classified elsewhere —*see* category
    G59
  intercostal G58.0
  lower limb G57.9-
    causalgia —*see* Causalgia, lower limb
    femoral nerve —*see* Lesion, nerve,
      femoral
    meralgia paresthetica G57.1-
    plantar nerve —*see* Lesion, nerve, plantar
    popliteal nerve —*see* Lesion, nerve,
      popliteal
    sciatic nerve —*see* Lesion, nerve, sciatic
    specified NEC G57.8-
    tarsal tunnel syndrome —*see* Syndrome,
      tarsal tunnel
  median nerve —*see* Lesion, nerve, median
  multiplex G58.7
  obturator nerve G57.8-
  popliteal nerve —*see* Lesion, nerve,
    popliteal
  radial nerve —*see* Lesion, nerve, radial
  saphenous nerve G57.8-
  specified NEC G58.8
  tarsal tunnel syndrome —*see* Syndrome,
    tarsal tunnel
  tuberculous A17.83
  ulnar nerve —*see* Lesion, nerve, ulnar
  upper limb G56.9-
    carpal tunnel syndrome —*see* Syndrome,
      carpal tunnel
    causalgia —*see* Causalgia
    median nerve —*see* Lesion, nerve, median
    radial nerve —*see* Lesion, nerve, radial
    specified site NEC G56.8-
    ulnar nerve —*see* Lesion, nerve, ulnar
Mononucleosis, infectious B27.90
  with
    complication NEC B27.99
    meningitis B27.92
    polyneuropathy B27.91
  cytomegaloviral B27.10
    with
      complication NEC B27.19
      meningitis B27.12
      polyneuropathy B27.11
  Epstein-Barr (virus) B27.00
    with
      complication NEC B27.09
      meningitis B27.02
      polyneuropathy B27.01
  gammaherpesviral B27.00
    with
      complication NEC B27.09
      meningitis B27.02
      polyneuropathy B27.01

Mononucleosis, infectious *(Continued)*
  specified NEC B27.80
    with
      complication NEC B27.89
      meningitis B27.82
      polyneuropathy B27.81
Monoplegia G83.3-
  congenital (cerebral) G80.8
    spastic G80.1
  embolic (current episode) I63.4- ◄▥
  following
    cerebrovascular disease
      cerebral infarction
        lower limb I69.34-
        upper limb I69.33-
      intracerebral hemorrhage
        lower limb I69.14-
        upper limb I69.13-
      lower limb I69.94-
      nontraumatic intracranial hemorrhage
        NEC
        lower limb I69.24-
        upper limb I69.23-
      specified disease NEC
        lower limb I69.84-
        upper limb I69.83-
      stroke NOS
        lower limb I69.34-
        upper limb I69.33-
      subarachnoid hemorrhage
        lower limb I69.04-
        upper limb I69.03-
      upper limb I69.93-
  hysterical (transient) F44.4
  lower limb G83.1-
  psychogenic (conversion reaction) F44.4
  thrombotic (current episode) I63.3- ◄▥
  transient R29.818
  upper limb G83.2-
Monorchism, monorchidism Q55.0
Monosomy —*see also* Deletion, chromosome
    Q93.9
  specified NEC Q93.89
  whole chromosome
    meiotic nondisjunction Q93.0
    mitotic nondisjunction Q93.1
    mosaicism Q93.1
  X Q96.9
Monster, monstrosity (single) Q89.7
  acephalic Q00.0
  twin Q89.4
Monteggia's fracture (-dislocation) S52.27-
Mooren's ulcer (cornea) —*see* Ulcer, cornea,
    Mooren's
Moore's syndrome —*see* Epilepsy, specified
    NEC
Mooser-Neill reaction A75.2
Mooser's bodies A75.2
Morbidity not stated or unknown R69
Morbilli —*see* Measles
Morbus —*see also* Disease
  angelicus, anglorum E55.0
  Beigel B36.2
  caducus —*see* Epilepsy
  celiacus K90.0
  comitialis —*see* Epilepsy
  cordis —*see also* Disease, heart I51.9
    valvulorum —*see* Endocarditis
  coxae senilis M16.9
    tuberculous A18.02
  hemorrhagicus neonatorum P53
  maculosus neonatorum P54.5
Morel (-Stewart)(-Morgagni) **syndrome** M85.2
Morel-Kraepelin disease —*see* Schizophrenia
Morel-Moore syndrome M85.2
Morgagni's
  cyst, organ, hydatid, or appendage
    female Q50.5
    male (epididymal) Q55.4
      testicular Q55.29
  syndrome M85.2

Morgagni-Stewart-Morel syndrome M85.2
Morgagni-Stokes-Adams syndrome I45.9
Morgagni-Turner (-Albright) syndrome Q96.9
Moria F07.0
Moron (I.Q. 50-69) F70
Morphea L94.0
Morphinism (without remission) F11.20
  with remission F11.21
Morphinomania (without remission) F11.20
  with remission F11.21
Morquio (-Ullrich)(-Brailsford) disease or
  syndrome —see Mucopolysaccharidosis
Mortification (dry) (moist) —see Gangrene
Morton's metatarsalgia (neuralgia)(neuroma)
  (syndrome) G57.6
Morvan's disease or syndrome G60.8
Mosaicism, mosaic (autosomal) (chromosomal)
  45,X/46,XX Q96.3
  45,X/other cell lines NEC with abnormal sex
      chromosome Q96.4
  sex chromosome
    female Q97.8
    lines with various numbers of X
      chromosomes Q97.2
    male Q98.7
  XY Q96.3
Moschowitz' disease M31.1
Mother yaw A66.0
Motion sickness (from travel, any vehicle)
  (from roundabouts or swings) T75.3
Mottled, mottling, teeth (enamel) (endemic)
  (nonendemic) K00.3
Mounier-Kuhn syndrome Q32.4
  with bronchiectasis J47.9
    exacerbation (acute) J47.1
    lower respiratory infection J47.0
  acquired J98.09
    with bronchiectasis J47.9
      with
        exacerbation (acute) J47.1
        lower respiratory infection J47.0
Mountain
  sickness T70.29
    with polycythemia , acquired (acute) D75.1
  tick fever A93.2
Mouse, joint —see Loose, body, joint
  knee M23.4-
Mouth —see condition
Movable
  coccyx —see subcategory M53.2
  kidney N28.89
    congenital Q63.8
  spleen D73.89
Movements, dystonic R25.8
Moyamoya disease I67.5
MRSA (Methicillin resistant Staphylococcus
  aureus)
  infection A49.02
    as the cause of diseases classified
      elsewhere B95.62
  sepsis A41.02
MSSA (Methicillin susceptible Staphylococcus
  aureus)
  infection A49.01
    as the cause of diseases classified
      elsewhere B95.61
  sepsis A41.01
Mucha-Habermann disease L41.0
Mucinosis (cutaneous) (focal) (papular)
  (reticular erythematous) (skin) L98.5
  oral K13.79
Mucocele
  appendix K38.8
  buccal cavity K13.79
  gallbladder K82.1
  lacrimal sac, chronic H04.43-
  nasal sinus J34.1
  nose J34.1
  salivary gland (any) K11.6
  sinus (accessory) (nasal) J34.1
  turbinate (bone) (middle) (nasal) J34.1
  uterus N85.8

Mucolipidosis
  I E77.1
  II, III E77.0
  IV E75.11
Mucopolysaccharidosis E76.3
  beta-gluduronidase deficiency E76.29
  cardiopathy E76.3 [152]
  Hunter's syndrome E76.1
  Hurler's syndrome E76.01
  Hurler-Scheie syndrome E76.02
  Maroteaux-Lamy syndrome E76.29
  Morquio syndrome E76.219
    A E76.210
    B E76.211
    classic E76.210
  Sanfilippo syndrome E76.22
  Scheie's syndrome E76.03
  specified NEC E76.29
  type
    I
      Hurler's syndrome E76.01
      Hurler-Scheie syndrome E76.02
      Scheie's syndrome E76.03
    II E76.1
    III E76.22
    IV E76.219
    IVA E76.210
    IVB E76.211
    VI E76.29
    VII E76.29
Mucormycosis B46.5
  cutaneous B46.3
  disseminated B46.4
  gastrointestinal B46.2
  generalized B46.4
  pulmonary B46.0
  rhinocerebral B46.1
  skin B46.3
  subcutaneous B46.3
Mucositis (ulcerative) K12.30
  due to drugs NEC K12.32
  gastrointestinal K92.81
  mouth (oral) (oropharyngeal) K12.30
    due to antineoplastic therapy K12.31
    due to drugs NEC K12.32
    due to radiation K12.33
    specified NEC K12.39
    viral K12.39
  nasal J34.81
  oral cavity —see Mucositis, mouth
  oral soft tissues —see Mucositis, mouth
  vagina and vulva N76.81
Mucositis necroticans agranulocytica —see
  Agranulocytosis
Mucous —see also condition
  patches (syphilitic) A51.39
    congenital A50.07
Mucoviscidosis E84.9
  with meconium obstruction E84.11
Mucus
  asphyxia or suffocation —see Asphyxia,
    mucus
  in stool R19.5
  plug —see Asphyxia, mucus
Muguet B37.0
Mulberry molars (congenital syphilis)
  A50.52
Müllerian mixed tumor
  specified site —see Neoplasm, malignant, by
    site
  unspecified site C54.9
Multicystic kidney (development) Q61.4
Multiparity (grand) Z64.1
  affecting management of pregnancy, labor
    and delivery (supervision only)
    O09.4-
  requiring contraceptive management —see
    Contraception
Multipartita placenta O43.19-
Multiple, multiplex —see also condition
  digits (congenital) Q69.9

Multiple, multiplex (Continued)
  endocrine neoplasia —see Neoplasia,
    endocrine, multiple [MEN]
  personality F44.81
Mumps B26.9
  arthritis B26.85
  complication NEC B26.89
  encephalitis B26.2
  hepatitis B26.81
  meningitis (aseptic) B26.1
  meningoencephalitis B26.2
  myocarditis B26.82
  oophoritis B26.89
  orchitis B26.0
  pancreatitis B26.3
  polyneuropathy B26.84
Mumu —see also Infestation, filarial B74.9
  [N51]
Münchhausen's syndrome —see Disorder,
  factitious
Münchmeyer's syndrome —see Myositis,
  ossificans, progressiva
Mural —see condition
Murmur (cardiac) (heart) (organic) R01.1
  abdominal R19.15
  aortic (valve) —see Endocarditis, aortic
  benign R01.0
  diastolic —see Endocarditis
  Flint I35.1
  functional R01.0
  Graham Steell I37.1
  innocent R01.0
  mitral (valve) —see Insufficiency, mitral
  nonorganic R01.0
  presystolic, mitral —see Insufficiency, mitral
  pulmonic (valve) I37.8
  systolic R01.1 ◀▥
  tricuspid (valve) I07.9
  valvular —see Endocarditis
Murri's disease (intermittent hemoglobinuria)
  D59.6
Muscle, muscular —see also condition
  carnitine (palmityltransferase) deficiency
    E71.314
Musculoneuralgia —see Neuralgia
Mushroom-workers' (pickers') disease or lung
  J67.5
Mushrooming hip —see Derangement, joint,
  specified NEC, hip
Mutation (s)
  factor V Leiden D68.51
  surfactant, of lung J84.83
  prothrombin gene D68.52
Mutism —see also Aphasia
  deaf (acquired) (congenital) NEC H91.3
  elective (adjustment reaction) (childhood)
    F94.0
  hysterical F44.4
  selective (childhood) F94.0
MVD (microvillus inclusion disease) Q43.8
MVID (microvillus inclusion disease) Q43.8
Myalgia M79.1
  epidemic (cervical) B33.0
  traumatic NEC T14.8
Myasthenia G70.9
  congenital G70.2
  cordis —see Failure, heart
  developmental G70.2
  gravis G70.00
    with exacerbation (acute) G70.01
    in crisis G70.01
    neonatal, transient P94.0
    pseudoparalytica G70.00
      with exacerbation (acute) G70.01
      in crisis G70.01
  stomach, psychogenic F45.8
  syndrome
    in
      diabetes mellitus —see E08-E13 with .44
      neoplastic disease —see also Neoplasm
        D49.9 [G73.3]

◀ New   ◀▥ Revised   ~~deleted~~ Deleted

Myasthenia (Continued)
  syndrome (Continued)
    in (Continued)
      pernicious anemia D51.0 [G73.3]
      thyrotoxicosis E05.90 [G73.3]
        with thyroid storm E05.91 [G73.3]
Myasthenic M62.81
Mycelium infection B49
Mycetismus —see Poisoning, food, noxious,
  mushroom
Mycetoma B47.9
  actinomycotic B47.1
  bone (mycotic) B47.9 [M90.80]
  eumycotic B47.0
  foot B47.9
    actinomycotic B47.1
    mycotic B47.0
  madurae NEC B47.9
    mycotic B47.0
  maduromycotic B47.0
  mycotic B47.0
  nocardial B47.1
Mycobacteriosis —see Mycobacterium
Mycobacterium, mycobacterial (infection)
  A31.9
  anonymous A31.9
  atypical A31.9
    cutaneous A31.1
    pulmonary A31.0
      tuberculous —see Tuberculosis,
        pulmonary
    specified site NEC A31.8
  avium (intracellulare complex) A31.0
  balnei A31.1
  Battey A31.0
  chelonei A31.8
  cutaneous A31.1
  extrapulmonary systemic A31.8
  fortuitum A31.8
  intracellulare (Battey bacillus) A31.0
  kakaferifu A31.8
  kansasii (yellow bacillus) A31.0
  kasongo A31.8
  leprae —see also Leprosy A30.9
  luciflavum A31.1
  marinum (M. balnei) A31.1
  nonspecific —see Mycobacterium, atypical
  pulmonary (atypical) A31.0
    tuberculous —see Tuberculosis,
      pulmonary
  scrofulaceum A31.8
  simiae A31.8
  systemic, extrapulmonary A31.8
  szulgai A31.8
  terrae A31.8
  triviale A31.8
  tuberculosis (human, bovine) —see
    Tuberculosis
  ulcerans A31.1
  xenopi A31.8
Mycoplasma (M.) pneumoniae, as cause of
  disease classified elsewhere B96.0
Mycosis, mycotic B49
  cutaneous NEC B36.9
  ear B36.9 ◀▥
    in ◀
      aspergillosis B44.89 ◀
      candidiasis B37.84 ◀
      moniliasis B37.84 ◀
  fungoides (extranodal) (solid organ)
    C84.0-
  mouth B37.0
  nails B35.1
  opportunistic B48.8
  skin NEC B36.9
  specified NEC B48.8
  stomatitis B37.0
  vagina, vaginitis (candidal) B37.3
Mydriasis (pupil) H57.04
Myelatelia Q06.1
Myelinolysis, pontine, central G37.2

Myelitis (acute) (ascending) (childhood)
    (chronic) (descending) (diffuse)
    (disseminated) (idiopathic) (pressure)
    (progressive) (spinal cord) (subacute) —see
    also Encephalitis G04.91
  herpes simplex B00.82
  herpes zoster B02.24
  in diseases classified elsewhere G05.4
  necrotizing, subacute G37.4
  optic neuritis in G36.0
  postchickenpox B01.12
  postherpetic B02.24
  postimmunization G04.02
  postinfectious NEC G04.89
  postvaccinal G04.02
  specified NEC G04.89
  syphilitic (transverse) A52.14
  toxic G92
  transverse (in demyelinating diseases of
    central nervous system) G37.3
  tuberculous A17.82
  varicella B01.12
Myeloblastic —see condition
Myeloblastoma
  granular cell —see also Neoplasm, connective
    tissue
    malignant —see Neoplasm, connective
      tissue, malignant
  tongue D10.1
Myelocele —see Spina bifida
Myelocystocele —see Spina bifida
Myelocytic —see condition
Myelodysplasia D46.9
  specified NEC D46.Z
  spinal cord (congenital) Q06.1
Myelodysplastic syndrome D46.9
  with
    5q deletion D46.C
    isolated del (5q) chromosomal abnormality
      C46.C
  specified NEC D46.Z
Myeloencephalitis —see Encephalitis
Myelofibrosis D75.81
  with myeloid metaplasia D47.4
  acute C94.4-
  idiopathic (chronic) D47.4
  primary D47.1
  secondary D75.81
    in myeloproliferative disease D47.4
Myelogenous —see condition
Myeloid —see condition
Myelokathexis D70.9
Myeloleukodystrophy E75.29
Myelolipoma —see Lipoma
Myeloma (multiple) C90.0-
  monostotic C90.3
    plasma cell C90.0-
  plasma cell C90.0-
  solitary —see also Plasmacytoma, solitary
    C90.3-
Myelomalacia G95.89
Myelomatosis C90.0-
Myelomeningitis —see Meningoencephalitis
Myelomeningocele (spinal cord) —see Spina
  bifida
Myelo-osteo-musculodysplasia hereditaria
  Q79.8
Myelopathic
  anemia D64.89
  muscle atrophy —see Atrophy, muscle, spinal
  pain syndrome G89.0
Myelopathy (spinal cord) G95.9
  drug-induced G95.89
  in (due to)
    degeneration or displacement,
      intervertebral disc NEC —see
      Disorder, disc, with, myelopathy
    infection —see Encephalitis
    intervertebral disc disorder —see also
      Disorder, disc, with, myelopathy
    mercury —see subcategory T56.1

Myelopathy (Continued)
  in (due to) (Continued)
    neoplastic disease —see also Neoplasm
      D49.9 [G99.2]
    pernicious anemia D51.0 [G99.2]
    spondylosis —see Spondylosis, with
      myelopathy NEC
  necrotic (subacute) (vascular) G95.19
  radiation-induced G95.89
  spondylogenic NEC —see Spondylosis, with
    myelopathy NEC
  toxic G95.89
  transverse, acute G37.3
  vascular G95.19
  vitamin B12 E53.8 [G32.0]
Myelophthisis D61.82
Myeloradiculitis G04.91
Myeloradiculodysplasia (spinal)
  Q06.1
Myelosarcoma C92.3-
Myelosclerosis D75.89
  with myeloid metaplasia D47.4
  disseminated, of nervous system
    G35
  megakaryocytic D47.4
    with myeloid metaplasia D47.4
Myelosis
  acute C92.0-
  aleukemic C92.9-
  chronic D47.1
  erythremic (acute) C94.0-
  megakaryocytic C94.2-
  nonleukemic D72.828
  subacute C92.9-
Myiasis (cavernous) B87.9
  aural B87.4
  creeping B87.0
  cutaneous B87.0
  dermal B87.0
  ear (external) (middle) B87.4
  eye B87.2
  genitourinary B87.81
  intestinal B87.82
  laryngeal B87.3
  nasopharyngeal B87.3
  ocular B87.2
  orbit B87.2
  skin B87.0
  specified site NEC B87.89
  traumatic B87.1
  wound B87.1
Myoadenoma, prostate —see Hyperplasia,
  prostate
Myoblastoma
  granular cell —see also Neoplasm, connective
    tissue, benign
    malignant —see Neoplasm, connective
      tissue, malignant
  tongue D10.1
Myocardial —see condition
Myocardiopathy (congestive) (constrictive)
    (familial) (hypertrophic nonobstructive)
    (idiopathic) (infiltrative) (obstructive)
    (primary) (restrictive) (sporadic) —see also
    Cardiomyopathy I42.9
  alcoholic I42.6
  cobalt-beer I42.6
  glycogen storage E74.02 [I43]
  hypertrophic obstructive I42.1
  in (due to)
    beriberi E51.12
    cardiac glycogenosis E74.02 [I43]
    Friedreich's ataxia G11.1 [I43]
    myotonia atrophica G71.11 [I43]
    progressive muscular dystrophy G71.0
      [I43]
  obscure (African) I42.8
  secondary I42.9
  thyrotoxic E05.90 [I43]
    with storm E05.91 [I43]
  toxic NEC I42.7

Myocarditis (with arteriosclerosis) (chronic)
   (fibroid) (interstitial) (old) (progressive)
   (senile) I51.4
  with
    rheumatic fever (conditions in I00) I09.0
      active —see Myocarditis, acute,
        rheumatic
      inactive or quiescent (with chorea) I09.0
  active I40.9
    rheumatic I01.2
      with chorea (acute) (rheumatic)
        (Sydenham's) I02.0
  acute or subacute (interstitial) I40.9
    due to
      streptococcus (beta-hemolytic) I01.2
    idiopathic I40.1
    rheumatic I01.2
      with chorea (acute) (rheumatic)
        (Sydenham's) I02.0
    specified NEC I40.8
  aseptic of newborn B33.22
  bacterial (acute) I40.0
  Coxsackie (virus) B33.22
  diphtheritic A36.81
  eosinophilic I40.1
  epidemic of newborn (Coxsackie) B33.22
  Fiedler's (acute) (isolated) I40.1
  giant cell (acute) (subacute) I40.1
  gonococcal A54.83
  granulomatous (idiopathic) (isolated)
    (nonspecific) I40.1
  hypertensive —see Hypertension, heart
  idiopathic (granulomatous) I40.1
  in (due to)
    diphtheria A36.81
    epidemic louse-borne typhus A75.0 [I41]
    Lyme disease A69.29
    sarcoidosis D86.85
    scarlet fever A38.1
    toxoplasmosis (acquired) B58.81
    typhoid A01.02
    typhus NEC A75.9 [I41]
  infective I40.0
  influenzal —see Influenza, with, myocarditis
  isolated (acute) I40.1
  meningococcal A39.52
  mumps B26.82
  nonrheumatic, active I40.9
  parenchymatous I40.9
  pneumococcal I40.0
  rheumatic (chronic) (inactive) (with chorea)
    I09.0
    active or acute I01.2
      with chorea (acute) (rheumatic)
        (Sydenham's) I02.0
  rheumatoid —see Rheumatoid, carditis
  septic I40.0
  staphylococcal I40.0
  suppurative I40.0
  syphilitic (chronic) A52.06
  toxic I40.8
    rheumatic —see Myocarditis, acute,
      rheumatic
  tuberculous A18.84
  typhoid A01.02
  valvular —see Endocarditis
  virus, viral I40.0
    of newborn (Coxsackie) B33.22
Myocardium, myocardial —see condition
Myocardosis —see Cardiomyopathy
Myoclonus, myoclonic, myoclonia (familial)
  (essential) (multifocal) (simplex) G25.3
  drug-induced G25.3
  epilepsy —see also Epilepsy, generalized,
    specified NEC G40.4-
    familial (progressive) G25.3
  epileptica G40.409
    with status epilepticus G40.401
  facial G51.3
  familial progressive G25.3
  Friedreich's G25.3

Myoclonus, myoclonic, myoclonia (Continued)
  jerks G25.3
  massive G25.3
  palatal G25.3
  pharyngeal G25.3
Myocytolysis I51.5
Myodiastasis —see Diastasis, muscle
Myoendocarditis —see Endocarditis
Myoepithelioma —see Neoplasm, benign, by
  site
Myofasciitis (acute) —see Myositis
Myofibroma —see also Neoplasm, connective
  tissue, benign
  uterus (cervix) (corpus) —see Leiomyoma
Myofibromatosis D48.1
  infantile Q89.8
Myofibrosis M62.89
  heart —see Myocarditis
  scapulohumeral —see Lesion, shoulder,
    specified NEC
Myofibrositis M79.7
  scapulohumeral —see Lesion, shoulder,
    specified NEC
Myoglobulinuria, myoglobinuria (primary)
  R82.1
Myokymia, facial G51.4
Myolipoma —see Lipoma
Myoma —see also Neoplasm, connective tissue,
  benign
  malignant —see Neoplasm, connective tissue,
    malignant
  prostate D29.1
  uterus (cervix) (corpus) —see Leiomyoma
Myomalacia M62.89
Myometritis —see Endometritis
Myometrium —see condition
Myonecrosis, clostridial A48.0
Myopathy G72.9
  acute
    necrotizing G72.81
    quadriplegic G72.81
  alcoholic G72.1
  benign congenital G71.2
  central core G71.2
  centronuclear G71.2
  congenital (benign) G71.2
  critical illness G72.81
  distal G71.0
  drug-induced G72.0
  endocrine NEC E34.9 [G73.7]
  extraocular muscles H05.82-
  facioscapulohumeral G71.0
  hereditary G71.9
    specified NEC G71.8
  immune NEC G72.49
  in (due to)
    Addison's disease E27.1 [G73.7]
    alcohol G72.1
    amyloidosis E85.0 [G73.7]
    cretinism E00.9 [G73.7]
    Cushing's syndrome E24.9 [G73.7]
    drugs G72.0
    endocrine disease NEC E34.9 [G73.7]
    giant cell arteritis M31.6 [G73.7]
    glycogen storage disease E74.00 [G73.7]
    hyperadrenocorticism E24.9 [G73.7]
    hyperparathyroidism NEC E21.3 [G73.7]
    hypoparathyroidism E20.9 [G73.7]
    hypopituitarism E23.0 [G73.7]
    hypothyroidism E03.9 [G73.7]
    infectious disease NEC B99 [G73.7]
    lipid storage disease E75.6 [G73.7]
    metabolic disease NEC E88.9 [G73.7]
    myxedema E03.9 [G73.7]
    parasitic disease NEC B89 [G73.7]
    polyarteritis nodosa M30.0 [G73.7]
    rheumatoid arthritis —see Rheumatoid,
      myopathy
    sarcoidosis D86.87
    scleroderma M34.82
    sicca syndrome M35.03

Myopathy (Continued)
  in (due to) (Continued)
    Sjögren's syndrome M35.03
    systemic lupus erythematosus M32.19
    thyrotoxicosis (hyperthyroidism) E05.90
      [G73.7]
      with thyroid storm E05.91 [G73.7]
    toxic agent NEC G72.2
  inflammatory NEC G72.49
  intensive care (ICU) G72.81
  limb-girdle G71.0
  mitochondrial NEC G71.3
  myotubular G71.2
  mytonic, proximal (PROMM) G71.11
  nemaline G71.2
  ocular G71.0
  oculopharyngeal G71.0
  of critical illness G72.81
  primary G71.9
    specified NEC G71.8
  progressive NEC G72.89
  proximal myotonic (PROMM) G71.11
  rod G71.2
  scapulohumeral G71.0
  specified NEC G72.89
  toxic G72.2
Myopericarditis —see also Pericarditis
  chronic rheumatic I09.2
Myopia (axial) (congenital) H52.1-
  degenerative (malignant) H44.2-
  malignant H44.2-
  pernicious H44.2-
  progressive high (degenerative) H44.2-
Myosarcoma —see Neoplasm, connective tissue,
  malignant
Myosis (pupil) H57.03
  stromal (endolymphatic) D39.0
Myositis M60.9
  clostridial A48.0
  due to posture —see Myositis, specified type
    NEC
  epidemic B33.0
  fibrosa or fibrous (chronic), Volkmann's
    T79.6
  foreign body granuloma —see Granuloma,
    foreign body
  in (due to)
    bilharziasis B65.9 [M63.8-]
    cysticercosis B69.81
    leprosy A30.9 [M63.8-]
    mycosis B49 [M63.8-]
    sarcoidosis D86.87
    schistosomiasis B65.9 [M63.8-]
    syphilis
      late A52.78
      secondary A51.49
    toxoplasmosis (acquired) B58.82
    trichinellosis B75 [M63.8-]
    tuberculosis A18.09
  inclusion body [IBM] G72.41
  infective M60.009
    arm M60.002
      left M60.001
      right M60.000
    leg M60.005
      left M60.004
      right M60.003
    lower limb M60.005
      ankle M60.07-
      foot M60.07-
      lower leg M60.06-
      thigh M60.05-
      toe M60.07-
    multiple sites M60.09
    specified site NEC M60.08
    upper limb M60.002
      finger M60.04-
      forearm M60.03-
      hand M60.04-
      shoulder region M60.01-
      upper arm M60.02-

◀ New   ◀║║ Revised   ~~deleted~~ Deleted

M

Myosagitis *(Continued)*
interstitial M60.10
  ankle M60.17-
  foot M60.17-
  forearm M60.13-
  hand M60.14-
  lower leg M60.16-
  multiple sites M60.19
  shoulder region M60.11-
  specified site NEC M60.18
  thigh M60.15-
  upper arm M60.12-
mycotic B49 *[M63.8-]*
ossificans or ossifying (circumscripta) —*see also* Ossification, muscle, specified NEC
  in (due to)
    burns M61.30
      ankle M61.37-
      foot M61.37-
      forearm M61.33-
      hand M61.34-
      lower leg M61.36-
      multiple sites M61.39
      pelvic region M61.35-
      shoulder region M61.31-
      specified site NEC M61.38
      thigh M61.35-
      upper arm M61.32-
    quadriplegia or paraplegia M61.20
      ankle M61.27-
      foot M61.27-
      forearm M61.23-
      hand M61.24-
      lower leg M61.26-
      multiple sites M61.29
      pelvic region M61.25-
      shoulder region M61.21-
      specified site NEC M61.28
      thigh M61.25-
      upper arm M61.22-
  progressiva M61.10
    ankle M61.17-
    finger M61.14-
    foot M61.17-
    forearm M61.13-
    hand M61.14-
    lower leg M61.16-

Myositis *(Continued)*
  ossificans or ossifying *(Continued)*
    progressiva *(Continued)*
      multiple sites M61.19
      pelvic region M61.15-
      shoulder region M61.11-
      specified site NEC M61.18
      thigh M61.15-
      toe M61.17-
      upper arm M61.12-
    traumatica M61.00
      ankle M61.07-
      foot M61.07-
      forearm M61.03-
      hand M61.04-
      lower leg M61.06-
      multiple sites M61.09
      pelvic region M61.05-
      shoulder region M61.01-
      specified site NEC M61.08
      thigh M61.05-
      upper arm M61.02-
    purulent —*see* Myositis, infective
    specified type NEC M60.80
      ankle M60.87-
      foot M60.87-
      forearm M60.83-
      hand M60.84-
      lower leg M60.86-
      multiple sites M60.89
      pelvic region M60.85-
      shoulder region M60.81-
      specified site NEC M60.88
      thigh M60.85-
      upper arm M60.82-
    suppurative —*see* Myositis, infective
    traumatic (old) —*see* Myositis, specified type NEC
Myospasia impulsiva F95.2
Myotonia (acquisita) (intermittens) M62.89
  atrophica G71.11
  chondrodystrophic G71.13
  congenita (acetazolamide responsive) (dominant) (recessive) G71.12
  drug-induced G71.14
  dystrophica G71.11
  fluctuans G71.19

Myotonia *(Continued)*
  levior G71.12
  permanens G71.19
  symptomatic G71.19
Myotonic pupil —*see* Anomaly, pupil, function, tonic pupil
Myriapodiasis B88.2
Myringitis H73.2-
  with otitis media —*see* Otitis, media
  acute H73.00-
    bullous H73.01-
    specified NEC H73.09-
  bullous —*see* Myringitis, acute, bullous
  chronic H73.1-
Mysophobia F40.228
Mytilotoxism —*see* Poisoning, fish
Myxadenitis labialis K13.0
Myxedema (adult) (idiocy) (infantile) (juvenile) —*see also* Hypothyroidism E03.9
  circumscribed E05.90
    with storm E05.91
  coma E03.5
  congenital E00.1
  cutis L98.5
  localized (pretibial) E05.90
    with storm E05.91
  papular L98.5
Myxochondrosarcoma —*see* Neoplasm, cartilage, malignant
Myxofibroma —*see* Neoplasm, connective tissue, benign
  odontogenic —*see* Cyst, calcifying odontogenic
Myxofibrosarcoma —*see* Neoplasm, connective tissue, malignant
Myxolipoma D17.9
Myxoliposarcoma —*see* Neoplasm, connective tissue, malignant
Myxoma —*see also* Neoplasm, connective tissue, benign
  nerve sheath —*see* Neoplasm, nerve, benign
  odontogenic —*see* Cyst, calcifying odontogenic
Myxosarcoma —*see* Neoplasm, connective tissue, malignant

N

Naegeli's
  disease Q82.8
  leukemia, monocytic C93.1-
Naegleriasis (with meningoencephalitis) B60.2
Naffziger's syndrome G54.0
Naga sore —*see* Ulcer, skin
Nägele's pelvis M95.5
  with disproportion (fetopelvic) O33.0
    causing obstructed labor O65.0
Nail —*see also* condition
  biting F98.8
  patella syndrome Q87.2
Nanism, nanosomia —*see* Dwarfism
Nanophyetiasis B66.8
Nanukayami A27.89
Napkin rash L22
Narcolepsy G47.419
  with cataplexy G47.411
  in conditions classified elsewhere G47.429
    with cataplexy G47.421
Narcosis R06.89
Narcotism —*see* Dependence
NARP (Neuropathy, Ataxia and Retinitis pigmentosa) syndrome E88.49
Narrow
  anterior chamber angle H40.03-
  gingival width (of periodontal soft tissue) K05.5 ◄
  pelvis —*see* Contraction, pelvis
Narrowing —*see also* Stenosis
  artery I77.1
    auditory, internal I65.8
    basilar —*see* Occlusion, artery, basilar
    carotid —*see* Occlusion, artery, carotid
    cerebellar —*see* Occlusion, artery, cerebellar
    cerebral —*see* Occlusion artery, cerebral
    choroidal —*see* Occlusion, artery, cerebral, specified NEC
    communicating posterior —*see* Occlusion, artery, cerebral, specified NEC
    coronary —*see also* Disease, heart, ischemic, atherosclerotic
      congenital Q24.5
        syphilitic A50.54 [I52]
      due to syphilis NEC A52.06
    hypophyseal —*see* Occlusion, artery, cerebral, specified NEC
    pontine —*see* Occlusion, artery, cerebral, specified NEC
    precerebral —*see* Occlusion, artery, precerebral
    vertebral —*see* Occlusion, artery, vertebral
  auditory canal (external) —*see* Stenosis, external ear canal
  eustachian tube —*see* Obstruction, eustachian tube
  eyelid —*see* Disorder, eyelid function
  larynx J38.6
  mesenteric artery —*see also* Ischemia, intestine, acute K55.059 ◄▥
  palate M26.89
  palpebral fissure —*see* Disorder, eyelid function
  ureter N13.5
    with infection N13.6
  urethra —*see* Stricture, urethra
Narrowness, abnormal, eyelid Q10.3
Nasal —*see* condition
Nasolachrymal, nasolacrimal —*see* condition
Nasopharyngeal —*see also* condition
  pituitary gland Q89.2
  torticollis M43.6
Nasopharyngitis (acute) (infective) (streptococcal) (subacute) J00
  chronic (suppurative) (ulcerative) J31.1
Nasopharynx, nasopharyngeal —*see* condition
Natal tooth, teeth K00.6

Nausea (without vomiting) R11.0
  with vomiting R11.2
  gravidarum —*see* Hyperemesis, gravidarum
  marina T75.3
  navalis T75.3
Navel —*see* condition
Neapolitan fever —*see* Brucellosis
Near drowning T75.1
Nearsightedness —*see* Myopia
Near-syncope R55
Nebula, cornea —*see* Opacity, cornea
Necator americanus infestation B76.1
Necatoriasis B76.1
Neck —*see* condition
Necrobiosis R68.89
  lipoidica NEC L92.1
    with diabetes —*see* E08-E13 with .620
Necrolysis, toxic epidermal L51.2
  due to drug
    correct substance properly administered — *see* Table of Drugs and Chemicals, by drug, adverse effect
    overdose or wrong substance given or taken —*see* Table of Drugs and Chemicals, by drug, poisoning
Necrophilia F65.89
Necrosis, necrotic (ischemic) —*see also* Gangrene
  adrenal (capsule) (gland) E27.49
  amputation stump (surgical) (late) T87.50
    arm T87.5-
    leg T87.5-
  antrum J32.0
  aorta (hyaline) —*see also* Aneurysm, aorta
    cystic medial —*see* Dissection, aorta
  artery I77.5
  bladder (aseptic) (sphincter) N32.89
  bone —*see also* Osteonecrosis M87.9
    aseptic or avascular —*see* Osteonecrosis idiopathic M87.00
    ethmoid J32.2
    jaw M27.2
    tuberculous —*see* Tuberculosis, bone
  brain I67.89
  breast (aseptic) (fat) (segmental) N64.1
  bronchus J98.09
  central nervous system NEC I67.89
  cerebellar I67.89
  cerebral I67.89
  colon —*see also* Infarct, intestine K55.049 ◄▥
  cornea H18.89- ◄▥
  cortical (acute) (renal) N17.1
  cystic medial (aorta) —*see* Dissection, aorta
  dental pulp K04.1
  esophagus K22.8
  ethmoid (bone) J32.2
  eyelid —*see* Disorder, eyelid, degenerative
  fat, fatty (generalized) —*see also* Disorder, soft tissue, specified type NEC
    abdominal wall K65.4
    breast (aseptic) (segmental) N64.1
    localized —*see* Degeneration, by site, fatty
    mesentery K65.4
    omentum K65.4
    pancreas K86.89 ◄▥
    peritoneum K65.4
    skin (subcutaneous), newborn P83.0
    subcutaneous, due to birth injury P15.6
  gallbladder —*see* Cholecystitis, acute
  heart —*see* Infarct, myocardium
  hip, aseptic or avascular —*see* Osteonecrosis, by type, femur
  intestine (acute) (hemorrhagic) (massive) — *see also* Infarct, intestine K55.069 ◄▥
  jaw M27.2
  kidney (bilateral) N28.0
    acute N17.9
    cortical (acute) (bilateral) N17.1
      with ectopic or molar pregnancy O08.4
    medullary (bilateral) (in acute renal failure) (papillary) N17.2

Necrosis, necrotic (*Continued*)
  kidney (*Continued*)
    papillary (bilateral) (in acute renal failure) N17.2
    tubular N17.0
      with ectopic or molar pregnancy O08.4
      complicating
        abortion —*see* Abortion, by type, complicated by, tubular necrosis
        ectopic or molar pregnancy O08.4
        pregnancy —*see* Pregnancy, complicated by, diseases of, specified type or system NEC
      following ectopic or molar pregnancy O08.4
      traumatic T79.5
  larynx J38.7
  liver (with hepatic failure) (cell) —*see* Failure, hepatic
  hemorrhagic, central K76.2
  lung J85.0
  lymphatic gland —*see* Lymphadenitis, acute
  mammary gland (fat) (segmental) N64.1
  mastoid (chronic) —*see* Mastoiditis, chronic
  medullary (acute) (renal) N17.2
  mesentery —*see also* Infarct, intestine K55.069 ◄▥
    fat K65.4
  mitral valve —*see* Insufficiency, mitral
  myocardium, myocardial —*see* Infarct, myocardium
  nose J34.0
  omentum (with mesenteric infarction) —*see also* Infarct, intestine K55.069 ◄▥
    fat K65.4
  orbit, orbital —*see* Osteomyelitis, orbit
  ossicles, ear —*see* Abnormal, ear ossicles
  ovary N70.92
  pancreas (aseptic) (duct) (fat) K86.89 ◄▥
    acute (infective) —*see* Pancreatitis, acute
    infective —*see* Pancreatitis, acute
  papillary (acute) (renal) N17.2
  perineum N90.89
  peritoneum (with mesenteric infarction) —*see also* Infarct, intestine K55.069 ◄▥
    fat K65.4
  pharynx J02.9
    in granulocytopenia —*see* Neutropenia
    Vincent's A69.1
  phosphorus —*see* subcategory T54.2
  pituitary (gland) E23.0 ◄▥
    postpartum O99.285 ◄
    Sheehan O99.285 ◄
  pressure —*see* Ulcer, pressure, by site
  pulmonary J85.0
  pulp (dental) K04.1
  radiation —*see* Necrosis, by site
  radium —*see* Necrosis, by site
  renal —*see* Necrosis, kidney
  sclera H15.89
  scrotum N50.89 ◄▥
  skin or subcutaneous tissue NEC I96
  spine, spinal (column) —*see also* Osteonecrosis, by type, vertebra
    cord G95.19
  spleen D73.5
  stomach K31.89
  stomatitis (ulcerative) A69.0
  subcutaneous fat, newborn P83.8
  subendocardial (acute) I21.4
    chronic I25.89
  suprarenal (capsule) (gland) E27.49
  testis N50.89 ◄▥
  thymus (gland) E32.8
  tonsil J35.8
  trachea J39.8
  tuberculous NEC —*see* Tuberculosis
  tubular (acute) (anoxic) (renal) (toxic) N17.0
    postprocedural N99.0
  vagina N89.8

◄ New   ◄▥ Revised   ~~deleted~~ Deleted

Nephritis, nephritic *(Continued)*
  rapidly progressive *(Continued)*
    with *(Continued)*
      diffuse *(Continued)*
        membranous glomerulonephritis N01.2
        mesangial proliferative glomerulonephritis N01.3
        mesangiocapillary glomerulonephritis N01.5
        focal and segmental glomerular lesions N01.1
        minor glomerular abnormality N01.0
        specified morphological changes NEC N01.8
  salt losing or wasting NEC N28.89
  saturnine N14.3
  sclerosing, diffuse N05.8
  septic —*see* Nephritis, tubulo-interstitial
  specified pathology NEC —*see also* N00-N07
    with fourth character .8 N05.8
  subacute N01.9
  suppurative —*see* Nephritis, tubulo-interstitial
  syphilitic (late) A52.75
    congenital A50.59 *[N08]*
    early (secondary) A51.44
  toxic —*see* Nephropathy, toxic
  tubal, tubular —*see* Nephritis, tubulo-interstitial
  tuberculous A18.11
  tubulo-interstitial (in) N12
    acute (infectious) N10
    chronic (infectious) N11.9
      nonobstructive N11.8
        reflux-associated N11.0
      obstructive N11.1
      specified NEC N11.8
    due to
      brucellosis A23.9 *[N16]*
      cryoglobulinemia D89.1 *[N16]*
      glycogen storage disease E74.00 *[N16]*
      Sjögren's syndrome M35.04
  vascular —*see* Hypertension, kidney
  war N00.9
Nephroblastoma (epithelial) (mesenchymal) C64-
Nephrocalcinosis E83.59 *[N29]*
Nephrocystitis, pustular —*see* Nephritis, tubulo-interstitial
Nephrolithiasis (congenital) (pelvis) (recurrent) —*see also* Calculus, kidney
Nephroma C64-
  mesoblastic D41.0-
Nephronephritis —*see* Nephrosis
Nephronophthisis Q61.5
Nephropathia epidemica A98.5
Nephropathy —*see also* Nephritis N28.9
  with
    edema —*see* Nephrosis
    glomerular lesion —*see* Glomerulonephritis
  amyloid, hereditary E85.0
  analgesic N14.0
    with medullary necrosis, acute N17.2
  Balkan (endemic) N15.0
  chemical —*see* Nephropathy, toxic
  diabetic —*see* E08-E13 with .21
  drug-induced N14.2
    specified NEC N14.1
  focal and segmental hyalinosis or sclerosis N02.1
  heavy metal-induced N14.3
  hereditary NEC N07.9
    with
      dense deposit disease N07.6
      diffuse
        crescentic glomerulonephritis N07.7
        endocapillary proliferative glomerulonephritis N07.4

Nephropathy *(Continued)*
  hereditary NEC *(Continued)*
    with *(Continued)*
      diffuse *(Continued)*
        membranous glomerulonephritis N07.2
        mesangial proliferative glomerulonephritis N07.3
        mesangiocapillary glomerulonephritis N07.5
        focal and segmental glomerular lesions N07.1
        minor glomerular abnormality N07.0
        specified morphological changes NEC N07.8
  hypercalcemic N25.89
  hypertensive —*see* Hypertension, kidney
  hypokalemic (vacuolar) N25.89
  IgA N02.8
    with glomerular lesion N02.9
      focal and segmental hyalinosis or sclerosis N02.1
      membranoproliferative (diffuse) N02.5
      membranous (diffuse) N02.2
      mesangial proliferative (diffuse) N02.3
      mesangiocapillary (diffuse) N02.5
      proliferative NEC N02.8
      specified pathology NEC N02.8
  lead N14.3
  membranoproliferative (diffuse) N02.5
  membranous (diffuse) N02.2
  mesangial (IgA/IgG) —*see* Nephropathy, IgA
    proliferative (diffuse) N02.3
  mesangiocapillary (diffuse) N02.5
  obstructive N13.8
  phenacetin N17.2
  phosphate-losing N25.0
  potassium depletion N25.89
  pregnancy-related O26.83-
  proliferative NEC (*see also* N00-N07 with fourth character .8) N05.8
  protein-losing N25.89
  saturnine N14.3
  sickle-cell D57.- *[N08]*
  toxic NEC N14.4
    due to
      drugs N14.2
        analgesic N14.0
        specified NEC N14.1
      heavy metals N14.3
  vasomotor N17.0
  water-losing N25.89
Nephroptosis N28.83
Nephropyosis —*see* Abscess, kidney
Nephrorrhagia N28.89
Nephrosclerosis (arteriolar) (arteriosclerotic) (chronic) (hyaline) —*see also* Hypertension, kidney
  hyperplastic —*see* Hypertension, kidney
  senile N26.9
Nephrosis, nephrotic (Epstein's) (syndrome) (congenital) N04.9
  with
    foot process disease N04.9
    glomerular lesion N04.1
    hypocomplementemic N04.5
  acute N04.9
  anoxic —*see* Nephrosis, tubular
  chemical —*see* Nephrosis, tubular
  cholemic K76.7
  diabetic —*see* E08-E13 with .21
  Finnish type (congenital) Q89.8
  hemoglobin N10
  hemoglobinuric —*see* Nephrosis, tubular
  in
    amyloidosis E85.4 *[N08]*
    diabetes mellitus —*see* E08-E13 with .21
    epidemic hemorrhagic fever A98.5
    malaria (malariae) B52.0
  ischemic —*see* Nephrosis, tubular
  lipoid N04.9

Nephrosis, nephrotic *(Continued)*
  lower nephron —*see* Nephrosis, tubular
  malarial (malariae) B52.0
  minimal change N04.0
  myoglobin N10
  necrotizing —*see* Nephrosis, tubular
  osmotic (sucrose) N25.89
  radiation N04.9
  syphilitic (late) A52.75
  toxic —*see* Nephrosis, tubular
  tubular (acute) N17.0
    postprocedural N99.0
    radiation N04.9
Nephrosonephritis, hemorrhagic (endemic) A98.5
Nephrostomy
  attention to Z43.6
  status Z93.6
Nerve —*see also* condition
  injury —*see* Injury, nerve, by body site
Nerves R45.0
Nervous —*see also* condition R45.0
  heart F45.8
  stomach F45.8
  tension R45.0
Nervousness R45.0
Nesidioblastoma
  pancreas D13.7
  specified site NEC —*see* Neoplasm, benign, by site
  unspecified site D13.7
Nettleship's syndrome Q82.2
Neumann's disease or syndrome L10.1
Neuralgia, neuralgic (acute) M79.2
  accessory (nerve) G52.8
  acoustic (nerve) —*see* subcategory H93.3
  auditory (nerve) —*see* subcategory H93.3
  ciliary G44.009
    intractable G44.001
    not intractable G44.009
  cranial
    nerve —*see also* Disorder, nerve, cranial
      fifth or trigeminal —*see* Neuralgia, trigeminal
    postherpetic, postzoster B02.29
  ear —*see* subcategory H92.0
  facialis vera G51.1
  Fothergill's —*see* Neuralgia, trigeminal
  glossopharyngeal (nerve) G52.1
  Horton's G44.099
    intractable G44.091
    not intractable G44.099
  Hunt's B02.21
  hypoglossal (nerve) G52.3
  infraorbital —*see* Neuralgia, trigeminal
  malarial —*see* Malaria
  migrainous G44.009
    intractable G44.001
    not intractable G44.009
  Morton's G57.6-
  nerve, cranial —*see* Disorder, nerve, cranial
  nose G52.0
  occipital M54.81
  olfactory G52.0
  penis N48.9
  perineum R10.2
  postherpetic NEC B02.29
    trigeminal B02.22
  pubic region R10.2
  scrotum R10.2
  Sluder's G44.89
  specified nerve NEC G58.8
  spermatic cord R10.2
  sphenopalatine (ganglion) G90.09
  trifacial —*see* Neuralgia, trigeminal
  trigeminal G50.0
    postherpetic, postzoster B02.22
  vagus (nerve) G52.2
  writer's F48.8
    organic G25.89

◀ New ◀◀ Revised ~~deleted~~ Deleted

Neurapraxia —*see* Injury, nerve
Neurasthenia F48.8
  cardiac F45.8
  gastric F45.8
  heart F45.8
Neurilemmoma —*see also* Neoplasm, nerve, benign
  acoustic (nerve) D33.3
  malignant —*see also* Neoplasm, nerve, malignant
    acoustic (nerve) C72.4
Neurilemmosarcoma —*see* Neoplasm, nerve, malignant
Neurinoma —*see* Neoplasm, nerve, benign
Neurinomatosis —*see* Neoplasm, nerve, uncertain behavior
Neuritis (rheumatoid) M79.2
  abducens (nerve) —*see* Strabismus, paralytic, sixth nerve
  accessory (nerve) G52.8
  acoustic (nerve) —*see also* subcategory H93.3
    in (due to)
      infectious disease NEC B99 [H94.0-]
      parasitic disease NEC B89 [H94.0-]
      syphilitic A52.15
  alcoholic G62.1
    with psychosis —*see* Psychosis, alcoholic
  amyloid, any site E85.4 [G63]
  auditory (nerve) —*see* subcategory H93.3
  brachial —*see* Radiculopathy
    due to displacement, intervertebral disc —*see* Disorder, disc, cervical, with neuritis
  cranial nerve
    due to Lyme disease A69.22
    eighth or acoustic or auditory —*see* subcategory H93.3
    eleventh or accessory G52.8
    fifth or trigeminal G51.0
    first or olfactory G52.0
    fourth or trochlear —*see* Strabismus, paralytic, fourth nerve
    second or optic —*see* Neuritis, optic
    seventh or facial G51.8
      newborn (birth injury) P11.3
    sixth or abducent —*see* Strabismus, paralytic, sixth nerve
    tenth or vagus G52.2
    third or oculomotor —*see* Strabismus, paralytic, third nerve
    twelfth or hypoglossal G52.3
  Déjérine-Sottas G60.0
  diabetic (mononeuropathy) —*see* E08-E13 with .41
    polyneuropathy —*see* E08-E13 with .42
  due to
    beriberi E51.11
    displacement, prolapse or rupture, intervertebral disc —*see* Disorder, disc, with, radiculopathy
    herniation, nucleus pulposus M51.9 [G55]
  endemic E51.11
  facial G51.8
    newborn (birth injury) P11.3
  general —*see* Polyneuropathy
  geniculate ganglion G51.1
    due to herpes (zoster) B02.21
  gouty —*see also* Gout, by type M10.9 [G63] ◀▥
  hypoglossal (nerve) G52.3
  ilioinguinal (nerve) G57.9-
  infectious (multiple) NEC G61.0
  interstitial hypertrophic progressive G60.0
  lumbar M54.16
  lumbosacral M54.17
  multiple —*see also* Polyneuropathy
    endemic E51.11
    infective, acute G61.0
  multiplex endemica E51.11
  nerve root —*see* Radiculopathy
  oculomotor (nerve) —*see* Strabismus, paralytic, third nerve

Neuritis (*Continued*)
  olfactory nerve G52.0
  optic (nerve) (hereditary) (sympathetic) H46.9
    with demyelination G36.0
    in myelitis G36.0
    nutritional H46.2
    papillitis —*see* Papillitis, optic
    retrobulbar H46.1-
    specified type NEC H46.8
    toxic H46.3
  peripheral (nerve) G62.9
    multiple —*see* Polyneuropathy
    single —*see* Mononeuritis
  pneumogastric (nerve) G52.2
  postherpetic, postzoster B02.29
  progressive hypertrophic interstitial G60.0
  retrobulbar —*see also* Neuritis, optic, retrobulbar
    in (due to)
      late syphilis A52.15
      meningococcal infection A39.82
      meningococcal A39.82
      syphilitic A52.15
  sciatic (nerve) —*see also* Sciatica
    due to displacement of intervertebral disc —*see* Disorder, disc, with, radiculopathy
  serum —*see also* Reaction, serum T80.69
  shoulder-girdle G54.5
  specified nerve NEC G58.8
  spinal (nerve) root —*see* Radiculopathy
  syphilitic A52.15
  thenar (median) G56.1-
  thoracic M54.14
  toxic NEC G62.2
  trochlear (nerve) —*see* Strabismus, paralytic, fourth nerve
  vagus (nerve) G52.2
Neuroastrocytoma —*see* Neoplasm, uncertain behavior, by site
Neuroavitaminosis E56.9 [G99.8]
Neuroblastoma
  olfactory C30.0
  specified site —*see* Neoplasm, malignant, by site
  unspecified site C74.90
Neurochorioretinitis —*see* Chorioretinitis
Neurocirculatory asthenia F45.8
Neurocysticercosis B69.0
Neurocytoma —*see* Neoplasm, benign, by site
Neurodermatitis (circumscribed) (circumscripta) (local) L28.0
  atopic L20.81
  diffuse (Brocq) L20.81
  disseminated L20.81
Neuroencephalomyelopathy, optic G36.0
Neuroepithelioma —*see also* Neoplasm, malignant, by site
  olfactory C30.0
Neurofibroma —*see also* Neoplasm, nerve, benign
  melanotic —*see* Neoplasm, nerve, benign
  multiple —*see* Neurofibromatosis
  plexiform —*see* Neoplasm, nerve, benign
Neurofibromatosis (multiple) (nonmalignant) Q85.00
  acoustic Q85.02
  malignant —*see* Neoplasm, nerve, malignant
  specified NEC Q85.09
  type 1 (von Recklinghausen) Q85.01
  type 2 Q85.02
Neurofibrosarcoma —*see* Neoplasm, nerve, malignant
Neurogenic —*see also* condition
  bladder (*see also* Dysfunction, bladder, neuromuscular) N31.9
    cauda equina syndrome G83.4
  bowel NEC K59.2
  heart F45.8
Neuroglioma —*see* Neoplasm, uncertain behavior, by site

Neurolabyrinthitis (of Dix and Hallpike) —*see* Neuronitis, vestibular
Neurolathyrism —*see* Poisoning, food, noxious, plant
Neuroleprosy A30.9
Neuroma —*see also* Neoplasm, nerve, benign
  acoustic (nerve) D33.3
  amputation (stump) (traumatic) (surgical complication) (late) T87.3-
    arm T87.3-
    leg T87.3-
  digital (toe) G57.6-
  interdigital G58.8 ◀▥
    lower limb toe G57.8- ◀▥
    upper limb G56.8-
  intermetatarsal G57.8-
  Morton's G57.6-
  nonneoplastic
    arm G56.9-
    leg G57.9-
    lower extremity G57.9-
    upper extremity G56.9-
  optic (nerve) D33.3
  plantar G57.6-
  plexiform —*see* Neoplasm, nerve, benign
  surgical (nonneoplastic)
    arm G56.9-
    leg G57.9-
    lower extremity G57.9-
    upper extremity G56.9-
Neuromyalgia —*see* Neuralgia
Neuromyasthenia (epidemic) (postinfectious) G93.3
Neuromyelitis G36.9
  ascending G61.0
  optica G36.0
Neuromyopathy G70.9
  paraneoplastic D49.9 [G13.0]
Neuromyotonia (Isaacs) G71.19
Neuronevus —*see* Nevus
Neuronitis G58.9
  ascending (acute) G57.2-
  vestibular H81.2-
Neuroparalytic —*see* condition
Neuropathy, neuropathic G62.9
  acute motor G62.81
  alcoholic G62.1
    with psychosis —*see* Psychosis, alcoholic
  arm G56.9-
  autonomic, peripheral —*see* Neuropathy, peripheral, autonomic
  axillary G56.9-
  bladder N31.9
    atonic (motor) (sensory) N31.2
    autonomous N31.2
    flaccid N31.2
    nonreflex N31.2
    reflex N31.1
    uninhibited N31.0
  brachial plexus G54.0
  cervical plexus G54.2
  chronic
    progressive segmentally demyelinating G62.89
    relapsing demyelinating G62.89
  Déjérine-Sottas G60.0
  diabetic —*see* E08-E13 with .40
    mononeuropathy —*see* E08-E13 with .41
    polyneuropathy —*see* E08-E13 with .42
  entrapment G58.9
    iliohypogastric nerve G57.8-
    ilioinguinal nerve G57.8-
    lateral cutaneous nerve of thigh G57.1-
    median nerve G56.0-
    obturator nerve G57.8-
    peroneal nerve G57.3-
    posterior tibial nerve G57.5-
    saphenous nerve G57.8-
    ulnar nerve G56.2-

Neuropathy, neuropathic (Continued)
  facial nerve G51.9
  hereditary G60.9
    motor and sensory (types I-IV) G60.0
    sensory G60.8
    specified NEC G60.8
  hypertrophic G60.0
    Charcot-Marie-Tooth G60.0
    Déjérine-Sottas G60.0
    interstitial progressive G60.0
    of infancy G60.0
    Refsum G60.1
  idiopathic G60.9
    progressive G60.3
    specified NEC G60.8
  in association with hereditary ataxia G60.2
  intercostal G58.0
  ischemic —see Disorder, nerve
  Jamaica (ginger) G62.2
  leg NEC G57.9-
  lower extremity G57.9-
  lumbar plexus G54.1
  median nerve G56.1-
  motor and sensory —see also Polyneuropathy
    hereditary (types I-IV) G60.0
  multifocal motor (MMN) G61.82 ◀
  multiple (acute) (chronic) —see
    Polyneuropathy
  optic (nerve) —see also Neuritis, optic
    ischemic H47.01-
  paraneoplastic (sensorial) (Denny Brown)
    D49.9 [G13.0]
  peripheral (nerve) —see also Polyneuropathy
    G62.9
    autonomic G90.9
      idiopathic G90.09
      in (due to)
        amyloidosis E85.4 [G99.0]
        diabetes mellitus —see E08-E13 with
          .43
        endocrine disease NEC E34.9 [G99.0]
        gout M10.00 [G99.0]
        hyperthyroidism E05.90 [G99.0]
          with thyroid storm E05.91 [G99.0]
        metabolic disease NEC E88.9 [G99.0]
    idiopathic G60.9
      progressive G60.3
    in (due to)
      antitetanus serum G62.0
      arsenic G62.2
      drugs NEC G62.0
      lead G62.2
      organophosphate compounds G62.2
      toxic agent NEC G62.2
  plantar nerves G57.6-
  progressive
    hypertrophic interstitial G60.0
    inflammatory G62.81
  radicular NEC —see Radiculopathy
  sacral plexus G54.1
  sciatic G57.0-
  serum G61.1
  toxic NEC G62.2
  trigeminal sensory G50.8
  ulnar nerve G56.2-
  uremic N18.9 [G63]
  vitamin B12 E53.8 [G63]
    with anemia (pernicious) D51.0 [G63]
    due to dietary deficiency D51.3 [G63]
Neurophthisis —see also Disorder, nerve
  peripheral, diabetic —see E08-E13 with .42
Neuroretinitis —see Chorioretinitis
Neuroretinopathy, hereditary optic H47.22
Neurosarcoma —see Neoplasm, nerve, malignant
Neurosclerosis —see Disorder, nerve
Neurosis, neurotic F48.9
  anankastic F42.8 ◀▦
  anxiety (state) F41.1
    panic type F41.0
  asthenic F48.8
  bladder F45.8

Neurosis, neurotic (Continued)
  cardiac (reflex) F45.8
  cardiovascular F45.8
  character F60.9
  colon F45.8
  compensation F68.1
  compulsive, compulsion F42.8 ◀▦
  conversion F44.9
  craft F48.8
  cutaneous F45.8
  depersonalization F48.1
  depressive (reaction) (type) F34.1
  environmental F48.8
  excoriation L98.1
  fatigue F48.8
  functional —see Disorder, somatoform
  gastric F45.8
  gastrointestinal F45.8
  heart F45.8
  hypochondriacal F45.21
  hysterical F44.9
  incoordination F45.8
    larynx F45.8
    vocal cord F45.8
  intestine F45.8
  larynx (sensory) F45.8
    hysterical F44.4
  mixed NEC F48.8
  musculoskeletal F45.8
  obsessional F42.8 ◀▦
  obsessive-compulsive F42.8 ◀▦
  occupational F48.8
  ocular NEC F45.8
  organ —see Disorder, somatoform
  pharynx F45.8
  phobic F40.9
  posttraumatic (situational) F43.10
    acute F43.11
    chronic F43.12
  psychasthenic (type) F48.8
  railroad F48.8
  rectum F45.8
  respiratory F45.8
  rumination F45.8
  sexual F65.9
  situational F48.8
  social F40.10
    generalized F40.11
  specified type NEC F48.8
  state F48.9
    with depersonalization episode F48.1
  stomach F45.8
  traumatic F43.10
    acute F43.11
    chronic F43.12
  vasomotor F45.8
  visceral F45.8
  war F48.8
Neurospongioblastosis diffusa Q85.1
Neurosyphilis (arrested) (early) (gumma) (late)
    (latent) (recurrent) (relapse) A52.3
  with ataxia (cerebellar) (locomotor) (spastic)
    (spinal) A52.19
  aneurysm (cerebral) A52.05
  arachnoid (adhesive) A52.13
  arteritis (any artery) (cerebral) A52.04
  asymptomatic A52.2
  congenital A50.40
  dura (mater) A52.13
  general paresis A52.17
  hemorrhagic A52.05
  juvenile (asymptomatic) (meningeal)
    A50.40
  leptomeninges (aseptic) A52.13
  meningeal, meninges (adhesive) A52.13
  meningitis A52.13
  meningovascular (diffuse) A52.13
  optic atrophy A52.15
  parenchymatous (degenerative) A52.19
  paresis, paretic A52.17
    juvenile A50.45

Neurosyphilis (Continued)
  remission in (sustained) A52.3
  serological (without symptoms) A52.2
  specified nature or site NEC A52.19
  tabes, tabetic (dorsalis) A52.11
    juvenile A50.45
  taboparesis A52.17
    juvenile A50.45
  thrombosis (cerebral) A52.05
  vascular (cerebral) NEC A52.05
Neurothekeoma —see Neoplasm, nerve, benign
Neurotic —see Neurosis
Neurotoxemia —see Toxemia
Neutroclusion M26.211
Neutropenia, neutropenic (chronic) (genetic)
    (idiopathic) (immune) (infantile)
    (malignant) (pernicious) (splenic) D70.9
  congenital (primary) D70.0
  cyclic D70.4
  cytoreductive cancer chemotherapy sequela
    D70.1
  drug-induced D70.2
    due to cytoreductive cancer chemotherapy
      D70.1
  due to infection D70.3
  fever D70.9
  neonatal, transitory (isoimmune) (maternal
    transfer) P61.5
  periodic D70.4
  secondary (cyclic) (periodic) (splenic) D70.4
    drug-induced D70.2
    due to cytoreductive cancer
      chemotherapy D70.1
  toxic D70.8
Neutrophilia, hereditary giant D72.0
Nevocarcinoma —see Melanoma
Nevus D22.9
  achromic —see Neoplasm, skin, benign
  amelanotic —see Neoplasm, skin, benign
  angiomatous D18.00
    intra-abdominal D18.03
    intracranial D18.02
    skin D18.01
    specified site NEC D18.09
  araneus I78.1
  balloon cell —see Neoplasm, skin, benign
  bathing trunk D48.5
  blue —see Neoplasm, skin, benign
    cellular —see Neoplasm, skin, benign
    giant —see Neoplasm, skin, benign
    Jadassohn's —see Neoplasm, skin, benign
    malignant —see Melanoma
  capillary D18.00
    intra-abdominal D18.03
    intracranial D18.02
    skin D18.01
    specified site NEC D18.09
  cavernous D18.00
    intra-abdominal D18.03
    intracranial D18.02
    skin D18.01
    specified site NEC D18.09
  cellular —see Neoplasm, skin, benign
    blue —see Neoplasm, skin, benign
  choroid D31.3-
  comedonicus Q82.5
  conjunctiva D31.0-
  dermal —see Neoplasm, skin, benign
    with epidermal nevus —see Neoplasm,
      skin, benign
  dysplastic —see Neoplasm, skin, benign
  eye D31.9-
  flammeus Q82.5
  hemangiomatous D18.00
    intra-abdominal D18.03
    intracranial D18.02
    skin D18.01
    specified site NEC D18.09
  iris D31.4-
  lacrimal gland D31.5-
  lymphatic D18.1

Nevus (Continued)
  magnocellular
    specified site —see Neoplasm, benign, by
      site
    unspecified site D31.40
  malignant —see Melanoma
  meaning hemangioma D18.00
    intra-abdominal D18.03
    intracranial D18.02
    skin D18.01
    specified site NEC D18.09
  mouth (mucosa) D10.30
    specified site NEC D10.39
    white sponge Q38.6
  multiplex Q85.1
  non-neoplastic I78.1
  oral mucosa D10.30
    specified site NEC D10.39
    white sponge Q38.6
  orbit D31.6-
  pigmented
    giant —see also Neoplasm, skin, uncertain
      behavior D48.5
    malignant melanoma in —see Melanoma
  portwine Q82.5
  retina D31.2-
  retrobulbar D31.6-
  sanguineous Q82.5
  senile I78.1
  skin D22.9
    abdominal wall D22.5
    ala nasi D22.39
    ankle D22.7-
    anus, anal D22.5
    arm D22.6-
    auditory canal (external) D22.2-
    auricle (ear) D22.2-
    auricular canal (external) D22.2-
    axilla, axillary fold D22.5
    back D22.5
    breast D22.5
    brow D22.39
    buttock D22.5
    canthus (eye) D22.1-
    cheek (external) D22.39
    chest wall D22.5
    chin D22.39
    ear (external) D22.2-
    external meatus (ear) D22.2-
    eyebrow D22.39
    eyelid (lower) (upper) D22.1-
    face D22.30
      specified NEC D22.39
    female genital organ (external) NEC D28.0
    finger D22.6-
    flank D22.5
    foot D22.7-
    forearm D22.6-
    forehead D22.39
    foreskin D29.0
    genital organ (external) NEC
      female D28.0
      male D29.9
    gluteal region D22.5
    groin D22.5
    hand D22.6-
    heel D22.7-
    helix D22.2-
    hip D22.7-
    interscapular region D22.5
    jaw D22.39
    knee D22.7-
    labium (majus) (minus) D28.0
    leg D22.7-
    lip (lower) (upper) D22.0
    lower limb D22.7-
    male genital organ (external) D29.9
    nail D22.9
      finger D22.6-
      toe D22.7-
    nasolabial groove D22.39
    nates D22.5

Nevus (Continued)
  skin (Continued)
    neck D22.4
    nose (external) D22.39
    palpebra D22.1-
    penis D29.0
    perianal skin D22.5
    perineum D22.5
    pinna D22.2-
    popliteal fossa or space D22.7-
    prepuce D29.0
    pudendum D28.0
    scalp D22.4
    scrotum D29.4
    shoulder D22.6-
    submammary fold D22.5
    temple D22.39
    thigh D22.7-
    toe D22.7-
    trunk NEC D22.5
    umbilicus D22.5
    upper limb D22.6-
    vulva D28.0
  specified site NEC —see Neoplasm, benign,
    by site
  spider I78.1
  stellar I78.1
  strawberry Q82.5
  Sutton's —see Neoplasm, skin, benign
  unius lateris Q82.5
  Unna's Q82.5
  vascular Q82.5
  verrucous Q82.5
Newborn (infant) (liveborn) (singleton) Z38.2
  abstinence syndrome P96.1
  acne L70.4
  affected by ◄▥▥
    abnormalities of membranes P02.9
      specified NEC P02.8
    abruptio placenta P02.1
    amino-acid metabolic disorder, transitory
      P74.8
    amniocentesis (while in utero) P00.6
    amnionitis P02.7
    apparent life threatening event (ALTE)
      R68.13
    bleeding (into)
      cerebral cortex P52.22
      germinal matrix P52.0
      ventricles P52.1
    breech delivery P03.0
    cardiac arrest P29.81
    cardiomyopathy I42.8
      congenital I42.4
    cerebral ischemia P91.0
    Cesarean delivery P03.4
    chemotherapy agents P04.1
    chorioamnionitis P02.7
    cocaine (crack) P04.41
    complications of labor and delivery P03.9
      specified NEC P03.89
    compression of umbilical cord NEC P02.5
    contracted pelvis P03.1
    delivery P03.9
      Cesarean P03.4
      forceps P03.2
      vacuum extractor P03.3
    entanglement (knot) in umbilical cord
      P02.5
    environmental chemicals P04.6
    fetal (intrauterine)
      growth retardation P05.9
      malnutrition not light or small for
        gestational age P05.2
    forceps delivery P03.2
    heart rate abnormalities
      bradycardia P29.12
      intrauterine P03.819
        before onset of labor P03.810
        during labor P03.811
      tachycardia P29.11

Newborn (Continued)
  affected by (Continued)
    hemorrhage (antepartum) P02.1
      cerebellar (nontraumatic) P52.6
      intracerebral (nontraumatic) P52.4
      intracranial (nontraumatic) P52.9
        specified NEC P52.8
      intraventricular (nontraumatic) P52.3
        grade 1 P52.0
        grade 2 P52.1
        grade 3 P52.21
        grade 4 P52.22
      posterior fossa (nontraumatic) P52.6
      subarachnoid (nontraumatic) P52.5
      subependymal P52.0
        with intracerebral extension P52.22
        with intraventricular extension P52.1
          with enlargment of ventricles
            P52.21
        without intraventricular extension
          P52.0
    hypoxic ischemic encephalopathy [HIE]
      P91.60
      mild P91.61
      moderate P91.62
      severe P91.63
    induction of labor P03.89
    intestinal perforation P78.0
    intrauterine (fetal) blood loss P50.9
      due to (from)
        cut end of co-twin cord P50.5
        hemorrhage into
          co-twin P50.3
            maternal circulation P50.4
          placenta P50.2
          ruptured cord blood P50.1
          vasa previa P50.0
      specified NEC P50.8
    intrauterine (fetal) hemorrhage P50.9
    intrauterine (in utero) procedure P96.5
    malpresentation (malposition) NEC P03.1
    maternal (complication of) (use of)
      alcohol P04.3
      analgesia (maternal) P04.0
      anesthesia (maternal) P04.0
      blood loss P02.1
      circulatory disease P00.3
      condition P00.9
        specified NEC P00.89
      delivery P03.9
        Cesarean P03.4
        forceps P03.2
        vacuum extractor P03.3
      diabetes mellitus (pre-existing) P70.1
      disorder P00.9
        specified NEC P00.89
      drugs (addictive) (illegal) NEC P04.49
      ectopic pregnancy P01.4
      gestational diabetes P70.0
      hemorrhage P02.1
      hypertensive disorder P00.0
      incompetent cervix P01.0
      infectious disease P00.2
      injury P00.5
      labor and delivery P03.9
      malpresentation before labor P01.7
      maternal death P01.6
      medical procedure P00.7
      medication P04.1
      multiple pregnancy P01.5
      nutritional disorder P00.4
      oligohydramnios P01.2
      parasitic disease P00.2
      periodontal disease P00.81
      placenta previa P02.0
      polyhydramnios P01.3
      precipitate delivery P03.5
      pregnancy P01.9
        specified P01.8
      premature rupture of membranes P01.1
      renal disease P00.1

Newborn *(Continued)*
  affected by *(Continued)*
    maternal *(Continued)*
      respiratory disease P00.3
      surgical procedure P00.6
      urinary tract disease P00.1
      uterine contraction (abnormal) P03.6
    meconium peritonitis P78.0
    medication (legal) (maternal use)
      (prescribed) P04.1
    membrane abnormalities P02.9
      specified NEC P02.8
    membranitis P02.7
    methamphetamine (s) P04.49
    mixed metabolic and respiratory acidosis
      P84
    neonatal abstinence syndrome P96.1
    noxious substances transmitted via
      placenta or breast milk P04.9
      specified NEC P04.8
    nutritional supplements P04.5
    placenta previa P02.0
    placental
      abnormality (functional)
        (morphological) P02.20
        specified NEC P02.29
      dysfunction P02.29
      infarction P02.29
      insufficiency P02.29
      separation NEC P02.1
      transfusion syndromes P02.3
    placentitis P02.7
    precipitate delivery P03.5
    prolapsed cord P02.4
    respiratory arrest P28.81
    slow intrauterine growth P05.9
    tobacco P04.2
    twin to twin transplacental transfusion
      P02.3
    umbilical cord (tightly) around neck P02.5
    umbilical cord condition P02.60
      short cord P02.69
      specified NEC P02.69
    uterine contractions (abnormal) P03.6
    vasa previa P02.69
      from intrauterine blood loss P50.0
  apnea P28.4 ◀▥
    obstructive P28.4
    primary P28.3
    ~~specified P28.4~~
    sleep (central) (obstructive) (primary)
      P28.3 ◀
  born in hospital Z38.00
    by cesarean Z38.01
  born outside hospital Z38.1
  breast buds P96.89
  breast engorgement P83.4
  check-up —*see* Newborn, examination
  convulsion P90
  dehydration P74.1
  examination
    8 to 28 days old Z00.111
    under 8 days old Z00.110
  fever P81.9
    environmentally-induced P81.0
  hyperbilirubinemia P59.9
    of prematurity P59.0
  hypernatremia P74.2
  hyponatremia P74.2
  infection P39.9
    candidal P37.5
    specified NEC P39.8
    urinary tract P39.3
  jaundice P59.9 ◀▥
    due to
      breast milk inhibitor P59.3
      hepatocellular damage P59.20
        specified NEC P59.29
      preterm delivery P59.0
    of prematurity P59.0
    specified NEC P59.8

Newborn *(Continued)*
  late metabolic acidosis P74.0
  mastitis P39.0
    infective P39.0
    noninfective P83.4
  multiple born NEC Z38.8
    born in hospital Z38.68
      by cesarean Z38.69
    born outside hospital Z38.7
  omphalitis P38.9
    with mild hemorrhage P38.1
    without hemorrhage P38.9
  post-term P08.21
  prolonged gestation (over 42 completed
    weeks) P08.22
  quadruplet Z38.8
    born in hospital Z38.63
      by cesarean Z38.64
    born outside hospital Z38.7
  quintuplet Z38.8
    born in hospital Z38.65
      by cesarean Z38.66
    born outside hospital Z38.7
  seizure P90
  sepsis (congenital) P36.9
    due to
      anaerobes NEC P36.5
      Escherichia coli P36.4
      Staphylococcus P36.30
        aureus P36.2
        specified NEC P36.39
      Streptococcus P36.10
        group B P36.0
        specified NEC P36.19
      specified NEC P36.8
  triplet Z38.8
    born in hospital Z38.61
      by cesarean Z38.62
    born outside hospital Z38.7
  twin Z38.5
    born in hospital Z38.30
      by cesarean Z38.31
    born outside hospital Z38.4
  vomiting P92.09
    bilious P92.01
  weight check Z00.111
Newcastle conjunctivitis or disease B30.8
Nezelof's syndrome (pure alymphocytosis)
  D81.4
Niacin (amide) deficiency E52
Nicolas (-Durand)-Favre disease A55
Nicotine —*see* Tobacco
Nicotinic acid deficiency E52
Niemann-Pick disease or syndrome E75.249
  specified NEC E75.248
  type
    A E75.240
    B E75.241
    C E75.242
    D E75.243
Night
  blindness —*see* Blindness, night
  sweats R61
  terrors (child) F51.4
Nightmares (REM sleep type) F51.5
NIHSS (National Institutes of Health Stroke
  Scale) score R29.7- ◀
Nipple —*see* condition
Nisbet's chancre A57
Nishimoto (-Takeuchi) disease I67.5
Nitritoid crisis or reaction —*see* Crisis, nitritoid
Nitrosohemoglobinemia D74.8
Njovera A65
Nocardiosis, nocardiasis A43.9
  cutaneous A43.1
  lung A43.0
  pneumonia A43.0
  pulmonary A43.0
  specified site NEC A43.8
Nocturia R35.1
  psychogenic F45.8

Nocturnal —*see* condition
Nodal rhythm I49.8
Node (s) —*see also* Nodule
  Bouchard's (with arthropathy) M15.2
  Haygarth's M15.8
  Heberden's (with arthropathy) M15.1
  larynx J38.7
  lymph —*see* condition
  milker's B08.03
  Osler's I33.0
  Schmorl's —*see* Schmorl's disease
  singer's J38.2
  teacher's J38.2
  tuberculous —*see* Tuberculosis, lymph
    gland
  vocal cord J38.2
Nodule (s), nodular
  actinomycotic —*see* Actinomycosis
  breast NEC N63
  colloid (cystic), thyroid E04.1
  cutaneous —*see* Swelling, localized
  endometrial (stromal) D26.1
  Haygarth's M15.8
  inflammatory —*see* Inflammation
  juxta-articular
    syphilitic A52.77
    yaws A66.7
  larynx J38.7
  lung, solitary (subsegmental branch of the
    bronchial tree) R91.1
    multiple R91.8
  milker's B08.03
  prostate N40.2
    with lower urinary tract symptoms (LUTS)
      N40.3
    without lower urinary tract symptoms
      (LUTS) N40.2
  pulmonary, solitary (subsegmental branch of
    the bronchial tree) R91.1
  retrocardiac R09.89
  rheumatoid M06.30
    ankle M06.37-
    elbow M06.32-
    foot joint M06.37-
    hand joint M06.34-
    hip M06.35-
    knee M06.36-
    multiple site M06.39
    shoulder M06.31-
    vertebra M06.38
    wrist M06.33-
  scrotum (inflammatory) N49.2
  singer's J38.2
  solitary, lung (subsegmental branch of the
    bronchial tree) R91.1
    multiple R91.8
  subcutaneous —*see* Swelling, localized
  teacher's J38.2
  thyroid (cold) (gland) (nontoxic) E04.1
    with thyrotoxicosis E05.20
      with thyroid storm E05.21
    toxic or with hyperthyroidism E05.20
      with thyroid storm E05.21
  vocal cord J38.2
Noma (gangrenous) (hospital) (infective)
  A69.0
  auricle I96
  mouth A69.0
  pudendi N76.89
  vulvae N76.89
Nomad, nomadism Z59.0
NOMID (neonatal onset multisystemic
  inflammatory disorder) M04.2 ◀
Nonautoimmune hemolytic anemia
  D59.4
  drug-induced D59.2
Nonclosure —*see also* Imperfect, closure
  ductus arteriosus (Botallo's) Q25.0
  foramen
    botalli Q21.1
    ovale Q21.1

Noncompliance Z91.19
  with
    dialysis Z91.15
    dietary regimen Z91.11
    medical treatment Z91.19
    medication regimen NEC Z91.14
      underdosing —*see also* Table of Drugs
        and Chemicals, categories T36-T50,
        with final character 6 Z91.14
      intentional NEC Z91.128
        due to financial hardship of patient
          Z91.120
      unintentional NEC Z91.138
        due to patient's age related debility
          Z91.130
    renal dialysis Z91.15
Nondescent (congenital) —*see also* Malposition,
    congenital
  cecum Q43.3
  colon Q43.3
  testicle Q53.9
    bilateral Q53.20
      abdominal Q53.21
      perineal Q53.22
    unilateral Q53.10
      abdominal Q53.11
      perineal Q53.12
Nondevelopment
  brain Q02
    part of Q04.3
  heart Q24.8
  organ or site, congenital NEC —*see*
    Hypoplasia
Nonengagement
  head NEC O32.4
    in labor, causing obstructed labor O64.8
Nonexanthematous tick fever A93.2
Nonexpansion, lung (newborn) P28.0
Nonfunctioning
  cystic duct —*see also* Disease, gallbladder
    K82.8
  gallbladder —*see also* Disease, gallbladder
    K82.8
  kidney N28.9
  labyrinth —*see* subcategory H83.2

Non-Hodgkin lymphoma NEC —*see*
    Lymphoma, non-Hodgkin
Nonimplantation, ovum N97.2
Noninsufflation, fallopian tube N97.1
Non-ketotic hyperglycinemia E72.51
Nonne-Milroy syndrome Q82.0
Nonovulation N97.0
Nonpatent fallopian tube N97.1
Nonpneumatization, lung NEC P28.0
Nonrotation —*see* Malrotation
Nonsecretion, urine —*see* Anuria
Nonunion
  fracture —*see* Fracture, by site
  joint, following fusion or arthrodesis
    M96.0 ◀
  organ or site, congenital NEC —*see* Imperfect,
    closure
  symphysis pubis, congenital Q74.2
Nonvisualization, gallbladder R93.2
Nonvital, nonvitalized tooth K04.99
Non-working side interference
    M26.56
Noonan's syndrome Q87.1
Normocytic anemia (infectional) due to blood
    loss (chronic) D50.0
  acute D62
Norrie's disease (congenital) Q15.8
North American blastomycosis B40.9
Norwegian itch B86
Nose, nasal —*see* condition
Nosebleed R04.0
Nose-picking F98.8
Nosomania F45.21
Nosophobia F45.22
Nostalgia F43.20
Notch of iris Q13.2
Notching nose, congenital (tip)
    Q30.2
Nothnagel's
  syndrome —*see* Strabismus, paralytic, third
    nerve
  vasomotor acroparesthesia I73.89
Novy's relapsing fever A68.9
  louse-borne A68.0
  tick-borne A68.1

Noxious
  foodstuffs, poisoning by —*see* Poisoning,
    food, noxious, plant
  substances transmitted through placenta or
    breast milk P04.9
Nucleus pulposus —*see* condition
Numbness R20.0
Nuns' knee —*see* Bursitis, prepatellar
Nursemaid's elbow S53.03-
Nutcracker esophagus K22.4
Nutmeg liver K76.1
Nutrient element deficiency E61.9
  specified NEC E61.8
Nutrition deficient or insufficient —*see also*
    Malnutrition E46
  due to
    insufficient food T73.0
    lack of
      care (child) T76.02
        adult T76.01
      food T73.0
Nutritional stunting E45
Nyctalopia (night blindness) —*see* Blindness,
    night
Nycturia R35.1
  psychogenic F45.8
Nymphomania F52.8
Nystagmus H55.00
  benign paroxysmal —*see* Vertigo, benign
    paroxysmal
  central positional H81.4-
  congenital H55.01
  dissociated H55.04
  latent H55.02
  miners' H55.09
  positional
    benign paroxysmal H81.4-
    central H81.4-
  specified form NEC H55.09
  visual deprivation H55.03

O

Obermeyer's relapsing fever (European)
A68.0
Obesity E66.9
~~with alveolar hyperventilation E66.2~~
  with alveolar hypoventilation E66.2 ◄
  adrenal E27.8
  complicating
    childbirth O99.214
    pregnancy O99.21-
    puerperium O99.215
  constitutional E66.8
  dietary counseling and surveillance Z71.3
  drug-induced E66.1
  due to
    drug E66.1
    excess calories E66.09
      morbid E66.01
      severe E66.01
  endocrine E66.8
  endogenous E66.8
  exogenous E66.09 ◄
  familial E66.8
  glandular E66.8
  hypothyroid —see Hypothyroidism
  hypoventilation syndrome (OHS)
      E66.2 ◄
  morbid E66.01
    ~~with alveolar hypoventilation E66.2~~
    with ◄
      alveolar hypoventilation E66.2 ◄
      obesity hypoventilation syndrome
          (OHS) E66.2 ◄
    due to excess calories E66.01
  nutritional E66.09
  pituitary E23.6
  severe E66.01
  specified type NEC E66.8
Oblique —see condition
Obliteration
  appendix (lumen) K38.8
  artery I77.1
  bile duct (noncalculous) K83.1
  common duct (noncalculous) K83.1
  cystic duct —see Obstruction, gallbladder
  disease, arteriolar I77.1
  endometrium N85.8
  eye, anterior chamber —see Disorder, globe,
      hypotony
  fallopian tube N97.1
  lymphatic vessel I89.0
    due to mastectomy I97.2
  organ or site, congenital NEC —see Atresia,
      by site
  ureter N13.5
    with infection N13.6
  urethra —see Stricture, urethra
  vein I87.8
  vestibule (oral) K08.89 ◄⼿
Observation (following) (for) (without need for
      further medical care) Z04.9
  accident NEC Z04.3
    at work Z04.2
    transport Z04.1
  adverse effect of drug Z03.6
  alleged rape or sexual assault (victim),
      ruled out
    adult Z04.41
    child Z04.42
  criminal assault Z04.8
  development state
    adolescent Z00.3
    period of rapid growth in childhood Z00.2
    puberty Z00.3
  disease, specified NEC Z03.89
  following work accident Z04.2
  growth and development state —see
      Observation, development state
  injuries (accidental) NEC —see also
      Observation, accident

Observation (Continued)
  newborn (for) ◄⼿
    suspected condition, related to exposure
        from the mother or birth process —
        see Newborn, affected by,
        maternal ◄
    ruled out Z05.9 ◄
      cardiac Z05.0 ◄
      connective tissue Z05.73 ◄
      gastrointestinal Z05.5 ◄
      genetic Z05.41 ◄
      genitourinary Z05.6 ◄
      immunologic Z05.43 ◄
      infectious Z05.1 ◄
      metabolic Z05.42 ◄
      musculoskeletal Z05.72 ◄
      neurological Z05.2 ◄
      respiratory Z05.3 ◄
      skin and subcutaneous tissue
          Z05.71 ◄
      specified condition NEC
          Z05.8 ◄
  postpartum
    immediately after delivery Z39.0
    routine follow-up Z39.2
  pregnancy (normal) (without complication)
      Z34.9-
    high risk O09.9-
  suicide attempt, alleged NEC Z03.89
    self-poisoning Z03.6
  suspected, ruled out —see also Suspected
      condition, ruled out
    abuse, physical
      adult Z04.71
      child Z04.72
    accident at work Z04.2
    adult battering victim Z04.71
    child battering victim Z04.72
    condition NEC Z03.89
      newborn —see also Observation,
          newborn (for), suspected condition,
          ruled out Z05.9 ◄⼿
    drug poisoning or adverse effect
        Z03.6
    exposure (to)
      anthrax Z03.810
      biological agent NEC Z03.818
    inflicted injury NEC Z04.8
    suicide attempt, alleged Z03.89
      self-poisoning Z03.6
    toxic effects from ingested substance (drug)
        (poison) Z03.6
  toxic effects from ingested substance (drug)
      (poison) Z03.6
Obsession, obsessional state F42.8 ◄⼿
  mixed thoughts and acts F42.2 ◄
Obsessive-compulsive neurosis or reaction
    F42.8 ◄⼿
Obstetric embolism, septic —see Embolism,
    obstetric, septic
Obstetrical trauma (complicating delivery)
    O71.9
  with or following ectopic or molar pregnancy
      O08.6
  specified type NEC O71.89
Obstipation —see Constipation
Obstruction, obstructed, obstructive
  airway J98.8
    with
      allergic alveolitis J67.9
      asthma J45.909
        with
          exacerbation (acute) J45.901
          status asthmaticus J45.902
      bronchiectasis J47.9
        with
          exacerbation (acute) J47.1
          lower respiratory infection
              J47.0
      bronchitis (chronic) J44.9
      emphysema J43.9

Obstruction, obstructed, obstructive
    (Continued)
  airway (Continued)
    chronic J44.9
      with
        allergic alveolitis —see Pneumonitis,
            hypersensitivity
        bronchiectasis J47.9
          with
            exacerbation (acute) J47.1
            lower respiratory infection J47.0
    due to
      foreign body —see Foreign body, by site,
          causing asphyxia
      inhalation of fumes or vapors J68.9
      laryngospasm J38.5
  ampulla of Vater K83.1
  aortic (heart) (valve) —see Stenosis, aortic
  aortoiliac I74.09
  aqueduct of Sylvius G91.1
    congenital Q03.0
      with spina bifida —see Spina bifida, by
          site, with hydrocephalus
  Arnold-Chiari —see Arnold-Chiari disease
  artery (see also Embolism, artery) I74.9
    basilar (complete) (partial) —see Occlusion,
        artery, basilar
    carotid (complete) (partial) —see Occlusion,
        artery, carotid
    cerebellar —see Occlusion, artery, cerebellar
    cerebral (anterior) (middle) (posterior) —
        see Occlusion, artery, cerebral
    precerebral —see Occlusion, artery,
        precerebral
    renal N28.0
    retinal NEC —see Occlusion, artery, retina
    stent —see Restenosis, stent ◄
    vertebral (complete) (partial) —see
        Occlusion, artery, vertebral
  band (intestinal) K56.69
  bile duct or passage (common) (hepatic)
      (noncalculous) K83.1
    with calculus K80.51
    congenital (causing jaundice) Q44.3
  biliary (duct) (tract) K83.1
    gallbladder K82.0
  bladder-neck (acquired) N32.0
    congenital Q64.31
    due to hyperplasia (hypertrophy) of
        prostate —see Hyperplasia, prostate
  bowel —see Obstruction, intestine
  bronchus J98.09
  canal, ear —see Stenosis, external ear canal
  cardia K22.2
  caval veins (inferior) (superior) I87.1
  cecum —see Obstruction, intestine
  circulatory I99.8
  colon —see Obstruction, intestine
  common duct (noncalculous) K83.1
  coronary (artery) —see Occlusion, coronary
  cystic duct —see also Obstruction, gallbladder
    with calculus K80.21
  device, implant or graft —see also
      Complications, by site and type,
      mechanical T85.698
    arterial graft NEC —see Complication,
        cardiovascular device, mechanical,
        vascular
    catheter NEC T85.628
      cystostomy T83.090
      dialysis (renal) T82.49
        intraperitoneal T85.691
      Hopkins T83.098 ◄
      ileostomy T83.098 ◄
      infusion NEC T82.594
        spinal (epidural) (subdural) T85.690
      nephrostomy T83.092 ◄
      urethral indwelling T83.091 ◄
      urinary T83.098 ◄
      ~~urinary, indwelling T83.098~~
      urostomy T83.098 ◄

◄ New   ◄⼿ Revised   ~~deleted~~ Deleted

Obstruction, obstructed, obstructive
(Continued)
device, implant or graft (Continued)
  due to infection T85.79
  gastrointestinal —see Complications,
    prosthetic device, mechanical,
    gastrointestinal device
  genital NEC T83.498
    intrauterine contraceptive device T83.39
    penile prosthesis (cylinder) (implanted)
      (pump) (resevoir) T83.490 ◄▥
    testicular prosthesis T83.491 ◄
  heart NEC —see Complication,
    cardiovascular device, mechanical
  joint prosthesis —see Complications, joint
    prosthesis, mechanical, specified
    NEC, by site
  orthopedic NEC —see Complication,
    orthopedic, device, mechanical
  specified NEC T85.628
  urinary NEC —see also Complication,
    genitourinary, device, urinary,
    mechanical
    graft T83.29
  vascular NEC —see Complication,
    cardiovascular device, mechanical
  ventricular intracranial shunt T85.09
due to foreign body accidentally left in
  operative wound T81.529
duodenum K31.5
ejaculatory duct N50.89 ◄▥
esophagus K22.2
eustachian tube (complete) (partial) H68.10-
  cartilagenous (extrinsic) H68.13-
    intrinsic H68.12-
  osseous H68.11-
fallopian tube (bilateral) N97.1
fecal K56.41
  with hernia —see Hernia, by site, with
    obstruction
foramen of Monro (congenital) Q03.8
  with spina bifida —see Spina bifida,
    by site, with hydrocephalus
foreign body —see Foreign body
gallbladder K82.0
  with calculus, stones K80.21
  congenital Q44.1
gastric outlet K31.1
gastrointestinal —see Obstruction, intestine
hepatic K76.89
  duct (noncalculous) K83.1
hepatobiliary K83.1
ileum —see Obstruction, intestine
iliofemoral (artery) I74.5
intestine K56.60
  with
    adhesions (intestinal) (peritoneal) K56.5
  adynamic K56.0
  by gallstone K56.3
  congenital (small) Q41.9
    large Q42.9
      specified part NEC Q42.8
  neurogenic K56.0
    Hirschsprung's disease or megacolon
      Q43.1
  newborn P76.9
    due to
      fecaliths P76.8
      inspissated milk P76.2
      meconium (plug) P76.0
        in mucoviscidosis E84.11
      specified NEC P76.8
  postoperative K91.3
  reflex K56.0
  specified NEC K56.69
  volvulus K56.2
intracardiac ball valve prosthesis T82.09
jejunum —see Obstruction, intestine
joint prosthesis —see Complications, joint
  prosthesis, mechanical, specified NEC,
  by site

Obstruction, obstructed, obstructive
(Continued)
kidney (calices) N28.89
labor —see Delivery
lacrimal (passages) (duct)
  by
    dacryolith —see Dacryolith
    stenosis —see Stenosis, lacrimal
  congenital Q10.5
  neonatal H04.53-
lacrimonasal duct —see Obstruction,
  lacrimal
lacteal, with steatorrhea K90.2
laryngitis —see Laryngitis
larynx NEC J38.6
  congenital Q31.8
lung J98.4
  disease, chronic J44.9
lymphatic I89.0
meconium (plug)
  newborn P76.0
    due to fecaliths P76.0
    in mucoviscidosis E84.11
mitral —see Stenosis, mitral
nasal J34.89
nasolacrimal duct —see also Obstruction,
  lacrimal
  congenital Q10.5
nasopharynx J39.2
nose J34.89
organ or site, congenital NEC —see Atresia,
  by site
pancreatic duct K86.89 ◄▥
parotid duct or gland K11.8
pelviureteral junction N13.5
  with hydronephrosis N13.0 ◄
  congenital Q62.39
pharynx J39.2
portal (circulation) (vein) I81
prostate —see also Hyperplasia, prostate
  valve (urinary) N32.0
pulmonary valve (heart) I37.0
pyelonephritis (chronic) N11.1
pylorus
  adult K31.1
  congenital or infantile Q40.0
rectosigmoid —see Obstruction,
  intestine
rectum K62.4
renal N28.89
  outflow N13.8
  pelvis, congenital Q62.39
respiratory J98.8
  chronic J44.9
retinal (vessels) H34.9
salivary duct (any) K11.8
  with calculus K11.5
sigmoid —see Obstruction, intestine
sinus (accessory) (nasal) J34.89
Stensen's duct K11.8
stomach NEC K31.89
  acute K31.0
  congenital Q40.2
  due to pylorospasm K31.3
submandibular duct K11.8
submaxillary gland K11.8
  with calculus K11.5
thoracic duct I89.0
thrombotic —see Thrombosis
trachea J39.8
tracheostomy airway J95.03
tricuspid (valve) —see Stenosis, tricuspid
upper respiratory, congenital Q34.8
ureter (functional) (pelvic junction) NEC
  N13.5
  with
    hydronephrosis N13.1
      with infection N13.6
    pyelonephritis (chronic) N11.1
  congenital Q62.39
  due to calculus —see Calculus, ureter

Obstruction, obstructed, obstructive
(Continued)
urethra NEC N36.8
  congenital Q64.39
urinary (moderate) N13.9
  due to hyperplasia (hypertrophy) of
    prostate —see Hyperplasia, prostate
  organ or tract (lower) N13.9
  prostatic valve N32.0
  specified NEC N13.8
uropathy N13.9
uterus N85.8
vagina N89.5
valvular —see Endocarditis
vein, venous I87.1
  caval (inferior) (superior) I87.1
  thrombotic —see Thrombosis
vena cava (inferior) (superior) I87.1
vesical NEC N32.0
vesicourethral orifice N32.0
  congenital Q64.31
vessel NEC I99.8
  stent —see Restenosis, stent ◄
Obturator —see condition
Occlusal wear, teeth K03.0
Occlusio pupillae —see Membrane, pupillary
Occlusion, occluded
anus K62.4
  congenital Q42.3
    with fistula Q42.2
aortoiliac (chronic) I74.09
aqueduct of Sylvius G91.1
  congenital Q03.0
    with spina bifida —see Spina bifida, by
      site, with hydrocephalus
artery —see also Embolism, artery I74.9
  auditory, internal I65.8
  basilar I65.1
    with
      infarction I63.22
      due to
        embolism I63.12
        thrombosis I63.02
  brain or cerebral I66.9
    with infarction (due to) I63.5- ◄▥
      embolism I63.4- ◄▥
      thrombosis I63.3- ◄▥
  carotid I65.2-
    with
      infarction I63.23-
      due to
        embolism I63.13-
        thrombosis I63.03-
  cerebellar (anterior inferior) (posterior
    inferior) (superior) I66.3
    with infarction I63.54-
      due to
        embolism I63.44-
        thrombosis I63.34-
  cerebral I66.9
    with infarction I63.50
      due to
        embolism I63.40
          specified NEC I63.49
        thrombosis I63.30
          specified NEC I63.39
    anterior I66.1-
      with infarction I63.52-
        due to
          embolism I63.42-
          thrombosis I63.32-
    middle I66.0-
      with infarction I63.51-
        due to
          embolism I63.41-
          thrombosis I63.31-
    posterior I66.2-
      with infarction I63.53-
        due to
          embolism I63.43-
          thrombosis I63.33-

Occlusion, occluded *(Continued)*
  artery *(Continued)*
    cerebral *(Continued)*
      specified NEC I66.8
        with infarction I63.59
          due to
            embolism I63.4- ◀▥
            thrombosis I63.3- ◀▥
    choroidal (anterior) —*see* Occlusion,
      artery, cerebral, specified NEC
    communicating posterior —*see*
      Occlusion, artery, precerebral,
      specified NEC
    complete
      coronary I25.82
      extremities I70.92
    coronary (acute) (thrombotic) (without
      myocardial infarction) I24.0
      with myocardial infarction —*see*
        Infarction, myocardium
      chronic total I25.82
      complete I25.82
      healed or old I25.2
      total (chronic) I25.82
    hypophyseal —*see* Occlusion, artery,
      precerebral, specified NEC
    iliac I74.5
    lower extremities due to stenosis or
      stricture I77.1
    mesenteric (embolic) (thrombotic) —*see also*
      Infarct, intestine K55.069 ◀▥
    perforating —*see* Occlusion, artery,
      cerebral, specified NEC
    peripheral I77.9
      thrombotic or embolic I74.4
    pontine —*see* Occlusion, artery, cerebral,
      specified NEC
    precerebral I65.9
      with infarction I63.20
        due to
          embolism I63.10
            specified NEC I63.19
          thrombosis I63.00
            specified NEC I63.09
        specified NEC I63.29
      basilar —*see* Occlusion, artery, basilar
      carotid —*see* Occlusion, artery, carotid
      puerperal O88.23
      specified NEC I65.8
        with infarction I63.29
          due to
            embolism I63.19
            thrombosis I63.00
      vertebral —*see* Occlusion, artery,
        vertebral
    renal N28.0
    retinal
      branch H34.23-
      central H34.1-
      partial H34.21-
      transient H34.0-
    spinal —*see* Occlusion, artery, precerebral,
      vertebral
    total (chronic)
      coronary I25.82
      extremities I70.92
    vertebral I65.0-
      with
        infarction I63.21-
          due to
            embolism I63.11-
            thrombosis I63.01-
  basilar artery —*see* Occlusion, artery, basilar
  bile duct (common) (hepatic) (noncalculous)
    K83.1
  bowel —*see* Obstruction, intestine
  carotid (artery) (common) (internal) —*see*
    Occlusion, artery, carotid
  centric (of teeth) M26.59
    maximum intercuspation discrepancy
      M26.55

Occlusion, occluded *(Continued)*
  cerebellar (artery) —*see* Occlusion, artery,
    cerebellar
  cerebral (artery) —*see* Occlusion, artery,
    cerebral
  cerebrovascular —*see also* Occlusion, artery,
    cerebral
    with infarction I63.5- ◀▥
  cervical canal —*see* Stricture, cervix
  cervix (uteri) —*see* Stricture, cervix
  choanal Q30.0
  choroidal (artery) —*see* Occlusion, artery,
    precerebral, specified NEC
  colon —*see* Obstruction, intestine
  communicating posterior artery —*see*
    Occlusion, artery, precerebral, specified
    NEC
  coronary (artery) (vein) (thrombotic) —*see*
    also Infarct, myocardium
    chronic total I25.82
    healed or old I25.2
    not resulting in infarction I24.0
    total (chronic) I25.82
  cystic duct —*see* Obstruction, gallbladder
  embolic —*see* Embolism
  fallopian tube N97.1
    congenital Q50.6
  gallbladder —*see also* Obstruction,
    gallbladder
    congenital (causing jaundice) Q44.1
  gingiva, traumatic K06.2
  hymen N89.6
    congenital Q52.3
  hypophyseal (artery) —*see* Occlusion, artery,
    precerebral, specified NEC
  iliac artery I74.5
  intestine —*see* Obstruction, intestine
  lacrimal passages —*see* Obstruction, lacrimal
  lung J98.4
  lymph or lymphatic channel I89.0
  mammary duct N64.89
  mesenteric artery (embolic) (thrombotic) —
    see also Infarct, intestine K55.069 ◀▥
  nose J34.89
    congenital Q30.0
  organ or site, congenital NEC —*see* Atresia,
    by site
  oviduct N97.1
    congenital Q50.6
  peripheral arteries
    due to stricture or stenosis I77.1
    upper extremity I74.2
  pontine (artery) —*see* Occlusion, artery,
    precerebral, specified NEC
  posterior lingual, of mandibular teeth M26.29
  precerebral artery —*see* Occlusion, artery,
    precerebral
  punctum lacrimale —*see* Obstruction,
    lacrimal
  pupil —*see* Membrane, pupillary
  pylorus, adult —*see also* Stricture, pylorus
    K31.1
  renal artery N28.0
  retina, retinal
    artery —*see* Occlusion, artery, retinal
    vein (central) H34.81-
      engorgement H34.82-
      tributary H34.83-
    vessels H34.9
  spinal artery —*see* Occlusion, artery,
    precerebral, vertebral
  teeth (mandibular) (posterior lingual) M26.29
  thoracic duct I89.0
  thrombotic —*see* Thrombosis, artery
  traumatic
    edentulous (alveolar) ridge K06.2
    gingiva K06.2
    periodontal K05.5
  tubal N97.1
  ureter (complete) (partial) N13.5
    congenital Q62.10

Occlusion, occluded *(Continued)*
  ureteropelvic junction N13.5
    congenital Q62.11
  ureterovesical orifice N13.5
    congenital Q62.12
  urethra —*see* Stricture, urethra
  uterus N85.8
  vagina N89.5
  vascular NEC I99.8
  vein —*see* Thrombosis
    retinal —*see* Occlusion, retinal, vein
  vena cava (inferior) (superior) —*see*
    Embolism, vena cava
  ventricle (brain) NEC G91.1
  vertebral (artery) —*see* Occlusion, artery,
    vertebral
  vessel (blood) I99.8
  vulva N90.5
Occult
  blood in feces (stools) R19.5
Occupational
  problems NEC Z56.89
Ochlophobia —*see* Agoraphobia
Ochronosis (endogenous) E70.29
Ocular muscle —*see* condition
Oculogyric crisis or disturbance H51.8
  psychogenic F45.8
Oculomotor syndrome H51.9
Oculopathy
  syphilitic NEC A52.71
    congenital
      early A50.01
      late A50.30
    early (secondary) A51.43
    late A52.71
Oddi's sphincter spasm K83.4
Odontalgia K08.89 ◀▥
Odontoameloblastoma —*see* Cyst, calcifying
  odontogenic
Odontoclasia K03.89
Odontodysplasia, regional K00.4
Odontogenesis imperfecta K00.5
Odontoma (ameloblastic) (complex)
  (compound) (fibroameloblastic) —*see* Cyst,
  calcifying odontogenic
Odontomyelitis (closed) (open) K04.01 ◀▥
  irreversible K04.02 ◀
  reversible K04.01 ◀
Odontorrhagia K08.89 ◀▥
Odontosarcoma, ameloblastic C41.1
  upper jaw (bone) C41.0
Oestriasis —*see* Myiasis
Oguchi's disease H53.63
Ohara's disease —*see* Tularemia
OHS (obesity hypoventilation syndrome)
  E66.2 ◀
Oidiomycosis —*see* Candidiasis
Oidium albicans infection —*see* Candidiasis
Old (previous) myocardial infarction
  I25.2
Old age (without mention of debility) R54-
  dementia F03
Olfactory —*see* condition
Oligemia —*see* Anemia
Oligoastrocytoma
  specified site —*see* Neoplasm, malignant,
    by site
  unspecified site C71.9
Oligocythemia D64.9
Oligodendroblastoma
  specified site —*see* Neoplasm, malignant
  unspecified site C71.9
Oligodendroglioma
  anaplastic type
    specified site —*see* Neoplasm, malignant,
      by site
    unspecified site C71.9
  specified site —*see* Neoplasm, malignant,
    by site
  unspecified site C71.9
Oligodontia —*see* Anodontia

◀ New   ◀▥ Revised   ~~deleted~~ Deleted

Oligoencephalon Q02
Oligohidrosis L74.4
Oligohydramnios O41.0-
Oligohydrosis L74.4
Oligomenorrhea N91.5
  primary N91.3
  secondary N91.4
Oligophrenia —see also Disability, intellectual
  phenylpyruvic E70.0
Oligospermia N46.11
  due to
    drug therapy N46.121
    efferent duct obstruction N46.123
    infection N46.122
    radiation N46.124
    specified cause NEC N46.129
    systemic disease N46.125
Oligotrichia —see Alopecia
Oliguria R34
  with, complicating or following ectopic or
    molar pregnancy O08.4
  postprocedural N99.0
Ollier's disease Q78.4
Omenotocele —see Hernia, abdomen, specified
  site NEC
Omentitis —see Peritonitis
Omentum, omental —see condition
Omphalitis (congenital) (newborn) P38.9
  with mild hemorrhage P38.1
  without hemorrhage P38.9
  not of newborn L08.82
  tetanus A33
Omphalocele Q79.2
Omphalomesenteric duct, persistent
  Q43.0
Omphalorrhagia, newborn P51.9
Omsk hemorrhagic fever A98.1
Onanism (excessive) F98.8
Onchocerciasis, onchocercosis B73.1
  with
    eye disease B73.00
      endophthalmitis B73.01
      eyelid B73.09
      glaucoma B73.02
      specified NEC B73.09
    eye NEC B73.00
    eyelid B73.09
Oncocytoma —see Neoplasm, benign, by site
Oncovirus, as cause of disease classified
  elsewhere B97.32
Ondine's curse —see Apnea, sleep
Oneirophrenia F23
Onychauxis L60.2
  congenital Q84.5
Onychia —see also Cellulitis, digit
  with lymphangitis —see Lymphangitis, acute,
    digit
  candidal B37.2
  dermatophytic B35.1
Onychitis —see also Cellulitis, digit
  with lymphangitis —see Lymphangitis, acute,
    digit
Onychocryptosis L60.0
Onychodystrophy L60.3
  congenital Q84.6
Onychogryphosis, onychogryposis L60.2
Onycholysis L60.1
Onychomadesis L60.8
Onychomalacia L60.3
Onychomycosis (finger) (toe) B35.1
Onycho-osteodysplasia Q87.2 ◀▥
Onychophagia F98.8
Onychophosis L60.8
Onychoptosis L60.8
Onychorrhexis L60.3
  congenital Q84.6
Onychoschizia L60.3
Onyxis (finger) (toe) L60.0
Onyxitis —see also Cellulitis, digit
  with lymphangitis —see Lymphangitis, acute,
    digit

Oophoritis (cystic) (infectional) (interstitial)
  N70.92
  with salpingitis N70.93
  acute N70.02
    with salpingitis N70.03
  chronic N70.12
    with salpingitis N70.13
  complicating abortion —see Abortion, by
    type, complicated by, oophoritis
Oophorocele N83.4- ◀▥
Opacity, opacities
  cornea H17.-
    central H17.1-
    congenital Q13.3
    degenerative —see Degeneration, cornea
    hereditary —see Dystrophy, cornea
    inflammatory —see Keratitis
    minor H17.81-
    peripheral H17.82-
    sequelae of trachoma (healed) B94.0
    specified NEC H17.89
  enamel (teeth) (fluoride) (nonfluoride)
    K00.3
  lens —see Cataract
  snowball —see Deposit, crystalline
  vitreous (humor) NEC H43.39-
    congenital Q14.0
    membranes and strands H43.31-
Opalescent dentin (hereditary) K00.5
Open, opening
  abnormal, organ or site, congenital —see
    Imperfect, closure
  angle with
    borderline
      findings
        high risk H40.02-
        low risk H40.01-
      intraocular pressure H40.00-
    cupping of discs H40.01-
    glaucoma (primary) —see Glaucoma, open
      angle
  bite
    anterior M26.220
    posterior M26.221
  false —see Imperfect, closure
  margin on tooth restoration K08.51
  restoration margins of tooth K08.51
  wound —see Wound, open
Operational fatigue F48.8
Operative —see condition
Operculitis —see Periodontitis
Operculum —see Break, retina
Ophiasis L63.2
Ophthalmia —see also Conjunctivitis H10.9
  actinic rays —see Photokeratitis
  allergic (acute) —see Conjunctivitis, acute,
    atopic
  blennorrhagic (gonococcal) (neonatorum)
    A54.31
  diphtheritic A36.86
  Egyptian A71.1
  electrica —see Photokeratitis
  gonococcal (neonatorum) A54.31
  metastatic —see Endophthalmitis, purulent
  migraine —see Migraine, ophthalmoplegic
  neonatorum, newborn P39.1
    gonococcal A54.31
  nodosa H16.24-
  purulent —see Conjunctivitis, acute,
    mucopurulent
  spring —see Conjunctivitis, acute, atopic
  sympathetic —see Uveitis, sympathetic
Ophthalmitis —see Ophthalmia
Ophthalmocele (congenital) Q15.8
Ophthalmoneuromyelitis G36.0
Ophthalmoplegia —see also Strabismus,
  paralytic
  anterior internuclear —see Ophthalmoplegia,
    internuclear
  ataxia-areflexia G61.0
  diabetic —see E08-E13 with .39

Ophthalmoplegia (Continued)
  exophthalmic E05.00
    with thyroid storm E05.01
  external H49.88-
    progressive H49.4-
      with pigmentary retinopathy —see
        Kearns-Sayre syndrome
    total H49.3-
  internal (complete) (total) H52.51-
  internuclear H51.2-
  migraine —see Migraine, ophthalmoplegic
  Parinaud's H49.88-
  progressive external —see Ophthalmoplegia,
    external, progressive
  supranuclear, progressive G23.1
  total (external) —see Ophthalmoplegia,
    external, total
Opioid (s)
  abuse —see Abuse, drug, opioids
  dependence —see Dependence, drug, opioids
  induced, without use disorder ◀
    anxiety disorder F11.988 ◀
    delirium F11.921 ◀
    depressive disorder F11.94 ◀
    sexual dysfunction F11.981 ◀
    sleep disorder F11.982 ◀
Opisthognathism M26.09
Opisthorchiasis (felineus) (viverrini) B66.0
Opitz' disease D73.2
Opiumism —see Dependence, drug, opioid
Oppenheim's disease G70.2
Oppenheim-Urbach disease (necrobiosis
  lipoidica diabeticorum) —see E08-E13 with
  .620
Optic nerve —see condition
Orbit —see condition
Orchioblastoma C62.9-
Orchitis (gangrenous) (nonspecific) (septic)
  (suppurative) N45.2
  blennorrhagic (gonococcal) (acute) (chronic)
    A54.23
  chlamydial A56.19
  filarial —see also Infestation, filarial B74.9
    [N51]
  gonococcal (acute) (chronic) A54.23
  mumps B26.0
  syphilitic A52.76
  tuberculous A18.15
Orf (virus disease) B08.02
Organic —see also condition
  brain syndrome F09
  heart —see Disease, heart
  mental disorder F09
  psychosis F09
Orgasm
  anejaculatory N53.13
Oriental
  bilharziasis B65.2
  schistosomiasis B65.2
Orifice —see condition
Origin of both great vessels from right
  ventricle Q20.1
Ormond's disease (with ureteral obstruction)
  N13.5
  with infection N13.6
Ornithine metabolism disorder E72.4
Ornithinemia (Type I) (Type II) E72.4
Ornithosis A70
Orotaciduria, oroticaciduria (congenital)
  (hereditary) (pyrimidine deficiency) E79.8
  anemia D53.0
Orthodontics
  adjustment Z46.4
  fitting Z46.4
Orthopnea R06.01
Orthopoxvirus B08.09
  specified NEC B08.09
Os, uterus —see condition
Osgood-Schlatter disease or
  osteochondrosis —see Osteochondrosis,
  juvenile, tibia

Osler (-Weber)-Rendu disease I78.0
Osler's nodes I33.0
Osmidrosis L75.0
Osseous —*see* condition
Ossification
 artery —*see* Arteriosclerosis
 auricle (ear) —*see* Disorder, pinna, specified
  type NEC
 bronchial J98.09
 cardiac —*see* Degeneration, myocardial
 cartilage (senile) —*see* Disorder, cartilage,
  specified type NEC
 coronary (artery) —*see* Disease, heart,
  ischemic, atherosclerotic
 diaphragm J98.6
 ear, middle —*see* Otosclerosis
 falx cerebri G96.19
 fontanel, premature Q75.0
 heart —*see also* Degeneration, myocardial
  valve —*see* Endocarditis
 larynx J38.7
 ligament —*see* Disorder, tendon, specified
  type NEC
  posterior longitudinal —*see*
   Spondylopathy, specified NEC
 meninges (cerebral) (spinal) G96.19
 multiple, eccentric centers —*see* Disorder,
  bone, development or growth
 muscle —*see also* Calcification, muscle
  due to burns —*see* Myositis, ossificans, in,
   burns
  paralytic —*see* Myositis, ossificans, in,
   quadriplegia
  progressive —*see* Myositis, ossificans,
   progressiva
  specified NEC M61.50
   ankle M61.57-
   foot M61.57-
   forearm M61.53-
   hand M61.54-
   lower leg M61.56-
   multiple sites M61.59
   pelvic region M61.55-
   shoulder region M61.51-
   specified site NEC M61.58
   thigh M61.55-
   upper arm M61.52-
  traumatic —*see* Myositis, ossificans,
   traumatica
 myocardium, myocardial —*see* Degeneration,
  myocardial
 penis N48.89
 periarticular —*see* Disorder, joint, specified
  type NEC
 pinna —*see* Disorder, pinna, specified type
  NEC
 rider's bone —*see* Ossification, muscle,
  specified NEC
 sclera H15.89
 subperiosteal, post-traumatic M89.8X-
 tendon —*see* Disorder, tendon, specified
  type NEC
 trachea J39.8
 tympanic membrane —*see* Disorder,
  tympanic membrane, specified
  NEC
 vitreous (humor) —*see* Deposit,
  crystalline
Osteitis —*see also* Osteomyelitis
 alveolar M27.3
 condensans M85.30
  ankle M85.37-
  foot M85.37-
  forearm M85.33-
  hand M85.34-
  lower leg M85.36-
  multiple site M85.39
  neck M85.38
  rib M85.38
  shoulder M85.31-
  skull M85.38

Osteitis (*Continued*)
 condensans (*Continued*)
  specified site NEC M85.38
  thigh M85.35-
  toe M85.37-
  upper arm M85.32-
  vertebra M85.38
 deformans M88.9
  in (due to)
   malignant neoplasm of bone
    C41.9 [*M90.60*]
   neoplastic disease —*see also* Neoplasm
    D49.9 [*M90.60*]
    carpus D49.9 [*M90.64-*]
    clavicle D49.9 [*M90.61-*]
    femur D49.9 [*M90.65-*]
    fibula D49.9 [*M90.66-*]
    finger D49.9 [*M90.64-*]
    humerus D49.9 [*M90.62-*]
    ilium D49.9 [*M90.65-*]
    ischium D49.9 [*M90.65-*]
    metacarpus D49.9 [*M90.64-*]
    metatarsus D49.9 [*M90.67-*]
    multiple sites D49.9 [*M90.69*]
    neck D49.9 [*M90.68*]
    radius D49.9 [*M90.63-*]
    rib D49.9 [*M90.68*]
    scapula D49.9 [*M90.61-*]
    skull D49.9 [*M90.68*]
    tarsus D49.9 [*M90.67-*]
    tibia D49.9 [*M90.66-*]
    toe D49.9 [*M90.67-*]
    ulna D49.9 [*M90.63-*]
    vertebra D49.9 [*M90.68*]
  skull M88.0
  specified NEC —*see* Paget's disease, bone,
   by site
  vertebra M88.1
 due to yaws A66.6
 fibrosa NEC —*see* Cyst, bone, by site
  circumscripta —*see* Dysplasia, fibrous,
   bone NEC
  cystica (generalisata) E21.0
  disseminata Q78.1
  osteoplastica E21.0
 fragilitans Q78.0
 Garr's (sclerosing) —*see* Osteomyelitis,
  specified type NEC
 jaw (acute) (chronic) (lower) (suppurative)
  (upper) M27.2
 parathyroid E21.0
 petrous bone (acute) (chronic) —*see* Petrositis
 sclerotic, nonsuppurative —*see* Osteomyelitis,
  specified type NEC
 tuberculosa A18.09
  cystica D86.89
  multiplex cystoides D86.89
Osteoarthritis M19.90
 ankle M19.07-
 elbow M19.02-
 foot joint M19.07-
 generalized M15.9
  erosive M15.4
  primary M15.0
  specified NEC M15.8
 hand joint M19.04-
  first carpometacarpal joint M18.9-
 hip M16.1-
  bilateral M16.0
  due to hip dysplasia (unilateral)
   M16.3-
   bilateral M16.2
 interphalangeal
  distal (Heberden) M15.1
  proximal (Bouchard) M15.2
 knee M17.9-
  bilateral M17.0
 post-traumatic NEC M19.92
  ankle M19.17-
  elbow M19.12-
  foot joint M19.17-

Osteoarthritis (*Continued*)
 post-traumatic NEC (*Continued*)
  hand joint M19.14-
   first carpometacarpal joint M18.3-
    bilateral M18.2
  hip M16.5-
   bilateral M16.4
  knee M17.3-
   bilateral M17.2
  shoulder M19.11-
  wrist M19.13-
 primary M19.91
  ankle M19.07-
  elbow M19.02-
  foot joint M19.07-
  hand joint M19.04-
   first carpometacarpal joint M18.1-
    bilateral M18.0
  hip M16.1-
   bilateral M16.0
  knee M17.1-
   bilateral M17.0
  shoulder M19.01-
  spine —*see* Spondylosis
  wrist M19.03-
 secondary M19.93
  ankle M19.27-
  elbow M19.22-
  foot joint M19.27-
  hand joint M19.24-
   first carpometacarpal joint M18.5-
    bilateral M18.4
  hip M16.7
   bilateral M16.6
  knee M17.5
   bilateral M17.4
  multiple M15.3
  shoulder M19.21-
  spine —*see* Spondylosis
  wrist M19.23-
 shoulder M19.01-
 spine —*see* Spondylosis
 wrist M19.03-
Osteoarthropathy (hypertrophic) M19.90
 ankle —*see* Osteoarthritis, primary, ankle
 elbow —*see* Osteoarthritis, primary, elbow
 foot joint —*see* Osteoarthritis, primary, foot
 hand joint —*see* Osteoarthritis, primary, hand
  joint
 knee joint —*see* Osteoarthritis, primary, knee
 multiple site —*see* Osteoarthritis, primary,
  multiple joint
 pulmonary —*see also* Osteoarthropathy,
  specified type NEC
  hypertrophic —*see* Osteoarthropathy,
   hypertrophic, specified type NEC
 secondary —*see* Osteoarthropathy, specified
  type NEC
 secondary hypertrophic —*see*
  Osteoarthropathy, specified type NEC
 shoulder —*see* Osteoarthritis, primary,
  shoulder
 specified joint NEC —*see* Osteoarthritis,
  primary, specified joint NEC
 specified type NEC M89.40
  carpus M89.44-
  clavicle M89.41-
  femur M89.45-
  fibula M89.46-
  finger M89.44-
  humerus M89.42-
  ilium M89.459
  ischium M89.459
  metacarpus M89.44-
  metatarsus M89.47-
  multiple sites M89.49
  neck M89.48
  radius M89.43-
  rib M89.48
  scapula M89.41-
  skull M89.48

◄ New ◄▥ Revised ~~deleted~~ Deleted

Osteoarthropathy (Continued)
  specified type NEC (Continued)
    tarsus M89.47-
    tibia M89.46-
    toe M89.47-
    ulna M89.43-
    vertebra M89.48
  spine —see Spondylosis
  wrist —see Osteoarthritis, primary, wrist
Osteoarthrosis (degenerative) (hypertrophic)
    (joint) —see also Osteoarthritis
  deformans alkaptonurica E70.29 [M36.8]
  erosive M15.4
  generalized M15.9
    primary M15.0
  polyarticular M15.9
  spine —see Spondylosis
Osteoblastoma —see Neoplasm, bone, benign
  aggressive —see Neoplasm, bone, uncertain
    behavior
Osteochondroarthrosis deformans
    endemica —see Disease, Kaschin-Beck
Osteochondritis —see also Osteochondropathy,
    by site
  Brailsford's —see Osteochondrosis, juvenile,
    radius
  dissecans M93.20
    ankle M93.27-
    elbow M93.22-
    foot M93.27-
    hand M93.24-
    hip M93.25-
    knee M93.26-
    multiple sites M93.29
    shoulder joint M93.21-
    specified site NEC M93.28
    wrist M93.23-
  juvenile M92.9
    patellar —see Osteochondrosis, juvenile,
      patella
  syphilitic (congenital) (early) A50.02
    [M90.80]
    ankle A50.02 [M90.87-]
    elbow A50.02 [M90.82-]
    foot A50.02 [M90.87-]
    forearm A50.02 [M90.83-]
    hand A50.02 [M90.84-]
    hip A50.02 [M90.85-]
    knee A50.02 [M90.86-]
    multiple sites A50.02 [M90.89]
    shoulder joint A50.02 [M90.81-]
    specified site NEC A50.02 [M90.88]
Osteochondrodysplasia Q78.9
  with defects of growth of tubular bones and
    spine Q77.9
    specified NEC Q77.8
  specified NEC Q78.8
Osteochondrodystrophy E78.9
Osteochondrolysis —see Osteochondritis,
    dissecans
Osteochondroma —see Neoplasm, bone, benign
Osteochondromatosis D48.0
  syndrome Q78.4
Osteochondromyxosarcoma —see Neoplasm,
    bone, malignant
Osteochondropathy M93.90
  ankle M93.97-
  elbow M93.92-
  foot M93.97-
  hand M93.94-
  hip M93.95-
  Kienböck's disease of adults M93.1
  knee M93.96-
  multiple joints M93.99
  osteochondritis dissecans —see
    Osteochondritis, dissecans
  osteochondrosis —see Osteochondrosis
  shoulder region M93.91-
  slipped upper femoral epiphysis —see
    Slipped, epiphysis, upper femoral
  specified joint NEC M93.98

Osteochondropathy (Continued)
  specified type NEC M93.80
    ankle M93.87-
    elbow M93.82-
    foot M93.87-
    hand M93.84-
    hip M93.85-
    knee M93.86-
    multiple joints M93.89
    shoulder region M93.81-
    specified joint NEC M93.88
    wrist M93.83-
  syphilitic, congenital
    early A50.02 [M90.80]
    late A50.56 [M90.80]
  wrist M93.93-
Osteochondrosarcoma —see Neoplasm, bone,
    malignant
Osteochondrosis —see also Osteochondropathy,
    by site
  acetabulum (juvenile) M91.0
  adult —see Osteochondropathy, specified
    type NEC, by site
  astragalus (juvenile) —see Osteochondrosis,
    juvenile, tarsus
  Blount's —see Osteochondrosis, juvenile, tibia
  Buchanan's M91.0
  Burns' —see Osteochondrosis, juvenile, ulna
  calcaneus (juvenile) —see Osteochondrosis,
    juvenile, tarsus
  capitular epiphysis (femur) (juvenile) —see
    Legg-Calvé-Perthes disease
  carpal (juvenile) (lunate) (scaphoid) —see
    Osteochondrosis, juvenile, hand, carpal
    lunate
    adult M93.1
  coxae juvenilis —see Legg-Calvé-Perthes
    disease
  deformans juvenilis, coxae —see Legg-Calvé-
    Perthes disease
  Diaz's —see Osteochondrosis, juvenile,
    tarsus
  dissecans (knee) (shoulder) —see
    Osteochondritis, dissecans
  femoral capital epiphysis (juvenile) —see
    Legg-Calvé-Perthes disease
  femur (head), juvenile —see Legg-Calvé-
    Perthes disease
  fibula (juvenile) —see Osteochondrosis,
    juvenile, fibula
  foot NEC (juvenile) M92.8
  Freiberg's —see Osteochondrosis, juvenile,
    metatarsus
  Haas' (juvenile) —see Osteochondrosis,
    juvenile, humerus
  Haglund's —see Osteochondrosis, juvenile,
    tarsus
  hip (juvenile) —see Legg-Calvé-Perthes
    disease
  humerus (capitulum) (head) (juvenile) —see
    Osteochondrosis, juvenile, humerus
  ilium, iliac crest (juvenile) M91.0
  ischiopubic synchondrosis M91.0
  Iselin's —see Osteochondrosis, juvenile,
    metatarsus
  juvenile, juvenilis M92.9
    after congenital dislocation of hip
      reduction —see Osteochondrosis,
      juvenile, hip, specified NEC
    arm —see Osteochondrosis, juvenile, upper
      limb NEC
    capitular epiphysis (femur) —see Legg-
      Calvé-Perthes disease
    clavicle, sternal epiphysis —see
      Osteochondrosis, juvenile, upper
      limb NEC
    coxae —see Legg-Calvé-Perthes
      disease
    deformans M92.9
    fibula M92.5-
    foot NEC M92.8

Osteochondrosis (Continued)
  juvenile, juvenilis (Continued)
    hand M92.20-
      carpal lunate M92.21-
      metacarpal head M92.22-
      specified site NEC M92.29-
    head of femur —see Legg-Calvé-Perthes
      disease
    hip and pelvis M91.9-
      coxa plana —see Coxa, plana
      femoral head —see Legg-Calvé-Perthes
        disease
      pelvis M91.0
      pseudocoxalgia —see Pseudocoxalgia
      specified NEC M91.8-
    humerus M92.0-
    limb
      lower NEC M92.8
      upper NEC —see Osteochondrosis,
        juvenile, upper limb NEC
    medial cuneiform bone —see
      Osteochondrosis, juvenile, tarsus
    metatarsus M92.7-
    patella M92.4-
    radius M92.1-
    specified site NEC M92.8
    spine M42.00
      cervical region M42.02
      cervicothoracic region M42.03
      lumbar region M42.06
      lumbosacral region M42.07
      multiple sites M42.09
      occipito-atlanto-axial region M42.01
      sacrococcygeal region M42.08
      thoracic region M42.04
      thoracolumbar region M42.05
    tarsus M92.6-
    tibia M92.5-
    ulna M92.1-
    upper limb NEC M92.3-
    vertebra (body) (epiphyseal plates)
      (Calvé's) (Scheuermann's) —see
      Osteochondrosis, juvenile, spine
  Kienböck's —see Osteochondrosis, juvenile,
    hand, carpal lunate
    adult M93.1
  Köhler's
    patellar —see Osteochondrosis, juvenile,
      patella
    tarsal navicular —see Osteochondrosis,
      juvenile, tarsus
  Legg-Perthes (-Calvé's) (-Waldenström) —see
    Legg-Calvé-Perthes disease
  limb
    lower NEC (juvenile) M92.8
    upper NEC (juvenile) —see
      Osteochondrosis, juvenile, upper
      limb NEC
  lunate bone (carpal) (juvenile) —see also
    Osteochondrosis, juvenile, hand, carpal
    lunate
    adult M93.1
  Mauclaire's —see Osteochondrosis, juvenile,
    hand, metacarpal
  metacarpal (head) (juvenile) —see
    Osteochondrosis, juvenile, hand,
    metacarpal
  metatarsus (fifth) (head) (juvenile)
    (second) —see Osteochondrosis,
    juvenile, metatarsus
  navicular (juvenile) —see Osteochondrosis,
    juvenile, tarsus
  os
    calcis (juvenile) —see Osteochondrosis,
      juvenile, tarsus
    tibiale externum (juvenile) —see
      Osteochondrosis, juvenile, tarsus
  Osgood-Schlatter —see Osteochondrosis,
    juvenile, tibia
  Panner's —see Osteochondrosis, juvenile,
    humerus

◀ New ◀▥ Revised ~~deleted~~ Deleted

Osteomyelitis (Continued)
chronic (Continued)
  hematogenous NEC (Continued)
    multifocal (Continued)
      skull M86.38
      tarsus M86.37-
      tibia M86.36-
      toe M86.37-
      ulna M86.33-
      vertebra —see Osteomyelitis, vertebra
    multiple sites M86.59
    neck M86.58
    orbit H05.02-
    petrous bone —see Petrositis
    radius M86.53-
    rib M86.58
    scapula M86.51-
    skull M86.58
    tarsus M86.57-
    tibia M86.56-
    toe M86.57-
    ulna M86.53-
    vertebra —see Osteomyelitis, vertebra
  humerus M86.62-
  ilium M86.659
  ischium M86.659
  mandible M27.2
  metacarpus M86.64-
  metatarsus M86.67-
  multifocal —see Osteomyelitis, chronic,
    hematogenous, multifocal
  multiple sites M86.69
  neck M86.68
  orbit H05.02-
  petrous bone —see Petrositis
  radius M86.63-
  rib M86.68
  scapula M86.61-
  skull M86.68
  tarsus M86.67-
  tibia M86.66-
  toe M86.67-
  ulna M86.63-
  vertebra —see Osteomyelitis, vertebra
echinococcal B67.2
Garr's —see Osteomyelitis, specified type
  NEC
in diabetes mellitus —see E08-E13 with .69 ◄
jaw (acute) (chronic) (lower) (neonatal)
  (suppurative) (upper) M27.2
nonsuppurating —see Osteomyelitis,
  specified type NEC
orbit H05.02-
petrous bone —see Petrositis
Salmonella (arizonae) (cholerae-suis)
  (enteritidis) (typhimurium) A02.24
sclerosing, nonsuppurative —see
  Osteomyelitis, specified type NEC
specified type NEC —see also subcategory
  M86.8X-
  mandible M27.2
  orbit H05.02-
  petrous bone —see Petrositis
  vertebra —see Osteomyelitis, vertebra
subacute M86.20
  carpus M86.24-
  clavicle M86.21-
  femur M86.25-
  fibula M86.26-
  finger M86.24-
  humerus M86.22-
  mandible M27.2
  metacarpus M86.24-
  metatarsus M86.27-
  multiple sites M86.29
  neck M86.28
  orbit H05.02-
  petrous bone —see Petrositis
  radius M86.23-
  rib M86.28
  scapula M86.21-

Osteomyelitis (Continued)
subacute (Continued)
  skull M86.28
  tarsus M86.27-
  tibia M86.26-
  toe M86.27-
  ulna M86.23-
  vertebra —see Osteomyelitis, vertebra
syphilitic A52.77
  congenital (early) A50.02 [M90.80]
tuberculous —see Tuberculosis, bone
typhoid A01.05
vertebra M46.20
  cervical region M46.22
  cervicothoracic region M46.23
  lumbar region M46.26
  lumbosacral region M46.27
  occipito-atlanto-axial region
    M46.21
  sacrococcygeal region M46.28
  thoracic region M46.24
  thoracolumbar region M46.25
Osteomyelofibrosis D47.4 ◄▥
Osteomyelosclerosis D75.89
Osteonecrosis M87.9
  due to
    drugs —see Osteonecrosis, secondary, due
      to, drugs
    trauma —see Osteonecrosis, secondary, due
      to, trauma
  idiopathic aseptic M87.00
    ankle M87.07-
    carpus M87.03-
    clavicle M87.01-
    femur M87.05-
    fibula M87.06-
    finger M87.04-
    humerus M87.02-
    ilium M87.050
    ischium M87.050
    metacarpus M87.04-
    metatarsus M87.07-
    multiple sites M87.09
    neck M87.08
    pelvis M87.050
    radius M87.03-
    rib M87.08
    scapula M87.01-
    skull M87.08
    tarsus M87.07-
    tibia M87.06-
    toe M87.07-
    ulna M87.03-
    vertebra M87.08
  secondary NEC M87.30
    carpus M87.33-
    clavicle M87.31-
    due to
      drugs M87.10
        carpus M87.13-
        clavicle M87.11-
        femur M87.15-
        fibula M87.16-
        finger M87.14-
        humerus M87.12-
        ilium M87.159
        ischium M87.159
        jaw M87.180
        metacarpus M87.14-
        metatarsus M87.17-
        multiple sites M87.19
        neck M87.18
        radius M87.13-
        rib M87.18
        scapula M87.11-
        skull M87.18
        tarsus M87.17-
        tibia M87.16-
        toe M87.17-
        ulna M87.13-
        vertebra M87.18

Osteonecrosis (Continued)
secondary NEC (Continued)
  due to (Continued)
    hemoglobinopathy NEC D58.2
      [M90.50]
      carpus D58.2 [M90.54-]
      clavicle D58.2 [M90.51-]
      femur D58.2 [M90.55-]
      fibula D58.2 [M90.56-]
      finger D58.2 [M90.54-]
      humerus D58.2 [M90.52-]
      ilium D58.2 [M90.55-]
      ischium D58.2 [M90.55-]
      metacarpus D58.2 [M90.54-]
      metatarsus D58.2 [M90.57-]
      multiple sites D58.2 [M90.58]
      neck D58.2 [M90.58]
      radius D58.2 [M90.53-]
      rib D58.2 [M90.58]
      scapula D58.2 [M90.51-]
      skull D58.2 [M90.58]
      tarsus D58.2 [M90.57-]
      tibia D58.2 [M90.56-]
      toe D58.2 [M90.57-]
      ulna D58.2 [M90.53-]
      vertebra D58.2 [M90.58]
    trauma (previous) M87.20
      carpus M87.23-
      clavicle M87.21-
      femur M87.25-
      fibula M87.26-
      finger M87.24-
      humerus M87.22-
      ilium M87.25-
      ischium M87.25-
      metacarpus M87.24-
      metatarsus M87.27-
      multiple sites M87.29
      neck M87.28
      radius M87.23-
      rib M87.28
      scapula M87.21-
      skull M87.28
      tarsus M87.27-
      tibia M87.26-
      toe M87.27-
      ulna M87.23-
      vertebra M87.28
  femur M87.35-
  fibula M87.36-
  finger M87.34-
  humerus M87.32
  ilium M87.350
  in
    caisson disease T70.3 [M90.50]
      carpus T70.3 [M90.54-]
      clavicle T70.3 [M90.51-]
      femur T70.3 [M90.55-]
      fibula T70.3 [M90.56-]
      finger T70.3 [M90.54-]
      humerus T70.3 [M90.52-]
      ilium T70.3 [M90.55-]
      ischium T70.3 [M90.55-]
      metacarpus T70.3 [M90.54-]
      metatarsus T70.3 [M90.57-]
      multiple sites T70.3 [M90.59]
      neck T70.3 [M90.58]
      radius T70.3 [M90.53-]
      rib T70.3 [M90.58]
      scapula T70.3 [M90.51-]
      skull T70.3 [M90.58]
      tarsus T70.3 [M90.57-]
      tibia T70.3 [M90.56-]
      toe T70.3 [M90.57-]
      ulna T70.3 [M90.53-]
      vertebra T70.3 [M90.58]
  ischium M87.350
  metacarpus M87.34-
  metatarsus M87.37-
  multiple site M87.39
  neck M87.38

Osteonecrosis (Continued)
  secondary NEC (Continued)
    radius M87.33-
    rib M87.38
    scapula M87.319
    skull M87.38
    tarsus M87.379
    tibia M87.366
    toe M87.379
    ulna M87.33-
    vertebra M87.38
  specified type NEC M87.80
    carpus M87.83-
    clavicle M87.81-
    femur M87.85-
    fibula M87.86-
    finger M87.84-
    humerus M87.82-
    ilium M87.85-
    ischium M87.85-
    metacarpus M87.84-
    metatarsus M87.87-
    multiple sites M87.89
    neck M87.88
    radius M87.83-
    rib M87.88-
    scapula M87.81-
    skull M87.88
    tarsus M87.87-
    tibia M87.86-
    toe M87.87-
    ulna M87.83-
    vertebra M87.88
Osteo-onycho-arthro-dysplasia Q87.2 ◀▥
Osteo-onychodysplasia, hereditary Q87.2 ◀▥
Osteopathia condensans disseminata Q78.8
Osteopathy —see also Osteomyelitis,
    Osteonecrosis, Osteoporosis
  after poliomyelitis M89.60
    carpus M89.64-
    clavicle M89.61-
    femur M89.65-
    fibula M89.66-
    finger M89.64-
    humerus M89.62-
    ilium M89.659
    ischium M89.659
    metacarpus M89.64-
    metatarsus M89.67-
    multiple sites M89.69
    neck M89.68
    radius M89.63-
    rib M89.68
    scapula M89.61-
    skull M89.68
    tarsus M89.67-
    tibia M89.66-
    toe M89.67-
    ulna M89.63-
    vertebra M89.68
  in (due to)
    renal osteodystrophy N25.0
    specified diseases classified elsewhere —
      see subcategory M90.8
Osteopenia M85.8-
  borderline M85.8-
Osteoperiostitis —see Osteomyelitis, specified
    type NEC
Osteopetrosis (familial) Q78.2
Osteophyte M25.70
  ankle M25.77-
  elbow M25.72-
  foot joint M25.77-
  hand joint M25.74-
  hip M25.75-
  knee M25.76-
  shoulder M25.71-
  spine M25.78
  vertebrae M25.78
  wrist M25.73-
Osteopoikilosis Q78.8

Osteoporosis (female) (male) M81.0
  with current pathological fracture M80.00
  age-related M81.0
    with current pathologic fracture M80.00
      carpus M80.04-
      clavicle M80.01-
      fibula M80.06-
      finger M80.04-
      humerus M80.02-
      ilium M80.05-
      ischium M80.05-
      metacarpus M80.04-
      metatarsus M80.07-
      pelvis M80.05-
      radius M80.03-
      scapula M80.01-
      tarsus M80.07-
      tibia M80.06-
      toe M80.07-
      ulna M80.03-
      vertebra M80.08
  disuse M81.8
    with current pathological fracture M80.80
      carpus M80.84-
      clavicle M80.81-
      fibula M80.86-
      finger M80.84-
      humerus M80.82-
      ilium M80.85-
      ischium M80.85-
      metacarpus M80.84-
      metatarsus M80.87-
      pelvis M80.85-
      radius M80.83-
      scapula M80.81-
      tarsus M80.87-
      tibia M80.86-
      toe M80.87-
      ulna M80.83-
      vertebra M80.88
  drug-induced —see Osteoporosis, specified
    type NEC
  idiopathic —see Osteoporosis, specified type
    NEC
  involutional —see Osteoporosis, age-related
  Lequesne M81.6
  localized M81.6
  postmenopausal M81.0
    with pathological fracture M80.00
      carpus M80.04-
      clavicle M80.01-
      fibula M80.06-
      finger M80.04-
      humerus M80.02-
      ilium M80.05-
      ischium M80.05-
      metacarpus M80.04-
      metatarsus M80.07-
      pelvis M80.05-
      radius M80.03-
      scapula M80.01-
      tarsus M80.07-
      tibia M80.06-
      toe M80.07-
      ulna M80.03-
      vertebra M80.08
  postoophorectomy —see Osteoporosis,
    specified type NEC
  postsurgical malabsorption —see
    Osteoporosis, specified type NEC
  post-traumatic —see Osteoporosis, specified
    type NEC
  senile —see Osteoporosis, age-related
  specified type NEC M81.8
    with pathological fracture M80.80
      carpus M80.84-
      clavicle M80.81-
      fibula M80.86-
      finger M80.84-
      humerus M80.82-
      ilium M80.85-

Osteoporosis (Continued)
  specified type NEC (Continued)
    with pathological fracture (Continued)
      ischium M80.85-
      metacarpus M80.84-
      metatarsus M80.87-
      pelvis M80.85-
      radius M80.83-
      scapula M80.81-
      tarsus M80.87-
      tibia M80.86-
      toe M80.87-
      ulna M80.83-
      vertebra M80.88
Osteopsathyrosis (idiopathica) Q78.0
Osteoradionecrosis, jaw (acute) (chronic)
  (lower) (suppurative) (upper)
  M27.2
Osteosarcoma (any form) —see Neoplasm,
  bone, malignant
Osteosclerosis Q78.2
  acquired M85.8-
  congenita Q77.4
  fragilitas (generalisata) Q78.2
  myelofibrosis D75.81
Osteosclerotic anemia D64.89
Osteosis
  cutis L94.2
  renal fibrocystic N25.0
Österreicher-Turner syndrome Q87.2
Ostium
  atrioventriculare commune Q21.2
  primum (arteriosum) (defect) (persistent)
    Q21.2
  secundum (arteriosum) (defect) (patent)
    (persistent) Q21.1
Ostrum-Furst syndrome Q75.8
Otalgia —see subcategory H92.0
Otitis (acute) H66.90
  with effusion —see also Otitis, media,
    nonsuppurative
    purulent —see Otitis, media, suppurative
  adhesive —see subcategory H74.1
  chronic —see also Otitis, media, chronic
    with effusion —see also Otitis, media,
      nonsuppurative, chronic
  externa H60.9-
    abscess —see Abscess, ear, external
    acute (noninfective) H60.50-
      actinic H60.51-
      chemical H60.52-
      contact H60.53-
      eczematoid H60.54-
      infective —see Otitis, externa, infective
      reactive H60.55-
      specified NEC H60.59-
    cellulitis —see Cellulitis, ear
    chronic H60.6-
    diffuse —see Otitis, externa, infective, diffuse
    hemorrhagic —see Otitis, externa, infective,
      hemorrhagic
    in (due to)
      aspergillosis B44.89
      candidiasis B37.84
      erysipelas A46 [H62.40]
      herpes (simplex) virus infection B00.1
        zoster B02.8
      impetigo L01.00 [H62.40]
      infectious disease NEC B99 [H62.4-]
      mycosis NEC B36.9 [H62.40]
      parasitic disease NEC B89 [H62.40]
      viral disease NEC B34.9 [H62.40]
      zoster B02.8
    infective NEC H60.39-
      abscess —see Abscess, ear, external
      cellulitis —see Cellulitis, ear
      diffuse H60.31-
      hemorrhagic H60.32-
      swimmer's ear —see Swimmer's, ear
    malignant H60.2-
    ~~mycotic B36.9 [H62.40]~~

◀ New   ▥ Revised   ~~deleted~~ Deleted

Otitis (Continued)
  externa (Continued)
    mycotic NEC B36.9 [H62.40] ◀
      in ◀
        aspergillosis B44.89 ◀
        candidiasis B37.84 ◀
        moniliasis B37.84 ◀
    necrotizing —see Otitis, externa, malignant
    Pseudomonas aeruginosa —see Otitis, externa, malignant
    reactive —see Otitis, externa, acute, reactive
    specified NEC —see subcategory H60.8
    tropical B36.8
    tropical NEC B36.9 [H62.40] ◀
      in ◀
        aspergillosis B44.89 ◀
        candidiasis B37.84 ◀
        moniliasis B37.84 ◀
  insidiosa —see Otosclerosis
  interna —see subcategory H83.0
  media (hemorrhagic) (staphylococcal) (streptococcal) H66.9-
    with effusion (nonpurulent) —see Otitis, media, nonsuppurative
    acute, subacute H66.90
      allergic —see Otitis, media, nonsuppurative, acute, allergic
      exudative —see Otitis, media, suppurative, acute ◀▥
      mucoid —see Otitis, media, nonsuppurative, acute
      necrotizing —see also Otitis, media, suppurative, acute
        in
          measles B05.3
          scarlet fever A38.0
      nonsuppurative NEC —see Otitis, media, nonsuppurative, acute
      purulent —see Otitis, media, suppurative, acute
      sanguinous —see Otitis, media, nonsuppurative, acute
      secretory —see Otitis, media, nonsuppurative, acute, serous
      seromucinous —see Otitis, media, nonsuppurative, acute
      serous —see Otitis, media, nonsuppurative, acute, serous
      suppurative —see Otitis, media, suppurative, acute
    allergic —see Otitis, media, nonsuppurative
    catarrhal —see Otitis, media, nonsuppurative
    chronic H66.90
      with effusion (nonpurulent) —see Otitis, media, nonsuppurative, chronic
      allergic —see Otitis, media, nonsuppurative, chronic, allergic
      benign suppurative —see Otitis, media, suppurative, chronic, tubotympanic
      catarrhal —see Otitis, media, nonsuppurative, chronic, serous
      exudative —see Otitis, media, suppurative, chronic ◀▥
      mucinous —see Otitis, media, nonsuppurative, chronic, mucoid
      mucoid —see Otitis, media, nonsuppurative, chronic, mucoid
      nonsuppurative NEC —see Otitis, media, nonsuppurative, chronic
      purulent —see Otitis, media, suppurative, chronic
      secretory —see Otitis, media, nonsuppurative, chronic, mucoid
      seromucinous —see Otitis, media, nonsuppurative, chronic
      serous —see Otitis, media, nonsuppurative, chronic, serous
      suppurative —see Otitis, media, suppurative, chronic

Otitis (Continued)
  media (Continued)
    chronic (Continued)
      transudative —see Otitis, media, nonsuppurative, chronic, mucoid
    exudative —see Otitis, media, nonsuppurative
    in (due to) (with)
      influenza —see Influenza, with, otitis media
      measles B05.3
      scarlet fever A38.0
      tuberculosis A18.6
      viral disease NEC B34.- [H67.-]
    mucoid —see Otitis, media, nonsuppurative
    nonsuppurative H65.9-
      acute or subacute NEC H65.19-
        allergic H65.11-
          recurrent H65.11-
        recurrent H65.19-
        secretory —see Otitis, media, nonsuppurative, serous
        serous H65.0-
          recurrent H65.0-
      chronic H65.49-
        allergic H65.41-
        mucoid H65.3-
        serous H65.2-
      postmeasles B05.3
      purulent —see Otitis, media, suppurative
      secretory —see Otitis, media, nonsuppurative
      seromucinous —see Otitis, media, nonsuppurative
      serous —see Otitis, media, nonsuppurative
    suppurative H66.4-
      acute H66.00-
        with rupture of ear drum H66.01-
        recurrent H66.00-
          with rupture of ear drum H66.01-
      chronic —see also subcategory H66.3
        atticoantral H66.2-
        benign —see Otitis, media, suppurative, chronic, tubotympanic
        tubotympanic H66.1-
    transudative —see Otitis, media, nonsuppurative
    tuberculous A18.6
Otocephaly Q18.2
Otolith syndrome —see subcategory H81.8
Otomycosis (diffuse) NEC B36.9 [H62.40]
  in
    aspergillosis B44.89
    candidiasis B37.84
    moniliasis B37.84
Otoporosis —see Otosclerosis
Otorrhagia (nontraumatic) H92.2-
  traumatic - code by Type of injury
Otorrhea H92.1-
  cerebrospinal G96.0
Otosclerosis (general) H80.9-
  cochlear (endosteal) H80.2-
  involving
    otic capsule —see Otosclerosis, cochlear
    oval window
      nonobliterative H80.0-
      obliterative H80.1-
    round window —see Otosclerosis, cochlear
  nonobliterative —see Otosclerosis, involving, oval window, nonobliterative
  obliterative —see Otosclerosis, involving, oval window, obliterative
  specified NEC H80.8-
Otospongiosis —see Otosclerosis
Otto's disease or pelvis M24.7
Outcome of delivery Z37.9
  multiple births Z37.9
    all liveborn Z37.50
      quadruplets Z37.52
      quintuplets Z37.53

Outcome of delivery (Continued)
  multiple births (Continued)
    all liveborn (Continued)
      sextuplets Z37.54
      specified number NEC Z37.59
      triplets Z37.51
    all stillborn Z37.7
    some liveborn Z37.60
      quadruplets Z37.62
      quintuplets Z37.63
      sextuplets Z37.64
      specified number NEC Z37.69
      triplets Z37.61
    single NEC Z37.9
      liveborn Z37.0
      stillborn Z37.1
    twins NEC Z37.9
      both liveborn Z37.2
      both stillborn Z37.4
      one liveborn, one stillborn Z37.3
Outlet —see condition
Ovalocytosis (congenital) (hereditary) —see Elliptocytosis
Ovarian —see Condition
Ovariocele N83.4- ◀▥
Ovaritis (cystic) —see Oophoritis
Ovary, ovarian —see also condition
  resistant syndrome E28.39
  vein syndrome N13.8
Overactive —see also Hyperfunction
  adrenal cortex NEC E27.0
  bladder N32.81
  hypothalamus E23.3
  thyroid —see Hyperthyroidism
Overactivity R46.3
  child —see Disorder, attention-deficit hyperactivity
Overbite (deep) (excessive) (horizontal) (vertical) M26.29
Overbreathing —see Hyperventilation
Overconscientious personality F60.5
Overdevelopment —see Hypertrophy
Overdistension —see Distension
Overdose, overdosage (drug) —see Table of Drugs and Chemicals, by drug, poisoning
Overeating R63.2
  nonorganic origin F50.89 ◀▥
  psychogenic F50.89 ◀▥
Overexertion (effects) (exhaustion) T73.3
Overexposure (effects) T73.9
  exhaustion T73.2
Overfeeding —see Overeating
  newborn P92.4
Overfill, endodontic M27.52
Overgrowth, bone —see Hypertrophy, bone
Overhanging of dental restorative material (unrepairable) K08.52
Overheated (places) (effects) —see Heat
Overjet (excessive horizontal) M26.23
Overlaid, overlying (suffocation) —see Asphyxia, traumatic, due to mechanical threat
Overlap, excessive horizontal (teeth) M26.23
Overl apping toe (acquired) —see also Deformity, toe, specified NEC
  congenital (fifth toe) Q66.89
Overload
  circulatory, due to transfusion (blood) (blood components) (TACO) E87.71
  fluid E87.70
    due to transfusion (blood) (blood components) E87.71
    specified NEC E87.79
  iron, due to repeated red blood cell transfusions E83.111
  potassium (K) E87.5
  sodium (Na) E87.0
Overnutrition —see Hyperalimentation
Overproduction —see also Hypersecretion
  ACTH E27.0
  catecholamine E27.5
  growth hormone E22.0

Overprotection, child by parent Z62.1
Overriding
   aorta Q25.49 ◀▥
   finger (acquired) —*see* Deformity, finger
      congenital Q68.1
   toe (acquired) —*see also* Deformity, toe,
      specified NEC
      congenital Q66.89
Overstrained R53.83
   heart —*see* Hypertrophy, cardiac

Overuse, muscle NEC
   M70.8-
Overweight E66.3
Overworked R53.83
Oviduct —*see* condition
Ovotestis Q56.0
Ovulation (cycle)
   failure or lack of N97.0
   pain N94.0
Ovum —*see* condition

Owren's disease or syndrome (parahemophilia)
   D68.2
Ox heart —*see* Hypertrophy, cardiac
Oxalosis E72.53
Oxaluria E72.53
Oxycephaly, oxycephalic Q75.0
   syphilitic, congenital A50.02
Oxyuriasis B80
Oxyuris vermicularis (infestation) B80
Ozena J31.0

P

Pachyderma, pachydermia L85.9
　larynx (verrucosa) J38.7
Pachydermatocele (congenital) Q82.8
Pachydermoperiostosis —see also
　　Osteoarthropathy, hypertrophic, specified
　　type NEC
　clubbed nail M89.40 [L62]
Pachygyria Q04.3
Pachymeningitis (adhesive) (basal) (brain)
　　(cervical) (chronic) (circumscribed)
　　(external) (fibrous) (hemorrhagic)
　　(hypertrophic) (internal) (purulent)
　　(spinal) (suppurative) —see Meningitis
Pachyonychia (congenital) Q84.5
Pacinian tumor —see Neoplasm, skin, benign
Pad, knuckle or Garrod's M72.1
Paget-Schroetter syndrome I82.890
Paget's disease
　with infiltrating duct carcinoma —see
　　Neoplasm, breast, malignant
　bone M88.9
　　carpus M88.84-
　　clavicle M88.81-
　　femur M88.85-
　　fibula M88.86-
　　finger M88.84-
　　humerus M88.82-
　　ilium M88.85-
　　in neoplastic disease —see Osteitis,
　　　deformans, in neoplastic disease
　　ischium M88.85-
　　metacarpus M88.84-
　　metatarsus M88.87-
　　multiple sites M88.89
　　neck M88.88
　　radius M88.83-
　　rib M88.88
　　scapula M88.81-
　　skull M88.0
　　tarsus M88.87-
　　tibia M88.86-
　　toe M88.87-
　　ulna M88.83-
　　vertebra M88.88
　breast (female) C50.01-
　　male C50.02-
　extramammary —see also Neoplasm, skin,
　　malignant
　　anus C21.0
　　　margin C44.590
　　　skin C44.590
　intraductal carcinoma —see Neoplasm,
　　breast, malignant
　malignant —see Neoplasm, skin, malignant
　　breast (female) C50.01-
　　　male C50.02-
　　unspecified site (female) C50.01-
　　　male C50.02-
　mammary —see Paget's disease, breast
　nipple —see Paget's disease, breast
　osteitis deformans —see Paget's disease, bone
Pain(s) —see also Painful R52
　abdominal R10.9
　　colic R10.83
　　generalized R10.84
　　　with acute abdomen R10.0
　　lower R10.30
　　　left quadrant R10.32
　　　pelvic or perineal R10.2
　　　periumbilical R10.33
　　　right quadrant R10.31
　　rebound —see Tenderness, abdominal,
　　　rebound
　　severe with abdominal rigidity R10.0
　　tenderness —see Tenderness, abdominal
　　upper R10.10
　　　epigastric R10.13
　　　left quadrant R10.12
　　　right quadrant R10.11

Pain (Continued)
　acute R52
　　due to trauma G89.11
　　neoplasm related G89.3
　　postprocedural NEC G89.18
　　post-thoracotomy G89.12
　　specified by site — code to Pain, by site
　adnexa (uteri) R10.2
　anginoid —see Pain, precordial
　anus K62.89
　arm —see Pain, limb, upper
　axillary (axilla) M79.62-
　back (postural) M54.9
　bladder R39.89
　　associated with micturition —see
　　　Micturition, painful
　　chronic R39.82 ◀
　bone —see Disorder, bone, specified type
　　NEC
　breast N64.4
　broad ligament R10.2
　cancer associated (acute) (chronic) G89.3
　cecum —see Pain, abdominal
　cervicobrachial M53.1
　chest (central) R07.9
　　anterior wall R07.89
　　atypical R07.89
　　ischemic I20.9
　　musculoskeletal R07.89
　　non-cardiac R07.89
　　on breathing R07.1
　　pleurodynia R07.81
　　precordial R07.2
　　wall (anterior) R07.89
　chronic G89.29
　　associated with significant psychosocial
　　　dysfunction G89.4
　　due to trauma G89.21
　　neoplasm related G89.3
　　postoperative NEC G89.28
　　postprocedural NEC G89.28
　　post-thoracotomy G89.22
　　specified NEC G89.29
　coccyx M53.3
　colon —see Pain, abdominal
　coronary —see Angina
　costochondral R07.1
　diaphragm R07.1
　due to cancer G89.3
　due to device, implant or graft —see also
　　Complications, by site and type,
　　　specified NEC T85.848 ◀▥
　　arterial graft NEC T82.848
　　breast (implant) T85.848 ◀▥
　　catheter NEC T85.848 ◀▥
　　　dialysis (renal) T82.848
　　　　intraperitoneal T85.848 ◀▥
　　　infusion NEC T82.848
　　　　spinal (epidural) (subdural) T85.840 ◀▥
　　　urinary (indwelling) T83.84
　　electronic (electrode) (pulse generator)
　　　(stimulator)
　　　bone T84.84
　　　cardiac T82.847
　　　nervous system (brain) (peripheral
　　　　nerve) (spinal) T85.840 ◀▥
　　　urinary T83.84
　　fixation, internal (orthopedic) NEC T84.84
　　gastrointestinal (bile duct) (esophagus)
　　　T85.848 ◀▥
　　genital NEC T83.84
　　heart NEC T82.847
　　infusion NEC T85.848 ◀▥
　　joint prosthesis T84.84
　　ocular (corneal graft) (orbital implant)
　　　NEC T85.848 ◀▥
　　orthopedic NEC T84.84
　　specified NEC T85.848 ◀▥
　　urinary NEC T83.84
　　vascular NEC T82.848
　　ventricular intracranial shunt T85.840 ◀▥

Pain (Continued)
　due to malignancy (primary) (secondary)
　　G89.3
　ear —see subcategory H92.0
　epigastric, epigastrium R10.13
　eye —see Pain, ocular
　face, facial R51
　　atypical G50.1
　female genital organs NEC N94.89
　finger —see Pain, limb, upper
　flank —see Pain, abdominal
　foot —see Pain, limb, lower
　gallbladder K82.9
　gas (intestinal) R14.1
　gastric —see Pain, abdominal
　generalized NOS R52
　genital organ
　　female N94.89
　　male N50.89 ◀▥
　groin —see Pain, abdominal, lower
　hand —see Pain, limb, upper
　head —see Headache
　heart —see Pain, precordial
　infra-orbital —see Neuralgia, trigeminal
　intercostal R07.82
　intermenstrual N94.0
　jaw R68.84
　joint M25.50
　　ankle M25.57-
　　elbow M25.52-
　　finger M25.54- ◀▥
　　foot M25.57-
　　hand M25.54- ◀▥
　　hip M25.55-
　　knee M25.56-
　　shoulder M25.51-
　　toe M25.57-
　　wrist M25.53-
　kidney N23
　laryngeal R07.0
　leg —see Pain, limb, lower
　limb M79.609
　　lower M79.60-
　　　foot M79.67-
　　　lower leg M79.66-
　　　thigh M79.65-
　　　toe M79.67-
　　upper M79.60-
　　　axilla M79.62-
　　　finger M79.64-
　　　forearm M79.63-
　　　hand M79.64-
　　　upper arm M79.62-
　loin M54.5
　low back M54.5
　lumbar region M54.5
　mandibular R68.84
　mastoid —see subcategory H92.0
　maxilla R68.84
　menstrual —see also Dysmenorrhea N94.6
　metacarpophalangeal (joint) —see Pain, joint,
　　hand
　metatarsophalangeal (joint) —see Pain, joint,
　　foot
　mouth K13.79
　muscle —see Myalgia
　musculoskeletal —see also Pain, by site M79.1
　myofascial M79.1
　nasal J34.89
　nasopharynx J39.2
　neck NEC M54.2
　nerve NEC —see Neuralgia
　neuromuscular —see Neuralgia
　nose J34.89
　ocular H57.1-
　ophthalmic —see Pain, ocular
　orbital region —see Pain, ocular
　ovary N94.89
　over heart —see Pain, precordial
　ovulation N94.0
　pelvic (female) R10.2

Pain *(Continued)*
  penis N48.89
  pericardial —*see* Pain, precordial
  perineal, perineum R10.2
  pharynx J39.2
  pleura, pleural, pleuritic R07.81
  postoperative NOS G89.18
  postprocedural NOS G89.18
  post-thoracotomy G89.12
  precordial (region) R07.2
  premenstrual N94.3
  psychogenic (persistent) (any site) F45.41
  radicular (spinal) —*see* Radiculopathy
  rectum K62.89
  respiration R07.1
  retrosternal R07.2
  rheumatoid, muscular —*see* Myalgia
  rib R07.81
  root (spinal) —*see* Radiculopathy
  round ligament (stretch) R10.2
  sacroiliac M53.3
  sciatic —*see* Sciatica
  scrotum N50.82 ◀▥
  seminal vesicle N50.89 ◀▥
  shoulder M25.51-
  spermatic cord N50.89 ◀▥
  spinal root —*see* Radiculopathy
  spine M54.9
    cervical M54.2
    low back M54.5
      with sciatica M54.4-
    thoracic M54.6
  stomach —*see* Pain, abdominal
  substernal R07.2
  temporomandibular (joint) M26.62- ◀▥
  testis N50.81- ◀▥
  thoracic spine M54.6
    with radicular and visceral pain
        M54.14
  throat R07.0
  tibia —*see* Pain, limb, lower
  toe —*see* Pain, limb, lower
  tongue K14.6
  tooth K08.89 ◀▥
  trigeminal —*see* Neuralgia, trigeminal
  tumor associated G89.3
  ureter N23
  urinary (organ) (system) N23
  uterus NEC N94.89
  vagina R10.2
  vertebrogenic (syndrome) M54.89
  vesical R39.89
    associated with micturition —*see*
        Micturition, painful
  vulva R10.2
Painful —*see also* Pain
  coitus
    female N94.10 ◀▥
    male N53.12
    psychogenic F52.6
  ejaculation (semen) N53.12
    psychogenic F52.6
  erection —*see* Priapism
  feet syndrome E53.8
  joint replacement (hip) (knee) T84.84
  menstruation —*see* Dysmenorrhea
    psychogenic F45.8
  micturition —*see* Micturition, painful
  respiration R07.1
  scar NEC L90.5
  wire sutures T81.89
Painter's colic —*see* subcategory T56.0
Palate —*see* condition
Palatoplegia K13.79
Palatoschisis —*see* Cleft, palate
Palilalia R48.8
Palliative care Z51.5
Pallor R23.1
  optic disc, temporal —*see* Atrophy, optic
Palmar —*see also* condition
  fascia —*see* condition

Palpable
  cecum K63.89
  kidney N28.89
  ovary N83.8
  prostate N42.9
  spleen —*see* Splenomegaly
Palpitations (heart) R00.2
  psychogenic F45.8
Palsy —*see also* Paralysis G83.9
  atrophic diffuse (progressive) G12.22
  Bell's —*see also* Palsy, facial
    newborn P11.3
  brachial plexus NEC G54.0
    newborn (birth injury) P14.3
  brain —*see* Palsy, cerebral
  bulbar (progressive) (chronic) G12.22
    of childhood (Fazio-Londe) G12.1
    pseudo NEC G12.29
    supranuclear (progressive) G23.1
  cerebral (congenital) G80.9
    ataxic G80.4
    athetoid G80.3
      choreathetoid G80.3
    diplegic G80.8
      spastic G80.1
    dyskinetic G80.3
      athetoid G80.3
      choreathetoid G80.3
      distonic G80.3
    dystonic G80.3
    hemiplegic G80.8
      spastic G80.2
    mixed G80.8
    monoplegic G80.8
      spastic G80.1
    paraplegic G80.8
      spastic G80.1
    quadriplegic G80.8
      spastic G80.0
    spastic G80.1
      diplegic G80.1
      hemiplegic G80.2
      monoplegic G80.1
      quadriplegic G80.0
      specified NEC G80.1
      tetrapelgic G80.0
    specified NEC G80.8
    syphilitic A52.12
      congenital A50.49
    tetraplegic G80.8
      spastic G80.0
  cranial nerve —*see also* Disorder, nerve,
      cranial
    multiple G52.7
      in
        infectious disease B99 *[G53]*
        neoplastic disease —*see also* Neoplasm
            D49.9 *[G53]*
        parasitic disease B89 *[G53]*
        sarcoidosis D86.82
  creeping G12.22
  diver's T70.3
  Erb's P14.0
  facial G51.0
    newborn (birth injury) P11.3
  glossopharyngeal G52.1
  Klumpke (-Déjérine) P14.1
  lead —*see* subcategory T56.0
  median nerve (tardy) G56.1-
  nerve G58.9
    specified NEC G58.8
  peroneal nerve (acute) (tardy) G57.3-
  progressive supranuclear G23.1
  pseudobulbar NEC G12.29
  radial nerve (acute) G56.3-
  seventh nerve —*see also* Palsy, facial
    newborn P11.3
  shaking —*see* Parkinsonism
  spastic (cerebral) (spinal) G80.1
  ulnar nerve (tardy) G56.2-
  wasting G12.29

Paludism —*see* Malaria
Panangiitis M30.0
Panaris, panaritium —*see also* Cellulitis, digit
  with lymphangitis —*see* Lymphangitis, acute,
      digit
Panarteritis nodosa M30.0
  brain or cerebral I67.7
Pancake heart R93.1
  with cor pulmonale (chronic) I27.81
Pancarditis (acute) (chronic) I51.89
  rheumatic I09.89
    active or acute I01.8
Pancoast's syndrome or tumor C34.1-
Pancolitis, ulcerative (chronic) K51.00
  with
    abscess K51.014
    complication K51.019
    fistula K51.013
    obstruction K51.012
    rectal bleeding K51.011
    specified complication NEC K51.018
Pancreas, pancreatic —*see* condition
Pancreatitis (annular) (apoplectic) (calcareous)
    (edematous) (hemorrhagic) (malignant)
    (recurrent) (subacute) (suppurative)
    K85.90 ◀▥
  with necrosis (uninfected) K85.91 ◀
    infected K85.92 ◀
  acute (without necrosis or infection)
      K85.90 ◀▥
    with necrosis (uninfected) K85.91 ◀
      infected K85.92 ◀
    alcohol induced (without necrosis or
        infection) K85.20 ◀▥
      with necrosis (uninfected) K85.21 ◀
        infected K85.22 ◀
    biliary (without necrosis or infection)
        K85.10 ◀▥
      with necrosis (uninfected) K85.11 ◀
        infected K85.12 ◀
    drug induced (without necrosis or
        infection) K85.30 ◀▥
      with necrosis (uninfected) K85.31 ◀
        infected K85.32 ◀
    gallstone (without necrosis or infection)
        K85.10 ◀▥
      with necrosis (uninfected) K85.11 ◀
        infected K85.12 ◀
    idiopathic (without necrosis or infection)
        K85.00 ◀▥
      with necrosis (uninfected) K85.01 ◀
        infected K85.02 ◀
    specified NEC (without necrosis or
        infection) K85.80 ◀▥
      with necrosis (uninfected)
          K85.81 ◀
        infected K85.82 ◀
  chronic (infectious) K86.1
    alcohol-induced K86.0
    recurrent K86.1
    relapsing K86.1
  cystic (chronic) K86.1
  cytomegaloviral B25.2
  fibrous (chronic) K86.1
  gallstone (without necrosis or infection)
      K85.10 ◀▥
    with necrosis (uninfected)
        K85.11 ◀
      infected K85.12 ◀
  gangrenous —*see* Pancreatitis, acute ◀▥
  interstitial (chronic) K86.1
    acute —*see also* Pancreatitis, acute
        K85.80 ◀▥
  mumps B26.3
  recurrent (chronic) K86.1
  relapsing, chronic K86.1
  syphilitic A52.74
Pancreatoblastoma —*see* Neoplasm, pancreas,
    malignant
Pancreolithiasis K86.89 ◀▥
Pancytolysis D75.89

◀ New   ◀▥ Revised   ~~deleted~~ Deleted

Pancytopenia (acquired) D61.818
  with
    malformations D61.09
    myelodysplastic syndrome —*see*
      Syndrome, myelodysplastic
    antineoplastic chemotherapy induced
      D61.810
  congenital D61.09
  drug-induced NEC D61.811
Panencephalitis, subacute, sclerosing
  A81.1
Panhematopenia D61.9
  congenital D61.09
  constitutional D61.09
  splenic, primary D73.1
Panhemocytopenia D61.9
  congenital D61.09
  constitutional D61.09
Panhypogonadism E29.1
Panhypopituitarism E23.0
  prepubertal E23.0
Panic (attack) (state) F41.0
  reaction to exceptional stress (transient)
    F43.0
Panmyelopathy, familial, constitutional
  D61.09
Panmyelophthisis D61.82
  congenital D61.09
Panmyelosis (acute) (with myelofibrosis)
  C94.4-
Panner's disease —*see* Osteochondrosis,
  juvenile, humerus
Panneuritis endemica E51.11
Panniculitis (nodular) (nonsuppurative) M79.3
  back M54.00
    cervical region M54.02
    cervicothoracic region M54.03
    lumbar region M54.06
    lumbosacral region M54.07
    multiple sites M54.09
    occipito-atlanto-axial region M54.01
    sacrococcygeal region M54.08
    thoracic region M54.04
    thoracolumbar region M54.05
  lupus L93.2
  mesenteric K65.4
  neck M54.02
    cervicothoracic region M54.03
    occipito-atlanto-axial region M54.01
  relapsing M35.6
Panniculus adiposus (abdominal) E65
Pannus (allergic) (cornea) (degenerativus)
  (keratic) H16.42-
  abdominal (symptomatic) E65
  trachomatosus, trachomatous (active) A71.1
Panophthalmitis H44.01-
Pansinusitis (chronic) (hyperplastic)
  (nonpurulent) (purulent) J32.4
  acute J01.40
    recurrent J01.41
  tuberculous A15.8
Panuveitis (sympathetic) H44.11-
Panvalvular disease I08.9
  specified NEC I08.8
PAPA (pyogenic arthritis, pyoderma
  gangrenosum, and acne syndrome)
  M04.8 ◀
Papanicolaou smear, cervix Z12.4
  as part of routine gynecological examination
    Z01.419
    with abnormal findings Z01.411
  for suspected neoplasm Z12.4
  nonspecific abnormal finding R87.619
  routine Z01.419
    with abnormal findings Z01.411
Papilledema (choked disc) H47.10
  associated with
    decreased ocular pressure H47.12
    increased intracranial pressure H47.11
    retinal disorder H47.13
  Foster-Kennedy syndrome H47.14-

Papillitis H46.00
  anus K62.89
  chronic lingual K14.4
  necrotizing, kidney N17.2
  optic H46.0-
  rectum K62.89
  renal, necrotizing N17.2
  tongue K14.0
Papilloma —*see also* Neoplasm, benign,
  by site
  acuminatum (female) (male) (anogenital)
    A63.0
  basal cell L82.1 ◀
    inflamed L82.0 ◀
  benign pinta (primary) A67.0
  bladder (urinary) (transitional cell) D41.4
  choroid plexus (lateral ventricle) (third
    ventricle) D33.0
    anaplastic C71.5
    fourth ventricle D33.1
    malignant C71.5
  renal pelvis (transitional cell) D41.1-
    benign D30.1-
  Schneiderian
    specified site —*see* Neoplasm, benign, by
      site
    unspecified site D14.0
  serous surface
    borderline malignancy
      specified site —*see* Neoplasm, uncertain
        behavior, by site
      unspecified site D39.10
    specified site —*see* Neoplasm, benign, by
      site
    unspecified site D27.9
  transitional (cell)
    bladder (urinary) D41.4
    inverted type —*see* Neoplasm, uncertain
      behavior, by site
    renal pelvis D41.1-
    ureter D41.2-
  ureter (transitional cell) D41.2-
    benign D30.2-
  urothelial —*see* Neoplasm, uncertain
    behavior, by site
  villous —*see* Neoplasm, uncertain behavior,
    by site
    adenocarcinoma in —*see* Neoplasm,
      malignant, by site
    in situ —*see* Neoplasm, in situ
  yaws, plantar or palmar A66.1
Papillomata, multiple, of yaws A66.1
Papillomatosis —*see also* Neoplasm, benign,
  by site
  confluent and reticulated L83
  cystic, breast —*see* Mastopathy, cystic
  ductal, breast —*see* Mastopathy, cystic
  intraductal (diffuse) —*see* Neoplasm, benign,
    by site
  subareolar duct D24-
Papillomavirus, as cause of disease classified
  elsewhere B97.7
Papillon-Léage and Psaume syndrome
  Q87.0
Papule (s) R23.8
  carate (primary) A67.0
  fibrous, of nose D22.39
  Gottron's L94.4
  pinta (primary) A67.0
Papulosis
  lymphomatoid C86.6
  malignant I77.89
Papyraceous fetus O31.0-
Para-albuminemia E88.09
Paracephalus Q89.7
Parachute mitral valve Q23.2
Paracoccidioidomycosis B41.9
  disseminated B41.7
  generalized B41.7
  mucocutaneous-lymphangitic B41.8
  pulmonary B41.0

Paracoccidioidomycosis *(Continued)*
  specified NEC B41.8
  visceral B41.8
Paradentosis K05.4
Paraffinoma T88.8
Paraganglioma D44.7
  adrenal D35.0-
    malignant C74.1-
  aortic body D44.7
    malignant C75.5
  carotid body D44.6
    malignant C75.4
  chromaffin —*see also* Neoplasm, benign, by
    site
    malignant —*see* Neoplasm, malignant, by
      site
  extra-adrenal D44.7
    malignant C75.5
      specified site —*see* Neoplasm,
        malignant, by site
      unspecified site C75.5
    specified site —*see* Neoplasm, uncertain
      behavior, by site
    unspecified site D44.7
  gangliocytic D13.2
    specified site —*see* Neoplasm, benign, by
      site
    unspecified site D13.2
  glomus jugulare D44.7
    malignant C75.5
  jugular D44.7
  malignant C75.5
    specified site —*see* Neoplasm, malignant,
      by site
    unspecified site C75.5
  nonchromaffin D44.7
    malignant C75.5
      specified site —*see* Neoplasm,
        malignant, by site
      unspecified site C75.5
    specified site —*see* Neoplasm, uncertain
      behavior, by site
    unspecified site D44.7
  parasympathetic D44.7
    specified site —*see* Neoplasm, uncertain
      behavior, by site
    unspecified site D44.7
  specified site —*see* Neoplasm, uncertain
    behavior, by site
  sympathetic D44.7
    specified site —*see* Neoplasm, uncertain
      behavior, by site
    unspecified site D44.7
  unspecified site D44.7
Parageusia R43.2
  psychogenic F45.8
Paragonimiasis B66.4
Paragranuloma, Hodgkin —*see*
  Lymphoma, Hodgkin, classical,
  specified NEC
Parahemophilia —*see also* Defect, coagulation
  D68.2
Parakeratosis R23.4
  variegata L41.0
Paralysis, paralytic (complete) (incomplete)
  G83.9
  with
    syphilis A52.17
  abducens, abducent (nerve) —*see* Strabismus,
    paralytic, sixth nerve
  abductor, lower extremity G57.9-
  accessory nerve G52.8
  accommodation —*see also* Paresis, of
    accommodation
    hysterical F44.89
  acoustic nerve (except Deafness) —*see*
    subcategory H93.3
  agitans —*see also* Parkinsonism G20
    arteriosclerotic G21.4
  alternating (oculomotor) G83.89
  amyotrophic G12.21

Paralysis, paralytic *(Continued)*
  ankle G57.9-
  anus (sphincter) K62.89
  arm —*see* Monoplegia, upper limb
  ascending (spinal), acute G61.0
  association G12.29
  asthenic bulbar G70.00
    with exacerbation (acute) G70.01
    in crisis G70.01
  ataxic (hereditary) G11.9
    general (syphilitic) A52.17
  atrophic G58.9
    infantile, acute —*see* Poliomyelitis, paralytic
    progressive G12.22
    spinal (acute) —*see* Poliomyelitis, paralytic
  axillary G54.0
  Babinski-Nageotte's G83.89
  Bell's G51.0
    newborn P11.3
  Benedikt's G46.3
  birth injury P14.9
    spinal cord P11.5
  bladder (neurogenic) (sphincter)
    N31.2
  bowel, colon or intestine K56.0
  brachial plexus G54.0
    birth injury P14.3
    newborn (birth injury) P14.3
  brain G83.9
    diplegia G83.0
    triplegia G83.89
  bronchial J98.09
  Brown-Séquard G83.81
  bulbar (chronic) (progressive) G12.22
    infantile —*see* Poliomyelitis, paralytic
    poliomyelitic —*see* Poliomyelitis, paralytic
    pseudo G12.29
  bulbospinal G70.00
    with exacerbation (acute) G70.01
    in crisis G70.01
  cardiac —*see also* Failure, heart I50.9
  cerebrocerebellar, diplegic G80.1
  cervical
    plexus G54.2
    sympathetic G90.09
  Céstan-Chenais G46.3
  Charcot-Marie-Tooth type G60.0
  Clark's G80.9
  colon K56.0
  compressed air T70.3
  compression
    arm G56.9-
    leg G57.9-
    lower extremity G57.9-
    upper extremity G56.9-
  congenital (cerebral) —*see* Palsy, cerebral
  conjugate movement (gaze) (of eye) H51.0
    cortical (nuclear) (supranuclear) H51.0
  cordis —*see* Failure, heart
  cranial or cerebral nerve G52.9
  creeping G12.22
  crossed leg G83.89
  crutch —*see* Injury, brachial plexus
  deglutition R13.0
    hysterical F44.4
  dementia A52.17
  descending (spinal) NEC G12.29
  diaphragm (flaccid) J98.6
    due to accidental dissection of phrenic
      nerve during procedure —*see*
      Puncture, accidental complicating
      surgery
  digestive organs NEC K59.8
  diplegic —*see* Diplegia
  divergence (nuclear) H51.8
  diver's T70.3
  Duchenne's
    birth injury P14.0
    due to or associated with
      motor neuron disease G12.22
      muscular dystrophy G71.0

Paralysis, paralytic *(Continued)*
  due to intracranial or spinal birth injury —*see*
    Palsy, cerebral
  embolic (current episode) I63.4- ◀▥
  Erb (-Duchenne) (birth) (newborn) P14.0
  Erb's syphilitic spastic spinal A52.17
  esophagus K22.8
  eye muscle (extrinsic) H49.9
    intrinsic —*see also* Paresis, of
      accommodation
  facial (nerve) G51.0
    birth injury P11.3
    congenital P11.3
    following operation NEC —*see* Puncture,
      accidental complicating surgery
    newborn (birth injury) P11.3
  familial (recurrent) (periodic) G72.3
    spastic G11.4
  fauces J39.2
  finger G56.9-
  gait R26.1
  gastric nerve (nondiabetic) G52.2
  gaze, conjugate H51.0
  general (progressive) (syphilitic) A52.17
    juvenile A50.45
  glottis J38.00
    bilateral J38.02
    unilateral J38.01
  gluteal G54.1
  Gubler (-Millard) G46.3
  hand —*see* Monoplegia, upper limb
  heart —*see* Arrest, cardiac
  hemiplegic —*see* Hemiplegia
  hyperkalemic periodic (familial) G72.3
  hypoglossal (nerve) G52.3
  hypokalemic periodic G72.3
  hysterical F44.4
  ileus K56.0
  infantile —*see also* Poliomyelitis, paralytic
    A80.30
    bulbar —*see* Poliomyelitis, paralytic
    cerebral —*see* Palsy, cerebral
    spastic —*see* Palsy, cerebral, spastic
  infective —*see* Poliomyelitis, paralytic
  inferior nuclear G83.9
  internuclear —*see* Ophthalmoplegia,
    internuclear
  intestine K56.0
  iris H57.09
    due to diphtheria (toxin) A36.89
  ischemic, Volkmann's (complicating trauma)
    T79.6
  Jackson's G83.89
  jake —*see* Poisoning, food, noxious, plant
  Jamaica ginger (jake) G62.2
  juvenile general A50.45
  Klumpke (-Déjérine) (birth) (newborn) P14.1
  labioglossal (laryngeal) (pharyngeal) G12.29
  Landry's G61.0
  laryngeal nerve (recurrent) (superior)
    (unilateral) J38.00
    bilateral J38.02
    unilateral J38.01
  larynx J38.00
    bilateral J38.02
    due to diphtheria (toxin) A36.2
    unilateral J38.01
  lateral G12.21
  lead —*see* subcategory T56.0
  left side —*see* Hemiplegia
  leg G83.1-
    both —*see* Paraplegia
    crossed G83.89
    hysterical F44.4
    psychogenic F44.4
    transient or transitory R29.818
      traumatic NEC —*see* Injury, nerve, leg
  levator palpebrae superioris —*see*
    Blepharoptosis, paralytic
  limb —*see* Monoplegia
  lip K13.0

Paralysis, paralytic *(Continued)*
  Lissauer's A52.17
  lower limb —*see* Monoplegia, lower
    limb
    both —*see* Paraplegia
  lung J98.4
  median nerve G56.1-
  medullary (tegmental) G83.89
  mesencephalic NEC G83.89
    tegmental G83.89
  middle alternating G83.89
  Millard-Gubler-Foville G46.3
  monoplegic —*see* Monoplegia
  motor G83.9
  muscle, muscular NEC G72.89
    due to nerve lesion G58.9
    eye (extrinsic) H49.9
      intrinsic —*see* Paresis, of
        accommodation
      oblique —*see* Strabismus, paralytic,
        fourth nerve
    iris sphincter H21.9
    ischemic (Volkmann's) (complicating
      trauma) T79.6
    progressive G12.21
    pseudohypertrophic G71.0
  musculocutaneous nerve G56.9-
  musculospiral G56.9-
  nerve —*see also* Disorder, nerve
    abducent —*see* Strabismus, paralytic, sixth
      nerve
    accessory G52.8
    auditory (except Deafness) —*see*
      subcategory H93.3
    birth injury P14.9
    cranial or cerebral G52.9
    facial G51.0
      birth injury P11.3
      congenital P11.3
      newborn (birth injury) P11.3
    fourth or trochlear —*see* Strabismus,
      paralytic, fourth nerve
    newborn (birth injury) P14.9
    oculomotor —*see* Strabismus, paralytic,
      third nerve
    phrenic (birth injury) P14.2
    radial G56.3-
    seventh or facial G51.0
      newborn (birth injury) P11.3
    sixth or abducent —*see* Strabismus,
      paralytic, sixth nerve
    syphilitic A52.15
    third or oculomotor —*see* Strabismus,
      paralytic, third nerve
    trigeminal G50.9
    trochlear —*see* Strabismus, paralytic,
      fourth nerve
    ulnar G56.2-
  normokalemic periodic G72.3
  ocular H49.9
    alternating G83.89
  oculofacial, congenital (Moebius) Q87.0
  oculomotor (external bilateral) (nerve) —*see*
    Strabismus, paralytic, third nerve
  palate (soft) K13.79
  paratrigeminal G50.9
  periodic (familial) (hyperkalemic)
    (hypokalemic) (myotonic)
    (normokalemic) (potassium sensitive)
    (secondary) G72.3
  peripheral autonomic nervous system —*see*
    Neuropathy, peripheral, autonomic
  peroneal (nerve) G57.3-
  pharynx J39.2
  phrenic nerve G56.8-
  plantar nerve (s) G57.6-
  pneumogastric nerve G52.2
  poliomyelitis (current) —*see* Poliomyelitis,
    paralytic
  popliteal nerve G57.3-
  postepileptic transitory G83.84

◀ New   ◀▥ Revised   ~~deleted~~ Deleted

Paralysis, paralytic (Continued)
  progressive (atrophic) (bulbar) (spinal)
      G12.22
    general A52.17
    infantile acute —see Poliomyelitis, paralytic
    supranuclear G23.1
  pseudobulbar G12.29
  pseudohypertrophic (muscle) G71.0
  psychogenic F44.4
  quadriceps G57.9-
  quadriplegic —see Tetraplegia
  radial nerve G56.3-
  rectus muscle (eye) H49.9
  recurrent isolated sleep G47.53
  respiratory (muscle) (system) (tract) R06.81
    center NEC G93.89
    congenital P28.89
    newborn P28.89
  right side —see Hemiplegia
  saturnine —see subcategory T56.0
  sciatic nerve G57.0-
  senile G83.9
  shaking —see Parkinsonism
  shoulder G56.9-
  sleep, recurrent isolated G47.53
  spastic G83.9
    cerebral —see Palsy, cerebral, spastic
    congenital (cerebral) —see Palsy, cerebral,
        spastic
    familial G11.4
    hereditary G11.4
    quadriplegic G80.0
    syphilitic (spinal) A52.17
  sphincter, bladder —see Paralysis, bladder
  spinal (cord) G83.9
    accessory nerve G52.8
    acute —see Poliomyelitis, paralytic
    ascending acute G61.0
    atrophic (acute) —see also Poliomyelitis,
        paralytic
      spastic, syphilitic A52.17
    congenital NEC —see Palsy, cerebral
    hereditary G95.89
    infantile —see Poliomyelitis, paralytic
    progressive G12.21
    sequelae NEC G83.89
  sternomastoid G52.8
  stomach K31.84
    diabetic —see Diabetes, by type, with
        gastroparesis
    nerve G52.2
      diabetic —see Diabetes, by type, with
          gastroparesis
  stroke —see Infarct, brain
  subcapsularis G56.8-
  supranuclear (progressive) G23.1
  sympathetic G90.8
    cervical G90.09
    nervous system —see Neuropathy,
        peripheral, autonomic
  syndrome G83.9
    specified NEC G83.89
  syphilitic spastic spinal (Erb's) A52.17
  thigh G57.9-
  throat J39.2
    diphtheritic A36.0
    muscle J39.2
  thrombotic (current episode) I63.3- ◀▥
  thumb G56.9-
  tick —see Toxicity, venom, arthropod,
      specified NEC
  Todd's (postepileptic transitory paralysis)
      G83.84
  toe G57.6-
  tongue K14.8
  transient R29.5
    arm or leg NEC R29.818
    traumatic NEC —see Injury, nerve
  trapezius G52.8
  traumatic, transient NEC —see Injury,
      nerve

Paralysis, paralytic (Continued)
  trembling —see Parkinsonism
  triceps brachii G56.9-
  trigeminal nerve G50.9
  trochlear (nerve) —see Strabismus, paralytic,
      fourth nerve
  ulnar nerve G56.2-
  upper limb —see Monoplegia, upper limb
  uremic N18.9 [G99.8]
  uveoparotitic D86.89
  uvula K13.79
    postdiphtheritic A36.0
  vagus nerve G52.2
  vasomotor NEC G90.8
  velum palati K13.79
  vesical —see Paralysis, bladder
  vestibular nerve (except Vertigo) —see
      subcategory H93.3
  vocal cords J38.00
    bilateral J38.02
    unilateral J38.01
  Volkmann's (complicating trauma)
      T79.6
  wasting G12.29
  Weber's G46.3
  wrist G56.9-
Paramedial urethrovesical orifice
    Q64.79
Paramenia N92.6
Parametritis —see also Disease, pelvis,
    inflammatory N73.2
  acute N73.0
  complicating abortion —see Abortion, by
      type, complicated by, parametritis
Parametrium, parametric —see condition
Paramnesia —see Amnesia
Paramolar K00.1
Paramyloidosis E85.8
Paramyoclonus multiplex G25.3
Paramyotonia (congenita) G71.19
Parangi —see Yaws
Paranoia (querulans) F22
  senile F03
Paranoid
  dementia (senile) F03
    praecox —see Schizophrenia
  personality F60.0
  psychosis (climacteric) (involutional)
      (menopausal) F22
    psychogenic (acute) F23
    senile F03
  reaction (acute) F23
    chronic F22
  schizophrenia F20.0
  state (climacteric) (involutional)
      (menopausal) (simple) F22
    senile F03
  tendencies F60.0
  traits F60.0
  trends F60.0
  type, psychopathic personality F60.0
Paraparesis —see Paraplegia
Paraphasia R47.02
Paraphilia F65.9
Paraphimosis (congenital) N47.2
  chancroidal A57
Paraphrenia, paraphrenic (late) F22
  schizophrenia F20.0
Paraplegia (lower) G82.20
  ataxic —see Degeneration, combined, spinal
      cord
  complete G82.21
  congenital (cerebral) G80.8
    spastic G80.1
  familial spastic G11.4
  functional (hysterical) F44.4
  hereditary, spastic G11.4
  hysterical F44.4
  incomplete G82.22
  Pott's A18.01
  psychogenic F44.4

Paraplegia (Continued)
  spastic
    Erb's spinal, syphilitic A52.17
    hereditary G11.4
    tropical G04.1
  syphilitic (spastic) A52.17
  tropical spastic G04.1
Parapoxvirus B08.60
  specified NEC B08.69
Paraproteinemia D89.2
  benign (familial) D89.2
  monoclonal D47.2
  secondary to malignant disease D47.2
Parapsoriasis L41.9
  en plaques L41.4
  guttata L41.1
  large plaque L41.4
  retiform, retiformis L41.5
  small plaque L41.3
  specified NEC L41.8
  varioliformis (acuta) L41.0
Parasitic —see also condition
  disease NEC B89
  stomatitis B37.0
  sycosis (beard) (scalp) B35.0
  twin Q89.4
Parasitism B89
  intestinal B82.9
  skin B88.9
  specified —see Infestation
Parasitophobia F40.218
Parasomnia G47.50
  due to
    alcohol
      abuse F10.182
      dependence F10.282
      use F10.982
    amphetamines
      abuse F15.182
      dependence F15.282
      use F15.982
    caffeine
      abuse F15.182
      dependence F15.282
      use F15.982
    cocaine
      abuse F14.182
      dependence F14.282
      use F14.982
    drug NEC
      abuse F19.182
      dependence F19.282
      use F19.982
    opioid
      abuse F11.182
      dependence F11.282
      use F11.982
    psychoactive substance NEC
      abuse F19.182
      dependence F19.282
      use F19.982
    sedative, hypnotic, or anxiolytic
      abuse F13.182
      dependence F13.282
      use F13.982
    stimulant NEC
      abuse F15.182
      dependence F15.282
      use F15.982
  in conditions classified elsewhere G47.54
  nonorganic origin F51.8
  organic G47.50
  specified NEC G47.59
Paraspadias Q54.9
Paraspasmus facialis G51.8
Parasuicide (attempt)
  history of (personal) Z91.5
    in family Z81.8
Parathyroid gland —see condition
Parathyroid tetany E20.9
Paratrachoma A74.0

Paratyphilitis —*see* Appendicitis
Paratyphoid (fever) —*see* Fever, paratyphoid
Paratyphus —*see* Fever, paratyphoid
Paraurethral duct Q64.79
  nonorganic origin F51.5
Paraurethritis —*see also* Urethritis
  gonococcal (acute) (chronic) (with abscess)
    A54.1
Paravaccinia NEC B08.04
Paravaginitis —*see* Vaginitis
Parencephalitis —*see also* Encephalitis
  sequelae G09
Parent-child conflict —*see* Conflict, parent-child
  estrangement NEC Z62.890
Paresis —*see also* Paralysis
  accommodation —*see* Paresis, of
    accommodation
  Bernhardt's G57.1-
  bladder (sphincter) —*see also* Paralysis, bladder
    tabetic A52.17
  bowel, colon or intestine K56.0
  extrinsic muscle, eye H49.9
  general (progressive) (syphilitic) A52.17
    juvenile A50.45
  heart —*see* Failure, heart
  insane (syphilitic) A52.17
  juvenile (general) A50.45
  of accommodation H52.52-
  peripheral progressive (idiopathic) G60.3
  pseudohypertrophic G71.0
  senile G83.9
  syphilitic (general) A52.17
    congenital A50.45
  vesical NEC N31.2
Paresthesia —*see also* Disturbance, sensation
  Bernhardt G57.1-
Paretic —*see* condition
Parinaud's
  conjunctivitis H10.89
  oculoglandular syndrome H10.89
  ophthalmoplegia H49.88
Parkinsonism (idiopathic) (primary) G20
  with neurogenic orthostatic hypotension
    (symptomatic) G90.3
  arteriosclerotic G21.4
  dementia G31.83 *[F02.80]*
    with behavioral disturbance G31.83
      [F02.81]
  due to
    drugs NEC G21.19
      neuroleptic G21.11
  neuroleptic induced G21.11
  postencephalitic G21.3
  secondary G21.9
    due to
      arteriosclerosis G21.4
      drugs NEC G21.19
        neuroleptic G21.11
      encephalitis G21.3
      external agents NEC G21.2
      syphilis A52.19
    specified NEC G21.8
  syphilitic A52.19
  treatment-induced NEC G21.19
  vascular G21.4
Parkinson's disease, syndrome or tremor —*see*
  Parkinsonism
Parodontitis —*see* Periodontitis
Parodontosis K05.4
Paronychia —*see also* Cellulitis, digit
  with lymphangitis —*see* Lymphangitis, acute,
    digit
  candidal (chronic) B37.2
  tuberculous (primary) A18.4
Parorexia (psychogenic) F50.89 ◀▥
Parosmia R43.1
  psychogenic F45.8
Parotid gland —*see* condition
Parotitis, parotiditis (allergic) (nonspecific
  toxic) (purulent) (septic) (suppurative) —
  see also Sialoadenitis

Parotitis, parotiditis *(Continued)*
  epidemic —*see* Mumps
  infectious —*see* Mumps
  postoperative K91.89
  surgical K91.89
Parrot fever A70
Parrot's disease (early congenital syphilitic
  pseudoparalysis) A50.02
Parry-Romberg syndrome G51.8
Parry's disease or syndrome E05.00
  with thyroid storm E05.01
Pars planitis —*see* Cyclitis
Parsonage (-Aldren)-Turner syndrome G54.5
Parson's disease (exophthalmic goiter) E05.00
  with thyroid storm E05.01
Particolored infant Q82.8
Parturition —*see* Delivery
Parulis K04.7
  with sinus K04.6
Parvovirus, as cause of disease classified
  elsewhere B97.6
Pasini and Pierini's atrophoderma L90.3
Passage
  false, urethra N36.5
  meconium (newborn) during delivery
    P03.82
  of sounds or bougies —*see* Attention to,
    artificial, opening
Passive —*see* condition
  smoking Z77.22
Pasteurella septica A28.0
Pasteurellosis —*see* Infection, Pasteurella
PAT (paroxysmal atrial tachycardia) I47.1
Patau's syndrome —*see* Trisomy, 13
Patches
  mucous (syphilitic) A51.39
    congenital A50.07
  smokers' (mouth) K13.24
Patellar —*see* condition
Patent —*see also* Imperfect, closure
  canal of Nuck Q52.4
  cervix N88.3
  ductus arteriosus or Botallo's Q25.0
  foramen
    botalli Q21.1
    ovale Q21.1
  interauricular septum Q21.1
  interventricular septum Q21.0
  omphalomesenteric duct Q43.0
  os (uteri) —*see* Patent, cervix
  ostium secundum Q21.1
  urachus Q64.4
  vitelline duct Q43.0
Paterson (-Brown)(-Kelly) syndrome or web
  D50.1
Pathologic, pathological —*see also* condition
  asphyxia R09.01
  fire-setting F63.1
  gambling F63.0
  ovum O02.0
  resorption, tooth K03.3
  stealing F63.2
Pathology (of) —*see* Disease
  periradicular, associated with previous
    endodontic treatment NEC M27.59
Pattern, sleep-wake, irregular G47.23
Patulous —*see also* Imperfect, closure
  (congenital)
  alimentary tract Q45.8
    lower Q43.8
    upper Q40.8
  eustachian tube H69.0-
Pause, sinoatrial I49.5
Paxton's disease B36.2
Pearl (s)
  enamel K00.2
  Epstein's K09.8
Pearl-worker's disease —*see* Osteomyelitis,
  specified type NEC
Pectenosis K62.4
Pectoral —*see* condition

Pectus
  carinatum (congenital) Q67.7
    acquired M95.4
    rachitic sequelae (late effect) E64.3
  excavatum (congenital) Q67.6
    acquired M95.4
    rachitic sequelae (late effect) E64.3
  recurvatum (congenital) Q67.6
Pedatrophia E41
Pederosis F65.4
Pediculosis (infestation) B85.2
  capitis (head-louse) (any site) B85.0
  corporis (body-louse) (any site) B85.1
  eyelid B85.0
  mixed (classifiable to more than one of the
    titles B85.0-B85.3) B85.4
  pubis (pubic louse) (any site) B85.3
  vestimenti B85.1
  vulvae B85.3
Pediculus (infestation) —*see* Pediculosis
Pedophilia F65.4
Peg-shaped teeth K00.2
Pelade —*see* Alopecia, areata
Pelger-Huët anomaly or syndrome D72.0
Peliosis (rheumatica) D69.0
  hepatis K76.4
    with toxic liver disease K71.8
Pelizaeus-Merzbacher disease E75.29
Pellagra (alcoholic) (with polyneuropathy) E52
Pellagra-cerebellar-ataxia-renal aminoaciduria
  syndrome E72.02
Pellegrini (-Stieda) disease or syndrome —*see*
  Bursitis, tibial collateral
Pellizzi's syndrome E34.8
Pel's crisis A52.11
Pelvic —*see also* condition
  examination (periodic) (routine) Z01.419
    with abnormal findings Z01.411
  kidney, congenital Q63.2
Pelviolithiasis —*see* Calculus, kidney
Pelviperitonitis —*see also* Peritonitis, pelvic
  gonococcal A54.24
  puerperal O85
Pelvis —*see* condition or type
Pemphigoid L12.9
  benign, mucous membrane L12.1
  bullous L12.0
  cicatricial L12.1
  juvenile L12.2
  ocular L12.1
  specified NEC L12.8
Pemphigus L10.9
  benign familial (chronic) Q82.8
  Brazilian L10.3
  circinatus L13.0
  conjunctiva L12.1
  drug-induced L10.5
  erythematosus L10.4
  foliaceus L10.2
  gangrenous —*see* Gangrene
  neonatorum L01.03
  ocular L12.1
  paraneoplastic L10.81
  specified NEC L10.89
  syphilitic (congenital) A50.06
  vegetans L10.1
  vulgaris L10.0
  wildfire L10.3
Pendred's syndrome E07.1
Pendulous
  abdomen, in pregnancy —*see* Pregnancy,
    complicated by, abnormal, pelvic organs
    or tissues NEC
  breast N64.89
Penetrating wound —*see also* Puncture
  with internal injury —*see* Injury, by site
  eyeball —*see* Puncture, eyeball
  orbit (with or without foreign body) —*see*
    Puncture, orbit
  uterus by instrument with or following
    ectopic or molar pregnancy O08.6

◀ New   ◀▥ Revised   ~~deleted~~ Deleted

Penicillosis B48.4
Penis —see condition
Penitis N48.29
Pentalogy of Fallot Q21.8
Pentasomy X syndrome Q97.1
Pentosuria (essential) E74.8
Percreta placenta O43.23-
Peregrinating patient —see Disorder, factitious
Perforation, perforated (nontraumatic) (of)
    accidental during procedure (blood vessel)
        (nerve) (organ) —see Complication,
        accidental puncture or laceration
    antrum —see Sinusitis, maxillary
    appendix K35.2
        with localized peritonitis K35.3 ◄
    atrial septum, multiple Q21.1
    attic, ear —see Perforation, tympanum, attic
    bile duct (common) (hepatic) K83.2
        cystic K82.2
    bladder (urinary)
        with or following ectopic or molar
            pregnancy O08.6
        obstetrical trauma O71.5
        traumatic S37.29
            at delivery O71.5
    bowel K63.1
        with or following ectopic or molar
            pregnancy O08.6
        newborn P78.0
        obstetrical trauma O71.5
        traumatic —see Laceration, intestine
    broad ligament N83.8
        with or following ectopic or molar
            pregnancy O08.6
        obstetrical trauma O71.6
    by
        device, implant or graft —see also
            Complications, by site and type,
            mechanical T85.628
        arterial graft NEC —see Complication,
            cardiovascular device, mechanical,
            vascular
        breast (implant) T85.49
        catheter NEC T85.698
            cystostomy T83.090
            dialysis (renal) T82.49
                intraperitoneal T85.691
            infusion NEC T82.594
                spinal (epidural) (subdural) T85.690
            urinary —see also Complications,
                catheter, urinary T83.098 ◄
        electronic (electrode) (pulse generator)
            (stimulator)
            bone T84.390
            cardiac T82.199
                electrode T82.190
                pulse generator T82.191
                specified type NEC T82.198
            nervous system —see Complication,
                prosthetic device, mechanical,
                electronic nervous system
                stimulator
            urinary —see Complication,
                genitourinary, device, urinary,
                mechanical
        fixation, internal (orthopedic) NEC —see
            Complication, fixation device,
            mechanical
        gastrointestinal —see Complications,
            prosthetic device, mechanical,
            gastrointestinal device
        genital NEC T83.498
            intrauterine contraceptive device
                T83.39
            penile prosthesis T83.490
        heart NEC —see Complication,
            cardiovascular device,
            mechanical
        joint prosthesis —see Complications,
            joint prosthesis, mechanical,
            specified NEC, by site

Perforation, perforated (Continued)
    by (Continued)
        urinary (Continued)
            ocular NEC —see Complications,
                prosthetic device, mechanical,
                ocular device
            orthopedic NEC —see Complication,
                orthopedic, device, mechanical
            specified NEC T85.628
            urinary NEC —see also Complication,
                genitourinary, device, urinary,
                mechanical
                graft T83.29
                urinary, indwelling T83.098
            vascular NEC —see Complication,
                cardiovascular device, mechanical
            ventricular intracranial shunt T85.09
        foreign body left accidentally in
            operative wound T81.539
        instrument (any) during a procedure,
            accidental —see Puncture, accidental
            complicating surgery
    cecum K35.2
        with localized peritonitis K35.3 ◄
    cervix (uteri) N88.8
        with or following ectopic or molar
            pregnancy O08.6
        obstetrical trauma O71.3
    colon K63.1
        newborn P78.0
        obstetrical trauma O71.5
        traumatic —see Laceration, intestine, large
    common duct (bile) K83.2
    cornea (due to ulceration) —see Ulcer,
        cornea, perforated
    cystic duct K82.2
    diverticulum (intestine) K57.80
        with bleeding K57.81
        large intestine K57.20
            with
                bleeding K57.21
                small intestine K57.40
                    with bleeding K57.41
        small intestine K57.00
            with
                bleeding K57.01
                large intestine K57.40
                    with bleeding K57.41
    ear drum —see Perforation, tympanum
    esophagus K22.3
    ethmoidal sinus —see Sinusitis, ethmoidal
    frontal sinus —see Sinusitis, frontal
    gallbladder K82.2
    heart valve —see Endocarditis
    ileum K63.1
        newborn P78.0
        obstetrical trauma O71.5
        traumatic —see Laceration, intestine, small
    instrumental, surgical (accidental) (blood
        vessel) (nerve) (organ) —see Puncture,
        accidental complicating surgery
    intestine NEC K63.1
        with ectopic or molar pregnancy O08.6
        newborn P78.0
        obstetrical trauma O71.5
        traumatic —see Laceration, intestine
        ulcerative NEC K63.1
            newborn P78.0
    jejunum, jejunal K63.1
        obstetrical trauma O71.5
        traumatic —see Laceration, intestine, small
        ulcer —see Ulcer, gastrojejunal, with
            perforation
    joint prosthesis —see Complications, joint
        prosthesis, mechanical, specified NEC,
        by site
    mastoid (antrum) (cell) —see Disorder,
        mastoid, specified NEC
    maxillary sinus —see Sinusitis, maxillary
    membrana tympani —see Perforation,
        tympanum

Perforation, perforated (Continued)
    nasal
        septum J34.89
            congenital Q30.3
            syphilitic A52.73
        sinus J34.89
            congenital Q30.8
            due to sinusitis —see Sinusitis
    palate —see also Cleft, palate Q35.9
        syphilitic A52.79
    palatine vault —see also Cleft, palate, hard
        Q35.1
        syphilitic A52.79
            congenital A50.59
    pars flaccida (ear drum) —see Perforation,
        tympanum, attic
    pelvic
        floor S31.030
            with
                ectopic or molar pregnancy O08.6
                penetration into retroperitoneal space
                    S31.031
                retained foreign body S31.040
                    with penetration into
                        retroperitoneal space S31.041
            following ectopic or molar pregnancy
                O08.6
            obstetrical trauma O70.1
        organ S37.99
            adrenal gland S37.818
            bladder —see Perforation, bladder
            fallopian tube S37.599
                bilateral S37.592
                unilateral S37.591
            kidney S37.09-
            obstetrical trauma O71.5
            ovary S37.499
                bilateral S37.492
                unilateral S37.491
            prostate S37.828
            specified organ NEC S37.898
            ureter —see Perforation, ureter
            urethra —see Perforation, urethra
            uterus —see Perforation, uterus
    perineum —see Laceration, perineum
    pharynx J39.2
    rectum K63.1
        newborn P78.0
        obstetrical trauma O71.5
        traumatic S36.63
    root canal space due to endodontic treatment
        M27.51
    sigmoid K63.1
        newborn P78.0
        obstetrical trauma O71.5
        traumatic S36.533
    sinus (accessory) (chronic) (nasal) J34.89
    sphenoidal sinus —see Sinusitis, sphenoidal
    surgical (accidental) (by instrument) (blood
        vessel) (nerve) (organ) —see Puncture,
        accidental complicating surgery
    traumatic
        external —see Puncture
        eye —see Puncture, eyeball
        internal organ —see Injury, by site
    tympanum, tympanic (membrane) (persistent
        post-traumatic) (postinflammatory)
        H72.9-
        attic H72.1-
            multiple —see Perforation, tympanum,
                multiple
            total —see Perforation, tympanum, total
        central H72.0-
            multiple —see Perforation, tympanum,
                multiple
            total —see Perforation, tympanum, total
        marginal NEC —see subcategory H72.2
        multiple H72.81-
        pars flaccida —see Perforation, tympanum,
            attic
        total H72.82-
        traumatic, current episode S09.2-

Perforation, perforated *(Continued)*
   typhoid, gastrointestinal —*see* Typhoid
   ulcer —*see* Ulcer, by site, with perforation
   ureter N28.89
      traumatic S37.19
   urethra N36.8
      with ectopic or molar pregnancy O08.6
      following ectopic or molar pregnancy
         O08.6
      obstetrical trauma O71.5
      traumatic S37.39
         at delivery O71.5
   uterus
      with ectopic or molar pregnancy O08.6
      by intrauterine contraceptive device T83.39
      following ectopic or molar pregnancy
         O08.6
      obstetrical trauma O71.1
      traumatic S37.69
         obstetric O71.1
   uvula K13.79
      syphilitic A52.79
   vagina
      obstetrical trauma O71.4
      other trauma - see Puncture, vagina
Periadenitis mucosa necrotica recurrens K12.0
Periappendicitis (acute) —*see* Appendicitis
Periarteritis nodosa (disseminated) (infectious)
      (necrotizing) M30.0
Periarthritis (joint) —*see also* Enthesopathy
   Duplay's M75.0-
   gonococcal A54.42
   humeroscapularis —*see* Capsulitis, adhesive
   scapulohumeral —*see* Capsulitis, adhesive
   shoulder —*see* Capsulitis, adhesive
   wrist M77.2-
Periarthrosis (angioneural) —*see*
      Enthesopathy
Pericapsulitis, adhesive (shoulder) —*see*
      Capsulitis, adhesive
Pericarditis (with decompensation) (with
      effusion) I31.9
   with rheumatic fever (conditions in I00)
      active —*see* Pericarditis, rheumatic
      inactive or quiescent I09.2
   acute (hemorrhagic) (nonrheumatic) (Sicca)
         I30.9
      with chorea (acute) (rheumatic)
         (Sydenham's) I02.0
      benign I30.8
      nonspecific I30.0
      rheumatic I01.0
         with chorea (acute) (Sydenham's)
            I02.0
   adhesive or adherent (chronic) (external)
         (internal) I31.0
   acute —*see* Pericarditis, acute
      rheumatic I09.2
   bacterial (acute) (subacute) (with serous or
         seropurulent effusion) I30.1
   calcareous I31.1
   cholesterol (chronic) I31.8
      acute I30.9
   chronic (nonrheumatic) I31.9
      rheumatic I09.2
   constrictive (chronic) I31.1
   coxsackie B33.23
   fibrinocaseous (tuberculous) A18.84
   fibrinopurulent I30.1
   fibrinous I30.8
   fibrous I31.0
   gonococcal A54.83
   idiopathic I30.0
   in systemic lupus erythematosus M32.12
   infective I30.1
   meningococcal A39.53
   neoplastic (chronic) I31.8
      acute I30.9
   obliterans, obliterating I31.0
   plastic I31.0
   pneumococcal I30.1

Pericarditis *(Continued)*
   postinfarction I24.1
   purulent I30.1
   rheumatic (active) (acute) (with effusion)
         (with pneumonia) I01.0
      with chorea (acute) (rheumatic)
         (Sydenham's) I02.0
      chronic or inactive (with chorea) I09.2
   rheumatoid —*see* Rheumatoid, carditis
   septic I30.1
   serofibrinous I30.8
   staphylococcal I30.1
   streptococcal I30.1
   suppurative I30.1
   syphilitic A52.06
   tuberculous A18.84
   uremic N18.9 *[I32]*
   viral I30.1
Pericardium, pericardial —*see* condition
Pericellulitis —*see* Cellulitis
Pericementitis (chronic) (suppurative) —*see also*
      Periodontitis
   acute K05.20
      generalized —*see* Peridontitis, aggressive,
         generalized ◄▥
      localized —*see* Peridontitis, aggressive,
         localized ◄▥
Perichondritis
   auricle —*see* Perichondritis, ear
   bronchus J98.09
   ear (external) H61.00-
      acute H61.01-
      chronic H61.02-
   external auditory canal —*see* Perichondritis,
      ear
   larynx J38.7
      syphilitic A52.73
      typhoid A01.09
   nose J34.89
   pinna —*see* Perichondritis, ear
   trachea J39.8
Periclasia K05.4
Pericoronitis —*see* Periodontitis
Pericystitis N30.90
   with hematuria N30.91
Peridiverticulitis (intestine) K57.92
   cecum —*see* Diverticulitis, intestine, large
   colon —*see* Diverticulitis, intestine, large
   duodenum —*see* Diverticulitis, intestine,
      small
   intestine —*see* Diverticulitis, intestine
   jejunum —*see* Diverticulitis, intestine, small
   rectosigmoid —*see* Diverticulitis, intestine,
      large
   rectum —*see* Diverticulitis, intestine, large
   sigmoid —*see* Diverticulitis, intestine, large
Periendocarditis —*see* Endocarditis
Periepididymitis N45.1
Perifolliculitis L01.02
   abscedens, caput, scalp L66.3
   capitis, abscedens (et suffodiens) L66.3
   superficial pustular L01.02
Perihepatitis K65.8
Perilabyrinthitis (acute) —*see* subcategory H83.0
Perimeningitis —*see* Meningitis
Perimetritis —*see* Endometritis
Perimetrosalpingitis —*see* Salpingo-oophoritis
Perineocele N81.81
Perinephric, perinephritic —*see* condition
Perinephritis —*see also* Infection, kidney
   purulent —*see* Abscess, kidney
Perineum, perineal —*see* condition
Perineuritis NEC —*see* Neuralgia
Periodic —*see* condition
Periodontitis (chronic) (complex) (compound)
      (local) (simplex) K05.30
   acute K05.20
      generalized K05.229 ◄▥
         moderate K05.222 ◄
         severe K05.223 ◄
         slight K05.221 ◄

Periodontitis *(Continued)*
   acute *(Continued)*
      localized K05.219 ◄▥
         moderate K05.212 ◄
         severe K05.213 ◄
         slight K05.211 ◄
   apical K04.5
      acute (pulpal origin) K04.4
   generalized K05.329 ◄▥
      moderate K05.322 ◄
      severe K05.323 ◄
      slight K05.321 ◄
   localized K05.319 ◄▥
      moderate K05.312 ◄
      severe K05.313 ◄
      slight K05.311 ◄
Periodontoclasia K05.4
Periodontosis (juvenile) K05.4
Periods —*see also* Menstruation
   heavy N92.0
   irregular N92.6
   shortened intervals (irregular) N92.1
Perionychia —*see also* Cellulitis, digit
   with lymphangitis —*see* Lymphangitis, acute,
      digit
Perioophoritis —*see* Salpingo-oophoritis
Periorchitis N45.2
Periosteum, periosteal —*see* condition
Periostitis (albuminosa) (circumscribed)
      (diffuse) (infective) (monomelic) —*see also*
      Osteomyelitis
   alveolar M27.3
   alveolodental M27.3
   dental M27.3
   gonorrheal A54.43
   jaw (lower) (upper) M27.2
   orbit H05.03-
   syphilitic A52.77
      congenital (early) A50.02 *[M90.80]*
      secondary A51.46
   tuberculous —*see* Tuberculosis, bone
   yaws (hypertrophic) (early) (late) A66.6
      [M90.80]
Periostosis (hyperplastic) —*see also* Disorder,
      bone, specified type NEC
   with osteomyelitis —*see* Osteomyelitis,
      specified type NEC
Peripartum
   cardiomyopathy O90.3
Periphlebitis —*see* Phlebitis
Periproctitis K62.89
Periprostatitis —*see* Prostatitis
Perirectal —*see* condition
Perirenal —*see* condition
Perisalpingitis —*see* Salpingo-oophoritis
Perisplenitis (infectional) D73.89
Peristalsis, visible or reversed R19.2
Peritendinitis —*see* Enthesopathy
Peritoneum, peritoneal —*see* condition
Peritonitis (adhesive) (bacterial) (fibrinous)
      (hemorrhagic) (idiopathic) (localized)
      (perforative) (primary) (with adhesions)
      (with effusion) K65.9
   with or following
      abscess K65.1
      appendicitis K35.3 ◄▥
         with perforation or rupture K35.2
         generalized K35.2
         localized K35.3
      diverticular disease (intestine) K57.80
         with bleeding K57.81
      ectopic or molar pregnancy O08.0
      large intestine K57.20
         with
            bleeding K57.21
            small intestine K57.40
               with bleeding K57.41
      small intestine K57.00
         with
            bleeding K57.01
            large intestine K57.40
               with bleeding K57.41

Peritonitis *(Continued)*
  acute (generalized) K65.0
  aseptic T81.61
  bile, biliary K65.3
  chemical T81.61
  chlamydial A74.81
  chronic proliferative K65.8
  complicating abortion —*see* Abortion, by
      type, complicated by, pelvic peritonitis
  congenital P78.1
  diaphragmatic K65.0
  diffuse K65.0
  diphtheritic A36.89
  disseminated K65.0
  due to
    bile K65.3
    foreign
      body or object accidentally left during
          a procedure (instrument) (sponge)
          (swab) T81.599
      substance accidentally left during a
          procedure (chemical) (powder)
          (talc) T81.61
    talc T81.61
    urine K65.8
  eosinophilic K65.8
    acute K65.0
  fibrocaseous (tuberculous) A18.31
  fibropurulent K65.0
  following ectopic or molar pregnancy
      O08.0
  general (ized) K65.0
  gonococcal A54.85
  meconium (newborn) P78.0
  neonatal P78.1
    meconium P78.0
  pancreatic K65.0
  paroxysmal, familial E85.0
    benign E85.0
  pelvic
    female N73.5
      acute N73.3
      chronic N73.4
        with adhesions N73.6
    male K65.0
  periodic, familial E85.0
  proliferative, chronic K65.8
  puerperal, postpartum, childbirth O85
  purulent K65.0
  septic K65.0
  specified NEC K65.8
  spontaneous bacterial K65.2
  subdiaphragmatic K65.0
  subphrenic K65.0
  suppurative K65.0
  syphilitic A52.74
    congenital (early) A50.08 *[K67]*
  talc T81.61
  tuberculous A18.31
  urine K65.8
Peritonsillar —*see* condition
Peritonsillitis J36
Perityphlitis K37
Periureteritis N28.89
Periurethral —*see* condition
Periurethritis (gangrenous) —*see* Urethritis
Periuterine —*see* condition
Perivaginitis —*see* Vaginitis
Perivasculitis, retinal H35.06-
Perivasitis (chronic) N49.1
Perivesiculitis (seminal) —*see* Vesiculitis
Perlèche NEC K13.0
  due to
    candidiasis B37.83
    moniliasis B37.83
    riboflavin deficiency E53.0
    vitamin B2 (riboflavin) deficiency E53.0
Pernicious —*see* condition
Pernio, perniosis T69.1
Perpetrator (of abuse) —*see* Index to External
    Causes of Injury, Perpetrator

Persecution
  delusion F22
  social Z60.5
Perseveration (tonic) R48.8
Persistence, persistent (congenital)
  anal membrane Q42.3
    with fistula Q42.2
  arteria stapedia Q16.3
  atrioventricular canal Q21.2
  branchial cleft Q18.0
  bulbus cordis in left ventricle Q21.8
  canal of Cloquet Q14.0
  capsule (opaque) Q12.8
  cilioretinal artery or vein Q14.8
  cloaca Q43.7
  communication —*see* Fistula, congenital
  convolutions
    aortic arch Q25.46 ◀▥
    fallopian tube Q50.6
    oviduct Q50.6
    uterine tube Q50.6
  double aortic arch Q25.45 ◀▥
  ductus arteriosus (Botalli) Q25.0
  fetal
    circulation P29.3
    form of cervix (uteri) Q51.828
    hemoglobin, hereditary (HPFH) D56.4
  foramen
    Botalli Q21.1
    ovale Q21.1
  Gartner's duct Q52.4
  hemoglobin, fetal (hereditary) (HPFH)
      D56.4
  hyaloid
    artery (generally incomplete) Q14.0
    system Q14.8
  hymen, in pregnancy or childbirth —*see*
      Pregnancy, complicated by, abnormal,
      vulva
  lanugo Q84.2
  left
    posterior cardinal vein Q26.8
    root with right arch of aorta Q25.49 ◀▥
    superior vena cava Q26.1
  Meckel's diverticulum Q43.0
    malignant —*see* Table of Neoplasms, small
        intestine, malignant
  mucosal disease (middle ear) —*see*
      Otitis, media, suppurative, chronic,
      tubotympanic
  nail (s), anomalous Q84.6
  omphalomesenteric duct Q43.0
  organ or site not listed —*see* Anomaly, by site
  ostium
    atrioventriculare commune Q21.2
    primum Q21.2
    secundum Q21.1
  ovarian rests in fallopian tube Q50.6
  pancreatic tissue in intestinal tract Q43.8
  primary (deciduous)
    teeth K00.6
    vitreous hyperplasia Q14.0
  pupillary membrane Q13.89
  rhesus (Rh)titer —*see* Complication (s),
      transfusion, incompatibility reaction,
      Rh (factor)
  right aortic arch Q25.47 ◀▥
  sinus
    urogenitalis
      female Q52.8
      male Q55.8
    venosus with imperfect incorporation in
        right auricle Q26.8
  thymus (gland) (hyperplasia) E32.0
  thyroglossal duct Q89.2
  thyrolingual duct Q89.2
  truncus arteriosus or communis Q20.0
  tunica vasculosa lentis Q12.2
  umbilical sinus Q64.4
  urachus Q64.4
  vitelline duct Q43.0

Person (with)
  admitted for clinical research, as a control
      subject (normal comparison)
      (participant) Z00.6
  awaiting admission to adequate facility
      elsewhere Z75.1
  concern (normal) about sick person in family
      Z63.6
  consulting on behalf of another Z71.0
  feigning illness Z76.5
  living (in)
    without
      adequate housing (heating) (space)
          Z59.1
      housing (permanent) (temporary)
          Z59.0
      person able to render necessary care
          Z74.2
      shelter Z59.0
    alone Z60.2
    boarding school Z59.3
    residential institution Z59.3
  on waiting list Z75.1
  sick or handicapped in family Z63.6
Personality (disorder) F60.9
  accentuation of traits (type A pattern) Z73.1
  affective F34.0
  aggressive F60.3
  amoral F60.2
  anacastic, anankastic F60.5
  antisocial F60.2
  anxious F60.6
  asocial F60.2
  asthenic F60.7
  avoidant F60.6
  borderline F60.3
  change due to organic condition (enduring)
      F07.0
  compulsive F60.5
  cycloid F34.0
  cyclothymic F34.0
  dependent F60.7
  depressive F34.1
  dissocial F60.2
  dual F44.81
  eccentric F60.89
  emotionally unstable F60.3
  expansive paranoid F60.0
  explosive F60.3
  fanatic F60.0
  haltlose type F60.89
  histrionic F60.4
  hyperthymic F34.0
  hypothymic F34.1
  hysterical F60.4
  immature F60.89
  inadequate F60.7
  labile (emotional) F60.3
  mixed (nonspecific) F60.89 ◀▥
  morally defective F60.2
  multiple F44.81
  narcissistic F60.81
  obsessional F60.5
  obsessive (-compulsive) F60.5
  organic F07.0
  overconscientious F60.5
  paranoid F60.0
  passive (-dependent) F60.7
  passive-aggressive F60.89
  pathologic F60.9
  pattern defect or disturbance F60.9
  pseudopsychopathic (organic) F07.0
  pseudoretarded (organic) F07.0
  psychoinfantile F60.4
  psychoneurotic NEC F60.89
  psychopathic F60.2
  querulant F60.0
  sadistic F60.89
  schizoid F60.1
  self-defeating F60.7
  sensitive paranoid F60.0

Personality *(Continued)*
  sociopathic (amoral) (antisocial) (asocial)
    (dissocial) F60.2
  specified NEC F60.89
  type A Z73.1
  unstable (emotional) F60.3
Perthes' disease —*see* Legg-Calvé-Perthes
  disease
Pertussis *(see also* Whooping cough) A37.90
Perversion, perverted
  appetite F50.89 ◀
    psychogenic F50.89 ◀
  function
    pituitary gland E23.2
      posterior lobe E22.2
  sense of smell and taste R43.8
    psychogenic F45.8
  sexual —*see* Deviation, sexual
Pervious, congenital —*see also* Imperfect,
  closure
  ductus arteriosus Q25.0
Pes (congenital) —*see also* Talipes
  acquired —*see also* Deformity, limb, foot,
    specified NEC
    planus —*see* Deformity, limb, flat foot
  adductus Q66.89
  cavus Q66.7
  deformity NEC, acquired —*see* Deformity,
    limb, foot, specified NEC
  planus (acquired) (any degree) —*see also*
    Deformity, limb, flat foot
    rachitic sequelae (late effect) E64.3
  valgus Q66.6
Pest, pestis —*see* Plague
Petechia, petechiae R23.3
  newborn P54.5
Petechial typhus A75.9
Peter's anomaly Q13.4
Petit mal seizure —*see* Epilepsy, generalized,
  specified NEC
Petit's hernia —*see* Hernia, abdomen, specified
  site NEC
Petrellidosis B48.2
Petrositis H70.20-
  acute H70.21-
  chronic H70.22-
Peutz-Jeghers disease or syndrome Q85.8
Peyronie's disease N48.6
PFAPA (periodic fever, aphthous stomatitis,
  pharyngitis, and adenopathy syndrome)
  M04.8 ◀
Pfeiffer's disease —*see* Mononucleosis,
  infectious
Phagedena (dry) (moist) (sloughing) —*see also*
  Gangrene
  geometric L88
  penis N48.29
  tropical —*see* Ulcer, skin
  vulva N76.6
Phagedenic —*see* condition
Phakoma H35.89
Phakomatosis —*see also* specific eponymous
  syndromes Q85.9
  Bourneville's Q85.1
  specified NEC Q85.8
Phantom limb syndrome (without pain)
  G54.7
  with pain G54.6
Pharyngeal pouch syndrome D82.1
Pharyngitis (acute) (catarrhal) (gangrenous)
  (infective) (malignant) (membranous)
  (phlegmonous) (pseudomembranous)
  (simple) (subacute) (suppurative)
  (ulcerative) (viral) J02.9
  with influenza, flu, or grippe —*see* Influenza,
    with, pharyngitis
  aphthous B08.5
  atrophic J31.2
  chlamydial A56.4
  chronic (atrophic) (granular) (hypertrophic)
    J31.2

Pharyngitis *(Continued)*
  coxsackievirus B08.5
  diphtheritic A36.0
  enteroviral vesicular B08.5
  follicular (chronic) J31.2
  fusospirochetal A69.1
  gonococcal A54.5
  granular (chronic) J31.2
  herpesviral B00.2
  hypertrophic J31.2
  infectional, chronic J31.2
  influenzal —*see* Influenza, with, respiratory
    manifestations NEC
  lymphonodular, acute (enteroviral) B08.8
  pneumococcal J02.8
  purulent J02.9
  putrid J02.9
  septic J02.0
  sicca J31.2
  specified organism NEC J02.8
  staphylococcal J02.8
  streptococcal J02.0
  syphilitic, congenital (early) A50.03
  tuberculous A15.8
  vesicular, enteroviral B08.5
  viral NEC J02.8
Pharyngoconjunctivitis, viral B30.2
Pharyngolaryngitis (acute) J06.0
  chronic J37.0
Pharyngoplegia J39.2
Pharyngotonsillitis, herpesviral B00.2
Pharyngotracheitis, chronic J42
Pharynx, pharyngeal —*see* condition
Phencyclidine-induced ◀
  anxiety disorder F16.980 ◀
  bipolar and related disorder F16.94 ◀
  depressive disorder F16.94 ◀
  psychotic disorder F16.959 ◀
Phenomenon
  Arthus' —*see* Arthus' phenomenon
  jaw-winking Q07.8
  lupus erythematosus (LE) cell M32.9
  Raynaud's (secondary) I73.00
    with gangrene I73.01
  vasomotor R55
  vasospastic I73.9
  vasovagal R55
  Wenckebach's I44.1
Phenylketonuria E70.1
  classical E70.0
  maternal E70.1
Pheochromoblastoma
  specified site —*see* Neoplasm, malignant, by
    site
  unspecified site C74.10
Pheochromocytoma
  malignant
    specified site —*see* Neoplasm, malignant,
      by site
    unspecified site C74.10
  specified site —*see* Neoplasm, benign, by site
  unspecified site D35.00
Pheohyphomycosis —*see* Chromomycosis
Pheomycosis —*see* Chromomycosis
Phimosis (congenital) (due to infection) N47.1
  chancroidal A57
Phlebectasia —*see also* Varix
  congenital Q27.4
Phlebitis (infective) (pyemic) (septic)
  (suppurative) I80.9
  antepartum —*see* Thrombophlebitis,
    antepartum
  blue —*see* Phlebitis, leg, deep
  breast, superficial I80.8
  cavernous (venous) sinus —*see* Phlebitis,
    intracranial (venous) sinus
  cerebral (venous) sinus —*see* Phlebitis,
    intracranial (venous) sinus
  chest wall, superficial I80.8
  cranial (venous) sinus —*see* Phlebitis,
    intracranial (venous) sinus

Phlebitis *(Continued)*
  deep (vessels) —*see* Phlebitis, leg, deep
  due to implanted device —*see* Complications,
    by site and type, specified NEC
  during or resulting from a procedure
    T81.72
  femoral vein (superficial) I80.1-
  femoropopliteal vein I80.0-
  gestational —*see* Phlebopathy, gestational
  hepatic veins I80.8
  iliofemoral —*see* Phlebitis, femoral vein
  intracranial (venous) sinus (any) G08
    nonpyogenic I67.6
  intraspinal venous sinuses and veins G08
    nonpyogenic G95.19
  lateral (venous) sinus —*see* Phlebitis,
    intracranial (venous) sinus
  leg I80.3
    antepartum —*see* Thrombophlebitis,
      antepartum
    deep (vessels) NEC I80.20-
      iliac I80.21-
      popliteal vein I80.22-
      specified vessel NEC I80.29-
      tibial vein I80.23-
    femoral vein (superficial) I80.1-
    superficial (vessels) I80.0-
  longitudinal sinus —*see* Phlebitis, intracranial
    (venous) sinus
  lower limb —*see* Phlebitis, leg
  migrans, migrating (superficial) I82.1
  pelvic
    with ectopic or molar pregnancy O08.0
    following ectopic or molar pregnancy
      O08.0
    puerperal, postpartum O87.1
  popliteal vein —*see* Phlebitis, leg, deep,
    popliteal
  portal (vein) K75.1
  postoperative T81.72
  pregnancy —*see* Thrombophlebitis,
    antepartum
  puerperal, postpartum, childbirth O87.0
    deep O87.1
    pelvic O87.1
    superficial O87.0
  retina —*see* Vasculitis, retina
  saphenous (accessory) (great) (long)
    (small) —*see* Phlebitis, leg, superficial
  sinus (meninges) —*see* Phlebitis, intracranial
    (venous) sinus
  specified site NEC I80.8
  syphilitic A52.09
  tibial vein —*see* Phlebitis, leg, deep, tibial
  ulcerative I80.9
    leg —*see* Phlebitis, leg
  umbilicus I80.8
  uterus (septic) —*see* Endometritis
  varicose (leg) (lower limb) —*see* Varix, leg,
    with, inflammation
Phlebofibrosis I87.8
Phleboliths I87.8
Phlebopathy
  gestational O22.9-
  puerperal O87.9
Phlebosclerosis I87.8
Phlebothrombosis —*see also* Thrombosis
  antepartum —*see* Thrombophlebitis,
    antepartum
  pregnancy —*see* Thrombophlebitis,
    antepartum
  puerperal —*see* Thrombophlebitis,
    puerperal
Phlebotomus fever A93.1
Phlegmasia
  alba dolens O87.1
    nonpuerperal —*see* Phlebitis, femoral
      vein
  cerulea dolens —*see* Phlebitis, leg, deep
Phlegmon —*see* Abscess
Phlegmonous —*see* condition

◀ New   ◀▦ Revised   ~~deleted~~ Deleted

P

Phlyctenulosis (allergic) (keratoconjunctivitis) (nontuberculous) —see also Keratoconjunctivitis
  cornea —see Keratoconjunctivitis
  tuberculous A18.52
Phobia, phobic F40.9
  animal F40.218
    spiders F40.210
  examination F40.298
  reaction F40.9
  simple F40.298
  social F40.10
    generalized F40.11
  specific (isolated) F40.298
    animal F40.218
      spiders F40.210
    blood F40.230
    injection F40.231
    injury F40.233
    men F40.290
    natural environment F40.228
      thunderstorms F40.220
    situational F40.248
      bridges F40.242
      closed in spaces F40.240
      flying F40.243
      heights F40.241
    specified focus NEC F40.298
    transfusion F40.231
    women F40.291
  specified NEC F40.8
    medical care NEC F40.232
  state F40.9
Phocas' disease —see Mastopathy, cystic
Phocomelia Q73.1
  lower limb —see Agenesis, leg, with foot present
  upper limb —see Agenesis, arm, with hand present
Phoria H50.50
Phosphate-losing tubular disorder N25.0
Phosphatemia E83.39
Phosphaturia E83.39
Photodermatitis (sun) L56.8
  chronic L57.8
  due to drug L56.8
  light other than sun L59.8
Photokeratitis H16.13-
Photophobia H53.14-
Photophthalmia —see Photokeratitis
Photopsia H53.19
Photoretinitis —see Retinopathy, solar
Photosensitivity, photosensitization (sun) skin L56.8
  light other than sun L59.8
Phrenitis —see Encephalitis
Phrynoderma (vitamin A deficiency) E50.8
Phthiriasis (pubis) B85.3
  with any infestation classifiable to B85.0-B85.2 B85.4
Phthirus infestation —see Phthiriasis
Phthisis —see also Tuberculosis
  bulbi (infectional) —see Disorder, globe, degenerated condition, atrophy
  eyeball (due to infection) —see Disorder, globe, degenerated condition, atrophy
Phycomycosis —see Zygomycosis
Physalopteriasis B81.8
Physical restraint status Z78.1
Phytobezoar T18.9
  intestine T18.3
  stomach T18.2
Pian —see Yaws
Pianoma A66.1
Pica F50.89 ◀▥
  in adults F50.89 ◀▥
  infant or child F98.3
Picking, nose F98.8
Pick-Niemann disease —see Niemann-Pick disease or syndrome

Pick's
  cerebral atrophy G31.01 [F02.80]
    with behavioral disturbance G31.01 [F02.81]
  disease or syndrome (brain) G31.01 [F02.80]
    with behavioral disturbance G31.01 [F02.81]
    brain G31.01 [F02.80] ◀
      with behavioral disturbance G31.01 [F02.81] ◀
    pericardium (pericardial pseudocirrhosis of liver) I31.1 ◀
  syndrome ◀
    brain G31.01 [F02.80] ◀
      with behavioral disturbance G31.01 [F02.81] ◀
    of heart (pericardial pseudocirrhosis of liver) I31.1 ◀
Pickwickian syndrome E66.2
Piebaldism E70.39
Piedra (beard) (scalp) B36.8
  black B36.3
  white B36.2
Pierre Robin deformity or syndrome Q87.0
Pierson's disease or osteochondrosis M91.0
Pig-bel A05.2
Pigeon
  breast or chest (acquired) M95.4
    congenital Q67.7
    rachitic sequelae (late effect) E64.3
  breeder's disease or lung J67.2
  fancier's disease or lung J67.2
  toe —see Deformity, toe, specified NEC
Pigmentation (abnormal) (anomaly) L81.9
  conjunctiva H11.13-
  cornea (anterior) H18.01-
    posterior H18.05-
    stromal H18.06-
  diminished melanin formation NEC L81.6
  iron L81.8
  lids, congenital Q82.8
  limbus corneae —see Pigmentation, cornea
  metals L81.8
  optic papilla, congenital Q14.2
  retina, congenital (grouped) (nevoid) Q14.1
  scrotum, congenital Q82.8
  tattoo L81.8
Piles —see also Hemorrhoids K64.9
Pili
  annulati or torti (congenital) Q84.1
  incarnati L73.1
Pill roller hand (intrinsic) —see Parkinsonism
Pilomatrixoma —see Neoplasm, skin, benign
  malignant —see Neoplasm, skin, malignant
Pilonidal —see condition
Pimple R23.8
PIN —see Neoplasia, intraepithelial, prostate ◀
Pinched nerve —see Neuropathy, entrapment
Pindborg tumor —see Cyst, calcifying odontogenic
Pineal body or gland —see condition
Pinealoblastoma C75.3
Pinealoma D44.5
  malignant C75.3
Pineoblastoma C75.3
Pineocytoma D44.5
Pinguecula H11.15-
Pingueculitis H10.81-
Pinhole meatus —see also Stricture, urethra N35.9
Pink
  disease —see subcategory T56.1
  eye —see Conjunctivitis, acute, mucopurulent
Pinkus' disease (lichen nitidus) L44.1
Pinpoint
  meatus —see Stricture, urethra
  os (uteri) —see Stricture, cervix
Pins and needles R20.2
Pinta A67.9
  cardiovascular lesions A67.2
  chancre (primary) A67.0

Pinta (Continued)
  erythematous plaques A67.1
  hyperchromic lesions A67.1
  hyperkeratosis A67.1
  lesions A67.9
    cardiovascular A67.2
    hyperchromic A67.1
    intermediate A67.1
    late A67.2
    mixed A67.3
    primary A67.0
    skin (achromic) (cicatricial) (dyschromic) A67.2
      hyperchromic A67.1
      mixed (achromic and hyperchromic) A67.3
  papule (primary) A67.0
  skin lesions (achromic) (cicatricial) (dyschromic) A67.2
    hyperchromic A67.1
    mixed (achromic and hyperchromic) A67.3
  vitiligo A67.2
Pintids A67.1
Pinworm (disease) (infection) (infestation) B80
Piroplasmosis B60.0
Pistol wound —see Gunshot wound
Pitchers' elbow —see Derangement, joint, specified type NEC, elbow
Pithecoid pelvis Q74.2
  with disproportion (fetopelvic) O33.0
    causing obstructed labor O65.0
Pithiatism F48.8
Pitted —see Pitting
Pitting —see also Edema R60.9
  lip R60.0
  nail L60.8
  teeth K00.4
Pituitary gland —see condition
Pituitary-snuff-taker's disease J67.8
Pityriasis (capitis) L21.0
  alba L30.5
  circinata (et maculata) L42
  furfuracea L21.0
  Hebra's L26
  lichenoides L41.0
    chronica L41.1
    et varioliformis (acuta) L41.0
  maculata (et circinata) L30.5
  nigra B36.1
  pilaris, Hebra's L44.0
  rosea L42
  rotunda L44.8
  rubra (Hebra) pilaris L44.0
  simplex L30.5
  specified type NEC L30.5
  streptogenes L30.5
  versicolor (scrotal) B36.0
Placenta, placental —see Pregnancy, complicated by (care of) (management affected by), specified condition
Placentitis O41.14-
Plagiocephaly Q67.3
Plague A20.9
  abortive A20.8
  ambulatory A20.8
  asymptomatic A20.8
  bubonic A20.0
  cellulocutaneous A20.1
  cutaneobubonic A20.1
  lymphatic gland A20.0
  meningitis A20.3
  pharyngeal A20.8
  pneumonic (primary) (secondary) A20.2
  pulmonary, pulmonic A20.2
  septicemic A20.7
  tonsillar A20.8
    septicemic A20.7
Planning, family
  contraception Z30.9
  procreation Z31.69

Plaque (s)
  artery, arterial —*see* Arteriosclerosis
  calcareous —*see* Calcification
  coronary, lipid rich I25.83
  epicardial I31.8
  erythematous, of pinta A67.1
  Hollenhorst's —*see* Occlusion, artery,
    retina
  lipid rich, coronary I25.83
  pleural (without asbestos) J92.9
    with asbestos J92.0
  tongue K13.29
Plasmacytoma C90.3-
  extramedullary C90.2-
  medullary C90.0-
  solitary C90.3-
Plasmacytopenia D72.818
Plasmacytosis D72.822
Plaster ulcer —*see* Ulcer, pressure, by site
Plateau iris syndrome (post-iridectomy)
    (postprocedural) (without glaucoma)
    H21.82
  with glaucoma H40.22-
Platybasia Q75.8
Platyonychia (congenital) Q84.6
  acquired L60.8
Platypelloid pelvis M95.5
  with disproportion (fetopelvic) O33.0
    causing obstructed labor O65.0
  congenital Q74.2
Platyspondylisis Q76.49
Plaut (-Vincent) disease —*see also* Vincent's
    A69.1
Plethora R23.2
  newborn P61.1
Pleura, pleural —*see* condition
Pleuralgia R07.81
Pleurisy (acute) (adhesive) (chronic) (costal)
    (diaphragmatic) (double) (dry) (fibrinous)
    (fibrous) (interlobar) (latent) (plastic)
    (primary) (residual) (sicca) (sterile)
    (subacute) (unresolved) R09.1
  with
    adherent pleura J86.0
    effusion J90
      chylous, chyliform J94.0
      tuberculous (non primary)
        A15.6
        primary (progressive) A15.7
      tuberculosis —*see* Pleurisy, tuberculous
        (non primary)
  encysted —*see* Pleurisy, with effusion
  exudative —*see* Pleurisy, with effusion
  fibrinopurulent, fibropurulent —*see*
    Pyothorax
  hemorrhagic —*see* Hemothorax
  pneumococcal J90
  purulent —*see* Pyothorax
  septic —*see* Pyothorax
  serofibrinous —*see* Pleurisy, with effusion
  seropurulent —*see* Pyothorax
  serous —*see* Pleurisy, with effusion
  staphylococcal J86.9
  streptococcal J90
  suppurative —*see* Pyothorax
  traumatic (post) (current) —*see* Injury,
    intrathoracic, pleura
  tuberculous (with effusion) (non primary)
    A15.6
    primary (progressive) A15.7
Pleuritis sicca —*see* Pleurisy
Pleurobronchopneumonia —*see* Pneumonia,
    broncho
Pleurodynia R07.81
  epidemic B33.0
  viral B33.0
Pleuropericarditis —*see also* Pericarditis
  acute I30.9
Pleuropneumonia (acute) (bilateral) (double)
    (septic) —*see also* Pneumonia J18.8
  chronic —*see* Fibrosis, lung

Pleuro-pneumonia-like-organism (PPLO),
    as cause of disease classified elsewhere
    B96.0
Pleurorrhea —*see* Pleurisy, with effusion
Plexitis, brachial G54.0
Plica
  polonica B85.0
  syndrome, knee M67.5
  tonsil J35.8
Plicated tongue K14.5
Plug
  bronchus NEC J98.09
  meconium (newborn) NEC syndrome P76.0
  mucus —*see* Asphyxia, mucus
Plumbism —*see* subcategory T56.0
Plummer's disease E05.20
  with thyroid storm E05.21
Plummer-Vinson syndrome D50.1
Pluricarential syndrome of infancy E40
Plus (and minus) hand (intrinsic) —*see*
    Deformity, limb, specified type NEC,
    forearm
Pneumathemia —*see* Air, embolism
Pneumatic hammer (drill) syndrome T75.21
Pneumatocele (lung) J98.4
  intracranial G93.89
  tension J44.9
Pneumatosis
  cystoides intestinalis K63.89
  intestinalis K63.89
  peritonei K66.8
Pneumaturia R39.89
Pneumoblastoma —*see* Neoplasm, lung,
    malignant
Pneumocephalus G93.89
Pneumococcemia A40.3
Pneumococcus, pneumococcal —*see* condition
Pneumoconiosis (due to) (inhalation of) J64
  with tuberculosis (any type in A15) J65
  aluminum J63.0
  asbestos J61
  bagasse, bagassosis J67.1
  bauxite J63.1
  beryllium J63.2
  coal miners' (simple) J60
  coalworkers' (simple) J60
  collier's J60
  cotton dust J66.0
  diatomite (diatomaceous earth) J62.8
  dust
    inorganic NEC J63.6
    lime J62.8
    marble J62.8
    organic NEC J66.8
  fumes or vapors (from silo) J68.9
  graphite J63.3
  grinder's J62.8
  kaolin J62.8
  mica J62.8
  millstone maker's J62.8
  mineral fibers NEC J61
  miner's J60
  moldy hay J67.0
  potter's J62.8
  rheumatoid —*see* Rheumatoid, lung
  sandblaster's J62.8
  silica, silicate NEC J62.8
    with carbon J60
  stonemason's J62.8
  talc (dust) J62.0
Pneumocystis carinii pneumonia B59
Pneumocystis jiroveci (pneumonia) B59
Pneumocystosis (with pneumonia) B59
Pneumohemopericardium I31.2
Pneumohemothorax J94.2
  traumatic S27.2
Pneumohydropericardium —*see* Pericarditis
Pneumohydrothorax —*see* Hydrothorax
Pneumomediastinum J98.2
  congenital or perinatal P25.2
Pneumomycosis B49 *[J99]*

Pneumonia (acute) (double) (migratory)
    (purulent) (septic) (unresolved) J18.9
  with
    influenza —*see* Influenza, with, pneumonia
    lung abscess J85.1
      due to specified organism —*see*
        Pneumonia, in (due to)
  adenoviral J12.0
  adynamic J18.2
  alba A50.04
  allergic (eosinophilic) J82
  alveolar —*see* Pneumonia, lobar
  anaerobes J15.8
  anthrax A22.1
  apex, apical —*see* Pneumonia, lobar
  Ascaris B77.81
  aspiration J69.0
    due to
      aspiration of microorganisms
        bacterial J15.9
        viral J12.9
      food (regurgitated) J69.0
      gastric secretions J69.0
      milk (regurgitated) J69.0
      oils, essences J69.1
      solids, liquids NEC J69.8
      vomitus J69.0
    newborn P24.81
      amniotic fluid (clear) P24.11
      blood P24.21
      food (regurgitated) P24.31
      liquor (amnii) P24.11
      meconium P24.01
      milk P24.31
      mucus P24.11
      specified NEC P24.81
      stomach contents P24.31
    postprocedural J95.4
  atypical NEC J18.9
  bacillus J15.9
    specified NEC J15.8
  bacterial J15.9
    specified NEC J15.8
  Bacteroides (fragilis) (oralis)
    (melaninogenicus) J15.8
  basal, basic, basilar —*see* Pneumonia, by type
  bronchiolitis obliterans organized (BOOP)
    J84.89
  broncho-, bronchial (confluent) (croupous)
    (diffuse) (disseminated) (hemorrhagic)
    (involving lobes) (lobar) (terminal) J18.0
  allergic (eosinophilic) J82
  aspiration —*see* Pneumonia, aspiration
  bacterial J15.9
    specified NEC J15.8
  chronic —*see* Fibrosis, lung
  diplococcal J13
  Eaton's agent J15.7
  Escherichia coli (E. coli) J15.5
  Friedländer's bacillus J15.0
  Hemophilus influenzae J14
  hypostatic J18.2
  inhalation (*see also* Pneumonia, aspiration
    due to fumes or vapors (chemical) J68.0
    of oils or essences J69.1
  Klebsiella (pneumoniae) J15.0
  lipid, lipoid J69.1
    endogenous J84.89
  Mycoplasma (pneumoniae) J15.7
  pleuro-pneumonia-like-organisms (PPLO)
    J15.7
  pneumococcal J13
  Proteus J15.6
  Pseudomonas J15.1
  Serratia marcescens J15.6
  specified organism NEC J16.8
  staphylococcal —*see* Pneumonia,
    staphylococcal
  streptococcal NEC J15.4
    group B J15.3
    pneumoniae J13
  viral, virus —*see* Pneumonia, viral

◀ New   ◀▥ Revised   ~~deleted~~ Deleted

Pneumonia (Continued)
  Butyrivibrio (fibriosolvens) J15.8
  Candida B37.1
  caseous —see Tuberculosis, pulmonary
  catarrhal —see Pneumonia, broncho
  chlamydial J16.0
    congenital P23.1
  cholesterol J84.89
  cirrhotic (chronic) —see Fibrosis, lung
  Clostridium (haemolyticum) (novyi) J15.8
  confluent —see Pneumonia, broncho
  congenital (infective) P23.9
    due to
      bacterium NEC P23.6
      Chlamydia P23.1
      Escherichia coli P23.4
      Haemophilus influenzae P23.6
      infective organism NEC P23.8
      Klebsiella pneumoniae P23.6
      Mycoplasma P23.6
      Pseudomonas P23.5
      Staphylococcus P23.2
      Streptococcus (except group B) P23.6
        group B P23.3
      viral agent P23.0
    specified NEC P23.8
  croupous —see Pneumonia, lobar
  cryptogenic organizing J84.116
  cytomegalic inclusion B25.0
  cytomegaloviral B25.0
  deglutition —see Pneumonia, aspiration
  desquamative interstitial J84.117
  diffuse —see Pneumonia, broncho
  diplococcal, diplococcus (broncho-) (lobar)
    J13
  disseminated (focal) —see Pneumonia,
    broncho
  Eaton's agent J15.7
  embolic, embolism —see Embolism,
    pulmonary
  Enterobacter J15.6
  eosinophilic J82
  Escherichia coli (E. coli) J15.5
  Eubacterium J15.8
  fibrinous —see Pneumonia, lobar
  fibroid, fibrous (chronic) —see Fibrosis, lung
  Friedländer's bacillus J15.0
  Fusobacterium (nucleatum) J15.8
  gangrenous J85.0
  giant cell (measles) B05.2
  gonococcal A54.84
  gram-negative bacteria NEC J15.6
    anaerobic J15.8
  Hemophilus influenzae (broncho) (lobar) J14
  human metapneumovirus J12.3
  hypostatic (broncho) (lobar) J18.2
  in (due to)
    actinomycosis A42.0
    adenovirus J12.0
    anthrax A22.1
    ascariasis B77.81
    aspergillosis B44.9
    Bacillus anthracis A22.1
    Bacterium anitratum J15.6
    candidiasis B37.1
    chickenpox B01.2
    Chlamydia J16.0
      neonatal P23.1
    coccidioidomycosis B38.2
      acute B38.0
      chronic B38.1
    cytomegalovirus disease B25.0
    Diplococcus (pneumoniae) J13
    Eaton's agent J15.7
    Enterobacter J15.6
    Escherichia coli (E. coli) J15.5
    Friedländer's bacillus J15.0
    fumes and vapors (chemical) (inhalation)
      J68.0
    gonorrhea A54.84
    Hemophilus influenzae (H. influenzae) J14

Pneumonia (Continued)
  in (Continued)
    Herellea J15.6
    histoplasmosis B39.2
      acute B39.0
      chronic B39.1
    human metapneumovirus J12.3
    Klebsiella (pneumoniae) J15.0
    measles B05.2
    Mycoplasma (pneumoniae) J15.7
    nocardiosis, nocardiasis A43.0
    ornithosis A70
    parainfluenza virus J12.2
    pleuro-pneumonia-like-organism (PPLO)
      J15.7
    pneumococcus J13
    pneumocystosis (Pneumocystis carinii)
      (Pneumocystis jiroveci) B59
    Proteus J15.6
    Pseudomonas NEC J15.1
      pseudomallei A24.1
    psittacosis A70
    Q fever A78
    respiratory syncytial virus J12.1
    rheumatic fever I00 [J17]
    rubella B06.81
    Salmonella (infection) A02.22
      typhi A01.03
    schistosomiasis B65.9 [J17]
    Serratia marcescens J15.6
    specified
      bacterium NEC J15.8
      organism NEC J16.8
      spirochetal NEC A69.8
    Staphylococcus J15.20
      aureus (methicillin susceptible) (MSSA)
        J15.211
        methicillin resistant (MRSA)
          J15.212
      specified NEC J15.29
    Streptococcus J15.4
      group B J15.3
      pneumoniae J13
      specified NEC J15.4
    toxoplasmosis B58.3
    tularemia A21.2
    typhoid (fever) A01.03
    varicella B01.2
    virus —see Pneumonia, viral
    whooping cough A37.91
      due to
        Bordetella parapertussis A37.11
        Bordetella pertussis A37.01
        specified NEC A37.81
    Yersinia pestis A20.2
  inhalation of food or vomit —see Pneumonia,
    aspiration
  interstitial J84.9
    chronic J84.111
    desquamative J84.117
    due to
      collagen vascular disease J84.17
      known underlying cause J84.17
    idiopathic NOS J84.111
    in disease classified elsewhere J84.17
    lymphocytic (due to collagen vascular
      disease) (in diseases classified
      elsewhere) J84.17
    lymphoid J84.2
    non-specific J84.89
      due to
        collagen vascular disease J84.17
        known underlying cause J84.17
      idiopathic J84.113
      in diseases classified elsewhere J84.17
    plasma cell B59
    pseudomonas J15.1
    usual J84.112
      due to collagen vascular disease J84.17
      idiopathic J84.112
      in diseases classified elsewhere J84.17

Pneumonia (Continued)
  Klebsiella (pneumoniae) J15.0
  lipid, lipoid (exogenous) J69.1
    endogenous J84.89
  lobar (disseminated) (double) (interstitial)
    J18.1
    bacterial J15.9
      specified NEC J15.8
    chronic —see Fibrosis, lung
    Escherichia coli (E. coli) J15.5
    Friedländer's bacillus J15.0
    Hemophilus influenzae J14
    hypostatic J18.2
    Klebsiella (pneumoniae) J15.0
    pneumococcal J13
    Proteus J15.6
    Pseudomonas J15.1
    specified organism NEC J16.8
    staphylococcal —see Pneumonia,
      staphylococcal
    streptococcal NEC J15.4
    Streptococcus pneumoniae J13
    viral, virus —see Pneumonia, viral
  lobular —see Pneumonia, broncho
  Löffler's J82
  lymphoid interstitial J84.2
  massive —see Pneumonia, lobar
  meconium P24.01
  MRSA (Methicillin resistant Staphylococcus
    aureus) J15.212 ◀
  MSSA (methicillin susceptible Staphylococcus
    aureus) J15.211
  multilobar —see Pneumonia, by type
  Mycoplasma (pneumoniae) J15.7
  necrotic J85.0
  neonatal P23.9
    aspiration —see Aspiration, by substance,
      with pneumonia
  nitrogen dioxide J68.0 ◀▥
  organizing J84.89
    due to
      collagen vascular disease J84.17
      known underlying cause J84.17
    in diseases classified elsewhere
      J84.17
  orthostatic J18.2
  parainfluenza virus J12.2
  parenchymatous —see Fibrosis, lung
  passive J18.2
  patchy —see Pneumonia, broncho
  Peptococcus J15.8
  Peptostreptococcus J15.8
  plasma cell (of infants) B59
  pleurolobar —see Pneumonia, lobar
  pleuro-pneumonia-like organism (PPLO)
    J15.7
  pneumococcal (broncho) (lobar) J13
  Pneumocystis (carinii) (jiroveci) B59
  postinfectional NEC B99 [J17]
  postmeasles B05.2
  Proteus J15.6
  Pseudomonas J15.1
  psittacosis A70
  radiation J70.0
  respiratory syncytial virus J12.1
  resulting from a procedure J95.89
  rheumatic I00 [J17]
  Salmonella (arizonae) (cholerae-suis)
    (enteritidis) (typhimurium)
    A02.22
    typhi A01.03
    typhoid fever A01.03
  SARS-associated coronavirus J12.81
  segmented, segmental —see Pneumonia,
    broncho-
  Serratia marcescens J15.6
  specified NEC J18.8
    bacterium NEC J15.8
    organism NEC J16.8
    virus NEC J12.89
  spirochetal NEC A69.8

Pneumonia *(Continued)*
staphylococcal (broncho) (lobar) J15.20
aureus (methicillin susceptible) (MSSA)
J15.211
methicillin resistant (MRSA) J15.212
specified NEC J15.29
static, stasis J18.2
streptococcal NEC (broncho) (lobar) J15.4
group
A J15.4
B J15.3
specified NEC J15.4
Streptococcus pneumoniae J13
syphilitic, congenital (early) A50.04
traumatic (complication) (early) (secondary)
T79.8
tuberculous (any) —*see* Tuberculosis,
pulmonary
tularemic A21.2
varicella B01.2
Veillonella J15.8
ventilator associated J95.851
viral, virus (broncho) (interstitial) (lobar) J12.9
adenoviral J12.0
congenital P23.0
human metapneumovirus J12.3
parainfluenza J12.2
respiratory syncytial J12.1
SARS-associated coronavirus J12.81
specified NEC J12.89
white (congenital) A50.04
Pneumonic —*see* condition
Pneumonitis (acute) (primary) —*see also*
Pneumonia
air-conditioner J67.7
allergic (due to) J67.9
organic dust NEC J67.8
red cedar dust J67.8
sequoiosis J67.8
wood dust J67.8
aspiration J69.0
due to
anesthesia J95.4
during
labor and delivery O74.0
pregnancy O29.01-
puerperium O89.01
fumes or gases J68.0
obstetric O74.0
chemical (due to gases, fumes or vapors)
(inhalation) J68.0
due to anesthesia J95.4
cholesterol J84.89
chronic —*see* Fibrosis, lung
congenital rubella P35.0
crack (cocaine) J68.0
due to
beryllium J68.0
cadmium J68.0
crack (cocaine) J68.0
detergent J69.8
fluorocarbon-polymer J68.0
food, vomit (aspiration) J69.0
fumes or vapors J68.0
gases, fumes or vapors (inhalation) J68.0
inhalation
blood J69.8
essences J69.1
food (regurgitated), milk, vomit
J69.0
oils, essences J69.1
saliva J69.0
solids, liquids NEC J69.8
manganese J68.0
nitrogen dioxide J68.0
oils, essences J69.1
solids, liquids NEC J69.8
toxoplasmosis (acquired) B58.3
congenital P37.1
vanadium J68.0
ventilator J95.851

Pneumonitis *(Continued)*
eosinophilic J82
hypersensitivity J67.9
air conditioner lung J67.7
bagassosis J67.1
bird fancier's lung J67.2
farmer's lung J67.0
maltworker's lung J67.4
maple bark-stripper's lung J67.6
mushroom worker's lung J67.5
specified organic dust NEC J67.8
suberosis J67.3
interstitial (chronic) J84.89
acute J84.114
lymphoid J84.2
non-specific J84.89
idiopathic J84.113
lymphoid, interstitial J84.2
meconium P24.01
postanesthetic J95.4
correct substance properly administered —
see Table of Drugs and Chemcials, by
drug, adverse effect
in labor and delivery O74.0
in pregnancy O29.01-
obstetric O74.0
overdose or wrong substance given or taken
(by accident) —*see* Table of Drugs and
Chemicals, by drug, poisoning
postpartum, puerperal O89.01
postoperative J95.4
obstetric O74.0
radiation J70.0
rubella, congenital P35.0
ventilation (air-conditioning) J67.7
ventilator associated J95.851
wood-dust J67.8
Pneumonoconiosis —*see* Pneumoconiosis
Pneumoparotid K11.8
Pneumopathy NEC J98.4
alveolar J84.09
due to organic dust NEC J66.8
parietoalveolar J84.09
Pneumopericarditis —*see also* Pericarditis
acute I30.9
Pneumopericardium —*see also* Pericarditis
congenital P25.3
newborn P25.3
traumatic (post) —*see* Injury, heart
Pneumophagia (psychogenic) F45.8
Pneumopleurisy, pneumopleuritis —*see also*
Pneumonia J18.8
Pneumopyopericardium I30.1
Pneumopyothorax —*see* Pyopneumothorax
with fistula J86.0
Pneumorrhagia —*see also* Hemorrhage, lung
tuberculous —*see* Tuberculosis, pulmonary
Pneumothorax NOS J93.9
acute J93.83
chronic J93.81
congenital P25.1
perinatal period P25.1
postprocedural J95.811
specified NEC J93.83
spontaneous NOS J93.83
newborn P25.1
primary J93.11
secondary J93.12
tension J93.0
tense valvular, infectional J93.0
tension (spontaneous) J93.0
traumatic S27.0
with hemothorax S27.2
tuberculous —*see* Tuberculosis, pulmonary
Podagra —*see also* Gout M10.9
Podencephalus Q01.9
Poikilocytosis R71.8
Poikiloderma L81.6
Civatte's L57.3
congenital Q82.8
vasculare atrophicans L94.5

Poikilodermatomyositis M33.10
with
myopathy M33.12
respiratory involvement M33.11
specified organ involvement NEC M33.19
Pointed ear (congenital) Q17.3
Poison ivy, oak, sumac or other plant
dermatitis (allergic) (contact) L23.7
Poisoning (acute) —*see also* Table of Drugs and
Chemicals
algae and toxins T65.82-
Bacillus B (aertrycke) (cholerae (suis))
(paratyphosus) (suipestifer) A02.9
botulinus A05.1
bacterial toxins A05.9
berries, noxious —*see* Poisoning, food,
noxious, berries
botulism A05.1
ciguatera fish T61.0-
Clostridium botulinum A05.1
death-cap (Amanita phalloides) (Amanita
verna) —*see* Poisoning, food, noxious,
mushrooms
drug —*see* Table of Drugs and Chemicals, by
drug, poisoning
epidemic, fish (noxious) —*see* Poisoning,
seafood
bacterial A05.9
fava bean D55.0
fish (noxious) T61.9-
bacterial —*see* Intoxication, foodborne, by
agent
ciguatera fish —*see* Poisoning, ciguatera
fish
scombroid fish —*see* Poisoning, scombroid
fish
specified type NEC T61.77-
food (acute) (diseased) (infected) (noxious)
NEC T62.9-
bacterial —*see* Intoxication, foodborne, by
agent
due to
Bacillus (aertrycke) (choleraesuis)
(paratyphosus) (suipestifer)
A02.9
botulinus A05.1
Clostridium (perfringens) (Welchii)
A05.2
salmonella (aertrycke) (callinarum)
(choleraesuis) (enteritidis)
(paratyphi) (suipestifer) A02.9
with
gastroenteritis A02.0
sepsis A02.1
staphylococcus A05.0
Vibrio
parahaemolyticus A05.3
vulnificus A05.5
noxious or naturally toxic T62.9-
berries —*see* subcategory T62.1-
fish —*see* Poisoning, seafood
mushrooms —*see* subcategory T62.0X-
plants NEC —*see* subcategory T62.2X-
seafood —*see* Poisoning, seafood
specified NEC —*see* subcategory T62.8X-
ichthyotoxism —*see* Poisoning, seafood
kreotoxism, food A05.9
latex T65.81-
lead T56.0-
mushroom —*see* Poisoning, food, noxious,
mushroom
mussels —*see also* Poisoning, shellfish
bacterial —*see* Intoxication, foodborne, by
agent
nicotine (tobacco) T65.2-
noxious foodstuffs —*see* Poisoning, food,
noxious
plants, noxious —*see* Poisoning, food,
noxious, plants NEC
ptomaine —*see* Poisoning, food
radiation J70.0

◀ New ◀◀◀ Revised ~~deleted~~ Deleted

Poisoning (Continued)
  Salmonella (arizonae) (cholerae-suis) (enteritidis) (typhimurium) A02.9
  scombroid fish T61.1-
  seafood (noxious) T61.9-
    bacterial —see Intoxication, foodborne, by agent
    fish —see Poisoning, fish
    shellfish —see Poisoning, shellfish
    specified NEC —see subcategory T61.8X-
  shellfish (amnesic) (azaspiracid) (diarrheic) (neurotoxic) (noxious) (paralytic) T61.78-
    bacterial —see Intoxication, foodborne, by agent
    ciguatera mollusk —see Poisoning, ciguatera fish
  specified substance NEC T65.891
  Staphylococcus, food A05.0
  tobacco (nicotine) T65.2-
  water E87.79
Poker spine —see Spondylitis, ankylosing
Poland syndrome Q79.8
Polioencephalitis (acute) (bulbar) A80.9
  inferior G12.22
  influenzal —see Influenza, with, encephalopathy
  superior hemorrhagic (acute) (Wernicke's) E51.2
  Wernicke's E51.2
Polioencephalomyelitis (acute) (anterior) A80.9
  with beriberi E51.2
Polioencephalopathy, superior hemorrhagic E51.2
  with
    beriberi E51.11
    pellagra E52
Poliomeningoencephalitis —see Meningoencephalitis
Poliomyelitis (acute) (anterior) (epidemic) A80.9
  with paralysis (bulbar) —see Poliomyelitis, paralytic
  abortive A80.4
  ascending (progressive) —see Poliomyelitis, paralytic
  bulbar (paralytic) —see Poliomyelitis, paralytic
  congenital P35.8
  nonepidemic A80.9
  nonparalytic A80.4
  paralytic A80.30
    specified NEC A80.39
    vaccine-associated A80.0
    wild virus
      imported A80.1
      indigenous A80.2
  spinal, acute A80.9
Poliosis (eyebrow) (eyelashes) L67.1
  circumscripta, acquired L67.1
Pollakiuria R35.0
  psychogenic F45.8
Pollinosis J30.1
Pollitzer's disease L73.2
Polyadenitis —see also Lymphadenitis
  malignant A20.0
Polyalgia M79.89
Polyangiitis M30.0
  microscopic M31.7
  overlap syndrome M30.8
Polyarteritis
  microscopic M31.7
  nodosa M30.0
    with lung involvement M30.1
    juvenile M30.2
    related condition NEC M30.8
Polyarthralgia —see Pain, joint
Polyarthritis, polyarthropathy —see also Arthritis M13.0
  due to or associated with other specified conditions —see Arthritis

Polyarthritis, polyarthropathy (Continued)
  epidemic (Australian) (with exanthema) B33.1
  infective —see Arthritis, pyogenic or pyemic
  inflammatory M06.4
  juvenile (chronic) (seronegative) M08.3
  migratory —see Fever, rheumatic
  rheumatic, acute —see Fever, rheumatic
Polyarthrosis M15.9
  post-traumatic M15.3
  primary M15.0
  specified NEC M15.8
Polycarential syndrome of infancy E40
Polychondritis (atrophic) (chronic) —see also Disorder, cartilage, specified type NEC
  relapsing M94.1
Polycoria Q13.2
Polycystic (disease)
  degeneration, kidney Q61.3
    autosomal dominant (adult type) Q61.2
    autosomal recessive (infantile type) NEC Q61.19
  kidney Q61.3
    autosomal
      dominant Q61.2
      recessive NEC Q61.19
    autosomal dominant (adult type) Q61.2
    autosomal recessive (childhood type) NEC Q61.19
    infantile type NEC Q61.19
  liver Q44.6
  lung J98.4
    congenital Q33.0
  ovary, ovaries E28.2
  spleen Q89.09
Polycythemia (secondary) D75.1
  acquired D75.1
  benign (familial) D75.0
  due to
    donor twin P61.1
    erythropoietin D75.1
    fall in plasma volume D75.1
    high altitude D75.1
    maternal-fetal transfusion P61.1
    stress D75.1
  emotional D75.1
  erythropoietin D75.1
  familial (benign) D75.0
  Gaisböck's (hypertonica) D75.1
  high altitude D75.1
  hypertonica D75.1
  hypoxemic D75.1
  neonatorum P61.1
  nephrogenous D75.1
  relative D75.1
  secondary D75.1
  spurious D75.1
  stress D75.1
  vera D45
Polycytosis cryptogenica D75.1
Polydactylism, polydactyly Q69.9
  toes Q69.2
Polydipsia R63.1
Polydystrophy, pseudo-Hurler E77.0
Polyembryoma —see Neoplasm, malignant, by site
Polyglandular
  deficiency E31.0
  dyscrasia E31.9
  dysfunction E31.9
  syndrome E31.8
Polyhydramnios O40.-
Polymastia Q83.1
Polymenorrhea N92.0
Polymyalgia M35.3
  arteritica, giant cell M31.5
  rheumatica M35.3
    with giant cell arteritis M31.5

Polymyositis (acute) (chronic) (hemorrhagic) M33.20
  with
    myopathy M33.22
    respiratory involvement M33.21
    skin involvement —see Dermatopolymyositis
    specified organ involvement NEC M33.29
  ossificans (generalisata) (progressiva) —see Myositis, ossificans, progressiva
Polyneuritis, polyneuritic —see also Polyneuropathy
  acute (post-)infective G61.0
  alcoholic G62.1
  cranialis G52.7
  demyelinating, chronic inflammatory (CIDP) G61.81
  diabetic —see Diabetes, polyneuropathy
  diphtheritic A36.83
  due to lack of vitamin NEC E56.9 [G63]
  endemic E51.11
  erythredema —see subcategory T56.1
  febrile, acute G61.0
  hereditary ataxic G60.1
  idiopathic, acute G61.0
  infective (acute) G61.0
  inflammatory, chronic demyelinating (CIDP) G61.81
  nutritional E63.9 [G63]
  postinfective (acute) G61.0
  specified NEC G62.89
Polyneuropathy (peripheral) G62.9
  alcoholic G62.1
  amyloid (Portuguese) E85.1 [G63]
  arsenical G62.2
  critical illness G62.81
  demyelinating, chronic inflammatory (CIDP) G61.81
  diabetic —see Diabetes, polyneuropathy
  drug-induced G62.0
  hereditary G60.9
    specified NEC G60.8
  idiopathic G60.9
    progressive G60.3
  in (due to)
    alcohol G62.1
      sequelae G65.2
    amyloidosis, familial (Portuguese) E85.1 [G63]
    antitetanus serum G61.1
    arsenic G62.2
      sequelae G65.2
    avitaminosis NEC E56.9 [G63]
    beriberi E51.11
    collagen vascular disease NEC M35.9 [G63]
    deficiency (of)
      B (-complex) vitamins E53.9 [G63]
      vitamin B6 E53.1 [G63]
    diabetes —see Diabetes, polyneuropathy
    diphtheria A36.83
    drug or medicament G62.0
      correct substance properly administered —see Table of Drugs and Chemicals, by drug, adverse effect
      overdose or wrong substance given or taken —see Table of Drugs and Chemicals, by drug, poisoning
    endocrine disease NEC E34.9 [G63]
    herpes zoster B02.23
    hypoglycemia E16.2 [G63]
    infectious
      disease NEC B99 [G63]
      mononucleosis B27.91
    lack of vitamin NEC E56.9 [G63]
    lead G62.2
      sequelae G65.2
    leprosy A30.9 [G63]
    Lyme disease A69.22
    metabolic disease NEC E88.9 [G63]
    microscopic polyangiitis M31.7 [G63]

Polyneuropathy (Continued)
  in (Continued)
    mumps B26.84
    neoplastic disease —see also Neoplasm
      D49.9 [G63]
    nutritional deficiency NEC E63.9 [G63]
    organophosphate compounds G62.2
      sequelae G65.2
    parasitic disease NEC B89 [G63]
    pellagra E52 [G63]
    polyarteritis nodosa M30.0
    porphyria E80.20 [G63]
    radiation G62.82
    rheumatoid arthritis —see Rheumatoid,
      polyneuropathy
    sarcoidosis D86.89
    serum G61.1
    syphilis (late) A52.15
      congenital A50.43
    systemic
      connective tissue disorder M35.9
        [G63]
      lupus erythematosus M32.19
    toxic agent NEC G62.2
      sequelae G65.2
    triorthocresyl phosphate G62.2
      sequelae G65.2
    tuberculosis A17.89
    uremia N18.9 [G63]
    vitamin B12 deficiency E53.8 [G63]
      with anemia (pernicious) D51.0
        [G63]
        due to dietary deficiency D51.3
          [G63]
    zoster B02.23
  inflammatory G61.9
    chronic demyelinating (CIDP) G61.81
    sequelae G65.1
    specified NEC G61.89
  lead G62.2
    sequelae G65.2
  nutritional NEC E63.9 [G63]
  postherpetic (zoster) B02.23
  progressive G60.3
  radiation-induced G62.82
  sensory (hereditary) (idiopathic) G60.8
  specified NEC G62.89
  syphilitic (late) A52.15
    congenital A50.43
Polyopia H53.8
Polyorchism, polyorchidism Q55.21
Polyosteoarthritis —see also Osteoarthritis,
  generalized M15.9-
  post-traumatic M15.3
  specified NEC M15.8
Polyostotic fibrous dysplasia Q78.1
Polyotia Q17.0
Polyp, polypus
  accessory sinus J33.8
  adenocarcinoma in —see Neoplasm,
    malignant, by site
  adenocarcinoma in situ in —see Neoplasm, in
    situ, by site
  adenoid tissue J33.0
  adenomatous —see also Neoplasm, benign,
    by site
    adenocarcinoma in —see Neoplasm,
      malignant, by site
    adenocarcinoma in situ in —see Neoplasm,
      in situ, by site
    carcinoma in —see Neoplasm, malignant,
      by site
    carcinoma in situ in —see Neoplasm, in
      situ, by site
    multiple —see Neoplasm, benign
      adenocarcinoma in —see Neoplasm,
        malignant, by site
      adenocarcinoma in situ in —see
        Neoplasm, in situ, by site
  antrum J33.8
  anus, anal (canal) K62.0

Polyp, polypus (Continued)
  Bartholin's gland N84.3
  bladder D41.4
  carcinoma in —see Neoplasm, malignant, by
    site
  carcinoma in situ in —see Neoplasm, in situ,
    by site
  cecum D12.0
  cervix (uteri) N84.1
    in pregnancy or childbirth —see Pregnancy,
      complicated by, abnormal, cervix
    mucous N84.1
    nonneoplastic N84.1
  choanal J33.0
  cholesterol K82.4
  clitoris N84.3
  colon K63.5
    adenomatous D12.6
    ascending D12.2
    cecum D12.0
    descending D12.4
    inflammatory K51.40
      with
        abscess K51.414
        complication K51.419
          specified NEC K51.418
        fistula K51.413
        intestinal obstruction K51.412
        rectal bleeding K51.411
    sigmoid D12.5
    transverse D12.3
  corpus uteri N84.0
  dental K04.01 ◄▥
    irreversible K04.02 ◄
    reversible K04.01 ◄
  duodenum K31.7
  ear (middle) H74.4-
  endometrium N84.0
  ethmoidal (sinus) J33.8
  fallopian tube N84.8
  female genital tract N84.9
    specified NEC N84.8
  frontal (sinus) J33.8
  gallbladder K82.4
  gingiva, gum K06.8
  labia, labium (majus) (minus) N84.3
  larynx (mucous) J38.1
    adenomatous D14.1
  malignant —see Neoplasm, malignant, by site
  maxillary (sinus) J33.8
  middle ear —see Polyp, ear (middle)
  myometrium N84.0
  nares
    anterior J33.9
    posterior J33.0
  nasal (mucous) J33.9
    cavity J33.0
    septum J33.0
  nasopharyngeal J33.0
  nose (mucous) J33.9
  oviduct N84.8
  pharynx J39.2
  placenta O90.89
  prostate —see Enlargement, enlarged,
    prostate
  pudenda, pudendum N84.3
  pulpal (dental) K04.01 ◄▥
    irreversible K04.02 ◄
    reversible K04.01 ◄
  rectum (nonadenomatous) K62.1
    adenomatous —see Polyp, adenomatous
  septum (nasal) J33.0
  sinus (accessory) (ethmoidal) (frontal)
    (maxillary) (sphenoidal) J33.8
  sphenoidal (sinus) J33.8
  stomach K31.7
    adenomatous D13.1
  tube, fallopian N84.8
  turbinate, mucous membrane J33.8
  umbilical, newborn P83.6
  ureter N28.89

Polyp, polypus (Continued)
  urethra N36.2
  uterus (body) (corpus) (mucous) N84.0
    cervix N84.1
    in pregnancy or childbirth —see Pregnancy,
      complicated by, tumor, uterus
  vagina N84.2
  vocal cord (mucous) J38.1
  vulva N84.3
Polyphagia R63.2
Polyploidy Q92.7
Polypoid —see condition
Polyposis —see also Polyp
  coli (adenomatous) D12.6
    adenocarcinoma in C18.9
    adenocarcinoma in situ in —see Neoplasm,
      in situ, by site
    carcinoma in C18.9
  colon (adenomatous) D12.6
  familial D12.6
    adenocarcinoma in situ in —see Neoplasm,
      in situ, by site
  intestinal (adenomatous) D12.6
  malignant lymphomatous C83.1
  multiple, adenomatous —see also Neoplasm,
    benign D36.9
Polyradiculitis —see Polyneuropathy
Polyradiculoneuropathy (acute) (postinfective)
  (segmentally demyelinating) G61.0
Polyserositis
  due to pericarditis I31.1
  pericardial I31.1
  periodic, familial E85.0
  tuberculous A19.9
    acute A19.1
    chronic A19.8
Polysplenia syndrome Q89.09
Polysyndactyly —see also Syndactylism,
  syndactyly Q70.4
Polytrichia L68.3
Polyunguia Q84.6
Polyuria R35.8
  nocturnal R35.1
  psychogenic F45.8
Pompe's disease (glycogen storage) E74.02
Pompholyx L30.1
Poncet's disease (tuberculous rheumatism)
  A18.09
Pond fracture —see Fracture, skull
Ponos B55.0
Pons, pontine —see condition
Poor
  aesthetic of existing restoration of tooth
    K08.56
  contractions, labor O62.2
  gingival margin to tooth restoration K08.51
  personal hygiene R46.0
  prenatal care, affecting management of
    pregnancy —see Pregnancy, complicated
    by, insufficient, prenatal care
  sucking reflex (newborn) R29.2
  urinary stream R39.12
  vision NEC H54.7
Poradenitis, nostras inguinalis or venerea A55
Porencephaly (congenital) (developmental)
  (true) Q04.6
  acquired G93.0
  nondevelopmental G93.0
  traumatic (post) F07.89
Porocephaliasis B88.8
Porokeratosis Q82.8
Poroma, eccrine —see Neoplasm, skin, benign
Porphyria (South African) E80.20
  acquired E80.20
  acute intermittent (hepatic) (Swedish) E80.21
  cutanea tarda (hereditary) (symptomatic)
    E80.1
  due to drugs E80.20
    correct substance properly administered —
      see Table of Drugs and Chemicals, by
      drug, adverse effect

◄ New   ◄▥ Revised   ~~deleted~~ Deleted

Porphyria (Continued)
 due to (Continued)
  overdose or wrong substance given or
   taken —see Table of Drugs and
   Chemicals, by drug, poisoning
  erythropoietic (congenital) (hereditary)
   E80.0
   hepatocutaneous type E80.1
   secondary E80.20
   toxic NEC E80.20
   variegata E80.20
Porphyrinuria —see Porphyria
Porphyruria —see Porphyria
Portal —see condition
Port wine nevus, mark, or stain Q82.5
Posadas-Wernicke disease B38.9
Positive
 culture (nonspecific)
  blood R78.81
  bronchial washings R84.5
  cerebrospinal fluid R83.5
  cervix uteri R87.5
  nasal secretions R84.5
  nipple discharge R89.5
  nose R84.5
   staphylococcus (Methicillin susceptible)
    Z22.321
    Methicillin resistant Z22.322
  peritoneal fluid R85.5
  pleural fluid R84.5
  prostatic secretions R86.5
  saliva R85.5
  seminal fluid R86.5
  sputum R84.5
  synovial fluid R89.5
  throat scrapings R84.5
  urine R82.79 ◀▥
  vagina R87.5
  vulva R87.5
  wound secretions R89.5
 PPD (skin test) R76.11
 serology for syphilis A53.0
  with signs or symptoms - code as Syphilis,
   by site and stage
  false R76.8
 skin test, tuberculin (without active
  tuberculosis) R76.11
 test, human immunodeficiency virus (HIV)
  R75
 VDRL A53.0
  with signs or symptoms - code by site and
   stage under Syphilis A53.9
 Wassermann reaction A53.0
Postcardiotomy syndrome I97.0
Postcaval ureter Q62.62
Postcholecystectomy syndrome K91.5
Postclimacteric bleeding N95.0
Postcommissurotomy syndrome I97.0
Postconcussional syndrome F07.81
Postcontusional syndrome F07.81
Postcricoid region —see condition
Post-dates (40-42 weeks) (pregnancy) (mother)
 O48.0
 more than 42 weeks gestation O48.1
Postencephalitic syndrome F07.89
Posterior —see condition
Posterolateral sclerosis (spinal cord) —see
 Degeneration, combined
Postexanthematous —see condition
Postfebrile —see condition
Postgastrectomy dumping syndrome K91.1
Posthemiplegic chorea —see Monoplegia
Posthemorrhagic anemia (chronic) D50.0
 acute D62
 newborn P61.3
Postherpetic neuralgia (zoster) B02.29
 trigeminal B02.22
Posthitis N47.7
Postimmunization complication or reaction —
 see Complications, vaccination
Postinfectious —see condition

Postlaminectomy syndrome NEC M96.1
Postleukotomy syndrome F07.0
Postmastectomy lymphedema (syndrome) I97.2
Postmaturity, postmature (over 42 weeks)
 maternal (over 42 weeks gestation) O48.1
 newborn P08.22
Postmeasles complication NEC —see also
 condition B05.89
Postmenopausal
 endometrium (atrophic) N95.8
  suppurative —see also Endometritis N71.9
 osteoporosis —see Osteoporosis,
  postmenopausal
Postnasal drip R09.82
 due to
  allergic rhinitis —see Rhinitis, allergic
  common cold J00
  gastroesophageal reflux —see Reflux,
   gastroesophageal
  nasopharyngitis —see Nasopharyngitis
  other know condition — code to condition
  sinusitis —see Sinusitis
Postnatal —see condition
Postoperative (postprocedural) —see
 Complication, postoperative
 pneumothorax, therapeutic Z98.3
 state NEC Z98.890 ◀▥
Postpancreatectomy hyperglycemia E89.1
Postpartum —see Puerperal
Postphlebitic syndrome —see Syndrome,
 postthrombotic
Postpolio (myelitic) syndrome G14
Postpoliomyelitic —see also condition
 osteopathy —see Osteopathy, after
  poliomyelitis
Postprocedural —see also Postoperative
 hypoinsulinemia E89.1
Postschizophrenic depression F32.89 ◀▥
Postsurgery status —see also Status (post)
 pneumothorax, therapeutic Z98.3
Post-term (40-42 weeks) (pregnancy) (mother)
 O48.0
 infant P08.21
 more than 42 weeks gestation (mother) O48.1
Post-traumatic brain syndrome, nonpsychotic
 F07.81
Post-typhoid abscess A01.09
Postures, hysterical F44.2
Postvaccinal reaction or complication —see
 Complications, vaccination
Postvalvulotomy syndrome I97.0
Potain's
 disease (pulmonary edema) —see Edema,
  lung
 syndrome (gastrectasis with dyspepsia) K31.0
Potter's
 asthma J62.8
 facies Q60.6
 lung J62.8
 syndrome (with renal agenesis) Q60.6
Pott's
 curvature (spinal) A18.01
 disease or paraplegia A18.01
 spinal curvature A18.01
 tumor, puffy —see Osteomyelitis, specified
  type NEC
Pouch
 bronchus Q32.4
 Douglas' —see condition
 esophagus, esophageal, congenital Q39.6
  acquired K22.5
 gastric K31.4
 Hartmann's K82.8
 pharynx, pharyngeal (congenital) Q38.7
Pouchitis K91.850
Poultrymen's itch B88.0
Poverty NEC Z59.6
 extreme Z59.5
Poxvirus NEC B08.8
Prader-Willi syndrome Q87.1
Preauricular appendage or tag Q17.0

Prebetalipoproteinemia (acquired) (essential)
 (familial) (hereditary) (primary)
 (secondary) E78.1
 with chylomicronemia E78.3
Precipitate labor or delivery O62.3
Preclimacteric bleeding (menorrhagia) N92.4
Precocious
 adrenarche E30.1
 menarche E30.1
 menstruation E30.1
 pubarche E30.1
 puberty E30.1
  central E22.8
 sexual development NEC E30.1
 thelarche E30.8
Precocity, sexual (constitutional) (cryptogenic)
 (female) (idiopathic) (male) E30.1
 with adrenal hyperplasia E25.9
  congenital E25.0
Precordial pain R07.2
Predeciduous teeth K00.2
Prediabetes, prediabetic R73.03 ◀▥
 complicating
  pregnancy —see Pregnancy, complicated
   by, diseases of, specified type or
   system NEC
  puerperium O99.89
Predislocation status of hip at birth Q65.6
Pre-eclampsia O14.9-
 with pre-existing hypertension —see
  Hypertension, complicating pregnancy,
  pre-existing, with, pre-eclampsia
 complicating ◀
  childbirth O14.94 ◀
  puerperium O14.95 ◀
 mild O14.0-
  complicating ◀
   childbirth O14.04 ◀
   puerperium O14.05 ◀
 moderate O14.0-
  complicating ◀
   childbirth O14.04 ◀
   puerperium O14.05 ◀
 severe O14.1-
  with hemolysis, elevated liver enzymes
   and low platelet count (HELLP)
   O14.2-
  complicating ◀
   childbirth O14.24 ◀
   puerperium O14.25 ◀
  complicating ◀
   childbirth O14.14 ◀
   puerperium O14.15 ◀
Pre-eruptive color change, teeth, tooth
 K00.8
Pre-excitation atrioventricular conduction
 I45.6
Preglaucoma H40.00-
Pregnancy (single) (uterine) —see also Delivery
 and Puerperal

Note: The Tabular must be reviewed for
assignment of the appropriate character
indicating the trimester of the pregnancy

Note: The Tabular must be reviewed for
assignment of appropriate seventh character
for multiple gestation codes in Chapter 15

 abdominal (ectopic) O00.00 ◀▥
  with intrauterine pregnancy O00.01 ◀
  with viable fetus O36.7-
 ampullar O00.10 ◀▥
  with intrauterine pregnancy O00.11 ◀
 biochemical O02.81
 broad ligament O00.80 ◀▥
  with intrauterine pregnancy O00.81 ◀
 cervical O00.80 ◀▥
  with intrauterine pregnancy O00.81 ◀
 chemical O02.81
 complicated NOS O26.9-

Pregnancy *(Continued)*
  complicated by (care of) (management
      affected by)
    abnormal, abnormality
      cervix O34.4-
        causing obstructed labor O65.5
      cord (umbilical) O69.9
      findings on antenatal screening of
          mother O28.9
        biochemical O28.1
        chromosomal O28.5
        cytological O28.2
        genetic O28.5
        hematological O28.0
        radiological O28.4
        specified NEC O28.8
        ultrasonic O28.3
      glucose (tolerance) NEC O99.810
      pelvic organs O34.9-
        specified NEC O34.8-
          causing obstructed labor O65.5
      pelvis (bony) (major) NEC O33.0
      perineum O34.7-
      position
        placenta O44.0- ◀▥
          without hemorrhage O44.0-
          with hemorrhage O44.1- ◀
        uterus O34.59-
      uterus O34.59-
        causing obstructed labor O65.5
        congenital O34.0-
      vagina O34.6-
        causing obstructed labor O65.5
      vulva O34.7-
        causing obstructed labor O65.5
    abruptio placentae —*see* Abruptio
        placentae
    abscess or cellulitis
      bladder O23.1-
      breast O91.11-
      genital organ or tract O23.9-
    abuse
      physical O9A.31-
      psychological O9A.51-
      sexual O9A.41-
    adverse effect anesthesia O29.9-
      aspiration pneumonitis O29.01-
      cardiac arrest O29.11-
      cardiac complication NEC O29.19-
      cardiac failure O29.12-
      central nervous system complication
          NEC O29.29-
      cerebral anoxia O29.21-
      failed or difficult intubation O29.6-
      inhalation of stomach contents or
          secretions NOS O29.01-
      local, toxic reaction O29.3X
      Mendelson's syndrome O29.01-
      pressure collapse of lung O29.02-
      pulmonary complications NEC O29.09-
      specified NEC O29.8X
      spinal and epidural type NEC O29.5X
        induced headache O29.4-
    albuminuria —*see also* Proteinuria,
        gestational O12.1- ◀▥
    alcohol use O99.31-
    amnionitis O41.12-
    anaphylactoid syndrome of pregnancy
        O88.01-
    anemia (conditions in D50-D64) (pre-
        existing) O99.01-
      complicating the puerperium O99.03
    antepartum hemorrhage O46.9-
      with coagulation defect —*see*
          Hemorrhage, antepartum, with
          coagulation defect
      specified NEC O46.8X-
    appendicitis O99.61-
    atrophy (yellow) (acute) liver (subacute)
        O26.61-
    bariatric surgery status O99.84- ◀▥

Pregnancy *(Continued)*
  complicated by *(Continued)*
    bicornis or bicornuate uterus O34.0- ◀▥
    biliary tract problems O26.61-
    breech presentation O32.1
    cardiovascular diseases (conditions in
        I00-I09, I20-I52, I70-I99) O99.41-
    cerebrovascular disorders (conditions in
        I60-I69) O99.41-
    cervical shortening O26.87-
    cervicitis O23.51-
    chloasma (gravidarum) O26.89-
    cholecystitis O99.61-
    cholestasis (intrahepatic) O26.61-
    chorioamnionitis O41.12-
    circulatory system disorder (conditions in
        I00-I09, I20-I99, O99.41-)
    compound presentation O32.6
    conjoined twins O30.02-
    connective system disorders (conditions in
        M00-M99) O99.89
    contracted pelvis (general) O33.1
      inlet O33.2
      outlet O33.3
    convulsions (eclamptic) (uremic) —*see also*
        Eclampsia O15.9-
    cracked nipple O92.11-
    cystitis O23.1-
    cystocele O34.8-
    death of fetus (near term) O36.4
      early pregnancy O02.1
      of one fetus or more in multiple
          gestation O31.2-
    deciduitis O41.14-
    decreased fetal movement O36.81-
    dental problems O99.61-
    diabetes (mellitus) O24.91-
      gestational (pregnancy induced) —*see*
          Diabetes, gestational
      pre-existing O24.31-
        specified NEC O24.81-
        type 1 O24.01-
        type 2 O24.11-
    digestive system disorders (conditions in
        K00-K93) O99.61-
      biliary tract O26.61-
      blood NEC (conditions in D65-D77)
          O99.11-
      liver O26.61-
      specified NEC O99.89
    disorders of —*see* Pregnancy, complicated
        by, specified body system disorder
      amniotic fluid and membranes O41.9-
        specified NEC O41.8X-
      biliary tract O26.61-
      ear and mastoid process (conditions in
          H60-H95) O99.89
      eye and adnexa (conditions in H00-H59)
          O99.89
      liver O26.61-
      skin (conditions in L00-L99) O99.71-
      specified NEC O99.89
    displacement, uterus NEC O34.59-
      causing obstructed labor O65.5
    disproportion (due to) O33.9
      fetal deformities NEC O33.7
      fetal (ascites) (hydrops)
          (meningomyelocele) (sacral
          teratoma) (tumor) deformities NEC
          O33.7 ◀
      generally contracted pelvis O33.1
      hydrocephalic fetus O33.6
      inlet contraction of pelvis O33.2
      mixed maternal and fetal origin O33.4
      specified NEC O33.8
    double uterus O34.0- ◀▥
      causing obstructed labor O65.5
    drug use (conditions in F11-F19)
        O99.32-

Pregnancy *(Continued)*
  complicated by *(Continued)*
    eclampsia, eclamptic (coma) (convulsions)
        (delirium) (nephritis) (uremia) (*see
        also* Eclampsia) O15-
    ectopic pregnancy —*see* Pregnancy, ectopic
    edema O12.0-
      with
        gestational hypertension, mild —*see
            also* Pre-eclampsia O14.0-
        proteinuria O12.2-
    effusion, amniotic fluid —*see* Pregnancy,
        complicated by, premature rupture of
        membranes
    elderly
      multigravida O09.52-
      primigravida O09.51-
    embolism —*see also* Embolism, obstetric,
        pregnancy O88.-
    endocrine diseases NEC O99.28-
    endometritis O86.12
    excessive weight gain O26.0-
    exhaustion O26.81-
      during labor and delivery O75.81
    face presentation O32.3
    failed induction of labor O61.9
    failed or difficult intubation for anesthesia
        O29.6-
      instrumental O61.1
      mechanical O61.1
      medical O61.0
      specified NEC O61.8
      surgical O61.1
    false labor (pains) O47.9
      at or after 37 completed weeks of
          pregnancy O47.1
      before 37 completed weeks of pregnancy
          O47.0-
    fatigue O26.81-
      during labor and delivery O75.81
    fatty metamorphosis of liver O26.61-
    female genital mutilation O34.8- *[N90.81-]*
    fetal (maternal care for)
      abnormality or damage O35.9
        acid-base balance O68
        specified type NEC O35.8
      acidemia O68
      acidosis O68
      alkalosis O68
      anemia and thrombocytopenia O36.82-
      anencephaly O35.0
      chromosomal abnormality (conditions in
          Q90-Q99) O35.1
      conjoined twins O30.02-
      damage from
        amniocentesis O35.7
        biopsy procedures O35.7
        drug addiction O35.5
        hematological investigation O35.7
        intrauterine contraceptive device
            O35.7
        maternal
          alcohol addiction O35.4
          cytomegalovirus infection O35.3
          disease NEC O35.8
          drug addiction O35.5
          listeriosis O35.8
          rubella O35.3
          toxoplasmosis O35.8
          viral infection O35.3
        medical procedure NEC O35.7
        radiation O35.6
      death (near term) O36.4
        early pregnancy O02.1
      decreased movement O36.81-
      disproportion due to deformity (fetal)
          O33.7
      excessive growth (large for dates) O36.6-
      growth retardation O36.59-
        light for dates O36.59-
        small for dates O36.59-

◀ New   ◀▥ Revised   ~~deleted~~ Deleted

Pregnancy *(Continued)*
  complicated by *(Continued)*
    fetal *(Continued)*
      heart rate irregularity (bradycardia)
          (decelerations) (tachycardia) O76
      hereditary disease O35.2
      hydrocephalus O35.0
      intrauterine death O36.4
      poor growth O36.59-
        light for dates O36.59-
        small for dates O36.59-
      problem O36.9-
        specified NEC O36.89-
      reduction (elective) O31.3-
      selective termination O31.3-
      spina bifida O35.0
      thrombocytopenia O36.82-
    fibroid (tumor) (uterus) O34.1-
    fissure of nipple O92.11-
    gallstones O99.61-
    gastric banding status O99.84-
    gastric bypass status O99.84-
    genital herpes (asymptomatic) (history of)
        (inactive) O98.51-
    genital tract infection O23.9-
    glomerular diseases (conditions in
        N00-N07) O26.83-
      with hypertension, pre-existing —*see*
          Hypertension, complicating,
          pregnancy, pre-existing, with, renal
          disease
    gonorrhea O98.21-
    grand multiparity O09.4
    habitual aborter —*see* Pregnancy,
        complicated by, recurrent pregnancy
        loss
    HELLP syndrome (hemolysis, elevated
        liver enzymes and low platelet count)
        O14.2-
    hemorrhage
      antepartum —*see* Hemorrhage,
          antepartum
      before 20 completed weeks gestation
          O20.9
        specified NEC O20.8
      due to premature separation, placenta —
          see also Abruptio placentae O45.9-
      early O20.9
        specified NEC O20.8
      threatened abortion O20.0
    hemorrhoids O22.4-
    hepatitis (viral) O98.41-
    herniation of uterus O34.59-
    high
      head at term O32.4
      risk —*see* Supervision (of) (for), high-risk
    history of in utero procedure during
        previous pregnancy O09.82-
    HIV O98.71-
    human immunodeficiency virus (HIV)
        disease O98.71-
    hydatidiform mole —*see also* Mole,
        hydatidiform O01.9-
    hydramnios O40.-
    hydrocephalic fetus (disproportion) O33.6
    hydrops
      amnii O40.-
      fetalis O36.2-
        associated with isoimmunization —*see
            also* Pregnancy, complicated by,
            isoimmunization O36.11-
    hydrorrhea O42.90
    hyperemesis (gravidarum) (mild) —*see also*
        Hyperemesis, gravidarum O21.0-
    hypertension —*see* Hypertension,
        complicating pregnancy
    hypertensive
      heart and renal disease, pre-existing —
          see Hypertension, complicating,
          pregnancy, pre-existing, with, heart
          disease, with renal disease

Pregnancy *(Continued)*
  complicated by *(Continued)*
    hypertensive *(Continued)*
      heart disease, pre-existing —*see*
          Hypertension, complicating,
          pregnancy, pre-existing, with, heart
          disease
      renal disease, pre-existing —*see*
          Hypertension, complicating,
          pregnancy, pre-existing, with, renal
          disease
    hypotension O26.5-
    immune disorders NEC (conditions in
        D80-D89) O99.11-
    incarceration, uterus O34.51-
    incompetent cervix O34.3-
    inconclusive fetal viability O36.80
    infection (s) O98.91-
      amniotic fluid or sac O41.10-
      bladder O23.1-
      carrier state NEC O99.830
        streptococcus B O99.820
      genital organ or tract O23.9-
        specified NEC O23.59-
      genitourinary tract O23.9-
      gonorrhea O98.21-
      hepatitis (viral) O98.41-
      HIV O98.71-
      human immunodeficiency virus (HIV)
          O98.71-
      kidney O23.0-
      nipple O91.01-
      parasitic disease O98.91-
        specified NEC O98.81-
      protozoal disease O98.61-
      sexually transmitted NEC O98.31-
      specified type NEC O98.81-
      syphilis O98.11-
      tuberculosis O98.01-
      urethra O23.2-
      urinary (tract) O23.4-
        specified NEC O23.3-
      viral disease O98.51-
    injury or poisoning (conditions in S00-T88)
        O9A.21-
      due to abuse
        physical O9A.31-
        psychological O9A.51-
        sexual O9A.41-
    insufficient
      prenatal care O09.3-
      weight gain O26.1-
    insulin resistance O26.89
    intrauterine fetal death (near term) O36.4
      early pregnancy O02.1
      multiple gestation (one fetus or more)
          O31.2-
    isoimmunization O36.11-
      anti-A sensitization O36.11-
      anti-B sensitization O36.19-
      Rh O36.09-
        anti-D antibody O36.01-
      specified NEC O36.19-
    laceration of uterus NEC O71.81
    malformation
      placenta, placental (vessel) O43.10-
        specified NEC O43.19-
      uterus (congenital) O34.0-
    malnutrition (conditions in E40-E46)
        O25.1-
    maternal hypotension syndrome O26.5-
    mental disorders (conditions in F01-F09,
        F20-F99) O99.34-
      alcohol use O99.31-
      drug use O99.32-
      smoking O99.33-
    mentum presentation O32.3
    metabolic disorders O99.28-
    missed
      abortion O02.1
      delivery O36.4

Pregnancy *(Continued)*
  complicated by *(Continued)*
    multiple gestations O30.9-
      conjoined twins O30.02-
      quadruplet —*see* Pregnancy, quadruplet
      specified complication NEC O31.8X-
      specified number of multiples NEC —*see*
          Pregnancy, multiple (gestation),
          specified NEC
      triplet —*see* Pregnancy, triplet
      twin —*see* Pregnancy, twin
    musculoskeletal condition (conditions is
        M00-M99) O99.89
    necrosis, liver (conditions in K72) O26.61-
    neoplasm
      benign
        cervix O34.4-
        corpus uteri O34.1-
        uterus O34.1-
      malignant O9A.11-
    nephropathy NEC O26.83-
    nervous system condition (conditions in
        G00-G99) O99.35-
    nutritional diseases NEC O99.28-
    obesity (pre-existing) O99.21-
    obesity surgery status O99.84-
    oblique lie or presentation O32.2
    older mother —*see* Pregnancy, complicated
        by, elderly
    oligohydramnios O41.0-
      with premature rupture of
          membranes —*see also* Pregnancy,
          complicated by, premature rupture
          of membranes O42-
    onset (spontaneous) of labor after 37
        completed weeks of gestation but
        before 39 completed weeks gestation,
        with delivery by (planned) cesarean
        section O75.82
    oophoritis O23.52-
    overdose, drug —*see also* Table of Drugs
        and Chemicals, by drug, poisoning
        O9A.21-
    oversize fetus O33.5
    papyraceous fetus O31.0-
    pelvic inflammatory disease O99.89
    periodontal disease O99.61-
    peripheral neuritis O26.82-
    peritoneal (pelvic) adhesions O99.89
    phlebitis O22.9-
    phlebopathy O22.9-
    phlebothrombosis (superficial) O22.2-
      deep O22.3-
    placenta accreta O43.21-
    placenta increta O43.22-
    placenta percreta O43.23-
    placenta previa O44.0- ◀▥▥
      complete O44.0- ◀
        with hemorrhage O44.1- ◀
      marginal O44.2- ◀
        with hemorrhage O44.3- ◀
      partial O44.2- ◀
        with hemorrhage O44.3- ◀
        without hemorrhage O44.0-
    placental disorder O43.9-
      specified NEC O43.89-
    placental dysfunction O43.89-
    placental infarction O43.81-
    placental insufficiency O36.51-
    placental transfusion syndromes
      fetomaternal O43.01-
      fetus to fetus O43.02-
      maternofetal O43.01-
    placentitis O41.14-
    pneumonia O99.51-
    poisoning —*see also* Table of Drugs and
        Chemicals O9A.21-
    polyhydramnios O40-
    polymorphic eruption of pregnancy
        O26.86
    poor obstetric history NEC O09.29-

Pregnancy *(Continued)*
   complicated by *(Continued)*
      postmaturity (post-term) (40 to 42 weeks)
        O48.0
        more than 42 completed weeks gestation
          (prolonged) O48.1
      pre-eclampsia O14.9-
        mild O14.0-
        moderate O14.0-
        severe O14.1-
          with hemolysis, elevated liver
             enzymes and low platelet count
             (HELLP) O14.2-
      premature labor —*see* Pregnancy,
        complicated by, preterm labor
      premature rupture of membranes O42.90
        full-term, unspecified as to length of
          time between rupture and onset of
          labor O42.92 ◀
        with onset of labor
          within 24 hours O42.00
            after 37 weeks gestation O42.02
            at or after 37 weeks gestation, onset
              of labor within 24 hours of
              rupture O42.02 ◀
            pre-term (before 37 completed
              weeks of gestation) O42.01-
          after 24 hours O42.10
            after 37 weeks gestation O42.12
            at or after 37 weeks gestation, onset
              of labor more than 24 hours
              following rupture O42.12 ◀
            pre-term (before 37 completed
               weeks of gestation) O42.11-
          after 37 weeks gestation O42.92
          at or after 37 weeks gestation,
            unspecified as to length of time
            between rupture and onset of labor
            O42.92 ◀
          full-term O42.92
         pre-term (before 37 completed weeks of
           gestation) O42.91-
      premature separation of placenta —*see also*
        Abruptio placentae O45.9-
      presentation, fetal —*see* Delivery,
        complicated by, malposition
      preterm delivery O60.10
      preterm labor
        with delivery O60.10
          preterm O60.10
          term O60.20
        second trimester
          with preterm delivery
            second trimester O60.12
            third trimester O60.13
          with term delivery O60.22
          without delivery O60.02
        third trimester
          with term delivery O60.23
          with third trimester preterm delivery
           O60.14
          without delivery O60.03
        without delivery O60.00
          second trimester O60.02
          third trimester O60.03
      previous history of —*see* Pregnancy,
        supervision of, high-risk
      prolapse, uterus O34.52-
      proteinuria (gestational) —*see also*
        Proteinuria, gestational O12.1- ◀▥
        with edema O12.2-
      pruritic urticarial papules and plaques of
        pregnancy (PUPPP) O26.86
      pruritus (neurogenic) O26.89-
      psychosis or psychoneurosis (puerperal)
        F53
      ptyalism O26.89-
      PUPPP (pruritic urticarial papules and
        plaques of pregnancy) O26.86
      pyelitis O23.0-
      recurrent pregnancy loss O26.2-

Pregnancy *(Continued)*
   complicated by *(Continued)*
      renal disease or failure NEC O26.83-
        with secondary hypertension, pre-
          existing —*see* Hypertension,
          complicating, pregnancy, pre-
          existing, secondary
        hypertensive, pre-existing —*see*
          Hypertension, complicating,
          pregnancy, pre-existing, with, renal
          disease
      respiratory condition (conditions in
        J00-J99) O99.51-
      retained, retention
        dead ovum O02.0
        intrauterine contraceptive device
          O26.3-
      retroversion, uterus O34.53-
      Rh immunization, incompatibility or
        sensitization NEC O36.09-
        anti-D antibody O36.01-
      rupture
        amnion (premature) —*see also*
          Pregnancy, complicated by,
          premature rupture of membranes
          O42-
        membranes (premature) —*see also*
          Pregnancy, complicated by,
          premature rupture of membranes
          O42-
        uterus (during labor) O71.1
          before onset of labor O71.0-
      salivation (excessive) O26.89-
      salpingitis O23.52-
      salpingo-oophoritis O23.52-
      sepsis (conditions in A40, A41) O98.81-
      size date discrepancy (uterine) O26.84-
      skin condition (conditions in L00-L99)
        O99.71-
      smoking (tobacco) O99.33-
      social problem O09.7-
      specified condition NEC O26.89-
      spotting O26.85-
      streptococcus B carrier state O99.820
      streptococcus group B (GBS) carrier state
        O99.820 ◀
      subluxation of symphysis (pubis) O26.71-
      syphilis (conditions in A50-A53) O98.11-
      threatened
        abortion O20.0
        labor O47.9
          at or after 37 completed weeks of
            gestation O47.1
          before 37 completed weeks of
            gestation O47.0-
      thrombophlebitis (superficial) O22.2-
      thrombosis O22.9-
        cerebral venous O22.5-
        cerebrovenous sinus O22.5-
        deep O22.3-
      tobacco use disorder (smoking) O99.33- ◀
      torsion of uterus O34.59-
      toxemia O14.9-
      transverse lie or presentation O32.2
      tuberculosis (conditions in A15-A19) O98.01-
      tumor (benign)
        cervix O34.4-
          malignant O9A.11-
        uterus O34.1-
      unstable lie O32.0
      upper respiratory infection O99.51-
      urethritis O23.2-
      uterine size date discrepancy O26.84-
      vaginitis or vulvitis O23.59-
      varicose veins (lower extremities) O22.0-
        genitals O22.1-
        legs O22.0-
        perineal O22.1-
        vaginal or vulval O22.1-
      venereal disease NEC (conditions in A63.8)
        O98.31-

Pregnancy *(Continued)*
   complicated by *(Continued)*
      venous disorders O22.9-
        specified NEC O22.8X-
      very young mother —*see* Pregnancy,
        complicated by, young mother
      viral diseases (conditions in A80-B09,
        B25-B34) O98.51-
      vomiting O21.9
        due to diseases classified elsewhere O21.8
        hyperemesis gravidarum (mild) —*see*
          also Hyperemesis, gravidarum
          O21.0-
        late (occurring after 20 weeks of
          gestation) O21.2
      young mother
        multigravida O09.62-
        primigravida O09.61-
   concealed O09.3-
   continuing following
      elective fetal reduction of one or more fetus
        O31.3-
      intrauterine death of one or more fetus
        O31.2-
      spontaneous abortion of one or more fetus
        O31.1-
   cornual O00.80 ◀▥
      with intrauterine pregnancy O00.81 ◀
   ectopic (ruptured) O00.90 ◀▥
      with intrauterine pregnancy O00.91 ◀
      abdominal O00.00 ◀▥
        with viable fetus O36.7-
        with ◀
          intrauterine pregnancy O00.01 ◀
          viable fetus O36.7- ◀
      cervical O00.80 ◀▥
        with intrauterine pregnancy O00.81 ◀
   complicated (by) O08.9
      afibrinogenemia O08.1
      cardiac arrest O08.81
      chemical damage of pelvic organ (s)
        O08.6
      circulatory collapse O08.3
      defibrination syndrome O08.1
      electrolyte imbalance O08.5
      embolism (amniotic fluid) (blood clot)
        (pulmonary) (septic) O08.2
      endometritis O08.0
      genital tract and pelvic infection O08.0
      hemorrhage (delayed) (excessive) O08.1
      infection
        genital tract or pelvic O08.0
        kidney 008.83
        urinary tract O08.83
      intravascular coagulation O08.1
      laceration of pelvic organ (s)
        O08.6
      metabolic disorder O08.5
      oliguria O08.4
      oophoritis O08.0
      parametritis O08.0
      pelvic peritonitis O08.0
      perforation of pelvic organ (s)
        O08.6
      renal failure or shutdown O08.4
      salpingitis or salpingo-oophoritis
        O08.0
      sepsis O08.82
      shock O08.83
        septic O08.82
      specified condition NEC O08.89
      tubular necrosis (renal) O08.4
      uremia O08.4
      urinary infection O08.83
      venous complication NEC O08.7
        embolism O08.2
   cornual O00.80 ◀▥
      with intrauterine pregnancy O00.81 ◀
   intraligamentous O00.80 ◀▥
      with intrauterine pregnancy
        O00.81 ◀

◀ New   ◀▥ Revised   ~~deleted~~ Deleted

Pregnancy *(Continued)*
  complicated by *(Continued)*
    mural O00.80 ◀▥
      with intrauterine pregnancy O00.81 ◀
    ovarian O00.20 ▥
      with intrauterine pregnancy O00.21 ◀
    specified site NEC O00.80 ◀▥
      with intrauterine pregnancy O00.81 ◀
    tubal (ruptured) O00.10 ◀▥
      with intrauterine pregnancy O00.11 ◀
  examination (normal) Z34.9-
    first Z34.0-
    high-risk —*see* Pregnancy, supervision of,
      high-risk
    specified Z34.8-
  extrauterine —*see* Pregnancy, ectopic
  fallopian O00.10 ▥
    with intrauterine pregnancy O00.11 ◀
  false F45.8
  gestational carrier Z33.3 ◀
  hidden O09.3-
  high-risk —*see* Pregnancy, supervision of,
    high-risk
  incidental finding Z33.1
  interstitial O00.80 ◀▥
    with intrauterine pregnancy O00.81 ◀
  intraligamentous O00.80 ◀▥
    with intrauterine pregnancy O00.81 ◀
  intramural O00.80 ◀▥
    with intrauterine pregnancy O00.81 ◀
  intraperitoneal O00.00 ◀▥
    with intrauterine pregnancy O00.01 ◀
  isthmian O00.10 ◀▥
    with intrauterine pregnancy O00.11 ◀
  mesometric (mural) O00.80 ◀▥
    with intrauterine pregnancy O00.81 ◀
  molar NEC O02.0
    complicated (by) O08.9
      afibrinogenemia O08.1
      cardiac arrest O08.81
      chemical damage of pelvic organ (s)
        O08.6
      circulatory collapse O08.3
      defibrination syndrome O08.1
      electrolyte imbalance O08.5
      embolism (amniotic fluid) (blood clot)
        (pulmonary) (septic) O08.2
      endometritis O08.0
      genital tract and pelvic infection
        O08.0
      hemorrhage (delayed) (excessive)
        O08.1
      infection
        genital tract or pelvic O08.0
        kidney O08.83
        urinary tract O08.83
      intravascular coagulation O08.1
      laceration of pelvic organ (s)
        O08.6
      metabolic disorder O08.5
      oliguria O08.4
      oophoritis O08.0
      parametritis O08.0
      pelvic peritonitis O08.0
      perforation of pelvic organ (s) O08.6
      renal failure or shutdown O08.4
      salpingitis or salpingo-oophoritis O08.0
      sepsis O08.82
      shock O08.3
        septic O08.82
      specified condition NEC O08.89
      tubular necrosis (renal) O08.4
      uremia O08.4
      urinary infection O08.83
      venous complication NEC O08.7
        embolism O08.2
  hydatidiform —*see also* Mole, hydatidiform
    O01.9-
  multiple (gestation) O30.9-
    greater than quadruplets —*see* Pregnancy,
      multiple (gestation), specified NEC

Pregnancy *(Continued)*
  multiple (gestation) *(Continued)*
    specified NEC O30.80-
      with
        two or more monoamniotic fetuses
          O30.82-
        two or more monochorionic fetuses
          O30.81-
      two or more monoamniotic fetuses
        O30.82-
      two or more monochorionic fetuses
        O30.81-
      unable to determine number of placenta
        and number of amniotic sacs
        O30.89-
      unspecified number of placenta and
        unspecified number of amniotic
        sacs O30.80-
    mural O00.80 ◀▥
      with intrauterine pregnancy O00.81 ◀
    normal (supervision of) Z34.9-
      first Z34.0-
      high-risk —*see* Pregnancy, supervision of,
        high-risk
      specified Z34.8-
    ovarian O00.20 ▥
      with intrauterine pregnancy O00.21 ◀
    postmature (40 to 42 weeks) O48.0
      more than 42 weeks gestation O48.1
    post-term (40 to 42 weeks) O48.0
    prenatal care only Z34.9-
      first Z34.0-
      high-risk —*see* Pregnancy, supervision of,
        high-risk
      specified Z34.8-
    prolonged (more than 42 weeks gestation)
      O48.1
    quadruplet O30.20-
      with
        two or more monoamniotic fetuses
          O30.22-
        two or more monochorionic fetuses
          O30.21-
      two or more monoamniotic fetuses
        O30.22-
      two or more monochorionic fetuses
        O30.21-
      unable to determine number of placenta
        and number of amniotic sacs O30.29-
      unspecified number of placenta and
        unspecified number of amniotic sacs
        O30.20-
    quintuplet —*see* Pregnancy, multiple
      (gestation), specified NEC
    sextuplet —*see* Pregnancy, multiple
      (gestation), specified NEC
  supervision of
    concealed pregnancy O09.3-
    elderly mother
      multigravida O09.52-
      primigravida O09.51-
    hidden pregnancy O09.3-
    high-risk O09.9-
      due to (history of)
        ectopic pregnancy O09.1-
        elderly —*see* Pregnancy, supervision,
          elderly mother
        grand multiparity O09.4
        infertility O09.0-
        insufficient prenatal care O09.3-
        in utero procedure during previous
          pregnancy O09.82-
        in vitro fertilization O09.81-
        molar pregnancy O09.A- ◀▥
        multiple previous pregnancies O09.4-
        older mother —*see* Pregnancy,
          supervision of, elderly mother
        poor reproductive or obstetric history
          NEC O09.29-
        pre-term labor O09.21-
        previous
          neonatal death O09.29-

Pregnancy *(Continued)*
  supervision of *(Continued)*
    high-risk *(Continued)*
      due to *(Continued)*
        social problems O09.7-
        specified NEC O09.89-
        very young mother —*see* Pregnancy,
          supervision, young mother
      resulting from in vitro fertilization
        O09.81-
    normal Z34.9-
      first Z34.0-
      specified NEC Z34.8-
    young mother
      multigravida O09.62-
      primigravida O09.61-
  triplet O30.10-
    with
      two or more monoamniotic fetuses
        O30.12-
      two or more monochorionic fetuses
        O30.11-
    two or more monoamniotic fetuses O30.12-
    two or more monochorionic fetuses O30.11-
    unable to determine number of placenta
      and number of amniotic sacs O30.19-
    unspecified number of placenta and
      unspecified number of amniotic sacs
      O30.10-
  tubal (with abortion) (with rupture) O00.10 ◀▥
    with intrauterine pregnancy O00.11 ◀
  twin O30.00-
    conjoined O30.02-
    dichorionic/diamniotic (two placenta, two
      amniotic sacs) O30.04-
    monochorionic/diamniotic (one placenta,
      two amniotic sacs) O30.03-
    monochorionic/monoamniotic (one
      placenta, one amniotic sac) O30.01-
    unable to determine number of placenta
      and number of amniotic sacs O30.09-
    unspecified number of placenta and
      unspecified number of amniotic sacs
      O30.00-
  unwanted Z64.0
  weeks of gestation
    8 weeks Z3A.08
    9 weeks Z3A.09
    10 weeks Z3A.10
    11 weeks Z3A.11
    12 weeks Z3A.12
    13 weeks Z3A.13
    14 weeks Z3A.14
    15 weeks Z3A.15
    16 weeks Z3A.16
    17 weeks Z3A.17
    18 weeks Z3A.18
    19 weeks Z3A.19
    20 weeks Z3A.20
    21 weeks Z3A.21
    22 weeks Z3A.22
    23 weeks Z3A.23
    24 weeks Z3A.24
    25 weeks Z3A.25
    26 weeks Z3A.26
    27 weeks Z3A.27
    28 weeks Z3A.28
    29 weeks Z3A.29
    30 weeks Z3A.30
    31 weeks Z3A.31
    32 weeks Z3A.32
    33 weeks Z3A.33
    34 weeks Z3A.34
    35 weeks Z3A.35
    36 weeks Z3A.36
    37 weeks Z3A.37
    38 weeks Z3A.38
    39 weeks Z3A.39
    40 weeks Z3A.40
    41 weeks Z3A.41
    42 weeks Z3A.42

Pregnancy *(Continued)*
  weeks of gestation *(Continued)*
    greater than 42 weeks Z3A.49
    less than 8 weeks Z3A.01
    not specified Z3A.00
Preiser's disease —*see* Osteonecrosis,
    secondary, due to, trauma, metacarpus
Pre-kwashiorkor —*see* Malnutrition, severe
Preleukemia (syndrome) D46.9
Preluxation, hip, congenital Q65.6
Premature —*see also* condition
  adrenarche E27.0
  aging E34.8
  beats I49.40
    atrial I49.1
    auricular I49.1
    supraventricular I49.1
  birth NEC —*see* Preterm, newborn
  closure, foramen ovale Q21.8
  contraction
    atrial I49.1
    atrioventricular I49.49
    auricular I49.1
    auriculoventricular I49.2
    heart (extrasystole) I49.49
    junctional I49.2
    ventricular I49.3
  delivery —*see also* Pregnancy, complicated by,
    preterm labor O60.10
  ejaculation F52.4
  infant NEC —*see* Preterm, newborn
    light-for-dates —*see* Light for dates
  labor —*see* Pregnancy, complicated by,
    preterm labor
  lungs P28.0
  menopause E28.319
    asymptomatic E28.319
    symptomatic E28.310
  newborn
    extreme (less than 28 completed weeks) —
      see Immaturity, extreme
    less than 37 completed weeks —*see*
      Preterm, newborn
  puberty E30.1
  rupture membranes or amnion —*see*
    Pregnancy, complicated by, premature
    rupture of membranes
  senility E34.8
  thelarche E30.8
  ventricular systole I49.3
Prematurity NEC (less than 37 completed
  weeks) —*see* Preterm, newborn
  extreme (less than 28 completed weeks) —*see*
    Immaturity, extreme
Premenstrual
  dysphoric disorder (PMDD) F32.81 ◀▥
  tension (syndrome) N94.3
Premolarization, cuspids K00.2
Prenatal
  care, normal pregnancy —*see* Pregnancy,
    normal
  screening of mother Z36
  teeth K00.6
Preparatory care for subsequent treatment
  NEC
  for dialysis Z49.01
    peritoneal Z49.02
Prepartum —*see* condition
Preponderance, left or right ventricular I51.7
Prepuce —*see* condition
PRES (posterior reversible encephalopathy
  syndrome) I67.83
Presbycardia R54
Presbycusis, presbyacusia H91.1-
Presbyesophagus K22.8
Presbyophrenia F03
Presbyopia H52.4
Prescription of contraceptives (initial) Z30.019
  barrier Z30.018 ◀
  diaphragm Z30.018 ◀
  emergency (postcoital) Z30.012

Prescription of contraceptives *(Continued)*
  implantable subdermal Z30.017 ◀▥
  injectable Z30.013
  intrauterine contraceptive device Z30.014
  pills Z30.011
  postcoital (emergency) Z30.012
  repeat Z30.40
    barrier Z30.49 ◀
    diaphragm Z30.49 ◀
    implantable subdermal Z30.46 ◀▥
    injectable Z30.42
    pills Z30.41
    specified type NEC Z30.49
    transdermal patch hormonal Z30.45 ◀
    vaginal ring hormonal Z30.44 ◀
  specified type NEC Z30.018
    transdermal patch hormonal Z30.016 ◀
    vaginal ring hormonal Z30.015 ◀
Presence (of)
  ankle-joint implant (functional) (prosthesis)
    Z96.66-
  aortocoronary (bypass) graft Z95.1
  arterial-venous shunt (dialysis) Z99.2
  artificial
    eye (globe) Z97.0
    heart (fully implantable) (mechanical)
      Z95.812
      valve Z95.2
    larynx Z96.3
    lens (intraocular) Z96.1
    limb (complete) (partial) Z97.1-
      arm Z97.1-
        bilateral Z97.15
      leg Z97.1-
        bilateral Z97.16
  audiological implant (functional) Z96.29
  bladder implant (functional) Z96.0
  bone
    conduction hearing device Z96.29
    implant (functional) NEC Z96.7
    joint (prosthesis) —*see* Presence, joint
      implant
  cardiac
    defibrillator (functional) (with synchronous
      cardiac pacemaker)Z95.810
    implant or graft Z95.9
      specified type NEC Z95.818
    pacemaker Z95.0
    resynchronization therapy ◀
      defibrillator Z95.810 ◀
      pacemaker Z95.0 ◀
  cerebrospinal fluid drainage device Z98.2
  cochlear implant (functional) Z96.21
  contact lens (es) Z97.3
  coronary artery graft or prosthesis Z95.5
  CRT-D (cardiac resynchronization therapy
    defibrillator) Z95.810 ◀
  CRT-P (cardiac resynchronization therapy
    pacemaker) Z95.0 ◀
  cardioverter-defibrillator (ICD) Z95.810 ◀
  CSF shunt Z98.2
  dental prosthesis device Z97.2
  dentures Z97.2
  device (external) NEC Z97.8
    cardiac NEC Z95.818
    heart assist Z95.811
    implanted (functional) Z96.9
      specified NEC Z96.89
    prosthetic Z97.8
  ear implant Z96.20
    cochlear implant Z96.21
    myringotomy tube Z96.22
    specified type NEC Z96.29
  elbow-joint implant (functional) (prosthesis)
    Z96.62-
  endocrine implant (functional) NEC Z96.49
  eustachian tube stent or device (functional)
    Z96.29
  external hearing-aid or device Z97.4
  finger-joint implant (functional) (prosthetic)
    Z96.69-

Presence *(Continued)*
  functional implant Z96.9
    specified NEC Z96.89
  graft
    cardiac NEC Z95.818
    vascular NEC Z95.828
  hearing-aid or device (external) Z97.4
    implant (bone) (cochlear) (functional)
      Z96.21
  heart assist device Z95.811
  heart valve implant (functional) Z95.2
    prosthetic Z95.2
    specified type NEC Z95.4
    xenogenic Z95.3
  hip-joint implant (functional) (prosthesis)
    Z96.64-
  ICD (cardioverter-defibrillator) Z95.810 ◀
  implanted device (artificial) (functional)
    (prosthetic) Z96.9
    automatic cardiac defibrillator (with
      synchronous cardiac pacemaker)
      Z95.810
    cardiac pacemaker Z95.0
    cochlear Z96.21
    dental Z96.5
    heart Z95.812
    heart valve Z95.2
      prosthetic Z95.2
      specified NEC Z95.4
      xenogenic Z95.3
    insulin pump Z96.41
    intraocular lens Z96.1
    joint Z96.60
      ankle Z96.66-
      elbow Z96.62-
      finger Z96.69-
      hip Z96.64-
      knee Z96.65-
      shoulder Z96.61-
      specified NEC Z96.698
      wrist Z96.63-
    larynx Z96.3
    myringotomy tube Z96.22
    otological Z96.20
      cochlear Z96.21
      eustachian stent Z96.29
      myringotomy Z96.22
      specified NEC Z96.29
      stapes Z96.29
    skin Z96.81
    skull plate Z96.7
    specified NEC Z96.89
    urogenital Z96.0
  insulin pump (functional) Z96.41
  intestinal bypass or anastomosis Z98.0
  intraocular lens (functional) Z96.1
  intrauterine contraceptive device (IUD) Z97.5
  intravascular implant (functional) (prosthetic)
    NEC Z95.9
    coronary artery Z95.5
    defibrillator (with synchronous cardiac
      pacemaker) Z95.810
    peripheral vessel (with angioplasty)
      Z95.820
  joint implant (prosthetic) (any) Z96.60
    ankle —*see* Presence, ankle joint implant
    elbow —*see* Presence, elbow joint implant
    finger —*see* Presence, finger joint implant
    hip —*see* Presence, hip joint implant
    knee —*see* Presence, knee joint implant
    shoulder —*see* Presence, shoulder joint
      implant
    specified joint NEC Z96.698
    wrist —*see* Presence, wrist joint implant
  knee-joint implant (functional) (prosthesis)
    Z96.65-
  laryngeal implant (functional) Z96.3
  mandibular implant (dental) Z96.5
  myringotomy tube (s) Z96.22
  orthopedic-joint implant (prosthetic) (any) —
    see Presence, joint implant

◀ New   ◀▥ Revised   ~~deleted~~ Deleted

Presence *(Continued)*
  otological implant (functional) Z96.29
  shoulder-joint implant (functional)
      (prosthesis) Z96.61-
  skull-plate implant Z96.7
  spectacles Z97.3
  stapes implant (functional) Z96.29
  systemic lupus erythematosus [SLE] inhibitor
      D68.62
  tendon implant (functional) (graft) Z96.7
  tooth root (s) implant Z96.5
  ureteral stent Z96.0
  urethral stent Z96.0
  urogenital implant (functional) Z96.0
  vascular implant or device Z95.9
      access port device Z95.828
      specified type NEC Z95.828
  wrist-joint implant (functional) (prosthesis)
      Z96.63-
Presenile —*see also* condition
  dementia F03
  premature aging E34.8
Presentation, fetal —*see* Delivery, complicated
      by, malposition
Prespondylolisthesis (congenital) Q76.2
Pressure
  area, skin —*see* Ulcer, pressure, by site
  brachial plexus G54.0
  brain G93.5
      injury at birth NEC P11.1
  cerebral —*see* Pressure, brain
  chest R07.89
  cone, tentorial G93.5
  hyposystolic —*see also* Hypotension
      incidental reading, without diagnosis of
          hypotension R03.1
  increased
      intracranial (benign) G93.2
          injury at birth P11.0
      intraocular H40.05-
  lumbosacral plexus G54.1
  mediastinum J98.59 ◀▥
  necrosis (chronic) —*see* Ulcer, pressure,
      by site
  parental, inappropriate (excessive) Z62.6
  sore (chronic) —*see* Ulcer, pressure,
      by site
  spinal cord G95.20
  ulcer (chronic) —*see* Ulcer, pressure,
      by site
  venous, increased I87.8
Pre-syncope R55
Preterm
  delivery (*see also* Pregnancy, complicated by,
      preterm labor) O60.10
  labor —*see* Pregnancy, complicated by,
      preterm labor
  newborn (infant) P07.30
      gestational age
          28 completed weeks (28 weeks, 0 days
              through 28 weeks, 6 days) P07.31
          29 completed weeks (29 weeks, 0 days
              through 29 weeks, 6 days) P07.32
          30 completed weeks (30 weeks, 0 days
              through 30 weeks, 6 days) P07.33
          31 completed weeks (31 weeks, 0 days
              through 31 weeks, 6 days) P07.34
          32 completed weeks (32 weeks, 0 days
              through 32 weeks, 6 days) P07.35
          33 completed weeks (33 weeks, 0 days
              through 33 weeks, 6 days) P07.36
          34 completed weeks (34 weeks, 0 days
              through 34 weeks, 6 days) P07.37
          35 completed weeks (35 weeks, 0 days
              through 35 weeks, 6 days) P07.38
          36 completed weeks (36 weeks, 0 days
              through 36 weeks, 6 days) P07.39
Previa
  placenta (total) (without hemorrhage)
      O44.0- ◀▥
      ~~without hemorrhage O44.0-~~

Previa *(Continued)*
  placenta *(Continued)*
      with hemorrhage O44.1- ◀
      complete O44.0- ◀
          with hemorrhage O44.1- ◀
      low —*see also* Delivery, complicated, by,
          placenta, low O44.4- ◀
          with hemorrhage O44.5- ◀
      marginal O44.2- ◀
          with hemorrhage O44.3- ◀
      partial O44.2- ◀
          with hemorrhage O44.3- ◀
  vasa O69.4
Priapism N48.30
  due to
      disease classified elsewhere N48.32
      drug N48.33
      specified cause NEC N48.39
      trauma N48.31
Prickling sensation (skin) R20.2
Prickly heat L74.0
Primary —*see* condition
Primigravida
  elderly, affecting management of pregnancy,
      labor and delivery (supervision only) —
      see Pregnancy, complicated by, elderly,
      primigravida
  older, affecting management of pregnancy,
      labor and delivery (supervision only) —
      see Pregnancy, complicated by, elderly,
      primigravida
  very young, affecting management of
      pregnancy, labor and delivery
      (supervision only) —*see* Pregnancy,
      complicated by, young mother,
      primigravida
Primipara
  elderly, affecting management of pregnancy,
      labor and delivery (supervision only) —
      see Pregnancy, complicated by, elderly,
      primigravida
  older, affecting management of pregnancy,
      labor and delivery (supervision only) —
      see Pregnancy, complicated by, elderly,
      primigravida
  very young, affecting management of
      pregnancy, labor and delivery
      (supervision only) —*see* Pregnancy,
      complicated by, young mother,
      primigravida
Primus varus (bilateral) Q66.2
PRIND (Prolonged reversible ischemic
      neurologic deficit) I63.9
Pringle's disease (tuberous sclerosis) Q85.1
Prinzmetal angina I20.1
Prizefighter ear —*see* Cauliflower ear
Problem (with) (related to)
  academic Z55.8
  acculturation Z60.3
  adjustment (to)
      change of job Z56.1
      life-cycle transition Z60.0
      pension Z60.0
      retirement Z60.0
  adopted child Z62.821
  alcoholism in family Z63.72
  atypical parenting situation Z62.9
  bankruptcy Z59.8
  behavioral (adult) F69
      drug seeking Z76.5 ◀▥
  birth of sibling affecting child Z62.898
  care (of)
      provider dependency Z74.9
          specified NEC Z74.8
      sick or handicapped person in family or
          household Z63.6
  child
      abuse (affecting the child) —*see*
          Maltreatment, child
      custody or support proceedings Z65.3
      in care of non-parental family member
          Z62.21

Problem *(Continued)*
  child *(Continued)*
      in foster care Z62.21
      in welfare custody Z62.21
      living in orphanage or group home Z62.22
  child-rearing Z62.9
      specified NEC Z62.898
  communication (developmental) F80.9
  conflict or discord (with)
      boss Z56.4
      classmates Z55.4
      counselor Z64.4
      employer Z56.4
      family Z63.9
          specified NEC Z63.8
      probation officer Z64.4
      social worker Z64.4
      teachers Z55.4
      workmates Z56.4
  conviction in legal proceedings Z65.0
      with imprisonment Z65.1
  counselor Z64.4
  creditors Z59.8
  digestive K92.9
  drug addict in family Z63.72
  ear —*see* Disorder, ear
  economic Z59.9
      affecting care Z59.9
      specified NEC Z59.8
  education Z55.9
      specified NEC Z55.8
  employment Z56.9
      change of job Z56.1
      discord Z56.4
      environment Z56.5
      sexual harassment Z56.81
      specified NEC Z56.89
      stress NEC Z56.6
      stressful schedule Z56.3
      threat of job loss Z56.2
      unemployment Z56.0
  enuresis, child F98.0
  eye H57.9
  failed examinations (school) Z55.2
  falling Z91.81
  family —*see also* Disruption, family Z63.9-
      specified NEC Z63.8
  feeding (elderly) (infant) R63.3
      newborn P92.9
          breast P92.5
          overfeeding P92.4
          slow P92.2
          specified NEC P92.8
          underfeeding P92.3
      nonorganic F50.89 ◀▥
  finance Z59.9
      specified NEC Z59.8
  foreclosure on loan Z59.8
  foster child Z62.822
  frightening experience (s) in childhood
      Z62.898
  genital NEC
      female N94.9
      male N50.9
  health care Z75.9
      specified NEC Z75.8
  hearing —*see* Deafness
  homelessness Z59.0
  housing Z59.9
      inadequate Z59.1
      isolated Z59.8
      specified NEC Z59.8
  identity (of childhood) F93.8
  illegitimate pregnancy (unwanted) Z64.0
  illiteracy Z55.0
  impaired mobility Z74.09
  imprisonment or incarceration Z65.1
  inadequate teaching affecting education
      Z55.8
  inappropriate (excessive) parental pressure
      Z62.6

Problem (*Continued*)
- influencing health status NEC Z78.9
- in-law Z63.1
- institutionalization, affecting child Z62.22
- intrafamilial communication Z63.8
- jealousy, child F93.8
- landlord Z59.2
- language (developmental) F80.9
- learning (developmental) F81.9
- legal Z65.3
  - conviction without imprisonment Z65.0
  - imprisonment Z65.1
  - release from prison Z65.2
- life-management Z73.9
  - specified NEC Z73.89
- life-style Z72.9
  - gambling Z72.6
  - high-risk sexual behavior (heterosexual) Z72.51
    - bisexual Z72.53
    - homosexual Z72.52
  - inappropriate eating habits Z72.4
  - self-damaging behavior NEC Z72.89
  - specified NEC Z72.89
  - tobacco use Z72.0
- literacy Z55.9
  - low level Z55.0
  - specified NEC Z55.8
- living alone Z60.2
- lodgers Z59.2
- loss of love relationship in childhood Z62.898
- marital Z63.0
  - involving
    - divorce Z63.5
    - estrangement Z63.5
    - gender identity F66
- mastication K08.89 ◀▥
- medical
  - care, within family Z63.6
  - facilities Z75.9
    - specified NEC Z75.8
- mental F48.9
- multiparity Z64.1
- negative life events in childhood Z62.9
  - altered pattern of family relationships Z62.898
  - frightening experience Z62.898
  - loss of
    - love relationship Z62.898
    - self-esteem Z62.898
  - physical abuse (alleged) —*see* Maltreatment, child
  - removal from home Z62.29
  - specified event NEC Z62.898
- neighbor Z59.2
- neurological NEC R29.818
- new step-parent affecting child Z62.898
- none (feared complaint unfounded) Z71.1
- occupational NEC Z56.89
- parent-child —*see* Conflict, parent-child
- personal hygiene Z91.89
- personality F69
- phase-of-life transition, adjustment Z60.0
- presence of sick or disabled person in family or household Z63.79
  - needing care Z63.6
- primary support group (family) Z63.9
  - specified NEC Z63.8
- probation officer Z64.4
- psychiatric F99
- psychosexual (development) F66
- psychosocial Z65.9
  - specified NEC Z65.8
- relationship Z63.9
  - childhood F93.8
- release from prison Z65.2
- removal from home affecting child Z62.29

Problem (*Continued*)
- seeking and accepting known hazardous and harmful
  - behavioral or psychological interventions Z65.8
  - chemical, nutritional or physical interventions Z65.8
- sexual function (nonorganic) F52.9
- sight H54.7
- sleep disorder, child F51.9
- smell —*see* Disturbance, sensation, smell
- social
  - environment Z60.9
    - specified NEC Z60.8
  - exclusion and rejection Z60.4
  - worker Z64.4
- speech R47.9
  - developmental F80.9
  - specified NEC R47.89
- swallowing —*see* Dysphagia
- taste —*see* Disturbance, sensation, taste
- tic, child F95.0
- underachievement in school Z55.3
- unemployment Z56.0
  - threatened Z56.2
- unwanted pregnancy Z64.0
- upbringing Z62.9
  - specified NEC Z62.898
- urinary N39.9
- voice production R47.89
- work schedule (stressful) Z56.3

Procedure (surgical)
- converted ◀
  - arthroscopic to open Z53.33 ◀
  - laparoscopic to open Z53.31 ◀
  - specified procedure NEC to open Z53.39 ◀
  - thoracoscopic to open Z53.32 ◀
- for purpose other than remedying health state Z41.9
  - specified NEC Z41.8
- not done Z53.9
  - because of
    - administrative reasons Z53.8
    - contraindication Z53.09
      - smoking Z53.01
    - patient's decision Z53.20
      - for reasons of belief or group pressure Z53.1
      - left against medical advice (AMA) Z53.21
      - specified reason NEC Z53.29
    - specified reason NEC Z53.8

Procidentia (uteri) N81.3

Proctalgia K62.89
- fugax K59.4
- spasmodic K59.4

Proctitis K62.89
- amebic (acute) A06.0
- chlamydial A56.3
- gonococcal A54.6
- granulomatous —*see* Enteritis, regional, large intestine
- herpetic A60.1
- radiation K62.7
- tuberculous A18.32
- ulcerative (chronic) K51.20
  - with
    - complication K51.219
      - abscess K51.214
      - fistula K51.213
      - obstruction K51.212
      - rectal bleeding K51.211
      - specified NEC K51.218

Proctocele
- female (without uterine prolapse) N81.6
  - with uterine prolapse N81.2
    - complete N81.3
- male K62.3

Proctocolitis, mucosal —*see* Rectosigmoiditis, ulcerative

Proctocolitis ◀
- food-induced eosinophilic K52.82 ◀
- food protein-induced K52.82 ◀
- milk protein-induced K52.82 ◀
- mucosal —*see* Rectosigmoiditis, ulcerative ◀

Proctoptosis K62.3

Proctorrhagia K62.5

Proctosigmoiditis K63.89
- ulcerative (chronic) —*see* Rectosigmoiditis, ulcerative

Proctospasm K59.4
- psychogenic F45.8

Profichet's disease —*see* Disorder, soft tissue, specified type NEC

Progeria E34.8

Prognathism (mandibular) (maxillary) M26.19

Progonoma (melanotic) —*see* Neoplasm, benign, by site

Progressive —*see* condition

Prolactinoma
- specified site —*see* Neoplasm, benign, by site
- unspecified site D35.2

Prolapse, prolapsed
- anus, anal (canal) (sphincter) K62.2
- arm or hand O32.2
  - causing obstructed labor O64.4
- bladder (mucosa) (sphincter) (acquired)
  - congenital Q79.4
  - female —*see* Cystocele
  - male N32.89
- breast implant (prosthetic) T85.49
- cecostomy K94.09
- cecum K63.4
- cervix, cervical (hypertrophied) N81.2
  - anterior lip, obstructing labor O65.5
  - congenital Q51.828
  - postpartal, old N81.2
  - stump N81.85
- ciliary body (traumatic) —*see* Laceration, eye(ball), with prolapse or loss of interocular tissue
- colon (pedunculated) K63.4
- colostomy K94.09
- disc (intervertebral) —*see* Displacement, intervertebral disc
- eye implant (orbital) T85.398
  - lens (ocular) —*see* Complications, intraocular lens
- fallopian tube N83.4- ◀▥
- gastric (mucosa) K31.89
- genital, female N81.9
  - specified NEC N81.89
- globe, nontraumatic —*see* Luxation, globe
- ileostomy bud K94.19
- intervertebral disc —*see* Displacement, intervertebral disc
- intestine (small) K63.4
- iris (traumatic) —*see* Laceration, eye(ball), with prolapse or loss of interocular tissue
  - nontraumatic H21.89
- kidney N28.83
  - congenital Q63.2
- laryngeal muscles or ventricle J38.7
- liver K76.89
- meatus urinarius N36.8
- mitral (valve) I34.1
- ocular lens implant —*see* Complications, intraocular lens
- organ or site, congenital NEC —*see* Malposition, congenital
- ovary N83.4- ◀▥
- pelvic floor, female N81.89
- perineum, female N81.89
- rectum (mucosa) (sphincter) K62.3
  - due to trichuris trichuria B79
- spleen D73.89
- stomach K31.89
- umbilical cord
  - complicating delivery O69.0

◀ New   ◀▥ Revised   ~~deleted~~ Deleted

Prolapse, prolapsed *(Continued)*
 urachus, congenital Q64.4
 ureter N28.89
  with obstruction N13.5
   with infection N13.6
 ureterovesical orifice N28.89
 urethra (acquired) (infected) (mucosa)
   N36.8
  congenital Q64.71
 urinary meatus N36.8
  congenital Q64.72
 uterovaginal N81.4
  complete N81.3
  incomplete N81.2
 uterus (with prolapse of vagina) N81.4
  complete N81.3
  congenital Q51.818
  first degree N81.2
  in pregnancy or childbirth —*see*
    Pregnancy, complicated by,
    abnormal, uterus
  incomplete N81.2
  postpartal (old) N81.4
  second degree N81.2
  third degree N81.3
 uveal (traumatic) —*see* Laceration, eye(ball),
   with prolapse or loss of interocular
   tissue
 vagina (anterior) (wall) —*see* Cystocele
  with prolapse of uterus N81.4
   complete N81.3
   incomplete N81.2
  posterior wall N81.6
  posthysterectomy N99.3
 vitreous (humor) H43.0-
  in wound —*see* Laceration, eye(ball), with
    prolapse or loss of interocular tissue
 womb —*see* Prolapse, uterus
Prolapsus, female N81.9
 specified NEC N81.89
Proliferation (s)
 primary cutaneous CD30-positive large T-cell
   C86.6
 prostate, atypical small acinar N42.32 ◀
Proliferative —*see* condition
Prolonged, prolongation (of)
 bleeding (time) (idiopathic) R79.1
 coagulation (time) R79.1
 gestation (over 42 completed weeks)
  mother O48.1
  newborn P08.22
 interval I44.0
 labor O63.9
  first stage O63.0
  second stage O63.1
 partial thromboplastin time (PTT) R79.1
 pregnancy (more than 42 weeks gestation)
   O48.1
 prothrombin time R79.1
 QT interval I45.81
 uterine contractions in labor O62.4
Prominence, prominent
 with disproportion (fetopelvic) O33.0
  causing obstructed labor O65.0
 auricle (congenital) (ear) Q17.5
 ischial spine or sacral promontory
 nose (congenital) acquired M95.0
Promiscuity —*see* High, risk, sexual behavior
Pronation
 ankle —*see* Deformity, limb, foot, specified
   NEC
 foot —*see also* Deformity, limb, foot, specified
   NEC
  congenital Q74.2
Prophylactic
 administration of
  antibiotics, long-term Z79.2
   short-term use - omit code
  drug —*see also* Long-term (current) drug
    therapy (use of) Z79.899-
  medication Z79.899

Prophylactic *(Continued)*
 organ removal (for neoplasia management)
   Z40.00
  breast Z40.01
  ovary Z40.02
  specified site NEC Z40.09
 surgery Z40.9
  for risk factors related to malignant
    neoplasm —*see* Prophylactic, organ
    removal
  specified NEC Z40.8
 vaccination Z23
Propionic acidemia E71.121
Proptosis (ocular) —*see also* Exophthalmos
 thyroid —*see* Hyperthyroidism, with goiter
Prosecution, anxiety concerning Z65.3
Prosopagnosia R48.3
Prostadynia N42.81
Prostate, prostatic —*see* condition
Prostatism —*see* Hyperplasia, prostate
Prostatitis (congestive) (suppurative) (with
   cystitis) N41.9
 acute N41.0
 cavitary N41.8
 chronic N41.1
 diverticular N41.8
 due to Trichomonas (vaginalis) A59.02
 fibrous N41.1
 gonococcal (acute) (chronic) A54.22
 granulomatous N41.4
 hypertrophic N41.1
 subacute N41.1
 trichomonal A59.02
 tuberculous A18.14
Prostatocystitis N41.3
Prostatorrhea N42.89
Prostatosis N42.82
Prostration R53.83
 heat —*see also* Heat, exhaustion
  anhydrotic T67.3
  due to
   salt (and water) depletion T67.4
   water depletion T67.3
 nervous F48.8
 senile R54
Protanomaly (anomalous trichromat) H53.54
Protanopia (complete) (incomplete) H53.54
Protection (against) (from) —*see* Prophylactic
Protein
 deficiency NEC —*see* Malnutrition
 malnutrition —*see* Malnutrition
 sickness —*see also* Reaction, serum T80.69
Proteinemia R77.9
Proteinosis
 alveolar (pulmonary) J84.01
 lipid or lipoid (of Urbach) E78.89
Proteinuria R80.9
 Bence Jones R80.3
 complicating pregnancy —*see* Proteinuria,
   gestational
 gestational ◀▥
  with edema O12.2-
  complicating ◀
   childbirth O12.14 ◀
   pregnancy O12.1- ◀
    with edema O12.2- ◀
   puerperium O12.15 ◀
 idiopathic R80.0
 isolated R80.0
  with glomerular lesion N06.9
   dense deposit disease N06.6
   diffuse
    crescentic glomerulonephritis
      N06.7
    endocapillary proliferative
      glomerulonephritis N06.4
    mesangiocapillary glomerulonephritis
      N06.5
   focal and segmental hyalinosis or
     sclerosis N06.1
   membranous (diffuse) N06.2

Proteinuria *(Continued)*
 isolated *(Continued)*
  with glomerular lesion *(Continued)*
   mesangial proliferative (diffuse) N06.3
   minimal change N06.0
   specified pathology NEC N06.8
 orthostatic R80.2
  with glomerular lesion —*see* Proteinuria,
    isolated, with glomerular lesion
 persistent R80.1
  with glomerular lesion —*see* Proteinuria,
    isolated, with glomerular lesion
 postural R80.2
  with glomerular lesion —*see* Proteinuria,
    isolated, with glomerular lesion
 pre-eclamptic —*see* Pre-eclampsia
 puerperal O12.15 ◀
 specified type NEC R80.8
Proteolysis, pathologic D65
Proteus (mirabilis) (morganii), as cause of
  disease classified elsewhere B96.4
Prothrombin gene mutation D68.52
Protoporphyria, erythropoietic E80.0
Protozoal —*see also* condition
 disease B64
 specified NEC B60.8
Protrusion, protrusio
 acetabuli M24.7
 acetabulum (into pelvis) M24.7
 device, implant or graft —*see also*
   Complications, by site and type,
   mechanical T85.698
  arterial graft NEC —*see* Complication,
    cardiovascular device, mechanical,
    vascular
  breast (implant) T85.49
  catheter NEC T85.698
   cystostomy T83.090
   dialysis (renal) T82.49
    intraperitoneal T85.691
   infusion NEC T82.594
    spinal (epidural) (subdural)
      T85.690
   urinary, indwelling T83.098
   urinary —*see also* Complications,
     catheter, urinary T83.098 ◀
  electronic (electrode) (pulse generator)
    (stimulator)
   bone T84.390
   nervous system —*see* Complication,
     prosthetic device, mechanical,
     electronic nervous system
     stimulator
  fixation, internal (orthopedic) NEC —*see*
    Complication, fixation device,
    mechanical
  gastrointestinal —*see* Complications,
    prosthetic device, mechanical,
    gastrointestinal device
  genital NEC T83.498
   intrauterine contraceptive device
     T83.39
   penile prosthesis (cylinder) (implanted)
     (pump) (resevoir) T83.490 ◀▥
   testicular prosthesis T83.491 ◀
  heart NEC —*see* Complication,
    cardiovascular device, mechanical
  joint prosthesis —*see* Complications, joint
    prosthesis, mechanical, specified
    NEC, by site
  ocular NEC —*see* Complications, prosthetic
    device, mechanical, ocular device
  orthopedic NEC —*see* Complication,
    orthopedic, device, mechanical
  specified NEC T85.628
  urinary NEC —*see also* Complication,
    genitourinary, device, urinary,
    mechanical
   graft T83.29
  vascular NEC —*see* Complication,
    cardiovascular device, mechanical

Protrusion, protrusio *(Continued)*
  device, implant or graft *(Continued)*
    ventricular intracranial shunt T85.09
  intervertebral disc —*see* Displacement,
    intervertebral disc
  joint prosthesis —*see* Complications, joint
    prosthesis, mechanical, specified NEC,
    by site
  nucleus pulposus —*see* Displacement,
    intervertebral disc
Prune belly (syndrome) Q79.4
Prurigo (ferox) (gravis) (Hebrae) (Hebra's)
  (mitis) (simplex) L28.2
  Besnier's L20.0
  estivalis L56.4
  nodularis L28.1
  psychogenic F45.8
Pruritus, pruritic (essential) L29.9
  ani, anus L29.0
    psychogenic F45.8
  anogenital L29.3
    psychogenic F45.8
  due to onchocerca volvulus B73.1
  gravidarum —*see* Pregnancy, complicated by,
    specified pregnancy-related condition
    NEC
  hiemalis L29.8
  neurogenic (any site) F45.8
  perianal L29.0
  psychogenic (any site) F45.8
  scroti, scrotum L29.1
    psychogenic F45.8
  senile, senilis L29.8
  specified NEC L29.8
    psychogenic F45.8
  Trichomonas A59.9
  vulva, vulvae L29.2
    psychogenic F45.8
Pseudarthrosis, pseudoarthrosis (bone) —*see*
    Nonunion, fracture
  clavicle, congenital Q74.0
  joint, following fusion or arthrodesis
    M96.0
Pseudoaneurysm —*see* Aneurysm
Pseudoangina (pectoris) —*see* Angina
Pseudoangioma I81
Pseudoarteriosus Q28.8
Pseudoarthrosis —*see* Pseudarthrosis
Pseudobulbar affect (PBA) F48.2
Pseudochromhidrosis L67.8
Pseudocirrhosis, liver, pericardial I31.1
Pseudocowpox B08.03
Pseudocoxalgia M91.3-
Pseudocroup J38.5
Pseudo-Cushing's syndrome, alcohol-induced
    E24.4
Pseudocyesis F45.8
Pseudocyst
  lung J98.4
  pancreas K86.3
  retina —*see* Cyst, retina
Pseudoelephantiasis neuroarthritica Q82.0
Pseudoexfoliation, capsule (lens) —*see*
    Cataract, specified NEC
Pseudofolliculitis barbae L73.1
Pseudoglioma H44.89
Pseudohemophilia (Bernuth's) (hereditary)
    (type B) D68.0
  Type A D69.8
  vascular D69.8
Pseudohermaphroditism Q56.3
  adrenal E25.8
  female Q56.2
    with adrenocortical disorder E25.8
    without adrenocortical disorder Q56.2
    adrenal, congenital E25.0
    adrenal (congenital) E25.0 ◀
  male Q56.1
    with
      adrenocortical disorder E25.8
      androgen resistance E34.51

Pseudohermaphroditism *(Continued)*
  male *(Continued)*
    with *(Continued)*
      cleft scrotum Q56.1
      feminizing testis E34.51
      5-alpha-reductase deficiency E29.1
    without gonadal disorder Q56.1
    adrenal E25.8
Pseudo-Hurler's polydystrophy E77.0
Pseudohydrocephalus G93.2
Pseudohypertrophic muscular dystrophy
    (Erb's) G71.0
Pseudohypertrophy, muscle G71.0
Pseudohypoparathyroidism E20.1
Pseudoinsomnia F51.03
Pseudoleukemia, infantile D64.89
Pseudomembranous —*see* condition
Pseudomeningocele (cerebral) (infective) (post-
    traumatic) G96.19
  postprocedural (spinal) G97.82
Pseudomenses (newborn) P54.6
Pseudomenstruation (newborn) P54.6
Pseudomonas
  aeruginosa, as cause of disease classified
    elsewhere B96.5
  mallei infection A24.0
    as cause of disease classified elsewhere
      B96.5
  pseudomallei, as cause of disease classified
    elsewhere B96.5
Pseudomyotonia G71.19
Pseudomyxoma peritonei C78.6
Pseudoneuritis, optic (nerve) (disc) (papilla),
    congenital Q14.2
Pseudo-obstruction intestine (acute) (chronic)
    (idiopathic) (intermittent secondary)
    (primary) K59.8
Pseudopapilledema H47.33-
  congenital Q14.2
Pseudoparalysis
  arm or leg R29.818
  atonic, congenital P94.2
Pseudopelade L66.0
Pseudophakia Z96.1
Pseudopolyarthritis, rhizomelic M35.3
Pseudopolycythemia D75.1
Pseudopseudohypoparathyroidism
    E20.1
Pseudopterygium H11.81-
Pseudoptosis (eyelid) —*see* Blepharochalasis
Pseudopuberty, precocious
  female heterosexual E25.8
  male isosexual E25.8
Pseudorickets (renal) N25.0
Pseudorubella B08.20
Pseudosclerema, newborn P83.8
Pseudosclerosis (brain)
  Jakob's —*see* Creutzfeldt-Jakob disease or
    syndrome
  of Westphal (Strüümpell) E83.01
  spastic —*see* Creutzfeldt-Jakob disease or
    syndrome
Pseudotetanus —*see* Convulsions
Pseudotetany R29.0
  hysterical F44.5
Pseudotruncus arteriosus Q25.49 ◀▥
Pseudotuberculosis A28.2
  enterocolitis A04.8
  pasteurella (infection) A28.0
Pseudotumor
  cerebri G93.2
  orbital H05.11-
Pseudoxanthoma elasticum Q82.8
Psilosis (sprue) (tropical) K90.1
  nontropical K90.0
Psittacosis A70
Psoitis M60.88
Psoriasis L40.9
  arthropathic L40.50
    arthritis mutilans L40.52
    distal interphalangeal L40.51

Psoriasis *(Continued)*
  arthropathic *(Continued)*
    juvenile L40.54
    other specified L40.59
    spondylitis L40.53
  buccal K13.29
  flexural L40.8
  guttate L40.4
  mouth K13.29
  nummular L40.0
  plaque L40.0
  psychogenic F54
  pustular (generalized) L40.1
    palmaris et plantaris L40.3
  specified NEC L40.8
  vulgaris L40.0
Psychasthenia F48.8
Psychiatric disorder or problem F99
Psychogenic —*see also* condition
  factors associated with physical conditions
    F54
Psychological and behavioral factors affecting
    medical condition F59
Psychoneurosis, psychoneurotic —*see also*
    Neurosis
  anxiety (state) F41.1
  depersonalization F48.1
  hypochondriacal F45.21
  hysteria F44.9
  neurasthenic F48.8
  personality NEC F60.89
Psychopathy, psychopathic
  affectionless F94.2
  autistic F84.5
  constitution, post-traumatic F07.81
  personality —*see* Disorder, personality
  sexual —*see* Deviation, sexual
  state F60.2
Psychosexual identity disorder of childhood
    F64.2
Psychosis, psychotic F29
  acute (transient) F23
    hysterical F44.9
  affective —*see* Disorder, mood
  alcoholic F10.959
    with
      abuse F10.159
      anxiety disorder F10.980
        with
          abuse F10.180
          dependence F10.280
      delirium tremens F10.231
      delusions F10.950
        with
          abuse F10.150
          dependence F10.250
      dementia F10.97
        with dependence F10.27
      dependence F10.259
      hallucinosis F10.951
        with
          abuse F10.151
          dependence F10.251
      mood disorder F10.94
        with
          abuse F10.14
          dependence F10.24
      paranoia F10.950
        with
          abuse F10.150
          dependence F10.250
      persisting amnesia F10.96
        with dependence F10.26
    amnestic confabulatory F10.96
      with dependence F10.26
    delirium tremens F10.231
    Korsakoff's, Korsakov's, Korsakow's F10.26
    paranoid type F10.950
      with
        abuse F10.150
        dependence F10.250

Psychosis, psychotic (Continued)
anergastic —see Psychosis, organic
arteriosclerotic (simple type) (uncomplicated)
   F01.50
   with behavioral disturbance F01.51
childhood F84.0
   atypical F84.8
climacteric —see Psychosis, involutional
confusional F29
   acute or subacute F05
   reactive F23
cycloid F23
depressive —see Disorder, depressive
disintegrative (childhood) F84.3
drug-induced —see F11-F19 with .x59
   paranoid and hallucinatory states —see
      F11-F19 with .x50 or .x51
due to or associated with
   addiction, drug —see F11-F19 with .X59
   dependence
      alcohol F10.259
      drug —see F11-F19 with .x59
   epilepsy F06.8
   Huntington's chorea F06.8
   ischemia, cerebrovascular (generalized)
      F06.8
   multiple sclerosis F06.8
   physical disease F06.8
   presenile dementia F03
   senile dementia F03
   vascular disease (arteriosclerotic) (cerebral)
      F01.50
      with behavioral disturbance F01.51
epileptic F06.8
episode F23
   due to or associated with physical
      condition F06.8
exhaustive F43.0
hallucinatory, chronic F28
hypomanic F30.8
hysterical (acute) F44.9
induced F24
infantile F84.0
   atypical F84.8
infective (acute) (subacute) F05
involutional F28
   depressive —see Disorder, depressive
   melancholic —see Disorder, depressive
   paranoid (state) F22
Korsakoff's, Korsakov's, Korsakow's
   (nonalcoholic) F04
   alcoholic F10.96
      in dependence F10.26
   induced by other psychoactive
      substance —see categories F11-F19
      with .x5x
mania, manic (single episode) F30.2
   recurrent type F31.89
manic-depressive —see Disorder, bipolar ◀▥
menopausal —see Psychosis, involutional
mixed schizophrenic and affective F25.8
multi-infarct (cerebrovascular) F01.50
   with behavioral disturbance F01.51
nonorganic F29
   specified NEC F28
organic F09
   due to or associated with
      arteriosclerosis (cerebral) —see
         Psychosis, arteriosclerotic
      cerebrovascular disease,
         arteriosclerotic —see Psychosis,
         arteriosclerotic
      childbirth —see Psychosis, puerperal
      Creutzfeldt-Jakob disease or
         syndrome —see Creutzfeldt-Jakob
         disease or syndrome
      dependence, alcohol F10.259
      disease
         alcoholic liver F10.259
         brain, arteriosclerotic —see Psychosis,
            arteriosclerotic

Psychosis, psychotic (Continued)
organic (Continued)
   due to or associated with (Continued)
      disease (Continued)
         cerebrovascular F01.50
            with behavioral disturbance
               F01.51
         Creutzfeldt-Jakob —see Creutzfeldt-
            Jakob disease or syndrome
         endocrine or metabolic F06.8
            acute or subacute F05
         liver, alcoholic F10.259
      epilepsy transient (acute) F05
      infection
         brain (intracranial) F06.8
            acute or subacute F05
      intoxication
         alcoholic (acute) F10.259
         drug F19 with .X59 F11-
      ischemia, cerebrovascular (generalized) —
         see Psychosis, arteriosclerotic
      puerperium —see Psychosis, puerperal
      trauma, brain (birth) (from electric
         current) (surgical) F06.8
         acute or subacute F05
   infective F06.8
      acute or subacute F05
   post-traumatic F06.8
      acute or subacute F05
paranoiac F22
paranoid (climacteric) (involutional)
   (menopausal) F22
   psychogenic (acute) F23
   schizophrenic F20.0
   senile F03
postpartum F53
presbyophrenic (type) F03
presenile F03
psychogenic (paranoid) F23
   depressive F32.3
puerperal F53
   specified type —see Psychosis, by type
reactive (brief) (transient) (emotional stress)
   (psychological trauma) F23
   depressive F32.3
      recurrent F33.3
   excitative type F30.8
schizoaffective F25.9
   depressive type F25.1
   manic type F25.0
schizophrenia, schizophrenic —see
   Schizophrenia
schizophrenia-like, in epilepsy F06.2
schizophreniform F20.81
   affective type F25.9
   brief F23
   confusional type F23
   depressive type F25.1
   manic type F25.0
   mixed type F25.0
senile NEC F03
   depressed or paranoid type F03
   simple deterioration F03
   specified type — code to condition
shared F24
situational (reactive) F23
symbiotic (childhood) F84.3
symptomatic F09
Psychosomatic —see Disorder, psychosomatic
Psychosyndrome, organic F07.9
Psychotic episode due to or associated with
   physical condition F06.8
Pterygium (eye) H11.00-
   amyloid H11.01-
   central H11.02-
   colli Q18.3
   double H11.03-
   peripheral
      progressive H11.05-
      stationary H11.04-
   recurrent H11.06-

Ptilosis (eyelid) —see Madarosis
Ptomaine (poisoning) —see Poisoning, food
Ptosis —see also Blepharoptosis
   adiposa (false) —see Blepharoptosis
   breast N64.81
   cecum K63.4
   colon K63.4
   congenital (eyelid) Q10.0
      specified site NEC —see Anomaly, by site
   eyelid —see Blepharoptosis
      congenital Q10.0
   gastric K31.89
   intestine K63.4
   kidney N28.83
   liver K76.89
   renal N28.83
   splanchnic K63.4
   spleen D73.89
   stomach K31.89
   viscera K63.4
PTP D69.51
Ptyalism (periodic) K11.7
   hysterical F45.8
   pregnancy —see Pregnancy, complicated by,
      specified pregnancy-related condition
      NEC
   psychogenic F45.8
Ptyalolithiasis K11.5
Pubarche, precocious E30.1
Pubertas praecox E30.1
Puberty (development state) Z00.3
   bleeding (excessive) N92.2
   delayed E30.0
   precocious (constitutional) (cryptogenic)
      (idiopathic) E30.1
      central E22.8
      due to
         ovarian hyperfunction E28.1
            estrogen E28.0
         testicular hyperfunction E29.0
   premature E30.1
      due to
         adrenal cortical hyperfunction E25.8
         pineal tumor E34.8
         pituitary (anterior) hyperfunction E22.8
Puckering, macula —see Degeneration, macula,
   puckering
Pudenda, pudendum —see condition
Puente's disease (simple glandular cheilitis)
   K13.0
Puerperal, puerperium (complicated by,
   complications)
   abnormal glucose (tolerance test) O99.815
   abscess
      areola O91.02
         associated with lactation O91.03
      Bartholin's gland O86.19
      breast O91.12
         associated with lactation O91.13
      cervix (uteri) O86.11
      genital organ NEC O86.19
      kidney O86.21
      mammary O91.12
         associated with lactation O91.13
      nipple O91.02
         associated with lactation O91.03
      peritoneum O85
      subareolar O91.12
         associated with lactation O91.13
      urinary tract —see Puerperal, infection,
         urinary
      uterus O86.12
      vagina (wall) O86.13
      vaginorectal O86.13
      vulvovaginal gland O86.13
   adnexitis O86.19
   afibrinogenemia, or other coagulation defect
      O72.3
   albuminuria (acute) (subacute) —see
      Proteinuria, gestational
   alcohol use O99.315

Puerperal, puerperium (Continued)
  anemia O90.81
    pre-existing (pre-pregnancy) O99.03
  anesthetic death O89.8
  apoplexy O99.43
  bariatric surgery status O99.845
  blood disorder NEC O99.13
  blood dyscrasia O72.3
  cardiomyopathy O90.3
  cerebrovascular disorder (conditions in
    I60-I69) O99.43
  cervicitis O86.11
  circulatory system disorder O99.43
  coagulopathy (any) O72.3
  complications O90.9
    specified NEC O90.89
  convulsions —see Eclampsia
  cystitis O86.22
  cystopyelitis O86.29
  delirium NEC F05
  diabetes O24.93
    gestational —see Puerperal, gestational
      diabetes
    pre-existing O24.33
      specified NEC O24.83
      type 1 O24.03
      type 2 O24.13
  digestive system disorder O99.63
  disease O90.9
    breast NEC O92.29
    cerebrovascular (acute) O99.43
    nonobstetric NEC O99.89
    tubo-ovarian O86.19
    Valsuani's O99.03
  disorder O90.9
    biliary tract O26.63
    lactation O92.70
    liver O26.63
    nonobstetric NEC O99.89
  disruption
    cesarean wound O90.0
    episiotomy wound O90.1
    perineal laceration wound O90.1
  drug use O99.325
  eclampsia (with pre-existing hypertension)
    O15.2
  embolism (pulmonary) (blood clot) —see
    Embolism, obstetric, puerperal
  endocrine, nutritional or metabolic disease
    NEC O99.285
  endophlebitis —see Puerperal, phlebitis
  endotrachelitis O86.11
  failure
    lactation (complete) O92.3
      partial O92.4
    renal, acute O90.4
  fever (of unknown origin) O86.4
    septic O85
  fissure, nipple O92.12
    associated with lactation O92.13
  fistula
    breast (due to mastitis) O91.12
      associated with lactation O91.13
    nipple O91.02
      associated with lactation O91.03
  galactophoritis O91.22
    associated with lactation O91.23
  galactorrhea O92.6
  gastric banding status O99.845
  gastric bypass status O99.845
  gastrointestinal disease NEC O99.63
  gestational diabetes O24.439
    diet controlled O24.430
    insulin (and diet) controlled
      O24.434
  gestational ◄
    diabetes O24.439 ◄
      diet controlled O24.430 ◄
      insulin (and diet) controlled O24.434 ◄
      oral drug controlled (antidiabetic)
        (hypoglycemic) O24.435 ◄

Puerperal, puerperium (Continued)
  gestational (Continued)
    edema O12.05 ◄
      with proteinuria O12.25 ◄
    proteinuria O12.15 ◄
  gonorrhea O98.23
  hematoma, subdural O99.43
  hemiplegia, cerebral O99.355-
    due to cerebrovascular disorder
      O99.43
  hemorrhage O72.1
    brain O99.43
    bulbar O99.43
    cerebellar O99.43
    cerebral O99.43
    cortical O99.43
    delayed or secondary O72.2
    extradural O99.43
    internal capsule O99.43
    intracranial O99.43
    intrapontine O99.43
    meningeal O99.43
    pontine O99.43
    retained placenta O72.0
    subarachnoid O99.43
    subcortical O99.43
    subdural O99.43
    third stage O72.0
    uterine, delayed O72.2
    ventricular O99.43
  hemorrhoids O87.2
  hepatorenal syndrome O90.4
  hypertension —see Hypertension,
    complicating, puerperium
  hypertrophy, breast O92.29
  induration breast (fibrous) O92.29
  infection O86.4
    cervix O86.11
    generalized O85
    genital tract NEC O86.19
      obstetric surgical wound O86.0
    kidney (bacillus coli) O86.21
    maternal O98.93
      carrier state NEC O99.835
      gonorrhea O98.23
      human immunodeficiency virus (HIV)
        O98.73
      protozoal O98.63
      sexually transmitted NEC O98.33
      specified NEC O98.83
      streptococcus B carrier state
        O99.825
      streptococcus group B (GBS) carrier state
        O99.825 ◄
      syphilis O98.13
      tuberculosis O98.03
      viral hepatitis O98.43
      viral NEC O98.53
    nipple O91.02
      associated with lactation O91.03
    peritoneum O85
    renal O86.21
    specified NEC O86.89
    urinary (asymptomatic) (tract) NEC O86.20
      bladder O86.22
      kidney O86.21
      specified site NEC O86.29
      urethra O86.22
    vagina O86.13
    vein —see Puerperal, phlebitis
  ischemia, cerebral O99.43
  lymphangitis O86.89
    breast O91.22
      associated with lactation O91.23
  malignancy O9A.13
  malnutrition O25.3
  mammillitis O91.02
    associated with lactation O91.03
  mammitis O91.22
    associated with lactation O91.23
  mania F30.8

Puerperal, puerperium (Continued)
  mastitis O91.22
    associated with lactation O91.23
    purulent O91.12
      associated with lactation O91.13
  melancholia —see Disorder, depressive
  mental disorder NEC O99.345
  metroperitonitis O85
  metrorrhagia —see Hemorrhage, postpartum
  metrosalpingitis O86.19
  metrovaginitis O86.13
  milk leg O87.1
  monoplegia, cerebral O99.43
  mood disturbance O90.6
  necrosis, liver (acute) (subacute) (conditions
    in subcategory K72.0) O26.63 ◄▥
    with renal failure O90.4
  nervous system disorder O99.355
  neuritis O90.89
  obesity (pre-existing prior to pregnancy)
    O99.215
  obesity surgery status O99.845
  occlusion, precerebral artery O99.43
  paralysis
    bladder (sphincter) O90.89
    cerebral O99.43
  paralytic stroke O99.43
  parametritis O85
  paravaginitis O86.13
  pelviperitonitis O85
  perimetritis O86.12
  perimetrosalpingitis O86.19
  perinephritis O86.21
  periphlebitis —see Puerperal phlebitis
  peritoneal infection O85
  peritonitis (pelvic) O85
  perivaginitis O86.13
  phlebitis O87.0
    deep O87.1
    pelvic O87.1
    superficial O87.0
  phlebothrombosis, deep O87.1
  phlegmasia alba dolens O87.1
  placental polyp O90.89
  pneumonia, embolic —see Embolism,
    obstetric, puerperal
  pre-eclampsia —see Pre-eclampsia
  psychosis F53
  pyelitis O86.21
  pyelocystitis O86.29
  pyelonephritis O86.21
  pyelonephrosis O86.21
  pyemia O85
  pyocystitis O86.29
  pyohemia O85
  pyometra O86.12
  pyonephritis O86.21
  pyosalpingitis O86.19
  pyrexia (of unknown origin) O86.4
  renal
    disease NEC O90.89
    failure O90.4
  respiratory disease NEC O99.53
  retention
    decidua —see Retention, decidua
    placenta O72.0
    secundines —see Retention,
      secundines
  retrated nipple O92.02
  salpingo-ovaritis O86.19
  salpingoperitonitis O85
  secondary perineal tear O90.1
  sepsis O85
  sepsis (pelvic) O85
  septic thrombophlebitis O86.81
  skin disorder NEC O99.73
  specified condition NEC O99.89
  stroke O99.43
  subinvolution (uterus) O90.89
  subluxation of symphysis (pubis)
    O26.73

◄ New   ◄▥ Revised   deleted Deleted

Puerperal, puerperium (Continued)
  suppuration —see Puerperal, abscess
  tetanus A34
  thelitis O91.02
    associated with lactation O91.03
  thrombocytopenia O72.3
  thrombophlebitis (superficial) O87.0
    deep O87.1
    pelvic O87.1
    septic O86.81
  thrombosis (venous) —see Thrombosis,
    puerperal
  thyroiditis O90.5
  toxemia (eclamptic) (pre-eclamptic)
    (with convulsions) O15.2
  trauma, non-obstetric O9A.23
    caused by abuse (physical) (suspected)
      O9A.33
      confirmed O9A.33
      psychological (suspected) O9A.53
        confirmed O9A.53
      sexual (suspected) O9A.43
        confirmed O9A.43
  uremia (due to renal failure)
    O90.4
  urethritis O86.22
  vaginitis O86.13
  varicose veins (legs) O87.4
    vulva or perineum O87.8
  venous O87.9
  vulvitis O86.19
  vulvovaginitis O86.13
  white leg O87.1
Puerperium —see Puerperal
Pulmolithiasis J98.4
Pulmonary —see condition
Pulpitis (acute) (anachoretic) (chronic)
    (hyperplastic) (putrescent) (suppurative)
    (ulcerative) K04.01 ◀▥
  irreversible K04.02 ◀▥
  reversible K04.01 ◀▥
Pulpless tooth K04.99
Pulse
  alternating R00.8
  bigeminal R00.8
  fast R00.0
  feeble, rapid due to shock following injury
    T79.4
  rapid R00.0
  weak R09.89
Pulsus alternans or trigeminus R00.8
Punch drunk F07.81
Punctum lacrimale occlusion —see Obstruction,
    lacrimal
Puncture
  abdomen, abdominal
    wall S31.139
      with
        foreign body S31.149
        penetration into peritoneal cavity
          S31.639
          with foreign body S31.649
      epigastric region S31.132
        with
          foreign body S31.142
          penetration into peritoneal cavity
            S31.632
            with foreign body S31.642
      left
        lower quadrant S31.134
          with
            foreign body S31.144
            penetration into peritoneal cavity
              S31.634
              with foreign body S31.644
        upper quadrant S31.131
          with
            foreign body S31.141
            penetration into peritoneal cavity
              S31.631
              with foreign body S31.641

Puncture (Continued)
  abdomen, abdominal (Continued)
    wall (Continued)
      periumbilic region S31.135
        with
          foreign body S31.145
          penetration into peritoneal cavity
            S31.635
            with foreign body S31.645
      right
        lower quadrant S31.133
          with
            foreign body S31.143
            penetration into peritoneal cavity
              S31.633
              with foreign body S31.643
        upper quadrant S31.130
          with
            foreign body S31.140
            penetration into peritoneal cavity
              S31.630
              with foreign body S31.640
  accidental, complicating surgery —see
      Complication, accidental puncture or
      laceration
  alveolar (process) —see Puncture, oral cavity
  ankle S91.039
    with
      foreign body S91.049
    left S91.032
      with
        foreign body S91.042
    right S91.031
      with
        foreign body S91.041
  anus S31.833
    with foreign body S31.834
  arm (upper) S41.139
    with foreign body S41.149
    left S41.132
      with foreign body S41.142
    lower —see Puncture, forearm
    right S41.131
      with foreign body S41.141
  auditory canal (external) (meatus) —see
      Puncture, ear
  auricle, ear —see Puncture, ear
  axilla —see Puncture, arm
  back —see also Puncture, thorax, back
    lower S31.030
      with
        foreign body S31.040
          with penetration into
            retroperitoneal space S31.041
        penetration into retroperitoneal space
          S31.031
  bladder (traumatic) S37.29
    nontraumatic N32.89
  breast S21.039
    with foreign body S21.049
    left S21.032
      with foreign body S21.042
    right S21.031
      with foreign body S21.041
  buttock S31.803
    with foreign body S31.804
    left S31.823
      with foreign body S31.824
    right S31.813
      with foreign body S31.814
  by
    device, implant or graft —see
        Complications, by site and type,
        mechanical
    foreign body left accidentally in operative
        wound T81.539
    instrument (any) during a procedure,
        accidental —see Puncture, accidental
        complicating surgery
  calf —see Puncture, leg
  canaliculus lacrimalis —see Puncture, eyelid

Puncture (Continued)
  canthus, eye —see Puncture, eyelid
  cervical esophagus S11.23
    with foreign body S11.24
  cheek (external) S01.439
    with foreign body S01.449
    internal —see Puncture, oral cavity
    left S01.432
      with foreign body S01.442
    right S01.431
      with foreign body S01.441
  chest wall —see Puncture, thorax
  chin —see Puncture, head, specified site NEC
  clitoris —see Puncture, vulva
  costal region —see Puncture, thorax
  digit (s)
    foot —see Puncture, toe
    hand —see Puncture, finger
  ear (canal) (external) S01.339
    with foreign body S01.349
    drum S09.2-
    left S01.332
      with foreign body S01.342
    right S01.331
      with foreign body S01.341
  elbow S51.039
    with
      foreign body S51.049
    left S51.032
      with
        foreign body S51.042
    right S51.031
      with
        foreign body S51.041
  epididymis —see Puncture, testis
  epigastric region —see Puncture, abdomen,
      wall, epigastric
  epiglottis S11.83
    with foreign body S11.84
  esophagus
    cervical S11.23
      with foreign body S11.24
    thoracic S27.818
  eyeball S05.6-
    with foreign body S05.5-
  eyebrow —see Puncture, eyelid
  eyelid S01.13-
    with foreign body S01.14-
    left S01.132
      with foreign body S01.142
    right S01.131
      with foreign body S01.141
  face NEC —see Puncture, head, specified site
      NEC
  finger (s) S61.239
    with
      damage to nail S61.339
        with
          foreign body S61.349
      foreign body S61.249
    index S61.238
      with
        damage to nail S61.338
          with
            foreign body S61.348
        foreign body S61.248
      left S61.231
        with
          damage to nail S61.331
            with
              foreign body S61.341
          foreign body S61.241
      right S61.230
        with
          damage to nail S61.330
            with
              foreign body S61.340
          foreign body S61.240
    little S61.238
      with
        damage to nail S61.338

Puncture *(Continued)*
  finger *(Continued)*
    with *(Continued)*
      with *(Continued)*
        damage to nail *(Continued)*
          with
            foreign body S61.348
          foreign body S61.248
        left S61.237
          with
            damage to nail S61.337
              with
                foreign body S61.347
            foreign body S61.247
        right S61.236
          with
            damage to nail S61.336
              with
                foreign body S61.346
            foreign body S61.246
      middle S61.238
        with
          damage to nail S61.338
            with
              foreign body S61.348
          foreign body S61.248
        left S61.233
          with
            damage to nail S61.333
              with
                foreign body S61.343
            foreign body S61.243
        right S61.232
          with
            damage to nail S61.332
              with
                foreign body S61.342
            foreign body S61.242
      ring S61.238
        with
          damage to nail S61.338
            with
              foreign body S61.348
          foreign body S61.248
        left S61.235
          with
            damage to nail S61.335
              with
                foreign body S61.345
            foreign body S61.245
        right S61.234
          with
            damage to nail S61.334
              with
                foreign body S61.344
            foreign body S61.244
  flank S31.139
    with foreign body S31.149
  foot (except toe (s) alone) S91.339
    with foreign body S91.349
    left S91.332
      with foreign body S91.342
    right S91.331
      with foreign body S91.341
    toe —*see* Puncture, toe
  forearm S51.839
    with
      foreign body S51.849
    elbow only —*see* Puncture, elbow
    left S51.832
      with
        foreign body S51.842
    right S51.831
      with
        foreign body S51.841
  forehead —*see* Puncture, head, specified site
    NEC
  genital organs, external
    female S31.532
      with foreign body S31.542
      vagina —*see* Puncture, vagina
      vulva —*see* Puncture, vulva

Puncture *(Continued)*
  genital organs, external *(Continued)*
    male S31.531
      with foreign body S31.541
      penis —*see* Puncture, penis
      scrotum —*see* Puncture, scrotum
      testis —*see* Puncture, testis
  groin —*see* Puncture, abdomen, wall
  gum —*see* Puncture, oral cavity
  hand S61.439
    with
      foreign body S61.449
    finger —*see* Puncture, finger
    left S61.432
      with
        foreign body S61.442
    right S61.431
      with
        foreign body S61.441
    thumb —*see* Puncture, thumb
  head S01.93
    with foreign body S01.94
    cheek —*see* Puncture, cheek
    ear —*see* Puncture, ear
    eyelid —*see* Puncture, eyelid
    lip —*see* Puncture, oral cavity
    nose —*see* Puncture, nose
    oral cavity —*see* Puncture, oral cavity
    scalp S01.03
      with foreign body S01.04
    specified site NEC S01.83
      with foreign body S01.84
    temporomandibular area —*see* Puncture,
      cheek
  heart S26.99
    with hemopericardium S26.09
    without hemopericardium S26.19
  heel —*see* Puncture, foot
  hip S71.039
    with foreign body S71.049
    left S71.032
      with foreign body S71.042
    right S71.031
      with foreign body S71.041
  hymen —*see* Puncture, vagina
  hypochondrium —*see* Puncture, abdomen,
    wall
  hypogastric region —*see* Puncture, abdomen,
    wall
  inguinal region —*see* Puncture, abdomen,
    wall
  instep —*see* Puncture, foot
  internal organs —*see* Injury, by site
  interscapular region —*see* Puncture, thorax,
    back
  intestine
    large
      colon S36.599
        ascending S36.590
        descending S36.592
        sigmoid S36.593
        specified site NEC S36.598
        transverse S36.591
      rectum S36.69
    small S36.499
      duodenum S36.490
      specified site NEC S36.498
  intra-abdominal organ S36.99
    gallbladder S36.128
    intestine —*see* Puncture, intestine
    liver S36.118
    pancreas —*see* Puncture, pancreas
    peritoneum S36.81
    specified site NEC S36.898
    spleen S36.09
    stomach S36.39
  jaw —*see* Puncture, head, specified site NEC
  knee S81.039
    with foreign body S81.049
    left S81.032
      with foreign body S81.042

Puncture *(Continued)*
  knee *(Continued)*
    right S81.031
      with foreign body S81.041
    labium (majus) (minus) —*see* Puncture,
      vulva
    lacrimal duct —*see* Puncture, eyelid
  larynx S11.013
    with foreign body S11.014
  leg (lower) S81.839
    with foreign body S81.849
    foot —*see* Puncture, foot
    knee —*see* Puncture, knee
    left S81.832
      with foreign body S81.842
    right S81.831
      with foreign body S81.841
    upper —*see* Puncture, thigh
  lip S01.531
    with foreign body S01.541
  loin —*see* Puncture, abdomen, wall
  lower back —*see* Puncture, back, lower
  lumbar region —*see* Puncture, back, lower
  malar region —*see* Puncture, head, specified
    site NEC
  mammary —*see* Puncture, breast
  mastoid region —*see* Puncture, head,
    specified site NEC
  mouth —*see* Puncture, oral cavity
  nail
    finger —*see* Puncture, finger, with damage
      to nail
    toe —*see* Puncture, toe, with damage to
      nail
  nasal (septum) (sinus) —*see* Puncture, nose
  nasopharynx —*see* Puncture, head, specified
    site NEC
  neck S11.93
    with foreign body S11.94
    involving
      cervical esophagus —*see* Puncture,
        cervical esophagus
      larynx —*see* Puncture, larynx
      pharynx —*see* Puncture, pharynx
      thyroid gland —*see* Puncture, thyroid
        gland
      trachea —*see* Puncture, trachea
    specified site NEC S11.83
      with foreign body S11.84
  nose (septum) (sinus) S01.23
    with foreign body S01.24
  ocular —*see* Puncture, eyeball - oral cavity
    S01.532
    with foreign body S01.542
  orbit S05.4-
  palate —*see* Puncture, oral cavity
  palm —*see* Puncture, hand
  pancreas S36.299
    body S36.291
    head S36.290
    tail S36.292
  pelvis —*see* Puncture, back, lower
  penis S31.23
    with foreign body S31.24
  perineum
    female S31.43
      with foreign body S31.44
    male S31.139
      with foreign body S31.149
  periocular area (with or without lacrimal
    passages) —*see* Puncture, eyelid
  phalanges
    finger —*see* Puncture, finger
    toe —*see* Puncture, toe
  pharynx S11.23
    with foreign body S11.24
  pinna —*see* Puncture, ear
  popliteal space —*see* Puncture, knee
  prepuce —*see* Puncture, penis
  pubic region S31.139
    with foreign body S31.149

◄ New   ◄▥ Revised   ~~deleted~~ Deleted

Puncture *(Continued)*
  pudendum —*see* Puncture, genital organs, external
  rectovaginal septum —*see* Puncture, vagina
  sacral region —*see* Puncture, back, lower
  sacroiliac region —*see* Puncture, back, lower
  salivary gland —*see* Puncture, oral cavity
  scalp S01.03
    with foreign body S01.04
  scapular region —*see* Puncture, shoulder
  scrotum S31.33
    with foreign body S31.34
  shin —*see* Puncture, leg
  shoulder S41.039
    with foreign body S41.049
    left S41.032
      with foreign body S41.042
    right S41.031
      with foreign body S41.041
  spermatic cord —*see* Puncture, testis
  sternal region —*see* Puncture, thorax, front
  submaxillary region —*see* Puncture, head, specified site NEC
  submental region —*see* Puncture, head, specified site NEC
  subungual
    finger (s) —*see* Puncture, finger, with damage to nail
    toe —*see* Puncture, toe, with damage to nail
  supraclavicular fossa —*see* Puncture, neck, specified site NEC
  temple, temporal region —*see* Puncture, head, specified site NEC
  temporomandibular area —*see* Puncture, cheek
  testis S31.33
    with foreign body S31.34
  thigh S71.139
    with foreign body S71.149
    left S71.132
      with foreign body S71.142
    right S71.131
      with foreign body S71.141
  thorax, thoracic (wall) S21.93
    with foreign body S21.94
    back S21.23-
      with
        foreign body S21.24-
          with penetration S21.44
        penetration S21.43
    breast —*see* Puncture, breast
    front S21.13-
      with
        foreign body S21.14-
          with penetration S21.34
        penetration S21.33
  throat —*see* Puncture, neck
  thumb S61.039
    with
      damage to nail S61.139
        with
          foreign body S61.149
      foreign body S61.049
    left S61.032
      with
        damage to nail S61.132
          with
            foreign body S61.142
        foreign body S61.042
    right S61.031
      with
        damage to nail S61.131
          with
            foreign body S61.141
        foreign body S61.041

Puncture *(Continued)*
  thyroid gland S11.13
    with foreign body S11.14
  toe (s) S91.139
    with
      damage to nail S91.239
        with
          foreign body S91.249
      foreign body S91.149
    great S91.133
      with
        damage to nail S91.233
          with
            foreign body S91.243
        foreign body S91.143
    left S91.132
      with
        damage to nail S91.232
          with
            foreign body S91.242
        foreign body S91.142
    right S91.131
      with
        damage to nail S91.231
          with
            foreign body S91.241
        foreign body S91.141
    lesser S91.136
      with
        damage to nail S91.236
          with
            foreign body S91.246
        foreign body S91.146
      left S91.135
        with
          damage to nail S91.235
            with
              foreign body S91.245
          foreign body S91.145
      right S91.134
        with
          damage to nail S91.234
            with
              foreign body S91.244
          foreign body S91.144
  tongue —*see* Puncture, oral cavity
  trachea S11.023
    with foreign body S11.024
  tunica vaginalis —*see* Puncture, testis
  tympanum, tympanic membrane S09.2-
  umbilical region S31.135
    with foreign body S31.145
  uvula —*see* Puncture, oral cavity
  vagina S31.43
    with foreign body S31.44
  vocal cords S11.033
    with foreign body S11.034
  vulva S31.43
    with foreign body S31.44
  wrist S61.539
    with
      foreign body S61.549
    left S61.532
      with
        foreign body S61.542
    right S61.531
      with
        foreign body S61.541
PUO (pyrexia of unknown origin) R50.9
Pupillary membrane (persistent) Q13.89
Pupillotonia —*see* Anomaly, pupil, function, tonic pupil
Purpura D69.2
  abdominal D69.0
  allergic D69.0
  anaphylactoid D69.0
  annularis telangiectodes L81.7
  arthritic D69.0
  autoerythrocyte sensitization D69.2
  autoimmune D69.0

Purpura *(Continued)*
  bacterial D69.0
  Bateman's (senile) D69.2
  capillary fragility (hereditary) (idiopathic) D69.8
  cryoglobulinemic D89.1
  Devil's pinches D69.2
  fibrinolytic —*see* Fibrinolysis
  fulminans, fulminous D65
  gangrenous D65
  hemorrhagic, hemorrhagica D69.3
    not due to thrombocytopenia D69.0
  Henoch (-Schönlein) (allergic) D69.0
  hypergammaglobulinemic (benign) (Waldenström's) D89.0
  idiopathic (thrombocytopenic) D69.3
    nonthrombocytopenic D69.0
  immune thrombocytopenic D69.3
  infectious D69.0
  malignant D69.0
  neonatorum P54.5
  nervosa D69.0
  newborn P54.5
  nonthrombocytopenic D69.2
    hemorrhagic D69.0
    idiopathic D69.0
  nonthrombopenic D69.2
  peliosis rheumatica D69.0
  posttransfusion (post-transfusion) (from (fresh) whole blood or blood products) D69.51
  primary D69.49
  red cell membrane sensitivity D69.2
  rheumatica D69.0
  Schönlein (-Henoch) (allergic) D69.0
  scorbutic E54 *[D77]*
  senile D69.2
  simplex D69.2
  symptomatica D69.0
  telangiectasia annularis L81.7
  thrombocytopenic D69.49
    congenital D69.42
    hemorrhagic D69.3
    hereditary D69.42
    idiopathic D69.3
    immune D69.3
    neonatal, transitory P61.0
    thrombotic M31.1
  thrombohemolytic —*see* Fibrinolysis
  thrombolytic —*see* Fibrinolysis
  thrombopenic D69.49
  thrombotic, thrombocytopenic M31.1
  toxic D69.0
  vascular D69.0
  visceral symptoms D69.0
Purpuric spots R23.3
Purulent —*see* condition
Pus
  in
    stool R19.5
    urine N39.0
  tube (rupture) —*see* Salpingo-oophoritis
Pustular rash L08.0
Pustule (nonmalignant) L08.9
  malignant A22.0
Pustulosis palmaris et plantaris L40.3
Putnam (-Dana) disease or syndrome —*see* Degeneration, combined
Putrescent pulp (dental) K04.1
Pyarthritis, pyarthrosis —*see* Arthritis, pyogenic or pyemic
  tuberculous —*see* Tuberculosis, joint
Pyelectasis —*see* Hydronephrosis
Pyelitis (congenital) (uremic) —*see also* Pyelonephritis
  with
    calculus —*see* category N20
      with hydronephrosis N13.2
    contracted kidney N11.9

Pyelitis *(Continued)*
  acute N10
  chronic N11.9
    with calculus —*see* category N20
      with hydronephrosis N13.2
    cystica N28.84
    puerperal (postpartum) O86.21
    tuberculous A18.11
Pyelocystitis —*see* Pyelonephritis
Pyelonephritis —*see also* Nephritis,
    tubulo-interstitial
  with
    calculus —*see* category N20
      with hydronephrosis N13.2
    contracted kidney N11.9
  acute N10
  calculous —*see* category N20
    with hydronephrosis N13.2
  chronic N11.9
    with calculus —*see* category N20
      with hydronephrosis N13.2
    associated with ureteral obstruction or
      stricture N11.1
    nonobstructive N11.8
      with reflux (vesicoureteral) N11.0
    obstructive N11.1
    specified NEC N11.8
  in (due to)
    brucellosis A23.9 *[N16]*
    cryoglobulinemia (mixed) D89.1 *[N16]*
    cystinosis E72.04
    diphtheria A36.84
    glycogen storage disease E74.09 *[N16]*
    leukemia NEC C95.9- *[N16]*
    lymphoma NEC C85.90 *[N16]*
    multiple myeloma C90.0- *[N16]*
    obstruction N11.1
    Salmonella infection A02.25
    sarcoidosis D86.84
    sepsis A41.9 *[N16]*
    Sjögren's disease M35.04
    toxoplasmosis B58.83
    transplant rejection T86.91 *[N16]*
    Wilson's disease E83.01 *[N16]*
  nonobstructive N12
    with reflux (vesicoureteral) N11.0
    chronic N11.8
  syphilitic A52.75

Pyelonephrosis (obstructive) N11.1
  chronic N11.9
Pyelophlebitis I80.8
Pyeloureteritis cystica N28.85
Pyemia, pyemic (fever) (infection) (purulent) —
    see also Sepsis
  joint —*see* Arthritis, pyogenic or pyemic
  liver K75.1
  pneumococcal A40.3
  portal K75.1
  postvaccinal T88.0
  puerperal, postpartum, childbirth O85
  specified organism NEC A41.89
  tuberculous —*see* Tuberculosis, miliary
Pygopagus Q89.4
Pyknoepilepsy (idiopathic) —*see* Pyknolepsy
Pyknolepsy G40.A09
  intractable G40.A19
    with status epilepticus G40.A11
    without status epilepticus G40.A19
  not intractable G40.A09
    with status epilepticus G40.A01
    without status epilepticus G40.A09
Pylephlebitis K75.1
Pyle's syndrome Q78.5
Pylethrombophlebitis K75.1
Pylethrombosis K75.1
Pyloritis K29.90
  with bleeding K29.91
Pylorospasm (reflex) NEC K31.3
  congenital or infantile Q40.0
  neurotic F45.8
  newborn Q40.0
  psychogenic F45.8
Pylorus, pyloric —*see* condition
Pyoarthrosis —*see* Arthritis, pyogenic or
    pyemic
Pyocele
  mastoid —*see* Mastoiditis, acute
  sinus (accessory) —*see* Sinusitis
  turbinate (bone) J32.9
  urethra —*see also* Urethritis N34.0
Pyocolpos —*see* Vaginitis
Pyocystitis N30.80
  with hematuria N30.81
Pyoderma, pyodermia L08.0
  gangrenosum L88
  newborn P39.4

Pyoderma, pyodermia *(Continued)*
  phagedenic L88
  vegetans L08.81
Pyodermatitis L08.0
  vegetans L08.81
Pyogenic —*see* condition
Pyohydronephrosis N13.6
Pyometra, pyometrium, pyometritis —*see*
    Endometritis
Pyomyositis (tropical) —*see* Myositis,
    infective
Pyonephritis N12
Pyonephrosis N13.6
  tuberculous A18.11
Pyo-oophoritis —*see* Salpingo-oophoritis
Pyo-ovarium —*see* Salpingo-oophoritis
Pyopericarditis, pyopericardium
    I30.1
Pyophlebitis —*see* Phlebitis
Pyopneumopericardium I30.1
Pyopneumothorax (infective) J86.9
  with fistula J86.0
  tuberculous NEC A15.6
Pyosalpinx, pyosalpingitis —*see also*
    Salpingo-oophoritis
Pyothorax J86.9
  with fistula J86.0
  tuberculous NEC A15.6
Pyoureter N28.89
  tuberculous A18.11
Pyramidopallidonigral syndrome
    G20
Pyrexia (of unknown origin) R50.9
  atmospheric T67.0
  during labor NEC O75.2
  heat T67.0
  newborn P81.9
    environmentally-induced P81.0
  persistent R50.9
  puerperal O86.4
Pyroglobulinemia NEC E88.09
Pyromania F63.1
Pyrosis R12
Pyuria (bacterial) N39.0

◄ New   ◄⊪ Revised   ~~deleted~~ Deleted

Q

Q fever A78
 with pneumonia A78
Quadricuspid aortic valve Q23.8
Quadrilateral fever A78
Quadriparesis —*see* Quadriplegia
 meaning muscle weakness M62.81
Quadriplegia G82.50-
 complete
  C1-C4 level G82.51
  C5-C7 level G82.53
 congenital (cerebral) (spinal) G80.8
  spastic G80.0

Quadriplegia (*Continued*)
 embolic (current episode) I63.4- ◀▥
 functional R53.2
 incomplete
  C1-C4 level G82.52
  C5-C7 level G82.54
 thrombotic (current episode) I63.3- ◀▥
 traumatic — code to injury with seventh
  character S
  current episode —*see* Injury, spinal (cord),
   cervical
Quadruplet, pregnancy —*see* Pregnancy,
 quadruplet
Quarrelsomeness F60.3

Queensland fever A77.3
Quervain's disease M65.4
 thyroid E06.1
Queyrat's erythroplasia D07.4
 penis D07.4
 specified site —*see* Neoplasm, skin,
  in situ
 unspecified site D07.4
Quincke's disease or edema T78.3
 hereditary D84.1
Quinsy (gangrenous) J36
Quintan fever A79.0
Quintuplet, pregnancy —*see* Pregnancy,
 quintuplet

R

Rabbit fever —see Tularemia
Rabies A82.9
  contact Z20.3
  exposure to Z20.3
  inoculation reaction —see Complications,
    vaccination
  sylvatic A82.0
  urban A82.1
Rachischisis —see Spina bifida
Rachitic —see also condition
  deformities of spine (late effect) (sequelae)
    E64.3
  pelvis (late effect) (sequelae) E64.3
    with disproportion (fetopelvic) O33.0
      causing obstructed labor O65.0
Rachitis, rachitism (acute) (tarda) —see also
    Rickets
  renalis N25.0
  sequelae E64.3
Radial nerve —see condition
Radiation
  burn —see Burn
  effects NOS T66
  sickness NOS T66
  therapy, encounter for Z51.0
Radiculitis (pressure) (vertebrogenic) —see
    Radiculopathy
Radiculomyelitis —see also Encephalitis
  toxic, due to
    Clostridium tetani A35
    Corynebacterium diphtheriae A36.82
Radiculopathy M54.10
  cervical region M54.12
  cervicothoracic region M54.13
  due to
    disc disorder
      C3 M50.11
      C4 M50.11
      C5 M50.121 ◄
      C6 M50.122 ◄
      C7 M50.123 ◄
      C8 M50.13
    displacement of intervertebral disc —see
      Disorder, disc, with, radiculopathy
  leg M54.1-
  lumbar region M54.16
  lumbosacral region M54.17
  occipito-atlanto-axial region M54.11
  postherpetic B02.29
  sacrococcygeal region M54.18
  syphilitic A52.11
  thoracic region (with visceral pain)
    M54.14
  thoracolumbar region M54.15
Radiodermal burns (acute, chronic, or
    occupational) —see Burn
Radiodermatitis L58.9
  acute L58.0
  chronic L58.1
Radiotherapy session Z51.0
RAEB (refractory anemia with excess blasts)
    D46.2- ◄
Rage, meaning rabies —see Rabies
Ragpicker's disease A22.1
Ragsorter's disease A22.1
Raillietiniasis B71.8
Railroad neurosis F48.8
Railway spine F48.8
Raised —see also Elevated
  antibody titer R76.0
Rake teeth, tooth M26.39
Rales R09.89
Ramifying renal pelvis Q63.8
Ramsay-Hunt disease or syndrome —see also
    Hunt's disease B02.21
  meaning dyssynergia cerebellaris myoclonica
    G11.1
Ranula K11.6
  congenital Q38.4

Rape
  adult
    confirmed T74.21
    suspected T76.21
  alleged, observation or examination, ruled out
    adult Z04.41
    child Z04.42
  child
    confirmed T74.22
    suspected T76.22
Rapid
  feeble pulse, due to shock, following injury
    T79.4
  heart (beat) R00.0
    psychogenic F45.8
  second stage (delivery) O62.3
  time-zone change syndrome —see Disorder,
    sleep, circadian rhythm, psychogenic
Rarefaction, bone —see Disorder, bone, density
    and structure, specified NEC
Rash (toxic) R21
  canker A38.9
  diaper L22
  drug (internal use) L27.0
    contact —see also Dermatitis, due to, drugs,
      external L25.1
  following immunization T88.1
  food —see Dermatitis, due to, food
  heat L74.0
  napkin (psoriasiform) L22
  nettle —see Urticaria
  pustular L08.0
  rose R21
    epidemic B06.9
  scarlet A38.9
  serum —see also Reaction, serum T80.69
  wandering tongue K14.1
Rasmussen aneurysm —see Tuberculosis,
    pulmonary
Rasmussen encephalitis G04.81
Rat-bite fever A25.9
  due to Streptobacillus moniliformis A25.1
  spirochetal (morsus muris) A25.0
Rathke's pouch tumor D44.3
Raymond (-Céstan) syndrome I65.8
Raynaud's disease, phenomenon or syndrome
    (secondary) I73.00
  with gangrene (symmetric) I73.01
RDS (newborn) (type I) P22.0
  type II P22.1
Reaction —see also Disorder
  adaptation —see Disorder, adjustment
  adjustment (anxiety) (conduct disorder)
    (depressiveness) (distress) —see
      Disorder, adjustment
    with
      mutism, elective (child) (adolescent) F94.0
  adverse
    food (any) (ingested) NEC T78.1
      anaphylactic —see Shock, anaphylactic,
        due to food
  anaphylactoid —see Shock, anaphylactic
  affective —see Disorder, mood
  allergic —see Allergy
  anaphylactic —see Shock, anaphylactic
  anesthesia —see Anesthesia, complication
  antitoxin (prophylactic) (therapeutic) —see
    Complications, vaccination
  anxiety F41.1
  Arthus —see Arthus' phenomenon
  asthenic F48.8
  combat and operational stress F43.0
  compulsive F42.8 ◄═
  conversion F44.9
  crisis, acute F43.0
  deoxyribonuclease (DNA) (DNase)
    hypersensitivity D69.2
  depressive (single episode) F32.9
    affective (single episode) F31.4
      recurrent episode F33.9
    neurotic F34.1
    psychoneurotic F34.1

Reaction (Continued)
  depressive (Continued)
    psychotic F32.3
    recurrent —see Disorder, depressive,
      recurrent
  dissociative F44.9
  drug NEC T88.7
    addictive —see Dependence, drug
      transmitted via placenta or breast
        milk —see Absorption, drug,
          addictive, through placenta
    allergic —see Allergy, drug
    lichenoid L43.2
    newborn P93.8
      gray baby syndrome P93.0
    overdose or poisoning (by accident) —see
      Table of Drugs and Chemicals, by
        drug, poisoning
    photoallergic L56.1
    phototoxic L56.0
    withdrawal —see Dependence, by drug,
      with, withdrawal
      infant of dependent mother P96.1
      newborn P96.1
    wrong substance given or taken (by
      accident) —see Table of Drugs and
        Chemicals, by drug, poisoning
  fear F40.9
    child (abnormal) F93.8
  febrile nonhemolytic transfusion (FNHTR)
    R50.84
  fluid loss, cerebrospinal G97.1
  foreign
    body NEC —see Granuloma, foreign body
      in operative wound (inadvertently
        left) —see Foreign body,
          accidentally left during a
            procedure
    substance accidentally left during a
      procedure (chemical) (powder) (talc)
        T81.60
      aseptic peritonitis T81.61
      body or object (instrument) (sponge)
        (swab) —see Foreign body,
          accidentally left during a
            procedure
      specified reaction NEC T81.69
  grief —see Disorder, adjustment
  Herxheimer's R68.89
  hyperkinetic —see Hyperkinesia
  hypochondriacal F45.20
  hypoglycemic, due to insulin E16.0
    with coma (diabetic) —see Diabetes, coma
      nondiabetic E15
    therapeutic misadventure —see
      subcategory T38.3
  hypomanic F30.8
  hysterical F44.9
  immunization —see Complications, vaccination
  incompatibility
    ABO blood group (infusion) (transfusion) —
      see Complication (s), transfusion,
        incompatibility reaction, ABO
      delayed serologic T80.39
    minor blood group (Duffy) (E) (K(ell))
      (Kidd) (Lewis) (M) (N) (P) (S) T80.89
    Rh (factor) (infusion) (transfusion) —see
      Complication (s), transfusion,
        incompatibility reaction, Rh (factor)
  inflammatory —see Infection
  infusion —see Complications, infusion
  inoculation (immune serum) —see
    Complications, vaccination
  insulin T38.3-
  involutional psychotic —see Disorder,
    depressive
  leukemoid D72.823
    basophilic D72.823
    lymphocytic D72.823
    monocytic D72.823
    myelocytic D72.823
    neutrophilic D72.823

◄ New   ◄═ Revised   ~~deleted~~ Deleted

Reaction *(Continued)*
  LSD (acute)
    due to drug abuse —*see* Abuse, drug,
      hallucinogen
    due to drug dependence —*see* Dependence,
      drug, hallucinogen
  lumbar puncture G97.1
  manic-depressive —*see* Disorder, bipolar
  neurasthenic F48.8
  neurogenic —*see* Neurosis
  neurotic F48.9
  neurotic-depressive F34.1
  nitritoid —*see* Crisis, nitritoid - obsessive-
    compulsive F42
  nonspecific
    to
      cell mediated immunity measurement
        of gamma interferon antigen
        response without active
        tuberculosis R76.12
      QuantiFERON-TB test (QFT) without
        active tuberculosis R76.12
      tuberculin test —*see also* Reaction,
        tuberculin skin test R76.11
  obsessive-compulsive F42.8 ◀▥
  organic, acute or subacute —*see* Delirium
  paranoid (acute) F23
    chronic F22
    senile F03
  passive dependency F60.7
  phobic F40.9
  post-traumatic stress, uncomplicated
    Z73.3
  psychogenic F99
  psychoneurotic —*see also* Neurosis
    compulsive F42.8 ◀▥
    depersonalization F48.1
    depressive F34.1
    hypochondriacal F45.20
    neurasthenic F48.8
    obsessive F42.8 ◀▥
  psychophysiologic —*see* Disorder,
    somatoform
  psychosomatic —*see* Disorder, somatoform
  psychotic —*see* Psychosis
  scarlet fever toxin —*see* Complications,
    vaccination
  schizophrenic F23
    acute (brief) (undifferentiated) F23
    latent F21
    undifferentiated (acute) (brief) F23
  serological for syphilis —*see* Serology for
    syphilis
  serum T80.69
    anaphylactic (immediate) —*see also* Shock,
      anaphylactic T80.59
    specified reaction NEC
      due to
        administration of blood and blood
          products T80.61
        immunization T80.62
        serum specified NEC T80.69
        vaccination T80.62
  situational —*see* Disorder, adjustment
  somatization —*see* Disorder, somatoform
  spinal puncture G97.1
  stress (severe) F43.9
    acute (agitation) ("daze") (disorientation)
      (disturbance of consciousness) (flight
      reaction) (fugue) F43.0
    specified NEC F43.8
  surgical procedure —*see* Complications,
    surgical procedure
  tetanus antitoxin —*see* Complications,
    vaccination
  toxic, to local anesthesia T81.59 ◀▥
    in labor and delivery O74.4
    in pregnancy O29.3X-
    postpartum, puerperal O89.3
  toxin-antitoxin —*see* Complications,
    vaccination

Reaction *(Continued)*
  transfusion (blood) (bone marrow)
    (lymphocytes) (allergic) —*see*
    Complications, transfusion
  tuberculin skin test, abnormal R76.11
  vaccination (any) —*see* Complications,
    vaccination
  withdrawing, child or adolescent F93.8
Reactive airway disease —*see* Asthma
Reactive depression —*see* Reaction, depressive
Rearrangement
  chromosomal
    balanced (in) Q95.9
      abnormal individual (autosomal) Q95.2
      non-sex (autosomal) chromosomes
        Q95.2
      sex/non-sex chromosomes Q95.3
      specified NEC Q95.8
Recalcitrant patient —*see* Noncompliance
Recanalization, thrombus —*see* Thrombosis
Recession, receding
  chamber angle (eye) H21.55-
  chin M26.09
  gingival (generalized) (localized)
    (postinfective) (postoperative) K06.00 ◀▥
    Miller Class I K06.01 ◀
    Miller Class II K06.02 ◀
    Miller Class III K06.03 ◀
    Miller Class IV K06.04 ◀
Recklinghausen's disease Q85.01
  bones E21.0
Reclus' disease (cystic) —*see* Mastopathy, cystic
Recrudescent typhus (fever) A75.1
Recruitment, auditory H93.21-
Rectalgia K62.89
Rectitis K62.89
Rectocele
  female (without uterine prolapse) N81.6
    with uterine prolapse N81.4
      incomplete N81.2
  in pregnancy —*see* Pregnancy, complicated
    by, abnormal, pelvic organs or tissues
    NEC
  male K62.3
Rectosigmoid junction —*see* condition
Rectosigmoiditis K63.89
  ulcerative (chronic) K51.30
    with
      complication K51.319
        abscess K51.314
        fistula K51.313
        obstruction K51.312
        rectal bleeding K51.311
        specified NEC K51.318
Rectourethral —*see* condition
Rectovaginal —*see* condition
Rectovesical —*see* condition
Rectum, rectal —*see* condition
Recurrent —*see* condition
  pregnancy loss —*see* Loss (of), pregnancy,
    recurrent
Red bugs B88.0
Red-cedar lung or pneumonitis J67.8
Red tide —*see also* Table of Drugs and
  Chemicals T65.82-
Reduced
  mobility Z74.09
  ventilatory or vital capacity R94.2
Redundant, redundancy
  anus (congenital) Q43.8
  clitoris N90.89
  colon (congenital) Q43.8
  foreskin (congenital) N47.8
  intestine (congenital) Q43.8
  labia N90.69 ◀▥
  organ or site, congenital NEC —*see* Accessory
  panniculus (abdominal) E65
  prepuce (congenital) N47.8
  pylorus K31.89
  rectum (congenital) Q43.8
  scrotum N50.89 ◀▥

Redundant, redundancy *(Continued)*
  sigmoid (congenital) Q43.8
  skin L98.7 ◀▥
    ~~eyelids —*see* Blepharochalasis~~
    and subcutaneous tissue L98.7 ◀
    of face L57.4 ◀
    eyelids —*see* Blepharochalasis ◀
  stomach K31.89
Reduplication —*see* Duplication
Reflex R29.2
  hyperactive gag J39.2
  pupillary, abnormal —*see* Anomaly, pupil,
    function
  vasoconstriction I73.9
  vasovagal R55
Reflux K21.9
  acid K21.9
  esophageal K21.9
    with esophagitis K21.0
    newborn P78.83
  gastroesophageal K21.9
    with esophagitis K21.0
  mitral —*see* Insufficiency, mitral
  ureteral —*see* Reflux, vesicoureteral
  vesicoureteral (with scarring) N13.70
    with
      nephropathy N13.729
        with hydroureter N13.739
          bilateral N13.732
          unilateral N13.731
        without hydroureter N13.729
          bilateral N13.722
          unilateral N13.721
        bilateral N13.722
        unilateral N13.721
      pyelonephritis (chronic) N11.0
    without nephropathy N13.71
    congenital Q62.7
Reforming, artificial openings —*see* Attention
  to, artificial, opening
Refractive error —*see* Disorder, refraction
Refsum's disease or syndrome G60.1
Refusal of
  food, psychogenic F50.89 ◀▥
  treatment (because of) Z53.20
    left against medical advice (AMA) Z53.21
    patient's decision NEC Z53.29
    reasons of belief or group pressure Z53.1
Regional —*see* condition
Regurgitation R11.10
  aortic (valve) —*see* Insufficiency, aortic
  food —*see also* Vomiting
    with reswallowing —*see* Rumination
    newborn P92.1
  gastric contents —*see* Vomiting
  heart —*see* Endocarditis
  mitral (valve) —*see* Insufficiency, mitral
    congenital Q23.3
  myocardial —*see* Endocarditis
  pulmonary (valve) (heart) I37.1
    congenital Q22.2
    syphilitic A52.03
  tricuspid —*see* Insufficiency, tricuspid
  valve, valvular —*see* Endocarditis
    congenital Q24.8
  vesicoureteral —*see* Reflux, vesicoureteral
Reichmann's disease or syndrome K31.89
Reifenstein syndrome E34.52
~~Reinsertion, contraceptive device Z30.433~~
Reinsertion ◀
  implantable subdermal contraceptive Z30.46 ◀
  intrauterine contraceptive device Z30.433 ◀
Reiter's disease, syndrome, or urethritis
  M02.30
  ankle M02.37-
  elbow M02.32-
  foot joint M02.37-
  hand joint M02.34-
  hip M02.35-
  knee M02.36-
  multiple site M02.39

Reiter's disease, syndrome, or urethritis
(Continued)
  shoulder M02.31-
  vertebra M02.38
  wrist M02.33-
Rejection
  food, psychogenic F50.89 ◄▥
  transplant T86.91
    bone T86.830
      marrow T86.01
    cornea T86.840
    heart T86.21
      with lung (s) T86.31
    intestine T86.850
    kidney T86.11
    liver T86.41
    lung (s) T86.810
      with heart T86.31
    organ (immune or nonimmune cause)
      T86.91
    pancreas T86.890
    skin (allograft) (autograft) T86.820
    specified NEC T86.890
    stem cell (peripheral blood) (umbilical
      cord) T86.5
Relapsing fever A68.9
  Carter's (Asiatic) A68.1
  Dutton's (West African) A68.1
  Koch's A68.9
  louse-borne (epidemic) A68.0
  Novy's (American) A68.1
  Obermeyers's (European) A68.0
  Spirillum A68.9
  tick-borne (endemic) A68.1
Relationship
  occlusal
    open anterior M26.220
    open posterior M26.221
Relaxation
  anus (sphincter) K62.89
    psychogenic F45.8
  arch (foot) —see also Deformity, limb, flat
    foot
  back ligaments —see Instability, joint,
    spine
  bladder (sphincter) N31.2
  cardioesophageal K21.9
  cervix —see Incompetency, cervix
  diaphragm J98.6
  joint (capsule) (ligament) (paralytic) —see
    Flail, joint
    congenital NEC Q74.8
  lumbosacral (joint) —see subcategory M53.2
  pelvic floor N81.89
  perineum N81.89
  posture R29.3
  rectum (sphincter) K62.89
  sacroiliac (joint) —see subcategory M53.2
  scrotum N50.89 ◄▥
  urethra (sphincter) N36.44
  vesical N31.2
Release from prison, anxiety concerning
  Z65.2
Remains
  canal of Cloquet Q14.0
  capsule (opaque) Q14.8
Remittent fever (malarial) B54
Remnant
  canal of Cloquet Q14.0
  capsule (opaque) Q14.8
  cervix, cervical stump (acquired)
    (postoperative) N88.8
  cystic duct, postcholecystectomy K91.5
  fingernail L60.8
    congenital Q84.6
  meniscus, knee —see Derangement, knee,
    meniscus, specified NEC
  thyroglossal duct Q89.2
  tonsil J35.8
    infected (chronic) J35.01
  urachus Q64.4

Removal (from) (of)
  artificial
    arm Z44.00-
      complete Z44.01-
      partial Z44.02-
    eye Z44.2-
    leg Z44.10-
      complete Z44.11-
      partial Z44.12-
  breast implant Z45.81
  cardiac pulse generator (battery) (end-of-life)
    Z45.010
  catheter (urinary) (indwelling) Z46.6
    from artificial opening —see Attention to,
      artificial, opening
    non-vascular Z46.82
    vascular NEC Z45.2
  device Z46.9
    contraceptive Z30.432
      implantable subdermal Z30.46 ◄
    implanted NEC Z45.89
    specified NEC Z46.89
  drains Z48.03
  dressing (nonsurgical) Z48.00
    surgical Z48.01
  external
    fixation device — code to fracture with
      seventh character D
    prosthesis, prosthetic device Z44.9
      breast Z44.3-
      specified NEC Z44.8
  home in childhood (to foster home or
    institution) Z62.29
  ileostomy Z43.2
  insulin pump Z46.81
  myringotomy device (stent) (tube) Z45.82
  nervous system device NEC Z46.2
    brain neuropacemaker Z46.2
    visual substitution device Z46.2
      implanted Z45.31
  non-vascular catheter Z46.82
  organ, prophylactic (for neoplasia
    management) —see Prophylactic, organ
    removal
  orthodontic device Z46.4
  staples Z48.02
  stent
    ureteral Z46.6
  suture Z48.02
  urinary device Z46.6
  vascular access device or catheter Z45.2
Ren
  arcuatus Q63.1
  mobile, mobilis N28.89
    congenital Q63.8
  unguliformis Q63.1
Renal —see condition
Rendu-Osler-Weber disease or syndrome
  I78.0
Reninoma D41.0-
Renon-Delille syndrome E23.3
Reovirus, as cause of disease classified
  elsewhere B97.5
Repeated falls NEC R29.6
Replaced chromosome by dicentric ring
  Q93.2
Replacement by artificial or mechanical device
  or prosthesis of
  bladder Z96.0
  blood vessel NEC Z95.828
  bone NEC Z96.7
  cochlea Z96.21
  coronary artery Z95.5
  eustachian tube Z96.29
  eye globe Z97.0
  heart Z95.812
    valve Z95.2
      prosthetic Z95.2
      specified NEC Z95.4
      xenogenic Z95.3
  intestine Z96.89

Replacement by artificial or mechanical device
  or prosthesis of (Continued)
  joint Z96.60
    hip —see Presence, hip joint implant
    knee —see Presence, knee joint implant
    specified site NEC Z96.698
  larynx Z96.3
  lens Z96.1
  limb (s) —see Presence, artificial, limb
  mandible NEC (for tooth root implant (s))
    Z96.5
  organ NEC Z96.89
  peripheral vessel NEC Z95.828
  stapes Z96.29
  teeth Z97.2
  tendon Z96.7
  tissue NEC Z96.89
  tooth root (s) Z96.5
  vessel NEC Z95.828
    coronary (artery) Z95.5
Request for expert evidence Z04.8
Reserve, decreased or low
  cardiac —see Disease, heart
  kidney N28.89
Residual —see also condition
  ovary syndrome N99.83
  state, schizophrenic F20.5
  urine R39.198 ◄▥
Resistance, resistant (to)
  activated protein C D68.51
  complicating pregnancy O26.89
  insulin E88.81
  organism (s)
    to
      drug Z16.30 ◄▥
        aminoglycosides Z16.29
        amoxicillin Z16.11
        ampicillin Z16.11
        antibiotic (s) Z16.20
          multiple Z16.24
          specified NEC Z16.29
        antifungal Z16.32
        antimicrobial (single) Z16.30
          multiple Z16.35
          specified NEC Z16.39
        antimycobacterial (single) Z16.341
          multiple Z16.342
        antimycobacterial (single)
          Z16.341 ◄
          multiple Z16.342 ◄
        antiparasitic Z16.31
        antiviral Z16.33
        beta lactam antibiotics Z16.10
          specified NEC Z16.19
        cephalosporins Z16.19
        extended beta lactamase (ESBL)
          Z16.12
        fluoroquinolones Z16.23
        macrolides Z16.29
        methicillin —see MRSA
        multiple drugs (MDRO)
          antibiotics Z16.24
          antimicrobial Z16.35 ◄
          antimycobacterials
            Z16.342 ◄
        penicillins Z16.11
        quinine (and related compounds)
          Z16.31
        quinolones Z16.23
        sulfonamides Z16.29
        tetracyclines Z16.29
        tuberculostatics (single) Z16.341
          multiple Z16.342
        vancomycin Z16.21
          related antibiotics Z16.22
  thyroid hormone E07.89
Resorption
  dental (roots) K03.3
    alveoli M26.79
  teeth (external) (internal) (pathological)
    (roots) K03.3

◄ New   ◄▥ Revised   ~~deleted~~ Deleted

Respiration
  Cheyne-Stokes R06.3
  decreased due to shock, following injury
      T79.4
  disorder of, psychogenic F45.8
  insufficient, or poor R06.89
      newborn P28.5
  painful R07.1
  sighing, psychogenic F45.8
Respiratory —see also condition
  distress syndrome (newborn) (type I)
      P22.0
      type II P22.1
  syncytial virus, as cause of disease classified
      elsewhere B97.4
Respite care Z75.5
Response (drug)
  photoallergic L56.1
  phototoxic L56.0
Restenosis ◀
  stent ◀
    vascular ◀
      end stent ◀
        adjacent to stent —see
            Arteriosclerosis ◀
        within the stent ◀
          coronary T82.855 ◀
          peripheral T82.856 ◀
      in stent ◀
        coronary vessel T82.855 ◀
        peripheral vessel T82.856 ◀
Restless legs (syndrome) G25.81
Restlessness R45.1
Restoration (of)
  dental
    aesthetically inadequate or displeasing
        K08.56
    defective K08.50
        specified NEC K08.59
    failure of marginal integrity K08.51
    failure of periodontal anatomical intergrity
        K08.54
  organ continuity from previous sterilization
      (tuboplasty) (vasoplasty) Z31.0
    aftercare Z31.42
  tooth (existing)
    contours biologically incompatible with
        oral health K08.54
    open margins K08.51
    overhanging K08.52
    poor aesthetic K08.56
    poor gingival margins K08.51
  unsatisfactory, of tooth K08.50
    specified NEC K08.59
Restorative material (dental)
  allergy to K08.55
  fractured K08.539
    with loss of material K08.531
    without loss of material K08.530
  unrepairable overhanging of K08.52
Restriction of housing space Z59.1
Rests, ovarian, in fallopian tube Q50.6
Restzustand (schizophrenic) F20.5
Retained —see also Retention
  cholelithiasis following cholecystectomy
      K91.86
  foreign body fragments (type of) Z18.9
    acrylics Z18.2
    animal quill (s) or spines Z18.31
    cement Z18.83
    concrete Z18.83
    crystalline Z18.83
    depleted isotope Z18.09
    depleted uranium Z18.01
    diethylhexylphthalates Z18.2
    glass Z18.81
    isocyanate Z18.2
    magnetic metal Z18.11
    metal Z18.10
    nonmagnetic metal Z18.12
    nontherapeutic radioactive Z18.09

Retained (Continued)
  foreign body fragments (Continued)
    organic NEC Z18.39
    plastic Z18.2
    quill (s) (animal) Z18.31
    radioactive (nontherapeutic) NEC
        Z18.09
    specified NEC Z18.89
    spine (s) (animal) Z18.31
    stone Z18.83
    tooth (teeth) Z18.32
    wood Z18.33
  fragments (type of) Z18.9
    acrylics Z18.2
    animal quill (s) or spines Z18.31
    cement Z18.83
    concrete Z18.83
    crystalline Z18.83
    depleted isotope Z18.09
    depleted uranium Z18.01
    diethylhexylphthalates Z18.2
    glass Z18.81
    isocyanate Z18.2
    magnetic metal Z18.11
    metal Z18.10
    nonmagnectic metal Z18.12
    nontherapeutic radioactive Z18.09
    organic NEC Z18.39
    plastic Z18.2
    quill (s) (animal) Z18.31
    radioactive (nontherapeutic) NEC
        Z18.09
    specified NEC Z18.89
    spine (s) (animal) Z18.31
    stone Z18.83
    tooth (teeth) Z18.32
    wood Z18.33
  gallstones, following cholecystectomy K91.86
Retardation
  development, developmental, specific —see
      Disorder, developmental
  endochondral bone growth —see Disorder,
      bone, development or growth
  growth R62.50
    due to malnutrition E45
  mental —see Disability, intellectual
  motor function, specific F82
  physical (child) R62.52
    due to malnutrition E45
  reading (specific) F81.0
  spelling (specific) (without reading disorder)
      F81.81
Retching —see Vomiting
Retention —see also Retained
  bladder —see Retention, urine
  carbon dioxide E87.2
  cholelithiasis following cholecystectomy
      K91.86
  cyst —see Cyst
  dead
    fetus (at or near term) (mother) O36.4
      early fetal death O02.1
    ovum O02.0
  decidua (fragments) (following delivery)
      (with hemorrhage) O72.2
    without hemorrhage O73.1
  deciduous tooth K00.6
  dental root K08.3
  fecal —see Constipation
  fetus
    dead O36.4
      early O02.1
  fluid R60.9
  foreign body —see also Foreign body, retained
    current trauma - code as Foreign body, by
        site or type
  gallstones, following cholecystectomy K91.86
  gastric K31.89
  intrauterine contraceptive device, in
      pregnancy —see Pregnancy, complicated
      by, retention, intrauterine device

Retention (Continued)
  membranes (complicating delivery) (with
      hemorrhage) O72.2
    with abortion —see Abortion, by type
    without hemorrhage O73.1
  meniscus —see Derangement, meniscus
  menses N94.89
  milk (puerperal, postpartum) O92.79
  nitrogen, extrarenal R39.2
  ovary syndrome N99.83
  placenta (total) (with hemorrhage) O72.0
    without hemorrhage O73.0
    portions or fragments (with hemorrhage)
        O72.2
      without hemorrhage O73.1
  products of conception
    early pregnancy (dead fetus) O02.1
    following
      delivery (with hemorrhage) O72.2
        without hemorrhage O73.1
    secundines (following delivery) (with
        hemorrhage) O72.0
      without hemorrhage O73.0
    complicating puerperium (delayed
        hemorrhage) O72.2
    partial O72.2
      without hemorrhage O73.1
  smegma, clitoris N90.89
  urine R33.9
    drug-induced R33.0
    due to hyperplasia (hypertrophy) of
        prostate —see Hyperplasia, prostate
    organic R33.8
      drug-induced R33.0
    psychogenic F45.8
    specified NEC R33.8
  water (in tissues) —see Edema
Reticular erythematous mucinosis L98.5
Reticulation, dust —see Pneumoconiosis
Reticulocytosis R70.1
Reticuloendotheliosis
  acute infantile C96.0
  leukemic C91.4-
  malignant C96.9
  nonlipid C96.0
Reticulohistiocytoma (giant-cell) D76.3
Reticuloid, actinic L57.1
Reticulosis (skin)
  acute of infancy C96.0
  hemophagocytic, familial D76.1
  histiocytic medullary C96.A ◀▥
  lipomelanotic I89.8
  malignant (midline) C86.0
  nonlipid C96.0
  polymorphic C86.0
  Sézary —see Sézary disease
Retina, retinal —see also condition
  dark area D49.81
Retinitis —see also Inflammation, chorioretinal
  albuminurica N18.9 [H32]
  diabetic —see Diabetes, retinitis
  disciformis —see Degeneration, macula
  focal —see Inflammation, chorioretinal,
      focal
  gravidarum —see Pregnancy, complicated by,
      specified pregnancy-related condition
      NEC
  juxtapapillaris —see Inflammation,
      chorioretinal, focal, juxtapapillary
  luetic —see Retinitis, syphilitic
  pigmentosa H35.52
  proliferans —see Disorder, globe,
      degenerative, specified type NEC
  proliferating —see Disorder, globe,
      degenerative, specified type NEC
  renal N18.9 [H32]
  syphilitic (early) (secondary) A51.43
    central, recurrent A52.71
    congenital (early) A50.01 [H32]
    late A52.71
  tuberculous A18.53

Retinoblastoma C69.2-
  differentiated C69.2-
  undifferentiated C69.2-
Retinochoroiditis —see also Inflammation,
    chorioretinal
  disseminated —see Inflammation,
      chorioretinal, disseminated
    syphilitic A52.71
  focal —see Inflammation, chorioretinal
  juxtapapillaris —see Inflammation,
      chorioretinal, focal, juxtapapillary
Retinopathy (background) H35.00
  arteriosclerotic I70.8 [H35.0-]
  atherosclerotic I70.8 [H35.0-]
  central serous —see Chorioretinopathy,
      central serous
  Coats H35.02-
  diabetic —see Diabetes, retinopathy
  exudative H35.02-
  hypertensive H35.03-
  in (due to)
    diabetes —see Diabetes, retinopathy
  sickle-cell disorders D57.- [H36]
  of prematurity H35.10-
    stage 0 H35.11-
    stage 1 H35.12-
    stage 2 H35.13-
    stage 3 H35.14-
    stage 4 H35.15-
    stage 5 H35.16-
  pigmentary, congenital —see Dystrophy,
      retina
  proliferative NEC H35.2-
    diabetic —see Diabetes, retinopathy,
        proliferative
    sickle-cell D57.- [H36]
  solar H31.02-
Retinoschisis H33.10-
  congenital Q14.1
  specified type NEC H33.19-
Retortamoniasis A07.8
Retractile testis Q55.22
Retraction
  cervix —see Retroversion, uterus
  drum (membrane) —see Disorder, tympanic
      membrane, specified NEC
  finger —see Deformity, finger
  lid H02.539
    left H02.536
      lower H02.535
      upper H02.534
    right H02.533
      lower H02.532
      upper H02.531
  lung J98.4
  mediastinum J98.59 ◀▥
  nipple N64.53
    associated with
      lactation O92.03
      pregnancy O92.01-
      puerperium O92.02
    congenital Q83.8
  palmar fascia M72.0
  pleura —see Pleurisy
  ring, uterus (Bandl's) (pathological) O62.4
  sternum (congenital) Q76.7
    acquired M95.4
  uterus —see Retroversion, uterus
  valve (heart) —see Endocarditis
Retrobulbar —see condition
Retrocecal —see condition
Retrocession —see Retroversion
Retrodisplacement —see Retroversion
Retroflection, retroflexion —see Retroversion
Retrognathia, retrognathism (mandibular)
    (maxillary) M26.19
Retrograde menstruation N92.5
Retroperineal —see condition
Retroperitoneal —see condition
Retroperitonitis K68.9
Retropharyngeal —see condition

Retroplacental —see condition
Retroposition —see Retroversion
Retroprosthetic membrane T85.398
Retrosternal thyroid (congenital) Q89.2
Retroversion, retroverted
  cervix —see Retroversion, uterus
  female NEC —see Retroversion, uterus
  iris H21.89
  testis (congenital) Q55.29
  uterus (acquired) (acute) (any
      degree) (asymptomatic) (cervix)
      (postinfectional) (postpartal, old) N85.4
    congenital Q51.818
    in pregnancy O34.53-
Retrovirus, as cause of disease classified
    elsewhere B97.30
  human
    immunodeficiency, type 2 (HIV 2) B97.35
    T-cell lymphotropic
      type I (HTLV-I) B97.33
      type II (HTLV-II) B97.34
  lentivirus B97.31
  oncovirus B97.32
  specified NEC B97.39
Retrusion, premaxilla (developmental) M26.09
Rett's disease or syndrome F84.2
Reverse peristalsis R19.2
Reye's syndrome G93.7
Rh (factor)
  hemolytic disease (newborn) P55.0
  incompatibility, immunization or
      sensitization
    affecting management of pregnancy NEC
        O36.09-
      anti-D antibody O36.01-
    newborn P55.0
    transfusion reaction —see Complication (s),
        transfusion, incompatibility reaction,
        Rh (factor)
  negative mother affecting newborn P55.0
  titer elevated —see Complication (s),
      transfusion, incompatibility reaction,
      Rh (factor)
  transfusion reaction —see Complication (s),
      transfusion, incompatibility reaction,
      Rh (factor)
Rhabdomyolysis (idiopathic) NEC M62.82
  traumatic T79.6
Rhabdomyoma —see also Neoplasm, connective
    tissue, benign
  adult —see Neoplasm, connective tissue,
      benign
  fetal —see Neoplasm, connective tissue, benign
  glycogenic —see Neoplasm, connective tissue,
      benign
Rhabdomyosarcoma (any type) —see
    Neoplasm, connective tissue, malignant
Rhabdosarcoma —see Rhabdomyosarcoma
Rhesus (factor) incompatibility —see Rh,
    incompatibility
Rheumatic (acute) (subacute) (chronic)
  adherent pericardium I09.2
  coronary arteritis I01.9
  degeneration, myocardium I09.0
  fever (acute) —see Fever, rheumatic
  heart —see Disease, heart, rheumatic
  myocardial degeneration —see Degeneration,
      myocardium
  myocarditis (chronic) (inactive) (with chorea)
      I09.0
    with chorea (acute) (rheumatic)
        (Sydenham's) I02.0
    active or acute I01.2
  pancarditis, acute I01.8
    with chorea (acute (rheumatic)
        Sydenham's) I02.0
  pericarditis (active) (acute) (with effusion)
      (with pneumonia) I01.0
    with chorea (acute) (rheumatic)
        (Sydenham's) I02.0
    chronic or inactive I09.2

Rheumatic (Continued)
  pneumonia I00 [J17]
  torticollis M43.6
  typhoid fever A01.09
Rheumatism (articular) (neuralgic)
    (nonarticular) M79.0
  gout —see Arthritis, rheumatoid
  intercostal, meaning Tietze's disease M94.0
  palindromic (any site) M12.30
    ankle M12.37-
    elbow M12.32-
    foot joint M12.37-
    hand joint M12.34-
    hip M12.35-
    knee M12.36-
    multiple site M12.39
    shoulder M12.31-
    specified joint NEC M12.38
    vertebrae M12.38
    wrist M12.33-
  sciatic M54.4-
Rheumatoid —see also condition
  arthritis —see also Arthritis, rheumatoid
    with involvement of organs NEC M05.60
      ankle M05.67-
      elbow M05.62-
      foot joint M05.67-
      hand joint M05.64-
      hip M05.65-
      knee M05.66-
      multiple site M05.69
      shoulder M05.61-
      vertebra —see Spondylitis, ankylosing
      wrist M05.63-
    seronegative —see Arthritis, rheumatoid,
        seronegative
    seropositive —see Arthritis, rheumatoid,
        seropositive
  carditis M05.30
    ankle M05.37-
    elbow M05.32-
    foot joint M05.37-
    hand joint M05.34-
    hip M05.35-
    knee M05.36-
    multiple site M05.39
    shoulder M05.31-
    vertebra —see Spondylitis, ankylosing
    wrist M05.33-
  endocarditis —see Rheumatoid, carditis
  lung (disease) M05.10
    ankle M05.17-
    elbow M05.12-
    foot joint M05.17-
    hand joint M05.14-
    hip M05.15-
    knee M05.16-
    multiple site M05.19
    shoulder M05.11-
    vertebra —see Spondylitis, ankylosing
    wrist M05.13-
  myocarditis —see Rheumatoid, carditis
  myopathy M05.40
    ankle M05.47-
    elbow M05.42-
    foot joint M05.47-
    hand joint M05.44-
    hip M05.45-
    knee M05.46-
    multiple site M05.49
    shoulder M05.41-
    vertebra —see Spondylitis, ankylosing
    wrist M05.43-
  pericarditis —see Rheumatoid, carditis
  polyarthritis —see Arthritis, rheumatoid
  polyneuropathy M05.50
    ankle M05.57-
    elbow M05.52-
    foot joint M05.57-
    hand joint M05.54-
    hip M05.55-

◀ New   ◀▥ Revised   ~~deleted~~ Deleted

Rheumatoid *(Continued)*
  polyneuropathy *(Continued)*
    knee M05.56-
    multiple site M05.59
    shoulder M05.51-
    vertebra —*see* Spondylitis, ankylosing
    wrist M05.53-
  vasculitis M05.20
    ankle M05.27-
    elbow M05.22-
    foot joint M05.27-
    hand joint M05.24-
    hip M05.25-
    knee M05.26-
    multiple site M05.29
    shoulder M05.21-
    vertebra —*see* Spondylitis, ankylosing
    wrist M05.23-
Rhinitis (atrophic) (catarrhal) (chronic)
    (croupous) (fibrinous) (granulomatous)
    (hyperplastic) (hypertrophic)
    (membranous) (obstructive) (purulent)
    (suppurative) (ulcerative) J31.0
  with
    sore throat —*see* Nasopharyngitis
  acute J00
  allergic J30.9
    with asthma J45.909
      with
        exacerbation (acute) J45.901
          status asthmaticus J45.902
    due to
      food J30.5
      pollen J30.1
    nonseasonal J30.89
    perennial J30.89
    seasonal NEC J30.2
    specified NEC J30.89
  infective J00
  pneumococcal J00
  syphilitic A52.73
    congenital A50.05 *[J99]*
  tuberculous A15.8
  vasomotor J30.0
Rhinoantritis (chronic) —*see* Sinusitis,
    maxillary
Rhinodacryolith —*see* Dacryolith
Rhinolith (nasal sinus) J34.89
Rhinomegaly J34.89
Rhinopharyngitis (acute) (subacute) —*see also*
    Nasopharyngitis
  chronic J31.1
  destructive ulcerating A66.5
  mutilans A66.5
Rhinophyma L71.1
Rhinorrhea J34.89
  cerebrospinal (fluid) G96.0
  paroxysmal —*see* Rhinitis, allergic
  spasmodic —*see* Rhinitis, allergic
Rhinosalpingitis —*see* Salpingitis, eustachian
Rhinoscleroma A48.8
Rhinosporidiosis B48.1
Rhinovirus infection NEC B34.8
Rhizomelic chondrodysplasia punctata
    E71.540
Rhythm
  atrioventricular nodal I49.8
  disorder I49.9
    coronary sinus I49.8
    ectopic I49.8
    nodal I49.8
  escape I49.9
  heart, abnormal I49.9
  idioventricular I44.2
  nodal I49.8
  sleep, inversion G47.2-
    nonorganic origin —*see* Disorder, sleep,
      circadian rhythm, psychogenic
Rhytidosis facialis L98.8
Rib —*see also* condition
  cervical Q76.5

Riboflavin deficiency E53.0
Rice bodies —*see also* Loose, body, joint
    knee M23.4-
Richter syndrome —*see* Leukemia, chronic
    lymphocytic, B-cell type
Richter's hernia —*see* Hernia, abdomen, with
    obstruction
Ricinism —*see* Poisoning, food, noxious,
    plant
Rickets (active) (acute) (adolescent) (chest
    wall) (congenital) (current) (infantile)
    (intestinal) E55.0
  adult —*see* Osteomalacia
  celiac K90.0
  hypophosphatemic with nephrotic-glycosuric
    dwarfism E72.09
  inactive E64.3
  kidney N25.0
  renal N25.0
  sequelae, any E64.3
  vitamin-D-resistant E83.31 *[M90.80]*
Rickettsial disease A79.9
  specified type NEC A79.89
Rickettsialpox (Rickettsia akari) A79.1
Rickettsiosis A79.9
  due to
    Ehrlichia sennetsu A79.81
    Rickettsia akari (rickettsialpox) A79.1
  specified type NEC A79.89
  tick-borne A77.9
  vesicular A79.1
Rider's bone —*see* Ossification, muscle,
    specified NEC
Ridge, alveolus —*see also* condition
  flabby K06.8
Ridged ear, congenital Q17.3
Riedel's
  lobe, liver Q44.7
  struma, thyroiditis or disease E06.5
Rieger's anomaly or syndrome Q13.81
Riehl's melanosis L81.4
Rietti-Greppi-Micheli anemia D56.9
Rieux's hernia —*see* Hernia, abdomen, specified
    site NEC
Riga (-Fede) **disease** K14.0
Riggs' disease —*see* Periodontitis
Right aortic arch Q25.47 ◀
Right middle lobe syndrome J98.11
Rigid, rigidity —*see also* condition
  abdominal R19.30
    with severe abdominal pain R10.0
    epigastric R19.36
    generalized R19.37
    left lower quadrant R19.34
    left upper quadrant R19.32
    periumbilic R19.35
    right lower quadrant R19.33
    right upper quadrant R19.31
  articular, multiple, congenital Q68.8
  cervix (uteri) in pregnancy —*see* Pregnancy,
    complicated by, abnormal, cervix
  hymen (acquired) (congenital) N89.6
  nuchal R29.1
  pelvic floor in pregnancy —*see* Pregnancy,
    complicated by, abnormal, pelvic organs
    or tissues NEC
  perineum or vulva in pregnancy —*see*
    Pregnancy, complicated by, abnormal,
    vulva
  spine —*see* Dorsopathy, specified NEC
  vagina in pregnancy —*see* Pregnancy,
    complicated by, abnormal, vagina
Rigors R68.89
  with fever R50.9
Riley-Day syndrome G90.1
RIND (reversible ischemic neurologic deficit)
    I63.9
Ring (s)
  aorta (vascular) Q25.45 ◀▥
  Bandl's O62.4
  contraction, complicating delivery O62.4

Ring (s) *(Continued)*
  esophageal, lower (muscular) K22.2
  Fleischer's (cornea) H18.04-
  hymenal, tight (acquired) (congenital) N89.6
  Kayser-Fleischer (cornea) H18.04-
  retraction, uterus, pathological O62.4
  Schatzki's (esophagus) (lower) K22.2
    congenital Q39.3
  Soemmerring's —*see* Cataract, secondary
  vascular (congenital) Q25.8
    aorta Q25.45 ◀▥
Ringed hair (congenital) Q84.1
Ringworm B35.9
  beard B35.0
  black dot B35.0
  body B35.4
  Burmese B35.5
  corporeal B35.4
  foot B35.3
  groin B35.6
  hand B35.2
  honeycomb B35.0
  nails B35.1
  perianal (area) B35.6
  scalp B35.0
  specified NEC B35.8
  Tokelau B35.5
Rise, venous pressure I87.8
Rising, PSA following treatment for malignant
    neoplasm of prostate R97.21 ◀
Risk, suicidal
  meaning personal history of attempted
    suicide Z91.5
  meaning suicidal ideation —*see* Ideation,
    suicidal
Ritter's disease L00
Rivalry, sibling Z62.891
Rivalta's disease A42.2
River blindness B73.01
Robert's pelvis Q74.2
  with disproportion (fetopelvic) O33.0
    causing obstructed labor O65.0
Robin (-Pierre) **syndrome** Q87.0
Robinow-Silvermann-Smith syndrome Q87.1
Robinson's (hidrotic) **ectodermal dysplasia or**
    syndrome Q82.4
Robles' disease B73.01
Rocky Mountain (spotted) **fever** A77.0
Roetheln —*see* Rubella
Roger's disease Q21.0
Rokitansky-Aschoff sinuses (gallbladder) K82.8
Rolando's fracture (displaced) S62.22-
  nondisplaced S62.22-
Romano-Ward (prolonged QT interval)
    syndrome I45.81
Romberg's disease or syndrome G51.8
Roof, mouth —*see* condition
Rosacea L71.9
  acne L71.9
  keratitis L71.8
  specified NEC L71.8
Rosary, rachitic E55.0
Rose
  cold J30.1
  fever J30.1
  rash R21
    epidemic B06.9
Rosenbach's erysipeloid A26.0
Rosenthal's disease or syndrome D68.1
Roseola B09
  infantum B08.20
    due to human herpesvirus 6 B08.21
    due to human herpesvirus 7 B08.22
Ross River disease or fever B33.1
Rossbach's disease K31.89
  psychogenic F45.8
Rostan's asthma (cardiac) —*see* Failure,
    ventricular, left
Rotation
  anomalous, incomplete or insufficient,
    intestine Q43.3

Rotation *(Continued)*
  cecum (congenital) Q43.3
  colon (congenital) Q43.3
  spine, incomplete or insufficient —*see*
    Dorsopathy, deforming, specified NEC
  tooth, teeth, fully erupted M26.35
  vertebra, incomplete or insufficient —*see*
    Dorsopathy, deforming, specified NEC
Rotes Quérol disease or syndrome —*see*
  Hyperostosis, ankylosing
Roth (-Bernhardt) disease or syndrome —*see*
  Meralgia paraesthetica
Rothmund (-Thomson) syndrome Q82.8
Rotor's disease or syndrome E80.6
Round
  back (with wedging of vertebrae) —*see*
    Kyphosis
  sequelae (late effect) of rickets E64.3
  worms (large) (infestation) NEC B82.0
    Ascariasis —*see also* Ascariasis B77.9
Roussy-Lévy syndrome G60.0
Rubella (German measles) B06.9
  complication NEC B06.09
    neurological B06.00
  congenital P35.0
  contact Z20.4
  exposure to Z20.4
  maternal
    care for (suspected) damage to fetus O35.3
    manifest rubella in infant P35.0
    suspected damage to fetus affecting
      management of pregnancy O35.3
  specified complications NEC B06.89
Rubeola (meaning measles) —*see* Measles
  meaning rubella —*see* Rubella
Rubeosis, iris —*see* Disorder, iris, vascular
Rubinstein-Taybi syndrome Q87.2
Rudimentary (congenital) —*see also* Agenesis
  arm —*see* Defect, reduction, upper limb
  bone Q79.9
  cervix uteri Q51.828
  eye Q11.2
  lobule of ear Q17.3
  patella Q74.1
  respiratory organs in thoracopagus Q89.4
  tracheal bronchus Q32.4
  uterus Q51.818
    in male Q56.1
  vagina Q52.0
Ruled out condition —*see* Observation,
  suspected
Rumination R11.10
  with nausea R11.2
  disorder of infancy F98.21
  neurotic F42.8 ◀▥
  newborn P92.1
  obsessional F42.8 ◀▥
  psychogenic F42.8 ◀▥
Runeberg's disease D51.0
Runny nose R09.89
Rupia (syphilitic) A51.39
  congenital A50.06
  tertiary A52.79
Rupture, ruptured
  abscess (spontaneous) - code by site under
    Abscess
  aneurysm —*see* Aneurysm
  anus (sphincter) —*see* Laceration, anus
  aorta, aortic I71.8
    abdominal I71.3
    arch I71.1
    ascending I71.1
    descending I71.8
      abdominal I71.3
      thoracic I71.1
    syphilitic A52.01
    thoracoabdominal I71.5
    thorax, thoracic I71.1
    transverse I71.1
    traumatic —*see* Injury, aorta, laceration,
      major

Rupture, ruptured *(Continued)*
  aorta, aortic *(Continued)*
    valve or cusp —*see also* Endocarditis, aortic
      I35.8
  appendix (with peritonitis) K35.2
    with localized peritonitis K35.3 ◀
  arteriovenous fistula, brain I60.8
  artery I77.2
    brain —*see* Hemorrhage, intracranial,
      intracerebral
    coronary —*see* Infarct, myocardium
    heart —*see* Infarct, myocardium
    pulmonary I28.8
    traumatic (complication) —*see* Injury,
      blood vessel
  bile duct (common) (hepatic) K83.2
    cystic K82.2
  bladder (sphincter) (nontraumatic)
    (spontaneous) N32.89
    following ectopic or molar pregnancy
      O08.6
    obstetrical trauma O71.5
    traumatic S37.29
  blood vessel —*see also* Hemorrhage
    brain —*see* Hemorrhage, intracranial,
      intracerebral
    heart —*see* Infarct, myocardium
    traumatic (complication) —*see* Injury,
      blood vessel, laceration, major, by site
  bone —*see* Fracture
  bowel (nontraumatic) K63.1
  brain
    aneurysm (congenital) —*see also*
      Hemorrhage, intracranial,
      subarachnoid
      syphilitic A52.05
    hemorrhagic —*see* Hemorrhage,
      intracranial, intracerebral
  capillaries I78.8
  cardiac (auricle) (ventricle) (wall) I23.3
    with hemopericardium I23.0
    infectional I40.9
    traumatic —*see* Injury, heart
  cartilage (articular) (current) —*see also* Sprain
    knee S83.3-
    semilunar —*see* Tear, meniscus
  cecum (with peritonitis) K65.0
    with peritoneal abscess K35.3
    traumatic S36.598
  celiac artery, traumatic —*see* Injury, blood
    vessel, celiac artery, laceration, major
  cerebral aneurysm (congenital) (*see*
    Hemorrhage, intracranial,
    subarachnoid)
  cervix (uteri)
    with ectopic or molar pregnancy O08.6
    following ectopic or molar pregnancy
      O08.6
    obstetrical trauma O71.3
    traumatic S37.69
  chordae tendineae NEC I51.1
    concurrent with acute myocardial
      infarction —*see* Infarct, myocardium
    following acute myocardial infarction
      (current complication) I23.4
  choroid (direct) (indirect) (traumatic) H31.32-
  circle of Willis I60.6
  colon (nontraumatic) K63.1
    traumatic —*see* Injury, intestine, large
  cornea (traumatic) —*see* Injury, eye, laceration
  coronary (artery) (thrombotic) —*see* Infarct,
    myocardium
  corpus luteum (infected) (ovary) N83.1- ◀▥
  cyst —*see* Cyst
  cystic duct K82.2
  Descemet's membrane —*see* Change, corneal
    membrane, Descemet's, rupture
    traumatic —*see* Injury, eye, laceration
  diaphragm, traumatic —*see* Injury,
    intrathoracic, diaphragm
  disc —*see* Rupture, intervertebral disc

Rupture, ruptured *(Continued)*
  diverticulum (intestine) K57.80
    with bleeding K57.81
    bladder N32.3
    large intestine K57.20
      with
        bleeding K57.21
        small intestine K57.40
          with bleeding K57.41
      small intestine K57.00
      with
        bleeding K57.01
        large intestine K57.40
          with bleeding K57.41
  duodenal stump K31.89
  ear drum (nontraumatic) —*see also*
    Perforation, tympanum
    traumatic S09.2-
      due to blast injury —*see* Injury, blast, ear
  esophagus K22.3
  eye (without prolapse or loss of intraocular
    tissue) —*see* Injury, eye, laceration
  fallopian tube NEC (nonobstetric)
    (nontraumatic) N83.8
    due to pregnancy O00.10 ◀▥
      with intrauterine pregnancy O00.11 ◀
  fontanel P13.1
  gallbladder K82.2
    traumatic S36.128
  gastric —*see also* Rupture, stomach
    vessel K92.2
  globe (eye) (traumatic) —*see* Injury, eye,
    laceration
  graafian follicle (hematoma) N83.0- ◀▥
  heart —*see* Rupture, cardiac
  hymen (nontraumatic) (nonintentional)
    N89.8
  internal organ, traumatic —*see* Injury,
    by site
  intervertebral disc —*see* Displacement,
    intervertebral disc
    traumatic —*see* Rupture, traumatic,
      intervertebral disc
  intestine NEC (nontraumatic) K63.1
    traumatic —*see* Injury, intestine
  iris —*see also* Abnormality, pupillary
    traumatic —*see* Injury, eye, laceration
  joint capsule, traumatic —*see* Sprain
  kidney (traumatic) S37.06-
    birth injury P15.8
    nontraumatic N28.89
  lacrimal duct (traumatic) —*see* Injury, eye,
    specified site NEC
  lens (cataract) (traumatic) —*see* Cataract,
    traumatic
  ligament, traumatic —*see* Rupture, traumatic,
    ligament, by site
  liver S36.116
    birth injury P15.0
  lymphatic vessel I89.8
  marginal sinus (placental) (with
    hemorrhage) —*see* Hemorrhage,
    antepartum, specified cause NEC
  membrana tympani (nontraumatic) —*see*
    Perforation, tympanum
  membranes (spontaneous)
    artificial
      delayed delivery following O75.5
    delayed delivery following —*see*
      Pregnancy, complicated by,
      premature rupture of membranes
  meningeal artery I60.8
  meniscus (knee) —*see also* Tear, meniscus
    old —*see* Derangement, meniscus
    site other than knee - code as Sprain
  mesenteric artery, traumatic —*see* Injury,
    mesenteric, artery, laceration, major
  mesentery (nontraumatic) K66.8
    traumatic —*see* Injury, intra-abdominal,
      specified, site NEC
  mitral (valve) I34.8

◀ New   ◀▥ Revised   ~~deleted~~ Deleted

Rupture, ruptured *(Continued)*
  muscle (traumatic) —*see also* Strain
    diastasis —*see* Diastasis, muscle
    nontraumatic M62.10
      ankle M62.17-
      foot M62.17-
      forearm M62.13-
      hand M62.14-
      lower leg M62.16-
      pelvic region M62.15-
      shoulder region M62.11-
      specified site NEC M62.18
      thigh M62.15-
      upper arm M62.12-
    traumatic —*see* Strain, by site
  musculotendinous junction NEC,
      nontraumatic —*see* Rupture, tendon,
      spontaneous
  mycotic aneurysm causing cerebral
      hemorrhage —*see* Hemorrhage,
      intracranial, subarachnoid
  myocardium, myocardial —*see* Rupture,
      cardiac
    traumatic —*see* Injury, heart
  nontraumatic, meaning hernia —*see* Hernia
  obstructed —*see* Hernia, by site, obstructed
  operation wound —*see* Disruption, wound,
      operation
  ovary, ovarian N83.8
    corpus luteum cyst N83.1- ◀▥
    follicle (graafian) N83.0- ◀▥
  oviduct (nonobstetric) (nontraumatic)
      N83.8
    due to pregnancy O00.10 ◀▥
      with intrauterine pregnancy
        O00.11 ◀
  pancreas (nontraumatic) K86.89 ◀▥
    traumatic S36.299
  papillary muscle NEC I51.2
    following acute myocardial infarction
        (current complication) I23.5
  pelvic
    floor, complicating delivery O70.1
    organ NEC, obstetrical trauma O71.5
  perineum (nonobstetric) (nontraumatic)
      N90.89
    complicating delivery —*see* Delivery,
        complicated, by, laceration, anus
        (sphincter)
  postoperative wound —*see* Disruption,
      wound, operation
  prostate (traumatic) S37.828
  pulmonary
    artery I28.8
    valve (heart) I37.8
    vein I28.8
    vessel I28.8
  pus tube —*see* Salpingitis
  pyosalpinx —*see* Salpingitis
  rectum (nontraumatic) K63.1
    traumatic S36.69
  retina, retinal (traumatic) (without
      detachment) —*see also* Break, retina
    with detachment —*see* Detachment, retina,
        with retinal, break
  rotator cuff (nontraumatic) M75.10-
    complete M75.12-
    incomplete M75.11-
  sclera —*see* Injury, eye, laceration
  sigmoid (nontraumatic) K63.1
    traumatic S36.593
  spinal cord —*see also* Injury, spinal cord, by
      region
    due to injury at birth P11.5
    newborn (birth injury) P11.5
  spleen (traumatic) S36.09
    birth injury P15.1
    congenital (birth injury) P15.1
    due to P. vivax malaria B51.0
    nontraumatic D73.5
    spontaneous D73.5

Rupture, ruptured *(Continued)*
  splenic vein R58
    traumatic —*see* Injury, blood vessel,
        splenic vein
  stomach (nontraumatic) (spontaneous)
      K31.89
    traumatic S36.39
  supraspinatus (complete) (incomplete)
      (nontraumatic) —*see* Tear, rotator
      cuff
  symphysis pubis
    obstetric O71.6
    traumatic S33.4
  synovium (cyst) M66.10
    ankle M66.17-
    elbow M66.12-
    finger M66.14-
    foot M66.17-
    forearm M66.13-
    hand M66.14-
    pelvic region M66.15-
    shoulder region M66.11-
    specified site NEC M66.18
    thigh M66.15-
    toe M66.17-
    upper arm M66.12-
    wrist M66.13-
  tendon (traumatic) —*see* Strain
    nontraumatic (spontaneous) M66.9
      ankle M66.87-
      extensor M66.20
        ankle M66.27-
        foot M66.27-
        forearm M66.23-
        hand M66.24-
        lower leg M66.26-
        multiple sites M66.29
        pelvic region M66.25-
        shoulder region M66.21-
        specified site NEC M66.28
        thigh M66.25-
        upper arm M66.22-
      flexor M66.30
        ankle M66.37-
        foot M66.37-
        forearm M66.33-
        hand M66.34-
        lower leg M66.36-
        multiple sites M66.39
        pelvic region M66.35-
        shoulder region M66.31-
        specified site NEC M66.38
        thigh M66.35-
        upper arm M66.32-
      foot M66.87-
      forearm M66.83-
      hand M66.84-
      lower leg M66.86-
      multiple sites M66.89
      pelvic region M66.85-
      shoulder region M66.81-
      specified
        site NEC M66.88
        tendon M66.80
      thigh M66.85-
      upper arm M66.82-
  thoracic duct I89.8
  tonsil J35.8
  traumatic
    aorta —*see* Injury, aorta, laceration,
        major
    diaphragm —*see* Injury, intrathoracic,
        diaphragm
    external site —*see* Wound, open,
        by site
    eye —*see* Injury, eye, laceration
    internal organ —*see* Injury, by site
    intervertebral disc
      cervical S13.0
      lumbar S33.0
      thoracic S23.0

Rupture, ruptured *(Continued)*
  traumatic *(Continued)*
    kidney S37.06-
    ligament —*see also* Sprain
      ankle —*see* Sprain, ankle
      carpus —*see* Rupture, traumatic,
          ligament, wrist
      collateral (hand) —*see* Rupture,
          traumatic, ligament, finger,
          collateral
      finger (metacarpophalangeal)
          (interphalangeal) S63.40-
        collateral S63.41-
          index S63.41-
          little S63.41-
          middle S63.41-
          ring S63.41-
        index S63.40-
        little S63.40-
        middle S63.40-
        palmar S63.42-
          index S63.42-
          little S63.42-
          middle S63.42-
          ring S63.42-
        ring S63.40-
        specified site NEC S63.499
          index S63.49-
          little S63.49-
          middle S63.49-
          ring S63.49-
        volar plate S63.43-
          index S63.43-
          little S63.43-
          middle S63.43-
          ring S63.43-
      foot —*see* Sprain, foot
      radial collateral S53.2-
      radiocarpal —*see* Rupture, traumatic,
          ligament, wrist, radiocarpal
      ulnar collateral S53.3-
      ulnocarpal —*see* Rupture, traumatic,
          ligament, wrist, ulnocarpal
      wrist S63.30-
        collateral S63.31-
        radiocarpal S63.32-
        specified site NEC S63.39-
        ulnocarpal (palmar) S63.33-
    liver S36.116
    membrana tympani —*see* Rupture, ear
        drum, traumatic
    muscle or tendon —*see* Strain
    myocardium —*see* Injury, heart
    pancreas S36.299
    rectum S36.69
    sigmoid S36.593
    spleen S36.09
    stomach S36.39
    symphysis pubis S33.4
    tympanum, tympanic (membrane) —*see*
        Rupture, ear drum, traumatic
    ureter S37.19
    uterus S37.69
    vagina —*see* Injury, vagina
    vena cava —*see* Injury, vena cava,
        laceration, major
  tricuspid (heart) (valve) I07.8
  tube, tubal (nonobstetric) (nontraumatic)
      N83.8
    abscess —*see* Salpingitis
    due to pregnancy O00.10 ◀▥
      with intrauterine pregnancy O00.11 ◀
  tympanum, tympanic (membrane)
      (nontraumatic) —*see also* Perforation,
      tympanic membrane H72.9-
    traumatic —*see* Rupture, ear drum,
        traumatic
  umbilical cord, complicating delivery
      O69.89
  ureter (traumatic) S37.19
    nontraumatic N28.89

Rupture, ruptured *(Continued)*
   urethra (nontraumatic) N36.8
      with ectopic or molar pregnancy
         O08.6
      following ectopic or molar pregnancy
         O08.6
      obstetrical trauma O71.5
      traumatic S37.39
   uterosacral ligament (nonobstetric)
         (nontraumatic) N83.8
   uterus (traumatic) S37.69
      before labor O71.0-
      during or after labor O71.1

Rupture, ruptured *(Continued)*
   uterus *(Continued)*
      nonpuerperal, nontraumatic N85.8
      pregnant (during labor) O71.1
         before labor O71.0-
   vagina —*see* Injury, vagina
   valve, valvular (heart) —*see* Endocarditis
   varicose vein —*see* Varix
   varix —*see* Varix
   vena cava R58
      traumatic —*see* Injury, vena cava,
         laceration, major
   vesical (urinary) N32.89

Rupture, ruptured *(Continued)*
   vessel (blood) R58
      pulmonary I28.8
      traumatic —*see* Injury, blood vessel
   viscus R19.8
   vulva complicating delivery O70.0
Russell-Silver syndrome Q87.1
Russian spring-summer type encephalitis
   A84.0
Rust's disease (tuberculous cervical spondylitis)
   A18.01
Ruvalcaba-Myhre-Smith syndrome E71.440
Rytand-Lipsitch syndrome I44.2

◀ New   ◀▥ Revised   ~~deleted~~ Deleted

S

Saber, sabre shin or tibia (syphilitic) A50.56 [M90.8-]
Sac lacrimal —see condition
Saccharomyces infection B37.9
Saccharopinuria E72.3
Saccular —see condition
Sacculation
  aorta (nonsyphilitic) —see Aneurysm, aorta
  bladder N32.3
  intralaryngeal (congenital) (ventricular) Q31.3
  larynx (congenital) (ventricular) Q31.3
  organ or site, congenital —see Distortion
  pregnant uterus —see Pregnancy, complicated by, abnormal, uterus
  ureter N28.89
  urethra N36.1
  vesical N32.3
Sachs' amaurotic familial idiocy or disease E75.02
Sachs-Tay disease E75.02
Sacks-Libman disease M32.11
Sacralgia M53.3
Sacralization Q76.49
Sacrodynia M53.3
Sacroiliac joint —see condition
Sacroiliitis NEC M46.1
Sacrum —see condition
Saddle
  back —see Lordosis
  embolus
    abdominal aorta I74.01
    pulmonary artery I26.92
      with acute cor pulmonale I26.02
  injury — code to condition
  nose M95.0
    due to syphilis A50.57
Sadism (sexual) F65.52
Sadness, postpartal O90.6
Sadomasochism F65.50
Saemisch's ulcer (cornea) —see Ulcer, cornea, central
Sagging ◀
  skin and subcutaneous tissue (following bariatric surgery weight loss) (following dietary weight loss) L98.7 ◀
Sahib disease B55.0
Sailors' skin L57.8
Saint
  Anthony's fire —see Erysipelas
  triad —see Hernia, diaphragm
  Vitus' dance —see Chorea, Sydenham's
Salaam
  attack (s) —see Epilepsy, spasms
  tic R25.8
Salicylism
  abuse F55.8
  overdose or wrong substance given —see Table of Drugs and Chemicals, by drug, poisoning
Salivary duct or gland —see condition
Salivation, excessive K11.7
Salmonella —see Infection, Salmonella
Salmonellosis A02.0
Salpingitis (catarrhal) (fallopian tube) (nodular) (pseudofollicular) (purulent) (septic) N70.91
  with oophoritis N70.93
  acute N70.01
    with oophoritis N70.03
  chlamydial A56.11
  chronic N70.11
    with oophoritis N70.13
  complicating abortion —see Abortion, by type, complicated by, salpingitis
  ear —see Salpingitis, eustachian
  eustachian (tube) H68.00-
    acute H68.01-
    chronic H68.02-

Salpingitis (Continued)
  follicularis N70.11
    with oophoritis N70.13
  gonococcal (acute) (chronic) A54.24
  interstitial, chronic N70.11
    with oophoritis N70.13
  isthmica nodosa N70.11
    with oophoritis N70.13
  specific (gonococcal) (acute) (chronic) A54.24
  tuberculous (acute) (chronic) A18.17
  venereal (gonococcal) (acute) (chronic) A54.24
Salpingocele N83.4- ◀▥
Salpingo-oophoritis (catarrhal) (purulent) (ruptured) (septic) (suppurative) N70.93
  acute N70.03
    with ectopic or molar pregnancy O08.0
    following ectopic or molar pregnancy O08.0
    gonococcal A54.24
  chronic N70.13
  following ectopic or molar pregnancy O08.0
  gonococcal (acute) (chronic) A54.24
  puerperal O86.19
  specific (gonococcal) (acute) (chronic) A54.24
  subacute N70.03
  tuberculous (acute) (chronic) A18.17
  venereal (gonococcal) (acute) (chronic) A54.24
Salpingo-ovaritis —see Salpingo-oophoritis
Salpingoperitonitis —see Salpingo-oophoritis
Salzmann's nodular dystrophy —see Degeneration, cornea, nodular
Sampson's cyst or tumor N80.1
San Joaquin (Valley) fever B38.0
Sandblaster's asthma, lung or pneumoconiosis J62.8
Sander's disease (paranoia) F22
Sandfly fever A93.1
Sandhoff's disease E75.01
Sanfilippo (Type B) (Type C) (Type D) syndrome E76.22
Sanger-Brown ataxia G11.2
Sao Paulo fever or typhus A77.0
Saponification, mesenteric K65.8
Sarcocele (benign)
  syphilitic A52.76
    congenital A50.59
Sarcocystosis A07.8
Sarcoepiplocele —see Hernia
Sarcoepiplomphalocele Q79.2
Sarcoid —see also Sarcoidosis
  arthropathy D86.86
  Boeck's D86.9
  Darier-Roussy D86.3
  iridocyclitis D86.83
  meningitis D86.81
  myocarditis D86.85
  myositis D86.87
  pyelonephritis D86.84
  Spiegler-Fendt L08.89
Sarcoidosis D86.9
  with
    cranial nerve palsies D86.82
    hepatic granuloma D86.89
    polyarthritis D86.86
    tubulo-interstitial nephropathy D86.84
  combined sites NEC D86.89
  lung D86.0
    and lymph nodes D86.2
  lymph nodes D86.1
    and lung D86.2
  meninges D86.81
  skin D86.3
  specified type NEC D86.89
Sarcoma (of) —see also Neoplasm, connective tissue, malignant
  alveolar soft part —see Neoplasm, connective tissue, malignant
  ameloblastic C41.1
    upper jaw (bone) C41.0
  botryoid —see Neoplasm, connective tissue, malignant

Sarcoma (Continued)
  botryoides —see Neoplasm, connective tissue, malignant
  cerebellar C71.6
    circumscribed (arachnoidal) C71.6
  circumscribed (arachnoidal) cerebellar C71.6
  clear cell —see also Neoplasm, connective tissue, malignant
    kidney C64.-
  dendritic cells (accessory cells) C96.4
  embryonal —see Neoplasm, connective tissue, malignant
  endometrial (stromal) C54.1
    isthmus C54.0
  epithelioid (cell) —see Neoplasm, connective tissue, malignant
  Ewing's —see Neoplasm, bone, malignant
  follicular dendritic cell C96.4
  germinoblastic (diffuse) —see Lymphoma, diffuse, large cell
    follicular —see Lymphoma, follicular, specified NEC
  giant cell (except of bone) —see also Neoplasm, connective tissue, malignant
    bone —see Neoplasm, bone, malignant
  glomoid —see Neoplasm, connective tissue, malignant
  granulocytic C92.3-
  hemangioendothelial —see Neoplasm, connective tissue, malignant
  hemorrhagic, multiple —see Sarcoma, Kaposi's
  histiocytic C96.A
  Hodgkin —see Lymphoma, Hodgkin
  immunoblastic (diffuse) —see Lymphoma, diffuse large cell
  interdigitating dendritic cell C96.4
  Kaposi's
    colon C46.4
    connective tissue C46.1
    gastrointestinal organ C46.4
    lung C46.5-
    lymph node (s) C46.3
    palate (hard) (soft) C46.2
    rectum C46.4
    skin C46.0
    specified site NEC C46.7
    stomach C46.4
    unspecified site C46.9
  Kupffer cell C22.3
  Langerhans cell C96.4
  leptomeningeal —see Neoplasm, meninges, malignant
  liver NEC C22.4
  lymphangioendothelial —see Neoplasm, connective tissue, malignant
  lymphoblastic —see Lymphoma, lymphoblastic (diffuse)
  lymphocytic —see Lymphoma, small cell B-cell
  mast cell C96.2
  melanotic —see Melanoma
  meningeal —see Neoplasm, meninges, malignant
  meningothelial —see Neoplasm, meninges, malignant
  mesenchymal —see also Neoplasm, connective tissue, malignant
    mixed —see Neoplasm, connective tissue, malignant
  mesothelial —see Mesothelioma
  monstrocellular
    specified site —see Neoplasm, malignant, by site
    unspecified site C71.9
  myeloid C92.3-
  neurogenic —see Neoplasm, nerve, malignant
  odontogenic C41.1
    upper jaw (bone) C41.0

Sarcoma *(Continued)*
  osteoblastic —*see* Neoplasm, bone,
    malignant
  osteogenic —*see also* Neoplasm, bone,
    malignant
    juxtacortical —*see* Neoplasm, bone,
      malignant
    periosteal —*see* Neoplasm, bone,
      malignant
  periosteal —*see also* Neoplasm, bone,
    malignant
    osteogenic —*see* Neoplasm, bone,
      malignant
  pleomorphic cell —*see* Neoplasm, connective
    tissue, malignant
  reticulum cell (diffuse) —*see* Lymphoma,
    diffuse large cell
    nodular —*see* Lymphoma, follicular
    pleomorphic cell type —*see* Lymphoma,
      diffuse large cell
  rhabdoid —*see* Neoplasm, malignant, by site
  round cell —*see* Neoplasm, connective tissue,
    malignant
  small cell —*see* Neoplasm, connective tissue,
    malignant
  soft tissue —*see* Neoplasm, connective tissue,
    malignant
  spindle cell —*see* Neoplasm, connective
    tissue, malignant
  stromal (endometrial) C54.1
    isthmus C54.0
  synovial —*see also* Neoplasm, connective
    tissue, malignant
    biphasic —*see* Neoplasm, connective tissue,
      malignant
    epithelioid cell —*see* Neoplasm, connective
      tissue, malignant
    spindle cell —*see* Neoplasm, connective
      tissue, malignant
Sarcomatosis
  meningeal —*see* Neoplasm, meninges,
    malignant
  specified site NEC —*see* Neoplasm,
    connective tissue, malignant
  unspecified site C80.1
Sarcopenia (age-related) M62.84 ◀
Sarcosinemia E72.59
Sarcosporidiosis (intestinal) A07.8
Satiety, early R68.81
Saturnine —*see* condition
Saturnism
  overdose or wrong substance given or
    taken —*see* Table of Drugs and
    Chemicals, by drug, poisoning
Satyriasis F52.8
Sauriasis —*see* Ichthyosis
SBE (subacute bacterial endocarditis) I33.0
Scabies (any site) B86
Scabs R23.4
Scaglietti-Dagnini syndrome E22.0
Scald —*see* Burn
Scalenus anticus (anterior) syndrome G54.0
Scales R23.4
Scaling, skin R23.4
Scalp —*see* condition
Scapegoating affecting child Z62.3
Scaphocephaly Q75.0
Scapulalgia M89.8X1
Scapulohumeral myopathy G71.0
Scar, scarring —*see also* Cicatrix L90.5
  adherent L90.5
  atrophic L90.5
  cervix
    in pregnancy or childbirth —*see* Pregnancy,
      complicated by, abnormal cervix
  cheloid L91.0
  chorioretinal H31.00-
    posterior pole macula H31.01-
    postsurgical H59.81-
    solar retinopathy H31.02-
    specified type NEC H31.09-

Scar, scarring *(Continued)*
  choroid —*see* Scar, chorioretinal
  conjunctiva H11.24-
  cornea H17.9
    xerophthalmic —*see also* Opacity, cornea
      vitamin A deficiency E50.6
  duodenum, obstructive K31.5
  hypertrophic L91.0
  keloid L91.0
  labia N90.89
  lung (base) J98.4
  macula —*see* Scar, chorioretinal, posterior
    pole
  muscle M62.89
  myocardium, myocardial I25.2
  painful L90.5
  posterior pole (eye) —*see* Scar, chorioretinal,
    posterior pole
  retina —*see* Scar, chorioretinal
  trachea J39.8
  transmural uterine, in pregnancy O34.29 ◀
  uterus N85.8
    in pregnancy O34.29
  vagina N89.8
    postoperative N99.2
  vulva N90.89
Scarabiasis B88.2
Scarlatina (anginosa) (maligna) (ulcerosa)
  A38.9
  myocarditis (acute) A38.1
    old —*see* Myocarditis
  otitis media A38.0
Scarlet fever (albuminuria) (angina) A38.9
Schamberg's disease (progressive pigmentary
  dermatosis) L81.7
Schatzki's ring (acquired) (esophagus) (lower)
  K22.2
  congenital Q39.3
Schaufenster krankheit I20.8
Schaumann's
  benign lymphogranulomatosis D86.1
  disease or syndrome —*see* Sarcoidosis
Scheie's syndrome E76.03
Schenck's disease B42.1
Scheuermann's disease or osteochondrosis —
  see Osteochondrosis, juvenile, spine
Schilder (-Flatau) disease G37.0
Schilling-type monocytic leukemia C93.0-
Schimmelbusch's disease, cystic mastitis, or
  hyperplasia —*see* Mastopathy, cystic
Schistosoma infestation —*see* Infestation,
  Schistosoma
Schistosomiasis B65.9
  with muscle disorder B65.9 *[M63.80]*
    ankle B65.9 *[M63.87-]*
    foot B65.9 *[M63.87-]*
    forearm B65.9 *[M63.83-]*
    hand B65.9 *[M63.84-]*
    lower leg B65.9 *[M63.86-]*
    multiple sites B65.9 *[M63.89]*
    pelvic region B65.9 *[M63.85-]*
    shoulder region B65.9 *[M63.81-]*
    specified site NEC B65.9 *[M63.88]*
    thigh B65.9 *[M63.85-]*
    upper arm B65.9 *[M63.82-]*
  Asiatic B65.2
  bladder B65.0
  chestermani B65.8
  colon B65.1
  cutaneous B65.3
  due to
    S. haematobium B65.0
    S. japonicum B65.2
    S. mansoni B65.1
    S. mattheii B65.8
  Eastern B65.2
  genitourinary tract B65.0
  intestinal B65.1
  lung NEC B65.9 *[J99]*
    pneumonia B65.9 *[J17]*
  Manson's (intestinal) B65.1

Schistosomiasis *(Continued)*
  oriental B65.2
  pulmonary NEC B65.9 *[J99]*
    pneumonia B65.9
  Schistosoma
    haematobium B65.0
    japonicum B65.2
    mansoni B65.1
  specified type NEC B65.8
  urinary B65.0
  vesical B65.0
Schizencephaly Q04.6
Schizoaffective psychosis F25.9
Schizodontia K00.2
Schizoid personality F60.1
Schizophrenia, schizophrenic F20.9
  acute (brief) (undifferentiated) F23
  atypical (form) F20.3
  borderline F21
  catalepsy F20.2
  catatonic (type) (excited) (withdrawn) F20.2
  cenesthopathic, cenesthesiopathic F20.89
  childhood type F84.5
  chronic undifferentiated F20.5
  cyclic F25.0
  disorganized (type) F20.1
  flexibilitas cerea F20.2
  hebephrenic (type) F20.1
  incipient F21
  latent F21
  negative type F20.5
  paranoid (type) F20.0
  paraphrenic F20.0
  post-psychotic depression F32.89 ◀||||
  prepsychotic F21
  prodromal F21
  pseudoneurotic F21
  pseudopsychopathic F21
  reaction F23
  residual (state) (type) F20.5
  restzustand F20.5
  schizoaffective (type) —*see* Psychosis,
    schizoaffective
  simple (type) F20.89
  simplex F20.89
  specified type NEC F20.89
  stupor F20.2
  syndrome of childhood F84.5
  undifferentiated (type) F20.3
    chronic F20.5
Schizothymia (persistent) F60.1
Schlatter-Osgood disease or
  osteochondrosis —*see* Osteochondrosis,
  juvenile, tibia
Schlatter's tibia —*see* Osteochondrosis,
  juvenile, tibia
Schmidt's syndrome (polyglandular,
  autoimmune) E31.0
Schmincke's carcinoma or tumor —*see*
  Neoplasm, nasopharynx, malignant
Schmitz (-Stutzer) dysentery A03.0
Schmorl's disease or nodes
  lumbar region M51.46
  lumbosacral region M51.47
  sacrococcygeal region M53.3
  thoracic region M51.44
  thoracolumbar region M51.45
Schneiderian
  papilloma —*see* Neoplasm, nasopharynx
    benign
      specified site —*see* Neoplasm, benign, by
        site
      unspecified site D14.0
    specified site —*see* Neoplasm, malignant, by
      site
    unspecified site C30.0
Scholte's syndrome (malignant carcinoid) E34.0
Scholz (-Bielchowsky-Henneberg) disease or
  syndrome E75.25
Schönlein (-Henoch) disease or purpura
  (primary) (rheumatic) D69.0

◀ New   ◀|||| Revised   ~~deleted~~ Deleted

Schottmuller's disease A01.4
Schroeder's syndrome (endocrine hypertensive) E27.0
Schüller-Christian disease or syndrome C96.5
Schultze's type acroparesthesia, simple I73.89
Schultz's disease or syndrome —*see* Agranulocytosis
Schwalbe-Ziehen-Oppenheim disease G24.1
Schwannoma —*see also* Neoplasm, nerve, benign
 malignant —*see also* Neoplasm, nerve, malignant
  with rhabdomyoblastic differentiation — *see* Neoplasm, nerve, malignant
 melanocytic —*see* Neoplasm, nerve, benign
 pigmented —*see* Neoplasm, nerve, benign
Schwannomatosis Q85.03
Schwartz (-Jampel) syndrome G71.13
Schwartz-Bartter syndrome E22.2
Schweniger-Buzzi anetoderma L90.1
Sciatic —*see* condition
Sciatica (infective)
 with lumbago M54.4-
  due to intervertebral disc disorder —*see* Disorder, disc, with, radiculopathy
 due to displacement of intervertebral disc (with lumbago) —*see* Disorder, disc, with, radiculopathy
 wallet M54.3-
Scimitar syndrome Q26.8
Sclera —*see* condition
Sclerectasia H15.84-
Scleredema
 adultorum —*see* Sclerosis, systemic
 Buschke's —*see* Sclerosis, systemic
 newborn P83.0
Sclerema (adiposum) (edematosum) (neonatorum) (newborn) P83.0
 adultorum —*see* Sclerosis, systemic
Scleriasis —*see* Scleroderma
Scleritis H15.00-
 with corneal involvement H15.04-
 anterior H15.01-
 brawny H15.02-
 in (due to) zoster B02.34
 posterior H15.03-
 specified type NEC H15.09-
 syphilitic A52.71
 tuberculous (nodular) A18.51
Sclerochoroiditis H31.8
Scleroconjunctivitis —*see* Scleritis
Sclerocystic ovary syndrome E28.2
Sclerodactyly, sclerodactylia L94.3
Scleroderma, sclerodermia (acrosclerotic) (diffuse) (generalized) (progressive) (pulmonary) —*see also* Sclerosis, systemic M34.9-
 circumscribed L94.0
 linear L94.1
 localized L94.0
 newborn P83.8
 systemic M34.9
Sclerokeratitis H16.8
 tuberculous A18.52
Scleroma nasi A48.8
Scleromalacia (perforans) H15.05-
Scleromyxedema L98.5
Sclérose en plaques G35
Sclerosis, sclerotic
 adrenal (gland) E27.8
 Alzheimer's —*see* Disease, Alzheimer's
 amyotrophic (lateral) G12.21
 aorta, aortic I70.0
  valve —*see* Endocarditis, aortic
 artery, arterial, arteriolar, arteriovascular — *see* Arteriosclerosis
 ascending multiple G35
 brain (generalized) (lobular) G37.9
  artery, arterial I67.2
  diffuse G37.0
  disseminated G35

Sclerosis, sclerotic *(Continued)*
 brain *(Continued)*
  insular G35
  Krabbe's E75.23
  miliary G35
  multiple G35
  presenile (Alzheimer's) —*see* Disease, Alzheimer's, early onset
  senile (arteriosclerotic) I67.2
  stem, multiple G35
  tuberous Q85.1
 bulbar, multiple G35
 bundle of His I44.39
 cardiac —*see* Disease, heart, ischemic, atherosclerotic
 cardiorenal —*see* Hypertension, cardiorenal
 cardiovascular —*see also* Disease, cardiovascular
  renal —*see* Hypertension, cardiorenal
 cerebellar —*see* Sclerosis, brain
 cerebral —*see* Sclerosis, brain
 cerebrospinal (disseminated) (multiple) G35
 cerebrovascular I67.2
 choroid —*see* Degeneration, choroid
 combined (spinal cord) —*see also* Degeneration, combined
  multiple G35
 concentric (Balo) G37.5
 cornea —*see* Opacity, cornea
 coronary (artery) I25.10
  with angina pectoris —*see* Arteriosclerosis, coronary (artery),
 corpus cavernosum
  female N90.89
  male N48.6
 diffuse (brain) (spinal cord) G37.0
 disseminated G35
 dorsal G35
 dorsolateral (spinal cord) —*see* Degeneration, combined
 endometrium N85.5
 extrapyramidal G25.9
 eye, nuclear (senile) —*see* Cataract, senile, nuclear
 focal and segmental (glomerular) —*see also* N00-N07 with fourth character .1 N05.1
 Friedreich's (spinal cord) G11.1
 funicular (spermatic cord) N50.89 ◄▥
 general (vascular) —*see* Arteriosclerosis
 gland (lymphatic) I89.8
 hepatic K74.1
  alcoholic K70.2
 hereditary
  cerebellar G11.9
  spinal (Friedreich's ataxia) G11.1
 hippocampal G93.81
 insular G35
 kidney —*see* Sclerosis, renal
 larynx J38.7
 lateral (amyotrophic) (descending) (primary) (spinal) G12.21
 lens, senile nuclear —*see* Cataract, senile, nuclear
 liver K74.1
  with fibrosis K74.2
   alcoholic K70.2
  alcoholic K70.2
  cardiac K76.1
 lung —*see* Fibrosis, lung
 mastoid —*see* Mastoiditis, chronic
 mesial temporal G93.81
 mitral I05.8
 Mönckeberg's (medial) —*see* Arteriosclerosis, extremities
 multiple (brain stem) (cerebral) (generalized) (spinal cord) G35
 myocardium, myocardial —*see* Disease, heart, ischemic, atherosclerotic
 nuclear (senile), eye —*see* Cataract, senile, nuclear

Sclerosis, sclerotic *(Continued)*
 ovary N83.8
 pancreas K86.89 ◄▥
 penis N48.6
 peripheral arteries —*see* Arteriosclerosis, extremities
 plaques G35
 pluriglandular E31.8
 polyglandular E31.8
 posterolateral (spinal cord) —*see* Degeneration, combined
 presenile (Alzheimer's) —*see* Disease, Alzheimer's, early onset
 primary, lateral G12.29
 progressive, systemic M34.0
 pulmonary —*see* Fibrosis, lung
  artery I27.0
  valve (heart) —*see* Endocarditis, pulmonary
 renal N26.9
  with
   cystine storage disease E72.09
   hypertensive heart disease (conditions in I11) —*see* Hypertension, cardiorenal
   arteriolar (hyaline) (hyperplastic) —*see* Hypertension, kidney
 retina (senile) (vascular) H35.00
 senile (vascular) —*see* Arteriosclerosis
 spinal (cord) (progressive) G95.89
  ascending G61.0
  combined —*see also* Degeneration, combined
   multiple G35
   syphilitic A52.11
  disseminated G35
  dorsolateral —*see* Degeneration, combined
  hereditary (Friedreich's) (mixed form) G11.1
  lateral (amyotrophic) G12.21
  multiple G35
  posterior (syphilitic) A52.11
 stomach K31.89
 subendocardial, congenital I42.4
 systemic M34.9
  with
   lung involvement M34.81
   myopathy M34.82
   polyneuropathy M34.83
  drug-induced M34.2
  due to chemicals NEC M34.2
  progressive M34.0
  specified NEC M34.89
 temporal (mesial) G93.81
 tricuspid (heart) (valve) I07.8
 tuberous (brain) Q85.1
 tympanic membrane —*see* Disorder, tympanic membrane, specified NEC
 valve, valvular (heart) —*see* Endocarditis
 vascular —*see* Arteriosclerosis
 vein I87.8
Scoliosis (acquired) (postural) M41.9
 adolescent (idiopathic) —*see* Scoliosis, idiopathic, adolescent ◄▥
 congenital Q67.5
  due to bony malformation Q76.3
  failure of segmentation (hemivertebra) Q76.3
  hemivertebra fusion Q76.3
  postural Q67.5
 idiopathic M41.20
  adolescent M41.129
   cervical region M41.122
   cervicothoracic region M41.123
   lumbar region M41.126
   lumbosacral region M41.127
   thoracic region M41.124
   thoracolumbar region M41.125
  cervical region M41.22
  cervicothoracic region M41.23

Scoliosis (Continued)
    idiopathic (Continued)
        infantile M41.00
            cervical region M41.02
            cervicothoracic region M41.03
            lumbar region M41.06
            lumbosacral region M41.07
            sacrococcygeal region M41.08
            thoracic region M41.04
            thoracolumbar region M41.05
        juvenile M41.119
            cervical region M41.112
            cervicothoracic region M41.113
            lumbar region M41.116
            lumbosacral region M41.117
            thoracic region M41.114
            thoracolumbar region M41.115
        lumbar region M41.26
        lumbosacral region M41.27
        thoracic region M41.24
        thoracolumbar region M41.25
    infantile —see Scoliosis, idiopathic,
        infantile ◄
    neuromuscular M41.40
        cervical region M41.42
        cervicothoracic region M41.43
        lumbar region M41.46
        lumbosacral region M41.47
        occipito-atlanto-axial region M41.41
        thoracic region M41.44
        thoracolumbar region M41.45
    paralytic —see Scoliosis, neuromuscular
    postradiation therapy M96.5
    rachitic (late effect or sequelae) E64.3
        [M49.80]
        cervical region E64.3 [M49.82]
        cervicothoracic region E64.3 [M49.83]
        lumbar region E64.3 [M49.86]
        lumbosacral region E64.3 [M49.87]
        multiple sites E64.3 [M49.89]
        occipito-atlanto-axial region E64.3
            [M49.81]
        sacrococcygeal region E64.3 [M49.88]
        thoracic region E64.3 [M49.84]
        thoracolumbar region E64.3 [M49.85]
    sciatic M54.4-
    secondary (to) NEC M41.50
        cerebral palsy, Friedreich's ataxia,
            poliomyelitis, neuromuscular
            disorders —see Scoliosis,
            neuromuscular
        cervical region M41.52
        cervicothoracic region M41.53
        lumbar region M41.56
        lumbosacral region M41.57
        thoracic region M41.54
        thoracolumbar region M41.55
    specified form NEC M41.80
        cervical region M41.82
        cervicothoracic region M41.83
        lumbar region M41.86
        lumbosacral region M41.87
        thoracic region M41.84
        thoracolumbar region M41.85
    thoracogenic M41.30
        thoracic region M41.34
        thoracolumbar region M41.35
    tuberculous A18.01
Scoliotic pelvis
    with disproportion (fetopelvic) O33.0
        causing obstructed labor O65.0
Scorbutus, scorbutic —see also Scurvy
    anemia D53.2
Score, NIHSS (National Institutes of Health
    Stroke Scale) R29.7- ◄
Scotoma (arcuate) (Bjerrum) (central) (ring) —
    see also Defect, visual field, localized,
    scotoma
    scintillating H53.19
Scratch —see Abrasion
Scratchy throat R09.89

Screening (for) Z13.9
    alcoholism Z13.89
    anemia Z13.0
    anomaly, congenital Z13.89
    antenatal, of mother Z36
    arterial hypertension Z13.6
    arthropod-borne viral disease NEC Z11.59
    bacteriuria, asymptomatic Z13.89
    behavioral disorder Z13.89
    brain injury, traumatic Z13.850
    bronchitis, chronic Z13.83
    brucellosis Z11.2
    cardiovascular disorder Z13.6
    cataract Z13.5
    chlamydial diseases Z11.8
    cholera Z11.0
    chromosomal abnormalities (nonprocreative)
        NEC Z13.79
    colonoscopy Z12.11
    congenital
        dislocation of hip Z13.89
        eye disorder Z13.5
        malformation or deformation Z13.89
    contamination NEC Z13.88
    cystic fibrosis Z13.228
    dengue fever Z11.59
    dental disorder Z13.84
    depression Z13.89
    developmental handicap Z13.42 ◄▥
        in early childhood Z13.42 ◄▥
        infant Z13.41 ◄
    diabetes mellitus Z13.1
    diphtheria Z11.2
    disability, intellectual Z13.42 ◄▥
        infant Z13.41 ◄
    disease or disorder Z13.9
        bacterial NEC Z11.2
            intestinal infectious Z11.0
            respiratory tuberculosis Z11.1
        blood or blood-forming organ Z13.0
        cardiovascular Z13.6
        Chagas' Z11.6
        chlamydial Z11.8
        dental Z13.89
        developmental Z13.42 ◄▥
            in child Z13.42 ◄
            infant Z13.41 ◄
        digestive tract NEC Z13.818
            lower GI Z13.811
            upper GI Z13.810
        ear Z13.5
        endocrine Z13.29
        eye Z13.5
        genitourinary Z13.89
        heart Z13.6
        human immunodeficiency virus (HIV)
            infection Z11.4
        immunity Z13.0
        infection
            intestinal Z11.0
                specified NEC Z11.6
        infectious Z11.9
        mental Z13.89
        metabolic Z13.228
        neurological Z13.89
        nutritional Z13.21
            metabolic Z13.228
                lipoid disorders Z13.220
        protozoal Z11.6
            intestinal Z11.0
        respiratory Z13.83
        rheumatic Z13.828
        rickettsial Z11.8
        sexually-transmitted NEC Z11.3
            human immunodeficiency virus (HIV)
                Z11.4
        sickle-cell (trait) Z13.0
        skin Z13.89
        specified NEC Z13.89
        spirochetal Z11.8
        thyroid Z13.29

Screening (Continued)
    disease or disorder (Continued)
        vascular Z13.6
        venereal Z11.3
        viral NEC Z11.59
            human immunodeficiency virus (HIV)
                Z11.4
            intestinal Z11.0
    elevated titer Z13.89
    emphysema Z13.83
    encephalitis, viral (mosquito- or tick-borne)
        Z11.59
    exposure to contaminants (toxic) Z13.88
    fever
        dengue Z11.59
        hemorrhagic Z11.59
        yellow Z11.59
    filariasis Z11.6
    galactosemia Z13.228
    gastrointestinal condition Z13.818
    genetic (nonprocreative)- for procreative
        management —see Testing, genetic, for
        procreative management
        disease carrier status (nonprocreative)
            Z13.71
        specified NEC (nonprocreative) Z13.79
    genitourinary condition Z13.89
    glaucoma Z13.5
    gonorrhea Z11.3
    gout Z13.89
    helminthiasis (intestinal) Z11.6
    hematopoietic malignancy Z12.89
    hemoglobinopathies NEC Z13.0
    hemorrhagic fever Z11.59
    Hodgkin disease Z12.89
    human immunodeficiency virus (HIV)
        Z11.4
    human papillomavirus Z11.51
    hypertension Z13.6
    immunity disorders Z13.0
    infection
        mycotic Z11.8
        parasitic Z11.8
    ingestion of radioactive substance Z13.88
    intellectual disability Z13.42 ◄▥
        infant Z13.41 ◄
    intestinal
        helminthiasis Z11.6
        infectious disease Z11.0
    leishmaniasis Z11.6
    leprosy Z11.2
    leptospirosis Z11.8
    leukemia Z12.89
    lymphoma Z12.89
    malaria Z11.6
    malnutrition Z13.29
        metabolic Z13.228
        nutritional Z13.21
    measles Z11.59
    mental disorder Z13.89
    metabolic errors, inborn Z13.228
    multiphasic Z13.89
    musculoskeletal disorder Z13.828
        osteoporosis Z13.820
    mycoses Z11.8
    myocardial infarction (acute) Z13.6
    neoplasm (malignant) (of) Z12.9
        bladder Z12.6
        blood Z12.89
        breast Z12.39
            routine mammogram Z12.31
        cervix Z12.4
        colon Z12.11
        genitourinary organs NEC Z12.79
            bladder Z12.6
            cervix Z12.4
            ovary Z12.73
            prostate Z12.5
            testis Z12.71
            vagina Z12.72
        hematopoietic system Z12.89

◄ New   ◄▥ Revised   ~~deleted~~ Deleted

Screening *(Continued)*
  neoplasm *(Continued)*
    intestinal tract Z12.10
      colon Z12.11
      rectum Z12.12
      small intestine Z12.13
    lung Z12.2
    lymph (glands) Z12.89
    nervous system Z12.82
    oral cavity Z12.81
    prostate Z12.5
    rectum Z12.12
    respiratory organs Z12.2
    skin Z12.83
    small intestine Z12.13
    specified site NEC Z12.89
    stomach Z12.0
  nephropathy Z13.89
  nervous system disorders NEC Z13.858
  neurological condition Z13.89
  osteoporosis Z13.820
  parasitic infestation Z11.9
    specified NEC Z11.8
  phenylketonuria Z13.228
  plague Z11.2
  poisoning (chemical) (heavy metal)
    Z13.88
  poliomyelitis Z11.59
  postnatal, chromosomal abnormalities
    Z13.89
  prenatal, of mother Z36
  protozoal disease Z11.6
    intestinal Z11.0
  pulmonary tuberculosis Z11.1
  radiation exposure Z13.88
  respiratory condition Z13.83
  respiratory tuberculosis Z11.1
  rheumatoid arthritis Z13.828
  rubella Z11.59
  schistosomiasis Z11.6
  sexually-transmitted disease NEC Z11.3
    human immunodeficiency virus (HIV)
      Z11.4
  sickle-cell disease or trait Z13.0
  skin condition Z13.89
  sleeping sickness Z11.6
  special Z13.9
    specified NEC Z13.89
  syphilis Z11.3
  tetanus Z11.2
  trachoma Z11.8
  traumatic brain injury Z13.850
  trypanosomiasis Z11.6
  tuberculosis, respiratory Z11.1
  venereal disease Z11.3
  viral encephalitis (mosquito- or tick-borne)
    Z11.59
  whooping cough Z11.2
  worms, intestinal Z11.6
  yaws Z11.8
  yellow fever Z11.59
Scrofula, scrofulosis (tuberculosis of cervical
  lymph glands) A18.2
Scrofulide (primary) (tuberculous) A18.4
Scrofuloderma, scrofulodermia (any site)
  (primary) A18.4
Scrofulosus lichen (primary) (tuberculous)
  A18.4
Scrofulous —*see* condition
Scrotal tongue K14.5
Scrotum —*see* condition
Scurvy, scorbutic E54
  anemia D53.2
  gum E54
  infantile E54
  rickets E55.0 [M90.80]
Sealpox B08.62
Seasickness T75.3
Seatworm (infection) (infestation) B80
Sebaceous —*see also* condition
  cyst —*see* Cyst, sebaceous

Seborrhea, seborrheic L21.9
  capillitii R23.8
  capitis L21.0
  dermatitis L21.9
    infantile L21.1
  eczema L21.9
    infantile L21.1
  sicca L21.0
Seckel's syndrome Q87.1
Seclusion, pupil —*see* Membrane, pupillary
Second hand tobacco smoke exposure (acute)
  (chronic) Z77.22
  in the perinatal period P96.81
Secondary
  dentin (in pulp) K04.3
  neoplasm, secondaries —*see* Table of
    Neoplasms, secondary
Secretion
  antidiuretic hormone, inappropriate E22.2
  catecholamine, by pheochromocytoma E27.5
  hormone
    antidiuretic, inappropriate (syndrome)
      E22.2
    by
      carcinoid tumor E34.0
      pheochromocytoma E27.5
    ectopic NEC E34.2
  urinary
    excessive R35.8
    suppression R34
Section
  nerve, traumatic —*see* Injury, nerve
Sedative, hypnotic, or anxiolytic-induced ◀
  anxiety disorder F13.980 ◀
  bipolar and related disorder F13.94 ◀
  delirium F13.921 ◀
  depressive disorder F13.94 ◀
  major neurocognitive disorder F13.97 ◀
  mild neurocognitive disorder F13.988 ◀
  psychotic disorder F13.959 ◀
  sexual dysfunction F13.981 ◀
  sleep disorder F13.982 ◀
Segmentation, incomplete (congenital) —*see*
  also Fusion
  bone NEC Q78.8
  lumbosacral (joint) (vertebra) Q76.49
Seitelberger's syndrome (infantile neuraxonal
  dystrophy) G31.89
Seizure(s) —*see also* Convulsions R56.9
  akinetic —*see* Epilepsy, generalized, specified
    NEC
  atonic —*see* Epilepsy, generalized, specified
    NEC
  autonomic (hysterical) F44.5
  convulsive —*see* Convulsions
  cortical (focal) (motor) —*see* Epilepsy,
    localization-related, symptomatic, with
    simple partial seizures
  disorder —*see also* Epilepsy G40.909
  due to stroke —*see* Sequelae (of), disease,
    cerebrovascular, by type, specified NEC
  epileptic —*see* Epilepsy
  febrile (simple) R56.00
    with status epilepticus G40.901
    complex (atypical) (complicated) R56.01
      with status epilepticus G40.901
  grand mal G40.409
    intractable G40.419
      with status epilepticus G40.411
      without status epilepticus G40.419
    not intractable G40.409
      with status epilepticus G40.401
      without status epilepticus G40.409
  heart —*see* Disease, heart
  hysterical F44.5
  intractable G40.919
    with status epilepticus G40.911
  Jacksonian (focal) (motor type) (sensory
    type) —*see* Epilepsy, localization-
    related, symptomatic, with simple
    partial seizures

Seizure *(Continued)*
  newborn P90
  nonspecific epileptic
    atonic —*see* Epilepsy, generalized, specified
      NEC
    clonic —*see* Epilepsy, generalized, specified
      NEC
    myoclonic —*see* Epilepsy, generalized,
      specified NEC
    tonic —*see* Epilepsy, generalized, specified
      NEC
    tonic-clonic —*see* Epilepsy, generalized,
      specified NEC
  partial, developing into secondarily
    generalized seizures
    complex —*see* Epilepsy, localization-
      related, symptomatic, with complex
      partial seizures
    simple —*see* Epilepsy, localization-related,
      symptomatic, with simple partial
      seizures
  petit mal G40.409
    intractable G40.419
      with status epilepticus G40.411
      without status epilepticus G40.419
    not intractable G40.409
      with status epilepticus G40.401
      without status epilepticus G40.409
  post traumatic R56.1
  recurrent G40.909
  specified NEC G40.89
  uncinate —*see* Epilepsy, localization-related,
    symptomatic, with complex partial
    seizures
Selenium deficiency, dietary E59
Self-damaging behavior (life-style) Z72.89
Self-harm (attempted)
  history (personal) Z91.5
    in family Z81.8
Self-mutilation (attempted)
  history (personal) Z91.5
    in family Z81.8
Self-poisoning
  history (personal) Z91.5
    in family Z81.8
  observation following (alleged) attempt Z03.6
Semicoma R40.1
Seminal vesiculitis N49.0
Seminoma C62.9-
  specified site —*see* Neoplasm, malignant, by
    site
Senear-Usher disease or syndrome L10.4
Senectus R54
Senescence (without mention of psychosis)
  R54
Senile, senility —*see also* condition R41.81
  with
    acute confusional state F05
    mental changes NOS F03
    psychosis NEC —*see* Psychosis, senile
  asthenia R54
  cervix (atrophic) N88.8
  debility R54
  endometrium (atrophic) N85.8
  fallopian tube (atrophic) —*see* Atrophy,
    fallopian tube
  heart (failure) R54
  ovary (atrophic) —*see* Atrophy, ovary
  premature E34.8
  vagina, vaginitis (atrophic) N95.2
  wart L82.1
Sensation
  burning (skin) R20.8
    tongue K14.6
  loss of R20.8
  prickling (skin) R20.2
  tingling (skin) R20.2
Sense loss
  smell —*see* Disturbance, sensation, smell
  taste —*see* Disturbance, sensation, taste
  touch R20.8

Sensibility disturbance (cortical) (deep)
(vibratory) R20.9
Sensitive, sensitivity —see also Allergy
carotid sinus G90.01
child (excessive) F93.8
cold, autoimmune D59.1
dentin K03.89
gluten (non-celiac) K90.41 ◀
latex Z91.040
methemoglobin D74.8
tuberculin, without clinical or radiological
symptoms R76.11
visual
glare H53.71
impaired contrast H53.72
Sensitiver Beziehungswahn F22
Sensitization, auto-erythrocytic D69.2
Separation
anxiety, abnormal (of childhood) F93.0
apophysis, traumatic - code as Fracture, by
site
choroid —see Detachment, choroid
epiphysis, epiphyseal
nontraumatic —see also
Osteochondropathy, specified type
NEC
upper femoral —see Slipped, epiphysis,
upper femoral
traumatic - code as Fracture, by site
fracture —see Fracture
infundibulum cardiac from right ventricle by
a partition Q24.3
joint (traumatic) (current) - code by site under
Dislocation
pubic bone, obstetrical trauma O71.6
retina, retinal —see Detachment, retina
symphysis pubis, obstetrical trauma O71.6
tracheal ring, incomplete, congenital Q32.1
Sepsis (generalized) (unspecified organism)
A41.9
with
organ dysfunction (acute) (multiple) R65.20
with septic shock R65.21
actinomycotic A42.7
adrenal hemorrhage syndrome
(meningococcal) A39.1
anaerobic A41.4
Bacillus anthracis A22.7
Brucella —see also Brucellosis A23.9
candidal B37.7
cryptogenic A41.9
due to device, implant or graft T85.79
arterial graft NEC T82.7
breast (implant) T85.79
catheter NEC T85.79
dialysis (renal) T82.7
intraperitoneal T85.71
infusion NEC T82.7
spinal (cranial) (epidural) (intrathecal)
(spinal) (subarachnoid)
(subdural) T85.735 ◀▥
urethral indwelling T83.511 ◀
urinary T83.518 ◀▥
ectopic or molar pregnancy O08.82
electronic (electrode) (pulse generator)
(stimulator)
bone T84.7
cardiac T82.7
nervous system T85.738 ◀▥
brain T85.731 ◀
neurostimulator generator T85.734 ◀
peripheral nerve T85.732 ◀
spinal cord T85.733 ◀
urinary T83.590 ◀▥
fixation, internal (orthopedic) —see
Complication, fixation device,
infection
gastrointestinal (bile duct) (esophagus)
T85.79
neurostimulator electrode (lead)
T85.732 ◀

Sepsis (Continued)
due to device, implant or graft (Continued)
genital T83.69 ◀▥
heart NEC T82.7
valve (prosthesis) T82.6
graft T82.7
joint prosthesis —see Complication, joint
prosthesis, infection
ocular (corneal graft) (orbital implant)
T85.79
orthopedic NEC T84.7
fixation device, internal —see
Complication, fixation device,
infection
specified NEC T85.79
vascular T82.7
ventricular intracranial shunt T85.79
ventricular intracranial (communicating)
shunt T85.730 ◀
during labor O75.3
Enterococcus A41.81
Erysipelothrix (rhusiopathiae) (erysipeloid)
A26.7
Escherichia coli (E. coli) A41.5
extraintestinal yersiniosis A28.2
following
abortion (subsequent episode) O08.0
current episode —see Abortion
ectopic or molar pregnancy O08.82
immunization T88.0
infusion, therapeutic injection or
transfusion NEC T80.29
gangrenous A41.9
gonococcal A54.86
Gram-negative (organism) A41.5
anaerobic A41.4
Haemophilus influenzae A41.3
herpesviral B00.7
intra-abdominal K65.1
intraocular —see Endophthalmitis, purulent
Listeria monocytogenes A32.7
localized — code to specific localized
infection
in operation wound T81.49 ◀▥
skin —see Abscess
malleus A24.0
melioidosis A24.1
meningeal —see Meningitis
meningococcal A39.4
acute A39.2
chronic A39.3
MSSA (Methicillin susceptible
Staphylococcus aureus) A41.01
newborn P36.9
due to
anaerobes NEC P36.5
Escherichia coli P36.4
Staphylococcus P36.30
aureus P36.2
specified NEC P36.39
Streptococcus P36.10
group B P36.0
specified NEC P36.19
specified NEC P36.8
Pasteurella multocida A28.0
pelvic, puerperal, postpartum, childbirth O85
pneumococcal A40.3
postprocedural T81.49 ◀▥
puerperal, postpartum, childbirth (pelvic)
O85
Salmonella (arizonae) (cholerae-suis)
(enteritidis) (typhimurium) A02.1
severe R65.20
with septic shock R65.21
Shigella (see also Dysentery, bacillary) A03.9
skin, localized —see Abscess
specified organism NEC A41.89
Staphylococcus, staphylococcal A41.2
aureus (methicillin susceptible) (MSSA)
A41.01
methicillin resistant (MRSA) A41.02

Sepsis (Continued)
Staphylococcus, staphylococcal (Continued)
coagulase-negative A41.1
specified NEC A41.1
Streptococcus, streptococcal A40.9
agalactiae A40.1
group
A A40.0
B A40.1
D A41.81
neonatal P36.10
group B P36.0
specified NEC P36.19
pneumoniae A40.3
pyogenes A40.0
specified NEC A40.8
tracheostomy stoma J95.02
tularemic A21.7
umbilical, umbilical cord (newborn) —see
Sepsis, newborn
Yersinia pestis A20.7
Septate —see Septum
Septic —see condition
arm —see Cellulitis, upper limb
with lymphangitis —see Lymphangitis,
acute, upper limb
embolus —see Embolism
finger —see Cellulitis, digit
with lymphangitis —see Lymphangitis,
acute, digit
foot —see Cellulitis, lower limb
with lymphangitis —see Lymphangitis,
acute, lower limb
gallbladder (acute) K81.0
hand —see Cellulitis, upper limb
with lymphangitis —see Lymphangitis,
acute, upper limb
joint —see Arthritis, pyogenic or pyemic
leg —see Cellulitis, lower limb
with lymphangitis —see Lymphangitis,
acute, lower limb
nail —see also Cellulitis, digit
with lymphangitis —see Lymphangitis,
acute, digit
sore —see also Abscess
throat J02.0
streptococcal J02.0
spleen (acute) D73.89
teeth, tooth (pulpal origin) K04.4
throat —see Pharyngitis
thrombus —see Thrombosis
toe —see Cellulitis, digit
with lymphangitis —see Lymphangitis,
acute, digit
tonsils, chronic J35.01
with adenoiditis J35.03
uterus —see Endometritis
Septicemia A41.9
meaning sepsis —see Sepsis
Septum, septate (congenital) —see also
Anomaly, by site
anal Q42.3
with fistula Q42.2
aqueduct of Sylvius Q03.0
with spina bifida —see Spina bifida, by site,
with hydrocephalus
uterus (complete) (partial) Q51.2
vagina Q52.10
in pregnancy —see Pregnancy, complicated
by, abnormal vagina
causing obstructed labor
O65.5
longitudinal Q52.129 ◀▥
microperforate ◀
left side Q52.124 ◀
right side Q52.123 ◀
nonobstruction Q52.120 ◀
obstructing Q52.129 ◀
left side Q52.122 ◀
right side Q52.121 ◀
transverse Q52.11

◀ New   ◀▥ Revised   ~~deleted~~ Deleted

Sequelae *(Continued)*
  viral
    encephalitis B94.1
    hepatitis B94.2
  vitamin deficiency NEC E64.8
    A E64.1
    B E64.8
    C E64.2
  wound, open — code to injury with seventh
    character S
Sequestration —*see also* Sequestrum
  disk —*see* Displacement, intervertebral
    disk ◄
  lung, congenital Q33.2
Sequestrum
  bone —*see* Osteomyelitis, chronic
  dental M27.2
  jaw bone M27.2
  orbit —*see* Osteomyelitis, orbit
  sinus (accessory) (nasal) —*see* Sinusitis
Sequoiosis lung or pneumonitis J67.8
Serology for syphilis
  doubtful
    with signs or symptoms - code by site and
      stage under Syphilis
    follow-up of latent syphilis —*see* Syphilis,
      latent
  negative, with signs or symptoms — code by
    site and stage under Syphilis
  positive A53.0
    with signs or symptoms - code by site and
      stage under Syphilis
  reactivated A53.0
Seroma —*see also* Hematoma
  postprocedural —*see* Complication,
    postprocedural, seroma ◄
  traumatic, secondary and recurrent
    T79.2
Seropurulent —*see* condition
Serositis, multiple K65.8
  pericardial I31.1
  peritoneal K65.8
Serous —*see* condition
Sertoli cell
  adenoma
    specified site —*see* Neoplasm, benign, by
      site
    unspecified site
      female D27.9
      male D29.20
  carcinoma
    specified site —*see* Neoplasm, malignant,
      by site
    unspecified site (male) C62.9-
      female C56.9
  tumor
    with lipid storage
      specified site —*see* Neoplasm, benign,
        by site
      unspecified site
        female D27.9
        male D29.20
    specified site —*see* Neoplasm, benign, by
      site
    unspecified site
      female D27.9
      male D29.20
Sertoli-Leydig cell tumor —*see* Neoplasm,
  benign, by site
  specified site —*see* Neoplasm, benign,
    by site
  unspecified site
    female D27.9
    male D29.20
Serum
  allergy, allergic reaction —*see also* Reaction,
    serum T80.69
    shock —*see also* Shock, anaphylactic T80.59
  arthritis —*see also* Reaction, serum T80.69
  complication or reaction NEC —*see also*
    Reaction, serum T80.69

Serum *(Continued)*
  disease NEC —*see also* Reaction, serum
    T80.69
  hepatitis —*see also* Hepatitis, viral, type B
    carrier (suspected) of B18.1 ◄▥
  intoxication —*see also* Reaction, serum T80.69
  neuritis —*see also* Reaction, serum T80.69
  neuropathy G61.1
  poisoning NEC —*see also* Reaction, serum
    T80.69
  rash NEC —*see also* Reaction, serum T80.69
  reaction NEC —*see also* Reaction, serum
    T80.69
  sickness NEC —*see also* Reaction, serum
    T80.69
  urticaria —*see also* Reaction, serum T80.69
Sesamoiditis M25.8-
Sever's disease or osteochondrosis —*see*
  Osteochondrosis, juvenile, tarsus
Severe sepsis R65.20
  with septic shock R65.21
Sex
  chromosome mosaics Q97.8
    lines with various numbers of
      X chromosomes Q97.2
  education Z70.8
  reassignment surgery status Z87.890
Sextuplet pregnancy —*see* Pregnancy,
  sextuplet
Sexual
  function, disorder of (psychogenic) F52.9
  immaturity (female) (male) E30.0
  impotence (psychogenic) organic origin
    NEC —*see* Dysfunction, sexual, male
  precocity (constitutional) (cryptogenic)
    (female) (idiopathic) (male) E30.1
Sexuality, pathologic —*see* Deviation, sexual
Sézary disease C84.1-
Shadow, lung R91.8
Shaking palsy or paralysis —*see* Parkinsonism
Shallowness, acetabulum —*see* Derangement,
  joint, specified type NEC, hip
Shaver's disease J63.1
Sheath (tendon) —*see* condition
Sheathing, retinal vessels H35.01-
Shedding
  nail L60.8
  premature, primary (deciduous) teeth
    K00.6
Sheehan's disease or syndrome E23.0
Shelf, rectal K62.89
Shell teeth K00.5
Shellshock (current) F43.0
  lasting state —*see* Disorder, post-traumatic
    stress
Shield kidney Q63.1
Shift
  auditory threshold (temporary) H93.24-
  mediastinal R93.8
Shifting sleep-work schedule (affecting sleep)
  G47.26
Shiga (-Kruse) dysentery A03.0
Shiga's bacillus A03.0
Shigella (dysentery) —*see* Dysentery, bacillary
Shigellosis A03.9
  Group A A03.0
  Group B A03.1
  Group C A03.2
  Group D A03.3
Shin splints S86.89
Shingles —*see* Herpes, zoster
Shipyard disease or eye B30.0
Shirodkar suture, in pregnancy —*see*
  Pregnancy, complicated by, incompetent
  cervix
Shock R57.9
  with ectopic or molar pregnancy O08.3
  adrenal (cortical) (Addisonian) E27.2
  adverse food reaction (anaphylactic) —*see*
    Shock, anaphylactic, due to food
  allergic —*see* Shock, anaphylactic

Shock *(Continued)*
  anaphylactic T78.2
    chemical —*see* Table of Drugs and
      Chemicals
    due to drug or medicinal substance
      correct substance properly administered
        T88.6
      overdose or wrong substance given or
        taken (by accident) —*see* Table of
        Drugs and Chemicals, by drug,
        poisoning
    due to food (nonpoisonous) T78.00
      additives T78.06
      dairy products T78.07
      eggs T78.08
      fish T78.03
        shellfish T78.02
      fruit T78.04
      milk T78.07
      nuts T78.05
        multiple types T78.05 ◄
        peanuts T78.01
      peanuts T78.01
      seeds T78.05
      specified type NEC T78.09
      vegetable T78.04
    following sting (s) —*see* Venom
    immunization T80.52
    serum T80.59
      blood and blood products T80.51
      immunization T80.52
      specified NEC T80.59
      vaccination T80.52
  anaphylactoid —*see* Shock, anaphylactic
  anesthetic
    correct substance properly administered
      T88.2
    overdose or wrong substance given or
      taken —*see* Table of Drugs and
      Chemicals, by drug, poisoning
    specified anesthetic —*see* Table of
      Drugs and Chemicals, by drug,
      poisoning
  cardiogenic R57.0
  chemical substance —*see* Table of Drugs and
    Chemicals
  complicating ectopic or molar pregnancy O08.3
  culture —*see* Disorder, adjustment
  drug
    due to correct substance properly
      administered T88.6
    overdose or wrong substance given or
      taken (by accident) —*see* Table of
      Drugs and Chemicals, by drug,
      poisoning
  during or after labor and delivery O75.1
  electric T75.4
    (taser) T75.4
  endotoxic R65.21
    postprocedural (resulting from a
      procedure, not elsewhere classified)
      T81.12 ◄▥
  following
    ectopic or molar pregnancy O08.3
    injury (immediate) (delayed) T79.4
    labor and delivery O75.1
  food (anaphylactic) —*see* Shock, anaphylactic,
    due to food
  from electroshock gun (taser) T75.4
  gram-negative R65.21
    postprocedural (resulting from a
      procedure, not elsewhere classified)
      T81.12 ◄▥
  hematologic R57.8
  hemorrhagic
    surgery (intraoperative) (postoperative)
      T81.19
    trauma T79.4
  hypovolemic R57.1
    surgical T81.19
    traumatic T79.4

Shock (*Continued*)
  insulin E15
    therapeutic misadventure —*see*
      subcategory T38.3
  kidney N17.Ø
    traumatic (following crushing) T79.5
  lightning T75.Ø1
  liver K72.ØØ ◄
  lung J8Ø
  obstetric O75.1
    with ectopic or molar pregnancy OØ8.3
    following ectopic or molar pregnancy
      OØ8.3
  pleural (surgical) T81.19
    due to trauma T79.4
  postprocedural (postoperative) T81.1Ø
    with ectopic or molar pregnancy OØ8.3
    cardiogenic T81.11
    endotoxic T81.12
    following ectopic or molar pregnancy OØ8.3
    gram-negative T81.12
    hypovolemic T81.19
    septic T81.12
    specified type NEC T81.19
  psychic F43.Ø
  septic (due to severe sepsis) R65.21
  specified NEC R57.8
  surgical T81.1Ø
  taser gun (taser) T75.4
  therapeutic misadventure NEC T81.1Ø
  thyroxin
    overdose or wrong substance given or
      taken —*see* Table of Drugs and
      Chemicals, by drug, poisoning
  toxic, syndrome A48.3
  transfusion —*see* Complications, transfusion
  traumatic (immediate) (delayed) T79.4
Shoemaker's chest M95.4
Short, shortening, shortness
  arm (acquired) —*see also* Deformity, limb,
    unequal length
    congenital Q71.81-
    forearm —*see* Deformity, limb, unequal
      length
  bowel syndrome K91.2
  breath RØ6.Ø2
  cervical (complicating pregnancy) O26.87-
    non-gravid uterus N88.3
  common bile duct, congenital Q44.5
  cord (umbilical), complicating delivery O69.3
  cystic duct, congenital Q44.5
  esophagus (congenital) Q39.8
  femur (acquired) —*see* Deformity, limb,
    unequal length, femur
    congenital —*see* Defect, reduction, lower
      limb, longitudinal, femur
  frenum, frenulum, linguae (congenital) Q38.1
  hip (acquired) —*see also* Deformity, limb,
    unequal length
    congenital Q65.89
  leg (acquired) —*see also* Deformity, limb,
    unequal length
    congenital Q72.81-
    lower leg —*see also* Deformity, limb,
      unequal length
  limbed stature, with immunodeficiency D82.2
  lower limb (acquired) —*see also* Deformity,
    limb, unequal length
    congenital Q72.81-
  organ or site, congenital NEC —*see* Distortion
  palate, congenital Q38.5
  radius (acquired) —*see also* Deformity, limb,
    unequal length
    congenital —*see* Defect, reduction, upper
      limb, longitudinal, radius
  rib syndrome Q77.2
  stature (child) (hereditary) (idiopathic) NEC
    R62.52
    constitutional E34.3
    due to endocrine disorder E34.3
    Laron-type E34.3

Short, shortening, shortness (*Continued*)
  tendon —*see also* Contraction, tendon
    with contracture of joint —*see* Contraction,
      joint
    Achilles (acquired) M67.Ø-
      congenital Q66.89
    congenital Q79.8
    thigh (acquired) —*see also* Deformity, limb,
      unequal length, femur
      congenital —*see* Defect, reduction, lower
        limb, longitudinal, femur
    tibialis anterior (tendon) —*see* Contraction,
      tendon
  umbilical cord
    complicating delivery O69.3
  upper limb, congenital —*see* Defect,
    reduction, upper limb, specified type
    NEC
  urethra N36.8
  uvula, congenital Q38.5
  vagina (congenital) Q52.4
Shortsightedness —*see* Myopia
Shoshin (acute fulminating beriberi) E51.11
Shoulder —*see* condition
Shovel-shaped incisors KØØ.2
Shower, thromboembolic —*see* Embolism
Shunt
  arterial-venous (dialysis) Z99.2
  arteriovenous, pulmonary (acquired) I28.Ø
    congenital Q25.72
  cerebral ventricle (communicating) in situ
    Z98.2
  surgical, prosthetic, with complications —*see*
    Complications, cardiovascular, device
    or implant Shutdown, renal N28.9
Shutdown, renal N28.9
Shy-Drager syndrome G9Ø.3
Sialadenitis, sialadenosis (any gland) (chronic)
  (periodic) (suppurative) —*see* Sialoadenitis
Sialectasia K11.8
Sialidosis E77.1
Sialitis, silitis (any gland) (chronic)
  (suppurative) —*see* Sialoadenitis
Sialoadenitis (any gland) (periodic)
  (suppurative) K11.2Ø
  acute K11.21
    recurrent K11.22
  chronic K11.23
Sialoadenopathy K11.9
Sialoangitis —*see* Sialoadenitis
Sialodochitis (fibrinosa) —*see* Sialoadenitis
Sialodocholithiasis K11.5
Sialolithiasis K11.5
Sialometaplasia, necrotizing K11.8
Sialorrhea —*see also* Ptyalism
  periodic —*see* Sialoadenitis
Sialosis K11.7
Siamese twin Q89.4
Sibling rivalry Z62.891
Sicard's syndrome G52.7
Sicca syndrome M35.ØØ
  with
    keratoconjunctivitis M35.Ø1
    lung involvement M35.Ø2
    myopathy M35.Ø3
    renal tubulo-interstitial disorders M35.Ø4
  specified organ involvement NEC M35.Ø9
Sick R69
  or handicapped person in family Z63.79
    needing care at home Z63.6
  sinus (syndrome) I49.5
Sick-euthyroid syndrome EØ7.81
Sickle-cell
  anemia —*see* Disease, sickle-cell
  trait D57.3
Sicklemia —*see also* Disease, sickle-cell
  trait D57.3
Sickness
  air (travel) T75.3
  airplane T75.3
  alpine T7Ø.29

Sickness (*Continued*)
  altitude T7Ø.2Ø
  Andes T7Ø.29
  aviator's T7Ø.29
  balloon T7Ø.29
  car T75.3
  compressed air T7Ø.3
  decompression T7Ø.3
  green D5Ø.8
  milk —*see* Poisoning, food, noxious
  motion T75.3
  mountain T7Ø.29
    acute D75.1
  protein —*see also* Reaction, serum T8Ø.69
  radiation T66
  roundabout (motion) T75.3
  sea T75.3
  serum NEC —*see also* Reaction, serum T8Ø.69
  sleeping (African) B56.9
    by Trypanosoma B56.9
      brucei
        gambiense B56.Ø
        rhodesiense B56.1
    East African B56.1
    Gambian B56.Ø
    Rhodesian B56.1
    West African B56.Ø
  swing (motion) T75.3
  train (railway) (travel) T75.3
  travel (any vehicle) T75.3
Sideropenia —*see* Anemia, iron deficiency
Siderosilicosis J62.8
Siderosis (lung) J63.4
  eye (globe) —*see* Disorder, globe,
    degenerative, siderosis
Siemens' syndrome (ectodermal dysplasia) Q82.8
Sighing RØ6.89
  psychogenic F45.8
Sigmoid —*see also* condition
  flexure —*see* condition
  kidney Q63.1
Sigmoiditis —*see also* Enteritis K52.9
  infectious AØ9
  noninfectious K52.9
Silfversköld's syndrome Q78.9
Silicosiderosis J62.8
Silicosis, silicotic (simple) (complicated) J62.8
  with tuberculosis J65
Silicotuberculosis J65
Silo-fillers' disease J68.8
  bronchitis J68.Ø
  pneumonitis J68.Ø
  pulmonary edema J68.1
Silver's syndrome Q87.1
Simian malaria B53.1
Simmonds' cachexia or disease E23.Ø
Simons' disease or syndrome (progressive
  lipodystrophy) E88.1
Simple, simplex —*see* condition
Simulation, conscious (of illness) Z76.5
Simultanagnosia (asimultagnosia) R48.3
Sin Nombre virus disease (Hantavirus)
  (cardio)-pulmonary syndrome) B33.4
Sinding-Larsen disease or osteochondrosis —
  see Osteochondrosis, juvenile, patella
Singapore hemorrhagic fever A91
Singer's node or nodule J38.2
Single
  atrium Q21.2
  coronary artery Q24.5
  umbilical artery Q27.Ø
  ventricle Q2Ø.4
Singultus RØ6.6
  epidemicus B33.Ø
Sinus —*see also* Fistula
  abdominal K63.89
  arrest I45.5
  arrhythmia I49.8
  bradycardia RØØ.1
  branchial cleft (internal) (external) Q18.Ø
  coccygeal —*see* Sinus, pilonidal

Sinus *(Continued)*
  dental K04.6
  dermal (congenital) Q06.8
    with abscess Q06.8
    coccygeal, pilonidal —*see* Sinus,
      coccygeal
  infected, skin NEC L08.89
  marginal, ruptured or bleeding —*see*
    Hemorrhage, antepartum, specified
    cause NEC
  medial, face and neck Q18.8
  pause I45.5
  pericranii Q01.9
  pilonidal (infected) (rectum) L05.92
    with abscess L05.02
  preauricular Q18.1
  rectovaginal N82.3
  Rokitansky-Aschoff (gallbladder) K82.8
  sacrococcygeal (dermoid) (infected) —*see*
    Sinus, pilonidal
  tachycardia R00.0
    paroxysmal I47.1
  tarsi syndrome M25.57- ◄▥
  testis N50.89 ◄▥
  tract (postinfective) —*see* Fistula
  urachus Q64.4
Sinusitis (accessory) (chronic) (hyperplastic)
  (nasal) (nonpurulent) (purulent) J32.9
  acute J01.90
    ethmoidal J01.20
      recurrent J01.21
    frontal J01.10
      recurrent J01.11
    involving more than one sinus, other than
      pansinusitis J01.80
        recurrent J01.81
    maxillary J01.00
      recurrent J01.01
    pansinusitis J01.40
      recurrent J01.41
    recurrent J01.91
    specified NEC J01.80
      recurrent J01.81
    sphenoidal J01.30
      recurrent J01.31
  allergic —*see* Rhinitis, allergic
  due to high altitude T70.1
  ethmoidal J32.2
    acute J01.20
      recurrent J01.21
  frontal J32.1
    acute J01.10
      recurrent J01.11
  influenzal —*see* Influenza, with, respiratory
    manifestations NEC
  involving more than one sinus but not
    pansinusitis J32.8
    acute J01.80
      recurrent J01.81
  maxillary J32.0
    acute J01.00
      recurrent J01.01
  sphenoidal J32.3
    acute J01.30
      recurrent J01.31
  tuberculous, any sinus A15.8
Sinusitis-bronchiectasis-situs inversus
  (syndrome) (triad) Q89.3
Sipple's syndrome E31.22
Sirenomelia (syndrome) Q87.2
Siriasis T67.0
Sirkari's disease B55.0
Siti A65
Situation, psychiatric F99
Situational
  disturbance (transient) —*see* Disorder,
    adjustment
    acute F43.0
  maladjustment —*see* Disorder, adjustment
  reaction —*see* Disorder, adjustment
    acute F43.0

Situs inversus or transversus (abdominalis)
  (thoracis) Q89.3
Sixth disease B08.20
  due to human herpesvirus 6 B08.21
  due to human herpesvirus 7 B08.22
Sjögren-Larsson syndrome Q87.1
Sjögren's syndrome or disease —*see* Sicca
  syndrome
Skeletal —*see* condition
Skene's gland —*see* condition
Skenitis —*see* Urethritis
Skerljevo A65
Skevas-Zerfus disease —*see* Toxicity, venom,
  marine animal, sea anemone
Skin —*see also* condition
  clammy R23.1
  donor —*see* Donor, skin
  hidebound M35.9
Slate-dressers' or slate-miners' lung J62.8
Sleep
  apnea —*see* Apnea, sleep
  deprivation Z72.820
  disorder or disturbance G47.9
    child F51.9
    nonorganic origin F51.9
    specified NEC G47.8
  disturbance G47.9
    nonorganic origin F51.9
  drunkenness F51.9
  rhythm inversion G47.2-
  terrors F51.4
  walking F51.3
    hysterical F44.89
Sleep hygiene
  abuse Z72.821
  inadequate Z72.821
  poor Z72.821
Sleeping sickness —*see* Sickness, sleeping
Sleeplessness —*see* Insomnia
  menopausal N95.11
Sleep-wake schedule disorder G47.20
Slim disease (in HIV infection) B20
Slipped, slipping
  epiphysis (traumatic) —*see also*
    Osteochondropathy, specified type
    NEC
    capital femoral (traumatic)
      acute (on chronic) S79.01-
    current traumatic - code as Fracture, by site
    upper femoral (nontraumatic) M93.00-
      acute M93.01-
        on chronic M93.03-
      chronic M93.02-
  intervertebral disc —*see* Displacement,
    intervertebral disc
  ligature, umbilical P51.8
  patella —*see* Disorder, patella, derangement
    NEC
  rib M89.8X8
  sacroiliac joint —*see* subcategory M53.2
  tendon —*see* Disorder, tendon
  ulnar nerve, nontraumatic —*see* Lesion,
    nerve, ulnar
  vertebra NEC —*see* Spondylolisthesis
Slocumb's syndrome E27.0
Sloughing (multiple) (phagedena) (skin) —*see*
  also Gangrene
  abscess —*see* Abscess
  appendix K38.8
  fascia —*see* Disorder, soft tissue, specified
    type NEC
  scrotum N50.89 ◄▥
  tendon —*see* Disorder, tendon
  transplanted organ —*see* Rejection, transplant
  ulcer —*see* Ulcer, skin
Slow
  feeding, newborn P92.2
  flow syndrome, coronary I20.8
  heart(beat) R00.1
Slowing, urinary stream R39.198 ◄▥
Sluder's neuralgia (syndrome) G44.89

Slurred, slurring speech R47.81
Small (ness)
  for gestational age —*see* Small for dates
  introitus, vagina N89.6
  kidney (unknown cause) N27.9
    bilateral N27.1
    unilateral N27.0
  ovary (congenital) Q50.39
  pelvis
    with disproportion (fetopelvic) O33.1
      causing obstructed labor O65.1
  uterus N85.8
  white kidney N03.9
Small-and-light-for-dates —*see* Small for
  dates
Small-for-dates (infant) P05.10
  with weight of
    499 grams or less P05.11
    500-749 grams P05.12
    750-999 grams P05.13
    1000-1249 grams P05.14
    1250-1499 grams P05.15
    1500-1749 grams P05.16
    1750-1999 grams P05.17
    2000-2499 grams P05.18
    2500 grams and over P05.19 ◄
  specified NEC P05.19 ◄
Smallpox B03
Smearing, fecal R15.1
Smith-Lemli-Opitz syndrome E78.72
Smith's fracture S52.54-
Smoker —*see* Dependence, drug, nicotine
Smoker's
  bronchitis J41.0
  cough J41.0
  palate K13.24
  throat J31.2
  tongue K13.24
Smoking
  passive Z77.22
Smothering spells R06.81
Snaggle teeth, tooth M26.39
Snapping
  finger —*see* Trigger finger
  hip —*see* Derangement, joint, specified type
    NEC, hip
    involving the iliotiblial band M76.3-
  knee —*see* Derangement, knee
    involving the iliotibial band M76.3-
Sneddon-Wilkinson disease or syndrome (subcorneal pustular dermatosis) L13.1
Sneezing (intractable) R06.7
Sniffing
  cocaine
    abuse —*see* Abuse, drug, cocaine
    dependence —*see* Dependence, drug,
      cocaine
  gasoline
    abuse —*see* Abuse, drug, inhalant
    dependence —*see* Dependence, drug,
      inhalant
  glue (airplane)
    abuse —*see* Abuse, drug, inhalant
    drug dependence —*see* Dependence, drug,
      inhalant
Sniffles
  newborn P28.89
Snoring R06.83
Snow blindness —*see* Photokeratitis
Snuffles (non-syphilitic) R06.5
  newborn P28.89
  syphilitic (infant) A50.05 [J99]
Social
  exclusion Z60.4
    due to discrimination or persecution
      (perceived) Z60.5
  migrant Z59.0
    acculturation difficulty Z60.3
  rejection Z60.4
    due to discrimination or persecution
      Z60.5

◄ New   ◄▥ Revised   ~~deleted~~ Deleted

Social *(Continued)*
  role conflict NEC Z73.5
  skills inadequacy NEC Z73.4
  transplantation Z60.3
Sodoku A25.0
Soemmerring's ring —*see* Cataract, secondary
Soft —*see also* condition
  nails L60.3
Softening
  bone —*see* Osteomalacia
  brain (necrotic) (progressive) G93.89
    congenital Q04.8
    embolic I63.4- ◀▥
    hemorrhagic —*see* Hemorrhage,
      intracranial, intracerebral
    occlusive I63.5- ◀▥
    thrombotic I63.3- ◀▥
  cartilage M94.2-
    patella M22.4-
  cerebellar —*see* Softening, brain
  cerebral —*see* Softening, brain
  cerebrospinal —*see* Softening, brain
  myocardial, heart —*see* Degeneration,
    myocardial
  spinal cord G95.89
  stomach K31.89
Soldier's
  heart F45.8
  patches I31.0
Solitary
  cyst, kidney N28.1
  kidney, congenital Q60.0
Solvent abuse —*see* Abuse, drug, inhalant
  dependence —*see* Dependence, drug,
    inhalant
Somatization reaction, somatic reaction —*see*
  Disorder, somatoform
Somnambulism F51.3
  hysterical F44.89
Somnolence R40.0
  nonorganic origin F51.11
Sonne dysentery A03.3
Soor B37.0
Sore
  bed —*see* Ulcer, pressure, by site
  chiclero B55.1
  Delhi B55.1
  desert —*see* Ulcer, skin
  eye H57.1-
  Lahore B55.1
  mouth K13.79
    canker K12.0
  muscle M79.1
  Naga —*see* Ulcer, skin
  of skin —*see* Ulcer, skin - oriental B55.1
  pressure —*see* Ulcer, pressure, by site
  skin L98.9
  soft A57
  throat (acute) —*see also* Pharyngitis
    with influenza, flu, or grippe —*see*
      Influenza, with, respiratory
      manifestations NEC
    chronic J31.2
    coxsackie (virus) B08.5
    diphtheritic A36.0
    herpesviral B00.2
    influenzal —*see* Influenza, with, respiratory
      manifestations NEC
    septic J02.0
    streptococcal (ulcerative) J02.0
    viral NEC J02.8
      coxsackie B08.5
  tropical —*see* Ulcer, skin
  veldt —*see* Ulcer, skin
Soto's syndrome (cerebral gigantism) Q87.3
South African cardiomyopathy syndrome I42.8
Southeast Asian hemorrhagic fever A91
Spacing
  abnormal, tooth, teeth, fully erupted M26.30
  excessive, tooth, fully erupted M26.32
Spade-like hand (congenital) Q68.1

Spading nail L60.8
  congenital Q84.6
Spanish collar N47.1
Sparganosis B70.1
Spasm (s), spastic, spasticity —*see also*
    condition R25.2
  accommodation —*see* Spasm, of
    accommodation
  ampulla of Vater K83.4
  anus, ani (sphincter) (reflex) K59.4
    psychogenic F45.8
  artery I73.9
    cerebral G45.9
  Bell's G51.3
  bladder (sphincter, external or internal) N32.89
    psychogenic F45.8
  bronchus, bronchiole J98.01
  cardia K22.0
  cardiac I20.1
  carpopedal —*see* Tetany
  cerebral (arteries) (vascular) G45.9
  cervix, complicating delivery O62.4
  ciliary body (of accommodation) —*see* Spasm,
    of accommodation
  colon —*see also* Irritable, bowel K58.9 ◀▥
    with diarrhea K58.0
    psychogenic F45.8
  common duct K83.8
  compulsive —*see* Tic
  conjugate H51.8
  coronary (artery) I20.1
  diaphragm (reflex) R06.6
    epidemic B33.0
    psychogenic F45.8
  duodenum K59.8
  epidemic diaphragmatic (transient) B33.0
  esophagus (diffuse) K22.4
    psychogenic F45.8
  facial G51.3
  fallopian tube N83.8
  gastrointestinal (tract) K31.89
    psychogenic F45.8
  glottis J38.5
    hysterical F44.4
    psychogenic F45.8
      conversion reaction F44.4
    reflex through recurrent laryngeal nerve
      J38.5
  habit —*see* Tic
  heart I20.1
  hemifacial (clonic) G51.3
  hourglass —*see* Contraction, hourglass
  hysterical F44.4
  infantile —*see* Epilepsy, spasms
  inferior oblique, eye H51.8
  intestinal —*see also* Syndrome, irritable bowel
    K58.9
    psychogenic F45.8
  larynx, laryngeal J38.5
    hysterical F44.4
    psychogenic F45.8
      conversion reaction F44.4
  levator palpebrae superioris —*see* Disorder,
    eyelid function
  muscle NEC M62.838
    back M62.830
  nerve, trigeminal G51.0
  nervous F45.8
  nodding F98.4
  occupational F48.8
  oculogyric H51.8
    psychogenic F45.8
  of accommodation H52.53-
  ophthalmic artery —*see* Occlusion, artery,
    retina
  perineal, female N94.89
  peroneo-extensor —*see also* Deformity, limb,
    flat foot
  pharynx (reflex) J39.2
    hysterical F45.8
    psychogenic F45.8

Spasm (s), spastic, spasticity *(Continued)*
  psychogenic F45.8
  pylorus NEC K31.3
    adult hypertrophic K31.89
    congenital or infantile Q40.0
    psychogenic F45.8
  rectum (sphincter) K59.4
    psychogenic F45.8
  retinal (artery) —*see* Occlusion, artery, retina
  sigmoid —*see also* Syndrome, irritable bowel
    K58.9
    psychogenic F45.8
  sphincter of Oddi K83.4
  stomach K31.89
    neurotic F45.8
  throat J39.2
    hysterical F45.8
    psychogenic F45.8
  tic F95.9
    chronic F95.1
    transient of childhood F95.0
  tongue K14.8
  torsion (progressive) G24.1
  trigeminal nerve —*see* Neuralgia, trigeminal
  ureter N13.5
  urethra (sphincter) N35.9
  uterus N85.8
    complicating labor O62.4
  vagina N94.2
    psychogenic F52.5
  vascular I73.9
  vasomotor I73.9
  vein NEC I87.8
  viscera —*see* Pain, abdominal
Spasmodic —*see* condition
Spasmophilia —*see* Tetany
Spasmus nutans F98.4
Spastic, spasticity —*see also* Spasm
  child (cerebral) (congenital) (paralysis) G80.1
Speaker's throat R49.8
Specific, specified —*see* condition
Speech
  defect, disorder, disturbance, impediment
    R47.9
    psychogenic, in childhood and adolescence
      F98.8
    slurring R47.81
    specified NEC R47.89
Spencer's disease A08.19
Spens' syndrome (syncope with heart block)
    I45.9
Sperm counts (fertility testing) Z31.41
  postvasectomy Z30.8
  reversal Z31.42
Spermatic cord —*see* condition
Spermatocele N43.40
  congenital Q55.4
  multiple N43.42
  single N43.41
Spermatocystitis N49.0
Spermatocytoma C62.9-
  specified site —*see* Neoplasm, malignant, by
    site
Spermatorrhea N50.89 ◀▥
Sphacelus —*see* Gangrene
Sphenoidal —*see* condition
Sphenoiditis (chronic) —*see* Sinusitis,
    sphenoidal
Sphenopalatine ganglion neuralgia G90.09
Sphericity, increased, lens (congenital)
    Q12.4
Spherocytosis (congenital) (familial)
    (hereditary) D58.0
  hemoglobin disease D58.0
  sickle-cell (disease) D57.8-
Spherophakia Q12.4
Sphincter —*see* condition
Sphincteritis, sphincter of Oddi —*see*
    Cholangitis
Sphingolipidosis E75.3
  specified NEC E75.29

Sphingomyelinosis E75.3
Spicule tooth K00.2
Spider
  bite —see Toxicity, venom, spider
  fingers —see Syndrome, Marfan's
  nevus I78.1
  toes —see Syndrome, Marfan's
  vascular I78.1
Spiegler-Fendt
  benign lymphocytoma L98.8
  sarcoid L08.89
Spielmeyer-Vogt disease E75.4
Spina bifida (aperta) Q05.9
  with hydrocephalus NEC Q05.4
  cervical Q05.5
    with hydrocephalus Q05.0
  dorsal Q05.6
    with hydrocephalus Q05.1
  lumbar Q05.7
    with hydrocephalus Q05.2
  lumbosacral Q05.7
    with hydrocephalus Q05.2
  occulta Q76.0
  sacral Q05.8
    with hydrocephalus Q05.3
  thoracic Q05.6
    with hydrocephalus Q05.1
  thoracolumbar Q05.6
    with hydrocephalus Q05.1
Spindle, Krukenberg's —see Pigmentation,
    cornea, posterior
Spine, spinal —see condition
Spiradenoma (eccrine) —see Neoplasm, skin,
    benign
Spirillosis A25.0
Spirillum
  minus A25.0
  obermeieri infection A68.0
Spirochetal —see condition
Spirochetosis A69.9
  arthritic, arthritica A69.9
  bronchopulmonary A69.8
  icterohemorrhagic A27.0
  lung A69.8
Spirometrosis B70.1
Spitting blood —see Hemoptysis
Splanchnoptosis K63.4
Spleen, splenic —see condition
Splenectasis —see Splenomegaly
Splenitis (interstitial) (malignant) (nonspecific)
    D73.89
  malarial —see also Malaria B54 [D77]
  tuberculous A18.85
Splenocele D73.89
Splenomegaly, splenomegalia (Bengal)
    (cryptogenic) (idiopathic) (tropical) R16.1
  with hepatomegaly R16.2
  cirrhotic D73.2
  congenital Q89.09
  congestive, chronic D73.2
  Egyptian B65.1
  Gaucher's E75.22
  malarial —see also Malaria B54 [D77]
  neutropenic D73.81
  Niemann-Pick —see Niemann-Pick disease or
      syndrome
  siderotic D73.2
  syphilitic A52.79
    congenital (early) A50.08 [D77]
Splenopathy D73.9
Splenoptosis D73.89
Splenosis D73.89
Splinter —see Foreign body, superficial, by site
Split, splitting
  foot Q72.7-
  hand Q71.6 ◄
  heart sounds R01.2
  lip, congenital —see Cleft, lip
  nails L60.3
  urinary stream R39.13
Spondylarthrosis —see Spondylosis

Spondylitis (chronic) —see also Spondylopathy,
    inflammatory
  ankylopoietica —see Spondylitis, ankylosing
  ankylosing (chronic) M45.9
    with lung involvement M45.9 [J99]
    cervical region M45.2
    cervicothoracic region M45.3
    juvenile M08.1
    lumbar region M45.6
    lumbosacral region M45.7
    multiple sites M45.0
    occipito-atlanto-axial region M45.1
    sacrococcygeal region M45.8
    thoracic region M45.4
    thoracolumbar region M45.5
  atrophic (ligamentous) —see Spondylitis,
      ankylosing
  deformans (chronic) —see Spondylosis
  gonococcal A54.41
  gouty —see also Gout, by type, vertebrae
    M10.08 ◄▥
  in (due to)
    brucellosis A23.9 [M49.80]
      cervical region A23.9 [M49.82]
      cervicothoracic region A23.9 [M49.83]
      lumbar region A23.9 [M49.86]
      lumbosacral region A23.9 [M49.87]
      multiple sites A23.9 [M49.89]
      occipito-atlanto-axial region A23.9
          [M49.81]
      sacrococcygeal region A23.9 [M49.88]
      thoracic region A23.9 [M49.84]
      thoracolumbar region A23.9 [M49.85]
    enterobacteria —see also subcategory M49.8
        A04.9
    tuberculosis A18.01
  infectious NEC —see Spondylopathy,
      infective
  juvenile ankylosing (chronic) M08.1
  Kümmell's —see Spondylopathy, traumatic
  Marie-Strümpell —see Spondylitis,
      ankylosing
  muscularis —see Spondylopathy, specified
      NEC
  psoriatic L40.53
  rheumatoid —see Spondylitis, ankylosing
  rhizomelica —see Spondylitis, ankylosing
  sacroiliac NEC M46.1
  senescent, senile —see Spondylosis
  traumatic (chronic) or post-traumatic —see
      Spondylopathy, traumatic
  tuberculous A18.01
  typhosa A01.05
Spondylolisthesis (acquired) (degenerative)
    M43.10
  with disproportion (fetopelvic) O33.0
    causing obstructed labor O65.0
  cervical region M43.12
  cervicothoracic region M43.13
  congenital Q76.2
  lumbar region M43.16
  lumbosacral region M43.17
  multiple sites M43.19
  occipito-atlanto-axial region M43.11
  sacrococcygeal region M43.18
  thoracic region M43.14
  thoracolumbar region M43.15
  traumatic (old) M43.10
    acute
      fifth cervical (displaced) S12.430
        nondisplaced S12.431
        specified type NEC (displaced)
            S12.450
          nondisplaced S12.451
        type III S12.44
      fourth cervical (displaced) S12.330
        nondisplaced S12.331
        specified type NEC (displaced)
            S12.350
          nondisplaced S12.351
        type III S12.34

Spondylolisthesis (Continued)
  traumatic (Continued)
    acute (Continued)
      second cervical (displaced) S12.130
        nondisplaced S12.131
        specified type NEC (displaced)
            S12.150
          nondisplaced S12.151
        type III S12.14
      seventh cervical (displaced) S12.630
        nondisplaced S12.631
        specified type NEC (displaced)
            S12.650
          nondisplaced S12.651
        type III S12.64
      sixth cervical (displaced) S12.530
        nondisplaced S12.531
        specified type NEC (displaced)
            S12.550
          nondisplaced S12.551
        type III S12.54
      third cervical (displaced) S12.230
        nondisplaced S12.231
        specified type NEC (displaced)
            S12.250
          nondisplaced S12.251
        type III S12.24
Spondylolysis (acquired) M43.00
  cervical region M43.02
  cervicothoracic region M43.03
  congenital Q76.2
  lumbar region M43.06
  lumbosacral region M43.07
    with disproportion (fetopelvic) O33.0
      causing obstructed labor O65.8
  multiple sites M43.09
  occipito-atlanto-axial region M43.01
  sacrococcygeal region M43.08
  thoracic region M43.04
  thoracolumbar region M43.05
Spondylopathy M48.9
  infective NEC M46.50
    cervical region M46.52
    cervicothoracic region M46.53
    lumbar region M46.56
    lumbosacral region M46.57
    multiple sites M46.59
    occipito-atlanto-axial region M46.51
    sacrococcygeal region M46.58
    thoracic region M46.54
    thoracolumbar region M46.55
  inflammatory M46.90
    cervical region M46.92
    cervicothoracic region M46.93
    lumbar region M46.96
    lumbosacral region M46.97
    multiple sites M46.99
    occipito-atlanto-axial region M46.91
    sacrococcygeal region M46.98
    specified type NEC M46.80
      cervical region M46.82
      cervicothoracic region M46.83
      lumbar region M46.86
      lumbosacral region M46.87
      multiple sites M46.89
      occipito-atlanto-axial region M46.81
      sacrococcygeal region M46.88
      thoracic region M46.84
      thoracolumbar region M46.85
    thoracic region M46.94
    thoracolumbar region M46.95
  neuropathic, in
    syringomyelia and syringobulbia G95.0
    tabes dorsalis A52.11
  specified NEC —see subcategory M48.8
  traumatic M48.30
    cervical region M48.32
    cervicothoracic region M48.33
    lumbar region M48.36
    lumbosacral region M48.37
    occipito-atlanto-axial region M48.31

◄ New   ◄▥ Revised   ~~deleted~~ Deleted

Spondylopathy (Continued)
    traumatic (Continued)
        sacrococcygeal region M48.38
        thoracic region M48.34
        thoracolumbar region M48.35
Spondylosis M47.9
    with
        disproportion (fetopelvic) O33.0
            causing obstructed labor O65.0
        myelopathy NEC M47.10
            cervical region M47.12
            cervicothoracic region M47.13
            lumbar region M47.16
            occipito-atlanto-axial region
                M47.11
            thoracic region M47.14
            thoracolumbar region M47.15
        radiculopathy M47.20
            cervical region M47.22
            cervicothoracic region M47.23
            lumbar region M47.26
            lumbosacral region M47.27
            occipito-atlanto-axial region
                M47.21
            sacrococcygeal region M47.28
            thoracic region M47.24
            thoracolumbar region M47.25
    without myelopathy or radiculopathy
        M47.819
        cervical region M47.812
        cervicothoracic region M47.813
        lumbar region M47.816
        lumbosacral region M47.817
        occipito-atlanto-axial region M47.811
        sacrococcygeal region M47.818
        thoracic region M47.814
        thoracolumbar region M47.815
    specified NEC M47.899
        cervical region M47.892
        cervicothoracic region M47.893
        lumbar region M47.896
        lumbosacral region M47.897
        occipito-atlanto-axial region M47.891
        sacrococcygeal region M47.898
        thoracic region M47.894
        thoracolumbar region M47.895
    traumatic —see Spondylopathy, traumatic
Sponge
    inadvertently left in operation wound —see
        Foreign body, accidentally left during a
        procedure
    kidney (medullary) Q61.5
Sponge-diver's disease —see Toxicity, venom,
    marine animal, sea anemone
Spongioblastoma (any type) —see Neoplasm,
    malignant, by site
    specified site —see Neoplasm, malignant, by
        site
    unspecified site C71.9
Spongioneuroblastoma —see Neoplasm,
    malignant, by site
Spontaneous —see also condition
    fracture (cause unknown) —see Fracture,
        pathological
Spoon nail L60.3
    congenital Q84.6
Sporadic —see condition
Sporothrix schenckii infection —see
    Sporotrichosis
Sporotrichosis B42.9
    arthritis B42.82
    disseminated B42.7
    generalized B42.7
    lymphocutaneous (fixed) (progressive)
        B42.1
    pulmonary B42.0
    specified NEC B42.89
Spots, spotting (in) (of)
    Bitot's —see also Pigmentation, conjunctiva
        in the young child E50.1
        vitamin A deficiency E50.1

Spots, spotting (Continued)
    café, au lait L81.3
    Cayenne pepper I78.1
    cotton wool, retina —see Occlusion, artery,
        retina
    de Morgan's (senile angiomas) I78.1
    Fuchs' black (myopic) H44.2-
    intermenstrual (regular) N92.0
        irregular N92.1
    Koplik's B05.9
    liver L81.4
    pregnancy O26.85-
    purpuric R23.3
    ruby I78.1
Spotted fever —see Fever, spotted N92.3
Sprain (joint) (ligament)
    acromioclavicular joint or ligament S43.5-
    ankle S93.40-
        calcaneofibular ligament S93.41-
        deltoid ligament S93.42-
        internal collateral ligament —see Sprain,
            ankle, specified ligament NEC
        specified ligament NEC S93.49-
        talofibular ligament —see Sprain, ankle,
            specified ligament NEC
        tibiofibular ligament S93.43-
    anterior longitudinal, cervical S13.4
    atlas, atlanto-axial, atlanto-occipital S13.4
    breast bone —see Sprain, sternum
    calcaneofibular —see Sprain, ankle
    carpal —see Sprain, wrist
    carpometacarpal —see Sprain, hand, specified
        site NEC
    cartilage
        costal S23.41
        semilunar (knee) —see Sprain, knee,
            specified site NEC
            with current tear —see Tear, meniscus
        thyroid region S13.5
        xiphoid —see Sprain, sternum
    cervical, cervicodorsal, cervicothoracic
        S13.4
    chondrosternal S23.421
    coracoclavicular S43.8-
    coracohumeral S43.41-
    coronary, knee —see Sprain, knee, specified
        site NEC
    costal cartilage S23.41
    cricoarytenoid articulation or ligament S13.5
    cricothyroid articulation S13.5
    cruciate, knee —see Sprain, knee, cruciate
    deltoid, ankle —see Sprain, ankle
    dorsal (spine) S23.3
    elbow S53.40-
        radial collateral ligament S53.43-
        radiohumeral S53.41-
        rupture
            radial collateral ligament —see Rupture,
                traumatic, ligament, radial
                collateral
            ulnar collateral ligament —see Rupture,
                traumatic, ligament, ulnar
                collateral
        specified type NEC S53.49-
        ulnar collateral ligament S53.44-
        ulnohumeral S53.42-
    femur, head —see Sprain, hip
    fibular collateral, knee —see Sprain, knee,
        collateral
    fibulocalcaneal —see Sprain, ankle
    finger (s) S63.61-
        index S63.61-
        interphalangeal (joint) S63.63-
            index S63.63-
            little S63.63-
            middle S63.63-
            ring S63.63-
        little S63.61-
        metacarpophalangeal (joint) S63.65-
        middle S63.61-
        ring S63.61-

Sprain (Continued)
    finger (s) (Continued)
        specified site NEC S63.69-
            index S63.69-
            little S63.69-
            middle S63.69-
            ring S63.69-
    foot S93.60-
        specified ligament NEC S93.69-
        tarsal ligament S93.61-
        tarsometatarsal ligament S93.62-
        toe —see Sprain, toe
    hand S63.9-
        finger —see Sprain, finger
        specified site NEC —see subcategory S63.8
        thumb —see Sprain, thumb
    head S03.9
    hip S73.10-
        iliofemoral ligament S73.11-
        ischiocapsular (ligament) S73.12-
        specified NEC S73.19-
    iliofemoral —see Sprain, hip
    innominate
        acetabulum —see Sprain, hip
        sacral junction S33.6
    internal
        collateral, ankle —see Sprain, ankle
        semilunar cartilage —see Sprain, knee,
            specified site NEC
    interphalangeal
        finger —see Sprain, finger, interphalangeal
            (joint)
        toe —see Sprain, toe, interphalangeal joint
    ischiocapsular —see Sprain, hip
    ischiofemoral —see Sprain, hip
    jaw (articular disc) (cartilage) (meniscus)
        S03.4- ◄▥
        old M26.69
    knee S83.9-
        collateral ligament S83.40-
            lateral (fibular) S83.42-
            medial (tibial) S83.41-
        cruciate ligament S83.50-
            anterior S83.51-
            posterior S83.52-
        lateral (fibular) collateral ligament S83.42-
        medial (tibial) collateral ligament S83.41-
        patellar ligament S76.11-
        specified site NEC S83.8X-
        superior tibiofibular joint (ligament) S83.6-
    lateral collateral, knee —see Sprain, knee,
        collateral
    lumbar (spine) S33.5
    lumbosacral S33.9
    mandible (articular disc) S03.4- ◄▥
        old M26.69
    medial collateral, knee —see Sprain, knee,
        collateral
    meniscus
        jaw S03.4- ◄▥
            old M26.69
        knee —see Sprain, knee, specified site NEC
            with current tear —see Tear, meniscus
            old —see Derangement, knee,
                meniscus, due to old tear
        mandible S03.4- ◄▥
            old M26.69
    metacarpal (distal) (proximal) —see Sprain,
        hand, specified site NEC
    metacarpophalangeal —see Sprain, finger,
        metacarpophalangeal (joint)
    metatarsophalangeal —see Sprain, toe,
        metatarsophalangeal joint
    midcarpal —see Sprain, hand, specified site
        NEC
    midtarsal —see Sprain, foot, specified site
        NEC
    neck S13.9
        anterior longitudinal cervical ligament
            S13.4
        atlanto-axial joint S13.4

Sprain *(Continued)*
  neck *(Continued)*
    atlanto-occipital joint S13.4
    cervical spine S13.4
    cricoarytenoid ligament S13.5
    cricothyroid ligament S13.5
    specified site NEC S13.8
    thyroid region (cartilage) S13.5
  nose S03.8
  orbicular, hip —*see* Sprain, hip
  patella —*see* Sprain, knee, specified site NEC
  patellar ligament S76.11-
  pelvis NEC S33.8
  phalanx
    finger —*see* Sprain, finger
    toe —*see* Sprain, toe
  pubofemoral —*see* Sprain, hip
  radiocarpal —*see* Sprain, wrist
  radiohumeral —*see* Sprain, elbow
  radius, collateral —*see* Rupture, traumatic,
    ligament, radial collateral
  rib (cage) S23.41
  rotator cuff (capsule) S43.42-
  sacroiliac (region)
    chronic or old —*see* subcategory M53.2
    joint S33.6
  scaphoid (hand) —*see* Sprain, hand, specified
    site NEC
  scapula (r) —*see* Sprain, shoulder girdle,
    specified site NEC
  semilunar cartilage (knee) —*see* Sprain, knee,
    specified site NEC
    with current tear —*see* Tear, meniscus
      old —*see* Derangement, knee, meniscus,
        due to old tear
  shoulder joint S43.40-
    acromioclavicular joint (ligament) —*see*
      Sprain, acromioclavicular joint
    blade —*see* Sprain, shoulder, girdle,
      specified site NEC
    coracoclavicular joint (ligament) —*see*
      Sprain, coracoclavicular joint
    coracohumeral ligament —*see* Sprain,
      coracohumeral joint
    girdle S43.9-
      specified site NEC S43.8-
    rotator cuff —*see* Sprain, rotator cuff
    specified site NEC S43.49-
    sternoclavicular joint (ligament) —*see*
      Sprain, sternoclavicular joint
  spine
    cervical S13.4
    lumbar S33.5
    thoracic S23.3
  sternoclavicular joint S43.6-
  sternum S23.429
    chondrosternal joint S23.421
    specified site NEC S23.428
    sternoclavicular (joint) (ligament)
      S23.420
  symphysis
    jaw S03.4- ◀▥
      old M26.69
    mandibular S03.4- ◀▥
      old M26.69
  talofibular —*see* Sprain, ankle
  tarsal —*see* Sprain, foot, specified site NEC
  tarsometatarsal —*see* Sprain, foot, specified
    site NEC
  temporomandibular S03.4- ◀▥
    old M26.69
  thorax S23.9
    ribs S23.41
    specified site NEC S23.8
    spine S23.3
    sternum —*see* Sprain, sternum
  thumb S63.60-
    interphalangeal (joint) S63.62-
    metacarpophalangeal (joint) S63.64-
    specified site NEC S63.68-
  thyroid cartilage or region S13.5

Sprain *(Continued)*
  tibia (proximal end) —*see* Sprain, knee,
    specified site NEC
  tibial collateral, knee —*see* Sprain, knee,
    collateral
  tibiofibular
    distal —*see* Sprain, ankle
    superior —*see* Sprain, knee, specified site
      NEC
  toe (s) S93.50-
    great S93.50-
      interphalangeal joint S93.51-
        great S93.51-
        lesser S93.51-
    lesser S93.50-
    metatarsophalangeal joint S93.52-
      great S93.52-
      lesser S93.52-
  ulna, collateral —*see* Rupture, traumatic,
    ligament, ulnar collateral
  ulnohumeral —*see* Sprain, elbow
  wrist S63.50-
    carpal S63.51-
    radiocarpal S63.52-
    specified site NEC S63.59-
  xiphoid cartilage —*see* Sprain, sternum
Sprengel's deformity (congenital) Q74.0
Sprue (tropical) K90.1
  celiac K90.0
  idiopathic K90.49 ◀▥
  meaning thrush B37.0
  nontropical K90.0
Spur, bone —*see also* Enthesopathy
  calcaneal M77.3-
  iliac crest M76.2-
  nose (septum) J34.89
Spurway's syndrome Q78.0
Sputum
  abnormal (amount) (color) (odor) (purulent)
    R09.3
  blood-stained R04.2
  excessive (cause unknown) R09.3
Squamous —*see also* condition
  epithelium in
    cervical canal (congenital) Q51.828
    uterine mucosa (congenital) Q51.818
Squashed nose M95.0
  congenital Q67.4
Squeeze, diver's T70.3
Squint —*see also* Strabismus
  accommodative —*see* Strabismus, convergent
    concomitant
St. Hubert's disease A82.9
Stab —*see also* Laceration
  internal organs —*see* Injury, by site
Stafne's cyst or cavity M27.0
Staggering gait R26.0
  hysterical F44.4
Staghorn calculus —*see* Calculus, kidney
Stähli's line (cornea) (pigment) —*see*
  Pigmentation, cornea, anterior
Stain, staining
  meconium (newborn) P96.83
  port wine Q82.5
  tooth, teeth (hard tissues) (extrinsic) K03.6
    due to
      accretions K03.6
      deposits (betel) (black) (green) (materia
        alba) (orange) (soft) (tobacco) K03.6
      metals (copper) (silver) K03.7
      nicotine K03.6
      pulpal bleeding K03.7
      tobacco K03.6
    intrinsic K00.8
Stammering —*see also* Disorder, fluency F80.81
Standstill
  auricular I45.5
  cardiac —*see* Arrest, cardiac
  sinoatrial I45.5
  ventricular —*see* Arrest, cardiac
Stannosis J63.5

Stanton's disease —*see* Melioidosis
Staphylitis (acute) (catarrhal) (chronic)
  (gangrenous) (membranous) (suppurative)
  (ulcerative) K12.2
Staphylococcal scalded skin syndrome L00
Staphylococcemia A41.2
Staphylococcus, staphylococcal —*see also*
  condition
  as cause of disease classified elsewhere
    B95.8
    aureus (methicillin susceptible) (MSSA)
      B95.61
      methicillin resistant (MRSA) B95.62
  specified NEC, as cause of disease classified
    elsewhere B95.7
Staphyloma (sclera)
  cornea H18.72-
  equatorial H15.81-
  localized (anterior) H15.82-
  posticum H15.83-
  ring H15.85-
Stargardt's disease —*see* Dystrophy, retina
Starvation (inanition) (due to lack of food)
  T73.0
  edema —*see* Malnutrition, severe
Stasis
  bile (noncalculous) K83.1
  bronchus J98.09
    with infection —*see* Bronchitis
  cardiac —*see* Failure, heart, congestive
  cecum K59.8
  colon K59.8
  dermatitis I87.2 ◀▥
    with ◀
      varicose ulcer —*see* Varix, leg, with ulcer,
        with inflammation ◀
      varicose veins —*see* Varix, leg, with,
        inflammation ◀
      due to postthrombotic syndrome —*see*
        Syndrome, postthrombotic ◀
  duodenal K31.5
  eczema —*see* Varix, leg, with, inflammation
  edema —*see* Hypertension, venous (chronic),
    idiopathic
  foot T69.0-
  ileocecal coil K59.8
  ileum K59.8
  intestinal K59.8
  jejunum K59.8
  kidney N19
  liver (cirrhotic) K76.1
  lymphatic I89.8
  pneumonia J18.2
  pulmonary —*see* Edema, lung
  rectal K59.8
  renal N19
    tubular N17.0
  ulcer —*see* Varix, leg, with, ulcer
    without varicose veins I87.2
  urine —*see* Retention, urine
  venous I87.8
State (of)
  affective and paranoid, mixed, organic
    psychotic F06.8
  agitated R45.1
    acute reaction to stress F43.0
  anxiety (neurotic) F41.1
  apprehension F41.1
  burn-out Z73.0
  climacteric, female Z78.0
    symptomatic N95.1
  compulsive F42.8 ◀▥
    mixed with obsessional thoughts F42.2 ◀▥
  confusional (psychogenic) F44.89
    acute —*see also* Delirium
      with
        arteriosclerotic dementia F01.50
          with behavioral disturbance
            F01.51
        senility or dementia F05
      alcoholic F10.231

◀ New   ◀▥ Revised   ~~deleted~~ Deleted

State (Continued)
  confusional (psychogenic) (Continued)
    epileptic F05
    reactive (from emotional stress,
      psychological trauma) F44.89
    subacute —see Delirium
  convulsive —see Convulsions
  crisis F43.0
  depressive F32.9
    neurotic F34.1
  dissociative F44.9
  emotional shock (stress) R45.7
  hypercoagulation —see Hypercoagulable
  locked-in G83.5
  menopausal Z78.0
    symptomatic N95.1
  neurotic F48.9
    with depersonalization F48.1
  obsessional F42.8 ◀▥
  oneiroid (schizophrenia-like) F23
  organic
    hallucinatory (nonalcoholic) F06.0
    paranoid (-hallucinatory) F06.2
  panic F41.0
  paranoid F22
    climacteric F22
    involutional F22
    menopausal F22
    organic F06.2
    senile F03
    simple F22
  persistent vegetative R40.3
  phobic F40.9
  postleukotomy F07.0
  ~~pregnant, incidental Z33.1~~
  pregnant ◀
    gestational carrier Z33.3 ◀
    incidental Z33.1 ◀
  psychogenic, twilight F44.89
  psychopathic (constitutional) F60.2
  psychotic, organic —see also Psychosis,
    organic
    mixed paranoid and affective F06.8
    senile or presenile F03
    transient NEC F06.8
      with
        depression F06.31
        hallucinations F06.0
  residual schizophrenic F20.5
  restlessness R45.1
  stress (emotional) R45.7
  tension (mental) F48.9
    specified NEC F48.8
  transient organic psychotic NEC F06.8
    depressive type F06.31
    hallucinatory type F06.0 ◀▥
  twilight
    epileptic F05
    psychogenic F44.89
  vegetative, persistent R40.3
  vital exhaustion Z73.0
  withdrawal —see Withdrawal, state
Status (post) —see also Presence (of)
  absence, epileptic —see Epilepsy, by type,
    with status epilepticus
  administration of tPA (rtPA) in a different
    facility within the last 24 hours prior to
    admission to the current facility
    Z92.82
  adrenalectomy (unilateral) (bilateral) E89.6
  anastomosis Z98.0
  anginosus I20.9
  angioplasty (peripheral) Z98.62
    with implant Z95.820
    coronary artery Z98.61
      with implant Z95.5
  aortocoronary bypass Z95.1
  arthrodesis Z98.1
  artificial opening (of) Z93.9
    gastrointestinal tract Z93.4
    specified NEC Z93.8

Status (Continued)
  artificial opening (of) (Continued)
    urinary tract Z93.6
    vagina Z93.8
  asthmaticus —see Asthma, by type, with
    status asthmaticus
  awaiting organ transplant Z76.82
  bariatric surgery Z98.84
  bed confinement Z74.01
  bleb, filtering (vitreous), after glaucoma
    surgery Z98.83
  breast implant Z98.82
    removal Z98.86
  cataract extraction Z98.4-
  cholecystectomy Z90.49
  clitorectomy N90.811
    with excision of labia minora N90.812
  colectomy (complete) (partial) Z90.49
  colonization —see Carrier (suspected) of
  colostomy Z93.3
  convulsivus idiopathicus —see Epilepsy, by
    type, with status epilepticus
  coronary artery angioplasty —see Status,
    angioplasty, coronary artery
  cystectomy (urinary bladder) Z90.6
  cystostomy Z93.50
    appendico-vesicostomy Z93.52
    cutaneous Z93.51
    specified NEC Z93.59
  delinquent immunization Z28.3
  dental Z98.818
    crown Z98.811
    fillings Z98.811
    restoration Z98.811
    sealant Z98.810
    specified NEC Z98.818
  deployment (current) (military) Z56.82
  dialysis (hemodialysis) (peritoneal) Z99.2
  do not resuscitate (DNR) Z66
  donor —see Donor
  embedded fragments —see Retained, foreign
    body fragments (type of)
  embedded splinter —see Retained, foreign
    body fragments (type of)
  enterostomy Z93.4
  epileptic, epilepticus —see also Epilepsy, by
    type, with status epilepticus G40.901
  estrogen receptor
    negative Z17.1
    positive Z17.0
  female genital cutting —see Female genital
    mutilation status
  female genital mutilation —see Female genital
    mutilation status
  filtering (vitreous) bleb after glaucoma
    surgery Z98.83
  gastrectomy (complete) (partial) Z90.3
  gastric banding Z98.84
  gastric bypass for obesity Z98.84
  gastrostomy Z93.1
  human immunodeficiency virus (HIV)
    infection, asymptomatic Z21
  hysterectomy (complete) (total) Z90.710
    partial (with remaining cervical stump)
      Z90.711
  ileostomy Z93.2
  implant
    breast Z98.82
  infibulation N90.813
  intestinal bypass Z98.0
  jejunostomy Z93.4
  lapsed immunization schedule Z28.3
  laryngectomy Z90.02
  lymphaticus E32.8
  malignancy ◀
    castrate resistant prostate Z19.2 ◀
    hormone resistant Z19.2 ◀
    hormone sensitive Z19.1 ◀
  marmoratus G80.3
  mastectomy (unilateral) (bilateral)
    Z90.1-

Status (Continued)
  military deployment status (current) Z56.82
    in theater or in support of military war,
      peacekeeping and humanitarian
      operations Z56.82
  nephrectomy (unilateral) (bilateral) Z90.5
  nephrostomy Z93.6
  obesity surgery Z98.84
  oophorectomy
    bilateral Z90.722
    unilateral Z90.721
  organ replacement
    by artificial or mechanical device or
      prosthesis of
      artery Z95.828
      bladder Z96.0
      blood vessel Z95.828
      breast Z97.8
      eye globe Z97.0
      heart Z95.812
        valve Z95.2
      intestine Z97.8
      joint Z96.60
        hip —see Presence, hip joint implant
        knee —see Presence, knee joint
          implant
        specified site NEC Z96.698
      kidney Z97.8
      larynx Z96.3
      lens Z96.1
      limbs —see Presence, artificial, limb
      liver Z97.8
      lung Z97.8
      pancreas Z97.8
    by organ transplant (heterologous)
      (homologous) —see Transplant
  pacemaker
    brain Z96.89
    cardiac Z95.0
    specified NEC Z96.89
  pancreatectomy Z90.410
    complete Z90.410
    partial Z90.411
    total Z90.410
  pneumonectomy (complete) (partial) Z90.2
  pneumothorax, therapeutic Z98.3
  postcommotio cerebri F07.81
  postoperative (postprocedural) NEC
    Z98.890 ◀▥
    breast implant Z98.82
    dental Z98.818
      crown Z98.811
      fillings Z98.811
      restoration Z98.811
      sealant Z98.810
      specified NEC Z98.818
    pneumothorax, therapeutic Z98.3
    uterine scar Z98.891 ◀
  postpartum (routine follow-up) Z39.2
    care immediately after delivery Z39.0
  postsurgical (postprocedural) NEC
    Z98.890 ◀▥
    pneumothorax, therapeutic Z98.3
  pregnancy, incidental Z33.1
  prosthesis coronary angioplasty Z95.5
  pseudophakia Z96.1
  renal dialysis (hemodialysis) (peritoneal)
    Z99.2
  retained foreign body —see Retained, foreign
    body fragments (type of)
  reversed jejunal transposition (for bypass
    Z98.0
  salpingo-oophorectomy
    bilateral Z90.722
    unilateral Z90.721
  sex reassignment surgery status Z87.890
  shunt
    arteriovenous (for dialysis) Z99.2
    cerebrospinal fluid Z98.2
    ventricular (communicating) (for
      drainage) Z98.2

Status *(Continued)*
    splenectomy Z90.81
    thymicolymphaticus E32.8
    thymicus E32.8
    thymolymphaticus E32.8
    thyroidectomy (hypothyroidism) E89.0
    tooth (teeth) extraction —*see also* Absence,
        teeth, acquired K08.409
    tPA (rtPA) administration in a different
        facility within the last 24 hours prior to
        admission to current facility Z92.82
    tracheostomy Z93.0
    transplant —*see* Transplant
        organ removed Z98.85
    tubal ligation Z98.51
    underimmunization Z28.3
    ureterostomy Z93.6
    urethrostomy Z93.6
    vagina, artificial Z93.8
    vasectomy Z98.52
    wheelchair confinement Z99.3
Stealing
    child problem F91.8
        in company with others Z72.810
    pathological (compulsive) F63.2
Steam burn —*see* Burn
Steatocystoma multiplex L72.2
Steatohepatitis (nonalcoholic) (NASH)
    K75.81
Steatoma L72.3
    eyelid (cystic) —*see* Dermatosis, eyelid
        infected —*see* Hordeolum
Steatorrhea (chronic) K90.9 ◄▥
    with lacteal obstruction K90.2
    idiopathic (adult) (infantile) K90.9 ◄▥
    pancreatic K90.3
    primary K90.0
    tropical K90.1
Steatosis E88.89
    heart —*see* Degeneration, myocardial
    kidney N28.89
    liver NEC K76.0
Steele-Richardson-Olszewski disease or
    syndrome G23.1
Steinbrocker's syndrome G90.8
Steinert's disease G71.11
Stein-Leventhal syndrome E28.2
Stein's syndrome E28.2
STEMI —*see also* - Infarct, myocardium, ST
    elevation I21.3
Stenocardia I20.8
Stenocephaly Q75.8
Stenosis, stenotic (cicatricial) —*see also*
    Stricture
    ampulla of Vater K83.1
    anus, anal (canal) (sphincter) K62.4
        and rectum K62.4
        congenital Q42.3
            with fistula Q42.2
    aorta (ascending) (supraventricular)
        (congenital) Q25.1 ◄▥
        arteriosclerotic I70.0
        calcified I70.0
        supravalvular Q25.3 ◄
    aortic (valve) I35.0
        with insufficiency I35.2
        congenital Q23.0
        rheumatic I06.0
            with
                incompetency, insufficiency or
                    regurgitation I06.2
                    with mitral (valve) disease I08.0
                        with tricuspid (valve) disease
                            I08.3
                    mitral (valve) disease I08.0
                        with tricuspid (valve) disease
                            I08.3
                    tricuspid (valve) disease I08.2
                        with mitral (valve) disease I08.3
        specified cause NEC I35.0
        syphilitic A52.03

Stenosis, stenotic *(Continued)*
    aqueduct of Sylvius (congenital) Q03.0
        with spina bifida —*see* Spina bifida,
            by site, with hydrocephalus
        acquired G91.1
    artery NEC —*see also* Arteriosclerosis
        I77.1
        celiac I77.4
        cerebral —*see* Occlusion, artery, cerebral
        extremities —*see* Arteriosclerosis,
            extremities
        precerebral —*see* Occlusion, artery,
            precerebral
        pulmonary (congenital) Q25.6
            acquired I28.8
        renal I70.1
        stent ◄
            coronary T82.855 ◄
            peripheral T82.856 ◄
    bile duct (common) (hepatic) K83.1
        congenital Q44.3
    bladder-neck (acquired) N32.0
        congenital Q64.31
    brain G93.89
    bronchus J98.09
        congenital Q32.3
        syphilitic A52.72
    cardia (stomach) K22.2
        congenital Q39.3
    cardiovascular —*see* Disease, cardiovascular
    caudal M48.08
    cervix, cervical (canal) N88.2
        congenital Q51.828
        in pregnancy or childbirth —*see* Pregnancy,
            complicated by, abnormal cervix
    colon —*see also* Obstruction, intestine
        congenital Q42.9
            specified NEC Q42.8
    colostomy K94.03
    common (bile) duct K83.1
        congenital Q44.3
    coronary (artery) —*see* Disease, heart,
        ischemic, atherosclerotic
    cystic duct —*see* Obstruction, gallbladder
    due to presence of device, implant or
            graft —*see also* Complications, by site
            and type, specified NEC T85.858 ◄▥
        arterial graft NEC T82.858
        breast (implant) T85.858 ◄▥
        catheter T85.858 ◄▥
            dialysis (renal) T82.858
                intraperitoneal T85.858 ◄▥
            infusion NEC T82.858
                spinal (epidural) (subdural)
                    T85.850 ◄▥
            urinary (indwelling) T83.85
        fixation, internal (orthopedic) NEC
            T84.85
        gastrointestinal (bile duct) (esophagus)
            T85.858 ◄▥
        genital NEC T83.85
        heart NEC T82.857
        joint prosthesis T84.85
        ocular (corneal graft) (orbital implant)
            NEC T85.858 ◄▥
        orthopedic NEC T84.85
        specified NEC T85.858 ◄▥
        urinary NEC T83.85
        vascular NEC T82.858
        ventricular intracranial shunt T85.850 ◄▥
    duodenum K31.5
        congenital Q41.0
    ejaculatory duct NEC N50.89 ◄▥
    endocervical os —*see* Stenosis, cervix
    enterostomy K94.13
    esophagus K22.2
        congenital Q39.3
        syphilitic A52.79
            congenital A50.59 [K23]
    eustachian tube —*see* Obstruction, eustachian
        tube

Stenosis, stenotic *(Continued)*
    external ear canal (acquired) H61.30-
        congenital Q16.1
        due to
            inflammation H61.32-
            trauma H61.31-
        postprocedural H95.81-
        specified cause NEC H61.39-
    gallbladder —*see* Obstruction,
        gallbladder
    glottis J38.6
    heart valve (congenital) Q24.8
        aortic Q23.0
        mitral Q23.2
        pulmonary Q22.1
        tricuspid Q22.4
    hepatic duct K83.1
    hymen N89.6
    hypertrophic subaortic (idiopathic) I42.1
    ileum K56.69
        congenital Q41.2
    infundibulum cardia Q24.3
    intervertebral foramina —*see also* Lesion,
            biomechanical, specified NEC
        connective tissue M99.79
            abdomen M99.79
            cervical region M99.71
            cervicothoracic M99.71
            head region M99.70
            lumbar region M99.73
            lumbosacral M99.73
            occipitocervical M99.70
            sacral region M99.74
            sacrococcygeal M99.74
            sacroiliac M99.74
            specified NEC M99.79
            thoracic region M99.72
            thoracolumbar M99.72
        disc M99.79
            abdomen M99.79
            cervical region M99.71
            cervicothoracic M99.71
            head region M99.70
            lower extremity M99.76
            lumbar region M99.73
            lumbosacral M99.73
            occipitocervical M99.70
            pelvic M99.75
            rib cage M99.78
            sacral region M99.74
            sacrococcygeal M99.74
            sacroiliac M99.74
            specified NEC M99.79
            thoracic region M99.72
            thoracolumbar M99.72
            upper extremity M99.77
        osseous M99.69
            abdomen M99.69
            cervical region M99.61
            cervicothoracic M99.61
            head region M99.60
            lower extremity M99.66
            lumbar region M99.63
            lumbosacral M99.63
            occipitocervical M99.60
            pelvic M99.65
            rib cage M99.68
            sacral region M99.64
            sacrococcygeal M99.64
            sacroiliac M99.64
            specified NEC M99.69
            thoracic region M99.62
            thoracolumbar M99.62
            upper extremity M99.67
        subluxation —*see* Stenosis, intervertebral
            foramina, osseous
    intestine —*see also* Obstruction, intestine
        congenital (small) Q41.9
            large Q42.9
                specified NEC Q42.8
            specified NEC Q41.8

◄ New   ◄▥ Revised   ~~deleted~~ Deleted

Stenosis, stenotic (Continued)
  jejunum K56.69
    congenital Q41.1
  lacrimal (passage)
    canaliculi H04.54-
    congenital Q10.5
    duct H04.55-
    punctum H04.56-
    sac H04.57-
  lacrimonasal duct —see Stenosis, lacrimal, duct
    congenital Q10.5
  larynx J38.6
    congenital NEC Q31.8
      subglottic Q31.1
    syphilitic A52.73
      congenital A50.59 [J99]
  mitral (chronic) (inactive) (valve) I05.0
    with
      aortic valve disease I08.0
      incompetency, insufficiency or regurgitation I05.2
    active or acute I01.1
      with rheumatic or Sydenham's chorea I02.0
    congenital Q23.2
    specified cause, except rheumatic I34.2
    syphilitic A52.03
  myocardium, myocardial —see also Degeneration, myocardial
    hypertrophic subaortic (idiopathic) I42.1
  nares (anterior) (posterior) J34.89
    congenital Q30.0
  nasal duct —see also Stenosis, lacrimal, duct
    congenital Q10.5
  nasolacrimal duct —see also Stenosis, lacrimal, duct
    congenital Q10.5
  neural canal —see also Lesion, biomechanical, specified NEC
    connective tissue M99.49
      abdomen M99.49
      cervical region M99.41
      cervicothoracic M99.41
      head region M99.40
      lower extremity M99.46
      lumbar region M99.43
      lumbosacral M99.43
      occipitocervical M99.40
      pelvic M99.45
      rib cage M99.48
      sacral region M99.44
      sacrococcygeal M99.44
      sacroiliac M99.44
      specified NEC M99.49
      thoracic region M99.42
      thoracolumbar M99.42
      upper extremity M99.47
    intervertebral disc M99.59
      abdomen M99.59
      cervical region M99.51
      cervicothoracic M99.51
      head region M99.50
      lower extremity M99.56
      lumbar region M99.53
      lumbosacral M99.53
      occipitocervical M99.50
      pelvic M99.55
      rib cage M99.58
      sacral region M99.54
      sacrococcygeal M99.54
      sacroiliac M99.54
      specified NEC M99.59
      thoracic region M99.52
      thoracolumbar M99.52
      upper extremity M99.57
    osseous M99.39
      abdomen M99.39
      cervical region M99.31
      cervicothoracic M99.31
      head region M99.30

Stenosis, stenotic (Continued)
  neural canal (Continued)
    osseous (Continued)
      lower extremity M99.36
      lumbar region M99.33
      lumbosacral M99.33
      occipitocervical M99.30
      pelvic M99.35
      rib cage M99.38
      sacral region M99.34
      sacrococcygeal M99.34
      sacroiliac M99.34
      specified NEC M99.39
      thoracic region M99.32
      thoracolumbar M99.32
      upper extremity M99.37
    subluxation M99.29
      cervical region M99.21
      cervicothoracic M99.21
      head region M99.20
      lower extremity M99.26
      lumbar region M99.23
      lumbosacral M99.23
      occipitocervical M99.20
      pelvic M99.25
      rib cage M99.28
      sacral region M99.24
      sacrococcygeal M99.24
      sacroiliac M99.24
      specified NEC M99.29
      thoracic region M99.22
      thoracolumbar M99.22
      upper extremity M99.27
  organ or site, congenital NEC —see Atresia, by site
  papilla of Vater K83.1
  pulmonary (artery) (congenital) Q25.6
    with ventricular septal defect, transposition of aorta, and hypertrophy of right ventricle Q21.3
    acquired I28.8
    in tetralogy of Fallot Q21.3
    infundibular Q24.3
    subvalvular Q24.3
    supravalvular Q25.6
    valve I37.0
      with insufficiency I37.2
      congenital Q22.1
      rheumatic I09.89
        with aortic, mitral or tricuspid (valve) disease I08.8
    vein, acquired I28.8
    vessel NEC I28.8
  pulmonic (congenital) Q22.1
    infundibular Q24.3
    subvalvular Q24.3
  pylorus (hypertrophic) (acquired) K31.1
    adult K31.1
    congenital Q40.0
    infantile Q40.0
  rectum (sphincter) —see Stricture, rectum
  renal artery I70.1
    congenital Q27.1
  salivary duct (any) K11.8
  sphincter of Oddi K83.1
  spinal M48.00
    cervical region M48.02
    cervicothoracic region M48.03
    lumbar region M48.06
    lumbosacral region M48.07
    occipito-atlanto-axial region M48.01
    sacrococcygeal region M48.08
    thoracic region M48.04
    thoracolumbar region M48.05
  stent ◄
    vascular ◄
      end stent ◄
        adjacent to stent —see Arteriosclerosis ◄

Stenosis, stenotic (Continued)
  stent (Continued)
    vascular (Continued)
      end stent (Continued)
        within the stent ◄
          coronary T82.855 ◄
          peripheral T82.856 ◄
      in stent ◄
        coronary vessel T82.855 ◄
        peripheral vessel T82.856 ◄
  stomach, hourglass K31.2
  subaortic (congenital) Q24.4
    hypertrophic (idiopathic) I42.1
  subglottic J38.6
    congenital Q31.1
    postprocedural J95.5
  trachea J39.8
    congenital Q32.1
    syphilitic A52.73
    tuberculous NEC A15.5
  tracheostomy J95.03
  tricuspid (valve) I07.0
    with
      aortic (valve) disease I08.2
      incompetency, insufficiency or regurgitation I07.2
        with aortic (valve) disease I08.2
          with mitral (valve) disease I08.3
      mitral (valve) disease I08.1
        with aortic (valve) disease I08.3
    congenital Q22.4
    nonrheumatic I36.0
      with insufficiency I36.2
  tubal N97.1
  ureter —see Atresia, ureter
  ureteropelvic junction, congenital Q62.11
  ureterovesical orifice, congenital Q62.12
  urethra (valve) —see also Stricture, urethra
    congenital Q64.32
  urinary meatus, congenital Q64.33
  vagina N89.5
    congenital Q52.4
    in pregnancy —see Pregnancy, complicated by, abnormal vagina
      causing obstructed labor O65.5
  valve (cardiac) (heart) —see also Endocarditis I38
    congenital Q24.8
      aortic Q23.0
      mitral Q23.2
      pulmonary Q22.1
      tricuspid Q22.4
  vena cava (inferior) (superior) I87.1
    congenital Q26.0
  vesicourethral orifice Q64.31
  vulva N90.5
Stent jail T82.897
Stercolith (impaction) K56.41
  appendix K38.1
Stercoraceous, stercoral ulcer K63.3
  anus or rectum K62.6
Stereotypies NEC F98.4
Sterility —see Infertility
Sterilization —see Encounter (for), sterilization
Sternalgia —see Angina
Sternopagus Q89.4
Sternum bifidum Q76.7
Steroid
  effects (adverse) (adrenocortical) (iatrogenic)
    cushingoid E24.2
      correct substance properly administered —see Table of Drugs and Chemicals, by drug, adverse effect
      overdose or wrong substance given or taken —see Table of Drugs and Chemicals, by drug, poisoning

Steroid *(Continued)*
  effects *(Continued)*
    diabetes —*see* category E09
      correct substance properly
        administered —*see* Table of Drugs
        and Chemicals, by drug, adverse
        effect
      overdose or wrong substance given or
        taken —*see* Table of Drugs and
        Chemicals, by drug, poisoning
    fever R50.2
    insufficiency E27.3
      correct substance properly
        administered —*see* Table of Drugs
        and Chemicals, by drug, adverse
        effect
      overdose or wrong substance given or
        taken —*see* Table of Drugs and
        Chemicals, by drug, poisoning
    responder H40.04-
Stevens-Johnson disease or syndrome L51.1
  toxic epidermal necrolysis overlap L51.3
Stewart-Morel syndrome M85.2
Sticker's disease B08.3
Sticky eye —*see* Conjunctivitis, acute,
  mucopurulent
Stieda's disease —*see* Bursitis, tibial collateral
Stiff neck —*see* Torticollis
Stiff-man syndrome G25.82
Stiffness, joint NEC M25.60-
  ankle M25.67-
  ankylosis —*see* Ankylosis, joint
  contracture —*see* Contraction, joint
  elbow M25.62-
  foot M25.67-
  hand M25.64-
  hip M25.65-
  knee M25.66-
  shoulder M25.61-
  wrist M25.63-
Stigmata congenital syphilis A50.59
Stillbirth P95
Still-Felty syndrome —*see* Felty's syndrome
Still's disease or syndrome (juvenile) M08.20
  adult-onset M06.1
  ankle M08.27-
  elbow M08.22-
  foot joint M08.27-
  hand joint M08.24-
  hip M08.25-
  knee M08.26-
  multiple site M08.29
  shoulder M08.21-
  vertebra M08.28
  wrist M08.23-
Stimulation, ovary E28.1
Sting (venomous) (with allergic or anaphylactic
  shock) —*see* Table of Drugs and
  Chemicals, by animal or substance,
  poisoning
Stippled epiphyses Q78.8
Stitch
  abscess T81.48 ◀▥
  burst (in operation wound) —*see* Disruption,
    wound, operation
Stokes-Adams disease or syndrome I45.9
Stokes' disease E05.00
  with thyroid storm E05.01
Stokvis (-Talma) disease D74.8
Stoma malfunction
  colostomy K94.03
  enterostomy K94.13
  gastrostomy K94.23
  ileostomy K94.13
  tracheostomy J95.03
Stomach —*see* condition
Stomatitis (denture) (ulcerative) K12.1
  angular K13.0
    due to dietary or vitamin deficiency E53.0
  aphthous K12.0
  bovine B08.61

Stomatitis *(Continued)*
  candidal B37.0
  catarrhal K12.1
  diphtheritic A36.89
  due to
    dietary deficiency E53.0
    thrush B37.0
    vitamin deficiency
      B group NEC E53.9
      B2 (riboflavin) E53.0
  epidemic B08.8
  epizootic B08.8
  follicular K12.1
  gangrenous A69.0
  Geotrichum B48.3
  herpesviral, herpetic B00.2
  herpetiformis K12.0
  malignant K12.1
  membranous acute K12.1
  monilial B37.0
  mycotic B37.0
  necrotizing ulcerative A69.0
  parasitic B37.0
  septic K12.1
  spirochetal A69.1
  suppurative (acute) K12.2
  ulceromembranous A69.1
  vesicular K12.1
    with exanthem (enteroviral)
      B08.4
    virus disease A93.8
  Vincent's A69.1
Stomatocytosis D58.8
Stomatomycosis B37.0
Stomatorrhagia K13.79
Stone (s) —*see also* Calculus
  bladder (diverticulum) N21.0
  cystine E72.09
  heart syndrome I50.1
  kidney N20.0
  prostate N42.0
  pulpal (dental) K04.2
  renal N20.0
  salivary gland or duct (any) K11.5
  urethra (impacted) N21.1
  urinary (duct) (impacted) (passage)
    N20.9
    bladder (diverticulum) N21.0
    lower tract N21.9
    specified NEC N21.8
  xanthine E79.8 [N22]
Stonecutter's lung J62.8
Stonemason's asthma, disease, lung or
  pneumoconiosis J62.8
Stoppage
  heart —*see* Arrest, cardiac
  urine —*see* Retention, urine
Storm, thyroid —*see* Thyrotoxicosis
Strabismus (congenital) (nonparalytic)
  H50.9
  concomitant H50.40
    convergent —*see* Strabismus, convergent
      concomitant
    divergent —*see* Strabismus, divergent
      concomitant
  convergent concomitant H50.00
    accommodative component H50.43
    alternating H50.05
      with
        A pattern H50.06
        specified nonconcomitances NEC
          H50.08
        V pattern H50.07
    monocular H50.01-
      with
        A pattern H50.02-
        specified nonconcomitances NEC
          H50.04-
        V pattern H50.03-
    intermittent H50.31-
      alternating H50.32

Strabismus *(Continued)*
  cyclotropia H50.41 ◀▥
  divergent concomitant H50.10
    alternating H50.15
      with
        A pattern H50.16
        specified noncomitances NEC
          H50.18
        V pattern H50.17
    monocular H50.11-
      with
        A pattern H50.12-
        specified noncomitances NEC
          H50.14-
        V pattern H50.13-
    intermittent H50.33-
      alternating H50.34
  Duane's syndrome H50.81-
  due to adhesions, scars H50.69
  heterophoria H50.50
    alternating H50.55
    cyclophoria H50.54
    esophoria H50.51
    exophoria H50.52
    vertical H50.53
  heterotropia H50.40
    intermittent H50.30
  hypertropia H50.2-
  hypotropia —*see* Hypertropia
  latent H50.50
  mechanical H50.60
    Brown's sheath syndrome H50.61-
    specified type NEC H50.69
  monofixation syndrome H50.42
  paralytic H49.9
    abducens nerve H49.2-
    fourth nerve H49.1-
    Kearns-Sayre syndrome H49.81-
    ophthalmoplegia (external)
      progressive H49.4-
        with pigmentary retinopathy H49.81-
      total H49.3-
    sixth nerve H49.2-
    specified type NEC H49.88-
    third nerve H49.0-
    trochlear nerve H49.1-
  specified type NEC H50.89
  vertical H50.2-
Strain
  back S39.012
  cervical S16.1
  eye NEC —*see* Disturbance, vision, subjective
  heart —*see* Disease, heart
  low back S39.012
  mental NOS Z73.3
    work-related Z56.6
  muscle (tendon) —*see* Injury, muscle, by site,
    strain
  neck S16.1
  physical NOS Z73.3
    work-related Z56.6
  postural —*see also* Disorder, soft tissue, due
    to use
  psychological NEC Z73.3
  tendon —*see* Injury, muscle, by site, strain
Straining, on urination R39.16
Strand, vitreous —*see* Opacity, vitreous,
  membranes and strands
Strangulation, strangulated —*see also*
  Asphyxia, traumatic
  appendix K38.8
  bladder-neck N32.0
  bowel or colon K56.2
  food or foreign body —*see* Foreign body, by
    site
  hemorrhoids —*see* Hemorrhoids, with
    complication
  hernia —*see also* Hernia, by site, with
    obstruction
    with gangrene —*see* Hernia, by site, with
      gangrene

◀ New   ◀▥ Revised   ~~deleted~~ Deleted

Strangulation, strangulated (*Continued*)
  intestine (large) (small) K56.2
    with hernia —*see also* Hernia, by site, with obstruction
      with gangrene —*see* Hernia, by site, with gangrene
  mesentery K56.2
  mucus —*see* Asphyxia, mucus
  omentum K56.2
  organ or site, congenital NEC —*see* Atresia, by site
  ovary —*see* Torsion, ovary
  penis N48.89
    foreign body T19.4
  rupture —*see* Hernia, by site, with obstruction
  stomach due to hernia —*see also* Hernia, by site, with obstruction
    with gangrene —*see* Hernia, by site, with gangrene
  vesicourethral orifice N32.0
Strangury R30.0
Straw itch B88.0
Strawberry
  gallbladder K82.4
  mark Q82.5
  tongue (red) (white) K14.3
Streak (s)
  macula, angioid H35.33
  ovarian Q50.32
Strephosymbolia F81.0
  secondary to organic lesion R48.8
Streptobacillary fever A25.1
Streptobacillosis A25.1
Streptobacillus moniliformis A25.1
Streptococcus, streptococcal —*see also* condition
  as cause of disease classified elsewhere B95.5
  group
    A, as cause of disease classified elsewhere B95.0
    B, as cause of disease classified elsewhere B95.1
    D, as cause of disease classified elsewhere B95.2
  pneumoniae, as cause of disease classified elsewhere B95.3
  specified NEC, as cause of disease classified elsewhere B95.4
Streptomycosis B47.1
Streptotrichosis A48.8
Stress F43.9
  family —*see* Disruption, family
  fetal P84
    complicating pregnancy O77.9
      due to drug administration O77.1
  mental NEC Z73.3
    work-related Z56.6
  physical NEC Z73.3
    work-related Z56.6
  polycythemia D75.1
  reaction —*see also* Reaction, stress F43.9
  work schedule Z56.3
Stretching, nerve —*see* Injury, nerve
Striae albicantes, atrophicae or distensae (cutis) L90.6
Stricture —*see also* Stenosis
  ampulla of Vater K83.1
  anus (sphincter) K62.4
    congenital Q42.3
      with fistula Q42.2
    infantile Q42.3
      with fistula Q42.2
  aorta (ascending) (congenital) Q25.1 ◀
    arteriosclerotic I70.0
    calcified I70.0
    supravalvular, congenital Q25.3
  aortic (valve) —*see* Stenosis, aortic
  aqueduct of Sylvius (congenital) Q03.0
    with spina bifida —*see* Spina bifida, by site, with hydrocephalus
    acquired G91.1

Stricture (*Continued*)
  artery I77.1
    basilar —*see* Occlusion, artery, basilar
    carotid —*see* Occlusion, artery, carotid
    celiac I77.4
    congenital (peripheral) Q27.8
      cerebral Q28.3
      coronary Q24.5
      digestive system Q27.8
      lower limb Q27.8
      retinal Q14.1
      specified site NEC Q27.8
      umbilical Q27.0
      upper limb Q27.8
    coronary —*see* Disease, heart, ischemic, atherosclerotic
      congenital Q24.5
    precerebral —*see* Occlusion, artery, precerebral
    pulmonary (congenital) Q25.6
      acquired I28.8
    renal I70.1
    vertebral —*see* Occlusion, artery, vertebral
  auditory canal (external) (congenital)
    acquired —*see* Stenosis, external ear canal
  bile duct (common) (hepatic) K83.1
    congenital Q44.3
    postoperative K91.89
  bladder N32.89
    neck N32.0
  bowel —*see* Obstruction, intestine
  brain G93.89
  bronchus J98.09
    congenital Q32.3
    syphilitic A52.72
  cardia (stomach) K22.2
    congenital Q39.3
  cardiac —*see also* Disease, heart
    orifice (stomach) K22.2
  cecum —*see* Obstruction, intestine
  cervix, cervical (canal) N88.2
    congenital Q51.828
    in pregnancy —*see* Pregnancy, complicated by, abnormal cervix
      causing obstructed labor O65.5
  colon —*see also* Obstruction, intestine
    congenital Q42.9
      specified NEC Q42.8
  colostomy K94.03
  common (bile) duct K83.1
  coronary (artery) —*see* Disease, heart, ischemic, atherosclerotic
  cystic duct —*see* Obstruction, gallbladder
  digestive organs NEC, congenital Q45.8
  duodenum K31.5
    congenital Q41.0
  ear canal (external) (congenital) Q16.1
    acquired —*see* Stricture, auditory canal, acquired
  ejaculatory duct N50.89 ◀▥
  enterostomy K94.13
  esophagus K22.2
    congenital Q39.3
    syphilitic A52.79
      congenital A50.59 [*K23*]
  eustachian tube —*see also* Obstruction, eustachian tube
    congenital Q17.8
  fallopian tube N97.1
    gonococcal A54.24
    tuberculous A18.17
  gallbladder —*see* Obstruction, gallbladder
  glottis J38.6
  heart —*see also* Disease, heart
    valve (*see also* Endocarditis) I38
      aortic Q23.0
      mitral Q23.4
      pulmonary Q22.1
      tricuspid Q22.4
  hepatic duct K83.1
  hourglass, of stomach K31.2

Stricture (*Continued*)
  hymen N89.6
  hypopharynx J39.2
  ileum K56.69
    congenital Q41.2
  intestine —*see also* Obstruction, intestine
    congenital (small) Q41.9
      large Q42.9
        specified NEC Q42.8
      specified NEC Q41.8
    ischemic K55.1
  jejunum K56.69
    congenital Q41.1
  lacrimal passages —*see also* Stenosis, lacrimal
    congenital Q10.5
  larynx J38.6
    congenital NEC Q31.8
      subglottic Q31.1
    syphilitic A52.73
      congenital A50.59 [*J99*]
  meatus
    ear (congenital) Q16.1
      acquired —*see* Stricture, auditory canal, acquired
    osseous (ear) (congenital) Q16.1
      acquired —*see* Stricture, auditory canal, acquired
    urinarius —*see also* Stricture, urethra
      congenital Q64.33
  mitral (valve) —*see* Stenosis, mitral
  myocardium, myocardial I51.5
    hypertrophic subaortic (idiopathic) I42.1
  nares (anterior) (posterior) J34.89
    congenital Q30.0
  nasal duct —*see also* Stenosis, lacrimal, duct
    congenital Q10.5
  nasolacrimal duct —*see also* Stenosis, lacrimal, duct
    congenital Q10.5
  nasopharynx J39.2
    syphilitic A52.73
  nose J34.89
    congenital Q30.0
  nostril (anterior) (posterior) J34.89
    congenital Q30.0
    syphilitic A52.73
      congenital A50.59 [*J99*]
  organ or site, congenital NEC —*see* Atresia, by site
  os uteri —*see* Stricture, cervix
  osseous meatus (ear) (congenital) Q16.1
    acquired —*see* Stricture, auditory canal, acquired
  oviduct —*see* Stricture, fallopian tube
  pelviureteric junction (congenital) Q62.11
    acquired, with hydronephrosis N13.0 ◀
  penis, by foreign body T19.4
  pharynx J39.2
  prostate N42.89
  pulmonary, pulmonic
    artery (congenital) Q25.6
      acquired I28.8
      noncongenital I28.8
    infundibulum (congenital) Q24.3
    valve I37.0
      congenital Q22.1
    vein, acquired I28.8
    vessel NEC I28.8
  punctum lacrimale —*see also* Stenosis, lacrimal, punctum
    congenital Q10.5
  pylorus (hypertrophic) K31.1
    adult K31.1
    congenital Q40.0
    infantile Q40.0
  rectosigmoid K56.69
  rectum (sphincter) K62.4
    congenital Q42.1
      with fistula Q42.0

Stricture *(Continued)*
  rectum (sphincter) *(Continued)*
    due to
      chlamydial lymphogranuloma A55
      irradiation K91.89
      lymphogranuloma venereum A55
    gonococcal A54.6
    inflammatory (chlamydial) A55
    syphilitic A52.74
    tuberculous A18.32
  renal artery I70.1
    congenital Q27.1
  salivary duct or gland (any) K11.8
  sigmoid (flexure) —*see* Obstruction, intestine
  spermatic cord N50.89
  stoma (following) (of)
    colostomy K94.03
    enterostomy K94.13
    gastrostomy K94.23
    ileostomy K94.13
    tracheostomy J95.03
  stomach K31.89
    congenital Q40.2
    hourglass K31.2
  subaortic Q24.4
    hypertrophic (acquired) (idiopathic) I42.1
  subglottic J38.6
  syphilitic NEC A52.79
  trachea J39.8
    congenital Q32.1
    syphilitic A52.73
    tuberculous NEC A15.5
  tracheostomy J95.03
  tricuspid (valve) —*see* Stenosis, tricuspid
  tunica vaginalis N50.89
  ureter (postoperative) N13.5
    with
      hydronephrosis N13.1
        with infection N13.6
      pyelonephritis (chronic) N11.1
    congenital —*see* Atresia, ureter
    tuberculous A18.11
  ureteropelvic junction (congenital) Q62.11
    acquired, with hydronephrosis N13.0
  ureterovesical orifice N13.5
    with infection N13.6
  urethra (organic) (spasmodic) N35.9
    associated with schistosomiasis B65.0 [N37]
    congenital Q64.39
      valvular (posterior) Q64.2
    due to
      infection —*see* Stricture, urethra, postinfective
      trauma —*see* Stricture, urethra, post-traumatic
    gonococcal, gonorrheal A54.01
    infective NEC —*see* Stricture, urethra, postinfective
    late effect (sequelae) of injury —*see* Stricture, urethra, post-traumatic
    postcatheterization —*see* Stricture, urethra, postprocedural
    postinfective NEC
      female N35.12
      male N35.119
        anterior urethra N35.114
        bulbous urethra N35.112
        meatal N35.111
        membranous urethra N35.113
    postobstetric N35.021
    postoperative —*see* Stricture, urethra, postprocedural
    postprocedural
      female N99.12
      male N99.114
        ~~anterior urethra N99.113~~
        anterior bulbous urethra N99.113
        bulbous urethra N99.111
        fossa navicularis N99.115
        meatal N99.110
        membranous urethra N99.112

Stricture *(Continued)*
  urethra (organic) (spasmodic) *(Continued)*
    post-traumatic
      female N35.028
        due to childbirth N35.021
      male N35.014
        anterior urethra N35.013
        bulbous urethra N35.011
        meatal N35.010
        membranous urethra N35.012
    sequela (late effect) of
      childbirth N35.021
      injury —*see* Stricture, urethra, post-traumatic
    specified cause NEC N35.8
    syphilitic A52.76
    traumatic —*see* Stricture, urethra, post-traumatic
    valvular (posterior), congenital Q64.2
  urinary meatus —*see* Stricture, urethra
  uterus, uterine (synechiae) N85.6
    os (external) (internal) —*see* Stricture, cervix
  vagina (outlet) —*see* Stenosis, vagina
  valve (cardiac) (heart) —*see also* Endocarditis
    congenital
      aortic Q23.0
      mitral Q23.2
      pulmonary Q22.1
      tricuspid Q22.4
  vas deferens N50.89
    congenital Q55.4
  vein I87.1
  vena cava (inferior) (superior) NEC I87.1
    congenital Q26.0
  vesicourethral orifice N32.0
    congenital Q64.31
  vulva (acquired) N90.5
Stridor R06.1
  congenital (larynx) P28.89
Stridulous —*see* condition
Stroke (apoplectic) (brain) (embolic) (ischemic) (paralytic) (thrombotic) I63.9
  epileptic —*see* Epilepsy
  heat T67.0
  in evolution I63.9
  intraoperative
    during cardiac surgery I97.810
    during other surgery I97.811
  lightning —*see* Lightning
  meaning
    cerebral hemorrhage — code to Hemorrhage, intracranial
    cerebral infarction — code to Infarction, cerebral
  postprocedural
    following cardiac surgery I97.820
    following other surgery I97.821
  unspecified (NOS) I63.9
Stromatosis, endometrial D39.0
Strongyloidiasis, strongyloidosis B78.9
  cutaneous B78.1
  disseminated B78.7
  intestinal B78.0
Strophulus pruriginosus L28.2
Struck by lightning —*see* Lightning
Struma —*see also* Goiter
  Hashimoto E06.3
  lymphomatosa E06.3
  nodosa (simplex) E04.9
    endemic E01.2
      multinodular E01.1
    multinodular E04.2
      iodine-deficiency related E01.1
    toxic or with hyperthyroidism E05.20
      with thyroid storm E05.21
      multinodular E05.20
        with thyroid storm E05.21
      uninodular E05.10
        with thyroid storm E05.11

Struma *(Continued)*
  nodosa (simplex) *(Continued)*
    toxicosa E05.20
      with thyroid storm E05.21
      multinodular E05.20
        with thyroid storm E05.21
      uninodular E05.10
        with thyroid storm E05.11
    uninodular E04.1
  ovarii D27.-
  Riedel's E06.5
Strumipriva cachexia E03.4
Strümpell-Marie spine —*see* Spondylitis, ankylosing
Strümpell-Westphal pseudosclerosis E83.01
Stuart deficiency disease (factor X) D68.2
Stuart-Prower factor deficiency (factor X) D68.2
Student's elbow —*see* Bursitis, elbow, olecranon
Stump —*see* Amputation
Stunting, nutritional E45
Stupor (catatonic) R40.1
  depressive (single episode) F32.89
    recurrent episode F33.8
  dissociative F44.2
  manic F30.2
  manic-depressive F31.89
  psychogenic (anergic) F44.2
  reaction to exceptional stress (transient) F43.0
Sturge (-Weber) (-Dimitri) (-Kalischer) disease or syndrome Q85.8
Stuttering F80.81
  adult onset F98.5
  childhood onset F80.81
  following cerebrovascular disease — *see* Disorder, fluency, following cerebrovascular disease
  in conditions classified elsewhere R47.82
Sty, stye (external) (internal) (meibomian) (zeisian) —*see* Hordeolum
Subacidity, gastric K31.89
  psychogenic F45.8
Subacute —*see* condition
Subarachnoid —*see* condition
Subcortical —*see* condition
Subcostal syndrome, nerve compression —*see* Mononeuropathy, upper limb, specified site NEC
Subcutaneous, subcuticular —*see* condition
Subdural —*see* condition
Subendocardium —*see* condition
Subependymoma
  specified site —*see* Neoplasm, uncertain behavior, by site
  unspecified site D43.2
Suberosis J67.3
Subglossitis —*see* Glossitis
Subhemophilia D66
Subinvolution
  breast (postlactational) (postpuerperal) N64.89
  puerperal O90.89
  uterus (chronic) (nonpuerperal) N85.3
    puerperal O90.89
Sublingual —*see* condition
Sublinguitis —*see* Sialoadenitis
Subluxatable hip Q65.6
Subluxation —*see also* Dislocation
  acromioclavicular S43.11-
  ankle S93.0-
  atlantoaxial, recurrent M43.4
    with myelopathy M43.3
  carpometacarpal (joint) NEC S63.05-
    thumb S63.04-
  complex, vertebral —*see* Complex, subluxation
  congenital —*see also* Malposition, congenital
    hip —*see* Dislocation, hip, congenital, partial

Subluxation (Continued)
congenital (Continued)
joint (excluding hip)
lower limb Q68.8
shoulder Q68.8
upper limb Q68.8
elbow (traumatic) S53.10-
anterior S53.11-
lateral S53.14-
medial S53.13-
posterior S53.12-
specified type NEC S53.19-
finger S63.20-
index S63.20-
interphalangeal S63.22-
distal S63.24-
index S63.24-
little S63.24-
middle S63.24-
ring S63.24-
index S63.22-
little S63.22-
middle S63.22-
proximal S63.23-
index S63.23-
little S63.23-
middle S63.23-
ring S63.23-
ring S63.22-
little S63.20-
metacarpophalangeal S63.21-
index S63.21-
little S63.21-
middle S63.21-
ring S63.21-
middle S63.20-
ring S63.20-
foot S93.30-
specified site NEC S93.33-
tarsal joint S93.31-
tarsometatarsal joint S93.32-
toe —see Subluxation, toe
hip S73.00-
anterior S73.03-
obturator S73.02-
central S73.04-
posterior S73.01-
interphalangeal (joint)
finger S63.22-
distal joint S63.24-
index S63.24-
little S63.24-
middle S63.24-
ring S63.24-
index S63.22-
little S63.22-
middle S63.22-
proximal joint S63.23-
index S63.23-
little S63.23-
middle S63.23-
ring S63.23-
ring S63.22-
thumb S63.12-
distal joint S63.14-
proximal joint S63.13-
toe S93.13-
great S93.13-
lesser S93.13-
joint prosthesis —see Complications, joint
prosthesis, mechanical, displacement,
by site
knee S83.10-
cap —see Subluxation, patella
patella —see Subluxation, patella
proximal tibia
anteriorly S83.11-
laterally S83.14-
medially S83.13-
posteriorly S83.12-
specified type NEC S83.19-

Subluxation (Continued)
lens —see Dislocation, lens, partial
ligament, traumatic —see Sprain, by site
metacarpal (bone)
proximal end S63.06-
metacarpophalangeal (joint)
finger S63.21-
index S63.21-
little S63.21-
middle S63.21-
ring S63.21-
thumb S63.11-
metatarsophalangeal joint S93.14-
great toe S93.14-
lesser toe S93.14-
midcarpal (joint) S63.03-
patella S83.00-
lateral S83.01-
recurrent (nontraumatic) —see Dislocation,
patella, recurrent, incomplete
specified type NEC S83.09-
pathological —see Dislocation, pathological
radial head S53.00-
anterior S53.01-
nursemaid's elbow S53.03-
posterior S53.02-
specified type NEC S53.09-
radiocarpal (joint) S63.02-
radioulnar (joint)
distal S63.01-
proximal —see Subluxation, elbow
shoulder
congenital Q68.8
girdle S43.30-
scapula S43.31-
specified site NEC S43.39-
traumatic S43.00-
anterior S43.01-
inferior S43.03-
posterior S43.02-
specified type NEC S43.08-
sternoclavicular (joint) S43.20-
anterior S43.21-
posterior S43.22-
symphysis (pubis)
thumb S63.103
interphalangeal joint —see Subluxation,
interphalangeal (joint), thumb
metacarpophalangeal joint —see
Subluxation, metacarpophalangeal
(joint), thumb
toe (s) S93.10-
great S93.10-
interphalangeal joint S93.13-
metatarsophalangeal joint S93.14-
interphalangeal joint S93.13-
lesser S93.10-
interphalangeal joint S93.13-
metatarsophalangeal joint S93.14-
metatarsophalangeal joint S93.149
ulnohumeral joint —see Subluxation,
elbow
vertebral
recurrent NEC —see subcategory
M43.5
traumatic
cervical S13.100
atlantoaxial joint S13.120
atlantooccipital joint S13.110
atloidooccipital joint S13.110
joint between
C0 and C1 S13.110
C1 and C2 S13.120
C2 and C3 S13.130
C3 and C4 S13.140
C4 and C5 S13.150
C5 and C6 S13.160
C6 and C7 S13.170
C7 and T1 S13.180
occipitoatloid joint
S13.110

Subluxation (Continued)
vertebral (Continued)
traumatic (Continued)
lumbar S33.100
joint between
L1 and L2 S33.110
L2 and L3 S33.120
L3 and L4 S33.130
L4 and L5 S33.140
thoracic S23.100
joint between
T1 and T2 S23.110
T2 and T3 S23.120
T3 and T4 S23.122
T4 and T5 S23.130
T5 and T6 S23.132
T6 and T7 S23.140
T7 and T8 S23.142
T8 and T9 S23.150
T9 and T10 S23.152
T10 and T11 S23.160
T11 and T12 S23.162
T12 and L1 S23.170
ulna
distal end S63.07-
proximal end —see Subluxation, elbow
wrist (carpal bone) S63.00-
carpometacarpal joint —see Subluxation,
carpometacarpal (joint)
distal radioulnar joint —see Subluxation,
radioulnar (joint), distal
metacarpal bone, proximal —see
Subluxation, metacarpal (bone),
proximal end
midcarpal —see Subluxation, midcarpal
(joint)
radiocarpal joint —see Subluxation,
radiocarpal (joint)
recurrent —see Dislocation, recurrent, wrist
specified site NEC S63.09-
ulna —see Subluxation, ulna, distal end
Submaxillary —see condition
Submersion (fatal) (nonfatal) T75.1
Submucous —see condition
Subnormal, subnormality
accommodation (old age) H52.4
mental —see Disability, intellectual
temperature (accidental) T68
Subphrenic —see condition
Subscapular nerve —see condition
Subseptus uterus Q51.2
Subsiding appendicitis K36
Substance (other psychoactive) -induced ◄
anxiety disorder F19.980 ◄
bipolar and related disorder F19.94 ◄
delirium F19.921 ◄
depressive disorder F19.94 ◄
major neurocognitive disorder F19.97 ◄
mild neurocognitive disorder F19.988 ◄
obsessive-compulsive and related disorder
F19.988 ◄
psychotic disorder F19.959 ◄
sexual dysfunction F19.981 ◄
sleep disorder F19.982 ◄
Substernal thyroid E04.9
congenital Q89.2
Substitution disorder F44.9
Subtentorial —see condition
Subthyroidism (acquired) —see also
Hypothyroidism
congenital E03.1
Succenturiate placenta O43.19-
Sucking thumb, child (excessive) F98.8
Sudamen, sudamina L74.1
Sudanese kala-azar B55.0
Sudden
hearing loss —see Deafness, sudden
heart failure —see Failure, heart
Sudeck's atrophy, disease, or syndrome —see
Algoneurodystrophy
Suffocation —see Asphyxia, traumatic

S

Sugar
  blood
    high (transient) R73.9
    low (transient) E16.2
  in urine R81
Suicide, suicidal (attempted) T14.91
  by poisoning —see Table of Drugs and
      Chemicals
  history of (personal) Z91.5
    in family Z81.8
  ideation —see Ideation, suicidal
  risk
    meaning personal history of attempted
        suicide Z91.5
    meaning suicidal ideation —see Ideation,
        suicidal
  tendencies
    meaning personal history of attempted
        suicide Z91.5
    meaning suicidal ideation —see Ideation,
        suicidal
  trauma —see nature of injury by site
Suipestifer infection —see Infection, salmonella
Sulfhemoglobinemia, sulphemoglobinemia
    (acquired) (with methemoglobinemia)
    D74.8
Sumatran mite fever A75.3
Summer —see condition
Sunburn L55.9
  due to ◀
    tanning bed (acute) L56.8 ◀
      chronic L57.8 ◀
    ultraviolet radiation (acute) L56.8 ◀
      chronic L57.8 ◀
  first degree L55.0
  second degree L55.1
  third degree L55.2
SUNCT (short lasting unilateral neuralgiform
      headache with conjunctival injection and
      tearing) G44.059
  intractable G44.051
  not intractable G44.059
Sunken acetabulum —see Derangement, joint,
    specified type NEC, hip
Sunstroke T67.0
Superfecundation —see Pregnancy,
    multiple
Superfetation —see Pregnancy, multiple
Superinvolution (uterus) N85.8
Supernumerary (congenital)
  aortic cusps Q23.8
  auditory ossicles Q16.3
  bone Q79.8
  breast Q83.1
  carpal bones Q74.0
  cusps, heart valve NEC Q24.8
    aortic Q23.8
    mitral Q23.2
    pulmonary Q22.3
  digit (s) Q69.9
  ear (lobule) Q17.0
  fallopian tube Q50.6
  finger Q69.0
  hymen Q52.4
  kidney Q63.0
  lacrimonasal duct Q10.6
  lobule (ear) Q17.0
  mitral cusps Q23.2
  muscle Q79.8
  nipple (s) Q83.3
  organ or site not listed —see Accessory
    ossicles, auditory Q16.3
  ovary Q50.31
  oviduct Q50.6
  pulmonary, pulmonic cusps Q22.3
  rib Q76.6
    cervical or first (syndrome) Q76.5
  roots (of teeth) K00.2
  spleen Q89.09
  tarsal bones Q74.2
  teeth K00.1

Supernumerary (Continued)
  testis Q55.29
  thumb Q69.1
  toe Q69.2
  uterus Q51.2
  vagina Q52.1
  vertebra Q76.49
Supervision (of)
  contraceptive —see Prescription,
      contraceptives
  dietary (for) Z71.3
    allergy (food) Z71.3
    colitis Z71.3
    diabetes mellitus Z71.3
    food allergy or intolerance Z71.3
    gastritis Z71.3
    hypercholesterolemia Z71.3
    hypoglycemia Z71.3
    intolerance (food) Z71.3
    obesity Z71.3
    specified NEC Z71.3
  healthy infant or child Z76.2
    foundling Z76.1
  high-risk pregnancy —see Pregnancy,
      complicated by, high, risk
  lactation Z39.1
  pregnancy —see Pregnancy, supervision of
Supplemental teeth K00.1
Suppression
  binocular vision H53.34
  lactation O92.5
  menstruation N94.89
  ovarian secretion E28.39
  renal N28.9
  urine, urinary secretion R34
Suppuration, suppurative —see also condition
  accessory sinus (chronic) —see Sinusitis
  adrenal gland
  antrum (chronic) —see Sinusitis, maxillary
  bladder —see Cystitis
  brain G06.0
    sequelae G09
  breast N61.1 ◀⊪
    puerperal, postpartum or gestational —see
        Mastitis, obstetric, purulent
  dental periosteum M27.3
  ear (middle) —see also Otitis, media
    external NEC —see Otitis, externa,
        infective
    internal —see subcategory H83.0
  ethmoidal (chronic) (sinus) —see Sinusitis,
      ethmoidal
  fallopian tube —see Salpingo-oophoritis
  frontal (chronic) (sinus) —see Sinusitis,
      frontal
  gallbladder (acute) K81.0
  gum K05.20
    generalized —see Peridontitis, aggressive,
        generalized ◀⊪
    localized —see Peridontitis, aggressive,
        localized ◀⊪
  intracranial G06.0
  joint —see Arthritis, pyogenic or pyemic
  labyrinthine —see subcategory H83.0
  lung —see Abscess, lung
  mammary gland N61.1 ◀⊪
    puerperal, postpartum O91.12
      associated with lactation O91.13
  maxilla, maxillary M27.2
    sinus (chronic) —see Sinusitis, maxillary
  muscle —see Myositis, infective
  nasal sinus (chronic) —see Sinusitis
  pancreas, acute —see also Pancreatitis, acute
      K85.80 ◀⊪
  parotid gland —see Sialoadenitis
  pelvis, pelvic
    female —see Disease, pelvis, inflammatory
    male K65.0
  pericranial —see Osteomyelitis
  salivary duct or gland (any) —see
      Sialoadenitis

Suppuration, suppurative (Continued)
  sinus (accessory) (chronic) (nasal) —see
      Sinusitis
  sphenoidal sinus (chronic) —see Sinusitis,
      sphenoidal
  thymus (gland) E32.1
  thyroid (gland) E06.0
  tonsil —see Tonsillitis
  uterus —see Endometritis
Supraeruption of tooth (teeth) M26.34
Supraglottitis J04.30
  with obstruction J04.31
Suprarenal (gland) —see condition
Suprascapular nerve —see condition
Suprasellar —see condition
Surfer's knots or nodules S89.8-
Surgical
  emphysema T81.82
  procedures, complication or misadventure —
      see Complications, surgical procedures
  shock T81.10
Surveillance (of) (for) —see also Observation
  alcohol abuse Z71.41
  contraceptive —see Prescription,
      contraceptives
  dietary Z71.3
  drug abuse Z71.51
Susceptibility to disease, genetic Z15.89
  malignant neoplasm Z15.09
    breast Z15.01
    endometrium Z15.04
    ovary Z15.02
    prostate Z15.03
    specified NEC Z15.09
  multiple endocrine neoplasia Z15.81
Suspected condition, ruled out —see also
    Observation, suspected
  amniotic cavity and membrane Z03.71
  cervical shortening Z03.75
  fetal anomaly Z03.73
  fetal growth Z03.74
  maternal and fetal conditions NEC Z03.79
  newborn —see also Observation, newborn,
      suspected condition ruled out Z05.9 ◀
  oligohydramnios Z03.71
  placental problem Z03.72
  polyhydramnios Z03.71
Suspended uterus
  in pregnancy or childbirth —see Pregnancy,
      complicated by, abnormal uterus
Sutton's nevus D22.9
Suture
  burst (in operation wound) T81.31
    external operation wound T81.31
    internal operation wound T81.32
  inadvertently left in operation wound —see
      Foreign body, accidentally left during a
      procedure
  removal Z48.02
Swab inadvertently left in operation wound —
    see Foreign body, accidentally left during
    a procedure
Swallowed, swallowing
  difficulty —see Dysphagia
  foreign body —see Foreign body, alimentary
      tract
Swan-neck deformity (finger) —see Deformity,
    finger, swan-neck
Swearing, compulsive F42.8 ◀⊪
  in Gilles de la Tourette's syndrome F95.2
Sweat, sweats
  fetid L75.0
  night R61
Sweating, excessive R61
Sweeley-Klionsky disease E75.21
Sweet's disease or dermatosis L98.2
Swelling (of) R60.9
  abdomen, abdominal (not referable to any
      particular organ) —see Mass,
      abdominal
  ankle —see Effusion, joint, ankle

◀ New   ◀⊪ Revised   ~~deleted~~ Deleted

Swelling *(Continued)*
  arm M79.89
    forearm M79.89
  breast N63
  Calabar B74.3
  cervical gland R59.0
  chest, localized R22.2
  ear H93.8-
  extremity (lower) (upper) —*see* Disorder, soft
      tissue, specified type NEC
  finger M79.89
  foot M79.89
  glands R59.9
    generalized R59.1
    localized R59.0
  hand M79.89
  head (localized) R22.0
  inflammatory —*see* Inflammation
  intra-abdominal —*see* Mass, abdominal
  joint —*see* Effusion, joint
  leg M79.89
    lower M79.89
  limb —*see* Disorder, soft tissue, specified type
      NEC
  localized (skin) R22.9
    chest R22.2
    head R22.0
    limb
      lower —*see* Mass, localized, limb,
          lower
      upper —*see* Mass, localized, limb,
          upper
    neck R22.1
    trunk R22.2
  neck (localized) R22.1
  pelvic —*see* Mass, abdominal
  scrotum N50.89 ◀▥
  splenic —*see* Splenomegaly
  testis N50.89 ◀▥
  toe M79.89
  umbilical R19.09
  wandering, due to Gnathostoma
      (spinigerum) B83.1
  white —*see* Tuberculosis, arthritis
Swift (-Feer) disease
  overdose or wrong substance given or
      taken —*see* Table of Drugs and
      Chemicals, by drug, poisoning
Swimmer's
  cramp T75.1
  ear H60.33-
  itch B65.3
Swimming in the head R42
Swollen —*see* Swelling
Swyer syndrome Q99.1
Sycosis L73.8
  barbae (not parasitic) L73.8
  contagiosa (mycotic) B35.0
  lupoides L73.8
  mycotic B35.0
  parasitic B35.0
  vulgaris L73.8
Sydenham's chorea —*see* Chorea, Sydenham's
Sylvatic yellow fever A95.0
Sylvest's disease B33.0
Symblepharon H11.23-
  congenital Q10.3
Symond's syndrome G93.2
Sympathetic —*see* condition
Sympatheticotonia G90.8
Sympathicoblastoma
  specified site —*see* Neoplasm, malignant, by
      site
  unspecified site C74.90
Sympathogonioma —*see* Sympathicoblastoma
Symphalangy (fingers) (toes) Q70.9
Symptoms NEC R68.89
  breast NEC N64.59
  development NEC R63.8
  factitious, self-induced —*see* Disorder,
      factitious

Symptoms NEC *(Continued)*
  genital organs, female R10.2
  involving
    abdomen NEC R19.8
    appearance NEC R46.89
    awareness R41.9
      altered mental status R41.82
      amnesia —*see* Amnesia
      borderline intellectual functioning
          R41.83
      coma —*see* Coma
      disorientation R41.0
      neurologic neglect syndrome R41.4
      senile cognitive decline R41.81
      specified symptom NEC R41.89
    behavior NEC R46.89
    cardiovascular system NEC R09.89
    chest NEC R09.89
    circulatory system NEC R09.89
    cognitive functions R41.9
      altered mental status R41.82
      amnesia —*see* Amnesia
      borderline intellectual functioning
          R41.83
      coma —*see* Coma
      disorientation R41.0
      neurologic neglect syndrome R41.4
      senile cognitive decline R41.81
      specified symptom NEC R41.89
    development NEC R62.50
    digestive system NEC R19.8
    emotional state NEC R45.89
      emotional lability R45.86
    food and fluid intake R63.8
    general perceptions and sensations
        R44.9
      specified NEC R44.8
    musculoskeletal system R29.91
      specified NEC R29.898
    nervous system R29.90
      specified NEC R29.818
    pelvis NEC R19.8
    respiratory system NEC R09.89
    skin and integument R23.9
    urinary system R39.9
  menopausal N95.1
  metabolism NEC R63.8
  neurotic F48.8
  of infancy R68.19
  pelvis NEC, female R10.2
  skin and integument NEC R23.9
  subcutaneous tissue NEC R23.9
Sympus Q74.2
Syncephalus Q89.4
Synchondrosis
  abnormal (congenital) Q78.8
  ischiopubic M91.0
Synchysis (scintillans) (senile) (vitreous body)
    H43.89
Syncope (near) (pre-) R55
  anginosa I20.8
  bradycardia R00.1
  cardiac R55
  carotid sinus G90.01
  due to spinal (lumbar) puncture G97.1
  heart R55
  heat T67.1
  laryngeal R05
  psychogenic F48.8
  tussive R05
  vasoconstriction R55
  vasodepressor R55
  vasomotor R55
  vasovagal R55
Syndactylism, syndactyly Q70.9
  complex (with synostosis)
    fingers Q70.0-
    toes Q70.2-
  simple (without synostosis)
    fingers Q70.1-
    toes Q70.3-

Syndrome —*see also* Disease
  5q minus NOS D46.C
  48,XXXX Q97.1
  49,XXXXX Q97.1
  abdominal
    acute R10.0
    muscle deficiency Q79.4
  abnormal innervation H02.519
    left H02.516
      lower H02.515
      upper H02.514
    right H02.513
      lower H02.512
      upper H02.511
  abstinence, neonatal P96.1
  acid pulmonary aspiration, obstetric O74.0
  acquired immunodeficiency —*see* Human,
      immunodeficiency virus (HIV)
      disease
  acute abdominal R10.0
  acute respiratory distress (adult) (child) J80
    idiopathic J84.114 ◀
  Adair-Dighton Q78.0
  Adams-Stokes (-Morgagni) I45.9
  adiposogenital E23.6
  adrenal
    hemorrhage (meningococcal) A39.1
    meningococcic A39.1
  adrenocortical —*see* Cushing's, syndrome
  adrenogenital E25.9
    congenital, associated with enzyme
        deficiency E25.0
  afferent loop NEC K91.89
  Alagille's Q44.7
  alcohol withdrawal (without convulsions) —
      see Dependence, alcohol, with,
      withdrawal
  Alder's D72.0
  Aldrich (-Wiskott) D82.0
  alien hand R41.4
  Alport Q87.81
  alveolar hypoventilation E66.2
  alveolocapillary block J84.10
  amnesic, amnestic (confabulatory) (due to) —
      see Disorder, amnesic
  amyostatic (Wilson's disease) E83.01
  androgen insensitivity E34.50
    complete E34.51
    partial E34.52
  androgen resistance (*see also* Syndrome,
      androgen insensitivity) E34.50
  Angelman Q93.5
  anginal —*see* Angina
  ankyloglossia superior Q38.1
  anterior
    chest wall R07.89
    cord G83.82
    spinal artery G95.19
      compression M47.019
        cervical region M47.012
        cervicothoracic region M47.013
        lumbar region M47.016
        occipito-atlanto-axial region M47.011
        thoracic region M47.014
        thoracolumbar region M47.015
    tibial M76.81-
  antibody deficiency D80.9
    agammaglobulinemic D80.1
      hereditary D80.0
    congenital D80.0
    hypogammaglobulinemic D80.1
      hereditary D80.0
  anticardiolipin (-antibody) D68.61
  antiphospholipid (-antibody) D68.61
  aortic
    arch M31.4
    bifurcation I74.09
  aortomesenteric duodenum occlusion K31.5
  apical ballooning (transient left ventricular)
      I51.81
  arcuate ligament I77.4

Syndrome *(Continued)*
- argentaffin, argintaffinoma E34.0
- Arnold-Chiari —*see* Arnold-Chiari disease
- Arrillaga-Ayerza I27.0
- arterial tortuosity Q87.82 ◀
- arteriovenous steal T82.898- ◀
- Asherman's N85.6
- aspiration, of newborn —*see* Aspiration, by substance, with pneumonia
  - meconium P24.01
- ataxia-telangiectasia G11.3
- auriculotemporal G50.8
- autoerythrocyte sensitization (Gardner-Diamond) D69.2
- autoimmune lymphoproliferative [ALPS] D89.82
- autoimmune polyglandular E31.0
- autoinflammatory M04.9 ◀
  - specified type NEC M04.8 ◀
- autosomal —*see* Abnormal, autosomes
- Avellis' G46.8
- Ayerza (-Arrillaga) I27.0
- Babinski-Nageotte G83.89
- Bakwin-Krida Q78.5 ◀█
- bare lymphocyte D81.6
- Barré-Guillain G61.0
- Barré-Liéou M53.0
- Barrett's —*see* Barrett's, esophagus
- Barsony-Polgar K22.4
- Barsony-Teschendorf K22.4
- Barth E78.71
- Bartter's E26.81
- basal cell nevus Q87.89
- Basedow's E05.00
  - with thyroid storm E05.01
- basilar artery G45.0
- Batten-Steinert G71.11
- battered
  - baby or child —*see* Maltreatment, child, physical abuse
  - spouse —*see* Maltreatment, adult, physical abuse
- Beals Q87.40
- Beau's I51.5
- Beck's I65.8
- Benedikt's G46.3
- Béquez César (-Steinbrinck-Chédiak-Higashi) D70.330
- Bernhardt-Roth —*see* Meralgia paresthetica
- Bernheim's I50.9
- big spleen D73.1
- bilateral polycystic ovarian E28.2
- Bing-Horton's —*see* Horton's headache
- Birt-Hogg-Dube syndrome Q87.89
- Björck (-Thorsen) E34.0
- black
  - lung J60
  - widow spider bite —*see* Toxicity, venom, spider, black widow
- Blackfan-Diamond D61.01
- Blau M04.8 ◀
- blind loop K90.2
  - congenital Q43.8
  - postsurgical K91.2
- blue sclera Q78.0
- blue toe I75.02-
- Boder-Sedgewick G11.3
- Boerhaave's K22.3
- Borjeson Forssman Lehmann Q89.8
- Bouillaud's I01.9
- Bourneville (-Pringle) Q85.1
- Bouveret (-Hoffman) I47.9
- brachial plexus G54.0
- bradycardia-tachycardia I49.5
- brain (nonpsychotic) F09
  - with psychosis, psychotic reaction F09
  - acute or subacute —*see* Delirium
  - congenital —*see* Disability, intellectual
  - organic F09
    - post-traumatic (nonpsychotic) F07.81
      - psychotic F09

Syndrome *(Continued)*
- brain (nonpsychotic) *(Continued)*
  - personality change F07.0
  - postcontusional F07.81
  - post-traumatic, nonpsychotic F07.81
  - psycho-organic F09
  - psychotic F06.8
- brain stem stroke G46.3
- Brandt's (acrodermatitis enteropathica) E83.2
- broad ligament laceration N83.8
- Brock's J98.11
- bronze baby P83.8
- Brown-Sequard G83.81
- bubbly lung P27.0
- Buchem's M85.2
- Budd-Chiari I82.0
- bulbar (progressive) G12.22
- Bürger-Grütz E78.3
- Burke's K86.89 ◀█
- Burnett's (milk-alkali) E83.52
- burning feet E53.9
- Bywaters' T79.5
- Call-Fleming I67.841
- carbohydrate-deficient glycoprotein (CDGS) E77.8
- carcinogenic thrombophlebitis I82.1
- carcinoid E34.0
- cardiac asthma I50.1
- cardiacos negros I27.0
- cardiofaciocutaneous Q87.89
- cardiopulmonary-obesity E66.2
- cardiorenal —*see* Hypertension, cardiorenal
- cardiorespiratory distress (idiopathic), newborn P22.0
- cardiovascular renal —*see* Hypertension, cardiorenal
- carotid
  - artery (hemispheric) (internal) G45.1
  - body G90.01
  - sinus G90.01
- carpal tunnel G56.0-
- Cassidy (-Scholte) E34.0
- cat-cry Q93.4
- cat eye Q92.8
- cauda equina G83.4
- causalgia —*see* Causalgia
- celiac K90.0
  - artery compression I77.4
  - axis I77.4
- central pain G89.0
- cerebellar
  - hereditary G11.9
  - stroke G46.4
- cerebellomedullary malformation —*see* Spina bifida
- cerebral
  - artery
    - anterior G46.1
    - middle G46.0
    - posterior G46.2
  - gigantism E22.0
- cervical (root) M53.1
  - disc —*see* Disorder, disc, cervical, with neuritis
  - fusion Q76.1
  - posterior, sympathicus M53.0
  - rib Q76.5
  - sympathetic paralysis G90.2
- cervicobrachial (diffuse) M53.1
- cervicocranial M53.0
- cervicodorsal outlet G54.2
- cervicothoracic outlet G54.0
- Céstan (-Raymond) I65.8
- Charcot's (angina cruris) (intermittent claudication) I73.9
- Charcot-Weiss-Baker G90.09
- CHARGE Q89.8
- Chédiak-Higashi (-Steinbrinck) E70.330
- chest wall R07.1
- Chiari's (hepatic vein thrombosis) I82.0
- Chilaiditi's Q43.3

Syndrome *(Continued)*
- child maltreatment —*see* Maltreatment, child
- chondrocostal junction M94.0
- chondroectodermal dysplasia Q77.6
- chromosome 4 short arm deletion Q93.3
- chromosome 5 short arm deletion Q93.4
- chronic
  - infantile neurological, cutaneous and articular (CINCA) M04.2 ◀
  - pain G89.4
  - personality F68.8
- Clarke-Hadfield K86.89 ◀█
- Clerambault's automatism G93.89
- Clouston's (hidrotic ectodermal dysplasia) Q82.4
- clumsiness, clumsy child F82
- cluster headache G44.009
  - intractable G44.001
  - not intractable G44.009
- Coffin-Lowry Q89.8
- cold injury (newborn) P80.0
- combined immunity deficiency D81.9
- compartment (deep) (posterior) (traumatic) T79.A0
  - abdomen T79.A3
  - lower extremity (hip, buttock, thigh, leg, foot, toes) T79.A2
  - nontraumatic
    - abdomen M79.A3
    - lower extremity (hip, buttock, thigh, leg, foot, toes) M79.A2-
    - specified site NEC M79.A9
    - upper extremity (shoulder, arm, forearm, wrist, hand, fingers) M79.A1-
  - postprocedural —*see* Syndrome compartment, nontraumatic
  - specified site NEC T79.A9
  - upper extremity (shoulder, arm, forearm, wrist, hand, fingers) T79.A1
- complex regional pain —*see* Syndrome, pain, complex regional
- compression T79.5
  - anterior spinal —*see* Syndrome, anterior, spinal artery, compression
  - cauda equina G83.4
  - celiac artery I77.4
  - vertebral artery M47.029
    - cervical region M47.022
    - occipito-atlanto-axial region M47.021
- concussion F07.81
- congenital
  - affecting multiple systems NEC Q87.89
  - central alveolar hypoventilation G47.35
  - facial diplegia Q87.0
  - muscular hypertrophy-cerebral Q87.89
  - oculo-auriculovertebral Q87.0
  - oculofacial diplegia (Moebius) Q87.0
  - rubella (manifest) P35.0
- congestion-fibrosis (pelvic), female N94.89
- congestive dysmenorrhea N94.6
- Conn's E26.01
- connective tissue M35.9
  - overlap NEC M35.1
- conus medullaris G95.81
- cord
  - anterior G83.82
  - posterior G83.83
- coronary
  - acute NEC I24.9
  - insufficiency or intermediate I20.0
  - slow flow I20.8
- Costen's (complex) M26.69
- costochondral junction M94.0
- costoclavicular G54.0
- costovertebral E22.0
- Cowden Q85.8
- craniovertebral M53.0
- Creutzfeldt-Jakob —*see* Creutzfeldt-Jakob disease or syndrome
- cri-du-chat Q93.4

◀ New ◀█ Revised ~~deleted~~ Deleted

Syndrome *(Continued)*
  crib death R99
  cricopharyngeal —*see* Dysphagia
  croup J05.0
  CRPS I —*see* Syndrome, pain, complex
      regional I
  crush T79.5
  cubital tunnel —*see* Lesion, nerve, ulnar
  Curschmann (-Batten) (-Steinert) G71.11
  Cushing's E24.9
    alcohol-induced E24.4
    drug-induced E24.2
    due to
      alcohol
        drugs E24.2
      ectopic ACTH E24.3
      overproduction of pituitary ACTH E24.0
    overdose or wrong substance given or
        taken —*see* Table of Drugs and
        Chemicals, by drug, poisoning
    pituitary-dependent E24.0
    specified type NEC E24.8
  cryopyrin-associated periodic M04.2 ◄
  cryptophthalmos Q87.0
  cystic duct stump K91.5
  Dana-Putnam D51.0
  Danbolt (-Cross) (acrodermatitis
      enteropathica) E83.2
  Dandy-Walker Q03.1
    with spina bifida Q07.01
  Danlos' Q79.6 ◄▥
  defibrination —*see also* Fibrinolysis
    with
      antepartum hemorrhage —*see*
          Hemorrhage, antepartum, with
          coagulation defect
      intrapartum hemorrhage —*see*
          Hemorrhage, complicating,
          delivery
    newborn P60
    postpartum O72.3
  Degos' I77.8
  Déjérine-Roussy G89.0
  delayed sleep phase G47.21
  demyelinating G37.9
  dependence —*see* F10-F19 with fourth
      character .2
  depersonalization (-derealization) F48.1
  De Quervain E34.51
  de Toni-Fanconi (-Debré) E72.09
    with cystinosis E72.04
  diabetes mellitus-hypertension-nephrosis —
      see Diabetes, nephrosis
  diabetes mellitus in newborn infant P70.2
  diabetes-nephrosis —*see* Diabetes, nephrosis
  diabetic amyotrophy —*see* Diabetes,
      amyotrophy
  dialysis associated steal T82.898- ◄
  Diamond-Blackfan D61.01
  Diamond-Gardener D69.2
  DIC (diffuse or disseminated intravascular
      coagulopathy) D65
  di George's D82.1
  Dighton's Q78.0
  disequilibrium E87.8
  Döhle body-panmyelopathic D72.0
  dorsolateral medullary G46.4
  double athetosis G80.3
  Down (*see also* Down syndrome) Q90.9
  Dresbach's (elliptocytosis) D58.1
  Dressler's (postmyocardial infarction) I24.1
    postcardiotomy I97.0
  drug withdrawal, infant of dependent mother
      P96.1
  dry eye H04.12-
  due to abnormality
    chromosomal Q99.9
      sex
        female phenotype Q97.9
        male phenotype Q98.9
      specified NEC Q99.8

Syndrome *(Continued)*
  dumping (postgastrectomy) K91.1
    nonsurgical K31.89
  Dupré's (meningism) R29.1
  dysmetabolic X E88.81
  dyspraxia, developmental F82
  Eagle-Barrett Q79.4
  Eaton-Lambert —*see* Syndrome,
      Lambert-Eaton
  Ebstein's Q22.5
  ectopic ACTH E24.3
  eczema-thrombocytopenia D82.0
  Eddowes' Q78.0
  effort (psychogenic) F45.8
  Ehlers-Danlos Q79.6
  Eisenmenger's I27.89
  Ekman's Q78.0
  electric feet E53.8
  Ellis-van Creveld Q77.6
  empty nest Z60.0
  endocrine-hypertensive E27.0
  entrapment —*see* Neuropathy,
      entrapment
  eosinophilia-myalgia M35.8
  epileptic —*see also* Epilepsy, by type
    absence G40.A09
      intractable G40.A19
        with status epilepticus G40.A11
        without status epilepticus G40.A19
      not intractable G40.A09
        with status epilepticus G40.A01
        without status epilepticus G40.A09
  Erdheim-Chester (ECD) E88.89
  Erdheim's E22.0
  erythrocyte fragmentation D59.4
  Evans D69.41
  exhaustion F48.8
  extrapyramidal G25.9
    specified NEC G25.89
  eye retraction —*see* Strabismus
  eyelid-malar-mandible Q87.0
  Faber's D50.9
  facial pain, paroxysmal G50.0
  Fallot's Q21.3
  familial cold autoinflammatory M04.2 ◄
  familial eczema-thrombocytopenia (Wiskott-
      Aldrich) D82.0
  Fanconi (-de Toni) (-Debré) E72.09
    with cystinosis E72.04
  Fanconi's (anemia) (congenital pancytopenia)
      D61.09
  fatigue
    chronic R53.82
    psychogenic F48.8
  faulty bowel habit K59.39 ◄▥
  Feil-Klippel (brevicollis) Q76.1
  Felty's —*see* Felty's syndrome
  fertile eunuch E23.0
  fetal
    alcohol (dysmorphic) Q86.0
    hydantoin Q86.1
  Fiedler's I40.1
  first arch Q87.0
  fish odor E72.8
  Fisher's G61.0
  Fitzhugh-Curtis
    due to
      Chlamydia trachomatis A74.81
      Neisseria gonorrhorea (gonococcal
          peritonitis) A54.85
  Fitz's —*see also* Pancreatitis, acute K85.80 ◄▥
  Flajani (-Basedow) E05.00
    with thyroid storm E05.01
  flatback —*see* Flatback syndrome
  floppy
    baby P94.2
    iris (intraoeprative) (IFIS) H21.81
    mitral valve I34.1
  flush E34.0
  Foix-Alajouanine G95.19
  Fong's Q87.2 ◄▥

Syndrome *(Continued)*
  food protein-induced enterocolitis K52.21 ◄
  foramen magnum G93.5
  Foster-Kennedy H47.14-
  Foville's (peduncular) G46.3
  fragile X Q99.2
  Franceschetti Q75.4
  Frey's
    auriculotemporal G50.8
    hyperhidrosis L74.52
  Friderichsen-Waterhouse A39.1
  Froin's G95.89
  frontal lobe F07.0
  Fukuhara E88.49
  functional
    bowel K59.9
    prepubertal castrate E29.1
  Gaisböck's D75.1
  ganglion (basal ganglia brain) G25.9
    geniculi G51.1
  Gardner-Diamond D69.2
  gastroesophageal
    junction K22.0
    laceration-hemorrhage K22.6
  gastrojejunal loop obstruction K91.89
  Gee-Herter-Heubner K90.0
  Gelineau's G47.419
    with cataplexy G47.411
  genito-anorectal A55
  Gerstmann-Sträussler-Scheinker (GSS)
      A81.82
  Gianotti-Crosti L44.4
  giant platelet (Bernard-Soulier) D69.1
  Gilles de la Tourette's F95.2
  goiter-deafness E07.1
  Goldberg Q89.8
  Goldberg-Maxwell E34.51
  Good's D83.8
  Gopalan' (burning feet) E53.8
  Gorlin's Q87.89
  Gougerot-Blum L81.7
  Gouley's I31.1
  Gower's R55
  gray or grey (newborn) P93.0
    platelet D69.1
  Gubler-Millard G46.3
  Guillain-Barré (-Strohl) G61.0
  gustatory sweating G50.8
  Hadfield-Clarke K86.89 ◄▥
  hair tourniquet —*see* Constriction, external,
      by site
  Hamman's J98.19
  hand-foot L27.1
  hand-shoulder G90.8
  hantavirus (cardio)-pulmonary (HPS) (HCPS)
      B33.4
  happy puppet Q93.5
  Harada's H30.81-
  Hayem-Faber D50.9
  headache NEC G44.89
    complicated NEC G44.59
  Heberden's I20.8
  Hedinger's E34.0
  Hegglin's D72.0
  HELLP (hemolysis, elevated liver enzymes
      and low platelet count) O14.2-
    complicating ◄
      childbirth O14.24 ◄
        puerperium O14.25 ◄
  hemolytic-uremic D59.3
  hemophagocytic, infection-associated
      D76.2
  Henoch-Schönlein D69.0
  hepatic flexure K59.8
  hepatopulmonary K76.81
  hepatorenal K76.7
    following delivery O90.4
    postoperative or postprocedural K91.83
    postpartum, puerperal O90.4
  hepatourologic K76.7
  Herter (-Gee) (nontropical sprue) K90.0

Syndrome (Continued)
  Heubner-Herter K90.0
  Heyd's K76.7
  Hilger's G90.09
  histamine-like (fish poisoning) —see
    Poisoning, fish
  histiocytic D76.3
  histiocytosis NEC D76.3
  HIV infection, acute B20
  Hoffmann-Werdnig G12.0
  Hollander-Simons E88.1
  Hoppe-Goldflam G70.00
    with exacerbation (acute) G70.01
    in crisis G70.01
  Horner's G90.2
  hungry bone E83.81
  hunterian glossitis D51.0
  Hutchinson's triad A50.53
  hyperabduction G54.0
  hyperammonemia-hyperornithinemia-
    homocitrullinemia E72.4
  hypereosinophilic (idiopathic) D72.1
  hyperimmunoglobulin D M04.1 ◄
  hyperimmunoglobulin E (IgE) D82.4
  hyperkalemic E87.5
  hyperkinetic —see Hyperkinesia
  hypermobility M35.7
  hypernatremia E87.0
  hyperosmolarity E87.0
  hyperperfusion G97.82
  hypersplenic D73.1
  hypertransfusion, newborn P61.1
  hyperventilation F45.8
  hyperviscosity (of serum)
    polycythemic D75.1
    sclerothymic D58.8
  hypoglycemic (familial) (neonatal) E16.2
  hypokalemic E87.6
  hyponatremic E87.1
  hypopituitarism E23.0
  hypoplastic left-heart Q23.4
  hypopotassemia E87.6
  hyposmolality E87.1
  hypotension, maternal O26.5-
  hypothenar hammer I73.89
  hypoventilation, obesity (OHS) E66.2 ◄
  ICF (intravascular coagulation-fibrinolysis)
    D65
  idiopathic
    cardiorespiratory distress, newborn P22.0
    nephrotic (infantile) N04.9
  iliotibial band M76.3-
  immobility, immobilization (paraplegic) M62.3
  immune reconstitution D89.3
  immune reconstitution inflammatory [IRIS]
    D89.3
  immunity deficiency, combined D81.9
  immunodeficiency
    acquired —see Human, immunodeficiency
      virus (HIV) disease
    combined D81.9
  impending coronary I20.0
  impingement, shoulder M75.4-
  inappropriate secretion of antidiuretic
    hormone E22.2
  infant
    gestational diabetes P70.0
    of diabetic mother P70.1
  infantilism (pituitary) E23.0
  inferior vena cava I87.1
  inspissated bile (newborn) P59.1
  institutional (childhood) F94.2
  insufficient sleep F51.12
  intermediate coronary (artery) I20.0
  interspinous ligament —see Spondylopathy,
    specified NEC
  intestinal
    carcinoid E34.0
    knot K56.2
  intravascular coagulation-fibrinolysis (ICF)
    D65

Syndrome (Continued)
  iodine-deficiency, congenital E00.9
    type
      mixed E00.2
      myxedematous E00.1
      neurological E00.0
  IRDS (idiopathic respiratory distress,
    newborn) P22.0
  irritable
    bowel K58.9
      with diarrhea K58.0
      with ◄
        constipation K58.1 ◄
        diarrhea K58.0 ◄
      mixed K58.2 ◄
      psychogenic F45.8
      specified NEC K58.8 ◄
    heart (psychogenic) F45.8
    weakness F48.8
  ischemic bowel (transient) K55.9
    chronic K55.1
    due to mesenteric artery insufficiency
      K55.1
  ischemic ◄
    bowel (transient) K55.9 ◄
      chronic K55.1 ◄
      due to mesenteric artery insufficiency
        K55.1 ◄
    steal T82.898 ◄
  IVC (intravascular coagulopathy) D65
  Ivemark's Q89.01
  Jaccoud's —see Arthropathy, postrheumatic,
    chronic
  Jackson's G83.89
  Jakob-Creutzfeldt —see Creutzfeldt-Jakob
    disease or syndrome
  jaw-winking Q07.8
  Jervell-Lange-Nielsen I45.81
  jet lag G47.25
  Job's D71
  Joseph-Diamond-Blackfan D61.01
  jugular foramen G52.7
  Kabuki Q89.8
  Kanner's (autism) F84.0
  Kartagener's Q89.3
  Kelly's D50.1
  Kimmelstiel-Wilson —see Diabetes, specified
    type, with Kimmelstiel-Wilson disease
  Klein (e)-Levine G47.13
  Klippel-Feil (brevicollis) Q76.1
  Köhler-Pellegrini-Steida —see Bursitis, tibial
    collateral
  König's K59.8
  Korsakoff (-Wernicke) (nonalcoholic) F04
    alcoholic F10.26
  Kostmann's D70.0
  Krabbe's congenital muscle hypoplasia Q79.8
  labyrinthine —see subcategory H83.2
  lacunar NEC G46.7
  Lambert-Eaton G70.80
    in
      neoplastic disease G73.1
      specified disease NEC G70.81
  Landau-Kleffner —see Epilepsy, specified
    NEC
  Larsen's Q74.8
  lateral
    cutaneous nerve of thigh G57.1-
    medullary G46.4
  Launois' E22.0
  lazy
    leukocyte D70.8
    posture M62.3
  Lemiere I80.8
  Lennox-Gastaut G40.812
    intractable G40.814
      with status epilepticus G40.813
      without status epilepticus G40.814
    not intractable G40.812
      with status epilepticus G40.811
      without status epilepticus G40.812

Syndrome (Continued)
  lenticular, progressive E83.01
  Leopold-Levi's E05.90
  Lev's I44.2
  Li-Fraumeni Z15.01
  Lichtheim's D51.0
  Lightwood's N25.89
  Lignac (de Toni) (-Fanconi) (-Debré) E72.09
    with cystinosis E72.04
  Likoff's I20.8
  limbic epilepsy personality F07.0
  liver-kidney K76.7
  lobotomy F07.0
  Loffler's J82
  long arm 18 or 21 deletion Q93.89
  long QT I45.81
  Louis-Barré G11.3
  low
    atmospheric pressure T70.29
    back M54.5
    output (cardiac) I50.9
  lower radicular, newborn (birth injury) P14.8
  Luetscher's (dehydration) E86.0
  Lupus anticoagulant D68.62
  Lutembacher's Q21.1
  macrophage activation D76.1
    due to infection D76.2
  magnesium-deficiency R29.0
  Majeed M04.8 ◄
  Mal de Debarquement R42
  malabsorption K90.9
    postsurgical K91.2
  malformation, congenital, due to
    alcohol Q86.0
    exogenous cause NEC Q86.8
    hydantoin Q86.1
    warfarin Q86.2
  malignant
    carcinoid E34.0
    neuroleptic G21.0
  Mallory-Weiss K22.6
  mandibulofacial dysostosis Q75.4
  manic-depressive —see Disorder, bipolar ◄≡
  maple-syrup-urine E71.0
  Marable's I77.4
  Marfan's Q87.40
    with
      cardiovascular manifestations Q87.418
        aortic dilation Q87.410
      ocular manifestations Q87.42
      skeletal manifestations Q87.43
  Marie's (acromegaly) E22.0
  mast cell activation —see Activation, mast
    cell ◄
  maternal hypotension —see Syndrome,
    hypotension, maternal
  May (-Hegglin) D72.0
  McArdle (-Schmidt) (-Pearson) E74.04
  McQuarrie's E16.2
  meconium plug (newborn) P76.0
  median arcuate ligament I77.4
  Meekeren-Ehlers-Danlos Q79.6
  megavitamin-B6 E67.2
  Meige G24.4
  MELAS E88.41
  Mendelson's O74.0
  MERRF (myoclonic epilepsy associated with
    ragged-red fibers) E88.42
  mesenteric
    artery (superior) K55.1
    vascular insufficiency K55.1
  metabolic E88.81
  metastatic carcinoid E34.0
  micrognathia-glossoptosis Q87.0
  midbrain NEC G93.89
  middle lobe (lung) J98.19
  middle radicular G54.0
  migraine —see also Migraine G43.909-
  Mikulicz' K11.8
  milk-alkali E83.52
  Millard-Gubler G46.3

◄ New   ◄≡ Revised   ~~deleted~~ Deleted

Syndrome *(Continued)*
  Miller-Dieker Q93.88
  Miller-Fisher G61.0
  Minkowski-Chauffard D58.0
  Mirizzi's K83.1
  MNGIE (Mitochondrial Neurogastrointestinal
    Encephalopathy) E88.49
  Möbius, ophthalmoplegic migraine —*see*
    Migraine, ophthalmoplegic
  monofixation H50.42
  Morel-Moore M85.2
  Morel-Morgagni M85.2
  Morgagni (-Morel) (-Stewart) M85.2
  Morgagni-Adams-Stokes I45.9
  Mounier-Kuhn Q32.4
    with bronchiectasis J47.9
      with
        exacerbation (acute) J47.1
        lower respiratory infection J47.0
    acquired J98.09
      with bronchiectasis J47.9
        with
          exacerbation (acute) J47.1
          lower respiratory infection J47.0
  Muckle-Wells M04.2 ◄
  mucocutaneous lymph node (acute febrile)
    (MCLS) M30.3
  multiple endocrine neoplasia (MEN) —*see*
    Neoplasia, endocrine, multiple (MEN}
  multiple operations —*see* Disorder, factitious
  myasthenic G70.9
    in
      diabetes mellitus —*see* Diabetes,
        amyotrophy
      endocrine disease NEC E34.9 *[G73.3]*
      neoplastic disease —*see also* Neoplasm
        D49.9 *[G73.3]*
      thyrotoxicosis (hyperthyroidism) E05.90
        [G73.3]
        with thyroid storm E05.91 *[G73.3]*
  myelodysplastic D46.9
    with
      5q deletion D46.C
      isolated del (5q) chromosomal
        abnormality D46.C
    lesions, low grade D46.20
    specified NEC D46.Z
  myelopathic pain G89.0
  myeloproliferative (chronic) D47.1
  myofascial pain M79.1
  Naffziger's G54.0
  nail patella Q87.2
  NARP (Neuropathy, Ataxia and Retinitis
    pigmentosa) E88.49
  neonatal abstinence P96.1
  nephritic —*see also* Nephritis
    with edema —*see* Nephrosis
    acute N00.9
    chronic N03.9
    rapidly progressive N01.9
  nephrotic (congenital) —*see also* Nephrosis
    N04.9
    with
      dense deposit disease N04.6
      diffuse
        crescentic glomerulonephritis
          N04.7
        endocapillary proliferative
          glomerulonephritis N04.4
        membranous glomerulonephritis
          N04.2
        mesangial proliferative
          glomerulonephritis N04.3
        mesangiocapillary glomerulonephritis
          N04.5
      focal and segmental glomerular lesions
        N04.1
      minor glomerular abnormality N04.0
      specified morphological changes NEC
        N04.8
    diabetic —*see* Diabetes, nephrosis

Syndrome *(Continued)*
  neurologic neglect R41.4
  Nezelof's D81.4
  Nonne-Milroy-Meige Q82.0
  Nothnagel's vasomotor acroparesthesia
    I73.89
  obesity hypoventilation (OHS) E66.2 ◄
  oculomotor H51.9
  ophthalmoplegia-cerebellar ataxia —*see*
    Strabismus, paralytic, third nerve
  oral allergy T78.1 ◄
  oral-facial-digital Q87.0
  organic
    affective F06.30
    amnesic (not alcohol- or drug-induced) F04
    brain F09
    depressive F06.31
    hallucinosis F06.0
    personality F07.0
  Ormond's N13.5
  oro-facial-digital Q87.0
  os trigonum Q68.8
  Osler-Weber-Rendu I78.0
  osteoporosis-osteomalacia M83.8
  Osterreicher-Turner Q87.2 ◄▥
  otolith —*see* subcategory H81.8
  oto-palatal-digital Q87.0
  outlet (thoracic) G54.0
  ovary
    polycystic E28.2
    resistant E28.39
    sclerocystic E28.2
  Owren's D68.2
  Paget-Schroetter I82.890
  pain —*see also* Pain
    complex regional I G90.50
      lower limb G90.52-
      specified site NEC G90.59
      upper limb G90.51-
    complex regional II —*see* Causalgia
  painful
    bruising D69.2
    feet E53.8
    prostate N42.81
  paralysis agitans —*see* Parkinsonism
  paralytic G83.9
    specified NEC G83.89
  Parinaud's H51.0
  parkinsonian —*see* Parkinsonism
  Parkinson's —*see* Parkinsonism
  paroxysmal facial pain G50.0
  Parry's E05.00
    with thyroid storm E05.01
  Parsonage (-Aldren)-Turner G54.5
  patella clunk M25.86-
  Paterson (-Brown) (-Kelly) D50.1
  pectoral girdle I77.89
  pectoralis minor I77.89
  Pelger-Huet D72.0
  pellagra-cerebellar ataxia-renal
    aminoaciduria E72.02
  pellagroid E52
  Pellegrini-Stieda —*see* Bursitis, tibial
    collateral
  pelvic congestion-fibrosis, female N94.89
  penta X Q97.1
  peptic ulcer —*see* Ulcer, peptic
  perabduction I77.89
  periodic fever M04.1 ◄
  periodic fever, aphthous stomatitis,
    pharyngitis, and adenopathy [PFAPA]
    M04.8 ◄
  periodic headache, in adults and children —
    see Headache, periodic syndromes in
    adults and children
  periurethral fibrosis N13.5
  phantom limb (without pain) G54.7
    with pain G54.6
  pharyngeal pouch D82.1
  Pick's —*see* Disease, Pick's ◄▥
  Pickwickian E66.2

Syndrome *(Continued)*
  PIE (pulmonary infiltration with
    eosinophilia) J82
  pigmentary pallidal degeneration
    (progressive) G23.0
  pineal E34.8
  pituitary E22.0
  placental transfusion —*see* Pregnancy,
    complicated by, placental transfusion
    syndromes
  plantar fascia M72.2
  plateau iris (post-iridectomy)
    (postprocedural) H21.82
  Plummer-Vinson D50.1
  pluricarential of infancy E40
  plurideficiency E40
  pluriglandular (compensatory) E31.8
    autoimmune E31.0
  pneumatic hammer T75.21
  polyangiitis overlap M30.8
  polycarential of infancy E40
  polyglandular E31.8
    autoimmune E31.0
  polysplenia Q89.09
  pontine NEC G93.89
  popliteal
    artery entrapment I77.89
    web Q87.89
  postcardiac injury
    postcardiotomy I97.0
    postmyocardial infarction I24.1
  postcardiotomy I97.0
  post chemoembolization — code to
    associated conditions
  postcholecystectomy K91.5
  postcommissurotomy I97.0
  postconcussional F07.81
  postcontusional F07.81
  postencephalitic F07.89
  posterior
    cervical sympathetic M53.0
    cord G83.83
    fossa compression G93.5
    reversible encephalopathy (PRES) I67.83
  postgastrectomy (dumping) K91.1
  postgastric surgery K91.1
  postinfarction I24.1
  postlaminectomy NEC M96.1
  postleukotomy F07.0
  postmastectomy lymphedema I97.2
  postmyocardial infarction I24.1
  postoperative NEC T81.9
    blind loop K90.2
  postpartum panhypopituitary (Sheehan)
    E23.0
  postpolio (myelitic) G14
  postthrombotic I87.009
    with
      inflammation I87.02-
        with ulcer I87.03-
      specified complication NEC I87.09-
      ulcer I87.01-
        with inflammation I87.03-
    asymptomatic I87.00-
  postvagotomy K91.1
  postvalvulotomy I97.0
  postviral NEC G93.3
    fatigue G93.3
  Potain's K31.0
  potassium intoxication E87.5
  precerebral artery (multiple) (bilateral)
    G45.2
  preinfarction I20.0
  preleukemic D46.9
  premature senility E34.8
  premenstrual dysphoric F32.89 ◄▥
  premenstrual tension N94.3
  Prinzmetal-Massumi R07.1
  prune belly Q79.4
  pseudocarpal tunnel (sublimis) —*see*
    Syndrome, carpal tunnel

Syndrome *(Continued)*
  pseudoparalytica G70.00
    with exacerbation (acute) G70.01
    in crisis G70.01
  pseudo -Turner's Q87.1
  psycho-organic (nonpsychotic severity) F07.9
    acute or subacute F05
    depressive type F06.31
    hallucinatory type F06.0
    nonpsychotic severity F07.0
    specified NEC F07.89
  pulmonary
    arteriosclerosis I27.0
    dysmaturity (Wilson-Mikity) P27.0
    hypoperfusion (idiopathic) P22.0
    renal (hemorrhagic) (Goodpasture's) M31.0
  pure
    motor lacunar G46.5
    sensory lacunar G46.6
  Putnam-Dana D51.0
  pyogenic arthritis, pyoderma gangrenosum, and acne [PAPA] M04.8 ◄
  pyramidopallidonigral G20
  pyriformis —*see* Lesion, nerve, sciatic
  QT interval prolongation I45.81
  radicular NEC —*see* Radiculopathy
    upper limbs, newborn (birth injury) P14.3
  rapid time-zone change G47.25
  Rasmussen G04.81
  Raymond (-Céstan) I65.8
  Raynaud's I73.00
    with gangrene I73.01
  RDS (respiratory distress syndrome, newborn) P22.0
  reactive airways dysfunction J68.3
  Refsum's G60.1
  Reifenstein E34.52
  renal glomerulohyalinosis-diabetic —*see* Diabetes, nephrosis
  Rendu-Osler-Weber I78.0
  residual ovary N99.83
  resistant ovary E28.39
  respiratory
    distress
      acute J80
        adult J80
        child J80
        idiopathic J84.114 ◄
      newborn (idiopathic) (type I) P22.0
        type II P22.1
  restless legs G25.81
  retinoblastoma (familial) C69.2
  retroperitoneal fibrosis N13.5
  retroviral seroconversion (acute) Z21
  Reye's G93.7
  Richter —*see* Leukemia, chronic lymphocytic, B-cell type
  Ridley's I50.1
  right
    heart, hypoplastic Q22.6
    ventricular obstruction —*see* Failure, heart, congestive
  Romano-Ward (prolonged QT interval) I45.81
  rotator cuff, shoulder —*see also* Tear, rotator cuff M75.10-
  Rotes Quérol —*see* Hyperostosis, ankylosing
  Roth —*see* Meralgia paresthetica
  rubella (congenital) P35.0
  Ruvalcaba-Myhre-Smith E71.440
  Rytand-Lipsitch I44.2
  salt
    depletion E87.1
      due to heat NEC T67.8
        causing heat exhaustion or prostration T67.4
    low E87.1
  salt-losing N28.89
  Scaglietti-Dagnini E22.0
  scalenus anticus (anterior) G54.0
  scapulocostal —*see* Mononeuropathy, upper limb, specified site NEC

Syndrome *(Continued)*
  scapuloperoneal G71.0
  schizophrenic, of childhood NEC F84.5
  Schnitzler D47.2
  Scholte's E34.0
  Schroeder's E27.0
  Schüller-Christian C96.5
  Schwachman's —*see* Syndrome, Shwachman's
  Schwartz (-Jampel) G71.13
  Schwartz-Bartter E22.2
  scimitar Q26.8
  sclerocystic ovary E28.2
  Seitelberger's G31.89
  septicemic adrenal hemorrhage A39.1
  seroconversion, retroviral (acute) Z21
  serous meningitis G93.2
  severe acute respiratory (SARS) J12.81
  shaken infant T74.4
  shock (traumatic) T79.4
    kidney N17.0
      following crush injury T79.5
    toxic A48.3
  shock-lung J80
  Shone's — code to specific anomalies
  short
    bowel K91.2
    rib Q77.2
  shoulder-hand —*see* Algoneurodystrophy
  Shwachman's D70.4
  sicca —*see* Sicca syndrome
  sick
    cell E87.1
    sinus I49.5
  sick-euthyroid E07.81
  sideropenic D50.1
  Siemens' ectodermal dysplasia Q82.4
  Silfversköld's Q78.9
  Simons' E88.1
  sinus tarsi M25.57- ◄
  sinusitis-bronchiectasis-situs inversus Q89.3
  Sipple's E31.22
  sirenomelia Q87.2
  Slocumb's E27.0
  slow flow, coronary I20.8
  Sluder's G44.89
  Smith-Magenis Q93.88
  Sneddon-Wilkinson L13.1
  Sotos' Q87.3 ◄
  South African cardiomyopathy I42.8
  spasmodic
    upward movement, eyes H51.8
    winking F95.8
  Spen's I45.9
  splenic
    agenesis Q89.01
    flexure K59.8
    neutropenia D73.81
  Spurway's Q78.0
  staphylococcal scalded skin L00
  steal ◄
    arteriovenous T82.898- ◄
    ischemic T82.898- ◄
    subclavian G45.8 ◄
  Stein-Leventhal E28.2
  Stein's E28.2
  Stevens-Johnson syndrome L51.1
    toxic epidermal necrolysis overlap L51.3
  Stewart-Morel M85.2
  Stickler Q89.8
  stiff baby Q89.8
  stiff man G25.82
  Still-Felty —*see* Felty's syndrome
  Stokes (-Adams) I45.9
  stone heart I50.1
  straight back, congenital Q76.49
  subclavian steal G45.8
  subcoracoid-pectoralis minor G54.0
  subcostal nerve compression I77.89
  subphrenic interposition Q43.3

Syndrome *(Continued)*
  superior
    cerebellar artery I63.8
    mesenteric artery K55.1
    semi-circular canal dehiscence H83.8X-
    vena cava I87.1
  supine hypotensive (maternal) —*see* Syndrome, hypotension, maternal
  suprarenal cortical E27.0
  supraspinatus —*see also* Tear, rotator cuff M75.10-
  Susac G93.49
  swallowed blood P78.2
  sweat retention L74.0
  Swyer Q99.1
  Symond's G93.2
  sympathetic
    cervical paralysis G90.2
    pelvic, female N94.89
  systemic inflammatory response (SIRS), of non-infectious origin (without organ dysfunction) R65.10
    with acute organ dysfunction R65.11
  tachycardia-bradycardia I49.5
  takotsubo I51.81
  TAR (thrombocytopenia with absent radius) Q87.2
  tarsal tunnel G57.5-
  teething K00.7
  tegmental G93.89
  telangiectasic-pigmentation-cataract Q82.8
  temporal pyramidal apex —*see* Otitis, media, suppurative, acute
  temporomandibular joint-pain-dysfunction M26.62- ◄
  Terry's H44.2-
  testicular feminization —*see also* Syndrome, androgen insensitivity E34.51
  thalamic pain (hyperesthetic) G89.0
  thoracic outlet (compression) G54.0
  Thorson-Björck E34.0
  thrombocytopenia with absent radius (TAR) Q87.2
  thyroid-adrenocortical insufficiency E31.0
  tibial
    anterior M76.81-
    posterior M76.82-
  Tietze's M94.0
  time-zone (rapid) G47.25
  Toni-Fanconi E72.09
    with cystinosis E72.04
  Touraine's Q79.8
  tourniquet —*see* Constriction, external, by site
  toxic shock A48.3
  transient left ventricular apical ballooning I51.81
  traumatic vasospastic T75.22
  Treacher Collins Q75.4
  triple X, female Q97.0
  trisomy Q92.9
    13 Q91.7
      meiotic nondisjunction Q91.4
      mitotic nondisjunction Q91.5
      mosaicism Q91.5
      translocation Q91.6
    18 Q91.3
      meiotic nondisjunction Q91.0
      mitotic nondisjunction Q91.1
      mosaicism Q91.1
      translocation Q91.2
    20 (q)(p) Q92.8
    21 Q90.9
      meiotic nondisjunction Q90.0
      mitotic nondisjunction Q90.1
      mosaicism Q90.1
      translocation Q90.2
    22 Q92.8
  tropical wet feet T69.0-
  Trousseau's I82.1

Syndrome *(Continued)*
 tumor lysis (following antineoplastic
  chemotherapy) (spontaneous) NEC
  E88.3
 tumor necrosis factor receptor associated
  periodic (TRAPS) M04.1 ◀
 Twiddler's (due to)
  automatic implantable defibrillator
   T82.198
  cardiac pacemaker T82.198
 Unverricht (-Lundborg) —*see* Epilepsy,
  generalized, idiopathic
 upward gaze H51.8
 uremia, chronic —*see also* Disease, kidney,
  chronic N18.9
 urethral N34.3
 urethro-oculo-articular —*see* Reiter's disease
 urohepatic K76.7
 vago-hypoglossal G52.7
 van Buchem's M85.2
 van der Hoeve's Q78.0
 vascular NEC in cerebrovascular disease
  G46.8
 vasoconstriction, reversible cerebrovascular
  I67.841
 vasomotor I73.9
 vasospastic (traumatic) T75.22
 vasovagal R55
 VATER Q87.2
 velo-cardio-facial Q93.81
 vena cava (inferior) (superior) (obstruction)
  I87.1
 vertebral
  artery G45.0
   compression —*see* Syndrome, anterior,
    spinal artery, compression
  steal G45.0
 vertebro-basilar artery G45.0
 vertebrogenic (pain) M54.89
 vertiginous —*see* Disorder, vestibular
  function
 Vinson-Plummer D50.1
 virus B34.9
 visceral larva migrans B83.0
 visual disorientation H53.8
 vitamin B6 deficiency E53.1
 vitreal corneal H59.01-
 vitreous (touch) H59.01-
 Vogt-Koyanagi H20.82-
 Volkmann's T79.6
 von Schroetter's I82.890
 von Willebrand (-Jürgen) D68.0
 Waldenström-Kjellberg D50.1
 Wallenberg's G46.3
 water retention E87.79
 Waterhouse (-Friderichsen) A39.1
 Weber-Gubler G46.3
 Weber-Leyden G46.3
 Weber's G46.3
 Wegener's M31.30
  with
   kidney involvement M31.31
   lung involvement M31.30
    with kidney involvement M31.31
 Weingarten's (tropical eosinophilia) J82
 Weiss-Baker G90.09
 Werdnig-Hoffman G12.0
 Wermer's E31.21
 Werner's E34.8
 Wernicke-Korsakoff (nonalcoholic) F04
  alcoholic F10.26
 West's —*see* Epilepsy, spasms
 Westphal-Strümpell E83.01
 wet
  feet (maceration) (tropical) T69.0-
  lung, newborn P22.1
 whiplash S13.4
 whistling face Q87.0
 Wilkie's K55.1
 Wilkinson-Sneddon L13.1
 Willebrand (-Jürgens) D68.0

Syndrome *(Continued)*
 Wilson's (hepatolenticular degeneration)
  E83.01
 Wiskott-Aldrich D82.0
 withdrawal —*see* Withdrawal, state
  drug
   infant of dependent mother P96.1
   therapeutic use, newborn P96.2
 Woakes' (ethmoiditis) J33.1
 Wright's (hyperabduction) I77.89
 X I20.9
 XXXX Q97.1
 XXXXX Q97.1
 XXXXY Q98.1
 XXY Q98.0
 yellow nail L60.5
 Zahorsky's B08.5
 Zellweger syndrome E71.510
 Zellweger-like syndrome E71.541
Synechia (anterior) (iris) (posterior) (pupil) —
 see also Adhesions, iris
 intra-uterine (traumatic) N85.6
Synesthesia R20.8
Syngamiasis, syngamosis B83.3
Synodontia K00.2
Synorchidism, synorchism Q55.1
Synostosis (congenital) Q78.8
 astragalo-scaphoid Q74.2
 radioulnar Q74.0
Synovial sarcoma —*see* Neoplasm, connective
 tissue, malignant
Synovioma (malignant) —*see also* Neoplasm,
 connective tissue, malignant
 benign —*see* Neoplasm, connective tissue,
  benign
Synoviosarcoma —*see* Neoplasm, connective
 tissue, malignant
Synovitis —*see also* Tenosynovitis M65.9 ◀▥
 crepitant
  hand M70.0-
  wrist M70.03-
 gonococcal A54.49
 gouty —*see* Gout ◀▥
 in (due to)
  crystals M65.8-
  gonorrhea A54.49
  syphilis (late) A52.78
  use, overuse, pressure —*see* Disorder, soft
   tissue, due to use
 infective NEC —*see* Tenosynovitis, infective
  NEC
 specified NEC —*see* Tenosynovitis, specified
  type NEC
 syphilitic A52.78
  congenital (early) A50.02
 toxic —*see* Synovitis, transient
 transient M67.3-
  ankle M67.37-
  elbow M67.32-
  foot joint M67.37-
  hand joint M67.34-
  hip M67.35-
  knee M67.36-
  multiple site M67.39
  pelvic region M67.35-
  shoulder M67.31-
  specified joint NEC M67.38
  wrist M67.33-
 traumatic, current —*see* Sprain
 tuberculous —*see* Tuberculosis, synovitis
 villonodular (pigmented) M12.2-
  ankle M12.27-
  elbow M12.22-
  foot joint M12.27-
  hand joint M12.24-
  hip M12.25-
  knee M12.26-
  multiple site M12.29
  pelvic region M12.25-
  shoulder M12.21-
  specified joint NEC M12.28

Synovitis *(Continued)*
 villonodular (pigmented) *(Continued)*
  vertebrae M12.28
  wrist M12.23-
Syphilid A51.39
 congenital A50.06
 newborn A50.06
 tubercular (late) A52.79
Syphilis, syphilitic (acquired) A53.9
 abdomen (late) A52.79
 acoustic nerve A52.15
 adenopathy (secondary) A51.49
 adrenal (gland) (with cortical hypofunction)
  A52.79
 age under 2 years NOS —*see also* Syphilis,
  congenital, early
  acquired A51.9
 alopecia (secondary) A51.32
 anemia (late) A52.79 *[D63.8]*
 aneurysm (aorta) (ruptured) A52.01
  central nervous system A52.05
  congenital A50.54 *[I79.0]*
 anus (late) A52.74
  primary A51.1
  secondary A51.39
 aorta (arch) (abdominal) (thoracic) A52.02
  aneurysm A52.01
 aortic (insufficiency) (regurgitation)
  (stenosis)A52.03
  aneurysm A52.01
 arachnoid (adhesive) (cerebral) (spinal) A52.13
 asymptomatic —*see* Syphilis, latent
 ataxia (locomotor) A52.11
 atrophoderma maculatum A51.39
 auricular fibrillation A52.06
 bladder (late) A52.76
 bone A52.77
  secondary A51.46
 brain A52.17
 breast (late) A52.79
 bronchus (late) A52.72
 bubo (primary) A51.0
 bulbar palsy A52.19
 bursa (late) A52.78
 cardiac decompensation A52.06
 cardiovascular A52.00
 central nervous system (late) (recurrent)
  (relapse) (tertiary) A52.3
  with
   ataxia A52.11
   general paralysis A52.17
    juvenile A50.45
   paresis (general) A52.17
    juvenile A50.45
   tabes (dorsalis) A52.11
    juvenile A50.45
   taboparesis A52.17
    juvenile A50.45
  aneurysm A52.05
  congenital A50.40
  juvenile A50.40
  remission in (sustained) A52.3
  serology doubtful, negative, or positive
   A52.3
  specified nature or site NEC A52.19
  vascular A52.05
 cerebral A52.17
  meningovascular A52.13
  nerves (multiple palsies) A52.15
  sclerosis A52.17
  thrombosis A52.05
 cerebrospinal (tabetic type) A52.12
 cerebrovascular A52.05
 cervix (late) A52.76
 chancre (multiple) A51.0
  extragenital A51.2
  Rollet's A51.0
 Charcot's joint A52.16
 chorioretinitis A51.43
  congenital A50.01
  late A52.71
  prenatal A50.01

Syphilis, syphilitic (Continued)
  choroiditis —see Syphilitic chorioretinitis
  choroidoretinitis —see Syphilitic
      chorioretinitis
  ciliary body (secondary) A51.43
      late A52.71
  colon (late) A52.74
  combined spinal sclerosis A52.11
  condyloma (latum) A51.31
  congenital A50.9
      with
          paresis (general) A50.45
          tabes (dorsalis) A50.45
          taboparesis A50.45
      chorioretinitis, choroiditis A50.01 [H32]
      early, or less than 2 years after birth NEC
          A50.2
          with manifestations —see Syphilis,
              congenital, early, symptomatic
          latent (without manifestations) A50.1
              negative spinal fluid test A50.1
              serology positive A50.1
          symptomatic A50.09
              cutaneous A50.06
              mucocutaneous A50.07
              oculopathy A50.01
              osteochondropathy A50.02
              pharyngitis A50.03
              pneumonia A50.04
              rhinitis A50.05
              visceral A50.08
      interstitial keratitis A50.31
      juvenile neurosyphilis A50.45
      late, or 2 years or more after birth NEC
          A50.7
          chorioretinitis, choroiditis A50.32
          interstitial keratitis A50.31
          juvenile neurosyphilis A50.45
          latent (without manifestations) A50.6
              negative spinal fluid test A50.6
              serology positive A50.6
          symptomatic or with manifestations
              NEC A50.59
              arthropathy A50.55
              cardiovascular A50.54
              Clutton's joints A50.51
              Hutchinson's teeth A50.52
              Hutchinson's triad A50.53
              osteochondropathy A50.56
              saddle nose A50.57
  conjugal A53.9
      tabes A52.11
  conjunctiva (late) A52.71
  contact Z20.2
  cord bladder A52.19
  cornea, late A52.71
  coronary (artery) (sclerosis) A52.06
  coryza, congenital A50.05
  cranial nerve A52.15
      multiple palsies A52.15
  cutaneous —see Syphilis, skin
  dacryocystitis (late) A52.71
  degeneration, spinal cord A52.12
  dementia paralytica A52.17
      juvenilis A50.45
  destruction of bone A52.77
  dilatation, aorta A52.01
  due to blood transfusion A53.9
  dura mater A52.13
  ear A52.79
      inner A52.79
          nerve (eighth) A52.15
          neurorecurrence A52.15
  early A51.9
      cardiovascular A52.00
      central nervous system A52.3
      latent (without manifestations) (less than 2
          years after infection) A51.5
          negative spinal fluid test A51.5
          serological relapse after treatment A51.5
          serology positive A51.5

Syphilis, syphilitic (Continued)
  early (Continued)
      relapse (treated, untreated) A51.9
      skin A51.39
      symptomatic A51.9
          extragenital chancre A51.2
          primary, except extragenital chancre
              A51.0
          secondary —see also Syphilis, secondary
              A51.39
              relapse (treated, untreated) A51.49
      ulcer A51.39
  eighth nerve (neuritis) A52.15
  endemic A65
  endocarditis A52.03
      aortic A52.03
      pulmonary A52.03
  epididymis (late) A52.76
  epiglottis (late) A52.73
  epiphysitis (congenital) (early) A50.02
  episcleritis (late) A52.71
  esophagus A52.79
  eustachian tube A52.73
  exposure to Z20.2
  eye A52.71
  eyelid (late) (with gumma) A52.71
  fallopian tube (late) A52.76
  fracture A52.77
  gallbladder (late) A52.74
  gastric (polyposis) (late) A52.74
  general A53.9
      paralysis A52.17
          juvenile A50.45
  genital (primary) A51.0
  glaucoma A52.71
  gumma NEC A52.79
      cardiovascular system A52.00
      central nervous system A52.3
      congenital A50.59
  heart (block) (decompensation) (disease)
      (failure) A52.06 [I52]
      valve NEC A52.03
  hemianesthesia A52.19
  hemianopsia A52.71
  hemiparesis A52.17
  hemiplegia A52.17
  hepatic artery A52.09
  hepatis A52.74
  hepatomegaly, congenital A50.08
  hereditaria tarda —see Syphilis, congenital,
      late
  hereditary —see Syphilis, congenital
  Hutchinson's teeth A50.52
  hyalitis A52.71
  inactive —see Syphilis, latent
  infantum —see Syphilis, congenital
  inherited —see Syphilis, congenital
  internal ear A52.79
  intestine (late) A52.74
  iris, iritis (secondary) A51.43
      late A52.71
  joint (late) A52.77
  keratitis (congenital) (interstitial) (late) A50.31
  kidney (late) A52.75
  lacrimal passages (late) A52.71
  larynx (late) A52.73
  late A52.9
      cardiovascular A52.00
      central nervous system A52.3
      kidney A52.75
      latent or 2 years or more after infection
          (without manifestations) A52.8
          negative spinal fluid test A52.8
          serology positive A52.8
      paresis A52.17
      specified site NEC A52.79
      symptomatic or with manifestations A52.79
      tabes A52.11
  latent A53.0
      with signs or symptoms - code by site and
          stage under Syphilis

Syphilis, syphilitic (Continued)
  latent (Continued)
      central nervous system A52.2
      date of infection unspecified A53.0
      early, or less than 2 years after infection
          A51.5
      follow-up of latent syphilis A53.0
          date of infection unspecified A53.0
          late, or 2 years or more after infection
              A52.8
      late, or 2 years or more after infection
          A52.8
      positive serology (only finding) A53.0
          date of infection unspecified A53.0
          early, or less than 2 years after infection
              A51.5
          late, or 2 years or more after infection
              A52.8
  lens (late) A52.71
  leukoderma A51.39
      late A52.79
  lienitis A52.79
  lip A51.39
      chancre (primary) A51.2
      late A52.79
  Lissauer's paralysis A52.17
  liver A52.74
  locomotor ataxia A52.11
  lung A52.72
  lymph gland (early) (secondary) A51.49
      late A52.79
  lymphadenitis (secondary) A51.49
  macular atrophy of skin A51.39
      striated A52.79
  mediastinum (late) A52.73
  meninges (adhesive) (brain) (spinal cord)
      A52.13
  meningitis A52.13
      acute (secondary) A51.41
      congenital A50.41
  meningoencephalitis A52.14
  meningovascular A52.13
      congenital A50.41
  mesarteritis A52.09
      brain A52.04
  middle ear A52.77
  mitral stenosis A52.03
  monoplegia A52.17
  mouth (secondary) A51.39
      late A52.79
  mucocutaneous (secondary) A51.39
      late A52.79
  mucous
      membrane (secondary) A51.39
          late A52.79
      patches A51.39
          congenital A50.07
  mulberry molars A50.52
  muscle A52.78
  myocardium A52.06
  nasal sinus (late) A52.73
  neonatorum —see Syphilis, congenital
  nephrotic syndrome (secondary)
      A51.44
  nerve palsy (any cranial nerve) A52.15
      multiple A52.15
  nervous system, central A52.3
  neuritis A52.15
      acoustic A52.15
  neurorecidive of retina A52.19
  neuroretinitis A52.19
  newborn —see Syphilis, congenital
  nodular superficial (late) A52.79
  nonvenereal A65
  nose (late) A52.73
      saddle back deformity A50.57
  occlusive arterial disease A52.09
  oculopathy A52.71
  ophthalmic (late) A52.71
  optic nerve (atrophy) (neuritis) (papilla)
      A52.15

◀ New   ◀▦ Revised   ~~deleted~~ Deleted

Syphilis, syphilitic (Continued)
orbit (late) A52.71
organic A53.9
osseous (late) A52.77
osteochondritis (congenital) (early) A50.02
[M90.80]
osteoporosis A52.77
ovary (late) A52.76
oviduct (late) A52.76
palate (late) A52.79
pancreas (late) A52.74
paralysis A52.17
general A52.17
juvenile A50.45
paresis (general) A52.17
juvenile A50.45
paresthesia A52.19
Parkinson's disease or syndrome A52.19
paroxysmal tachycardia A52.06
pemphigus (congenital) A50.06
penis (chancre) A51.0
late A52.76
pericardium A52.06
perichondritis, larynx (late) A52.73
periosteum (late) A52.77
congenital (early) A50.02 [M90.80]
early (secondary) A51.46
peripheral nerve A52.79
petrous bone (late) A52.77
pharynx (late) A52.73
secondary A51.39
pituitary (gland) A52.79
pleura (late) A52.73
pneumonia, white A50.04
pontine lesion A52.17
portal vein A52.09
primary A51.0
anal A51.1
and secondary —see Syphilis, secondary
central nervous system A52.3
extragenital chancre NEC A51.2
fingers A51.2
genital A51.0
lip A51.2
specified site NEC A51.2
tonsils A51.2
prostate (late) A52.76
ptosis (eyelid) A52.71
pulmonary (late) A52.72
artery A52.09
pyelonephritis (late) A52.75
recently acquired, symptomatic A51.9
rectum (late) A52.74
respiratory tract (late) A52.73
retina, late A52.71
retrobulbar neuritis A52.15
salpingitis A52.76
sclera (late) A52.71
sclerosis
cerebral A52.17
coronary A52.06
multiple A52.11
scotoma (central) A52.71
scrotum (late) A52.76

Syphilis, syphilitic (Continued)
secondary (and primary) A51.49
adenopathy A51.49
anus A51.39
bone A51.46
chorioretinitis, choroiditis A51.43
hepatitis A51.45
liver A51.45
lymphadenitis A51.49
meningitis (acute) A51.41
mouth A51.39
mucous membranes A51.39
periosteum, periostitis A51.46
pharynx A51.39
relapse (treated, untreated) A51.49
skin A51.39
specified form NEC A51.49
tonsil A51.39
ulcer A51.39
viscera NEC A51.49
vulva A51.39
seminal vesicle (late) A52.76
seronegative with signs or symptoms - code
by site and stage under Syphilis
seropositive
with signs or symptoms - code by site and
stage under Syphilis
follow-up of latent syphilis —see Syphilis,
latent
only finding —see Syphilis, latent
seventh nerve (paralysis) A52.15
sinus, sinusitis (late) A52.73
skeletal system A52.77
skin (with ulceration) (early) (secondary)
A51.39
late or tertiary A52.79
small intestine A52.74
spastic spinal paralysis A52.17
spermatic cord (late) A52.76
spinal (cord) A52.12
spleen A52.79
splenomegaly A52.79
spondylitis A52.77
staphyloma A52.71
stigmata (congenital) A50.59
stomach A52.74
synovium A52.78
tabes dorsalis (late) A52.11
juvenile A50.45
tabetic type A52.11
juvenile A50.45
taboparesis A52.17
juvenile A50.45
tachycardia A52.06
tendon (late) A52.78
tertiary A52.9
with symptoms NEC A52.79
cardiovascular A52.00
central nervous system A52.3
multiple NEC A52.79
specified site NEC A52.79
testis A52.76
thorax A52.73
throat A52.73

Syphilis, syphilitic (Continued)
thymus (gland) (late) A52.79
thyroid (late) A52.79
tongue (late) A52.79
tonsil (lingual) (late) A52.73
primary A51.2
secondary A51.39
trachea (late) A52.73
tunica vaginalis (late) A52.76
ulcer (any site) (early) (secondary)
A51.39
late A52.79
perforating A52.79
foot A52.11
urethra (late) A52.76
urogenital (late) A52.76
uterus (late) A52.76
uveal tract (secondary) A51.43
late A52.71
uveitis (secondary) A51.43
late A52.71
uvula (late) (perforated) A52.79
vagina A51.0
late A52.76
valvulitis NEC A52.03
vascular A52.00
brain (cerebral) A52.05
ventriculi A52.74
vesicae urinariae (late) A52.76
viscera (abdominal) (late) A52.74
secondary A51.49
vitreous (opacities) (late) A52.71
hemorrhage A52.71
vulva A51.0
late A52.76
secondary A51.39
Syphiloma A52.79
cardiovascular system A52.00
central nervous system A52.3
circulatory system A52.00
congenital A50.59
Syphilophobia F45.29
Syringadenoma —see also Neoplasm, skin,
benign
papillary —see Neoplasm, skin, benign
Syringobulbia G95.0
Syringocystadenoma —see Neoplasm, skin,
benign
papillary —see Neoplasm, skin, benign
Syringoma —see also Neoplasm, skin, benign
chondroid —see Neoplasm, skin, benign
Syringomyelia G95.0
Syringomyelitis —see Encephalitis
Syringomyelocele —see Spina bifida
Syringopontia G95.0
System, systemic —see also condition
disease, combined —see Degeneration,
combined
inflammatory response syndrome (SIRS) of
non-infectious origin (without organ
dysfunction) R65.10
with acute organ dysfunction R65.11
lupus erythematosus M32.9
inhibitor present D68.62

T

Tabacism, tabacosis, tabagism —see also
    Poisoning, tobacco
    meaning dependence (without remission)
        F17.200
        with
            disorder F17.299
                remission F17.211
                specified disorder NEC F17.298
            withdrawal F17.203
Tabardillo A75.9
    flea-borne A75.2
    louse-borne A75.0
Tabes, tabetic A52.10
    with
        central nervous system syphilis A52.10
        Charcot's joint A52.16
        cord bladder A52.19
        crisis, viscera (any) A52.19
        paralysis, general A52.17
        paresis (general) A52.17
        perforating ulcer (foot) A52.19
    arthropathy (Charcot) A52.16
    bladder A52.19
    bone A52.11
    cerebrospinal A52.12
    congenital A50.45
    conjugal A52.10
    dorsalis A52.11
        juvenile A50.49
    juvenile A50.49
    latent A52.19
    mesenterica A18.39
    paralysis, insane, general A52.17
    spasmodic A52.17
    syphilis (cerebrospinal) A52.12
Taboparalysis A52.17
Taboparesis (remission) A52.17
    juvenile A50.45
TAC (trigeminal autonomic cephalgia) NEC
    G44.099
    intractable G44.091
    not intractable G44.099
Tache noir S60.22-
Tachyalimentation K91.2
Tachyarrhythmia, tachyrhythmia —see
    Tachycardia
Tachycardia R00.0
    atrial (paroxysmal) I47.1
    auricular I47.1
    AV nodal re-entry (re-entrant) I47.1
    junctional (paroxysmal) I47.1
    newborn P29.11
    nodal (paroxysmal) I47.1
    non-paroxysmal AV nodal I45.89
    paroxysmal (sustained) (nonsustained)
        I47.9
        with sinus bradycardia I49.5
        atrial (PAT) I47.1
        atrioventricular (AV) (re-entrant) I47.1
            psychogenic F54
        junctional I47.1
            ectopic I47.1
        nodal I47.1
        psychogenic (atrial) (supraventricular)
            (ventricular) F54
        supraventricular (sustained) I47.1
            psychogenic F54
        ventricular I47.2
            psychogenic F54
    psychogenic F45.8
    sick sinus I49.5
    sinoauricular NOS R00.0
        paroxysmal I47.1
    sinus [sinusal] NOS R00.0
        paroxysmal I47.1
    supraventricular I47.1
    ventricular (paroxysmal) (sustained) I47.2
        psychogenic F54
Tachygastria K31.89

Tachypnea R06.82
    hysterical F45.8
    newborn (idiopathic) (transitory) P22.1
    psychogenic F45.8
    transitory, of newborn P22.1
TACO (transfusion associated circulatory
    overload) E87.71
Taenia (infection) (infestation) B68.9
    diminuta B71.0
    echinococcal infestation B67.90
    mediocanellata B68.1
    nana B71.0
    saginata B68.1
    solium (intestinal form) B68.0
        larval form —see Cysticercosis
Taeniasis (intestine) —see Taenia
Tag (hypertrophied skin) (infected) L91.8
    adenoid J35.8
    anus K64.4
        hemorrhoidal K64.4
    hymen N89.8
    perineal N90.89
    preauricular Q17.0
    sentinel K64.4
    skin L91.8
        accessory (congenital) Q82.8
        anus K64.4
        congenital Q82.8
        preauricular Q17.0
    tonsil J35.8
    urethra, urethral N36.8
    vulva N90.89
Tahyna fever B33.8
Takahara's disease E80.3
Takayasu's disease or syndrome M31.4
Talcosis (pulmonary) J62.0
Talipes (congenital) Q66.89
    acquired, planus —see Deformity, limb, flat
        foot
    asymmetric Q66.89
    calcaneovalgus Q66.4
    calcaneovarus Q66.1
    calcaneus Q66.89
    cavus Q66.7
    equinovalgus Q66.6
    equinovarus Q66.0
    equinus Q66.89
    percavus Q66.7
    planovalgus Q66.6
    planus (acquired) (any degree) —see also
        Deformity, limb, flat foot
        congenital Q66.5-
        due to rickets (sequelae) E64.3
    valgus Q66.6
    varus Q66.3
Tall stature, constitutional E34.4
Talma's disease M62.89
Talon noir S90.3-
    hand S60.22-
    heel S90.3-
    toe S90.1-
Tamponade, heart I31.4
Tanapox (virus disease) B08.71
Tangier disease E78.6
Tantrum, child problem F91.8
Tapeworm (infection) (infestation) —see
    Infestation, tapeworm
Tapia's syndrome G52.7
TAR (thrombocytopenia with absent radius)
    syndrome Q87.2
Tarral-Besnier disease L44.0
Tarsal tunnel syndrome —see Syndrome, tarsal
    tunnel
Tarsalgia —see Pain, limb, lower
Tarsitis (eyelid) H01.8
    syphilitic A52.71
    tuberculous A18.4
Tartar (teeth) (dental calculus) K03.6
Tattoo (mark) L81.8
Tauri's disease E74.09
Taurodontism K00.2

Taussig-Bing syndrome Q20.1
Taybi's syndrome Q87.2
Tay-Sachs amaurotic familial idiocy or disease
    E75.02
TBI (traumatic brain injury) S06.9 ◀▥
Teacher's node or nodule J38.2
Tear, torn (traumatic) —see also Laceration
    with abortion —see Abortion
    annular fibrosis M51.35
    anus, anal (sphincter) S31.831
        complicating delivery
            with third degree perineal laceration —
                see also Delivery, complicated, by,
                laceration, perineum, third degree
                O70.20 ◀▥
                with mucosa O70.3
            without third degree perineal laceration
                O70.4
        nontraumatic (healed) (old) K62.81
    articular cartilage, old —see Derangement,
        joint, articular cartilage, by site
    bladder
        with ectopic or molar pregnancy O08.6
        following ectopic or molar pregnancy
            O08.6
        obstetrical O71.5
        traumatic —see Injury, bladder
    bowel
        with ectopic or molar pregnancy O08.6
        following ectopic or molar pregnancy
            O08.6
        obstetrical trauma O71.5
    broad ligament
        with ectopic or molar pregnancy O08.6
        following ectopic or molar pregnancy O08.6
        obstetrical trauma O71.6
    bucket handle (knee) (meniscus) —see Tear,
        meniscus
    capsule, joint —see Sprain
    cartilage —see also Sprain
        articular, old —see Derangement, joint,
            articular cartilage, by site
    cervix
        with ectopic or molar pregnancy O08.6
        following ectopic or molar pregnancy
            O08.6
        obstetrical trauma (current) O71.3
        old N88.1
        traumatic —see Injury, uterus
    dural G97.41
        nontraumatic G96.11
    internal organ —see Injury, by site
    knee cartilage
        articular (current) S83.3-
        old —see Derangement, knee, meniscus,
            due to old tear
    ligament —see Sprain
    meniscus (knee) (current injury) S83.209
        bucket-handle S83.20-
        lateral
            bucket-handle S83.25-
            complex S83.27-
            peripheral S83.26-
            specified type NEC S83.28-
        medial
            bucket-handle S83.21-
            complex S83.23-
            peripheral S83.22-
            specified type NEC S83.24-
        old —see Derangement, knee, meniscus,
            due to old tear
        site other than knee - code as Sprain
        specified type NEC S83.20-
    muscle —see Strain
    pelvic
        floor, complicating delivery O70.1
        organ NEC, obstetrical trauma O71.5
            with ectopic or molar pregnancy O08.6
            following ectopic or molar pregnancy
                O08.6
    perineal, secondary O90.1

◀ New   ◀▥ Revised   ~~deleted~~ Deleted

Tear, torn *(Continued)*
  periurethral tissue, obstetrical trauma O71.82
    with ectopic or molar pregnancy O08.6
    following ectopic or molar pregnancy O08.6
  rectovaginal septum —*see* Laceration, vagina
  retina, retinal (without detachment) (horseshoe) —*see also* Break, retina, horseshoe
    with detachment —*see* Detachment, retina, with retinal, break
  rotator cuff (nontraumatic) M75.10-
    complete M75.12-
    incomplete M75.11-
    traumatic S46.01-
      capsule S43.42-
  semilunar cartilage, knee —*see* Tear, meniscus
  supraspinatus (complete) (incomplete) (nontraumatic) —*see also* Tear, rotator cuff M75.10-
  tendon —*see* Strain
  tentorial, at birth P10.4
  umbilical cord
    complicating delivery O69.89
  urethra
    with ectopic or molar pregnancy O08.6
    following ectopic or molar pregnancy O08.6
    obstetrical trauma O71.5
  uterus —*see* Injury, uterus
  vagina —*see* Laceration, vagina
  vessel, from catheter —*see* Puncture, accidental complicating surgery
  vulva, complicating delivery O70.0
Tear-stone —*see* Dacryolith
Teeth —*see also* condition
  grinding
    psychogenic F45.8
    sleep related G47.63
Teething (syndrome) K00.7
Telangiectasia, telangiectasis (verrucous) I78.1
  ataxic (cerebellar) (Louis-Bar) G11.3
  familial I78.0
  hemorrhagic, hereditary (congenital) (senile) I78.0
  hereditary, hemorrhagic (congenital) (senile) I78.0
  juxtafoveal H35.07-
  macular H35.07-
  parafoveal H35.07-
  retinal (idiopathic) (juxtafoveal) (macular) (parafoveal) H35.07-
  spider I78.1
Telephone scatologia F65.89
Telescoped bowel or intestine K56.1
  congenital Q43.8
Temperature
  body, high (of unknown origin) R50.9
  cold, trauma from T69.9
    newborn P80.0
    specified effect NEC T69.8
Temple —*see* condition
Temporal —*see* condition
Temporomandibular joint pain-dysfunction syndrome M26.62- ◀━
Temporosphenoidal —*see* condition
Tendency
  bleeding —*see* Defect, coagulation
  suicide
    meaning personal history of attempted suicide Z91.5
    meaning suicidal ideation —*see* Ideation, suicidal
  to fall R29.6
Tenderness, abdominal R10.819
  epigastric R10.816
  generalized R10.817
  left lower quadrant R10.814
  left upper quadrant R10.812
  periumbilic R10.815

Tenderness, abdominal *(Continued)*
  rebound R10.829
    epigastric R10.826
    generalized R10.827
    left lower quadrant R10.824
    left upper quadrant R10.822
    periumbilic R10.825
    right lower quadrant R10.823
    right upper quadrant R10.821
  right lower quadrant R10.813
  right upper quadrant R10.811
Tendinitis, tendonitis —*see also* Enthesopathy
  Achilles M76.6-
  adhesive —*see* Tenosynovitis, specified type NEC
    shoulder —*see* Capsulitis, adhesive
  bicipital M75.2-
  calcific M65.2-
    ankle M65.27-
    foot M65.27-
    forearm M65.23-
    hand M65.24-
    lower leg M65.26-
    multiple sites M65.29
    pelvic region M65.25-
    shoulder M75.3-
    specified site NEC M65.28
    thigh M65.25-
    upper arm M65.22-
  due to use, overuse, pressure —*see also* Disorder, soft tissue, due to use
    specified NEC —*see* Disorder, soft tissue, due to use, specified NEC
  gluteal M76.0-
  patellar M76.5-
  peroneal M76.7-
  psoas M76.1-
  tibial (posterior) M76.82-
    anterior M76.81-
  trochanteric —*see* Bursitis, hip, trochanteric
Tendon —*see* condition
Tendosynovitis —*see* Tenosynovitis
Tenesmus (rectal) R19.8
  vesical R30.1
Tennis elbow —*see* Epicondylitis, lateral
Tenonitis —*see also* Tenosynovitis
  eye (capsule) H05.04-
Tenontosynovitis —*see* Tenosynovitis
Tenontothecitis —*see* Tenosynovitis
Tenophyte —*see* Disorder, synovium, specified type NEC
Tenosynovitis —*see also* Synovitis M65.9
  adhesive —*see* Tenosynovitis, specified type NEC
    shoulder —*see* Capsulitis, adhesive
  bicipital (calcifying) —*see* Tendinitis, bicipital
  gonococcal A54.49
  in (due to)
    crystals M65.8-
    gonorrhea A54.49
    syphilis (late) A52.78
    use, overuse, pressure —*see also* Disorder, soft tissue, due to use
      specified NEC —*see* Disorder, soft tissue, due to use, specified NEC
  infective NEC M65.1-
    ankle M65.17-
    foot M65.17-
    forearm M65.13-
    hand M65.14-
    lower leg M65.16-
    multiple sites M65.19
    pelvic region M65.15-
    shoulder region M65.11-
    specified site NEC M65.18
    thigh M65.15-
    upper arm M65.12-
  radial styloid M65.4
  shoulder region M65.81-
    adhesive —*see* Capsulitis, adhesive

Tenosynovitis *(Continued)*
  specified type NEC M65.88-
    ankle M65.87-
    foot M65.87-
    forearm M65.83-
    hand M65.84-
    lower leg M65.86-
    multiple sites M65.89
    pelvic region M65.85-
    shoulder region M65.81-
    specified site NEC M65.88
    thigh M65.85-
    upper arm M65.82-
  tuberculous —*see* Tuberculosis, tenosynovitis
Tenovaginitis —*see* Tenosynovitis
Tension
  arterial, high —*see also* Hypertension
    without diagnosis of hypertension R03.0
  headache G44.209
    intractable G44.201
    not intractable G44.209
  nervous R45.0
  pneumothorax J93.0
  premenstrual N94.3
  state (mental) F48.9
Tentorium —*see* condition
Teratencephalus Q89.8
Teratism Q89.7
Teratoblastoma (malignant) —*see* Neoplasm, malignant, by site
Teratocarcinoma —*see also* Neoplasm, malignant, by site
  liver C22.7
Teratoma (solid) —*see also* Neoplasm, uncertain behavior, by site
  with embryonal carcinoma, mixed —*see* Neoplasm, malignant, by site
  with malignant transformation —*see* Neoplasm, malignant, by site
  adult (cystic) —*see* Neoplasm, benign, by site
  benign —*see* Neoplasm, benign, by site
  combined with choriocarcinoma —*see* Neoplasm, malignant, by site
  cystic (adult) —*see* Neoplasm, benign, by site
  differentiated —*see* Neoplasm, benign, by site
  embryonal —*see also* Neoplasm, malignant, by site
    liver C22.7
  immature —*see* Neoplasm, malignant, by site
  liver C22.7
    adult, benign, cystic, differentiated type or mature D13.4
  malignant —*see also* Neoplasm, malignant, by site
    anaplastic —*see* Neoplasm, malignant, by site
    intermediate —*see* Neoplasm, malignant, by site
    specified site —*see* Neoplasm, malignant, by site
    unspecified site C62.90
    undifferentiated —*see* Neoplasm, malignant, by site
  mature —*see* Neoplasm, uncertain behavior, by site
  malignant —*see* Neoplasm, by site, malignant, by site
  ovary D27.-
    embryonal, immature or malignant C56-
  solid —*see* Neoplasm, uncertain behavior, by site
  testis C62.9-
    adult, benign, cystic, differentiated type or mature D29.2-
    scrotal C62.1-
    undescended C62.0-
Termination
  anomalous —*see also* Malposition, congenital
    right pulmonary vein Q26.3
  pregnancy, elective Z33.2

Ternidens diminutus infestation B81.8
Ternidensiasis B81.8
Terror (s) night (child) F51.4
Terrorism, victim of Z65.4
Terry's syndrome H44.2-
Tertiary —see condition
Test, tests, testing (for)
 adequacy (for dialysis)
  hemodialysis Z49.31
  peritoneal Z49.32
 blood pressure Z01.30
  abnormal reading —see Blood, pressure
 blood typing Z01.83
  Rh typing Z01.83
 blood-alcohol Z04.8
  positive —see Findings, abnormal, in blood
 blood-drug Z04.8
  positive —see Findings, abnormal, in blood
 cardiac pulse generator (battery) Z45.010
 fertility Z31.41
 genetic
  disease carrier status for procreative management
   female Z31.430
   male Z31.440
  male partner of patient with recurrent pregnancy loss Z31.441
  procreative management NEC
   female Z31.438
   male Z31.448
 hearing Z01.10
  with abnormal findings NEC Z01.118
 HIV (human immunodeficiency virus)
  nonconclusive (in infants) R75
  positive Z21
  seropositive Z21
 immunity status Z01.84
 intelligence NEC Z01.89
 laboratory (as part of a general medical examination) Z00.00
  with abnormal finding Z00.01
  for medicolegal reason NEC Z04.8
 male partner of patient with recurrent pregnancy loss Z31.441
 Mantoux (for tuberculosis) Z11.1
  abnormal result R76.11
 pregnancy, positive first pregnancy —see Pregnancy, normal, first
 procreative Z31.49
  fertility Z31.41
 skin, diagnostic
  allergy Z01.82
   special screening examination —see Screening, by name of disease
  Mantoux Z11.1
  tuberculin Z11.1
 specified NEC Z01.89
 tuberculin Z11.1
  abnormal result R76.11
 vision Z01.00
  with abnormal findings Z01.01
 Wassermann Z11.3
  positive —see Serology for syphilis, positive
Testicle, testicular, testis —see also condition
 feminization syndrome —see also Syndrome, androgen insensitivity E34.51
 migrans Q55.29
Tetanus, tetanic (cephalic) (convulsions) A35
 with
  abortion A34
  ectopic or molar pregnancy O08.0
 following ectopic or molar pregnancy O08.0
 inoculation reaction (due to serum) —see Complications, vaccination
 neonatorum A33
 obstetrical A34
 puerperal, postpartum, childbirth A34

Tetany (due to) R29.0
 alkalosis E87.3
 associated with rickets E55.0
 convulsions R29.0
  hysterical F44.5
 functional (hysterical) F44.5
 hyperkinetic R29.0
  hysterical F44.5
 hyperpnea R06.4
  hysterical F44.5
  psychogenic F45.8
 hyperventilation —see also Hyperventilation R06.4
  hysterical F44.5
 neonatal (without calcium or magnesium deficiency) P71.3
 parathyroid (gland) E20.9
 parathyroprival E89.2
 post- (para)thyroidectomy E89.2
 postoperative E89.2
 pseudotetany R29.0
 psychogenic (conversion reaction) F44.5
Tetralogy of Fallot Q21.3
Tetraplegia (chronic) —see also Quadriplegia G82.50-
Thailand hemorrhagic fever A91
Thalassanemia —see Thalassemia
Thalassemia (anemia) (disease) D56.9
 with other hemoglobinopathy D56.8
 alpha (major) (severe) (triple gene defect) D56.0
  minor D56.3
  silent carrier D56.3
  trait D56.3
 beta (severe) D56.1
  homozygous D56.1
  major D56.1
  minor D56.3
  trait D56.3
 delta-beta (homozygous) D56.2
  minor D56.3
  trait D56.3
 dominant D56.8
 hemoglobin
  C D56.8
  E-beta D56.5
 intermedia D56.1
 major D56.1
 minor D56.3
 mixed D56.8
 sickle-cell —see Disease, sickle-cell, thalassemia
 specified type NEC D56.8
 trait D56.3
 variants D56.8
Thanatophoric dwarfism or short stature Q77.1
Thaysen-Gee disease (nontropical sprue) K90.0
Thaysen's disease K90.0
Thecoma D27-
 luteinized D27-
 malignant C56-
Thelarche, premature E30.8
Thelaziasis B83.8
Thelitis N61.0 ◀▥
 puerperal, postpartum or gestational —see Infection, nipple
Therapeutic —see condition
Therapy
 drug, long-term (current) (prophylactic)
  agents affecting estrogen receptors and estrogen levels NEC Z79.818
  anastrozole (Arimidex) Z79.811
  antibiotics Z79.2
   short-term use - omit code
  anticoagulants Z79.01
  anti-inflammatory Z79.1
  antiplatelet Z79.02
  antithrombotics Z79.02
  aromatase inhibitors Z79.811
  aspirin Z79.82
  birth control pill or patch Z79.3

Therapy (Continued)
 drug, long-term (Continued)
  bisphosphonates Z79.83
  contraceptive, oral Z79.3
  drug, specified NEC Z79.899
  estrogen receptor downregulators Z79.818
  Evista Z79.810
  exemestane (Aromasin) Z79.811
  Fareston Z79.810
  fulvestrant (Faslodex) Z79.818
  gonadotropin-releasing hormone (GnRH) agonist Z79.818
  goserelin acetate (Zoladex) Z79.818
  hormone replacement (postmenopausal) Z79.890
  insulin Z79.4
  letrozole (Femara) Z79.811
  leuprolide acetate (leuprorelin) (Lupron) Z79.818
  megestrol acetate (Megace) Z79.818
  methadone
   for pain management Z79.891
   maintenance therapy F11.20
  Nolvadex Z79.810
  opiate analgesic Z79.891
  oral contraceptive Z79.3
  raloxifene (Evista) Z79.810
  selective estrogen receptor modulators (SERMs) Z79.810
  short term - omit code
  steroids
   inhaled Z79.51
   systemic Z79.52
  tamoxifen (Nolvadex) Z79.810
  toremifene (Fareston) Z79.810
Thermic —see condition
Thermography (abnormal) —see also Abnormal, diagnostic imaging R93.8
 breast R92.8
Thermoplegia T67.0
Thesaurismosis, glycogen —see Disease, glycogen storage
Thiamin deficiency E51.9
 specified NEC E51.8
Thiaminic deficiency with beriberi E51.11
Thibierge-Weissenbach syndrome —see Sclerosis, systemic
Thickening
 bone —see Hypertrophy, bone
 breast N64.59
 endometrium R93.8
 epidermal L85.9
  specified NEC L85.8
 hymen N89.6
 larynx J38.7
 nail L60.2
  congenital Q84.5
 periosteal —see Hypertrophy, bone
 pleura J92.9
  with asbestos J92.0
 skin R23.4
 subepiglottic J38.7
 tongue K14.8
 valve, heart —see Endocarditis
Thigh —see condition
Thinning vertebra —see Spondylopathy, specified NEC
Thirst, excessive R63.1
 due to deprivation of water T73.1
Thomsen disease G71.12
Thoracic —see also condition
 kidney Q63.2
 outlet syndrome G54.0
Thoracogastroschisis (congenital) Q79.8
Thoracopagus Q89.4
Thorax —see condition
Thorn's syndrome N28.89
Thorson-Björck syndrome E34.0
Threadworm (infection) (infestation) B80

◀ New   ◀▥ Revised   ~~deleted~~ Deleted

Threatened
abortion O20.0
  with subsequent abortion O03.9
job loss, anxiety concerning Z56.2
labor (without delivery) O47.9
  ~~after 37 completed weeks of gestation O47.1~~
  at or after 37 completed weeks of gestation O47.1 ◀
  before 37 completed weeks of gestation O47.0-
loss of job, anxiety concerning Z56.2
miscarriage O20.0
unemployment, anxiety concerning Z56.2
Three-day fever A93.1
Threshers' lung J67.0
Thrix annulata (congenital) Q84.1
Throat —see condition
Thrombasthenia (Glanzmann) (hemorrhagic) (hereditary) D69.1
Thromboangiitis I73.1
obliterans (general) I73.1
  cerebral I67.89
  vessels
    brain I67.89
    spinal cord I67.89
Thromboarteritis —see Arteritis
Thromboasthenia (Glanzmann) (hemorrhagic) (hereditary) D69.1
Thrombocytasthenia (Glanzmann) D69.1
Thrombocythemia (essential) (hemorrhagic) (idiopathic) (primary) D47.3
Thrombocytopathy (dystrophic) (granulopenic) D69.1
Thrombocytopenia, thrombocytopenic D69.6
with absent radius (TAR) Q87.2
congenital D69.42
dilutional D69.59
due to
  drugs D69.59
  extracorporeal circulation of blood D69.59
  (massive)blood transfusion D69.59
  platelet alloimmunization D69.59
essential D69.3
heparin induced (HIT) D75.82
hereditary D69.42
idiopathic D69.3
neonatal, transitory P61.0
  due to
    exchange transfusion P61.0
    idiopathic maternal thrombocytopenia P61.0
    isoimmunization P61.0
primary NEC D69.49
  idiopathic D69.3
puerperal, postpartum O72.3
secondary D69.59
transient neonatal P61.0
Thrombocytosis, essential D47.3
primary D47.3
Thromboembolism —see Embolism
Thrombopathy (Bernard-Soulier) D69.1
constitutional D68.0
Willebrand-Jurgens D68.0
Thrombopenia —see Thrombocytopenia
Thrombophilia D68.59
primary NEC D68.59
secondary NEC D68.69
specified NEC D68.69
Thrombophlebitis I80.9
antepartum O22.2-
  deep O22.3-
  superficial O22.2-
cavernous (venous) sinus G08
complicating pregnancy O22.5-
nonpyogenic I67.6
cerebral (sinus) (vein) G08
  nonpyogenic I67.6
  sequelae G09
due to implanted device —see Complications, by site and type, specified NEC

Thrombophlebitis (Continued)
during or resulting from a procedure NEC T81.72
femoral vein (superficial) I80.1-
femoropopliteal vein I80.0-
hepatic (vein) I80.8
idiopathic, recurrent I82.1
iliofemoral I80.1-
intracranial venous sinus (any) G08
  nonpyogenic I67.6
  sequelae G09
intraspinal venous sinuses and veins G08
  nonpyogenic G95.19
lateral (venous) sinus G08
  nonpyogenic I67.6
leg I80.299
  superficial I80.0-
longitudinal (venous) sinus G08
  nonpyogenic I67.6
lower extremity I80.299
migrans, migrating I82.1
pelvic
  with ectopic or molar pregnancy O08.0
  following ectopic or molar pregnancy O08.0
  puerperal O87.1
popliteal vein —see Phlebitis, leg, deep, popliteal
portal (vein) K75.1
postoperative T81.72
pregnancy —see Thrombophlebitis, antepartum
puerperal, postpartum, childbirth O87.0
  deep O87.1
  pelvic O87.1
  septic O86.81
  superficial O87.0
saphenous (greater) (lesser) I80.0-
sinus (intracranial) G08
  nonpyogenic I67.6
specified site NEC I80.8
tibial vein I80.23-
Thrombosis, thrombotic (bland) (multiple) (progressive) (silent) (vessel) I82.90
anal K64.5
antepartum —see Thrombophlebitis, antepartum
aorta, aortic I74.10
  abdominal I74.09
    saddle I74.01
  bifurcation I74.09
  saddle I74.01
  specified site NEC I74.19
  terminal I74.09
  thoracic I74.11
  valve —see Endocarditis, aortic
apoplexy I63.3- ◀
artery, arteries (postinfectional) I74.9
  auditory, internal —see Occlusion, artery, precerebral, specified NEC
  basilar —see Occlusion, artery, basilar
  carotid (common) (internal) —see Occlusion, artery, carotid
  cerebellar (anterior inferior) (posterior inferior) (superior) —see Occlusion, artery, cerebellar
  cerebral —see Occlusion, artery, cerebral
  choroidal (anterior) —see Occlusion, artery, cerebral, specified NEC
  communicating, posterior —see Occlusion, artery, cerebral, specified NEC
  coronary —see also Infarct, myocardium
    not resulting in infarction I24.0
  hepatic I74.8
  hypophyseal —see Occlusion, artery, cerebral, specified NEC
  iliac I74.5
  limb I74.4
    lower I74.3
    upper I74.2

Thrombosis, thrombotic (Continued)
artery, arteries (Continued)
  meningeal, anterior or posterior —see Occlusion, artery, cerebral, specified NEC
  mesenteric (with gangrene) —see also Infarct, intestine K55.069 ◀
  ophthalmic —see Occlusion, artery, retina
  pontine —see Occlusion, artery, cerebral, specified NEC
  precerebral —see Occlusion, artery, precerebral
  pulmonary (iatrogenic) —see Embolism, pulmonary
  renal N28.0
  retinal —see Occlusion, artery, retina
  spinal, anterior or posterior G95.11
  traumatic NEC T14.8
  vertebral —see Occlusion, artery, vertebral
atrium, auricular —see also Infarct, myocardium
  following acute myocardial infarction (current complication) I23.6
  not resulting in infarction I51.3 ◀
basilar (artery) —see Occlusion, artery, basilar
brain (artery) (stem) —see also Occlusion, artery, cerebral
  due to syphilis A52.05
  puerperal O99.43
  sinus —see Thrombosis, intracranial venous sinus
capillary I78.8
cardiac —see also Infarct, myocardium
  not resulting in infarction I51.3 ◀
  valve —see Endocarditis
carotid (artery) (common) (internal) —see Occlusion, artery, carotid
cavernous (venous) sinus —see Thrombosis, intracranial venous sinus
cerebellar artery (anterior inferior) (posterior inferior) (superior) I66.3
cerebral (artery) —see Occlusion, artery, cerebral
cerebrovenous sinus —see also Thrombosis, intracranial venous sinus
  puerperium O87.3
chronic I82.91
coronary (artery) (vein) —see also Infarct, myocardium
  not resulting in infarction I24.0
corpus cavernosum N48.89
cortical I66.9
deep —see Embolism, vein, lower extremity
due to device, implant or graft —see also Complications, by site and type, specified NEC T85.868 ◀
  arterial graft NEC T82.868
  breast (implant) T85.868 ◀
  catheter NEC T85.868 ◀
    dialysis (renal) T82.868
      intraperitoneal T85.868 ◀
    infusion NEC T82.868
      spinal (epidural) (subdural) T85.860 ◀
    urinary (indwelling) T83.86
  electronic (electrode) (pulse generator) (stimulator)
    bone T84.86
    cardiac T82.867
    nervous system (brain) (peripheral nerve) (spinal) T85.860 ◀
    urinary T83.86
  fixation, internal (orthopedic) NEC T84.86
  gastrointestinal (bile duct) (esophagus) T85.868 ◀
  genital NEC T83.86
  heart T82.867
  joint prosthesis T84.86
  ocular (corneal graft) (orbital implant) NEC T85.868 ◀
  orthopedic NEC T84.86

Thrombosis, thrombotic *(Continued)*
  due to device, implant or graft *(Continued)*
    specified NEC T85.868 ◀▥
    urinary NEC T83.86
    vascular NEC T82.868
    ventricular intracranial shunt T85.860 ◀▥
  during the puerperium —*see* Thrombosis,
    puerperal
  endocardial —*see also* Infarct, myocardium
    not resulting in infarction I51.3 ◀▥
  eye —*see* Occlusion, retina
  genital organ
    female NEC N94.89
      pregnancy —*see* Thrombophlebitis,
        antepartum
    male N50.1
  gestational —*see* Phlebopathy, gestational
  heart (chamber) —*see also* Infarct,
    myocardium
    not resulting in infarction I51.3 ◀▥
  hepatic (vein) I82.0
    artery I74.8
  history (of) Z86.718
  intestine (with gangrene) —*see also* Infarct,
    intestine K55.069 ◀▥
  intracardiac NEC (apical) (atrial) (auricular)
    (ventricular) (old) I51.3
  intracranial (arterial) I66.9
    venous sinus (any) G08
      nonpyogenic origin I67.6
      puerperium O87.3
  intramural —*see also* Infarct, myocardium
    not resulting in infarction I51.3 ◀▥
  intraspinal venous sinuses and veins
    G08
    nonpyogenic G95.19
  kidney (artery) N28.0
  lateral (venous) sinus —*see* Thrombosis,
    intracranial venous sinus
  leg —*see* Thrombosis, vein, lower
    extremity
    arterial I74.3
  liver (venous) I82.0
    artery I74.8
    portal vein I81
  longitudinal (venous) sinus —*see* Thrombosis,
    intracranial venous sinus
  lower limb —*see* Thrombosis, vein, lower
    extremity
  lung (iatrogenic) (postoperative) —*see*
    Embolism, pulmonary
  meninges (brain) (arterial) I66.8
  mesenteric (artery) (with gangrene) —*see also*
    Infarct, intestine K55.069 ◀▥
    vein (inferior) (superior) I81
  mitral I34.8
  mural —*see also* Infarct, myocardium
    due to syphilis A52.06
    not resulting in infarction I51.3 ◀▥
  omentum (with gangrene) —*see also* Infarct,
    intestine K55.069 ◀▥
  ophthalmic —*see* Occlusion, retina
  pampiniform plexus (male) N50.1
  parietal —*see also* Infarct, myocardium
    not resulting in infarction I24.0
  penis, superficial vein N48.81
  perianal venous K64.5
  peripheral arteries I74.4
    upper I74.2
  personal history (of) Z86.718
  portal I81
    due to syphilis A52.09
  precerebral artery —*see* Occlusion, artery,
    precerebral
  puerperal, postpartum O87.0
    brain (artery) O99.43
      venous (sinus) O87.3
    cardiac O99.43
    cerebral (artery) O99.43
      venous (sinus) O87.3
    superficial O87.0

Thrombosis, thrombotic *(Continued)*
  pulmonary (artery) (iatrogenic)
    (postoperative) (vein) —*see* Embolism,
    pulmonary
  renal (artery) N28.0
    vein I82.3
  resulting from presence of device, implant or
    graft —*see* Complications, by site and
    type, specified NEC
  retina, retinal —*see* Occlusion, retina
  scrotum N50.1
  seminal vesicle N50.1
  sigmoid (venous) sinus —*see* Thrombosis,
    intracranial venous sinus
  sinus, intracranial (any) —*see* Thrombosis,
    intracranial venous sinus
  specified site NEC I82.890
    chronic I82.891
  spermatic cord N50.1
  spinal cord (arterial) G95.11
    due to syphilis A52.09
    pyogenic origin G06.1
  spleen, splenic D73.5
    artery I74.8
  testis N50.1
  traumatic NEC T14.8
  tricuspid I07.8
  tumor —*see* Neoplasm, by site
  tunica vaginalis N50.1
  umbilical cord (vessels), complicating
    delivery O69.5
  vas deferens N50.1
  vein (acute) I82.90
    antecubital I82.61-
      chronic I82.71-
    axillary I82.A1-
      chronic I82.A2-
    basilic I82.61-
      chronic I82.71-
    brachial I82.62-
      chronic I82.72-
    brachiocephalic (innominate) I82.290
      chronic I82.291
    cerebral, nonpyogenic I67.6
    cephalic I82.61-
      chronic I82.71-
    chronic I82.91
    deep (DVT) I82.40-
      calf I82.4Z-
        chronic I82.5Z-
      lower leg I82.4Z-
        chronic I82.5Z-
      thigh I82.4Y-
        chronic I82.5Y-
      upper leg I82.4Y
        chronic I82.5y-
    femoral I82.41-
      chronic I82.51-
    iliac (iliofemoral) I82.42-
      chronic I82.52-
    innominate I82.290
      chronic I82.291
    internal jugular I82.C1-
      chronic I82.C2-
    lower extremity
      deep I82.40-
        chronic I82.50-
        specified NEC I82.49-
          chronic NEC I82.59-
      distal
        deep I82.4Z-
      proximal
        deep I82.4Y-
          chronic I82.5Y-
      superficial I82.81-
    perianal K64.5
    popliteal I82.43-
      chronic I82.53-
    radial I82.62-
      chronic I82.72-
    renal I82.3

Thrombosis, thrombotic *(Continued)*
  vein *(Continued)*
    saphenous (greater) (lesser) I82.81-
    specified NEC I82.890
      chronic NEC I82.891
    subclavian I82.B1-
      chronic I82.B2-
    thoracic NEC I82.290
      chronic I82.291
    tibial I82.44-
      chronic I82.54-
    ulnar I82.62-
      chronic I82.72-
    upper extremity I82.60-
      chronic I82.70-
      deep I82.62-
        chronic I82.72-
      superficial I82.61-
        chronic I82.71-
  vena cava
    inferior I82.220
      chronic I82.221
    superior I82.210
      chronic I82.211
  venous, perianal K64.5
  ventricle —*see also* Infarct, myocardium
    following acute myocardial infarction
      (current complication) I23.6
    not resulting in infarction I24.0
Thrombus —*see* Thrombosis
Thrush —*see also* Candidiasis
  newborn P37.5
  oral B37.0
  vaginal B37.3
Thumb —*see also* condition
  sucking (child problem) F98.8
Thymitis E32.8
Thymoma (benign) D15.0
  malignant C37
Thymus, thymic (gland) —*see* condition
Thyrocele —*see* Goiter
Thyroglossal —*see also* condition
  cyst Q89.2
  duct, persistent Q89.2
Thyroid (gland) (body) —*see also* condition
  hormone resistance E07.89
  lingual Q89.2
  nodule (cystic) (nontoxic) (single) E04.1
Thyroiditis E06.9
  acute (nonsuppurative) (pyogenic)
    (suppurative) E06.0
  autoimmune E06.3
  chronic (nonspecific) (sclerosing) E06.5
    with thyrotoxicosis, transient E06.2
    fibrous E06.5
    lymphadenoid E06.3
    lymphocytic E06.3
    lymphoid E06.3
  de Quervain's E06.1
  drug-induced E06.4
  fibrous (chronic) E06.5
  giant-cell (follicular) E06.1
  granulomatous (de Quervain) (subacute)
    E06.1
  Hashimoto's (struma lymphomatosa) E06.3
  iatrogenic E06.4
  ligneous E06.5
  lymphocytic (chronic) E06.3
  lymphoid E06.3
  lymphomatous E06.3
  nonsuppurative E06.1
  postpartum, puerperal O90.5
  pseudotuberculous E06.1
  pyogenic E06.0
  radiation E06.4
  Riedel's E06.5
  subacute (granulomatous) E06.1
  suppurative E06.0
  tuberculous A18.81
  viral E06.1
  woody E06.5

◀ New   ◀▥ Revised   ~~deleted~~ Deleted

Thyrolingual duct, persistent Q89.2
Thyromegaly E01.0
Thyrotoxic
  crisis —*see* Thyrotoxicosis
  heart disease or failure —*see also*
      Thyrotoxicosis E05.90 [I43]
    with thyroid storm E05.91 [I43]
  storm —*see* Thyrotoxicosis
Thyrotoxicosis (recurrent) E05.90
  with
    goiter (diffuse) E05.00
      with thyroid storm E05.01
      adenomatous uninodular E05.10
        with thyroid storm E05.11
      multinodular E05.20
        with thyroid storm E05.21
      nodular E05.20
        with thyroid storm E05.21
      uninodular E05.10
        with thyroid storm E05.11
    infiltrative
      dermopathy E05.00
        with thyroid storm E05.01
      ophthalmopathy E05.00
        with thyroid storm E05.01
    single thyroid nodule E05.10
      with thyroid storm E05.11
    thyroid storm E05.91
  due to
    ectopic thyroid nodule or tissue E05.30
      with thyroid storm E05.31
    ingestion of (excessive) thyroid material
        E05.40
      with thyroid storm E05.41
    overproduction of thyroid-stimulating
        hormone E05.80
      with thyroid storm E05.81
    specified cause NEC E05.80
      with thyroid storm E05.81
  factitia E05.40
    with thyroid storm E05.41
  heart E05.90 [I43]
    with thyroid storm E05.91 [I43]
    failure E05.90 [I43]
  neonatal (transient) P72.1
  transient with chronic thyroiditis E06.2
Tibia vara —*see* Osteochondrosis, juvenile, tibia
Tic (disorder) F95.9
  breathing F95.8
  child problem F95.0
  compulsive F95.1
  de la Tourette F95.2
  degenerative (generalized) (localized) G25.69
    facial G25.69
  disorder
    chronic
      motor F95.1
      vocal F95.1
    combined vocal and multiple motor F95.2
    transient F95.0
  douloureux G50.0
    atypical G50.1
    postherpetic, postzoster B02.22
  drug-induced G25.61
  eyelid F95.8
  habit F95.9
    chronic F95.1
    transient of childhood F95.0
  lid, transient of childhood F95.0
  motor-verbal F95.2
  occupational F48.8
  orbicularis F95.8
    transient of childhood F95.0
  organic origin G25.69
  postchoreic G25.69
  provisional F95.0 ◀
  psychogenic, compulsive F95.1
  salaam R25.8
  spasm (motor or vocal) F95.9
    chronic F95.1
    transient of childhood F95.0
  specified NEC F95.8

Tick-borne —*see* condition
Tietze's disease or syndrome M94.0
Tight, tightness
  anus K62.89
  chest R07.89
  fascia (lata) M62.89
  foreskin (congenital) N47.1
  hymen, hymenal ring N89.6
  introitus (acquired) (congenital) N89.6
  rectal sphincter K62.89
  tendon —*see* Short, tendon
  urethral sphincter N35.9
Tilting vertebra —*see* Dorsopathy, deforming,
    specified NEC
Timidity, child F93.8
Tin-miner's lung J63.5
Tinea (intersecta) (tarsi) B35.9
  amiantacea L44.8
  asbestina B35.0
  barbae B35.0
  beard B35.0
  black dot B35.0
  blanca B36.2
  capitis B35.0
  corporis B35.4
  cruris B35.6
  flava B36.0
  foot B35.3
  furfuracea B36.0
  imbricata (Tokelau) B35.5
  kerion B35.0
  manuum B35.2
  microsporic —*see* Dermatophytosis
  nigra B36.1
  nodosa —*see* Piedra
  pedis B35.3
  scalp B35.0
  specified site NEC B35.8
  sycosis B35.0
  tonsurans B35.0
  trichophytic —*see* Dermatophytosis
  unguium B35.1
  versicolor B36.0
Tingling sensation (skin) R20.2
~~Tinnitus (audible) (aurium) (subjective) —see~~
  ~~subcategory H93.1~~
Tinnitus NOS H93.1- ◀
  audible H93.1- ◀
  aurium H93.1- ◀
  pulsatile H93.A- ◀
  subjective H93.1- ◀
Tipped tooth (teeth) M26.33
Tipping
  pelvis M95.5
    with disproportion (fetopelvic) O33.0
      causing obstructed labor O65.0
  tooth (teeth), fully erupted M26.33
Tiredness R53.83
Tissue —*see* condition
Tobacco (nicotine)
  abuse —*see* Tobacco, use ◀
  dependence —*see* Dependence, drug, nicotine
  harmful use Z72.0
  heart —*see* Tobacco, toxic effect
  maternal use, affecting newborn P04.2
  toxic effect —*see* Table of Drugs and
      Chemicals, by substance, poisoning
    chewing tobacco —*see* Table of Drugs
        and Chemicals, by substance,
        poisoning
    cigarettes —*see* Table of Drugs and
        Chemicals, by substance, poisoning
  use Z72.0
    complicating
      childbirth O99.334
      pregnancy O99.33-
      puerperium O99.335
    counseling and surveillance Z71.6
    history Z87.891 ◀
  withdrawal state —*see also* Dependence,
      drug, nicotine F17.203 ◀▦

Tocopherol deficiency E56.0
Todd's
  cirrhosis K74.3
  paralysis (postepileptic) (transitory) G83.84
Toe —*see* condition
Toilet, artificial opening —*see* Attention to,
    artificial, opening
Tokelau (ringworm) B35.5
Tollwut —*see* Rabies
Tommaselli's disease R31.9
  correct substance properly administered —*see*
      Table of Drugs and Chemicals, by drug,
      adverse effect
  overdose or wrong substance given or
      taken —*see* Table of Drugs and
      Chemicals, by drug, poisoning
Tongue —*see also* condition
  tie Q38.1
Tonic pupil —*see* Anomaly, pupil, function,
    tonic pupil
Toni-Fanconi syndrome (cystinosis) E72.09
  with cystinosis E72.04
Tonsil —*see* condition
Tonsillitis (acute) (catarrhal) (croupous)
    (follicular) (gangrenous) (infective)
    (lacunar) (lingual) (malignant)
    (membranous) (parenchymatous)
    (phlegmonous) (pseudomembranous)
    (purulent) (septic) (subacute)
    (suppurative) (toxic) (ulcerative)
    (vesicular) (viral) J03.90
  chronic J35.01
    with adenoiditis J35.03
  diphtheritic A36.0
  hypertrophic J35.01
    with adenoiditis J35.03
  recurrent J03.91
  specified organism NEC J03.80
    recurrent J03.81
  staphylococcal J03.80
    recurrent J03.81
  streptococcal J03.00
    recurrent J03.01
  tuberculous A15.8
  Vincent's A69.1
Tooth, teeth —*see* condition
Toothache K08.89 ◀▦
Topagnosis R20.8
Tophi —*see* Gout, chronic
TORCH infection —*see* Infection, congenital
  without active infection P00.2
Torn —*see* Tear
Tornwaldt's cyst or disease J39.2
Torsion
  accessory tube —*see* Torsion, fallopian tube
  adnexa (female) —*see* Torsion, fallopian tube
  aorta, acquired I77.1
  appendix epididymis N44.04
  appendix testis N44.03
  bile duct (common) (hepatic) K83.8
    congenital Q44.5
  bowel, colon or intestine K56.2
  cervix —*see* Malposition, uterus
  cystic duct K82.8
  dystonia —*see* Dystonia, torsion
  epididymis (appendix) N44.04
  fallopian tube N83.52- ◀▦
    with ovary N83.53
  gallbladder K82.8
    congenital Q44.1
  hydatid of Morgagni
    female N83.52- ◀▦
    male N44.03
  kidney (pedicle) (leading to infarction) N28.0
  Meckel's diverticulum (congenital) Q43.0
    malignant —*see* Table of Neoplasms, small
        intestine, malignant
  mesentery K56.2
  omentum K56.2
  organ or site, congenital NEC —*see* Anomaly,
      by site

Torsion *(Continued)*
  ovary (pedicle) N83.51- ◄▥
    with fallopian tube N83.53
    congenital Q50.2
  oviduct —*see* Torsion, fallopian tube
  penis (acquired) N48.82
    congenital Q55.63
  spasm —*see* Dystonia, torsion
  spermatic cord N44.02
    extravaginal N44.01
    intravaginal N44.02
  spleen D73.5
  testis, testicle N44.00
    appendix N44.03
  tibia —*see* Deformity, limb, specified type
    NEC, lower leg
  uterus —*see* Malposition, uterus
Torticollis (intermittent) (spastic) M43.6
  congenital (sternomastoid) Q68.0
  due to birth injury P15.8
  hysterical F44.4
  ocular R29.891
  psychogenic F45.8
    conversion reaction F44.4
  rheumatic M43.6
  rheumatoid M06.88
  spasmodic G24.3
  traumatic, current S13.4
Tortipelvis G24.1
Tortuous
  aortic arch Q25.46 ◄
  artery I77.1
  organ or site, congenital NEC —*see* Distortion
  retinal vessel, congenital Q14.1
  ureter N13.8
  urethra N36.8
  vein —*see* Varix
Torture, victim of Z65.4
Torula, torular (histolytica) (infection) —*see*
  Cryptococcosis
Torulosis —*see* Cryptococcosis
Torus (mandibularis) (palatinus) M27.0
  fracture —*see* Fracture, by site, torus
Touraine's syndrome Q79.8
Tourette's syndrome F95.2
Tourniquet syndrome —*see* Constriction,
  external, by site
Tower skull Q75.0
  with exophthalmos Q87.0
Toxemia R68.89
  bacterial —*see* Sepsis
  burn —*see* Burn
  eclamptic (with pre-existing hypertension) —
    see Eclampsia
  erysipelatous —*see* Erysipelas
  fatigue R68.89
  food —*see* Poisoning, food
  gastrointestinal K52.1
  intestinal K52.1
  kidney —*see* Uremia
  malarial —*see* Malaria
  myocardial —*see* Myocarditis, toxic
  of pregnancy —*see* Pre-eclampsia
  pre-eclamptic —*see* Pre-eclampsia
  small intestine K52.1
  staphylococcal, due to food A05.0
  stasis R68.89
  uremic —*see* Uremia
  urinary —*see* Uremia
Toxemica cerebropathia psychica
  (nonalcoholic) F04
  alcoholic —*see* Alcohol, amnestic disorder
Toxic (poisoning) —*see also* condition T65.91
  effect —*see* Table of Drugs and Chemicals, by
    substance, poisoning
  shock syndrome A48.3
  thyroid (gland) —*see* Thyrotoxicosis
Toxicemia —*see* Toxemia
Toxicity —*see* Table of Drugs and Chemicals, by
  substance, poisoning
  fava bean D55.0

Toxic *(Continued)*
  food, noxious —*see* Poisoning, food
  from drug or nonmedicinal substance —*see*
    Table of Drugs and Chemicals, by drug
Toxicosis —*see also* Toxemia
  capillary, hemorrhagic D69.0
Toxinfection, gastrointestinal K52.1
Toxocariasis B83.0
Toxoplasma, toxoplasmosis (acquired) B58.9
  with
    hepatitis B58.1
    meningoencephalitis B58.2
    ocular involvement B58.00
    other organ involvement B58.89
    pneumonia, pneumonitis B58.3
  congenital (acute) (subacute) (chronic) P37.1
  maternal, manifest toxoplasmosis in infant
    (acute) (subacute) (chronic) P37.1
tPA (rtPA) administation in a different facility
  within the last 24 hours prior to admission
  to current facility Z92.82
Trabeculation, bladder N32.89
Trachea —*see* condition
Tracheitis (catarrhal) (infantile) (membranous)
  (plastic) (septal) (suppurative) (viral)
  J04.10
  with
    bronchitis (15 years of age and above) J40
      acute or subacute —*see* Bronchitis, acute
      chronic J42
      tuberculous NEC A15.5
      under 15 years of age J20.9
    laryngitis (acute) J04.2
      chronic J37.1
      tuberculous NEC A15.5
  acute J04.10
    with obstruction J04.11
  chronic J42
    with
      bronchitis (chronic) J42
      laryngitis (chronic) J37.1
  diphtheritic (membranous) A36.89
  due to external agent —*see* Inflammation,
    respiratory, upper, due to
  syphilitic A52.73
  tuberculous A15.5
Trachelitis (nonvenereal) —*see* Cervicitis
Tracheobronchial —*see* condition
Tracheobronchitis (15 years of age and
  above) —*see also* Bronchitis
  due to
    Bordetella bronchiseptica A37.80
      with pneumonia A37.81
    Francisella tularensis A21.8
Tracheobronchomegaly Q32.4
  with bronchiectasis J47.9
    with
      exacerbation (acute) J47.1
      lower respiratory infection J47.0
  acquired J98.09
    with bronchiectasis J47.9
      with
        exacerbation (acute) J47.1
        lower respiratory infection J47.0
Tracheobronchopneumonitis —*see* Pneumonia,
  broncho-
Tracheocele (external) (internal) J39.8
  congenital Q32.1
Tracheomalacia J39.8
  congenital Q32.0
Tracheopharyngitis (acute) J06.9
  chronic J42
  due to external agent —*see* Inflammation,
    respiratory, upper, due to
Tracheostenosis J39.8
Tracheostomy
  complication —*see* Complication,
    tracheostomy
  status Z93.0
    attention to Z43.0
    malfunctioning J95.03

Trachoma, trachomatous A71.9
  active (stage) A71.1
  contraction of conjunctiva A71.1
  dubium A71.0
  healed or sequelae B94.0
  initial (stage) A71.0
  pannus A71.1
  Türck's J37.0
Traction, vitreomacular H43.82-
Train sickness T75.3
Trait (s)
  Hb-S D57.3
  hemoglobin
    abnormal NEC D58.2
      with thalassemia D56.3
    C —*see* Disease, hemoglobin C
    S (Hb-S) D57.3
  Lepore D56.3
  personality, accentuated Z73.1
  sickle-cell D57.3
    with elliptocytosis or spherocytosis D57.3
  type A personality Z73.1
Tramp Z59.0
Trance R41.89
  hysterical F44.89
Transaminasemia R74.0
Transection
  abdomen (partial) S38.3
  aorta (incomplete) —*see also* Injury, aorta
    complete —*see* Injury, aorta, laceration,
      major
  carotid artery (incomplete) —*see also* Injury,
    blood vessel, carotid, laceration
    complete —*see* Injury, blood vessel, carotid,
      laceration, major
  celiac artery (incomplete) S35.211
    branch (incomplete) S35.291
      complete S35.292
    complete S35.212
  innominate
    artery (incomplete) —*see also* Injury, blood
      vessel, thoracic, innominate, artery,
      laceration
      complete —*see* Injury, blood vessel,
        thoracic, innominate, artery,
        laceration, major
    vein (incomplete) —*see also* Injury, blood
      vessel, thoracic, innominate, vein,
      laceration
      complete —*see* Injury, blood vessel,
        thoracic, innominate, vein,
        laceration, major
  jugular vein (external) (incomplete) —*see
    also* Injury, blood vessel, jugular vein,
    laceration
    complete —*see* Injury, blood vessel, jugular
      vein, laceration, major
    internal (incomplete) —*see also* Injury,
      blood vessel, jugular vein, internal,
      laceration
      complete —*see* Injury, blood vessel,
        jugular vein, internal, laceration,
        major
  mesenteric artery (incomplete) —*see also*
    Injury, mesenteric, artery, laceration
    complete —*see* Injury, mesenteric artery,
      laceration, major
  pulmonary vessel (incomplete) —*see
    also* Injury, blood vessel, thoracic,
    pulmonary, laceration
    complete —*see* Injury, blood vessel,
      thoracic, pulmonary, laceration, major
  subclavian —*see* Transection, innominate
  vena cava (incomplete) —*see also* Injury, vena
    cava
    complete —*see* Injury, vena cava,
      laceration, major
  vertebral artery (incomplete) —*see also* Injury,
    blood vessel, vertebral, laceration
    complete —*see* Injury, blood vessel,
      vertebral, laceration, major

◄ New   ◄▥ Revised   ~~deleted~~ Deleted

Transfusion
  associated (red blood cell) hemochromatosis
      E83.111
  blood
    ABO incompatible —*see* Complication (s),
        transfusion, incompatibility reaction,
        ABO
    minor blood group (Duffy) (E) (K(ell))
        (Kidd) (Lewis) (M) (N) (P) (S)
        T80.89
    reaction or complication —*see*
        Complications, transfusion
  fetomaternal (mother) —*see* Pregnancy,
      complicated by, placenta, transfusion
      syndrome
  maternofetal (mother) —*see* Pregnancy,
      complicated by, placenta, transfusion
      syndrome
  placental (syndrome) (mother) —*see*
      Pregnancy, complicated by, placenta,
      transfusion syndrome
  reaction (adverse) —*see* Complications,
      transfusion
  related acute lung injury (TRALI) J95.84
  twin-to-twin —*see* Pregnancy, complicated by,
      placenta, transfusion syndrome, fetus
      to fetus
Transient (meaning homeless) —*see also*
      condition Z59.0
Translocation
  balanced autosomal Q95.9
    in normal individual Q95.0
  chromosomes NEC Q99.8
    balanced and insertion in normal
        individual Q95.0
  Down's syndrome Q90.2
  trisomy
      13 Q91.6
      18 Q91.2
      21 Q90.2
Translucency, iris —*see* Degeneration, iris
Transmission of chemical substances through
      the placenta —*see* Absorption, chemical,
      through placenta
Transparency, lung, unilateral J43.0
Transplant (ed) (status) Z94.9
  awaiting organ Z76.82
  bone Z94.6
    marrow Z94.81
  candidate Z76.82
  complication —*see* Complication, transplant
  cornea Z94.7
  heart Z94.1
    and lung (s) Z94.3
    valve Z95.2
      prosthetic Z95.2
      specified NEC Z95.4
      xenogenic Z95.3
  intestine Z94.82
  kidney Z94.0
  liver Z94.4
  lung (s) Z94.2
    and heart Z94.3
  organ (failure) (infection) (rejection)Z94.9
    removal status Z98.85
  pancreas Z94.83
  skin Z94.5
  social Z60.3
  specified organ or tissue NEC Z94.89
  stem cells Z94.84
  tissue Z94.9
Transplants, ovarian, endometrial N80.1
Transposed —*see* Transposition
Transposition (congenital) —*see also*
      Malposition, congenital
  abdominal viscera Q89.3
  aorta (dextra) Q20.3
  appendix Q43.8
  colon Q43.8
  corrected Q20.5
  great vessels (complete) (partial) Q20.3

Transposition (*Continued*)
  heart Q24.0
    with complete transposition of viscera
        Q89.3
  intestine (large) (small) Q43.8
  reversed jejunal (for bypass) (status) Z98.0
  scrotum Q55.23
  stomach Q40.2
    with general transposition of viscera
        Q89.3
  tooth, teeth, fully erupted M26.30
  vessels, great (complete) (partial) Q20.3
  viscera (abdominal) (thoracic) Q89.3
Transsexualism F64.0 ◀⃥
Transverse —*see also* condition
  arrest (deep), in labor O64.0
  lie (mother) O32.2
    causing obstructed labor O64.8
Transvestism, transvestitism (dual-role)
      F64.1
  fetishistic F65.1
Trapped placenta (with hemorrhage) O72.0
  without hemorrhage O73.0
TRAPS (tumor necrosis factor receptor
      associated periodic syndrome) M04.1 ◀
Trauma, traumatism —*see also* Injury
  acoustic —*see* subcategory H83.3
  birth —*see* Birth, injury
  complicating ectopic or molar pregnancy
      O08.6
  during delivery O71.9
  following ectopic or molar pregnancy O08.6
  obstetric O71.9
    specified NEC O71.89
  occlusal ◀
    primary K08.81 ◀
    secondary K08.82 ◀
Traumatic —*see also* condition
  brain injury S06.9 ◀⃥
Treacher Collins syndrome Q75.4
Treitz's hernia —*see* Hernia, abdomen, specified
      site NEC
Trematode infestation —*see* Infestation, fluke
Trematodiasis —*see* Infestation, fluke
Trembling paralysis —*see* Parkinsonism
Tremor (s) R25.1
  drug induced G25.1
  essential (benign) G25.0
  familial G25.0
  hereditary G25.0
  hysterical F44.4
  intention G25.2
  medication induced postural G25.1
  mercurial —*see* subcategory T56.1
  Parkinson's —*see* Parkinsonism
  psychogenic (conversion reaction) F44.4
  senilis R54
  specified type NEC G25.2
Trench
  fever A79.0
  foot —*see* Immersion, foot
  mouth A69.1
Treponema pallidum infection —*see* Syphilis
Treponematosis
  due to
    T. pallidum —*see* Syphilis
    T. pertenue —*see* Yaws
Triad
  Hutchinson's (congenital syphilis) A50.53
  Kartagener's Q89.3
  Saint's —*see* Hernia, diaphragm
Trichiasis (eyelid) H02.059
  with entropion —*see* Entropion
  left H02.056
    lower H02.055
    upper H02.054
  right H02.053
    lower H02.052
    upper H02.051
Trichinella spiralis (infection) (infestation)
      B75

Trichinellosis, trichiniasis, trichinelliasis,
      trichinosis B75
  with muscle disorder B75 *[M63.80]*
    ankle B75 *[M63.87-]*
    foot B75 *[M63.87-]*
    forearm B75 *[M63.83-]*
    hand B75 *[M63.84-]*
    lower leg B75 *[M63.86-]*
    multiple sites B75 *[M63.89]*
    pelvic region B75 *[M63.85-]*
    shoulder region B75 *[M63.81-]*
    specified site NEC B75 *[M63.88]*
    thigh B75 *[M63.85-]*
    upper arm B75 *[M63.82-]*
Trichobezoar T18.9
  intestine T18.3
  stomach T18.2
Trichocephaliasis, trichocephalosis B79
Trichocephalus infestation B79
Trichoclasis L67.8
Trichoepithelioma —*see also* Neoplasm, skin,
      benign
  malignant —*see* Neoplasm, skin, malignant
Trichofolliculoma —*see* Neoplasm, skin,
      benign
Tricholemmoma —*see* Neoplasm, skin,
      benign
Trichomoniasis A59.9
  bladder A59.03
  cervix A59.09
  intestinal A07.8
  prostate A59.02
  seminal vesicles A59.09
  specified site NEC A59.8
  urethra A59.03
  urogenitalis A59.00
  vagina A59.01
  vulva A59.01
Trichomycosis
  axillaris A48.8
  nodosa, nodularis B36.8
Trichonodosis L67.8
Trichophytid, trichophyton infection —*see*
      Dermatophytosis
Trichophytobezoar T18.9
  intestine T18.3
  stomach T18.2
Trichophytosis —*see* Dermatophytosis
Trichoptilosis L67.8
Trichorrhexis (nodosa) (invaginata) L67.0
Trichosis axillaris A48.8
Trichosporosis nodosa B36.2
Trichostasis spinulosa (congenital) Q84.1
Trichostrongyliasis, trichostrongylosis (small
      intestine) B81.2
Trichostrongylus infection B81.2
Trichotillomania F63.3
Trichromat, trichromatopsia, anomalous
      (congenital) H53.55
Trichuriasis B79
Trichuris trichiura (infection) (infestation) (any
      site) B79
Tricuspid (valve) —*see* condition
Trifid —*see also* Accessory
  kidney (pelvis) Q63.8
  tongue Q38.3
Trigeminal neuralgia —*see* Neuralgia,
      trigeminal
Trigeminy R00.8
Trigger finger (acquired) M65.30
  congenital Q74.0
  index finger M65.32-
  little finger M65.35-
  middle finger M65.33-
  ring finger M65.34-
  thumb M65.31-
Trigonitis (bladder) (chronic)
      (pseudomembranous) N30.30
  with hematuria N30.31
Trigonocephaly Q75.0
Trilocular heart —*see* Cor triloculare

Trimethylaminuria E72.52
Tripartite placenta O43.19-
Triphalangeal thumb Q74.0
Triple —see also Accessory
  kidneys Q63.0
  uteri Q51.818
  X, female Q97.0
Triplegia G83.89
  congenital G80.8
Triplet (newborn) —see also Newborn, triplet
  complicating pregnancy —see Pregnancy,
    triplet
Triplication —see Accessory
Triploidy Q92.7
Trismus R25.2
  neonatorum A33
  newborn A33
Trisomy (syndrome) Q92.9
  13 (partial) Q91.7
    meiotic nondisjunction Q91.4
    mitotic nondisjunction Q91.5
    mosaicism Q91.5
    translocation Q91.6
  18 (partial) Q91.3
    meiotic nondisjunction Q91.0
    mitotic nondisjunction Q91.1
    mosaicism Q91.1
    translocation Q91.2
  20 Q92.8
  21 (partial) Q90.9
    meiotic nondisjunction Q90.0
    mitotic nondisjunction Q90.1
    mosaicism Q90.1
    translocation Q90.2
  22 Q92.8
  autosomes Q92.9
  chromosome specified NEC Q92.8
    partial Q92.2
      due to unbalanced translocation Q92.5
    specified NEC Q92.8
    whole (nonsex chromosome)
      meiotic nondisjunction Q92.0
      mitotic nondisjunction Q92.1
      mosaicism Q92.1
  due to
    dicentrics —see Extra, marker
      chromosomes
    extra rings —see Extra, marker
      chromosomes
    isochromosomes —see Extra, marker
      chromosomes
  specified NEC Q92.8
  whole chromosome Q92.9
    meiotic nondisjunction Q92.0
    mitotic nondisjunction Q92.1
    mosaicism Q92.1
    partial Q92.9
    specified NEC Q92.8
Tritanomaly, tritanopia H53.55
Trombiculosis, trombiculiasis, trombidiosis
  B88.0
Trophedema (congenital) (hereditary) Q82.0
Trophoblastic disease —see also Mole,
  hydatidiform O01.9
Tropholymphedema Q82.0
Trophoneurosis NEC G96.8
  disseminated M34.9
Tropical —see condition
Trouble —see also Disease
  heart —see Disease, heart
  kidney —see Disease, renal
  nervous R45.0
  sinus —see Sinusitis
Trousseau's syndrome (thrombophlebitis
  migrans) I82.1
Truancy, childhood
  from school Z72.810
Truncus
  arteriosus (persistent) Q20.0
  communis Q20.0
Trunk —see condition

Trypanosomiasis
  African B56.9
    by Trypanosoma brucei
      gambiense B56.0
      rhodesiense B56.1
    American —see Chagas' disease
    Brazilian —see Chagas' disease
    by Trypanosoma
      brucei gambiense B56.0
      brucei rhodesiense B56.1
      cruzi —see Chagas' disease
      gambiensis, Gambian B56.0
      rhodesiensis, Rhodesian B56.1
    South American —see Chagas' disease
    where
      African trypanosomiasis is prevalent B56.9
      Chagas' disease is prevalent B57.2
T-shaped incisors K00.2
Tsutsugamushi (disease) (fever) A75.3
Tube, tubal, tubular —see condition
Tubercle —see also Tuberculosis
  brain, solitary A17.81
  Darwin's Q17.8
  Ghon, primary infection A15.7
Tuberculid, tuberculide (indurating,
  subcutaneous) (lichenoid) (miliary)
  (papulonecrotic) (primary) (skin) A18.4
Tuberculoma —see also Tuberculosis
  brain A17.81
  meninges (cerebral) (spinal) A17.1
  spinal cord A17.81
Tuberculosis, tubercular, tuberculous
  (calcification) (calcified) (caseous)
  (chromogenic acid-fast bacilli)
  (degeneration) (fibrocaseous) (fistula)
  (interstitial) (isolated circumscribed
  lesions) (necrosis) (parenchymatous)
  (ulcerative) A15.9
  with pneumoconiosis (any condition in
    J60-J64) J65
  abdomen (lymph gland) A18.39
  abscess (respiratory) A15.9
    bone A18.03
      hip A18.02
      knee A18.02
      sacrum A18.01
      specified site NEC A18.03
      spinal A18.01
      vertebra A18.01
    brain A17.81
    breast A18.89
    Cowper's gland A18.15
    dura (mater) (cerebral) (spinal) A17.81
    epidural (cerebral) (spinal) A17.81
    female pelvis A18.17
    frontal sinus A15.8
    genital organs NEC A18.10
    genitourinary A18.10
    gland (lymphatic) —see Tuberculosis,
      lymph gland
    hip A18.02
    intestine A18.32
    ischiorectal A18.32
    joint NEC A18.02
      hip A18.02
      knee A18.02
      specified NEC A18.02
      vertebral A18.01
    kidney A18.11
    knee A18.02
    latent R76.11
    lumbar (spine) A18.01
    lung —see Tuberculosis, pulmonary
    meninges (cerebral) (spinal) A17.0
    muscle A18.09
    perianal (fistula) A18.32
    perinephritic A18.11
    perirectal A18.32
    rectum A18.32
    retropharyngeal A15.8
    sacrum A18.01

Tuberculosis, tubercular, tuberculous
  (Continued)
  abscess (Continued)
    scrofulous A18.2
    scrotum A18.15
    skin (primary) A18.4
    spinal cord A17.81
    spine or vertebra (column) A18.01
    subdiaphragmatic A18.31
    testis A18.15
    urinary A18.13
    uterus A18.17
  accessory sinus —see Tuberculosis, sinus
  Addison's disease A18.7
  adenitis —see Tuberculosis, lymph gland
  adenoids A15.8
  adenopathy —see Tuberculosis, lymph gland
  adherent pericardium A18.84
  adnexa (uteri) A18.17
  adrenal (capsule) (gland) A18.7
  alimentary canal A18.32
  anemia A18.89
  ankle (joint) (bone) A18.02
  anus A18.32
  apex, apical —see Tuberculosis, pulmonary
  appendicitis, appendix A18.32
  arachnoid A17.0
  artery, arteritis A18.89
    cerebral A18.89
  arthritis (chronic) (synovial) A18.02
    spine or vertebra (column) A18.01
  articular —see Tuberculosis, joint
  ascites A18.31
  asthma —see Tuberculosis, pulmonary
  axilla, axillary (gland) A18.2
  bladder A18.12
  bone A18.03
    hip A18.02
    knee A18.02
    limb NEC A18.03
    sacrum A18.01
    spine or vertebral column A18.01
  bowel (miliary) A18.32
  brain A17.81
  breast A18.89
  broad ligament A18.17
  bronchi, bronchial, bronchus A15.5
    ectasia, ectasis (bronchiectasis) —see
      Tuberculosis, pulmonary
    fistula A15.5
      primary (progressive) A15.7
    gland or node A15.4
      primary (progressive) A15.7
    lymph gland or node A15.4
      primary (progressive) A15.7
  bronchiectasis —see Tuberculosis, pulmonary
  bronchitis A15.5
  bronchopleural A15.6
  bronchopneumonia, bronchopneumonic —see
    Tuberculosis, pulmonary
  bronchorrhagia A15.5
  bronchotracheal A15.5
  bronze disease A18.7
  buccal cavity A18.83
  bulbourethral gland A18.15
  bursa A18.09
  cachexia A15.9
  cardiomyopathy A18.84
  caries —see Tuberculosis, bone
  cartilage A18.02
    intervertebral A18.01
  catarrhal —see Tuberculosis, respiratory
  cecum A18.32
  cellulitis (primary) A18.4
  cerebellum A17.81
  cerebral, cerebrum A17.81
  cerebrospinal A17.81
    meninges A17.0
  cervical (lymph gland or node) A18.2
  cervicitis, cervix (uteri) A18.16
  chest —see Tuberculosis, respiratory

◀ New   ◀▥ Revised   ~~deleted~~ Deleted

Tuberculosis, tubercular, tuberculous
(Continued)
chorioretinitis A18.53
choroid, choroiditis A18.53
ciliary body A18.54
colitis A18.32
collier's J65
colliquativa (primary) A18.4
colon A18.32
complex, primary A15.7
congenital P37.0
conjunctiva A18.59
connective tissue (systemic) A18.89
contact Z20.1
cornea (ulcer) A18.52
Cowper's gland A18.15
coxae A18.02
coxalgia A18.02
cul-de-sac of Douglas A18.17
curvature, spine A18.01
cutis (colliquativa) (primary) A18.4
cyst, ovary A18.18
cystitis A18.12
dactylitis A18.03
diarrhea A18.32
diffuse —see Tuberculosis, miliary
digestive tract A18.32
disseminated —see Tuberculosis, miliary
duodenum A18.32
dura (mater) (cerebral) (spinal) A17.0
    abscess (cerebral) (spinal) A17.81
dysentery A18.32
ear (inner) (middle) A18.6
    bone A18.03
    external (primary) A18.4
    skin (primary) A18.4
elbow A18.02
emphysema —see Tuberculosis, pulmonary
empyema A15.6
encephalitis A17.82
endarteritis A18.89
endocarditis A18.84
    aortic A18.84
    mitral A18.84
    pulmonary A18.84
    tricuspid A18.84
endocrine glands NEC A18.82
endometrium A18.17
enteric, enterica, enteritis A18.32
enterocolitis A18.32
epididymis, epididymitis A18.15
epidural abscess (cerebral) (spinal) A17.81
epiglottis A15.5
episcleritis A18.51
erythema (induratum) (nodosum) (primary)
    A18.4
esophagus A18.83
eustachian tube A18.6
exposure (to) Z20.1
exudative —see Tuberculosis, pulmonary
eye A18.50
eyelid (primary) (lupus) A18.4
fallopian tube (acute) (chronic) A18.17
fascia A18.09
fauces A15.8
female pelvic inflammatory disease A18.17
finger A18.03
first infection A15.7
gallbladder A18.83
ganglion A18.09
gastritis A18.83
gastrocolic fistula A18.32
gastroenteritis A18.32
gastrointestinal tract A18.32
general, generalized —see Tuberculosis,
    miliary
genital organs A18.10
genitourinary A18.10
genu A18.02
glandula suprarenalis A18.7
glandular, general A18.2

Tuberculosis, tubercular, tuberculous
(Continued)
glottis A15.5
grinder's J65
gum A18.83
hand A18.03
heart A18.84
hematogenous —see Tuberculosis, miliary
hemoptysis —see Tuberculosis, pulmonary
hemorrhage NEC —see Tuberculosis,
    pulmonary
hemothorax A15.6
hepatitis A18.83
hilar lymph nodes A15.4
    primary (progressive) A15.7
hip (joint) (disease) (bone) A18.02
hydropneumothorax A15.6
hydrothorax A15.6
hypoadrenalism A18.7
hypopharynx A15.8
ileocecal (hyperplastic) A18.32
ileocolitis A18.32
ileum A18.32
iliac spine (superior) A18.03
immunological findings only A15.7
indurativa (primary) A18.4
infantile A15.7
infection A15.9
    without clinical manifestations A15.7
infraclavicular gland A18.2
inguinal gland A18.2
inguinalis A18.2
intestine (any part) A18.32
iridocyclitis A18.54
iris, iritis A18.54
ischiorectal A18.32
jaw A18.03
jejunum A18.32
joint A18.02
    vertebral A18.01
keratitis (interstitial) A18.52
keratoconjunctivitis A18.52
kidney A18.11
knee (joint) A18.02
kyphosis, kyphoscoliosis A18.01
laryngitis A15.5
larynx A15.5
latent R76.11
leptomeninges, leptomeningitis (cerebral)
    (spinal) A17.0
lichenoides (primary) A18.4
linguae A18.83
lip A18.83
liver A18.83
lordosis A18.01
lung —see Tuberculosis, pulmonary
lupus vulgaris A18.4
lymph gland or node (peripheral) A18.2
    abdomen A18.39
    bronchial A15.4
        primary (progressive) A15.7
    cervical A18.2
    hilar A15.4
        primary (progressive) A15.7
    intrathoracic A15.4
        primary (progressive) A15.7
    mediastinal A15.4
        primary (progressive) A15.7
    mesenteric A18.39
    retroperitoneal A18.39
    tracheobronchial A15.4
        primary (progressive) A15.7
lymphadenitis —see Tuberculosis, lymph
    gland
lymphangitis —see Tuberculosis, lymph
    gland
lymphatic (gland) (vessel) —see Tuberculosis,
    lymph gland
mammary gland A18.89
marasmus A15.9
mastoiditis A18.03

Tuberculosis, tubercular, tuberculous
(Continued)
mediastinal lymph gland or node
    A15.4
    primary (progressive) A15.7
mediastinitis A15.8
    primary (progressive) A15.7
mediastinum A15.8
    primary (progressive) A15.7
medulla A17.81
melanosis, Addisonian A18.7
meninges, meningitis (basilar) (cerebral)
    (cerebrospinal) (spinal) A17.0
meningoencephalitis A17.82
mesentery, mesenteric (gland or node)
    A18.39
miliary A19.9
    acute A19.2
        multiple sites A19.1
        single specified site A19.0
    chronic A19.8
    specified NEC A19.8
millstone makers' J65
miner's J65
molder's J65
mouth A18.83
multiple A19.9
    acute A19.1
    chronic A19.8
muscle A18.09
myelitis A17.82
myocardium, myocarditis A18.84
nasal (passage) (sinus) A15.8
nasopharynx A15.8
neck gland A18.2
nephritis A18.11
nerve (mononeuropathy) A17.83
nervous system A17.9
nose (septum) A15.8
ocular A18.50
omentum A18.31
oophoritis (acute) (chronic) A18.17
optic (nerve trunk) (papilla) A18.59
orbit A18.59
orchitis A18.15
organ, specified NEC A18.89
osseous —see Tuberculosis, bone
osteitis —see Tuberculosis, bone
osteomyelitis —see Tuberculosis, bone
otitis media A18.6
ovary, ovaritis (acute) (chronic) A18.17
oviduct (acute) (chronic) A18.17
pachymeningitis A17.0
palate (soft) A18.83
pancreas A18.83
papulonecrotic (a) (primary) A18.4
parathyroid glands A18.82
paronychia (primary) A18.4
parotid gland or region A18.83
pelvis (bony) A18.03
penis A18.15
peribronchitis A15.5
pericardium, pericarditis A18.84
perichondritis, larynx A15.5
periostitis —see Tuberculosis, bone
perirectal fistula A18.32
peritoneum NEC A18.31
peritonitis A18.31
pharynx, pharyngitis A15.8
phlyctenulosis (keratoconjunctivitis) A18.52
phthisis NEC —see Tuberculosis, pulmonary
pituitary gland A18.82
pleura, pleural, pleurisy, pleuritis (fibrinous)
    (obliterative) (purulent) (simple plastic)
    (with effusion) A15.6
    primary (progressive) A15.7
pneumonia, pneumonic —see Tuberculosis,
    pulmonary
pneumothorax (spontaneous) (tense
    valvular) —see Tuberculosis, pulmonary
polyneuropathy A17.89

Tuberculosis, tubercular, tuberculous
(Continued)
polyserositis A19.9
acute A19.1
chronic A19.8
potter's J65
prepuce A18.15
primary (complex) A15.7
proctitis A18.32
prostate, prostatitis A18.14
pulmonalis —see Tuberculosis, pulmonary
pulmonary (cavitated) (fibrotic) (infiltrative)
(nodular) A15.0
childhood type or first infection A15.7
primary (complex) A15.7
pyelitis A18.11
pyelonephritis A18.11
pyemia —see Tuberculosis, miliary
pyonephrosis A18.11
pyopneumothorax A15.6
pyothorax A15.6
rectum (fistula) (with abscess) A18.32
reinfection stage —see Tuberculosis,
pulmonary
renal A18.11
renis A18.11
respiratory A15.9
primary A15.7
specified site NEC A15.8
retina, retinitis A18.53
retroperitoneal (lymph gland or node)
A18.39
rheumatism NEC A18.09
rhinitis A15.8
sacroiliac (joint) A18.01
sacrum A18.01
salivary gland A18.83
salpingitis (acute) (chronic) A18.17
sandblaster's J65
sclera A18.51
scoliosis A18.01
scrofulous A18.2
scrotum A18.15
seminal tract or vesicle A18.15
senile A15.9
septic —see Tuberculosis, miliary
shoulder (joint) A18.02
blade A18.03
sigmoid A18.32
sinus (any nasal) A15.8
bone A18.03
epididymis A18.15
skeletal NEC A18.03
skin (any site) (primary) A18.4
small intestine A18.32
soft palate A18.83
spermatic cord A18.15
spine, spinal (column) A18.01
cord A17.81
medulla A17.81
membrane A17.0
meninges A17.0
spleen, splenitis A18.85
spondylitis A18.01
sternoclavicular joint A18.02
stomach A18.83
stonemason's J65
subcutaneous tissue (cellular) (primary)
A18.4
subcutis (primary) A18.4
subdeltoid bursa A18.83
submaxillary (region) A18.83
supraclavicular gland A18.2
suprarenal (capsule) (gland) A18.7
swelling, joint —see also category M01 (see also
Tuberculosis, joint) A18.02
symphysis pubis A18.02
synovitis A18.09
articular A18.02
spine or vertebra A18.01
systemic —see Tuberculosis, miliary

Tuberculosis, tubercular, tuberculous
(Continued)
tarsitis A18.4
tendon (sheath) —see Tuberculosis,
tenosynovitis
tenosynovitis A18.09
spine or vertebra A18.01
testis A18.15
throat A15.8
thymus gland A18.82
thyroid gland A18.81
tongue A18.83
tonsil, tonsillitis A15.8
trachea, tracheal A15.5
lymph gland or node A15.4
primary (progressive) A15.7
tracheobronchial A15.5
lymph gland or node A15.4
primary (progressive) A15.7
tubal (acute) (chronic) A18.17
tunica vaginalis A18.15
ulcer (skin) (primary) A18.4
bowel or intestine A18.32
specified NEC - code under Tuberculosis,
by site
unspecified site A15.9
ureter A18.11
urethra, urethral (gland) A18.13
urinary organ or tract A18.13
uterus A18.17
uveal tract A18.54
uvula A18.83
vagina A18.18
vas deferens A18.15
verruca, verrucosa (cutis) (primary) A18.4
vertebra (column) A18.01
vesiculitis A18.15
vulva A18.18
wrist (joint) A18.02
Tuberculum
Carabelli —see Note at K00.2
occlusal —see Note at K00.2
paramolare K00.2
Tuberosity, enitre maxillary M26.07
Tuberous sclerosis (brain) Q85.1
Tubo-ovarian —see condition
Tuboplasty, after previous sterilization
Z31.0
aftercare Z31.42
Tubotympanitis, catarrhal (chronic) —see Otitis,
media, nonsuppurative, chronic, serous
Tularemia A21.9
with
conjunctivitis A21.1
pneumonia A21.2
abdominal A21.3
bronchopneumonic A21.2
conjunctivitis A21.1
cryptogenic A21.3
enteric A21.3
gastrointestinal A21.3
generalized A21.7
ingestion A21.3
intestinal A21.3
oculoglandular A21.1
ophthalmic A21.1
pneumonia (any), pneumonic A21.2
pulmonary A21.2
sepsis A21.7
specified NEC A21.8
typhoidal A21.7
ulceroglandular A21.0
Tularensis conjunctivitis A21.1
Tumefaction —see also Swelling
liver —see Hypertrophy, liver
Tumor —see also Neoplasm, unspecified
behavior, by site
acinar cell —see Neoplasm, uncertain
behavior, by site
acinic cell —see Neoplasm, uncertain
behavior, by site

Tumor (Continued)
adenocarcinoid —see Neoplasm, malignant,
by site
adenomatoid —see also Neoplasm, benign,
by site
odontogenic —see Cyst, calcifying
odontogenic
adnexal (skin) —see Neoplasm, skin, benign,
by site
adrenal
cortical (benign) D35.0-
malignant C74.0-
rest —see Neoplasm, benign, by site
alpha-cell
malignant
pancreas C25.4
specified site NEC —see Neoplasm,
malignant, by site
unspecified site C25.4
pancreas D13.7
specified site NEC —see Neoplasm, benign,
by site
unspecified site D13.7
aneurysmal —see Aneurysm
aortic body D44.7
malignant C75.5
Askin's —see Neoplasm, connective tissue,
malignant
basal cell —see also Neoplasm, skin, uncertain
behavior D48.5
Bednar —see Neoplasm, skin, malignant
benign (unclassified) —see Neoplasm, benign,
by site
beta-cell
malignant
pancreas C25.4
specified site NEC —see Neoplasm,
malignant, by site
unspecified site C25.4
pancreas D13.7
specified site NEC —see Neoplasm, benign,
by site
unspecified site D13.7
Brenner D27.9
borderline malignancy D39.1-
malignant C56-
proliferating D39.1
bronchial alveolar, intravascular D38.1
Brooke's —see Neoplasm, skin, benign
brown fat —see Lipoma
Burkitt —see Lymphoma, Burkitt
calcifying epithelial odontogenic —see Cyst,
calcifying odontogenic
carcinoid
benign D3A.00
appendix D3A.020
ascending colon D3A.022
bronchus (lung) D3A.090
cecum D3A.021
colon D3A.029
descending colon D3A.024
duodenum D3A.010
foregut NOS D3A.094
hindgut NOS D3A.096
ileum D3A.012
jejunum D3A.011
kidney D3A.093
large intestine D3A.029
lung (bronchus) D3A.090
midgut NOS D3A.095
rectum D3A.026
sigmoid colon D3A.025
small intestine D3A.019
specified NEC D3A.098
stomach D3A.092
thymus D3A.091
transverse colon D3A.023
malignant C7A.00
appendix C7A.020
ascending colon C7A.022
bronchus (lung) C7A.090

◀ New   ◀|||| Revised   ~~deleted~~ Deleted

Tumor *(Continued)*
  carcinoid *(Continued)*
    malignant *(Continued)*
      cecum C7A.021
      colon C7A.029
      descending colon C7A.024
      duodenum C7A.010
      foregut NOS C7A.094
      hindgut NOS C7A.096
      ileum C7A.012
      jejunum C7A.011
      kidney C7A.093
      large intestine C7A.029
      lung (bronchus) C7A.090
      midgut NOS C7A.095
      rectum C7A.026
      sigmoid colon C7A.025
      small intestine C7A.019
      specified NEC C7A.098
      stomach C7A.092
      thymus C7A.091
      transverse colon C7A.023
    mesentary metastasis C7B.04
    secondary C7B.00
      bone C7B.03
      distant lymph nodes C7B.01
      liver C7B.02
      peritoneum C7B.04
      specified NEC C7B.09
  carotid body D44.6
    malignant C75.4
  cells —*see also* Neoplasm, unspecified behavior, by site
    benign —*see* Neoplasm, benign, by site
    malignant —*see* Neoplasm, malignant, by site
    uncertain whether benign or malignant —*see* Neoplasm, uncertain behavior, by site
  cervix, in pregnancy or childbirth —*see* Pregnancy, complicated by, tumor, cervix
  chondromatous giant cell —*see* Neoplasm, bone, benign
  chromaffin —*see also* Neoplasm, benign, by site
    malignant —*see* Neoplasm, malignant, by site
  Cock's peculiar L72.3
  Codman's —*see* Neoplasm, bone, benign
  dentigerous, mixed —*see* Cyst, calcifying odontogenic
  dermoid —*see* Neoplasm, benign, by site
    with malignant transformation C56-
  desmoid (extra-abdominal) —*see also* Neoplasm, connective tissue, uncertain behavior
    abdominal —*see* Neoplasm, connective tissue, uncertain behavior
  embolus —*see* Neoplasm, secondary, by site
  embryonal (mixed) —*see also* Neoplasm, uncertain behavior, by site
    liver C22.7
  endodermal sinus
    specified site —*see* Neoplasm, malignant, by site
    unspecified site
      female C56.-
      male C62.90
  epithelial
    benign —*see* Neoplasm, benign, by site
    malignant —*see* Neoplasm, malignant, by site
  Ewing's —*see* Neoplasm, bone, malignant, by site
  fatty —*see* Lipoma
  fibroid —*see* Leiomyoma

Tumor *(Continued)*
  G cell
    malignant
      pancreas C25.4
      specified site NEC —*see* Neoplasm, malignant, by site
      unspecified site C25.4
    specified site —*see* Neoplasm, uncertain behavior, by site
    unspecified site D37.8
  germ cell —*see also* Neoplasm, malignant, by site
    mixed —*see* Neoplasm, malignant, by site
  ghost cell, odontogenic —*see* Cyst, calcifying odontogenic
  giant cell —*see also* Neoplasm, uncertain behavior, by site
    bone D48.0
      malignant —*see* Neoplasm, bone, malignant
    chondromatous —*see* Neoplasm, bone, benign
    malignant —*see* Neoplasm, malignant, by site
    soft parts —*see* Neoplasm, connective tissue, uncertain behavior
      malignant —*see* Neoplasm, connective tissue, malignant
  glomus D18.00
    intra-abdominal D18.03
    intracranial D18.02
    jugulare D44.7
      malignant C75.5
    skin D18.01
    specified site NEC D18.09
  gonadal stromal —*see* Neoplasm, uncertain behavior, by site
  granular cell —*see also* Neoplasm, connective tissue, benign
    malignant —*see* Neoplasm, connective tissue, malignant
  granulosa cell D39.1-
    juvenile D39.1-
    malignant C56-
  granulosa cell-theca cell D39.1-
    malignant C56-
  Grawitz's C64-
  hemorrhoidal —*see* Hemorrhoids
  hilar cell D27-
  hilus cell D27-
  Hurthle cell (benign) D34
    malignant C73
  hydatid —*see* Echinococcus
  hypernephroid —*see also* Neoplasm, uncertain behavior, by site
  interstitial cell —*see also* Neoplasm, uncertain behavior, by site
    benign —*see* Neoplasm, benign, by site
    malignant —*see* Neoplasm, malignant, by site
  intravascular bronchial alveolar D38.1
  islet cell —*see* Neoplasm, benign, by site
    malignant —*see* Neoplasm, malignant, by site
      pancreas C25.4
      specified site NEC —*see* Neoplasm, malignant, by site
      unspecified site C25.4
    pancreas D13.7
    specified site NEC —*see* Neoplasm, benign, by site
    unspecified site D13.7
  juxtaglomerular D41.0-
  Klatskin's C24.0
  Krukenberg's C79.6-
  Leydig cell —*see* Neoplasm, uncertain behavior, by site
    benign —*see* Neoplasm, benign, by site
      specified site —*see* Neoplasm, benign, by site

Tumor *(Continued)*
  Leydig cell *(Continued)*
    benign *(Continued)*
      unspecified site
        female D27.9
        male D29.20
    malignant —*see* Neoplasm, malignant, by site
      specified site —*see* Neoplasm, malignant, by site
      unspecified site
        female C56.9
        male C62.90
    specified site —*see* Neoplasm, uncertain behavior, by site
    unspecified site
      female D39.10
      male D40.10
  lipid cell, ovary D27-
  lipoid cell, ovary D27-
  malignant —*see also* Neoplasm, malignant, by site C80.1
    fusiform cell (type) C80.1
    giant cell (type) C80.1
    localized, plasma cell —*see* Plasmacytoma, solitary
    mixed NEC C80.1
    small cell (type) C80.1
    spindle cell (type) C80.1
    unclassified C80.1
  mast cell D47.0
    malignant C96.2
  melanotic, neuroectodermal —*see* Neoplasm, benign, by site
  Merkel cell —*see* Carcinoma, Merkel cell
  mesenchymal
    malignant —*see* Neoplasm, connective tissue, malignant
    mixed —*see* Neoplasm, connective tissue, uncertain behavior
  mesodermal, mixed —*see also* Neoplasm, malignant, by site
    liver C22.4
  mesonephric —*see also* Neoplasm, uncertain behavior, by site
    malignant —*see* Neoplasm, malignant, by site
  metastatic
    from specified site —*see* Neoplasm, malignant, by site
    of specified site —*see* Neoplasm, malignant, by site
    to specified site —*see* Neoplasm, secondary, by site
  mixed NEC —*see also* Neoplasm, benign, by site
    malignant —*see* Neoplasm, malignant, by site
  mucinous of low malignant potential
    specified site —*see* Neoplasm, malignant, by site
    unspecified site C56.9
  mucocarcinoid
    specified site —*see* Neoplasm, malignant, by site
    unspecified site C18.1
  mucoepidermoid —*see* Neoplasm, uncertain behavior, by site
  Müllerian, mixed
    specified site —*see* Neoplasm, malignant, by site
    unspecified site C54.9
  myoepithelial —*see* Neoplasm, benign, by site
  neuroectodermal (peripheral) —*see* Neoplasm, malignant, by site
  primitive
    specified site —*see* Neoplasm, malignant, by site
    unspecified site C71.9

Tumor (Continued)
 neuroendocrine D3A.8
  malignant poorly differentiated C7A.1
  secondary NEC C7B.8
  specified NEC C7A.8
 neurogenic olfactory C30.0
 nonencapsulated sclerosing C73
 odontogenic (adenomatoid) (benign)
     (calcifying epithelial) (keratocystic)
     (squamous) —see Cyst, calcifying
     odontogenic
  malignant C41.1
   upper jaw (bone) C41.0
 ovarian stromal D39.1-
 ovary, in pregnancy —see Pregnancy,
     complicated by
 pacinian —see Neoplasm, skin, benign
 Pancoast's —see Pancoast's syndrome
 papillary —see also Papilloma
  cystic D37.9
   mucinous of low malignant potential C56-
    specified site —see Neoplasm,
       malignant, by site
    unspecified site C56.9
   serous of low malignant potential
    specified site —see Neoplasm,
       malignant, by site
    unspecified site C56.9
 pelvic, in pregnancy or childbirth —see
     Pregnancy, complicated by
 phantom F45.8
 phyllodes D48.6-
  benign D24-
  malignant —see Neoplasm, breast,
     malignant
 Pindborg —see Cyst, calcifying odontogenic
 placental site trophoblastic D39.2
 plasma cell (malignant) (localized) —see
     Plasmacytoma, solitary
 polyvesicular vitelline
  specified site —see Neoplasm, malignant,
     by site
  unspecified site
   female C56.9
   male C62.90
 Pott's puffy —see Osteomyelitis, specified
     NEC
 Rathke's pouch D44.3
 retinal anlage —see Neoplasm, benign, by site
 salivary gland type, mixed —see Neoplasm,
     salivary gland, benign
  malignant —see Neoplasm, salivary gland,
     malignant
 Sampson's N80.1
 Schmincke's —see Neoplasm, nasopharynx,
     malignant
 sclerosing stromal D27-
 sebaceous —see Cyst, sebaceous
 secondary —see Neoplasm, secondary, by site
  carcinoid C7B.00
   bone C7B.03
   distant lymph nodes C7B.01
   liver C7B.02
   peritoneum C7B.04
   specified NEC C7B.09
  neuroendocrine NEC C7B.8
 serous of low malignant potential
  specified site —see Neoplasm, malignant,
     by site
  unspecified site C56.9
 Sertoli cell —see Neoplasm, benign, by site
  with lipid storage
   specified site —see Neoplasm, benign,
      by site
   unspecified site
    female D27.9
    male D29.20
  specified site —see Neoplasm, benign, by site
  unspecified site
   female D27.9
   male D29.20

Tumor (Continued)
 Sertoli-Leydig cell —see Neoplasm, benign,
     by site
  specified site —see Neoplasm, benign, by
     site
  unspecified site
   female D27.9
   male D29.20
 sex cord(-stromal) —see Neoplasm, uncertain
     behavior, by site
  with annular tubules D39.1-
 skin appendage —see Neoplasm, skin,
     benign
 smooth muscle —see Neoplasm, connective
     tissue, uncertain behavior
 soft tissue
  benign —see Neoplasm, connective tissue,
     benign
  malignant —see Neoplasm, connective
     tissue, malignant
 sternomastoid (congenital) Q68.0
 stromal
  endometrial D39.0
  gastric D48.1
   benign D21.4
   malignant C16.9
   uncertain behavior D48.1
  gastrointestinal C49.A- ◀▥
   benign D21.4
   esophagus C49.A1 ◀
   large intestine C49.A4 ◀
   malignant C49.A0 ◀▥
    colon C49.A4 ◀
    duodenum C49.A3 ◀
    esophagus C49.A1 ◀
    ileum C49.A3 ◀
    jejunum C49.A3 ◀
    Meckel diverticulum C49.A3 ◀
    large intestine C49.A4 ◀
    omentum C49.A9 ◀
    peritoneum C49.A9 ◀
    rectum C49.A5 ◀
    small intestine C49.A3 ◀
    specified site NEC C49.A9 ◀
    stomach C49.A2 ◀
   large intestine C49.A4 ◀
   rectum C49.A5 ◀
   small intestine C49.A3 ◀
   specified site NEC C49.A9 ◀
   stomach C49.A2 ◀
   uncertain behavior D48.1
  intestine
   benign D21.4
   malignant ◀▥
    large C49.A4 ◀
    small C49.A3 ◀
   uncertain behavior D48.1
  ovarian D39.1-
  stomach C49.A2 ◀▥
   benign D21.4
   malignant C49.A2 ◀▥
   uncertain behavior D48.1
 sweat gland —see also Neoplasm, skin,
     uncertain behavior
  benign —see Neoplasm, skin, benign
  malignant —see Neoplasm, skin, malignant
 syphilitic, brain A52.17
 testicular D40.10
 testicular stromal D40.1-
 theca cell D27.-
 theca cell-granulosa cell D39.1-
 Triton, malignant —see Neoplasm, nerve,
     malignant
 trophoblastic, placental site D39.2
 turban D23.4
 uterus (body), in pregnancy or childbirth —
     see Pregnancy, complicated by, tumor,
     uterus
 vagina, in pregnancy or childbirth —see
     Pregnancy, complicated by
 varicose —see Varix

Tumor (Continued)
 von Recklinghausen's —see
     Neurofibromatosis
 vulva or perineum, in pregnancy or
     childbirth —see Pregnancy, complicated
     by
  causing obstructed labor O65.5
 Warthin's —see Neoplasm, salivary gland,
     benign
 Wilms' C64-
  yolk sac —see Neoplasm, malignant, by site
   specified site —see Neoplasm, malignant,
      by site
   unspecified site
    female C56.9
    male C62.90
Tumor lysis syndrome (following
    antineoplastic chemotherapy)
    (spontaneous) NEC E88.3
Tumorlet —see Neoplasm, uncertain behavior,
    by site
Tungiasis B88.1
Tunica vasculosa lentis Q12.2
Turban tumor D23.4
Türck's trachoma J37.0
Turner-Kieser syndrome Q87.2 ◀▥
Turner-like syndrome Q87.1
Turner's
 hypoplasia (tooth) K00.4
 syndrome Q96.9
  specified NEC Q96.8
 tooth K00.4
Turner-Ullrich syndrome Q96.9
Tussis convulsiva —see Whooping cough
Twiddler's syndrome (due to)
 automatic implantable defibrillator T82.198
 cardiac pacemaker T82.198
Twilight state
 epileptic F05
 psychogenic F44.89
Twin (newborn) —see also Newborn, twin
 conjoined Q89.4
 pregnancy —see Pregnancy, twin, conjoined
Twinning, teeth K00.2
Twist, twisted
 bowel, colon or intestine K56.2
 hair (congenital) Q84.1
 mesentery K56.2
 omentum K56.2
 organ or site, congenital NEC —see Anomaly,
     by site
 ovarian pedicle —see Torsion, ovary
Twitching R25.3
Tylosis (acquired) L84
 buccalis K13.29
 linguae K13.29
 palmaris et plantaris (congenital) (inherited)
     Q82.8
  acquired L85.1
Tympanism R14.0
Tympanites (abdominal) (intestinal) R14.0
Tympanitis —see Myringitis
Tympanosclerosis —see subcategory H74.0
Tympanum —see condition
Tympany
 abdomen R14.0
 chest R09.89
Type A behavior pattern Z73.1
Typhlitis —see Appendicitis
Typhoenteritis —see Typhoid
Typhoid (abortive) (ambulant) (any site)
     (clinical) (fever) (hemorrhagic) (infection)
     (intermittent) (malignant) (rheumatic)
     (Widal negative) A01.00
 with pneumonia A01.03
 abdominal A01.09
 arthritis A01.04
 carrier (suspected) of Z22.0
 cholecystitis (current) A01.09
 endocarditis A01.02
 heart involvement A01.02

◀ New   ◀▥ Revised   ~~deleted~~ Deleted

Typhoid (*Continued*)
  inoculation reaction —*see* Complications, vaccination
  meningitis A01.01
  mesenteric lymph nodes A01.09
  myocarditis A01.02
  osteomyelitis A01.05
  perichondritis, larynx A01.09
  pneumonia A01.03
  specified NEC A01.09
  spine A01.05
  ulcer (perforating) A01.09
Typhomalaria (fever) —*see* Malaria
Typhomania A01.00
Typhoperitonitis A01.09
Typhus (fever) A75.9
  abdominal, abdominalis —*see* Typhoid
  African tick A77.1
  amarillic A95.9
  brain A75.9 [G94]

Typhus (*Continued*)
  cerebral A75.9 [G94]
  classical A75.0
  due to Rickettsia
    prowazekii A75.0
      recrudescent A75.1
    tsutsugamushi A75.3
    typhi A75.2
  endemic (flea-borne) A75.2
  epidemic (louse-borne) A75.0
  exanthematic NEC A75.0
  exanthematicus SAI A75.0
    brillii SAI A75.1
    mexicanus SAI A75.2
    typhus murinus A75.2
  flea-borne A75.2
  India tick A77.1
  Kenya (tick) A77.1
  louse-borne A75.0
  Mexican A75.2

Typhus (*Continued*)
  mite-borne A75.3
  murine A75.2
  North Asian tick-borne A77.2
  petechial A75.9
  Queensland tick A77.3
  rat A75.2
  recrudescent A75.1
  recurrens —*see* Fever, relapsing
  Sao Paulo A77.0
  scrub (China) (India) (Malaysia) (New Guinea) A75.3
  shop (of Malaysia) A75.2
  Siberian tick A77.2
  tick-borne A77.9
  tropical (mite-borne) A75.3
Tyrosinemia E70.21
  newborn, transitory P74.5
Tyrosinosis E70.21
Tyrosinuria E70.29

U

Uhl's anomaly or disease Q24.8
Ulcer, ulcerated, ulcerating, ulceration, ulcerative
  alveolar process M27.3
  amebic (intestine) A06.1
    skin A06.7
  anastomotic —see Ulcer, gastrojejunal
  anorectal K62.6
  antral —see Ulcer, stomach
  anus (sphincter) (solitary) K62.6
  aorta —see Aneurysm
  aphthous (oral) (recurrent) K12.0
    genital organ (s)
      female N76.6
      male N50.89 ◀▥
  artery I77.2
  atrophic —see Ulcer, skin
    decubitus —see Ulcer, pressure, by site
  back L98.429
    with
      bone necrosis L98.424
      exposed fat layer L98.422
      muscle necrosis L98.423
      skin breakdown only L98.421
  Barrett's (esophagus) K22.10
    with bleeding K22.11
  bile duct (common) (hepatic) K83.8
  bladder (solitary) (sphincter) NEC N32.89
    bilharzial B65.9 [N33]
    in schistosomiasis (bilharzial) B65.9 [N33]
    submucosal —see Cystitis, interstitial
    tuberculous A18.12
  bleeding K27.4
  bone —see Osteomyelitis, specified type NEC
  bowel —see Ulcer, intestine
  breast N61.1 ◀▥
  bronchus J98.09
  buccal (cavity) (traumatic) K12.1
  Buruli A31.1
  buttock L98.419
    with
      bone necrosis L98.414
      exposed fat layer L98.412
      muscle necrosis L98.413
      skin breakdown only L98.411
  cancerous —see Neoplasm, malignant, by site
  cardia K22.10
    with bleeding K22.11
  cardioesophageal (peptic) K22.10
    with bleeding K22.11
  cecum —see Ulcer, intestine
  cervix (uteri) (decubitus) (trophic) N86
    with cervicitis N72
  chancroidal A57
  chiclero B55.1
  chronic (cause unknown) —see Ulcer, skin
  Cochin-China B55.1
  colon —see Ulcer, intestine
  conjunctiva H10.89
  cornea H16.00-
    with hypopyon H16.03-
    central H16.01-
    dendritic (herpes simplex) B00.52
    marginal H16.04-
    Mooren's H16.05-
    mycotic H16.06-
    perforated H16.07-
    ring H16.02-
    tuberculous (phlyctenular) A18.52
  corpus cavernosum (chronic) N48.5
  crural —see Ulcer, lower limb
  Curling's —see Ulcer, peptic, acute
  Cushing's —see Ulcer, peptic, acute
  cystic duct K82.8
  cystitis (interstitial) —see Cystitis, interstitial
  decubitus —see Ulcer, pressure, by site
  dendritic, cornea (herpes simplex) B00.52
  diabetes, diabetic —see Diabetes, ulcer
  Dieulafoy's K25.0

Ulcer, ulcerated, ulcerating, ulceration, ulcerative (Continued)
  due to
    infection NEC —see Ulcer, skin
    radiation NEC L59.8
    trophic disturbance (any region) —see Ulcer, skin
    X-ray L58.1
  duodenum, duodenal (eroded) (peptic) K26.9
    with
      hemorrhage K26.4
        and perforation K26.6
      perforation K26.5
    acute K26.3
      with
        hemorrhage K26.0
          and perforation K26.2
        perforation K26.1
    chronic K26.7
      with
        hemorrhage K26.4
          and perforation K26.6
        perforation K26.5
  dysenteric A09
  elusive —see Cystitis, interstitial
  endocarditis (acute) (chronic) (subacute) I28.8
  epiglottis J38.7
  esophagus (peptic) K22.10
    with bleeding K22.11
    due to
      aspirin K22.10
        with bleeding K22.11
      gastrointestinal reflux disease K21.0
      ingestion of chemical or medicament K22.10
        with bleeding K22.11
    fungal K22.10
      with bleeding K22.11
    infective K22.10
      with bleeding K22.11
    varicose —see Varix, esophagus
  eyelid (region) H01.8
  fauces J39.2
  Fenwick (-Hunner) (solitary) —see Cystitis, interstitial
  fistulous —see Ulcer, skin
  foot (indolent) (trophic) —see Ulcer, lower limb
  frambesial, initial A66.0
  frenum (tongue) K14.0
  gallbladder or duct K82.8
  gangrenous —see Gangrene
  gastric —see Ulcer, stomach
  gastrocolic —see Ulcer, gastrojejunal
  gastroduodenal —see Ulcer, peptic
  gastroesophageal —see Ulcer, stomach
  gastrointestinal —see Ulcer, gastrojejunal
  gastrojejunal (peptic) K28.9
    with
      hemorrhage K28.4
        and perforation K28.6
      perforation K28.5
    acute K28.3
      with
        hemorrhage K28.0
          and perforation K28.2
        perforation K28.1
    chronic K28.7
      with
        hemorrhage K28.4
          and perforation K28.6
        perforation K28.5
  gastrojejunocolic —see Ulcer, gastrojejunal
  gingiva K06.8
  gingivitis K05.10
    nonplaque induced K05.11
    plaque induced K05.10
  glottis J38.7
  granuloma of pudenda A58
  gum K06.8
  gumma, due to yaws A66.4

Ulcer, ulcerated, ulcerating, ulceration, ulcerative (Continued)
  heel —see Ulcer, lower limb
  hemorrhoid —see also Hemorrhoids, by degree K64.8
  Hunner's —see Cystitis, interstitial
  hypopharynx J39.2
  hypopyon (chronic) (subacute) —see Ulcer, cornea, with hypopyon
  hypostaticum —see Ulcer, varicose
  ileum —see Ulcer, intestine
  intestine, intestinal K63.3
    with perforation K63.1
    amebic A06.1
    duodenal —see Ulcer, duodenum
    granulocytopenic (with hemorrhage) —see Neutropenia
    marginal —see Ulcer, gastrojejunal
    perforating K63.1
      newborn P78.0
    primary, small intestine K63.3
    rectum K62.6
    stercoraceous, stercoral K63.3
    tuberculous A18.32
    typhoid (fever) —see Typhoid
    varicose I86.8
  jejunum, jejunal —see Ulcer, gastrojejunal
  keratitis —see Ulcer, cornea
  knee —see Ulcer, lower limb
  labium (majus) (minus) N76.6
  laryngitis —see Laryngitis
  larynx (aphthous) (contact) J38.7
    diphtheritic A36.2
  leg —see Ulcer, lower limb
  lip K13.0
  Lipschütz's N76.6
  lower limb (atrophic) (chronic) (neurogenic) (perforating) (pyogenic) (trophic) (tropical) L97.909
    with
      bone necrosis L97.904
      exposed fat layer L97.902
      muscle necrosis L97.903
      skin breakdown only L97.901
    ankle L97.309
      with
        bone necrosis L97.304
        exposed fat layer L97.302
        muscle necrosis L97.303
        skin breakdown only L97.301
      left L97.329
        with
          bone necrosis L97.324
          exposed fat layer L97.322
          muscle necrosis L97.323
          skin breakdown only L97.321
      right L97.319
        with
          bone necrosis L97.314
          exposed fat layer L97.312
          muscle necrosis L97.313
          skin breakdown only L97.311
    calf L97.209
      with
        bone necrosis L97.204
        exposed fat layer L97.202
        muscle necrosis L97.203
        skin breakdown only L97.201
      left L97.229
        with
          bone necrosis L97.224
          exposed fat layer L97.222
          muscle necrosis L97.223
          skin breakdown only L97.221
      right L97.219
        with
          bone necrosis L97.214
          exposed fat layer L97.212
          muscle necrosis L97.213
          skin breakdown only L97.211
    decubitus —see Ulcer, pressure, by site

◀ New   ◀▥ Revised   ~~deleted~~ Deleted

Ulcer, ulcerated, ulcerating, ulceration, ulcerative (Continued)
  lower limb (Continued)
    foot specified NEC L97.509
      with
        bone necrosis L97.504
        exposed fat layer L97.502
        muscle necrosis L97.503
        skin breakdown only L97.501
      left L97.529
        with
          bone necrosis L97.524
          exposed fat layer L97.522
          muscle necrosis L97.523
          skin breakdown only L97.521
      right L97.519
        with
          bone necrosis L97.514
          exposed fat layer L97.512
          muscle necrosis L97.513
          skin breakdown only L97.511
    heel L97.409
      with
        bone necrosis L97.404
        exposed fat layer L97.402
        muscle necrosis L97.403
        skin breakdown only L97.401
      left L97.429
        with
          bone necrosis L97.424
          exposed fat layer L97.422
          muscle necrosis L97.423
          skin breakdown only L97.421
      right L97.419
        with
          bone necrosis L97.414
          exposed fat layer L97.412
          muscle necrosis L97.413
          skin breakdown only L97.411
    left L97.929
      with
        bone necrosis L97.924
        exposed fat layer L97.922
        muscle necrosis L97.923
        skin breakdown only L97.921
    lower leg NOS L97.909
      with
        bone necrosis L97.904
        exposed fat layer L97.902
        muscle necrosis L97.903
        skin breakdown only L97.901
      left L97.929
        with
          bone necrosis L97.924
          exposed fat layer L97.922
          muscle necrosis L97.923
          skin breakdown only L97.921
      right L97.919
        with
          bone necrosis L97.914
          exposed fat layer L97.912
          muscle necrosis L97.913
          skin breakdown only L97.911
    specified site NEC L97.809
      with
        bone necrosis L97.804
        exposed fat layer L97.802
        muscle necrosis L97.803
        skin breakdown only L97.801
      left L97.829
        with
          bone necrosis L97.824
          exposed fat layer L97.822
          muscle necrosis L97.823
          skin breakdown only L97.821
      right L97.819
        with
          bone necrosis L97.814
          exposed fat layer L97.812
          muscle necrosis L97.813
          skin breakdown only L97.811

Ulcer, ulcerated, ulcerating, ulceration, ulcerative (Continued)
  lower limb (Continued)
    midfoot L97.409
      with
        bone necrosis L97.404
        exposed fat layer L97.402
        muscle necrosis L97.403
        skin breakdown only L97.401
      left L97.429
        with
          bone necrosis L97.424
          exposed fat layer L97.422
          muscle necrosis L97.423
          skin breakdown only L97.421
      right L97.419
        with
          bone necrosis L97.414
          exposed fat layer L97.412
          muscle necrosis L97.413
          skin breakdown only L97.411
    right L97.919
      with
        bone necrosis L97.914
        exposed fat layer L97.912
        muscle necrosis L97.913
        skin breakdown only L97.911
    thigh L97.109
      with
        bone necrosis L97.104
        exposed fat layer L97.102
        muscle necrosis L97.103
        skin breakdown only L97.101
      left L97.129
        with
          bone necrosis L97.124
          exposed fat layer L97.122
          muscle necrosis L97.123
          skin breakdown only L97.121
      right L97.119
        with
          bone necrosis L97.114
          exposed fat layer L97.112
          muscle necrosis L97.113
          skin breakdown only L97.111
    toe L97.509
      with
        bone necrosis L97.504
        exposed fat layer L97.502
        muscle necrosis L97.503
        skin breakdown only L97.501
      left L97.529
        with
          bone necrosis L97.524
          exposed fat layer L97.522
          muscle necrosis L97.523
          skin breakdown only L97.521
      right L97.519
        with
          bone necrosis L97.514
          exposed fat layer L97.512
          muscle necrosis L97.513
          skin breakdown only L97.511
  leprous A30.1
  syphilitic A52.19
  varicose —see Varix, leg, with, ulcer
  luetic —see Ulcer, syphilitic
  lung J98.4
    tuberculous —see Tuberculosis, pulmonary
  malignant —see Neoplasm, malignant, by site
  marginal NEC —see Ulcer, gastrojejunal
  meatus (urinarius) N34.2
  Meckel's diverticulum Q43.0
    malignant —see Table of Neoplasms, small intestine, malignant
  Meleney's (chronic undermining) —see Ulcer, skin
  Mooren's (cornea) —see Ulcer, cornea, Mooren's
  mycobacterial (skin) A31.1
  nasopharynx J39.2

Ulcer, ulcerated, ulcerating, ulceration, ulcerative (Continued)
  neck, uterus N86
  neurogenic NEC —see Ulcer, skin
  nose, nasal (passage) (infective) (septum) J34.0
    skin —see Ulcer, skin
    spirochetal A69.8
    varicose (bleeding) I86.8
  oral mucosa (traumatic) K12.1
  palate (soft) K12.1
  penis (chronic) N48.5
  peptic (site unspecified) K27.9
    with
      hemorrhage K27.4
        and perforation K27.6
      perforation K27.5
    acute K27.3
      with
        hemorrhage K27.0
          and perforation K27.2
        perforation K27.1
    chronic K27.7
      with
        hemorrhage K27.4
          and perforation K27.6
        perforation K27.5
    esophagus K22.10
      with bleeding K22.11
    newborn P78.82
  perforating K27.5
    skin —see Ulcer, skin
  peritonsillar J35.8
  phagedenic (tropical) —see Ulcer, skin
  pharynx J39.2
  phlebitis —see Phlebitis
  plaster —see Ulcer, pressure, by site
  popliteal space —see Ulcer, lower limb
  postpyloric —see Ulcer, duodenum
  prepuce N47.7
  prepyloric —see Ulcer, stomach
  pressure (pressure area) L89.9-
    ankle L89.5-
    back L89.1-
    buttock L89.3-
    coccyx L89.15-
    contiguous site of back, buttock, hip L89.4-
    elbow L89.0-
    face L89.81-
    head L89.81-
    heel L89.6-
    hip L89.2-
    sacral region (tailbone) L89.15-
    specified site NEC L89.89-
    stage 1 (healing) (pre-ulcer skin changes limited to persistent focal edema)
      ankle L89.5-
      back L89.1-
      buttock L89.3-
      coccyx L89.15-
      contiguous site of back, buttock, hip L89.4-
      elbow L89.0-
      face L89.81-
      head L89.81-
      heel L89.6-
      hip L89.2-
      sacral region (tailbone) L89.15-
      specified site NEC L89.89-
    stage 2 (healing) (abrasion, blister, partial thickness skin loss involving epidermis and/or dermis)
      ankle L89.5-
      back L89.1-
      buttock L89.3-
      coccyx L89.15-
      contiguous site of back, buttock, hip L89.4-
      elbow L89.0-
      face L89.81-
      head L89.81-

Ulcer, ulcerated, ulcerating, ulceration,
    ulcerative (Continued)
  pressure (Continued)
    stage 2 (Continued)
      heel L89.6-
      hip L89.2-
      sacral region (tailbone) L89.15-
      specified site NEC L89.89-
    stage 3 (healing) (full thickness skin loss
        involving damage or necrosis of
        subcutaneous tissue)
      ankle L89.5-
      back L89.1-
      buttock L89.3-
      coccyx L89.15-
      contiguous site of back, buttock, hip
        L89.4-
      elbow L89.0-
      face L89.81-
      head L89.81-
      heel L89.6-
      hip L89.2-
      sacral region (tailbone) L89.15-
      specified site NEC L89.89-
    stage 4 (healing) (necrosis of soft tissues
        through to underlying muscle,
        tendon, or bone)
      ankle L89.5-
      back L89.1-
      buttock L89.3-
      coccyx L89.15-
      contiguous site of back, buttock, hip
        L89.4-
      elbow L89.0-
      face L89.81-
      head L89.81-
      heel L89.6-
      hip L89.2-
      sacral region (tailbone) L89.15-
      specified site NEC L89.89-
    unspecified stage
      ankle L89.5-
      back L89.1-
      buttock L89.3-
      coccyx L89.15-
      contiguous site of back, buttock, hip
        L89.4-
      elbow L89.0-
      face L89.81-
      head L89.81-
      heel L89.6-
      hip L89.2-
      sacral region (tailbone) L89.15-
      specified site NEC L89.89-
    unstageable
      ankle L89.5-
      back L89.1-
      buttock L89.3-
      coccyx L89.15-
      contiguous site of back, buttock, hip
        L89.4-
      elbow L89.0-
      face L89.81-
      head L89.81-
      heel L89.6-
      hip L89.2-
      sacral region (tailbone) L89.15-
      specified site NEC L89.89-
  primary of intestine K63.3
    with perforation K63.1
  prostate N41.9
  pyloric —see Ulcer, stomach
  rectosigmoid K63.3
    with perforation K63.1
  rectum (sphincter) (solitary) K62.6
    stercoraceous, stercoral K62.6
  retina —see Inflammation, chorioretinal
  rodent —see also Neoplasm, skin,
      malignant
  sclera —see Scleritis
  scrofulous (tuberculous) A18.2

Ulcer, ulcerated, ulcerating, ulceration,
    ulcerative (Continued)
  scrotum N50.89 ◂▥
    tuberculous A18.15
    varicose I86.1
  seminal vesicle N50.89 ◂▥
  sigmoid —see Ulcer, intestine
  skin (atrophic) (chronic) (neurogenic)
      (non-healing) (perforating) (pyogenic)
      (trophic) (tropical) L98.499
    with gangrene —see Gangrene
    amebic A06.7
    back —see Ulcer, back
    buttock —see Ulcer, buttock
    decubitus —see Ulcer, pressure
    lower limb —see Ulcer, lower limb
    mycobacterial A31.1
    specified site NEC L98.499
      with
        bone necrosis L98.494
        exposed fat layer L98.492
        muscle necrosis L98.493
        skin breakdown only L98.491
    tuberculous (primary) A18.4
    varicose —see Ulcer, varicose
  sloughing —see Ulcer, skin
  solitary, anus or rectum (sphincter)
      K62.6
  sore throat J02.9
    streptococcal J02.0
  spermatic cord N50.89 ◂▥
  spine (tuberculous) A18.01
  stasis (venous) —see Varix, leg, with,
      ulcer
    without varicose veins I87.2
  stercoraceous, stercoral K63.3
    with perforation K63.1
    anus or rectum K62.6
  stoma, stomal —see Ulcer, gastrojejunal
  stomach (eroded) (peptic) (round)
      K25.9
    with
      hemorrhage K25.4
        and perforation K25.6
      perforation K25.5
    acute K25.3
      with
        hemorrhage K25.0
          and perforation K25.2
        perforation K25.1
    chronic K25.7
      with
        hemorrhage K25.4
          and perforation K25.6
        perforation K25.5
  stomal —see Ulcer, gastrojejunal
  stomatitis K12.1
  stress —see Ulcer, peptic
  strumous (tuberculous) A18.2
  submucosal, bladder —see Cystitis,
      interstitial
  syphilitic (any site) (early) (secondary)
      A51.39
    late A52.79
    perforating A52.79
      foot A52.11
  testis N50.89 ◂▥
  thigh —see Ulcer, lower limb
  throat J39.2
    diphtheritic A36.0
  toe —see Ulcer, lower limb
  tongue (traumatic) K14.0
  tonsil J35.8
    diphtheritic A36.0
  trachea J39.8
  trophic —see Ulcer, skin
  tropical —see Ulcer, skin
  tuberculous —see Tuberculosis, ulcer
  tunica vaginalis N50.89 ◂▥
  turbinate J34.89
  typhoid (perforating) —see Typhoid

Ulcer, ulcerated, ulcerating, ulceration,
    ulcerative (Continued)
  unspecified site —see Ulcer, skin
  urethra (meatus) —see Urethritis
  uterus N85.8
    cervix N86
      with cervicitis N72
    neck N86
      with cervicitis N72
  vagina N76.5
    in Behçet's disease M35.2 [N77.0]
    pessary N89.8
  valve, heart I33.0
  varicose (lower limb, any part) —see also
      Varix, leg, with, ulcer
    broad ligament I86.2
    esophagus —see Varix, esophagus
    inflamed or infected —see Varix, leg, with,
        ulcer, with inflammation
    nasal septum I86.8
    perineum I86.3
    scrotum I86.1
    specified site NEC I86.8
    sublingual I86.0
    vulva I86.3
  vas deferens N50.89 ◂▥
  vulva (acute) (infectional) N76.6
    in (due to)
      Behçet's disease M35.2 [N77.0]
      herpesviral (herpes simplex) infection
          A60.04
      tuberculosis A18.18
  vulvobuccal, recurring N76.6
  X-ray L58.1
  yaws A66.4
Ulcerosa scarlatina A38.8
Ulcus —see also Ulcer
  cutis tuberculosum A18.4
  duodeni —see Ulcer, duodenum
  durum (syphilitic) A51.0
    extragenital A51.2
  gastrojejunale —see Ulcer, gastrojejunal
  hypostaticum —see Ulcer, varicose
  molle (cutis) (skin) A57
  serpens corneae —see Ulcer, cornea, central
  ventriculi —see Ulcer, stomach
Ulegyria Q04.8
Ulerythema
  ophryogenes, congenital Q84.2
  sycosiforme L73.8
Ullrich(-Bonnevie)(-Turner) syndrome —see
    also Turner's syndrome Q87.1 ◂▥
Ullrich-Feichtiger syndrome Q87.0
Ulnar —see condition
Ulorrhagia, ulorrhea K06.8
Umbilicus, umbilical —see condition
Unacceptable
  contours of tooth K08.54
  morphology of tooth K08.54
Unavailability (of)
  bed at medical facility Z75.1
  health service-related agencies Z75.4
  medical facilities (at) Z75.3
    due to
      investigation by social service agency
          Z75.2
      lack of services at home Z75.0
      remoteness from facility Z75.3
      waiting list Z75.1
    home Z75.0
    outpatient clinic Z75.3
  schooling Z55.1
  social service agencies Z75.4
Uncinaria americana infestation B76.1
Uncinariasis B76.9
Uncongenial work Z56.5
Unconscious (ness) —see Coma
Underachievement in school Z55.3
Underdevelopment —see also Undeveloped
  nose Q30.1
  sexual E30.0

Underdosing —*see also* Table of Drugs and
   Chemicals, categories T36-T50, with final
   character 6 Z91.14
   intentional NEC Z91.128
      due to financial hardship of patient
      Z91.120
   unintentional NEC Z91.138
      due to patient's age related debility
      Z91.130
Underfeeding, newborn P92.3
Underfill, endodontic M27.53
Underimmunization status Z28.3
Undernourishment —*see* Malnutrition
Undernutrition —*see* Malnutrition
Under observation —*see* Observation
Underweight R63.6
   for gestational age —*see* Light for dates
Underwood's disease P83.0
Undescended —*see also* Malposition, congenital
   cecum Q43.3
   colon Q43.3
   testicle —*see* Cryptorchid
Undeveloped, undevelopment —*see also*
      Hypoplasia
   brain (congenital) Q02
   cerebral (congenital) Q02
   heart Q24.8
   lung Q33.6
   testis E29.1
   uterus E30.0
Undiagnosed (disease) R69
Undulant fever —*see* Brucellosis
Unemployment, anxiety concerning Z56.0
   threatened Z56.2
Unequal length (acquired) (limb) —*see also*
      Deformity, limb, unequal length
   leg —*see also* Deformity, limb, unequal
      length
   congenital Q72.9-
Unextracted dental root K08.3
Unguis incarnatus L60.0
Unhappiness R45.2
Unicornate uterus Q51.4
Unilateral —*see also* condition
   development, breast N64.89
   organ or site, congenital NEC —*see* Agenesis,
      by site
Unilocular heart Q20.8
Union, abnormal —*see also* Fusion
   larynx and trachea Q34.8
Universal mesentery Q43.3
Unrepairable overhanging of dental
   restorative materials K08.52
Unsatisfactory
   restoration of tooth K08.50
      specified NEC K08.59
   sample of cytologic smear
      anus R85.615
      cervix R87.615
      vagina R87.625
   surroundings Z59.1
   work Z56.5
Unsoundness of mind —*see* Psychosis
Unstable
   back NEC —*see* Instability, joint, spine
   hip (congenital) Q65.6
      acquired —*see* Derangement, joint,
         specified type NEC, hip
   joint —*see* Instability, joint
      secondary to removal of joint prosthesis
         M96.89
   lie (mother) O32.0
   lumbosacral joint (congenital)
      acquired —*see* subcategory M53.2
   sacroiliac —*see* subcategory M53.2
   spine NEC —*see* Instability, joint, spine
Unsteadiness on feet R26.81
Untruthfulness, child problem F91.8
Unverricht(-Lundborg) disease or epilepsy —
   see Epilepsy, generalized, idiopathic
Unwanted pregnancy Z64.0

Upbringing, institutional Z62.22
   away from parents NEC Z62.29
   in care of non-parental family member Z62.21
   in foster care Z62.21
   in orphanage or group home Z62.22
   in welfare custody Z62.21
Upper respiratory —*see* condition
Upset
   gastric K30
   gastrointestinal K30
      psychogenic F45.8
   intestinal (large) (small) K59.9
      psychogenic F45.8
   menstruation N93.9
   mental F48.9
   stomach K30
      psychogenic F45.8
Urachus —*see also* condition
   patent or persistent Q64.4
Urbach-Oppenheim disease (necrobiosis
      lipoidica diabeticorum) —*see* E08-E13 with
      .620
Urbach's lipoid proteinosis E78.89
Urbach-Wiethe disease E78.89
Urban yellow fever A95.1
Urea
   blood, high —*see* Uremia
   cycle metabolism disorder —*see* Disorder,
      urea cycle metabolism
Uremia, uremic N19
   with
      ectopic or molar pregnancy O08.4
      polyneuropathy N18.9 *[G63]*
   chronic —*see also* Disease, kidney, chronic
      N18.9
      due to hypertension —*see* Hypertensive,
         kidney
   complicating
      ectopic or molar pregnancy O08.4
   congenital P96.0
   extrarenal R39.2
   following ectopic or molar pregnancy O08.4
   newborn P96.0
   prerenal R39.2
Ureter, ureteral —*see* condition
Ureteralgia N23
Ureterectasis —*see* Hydroureter
Ureteritis N28.89
   cystica N28.86
   due to calculus N20.1
      with calculus, kidney N20.2
         with hydronephrosis N13.2
   gonococcal (acute) (chronic) A54.21
   nonspecific N28.89
Ureterocele N28.89
   congenital (orthotopic) Q62.31
      ectopic Q62.32
Ureterolith, ureterolithiasis —*see* Calculus,
   ureter
Ureterostomy
   attention to Z43.6
   status Z93.6
Urethra, urethral —*see* condition
Urethralgia R39.89
Urethritis (anterior) (posterior) N34.2
   calculous N21.1
   candidal B37.41
   chlamydial A56.01
   diplococcal (gonococcal) A54.01
      with abscess (accessory gland)
         (periurethral) A54.1
   gonococcal A54.01
      with abscess (accessory gland)
         (periurethral) A54.1
   nongonococcal N34.1
      Reiter's —*see* Reiter's disease
   nonspecific N34.1
   nonvenereal N34.1
   postmenopausal N34.2
   puerperal O86.22
   Reiter's —*see* Reiter's disease

Urethritis (Continued)
   specified NEC N34.2
   trichomonal or due to Trichomonas
      (vaginalis) A59.03
Urethrocele N81.0
   with
      cystocele —*see* Cystocele
      prolapse of uterus —*see* Prolapse, uterus
Urethrolithiasis (with colic or infection) N21.1
Urethrorectal —*see* condition
Urethrorrhagia N36.8
Urethrorrhea R36.9
Urethrostomy
   attention to Z43.6
   status Z93.6
Urethrotrigonitis —*see* Trigonitis
Urethrovaginal —*see* condition
Urgency
   fecal R15.2
   hypertensive —*see* Hypertension
   urinary N39.15 ◄‖‖
Urhidrosis, uridrosis L74.8
Uric acid in blood (increased) E79.0
Uricacidemia (asymptomatic) E79.0
Uricemia (asymptomatic) E79.0
Uricosuria R82.99
Urinary —*see* condition
Urination
   frequent R35.0
   painful R30.9
Urine
   blood in —*see* Hematuria
   discharge, excessive R35.8
   enuresis, nonorganic origin F98.0
   extravasation R39.0
   frequency R35.0
   incontinence R32
      nonorganic origin F98.0
   intermittent stream R39.198 ◄‖‖
   pus in N39.0
   retention or stasis R33.9
      organic R33.8
         drug-induced R33.0
      psychogenic F45.8
   secretion
      deficient R34
      excessive R35.8
      frequency R35.0
   stream
      intermittent R39.198 ◄‖‖
      slowing R39.198 ◄‖‖
      splitting R39.13
      weak R39.12
Urinemia —*see* Uremia
Urinoma, urethra N36.8
Uroarthritis, infectious (Reiter's) —*see* Reiter's
   disease
Urodialysis R34
Urolithiasis —*see* Calculus, urinary
Uronephrosis —*see* Hydronephrosis
Uropathy N39.9
   obstructive N13.9
      specified NEC N13.8
   reflux N13.9
      specified NEC N13.8
   vesicoureteral reflux-associated —*see* Reflux,
      vesicoureteral
Urosepsis — code to condition
Urticaria L50.9
   with angioneurotic edema T78.3
      hereditary D84.1
   allergic L50.0
   cholinergic L50.5
   chronic L50.8
   cold, familial L50.2
   contact L50.6
   dermatographic L50.3
   due to
      cold or heat L50.2
      drugs L50.0
      food L50.0

Urticaria (Continued)
  due to (Continued)
    inhalants L50.0
    plants L50.6
    serum —see also Reaction, serum T80.69
  factitial L50.3
  familial cold M04.2 ◀
  giant T78.3
    hereditary D84.1
  gigantea T78.3
  idiopathic L50.1
  larynx T78.3
    hereditary D84.1
  neonatorum P83.8
  nonallergic L50.1
  papulosa (Hebra) L28.2
  pigmentosa Q82.2
  recurrent periodic L50.8
  serum —see also Reaction, serum T80.69
  solar L56.3
  specified type NEC L50.8
  thermal (cold) (heat) L50.2
  vibratory L50.4
  xanthelasmoidea Q82.2
Use (of)
  alcohol Z72.89 ◀⫶⫶
    with sleep disorder F10.982
    with ◀
      intoxication F10.929 ◀
      sleep disorder F10.982 ◀
    harmful —see Abuse, alcohol
  amphetamines —see Use, stimulant NEC
  caffeine —see Use, stimulant NEC
  cannabis F12.90
    with
      anxiety disorder F12.980
      intoxication F12.929
        with
          delirium F12.921
          perceptual disturbance F12.922
        uncomplicated F12.920
      other specified disorder F12.988
      psychosis F12.959
        delusions F12.950
        hallucinations F12.951
      unspecified disorder F12.99
  cocaine F14.90
    with
      anxiety disorder F14.980
      intoxication F14.929
        with
          delirium F14.921
          perceptual disturbance F14.922
        uncomplicated F14.920
      other specified disorder F14.988
      psychosis F14.959
        delusions F14.950
        hallucinations F14.951
      sexual dysfunction F14.981
      sleep disorder F14.982
      unspecified disorder F14.99
    harmful —see Abuse, drug, cocaine
  drug (s) NEC F19.90
    with sleep disorder F19.982
    harmful —see Abuse, drug, by type
  hallucinogen NEC F16.90
    with
      anxiety disorder F16.980
      intoxication F16.929
        with
          delirium F16.921
        uncomplicated F16.920
      mood disorder F16.94
      other specified disorder F16.988

Use (Continued)
  hallucinogen NEC (Continued)
    with (Continued)
      perception disorder (flashbacks) F16.983
      psychosis F16.959
        delusions F16.950
        hallucinations F16.951
      unspecified disorder F16.99
    harmful —see Abuse, drug, hallucinogen
      NEC
  inhalants F18.90
    with
      anxiety disorder F18.980
      intoxication F18.929
        with delirium F18.921
        uncomplicated F18.920
      mood disorder F18.94
      other specified disorder F18.988
      persisting dementia F18.97
      psychosis F18.959
        delusions F18.950
        hallucinations F18.951
      unspecified disorder F18.99
    harmful —see Abuse, drug, inhalant
  methadone —see Use, opioid ◀⫶⫶
  nonprescribed drugs F19.90
    harmful —see Abuse, non-psychoactive
      substance
  opioid F11.90
    with
      disorder F11.99
        mood F11.94
        sleep F11.982
        specified type NEC F11.988
      intoxication F11.929
        with
          delirium F11.921
          perceptual disturbance
            F11.922
        uncomplicated F11.920
      withdrawal F11.93
    harmful —see Abuse, drug, opioid
  patent medicines F19.90
    harmful —see Abuse, non-psychoactive
      substance
  psychoactive drug NEC F19.90
    with
      anxiety disorder F19.980
      intoxication F19.929
        with
          delirium F19.921
          perceptual disturbance
            F19.922
        uncomplicated F19.920
      mood disorder F19.94
      other specified disorder F19.988
      persisting
        amnestic disorder F19.96
        dementia F19.97
      psychosis F19.959
        delusions F19.950
        hallucinations F19.951
      sexual dysfunction F19.981
      sleep disorder F19.982
      unspecified disorder F19.99
      withdrawal F19.939
        with
          delirium F19.931
          perceptual disturbance
            F19.932
        uncomplicated F19.930
    harmful —see Abuse, drug NEC,
      psychoactive NEC

Use (Continued)
  sedative, hypnotic, or anxiolytic F13.90
    with
      anxiety disorder F13.980
      intoxication F13.929
        with
          delirium F13.921
        uncomplicated F13.920
      other specified disorder F13.988
      persisting
        amnestic disorder F13.96
        dementia F13.97
      psychosis F13.959
        delusions F13.950
        hallucinations F13.951
      sexual dysfunction F13.981
      sleep disorder F13.982
      unspecified disorder F13.99
    harmful —see Abuse, drug, sedative,
      hypnotic, or anxiolytic
  stimulant NEC F15.90
    with
      anxiety disorder F15.980
      intoxication F15.929
        with
          delirium F15.921
          perceptual disturbance F15.922
        uncomplicated F15.920
      mood disorder F15.94
      other specified disorder F15.988
      psychosis F15.959
        delusions F15.950
        hallucinations F15.951
      sexual dysfunction F15.981
      sleep disorder F15.982
      unspecified disorder F15.99
      withdrawal F15.93
    harmful —see Abuse, drug, stimulant NEC
  tobacco Z72.0
    with dependence —see Dependence, drug,
      nicotine
  volatile solvents —see also Use, inhalant
    F18.90
    harmful —see Abuse, drug, inhalant
Usher-Senear disease or syndrome L10.4
Uta B55.1
Uteromegaly N85.2
Uterovaginal —see condition
Uterovesical —see condition
Uveal —see condition
Uveitis (anterior) —see also Iridocyclitis
  acute —see Iridocyclitis, acute
  chronic —see Iridocyclitis, chronic
  due to toxoplasmosis (acquired) B58.09
    congenital P37.1
  granulomatous —see Iridocyclitis, chronic
  heterochromic —see Cyclitis, Fuchs'
    heterochromic
  lens-induced —see Iridocyclitis, lens-induced
  posterior —see Chorioretinitis
  sympathetic H44.13-
  syphilitic (secondary) A51.43
    congenital (early) A50.01
    late A52.71
  tuberculous A18.54
Uveoencephalitis —see Inflammation,
  chorioretinal
Uveokeratitis —see Iridocyclitis
Uveoparotitis D86.89
Uvula —see condition
Uvulitis (acute) (catarrhal) (chronic)
  (membranous) (suppurative) (ulcerative)
  K12.2

V

Vaccination (prophylactic)
  complication or reaction —*see* Complications, vaccination
  delayed Z28.9
  encounter for Z23
  not done —*see* Immunization, not done, because (of)
Vaccinia (generalized) (localized) T88.1
  without vaccination B08.011
  congenital P35.8
Vacuum, in sinus (accessory) (nasal) J34.89
Vagabond, vagabondage Z59.0
Vagabond's disease B85.1
Vagina, vaginal —*see* condition
Vaginalitis (tunica) (testis) N49.1
Vaginismus (reflex) N94.2
  functional F52.5
  nonorganic F52.5
  psychogenic F52.5
  secondary N94.2
Vaginitis (acute) (circumscribed) (diffuse) (emphysematous) (nonvenereal) (ulcerative) N76.0
  with ectopic or molar pregnancy O08.0
  amebic A06.82
  atrophic, postmenopausal N95.2
  bacterial N76.0
  blennorrhagic (gonococcal) A54.02
  candidal B37.3
  chlamydial A56.02
  chronic N76.1
  due to Trichomonas (vaginalis) A59.01
  following ectopic or molar pregnancy O08.0
  gonococcal A54.02
    with abscess (accessory gland) (periurethral) A54.1
  granuloma A58
  in (due to)
    candidiasis B37.3
    herpesviral (herpes simplex) infection A60.04
    pinworm infection B80 [N77.1]
  monilial B37.3
  mycotic (candidal) B37.3
  postmenopausal atrophic N95.2
  puerperal (postpartum) O86.13
  senile (atrophic) N95.2
  subacute or chronic N76.1
  syphilitic (early) A51.0
    late A52.76
  trichomonal A59.01
  tuberculous A18.18
Vaginosis —*see* Vaginitis
Vagotonia G52.2
Vagrancy Z59.0
VAIN —*see* Neoplasia, intraepithelial, vagina
Vallecula —*see* condition
Valley fever B38.0
Valsuani's disease —*see* Anemia, obstetric
Valve, valvular (formation) —*see also* condition
  cerebral ventricle (communicating) in situ Z98.2
  cervix, internal os Q51.828
  congenital NEC —*see* Atresia, by site
  ureter (pelvic junction) (vesical orifice) Q62.39
  urethra (congenital) (posterior) Q64.2
Valvulitis (chronic) —*see* Endocarditis
Valvulopathy —*see* Endocarditis
Van Bogaert's leukoencephalopathy (sclerosing) (subacute) A81.1
Van Bogaert-Scherer-Epstein disease or syndrome E75.5
Van Buchem's syndrome M85.2
Van Creveld-von Gierke disease E74.01
Van der Hoeve (-de Kleyn) syndrome Q78.0
Van der Woude's syndrome Q38.0
Van Neck's disease or osteochondrosis M91.0
Vanishing lung J44.9

Vapor asphyxia or suffocation T59.9
  specified agent —*see* Table of Drugs and Chemicals
Variance, lethal ball, prosthetic heart valve T82.09
Variants, thalassemic D56.8
Variations in hair color L67.1
Varicella B01.9
  with
    complications NEC B01.89
    encephalitis B01.11
    encephalomyelitis B01.11
    meningitis B01.0
    myelitis B01.12
    pneumonia B01.2
  congenital P35.8
Varices —*see* Varix
Varicocele (scrotum) (thrombosed) I86.1
  ovary I86.2
  perineum I86.3
  spermatic cord (ulcerated) I86.1
Varicose
  aneurysm (ruptured) I77.0
  dermatitis —*see* Varix, leg, with, inflammation
  eczema —*see* Varix, leg, with, inflammation
  phlebitis —*see* Varix, with, inflammation
  tumor —*see* Varix
  ulcer (lower limb, any part) —*see also* Varix, leg, with, ulcer
    anus —*see also* Hemorrhoids K64.8
    esophagus —*see* Varix, esophagus
    inflamed or infected —*see* Varix, leg, with, ulcer, with inflammation
    nasal septum I86.8
    perineum I86.3
    scrotum I86.1
    specified site NEC I86.8
  vein —*see* Varix
  vessel —*see* Varix, leg
Varicosis, varicosities, varicosity —*see* Varix
Variola (major) (minor) B03
Varioloid B03
Varix (lower limb) (ruptured) I83.90
  with
    edema I83.899
    inflammation I83.10
      with ulcer (venous) I83.209
    pain I83.819
    specified complication NEC I83.899
    stasis dermatitis I83.10
      with ulcer (venous) I83.209
    swelling I83.899
    ulcer I83.009
      with inflammation I83.209
  aneurysmal I77.0
  asymptomatic I83.9-
  bladder I86.2
  broad ligament I86.2
  complicating
    childbirth (lower extremity) O87.4
      anus or rectum O87.2
      genital (vagina, vulva or perineum) O87.8
    pregnancy (lower extremity) O22.0-
      anus or rectum O22.4-
      genital (vagina, vulva or perineum) O22.1-
    puerperium (lower extremity) O87.4
      anus or rectum O87.2
      genital (vagina, vulva, perineum) O87.8
  congenital (any site) Q27.8
  esophagus (idiopathic) (primary) (ulcerated) I85.00
    bleeding I85.01
    congenital Q27.8
    in (due to)
      alcoholic liver disease I85.10
        bleeding I85.11
      cirrhosis of liver I85.10
        bleeding I85.11

Varix (Continued)
  esophagus (Continued)
    in (Continued)
      portal hypertension I85.10
        bleeding I85.11
      schistosomiasis I85.10
        bleeding I85.11
      toxic liver disease I85.10
        bleeding I85.11
    secondary I85.10
      bleeding I85.11
  gastric I86.4
  inflamed or infected I83.10
    ulcerated I83.209
  labia (majora) I86.3
  leg (asymptomatic) I83.90
    with
      edema I83.899
      inflammation I83.10
        with ulcer —*see* Varix, leg, with, ulcer, with inflammation by site
      pain I83.819
      specified complication NEC I83.899
      swelling I83.899
      ulcer I83.009
        with inflammation I83.209
        ankle I83.003
          with inflammation I83.203
        calf I83.002
          with inflammation I83.202
        foot NEC I83.005
          with inflammation I83.205
        heel I83.004
          with inflammation I83.204
        lower leg NEC I83.008
          with inflammation I83.208
        midfoot I83.004
          with inflammation I83.204
        thigh I83.001
          with inflammation I83.201
    bilateral (asymptomatic) I83.93
      with
        edema I83.893
        pain I83.813
        specified complication NEC I83.893
        swelling I83.893
        ulcer I83.009
          with inflammation I83.209
    left (asymptomatic) I83.92
      with
        edema I83.892
        inflammation I83.12
          with ulcer —*see* Varix, leg, with, ulcer, with inflammation by site
        pain I83.812
        specified complication NEC I83.892
        swelling I83.892
        ulcer I83.029
          with inflammation I83.229
          ankle I83.023
            with inflammation I83.223
          calf I83.022
            with inflammation I83.222
          foot NEC I83.025
            with inflammation I83.225
          heel I83.024
            with inflammation I83.224
          lower leg NEC I83.028
            with inflammation I83.228
          midfoot I83.024
            with inflammation I83.224
          thigh I83.021
            with inflammation I83.221
    right (asymptomatic) I83.91
      with
        edema I83.891
        inflammation I83.11
          with ulcer —*see* Varix, leg, with, ulcer, with inflammation by site

Varix (Continued)
  leg (Continued)
    right (Continued)
      with (Continued)
        pain I83.811
        specified complication NEC I83.891
        swelling I83.891
        ulcer I83.019
          with inflammation I83.219
          ankle I83.013
            with inflammation I83.213
          calf I83.012
            with inflammation I83.212
          foot NEC I83.015
            with inflammation I83.215
          heel I83.014
            with inflammation I83.214
          lower leg NEC I83.018
            with inflammation I83.218
          midfoot I83.014
            with inflammation I83.214
          thigh I83.011
            with inflammation I83.211
  nasal septum I86.8
  orbit I86.8
    congenital Q27.8
  ovary I86.2
  papillary I78.1
  pelvis I86.2
  perineum I86.3
  pharynx I86.8
  placenta O43.89-
  renal papilla I86.8
  retina H35.09
  scrotum (ulcerated) I86.1
  sigmoid colon I86.8
  specified site NEC I86.8
  spinal (cord) (vessels) I86.8
  spleen, splenic (vein) (with phlebolith) I86.8
  stomach I86.4
  sublingual I86.0
  ulcerated I83.009
    inflamed or infected I83.209
  uterine ligament I86.2
  vagina I86.8
  vocal cord I86.8
  vulva I86.3
Vas deferens —see condition
Vas deferentitis N49.1
Vasa previa O69.4
  hemorrhage from, affecting newborn P50.0
Vascular —see also condition
  loop on optic papilla Q14.2
  spasm I73.9
  spider I78.1
Vascularization, cornea —see Neovascularization, cornea
Vasculitis I77.6
  allergic D69.0
  cryoglobulinemic D89.1
  disseminated I77.6
  hypocomplementemic M31.8
  kidney I77.89
  livedoid L95.0
  nodular L95.8
  retina H35.06-
  rheumatic —see Fever, rheumatic
  rheumatoid —see Rheumatoid, vasculitis
  skin (limited to) L95.9
    specified NEC L95.8
Vasculopathy, necrotizing M31.9
  cardiac allograft T86.290
  specified NEC M31.8
Vasitis (nodosa) N49.1
  tuberculous A18.15
Vasodilation I73.9
Vasomotor —see condition
Vasoplasty, after previous sterilization Z31.0
  aftercare Z31.42

Vasospasm (vasoconstriction) I73.9
  cerebral (cerebrovascular) (artery) I67.848
    reversible I67.841
  coronary I20.1
  nerve
    arm —see Mononeuropathy, upper limb
    brachial plexus G54.0
    cervical plexus G54.2
    leg —see Mononeuropathy, lower limb
  peripheral NOS I73.9
  retina (artery) —see Occlusion, artery, retina
Vasospastic —see condition
Vasovagal attack (paroxysmal) R55
  psychogenic F45.8
VATER syndrome Q87.2
Vater's ampulla —see condition
Vegetation, vegetative
  adenoid (nasal fossa) J35.8
  endocarditis (acute) (any valve) (subacute) I33.0
  heart (mycotic) (valve) I33.0
Veil
  Jackson's Q43.3
Vein, venous —see condition
Veldt sore —see Ulcer, skin
Velpeau's hernia —see Hernia, femoral
Venereal
  bubo A55
  disease A64
  granuloma inguinale A58
  lymphogranuloma (Durand-Nicolas-Favre) A55
Venofibrosis I87.8
Venom, venomous —see Table of Drugs and Chemicals, by animal or substance, poisoning
Venous —see condition
Ventilator lung, newborn P27.8
Ventral —see condition
Ventricle, ventricular —see also condition
  escape I49.3
  inversion Q20.5
Ventriculitis (cerebral) —see also Encephalitis G04.90
Ventriculostomy status Z98.2
Vernet's syndrome G52.7
Verneuil's disease (syphilitic bursitis) A52.78
Verruca (due to HPV) (filiformis) (simplex) (viral) (vulgaris) B07.9
  acuminata A63.0
  necrogenica (primary) (tuberculosa) A18.4
  plana B07.8
  plantaris B07.0
  seborrheica L82.1
    inflamed L82.0
  senile (seborrheic) L82.1
    inflamed L82.0
  tuberculosa (primary) A18.4
  venereal A63.0
Verrucosities —see Verruca
Verruga peruana, peruviana A44.1
Version
  with extraction
  cervix —see Malposition, uterus
  uterus (postinfectional) (postpartal, old) —see Malposition, uterus
Vertebra, vertebral —see condition
Vertical talus (congenital) Q66.80
  left foot Q66.82
  right foot Q66.81
Vertigo R42
  auditory —see Vertigo, aural
  aural H81.31-
  benign paroxysmal (positional) H81.1-
  central (origin) H81.4-
  cerebral H81.4-
  Dix and Hallpike (epidemic) —see Neuronitis, vestibular
  due to infrasound T75.23

Vertigo (Continued)
  epidemic A88.1
    Dix and Hallpike —see Neuronitis, vestibular
    Pedersen's —see Neuronitis, vestibular
    vestibular neuronitis —see Neuronitis, vestibular
  hysterical F44.89
  infrasound T75.23
  labyrinthine —see subcategory H81.0
  laryngeal R05
  malignant positional H81.4-
  Ménière's —see subcategory H81.40
  menopausal N95.11
  otogenic —see Vertigo, aural
  paroxysmal positional, benign —see Vertigo, benign paroxysmal
  Pedersen's (epidemic) —see Neuronitis, vestibular
  peripheral NEC H81.39-
  positional
    benign paroxysmal —see Vertigo, benign paroxysmal
    malignant H81.4-
Very-low-density-lipoprotein-type (VLDL) hyperlipoproteinemia E78.1
Vesania —see Psychosis
Vesical —see condition
Vesicle
  cutaneous R23.8
  seminal —see condition
  skin R23.8
Vesicocolic —see condition
Vesicoperineal —see condition
Vesicorectal —see condition
Vesicourethrorectal —see condition
Vesicovaginal —see condition
Vesicular —see condition
Vesiculitis (seminal) N49.0
  amebic A06.82
  gonorrheal (acute) (chronic) A54.23
  trichomonal A59.09
  tuberculous A18.15
Vestibulitis (ear) —see also subcategory H83.0
  nose (external) J34.89
  vulvar N94.810
Vestibulopathy, acute peripheral (recurrent) —see Neuronitis, vestibular
Vestige, vestigial —see also Persistence
  branchial Q18.0
  structures in vitreous Q14.0
Vibration
  adverse effects T75.20
    pneumatic hammer syndrome T75.21
    specified effect NEC T75.29
    vasospastic syndrome T75.22
    vertigo from infrasound T75.23
  exposure (occupational) Z57.7
  vertigo T75.23
Vibriosis A28.9
Victim (of)
  crime Z65.4
  disaster Z65.5
  terrorism Z65.4
  torture Z65.4
  war Z65.5
Vidal's disease L28.0
Villaret's syndrome G52.7
Villous —see condition
VIN —see Neoplasia, intraepithelial, vulva
Vincent's infection (angina) (gingivitis) A69.1
  stomatitis NEC A69.1
Vinson-Plummer syndrome D50.1
Violence, physical R45.6
Viosterol deficiency —see Deficiency, calciferol
Vipoma —see Neoplasm, malignant, by site
Viremia B34.9
Virilism (adrenal) E25.9
  congenital E25.0
Virilization (female) (suprarenal) E25.9
  congenital E25.0
  isosexual E28.2

Virulent bubo A57
Virus, viral —*see also* condition
  as cause of disease classified elsewhere
    B97.89
  cytomegalovirus B25.9
  human immunodeficiency (HIV) —*see*
    Human, immunodeficiency virus (HIV)
    disease
  infection —*see* Infection, virus
  specified NEC B34.8
  ~~swine influenza (viruses that normally cause~~
    ~~infections in pigs) (see also Influenza,~~
    ~~due to, identified novel influenza A~~
    ~~virus) J09.X2~~
  swine influenza (viruses that normally cause
    infections in pigs) —*see also* Influenza,
    due to, identified novel influenza A
    virus J09.X2 ◄
  West Nile (fever) A92.30
    with
      complications NEC A92.39
      cranial nerve disorders A92.32
      encephalitis A92.31
      encephalomyelitis A92.31
      neurologic manifestation NEC A92.32
      optic neuritis A92.32
      polyradiculitis A92.32
Viscera, visceral —*see* condition
Visceroptosis K63.4
Visible peristalsis R19.2
Vision, visual
  binocular, suppression H53.34
  blurred, blurring H53.8
    hysterical F44.6
  defect, defective NEC H54.7
  disorientation (syndrome) H53.8
  disturbance H53.9
    hysterical F44.6
  double H53.2
  examination Z01.00
    with abnormal findings Z01.01
  field, limitation (defect) —*see* Defect, visual
    field
  hallucinations R44.1
  halos H53.19
  loss —*see* Loss, vision
    sudden —*see* Disturbance, vision,
      subjective, loss, sudden
  low (both eyes) —*see* Low, vision
  perception, simultaneous without fusion
    H53.33
Vitality, lack or want of R53.83
  newborn P96.89
Vitamin deficiency —*see* Deficiency, vitamin
Vitelline duct, persistent Q43.0
Vitiligo L80
  eyelid H02.739
    left H02.736
      lower H02.735
      upper H02.734

Vitiligo (*Continued*)
  eyelid (*Continued*)
    right H02.733
      lower H02.732
      upper H02.731
  pinta A67.2
  vulva N90.89
Vitreal corneal syndrome H59.01-
Vitreoretinopathy, proliferative —*see also*
    Retinopathy, proliferative
  with retinal detachment —*see* Detachment,
    retina, traction
Vitreous —*see also* condition
  touch syndrome —*see* Complication,
    postprocedural, following cataract
    surgery
Vocal cord —*see* condition
Vogt-Koyanagi syndrome H20.82-
Vogt's disease or syndrome G80.3
Vogt-Spielmeyer amaurotic idiocy or disease
    E75.4
Voice
  change R49.9
    specified NEC R49.8
  loss —*see* Aphonia
Volhynian fever A79.0
Volkmann's ischemic contracture or paralysis
    (complicating trauma) T79.6
Volvulus (bowel) (colon) (intestine) K56.2 ◄⁣▥
  with perforation K56.2
  congenital Q43.8
  duodenum K31.5 ◄
  fallopian tube —*see* Torsion, fallopian
    tube
  oviduct —*see* Torsion, fallopian tube
  stomach (due to absence of gastrocolic
    ligament) K31.89
Vomiting R11.10
  with nausea R11.2
  without nausea R11.11
  asphyxia —*see* Foreign body, by site, causing
    asphyxia, gastric contents
  bilious (cause unknown) R11.14
    following gastro-intestinal surgery
      K91.0
    in newborn P92.01
  blood —*see* Hematemesis
  causing asphyxia, choking, or suffocation —
    see Foreign body, by site
  cyclical G43.A0
    with refractory migraine G43.A1
    intractable G43.A1
    not intractable G43.A0
    psychogenic F50.89 ◄⁣▥
    without refractory migraine G43.A0
  fecal mater R11.13
  following gastrointestinal surgery
    K91.0
    psychogenic F50.89 ◄⁣▥

Vomiting (*Continued*)
  functional K31.89
  hysterical F50.89 ◄⁣▥
  nervous F50.89 ◄⁣▥
  neurotic F50.89 ◄⁣▥
  newborn NEC P92.09
    bilious P92.01
  periodic R11.10
    psychogenic F50.89 ◄⁣▥
  projectile R11.12
  psychogenic F50.89 ◄⁣▥
  uremic —*see* Uremia
Vomito negro —*see* Fever, yellow
Von Bezold's abscess —*see* Mastoiditis,
    acute
Von Economo-Cruchet disease A85.8
Von Eulenburg's disease G71.19
Von Gierke's disease E74.01
Von Hippel (-Lindau) disease or syndrome
    Q85.8
Von Jaksch's anemia or disease D64.89
Von Recklinghausen
  disease (neurofibromatosis) Q85.01
    bones E21.0
Von Schroetter's syndrome I82.890
Von Willebrand (-Jurgens)(-Minot) disease or
    syndrome D68.0
Von Zumbusch's disease L40.1
Voyeurism F65.3
Vrolik's disease Q78.0
Vulva —*see* condition
Vulvismus N94.2
Vulvitis (acute) (allergic) (atrophic)
    (hypertrophic) (intertriginous) (senile)
    N76.2
  with ectopic or molar pregnancy O08.0
  adhesive, congenital Q52.79
  blennorrhagic (gonococcal) A54.02
  candidal B37.3
  chlamydial A56.02
  due to Haemophilus ducreyi A57
  following ectopic or molar pregnancy
    O08.0
  gonococcal A54.02
    with abscess (accessory gland)
      (periurethral) A54.1
  herpesviral A60.04
  leukoplakic N90.4
  monilial B37.3
  puerperal (postpartum) O86.19
  subacute or chronic N76.3
  syphilitic (early) A51.0
    late A52.76
  trichomonal A59.01
  tuberculous A18.18
Vulvodynia N94.819
  specified NEC N94.818
Vulvorectal —*see* condition
Vulvovaginitis (acute) —*see* Vaginitis

W

Waiting list, person on Z75.1
  for organ transplant Z76.82
  undergoing social agency investigation Z75.2
Waldenström
  hypergammaglobulinemia D89.0
  syndrome or macroglobulinemia C88.0
Waldenström-Kjellberg syndrome D50.1
Walking
  difficulty R26.2
    psychogenic F44.4
  sleep F51.3
    hysterical F44.89
Wall, abdominal —see condition
Wallenberg's disease or syndrome G46.3
Wallgren's disease I87.8
Wandering
  gallbladder, congenital Q44.1
  in diseases classified elsewhere Z91.83
  kidney, congenital Q63.8
  organ or site, congenital NEC —see
    Malposition, congenital, by site
  pacemaker (heart) I49.8
  spleen D73.89
War neurosis F48.8
Wart (due to HPV) (filiform) (infectious) (viral)
    B07.9
  anogenital region (venereal) A63.0
  common B07.8
  external genital organs (venereal) A63.0
  flat B07.8
  Hassal-Henle's (of cornea) H18.49
  Peruvian A44.1
  plantar B07.0
  prosector (tuberculous) A18.4
  seborrheic L82.1
    inflamed L82.0
  senile (seborrheic) L82.1
    inflamed L82.0
  tuberculous A18.4
  venereal A63.0
Warthin's tumor —see Neoplasm, salivary
    gland, benign
Wassilieff's disease A27.0
Wasting
  disease R64
    due to malnutrition E41
  extreme (due to malnutrition) E41
  muscle NEC —see Atrophy, muscle
Water
  clefts (senile cataract) —see Cataract, senile,
    incipient
  deprivation of T73.1
  intoxication E87.79
  itch B76.9
  lack of T73.1
  loading E87.70
  on
    brain —see Hydrocephalus
    chest J94.8
  poisoning E87.79
Waterbrash R12
Waterhouse(-Friderichsen) syndrome or
    disease (meningococcal) A39.1
Water-losing nephritis N25.89
Watermelon stomach K31.819
  with hemorrhage K31.811
  without hemorrhage K31.819
Watsoniasis B66.8
Wax in ear —see Impaction, cerumen
Weak, weakening, weakness (generalized)
    R53.1
  arches (acquired) —see also Deformity, limb,
    flat foot
  bladder (sphincter) R32
  facial R29.810
    following
      cerebrovascular disease I69.992
        cerebral infarction I69.392
        intracerebral hemorrhage I69.192

Weak, weakening, weakness (Continued)
  facial (Continued)
    following (Continued)
      cerebrovascular disease (Continued)
        nontraumatic intracranial hemorrhage
          NEC I69.292
        specified disease NEC I69.892
        stroke I69.392
        subarachnoid hemorrhage I69.092
  foot (double) —see Weak, arches
  heart, cardiac —see Failure, heart
  mind F70
  muscle M62.81
  myocardium —see Failure, heart
  newborn P96.89
  pelvic fundus N81.89
  pubocervical tissue N81.82
  rectovaginal tissue N81.83
  senile R54
  urinary stream R39.12
  valvular —see Endocarditis
Wear, worn (with normal or routine use)
  articular bearing surface of internal joint
    prosthesis —see Complications, joint
    prosthesis, mechanical, wear of articular
    bearing surfaces, by site
  device, implant or graft —see Complications,
    by site, mechanical complication
  tooth, teeth (approximal) (hard tissues)
    (interproximal) (occlusal) K03.0
Weather, weathered
  effects of
    cold T69.9
      specified effect NEC T69.8
    hot —see Heat
  skin L57.8
Weaver's syndrome Q87.3
Web, webbed (congenital)
  duodenal Q43.8
  esophagus Q39.4
  fingers Q70.1
  larynx (glottic) (subglottic) Q31.0
  neck (pterygium colli) Q18.3
  Paterson-Kelly D50.1
  popliteal syndrome Q87.89
  toes Q70.3
Weber-Christian disease M35.6
Weber-Cockayne syndrome (epidermolysis
    bullosa) Q81.8
Weber-Gubler syndrome G46.3
Weber-Leyden syndrome G46.3
Weber-Osler syndrome I78.0
Weber's paralysis or syndrome G46.3
Wedge-shaped or wedging vertebra —see
    Collapse, vertebra NEC
Wegener's granulomatosis or syndrome
    M31.30
  with
    kidney involvement M31.31
    lung involvement M31.30
      with kidney involvement M31.31
Wegner's disease A50.02
Weight
  1000-2499 grams at birth (low) —see Low,
    birthweight
  999 grams or less at birth (extremely low) —
    see Low, birthweight, extreme
  and length below 10th percentile for
    gestational age P05.1- ◀
  below but length above 10th percentile for
    gestational age P05.0- ◀
  gain (abnormal) (excessive) R63.5
    in pregnancy —see Pregnancy, complicated
      by, excessive weight gain
    low —see Pregnancy, complicated by,
      insufficient, weight gain
  loss (abnormal) (cause unknown) R63.4
Weightlessness (effect of) T75.82
Weil (l)-Marchesani syndrome Q87.1
Weil's disease A27.0
Weingarten's syndrome J82

Weir Mitchell's disease I73.81
Weiss-Baker syndrome G90.09
Wells' disease L98.3
Wen —see Cyst, sebaceous
Wenckebach's block or phenomenon I44.1
Werdnig-Hoffmann syndrome (muscular
    atrophy) G12.0
Werlhof's disease D69.3
Werner-His disease A79.0
Wermer's disease or syndrome E31.21
Werner's disease or syndrome E34.8
Wernicke-Korsakoff's syndrome or psychosis
    (alcoholic) F10.96
  with dependence F10.26
  drug-induced
    due to drug abuse —see Abuse, drug, by
      type, with amnestic disorder
    due to drug dependence —see Dependence,
      drug, by type, with amnestic disorder
  nonalcoholic F04
Wernicke-Posadas disease B38.9
Wernicke's
  developmental aphasia F80.2
  disease or syndrome E51.2
  encephalopathy E51.2
  polioencephalitis, superior E51.2
West African fever B50.8
Westphal-Strümpell syndrome E83.01
West's syndrome —see Epilepsy, spasms
Wet
  feet, tropical (maceration) (syndrome) —see
    Immersion, foot
  lung (syndrome), newborn P22.1
Wharton's duct —see condition
Wheal —see Urticaria
Wheezing R06.2
Whiplash injury S13.4
Whipple's disease —see also subcategory
    M14.8- K90.81
Whipworm (disease) (infection) (infestation)
    B79
Whistling face Q87.0
White —see also condition
  kidney, small N03.9
  leg, puerperal, postpartum, childbirth O87.1
  mouth B37.0
  patches of mouth K13.29
  spot lesions, teeth
    chewing surface K02.51
    pit and fissure surface K02.51
    smooth surface K02.61
Whitehead L70.0
Whitlow —see also Cellulitis, digit
  with lymphangitis —see Lymphangitis, acute,
    digit
  herpesviral B00.89
Whitmore's disease or fever —see Melioidosis
Whooping cough A37.90
  with pneumonia A37.91
    due to Bordetella
      bronchiseptica A37.81
      parapertussis A37.11
      pertussis A37.01
    specified organism NEC A37.81
  due to
    Bordetella
      bronchiseptica A37.80
        with pneumonia A37.81
      parapertussis A37.10
        with pneumonia A37.11
      pertussis A37.00
        with pneumonia A37.01
    specified NEC A37.80
      with pneumonia A37.81
Wichman's asthma J38.5
Wide cranial sutures, newborn P96.3
Widening aorta —see Ectasia, aorta
  with aneurysm —see Aneurysm, aorta
Wilkie's disease or syndrome K55.1
Wilkinson-Sneddon disease or syndrome
    L13.1

◀ New   ◀▥ Revised   ~~deleted~~ Deleted

Willebrand (-Jürgens) thrombopathy D68.0
Willige-Hunt disease or syndrome G23.1
Wilms' tumor C64-
Wilson-Mikity syndrome P27.0
Wilson's
  disease or syndrome E83.01
  hepatolenticular degeneration E83.01
  lichen ruber L43.9
Window —see also Imperfect, closure
  aorticopulmonary Q21.4
Winter —see condition
Wiskott-Aldrich syndrome D82.0
Withdrawal state —see also Dependence, drug
    by type, with withdrawal
  alcohol ◀
    with perceptual disturbances F10.232 ◀
    without perceptual disturbances F10.239 ◀
  caffeine F15.93 ◀
  cannabis F12.288 ◀
  newborn
    correct therapeutic substance properly
      administered P96.2
    infant of dependent mother P96.1
    therapeutic substance, neonatal P96.2
Witts' anemia D50.8
Witzelsucht F07.0
Woakes' ethmoiditis or syndrome J33.1
Wolff-Hirschorn syndrome Q93.3
Wolff-Parkinson-White syndrome I45.6
Wolhynian fever A79.0
Wolman's disease E75.5
Wood lung or pneumonitis J67.8
Woolly, wooly hair (congenital) (nevus) Q84.1
Woolsorter's disease A22.1
Word
  blindness (congenital) (developmental) F81.0
  deafness (congenital) (developmental) H93.25
Worm (s) (infection) (infestation) —see also
    Infestation, helminth
  guinea B72
  in intestine NEC B82.0
Worm-eaten soles A66.3
Worn out —see Exhaustion
  cardiac
    defibrillator (with synchronous cardiac
      pacemaker) Z45.02
    pacemaker
      battery Z45.010
      lead Z45.018
  device, implant or graft —see Complications,
    by site, mechanical
Worried well Z71.1
Worries R45.82
Wound, open
  abdomen, abdominal
    wall S31.109
      with penetration into peritoneal cavity
        S31.609
      bite —see Bite, abdomen, wall
      epigastric region S31.102
        with penetration into peritoneal cavity
          S31.602
        bite —see Bite, abdomen, wall,
          epigastric region
        laceration —see Laceration, abdomen,
          wall, epigastric region
        puncture —see Puncture, abdomen,
          wall, epigastric region
      laceration —see Laceration, abdomen,
        wall
      left
        lower quadrant S31.104
          with penetration into peritoneal
            cavity S31.604
          bite —see Bite, abdomen, wall, left,
            lower quadrant
          laceration —see Laceration,
            abdomen, wall, left, lower
            quadrant
          puncture —see Puncture, abdomen,
            wall, left, lower quadrant

Wound, open (Continued)
  abdomen, abdominal (Continued)
    wall (Continued)
      left (Continued)
        upper quadrant S31.101
          with penetration into peritoneal
            cavity S31.601
          bite —see Bite, abdomen, wall, left,
            upper quadrant
          laceration —see Laceration,
            abdomen, wall, left, upper
            quadrant
          puncture —see Puncture, abdomen,
            wall, left, upper quadrant
        periumbilic region S31.105
          with penetration into peritoneal cavity
            S31.605
          bite —see Bite, abdomen, wall,
            periumbilic region
          laceration —see Laceration, abdomen,
            wall, periumbilic region
          puncture —see Puncture, abdomen,
            wall, periumbilic region
        puncture —see Puncture, abdomen, wall
      right
        lower quadrant S31.103
          with penetration into peritoneal
            cavity S31.603
          bite —see Bite, abdomen, wall, right,
            lower quadrant
          laceration —see Laceration,
            abdomen, wall, right, lower
            quadrant
          puncture —see Puncture, abdomen,
            wall, right, lower quadrant
        upper quadrant S31.100
          with penetration into peritoneal
            cavity S31.600
          bite —see Bite, abdomen, wall, right,
            upper quadrant
          laceration —see Laceration,
            abdomen, wall, right, upper
            quadrant
          puncture —see Puncture, abdomen,
            wall, right, upper quadrant
    alveolar (process) —see Wound, open, oral
      cavity
    ankle S91.00-
      bite —see Bite, ankle
      laceration —see Laceration, ankle
      puncture —see Puncture, ankle
    antecubital space —see Wound, open, elbow
    anterior chamber, eye —see Wound, open,
      ocular
    anus S31.839
      bite S31.835
      laceration —see Laceration, anus
      puncture —see Puncture, anus
    arm (upper) S41.10-
      with amputation —see Amputation,
        traumatic, arm
      bite —see Bite, arm
      forearm —see Wound, open, forearm
      laceration —see Laceration, arm
      puncture —see Puncture, arm
    auditory canal (external) (meatus) —see
      Wound, open, ear
    auricle, ear —see Wound, open, ear
    axilla —see Wound, open, arm
    back —see also Wound, open, thorax, back
      lower S31.000
        with penetration into retroperitoneal
          space S31.001
        bite —see Bite, back, lower
        laceration —see Laceration, back, lower
        puncture —see Puncture, back, lower
    bite —see Bite
    blood vessel —see Injury, blood vessel
    breast S21.00-
      with amputation —see Amputation,
        traumatic, breast

Wound, open (Continued)
  breast (Continued)
    bite —see Bite, breast
    laceration —see Laceration, breast
    puncture —see Puncture, breast
  buttock S31.809
    bite —see Bite, buttock
    laceration —see Laceration, buttock
    left S31.829
    puncture —see Puncture, buttock
    right S31.819
  calf —see Wound, open, leg
  canaliculus lacrimalis —see Wound, open,
    eyelid
  canthus, eye —see Wound, open, eyelid
  cervical esophagus S11.20
    bite S11.25
    laceration —see Laceration, esophagus,
      traumatic, cervical
    puncture —see Puncture, cervical esophagus
  cheek (external) S01.40-
    bite —see Bite, cheek
    internal —see Wound, open, oral cavity
    laceration —see Laceration, cheek
    puncture —see Puncture, cheek
  chest wall —see Wound, open, thorax
  chin —see Wound, open, head, specified site
    NEC
  choroid —see Wound, open, ocular
  ciliary body (eye) —see Wound, open, ocular
  clitoris S31.40
    with amputation —see Amputation,
      traumatic, clitoris
    bite S31.45
    laceration —see Laceration, vulva
    puncture —see Puncture, vulva
  conjunctiva —see Wound, open, ocular
  cornea —see Wound, open, ocular
  costal region —see Wound, open, thorax
  Descemet's membrane —see Wound, open,
    ocular
  digit (s)
    foot —see Wound, open, toe
    hand —see Wound, open, finger
  ear (canal) (external) S01.30-
    with amputation —see Amputation,
      traumatic, ear
    bite —see Bite, ear
    drum S09.2-
    laceration —see Laceration, ear
    puncture —see Puncture, ear
  elbow S51.00-
    bite —see Bite, elbow
    laceration —see Laceration, elbow
    puncture —see Puncture, elbow
  epididymis —see Wound, open, testis
  epigastric region S31.102
    with penetration into peritoneal cavity
      S31.602
    bite —see Bite, abdomen, wall, epigastric
      region
    laceration —see Laceration, abdomen, wall,
      epigastric region
    puncture —see Puncture, abdomen, wall,
      epigastric region
  epiglottis —see Wound, open, neck, specified
    site NEC
  esophagus (thoracic) S27.819
    cervical —see Wound, open, cervical
      esophagus
    laceration S27.813
    specified type NEC S27.818
  eye —see Wound, open, ocular
  eyeball —see Wound, open, ocular
  eyebrow —see Wound, open, eyelid
  eyelid S01.10-
    bite —see Bite, eyelid
    laceration —see Laceration, eyelid
    puncture —see Puncture, eyelid
  face NEC —see Wound, open, head, specified
    site NEC

◄ New   ◄▮▮▮ Revised   ~~deleted~~ Deleted

Wound, open (Continued)
  oral cavity S01.502
    bite S01.552
    laceration —see Laceration, oral cavity
    puncture —see Puncture, oral cavity
  orbit —see Wound, open, ocular, orbit
  palate —see Wound, open, oral cavity
  palm —see Wound, open, hand
  pelvis, pelvic —see also Wound, open, back,
    lower
    girdle —see Wound, open, hip
  penetrating —see Puncture, by site
  penis S31.20
    with amputation —see Amputation,
      traumatic, penis
    bite S31.25
    laceration —see Laceration, penis
    puncture —see Puncture, penis
  perineum
    bite —see Bite, perineum
    female S31.502
    laceration —see Laceration, perineum
    male S31.501
    puncture —see Puncture, perineum
  periocular area (with or without lacrimal
    passages) —see Wound, open, eyelid
  periumbilic region S31.105
    with penetration into peritoneal cavity
      S31.605
    bite —see Bite, abdomen, wall, periumbilic
      region
    laceration —see Laceration, abdomen, wall,
      periumbilic region
    puncture —see Puncture, abdomen, wall,
      periumbilic region
  phalanges
    finger —see Wound, open, finger
    toe —see Wound, open, toe
  pharynx S11.20
  pinna —see Wound, open, ear
  popliteal space —see Wound, open, knee
  prepuce —see Wound, open, penis
  pubic region —see Wound, open, back,
    lower
  pudendum —see Wound, open, genital
    organs, external
  puncture wound —see Puncture
  rectovaginal septum —see Wound, open,
    vagina
  right
    lower quadrant S31.103
      with penetration into peritoneal cavity
        S31.603
      bite —see Bite, abdomen, wall, right,
        lower quadrant
      laceration —see Laceration, abdomen,
        wall, right, lower quadrant
      puncture —see Puncture, abdomen, wall,
        right, lower quadrant
    upper quadrant S31.100
      with penetration into peritoneal cavity
        S31.600
      bite —see Bite, abdomen, wall, right,
        upper quadrant
      laceration —see Laceration, abdomen,
        wall, right, upper quadrant
      puncture —see Puncture, abdomen, wall,
        right, upper quadrant
  sacral region —see Wound, open, back,
    lower
  sacroiliac region —see Wound, open, back,
    lower
  salivary gland —see Wound, open, oral
    cavity

Wound, open (Continued)
  scalp S01.00
    bite S01.05
    laceration —see Laceration, scalp
    puncture —see Puncture, scalp
  scalpel, newborn (birth injury) P15.8
  scapular region —see Wound, open, shoulder
  sclera —see Wound, open, ocular
  scrotum S31.30
    with amputation —see Amputation,
      traumatic, scrotum
    bite S31.35
    laceration —see Laceration, scrotum
    puncture —see Puncture, scrotum
  shin —see Wound, open, leg
  shoulder S41.00-
    with amputation —see Amputation,
      traumatic, arm
    bite —see Bite, shoulder
    laceration —see Laceration, shoulder
    puncture —see Puncture, shoulder
  skin NOS T14.8
  spermatic cord —see Wound, open, testis
  sternal region —see Wound, open, thorax,
    front wall
  submaxillary region —see Wound, open,
    head, specified site NEC
  submental region —see Wound, open, head,
    specified site NEC
  subungual
    finger (s) —see Wound, open, finger
    toe (s) —see Wound, open, toe
  supraclavicular region —see Wound, open,
    neck, specified site NEC
  temple, temporal region —see Wound, open,
    head, specified site NEC
  temporomandibular area —see Wound, open,
    cheek
  testis S31.30
    with amputation —see Amputation,
      traumatic, testes
    bite S31.35
    laceration —see Laceration, testis
    puncture —see Puncture, testis
  thigh S71.10-
    with amputation —see Amputation,
      traumatic, hip
    bite —see Bite, thigh
    laceration —see Laceration, thigh
    puncture —see Puncture, thigh
  thorax, thoracic (wall) S21.90
    back S21.20-
      with penetration S21.40
    bite —see Bite, thorax
    breast —see Wound, open, breast
    front S21.10-
      with penetration S21.30
    laceration —see Laceration, thorax
    puncture —see Puncture, thorax
  throat —see Wound, open, neck
  thumb S61.009
    with
      amputation —see Amputation,
        traumatic, thumb
      damage to nail S61.109
    bite —see Bite, thumb
    laceration —see Laceration, thumb
    left S61.002
      with
        damage to nail S61.102
    puncture —see Puncture, thumb
    right S61.001
      with
        damage to nail S61.101

Wound, open (Continued)
  thyroid (gland) —see Wound, open, neck,
    thyroid
  toe (s) S91.109
    with
      amputation —see Amputation,
        traumatic, toe
      damage to nail S91.209
    bite —see Bite, toe
    great S91.103
      with
        damage to nail S91.203
      left S91.102
        with
          damage to nail S91.202
      right S91.101
        with
          damage to nail S91.201
    laceration —see Laceration, toe
    lesser S91.106
      with
        damage to nail S91.206
      left S91.105
        with
          damage to nail S91.205
      right S91.104
        with
          damage to nail S91.204
    puncture —see Puncture, toe
  tongue —see Wound, open, oral cavity
  trachea (cervical region) —see Wound, open,
    neck, trachea
  tunica vaginalis —see Wound, open, testis
  tympanum, tympanic membrane S09.2-
    laceration —see Laceration, ear, drum
    puncture —see Puncture, tympanum
  umbilical region —see Wound, open,
    abdomen, wall, periumbilic region
  uvula —see Wound, open, oral cavity
  vagina S31.40
    bite S31.45
    laceration —see Laceration, vagina
    puncture —see Puncture, vagina
  vitreous (humor) —see Wound, open,
    ocular
  vocal cord S11.039
    bite —see Bite, vocal cord
    laceration S11.031
      with foreign body S11.032
    puncture S11.033
      with foreign body S11.034
  vulva S31.40
    with amputation —see Amputation,
      traumatic, vulva
    bite S31.45
    laceration —see Laceration, vulva
    puncture —see Puncture, vulva
  wrist S61.50-
    bite —see Bite, wrist
    laceration —see Laceration, wrist
    puncture —see Puncture, wrist
Wound, superficial —see Injury (see also
  specified injury type)
Wright's syndrome G54.0
Wrist —see condition
Wrong drug (by accident) (given in error) —
  see Table of Drugs and Chemicals, by
  drug, poisoning
Wry neck —see Torticollis
Wuchereria (bancrofti) infestation B74.0
Wuchereriasis B74.0
Wuchernde Struma Langhans C73

X

Xanthelasma (eyelid) (palpebrarum) H02.60
  left H02.66
    lower H02.65
    upper H02.64
  right H02.63
    lower H02.62
    upper H02.61
Xanthelasmatosis (essential) E78.2
Xanthinuria, hereditary E79.8
Xanthoastrocytoma
  specified site —*see* Neoplasm, malignant, by
    site
  unspecified site C71.9
Xanthofibroma —*see* Neoplasm, connective
    tissue, benign
Xanthogranuloma D76.3
Xanthoma (s), xanthomatosis (primary)
    (familial) (hereditary) E75.5
  with
    hyperlipoproteinemia
      Type I E78.3
      Type III E78.2
      Type IV E78.1
      Type V E78.3
  bone (generalisata) C96.5
  cerebrotendinous E75.5
  cutaneotendinous E75.5

Xanthoma (s), xanthomatosis (*Continued*)
  disseminatum (skin) E78.2
  eruptive E78.2
  hypercholesterinemic E78.00 ◀▥▥
  hypercholesterolemic E78.00 ◀▥▥
  hyperlipidemic E78.5
  joint E75.5
  multiple (skin) E78.2
  tendon (sheath) E75.5
  tuberosum E78.2
  tuberous E78.2
  tubo-eruptive E78.2
  verrucous, oral mucosa K13.4
Xanthosis R23.8
Xenophobia F40.10
Xeroderma —*see also* Ichthyosis
  acquired L85.0
    eyelid H01.149
      left H01.146
        lower H01.145
        upper H01.144
      right H01.143
        lower H01.142
        upper H01.141
  pigmentosum Q82.1
  vitamin A deficiency E50.8
Xerophthalmia (vitamin A deficiency) E50.7
  unrelated to vitamin A deficiency —*see*
    Keratoconjunctivitis

Xerosis
  conjunctiva H11.14-
    with Bitot's spots —*see also* Pigmentation,
      conjunctiva
      vitamin A deficiency E50.1
    vitamin A deficiency E50.0
  cornea H18.89-
    with ulceration —*see* Ulcer, cornea
      vitamin A deficiency E50.3
    vitamin A deficiency E50.2
  cutis L85.3
  skin L85.3
Xerostomia K11.7
Xiphopagus Q89.4
XO syndrome Q96.9
X-ray (of)
  abnormal findings —*see* Abnormal,
    diagnostic imaging
  breast (mammogram) (routine) Z12.31
  chest
    routine (as part of a general medical
      examination) Z00.00
    with abnormal findings Z00.01
  routine (as part of a general medical
    examination) Z00.00
  with abnormal findings Z00.01
XXXXY syndrome Q98.1
XXY syndrome Q98.0

◀ New   ◀▥▥ Revised   ~~deleted~~ Deleted

Y

Yaba pox virus disease B08.72
Yatapoxvirus B08.70
  specified NEC B08.79
Yawning R06.89
  psychogenic F45.8
Yaws A66.9
  bone lesions A66.6
  butter A66.1
  chancre A66.0
  cutaneous, less than five years after infection
      A66.2
  early (cutaneous) (macular) (maculopapular)
      (micropapular) (papular) A66.2
    frambeside A66.2
    skin lesions NEC A66.2
  eyelid A66.2
  ganglion A66.6
  gangosis, gangosa A66.5
  gumma, gummata A66.4
    bone A66.6
  gummatous
    frambeside A66.4
    osteitis A66.6
    periostitis A66.6
  hydrarthrosis —*see also* subcategory
      M14.8- A66.6
  hyperkeratosis (early) (late) A66.3

Yaws *(Continued)*
    initial lesions A66.0
    joint lesions —*see also* subcategory
        M14.8- A66.6
    juxta-articular nodules A66.7
    late nodular (ulcerated) A66.4
    latent (without clinical manifestations) (with
        positive serology) A66.8
    mother A66.0
    mucosal A66.7
    multiple papillomata A66.1
    nodular, late (ulcerated) A66.4
    osteitis A66.6
    papilloma, plantar or palmar A66.1
    periostitis (hypertrophic) A66.6
    specified NEC A66.7
    ulcers A66.4
    wet crab A66.1
Yeast infection —*see also* Candidiasis B37.9
Yellow
    atrophy (liver) —*see* Failure, hepatic
    fever —*see* Fever, yellow
    jack —*see* Fever, yellow
    jaundice —*see* Jaundice
    nail syndrome L60.5
Yersiniosis —*see also* Infection, Yersinia
    extraintestinal A28.2
    intestinal A04.6

Z

Zahorsky's syndrome (herpangina) B08.5
Zellweger's syndrome Q87.89
Zenker's diverticulum (esophagus) K22.5
Ziehen-Oppenheim disease G24.1
Zieve's syndrome K70.0
Zika NOS A92.5 ◀
Zinc
    deficiency, dietary E60
    metabolism disorder E83.2
Zollinger-Ellison syndrome E16.4
Zona —*see* Herpes, zoster
Zoophobia F40.218
Zoster (herpes) —*see* Herpes, zoster
Zygomycosis B46.9
    specified NEC B46.8
Zymotic —*see* condition

ICD-10-CM
Table of Neoplasms

ICD-10-CM
Table of Neoplasms

The list below gives the code numbers for neoplasms by anatomical site. For each site there are six possible code numbers according to whether the neoplasm in question is malignant, benign, in situ, of uncertain behavior, or of unspecified nature. The description of the neoplasm will often indicate which of the six columns is appropriate; e.g., malignant melanoma of skin, benign fibroadenoma of breast, carcinoma in situ of cervix uteri.

Where such descriptors are not present, the remainder of the Index should be consulted where guidance is given to the appropriate column for each morphological (histological) variety listed; e.g., Mesonephroma — *see Neoplasm, malignant;* Embryoma — *see also Neoplasm, uncertain behavior;* Disease, Bowen's — *see Neoplasm, skin, in situ.* However, the guidance in the Index can be overridden if one of the descriptors mentioned above is present; e.g., malignant adenoma of colon is coded to C18.9 and not to D12.6 as the adjective "Malignant" overrides the Index entry 'Adenoma — *see also Neoplasm, benign.*'

Codes listed with a dash -, following the code have a required additional character for laterality. The Tablular must be reviewed for the complete code.

	Malignant Primary	Malignant Secondary	Ca in situ	Benign	Uncertain Behavior	Unspecified Behavior
Neoplasm, neoplastic	C80.1	C79.9	D09.9	D36.9	D48.9	D49.9
abdomen, abdominal	C76.2	C79.8-	D09.8	D36.7	D48.7	D49.89
cavity	C76.2	C79.8-	D09.8	D36.7	D48.7	D49.89
organ	C76.2	C79.8-	D09.8	D36.7	D48.7	D49.89
viscera	C76.2	C79.8-	D09.8	D36.7	D48.7	D49.89
wall — *see also Neoplasm, abdomen, wall, skin*	C44.509	C79.2-	D04.5	D23.5	D48.5	D49.2
connective tissue	C49.4	C79.8-	—	D21.4	D48.1	D49.2
skin	C44.509					
basal cell carcinoma	C44.519	—	—	—	—	—
specified type NEC	C44.599	—	—	—	—	—
squamous cell carcinoma	C44.529	—	—	—	—	—
abdominopelvic	C76.8	C79.8-	—	D36.7	D48.7	D49.89
accessory sinus — *see Neoplasm, sinus*						
acoustic nerve	C72.4-	C79.49	—	D33.3	D43.3	D49.7
adenoid (pharynx) (tissue)	C11.1	C79.89	D00.08	D10.6	D37.05	D49.0
adipose tissue — *see also Neoplasm, connective tissue*	C49.4	C79.89	—	D21.9	D48.1	D49.2
adnexa (uterine)	C57.4	C79.89	D07.39	D28.7	D39.8	D49.59
adrenal	C74.9-	C79.7-	D09.3	D35.0-	D44.1-	D49.7
capsule	C74.9-	C79.7-	D09.3	D35.0-	D44.1-	D49.7
cortex	C74.0-	C79.7-	D09.3	D35.0-	D44.1-	D49.7
gland	C74.9-	C79.7-	D09.3	D35.0-	D44.1-	D49.7
medulla	C74.1-	C79.7-	D09.3	D35.0-	D44.1-	D49.7
ala nasi (external) — *see also Neoplasm, skin, nose*	C44.301	C79.2	D04.39	D23.39	D48.5	D49.2

	Malignant Primary	Malignant Secondary	Ca in situ	Benign	Uncertain Behavior	Unspecified Behavior
alimentary canal or tract NEC	C26.9	C78.80	D01.9	D13.9	D37.9	D49.0
alveolar	C03.9	C79.89	D00.03	D10.39	D37.09	D49.0
mucosa	C03.9	C79.89	D00.03	D10.39	D37.09	D49.0
lower	C03.1	C79.89	D00.03	D10.39	D37.09	D49.0
upper	C03.0	C79.89	D00.03	D10.39	D37.09	D49.0
ridge or process	C41.1	C79.51	—	D16.5-	D48.0	D49.2
carcinoma	C03.9	C79.8-	—	—	—	—
lower	C03.1	C79.8-	—	—	—	—
upper	C03.0	C79.8-	—	—	—	—
lower	C41.1	C79.51	—	D16.5-	D48.0	D49.2
mucosa	C03.9	C79.89	D00.03	D10.39	D37.09	D49.0
lower	C03.1	C79.89	D00.03	D10.39	D37.09	D49.0
upper	C03.0	C79.89	D00.03	D10.39	D37.09	D49.0
upper	C41.0	C79.51	—	D16.4-	D48.0	D49.2
sulcus	C06.1	C79.89	D00.02	D10.39	D37.09	D49.0
alveolus	C03.9	C79.89	D00.03	D10.39	D37.09	D49.0
lower	C03.1	C79.89	D00.03	D10.39	D37.09	D49.0
upper	C03.0	C79.89	D00.03	D10.39	D37.09	D49.0
ampulla of Vater	C24.1	C78.89	D01.5	D13.5	D37.6	D49.0
ankle NEC	C76.5-	C79.89	D04.7-	D36.7	D48.7	D49.89
anorectum, anorectal (junction)	C21.8	C78.5	D01.3	D12.9	D37.8	D49.0
antecubital fossa or space	C76.4-	C79.89	D04.6-	D36.7	D48.7	D49.89
antrum (Highmore) (maxillary)	C31.0	C78.39	D02.3	D14.0	D38.5	D49.1
pyloric	C16.3	C78.89	D00.2	D13.1	D37.1	D49.0
tympanicum	C30.1	C78.39	D02.3	D14.0	D38.5	D49.1
anus, anal	C21.0	C78.5	D01.3	D12.9	D37.8	D49.0
canal	C21.1	C78.5	D01.3	D12.9	D37.8	D49.0
cloacogenic zone	C21.2	C78.5	D01.3	D12.9	D37.8	D49.0
margin — *see also Neoplasm, anus, skin*	C44.500	C79.2	D04.5	D23.5	D48.5	D49.2
overlapping lesion with rectosigmoid junction or rectum	C21.8					
skin	C44.500	C79.2	D04.5	D23.5	D48.5	D49.2
basal cell carcinoma	C44.510	—	—	—	—	—
specified type NEC	C44.590	—	—	—	—	—
squamous cell carcinoma	C44.520	—	—	—	—	—
sphincter	C21.1	C78.5	D01.3	D12.9	D37.8	D49.0
aorta (thoracic)	C49.3	C79.89	—	D21.3	D48.1	D49.2
abdominal	C49.4	C79.89	—	D21.4	D48.1	D49.2
aortic body	C75.5	C79.89	—	D35.6	D44.7	D49.7
aponeurosis	C49.9	C79.89	—	D21.9	D48.1	D49.2
palmar	C49.1-	C79.89	—	D21.1-	D48.1	D49.2
plantar	C49.2-	C79.89	—	D21.2-	D48.1	D49.2

TABLE OF NEOPLASMS

	Malignant Primary	Malignant Secondary	Ca in situ	Benign	Uncertain Behavior	Unspecified Behavior
appendix	C18.1	C78.5	D01.0	D12.1	D37.3	D49.0
arachnoid	C70.9	C79.49	—	D32.9	D42.9	D49.7
cerebral	C70.0	C79.32	—	D32.0	D42.0	D49.7
spinal	C70.1	C79.49	—	D32.1	D42.1	D49.7
areola	C50.0-	C79.81	D05.-	D24.-	D48.6-	D49.3
arm NEC	C76.4-	C79.89	D04.6-	D36.7	D48.7	D49.89
artery — see Neoplasm, connective tissue						
aryepiglottic fold	C13.1	C79.89	D00.08	D10.7	D37.05	D49.0
hypopharyngeal aspect	C13.1	C79.89	D00.08	D10.7	D37.05	D49.0
laryngeal aspect	C32.1	C78.39	D02.0	D14.1	D38.0	D49.1
marginal zone	C13.1	C79.89	D00.08	D10.7	D37.05	D49.0
arytenoid (cartilage)	C32.3	C78.39	D02.0	D14.1	D38.0	D49.1
fold — see Neoplasm, aryepiglottic						
associated with transplanted organ	C80.2	—	—	—	—	—
atlas	C41.2	C79.51	—	D16.6	D48.0	D49.2
atrium, cardiac	C38.0	C79.89	—	D15.1	D48.7	D49.89
auditory						
canal (external) (skin)	C44.20-	C79.2	D04.2-	D23.2-	D48.5	D49.2
internal	C30.1	C78.39	D02.3	D14.0	D38.5	D49.1
nerve	C72.4-	C79.49	—	D33.3	D43.3	D49.7
tube	C30.1	C78.39	D02.3	D14.0	D38.5	D49.1
opening	C11.2	C79.89	D00.08	D10.6	D37.05	D49.0
auricle, ear — see also Neoplasm, skin, ear	C44.20-	C79.2	D04.2-	D23.2-	D48.5	D49.2
auricular canal (external) — see also Neoplasm, skin, ear	C44.20-	C79.2	D04.2-	D23.2-	D48.5	D49.2
internal	C30.1	C78.39	D02.3	D14.0	D38.5	D49.2
autonomic nerve or nervous system NEC (see Neoplasm, nerve, peripheral)						
axilla, axillary	C76.1	C79.89	D09.8	D36.7	D48.7	D49.89
fold — see also Neoplasm, skin, trunk	C44.509	C79.2	D04.5	D23.5	D48.5	D49.2
back NEC	C76.8	C79.89	D04.5	D36.7	D48.7	D49.89
Bartholin's gland	C51.0	C79.82	D07.1	D28.0	D39.8	D49.59
basal ganglia	C71.0	C79.31	—	D33.0	D43.0	D49.6
basis pedunculi	C71.7	C79.31	—	D33.1	D43.1	D49.6
bile or biliary (tract)	C24.9	C78.89	D01.5	D13.5	D37.6	D49.0
canaliculi (biliferi) (intrahepatic)	C22.1	C78.7	D01.5	D13.4	D37.6	D49.0
canals, interlobular	C22.1	C78.89	D01.5	D13.4	D37.6	D49.0

	Malignant Primary	Malignant Secondary	Ca in situ	Benign	Uncertain Behavior	Unspecified Behavior
bile or biliary (Continued)						
duct or passage (common) (cystic) (extrahepatic)	C24.0	C78.89	D01.5	D13.5	D37.6	D49.0
interlobular	C22.1	C78.89	D01.5	D13.4	D37.6	D49.0
intrahepatic	C22.1	C78.7	D01.5	D13.4	D37.6	D49.0
and extrahepatic	C24.8	C78.89	D01.5	D13.5	D37.6	D49.0
bladder (urinary)	C67.9	C79.11	D09.0	D30.3	D41.4	D49.4
dome	C67.1	C79.11	D09.0	D30.3	D41.4	D49.4
neck	C67.5	C79.11	D09.0	D30.3	D41.4	D49.4
orifice	C67.9	C79.11	D09.0	D30.3	D41.4	D49.4
ureteric	C67.6	C79.11	D09.0	D30.3	D41.4	D49.4
urethral	C67.5	C79.11	D09.0	D30.3	D41.4	D49.4
overlapping lesion	C67.8	—	—	—	—	—
sphincter	C67.8	C79.11	D09.0	D30.3	D41.4	D49.4
trigone	C67.0	C79.11	D09.0	D30.3	D41.4	D49.4
urachus	C67.7	C79.11	D09.0	D30.3	D41.4	D49.4
wall	C67.9	C79.11	D09.0	D30.3	D41.4	D49.4
anterior	C67.3	C79.11	D09.0	D30.3	D41.4	D49.4
lateral	C67.2	C79.11	D09.0	D30.3	D41.4	D49.4
posterior	C67.4	C79.11	D09.0	D30.3	D41.4	D49.4
blood vessel — see Neoplasm, connective tissue						
bone (periosteum)	C41.9	C79.51	—	D16.9-	D48.0	D49.2
acetabulum	C41.4	C79.51	—	D16.8-	D48.0	D49.2
ankle	C40.3-	C79.51	—	D16.3-	—	—
arm NEC	C40.0-	C79.51	—	D16.0-	—	—
astragalus	C40.3-	C79.51	—	D16.3-	—	—
atlas	C41.2	C79.51	—	D16.6-	D48.0	D49.2
axis	C41.2	C79.51	—	D16.6-	D48.0	D49.2
back NEC	C41.2	C79.51	—	D16.6-	D48.0	D49.2
calcaneus	C40.3-	C79.51	—	D16.3-	—	—
calvarium	C41.0	C79.51	—	D16.4-	D48.0	D49.2
carpus (any)	C40.1-	C79.51	—	D16.1-	—	—
cartilage NEC	C41.9	C79.51	—	D16.9-	D48.0	D49.2
clavicle	C41.3	C79.51	—	D16.7-	D48.0	D49.2
clivus	C41.0	C79.51	—	D16.4-	D48.0	D49.2
coccygeal vertebra	C41.4	C79.51	—	D16.8-	D48.0	D49.2
coccyx	C41.4	C79.51	—	D16.8-	D48.0	D49.2
costal cartilage	C41.3	C79.51	—	D16.7-	D48.0	D49.2
costovertebral joint	C41.3	C79.51	—	D16.7-	D48.0	D49.2
cranial	C41.0	C79.51	—	D16.4-	D48.0	D49.2
cuboid	C40.3-	C79.51	—	D16.3-	—	—
cuneiform	C41.9	C79.51	—	D16.9-	D48.0	D49.2
elbow	C40.0-	C79.51	—	D16.0-	—	—

◀ New   ◀▦ Revised   ~~deleted~~ Deleted

	Malignant Primary	Malignant Secondary	Ca in situ	Benign	Uncertain Behavior	Unspecified Behavior
bone *(Continued)*						
ethmoid (labyrinth)	C41.0	C79.51	—	D16.4-	D48.0	D49.2
face	C41.0	C79.51	—	D16.4-	D48.0	D49.2
femur (any part)	C40.2-	C79.51	—	D16.2-	—	—
fibula (any part)	C40.2-	C79.51	—	D16.2-	—	—
finger (any)	C40.1-	C79.51	—	D16.1-	—	—
foot	C40.3-	C79.51	—	D16.3-	—	—
forearm	C40.0-	C79.51	—	D16.0-	—	—
frontal	C41.0	C79.51	—	D16.4-	D48.0	D49.2
hand	C40.1-	C79.51	—	D16.1-	—	—
heel	C40.3-	C79.51	—	D16.3-	—	—
hip	C41.4	C79.51	—	D16.8	D48.0	D49.2
humerus (any part)	C40.0-	C79.51	—	D16.0-	—	—
hyoid	C41.0	C79.51	—	D16.4-	D48.0	D49.2
ilium	C41.4	C79.51	—	D16.8	D48.0	D49.2
innominate	C41.4	C79.51	—	D16.8	D48.0	D49.2
intervertebral cartilage or disc	C41.2	C79.51	—	D16.6	D48.0	D49.2
ischium	C41.4	C79.51	—	D16.8	D48.0	D49.2
jaw (lower)	C41.1	C79.51	—	D16.5-	D48.0	D49.2
knee	C40.2-	C79.51	—	D16.2-	—	—
leg NEC	C40.2-	C79.51	—	D16.2-	—	—
limb NEC	C40.9-	C79.51	—	D16.9-	—	—
lower (long bones)	C40.2-	C79.51	—	D16.2-	—	—
short bones	C40.3-	C79.51	—	D16.3-	—	—
upper (long bones)	C40.0-	C79.51	—	D16.0-	—	—
short bones	C40.1-	C79.51	—	D16.1-	—	—
malar	C41.0	C79.51	—	D16.4-	D48.0	D49.2
mandible	C41.1	C79.51	—	D16.5-	D48.0	D49.2
marrow NEC (any bone)	C96.9	C79.52	—	—	D47.9	D49.89
mastoid	C41.0	C79.51	—	D16.4-	D48.0	D49.2
maxilla, maxillary (superior)	C41.0	C79.51	—	D16.4-	D48.0	D49.2
inferior	C41.1	C79.51	—	D16.5-	D48.0	D49.2
metacarpus (any)	C40.1-	C79.51	—	D16.1-	—	—
metatarsus (any)	C40.3-	C79.51	—	D16.3-	—	—
overlapping sites	C40.8-	—	—	—	—	—
navicular						
ankle	C40.3-	C79.51	—	—	—	—
hand	C40.1-	C79.51	—	—	—	—
nose, nasal	C41.0	C79.51	—	D16.4-	D48.0	D49.2
occipital	C41.0	C79.51	—	D16.4-	D48.0	D49.2
orbit	C41.0	C79.51	—	D16.4-	D48.0	D49.2
parietal	C41.0	C79.51	—	D16.4-	D48.0	D49.2
patella	C40.2-	C79.51	—	—	—	—
pelvic	C41.4	C79.51	—	D16.8	D48.0	D49.2
bone *(Continued)*						
phalanges						
foot	C40.3-	C79.51	—	—	—	—
hand	C40.1-	C79.51	—	—	—	—
pubic	C41.4	C79.51	—	D16.8	D48.0	D49.2
radius (any part)	C40.0-	C79.51	—	D16.0-	—	—
rib	C41.3	C79.51	—	D16.7	D48.0	D49.2
sacral vertebra	C41.4	C79.51	—	D16.8	D48.0	D49.2
sacrum	C41.4	C79.51	—	D16.8	D48.0	D49.2
scaphoid				—	—	—
of ankle	C40.3-	C79.51	—	—	—	—
of hand	C40.1-	C79.51	—	—	—	—
scapula (any part)	C40.0-	C79.51	—	D16.0-	—	—
sella turcica	C41.0	C79.51	—	D16.4-	D48.0	D49.2
shoulder	C40.0-	C79.51	—	D16.0-	—	—
skull	C41.0	C79.51	—	D16.4-	D48.0	D49.2
sphenoid	C41.0	C79.51	—	D16.4-	D48.0	D49.2
spine, spinal (column)	C41.2	C79.51	—	D16.6	D48.0	D49.2
coccyx	C41.4	C79.51	—	D16.8	D48.0	D49.2
sacrum	C41.4	C79.51	—	D16.8	D48.0	D49.2
sternum	C41.3	C79.51	—	D16.7	D48.0	D49.2
tarsus (any)	C40.3-	C79.51	—	—	—	—
temporal	C41.0	C79.51	—	D16.4-	D48.0	D49.2
thumb	C40.1-	C79.51	—	—	—	—
tibia (any part)	C40.2-	C79.51	—	—	—	—
toe (any)	C40.3-	C79.51	—	—	—	—
trapezium	C40.1-	C79.51	—	—	—	—
trapezoid	C40.1-	C79.51	—	—	—	—
turbinate	C41.0	C79.51	—	D16.4-	D48.0	D49.2
ulna (any part)	C40.0-	C79.51	—	D16.0-	—	—
unciform	C40.1-	C79.51	—	—	—	—
vertebra (column)	C41.2	C79.51	—	D16.6	D48.0	D49.2
coccyx	C41.4	C79.51	—	D16.8	D48.0	D49.2
sacrum	C41.4	C79.51	—	D16.8	D48.0	D49.2
vomer	C41.0	C79.51	—	D16.4-	D48.0	D49.2
wrist	C40.1-	C79.51	—	—	—	—
xiphoid process	C41.3	C79.51	—	D16.7	D48.0	D49.2
zygomatic	C41.0	C79.51	—	D16.4-	D48.0	D49.2
book-leaf (mouth)	C06.89	C79.89	D00.00	D10.39	D37.09	D49.0
bowel — *see Neoplasm, intestine*						
brachial plexus	C47.1-	C79.89	—	D36.12	D48.2	D49.2
brain NEC	C71.9	C79.31	—	D33.2	D43.2	D49.6
basal ganglia	C71.0	C79.31	—	D33.0	D43.0	D49.6
cerebellopontine angle	C71.6	C79.31	—	D33.1	D43.1	D49.6

◀ New ◀▦ Revised ~~deleted~~ Deleted

TABLE OF NEOPLASMS

	Malignant Primary	Malignant Secondary	Ca in situ	Benign	Uncertain Behavior	Unspecified Behavior
brain NEC *(Continued)*						
cerebellum NOS	C71.6	C79.31	—	D33.1	D43.1	D49.6
cerebrum	C71.0	C79.31	—	D33.0	D43.0	D49.6
choroid plexus	C71.7	C79.31	—	D33.1	D43.1	D49.6
corpus callosum	C71.8	C79.31	—	D33.2	D43.2	D49.6
corpus striatum	C71.0	C79.31	—	D33.0	D43.0	D49.6
cortex (cerebral)	C71.0	C79.31	—	D33.0	D43.0	D49.6
frontal lobe	C71.1	C79.31	—	D33.0	D43.0	D49.6
globus pallidus	C71.0	C79.31	—	D33.0	D43.0	D49.6
hippocampus	C71.2	C79.31	—	D33.0	D43.0	D49.6
hypothalamus	C71.0	C79.31	—	D33.0	D43.0	D49.6
internal capsule	C71.0	C79.31	—	D33.0	D43.0	D49.6
medulla oblongata	C71.7	C79.31	—	D33.1	D43.1	D49.6
meninges	C70.0	C79.32	—	D32.0	D42.0	D49.7
midbrain	C71.7	C79.31	—	D33.1	D43.1	D49.6
occipital lobe	C71.4	C79.31	—	D33.0	D43.0	D49.6
overlapping lesion	C71.8	C79.31	—	—	—	—
parietal lobe	C71.3	C79.31	—	D33.0	D43.0	D49.6
peduncle	C71.7	C79.31	—	D33.1	D43.1	D49.6
pons	C71.7	C79.31	—	D33.1	D43.1	D49.6
stem	C71.7	C79.31	—	D33.1	D43.1	D49.6
tapetum	C71.8	C79.31	—	D33.2	D43.2	D49.6
temporal lobe	C71.2	C79.31	—	D33.0	D43.0	D49.6
thalamus	C71.0	C79.31	—	D33.0	D43.0	D49.6
uncus	C71.2	C79.31	—	D33.0	D43.0	D49.6
ventricle (floor)	C71.5	C79.31	—	D33.0	D43.0	D49.6
fourth	C71.7	C79.31	—	D33.1	D43.1	D49.6
branchial (cleft) (cyst) (vestiges)	C10.4	C79.89	D00.08	D10.5	D37.05	D49.0
breast (connective tissue) (glandular tissue) (soft parts)	C50.9-	C79.81	D05.-	D24.-	D48.6-	D49.3
areola	C50.0-	C79.81	D05.-	D24.-	D48.6-	D49.3
axillary tail	C50.6-	C79.81	D05.-	D24.-	D48.6-	D49.3
central portion	C50.1-	C79.81	D05.-	D24.-	D48.6-	D49.3
inner	C50.8-	C79.81	D05.-	D24.-	D48.6-	D49.3
lower	C50.8-	C79.81	D05.-	D24.-	D48.6-	D49.3
lower-inner quadrant	C50.3-	C79.81	D05.-	D24.-	D48.6-	D49.3
lower-outer quadrant	C50.5-	C79.81	D05.-	D24.-	D48.6-	D49.3
mastectomy site (skin) — *see also Neoplasm, breast, skin*	C44.501	C79.2				
specified as breast tissue	C50.8-	C79.81		—	—	—
midline	C50.8-	C79.81	D05.-	D24.-	D48.6-	D49.3
nipple	C50.0-	C79.81	D05.-	D24.-	D48.6-	D49.3
outer	C50.8-	C79.81	D05.-	D24.-	D48.6-	D49.3
overlapping lesion	C50.8-	—	—	—	—	—

	Malignant Primary	Malignant Secondary	Ca in situ	Benign	Uncertain Behavior	Unspecified Behavior
breast *(Continued)*						
skin	C44.501	C79.2	D04.5	D23.5	D48.5	D49.2
basal cell carcinoma	C44.511	—	—	—	—	—
specified type NEC	C44.591	—	—	—	—	—
squamous cell carcinoma	C44.521	—	—	—	—	—
tail (axillary)	C50.6-	C79.81	D05.-	D24.-	D48.6-	D49.3
upper	C50.8-	C79.81	D05.-	D24.-	D48.6-	D49.3
upper-inner quadrant	C50.2-	C79.81	D05.-	D24.-	D48.6-	D49.3
upper-outer quadrant	C50.4-	C79.81	D05.-	D24.-	D48.6-	D49.3
broad ligament	C57.1	C79.82	D07.39	D28.2	D39.8	D49.59 ◀▬
bronchiogenic, bronchogenic (lung)	C34.9-	C78.0-	D02.2-	D14.3-	D38.1	D49.1
bronchiole	C34.9-	C78.0-	D02.2-	D14.3-	D38.1	D49.1
bronchus	C34.9-	C78.0-	D02.2-	D14.3-	D38.1	D49.1
carina	C34.0-	C78.0-	D02.2-	D14.3-	D38.1	D49.1
lower lobe of lung	C34.3-	C78.0-	D02.2-	D14.3-	D38.1	D49.1
main	C34.0-	C78.0-	D02.2-	D14.3-	D38.1	D49.1
middle lobe of lung	C34.2	C78.0-	D02.21	D14.31	D38.1	D49.1
overlapping lesion	C34.8-	—	—	—	—	—
upper lobe of lung	C34.1-	C78.0-	D02.2-	D14.3-	D38.1	D49.1
brow	C44.309	C79.2	D04.39	D23.39	D48.5	D49.2
basal cell carcinoma	C44.319	—	—	—	—	—
specified type NEC	C44.399	—	—	—	—	—
squamous cell carcinoma	C44.329	—	—	—	—	—
buccal (cavity)	C06.9	C79.89	D00.00	D10.39	D37.09	D49.0
commissure	C06.0	C79.89	D00.02	D10.39	D37.09	D49.0
groove (lower) (upper)	C06.1	C79.89	D00.02	D10.39	D37.09	D49.0
mucosa	C06.0	C79.89	D00.02	D10.39	D37.09	D49.0
sulcus (lower) (upper)	C06.1	C79.89	D00.02	D10.39	D37.09	D49.0
bulbourethral gland	C68.0	C79.19	D09.19	D30.4	D41.3	D49.59 ◀▬
bursa — *see Neoplasm, connective tissue*						
buttock NEC	C76.3	C79.89	D04.5	D36.7	D48.7	D49.89
calf	C76.5-	C79.89	D04.7-	D36.7	D48.7	D49.89
calvarium	C41.0	C79.51	—	D16.4-	D48.0	D49.2
calyx, renal	C65.-	C79.0-	D09.19	D30.1-	D41.1-	D49.51- ◀▬
canal						
anal	C21.1	C78.5	D01.3	D12.9	D37.8	D49.0
auditory (external) — *see also Neoplasm, skin, ear*	C44.20-	C79.2	D04.2-	D23.2-	D48.5	D49.2
auricular (external) — *see also Neoplasm, skin, ear*	C44.20-	C79.2	D04.2-	D23.2-	D48.5	D49.2
canaliculi, biliary (biliferi) (intrahepatic)	C22.1	C78.7	D01.5	D13.4	D37.6	D49.0

◀ New   ◀▬ Revised   ~~deleted~~ Deleted

	Malignant Primary	Malignant Secondary	Ca in situ	Benign	Uncertain Behavior	Unspecified Behavior
canthus (eye) (inner) (outer)	C44.10-	C79.2	D04.1-	D23.1-	D48.5	D49.2
basal cell carcinoma	C44.11-	—	—	—	—	—
specified type NEC	C44.19-	—	—	—	—	—
squamous cell carcinoma	C44.12-	—	—	—	—	—
capillary — see Neoplasm, connective tissue						
caput coli	C18.0	C78.5	D01.0	D12.0	D37.4	D49.0
carcinoid — see Tumor, carcinoid						
cardia (gastric)	C16.0	C78.89	D00.2	D13.1	D37.1	D49.0
cardiac orifice (stomach)	C16.0	C78.89	D00.2	D13.1	D37.1	D49.0
cardio-esophageal junction	C16.0	C78.89	D00.2	D13.1	D37.1	D49.0
cardio-esophagus	C16.0	C78.89	D00.2	D13.1	D37.1	D49.0
carina (bronchus)	C34.0-	C78.0-	D02.2-	D14.3-	D38.1	D49.1
carotid (artery)	C49.0	C79.89	—	D21.0	D48.1	D49.2
body	C75.4	C79.89	—	D35.5	D44.6	D49.7
carpus (any bone)	C40.1-	C79.51	—	D16.1-	—	—
cartilage (articular) (joint) NEC — see also Neoplasm, bone	C41.9	C79.51		D16.9-	D48.0	D49.2
arytenoid	C32.3	C78.39	D02.0	D14.1	D38.0	D49.1
auricular	C49.0	C79.89	—	D21.0	D48.1	D49.2
bronchi	C34.0-	C78.39	—	D14.3-	D38.1	D49.1
costal	C41.3	C79.51	—	D16.7	D48.0	D49.2
cricoid	C32.3	C78.39	D02.0	D14.1	D38.0	D49.1
cuneiform	C32.3	C78.39	D02.0	D14.1	D38.0	D49.1
ear (external)	C49.0	C79.89	—	D21.0	D48.1	D49.2
ensiform	C41.3	C79.51	—	D16.7	D48.0	D49.2
epiglottis	C32.1	C78.39	D02.0	D14.1	D38.0	D49.1
anterior surface	C10.1	C79.89	D00.08	D10.5	D37.05	D49.0
eyelid	C49.0	C79.89	—	D21.0	D48.1	D49.2
intervertebral	C41.2	C79.51	—	D16.6	D48.0	D49.2
larynx, laryngeal	C32.3	C78.39	D02.0	D14.1	D38.0	D49.1
nose, nasal	C30.0	C78.39	D02.3	D14.0	D38.5	D49.1
pinna	C49.0	C79.89	—	D21.0	D48.1	D49.2
rib	C41.3	C79.51	—	D16.7	D48.0	D49.2
semilunar (knee)	C40.2-	C79.51	—	D16.2-	D48.0	D49.2
thyroid	C32.3	C78.39	D02.0	D14.1	D38.0	D49.1
trachea	C33	C78.39	D02.1	D14.2	D38.1	D49.1
cauda equina	C72.1	C79.49	—	D33.4	D43.4	D49.7
cavity						
buccal	C06.9	C79.89	D00.00	D10.30	D37.09	D49.0
nasal	C30.0	C78.39	D02.3	D14.0	D38.5	D49.1
oral	C06.9	C79.89	D00.00	D10.30	D37.09	D49.0
peritoneal	C48.2	C78.6	—	D20.1	D48.4	D49.0
tympanic	C30.1	C78.39	D02.3	D14.0	D38.5	D49.1

	Malignant Primary	Malignant Secondary	Ca in situ	Benign	Uncertain Behavior	Unspecified Behavior
cecum	C18.0	C78.5	D01.0	D12.0	D37.4	D49.0
central nervous system	C72.9	C79.40	—	—	—	—
cerebellopontine (angle)	C71.6	C79.31	—	D33.1	D43.1	D49.6
cerebellum, cerebellar	C71.6	C79.31		D33.1	D43.1	D49.6
cerebrum, cerebral (cortex) (hemisphere) (white matter)	C71.0	C79.31	—	D33.0	D43.0	D49.6
meninges	C70.0	C79.32		D32.0	D42.0	D49.7
peduncle	C71.7	C79.31		D33.1	D43.1	D49.6
ventricle	C71.5	C79.31		D33.0	D43.0	D49.6
fourth	C71.7	C79.31		D33.1	D43.1	D49.6
cervical region	C76.0	C79.89	D09.8	D36.7	D48.7	D49.89
cervix (cervical) (uteri) (uterus)	C53.9	C79.82	D06.9	D26.0	D39.0	D49.59 ◀
canal	C53.0	C79.82	D06.0	D26.0	D39.0	D49.59 ◀
endocervix (canal) (gland)	C53.0	C79.82	D06.0	D26.0	D39.0	D49.59 ◀
exocervix	C53.1	C79.82	D06.1	D26.0	D39.0	D49.59 ◀
external os	C53.1	C79.82	D06.1	D26.0	D39.0	D49.59 ◀
internal os	C53.0	C79.82	D06.0	D26.0	D39.0	D49.59 ◀
nabothian gland	C53.0	C79.82	D06.0	D26.0	D39.0	D49.59 ◀
overlapping lesion	C53.8	—	—	—	—	—
squamocolumnar junction	C53.8	C79.82	D06.7	D26.0	D39.0	D49.59 ◀
stump	C53.8	C79.82	D06.7	D26.0	D39.0	D49.59 ◀
cheek	C76.0	C79.89	D09.8	D36.7	D48.7	D49.89
external	C44.309	C79.2	D04.39	D23.39	D48.5	D49.2
basal cell carcinoma	C44.319	—	—	—	—	—
specified type NEC	C44.399	—	—	—	—	—
squamous cell carcinoma	C44.329	—	—	—	—	—
inner aspect	C06.0	C79.89	D00.02	D10.39	D37.09	D49.0
internal	C06.0	C79.89	D00.02	D10.39	D37.09	D49.0
mucosa	C06.0	C79.89	D00.02	D10.39	D37.09	D49.0
chest (wall) NEC	C76.1	C79.89	D09.8	D36.7	D48.7	D49.89
chiasma opticum	C72.3-	C79.49	—	D33.3	D43.3	D49.7
chin	C44.309	C79.2	D04.39	D23.39	D48.5	D49.2
basal cell carcinoma	C44.319	—	—	—	—	—
specified type NEC	C44.399	—	—	—	—	—
squamous cell carcinoma	C44.329	—	—	—	—	—
choana	C11.3	C79.89	D00.08	D10.6	D37.05	D49.0
cholangiole	C22.1	C78.89	D01.5	D13.4	D37.6	D49.0
choledochal duct	C24.0	C78.89	D01.5	D13.5	D37.6	D49.0
choroid	C69.3-	C79.49	D09.2-	D31.3-	D48.7	D49.81
plexus	C71.5	C79.31	—	D33.0	D43.0	D49.6
ciliary body	C69.4-	C79.49	D09.2-	D31.4-	D48.7	D49.89
clavicle	C41.3	C79.51	—	D16.7	D48.0	D49.2
clitoris	C51.2	C79.82	D07.1	D28.0	D39.8	D49.59 ◀
clivus	C41.0	C79.51	—	D16.4-	D48.0	D49.2

TABLE OF NEOPLASMS

	Malignant Primary	Malignant Secondary	Ca in situ	Benign	Uncertain Behavior	Unspecified Behavior
cloacogenic zone	C21.2	C78.5	D01.3	D12.9	D37.8	D49.0
coccygeal						
body or glomus	C49.5	C79.89	—	D21.5	D48.1	D49.2
vertebra	C41.4	C79.51	—	D16.8	D48.0	D49.2
coccyx	C41.4	C79.51	—	D16.8	D48.0	D49.2
colon — *see also Neoplasm, intestine, large*	C18.9	C78.5	—	—	—	—
with rectum	C19	C78.5	D01.1	D12.7	D37.5	D49.0
column, spinal — *see Neoplasm, spine*						
columnella — *see also Neoplasm, skin, face*	C44.390	C79.2	D04.39	D23.39	D48.5	D49.2
commissure						
labial, lip	C00.6	C79.89	D00.01	D10.39	D37.01	D49.0
laryngeal	C32.0	C78.39	D02.0	D14.1	D38.0	D49.1
common (bile) duct	C24.0	C78.89	D01.5	D13.5	D37.6	D49.0
concha — *see also Neoplasm, skin, ear*	C44.20-	C79.2	D04.2-	D23.2-	D48.5	D49.2
nose	C30.0	C78.39	D02.3	D14.0	D38.5	D49.1
conjunctiva	C69.0-	C79.49	D09.2-	D31.0-	D48.7	D49.89
connective tissue NEC	C49.9	C79.89	—	D21.9	D48.1	D49.2

Note: For neoplasms of connective tissue (blood vessel, bursa, fascia, ligament, muscle, peripheral nerves, sympathetic and parasympathetic nerves and ganglia, synovia, tendon, etc.) or of morphological types that indicate connective tissue, code according to the list under "Neoplasm, connective tissue". For sites that do not appear in this list, code to neoplasm of that site; e.g., fibrosarcoma, pancreas (C25.9)

Note: Morphological types that indicate connective tissue appear in their proper place in the alphabetic index with the instruction "*see Neoplasm, connective tissue ....*"

	Malignant Primary	Malignant Secondary	Ca in situ	Benign	Uncertain Behavior	Unspecified Behavior
abdomen	C49.4	C79.89	—	D21.4	D48.1	D49.2
abdominal wall	C49.4	C79.89	—	D21.4	D48.1	D49.2
ankle	C49.2-	C79.89	—	D21.2-	D48.1	D49.2
antecubital fossa or space	C49.1-	C79.89	—	D21.1-	D48.1	D49.2
arm	C49.1-	C79.89	—	D21.1-	D48.1	D49.2
auricle (ear)	C49.0	C79.89	—	D21.0	D48.1	D49.2
axilla	C49.3	C79.89	—	D21.3	D48.1	D49.2
back	C49.6	C79.89	—	D21.6	D48.1	D49.2
breast — *see Neoplasm, breast*						
buttock	C49.5	C79.89	—	D21.5	D48.1	D49.2
calf	C49.2-	C79.89	—	D21.2-	D48.1	D49.2
cervical region	C49.0	C79.89	—	D21.0	D48.1	D49.2
cheek	C49.0	C79.89	—	D21.0	D48.1	D49.2
chest (wall)	C49.3	C79.89	—	D21.3	D48.1	D49.2
chin	C49.0	C79.89	—	D21.0	D48.1	D49.2

	Malignant Primary	Malignant Secondary	Ca in situ	Benign	Uncertain Behavior	Unspecified Behavior
connective tissue NEC *(Continued)*						
diaphragm	C49.3	C79.89	—	D21.3	D48.1	D49.2
ear (external)	C49.0	C79.89	—	D21.0	D48.1	D49.2
elbow	C49.1-	C79.89	—	D21.1-	D48.1	D49.2
extrarectal	C49.5	C79.89	—	D21.5	D48.1	D49.2
extremity	C49.9	C79.89	—	D21.9	D48.1	D49.2
lower	C49.2-	C79.89	—	D21.2-	D48.1	D49.2
upper	C49.1-	C79.89	—	D21.1-	D48.1	D49.2
eyelid	C49.0	C79.89	—	D21.0	D48.1	D49.2
face	C49.0	C79.89	—	D21.0	D48.1	D49.2
finger	C49.1-	C79.89	—	D21.1-	D48.1	D49.2
flank	C49.6	C79.89	—	D21.6	D48.1	D49.2
foot	C49.2-	C79.89	—	D21.2-	D48.1	D49.2
forearm	C49.1-	C79.89	—	D21.1-	D48.1	D49.2
forehead	C49.0	C79.89	—	D21.0	D48.1	D49.2
gastric	C49.4	C79.89	—	D21.4	D48.1	D49.2
gastrointestinal	C49.4	C79.89	—	D21.4	D48.1	D49.2
gluteal region	C49.5	C79.89	—	D21.5	D48.1	D49.2
great vessels NEC	C49.3	C79.89	—	D21.3	D48.1	D49.2
groin	C49.5	C79.89	—	D21.5	D48.1	D49.2
hand	C49.1-	C79.89	—	D21.1-	D48.1	D49.2
head	C49.0	C79.89	—	D21.0	D48.1	D49.2
heel	C49.2-	C79.89	—	D21.2-	D48.1	D49.2
hip	C49.2-	C79.89	—	D21.2-	D48.1	D49.2
hypochondrium	C49.4	C79.89	—	D21.4	D48.1	D49.2
iliopsoas muscle	C49.5	C79.89	—	D21.5	D48.1	D49.2
infraclavicular region	C49.3	C79.89	—	D21.3	D48.1	D49.2
inguinal (canal) (region)	C49.5	C79.89	—	D21.5	D48.1	D49.2
intestinal	C49.4	C79.89	—	D21.4	D48.1	D49.2
intrathoracic	C49.3	C79.89	—	D21.3	D48.1	D49.2
ischiorectal fossa	C49.5	C79.89	—	D21.5	D48.1	D49.2
jaw	C03.9	C79.89	D00.03	D10.39	D48.1	D49.0
knee	C49.2-	C79.89	—	D21.2-	D48.1	D49.2
leg	C49.2-	C79.89	—	D21.2-	D48.1	D49.2
limb NEC	C49.9	C79.89	—	D21.9	D48.1	D49.2
lower	C49.2-	C79.89	—	D21.2-	D48.1	D49.2
upper	C49.1-	C79.89	—	D21.1-	D48.1	D49.2
nates	C49.5	C79.89	—	D21.5	D48.1	D49.2
neck	C49.0	C79.89	—	D21.0	D48.1	D49.2
orbit	C69.6-	C79.49	D09.2-	D31.6-	D48.1	D49.89
overlapping lesion	C49.8	—	—	—	—	—
pararectal	C49.5	C79.89	—	D21.5	D48.1	D49.2
para-urethral	C49.5	C79.89	—	D21.5	D48.1	D49.2
paravaginal	C49.5	C79.89	—	D21.5	D48.1	D49.2

◄ New   ⇐ Revised   ~~deleted~~ Deleted

	Malignant Primary	Malignant Secondary	Ca in situ	Benign	Uncertain Behavior	Unspecified Behavior
connective tissue NEC *(Continued)*						
pelvis (floor)	C49.5	C79.89	—	D21.5	D48.1	D49.2
pelvo-abdominal	C49.8	C79.89	—	D21.6	D48.1	D49.2
perineum	C49.5	C79.89	—	D21.5	D48.1	D49.2
perirectal (tissue)	C49.5	C79.89	—	D21.5	D48.1	D49.2
periurethral (tissue)	C49.5	C79.89	—	D21.5	D48.1	D49.2
popliteal fossa or space	C49.2-	C79.89	—	D21.2-	D48.1	D49.2
presacral	C49.5	C79.89	—	D21.5	D48.1	D49.2
psoas muscle	C49.4	C79.89	—	D21.4	D48.1	D49.2
pterygoid fossa	C49.0	C79.89	—	D21.0	D48.1	D49.2
rectovaginal septum or wall	C49.5	C79.89	—	D21.5	D48.1	D49.2
rectovesical	C49.5	C79.89	—	D21.5	D48.1	D49.2
retroperitoneum	C48.0	C78.6	—	D20.0	D48.3	D49.0
sacrococcygeal region	C49.5	C79.89	—	D21.5	D48.1	D49.2
scalp	C49.0	C79.89	—	D21.0	D48.1	D49.2
scapular region	C49.3	C79.89	—	D21.3	D48.1	D49.2
shoulder	C49.1-	C79.89	—	D21.1-	D48.1	D49.2
skin (dermis) NEC — *see also Neoplasm, skin, by site*	C44.90	C79.2	D04.9	D23.9	D48.5	D49.2
stomach	C49.4	C79.89	—	D21.4	D48.1	D49.2
submental	C49.0	C79.89	—	D21.0	D48.1	D49.2
supraclavicular region	C49.0	C79.89	—	D21.0	D48.1	D49.2
temple	C49.0	C79.89	—	D21.0	D48.1	D49.2
temporal region	C49.0	C79.89	—	D21.0	D48.1	D49.2
thigh	C49.2-	C79.89	—	D21.2-	D48.1	D49.2
thoracic (duct) (wall)	C49.3	C79.89	—	D21.3	D48.1	D49.2
thorax	C49.3	C79.89	—	D21.3	D48.1	D49.2
thumb	C49.1-	C79.89	—	D21.1-	D48.1	D49.2
toe	C49.2-	C79.89	—	D21.2-	D48.1	D49.2
trunk	C49.6	C79.89	—	D21.6	D48.1	D49.2
umbilicus	C49.4	C79.89	—	D21.4	D48.1	D49.2
vesicorectal	C49.5	C79.89	—	D21.5	D48.1	D49.2
wrist	C49.1-	C79.89	—	D21.1-	D48.1	D49.2
conus medullaris	C72.0	C79.49	—	D33.4	D43.4	D49.7
cord (true) (vocal)	C32.0	C78.39	D02.0	D14.1	D38.0	D49.1
false	C32.1	C78.39	D02.0	D14.1	D38.0	D49.1
spermatic	C63.1-	C79.82	D07.69	D29.8	D40.8	D49.59
spinal (cervical) (lumbar) (thoracic)	C72.0	C79.49	—	D33.4	D43.4	D49.7
cornea (limbus)	C69.1-	C79.49	D09.2-	D31.1-	D48.7	D49.89
corpus						
albicans	C56.-	C79.6-	D07.39	D27.-	D39.1-	D49.59
callosum, brain	C71.0	C79.31	—	D33.2	D43.2	D49.6
cavernosum	C60.2	C79.82	D07.4	D29.0	D40.8	D49.59

	Malignant Primary	Malignant Secondary	Ca in situ	Benign	Uncertain Behavior	Unspecified Behavior
corpus *(Continued)*						
gastric	C16.2	C78.89	D00.2	D13.1	D37.1	D49.0
overlapping sites	C54.8	—				
penis	C60.2	C79.82	D07.4	D29.0	D40.8	D49.59
striatum, cerebrum	C71.0	C79.31	—	D33.0	D43.0	D49.6
uteri	C54.9	C79.82	D07.0	D26.1	D39.0	D49.59
isthmus	C54.0	C79.82	D07.0	D26.1	D39.0	D49.59
cortex						
adrenal	C74.0-	C79.7-	D09.3	D35.0-	D44.1-	D49.7
cerebral	C71.0	C79.31	—	D33.0	D43.0	D49.6
costal cartilage	C41.3	C79.51	—	D16.7	D48.0	D49.2
costovertebral joint	C41.3	C79.51	—	D16.7	D48.0	D49.2
Cowper's gland	C68.0	C79.19	D09.19	D30.4	D41.3	D49.59
cranial (fossa, any)	C71.9	C79.31	—	D33.2	D43.2	D49.6
meninges	C70.0	C79.32	—	D32.0	D42.0	D49.7
nerve	C72.50	C79.49	—	D33.3	D43.3	D49.7
specified NEC	C72.59	C79.49	—	D33.3	D43.3	D49.7
craniobuccal pouch	C75.2	C79.89	D09.3	D35.2	D44.3	D49.7
craniopharyngeal (duct) (pouch)	C75.2	C79.89	D09.3	D35.3	D44.4	D49.7
cricoid	C13.0	C79.89	D00.08	D10.7	D37.05	D49.0
cartilage	C32.3	C78.39	D02.0	D14.1	D38.0	D49.1
cricopharynx	C13.0	C79.89	D00.08	D10.7	D37.05	D49.0
crypt of Morgagni	C21.8	C78.5	D01.3	D12.9	D37.8	D49.0
crystalline lens	C69.4-	C79.49	D09.2-	D31.4-	D48.7	D49.89
cul-de-sac (Douglas')	C48.1	C78.6	—	D20.1	D48.4	D49.0
cuneiform cartilage	C32.3	C78.39	D02.0	D14.1	D38.0	D49.1
cutaneous — *see Neoplasm, skin*						
cutis — *see Neoplasm, skin*						
cystic (bile) duct (common)	C24.0	C78.89	D01.5	D13.5	D37.6	D49.0
dermis — *see Neoplasm, skin*						
diaphragm	C49.3	C79.89	—	D21.3	D48.1	D49.2
digestive organs, system, tube, or tract NEC	C26.9	C78.89	D01.9	D13.9	D37.9	D49.0
disc, intervertebral	C41.2	C79.51	—	D16.6	D48.0	D49.2
disease, generalized	C80.0	—	—	—	—	—
disseminated	C80.0	—	—	—	—	—
Douglas' cul-de-sac or pouch	C48.1	C78.6	—	D20.1	D48.4	D49.0
duodenojejunal junction	C17.8	C78.4	D01.49	D13.39	D37.2	D49.0
duodenum	C17.0	C78.4	D01.49	D13.2	D37.2	D49.0
dura (cranial) (mater)	C70.9	C79.49	—	D32.9	D42.9	D49.7
cerebral	C70.0	C79.32	—	D32.0	D42.0	D49.7
spinal	C70.1	C79.49	—	D32.1	D42.1	D49.7

◀ New ◀▬ Revised ~~deleted~~ Deleted

TABLE OF NEOPLASMS

	Malignant Primary	Malignant Secondary	Ca in situ	Benign	Uncertain Behavior	Unspecified Behavior
ear (external) — *see also Neoplasm, skin, ear*	C44.20-	C79.2	D04.2-	D23.2-	D48.5	D49.2
auricle or auris — *see also Neoplasm, skin, ear*	C44.20-	C79.2	D04.2-	D23.2-	D48.5	D49.2
canal, external — *see also Neoplasm, skin, ear*	C44.20-	C79.2	D04.2-	D23.2-	D48.5	D49.2
cartilage	C49.0	C79.89	—	D21.0	D48.1	D49.2
external meatus — *see also Neoplasm, skin, ear*	C44.20-	C79.2	D04.2-	D23.2-	D48.5	D49.2
inner	C30.1	C78.39	D02.3	D14.0	D38.5	D49.1
lobule — *see also Neoplasm, skin, ear*	C44.20-	C79.2	D04.2-	D23.2-	D48.5	D49.2
middle	C30.1	C78.39	D02.3	D14.0	D38.5	D49.1
overlapping lesion with accessory sinuses	C31.8	—	—	—	—	—
skin	C44.20-	C79.2	D04.2-	D23.2-	D48.5	D49.2
basal cell carcinoma	C44.21-	—	—	—	—	—
specified type NEC	C44.29-	—	—	—	—	—
squamous cell carcinoma	C44.22-	—	—	—	—	—
earlobe	C44.20-	C79.2	D04.2-	D23.2-	D48.5	D49.2
basal cell carcinoma	C44.21-	—	—	—	—	—
specified type NEC	C44.29-	—	—	—	—	—
squamous cell carcinoma	C44.22-	—	—	—	—	—
ejaculatory duct	C63.7	C79.82	D07.69	D29.8	D40.8	D49.59
elbow NEC	C76.4-	C79.89	D04.6-	D36.7	D48.7	D49.89
endocardium	C38.0	C79.89	—	D15.1	D48.7	D49.89
endocervix (canal) (gland)	C53.0	C79.82	D06.0	D26.0	D39.0	D49.59
endocrine gland NEC	C75.9	C79.89	D09.3	D35.9	D44.9	D49.7
pluriglandular	C75.8	C79.89	D09.3	D35.7	D44.9	D49.7
endometrium (gland) (stroma)	C54.1	C79.82	D07.0	D26.1	D39.0	D49.59
ensiform cartilage	C41.3	C79.51	—	D16.7	D48.0	D49.2
enteric — *see Neoplasm, intestine*						
ependyma (brain)	C71.5	C79.31	—	D33.0	D43.0	D49.6
fourth ventricle	C71.7	C79.31	—	D33.1	D43.1	D49.6
epicardium	C38.0	C79.89	—	D15.1	D48.7	D49.89
epididymis	C63.0-	C79.82	D07.69	D29.3-	D40.8	D49.59
epidural	C72.9	C79.49	—	D33.9	D43.9	D49.7
epiglottis	C32.1	C78.39	D02.0	D14.1	D38.0	D49.1
anterior aspect or surface	C10.1	C79.89	D00.08	D10.5	D37.05	D49.0
cartilage	C32.3	C78.39	D02.0	D14.1	D38.0	D49.1
free border (margin)	C10.1	C79.89	D00.08	D10.5	D37.05	D49.0
junctional region	C10.8	C79.89	D00.08	D10.5	D37.05	D49.0
posterior (laryngeal) surface	C32.1	C78.39	D02.0	D14.1	D38.0	D49.1
suprahyoid portion	C32.1	C78.39	D02.0	D14.1	D38.0	D49.1

	Malignant Primary	Malignant Secondary	Ca in situ	Benign	Uncertain Behavior	Unspecified Behavior
esophagogastric junction	C16.0	C78.89	D00.2	D13.1	D37.1	D49.0
esophagus	C15.9	C78.89	D00.1	D13.0	D37.8	D49.0
abdominal	C15.5	C78.89	D00.1	D13.0	D37.8	D49.0
cervical	C15.3	C78.89	D00.1	D13.0	D37.8	D49.0
distal (third)	C15.5	C78.89	D00.1	D13.0	D37.8	D49.0
lower (third)	C15.5	C78.89	D00.1	D13.0	D37.8	D49.0
middle (third)	C15.4	C78.89	D00.1	D13.0	D37.8	D49.0
overlapping lesion	C15.8	—	—	—	—	—
proximal (third)	C15.3	C78.89	D00.1	D13.0	D37.8	D49.0
thoracic	C15.4	C78.89	D00.1	D13.0	D37.8	D49.0
upper (third)	C15.3	C78.89	D00.1	D13.0	D37.8	D49.0
ethmoid (sinus)	C31.1	C78.39	D02.3	D14.0	D38.5	D49.1
bone or labyrinth	C41.0	C79.51	—	D16.4-	D48.0	D49.2
eustachian tube	C30.1	C78.39	D02.3	D14.0	D38.5	D49.1
exocervix	C53.1	C79.82	D06.1	D26.0	D39.0	D49.59
external						
meatus (ear) — *see also Neoplasm, skin, ear*	C44.20-	C79.2	D04.2-	D23.2-	D48.5	D49.2
os, cervix uteri	C53.1	C79.82	D06.1	D26.0	D39.0	D49.59
extradural	C72.9	C79.49	—	D33.9	D43.9	D49.7
extrahepatic (bile) duct	C24.0	C78.89	D01.5	D13.5	D37.6	D49.0
overlapping lesion with gallbladder	C24.8	—	—	—	—	—
extraocular muscle	C69.6-	C79.49	D09.2-	D31.6-	D48.7	D49.89
extrarectal	C76.3	C79.89	D09.8	D36.7	D48.7	D49.89
extremity	C76.8	C79.89	D04.8	D36.7	D48.7	D49.89
lower	C76.5-	C79.89	D04.7-	D36.7	D48.7	D49.89
upper	C76.4-	C79.89	D04.6-	D36.7	D48.7	D49.89
eye NEC	C69.9-	C79.49	D09.2	D31.9	D48.7	D49.89
overlapping sites	C69.8	—	—	—	—	—
eyeball	C69.9-	C79.49	D09.2-	D31.9-	D48.7	D49.89
eyebrow	C44.309	C79.2	D04.39	D23.39	D48.5	D49.2
basal cell carcinoma	C44.319	—	—	—	—	—
specified type NEC	C44.399	—	—	—	—	—
squamous cell carcinoma	C44.329	—	—	—	—	—
eyelid (lower) (skin) (upper)	C44.10-	—	—	—	—	—
basal cell carcinoma	C44.11-	—	—	—	—	—
cartilage	C49.0	C79.89	—	D21.0	D48.1	D49.2
specified type NEC	C44.19-	—	—	—	—	—
squamous cell carcinoma	C44.12-	—	—	—	—	—
face NEC	C76.0	C79.89	D04.39	D36.7	D48.7	D49.89
fallopian tube (accessory)	C57.0-	C79.82	D07.39	D28.2	D39.8	D49.59
falx (cerebella) (cerebri)	C70.0	C79.32	—	D32.0	D42.0	D49.7

◀ New ⬅ Revised ~~deleted~~ Deleted

	Malignant Primary	Malignant Secondary	Ca in situ	Benign	Uncertain Behavior	Unspecified Behavior
fascia — *see also* Neoplasm, connective tissue						
palmar	C49.1-	C79.89	—	D21.1-	D48.1	D49.2
plantar	C49.2-	C79.89	—	D21.2-	D48.1	D49.2
fatty tissue — *see* Neoplasm, connective tissue						
fauces, faucial NEC	C10.9	C79.89	D00.08	D10.5	D37.05	D49.0
pillars	C09.1	C79.89	D00.08	D10.5	D37.05	D49.0
tonsil	C09.9	C79.89	D00.08	D10.4	D37.05	D49.0
femur (any part)	C40.2-	—		D16.2-	—	—
fetal membrane	C58	C79.82	D07.0	D26.7	D39.2	D49.59
fibrous tissue — *see* Neoplasm, connective tissue						
fibula (any part)	C40.2-	C79.51	—	D16.2-	—	—
filum terminale	C72.0	C79.49	—	D33.4	D43.4	D49.7
finger NEC	C76.4-	C79.89	D04.6-	D36.7	D48.7	D49.89
flank NEC	C76.8	C79.89	D04.5	D36.7	D48.7	D49.89
follicle, nabothian	C53.0	C79.82	D06.0	D26.0	D39.0	D49.59
foot NEC	C76.5-	C79.89	D04.7-	D36.7	D48.7	D49.89
forearm NEC	C76.4-	C79.89	D04.6-	D36.7	D48.7	D49.89
forehead (skin)	C44.309	C79.2	D04.39	D23.39	D48.5	D49.2
basal cell carcinoma	C44.319	—	—	—	—	—
specified type NEC	C44.399	—	—	—	—	—
squamous cell carcinoma	C44.329	—	—	—	—	—
foreskin	C60.0	C79.82	D07.4	D29.0	D40.8	D49.59
fornix						
pharyngeal	C11.3	C79.89	D00.08	D10.6	D37.05	D49.0
vagina	C52	C79.82	D07.2	D28.1	D39.8	D49.59
fossa (of)						
anterior (cranial)	C71.9	C79.31	—	D33.2	D43.2	D49.6
cranial	C71.9	C79.31	—	D33.2	D43.2	D49.6
ischiorectal	C76.3	C79.89	D09.8	D36.7	D48.7	D49.89
middle (cranial)	C71.9	C79.31	—	D33.2	D43.2	D49.6
piriform	C12	C79.89	D00.08	D10.7	D37.05	D49.0
pituitary	C75.1	C79.89	D09.3	D35.2	D44.3	D49.7
posterior (cranial)	C71.9	C79.31	—	D33.2	D43.2	D49.6
pterygoid	C49.0	C79.89	—	D21.0	D48.1	D49.2
pyriform	C12	C79.89	D00.08	D10.7	D37.05	D49.0
Rosenmuller	C11.2	C79.89	D00.08	D10.6	D37.05	D49.0
tonsillar	C09.0	C79.89	D00.08	D10.5	D37.05	D49.0
fourchette	C51.9	C79.82	D07.1	D28.0	D39.8	D49.59
frenulum						
labii — *see* Neoplasm, lip, internal						
linguae	C02.2	C79.89	D00.07	D10.1	D37.02	D49.0

	Malignant Primary	Malignant Secondary	Ca in situ	Benign	Uncertain Behavior	Unspecified Behavior
frontal						
bone	C41.0	C79.51	—	D16.4-	D48.0	D49.2
lobe, brain	C71.1	C79.31	—	D33.0	D43.0	D49.6
pole	C71.1	C79.31	—	D33.0	D43.0	D49.6
sinus	C31.2	C78.39	D02.3	D14.0	D38.5	D49.1
fundus						
stomach	C16.1	C78.89	D00.2	D13.1	D37.1	D49.0
uterus	C54.3	C79.82	D07.0	D26.1	D39.0	D49.59
gall duct (extrahepatic)	C24.0	C78.89	D01.5	D13.5	D37.6	D49.0
intrahepatic	C22.1	C78.7	D01.5	D13.4	D37.6	D49.0
gallbladder	C23	C78.89	D01.5	D13.5	D37.6	D49.0
overlapping lesion with extrahepatic bile ducts	C24.8	—	—	—	—	—
ganglia — *see also* Neoplasm, nerve, peripheral	C47.9	C79.89	—	D36.10	D48.2	D49.2
basal	C71.0	C79.31	—	D33.0	D43.0	D49.6
cranial nerve	C72.50	C79.49	—	D33.3	D43.3	D49.7
Gartner's duct	C52	C79.82	D07.2	D28.1	D39.8	D49.59
gastric — *see* Neoplasm, stomach						
gastrocolic	C26.9	C78.89	D01.9	D13.9	D37.9	D49.0
gastroesophageal junction	C16.0	C78.89	D00.2	D13.1	D37.1	D49.0
gastrointestinal (tract) NEC	C26.9	C78.89	D01.9	D13.9	D37.9	D49.0
generalized	C80.0	—	—	—	—	—
genital organ or tract						
female NEC	C57.9	C79.82	D07.30	D28.9	D39.9	D49.59
overlapping lesion	C57.8	—	—	—	—	—
specified site NEC	C57.7	C79.82	D07.39	D28.7	D39.8	D49.59
male NEC	C63.9	C79.82	D07.60	D29.9	D40.9	D49.59
overlapping lesion	C63.8	—	—	—	—	—
specified site NEC	C63.7	C79.82	D07.69	D29.8	D40.8	D49.59
genitourinary tract						
female	C57.9	C79.82	D07.30	D28.9	D39.9	D49.59
male	C63.9	C79.82	D07.60	D29.9	D40.9	D49.59
gingiva (alveolar) (marginal)	C03.9	C79.89	D00.03	D10.39	D37.09	D49.0
lower	C03.1	C79.89	D00.03	D10.39	D37.09	D49.0
mandibular	C03.1	C79.89	D00.03	D10.39	D37.09	D49.0
maxillary	C03.0	C79.89	D00.03	D10.39	D37.09	D49.0
upper	C03.0	C79.89	D00.03	D10.39	D37.09	D49.0
gland, glandular (lymphatic) (system) — *see also* Neoplasm, lymph gland						
endocrine NEC	C75.9	C79.89	D09.3	D35.9	D44.9	D49.7
salivary — *see* Neoplasm, salivary gland						

◀ New   ◀ Revised   ~~deleted~~ Deleted

TABLE OF NEOPLASMS

	Malignant Primary	Malignant Secondary	Ca in situ	Benign	Uncertain Behavior	Unspecified Behavior
glans penis	C60.1	C79.82	D07.4	D29.0	D40.8	D49.59
globus pallidus	C71.0	C79.31	—	D33.0	D43.0	D49.6
glomus						
coccygeal	C49.5	C79.89	—	D21.5	D48.1	D49.2
jugularis	C75.5	C79.89	—	D35.6	D44.7	D49.7
glosso-epiglottic fold(s)	C10.1	C79.89	D00.08	D10.5	D37.05	D49.0
glossopalatine fold	C09.1	C79.89	D00.08	D10.5	D37.05	D49.0
glossopharyngeal sulcus	C09.0	C79.89	D00.08	D10.5	D37.05	D49.0
glottis	C32.0	C78.39	D02.0	D14.1	D38.0	D49.1
gluteal region	C76.3	C79.89	D04.5	D36.7	D48.7	D49.89
great vessels NEC	C49.3	C79.89	—	D21.3	D48.1	D49.2
groin NEC	C76.3	C79.89	D04.5	D36.7	D48.7	D49.89
gum	C03.9	C79.89	D00.03	D10.39	D37.09	D49.0
lower	C03.1	C79.89	D00.03	D10.39	D37.09	D49.0
upper	C03.0	C79.89	D00.03	D10.39	D37.09	D49.0
hand NEC	C76.4-	C79.89	D04.6-	D36.7	D48.7	D49.89
head NEC	C76.0	C79.89	D04.4	D36.7	D48.7	D49.89
heart	C38.0	C79.89	—	D15.1	D48.7	D49.89
heel NEC	C76.5-	C79.89	D04.7-	D36.7	D48.7	D49.89
helix — see also Neoplasm, skin, ear	C44.20-	C79.2	D04.2-	D23.2-	D48.5	D49.2
hematopoietic, hemopoietic tissue NEC	C96.9	—	—	—	—	—
specified NEC	C96.Z	—	—	—	—	—
hemisphere, cerebral	C71.0	C79.31	—	D33.0	D43.0	D49.6
hemorrhoidal zone	C21.1	C78.5	D01.3	D12.9	D37.8	D49.0
hepatic — see also Index to disease, by histology	C22.9	C78.7	D01.5	D13.4	D37.6	D49.0
duct (bile)	C24.0	C78.89	D01.5	D13.5	D37.6	D49.0
flexure (colon)	C18.3	C78.5	D01.0	D12.3	D37.4	D49.0
primary	C22.8	C78.7	D01.5	D13.4	D37.6	D49.0
hepatobiliary	C24.9	C79.89	D01.5	D13.5	D37.6	D49.0
hepatoblastoma	C22.2	C78.7	D01.5	D13.4	D37.6	D49.0
hepatoma	C22.0	C78.7	D01.5	D13.4	D37.6	D49.0
hilus of lung	C34.0-	C78.0-	D02.2-	D14.3-	D38.1	D49.1
hip NEC	C76.5-	C79.89	D04.7-	D36.7	D48.7	D49.89
hippocampus, brain	C71.2	C79.31	—	D33.0	D43.0	D49.6
humerus (any part)	C40.0-	C79.51	—	D16.0-	—	—
hymen	C52	C79.82	D07.2	D28.1	D39.8	D49.59
hypopharynx, hypopharyngeal NEC	C13.9	C79.89	D00.08	D10.7	D37.05	D49.0
overlapping lesion	C13.8	—	—	—	—	—
postcricoid region	C13.0	C79.89	D00.08	D10.7	D37.05	D49.0
posterior wall	C13.2	C79.89	D00.08	D10.7	D37.05	D49.0
pyriform fossa (sinus)	C12	C79.89	D00.08	D10.7	D37.05	D49.0
hypophysis	C75.1	C79.89	D09.3	D35.2	D44.3	D49.7

	Malignant Primary	Malignant Secondary	Ca in situ	Benign	Uncertain Behavior	Unspecified Behavior
hypothalamus	C71.0	C79.31	—	D33.0	D43.0	D49.6
ileocecum, ileocecal (coil) (junction) (valve)	C18.0	C78.5	D01.0	D12.0	D37.4	D49.0
ileum	C17.2	C78.4	D01.49	D13.39	D37.2	D49.0
ilium	C41.4	C79.51	—	D16.8	D48.0	D49.2
immunoproliferative NEC	C88.9	—	—	—	—	—
infraclavicular (region)	C76.1	C79.89	D04.5	D36.7	D48.7	D49.89
inguinal (region)	C76.3	C79.89	D04.5	D36.7	D48.7	D49.89
insula	C71.0	C79.31	—	D33.0	D43.0	D49.6
insular tissue (pancreas)	C25.4	C78.89	D01.7	D13.7	D37.8	D49.0
brain	C71.0	C79.31	—	D33.0	D43.0	D49.6
interarytenoid fold	C13.1	C79.89	D00.08	D10.7	D37.05	D49.0
hypopharyngeal aspect	C13.1	C79.89	D00.08	D10.7	D37.05	D49.0
laryngeal aspect	C32.1	C78.39	D02.0	D14.1	D38.0	D49.1
marginal zone	C13.1	C79.89	D00.08	D10.7	D37.05	D49.0
interdental papillae	C03.9	C79.89	D00.03	D10.39	D37.09	D49.0
lower	C03.1	C79.89	D00.03	D10.39	D37.09	D49.0
upper	C03.0	C79.89	D00.03	D10.39	D37.09	D49.0
internal						
capsule	C71.0	C79.31	—	D33.0	D43.0	D49.6
os (cervix)	C53.0	C79.82	D06.0	D26.0	D39.0	D49.59
intervertebral cartilage or disc	C41.2	C79.51	—	D16.6	D48.0	D49.2
intestine, intestinal	C26.0	C78.80	D01.40	D13.9	D37.8	D49.0
large	C18.9	C78.5	D01.0	D12.6	D37.4	D49.0
appendix	C18.1	C78.5	D01.0	D12.1	D37.3	D49.0
caput coli	C18.0	C78.5	D01.0	D12.0	D37.4	D49.0
cecum	C18.0	C78.5	D01.0	D12.0	D37.4	D49.0
colon	C18.9	C78.5	D01.0	D12.6	D37.4	D49.0
and rectum	C19	C78.5	D01.1	D12.7	D37.5	D49.0
ascending	C18.2	C78.5	D01.0	D12.2	D37.4	D49.0
caput	C18.0	C78.5	D01.0	D12.0	D37.4	D49.0
descending	C18.6	C78.5	D01.0	D12.4	D37.4	D49.0
distal	C18.6	C78.5	D01.0	D12.4	D37.4	D49.0
left	C18.6	C78.5	D01.0	D12.4	D37.4	D49.0
overlapping lesion	C18.8	—	—	—	—	—
pelvic	C18.7	C78.5	D01.0	D12.5	D37.4	D49.0
right	C18.2	C78.5	D01.0	D12.2	D37.4	D49.0
sigmoid (flexure)	C18.7	C78.5	D01.0	D12.5	D37.4	D49.0
transverse	C18.4	C78.5	D01.0	D12.3	D37.4	D49.0
hepatic flexure	C18.3	C78.5	D01.0	D12.3	D37.4	D49.0
ileocecum, ileocecal (coil) (valve)	C18.0	C78.5	D01.0	D12.0	D37.4	D49.0
overlapping lesion	C18.8	—	—	—	—	—

◄ New ⇐ Revised ~~deleted~~ Deleted

	Malignant Primary	Malignant Secondary	Ca in situ	Benign	Uncertain Behavior	Unspecified Behavior
intestine, intestinal *(Continued)*						
large *(Continued)*						
sigmoid flexure (lower) (upper)	C18.7	C78.5	D01.0	D12.5	D37.4	D49.0
splenic flexure	C18.5	C78.5	D01.0	D12.3	D37.4	D49.0
small	C17.9	C78.4	D01.40	D13.30	D37.2	D49.0
duodenum	C17.0	C78.4	D01.49	D13.2	D37.2	D49.0
ileum	C17.2	C78.4	D01.49	D13.39	D37.2	D49.0
jejunum	C17.1	C78.4	D01.49	D13.39	D37.2	D49.0
overlapping lesion	C17.8	—	—	—	—	—
tract NEC	C26.0	C78.89	D01.40	D13.9	D37.8	D49.0
intra-abdominal	C76.2	C79.89	D09.8	D36.7	D48.7	D49.89
intracranial NEC	C71.9	C79.31	—	D33.2	D43.2	D49.6
intrahepatic (bile) duct	C22.1	C78.7	D01.5	D13.4	D37.6	D49.0
intraocular	C69.9-	C79.49	D09.2-	D31.9-	D48.7	D49.89
intraorbital	C69.6-	C79.49	D09.2-	D31.6-	D48.7	D49.89
intrasellar	C75.1	C79.89	D09.3	D35.2	D44.3	D49.7
intrathoracic (cavity) (organs)	C76.1	C79.89	D09.8	D15.9	D48.7	D49.89
specified NEC	C76.1	C79.89	D09.8	D15.7	—	—
iris	C69.4-	C79.49	D09.2-	D31.4-	D48.7	D49.89
ischiorectal (fossa)	C76.3	C79.89	D09.8	D36.7	D48.7	D49.89
ischium	C41.4	C79.51	—	D16.8	D48.0	D49.2
island of Reil	C71.0	C79.31	—	D33.0	D43.0	D49.6
islands or islets of Langerhans	C25.4	C78.89	D01.7	D13.7	D37.8	D49.0
isthmus uteri	C54.0	C79.82	D07.0	D26.1	D39.0	D49.59
jaw	C76.0	C79.89	D09.8	D36.7	D48.7	D49.89
bone	C41.1	C79.51	—	D16.5-	D48.0	D49.2
lower	C41.1	C79.51	—	D16.5-	—	—
upper	C41.0	C79.51	—	D16.4-	—	—
carcinoma (any type) (lower) (upper)	C76.0	C79.89	—	—	—	—
skin — *see also Neoplasm, skin, face*	C44.309	C79.2	D04.39	D23.39	D48.5	D49.2
soft tissues	C03.9	C79.89	D00.03	D10.39	D37.09	D49.0
lower	C03.1	C79.89	D00.03	D10.39	D37.09	D49.0
upper	C03.0	C79.89	D00.03	D10.39	D37.09	D49.0
jejunum	C17.1	C78.4	D01.49	D13.39	D37.2	D49.0
joint NEC — *see also Neoplasm, bone*	C41.9	C79.51	—	D16.9-	D48.0	D49.2
acromioclavicular	C40.0-	C79.51	—	D16.0-	—	—
bursa or synovial membrane — *see Neoplasm, connective tissue*						
costovertebral	C41.3	C79.51	—	D16.7	D48.0	D49.2
sternocostal	C41.3	C79.51	—	D16.7	D48.0	D49.2
temporomandibular	C41.1	C79.51	—	D16.5-	D48.0	D49.2

	Malignant Primary	Malignant Secondary	Ca in situ	Benign	Uncertain Behavior	Unspecified Behavior
junction						
anorectal	C21.8	C78.5	D01.3	D12.9	D37.8	D49.0
cardioesophageal	C16.0	C78.89	D00.2	D13.1	D37.1	D49.0
esophagogastric	C16.0	C78.89	D00.2	D13.1	D37.1	D49.0
gastroesophageal	C16.0	C78.89	D00.2	D13.1	D37.1	D49.0
hard and soft palate	C05.9	C79.89	D00.00	D10.39	D37.09	D49.0
ileocecal	C18.0	C78.5	D01.0	D12.0	D37.4	D49.0
pelvirectal	C19	C78.5	D01.1	D12.7	D37.5	D49.0
pelviureteric	C65.-	C79.0-	D09.19	D30.1-	D41.1-	D49.59 ◀
rectosigmoid	C19	C78.5	D01.1	D12.7	D37.5	D49.0
squamocolumnar, of cervix	C53.8	C79.82	D06.7	D26.0	D39.0	D49.59 ◀
Kaposi's sarcoma — *see Kaposi's, sarcoma*						
kidney (parenchymal)	C64.-	C79.0-	D09.19	D30.0-	D41.0-	D49.51- ◀
calyx	C65.-	C79.0-	D09.19	D30.1-	D41.1-	D49.51- ◀
hilus	C65.-	C79.0-	D09.19	D30.1-	D41.1-	D49.51- ◀
pelvis	C65.-	C79.0-	D09.19	D30.1-	D41.1-	D49.51- ◀
knee NEC	C76.5-	C79.89	D04.7-	D36.7	D48.7	D49.89
labia (skin)	C51.9	C79.82	D07.1	D28.0	D39.8	D49.59 ◀
majora	C51.0	C79.82	D07.1	D28.0	D39.8	D49.59 ◀
minora	C51.1	C79.82	D07.1	D28.0	D39.8	D49.59 ◀
labial — *see also Neoplasm, lip*	C00.9	C79.89	D00.01	D10.0	D37.01	D49.0
sulcus (lower) (upper)	C06.1	C79.89	D00.02	D10.39	D37.09	D49.0
labium (skin)	C51.9	C79.82	D07.1	D28.0	D39.8	D49.59 ◀
majus	C51.0	C79.82	D07.1	D28.0	D39.8	D49.59 ◀
minus	C51.1	C79.82	D07.1	D28.0	D39.8	D49.59 ◀
lacrimal						
canaliculi	C69.5-	C79.49	D09.2-	D31.5-	D48.7	D49.89
duct (nasal)	C69.5-	C79.49	D09.2-	D31.5-	D48.7	D49.89
gland	C69.5-	C79.49	D09.2-	D31.5-	D48.7	D49.89
punctum	C69.5-	C79.49	D09.2-	D31.5-	D48.7	D49.89
sac	C69.5-	C79.49	D09.2-	D31.5-	D48.7	D49.89
Langerhans, islands or islets	C25.4	C78.89	D01.7	D13.7	D37.8	D49.0
laryngopharynx	C13.9	C79.89	D00.08	D10.7	D37.05	D49.0
larynx, laryngeal NEC	C32.9	C78.39	D02.0	D14.1	D38.0	D49.1
aryepiglottic fold	C32.1	C78.39	D02.0	D14.1	D38.0	D49.1
cartilage (arytenoid) (cricoid) (cuneiform) (thyroid)	C32.3	C78.39	D02.0	D14.1	D38.0	D49.1
commissure (anterior) (posterior)	C32.0	C78.39	D02.0	D14.1	D38.0	D49.1
extrinsic NEC	C32.1	C78.39	D02.0	D14.1	D38.0	D49.1
meaning hypopharynx	C13.9	C79.89	D00.08	D10.7	D37.05	D49.0
interarytenoid fold	C32.1	C78.39	D02.0	D14.1	D38.0	D49.1
intrinsic	C32.0	C78.39	D02.0	D14.1	D38.0	D49.1

	Malignant Primary	Malignant Secondary	Ca in situ	Benign	Uncertain Behavior	Unspecified Behavior
larynx, laryngeal NEC *(Continued)*						
overlapping lesion	C32.8	—	—	—	—	—
ventricular band	C32.1	C78.39	D02.0	D14.1	D38.0	D49.1
leg NEC	C76.5-	C79.89	D04.7-	D36.7	D48.7	D49.89
lens, crystalline	C69.4-	C79.49	D09.2-	D31.4-	D48.7	D49.89
lid (lower) (upper)	C44.10-	C79.2	D04.1-	D23.1-	D48.5	D49.2
basal cell carcinoma	C44.11-	—	—	—	—	—
specified type NEC	C44.19-	—	—	—	—	—
squamous cell carcinoma	C44.12-	—	—	—	—	—
ligament — *see also Neoplasm, connective tissue*						
broad	C57.1	C79.82	D07.39	D28.2	D39.8	D49.59 ◄▥
Mackenrodt's	C57.7	C79.82	D07.39	D28.7	D39.8	D49.59 ◄▥
non-uterine — *see Neoplasm, connective tissue*						
round	C57.2	C79.82	—	D28.2	D39.8	D49.59 ◄▥
sacro-uterine	C57.3	C79.82	—	D28.2	D39.8	D49.59 ◄▥
uterine	C57.3	C79.82	—	D28.2	D39.8	D49.59 ◄▥
utero-ovarian	C57.7	C79.82	D07.39	D28.2	D39.8	D49.59 ◄▥
uterosacral	C57.3	C79.82	—	D28.2	D39.8	D49.59 ◄▥
limb	C76.8	C79.89	D04.8	D36.7	D48.7	D49.89
lower	C76.5-	C79.89	D04.7-	D36.7	D48.7	D49.89
upper	C76.4-	C79.89	D04.6-	D36.7	D48.7	D49.89
limbus of cornea	C69.1-	C79.49	D09.2-	D31.1-	D48.7	D49.89
lingual NEC — *see also Neoplasm, tongue*	C02.9	C79.89	D00.07	D10.1	D37.02	D49.0
lingula, lung	C34.1-	C78.0-	D02.2-	D14.3-	D38.1	D49.1
lip	C00.9	C79.89	D00.01	D10.0	D37.01	D49.0
buccal aspect — *see Neoplasm, lip, internal*						
commissure	C00.6	C79.89	D00.01	D10.0	D37.01	D49.0
external	C00.2	C79.89	D00.01	D10.0	D37.01	D49.0
lower	C00.1	C79.89	D00.01	D10.0	D37.01	D49.0
upper	C00.0	C79.89	D00.01	D10.0	D37.01	D49.0
frenulum — *see Neoplasm, lip, internal*						
inner aspect — *see Neoplasm, lip, internal*						
internal	C00.5	C79.89	D00.01	D10.0	D37.01	D49.0
lower	C00.4	C79.89	D00.01	D10.0	D37.01	D49.0
upper	C00.3	C79.89	D00.01	D10.0	D37.01	D49.0
lipstick area	C00.2	C79.89	D00.01	D10.0	D37.01	D49.0
lower	C00.1	C79.89	D00.01	D10.0	D37.01	D49.0
upper	C00.0	C79.89	D00.01	D10.0	D37.01	D49.0

	Malignant Primary	Malignant Secondary	Ca in situ	Benign	Uncertain Behavior	Unspecified Behavior
lip *(Continued)*						
lower	C00.1	C79.89	D00.01	D10.0	D37.01	D49.0
internal	C00.4	C79.89	D00.01	D10.0	D37.01	D49.0
mucosa — *see Neoplasm, lip, internal*						
oral aspect — *see Neoplasm, lip, internal*						
overlapping lesion	C00.8	—	—	—	—	—
with oral cavity or pharynx	C14.8	—	—	—	—	—
skin (commissure) (lower) (upper)	C44.00	C79.2	D04.0	D23.0	D48.5	D49.2
basal cell carcinoma	C44.01	—	—	—	—	—
specified type NEC	C44.09	—	—	—	—	—
squamous cell carcinoma	C44.02	—	—	—	—	—
upper	C00.0	C79.89	D00.01	D10.0	D37.01	D49.0
internal	C00.3	C79.89	D00.01	D10.0	D37.01	D49.0
vermilion border	C00.2	C79.89	D00.01	D10.0	D37.01	D49.0
lower	C00.1	C79.89	D00.01	D10.0	D37.01	D49.0
upper	C00.0	C79.89	D00.01	D10.0	D37.01	D49.0
lipomatous — *see Lipoma, by site*						
liver — *see also Index to disease, by histology*	C22.9	C78.7	D01.5	D13.4	D37.6	D49.0
primary	C22.8	C78.7	D01.5	D13.4	D37.6	D49.0
lumbosacral plexus	C47.5	C79.89	—	D36.16	D48.2	D49.2
lung	C34.9-	C78.0-	D02.2-	D14.3-	D38.1	D49.1
azygos lobe	C34.1-	C78.0-	D02.2-	D14.3-	D38.1	D49.1
carina	C34.0-	C78.0-	D02.2-	D14.3-	D38.1	D49.1
hilus	C34.0-	C78.0-	D02.2-	D14.3-	D38.1	D49.1
lingula	C34.1-	C78.0-	D02.2-	D14.3-	D38.1	D49.1
lobe NEC	C34.9-	C78.0-	D02.2-	D14.3-	D38.1	D49.1
lower lobe	C34.3-	C78.0-	D02.2-	D14.3-	D38.1	D49.1
main bronchus	C34.0-	C78.0-	D02.2-	D14.3-	D38.1	D49.1
mesothelioma — *see Mesothelioma*						
middle lobe	C34.2	C78.0-	D02.21	D14.31	D38.1	D49.1
overlapping lesion	C34.8-	—	—	—	—	—
upper lobe	C34.1-	C78.0-	D02.2-	D14.3-	D38.1	D49.1
lymph, lymphatic channel NEC	C49.9	C79.89	—	D21.9	D48.1	D49.2
gland (secondary)	—	C77.9	—	D36.0	D48.7	D49.89
abdominal	—	C77.2	—	D36.0	D48.7	D49.89
aortic	—	C77.2	—	D36.0	D48.7	D49.89
arm	—	C77.3	—	D36.0	D48.7	D49.89
auricular (anterior) (posterior)	—	C77.0	—	D36.0	D48.7	D49.89

◄ New ◄▥ Revised ~~deleted~~ Deleted

	Malignant Primary	Malignant Secondary	Ca in situ	Benign	Uncertain Behavior	Unspecified Behavior
lymph, lymphatic channel NEC *(Continued)*						
gland *(Continued)*						
axilla, axillary	—	C77.3	—	D36.0	D48.7	D49.89
brachial	—	C77.3	—	D36.0	D48.7	D49.89
bronchial	—	C77.1	—	D36.0	D48.7	D49.89
bronchopulmonary	—	C77.1	—	D36.0	D48.7	D49.89
celiac	—	C77.2	—	D36.0	D48.7	D49.89
cervical	—	C77.0	—	D36.0	D48.7	D49.89
cervicofacial	—	C77.0	—	D36.0	D48.7	D49.89
Cloquet	—	C77.4	—	D36.0	D48.7	D49.89
colic	—	C77.2	—	D36.0	D48.7	D49.89
common duct	—	C77.2	—	D36.0	D48.7	D49.89
cubital	—	C77.3	—	D36.0	D48.7	D49.89
diaphragmatic	—	C77.1	—	D36.0	D48.7	D49.89
epigastric, inferior	—	C77.1	—	D36.0	D48.7	D49.89
epitrochlear	—	C77.3	—	D36.0	D48.7	D49.89
esophageal	—	C77.1	—	D36.0	D48.7	D49.89
face	—	C77.0	—	D36.0	D48.7	D49.89
femoral	—	C77.4	—	D36.0	D48.7	D49.89
gastric	—	C77.2	—	D36.0	D48.7	D49.89
groin	—	C77.4	—	D36.0	D48.7	D49.89
head	—	C77.0	—	D36.0	D48.7	D49.89
hepatic	—	C77.2	—	D36.0	D48.7	D49.89
hilar (pulmonary)	—	C77.1	—	D36.0	D48.7	D49.89
splenic	—	C77.2	—	D36.0	D48.7	D49.89
hypogastric	—	C77.5	—	D36.0	D48.7	D49.89
ileocolic	—	C77.2	—	D36.0	D48.7	D49.89
iliac	—	C77.5	—	D36.0	D48.7	D49.89
infraclavicular	—	C77.3	—	D36.0	D48.7	D49.89
inguina, inguinal	—	C77.4	—	D36.0	D48.7	D49.89
innominate	—	C77.1	—	D36.0	D48.7	D49.89
intercostal	—	C77.1	—	D36.0	D48.7	D49.89
intestinal	—	C77.2	—	D36.0	D48.7	D49.89
intrabdominal	—	C77.2	—	D36.0	D48.7	D49.89
intrapelvic	—	C77.5	—	D36.0	D48.7	D49.89
intrathoracic	—	C77.1	—	D36.0	D48.7	D49.89
jugular	—	C77.0	—	D36.0	D48.7	D49.89
leg	—	C77.4	—	D36.0	D48.7	D49.89
limb						
lower	—	C77.4	—	D36.0	D48.7	D49.89
upper	—	C77.3	—	D36.0	D48.7	D49.89
lower limb	—	C77.4	—	D36.0	D48.7	D49.89
lumbar	—	C77.2	—	D36.0	D48.7	D49.89

	Malignant Primary	Malignant Secondary	Ca in situ	Benign	Uncertain Behavior	Unspecified Behavior
lymph, lymphatic channel NEC *(Continued)*						
gland *(Continued)*						
mandibular	—	C77.0	—	D36.0	D48.7	D49.89
mediastinal	—	C77.1	—	D36.0	D48.7	D49.89
mesenteric (inferior) (superior)	—	C77.2	—	D36.0	D48.7	D49.89
midcolic	—	C77.2	—	D36.0	D48.7	D49.89
multiple sites in categories C77.0 - C77.5	—	C77.8	—	D36.0	D48.7	D49.89
neck	—	C77.0	—	D36.0	D48.7	D49.89
obturator	—	C77.5	—	D36.0	D48.7	D49.89
occipital	—	C77.0	—	D36.0	D48.7	D49.89
pancreatic	—	C77.2	—	D36.0	D48.7	D49.89
para-aortic	—	C77.2	—	D36.0	D48.7	D49.89
paracervical	—	C77.5	—	D36.0	D48.7	D49.89
parametrial	—	C77.5	—	D36.0	D48.7	D49.89
parasternal	—	C77.1	—	D36.0	D48.7	D49.89
parotid	—	C77.0	—	D36.0	D48.7	D49.89
pectoral	—	C77.3	—	D36.0	D48.7	D49.89
pelvic	—	C77.5	—	D36.0	D48.7	D49.89
peri-aortic	—	C77.2	—	D36.0	D48.7	D49.89
peripancreatic	—	C77.2	—	D36.0	D48.7	D49.89
popliteal	—	C77.4	—	D36.0	D48.7	D49.89
porta hepatis	—	C77.2	—	D36.0	D48.7	D49.89
portal	—	C77.2	—	D36.0	D48.7	D49.89
preauricular	—	C77.0	—	D36.0	D48.7	D49.89
prelaryngeal	—	C77.0	—	D36.0	D48.7	D49.89
presymphysial	—	C77.5	—	D36.0	D48.7	D49.89
pretracheal	—	C77.0	—	D36.0	D48.7	D49.89
primary (any site) NEC	C96.9	—	—	—	—	—
pulmonary (hiler)	—	C77.1	—	D36.0	D48.7	D49.89
pyloric	—	C77.2	—	D36.0	D48.7	D49.89
retroperitoneal	—	C77.2	—	D36.0	D48.7	D49.89
retropharyngeal	—	C77.0	—	D36.0	D48.7	D49.89
Rosenmuller's	—	C77.4	—	D36.0	D48.7	D49.89
sacral	—	C77.5	—	D36.0	D48.7	D49.89
scalene	—	C77.0	—	D36.0	D48.7	D49.89
site NEC	—	C77.9	—	D36.0	D48.7	D49.89
splenic (hilar)	—	C77.2	—	D36.0	D48.7	D49.89
subclavicular	—	C77.3	—	D36.0	D48.7	D49.89
subinguinal	—	C77.4	—	D36.0	D48.7	D49.89
sublingual	—	C77.0	—	D36.0	D48.7	D49.89
submandibular	—	C77.0	—	D36.0	D48.7	D49.89

◀ New ◀▦ Revised ~~deleted~~ Deleted

TABLE OF NEOPLASMS

	Malignant Primary	Malignant Secondary	Ca in situ	Benign	Uncertain Behavior	Unspecified Behavior
lymph, lymphatic channel NEC *(Continued)*						
gland *(Continued)*						
submaxillary	—	C77.0	—	D36.0	D48.7	D49.89
submental	—	C77.0	—	D36.0	D48.7	D49.89
subscapular	—	C77.3	—	D36.0	D48.7	D49.89
supraclavicular	—	C77.0	—	D36.0	D48.7	D49.89
thoracic	—	C77.1	—	D36.0	D48.7	D49.89
tibial	—	C77.4	—	D36.0	D48.7	D49.89
tracheal	—	C77.1	—	D36.0	D48.7	D49.89
tracheobronchial	—	C77.1	—	D36.0	D48.7	D49.89
upper limb	—	C77.3	—	D36.0	D48.7	D49.89
Virchow's	—	C77.0	—	D36.0	D48.7	D49.89
node — *see also Neoplasm, lymph gland*						
primary NEC	C96.9	—	—	—	—	—
vessel — *see also Neoplasm, connective tissue*	C49.9	C79.89	—	D21.9	D48.1	D49.2
Mackenrodt's ligament	C57.7	C79.82	D07.39	D28.7	D39.8	D49.59
malar	C41.0	C79.51	—	D16.4-	D48.0	D49.2
region — *see Neoplasm, cheek*						
mammary gland — *see Neoplasm, breast*						
mandible	C41.1	C79.51	—	D16.5-	D48.0	D49.2
alveolar						
mucosa (carcinoma)	C03.1	C79.89	D00.03	D10.39	D37.09	D49.0
ridge or process	C41.1	C79.51	—	D16.5-	D48.0	D49.2
marrow (bone) NEC	C96.9	C79.52	—	—	D47.9	D49.89
mastectomy site (skin) — *see also Neoplasm, breast, skin*	C44.501	C79.2	—	—	—	—
specified as breast tissue	C50.8-	C79.81	—	—	—	—
mastoid (air cells) (antrum) (cavity)	C30.1	C78.39	D02.3	D14.0	D38.5	D49.1
bone or process	C41.0	C79.51	—	D16.4-	D48.0	D49.2
maxilla, maxillary (superior)	C41.0	C79.51	—	D16.4-	D48.0	D49.2
alveolar						
mucosa	C03.0	C79.89	D00.03	D10.39	D37.09	D49.0
ridge or process (carcinoma)	C41.0	C79.51	—	D16.4-	D48.0	D49.2
antrum	C31.0	C78.39	D02.3	D14.0	D38.5	D49.1
carcinoma	C03.0	C79.51	—	—	—	—
inferior — *see Neoplasm, mandible*						
sinus	C31.0	C78.39	D02.3	D14.0	D38.5	D49.1
meatus external (ear) — *see also Neoplasm, skin, ear*	C44.20-	C79.2	D04.2-	D23.2-	D48.5	D49.2
Meckel diverticulum, malignant	C17.3	C78.4	D01.49	D13.39	D37.2	D49.0
mediastinum, mediastinal	C38.3	C78.1	—	D15.2	D38.3	D49.89
anterior	C38.1	C78.1	—	D15.2	D38.3	D49.89
posterior	C38.2	C78.1	—	D15.2	D38.3	D49.89
medulla						
adrenal	C74.1-	C79.7-	D09.3	D35.0-	D44.1-	D49.7
oblongata	C71.7	C79.31	—	D33.1	D43.1	D49.6
meibomian gland	C44.10-	C79.2	D04.1-	D23.1-	D48.5	D49.2
basal cell carcinoma	C44.11-	—	—	—	—	—
specified type NEC	C44.19-	—	—	—	—	—
squamous cell carcinoma	C44.12-	—	—	—	—	—
melanoma — *see Melanoma*						
meninges	C70.9	C79.49	—	D32.9	D42.9	D49.7
brain	C70.0	C79.32	—	D32.0	D42.0	D49.7
cerebral	C70.0	C79.32	—	D32.0	D42.0	D49.7
crainial	C70.0	C79.32	—	D32.0	D42.0	D49.7
intracranial	C70.0	C79.32	—	D32.0	D42.0	D49.7
spinal (cord)	C70.1	C79.49	—	D32.1	D42.1	D49.7
meniscus, knee joint (lateral) (medial)	C40.2-	C79.51	—	D16.2-	D48.0	D49.2
Merkel cell — *see Carcinoma, Merkel cell*						
mesentery, mesenteric	C48.1	C78.6	—	D20.1	D48.4	D49.0
mesoappendix	C48.1	C78.6	—	D20.1	D48.4	D49.0
mesocolon	C48.1	C78.6	—	D20.1	D48.4	D49.0
mesopharynx — *see Neoplasm, oropharynx*						
mesosalpinx	C57.1	C79.82	D07.39	D28.2	D39.8	D49.59
mesothelial tissue — *see Mesothelioma*						
mesothelioma — *see Mesothelioma*						
mesovarium	C57.1	C79.82	D07.39	D28.2	D39.8	D49.59
metacarpus (any bone)	C40.1-	C79.51	—	D16.1-	—	—
metastatic NEC — *see also Neoplasm, by site, secondary*	—	C79.9	—	—	—	—
metatarsus (any bone)	C40.3-	C79.51	—	D16.3-	—	—
midbrain	C71.7	C79.31	—	D33.1	D43.1	D49.6
milk duct — *see Neoplasm, breast*						
mons						
pubis	C51.9	C79.82	D07.1	D28.0	D39.8	D49.59
veneris	C51.9	C79.82	D07.1	D28.0	D39.8	D49.59
motor tract	C72.9	C79.49	—	D33.9	D43.9	D49.7
brain	C71.9	C79.31	—	D33.2	D43.2	D49.6
cauda equina	C72.1	C79.49	—	D33.4	D43.4	D49.7
spinal	C72.0	C79.49	—	D33.4	D43.4	D49.7

◀ New   ⬅ Revised   ~~deleted~~ Deleted

	Malignant Primary	Malignant Secondary	Ca in situ	Benign	Uncertain Behavior	Unspecified Behavior
mouth	C06.9	C79.89	D00.00	D10.30	D37.09	D49.0
book-leaf	C06.89	C79.89	—	—	—	—
floor	C04.9	C79.89	D00.06	D10.2	D37.09	D49.0
anterior portion	C04.0	C79.89	D00.06	D10.2	D37.09	D49.0
lateral portion	C04.1	C79.89	D00.06	D10.2	D37.09	D49.0
overlapping lesion	C04.8	—	—	—	—	—
overlapping NEC	C06.80	—	—	—	—	—
roof	C05.9	C79.89	D00.00	D10.39	D37.09	D49.0
specified part NEC	C06.89	C79.89	D00.00	D10.39	D37.09	D49.0
vestibule	C06.1	C79.89	D00.00	D10.39	D37.09	D49.0
mucosa						
alveolar (ridge or process)	C03.9	C79.89	D00.03	D10.39	D37.09	D49.0
lower	C03.1	C79.89	D00.03	D10.39	D37.09	D49.0
upper	C03.0	C79.89	D00.03	D10.39	D37.09	D49.0
buccal	C06.0	C79.89	D00.02	D10.39	D37.09	D49.0
cheek	C06.0	C79.89	D00.02	D10.39	D37.09	D49.0
lip — see Neoplasm, lip, internal						
nasal	C30.0	C78.39	D02.3	D14.0	D38.5	D49.1
oral	C06.0	C79.89	D00.02	D10.39	D37.09	D49.0
Mullerian duct						
female	C57.7	C79.82	D07.39	D28.7	D39.8	D49.59 ◀
male	C63.7	C79.82	D07.69	D29.8	D40.8	D49.59 ◀
muscle — see also Neoplasm, connective tissue						
extraocular	C69.6-	C79.49	D09.2-	D31.6-	D48.7	D49.89
myocardium	C38.0	C79.89	—	D15.1	D48.7	D49.89
myometrium	C54.2	C79.82	D07.0	D26.1	D39.0	D49.59 ◀
myopericardium	C38.0	C79.89	—	D15.1	D48.7	D49.89
nabothian gland (follicle)	C53.0	C79.82	D06.0	D26.0	D39.0	D49.59 ◀
nail — see also Neoplasm, skin, limb	C44.90	C79.2	D04.9	D23.9	D48.5	D49.2
finger — see also Neoplasm, skin, limb, upper	C44.60-	C79.2	D04.6-	D23.6-	D48.5	D49.2
toe — see also Neoplasm, skin, limb, lower	C44.70-	C79.2	D04.7-	D23.7-	D48.5	D49.2
nares, naris (anterior) (posterior)	C30.0	C78.39	D02.3	D14.0	D38.5	D49.1
nasal — see Neoplasm, nose						
nasolabial groove — see also Neoplasm, skin, face	C44.309	C79.2	D04.39	D23.39	D48.5	D49.2
nasolacrimal duct	C69.5-	C79.49	D09.2-	D31.5-	D48.7	D49.89
nasopharynx, nasopharyngeal	C11.9	C79.89	D00.08	D10.6	D37.05	D49.0
floor	C11.3	C79.89	D00.08	D10.6	D37.05	D49.0
overlapping lesion	C11.8	—	—	—	—	—
roof	C11.0	C79.89	D00.08	D10.6	D37.05	D49.0

	Malignant Primary	Malignant Secondary	Ca in situ	Benign	Uncertain Behavior	Unspecified Behavior
nasopharynx, nasopharyngeal (Continued)						
wall	C11.9	C79.89	D00.08	D10.6	D37.05	D49.0
anterior	C11.3	C79.89	D00.08	D10.6	D37.05	D49.0
lateral	C11.2	C79.89	D00.08	D10.6	D37.05	D49.0
posterior	C11.1	C79.89	D00.08	D10.6	D37.05	D49.0
superior	C11.0	C79.89	D00.08	D10.6	D37.05	D49.0
nates — see also Neoplasm, skin, trunk	C44.509	C79.2	D04.5	D23.5	D48.5	D49.2
neck NEC	C76.0	C79.89	D09.8	D36.7	D48.7	D49.89
skin	C44.40	—	—	—	—	—
basal cell carcinoma	C44.41	—	—	—	—	—
specified type NEC	C44.49	—	—	—	—	—
squamous cell carcinoma	C44.42	—	—	—	—	—
nerve (ganglion)	C47.9	C79.89	—	D36.10	D48.2	D49.2
abducens	C72.59	C79.49	—	D33.3	D43.3	D49.7
accessory (spinal)	C72.59	C79.49	—	D33.3	D43.3	D49.7
acoustic	C72.4-	C79.49	—	D33.3	D43.3	D49.7
auditory	C72.4-	C79.49	—	D33.3	D43.3	D49.7
autonomic NEC — see also Neoplasm, nerve, peripheral	C47.9	C79.89	—	D36.10	D48.2	D49.2
brachial	C47.1-	C79.89	—	D36.12	D48.2	D49.2
cranial	C72.50	C79.49	—	D33.3	D43.3	D49.7
specified NEC	C72.59	C79.49	—	D33.3	D43.3	D49.7
facial	C72.59	C79.49	—	D33.3	D43.3	D49.7
femoral	C47.2-	C79.89	—	D36.13	D48.2	D49.2
ganglion NEC — see also Neoplasm, nerve, peripheral	C47.9	C79.89	—	D36.10	D48.2	D49.2
glossopharyngeal	C72.59	C79.49	—	D33.3	D43.3	D49.7
hypoglossal	C72.59	C79.49	—	D33.3	D43.3	D49.7
intercostal	C47.3	C79.89	—	D36.14	D48.2	D49.2
lumbar	C47.6	C79.89	—	D36.17	D48.2	D49.2
median	C47.1-	C79.89	—	D36.12	D48.2	D49.2
obturator	C47.2-	C79.89	—	D36.13	D48.2	D49.2
oculomotor	C72.59	C79.49	—	D33.3	D43.3	D49.7
olfactory	C47.2-	C79.49	—	D33.3	D43.3	D49.7
optic	C72.3-	C79.49	—	D33.3	D43.3	D49.7
parasympathetic NEC	C47.9	C79.89	—	D36.10	D48.2	D49.2
peripheral NEC	C47.9	C79.89	—	D36.10	D48.2	D49.2
abdomen	C47.4	C79.89	—	D36.15	D48.2	D49.2
abdominal wall	C47.4	C79.89	—	D36.15	D48.2	D49.2
ankle	C47.2-	C79.89	—	D36.13	D48.2	D49.2

nerve *(Continued)*	Malignant Primary	Malignant Secondary	Ca in situ	Benign	Uncertain Behavior	Unspecified Behavior
peripheral NEC *(Continued)*						
antecubital fossa or space	C47.1-	C79.89	—	D36.12	D48.2	D49.2
arm	C47.1-	C79.89	—	D36.12	D48.2	D49.2
auricle (ear)	C47.0	C79.89	—	D36.11	D48.2	D49.2
axilla	C47.3	C79.89	—	D36.12	D48.2	D49.2
back	C47.6	C79.89	—	D36.17	D48.2	D49.2
buttock	C47.5	C79.89	—	D36.16	D48.2	D49.2
calf	C47.2-	C79.89	—	D36.13	D48.2	D49.2
cervical region	C47.0	C79.89	—	D36.11	D48.2	D49.2
cheek	C47.0	C79.89	—	D36.11	D48.2	D49.2
chest (wall)	C47.3	C79.89	—	D36.14	D48.2	D49.2
chin	C47.0	C79.89	—	D36.11	D48.2	D49.2
ear (external)	C47.0	C79.89	—	D36.11	D48.2	D49.2
elbow	C47.1-	C79.89	—	D36.12	D48.2	D49.2
extrarectal	C47.5	C79.89	—	D36.16	D48.2	D49.2
extremity	C47.9	C79.89	—	D36.10	D48.2	D49.2
lower	C47.2-	C79.89	—	D36.13	D48.2	D49.2
upper	C47.1-	C79.89	—	D36.12	D48.2	D49.2
eyelid	C47.0	C79.89	—	D36.11	D48.2	D49.2
face	C47.0	C79.89	—	D36.11	D48.2	D49.2
finger	C47.1-	C79.89	—	D36.12	D48.2	D49.2
flank	C47.6	C79.89	—	D36.17	D48.2	D49.2
foot	C47.2-	C79.89	—	D36.13	D48.2	D49.2
forearm	C47.1-	C79.89	—	D36.12	D48.2	D49.2
forehead	C47.0	C79.89	—	D36.11	D48.2	D49.2
gluteal region	C47.5	C79.89	—	D36.16	D48.2	D49.2
groin	C47.5	C79.89	—	D36.16	D48.2	D49.2
hand	C47.1-	C79.89	—	D36.12	D48.2	D49.2
head	C47.0	C79.89	—	D36.11	D48.2	D49.2
heel	C47.2-	C79.89	—	D36.13	D48.2	D49.2
hip	C47.2-	C79.89	—	D36.13	D48.2	D49.2
infraclavicular region	C47.3	C79.89	—	D36.14	D48.2	D49.2
inguinal (canal) (region)	C47.5	C79.89	—	D36.16	D48.2	D49.2
intrathoracic	C47.3	C79.89	—	D36.14	D48.2	D49.2
ischiorectal fossa	C47.5	C79.89	—	D36.16	D48.2	D49.2
knee	C47.2-	C79.89	—	D36.13	D48.2	D49.2
leg	C47.2-	C79.89	—	D36.13	D48.2	D49.2
limb NEC	C47.9	C79.89	—	D36.10	D48.2	D49.2
lower	C47.2-	C79.89	—	D36.13	D48.2	D49.2
upper	C47.1-	C79.89	—	D36.12	D48.2	D49.2
nates	C47.5	C79.89	—	D36.16	D48.2	D49.2
neck	C47.0	C79.89	—	D36.11	D48.2	D49.2
orbit	C69.6-	C79.49	—	D31.6-	D48.7	D49.2

nerve *(Continued)*	Malignant Primary	Malignant Secondary	Ca in situ	Benign	Uncertain Behavior	Unspecified Behavior
peripheral NEC *(Continued)*						
pararectal	C47.5	C79.89	—	D36.16	D48.2	D49.2
paraurethral	C47.5	C79.89	—	D36.16	D48.2	D49.2
paravaginal	C47.5	C79.89	—	D36.16	D48.2	D49.2
pelvis (floor)	C47.5	C79.89	—	D36.16	D48.2	D49.2
pelvoabdominal	C47.8	C79.89	—	D36.17	D48.2	D49.2
perineum	C47.5	C79.89	—	D36.16	D48.2	D49.2
perirectal (tissue)	C47.5	C79.89	—	D36.16	D48.2	D49.2
periurethral (tissue)	C47.5	C79.89	—	D36.16	D48.2	D49.2
popliteal fossa or space	C47.2-	C79.89	—	D36.13	D48.2	D49.2
presacral	C47.5	C79.89	—	D36.16	D48.2	D49.2
pterygoid fossa	C47.0	C79.89	—	D36.11	D48.2	D49.2
rectovaginal septum or wall	C47.5	C79.89	—	D36.16	D48.2	D49.2
rectovesical	C47.5	C79.89	—	D36.16	D48.2	D49.2
sacrococcygeal region	C47.5	C79.89	—	D36.16	D48.2	D49.2
scalp	C47.0	C79.89	—	D36.11	D48.2	D49.2
scapular region	C47.3	C79.89	—	D36.14	D48.2	D49.2
shoulder	C47.1-	C79.89	—	D36.12	D48.2	D49.2
submental	C47.0	C79.89	—	D36.11	D48.2	D49.2
supraclavicular region	C47.0	C79.89	—	D36.11	D48.2	D49.2
temple	C47.0	C79.89	—	D36.11	D48.2	D49.2
temporal region	C47.0	C79.89	—	D36.11	D48.2	D49.2
thigh	C47.2-	C79.89	—	D36.13	D48.2	D49.2
thoracic (duct) (wall)	C47.3	C79.89	—	D36.14	D48.2	D49.2
thorax	C47.3	C79.89	—	D36.14	D48.2	D49.2
thumb	C47.1-	C79.89	—	D36.12	D48.2	D49.2
toe	C47.2-	C79.89	—	D36.13	D48.2	D49.2
trunk	C47.6	C79.89	—	D36.17	D48.2	D49.2
umbilicus	C47.4	C79.89	—	D36.15	D48.2	D49.2
vesicorectal	C47.5	C79.89	—	D36.16	D48.2	D49.2
wrist	C47.1-	C79.89	—	D36.12	D48.2	D49.2
radial	C47.1-	C79.89	—	D36.12	D48.2	D49.2
sacral	C47.5	C79.89	—	D36.16	D48.2	D49.2
sciatic	C47.2-	C79.89	—	D36.13	D48.2	D49.2
spinal NEC	C47.9	C79.89	—	D36.10	D48.2	D49.2
accessory	C72.59	C79.49	—	D33.3	D43.3	D49.7
sympathetic NEC—*see also* Neoplasm, nerve, peripheral	C47.9	C79.89	—	D36.10	D48.2	D49.2
trigeminal	C72.59	C79.49	—	D33.3	D43.3	D49.7
trochlear	C72.59	C79.49	—	D33.3	D43.3	D49.7
ulnar	C47.1-	C79.89	—	D36.12	D48.2	D49.2
vagus	C72.59	C79.49	—	D33.3	D43.3	D49.7

◄ New   ◄▥ Revised   ~~deleted~~ Deleted

	Malignant Primary	Malignant Secondary	Ca in situ	Benign	Uncertain Behavior	Unspecified Behavior
nervous system (central)	C72.9	C79.40	—	D33.9	D43.9	D49.7
autonomic — see Neoplasm, nerve, peripheral						
parasympathetic — see Neoplasm, nerve, peripheral						
specified site NEC	—	C79.49	—	D33.7	D43.8	—
sympathetic — see Neoplasm, nerve, peripheral						
nevus — see Nevus						
nipple	C50.0-	C79.81	D05.-	D24.-	—	—
nose, nasal	C76.0	C79.89	D09.8	D36.7	D48.7	D49.89
ala (external) (nasi) — see also Neoplasm, nose, skin	C44.301	C79.2	D04.39	D23.39	D48.5	D49.2
bone	C41.0	C79.51	—	D16.4-	D48.0	D49.2
cartilage	C30.0	C78.39	D02.3	D14.0	D38.5	D49.1
cavity	C30.0	C78.39	D02.3	D14.0	D38.5	D49.1
choana	C11.3	C79.89	D00.08	D10.6	D37.05	D49.0
external (skin) — see also Neoplasm, nose, skin	C44.301	C79.2	D04.39	D23.39	D48.5	D49.2
fossa	C30.0	C78.39	D02.3	D14.0	D38.5	D49.1
internal	C30.0	C78.39	D02.3	D14.0	D38.5	D49.1
mucosa	C30.0	C78.39	D02.3	D14.0	D38.5	D49.1
septum	C30.0	C78.39	D02.3	D14.0	D38.5	D49.1
posterior margin	C11.3	C79.89	D00.08	D10.6	D37.05	D49.0
sinus — see Neoplasm, sinus						
skin	C44.301	C79.2	D04.39	D23.39	D48.5	D49.2
basal cell carcinoma	C44.311	—	—	—	—	—
specified type NEC	C44.391	—	—	—	—	—
squamous cell carcinoma	C44.321	—	—	—	—	—
turbinate (mucosa)	C30.0	C78.39	D02.3	D14.0	D38.5	D49.1
bone	C41.0	C79.51	—	D16.4-	D48.0	D49.2
vestibule	C30.0	C78.39	D02.3	D14.0	D38.5	D49.1
nostril	C30.0	C78.39	D02.3	D14.0	D38.5	D49.1
nucleus pulposus	C41.2	C79.51	—	D16.6	D48.0	D49.2
occipital						
bone	C41.0	C79.51	—	D16.4-	D48.0	D49.2
lobe or pole, brain	C71.4	C79.31	—	D33.0	D43.0	D49.6
odontogenic — see Neoplasm, jaw bone						
olfactory nerve or bulb	C72.2-	C79.49	—	D33.3	D43.3	D49.7
olive (brain)	C71.7	C79.31	—	D33.1	D43.1	D49.6
omentum	C48.1	C78.6	—	D20.1	D48.4	D49.0
operculum (brain)	C71.0	C79.31	—	D33.0	D43.0	D49.6
optic nerve, chiasm, or tract	C72.3-	C79.49	—	D33.3	D43.3	D49.7
oral (cavity)	C06.9	C79.89	D00.00	D10.30	D37.09	D49.0
ill-defined	C14.8	C79.89	D00.00	D10.30	D37.09	D49.0
mucosa	C06.0	C79.89	D00.02	D10.39	D37.09	D49.0
orbit	C69.6-	C79.49	D09.2-	D31.6-	D48.7	D49.89
autonomic nerve	C69.6-	C79.49	—	D31.6-	D48.7	D49.2
bone	C41.0	C79.51	—	D16.4-	D48.0	D49.2
eye	C69.6-	C79.49	D09.2-	D31.6-	D48.7	D49.89
peripheral nerves	C69.6-	C79.49	—	D31.6-	D48.7	D49.2
soft parts	C69.6-	C79.49	D09.2-	D31.6-	D48.7	D49.89
organ of Zuckerkandl	C75.5	C79.89	—	D35.6	D44.7	D49.7
oropharynx	C10.9	C79.89	D00.08	D10.5	D37.05	D49.0
branchial cleft (vestige)	C10.4	C79.89	D00.08	D10.5	D37.05	D49.0
junctional region	C10.8	C79.89	D00.08	D10.5	D37.05	D49.0
lateral wall	C10.2	C79.89	D00.08	D10.5	D37.05	D49.0
overlapping lesion	C10.8	—	—	—	—	—
pillars or fauces	C09.1	C79.89	D00.08	D10.5	D37.05	D49.0
posterior wall	C10.3	C79.89	D00.08	D10.5	D37.05	D49.0
vallecula	C10.0	C79.89	D00.08	D10.5	D37.05	D49.0
os						
external	C53.1	C79.82	D06.1	D26.0	D39.0	D49.59
internal	C53.0	C79.82	D06.0	D26.0	D39.0	D49.59
ovary	C56.-	C79.6-	D07.39	D27.-	D39.1-	D49.59
oviduct	C57.0-	C79.82	D07.39	D28.2	D39.8	D49.59
palate	C05.9	C79.89	D00.00	D10.39	D37.09	D49.0
hard	C05.0	C79.89	D00.05	D10.39	D37.09	D49.0
junction of hard and soft palate	C05.9	C79.89	D00.00	D10.39	D37.09	D49.0
overlapping lesions	C05.8	—	—	—	—	—
soft	C05.1	C79.89	D00.04	D10.39	D37.09	D49.0
nasopharyngeal surface	C11.3	C79.89	D00.08	D10.6	D37.05	D49.0
posterior surface	C11.3	C79.89	D00.08	D10.6	D37.05	D49.0
superior surface	C11.3	C79.89	D00.08	D10.6	D37.05	D49.0
palatoglossal arch	C09.1	C79.89	D00.00	D10.5	D37.09	D49.0
palatopharyngeal arch	C09.1	C79.89	D00.00	D10.5	D37.09	D49.0
pallium	C71.0	C79.31	—	D33.0	D43.0	D49.6
palpebra	C44.10-	C79.2	D04.1-	D23.1-	D48.5	D49.2
basal cell carcinoma	C44.11-	—	—	—	—	—
specified type NEC	C44.19-	—	—	—	—	—
squamous cell carcinoma	C44.12-	—	—	—	—	—
pancreas	C25.9	C78.89	D01.7	D13.6	D37.8	D49.0
body	C25.1	C78.89	D01.7	D13.6	D37.8	D49.0
duct (of Santorini) (of Wirsung)	C25.3	C78.89	D01.7	D13.6	D37.8	D49.0
ectopic tissue	C25.7	C78.89	—	D13.6	D37.8	D49.0
head	C25.0	C78.89	D01.7	D13.6	D37.8	D49.0

◄ New ◄▥ Revised ~~deleted~~ Deleted

	Malignant Primary	Malignant Secondary	Ca in situ	Benign	Uncertain Behavior	Unspecified Behavior
pancreas *(Continued)*						
islet cells	C25.4	C78.89	D01.7	D13.7	D37.8	D49.0
neck	C25.7	C78.89	D01.7	D13.6	D37.8	D49.0
overlapping lesion	C25.8	—	—	—	—	—
tail	C25.2	C78.89	D01.7	D13.6	D37.8	D49.0
para-aortic body	C75.5	C79.89	—	D35.6	D44.7	D49.7
paraganglion NEC	C75.5	C79.89	—	D35.6	D44.7	D49.7
parametrium	C57.3	C79.82	—	D28.2	D39.8	D49.59
paranephric	C48.0	C78.6	—	D20.0	D48.3	D49.0
pararectal	C76.3	C79.89	—	D36.7	D48.7	D49.89
parasagittal (region)	C76.0	C79.89	D09.8	D36.7	D48.7	D49.89
parasellar	C72.9	C79.49	—	D33.9	D43.8	D49.7
parathyroid (gland)	C75.0	C79.89	D09.3	D35.1	D44.2	D49.7
paraurethral	C76.3	C79.89	—	D36.7	D48.7	D49.89
gland	C68.1	C79.19	D09.19	D30.8	D41.8	D49.59
paravaginal	C76.3	C79.89	—	D36.7	D48.7	D49.89
parenchyma, kidney	C64.-	C79.0-	D09.19	D30.0-	D41.0-	D49.51-
parietal						
bone	C41.0	C79.51	—	D16.4-	D48.0	D49.2
lobe, brain	C71.3	C79.31	—	D33.0	D43.0	D49.6
paroophoron	C57.1	C79.82	D07.39	D28.2	D39.8	D49.59
parotid (duct) (gland)	C07	C79.89	D00.00	D11.0	D37.030	D49.0
parovarium	C57.1	C79.82	D07.39	D28.2	D39.8	D49.59
patella	C40.20	C79.51	—	—	—	—
peduncle, cerebral	C71.7	C79.31	—	D33.1	D43.1	D49.6
pelvirectal junction	C19	C78.5	D01.1	D12.7	D37.5	D49.0
pelvis, pelvic NEC	C76.3	C79.89	D09.8	D36.7	D48.7	D49.89
bone	C41.4	C79.51	—	D16.8	D48.0	D49.2
floor	C76.3	C79.89	D09.8	D36.7	D48.7	D49.89
renal	C65.-	C79.0-	D09.19	D30.1-	D41.1-	D49.51-
viscera	C76.3	C79.89	D09.8	D36.7	D48.7	D49.89
wall	C76.3	C79.89	D09.8	D36.7	D48.7	D49.89
pelvo-abdominal	C76.8	C79.89	D09.8	D36.7	D48.7	D49.89
penis	C60.9	C79.82	D07.4	D29.0	D40.8	D49.59
body	C60.2	C79.82	D07.4	D29.0	D40.8	D49.59
corpus (cavernosum)	C60.2	C79.82	D07.4	D29.0	D40.8	D49.59
glans	C60.1	C79.82	D07.4	D29.0	D40.8	D49.59
overlapping sites	C60.8	—	—	—	—	—
skin NEC	C60.9	C79.82	D07.4	D29.0	D40.8	D49.59
periadrenal (tissue)	C48.0	C78.6	—	D20.0	D48.3	D49.0
perianal (skin) — *see also* Neoplasm, anus, skin	C44.500	C79.2	D04.5	D23.5	D48.5	D49.2
pericardium	C38.0	C79.89	—	D15.1	D48.7	D49.89
perinephric	C48.0	C78.6	—	D20.0	D48.3	D49.0

	Malignant Primary	Malignant Secondary	Ca in situ	Benign	Uncertain Behavior	Unspecified Behavior
perineum	C76.3	C79.89	D09.8	D36.7	D48.7	D49.89
periodontal tissue NEC	C03.9	C79.89	D00.03	D10.39	D37.09	D49.0
periosteum — *see Neoplasm, bone*						
peripancreatic	C48.0	C78.6	—	D20.0	D48.3	D49.0
peripheral nerve NEC	C47.9	C79.89	—	D36.10	D48.2	D49.2
perirectal (tissue)	C76.3	C79.89	—	D36.7	D48.7	D49.89
perirenal (tissue)	C48.0	C78.6	—	D20.0	D48.3	D49.0
peritoneum, peritoneal (cavity)	C48.2	C78.6	—	D20.1	D48.4	D49.0
benign mesothelial tissue — *see Mesothelioma, benign*						
overlapping lesion	C48.8	—	—	—	—	—
with digestive organs	C26.9	—	—	—	—	—
parietal	C48.1	C78.6	—	D20.1	D48.4	D49.0
pelvic	C48.1	C78.6	—	D20.1	D48.4	D49.0
specified part NEC	C48.1	C78.6	—	D20.1	D48.4	D49.0
peritonsillar (tissue)	C76.0	C79.89	D09.8	D36.7	D48.7	D49.89
periurethral tissue	C76.3	C79.89	—	D36.7	D48.7	D49.89
phalanges						
foot	C40.3-	C79.51	—	D16.3-	—	—
hand	C40.1-	C79.51	—	D16.1-	—	—
pharynx, pharyngeal	C14.0	C79.89	D00.08	D10.9	D37.05	D49.0
bursa	C11.1	C79.89	D00.08	D10.6	D37.05	D49.0
fornix	C11.3	C79.89	D00.08	D10.6	D37.05	D49.0
recess	C11.2	C79.89	D00.08	D10.6	D37.05	D49.0
region	C14.0	C79.89	D00.08	D10.9	D37.05	D49.0
tonsil	C11.1	C79.89	D00.08	D10.6	D37.05	D49.0
wall (lateral) (posterior)	C14.0	C79.89	D00.08	D10.9	D37.05	D49.0
pia mater	C70.9	C79.40	—	D32.9	D42.9	D49.7
cerebral	C70.0	C79.32	—	D32.0	D42.0	D49.7
cranial	C70.0	C79.32	—	D32.0	D42.0	D49.7
spinal	C70.1	C79.49	—	D32.1	D42.1	D49.7
pillars of fauces	C09.1	C79.89	D00.08	D10.5	D37.05	D49.0
pineal (body) (gland)	C75.3	C79.89	D09.3	D35.4	D44.5	D49.7
pinna (ear) NEC — *see also* Neoplasm, skin, ear	C44.20-	C79.2	D04.2-	D23.2-	D48.5	D49.2
piriform fossa or sinus	C12	C79.89	D00.08	D10.7	D37.05	D49.0
pituitary (body) (fossa) (gland) (lobe)	C75.1	C79.89	D09.3	D35.2	D44.3	D49.7
placenta	C58	C79.82	D07.0	D26.7	D39.2	D49.59
pleura, pleural (cavity)	C38.4	C78.2	—	D19.0	D38.2	D49.1
overlapping lesion with heart or mediastinum	C38.8	—	—	—	—	—
parietal	C38.4	C78.2	—	D19.0	D38.2	D49.1
visceral	C38.4	C78.2	—	D19.0	D38.2	D49.1

◀ New ◀▦ Revised ~~deleted~~ Deleted

	Malignant Primary	Malignant Secondary	Ca in situ	Benign	Uncertain Behavior	Unspecified Behavior
plexus						
brachial	C47.1-	C79.89	—	D36.12	D48.2	D49.2
cervical	C47.0	C79.89	—	D36.11	D48.2	D49.2
choroid	C71.5	C79.31	—	D33.0	D43.0	D49.6
lumbosacral	C47.5	C79.89	—	D36.16	D48.2	D49.2
sacral	C47.5	C79.89	—	D36.16	D48.2	D49.2
pluriendocrine	C75.8	C79.89	D09.3	D35.7	D44.9	D49.7
pole						
frontal	C71.1	C79.31	—	D33.0	D43.0	D49.6
occipital	C71.4	C79.31	—	D33.0	D43.0	D49.6
pons (varolii)	C71.7	C79.31	—	D33.1	D43.1	D49.6
popliteal fossa or space	C76.5-	C79.89	D04.7-	D36.7	D48.7	D49.89
postcricoid (region)	C13.0	C79.89	D00.08	D10.7	D37.05	D49.0
posterior fossa (cranial)	C71.9	C79.31	—	D33.2	D43.2	D49.6
postnasal space	C11.9	C79.89	D00.08	D10.6	D37.05	D49.0
prepuce	C60.0	C79.82	D07.4	D29.0	D40.8	D49.59
prepylorus	C16.4	C78.89	D00.2	D13.1	D37.1	D49.0
presacral (region)	C76.3	C79.89	—	D36.7	D48.7	D49.89
prostate (gland)	C61	C79.82	D07.5	D29.1	D40.0	D49.59
utricle	C68.0	C79.19	D09.19	D30.4	D41.3	D49.59
pterygoid fossa	C49.0	C79.89	—	D21.0	D48.1	D49.2
pubic bone	C41.4	C79.51	—	D16.8	D48.0	D49.2
pudenda, pudendum (female)	C51.9	C79.82	D07.1	D28.0	D39.8	D49.59
pulmonary — *see also Neoplasm, lung*	C34.9-	C78.0-	D02.2-	D14.3-	D38.1	D49.1
putamen	C71.0	C79.31	—	D33.0	D43.0	D49.6
pyloric						
antrum	C16.3	C78.89	D00.2	D13.1	D37.1	D49.0
canal	C16.4	C78.89	D00.2	D13.1	D37.1	D49.0
pylorus	C16.4	C78.89	D00.2	D13.1	D37.1	D49.0
pyramid (brain)	C71.7	C79.31	—	D33.1	D43.1	D49.6
pyriform fossa or sinus	C12	C79.89	D00.08	D10.7	D37.05	D49.0
radius (any part)	C40.0-	C79.51	—	D16.0-	—	—
Rathke's pouch	C75.1	C79.89	D09.3	D35.2	D44.3	D49.7
rectosigmoid (junction)	C19	C78.5	D01.1	D12.7	D37.5	D49.0
overlapping lesion with anus or rectum	C21.8	—	—	—	—	—
rectouterine pouch	C48.1	C78.6	—	D20.1	D48.4	D49.0
rectovaginal septum or wall	C76.3	C79.89	D09.8	D36.7	D48.7	D49.89
rectovesical septum	C76.3	C79.89	D09.8	D36.7	D48.7	D49.89
rectum (ampulla)	C20	C78.5	D01.2	D12.8	D37.5	D49.0
and colon	C19	C78.5	D01.1	D12.7	D37.5	D49.0
overlapping lesion with anus or rectosigmoid junction	C21.8	—	—	—	—	—
renal	C64.-	C79.0-	D09.19	D30.0-	D41.0-	D49.51-
calyx	C65.-	C79.0-	D09.19	D30.1-	D41.1-	D49.51-
hilus	C65.-	C79.0-	D09.19	D30.1-	D41.1-	D49.51-
parenchyma	C64.-	C79.0-	D09.19	D30.0-	D41.0-	D49.51-
pelvis	C65.-	C79.0-	D09.19	D30.1-	D41.1-	D49.51-
respiratory						
organs or system NEC	C39.9	C78.30	D02.4	D14.4	D38.6	D49.1
tract NEC	C39.9	C78.30	D02.4	D14.4	D38.5	D49.1
upper	C39.0	C78.30	D02.4	D14.4	D38.5	D49.1
retina	C69.2-	C79.49	D09.2-	D31.2-	D48.7	D49.81
retrobulbar	C69.6-	C79.49	—	D31.6-	D48.7	D49.89
retrocecal	C48.0	C78.6	—	D20.0	D48.3	D49.0
retromolar (area) (triangle) (trigone)	C06.2	C79.89	D00.00	D10.39	D37.09	D49.0
retro-orbital	C76.0	C79.89	D09.8	D36.7	D48.7	D49.89
retroperitoneal (space) (tissue)	C48.0	C78.6	—	D20.0	D48.3	D49.0
retroperitoneum	C48.0	C78.6	—	D20.0	D48.3	D49.0
retropharyngeal	C14.0	C79.89	D00.08	D10.9	D37.05	D49.0
retrovesical (septum)	C76.3	C79.89	D09.8	D36.7	D48.7	D49.89
rhinencephalon	C71.0	C79.31	—	D33.0	D43.0	D49.6
rib	C41.3	C79.51	—	D16.7	D48.0	D49.2
Rosenmuller's fossa	C11.2	C79.89	D00.08	D10.6	D37.05	D49.0
round ligament	C57.2	C79.82	—	D28.2	D39.8	D49.59
sacrococcyx, sacrococcygeal	C41.4	C79.51	—	D16.8	D48.0	D49.2
region	C76.3	C79.89	D09.8	D36.7	D48.7	D49.89
sacrouterine ligament	C57.3	C79.82	—	D28.2	D39.8	D49.59
sacrum, sacral (vertebra)	C41.4	C79.51	—	D16.8	D48.0	D49.2
salivary gland or duct (major)	C08.9	C79.89	D00.00	D11.9	D37.039	D49.0
minor NEC	C06.9	C79.89	D00.00	D10.39	D37.04	D49.0
overlapping lesion	C08.9	—	—	—	—	—
parotid	C07	C79.89	D00.00	D11.0	D37.030	D49.0
pluriglandular	C08.9	C79.89	D00.00	D11.9	D37.039	D49.0
sublingual	C08.1	C79.89	D00.00	D11.7	D37.031	D49.0
submandibular	C08.0	C79.89	D00.00	D11.7	D37.032	D49.0
submaxillary	C08.0	C79.89	D00.00	D11.7	D37.032	D49.0
salpinx (uterine)	C57.0-	C79.82	D07.39	D28.2	D39.8	D49.59
Santorini's duct	C25.3	C78.89	D01.7	D13.6	D37.8	D49.0
scalp	C44.40	C79.2	D04.4	D23.4	D48.5	D49.2
basal cell carcinoma	C44.41	—	—	—	—	—
specified type NEC	C44.49	—	—	—	—	—
squamous cell carcinoma	C44.42	—	—	—	—	—
scapula (any part)	C40.0-	C79.51	—	D16.0-	—	—
scapular region	C76.1	C79.89	D09.8	D36.7	D48.7	D49.89

◀ New   ⬅ Revised   ~~deleted~~ Deleted

TABLE OF NEOPLASMS

	Malignant Primary	Malignant Secondary	Ca in situ	Benign	Uncertain Behavior	Unspecified Behavior
scar NEC — see also Neoplasm, skin, by site	C44.90	C79.2	D04.9	D23.9	D48.5	D49.2
sciatic nerve	C47.2-	C79.89	—	D36.13	D48.2	D49.2
sclera	C69.4-	C79.49	D09.2-	D31.4-	D48.7	D49.89
scrotum (skin)	C63.2	C79.82	D07.61	D29.4	D40.8	D49.59
sebaceous gland — see Neoplasm, skin						
sella turcica	C75.1	C79.89	D09.3	D35.2	D44.3	D49.7
bone	C41.0	C79.51	—	D16.4-	D48.0	D49.2
semilunar cartilage (knee)	C40.2-	C79.51	—	D16.2-	D48.0	D49.2
seminal vesicle	C63.7	C79.82	D07.69	D29.8	D40.8	D49.59
septum						
nasal	C30.0	C78.39	D02.3	D14.0	D38.5	D49.1
posterior margin	C11.3	C79.89	D00.08	D10.6	D37.05	D49.0
rectovaginal	C76.3	C79.89	D09.8	D36.7	D48.7	D49.89
rectovesical	C76.3	C79.89	D09.8	D36.7	D48.7	D49.89
urethrovaginal	C57.9	C79.82	D07.30	D28.9	D39.9	D49.59
vesicovaginal	C57.9	C79.82	D07.30	D28.9	D39.9	D49.59
shoulder NEC	C76.4-	C79.89	D04.6-	D36.7	D48.7	D49.89
sigmoid flexure (lower) (upper)	C18.7	C78.5	D01.0	D12.5	D37.4	D49.0
sinus (accessory)	C31.9	C78.39	D02.3	D14.0	D38.5	D49.1
bone (any)	C41.0	C79.51	—	D16.4-	D48.0	D49.2
ethmoidal	C31.1	C78.39	D02.3	D14.0	D38.5	D49.1
frontal	C31.2	C78.39	D02.3	D14.0	D38.5	D49.1
maxillary	C31.0	C78.39	D02.3	D14.0	D38.5	D49.1
nasal, paranasal NEC	C31.9	C78.39	D02.3	D14.0	D38.5	D49.1
overlapping lesion	C31.8	—	—	—	—	—
pyriform	C12	C79.89	D00.08	D10.7	D37.05	D49.0
sphenoid	C31.3	C78.39	D02.3	D14.0	D38.5	D49.1
skeleton, skeletal NEC	C41.9	C79.51	—	D16.9-	D48.0	D49.2
Skene's gland	C68.1	C79.19	D09.19	D30.8	D41.8	D49.59
skin NOS	C44.90	C79.2	D04.9	D23.9	D48.5	D49.2
abdominal wall	C44.509	C79.2	D04.5	D23.5	D48.5	D49.2
basal cell carcinoma	C44.519	—	—	—	—	—
specified type NEC	C44.599	—	—	—	—	—
squamous cell carcinoma	C44.529	—	—	—	—	—
ala nasi — see also Neoplasm, nose, skin	C44.301	C79.2	D04.39	D23.39	D48.5	D49.2
ankle — see also Neoplasm, skin, limb, lower	C44.70-	C79.2	D04.7-	D23.7-	D48.5	D49.2
antecubital space — see also Neoplasm, skin, limb, upper	C44.60-	C79.2	D04.6-	D23.6-	D48.5	D49.2

	Malignant Primary	Malignant Secondary	Ca in situ	Benign	Uncertain Behavior	Unspecified Behavior
skin NOS (Continued)						
anus	C44.500	C79.2	D04.5	D23.5	D48.5	D49.2
basal cell carcinoma	C44.510	—	—	—	—	—
specified type NEC	C44.590	—	—	—	—	—
squamous cell carcinoma	C44.520	—	—	—	—	—
arm — see also Neoplasm, skin, limb, upper	C44.60-	C79.2	D04.6-	D23.6-	D48.5	D49.2
auditory canal (external) — see also Neoplasm, skin, ear	C44.20-	C79.2	D04.2-	D23.2-	D48.5	D49.2
auricle (ear) — see also Neoplasm, skin, ear	C44.20-	C79.2	D04.2-	D23.2-	D48.5	D49.2
auricular canal (external) — see also Neoplasm, skin, ear	C44.20-	C79.2	D04.2-	D23.2-	D48.5	D49.2
axilla, axillary fold — see also Neoplasm, skin, trunk	C44.509	C79.2	D04.5	D23.5	D48.5	D49.2
back — see also Neoplasm, skin, trunk	C44.509	C79.2	D04.5	D23.5	D48.5	D49.2
basal cell carcinoma	C44.91					
breast	C44.501	C79.2	D04.5	D23.5	D48.5	D49.2
basal cell carcinoma	C44.511	—	—	—	—	—
specified type NEC	C44.591	—	—	—	—	—
squamous cell carcinoma	C44.521	—	—	—	—	—
brow — see also Neoplasm, skin, face	C44.309	C79.2	D04.39	D23.39	D48.5	D49.2
buttock — see also Neoplasm, skin, trunk	C44.509	C79.2	D04.5	D23.5	D48.5	D49.2
calf — see also Neoplasm, skin, limb, lower	C44.70-	C79.2	D04.7-	D23.7-	D48.5	D49.2
canthus (eye) (inner) (outer)	C44.10-	C79.2	D04.1-	D23.1-	D48.5	D49.2
basal cell carcinoma	C44.11-	—	—	—	—	—
specified type NEC	C44.19-	—	—	—	—	—
squamous cell carcinoma	C44.12-	—	—	—	—	—
cervical region — see also Neoplasm, skin, neck	C44.40	C79.2	D04.4	D23.4	D48.5	D49.2
cheek (external) — see also Neoplasm, skin, face	C44.309	C79.2	D04.39	D23.39	D48.5	D49.2
chest (wall) — see also Neoplasm, skin, trunk	C44.509	C79.2	D04.5	D23.5	D48.5	D49.2
chin — see also Neoplasm, skin, face	C44.309	C79.2	D04.39	D23.39	D48.5	D49.2
clavicular area — see also Neoplasm, skin, trunk	C44.509	C79.2	D04.5	D23.5	D48.5	D49.2
clitoris	C51.2	C79.82	D07.1	D28.0	D39.8	D49.59
columnella — see also Neoplasm, skin, face	C44.309	C79.2	D04.39	D23.39	D48.5	D49.2

◀ New   ⬅ Revised   ~~deleted~~ Deleted

TABLE OF NEOPLASMS

	Malignant Primary	Malignant Secondary	Ca in situ	Benign	Uncertain Behavior	Unspecified Behavior
skin NOS *(Continued)*						
concha — *see also Neoplasm, skin, ear*	C44.20-	C79.2	D04.2-	D23.2-	D48.5	D49.2
ear (external)	C44.20-	C79.2	D04.2-	D23.2-	D48.5	D49.2
basal cell carcinoma	C44.21-	—	—	—	—	—
specified type NEC	C44.29-	—	—	—	—	—
squamous cell carcinoma	C44.22-	—	—	—	—	—
elbow — *see also Neoplasm, skin, limb, upper*	C44.60-	C79.2	D04.6-	D23.6-	D48.5	D49.2
eyebrow — *see also Neoplasm, skin, face*	C44.309	C79.2	D04.39	D23.39	D48.5	D49.2
eyelid	C44.10-	C79.2	D04.1-	D23.1-	D48.5	D49.2
basal cell carcinoma	C44.11-	—	—	—	—	—
specified type NEC	C44.19-	—	—	—	—	—
squamous cell carcinoma	C44.12-	—	—	—	—	—
face NOS	C44.300	C79.2	D04.30	D23.30	D48.5	D49.2
basal cell carcinoma	C44.310	—	—	—	—	—
specified type NEC	C44.390	—	—	—	—	—
squamous cell carcinoma	C44.320	—	—	—	—	—
female genital organs (external)	C51.9	C79.82	D07.1	D28.0	D39.8	D49.59
clitoris	C51.2	C79.82	D07.1	D28.0	D39.8	D49.59
labium NEC	C51.9	C79.82	D07.1	D28.0	D39.8	D49.59
majus	C51.0	C79.82	D07.1	D28.0	D39.8	D49.59
minus	C51.1	C79.82	D07.1	D28.0	D39.8	D49.59
pudendum	C51.9	C79.82	D07.1	D28.0	D39.8	D49.59
vulva	C51.9	C79.82	D07.1	D28.0	D39.8	D49.59
finger — *see also Neoplasm, skin, limb, upper*	C44.60-	C79.2	D04.6-	D23.6-	D48.5	D49.2
flank — *see also Neoplasm, skin, trunk*	C44.509	C79.2	D04.5	D23.5	D48.5	D49.2
foot — *see also Neoplasm, skin, limb, lower*	C44.70-	C79.2	D04.7-	D23.7-	D48.5	D49.2
forearm — *see also Neoplasm, skin, limb, upper*	C44.60-	C79.2	D04.6-	D23.6-	D48.5	D49.2
forehead — *see also Neoplasm, skin, face*	C44.309	C79.2	D04.39	D23.39	D48.5	D49.2
glabella — *see also Neoplasm, skin, face*	C44.309	C79.2	D04.39	D23.39	D48.5	D49.2
gluteal region — *see also Neoplasm, skin, trunk*	C44.509	C79.2	D04.5	D23.5	D48.5	D49.2
groin — *see also Neoplasm, skin, trunk*	C44.509	C79.2	D04.5	D23.5	D48.5	D49.2
hand — *see also Neoplasm, skin, limb, upper*	C44.60-	C79.2	D04.6-	D23.6-	D48.5	D49.2

	Malignant Primary	Malignant Secondary	Ca in situ	Benign	Uncertain Behavior	Unspecified Behavior
skin NOS *(Continued)*						
head NEC — *see also Neoplasm, skin, scalp*	C44.40	C79.2	D04.4	D23.4	D48.5	D49.2
heel — *see also Neoplasm, skin, limb, lower*	C44.70-	C79.2	D04.7-	D23.7-	D48.5	D49.2
helix — *see also Neoplasm, skin, ear*	C44.20-	C79.2	D04.2-	D23.2-	D48.5	D49.2
hip — *see also Neoplasm, skin, limb, lower*	C44.70-	C79.2	D04.7-	D23.7-	D48.5	D49.2
infraclavicular region — *see also Neoplasm, skin, trunk*	C44.509	C79.2	D04.5	D23.5	D48.5	D49.2
inguinal region — *see also Neoplasm, skin, trunk*	C44.509	C79.2	D04.5	D23.5	D48.5	D49.2
jaw — *see also Neoplasm, skin, face*	C44.309	C79.2	D04.39	D23.39	D48.5	D49.2
Kaposi's sarcoma — *see Kaposi's, sarcoma, skin*						
knee — *see also Neoplasm, skin, limb, lower*	C44.70-	C79.2	D04.7-	D23.7-	D48.5	D49.2
labia						
majora	C51.0	C79.82	D07.1	D28.0	D39.8	D49.59
minora	C51.1	C79.82	D07.1	D28.0	D39.8	D49.59
leg — *see also Neoplasm, skin, limb, lower*	C44.70-	C79.2	D04.7-	D23.7-	D48.5	D49.2
lid (lower) (upper)	C44.10-	C79.2	D04.1-	D23.1-	D48.5	D49.2
basal cell carcinoma	C44.11-	—	—	—	—	—
specified type NEC	C44.19-	—	—	—	—	—
squamous cell carcinoma	C44.12-	—	—	—	—	—
limb NEC	C44.90	C79.2	D04.9	D23.9	D48.5	D49.2
basal cell carcinoma	C44.91					
lower	C44.70-	C79.2	D04.7-	D23.7-	D48.5	D49.2
basal cell carcinoma	C44.71-	—	—	—	—	—
specified type NEC	C44.79-	—	—	—	—	—
squamous cell carcinoma	C44.72-	—	—	—	—	—
upper	C44.60-	C79.2	D04.6-	D23.6-	D48.5	D49.2
basal cell carcinoma	C44.61-	—	—	—	—	—
specified type NEC	C44.69-	—	—	—	—	—
squamous cell carcinoma	C44.62-	—	—	—	—	—
lip (lower) (upper)	C44.00	C79.2	D04.0	D23.0	D48.5	D49.2
basal cell carcinoma	C44.01	—	—	—	—	—
specified type NEC	C44.09	—	—	—	—	—
squamous cell carcinoma	C44.02	—	—	—	—	—

◄ New   ◀▥ Revised   ~~deleted~~ Deleted

TABLE OF NEOPLASMS

skin NOS (Continued)	Malignant Primary	Malignant Secondary	Ca in situ	Benign	Uncertain Behavior	Unspecified Behavior
male genital organs	C63.9	C79.82	D07.60	D29.9	D40.8	D49.59
penis	C60.9	C79.82	D07.4	D29.0	D40.8	D49.59
prepuce	C60.0	C79.82	D07.4	D29.0	D40.8	D49.59
scrotum	C63.2	C79.82	D07.61	D29.4	D40.8	D49.59
mastectomy site (skin) — see also Neoplasm, skin, breast	C44.501	C79.2	—	—	—	—
specified as breast tissue	C50.8-	C79.81	—	—	—	—
meatus, acoustic (external) — see also Neoplasm, skin, ear	C44.20-	C79.2	D04.2-	D23.2-	D48.5	D49.2
melanotic — see Melanoma						
Merkel cell — see Carcinoma, Merkel cell						
nates — see also Neoplasm, skin, trunk	C44.509	C79.2	D04.5	D23.5	D48.5	D49.2
neck	C44.40	C79.2	D04.4	D23.4	D48.5	D49.2
basal cell carcinoma	C44.41	—	—	—	—	—
specified type NEC	C44.49	—	—	—	—	—
squamous cell carcinoma	C44.42	—	—	—	—	—
nevus — see Nevus, skin						
nose (external) — see also Neoplasm, nose, skin	C44.301	C79.2	D04.39	D23.39	D48.5	D49.2
overlapping lesion	C44.80	—	—	—	—	—
basal cell carcinoma	C44.81	—	—	—	—	—
specified type NEC	C44.89	—	—	—	—	—
squamous cell carcinoma	C44.82	—	—	—	—	—
palm — see also Neoplasm, skin, limb, upper	C44.60-	C79.2	D04.6-	D23.6-	D48.5	D49.2
palpebra	C44.10-	C79.2	D04.1-	D23.1-	D48.5	D49.2
basal cell carcinoma	C44.11-	—	—	—	—	—
specified type NEC	C44.19-	—	—	—	—	—
squamous cell carcinoma	C44.12-	—	—	—	—	—
penis NEC	C60.9	C79.82	D07.4	D29.0	D40.8	D49.59
perianal — see also Neoplasm, skin, anus	C44.500	C79.2	D04.5	D23.5	D48.5	D49.2
perineum — see also Neoplasm, skin, anus	C44.500	C79.2	D04.5	D23.5	D48.5	D49.2
pinna — see also Neoplasm, skin, ear	C44.20-	C79.2	D04.2-	D23.2-	D48.5	D49.2
plantar — see also Neoplasm, skin, limb, lower	C44.70-	C79.2	D04.7-	D23.7-	D48.5	D49.2
popliteal fossa or space — see also Neoplasm, skin, limb, lower	C44.70-	C79.2	D04.7-	D23.7-	D48.5	D49.2
prepuce	C60.0	C79.82	D07.4	D29.0	D40.8	D49.59

skin NOS (Continued)	Malignant Primary	Malignant Secondary	Ca in situ	Benign	Uncertain Behavior	Unspecified Behavior
pubes — see also Neoplasm, skin, trunk	C44.509	C79.2	D04.5	D23.5	D48.5	D49.2
sacrococcygeal region — see also Neoplasm, skin, trunk	C44.509	C79.2	D04.5	D23.5	D48.5	D49.2
scalp	C44.40	C79.2	D04.4	D23.4	D48.5	D49.2
basal cell carcinoma	C44.41	—	—	—	—	—
specified type NEC	C44.49	—	—	—	—	—
squamous cell carcinoma	C44.42	—	—	—	—	—
scapular region — see also Neoplasm, skin, trunk	C44.509	C79.2	D04.5	D23.5	D48.5	D49.2
scrotum	C63.2	C79.82	D07.61	D29.4	D40.8	D49.59
shoulder — see also Neoplasm, skin, limb, upper	C44.60-	C79.2	D04.6-	D23.6-	D48.5	D49.2
sole (foot) — see also Neoplasm, skin, limb, lower	C44.70-	C79.2	D04.7-	D23.7-	D48.5	D49.2
specified sites NEC	C44.80	C79.2	D04.8	D23.9	D48.5	D49.2
basal cell carcinoma	C44.81	—	—	—	—	—
specified type NEC	C44.89	—	—	—	—	—
squamous cell carcinoma	C44.82	—	—	—	—	—
specified type NEC	C44.99	—	—	—	—	—
squamous cell carcinoma	C44.92	—	—	—	—	—
submammary fold — see also Neoplasm, skin, trunk	C44.509	C79.2	D04.5	D23.5	D48.5	D49.2
supraclavicular region — see also Neoplasm, skin, neck	C44.40	C79.2	D04.4	D23.4	D48.5	D49.2
temple — see also Neoplasm, skin, face	C44.309	C79.2	D04.39	D23.39	D48.5	D49.2
thigh — see also Neoplasm, skin, limb, lower	C44.70-	C79.2	D04.7-	D23.7-	D48.5	D49.2
thoracic wall — see also Neoplasm, skin, trunk	C44.509	C79.2	D04.5	D23.5	D48.5	D49.2
thumb — see also Neoplasm, skin, limb, upper	C44.60-	C79.2	D04.6-	D23.6-	D48.5	D49.2
toe — see also Neoplasm, skin, limb, lower	C44.70-	C79.2	D04.7-	D23.7-	D48.5	D49.2
tragus — see also Neoplasm, skin, ear	C44.20-	C79.2	D04.2-	D23.2-	D48.5	D49.2
trunk	C44.509	C79.2	D04.5	D23.5	D48.5	D49.2
basal cell carcinoma	C44.519	—	—	—	—	—
specified type NEC	C44.599	—	—	—	—	—
squamous cell carcinoma	C44.529	—	—	—	—	—
umbilicus — see also Neoplasm, skin, trunk	C44.509	C79.2	D04.5	D23.5	D48.5	D49.2

◀ New ◀▪▪▪ Revised ~~deleted~~ Deleted

	Malignant Primary	Malignant Secondary	Ca in situ	Benign	Uncertain Behavior	Unspecified Behavior
skin NOS *(Continued)*						
vulva	C51.9	C79.82	D07.1	D28.0	D39.8	D49.59
overlapping lesion	C51.8	—	—	—	—	—
wrist — *see also Neoplasm, skin, limb, upper*	C44.60-	C79.2	D04.6-	D23.6-	D48.5	D49.2
skull	C41.0	C79.51	—	D16.4-	D48.0	D49.2
soft parts or tissues — *see Neoplasm, connective tissue*						
specified site NEC	C76.8	C79.89	D09.8	D36.7	D48.7	D49.89
spermatic cord	C63.1-	C79.82	D07.69	D29.8	D40.8	D49.59
sphenoid	C31.3	C78.39	D02.3	D14.0	D38.5	D49.1
bone	C41.0	C79.51	—	D16.4-	D48.0	D49.2
sinus	C31.3	C78.39	D02.3	D14.0	D38.5	D49.1
sphincter						
anal	C21.1	C78.5	D01.3	D12.9	D37.8	D49.0
of Oddi	C24.0	C78.89	D01.5	D13.5	D37.6	D49.0
spine, spinal (column)	C41.2	C79.51	—	D16.6	D48.0	D49.2
bulb	C71.7	C79.31		D33.1	D43.1	D49.6
coccyx	C41.4	C79.51	—	D16.8	D48.0	D49.2
cord (cervical) (lumbar) (sacral) (thoracic)	C72.0	C79.49	—	D33.4	D43.4	D49.7
dura mater	C70.1	C79.49		D32.1	D42.1	D49.7
lumbosacral	C41.2	C79.51	—	D16.6	D48.0	D49.2
marrow NEC	C96.9	C79.52	—	—	D47.9	D49.89
membrane	C70.1	C79.49		D32.1	D42.1	D49.7
meninges	C70.1	C79.49		D32.1	D42.1	D49.7
nerve (root)	C47.9	C79.89	—	D36.10	D48.2	D49.2
pia mater	C70.1	C79.49		D32.1	D42.1	D49.7
root	C47.9	C79.89		D36.10	D48.2	D49.2
sacrum	C41.4	C79.51	—	D16.8	D48.0	D49.2
spleen, splenic NEC	C26.1	C78.89	D01.7	D13.9	D37.8	D49.0
flexure (colon)	C18.5	C78.5	D01.0	D12.3	D37.4	D49.0
stem, brain	C71.7	C79.31	—	D33.1	D43.1	D49.6
Stensen's duct	C07	C79.89	D00.00	D11.0	D37.030	D49.0
sternum	C41.3	C79.51		D16.7	D48.0	D49.2
stomach	C16.9	C78.89	D00.2	D13.1	D37.1	D49.0
antrum (pyloric)	C16.3	C78.89	D00.2	D13.1	D37.1	D49.0
body	C16.2	C78.89	D00.2	D13.1	D37.1	D49.0
cardia	C16.0	C78.89	D00.2	D13.1	D37.1	D49.0
cardiac orifice	C16.0	C78.89	D00.2	D13.1	D37.1	D49.0
corpus	C16.2	C78.89	D00.2	D13.1	D37.1	D49.0
fundus	C16.1	C78.89	D00.2	D13.1	D37.1	D49.0
greater curvature NEC	C16.6	C78.89	D00.2	D13.1	D37.1	D49.0
lesser curvature NEC	C16.5	C78.89	D00.2	D13.1	D37.1	D49.0

	Malignant Primary	Malignant Secondary	Ca in situ	Benign	Uncertain Behavior	Unspecified Behavior
stomach *(Continued)*						
overlapping lesion	C16.8	—	—	—	—	—
prepylorus	C16.4	C78.89	D00.2	D13.1	D37.1	D49.0
pylorus	C16.4	C78.89	D00.2	D13.1	D37.1	D49.0
wall NEC	C16.9	C78.89	D00.2	D13.1	D37.1	D49.0
anterior NEC	C16.8	C78.89	D00.2	D13.1	D37.1	D49.0
posterior NEC	C16.8	C78.89	D00.2	D13.1	D37.1	D49.0
stroma, endometrial	C54.1	C79.82	D07.0	D26.1	D39.0	D49.59
stump, cervical	C53.8	C79.82	D06.7	D26.0	D39.0	D49.59
subcutaneous (nodule) (tissue) NEC — *see Neoplasm, connective tissue*						
subdural	C70.9	C79.32	—	D32.9	D42.9	D49.7
subglottis, subglottic	C32.2	C78.39	D02.0	D14.1	D38.0	D49.1
sublingual	C04.9	C79.89	D00.06	D10.2	D37.09	D49.0
gland or duct	C08.1	C79.89	D00.00	D11.7	D37.031	D49.0
submandibular gland	C08.0	C79.89	D00.00	D11.7	D37.032	D49.0
submaxillary gland or duct	C08.0	C79.89	D00.00	D11.7	D37.032	D49.0
submental	C76.0	C79.89	D09.8	D36.7	D48.7	D49.89
subpleural	C34.9-	C78.0-	D02.2-	D14.3-	D38.1	D49.1
substernal	C38.1	C78.1		D15.2	D38.3	D49.89
sudoriferous, sudoriparous gland, site unspecified	C44.90	C79.2	D04.9	D23.9	D48.5	D49.2
specified site — *see Neoplasm, skin*						
supraclavicular region	C76.0	C79.89	D09.8	D36.7	D48.7	D49.89
supraglottis	C32.1	C78.39	D02.0	D14.1	D38.0	D49.1
suprarenal	C74.9-	C79.7-	D09.3	D35.0-	D44.1-	D49.7
capsule	C74.9-	C79.7-	D09.3	D35.0-	D44.1-	D49.7
cortex	C74.0-	C79.7-	D09.3	D35.0-	D44.1-	D49.7
gland	C74.9-	C79.7-	D09.3	D35.0-	D44.1-	D49.7
medulla	C74.1-	C79.7-	D09.3	D35.0-	D44.1-	D49.7
suprasellar (region)	C71.9	C79.31	—	D33.2	D43.2	D49.6
supratentorial (brain) NEC	C71.0	C79.31	—	D33.0	D43.0	D49.6
sweat gland (apocrine) (eccrine), site unspecified	C44.90	C79.2	D04.9	D23.9	D48.5	D49.2
specified site — *see Neoplasm, skin*						
sympathetic nerve or nervous system NEC	C47.9	C79.89	—	D36.10	D48.2	D49.2
symphysis pubis	C41.4	C79.51	—	D16.8	D48.0	D49.2
synovial membrane — *see Neoplasm, connective tissue*						
tapetum, brain	C71.8	C79.31	—	D33.2	D43.2	D49.6

TABLE OF NEOPLASMS

TABLE OF NEOPLASMS

	Malignant Primary	Malignant Secondary	Ca in situ	Benign	Uncertain Behavior	Unspecified Behavior
tarsus (any bone)	C40.3-	C79.51	—	D16.3-	—	—
temple (skin) — see also Neoplasm, skin, face	C44.309	C79.2	D04.39	D23.39	D48.5	D49.2
temporal						
bone	C41.0	C79.51	—	D16.4-	D48.0	D49.2
lobe or pole	C71.2	C79.31	—	D33.0	D43.0	D49.6
region	C76.0	C79.89	D09.8	D36.7	D48.7	D49.89
skin — see also Neoplasm, skin, face	C44.309	C79.2	D04.39	D23.39	D48.5	D49.2
tendon (sheath) — see Neoplasm, connective tissue						
tentorium (cerebelli)	C70.0	C79.32	—	D32.0	D42.0	D49.7
testis, testes	C62.9-	C79.82	D07.69	D29.2-	D40.1-	D49.59
descended	C62.1-	C79.82	D07.69	D29.2-	D40.1-	D49.59
ectopic	C62.0-	C79.82	D07.69	D29.2-	D40.1-	D49.59
retained	C62.0-	C79.82	D07.69	D29.2-	D40.1-	D49.59
scrotal	C62.1-	C79.82	D07.69	D29.2-	D40.1-	D49.59
undescended	C62.0-	C79.82	D07.69	D29.2-	D40.1-	D49.59
unspecified whether descended or undescended	C62.9-	C79.82	D07.69	D29.2-	D40.1-	D49.59
thalamus	C71.0	C79.31	—	D33.0	D43.0	D49.6
thigh NEC	C76.5-	C79.89	D04.7-	D36.7	D48.7	D49.89
thorax, thoracic (cavity) (organs NEC)	C76.1	C79.89	D09.8	D36.7	D48.7	D49.89
duct	C49.3	C79.89	—	D21.3	D48.1	D49.2
wall NEC	C76.1	C79.89	D09.8	D36.7	D48.7	D49.89
throat	C14.0	C79.89	D00.08	D10.9	D37.05	D49.0
thumb NEC	C76.4-	C79.89	D04.6-	D36.7	D48.7	D49.89
thymus (gland)	C37	C79.89	D09.3	D15.0	D38.4	D49.89
thyroglossal duct	C73	C79.89	D09.3	D34	D44.0	D49.7
thyroid (gland)	C73	C79.89	D09.3	D34	D44.0	D49.7
cartilage	C32.3	C78.39	D02.0	D14.1	D38.0	D49.1
tibia (any part)	C40.2-	C79.51	—	D16.2-	—	—
toe NEC	C76.5-	C79.89	D04.7-	D36.7	D48.7	D49.89
tongue	C02.9	C79.89	D00.07	D10.1	D37.02	D49.0
anterior (two-thirds) NEC	C02.3	C79.89	D00.07	D10.1	D37.02	D49.0
dorsal surface	C02.0	C79.89	D00.07	D10.1	D37.02	D49.0
ventral surface	C02.2	C79.89	D00.07	D10.1	D37.02	D49.0
base (dorsal surface)	C01	C79.89	D00.07	D10.1	D37.02	D49.0
border (lateral)	C02.1	C79.89	D00.07	D10.1	D37.02	D49.0
dorsal surface NEC	C02.0	C79.89	D00.07	D10.1	D37.02	D49.0
fixed part NEC	C01	C79.89	D00.07	D10.1	D37.02	D49.0
foreamen cecum	C02.0	C79.89	D00.07	D10.1	D37.02	D49.0
frenulum linguae	C02.2	C79.89	D00.07	D10.1	D37.02	D49.0

	Malignant Primary	Malignant Secondary	Ca in situ	Benign	Uncertain Behavior	Unspecified Behavior
tongue (Continued)						
junctional zone	C02.8	C79.89	D00.07	D10.1	D37.02	D49.0
margin (lateral)	C02.1	C79.89	D00.07	D10.1	D37.02	D49.0
midline NEC	C02.0	C79.89	D00.07	D10.1	D37.02	D49.0
mobile part NEC	C02.3	C79.89	D00.07	D10.1	D37.02	D49.0
overlapping lesion	C02.8	—	—	—	—	—
posterior (third)	C01	C79.89	D00.07	D10.1	D37.02	D49.0
root	C01	C79.89	D00.07	D10.1	D37.02	D49.0
surface (dorsal)	C02.0	C79.89	D00.07	D10.1	D37.02	D49.0
base	C01	C79.89	D00.07	D10.1	D37.02	D49.0
ventral	C02.2	C79.89	D00.07	D10.1	D37.02	D49.0
tip	C02.1	C79.89	D00.07	D10.1	D37.02	D49.0
tonsil	C02.4	C79.89	D00.07	D10.1	D37.02	D49.0
tonsil	C09.9	C79.89	D00.08	D10.4	D37.05	D49.0
fauces, faucial	C09.9	C79.89	D00.08	D10.4	D37.05	D49.0
lingual	C02.4	C79.89	D00.07	D10.1	D37.02	D49.0
overlapping sites	C09.8	—	—	—	—	—
palatine	C09.9	C79.89	D00.08	D10.4	D37.05	D49.0
pharyngeal	C11.1	C79.89	D00.08	D10.6	D37.05	D49.0
pillar (anterior) (posterior)	C09.1	C79.89	D00.08	D10.5	D37.05	D49.0
tonsillar fossa	C09.0	C79.89	D00.08	D10.5	D37.05	D49.0
tooth socket NEC	C03.9	C79.89	D00.03	D10.39	D37.09	D49.0
trachea (cartilage) (mucosa)	C33	C78.39	D02.1	D14.2	D38.1	D49.1
overlapping lesion with bronchus or lung	C34.8-	—	—	—	—	—
tracheobronchial	C34.8-	C78.39	D02.1	D14.2	D38.1	D49.1
overlapping lesion with lung	C34.8-	—	—	—	—	—
tragus — see also Neoplasm, skin, ear	C44.20-	C79.2	D04.2-	D23.2-	D48.5	D49.2
trunk NEC	C76.8	C79.89	D04.5	D36.7	D48.7	D49.89
tubo-ovarian	C57.8	C79.82	D07.39	D28.7	D39.8	D49.59
tunica vaginalis	C63.7	C79.82	D07.69	D29.8	D40.8	D49.59
turbinate (bone)	C41.0	C79.51	—	D16.4-	D48.0	D49.2
nasal	C30.0	C78.39	D02.3	D14.0	D38.5	D49.1
tympanic cavity	C30.1	C78.39	D02.3	D14.0	D38.5	D49.1
ulna (any part)	C40.0-	C79.51	—	D16.0-	—	—
umbilicus, umbilical — see also Neoplasm, skin, trunk	C44.509	C79.2	D04.5	D23.5	D48.5	D49.2
uncus, brain	C71.2	C79.31	—	D33.0	D43.0	D49.6
unknown site or unspecified	C80.1	C79.9	D09.9	D36.9	D48.9	D49.9
urachus	C67.7	C79.11	D09.0	D30.3	D41.4	D49.4
ureter, ureteral	C66.-	C79.19	D09.19	D30.2-	D41.2-	D49.59
orifice (bladder)	C67.6	C79.11	D09.0	D30.3	D41.4	D49.4
ureter-bladder (junction)	C67.6	C79.11	D09.0	D30.3	D41.4	D49.4

◄ New   ◄━ Revised   ~~deleted~~ Deleted

	Malignant Primary	Malignant Secondary	Ca in situ	Benign	Uncertain Behavior	Unspecified Behavior
urethra, urethral (gland)	C68.0	C79.19	D09.19	D30.4	D41.3	D49.59 ◄
orifice, internal	C67.5	C79.11	D09.0	D30.3	D41.4	D49.4
urethrovaginal (septum)	C57.9	C79.82	D07.30	D28.9	D39.8	D49.59 ◄
urinary organ or system	C68.9	C79.10	D09.10	D30.9	D41.9	D49.59 ◄
bladder — see Neoplasm, bladder						
overlapping lesion	C68.8	—	—	—	—	—
specified sites NEC	C68.8	C79.19	D09.19	D30.8	D41.8	D49.59 ◄
utero-ovarian	C57.8	C79.82	D07.39	D28.7	D39.8	D49.59 ◄
ligament	C57.1	C79.82	D07.39	D28.2	D39.8	D49.59 ◄
uterosacral ligament	C57.3	C79.82	—	D28.2	D39.8	D49.59 ◄
uterus, uteri, uterine	C55	C79.82	D07.0	D26.9	D39.0	D49.59 ◄
adnexa NEC	C57.4	C79.82	D07.39	D28.7	D39.8	D49.59 ◄
body	C54.9	C79.82	D07.0	D26.1	D39.0	D49.59 ◄
cervix	C53.9	C79.82	D06.9	D26.0	D39.0	D49.59 ◄
cornu	C54.9	C79.82	D07.0	D26.1	D39.0	D49.59 ◄
corpus	C54.9	C79.82	D07.0	D26.1	D39.0	D49.59 ◄
endocervix (canal) (gland)	C53.0	C79.82	D06.0	D26.0	D39.0	D49.59 ◄
endometrium	C54.1	C79.82	D07.0	D26.1	D39.0	D49.59 ◄
exocervix	C53.1	C79.82	D06.1	D26.0	D39.0	D49.59 ◄
external os	C53.1	C79.82	D06.1	D26.0	D39.0	D49.59 ◄
fundus	C54.3	C79.82	D07.0	D26.1	D39.0	D49.59 ◄
internal os	C53.0	C79.82	D06.0	D26.0	D39.0	D49.59 ◄
isthmus	C54.0	C79.82	D07.0	D26.1	D39.0	D49.59 ◄
ligament	C57.3	C79.82	—	D28.2	D39.8	D49.59 ◄
broad	C57.1	C79.82	D07.39	D28.2	D39.8	D49.59 ◄
round	C57.2	C79.82	—	D28.2	D39.8	D49.59 ◄
lower segment	C54.0	C79.82	D07.0	D26.1	D39.0	D49.59 ◄
myometrium	C54.2	C79.82	D07.0	D26.1	D39.0	D49.59 ◄
overlapping sites	C54.8	—	—	—	—	—
squamocolumnar junction	C53.8	C79.82	D06.7	D26.0	D39.0	D49.59 ◄
tube	C57.0-	C79.82	D07.39	D28.2	D39.8	D49.59 ◄
utricle, prostatic	C68.0	C79.19	D09.19	D30.4	D41.3	D49.59 ◄
uveal tract	C69.4-	C79.49	D09.2-	D31.4-	D48.7	D49.89
uvula	C05.2	C79.89	D00.04	D10.39	D37.09	D49.0
vagina, vaginal (fornix) (vault) (wall)	C52	C79.82	D07.2	D28.1	D39.8	D49.59 ◄
vaginovesical	C57.9	C79.82	D07.30	D28.9	D39.9	D49.59 ◄
septum	C57.9	C79.82	D07.30	D28.9	D39.9	D49.59 ◄
vallecula (epiglottis)	C10.0	C79.89	D00.08	D10.5	D37.05	D49.0
vas deferens	C63.1-	C79.82	D07.69	D29.8	D40.8	D49.59 ◄
vascular — see Neoplasm, connective tissue						

	Malignant Primary	Malignant Secondary	Ca in situ	Benign	Uncertain Behavior	Unspecified Behavior
Vater's ampulla	C24.1	C78.89	D01.5	D13.5	D37.6	D49.0
vein, venous — see Neoplasm, connective tissue						
vena cava (abdominal) (inferior)	C49.4	C79.89	—	D21.4	D48.1	D49.2
superior	C49.3	C79.89	—	D21.3	D48.1	D49.2
ventricle (cerebral) (floor) (lateral) (third)	C71.5	C79.31		D33.0	D43.0	D49.6
cardiac (left) (right)	C38.0	C79.89	—	D15.1	D48.7	D49.89
fourth	C71.7	C79.31		D33.1	D43.1	D49.6
ventricular band of larynx	C32.1	C78.39	D02.0	D14.1	D38.0	D49.1
ventriculus — see Neoplasm, stomach						
vermillion border — see Neoplasm, lip						
vermis, cerebellum	C71.6	C79.31	—	D33.1	D43.1	D49.6
vertebra (column)	C41.2	C79.51	—	D16.6	D48.0	D49.2
coccyx	C41.4	C79.51	—	D16.8-	D48.0	D49.2
marrow NEC	C96.9	C79.52	—	D47.9	D49.89	
sacrum	C41.4	C79.51	—	D16.8-	D48.0	D49.2
vesical — see Neoplasm, bladder						
vesicle, seminal	C63.7	C79.82	D07.69	D29.8	D40.8	D49.59
vesicocervical tissue	C57.9	C79.82	D07.30	D28.9	D39.9	D49.59
vesicorectal	C76.3	C79.82	D09.8	D36.7	D48.7	D49.89
vesicovaginal	C57.9	C79.82	D07.30	D28.9	D39.9	D49.59 ◄
septum	C57.9	C79.82	D07.30	D28.9	D39.8	D49.59 ◄
vessel (blood) — see Neoplasm, connective tissue						
vestibular gland, greater	C51.0	C79.82	D07.1	D28.0	D39.8	D49.59 ◄
vestibule						
mouth	C06.1	C79.89	D00.00	D10.39	D37.09	D49.0
nose	C30.0	C78.39	D02.3	D14.0	D38.5	D49.1
Virchow's gland	C77.0	C77.0	—	D36.0	D48.7	D49.89
viscera NEC	C76.8	C79.89	D09.8	D36.7	D48.7	D49.89
vocal cords (true)	C32.0	C78.39	D02.0	D14.1	D38.0	D49.1
false	C32.1	C78.39	D02.0	D14.1	D38.0	D49.1
vomer	C41.0	C79.51	—	D16.4-	D48.0	D49.2
vulva	C51.9	C79.82	D07.1	D28.0	D39.8	D49.59 ◄
vulvovaginal gland	C51.0	C79.82	D07.1	D28.0	D39.8	D49.59 ◄
Waldeyer's ring	C14.2	C79.89	D00.08	D10.9	D37.05	D49.0
Wharton's duct	C08.0	C79.89	D00.00	D11.7	D37.032	D49.0
white matter (central) (cerebral)	C71.0	C79.31	—	D33.0	D43.0	D49.6
windpipe	C33	C78.39	D02.1	D14.2	D38.1	D49.1

TABLE OF NEOPLASMS

◄ New   ⟵ Revised   ~~deleted~~ Deleted

	Malignant Primary	Malignant Secondary	Ca in situ	Benign	Uncertain Behavior	Unspecified Behavior
Wirsung's duct	C25.3	C78.89	D01.7	D13.6	D37.8	D49.0
wolffian (body) (duct)						
female	C57.7	C79.82	D07.39	D28.7	D39.8	D49.59
male	C63.7	C79.82	D07.69	D29.8	D40.8	D49.59

	Malignant Primary	Malignant Secondary	Ca in situ	Benign	Uncertain Behavior	Unspecified Behavior
womb — see Neoplasm, uterus						
wrist NEC	C76.4-	C79.89	D04.6-	D36.7	D48.7	D49.89
xiphoid process	C41.3	C79.51	—	D16.7	D48.0	D49.2
Zuckerkandl organ	C75.5	C79.89	—	D35.6	D44.7	D49.7

◀ New   ⬅ Revised   ~~deleted~~ Deleted

TABLE OF NEOPLASMS

ICD-10-CM
Table of Drugs and Chemicals

TOD

ICD-10-CM
Table of Drugs and Chemicals

Substance	Poisoning, Accidental (Unintentional)	Poisoning, Intentional Self-Harm	Poisoning, Assault	Poisoning, Undetermined	Adverse Effect	Underdosing
#						
1-propanol	T51.3X1	T51.3X2	T51.3X3	T51.3X4	—	—
2-propanol	T51.2X1	T51.2X2	T51.2X3	T51.2X4	—	—
2,4-D (dichlorophen-oxyacetic acid)	T60.3X1	T60.3X2	T60.3X3	T60.3X4	—	—
2,4-toluene diisocyanate	T65.0X1	T65.0X2	T65.0X3	T65.0X4	—	—
2,4,5-T (trichloro-phenoxyacetic acid)	T60.1X1	T60.1X2	T60.1X3	T60.1X4	—	—
14-hydroxydihydro-morphinone	T40.2X1	T40.2X2	T40.2X3	T40.2X4	T40.2X5	T40.2X6
A						
ABOB	T37.5X1	T37.5X2	T37.5X3	T37.5X4	T37.5X5	T37.5X6
Abrine	T62.2X1	T62.2X2	T62.2X3	T62.2X4	—	—
Abrus (seed)	T62.2X1	T62.2X2	T62.2X3	T62.2X4	—	—
Absinthe	T51.0X1	T51.0X2	T51.0X3	T51.0X4	—	—
beverage	T51.0X1	T51.0X2	T51.0X3	T51.0X4	—	—
Acaricide	T60.8X1	T60.8X2	T60.8X3	T60.8X4	—	—
Acebutolol	T44.7X1	T44.7X2	T44.7X3	T44.7X4	T44.7X5	T44.7X6
Acecarbromal	T42.6X1	T42.6X2	T42.6X3	T42.6X4	T42.6X5	T42.6X6
Aceclidine	T44.1X1	T44.1X2	T44.1X3	T44.1X4	T44.1X5	T44.1X6
Acedapsone	T37.0X1	T37.0X2	T37.0X3	T37.0X4	T37.0X5	T37.0X6
Acefylline piperazine	T48.6X1	T48.6X2	T48.6X3	T48.6X4	T48.6X5	T48.6X6
Acemorphan	T40.2X1	T40.2X2	T40.2X3	T40.2X4	T40.2X5	T40.2X6
Acenocoumarin	T45.511	T45.512	T45.513	T45.514	T45.515	T45.516
Acenocoumarol	T45.511	T45.512	T45.513	T45.514	T45.515	T45.516
Acepifylline	T48.6X1	T48.6X2	T48.6X3	T48.6X4	T48.6X5	T48.6X6
Acepromazine	T43.3X1	T43.3X2	T43.3X3	T43.3X4	T43.3X5	T43.3X6
Acesulfamethoxypyridazine	T37.0X1	T37.0X2	T37.0X3	T37.0X4	T37.0X5	T37.0X6
Acetal	T52.8X1	T52.8X2	T52.8X3	T52.8X4	—	—
Acetaldehyde (vapor)	T52.8X1	T52.8X2	T52.8X3	T52.8X4	—	—
liquid	T65.891	T65.892	T65.893	T65.894	—	—
P-Acetamidophenol	T39.1X1	T39.1X2	T39.1X3	T39.1X4	T39.1X5	T39.1X6
Acetaminophen	T39.1X1	T39.1X2	T39.1X3	T39.1X4	T39.1X5	T39.1X6
Acetaminosalol	T39.1X1	T39.1X2	T39.1X3	T39.1X4	T39.1X5	T39.1X6
Acetanilide	T39.1X1	T39.1X2	T39.1X3	T39.1X4	T39.1X5	T39.1X6
Acetarsol	T37.3X1	T37.3X2	T37.3X3	T37.3X4	T37.3X5	T37.3X6
Acetazolamide	T50.2X1	T50.2X2	T50.2X3	T50.2X4	T50.2X5	T50.2X6
Acetiamine	T45.2X1	T45.2X2	T45.2X3	T45.2X4	T45.2X5	T45.2X6
Acetic						
acid	T54.2X1	T54.2X2	T54.2X3	T54.2X4	—	—
with sodium acetate (ointment)	T49.3X1	T49.3X2	T49.3X3	T49.3X4	T49.3X5	T49.3X6

Substance	Poisoning, Accidental (Unintentional)	Poisoning, Intentional Self-Harm	Poisoning, Assault	Poisoning, Undetermined	Adverse Effect	Underdosing
Acetic *(Continued)*						
acid *(Continued)*						
ester (solvent) (vapor)	T52.8X1	T52.8X2	T52.8X3	T52.8X4	—	—
irrigating solution	T50.3X1	T50.3X2	T50.3X3	T50.3X4	T50.3X5	T50.3X6
medicinal (lotion)	T49.2X1	T49.2X2	T49.2X3	T49.2X4	T49.2X5	T49.2X6
anhydride	T65.891	T65.892	T65.893	T65.894	—	—
ether (vapor)	T52.8X1	T52.8X2	T52.8X3	T52.8X4	—	—
Acetohexamide	T38.3X1	T38.3X2	T38.3X3	T38.3X4	T38.3X5	T38.3X6
Acetohydroxamic acid	T50.991	T50.992	T50.993	T50.994	T50.995	T50.996
Acetomenaphthone	T45.7X1	T45.7X2	T45.7X3	T45.7X4	T45.7X5	T45.7X6
Acetomorphine	T40.1X1	T40.1X2	T40.1X3	T40.1X4	—	—
Acetone (oils)	T52.4X1	T52.4X2	T52.4X3	T52.4X4	—	—
chlorinated	T52.4X1	T52.4X2	T52.4X3	T52.4X4	—	—
vapor	T52.4X1	T52.4X2	T52.4X3	T52.4X4	—	—
Acetonitrile	T52.8X1	T52.8X2	T52.8X3	T52.8X4	—	—
Acetophenazine	T43.3X1	T43.3X2	T43.3X3	T43.3X4	T43.3X5	T43.3X6
Acetophenetedin	T39.1X1	T39.1X2	T39.1X3	T39.1X4	T39.1X5	T39.1X6
Acetophenone	T52.4X1	T52.4X2	T52.4X3	T52.4X4	—	—
Acetorphine	T40.2X1	T40.2X2	T40.2X3	T40.2X4	—	—
Acetosulfone (sodium)	T37.1X1	T37.1X2	T37.1X3	T37.1X4	T37.1X5	T37.1X6
Acetrizoate (sodium)	T50.8X1	T50.8X2	T50.8X3	T50.8X4	T50.8X5	T50.8X6
Acetylcarbromal	T42.6X1	T42.6X2	T42.6X3	T42.6X4	T42.6X5	T42.6X6
Acetrizoic acid	T50.8X1	T50.8X2	T50.8X3	T50.8X4	T50.8X5	T50.8X6
Acetyl						
bromide	T53.6X1	T53.6X2	T53.6X3	T53.6X4	—	—
chloride	T53.6X1	T53.6X2	T53.6X3	T53.6X4	—	—
Acetylcholine						
chloride	T44.1X1	T44.1X2	T44.1X3	T44.1X4	T44.1X5	T44.1X6
derivative	T44.1X1	T44.1X2	T44.1X3	T44.1X4	T44.1X5	T44.1X6
Acetylcysteine	T48.4X1	T48.4X2	T48.4X3	T48.4X4	T48.4X5	T48.4X6
Acetyldigitoxin	T46.0X1	T46.0X2	T46.0X3	T46.0X4	T46.0X5	T46.0X6
Acetyldigoxin	T46.0X1	T46.0X2	T46.0X3	T46.0X4	T46.0X5	T46.0X6
Acetyldihydrocodeine	T40.2X1	T40.2X2	T40.2X3	T40.2X4	—	—
Acetyldihydrocodeinone	T40.2X1	T40.2X2	T40.2X3	T40.2X4	—	—
Acetylene (gas)	T59.891	T59.892	T59.893	T59.894	—	—
dichloride	T53.6X1	T53.6X2	T53.6X3	T53.6X4	—	—
incomplete combustion of	T58.11	T58.12	T58.13	T58.14	—	—
industrial	T59.891	T59.892	T59.893	T59.894	—	—
tetrachloride	T53.6X1	T53.6X2	T53.6X3	T53.6X4	—	—
vapor	T53.6X1	T53.6X2	T53.6X3	T53.6X4	—	—
Acetylphenylhydrazine	T39.8X1	T39.8X2	T39.8X3	T39.8X4	T39.8X5	T39.8X6
Acetylpheneturide	T42.6X1	T42.6X2	T42.6X3	T42.6X4	T42.6X5	T42.6X6

TABLE OF DRUGS AND CHEMICALS

TABLE OF DRUGS AND CHEMICALS

Substance	Poisoning, Accidental (Unintentional)	Poisoning, Intentional Self-Harm	Poisoning, Assault	Poisoning, Undetermined	Adverse Effect	Underdosing
Acetylsalicylic acid (salts)	T39.Ø11	T39.Ø12	T39.Ø13	T39.Ø14	T39.Ø15	T39.Ø16
enteric coated	T39.Ø11	T39.Ø12	T39.Ø13	T39.Ø14	T39.Ø15	T39.Ø16
Acetylsulfamethoxypyridazine	T37.ØX1	T37.ØX2	T37.ØX3	T37.ØX4	T37.ØX5	T37.ØX6
Achromycin	T36.4X1	T36.4X2	T36.4X3	T36.4X4	T36.4X5	T36.4X6
ophthalmic preparation	T49.5X1	T49.5X2	T49.5X3	T49.5X4	T49.5X5	T49.5X6
topical NEC	T49.ØX1	T49.ØX2	T49.ØX3	T49.ØX4	T49.ØX5	T49.ØX6
Aciclovir	T37.5X1	T37.5X2	T37.5X3	T37.5X4	T37.5X5	T37.5X6
Acid (corrosive) NEC	T54.2X1	T54.2X2	T54.2X3	T54.2X4	—	—
Acidifying agent NEC	T50.9Ø1	T50.9Ø2	T50.9Ø3	T50.9Ø4	T50.9Ø5	T50.9Ø6
Acipimox	T46.6X1	T46.6X2	T46.6X3	T46.6X4	T46.6X5	T46.6X6
Acitretin	T50.991	T50.992	T50.993	T50.994	T50.995	T50.996
Aclarubicin	T45.1X1	T45.1X2	T45.1X3	T45.1X4	T45.1X5	T45.1X6
Aclatonium napadisilate	T48.1X1	T48.1X2	T48.1X3	T48.1X4	T48.1X5	T48.1X6
Aconite (wild)	T46.991	T46.992	T46.993	T46.994	T46.995	T46.996
Aconitine	T46.991	T46.992	T46.993	T46.994	T46.995	T46.996
Aconitum ferox	T46.991	T46.992	T46.993	T46.994	T46.995	T46.996
Acridine	T65.6X1	T65.6X2	T65.6X3	T65.6X4	—	—
vapor	T59.891	T59.892	T59.893	T59.894	—	—
Acriflavine	T37.91	T37.92	T37.93	T37.94	T37.95	T37.96
Acriflavinium chloride	T49.ØX1	T49.ØX2	T49.ØX3	T49.ØX4	T49.ØX5	T49.ØX6
Acrinol	T49.ØX1	T49.ØX2	T49.ØX3	T49.ØX4	T49.ØX5	T49.ØX6
Acrisorcin	T49.ØX1	T49.ØX2	T49.ØX3	T49.ØX4	T49.ØX5	T49.ØX6
Acrivastine	T45.ØX1	T45.ØX2	T45.ØX3	T45.ØX4	T45.ØX5	T45.ØX6
Acrolein (gas)	T59.891	T59.892	T59.893	T59.894	—	—
liquid	T54.1X1	T54.1X2	T54.1X3	T54.1X4	—	—
Acrylamide	T65.891	T65.892	T65.893	T65.894	—	—
Acrylic resin	T49.3X1	T49.3X2	T49.3X3	T49.3X4	T49.3X5	T49.3X6
Acrylonitrile	T65.891	T65.892	T65.893	T65.894	—	—
Actaea spicata	T62.2X1	T62.2X2	T62.2X3	T62.2X4	—	—
berry	T62.1X1	T62.1X2	T62.1X3	T62.1X4	—	—
Acterol	T37.3X1	T37.3X2	T37.3X3	T37.3X4	T37.3X5	T37.3X6
ACTH	T38.811	T38.812	T38.813	T38.814	T38.815	T38.816
Actinomycin C	T45.1X1	T45.1X2	T45.1X3	T45.1X4	T45.1X5	T45.1X6
Actinomycin D	T45.1X1	T45.1X2	T45.1X3	T45.1X4	T45.1X5	T45.1X6
Activated charcoal — see also Charcoal, medicinal	T47.6X1	T47.6X2	T47.6X3	T47.6X4	T47.6X5	T47.6X6
Acyclovir	T37.5X1	T37.5X2	T37.5X3	T37.5X4	T37.5X5	T37.5X6
Adenine	T45.2X1	T45.2X2	T45.2X3	T45.2X4	T45.2X5	T45.2X6
arabinoside	T37.5X1	T37.5X2	T37.5X3	T37.5X4	T37.5X5	T37.5X6
Adenosine (phosphate)	T46.2X1	T46.2X2	T46.2X3	T46.2X4	T46.2X5	T46.2X6
ADH	T38.891	T38.892	T38.893	T38.894	T38.895	T38.896
Adhesive NEC	T65.891	T65.892	T65.893	T65.894	—	—

Substance	Poisoning, Accidental (Unintentional)	Poisoning, Intentional Self-Harm	Poisoning, Assault	Poisoning, Undetermined	Adverse Effect	Underdosing
Adicillin	T36.ØX1	T36.ØX2	T36.ØX3	T36.ØX4	T36.ØX5	T36.ØX6
Adiphenine	T44.3X1	T44.3X2	T44.3X3	T44.3X4	T44.3X5	T44.3X6
Adipiodone	T50.8X1	T50.8X2	T50.8X3	T50.8X4	T50.8X5	T50.8X6
Adjunct, pharmaceutical	T50.9Ø1	T50.9Ø2	T50.9Ø3	T50.9Ø4	T50.9Ø5	T50.9Ø6
Adrenal (extract, cortex or medulla) (glucocorticoids) (hormones) (mineralo corticoids)	T38.ØX1	T38.ØX2	T38.ØX3	T38.ØX4	T38.ØX5	T38.ØX6
ENT agent	T49.6X1	T49.6X2	T49.6X3	T49.6X4	T49.6X5	T49.6X6
ophthalmic preparation	T49.5X1	T49.5X2	T49.5X3	T49.5X4	T49.5X5	T49.5X6
topical NEC	T49.ØX1	T49.ØX2	T49.ØX3	T49.ØX4	T49.ØX5	T49.ØX6
Adrenaline	T44.5X1	T44.5X2	T44.5X3	T44.5X4	T44.5X5	T44.5X6
Adrenalin — see Adrenaline						
Adrenergic NEC	T44.9Ø1	T44.9Ø2	T44.9Ø3	T44.9Ø4	T44.9Ø5	T44.9Ø6
blocking agent NEC	T44.8X1	T44.8X2	T44.8X3	T44.8X4	T44.8X5	T44.8X6
beta, heart	T44.7X1	T44.7X2	T44.7X3	T44.7X4	T44.7X5	T44.7X6
specified NEC	T44.991	T44.992	T44.993	T44.994	T44.995	T44.996
Adrenochrome						
(mono) semicarbazone	T46.991	T46.992	T46.993	T46.994	T46.995	T46.996
derivative	T46.991	T46.992	T46.993	T46.994	T46.995	T46.996
Adrenocorticotrophic hormone	T38.811	T38.812	T38.813	T38.814	T38.815	T38.816
Adrenocorticotrophin	T38.811	T38.812	T38.813	T38.814	T38.815	T38.816
Adriamycin	T45.1X1	T45.1X2	T45.1X3	T45.1X4	T45.1X5	T45.1X6
Aerosol spray NEC	T65.91	T65.92	T65.93	T65.94	—	—
Aerosporin	T36.8X1	T36.8X2	T36.8X3	T36.8X4	T36.8X5	T36.8X6
ENT agent	T49.6X1	T49.6X2	T49.6X3	T49.6X4	T49.6X5	T49.6X6
ophthalmic preparation	T49.5X1	T49.5X2	T49.5X3	T49.5X4	T49.5X5	T49.5X6
topical NEC	T49.ØX1	T49.ØX2	T49.ØX3	T49.ØX4	T49.ØX5	T49.ØX6
Aethusa cynapium	T62.2X1	T62.2X2	T62.2X3	T62.2X4	—	—
Afghanistan black	T40.7X1	T40.7X2	T40.7X3	T40.7X4	T40.7X5	T40.7X6
Aflatoxin	T64.Ø1	T64.Ø2	T64.Ø3	T64.Ø4		
Afloqualone	T42.8X1	T42.8X2	T42.8X3	T42.8X4	T42.8X5	T42.8X6
African boxwood	T62.2X1	T62.2X2	T62.2X3	T62.2X4	—	—
Agar	T47.4X1	T47.4X2	T47.4X3	T47.4X4	T47.4X5	T47.4X6
Agonist						
predominantly						
alpha-adrenoreceptor	T44.4X1	T44.4X2	T44.4X3	T44.4X4	T44.4X5	T44.4X6
beta-adrenoreceptor	T44.5X1	T44.5X2	T44.5X3	T44.5X4	T44.5X5	T44.5X6
Agricultural agent NEC	T65.91	T65.92	T65.93	T65.94	—	—
Agrypnal	T42.3X1	T42.3X2	T42.3X3	T42.3X4	T42.3X5	T42.3X6
AHLG	T50.Z11	T50.Z12	T50.Z13	T50.Z14	T50.Z15	T50.Z16
Air contaminant(s), source/type NOS	T65.91	T65.92	T65.93	T65.94	—	—

◀ New   ◀▪▪ Revised   ~~deleted~~ Deleted

Substance	External Cause (T-Code) Poisoning, Accidental (Unintentional)	Poisoning, Intentional Self-Harm	Poisoning, Assault	Poisoning, Undetermined	Adverse Effect	Underdosing
Ajmaline	T46.2X1	T46.2X2	T46.2X3	T46.2X4	T46.2X5	T46.2X6
Akritoin	T37.8X1	T37.8X2	T37.8X3	T37.8X4	T37.8X5	T37.8X6
Akee	T62.1X1	T62.1X2	T62.1X3	T62.1X4	—	—
Akrinol	T49.0X1	T49.0X2	T49.0X3	T49.0X4	T49.0X5	T49.0X6
Alacepril	T46.4X1	T46.4X2	T46.4X3	T46.4X4	T46.4X5	T46.4X6
Alantolactone	T37.4X1	T37.4X2	T37.4X3	T37.4X4	T37.4X5	T37.4X6
Albamycin	T36.8X1	T36.8X2	T36.8X3	T36.8X4	T36.8X5	T36.8X6
Albendazole	T37.4X1	T37.4X2	T37.4X3	T37.4X4	T37.4X5	T37.4X6
Albumin						
bovine	T45.8X1	T45.8X2	T45.8X3	T45.8X4	T45.8X5	T45.8X6
human serum	T45.8X1	T45.8X2	T45.8X3	T45.8X4	T45.8X5	T45.8X6
salt-poor	T45.8X1	T45.8X2	T45.8X3	T45.8X4	T45.8X5	T45.8X6
normal human serum	T45.8X1	T45.8X2	T45.8X3	T45.8X4	T45.8X5	T45.8X6
Albuterol	T48.6X1	T48.6X2	T48.6X3	T48.6X4	T48.6X5	T48.6X6
Albutoin	T42.0X1	T42.0X2	T42.0X3	T42.0X4	T42.0X5	T42.0X6
Alclometasone	T49.0X1	T49.0X2	T49.0X3	T49.0X4	T49.0X5	T49.0X6
Alcohol	T51.91	T51.92	T51.93	T51.94	—	—
absolute	T51.0X1	T51.0X2	T51.0X3	T51.0X4	—	—
beverage	T51.0X1	T51.0X2	T51.0X3	T51.0X4	—	—
allyl	T51.8X1	T51.8X2	T51.8X3	T51.8X4	—	—
amyl	T51.3X1	T51.3X2	T51.3X3	T51.3X4	—	—
antifreeze	T51.1X1	T51.1X2	T51.1X3	T51.1X4	—	—
beverage	T51.0X1	T51.0X2	T51.0X3	T51.0X4	—	—
butyl	T51.3X1	T51.3X2	T51.3X3	T51.3X4	—	—
dehydrated	T51.0X1	T51.0X2	T51.0X3	T51.0X4	—	—
beverage	T51.0X1	T51.0X2	T51.0X3	T51.0X4	—	—
denatured	T51.0X1	T51.0X2	T51.0X3	T51.0X4	—	—
deterrent NEC	T50.6X1	T50.6X2	T50.6X3	T50.6X4	T50.6X5	T50.6X6
diagnostic (gastric function)	T50.8X1	T50.8X2	T50.8X3	T50.8X4	T50.8X5	T50.8X6
ethyl	T51.0X1	T51.0X2	T51.0X3	T51.0X4	—	—
beverage	T51.0X1	T51.0X2	T51.0X3	T51.0X4	—	—
grain	T51.0X1	T51.0X2	T51.0X3	T51.0X4	—	—
beverage	T51.0X1	T51.0X2	T51.0X3	T51.0X4	—	—
industrial	T51.0X1	T51.0X2	T51.0X3	T51.0X4	—	—
isopropyl	T51.2X1	T51.2X2	T51.2X3	T51.2X4	—	—
methyl	T51.1X1	T51.1X2	T51.1X3	T51.1X4	—	—
preparation for consumption	T51.0X1	T51.0X2	T51.0X3	T51.0X4	—	—
propyl	T51.3X1	T51.3X2	T51.3X3	T51.3X4	—	—
secondary	T51.2X1	T51.2X2	T51.2X3	T51.2X4	—	—
radiator	T51.1X1	T51.1X2	T51.1X3	T51.1X4	—	—
rubbing	T51.2X1	T51.2X2	T51.2X3	T51.2X4	—	—
specified type NEC	T51.8X1	T51.8X2	T51.8X3	T51.8X4	—	—

Substance	External Cause (T-Code) Poisoning, Accidental (Unintentional)	Poisoning, Intentional Self-Harm	Poisoning, Assault	Poisoning, Undetermined	Adverse Effect	Underdosing
Alcohol *(Continued)*						
surgical	T51.0X1	T51.0X2	T51.0X3	T51.0X4	—	—
vapor (from any type of Alcohol)	T59.891	T59.892	T59.893	T59.894	—	—
wood	T51.1X1	T51.1X2	T51.1X3	T51.1X4	—	—
Alcuronium (chloride)	T48.1X1	T48.1X2	T48.1X3	T48.1X4	T48.1X5	T48.1X6
Aldactone	T50.0X1	T50.0X2	T50.0X3	T50.0X4	T50.0X5	T50.0X6
Aldesulfone sodium	T37.1X1	T37.1X2	T37.1X3	T37.1X4	T37.1X5	T37.1X6
Aldicarb	T60.0X1	T60.0X2	T60.0X3	T60.0X4	—	—
Aldomet	T46.5X1	T46.5X2	T46.5X3	T46.5X4	T46.5X5	T46.5X6
Aldosterone	T50.0X1	T50.0X2	T50.0X3	T50.0X4	T50.0X5	T50.0X6
Aldrin (dust)	T60.1X1	T60.1X2	T60.1X3	T60.1X4	—	—
Aleve — *see Naproxen*						
Alexitol sodium	T47.1X1	T47.1X2	T47.1X3	T47.1X4	T47.1X5	T47.1X6
Alfacalcidol	T45.2X1	T45.2X2	T45.2X3	T45.2X4	T45.2X5	T45.2X6
Alfadolone	T41.1X1	T41.1X2	T41.1X3	T41.1X4	T41.1X5	T41.1X6
Alfaxalone	T41.1X1	T41.1X2	T41.1X3	T41.1X4	T41.1X5	T41.1X6
Alfentanil	T40.4X1	T40.4X2	T40.4X3	T40.4X4	T40.4X5	T40.4X6
Alfuzosin (hydrochloride)	T44.8X1	T44.8X2	T44.8X3	T44.8X4	T44.8X5	T44.8X6
Algae (harmful) (toxin)	T65.821	T65.822	T65.823	T65.824	—	—
Algeldrate	T47.1X1	T47.1X2	T47.1X3	T47.1X4	T47.1X5	T47.1X6
Algin	T47.8X1	T47.8X2	T47.8X3	T47.8X4	T47.8X5	T47.8X6
Alglucerase	T45.3X1	T45.3X2	T45.3X3	T45.3X4	T45.3X5	T45.3X6
Alidase	T45.3X1	T45.3X2	T45.3X3	T45.3X4	T45.3X5	T45.3X6
Alimemazine	T43.3X1	T43.3X2	T43.3X3	T43.3X4	T43.3X5	T43.3X6
Aliphatic thiocyanates	T65.0X1	T65.0X2	T65.0X3	T65.0X4	—	—
Alizapride	T45.0X1	T45.0X2	T45.0X3	T45.0X4	T45.0X5	T45.0X6
Alkali (caustic)	T54.3X1	T54.3X2	T54.3X3	T54.3X4	—	—
Alkalizing agent NEC	T50.901	T50.902	T50.903	T50.904	T50.905	T50.906
Alkaline antiseptic solution (aromatic)	T49.6X1	T49.6X2	T49.6X3	T49.6X4	T49.6X5	T49.6X6
Alkalinizing agents (medicinal)	T50.901	T50.902	T50.903	T50.904	T50.905	T50.906
Alka-seltzer	T39.011	T39.012	T39.013	T39.014	T39.015	T39.016
Alkavervir	T46.5X1	T46.5X2	T46.5X3	T46.5X4	T46.5X5	T46.5X6
Alkonium (bromide)	T49.0X1	T49.0X2	T49.0X3	T49.0X4	T49.0X5	T49.0X6
Alkylating drug NEC	T45.1X1	T45.1X2	T45.1X3	T45.1X4	T45.1X5	T45.1X6
antimyeloproliferative	T45.1X1	T45.1X2	T45.1X3	T45.1X4	T45.1X5	T45.1X6
lymphatic	T45.1X1	T45.1X2	T45.1X3	T45.1X4	T45.1X5	T45.1X6
Alkylisocyanate	T65.0X1	T65.0X2	T65.0X3	T65.0X4	—	—
Allantoin	T49.411	T49.412	T49.413	T49.414	T49.415	T49.416
Allegron	T43.0X1	T43.0X2	T43.0X3	T43.0X4	T43.0X5	T43.0X6
Allethrin	T49.0X1	T49.0X2	T49.0X3	T49.0X4	T49.0X5	T49.0X6
Allobarbital	T42.3X1	T42.3X2	T42.3X3	T42.3X4	T42.3X5	T42.3X6

◀ New ◀▪▪ Revised ~~deleted~~ Deleted

TABLE OF DRUGS AND CHEMICALS

Substance	External Cause (T-Code)					
	Poisoning, Accidental (Unintentional)	Poisoning, Intentional Self-Harm	Poisoning, Assault	Poisoning, Undetermined	Adverse Effect	Underdosing
Allopurinol	T50.4X1	T50.4X2	T50.4X3	T50.4X4	T50.4X5	T50.4X6
Allyl						
alcohol	T51.8X1	T51.8X2	T51.8X3	T51.8X4	—	—
disulfide	T46.6X1	T46.6X2	T46.6X3	T46.6X4	T46.6X5	T46.6X6
Allylestrenol	T38.5X1	T38.5X2	T38.5X3	T38.5X4	T38.5X5	T38.5X6
Allylisopropylacetylurea	T42.6X1	T42.6X2	T42.6X3	T42.6X4	T42.6X5	T42.6X6
Allylisopropylmalonylurea	T42.3X1	T42.3X2	T42.3X3	T42.3X4	T42.3X5	T42.3X6
Allylthiourea	T49.3X1	T49.3X2	T49.3X3	T49.3X4	T49.3X5	T49.3X6
Allyltribromide	T42.6X1	T42.6X2	T42.6X3	T42.6X4	T42.6X5	T42.6X6
Allypropymal	T42.3X1	T42.3X2	T42.3X3	T42.3X4	T42.3X5	T42.3X6
Almagate	T47.1X1	T47.1X2	T47.1X3	T47.1X4	T47.1X5	T47.1X6
Almasilate	T47.1X1	T47.1X2	T47.1X3	T47.1X4	T47.1X5	T47.1X6
Almitrine	T50.7X1	T50.7X2	T50.7X3	T50.7X4	T50.7X5	T50.7X6
Aloes	T47.2X1	T47.2X2	T47.2X3	T47.2X4	T47.2X5	T47.2X6
Aloglutamol	T47.1X1	T47.1X2	T47.1X3	T47.1X4	T47.1X5	T47.1X6
Aloin	T47.2X1	T47.2X2	T47.2X3	T47.2X4	T47.2X5	T47.2X6
Aloxidone	T42.2X1	T42.2X2	T42.2X3	T42.2X4	T42.2X5	T42.2X6
Alpha						
acetyldigoxin	T46.0X1	T46.0X2	T46.0X3	T46.0X4	T46.0X5	T46.0X6
adrenergic blocking drug	T44.6X1	T44.6X2	T44.6X3	T44.6X4	T44.6X5	T44.6X6
amylase	T45.3X1	T45.3X2	T45.3X3	T45.3X4	T45.3X5	T45.3X6
tocoferol (acetate)	T45.2X1	T45.2X2	T45.2X3	T45.2X4	T45.2X5	T45.2X6
tocopherol	T45.2X1	T45.2X2	T45.2X3	T45.2X4	T45.2X5	T45.2X6
Alphadolone	T41.1X1	T41.1X2	T41.1X3	T41.1X4	T41.1X5	T41.1X6
Alphaprodine	T40.4X1	T40.4X2	T40.4X3	T40.4X4	T40.4X5	T40.4X6
Alphaxalone	T41.1X1	T41.1X2	T41.1X3	T41.1X4	T41.1X5	T41.1X6
Alprazolam	T42.4X1	T42.4X2	T42.4X3	T42.4X4	T42.4X5	T42.4X6
Alprenolol	T44.7X1	T44.7X2	T44.7X3	T44.7X4	T44.7X5	T44.7X6
Alprostadil	T46.7X1	T46.7X2	T46.7X3	T46.7X4	T46.7X5	T46.7X6
Alsactide	T38.811	T38.812	T38.813	T38.814	T38.815	T38.816
Alseroxylon	T46.5X1	T46.5X2	T46.5X3	T46.5X4	T46.5X5	T46.5X6
Alteplase	T45.611	T45.612	T45.613	T45.614	T45.615	T45.616
Altizide	T50.2X1	T50.2X2	T50.2X3	T50.2X4	T50.2X5	T50.2X6
Altretamine	T45.1X1	T45.1X2	T45.1X3	T45.1X4	T45.1X5	T45.1X6
Alum (medicinal)	T49.4X1	T49.4X2	T49.4X3	T49.4X4	T49.4X5	T49.4X6
nonmedicinal (ammonium) (potassium)	T56.891	T56.892	T56.893	T56.894	—	—
Aluminium, aluminum						
acetate	T49.2X1	T49.2X2	T49.2X3	T49.2X4	T49.2X5	T49.2X6
solution	T49.0X1	T49.0X2	T49.0X3	T49.0X4	T49.0X5	T49.0X6
aspirin	T39.011	T39.012	T39.013	T39.014	T39.015	T39.016
bis (acetylsalicylate)	T39.011	T39.012	T39.013	T39.014	T39.015	T39.016

Substance	External Cause (T-Code)					
	Poisoning, Accidental (Unintentional)	Poisoning, Intentional Self-Harm	Poisoning, Assault	Poisoning, Undetermined	Adverse Effect	Underdosing
Aluminium, aluminum *(Continued)*						
carbonate (gel, basic)	T47.1X1	T47.1X2	T47.1X3	T47.1X4	T47.1X5	T47.1X6
chlorhydroxide-complex	T47.1X1	T47.1X2	T47.1X3	T47.1X4	T47.1X5	T47.1X6
chloride	T49.2X1	T49.2X2	T49.2X3	T49.2X4	T49.2X5	T49.2X6
clofibrate	T46.6X1	T46.6X2	T46.6X3	T46.6X4	T46.6X5	T46.6X6
diacetate	T49.2X1	T49.2X2	T49.2X3	T49.2X4	T49.2X5	T49.2X6
glycinate	T47.1X1	T47.1X2	T47.1X3	T47.1X4	T47.1X5	T47.1X6
hydroxide (gel)	T47.1X1	T47.1X2	T47.1X3	T47.1X4	T47.1X5	T47.1X6
hydroxide-magnesium carb. gel	T47.1X1	T47.1X2	T47.1X3	T47.1X4	T47.1X5	T47.1X6
magnesium silicate	T47.1X1	T47.1X2	T47.1X3	T47.1X4	T47.1X5	T47.1X6
nicotinate	T46.7X1	T46.7X2	T46.7X3	T46.7X4	T46.7X5	T46.7X6
ointment (surgical) (topical)	T49.3X1	T49.3X2	T49.3X3	T49.3X4	T49.3X5	T49.3X6
phosphate	T47.1X1	T47.1X2	T47.1X3	T47.1X4	T47.1X5	T47.1X6
salicylate	T39.091	T39.092	T39.093	T39.094	T39.095	T39.096
silicate	T47.1X1	T47.1X2	T47.1X3	T47.1X4	T47.1X5	T47.1X6
sodium silicate	T47.1X1	T47.1X2	T47.1X3	T47.1X4	T47.1X5	T47.1X6
subacetate	T49.2X1	T49.2X2	T49.2X3	T49.2X4	T49.2X5	T49.2X6
sulfate	T49.0X1	T49.0X2	T49.0X3	T49.0X4	T49.0X5	T49.0X6
tannate	T47.6X1	T47.6X2	T47.6X3	T47.6X4	T47.6X5	T47.6X6
topical NEC	T49.3X1	T49.3X2	T49.3X3	T49.3X4	T49.3X5	T49.3X6
Alurate	T42.3X1	T42.3X2	T42.3X3	T42.3X4	T42.3X5	T42.3X6
Alverine	T44.3X1	T44.3X2	T44.3X3	T44.3X4	T44.3X5	T44.3X6
Alvodine	T40.2X1	T40.2X2	T40.2X3	T40.2X4	T40.2X5	T40.2X6
Amanita phalloides	T62.0X1	T62.0X2	T62.0X3	T62.0X4	—	—
Amanitine	T62.0X1	T62.0X2	T62.0X3	T62.0X4	—	—
Amantadine	T42.8X1	T42.8X2	T42.8X3	T42.8X4	T42.8X5	T42.8X6
Ambazone	T49.6X1	T49.6X2	T49.6X3	T49.6X4	T49.6X5	T49.6X6
Ambenonium (chloride)	T44.0X1	T44.0X2	T44.0X3	T44.0X4	T44.0X5	T44.0X6
Ambroxol	T48.4X1	T48.4X2	T48.4X3	T48.4X4	T48.4X5	T48.4X6
Ambuphylline	T48.6X1	T48.6X2	T48.6X3	T48.6X4	T48.6X5	T48.6X6
Ambutonium bromide	T44.3X1	T44.3X2	T44.3X3	T44.3X4	T44.3X5	T44.3X6
Amcinonide	T49.0X1	T49.0X2	T49.0X3	T49.0X4	T49.0X5	T49.0X6
Amdinocilline	T36.0X1	T36.0X2	T36.0X3	T36.0X4	T36.0X5	T36.0X6
Ametazole	T50.8X1	T50.8X2	T50.8X3	T50.8X4	T50.8X5	T50.8X6
Amethocaine	T41.3X1	T41.3X2	T41.3X3	T41.3X4	T41.3X5	T41.3X6
regional	T41.3X1	T41.3X2	T41.3X3	T41.3X4	T41.3X5	T41.3X6
spinal	T41.3X1	T41.3X2	T41.3X3	T41.3X4	T41.3X5	T41.3X6
Amethopterin	T45.1X1	T45.1X2	T45.1X3	T45.1X4	T45.1X5	T45.1X6
Amezinium metilsulfate	T44.991	T44.992	T44.993	T44.994	T44.995	T44.996
Amfebutamone	T43.291	T43.292	T43.293	T43.294	T43.295	T43.296
Amfepramone	T50.5X1	T50.5X2	T50.5X3	T50.5X4	T50.5X5	T50.5X6

◄ New ⬅ Revised ~~deleted~~ Deleted

Substance	External Cause (T-Code) Poisoning, Accidental (Unintentional)	Poisoning, Intentional Self-Harm	Poisoning, Assault	Poisoning, Undetermined	Adverse Effect	Underdosing
Amfetamine	T43.621	T43.622	T43.623	T43.624	T43.625	T43.626
Amfetaminil	T43.621	T43.622	T43.623	T43.624	T43.625	T43.626
Amfomycin	T36.8X1	T36.8X2	T36.8X3	T36.8X4	T36.8X5	T36.8X6
Amidefrine mesilate	T48.5X1	T48.5X2	T48.5X3	T48.5X4	T48.5X5	T48.5X6
Amidone	T40.3X1	T40.3X2	T40.3X3	T40.3X4	T40.3X5	T40.3X6
Amidopyrine	T39.2X1	T39.2X2	T39.2X3	T39.2X4	T39.2X5	T39.2X6
Amidotrizoate	T50.8X1	T50.8X2	T50.8X3	T50.8X4	T50.8X5	T50.8X6
Amiflamine	T43.1X1	T43.1X2	T43.1X3	T43.1X4	T43.1X5	T43.1X6
Amikacin	T36.5X1	T36.5X2	T36.5X3	T36.5X4	T36.5X5	T36.5X6
Amikhelline	T46.3X1	T46.3X2	T46.3X3	T46.3X4	T46.3X5	T46.3X6
Amiloride	T50.2X1	T50.2X2	T50.2X3	T50.2X4	T50.2X5	T50.2X6
Aminacrine	T49.0X1	T49.0X2	T49.0X3	T49.0X4	T49.0X5	T49.0X6
Amineptine	T43.011	T43.012	T43.013	T43.014	T43.015	T43.016
Aminitrozole	T37.3X1	T37.3X2	T37.3X3	T37.3X4	T37.3X5	T37.3X6
Aminoacetic acid (derivatives)	T50.3X1	T50.3X2	T50.3X3	T50.3X4	T50.3X5	T50.3X6
Amino acids	T50.3X1	T50.3X2	T50.3X3	T50.3X4	T50.3X5	T50.3X6
Aminoacridine	T49.0X1	T49.0X2	T49.0X3	T49.0X4	T49.0X5	T49.0X6
Aminobenzoic acid (-p)	T49.3X1	T49.3X2	T49.3X3	T49.3X4	T49.3X5	T49.3X6
4-Aminobutyric acid	T43.8X1	T43.8X2	T43.8X3	T43.8X4	T43.8X5	T43.8X6
Aminocaproic acid	T45.621	T45.622	T45.623	T45.624	T45.625	T45.626
Aminofenazone	T39.2X1	T39.2X2	T39.2X3	T39.2X4	T39.2X5	T39.2X6
Aminoethylisothiourium	T45.8X1	T45.8X2	T45.8X3	T45.8X4	T45.8X5	T45.8X6
Aminoglutethimide	T45.1X1	T45.1X2	T45.1X3	T45.1X4	T45.1X5	T45.1X6
Aminohippuric acid	T50.8X1	T50.8X2	T50.8X3	T50.8X4	T50.8X5	T50.8X6
Aminomethylbenzoic acid	T45.691	T45.692	T45.693	T45.694	T45.695	T45.696
Aminometradine	T50.2X1	T50.2X2	T50.2X3	T50.2X4	T50.2X5	T50.2X6
Aminopentamide	T44.3X1	T44.3X2	T44.3X3	T44.3X4	T44.3X5	T44.3X6
Aminophenazone	T39.2X1	T39.2X2	T39.2X3	T39.2X4	T39.2X5	T39.2X6
Aminophenol	T54.0X1	T54.0X2	T54.0X3	T54.0X4	—	—
4-Aminophenol derivatives	T39.1X1	T39.1X2	T39.1X3	T39.1X4	T39.1X5	T39.1X6
Aminophenylpyridone	T43.591	T43.592	T43.593	T43.594	T43.595	T43.596
Aminophylline	T48.6X1	T48.6X2	T48.6X3	T48.6X4	T48.6X5	T48.6X6
Aminopterin sodium	T45.1X1	T45.1X2	T45.1X3	T45.1X4	T45.1X5	T45.1X6
Aminopyrine	T39.2X1	T39.2X2	T39.2X3	T39.2X4	T39.2X5	T39.2X6
8-Aminoquinoline drugs	T37.2X1	T37.2X2	T37.2X3	T37.2X4	T37.2X5	T37.2X6
Aminorex	T50.5X1	T50.5X2	T50.5X3	T50.5X4	T50.5X5	T50.5X6
Aminosalicylic acid	T37.1X1	T37.1X2	T37.1X3	T37.1X4	T37.1X5	T37.1X6
Aminosalylum	T37.1X1	T37.1X2	T37.1X3	T37.1X4	T37.1X5	T37.1X6
Amiodarone	T46.2X1	T46.2X2	T46.2X3	T46.2X4	T46.2X5	T46.2X6
Amiphenazole	T50.7X1	T50.7X2	T50.7X3	T50.7X4	T50.7X5	T50.7X6
Amiquinsin	T46.5X1	T46.5X2	T46.5X3	T46.5X4	T46.5X5	T46.5X6
Amisometradine	T50.2X1	T50.2X2	T50.2X3	T50.2X4	T50.2X5	T50.2X6

Substance	External Cause (T-Code) Poisoning, Accidental (Unintentional)	Poisoning, Intentional Self-Harm	Poisoning, Assault	Poisoning, Undetermined	Adverse Effect	Underdosing
Amisulpride	T43.591	T43.592	T43.593	T43.594	T43.595	T43.596
Amitriptyline	T43.021	T43.022	T43.023	T43.024	T43.025	T43.026
Amitriptylinoxide	T43.021	T43.022	T43.023	T43.024	T43.025	T43.026
Amlexanox	T48.6X1	T48.6X2	T48.6X3	T48.6X4	T48.6X5	T48.6X6
Ammonia (fumes) (gas) (vapor)	T59.891	T59.892	T59.893	T59.894	—	—
aromatic spirit	T48.991	T48.992	T48.993	T48.994	T48.995	T48.996
liquid (household)	T54.3X1	T54.3X2	T54.3X3	T54.3X4		
Ammoniated mercury	T49.0X1	T49.0X2	T49.0X3	T49.0X4	T49.0X5	T49.0X6
Ammonium						
acid tartrate	T49.5X1	T49.5X2	T49.5X3	T49.5X4	T49.5X5	T49.5X6
bromide	T42.6X1	T42.6X2	T42.6X3	T42.6X4	T42.6X5	T42.6X6
carbonate	T54.3X1	T54.3X2	T54.3X3	T54.3X4	—	—
chloride	T50.991	T50.992	T50.993	T50.994	T50.995	T50.996
expectorant	T48.4X1	T48.4X2	T48.4X3	T48.4X4	T48.4X5	T48.4X6
compounds (household) NEC	T54.3X1	T54.3X2	T54.3X3	T54.3X4	—	—
fumes (any usage)	T59.891	T59.892	T59.893	T59.894	—	—
industrial	T54.3X1	T54.3X2	T54.3X3	T54.3X4	—	—
ichthyosulronate	T49.4X1	T49.4X2	T49.4X3	T49.4X4	T49.4X5	T49.4X6
mandelate	T37.91	T37.92	T37.93	T37.94	T37.95	T37.96
sulfamate	T60.3X1	T60.3X2	T60.3X3	T60.3X4	—	—
sulfonate resin	T47.8X1	T47.8X2	T47.8X3	T47.8X4	T47.8X5	T47.8X6
Amobarbital (sodium)	T42.3X1	T42.3X2	T42.3X3	T42.3X4	T42.3X5	T42.3X6
Amodiaquine	T37.2X1	T37.2X2	T37.2X3	T37.2X4	T37.2X5	T37.2X6
Amopyroquin(e)	T37.2X1	T37.2X2	T37.2X3	T37.2X4	T37.2X5	T37.2X6
Amoxapine	T43.011	T43.012	T43.013	T43.014	T43.015	T43.016
Amoxicillin	T36.0X1	T36.0X2	T36.0X3	T36.0X4	T36.0X5	T36.0X6
Amperozide	T43.591	T43.592	T43.593	T43.594	T43.595	T43.596
Amphenidone	T43.591	T43.592	T43.593	T43.594	T43.595	T43.596
Amphetamine NEC	T43.621	T43.622	T43.623	T43.624	T43.625	T43.626
Amphomycin	T36.8X1	T36.8X2	T36.8X3	T36.8X4	T36.8X5	T36.8X6
Amphotalide	T37.4X1	T37.4X2	T37.4X3	T37.4X4	T37.4X5	T37.4X6
Amphotericin B	T36.7X1	T36.7X2	T36.7X3	T36.7X4	T36.7X5	T36.7X6
topical	T49.0X1	T49.0X2	T49.0X3	T49.0X4	T49.0X5	T49.0X6
Ampicillin	T36.0X1	T36.0X2	T36.0X3	T36.0X4	T36.0X5	T36.0X6
Amprotropine	T44.3X1	T44.3X2	T44.3X3	T44.3X4	T44.3X5	T44.3X6
Amsacrine	T45.1X1	T45.1X2	T45.1X3	T45.1X4	T45.1X5	T45.1X6
Amygdaline	T62.2X1	T62.2X2	T62.2X3	T62.2X4	—	—
Amyl						
acetate	T52.8X1	T52.8X2	T52.8X3	T52.8X4	—	—
vapor	T59.891	T59.892	T59.893	T59.894	—	—
alcohol	T51.3X1	T51.3X2	T51.3X3	T51.3X4	—	—
chloride	T53.6X1	T53.6X2	T53.6X3	T53.6X4	—	—

◀ New ◀ Revised ~~deleted~~ Deleted

TABLE OF DRUGS AND CHEMICALS

Substance	External Cause (T-Code)					
	Poisoning, Accidental (Unintentional)	Poisoning, Intentional Self-Harm	Poisoning, Assault	Poisoning, Undetermined	Adverse Effect	Underdosing
Amyl *(Continued)*						
formate	T52.8X1	T52.8X2	T52.8X3	T52.8X4	—	—
nitrite	T46.3X1	T46.3X2	T46.3X3	T46.3X4	T46.3X5	T46.3X6
propionate	T65.891	T65.892	T65.893	T65.894	—	—
Amylase	T47.5X1	T47.5X2	T47.5X3	T47.5X4	T47.5X5	T47.5X6
Amyleine, regional	T41.3X1	T41.3X2	T41.3X3	T41.3X4	T41.3X5	T41.3X6
Amylene						
dichloride	T53.6X1	T53.6X2	T53.6X3	T53.6X4	—	—
hydrate	T51.3X1	T51.3X2	T51.3X3	T51.3X4	—	—
Amylmetacresol	T49.6X1	T49.6X2	T49.6X3	T49.6X4	T49.6X5	T49.6X6
Amylobarbitone	T42.3X1	T42.3X2	T42.3X3	T42.3X4	T42.3X5	T42.3X6
Amylocaine, regional	T41.3X1	T41.3X2	T41.3X3	T41.3X4	T41.3X5	T41.3X6
infiltration (subcutaneous)	T41.3X1	T41.3X2	T41.3X3	T41.3X4	T41.3X5	T41.3X6
nerve block (peripheral) (plexus)	T41.3X1	T41.3X2	T41.3X3	T41.3X4	T41.3X5	T41.3X6
spinal	T41.3X1	T41.3X2	T41.3X3	T41.3X4	T41.3X5	T41.3X6
topical (surface)	T41.3X1	T41.3X2	T41.3X3	T41.3X4	T41.3X5	T41.3X6
Amylopectin	T47.6X1	T47.6X2	T47.6X3	T47.6X4	T47.6X5	T47.6X6
Amytal (sodium)	T42.3X1	T42.3X2	T42.3X3	T42.3X4	T42.3X5	T42.3X6
Anabolic steroid	T38.7X1	T38.7X2	T38.7X3	T38.7X4	T38.7X5	T38.7X6
Analeptic NEC	T50.7X1	T50.7X2	T50.7X3	T50.7X4	T50.7X5	T50.7X6
Analgesic	T39.91	T39.92	T39.93	T39.94	T39.95	T39.96
anti-inflammatory NEC	T39.91	T39.92	T39.93	T39.94	T39.95	T39.96
propionic acid derivative	T39.311	T39.312	T39.313	T39.314	T39.315	T39.316
antirheumatic NEC	T39.4X1	T39.4X2	T39.4X3	T39.4X4	T39.4X5	T39.4X6
aromatic NEC	T39.1X1	T39.1X2	T39.1X3	T39.1X4	T39.1X5	T39.1X6
narcotic NEC	T40.601	T40.602	T40.603	T40.604	T40.605	T40.606
combination	T40.601	T40.602	T40.603	T40.604	T40.605	T40.606
obstetric	T40.601	T40.602	T40.603	T40.604	T40.605	T40.606
non-narcotic NEC	T39.91	T39.92	T39.93	T39.94	T39.95	T39.96
combination	T39.91	T39.92	T39.93	T39.94	T39.95	T39.96
pyrazole	T39.2X1	T39.2X2	T39.2X3	T39.2X4	T39.2X5	T39.2X6
specified NEC	T39.8X1	T39.8X2	T39.8X3	T39.8X4	T39.8X5	T39.8X6
Analgin	T39.2X1	T39.2X2	T39.2X3	T39.2X4	T39.2X5	T39.2X6
Anamirta cocculus	T62.1X1	T62.1X2	T62.1X3	T62.1X4	—	—
Ancillin	T36.0X1	T36.0X2	T36.0X3	T36.0X4	T36.0X5	T36.0X6
Ancrod	T45.691	T45.692	T45.693	T45.694	T45.695	T45.696
Androgen	T38.7X1	T38.7X2	T38.7X3	T38.7X4	T38.7X5	T38.7X6
Androgen-estrogen mixture	T38.7X1	T38.7X2	T38.7X3	T38.7X4	T38.7X5	T38.7X6
Androstalone	T38.7X1	T38.7X2	T38.7X3	T38.7X4	T38.7X5	T38.7X6
Androstanolone	T38.7X1	T38.7X2	T38.7X3	T38.7X4	T38.7X5	T38.7X6
Androsterone	T38.7X1	T38.7X2	T38.7X3	T38.7X4	T38.7X5	T38.7X6

Substance	External Cause (T-Code)					
	Poisoning, Accidental (Unintentional)	Poisoning, Intentional Self-Harm	Poisoning, Assault	Poisoning, Undetermined	Adverse Effect	Underdosing
Anemone pulsatilla	T62.2X1	T62.2X2	T62.2X3	T62.2X4	—	—
Anesthesia						
caudal	T41.3X1	T41.3X2	T41.3X3	T41.3X4	T41.3X5	T41.3X6
endotracheal	T41.0X1	T41.0X2	T41.0X3	T41.0X4	T41.0X5	T41.0X6
epidural	T41.3X1	T41.3X2	T41.3X3	T41.3X4	T41.3X5	T41.3X6
inhalation	T41.0X1	T41.0X2	T41.0X3	T41.0X4	T41.0X5	T41.0X6
local	T41.3X1	T41.3X2	T41.3X3	T41.3X4	T41.3X5	T41.3X6
mucosal	T41.3X1	T41.3X2	T41.3X3	T41.3X4	T41.3X5	T41.3X6
muscle relaxation	T48.1X1	T48.1X2	T48.1X3	T48.1X4	T48.1X5	T48.1X6
nerve blocking	T41.3X1	T41.3X2	T41.3X3	T41.3X4	T41.3X5	T41.3X6
plexus blocking	T41.3X1	T41.3X2	T41.3X3	T41.3X4	T41.3X5	T41.3X6
potentiated	T41.201	T41.202	T41.203	T41.204	T41.205	T41.206
rectal	T41.201	T41.202	T41.203	T41.204	T41.205	T41.206
general	T41.201	T41.202	T41.203	T41.204	T41.205	T41.206
local	T41.3X1	T41.3X2	T41.3X3	T41.3X4	T41.3X5	T41.3X6
regional	T41.3X1	T41.3X2	T41.3X3	T41.3X4	T41.3X5	T41.3X6
surface	T41.3X1	T41.3X2	T41.3X3	T41.3X4	T41.3X5	T41.3X6
Anesthetic NEC— *see also Anesthesia*	T41.41	T41.42	T41.43	T41.44	T41.45	T41.46
with muscle relaxant	T41.201	T41.202	T41.203	T41.204	T41.205	T41.206
general	T41.201	T41.202	T41.203	T41.204	T41.205	T41.206
local	T41.3X1	T41.3X2	T41.3X3	T41.3X4	T41.3X5	T41.3X6
gaseous NEC	T41.0X1	T41.0X2	T41.0X3	T41.0X4	T41.0X5	T41.0X6
general NEC	T41.201	T41.202	T41.203	T41.204	T41.205	T41.206
halogenated hydrocarbon derivatives NEC	T41.0X1	T41.0X2	T41.0X3	T41.0X4	T41.0X5	T41.0X6
infiltration NEC	T41.3X1	T41.3X2	T41.3X3	T41.3X4	T41.3X5	T41.3X6
intravenous NEC	T41.1X1	T41.1X2	T41.1X3	T41.1X4	T41.1X5	T41.1X6
local NEC	T41.3X1	T41.3X2	T41.3X3	T41.3X4	T41.3X5	T41.3X6
rectal	T41.201	T41.202	T41.203	T41.204	T41.205	T41.206
general	T41.201	T41.202	T41.203	T41.204	T41.205	T41.206
local	T41.3X1	T41.3X2	T41.3X3	T41.3X4	T41.3X5	T41.3X6
regional NEC	T41.3X1	T41.3X2	T41.3X3	T41.3X4	T41.3X5	T41.3X6
spinal NEC	T41.3X1	T41.3X2	T41.3X3	T41.3X4	T41.3X5	T41.3X6
thiobarbiturate	T41.1X1	T41.1X2	T41.1X3	T41.1X4	T41.1X5	T41.1X6
topical	T41.3X1	T41.3X2	T41.3X3	T41.3X4	T41.3X5	T41.3X6
Aneurine	T45.2X1	T45.2X2	T45.2X3	T45.2X4	T45.2X5	T45.2X6
Angio-Conray	T50.8X1	T50.8X2	T50.8X3	T50.8X4	T50.8X5	T50.8X6
Angiotensin	T44.5X1	T44.5X2	T44.5X3	T44.5X4	T44.5X5	T44.5X6
Angiotensinamide	T44.991	T44.992	T44.993	T44.994	T44.995	T44.996
Anhydrohydroxy-progesterone	T38.5X1	T38.5X2	T38.5X3	T38.5X4	T38.5X5	T38.5X6
Anhydron	T50.2X1	T50.2X2	T50.2X3	T50.2X4	T50.2X5	T50.2X6
Anileridine	T40.4X1	T40.4X2	T40.4X3	T40.4X4	T40.4X5	T40.4X6

◀ New ◀━ Revised ~~deleted~~ Deleted

Substance	External Cause (T-Code) Poisoning, Accidental (Unintentional)	Poisoning, Intentional Self-Harm	Poisoning, Assault	Poisoning, Undetermined	Adverse Effect	Underdosing
Aniline (dye) (liquid)	T65.3X1	T65.3X2	T65.3X3	T65.3X4	—	—
analgesic	T39.1X1	T39.1X2	T39.1X3	T39.1X4	T39.1X5	T39.1X6
derivatives, therapeutic NEC	T39.1X1	T39.1X2	T39.1X3	T39.1X4	T39.1X5	T39.1X6
vapor	T65.3X1	T65.3X2	T65.3X3	T65.3X4	—	—
Anise oil	T47.5X1	T47.5X2	T47.5X3	T47.5X4	T47.5X5	T47.5X6
Aniscoropine	T44.3X1	T44.3X2	T44.3X3	T44.3X4	T44.3X5	T44.3X6
Anisidine	T65.3X1	T65.3X2	T65.3X3	T65.3X4	—	—
Anisindione	T45.511	T45.512	T45.513	T45.514	T45.515	T45.516
Anisotropine methyl-bromide	T44.3X1	T44.3X2	T44.3X3	T44.3X4	T44.3X5	T44.3X6
Anistreplase	T45.611	T45.612	T45.613	T45.614	T45.615	T45.616
Anorexiant (central)	T50.5X1	T50.5X2	T50.5X3	T50.5X4	T50.5X5	T50.5X6
Anorexic agents	T50.5X1	T50.5X2	T50.5X3	T50.5X4	T50.5X5	T50.5X6
Ansamycin	T36.6X1	T36.6X2	T36.6X3	T36.6X4	T36.6X5	T36.6X6
Ant (bite) (sting)	T63.421	T63.422	T63.423	T63.424	—	—
Antabuse	T50.6X1	T50.6X2	T50.6X3	T50.6X4	T50.6X5	T50.6X6
Ant poison — see Insecticide						
Antacid NEC	T47.1X1	T47.1X2	T47.1X3	T47.1X4	T47.1X5	T47.1X6
Antagonist						
Aldosterone	T50.0X1	T50.0X2	T50.0X3	T50.0X4	T50.0X5	T50.0X6
alpha-adrenoreceptor	T44.6X1	T44.6X2	T44.6X3	T44.6X4	T44.6X5	T44.6X6
anticoagulant	T45.7X1	T45.7X2	T45.7X3	T45.7X4	T45.7X5	T45.7X6
beta-adrenoreceptor	T44.7X1	T44.7X2	T44.7X3	T44.7X4	T44.7X5	T44.7X6
extrapyramidal NEC	T44.3X1	T44.3X2	T44.3X3	T44.3X4	T44.3X5	T44.3X6
folic acid	T45.1X1	T45.1X2	T45.1X3	T45.1X4	T45.1X5	T45.1X6
H2 receptor	T47.0X1	T47.0X2	T47.0X3	T47.0X4	T47.0X5	T47.0X6
heavy metal	T45.8X1	T45.8X2	T45.8X3	T45.8X4	T45.8X5	T45.8X6
narcotic analgesic	T50.7X1	T50.7X2	T50.7X3	T50.7X4	T50.7X5	T50.7X6
opiate	T50.7X1	T50.7X2	T50.7X3	T50.7X4	T50.7X5	T50.7X6
pyrimidine	T45.1X1	T45.1X2	T45.1X3	T45.1X4	T45.1X5	T45.1X6
serotonin	T46.5X1	T46.5X2	T46.5X3	T46.5X4	T46.5X5	T46.5X6
Antazolin(e)	T45.0X1	T45.0X2	T45.0X3	T45.0X4	T45.0X5	T45.0X6
Anterior pituitary hormone NEC	T38.811	T38.812	T38.813	T38.814	T38.815	T38.816
Anthelmintic NEC	T37.4X1	T37.4X2	T37.4X3	T37.4X4	T37.4X5	T37.4X6
Anthiolimine	T37.4X1	T37.4X2	T37.4X3	T37.4X4	T37.4X5	T37.4X6
Anthralin	T49.4X1	T49.4X2	T49.4X3	T49.4X4	T49.4X5	T49.4X6
Anthramycin	T45.1X1	T45.1X2	T45.1X3	T45.1X4	T45.1X5	T45.1X6
Antiadrenergic NEC	T44.8X1	T44.8X2	T44.8X3	T44.8X4	T44.8X5	T44.8X6
Antiallergic NEC	T45.0X1	T45.0X2	T45.0X3	T45.0X4	T45.0X5	T45.0X6
Anti-anemic (drug) (preparation)	T45.8X1	T45.8X2	T45.8X3	T45.8X4	T45.8X5	T45.8X6
Antiandrogen NEC	T38.6X1	T38.6X2	T38.6X3	T38.6X4	T38.6X5	T38.6X6
Antianxiety drug NEC	T43.501	T43.502	T43.503	T43.504	T43.505	T43.506
Antiaris toxicaria	T65.891	T65.892	T65.893	T65.894	—	—

Substance	External Cause (T-Code) Poisoning, Accidental (Unintentional)	Poisoning, Intentional Self-Harm	Poisoning, Assault	Poisoning, Undetermined	Adverse Effect	Underdosing
Antiarteriosclerotic drug	T46.6X1	T46.6X2	T46.6X3	T46.6X4	T46.6X5	T46.6X6
Antiasthmatic drug NEC	T48.6X1	T48.6X2	T48.6X3	T48.6X4	T48.6X5	T48.6X6
Antibiotic NEC	T36.91	T36.92	T36.93	T36.94	T36.95	T36.96
aminoglycoside	T36.5X1	T36.5X2	T36.5X3	T36.5X4	T36.5X5	T36.5X6
anticancer	T45.1X1	T45.1X2	T45.1X3	T45.1X4	T45.1X5	T45.1X6
antifungal	T36.7X1	T36.7X2	T36.7X3	T36.7X4	T36.7X5	T36.7X6
antimycobacterial	T36.5X1	T36.5X2	T36.5X3	T36.5X4	T36.5X5	T36.5X6
antineoplastic	T45.1X1	T45.1X2	T45.1X3	T45.1X4	T45.1X5	T45.1X6
cephalosporin (group)	T36.1X1	T36.1X2	T36.1X3	T36.1X4	T36.1X5	T36.1X6
chloramphenicol (group)	T36.2X1	T36.2X2	T36.2X3	T36.2X4	T36.2X5	T36.2X6
ENT	T49.6X1	T49.6X2	T49.6X3	T49.6X4	T49.6X5	T49.6X6
eye	T49.5X1	T49.5X2	T49.5X3	T49.5X4	T49.5X5	T49.5X6
fungicidal (local)	T49.0X1	T49.0X2	T49.0X3	T49.0X4	T49.0X5	T49.0X6
intestinal	T36.8X1	T36.8X2	T36.8X3	T36.8X4	T36.8X5	T36.8X6
b-lactam NEC	T36.1X1	T36.1X2	T36.1X3	T36.1X4	T36.1X5	T36.1X6
local	T49.0X1	T49.0X2	T49.0X3	T49.0X4	T49.0X5	T49.0X6
macrolides	T36.3X1	T36.3X2	T36.3X3	T36.3X4	T36.3X5	T36.3X6
polypeptide	T36.8X1	T36.8X2	T36.8X3	T36.8X4	T36.8X5	T36.8X6
specified NEC	T36.8X1	T36.8X2	T36.8X3	T36.8X4	T36.8X5	T36.8X6
tetracycline (group)	T36.4X1	T36.4X2	T36.4X3	T36.4X4	T36.4X5	T36.4X6
throat	T49.6X1	T49.6X2	T49.6X3	T49.6X4	T49.6X5	T49.6X6
Anticancer agents NEC	T45.1X1	T45.1X2	T45.1X3	T45.1X4	T45.1X5	T45.1X6
Anticholesterolemic drug NEC	T46.6X1	T46.6X2	T46.6X3	T46.6X4	T46.6X5	T46.6X6
Anticholinergic NEC	T44.3X1	T44.3X2	T44.3X3	T44.3X4	T44.3X5	T44.3X6
Anticholinesterase	T44.0X1	T44.0X2	T44.0X3	T44.0X4	T44.0X5	T44.0X6
organophosphorus	T44.0X1	T44.0X2	T44.0X3	T44.0X4	T44.0X5	T44.0X6
insecticide	T60.0X1	T60.0X2	T60.0X3	T60.0X4	—	—
nerve gas	T59.891	T59.892	T59.893	T59.894	—	—
reversible	T44.0X1	T44.0X2	T44.0X3	T44.0X4	T44.0X5	T44.0X6
ophthalmological	T49.5X1	T49.5X2	T49.5X3	T49.5X4	T49.5X5	T49.5X6
Anticoagulant NEC	T45.511	T45.512	T45.513	T45.514	T45.515	T45.516
Antagonist	T45.7X1	T45.7X2	T45.7X3	T45.7X4	T45.7X5	T45.7X6
Anti-common-cold drug NEC	T48.5X1	T48.5X2	T48.5X3	T48.5X4	T48.5X5	T48.5X6
Anticonvulsant	T42.71	T42.72	T42.73	T42.74	T42.75	T42.76
barbiturate	T42.3X1	T42.3X2	T42.3X3	T42.3X4	T42.3X5	T42.3X6
combination (with barbiturate)	T42.3X1	T42.3X2	T42.3X3	T42.3X4	T42.3X5	T42.3X6
hydantoin	T42.0X1	T42.0X2	T42.0X3	T42.0X4	T42.0X5	T42.0X6
hypnotic NEC	T42.6X1	T42.6X2	T42.6X3	T42.6X4	T42.6X5	T42.6X6
oxazolidinedione	T42.2X1	T42.2X2	T42.2X3	T42.2X4	T42.2X5	T42.2X6
pyrimidinedione	T42.6X1	T42.6X2	T42.6X3	T42.6X4	T42.6X5	T42.6X6
specified NEC	T42.6X1	T42.6X2	T42.6X3	T42.6X4	T42.6X5	T42.6X6
succinimide	T42.2X1	T42.2X2	T42.2X3	T42.2X4	T42.2X5	T42.2X6

Substance	Poisoning, Accidental (Unintentional)	Poisoning, Intentional Self-Harm	Poisoning, Assault	Poisoning, Undetermined	Adverse Effect	Underdosing
Anti-D immunoglobulin (human)	T50.Z11	T50.Z12	T50.Z13	T50.Z14	T50.Z15	T50.Z16
Antidepressant NEC	T43.201	T43.202	T43.203	T43.204	T43.205	T43.206
monoamine oxidase inhibitor	T43.1X1	T43.1X2	T43.1X3	T43.1X4	T43.1X5	T43.1X6
selective serotonin norepinephrine reuptake inhibitor	T43.211	T43.212	T43.213	T43.214	T43.215	T43.216
selective serotonin reuptake inhibitor	T43.221	T43.222	T43.223	T43.224	T43.225	T43.226
specified NEC	T43.291	T43.292	T43.293	T43.294	T43.295	T43.296
tetracyclic	T43.021	T43.022	T43.023	T43.024	T43.025	T43.026
triazolopyridine	T43.221	T43.222	T43.223	T43.224	T43.225	T43.226
tricyclic	T43.011	T43.012	T43.013	T43.014	T43.015	T43.016
Antidiabetic NEC	T38.3X1	T38.3X2	T38.3X3	T38.3X4	T38.3X5	T38.3X6
biguanide	T38.3X1	T38.3X2	T38.3X3	T38.3X4	T38.3X5	T38.3X6
and sulfonyl combined	T38.3X1	T38.3X2	T38.3X3	T38.3X4	T38.3X5	T38.3X6
combined	T38.3X1	T38.3X2	T38.3X3	T38.3X4	T38.3X5	T38.3X6
sulfonylurea	T38.3X1	T38.3X2	T38.3X3	T38.3X4	T38.3X5	T38.3X6
Antidiarrheal drug NEC	T47.6X1	T47.6X2	T47.6X3	T47.6X4	T47.6X5	T47.6X6
absorbent	T47.6X1	T47.6X2	T47.6X3	T47.6X4	T47.6X5	T47.6X6
Antidiphtheria serum	T50.Z11	T50.Z12	T50.Z13	T50.Z14	T50.Z15	T50.Z16
Antidiuretic hormone	T38.891	T38.892	T38.893	T38.894	T38.895	T38.896
Antidote NEC	T50.6X1	T50.6X2	T50.6X3	T50.6X4	T50.6X5	T50.6X6
heavy metal	T45.8X1	T45.8X2	T45.8X3	T45.8X4	T45.8X5	T45.8X6
Antidysrhythmic NEC	T46.2X1	T46.2X2	T46.2X3	T46.2X4	T46.2X5	T46.2X6
Antiemetic drug	T45.0X1	T45.0X2	T45.0X3	T45.0X4	T45.0X5	T45.0X6
Antiepilepsy agent	T42.71	T42.72	T42.73	T42.74	T42.75	T42.76
combination	T42.5X1	T42.5X2	T42.5X3	T42.5X4	T42.5X5	T42.5X6
mixed	T42.5X1	T42.5X2	T42.5X3	T42.5X4	T42.5X5	T42.5X6
specified, NEC	T42.6X1	T42.6X2	T42.6X3	T42.6X4	T42.6X5	T42.6X6
Antiestrogen NEC	T38.6X1	T38.6X2	T38.6X3	T38.6X4	T38.6X5	T38.6X6
Antifertility pill	T38.4X1	T38.4X2	T38.4X3	T38.4X4	T38.4X5	T38.4X6
Antifibrinolytic drug	T45.621	T45.622	T45.623	T45.624	T45.625	T45.626
Antifilarial drug	T37.4X1	T37.4X2	T37.4X3	T37.4X4	T37.4X5	T37.4X6
Antiflatulent	T47.5X1	T47.5X2	T47.5X3	T47.5X4	T47.5X5	T47.5X6
Antifreeze	T65.91	T65.92	T65.93	T65.94	—	—
alcohol	T51.1X1	T51.1X2	T51.1X3	T51.1X4	—	—
ethylene glycol	T51.8X1	T51.8X2	T51.8X3	T51.8X4	—	—
Antifungal						
antibiotic (systemic)	T36.7X1	T36.7X2	T36.7X3	T36.7X4	T36.7X5	T36.7X6
anti-infective NEC	T37.91	T37.92	T37.93	T37.94	T37.95	T37.96
disinfectant, local	T49.0X1	T49.0X2	T49.0X3	T49.0X4	T49.0X5	T49.0X6
nonmedicinal (spray)	T60.3X1	T60.3X2	T60.3X3	T60.3X4	—	—
topical	T49.0X1	T49.0X2	T49.0X3	T49.0X4	T49.0X5	T49.0X6

Substance	Poisoning, Accidental (Unintentional)	Poisoning, Intentional Self-Harm	Poisoning, Assault	Poisoning, Undetermined	Adverse Effect	Underdosing
Anti-gastric-secretion drug NEC	T47.1X1	T47.1X2	T47.1X3	T47.1X4	T47.1X5	T47.1X6
Antigonadotrophin NEC	T38.6X1	T38.6X2	T38.6X3	T38.6X4	T38.6X5	T38.6X6
Antihallucinogen	T43.501	T43.502	T43.503	T43.504	T43.505	T43.506
Antihelmintics	T37.4X1	T37.4X2	T37.4X3	T37.4X4	T37.4X5	T37.4X6
Antihemophilic						
factor	T45.8X1	T45.8X2	T45.8X3	T45.8X4	T45.8X5	T45.8X6
fraction	T45.8X1	T45.8X2	T45.8X3	T45.8X4	T45.8X5	T45.8X6
globulin concentrate	T45.7X1	T45.7X2	T45.7X3	T45.7X4	T45.7X5	T45.7X6
human plasma	T45.8X1	T45.8X2	T45.8X3	T45.8X4	T45.8X5	T45.8X6
plasma, dried	T45.7X1	T45.7X2	T45.7X3	T45.7X4	T45.7X5	T45.7X6
Antihemorrhoidal preparation	T49.2X1	T49.2X2	T49.2X3	T49.2X4	T49.2X5	T49.2X6
Antiheparin drug	T45.7X1	T45.7X2	T45.7X3	T45.7X4	T45.7X5	T45.7X6
Antihistamine	T45.0X1	T45.0X2	T45.0X3	T45.0X4	T45.0X5	T45.0X6
Antihookworm drug	T37.4X1	T37.4X2	T37.4X3	T37.4X4	T37.4X5	T37.4X6
Anti-human lymphocytic globulin	T50.Z11	T50.Z12	T50.Z13	T50.Z14	T50.Z15	T50.Z16
Antihyperlipidemic drug	T46.6X1	T46.6X2	T46.6X3	T46.6X4	T46.6X5	T46.6X6
Antihypertensive drug NEC	T46.5X1	T46.5X2	T46.5X3	T46.5X4	T46.5X5	T46.5X6
Anti-infective NEC	T37.91	T37.92	T37.93	T37.94	T37.95	T37.96
anthelmintic	T37.4X1	T37.4X2	T37.4X3	T37.4X4	T37.4X5	T37.4X6
antibiotics	T36.91	T36.92	T36.93	T36.94	T36.95	T36.96
specified NEC	T36.8X1	T36.8X2	T36.8X3	T36.8X4	T36.8X5	T36.8X6
antimalarial	T37.2X1	T37.2X2	T37.2X3	T37.2X4	T37.2X5	T37.2X6
antimycobacterial NEC	T37.1X1	T37.1X2	T37.1X3	T37.1X4	T37.1X5	T37.1X6
antibiotics	T36.5X1	T36.5X2	T36.5X3	T36.5X4	T36.5X5	T36.5X6
antiprotozoal NEC	T37.3X1	T37.3X2	T37.3X3	T37.3X4	T37.3X5	T37.3X6
blood	T37.2X1	T37.2X2	T37.2X3	T37.2X4	T37.2X5	T37.2X6
antiviral	T37.5X1	T37.5X2	T37.5X3	T37.5X4	T37.5X5	T37.5X6
arsenical	T37.8X1	T37.8X2	T37.8X3	T37.8X4	T37.8X5	T37.8X6
bismuth, local	T49.0X1	T49.0X2	T49.0X3	T49.0X4	T49.0X5	T49.0X6
ENT	T49.6X1	T49.6X2	T49.6X3	T49.6X4	T49.6X5	T49.6X6
eye NEC	T49.5X1	T49.5X2	T49.5X3	T49.5X4	T49.5X5	T49.5X6
heavy metals NEC	T37.8X1	T37.8X2	T37.8X3	T37.8X4	T37.8X5	T37.8X6
local NEC	T49.0X1	T49.0X2	T49.0X3	T49.0X4	T49.0X5	T49.0X6
specified NEC	T49.0X1	T49.0X2	T49.0X3	T49.0X4	T49.0X5	T49.0X6
mixed	T37.91	T37.92	T37.93	T37.94	T37.95	T37.96
ophthalmic preparation	T49.5X1	T49.5X2	T49.5X3	T49.5X4	T49.5X5	T49.5X6
topical NEC	T49.0X1	T49.0X2	T49.0X3	T49.0X4	T49.0X5	T49.0X6
Anti-inflammatory drug NEC	T49.0X1	T49.0X2	T49.0X3	T49.0X4	T49.0X5	T49.0X6
local	T49.0X1	T49.0X2	T49.0X3	T49.0X4	T49.0X5	T49.0X6
nonsteroidal NEC	T39.391	T39.392	T39.393	T39.394	T39.395	T39.396
propionic acid derivative	T39.311	T39.312	T39.313	T39.314	T39.315	T39.316
specified NEC	T39.391	T39.392	T39.393	T39.394	T39.395	T39.396

◀ New ◀━ Revised ~~deleted~~ Deleted

Substance	Poisoning, Accidental (Unintentional)	Poisoning, Intentional Self-Harm	Poisoning, Assault	Poisoning, Undetermined	Adverse Effect	Underdosing
Antikaluretic	T50.3X1	T50.3X2	T50.3X3	T50.3X4	T50.3X5	T50.3X6
Antiknock (tetraethyl lead)	T56.0X1	T56.0X2	T56.0X3	T56.0X4	—	—
Antilipemic drug NEC	T46.6X1	T46.6X2	T46.6X3	T46.6X4	T46.6X5	T46.6X6
Antimalarial	T37.2X1	T37.2X2	T37.2X3	T37.2X4	T37.2X5	T37.2X6
prophylactic NEC	T37.2X1	T37.2X2	T37.2X3	T37.2X4	T37.2X5	T37.2X6
pyrimidine derivative	T37.2X1	T37.2X2	T37.2X3	T37.2X4	T37.2X5	T37.2X6
Antimetabolite	T45.1X1	T45.1X2	T45.1X3	T45.1X4	T45.1X5	T45.1X6
Antimitotic agent	T45.1X1	T45.1X2	T45.1X3	T45.1X4	T45.1X5	T45.1X6
Antimony (compounds) (vapor) NEC	T56.891	T56.892	T56.893	T56.894	—	—
anti-infectives	T37.8X1	T37.8X2	T37.8X3	T37.8X4	T37.8X5	T37.8X6
dimercaptosuccinate	T37.3X1	T37.3X2	T37.3X3	T37.3X4	T37.3X5	T37.3X6
hydride	T56.891	T56.892	T56.893	T56.894	—	—
pesticide (vapor)	T60.8X1	T60.8X2	T60.8X3	T60.8X4	—	—
potassium (sodium) tartrate	T37.8X1	T37.8X2	T37.8X3	T37.8X4	T37.8X5	T37.8X6
sodium dimercaptosuccinate	T37.3X1	T37.3X2	T37.3X3	T37.3X4	T37.3X5	T37.3X6
tartrated	T37.8X1	T37.8X2	T37.8X3	T37.8X4	T37.8X5	T37.8X6
Antimuscarinic NEC	T44.3X1	T44.3X2	T44.3X3	T44.3X4	T44.3X5	T44.3X6
Antimycobacterial drug NEC	T37.1X1	T37.1X2	T37.1X3	T37.1X4	T37.1X5	T37.1X6
antibiotics	T36.5X1	T36.5X2	T36.5X3	T36.5X4	T36.5X5	T36.5X6
combination	T37.1X1	T37.1X2	T37.1X3	T37.1X4	T37.1X5	T37.1X6
Antinausea drug	T45.0X1	T45.0X2	T45.0X3	T45.0X4	T45.0X5	T45.0X6
Antinematode drug	T37.4X1	T37.4X2	T37.4X3	T37.4X4	T37.4X5	T37.4X6
Antineoplastic NEC	T45.1X1	T45.1X2	T45.1X3	T45.1X4	T45.1X5	T45.1X6
alkaloidal	T45.1X1	T45.1X2	T45.1X3	T45.1X4	T45.1X5	T45.1X6
antibiotics	T45.1X1	T45.1X2	T45.1X3	T45.1X4	T45.1X5	T45.1X6
combination	T45.1X1	T45.1X2	T45.1X3	T45.1X4	T45.1X5	T45.1X6
estrogen	T38.5X1	T38.5X2	T38.5X3	T38.5X4	T38.5X5	T38.5X6
steroid	T38.7X1	T38.7X2	T38.7X3	T38.7X4	T38.7X5	T38.7X6
Antiparasitic drug (systemic)	T37.91	T37.92	T37.93	T37.94	T37.95	T37.96
local	T49.0X1	T49.0X2	T49.0X3	T49.0X4	T49.0X5	T49.0X6
specified NEC	T37.8X1	T37.8X2	T37.8X3	T37.8X4	T37.8X5	T37.8X6
Antiparkinsonism drug NEC	T42.8X1	T42.8X2	T42.8X3	T42.8X4	T42.8X5	T42.8X6
Antiperspirant NEC	T49.2X1	T49.2X2	T49.2X3	T49.2X4	T49.2X5	T49.2X6
Antiphlogistic NEC	T39.4X1	T39.4X2	T39.4X3	T39.4X4	T39.4X5	T39.4X6
Antiplatyhelmintic drug	T37.4X1	T37.4X2	T37.4X3	T37.4X4	T37.4X5	T37.4X6
Antiprotozoal drug NEC	T37.3X1	T37.3X2	T37.3X3	T37.3X4	T37.3X5	T37.3X6
blood	T37.2X1	T37.2X2	T37.2X3	T37.2X4	T37.2X5	T37.2X6
local	T49.0X1	T49.0X2	T49.0X3	T49.0X4	T49.0X5	T49.0X6
Antipruritic drug NEC	T49.1X1	T49.1X2	T49.1X3	T49.1X4	T49.1X5	T49.1X6
Antipsychotic drug	T43.501	T43.502	T43.503	T43.504	T43.505	T43.506
specified NEC	T43.591	T43.592	T43.593	T43.594	T43.595	T43.596

Substance	Poisoning, Accidental (Unintentional)	Poisoning, Intentional Self-Harm	Poisoning, Assault	Poisoning, Undetermined	Adverse Effect	Underdosing
Antipyretic	T39.91	T39.92	T39.93	T39.94	T39.95	T39.96
specified NEC	T39.8X1	T39.8X2	T39.8X3	T39.8X4	T39.8X5	T39.8X6
Antipyrine	T39.2X1	T39.2X2	T39.2X3	T39.2X4	T39.2X5	T39.2X6
Antirabies hyperimmune serum	T50.Z11	T50.Z12	T50.Z13	T50.Z14	T50.Z15	T50.Z16
Antirheumatic NEC	T39.4X1	T39.4X2	T39.4X3	T39.4X4	T39.4X5	T39.4X6
Antirigidity drug NEC	T42.8X1	T42.8X2	T42.8X3	T42.8X4	T42.8X5	T42.8X6
Antischistosomal drug	T37.4X1	T37.4X2	T37.4X3	T37.4X4	T37.4X5	T37.4X6
Antiscorpion sera	T50.Z11	T50.Z12	T50.Z13	T50.Z14	T50.Z15	T50.Z16
Antiseborrheics	T49.4X1	T49.4X2	T49.4X3	T49.4X4	T49.4X5	T49.4X6
Antiseptics (external) (medicinal)	T49.0X1	T49.0X2	T49.0X3	T49.0X4	T49.0X5	T49.0X6
Antistine	T45.0X1	T45.0X2	T45.0X3	T45.0X4	T45.0X5	T45.0X6
Antitapeworm drug	T37.4X1	T37.4X2	T37.4X3	T37.4X4	T37.4X5	T37.4X6
Antitetanus immunoglobulin	T50.Z11	T50.Z12	T50.Z13	T50.Z14	T50.Z15	T50.Z16
Antithyroid drug NEC	T38.2X1	T38.2X2	T38.2X3	T38.2X4	T38.2X5	T38.2X6
Antitoxin	T50.Z11	T50.Z12	T50.Z13	T50.Z14	T50.Z15	T50.Z16
diphtheria	T50.Z11	T50.Z12	T50.Z13	T50.Z14	T50.Z15	T50.Z16
gas gangrene	T50.Z11	T50.Z12	T50.Z13	T50.Z14	T50.Z15	T50.Z16
tetanus	T50.Z11	T50.Z12	T50.Z13	T50.Z14	T50.Z15	T50.Z16
Antitoxin, any	T50.901	T50.902	T50.903	T50.904	T50.905	T50.906
Antitrichomonal drug	T37.3X1	T37.3X2	T37.3X3	T37.3X4	T37.3X5	T37.3X6
Antituberculars	T37.1X1	T37.1X2	T37.1X3	T37.1X4	T37.1X5	T37.1X6
antibiotics	T36.5X1	T36.5X2	T36.5X3	T36.5X4	T36.5X5	T36.5X6
Antitussive NEC	T48.3X1	T48.3X2	T48.3X3	T48.3X4	T48.3X5	T48.3X6
codeine mixture	T40.2X1	T40.2X2	T40.2X3	T40.2X4	T40.2X5	T40.2X6
opiate	T40.2X1	T40.2X2	T40.2X3	T40.2X4	T40.2X5	T40.2X6
Antivaricose drug	T46.8X1	T46.8X2	T46.8X3	T46.8X4	T46.8X5	T46.8X6
Antivenin, antivenom (sera)	T50.Z11	T50.Z12	T50.Z13	T50.Z14	T50.Z15	T50.Z16
crotaline	T50.Z11	T50.Z12	T50.Z13	T50.Z14	T50.Z15	T50.Z16
spider bite	T50.Z11	T50.Z12	T50.Z13	T50.Z14	T50.Z15	T50.Z16
Antivertigo drug	T45.0X1	T45.0X2	T45.0X3	T45.0X4	T45.0X5	T45.0X6
Antiviral drug NEC	T37.5X1	T37.5X2	T37.5X3	T37.5X4	T37.5X5	T37.5X6
eye	T49.5X1	T49.5X2	T49.5X3	T49.5X4	T49.5X5	T49.5X6
Antiwhipworm drug	T37.4X1	T37.4X2	T37.4X3	T37.4X4	T37.4X5	T37.4X6
Ant poisons—see Pesticides						
Antrol—see also by specific chemical substance	T60.91	T60.92	T60.93	T60.94	—	—
fungicide	T60.91	T60.92	T60.93	T60.94	—	—
ANTU (alpha naphthylthiourea)	T60.4X1	T60.4X2	T60.4X3	T60.4X4	—	—
Apalcillin	T36.0X1	T36.0X2	T36.0X3	T36.0X4	T36.0X5	T36.0X6
APC	T48.5X1	T48.5X2	T48.5X3	T48.5X4	T48.5X5	T48.5X6
Aplonidine	T44.4X1	T44.4X2	T44.4X3	T44.4X4	T44.4X5	T44.4X6
Apomorphine	T47.7X1	T47.7X2	T47.7X3	T47.7X4	T47.7X5	T47.7X6

◀ New ◀▬ Revised ~~deleted~~ Deleted

TABLE OF DRUGS AND CHEMICALS

Substance	External Cause (T-Code)					
	Poisoning, Accidental (Unintentional)	Poisoning, Intentional Self-Harm	Poisoning, Assault	Poisoning, Undetermined	Adverse Effect	Underdosing
Appetite depressants, central	T50.5X1	T50.5X2	T50.5X3	T50.5X4	T50.5X5	T50.5X6
Apraclonidine (hydrochloride)	T44.4X1	T44.4X2	T44.4X3	T44.4X4	T44.4X5	T44.4X6
Apresoline	T46.5X1	T46.5X2	T46.5X3	T46.5X4	T46.5X5	T46.5X6
Aprindine	T46.2X1	T46.2X2	T46.2X3	T46.2X4	T46.2X5	T46.2X6
Aprobarbital	T42.3X1	T42.3X2	T42.3X3	T42.3X4	T42.3X5	T42.3X6
Apronalide	T42.6X1	T42.6X2	T42.6X3	T42.6X4	T42.6X5	T42.6X6
Aprotinin	T45.621	T45.622	T45.623	T45.624	T45.625	T45.626
Aptocaine	T41.3X1	T41.3X2	T41.3X3	T41.3X4	T41.3X5	T41.3X6
Aqua fortis	T54.2X1	T54.2X2	T54.2X3	T54.2X4	—	—
Ara-A	T37.5X1	T37.5X2	T37.5X3	T37.5X4	T37.5X5	T37.5X6
Ara-C	T45.1X1	T45.1X2	T45.1X3	T45.1X4	T45.1X5	T45.1X6
Arachis oil	T49.3X1	T49.3X2	T49.3X3	T49.3X4	T49.3X5	T49.3X6
cathartic	T47.4X1	T47.4X2	T47.4X3	T47.4X4	T47.4X5	T47.4X6
Aralen	T37.2X1	T37.2X2	T37.2X3	T37.2X4	T37.2X5	T37.2X6
Arecoline	T44.1X1	T44.1X2	T44.1X3	T44.1X4	T44.1X5	T44.1X6
Arginine	T50.991	T50.992	T50.993	T50.994	T50.995	T50.996
glutamate	T50.991	T50.992	T50.993	T50.994	T50.995	T50.996
Argyrol	T49.0X1	T49.0X2	T49.0X3	T49.0X4	T49.0X5	T49.0X6
ENT agent	T49.6X1	T49.6X2	T49.6X3	T49.6X4	T49.6X5	T49.6X6
ophthalmic preparation	T49.5X1	T49.5X2	T49.5X3	T49.5X4	T49.5X5	T49.5X6
Aristocort	T38.0X1	T38.0X2	T38.0X3	T38.0X4	T38.0X5	T38.0X6
ENT agent	T49.6X1	T49.6X2	T49.6X3	T49.6X4	T49.6X5	T49.6X6
ophthalmic preparation	T49.5X1	T49.5X2	T49.5X3	T49.5X4	T49.5X5	T49.5X6
topical NEC	T49.0X1	T49.0X2	T49.0X3	T49.0X4	T49.0X5	T49.0X6
Aromatics, corrosive	T54.1X1	T54.1X2	T54.1X3	T54.1X4	—	—
disinfectants	T54.1X1	T54.1X2	T54.1X3	T54.1X4	—	—
Arsenate of lead	T57.0X1	T57.0X2	T57.0X3	T57.0X4	—	—
herbicide	T57.0X1	T57.0X2	T57.0X3	T57.0X4	—	—
Arsenic, arsenicals (compounds) (dust) (vapor) NEC	T57.0X1	T57.0X2	T57.0X3	T57.0X4	—	—
anti-infectives	T37.8X1	T37.8X2	T37.8X3	T37.8X4	T37.8X5	T37.8X6
pesticide (dust) (fumes)	T57.0X1	T57.0X2	T57.0X3	T57.0X4	—	—
Arsine (gas)	T57.0X1	T57.0X2	T57.0X3	T57.0X4	—	—
Arsphenamine (silver)	T37.8X1	T37.8X2	T37.8X3	T37.8X4	T37.8X5	T37.8X6
Arsthinol	T37.3X1	T37.3X2	T37.3X3	T37.3X4	T37.3X5	T37.3X6
Artane	T44.3X1	T44.3X2	T44.3X3	T44.3X4	T44.3X5	T44.3X6
Arthropod (venomous) NEC	T63.481	T63.482	T63.483	T63.484	—	—
Articaine	T41.3X1	T41.3X2	T41.3X3	T41.3X4	T41.3X5	T41.3X6
Asbestos	T57.8X1	T57.8X2	T57.8X3	T57.8X4	—	—
Ascaridole	T37.4X1	T37.4X2	T37.4X3	T37.4X4	T37.4X5	T37.4X6
Ascorbic acid	T45.2X1	T45.2X2	T45.2X3	T45.2X4	T45.2X5	T45.2X6
Asiaticoside	T49.0X1	T49.0X2	T49.0X3	T49.0X4	T49.0X5	T49.0X6
Asparaginase	T45.1X1	T45.1X2	T45.1X3	T45.1X4	T45.1X5	T45.1X6
Aspidium (oleoresin)	T37.4X1	T37.4X2	T37.4X3	T37.4X4	T37.4X5	T37.4X6
Aspirin (aluminum) (soluble)	T39.011	T39.012	T39.013	T39.014	T39.015	T39.016
Aspoxicillin	T36.0X1	T36.0X2	T36.0X3	T36.0X4	T36.0X5	T36.0X6
Astemizole	T45.0X1	T45.0X2	T45.0X3	T45.0X4	T45.0X5	T45.0X6
Astringent (local)	T49.2X1	T49.2X2	T49.2X3	T49.2X4	T49.2X5	T49.2X6
specified NEC	T49.2X1	T49.2X2	T49.2X3	T49.2X4	T49.2X5	T49.2X6
Astromicin	T36.5X1	T36.5X2	T36.5X3	T36.5X4	T36.5X5	T36.5X6
Ataractic drug NEC	T43.501	T43.502	T43.503	T43.504	T43.505	T43.506
Atenolol	T44.7X1	T44.7X2	T44.7X3	T44.7X4	T44.7X5	T44.7X6
Atonia drug, intestinal	T47.4X1	T47.4X2	T47.4X3	T47.4X4	T47.4X5	T47.4X6
Atophan	T50.4X1	T50.4X2	T50.4X3	T50.4X4	T50.4X5	T50.4X6
Atracurium besilate	T48.1X1	T48.1X2	T48.1X3	T48.1X4	T48.1X5	T48.1X6
Atropine	T44.3X1	T44.3X2	T44.3X3	T44.3X4	T44.3X5	T44.3X6
derivative	T44.3X1	T44.3X2	T44.3X3	T44.3X4	T44.3X5	T44.3X6
methonitrate	T44.3X1	T44.3X2	T44.3X3	T44.3X4	T44.3X5	T44.3X6
Attapulgite	T47.6X1	T47.6X2	T47.6X3	T47.6X4	T47.6X5	T47.6X6
Attenuvax	T50.991	T50.992	T50.993	T50.994	T50.995	T50.996
Auramine	T65.891	T65.892	T65.893	T65.894	—	—
dye	T65.6X1	T65.6X2	T65.6X3	T65.6X4	—	—
fungicide	T60.3X1	T60.3X2	T60.3X3	T60.3X4	—	—
Auranofin	T39.4X1	T39.4X2	T39.4X3	T39.4X4	T39.4X5	T39.4X6
Aurantiin	T46.991	T46.992	T46.993	T46.994	T46.995	T46.996
Aureomycin	T36.4X1	T36.4X2	T36.4X3	T36.4X4	T36.4X5	T36.4X6
ophthalmic preparation	T49.5X1	T49.5X2	T49.5X3	T49.5X4	T49.5X5	T49.5X6
topical NEC	T49.0X1	T49.0X2	T49.0X3	T49.0X4	T49.0X5	T49.0X6
Aurothioglucose	T39.4X1	T39.4X2	T39.4X3	T39.4X4	T39.4X5	T39.4X6
Aurothioglycanide	T39.4X1	T39.4X2	T39.4X3	T39.4X4	T39.4X5	T39.4X6
Aurothiomalate sodium	T39.4X1	T39.4X2	T39.4X3	T39.4X4	T39.4X5	T39.4X6
Aurotioprol	T39.4X1	T39.4X2	T39.4X3	T39.4X4	T39.4X5	T39.4X6
Automobile fuel	T52.0X1	T52.0X2	T52.0X3	T52.0X4	—	—
Autonomic nervous system agent NEC	T44.901	T44.902	T44.903	T44.904	T44.905	T44.906
Avlosulfon	T37.1X1	T37.1X2	T37.1X3	T37.1X4	T37.1X5	T37.1X6
Avomine	T42.6X1	T42.6X2	T42.6X3	T42.6X4	T42.6X5	T42.6X6
Axerophthol	T45.2X1	T45.2X2	T45.2X3	T45.2X4	T45.2X5	T45.2X6
Azacitidine	T45.1X1	T45.1X2	T45.1X3	T45.1X4	T45.1X5	T45.1X6
Azacyclonol	T43.591	T43.592	T43.593	T43.594	T43.595	T43.596
Azadirachta	T60.2X1	T60.2X2	T60.2X3	T60.2X4	—	—
Azanidazole	T37.3X1	T37.3X2	T37.3X3	T37.3X4	T37.3X5	T37.3X6
Azapetine	T46.7X1	T46.7X2	T46.7X3	T46.7X4	T46.7X5	T46.7X6
Azapropazone	T39.2X1	T39.2X2	T39.2X3	T39.2X4	T39.2X5	T39.2X6

◀ New ◀═ Revised ~~deleted~~ Deleted

Substance	Poisoning, Accidental (Unintentional)	Poisoning, Intentional Self-Harm	Poisoning, Assault	Poisoning, Undetermined	Adverse Effect	Underdosing
Azaribine	T45.1X1	T45.1X2	T45.1X3	T45.1X4	T45.1X5	T45.1X6
Azaserine	T45.1X1	T45.1X2	T45.1X3	T45.1X4	T45.1X5	T45.1X6
Azatadine	T45.0X1	T45.0X2	T45.0X3	T45.0X4	T45.0X5	T45.0X6
Azatepa	T45.1X1	T45.1X2	T45.1X3	T45.1X4	T45.1X5	T45.1X6
Azathioprine	T45.1X1	T45.1X2	T45.1X3	T45.1X4	T45.1X5	T45.1X6
Azelaic acid	T49.0X1	T49.0X2	T49.0X3	T49.0X4	T49.0X5	T49.0X6
Azelastine	T45.0X1	T45.0X2	T45.0X3	T45.0X4	T45.0X5	T45.0X6
Azidocillin	T36.0X1	T36.0X2	T36.0X3	T36.0X4	T36.0X5	T36.0X6
Azidothymidine	T37.5X1	T37.5X2	T37.5X3	T37.5X4	T37.5X5	T37.5X6
Azinphos (ethyl) (methyl)	T60.0X1	T60.0X2	T60.0X3	T60.0X4	—	—
Aziridine (chelating)	T54.1X1	T54.1X2	T54.1X3	T54.1X4	—	—
Azithromycin	T36.3X1	T36.3X2	T36.3X3	T36.3X4	T36.3X5	T36.3X6
Azlocillin	T36.01	T36.02	T36.03	T36.04	T36.05	T36.06
Azobenzene smoke	T65.3X1	T65.3X2	T65.3X3	T65.3X4	—	—
acaricide	T60.8X1	T60.8X2	T60.8X3	T60.8X4	—	—
Azosulfamide	T37.0X1	T37.0X2	T37.0X3	T37.0X4	T37.0X5	T37.0X6
AZT	T37.5X1	T37.5X2	T37.5X3	T37.5X4	T37.5X5	T37.5X6
Aztreonam	T36.1X1	T36.1X2	T36.1X3	T36.1X4	T36.1X5	T36.1X6
Azulfidine	T37.0X1	T37.0X2	T37.0X3	T37.0X4	T37.0X5	T37.0X6
Azuresin	T50.8X1	T50.8X2	T50.8X3	T50.8X4	T50.8X5	T50.8X6
B						
Bacampicillin	T36.0X1	T36.0X2	T36.0X3	T36.0X4	T36.0X5	T36.0X6
Bacillus						
lactobacillus	T47.8X1	T47.8X2	T47.8X3	T47.8X4	T47.8X5	T47.8X6
subtilis	T47.6X1	T47.6X2	T47.6X3	T47.6X4	T47.6X5	T47.6X6
Bacimycin	T49.0X1	T49.0X2	T49.0X3	T49.0X4	T49.0X5	T49.0X6
ophthalmic preparation	T49.5X1	T49.5X2	T49.5X3	T49.5X4	T49.5X5	T49.5X6
Bacitracin zinc	T49.0X1	T49.0X2	T49.0X3	T49.0X4	T49.0X5	T49.0X6
with neomycin	T49.0X1	T49.0X2	T49.0X3	T49.0X4	T49.0X5	T49.0X6
ENT agent	T49.6X1	T49.6X2	T49.6X3	T49.6X4	T49.6X5	T49.6X6
ophthalmic preparation	T49.5X1	T49.5X2	T49.5X3	T49.5X4	T49.5X5	T49.5X6
topical NEC	T49.0X1	T49.0X2	T49.0X3	T49.0X4	T49.0X5	T49.0X6
Baclofen	T42.8X1	T42.8X2	T42.8X3	T42.8X4	T42.8X5	T42.8X6
Baking soda	T50.991	T50.992	T50.993	T50.994	T50.995	T50.996
BAL	T45.8X1	T45.8X2	T45.8X3	T45.8X4	T45.8X5	T45.8X6
Bambuterol	T48.6X1	T48.6X2	T48.6X3	T48.6X4	T48.6X5	T48.6X6
Bamethan (sulfate)	T46.7X1	T46.7X2	T46.7X3	T46.7X4	T46.7X5	T46.7X6
Bamifylline	T48.6X1	T48.6X2	T48.6X3	T48.6X4	T48.6X5	T48.6X6
Bamipine	T45.0X1	T45.0X2	T45.0X3	T45.0X4	T45.0X5	T45.0X6
Baneberry — see Actaea spicata						
Banewort — see Belladonna						

Substance	Poisoning, Accidental (Unintentional)	Poisoning, Intentional Self-Harm	Poisoning, Assault	Poisoning, Undetermined	Adverse Effect	Underdosing
Barbenyl	T42.3X1	T42.3X2	T42.3X3	T42.3X4	T42.3X5	T42.3X6
Barbexaclone	T42.6X1	T42.6X2	T42.6X3	T42.6X4	T42.6X5	T42.6X6
Barbital	T42.3X1	T42.3X2	T42.3X3	T42.3X4	T42.3X5	T42.3X6
sodium	T42.3X1	T42.3X2	T42.3X3	T42.3X4	T42.3X5	T42.3X6
Barbitone	T42.3X1	T42.3X2	T42.3X3	T42.3X4	T42.3X5	T42.3X6
Barbiturate NEC	T42.3X1	T42.3X2	T42.3X3	T42.3X4	T42.3X5	T42.3X6
with tranquilizer	T42.3X1	T42.3X2	T42.3X3	T42.3X4	T42.3X5	T42.3X6
anesthetic (intravenous)	T41.1X1	T41.1X2	T41.1X3	T41.1X4	T41.1X5	T41.1X6
Barium (carbonate) (chloride) (sulfite)	T57.8X1	T57.8X2	T57.8X3	T57.8X4	—	—
diagnostic agent	T50.8X1	T50.8X2	T50.8X3	T50.8X4	T50.8X5	T50.8X6
pesticide	T60.4X1	T60.4X2	T60.4X3	T60.4X4	—	—
rodenticide	T60.4X1	T60.4X2	T60.4X3	T60.4X4	—	—
sulfate (medicinal)	T50.8X1	T50.8X2	T50.8X3	T50.8X4	T50.8X5	T50.8X6
Barrier cream	T49.3X1	T49.3X2	T49.3X3	T49.3X4	T49.3X5	T49.3X6
Basic fuchsin	T49.0X1	T49.0X2	T49.0X3	T49.0X4	T49.0X5	T49.0X6
Battery acid or fluid	T54.2X1	T54.2X2	T54.2X3	T54.2X4		
Bay rum	T51.8X1	T51.8X2	T51.8X3	T51.8X4	—	—
BCG (vaccine)	T50.A91	T50.A92	T50.A93	T50.A94	T50.A95	T50.A96
BCNU	T45.1X1	T45.1X2	T45.1X3	T45.1X4	T45.1X5	T45.1X6
Bearsfoot	T62.2X1	T62.2X2	T62.2X3	T62.2X4	—	—
Beclamide	T42.6X1	T42.6X2	T42.6X3	T42.6X4	T42.6X5	T42.6X6
Beclomethasone	T44.5X1	T44.5X2	T44.5X3	T44.5X4	T44.5X5	T44.5X6
Bee (sting) (venom)	T63.441	T63.442	T63.443	T63.444	—	—
Befunolol	T49.5X1	T49.5X2	T49.5X3	T49.5X4	T49.5X5	T49.5X6
Bekanamycin	T36.5X1	T36.5X2	T36.5X3	T36.5X4	T36.5X5	T36.5X6
Belladonna — see also Nightshade						
alkaloids	T44.3X1	T44.3X2	T44.3X3	T44.3X4	T44.3X5	T44.3X6
extract	T44.3X1	T44.3X2	T44.3X3	T44.3X4	T44.3X5	T44.3X6
herb	T44.3X1	T44.3X2	T44.3X3	T44.3X4	T44.3X5	T44.3X6
Bemegride	T50.7X1	T50.7X2	T50.7X3	T50.7X4	T50.7X5	T50.7X6
Benactyzine	T44.3X1	T44.3X2	T44.3X3	T44.3X4	T44.3X5	T44.3X6
Benadryl	T45.0X1	T45.0X2	T45.0X3	T45.0X4	T45.0X5	T45.0X6
Benaprizine	T44.3X1	T44.3X2	T44.3X3	T44.3X4	T44.3X5	T44.3X6
Benazepril	T46.4X1	T46.4X2	T46.4X3	T46.4X4	T46.4X5	T46.4X6
Bencyclane	T46.7X1	T46.7X2	T46.7X3	T46.7X4	T46.7X5	T46.7X6
Bendazol	T46.3X1	T46.3X2	T46.3X3	T46.3X4	T46.3X5	T46.3X6
Bendrofluazide	T50.2X1	T50.2X2	T50.2X3	T50.2X4	T50.2X5	T50.2X6
Bendroflumethiazide	T50.2X1	T50.2X2	T50.2X3	T50.2X4	T50.2X5	T50.2X6
Benemid	T50.4X1	T50.4X2	T50.4X3	T50.4X4	T50.4X5	T50.4X6
Benethamine penicillin	T36.0X1	T36.0X2	T36.0X3	T36.0X4	T36.0X5	T36.0X6
Benisone	T49.0X1	T49.0X2	T49.0X3	T49.0X4	T49.0X5	T49.0X6

◀ New   ◀▥ Revised   ~~deleted~~ Deleted

Substance	Poisoning, Accidental (Unintentional)	Poisoning, Intentional Self-Harm	Poisoning, Assault	Poisoning, Undetermined	Adverse Effect	Underdosing
Benexate	T47.1X1	T47.1X2	T47.1X3	T47.1X4	T47.1X5	T47.1X6
Benfluorex	T46.6X1	T46.6X2	T46.6X3	T46.6X4	T46.6X5	T46.6X6
Benfotiamine	T45.2X1	T45.2X2	T45.2X3	T45.2X4	T45.2X5	T45.2X6
Benomyl	T60.0X1	T60.0X2	T60.0X3	T60.0X4	—	—
Benoquin	T49.8X1	T49.8X2	T49.8X3	T49.8X4	T49.8X5	T49.8X6
Benoxinate	T41.3X1	T41.3X2	T41.3X3	T41.3X4	T41.3X5	T41.3X6
Benperidol	T43.4X1	T43.4X2	T43.4X3	T43.4X4	T43.4X5	T43.4X6
Benproperine	T48.3X1	T48.3X2	T48.3X3	T48.3X4	T48.3X5	T48.3X6
Benserazide	T42.8X1	T42.8X2	T42.8X3	T42.8X4	T42.8X5	T42.8X6
Bentazepam	T42.4X1	T42.4X2	T42.4X3	T42.4X4	T42.4X5	T42.4X6
Bentiromide	T50.8X1	T50.8X2	T50.8X3	T50.8X4	T50.8X5	T50.8X6
Bentonite	T49.3X1	T49.3X2	T49.3X3	T49.3X4	T49.3X5	T49.3X6
Benzalbutyramide	T46.6X1	T46.6X2	T46.6X3	T46.6X4	T46.6X5	T46.6X6
Benzalkonium (chloride)	T49.0X1	T49.0X2	T49.0X3	T49.0X4	T49.0X5	T49.0X6
ophthalmic preparation	T49.5X1	T49.5X2	T49.5X3	T49.5X4	T49.5X5	T49.5X6
Benzamine	T41.3X1	T41.3X2	T41.3X3	T41.3X4	T41.3X5	T41.3X6
lactate	T49.1X1	T49.1X2	T49.1X3	T49.1X4	T49.1X5	T49.1X6
Benzamidosalicylate (calcium)	T37.1X1	T37.1X2	T37.1X3	T37.1X4	T37.1X5	T37.1X6
Benzamphetamine	T50.5X1	T50.5X2	T50.5X3	T50.5X4	T50.5X5	T50.5X6
Benzapril hydrochloride	T46.5X1	T46.5X2	T46.5X3	T46.5X4	T46.5X5	T46.5X6
Benzathine benzylpenicillin	T36.0X1	T36.0X2	T36.0X3	T36.0X4	T36.0X5	T36.0X6
Benzathine penicillin	T36.0X1	T36.0X2	T36.0X3	T36.0X4	T36.0X5	T36.0X6
Benzatropine	T42.8X1	T42.8X2	T42.8X3	T42.8X4	T42.8X5	T42.8X6
Benzbromarone	T50.4X1	T50.4X2	T50.4X3	T50.4X4	T50.4X5	T50.4X6
Benzcarbimine	T45.1X1	T45.1X2	T45.1X3	T45.1X4	T45.1X5	T45.1X6
Benzedrex	T44.991	T44.992	T44.993	T44.994	T44.995	T44.996
Benzedrine (amphetamine)	T43.621	T43.622	T43.623	T43.624	T43.625	T43.626
Benzenamine	T65.3X1	T65.3X2	T65.3X3	T65.3X4	—	—
Benzene	T52.1X1	T52.1X2	T52.1X3	T52.1X4	—	—
homologues (acetyl) (dimethyl) (methyl) (solvent)	T52.2X1	T52.2X2	T52.2X3	T52.2X4	—	—
Benzethonium (chloride)	T49.0X1	T49.0X2	T49.0X3	T49.0X4	T49.0X5	T49.0X6
Benzfetamine	T50.5X1	T50.5X2	T50.5X3	T50.5X4	T50.5X5	T50.5X6
Benzhexol	T44.3X1	T44.3X2	T44.3X3	T44.3X4	T44.3X5	T44.3X6
Benzhydramine (chloride)	T45.0X1	T45.0X2	T45.0X3	T45.0X4	T45.0X5	T45.0X6
Benzidine	T65.891	T65.892	T65.893	T65.894	—	—
Benzilonium bromide	T44.3X1	T44.3X2	T44.3X3	T44.3X4	T44.3X5	T44.3X6
Benzimidazole	T60.3X1	T60.3X2	T60.3X3	T60.3X4	—	—
Benzin(e) — *see Ligroin*						
Benziodarone	T46.3X1	T46.3X2	T46.3X3	T46.3X4	T46.3X5	T46.3X6
Benznidazole	T37.3X1	T37.3X2	T37.3X3	T37.3X4	T37.3X5	T37.3X6
Benzocaine	T41.3X1	T41.3X2	T41.3X3	T41.3X4	T41.3X5	T41.3X6
Benzoctamine	T43.0X1	T43.0X2	T43.0X3	T43.0X4	T43.0X5	T43.0X6
Benzodiapin	T42.4X1	T42.4X2	T42.4X3	T42.4X4	T42.4X5	T42.4X6
Benzodiazepine NEC	T42.4X1	T42.4X2	T42.4X3	T42.4X4	T42.4X5	T42.4X6
Benzoic acid	T49.0X1	T49.0X2	T49.0X3	T49.0X4	T49.0X5	T49.0X6
with salicylic acid	T49.0X1	T49.0X2	T49.0X3	T49.0X4	T49.0X5	T49.0X6
Benzoin (tincture)	T48.5X1	T48.5X2	T48.5X3	T48.5X4	T48.5X5	T48.5X6
Benzol (benzene)	T52.1X1	T52.1X2	T52.1X3	T52.1X4	—	—
vapor	T52.0X1	T52.0X2	T52.0X3	T52.0X4	—	—
Benzomorphan	T40.2X1	T40.2X2	T40.2X3	T40.2X4	T40.2X5	T40.2X6
Benzonatate	T48.3X1	T48.3X2	T48.3X3	T48.3X4	T48.3X5	T48.3X6
Benzophenones	T49.3X1	T49.3X2	T49.3X3	T49.3X4	T49.3X5	T49.3X6
Benzopyrone	T46.991	T46.992	T46.993	T46.994	T46.995	T46.996
Benzothiadiazides	T50.2X1	T50.2X2	T50.2X3	T50.2X4	T50.2X5	T50.2X6
Benzoxonium chloride	T49.0X1	T49.0X2	T49.0X3	T49.0X4	T49.0X5	T49.0X6
Benzoyl peroxide	T49.0X1	T49.0X2	T49.0X3	T49.0X4	T49.0X5	T49.0X6
Benzoylpas calcium	T37.1X1	T37.1X2	T37.1X3	T37.1X4	T37.1X5	T37.1X6
Benzperidin	T43.591	T43.592	T43.593	T43.594	T43.595	T43.596
Benzperidol	T43.591	T43.592	T43.593	T43.594	T43.595	T43.596
Benzphetamine	T50.5X1	T50.5X2	T50.5X3	T50.5X4	T50.5X5	T50.5X6
Benzpyrinium bromide	T44.1X1	T44.1X2	T44.1X3	T44.1X4	T44.1X5	T44.1X6
Benzquinamide	T45.0X1	T45.0X2	T45.0X3	T45.0X4	T45.0X5	T45.0X6
Benzthiazide	T50.2X1	T50.2X2	T50.2X3	T50.2X4	T50.2X5	T50.2X6
Benztropine						
anticholinergic	T44.3X1	T44.3X2	T44.3X3	T44.3X4	T44.3X5	T44.3X6
antiparkinson	T42.8X1	T42.8X2	T42.8X3	T42.8X4	T42.8X5	T42.8X6
Benzydamine	T49.0X1	T49.0X2	T49.0X3	T49.0X4	T49.0X5	T49.0X6
Benzyl						
acetate	T52.8X1	T52.8X2	T52.8X3	T52.8X4	—	—
alcohol	T49.0X1	T49.0X2	T49.0X3	T49.0X4	T49.0X5	T49.0X6
benzoate	T49.0X1	T49.0X2	T49.0X3	T49.0X4	T49.0X5	T49.0X6
Benzoic acid	T49.0X1	T49.0X2	T49.0X3	T49.0X4	T49.0X5	T49.0X6
morphine	T40.2X1	T40.2X2	T40.2X3	T40.2X4	—	—
nicotinate	T46.6X1	T46.6X2	T46.6X3	T46.6X4	T46.6X5	T46.6X6
penicillin	T36.0X1	T36.0X2	T36.0X3	T36.0X4	T36.0X5	T36.0X6
Benzylhydrochlorthia-zide	T50.2X1	T50.2X2	T50.2X3	T50.2X4	T50.2X5	T50.2X6
Benzylpenicillin	T36.0X1	T36.0X2	T36.0X3	T36.0X4	T36.0X5	T36.0X6
Benzylthiouracil	T38.2X1	T38.2X2	T38.2X3	T38.2X4	T38.2X5	T38.2X6
Bephenium hydroxy-naphthoate	T37.4X1	T37.4X2	T37.4X3	T37.4X4	T37.4X5	T37.4X6
Bepridil	T46.1X1	T46.1X2	T46.1X3	T46.1X4	T46.1X5	T46.1X6
Bergamot oil	T65.891	T65.892	T65.893	T65.894	—	—
Bergapten	T50.991	T50.992	T50.993	T50.994	T50.995	T50.996
Berries, poisonous	T62.1X1	T62.1X2	T62.1X3	T62.1X4	—	—

◀ New ◀▥ Revised ~~deleted~~ Deleted

Substance	Poisoning, Accidental (Unintentional)	Poisoning, Intentional Self-Harm	Poisoning, Assault	Poisoning, Undetermined	Adverse Effect	Underdosing
Beryllium (compounds)	T56.7X1	T56.7X2	T56.7X3	T56.7X4	—	—
b-acetyldigoxin	T46.0X1	T46.0X2	T46.0X3	T46.0X4	T46.0X5	T46.0X6
beta adrenergic blocking agent, heart	T44.7X1	T44.7X2	T44.7X3	T44.7X4	T44.7X5	T44.7X6
b-benzalbutyramide	T46.6X1	T46.6X2	T46.6X3	T46.6X4	T46.6X5	T46.6X6
Betacarotene	T45.2X1	T45.2X2	T45.2X3	T45.2X4	T45.2X5	T45.2X6
b-eucaine	T49.1X1	T49.1X2	T49.1X3	T49.1X4	T49.1X5	T49.1X6
Beta-Chlor	T42.6X1	T42.6X2	T42.6X3	T42.6X4	T42.6X5	T42.6X6
b-galactosidase	T47.5X1	T47.5X2	T47.5X3	T47.5X4	T47.5X5	T47.5X6
Betahistine	T46.7X1	T46.7X2	T46.7X3	T46.7X4	T46.7X5	T46.7X6
Betaine	T47.5X1	T47.5X2	T47.5X3	T47.5X4	T47.5X5	T47.5X6
Betamethasone	T49.0X1	T49.0X2	T49.0X3	T49.0X4	T49.0X5	T49.0X6
topical	T49.0X1	T49.0X2	T49.0X3	T49.0X4	T49.0X5	T49.0X6
Betamicin	T36.8X1	T36.8X2	T36.8X3	T36.8X4	T36.8X5	T36.8X6
Betanidine	T46.5X1	T46.5X2	T46.5X3	T46.5X4	T46.5X5	T46.5X6
b-sitosterol(s)	T46.6X1	T46.6X2	T46.6X3	T46.6X4	T46.6X5	T46.6X6
Betaxolol	T44.7X1	T44.7X2	T44.7X3	T44.7X4	T44.7X5	T44.7X6
Betazole	T50.8X1	T50.8X2	T50.8X3	T50.8X4	T50.8X5	T50.8X6
Bethanechol	T44.1X1	T44.1X2	T44.1X3	T44.1X4	T44.1X5	T44.1X6
chloride	T44.1X1	T44.1X2	T44.1X3	T44.1X4	T44.1X5	T44.1X6
Bethanidine	T46.5X1	T46.5X2	T46.5X3	T46.5X4	T46.5X5	T46.5X6
Betoxycaine	T41.3X1	T41.3X2	T41.3X3	T41.3X4	T41.3X5	T41.3X6
Betula oil	T49.3X1	T49.3X2	T49.3X3	T49.3X4	T49.3X5	T49.3X6
Bevantolol	T44.7X1	T44.7X2	T44.7X3	T44.7X4	T44.7X5	T44.7X6
Bevonium metilsulfate	T44.3X1	T44.3X2	T44.3X3	T44.3X4	T44.3X5	T44.3X6
Bezafibrate	T46.6X1	T46.6X2	T46.6X3	T46.6X4	T46.6X5	T46.6X6
Bezitramide	T40.4X1	T40.4X2	T40.4X3	T40.4X4	T40.4X5	T40.4X6
BHA	T50.991	T50.992	T50.993	T50.994	T50.995	T50.996
Bhang	T40.7X1	T40.7X2	T40.7X3	T40.7X4	T40.7X5	T40.7X6
BHC (medicinal)	T49.0X1	T49.0X2	T49.0X3	T49.0X4	T49.0X5	T49.0X6
nonmedicinal (vapor)	T53.6X1	T53.6X2	T53.6X3	T53.6X4	—	—
Bialamicol	T37.3X1	T37.3X2	T37.3X3	T37.3X4	T37.3X5	T37.3X6
Bibenzonium bromide	T48.3X1	T48.3X2	T48.3X3	T48.3X4	T48.3X5	T48.3X6
Bibrocathol	T49.5X1	T49.5X2	T49.5X3	T49.5X4	T49.5X5	T49.5X6
Bichloride of mercury — see Mercury, chloride						
Bichromates (calcium) (potassium) (sodium) (crystals)	T57.8X1	T57.8X2	T57.8X3	T57.8X4	—	—
fumes	T56.2X1	T56.2X2	T56.2X3	T56.2X4	—	—
Biclotymol	T49.6X1	T49.6X2	T49.6X3	T49.6X4	T49.6X5	T49.6X6
Bicuculline	T50.7X1	T50.7X2	T50.7X3	T50.7X4	T50.7X5	T50.7X6
Bifemelane	T43.291	T43.292	T43.293	T43.294	T43.295	T43.296
Biguanide derivatives, oral	T38.3X1	T38.3X2	T38.3X3	T38.3X4	T38.3X5	T38.3X6

Substance	Poisoning, Accidental (Unintentional)	Poisoning, Intentional Self-Harm	Poisoning, Assault	Poisoning, Undetermined	Adverse Effect	Underdosing
Biligrafin	T50.8X1	T50.8X2	T50.8X3	T50.8X4	T50.8X5	T50.8X6
Bile salts	T47.5X1	T47.5X2	T47.5X3	T47.5X4	T47.5X5	T47.5X6
Bilopaque	T50.8X1	T50.8X2	T50.8X3	T50.8X4	T50.8X5	T50.8X6
Binifibrate	T46.6X1	T46.6X2	T46.6X3	T46.6X4	T46.6X5	T46.6X6
Binitrobenzol	T65.3X1	T65.3X2	T65.3X3	T65.3X4	—	—
Bioflavonoid(s)	T46.991	T46.992	T46.993	T46.994	T46.995	T46.996
Biological substance NEC	T50.901	T50.902	T50.903	T50.904	T50.905	T50.906
Biotin	T45.2X1	T45.2X2	T45.2X3	T45.2X4	T45.2X5	T45.2X6
Biperiden	T44.3X1	T44.3X2	T44.3X3	T44.3X4	T44.3X5	T44.3X6
Bisacodyl	T47.2X1	T47.2X2	T47.2X3	T47.2X4	T47.2X5	T47.2X6
Bisbentiamine	T45.2X1	T45.2X2	T45.2X3	T45.2X4	T45.2X5	T45.2X6
Bisbutiamine	T45.2X1	T45.2X2	T45.2X3	T45.2X4	T45.2X5	T45.2X6
Bisdequalinium (salts) (diacetate)	T49.6X1	T49.6X2	T49.6X3	T49.6X4	T49.6X5	T49.6X6
Bishydroxycoumarin	T45.511	T45.512	T45.513	T45.514	T45.515	T45.516
Bismarsen	T37.8X1	T37.8X2	T37.8X3	T37.8X4	T37.8X5	T37.8X6
Bismuth salts	T47.6X1	T47.6X2	T47.6X3	T47.6X4	T47.6X5	T47.6X6
aluminate	T47.1X1	T47.1X2	T47.1X3	T47.1X4	T47.1X5	T47.1X6
anti-infectives	T37.8X1	T37.8X2	T37.8X3	T37.8X4	T37.8X5	T37.8X6
formic iodide	T49.0X1	T49.0X2	T49.0X3	T49.0X4	T49.0X5	T49.0X6
glycolylarsenate	T49.0X1	T49.0X2	T49.0X3	T49.0X4	T49.0X5	T49.0X6
nonmedicinal (compounds) NEC	T65.91	T65.92	T65.93	T65.94	—	—
subcarbonate	T47.6X1	T47.6X2	T47.6X3	T47.6X4	T47.6X5	T47.6X6
subsalicylate	T37.8X1	T37.8X2	T37.8X3	T37.8X4	T37.8X5	T37.8X6
sulfarsphenamine	T37.8X1	T37.8X2	T37.8X3	T37.8X4	T37.8X5	T37.8X6
Bisoprolol	T44.7X1	T44.7X2	T44.7X3	T44.7X4	T44.7X5	T44.7X6
Bisoxatin	T47.2X1	T47.2X2	T47.2X3	T47.2X4	T47.2X5	T47.2X6
Bisulepin (hydrochloride)	T45.0X1	T45.0X2	T45.0X3	T45.0X4	T45.0X5	T45.0X6
Bithionol	T37.8X1	T37.8X2	T37.8X3	T37.8X4	T37.8X5	T37.8X6
anthelminthic	T37.4X1	T37.4X2	T37.4X3	T37.4X4	T37.4X5	T37.4X6
Bitolterol	T48.6X1	T48.6X2	T48.6X3	T48.6X4	T48.6X5	T48.6X6
Bitoscanate	T37.4X1	T37.4X2	T37.4X3	T37.4X4	T37.4X5	T37.4X6
Bitter almond oil	T62.8X1	T62.8X2	T62.8X3	T62.8X4	—	—
Bittersweet	T62.2X1	T62.2X2	T62.2X3	T62.2X4	—	—
Black						
flag	T60.91	T60.92	T60.93	T60.94	—	—
henbane	T62.2X1	T62.2X2	T62.2X3	T62.2X4	—	—
leaf (40)	T60.91	T60.92	T60.93	T60.94	—	—
widow spider (bite)	T63.311	T63.312	T63.313	T63.314	—	—
antivenin	T50.Z11	T50.Z12	T50.Z13	T50.Z14	T50.Z15	T50.Z16
Blast furnace gas (carbon monoxide from)	T58.8X1	T58.8X2	T58.8X3	T58.8X4	—	—
Bleach	T54.91	T54.92	T54.93	T54.94	—	—

TABLE OF DRUGS AND CHEMICALS

Substance	Poisoning, Accidental (Unintentional)	Poisoning, Intentional Self-Harm	Poisoning, Assault	Poisoning, Undetermined	Adverse Effect	Underdosing
Bleaching agent (medicinal)	T49.4X1	T49.4X2	T49.4X3	T49.4X4	T49.4X5	T49.4X6
Bleomycin	T45.1X1	T45.1X2	T45.1X3	T45.1X4	T45.1X5	T45.1X6
Blockain	T41.3X1	T41.3X2	T41.3X3	T41.3X4	T41.3X5	T41.3X6
infiltration (subcutaneous)	T41.3X1	T41.3X2	T41.3X3	T41.3X4	T41.3X5	T41.3X6
nerve block (peripheral) (plexus)	T41.3X1	T41.3X2	T41.3X3	T41.3X4	T41.3X5	T41.3X6
topical (surface)	T41.3X1	T41.3X2	T41.3X3	T41.3X4	T41.3X5	T41.3X6
Blockers, calcium channel	T46.1X1	T46.1X2	T46.1X3	T46.1X4	T46.1X5	T46.1X6
Blood (derivatives) (natural) (plasma) (whole)	T45.8X1	T45.8X2	T45.8X3	T45.8X4	T45.8X5	T45.8X6
dried	T45.8X1	T45.8X2	T45.8X3	T45.8X4	T45.8X5	T45.8X6
drug affecting NEC	T45.91	T45.92	T45.93	T45.94	T45.95	T45.96
expander NEC	T45.8X1	T45.8X2	T45.8X3	T45.8X4	T45.8X5	T45.8X6
fraction NEC	T45.8X1	T45.8X2	T45.8X3	T45.8X4	T45.8X5	T45.8X6
substitute (macromolecular)	T45.8X1	T45.8X2	T45.8X3	T45.8X4	T45.8X5	T45.8X6
Blue velvet	T40.2X1	T40.2X2	T40.2X3	T40.2X4	—	—
Bone meal	T62.8X1	T62.8X2	T62.8X3	T62.8X4	—	—
Bonine	T45.0X1	T45.0X2	T45.0X3	T45.0X4	T45.0X5	T45.0X6
Bopindolol	T44.7X1	T44.7X2	T44.7X3	T44.7X4	T44.7X5	T44.7X6
Boracic acid	T49.0X1	T49.0X2	T49.0X3	T49.0X4	T49.0X5	T49.0X6
ENT agent	T49.6X1	T49.6X2	T49.6X3	T49.6X4	T49.6X5	T49.6X6
ophthalmic preparation	T49.5X1	T49.5X2	T49.5X3	T49.5X4	T49.5X5	T49.5X6
Borane complex	T57.8X1	T57.8X2	T57.8X3	T57.8X4	—	—
Borate(s)	T57.8X1	T57.8X2	T57.8X3	T57.8X4	—	—
buffer	T50.991	T50.992	T50.993	T50.994	T50.995	T50.996
cleanser	T54.91	T54.92	T54.93	T54.94		
sodium	T57.8X1	T57.8X2	T57.8X3	T57.8X4	—	—
Borax (cleanser)	T54.91	T54.92	T54.93	T54.94		
Bordeaux mixture	T60.3X1	T60.3X2	T60.3X3	T60.3X4	—	—
Boric acid	T49.0X1	T49.0X2	T49.0X3	T49.0X4	T49.0X5	T49.0X6
ENT agent	T49.6X1	T49.6X2	T49.6X3	T49.6X4	T49.6X5	T49.6X6
ophthalmic preparation	T49.5X1	T49.5X2	T49.5X3	T49.5X4	T49.5X5	T49.5X6
Bornaprine	T44.3X1	T44.3X2	T44.3X3	T44.3X4	T44.3X5	T44.3X6
Boron	T57.8X1	T57.8X2	T57.8X3	T57.8X4	—	—
hydride NEC	T57.8X1	T57.8X2	T57.8X3	T57.8X4	—	—
fumes or gas	T57.8X1	T57.8X2	T57.8X3	T57.8X4	—	—
trifluoride	T59.891	T59.892	T59.893	T59.894	—	—
Botox	T48.291	T48.292	T48.293	T48.294	T48.295	T48.296
Botulinus anti-toxin (type A, B)	T50.Z11	T50.Z12	T50.Z13	T50.Z14	T50.Z15	T50.Z16
Brake fluid vapor	T59.891	T59.892	T59.893	T59.894	—	—
Brallobarbital	T42.3X1	T42.3X2	T42.3X3	T42.3X4	T42.3X5	T42.3X6
Bran (wheat)	T47.4X1	T47.4X2	T47.4X3	T47.4X4	T47.4X5	T47.4X6
Brass (fumes)	T56.891	T56.892	T56.893	T56.894	—	—

Substance	Poisoning, Accidental (Unintentional)	Poisoning, Intentional Self-Harm	Poisoning, Assault	Poisoning, Undetermined	Adverse Effect	Underdosing
Brasso	T52.0X1	T52.0X2	T52.0X3	T52.0X4	—	—
Bretylium tosilate	T46.2X1	T46.2X2	T46.2X3	T46.2X4	T46.2X5	T46.2X6
Brevital (sodium)	T41.1X1	T41.1X2	T41.1X3	T41.1X4	T41.1X5	T41.1X6
Brinase	T45.3X1	T45.3X2	T45.3X3	T45.3X4	T45.3X5	T45.3X6
British antilewisite	T45.8X1	T45.8X2	T45.8X3	T45.8X4	T45.8X5	T45.8X6
Brodifacoum	T60.4X1	T60.4X2	T60.4X3	T60.4X4	—	—
Bromal (hydrate)	T42.6X1	T42.6X2	T42.6X3	T42.6X4	T42.6X5	T42.6X6
Bromazepam	T42.4X1	T42.4X2	T42.4X3	T42.4X4	T42.4X5	T42.4X6
Bromazine	T45.0X1	T45.0X2	T45.0X3	T45.0X4	T45.0X5	T45.0X6
Brombenzylcyanide	T59.3X1	T59.3X2	T59.3X3	T59.3X4	—	—
Bromelains	T45.3X1	T45.3X2	T45.3X3	T45.3X4	T45.3X5	T45.3X6
Bromethalin	T60.4X1	T60.4X2	T60.4X3	T60.4X4	—	—
Bromhexine	T48.4X1	T48.4X2	T48.4X3	T48.4X4	T48.4X5	T48.4X6
Bromide salts	T42.6X1	T42.6X2	T42.6X3	T42.6X4	T42.6X5	T42.6X6
Bromindione	T45.511	T45.512	T45.513	T45.514	T45.515	T45.516
Bromine						
compounds (medicinal)	T42.6X1	T42.6X2	T42.6X3	T42.6X4	T42.6X5	T42.6X6
sedative	T42.6X1	T42.6X2	T42.6X3	T42.6X4	T42.6X5	T42.6X6
vapor	T59.891	T59.892	T59.893	T59.894	—	—
Bromisovalum	T42.6X1	T42.6X2	T42.6X3	T42.6X4	T42.6X5	T42.6X6
Bromisoval	T42.6X1	T42.6X2	T42.6X3	T42.6X4	T42.6X5	T42.6X6
Bromobenzylcyanide	T59.3X1	T59.3X2	T59.3X3	T59.3X4	—	—
Bromochlorosalicylani-lide	T49.0X1	T49.0X2	T49.0X3	T49.0X4	T49.0X5	T49.0X6
Bromocriptine	T42.8X1	T42.8X2	T42.8X3	T42.8X4	T42.8X5	T42.8X6
Bromodiphenhydramine	T45.0X1	T45.0X2	T45.0X3	T45.0X4	T45.0X5	T45.0X6
Bromoform	T42.6X1	T42.6X2	T42.6X3	T42.6X4	T42.6X5	T42.6X6
Bromophenol blue reagent	T50.991	T50.992	T50.993	T50.994	T50.995	T50.996
Bromopride	T47.8X1	T47.8X2	T47.8X3	T47.8X4	T47.8X5	T47.8X6
Bromosalicylchloranitide	T49.0X1	T49.0X2	T49.0X3	T49.0X4	T49.0X5	T49.0X6
Bromosalicylhydroxamic acid	T37.1X1	T37.1X2	T37.1X3	T37.1X4	T37.1X5	T37.1X6
Bromo-seltzer	T39.1X1	T39.1X2	T39.1X3	T39.1X4	T39.1X5	T39.1X6
Bromoxynil	T60.3X1	T60.3X2	T60.3X3	T60.3X4	—	—
Bromperidol	T43.4X1	T43.4X2	T43.4X3	T43.4X4	T43.4X5	T43.4X6
Brompheniramine	T45.0X1	T45.0X2	T45.0X3	T45.0X4	T45.0X5	T45.0X6
Bromsulfophthalein	T50.8X1	T50.8X2	T50.8X3	T50.8X4	T50.8X5	T50.8X6
Bromural	T42.6X1	T42.6X2	T42.6X3	T42.6X4	T42.6X5	T42.6X6
Bromvaletone	T42.6X1	T42.6X2	T42.6X3	T42.6X4	T42.6X5	T42.6X6
Bronchodilator NEC	T48.6X1	T48.6X2	T48.6X3	T48.6X4	T48.6X5	T48.6X6
Brotizolam	T42.4X1	T42.4X2	T42.4X3	T42.4X4	T42.4X5	T42.4X6
Brovincamine	T46.7X1	T46.7X2	T46.7X3	T46.7X4	T46.7X5	T46.7X6
Brown spider (bite) (venom)	T63.391	T63.392	T63.393	T63.394	—	—

◀ New   ⬅ Revised   ~~deleted~~ Deleted

Substance	External Cause (T-Code)					
	Poisoning, Accidental (Unintentional)	Poisoning, Intentional Self-Harm	Poisoning, Assault	Poisoning, Undetermined	Adverse Effect	Underdosing
Brown recluse spider (bite) (venom)	T63.331	T63.332	T63.333	T63.334	—	—
Broxaterol	T48.6X1	T48.6X2	T48.6X3	T48.6X4	T48.6X5	T48.6X6
Broxuridine	T45.1X1	T45.1X2	T45.1X3	T45.1X4	T45.1X5	T45.1X6
Broxyquinoline	T37.8X1	T37.8X2	T37.8X3	T37.8X4	T37.8X5	T37.8X6
Bruceine	T48.291	T48.292	T48.293	T48.294	T48.295	T48.296
Brucia	T62.2X1	T62.2X2	T62.2X3	T62.2X4	—	—
Brucine	T65.1X1	T65.1X2	T65.1X3	T65.1X4	—	—
Brunswick green — *see* Copper						
Bruten — *see* Ibuprofen						
Bryonia	T47.2X1	T47.2X2	T47.2X3	T47.2X4	T47.2X5	T47.2X6
Buclizine	T45.0X1	T45.0X2	T45.0X3	T45.0X4	T45.0X5	T45.0X6
Buclosamide	T49.0X1	T49.0X2	T49.0X3	T49.0X4	T49.0X5	T49.0X6
Budesonide	T44.5X1	T44.5X2	T44.5X3	T44.5X4	T44.5X5	T44.5X6
Budralazine	T46.5X1	T46.5X2	T46.5X3	T46.5X4	T46.5X5	T46.5X6
Bufferin	T39.011	T39.012	T39.013	T39.014	T39.015	T39.016
Buflomedil	T46.7X1	T46.7X2	T46.7X3	T46.7X4	T46.7X5	T46.7X6
Buformin	T38.3X1	T38.3X2	T38.3X3	T38.3X4	T38.3X5	T38.3X6
Bufotenine	T40.991	T40.992	T40.993	T40.994	—	—
Bufrolin	T48.6X1	T48.6X2	T48.6X3	T48.6X4	T48.6X5	T48.6X6
Bufylline	T48.6X1	T48.6X2	T48.6X3	T48.6X4	T48.6X5	T48.6X6
Bulk filler	T50.5X1	T50.5X2	T50.5X3	T50.5X4	T50.5X5	T50.5X6
cathartic	T47.4X1	T47.4X2	T47.4X3	T47.4X4	T47.4X5	T47.4X6
Bumetanide	T50.1X1	T50.1X2	T50.1X3	T50.1X4	T50.1X5	T50.1X6
Bunaftine	T46.2X1	T46.2X2	T46.2X3	T46.2X4	T46.2X5	T46.2X6
Bunamiodyl	T50.8X1	T50.8X2	T50.8X3	T50.8X4	T50.8X5	T50.8X6
Bunazosin	T44.6X1	T44.6X2	T44.6X3	T44.6X4	T44.6X5	T44.6X6
Bunitrolol	T44.7X1	T44.7X2	T44.7X3	T44.7X4	T44.7X5	T44.7X6
Buphenine	T46.7X1	T46.7X2	T46.7X3	T46.7X4	T46.7X5	T46.7X6
Bupivacaine	T41.3X1	T41.3X2	T41.3X3	T41.3X4	T41.3X5	T41.3X6
infiltration (subcutaneous)	T41.3X1	T41.3X2	T41.3X3	T41.3X4	T41.3X5	T41.3X6
nerve block (peripheral) (plexus)	T41.3X1	T41.3X2	T41.3X3	T41.3X4	T41.3X5	T41.3X6
spinal	T41.3X1	T41.3X2	T41.3X3	T41.3X4	T41.3X5	T41.3X6
Bupranolol	T44.7X1	T44.7X2	T44.7X3	T44.7X4	T44.7X5	T44.7X6
Buprenorphine	T40.4X1	T40.4X2	T40.4X3	T40.4X4	T40.4X5	T40.4X6
Bupropion	T43.291	T43.292	T43.293	T43.294	T43.295	T43.296
Burimamide	T47.1X1	T47.1X2	T47.1X3	T47.1X4	T47.1X5	T47.1X6
Buserelin	T38.891	T38.892	T38.893	T38.894	T38.895	T38.896
Buspirone	T43.591	T43.592	T43.593	T43.594	T43.595	T43.596
Busulfan, busulphan	T45.1X1	T45.1X2	T45.1X3	T45.1X4	T45.1X5	T45.1X6
Butabarbital (sodium)	T42.3X1	T42.3X2	T42.3X3	T42.3X4	T42.3X5	T42.3X6
Butabarbitone	T42.3X1	T42.3X2	T42.3X3	T42.3X4	T42.3X5	T42.3X6

Substance	External Cause (T-Code)					
	Poisoning, Accidental (Unintentional)	Poisoning, Intentional Self-Harm	Poisoning, Assault	Poisoning, Undetermined	Adverse Effect	Underdosing
Butabarpal	T42.3X1	T42.3X2	T42.3X3	T42.3X4	T42.3X5	T42.3X6
Butacaine	T41.3X1	T41.3X2	T41.3X3	T41.3X4	T41.3X5	T41.3X6
Butalamine	T46.7X1	T46.7X2	T46.7X3	T46.7X4	T46.7X5	T46.7X6
Butalbital	T42.3X1	T42.3X2	T42.3X3	T42.3X4	T42.3X5	T42.3X6
Butallylonal	T42.3X1	T42.3X2	T42.3X3	T42.3X4	T42.3X5	T42.3X6
Butamben	T41.3X1	T41.3X2	T41.3X3	T41.3X4	T41.3X5	T41.3X6
Butamirate	T48.3X1	T48.3X2	T48.3X3	T48.3X4	T48.3X5	T48.3X6
Butane (distributed in mobile container)	T59.891	T59.892	T59.893	T59.894	—	—
distributed through pipes	T59.891	T59.892	T59.893	T59.894	—	—
incomplete combustion	T58.11	T58.12	T58.13	T58.14	—	—
Butanilicaine	T41.3X1	T41.3X2	T41.3X3	T41.3X4	T41.3X5	T41.3X6
Butanol	T51.3X1	T51.3X2	T51.3X3	T51.3X4	—	—
Butanone, 2-butanone	T52.4X1	T52.4X2	T52.4X3	T52.4X4	—	—
Butantrone	T49.4X1	T49.4X2	T49.4X3	T49.4X4	T49.4X5	T49.4X6
Butaperazine	T43.3X1	T43.3X2	T43.3X3	T43.3X4	T43.3X5	T43.3X6
Butazolidin	T39.2X1	T39.2X2	T39.2X3	T39.2X4	T39.2X5	T39.2X6
Butetamate	T48.6X1	T48.6X2	T48.6X3	T48.6X4	T48.6X5	T48.6X6
Butethal	T42.3X1	T42.3X2	T42.3X3	T42.3X4	T42.3X5	T42.3X6
Butethamate	T44.3X1	T44.3X2	T44.3X3	T44.3X4	T44.3X5	T44.3X6
Buthalitone (sodium)	T41.1X1	T41.1X2	T41.1X3	T41.1X4	T41.1X5	T41.1X6
Butisol (sodium)	T42.3X1	T42.3X2	T42.3X3	T42.3X4	T42.3X5	T42.3X6
Butizide	T50.2X1	T50.2X2	T50.2X3	T50.2X4	T50.2X5	T50.2X6
Butobarbital	T42.3X1	T42.3X2	T42.3X3	T42.3X4	T42.3X5	T42.3X6
sodium	T42.3X1	T42.3X2	T42.3X3	T42.3X4	T42.3X5	T42.3X6
Butobarbitone	T42.3X1	T42.3X2	T42.3X3	T42.3X4	T42.3X5	T42.3X6
Butoconazole (nitrate)	T49.0X1	T49.0X2	T49.0X3	T49.0X4	T49.0X5	T49.0X6
Butorphanol	T40.4X1	T40.4X2	T40.4X3	T40.4X4	T40.4X5	T40.4X6
Butriptyline	T43.011	T43.012	T43.013	T43.014	T43.015	T43.016
Butropium bromide	T44.3X1	T44.3X2	T44.3X3	T44.3X4	T44.3X5	T44.3X6
Buttercups	T62.2X1	T62.2X2	T62.2X3	T62.2X4	—	—
Butter of antimony — *see* Antimony						
Butyl						
acetate (secondary)	T52.8X1	T52.8X2	T52.8X3	T52.8X4	—	—
alcohol	T51.3X1	T51.3X2	T51.3X3	T51.3X4	—	—
aminobenzoate	T41.3X1	T41.3X2	T41.3X3	T41.3X4	T41.3X5	T41.3X6
butyrate	T52.8X1	T52.8X2	T52.8X3	T52.8X4	—	—
carbinol	T51.3X1	T51.3X2	T51.3X3	T51.3X4	—	—
carbitol	T52.3X1	T52.3X2	T52.3X3	T52.3X4	—	—
cellosolve	T52.3X1	T52.3X2	T52.3X3	T52.3X4	—	—
chloral (hydrate)	T42.6X1	T42.6X2	T42.6X3	T42.6X4	T42.6X5	T42.6X6
formate	T52.8X1	T52.8X2	T52.8X3	T52.8X4	—	—

◀ New ◀|||| Revised ~~deleted~~ Deleted

TABLE OF DRUGS AND CHEMICALS

Substance	Poisoning, Accidental (Unintentional)	Poisoning, Intentional Self-Harm	Poisoning, Assault	Poisoning, Undetermined	Adverse Effect	Underdosing
External Cause (T-Code)						
Butyl *(Continued)*						
lactate	T52.8X1	T52.8X2	T52.8X3	T52.8X4	—	—
propionate	T52.8X1	T52.8X2	T52.8X3	T52.8X4	—	—
scopolamine bromide	T44.3X1	T44.3X2	T44.3X3	T44.3X4	T44.3X5	T44.3X6
thiobarbital sodium	T41.1X1	T41.1X2	T41.1X3	T41.1X4	T41.1X5	T41.1X6
Butylated hydroxy-anisole	T50.991	T50.992	T50.993	T50.994	T50.995	T50.996
Butylchloral hydrate	T42.6X1	T42.6X2	T42.6X3	T42.6X4	T42.6X5	T42.6X6
Butyltoluene	T52.2X1	T52.2X2	T52.2X3	T52.2X4	—	—
Butyn	T41.3X1	T41.3X2	T41.3X3	T41.3X4	T41.3X5	T41.3X6
Butyrophenone (-based tranquilizers)	T43.4X1	T43.4X2	T43.4X3	T43.4X4	T43.4X5	T43.4X6
C						
Cabergoline	T42.8X1	T42.8X2	T42.8X3	T42.8X4	T42.8X5	T42.8X6
Cacodyl, cacodylic acid	T57.0X1	T57.0X2	T57.0X3	T57.0X4	—	—
Cactinomycin	T45.1X1	T45.1X2	T45.1X3	T45.1X4	T45.1X5	T45.1X6
Cade oil	T49.4X1	T49.4X2	T49.4X3	T49.4X4	T49.4X5	T49.4X6
Cadexomer iodine	T49.0X1	T49.0X2	T49.0X3	T49.0X4	T49.0X5	T49.0X6
Cadmium (chloride) (fumes) (oxide)	T56.3X1	T56.3X2	T56.3X3	T56.3X4	—	—
sulfide (medicinal) NEC	T49.4X1	T49.4X2	T49.4X3	T49.4X4	T49.4X5	T49.4X6
Cadralazine	T46.5X1	T46.5X2	T46.5X3	T46.5X4	T46.5X5	T46.5X6
Caffeine	T43.611	T43.612	T43.613	T43.614	T43.615	T43.616
Calabar bean	T62.2X1	T62.2X2	T62.2X3	T62.2X4	—	—
Caladium seguinum	T62.2X1	T62.2X2	T62.2X3	T62.2X4	—	—
Calamine (lotion)	T49.3X1	T49.3X2	T49.3X3	T49.3X4	T49.3X5	T49.3X6
Calcifediol	T45.2X1	T45.2X2	T45.2X3	T45.2X4	T45.2X5	T45.2X6
Calciferol	T45.2X1	T45.2X2	T45.2X3	T45.2X4	T45.2X5	T45.2X6
Calcitonin	T50.991	T50.992	T50.993	T50.994	T50.995	T50.996
Calcitriol	T45.2X1	T45.2X2	T45.2X3	T45.2X4	T45.2X5	T45.2X6
Calcium	T50.3X1	T50.3X2	T50.3X3	T50.3X4	T50.3X5	T50.3X6
actylsalicylate	T39.011	T39.012	T39.013	T39.014	T39.015	T39.016
benzamidosalicylate	T37.1X1	T37.1X2	T37.1X3	T37.1X4	T37.1X5	T37.1X6
bromide	T42.6X1	T42.6X2	T42.6X3	T42.6X4	T42.6X5	T42.6X6
bromolactobionate	T42.6X1	T42.6X2	T42.6X3	T42.6X4	T42.6X5	T42.6X6
carbaspirin	T39.011	T39.012	T39.013	T39.014	T39.015	T39.016
carbimide	T50.6X1	T50.6X2	T50.6X3	T50.6X4	T50.6X5	T50.6X6
carbonate	T47.1X1	T47.1X2	T47.1X3	T47.1X4	T47.1X5	T47.1X6
chloride	T50.991	T50.992	T50.993	T50.994	T50.995	T50.996
anhydrous	T50.991	T50.992	T50.993	T50.994	T50.995	T50.996
cyanide	T57.8X1	T57.8X2	T57.8X3	T57.8X4	—	—
dioctyl sulfosuccinate	T47.4X1	T47.4X2	T47.4X3	T47.4X4	T47.4X5	T47.4X6
disodium edathamil	T45.8X1	T45.8X2		T45.8X4	T45.8X5	T45.8X6

Substance	Poisoning, Accidental (Unintentional)	Poisoning, Intentional Self-Harm	Poisoning, Assault	Poisoning, Undetermined	Adverse Effect	Underdosing
External Cause (T-Code)						
Calcium *(Continued)*						
disodium edetate	T45.8X1	T45.8X2	T45.8X3	T45.8X4	T45.8X5	T45.8X6
dobesilate	T46.991	T46.992	T46.993	T46.994	T46.995	T46.996
EDTA	T45.8X1	T45.8X2	T45.8X3	T45.8X4	T45.8X5	T45.8X6
ferrous citrate	T45.4X1	T45.4X2	T45.4X3	T45.4X4	T45.4X5	T45.4X6
folinate	T45.8X1	T45.8X2	T45.8X3	T45.8X4	T45.8X5	T45.8X6
glubionate	T50.3X1	T50.3X2	T50.3X3	T50.3X4	T50.3X5	T50.3X6
gluconate	T50.3X1	T50.3X2	T50.3X3	T50.3X4	T50.3X5	T50.3X6
gluconogalactogluconate	T50.3X1	T50.3X2	T50.3X3	T50.3X4	T50.3X5	T50.3X6
hydrate, hydroxide	T54.3X1	T54.3X2	T54.3X3	T54.3X4	—	—
hypochlorite	T54.3X1	T54.3X2	T54.3X3	T54.3X4	—	—
iodide	T48.4X1	T48.4X2	T48.4X3	T48.4X4	T48.4X5	T48.4X6
ipodate	T50.8X1	T50.8X2	T50.8X3	T50.8X4	T50.8X5	T50.8X6
lactate	T50.3X1	T50.3X2	T50.3X3	T50.3X4	T50.3X5	T50.3X6
leucovorin	T45.8X1	T45.8X2	T45.8X3	T45.8X4	T45.8X5	T45.8X6
mandelate	T37.91	T37.92	T37.93	T37.94	T37.95	T37.96
oxide	T54.3X1	T54.3X2	T54.3X3	T54.3X4	—	—
pantothenate	T45.2X1	T45.2X2	T45.2X3	T45.2X4	T45.2X5	T45.2X6
phosphate	T50.3X1	T50.3X2	T50.3X3	T50.3X4	T50.3X5	T50.3X6
salicylate	T39.091	T39.092	T39.093	T39.094	T39.095	T39.096
salts	T50.3X1	T50.3X2	T50.3X3	T50.3X4	T50.3X5	T50.3X6
Calculus-dissolving drug	T50.991	T50.992	T50.993	T50.994	T50.995	T50.996
Calomel	T49.0X1	T49.0X2	T49.0X3	T49.0X4	T49.0X5	T49.0X6
Caloric agent	T50.3X1	T50.3X2	T50.3X3	T50.3X4	T50.3X5	T50.3X6
Calusterone	T38.7X1	T38.7X2	T38.7X3	T38.7X4	T38.7X5	T38.7X6
Camazepam	T42.4X1	T42.4X2	T42.4X3	T42.4X4	T42.4X5	T42.4X6
Camomile	T49.0X1	T49.0X2	T49.0X3	T49.0X4	T49.0X5	T49.0X6
Camoquin	T37.2X1	T37.2X2	T37.2X3	T37.2X4	T37.2X5	T37.2X6
Camphor						
insecticide	T60.2X1	T60.2X2	T60.2X3	T60.2X4	—	—
medicinal	T49.8X1	T49.8X2	T49.8X3	T49.8X4	T49.8X5	T49.8X6
Camylofin	T44.3X1	T44.3X2	T44.3X3	T44.3X4	T44.3X5	T44.3X6
Cancer chemotherapy drug regimen	T45.1X1	T45.1X2	T45.1X3	T45.1X4	T45.1X5	T45.1X6
Candeptin	T49.0X1	T49.0X2	T49.0X3	T49.0X4	T49.0X5	T49.0X6
Candicidin	T49.0X1	T49.0X2	T49.0X3	T49.0X4	T49.0X5	T49.0X6
Cannabinol	T40.7X1	T40.7X2	T40.7X3	T40.7X4	T40.7X5	T40.7X6
Cannabis (derivatives)	T40.7X1	T40.7X2	T40.7X3	T40.7X4	T40.7X5	T40.7X6
Canned heat	T51.1X1	T51.1X2	T51.1X3	T51.1X4	—	—
Canrenoic acid	T50.0X1	T50.0X2	T50.0X3	T50.0X4	T50.0X5	T50.0X6
Canrenone	T50.0X1	T50.0X2	T50.0X3	T50.0X4	T50.0X5	T50.0X6
Cantharides, cantharidin, cantharis	T49.8X1	T49.8X2	T49.8X3	T49.8X4	T49.8X5	T49.8X6

◀ New   ◀▥ Revised   ~~deleted~~ Deleted

Substance	Poisoning, Accidental (Unintentional)	Poisoning, Intentional Self-Harm	Poisoning, Assault	Poisoning, Undetermined	Adverse Effect	Underdosing
Canthaxanthin	T50.991	T50.992	T50.993	T50.994	T50.995	T50.996
Capillary-active drug NEC	T46.901	T46.902	T46.903	T46.904	T46.905	T46.906
Capreomycin	T36.8X1	T36.8X2	T36.8X3	T36.8X4	T36.8X5	T36.8X6
Capsicum	T49.4X1	T49.4X2	T49.4X3	T49.4X4	T49.4X5	T49.4X6
Captafol	T60.3X1	T60.3X2	T60.3X3	T60.3X4	—	—
Captan	T60.3X1	T60.3X2	T60.3X3	T60.3X4	—	—
Captodiame, captodiamine	T43.591	T43.592	T43.593	T43.594	T43.595	T43.596
Captopril	T46.4X1	T46.4X2	T46.4X3	T46.4X4	T46.4X5	T46.4X6
Caramiphen	T44.3X1	T44.3X2	T44.3X3	T44.3X4	T44.3X5	T44.3X6
Carazolol	T44.7X1	T44.7X2	T44.7X3	T44.7X4	T44.7X5	T44.7X6
Carbachol	T44.1X1	T44.1X2	T44.1X3	T44.1X4	T44.1X5	T44.1X6
Carbacrylamine (resin)	T50.3X1	T50.3X2	T50.3X3	T50.3X4	T50.3X5	T50.3X6
Carbamate (insecticide)	T60.0X1	T60.0X2	T60.0X3	T60.0X4	—	—
Carbamate (sedative)	T42.6X1	T42.6X2	T42.6X3	T42.6X4	T42.6X5	T42.6X6
herbicide	T60.0X1	T60.0X2	T60.0X3	T60.0X4		
insecticide	T60.0X1	T60.0X2	T60.0X3	T60.0X4	—	—
Carbamazepine	T42.1X1	T42.1X2	T42.1X3	T42.1X4	T42.1X5	T42.1X6
Carbamide	T47.3X1	T47.3X2	T47.3X3	T47.3X4	T47.3X5	T47.3X6
peroxide	T49.0X1	T49.0X2	T49.0X3	T49.0X4	T49.0X5	T49.0X6
topical	T49.8X1	T49.8X2	T49.8X3	T49.8X4	T49.8X5	T49.8X6
Carbamylcholine chloride	T44.1X1	T44.1X2	T44.1X3	T44.1X4	T44.1X5	T44.1X6
Carbaril	T60.0X1	T60.0X2	T60.0X3	T60.0X4	—	—
Carbarsone	T37.3X1	T37.3X2	T37.3X3	T37.3X4	T37.3X5	T37.3X6
Carbaryl	T60.0X1	T60.0X2	T60.0X3	T60.0X4	—	—
Carbaspirin	T39.011	T39.012	T39.013	T39.014	T39.015	T39.016
Carbazochrome (salicylate) (sodium sulfonate)	T49.4X1	T49.4X2	T49.4X3	T49.4X4	T49.4X5	T49.4X6
Carbenicillin	T36.0X1	T36.0X2	T36.0X3	T36.0X4	T36.0X5	T36.0X6
Carbenoxolone	T47.1X1	T47.1X2	T47.1X3	T47.1X4	T47.1X5	T47.1X6
Carbetapentane	T48.3X1	T48.3X2	T48.3X3	T48.3X4	T48.3X5	T48.3X6
Carbethyl salicylate	T39.091	T39.092	T39.093	T39.094	T39.095	T39.096
Carbidopa (with levodopa)	T42.8X1	T42.8X2	T42.8X3	T42.8X4	T42.8X5	T42.8X6
Carbimazole	T38.2X1	T38.2X2	T38.2X3	T38.2X4	T38.2X5	T38.2X6
Carbinol	T51.1X1	T51.1X2	T51.1X3	T51.1X4	—	—
Carbinoxamine	T45.0X1	T45.0X2	T45.0X3	T45.0X4	T45.0X5	T45.0X6
Carbiphene	T39.8X1	T39.8X2	T39.8X3	T39.8X4	T39.8X5	T39.8X6
Carbitol	T52.3X1	T52.3X2	T52.3X3	T52.3X4	—	—
Carbocaine	T41.3X1	T41.3X2	T41.3X3	T41.3X4	T41.3X5	T41.3X6
infiltration (subcutaneous)	T41.3X1	T41.3X2	T41.3X3	T41.3X4	T41.3X5	T41.3X6
nerve block (peripheral) (plexus)	T41.3X1	T41.3X2	T41.3X3	T41.3X4	T41.3X5	T41.3X6
topical (surface)	T41.3X1	T41.3X2	T41.3X3	T41.3X4	T41.3X5	T41.3X6
Carbo medicinalis	T47.6X1	T47.6X2	T47.6X3	T47.6X4	T47.6X5	T47.6X6

Substance	Poisoning, Accidental (Unintentional)	Poisoning, Intentional Self-Harm	Poisoning, Assault	Poisoning, Undetermined	Adverse Effect	Underdosing
Carbomycin	T36.8X1	T36.8X2	T36.8X4	T36.8X4	T36.8X5	T36.8X6
Carbocisteine	T48.4X1	T48.4X2	T48.4X3	T48.4X4	T48.4X5	T48.4X6
Carbocromen	T46.3X1	T46.3X2	T46.3X3	T46.3X4	T46.3X5	T46.3X6
Carbol fuchsin	T49.0X1	T49.0X2	T49.0X3	T49.0X4	T49.0X5	T49.0X6
Carbolic acid — *see also* Phenol	T54.0X1	T54.0X2	T54.0X3	T54.0X4	—	—
Carbolonium (bromide)	T48.1X1	T48.1X2	T48.1X3	T48.1X4	T48.1X5	T48.1X6
Carbon						
bisulfide (liquid)	T65.4X1	T65.4X2	T65.4X3	T65.4X4		
vapor	T65.4X1	T65.4X2	T65.4X3	T65.4X4		
dioxide (gas)	T59.7X1	T59.7X2	T59.7X3	T59.7X4	—	—
medicinal	T41.5X1	T41.5X2	T41.5X3	T41.5X4	T41.5X5	T41.5X6
nonmedicinal	T59.7X1	T59.7X2	T59.7X3	T59.7X4		
snow	T49.4X1	T49.4X2	T49.4X3	T49.4X4	T49.4X5	T49.4X6
disulfide (liquid)	T65.4X1	T65.4X2	T65.4X3	T65.4X4		
vapor	T65.4X1	T65.4X2	T65.4X3	T65.4X4		
monoxide (from incomplete combustion)	T58.91	T58.92	T58.93	T58.94		
blast furnace gas	T58.8X1	T58.8X2	T58.8X3	T58.8X4	—	—
butane (distributed in mobile container)	T58.11	T58.12	T58.13	T58.14	—	—
distributed through pipes	T58.11	T58.12	T58.13	T58.14	—	—
charcoal fumes	T58.2X1	T58.2X2	T58.2X3	T58.2X4		
coal	T58.2X1	T58.2X2	T58.2X3	T58.2X4		
coke (in domestic stoves, fireplaces)	T58.2X1	T58.2X2	T58.2X3	T58.2X4		
gas (piped)	T58.11	T58.12	T58.13	T58.14	—	—
solid (in domestic stoves, fireplaces)	T58.2X1	T58.2X2	T58.2X3	T58.2X4	—	—
exhaust gas (motor) not in transit	T58.01	T58.02	T58.03	T58.04	—	—
combustion engine, any not in watercraft	T58.01	T58.02	T58.03	T58.04		
farm tractor, not in transit	T58.01	T58.02	T58.03	T58.04		
gas engine	T58.01	T58.02	T58.03	T58.04	—	—
motor pump	T58.01	T58.02	T58.03	T58.04	—	—
motor vehicle, not in transit	T58.01	T58.02	T58.03	T58.04	—	—
fuel (in domestic use)	T58.2X1	T58.2X2	T58.2X3	T58.2X4		
gas (piped)	T58.11	T58.12	T58.13	T58.14	—	—
in mobile container	T58.11	T58.12	T58.13	T58.14	—	—
utility	T58.11	T58.12	T58.13	T58.14		
in mobile container	T58.11	T58.12	T58.13	T58.14		
piped (natural)	T58.11	T58.12	T58.13	T58.14	—	—

◀ New   ◀▬ Revised   ~~deleted~~ Deleted

TABLE OF DRUGS AND CHEMICALS

	External Cause (T-Code)					
Substance	Poisoning, Accidental (Unintentional)	Poisoning, Intentional Self-Harm	Poisoning, Assault	Poisoning, Undetermined	Adverse Effect	Underdosing
Carbon (Continued)						
monoxide (Continued)						
illuminating gas	T58.11	T58.12	T58.13	T58.14	—	—
industrial fuels or gases, any	T58.8X1	T58.8X2	T58.8X3	T58.8X4	—	—
kerosene (in domestic stoves, fireplaces)	T58.2X1	T58.2X2	T58.2X3	T58.2X4	—	—
kiln gas or vapor	T58.8X1	T58.8X2	T58.8X3	T58.8X4	—	—
motor exhaust gas, not in transit	T58.01	T58.02	T58.03	T58.04	—	—
piped gas (manufactured) (natural)	T58.11	T58.12	T58.13	T58.14	—	—
producer gas	T58.8X1	T58.8X2	T58.8X3	T58.8X4	—	—
propane (distributed in mobile container)	T58.11	T58.12	T58.13	T58.14	—	—
distributed through pipes	T58.11	T58.12	T58.13	T58.14	—	—
specified source NEC	T58.8X1	T58.8X2	T58.8X3	T58.8X4	—	—
stove gas	T58.11	T58.12	T58.13	T58.14	—	—
piped	T58.11	T58.12	T58.13	T58.14	—	—
utility gas	T58.11	T58.12	T58.13	T58.14	—	—
piped	T58.11	T58.12	T58.13	T58.14	—	—
water gas	T58.11	T58.12	T58.13	T58.14	—	—
wood (in domestic stoves, fireplaces)	T58.2X1	T58.2X2	T58.2X3	T58.2X4	—	—
tetrachloride (vapor) NEC	T53.0X1	T53.0X2	T53.0X3	T53.0X4	—	—
liquid (cleansing agent) NEC	T53.0X1	T53.0X2	T53.0X3	T53.0X4	—	—
solvent	T53.0X1	T53.0X2	T53.0X3	T53.0X4	—	—
Carbonic acid gas	T59.7X1	T59.7X2	T59.7X3	T59.7X4	—	—
anhydrase inhibitor NEC	T50.2X1	T50.2X2	T50.2X3	T50.2X4	T50.2X5	T50.2X6
Carbophenothion	T60.0X1	T60.0X2	T60.0X3	T60.0X4	—	—
Carboplatin	T45.1X1	T45.1X2	T45.1X3	T45.1X4	T45.1X5	T45.1X6
Carboprost	T48.0X1	T48.0X2	T48.0X3	T48.0X4	T48.0X5	T48.0X6
Carboquone	T45.1X1	T45.1X2	T45.1X3	T45.1X4	T45.1X5	T45.1X6
Carbowax	T49.3X1	T49.3X2	T49.3X3	T49.3X4	T49.3X5	T49.3X6
Carboxymethyl-cellulose	T47.4X1	T47.4X2	T47.4X3	T47.4X4	T47.4X5	T47.4X6
S-Carboxymethyl-cysteine	T48.4X1	T48.4X2	T48.4X3	T48.4X4	T48.4X5	T48.4X6
Carbrital	T42.3X1	T42.3X2	T42.3X3	T42.3X4	T42.3X5	T42.3X6
Carbromal	T42.6X1	T42.6X2	T42.6X3	T42.6X4	T42.6X5	T42.6X6
Carbutamide	T38.3X1	T38.3X2	T38.3X3	T38.3X4	T38.3X5	T38.3X6
Carbuterol	T48.6X1	T48.6X2	T48.6X3	T48.6X4	T48.6X5	T48.6X6
Cardiac						
depressants	T46.2X1	T46.2X2	T46.2X3	T46.2X4	T46.2X5	T46.2X6
rhythm regulator	T46.2X1	T46.2X2	T46.2X3	T46.2X4	T46.2X5	T46.2X6
specified NEC	T46.2X1	T46.2X2	T46.2X3	T46.2X4	T46.2X5	T46.2X6

	External Cause (T-Code)					
Substance	Poisoning, Accidental (Unintentional)	Poisoning, Intentional Self-Harm	Poisoning, Assault	Poisoning, Undetermined	Adverse Effect	Underdosing
Cardiografin	T50.8X1	T50.8X2	T50.8X3	T50.8X4	T50.8X5	T50.8X6
Cardio-green	T50.8X1	T50.8X2	T50.8X3	T50.8X4	T50.8X5	T50.8X6
Cardiotonic (glycoside) NEC	T46.0X1	T46.0X2	T46.0X3	T46.0X4	T46.0X5	T46.0X6
Cardiovascular drug NEC	T46.901	T46.902	T46.903	T46.904	T46.905	T46.906
Cardrase	T50.2X1	T50.2X2	T50.2X3	T50.2X4	T50.2X5	T50.2X6
Carfusin	T49.0X1	T49.0X2	T49.0X3	T49.0X4	T49.0X5	T49.0X6
Carfecillin	T36.0X1	T36.0X2	T36.0X3	T36.0X4	T36.0X5	T36.0X6
Carfenazine	T43.3X1	T43.3X2	T43.3X3	T43.3X4	T43.3X5	T43.3X6
Carindacillin	T36.0X1	T36.0X2	T36.0X3	T36.0X4	T36.0X5	T36.0X6
Carisoprodol	T42.8X1	T42.8X2	T42.8X3	T42.8X4	T42.8X5	T42.8X6
Carmellose	T47.4X1	T47.4X2	T47.4X3	T47.4X4	T47.4X5	T47.4X6
Carminative	T47.5X1	T47.5X2	T47.5X3	T47.5X4	T47.5X5	T47.5X6
Carmofur	T45.1X1	T45.1X2	T45.1X3	T45.1X4	T45.1X5	T45.1X6
Carmustine	T45.1X1	T45.1X2	T45.1X3	T45.1X4	T45.1X5	T45.1X6
Carotene	T45.2X1	T45.2X2	T45.2X3	T45.2X4	T45.2X5	T45.2X6
Carphenazine	T43.3X1	T43.3X2	T43.3X3	T43.3X4	T43.3X5	T43.3X6
Carpipramine	T42.4X1	T42.4X2	T42.4X3	T42.4X4	T42.4X5	T42.4X6
Carprofen	T39.311	T39.312	T39.313	T39.314	T39.315	T39.316
Carpronium chloride	T44.3X1	T44.3X2	T44.3X3	T44.3X4	T44.3X5	T44.3X6
Carrageenan	T47.8X1	T47.8X2	T47.8X3	T47.8X4	T47.8X5	T47.8X6
Carteolol	T44.7X1	T44.7X2	T44.7X3	T44.7X4	T44.7X5	T44.7X6
Carter's Little Pills	T47.2X1	T47.2X2	T47.2X3	T47.2X4	T47.2X5	T47.2X6
Cascara (sagrada)	T47.2X1	T47.2X2	T47.2X3	T47.2X4	T47.2X5	T47.2X6
Cassava	T62.2X1	T62.2X2	T62.2X3	T62.2X4	—	—
Castellani's paint	T49.0X1	T49.0X2	T49.0X3	T49.0X4	T49.0X5	T49.0X6
Castor						
bean	T62.2X1	T62.2X2	T62.2X3	T62.2X4	—	—
oil	T47.2X1	T47.2X2	T47.2X3	T47.2X4	T47.2X5	T47.2X6
Catalase	T45.3X1	T45.3X2	T45.3X3	T45.3X4	T45.3X5	T45.3X6
Caterpillar (sting)	T63.431	T63.432	T63.433	T63.434	—	—
Catha (edulis) (tea)	T43.691	T43.692	T43.693	T43.694	—	—
Cathartic NEC	T47.4X1	T47.4X2	T47.4X3	T47.4X4	T47.4X5	T47.4X6
anthacene derivative	T47.2X1	T47.2X2	T47.2X3	T47.2X4	T47.2X5	T47.2X6
bulk	T47.4X1	T47.4X2	T47.4X3	T47.4X4	T47.4X5	T47.4X6
contact	T47.2X1	T47.2X2	T47.2X3	T47.2X4	T47.2X5	T47.2X6
emollient NEC	T47.4X1	T47.4X2	T47.4X3	T47.4X4	T47.4X5	T47.4X6
irritant NEC	T47.2X1	T47.2X2	T47.2X3	T47.2X4	T47.2X5	T47.2X6
mucilage	T47.4X1	T47.4X2	T47.4X3	T47.4X4	T47.4X5	T47.4X6
saline	T47.3X1	T47.3X2	T47.3X3	T47.3X4	T47.3X5	T47.3X6
vegetable	T47.2X1	T47.2X2	T47.2X3	T47.2X4	T47.2X5	T47.2X6
Cathine	T50.5X1	T50.5X2	T50.5X3	T50.5X4	T50.5X5	T50.5X6
Cathomycin	T36.8X1	T36.8X2	T36.8X3	T36.8X4	T36.8X5	T36.8X6

◄ New ◄▥ Revised ~~deleted~~ Deleted

Substance	Poisoning, Accidental (Unintentional)	Poisoning, Intentional Self-Harm	Poisoning, Assault	Poisoning, Undetermined	Adverse Effect	Underdosing
	External Cause (T-Code)					
Cation exchange resin	T50.3X1	T50.3X2	T50.3X3	T50.3X4	T50.3X5	T50.3X6
Caustic(s) NEC	T54.91	T54.92	T54.93	T54.94	—	—
alkali	T54.3X1	T54.3X2	T54.3X3	T54.3X4	—	—
hydroxide	T54.3X1	T54.3X2	T54.3X3	T54.3X4	—	—
potash	T54.3X1	T54.3X2	T54.3X3	T54.3X4	—	—
soda	T54.3X1	T54.3X2	T54.3X3	T54.3X4	—	—
specified NEC	T54.91	T54.92	T54.93	T54.94	—	—
Ceepryn	T49.0X1	T49.0X2	T49.0X3	T49.0X4	T49.0X5	T49.0X6
ENT agent	T49.6X1	T49.6X2	T49.6X3	T49.6X4	T49.6X5	T49.6X6
lozenges	T49.6X1	T49.6X2	T49.6X3	T49.6X4	T49.6X5	T49.6X6
Cefacetrile	T36.1X1	T36.1X2	T36.1X3	T36.1X4	T36.1X5	T36.1X6
Cefaclor	T36.1X1	T36.1X2	T36.1X3	T36.1X4	T36.1X5	T36.1X6
Cefadroxil	T36.1X1	T36.1X2	T36.1X3	T36.1X4	T36.1X5	T36.1X6
Cefalexin	T36.1X1	T36.1X2	T36.1X3	T36.1X4	T36.1X5	T36.1X6
Cefaloglycin	T36.1X1	T36.1X2	T36.1X3	T36.1X4	T36.1X5	T36.1X6
Cefaloridine	T36.1X1	T36.1X2	T36.1X3	T36.1X4	T36.1X5	T36.1X6
Cefalosporins	T36.1X1	T36.1X2	T36.1X3	T36.1X4	T36.1X5	T36.1X6
Cefalotin	T36.1X1	T36.1X2	T36.1X3	T36.1X4	T36.1X5	T36.1X6
Cefamandole	T36.1X1	T36.1X2	T36.1X3	T36.1X4	T36.1X5	T36.1X6
Cefamycin antibiotic	T36.1X1	T36.1X2	T36.1X3	T36.1X4	T36.1X5	T36.1X6
Cefapirin	T36.1X1	T36.1X2	T36.1X3	T36.1X4	T36.1X5	T36.1X6
Cefatrizine	T36.1X1	T36.1X2	T36.1X3	T36.1X4	T36.1X5	T36.1X6
Cefazedone	T36.1X1	T36.1X2	T36.1X3	T36.1X4	T36.1X5	T36.1X6
Cefazolin	T36.1X1	T36.1X2	T36.1X3	T36.1X4	T36.1X5	T36.1X6
Cefbuperazone	T36.1X1	T36.1X2	T36.1X3	T36.1X4	T36.1X5	T36.1X6
Cefetamet	T36.1X1	T36.1X2	T36.1X3	T36.1X4	T36.1X5	T36.1X6
Cefixime	T36.1X1	T36.1X2	T36.1X3	T36.1X4	T36.1X5	T36.1X6
Cefmenoxime	T36.1X1	T36.1X2	T36.1X3	T36.1X4	T36.1X5	T36.1X6
Cefmetazole	T36.1X1	T36.1X2	T36.1X3	T36.1X4	T36.1X5	T36.1X6
Cefminox	T36.1X1	T36.1X2	T36.1X3	T36.1X4	T36.1X5	T36.1X6
Cefonicid	T36.1X1	T36.1X2	T36.1X3	T36.1X4	T36.1X5	T36.1X6
Cefoperazone	T36.1X1	T36.1X2	T36.1X3	T36.1X4	T36.1X5	T36.1X6
Cefotaxime	T36.1X1	T36.1X2	T36.1X3	T36.1X4	T36.1X5	T36.1X6
Cefotetan	T36.1X1	T36.1X2	T36.1X3	T36.1X4	T36.1X5	T36.1X6
Cefotiam	T36.1X1	T36.1X2	T36.1X3	T36.1X4	T36.1X5	T36.1X6
Cefoxitin	T36.1X1	T36.1X2	T36.1X3	T36.1X4	T36.1X5	T36.1X6
Cefpimizole	T36.1X1	T36.1X2	T36.1X3	T36.1X4	T36.1X5	T36.1X6
Cefpiramide	T36.1X1	T36.1X2	T36.1X3	T36.1X4	T36.1X5	T36.1X6
Cefradine	T36.1X1	T36.1X2	T36.1X3	T36.1X4	T36.1X5	T36.1X6
Cefroxadine	T36.1X1	T36.1X2	T36.1X3	T36.1X4	T36.1X5	T36.1X6
Cefsulodin	T36.1X1	T36.1X2	T36.1X3	T36.1X4	T36.1X5	T36.1X6

Substance	Poisoning, Accidental (Unintentional)	Poisoning, Intentional Self-Harm	Poisoning, Assault	Poisoning, Undetermined	Adverse Effect	Underdosing
	External Cause (T-Code)					
Ceftazidime	T36.1X1	T36.1X2	T36.1X3	T36.1X4	T36.1X5	T36.1X6
Cefteram	T36.1X1	T36.1X2	T36.1X3	T36.1X4	T36.1X5	T36.1X6
Ceftezole	T36.1X1	T36.1X2	T36.1X3	T36.1X4	T36.1X5	T36.1X6
Ceftizoxime	T36.1X1	T36.1X2	T36.1X3	T36.1X4	T36.1X5	T36.1X6
Ceftriaxone	T36.1X1	T36.1X2	T36.1X3	T36.1X4	T36.1X5	T36.1X6
Cefuroxime	T36.1X1	T36.1X2	T36.1X3	T36.1X4	T36.1X5	T36.1X6
Cefuzonam	T36.1X1	T36.1X2	T36.1X3	T36.1X4	T36.1X5	T36.1X6
Celestone	T38.0X1	T38.0X2	T38.0X3	T38.0X4	T38.0X5	T38.0X6
topical	T49.0X1	T49.0X2	T49.0X3	T49.0X4	T49.0X5	T49.0X6
Celiprolol	T44.7X1	T44.7X2	T44.7X3	T44.7X4	T44.7X5	T44.7X6
Cellosolve	T52.91	T52.92	T52.93	T52.94	—	—
Cell stimulants and proliferants	T49.8X1	T49.8X2	T49.8X3	T49.8X4	T49.8X5	T49.8X6
Cellulose						
cathartic	T47.4X1	T47.4X2	T47.4X3	T47.4X4	T47.4X5	T47.4X6
hydroxyethyl	T47.4X1	T47.4X2	T47.4X3	T47.4X4	T47.4X5	T47.4X6
nitrates (topical)	T49.3X1	T49.3X2	T49.3X3	T49.3X4	T49.3X5	T49.3X6
oxidized	T49.4X1	T49.4X2	T49.4X3	T49.4X4	T49.4X5	T49.4X6
Centipede (bite)	T63.411	T63.412	T63.413	T63.414	—	—
Central nervous system						
depressants	T42.71	T42.72	T42.73	T42.74	T42.75	T42.76
anesthetic (general) NEC	T41.201	T41.202	T41.203	T41.204	T41.205	T41.206
gases NEC	T41.0X1	T41.0X2	T41.0X3	T41.0X4	T41.0X5	T41.0X6
intravenous	T41.1X1	T41.1X2	T41.1X3	T41.1X4	T41.1X5	T41.1X6
barbiturates	T42.3X1	T42.3X2	T42.3X3	T42.3X4	T42.3X5	T42.3X6
benzodiazepines	T42.4X1	T42.4X2	T42.4X3	T42.4X4	T42.4X5	T42.4X6
bromides	T42.6X1	T42.6X2	T42.6X3	T42.6X4	T42.6X5	T42.6X6
cannabis sativa	T40.7X1	T40.7X2	T40.7X3	T40.7X4	T40.7X5	T40.7X6
chloral hydrate	T42.6X1	T42.6X2	T42.6X3	T42.6X4	T42.6X5	T42.6X6
ethanol	T51.0X1	T51.0X2	T51.0X3	T51.0X4	—	—
hallucinogenics	T40.901	T40.902	T40.903	T40.904	T40.905	T40.906
hypnotics	T42.71	T42.72	T42.73	T42.74	T42.75	T42.76
specified NEC	T42.6X1	T42.6X2	T42.6X3	T42.6X4	T42.6X5	T42.6X6
muscle relaxants	T42.8X1	T42.8X2	T42.8X3	T42.8X4	T42.8X5	T42.8X6
paraldehyde	T42.6X1	T42.6X2	T42.6X3	T42.6X4	T42.6X5	T42.6X6
sedatives; sedative-hypnotics	T42.71	T42.72	T42.73	T42.74	T42.75	T42.76
mixed NEC	T42.6X1	T42.6X2	T42.6X3	T42.6X4	T42.6X5	T42.6X6
specified NEC	T42.6X1	T42.6X2	T42.6X3	T42.6X4	T42.6X5	T42.6X6
muscle-tone depressants	T42.8X1	T42.8X2	T42.8X3	T42.8X4	T42.8X5	T42.8X6
stimulants	T43.601	T43.602	T43.603	T43.604	T43.605	T43.606
amphetamines	T43.621	T43.622	T43.623	T43.624	T43.625	T43.626
analeptics	T50.7X1	T50.7X2	T50.7X3	T50.7X4	T50.7X5	T50.7X6

◀ New ◀▦ Revised ~~deleted~~ Deleted

TABLE OF DRUGS AND CHEMICALS

Substance	External Cause (T-Code)					
	Poisoning, Accidental (Unintentional)	Poisoning, Intentional Self-Harm	Poisoning, Assault	Poisoning, Undetermined	Adverse Effect	Underdosing
Central nervous system (Continued)						
stimulants (Continued)						
antidepressants	T43.2Ø1	T43.2Ø2	T43.2Ø3	T43.2Ø4	T43.2Ø5	T43.2Ø6
opiate antagonists	T5Ø.7X1	T5Ø.7X2	T5Ø.7X3	T5Ø.7X4	T5Ø.7X5	T5Ø.7X6
specified NEC	T43.691	T43.692	T43.693	T43.694	T43.695	T43.696
Cephalexin	T36.1X1	T36.1X2	T36.1X3	T36.1X4	T36.1X5	T36.1X6
Cephaloglycin	T36.1X1	T36.1X2	T36.1X3	T36.1X4	T36.1X5	T36.1X6
Cephaloridine	T36.1X1	T36.1X2	T36.1X3	T36.1X4	T36.1X5	T36.1X6
Cephalosporins	T36.1X1	T36.1X2	T36.1X3	T36.1X4	T36.1X5	T36.1X6
N (adicillin)	T36.ØX1	T36.ØX2	T36.ØX3	T36.ØX4	T36.ØX5	T36.ØX6
Cephalothin	T36.1X1	T36.1X2	T36.1X3	T36.1X4	T36.1X5	T36.1X6
Cephalotin	T36.1X1	T36.1X2	T36.1X3	T36.1X4	T36.1X5	T36.1X6
Cephradine	T36.1X1	T36.1X2	T36.1X3	T36.1X4	T36.1X5	T36.1X6
Cerbera (odallam)	T62.2X1	T62.2X2	T62.2X3	T62.2X4	—	—
Cerberin	T46.ØX1	T46.ØX2	T46.ØX3	T46.ØX4	T46.ØX5	T46.ØX6
Cerebral stimulants	T43.6Ø1	T43.6Ø2	T43.6Ø3	T43.6Ø4	T43.6Ø5	T43.6Ø6
psychotherapeutic	T43.6Ø1	T43.6Ø2	T43.6Ø3	T43.6Ø4	T43.6Ø5	T43.6Ø6
specified NEC	T43.691	T43.692	T43.693	T43.694	T43.695	T43.696
Cerium oxalate	T45.ØX1	T45.ØX2	T45.ØX3	T45.ØX4	T45.ØX5	T45.ØX6
Cerous oxalate	T45.ØX1	T45.ØX2	T45.ØX3	T45.ØX4	T45.ØX5	T45.ØX6
Ceruletide	T5Ø.8X1	T5Ø.8X2	T5Ø.8X3	T5Ø.8X4	T5Ø.8X5	T5Ø.8X6
Cetalkonium (chloride)	T49.ØX1	T49.ØX2	T49.ØX3	T49.ØX4	T49.ØX5	T49.ØX6
Cethexonium chloride	T49.ØX1	T49.ØX2	T49.ØX3	T49.ØX4	T49.ØX5	T49.ØX6
Cetiedil	T46.7X1	T46.7X2	T46.7X3	T46.7X4	T46.7X5	T46.7X6
Cetirizine	T45.ØX1	T45.ØX2	T45.ØX3	T45.ØX4	T45.ØX5	T45.ØX6
Cetomacrogol	T5Ø.991	T5Ø.992	T5Ø.993	T5Ø.994	T5Ø.995	T5Ø.996
Cetotiamine	T45.2X1	T45.2X2	T45.2X3	T45.2X4	T45.2X5	T45.2X6
Cetoxime	T45.ØX1	T45.ØX2	T45.ØX3	T45.ØX4	T45.ØX5	T45.ØX6
Cetraxate	T47.1X1	T47.1X2	T47.1X3	T47.1X4	T47.1X5	T47.1X6
Cetrimide	T49.ØX1	T49.ØX2	T49.ØX3	T49.ØX4	T49.ØX5	T49.ØX6
Cetrimonium (bromide)	T49.ØX1	T49.ØX2	T49.ØX3	T49.ØX4	T49.ØX5	T49.ØX6
Cetylpyridinium chloride	T49.ØX1	T49.ØX2	T49.ØX3	T49.ØX4	T49.ØX5	T49.ØX6
ENT agent	T49.6X1	T49.6X2	T49.6X3	T49.6X4	T49.6X5	T49.6X6
lozenges	T49.6X1	T49.6X2	T49.6X3	T49.6X4	T49.6X5	T49.6X6
Cevadillasee Sabadilla						
Cevitamic acid	T45.2X1	T45.2X2	T45.2X3	T45.2X4	T45.2X5	T45.2X6
Chalk, precipitated	T47.1X1	T47.1X2	T47.1X3	T47.1X4	T47.1X5	T47.1X6
Chamomile	T49.ØX1	T49.ØX2	T49.ØX3	T49.ØX4	T49.ØX5	T49.ØX6
Ch'an su	T46.ØX1	T46.ØX2	T46.ØX3	T46.ØX4	T46.ØX5	T46.ØX6
Charcoal	T47.6X1	T47.6X2	T47.6X3	T47.6X4	T47.6X5	T47.6X6
activated — see also Charcoal, medicinal	T47.6X1	T47.6X2	T47.6X3	T47.6X4	T47.6X5	T47.6X6

Substance	External Cause (T-Code)					
	Poisoning, Accidental (Unintentional)	Poisoning, Intentional Self-Harm	Poisoning, Assault	Poisoning, Undetermined	Adverse Effect	Underdosing
Charcoal (Continued)						
fumes (Carbon monoxide)	T58.2X1	T58.2X2	T58.2X3	T58.2X4	—	—
industrial	T58.8X1	T58.8X2	T58.8X3	T58.8X4	—	—
medicinal (activated)	T47.6X1	T47.6X2	T47.6X3	T47.6X4	T47.6X5	T47.6X6
antidiarrheal	T47.6X1	T47.6X2	T47.6X3	T47.6X4	T47.6X5	T47.6X6
poison control	T47.8X1	T47.8X2	T47.8X3	T47.8X4	T47.8X5	T47.8X6
specified use other than for diarrhea	T47.8X1	T47.8X2	T47.8X3	T47.8X4	T47.8X5	T47.8X6
topical	T49.8X1	T49.8X2	T49.8X3	T49.8X4	T49.8X5	T49.8X6
Chaulmosulfone	T37.1X1	T37.1X2	T37.1X3	T37.1X4	T37.1X5	T37.1X6
Chelating agent NEC	T5Ø.6X1	T5Ø.6X2	T5Ø.6X3	T5Ø.6X4	T5Ø.6X5	T5Ø.6X6
Chelidonium majus	T62.2X1	T62.2X2	T62.2X3	T62.2X4	—	—
Chemical substance NEC	T65.91	T65.92	T65.93	T65.94	—	—
Chenodeoxycholic acid	T47.5X1	T47.5X2	T47.5X3	T47.5X4	T47.5X5	T47.5X6
Chenodiol	T47.5X1	T47.5X2	T47.5X3	T47.5X4	T47.5X5	T47.5X6
Chenopodium	T37.4X1	T37.4X2	T37.4X3	T37.4X4	T37.4X5	T37.4X6
Cherry laurel	T62.2X1	T62.2X2	T62.2X3	T62.2X4	—	—
Chinidin(e)	T46.2X1	T46.2X2	T46.2X3	T46.2X4	T46.2X5	T46.2X6
Chiniofon	T37.8X1	T37.8X2	T37.8X3	T37.8X4	T37.8X5	T37.8X6
Chlophedianol	T48.3X1	T48.3X2	T48.3X3	T48.3X4	T48.3X5	T48.3X6
Chloral	T42.6X1	T42.6X2	T42.6X3	T42.6X4	T42.6X5	T42.6X6
derivative	T42.6X1	T42.6X2	T42.6X3	T42.6X4	T42.6X5	T42.6X6
hydrate	T42.6X1	T42.6X2	T42.6X3	T42.6X4	T42.6X5	T42.6X6
Chloralamide	T42.6X1	T42.6X2	T42.6X3	T42.6X4	T42.6X5	T42.6X6
Chloralodol	T42.6X1	T42.6X2	T42.6X3	T42.6X4	T42.6X5	T42.6X6
Chloralose	T6Ø.4X1	T6Ø.4X2	T6Ø.4X3	T6Ø.4X4	—	—
Chlorambucil	T45.1X1	T45.1X2	T45.1X3	T45.1X4	T45.1X5	T45.1X6
Chloramine	T57.8X1	T57.8X2	T57.8X3	T57.8X4	—	—
T	T49.ØX1	T49.ØX2	T49.ØX3	T49.ØX4	T49.ØX5	T49.ØX6
topical	T49.ØX1	T49.ØX2	T49.ØX3	T49.ØX4	T49.ØX5	T49.ØX6
Chloramphenicol	T36.2X1	T36.2X2	T36.2X3	T36.2X4	T36.2X5	T36.2X6
ENT agent	T49.6X1	T49.6X2	T49.6X3	T49.6X4	T49.6X5	T49.6X6
ophthalmic preparation	T49.5X1	T49.5X2	T49.5X3	T49.5X4	T49.5X5	T49.5X6
topical NEC	T49.ØX1	T49.ØX2	T49.ØX3	T49.ØX4	T49.ØX5	T49.ØX6
Chlorate (potassium) (sodium) NEC	T6Ø.3X1	T6Ø.3X2	T6Ø.3X3	T6Ø.3X4	—	—
herbicide	T6Ø.3X1	T6Ø.3X2	T6Ø.3X3	T6Ø.3X4	—	—
Chlorazanil	T5Ø.2X1	T5Ø.2X2	T5Ø.2X3	T5Ø.2X4	T5Ø.2X5	T5Ø.2X6
Chlorbenzene, chlorbenzol	T53.7X1	T53.7X2	T53.7X3	T53.7X4	—	—
Chlorbenzoxamine	T44.3X1	T44.3X2	T44.3X3	T44.3X4	T44.3X5	T44.3X6
Chlorbutol	T42.6X1	T42.6X2	T42.6X3	T42.6X4	T42.6X5	T42.6X6
Chlorcyclizine	T45.ØX1	T45.ØX2	T45.ØX3	T45.ØX4	T45.ØX5	T45.ØX6

◀ New   ⬅ Revised   ~~deleted~~ Deleted

Substance	Poisoning, Accidental (Unintentional)	Poisoning, Intentional Self-Harm	Poisoning, Assault	Poisoning, Undetermined	Adverse Effect	Underdosing
Chlordan(e) (dust)	T60.1X1	T60.1X2	T60.1X3	T60.1X4	—	—
Chlordantoin	T49.0X1	T49.0X2	T49.0X3	T49.0X4	T49.0X5	T49.0X6
Chlordiazepoxide	T42.4X1	T42.4X2	T42.4X3	T42.4X4	T42.4X5	T42.4X6
Chlordiethyl benzamide	T49.3X1	T49.3X2	T49.3X3	T49.3X4	T49.3X5	T49.3X6
Chloresium	T49.8X1	T49.8X2	T49.8X3	T49.8X4	T49.8X5	T49.8X6
Chlorethiazol	T42.6X1	T42.6X2	T42.6X3	T42.6X4	T42.6X5	T42.6X6
Chlorethyl — see Ethyl chloride						
Chloretone	T42.6X1	T42.6X2	T42.6X3	T42.6X4	T42.6X5	T42.6X6
Chlorex	T53.6X1	T53.6X2	T53.6X3	T53.6X4	—	—
insecticide	T60.1X1	T60.1X2	T60.1X3	T60.1X4	—	—
Chlorfenvinphos	T60.0X1	T60.0X2	T60.0X3	T60.0X4	—	—
Chlorhexadol	T42.6X1	T42.6X2	T42.6X3	T42.6X4	T42.6X5	T42.6X6
Chlorhexamide	T45.1X1	T45.1X2	T45.1X3	T45.1X4	T45.1X5	T45.1X6
Chlorhexidine	T49.0X1	T49.0X2	T49.0X3	T49.0X4	T49.0X5	T49.0X6
Chlorhydroxyquinolin	T49.0X1	T49.0X2	T49.0X3	T49.0X4	T49.0X5	T49.0X6
Chloride of lime (bleach)	T54.3X1	T54.3X2	T54.3X3	T54.3X4	—	—
Chlorimipramine	T43.011	T43.012	T43.013	T43.014	T43.015	T43.016
Chlorinated						
camphene	T53.6X1	T53.6X2	T53.6X3	T53.6X4	—	—
diphenyl	T53.7X1	T53.7X2	T53.7X3	T53.7X4	—	—
hydrocarbons NEC	T53.91	T53.92	T53.93	T53.94	—	—
solvents	T53.91	T53.92	T53.93	T53.94	—	—
lime (bleach)	T54.3X1	T54.3X2	T54.3X3	T54.3X4	—	—
and boric acid solution	T49.0X1	T49.0X2	T49.0X3	T49.0X4	T49.0X5	T49.0X6
naphthalene (insecticide)	T60.1X1	T60.1X2	T60.1X3	T60.1X4	—	—
industrial (non-pesticide)	T53.7X1	T53.7X2	T53.7X3	T53.7X4	—	—
pesticide NEC	T60.8X1	T60.8X2	T60.8X3	T60.8X4	—	—
soda — see also sodium hypochlorite						
solution	T49.0X1	T49.0X2	T49.0X3	T49.0X4	T49.0X5	T49.0X6
Chlorine (fumes) (gas)	T59.4X1	T59.4X2	T59.4X3	T59.4X4	—	—
bleach	T54.3X1	T54.3X2	T54.3X3	T54.3X4	—	—
compound gas NEC	T59.4X1	T59.4X2	T59.4X3	T59.4X4	—	—
disinfectant	T59.4X1	T59.4X2	T59.4X3	T59.4X4	—	—
releasing agents NEC	T59.4X1	T59.4X2	T59.4X3	T59.4X4	—	—
Chlorisondamine chloride	T46.991	T46.992	T46.993	T46.994	T46.995	T46.996
Chlormadinone	T38.5X1	T38.5X2	T38.5X3	T38.5X4	T38.5X5	T38.5X6
Chlormephos	T60.0X1	T60.0X2	T60.0X3	T60.0X4	—	—
Chlormerodrin	T50.2X1	T50.2X2	T50.2X3	T50.2X4	T50.2X5	T50.2X6
Chlormethiazole	T42.6X1	T42.6X2	T42.6X3	T42.6X4	T42.6X5	T42.6X6
Chlormethine	T45.1X1	T45.1X2	T45.1X3	T45.1X4	T45.1X5	T45.1X6
Chlormethylenecycline	T36.4X1	T36.4X2	T36.4X3	T36.4X4	T36.4X5	T36.4X6

Substance	Poisoning, Accidental (Unintentional)	Poisoning, Intentional Self-Harm	Poisoning, Assault	Poisoning, Undetermined	Adverse Effect	Underdosing
Chlormezanone	T42.6X1	T42.6X2	T42.6X3	T42.6X4	T42.6X5	T42.6X6
Chloroacetic acid	T60.3X1	T60.3X2	T60.3X3	T60.3X4	—	—
Chloroacetone	T59.3X1	T59.3X2	T59.3X3	T59.3X4	—	—
Chloroacetophenone	T59.3X1	T59.3X2	T59.3X3	T59.3X4	—	—
Chloroaniline	T53.7X1	T53.7X2	T53.7X3	T53.7X4	—	—
Chlorobenzene, chlorobenzol	T53.7X1	T53.7X2	T53.7X3	T53.7X4	—	—
Chlorobromomethane (fire extinguisher)	T53.6X1	T53.6X2	T53.6X3	T53.6X4	—	—
Chlorobutanol	T49.0X1	T49.0X2	T49.0X3	T49.0X4	T49.0X5	T49.0X6
Chlorocresol	T49.0X1	T49.0X2	T49.0X3	T49.0X4	T49.0X5	T49.0X6
Chlorodehydro-methyltestosterone	T38.7X1	T38.7X2	T38.7X3	T38.7X4	T38.7X5	T38.7X6
Chlorodinitrobenzene	T53.7X1	T53.7X2	T53.7X3	T53.7X4	—	—
dust or vapor	T53.7X1	T53.7X2	T53.7X3	T53.7X4	—	—
Chlorodiphenyl	T53.7X1	T53.7X2	T53.7X3	T53.7X4	—	—
Chloroethane — see Ethyl chloride						
Chloroethylene	T53.6X1	T53.6X2	T53.6X3	T53.6X4	—	—
Chlorofluorocarbons	T53.5X1	T53.5X2	T53.5X3	T53.5X4	—	—
Chloroform (fumes) (vapor)	T53.1X1	T53.1X2	T53.1X3	T53.1X4	—	—
anesthetic	T41.0X1	T41.0X2	T41.0X3	T41.0X4	T41.0X5	T41.0X6
solvent	T53.1X1	T53.1X2	T53.1X3	T53.1X4	—	—
water, concentrated	T41.0X1	T41.0X2	T41.0X3	T41.0X4	T41.0X5	T41.0X6
Chloroguanide	T37.2X1	T37.2X2	T37.2X3	T37.2X4	T37.2X5	T37.2X6
Chloromycetin	T36.2X1	T36.2X2	T36.2X3	T36.2X4	T36.2X5	T36.2X6
ENT agent	T49.6X1	T49.6X2	T49.6X3	T49.6X4	T49.6X5	T49.6X6
ophthalmic preparation	T49.5X1	T49.5X2	T49.5X3	T49.5X4	T49.5X5	T49.5X6
otic solution	T49.6X1	T49.6X2	T49.6X3	T49.6X4	T49.6X5	T49.6X6
topical NEC	T49.0X1	T49.0X2	T49.0X3	T49.0X4	T49.0X5	T49.0X6
Chloronitrobenzene	T53.7X1	T53.7X2	T53.7X3	T53.7X4	—	—
dust or vapor	T53.7X1	T53.7X2	T53.7X3	T53.7X4	—	—
Chlorophacinone	T60.4X1	T60.4X2	T60.4X3	T60.4X4	—	—
Chlorophenol	T53.7X1	T53.7X2	T53.7X3	T53.7X4	—	—
Chlorophenothane	T60.1X1	T60.1X2	T60.1X3	T60.1X4	—	—
Chlorophyll	T50.991	T50.992	T50.993	T50.994	T50.995	T50.996
Chloropicrin (fumes)	T53.6X1	T53.6X2	T53.6X3	T53.6X4	—	—
fumigant	T60.8X1	T60.8X2	T60.8X3	T60.8X4	—	—
fungicide	T60.3X1	T60.3X2	T60.3X3	T60.3X4	—	—
pesticide	T60.8X1	T60.8X2	T60.8X3	T60.8X4	—	—
Chloroprocaine	T41.3X1	T41.3X2	T41.3X3	T41.3X4	T41.3X5	T41.3X6
infiltration (subcutaneous)	T41.3X1	T41.3X2	T41.3X3	T41.3X4	T41.3X5	T41.3X6
nerve block (peripheral) (plexus)	T41.3X1	T41.3X2	T41.3X3	T41.3X4	T41.3X5	T41.3X6
spinal	T41.3X1	T41.3X2	T41.3X3	T41.3X4	T41.3X5	T41.3X6

TABLE OF DRUGS AND CHEMICALS

Substance	Poisoning, Accidental (Unintentional)	Poisoning, Intentional Self-Harm	Poisoning, Assault	Poisoning, Undetermined	Adverse Effect	Underdosing
Chloroptic	T49.5X1	T49.5X2	T49.5X3	T49.5X4	T49.5X5	T49.5X6
Chloropurine	T45.1X1	T45.1X2	T45.1X3	T45.1X4	T45.1X5	T45.1X6
Chloropyramine	T45.0X1	T45.0X2	T45.0X3	T45.0X4	T45.0X5	T45.0X6
Chloropyrifos	T60.0X1	T60.0X2	T60.0X3	T60.0X4	—	—
Chloropyrilene	T45.0X1	T45.0X2	T45.0X3	T45.0X4	T45.0X5	T45.0X6
Chloroquine	T37.2X1	T37.2X2	T37.2X3	T37.2X4	T37.2X5	T37.2X6
Chlorothalonil	T60.3X1	T60.3X2	T60.3X3	T60.3X4	—	—
Chlorothen	T45.0X1	T45.0X2	T45.0X3	T45.0X4	T45.0X5	T45.0X6
Chlorothiazide	T50.2X1	T50.2X2	T50.2X3	T50.2X4	T50.2X5	T50.2X6
Chlorothymol	T49.4X1	T49.4X2	T49.4X3	T49.4X4	T49.4X5	T49.4X6
Chlorotrianisene	T38.5X1	T38.5X2	T38.5X3	T38.5X4	T38.5X5	T38.5X6
Chlorovinyldichloro-arsine, not in war	T57.0X1	T57.0X2	T57.0X3	T57.0X4	—	—
Chloroxine	T49.4X1	T49.4X2	T49.4X3	T49.4X4	T49.4X5	T49.4X6
Chloroxylenol	T49.0X1	T49.0X2	T49.0X3	T49.0X4	T49.0X5	T49.0X6
Chlorphenamine	T45.0X1	T45.0X2	T45.0X3	T45.0X4	T45.0X5	T45.0X6
Chlorphenesin	T42.8X1	T42.8X2	T42.8X3	T42.8X4	T42.8X5	T42.8X6
topical (antifungal)	T49.0X1	T49.0X2	T49.0X3	T49.0X4	T49.0X5	T49.0X6
Chlorpheniramine	T45.0X1	T45.0X2	T45.0X3	T45.0X4	T45.0X5	T45.0X6
Chlorphenoxamine	T45.0X1	T45.0X2	T45.0X3	T45.0X4	T45.0X5	T45.0X6
Chlorphentermine	T50.5X1	T50.5X2	T50.5X3	T50.5X4	T50.5X5	T50.5X6
Chlorprocaine — see Chloroprocaine						
Chlorproguanil	T37.2X1	T37.2X2	T37.2X3	T37.2X4	T37.2X5	T37.2X6
Chlorpromazine	T43.3X1	T43.3X2	T43.3X3	T43.3X4	T43.3X5	T43.3X6
Chlorpropamide	T38.3X1	T38.3X2	T38.3X3	T38.3X4	T38.3X5	T38.3X6
Chlorprothixene	T43.4X1	T43.4X2	T43.4X3	T43.4X4	T43.4X5	T43.4X6
Chlorquinaldol	T49.0X1	T49.0X2	T49.0X3	T49.0X4	T49.0X5	T49.0X6
Chlorquinol	T49.0X1	T49.0X2	T49.0X3	T49.0X4	T49.0X5	T49.0X6
Chlortalidone	T50.2X1	T50.2X2	T50.2X3	T50.2X4	T50.2X5	T50.2X6
Chlortetracycline	T36.4X1	T36.4X2	T36.4X3	T36.4X4	T36.4X5	T36.4X6
Chlorthalidone	T50.2X1	T50.2X2	T50.2X3	T50.2X4	T50.2X5	T50.2X6
Chlorthiophos	T60.0X1	T60.0X2	T60.0X3	T60.0X4	—	—
Chlorotrianisene	T38.5X1	T38.5X2	T38.5X3	T38.5X4	T38.5X5	T38.5X6
Chlor-Trimeton	T45.0X1	T45.0X2	T45.0X3	T45.0X4	T45.0X5	T45.0X6
Chlorthion	T60.0X1	T60.0X2	T60.0X3	T60.0X4	—	—
Chlorzoxazone	T42.8X1	T42.8X2	T42.8X3	T42.8X4	T42.8X5	T42.8X6
Choke damp	T59.7X1	T59.7X2	T59.7X3	T59.7X4	—	—
Cholagogues	T47.5X1	T47.5X2	T47.5X3	T47.5X4	T47.5X5	T47.5X6
Cholebrine	T50.8X1	T50.8X2	T50.8X3	T50.8X4	T50.8X5	T50.8X6
Cholecalciferol	T45.2X1	T45.2X2	T45.2X3	T45.2X4	T45.2X5	T45.2X6
Cholecystokinin	T50.8X1	T50.8X2	T50.8X3	T50.8X4	T50.8X5	T50.8X6
Cholera vaccine	T50.A91	T50.A92	T50.A93	T50.A94	T50.A95	T50.A96

Substance	Poisoning, Accidental (Unintentional)	Poisoning, Intentional Self-Harm	Poisoning, Assault	Poisoning, Undetermined	Adverse Effect	Underdosing
Choleretic	T47.5X1	T47.5X2	T47.5X3	T47.5X4	T47.5X5	T47.5X6
Cholesterol-lowering agents	T46.6X1	T46.6X2	T46.6X3	T46.6X4	T46.6X5	T46.6X6
Cholestyramine (resin)	T46.6X1	T46.6X2	T46.6X3	T46.6X4	T46.6X5	T46.6X6
Cholic acid	T47.5X1	T47.5X2	T47.5X3	T47.5X4	T47.5X5	T47.5X6
Choline	T48.6X1	T48.6X2	T48.6X3	T48.6X4	T48.6X5	T48.6X6
chloride	T50.991	T50.992	T50.993	T50.994	T50.995	T50.996
dihydrogen citrate	T50.991	T50.992	T50.993	T50.994	T50.995	T50.996
salicylate	T39.091	T39.092	T39.093	T39.094	T39.095	T39.096
theophyllinate	T48.6X1	T48.6X2	T48.6X3	T48.6X4	T48.6X5	T48.6X6
Cholinergic (drug) NEC	T44.1X1	T44.1X2	T44.1X3	T44.1X4	T44.1X5	T44.1X6
muscle tone enhancer	T44.1X1	T44.1X2	T44.1X3	T44.1X4	T44.1X5	T44.1X6
organophosphorus	T44.0X1	T44.0X2	T44.0X3	T44.0X4	T44.0X5	T44.0X6
insecticide	T60.0X1	T60.0X2	T60.0X3	T60.0X4	—	—
nerve gas	T59.891	T59.892	T59.893	T59.894	—	—
trimethyl ammonium propanediol	T44.1X1	T44.1X2	T44.1X3	T44.1X4	T44.1X5	T44.1X6
Cholinesterase reactivator	T50.6X1	T50.6X2	T50.6X3	T50.6X4	T50.6X5	T50.6X6
Cholografin	T50.8X1	T50.8X2	T50.8X3	T50.8X4	T50.8X5	T50.8X6
Chorionic gonadotropin	T38.891	T38.892	T38.893	T38.894	T38.895	T38.896
Chromate	T56.2X1	T56.2X2	T56.2X3	T56.2X4	—	—
dust or mist	T56.2X1	T56.2X2	T56.2X3	T56.2X4	—	—
lead — see also lead	T56.0X1	T56.0X2	T56.0X3	T56.0X4	—	—
paint	T56.0X1	T56.0X2	T56.0X3	T56.0X4	—	—
Chromic						
acid	T56.2X1	T56.2X2	T56.2X3	T56.2X4	—	—
dust or mist	T56.2X1	T56.2X2	T56.2X3	T56.2X4	—	—
phosphate 32P	T45.1X1	T45.1X2	T45.1X3	T45.1X4	T45.1X5	T45.1X6
Chromium	T56.2X1	T56.2X2	T56.2X3	T56.2X4	—	—
compounds — see Chromate						
sesquioxide	T50.8X1	T50.8X2	T50.8X3	T50.8X4	T50.8X5	T50.8X6
Chromomycin A3	T45.1X1	T45.1X2	T45.1X3	T45.1X4	T45.1X5	T45.1X6
Chromonar	T46.3X1	T46.3X2	T46.3X3	T46.3X4	T46.3X5	T46.3X6
Chromyl chloride	T56.2X1	T56.2X2	T56.2X3	T56.2X4	—	—
Chrysarobin	T49.4X1	T49.4X2	T49.4X3	T49.4X4	T49.4X5	T49.4X6
Chrysazin	T47.2X1	T47.2X2	T47.2X3	T47.2X4	T47.2X5	T47.2X6
Chymar	T45.3X1	T45.3X2	T45.3X3	T45.3X4	T45.3X5	T45.3X6
ophthalmic preparation	T49.5X1	T49.5X2	T49.5X3	T49.5X4	T49.5X5	T49.5X6
Chymopapain	T45.3X1	T45.3X2	T45.3X3	T45.3X4	T45.3X5	T45.3X6
Chymotrypsin	T45.3X1	T45.3X2	T45.3X3	T45.3X4	T45.3X5	T45.3X6
ophthalmic preparation	T49.5X1	T49.5X2	T49.5X3	T49.5X4	T49.5X5	T49.5X6
Cianidanol	T50.991	T50.992	T50.993	T50.994	T50.995	T50.996
Cianopramine	T43.011	T43.012	T43.013	T43.014	T43.015	T43.016
Cibenzoline	T46.2X1	T46.2X2	T46.2X3	T46.2X4	T46.2X5	T46.2X6

◀ New   ◀▥ Revised   ~~deleted~~ Deleted

Substance	Poisoning, Accidental (Unintentional)	Poisoning, Intentional Self-Harm	Poisoning, Assault	Poisoning, Undetermined	Adverse Effect	Underdosing
Ciclacillin	T36.0X1	T36.0X2	T36.0X3	T36.0X4	T36.0X5	T36.0X6
Ciclobarbital — see Hexobarbital						
Ciclonicate	T46.7X1	T46.7X2	T46.7X3	T46.7X4	T46.7X5	T46.7X6
Ciclopirox (olamine)	T49.0X1	T49.0X2	T49.0X3	T49.0X4	T49.0X5	T49.0X6
Ciclosporin	T45.1X1	T45.1X2	T45.1X3	T45.1X4	T45.1X5	T45.1X6
Cicuta maculata or virosa	T62.2X1	T62.2X2	T62.2X3	T62.2X4	—	—
Cicutoxin	T62.2X1	T62.2X2	T62.2X3	T62.2X4	—	—
Cigarette lighter fluid	T52.0X1	T52.0X2	T52.0X3	T52.0X4	—	—
Cigarettes (tobacco)	T65.221	T65.222	T65.223	T65.224	—	—
Ciguatoxin	T61.01	T61.02	T61.03	T61.04	—	—
Cilazapril	T46.4X1	T46.4X2	T46.4X3	T46.4X4	T46.4X5	T46.4X6
Cimetidine	T47.0X1	T47.0X2	T47.0X3	T47.0X4	T47.0X5	T47.0X6
Cimetropium bromide	T44.3X1	T44.3X2	T44.3X3	T44.3X4	T44.3X5	T44.3X6
Cinchocaine	T41.3X1	T41.3X2	T41.3X3	T41.3X4	T41.3X5	T41.3X6
topical (surface)	T41.3X1	T41.3X2	T41.3X3	T41.3X4	T41.3X5	T41.3X6
Cinchona	T37.2X1	T37.2X2	T37.2X3	T37.2X4	T37.2X5	T37.2X6
Cinchonine alkaloids	T37.2X1	T37.2X2	T37.2X3	T37.2X4	T37.2X5	T37.2X6
Cinchophen	T50.4X1	T50.4X2	T50.4X3	T50.4X4	T50.4X5	T50.4X6
Cinepazide	T46.7X1	T46.7X2	T46.7X3	T46.7X4	T46.7X5	T46.7X6
Cinnamedrine	T48.5X1	T48.5X2	T48.5X3	T48.5X4	T48.5X5	T48.5X6
Cinnarizine	T45.0X1	T45.0X2	T45.0X3	T45.0X4	T45.0X5	T45.0X6
Cinoxacin	T37.8X1	T37.8X2	T37.8X3	T37.8X4	T37.8X5	T37.8X6
Ciprofibrate	T46.6X1	T46.6X2	T46.6X3	T46.6X4	T46.6X5	T46.6X6
Ciprofloxacin	T36.8X1	T36.8X2	T36.8X3	T36.8X4	T36.8X5	T36.8X6
Cisapride	T47.8X1	T47.8X2	T47.8X3	T47.8X4	T47.8X5	T47.8X6
Cisplatin	T45.1X1	T45.1X2	T45.1X3	T45.1X4	T45.1X5	T45.1X6
Citalopram	T43.221	T43.222	T43.223	T43.224	T43.225	T43.226
Citanest	T41.3X1	T41.3X2	T41.3X3	T41.3X4	T41.3X5	T41.3X6
infiltration (subcutaneous)	T41.3X1	T41.3X2	T41.3X3	T41.3X4	T41.3X5	T41.3X6
nerve block (peripheral) (plexus)	T41.3X1	T41.3X2	T41.3X3	T41.3X4	T41.3X5	T41.3X6
Citric acid	T47.5X1	T47.5X2	T47.5X3	T47.5X4	T47.5X5	T47.5X6
Citrovorum (factor)	T45.8X1	T45.8X2	T45.8X3	T45.8X4	T45.8X5	T45.8X6
Claviceps purpurea	T62.2X1	T62.2X2	T62.2X3	T62.2X4	—	—
Clavulanic acid	T36.1X1	T36.1X2	T36.1X3	T36.1X4	T36.1X5	T36.1X6
Cleaner, cleansing agent, type not specified	T65.891	T65.892	T65.893	T65.894	—	—
of paint or varnish	T52.91	T52.92	T52.93	T52.94		
specified type NEC	T65.891	T65.892	T65.893	T65.894	—	—
Clebopride	T47.8X1	T47.8X2	T47.8X3	T47.8X4	T47.8X5	T47.8X6
Clefamide	T37.3X1	T37.3X2	T37.3X3	T37.3X4	T37.3X5	T37.3X6
Clemastine	T45.0X1	T45.0X2	T45.0X3	T45.0X4	T45.0X5	T45.0X6
Clematis vitalba	T62.2X1	T62.2X2	T62.2X3	T62.2X4	—	—

Substance	Poisoning, Accidental (Unintentional)	Poisoning, Intentional Self-Harm	Poisoning, Assault	Poisoning, Undetermined	Adverse Effect	Underdosing
Clemizole	T45.0X1	T45.0X2	T45.0X3	T45.0X4	T45.0X5	T45.0X6
penicillin	T36.0X1	T36.0X2	T36.0X3	T36.0X4	T36.0X5	T36.0X6
Clenbuterol	T48.6X1	T48.6X2	T48.6X3	T48.6X4	T48.6X5	T48.6X6
Clidinium bromide	T44.3X1	T44.3X2	T44.3X3	T44.3X4	T44.3X5	T44.3X6
Clindamycin	T36.8X1	T36.8X2	T36.8X3	T36.8X4	T36.8X5	T36.8X6
Clinofibrate	T46.6X1	T46.6X2	T46.6X3	T46.6X4	T46.6X5	T46.6X6
Clioquinol	T37.8X1	T37.8X2	T37.8X3	T37.8X4	T37.8X5	T37.8X6
Cliradon	T40.2X1	T40.2X2	T40.2X3	T40.2X4	—	—
Clobazam	T42.4X1	T42.4X2	T42.4X3	T42.4X4	T42.4X5	T42.4X6
Clobenzorex	T50.5X1	T50.5X2	T50.5X3	T50.5X4	T50.5X5	T50.5X6
Clobetasol	T49.0X1	T49.0X2	T49.0X3	T49.0X4	T49.0X5	T49.0X6
Clobetasone	T49.0X1	T49.0X2	T49.0X3	T49.0X4	T49.0X5	T49.0X6
Clobutinol	T48.3X1	T48.3X2	T48.3X3	T48.3X4	T48.3X5	T48.3X6
Clocapramine	T43.0X1	T43.0X2	T43.0X3	T43.0X4	T43.0X5	T43.0X6
Clocortolone	T38.0X1	T38.0X2	T38.0X3	T38.0X4	T38.0X5	T38.0X6
Clodantoin	T49.0X1	T49.0X2	T49.0X3	T49.0X4	T49.0X5	T49.0X6
Clodronic acid	T50.991	T50.992	T50.993	T50.994	T50.995	T50.996
Clofazimine	T37.1X1	T37.1X2	T37.1X3	T37.1X4	T37.1X5	T37.1X6
Clofedanol	T48.3X1	T48.3X2	T48.3X3	T48.3X4	T48.3X5	T48.3X6
Clofenamide	T50.2X1	T50.2X2	T50.2X3	T50.2X4	T50.2X5	T50.2X6
Clofenotane	T49.0X1	T49.0X2	T49.0X3	T49.0X4	T49.0X5	T49.0X6
Clofezone	T39.2X1	T39.2X2	T39.2X3	T39.2X4	T39.2X5	T39.2X6
Clofibrate	T46.6X1	T46.6X2	T46.6X3	T46.6X4	T46.6X5	T46.6X6
Clofibride	T46.6X1	T46.6X2	T46.6X3	T46.6X4	T46.6X5	T46.6X6
Cloforex	T50.5X1	T50.5X2	T50.5X3	T50.5X4	T50.5X5	T50.5X6
Clomacran	T43.0X1	T43.0X2	T43.0X3	T43.0X4	T43.0X5	T43.0X6
Clomethiazole	T42.6X1	T42.6X2	T42.6X3	T42.6X4	T42.6X5	T42.6X6
Clometocillin	T36.0X1	T36.0X2	T36.0X3	T36.0X4	T36.0X5	T36.0X6
Clomifene	T38.5X1	T38.5X2	T38.5X3	T38.5X4	T38.5X5	T38.5X6
Clomiphene	T38.5X1	T38.5X2	T38.5X3	T38.5X4	T38.5X5	T38.5X6
Clomipramine	T43.011	T43.012	T43.013	T43.014	T43.015	T43.016
Clomocycline	T36.4X1	T36.4X2	T36.4X3	T36.4X4	T36.4X5	T36.4X6
Clonazepam	T42.4X1	T42.4X2	T42.4X3	T42.4X4	T42.4X5	T42.4X6
Clonidine	T46.5X1	T46.5X2	T46.5X3	T46.5X4	T46.5X5	T46.5X6
Clonixin	T39.8X1	T39.8X2	T39.8X3	T39.8X4	T39.8X5	T39.8X6
Clopamide	T50.2X1	T50.2X2	T50.2X3	T50.2X4	T50.2X5	T50.2X6
Clopenthixol	T43.4X1	T43.4X2	T43.4X3	T43.4X4	T43.4X5	T43.4X6
Cloperastine	T48.3X1	T48.3X2	T48.3X3	T48.3X4	T48.3X5	T48.3X6
Clophedianol	T48.3X1	T48.3X2	T48.3X3	T48.3X4	T48.3X5	T48.3X6
Cloponone	T36.2X1	T36.2X2	T36.2X3	T36.2X4	T36.2X5	T36.2X6
Cloprednol	T38.0X1	T38.0X2	T38.0X3	T38.0X4	T38.0X5	T38.0X6
Cloral betaine	T42.6X1	T42.6X2	T42.6X3	T42.6X4	T42.6X5	T42.6X6

External Cause (T-Code)

◀ New ◀▥ Revised ~~deleted~~ Deleted

TABLE OF DRUGS AND CHEMICALS

Substance	External Cause (T-Code)					
	Poisoning, Accidental (Unintentional)	Poisoning, Intentional Self-Harm	Poisoning, Assault	Poisoning, Undetermined	Adverse Effect	Underdosing
Cloramfenicol	T36.2X1	T36.2X2	T36.2X3	T36.2X4	T36.2X5	T36.2X6
Clorazepate (dipotassium)	T42.4X1	T42.4X2	T42.4X3	T42.4X4	T42.4X5	T42.4X6
Clorexolone	T50.2X1	T50.2X2	T50.2X3	T50.2X4	T50.2X5	T50.2X6
Clorox (bleach)	T54.91	T54.92	T54.93	T54.94	—	—
Clorfenamine	T45.0X1	T45.0X2	T45.0X3	T45.0X4	T45.0X5	T45.0X6
Clorgiline	T43.1X1	T43.1X2	T43.1X3	T43.1X4	T43.1X5	T43.1X6
Clorotepine	T44.3X1	T44.3X2	T44.3X3	T44.3X4	T44.3X5	T44.3X6
Clorprenaline	T48.6X1	T48.6X2	T48.6X3	T48.6X4	T48.6X5	T48.6X6
Clortermine	T50.5X1	T50.5X2	T50.5X3	T50.5X4	T50.5X5	T50.5X6
Clotiapine	T43.591	T43.592	T43.593	T43.594	T43.595	T43.596
Clotiazepam	T42.4X1	T42.4X2	T42.4X3	T42.4X4	T42.4X5	T42.4X6
Clotibric acid	T46.6X1	T46.6X2	T46.6X3	T46.6X4	T46.6X5	T46.6X6
Clotrimazole	T49.0X1	T49.0X2	T49.0X3	T49.0X4	T49.0X5	T49.0X6
Cloxacillin	T36.0X1	T36.0X2	T36.0X3	T36.0X4	T36.0X5	T36.0X6
Cloxazolam	T42.4X1	T42.4X2	T42.4X3	T42.4X4	T42.4X5	T42.4X6
Cloxiquine	T49.0X1	T49.0X2	T49.0X3	T49.0X4	T49.0X5	T49.0X6
Clozapine	T42.4X1	T42.4X2	T42.4X3	T42.4X4	T42.4X5	T42.4X6
Coagulant NEC	T45.7X1	T45.7X2	T45.7X3	T45.7X4	T45.7X5	T45.7X6
Coal (carbon monoxide from) — see also Carbon, monoxide, coal	T58.2X1	T58.2X2	T58.2X3	T58.2X4	—	—
oil — see Kerosene						
tar	T49.1X1	T49.1X2	T49.1X3	T49.1X4	T49.1X5	T49.1X6
fumes	T59.891	T59.892	T59.893	T59.894	—	—
medicinal (ointment)	T49.4X1	T49.4X2	T49.4X3	T49.4X4	T49.4X5	T49.4X6
analgesics NEC	T39.2X1	T39.2X2	T39.2X3	T39.2X4	T39.2X5	T39.2X6
naphtha (solvent)	T52.0X1	T52.0X2	T52.0X3	T52.0X4		
Cobalamine	T45.2X1	T45.2X2	T45.2X3	T45.2X4	T45.2X5	T45.2X6
Cobalt (nonmedicinal) (fumes) (industrial)	T56.891	T56.892	T56.893	T56.894		
medicinal (trace) (chloride)	T45.8X1	T45.8X2	T45.8X3	T45.8X4	T45.8X5	T45.8X6
Cobra (venom)	T63.041	T63.042	T63.043	T63.044		
Coca (leaf)	T40.5X1	T40.5X2	T40.5X3	T40.5X4	T40.5X5	T40.5X6
Cocaine	T40.5X1	T40.5X2	T40.5X3	T40.5X4	T40.5X5	T40.5X6
topical anesthetic	T41.3X1	T41.3X2	T41.3X3	T41.3X4	T41.3X5	T41.3X6
Cocarboxylase	T45.3X1	T45.3X2	T45.3X3	T45.3X4	T45.3X5	T45.3X6
Coccidioidin	T50.8X1	T50.8X2	T50.8X3	T50.8X4	T50.8X5	T50.8X6
Cocculus indicus	T62.1X1	T62.1X2	T62.1X3	T62.1X4		
Cochineal	T65.6X1	T65.6X2	T65.6X3	T65.6X4		
medicinal products	T50.991	T50.992	T50.993	T50.994	T50.995	T50.996
Codeine	T40.2X1	T40.2X2	T40.2X3	T40.2X4	T40.2X5	T40.2X6
Cod-liver oil	T45.2X1	T45.2X2	T45.2X3	T45.2X4	T45.2X5	T45.2X6

Substance	External Cause (T-Code)					
	Poisoning, Accidental (Unintentional)	Poisoning, Intentional Self-Harm	Poisoning, Assault	Poisoning, Undetermined	Adverse Effect	Underdosing
Coenzyme A	T50.991	T50.992	T50.993	T50.994	T50.995	T50.996
Coffee	T62.8X1	T62.8X2	T62.8X3	T62.8X4	—	—
Cogalactoisomerase	T50.991	T50.992	T50.993	T50.994	T50.995	T50.996
Cogentin	T44.3X1	T44.3X2	T44.3X3	T44.3X4	T44.3X5	T44.3X6
Coke fumes or gas (carbon monoxide)	T58.2X1	T58.2X2	T58.2X3	T58.2X4	—	—
industrial use	T58.8X1	T58.8X2	T58.8X3	T58.8X4	—	—
Colace	T47.4X1	T47.4X2	T47.4X3	T47.4X4	T47.4X5	T47.4X6
Colaspase	T45.1X1	T45.1X2	T45.1X3	T45.1X4	T45.1X5	T45.1X6
Colchicine	T50.4X1	T50.4X2	T50.4X3	T50.4X4	T50.4X5	T50.4X6
Colchicum	T62.2X1	T62.2X2	T62.2X3	T62.2X4	—	—
Cold cream	T49.3X1	T49.3X2	T49.3X3	T49.3X4	T49.3X5	T49.3X6
Colecalciferol	T45.2X1	T45.2X2	T45.2X3	T45.2X4	T45.2X5	T45.2X6
Colestipol	T46.6X1	T46.6X2	T46.6X3	T46.6X4	T46.6X5	T46.6X6
Colestyramine	T46.6X1	T46.6X2	T46.6X3	T46.6X4	T46.6X5	T46.6X6
Colimycin	T36.8X1	T36.8X2	T36.8X3	T36.8X4	T36.8X5	T36.8X6
Colistimethate	T36.8X1	T36.8X2	T36.8X3	T36.8X4	T36.8X5	T36.8X6
Colistin	T36.8X1	T36.8X2	T36.8X3	T36.8X4	T36.8X5	T36.8X6
sulfate (eye preparation)	T49.5X1	T49.5X2	T49.5X3	T49.5X4	T49.5X5	T49.5X6
Collagen	T50.991	T50.992	T50.993	T50.994	T50.995	T50.996
Collagenase	T49.4X1	T49.4X2	T49.4X3	T49.4X4	T49.4X5	T49.4X6
Collodion	T49.3X1	T49.3X2	T49.3X3	T49.3X4	T49.3X5	T49.3X6
Colocynth	T47.2X1	T47.2X2	T47.2X3	T47.2X4	T47.2X5	T47.2X6
Colophony adhesive	T49.3X1	T49.3X2	T49.3X3	T49.3X4	T49.3X5	T49.3X6
Colorant — see also Dye	T50.991	T50.992	T50.993	T50.994	T50.995	T50.996
Coloring matter — see Dye(s)						
Combustion gas (after combustion) — see Carbon, monoxide						
prior to combustion	T59.891	T59.892	T59.893	T59.894	—	—
Compazine	T43.3X1	T43.3X2	T43.3X3	T43.3X4	T43.3X5	T43.3X6
Compound						
42 (warfarin)	T60.4X1	T60.4X2	T60.4X3	T60.4X4	—	—
269 (endrin)	T60.1X1	T60.1X2	T60.1X3	T60.1X4	—	—
497 (dieldrin)	T60.1X1	T60.1X2	T60.1X3	T60.1X4	—	—
1080 (sodium fluoroacetate)	T60.4X1	T60.4X2	T60.4X3	T60.4X4	—	—
3422 (parathion)	T60.0X1	T60.0X2	T60.0X3	T60.0X4		
3911 (phorate)	T60.0X1	T60.0X2	T60.0X3	T60.0X4		
3956 (toxaphene)	T60.1X1	T60.1X2	T60.1X3	T60.1X4		
4049 (malathion)	T60.0X1	T60.0X2	T60.0X3	T60.0X4		
4069 (malathion)	T60.0X1	T60.0X2	T60.0X3	T60.0X4	—	—
4124 (dicapthon)	T60.0X1	T60.0X2	T60.0X3	T60.0X4	—	—

◄ New   ⬅ Revised   ~~deleted~~ Deleted

Substance	Poisoning, Accidental (Unintentional)	Poisoning, Intentional Self-Harm	Poisoning, Assault	Poisoning, Undetermined	Adverse Effect	Underdosing
Compound *(Continued)*						
E (cortisone)	T38.0X1	T38.0X2	T38.0X3	T38.0X4	T38.0X5	T38.0X6
F (hydrocortisone)	T38.0X1	T38.0X2	T38.0X3	T38.0X4	T38.0X5	T38.0X6
Congener, anabolic	T38.7X1	T38.7X2	T38.7X3	T38.7X4	T38.7X5	T38.7X6
Congo red	T50.8X1	T50.8X2	T50.8X3	T50.8X4	T50.8X5	T50.8X6
Coniine, conine	T62.2X1	T62.2X2	T62.2X3	T62.2X4	—	—
Conium (maculatum)	T62.2X1	T62.2X2	T62.2X3	T62.2X4	—	—
Conjugated estrogenic substances	T38.5X1	T38.5X2	T38.5X3	T38.5X4	T38.5X5	T38.5X6
Contac	T48.5X1	T48.5X2	T48.5X3	T48.5X4	T48.5X5	T48.5X6
Contact lens solution	T49.5X1	T49.5X2	T49.5X3	T49.5X4	T49.5X5	T49.5X6
Contraceptive (oral)	T38.4X1	T38.4X2	T38.4X3	T38.4X4	T38.4X5	T38.4X6
vaginal	T49.8X1	T49.8X2	T49.8X3	T49.8X4	T49.8X5	T49.8X6
Contrast medium, radiography	T50.8X1	T50.8X2	T50.8X3	T50.8X4	T50.8X5	T50.8X6
Convallaria glycosides	T46.0X1	T46.0X2	T46.0X3	T46.0X4	T46.0X5	T46.0X6
Convallaria majalis	T62.2X1	T62.2X2	T62.2X3	T62.2X4	—	—
berry	T62.1X1	T62.1X2	T62.1X3	T62.1X4	—	—
Copper (dust) (fumes) (nonmedicinal) NEC	T56.4X1	T56.4X2	T56.4X3	T56.4X4	—	—
arsenate, arsenite	T57.0X1	T57.0X2	T57.0X3	T57.0X4	—	—
insecticide	T60.2X1	T60.2X2	T60.2X3	T60.2X4	—	—
emetic	T47.7X1	T47.7X2	T47.7X3	T47.7X4	T47.7X5	T47.7X6
fungicide	T60.3X1	T60.3X2	T60.3X3	T60.3X4	—	—
gluconate	T49.0X1	T49.0X2	T49.0X3	T49.0X4	T49.0X5	T49.0X6
insecticide	T60.2X1	T60.2X2	T60.2X3	T60.2X4	—	—
medicinal (trace)	T45.8X1	T45.8X2	T45.8X3	T45.8X4	T45.8X5	T45.8X6
oleate	T49.0X1	T49.0X2	T49.0X3	T49.0X4	T49.0X5	T49.0X6
sulfate	T56.4X1	T56.4X2	T56.4X3	T56.4X4	—	—
cupric	T56.4X1	T56.4X2	T56.4X3	T56.4X4	—	—
fungicide	T60.3X1	T60.3X2	T60.3X3	T60.3X4	—	—
medicinal						
ear	T49.6X1	T49.6X2	T49.6X3	T49.6X4	T49.6X5	T49.6X6
emetic	T47.7X1	T47.7X2	T47.7X3	T47.7X4	T47.7X5	T47.7X6
eye	T49.5X1	T49.5X2	T49.5X3	T49.5X4	T49.5X5	T49.5X6
cuprous	T56.4X1	T56.4X2	T56.4X3	T56.4X4	—	—
fungicide	T60.3X1	T60.3X2	T60.3X3	T60.3X4	—	—
medicinal						
ear	T49.6X1	T49.6X2	T49.6X3	T49.6X4	T49.6X5	T49.6X6
emetic	T47.7X1	T47.7X2	T47.7X3	T47.7X4	T47.7X5	T47.7X6
eye	T49.5X1	T49.5X2	T49.5X3	T49.5X4	T49.5X5	T49.5X6
Copperhead snake (bite) (venom)	T63.061	T63.062	T63.063	T63.064	—	—
Coral (sting)	T63.691	T63.692	T63.693	T63.694	—	—
snake (bite) (venom)	T63.021	T63.022	T63.023	T63.024	—	—

Substance	Poisoning, Accidental (Unintentional)	Poisoning, Intentional Self-Harm	Poisoning, Assault	Poisoning, Undetermined	Adverse Effect	Underdosing
Corbadrine	T49.6X1	T49.6X2	T49.6X3	T49.6X4	T49.6X5	T49.6X6
Cordran	T49.0X1	T49.0X2	T49.0X3	T49.0X4	T49.0X5	T49.0X6
Cordite	T65.891	T65.892	T65.893	T65.894	—	—
vapor	T59.891	T59.892	T59.893	T59.894	—	—
Corn cures	T49.4X1	T49.4X2	T49.4X3	T49.4X4	T49.4X5	T49.4X6
Cornhusker's lotion	T49.3X1	T49.3X2	T49.3X3	T49.3X4	T49.3X5	T49.3X6
Corn starch	T49.3X1	T49.3X2	T49.3X3	T49.3X4	T49.3X5	T49.3X6
Coronary vasodilator NEC	T46.3X1	T46.3X2	T46.3X3	T46.3X4	T46.3X5	T46.3X6
Corrosive NEC	T54.91	T54.92	T54.93	T54.94		
acid NEC	T54.2X1	T54.2X2	T54.2X3	T54.2X4	—	—
aromatics	T54.1X1	T54.1X2	T54.1X3	T54.1X4	—	—
disinfectant	T54.1X1	T54.1X2	T54.1X3	T54.1X4	—	—
fumes NEC	T54.91	T54.92	T54.93	T54.94	—	—
specified NEC	T54.91	T54.92	T54.93	T54.94		
sublimate	T56.1X1	T56.1X2	T56.1X3	T56.1X4	—	—
Cortate	T38.0X1	T38.0X2	T38.0X3	T38.0X4	T38.0X5	T38.0X6
Cort-Dome	T38.0X1	T38.0X2	T38.0X3	T38.0X4	T38.0X5	T38.0X6
ENT agent	T49.6X1	T49.6X2	T49.6X3	T49.6X4	T49.6X5	T49.6X6
ophthalmic preparation	T49.5X1	T49.5X2	T49.5X3	T49.5X4	T49.5X5	T49.5X6
topical NEC	T49.0X1	T49.0X2	T49.0X3	T49.0X4	T49.0X5	T49.0X6
Cortef	T38.0X1	T38.0X2	T38.0X3	T38.0X4	T38.0X5	T38.0X6
ENT agent	T49.6X1	T49.6X2	T49.6X3	T49.6X4	T49.6X5	T49.6X6
ophthalmic preparation	T49.5X1	T49.5X2	T49.5X3	T49.5X4	T49.5X5	T49.5X6
topical NEC	T49.0X1	T49.0X2	T49.0X3	T49.0X4	T49.0X5	T49.0X6
Corticosteroid	T38.0X1	T38.0X2	T38.0X3	T38.0X4	T38.0X5	T38.0X6
ENT agent	T49.6X1	T49.6X2	T49.6X3	T49.6X4	T49.6X5	T49.6X6
mineral	T50.0X1	T50.0X2	T50.0X3	T50.0X4	T50.0X5	T50.0X6
ophthalmic	T49.5X1	T49.5X2	T49.5X3	T49.5X4	T49.5X5	T49.5X6
topical NEC	T49.0X1	T49.0X2	T49.0X3	T49.0X4	T49.0X5	T49.0X6
Corticotropin	T38.811	T38.812	T38.813	T38.814	T38.815	T38.816
Cortisol	T49.0X1	T49.0X2	T49.0X3	T49.0X4	T49.0X5	T49.0X6
ENT agent	T49.6X1	T49.6X2	T49.6X3	T49.6X4	T49.6X5	T49.6X6
ophthalmic preparation	T49.5X1	T49.5X2	T49.5X3	T49.5X4	T49.5X5	T49.5X6
topical NEC	T49.0X1	T49.0X2	T49.0X3	T49.0X4	T49.0X5	T49.0X6
Cortisone (acetate)	T38.0X1	T38.0X2	T38.0X3	T38.0X4	T38.0X5	T38.0X6
ENT agent	T49.6X1	T49.6X2	T49.6X3	T49.6X4	T49.6X5	T49.6X6
ophthalmic preparation	T49.5X1	T49.5X2	T49.5X3	T49.5X4	T49.5X5	T49.5X6
topical NEC	T49.0X1	T49.0X2	T49.0X3	T49.0X4	T49.0X5	T49.0X6
Cortivazol	T38.0X1	T38.0X2	T38.0X3	T38.0X4	T38.0X5	T38.0X6
Cortogen	T38.0X1	T38.0X2	T38.0X3	T38.0X4	T38.0X5	T38.0X6
ENT agent	T49.6X1	T49.6X2	T49.6X3	T49.6X4	T49.6X5	T49.6X6
ophthalmic preparation	T49.5X1	T49.5X2	T49.5X3	T49.5X4	T49.5X5	T49.5X6

◄ New   ◄▥ Revised   ~~deleted~~ Deleted

Substance	External Cause (T-Code)					
	Poisoning, Accidental (Unintentional)	Poisoning, Intentional Self-Harm	Poisoning, Assault	Poisoning, Undetermined	Adverse Effect	Underdosing
Cortone	T38.0X1	T38.0X2	T38.0X3	T38.0X4	T38.0X5	T38.0X6
ENT agent	T49.6X1	T49.6X2	T49.6X3	T49.6X4	T49.6X5	T49.6X6
ophthalmic preparation	T49.5X1	T49.5X2	T49.5X3	T49.5X4	T49.5X5	T49.5X6
Cortril	T38.0X1	T38.0X2	T38.0X3	T38.0X4	T38.0X5	T38.0X6
ENT agent	T49.6X1	T49.6X2	T49.6X3	T49.6X4	T49.6X5	T49.6X6
ophthalmic preparation	T49.5X1	T49.5X2	T49.5X3	T49.5X4	T49.5X5	T49.5X6
topical NEC	T49.0X1	T49.0X2	T49.0X3	T49.0X4	T49.0X5	T49.0X6
Corynebacterium parvum	T45.1X1	T45.1X2	T45.1X3	T45.1X4	T45.1X5	T45.1X6
Cosmetic preparation	T49.8X1	T49.8X2	T49.8X3	T49.8X4	T49.8X5	T49.8X6
Cosmetics	T49.8X1	T49.8X2	T49.8X3	T49.8X4	T49.8X5	T49.8X6
Cosyntropin	T38.811	T38.812	T38.813	T38.814	T38.815	T38.816
Cotarnine	T45.7X1	T45.7X2	T45.7X3	T45.7X4	T45.7X5	T45.7X6
Co-trimoxazole	T36.8X1	T36.8X2	T36.8X3	T36.8X4	T36.8X5	T36.8X6
Cottonseed oil	T49.3X1	T49.3X2	T49.3X3	T49.3X4	T49.3X5	T49.3X6
Cough mixture (syrup)	T48.4X1	T48.4X2	T48.4X3	T48.4X4	T48.4X5	T48.4X6
containing opiates	T40.2X1	T40.2X2	T40.2X3	T40.2X4	T40.2X5	T40.2X6
expectorants	T48.4X1	T48.4X2	T48.4X3	T48.4X4	T48.4X5	T48.4X6
Coumadin	T45.511	T45.512	T45.513	T45.514	T45.515	T45.516
rodenticide	T60.4X1	T60.4X2	T60.4X3	T60.4X4	—	—
Coumaphos	T60.0X1	T60.0X2	T60.0X3	T60.0X4	—	—
Coumarin	T45.511	T45.512	T45.513	T45.514	T45.515	T45.516
Coumetarol	T45.511	T45.512	T45.513	T45.514	T45.515	T45.516
Cowbane	T62.2X1	T62.2X2	T62.2X3	T62.2X4	—	—
Cozyme	T45.2X1	T45.2X2	T45.2X3	T45.2X4	T45.2X5	T45.2X6
Crack	T40.5X1	T40.5X2	T40.5X3	T40.5X4	—	—
Crataegus extract	T46.0X1	T46.0X2	T46.0X3	T46.0X4	T46.0X5	T46.0X6
Creolin	T54.1X1	T54.1X2	T54.1X3	T54.1X4	—	—
disinfectant	T54.1X1	T54.1X2	T54.1X3	T54.1X4	—	—
Creosol (compound)	T49.0X1	T49.0X2	T49.0X3	T49.0X4	T49.0X5	T49.0X6
Creosote (coal tar) (beechwood)	T49.0X1	T49.0X2	T49.0X3	T49.0X4	T49.0X5	T49.0X6
medicinal (expectorant)	T48.4X1	T48.4X2	T48.4X3	T48.4X4	T48.4X5	T48.4X6
syrup	T48.4X1	T48.4X2	T48.4X3	T48.4X4	T48.4X5	T48.4X6
Cresol(s)	T49.0X1	T49.0X2	T49.0X3	T49.0X4	T49.0X5	T49.0X6
and soap solution	T49.0X1	T49.0X2	T49.0X3	T49.0X4	T49.0X5	T49.0X6
Cresyl acetate	T49.0X1	T49.0X2	T49.0X3	T49.0X4	T49.0X5	T49.0X6
Cresylic acid	T49.0X1	T49.0X2	T49.0X3	T49.0X4	T49.0X5	T49.0X6
Crimidine	T60.4X1	T60.4X2	T60.4X3	T60.4X4	—	—
Croconazole	T37.8X1	T37.8X2	T37.8X3	T37.8X4	T37.8X5	T37.8X6
Cromoglicic acid	T48.6X1	T48.6X2	T48.6X3	T48.6X4	T48.6X5	T48.6X6
Cromolyn	T48.6X1	T48.6X2	T48.6X3	T48.6X4	T48.6X5	T48.6X6
Cromonar	T46.3X1	T46.3X2	T46.3X3	T46.3X4	T46.3X5	T46.3X6

Substance	External Cause (T-Code)					
	Poisoning, Accidental (Unintentional)	Poisoning, Intentional Self-Harm	Poisoning, Assault	Poisoning, Undetermined	Adverse Effect	Underdosing
Cropropamide	T39.8X1	T39.8X2	T39.8X3	T39.8X4	T39.8X5	T39.8X6
with crotethamide	T50.7X1	T50.7X2	T50.7X3	T50.7X4	T50.7X5	T50.7X6
Crotamiton	T49.0X1	T49.0X2	T49.0X3	T49.0X4	T49.0X5	T49.0X6
Crotethamide	T39.8X1	T39.8X2	T39.8X3	T39.8X4	T39.8X5	T39.8X6
with cropropamide	T50.7X1	T50.7X2	T50.7X3	T50.7X4	T50.7X5	T50.7X6
Croton (oil)	T47.2X1	T47.2X2	T47.2X3	T47.2X4	T47.2X5	T47.2X6
chloral	T42.6X1	T42.6X2	T42.6X3	T42.6X4	T42.6X5	T42.6X6
Crude oil	T52.0X1	T52.0X2	T52.0X3	T52.0X4	—	—
Cryogenine	T39.8X1	T39.8X2	T39.8X3	T39.8X4	T39.8X5	T39.8X6
Cryolite (vapor)	T60.1X1	T60.1X2	T60.1X3	T60.1X4	—	—
insecticide	T60.1X1	T60.1X2	T60.1X3	T60.1X4	—	—
Cryptenamine (tannates)	T46.5X1	T46.5X2	T46.5X3	T46.5X4	T46.5X5	T46.5X6
Crystal violet	T49.0X1	T49.0X2	T49.0X3	T49.0X4	T49.0X5	T49.0X6
Cuckoopint	T62.2X1	T62.2X2	T62.2X3	T62.2X4	—	—
Cumetharol	T45.511	T45.512	T45.513	T45.514	T45.515	T45.516
Cupric						
acetate	T60.3X1	T60.3X2	T60.3X3	T60.3X4	—	—
acetoarsenite	T57.0X1	T57.0X2	T57.0X3	T57.0X4	—	—
arsenate	T57.0X1	T57.0X2	T57.0X3	T57.0X4	—	—
gluconate	T49.0X1	T49.0X2	T49.0X3	T49.0X4	T49.0X5	T49.0X6
oleate	T49.0X1	T49.0X2	T49.0X3	T49.0X4	T49.0X5	T49.0X6
sulfate	T56.4X1	T56.4X2	T56.4X3	T56.4X4	—	—
Cuprous sulfate — see also Copper sulfate	T56.4X1	T56.4X2	T56.4X3	T56.4X4	—	—
Curare, curarine	T48.1X1	T48.1X2	T48.1X3	T48.1X4	T48.1X5	T48.1X6
Cyamemazine	T43.3X1	T43.3X2	T43.3X3	T43.3X4	T43.3X5	T43.3X6
Cyamopsis tetragono-loba	T46.6X1	T46.6X2	T46.6X3	T46.6X4	T46.6X5	T46.6X6
Cyanacetyl hydrazide	T37.1X1	T37.1X2	T37.1X3	T37.1X4	T37.1X5	T37.1X6
Cyanic acid (gas)	T59.891	T59.892	T59.893	T59.894	—	—
Cyanide(s) (compounds) (potassium) (sodium) NEC	T65.0X1	T65.0X2	T65.0X3	T65.0X4	—	—
dust or gas (inhalation) NEC	T57.3X1	T57.3X2	T57.3X3	T57.3X4	—	—
fumigant	T65.0X1	T65.0X2	T65.0X3	T65.0X4	—	—
hydrogen	T57.3X1	T57.3X2	T57.3X3	T57.3X4	—	—
mercuric — see Mercury						
pesticide (dust) (fumes)	T65.0X1	T65.0X2	T65.0X3	T65.0X4	—	—
Cyanoacrylate adhesive	T49.3X1	T49.3X2	T49.3X3	T49.3X4	T49.3X5	T49.3X6
Cyanocobalamin	T45.8X1	T45.8X2	T45.8X3	T45.8X4	T45.8X5	T45.8X6
Cyanogen (chloride) (gas) NEC	T59.891	T59.892	T59.893	T59.894	—	—
Cyclacillin	T36.0X1	T36.0X2	T36.0X3	T36.0X4	T36.0X5	T36.0X6
Cyclaine	T41.3X1	T41.3X2	T41.3X3	T41.3X4	T41.3X5	T41.3X6
Cyclamate	T50.991	T50.992	T50.993	T50.994	T50.995	T50.996

◀ New ◀≡ Revised ~~deleted~~ Deleted

Substance	Poisoning, Accidental (Unintentional)	Poisoning, Intentional Self-Harm	Poisoning, Assault	Poisoning, Undetermined	Adverse Effect	Underdosing
Cyclamen europaeum	T62.2X1	T62.2X2	T62.2X3	T62.2X4	—	—
Cyclandelate	T46.7X1	T46.7X2	T46.7X3	T46.7X4	T46.7X5	T46.7X6
Cyclazocine	T50.7X1	T50.7X2	T50.7X3	T50.7X4	T50.7X5	T50.7X6
Cyclizine	T45.0X1	T45.0X2	T45.0X3	T45.0X4	T45.0X5	T45.0X6
Cyclobarbital	T42.3X1	T42.3X2	T42.3X3	T42.3X4	T42.3X5	T42.3X6
Cyclobarbitone	T42.3X1	T42.3X2	T42.3X3	T42.3X4	T42.3X5	T42.3X6
Cyclobenzaprine	T48.1X1	T48.1X2	T48.1X3	T48.1X4	T48.1X5	T48.1X6
Cyclodrine	T44.3X1	T44.3X2	T44.3X3	T44.3X4	T44.3X5	T44.3X6
Cycloguanil embonate	T37.2X1	T37.2X2	T37.2X3	T37.2X4	T37.2X5	T37.2X6
Cycloheptadiene	T43.291	T43.292	T43.293	T43.294	T43.295	T43.296
Cyclohexane	T52.8X1	T52.8X2	T52.8X3	T52.8X4	—	—
Cyclohexanol	T51.8X1	T51.8X2	T51.8X3	T51.8X4	—	—
Cyclohexanone	T52.4X1	T52.4X2	T52.4X3	T52.4X4	—	—
Cycloheximide	T60.3X1	T60.3X2	T60.3X3	T60.3X4	—	—
Cyclohexyl acetate	T52.8X1	T52.8X2	T52.8X3	T52.8X4	—	—
Cycloleucin	T45.1X1	T45.1X2	T45.1X3	T45.1X4	T45.1X5	T45.1X6
Cyclomethycaine	T41.3X1	T41.3X2	T41.3X3	T41.3X4	T41.3X5	T41.3X6
Cyclopentamine	T44.4X1	T44.4X2	T44.4X3	T44.4X4	T44.4X5	T44.4X6
Cyclopenthiazide	T50.2X1	T50.2X2	T50.2X3	T50.2X4	T50.2X5	T50.2X6
Cyclopentolate	T44.3X1	T44.3X2	T44.3X3	T44.3X4	T44.3X5	T44.3X6
Cyclophosphamide	T45.1X1	T45.1X2	T45.1X3	T45.1X4	T45.1X5	T45.1X6
Cycloplegic drug	T49.5X1	T49.5X2	T49.5X3	T49.5X4	T49.5X5	T49.5X6
Cyclopropane	T41.291	T41.292	T41.293	T41.294	T41.295	T41.296
Cyclopyrabital	T39.8X1	T39.8X2	T39.8X3	T39.8X4	T39.8X5	T39.8X6
Cycloserine	T37.1X1	T37.1X2	T37.1X3	T37.1X4	T37.1X5	T37.1X6
Cyclosporin	T45.1X1	T45.1X2	T45.1X3	T45.1X4	T45.1X5	T45.1X6
Cyclothiazide	T50.2X1	T50.2X2	T50.2X3	T50.2X4	T50.2X5	T50.2X6
Cycrimine	T44.3X1	T44.3X2	T44.3X3	T44.3X4	T44.3X5	T44.3X6
Cyhalothrin	T60.1X1	T60.1X2	T60.1X3	T60.1X4	—	—
Cymarin	T46.0X1	T46.0X2	T46.0X3	T46.0X4	T46.0X5	T46.0X6
Cypermethrin	T60.1X1	T60.1X2	T60.1X3	T60.1X4	—	—
Cyphenothrin	T60.2X1	T60.2X2	T60.2X3	T60.2X4	—	—
Cyproheptadine	T45.0X1	T45.0X2	T45.0X3	T45.0X4	T45.0X5	T45.0X6
Cyprolidol	T43.291	T43.292	T43.293	T43.294	T43.295	T43.296
Cyproterone	T38.6X1	T38.6X2	T38.6X3	T38.6X4	T38.6X5	T38.6X6
Cysteamine	T50.6X1	T50.6X2	T50.6X3	T50.6X4	T50.6X5	T50.6X6
Cytarabine	T45.1X1	T45.1X2	T45.1X3	T45.1X4	T45.1X5	T45.1X6
Cytisus						
laburnum	T62.2X1	T62.2X2	T62.2X3	T62.2X4	—	—
scoparius	T62.2X1	T62.2X2	T62.2X3	T62.2X4	—	—
Cytochrome C	T47.5X1	T47.5X2	T47.5X3	T47.5X4	T47.5X5	T47.5X6
Cytomel	T38.1X1	T38.1X2	T38.1X3	T38.1X4	T38.1X5	T38.1X6

Substance	Poisoning, Accidental (Unintentional)	Poisoning, Intentional Self-Harm	Poisoning, Assault	Poisoning, Undetermined	Adverse Effect	Underdosing
Cytosine arabinoside	T45.1X1	T45.1X2	T45.1X3	T45.1X4	T45.1X5	T45.1X6
Cytoxan	T45.1X1	T45.1X2	T45.1X3	T45.1X4	T45.1X5	T45.1X6
Cytozyme	T45.7X1	T45.7X2	T45.7X3	T45.7X4	T45.7X5	T45.7X6
2,4-D	T60.3X1	T60.3X2	T60.3X3	T60.3X4	—	—
D						
Dacarbazine	T45.1X1	T45.1X2	T45.1X3	T45.1X4	T45.1X5	T45.1X6
Dactinomycin	T45.1X1	T45.1X2	T45.1X3	T45.1X4	T45.1X5	T45.1X6
DADPS	T37.1X1	T37.1X2	T37.1X3	T37.1X4	T37.1X5	T37.1X6
Dakin's solution	T49.0X1	T49.0X2	T49.0X3	T49.0X4	T49.0X5	T49.0X6
Dalapon (sodium)	T60.3X1	T60.3X2	T60.3X3	T60.3X4	—	—
Dalmane	T42.4X1	T42.4X2	T42.4X3	T42.4X4	T42.4X5	T42.4X6
Danazol	T38.6X1	T38.6X2	T38.6X3	T38.6X4	T38.6X5	T38.6X6
Danilone	T45.511	T45.512	T45.513	T45.514	T45.515	T45.516
Danthron	T47.2X1	T47.2X2	T47.2X3	T47.2X4	T47.2X5	T47.2X6
Dantrolene	T42.8X1	T42.8X2	T42.8X3	T42.8X4	T42.8X5	T42.8X6
Dantron	T47.2X1	T47.2X2	T47.2X3	T47.2X4	T47.2X5	T47.2X6
Daphne (gnidium) (mezereum)	T62.2X1	T62.2X2	T62.2X3	T62.2X4	—	—
berry	T62.1X1	T62.1X2	T62.1X3	T62.1X4	—	—
Dapsone	T37.1X1	T37.1X2	T37.1X3	T37.1X4	T37.1X5	T37.1X6
Daraprim	T37.2X1	T37.2X2	T37.2X3	T37.2X4	T37.2X5	T37.2X6
Darnel	T62.2X1	T62.2X2	T62.2X3	T62.2X4	—	—
Darvon	T39.8X1	T39.8X2	T39.8X3	T39.8X4	T39.8X5	T39.8X6
Daunomycin	T45.1X1	T45.1X2	T45.1X3	T45.1X4	T45.1X5	T45.1X6
Daunorubicin	T45.1X1	T45.1X2	T45.1X3	T45.1X4	T45.1X5	T45.1X6
DBI	T38.3X1	T38.3X2	T38.3X3	T38.3X4	T38.3X5	T38.3X6
D-Con	T60.91	T60.92	T60.93	T60.94	—	—
insecticide	T60.2X1	T60.2X2	T60.2X3	T60.2X4	—	—
rodenticide	T60.4X1	T60.4X2	T60.4X3	T60.4X4	—	—
DDAVP	T38.891	T38.892	T38.893	T38.894	T38.895	T38.896
DDE (bis(chlorophenyl)-dichloroethylene)	T60.2X1	T60.2X2	T60.2X3	T60.2X4	—	—
DDS	T37.1X1	T37.1X2	T37.1X3	T37.1X4	T37.1X5	T37.1X6
DDT (dust)	T60.1X1	T60.1X2	T60.1X3	T60.1X4	—	—
Deadly nightshade — see also Belladonna	T62.2X1	T62.2X2	T62.2X3	T62.2X4	—	—
berry	T62.1X1	T62.1X2	T62.1X3	T62.1X4	—	—
Deamino-D-arginine vasopressin	T38.891	T38.892	T38.893	T38.894	T38.895	T38.896
Deanol (aceglumate)	T50.991	T50.992	T50.993	T50.994	T50.995	T50.996
Debrisoquine	T46.5X1	T46.5X2	T46.5X3	T46.5X4	T46.5X5	T46.5X6
Decaborane	T57.8X1	T57.8X2	T57.8X3	T57.8X4	—	—
fumes	T59.891	T59.892	T59.893	T59.894	—	—

◀ New   ◀ Revised   ~~deleted~~ Deleted

Substance	Poisoning, Accidental (Unintentional)	Poisoning, Intentional Self-Harm	Poisoning, Assault	Poisoning, Undetermined	Adverse Effect	Underdosing
Decadron	T38.0X1	T38.0X2	T38.0X3	T38.0X4	T38.0X5	T38.0X6
ENT agent	T49.6X1	T49.6X2	T49.6X3	T49.6X4	T49.6X5	T49.6X6
ophthalmic preparation	T49.5X1	T49.5X2	T49.5X3	T49.5X4	T49.5X5	T49.5X6
topical NEC	T49.0X1	T49.0X2	T49.0X3	T49.0X4	T49.0X5	T49.0X6
Decahydronaphthalene	T52.8X1	T52.8X2	T52.8X3	T52.8X4	—	—
Decalin	T52.8X1	T52.8X2	T52.8X3	T52.8X4	—	—
Decamethonium (bromide)	T48.1X1	T48.1X2	T48.1X3	T48.1X4	T48.1X5	T48.1X6
Decholin	T47.5X1	T47.5X2	T47.5X3	T47.5X4	T47.5X5	T47.5X6
Declomycin	T36.4X1	T36.4X2	T36.4X3	T36.4X4	T36.4X5	T36.4X6
Decongestant, nasal (mucosa)	T48.5X1	T48.5X2	T48.5X3	T48.5X4	T48.5X5	T48.5X6
combination	T48.5X1	T48.5X2	T48.5X3	T48.5X4	T48.5X5	T48.5X6
Deet	T60.8X1	T60.8X2	T60.8X3	T60.8X4	—	—
Deferoxamine	T45.8X1	T45.8X2	T45.8X3	T45.8X4	T45.8X5	T45.8X6
Deflazacort	T38.0X1	T38.0X2	T38.0X3	T38.0X4	T38.0X5	T38.0X6
Deglycyrrhizinized extract of licorice	T48.4X1	T48.4X2	T48.4X3	T48.4X4	T48.4X5	T48.4X6
Dehydrocholic acid	T47.5X1	T47.5X2	T47.5X3	T47.5X4	T47.5X5	T47.5X6
Dehydroemetine	T37.3X1	T37.3X2	T37.3X3	T37.3X4	T37.3X5	T37.3X6
Dekalin	T52.8X1	T52.8X2	T52.8X3	T52.8X4	—	—
Delalutin	T38.5X1	T38.5X2	T38.5X3	T38.5X4	T38.5X5	T38.5X6
Delphinium	T62.2X1	T62.2X2	T62.2X3	T62.2X4	—	—
Deltasone	T38.0X1	T38.0X2	T38.0X3	T38.0X4	T38.0X5	T38.0X6
Deltra	T38.0X1	T38.0X2	T38.0X3	T38.0X4	T38.0X5	T38.0X6
Delvinal	T42.3X1	T42.3X2	T42.3X3	T42.3X4	T42.3X5	T42.3X6
Delorazepam	T42.4X1	T42.4X2	T42.4X3	T42.4X4	T42.4X5	T42.4X6
Deltamethrin	T60.1X1	T60.1X2	T60.1X3	T60.1X4	—	—
Demecarium (bromide)	T49.5X1	T49.5X2	T49.5X3	T49.5X4	T49.5X5	T49.5X6
Demeclocycline	T36.4X1	T36.4X2	T36.4X3	T36.4X4	T36.4X5	T36.4X6
Demecolcine	T45.1X1	T45.1X2	T45.1X3	T45.1X4	T45.1X5	T45.1X6
Demegestone	T38.5X1	T38.5X2	T38.5X3	T38.5X4	T38.5X5	T38.5X6
Demelanizing agents	T49.8X1	T49.8X2	T49.8X3	T49.8X4	T49.8X5	T49.8X6
Demephion -O and -S	T60.0X1	T60.0X2	T60.0X3	T60.0X4	—	—
Demerol	T40.2X1	T40.2X2	T40.2X3	T40.2X4	T40.2X5	T40.2X6
Demethylchlortetracycline	T36.4X1	T36.4X2	T36.4X3	T36.4X4	T36.4X5	T36.4X6
Demethyltetracycline	T36.4X1	T36.4X2	T36.4X3	T36.4X4	T36.4X5	T36.4X6
Demeton -O and -S	T60.0X1	T60.0X2	T60.0X3	T60.0X4	—	—
Demulcent (external)	T49.3X1	T49.3X2	T49.3X3	T49.3X4	T49.3X5	T49.3X6
specified NEC	T49.3X1	T49.3X2	T49.3X3	T49.3X4	T49.3X5	T49.3X6
Demulen	T38.4X1	T38.4X2	T38.4X3	T38.4X4	T38.4X5	T38.4X6
Denatured alcohol	T51.0X1	T51.0X2	T51.0X3	T51.0X4	—	—
Dendrid	T49.5X1	T49.5X2	T49.5X3	T49.5X4	T49.5X5	T49.5X6
Dental drug, topical application NEC	T49.7X1	T49.7X2	T49.7X3	T49.7X4	T49.7X5	T49.7X6

Substance	Poisoning, Accidental (Unintentional)	Poisoning, Intentional Self-Harm	Poisoning, Assault	Poisoning, Undetermined	Adverse Effect	Underdosing
Dentifrice	T49.7X1	T49.7X2	T49.7X3	T49.7X4	T49.7X5	T49.7X6
Deodorant spray (feminine hygiene)	T49.8X1	T49.8X2	T49.8X3	T49.8X4	T49.8X5	T49.8X6
Deoxycortone	T50.0X1	T50.0X2	T50.0X3	T50.0X4	T50.0X5	T50.0X6
2-Deoxy-5-fluorouridine	T45.1X1	T45.1X2	T45.1X3	T45.1X4	T45.1X5	T45.1X6
5-Deoxy-5-fluorouridine	T45.1X1	T45.1X2	T45.1X3	T45.1X4	T45.1X5	T45.1X6
Deoxyribonuclease (pancreatic)	T45.3X1	T45.3X2	T45.3X3	T45.3X4	T45.3X5	T45.3X6
Depilatory	T49.4X1	T49.4X2	T49.4X3	T49.4X4	T49.4X5	T49.4X6
Deprenalin	T42.8X1	T42.8X2	T42.8X3	T42.8X4	T42.8X5	T42.8X6
Deprenyl	T42.8X1	T42.8X2	T42.8X3	T42.8X4	T42.8X5	T42.8X6
Depressant, appetite	T50.5X1	T50.5X2	T50.5X3	T50.5X4	T50.5X5	T50.5X6
Depressant						
appetite, central	T50.5X1	T50.5X2	T50.5X3	T50.5X4	T50.5X5	T50.5X6
cardiac	T46.2X1	T46.2X2	T46.2X3	T46.2X4	T46.2X5	T46.2X6
central nervous system (anesthetic) — see also Central nervous system, depressants	T42.71	T42.72	T42.73	T42.74	T42.75	T42.76
general anesthetic	T41.201	T41.202	T41.203	T41.204	T41.205	T41.206
muscle tone	T42.8X1	T42.8X2	T42.8X3	T42.8X4	T42.8X5	T42.8X6
muscle tone, central	T42.8X1	T42.8X2	T42.8X3	T42.8X4	T42.8X5	T42.8X6
psychotherapeutic	T43.501	T43.502	T43.503	T43.504	T43.505	T43.506
Deptropine	T45.0X1	T45.0X2	T45.0X3	T45.0X4	T45.0X5	T45.0X6
Dequalinium (chloride)	T49.0X1	T49.0X2	T49.0X3	T49.0X4	T49.0X5	T49.0X6
Derris root	T60.2X1	T60.2X2	T60.2X3	T60.2X4	—	—
Deserpidine	T43.011	T43.012	T43.013	T43.014	T43.015	T43.016
Desferrioxamine	T45.8X1	T45.8X2	T45.8X3	T45.8X4	T45.8X5	T45.8X6
Desipramine	T43.0X1	T43.0X2	T43.0X3	T43.0X4	T43.0X5	T43.0X6
Deslanoside	T46.0X1	T46.0X2	T46.0X3	T46.0X4	T46.0X5	T46.0X6
Desloughing agent	T49.4X1	T49.4X2	T49.4X3	T49.4X4	T49.4X5	T49.4X6
Desmethylimipramine	T43.011	T43.012	T43.013	T43.014	T43.015	T43.016
Desmopressin	T38.891	T38.892	T38.893	T38.894	T38.895	T38.896
Desocodeine	T40.2X1	T40.2X2	T40.2X3	T40.2X4	T40.2X5	T40.2X6
Desogestrel	T38.5X1	T38.5X2	T38.5X3	T38.5X4	T38.5X5	T38.5X6
Desomorphine	T40.2X1	T40.2X2	T40.2X3	T40.2X4	—	—
Desonide	T49.0X1	T49.0X2	T49.0X3	T49.0X4	T49.0X5	T49.0X6
Desoximetasone	T49.0X1	T49.0X2	T49.0X3	T49.0X4	T49.0X5	T49.0X6
Desoxycorticosteroid	T50.0X1	T50.0X2	T50.0X3	T50.0X4	T50.0X5	T50.0X6
Desoxycortone	T50.0X1	T50.0X2	T50.0X3	T50.0X4	T50.0X5	T50.0X6
Desoxyephedrine	T43.621	T43.622	T43.623	T43.624	T43.625	T43.626
Detaxtran	T46.6X1	T46.6X2	T46.6X3	T46.6X4	T46.6X5	T46.6X6
Detergent	T49.2X1	T49.2X2	T49.2X3	T49.2X4	T49.2X5	T49.2X6
external medication	T49.2X1	T49.2X2	T49.2X3	T49.2X4	T49.2X5	T49.2X6
local	T49.2X1	T49.2X2	T49.2X3	T49.2X4	T49.2X5	T49.2X6

◀ New ◀▥ Revised ~~deleted~~ Deleted

Substance	Poisoning, Accidental (Unintentional)	Poisoning, Intentional Self-Harm	Poisoning, Assault	Poisoning, Undetermined	Adverse Effect	Underdosing
Detergent (Continued)						
medicinal	T49.2X1	T49.2X2	T49.2X3	T49.2X4	T49.2X5	T49.2X6
nonmedicinal	T55.1X1	T55.1X2	T55.1X3	T55.1X4	—	—
specified NEC	T55.1X1	T55.1X2	T55.1X3	T55.1X4	T55.1X5	T55.1X6
Deterrent, alcohol	T50.6X1	T50.6X2	T50.6X3	T50.6X4	T50.6X5	T50.6X6
Detoxifying agent	T50.6X1	T50.6X2	T50.6X3	T50.6X4	T50.6X5	T50.6X6
Detrothyronine	T38.1X1	T38.1X2	T38.1X3	T38.1X4	T38.1X5	T38.1X6
Dettol (external medication)	T49.0X1	T49.0X2	T49.0X3	T49.0X4	T49.0X5	T49.0X6
Dexamethasone	T38.0X1	T38.0X2	T38.0X3	T38.0X4	T38.0X5	T38.0X6
ENT agent	T49.6X1	T49.6X2	T49.6X3	T49.6X4	T49.6X5	T49.6X6
ophthalmic preparation	T49.5X1	T49.5X2	T49.5X3	T49.5X4	T49.5X5	T49.5X6
topical NEC	T49.0X1	T49.0X2	T49.0X3	T49.0X4	T49.0X5	T49.0X6
Dexamfetamine	T43.621	T43.622	T43.623	T43.624	T43.625	T43.626
Dexamphetamine	T43.621	T43.622	T43.623	T43.624	T43.625	T43.626
Dexbrompheniramine	T45.0X1	T45.0X2	T45.0X3	T45.0X4	T45.0X5	T45.0X6
Dexchlorpheniramine	T45.0X1	T45.0X2	T45.0X3	T45.0X4	T45.0X5	T45.0X6
Dexedrine	T43.621	T43.622	T43.623	T43.624	T43.625	T43.626
Dexetimide	T44.3X1	T44.3X2	T44.3X3	T44.3X4	T44.3X5	T44.3X6
Dexfenfluramine	T50.5X1	T50.5X2	T50.5X3	T50.5X4	T50.5X5	T50.5X6
Dexpanthenol	T45.2X1	T45.2X2	T45.2X3	T45.2X4	T45.2X5	T45.2X6
Dextran (40) (70) (150)	T45.8X1	T45.8X2	T45.8X3	T45.8X4	T45.8X5	T45.8X6
Dextriferron	T45.4X1	T45.4X2	T45.4X3	T45.4X4	T45.4X5	T45.4X6
Dextroamphetamine	T43.621	T43.622	T43.623	T43.624	T43.625	T43.626
Dextro calcium pantothenate	T45.2X1	T45.2X2	T45.2X3	T45.2X4	T45.2X5	T45.2X6
Dextromethorphan	T48.3X1	T48.3X2	T48.3X3	T48.3X4	T48.3X5	T48.3X6
Dextromoramide	T40.4X1	T40.4X2	T40.4X3	T40.4X4	—	—
topical	T49.8X1	T49.8X2	T49.8X3	T49.8X4	T49.8X5	T49.8X6
Dextro pantothenyl alcohol	T45.2X1	T45.2X2	T45.2X3	T45.2X4	T45.2X5	T45.2X6
Dextropropoxyphene	T40.4X1	T40.4X2	T40.4X3	T40.4X4	T40.4X5	T40.4X6
Dextrorphan	T40.2X1	T40.2X2	T40.2X3	T40.2X4	T40.2X5	T40.2X6
Dextrose	T50.3X1	T50.3X2	T50.3X3	T50.3X4	T50.3X5	T50.3X6
concentrated solution, intravenous	T46.8X1	T46.8X2	T46.8X3	T46.8X4	T46.8X5	T46.8X6
Dextrothyroxin	T38.1X1	T38.1X2	T38.1X3	T38.1X4	T38.1X5	T38.1X6
Dextrothyroxine sodium	T38.1X1	T38.1X2	T38.1X3	T38.1X4	T38.1X5	T38.1X6
DFP	T44.0X1	T44.0X2	T44.0X3	T44.0X4	T44.0X5	T44.0X6
DHE	T37.3X1	T37.3X2	T37.3X3	T37.3X4	T37.3X5	T37.3X6
45	T46.5X1	T46.5X2	T46.5X3	T46.5X4	T46.5X5	T46.5X6
Diabinese	T38.3X1	T38.3X2	T38.3X3	T38.3X4	T38.3X5	T38.3X6
Diacetone alcohol	T52.4X1	T52.4X2	T52.4X3	T52.4X4	—	—
Diacetyl monoxime	T50.991	T50.992	T50.993	T50.994	—	—
Diacetylmorphine	T40.1X1	T40.1X2	T40.1X3	T40.1X4		
Diachylon plaster	T49.4X1	T49.4X2	T49.4X3	T49.4X4	T49.4X5	T49.4X6
Diaethylstilboestrolum	T38.5X1	T38.5X2	T38.5X3	T38.5X4	T38.5X5	T38.5X6
Diagnostic agent NEC	T50.8X1	T50.8X2	T50.8X3	T50.8X4	T50.8X5	T50.8X6
Dial (soap)	T49.2X1	T49.2X2	T49.2X3	T49.2X4	T49.2X5	T49.2X6
sedative	T42.3X1	T42.3X2	T42.3X3	T42.3X4	T42.3X5	T42.3X6
Dialkyl carbonate	T52.91	T52.92	T52.93	T52.94	—	—
Diallylbarbituric acid	T42.3X1	T42.3X2	T42.3X3	T42.3X4	T42.3X5	T42.3X6
Diallymal	T42.3X1	T42.3X2	T42.3X3	T42.3X4	T42.3X5	T42.3X6
Dialysis solution (intraperitoneal)	T50.3X1	T50.3X2	T50.3X3	T50.3X4	T50.3X5	T50.3X6
Diaminodiphenylsulfone	T37.1X1	T37.1X2	T37.1X3	T37.1X4	T37.1X5	T37.1X6
Diamorphine	T40.1X1	T40.1X2	T40.1X3	T40.1X4	—	—
Diamox	T50.2X1	T50.2X2	T50.2X3	T50.2X4	T50.2X5	T50.2X6
Diamthazole	T49.0X1	T49.0X2	T49.0X3	T49.0X4	T49.0X5	T49.0X6
Dianthone	T47.2X1	T47.2X2	T47.2X3	T47.2X4	T47.2X5	T47.2X6
Diaphenylsulfone	T37.0X1	T37.0X2	T37.0X3	T37.0X4	T37.0X5	T37.0X6
Diasone (sodium)	T37.1X1	T37.1X2	T37.1X3	T37.1X4	T37.1X5	T37.1X6
Diastase	T47.5X1	T47.5X2	T47.5X3	T47.5X4	T47.5X5	T47.5X6
Diatrizoate	T50.8X1	T50.8X2	T50.8X3	T50.8X4	T50.8X5	T50.8X6
Diazepam	T42.4X1	T42.4X2	T42.4X3	T42.4X4	T42.4X5	T42.4X6
Diazinon	T60.0X1	T60.0X2	T60.0X3	T60.0X4	—	—
Diazomethane (gas)	T59.891	T59.892	T59.893	T59.894	—	—
Diazoxide	T46.5X1	T46.5X2	T46.5X3	T46.5X4	T46.5X5	T46.5X6
Dibekacin	T36.5X1	T36.5X2	T36.5X3	T36.5X4	T36.5X5	T36.5X6
Dibenamine	T44.6X1	T44.6X2	T44.6X3	T44.6X4	T44.6X5	T44.6X6
Dibenzepin	T43.011	T43.012	T43.013	T43.014	T43.015	T43.016
Dibenzheptropine	T45.0X1	T45.0X2	T45.0X3	T45.0X4	T45.0X5	T45.0X6
Dibenzyline	T44.6X1	T44.6X2	T44.6X3	T44.6X4	T44.6X5	T44.6X6
Diborane (gas)	T59.891	T59.892	T59.893	T59.894	—	—
Dibromochloropropane	T60.8X1	T60.8X2	T60.8X3	T60.8X4	—	—
Dibromodulcitol	T45.1X1	T45.1X2	T45.1X3	T45.1X4	T45.1X5	T45.1X6
Dibromoethane	T53.6X1	T53.6X2	T53.6X3	T53.6X4	—	—
Dibromomannitol	T45.1X1	T45.1X2	T45.1X3	T45.1X4	T45.1X5	T45.1X6
Dibromopropamidine isethionate	T49.0X1	T49.0X2	T49.0X3	T49.0X4	T49.0X5	T49.0X6
Dibrompropamidine	T49.0X1	T49.0X2	T49.0X3	T49.0X4	T49.0X5	T49.0X6
Dibucaine	T41.3X1	T41.3X2	T41.3X3	T41.3X4	T41.3X5	T41.3X6
topical (surface)	T41.3X1	T41.3X2	T41.3X3	T41.3X4	T41.3X5	T41.3X6
Dibunate sodium	T48.3X1	T48.3X2	T48.3X3	T48.3X4	T48.3X5	T48.3X6
Dibutoline sulfate	T44.3X1	T44.3X2	T44.3X3	T44.3X4	T44.3X5	T44.3X6
Dicamba	T60.3X1	T60.3X2	T60.3X3	T60.3X4	—	—
Dicapthon	T60.0X1	T60.0X2	T60.0X3	T60.0X4	—	—
Dichlobenil	T60.3X1	T60.3X2	T60.3X3	T60.3X4	—	—
Dichlone	T60.3X1	T60.3X2	T60.3X3	T60.3X4	—	—

TABLE OF DRUGS AND CHEMICALS

Substance	External Cause (T-Code) Poisoning, Accidental (Unintentional)	Poisoning, Intentional Self-Harm	Poisoning, Assault	Poisoning, Undetermined	Adverse Effect	Underdosing
Dichloralphenozone	T42.6X1	T42.6X2	T42.6X3	T42.6X4	T42.6X5	T42.6X6
Dichlorbenzidine	T65.3X1	T65.3X2	T65.3X3	T65.3X4	—	—
Dichlorhydrin	T52.8X1	T52.8X2	T52.8X3	T52.8X4	—	—
Dichlorhydroxyquinoline	T37.8X1	T37.8X2	T37.8X3	T37.8X4	T37.8X5	T37.8X6
Dichlorobenzene	T53.7X1	T53.7X2	T53.7X3	T53.7X4	—	—
Dichlorobenzyl alcohol	T49.6X1	T49.6X2	T49.6X3	T49.6X4	T49.6X5	T49.6X6
Dichlorodifluoromethane	T53.5X1	T53.5X2	T53.5X3	T53.5X4	—	—
Dichloroethane	T52.8X1	T52.8X2	T52.8X3	T52.8X4	—	—
Sym-Dichloroethyl ether	T53.6X1	T53.6X2	T53.6X3	T53.6X4	—	—
Dichloroethyl sulfide, not in war	T59.891	T59.892	T59.893	T59.894	—	—
Dichloroethylene	T53.6X1	T53.6X2	T53.6X3	T53.6X4	—	—
Dichloroformoxine, not in war	T59.891	T59.892	T59.893	T59.894	—	—
Dichlorohydrin, alpha-dichlorohydrin	T52.8X1	T52.8X2	T52.8X3	T52.8X4	—	—
Dichloromethane (solvent)	T53.4X1	T53.4X2	T53.4X3	T53.4X4	—	—
vapor	T53.4X1	T53.4X2	T53.4X3	T53.4X4	—	—
Dichloronaphthoquinone	T60.3X1	T60.3X2	T60.3X3	T60.3X4	—	—
Dichlorophen	T37.4X1	T37.4X2	T37.4X3	T37.4X4	T37.4X5	T37.4X6
2,4-Dichlorophenoxy-acetic acid	T60.3X1	T60.3X2	T60.3X3	T60.3X4	—	—
Dichloropropene	T60.3X1	T60.3X2	T60.3X3	T60.3X4	—	—
Dichloropropionic acid	T60.3X1	T60.3X2	T60.3X3	T60.3X4	—	—
Dichlorphenamide	T50.2X1	T50.2X2	T50.2X3	T50.2X4	T50.2X5	T50.2X6
Dichlorvos	T60.0X1	T60.0X2	T60.0X3	T60.0X4	—	—
Diclofenac	T39.391	T39.392	T39.393	T39.394	T39.395	T39.396
Diclofenamide	T50.2X1	T50.2X2	T50.2X3	T50.2X4	T50.2X5	T50.2X6
Diclofensine	T43.291	T43.292	T43.293	T43.294	T43.295	T43.296
Diclonixine	T39.8X1	T39.8X2	T39.8X3	T39.8X4	T39.8X5	T39.8X6
Dicloxacillin	T36.0X1	T36.0X2	T36.0X3	T36.0X4	T36.0X5	T36.0X6
Dicophane	T49.0X1	T49.0X2	T49.0X3	T49.0X4	T49.0X5	T49.0X6
Dicoumarol, dicoumarin, dicumarol	T45.511	T45.512	T45.513	T45.514	T45.515	T45.516
Dicrotophos	T60.0X1	T60.0X2	T60.0X3	T60.0X4	—	—
Dicyanogen (gas)	T65.0X1	T65.0X2	T65.0X3	T65.0X4	—	—
Dicyclomine	T44.3X1	T44.3X2	T44.3X3	T44.3X4	T44.3X5	T44.3X6
Dicycloverine	T44.3X1	T44.3X2	T44.3X3	T44.3X4	T44.3X5	T44.3X6
Dideoxycytidine	T37.5X1	T37.5X2	T37.5X3	T37.5X4	T37.5X5	T37.5X6
Dideoxyinosine	T37.5X1	T37.5X2	T37.5X3	T37.5X4	T37.5X5	T37.5X6
Dieldrin (vapor)	T60.1X1	T60.1X2	T60.1X3	T60.1X4	—	—
Diemal	T42.3X1	T42.3X2	T42.3X3	T42.3X4	T42.3X5	T42.3X6
Dienestrol	T38.5X1	T38.5X2	T38.5X3	T38.5X4	T38.5X5	T38.5X6
Dienoestrol	T38.5X1	T38.5X2	T38.5X3	T38.5X4	T38.5X5	T38.5X6
Dietetic drug NEC	T50.901	T50.902	T50.903	T50.904	T50.905	T50.906
Diethazine	T42.8X1	T42.8X2	T42.8X3	T42.8X4	T42.8X5	T42.8X6

Substance	External Cause (T-Code) Poisoning, Accidental (Unintentional)	Poisoning, Intentional Self-Harm	Poisoning, Assault	Poisoning, Undetermined	Adverse Effect	Underdosing
Diethyl						
barbituric acid	T42.3X1	T42.3X2	T42.3X3	T42.3X4	T42.3X5	T42.3X6
carbamazine	T37.4X1	T37.4X2	T37.4X3	T37.4X4	T37.4X5	T37.4X6
carbinol	T51.3X1	T51.3X2	T51.3X3	T51.3X4	—	—
carbonate	T52.8X1	T52.8X2	T52.8X3	T52.8X4	—	—
ether (vapor) — see also ether	T41.0X1	T41.0X2	T41.0X3	T41.0X4	T41.0X5	T41.0X6
oxide	T52.8X1	T52.8X2	T52.8X3	T52.8X4	—	—
propion	T50.5X1	T50.5X2	T50.5X3	T50.5X4	T50.5X5	T50.5X6
stilbestrol	T38.5X1	T38.5X2	T38.5X3	T38.5X4	T38.5X5	T38.5X6
toluamide (nonmedicinal)	T60.8X1	T60.8X2	T60.8X3	T60.8X4	—	—
medicinal	T49.3X1	T49.3X2	T49.3X3	T49.3X4	T49.3X5	T49.3X6
Diethylcarbamazine	T37.4X1	T37.4X2	T37.4X3	T37.4X4	T37.4X5	T37.4X6
Diethylene						
dioxide	T52.8X1	T52.8X2	T52.8X3	T52.8X4	—	—
glycol (monoacetate) (monobutyl ether) (monoethyl ether)	T52.3X1	T52.3X2	T52.3X3	T52.3X4	—	—
Diethylhexylphthalate	T65.891	T65.892	T65.893	T65.894	—	—
Diethylpropion	T50.5X1	T50.5X2	T50.5X3	T50.5X4	T50.5X5	T50.5X6
Diethylstilbestrol	T38.5X1	T38.5X2	T38.5X3	T38.5X4	T38.5X5	T38.5X6
Diethylstilboestrol	T38.5X1	T38.5X2	T38.5X3	T38.5X4	T38.5X5	T38.5X6
Diethylsulfone-diethylmethane	T42.6X1	T42.6X2	T42.6X3	T42.6X4	T42.6X5	T42.6X6
Diethyltoluamide	T49.0X1	T49.0X2	T49.0X3	T49.0X4	T49.0X5	T49.0X6
Diethyltryptamine (DET)	T40.991	T40.992	T40.993	T40.994	—	—
Difebarbamate	T42.3X1	T42.3X2	T42.3X3	T42.3X4	T42.3X5	T42.3X6
Difencloxazine	T40.2X1	T40.2X2	T40.2X3	T40.2X4	T40.2X5	T40.2X6
Difenidol	T45.0X1	T45.0X2	T45.0X3	T45.0X4	T45.0X5	T45.0X6
Difenoxin	T47.6X1	T47.6X2	T47.6X3	T47.6X4	T47.6X5	T47.6X6
Difetarsone	T37.3X1	T37.3X2	T37.3X3	T37.3X4	T37.3X5	T37.3X6
Diffusin	T45.3X1	T45.3X2	T45.3X3	T45.3X4	T45.3X5	T45.3X6
Diflorasone	T49.0X1	T49.0X2	T49.0X3	T49.0X4	T49.0X5	T49.0X6
Diflubenzuron	T60.1X1	T60.1X2	T60.1X3	T60.1X4	—	—
Diflos	T44.0X1	T44.0X2	T44.0X3	T44.0X4	T44.0X5	T44.0X6
Diflucortolone	T49.0X1	T49.0X2	T49.0X3	T49.0X4	T49.0X5	T49.0X6
Diflunisal	T39.091	T39.092	T39.093	T39.094	T39.095	T39.096
Difluoromethyldopa	T42.8X1	T42.8X2	T42.8X3	T42.8X4	T42.8X5	T42.8X6
Difluorophate	T44.0X1	T44.0X2	T44.0X3	T44.0X4	T44.0X5	T44.0X6
Digestant NEC	T47.5X1	T47.5X2	T47.5X3	T47.5X4	T47.5X5	T47.5X6
Digitalin(e)	T46.0X1	T46.0X2	T46.0X3	T46.0X4	T46.0X5	T46.0X6
Digitalis (leaf) (glycoside)	T46.0X1	T46.0X2	T46.0X3	T46.0X4	T46.0X5	T46.0X6
lanata	T46.0X1	T46.0X2	T46.0X3	T46.0X4	T46.0X5	T46.0X6
purpurea	T46.0X1	T46.0X2	T46.0X3	T46.0X4	T46.0X5	T46.0X6
Digitoxin	T46.0X1	T46.0X2	T46.0X3	T46.0X4	T46.0X5	T46.0X6

◀ New ◀◀ Revised ~~deleted~~ Deleted

Substance	Poisoning, Accidental (Unintentional)	Poisoning, Intentional Self-Harm	Poisoning, Assault	Poisoning, Undetermined	Adverse Effect	Underdosing
Digitoxose	T46.0X1	T46.0X2	T46.0X3	T46.0X4	T46.0X5	T46.0X6
Digoxin	T46.0X1	T46.0X2	T46.0X3	T46.0X4	T46.0X5	T46.0X6
Digoxine	T46.0X1	T46.0X2	T46.0X3	T46.0X4	T46.0X5	T46.0X6
Dihydralazine	T46.5X1	T46.5X2	T46.5X3	T46.5X4	T46.5X5	T46.5X6
Dihydrazine	T46.5X1	T46.5X2	T46.5X3	T46.5X4	T46.5X5	T46.5X6
Dihydrocodeinone	T40.2X1	T40.2X2	T40.2X3	T40.2X4	T40.2X5	T40.2X6
Dihydroergocornine	T46.7X1	T46.7X2	T46.7X3	T46.7X4	T46.7X5	T46.7X6
Dihydroergocristine (mesilate)	T46.7X1	T46.7X2	T46.7X3	T46.7X4	T46.7X5	T46.7X6
Dihydroergokryptine	T46.7X1	T46.7X2	T46.7X3	T46.7X4	T46.7X5	T46.7X6
Dihydroergotamine	T46.5X1	T46.5X2	T46.5X3	T46.5X4	T46.5X5	T46.5X6
Dihydroergotoxine	T46.7X1	T46.7X2	T46.7X3	T46.7X4	T46.7X5	T46.7X6
mesilate	T46.7X1	T46.7X2	T46.7X3	T46.7X4	T46.7X5	T46.7X6
Dihydrohydroxycodein-one	T40.2X1	T40.2X2	T40.2X3	T40.2X4	T40.2X5	T40.2X6
Dihydrohydroxymorphinone	T40.2X1	T40.2X2	T40.2X3	T40.2X4	T40.2X5	T40.2X6
Dihydroisocodeine	T40.2X1	T40.2X2	T40.2X3	T40.2X4	T40.2X5	T40.2X6
Dihydromorphine	T40.2X1	T40.2X2	T40.2X3	T40.2X4	—	—
Dihydromorphinone	T40.2X1	T40.2X2	T40.2X3	T40.2X4	T40.2X5	T40.2X6
Dihydrostreptomycin	T36.5X1	T36.5X2	T36.5X3	T36.5X4	T36.5X5	T36.5X6
Dihydrotachysterol	T45.2X1	T45.2X2	T45.2X3	T45.2X4	T45.2X5	T45.2X6
Dihydroxyaluminum aminoacetate	T47.1X1	T47.1X2	T47.1X3	T47.1X4	T47.1X5	T47.1X6
Dihydroxyaluminum sodium carbonate	T47.1X1	T47.1X2	T47.1X3	T47.1X4	T47.1X5	T47.1X6
Dihydroxyanthraquinone	T47.2X1	T47.2X2	T47.2X3	T47.2X4	T47.2X5	T47.2X6
Dihydroxycodeinone	T40.2X1	T40.2X2	T40.2X3	T40.2X4	T40.2X5	T40.2X6
Dihydroxypropyl theophylline	T50.2X1	T50.2X2	T50.2X3	T50.2X4	T50.2X5	T50.2X6
Diiodohydroxyquin	T37.8X1	T37.8X2	T37.8X3	T37.8X4	T37.8X5	T37.8X6
topical	T49.0X1	T49.0X2	T49.0X3	T49.0X4	T49.0X5	T49.0X6
Diiodohydroxyquinoline	T37.8X1	T37.8X2	T37.8X3	T37.8X4	T37.8X5	T37.8X6
Diiodotyrosine	T38.2X1	T38.2X2	T38.2X3	T38.2X4	T38.2X5	T38.2X6
Diisopromine	T44.3X1	T44.3X2	T44.3X3	T44.3X4	T44.3X5	T44.3X6
Diisopropylamine	T46.3X1	T46.3X2	T46.3X3	T46.3X4	T46.3X5	T46.3X6
Diisopropylfluorophosphonate	T44.0X1	T44.0X2	T44.0X3	T44.0X4	T44.0X5	T44.0X6
Dilantin	T42.0X1	T42.0X2	T42.0X3	T42.0X4	T42.0X5	T42.0X6
Dilaudid	T40.2X1	T40.2X2	T40.2X3	T40.2X4	T40.2X5	T40.2X6
Dilazep	T46.3X1	T46.3X2	T46.3X3	T46.3X4	T46.3X5	T46.3X6
Dill	T47.5X1	T47.5X2	T47.5X3	T47.5X4	T47.5X5	T47.5X6
Diloxanide	T37.3X1	T37.3X2	T37.3X3	T37.3X4	T37.3X5	T37.3X6
Diltiazem	T46.1X1	T46.1X2	T46.1X3	T46.1X4	T46.1X5	T46.1X6
Dimazole	T49.0X1	T49.0X2	T49.0X3	T49.0X4	T49.0X5	T49.0X6
Dimefline	T50.7X1	T50.7X2	T50.7X3	T50.7X4	T50.7X5	T50.7X6
Dimefox	T60.0X1	T60.0X2	T60.0X3	T60.0X4	—	—

Substance	Poisoning, Accidental (Unintentional)	Poisoning, Intentional Self-Harm	Poisoning, Assault	Poisoning, Undetermined	Adverse Effect	Underdosing
Dimemorfan	T48.3X1	T48.3X2	T48.3X3	T48.3X4	T48.3X5	T48.3X6
Dimenhydrinate	T45.0X1	T45.0X2	T45.0X3	T45.0X4	T45.0X5	T45.0X6
Dimercaprol (British anti-lewisite)	T45.8X1	T45.8X2	T45.8X3	T45.8X4	T45.8X5	T45.8X6
Dimercaptopropanol	T45.8X1	T45.8X2	T45.8X3	T45.8X4	T45.8X5	T45.8X6
Dimestrol	T38.5X1	T38.5X2	T38.5X3	T38.5X4	T38.5X5	T38.5X6
Dimetane	T45.0X1	T45.0X2	T45.0X3	T45.0X4	T45.0X5	T45.0X6
Dimethicone	T47.1X1	T47.1X2	T47.1X3	T47.1X4	T47.1X5	T47.1X6
Dimethindene	T45.0X1	T45.0X2	T45.0X3	T45.0X4	T45.0X5	T45.0X6
Dimethisoquin	T49.1X1	T49.1X2	T49.1X3	T49.1X4	T49.1X5	T49.1X6
Dimethisterone	T38.5X1	T38.5X2	T38.5X3	T38.5X4	T38.5X5	T38.5X6
Dimethoate	T60.0X1	T60.0X2	T60.0X3	T60.0X4	—	—
Dimethocaine	T41.3X1	T41.3X2	T41.3X3	T41.3X4	T41.3X5	T41.3X6
Dimethoxanate	T48.3X1	T48.3X2	T48.3X3	T48.3X4	T48.3X5	T48.3X6
Dimethyl						
arsine, arsinic acid	T57.0X1	T57.0X2	T57.0X3	T57.0X4	—	—
carbinol	T51.2X1	T51.2X2	T51.2X3	T51.2X4	—	—
carbonate	T52.8X1	T52.8X2	T52.8X3	T52.8X4	—	—
diguanide	T38.3X1	T38.3X2	T38.3X3	T38.3X4	T38.3X5	T38.3X6
ketone	T52.4X1	T52.4X2	T52.4X3	T52.4X4	—	—
vapor	T52.4X1	T52.4X2	T52.4X3	T52.4X4	—	—
meperidine	T40.2X1	T40.2X2	T40.2X3	T40.2X4	T40.2X5	T40.2X6
parathion	T60.0X1	T60.0X2	T60.0X3	T60.0X4	—	—
phthlate	T49.3X1	T49.3X2	T49.3X3	T49.3X4	T49.3X5	T49.3X6
polysiloxane	T47.8X1	T47.8X2	T47.8X3	T47.8X4	T47.8X5	T47.8X6
sulfate (fumes)	T59.891	T59.892	T59.893	T59.894	—	—
liquid	T65.891	T65.892	T65.893	T65.894	—	—
sulfoxide (nonmedicinal)	T52.8X1	T52.8X2	T52.8X3	T52.8X4	—	—
medicinal	T49.4X1	T49.4X2	T49.4X3	T49.4X4	T49.4X5	T49.4X6
tryptamine	T40.991	T40.992	T40.993	T40.994		
tubocurarine	T48.1X1	T48.1X2	T48.1X3	T48.1X4	T48.1X5	T48.1X6
Dimethylamine sulfate	T49.4X1	T49.4X2	T49.4X3	T49.4X4	T49.4X5	T49.4X6
Dimethylformamide	T52.8X1	T52.8X2	T52.8X3	T52.8X4	—	—
Dimethyltubocurarinium chloride	T48.1X1	T48.1X2	T48.1X3	T48.1X4	T48.1X5	T48.1X6
Dimeticone	T47.1X1	T47.1X2	T47.1X3	T47.1X4	T47.1X5	T47.1X6
Dimetilan	T60.0X1	T60.0X2	T60.0X3	T60.0X4	—	—
Dimetindene	T45.0X1	T45.0X2	T45.0X3	T45.0X4	T45.0X5	T45.0X6
Dimetotiazine	T43.3X1	T43.3X2	T43.3X3	T43.3X4	T43.3X5	T43.3X6
Dimorpholamine	T50.7X1	T50.7X2	T50.7X3	T50.7X4	T50.7X5	T50.7X6
Dimoxyline	T46.3X1	T46.3X2	T46.3X3	T46.3X4	T46.3X5	T46.3X6
Dinitrobenzene	T65.3X1	T65.3X2	T65.3X3	T65.3X4	—	—
vapor	T59.891	T59.892	T59.893	T59.894		

TABLE OF DRUGS AND CHEMICALS

Substance	Poisoning, Accidental (Unintentional)	Poisoning, Intentional Self-Harm	Poisoning, Assault	Poisoning, Undetermined	Adverse Effect	Underdosing
Dinitrobenzol	T65.3X1	T65.3X2	T65.3X3	T65.3X4	—	—
vapor	T59.891	T59.892	T59.893	T59.894	—	—
Dinitrobutylphenol	T65.3X1	T65.3X2	T65.3X3	T65.3X4	—	—
Dinitro (-ortho-)cresol (pesticide) (spray)	T65.3X1	T65.3X2	T65.3X3	T65.3X4	—	—
Dinitrocyclohexylphenol	T65.3X1	T65.3X2	T65.3X3	T65.3X4	—	—
Dinitrophenol	T65.3X1	T65.3X2	T65.3X3	T65.3X4	—	—
Dinoprost	T48.0X1	T48.0X2	T48.0X3	T48.0X4	T48.0X5	T48.0X6
Dinoprostone	T48.0X1	T48.0X2	T48.0X3	T48.0X4	T48.0X5	T48.0X6
Dinoseb	T60.3X1	T60.3X2	T60.3X3	T60.3X4	—	—
Dioctyl sulfosuccinate (calcium) (sodium)	T47.4X1	T47.4X2	T47.4X3	T47.4X4	T47.4X5	T47.4X6
Diodone	T50.8X1	T50.8X2	T50.8X3	T50.8X4	T50.8X5	T50.8X6
Diodoquin	T37.8X1	T37.8X2	T37.8X3	T37.8X4	T37.8X5	T37.8X6
Dionin	T40.2X1	T40.2X2	T40.2X3	T40.2X4	T40.2X5	T40.2X6
Diosmin	T46.991	T46.992	T46.993	T46.994	T46.995	T46.996
Dioxane	T52.8X1	T52.8X2	T52.8X3	T52.8X4	—	—
Dioxathion	T60.0X1	T60.0X2	T60.0X3	T60.0X4	—	—
Dioxin	T53.7X1	T53.7X2	T53.7X3	T53.7X4	—	—
Dioxopromethazine	T43.3X1	T43.3X2	T43.3X3	T43.3X4	T43.3X5	T43.3X6
Dioxyline	T46.3X1	T46.3X2	T46.3X3	T46.3X4	T46.3X5	T46.3X6
Dipentene	T52.8X1	T52.8X2	T52.8X3	T52.8X4	—	—
Diperodon	T41.3X1	T41.3X2	T41.3X3	T41.3X4	T41.3X5	T41.3X6
Diphacinone	T60.4X1	T60.4X2	T60.4X3	T60.4X4	—	—
Diphemanil	T44.3X1	T44.3X2	T44.3X3	T44.3X4	T44.3X5	T44.3X6
metilsulfate	T44.3X1	T44.3X2	T44.3X3	T44.3X4	T44.3X5	T44.3X6
Diphenadione	T45.511	T45.512	T45.513	T45.514	T45.515	T45.516
rodenticide	T60.4X1	T60.4X2	T60.4X3	T60.4X4	—	—
Diphenhydramine	T45.0X1	T45.0X2	T45.0X3	T45.0X4	T45.0X5	T45.0X6
Diphenidol	T45.0X1	T45.0X2	T45.0X3	T45.0X4	T45.0X5	T45.0X6
Diphenoxylate	T47.6X1	T47.6X2	T47.6X3	T47.6X4	T47.6X5	T47.6X6
Diphenylamine	T65.3X1	T65.3X2	T65.3X3	T65.3X4	—	—
Diphenylbutazone	T39.2X1	T39.2X2	T39.2X3	T39.2X4	T39.2X5	T39.2X6
Diphenylchloroarsine, not in war	T57.0X1	T57.0X2	T57.0X3	T57.0X4	—	—
Diphenylhydantoin	T42.0X1	T42.0X2	T42.0X3	T42.0X4	T42.0X5	T42.0X6
Diphenylmethane dye	T52.1X1	T52.1X2	T52.1X3	T52.1X4	—	—
Diphenylpyraline	T45.0X1	T45.0X2	T45.0X3	T45.0X4	T45.0X5	T45.0X6
Diphtheria						
antitoxin	T50.Z11	T50.Z12	T50.Z13	T50.Z14	T50.Z15	T50.Z16
toxoid	T50.A91	T50.A92	T50.A93	T50.A94	T50.A95	T50.A96
with tetanus toxoid	T50.A21	T50.A22	T50.A23	T50.A24	T50.A25	T50.A26
with pertussis component	T50.A11	T50.A12	T50.A13	T50.A14	T50.A15	T50.A16

Substance	Poisoning, Accidental (Unintentional)	Poisoning, Intentional Self-Harm	Poisoning, Assault	Poisoning, Undetermined	Adverse Effect	Underdosing
Diphtheria *(Continued)*						
vaccine (combination)	T50.A91	T50.A92	T50.A93	T50.A94	T50.A95	T50.A96
combination						
including pertussis	T50.A11	T50.A12	T50.A13	T50.A14	T50.A15	T50.A16
without pertussis	T50.A21	T50.A22	T50.A23	T50.A24	T50.A25	T50.A26
Diphylline	T50.2X1	T50.2X2	T50.2X3	T50.2X4	T50.2X5	T50.2X6
Dipipanone	T40.4X1	T40.4X2	T40.4X3	T40.4X4	—	—
Dipivefrine	T49.5X1	T49.5X2	T49.5X3	T49.5X4	T49.5X5	T49.5X6
Diplovax	T50.B91	T50.B92	T50.B93	T50.B94	T50.B95	T50.B96
Diprophylline	T50.2X1	T50.2X2	T50.2X3	T50.2X4	T50.2X5	T50.2X6
Dipropyline	T48.291	T48.292	T48.293	T48.294	T48.295	T48.296
Dipyridamole	T46.3X1	T46.3X2	T46.3X3	T46.3X4	T46.3X5	T46.3X6
Dipyrone	T39.2X1	T39.2X2	T39.2X3	T39.2X4	T39.2X5	T39.2X6
Diquat (dibromide)	T60.3X1	T60.3X2	T60.3X3	T60.3X4	—	—
Disinfectant	T65.891	T65.892	T65.893	T65.894	—	—
alkaline	T54.3X1	T54.3X2	T54.3X3	T54.3X4	—	—
aromatic	T54.1X1	T54.1X2	T54.1X3	T54.1X4	—	—
intestinal	T37.8X1	T37.8X2	T37.8X3	T37.8X4	T37.8X5	T37.8X6
Disipal	T42.8X1	T42.8X2	T42.8X3	T42.8X4	T42.8X5	T42.8X6
Disodium edetate	T50.6X1	T50.6X2	T50.6X3	T50.6X4	T50.6X5	T50.6X6
Disoprofol	T41.291	T41.292	T41.293	T41.294	T41.295	T41.296
Disopyramide	T46.2X1	T46.2X2	T46.2X3	T46.2X4	T46.2X5	T46.2X6
Distigmine (bromide)	T44.0X1	T44.0X2	T44.0X3	T44.0X4	T44.0X5	T44.0X6
Disulfamide	T50.2X1	T50.2X2	T50.2X3	T50.2X4	T50.2X5	T50.2X6
Disulfanilamide	T37.0X1	T37.0X2	T37.0X3	T37.0X4	T37.0X5	T37.0X6
Disulfiram	T50.6X1	T50.6X2	T50.6X3	T50.6X4	T50.6X5	T50.6X6
Disulfoton	T60.0X1	T60.0X2	T60.0X3	T60.0X4	—	—
Dithiazanine iodide	T37.4X1	T37.4X2	T37.4X3	T37.4X4	T37.4X5	T37.4X6
Dithiocarbamate	T60.0X1	T60.0X2	T60.0X3	T60.0X4	—	—
Dithranol	T49.4X1	T49.4X2	T49.4X3	T49.4X4	T49.4X5	T49.4X6
Diucardin	T50.2X1	T50.2X2	T50.2X3	T50.2X4	T50.2X5	T50.2X6
Diupres	T50.2X1	T50.2X2	T50.2X3	T50.2X4	T50.2X5	T50.2X6
Diuretic NEC	T50.2X1	T50.2X2	T50.2X3	T50.2X4	T50.2X5	T50.2X6
benzothiadiazine	T50.2X1	T50.2X2	T50.2X3	T50.2X4	T50.2X5	T50.2X6
carbonic acid anhydrase inhibitors	T50.2X1	T50.2X2	T50.2X3	T50.2X4	T50.2X5	T50.2X6
furfuryl NEC	T50.2X1	T50.2X2	T50.2X3	T50.2X4	T50.2X5	T50.2X6
loop (high-ceiling)	T50.1X1	T50.1X2	T50.1X3	T50.1X4	T50.1X5	T50.1X6
mercurial NEC	T50.2X1	T50.2X2	T50.2X3	T50.2X4	T50.2X5	T50.2X6
osmotic	T50.2X1	T50.2X2	T50.2X3	T50.2X4	T50.2X5	T50.2X6
purine NEC	T50.2X1	T50.2X2	T50.2X3	T50.2X4	T50.2X5	T50.2X6
saluretic NEC	T50.2X1	T50.2X2	T50.2X3	T50.2X4	T50.2X5	T50.2X6

◄ New ◄▌ Revised ~~deleted~~ Deleted

Substance	Poisoning, Accidental (Unintentional)	Poisoning, Intentional Self-Harm	Poisoning, Assault	Poisoning, Undetermined	Adverse Effect	Underdosing
Diuretic NEC *(Continued)*						
sulfonamide	T50.2X1	T50.2X2	T50.2X3	T50.2X4	T50.2X5	T50.2X6
thiazide NEC	T50.2X1	T50.2X2	T50.2X3	T50.2X4	T50.2X5	T50.2X6
xanthine	T50.2X1	T50.2X2	T50.2X3	T50.2X4	T50.2X5	T50.2X6
Diurgin	T50.2X1	T50.2X2	T50.2X3	T50.2X4	T50.2X5	T50.2X6
Diuril	T50.2X1	T50.2X2	T50.2X3	T50.2X4	T50.2X5	T50.2X6
Diuron	T60.3X1	T60.3X2	T60.3X3	T60.3X4	—	—
Divalproex	T42.6X1	T42.6X2	T42.6X3	T42.6X4	T42.6X5	T42.6X6
Divinyl ether	T41.0X1	T41.0X2	T41.0X3	T41.0X4	T41.0X5	T41.0X6
Dixanthogen	T49.0X1	T49.0X2	T49.0X3	T49.0X4	T49.0X5	T49.0X6
Dixyrazine	T43.3X1	T43.3X2	T43.3X3	T43.3X4	T43.3X5	T43.3X6
D-lysergic acid diethylamide	T40.8X1	T40.8X2	T40.8X3	T40.8X4	—	—
DMCT	T36.4X1	T36.4X2	T36.4X3	T36.4X4	T36.4X5	T36.4X6
DMSO — *see Dimethyl sulfoxide*						
DNBP	T60.3X1	T60.3X2	T60.3X3	T60.3X4	—	—
DNOC	T65.3X1	T65.3X2	T65.3X3	T65.3X4	—	—
DOCA	T38.0X1	T38.0X2	T38.0X3	T38.0X4	T38.0X5	T38.0X6
Dobutamine	T44.5X1	T44.5X2	T44.5X3	T44.5X4	T44.5X5	T44.5X6
Docusate sodium	T47.4X1	T47.4X2	T47.4X3	T47.4X4	T47.4X5	T47.4X6
Dodicin	T49.0X1	T49.0X2	T49.0X3	T49.0X4	T49.0X5	T49.0X6
Dofamium chloride	T49.0X1	T49.0X2	T49.0X3	T49.0X4	T49.0X5	T49.0X6
Dolophine	T40.3X1	T40.3X2	T40.3X3	T40.3X4	T40.3X5	T40.3X6
Doloxene	T39.8X1	T39.8X2	T39.8X3	T39.8X4	T39.8X5	T39.8X6
Domestic gas (after combustion) — *see Gas, utility*						
prior to combustion	T59.891	T59.892	T59.893	T59.894	—	—
Domiodol	T48.4X1	T48.4X2	T48.4X3	T48.4X4	T48.4X5	T48.4X6
Domiphen (bromide)	T49.0X1	T49.0X2	T49.0X3	T49.0X4	T49.0X5	T49.0X6
Domperidone	T45.0X1	T45.0X2	T45.0X3	T45.0X4	T45.0X5	T45.0X6
Dopa	T42.8X1	T42.8X2	T42.8X3	T42.8X4	T42.8X5	T42.8X6
Dopamine	T44.991	T44.992	T44.993	T44.994	T44.995	T44.996
Doriden	T42.6X1	T42.6X2	T42.6X3	T42.6X4	T42.6X5	T42.6X6
Dormiral	T42.3X1	T42.3X2	T42.3X3	T42.3X4	T42.3X5	T42.3X6
Dormison	T42.6X1	T42.6X2	T42.6X3	T42.6X4	T42.6X5	T42.6X6
Dornase	T48.4X1	T48.4X2	T48.4X3	T48.4X4	T48.4X5	T48.4X6
Dorsacaine	T41.3X1	T41.3X2	T41.3X3	T41.3X4	T41.3X5	T41.3X6
Dosulepin	T43.011	T43.012	T43.013	T43.014	T43.015	T43.016
Dothiepin	T43.011	T43.012	T43.013	T43.014	T43.015	T43.016
Doxantrazole	T48.6X1	T48.6X2	T48.6X3	T48.6X4	T48.6X5	T48.6X6
Doxapram	T50.7X1	T50.7X2	T50.7X3	T50.7X4	T50.7X5	T50.7X6
Doxazosin	T44.6X1	T44.6X2	T44.6X3	T44.6X4	T44.6X5	T44.6X6
Doxepin	T43.011	T43.012	T43.013	T43.014	T43.015	T43.016

Substance	Poisoning, Accidental (Unintentional)	Poisoning, Intentional Self-Harm	Poisoning, Assault	Poisoning, Undetermined	Adverse Effect	Underdosing
Doxifluridine	T45.1X1	T45.1X2	T45.1X3	T45.1X4	T45.1X5	T45.1X6
Doxorubicin	T45.1X1	T45.1X2	T45.1X3	T45.1X4	T45.1X5	T45.1X6
Doxycycline	T36.4X1	T36.4X2	T36.4X3	T36.4X4	T36.4X5	T36.4X6
Doxylamine	T45.0X1	T45.0X2	T45.0X3	T45.0X4	T45.0X5	T45.0X6
Dramamine	T45.0X1	T45.0X2	T45.0X3	T45.0X4	T45.0X5	T45.0X6
Drano (drain cleaner)	T54.3X1	T54.3X2	T54.3X3	T54.3X4	—	—
Dressing, live pulp	T49.7X1	T49.7X2	T49.7X3	T49.7X4	T49.7X5	T49.7X6
Drocode	T40.2X1	T40.2X2	T40.2X3	T40.2X4	T40.2X5	T40.2X6
Dromoran	T40.2X1	T40.2X2	T40.2X3	T40.2X4	T40.2X5	T40.2X6
Dromostanolone	T38.7X1	T38.7X2	T38.7X3	T38.7X4	T38.7X5	T38.7X6
Dronabinol	T40.7X1	T40.7X2	T40.7X3	T40.7X4	T40.7X5	T40.7X6
Droperidol	T43.591	T43.592	T43.593	T43.594	T43.595	T43.596
Dropropizine	T48.3X1	T48.3X2	T48.3X3	T48.3X4	T48.3X5	T48.3X6
Drostanolone	T38.7X1	T38.7X2	T38.7X3	T38.7X4	T38.7X5	T38.7X6
Drotaverine	T44.3X1	T44.3X2	T44.3X3	T44.3X4	T44.3X5	T44.3X6
Drotrecogin alfa	T45.511	T45.512	T45.513	T45.514	T45.515	T45.516
Drug NEC	T50.901	T50.902	T50.903	T50.904	T50.905	T50.906
specified NEC	T50.991	T50.992	T50.993	T50.994	T50.995	T50.996
DTIC	T45.1X1	T45.1X2	T45.1X3	T45.1X4	T45.1X5	T45.1X6
Duboisine	T44.3X1	T44.3X2	T44.3X3	T44.3X4	T44.3X5	T44.3X6
Dulcolax	T47.2X1	T47.2X2	T47.2X3	T47.2X4	T47.2X5	T47.2X6
Duponol (C) (EP)	T49.2X1	T49.2X2	T49.2X3	T49.2X4	T49.2X5	T49.2X6
Durabolin	T38.7X1	T38.7X2	T38.7X3	T38.7X4	T38.7X5	T38.7X6
Dyclone	T41.3X1	T41.3X2	T41.3X3	T41.3X4	T41.3X5	T41.3X6
Dyclonine	T41.3X1	T41.3X2	T41.3X3	T41.3X4	T41.3X5	T41.3X6
Dydrogesterone	T38.5X1	T38.5X2	T38.5X3	T38.5X4	T38.5X5	T38.5X6
Dye NEC	T65.6X1	T65.6X2	T65.6X3	T65.6X4	—	—
antiseptic	T49.0X1	T49.0X2	T49.0X3	T49.0X4	T49.0X5	T49.0X6
diagnostic agents	T50.8X1	T50.8X2	T50.8X3	T50.8X4	T50.8X5	T50.8X6
pharmaceutical NEC	T50.901	T50.902	T50.903	T50.904	T50.905	T50.906
Dyflos	T44.0X1	T44.0X2	T44.0X3	T44.0X4	T44.0X5	T44.0X6
Dymelor	T38.3X1	T38.3X2	T38.3X3	T38.3X4	T38.3X5	T38.3X6
Dynamite	T65.3X1	T65.3X2	T65.3X3	T65.3X4	—	—
fumes	T59.891	T59.892	T59.893	T59.894	—	—
Dyphylline	T44.3X1	T44.3X2	T44.3X3	T44.3X4	T44.3X5	T44.3X6
E						
Ear drug NEC	T49.6X1	T49.6X2	T49.6X3	T49.6X4	T49.6X5	T49.6X6
Ear preparations	T49.6X1	T49.6X2	T49.6X3	T49.6X4	T49.6X5	T49.6X6
Econazole	T49.0X1	T49.0X2	T49.0X3	T49.0X4	T49.0X5	T49.0X6
Ecothiopate iodide	T49.5X1	T49.5X2	T49.5X3	T49.5X4	T49.5X5	T49.5X6
Echothiophate, echothiopate, ecothiopate	T49.5X1	T49.5X2	T49.5X3	T49.5X4	T49.5X5	T49.5X6

TABLE OF DRUGS AND CHEMICALS

	External Cause (T-Code)					
Substance	Poisoning, Accidental (Unintentional)	Poisoning, Intentional Self-Harm	Poisoning, Assault	Poisoning, Undetermined	Adverse Effect	Underdosing
Ecstasy	T43.621	T43.622	T43.623	T43.624	T43.625	T43.626
Ectylurea	T42.6X1	T42.6X2	T42.6X3	T42.6X4	T42.6X5	T42.6X6
Edathamil disodium	T45.8X1	T45.8X2	T45.8X3	T45.8X4	T45.8X5	T45.8X6
Edecrin	T50.1X1	T50.1X2	T50.1X3	T50.1X4	T50.1X5	T50.1X6
Edetate, disodium (calcium)	T45.8X1	T45.8X2	T45.8X3	T45.8X4	T45.8X5	T45.8X6
Edoxudine	T49.5X1	T49.5X2	T49.5X3	T49.5X4	T49.5X5	T49.5X6
Edrophonium	T44.0X1	T44.0X2	T44.0X3	T44.0X4	T44.0X5	T44.0X6
chloride	T44.0X1	T44.0X2	T44.0X3	T44.0X4	T44.0X5	T44.0X6
EDTA	T50.6X1	T50.6X2	T50.6X3	T50.6X4	T50.6X5	T50.6X6
Eflornithine	T37.2X1	T37.2X2	T37.2X3	T37.2X4	T37.2X5	T37.2X6
Efloxate	T46.3X1	T46.3X2	T46.3X3	T46.3X4	T46.3X5	T46.3X6
Elase	T49.8X1	T49.8X2	T49.8X3	T49.8X4	T49.8X5	T49.8X6
Elastase	T47.5X1	T47.5X2	T47.5X3	T47.5X4	T47.5X5	T47.5X6
Elaterium	T47.2X1	T47.2X2	T47.2X3	T47.2X4	T47.2X5	T47.2X6
Elcatonin	T50.991	T50.992	T50.993	T50.994	T50.995	T50.996
Elder	T62.2X1	T62.2X2	T62.2X3	T62.2X4	—	—
berry (unripe)	T62.1X1	T62.1X2	T62.1X3	T62.1X4	—	—
Electrolyte balance drug	T50.3X1	T50.3X2	T50.3X3	T50.3X4	T50.3X5	T50.3X6
Electrolytes NEC	T50.3X1	T50.3X2	T50.3X3	T50.3X4	T50.3X5	T50.3X6
Electrolytic agent NEC	T50.3X1	T50.3X2	T50.3X3	T50.3X4	T50.3X5	T50.3X6
Elemental diet	T50.901	T50.902	T50.903	T50.904	T50.905	T50.906
Elliptinium acetate	T45.1X1	T45.1X2	T45.1X3	T45.1X4	T45.1X5	T45.1X6
Embramine	T45.0X1	T45.0X2	T45.0X3	T45.0X4	T45.0X5	T45.0X6
Emepronium (salts)	T44.3X1	T44.3X2	T44.3X3	T44.3X4	T44.3X5	T44.3X6
bromide	T44.3X1	T44.3X2	T44.3X3	T44.3X4	T44.3X5	T44.3X6
Emetic NEC	T47.7X1	T47.7X2	T47.7X3	T47.7X4	T47.7X5	T47.7X6
Emetine	T37.3X1	T37.3X2	T37.3X3	T37.3X4	T37.3X5	T37.3X6
Emollient NEC	T49.3X1	T49.3X2	T49.3X3	T49.3X4	T49.3X5	T49.3X6
Emorfazone	T39.8X1	T39.8X2	T39.8X3	T39.8X4	T39.8X5	T39.8X6
Emylcamate	T43.591	T43.592	T43.593	T43.594	T43.595	T43.596
Enalapril	T46.4X1	T46.4X2	T46.4X3	T46.4X4	T46.4X5	T46.4X6
Enalaprilat	T46.4X1	T46.4X2	T46.4X3	T46.4X4	T46.4X5	T46.4X6
Encainide	T46.2X1	T46.2X2	T46.2X3	T46.2X4	T46.2X5	T46.2X6
Endocaine	T41.3X1	T41.3X2	T41.3X3	T41.3X4	T41.3X5	T41.3X6
Endosulfan	T60.2X1	T60.2X2	T60.2X3	T60.2X4	—	—
Endothall	T60.3X1	T60.3X2	T60.3X3	T60.3X4	—	—
Endralazine	T46.5X1	T46.5X2	T46.5X3	T46.5X4	T46.5X5	T46.5X6
Endrin	T60.1X1	T60.1X2	T60.1X3	T60.1X4	—	—
Enflurane	T41.0X1	T41.0X2	T41.0X3	T41.0X4	T41.0X5	T41.0X6
Enhexymal	T42.3X1	T42.3X2	T42.3X3	T42.3X4	T42.3X5	T42.3X6
Enocitabine	T45.1X1	T45.1X2	T45.1X3	T45.1X4	T45.1X5	T45.1X6
Enovid	T38.4X1	T38.4X2	T38.4X3	T38.4X4	T38.4X5	T38.4X6

	External Cause (T-Code)					
Substance	Poisoning, Accidental (Unintentional)	Poisoning, Intentional Self-Harm	Poisoning, Assault	Poisoning, Undetermined	Adverse Effect	Underdosing
Enoxacin	T36.8X1	T36.8X2	T36.8X3	T36.8X4	T36.8X5	T36.8X6
Enoxaparin (sodium)	T45.511	T45.512	T45.513	T45.514	T45.515	T45.516
Enpiprazole	T43.591	T43.592	T43.593	T43.594	T43.595	T43.596
Enprofylline	T48.6X1	T48.6X2	T48.6X3	T48.6X4	T48.6X5	T48.6X6
Enprostil	T47.1X1	T47.1X2	T47.1X3	T47.1X4	T47.1X5	T47.1X6
ENT preparations (anti-infectives)	T49.6X1	T49.6X2	T49.6X3	T49.6X4	T49.6X5	T49.6X6
Enviomycin	T36.8X1	T36.8X2	T36.8X3	T36.8X4	T36.8X5	T36.8X6
Enzodase	T45.3X1	T45.3X2	T45.3X3	T45.3X4	T45.3X5	T45.3X6
Enzyme NEC	T45.3X1	T45.3X2	T45.3X3	T45.3X4	T45.3X5	T45.3X6
depolymerizing	T49.8X1	T49.8X2	T49.8X3	T49.8X4	T49.8X5	T49.8X6
fibrolytic	T45.3X1	T45.3X2	T45.3X3	T45.3X4	T45.3X5	T45.3X6
gastric	T47.5X1	T47.5X2	T47.5X3	T47.5X4	T47.5X5	T47.5X6
intestinal	T47.5X1	T47.5X2	T47.5X3	T47.5X4	T47.5X5	T47.5X6
local action	T49.4X1	T49.4X2	T49.4X3	T49.4X4	T49.4X5	T49.4X6
proteolytic	T49.4X1	T49.4X2	T49.4X3	T49.4X4	T49.4X5	T49.4X6
thrombolytic	T45.3X1	T45.3X2	T45.3X3	T45.3X4	T45.3X5	T45.3X6
EPAB	T41.3X1	T41.3X2	T41.3X3	T41.3X4	T41.3X5	T41.3X6
Epanutin	T42.0X1	T42.0X2	T42.0X3	T42.0X4	T42.0X5	T42.0X6
Ephedra	T44.991	T44.992	T44.993	T44.994	T44.995	T44.996
Ephedrine	T44.991	T44.992	T44.993	T44.994	T44.995	T44.996
Epichlorhydrin, epichlorohydrin	T52.8X1	T52.8X2	T52.8X3	T52.8X4	—	—
Epicillin	T36.0X1	T36.0X2	T36.0X3	T36.0X4	T36.0X5	T36.0X6
Epiestriol	T38.5X1	T38.5X2	T38.5X3	T38.5X4	T38.5X5	T38.5X6
Epilim — see Sodium valproate						
Epimestrol	T38.5X1	T38.5X2	T38.5X3	T38.5X4	T38.5X5	T38.5X6
Epinephrine	T44.5X1	T44.5X2	T44.5X3	T44.5X4	T44.5X5	T44.5X6
Epirubicin	T45.1X1	T45.1X2	T45.1X3	T45.1X4	T45.1X5	T45.1X6
Epitiostanol	T38.7X1	T38.7X2	T38.7X3	T38.7X4	T38.7X5	T38.7X6
Epitizide	T50.2X1	T50.2X2	T50.2X3	T50.2X4	T50.2X5	T50.2X6
EPN	T60.0X1	T60.0X2	T60.0X3	T60.0X4	—	—
EPO	T45.8X1	T45.8X2	T45.8X3	T45.8X4	T45.8X5	T45.8X6
Epoetin alpha	T45.8X1	T45.8X2	T45.8X3	T45.8X4	T45.8X5	T45.8X6
Epomediol	T50.991	T50.992	T50.993	T50.994	T50.995	T50.996
Epoprostenol	T45.521	T45.522	T45.523	T45.524	T45.525	T45.526
Epoxy resin	T65.891	T65.892	T65.893	T65.894	—	—
Eprazinone	T48.4X1	T48.4X2	T48.4X3	T48.4X4	T48.4X5	T48.4X6
Epsilon amino-caproic acid	T45.621	T45.622	T45.623	T45.624	T45.625	T45.626
Epsom salt	T47.3X1	T47.3X2	T47.3X3	T47.3X4	T47.3X5	T47.3X6
Eptazocine	T40.4X1	T40.4X2	T40.4X3	T40.4X4	T40.4X5	T40.4X6
Equanil	T43.591	T43.592	T43.593	T43.594	T43.595	T43.596
Equisetum	T62.2X1	T62.2X2	T62.2X3	T62.2X4	—	—
diuretic	T50.2X1	T50.2X2	T50.2X3	T50.2X4	T50.2X5	T50.2X6

◀ New ◀▦ Revised ~~deleted~~ Deleted

Substance	Poisoning, Accidental (Unintentional)	Poisoning, Intentional Self-Harm	Poisoning, Assault	Poisoning, Undetermined	Adverse Effect	Underdosing
Ergobasine	T48.0X1	T48.0X2	T48.0X3	T48.0X4	T48.0X5	T48.0X6
Ergocalciferol	T45.2X1	T45.2X2	T45.2X3	T45.2X4	T45.2X5	T45.2X6
Ergoloid mesylates	T46.7X1	T46.7X2	T46.7X3	T46.7X4	T46.7X5	T46.7X6
Ergometrine	T48.0X1	T48.0X2	T48.0X3	T48.0X4	T48.0X5	T48.0X6
Ergonovine	T48.0X1	T48.0X2	T48.0X3	T48.0X4	T48.0X5	T48.0X6
Ergot NEC	T64.81	T64.82	T64.83	T64.84	—	—
derivative	T48.0X1	T48.0X2	T48.0X3	T48.0X4	T48.0X5	T48.0X6
medicinal (alkaloids)	T48.0X1	T48.0X2	T48.0X3	T48.0X4	T48.0X5	T48.0X6
prepared	T48.0X1	T48.0X2	T48.0X3	T48.0X4	T48.0X5	T48.0X6
Ergotamine	T46.5X1	T46.5X2	T46.5X3	T46.5X4	T46.5X5	T46.5X6
Ergotocine	T48.0X1	T48.0X2	T48.0X3	T48.0X4	T48.0X5	T48.0X6
Ergotrate	T48.0X1	T48.0X2	T48.0X3	T48.0X4	T48.0X5	T48.0X6
Eritrityl tetranitrate	T46.3X1	T46.3X2	T46.3X3	T46.3X4	T46.3X5	T46.3X6
Erythrityl tetranitrate	T46.3X1	T46.3X2	T46.3X3	T46.3X4	T46.3X5	T46.3X6
Erythrol tetranitrate	T46.3X1	T46.3X2	T46.3X3	T46.3X4	T46.3X5	T46.3X6
Erythromycin (salts)	T36.3X1	T36.3X2	T36.3X3	T36.3X4	T36.3X5	T36.3X6
ophthalmic preparation	T49.5X1	T49.5X2	T49.5X3	T49.5X4	T49.5X5	T49.5X6
topical NEC	T49.0X1	T49.0X2	T49.0X3	T49.0X4	T49.0X5	T49.0X6
Erythropoietin	T45.8X1	T45.8X2	T45.8X3	T45.8X4	T45.8X5	T45.8X6
human	T45.8X1	T45.8X2	T45.8X3	T45.8X4	T45.8X5	T45.8X6
Escin	T46.991	T46.992	T46.993	T46.994	T46.995	T46.996
Esculin	T45.2X1	T45.2X2	T45.2X3	T45.2X4	T45.2X5	T45.2X6
Esculoside	T45.2X1	T45.2X2	T45.2X3	T45.2X4	T45.2X5	T45.2X6
ESDT (ether-soluble tar distillate)	T49.1X1	T49.1X2	T49.1X3	T49.1X4	T49.1X5	T49.1X6
Eserine	T49.5X1	T49.5X2	T49.5X3	T49.5X4	T49.5X5	T49.5X6
Esflurbiprofen	T39.311	T39.312	T39.313	T39.314	T39.315	T39.316
Eskabarb	T42.3X1	T42.3X2	T42.3X3	T42.3X4	T42.3X5	T42.3X6
Eskalith	T43.8X1	T43.8X2	T43.8X3	T43.8X4	T43.8X5	T43.8X6
Esmolol	T44.7X1	T44.7X2	T44.7X3	T44.7X4	T44.7X5	T44.7X6
Estanozolol	T38.7X1	T38.7X2	T38.7X3	T38.7X4	T38.7X5	T38.7X6
Estazolam	T42.4X1	T42.4X2	T42.4X3	T42.4X4	T42.4X5	T42.4X6
Estradiol	T38.5X1	T38.5X2	T38.5X3	T38.5X4	T38.5X5	T38.5X6
with testosterone	T38.7X1	T38.7X2	T38.7X3	T38.7X4	T38.7X5	T38.7X6
benzoate	T38.5X1	T38.5X2	T38.5X3	T38.5X4	T38.5X5	T38.5X6
Estramustine	T45.1X1	T45.1X2	T45.1X3	T45.1X4	T45.1X5	T45.1X6
Estriol	T38.5X1	T38.5X2	T38.5X3	T38.5X4	T38.5X5	T38.5X6
Estrogen	T38.5X1	T38.5X2	T38.5X3	T38.5X4	T38.5X5	T38.5X6
with progesterone	T38.5X1	T38.5X2	T38.5X3	T38.5X4	T38.5X5	T38.5X6
conjugated	T38.5X1	T38.5X2	T38.5X3	T38.5X4	T38.5X5	T38.5X6
Estrone	T38.5X1	T38.5X2	T38.5X3	T38.5X4	T38.5X5	T38.5X6
Estropipate	T38.5X1	T38.5X2	T38.5X3	T38.5X4	T38.5X5	T38.5X6

Substance	Poisoning, Accidental (Unintentional)	Poisoning, Intentional Self-Harm	Poisoning, Assault	Poisoning, Undetermined	Adverse Effect	Underdosing
Etacrynate sodium	T50.1X1	T50.1X2	T50.1X3	T50.1X4	T50.1X5	T50.1X6
Etacrynic acid	T50.1X1	T50.1X2	T50.1X3	T50.1X4	T50.1X5	T50.1X6
Etafedrine	T48.6X1	T48.6X2	T48.6X3	T48.6X4	T48.6X5	T48.6X6
Etafenone	T46.3X1	T46.3X2	T46.3X3	T46.3X4	T46.3X5	T46.3X6
Etambutol	T37.1X1	T37.1X2	T37.1X3	T37.1X4	T37.1X5	T37.1X6
Etamiphyllin	T48.6X1	T48.6X2	T48.6X3	T48.6X4	T48.6X5	T48.6X6
Etamivan	T50.7X1	T50.7X2	T50.7X3	T50.7X4	T50.7X5	T50.7X6
Etamsylate	T45.7X1	T45.7X2	T45.7X3	T45.7X4	T45.7X5	T45.7X6
Etebenecid	T50.4X1	T50.4X2	T50.4X3	T50.4X4	T50.4X5	T50.4X6
Ethacridine	T49.0X1	T49.0X2	T49.0X3	T49.0X4	T49.0X5	T49.0X6
Ethacrynic acid	T50.1X1	T50.1X2	T50.1X3	T50.1X4	T50.1X5	T50.1X6
Ethadione	T42.2X1	T42.2X2	T42.2X3	T42.2X4	T42.2X5	T42.2X6
Ethambutol	T37.1X1	T37.1X2	T37.1X3	T37.1X4	T37.1X5	T37.1X6
Ethamide	T50.2X1	T50.2X2	T50.2X3	T50.2X4	T50.2X5	T50.2X6
Ethamivan	T50.7X1	T50.7X2	T50.7X3	T50.7X4	T50.7X5	T50.7X6
Ethamsylate	T45.7X1	T45.7X2	T45.7X3	T45.7X4	T45.7X5	T45.7X6
Ethanol	T51.0X1	T51.0X2	T51.0X3	T51.0X4	—	—
beverage	T51.0X1	T51.0X2	T51.0X3	T51.0X4		
Ethanolamine oleate	T46.8X1	T46.8X2	T46.8X3	T46.8X4	T46.8X5	T46.8X6
Ethaverine	T44.3X1	T44.3X2	T44.3X3	T44.3X4	T44.3X5	T44.3X6
Ethchlorvynol	T42.6X1	T42.6X2	T42.6X3	T42.6X4	T42.6X5	T42.6X6
Ethebenecid	T50.4X1	T50.4X2	T50.4X3	T50.4X4	T50.4X5	T50.4X6
Ether (vapor)	T41.0X1	T41.0X2	T41.0X3	T41.0X4	T41.0X5	T41.0X6
anesthetic	T41.0X1	T41.0X2	T41.0X3	T41.0X4	T41.0X5	T41.0X6
divinyl	T41.0X1	T41.0X2	T41.0X3	T41.0X4	T41.0X5	T41.0X6
ethyl (medicinal)	T41.0X1	T41.0X2	T41.0X3	T41.0X4	T41.0X5	T41.0X6
nonmedicinal	T52.8X1	T52.8X2	T52.8X3	T52.8X4	—	—
petroleum—see Ligroin						
solvent	T52.8X1	T52.8X2	T52.8X3	T52.8X4	—	—
Ethiazide	T50.2X1	T50.2X2	T50.2X3	T50.2X4	T50.2X5	T50.2X6
Ethidium chloride (vapor)	T59.891	T59.892	T59.893	T59.894	—	—
Ethinamate	T42.6X1	T42.6X2	T42.6X3	T42.6X4	T42.6X5	T42.6X6
Ethinylestradiol, ethinyloestradiol	T38.5X1	T38.5X2	T38.5X3	T38.5X4	T38.5X5	T38.5X6
with						
levonorgestrel	T38.4X1	T38.4X2	T38.4X3	T38.4X4	T38.4X5	T38.4X6
norethisterone	T38.4X1	T38.4X2	T38.4X3	T38.4X4	T38.4X5	T38.4X6
Ethiodized oil (131 I)	T50.8X1	T50.8X2	T50.8X3	T50.8X4	T50.8X5	T50.8X6
Ethion	T60.0X1	T60.0X2	T60.0X3	T60.0X4	—	—
Ethionamide	T37.1X1	T37.1X2	T37.1X3	T37.1X4	T37.1X5	T37.1X6
Ethioniamide	T37.1X1	T37.1X2	T37.1X3	T37.1X4	T37.1X5	T37.1X6
Ethisterone	T38.5X1	T38.5X2	T38.5X3	T38.5X4	T38.5X5	T38.5X6
Ethobral	T42.3X1	T42.3X2	T42.3X3	T42.3X4	T42.3X5	T42.3X6

Substance	External Cause (T-Code)					
	Poisoning, Accidental (Unintentional)	Poisoning, Intentional Self-Harm	Poisoning, Assault	Poisoning, Undetermined	Adverse Effect	Underdosing
Ethocaine (infiltration) (topical)	T41.3X1	T41.3X2	T41.3X3	T41.3X4	T41.3X5	T41.3X6
nerve block (peripheral) (plexus)	T41.3X1	T41.3X2	T41.3X3	T41.3X4	T41.3X5	T41.3X6
spinal	T41.3X1	T41.3X2	T41.3X3	T41.3X4	T41.3X5	T41.3X6
Ethoheptazine	T40.4X1	T40.4X2	T40.4X3	T40.4X4	T40.4X5	T40.4X6
Ethopropazine	T44.3X1	T44.3X2	T44.3X3	T44.3X4	T44.3X5	T44.3X6
Ethosuximide	T42.2X1	T42.2X2	T42.2X3	T42.2X4	T42.2X5	T42.2X6
Ethotoin	T42.0X1	T42.0X2	T42.0X3	T42.0X4	T42.0X5	T42.0X6
Ethoxazene	T37.91	T37.92	T37.93	T37.94	T37.95	T37.96
Ethoxazorutoside	T46.991	T46.992	T46.993	T46.994	T46.995	T46.996
2-Ethoxyethanol	T52.3X1	T52.3X2	T52.3X3	T52.3X4	—	—
Ethoxzolamide	T50.2X1	T50.2X2	T50.2X3	T50.2X4	T50.2X5	T50.2X6
Ethyl						
acetate	T52.8X1	T52.8X2	T52.8X3	T52.8X4	—	—
alcohol	T51.0X1	T51.0X2	T51.0X3	T51.0X4		
beverage	T51.0X1	T51.0X2	T51.0X3	T51.0X4		
aldehyde (vapor)	T59.891	T59.892	T59.893	T59.894		
liquid	T52.8X1	T52.8X2	T52.8X3	T52.8X4	—	—
aminobenzoate	T41.3X1	T41.3X2	T41.3X3	T41.3X4	T41.3X5	T41.3X6
aminophenothiazine	T43.3X1	T43.3X2	T43.3X3	T43.3X4	T43.3X5	T43.3X6
benzoate	T52.8X1	T52.8X2	T52.8X3	T52.8X4	—	—
biscoumacetate	T45.511	T45.512	T45.513	T45.514	T45.515	T45.516
bromide (anesthetic)	T41.0X1	T41.0X2	T41.0X3	T41.0X4	T41.0X5	T41.0X6
carbamate	T45.1X1	T45.1X2	T45.1X3	T45.1X4	T45.1X5	T45.1X6
carbinol	T51.3X1	T51.3X2	T51.3X3	T51.3X4	—	—
carbonate	T52.8X1	T52.8X2	T52.8X3	T52.8X4	—	—
chaulmoograte	T37.1X1	T37.1X2	T37.1X3	T37.1X4	T37.1X5	T37.1X6
chloride (anesthetic)	T41.0X1	T41.0X2	T41.0X3	T41.0X4	T41.0X5	T41.0X6
anesthetic (local)	T41.3X1	T41.3X2	T41.3X3	T41.3X4	T41.3X5	T41.3X6
inhaled	T41.0X1	T41.0X2	T41.0X3	T41.0X4	T41.0X5	T41.0X6
local	T49.4X1	T49.4X2	T49.4X3	T49.4X4	T49.4X5	T49.4X6
solvent	T53.6X1	T53.6X2	T53.6X3	T53.6X4	—	—
dibunate	T48.3X1	T48.3X2	T48.3X3	T48.3X4	T48.3X5	T48.3X6
dichloroarsine (vapor)	T57.0X1	T57.0X2	T57.0X3	T57.0X4	—	—
estranol	T38.7X1	T38.7X2	T38.7X3	T38.7X4	T38.7X5	T38.7X6
ether — see also ether	T52.8X1	T52.8X2	T52.8X3	T52.8X4	—	—
formate NEC (solvent)	T52.0X1	T52.0X2	T52.0X3	T52.0X4	—	—
fumarate	T49.4X1	T49.4X2	T49.4X3	T49.4X4	T49.4X5	T49.4X6
hydroxyisobutyrate NEC (solvent)	T52.8X1	T52.8X2	T52.8X3	T52.8X4	—	—
iodoacetate	T59.3X1	T59.3X2	T59.3X3	T59.3X4	—	—
lactate NEC (solvent)	T52.8X1	T52.8X2	T52.8X3	T52.8X4	—	—
loflazepate	T42.4X1	T42.4X2	T42.4X3	T42.4X4	T42.4X5	T42.4X6

Substance	External Cause (T-Code)					
	Poisoning, Accidental (Unintentional)	Poisoning, Intentional Self-Harm	Poisoning, Assault	Poisoning, Undetermined	Adverse Effect	Underdosing
Ethyl *(Continued)*						
mercuric chloride	T56.1X1	T56.1X2	T56.1X3	T56.1X4	—	—
methylcarbinol	T51.8X1	T51.8X2	T51.8X3	T51.8X4	—	—
morphine	T40.2X1	T40.2X2	T40.2X3	T40.2X4	T40.2X5	T40.2X6
noradrenaline	T48.6X1	T48.6X2	T48.6X3	T48.6X4	T48.6X5	T48.6X6
oxybutyrate NEC (solvent)	T52.8X1	T52.8X2	T52.8X3	T52.8X4	—	—
Ethylene (gas)	T59.891	T59.892	T59.893	T59.894	—	—
anesthetic (general)	T41.0X1	T41.0X2	T41.0X3	T41.0X4	T41.0X5	T41.0X6
chlorohydrin	T52.8X1	T52.8X2	T52.8X3	T52.8X4	—	—
vapor	T53.6X1	T53.6X2	T53.6X3	T53.6X4	—	—
dichloride	T52.8X1	T52.8X2	T52.8X3	T52.8X4	—	—
vapor	T53.6X1	T53.6X2	T53.6X3	T53.6X4	—	—
dinitrate	T52.3X1	T52.3X2	T52.3X3	T52.3X4	—	—
glycol(s)	T52.8X1	T52.8X2	T52.8X3	T52.8X4	—	—
dinitrate	T52.3X1	T52.3X2	T52.3X3	T52.3X4	—	—
monobutyl ether	T52.3X1	T52.3X2	T52.3X3	T52.3X4	—	—
imine	T54.1X1	T54.1X2	T54.1X3	T54.1X4	—	—
oxide (fumigant) (nonmedicinal)	T59.891	T59.892	T59.893	T59.894	—	—
medicinal	T49.0X1	T49.0X2	T49.0X3	T49.0X4	T49.0X5	T49.0X6
Ethylenediamine theophylline	T48.6X1	T48.6X2	T48.6X3	T48.6X4	T48.6X5	T48.6X6
Ethylenediaminetetra-acetic acid	T50.6X1	T50.6X2	T50.6X3	T50.6X4	T50.6X5	T50.6X6
Ethylenedinitrilotetra-acetate	T50.6X1	T50.6X2	T50.6X3	T50.6X4	T50.6X5	T50.6X6
Ethylestrenol	T38.7X1	T38.7X2	T38.7X3	T38.7X4	T38.7X5	T38.7X6
Ethylhydroxycellulose	T47.4X1	T47.4X2	T47.4X3	T47.4X4	T47.4X5	T47.4X6
Ethylidene						
chloride NEC	T53.6X1	T53.6X2	T53.6X3	T53.6X4	—	—
diacetate	T60.3X1	T60.3X2	T60.3X3	T60.3X4	—	—
dicoumarin	T45.511	T45.512	T45.513	T45.514	T45.515	T45.516
dicoumarol	T45.511	T45.512	T45.513	T45.514	T45.515	T45.516
diethyl ether	T52.0X1	T52.0X2	T52.0X3	T52.0X4	—	—
Ethylmorphine	T40.2X1	T40.2X2	T40.2X3	T40.2X4	T40.2X5	T40.2X6
Ethylnorepinephrine	T48.6X1	T48.6X2	T48.6X3	T48.6X4	T48.6X5	T48.6X6
Ethylparachlorophen-oxyisobutyrate	T46.6X1	T46.6X2	T46.6X3	T46.6X4	T46.6X5	T46.6X6
Ethynodiol	T38.4X1	T38.4X2	T38.4X3	T38.4X4	T38.4X5	T38.4X6
with mestranol diacetate	T38.4X1	T38.4X2	T38.4X3	T38.4X4	T38.4X5	T38.4X6
Etidocaine	T41.3X1	T41.3X2	T41.3X3	T41.3X4	T41.3X5	T41.3X6
infiltration (subcutaneous)	T41.3X1	T41.3X2	T41.3X3	T41.3X4	T41.3X5	T41.3X6
nerve (peripheral) (plexus)	T41.3X1	T41.3X2	T41.3X3	T41.3X4	T41.3X5	T41.3X6
Etidronate	T50.991	T50.992	T50.993	T50.994	T50.995	T50.996
Etidronic acid (disodium salt)	T50.991	T50.992	T50.993	T50.994	T50.995	T50.996
Etifoxine	T42.6X1	T42.6X2	T42.6X3	T42.6X4	T42.6X5	T42.6X6

◄ New   ◄||| Revised   ~~deleted~~ Deleted

Substance	Poisoning, Accidental (Unintentional)	Poisoning, Intentional Self-Harm	Poisoning, Assault	Poisoning, Undetermined	Adverse Effect	Underdosing
Etilefrine	T44.4X1	T44.4X2	T44.4X3	T44.4X4	T44.4X5	T44.4X6
Etilfen	T42.3X1	T42.3X2	T42.3X3	T42.3X4	T42.3X5	T42.3X6
Etinodiol	T38.4X1	T38.4X2	T38.4X3	T38.4X4	T38.4X5	T38.4X6
Etiroxate	T46.6X1	T46.6X2	T46.6X3	T46.6X4	T46.6X5	T46.6X6
Etizolam	T42.4X1	T42.4X2	T42.4X3	T42.4X4	T42.4X5	T42.4X6
Etodolac	T39.391	T39.392	T39.393	T39.394	T39.395	T39.396
Etofamide	T37.3X1	T37.3X2	T37.3X3	T37.3X4	T37.3X5	T37.3X6
Etofibrate	T46.6X1	T46.6X2	T46.6X3	T46.6X4	T46.6X5	T46.6X6
Etofylline	T46.7X1	T46.7X2	T46.7X3	T46.7X4	T46.7X5	T46.7X6
clofibrate	T46.6X1	T46.6X2	T46.6X3	T46.6X4	T46.6X5	T46.6X6
Etoglucid	T45.1X1	T45.1X2	T45.1X3	T45.1X4	T45.1X5	T45.1X6
Etomidate	T41.1X1	T41.1X2	T41.1X3	T41.1X4	T41.1X5	T41.1X6
Etomide	T39.8X1	T39.8X2	T39.8X3	T39.8X4	T39.8X5	T39.8X6
Etomidoline	T44.3X1	T44.3X2	T44.3X3	T44.3X4	T44.3X5	T44.3X6
Etoposide	T45.1X1	T45.1X2	T45.1X3	T45.1X4	T45.1X5	T45.1X6
Etorphine	T40.2X1	T40.2X2	T40.2X3	T40.2X4	T40.2X5	T40.2X6
Etoval	T42.3X1	T42.3X2	T42.3X3	T42.3X4	T42.3X5	T42.3X6
Etozolin	T50.1X1	T50.1X2	T50.1X3	T50.1X4	T50.1X5	T50.1X6
Etretinate	T50.991	T50.992	T50.993	T50.994	T50.995	T50.996
Etryptamine	T43.691	T43.692	T43.693	T43.694	T43.695	T43.696
Etybenzatropine	T44.3X1	T44.3X2	T44.3X3	T44.3X4	T44.3X5	T44.3X6
Etynodiol	T38.4X1	T38.4X2	T38.4X3	T38.4X4	T38.4X5	T38.4X6
Eucaine	T41.3X1	T41.3X2	T41.3X3	T41.3X4	T41.3X5	T41.3X6
Eucalyptus oil	T49.7X1	T49.7X2	T49.7X3	T49.7X4	T49.7X5	T49.7X6
Eucatropine	T49.5X1	T49.5X2	T49.5X3	T49.5X4	T49.5X5	T49.5X6
Eucodal	T40.2X1	T40.2X2	T40.2X3	T40.2X4	T40.2X5	T40.2X6
Euneryl	T42.3X1	T42.3X2	T42.3X3	T42.3X4	T42.3X5	T42.3X6
Euphthalmine	T44.3X1	T44.3X2	T44.3X3	T44.3X4	T44.3X5	T44.3X6
Eurax	T49.0X1	T49.0X2	T49.0X3	T49.0X4	T49.0X5	T49.0X6
Euresol	T49.4X1	T49.4X2	T49.4X3	T49.4X4	T49.4X5	T49.4X6
Euthroid	T38.1X1	T38.1X2	T38.1X3	T38.1X4	T38.1X5	T38.1X6
Evans blue	T50.8X1	T50.8X2	T50.8X3	T50.8X4	T50.8X5	T50.8X6
Evipal	T42.3X1	T42.3X2	T42.3X3	T42.3X4	T42.3X5	T42.3X6
sodium	T41.1X1	T41.1X2	T41.1X3	T41.1X4	T41.1X5	T41.1X6
Evipan	T42.3X1	T42.3X2	T42.3X3	T42.3X4	T42.3X5	T42.3X6
sodium	T41.1X1	T41.1X2	T41.1X3	T41.1X4	T41.1X5	T41.1X6
Exalamide	T49.0X1	T49.0X2	T49.0X3	T49.0X4	T49.0X5	T49.0X6
Exalgin	T39.1X1	T39.1X2	T39.1X3	T39.1X4	T39.1X5	T39.1X6
Excipients, pharmaceutical	T50.901	T50.902	T50.903	T50.904	T50.905	T50.906
Exhaust gas (engine) (motor vehicle)	T58.01	T58.02	T58.03	T58.04	—	—
Ex-Lax (phenolphthalein)	T47.2X1	T47.2X2	T47.2X3	T47.2X4	T47.2X5	T47.2X6
Expectorant NEC	T48.4X1	T48.4X2	T48.4X3	T48.4X4	T48.4X5	T48.4X6

Substance	Poisoning, Accidental (Unintentional)	Poisoning, Intentional Self-Harm	Poisoning, Assault	Poisoning, Undetermined	Adverse Effect	Underdosing
Extended insulin zinc suspension	T38.3X1	T38.3X2	T38.3X3	T38.3X4	T38.3X5	T38.3X6
External medications (skin) (mucous membrane)	T49.91	T49.92	T49.93	T49.94	T49.95	T49.96
dental agent	T49.7X1	T49.7X2	T49.7X3	T49.7X4	T49.7X5	T49.7X6
ENT agent	T49.6X1	T49.6X2	T49.6X3	T49.6X4	T49.6X5	T49.6X6
ophthalmic preparation	T49.5X1	T49.5X2	T49.5X3	T49.5X4	T49.5X5	T49.5X6
specified NEC	T49.8X1	T49.8X2	T49.8X3	T49.8X4	T49.8X5	T49.8X6
Extrapyramidal antagonist NEC	T44.3X1	T44.3X2	T44.3X3	T44.3X4	T44.3X5	T44.3X6
Eye agents (anti-infective)	T49.5X1	T49.5X2	T49.5X3	T49.5X4	T49.5X5	T49.5X6
Eye drug NEC	T49.5X1	T49.5X2	T49.5X3	T49.5X4	T49.5X5	T49.5X6
F						
FAC (fluorouracil + doxorubicin + cyclophosphamide)	T45.1X1	T45.1X2	T45.1X3	T45.1X4	T45.1X5	T45.1X6
Factor						
I (fibrinogen)	T45.8X1	T45.8X2	T45.8X3	T45.8X4	T45.8X5	T45.8X6
III (thromboplastin)	T45.8X1	T45.8X2	T45.8X3	T45.8X4	T45.8X5	T45.8X6
VIII (antihemophilic Factor) (Concentrate)	T45.8X1	T45.8X2	T45.8X3	T45.8X4	T45.8X5	T45.8X6
IX complex	T45.7X1	T45.7X2	T45.7X3	T45.7X4	T45.7X5	T45.7X6
human	T45.8X1	T45.8X2	T45.8X3	T45.8X4	T45.8X5	T45.8X6
Famotidine	T47.0X1	T47.0X2	T47.0X3	T47.0X4	T47.0X5	T47.0X6
Fat suspension, intravenous	T50.991	T50.992	T50.993	T50.994	T50.995	T50.996
Fazadinium bromide	T48.1X1	T48.1X2	T48.1X3	T48.1X4	T48.1X5	T48.1X6
Febarbamate	T42.3X1	T42.3X2	T42.3X3	T42.3X4	T42.3X5	T42.3X6
Fecal softener	T47.4X1	T47.4X2	T47.4X3	T47.4X4	T47.4X5	T47.4X6
Fedrilate	T48.3X1	T48.3X2	T48.3X3	T48.3X4	T48.3X5	T48.3X6
Felodipine	T46.1X1	T46.1X2	T46.1X3	T46.1X4	T46.1X5	T46.1X6
Felypressin	T38.891	T38.892	T38.893	T38.894	T38.895	T38.896
Femoxetine	T43.221	T43.222	T43.223	T43.224	T43.225	T43.226
Fenalcomine	T46.3X1	T46.3X2	T46.3X3	T46.3X4	T46.3X5	T46.3X6
Fenamisal	T37.1X1	T37.1X2	T37.1X3	T37.1X4	T37.1X5	T37.1X6
Fenazone	T39.2X1	T39.2X2	T39.2X3	T39.2X4	T39.2X5	T39.2X6
Fenbendazole	T37.4X1	T37.4X2	T37.4X3	T37.4X4	T37.4X5	T37.4X6
Fenbutrazate	T50.5X1	T50.5X2	T50.5X3	T50.5X4	T50.5X5	T50.5X6
Fencamfamine	T43.691	T43.692	T43.693	T43.694	T43.695	T43.696
Fendiline	T46.1X1	T46.1X2	T46.1X3	T46.1X4	T46.1X5	T46.1X6
Fenetylline	T43.691	T43.692	T43.693	T43.694	T43.695	T43.696
Fenflumizole	T39.391	T39.392	T39.393	T39.394	T39.395	T39.396
Fenfluramine	T50.5X1	T50.5X2	T50.5X3	T50.5X4	T50.5X5	T50.5X6
Fenobarbital	T42.3X1	T42.3X2	T42.3X3	T42.3X4	T42.3X5	T42.3X6
Fenofibrate	T46.6X1	T46.6X2	T46.6X3	T46.6X4	T46.6X5	T46.6X6
Fenoprofen	T39.311	T39.312	T39.313	T39.314	T39.315	T39.316
Fenoterol	T48.6X1	T48.6X2	T48.6X3	T48.6X4	T48.6X5	T48.6X6

◀ New   ◀▥ Revised   ~~deleted~~ Deleted

Substance	Poisoning, Accidental (Unintentional)	Poisoning, Intentional Self-Harm	Poisoning, Assault	Poisoning, Undetermined	Adverse Effect	Underdosing
Fenoverine	T44.3X1	T44.3X2	T44.3X3	T44.3X4	T44.3X5	T44.3X6
Fenoxazoline	T48.5X1	T48.5X2	T48.5X3	T48.5X4	T48.5X5	T48.5X6
Fenproporex	T50.5X1	T50.5X2	T50.5X3	T50.5X4	T50.5X5	T50.5X6
Fenquizone	T50.2X1	T50.2X2	T50.2X3	T50.2X4	T50.2X5	T50.2X6
Fentanyl	T40.4X1	T40.4X2	T40.4X3	T40.4X4	T40.4X5	T40.4X6
Fentazin	T43.3X1	T43.3X2	T43.3X3	T43.3X4	T43.3X5	T43.3X6
Fenthion	T60.0X1	T60.0X2	T60.0X3	T60.0X4	—	—
Fenticlor	T49.0X1	T49.0X2	T49.0X3	T49.0X4	T49.0X5	T49.0X6
Fenylbutazone	T39.2X1	T39.2X2	T39.2X3	T39.2X4	T39.2X5	T39.2X6
Feprazone	T39.2X1	T39.2X2	T39.2X3	T39.2X4	T39.2X5	T39.2X6
Fer de lance (bite) (venom)	T63.061	T63.062	T63.063	T63.064	—	—
Ferric — see also Iron						
chloride	T45.4X1	T45.4X2	T45.4X3	T45.4X4	T45.4X5	T45.4X6
citrate	T45.4X1	T45.4X2	T45.4X3	T45.4X4	T45.4X5	T45.4X6
hydroxide						
colloidal	T45.4X1	T45.4X2	T45.4X3	T45.4X4	T45.4X5	T45.4X6
polymaltose	T45.4X1	T45.4X2	T45.4X3	T45.4X4	T45.4X5	T45.4X6
pyrophosphate	T45.4X1	T45.4X2	T45.4X3	T45.4X4	T45.4X5	T45.4X6
Ferritin	T45.4X1	T45.4X2	T45.4X3	T45.4X4	T45.4X5	T45.4X6
Ferrocholinate	T45.4X1	T45.4X2	T45.4X3	T45.4X4	T45.4X5	T45.4X6
Ferrodextrane	T45.4X1	T45.4X2	T45.4X3	T45.4X4	T45.4X5	T45.4X6
Ferropolimaler	T45.4X1	T45.4X2	T45.4X3	T45.4X4	T45.4X5	T45.4X6
Ferrous — see also Iron						
phosphate	T45.4X1	T45.4X2	T45.4X3	T45.4X4	T45.4X5	T45.4X6
salt	T45.4X1	T45.4X2	T45.4X3	T45.4X4	T45.4X5	T45.4X6
with folic acid	T45.4X1	T45.4X2	T45.4X3	T45.4X4	T45.4X5	T45.4X6
Ferrous fumerate, gluconate, lactate, salt NEC, sulfate (medicinal)	T45.4X1	T45.4X2	T45.4X3	T45.4X4	T45.4X5	T45.4X6
Ferrovanadium (fumes)	T59.891	T59.892	T59.893	T59.894	—	—
Ferrum — see Iron						
Fertilizers NEC	T65.891	T65.892	T65.893	T65.894	—	—
with herbicide mixture	T60.3X1	T60.3X2	T60.3X3	T60.3X4	—	—
Fetoxilate	T47.6X1	T47.6X2	T47.6X3	T47.6X4	T47.6X5	T47.6X6
Fiber, dietary	T47.4X1	T47.4X2	T47.4X3	T47.4X4	T47.4X5	T47.4X6
Fibrinogen (human)	T45.8X1	T45.8X2	T45.8X3	T45.8X4	T45.8X5	T45.8X6
Fibrinolysin (human)	T45.691	T45.692	T45.693	T45.694	T45.695	T45.696
Fibrinolysis						
affecting drug	T45.601	T45.602	T45.603	T45.604	T45.605	T45.606
inhibitor NEC	T45.621	T45.622	T45.623	T45.624	T45.625	T45.626
Fibrinolytic drug	T45.611	T45.612	T45.613	T45.614	T45.615	T45.616
Filix mas	T37.4X1	T37.4X2	T37.4X3	T37.4X4	T37.4X5	T37.4X6
Filtering cream	T49.3X1	T49.3X2	T49.3X3	T49.3X4	T49.3X5	T49.3X6

Substance	Poisoning, Accidental (Unintentional)	Poisoning, Intentional Self-Harm	Poisoning, Assault	Poisoning, Undetermined	Adverse Effect	Underdosing
Fiorinal	T39.011	T39.012	T39.013	T39.014	T39.015	T39.016
Firedamp	T59.891	T59.892	T59.893	T59.894	—	—
Fish, noxious, nonbacterial	T61.91	T61.92	T61.93	T61.94	—	—
ciguatera	T61.01	T61.02	T61.03	T61.04	—	—
scombroid	T61.11	T61.12	T61.13	T61.14	—	—
shell	T61.781	T61.782	T61.783	T61.784	—	—
specified NEC	T61.771	T61.772	T61.773	T61.774	—	—
Flagyl	T37.3X1	T37.3X2	T37.3X3	T37.3X4	T37.3X5	T37.3X6
Flavine adenine dinucleotide	T45.2X1	T45.2X2	T45.2X3	T45.2X4	T45.2X5	T45.2X6
Flavodic acid	T46.991	T46.992	T46.993	T46.994	T46.995	T46.996
Flavoxate	T44.3X1	T44.3X2	T44.3X3	T44.3X4	T44.3X5	T44.3X6
Flaxedil	T48.1X1	T48.1X2	T48.1X3	T48.1X4	T48.1X5	T48.1X6
Flaxseed (medicinal)	T49.3X1	T49.3X2	T49.3X3	T49.3X4	T49.3X5	T49.3X6
Flecainide	T46.2X1	T46.2X2	T46.2X3	T46.2X4	T46.2X5	T46.2X6
Fleroxacin	T36.8X1	T36.8X2	T36.8X3	T36.8X4	T36.8X5	T36.8X6
Floctafenine	T39.8X1	T39.8X2	T39.8X3	T39.8X4	T39.8X5	T39.8X6
Flomax	T44.6X1	T44.6X2	T44.6X3	T44.6X4	T44.6X5	T44.6X6
Flomoxef	T36.1X1	T36.1X2	T36.1X3	T36.1X4	T36.1X5	T36.1X6
Flopropione	T44.3X1	T44.3X2	T44.3X3	T44.3X4	T44.3X5	T44.3X6
Florantyrone	T47.5X1	T47.5X2	T47.5X3	T47.5X4	T47.5X5	T47.5X6
Floraquin	T37.8X1	T37.8X2	T37.8X3	T37.8X4	T37.8X5	T37.8X6
Florinef	T38.0X1	T38.0X2	T38.0X3	T38.0X4	T38.0X5	T38.0X6
ENT agent	T49.6X1	T49.6X2	T49.6X3	T49.6X4	T49.6X5	T49.6X6
ophthalmic preparation	T49.5X1	T49.5X2	T49.5X3	T49.5X4	T49.5X5	T49.5X6
topical NEC	T49.0X1	T49.0X2	T49.0X3	T49.0X4	T49.0X5	T49.0X6
Flowers of sulfur	T49.4X1	T49.4X2	T49.4X3	T49.4X4	T49.4X5	T49.4X6
Floxuridine	T45.1X1	T45.1X2	T45.1X3	T45.1X4	T45.1X5	T45.1X6
Fluanisone	T43.4X1	T43.4X2	T43.4X3	T43.4X4	T43.4X5	T43.4X6
Flubendazole	T37.4X1	T37.4X2	T37.4X3	T37.4X4	T37.4X5	T37.4X6
Fluclorolone acetonide	T49.0X1	T49.0X2	T49.0X3	T49.0X4	T49.0X5	T49.0X6
Flucloxacillin	T36.0X1	T36.0X2	T36.0X3	T36.0X4	T36.0X5	T36.0X6
Fluconazole	T37.8X1	T37.8X2	T37.8X3	T37.8X4	T37.8X5	T37.8X6
Flucytosine	T37.8X1	T37.8X2	T37.8X3	T37.8X4	T37.8X5	T37.8X6
Fludeoxyglucose (18F)	T50.8X1	T50.8X2	T50.8X3	T50.8X4	T50.8X5	T50.8X6
Fludiazepam	T42.4X1	T42.4X2	T42.4X3	T42.4X4	T42.4X5	T42.4X6
Fludrocortisone	T50.0X1	T50.0X2	T50.0X3	T50.0X4	T50.0X5	T50.0X6
ENT agent	T49.6X1	T49.6X2	T49.6X3	T49.6X4	T49.6X5	T49.6X6
ophthalmic preparation	T49.5X1	T49.5X2	T49.5X3	T49.5X4	T49.5X5	T49.5X6
topical NEC	T49.0X1	T49.0X2	T49.0X3	T49.0X4	T49.0X5	T49.0X6
Fludroxycortide	T49.0X1	T49.0X2	T49.0X3	T49.0X4	T49.0X5	T49.0X6
Flufenamic acid	T39.391	T39.392	T39.393	T39.394	T39.395	T39.396
Fluindione	T45.511	T45.512	T45.513	T45.514	T45.515	T45.516

◀ New   ◀▬ Revised   ~~deleted~~ Deleted

TABLE OF DRUGS AND CHEMICALS

Substance	Poisoning, Accidental (Unintentional)	Poisoning, Intentional Self-Harm	Poisoning, Assault	Poisoning, Undetermined	Adverse Effect	Underdosing
Flumequine	T37.8X1	T37.8X2	T37.8X3	T37.8X4	T37.8X5	T37.8X6
Flumethasone	T49.0X1	T49.0X2	T49.0X3	T49.0X4	T49.0X5	T49.0X6
Flumethiazide	T50.2X1	T50.2X2	T50.2X3	T50.2X4	T50.2X5	T50.2X6
Flumidin	T37.5X1	T37.5X2	T37.5X3	T37.5X4	T37.5X5	T37.5X6
Flunarizine	T46.7X1	T46.7X2	T46.7X3	T46.7X4	T46.7X5	T46.7X6
Flunidazole	T37.8X1	T37.8X2	T37.8X3	T37.8X4	T37.8X5	T37.8X6
Flunisolide	T48.6X1	T48.6X2	T48.6X3	T48.6X4	T48.6X5	T48.6X6
Flunitrazepam	T42.4X1	T42.4X2	T42.4X3	T42.4X4	T42.4X5	T42.4X6
Fluocinolone (acetonide)	T49.0X1	T49.0X2	T49.0X3	T49.0X4	T49.0X5	T49.0X6
Fluocinonide	T49.0X1	T49.0X2	T49.0X3	T49.0X4	T49.0X5	T49.0X6
Fluocortin (butyl)	T49.0X1	T49.0X2	T49.0X3	T49.0X4	T49.0X5	T49.0X6
Fluocortolone	T49.0X1	T49.0X2	T49.0X3	T49.0X4	T49.0X5	T49.0X6
Fluohydrocortisone	T38.0X1	T38.0X2	T38.0X3	T38.0X4	T38.0X5	T38.0X6
ENT agent	T49.6X1	T49.6X2	T49.6X3	T49.6X4	T49.6X5	T49.6X6
ophthalmic preparation	T49.5X1	T49.5X2	T49.5X3	T49.5X4	T49.5X5	T49.5X6
topical NEC	T49.0X1	T49.0X2	T49.0X3	T49.0X4	T49.0X5	T49.0X6
Fluonid	T49.0X1	T49.0X2	T49.0X3	T49.0X4	T49.0X5	T49.0X6
Fluopromazine	T43.3X1	T43.3X2	T43.3X3	T43.3X4	T43.3X5	T43.3X6
Fluoroacetate	T60.8X1	T60.8X2	T60.8X3	T60.8X4	—	—
Fluorescein	T50.8X1	T50.8X2	T50.8X3	T50.8X4	T50.8X5	T50.8X6
Fluorhydrocortisone	T50.0X1	T50.0X2	T50.0X3	T50.0X4	T50.0X5	T50.0X6
Fluoride (nonmedicinal) (pesticide) (sodium) NEC	T60.8X1	T60.8X2	T60.8X3	T60.8X4	—	—
hydrogen — *see Hydrofluoric acid*						
medicinal NEC	T50.991	T50.992	T50.993	T50.994	T50.995	T50.996
dental use	T49.7X1	T49.7X2	T49.7X3	T49.7X4	T49.7X5	T49.7X6
not pesticide NEC	T54.91	T54.92	T54.93	T54.94	—	—
stannous	T49.7X1	T49.7X2	T49.7X3	T49.7X4	T49.7X5	T49.7X6
Fluorinated corticosteroids	T38.0X1	T38.0X2	T38.0X3	T38.0X4	T38.0X5	T38.0X6
Fluorine (gas)	T59.5X1	T59.5X2	T59.5X3	T59.5X4		
salt — *see Fluoride(s)*						
Fluoristan	T49.7X1	T49.7X2	T49.7X3	T49.7X4	T49.7X5	T49.7X6
Fluormetholone	T49.0X1	T49.0X2	T49.0X3	T49.0X4	T49.0X5	T49.0X6
Fluoroacetate	T60.8X1	T60.8X2	T60.8X3	T60.8X4	—	—
Fluorocarbon monomer	T53.6X1	T53.6X2	T53.6X3	T53.6X4	—	—
Fluorocytosine	T37.8X1	T37.8X2	T37.8X3	T37.8X4	T37.8X5	T37.8X6
Fluorodeoxyuridine	T45.1X1	T45.1X2	T45.1X3	T45.1X4	T45.1X5	T45.1X6
Fluorometholone	T49.0X1	T49.0X2	T49.0X3	T49.0X4	T49.0X5	T49.0X6
ophthalmic preparation	T49.5X1	T49.5X2	T49.5X3	T49.5X4	T49.5X5	T49.5X6
Fluorophosphate insecticide	T60.0X1	T60.0X2	T60.0X3	T60.0X4	—	—
Fluorosol	T46.3X1	T46.3X2	T46.3X3	T46.3X4	T46.3X5	T46.3X6
Fluorouracil	T45.1X1	T45.1X2	T45.1X3	T45.1X4	T45.1X5	T45.1X6

Substance	Poisoning, Accidental (Unintentional)	Poisoning, Intentional Self-Harm	Poisoning, Assault	Poisoning, Undetermined	Adverse Effect	Underdosing
Fluorphenylalanine	T49.5X1	T49.5X2	T49.5X3	T49.5X4	T49.5X5	T49.5X6
Fluothane	T41.0X1	T41.0X2	T41.0X3	T41.0X4	T41.0X5	T41.0X6
Fluoxetine	T43.221	T43.222	T43.223	T43.224	T43.225	T43.226
Fluoxymesterone	T38.7X1	T38.7X2	T38.7X3	T38.7X4	T38.7X5	T38.7X6
Flupenthixol	T43.4X1	T43.4X2	T43.4X3	T43.4X4	T43.4X5	T43.4X6
Flupentixol	T43.4X1	T43.4X2	T43.4X3	T43.4X4	T43.4X5	T43.4X6
Fluphenazine	T43.3X1	T43.3X2	T43.3X3	T43.3X4	T43.3X5	T43.3X6
Fluprednidene	T49.0X1	T49.0X2	T49.0X3	T49.0X4	T49.0X5	T49.0X6
Fluprednisolone	T38.0X1	T38.0X2	T38.0X3	T38.0X4	T38.0X5	T38.0X6
Fluradoline	T39.8X1	T39.8X2	T39.8X3	T39.8X4	T39.8X5	T39.8X6
Flurandrenolide	T49.0X1	T49.0X2	T49.0X3	T49.0X4	T49.0X5	T49.0X6
Flurandrenolone	T49.0X1	T49.0X2	T49.0X3	T49.0X4	T49.0X5	T49.0X6
Flurazepam	T42.4X1	T42.4X2	T42.4X3	T42.4X4	T42.4X5	T42.4X6
Flurbiprofen	T39.311	T39.312	T39.313	T39.314	T39.315	T39.316
Flurobate	T49.0X1	T49.0X2	T49.0X3	T49.0X4	T49.0X5	T49.0X6
Flurotyl	T43.291	T43.292	T43.293	T43.294	T43.295	T43.296
Fluroxene	T41.0X1	T41.0X2	T41.0X3	T41.0X4	T41.0X5	T41.0X6
Fluspirilene	T43.591	T43.592	T43.593	T43.594	T43.595	T43.596
Flutamide	T38.6X1	T38.6X2	T38.6X3	T38.6X4	T38.6X5	T38.6X6
Flutazolam	T42.4X1	T42.4X2	T42.4X3	T42.4X4	T42.4X5	T42.4X6
Fluticasone propionate	T49.1X1	T49.1X2	T49.1X3	T49.1X4	T49.1X5	T49.1X6
Flutoprazepam	T42.4X1	T42.4X2	T42.4X3	T42.4X4	T42.4X5	T42.4X6
Flutropium bromide	T48.6X1	T48.6X2	T48.6X3	T48.6X4	T48.6X5	T48.6X6
Fluvoxamine	T43.221	T43.222	T43.223	T43.224	T43.225	T43.226
Folacin	T45.8X1	T45.8X2	T45.8X3	T45.8X4	T45.8X5	T45.8X6
Folic acid	T45.8X1	T45.8X2	T45.8X3	T45.8X4	T45.8X5	T45.8X6
with ferrous salt	T45.2X1	T45.2X2	T45.2X3	T45.2X4	T45.2X5	T45.2X6
antagonist	T45.1X1	T45.1X2	T45.1X3	T45.1X4	T45.1X5	T45.1X6
Folinic acid	T45.8X1	T45.8X2	T45.8X3	T45.8X4	T45.8X5	T45.8X6
Folium stramoniae	T48.6X1	T48.6X2	T48.6X3	T48.6X4	T48.6X5	T48.6X6
Follicle-stimulating hormone, human	T38.811	T38.812	T38.813	T38.814	T38.815	T38.816
Folpet	T60.3X1	T60.3X2	T60.3X3	T60.3X4	—	—
Fominoben	T48.3X1	T48.3X2	T48.3X3	T48.3X4	T48.3X5	T48.3X6
Food, foodstuffs, noxious, nonbacterial, NEC	T62.91	T62.92	T62.93	T62.94	—	—
berries	T62.1X1	T62.1X2	T62.1X3	T62.1X4		
fish — *see also Fish*	T61.91	T61.92	T61.93	T61.94		
mushrooms	T62.0X1	T62.0X2	T62.0X3	T62.0X4		
plants	T62.2X1	T62.2X2	T62.2X3	T62.2X4		
seafood	T61.91	T61.92	T61.93	T61.94		
specified NEC	T61.8X1	T61.8X2	T61.8X3	T61.8X4	—	—
seeds	T62.2X1	T62.2X2	T62.2X3	T62.2X4	—	—

◀ New   ◀ Revised   ~~deleted~~ Deleted

TABLE OF DRUGS AND CHEMICALS

Substance	External Cause (T-Code)					
	Poisoning, Accidental (Unintentional)	Poisoning, Intentional Self-Harm	Poisoning, Assault	Poisoning, Undetermined	Adverse Effect	Underdosing
Food, foodstuffs, noxious, nonbacterial, NEC *(Continued)*						
shellfish	T61.781	T61.782	T61.783	T61.784	—	—
specified NEC	T62.8X1	T62.8X2	T62.8X3	T62.8X4	—	—
Fool's parsley	T62.2X1	T62.2X2	T62.2X3	T62.2X4	—	—
Formaldehyde (solution), gas or vapor	T59.2X1	T59.2X2	T59.2X3	T59.2X4	—	—
fungicide	T60.3X1	T60.3X2	T60.3X3	T60.3X4	—	—
Formalin	T59.2X1	T59.2X2	T59.2X3	T59.2X4	—	—
fungicide	T60.3X1	T60.3X2	T60.3X3	T60.3X4	—	—
vapor	T59.2X1	T59.2X2	T59.2X3	T59.2X4	—	—
Formic acid	T54.2X1	T54.2X2	T54.2X3	T54.2X4	—	—
vapor	T59.891	T59.892	T59.893	T59.894	—	—
Foscarnet sodium	T37.5X1	T37.5X2	T37.5X3	T37.5X4	T37.5X5	T37.5X6
Fosfestrol	T38.5X1	T38.5X2	T38.5X3	T38.5X4	T38.5X5	T38.5X6
Fosfomycin	T36.8X1	T36.8X2	T36.8X3	T36.8X4	T36.8X5	T36.8X6
Fosfonet sodium	T37.5X1	T37.5X2	T37.5X3	T37.5X4	T37.5X5	T37.5X6
Fosinopril	T46.4X1	T46.4X2	T46.4X3	T46.4X4	T46.4X5	T46.4X6
sodium	T46.4X1	T46.4X2	T46.4X3	T46.4X4	T46.4X5	T46.4X6
Fowler's solution	T57.0X1	T57.0X2	T57.0X3	T57.0X4	—	—
Foxglove	T62.2X1	T62.2X2	T62.2X3	T62.2X4	—	—
Framycetin	T36.5X1	T36.5X2	T36.5X3	T36.5X4	T36.5X5	T36.5X6
Frangula	T47.2X1	T47.2X2	T47.2X3	T47.2X4	T47.2X5	T47.2X6
extract	T47.2X1	T47.2X2	T47.2X3	T47.2X4	T47.2X5	T47.2X6
Frei antigen	T50.8X1	T50.8X2	T50.8X3	T50.8X4	T50.8X5	T50.8X6
Freon	T53.5X1	T53.5X2	T53.5X3	T53.5X4	—	—
Fructose	T50.3X1	T50.3X2	T50.3X3	T50.3X4	T50.3X5	T50.3X6
Frusemide	T50.1X1	T50.1X2	T50.1X3	T50.1X4	T50.1X5	T50.1X6
FSH	T38.811	T38.812	T38.813	T38.814	T38.815	T38.816
Ftorafur	T45.1X1	T45.1X2	T45.1X3	T45.1X4	T45.1X5	T45.1X6
Fuel						
automobile	T52.0X1	T52.0X2	T52.0X3	T52.0X4	—	—
exhaust gas, not in transit	T58.01	T58.02	T58.03	T58.04	—	—
vapor NEC	T52.0X1	T52.0X2	T52.0X3	T52.0X4	—	—
gas (domestic use) — *see also Carbon, monoxide, fuel, utility*	T59.891	T59.892	T59.893	T59.894	—	—
utility	T59.891	T59.892	T59.893	T59.894	—	—
in mobile container	T59.891	T59.892	T59.893	T59.894	—	—
incomplete combustion of — *see Carbon, monoxide, fuel, utility*						
piped (natural)	T59.891	T59.892	T59.893	T59.894	—	—
industrial, incomplete combustion	T58.8X1	T58.8X2	T58.8X3	T58.8X4	—	—

Substance	External Cause (T-Code)					
	Poisoning, Accidental (Unintentional)	Poisoning, Intentional Self-Harm	Poisoning, Assault	Poisoning, Undetermined	Adverse Effect	Underdosing
Fugillin	T36.8X1	T36.8X2	T36.8X3	T36.8X4	T36.8X5	T36.8X6
Fulminate of mercury	T56.1X1	T56.1X2	T56.1X3	T56.1X4	—	—
Fulvicin	T36.7X1	T36.7X2	T36.7X3	T36.7X4	T36.7X5	T36.7X6
Fumadil	T36.8X1	T36.8X2	T36.8X3	T36.8X4	T36.8X5	T36.8X6
Fumagillin	T36.8X1	T36.8X2	T36.8X3	T36.8X4	T36.8X5	T36.8X6
Fumaric acid	T49.4X1	T49.4X2	T49.4X3	T49.4X4	T49.4X5	T49.4X6
Fumes (from)	T59.91	T59.92	T59.93	T59.94	—	—
carbon monoxide — *see Carbon, monoxide*						
charcoal (domestic use) — *see Charcoal, fumes*						
chloroform — *see Chloroform*						
coke (in domestic stoves, fireplaces) — *see Coke, fumes*						
corrosive NEC	T54.91	T54.92	T54.93	T54.94	—	—
ether — *see ether*						
freons	T53.5X1	T53.5X2	T53.5X3	T53.5X4	—	—
hydrocarbons	T59.891	T59.892	T59.893	T59.894	—	—
petroleum (liquefied)	T59.891	T59.892	T59.893	T59.894	—	—
distributed through pipes (pure or mixed with air)	T59.891	T59.892	T59.893	T59.894	—	—
lead — *see lead*						
metal — *see Metals, or the specified metal*						
nitrogen dioxide	T59.0X1	T59.0X2	T59.0X3	T59.0X4	—	—
pesticides — *see Pesticides*						
petroleum (liquefied)	T59.891	T59.892	T59.893	T59.894	—	—
distributed through pipes (pure or mixed with air)	T59.891	T59.892	T59.893	T59.894	—	—
polyester	T59.891	T59.892	T59.893	T59.894	—	—
specified source NEC — *see also substance specified*	T59.891	T59.892	T59.893	T59.894	—	—
sulfur dioxide	T59.1X1	T59.1X2	T59.1X3	T59.1X4	—	—
Fumigant NEC	T60.91	T60.92	T60.93	T60.94	—	—
Fungi, noxious, used as food	T62.0X1	T62.0X2	T62.0X3	T62.0X4	—	—
Fungicide NEC (nonmedicinal)	T60.3X1	T60.3X2	T60.3X3	T60.3X4	—	—
Fungizone	T36.7X1	T36.7X2	T36.7X3	T36.7X4	T36.7X5	T36.7X6
topical	T49.0X1	T49.0X2	T49.0X3	T49.0X4	T49.0X5	T49.0X6
Furacin	T49.0X1	T49.0X2	T49.0X3	T49.0X4	T49.0X5	T49.0X6
Furadantin	T37.91	T37.92	T37.93	T37.94	T37.95	T37.96
Furazolidone	T37.8X1	T37.8X2	T37.8X3	T37.8X4	T37.8X5	T37.8X6
Furazolium chloride	T49.0X1	T49.0X2	T49.0X3	T49.0X4	T49.0X5	T49.0X6
Furfural	T52.8X1	T52.8X2	T52.8X3	T52.8X4	—	—

◄ New   ◄ Revised   ~~deleted~~ Deleted

Substance	Poisoning, Accidental (Unintentional)	Poisoning, Intentional Self-Harm	Poisoning, Assault	Poisoning, Undetermined	Adverse Effect	Underdosing
	External Cause (T-Code)					
Furnace (coal burning) (domestic), gas from industrial	T58.2X1	T58.2X2	T58.2X3	T58.2X4	—	—
industrial	T58.8X1	T58.8X2	T58.8X3	T58.8X4	—	—
Furniture polish	T65.891	T65.892	T65.893	T65.894	—	—
Furosemide	T50.1X1	T50.1X2	T50.1X3	T50.1X4	T50.1X5	T50.1X6
Furoxone	T37.91	T37.92	T37.93	T37.94	T37.95	T37.96
Fursultiamine	T45.2X1	T45.2X2	T45.2X3	T45.2X4	T45.2X5	T45.2X6
Fusafungine	T36.8X1	T36.8X2	T36.8X3	T36.8X4	T36.8X5	T36.8X6
Fusel oil (any) (amyl) (butyl) (propyl), vapor	T51.3X1	T51.3X2	T51.3X3	T51.3X4	—	—
Fusidate (ethanolamine) (sodium)	T36.8X1	T36.8X2	T36.8X3	T36.8X4	T36.8X5	T36.8X6
Fusidic acid	T36.8X1	T36.8X2	T36.8X3	T36.8X4	T36.8X5	T36.8X6
Fytic acid, nonasodium	T50.6X1	T50.6X2	T50.6X3	T50.6X4	T50.6X5	T50.6X6
G						
GABA	T43.8X1	T43.8X2	T43.8X3	T43.8X4	T43.8X5	T43.8X6
Gadopentetic acid	T50.8X1	T50.8X2	T50.8X3	T50.8X4	T50.8X5	T50.8X6
Galactose	T50.3X1	T50.3X2	T50.3X3	T50.3X4	T50.3X5	T50.3X6
b-Galactosidase	T47.5X1	T47.5X2	T47.5X3	T47.5X4	T47.5X5	T47.5X6
Galantamine	T44.0X1	T44.0X2	T44.0X3	T44.0X4	T44.0X5	T44.0X6
Gallamine (triethiodide)	T48.1X1	T48.1X2	T48.1X3	T48.1X4	T48.1X5	T48.1X6
Gallium citrate	T50.991	T50.992	T50.993	T50.994	T50.995	T50.996
Gallopamil	T46.1X1	T46.1X2	T46.1X3	T46.1X4	T46.1X5	T46.1X6
Gamboge	T47.2X1	T47.2X2	T47.2X3	T47.2X4	T47.2X5	T47.2X6
Gamimune	T50.Z11	T50.Z12	T50.Z13	T50.Z14	T50.Z15	T50.Z16
Gamma-aminobutyric acid	T43.8X1	T43.8X2	T43.8X3	T43.8X4	T43.8X5	T43.8X6
Gamma-benzene hexachloride (medicinal)	T49.0X1	T49.0X2	T49.0X3	T49.0X4	T49.0X5	T49.0X6
nonmedicinal, vapor	T53.6X1	T53.6X2	T53.6X3	T53.6X4	—	—
Gamma-BHC (medicinal) — see also Gamma-benzene hexachloride	T49.0X1	T49.0X2	T49.0X3	T49.0X4	T49.0X5	T49.0X6
Gamma globulin	T50.Z11	T50.Z12	T50.Z13	T50.Z14	T50.Z15	T50.Z16
Gamulin	T50.Z11	T50.Z12	T50.Z13	T50.Z14	T50.Z15	T50.Z16
Ganciclovir (sodium)	T37.5X1	T37.5X2	T37.5X3	T37.5X4	T37.5X5	T37.5X6
Ganglionic blocking drug NEC	T44.2X1	T44.2X2	T44.2X3	T44.2X4	T44.2X5	T44.2X6
specified NEC	T44.2X1	T44.2X2	T44.2X3	T44.2X4	T44.2X5	T44.2X6
Ganja	T40.7X1	T40.7X2	T40.7X3	T40.7X4	T40.7X5	T40.7X6
Garamycin	T36.5X1	T36.5X2	T36.5X3	T36.5X4	T36.5X5	T36.5X6
ophthalmic preparation	T49.5X1	T49.5X2	T49.5X3	T49.5X4	T49.5X5	T49.5X6
topical NEC	T49.0X1	T49.0X2	T49.0X3	T49.0X4	T49.0X5	T49.0X6
Gardenal	T42.3X1	T42.3X2	T42.3X3	T42.3X4	T42.3X5	T42.3X6
Gardepanyl	T42.3X1	T42.3X2	T42.3X3	T42.3X4	T42.3X5	T42.3X6

Substance	Poisoning, Accidental (Unintentional)	Poisoning, Intentional Self-Harm	Poisoning, Assault	Poisoning, Undetermined	Adverse Effect	Underdosing
	External Cause (T-Code)					
Gas	T59.91	T59.92	T59.93	T59.94	—	—
acetylene	T59.891	T59.892	T59.893	T59.894	—	—
incomplete combustion of	T58.11	T58.12	T58.13	T58.14	—	—
air contaminants, source or type not specified	T59.91	T59.92	T59.93	T59.94	—	—
anesthetic	T41.0X1	T41.0X2	T41.0X3	T41.0X4	T41.0X5	T41.0X6
blast furnace	T58.8X1	T58.8X2	T58.8X3	T58.8X4	—	—
butane — see butane						
carbon monoxide — see Carbon, monoxide						
chlorine	T59.4X1	T59.4X2	T59.4X3	T59.4X4	—	—
coal	T58.2X1	T58.2X2	T58.2X3	T58.2X4	—	—
cyanide	T57.3X1	T57.3X2	T57.3X3	T57.3X4	—	—
dicyanogen	T65.0X1	T65.0X2	T65.0X3	T65.0X4	—	—
domestic — see Domestic gas	T57.91	T57.92	T57.93	T57.94	—	—
exhaust	T57.91	T57.92	T57.93	T57.94	—	—
from utility (for cooking, heating, or lighting) (after combustion) — see Carbon, monoxide, fuel, utility						
prior to combustion	T59.891	T59.892	T59.893	T59.894	—	—
from wood or coal-burning stove or fireplace	T57.91	T57.92	T57.93	T57.94	—	—
fuel (domestic use) (after combustion) — see also Carbon, monoxide, fuel	T57.91	T57.92	T57.93	T57.94	—	—
industrial use	T58.8X1	T58.8X2	T58.8X3	T58.8X4	—	—
prior to combustion	T59.891	T59.892	T59.893	T59.894	—	—
utility	T59.891	T59.892	T59.893	T59.894	—	—
in mobile container	T59.891	T59.892	T59.893	T59.894	—	—
incomplete combustion of — see Carbon, monoxide, fuel, utility						
piped (natural)	T59.891	T59.892	T59.893	T59.894	—	—
garage	T58.01	T58.02	T58.03	T58.04	—	—
hydrocarbon NEC	T59.891	T59.892	T59.893	T59.894	—	—
incomplete combustion of — see Carbon, monoxide, fuel, utility						
liquefied — see butane						
piped	T59.891	T59.892	T59.893	T59.894	—	—
hydrocyanic acid	T65.0X1	T65.0X2	T65.0X3	T65.0X4	—	—

◀ New ◀||| Revised ~~deleted~~ Deleted

Substance	External Cause (T-Code)					
	Poisoning, Accidental (Unintentional)	Poisoning, Intentional Self-Harm	Poisoning, Assault	Poisoning, Undetermined	Adverse Effect	Underdosing
Gas (Continued)						
illuminating (after combustion)	T58.11	T58.12	T58.13	T58.14	—	—
prior to combustion	T59.891	T59.892	T59.893	T59.894	—	—
incomplete combustion, any — see Carbon, monoxide						
kiln	T58.8X1	T58.8X2	T58.8X3	T58.8X4	—	—
lacrimogenic	T59.3X1	T59.3X2	T59.3X3	T59.3X4	—	—
liquefied petroleum — see butane						
marsh	T59.891	T59.892	T59.893	T59.894	—	—
motor exhaust, not in transit	T58.01	T58.02	T58.03	T58.04	—	—
mustard, not in war	T59.891	T59.892	T59.893	T59.894	—	—
natural	T59.891	T59.892	T59.893	T59.894	—	—
nerve, not in war	T59.91	T59.92	T59.93	T59.94	—	—
oil	T52.0X1	T52.0X2	T52.0X3	T52.0X4	—	—
petroleum (liquefied) (distributed in mobile containers)	T59.891	T59.892	T59.893	T59.894	—	—
piped (pure or mixed with air)	T59.891	T59.892	T59.893	T59.894	—	—
piped (manufactured) (natural) NEC	T59.891	T59.892	T59.893	T59.894	—	—
producer	T58.8X1	T58.8X2	T58.8X3	T58.8X4	—	—
propane — see propane						
refrigerant (chlorofluoro-carbon)	T53.5X1	T53.5X2	T53.5X3	T53.5X4	—	—
not chlorofluoro-carbon	T59.891	T59.892	T59.893	T59.894	—	—
sewer	T59.91	T59.92	T59.93	T59.94	—	—
specified source NEC	T59.91	T59.92	T59.93	T59.94	—	—
stove (after combustion)	T58.11	T58.12	T58.13	T58.14	—	—
tear	T59.3X1	T59.3X2	T59.3X3	T59.3X4	—	—
therapeutic	T41.5X1	T41.5X2	T41.5X3	T41.5X4	T41.5X5	T41.5X6
utility (for cooking, heating, or lighting) (piped) NEC	T59.891	T59.892	T59.893	T59.894	—	—
in mobile container	T59.891	T59.892	T59.893	T59.894	—	—
incomplete combustion of — see Carbon, monoxide, fuel, utilty						
piped (natural)	T59.891	T59.892	T59.893	T59.894	—	—
water	T58.11	T58.12	T58.13	T58.14	—	—
incomplete combustion of — see Carbon, monoxide, fuel, utility						

Substance	External Cause (T-Code)					
	Poisoning, Accidental (Unintentional)	Poisoning, Intentional Self-Harm	Poisoning, Assault	Poisoning, Undetermined	Adverse Effect	Underdosing
Gaseous substance — see Gas						
Gasoline	T52.0X1	T52.0X2	T52.0X3	T52.0X4	—	—
vapor	T52.0X1	T52.0X2	T52.0X3	T52.0X4	—	—
Gastric enzymes	T47.5X1	T47.5X2	T47.5X3	T47.5X4	T47.5X5	T47.5X6
Gastrografin	T50.8X1	T50.8X2	T50.8X3	T50.8X4	T50.8X5	T50.8X6
Gastrointestinal drug	T47.91	T47.92	T47.93	T47.94	T47.95	T47.96
biological	T47.8X1	T47.8X2	T47.8X3	T47.8X4	T47.8X5	T47.8X6
specified NEC	T47.8X1	T47.8X2	T47.8X3	T47.8X4	T47.8X5	T47.8X6
Gaultheria procumbens	T62.2X1	T62.2X2	T62.2X3	T62.2X4	—	—
Gelatin (intravenous)	T45.8X1	T45.8X2	T45.8X3	T45.8X4	T45.8X5	T45.8X6
absorbable (sponge)	T45.7X1	T45.7X2	T45.7X3	T45.7X4	T45.7X5	T45.7X6
Gefarnate	T44.3X1	T44.3X2	T44.3X3	T44.3X4	T44.3X5	T44.3X6
Gelfilm	T49.8X1	T49.8X2	T49.8X3	T49.8X4	T49.8X5	T49.8X6
Gelfoam	T45.7X1	T45.7X2	T45.7X3	T45.7X4	T45.7X5	T45.7X6
Gelsemine	T50.991	T50.992	T50.993	T50.994	T50.995	T50.996
Gelsemium (sempervirens)	T62.2X1	T62.2X2	T62.2X3	T62.2X4	—	—
Gemeprost	T48.0X1	T48.0X2	T48.0X3	T48.0X4	T48.0X5	T48.0X6
Gemfibrozil	T46.6X1	T46.6X2	T46.6X3	T46.6X4	T46.6X5	T46.6X6
Gemonil	T42.3X1	T42.3X2	T42.3X3	T42.3X4	T42.3X5	T42.3X6
Gentamicin	T36.5X1	T36.5X2	T36.5X3	T36.5X4	T36.5X5	T36.5X6
ophthalmic preparation	T49.5X1	T49.5X2	T49.5X3	T49.5X4	T49.5X5	T49.5X6
topical NEC	T49.0X1	T49.0X2	T49.0X3	T49.0X4	T49.0X5	T49.0X6
Gentian	T47.5X1	T47.5X2	T47.5X3	T47.5X4	T47.5X5	T47.5X6
violet	T49.0X1	T49.0X2	T49.0X3	T49.0X4	T49.0X5	T49.0X6
Gepefrine	T44.4X1	T44.4X2	T44.4X3	T44.4X4	T44.4X5	T44.4X6
Gestonorone caproate	T38.5X1	T38.5X2	T38.5X3	T38.5X4	T38.5X5	T38.5X6
Gexane	T49.0X1	T49.0X2	T49.0X3	T49.0X4	T49.0X5	T49.0X6
Gila monster (venom)	T63.111	T63.112	T63.113	T63.114	—	—
Ginger	T47.5X1	T47.5X2	T47.5X3	T47.5X4	T47.5X5	T47.5X6
Jamaica — see Jamaica, ginger						
Gitalin	T46.0X1	T46.0X2	T46.0X3	T46.0X4	T46.0X5	T46.0X6
amorphous	T46.0X1	T46.0X2	T46.0X3	T46.0X4	T46.0X5	T46.0X6
Gitaloxin	T46.0X1	T46.0X2	T46.0X3	T46.0X4	T46.0X5	T46.0X6
Gitoxin	T46.0X1	T46.0X2	T46.0X3	T46.0X4	T46.0X5	T46.0X6
Glafenine	T39.8X1	T39.8X2	T39.8X3	T39.8X4	T39.8X5	T39.8X6
Glandular extract (medicinal) NEC	T50.Z91	T50.Z92	T50.Z93	T50.Z94	T50.Z95	T50.Z96
Glaucarubin	T37.3X1	T37.3X2	T37.3X3	T37.3X4	T37.3X5	T37.3X6
Glibenclamide	T38.3X1	T38.3X2	T38.3X3	T38.3X4	T38.3X5	T38.3X6
Glibornuride	T38.3X1	T38.3X2	T38.3X3	T38.3X4	T38.3X5	T38.3X6
Gliclazide	T38.3X1	T38.3X2	T38.3X3	T38.3X4	T38.3X5	T38.3X6
Glimidine	T38.3X1	T38.3X2	T38.3X3	T38.3X4	T38.3X5	T38.3X6

◀ New ◀|||| Revised ~~deleted~~ Deleted

Substance	Poisoning, Accidental (Unintentional)	Poisoning, Intentional Self-Harm	Poisoning, Assault	Poisoning, Undetermined	Adverse Effect	Underdosing
Glipizide	T38.3X1	T38.3X2	T38.3X3	T38.3X4	T38.3X5	T38.3X6
Gliquidone	T38.3X1	T38.3X2	T38.3X3	T38.3X4	T38.3X5	T38.3X6
Glisolamide	T38.3X1	T38.3X2	T38.3X3	T38.3X4	T38.3X5	T38.3X6
Glisoxepide	T38.3X1	T38.3X2	T38.3X3	T38.3X4	T38.3X5	T38.3X6
Globin zinc insulin	T38.3X1	T38.3X2	T38.3X3	T38.3X4	T38.3X5	T38.3X6
Globulin						
antilymphocytic	T50.Z11	T50.Z12	T50.Z13	T50.Z14	T50.Z15	T50.Z16
antirhesus	T50.Z11	T50.Z12	T50.Z13	T50.Z14	T50.Z15	T50.Z16
antivenin	T50.Z11	T50.Z12	T50.Z13	T50.Z14	T50.Z15	T50.Z16
antiviral	T50.Z11	T50.Z12	T50.Z13	T50.Z14	T50.Z15	T50.Z16
Glucagon	T38.3X1	T38.3X2	T38.3X3	T38.3X4	T38.3X5	T38.3X6
Glucocorticoids	T38.0X1	T38.0X2	T38.0X4	T38.0X4	T38.0X5	T38.0X6
Glucocorticosteroid	T38.0X1	T38.0X2	T38.0X3	T38.0X4	T38.0X5	T38.0X6
Gluconic acid	T50.991	T50.992	T50.993	T50.994	T50.995	T50.996
Glucosamine sulfate	T39.4X1	T39.4X2	T39.4X3	T39.4X4	T39.4X5	T39.4X6
Glucose	T50.3X1	T50.3X2	T50.3X3	T50.3X4	T50.3X5	T50.3X6
with sodium chloride	T50.3X1	T50.3X2	T50.3X3	T50.3X4	T50.3X5	T50.3X6
Glucosulfone sodium	T37.1X1	T37.1X2	T37.1X3	T37.1X4	T37.1X5	T37.1X6
Glucurolactone	T47.8X1	T47.8X2	T47.8X3	T47.8X4	T47.8X5	T47.8X6
Glue NEC	T52.8X1	T52.8X2	T52.8X3	T52.8X4	—	—
Glutamic acid	T47.5X1	T47.5X2	T47.5X3	T47.5X4	T47.5X5	T47.5X6
Glutaral (medicinal)	T49.0X1	T49.0X2	T49.0X3	T49.0X4	T49.0X5	T49.0X6
nonmedicinal	T65.891	T65.892	T65.893	T65.894		
Glutaraldehyde (nonmedicinal)	T65.891	T65.892	T65.893	T65.894	—	
medicinal	T49.0X1	T49.0X2	T49.0X3	T49.0X4	T49.0X5	T49.0X6
Glutathione	T50.6X1	T50.6X2	T50.6X4	T50.6X4	T50.6X5	T50.6X6
Glutethimide	T42.6X1	T42.6X2	T42.6X3	T42.6X4	T42.6X5	T42.6X6
Glyburide	T38.3X1	T38.3X2	T38.3X3	T38.3X4	T38.3X5	T38.3X6
Glycerin	T47.4X1	T47.4X2	T47.4X3	T47.4X4	T47.4X5	T47.4X6
Glycerol	T47.4X1	T47.4X2	T47.4X3	T47.4X4	T47.4X5	T47.4X6
borax	T49.6X1	T49.6X2	T49.6X3	T49.6X4	T49.6X5	T49.6X6
intravenous	T50.3X1	T50.3X2	T50.3X3	T50.3X4	T50.3X5	T50.3X6
iodinated	T48.4X1	T48.4X2	T48.4X3	T48.4X4	T48.4X5	T48.4X6
Glycerophosphate	T50.991	T50.992	T50.993	T50.994	T50.995	T50.996
Glyceryl						
gualacolate	T48.4X1	T48.4X2	T48.4X3	T48.4X4	T48.4X5	T48.4X6
nitrate	T46.3X1	T46.3X2	T46.3X3	T46.3X4	T46.3X5	T46.3X6
triacetate (topical)	T49.0X1	T49.0X2	T49.0X3	T49.0X4	T49.0X5	T49.0X6
trinitrate	T46.3X1	T46.3X2	T46.3X3	T46.3X4	T46.3X5	T46.3X6
Glycine	T50.3X1	T50.3X2	T50.3X3	T50.3X4	T50.3X5	T50.3X6
Glyclopyramide	T38.3X1	T38.3X2	T38.3X3	T38.3X4	T38.3X5	T38.3X6
Glycobiarsol	T37.3X1	T37.3X2	T37.3X3	T37.3X4	T37.3X5	T37.3X6

Substance	Poisoning, Accidental (Unintentional)	Poisoning, Intentional Self-Harm	Poisoning, Assault	Poisoning, Undetermined	Adverse Effect	Underdosing
Glycols (ether)	T52.3X1	T52.3X2	T52.3X3	T52.3X4	—	—
Glyconiazide	T37.1X1	T37.1X2	T37.1X3	T37.1X4	T37.1X5	T37.1X6
Glycopyrrolate	T44.3X1	T44.3X2	T44.3X3	T44.3X4	T44.3X5	T44.3X6
Glycopyrronium	T44.3X1	T44.3X2	T44.3X3	T44.3X4	T44.3X5	T44.3X6
bromide	T44.3X1	T44.3X2	T44.3X3	T44.3X4	T44.3X5	T44.3X6
Glycoside, cardiac (stimulant)	T46.0X1	T46.0X2	T46.0X3	T46.0X4	T46.0X5	T46.0X6
Glycyclamide	T38.3X1	T38.3X2	T38.3X3	T38.3X4	T38.3X5	T38.3X6
Glycyrrhiza extract	T48.4X1	T48.4X2	T48.4X3	T48.4X4	T48.4X5	T48.4X6
Glycyrrhizic acid	T48.4X1	T48.4X2	T48.4X3	T48.4X4	T48.4X5	T48.4X6
Glycyrrhizinate potassium	T48.4X1	T48.4X2	T48.4X3	T48.4X4	T48.4X5	T48.4X6
Glymidine sodium	T38.3X1	T38.3X2	T38.3X3	T38.3X4	T38.3X5	T38.3X6
Glyphosate	T60.3X1	T60.3X2	T60.3X3	T60.3X4	—	—
Glyphylline	T48.6X1	T48.6X2	T48.6X3	T48.6X4	T48.6X5	T48.6X6
Gold						
colloidal (I98Au)	T45.1X1	T45.1X2	T45.1X3	T45.1X4	T45.1X5	T45.1X6
salts	T39.4X1	T39.4X2	T39.4X3	T39.4X4	T39.4X5	T39.4X6
Golden sulfide of antimony	T56.891	T56.892	T56.893	T56.894	—	—
Goldylocks	T62.2X1	T62.2X2	T62.2X3	T62.2X4	—	—
Gonadal tissue extract	T38.901	T38.902	T38.903	T38.904	T38.905	T38.906
female	T38.5X1	T38.5X2	T38.5X3	T38.5X4	T38.5X5	T38.5X6
male	T38.7X1	T38.7X2	T38.7X3	T38.7X4	T38.7X5	T38.7X6
Gonadorelin	T38.891	T38.892	T38.893	T38.894	T38.895	T38.896
Gonadotropin	T38.891	T38.892	T38.893	T38.894	T38.895	T38.896
chorionic	T38.891	T38.892	T38.893	T38.894	T38.895	T38.896
pituitary	T38.811	T38.812	T38.813	T38.814	T38.815	T38.816
Goserelin	T45.1X1	T45.1X2	T45.1X3	T45.1X4	T45.1X5	T45.1X6
Grain alcohol	T51.0X1	T51.0X2	T51.0X3	T51.0X4	—	—
Gramicidin	T49.0X1	T49.0X2	T49.0X3	T49.0X4	T49.0X5	T49.0X6
Granisetron	T45.0X1	T45.0X2	T45.0X3	T45.0X4	T45.0X5	T45.0X6
Gratiola officinalis	T62.2X1	T62.2X2	T62.2X3	T62.2X4	—	—
Grease	T65.891	T65.892	T65.893	T65.894	—	—
Green hellebore	T62.2X1	T62.2X2	T62.2X3	T62.2X4	—	—
Green soap	T49.2X1	T49.2X2	T49.2X3	T49.2X4	T49.2X5	T49.2X6
Grifulvin	T36.7X1	T36.7X2	T36.7X3	T36.7X4	T36.7X5	T36.7X6
Griseofulvin	T36.7X1	T36.7X2	T36.7X3	T36.7X4	T36.7X5	T36.7X6
Growth hormone	T38.811	T38.812	T38.813	T38.814	T38.815	T38.816
Guaiacol derivatives	T48.4X1	T48.4X2	T48.4X3	T48.4X4	T48.4X5	T48.4X6
Guaiac reagent	T50.991	T50.992	T50.993	T50.994	T50.995	T50.996
Guaifenesin	T48.4X1	T48.4X2	T48.4X3	T48.4X4	T48.4X5	T48.4X6
Guaimesal	T48.4X1	T48.4X2	T48.4X3	T48.4X4	T48.4X5	T48.4X6
Guaiphenesin	T48.4X1	T48.4X2	T48.4X3	T48.4X4	T48.4X5	T48.4X6
Guamecycline	T36.4X1	T36.4X2	T36.4X3	T36.4X4	T36.4X5	T36.4X6

◀ New   ◀▥ Revised   ~~deleted~~ Deleted

TABLE OF DRUGS AND CHEMICALS

TABLE OF DRUGS AND CHEMICALS

Substance	Poisoning, Accidental (Unintentional)	Poisoning, Intentional Self-Harm	Poisoning, Assault	Poisoning, Undetermined	Adverse Effect	Underdosing
Guanabenz	T46.5X1	T46.5X2	T46.5X3	T46.5X4	T46.5X5	T46.5X6
Guanacline	T46.5X1	T46.5X2	T46.5X3	T46.5X4	T46.5X5	T46.5X6
Guanadrel	T46.5X1	T46.5X2	T46.5X3	T46.5X4	T46.5X5	T46.5X6
Guanatol	T37.2X1	T37.2X2	T37.2X3	T37.2X4	T37.2X5	T37.2X6
Guanethidine	T46.5X1	T46.5X2	T46.5X3	T46.5X4	T46.5X5	T46.5X6
Guanfacine	T46.5X1	T46.5X2	T46.5X3	T46.5X4	T46.5X5	T46.5X6
Guano	T65.891	T65.892	T65.893	T65.894	—	—
Guanochlor	T46.5X1	T46.5X2	T46.5X3	T46.5X4	T46.5X5	T46.5X6
Guanoclor	T46.5X1	T46.5X2	T46.5X3	T46.5X4	T46.5X5	T46.5X6
Guanoctine	T46.5X1	T46.5X2	T46.5X3	T46.5X4	T46.5X5	T46.5X6
Guanoxabenz	T46.5X1	T46.5X2	T46.5X3	T46.5X4	T46.5X5	T46.5X6
Guanoxan	T46.5X1	T46.5X2	T46.5X3	T46.5X4	T46.5X5	T46.5X6
Guar gum (medicinal)	T46.6X1	T46.6X2	T46.6X3	T46.6X4	T46.6X5	T46.6X6
H						
Hachimycin	T36.7X1	T36.7X2	T36.7X3	T36.7X4	T36.7X5	T36.7X6
Hair						
dye	T49.4X1	T49.4X2	T49.4X3	T49.4X4	T49.4X5	T49.4X6
preparation NEC	T49.4X1	T49.4X2	T49.4X3	T49.4X4	T49.4X5	T49.4X6
Halazepam	T42.4X1	T42.4X2	T42.4X3	T42.4X4	T42.4X5	T42.4X6
Halcinolone	T49.0X1	T49.0X2	T49.0X3	T49.0X4	T49.0X5	T49.0X6
Halcinonide	T49.0X1	T49.0X2	T49.0X3	T49.0X4	T49.0X5	T49.0X6
Halethazole	T49.0X1	T49.0X2	T49.0X3	T49.0X4	T49.0X5	T49.0X6
Hallucinogen NEC	T40.901	T40.902	T40.903	T40.904	T40.905	T40.906
Halofantrine	T37.2X1	T37.2X2	T37.2X3	T37.2X4	T37.2X5	T37.2X6
Halofenate	T46.6X1	T46.6X2	T46.6X3	T46.6X4	T46.6X5	T46.6X6
Halometasone	T49.0X1	T49.0X2	T49.0X3	T49.0X4	T49.0X5	T49.0X6
Haloperidol	T43.4X1	T43.4X2	T43.4X3	T43.4X4	T43.4X5	T43.4X6
Haloprogin	T49.0X1	T49.0X2	T49.0X3	T49.0X4	T49.0X5	T49.0X6
Halotex	T49.0X1	T49.0X2	T49.0X3	T49.0X4	T49.0X5	T49.0X6
Halothane	T41.0X1	T41.0X2	T41.0X3	T41.0X4	T41.0X5	T41.0X6
Haloxazolam	T42.4X1	T42.4X2	T42.4X3	T42.4X4	T42.4X5	T42.4X6
Halquinols	T49.0X1	T49.0X2	T49.0X3	T49.0X4	T49.0X5	T49.0X6
Hamamelis	T49.2X1	T49.2X2	T49.2X3	T49.2X4	T49.2X5	T49.2X6
Haptendextran	T45.8X1	T45.8X2	T45.8X3	T45.8X4	T45.8X5	T45.8X6
Harmonyl	T46.5X1	T46.5X2	T46.5X3	T46.5X4	T46.5X5	T46.5X6
Hartmann's solution	T50.3X1	T50.3X2	T50.3X3	T50.3X4	T50.3X5	T50.3X6
Hashish	T40.7X1	T40.7X2	T40.7X3	T40.7X4	T40.7X5	T40.7X6
Hawaiian Woodrose seeds	T40.991	T40.992	T40.993	T40.994	—	—
HCB	T60.3X1	T60.3X2	T60.3X3	T60.3X4	—	—
HCH	T53.6X1	T53.6X2	T53.6X3	T53.6X4	—	—
medicinal	T49.0X1	T49.0X2	T49.0X3	T49.0X4	T49.0X5	T49.0X6

Substance	Poisoning, Accidental (Unintentional)	Poisoning, Intentional Self-Harm	Poisoning, Assault	Poisoning, Undetermined	Adverse Effect	Underdosing
HCN	T57.3X1	T57.3X2	T57.3X3	T57.3X4	—	—
Headache cures, drugs, powders NEC	T50.901	T50.902	T50.903	T50.904	T50.905	T50.906
Heavenly Blue (morning glory)	T40.991	T40.992	T40.993	T40.994	—	—
Heavy metal antidote	T45.8X1	T45.8X2	T45.8X3	T45.8X4	T45.8X5	T45.8X6
Hedaquinium	T49.0X1	T49.0X2	T49.0X3	T49.0X4	T49.0X5	T49.0X6
Hedge hyssop	T62.2X1	T62.2X2	T62.2X3	T62.2X4	—	—
Heet	T49.8X1	T49.8X2	T49.8X3	T49.8X4	T49.8X5	T49.8X6
Helium	T48.991	T48.992	T48.993	T48.994	T48.995	T48.996
Helenin	T37.4X1	T37.4X2	T37.4X3	T37.4X4	T37.4X5	T37.4X6
Hellebore (black) (green) (white)	T62.2X1	T62.2X2	T62.2X3	T62.2X4	—	—
Helium (nonmedicinal) NEC	T59.891	T59.892	T59.893	T59.894	—	—
medicinal	T48.991	T48.992	T48.993	T48.994	T48.995	T48.996
Hematin	T45.8X1	T45.8X2	T45.8X3	T45.8X4	T45.8X5	T45.8X6
Hematinic preparation	T45.8X1	T45.8X2	T45.8X3	T45.8X4	T45.8X5	T45.8X6
Hemlock	T62.2X1	T62.2X2	T62.2X3	T62.2X4	—	—
Hemostatic	T45.621	T45.622	T45.623	T45.624	T45.625	T45.626
drug, systemic	T45.621	T45.622	T45.623	T45.624	T45.625	T45.626
Hemostyptic	T49.4X1	T49.4X2	T49.4X3	T49.4X4	T49.4X5	T49.4X6
Henbane	T62.2X1	T62.2X2	T62.2X3	T62.2X4	—	—
Heparin (sodium)	T45.511	T45.512	T45.513	T45.514	T45.515	T45.516
action reverser	T45.7X1	T45.7X2	T45.7X3	T45.7X4	T45.7X5	T45.7X6
Heparin-fraction	T45.511	T45.512	T45.513	T45.514	T45.515	T45.516
Heparinoid (systemic)	T45.511	T45.512	T45.513	T45.514	T45.515	T45.516
Hepatic secretion stimulant	T47.8X1	T47.8X2	T47.8X3	T47.8X4	T47.8X5	T47.8X6
Hepatitis B						
immune globulin	T50.Z11	T50.Z12	T50.Z13	T50.Z14	T50.Z15	T50.Z16
vaccine	T50.B91	T50.B92	T50.B93	T50.B94	T50.B95	T50.B96
Hepronicate	T46.7X1	T46.7X2	T46.7X3	T46.7X4	T46.7X5	T46.7X6
Heptabarb	T42.3X1	T42.3X2	T42.3X3	T42.3X4	T42.3X5	T42.3X6
Heptabarbitone	T42.3X1	T42.3X2	T42.3X3	T42.3X4	T42.3X5	T42.3X6
Heptabarbital	T42.3X1	T42.3X2	T42.3X3	T42.3X4	T42.3X5	T42.3X6
Heptachlor	T60.1X1	T60.1X2	T60.1X3	T60.1X4	—	—
Heptalgin	T40.2X1	T40.2X2	T40.2X3	T40.2X4	T40.2X5	T40.2X6
Heptaminol	T46.3X1	T46.3X2	T46.3X3	T46.3X4	T46.3X5	T46.3X6
Herbicide NEC	T60.3X1	T60.3X2	T60.3X3	T60.3X4	—	—
Heroin	T40.1X1	T40.1X2	T40.1X3	T40.1X4	—	—
Herplex	T49.5X1	T49.5X2	T49.5X3	T49.5X4	T49.5X5	T49.5X6
HES	T45.8X1	T45.8X2	T45.8X3	T45.8X4	T45.8X5	T45.8X6
Hesperidin	T46.991	T46.992	T46.993	T46.994	T46.995	T46.996
Hetacillin	T36.0X1	T36.0X2	T36.0X3	T36.0X4	T36.0X5	T36.0X6

◀ New   ◀═ Revised   ~~deleted~~ Deleted

	External Cause (T-Code)					
Substance	Poisoning, Accidental (Unintentional)	Poisoning, Intentional Self-Harm	Poisoning, Assault	Poisoning, Undetermined	Adverse Effect	Underdosing
Hetastarch	T45.8X1	T45.8X2	T45.8X3	T45.8X4	T45.8X5	T45.8X6
HETP	T60.0X1	T60.0X2	T60.0X3	T60.0X4	—	—
Hexachlorobenzene (vapor)	T60.3X1	T60.3X2	T60.3X3	T60.3X4	—	—
Hexachlorocyclohexane	T53.6X1	T53.6X2	T53.6X3	T53.6X4	—	—
Hexachlorophene	T49.0X1	T49.0X2	T49.0X3	T49.0X4	T49.0X5	T49.0X6
Hexadiline	T46.3X1	T46.3X2	T46.3X3	T46.3X4	T46.3X5	T46.3X6
Hexadimethrine (bromide)	T45.7X1	T45.7X2	T45.7X3	T45.7X4	T45.7X5	T45.7X6
Hexadylamine	T46.3X1	T46.3X2	T46.3X3	T46.3X4	T46.3X5	T46.3X6
Hexaethyl tetraphosphate	T60.0X1	T60.0X2	T60.0X3	T60.0X4	—	—
Hexafluorenium bromide	T48.1X1	T48.1X2	T48.1X3	T48.1X4	T48.1X5	T48.1X6
Hexafluorodiethyl ether	T43.291	T43.292	T43.293	T43.294	T43.295	T43.296
Hexafluronium (bromide)	T48.1X1	T48.1X2	T48.1X3	T48.1X4	T48.1X5	T48.1X6
Hexahydrobenzol	T52.8X1	T52.8X2	T52.8X3	T52.8X4	—	—
Hexahydrocresol(s)	T51.8X1	T51.8X2	T51.8X3	T51.8X4	—	—
arsenide	T57.0X1	T57.0X2	T57.0X3	T57.0X4	—	—
arseniurated	T57.0X1	T57.0X2	T57.0X3	T57.0X4	—	—
cyanide	T57.3X1	T57.3X2	T57.3X3	T57.3X4	—	—
gas	T59.891	T59.892	T59.893	T59.894	—	—
Fluoride (liquid)	T57.8X1	T57.8X2	T57.8X3	T57.8X4	—	—
vapor	T59.891	T59.892	T59.893	T59.894	—	—
phophorated	T60.0X1	T60.0X2	T60.0X3	T60.0X4	—	—
sulfate	T57.8X1	T57.8X2	T57.8X3	T57.8X4	—	—
sulfide (gas)	T59.6X1	T59.6X2	T59.6X3	T59.6X4	—	—
arseniurated	T57.0X1	T57.0X2	T57.0X3	T57.0X4	—	—
sulfurated	T57.8X1	T57.8X2	T57.8X3	T57.8X4	—	—
Hexahydrophenol	T51.8X1	T51.8X2	T51.8X3	T51.8X4	—	—
Hexa-germ	T49.2X1	T49.2X2	T49.2X3	T49.2X4	T49.2X5	T49.2X6
Hexalen	T51.8X1	T51.8X2	T51.8X3	T51.8X4	—	—
Hexamethonium bromide	T44.2X1	T44.2X2	T44.2X3	T44.2X4	T44.2X5	T44.2X6
Hexamethylene	T52.8X1	T52.8X2	T52.8X3	T52.8X4	—	—
Hexamethylmelamine	T45.1X1	T45.1X2	T45.1X3	T45.1X4	T45.1X5	T45.1X6
Hexamidine	T49.0X1	T49.0X2	T49.0X3	T49.0X4	T49.0X5	T49.0X6
Hexamine (mandelate)	T37.8X1	T37.8X2	T37.8X3	T37.8X4	T37.8X5	T37.8X6
Hexanone, 2-hexanone	T52.4X1	T52.4X2	T52.4X3	T52.4X4	—	—
Hexanuorenium	T48.1X1	T48.1X2	T48.1X3	T48.1X4	T48.1X5	T48.1X6
Hexapropymate	T42.6X1	T42.6X2	T42.6X3	T42.6X4	T42.6X5	T42.6X6
Hexasonium iodide	T44.3X1	T44.3X2	T44.3X3	T44.3X4	T44.3X5	T44.3X6
Hexcarbacholine bromide	T48.1X1	T48.1X2	T48.1X3	T48.1X4	T48.1X5	T48.1X6
Hexemal	T42.3X1	T42.3X2	T42.3X3	T42.3X4	T42.3X5	T42.3X6
Hexestrol	T38.5X1	T38.5X2	T38.5X3	T38.5X4	T38.5X5	T38.5X6
Hexethal (sodium)	T42.3X1	T42.3X2	T42.3X3	T42.3X4	T42.3X5	T42.3X6
Hexetidine	T37.8X1	T37.8X2	T37.8X3	T37.8X4	T37.8X5	T37.8X6

	External Cause (T-Code)					
Substance	Poisoning, Accidental (Unintentional)	Poisoning, Intentional Self-Harm	Poisoning, Assault	Poisoning, Undetermined	Adverse Effect	Underdosing
Hexobarbital	T42.3X1	T42.3X2	T42.3X3	T42.3X4	T42.3X5	T42.3X6
rectal	T41.291	T41.292	T41.293	T41.294	T41.295	T41.296
sodium	T41.1X1	T41.1X2	T41.1X3	T41.1X4	T41.1X5	T41.1X6
Hexobendine	T46.3X1	T46.3X2	T46.3X3	T46.3X4	T46.3X5	T46.3X6
Hexocyclium	T44.3X1	T44.3X2	T44.3X3	T44.3X4	T44.3X5	T44.3X6
metilsulfate	T44.3X1	T44.3X2	T44.3X3	T44.3X4	T44.3X5	T44.3X6
Hexoestrol	T38.5X1	T38.5X2	T38.5X3	T38.5X4	T38.5X5	T38.5X6
Hexone	T52.4X1	T52.4X2	T52.4X3	T52.4X4	—	—
Hexoprenaline	T48.6X1	T48.6X2	T48.6X3	T48.6X4	T48.6X5	T48.6X6
Hexylcaine	T41.3X1	T41.3X2	T41.3X3	T41.3X4	T41.3X5	T41.3X6
Hexylresorcinol	T52.2X1	T52.2X2	T52.2X3	T52.2X4	—	—
HGH (human growth hormone)	T38.811	T38.812	T38.813	T38.814	T38.815	T38.816
Hinkle's pills	T47.2X1	T47.2X2	T47.2X3	T47.2X4	T47.2X5	T47.2X6
Histalog	T50.8X1	T50.8X2	T50.8X3	T50.8X4	T50.8X5	T50.8X6
Histamine (phosphate)	T50.8X1	T50.8X2	T50.8X3	T50.8X4	T50.8X5	T50.8X6
Histoplasmin	T50.8X1	T50.8X2	T50.8X3	T50.8X4	T50.8X5	T50.8X6
Holly berries	T62.2X1	T62.2X2	T62.2X3	T62.2X4	—	—
Homatropine	T44.3X1	T44.3X2	T44.3X3	T44.3X4	T44.3X5	T44.3X6
methylbromide	T44.3X1	T44.3X2	T44.3X3	T44.3X4	T44.3X5	T44.3X6
Homochlorcyclizine	T45.0X1	T45.0X2	T45.0X3	T45.0X4	T45.0X5	T45.0X6
Homosalate	T49.3X1	T49.3X2	T49.3X3	T49.3X4	T49.3X5	T49.3X6
Homo-tet	T50.Z11	T50.Z12	T50.Z13	T50.Z14	T50.Z15	T50.Z16
Hormone	T38.801	T38.802	T38.803	T38.804	T38.805	T38.806
adrenal cortical steroids	T38.0X1	T38.0X2	T38.0X3	T38.0X4	T38.0X5	T38.0X6
androgenic	T38.7X1	T38.7X2	T38.7X3	T38.7X4	T38.7X5	T38.7X6
anterior pituitary NEC	T38.811	T38.812	T38.813	T38.814	T38.815	T38.816
antidiabetic agents	T38.3X1	T38.3X2	T38.3X3	T38.3X4	T38.3X5	T38.3X6
antidiuretic	T38.891	T38.892	T38.893	T38.894	T38.895	T38.896
cancer therapy	T45.1X1	T45.1X2	T45.1X3	T45.1X4	T45.1X5	T45.1X6
follicle stimulating	T38.811	T38.812	T38.813	T38.814	T38.815	T38.816
gonadotropic	T38.891	T38.892	T38.893	T38.894	T38.895	T38.896
pituitary	T38.811	T38.812	T38.813	T38.814	T38.815	T38.816
growth	T38.811	T38.812	T38.813	T38.814	T38.815	T38.816
luteinizing	T38.811	T38.812	T38.813	T38.814	T38.815	T38.816
ovarian	T38.5X1	T38.5X2	T38.5X3	T38.5X4	T38.5X5	T38.5X6
oxytocic	T48.0X1	T48.0X2	T48.0X3	T48.0X4	T48.0X5	T48.0X6
parathyroid (derivatives)	T50.991	T50.992	T50.993	T50.994	T50.995	T50.996
pituitary (posterior) NEC	T38.891	T38.892	T38.893	T38.894	T38.895	T38.896
anterior	T38.811	T38.812	T38.813	T38.814	T38.815	T38.816
specified, NEC	T38.891	T38.892	T38.893	T38.894	T38.895	T38.896
thyroid	T38.1X1	T38.1X2	T38.1X3	T38.1X4	T38.1X5	T38.1X6
Hornet (sting)	T63.451	T63.452	T63.453	T63.454	—	—

◀ New   ◀ Revised   ~~deleted~~ Deleted

TABLE OF DRUGS AND CHEMICALS

Substance	External Cause (T-Code)					
	Poisoning, Accidental (Unintentional)	Poisoning, Intentional Self-Harm	Poisoning, Assault	Poisoning, Undetermined	Adverse Effect	Underdosing
Horse anti-human lymphocytic serum	T50.Z11	T50.Z12	T50.Z13	T50.Z14	T50.Z15	T50.Z16
Horticulture agent NEC	T65.91	T65.92	T65.93	T65.94	—	—
with pesticide	T60.91	T60.92	T60.93	T60.94	—	—
Human						
albumin	T45.8X1	T45.8X2	T45.8X3	T45.8X4	T45.8X5	T45.8X6
growth hormone (HGH)	T38.811	T38.812	T38.813	T38.814	T38.815	T38.816
immune serum	T50.Z11	T50.Z12	T50.Z13	T50.Z14	T50.Z15	T50.Z16
Hyaluronidase	T45.3X1	T45.3X2	T45.3X3	T45.3X4	T45.3X5	T45.3X6
Hyazyme	T45.3X1	T45.3X2	T45.3X3	T45.3X4	T45.3X5	T45.3X6
Hycodan	T40.2X1	T40.2X2	T40.2X3	T40.2X4	T40.2X5	T40.2X6
Hydantoin derivative NEC	T42.0X1	T42.0X2	T42.0X3	T42.0X4	T42.0X5	T42.0X6
Hydeltra	T38.0X1	T38.0X2	T38.0X3	T38.0X4	T38.0X5	T38.0X6
Hydergine	T44.6X1	T44.6X2	T44.6X3	T44.6X4	T44.6X5	T44.6X6
Hydrabamine penicillin	T36.0X1	T36.0X2	T36.0X3	T36.0X4	T36.0X5	T36.0X6
Hydralazine	T46.5X1	T46.5X2	T46.5X3	T46.5X4	T46.5X5	T46.5X6
Hydrargaphen	T49.0X1	T49.0X2	T49.0X3	T49.0X4	T49.0X5	T49.0X6
Hydrargyri amino-chloridum	T49.0X1	T49.0X2	T49.0X3	T49.0X4	T49.0X5	T49.0X6
Hydrastine	T48.291	T48.292	T48.293	T48.294	T48.295	T48.296
Hydrazine	T54.1X1	T54.1X2	T54.1X3	T54.1X4	—	—
monoamine oxidase inhibitors	T43.1X1	T43.1X2	T43.1X3	T43.1X4	T43.1X5	T43.1X6
Hydrazoic acid, azides	T54.2X1	T54.2X2	T54.2X3	T54.2X4	—	—
Hydriodic acid	T48.4X1	T48.4X2	T48.4X3	T48.4X4	T48.4X5	T48.4X6
Hydrocarbon gas	T59.891	T59.892	T59.893	T59.894		
incomplete combustion of — see Carbon, monoxide, fuel, utility						
liquefied (mobile container)	T59.891	T59.892	T59.893	T59.894	—	—
piped (natural)	T59.891	T59.892	T59.893	T59.894	—	—
Hydrochloric acid (liquid)	T54.2X1	T54.2X2	T54.2X3	T54.2X4	—	—
medicinal (digestant)	T47.5X1	T47.5X2	T47.5X3	T47.5X4	T47.5X5	T47.5X6
vapor	T59.891	T59.892	T59.893	T59.894	—	—
Hydrochlorothiazide	T50.2X1	T50.2X2	T50.2X3	T50.2X4	T50.2X5	T50.2X6
Hydrocodone	T40.2X1	T40.2X2	T40.2X3	T40.2X4	T40.2X5	T40.2X6
Hydrocortisone (derivatives)	T38.0X1	T38.0X2	T38.0X3	T38.0X4	T38.0X5	T38.0X6
aceponate	T49.0X1	T49.0X2	T49.0X3	T49.0X4	T49.0X5	T49.0X6
ENT agent	T49.6X1	T49.6X2	T49.6X3	T49.6X4	T49.6X5	T49.6X6
ophthalmic preparation	T49.5X1	T49.5X2	T49.5X3	T49.5X4	T49.5X5	T49.5X6
topical NEC	T49.0X1	T49.0X2	T49.0X3	T49.0X4	T49.0X5	T49.0X6
Hydrocortone	T38.0X1	T38.0X2	T38.0X3	T38.0X4	T38.0X5	T38.0X6
ENT agent	T49.6X1	T49.6X2	T49.6X3	T49.6X4	T49.6X5	T49.6X6
ophthalmic preparation	T49.5X1	T49.5X2	T49.5X3	T49.5X4	T49.5X5	T49.5X6
topical NEC	T49.0X1	T49.0X2	T49.0X3	T49.0X4	T49.0X5	T49.0X6

Substance	External Cause (T-Code)					
	Poisoning, Accidental (Unintentional)	Poisoning, Intentional Self-Harm	Poisoning, Assault	Poisoning, Undetermined	Adverse Effect	Underdosing
Hydrocyanic acid (liquid)	T57.3X1	T57.3X2	T57.3X3	T57.3X4	—	—
gas	T65.0X1	T65.0X2	T65.0X3	T65.0X4	—	—
Hydroflumethiazide	T50.2X1	T50.2X2	T50.2X3	T50.2X4	T50.2X5	T50.2X6
Hydrofluoric acid (liquid)	T54.2X1	T54.2X2	T54.2X3	T54.2X4	—	—
vapor	T59.891	T59.892	T59.893	T59.894	—	—
Hydrogen	T59.891	T59.892	T59.893	T59.894	—	—
arsenide	T57.0X1	T57.0X2	T57.0X3	T57.0X4	—	—
arseniureted	T57.0X1	T57.0X2	T57.0X3	T57.0X4	—	—
chloride	T57.8X1	T57.8X2	T57.8X3	T57.8X4	—	—
cyanide (salts)	T57.3X1	T57.3X2	T57.3X3	T57.3X4	—	—
gas	T57.3X1	T57.3X2	T57.3X3	T57.3X4	—	—
Fluoride	T59.5X1	T59.5X2	T59.5X3	T59.5X4	—	—
vapor	T59.5X1	T59.5X2	T59.5X3	T59.5X4	—	—
peroxide	T49.0X1	T49.0X2	T49.0X3	T49.0X4	T49.0X5	T49.0X6
phosphureted	T57.1X1	T57.1X2	T57.1X3	T57.1X4	—	—
sulfide	T59.6X1	T59.6X2	T59.6X3	T59.6X4	—	—
arseniureted	T57.0X1	T57.0X2	T57.0X3	T57.0X4	—	—
sulfureted	T59.6X1	T59.6X2	T59.6X3	T59.6X4	—	—
Hydromethylpyridine	T46.7X1	T46.7X2	T46.7X3	T46.7X4	T46.7X5	T46.7X6
Hydromorphinol	T40.2X1	T40.2X2	T40.2X3	T40.2X4	—	—
Hydromorphinone	T40.2X1	T40.2X2	T40.2X3	T40.2X4	T40.2X5	T40.2X6
Hydromorphone	T40.2X1	T40.2X2	T40.2X3	T40.2X4	T40.2X5	T40.2X6
Hydromox	T50.2X1	T50.2X2	T50.2X3	T50.2X4	T50.2X5	T50.2X6
Hydrophilic lotion	T49.3X1	T49.3X2	T49.3X3	T49.3X4	T49.3X5	T49.3X6
Hydroquinidine	T46.2X1	T46.2X2	T46.2X3	T46.2X4	T46.2X5	T46.2X6
Hydroquinone	T52.2X1	T52.2X2	T52.2X3	T52.2X4	—	—
vapor	T59.891	T59.892	T59.893	T59.894	—	—
Hydrosulfuric acid (gas)	T59.6X1	T59.6X2	T59.6X3	T59.6X4	—	—
Hydrotalcite	T47.1X1	T47.1X2	T47.1X3	T47.1X4	T47.1X5	T47.1X6
Hydrous wool fat	T49.3X1	T49.3X2	T49.3X3	T49.3X4	T49.3X5	T49.3X6
Hydroxide, caustic	T54.3X1	T54.3X2	T54.3X3	T54.3X4	—	—
Hydroxocobalamin	T45.8X1	T45.8X2	T45.8X3	T45.8X4	T45.8X5	T45.8X6
Hydroxyamphetamine	T49.5X1	T49.5X2	T49.5X3	T49.5X4	T49.5X5	T49.5X6
Hydroxycarbamide	T45.1X1	T45.1X2	T45.1X3	T45.1X4	T45.1X5	T45.1X6
Hydroxychloroquine	T37.8X1	T37.8X2	T37.8X3	T37.8X4	T37.8X5	T37.8X6
Hydroxydihydrocodeinone	T40.2X1	T40.2X2	T40.2X3	T40.2X4	T40.2X5	T40.2X6
Hydroxyestrone	T38.5X1	T38.5X2	T38.5X3	T38.5X4	T38.5X5	T38.5X6
Hydroxyethyl starch	T45.8X1	T45.8X2	T45.8X3	T45.8X4	T45.8X5	T45.8X6
Hydroxymethylpentanone	T52.4X1	T52.4X2	T52.4X3	T52.4X4	—	—
Hydroxyphenamate	T43.591	T43.592	T43.593	T43.594	T43.595	T43.596
Hydroxyphenylbutazone	T39.2X1	T39.2X2	T39.2X3	T39.2X4	T39.2X5	T39.2X6

◄ New   ◄= Revised   ~~deleted~~ Deleted

TABLE OF DRUGS AND CHEMICALS

	External Cause (T-Code)					
Substance	Poisoning, Accidental (Unintentional)	Poisoning, Intentional Self-Harm	Poisoning, Assault	Poisoning, Undetermined	Adverse Effect	Underdosing
Hydroxyprogesterone	T38.5X1	T38.5X2	T38.5X3	T38.5X4	T38.5X5	T38.5X6
caproate	T38.5X1	T38.5X2	T38.5X3	T38.5X4	T38.5X5	T38.5X6
Hydroxyquinoline (derivatives) NEC	T37.8X1	T37.8X2	T37.8X3	T37.8X4	T37.8X5	T37.8X6
Hydroxystilbamidine	T37.3X1	T37.3X2	T37.3X3	T37.3X4	T37.3X5	T37.3X6
Hydroxytoluene (nonmedicinal)	T54.0X1	T54.0X2	T54.0X3	T54.0X4	—	—
medicinal	T49.0X1	T49.0X2	T49.0X3	T49.0X4	T49.0X5	T49.0X6
Hydroxyurea	T45.1X1	T45.1X2	T45.1X3	T45.1X4	T45.1X5	T45.1X6
Hydroxyzine	T43.591	T43.592	T43.593	T43.594	T43.595	T43.596
Hyoscine	T44.3X1	T44.3X2	T44.3X3	T44.3X4	T44.3X5	T44.3X6
Hyoscyamine	T44.3X1	T44.3X2	T44.3X3	T44.3X4	T44.3X5	T44.3X6
Hyoscyamus	T44.3X1	T44.3X2	T44.3X3	T44.3X4	T44.3X5	T44.3X6
dry extract	T44.3X1	T44.3X2	T44.3X3	T44.3X4	T44.3X5	T44.3X6
Hypaque	T50.8X1	T50.8X2	T50.8X3	T50.8X4	T50.8X5	T50.8X6
Hypertussis	T50.Z11	T50.Z12	T50.Z13	T50.Z14	T50.Z15	T50.Z16
Hypnotic	T42.71	T42.72	T42.73	T42.74	T42.75	T42.76
anticonvulsant	T42.71	T42.72	T42.73	T42.74	T42.75	T42.76
specified NEC	T42.6X1	T42.6X2	T42.6X3	T42.6X4	T42.6X5	T42.6X6
Hypochlorite	T49.0X1	T49.0X2	T49.0X3	T49.0X4	T49.0X5	T49.0X6
Hypophysis, posterior	T38.891	T38.892	T38.893	T38.894	T38.895	T38.896
Hypotensive NEC	T46.5X1	T46.5X2	T46.5X3	T46.5X4	T46.5X5	T46.5X6
Hypromellose	T49.5X1	T49.5X2	T49.5X3	T49.5X4	T49.5X5	T49.5X6
I						
Ibacitabine	T37.5X1	T37.5X2	T37.5X3	T37.5X4	T37.5X5	T37.5X6
Ibopamine	T44.991	T44.992	T44.993	T44.994	T44.995	T44.996
Ibufenac	T39.311	T39.312	T39.313	T39.314	T39.315	T39.316
Ibuprofen	T39.311	T39.312	T39.313	T39.314	T39.315	T39.316
Ibuproxam	T39.311	T39.312	T39.313	T39.314	T39.315	T39.316
Ibuterol	T48.6X1	T48.6X2	T48.6X3	T48.6X4	T48.6X5	T48.6X6
Ichthammol	T49.0X1	T49.0X2	T49.0X3	T49.0X4	T49.0X5	T49.0X6
Ichthyol	T49.4X1	T49.4X2	T49.4X3	T49.4X4	T49.4X5	T49.4X6
Idarubicin	T45.1X1	T45.1X2	T45.1X3	T45.1X4	T45.1X5	T45.1X6
Idrocilamide	T42.8X1	T42.8X2	T42.8X3	T42.8X4	T42.8X5	T42.8X6
Ifenprodil	T46.7X1	T46.7X2	T46.7X3	T46.7X4	T46.7X5	T46.7X6
Ifosfamide	T45.1X1	T45.1X2	T45.1X3	T45.1X4	T45.1X5	T45.1X6
Iletin	T38.3X1	T38.3X2	T38.3X3	T38.3X4	T38.3X5	T38.3X6
Ilex	T62.2X1	T62.2X2	T62.2X3	T62.2X4	—	—
Illuminating gas (after combustion)	T58.11	T58.12	T58.13	T58.14	—	—
prior to combustion	T59.891	T59.892	T59.893	T59.894	—	—
Ilopan	T45.2X1	T45.2X2	T45.2X3	T45.2X4	T45.2X5	T45.2X6
Iloprost	T46.7X1	T46.7X2	T46.7X3	T46.7X4	T46.7X5	T46.7X6

	External Cause (T-Code)					
Substance	Poisoning, Accidental (Unintentional)	Poisoning, Intentional Self-Harm	Poisoning, Assault	Poisoning, Undetermined	Adverse Effect	Underdosing
Ilotycin	T36.3X1	T36.3X2	T36.3X3	T36.3X4	T36.3X5	T36.3X6
ophthalmic preparation	T49.5X1	T49.5X2	T49.5X3	T49.5X4	T49.5X5	T49.5X6
topical NEC	T49.0X1	T49.0X2	T49.0X3	T49.0X4	T49.0X5	T49.0X6
Imidazole-4-carboxamide	T45.1X1	T45.1X2	T45.1X3	T45.1X4	T45.1X5	T45.1X6
Imipenem	T36.0X1	T36.0X2	T36.0X3	T36.0X4	T36.0X5	T36.0X6
Imipramine	T43.011	T43.012	T43.013	T43.014	T43.015	T43.016
Iminostilbene	T42.1X1	T42.1X2	T42.1X3	T42.1X4	T42.1X5	T42.1X6
Immu-G	T50.Z11	T50.Z12	T50.Z13	T50.Z14	T50.Z15	T50.Z16
Immuglobin	T50.Z11	T50.Z12	T50.Z13	T50.Z14	T50.Z15	T50.Z16
Immune						
globulin	T50.Z11	T50.Z12	T50.Z13	T50.Z14	T50.Z15	T50.Z16
serum globulin	T50.Z11	T50.Z12	T50.Z13	T50.Z14	T50.Z15	T50.Z16
Immunoglobin human (intravenous) (normal)	T50.Z11	T50.Z12	T50.Z13	T50.Z14	T50.Z15	T50.Z16
unmodified	T50.Z11	T50.Z12	T50.Z13	T50.Z14	T50.Z15	T50.Z16
Immunosuppressive drug	T45.1X1	T45.1X2	T45.1X3	T45.1X4	T45.1X5	T45.1X6
Immu-tetanus	T50.Z11	T50.Z12	T50.Z13	T50.Z14	T50.Z15	T50.Z16
Indalpine	T43.221	T43.222	T43.223	T43.224	T43.225	T43.226
Indanazoline	T48.5X1	T48.5X2	T48.5X3	T48.5X4	T48.5X5	T48.5X6
Indandione (derivatives)	T45.511	T45.512	T45.513	T45.514	T45.515	T45.516
Indapamide	T46.5X1	T46.5X2	T46.5X3	T46.5X4	T46.5X5	T46.5X6
Indendione (derivatives)	T45.511	T45.512	T45.513	T45.514	T45.515	T45.516
Indenolol	T44.7X1	T44.7X2	T44.7X3	T44.7X4	T44.7X5	T44.7X6
Inderal	T44.7X1	T44.7X2	T44.7X3	T44.7X4	T44.7X5	T44.7X6
Indian						
hemp	T40.7X1	T40.7X2	T40.7X3	T40.7X4	T40.7X5	T40.7X6
tobacco	T62.2X1	T62.2X2	T62.2X3	T62.2X4	—	—
Indigo carmine	T50.8X1	T50.8X2	T50.8X3	T50.8X4	T50.8X5	T50.8X6
Indobufen	T45.521	T45.522	T45.523	T45.524	T45.525	T45.526
Indocin	T39.2X1	T39.2X2	T39.2X3	T39.2X4	T39.2X5	T39.2X6
Indocyanine green	T50.8X1	T50.8X2	T50.8X3	T50.8X4	T50.8X5	T50.8X6
Indometacin	T39.391	T39.392	T39.393	T39.394	T39.395	T39.396
Indomethacin	T39.391	T39.392	T39.393	T39.394	T39.395	T39.396
farnesil	T39.4X1	T39.4X2	T39.4X3	T39.4X4	T39.4X5	T39.4X6
Indoramin	T44.6X1	T44.6X2	T44.6X3	T44.6X4	T44.6X5	T44.6X6
Industrial						
alcohol	T51.0X1	T51.0X2	T51.0X3	T51.0X4	—	—
fumes	T59.891	T59.892	T59.893	T59.894	—	—
solvents (fumes) (vapors)	T52.91	T52.92	T52.93	T52.94	—	—
Influenza vaccine	T50.B91	T50.B92	T50.B93	T50.B94	T50.B95	T50.B96
Ingested substance NEC	T65.91	T65.92	T65.93	T65.94		
INH	T37.1X1	T37.1X2	T37.1X3	T37.1X4	T37.1X5	T37.1X6

◀ New   ◀▮▮ Revised   ~~deleted~~ Deleted

TABLE OF DRUGS AND CHEMICALS

Substance	Poisoning, Accidental (Unintentional)	Poisoning, Intentional Self-Harm	Poisoning, Assault	Poisoning, Undetermined	Adverse Effect	Underdosing
Inhalation, gas (noxious) — see Gas						
Inhibitor						
angiotensin-converting enzyme	T46.4X1	T46.4X2	T46.4X3	T46.4X4	T46.4X5	T46.4X6
carbonic anhydrase	T50.2X1	T50.2X2	T50.2X3	T50.2X4	T50.2X5	T50.2X6
fibrinolysis	T45.621	T45.622	T45.623	T45.624	T45.625	T45.626
monoamine oxidase NEC	T43.1X1	T43.1X2	T43.1X3	T43.1X4	T43.1X5	T43.1X6
hydrazine	T43.1X1	T43.1X2	T43.1X3	T43.1X4	T43.1X5	T43.1X6
postsynaptic	T43.8X1	T43.8X2	T43.8X3	T43.8X4	T43.8X5	T43.8X6
prothrombin synthesis	T45.511	T45.512	T45.513	T45.514	T45.515	T45.516
Ink	T65.891	T65.892	T65.893	T65.894	—	—
Inorganic substance NEC	T57.91	T57.92	T57.93	T57.94	—	—
Inosine pranobex	T37.5X1	T37.5X2	T37.5X3	T37.5X4	T37.5X5	T37.5X6
Inositol	T50.991	T50.992	T50.993	T50.994	T50.995	T50.996
nicotinate	T46.7X1	T46.7X2	T46.7X3	T46.7X4	T46.7X5	T46.7X6
Inproquone	T45.1X1	T45.1X2	T45.1X3	T45.1X4	T45.1X5	T45.1X6
Insect (sting), venomous	T63.481	T63.482	T63.483	T63.484	—	—
ant	T63.421	T63.422	T63.423	T63.424	—	—
bee	T63.441	T63.442	T63.443	T63.444	—	—
caterpillar	T63.431	T63.432	T63.433	T63.434	—	—
hornet	T63.451	T63.452	T63.453	T63.454	—	—
wasp	T63.461	T63.462	T63.463	T63.464	—	—
Insecticide NEC	T60.91	T60.92	T60.93	T60.94	—	—
carbamate	T60.0X1	T60.0X2	T60.0X3	T60.0X4	—	—
chlorinated	T60.1X1	T60.1X2	T60.1X3	T60.1X4	—	—
mixed	T60.91	T60.92	T60.93	T60.94	—	—
organochlorine	T60.1X1	T60.1X2	T60.1X3	T60.1X4	—	—
organophosphorus	T60.0X1	T60.0X2	T60.0X3	T60.0X4	—	—
Insular tissue extract	T38.3X1	T38.3X2	T38.3X3	T38.3X4	T38.3X5	T38.3X6
Insulin (amorphous) (globin) (isophane) (Lente) (NPH) (Semilente) (Ultralente)	T38.3X1	T38.3X2	T38.3X3	T38.3X4	T38.3X5	T38.3X6
defalan	T38.3X1	T38.3X2	T38.3X3	T38.3X4	T38.3X5	T38.3X6
human	T38.3X1	T38.3X2	T38.3X3	T38.3X4	T38.3X5	T38.3X6
injection, soluble	T38.3X1	T38.3X2	T38.3X3	T38.3X4	T38.3X5	T38.3X6
biphasic	T38.3X1	T38.3X2	T38.3X3	T38.3X4	T38.3X5	T38.3X6
intermediate acting	T38.3X1	T38.3X2	T38.3X3	T38.3X4	T38.3X5	T38.3X6
protamine zinc	T38.3X1	T38.3X2	T38.3X3	T38.3X4	T38.3X5	T38.3X6
slow acting	T38.3X1	T38.3X2	T38.3X3	T38.3X4	T38.3X5	T38.3X6
zinc						
protamine injection	T38.3X1	T38.3X2	T38.3X3	T38.3X4	T38.3X5	T38.3X6
suspension (amorphous) (crystalline)	T38.3X1	T38.3X2	T38.3X3	T38.3X4	T38.3X5	T38.3X6

Substance	Poisoning, Accidental (Unintentional)	Poisoning, Intentional Self-Harm	Poisoning, Assault	Poisoning, Undetermined	Adverse Effect	Underdosing
Interferon (alpha) (beta) (gamma)	T37.5X1	T37.5X2	T37.5X3	T37.5X4	T37.5X5	T37.5X6
Intestinal motility control drug	T47.6X1	T47.6X2	T47.6X3	T47.6X4	T47.6X5	T47.6X6
biological	T47.8X1	T47.8X2	T47.8X3	T47.8X4	T47.8X5	T47.8X6
Intranarcon	T41.1X1	T41.1X2	T41.1X3	T41.1X4	T41.1X5	T41.1X6
Intravenous						
amino acids	T50.991	T50.992	T50.993	T50.994	T50.995	T50.996
fat suspension	T50.991	T50.992	T50.993	T50.994	T50.995	T50.996
Inulin	T50.8X1	T50.8X2	T50.8X3	T50.8X4	T50.8X5	T50.8X6
Invert sugar	T50.3X1	T50.3X2	T50.3X3	T50.3X4	T50.3X5	T50.3X6
Inza — see Naproxen						
Iobenzamic acid	T50.8X1	T50.8X2	T50.8X3	T50.8X4	T50.8X5	T50.8X6
Iocarmic acid	T50.8X1	T50.8X2	T50.8X3	T50.8X4	T50.8X5	T50.8X6
Iocetamic acid	T50.8X1	T50.8X2	T50.8X3	T50.8X4	T50.8X5	T50.8X6
Iodamide	T50.8X1	T50.8X2	T50.8X3	T50.8X4	T50.8X5	T50.8X6
Iodide NEC — see also Iodine	T49.0X1	T49.0X2	T49.0X3	T49.0X4	T49.0X5	T49.0X6
mercury (ointment)	T49.0X1	T49.0X2	T49.0X3	T49.0X4	T49.0X5	T49.0X6
methylate	T49.0X1	T49.0X2	T49.0X3	T49.0X4	T49.0X5	T49.0X6
potassium (expectorant) NEC	T48.4X1	T48.4X2	T48.4X3	T48.4X4	T48.4X5	T48.4X6
Iodinated						
contrast medium	T50.8X1	T50.8X2	T50.8X3	T50.8X4	T50.8X5	T50.8X6
glycerol	T48.4X1	T48.4X2	T48.4X3	T48.4X4	T48.4X5	T48.4X6
human serum albumin (131I)	T50.8X1	T50.8X2	T50.8X3	T50.8X4	T50.8X5	T50.8X6
Iodine (antiseptic, external) (tincture) NEC	T49.0X1	T49.0X2	T49.0X3	T49.0X4	T49.0X5	T49.0X6
125 — see also Radiation sickness, and Exposure to radioactivce isotopes	T50.8X1	T50.8X2	T50.8X3	T50.8X4	T50.8X5	T50.8X6
therapeutic	T50.991	T50.992	T50.993	T50.994	T50.995	T50.996
131 — see also Radiation sickness, and Exposure to radioactivce isotopes	T50.8X1	T50.8X2	T50.8X3	T50.8X4	T50.8X5	T50.8X6
therapeutic	T38.2X1	T38.2X2	T38.2X3	T38.2X4	T38.2X5	T38.2X6
diagnostic	T50.8X1	T50.8X2	T50.8X3	T50.8X4	T50.8X5	T50.8X6
for thyroid conditions (antithyroid)	T38.2X1	T38.2X2	T38.2X3	T38.2X4	T38.2X5	T38.2X6
solution	T49.0X1	T49.0X2	T49.0X3	T49.0X4	T49.0X5	T49.0X6
vapor	T59.891	T59.892	T59.893	T59.894	—	—
Iodipamide	T50.8X1	T50.8X2	T50.8X3	T50.8X4	T50.8X5	T50.8X6
Iodized (poppy seed) oil	T50.8X1	T50.8X2	T50.8X3	T50.8X4	T50.8X5	T50.8X6
Iodobismitol	T37.8X1	T37.8X2	T37.8X3	T37.8X4	T37.8X5	T37.8X6
Iodochlorhydroxyquin	T37.8X1	T37.8X2	T37.8X3	T37.8X4	T37.8X5	T37.8X6
topical	T49.0X1	T49.0X2	T49.0X3	T49.0X4	T49.0X5	T49.0X6
Iodochlorhydroxyquino-line	T37.8X1	T37.8X2	T37.8X3	T37.8X4	T37.8X5	T37.8X6
Iodocholesterol (131I)	T50.8X1	T50.8X2	T50.8X3	T50.8X4	T50.8X5	T50.8X6

◀ New   ◀ Revised   deleted Deleted

Substance	Poisoning, Accidental (Unintentional)	Poisoning, Intentional Self-Harm	Poisoning, Assault	Poisoning, Undetermined	Adverse Effect	Underdosing
Iodoform	T49.0X1	T49.0X2	T49.0X3	T49.0X4	T49.0X5	T49.0X6
Iodohippuric acid	T50.8X1	T50.8X2	T50.8X3	T50.8X4	T50.8X5	T50.8X6
Iodopanoic acid	T50.8X1	T50.8X2	T50.8X3	T50.8X4	T50.8X5	T50.8X6
Iodophthalein (sodium)	T50.8X1	T50.8X2	T50.8X3	T50.8X4	T50.8X5	T50.8X6
Iodopyracet	T50.8X1	T50.8X2	T50.8X3	T50.8X4	T50.8X5	T50.8X6
Iodoquinol	T37.8X1	T37.8X2	T37.8X3	T37.8X4	T37.8X5	T37.8X6
Iodoxamic acid	T50.8X1	T50.8X2	T50.8X3	T50.8X4	T50.8X5	T50.8X6
Iofendylate	T50.8X1	T50.8X2	T50.8X3	T50.8X4	T50.8X5	T50.8X6
Ioglycamic acid	T50.8X1	T50.8X2	T50.8X3	T50.8X4	T50.8X5	T50.8X6
Iohexol	T50.8X1	T50.8X2	T50.8X3	T50.8X4	T50.8X5	T50.8X6
Ion exchange resin						
anion	T47.8X1	T47.8X2	T47.8X3	T47.8X4	T47.8X5	T47.8X6
cation	T50.3X1	T50.3X2	T50.3X3	T50.3X4	T50.3X5	T50.3X6
cholestyramine	T46.6X1	T46.6X2	T46.6X3	T46.6X4	T46.6X5	T46.6X6
intestinal	T47.8X1	T47.8X2	T47.8X3	T47.8X4	T47.8X5	T47.8X6
Iopamidol	T50.8X1	T50.8X2	T50.8X3	T50.8X4	T50.8X5	T50.8X6
Iopanoic acid	T50.8X1	T50.8X2	T50.8X3	T50.8X4	T50.8X5	T50.8X6
Iophenoic acid	T50.8X1	T50.8X2	T50.8X3	T50.8X4	T50.8X5	T50.8X6
Iopodate, sodium	T50.8X1	T50.8X2	T50.8X3	T50.8X4	T50.8X5	T50.8X6
Iopodic acid	T50.8X1	T50.8X2	T50.8X3	T50.8X4	T50.8X5	T50.8X6
Iopromide	T50.8X1	T50.8X2	T50.8X3	T50.8X4	T50.8X5	T50.8X6
Iopydol	T50.8X1	T50.8X2	T50.8X3	T50.8X4	T50.8X5	T50.8X6
Iotalamic acid	T50.8X1	T50.8X2	T50.8X3	T50.8X4	T50.8X5	T50.8X6
Iothalamate	T50.8X1	T50.8X2	T50.8X3	T50.8X4	T50.8X5	T50.8X6
Iothiouracil	T38.2X1	T38.2X2	T38.2X3	T38.2X4	T38.2X5	T38.2X6
Iotrol	T50.8X1	T50.8X2	T50.8X3	T50.8X4	T50.8X5	T50.8X6
Iotrolan	T50.8X1	T50.8X2	T50.8X3	T50.8X4	T50.8X5	T50.8X6
Iotroxate	T50.8X1	T50.8X2	T50.8X3	T50.8X4	T50.8X5	T50.8X6
Iotroxic acid	T50.8X1	T50.8X2	T50.8X3	T50.8X4	T50.8X5	T50.8X6
Ioversol	T50.8X1	T50.8X2	T50.8X3	T50.8X4	T50.8X5	T50.8X6
Ioxaglate	T50.8X1	T50.8X2	T50.8X3	T50.8X4	T50.8X5	T50.8X6
Ioxaglic acid	T50.8X1	T50.8X2	T50.8X3	T50.8X4	T50.8X5	T50.8X6
Ioxitalamic acid	T50.8X1	T50.8X2	T50.8X3	T50.8X4	T50.8X5	T50.8X6
Ipecac	T47.7X1	T47.7X2	T47.7X3	T47.7X4	T47.7X5	T47.7X6
Ipecacuanha	T48.4X1	T48.4X2	T48.4X3	T48.4X4	T48.4X5	T48.4X6
Ipodate, calcium	T50.8X1	T50.8X2	T50.8X3	T50.8X4	T50.8X5	T50.8X6
Ipral	T42.3X1	T42.3X2	T42.3X3	T42.3X4	T42.3X5	T42.3X6
Ipratropium (bromide)	T48.6X1	T48.6X2	T48.6X3	T48.6X4	T48.6X5	T48.6X6
Ipriflavone	T46.3X1	T46.3X2	T46.3X3	T46.3X4	T46.3X5	T46.3X6
Iprindole	T43.011	T43.012	T43.013	T43.014	T43.015	T43.016
Iproclozide	T43.1X1	T43.1X2	T43.1X3	T43.1X4	T43.1X5	T43.1X6
Iprofenin	T50.8X1	T50.8X2	T50.8X3	T50.8X4	T50.8X5	T50.8X6
Iproheptine	T49.2X1	T49.2X2	T49.2X3	T49.2X4	T49.2X5	T49.2X6
Iproniazid	T43.1X1	T43.1X2	T43.1X3	T43.1X4	T43.1X5	T43.1X6
Iproplatin	T45.1X1	T45.1X2	T45.1X3	T45.1X4	T45.1X5	T45.1X6
Iproveratril	T46.1X1	T46.1X2	T46.1X3	T46.1X4	T46.1X5	T46.1X6
Iron (compounds) (medicinal) NEC	T45.4X1	T45.4X2	T45.4X3	T45.4X4	T45.4X5	T45.4X6
ammonium	T45.4X1	T45.4X2	T45.4X3	T45.4X4	T45.4X5	T45.4X6
dextran injection	T45.4X1	T45.4X2	T45.4X3	T45.4X4	T45.4X5	T45.4X6
nonmedicinal	T56.891	T56.892	T56.893	T56.894	—	—
salts	T45.4X1	T45.4X2	T45.4X3	T45.4X4	T45.4X5	T45.4X6
sorbitex	T45.4X1	T45.4X2	T45.4X3	T45.4X4	T45.4X5	T45.4X6
sorbitol citric acid complex	T45.4X1	T45.4X2	T45.4X3	T45.4X4	T45.4X5	T45.4X6
Irrigating fluid (vaginal)	T49.8X1	T49.8X2	T49.8X3	T49.8X4	T49.8X5	T49.8X6
eye	T49.5X1	T49.5X2	T49.5X3	T49.5X4	T49.5X5	T49.5X6
Isepamicin	T36.5X1	T36.5X2	T36.5X3	T36.5X4	T36.5X5	T36.5X6
Isoaminile (citrate)	T48.3X1	T48.3X2	T48.3X3	T48.3X4	T48.3X5	T48.3X6
Isoamyl nitrite	T46.3X1	T46.3X2	T46.3X3	T46.3X4	T46.3X5	T46.3X6
Isobenzan	T60.1X1	T60.1X2	T60.1X3	T60.1X4	—	—
Isobutyl acetate	T52.8X1	T52.8X2	T52.8X3	T52.8X4	—	—
Isocarboxazid	T43.1X1	T43.1X2	T43.1X3	T43.1X4	T43.1X5	T43.1X6
Isoconazole	T49.0X1	T49.0X2	T49.0X3	T49.0X4	T49.0X5	T49.0X6
Isocyanate	T65.0X1	T65.0X2	T65.0X3	T65.0X4	—	—
Isoephedrine	T44.991	T44.992	T44.993	T44.994	T44.995	T44.996
Isoetarine	T48.6X1	T48.6X2	T48.6X3	T48.6X4	T48.6X5	T48.6X6
Isoethadione	T42.2X1	T42.2X2	T42.2X3	T42.2X4	T42.2X5	T42.2X6
Isoetharine	T44.5X1	T44.5X2	T44.5X3	T44.5X4	T44.5X5	T44.5X6
Isoflurane	T41.0X1	T41.0X2	T41.0X3	T41.0X4	T41.0X5	T41.0X6
Isoflurophate	T44.0X1	T44.0X2	T44.0X3	T44.0X4	T44.0X5	T44.0X6
Isomaltose, ferric complex	T45.4X1	T45.4X2	T45.4X3	T45.4X4	T45.4X5	T45.4X6
Isometheptene	T44.3X1	T44.3X2	T44.3X3	T44.3X4	T44.3X5	T44.3X6
Isoniazid	T37.1X1	T37.1X2	T37.1X3	T37.1X4	T37.1X5	T37.1X6
with						
rifampicin	T36.6X1	T36.6X2	T36.6X3	T36.6X4	T36.6X5	T36.6X6
thioacetazone	T37.1X1	T37.1X2	T37.1X3	T37.1X4	T37.1X5	T37.1X6
Isonicotinic acid hydrazide	T37.1X1	T37.1X2	T37.1X3	T37.1X4	T37.1X5	T37.1X6
Isonipecaine	T40.4X1	T40.4X2	T40.4X3	T40.4X4	T40.4X5	T40.4X6
Isopentaquine	T37.2X1	T37.2X2	T37.2X3	T37.2X4	T37.2X5	T37.2X6
Isophane insulin	T38.3X1	T38.3X2	T38.3X3	T38.3X4	T38.3X5	T38.3X6
Isophorone	T65.891	T65.892	T65.893	T65.894	—	—
Isophosphamide	T45.1X1	T45.1X2	T45.1X3	T45.1X4	T45.1X5	T45.1X6
Isopregnenone	T38.5X1	T38.5X2	T38.5X3	T38.5X4	T38.5X5	T38.5X6
Isoprenaline	T48.6X1	T48.6X2	T48.6X3	T48.6X4	T48.6X5	T48.6X6
Isopromethazine	T43.3X1	T43.3X2	T43.3X3	T43.3X4	T43.3X5	T43.3X6

◄ New ◄═ Revised ~~deleted~~ Deleted

TABLE OF DRUGS AND CHEMICALS

Substance	External Cause (T-Code)					
	Poisoning, Accidental (Unintentional)	Poisoning, Intentional Self-Harm	Poisoning, Assault	Poisoning, Undetermined	Adverse Effect	Underdosing
Isopropamide	T44.3X1	T44.3X2	T44.3X3	T44.3X4	T44.3X5	T44.3X6
iodide	T44.3X1	T44.3X2	T44.3X3	T44.3X4	T44.3X5	T44.3X6
Isopropanol	T51.2X1	T51.2X2	T51.2X3	T51.2X4	—	—
Isopropyl						
acetate	T52.8X1	T52.8X2	T52.8X3	T52.8X4	—	—
alcohol	T51.2X1	T51.2X2	T51.2X3	T51.2X4	—	—
medicinal	T49.4X1	T49.4X2	T49.4X3	T49.4X4	T49.4X5	T49.4X6
ether	T52.8X1	T52.8X2	T52.8X3	T52.8X4	—	—
Isopropylaminophena-zone	T39.2X1	T39.2X2	T39.2X3	T39.2X4	T39.2X5	T39.2X6
Isoproterenol	T48.6X1	T48.6X2	T48.6X3	T48.6X4	T48.6X5	T48.6X6
Isosorbide dinitrate	T46.3X1	T46.3X2	T46.3X3	T46.3X4	T46.3X5	T46.3X6
Isothipendyl	T45.0X1	T45.0X2	T45.0X3	T45.0X4	T45.0X5	T45.0X6
Isotretinoin	T50.991	T50.992	T50.993	T50.994	T50.995	T50.996
Isoxazolyl penicillin	T36.0X1	T36.0X2	T36.0X3	T36.0X4	T36.0X5	T36.0X6
Isoxicam	T39.391	T39.392	T39.393	T39.394	T39.395	T39.396
Isoxsuprine	T46.7X1	T46.7X2	T46.7X3	T46.7X4	T46.7X5	T46.7X6
Ispagula	T47.4X1	T47.4X2	T47.4X3	T47.4X4	T47.4X5	T47.4X6
husk	T47.4X1	T47.4X2	T47.4X3	T47.4X4	T47.4X5	T47.4X6
Isradipine	T46.1X1	T46.1X2	T46.1X3	T46.1X4	T46.1X5	T46.1X6
l-thyroxine sodium	T38.1X1	T38.1X2	T38.1X3	T38.1X4	T38.1X5	T38.1X6
Itraconazole	T37.8X1	T37.8X2	T37.8X3	T37.8X4	T37.8X5	T37.8X6
Itramin tosilate	T46.3X1	T46.3X2	T46.3X3	T46.3X4	T46.3X5	T46.3X6
Ivermectin	T37.4X1	T37.4X2	T37.4X3	T37.4X4	T37.4X5	T37.4X6
Izoniazid	T37.1X1	T37.1X2	T37.1X3	T37.1X4	T37.1X5	T37.1X6
with thioacetazone	T37.1X1	T37.1X2	T37.1X3	T37.1X4	T37.1X5	T37.1X6
J						
Jalap	T47.2X1	T47.2X2	T47.2X3	T47.2X4	T47.2X5	T47.2X6
Jamaica						
dogwood (bark)	T39.8X1	T39.8X2	T39.8X3	T39.8X4	T39.8X5	T39.8X6
ginger	T65.891	T65.892	T65.893	T65.894		
root	T62.2X1	T62.2X2	T62.2X3	T62.2X4	—	—
Jatropha	T62.2X1	T62.2X2	T62.2X3	T62.2X4		
curcas	T62.2X1	T62.2X2	T62.2X3	T62.2X4		
Jectofer	T45.4X1	T45.4X2	T45.4X3	T45.4X4	T45.4X5	T45.4X6
Jellyfish (sting)	T63.621	T63.622	T63.623	T63.624		
Jequirity (bean)	T62.2X1	T62.2X2	T62.2X3	T62.2X4		
Jimson weed (stramonium)	T62.2X1	T62.2X2	T62.2X3	T62.2X4		
seeds	T62.2X1	T62.2X2	T62.2X3	T62.2X4	—	—
Josamycin	T36.3X1	T36.3X2	T36.3X3	T36.3X4	T36.3X5	T36.3X6
Juniper tar	T49.1X1	T49.1X2	T49.1X3	T49.1X4	T49.1X5	T49.1X6

Substance	External Cause (T-Code)					
	Poisoning, Accidental (Unintentional)	Poisoning, Intentional Self-Harm	Poisoning, Assault	Poisoning, Undetermined	Adverse Effect	Underdosing
K						
Kallidinogenase	T46.7X1	T46.7X2	T46.7X3	T46.7X4	T46.7X5	T46.7X6
Kallikrein	T46.7X1	T46.7X2	T46.7X3	T46.7X4	T46.7X5	T46.7X6
Kanamycin	T36.5X1	T36.5X2	T36.5X3	T36.5X4	T36.5X5	T36.5X6
Kantrex	T36.5X1	T36.5X2	T36.5X3	T36.5X4	T36.5X5	T36.5X6
Kaolin	T47.6X1	T47.6X2	T47.6X3	T47.6X4	T47.6X5	T47.6X6
light	T47.6X1	T47.6X2	T47.6X3	T47.6X4	T47.6X5	T47.6X6
Karaya (gum)	T47.4X1	T47.4X2	T47.4X3	T47.4X4	T47.4X5	T47.4X6
Kebuzone	T39.2X1	T39.2X2	T39.2X3	T39.2X4	T39.2X5	T39.2X6
Kelevan	T60.1X1	T60.1X2	T60.1X3	T60.1X4	—	—
Kemithal	T41.1X1	T41.1X2	T41.1X3	T41.1X4	T41.1X5	T41.1X6
Kenacort	T38.0X1	T38.0X2	T38.0X3	T38.0X4	T38.0X5	T38.0X6
Keratolytic drug NEC	T49.4X1	T49.4X2	T49.4X3	T49.4X4	T49.4X5	T49.4X6
anthracene	T49.4X1	T49.4X2	T49.4X3	T49.4X4	T49.4X5	T49.4X6
Keratoplastic NEC	T49.4X1	T49.4X2	T49.4X3	T49.4X4	T49.4X5	T49.4X6
Kerosene, kerosine (fuel) (solvent) NEC	T52.0X1	T52.0X2	T52.0X3	T52.0X4	—	—
insecticide	T52.0X1	T52.0X2	T52.0X3	T52.0X4		
vapor	T52.0X1	T52.0X2	T52.0X3	T52.0X4	—	—
Ketamine	T41.291	T41.292	T41.293	T41.294	T41.295	T41.296
Ketazolam	T42.4X1	T42.4X2	T42.4X3	T42.4X4	T42.4X5	T42.4X6
Ketazon	T39.2X1	T39.2X2	T39.2X3	T39.2X4	T39.2X5	T39.2X6
Ketobemidone	T40.4X1	T40.4X2	T40.4X3	T40.4X4	—	—
Ketoconazole	T49.0X1	T49.0X2	T49.0X3	T49.0X4	T49.0X5	T49.0X6
Ketols	T52.4X1	T52.4X2	T52.4X3	T52.4X4	—	—
Ketone oils	T52.4X1	T52.4X2	T52.4X3	T52.4X4	—	—
Ketoprofen	T39.311	T39.312	T39.313	T39.314	T39.315	T39.316
Ketorolac	T39.8X1	T39.8X2	T39.8X3	T39.8X4	T39.8X5	T39.8X6
Ketotifen	T45.0X1	T45.0X2	T45.0X3	T45.0X4	T45.0X5	T45.0X6
Khat	T43.691	T43.692	T43.693	T43.694	—	—
Khellin	T46.3X1	T46.3X2	T46.3X3	T46.3X4	T46.3X5	T46.3X6
Khelloside	T46.3X1	T46.3X2	T46.3X3	T46.3X4	T46.3X5	T46.3X6
Kiln gas or vapor (carbon monoxide)	T58.8X1	T58.8X2	T58.8X3	T58.8X4		
Kitasamycin	T36.3X1	T36.3X2	T36.3X3	T36.3X4	T36.3X5	T36.3X6
Konsyl	T47.4X1	T47.4X2	T47.4X3	T47.4X4	T47.4X5	T47.4X6
Kosam seed	T62.2X1	T62.2X2	T62.2X3	T62.2X4		
Krait (venom)	T63.091	T63.092	T63.093	T63.094	—	—
Kwell (insecticide)	T60.1X1	T60.1X2	T60.1X3	T60.1X4	—	—
anti-infective (topical)	T49.0X1	T49.0X2	T49.0X3	T49.0X4	T49.0X5	T49.0X6

◀ New ◀||| Revised ~~deleted~~ Deleted

Substance	External Cause (T-Code)					
	Poisoning, Accidental (Unintentional)	Poisoning, Intentional Self-Harm	Poisoning, Assault	Poisoning, Undetermined	Adverse Effect	Underdosing
L						
Labetalol	T44.8X1	T44.8X2	T44.8X3	T44.8X4	T44.8X5	T44.8X6
Laburnum (seeds)	T62.2X1	T62.2X2	T62.2X3	T62.2X4	—	—
leaves	T62.2X1	T62.2X2	T62.2X3	T62.2X4	—	—
Lachesine	T49.5X1	T49.5X2	T49.5X3	T49.5X4	T49.5X5	T49.5X6
Lacidipine	T46.5X1	T46.5X2	T46.5X3	T46.5X4	T46.5X5	T46.5X6
Lacquer	T65.6X1	T65.6X2	T65.6X3	T65.6X4	—	—
Lacrimogenic gas	T59.3X1	T59.3X2	T59.3X3	T59.3X4	—	—
Lactated potassic saline	T50.3X1	T50.3X2	T50.3X3	T50.3X4	T50.3X5	T50.3X6
Lactic acid	T49.8X1	T49.8X2	T49.8X3	T49.8X4	T49.8X5	T49.8X6
Lactobacillus						
acidophilus	T47.6X1	T47.6X2	T47.6X3	T47.6X4	T47.6X5	T47.6X6
compound	T47.6X1	T47.6X2	T47.6X3	T47.6X4	T47.6X5	T47.6X6
bifidus, lyophilized	T47.6X1	T47.6X2	T47.6X3	T47.6X4	T47.6X5	T47.6X6
bulgaricus	T47.6X1	T47.6X2	T47.6X3	T47.6X4	T47.6X5	T47.6X6
sporogenes	T47.6X1	T47.6X2	T47.6X3	T47.6X4	T47.6X5	T47.6X6
Lactoflavin	T45.2X1	T45.2X2	T45.2X3	T45.2X4	T45.2X5	T45.2X6
Lactose (as excipient)	T50.901	T50.902	T50.903	T50.904	T50.905	T50.906
Lactuca (virosa) (extract)	T42.6X1	T42.6X2	T42.6X3	T42.6X4	T42.6X5	T42.6X6
Lactucarium	T42.6X1	T42.6X2	T42.6X3	T42.6X4	T42.6X5	T42.6X6
Lactulose	T47.3X1	T47.3X2	T47.3X3	T47.3X4	T47.3X5	T47.3X6
Laevo — see Levo-						
Lanatosides	T46.0X1	T46.0X2	T46.0X3	T46.0X4	T46.0X5	T46.0X6
Lanolin	T49.3X1	T49.3X2	T49.3X3	T49.3X4	T49.3X5	T49.3X6
Largactil	T43.3X1	T43.3X2	T43.3X3	T43.3X4	T43.3X5	T43.3X6
Larkspur	T62.2X1	T62.2X2	T62.2X3	T62.2X4	—	—
Laroxyl	T43.011	T43.012	T43.013	T43.014	T43.015	T43.016
Lassar's paste	T49.4X1	T49.4X2	T49.4X3	T49.4X4	T49.4X5	T49.4X6
Lasix	T50.1X1	T50.1X2	T50.1X3	T50.1X4	T50.1X5	T50.1X6
Latamoxef	T36.1X1	T36.1X2	T36.1X3	T36.1X4	T36.1X5	T36.1X6
Latex	T65.811	T65.812	T65.813	T65.814	—	—
Lathyrus (seed)	T62.2X1	T62.2X2	T62.2X3	T62.2X4	—	—
Laudanum	T40.0X1	T40.0X2	T40.0X3	T40.0X4	T40.0X5	T40.0X6
Laudexium	T48.1X1	T48.1X2	T48.1X3	T48.1X4	T48.1X5	T48.1X6
Laughing gas	T41.0X1	T41.0X2	T41.0X3	T41.0X4	T41.0X5	T41.0X6
Laurel, black or cherry	T62.2X1	T62.2X2	T62.2X3	T62.2X4	—	—
Laurolinium	T49.0X1	T49.0X2	T49.0X3	T49.0X4	T49.0X5	T49.0X6
Lauryl sulfoacetate	T49.2X1	T49.2X2	T49.2X3	T49.2X4	T49.2X5	T49.2X6

Substance	External Cause (T-Code)					
	Poisoning, Accidental (Unintentional)	Poisoning, Intentional Self-Harm	Poisoning, Assault	Poisoning, Undetermined	Adverse Effect	Underdosing
Laxative NEC	T47.4X1	T47.4X2	T47.4X3	T47.4X4	T47.4X5	T47.4X6
osmotic	T47.3X1	T47.3X2	T47.3X3	T47.3X4	T47.3X5	T47.3X6
saline	T47.3X1	T47.3X2	T47.3X3	T47.3X4	T47.3X5	T47.3X6
stimulant	T47.2X1	T47.2X2	T47.2X3	T47.2X4	T47.2X5	T47.2X6
L-dopa	T42.8X1	T42.8X2	T42.8X3	T42.8X4	T42.8X5	T42.8X6
Lead (dust) (fumes) (vapor) NEC	T56.0X1	T56.0X2	T56.0X3	T56.0X4	—	—
acetate	T49.2X1	T49.2X2	T49.2X3	T49.2X4	T49.2X5	T49.2X6
alkyl (fuel additive)	T56.0X1	T56.0X2	T56.0X3	T56.0X4	—	—
anti-infectives	T37.8X1	T37.8X2	T37.8X3	T37.8X4	T37.8X5	T37.8X6
antiknock compound (tetraethyl)	T56.0X1	T56.0X2	T56.0X3	T56.0X4	—	—
arsenate, arsenite (dust) (herbicide) (insecticide) (vapor)	T57.0X1	T57.0X2	T57.0X3	T57.0X4	—	—
carbonate	T56.0X1	T56.0X2	T56.0X3	T56.0X4	—	—
paint	T56.0X1	T56.0X2	T56.0X3	T56.0X4	—	—
chromate	T56.0X1	T56.0X2	T56.0X3	T56.0X4	—	—
paint	T56.0X1	T56.0X2	T56.0X3	T56.0X4	—	—
dioxide	T56.0X1	T56.0X2	T56.0X3	T56.0X4	—	—
inorganic	T56.0X1	T56.0X2	T56.0X3	T56.0X4	—	—
iodide	T56.0X1	T56.0X2	T56.0X3	T56.0X4	—	—
pigment (paint)	T56.0X1	T56.0X2	T56.0X3	T56.0X4	—	—
monoxide (dust)	T56.0X1	T56.0X2	T56.0X3	T56.0X4	—	—
paint	T56.0X1	T56.0X2	T56.0X3	T56.0X4	—	—
organic	T56.0X1	T56.0X2	T56.0X3	T56.0X4	—	—
oxide	T56.0X1	T56.0X2	T56.0X3	T56.0X4	—	—
paint	T56.0X1	T56.0X2	T56.0X3	T56.0X4	—	—
paint	T56.0X1	T56.0X2	T56.0X3	T56.0X4	—	—
salts	T56.0X1	T56.0X2	T56.0X3	T56.0X4	—	—
specified compound NEC	T56.0X1	T56.0X2	T56.0X3	T56.0X4	—	—
tetra-ethyl	T56.0X1	T56.0X2	T56.0X3	T56.0X4	—	—
Lebanese red	T40.7X1	T40.7X2	T40.7X3	T40.7X4	T40.7X5	T40.7X6
Lefetamine	T39.8X1	T39.8X2	T39.8X3	T39.8X4	T39.8X5	T39.8X6
Lenperone	T43.4X1	T43.4X2	T43.4X3	T43.4X4	T43.4X5	T43.4X6
Lente lietin (insulin)	T38.3X1	T38.3X2	T38.3X3	T38.3X4	T38.3X5	T38.3X6
Leptazol	T50.7X1	T50.7X2	T50.7X3	T50.7X4	T50.7X5	T50.7X6
Leptophos	T60.0X1	T60.0X2	T60.0X3	T60.0X4	—	—
Leritine	T40.2X1	T40.2X2	T40.2X3	T40.2X4	T40.2X5	T40.2X6
Letosteine	T48.4X1	T48.4X2	T48.4X3	T48.4X4	T48.4X5	T48.4X6
Letter	T38.1X1	T38.1X2	T38.1X3	T38.1X4	T38.1X5	T38.1X6
Lettuce opium	T42.6X1	T42.6X2	T42.6X3	T42.6X4	T42.6X5	T42.6X6
Leucinocaine	T41.3X1	T41.3X2	T41.3X3	T41.3X4	T41.3X5	T41.3X6

◄ New ◄▯ Revised ~~deleted~~ Deleted

Substance	Poisoning, Accidental (Unintentional)	Poisoning, Intentional Self-Harm	Poisoning, Assault	Poisoning, Undetermined	Adverse Effect	Underdosing
Leucocianidol	T46.991	T46.992	T46.993	T46.994	T46.995	T46.996
Leucovorin (factor)	T45.8X1	T45.8X2	T45.8X3	T45.8X4	T45.8X5	T45.8X6
Leukeran	T45.1X1	T45.1X2	T45.1X3	T45.1X4	T45.1X5	T45.1X6
Leuprolide	T38.891	T38.892	T38.893	T38.894	T38.895	T38.896
Levalbuterol	T48.6X1	T48.6X2	T48.6X3	T48.6X4	T48.6X5	T48.6X6
Levallorphan	T50.7X1	T50.7X2	T50.7X3	T50.7X4	T50.7X5	T50.7X6
Levamisole	T37.4X1	T37.4X2	T37.4X3	T37.4X4	T37.4X5	T37.4X6
Levanil	T42.6X1	T42.6X2	T42.6X3	T42.6X4	T42.6X5	T42.6X6
Levarterenol	T44.4X1	T44.4X2	T44.4X3	T44.4X4	T44.4X5	T44.4X6
Levdropropizine	T48.3X1	T48.3X2	T48.3X3	T48.3X4	T48.3X5	T48.3X6
Levobunolol	T49.5X1	T49.5X2	T49.5X3	T49.5X4	T49.5X5	T49.5X6
Levocabastine (hydrochloride)	T45.0X1	T45.0X2	T45.0X3	T45.0X4	T45.0X5	T45.0X6
Levocarnitine	T50.991	T50.992	T50.993	T50.994	T50.995	T50.996
Levodopa	T42.8X1	T42.8X2	T42.8X3	T42.8X4	T42.8X5	T42.8X6
with carbidopa	T42.8X1	T42.8X2	T42.8X3	T42.8X4	T42.8X5	T42.8X6
Levo-dromoran	T40.2X1	T40.2X2	T40.2X3	T40.2X4	T40.2X5	T40.2X6
Levoglutamide	T50.991	T50.992	T50.993	T50.994	T50.995	T50.996
Levoid	T38.1X1	T38.1X2	T38.1X3	T38.1X4	T38.1X5	T38.1X6
Levo-iso-methadone	T40.3X1	T40.3X2	T40.3X3	T40.3X4	T40.3X5	T40.3X6
Levomepromazine	T43.3X1	T43.3X2	T43.3X3	T43.3X4	T43.3X5	T43.3X6
Levonordefrin	T49.6X1	T49.6X2	T49.6X3	T49.6X4	T49.6X5	T49.6X6
Levonorgestrel	T38.4X1	T38.4X2	T38.4X3	T38.4X4	T38.4X5	T38.4X6
with ethinylestradiol	T38.5X1	T38.5X2	T38.5X3	T38.5X4	T38.5X5	T38.5X6
Levopromazine	T43.3X1	T43.3X2	T43.3X3	T43.3X4	T43.3X5	T43.3X6
Levoprome	T42.6X1	T42.6X2	T42.6X3	T42.6X4	T42.6X5	T42.6X6
Levopropoxyphene	T40.4X1	T40.4X2	T40.4X3	T40.4X4	T40.4X5	T40.4X6
Levopropylhexedrine	T50.5X1	T50.5X2	T50.5X3	T50.5X4	T50.5X5	T50.5X6
Levoproxyphylline	T48.6X1	T48.6X2	T48.6X3	T48.6X4	T48.6X5	T48.6X6
Levorphanol	T40.4X1	T40.4X2	T40.4X3	T40.4X4	T40.4X5	T40.4X6
Levothyroxine	T38.1X1	T38.1X2	T38.1X3	T38.1X4	T38.1X5	T38.1X6
sodium	T38.1X1	T38.1X2	T38.1X3	T38.1X4	T38.1X5	T38.1X6
Levsin	T44.3X1	T44.3X2	T44.3X3	T44.3X4	T44.3X5	T44.3X6
Levulose	T50.3X1	T50.3X2	T50.3X3	T50.3X4	T50.3X5	T50.3X6
Lewisite (gas), not in war	T57.0X1	T57.0X2	T57.0X3	T57.0X4	—	—
Librium	T42.4X1	T42.4X2	T42.4X3	T42.4X4	T42.4X5	T42.4X6
Lidex	T49.0X1	T49.0X2	T49.0X3	T49.0X4	T49.0X5	T49.0X6
Lidocaine	T41.3X1	T41.3X2	T41.3X3	T41.3X4	T41.3X5	T41.3X6
regional	T41.3X1	T41.3X2	T41.3X3	T41.3X4	T41.3X5	T41.3X6
spinal	T41.3X1	T41.3X2	T41.3X3	T41.3X4	T41.3X5	T41.3X6
Lidofenin	T50.8X1	T50.8X2	T50.8X3	T50.8X4	T50.8X5	T50.8X6
Lidoflazine	T46.1X1	T46.1X2	T46.1X3	T46.1X4	T46.1X5	T46.1X6
Lighter fluid	T52.0X1	T52.0X2	T52.0X3	T52.0X4	—	—

Substance	Poisoning, Accidental (Unintentional)	Poisoning, Intentional Self-Harm	Poisoning, Assault	Poisoning, Undetermined	Adverse Effect	Underdosing
Lignin hemicellulose	T47.6X1	T47.6X2	T47.6X3	T47.6X4	T47.6X5	T47.6X6
Lignocaine	T41.3X1	T41.3X2	T41.3X3	T41.3X4	T41.3X5	T41.3X6
regional	T41.3X1	T41.3X2	T41.3X3	T41.3X4	T41.3X5	T41.3X6
spinal	T41.3X1	T41.3X2	T41.3X3	T41.3X4	T41.3X5	T41.3X6
Ligroin(e) (solvent)	T52.0X1	T52.0X2	T52.0X3	T52.0X4	—	—
vapor	T59.891	T59.892	T59.893	T59.894	—	—
Ligustrum vulgare	T62.2X1	T62.2X2	T62.2X3	T62.2X4	—	—
Lily of the valley	T62.2X1	T62.2X2	T62.2X3	T62.2X4	—	—
Lime (chloride)	T54.3X1	T54.3X2	T54.3X3	T54.3X4	—	—
Limonene	T52.8X1	T52.8X2	T52.8X3	T52.8X4	—	—
Lincomycin	T36.8X1	T36.8X2	T36.8X3	T36.8X4	T36.8X5	T36.8X6
Lindane (insecticide) (nonmedicinal) (vapor)	T53.6X1	T53.6X2	T53.6X3	T53.6X4	—	—
medicinal	T49.0X1	T49.0X2	T49.0X3	T49.0X4	T49.0X5	T49.0X6
Liniments NEC	T49.91	T49.92	T49.93	T49.94	T49.95	T49.96
Linoleic acid	T46.6X1	T46.6X2	T46.6X3	T46.6X4	T46.6X5	T46.6X6
Linolenic acid	T46.6X1	T46.6X2	T46.6X3	T46.6X4	T46.6X5	T46.6X6
Linseed	T47.4X1	T47.4X2	T47.4X3	T47.4X4	T47.4X5	T47.4X6
Liothyronine	T38.1X1	T38.1X2	T38.1X3	T38.1X4	T38.1X5	T38.1X6
Liotrix	T38.1X1	T38.1X2	T38.1X3	T38.1X4	T38.1X5	T38.1X6
Lipancreatin	T47.5X1	T47.5X2	T47.5X3	T47.5X4	T47.5X5	T47.5X6
Lipo-alprostadil	T46.7X1	T46.7X2	T46.7X3	T46.7X4	T46.7X5	T46.7X6
Lipo-Lutin	T38.5X1	T38.5X2	T38.5X3	T38.5X4	T38.5X5	T38.5X6
Lipotropic drug NEC	T50.901	T50.902	T50.903	T50.904	T50.905	T50.906
Liquefied petroleum gases	T59.891	T59.892	T59.893	T59.894	—	—
piped (pure or mixed with air)	T59.891	T59.892	T59.893	T59.894	—	—
Liquid						
paraffin	T47.4X1	T47.4X2	T47.4X3	T47.4X4	T47.4X5	T47.4X6
petrolatum	T47.4X1	T47.4X2	T47.4X3	T47.4X4	T47.4X5	T47.4X6
topical	T49.3X1	T49.3X2	T49.3X3	T49.3X4	T49.3X5	T49.3X6
specified NEC	T65.891	T65.892	T65.893	T65.894	—	—
substance	T65.91	T65.92	T65.93	T65.94	—	—
Liquor creosolis compositus	T65.891	T65.892	T65.893	T65.894	—	—
Liquorice	T48.4X1	T48.4X2	T48.4X3	T48.4X4	T48.4X5	T48.4X6
extract	T47.8X1	T47.8X2	T47.8X3	T47.8X4	T47.8X5	T47.8X6
Lirugen	T50.991	T50.992	T50.993	T50.994	T50.995	T50.996
Lisinopril	T46.4X1	T46.4X2	T46.4X3	T46.4X4	T46.4X5	T46.4X6
Lisuride	T42.8X1	T42.8X2	T42.8X3	T42.8X4	T42.8X5	T42.8X6
Lithane	T43.8X1	T43.8X2	T43.8X3	T43.8X4	T43.8X5	T43.8X6
Lithium	T56.891	T56.892	T56.893	T56.894	—	—
gluconate	T43.591	T43.592	T43.593	T43.594	T43.595	T43.596
salts (carbonate)	T43.591	T43.592	T43.593	T43.594	T43.595	T43.596

New ◀ Revised ◀▥ ~~deleted~~ Deleted

	External Cause (T-Code)					
Substance	Poisoning, Accidental (Unintentional)	Poisoning, Intentional Self-Harm	Poisoning, Assault	Poisoning, Undetermined	Adverse Effect	Underdosing
Lithonate	T43.8X1	T43.8X2	T43.8X3	T43.8X4	T43.8X5	T43.8X6
Liver						
extract	T45.8X1	T45.8X2	T45.8X3	T45.8X4	T45.8X5	T45.8X6
for parenteral use	T45.8X1	T45.8X2	T45.8X3	T45.8X4	T45.8X5	T45.8X6
fraction 1	T45.8X1	T45.8X2	T45.8X3	T45.8X4	T45.8X5	T45.8X6
hydrolysate	T45.8X1	T45.8X2	T45.8X3	T45.8X4	T45.8X5	T45.8X6
Lizard (bite) (venom)	T63.121	T63.122	T63.123	T63.124	—	—
LMD	T45.8X1	T45.8X2	T45.8X3	T45.8X4	T45.8X5	T45.8X6
Lobelia	T62.2X1	T62.2X2	T62.2X3	T62.2X4	—	—
Lobeline	T50.7X1	T50.7X2	T50.7X3	T50.7X4	T50.7X5	T50.7X6
Local action drug NEC	T49.8X1	T49.8X2	T49.8X3	T49.8X4	T49.8X5	T49.8X6
Locorten	T49.0X1	T49.0X2	T49.0X3	T49.0X4	T49.0X5	T49.0X6
Lofepramine	T43.011	T43.012	T43.013	T43.014	T43.015	T43.016
Lolium temulentum	T62.2X1	T62.2X2	T62.2X3	T62.2X4	—	—
Lomotil	T47.6X1	T47.6X2	T47.6X3	T47.6X4	T47.6X5	T47.6X6
Lomustine	T45.1X1	T45.1X2	T45.1X3	T45.1X4	T45.1X5	T45.1X6
Lonidamine	T45.1X1	T45.1X2	T45.1X3	T45.1X4	T45.1X5	T45.1X6
Loperamide	T47.6X1	T47.6X2	T47.6X3	T47.6X4	T47.6X5	T47.6X6
Loprazolam	T42.4X1	T42.4X2	T42.4X3	T42.4X4	T42.4X5	T42.4X6
Lorajmine	T46.2X1	T46.2X2	T46.2X3	T46.2X4	T46.2X5	T46.2X6
Loratidine	T45.0X1	T45.0X2	T45.0X3	T45.0X4	T45.0X5	T45.0X6
Lorazepam	T42.4X1	T42.4X2	T42.4X3	T42.4X4	T42.4X5	T42.4X6
Lorcainide	T46.2X1	T46.2X2	T46.2X3	T46.2X4	T46.2X5	T46.2X6
Lormetazepam	T42.4X1	T42.4X2	T42.4X3	T42.4X4	T42.4X5	T42.4X6
Lotions NEC	T49.91	T49.92	T49.93	T49.94	T49.95	T49.96
Lotusate	T42.3X1	T42.3X2	T42.3X3	T42.3X4	T42.3X5	T42.3X6
Lovastatin	T46.6X1	T46.6X2	T46.6X3	T46.6X4	T46.6X5	T46.6X6
Loxapine	T43.591	T43.592	T43.593	T43.594	T43.595	T43.596
Lowila	T49.2X1	T49.2X2	T49.2X3	T49.2X4	T49.2X5	T49.2X6
Lozenges (throat)	T49.6X1	T49.6X2	T49.6X3	T49.6X4	T49.6X5	T49.6X6
LSD	T40.8X1	T40.8X2	T40.8X3	T40.8X4	—	—
L-Tryptophan — *see amino acid*						
Lubricant, eye	T49.5X1	T49.5X2	T49.5X3	T49.5X4	T49.5X5	T49.5X6
Lubricating oil NEC	T52.0X1	T52.0X2	T52.0X3	T52.0X4	—	—
Lucanthone	T37.4X1	T37.4X2	T37.4X3	T37.4X4	T37.4X5	T37.4X6
Luminal	T42.3X1	T42.3X2	T42.3X3	T42.3X4	T42.3X5	T42.3X6
Lung irritant (gas) NEC	T59.91	T59.92	T59.93	T59.94	—	—
Luteinizing hormone	T38.811	T38.812	T38.813	T38.814	T38.815	T38.816
Lutocylol	T38.5X1	T38.5X2	T38.5X3	T38.5X4	T38.5X5	T38.5X6
Lutromone	T38.5X1	T38.5X2	T38.5X3	T38.5X4	T38.5X5	T38.5X6
Lututrin	T48.291	T48.292	T48.293	T48.294	T48.295	T48.296
Lye (Concentrated)	T54.3X1	T54.3X2	T54.3X3	T54.3X4	—	—

	External Cause (T-Code)					
Substance	Poisoning, Accidental (Unintentional)	Poisoning, Intentional Self-Harm	Poisoning, Assault	Poisoning, Undetermined	Adverse Effect	Underdosing
Lygranum (skin test)	T50.8X1	T50.8X2	T50.8X3	T50.8X4	T50.8X5	T50.8X6
Lymecycline	T36.4X1	T36.4X2	T36.4X3	T36.4X4	T36.4X5	T36.4X6
Lymphogranuloma venereum antigen	T50.8X1	T50.8X2	T50.8X3	T50.8X4	T50.8X5	T50.8X6
Lynestrenol	T38.4X1	T38.4X2	T38.4X3	T38.4X4	T38.4X5	T38.4X6
Lypressin	T38.891	T38.892	T38.893	T38.894	T38.895	T38.896
Lyovac Sodium Edecrin	T50.1X1	T50.1X2	T50.1X3	T50.1X4	T50.1X5	T50.1X6
Lysergic acid diethylamide	T40.8X1	T40.8X2	T40.8X3	T40.8X4	—	—
Lysergide	T40.8X1	T40.8X2	T40.8X3	T40.8X4	—	—
Lysine vasopressin	T38.891	T38.892	T38.893	T38.894	T38.895	T38.896
Lysol	T54.1X1	T54.1X2	T54.1X3	T54.1X4	—	—
Lysozyme	T49.0X1	T49.0X2	T49.0X3	T49.0X4	T49.0X5	T49.0X6
Lytta (vitatta)	T49.8X1	T49.8X2	T49.8X3	T49.8X4	T49.8X5	T49.8X6
M						
Mace	T59.3X1	T59.3X2	T59.3X3	T59.3X4	—	—
Macrogol	T50.991	T50.992	T50.993	T50.994	T50.995	T50.996
Macrolide						
anabolic drug	T38.7X1	T38.7X2	T38.7X3	T38.7X4	T38.7X5	T38.7X6
antibiotic	T36.3X1	T36.3X2	T36.3X3	T36.3X4	T36.3X5	T36.3X6
Mafenide	T49.0X1	T49.0X2	T49.0X3	T49.0X4	T49.0X5	T49.0X6
Magaldrate	T47.1X1	T47.1X2	T47.1X3	T47.1X4	T47.1X5	T47.1X6
Magic mushroom	T40.991	T40.992	T40.993	T40.994	—	—
Magnamycin	T36.8X1	T36.8X2	T36.8X3	T36.8X4	T36.8X5	T36.8X6
Magnesia magma	T47.1X1	T47.1X2	T47.1X3	T47.1X4	T47.1X5	T47.1X6
Magnesium NEC	T56.891	T56.892	T56.893	T56.894	—	—
carbonate	T47.1X1	T47.1X2	T47.1X3	T47.1X4	T47.1X5	T47.1X6
citrate	T47.4X1	T47.4X2	T47.4X3	T47.4X4	T47.4X5	T47.4X6
hydroxide	T47.1X1	T47.1X2	T47.1X3	T47.1X4	T47.1X5	T47.1X6
oxide	T47.1X1	T47.1X2	T47.1X3	T47.1X4	T47.1X5	T47.1X6
peroxide	T49.0X1	T49.0X2	T49.0X3	T49.0X4	T49.0X5	T49.0X6
salicylate	T39.091	T39.092	T39.093	T39.094	T39.095	T39.096
silicofluoride	T50.3X1	T50.3X2	T50.3X3	T50.3X4	T50.3X5	T50.3X6
sulfate	T47.4X1	T47.4X2	T47.4X3	T47.4X4	T47.4X5	T47.4X6
thiosulfate	T45.0X1	T45.0X2	T45.0X3	T45.0X4	T45.0X5	T45.0X6
trisilicate	T47.1X1	T47.1X2	T47.1X3	T47.1X4	T47.1X5	T47.1X6
Malathion (medicinal)	T49.0X1	T49.0X2	T49.0X3	T49.0X4	T49.0X5	T49.0X6
insecticide	T60.0X1	T60.0X2	T60.0X3	T60.0X4	—	—
Male fern extract	T37.4X1	T37.4X2	T37.4X3	T37.4X4	T37.4X5	T37.4X6
M-AMSA	T45.1X1	T45.1X2	T45.1X3	T45.1X4	T45.1X5	T45.1X6
Mandelic acid	T37.8X1	T37.8X2	T37.8X3	T37.8X4	T37.8X5	T37.8X6
Manganese (dioxide) (salts)	T57.2X1	T57.2X2	T57.2X3	T57.2X4	—	—
medicinal	T50.991	T50.992	T50.993	T50.994	T50.995	T50.996

◀ New   ◀ Revised   ~~deleted~~ Deleted

Substance	Poisoning, Accidental (Unintentional)	Poisoning, Intentional Self-Harm	Poisoning, Assault	Poisoning, Undetermined	Adverse Effect	Underdosing
Mannitol	T47.3X1	T47.3X2	T47.3X3	T47.3X4	T47.3X5	T47.3X6
hexanitrate	T46.3X1	T46.3X2	T46.3X3	T46.3X4	T46.3X5	T46.3X6
Mannomustine	T45.1X1	T45.1X2	T45.1X3	T45.1X4	T45.1X5	T45.1X6
MAO inhibitors	T43.1X1	T43.1X2	T43.1X3	T43.1X4	T43.1X5	T43.1X6
Mapharsen	T37.8X1	T37.8X2	T37.8X3	T37.8X4	T37.8X5	T37.8X6
Maphenide	T49.0X1	T49.0X2	T49.0X3	T49.0X4	T49.0X5	T49.0X6
Maprotiline	T43.021	T43.022	T43.023	T43.024	T43.025	T43.026
Marcaine	T41.3X1	T41.3X2	T41.3X3	T41.3X4	T41.3X5	T41.3X6
infiltration (subcutaneous)	T41.3X1	T41.3X2	T41.3X3	T41.3X4	T41.3X5	T41.3X6
nerve block (peripheral) (plexus)	T41.3X1	T41.3X2	T41.3X3	T41.3X4	T41.3X5	T41.3X6
Marezine	T45.0X1	T45.0X2	T45.0X3	T45.0X4	T45.0X5	T45.0X6
Marihuana	T40.7X1	T40.7X2	T40.7X3	T40.7X4	T40.7X5	T40.7X6
Marijuana	T40.7X1	T40.7X2	T40.7X3	T40.7X4	T40.7X5	T40.7X6
Marine (sting)	T63.691	T63.692	T63.693	T63.694	—	—
animals (sting)	T63.691	T63.692	T63.693	T63.694	—	—
plants (sting)	T63.711	T63.712	T63.713	T63.714	—	—
Marplan	T43.1X1	T43.1X2	T43.1X3	T43.1X4	T43.1X5	T43.1X6
Marsh gas	T59.891	T59.892	T59.893	T59.894	—	—
Marsilid	T43.1X1	T43.1X2	T43.1X3	T43.1X4	T43.1X5	T43.1X6
Matulane	T45.1X1	T45.1X2	T45.1X3	T45.1X4	T45.1X5	T45.1X6
Mazindol	T50.5X1	T50.5X2	T50.5X3	T50.5X4	T50.5X5	T50.5X6
MCPA	T60.3X1	T60.3X2	T60.3X3	T60.3X4	—	—
MDMA	T43.621	T43.622	T43.623	T43.624	T43.625	T43.626
Meadow saffron	T62.2X1	T62.2X2	T62.2X3	T62.2X4	—	—
Measles virus vaccine (attenuated)	T50.B91	T50.B92	T50.B93	T50.B94	T50.B95	T50.B96
Meat, noxious	T62.8X1	T62.8X2	T62.8X3	T62.8X4	—	—
Meballymal	T42.3X1	T42.3X2	T42.3X3	T42.3X4	T42.3X5	T42.3X6
Mebanazine	T43.1X1	T43.1X2	T43.1X3	T43.1X4	T43.1X5	T43.1X6
Mebaral	T42.3X1	T42.3X2	T42.3X3	T42.3X4	T42.3X5	T42.3X6
Mebendazole	T37.4X1	T37.4X2	T37.4X3	T37.4X4	T37.4X5	T37.4X6
Mebeverine	T44.3X1	T44.3X2	T44.3X3	T44.3X4	T44.3X5	T44.3X6
Mebhydrolin	T45.0X1	T45.0X2	T45.0X3	T45.0X4	T45.0X5	T45.0X6
Mebumal	T42.3X1	T42.3X2	T42.3X3	T42.3X4	T42.3X5	T42.3X6
Mebutamate	T43.591	T43.592	T43.593	T43.594	T43.595	T43.596
Mecamylamine	T44.2X1	T44.2X2	T44.2X3	T44.2X4	T44.2X5	T44.2X6
Mechlorethamine	T45.1X1	T45.1X2	T45.1X3	T45.1X4	T45.1X5	T45.1X6
Mecillinam	T36.0X1	T36.0X2	T36.0X3	T36.0X4	T36.0X5	T36.0X6
Meclizine (hydrochloride)	T45.0X1	T45.0X2	T45.0X3	T45.0X4	T45.0X5	T45.0X6
Meclocycline	T36.4X1	T36.4X2	T36.4X3	T36.4X4	T36.4X5	T36.4X6
Meclofenamate	T39.391	T39.392	T39.393	T39.394	T39.395	T39.396
Meclofenamic acid	T39.391	T39.392	T39.393	T39.394	T39.395	T39.396

Substance	Poisoning, Accidental (Unintentional)	Poisoning, Intentional Self-Harm	Poisoning, Assault	Poisoning, Undetermined	Adverse Effect	Underdosing
Meclofenoxate	T43.691	T43.692	T43.693	T43.694	T43.695	T43.696
Meclozine	T45.0X1	T45.0X2	T45.0X3	T45.0X4	T45.0X5	T45.0X6
Mecobalamin	T45.8X1	T45.8X2	T45.8X3	T45.8X4	T45.8X5	T45.8X6
Mecoprop	T60.3X1	T60.3X2	T60.3X3	T60.3X4	—	—
Mecrilate	T49.3X1	T49.3X2	T49.3X3	T49.3X4	T49.3X5	T49.3X6
Mecysteine	T48.4X1	T48.4X2	T48.4X3	T48.4X4	T48.4X5	T48.4X6
Medazepam	T42.4X1	T42.4X2	T42.4X3	T42.4X4	T42.4X5	T42.4X6
Medicament NEC	T50.901	T50.902	T50.903	T50.904	T50.905	T50.906
Medinal	T42.3X1	T42.3X2	T42.3X3	T42.3X4	T42.3X5	T42.3X6
Medomin	T42.3X1	T42.3X2	T42.3X3	T42.3X4	T42.3X5	T42.3X6
Medrogestone	T38.5X1	T38.5X2	T38.5X3	T38.5X4	T38.5X5	T38.5X6
Medroxalol	T44.8X1	T44.8X2	T44.8X3	T44.8X4	T44.8X5	T44.8X6
Medroxyprogesterone acetate (depot)	T38.5X1	T38.5X2	T38.5X3	T38.5X4	T38.5X5	T38.5X6
Medrysone	T49.0X1	T49.0X2	T49.0X3	T49.0X4	T49.0X5	T49.0X6
Mefenamic acid	T39.391	T39.392	T39.393	T39.394	T39.395	T39.396
Mefenorex	T50.5X1	T50.5X2	T50.5X3	T50.5X4	T50.5X5	T50.5X6
Mefloquine	T37.2X1	T37.2X2	T37.2X3	T37.2X4	T37.2X5	T37.2X6
Mefruside	T50.2X1	T50.2X2	T50.2X3	T50.2X4	T50.2X5	T50.2X6
Megahallucinogen	T40.901	T40.902	T40.903	T40.904	T40.905	T40.906
Megestrol	T38.5X1	T38.5X2	T38.5X3	T38.5X4	T38.5X5	T38.5X6
Meglumine						
antimoniate	T37.8X1	T37.8X2	T37.8X3	T37.8X4	T37.8X5	T37.8X6
diatrizoate	T50.8X1	T50.8X2	T50.8X3	T50.8X4	T50.8X5	T50.8X6
iodipamide	T50.8X1	T50.8X2	T50.8X3	T50.8X4	T50.8X5	T50.8X6
iotroxate	T50.8X1	T50.8X2	T50.8X3	T50.8X4	T50.8X5	T50.8X6
MEK (methyl ethyl ketone)	T52.4X1	T52.4X2	T52.4X3	T52.4X4	—	—
Meladrazine	T44.3X1	T44.3X2	T44.3X3	T44.3X4	T44.3X5	T44.3X6
Meladinin	T49.3X1	T49.3X2	T49.3X3	T49.3X4	T49.3X5	T49.3X6
Melaleuca alternifolia oil	T49.0X1	T49.0X2	T49.0X3	T49.0X4	T49.0X5	T49.0X6
Melanizing agents	T49.3X1	T49.3X2	T49.3X3	T49.3X4	T49.3X5	T49.3X6
Melanocyte-stimulating hormone	T38.891	T38.892	T38.893	T38.894	T38.895	T38.896
Melarsonyl potassium	T37.3X1	T37.3X2	T37.3X3	T37.3X4	T37.3X5	T37.3X6
Melarsoprol	T37.3X1	T37.3X2	T37.3X3	T37.3X4	T37.3X5	T37.3X6
Melia azedarach	T62.2X1	T62.2X2	T62.2X3	T62.2X4	—	—
Melitracen	T43.011	T43.012	T43.013	T43.014	T43.015	T43.016
Mellaril	T43.3X1	T43.3X2	T43.3X3	T43.3X4	T43.3X5	T43.3X6
Meloxine	T49.3X1	T49.3X2	T49.3X3	T49.3X4	T49.3X5	T49.3X6
Melperone	T43.4X1	T43.4X2	T43.4X3	T43.4X4	T43.4X5	T43.4X6
Melphalan	T45.1X1	T45.1X2	T45.1X3	T45.1X4	T45.1X5	T45.1X6
Memantine	T43.8X1	T43.8X2	T43.8X3	T43.8X4	T43.8X5	T43.8X6

◀ New ◀▥ Revised ~~deleted~~ Deleted

	External Cause (T-Code)					
Substance	Poisoning, Accidental (Unintentional)	Poisoning, Intentional Self-Harm	Poisoning, Assault	Poisoning, Undetermined	Adverse Effect	Underdosing
Menadiol	T45.7X1	T45.7X2	T45.7X3	T45.7X4	T45.7X5	T45.7X6
sodium sulfate	T45.7X1	T45.7X2	T45.7X3	T45.7X4	T45.7X5	T45.7X6
Menadione	T45.7X1	T45.7X2	T45.7X3	T45.7X4	T45.7X5	T45.7X6
sodium bisulfite	T45.7X1	T45.7X2	T45.7X3	T45.7X4	T45.7X5	T45.7X6
Menaphthone	T45.7X1	T45.7X2	T45.7X3	T45.7X4	T45.7X5	T45.7X6
Menaquinone	T45.7X1	T45.7X2	T45.7X3	T45.7X4	T45.7X5	T45.7X6
Menatetrenone	T45.7X1	T45.7X2	T45.7X3	T45.7X4	T45.7X5	T45.7X6
Meningococcal vaccine	T50.A91	T50.A92	T50.A93	T50.A94	T50.A95	T50.A96
Menningovax (-AC) (-C)	T50.A91	T50.A92	T50.A93	T50.A94	T50.A95	T50.A96
Menotropins	T38.811	T38.812	T38.813	T38.814	T38.815	T38.816
Menthol	T48.5X1	T48.5X2	T48.5X3	T48.5X4	T48.5X5	T48.5X6
Mepacrine	T37.2X1	T37.2X2	T37.2X3	T37.2X4	T37.2X5	T37.2X6
Meparfynol	T42.6X1	T42.6X2	T42.6X3	T42.6X4	T42.6X5	T42.6X6
Mepartricin	T36.7X1	T36.7X2	T36.7X3	T36.7X4	T36.7X5	T36.7X6
Mepazine	T43.3X1	T43.3X2	T43.3X3	T43.3X4	T43.3X5	T43.3X6
Mepenzolate	T44.3X1	T44.3X2	T44.3X3	T44.3X4	T44.3X5	T44.3X6
bromide	T44.3X1	T44.3X2	T44.3X3	T44.3X4	T44.3X5	T44.3X6
Meperidine	T40.4X1	T40.4X2	T40.4X3	T40.4X4	T40.4X5	T40.4X6
Mephebarbital	T42.3X1	T42.3X2	T42.3X3	T42.3X4	T42.3X5	T42.3X6
Mephenamin(e)	T42.8X1	T42.8X2	T42.8X3	T42.8X4	T42.8X5	T42.8X6
Mephenesin	T42.8X1	T42.8X2	T42.8X3	T42.8X4	T42.8X5	T42.8X6
Mephenhydramine	T45.0X1	T45.0X2	T45.0X3	T45.0X4	T45.0X5	T45.0X6
Mephenoxalone	T42.8X1	T42.8X2	T42.8X3	T42.8X4	T42.8X5	T42.8X6
Mephentermine	T44.991	T44.992	T44.993	T44.994	T44.995	T44.996
Mephenytoin	T42.0X1	T42.0X2	T42.0X3	T42.0X4	T42.0X5	T42.0X6
with phenobarbital	T42.3X1	T42.3X2	T42.3X3	T42.3X4	T42.3X5	T42.3X6
Mephobarbital	T42.3X1	T42.3X2	T42.3X3	T42.3X4	T42.3X5	T42.3X6
Mephosfolan	T60.0X1	T60.0X2	T60.0X3	T60.0X4	—	—
Mepindolol	T44.7X1	T44.7X2	T44.7X3	T44.7X4	T44.7X5	T44.7X6
Mepiperphenidol	T44.3X1	T44.3X2	T44.3X3	T44.3X4	T44.3X5	T44.3X6
Mepitiostane	T38.7X1	T38.7X2	T38.7X3	T38.7X4	T38.7X5	T38.7X6
Mepivacaine	T41.3X1	T41.3X2	T41.3X3	T41.3X4	T41.3X5	T41.3X6
epidural	T41.3X1	T41.3X2	T41.3X3	T41.3X4	T41.3X5	T41.3X6
Meprednisone	T38.0X1	T38.0X2	T38.0X3	T38.0X4	T38.0X5	T38.0X6
Meprobam	T43.591	T43.592	T43.593	T43.594	T43.595	T43.596
Meprobamate	T43.591	T43.592	T43.593	T43.594	T43.595	T43.596
Meproscillarin	T46.0X1	T46.0X2	T46.0X3	T46.0X4	T46.0X5	T46.0X6
Meprylcaine	T41.3X1	T41.3X2	T41.3X3	T41.3X4	T41.3X5	T41.3X6
Meptazinol	T39.8X1	T39.8X2	T39.8X3	T39.8X4	T39.8X5	T39.8X6
Mepyramine	T45.0X1	T45.0X2	T45.0X3	T45.0X4	T45.0X5	T45.0X6
Mequitazine	T43.3X1	T43.3X2	T43.3X3	T43.3X4	T43.3X5	T43.3X6
Meralluride	T50.2X1	T50.2X2	T50.2X3	T50.2X4	T50.2X5	T50.2X6

	External Cause (T-Code)					
Substance	Poisoning, Accidental (Unintentional)	Poisoning, Intentional Self-Harm	Poisoning, Assault	Poisoning, Undetermined	Adverse Effect	Underdosing
Merbaphen	T50.2X1	T50.2X2	T50.2X3	T50.2X4	T50.2X5	T50.2X6
Merbromin	T49.0X1	T49.0X2	T49.0X3	T49.0X4	T49.0X5	T49.0X6
Mercaptobenzothiazole salts	T49.0X1	T49.0X2	T49.0X3	T49.0X4	T49.0X5	T49.0X6
Mercaptomerin	T50.2X1	T50.2X2	T50.2X3	T50.2X4	T50.2X5	T50.2X6
Mercaptopurine	T45.1X1	T45.1X2	T45.1X3	T45.1X4	T45.1X5	T45.1X6
Mercumatilin	T50.2X1	T50.2X2	T50.2X3	T50.2X4	T50.2X5	T50.2X6
Mercuramide	T50.2X1	T50.2X2	T50.2X3	T50.2X4	T50.2X5	T50.2X6
Mercurochrome	T49.0X1	T49.0X2	T49.0X3	T49.0X4	T49.0X5	T49.0X6
Mercurophylline	T50.2X1	T50.2X2	T50.2X3	T50.2X4	T50.2X5	T50.2X6
Mercury, mercurial, mercuric, mercurous (compounds) (cyanide) (fumes) (nonmedicinal) (vapor) NEC	T56.1X1	T56.1X2	T56.1X3	T56.1X4	—	—
ammoniated	T49.0X1	T49.0X2	T49.0X3	T49.0X4	T49.0X5	T49.0X6
anti-infective						
local	T49.0X1	T49.0X2	T49.0X3	T49.0X4	T49.0X5	T49.0X6
systemic	T37.8X1	T37.8X2	T37.8X3	T37.8X4	T37.8X5	T37.8X6
topical	T49.0X1	T49.0X2	T49.0X3	T49.0X4	T49.0X5	T49.0X6
chloride (ammoniated)	T49.0X1	T49.0X2	T49.0X3	T49.0X4	T49.0X5	T49.0X6
fungicide	T56.1X1	T56.1X2	T56.1X3	T56.1X4	—	—
diuretic NEC	T50.2X1	T50.2X2	T50.2X3	T50.2X4	T50.2X5	T50.2X6
fungicide	T56.1X1	T56.1X2	T56.1X3	T56.1X4	—	—
organic (fungicide)	T56.1X1	T56.1X2	T56.1X3	T56.1X4	—	—
oxide, yellow	T49.0X1	T49.0X2	T49.0X3	T49.0X4	T49.0X5	T49.0X6
Mersalyl	T50.2X1	T50.2X2	T50.2X3	T50.2X4	T50.2X5	T50.2X6
Merthiolate	T49.0X1	T49.0X2	T49.0X3	T49.0X4	T49.0X5	T49.0X6
ophthalmic preparation	T49.5X1	T49.5X2	T49.5X3	T49.5X4	T49.5X5	T49.5X6
Meruvax	T50.B91	T50.B92	T50.B93	T50.B94	T50.B95	T50.B96
Mesalazine	T47.8X1	T47.8X2	T47.8X3	T47.8X4	T47.8X5	T47.8X6
Mescal buttons	T40.991	T40.992	T40.993	T40.994	—	—
Mescaline	T40.991	T40.992	T40.993	T40.994	—	—
Mesna	T48.4X1	T48.4X2	T48.4X3	T48.4X4	T48.4X5	T48.4X6
Mesoglycan	T46.6X1	T46.6X2	T46.6X3	T46.6X4	T46.6X5	T46.6X6
Mesoridazine	T43.3X1	T43.3X2	T43.3X3	T43.3X4	T43.3X5	T43.3X6
Mestanolone	T38.7X1	T38.7X2	T38.7X3	T38.7X4	T38.7X5	T38.7X6
Mesterolone	T38.7X1	T38.7X2	T38.7X3	T38.7X4	T38.7X5	T38.7X6
Mestranol	T38.5X1	T38.5X2	T38.5X3	T38.5X4	T38.5X5	T38.5X6
Mesulergine	T42.8X1	T42.8X2	T42.8X3	T42.8X4	T42.8X5	T42.8X6
Mesulfen	T49.0X1	T49.0X2	T49.0X3	T49.0X4	T49.0X5	T49.0X6
Mesuximide	T42.2X1	T42.2X2	T42.2X3	T42.2X4	T42.2X5	T42.2X6
Metabutethamine	T41.3X1	T41.3X2	T41.3X3	T41.3X4	T41.3X5	T41.3X6
Metactesylacetate	T49.0X1	T49.0X2	T49.0X3	T49.0X4	T49.0X5	T49.0X6

TABLE OF DRUGS AND CHEMICALS

◀ New ◀◀ Revised ~~deleted~~ Deleted

Substance	Poisoning, Accidental (Unintentional)	Poisoning, Intentional Self-Harm	Poisoning, Assault	Poisoning, Undetermined	Adverse Effect	Underdosing
Metacycline	T36.4X1	T36.4X2	T36.4X3	T36.4X4	T36.4X5	T36.4X6
Metaldehyde (snail killer) NEC	T60.8X1	T60.8X2	T60.8X3	T60.8X4	—	—
Metals (heavy) (nonmedicinal)	T56.91	T56.92	T56.93	T56.94	—	—
dust, fumes, or vapor NEC	T56.91	T56.92	T56.93	T56.94	—	—
light NEC	T56.91	T56.92	T56.93	T56.94	—	—
dust, fumes, or vapor NEC	T56.91	T56.92	T56.93	T56.94	—	—
specified NEC	T56.891	T56.892	T56.893	T56.894	—	—
thallium	T56.811	T56.812	T56.813	T56.814	—	—
Metamfetamine	T43.621	T43.622	T43.623	T43.624	T43.625	T43.626
Metamizole sodium	T39.2X1	T39.2X2	T39.2X3	T39.2X4	T39.2X5	T39.2X6
Metampicillin	T36.0X1	T36.0X2	T36.0X3	T36.0X4	T36.0X5	T36.0X6
Metamucil	T47.4X1	T47.4X2	T47.4X3	T47.4X4	T47.4X5	T47.4X6
Metaphen	T49.0X1	T49.0X2	T49.0X3	T49.0X4	T49.0X5	T49.0X6
Metandienone	T38.7X1	T38.7X2	T38.7X3	T38.7X4	T38.7X5	T38.7X6
Metandrostenolone	T38.7X1	T38.7X2	T38.7X3	T38.7X4	T38.7X5	T38.7X6
Metaphos	T60.0X1	T60.0X2	T60.0X3	T60.0X4	—	—
Metapramine	T43.011	T43.012	T43.013	T43.014	T43.015	T43.016
Metaproterenol	T48.291	T48.292	T48.293	T48.294	T48.295	T48.296
Metaraminol	T44.4X1	T44.4X2	T44.4X3	T44.4X4	T44.4X5	T44.4X6
Metaxalone	T42.8X1	T42.8X2	T42.8X3	T42.8X4	T42.8X5	T42.8X6
Metenolone	T38.7X1	T38.7X2	T38.7X3	T38.7X4	T38.7X5	T38.7X6
Metergoline	T42.8X1	T42.8X2	T42.8X3	T42.8X4	T42.8X5	T42.8X6
Metescufylline	T46.991	T46.992	T46.993	T46.994	T46.995	T46.996
Metetoin	T42.0X1	T42.0X2	T42.0X3	T42.0X4	T42.0X5	T42.0X6
Metformin	T38.3X1	T38.3X2	T38.3X3	T38.3X4	T38.3X5	T38.3X6
Methacholine	T44.1X1	T44.1X2	T44.1X3	T44.1X4	T44.1X5	T44.1X6
Methacycline	T36.4X1	T36.4X2	T36.4X3	T36.4X4	T36.4X5	T36.4X6
Methadone	T40.3X1	T40.3X2	T40.3X3	T40.3X4	T40.3X5	T40.3X6
Methallenestril	T38.5X1	T38.5X2	T38.5X3	T38.5X4	T38.5X5	T38.5X6
Methallenoestril	T38.5X1	T38.5X2	T38.5X3	T38.5X4	T38.5X5	T38.5X6
Methamphetamine	T43.621	T43.622	T43.623	T43.624	T43.625	T43.626
Methampyrone	T39.2X1	T39.2X2	T39.2X3	T39.2X4	T39.2X5	T39.2X6
Methandienone	T38.7X1	T38.7X2	T38.7X3	T38.7X4	T38.7X5	T38.7X6
Methandriol	T38.7X1	T38.7X2	T38.7X3	T38.7X4	T38.7X5	T38.7X6
Methandrostenolone	T38.7X1	T38.7X2	T38.7X3	T38.7X4	T38.7X5	T38.7X6
Methane	T59.891	T59.892	T59.893	T59.894	—	—
Methanethiol	T59.891	T59.892	T59.893	T59.894	—	—
Methaniazide	T37.1X1	T37.1X2	T37.1X3	T37.1X4	T37.1X5	T37.1X6
Methanol (vapor)	T51.1X1	T51.1X2	T51.1X3	T51.1X4	—	—
Methantheline	T44.3X1	T44.3X2	T44.3X3	T44.3X4	T44.3X5	T44.3X6
Methanthelinium bromide	T44.3X1	T44.3X2	T44.3X3	T44.3X4	T44.3X5	T44.3X6
Methaphenilene	T45.0X1	T45.0X2	T45.0X3	T45.0X4	T45.0X5	T45.0X6

Substance	Poisoning, Accidental (Unintentional)	Poisoning, Intentional Self-Harm	Poisoning, Assault	Poisoning, Undetermined	Adverse Effect	Underdosing
Methapyrilene	T45.0X1	T45.0X2	T45.0X3	T45.0X4	T45.0X5	T45.0X6
Methaqualone (compound)	T42.6X1	T42.6X2	T42.6X3	T42.6X4	T42.6X5	T42.6X6
Metharbital	T42.3X1	T42.3X2	T42.3X3	T42.3X4	T42.3X5	T42.3X6
Methazolamide	T50.2X1	T50.2X2	T50.2X3	T50.2X4	T50.2X5	T50.2X6
Methdilazine	T43.3X1	T43.3X2	T43.3X3	T43.3X4	T43.3X5	T43.3X6
Methedrine	T43.621	T43.622	T43.623	T43.624	T43.625	T43.626
Methenamine (mandelate)	T37.8X1	T37.8X2	T37.8X3	T37.8X4	T37.8X5	T37.8X6
Methenolone	T38.7X1	T38.7X2	T38.7X3	T38.7X4	T38.7X5	T38.7X6
Methergine	T48.0X1	T48.0X2	T48.0X3	T48.0X4	T48.0X5	T48.0X6
Methetoin	T42.0X1	T42.0X2	T42.0X3	T42.0X4	T42.0X5	T42.0X6
Methiacil	T38.2X1	T38.2X2	T38.2X3	T38.2X4	T38.2X5	T38.2X6
Methicillin	T36.0X1	T36.0X2	T36.0X3	T36.0X4	T36.0X5	T36.0X6
Methimazole	T38.2X1	T38.2X2	T38.2X3	T38.2X4	T38.2X5	T38.2X6
Methiodal sodium	T50.8X1	T50.8X2	T50.8X3	T50.8X4	T50.8X5	T50.8X6
Methionine	T50.991	T50.992	T50.993	T50.994	T50.995	T50.996
Methisazone	T37.5X1	T37.5X2	T37.5X3	T37.5X4	T37.5X5	T37.5X6
Methisoprinol	T37.5X1	T37.5X2	T37.5X3	T37.5X4	T37.5X5	T37.5X6
Methitural	T42.3X1	T42.3X2	T42.3X3	T42.3X4	T42.3X5	T42.3X6
Methixene	T44.3X1	T44.3X2	T44.3X3	T44.3X4	T44.3X5	T44.3X6
Methobarbital, methobarbitone	T42.3X1	T42.3X2	T42.3X3	T42.3X4	T42.3X5	T42.3X6
Methocarbamol	T42.8X1	T42.8X2	T42.8X3	T42.8X4	T42.8X5	T42.8X6
skeletal muscle relaxant	T48.1X1	T48.1X2	T48.1X3	T48.1X4	T48.1X5	T48.1X6
Methohexital	T41.1X1	T41.1X2	T41.1X3	T41.1X4	T41.1X5	T41.1X6
Methohexitone	T41.1X1	T41.1X2	T41.1X3	T41.1X4	T41.1X5	T41.1X6
Methoin	T42.0X1	T42.0X2	T42.0X3	T42.0X4	T42.0X5	T42.0X6
Methopholine	T39.8X1	T39.8X2	T39.8X3	T39.8X4	T39.8X5	T39.8X6
Methopromazine	T43.3X1	T43.3X2	T43.3X3	T43.3X4	T43.3X5	T43.3X6
Methorate	T48.3X1	T48.3X2	T48.3X3	T48.3X4	T48.3X5	T48.3X6
Methoserpidine	T46.5X1	T46.5X2	T46.5X3	T46.5X4	T46.5X5	T46.5X6
Methotrexate	T45.1X1	T45.1X2	T45.1X3	T45.1X4	T45.1X5	T45.1X6
Methotrimeprazine	T43.3X1	T43.3X2	T43.3X3	T43.3X4	T43.3X5	T43.3X6
Methoxa-Dome	T49.3X1	T49.3X2	T49.3X3	T49.3X4	T49.3X5	T49.3X6
Methoxamine	T44.4X1	T44.4X2	T44.4X3	T44.4X4	T44.4X5	T44.4X6
Methoxsalen	T50.991	T50.992	T50.993	T50.994	T50.995	T50.996
Methoxyaniline	T65.3X1	T65.3X2	T65.3X3	T65.3X4	—	—
Methoxybenzyl penicillin	T36.0X1	T36.0X2	T36.0X3	T36.0X4	T36.0X5	T36.0X6
Methoxychlor	T53.7X1	T53.7X2	T53.7X3	T53.7X4	—	—
Methoxy-DDT	T53.7X1	T53.7X2	T53.7X3	T53.7X4	—	—
2-Methoxyethanol	T52.3X1	T52.3X2	T52.3X3	T52.3X4	—	—
Methoxyflurane	T41.0X1	T41.0X2	T41.0X3	T41.0X4	T41.0X5	T41.0X6
Methoxyphenamine	T48.6X1	T48.6X2	T48.6X3	T48.6X4	T48.6X5	T48.6X6
Methoxypromazine	T43.3X1	T43.3X2	T43.3X3	T43.3X4	T43.3X5	T43.3X6

◀ New ◀ Revised ~~deleted~~ Deleted

Substance	External Cause (T-Code)					
	Poisoning, Accidental (Unintentional)	Poisoning, Intentional Self-Harm	Poisoning, Assault	Poisoning, Undetermined	Adverse Effect	Underdosing
5-Methoxypsoralen (5-MOP)	T50.991	T50.992	T50.993	T50.994	T50.995	T50.996
8-Methoxypsoralen (8-MOP)	T50.991	T50.992	T50.993	T50.994	T50.995	T50.996
Methscopolamine bromide	T44.3X1	T44.3X2	T44.3X3	T44.3X4	T44.3X5	T44.3X6
Methsuximide	T42.2X1	T42.2X2	T42.2X3	T42.2X4	T42.2X5	T42.2X6
Methyclothiazide	T50.2X1	T50.2X2	T50.2X3	T50.2X4	T50.2X5	T50.2X6
Methyl						
acetate	T52.4X1	T52.4X2	T52.4X3	T52.4X4	—	—
acetone	T52.4X1	T52.4X2	T52.4X3	T52.4X4	—	—
acrylate	T65.891	T65.892	T65.893	T65.894	—	—
alcohol	T51.1X1	T51.1X2	T51.1X3	T51.1X4	—	—
aminophenol	T65.3X1	T65.3X2	T65.3X3	T65.3X4	—	—
amphetamine	T43.621	T43.622	T43.623	T43.624	T43.625	T43.626
androstanolone	T38.7X1	T38.7X2	T38.7X3	T38.7X4	T38.7X5	T38.7X6
atropine	T44.3X1	T44.3X2	T44.3X3	T44.3X4	T44.3X5	T44.3X6
benzene	T52.2X1	T52.2X2	T52.2X3	T52.2X4	—	—
benzoate	T52.8X1	T52.8X2	T52.8X3	T52.8X4	—	—
benzol	T52.2X1	T52.2X2	T52.2X3	T52.2X4	—	—
bromide (gas)	T59.891	T59.892	T59.893	T59.894	—	—
fumigant	T60.8X1	T60.8X2	T60.8X3	T60.8X4	—	—
butanol	T51.3X1	T51.3X2	T51.3X3	T51.3X4	—	—
carbinol	T51.1X1	T51.1X2	T51.1X3	T51.1X4	—	—
carbonate	T52.8X1	T52.8X2	T52.8X3	T52.8X4	—	—
CCNU	T45.1X1	T45.1X2	T45.1X3	T45.1X4	T45.1X5	T45.1X6
cellosolve	T52.91	T52.92	T52.93	T52.94	—	—
cellulose	T47.4X1	T47.4X2	T47.4X3	T47.4X4	T47.4X5	T47.4X6
chloride (gas)	T59.891	T59.892	T59.893	T59.894	—	—
chloroformate	T59.3X1	T59.3X2	T59.3X3	T59.3X4	—	—
cyclohexane	T52.8X1	T52.8X2	T52.8X3	T52.8X4	—	—
cyclohexanol	T51.8X1	T51.8X2	T51.8X3	T51.8X4	—	—
cyclohexanone	T52.8X1	T52.8X2	T52.8X3	T52.8X4	—	—
cyclohexyl acetate	T52.8X1	T52.8X2	T52.8X3	T52.8X4	—	—
demeton	T60.0X1	T60.0X2	T60.0X3	T60.0X4	—	—
dihydromorphinone	T40.2X1	T40.2X2	T40.2X3	T40.2X4	T40.2X5	T40.2X6
ergometrine	T48.0X1	T48.0X2	T48.0X3	T48.0X4	T48.0X5	T48.0X6
ergonovine	T48.0X1	T48.0X2	T48.0X3	T48.0X4	T48.0X5	T48.0X6
ethyl ketone	T52.4X1	T52.4X2	T52.4X3	T52.4X4	—	—
glucamine antimonate	T37.8X1	T37.8X2	T37.8X3	T37.8X4	T37.8X5	T37.8X6
hydrazine	T65.891	T65.892	T65.893	T65.894	—	—
iodide	T65.891	T65.892	T65.893	T65.894	—	—
isobutyl ketone	T52.4X1	T52.4X2	T52.4X3	T52.4X4	—	—
isothiocyanate	T60.3X1	T60.3X2	T60.3X3	T60.3X4	—	—
mercaptan	T59.891	T59.892	T59.893	T59.894	—	—

Substance	External Cause (T-Code)					
	Poisoning, Accidental (Unintentional)	Poisoning, Intentional Self-Harm	Poisoning, Assault	Poisoning, Undetermined	Adverse Effect	Underdosing
Methyl (Continued)						
morphine NEC	T40.2X1	T40.2X2	T40.2X3	T40.2X4	T40.2X5	T40.2X6
nicotinate	T49.4X1	T49.4X2	T49.4X3	T49.4X4	T49.4X5	T49.4X6
paraben	T49.0X1	T49.0X2	T49.0X3	T49.0X4	T49.0X5	T49.0X6
parafynol	T42.6X1	T42.6X2	T42.6X3	T42.6X4	T42.6X5	T42.6X6
parathion	T60.0X1	T60.0X2	T60.0X3	T60.0X4	—	—
peridol	T43.4X1	T43.4X2	T43.4X3	T43.4X4	T43.4X5	T43.4X6
phenidate	T43.631	T43.632	T43.633	T43.634	T43.635	T43.636
prednisolone	T38.0X1	T38.0X2	T38.0X3	T38.0X4	T38.0X5	T38.0X6
ENT agent	T49.6X1	T49.6X2	T49.6X3	T49.6X4	T49.6X5	T49.6X6
ophthalmic preparation	T49.5X1	T49.5X2	T49.5X3	T49.5X4	T49.5X5	T49.5X6
topical NEC	T49.0X1	T49.0X2	T49.0X3	T49.0X4	T49.0X5	T49.0X6
propylcarbinol	T51.3X1	T51.3X2	T51.3X3	T51.3X4	—	—
rosaniline NEC	T49.0X1	T49.0X2	T49.0X3	T49.0X4	T49.0X5	T49.0X6
salicylate	T49.2X1	T49.2X2	T49.2X3	T49.2X4	T49.2X5	T49.2X6
sulfate (fumes)	T59.891	T59.892	T59.893	T59.894	—	—
liquid	T52.8X1	T52.8X2	T52.8X3	T52.8X4	—	—
sulfonal	T42.6X1	T42.6X2	T42.6X3	T42.6X4	T42.6X5	T42.6X6
testosterone	T38.7X1	T38.7X2	T38.7X3	T38.7X4	T38.7X5	T38.7X6
thiouracil	T38.2X1	T38.2X2	T38.2X3	T38.2X4	T38.2X5	T38.2X6
Methylamphetamine	T43.621	T43.622	T43.623	T43.624	T43.625	T43.626
Methylated spirit	T51.1X1	T51.1X2	T51.1X3	T51.1X4	—	—
Methylatropine nitrate	T44.3X1	T44.3X2	T44.3X3	T44.3X4	T44.3X5	T44.3X6
Methylbenactyzium bromide	T44.3X1	T44.3X2	T44.3X3	T44.3X4	T44.3X5	T44.3X6
Methylbenzethonium chloride	T49.0X1	T49.0X2	T49.0X3	T49.0X4	T49.0X5	T49.0X6
Methylcellulose	T47.4X1	T47.4X2	T47.4X3	T47.4X4	T47.4X5	T47.4X6
laxative	T47.4X1	T47.4X2	T47.4X3	T47.4X4	T47.4X5	T47.4X6
Methylchlorophenoxy-acetic acid	T60.3X1	T60.3X2	T60.3X3	T60.3X4	—	—
Methyldopa	T46.5X1	T46.5X2	T46.5X3	T46.5X4	T46.5X5	T46.5X6
Methyldopate	T46.5X1	T46.5X2	T46.5X3	T46.5X4	T46.5X5	T46.5X6
Methylene						
blue	T50.6X1	T50.6X2	T50.6X3	T50.6X4	T50.6X5	T50.6X6
chloride or dichloride (solvent) NEC	T53.4X1	T53.4X2	T53.4X3	T53.4X4	—	—
Methylenedioxyamphet-amine	T43.621	T43.622	T43.623	T43.624	T43.625	T43.626
Methylenedioxymethamphetamine	T43.621	T43.622	T43.623	T43.624	T43.625	T43.626
Methylergometrine	T48.0X1	T48.0X2	T48.0X3	T48.0X4	T48.0X5	T48.0X6
Methylergonovine	T48.0X1	T48.0X2	T48.0X3	T48.0X4	T48.0X5	T48.0X6
Methylestrenolone	T38.5X1	T38.5X2	T38.5X3	T38.5X4	T38.5X5	T38.5X6
Methylethyl cellulose	T50.991	T50.992	T50.993	T50.994	T50.995	T50.996
Methylhexabital	T42.3X1	T42.3X2	T42.3X3	T42.3X4	T42.3X5	T42.3X6
Methylmorphine	T40.2X1	T40.2X2	T40.2X3	T40.2X4	T40.2X5	T40.2X6

◀ New ◀|||| Revised ~~deleted~~ Deleted

TABLE OF DRUGS AND CHEMICALS

Substance	External Cause (T-Code)					
	Poisoning, Accidental (Unintentional)	Poisoning, Intentional Self-Harm	Poisoning, Assault	Poisoning, Undetermined	Adverse Effect	Underdosing
Methylparaben (ophthalmic)	T49.5X1	T49.5X2	T49.5X3	T49.5X4	T49.5X5	T49.5X6
Methylparafynol	T42.6X1	T42.6X2	T42.6X3	T42.6X4	T42.6X5	T42.6X6
Methylpentynol, methylpenthynol	T42.6X1	T42.6X2	T42.6X3	T42.6X4	T42.6X5	T42.6X6
Methylphenidate	T43.631	T43.632	T43.633	T43.634	T43.635	T43.636
Methylphenobarbital	T42.3X1	T42.3X2	T42.3X3	T42.3X4	T42.3X5	T42.3X6
Methylpolysiloxane	T47.1X1	T47.1X2	T47.1X3	T47.1X4	T47.1X5	T47.1X6
Methylprednisolone — see Methyl, prednisolone						
Methylrosaniline	T49.0X1	T49.0X2	T49.0X3	T49.0X4	T49.0X5	T49.0X6
Methylrosanilinium chloride	T49.0X1	T49.0X2	T49.0X3	T49.0X4	T49.0X5	T49.0X6
Methyltestosterone	T38.7X1	T38.7X2	T38.7X3	T38.7X4	T38.7X5	T38.7X6
Methylthionine chloride	T50.6X1	T50.6X2	T50.6X3	T50.6X4	T50.6X5	T50.6X6
Methylthioninium chloride	T50.6X1	T50.6X2	T50.6X3	T50.6X4	T50.6X5	T50.6X6
Methylthiouracil	T38.2X1	T38.2X2	T38.2X3	T38.2X4	T38.2X5	T38.2X6
Methyprylon	T42.6X1	T42.6X2	T42.6X3	T42.6X4	T42.6X5	T42.6X6
Methysergide	T46.5X1	T46.5X2	T46.5X3	T46.5X4	T46.5X5	T46.5X6
Metiamide	T47.1X1	T47.1X2	T47.1X3	T47.1X4	T47.1X5	T47.1X6
Meticillin	T36.0X1	T36.0X2	T36.0X3	T36.0X4	T36.0X5	T36.0X6
Meticrane	T50.2X1	T50.2X2	T50.2X3	T50.2X4	T50.2X5	T50.2X6
Metildigoxin	T46.0X1	T46.0X2	T46.0X3	T46.0X4	T46.0X5	T46.0X6
Metipranolol	T49.5X1	T49.5X2	T49.5X3	T49.5X4	T49.5X5	T49.5X6
Metirosine	T46.5X1	T46.5X2	T46.5X3	T46.5X4	T46.5X5	T46.5X6
Metisazone	T37.5X1	T37.5X2	T37.5X3	T37.5X4	T37.5X5	T37.5X6
Metixene	T44.3X1	T44.3X2	T44.3X3	T44.3X4	T44.3X5	T44.3X6
Metizoline	T48.5X1	T48.5X2	T48.5X3	T48.5X4	T48.5X5	T48.5X6
Metoclopramide	T45.0X1	T45.0X2	T45.0X3	T45.0X4	T45.0X5	T45.0X6
Metofenazate	T43.3X1	T43.3X2	T43.3X3	T43.3X4	T43.3X5	T43.3X6
Metofoline	T39.8X1	T39.8X2	T39.8X3	T39.8X4	T39.8X5	T39.8X6
Metolazone	T50.2X1	T50.2X2	T50.2X3	T50.2X4	T50.2X5	T50.2X6
Metopon	T40.2X1	T40.2X2	T40.2X3	T40.2X4	T40.2X5	T40.2X6
Metoprine	T45.1X1	T45.1X2	T45.1X3	T45.1X4	T45.1X5	T45.1X6
Metoprolol	T44.7X1	T44.7X2	T44.7X3	T44.7X4	T44.7X5	T44.7X6
Metrifonate	T60.0X1	T60.0X2	T60.0X3	T60.0X4	—	—
Metrizamide	T50.8X1	T50.8X2	T50.8X3	T50.8X4	T50.8X5	T50.8X6
Metrizoic acid	T50.8X1	T50.8X2	T50.8X3	T50.8X4	T50.8X5	T50.8X6
Metronidazole	T37.8X1	T37.8X2	T37.8X3	T37.8X4	T37.8X5	T37.8X6
Metycaine	T41.3X1	T41.3X2	T41.3X3	T41.3X4	T41.3X5	T41.3X6
infiltration (subcutaneous)	T41.3X1	T41.3X2	T41.3X3	T41.3X4	T41.3X5	T41.3X6
nerve block (peripheral) (plexus)	T41.3X1	T41.3X2	T41.3X3	T41.3X4	T41.3X5	T41.3X6
topical (surface)	T41.3X1	T41.3X2	T41.3X3	T41.3X4	T41.3X5	T41.3X6
Metyrapone	T50.8X1	T50.8X2	T50.8X3	T50.8X4	T50.8X5	T50.8X6
Mevinphos	T60.0X1	T60.0X2	T60.0X3	T60.0X4	—	—

Substance	External Cause (T-Code)					
	Poisoning, Accidental (Unintentional)	Poisoning, Intentional Self-Harm	Poisoning, Assault	Poisoning, Undetermined	Adverse Effect	Underdosing
Mexazolam	T42.4X1	T42.4X2	T42.4X3	T42.4X4	T42.4X5	T42.4X6
Mexenone	T49.3X1	T49.3X2	T49.3X3	T49.3X4	T49.3X5	T49.3X6
Mexiletine	T46.2X1	T46.2X2	T46.2X3	T46.2X4	T46.2X5	T46.2X6
Mezereon	T62.2X1	T62.2X2	T62.2X3	T62.2X4	—	—
berries	T62.1X1	T62.1X2	T62.1X3	T62.1X4	—	—
Mezlocillin	T36.0X1	T36.0X2	T36.0X3	T36.0X4	T36.0X5	T36.0X6
Mianserin	T43.021	T43.022	T43.023	T43.024	T43.025	T43.026
Micatin	T49.0X1	T49.0X2	T49.0X3	T49.0X4	T49.0X5	T49.0X6
Miconazole	T49.0X1	T49.0X2	T49.0X3	T49.0X4	T49.0X5	T49.0X6
Micronomicin	T36.5X1	T36.5X2	T36.5X3	T36.5X4	T36.5X5	T36.5X6
Midazolam	T42.4X1	T42.4X2	T42.4X3	T42.4X4	T42.4X5	T42.4X6
Midecamycin	T36.3X1	T36.3X2	T36.3X3	T36.3X4	T36.3X5	T36.3X6
Mifepristone	T38.6X1	T38.6X2	T38.6X3	T38.6X4	T38.6X5	T38.6X6
Milk of magnesia	T47.1X1	T47.1X2	T47.1X3	T47.1X4	T47.1X5	T47.1X6
Millipede (tropical) (venomous)	T63.411	T63.412	T63.413	T63.414	—	—
Miltown	T43.591	T43.592	T43.593	T43.594	T43.595	T43.596
Milverine	T44.3X1	T44.3X2	T44.3X3	T44.3X4	T44.3X5	T44.3X6
Minaprine	T43.291	T43.292	T43.293	T43.294	T43.295	T43.296
Minaxolone	T41.291	T41.292	T41.293	T41.294	T41.295	T41.296
Mineral						
acids	T54.2X1	T54.2X2	T54.2X3	T54.2X4	—	—
oil (laxative) (medicinal)	T47.4X1	T47.4X2	T47.4X3	T47.4X4	T47.4X5	T47.4X6
emulsion	T47.2X1	T47.2X2	T47.2X3	T47.2X4	T47.2X5	T47.2X6
nonmedicinal	T52.0X1	T52.0X2	T52.0X3	T52.0X4	—	—
topical	T49.3X1	T49.3X2	T49.3X3	T49.3X4	T49.3X5	T49.3X6
salt NEC	T50.3X1	T50.3X2	T50.3X3	T50.3X4	T50.3X5	T50.3X6
spirits	T52.0X1	T52.0X2	T52.0X3	T52.0X4	—	—
Mineralocorticosteroid	T50.0X1	T50.0X2	T50.0X3	T50.0X4	T50.0X5	T50.0X6
Minocycline	T36.4X1	T36.4X2	T36.4X3	T36.4X4	T36.4X5	T36.4X6
Minoxidil	T46.7X1	T46.7X2	T46.7X3	T46.7X4	T46.7X5	T46.7X6
Miokamycin	T36.3X1	T36.3X2	T36.3X3	T36.3X4	T36.3X5	T36.3X6
Miotic drug	T49.5X1	T49.5X2	T49.5X3	T49.5X4	T49.5X5	T49.5X6
Mipafox	T60.0X1	T60.0X2	T60.0X3	T60.0X4	—	—
Mirex	T60.1X1	T60.1X2	T60.1X3	T60.1X4	—	—
Mirtazapine	T43.021	T43.022	T43.023	T43.024	T43.025	T43.026
Misonidazole	T37.3X1	T37.3X2	T37.3X3	T37.3X4	T37.3X5	T37.3X6
Misoprostol	T47.1X1	T47.1X2	T47.1X3	T47.1X4	T47.1X5	T47.1X6
Mithramycin	T45.1X1	T45.1X2	T45.1X3	T45.1X4	T45.1X5	T45.1X6
Mitobronitol	T45.1X1	T45.1X2	T45.1X3	T45.1X4	T45.1X5	T45.1X6
Mitoguazone	T45.1X1	T45.1X2	T45.1X3	T45.1X4	T45.1X5	T45.1X6
Mitolactol	T45.1X1	T45.1X2	T45.1X3	T45.1X4	T45.1X5	T45.1X6
Mitomycin	T45.1X1	T45.1X2	T45.1X3	T45.1X4	T45.1X5	T45.1X6

◀ New   ◀▥▥ Revised   ~~deleted~~ Deleted

Substance	Poisoning, Accidental (Unintentional)	Poisoning, Intentional Self-Harm	Poisoning, Assault	Poisoning, Undetermined	Adverse Effect	Underdosing
	External Cause (T-Code)					
Mitopodozide	T45.1X1	T45.1X2	T45.1X3	T45.1X4	T45.1X5	T45.1X6
Mitotane	T45.1X1	T45.1X2	T45.1X3	T45.1X4	T45.1X5	T45.1X6
Mitoxantrone	T45.1X1	T45.1X2	T45.1X3	T45.1X4	T45.1X5	T45.1X6
Mivacurium chloride	T48.1X1	T48.1X2	T48.1X3	T48.1X4	T48.1X5	T48.1X6
Miyari bacteria	T47.6X1	T47.6X2	T47.6X3	T47.6X4	T47.6X5	T47.6X6
Moclobemide	T43.1X1	T43.1X2	T43.1X3	T43.1X4	T43.1X5	T43.1X6
Moderil	T46.5X1	T46.5X2	T46.5X3	T46.5X4	T46.5X5	T46.5X6
Mofebutazone	T39.2X1	T39.2X2	T39.2X3	T39.2X4	T39.2X5	T39.2X6
Mogadon — see Nitrazepam						
Molindone	T43.591	T43.592	T43.593	T43.594	T43.595	T43.596
Molsidomine	T46.3X1	T46.3X2	T46.3X3	T46.3X4	T46.3X5	T46.3X6
Mometasone	T49.0X1	T49.0X2	T49.0X3	T49.0X4	T49.0X5	T49.0X6
Monistat	T49.0X1	T49.0X2	T49.0X3	T49.0X4	T49.0X5	T49.0X6
Monkshood	T62.2X1	T62.2X2	T62.2X3	T62.2X4	—	—
Monoamine oxidase inhibitor NEC	T43.1X1	T43.1X2	T43.1X3	T43.1X4	T43.1X5	T43.1X6
hydrazine	T43.1X1	T43.1X2	T43.1X3	T43.1X4	T43.1X5	T43.1X6
Monobenzone	T49.4X1	T49.4X2	T49.4X3	T49.4X4	T49.4X5	T49.4X6
Monochloroacetic acid	T60.3X1	T60.3X2	T60.3X3	T60.3X4	—	—
Monochlorobenzene	T53.7X1	T53.7X2	T53.7X3	T53.7X4	—	—
Monoethanolamine	T46.8X1	T46.8X2	T46.8X3	T46.8X4	T46.8X5	T46.8X6
oleate	T46.8X1	T46.8X2	T46.8X3	T46.8X4	T46.8X5	T46.8X6
Monooctanoin	T50.991	T50.992	T50.993	T50.994	T50.995	T50.996
Monophenylbutazone	T39.2X1	T39.2X2	T39.2X3	T39.2X4	T39.2X5	T39.2X6
Monosodium glutamate	T65.891	T65.892	T65.893	T65.894	—	—
Monosulfiram	T49.0X1	T49.0X2	T49.0X3	T49.0X4	T49.0X5	T49.0X6
Monoxide, carbon — see Carbon, monoxide	T57.91	T57.92	T57.93	T57.94		
Monoxidine hydrochloride	T46.1X1	T46.1X2	T46.1X3	T46.1X4	T46.1X5	T46.1X6
Monuron	T60.3X1	T60.3X2	T60.3X3	T60.3X4	—	—
Moperone	T43.4X1	T43.4X2	T43.4X3	T43.4X4	T43.4X5	T43.4X6
Mopidamol	T45.1X1	T45.1X2	T45.1X3	T45.1X4	T45.1X5	T45.1X6
MOPP (mechlorethamine + vincristine + prednisone + procarbazine)	T45.1X1	T45.1X2	T45.1X3	T45.1X4	T45.1X5	T45.1X6
Morfin	T40.2X1	T40.2X2	T40.2X3	T40.2X4	T40.2X5	T40.2X6
Morinamide	T37.1X1	T37.1X2	T37.1X3	T37.1X4	T37.1X5	T37.1X6
Morning glory seeds	T40.991	T40.992	T40.993	T40.994	—	—
Moroxydine	T37.5X1	T37.5X2	T37.5X3	T37.5X4	T37.5X5	T37.5X6
Morphazinamide	T37.1X1	T37.1X2	T37.1X3	T37.1X4	T37.1X5	T37.1X6
Morphine	T40.2X1	T40.2X2	T40.2X3	T40.2X4	T40.2X5	T40.2X6
antagonist	T50.7X1	T50.7X2	T50.7X3	T50.7X4	T50.7X5	T50.7X6
Morpholinylethylmorphine	T40.2X1	T40.2X2	T40.2X3	T40.2X4	—	—
Morsuximide	T42.2X1	T42.2X2	T42.2X3	T42.2X4	T42.2X5	T42.2X6

Substance	Poisoning, Accidental (Unintentional)	Poisoning, Intentional Self-Harm	Poisoning, Assault	Poisoning, Undetermined	Adverse Effect	Underdosing
	External Cause (T-Code)					
Mosapramine	T43.591	T43.592	T43.593	T43.594	T43.595	T43.596
Moth balls — see also Pesticides	T60.2X1	T60.2X2	T60.2X3	T60.2X4	—	—
naphthalene	T60.2X1	T60.2X2	T60.2X3	T60.2X4	—	—
paradichlorobenzene	T60.1X1	T60.1X2	T60.1X3	T60.1X4	—	—
Motor exhaust gas	T58.01	T58.02	T58.03	T58.04		
Mouthwash (antiseptic) (zinc chloride)	T49.6X1	T49.6X2	T49.6X3	T49.6X4	T49.6X5	T49.6X6
Moxastine	T45.0X1	T45.0X2	T45.0X3	T45.0X4	T45.0X5	T45.0X6
Moxaverine	T44.3X1	T44.3X2	T44.3X3	T44.3X4	T44.3X5	T44.3X6
Moxifensine	T43.291	T43.292	T43.293	T43.294	T43.295	T43.296
Moxisylyte	T46.7X1	T46.7X2	T46.7X3	T46.7X4	T46.7X5	T46.7X6
Mucilage, plant	T47.4X1	T47.4X2	T47.4X3	T47.4X4	T47.4X5	T47.4X6
Mucolytic drug	T48.4X1	T48.4X2	T48.4X3	T48.4X4	T48.4X5	T48.4X6
Mucomyst	T48.4X1	T48.4X2	T48.4X3	T48.4X4	T48.4X5	T48.4X6
Mucous membrane agents (external)	T49.91	T49.92	T49.93	T49.94	T49.95	T49.96
specified NEC	T49.8X1	T49.8X2	T49.8X3	T49.8X4	T49.8X5	T49.8X6
Mumps						
immune globulin (human)	T50.Z11	T50.Z12	T50.Z13	T50.Z14	T50.Z15	T50.Z16
skin test antigen	T50.8X1	T50.8X2	T50.8X3	T50.8X4	T50.8X5	T50.8X6
vaccine	T50.B91	T50.B92	T50.B93	T50.B94	T50.B95	T50.B96
Mumpsvax	T50.B91	T50.B92	T50.B93	T50.B94	T50.B95	T50.B96
Mupirocin	T49.0X1	T49.0X2	T49.0X3	T49.0X4	T49.0X5	T49.0X6
Muriatic acid — see Hydrochloric acid						
Muromonab-CD3	T45.1X1	T45.1X2	T45.1X3	T45.1X4	T45.1X5	T45.1X6
Muscle relaxant — see Relaxant, muscle						
Muscle-action drug NEC	T48.201	T48.202	T48.203	T48.204	T48.205	T48.206
Muscle affecting agents NEC	T48.201	T48.202	T48.203	T48.204	T48.205	T48.206
oxytocic	T48.0X1	T48.0X2	T48.0X3	T48.0X4	T48.0X5	T48.0X6
relaxants	T48.201	T48.202	T48.203	T48.204	T48.205	T48.206
central nervous system	T42.8X1	T42.8X2	T42.8X3	T42.8X4	T42.8X5	T42.8X6
skeletal	T48.1X1	T48.1X2	T48.1X3	T48.1X4	T48.1X5	T48.1X6
smooth	T44.3X1	T44.3X2	T44.3X3	T44.3X4	T44.3X5	T44.3X6
Muscle-tone depressant, central NEC	T42.8X1	T42.8X2	T42.8X3	T42.8X4	T42.8X5	T42.8X6
specified NEC	T42.8X1	T42.8X2	T42.8X3	T42.8X4	T42.8X5	T42.8X6
Mushroom, noxious	T62.0X1	T62.0X2	T62.0X3	T62.0X4	—	—
Mussel, noxious	T61.781	T61.782	T61.783	T61.784	—	—
Mustard (emetic)	T47.7X1	T47.7X2	T47.7X3	T47.7X4	T47.7X5	T47.7X6
black	T47.7X1	T47.7X2	T47.7X3	T47.7X4	T47.7X5	T47.7X6
gas, not in war	T59.91	T59.92	T59.93	T59.94	—	—
nitrogen	T45.1X1	T45.1X2	T45.1X3	T45.1X4	T45.1X5	T45.1X6

Substance	Poisoning, Accidental (Unintentional)	Poisoning, Intentional Self-Harm	Poisoning, Assault	Poisoning, Undetermined	Adverse Effect	Underdosing
External Cause (T-Code)						
Mustine	T45.1X1	T45.1X2	T45.1X3	T45.1X4	T45.1X5	T45.1X6
M-vac	T45.1X1	T45.1X2	T45.1X3	T45.1X4	T45.1X5	T45.1X6
Mycifradin	T36.5X1	T36.5X2	T36.5X3	T36.5X4	T36.5X5	T36.5X6
topical	T49.0X1	T49.0X2	T49.0X3	T49.0X4	T49.0X5	T49.0X6
Mycitracin	T36.8X1	T36.8X2	T36.8X3	T36.8X4	T36.8X5	T36.8X6
ophthalmic preparation	T49.5X1	T49.5X2	T49.5X3	T49.5X4	T49.5X5	T49.5X6
Mycostatin	T36.7X1	T36.7X2	T36.7X3	T36.7X4	T36.7X5	T36.7X6
topical	T49.0X1	T49.0X2	T49.0X3	T49.0X4	T49.0X5	T49.0X6
Mycotoxins	T64.81	T64.82	T64.83	T64.84	—	—
aflatoxin	T64.01	T64.02	T64.03	T64.04	—	—
specified NEC	T64.81	T64.82	T64.83	T64.84	—	—
Mydriacyl	T44.3X1	T44.3X2	T44.3X3	T44.3X4	T44.3X5	T44.3X6
Mydriatic drug	T49.5X1	T49.5X2	T49.5X3	T49.5X4	T49.5X5	T49.5X6
Myelobromal	T45.1X1	T45.1X2	T45.1X3	T45.1X4	T45.1X5	T45.1X6
Myleran	T45.1X1	T45.1X2	T45.1X3	T45.1X4	T45.1X5	T45.1X6
Myochrysin(e)	T39.2X1	T39.2X2	T39.2X3	T39.2X4	T39.2X5	T39.2X6
Myoneural blocking agents	T48.1X1	T48.1X2	T48.1X3	T48.1X4	T48.1X5	T48.1X6
Myralact	T49.0X1	T49.0X2	T49.0X3	T49.0X4	T49.0X5	T49.0X6
Myristica fragrans	T62.2X1	T62.2X2	T62.2X3	T62.2X4	—	—
Myristicin	T65.891	T65.892	T65.893	T65.894	—	—
Mysoline	T42.3X1	T42.3X2	T42.3X3	T42.3X4	T42.3X5	T42.3X6
N						
Nabilone	T40.7X1	T40.7X2	T40.7X3	T40.7X4	T40.7X5	T40.7X6
Nabumetone	T39.391	T39.392	T39.393	T39.394	T39.395	T39.396
Nadolol	T44.7X1	T44.7X2	T44.7X3	T44.7X4	T44.7X5	T44.7X6
Nafcillin	T36.0X1	T36.0X2	T36.0X3	T36.0X4	T36.0X5	T36.0X6
Nafoxidine	T38.6X1	T38.6X2	T38.6X3	T38.6X4	T38.6X5	T38.6X6
Naftazone	T46.991	T46.992	T46.993	T46.994	T46.995	T46.996
Naftidrofuryl (oxalate)	T46.7X1	T46.7X2	T46.7X3	T46.7X4	T46.7X5	T46.7X6
Naftifine	T49.0X1	T49.0X2	T49.0X3	T49.0X4	T49.0X5	T49.0X6
Nail polish remover	T52.91	T52.92	T52.93	T52.94	—	—
Nalbuphine	T40.4X1	T40.4X2	T40.4X3	T40.4X4	T40.4X5	T40.4X6
Naled	T60.0X1	T60.0X2	T60.0X3	T60.0X4	—	—
Nalidixic acid	T37.8X1	T37.8X2	T37.8X3	T37.8X4	T37.8X5	T37.8X6
Nalorphine	T50.7X1	T50.7X2	T50.7X3	T50.7X4	T50.7X5	T50.7X6
Naloxone	T50.7X1	T50.7X2	T50.7X3	T50.7X4	T50.7X5	T50.7X6
Naltrexone	T50.7X1	T50.7X2	T50.7X3	T50.7X4	T50.7X5	T50.7X6
Namenda	T43.8X1	T43.8X2	T43.8X3	T43.8X4	T43.8X5	T43.8X6
Nandrolone	T38.7X1	T38.7X2	T38.7X3	T38.7X4	T38.7X5	T38.7X6
Naphazoline	T48.5X1	T48.5X2	T48.5X3	T48.5X4	T48.5X5	T48.5X6

Substance	Poisoning, Accidental (Unintentional)	Poisoning, Intentional Self-Harm	Poisoning, Assault	Poisoning, Undetermined	Adverse Effect	Underdosing
External Cause (T-Code)						
Naphtha (painters') (petroleum)	T52.0X1	T52.0X2	T52.0X3	T52.0X4	—	—
solvent	T52.0X1	T52.0X2	T52.0X3	T52.0X4	—	—
vapor	T52.0X1	T52.0X2	T52.0X3	T52.0X4	—	—
Naphthalene (non-chlorinated)	T60.2X1	T60.2X2	T60.2X3	T60.2X4	—	—
chlorinated	T60.1X1	T60.1X2	T60.1X3	T60.1X4	—	—
vapor	T60.1X1	T60.1X2	T60.1X3	T60.1X4	—	—
insecticide or moth repellent	T60.2X1	T60.2X2	T60.2X3	T60.2X4	—	—
chlorinated	T60.1X1	T60.1X2	T60.1X3	T60.1X4	—	—
vapor	T60.2X1	T60.2X2	T60.2X3	T60.2X4	—	—
chlorinated	T60.1X1	T60.1X2	T60.1X3	T60.1X4	—	—
Naphthol	T65.891	T65.892	T65.893	T65.894	—	—
Naphthylamine	T65.891	T65.892	T65.893	T65.894	—	—
Naphthylthiourea (ANTU)	T60.4X1	T60.4X2	T60.4X3	T60.4X4	—	—
Naprosyn — see Naproxen						
Naproxen	T39.311	T39.312	T39.313	T39.314	T39.315	T39.316
Narcotic (drug)	T40.601	T40.602	T40.603	T40.604	T40.605	T40.606
analgesic NEC	T40.601	T40.602	T40.603	T40.604	T40.605	T40.606
antagonist	T50.7X1	T50.7X2	T50.7X3	T50.7X4	T50.7X5	T50.7X6
specified NEC	T40.691	T40.692	T40.693	T40.694	T40.695	T40.696
synthetic	T40.4X1	T40.4X2	T40.4X3	T40.4X4	T40.4X5	T40.4X6
Narcotine	T48.3X1	T48.3X2	T48.3X3	T48.3X4	T48.3X5	T48.3X6
Nardil	T43.1X1	T43.1X2	T43.1X3	T43.1X4	T43.1X5	T43.1X6
Nasal drug NEC	T49.6X1	T49.6X2	T49.6X3	T49.6X4	T49.6X5	T49.6X6
Natamycin	T49.0X1	T49.0X2	T49.0X3	T49.0X4	T49.0X5	T49.0X6
Natrium cyanide — see Cyanide(s)						
Natural gas	T59.891	T59.892	T59.893	T59.894	—	—
incomplete combustion	T57.91	T57.92	T57.93	T57.94	—	—
Natural						
blood (product)	T45.8X1	T45.8X2	T45.8X3	T45.8X4	T45.8X5	T45.8X6
gas (piped)	T59.891	T59.892	T59.893	T59.894	—	—
incomplete combustion	T58.11	T58.12	T58.13	T58.14	—	—
Nealbarbital	T42.3X1	T42.3X2	T42.3X3	T42.3X4	T42.3X5	T42.3X6
Nectadon	T48.3X1	T48.3X2	T48.3X3	T48.3X4	T48.3X5	T48.3X6
Nedocromil	T48.6X1	T48.6X2	T48.6X3	T48.6X4	T48.6X5	T48.6X6
Nefopam	T39.8X1	T39.8X2	T39.8X3	T39.8X4	T39.8X5	T39.8X6
Nematocyst (sting)	T63.691	T63.692	T63.693	T63.694	—	—
Nembutal	T42.3X1	T42.3X2	T42.3X3	T42.3X4	T42.3X5	T42.3X6
Nemonapride	T43.591	T43.592	T43.593	T43.594	T43.595	T43.596
Neoarsphenamine	T37.8X1	T37.8X2	T37.8X3	T37.8X4	T37.8X5	T37.8X6

◄ New ◄ Revised ~~deleted~~ Deleted

Substance	Poisoning, Accidental (Unintentional)	Poisoning, Intentional Self-Harm	Poisoning, Assault	Poisoning, Undetermined	Adverse Effect	Underdosing
Neocinchophen	T50.4X1	T50.4X2	T50.4X3	T50.4X4	T50.4X5	T50.4X6
Neomycin (derivatives)	T36.5X1	T36.5X2	T36.5X3	T36.5X4	T36.5X5	T36.5X6
with						
bacitracin	T49.0X1	T49.0X2	T49.0X3	T49.0X4	T49.0X5	T49.0X6
neostigmine	T44.0X1	T44.0X2	T44.0X3	T44.0X4	T44.0X5	T44.0X6
ENT agent	T49.6X1	T49.6X2	T49.6X3	T49.6X4	T49.6X5	T49.6X6
ophthalmic preparation	T49.5X1	T49.5X2	T49.5X3	T49.5X4	T49.5X5	T49.5X6
topical NEC	T49.0X1	T49.0X2	T49.0X3	T49.0X4	T49.0X5	T49.0X6
Neonal	T42.3X1	T42.3X2	T42.3X3	T42.3X4	T42.3X5	T42.3X6
Neoprontosil	T37.0X1	T37.0X2	T37.0X3	T37.0X4	T37.0X5	T37.0X6
Neosalvarsan	T37.8X1	T37.8X2	T37.8X3	T37.8X4	T37.8X5	T37.8X6
Neosilversalvarsan	T37.8X1	T37.8X2	T37.8X3	T37.8X4	T37.8X5	T37.8X6
Neosporin	T36.8X1	T36.8X2	T36.8X3	T36.8X4	T36.8X5	T36.8X6
ENT agent	T49.6X1	T49.6X2	T49.6X3	T49.6X4	T49.6X5	T49.6X6
opthalmic preparation	T49.5X1	T49.5X2	T49.5X3	T49.5X4	T49.5X5	T49.5X6
topical NEC	T49.0X1	T49.0X2	T49.0X3	T49.0X4	T49.0X5	T49.0X6
Neostigmine bromide	T44.0X1	T44.0X2	T44.0X3	T44.0X4	T44.0X5	T44.0X6
Neraval	T42.3X1	T42.3X2	T42.3X3	T42.3X4	T42.3X5	T42.3X6
Neravan	T42.3X1	T42.3X2	T42.3X3	T42.3X4	T42.3X5	T42.3X6
Nerium oleander	T62.2X1	T62.2X2	T62.2X3	T62.2X4	—	—
Nerve gas, not in war	T59.91	T59.92	T59.93	T59.94	—	—
Nesacaine	T41.3X1	T41.3X2	T41.3X3	T41.3X4	T41.3X5	T41.3X6
infiltration (subcutaneous)	T41.3X1	T41.3X2	T41.3X3	T41.3X4	T41.3X5	T41.3X6
nerve block (peripheral) (plexus)	T41.3X1	T41.3X2	T41.3X3	T41.3X4	T41.3X5	T41.3X6
Netilmicin	T36.5X1	T36.5X2	T36.5X3	T36.5X4	T36.5X5	T36.5X6
Neurobarb	T42.3X1	T42.3X2	T42.3X3	T42.3X4	T42.3X5	T42.3X6
Neuroleptic drug NEC	T43.501	T43.502	T43.503	T43.504	T43.505	T43.506
Neuromuscular blocking drug	T48.1X1	T48.1X2	T48.1X3	T48.1X4	T48.1X5	T48.1X6
Neutral insulin injection	T38.3X1	T38.3X2	T38.3X3	T38.3X4	T38.3X5	T38.3X6
Neutral spirits	T51.0X1	T51.0X2	T51.0X3	T51.0X4	—	—
beverage	T51.0X1	T51.0X2	T51.0X3	T51.0X4	—	—
Niacin	T46.7X1	T46.7X2	T46.7X3	T46.7X4	T46.7X5	T46.7X6
Niacinamide	T45.2X1	T45.2X2	T45.2X3	T45.2X4	T45.2X5	T45.2X6
Nialamide	T43.1X1	T43.1X2	T43.1X3	T43.1X4	T43.1X5	T43.1X6
Niaprazine	T42.6X1	T42.6X2	T42.6X3	T42.6X4	T42.6X5	T42.6X6
Nicametate	T46.7X1	T46.7X2	T46.7X3	T46.7X4	T46.7X5	T46.7X6
Nicardipine	T46.1X1	T46.1X2	T46.1X3	T46.1X4	T46.1X5	T46.1X6
Nicergoline	T46.7X1	T46.7X2	T46.7X3	T46.7X4	T46.7X5	T46.7X6
Nickel (carbonyl) (tetra-carbonyl) (fumes) (vapor)	T56.891	T56.892	T56.893	T56.894	—	—

Substance	Poisoning, Accidental (Unintentional)	Poisoning, Intentional Self-Harm	Poisoning, Assault	Poisoning, Undetermined	Adverse Effect	Underdosing
Nickelocene	T56.891	T56.892	T56.893	T56.894	—	—
Niclosamide	T37.4X1	T37.4X2	T37.4X3	T37.4X4	T37.4X5	T37.4X6
Nicofuranose	T46.7X1	T46.7X2	T46.7X3	T46.7X4	T46.7X5	T46.7X6
Nicomorphine	T40.2X1	T40.2X2	T40.2X3	T40.2X4	—	—
Nicorandil	T46.3X1	T46.3X2	T46.3X3	T46.3X4	T46.3X5	T46.3X6
Nicotiana (plant)	T62.2X1	T62.2X2	T62.2X3	T62.2X4		
Nicotinamide	T45.2X1	T45.2X2	T45.2X3	T45.2X4	T45.2X5	T45.2X6
Nicotine (insecticide) (spray) (sulfate) NEC	T60.2X1	T60.2X2	T60.2X3	T60.2X4	—	—
from tobacco	T65.291	T65.292	T65.293	T65.294	—	—
cigarettes	T65.221	T65.222	T65.223	T65.224	—	—
not insecticide	T65.291	T65.292	T65.293	T65.294	—	—
Nicotinic acid	T46.7X1	T46.7X2	T46.7X3	T46.7X4	T46.7X5	T46.7X6
Nicotinyl alcohol	T46.7X1	T46.7X2	T46.7X3	T46.7X4	T46.7X5	T46.7X6
Nicoumalone	T45.511	T45.512	T45.513	T45.514	T45.515	T45.516
Nifedipine	T46.1X1	T46.1X2	T46.1X3	T46.1X4	T46.1X5	T46.1X6
Nifenazone	T39.2X1	T39.2X2	T39.2X3	T39.2X4	T39.2X5	T39.2X6
Nifuraldezone	T37.91	T37.92	T37.93	T37.94	T37.95	T37.96
Nifuratel	T37.8X1	T37.8X2	T37.8X3	T37.8X4	T37.8X5	T37.8X6
Nifurtimox	T37.3X1	T37.3X2	T37.3X3	T37.3X4	T37.3X5	T37.3X6
Nifurtoinol	T37.8X1	T37.8X2	T37.8X3	T37.8X4	T37.8X5	T37.8X6
Nightshade, deadly (solanum) — see also Belladonna	T62.2X1	T62.2X2	T62.2X3	T62.2X4	—	—
berry	T62.1X1	T62.1X2	T62.1X3	T62.1X4	—	—
Nikethamide	T50.7X1	T50.7X2	T50.7X3	T50.7X4	T50.7X5	T50.7X6
Nilstat	T36.7X1	T36.7X2	T36.7X3	T36.7X4	T36.7X5	T36.7X6
topical	T49.0X1	T49.0X2	T49.0X3	T49.0X4	T49.0X5	T49.0X6
Nilutamide	T38.6X1	T38.6X2	T38.6X3	T38.6X4	T38.6X5	T38.6X6
Nimesulide	T39.391	T39.392	T39.393	T39.394	T39.395	T39.396
Nimetazepam	T42.4X1	T42.4X2	T42.4X3	T42.4X4	T42.4X5	T42.4X6
Nimodipine	T46.1X1	T46.1X2	T46.1X3	T46.1X4	T46.1X5	T46.1X6
Nimorazole	T37.3X1	T37.3X2	T37.3X3	T37.3X4	T37.3X5	T37.3X6
Nimustine	T45.1X1	T45.1X2	T45.1X3	T45.1X4	T45.1X5	T45.1X6
Niridazole	T37.4X1	T37.4X2	T37.4X3	T37.4X4	T37.4X5	T37.4X6
Nisentil	T40.2X1	T40.2X2	T40.2X3	T40.2X4	T40.2X5	T40.2X6
Nisoldipine	T46.1X1	T46.1X2	T46.1X3	T46.1X4	T46.1X5	T46.1X6
Nitramine	T65.3X1	T65.3X2	T65.3X3	T65.3X4	—	—
Nitrate, organic	T46.3X1	T46.3X2	T46.3X3	T46.3X4	T46.3X5	T46.3X6
Nitrazepam	T42.4X1	T42.4X2	T42.4X3	T42.4X4	T42.4X5	T42.4X6
Nitrefazole	T50.6X1	T50.6X2	T50.6X3	T50.6X4	T50.6X5	T50.6X6
Nitrendipine	T46.1X1	T46.1X2	T46.1X3	T46.1X4	T46.1X5	T46.1X6

◀ New   ◀▥ Revised   ~~deleted~~ Deleted

TABLE OF DRUGS AND CHEMICALS

TABLE OF DRUGS AND CHEMICALS

Substance	External Cause (T-Code)					
	Poisoning, Accidental (Unintentional)	Poisoning, Intentional Self-Harm	Poisoning, Assault	Poisoning, Undetermined	Adverse Effect	Underdosing
Nitric						
acid (liquid)	T54.2X1	T54.2X2	T54.2X3	T54.2X4	—	—
vapor	T59.891	T59.892	T59.893	T59.894	—	—
oxide (gas)	T59.0X1	T59.0X2	T59.0X3	T59.0X4	—	—
Nitrimidazine	T37.3X1	T37.3X2	T37.3X3	T37.3X4	T37.3X5	T37.3X6
Nitrite, amyl (medicinal) (vapor)	T46.3X1	T46.3X2	T46.3X3	T46.3X4	T46.3X5	T46.3X6
Nitroaniline	T65.3X1	T65.3X2	T65.3X3	T65.3X4	—	—
vapor	T59.891	T59.892	T59.893	T59.894	—	—
Nitrobenzene, nitrobenzol	T65.3X1	T65.3X2	T65.3X3	T65.3X4	—	—
vapor	T65.3X1	T65.3X2	T65.3X3	T65.3X4	—	—
Nitrocellulose	T65.891	T65.892	T65.893	T65.894	—	—
lacquer	T65.891	T65.892	T65.893	T65.894	—	—
Nitrodiphenyl	T65.3X1	T65.3X2	T65.3X3	T65.3X4	—	—
Nitrofural	T49.0X1	T49.0X2	T49.0X3	T49.0X4	T49.0X5	T49.0X6
Nitrofurantoin	T37.8X1	T37.8X2	T37.8X3	T37.8X4	T37.8X5	T37.8X6
Nitrofurazone	T49.0X1	T49.0X2	T49.0X3	T49.0X4	T49.0X5	T49.0X6
Nitrogen	T59.0X1	T59.0X2	T59.0X3	T59.0X4	—	—
mustard	T45.1X1	T45.1X2	T45.1X3	T45.1X4	T45.1X5	T45.1X6
Nitroglycerin, nitro-glycerol (medicinal)	T46.3X1	T46.3X2	T46.3X3	T46.3X4	T46.3X5	T46.3X6
nonmedicinal	T65.5X1	T65.5X2	T65.5X3	T65.5X4	—	—
fumes	T65.5X1	T65.5X2	T65.5X3	T65.5X4	—	—
Nitroglycol	T52.3X1	T52.3X2	T52.3X3	T52.3X4	—	—
Nitrohydrochloric acid	T54.2X1	T54.2X2	T54.2X3	T54.2X4	—	—
Nitromersol	T49.0X1	T49.0X2	T49.0X3	T49.0X4	T49.0X5	T49.0X6
Nitronaphthalene	T65.891	T65.892	T65.893	T65.894	—	—
Nitrophenol	T54.0X1	T54.0X2	T54.0X3	T54.0X4	—	—
Nitropropane	T52.8X1	T52.8X2	T52.8X3	T52.8X4	—	—
Nitroprusside	T46.5X1	T46.5X2	T46.5X3	T46.5X4	T46.5X5	T46.5X6
Nitrosodimethylamine	T65.3X1	T65.3X2	T65.3X3	T65.3X4	—	—
Nitrothiazol	T37.4X1	T37.4X2	T37.4X3	T37.4X4	T37.4X5	T37.4X6
Nitrotoluene, nitrotoluol	T65.3X1	T65.3X2	T65.3X3	T65.3X4	—	—
vapor	T65.3X1	T65.3X2	T65.3X3	T65.3X4	—	—
Nitrous						
acid (liquid)	T54.2X1	T54.2X2	T54.2X3	T54.2X4	—	—
fumes	T59.891	T59.892	T59.893	T59.894	—	—
ether spirit	T46.3X1	T46.3X2	T46.3X3	T46.3X4	T46.3X5	T46.3X6
oxide	T41.0X1	T41.0X2	T41.0X3	T41.0X4	T41.0X5	T41.0X6
Nitroxoline	T37.8X1	T37.8X2	T37.8X3	T37.8X4	T37.8X5	T37.8X6
Nitrozone	T49.0X1	T49.0X2	T49.0X3	T49.0X4	T49.0X5	T49.0X6
Nizatidine	T47.0X1	T47.0X2	T47.0X3	T47.0X4	T47.0X5	T47.0X6

Substance	External Cause (T-Code)					
	Poisoning, Accidental (Unintentional)	Poisoning, Intentional Self-Harm	Poisoning, Assault	Poisoning, Undetermined	Adverse Effect	Underdosing
Nizofenone	T43.8X1	T43.8X2	T43.8X3	T43.8X4	T43.8X5	T43.8X6
Noctec	T42.6X1	T42.6X2	T42.6X3	T42.6X4	T42.6X5	T42.6X6
Noludar	T42.6X1	T42.6X2	T42.6X3	T42.6X4	T42.6X5	T42.6X6
Noptil	T42.3X1	T42.3X2	T42.3X3	T42.3X4	T42.3X5	T42.3X6
Nomegestrol	T38.5X1	T38.5X2	T38.5X3	T38.5X4	T38.5X5	T38.5X6
Nomifensine	T43.291	T43.292	T43.293	T43.294	T43.295	T43.296
Nonoxinol	T49.8X1	T49.8X2	T49.8X3	T49.8X4	T49.8X5	T49.8X6
Nonylphenoxy (polyethoxy-ethanol)	T49.8X1	T49.8X2	T49.8X3	T49.8X4	T49.8X5	T49.8X6
Noptil	T42.3X1	T42.3X2	T42.3X3	T42.3X4	T42.3X5	T42.3X6
Noradrenaline	T44.4X1	T44.4X2	T44.4X3	T44.4X4	T44.4X5	T44.4X6
Noramidopyrine	T39.2X1	T39.2X2	T39.2X3	T39.2X4	T39.2X5	T39.2X6
methanesulfonate sodium	T39.2X1	T39.2X2	T39.2X3	T39.2X4	T39.2X5	T39.2X6
Norbormide	T60.4X1	T60.4X2	T60.4X3	T60.4X4	—	—
Nordazepam	T42.4X1	T42.4X2	T42.4X3	T42.4X4	T42.4X5	T42.4X6
Norepinephrine	T44.4X1	T44.4X2	T44.4X3	T44.4X4	T44.4X5	T44.4X6
Norethandrolone	T38.7X1	T38.7X2	T38.7X3	T38.7X4	T38.7X5	T38.7X6
Norethindrone	T38.4X1	T38.4X2	T38.4X3	T38.4X4	T38.4X5	T38.4X6
Norethisterone (acetate) (enantate)	T38.4X1	T38.4X2	T38.4X3	T38.4X4	T38.4X5	T38.4X6
with ethinylestradiol	T38.5X1	T38.5X2	T38.5X3	T38.5X4	T38.5X5	T38.5X6
Noretynodrel	T38.5X1	T38.5X2	T38.5X3	T38.5X4	T38.5X5	T38.5X6
Norfenefrine	T44.4X1	T44.4X2	T44.4X3	T44.4X4	T44.4X5	T44.4X6
Norfloxacin	T36.8X1	T36.8X2	T36.8X3	T36.8X4	T36.8X5	T36.8X6
Norgestrel	T38.4X1	T38.4X2	T38.4X3	T38.4X4	T38.4X5	T38.4X6
Norgestrienone	T38.4X1	T38.4X2	T38.4X3	T38.4X4	T38.4X5	T38.4X6
Norlestrin	T38.4X1	T38.4X2	T38.4X3	T38.4X4	T38.4X5	T38.4X6
Norlutin	T38.4X1	T38.4X2	T38.4X3	T38.4X4	T38.4X5	T38.4X6
Normal serum albumin (human), salt-poor	T45.8X1	T45.8X2	T45.8X3	T45.8X4	T45.8X5	T45.8X6
Normethandrone	T38.5X1	T38.5X2	T38.5X3	T38.5X4	T38.5X5	T38.5X6
Normison — see Benzodiazepines						
Normorphine	T40.2X1	T40.2X2	T40.2X3	T40.2X4	—	—
Norpseudoephedrine	T50.5X1	T50.5X2	T50.5X3	T50.5X4	T50.5X5	T50.5X6
Nortestosterone (furanpropionate)	T38.7X1	T38.7X2	T38.7X3	T38.7X4	T38.7X5	T38.7X6
Nortriptyline	T43.011	T43.012	T43.013	T43.014	T43.015	T43.016
Noscapine	T48.3X1	T48.3X2	T48.3X3	T48.3X4	T48.3X5	T48.3X6
Nose preparations	T49.6X1	T49.6X2	T49.6X3	T49.6X4	T49.6X5	T49.6X6
Novobiocin	T36.5X1	T36.5X2	T36.5X3	T36.5X4	T36.5X5	T36.5X6
Novocain (infiltration) (topical)	T41.3X1	T41.3X2	T41.3X3	T41.3X4	T41.3X5	T41.3X6
nerve block (peripheral) (plexus)	T41.3X1	T41.3X2	T41.3X3	T41.3X4	T41.3X5	T41.3X6
spinal	T41.3X1	T41.3X2	T41.3X3	T41.3X4	T41.3X5	T41.3X6

◀ New ◀▦ Revised ~~deleted~~ Deleted

	External Cause (T-Code)					
Substance	Poisoning, Accidental (Unintentional)	Poisoning, Intentional Self-Harm	Poisoning, Assault	Poisoning, Undetermined	Adverse Effect	Underdosing
Noxious foodstuff	T62.91	T62.92	T62.93	T62.94	—	—
specified NEC	T62.8X1	T62.8X2	T62.8X3	T62.8X4	—	—
Noxiptiline	T43.011	T43.012	T43.013	T43.014	T43.015	T43.016
Noxytiolin	T49.0X1	T49.0X2	T49.0X3	T49.0X4	T49.0X5	T49.0X6
NPH Iletin (insulin)	T38.3X1	T38.3X2	T38.3X3	T38.3X4	T38.3X5	T38.3X6
Numorphan	T40.2X1	T40.2X2	T40.2X3	T40.2X4	T40.2X5	T40.2X6
Nunol	T42.3X1	T42.3X2	T42.3X3	T42.3X4	T42.3X5	T42.3X6
Nupercaine (spinal anesthetic)	T41.3X1	T41.3X2	T41.3X3	T41.3X4	T41.3X5	T41.3X6
topical (surface)	T41.3X1	T41.3X2	T41.3X3	T41.3X4	T41.3X5	T41.3X6
Nutmeg oil (liniment)	T49.3X1	T49.3X2	T49.3X3	T49.3X4	T49.3X5	T49.3X6
Nutritional supplement	T50.901	T50.902	T50.903	T50.904	T50.905	T50.906
Nux vomica	T65.1X1	T65.1X2	T65.1X3	T65.1X4	—	—
Nydrazid	T37.1X1	T37.1X2	T37.1X3	T37.1X4	T37.1X5	T37.1X6
Nylidrin	T46.7X1	T46.7X2	T46.7X3	T46.7X4	T46.7X5	T46.7X6
Nystatin	T36.7X1	T36.7X2	T36.7X3	T36.7X4	T36.7X5	T36.7X6
topical	T49.0X1	T49.0X2	T49.0X3	T49.0X4	T49.0X5	T49.0X6
Nytol	T45.0X1	T45.0X2	T45.0X3	T45.0X4	T45.0X5	T45.0X6
O						
Obidoxime chloride	T50.6X1	T50.6X2	T50.6X3	T50.6X4	T50.6X5	T50.6X6
Octafonium (chloride)	T49.3X1	T49.3X2	T49.3X3	T49.3X4	T49.3X5	T49.3X6
Octamethyl pyrophos-phoramide	T60.0X1	T60.0X2	T60.0X3	T60.0X4	—	—
Octanoin	T50.991	T50.992	T50.993	T50.994	T50.995	T50.996
Octatropine methyl-bromide	T44.3X1	T44.3X2	T44.3X3	T44.3X4	T44.3X5	T44.3X6
Octotiamine	T45.2X1	T45.2X2	T45.2X3	T45.2X4	T45.2X5	T45.2X6
Octoxinol (9)	T49.8X1	T49.8X2	T49.8X3	T49.8X4	T49.8X5	T49.8X6
Octreotide	T38.991	T38.992	T38.993	T38.994	T38.995	T38.996
Octyl nitrite	T46.3X1	T46.3X2	T46.3X3	T46.3X4	T46.3X5	T46.3X6
Oestradiol	T38.5X1	T38.5X2	T38.5X3	T38.5X4	T38.5X5	T38.5X6
Oestriol	T38.5X1	T38.5X2	T38.5X3	T38.5X4	T38.5X5	T38.5X6
Oestrogen	T38.5X1	T38.5X2	T38.5X3	T38.5X4	T38.5X5	T38.5X6
Oestrone	T38.5X1	T38.5X2	T38.5X3	T38.5X4	T38.5X5	T38.5X6
Ofloxacin	T36.8X1	T36.8X2	T36.8X3	T36.8X4	T36.8X5	T36.8X6
Oil (of)	T65.891	T65.892	T65.893	T65.894	—	—
bitter almond	T62.8X1	T62.8X2	T62.8X3	T62.8X4	—	—
cloves	T49.7X1	T49.7X2	T49.7X3	T49.7X4	T49.7X5	T49.7X6
colors	T65.6X1	T65.6X2	T65.6X3	T65.6X4	—	—
fumes	T59.891	T59.892	T59.893	T59.894	—	—
lubricating	T52.0X1	T52.0X2	T52.0X3	T52.0X4	—	—
Niobe	T52.8X1	T52.8X2	T52.8X3	T52.8X4	—	—

	External Cause (T-Code)					
Substance	Poisoning, Accidental (Unintentional)	Poisoning, Intentional Self-Harm	Poisoning, Assault	Poisoning, Undetermined	Adverse Effect	Underdosing
Oil (of) *(Continued)*						
vitriol (liquid)	T54.2X1	T54.2X2	T54.2X3	T54.2X4	—	—
fumes	T54.2X1	T54.2X2	T54.2X3	T54.2X4	—	—
wintergreen (bitter) NEC	T49.3X1	T49.3X2	T49.3X3	T49.3X4	T49.3X5	T49.3X6
Oily preparation (for skin)	T49.3X1	T49.3X2	T49.3X3	T49.3X4	T49.3X5	T49.3X6
Ointment NEC	T49.3X1	T49.3X2	T49.3X3	T49.3X4	T49.3X5	T49.3X6
Olanzapine	T43.591	T43.592	T43.593	T43.594	T43.595	T43.596
Oleander	T62.2X1	T62.2X2	T62.2X3	T62.2X4	—	—
Oleandomycin	T36.3X1	T36.3X2	T36.3X3	T36.3X4	T36.3X5	T36.3X6
Oleandrin	T46.0X1	T46.0X2	T46.0X3	T46.0X4	T46.0X5	T46.0X6
Oleic acid	T46.6X1	T46.6X2	T46.6X3	T46.6X4	T46.6X5	T46.6X6
Oleovitamin A	T45.2X1	T45.2X2	T45.2X3	T45.2X4	T45.2X5	T45.2X6
Oleum ricini	T47.2X1	T47.2X2	T47.2X3	T47.2X4	T47.2X5	T47.2X6
Olive oil (medicinal) NEC	T47.4X1	T47.4X2	T47.4X3	T47.4X4	T47.4X5	T47.4X6
Olivomycin	T45.1X1	T45.1X2	T45.1X3	T45.1X4	T45.1X5	T45.1X6
Olsalazine	T47.8X1	T47.8X2	T47.8X3	T47.8X4	T47.8X5	T47.8X6
Omeprazole	T47.1X1	T47.1X2	T47.1X3	T47.1X4	T47.1X5	T47.1X6
OMPA	T60.0X1	T60.0X2	T60.0X3	T60.0X4	—	—
Ondansetron	T45.0X1	T45.0X2	T45.0X3	T45.0X4	T45.0X5	T45.0X6
Oncovin	T45.1X1	T45.1X2	T45.1X3	T45.1X4	T45.1X5	T45.1X6
Ophthaine	T41.3X1	T41.3X2	T41.3X3	T41.3X4	T41.3X5	T41.3X6
Ophthetic	T41.3X1	T41.3X2	T41.3X3	T41.3X4	T41.3X5	T41.3X6
Opiate NEC	T40.601	T40.602	T40.603	T40.604	T40.605	T40.606
antagonists	T50.7X1	T50.7X2	T50.7X3	T50.7X4	T50.7X5	T50.7X6
Opioid NEC	T40.2X1	T40.2X2	T40.2X3	T40.2X4	T40.2X5	T40.2X6
Opipramol	T43.011	T43.012	T43.013	T43.014	T43.015	T43.016
Opium alkaloids (total)	T40.0X1	T40.0X2	T40.0X3	T40.0X4	T40.0X5	T40.0X6
standardized powdered	T40.0X1	T40.0X2	T40.0X3	T40.0X4	T40.0X5	T40.0X6
tincture (camphorated)	T40.0X1	T40.0X2	T40.0X3	T40.0X4	T40.0X5	T40.0X6
Oracon	T38.4X1	T38.4X2	T38.4X3	T38.4X4	T38.4X5	T38.4X6
Oragrafin	T50.8X1	T50.8X2	T50.8X3	T50.8X4	T50.8X5	T50.8X6
Oral contraceptives	T38.4X1	T38.4X2	T38.4X3	T38.4X4	T38.4X5	T38.4X6
Oral rehydration salts	T50.3X1	T50.3X2	T50.3X3	T50.3X4	T50.3X5	T50.3X6
Orazamide	T50.991	T50.992	T50.993	T50.994	T50.995	T50.996
Orciprenaline	T48.291	T48.292	T48.293	T48.294	T48.295	T48.296
Organidin	T48.4X1	T48.4X2	T48.4X3	T48.4X4	T48.4X5	T48.4X6
Organonitrate NEC	T46.3X1	T46.3X2	T46.3X3	T46.3X4	T46.3X5	T46.3X6
Organophosphates	T60.0X1	T60.0X2	T60.0X3	T60.0X4	—	—
Orimune	T50.B91	T50.B92	T50.B93	T50.B94	T50.B95	T50.B96
Orinase	T38.3X1	T38.3X2	T38.3X3	T38.3X4	T38.3X5	T38.3X6
Ormeloxifene	T38.6X1	T38.6X2	T38.6X3	T38.6X4	T38.6X5	T38.6X6

TABLE OF DRUGS AND CHEMICALS

TABLE OF DRUGS AND CHEMICALS

Substance	External Cause (T-Code) Poisoning, Accidental (Unintentional)	Poisoning, Intentional Self-Harm	Poisoning, Assault	Poisoning, Undetermined	Adverse Effect	Underdosing
Ornidazole	T37.3X1	T37.3X2	T37.3X3	T37.3X4	T37.3X5	T37.3X6
Ornithine aspartate	T50.991	T50.992	T50.993	T50.994	T50.995	T50.996
Ornoprostil	T47.1X1	T47.1X2	T47.1X3	T47.1X4	T47.1X5	T47.1X6
Orphenadrine (hydrochloride)	T42.8X1	T42.8X2	T42.8X3	T42.8X4	T42.8X5	T42.8X6
Ortal (sodium)	T42.3X1	T42.3X2	T42.3X3	T42.3X4	T42.3X5	T42.3X6
Orthoboric acid	T49.0X1	T49.0X2	T49.0X3	T49.0X4	T49.0X5	T49.0X6
ENT agent	T49.6X1	T49.6X2	T49.6X3	T49.6X4	T49.6X5	T49.6X6
ophthalmic preparation	T49.5X1	T49.5X2	T49.5X3	T49.5X4	T49.5X5	T49.5X6
Orthocaine	T41.3X1	T41.3X2	T41.3X3	T41.3X4	T41.3X5	T41.3X6
Orthodichlorobenzene	T53.7X1	T53.7X2	T53.7X3	T53.7X4	—	—
Ortho-Novum	T38.4X1	T38.4X2	T38.4X3	T38.4X4	T38.4X5	T38.4X6
Orthotolidine (reagent)	T54.2X1	T54.2X2	T54.2X3	T54.2X4	—	—
Osmic acid (liquid)	T54.2X1	T54.2X2	T54.2X3	T54.2X4	—	—
fumes	T54.2X1	T54.2X2	T54.2X3	T54.2X4	—	—
Osmotic diuretics	T50.2X1	T50.2X2	T50.2X3	T50.2X4	T50.2X5	T50.2X6
Otilonium bromide	T44.3X1	T44.3X2	T44.3X3	T44.3X4	T44.3X5	T44.3X6
Otorhinolaryngological drug NEC	T49.6X1	T49.6X2	T49.6X3	T49.6X4	T49.6X5	T49.6X6
Ouabain(e)	T46.0X1	T46.0X2	T46.0X3	T46.0X4	T46.0X5	T46.0X6
Ovarian						
hormone	T38.5X1	T38.5X2	T38.5X3	T38.5X4	T38.5X5	T38.5X6
stimulant	T38.5X1	T38.5X2	T38.5X3	T38.5X4	T38.5X5	T38.5X6
Ovral	T38.4X1	T38.4X2	T38.4X3	T38.4X4	T38.4X5	T38.4X6
Ovulen	T38.4X1	T38.4X2	T38.4X3	T38.4X4	T38.4X5	T38.4X6
Oxacillin	T36.0X1	T36.0X2	T36.0X3	T36.0X4	T36.0X5	T36.0X6
Oxalic acid	T54.2X1	T54.2X2	T54.2X3	T54.2X4	—	—
ammonium salt	T50.991	T50.992	T50.993	T50.994	T50.995	T50.996
Oxamniquine	T37.4X1	T37.4X2	T37.4X3	T37.4X4	T37.4X5	T37.4X6
Oxanamide	T43.591	T43.592	T43.593	T43.594	T43.595	T43.596
Oxandrolone	T38.7X1	T38.7X2	T38.7X3	T38.7X4	T38.7X5	T38.7X6
Oxantel	T37.4X1	T37.4X2	T37.4X3	T37.4X4	T37.4X5	T37.4X6
Oxapium iodide	T44.3X1	T44.3X2	T44.3X3	T44.3X4	T44.3X5	T44.3X6
Oxaprotiline	T43.021	T43.022	T43.023	T43.024	T43.025	T43.026
Oxaprozin	T39.311	T39.312	T39.313	T39.314	T39.315	T39.316
Oxatomide	T45.0X1	T45.0X2	T45.0X3	T45.0X4	T45.0X5	T45.0X6
Oxazepam	T42.4X1	T42.4X2	T42.4X3	T42.4X4	T42.4X5	T42.4X6
Oxazimedrine	T50.5X1	T50.5X2	T50.5X3	T50.5X4	T50.5X5	T50.5X6
Oxazolam	T42.4X1	T42.4X2	T42.4X3	T42.4X4	T42.4X5	T42.4X6
Oxazolidine derivatives	T42.2X1	T42.2X2	T42.2X3	T42.2X4	T42.2X5	T42.2X6
Oxazolidinedione (derivative)	T42.2X1	T42.2X2	T42.2X3	T42.2X4	T42.2X5	T42.2X6
Ox bile extract	T47.5X1	T47.5X2	T47.5X3	T47.5X4	T47.5X5	T47.5X6
Oxcarbazepine	T42.1X1	T42.1X2	T42.1X3	T42.1X4	T42.1X5	T42.1X6
Oxedrine	T44.4X1	T44.4X2	T44.4X3	T44.4X4	T44.4X5	T44.4X6

Substance	External Cause (T-Code) Poisoning, Accidental (Unintentional)	Poisoning, Intentional Self-Harm	Poisoning, Assault	Poisoning, Undetermined	Adverse Effect	Underdosing
Oxeladin (citrate)	T48.3X1	T48.3X2	T48.3X3	T48.3X4	T48.3X5	T48.3X6
Oxendolone	T38.5X1	T38.5X2	T38.5X3	T38.5X4	T38.5X5	T38.5X6
Oxetacaine	T41.3X1	T41.3X2	T41.3X3	T41.3X4	T41.3X5	T41.3X6
Oxethazine	T41.3X1	T41.3X2	T41.3X3	T41.3X4	T41.3X5	T41.3X6
Oxetorone	T39.8X1	T39.8X2	T39.8X3	T39.8X4	T39.8X5	T39.8X6
Oxiconazole	T49.0X1	T49.0X2	T49.0X3	T49.0X4	T49.0X5	T49.0X6
Oxidizing agent NEC	T54.91	T54.92	T54.93	T54.94	—	—
Oxipurinol	T50.4X1	T50.4X2	T50.4X3	T50.4X4	T50.4X5	T50.4X6
Oxitriptan	T43.291	T43.292	T43.293	T43.294	T43.295	T43.296
Oxitropium bromide	T48.6X1	T48.6X2	T48.6X3	T48.6X4	T48.6X5	T48.6X6
Oxodipine	T46.1X1	T46.1X2	T46.1X3	T46.1X4	T46.1X5	T46.1X6
Oxolamine	T48.3X1	T48.3X2	T48.3X3	T48.3X4	T48.3X5	T48.3X6
Oxolinic acid	T37.8X1	T37.8X2	T37.8X3	T37.8X4	T37.8X5	T37.8X6
Oxomemazine	T43.3X1	T43.3X2	T43.3X3	T43.3X4	T43.3X5	T43.3X6
Oxophenarsine	T37.3X1	T37.3X2	T37.3X3	T37.3X4	T37.3X5	T37.3X6
Oxprenolol	T44.7X1	T44.7X2	T44.7X3	T44.7X4	T44.7X5	T44.7X6
Oxsoralen	T49.3X1	T49.3X2	T49.3X3	T49.3X4	T49.3X5	T49.3X6
Oxtriphylline	T48.6X1	T48.6X2	T48.6X3	T48.6X4	T48.6X5	T48.6X6
Oxybate sodium	T41.291	T41.292	T41.293	T41.294	T41.295	T41.296
Oxybuprocaine	T41.3X1	T41.3X2	T41.3X3	T41.3X4	T41.3X5	T41.3X6
Oxybutynin	T44.3X1	T44.3X2	T44.3X3	T44.3X4	T44.3X5	T44.3X6
Oxychlorosene	T49.0X1	T49.0X2	T49.0X3	T49.0X4	T49.0X5	T49.0X6
Oxycodone	T40.2X1	T40.2X2	T40.2X3	T40.2X4	T40.2X5	T40.2X6
Oxyfedrine	T46.3X1	T46.3X2	T46.3X3	T46.3X4	T46.3X5	T46.3X6
Oxygen	T41.5X1	T41.5X2	T41.5X3	T41.5X4	T41.5X5	T41.5X6
Oxylone	T49.0X1	T49.0X2	T49.0X3	T49.0X4	T49.0X5	T49.0X6
ophthalmic preparation	T49.5X1	T49.5X2	T49.5X3	T49.5X4	T49.5X5	T49.5X6
Oxymesterone	T38.7X1	T38.7X2	T38.7X3	T38.7X4	T38.7X5	T38.7X6
Oxymetazoline	T48.5X1	T48.5X2	T48.5X3	T48.5X4	T48.5X5	T48.5X6
Oxymetholone	T38.7X1	T38.7X2	T38.7X3	T38.7X4	T38.7X5	T38.7X6
Oxymorphone	T40.2X1	T40.2X2	T40.2X3	T40.2X4	T40.2X5	T40.2X6
Oxypertine	T43.591	T43.592	T43.593	T43.594	T43.595	T43.596
Oxyphenbutazone	T39.2X1	T39.2X2	T39.2X3	T39.2X4	T39.2X5	T39.2X6
Oxyphencyclimine	T44.3X1	T44.3X2	T44.3X3	T44.3X4	T44.3X5	T44.3X6
Oxyphenisatine	T47.2X1	T47.2X2	T47.2X3	T47.2X4	T47.2X5	T47.2X6
Oxyphenonium bromide	T44.3X1	T44.3X2	T44.3X3	T44.3X4	T44.3X5	T44.3X6
Oxypolygelatin	T45.8X1	T45.8X2	T45.8X3	T45.8X4	T45.8X5	T45.8X6
Oxyquinoline (derivatives)	T37.8X1	T37.8X2	T37.8X3	T37.8X4	T37.8X5	T37.8X6
Oxytetracycline	T36.4X1	T36.4X2	T36.4X3	T36.4X4	T36.4X5	T36.4X6
Oxytocic drug NEC	T48.0X1	T48.0X2	T48.0X3	T48.0X4	T48.0X5	T48.0X6
Oxytocin (synthetic)	T48.0X1	T48.0X2	T48.0X3	T48.0X4	T48.0X5	T48.0X6
Ozone	T59.891	T59.892	T59.893	T59.894	—	—

◀ New ◀▥ Revised ~~deleted~~ Deleted

Substance	Poisoning, Accidental (Unintentional)	Poisoning, Intentional Self-Harm	Poisoning, Assault	Poisoning, Undetermined	Adverse Effect	Underdosing
P						
PABA	T49.3X1	T49.3X2	T49.3X3	T49.3X4	T49.3X5	T49.3X6
Packed red cells	T45.8X1	T45.8X2	T45.8X3	T45.8X4	T45.8X5	T45.8X6
Padimate	T49.3X1	T49.3X2	T49.3X3	T49.3X4	T49.3X5	T49.3X6
Paint NEC	T65.6X1	T65.6X2	T65.6X3	T65.6X4	—	—
cleaner	T52.91	T52.92	T52.93	T52.94	—	—
fumes NEC	T59.891	T59.892	T59.893	T59.894	—	—
lead (fumes)	T56.0X1	T56.0X2	T56.0X3	T56.0X4	—	—
solvent NEC	T52.8X1	T52.8X2	T52.8X3	T52.8X4	—	—
stripper	T52.8X1	T52.8X2	T52.8X3	T52.8X4	—	—
Palfium	T40.2X1	T40.2X2	T40.2X3	T40.2X4	—	—
Palm kernel oil	T50.991	T50.992	T50.993	T50.994	T50.995	T50.996
Paludrine	T37.2X1	T37.2X2	T37.2X3	T37.2X4	T37.2X5	T37.2X6
PAM (pralidoxime)	T50.6X1	T50.6X2	T50.6X3	T50.6X4	T50.6X5	T50.6X6
Pamaquine (naphthoute)	T37.2X1	T37.2X2	T37.2X3	T37.2X4	T37.2X5	T37.2X6
Panadol	T39.1X1	T39.1X2	T39.1X3	T39.1X4	T39.1X5	T39.1X6
Pancreatic						
digestive secretion stimulant	T47.8X1	T47.8X2	T47.8X3	T47.8X4	T47.8X5	T47.8X6
dornase	T45.3X1	T45.3X2	T45.3X3	T45.3X4	T45.3X5	T45.3X6
Pancreatin	T47.5X1	T47.5X2	T47.5X3	T47.5X4	T47.5X5	T47.5X6
Pancrelipase	T47.5X1	T47.5X2	T47.5X3	T47.5X4	T47.5X5	T47.5X6
Pancuronium (bromide)	T48.1X1	T48.1X2	T48.1X3	T48.1X4	T48.1X5	T48.1X6
Pangamic acid	T45.2X1	T45.2X2	T45.2X3	T45.2X4	T45.2X5	T45.2X6
Panthenol	T45.2X1	T45.2X2	T45.2X3	T45.2X4	T45.2X5	T45.2X6
topical	T49.8X1	T49.8X2	T49.8X3	T49.8X4	T49.8X5	T49.8X6
Pantopon	T40.0X1	T40.0X2	T40.0X3	T40.0X4	T40.0X5	T40.0X6
Pantothenic acid	T45.2X1	T45.2X2	T45.2X3	T45.2X4	T45.2X5	T45.2X6
Panwarfin	T45.511	T45.512	T45.513	T45.514	T45.515	T45.516
Papain	T47.5X1	T47.5X2	T47.5X3	T47.5X4	T47.5X5	T47.5X6
digestant	T47.5X1	T47.5X2	T47.5X3	T47.5X4	T47.5X5	T47.5X6
Papaveretum	T40.0X1	T40.0X2	T40.0X3	T40.0X4	T40.0X5	T40.0X6
Papaverine	T44.3X1	T44.3X2	T44.3X3	T44.3X4	T44.3X5	T44.3X6
Para-acetamidophenol	T39.1X1	T39.1X2	T39.1X3	T39.1X4	T39.1X5	T39.1X6
Para-aminobenzoic acid	T49.3X1	T49.3X2	T49.3X3	T49.3X4	T49.3X5	T49.3X6
Para-aminophenol derivatives	T39.1X1	T39.1X2	T39.1X3	T39.1X4	T39.1X5	T39.1X6
Para-aminosalicylic acid	T37.1X1	T37.1X2	T37.1X3	T37.1X4	T37.1X5	T37.1X6
Paracetaldehyde	T42.6X1	T42.6X2	T42.6X3	T42.6X4	T42.6X5	T42.6X6
Paracetamol	T39.1X1	T39.1X2	T39.1X3	T39.1X4	T39.1X5	T39.1X6
Parachlorophenol (camphorated)	T49.0X1	T49.0X2	T49.0X3	T49.0X4	T49.0X5	T49.0X6
Paracodin	T40.2X1	T40.2X2	T40.2X3	T40.2X4	T40.2X5	T40.2X6
Paradione	T42.2X1	T42.2X2	T42.2X3	T42.2X4	T42.2X5	T42.2X6

Substance	Poisoning, Accidental (Unintentional)	Poisoning, Intentional Self-Harm	Poisoning, Assault	Poisoning, Undetermined	Adverse Effect	Underdosing
Paraffin(s) (wax)	T52.0X1	T52.0X2	T52.0X3	T52.0X4	—	—
liquid (medicinal)	T47.4X1	T47.4X2	T47.4X3	T47.4X4	T47.4X5	T47.4X6
nonmedicinal	T52.0X1	T52.0X2	T52.0X3	T52.0X4	—	—
Paraformaldehyde	T60.3X1	T60.3X2	T60.3X3	T60.3X4	—	—
Paraldehyde	T42.6X1	T42.6X2	T42.6X3	T42.6X4	T42.6X5	T42.6X6
Paramethadione	T42.2X1	T42.2X2	T42.2X3	T42.2X4	T42.2X5	T42.2X6
Paramethasone	T38.0X1	T38.0X2	T38.0X3	T38.0X4	T38.0X5	T38.0X6
acetate	T49.0X1	T49.0X2	T49.0X3	T49.0X4	T49.0X5	T49.0X6
Paraoxon	T60.0X1	T60.0X2	T60.0X3	T60.0X4	—	—
Paraquat	T60.3X1	T60.3X2	T60.3X3	T60.3X4	—	—
Parasympatholytic NEC	T44.3X1	T44.3X2	T44.3X3	T44.3X4	T44.3X5	T44.3X6
Parasympathomimetic drug NEC	T44.1X1	T44.1X2	T44.1X3	T44.1X4	T44.1X5	T44.1X6
Parathion	T60.0X1	T60.0X2	T60.0X3	T60.0X4	—	—
Parathormone	T50.991	T50.992	T50.993	T50.994	T50.995	T50.996
Parathyroid extract	T50.991	T50.992	T50.993	T50.994	T50.995	T50.996
Paratyphoid vaccine	T50.A91	T50.A92	T50.A93	T50.A94	T50.A95	T50.A96
Paredrine	T44.4X1	T44.4X2	T44.4X3	T44.4X4	T44.4X5	T44.4X6
Paregoric	T40.0X1	T40.0X2	T40.0X3	T40.0X4	T40.0X5	T40.0X6
Pargyline	T46.5X1	T46.5X2	T46.5X3	T46.5X4	T46.5X5	T46.5X6
Paris green	T57.0X1	T57.0X2	T57.0X3	T57.0X4	—	—
insecticide	T57.0X1	T57.0X2	T57.0X3	T57.0X4	—	—
Parnate	T43.1X1	T43.1X2	T43.1X3	T43.1X4	T43.1X5	T43.1X6
Paromomycin	T36.5X1	T36.5X2	T36.5X3	T36.5X4	T36.5X5	T36.5X6
Paroxypropione	T45.1X1	T45.1X2	T45.1X3	T45.1X4	T45.1X5	T45.1X6
Parzone	T40.2X1	T40.2X2	T40.2X3	T40.2X4	T40.2X5	T40.2X6
PAS	T37.1X1	T37.1X2	T37.1X3	T37.1X4	T37.1X5	T37.1X6
Pasiniazid	T37.1X1	T37.1X2	T37.1X3	T37.1X4	T37.1X5	T37.1X6
PBB (polybrominated biphenyls)	T65.891	T65.892	T65.893	T65.894	—	—
PCB	T65.891	T65.892	T65.893	T65.894	—	—
PCP						
meaning pentachlorophenol	T60.1X1	T60.1X2	T60.1X3	T60.1X4	—	—
fungicide	T60.3X1	T60.3X2	T60.3X3	T60.3X4	—	—
herbicide	T60.3X1	T60.3X2	T60.3X3	T60.3X4	—	—
insecticide	T60.1X1	T60.1X2	T60.1X3	T60.1X4	—	—
meaning phencyclidine	T40.991	T40.992	T40.993	T40.994		
Peach kernel oil (emulsion)	T47.4X1	T47.4X2	T47.4X3	T47.4X4	T47.4X5	T47.4X6
Peanut oil (emulsion) NEC	T47.4X1	T47.4X2	T47.4X3	T47.4X4	T47.4X5	T47.4X6
topical	T49.3X1	T49.3X2	T49.3X3	T49.3X4	T49.3X5	T49.3X6
Pearly Gates (morning glory seeds)	T40.991	T40.992	T40.993	T40.994		
Pecazine	T43.3X1	T43.3X2	T43.3X3	T43.3X4	T43.3X5	T43.3X6
Pectin	T47.6X1	T47.6X2	T47.6X3	T47.6X4	T47.6X5	T47.6X6

Substance	Poisoning, Accidental (Unintentional)	Poisoning, Intentional Self-Harm	Poisoning, Assault	Poisoning, Undetermined	Adverse Effect	Underdosing
Pefloxacin	T37.8X1	T37.8X2	T37.8X3	T37.8X4	T37.8X5	T37.8X6
Pegademase, bovine	T50.Z91	T50.Z92	T50.Z93	T50.Z94	T50.Z95	T50.Z96
Pelletierine tannate	T37.4X1	T37.4X2	T37.4X3	T37.4X4	T37.4X5	T37.4X6
Pemirolast (potassium)	T48.6X1	T48.6X2	T48.6X3	T48.6X4	T48.6X5	T48.6X6
Pemoline	T50.7X1	T50.7X2	T50.7X3	T50.7X4	T50.7X5	T50.7X6
Pempidine	T44.2X1	T44.2X2	T44.2X3	T44.2X4	T44.2X5	T44.2X6
Penamecillin	T36.0X1	T36.0X2	T36.0X3	T36.0X4	T36.0X5	T36.0X6
Penbutolol	T44.7X1	T44.7X2	T44.7X3	T44.7X4	T44.7X5	T44.7X6
Penethamate	T36.0X1	T36.0X2	T36.0X3	T36.0X4	T36.0X5	T36.0X6
Penfluridol	T43.591	T43.592	T43.593	T43.594	T43.595	T43.596
Penflutizide	T50.2X1	T50.2X2	T50.2X3	T50.2X4	T50.2X5	T50.2X6
Pengitoxin	T46.0X1	T46.0X2	T46.0X3	T46.0X4	T46.0X5	T46.0X6
Penicillamine	T50.6X1	T50.6X2	T50.6X3	T50.6X4	T50.6X5	T50.6X6
Penicillin (any)	T36.0X1	T36.0X2	T36.0X3	T36.0X4	T36.0X5	T36.0X6
Penicillinase	T45.3X1	T45.3X2	T45.3X3	T45.3X4	T45.3X5	T45.3X6
Penicilloyl polylysine	T50.8X1	T50.8X2	T50.8X3	T50.8X4	T50.8X5	T50.8X6
Penimepicycline	T36.4X1	T36.4X2	T36.4X3	T36.4X4	T36.4X5	T36.4X6
Pentachloroethane	T53.6X1	T53.6X2	T53.6X3	T53.6X4	—	—
Pentachloronaphthalene	T53.7X1	T53.7X2	T53.7X3	T53.7X4	—	—
Pentachlorophenol (pesticide)	T60.1X1	T60.1X2	T60.1X3	T60.1X4	—	—
fungicide	T60.3X1	T60.3X2	T60.3X3	T60.3X4	—	—
herbicide	T60.3X1	T60.3X2	T60.3X3	T60.3X4	—	—
insecticide	T60.1X1	T60.1X2	T60.1X3	T60.1X4	—	—
Pentaerythritol tetranitrate	T46.3X1	T46.3X2	T46.3X3	T46.3X4	T46.3X5	T46.3X6
Pentaerythritol	T46.3X1	T46.3X2	T46.3X3	T46.3X4	T46.3X5	T46.3X6
chloral	T42.6X1	T42.6X2	T42.6X3	T42.6X4	T42.6X5	T42.6X6
tetranitrate NEC	T46.3X1	T46.3X2	T46.3X3	T46.3X4	T46.3X5	T46.3X6
Pentagastrin	T50.8X1	T50.8X2	T50.8X3	T50.8X4	T50.8X5	T50.8X6
Pentalin	T53.6X1	T53.6X2	T53.6X3	T53.6X4	—	—
Pentamethonium bromide	T44.2X1	T44.2X2	T44.2X3	T44.2X4	T44.2X5	T44.2X6
Pentamidine	T37.3X1	T37.3X2	T37.3X3	T37.3X4	T37.3X5	T37.3X6
Pentanol	T51.3X1	T51.3X2	T51.3X3	T51.3X4	—	—
Pentapyrrolinium (bitartrate)	T44.2X1	T44.2X2	T44.2X3	T44.2X4	T44.2X5	T44.2X6
Pentaquine	T37.2X1	T37.2X2	T37.2X3	T37.2X4	T37.2X5	T37.2X6
Pentazocine	T40.4X1	T40.4X2	T40.4X3	T40.4X4	T40.4X5	T40.4X6
Pentetrazole	T50.7X1	T50.7X2	T50.7X3	T50.7X4	T50.7X5	T50.7X6
Penthienate bromide	T44.3X1	T44.3X2	T44.3X3	T44.3X4	T44.3X5	T44.3X6
Pentifylline	T46.7X1	T46.7X2	T46.7X3	T46.7X4	T46.7X5	T46.7X6
Pentobarbital	T42.3X1	T42.3X2	T42.3X3	T42.3X4	T42.3X5	T42.3X6
sodium	T42.3X1	T42.3X2	T42.3X3	T42.3X4	T42.3X5	T42.3X6
Pentobarbitone	T42.3X1	T42.3X2	T42.3X3	T42.3X4	T42.3X5	T42.3X6
Pentolonium tartrate	T44.2X1	T44.2X2	T44.2X3	T44.2X4	T44.2X5	T44.2X6
Pentosan polysulfate (sodium)	T39.8X1	T39.8X2	T39.8X3	T39.8X4	T39.8X5	T39.8X6
Pentostatin	T45.1X1	T45.1X2	T45.1X3	T45.1X4	T45.1X5	T45.1X6
Pentothal	T41.1X1	T41.1X2	T41.1X3	T41.1X4	T41.1X5	T41.1X6
Pentoxifylline	T46.7X1	T46.7X2	T46.7X3	T46.7X4	T46.7X5	T46.7X6
Pentoxyverine	T48.3X1	T48.3X2	T48.3X3	T48.3X4	T48.3X5	T48.3X6
Pentrinat	T46.3X1	T46.3X2	T46.3X3	T46.3X4	T46.3X5	T46.3X6
Pentylenetetrazole	T50.7X1	T50.7X2	T50.7X3	T50.7X4	T50.7X5	T50.7X6
Pentylsalicylamide	T37.1X1	T37.1X2	T37.1X3	T37.1X4	T37.1X5	T37.1X6
Pentymal	T42.3X1	T42.3X2	T42.3X3	T42.3X4	T42.3X5	T42.3X6
Peplomycin	T45.1X1	T45.1X2	T45.1X3	T45.1X4	T45.1X5	T45.1X6
Peppermint (oil)	T47.5X1	T47.5X2	T47.5X3	T47.5X4	T47.5X5	T47.5X6
Pepsin	T47.5X1	T47.5X2	T47.5X3	T47.5X4	T47.5X5	T47.5X6
digestant	T47.5X1	T47.5X2	T47.5X3	T47.5X4	T47.5X5	T47.5X6
Pepstatin	T47.1X1	T47.1X2	T47.1X3	T47.1X4	T47.1X5	T47.1X6
Peptavlon	T50.8X1	T50.8X2	T50.8X3	T50.8X4	T50.8X5	T50.8X6
Perazine	T43.3X1	T43.3X2	T43.3X3	T43.3X4	T43.3X5	T43.3X6
Percaine (spinal)	T41.3X1	T41.3X2	T41.3X3	T41.3X4	T41.3X5	T41.3X6
topical (surface)	T41.3X1	T41.3X2	T41.3X3	T41.3X4	T41.3X5	T41.3X6
Perchloroethylene	T53.3X1	T53.3X2	T53.3X3	T53.3X4	—	—
medicinal	T37.4X1	T37.4X2	T37.4X3	T37.4X4	T37.4X5	T37.4X6
vapor	T53.3X1	T53.3X2	T53.3X3	T53.3X4	—	—
Percodan	T40.2X1	T40.2X2	T40.2X3	T40.2X4	T40.2X5	T40.2X6
Percogesic — see also acetaminophen	T45.0X1	T45.0X2	T45.0X3	T45.0X4	T45.0X5	T45.0X6
Percorten	T38.0X1	T38.0X2	T38.0X3	T38.0X4	T38.0X5	T38.0X6
Pergolide	T42.8X1	T42.8X2	T42.8X3	T42.8X4	T42.8X5	T42.8X6
Pergonal	T38.811	T38.812	T38.813	T38.814	T38.815	T38.816
Perhexilene	T46.3X1	T46.3X2	T46.3X3	T46.3X4	T46.3X5	T46.3X6
Perhexiline (maleate)	T46.3X1	T46.3X2	T46.3X3	T46.3X4	T46.3X5	T46.3X6
Periactin	T45.0X1	T45.0X2	T45.0X3	T45.0X4	T45.0X5	T45.0X6
Periciazine	T43.3X1	T43.3X2	T43.3X3	T43.3X4	T43.3X5	T43.3X6
Periclor	T42.6X1	T42.6X2	T42.6X3	T42.6X4	T42.6X5	T42.6X6
Perindopril	T46.4X1	T46.4X2	T46.4X3	T46.4X4	T46.4X5	T46.4X6
Perisoxal	T39.8X1	T39.8X2	T39.8X3	T39.8X4	T39.8X5	T39.8X6
Peritrate	T46.3X1	T46.3X2	T46.3X3	T46.3X4	T46.3X5	T46.3X6
Peritoneal dialysis solution	T50.3X1	T50.3X2	T50.3X3	T50.3X4	T50.3X5	T50.3X6
Perlapine	T42.4X1	T42.4X2	T42.4X3	T42.4X4	T42.4X5	T42.4X6
Permanganate	T65.891	T65.892	T65.893	T65.894	—	—
Permethrin	T60.1X1	T60.1X2	T60.1X3	T60.1X4	—	—
Pernocton	T42.3X1	T42.3X2	T42.3X3	T42.3X4	T42.3X5	T42.3X6
Pernoston	T42.3X1	T42.3X2	T42.3X3	T42.3X4	T42.3X5	T42.3X6
Peronine	T40.2X1	T40.2X2	T40.2X3	T40.2X4	—	—
Perphenazine	T43.3X1	T43.3X2	T43.3X3	T43.3X4	T43.3X5	T43.3X6

◄ New ◄= Revised ~~deleted~~ Deleted

Substance	Poisoning, Accidental (Unintentional)	Poisoning, Intentional Self-Harm	Poisoning, Assault	Poisoning, Undetermined	Adverse Effect	Underdosing
Pertofrane	T43.011	T43.012	T43.013	T43.014	T43.015	T43.016
Pertussis						
immune serum (human)	T50.Z11	T50.Z12	T50.Z13	T50.Z14	T50.Z15	T50.Z16
vaccine (with diphtheria toxoid) (with tetanus toxoid)	T50.A11	T50.A12	T50.A13	T50.A14	T50.A15	T50.A16
Peruvian balsam	T49.0X1	T49.0X2	T49.0X3	T49.0X4	T49.0X5	T49.0X6
Peruvoside	T46.0X1	T46.0X2	T46.0X3	T46.0X4	T46.0X5	T46.0X6
Pesticide (dust) (fumes) (vapor) NEC	T60.91	T60.92	T60.93	T60.94	—	—
arsenic	T57.0X1	T57.0X2	T57.0X3	T57.0X4	—	—
chlorinated	T60.1X1	T60.1X2	T60.1X3	T60.1X4	—	—
cyanide	T65.0X1	T65.0X2	T65.0X3	T65.0X4	—	—
kerosene	T52.0X1	T52.0X2	T52.0X3	T52.0X4	—	—
mixture (of compounds)	T60.91	T60.92	T60.93	T60.94	—	—
naphthalene	T60.2X1	T60.2X2	T60.2X3	T60.2X4	—	—
organochlorine (compounds)	T60.1X1	T60.1X2	T60.1X3	T60.1X4	—	—
petroleum (distillate) (products) NEC	T60.8X1	T60.8X2	T60.8X3	T60.8X4	—	—
specified ingredient NEC	T60.8X1	T60.8X2	T60.8X3	T60.8X4	—	—
strychnine	T65.1X1	T65.1X2	T65.1X3	T65.1X4	—	—
thallium	T60.4X1	T60.4X2	T60.4X3	T60.4X4	—	—
Pethidine	T40.4X1	T40.4X2	T40.4X3	T40.4X4	T40.4X5	T40.4X6
Petrichloral	T42.6X1	T42.6X2	T42.6X3	T42.6X4	T42.6X5	T42.6X6
Petrol	T52.0X1	T52.0X2	T52.0X3	T52.0X4	—	—
vapor	T52.0X1	T52.0X2	T52.0X3	T52.0X4	—	—
Petrolatum	T49.3X1	T49.3X2	T49.3X3	T49.3X4	T49.3X5	T49.3X6
hydrophilic	T49.3X1	T49.3X2	T49.3X3	T49.3X4	T49.3X5	T49.3X6
liquid	T47.4X1	T47.4X2	T47.4X3	T47.4X4	T47.4X5	T47.4X6
topical	T49.3X1	T49.3X2	T49.3X3	T49.3X4	T49.3X5	T49.3X6
nonmedicinal	T52.0X1	T52.0X2	T52.0X3	T52.0X4	—	—
red veterinary	T49.3X1	T49.3X2	T49.3X3	T49.3X4	T49.3X5	T49.3X6
white	T49.3X1	T49.3X2	T49.3X3	T49.3X4	T49.3X5	T49.3X6
Petroleum (products) NEC	T52.0X1	T52.0X2	T52.0X3	T52.0X4	—	—
benzine(s) — see Ligroin						
ether — see Ligroin						
jelly — see Petrolatum						
naphtha — see Ligroin						
pesticide	T60.8X1	T60.8X2	T60.8X3	T60.8X4	—	—
solids	T52.0X1	T52.0X2	T52.0X3	T52.0X4	—	—
solvents	T52.0X1	T52.0X2	T52.0X3	T52.0X4	—	—
vapor	T52.0X1	T52.0X2	T52.0X3	T52.0X4	—	—
Peyote	T40.991	T40.992	T40.993	T40.994	—	—
Phanodorm, phanodorn	T42.3X1	T42.3X2	T42.3X3	T42.3X4	T42.3X5	T42.3X6

Substance	Poisoning, Accidental (Unintentional)	Poisoning, Intentional Self-Harm	Poisoning, Assault	Poisoning, Undetermined	Adverse Effect	Underdosing
Phanquinone	T37.3X1	T37.3X2	T37.3X3	T37.3X4	T37.3X5	T37.3X6
Phanquone	T37.3X1	T37.3X2	T37.3X3	T37.3X4	T37.3X5	T37.3X6
Pharmaceutical						
adjunct NEC	T50.901	T50.902	T50.903	T50.904	T50.905	T50.906
excipient NEC	T50.901	T50.902	T50.903	T50.904	T50.905	T50.906
sweetener	T50.901	T50.902	T50.903	T50.904	T50.905	T50.906
viscous agent	T50.901	T50.902	T50.903	T50.904	T50.905	T50.906
Phemitone	T42.3X1	T42.3X2	T42.3X3	T42.3X4	T42.3X5	T42.3X6
Phenacaine	T41.3X1	T41.3X2	T41.3X3	T41.3X4	T41.3X5	T41.3X6
Phenacemide	T42.6X1	T42.6X2	T42.6X3	T42.6X4	T42.6X5	T42.6X6
Phenacetin	T39.1X1	T39.1X2	T39.1X3	T39.1X4	T39.1X5	T39.1X6
Phenadoxone	T40.2X1	T40.2X2	T40.2X3	T40.2X4	—	—
Phenaglycodol	T43.591	T43.592	T43.593	T43.594	T43.595	T43.596
Phenantoin	T42.0X1	T42.0X2	T42.0X3	T42.0X4	T42.0X5	T42.0X6
Phenaphthazine reagent	T50.991	T50.992	T50.993	T50.994	T50.995	T50.996
Phenazocine	T40.4X1	T40.4X2	T40.4X3	T40.4X4	T40.4X5	T40.4X6
Phenazone	T39.2X1	T39.2X2	T39.2X3	T39.2X4	T39.2X5	T39.2X6
Phenazopyridine	T39.8X1	T39.8X2	T39.8X3	T39.8X4	T39.8X5	T39.8X6
Phenbenicillin	T36.0X1	T36.0X2	T36.0X3	T36.0X4	T36.0X5	T36.0X6
Phenbutrazate	T50.5X1	T50.5X2	T50.5X3	T50.5X4	T50.5X5	T50.5X6
Phencyclidine	T40.991	T40.992	T40.993	T40.994	T40.995	T40.996
Phendimetrazine	T50.5X1	T50.5X2	T50.5X3	T50.5X4	T50.5X5	T50.5X6
Phenelzine	T43.1X1	T43.1X2	T43.1X3	T43.1X4	T43.1X5	T43.1X6
Phenemal	T42.3X1	T42.3X2	T42.3X3	T42.3X4	T42.3X5	T42.3X6
Phenergan	T42.6X1	T42.6X2	T42.6X3	T42.6X4	T42.6X5	T42.6X6
Pheneticillin	T36.0X1	T36.0X2	T36.0X3	T36.0X4	T36.0X5	T36.0X6
Pheneturide	T42.6X1	T42.6X2	T42.6X3	T42.6X4	T42.6X5	T42.6X6
Phenformin	T38.3X1	T38.3X2	T38.3X3	T38.3X4	T38.3X5	T38.3X6
Phenglutarimide	T44.3X1	T44.3X2	T44.3X3	T44.3X4	T44.3X5	T44.3X6
Phenicarbazide	T39.8X1	T39.8X2	T39.8X3	T39.8X4	T39.8X5	T39.8X6
Phenindamine	T45.0X1	T45.0X2	T45.0X3	T45.0X4	T45.0X5	T45.0X6
Phenindione	T45.511	T45.512	T45.513	T45.514	T45.515	T45.516
Pheniprazine	T43.1X1	T43.1X2	T43.1X3	T43.1X4	T43.1X5	T43.1X6
Pheniramine	T45.0X1	T45.0X2	T45.0X3	T45.0X4	T45.0X5	T45.0X6
Phenisatin	T47.2X1	T47.2X2	T47.2X3	T47.2X4	T47.2X5	T47.2X6
Phenmetrazine	T50.5X1	T50.5X2	T50.5X3	T50.5X4	T50.5X5	T50.5X6
Phenobal	T42.3X1	T42.3X2	T42.3X3	T42.3X4	T42.3X5	T42.3X6
Phenobarbital	T42.3X1	T42.3X2	T42.3X3	T42.3X4	T42.3X5	T42.3X6
with						
mephenytoin	T42.3X1	T42.3X2	T42.3X3	T42.3X4	T42.3X5	T42.3X6
phenytoin	T42.3X1	T42.3X2	T42.3X3	T42.3X4	T42.3X5	T42.3X6
sodium	T42.3X1	T42.3X2	T42.3X3	T42.3X4	T42.3X5	T42.3X6

TABLE OF DRUGS AND CHEMICALS

Substance	External Cause (T-Code)					
	Poisoning, Accidental (Unintentional)	Poisoning, Intentional Self-Harm	Poisoning, Assault	Poisoning, Undetermined	Adverse Effect	Underdosing
Phenobarbitone	T42.3X1	T42.3X2	T42.3X3	T42.3X4	T42.3X5	T42.3X6
Phenobutiodil	T50.8X1	T50.8X2	T50.8X3	T50.8X4	T50.8X5	T50.8X6
Phenoctide	T49.0X1	T49.0X2	T49.0X3	T49.0X4	T49.0X5	T49.0X6
Phenol	T49.0X1	T49.0X2	T49.0X3	T49.0X4	T49.0X5	T49.0X6
disinfectant	T54.0X1	T54.0X2	T54.0X3	T54.0X4	—	—
in oil injection	T46.8X1	T46.8X2	T46.8X3	T46.8X4	T46.8X5	T46.8X6
medicinal	T49.1X1	T49.1X2	T49.1X3	T49.1X4	T49.1X5	T49.1X6
nonmedicinal NEC	T54.0X1	T54.0X2	T54.0X3	T54.0X4	—	—
pesticide	T60.8X1	T60.8X2	T60.8X3	T60.8X4	—	—
red	T50.8X1	T50.8X2	T50.8X3	T50.8X4	T50.8X5	T50.8X6
Phenolic preparation	T49.1X1	T49.1X2	T49.1X3	T49.1X4	T49.1X5	T49.1X6
Phenolphthalein	T47.2X1	T47.2X2	T47.2X3	T47.2X4	T47.2X5	T47.2X6
Phenolsulfonphthalein	T50.8X1	T50.8X2	T50.8X3	T50.8X4	T50.8X5	T50.8X6
Phenomorphan	T40.2X1	T40.2X2	T40.2X3	T40.2X4	—	—
Phenonyl	T42.3X1	T42.3X2	T42.3X3	T42.3X4	T42.3X5	T42.3X6
Phenoperidine	T40.4X1	T40.4X2	T40.4X3	T40.4X4	—	—
Phenopyrazone	T46.991	T46.992	T46.993	T46.994	T46.995	T46.996
Phenoquin	T50.4X1	T50.4X2	T50.4X3	T50.4X4	T50.4X5	T50.4X6
Phenothiazine (psychotropic) NEC	T43.3X1	T43.3X2	T43.3X3	T43.3X4	T43.3X5	T43.3X6
insecticide	T60.2X1	T60.2X2	T60.2X3	T60.2X4	—	—
Phenothrin	T49.0X1	T49.0X2	T49.0X3	T49.0X4	T49.0X5	T49.0X6
Phenoxybenzamine	T46.7X1	T46.7X2	T46.7X3	T46.7X4	T46.7X5	T46.7X6
Phenoxyethanol	T49.0X1	T49.0X2	T49.0X3	T49.0X4	T49.0X5	T49.0X6
Phenoxymethyl penicillin	T36.0X1	T36.0X2	T36.0X3	T36.0X4	T36.0X5	T36.0X6
Phenprobamate	T42.8X1	T42.8X2	T42.8X3	T42.8X4	T42.8X5	T42.8X6
Phenprocoumon	T45.511	T45.512	T45.513	T45.514	T45.515	T45.516
Phensuximide	T42.2X1	T42.2X2	T42.2X3	T42.2X4	T42.2X5	T42.2X6
Phentermine	T50.5X1	T50.5X2	T50.5X3	T50.5X4	T50.5X5	T50.5X6
Phenthicillin	T36.0X1	T36.0X2	T36.0X3	T36.0X4	T36.0X5	T36.0X6
Phentolamine	T46.7X1	T46.7X2	T46.7X3	T46.7X4	T46.7X5	T46.7X6
Phenyl						
butazone	T39.2X1	T39.2X2	T39.2X3	T39.2X4	T39.2X5	T39.2X6
enediamine	T65.3X1	T65.3X2	T65.3X3	T65.3X4	—	—
hydrazine	T65.3X1	T65.3X2	T65.3X3	T65.3X4	—	—
antineoplastic	T45.1X1	T45.1X2	T45.1X3	T45.1X4	T45.1X5	T45.1X6
mercuric compounds — see Mercury						
salicylate	T49.3X1	T49.3X2	T49.3X3	T49.3X4	T49.3X5	T49.3X6
Phenylalanine mustard	T45.1X1	T45.1X2	T45.1X3	T45.1X4	T45.1X5	T45.1X6
Phenylbutazone	T39.2X1	T39.2X2	T39.2X3	T39.2X4	T39.2X5	T39.2X6
Phenylenediamine	T65.3X1	T65.3X2	T65.3X3	T65.3X4	—	—
Phenylephrine	T44.4X1	T44.4X2	T44.4X3	T44.4X4	T44.4X5	T44.4X6

Substance	External Cause (T-Code)					
	Poisoning, Accidental (Unintentional)	Poisoning, Intentional Self-Harm	Poisoning, Assault	Poisoning, Undetermined	Adverse Effect	Underdosing
Phenylethylbiguanide	T38.3X1	T38.3X2	T38.3X3	T38.3X4	T38.3X5	T38.3X6
Phenylmercuric						
acetate	T49.0X1	T49.0X2	T49.0X3	T49.0X4	T49.0X5	T49.0X6
borate	T49.0X1	T49.0X2	T49.0X3	T49.0X4	T49.0X5	T49.0X6
nitrate	T49.0X1	T49.0X2	T49.0X3	T49.0X4	T49.0X5	T49.0X6
Phenylmethylbarbitone	T42.3X1	T42.3X2	T42.3X3	T42.3X4	T42.3X5	T42.3X6
Phenylpropanol	T47.5X1	T47.5X2	T47.5X3	T47.5X4	T47.5X5	T47.5X6
Phenylpropanolamine	T44.991	T44.992	T44.993	T44.994	T44.995	T44.996
Phenylsulfthion	T60.0X1	T60.0X2	T60.0X3	T60.0X4	—	—
Phenyltoloxamine	T45.0X1	T45.0X2	T45.0X3	T45.0X4	T45.0X5	T45.0X6
Phenyramidol, phenyramidon	T39.8X1	T39.8X2	T39.8X3	T39.8X4	T39.8X5	T39.8X6
Phenytoin	T42.0X1	T42.0X2	T42.0X3	T42.0X4	T42.0X5	T42.0X6
with Phenobarbital	T42.3X1	T42.3X2	T42.3X3	T42.3X4	T42.3X5	T42.3X6
pHisoHex	T49.2X1	T49.2X2	T49.2X3	T49.2X4	T49.2X5	T49.2X6
Pholcodine	T48.3X1	T48.3X2	T48.3X3	T48.3X4	T48.3X5	T48.3X6
Pholedrine	T46.991	T46.992	T46.993	T46.994	T46.995	T46.996
Phorate	T60.0X1	T60.0X2	T60.0X3	T60.0X4	—	—
Phosdrin	T60.0X1	T60.0X2	T60.0X3	T60.0X4	—	—
Phosfolan	T60.0X1	T60.0X2	T60.0X3	T60.0X4	—	—
Phosgene (gas)	T59.891	T59.892	T59.893	T59.894		
Phosphamidon	T60.0X1	T60.0X2	T60.0X3	T60.0X4	—	—
Phosphate	T65.891	T65.892	T65.893	T65.894		
laxative	T47.4X1	T47.4X2	T47.4X3	T47.4X4	T47.4X5	T47.4X6
organic	T60.0X1	T60.0X2	T60.0X3	T60.0X4		
solvent	T52.91	T52.92	T52.93	T52.94	—	—
tricresyl	T65.891	T65.892	T65.893	T65.894		
Phosphine	T57.1X1	T57.1X2	T57.1X3	T57.1X4		
fumigant	T57.1X1	T57.1X2	T57.1X3	T57.1X4		
Phospholine	T49.5X1	T49.5X2	T49.5X3	T49.5X4	T49.5X5	T49.5X6
Phosphoric acid	T54.2X1	T54.2X2	T54.2X3	T54.2X4		
Phosphorus (compound) NEC	T57.1X1	T57.1X2	T57.1X3	T57.1X4		
pesticide	T60.0X1	T60.0X2	T60.0X3	T60.0X4		
Phthalates	T65.891	T65.892	T65.893	T65.894		
Phthalic anhydride	T65.891	T65.892	T65.893	T65.894		
Phthalimidoglutarimide	T42.6X1	T42.6X2	T42.6X3	T42.6X4	T42.6X5	T42.6X6
Phthalylsulfathiazole	T37.0X1	T37.0X2	T37.0X3	T37.0X4	T37.0X5	T37.0X6
Phylloquinone	T45.7X1	T45.7X2	T45.7X3	T45.7X4	T45.7X5	T45.7X6
Physeptone	T40.3X1	T40.3X2	T40.3X3	T40.3X4	T40.3X5	T40.3X6
Physostigma venenosum	T62.2X1	T62.2X2	T62.2X3	T62.2X4	—	—
Physostigmine	T49.5X1	T49.5X2	T49.5X3	T49.5X4	T49.5X5	T49.5X6
Phytolacca decandra	T62.2X1	T62.2X2	T62.2X3	T62.2X4	—	—
berries	T62.1X1	T62.1X2	T62.1X3	T62.1X4	—	—

◀ New ◀ Revised deleted Deleted

Substance	Poisoning, Accidental (Unintentional)	Poisoning, Intentional Self-Harm	Poisoning, Assault	Poisoning, Undetermined	Adverse Effect	Underdosing
Phytomenadione	T45.7X1	T45.7X2	T45.7X3	T45.7X4	T45.7X5	T45.7X6
Phytonadione	T45.7X1	T45.7X2	T45.7X3	T45.7X4	T45.7X5	T45.7X6
Picoperine	T48.3X1	T48.3X2	T48.3X3	T48.3X4	T48.3X5	T48.3X6
Picosulfate (sodium)	T47.2X1	T47.2X2	T47.2X3	T47.2X4	T47.2X5	T47.2X6
Picric (acid)	T54.2X1	T54.2X2	T54.2X3	T54.2X4	—	—
Picrotoxin	T50.7X1	T50.7X2	T50.7X3	T50.7X4	T50.7X5	T50.7X6
Piketoprofen	T49.0X1	T49.0X2	T49.0X3	T49.0X4	T49.0X5	T49.0X6
Pilocarpine	T44.1X1	T44.1X2	T44.1X3	T44.1X4	T44.1X5	T44.1X6
Pilocarpus (jaborandi) extract	T44.1X1	T44.1X2	T44.1X3	T44.1X4	T44.1X5	T44.1X6
Pilsicainide (hydrochloride)	T46.2X1	T46.2X2	T46.2X3	T46.2X4	T46.2X5	T46.2X6
Pimaricin	T36.7X1	T36.7X2	T36.7X3	T36.7X4	T36.7X5	T36.7X6
Pimeclone	T50.7X1	T50.7X2	T50.7X3	T50.7X4	T50.7X5	T50.7X6
Pimelic ketone	T52.8X1	T52.8X2	T52.8X3	T52.8X4	—	—
Pimethixene	T45.0X1	T45.0X2	T45.0X3	T45.0X4	T45.0X5	T45.0X6
Piminodine	T40.2X1	T40.2X2	T40.2X3	T40.2X4	T40.2X5	T40.2X6
Pimozide	T43.591	T43.592	T43.593	T43.594	T43.595	T43.596
Pinacidil	T46.5X1	T46.5X2	T46.5X3	T46.5X4	T46.5X5	T46.5X6
Pinaverium bromide	T44.3X1	T44.3X2	T44.3X3	T44.3X4	T44.3X5	T44.3X6
Pinazepam	T42.4X1	T42.4X2	T42.4X3	T42.4X4	T42.4X5	T42.4X6
Pindolol	T44.7X1	T44.7X2	T44.7X3	T44.7X4	T44.7X5	T44.7X6
Pindone	T60.4X1	T60.4X2	T60.4X3	T60.4X4	—	—
Pine oil (disinfectant)	T65.891	T65.892	T65.893	T65.894	—	—
Pinkroot	T37.4X1	T37.4X2	T37.4X3	T37.4X4	T37.4X5	T37.4X6
Pipadone	T40.2X1	T40.2X2	T40.2X3	T40.2X4	—	—
Pipamazine	T45.0X1	T45.0X2	T45.0X3	T45.0X4	T45.0X5	T45.0X6
Pipamperone	T43.4X1	T43.4X2	T43.4X3	T43.4X4	T43.4X5	T43.4X6
Pipazetate	T48.3X1	T48.3X2	T48.3X3	T48.3X4	T48.3X5	T48.3X6
Pipemidic acid	T37.8X1	T37.8X2	T37.8X3	T37.8X4	T37.8X5	T37.8X6
Pipenzolate bromide	T44.3X1	T44.3X2	T44.3X3	T44.3X4	T44.3X5	T44.3X6
Piperacetazine	T43.3X1	T43.3X2	T43.3X3	T43.3X4	T43.3X5	T43.3X6
Piperacillin	T36.0X1	T36.0X2	T36.0X3	T36.0X4	T36.0X5	T36.0X6
Piperazine	T37.4X1	T37.4X2	T37.4X3	T37.4X4	T37.4X5	T37.4X6
estrone sulfate	T38.5X1	T38.5X2	T38.5X3	T38.5X4	T38.5X5	T38.5X6
Piper cubeba	T62.2X1	T62.2X2	T62.2X3	T62.2X4		
Piperidione	T48.3X1	T48.3X2	T48.3X3	T48.3X4	—	—
Piperidolate	T44.3X1	T44.3X2	T44.3X3	T44.3X4	T44.3X5	T44.3X6
Piperocaine	T41.3X1	T41.3X2	T41.3X3	T41.3X4	T41.3X5	T41.3X6
infiltration (subcutaneous)	T41.3X1	T41.3X2	T41.3X3	T41.3X4	T41.3X5	T41.3X6
nerve block (peripheral) (plexus)	T41.3X1	T41.3X2	T41.3X3	T41.3X4	T41.3X5	T41.3X6
topical (surface)	T41.3X1	T41.3X2	T41.3X3	T41.3X4	T41.3X5	T41.3X6
Piperonyl butoxide	T60.8X1	T60.8X2	T60.8X3	T60.8X4	—	—
Pipethanate	T44.3X1	T44.3X2	T44.3X3	T44.3X4	T44.3X5	T44.3X6

Substance	Poisoning, Accidental (Unintentional)	Poisoning, Intentional Self-Harm	Poisoning, Assault	Poisoning, Undetermined	Adverse Effect	Underdosing
Pipobroman	T45.1X1	T45.1X2	T45.1X3	T45.1X4	T45.1X5	T45.1X6
Pipofezine	T43.0X1	T43.0X2	T43.0X3	T43.0X4	T43.0X5	T43.0X6
Pipotiazine	T43.3X1	T43.3X2	T43.3X3	T43.3X4	T43.3X5	T43.3X6
Pipoxizine	T45.0X1	T45.0X2	T45.0X3	T45.0X4	T45.0X5	T45.0X6
Pipradrol	T43.691	T43.692	T43.693	T43.694	T43.695	T43.696
Piprinhydrinate	T45.0X1	T45.0X2	T45.0X3	T45.0X4	T45.0X5	T45.0X6
Pirarubicin	T45.1X1	T45.1X2	T45.1X3	T45.1X4	T45.1X5	T45.1X6
Pirazinamide	T37.1X1	T37.1X2	T37.1X3	T37.1X4	T37.1X5	T37.1X6
Pirbuterol	T48.6X1	T48.6X2	T48.6X3	T48.6X4	T48.6X5	T48.6X6
Pirenzepine	T47.1X1	T47.1X2	T47.1X3	T47.1X4	T47.1X5	T47.1X6
Piretanide	T50.1X1	T50.1X2	T50.1X3	T50.1X4	T50.1X5	T50.1X6
Piribedil	T42.8X1	T42.8X2	T42.8X3	T42.8X4	T42.8X5	T42.8X6
Piridoxilate	T46.3X1	T46.3X2	T46.3X3	T46.3X4	T46.3X5	T46.3X6
Piritramide	T40.4X1	T40.4X2	T40.4X3	T40.4X4	—	—
Pirlindole	T43.0X1	T43.0X2	T43.0X3	T43.0X4	T43.0X5	T43.0X6
Piromidic acid	T37.8X1	T37.8X2	T37.8X3	T37.8X4	T37.8X5	T37.8X6
Piroxicam	T39.391	T39.392	T39.393	T39.394	T39.395	T39.396
beta-cyclodextrin complex	T39.8X1	T39.8X2	T39.8X3	T39.8X4	T39.8X5	T39.8X6
Pirozadil	T46.6X1	T46.6X2	T46.6X3	T46.6X4	T46.6X5	T46.6X6
Piscidia (bark) (erythrina)	T39.8X1	T39.8X2	T39.8X3	T39.8X4	T39.8X5	T39.8X6
Pitch	T65.891	T65.892	T65.893	T65.894	—	—
Pitkin's solution	T41.3X1	T41.3X2	T41.3X3	T41.3X4	T41.3X5	T41.3X6
Pitocin	T48.0X1	T48.0X2	T48.0X3	T48.0X4	T48.0X5	T48.0X6
Pitressin (tannate)	T38.891	T38.892	T38.893	T38.894	T38.895	T38.896
Pituitary extracts (posterior)	T38.891	T38.892	T38.893	T38.894	T38.895	T38.896
anterior	T38.811	T38.812	T38.813	T38.814	T38.815	T38.816
Pituitrin	T38.891	T38.892	T38.893	T38.894	T38.895	T38.896
Pivampicillin	T36.0X1	T36.0X2	T36.0X3	T36.0X4	T36.0X5	T36.0X6
Pivmecillinam	T36.0X1	T36.0X2	T36.0X3	T36.0X4	T36.0X5	T36.0X6
Placental hormone	T38.891	T38.892	T38.893	T38.894	T38.895	T38.896
Placidyl	T42.6X1	T42.6X2	T42.6X3	T42.6X4	T42.6X5	T42.6X6
Plague vaccine	T50.A91	T50.A92	T50.A93	T50.A94	T50.A95	T50.A96
Plant						
food or fertilizer NEC	T65.891	T65.892	T65.893	T65.894	—	—
containing herbicide	T60.3X1	T60.3X2	T60.3X3	T60.3X4	—	—
noxious, used as food	T62.2X1	T62.2X2	T62.2X3	T62.2X4	—	—
berries	T62.1X1	T62.1X2	T62.1X3	T62.1X4	—	—
seeds	T62.2X1	T62.2X2	T62.2X3	T62.2X4	—	—
specified type NEC	T62.2X1	T62.2X2	T62.2X3	T62.2X4	—	—
Plasma	T45.8X1	T45.8X2	T45.8X3	T45.8X4	T45.8X5	T45.8X6
expander NEC	T45.8X1	T45.8X2	T45.8X3	T45.8X4	T45.8X5	T45.8X6
protein fraction (human)	T45.8X1	T45.8X2	T45.8X3	T45.8X4	T45.8X5	T45.8X6

◀ New ◀▥ Revised ~~deleted~~ Deleted

Substance	Poisoning, Accidental (Unintentional)	Poisoning, Intentional Self-Harm	Poisoning, Assault	Poisoning, Undetermined	Adverse Effect	Underdosing
Plasmanate	T45.8X1	T45.8X2	T45.8X3	T45.8X4	T45.8X5	T45.8X6
Plasminogen (tissue) activator	T45.611	T45.612	T45.613	T45.614	T45.615	T45.616
Plaster dressing	T49.3X1	T49.3X2	T49.3X3	T49.3X4	T49.3X5	T49.3X6
Plastic dressing	T49.3X1	T49.3X2	T49.3X3	T49.3X4	T49.3X5	T49.3X6
Plegicil	T43.3X1	T43.3X2	T43.3X3	T43.3X4	T43.3X5	T43.3X6
Plicamycin	T45.1X1	T45.1X2	T45.1X3	T45.1X4	T45.1X5	T45.1X6
Podophyllotoxin	T49.8X1	T49.8X2	T49.8X3	T49.8X4	T49.8X5	T49.8X6
Podophyllum (resin)	T49.4X1	T49.4X2	T49.4X3	T49.4X4	T49.4X5	T49.4X6
Poison NEC	T65.91	T65.92	T65.93	T65.94	—	—
Poisonous berries	T62.1X1	T62.1X2	T62.1X3	T62.1X4	—	—
Pokeweed (any part)	T62.2X1	T62.2X2	T62.2X3	T62.2X4	—	—
Poldine metilsulfate	T44.3X1	T44.3X2	T44.3X3	T44.3X4	T44.3X5	T44.3X6
Polidexide (sulfate)	T46.6X1	T46.6X2	T46.6X3	T46.6X4	T46.6X5	T46.6X6
Polidocanol	T46.8X1	T46.8X2	T46.8X3	T46.8X4	T46.8X5	T46.8X6
Poliomyelitis vaccine	T50.B91	T50.B92	T50.B93	T50.B94	T50.B95	T50.B96
Polish (car) (floor) (furniture) (metal) (porcelain) (silver)	T65.891	T65.892	T65.893	T65.894	—	—
abrasive	T65.891	T65.892	T65.893	T65.894	—	—
porcelain	T65.891	T65.892	T65.893	T65.894	—	—
Poloxalkol	T47.4X1	T47.4X2	T47.4X3	T47.4X4	T47.4X5	T47.4X6
Poloxamer	T47.4X1	T47.4X2	T47.4X3	T47.4X4	T47.4X5	T47.4X6
Polyaminostyrene resins	T50.3X1	T50.3X2	T50.3X3	T50.3X4	T50.3X5	T50.3X6
Polycarbophil	T47.4X1	T47.4X2	T47.4X3	T47.4X4	T47.4X5	T47.4X6
Polychlorinated biphenyl	T65.891	T65.892	T65.893	T65.894	—	—
Polycycline	T36.4X1	T36.4X2	T36.4X3	T36.4X4	T36.4X5	T36.4X6
Polyester fumes	T59.891	T59.892	T59.893	T59.894	—	—
Polyester resin hardener	T52.91	T52.92	T52.93	T52.94	—	—
fumes	T59.891	T59.892	T59.893	T59.894	—	—
Polyestradiol phosphate	T38.5X1	T38.5X2	T38.5X3	T38.5X4	T38.5X5	T38.5X6
Polyethanolamine alkyl sulfate	T49.2X1	T49.2X2	T49.2X3	T49.2X4	T49.2X5	T49.2X6
Polyethylene adhesive	T49.3X1	T49.3X2	T49.3X3	T49.3X4	T49.3X5	T49.3X6
Polyferose	T45.4X1	T45.4X2	T45.4X3	T45.4X4	T45.4X5	T45.4X6
Polygeline	T45.8X1	T45.8X2	T45.8X3	T45.8X4	T45.8X5	T45.8X6
Polymyxin	T36.8X1	T36.8X2	T36.8X3	T36.8X4	T36.8X5	T36.8X6
B	T36.8X1	T36.8X2	T36.8X3	T36.8X4	T36.8X5	T36.8X6
ENT agent	T49.6X1	T49.6X2	T49.6X3	T49.6X4	T49.6X5	T49.6X6
ophthalmic preparation	T49.5X1	T49.5X2	T49.5X3	T49.5X4	T49.5X5	T49.5X6
topical NEC	T49.0X1	T49.0X2	T49.0X3	T49.0X4	T49.0X5	T49.0X6
E sulfate (eye preparation)	T49.5X1	T49.5X2	T49.5X3	T49.5X4	T49.5X5	T49.5X6
Polynoxylin	T49.0X1	T49.0X2	T49.0X3	T49.0X4	T49.0X5	T49.0X6
Polyoestradiol phosphate	T38.5X1	T38.5X2	T38.5X3	T38.5X4	T38.5X5	T38.5X6
Polyoxymethyleneurea	T49.0X1	T49.0X2	T49.0X3	T49.0X4	T49.0X5	T49.0X6

Substance	Poisoning, Accidental (Unintentional)	Poisoning, Intentional Self-Harm	Poisoning, Assault	Poisoning, Undetermined	Adverse Effect	Underdosing
Polysilane	T47.8X1	T47.8X2	T47.8X3	T47.8X4	T47.8X5	T47.8X6
Polytetrafluoroethylene (inhaled)	T59.891	T59.892	T59.893	T59.894	—	—
Polythiazide	T50.2X1	T50.2X2	T50.2X3	T50.2X4	T50.2X5	T50.2X6
Polyvidone	T45.8X1	T45.8X2	T45.8X3	T45.8X4	T45.8X5	T45.8X6
Polyvinylpyrrolidone	T45.8X1	T45.8X2	T45.8X3	T45.8X4	T45.8X5	T45.8X6
Pontocaine (hydrochloride) (infiltration) (topical)	T41.3X1	T41.3X2	T41.3X3	T41.3X4	T41.3X5	T41.3X6
nerve block (peripheral) (plexus)	T41.3X1	T41.3X2	T41.3X3	T41.3X4	T41.3X5	T41.3X6
spinal	T41.3X1	T41.3X2	T41.3X3	T41.3X4	T41.3X5	T41.3X6
Porfiromycin	T45.1X1	T45.1X2	T45.1X3	T45.1X4	T45.1X5	T45.1X6
Posterior pituitary hormone NEC	T38.891	T38.892	T38.893	T38.894	T38.895	T38.896
Pot	T40.7X1	T40.7X2	T40.7X3	T40.7X4	T40.7X5	T40.7X6
Potash (caustic)	T54.3X1	T54.3X2	T54.3X3	T54.3X4	—	—
Potassic saline injection (lactated)	T50.3X1	T50.3X2	T50.3X3	T50.3X4	T50.3X5	T50.3X6
Potassium (salts) NEC	T50.3X1	T50.3X2	T50.3X3	T50.3X4	T50.3X5	T50.3X6
aminobenzoate	T45.8X1	T45.8X2	T45.8X3	T45.8X4	T45.8X5	T45.8X6
aminosalicylate	T37.1X1	T37.1X2	T37.1X3	T37.1X4	T37.1X5	T37.1X6
antimony 'tartrate'	T37.8X1	T37.8X2	T37.8X3	T37.8X4	T37.8X5	T37.8X6
arsenite (solution)	T57.0X1	T57.0X2	T57.0X3	T57.0X4	—	—
bichromate	T56.2X1	T56.2X2	T56.2X3	T56.2X4	—	—
bisulfate	T47.3X1	T47.3X2	T47.3X3	T47.3X4	T47.3X5	T47.3X6
bromide	T42.6X1	T42.6X2	T42.6X3	T42.6X4	T42.6X5	T42.6X6
canrenoate	T50.0X1	T50.0X2	T50.0X3	T50.0X4	T50.0X5	T50.0X6
carbonate	T54.3X1	T54.3X2	T54.3X3	T54.3X4	—	—
chlorate NEC	T65.891	T65.892	T65.893	T65.894	—	—
chloride	T50.3X1	T50.3X2	T50.3X3	T50.3X4	T50.3X5	T50.3X6
citrate	T50.991	T50.992	T50.993	T50.994	T50.995	T50.996
cyanide	T65.0X1	T65.0X2	T65.0X3	T65.0X4	—	—
ferric hexacyanoferrate (medicinal)	T50.6X1	T50.6X2	T50.6X3	T50.6X4	T50.6X5	T50.6X6
nonmedicinal	T65.891	T65.892	T65.893	T65.894	—	—
Fluoride	T57.8X1	T57.8X2	T57.8X3	T57.8X4	—	—
glucaldrate	T47.1X1	T47.1X2	T47.1X3	T47.1X4	T47.1X5	T47.1X6
hydroxide	T54.3X1	T54.3X2	T54.3X3	T54.3X4	—	—
iodate	T49.0X1	T49.0X2	T49.0X3	T49.0X4	T49.0X5	T49.0X6
iodide	T48.4X1	T48.4X2	T48.4X3	T48.4X4	T48.4X5	T48.4X6
nitrate	T57.8X1	T57.8X2	T57.8X3	T57.8X4	—	—
oxalate	T65.891	T65.892	T65.893	T65.894	—	—
perchlorate (nonmedicinal) NEC	T65.891	T65.892	T65.893	T65.894	—	—
antithyroid	T38.2X1	T38.2X2	T38.2X3	T38.2X4	T38.2X5	T38.2X6
medicinal	T38.2X1	T38.2X2	T38.2X3	T38.2X4	T38.2X5	T38.2X6

◀ New ◀◀ Revised ~~deleted~~ Deleted

Substance	Poisoning, Accidental (Unintentional)	Poisoning, Intentional Self-Harm	Poisoning, Assault	Poisoning, Undetermined	Adverse Effect	Underdosing
Permanganate (nonmedicinal)	T65.891	T65.892	T65.893	T65.894	—	—
medicinal	T49.0X1	T49.0X2	T49.0X3	T49.0X4	T49.0X5	T49.0X6
sulfate	T47.2X1	T47.2X2	T47.2X3	T47.2X4	T47.2X5	T47.2X6
Potassium-removing resin	T50.3X1	T50.3X2	T50.3X3	T50.3X4	T50.3X5	T50.3X6
Potassium-retaining drug	T50.3X1	T50.3X2	T50.3X3	T50.3X4	T50.3X5	T50.3X6
Povidone	T45.8X1	T45.8X2	T45.8X4	T45.8X4	T45.8X5	T45.8X6
iodine	T49.0X1	T49.0X2	T49.0X3	T49.0X4	T49.0X5	T49.0X6
Practolol	T44.7X1	T44.7X2	T44.7X3	T44.7X4	T44.7X5	T44.7X6
Prajmalium bitartrate	T46.2X1	T46.2X2	T46.2X3	T46.2X4	T46.2X5	T46.2X6
Pralidoxime (iodide)	T50.6X1	T50.6X2	T50.6X3	T50.6X4	T50.6X5	T50.6X6
chloride	T50.6X1	T50.6X2	T50.6X3	T50.6X4	T50.6X5	T50.6X6
Pramiverine	T44.3X1	T44.3X2	T44.3X3	T44.3X4	T44.3X5	T44.3X6
Pramocaine	T49.1X1	T49.1X2	T49.1X3	T49.1X4	T49.1X5	T49.1X6
Pramoxine	T49.1X1	T49.1X2	T49.1X3	T49.1X4	T49.1X5	T49.1X6
Prasterone	T38.7X1	T38.7X2	T38.7X3	T38.7X4	T38.7X5	T38.7X6
Pravastatin	T46.6X1	T46.6X2	T46.6X3	T46.6X4	T46.6X5	T46.6X6
Prazepam	T42.4X1	T42.4X2	T42.4X3	T42.4X4	T42.4X5	T42.4X6
Praziquantel	T37.4X1	T37.4X2	T37.4X3	T37.4X4	T37.4X5	T37.4X6
Prazitone	T43.291	T43.292	T43.293	T43.294	T43.295	T43.296
Prazosin	T44.6X1	T44.6X2	T44.6X3	T44.6X4	T44.6X5	T44.6X6
Prednicarbate	T49.0X1	T49.0X2	T49.0X3	T49.0X4	T49.0X5	T49.0X6
Prednimustine	T45.1X1	T45.1X2	T45.1X3	T45.1X4	T45.1X5	T45.1X6
Prednisolone	T38.0X1	T38.0X2	T38.0X3	T38.0X4	T38.0X5	T38.0X6
ENT agent	T49.6X1	T49.6X2	T49.6X3	T49.6X4	T49.6X5	T49.6X6
ophthalmic preparation	T49.5X1	T49.5X2	T49.5X3	T49.5X4	T49.5X5	T49.5X6
steaglate	T49.0X1	T49.0X2	T49.0X3	T49.0X4	T49.0X5	T49.0X6
topical NEC	T49.0X1	T49.0X2	T49.0X3	T49.0X4	T49.0X5	T49.0X6
Prednisone	T38.0X1	T38.0X2	T38.0X3	T38.0X4	T38.0X5	T38.0X6
Prednylidene	T38.0X1	T38.0X2	T38.0X3	T38.0X4	T38.0X5	T38.0X6
Pregnandiol	T38.5X1	T38.5X2	T38.5X3	T38.5X4	T38.5X5	T38.5X6
Pregneninolone	T38.5X1	T38.5X2	T38.5X3	T38.5X4	T38.5X5	T38.5X6
Preludin	T43.691	T43.692	T43.693	T43.694	T43.695	T43.696
Premarin	T38.5X1	T38.5X2	T38.5X3	T38.5X4	T38.5X5	T38.5X6
Premedication anesthetic	T41.201	T41.202	T41.203	T41.204	T41.205	T41.206
Prenalterol	T44.5X1	T44.5X2	T44.5X3	T44.5X4	T44.5X5	T44.5X6
Prenoxdiazine	T48.3X1	T48.3X2	T48.3X3	T48.3X4	T48.3X5	T48.3X6
Prenylamine	T46.3X1	T46.3X2	T46.3X3	T46.3X4	T46.3X5	T46.3X6
Preparation, local	T49.4X1	T49.4X2	T49.4X3	T49.4X4	T49.4X5	T49.4X6
Preparation H	T49.8X1	T49.8X2	T49.8X3	T49.8X4	T49.8X5	T49.8X6
Preservative (nonmedicinal)	T65.891	T65.892	T65.893	T65.894	—	—
medicinal	T50.901	T50.902	T50.903	T50.904	T50.905	T50.906
wood	T60.91	T60.92	T60.93	T60.94	—	—

Substance	Poisoning, Accidental (Unintentional)	Poisoning, Intentional Self-Harm	Poisoning, Assault	Poisoning, Undetermined	Adverse Effect	Underdosing
Prethcamide	T50.7X1	T50.7X2	T50.7X3	T50.7X4	T50.7X5	T50.7X6
Pride of China	T62.2X1	T62.2X2	T62.2X3	T62.2X4	—	—
Pridinol	T44.3X1	T44.3X2	T44.3X3	T44.3X4	T44.3X5	T44.3X6
Prifinium bromide	T44.3X1	T44.3X2	T44.3X3	T44.3X4	T44.3X5	T44.3X6
Prilocaine	T41.3X1	T41.3X2	T41.3X3	T41.3X4	T41.3X5	T41.3X6
infiltration (subcutaneous)	T41.3X1	T41.3X2	T41.3X3	T41.3X4	T41.3X5	T41.3X6
nerve block (peripheral) (plexus)	T41.3X1	T41.3X2	T41.3X3	T41.3X4	T41.3X5	T41.3X6
regional	T41.3X1	T41.3X2	T41.3X3	T41.3X4	T41.3X5	T41.3X6
Primaquine	T37.2X1	T37.2X2	T37.2X3	T37.2X4	T37.2X5	T37.2X6
Primidone	T42.6X1	T42.6X2	T42.6X3	T42.6X4	T42.6X5	T42.6X6
Primula (veris)	T62.2X1	T62.2X2	T62.2X3	T62.2X4	—	—
Prinadol	T40.2X1	T40.2X2	T40.2X3	T40.2X4	T40.2X5	T40.2X6
Priscol, Priscoline	T44.6X1	T44.6X2	T44.6X3	T44.6X4	T44.6X5	T44.6X6
Pristinamycin	T36.3X1	T36.3X2	T36.3X3	T36.3X4	T36.3X5	T36.3X6
Privet	T62.2X1	T62.2X2	T62.2X3	T62.2X4	—	—
berries	T62.1X1	T62.1X2	T62.1X3	T62.1X4	—	—
Privine	T44.4X1	T44.4X2	T44.4X3	T44.4X4	T44.4X5	T44.4X6
Pro-Banthine	T44.3X1	T44.3X2	T44.3X3	T44.3X4	T44.3X5	T44.3X6
Probarbital	T42.3X1	T42.3X2	T42.3X3	T42.3X4	T42.3X5	T42.3X6
Probenecid	T50.4X1	T50.4X2	T50.4X3	T50.4X4	T50.4X5	T50.4X6
Probucol	T46.6X1	T46.6X2	T46.6X3	T46.6X4	T46.6X5	T46.6X6
Procainamide	T46.2X1	T46.2X2	T46.2X3	T46.2X4	T46.2X5	T46.2X6
Procaine	T41.3X1	T41.3X2	T41.3X3	T41.3X4	T41.3X5	T41.3X6
benzylpenicillin	T36.0X1	T36.0X2	T36.0X3	T36.0X4	T36.0X5	T36.0X6
nerve block (periphreal) (plexus)	T41.3X1	T41.3X2	T41.3X3	T41.3X4	T41.3X5	T41.3X6
penicillin G	T36.0X1	T36.0X2	T36.0X3	T36.0X4	T36.0X5	T36.0X6
regional	T41.3X1	T41.3X2	T41.3X3	T41.3X4	T41.3X5	T41.3X6
spinal	T41.3X1	T41.3X2	T41.3X3	T41.3X4	T41.3X5	T41.3X6
Procalmidol	T43.591	T43.592	T43.593	T43.594	T43.595	T43.596
Procarbazine	T45.1X1	T45.1X2	T45.1X3	T45.1X4	T45.1X5	T45.1X6
Procaterol	T44.5X1	T44.5X2	T44.5X3	T44.5X4	T44.5X5	T44.5X6
Prochlorperazine	T43.3X1	T43.3X2	T43.3X3	T43.3X4	T43.3X5	T43.3X6
Procyclidine	T44.3X1	T44.3X2	T44.3X3	T44.3X4	T44.3X5	T44.3X6
Producer gas	T58.8X1	T58.8X2	T58.8X3	T58.8X4	—	—
Profadol	T40.4X1	T40.4X2	T40.4X3	T40.4X4	T40.4X5	T40.4X6
Profenamine	T44.3X1	T44.3X2	T44.3X3	T44.3X4	T44.3X5	T44.3X6
Profenil	T44.3X1	T44.3X2	T44.3X3	T44.3X4	T44.3X5	T44.3X6
Proflavine	T49.0X1	T49.0X2	T49.0X3	T49.0X4	T49.0X5	T49.0X6
Progabide	T42.6X1	T42.6X2	T42.6X3	T42.6X4	T42.6X5	T42.6X6
Progestin	T38.5X1	T38.5X2	T38.5X3	T38.5X4	T38.5X5	T38.5X6
oral contraceptive	T38.4X1	T38.4X2	T38.4X3	T38.4X4	T38.4X5	T38.4X6

◀ New ◀▥ Revised ~~deleted~~ Deleted

Substance	Poisoning, Accidental (Unintentional)	Poisoning, Intentional Self-Harm	Poisoning, Assault	Poisoning, Undetermined	Adverse Effect	Underdosing
Progesterone	T38.5X1	T38.5X2	T38.5X3	T38.5X4	T38.5X5	T38.5X6
Progestogen NEC	T38.5X1	T38.5X2	T38.5X3	T38.5X4	T38.5X5	T38.5X6
Progestone	T38.5X1	T38.5X2	T38.5X3	T38.5X4	T38.5X5	T38.5X6
Proglumide	T47.1X1	T47.1X2	T47.1X3	T47.1X4	T47.1X5	T47.1X6
Proguanil	T37.2X1	T37.2X2	T37.2X3	T37.2X4	T37.2X5	T37.2X6
Prolactin	T38.811	T38.812	T38.813	T38.814	T38.815	T38.816
Prolintane	T43.691	T43.692	T43.693	T43.694	T43.695	T43.696
Proloid	T38.1X1	T38.1X2	T38.1X3	T38.1X4	T38.1X5	T38.1X6
Proluton	T38.5X1	T38.5X2	T38.5X3	T38.5X4	T38.5X5	T38.5X6
Promacetin	T37.1X1	T37.1X2	T37.1X3	T37.1X4	T37.1X5	T37.1X6
Promazine	T43.3X1	T43.3X2	T43.3X3	T43.3X4	T43.3X5	T43.3X6
Promedol	T40.2X1	T40.2X2	T40.2X3	T40.2X4	—	—
Promegestone	T38.5X1	T38.5X2	T38.5X3	T38.5X4	T38.5X5	T38.5X6
Promethazine (teoclate)	T43.3X1	T43.3X2	T43.3X3	T43.3X4	T43.3X5	T43.3X6
Promin	T37.1X1	T37.1X2	T37.1X3	T37.1X4	T37.1X5	T37.1X6
Pronase	T45.3X1	T45.3X2	T45.3X3	T45.3X4	T45.3X5	T45.3X6
Pronestyl (hydrochloride)	T46.2X1	T46.2X2	T46.2X3	T46.2X4	T46.2X5	T46.2X6
Pronetalol	T44.7X1	T44.7X2	T44.7X3	T44.7X4	T44.7X5	T44.7X6
Prontosil	T37.0X1	T37.0X2	T37.0X3	T37.0X4	T37.0X5	T37.0X6
Propachlor	T60.3X1	T60.3X2	T60.3X3	T60.3X4	—	—
Propafenone	T46.2X1	T46.2X2	T46.2X3	T46.2X4	T46.2X5	T46.2X6
Propallylonal	T42.3X1	T42.3X2	T42.3X3	T42.3X4	T42.3X5	T42.3X6
Propamidine	T49.0X1	T49.0X2	T49.0X3	T49.0X4	T49.0X5	T49.0X6
Propane (distributed in mobile container)	T59.891	T59.892	T59.893	T59.894	—	—
distributed through pipes	T59.891	T59.892	T59.893	T59.894	—	—
incomplete combustion	T57.11	T57.12	T57.13	T57.14	—	—
Propanidid	T41.291	T41.292	T41.293	T41.294	T41.295	T41.296
Propanil	T60.3X1	T60.3X2	T60.3X3	T60.3X4	—	—
1-Propanol	T51.3X1	T51.3X2	T51.3X3	T51.3X4	—	—
2-Propanol	T51.2X1	T51.2X2	T51.2X3	T51.2X4	—	—
Propantheline	T44.3X1	T44.3X2	T44.3X3	T44.3X4	T44.3X5	T44.3X6
bromide	T44.3X1	T44.3X2	T44.3X3	T44.3X4	T44.3X5	T44.3X6
Proparacaine	T41.3X1	T41.3X2	T41.3X3	T41.3X4	T41.3X5	T41.3X6
Propatylnitrate	T46.3X1	T46.3X2	T46.3X3	T46.3X4	T46.3X5	T46.3X6
Propicillin	T36.0X1	T36.0X2	T36.0X3	T36.0X4	T36.0X5	T36.0X6
Propiolactone	T49.0X1	T49.0X2	T49.0X3	T49.0X4	T49.0X5	T49.0X6
Propiomazine	T45.0X1	T45.0X2	T45.0X3	T45.0X4	T45.0X5	T45.0X6
Propionaidehyde (medicinal)	T42.6X1	T42.6X2	T42.6X3	T42.6X4	T42.6X5	T42.6X6
Propionaldehyde (medicinal) ◀	T42.6X1	T42.6X2	T42.6X3	T42.6X4	T42.6X5	T42.6X6
Propionate (calcium) (sodium)	T49.0X1	T49.0X2	T49.0X3	T49.0X4	T49.0X5	T49.0X6
Propion gel	T49.0X1	T49.0X2	T49.0X3	T49.0X4	T49.0X5	T49.0X6

Substance	Poisoning, Accidental (Unintentional)	Poisoning, Intentional Self-Harm	Poisoning, Assault	Poisoning, Undetermined	Adverse Effect	Underdosing
Propitocaine	T41.3X1	T41.3X2	T41.3X3	T41.3X4	T41.3X5	T41.3X6
infiltration (subcutaneous)	T41.3X1	T41.3X2	T41.3X3	T41.3X4	T41.3X5	T41.3X6
nerve block (peripheral) (plexus)	T41.3X1	T41.3X2	T41.3X3	T41.3X4	T41.3X5	T41.3X6
Propofol	T41.291	T41.292	T41.293	T41.294	T41.295	T41.296
Propoxur	T60.0X1	T60.0X2	T60.0X3	T60.0X4	—	—
Propoxycaine	T41.3X1	T41.3X2	T41.3X3	T41.3X4	T41.3X5	T41.3X6
infiltration (subcutaneous)	T41.3X1	T41.3X2	T41.3X3	T41.3X4	T41.3X5	T41.3X6
nerve block (peripheral) (plexus)	T41.3X1	T41.3X2	T41.3X3	T41.3X4	T41.3X5	T41.3X6
topical (surface)	T41.3X1	T41.3X2	T41.3X3	T41.3X4	T41.3X5	T41.3X6
Propoxyphene	T40.4X1	T40.4X2	T40.4X3	T40.4X4	T40.4X5	T40.4X6
Propranolol	T44.7X1	T44.7X2	T44.7X3	T44.7X4	T44.7X5	T44.7X6
Propyl						
alcohol	T51.3X1	T51.3X2	T51.3X3	T51.3X4	—	—
carbinol	T51.3X1	T51.3X2	T51.3X3	T51.3X4	—	—
hexadrine	T44.4X1	T44.4X2	T44.4X3	T44.4X4	T44.4X5	T44.4X6
iodone	T50.8X1	T50.8X2	T50.8X3	T50.8X4	T50.8X5	T50.8X6
thiouracil	T38.2X1	T38.2X2	T38.2X3	T38.2X4	T38.2X5	T38.2X6
Propylaminophenothiazine	T43.3X1	T43.3X2	T43.3X3	T43.3X4	T43.3X5	T43.3X6
Propylene	T59.891	T59.892	T59.893	T59.894	—	—
Propylhexedrine	T48.5X1	T48.5X2	T48.5X3	T48.5X4	T48.5X5	T48.5X6
Propyliodone	T50.8X1	T50.8X2	T50.8X3	T50.8X4	T50.8X5	T50.8X6
Propylthiouracil	T38.2X1	T38.2X2	T38.2X3	T38.2X4	T38.2X5	T38.2X6
Propylparaben (ophthalmic)	T49.5X1	T49.5X2	T49.5X3	T49.5X4	T49.5X5	T49.5X6
Propyphenazone	T39.2X1	T39.2X2	T39.2X3	T39.2X4	T39.2X5	T39.2X6
Proquazone	T39.391	T39.392	T39.393	T39.394	T39.395	T39.396
Proscillaridin	T46.0X1	T46.0X2	T46.0X3	T46.0X4	T46.0X5	T46.0X6
Prostacyclin	T45.521	T45.522	T45.523	T45.524	T45.525	T45.526
Prostaglandin (I2)	T45.521	T45.522	T45.523	T45.524	T45.525	T45.526
E1	T46.7X1	T46.7X2	T46.7X3	T46.7X4	T46.7X5	T46.7X6
E2	T48.0X1	T48.0X2	T48.0X3	T48.0X4	T48.0X5	T48.0X6
F2 alpha	T48.0X1	T48.0X2	T48.0X3	T48.0X4	T48.0X5	T48.0X6
Prostigmin	T44.0X1	T44.0X2	T44.0X3	T44.0X4	T44.0X5	T44.0X6
Prosultiamine	T45.2X1	T45.2X2	T45.2X3	T45.2X4	T45.2X5	T45.2X6
Protamine sulfate	T45.7X1	T45.7X2	T45.7X3	T45.7X4	T45.7X5	T45.7X6
zinc insulin	T38.3X1	T38.3X2	T38.3X3	T38.3X4	T38.3X5	T38.3X6
Protease	T47.5X1	T47.5X2	T47.5X3	T47.5X4	T47.5X5	T47.5X6
Protectant, skin NEC	T49.3X1	T49.3X2	T49.3X3	T49.3X4	T49.3X5	T49.3X6
Protein hydrolysate	T50.991	T50.992	T50.993	T50.994	T50.995	T50.996
Prothiaden — see Dothiepin hydrochloride						
Prothionamide	T37.1X1	T37.1X2	T37.1X3	T37.1X4	T37.1X5	T37.1X6

◀ New   ◀◀ Revised   ~~deleted~~ Deleted

Substance	Poisoning, Accidental (Unintentional)	Poisoning, Intentional Self-Harm	Poisoning, Assault	Poisoning, Undetermined	Adverse Effect	Underdosing
Prothipendyl	T43.591	T43.592	T43.593	T43.594	T43.595	T43.596
Prothoate	T60.0X1	T60.0X2	T60.0X3	T60.0X4	—	—
Prothrombin						
activator	T45.7X1	T45.7X2	T45.7X3	T45.7X4	T45.7X5	T45.7X6
synthesis inhibitor	T45.511	T45.512	T45.513	T45.514	T45.515	T45.516
Protionamide	T37.1X1	T37.1X2	T37.1X3	T37.1X4	T37.1X5	T37.1X6
Protirelin	T38.891	T38.892	T38.893	T38.894	T38.895	T38.896
Protokylol	T48.6X1	T48.6X2	T48.6X3	T48.6X4	T48.6X5	T48.6X6
Protopam	T50.6X1	T50.6X2	T50.6X3	T50.6X4	T50.6X5	T50.6X6
Protoveratrine(s) (A) (B)	T46.5X1	T46.5X2	T46.5X3	T46.5X4	T46.5X5	T46.5X6
Protriptyline	T43.011	T43.012	T43.013	T43.014	T43.015	T43.016
Provera	T38.5X1	T38.5X2	T38.5X3	T38.5X4	T38.5X5	T38.5X6
Provitamin A	T45.2X1	T45.2X2	T45.2X3	T45.2X4	T45.2X5	T45.2X6
Proxibarbal	T42.3X1	T42.3X2	T42.3X3	T42.3X4	T42.3X5	T42.3X6
Proxymetacaine	T41.3X1	T41.3X2	T41.3X3	T41.3X4	T41.3X5	T41.3X6
Proxyphylline	T48.6X1	T48.6X2	T48.6X3	T48.6X4	T48.6X5	T48.6X6
Prozac — see Fluoxetine hydrochloride						
Prunus						
laurocerasus	T62.2X1	T62.2X2	T62.2X3	T62.2X4	—	—
virginiana	T62.2X1	T62.2X2	T62.2X3	T62.2X4	—	—
Prussian blue						
commercial	T65.891	T65.892	T65.893	T65.894	—	—
therapeutic	T50.6X1	T50.6X2	T50.6X3	T50.6X4	T50.6X5	T50.6X6
Prussic acid	T65.0X1	T65.0X2	T65.0X3	T65.0X4	—	—
vapor	T57.3X1	T57.3X2	T57.3X3	T57.3X4		
Pseudoephedrine	T44.991	T44.992	T44.993	T44.994	T44.995	T44.996
Psilocin	T40.991	T40.992	T40.993	T40.994	—	—
Psilocybin	T40.991	T40.992	T40.993	T40.994	—	—
Psilocybine	T40.991	T40.992	T40.993	T40.994	—	—
Psoralene (nonmedicinal)	T65.891	T65.892	T65.893	T65.894	—	—
Psoralens (medicinal)	T50.991	T50.992	T50.993	T50.994	T50.995	T50.996
PSP (phenolsulfonphthalein)	T50.8X1	T50.8X2	T50.8X3	T50.8X4	T50.8X5	T50.8X6
Psychodysleptic drug NEC	T40.901	T40.902	T40.903	T40.904	T40.905	T40.906
Psychostimulant	T43.601	T43.602	T43.603	T43.604	T43.605	T43.606
amphetamine	T43.621	T43.622	T43.623	T43.624	T43.625	T43.626
caffeine	T43.611	T43.612	T43.613	T43.614	T43.615	T43.616
methylphenidate	T43.631	T43.632	T43.633	T43.634	T43.635	T43.636
specified NEC	T43.691	T43.692	T43.693	T43.694	T43.695	T43.696
Psychotherapeutic drug NEC	T43.91	T43.92	T43.93	T43.94	T43.95	T43.96
antidepressants — see also Antidepressant	T43.201	T43.202	T43.203	T43.204	T43.205	T43.206

Substance	Poisoning, Accidental (Unintentional)	Poisoning, Intentional Self-Harm	Poisoning, Assault	Poisoning, Undetermined	Adverse Effect	Underdosing
Psychotherapeutic drug NEC (Continued)						
specified NEC	T43.8X1	T43.8X2	T43.8X3	T43.8X4	T43.8X5	T43.8X6
tranquilizers NEC	T43.501	T43.502	T43.503	T43.504	T43.505	T43.506
Psychotomimetic agents	T40.901	T40.902	T40.903	T40.904	T40.905	T40.906
Psychotropic drug NEC	T43.91	T43.92	T43.93	T43.94	T43.95	T43.96
specified NEC	T43.8X1	T43.8X2	T43.8X3	T43.8X4	T43.8X5	T43.8X6
Psyllium hydrophilic mucilloid	T47.4X1	T47.4X2	T47.4X3	T47.4X4	T47.4X5	T47.4X6
Pteroylglutamic acid	T45.8X1	T45.8X2	T45.8X3	T45.8X4	T45.8X5	T45.8X6
Pteroyltriglutamate	T45.1X1	T45.1X2	T45.1X3	T45.1X4	T45.1X5	T45.1X6
PTFE — see Polytetrafluoroethylene						
Pulp						
devitalizing paste	T49.7X1	T49.7X2	T49.7X3	T49.7X4	T49.7X5	T49.7X6
dressing	T49.7X1	T49.7X2	T49.7X3	T49.7X4	T49.7X5	T49.7X6
Pulsatilla	T62.2X1	T62.2X2	T62.2X3	T62.2X4	—	—
Pumpkin seed extract	T37.4X1	T37.4X2	T37.4X3	T37.4X4	T37.4X5	T37.4X6
Purex (bleach)	T54.91	T54.92	T54.93	T54.94	—	—
Purgative NEC — see also Cathartic	T47.4X1	T47.4X2	T47.4X3	T47.4X4	T47.4X5	T47.4X6
Purine analogue (antineoplastic)	T45.1X1	T45.1X2	T45.1X3	T45.1X4	T45.1X5	T45.1X6
Purine diuretics	T50.2X1	T50.2X2	T50.2X3	T50.2X4	T50.2X5	T50.2X6
Purinethol	T45.1X1	T45.1X2	T45.1X3	T45.1X4	T45.1X5	T45.1X6
PVP	T45.8X1	T45.8X2	T45.8X3	T45.8X4	T45.8X5	T45.8X6
Pyrabital	T39.8X1	T39.8X2	T39.8X3	T39.8X4	T39.8X5	T39.8X6
Pyramidon	T39.2X1	T39.2X2	T39.2X3	T39.2X4	T39.2X5	T39.2X6
Pyrantel	T37.4X1	T37.4X2	T37.4X3	T37.4X4	T37.4X5	T37.4X6
Pyrathiazine	T45.0X1	T45.0X2	T45.0X3	T45.0X4	T45.0X5	T45.0X6
Pyrazinamide	T37.1X1	T37.1X2	T37.1X3	T37.1X4	T37.1X5	T37.1X6
Pyrazinoic acid (amide)	T37.1X1	T37.1X2	T37.1X3	T37.1X4	T37.1X5	T37.1X6
Pyrazole (derivatives)	T39.2X1	T39.2X2	T39.2X3	T39.2X4	T39.2X5	T39.2X6
Pyrazolone analgesic NEC	T39.2X1	T39.2X2	T39.2X3	T39.2X4	T39.2X5	T39.2X6
Pyrethrin, pyrethrum (nonmedicinal)	T60.2X1	T60.2X2	T60.2X3	T60.2X4	—	—
Pyrethrum extract	T49.0X1	T49.0X2	T49.0X3	T49.0X4	T49.0X5	T49.0X6
Pyribenzamine	T45.0X1	T45.0X2	T45.0X3	T45.0X4	T45.0X5	T45.0X6
Pyridine	T52.8X1	T52.8X2	T52.8X3	T52.8X4		
aldoxime methiodide	T50.6X1	T50.6X2	T50.6X3	T50.6X4	T50.6X5	T50.6X6
aldoxime methyl chloride	T50.6X1	T50.6X2	T50.6X3	T50.6X4	T50.6X5	T50.6X6
vapor	T59.891	T59.892	T59.893	T59.894	—	—
Pyridium	T39.8X1	T39.8X2	T39.8X3	T39.8X4	T39.8X5	T39.8X6
Pyridostigmine bromide	T44.0X1	T44.0X2	T44.0X3	T44.0X4	T44.0X5	T44.0X6
Pyridoxal phosphate	T45.2X1	T45.2X2	T45.2X3	T45.2X4	T45.2X5	T45.2X6

TABLE OF DRUGS AND CHEMICALS

Substance	Poisoning, Accidental (Unintentional)	Poisoning, Intentional Self-Harm	Poisoning, Assault	Poisoning, Undetermined	Adverse Effect	Underdosing
Pyridoxine	T45.2X1	T45.2X2	T45.2X3	T45.2X4	T45.2X5	T45.2X6
Pyrilamine	T45.0X1	T45.0X2	T45.0X3	T45.0X4	T45.0X5	T45.0X6
Pyrimethamine	T37.2X1	T37.2X2	T37.2X3	T37.2X4	T37.2X5	T37.2X6
with sulfadoxine	T37.2X1	T37.2X2	T37.2X3	T37.2X4	T37.2X5	T37.2X6
Pyrimidine antagonist	T45.1X1	T45.1X2	T45.1X3	T45.1X4	T45.1X5	T45.1X6
Pyriminil	T60.4X1	T60.4X2	T60.4X3	T60.4X4	—	—
Pyrithione zinc	T49.4X1	T49.4X2	T49.4X3	T49.4X4	T49.4X5	T49.4X6
Pyrithyldione	T42.6X1	T42.6X2	T42.6X3	T42.6X4	T42.6X5	T42.6X6
Pyrogallic acid	T49.0X1	T49.0X2	T49.0X3	T49.0X4	T49.0X5	T49.0X6
Pyrogallol	T49.0X1	T49.0X2	T49.0X3	T49.0X4	T49.0X5	T49.0X6
Pyroxylin	T49.3X1	T49.3X2	T49.3X3	T49.3X4	T49.3X5	T49.3X6
Pyrrobutamine	T45.0X1	T45.0X2	T45.0X3	T45.0X4	T45.0X5	T45.0X6
Pyrrolizidine alkaloids	T62.8X1	T62.8X2	T62.8X3	T62.8X4	—	—
Pyrvinium chloride	T37.4X1	T37.4X2	T37.4X3	T37.4X4	T37.4X5	T37.4X6
PZI	T38.3X1	T38.3X2	T38.3X3	T38.3X4	T38.3X5	T38.3X6
Q						
Quaalude	T42.6X1	T42.6X2	T42.6X3	T42.6X4	T42.6X5	T42.6X6
Quarternary ammonium						
anti-infective	T49.0X1	T49.0X2	T49.0X3	T49.0X4	T49.0X5	T49.0X6
ganglion blocking	T44.2X1	T44.2X2	T44.2X3	T44.2X4	T44.2X5	T44.2X6
parasympatholytic	T44.3X1	T44.3X2	T44.3X3	T44.3X4	T44.3X5	T44.3X6
Quazepam	T42.4X1	T42.4X2	T42.4X3	T42.4X4	T42.4X5	T42.4X6
Quicklime	T54.3X1	T54.3X2	T54.3X3	T54.3X4	—	—
Quillaja extract	T48.4X1	T48.4X2	T48.4X3	T48.4X4	T48.4X5	T48.4X6
Quinacrine	T37.2X1	T37.2X2	T37.2X3	T37.2X4	T37.2X5	T37.2X6
Quinaglute	T46.2X1	T46.2X2	T46.2X3	T46.2X4	T46.2X5	T46.2X6
Quinalbarbital	T42.3X1	T42.3X2	T42.3X3	T42.3X4	T42.3X5	T42.3X6
Quinalbarbitone sodium	T42.3X1	T42.3X2	T42.3X3	T42.3X4	T42.3X5	T42.3X6
Quinalphos	T60.0X1	T60.0X2	T60.0X3	T60.0X4	—	—
Quinapril	T46.4X1	T46.4X2	T46.4X3	T46.4X4	T46.4X5	T46.4X6
Quinestradiol	T38.5X1	T38.5X2	T38.5X3	T38.5X4	T38.5X5	T38.5X6
Quinestradol	T38.5X1	T38.5X2	T38.5X3	T38.5X4	T38.5X5	T38.5X6
Quinestrol	T38.5X1	T38.5X2	T38.5X3	T38.5X4	T38.5X5	T38.5X6
Quinethazone	T50.2X1	T50.2X2	T50.2X3	T50.2X4	T50.2X5	T50.2X6
Quingestanol	T38.4X1	T38.4X2	T38.4X3	T38.4X4	T38.4X5	T38.4X6
Quinidine	T46.2X1	T46.2X2	T46.2X3	T46.2X4	T46.2X5	T46.2X6
Quinine	T37.2X1	T37.2X2	T37.2X3	T37.2X4	T37.2X5	T37.2X6
Quiniobine	T37.8X1	T37.8X2	T37.8X3	T37.8X4	T37.8X5	T37.8X6
Quinisocaine	T49.1X1	T49.1X2	T49.1X3	T49.1X4	T49.1X5	T49.1X6
Quinocide	T37.2X1	T37.2X2	T37.2X3	T37.2X4	T37.2X5	T37.2X6
Quinoline (derivatives) NEC	T37.8X1	T37.8X2	T37.8X3	T37.8X4	T37.8X5	T37.8X6

Substance	Poisoning, Accidental (Unintentional)	Poisoning, Intentional Self-Harm	Poisoning, Assault	Poisoning, Undetermined	Adverse Effect	Underdosing
Quinupramine	T43.011	T43.012	T43.013	T43.014	T43.015	T43.016
Quotane	T41.3X1	T41.3X2	T41.3X3	T41.3X4	T41.3X5	T41.3X6
R						
Rabies						
immune globulin (human)	T50.Z11	T50.Z12	T50.Z13	T50.Z14	T50.Z15	T50.Z16
vaccine	T50.B91	T50.B92	T50.B93	T50.B94	T50.B95	T50.B96
Racemoramide	T40.2X1	T40.2X2	T40.2X3	T40.2X4	—	—
Racemorphan	T40.2X1	T40.2X2	T40.2X3	T40.2X4	T40.2X5	T40.2X6
Racepinefrin	T44.5X1	T44.5X2	T44.5X3	T44.5X4	T44.5X5	T44.5X6
Raclopride	T43.591	T43.592	T43.593	T43.594	T43.595	T43.596
Radiator alcohol	T51.1X1	T51.1X2	T51.1X3	T51.1X4	—	—
Radioactive drug NEC	T50.8X1	T50.8X2	T50.8X3	T50.8X4	T50.8X5	T50.8X6
Radio-opaque (drugs) (materials)	T50.8X1	T50.8X2	T50.8X3	T50.8X4	T50.8X5	T50.8X6
Ramifenazone	T39.2X1	T39.2X2	T39.2X3	T39.2X4	T39.2X5	T39.2X6
Ramipril	T46.4X1	T46.4X2	T46.4X3	T46.4X4	T46.4X5	T46.4X6
Ranitidine	T47.0X1	T47.0X2	T47.0X3	T47.0X4	T47.0X5	T47.0X6
Ranunculus	T62.2X1	T62.2X2	T62.2X3	T62.2X4	—	—
Rat poison NEC	T60.4X1	T60.4X2	T60.4X3	T60.4X4	—	—
Rattlesnake (venom)	T63.011	T63.012	T63.013	T63.014	—	—
Raubasine	T46.7X1	T46.7X2	T46.7X3	T46.7X4	T46.7X5	T46.7X6
Raudixin	T46.5X1	T46.5X2	T46.5X3	T46.5X4	T46.5X5	T46.5X6
Rautensin	T46.5X1	T46.5X2	T46.5X3	T46.5X4	T46.5X5	T46.5X6
Rautina	T46.5X1	T46.5X2	T46.5X3	T46.5X4	T46.5X5	T46.5X6
Rautotal	T46.5X1	T46.5X2	T46.5X3	T46.5X4	T46.5X5	T46.5X6
Rauwiloid	T46.5X1	T46.5X2	T46.5X3	T46.5X4	T46.5X5	T46.5X6
Rauwoldin	T46.5X1	T46.5X2	T46.5X3	T46.5X4	T46.5X5	T46.5X6
Rauwolfia (alkaloids)	T46.5X1	T46.5X2	T46.5X3	T46.5X4	T46.5X5	T46.5X6
Razoxane	T45.1X1	T45.1X2	T45.1X3	T45.1X4	T45.1X5	T45.1X6
Realgar	T57.0X1	T57.0X2	T57.0X3	T57.0X4	—	—
Recombinant (R) — see specific protein						
Red blood cells, packed	T45.8X1	T45.8X2	T45.8X3	T45.8X4	T45.8X5	T45.8X6
Red squill (scilliroside)	T60.4X1	T60.4X2	T60.4X3	T60.4X4	—	—
Reducing agent, industrial NEC	T65.891	T65.892	T65.893	T65.894	—	—
Refrigerant gas (chlorofluoro-carbon)	T53.5X1	T53.5X2	T53.5X3	T53.5X4	—	—
not chlorofluoro-carbon	T59.891	T59.892	T59.893	T59.894	—	—
Regroton	T50.2X1	T50.2X2	T50.2X3	T50.2X4	T50.2X5	T50.2X6
Rehydration salts (oral)	T50.3X1	T50.3X2	T50.3X3	T50.3X4	T50.3X5	T50.3X6
Rela	T42.8X1	T42.8X2	T42.8X3	T42.8X4	T42.8X5	T42.8X6

◀ New ◀▒▒ Revised ~~deleted~~ Deleted

Substance	Poisoning, Accidental (Unintentional)	Poisoning, Intentional Self-Harm	Poisoning, Assault	Poisoning, Undetermined	Adverse Effect	Underdosing
Relaxant, muscle						
anesthetic	T48.1X1	T48.1X2	T48.1X3	T48.1X4	T48.1X5	T48.1X6
central nervous system	T42.8X1	T42.8X2	T42.8X3	T42.8X4	T42.8X5	T42.8X6
skeletal NEC	T48.1X1	T48.1X2	T48.1X3	T48.1X4	T48.1X5	T48.1X6
smooth NEC	T44.3X1	T44.3X2	T44.3X3	T44.3X4	T44.3X5	T44.3X6
Remoxipride	T43.591	T43.592	T43.593	T43.594	T43.595	T43.596
Renese	T50.2X1	T50.2X2	T50.2X3	T50.2X4	T50.2X5	T50.2X6
Renografin	T50.8X1	T50.8X2	T50.8X3	T50.8X4	T50.8X5	T50.8X6
Replacement solution	T50.3X1	T50.3X2	T50.3X3	T50.3X4	T50.3X5	T50.3X6
Reproterol	T48.6X1	T48.6X2	T48.6X3	T48.6X4	T48.6X5	T48.6X6
Rescinnamine	T46.5X1	T46.5X2	T46.5X3	T46.5X4	T46.5X5	T46.5X6
Reserpin(e)	T46.5X1	T46.5X2	T46.5X3	T46.5X4	T46.5X5	T46.5X6
Resorcin, resorcinol (nonmedicinal)	T65.891	T65.892	T65.893	T65.894	—	—
medicinal	T49.4X1	T49.4X2	T49.4X3	T49.4X4	T49.4X5	T49.4X6
Respaire	T48.4X1	T48.4X2	T48.4X3	T48.4X4	T48.4X5	T48.4X6
Respiratory drug NEC	T48.901	T48.902	T48.903	T48.904	T48.905	T48.906
antiasthmatic NEC	T48.6X1	T48.6X2	T48.6X3	T48.6X4	T48.6X5	T48.6X6
anti-common-cold NEC	T48.5X1	T48.5X2	T48.5X3	T48.5X4	T48.5X5	T48.5X6
expectorant NEC	T48.4X1	T48.4X2	T48.4X3	T48.4X4	T48.4X5	T48.4X6
stimulant	T48.901	T48.902	T48.903	T48.904	T48.905	T48.906
Retinoic acid	T49.0X1	T49.0X2	T49.0X3	T49.0X4	T49.0X5	T49.0X6
Retinol	T45.2X1	T45.2X2	T45.2X3	T45.2X4	T45.2X5	T45.2X6
Rh (D) immune globulin (human)	T50.Z11	T50.Z12	T50.Z13	T50.Z14	T50.Z15	T50.Z16
Rhodine	T39.011	T39.012	T39.013	T39.014	T39.015	T39.016
RhoGAM	T50.Z11	T50.Z12	T50.Z13	T50.Z14	T50.Z15	T50.Z16
Rhubarb						
dry extract	T47.2X1	T47.2X2	T47.2X3	T47.2X4	T47.2X5	T47.2X6
tincture, compound	T47.2X1	T47.2X2	T47.2X3	T47.2X4	T47.2X5	T47.2X6
Ribavirin	T37.5X1	T37.5X2	T37.5X3	T37.5X4	T37.5X5	T37.5X6
Riboflavin	T45.2X1	T45.2X2	T45.2X3	T45.2X4	T45.2X5	T45.2X6
Ribostamycin	T36.5X1	T36.5X2	T36.5X3	T36.5X4	T36.5X5	T36.5X6
Ricin	T62.2X1	T62.2X2	T62.2X3	T62.2X4	—	—
Ricinus communis	T62.2X1	T62.2X2	T62.2X3	T62.2X4	—	—
Rickettsial vaccine NEC	T50.A91	T50.A92	T50.A93	T50.A94	T50.A95	T50.A96
Rifabutin	T36.6X1	T36.6X2	T36.6X3	T36.6X4	T36.6X5	T36.6X6
Rifamide	T36.6X1	T36.6X2	T36.6X3	T36.6X4	T36.6X5	T36.6X6
Rifampicin	T36.6X1	T36.6X2	T36.6X3	T36.6X4	T36.6X5	T36.6X6
with isoniazid	T37.1X1	T37.1X2	T37.1X3	T37.1X4	T37.1X5	T37.1X6
Rifampin	T36.6X1	T36.6X2	T36.6X3	T36.6X4	T36.6X5	T36.6X6
Rifamycin	T36.6X1	T36.6X2	T36.6X3	T36.6X4	T36.6X5	T36.6X6
Rifaximin	T36.6X1	T36.6X2	T36.6X3	T36.6X4	T36.6X5	T36.6X6

Substance	Poisoning, Accidental (Unintentional)	Poisoning, Intentional Self-Harm	Poisoning, Assault	Poisoning, Undetermined	Adverse Effect	Underdosing
Rimantadine	T37.5X1	T37.5X2	T37.5X3	T37.5X4	T37.5X5	T37.5X6
Rimazolium metilsulfate	T39.8X1	T39.8X2	T39.8X3	T39.8X4	T39.8X5	T39.8X6
Rimifon	T37.1X1	T37.1X2	T37.1X3	T37.1X4	T37.1X5	T37.1X6
Rimiterol	T48.6X1	T48.6X2	T48.6X3	T48.6X4	T48.6X5	T48.6X6
Ringer (lactate) solution	T50.3X1	T50.3X2	T50.3X3	T50.3X4	T50.3X5	T50.3X6
Ristocetin	T36.8X1	T36.8X2	T36.8X3	T36.8X4	T36.8X5	T36.8X6
Ritalin	T43.631	T43.632	T43.633	T43.634	T43.635	T43.636
Ritodrine	T44.5X1	T44.5X2	T44.5X3	T44.5X4	T44.5X5	T44.5X6
Roach killer — *see Insecticide*						
Rociverine	T44.3X1	T44.3X2	T44.3X3	T44.3X4	T44.3X5	T44.3X6
Rocky Mountain spotted fever vaccine	T50.A91	T50.A92	T50.A93	T50.A94	T50.A95	T50.A96
Rodenticide NEC	T60.4X1	T60.4X2	T60.4X3	T60.4X4	—	—
Rohypnol	T42.4X1	T42.4X2	T42.4X3	T42.4X4	T42.4X5	T42.4X6
Rokitamycin	T36.3X1	T36.3X2	T36.3X3	T36.3X4	T36.3X5	T36.3X6
Rolaids	T47.1X1	T47.1X2	T47.1X3	T47.1X4	T47.1X5	T47.1X6
Rolitetracycline	T36.4X1	T36.4X2	T36.4X3	T36.4X4	T36.4X5	T36.4X6
Romilar	T48.3X1	T48.3X2	T48.3X3	T48.3X4	T48.3X5	T48.3X6
Ronifibrate	T46.6X1	T46.6X2	T46.6X3	T46.6X4	T46.6X5	T46.6X6
Rosaprostol	T47.1X1	T47.1X2	T47.1X3	T47.1X4	T47.1X5	T47.1X6
Rose bengal sodium (131I)	T50.8X1	T50.8X2	T50.8X3	T50.8X4	T50.8X5	T50.8X6
Rose water ointment	T49.3X1	T49.3X2	T49.3X3	T49.3X4	T49.3X5	T49.3X6
Rosoxacin	T37.8X1	T37.8X2	T37.8X3	T37.8X4	T37.8X5	T37.8X6
Rotenone	T60.2X1	T60.2X2	T60.2X3	T60.2X4	—	—
Rotoxamine	T45.0X1	T45.0X2	T45.0X3	T45.0X4	T45.0X5	T45.0X6
Rough-on-rats	T60.4X1	T60.4X2	T60.4X3	T60.4X4	—	—
Roxatidine	T47.0X1	T47.0X2	T47.0X3	T47.0X4	T47.0X5	T47.0X6
Roxithromycin	T36.3X1	T36.3X2	T36.3X3	T36.3X4	T36.3X5	T36.3X6
Rt-PA	T45.611	T45.612	T45.613	T45.614	T45.615	T45.616
Rubbing alcohol	T51.2X1	T51.2X2	T51.2X3	T51.2X4	—	—
Rubefacient	T49.4X1	T49.4X2	T49.4X3	T49.4X4	T49.4X5	T49.4X6
Rubella vaccine	T50.B91	T50.B92	T50.B93	T50.B94	T50.B95	T50.B96
Rubelogen	T50.B91	T50.B92	T50.B93	T50.B94	T50.B95	T50.B96
Rubeovax	T50.991	T50.992	T50.993	T50.994	T50.995	T50.996
Rubidium chloride Rb82	T50.8X1	T50.8X2	T50.8X3	T50.8X4	T50.8X5	T50.8X6
Rubidomycin	T45.1X1	T45.1X2	T45.1X3	T45.1X4	T45.1X5	T45.1X6
Rue	T62.2X1	T62.2X2	T62.2X3	T62.2X4	—	—
Rufocromomycin	T45.1X1	T45.1X2	T45.1X3	T45.1X4	T45.1X5	T45.1X6
Russel's viper venin	T45.7X1	T45.7X2	T45.7X3	T45.7X4	T45.7X5	T45.7X6
Ruta (graveolens)	T62.2X1	T62.2X2	T62.2X3	T62.2X4	—	—
Rutinum	T46.991	T46.992	T46.993	T46.994	T46.995	T46.996
Rutoside	T46.991	T46.992	T46.993	T46.994	T46.995	T46.996

◀ New   ◀▥ Revised   ~~deleted~~ Deleted

TABLE OF DRUGS AND CHEMICALS

TABLE OF DRUGS AND CHEMICALS

Substance	Poisoning, Accidental (Unintentional)	Poisoning, Intentional Self-Harm	Poisoning, Assault	Poisoning, Undetermined	Adverse Effect	Underdosing
S						
Sabadilla (plant)	T62.2X1	T62.2X2	T62.2X3	T62.2X4	—	—
pesticide	T60.2X1	T60.2X2	T60.2X3	T60.2X4	—	—
Saccharated iron oxide	T45.8X1	T45.8X2	T45.8X3	T45.8X4	T45.8X5	T45.8X6
Saccharin	T50.901	T50.902	T50.903	T50.904	T50.905	T50.906
Saccharomyces boulardii	T47.6X1	T47.6X2	T47.6X3	T47.6X4	T47.6X5	T47.6X6
Safflower oil	T46.6X1	T46.6X2	T46.6X3	T46.6X4	T46.6X5	T46.6X6
Safrazine	T43.1X1	T43.1X2	T43.1X3	T43.1X4	T43.1X5	T43.1X6
Salazosulfapyridine	T37.0X1	T37.0X2	T37.0X3	T37.0X4	T37.0X5	T37.0X6
Salbutamol	T48.6X1	T48.6X2	T48.6X3	T48.6X4	T48.6X5	T48.6X6
Salicylamide	T39.091	T39.092	T39.093	T39.094	T39.095	T39.096
Salicylate NEC	T39.091	T39.092	T39.093	T39.094	T39.095	T39.096
methyl	T49.3X1	T49.3X2	T49.3X3	T49.3X4	T49.3X5	T49.3X6
theobromine calcium	T50.2X1	T50.2X2	T50.2X3	T50.2X4	T50.2X5	T50.2X6
Salicylazosulfapyridine	T37.0X1	T37.0X2	T37.0X3	T37.0X4	T37.0X5	T37.0X6
Salicylhydroxamic acid	T49.0X1	T49.0X2	T49.0X3	T49.0X4	T49.0X5	T49.0X6
Salicylic acid	T49.4X1	T49.4X2	T49.4X3	T49.4X4	T49.4X5	T49.4X6
with benzoic acid	T49.4X1	T49.4X2	T49.4X3	T49.4X4	T49.4X5	T49.4X6
congeners	T39.091	T39.092	T39.093	T39.094	T39.095	T39.096
derivative	T39.091	T39.092	T39.093	T39.094	T39.095	T39.096
salts	T39.091	T39.092	T39.093	T39.094	T39.095	T39.096
Salinazid	T37.1X1	T37.1X2	T37.1X3	T37.1X4	T37.1X5	T37.1X6
Salmeterol	T48.6X1	T48.6X2	T48.6X3	T48.6X4	T48.6X5	T48.6X6
Salol	T49.3X1	T49.3X2	T49.3X3	T49.3X4	T49.3X5	T49.3X6
Salsalate	T39.091	T39.092	T39.093	T39.094	T39.095	T39.096
Salt substitute	T50.901	T50.902	T50.903	T50.904	T50.905	T50.906
Salt-replacing drug	T50.901	T50.902	T50.903	T50.904	T50.905	T50.906
Salt-retaining mineralocorticoid	T50.0X1	T50.0X2	T50.0X3	T50.0X4	T50.0X5	T50.0X6
Saluretic NEC	T50.2X1	T50.2X2	T50.2X3	T50.2X4	T50.2X5	T50.2X6
Saluron	T50.2X1	T50.2X2	T50.2X3	T50.2X4	T50.2X5	T50.2X6
Salvarsan 606 (neosilver) (silver)	T37.8X1	T37.8X2	T37.8X3	T37.8X4	T37.8X5	T37.8X6
Sambucus canadensis	T62.2X1	T62.2X2	T62.2X3	T62.2X4	—	—
berry	T62.1X1	T62.1X2	T62.1X3	T62.1X4	—	—
Sandril	T46.5X1	T46.5X2	T46.5X3	T46.5X4	T46.5X5	T46.5X6
Sanguinaria canadensis	T62.2X1	T62.2X2	T62.2X3	T62.2X4	—	—
Saniflush (cleaner)	T54.2X1	T54.2X2	T54.2X3	T54.2X4	—	—
Santonin	T37.4X1	T37.4X2	T37.4X3	T37.4X4	T37.4X5	T37.4X6
Santyl	T49.8X1	T49.8X2	T49.8X3	T49.8X4	T49.8X5	T49.8X6
Saralasin	T46.5X1	T46.5X2	T46.5X3	T46.5X4	T46.5X5	T46.5X6
Sarcolysin	T45.1X1	T45.1X2	T45.1X3	T45.1X4	T45.1X5	T45.1X6
Sarkomycin	T45.1X1	T45.1X2	T45.1X3	T45.1X4	T45.1X5	T45.1X6
Saroten	T43.011	T43.012	T43.013	T43.014	T43.015	T43.016

Substance	Poisoning, Accidental (Unintentional)	Poisoning, Intentional Self-Harm	Poisoning, Assault	Poisoning, Undetermined	Adverse Effect	Underdosing
Saturnine — *see* Lead						
Savin (oil)	T49.4X1	T49.4X2	T49.4X3	T49.4X4	T49.4X5	T49.4X6
Scammony	T47.2X1	T47.2X2	T47.2X3	T47.2X4	T47.2X5	T47.2X6
Scarlet red	T49.8X1	T49.8X2	T49.8X3	T49.8X4	T49.8X5	T49.8X6
Scheele's green	T57.0X1	T57.0X2	T57.0X3	T57.0X4	—	—
insecticide	T57.0X1	T57.0X2	T57.0X3	T57.0X4	—	—
Schizontozide (blood) (tissue)	T37.2X1	T37.2X2	T37.2X3	T37.2X4	T37.2X5	T37.2X6
Schradan	T60.0X1	T60.0X2	T60.0X3	T60.0X4	—	—
Schweinfurth green	T57.0X1	T57.0X2	T57.0X3	T57.0X4	—	—
insecticide	T57.0X1	T57.0X2	T57.0X3	T57.0X4	—	—
Scilla, rat poison	T60.4X1	T60.4X2	T60.4X3	T60.4X4	—	—
Scillaren	T60.4X1	T60.4X2	T60.4X3	T60.4X4	—	—
Sclerosing agent	T46.8X1	T46.8X2	T46.8X3	T46.8X4	T46.8X5	T46.8X6
Scombrotoxin	T61.11	T61.12	T61.13	T61.14	—	—
Scopolamine	T44.3X1	T44.3X2	T44.3X3	T44.3X4	T44.3X5	T44.3X6
Scopolia extract	T44.3X1	T44.3X2	T44.3X3	T44.3X4	T44.3X5	T44.3X6
Scouring powder	T65.891	T65.892	T65.893	T65.894		
Sea						
anemone (sting)	T63.631	T63.632	T63.633	T63.634		
cucumber (sting)	T63.691	T63.692	T63.693	T63.694		
snake (bite) (venom)	T63.091	T63.092	T63.093	T63.094		
urchin spine (puncture)	T63.691	T63.692	T63.693	T63.694		
Seafood	T61.91	T61.92	T61.93	T61.94		
specified NEC	T61.8X1	T61.8X2	T61.8X3	T61.8X4		
Secbutabarbital	T42.3X1	T42.3X2	T42.3X3	T42.3X4	T42.3X5	T42.3X6
Secbutabarbitone	T42.3X1	T42.3X2	T42.3X3	T42.3X4	T42.3X5	T42.3X6
Secnidazole	T37.3X1	T37.3X2	T37.3X3	T37.3X4	T37.3X5	T37.3X6
Secobarbital	T42.3X1	T42.3X2	T42.3X3	T42.3X4	T42.3X5	T42.3X6
Seconal	T42.3X1	T42.3X2	T42.3X3	T42.3X4	T42.3X5	T42.3X6
Secretin	T50.8X1	T50.8X2	T50.8X3	T50.8X4	T50.8X5	T50.8X6
Sedative NEC	T42.71	T42.72	T42.73	T42.74	T42.75	T42.76
mixed NEC	T42.6X1	T42.6X2	T42.6X3	T42.6X4	T42.6X5	T42.6X6
Sedormid	T42.6X1	T42.6X2	T42.6X3	T42.6X4	T42.6X5	T42.6X6
Seed disinfectant or dressing	T60.8X1	T60.8X2	T60.8X3	T60.8X4	—	—
Seeds (poisonous)	T62.2X1	T62.2X2	T62.2X3	T62.2X4	—	—
Selegiline	T42.8X1	T42.8X2	T42.8X3	T42.8X4	T42.8X5	T42.8X6
Selenium NEC	T56.891	T56.892	T56.893	T56.894	—	—
disulfide or sulfide	T49.4X1	T49.4X2	T49.4X3	T49.4X4	T49.4X5	T49.4X6
fumes	T59.891	T59.892	T59.893	T59.894	—	—
sulfide	T49.4X1	T49.4X2	T49.4X3	T49.4X4	T49.4X5	T49.4X6
Selenomethionine (75Se)	T50.8X1	T50.8X2	T50.8X3	T50.8X4	T50.8X5	T50.8X6
Selsun	T49.4X1	T49.4X2	T49.4X3	T49.4X4	T49.4X5	T49.4X6

◀ New　◀▥ Revised　~~deleted~~ Deleted

Substance	Poisoning, Accidental (Unintentional)	Poisoning, Intentional Self-Harm	Poisoning, Assault	Poisoning, Undetermined	Adverse Effect	Underdosing
Semustine	T45.1X1	T45.1X2	T45.1X3	T45.1X4	T45.1X5	T45.1X6
Senega syrup	T48.4X1	T48.4X2	T48.4X3	T48.4X4	T48.4X5	T48.4X6
Senna	T47.2X1	T47.2X2	T47.2X3	T47.2X4	T47.2X5	T47.2X6
Sennoside A+B	T47.2X1	T47.2X2	T47.2X3	T47.2X4	T47.2X5	T47.2X6
Septisol	T49.2X1	T49.2X2	T49.2X3	T49.2X4	T49.2X5	T49.2X6
Seractide	T38.811	T38.812	T38.813	T38.814	T38.815	T38.816
Serax	T42.4X1	T42.4X2	T42.4X3	T42.4X4	T42.4X5	T42.4X6
Serenesil	T42.6X1	T42.6X2	T42.6X3	T42.6X4	T42.6X5	T42.6X6
Serenium (hydrochloride)	T37.91	T37.92	T37.93	T37.94	T37.95	T37.96
Serepax — see Oxazepam						
Sermorelin	T38.891	T38.892	T38.893	T38.894	T38.895	T38.896
Sernyl	T41.1X1	T41.1X2	T41.1X3	T41.1X4	T41.1X5	T41.1X6
Serotonin	T50.991	T50.992	T50.993	T50.994	T50.995	T50.996
Serpasil	T46.5X1	T46.5X2	T46.5X3	T46.5X4	T46.5X5	T46.5X6
Serrapeptase	T45.3X1	T45.3X2	T45.3X3	T45.3X4	T45.3X5	T45.3X6
Serum						
antibotulinus	T50.Z11	T50.Z12	T50.Z13	T50.Z14	T50.Z15	T50.Z16
anticytotoxic	T50.Z11	T50.Z12	T50.Z13	T50.Z14	T50.Z15	T50.Z16
antidiphtheria	T50.Z11	T50.Z12	T50.Z13	T50.Z14	T50.Z15	T50.Z16
antimeningococcus	T50.Z11	T50.Z12	T50.Z13	T50.Z14	T50.Z15	T50.Z16
anti-Rh	T50.Z11	T50.Z12	T50.Z13	T50.Z14	T50.Z15	T50.Z16
anti-snake-bite	T50.Z11	T50.Z12	T50.Z13	T50.Z14	T50.Z15	T50.Z16
antitetanic	T50.Z11	T50.Z12	T50.Z13	T50.Z14	T50.Z15	T50.Z16
antitoxic	T50.Z11	T50.Z12	T50.Z13	T50.Z14	T50.Z15	T50.Z16
complement (inhibitor)	T45.8X1	T45.8X2	T45.8X3	T45.8X4	T45.8X5	T45.8X6
convalescent	T50.Z11	T50.Z12	T50.Z13	T50.Z14	T50.Z15	T50.Z16
hemolytic complement	T45.8X1	T45.8X2	T45.8X3	T45.8X4	T45.8X5	T45.8X6
immune (human)	T50.Z11	T50.Z12	T50.Z13	T50.Z14	T50.Z15	T50.Z16
protective NEC	T50.Z11	T50.Z12	T50.Z13	T50.Z14	T50.Z15	T50.Z16
Setastine	T45.0X1	T45.0X2	T45.0X3	T45.0X4	T45.0X5	T45.0X6
Setoperone	T43.591	T43.592	T43.593	T43.594	T43.595	T43.596
Sewer gas	T59.91	T59.92	T59.93	T59.94	—	—
Shampoo	T55.0X1	T55.0X2	T55.0X3	T55.0X4	—	—
Shellfish, noxious, nonbacterial	T61.781	T61.782	T61.783	T61.784	—	—
Sildenafil	T46.7X1	T46.7X2	T46.7X3	T46.7X4	T46.7X5	T46.7X6
Silibinin	T50.991	T50.992	T50.993	T50.994	T50.995	T50.996
Silicone NEC	T65.891	T65.892	T65.893	T65.894	—	—
medicinal	T49.3X1	T49.3X2	T49.3X3	T49.3X4	T49.3X5	T49.3X6
Silvadene	T49.0X1	T49.0X2	T49.0X3	T49.0X4	T49.0X5	T49.0X6
Silver	T49.0X1	T49.0X2	T49.0X3	T49.0X4	T49.0X5	T49.0X6
anti-infectives	T49.0X1	T49.0X2	T49.0X3	T49.0X4	T49.0X5	T49.0X6
arsphenamine	T37.8X1	T37.8X2	T37.8X3	T37.8X4	T37.8X5	T37.8X6
Silver (Continued)						
colloidal	T49.0X1	T49.0X2	T49.0X3	T49.0X4	T49.0X5	T49.0X6
nitrate	T49.0X1	T49.0X2	T49.0X3	T49.0X4	T49.0X5	T49.0X6
ophthalmic preparation	T49.5X1	T49.5X2	T49.5X3	T49.5X4	T49.5X5	T49.5X6
toughened (keratolytic)	T49.4X1	T49.4X2	T49.4X3	T49.4X4	T49.4X5	T49.4X6
nonmedicinal (dust)	T56.891	T56.892	T56.893	T56.894	—	—
protein	T49.5X1	T49.5X2	T49.5X3	T49.5X4	T49.5X5	T49.5X6
salvarsan	T37.8X1	T37.8X2	T37.8X3	T37.8X4	T37.8X5	T37.8X6
sulfadiazine	T49.4X1	T49.4X2	T49.4X3	T49.4X4	T49.4X5	T49.4X6
Silymarin	T50.991	T50.992	T50.993	T50.994	T50.995	T50.996
Simaldrate	T47.1X1	T47.1X2	T47.1X3	T47.1X4	T47.1X5	T47.1X6
Simazine	T60.3X1	T60.3X2	T60.3X3	T60.3X4	—	—
Simethicone	T47.1X1	T47.1X2	T47.1X3	T47.1X4	T47.1X5	T47.1X6
Simfibrate	T46.6X1	T46.6X2	T46.6X3	T46.6X4	T46.6X5	T46.6X6
Simvastatin	T46.6X1	T46.6X2	T46.6X3	T46.6X4	T46.6X5	T46.6X6
Sincalide	T50.8X1	T50.8X2	T50.8X3	T50.8X4	T50.8X5	T50.8X6
Sinequan	T43.011	T43.012	T43.013	T43.014	T43.015	T43.016
Singoserp	T46.5X1	T46.5X2	T46.5X3	T46.5X4	T46.5X5	T46.5X6
Sintrom	T45.511	T45.512	T45.513	T45.514	T45.515	T45.516
Sisomicin	T36.5X1	T36.5X2	T36.5X3	T36.5X4	T36.5X5	T36.5X6
Sitosterols	T46.6X1	T46.6X2	T46.6X3	T46.6X4	T46.6X5	T46.6X6
Skeletal muscle relaxants	T48.1X1	T48.1X2	T48.1X3	T48.1X4	T48.1X5	T48.1X6
Skin						
agents (external)	T49.91	T49.92	T49.93	T49.94	T49.95	T49.96
specified NEC	T49.8X1	T49.8X2	T49.8X3	T49.8X4	T49.8X5	T49.8X6
test antigen	T50.8X1	T50.8X2	T50.8X3	T50.8X4	T50.8X5	T50.8X6
Sleep-eze	T45.0X1	T45.0X2	T45.0X3	T45.0X4	T45.0X5	T45.0X6
Sleeping draught, pill	T42.71	T42.72	T42.73	T42.74	T42.75	T42.76
Smallpox vaccine	T50.B11	T50.B12	T50.B13	T50.B14	T50.B15	T50.B16
Smelter fumes NEC	T56.91	T56.92	T56.93	T56.94	—	—
Smog	T59.1X1	T59.1X2	T59.1X3	T59.1X4	—	—
Smoke NEC	T59.811	T59.812	T59.813	T59.814	—	—
Smooth muscle relaxant	T44.3X1	T44.3X2	T44.3X3	T44.3X4	T44.3X5	T44.3X6
Snail killer NEC	T60.8X1	T60.8X2	T60.8X3	T60.8X4	—	—
Snake venom or bite	T63.001	T63.002	T63.003	T63.004	—	—
hemocoagulase	T45.7X1	T45.7X2	T45.7X3	T45.7X4	T45.7X5	T45.7X6
Snuff	T65.211	T65.212	T65.213	T65.214	—	—
Soap (powder) (product)	T55.0X1	T55.0X2	T55.0X3	T55.0X4	—	—
enema	T47.4X1	T47.4X2	T47.4X3	T47.4X4	T47.4X5	T47.4X6
medicinal, soft	T49.2X1	T49.2X2	T49.2X3	T49.2X4	T49.2X5	T49.2X6
superfatted	T49.2X1	T49.2X2	T49.2X3	T49.2X4	T49.2X5	T49.2X6
Sobrerol	T48.4X1	T48.4X2	T48.4X3	T48.4X4	T48.4X5	T48.4X6

◀ New ◀‖ Revised ~~deleted~~ Deleted

Substance	External Cause (T-Code)					
	Poisoning, Accidental (Unintentional)	Poisoning, Intentional Self-Harm	Poisoning, Assault	Poisoning, Undetermined	Adverse Effect	Underdosing
Soda (caustic)	T54.3X1	T54.3X2	T54.3X3	T54.3X4	—	—
bicarb	T47.1X1	T47.1X2	T47.1X3	T47.1X4	T47.1X5	T47.1X6
chlorinated — *see Sodium, hypochlorite*						
Sodium						
acetosulfone	T37.1X1	T37.1X2	T37.1X3	T37.1X4	T37.1X5	T37.1X6
acetrizoate	T50.8X1	T50.8X2	T50.8X3	T50.8X4	T50.8X5	T50.8X6
acid phosphate	T50.3X1	T50.3X2	T50.3X3	T50.3X4	T50.3X5	T50.3X6
alginate	T47.8X1	T47.8X2	T47.8X3	T47.8X4	T47.8X5	T47.8X6
amidotrizoate	T50.8X1	T50.8X2	T50.8X3	T50.8X4	T50.8X5	T50.8X6
aminopterin	T45.1X1	T45.1X2	T45.1X3	T45.1X4	T45.1X5	T45.1X6
amylosulfate	T47.8X1	T47.8X2	T47.8X3	T47.8X4	T47.8X5	T47.8X6
amytal	T42.3X1	T42.3X2	T42.3X3	T42.3X4	T42.3X5	T42.3X6
antimony gluconate	T37.3X1	T37.3X2	T37.3X3	T37.3X4	T37.3X5	T37.3X6
arsenate	T57.0X1	T57.0X2	T57.0X3	T57.0X4	—	—
aurothiomalate	T39.4X1	T39.4X2	T39.4X3	T39.4X4	T39.4X5	T39.4X6
aurothiosulfate	T39.4X1	T39.4X2	T39.4X3	T39.4X4	T39.4X5	T39.4X6
barbiturate	T42.3X1	T42.3X2	T42.3X3	T42.3X4	T42.3X5	T42.3X6
basic phosphate	T47.4X1	T47.4X2	T47.4X3	T47.4X4	T47.4X5	T47.4X6
bicarbonate	T47.1X1	T47.1X2	T47.1X3	T47.1X4	T47.1X5	T47.1X6
bichromate	T57.8X1	T57.8X2	T57.8X3	T57.8X4	—	—
biphosphate	T50.3X1	T50.3X2	T50.3X3	T50.3X4	T50.3X5	T50.3X6
bisulfate	T65.891	T65.892	T65.893	T65.894	—	—
borate						
cleanser	T57.8X1	T57.8X2	T57.8X3	T57.8X4	—	—
eye	T49.5X1	T49.5X2	T49.5X3	T49.5X4	T49.5X5	T49.5X6
therapeutic	T49.8X1	T49.8X2	T49.8X3	T49.8X4	T49.8X5	T49.8X6
bromide	T42.6X1	T42.6X2	T42.6X3	T42.6X4	T42.6X5	T42.6X6
cacodylate (nonmedicinal) NEC	T50.8X1	T50.8X2	T50.8X3	T50.8X4	T50.8X5	T50.8X6
anti-infective	T37.8X1	T37.8X2	T37.8X3	T37.8X4	T37.8X5	T37.8X6
herbicide	T60.3X1	T60.3X2	T60.3X3	T60.3X4	—	—
calcium edetate	T45.8X1	T45.8X2	T45.8X3	T45.8X4	T45.8X5	T45.8X6
carbonate NEC	T54.3X1	T54.3X2	T54.3X3	T54.3X4	—	—
chlorate NEC	T65.891	T65.892	T65.893	T65.894	—	—
herbicide	T54.91	T54.92	T54.93	T54.94	—	—
chloride	T50.3X1	T50.3X2	T50.3X3	T50.3X4	T50.3X5	T50.3X6
with glucose	T50.3X1	T50.3X2	T50.3X3	T50.3X4	T50.3X5	T50.3X6
chromate	T65.891	T65.892	T65.893	T65.894	—	—
citrate	T50.991	T50.992	T50.993	T50.994	T50.995	T50.996
cromoglicate	T48.6X1	T48.6X2	T48.6X3	T48.6X4	T48.6X5	T48.6X6
cyanide	T65.0X1	T65.0X2	T65.0X3	T65.0X4	—	—
cyclamate	T50.3X1	T50.3X2	T50.3X3	T50.3X4	T50.3X5	T50.3X6

Substance	External Cause (T-Code)					
	Poisoning, Accidental (Unintentional)	Poisoning, Intentional Self-Harm	Poisoning, Assault	Poisoning, Undetermined	Adverse Effect	Underdosing
Sodium *(Continued)*						
dehydrocholate	T45.8X1	T45.8X2	T45.8X3	T45.8X4	T45.8X5	T45.8X6
diatrizoate	T50.8X1	T50.8X2	T50.8X3	T50.8X4	T50.8X5	T50.8X6
dibunate	T48.4X1	T48.4X2	T48.4X3	T48.4X4	T48.4X5	T48.4X6
dioctyl sulfosuccinate	T47.4X1	T47.4X2	T47.4X3	T47.4X4	T47.4X5	T47.4X6
dipantoyl ferrate	T45.8X1	T45.8X2	T45.8X3	T45.8X4	T45.8X5	T45.8X6
edetate	T45.8X1	T45.8X2	T45.8X3	T45.8X4	T45.8X5	T45.8X6
ethacrynate	T50.1X1	T50.1X2	T50.1X3	T50.1X4	T50.1X5	T50.1X6
feredetate	T45.8X1	T45.8X2	T45.8X3	T45.8X4	T45.8X5	T45.8X6
Fluoride — *see Fluoride*						
fluoroacetate (dust) (pesticide)	T60.4X1	T60.4X2	T60.4X3	T60.4X4	—	—
free salt	T50.3X1	T50.3X2	T50.3X3	T50.3X4	T50.3X5	T50.3X6
fusidate	T36.8X1	T36.8X2	T36.8X3	T36.8X4	T36.8X5	T36.8X6
glucaldrate	T47.1X1	T47.1X2	T47.1X3	T47.1X4	T47.1X5	T47.1X6
glucosulfone	T37.1X1	T37.1X2	T37.1X3	T37.1X4	T37.1X5	T37.1X6
glutamate	T45.8X1	T45.8X2	T45.8X3	T45.8X4	T45.8X5	T45.8X6
hydrogen carbonate	T50.3X1	T50.3X2	T50.3X3	T50.3X4	T50.3X5	T50.3X6
hydroxide	T54.3X1	T54.3X2	T54.3X3	T54.3X4	—	—
hypochlorite (bleach) NEC	T54.3X1	T54.3X2	T54.3X3	T54.3X4	—	—
disinfectant	T54.3X1	T54.3X2	T54.3X3	T54.3X4	—	—
medicinal (anti-infective) (external)	T49.0X1	T49.0X2	T49.0X3	T49.0X4	T49.0X5	T49.0X6
vapor	T54.3X1	T54.3X2	T54.3X3	T54.3X4	—	—
hyposulfite	T49.0X1	T49.0X2	T49.0X3	T49.0X4	T49.0X5	T49.0X6
indigotin disulfonate	T50.8X1	T50.8X2	T50.8X3	T50.8X4	T50.8X5	T50.8X6
iodide	T50.991	T50.992	T50.993	T50.994	T50.995	T50.996
I-131	T50.8X1	T50.8X2	T50.8X3	T50.8X4	T50.8X5	T50.8X6
therapeutic	T38.2X1	T38.2X2	T38.2X3	T38.2X4	T38.2X5	T38.2X6
iodohippurate (131I)	T50.8X1	T50.8X2	T50.8X3	T50.8X4	T50.8X5	T50.8X6
iopodate	T50.8X1	T50.8X2	T50.8X3	T50.8X4	T50.8X5	T50.8X6
iothalamate	T50.8X1	T50.8X2	T50.8X3	T50.8X4	T50.8X5	T50.8X6
iron edetate	T45.4X1	T45.4X2	T45.4X3	T45.4X4	T45.4X5	T45.4X6
lactate (compound solution)	T45.8X1	T45.8X2	T45.8X3	T45.8X4	T45.8X5	T45.8X6
lauryl (sulfate)	T49.2X1	T49.2X2	T49.2X3	T49.2X4	T49.2X5	T49.2X6
(L)-triiodothyronine	T38.1X1	T38.1X2	T38.1X3	T38.1X4	T38.1X5	T38.1X6
magnesium citrate	T50.991	T50.992	T50.993	T50.994	T50.995	T50.996
mersalate	T50.2X1	T50.2X2	T50.2X3	T50.2X4	T50.2X5	T50.2X6
metasilicate	T65.891	T65.892	T65.893	T65.894	—	—
metrizoate	T50.8X1	T50.8X2	T50.8X3	T50.8X4	T50.8X5	T50.8X6
monofluoroacetate (pesticide)	T60.1X1	T60.1X2	T60.1X3	T60.1X4	—	—
morrhuate	T46.8X1	T46.8X2	T46.8X3	T46.8X4	T46.8X5	T46.8X6
nafcillin	T36.0X1	T36.0X2	T36.0X3	T36.0X4	T36.0X5	T36.0X6

◀ New ◀◀ Revised ~~deleted~~ Deleted

Substance	External Cause (T-Code)					
	Poisoning, Accidental (Unintentional)	Poisoning, Intentional Self-Harm	Poisoning, Assault	Poisoning, Undetermined	Adverse Effect	Underdosing
Sodium *(Continued)*						
nitrate (oxidizing agent)	T65.891	T65.892	T65.893	T65.894	—	—
nitrite	T50.6X1	T50.6X2	T50.6X3	T50.6X4	T50.6X5	T50.6X6
nitroferricyanide	T46.5X1	T46.5X2	T46.5X3	T46.5X4	T46.5X5	T46.5X6
nitroprusside	T46.5X1	T46.5X2	T46.5X3	T46.5X4	T46.5X5	T46.5X6
oxalate	T65.891	T65.892	T65.893	T65.894	—	—
oxide/peroxide	T65.891	T65.892	T65.893	T65.894	—	—
oxybate	T41.291	T41.292	T41.293	T41.294	T41.295	T41.296
para-aminohippurate	T50.8X1	T50.8X2	T50.8X3	T50.8X4	T50.8X5	T50.8X6
perborate (nonmedicinal) NEC	T65.891	T65.892	T65.893	T65.894	—	—
medicinal	T49.0X1	T49.0X2	T49.0X3	T49.0X4	T49.0X5	T49.0X6
soap	T55.0X1	T55.0X2	T55.0X3	T55.0X4		
percarbonate — *see Sodium, perborate*						
pertechnetate Tc99m	T50.8X1	T50.8X2	T50.8X3	T50.8X4	T50.8X5	T50.8X6
phosphate						
cellulose	T45.8X1	T45.8X2	T45.8X3	T45.8X4	T45.8X5	T45.8X6
dibasic	T47.2X1	T47.2X2	T47.2X3	T47.2X4	T47.2X5	T47.2X6
monobasic	T47.2X1	T47.2X2	T47.2X3	T47.2X4	T47.2X5	T47.2X6
phytate	T50.6X1	T50.6X2	T50.6X3	T50.6X4	T50.6X5	T50.6X6
picosulfate	T47.2X1	T47.2X2	T47.2X3	T47.2X4	T47.2X5	T47.2X6
polyhydroxyaluminium monocarbonate	T47.1X1	T47.1X2	T47.1X3	T47.1X4	T47.1X5	T47.1X6
polystyrene sulfonate	T50.3X1	T50.3X2	T50.3X3	T50.3X4	T50.3X5	T50.3X6
propionate	T49.0X1	T49.0X2	T49.0X3	T49.0X4	T49.0X5	T49.0X6
propyl hydroxybenzoate	T50.991	T50.992	T50.993	T50.994	T50.995	T50.996
psylliate	T46.8X1	T46.8X2	T46.8X3	T46.8X4	T46.8X5	T46.8X6
removing resins	T50.3X1	T50.3X2	T50.3X3	T50.3X4	T50.3X5	T50.3X6
salicylate	T39.091	T39.092	T39.093	T39.094	T39.095	T39.096
salt NEC	T50.3X1	T50.3X2	T50.3X3	T50.3X4	T50.3X5	T50.3X6
selenate	T60.2X1	T60.2X2	T60.2X3	T60.2X4	—	—
stibogluconate	T37.3X1	T37.3X2	T37.3X3	T37.3X4	T37.3X5	T37.3X6
sulfate	T47.4X1	T47.4X2	T47.4X3	T47.4X4	T47.4X5	T47.4X6
sulfoxone	T37.1X1	T37.1X2	T37.1X3	T37.1X4	T37.1X5	T37.1X6
tetradecyl sulfate	T46.8X1	T46.8X2	T46.8X3	T46.8X4	T46.8X5	T46.8X6
thiopental	T41.1X1	T41.1X2	T41.1X3	T41.1X4	T41.1X5	T41.1X6
thiosalicylate	T39.091	T39.092	T39.093	T39.094	T39.095	T39.096
thiosulfate	T50.6X1	T50.6X2	T50.6X3	T50.6X4	T50.6X5	T50.6X6
tolbutamide	T38.3X1	T38.3X2	T38.3X3	T38.3X4	T38.3X5	T38.3X6
l-triiodothyronine	T38.1X1	T38.1X2	T38.1X3	T38.1X4	T38.1X5	T38.1X6
tyropanoate	T50.8X1	T50.8X2	T50.8X3	T50.8X4	T50.8X5	T50.8X6
valproate	T42.6X1	T42.6X2	T42.6X3	T42.6X4	T42.6X5	T42.6X6
versenate	T50.6X1	T50.6X2	T50.6X3	T50.6X4	T50.6X5	T50.6X6

Substance	External Cause (T-Code)					
	Poisoning, Accidental (Unintentional)	Poisoning, Intentional Self-Harm	Poisoning, Assault	Poisoning, Undetermined	Adverse Effect	Underdosing
Sodium-free salt	T50.901	T50.902	T50.903	T50.904	T50.905	T50.906
Sodium-removing resin	T50.3X1	T50.3X2	T50.3X3	T50.3X4	T50.3X5	T50.3X6
Soft soap	T55.0X1	T55.0X2	T55.0X3	T55.0X4	—	—
Solanine	T62.2X1	T62.2X2	T62.2X3	T62.2X4	—	—
berries	T62.1X1	T62.1X2	T62.1X3	T62.1X4	—	—
Solanum dulcamara	T62.2X1	T62.2X2	T62.2X3	T62.2X4	—	—
berries	T62.1X1	T62.1X2	T62.1X3	T62.1X4	—	—
Solapsone	T37.1X1	T37.1X2	T37.1X3	T37.1X4	T37.1X5	T37.1X6
Solar lotion	T49.3X1	T49.3X2	T49.3X3	T49.3X4	T49.3X5	T49.3X6
Solasulfone	T37.1X1	T37.1X2	T37.1X3	T37.1X4	T37.1X5	T37.1X6
Soldering fluid	T65.891	T65.892	T65.893	T65.894	—	—
Solid substance	T65.91	T65.92	T65.93	T65.94		
specified NEC	T65.891	T65.892	T65.893	T65.894		
Solvent, industrial NEC	T52.91	T52.92	T52.93	T52.94	—	—
naphtha	T52.0X1	T52.0X2	T52.0X3	T52.0X4	—	—
petroleum	T52.0X1	T52.0X2	T52.0X3	T52.0X4	—	—
specified NEC	T52.8X1	T52.8X2	T52.8X3	T52.8X4	—	—
Soma	T42.8X1	T42.8X2	T42.8X3	T42.8X4	T42.8X5	T42.8X6
Somatorelin	T38.891	T38.892	T38.893	T38.894	T38.895	T38.896
Somatostatin	T38.991	T38.992	T38.993	T38.994	T38.995	T38.996
Somatotropin	T38.811	T38.812	T38.813	T38.814	T38.815	T38.816
Somatrem	T38.811	T38.812	T38.813	T38.814	T38.815	T38.816
Somatropin	T38.811	T38.812	T38.813	T38.814	T38.815	T38.816
Sominex	T45.0X1	T45.0X2	T45.0X3	T45.0X4	T45.0X5	T45.0X6
Somnos	T42.6X1	T42.6X2	T42.6X3	T42.6X4	T42.6X5	T42.6X6
Somonal	T42.3X1	T42.3X2	T42.3X3	T42.3X4	T42.3X5	T42.3X6
Soneryl	T42.3X1	T42.3X2	T42.3X3	T42.3X4	T42.3X5	T42.3X6
Soothing syrup	T50.901	T50.902	T50.903	T50.904	T50.905	T50.906
Sopor	T42.6X1	T42.6X2	T42.6X3	T42.6X4	T42.6X5	T42.6X6
Soporific	T42.71	T42.72	T42.73	T42.74	T42.75	T42.76
Soporific drug	T42.71	T42.72	T42.73	T42.74	T42.75	T42.76
specified type NEC	T42.6X1	T42.6X2	T42.6X3	T42.6X4	T42.6X5	T42.6X6
Sorbide nitrate	T46.3X1	T46.3X2	T46.3X3	T46.3X4	T46.3X5	T46.3X6
Sorbitol	T47.4X1	T47.4X2	T47.4X3	T47.4X4	T47.4X5	T47.4X6
Sotalol	T44.7X1	T44.7X2	T44.7X3	T44.7X4	T44.7X5	T44.7X6
Sotradecol	T46.8X1	T46.8X2	T46.8X3	T46.8X4	T46.8X5	T46.8X6
Soysterol	T46.6X1	T46.6X2	T46.6X3	T46.6X4	T46.6X5	T46.6X6
Spacoline	T44.3X1	T44.3X2	T44.3X3	T44.3X4	T44.3X5	T44.3X6
Spanish fly	T49.8X1	T49.8X2	T49.8X3	T49.8X4	T49.8X5	T49.8X6
Sparine	T43.3X1	T43.3X2	T43.3X3	T43.3X4	T43.3X5	T43.3X6
Sparteine	T48.0X1	T48.0X2	T48.0X3	T48.0X4	T48.0X5	T48.0X6

◄ New   ◄ Revised   ~~deleted~~ Deleted

TABLE OF DRUGS AND CHEMICALS

Substance	Poisoning, Accidental (Unintentional)	Poisoning, Intentional Self-Harm	Poisoning, Assault	Poisoning, Undetermined	Adverse Effect	Underdosing
Spasmolytic						
anticholinergics	T44.3X1	T44.3X2	T44.3X3	T44.3X4	T44.3X5	T44.3X6
autonomic	T44.3X1	T44.3X2	T44.3X3	T44.3X4	T44.3X5	T44.3X6
bronchial NEC	T48.6X1	T48.6X2	T48.6X3	T48.6X4	T48.6X5	T48.6X6
quaternary ammonium	T44.3X1	T44.3X2	T44.3X3	T44.3X4	T44.3X5	T44.3X6
skeletal muscle NEC	T48.1X1	T48.1X2	T48.1X3	T48.1X4	T48.1X5	T48.1X6
Spectinomycin	T36.5X1	T36.5X2	T36.5X3	T36.5X4	T36.5X5	T36.5X6
Speed	T43.621	T43.622	T43.623	T43.624	T43.625	T43.626
Spermicide	T49.8X1	T49.8X2	T49.8X3	T49.8X4	T49.8X5	T49.8X6
Spider (bite) (venom)	T63.391	T63.392	T63.393	T63.394	—	—
antivenin	T50.Z11	T50.Z12	T50.Z13	T50.Z14	T50.Z15	T50.Z16
Spigelia (root)	T37.4X1	T37.4X2	T37.4X3	T37.4X4	T37.4X5	T37.4X6
Spindle inactivator	T50.4X1	T50.4X2	T50.4X3	T50.4X4	T50.4X5	T50.4X6
Spiperone	T43.4X1	T43.4X2	T43.4X3	T43.4X4	T43.4X5	T43.4X6
Spiramycin	T36.3X1	T36.3X2	T36.3X3	T36.3X4	T36.3X5	T36.3X6
Spirapril	T46.4X1	T46.4X2	T46.4X3	T46.4X4	T46.4X5	T46.4X6
Spirilene	T43.591	T43.592	T43.593	T43.594	T43.595	T43.596
Spirit(s) (neutral) NEC	T51.0X1	T51.0X2	T51.0X3	T51.0X4	—	—
beverage	T51.0X1	T51.0X2	T51.0X3	T51.0X4	—	—
industrial	T51.0X1	T51.0X2	T51.0X3	T51.0X4	—	—
mineral	T52.0X1	T52.0X2	T52.0X3	T52.0X4	—	—
of salt — see Hydrochloric acid						
surgical	T51.0X1	T51.0X2	T51.0X3	T51.0X4	—	—
Spironolactone	T50.0X1	T50.0X2	T50.0X3	T50.0X4	T50.0X5	T50.0X6
Spiroperidol	T43.4X1	T43.4X2	T43.4X3	T43.4X4	T43.4X5	T43.4X6
Sponge, absorbable (gelatin)	T45.7X1	T45.7X2	T45.7X3	T45.7X4	T45.7X5	T45.7X6
Sporostacin	T49.0X1	T49.0X2	T49.0X3	T49.0X4	T49.0X5	T49.0X6
Spray (aerosol)	T65.91	T65.92	T65.93	T65.94	—	—
cosmetic	T65.891	T65.892	T65.893	T65.894	—	—
medicinal NEC	T50.901	T50.902	T50.903	T50.904	T50.905	T50.906
pesticides — see Pesticides						
specified content — see specific substance						
Spurge flax	T62.2X1	T62.2X2	T62.2X3	T62.2X4	—	—
Spurges	T62.2X1	T62.2X2	T62.2X3	T62.2X4	—	—
Sputum viscosity-lowering drug	T48.4X1	T48.4X2	T48.4X3	T48.4X4	T48.4X5	T48.4X6
Squill	T46.0X1	T46.0X2	T46.0X3	T46.0X4	T46.0X5	T46.0X6
rat poison	T60.4X1	T60.4X2	T60.4X3	T60.4X4	—	—
Squirting cucumber (cathartic)	T47.2X1	T47.2X2	T47.2X3	T47.2X4	T47.2X5	T47.2X6
Stains	T65.6X1	T65.6X2	T65.6X3	T65.6X4	—	—
Stannous fluoride	T49.7X1	T49.7X2	T49.7X3	T49.7X4	T49.7X5	T49.7X6
Stanolone	T38.7X1	T38.7X2	T38.7X3	T38.7X4	T38.7X5	T38.7X6
Stanozolol	T38.7X1	T38.7X2	T38.7X3	T38.7X4	T38.7X5	T38.7X6
Staphisagria or stavesacre (pediculicide)	T49.0X1	T49.0X2	T49.0X3	T49.0X4	T49.0X5	T49.0X6
Starch	T50.901	T50.902	T50.903	T50.904	T50.905	T50.906
Stelazine	T43.3X1	T43.3X2	T43.3X3	T43.3X4	T43.3X5	T43.3X6
Stemetil	T43.3X1	T43.3X2	T43.3X3	T43.3X4	T43.3X5	T43.3X6
Stepronin	T48.4X1	T48.4X2	T48.4X3	T48.4X4	T48.4X5	T48.4X6
Sterculia	T47.4X1	T47.4X2	T47.4X3	T47.4X4	T47.4X5	T47.4X6
Sternutator gas	T59.891	T59.892	T59.893	T59.894	—	—
Steroid	T38.0X1	T38.0X2	T38.0X3	T38.0X4	T38.0X5	T38.0X6
anabolic	T38.7X1	T38.7X2	T38.7X3	T38.7X4	T38.7X5	T38.7X6
androgenic	T38.7X1	T38.7X2	T38.7X3	T38.7X4	T38.7X5	T38.7X6
antineoplastic, hormone	T38.7X1	T38.7X2	T38.7X3	T38.7X4	T38.7X5	T38.7X6
estrogen	T38.5X1	T38.5X2	T38.5X3	T38.5X4	T38.5X5	T38.5X6
ENT agent	T49.6X1	T49.6X2	T49.6X3	T49.6X4	T49.6X5	T49.6X6
ophthalmic preparation	T49.5X1	T49.5X2	T49.5X3	T49.5X4	T49.5X5	T49.5X6
topical NEC	T49.0X1	T49.0X2	T49.0X3	T49.0X4	T49.0X5	T49.0X6
Stibine	T56.891	T56.892	T56.893	T56.894	—	—
Stibogluconate	T37.3X1	T37.3X2	T37.3X3	T37.3X4	T37.3X5	T37.3X6
Stibophen	T37.4X1	T37.4X2	T37.4X3	T37.4X4	T37.4X5	T37.4X6
Stilbamidine (isetionate)	T37.3X1	T37.3X2	T37.3X3	T37.3X4	T37.3X5	T37.3X6
Stilbestrol	T38.5X1	T38.5X2	T38.5X3	T38.5X4	T38.5X5	T38.5X6
Stilboestrol	T38.5X1	T38.5X2	T38.5X3	T38.5X4	T38.5X5	T38.5X6
Stimulant						
central nervous system — see also Psychostimulant	T43.601	T43.602	T43.603	T43.604	T43.605	T43.606
analeptics	T50.7X1	T50.7X2	T50.7X3	T50.7X4	T50.7X5	T50.7X6
opiate antagonist	T50.7X1	T50.7X2	T50.7X3	T50.7X4	T50.7X5	T50.7X6
psychotherapeutic NEC — see also Psychotherapeutic drug	T43.601	T43.602	T43.603	T43.604	T43.605	T43.606
specified NEC	T43.691	T43.692	T43.693	T43.694	T43.695	T43.696
respiratory	T48.901	T48.902	T48.903	T48.904	T48.905	T48.906
Stone-dissolving drug	T50.901	T50.902	T50.903	T50.904	T50.905	T50.906
Storage battery (cells) (acid)	T54.2X1	T54.2X2	T54.2X3	T54.2X4	—	—
Stovaine	T41.3X1	T41.3X2	T41.3X3	T41.3X4	T41.3X5	T41.3X6
infiltration (subcutaneous)	T41.3X1	T41.3X2	T41.3X3	T41.3X4	T41.3X5	T41.3X6
nerve block (peripheral) (plexus)	T41.3X1	T41.3X2	T41.3X3	T41.3X4	T41.3X5	T41.3X6
spinal	T41.3X1	T41.3X2	T41.3X3	T41.3X4	T41.3X5	T41.3X6
topical (surface)	T41.3X1	T41.3X2	T41.3X3	T41.3X4	T41.3X5	T41.3X6
Stovarsal	T37.8X1	T37.8X2	T37.8X3	T37.8X4	T37.8X5	T37.8X6
Stove gas — see Gas, stove	T57.91	T57.92	T57.93	T57.94	—	—

New   Revised   ~~deleted~~ Deleted

	External Cause (T-Code)					
Substance	Poisoning, Accidental (Unintentional)	Poisoning, Intentional Self-Harm	Poisoning, Assault	Poisoning, Undetermined	Adverse Effect	Underdosing
Stoxil	T49.5X1	T49.5X2	T49.5X3	T49.5X4	T49.5X5	T49.5X6
Stramonium	T48.6X1	T48.6X2	T48.6X3	T48.6X4	T48.6X5	T48.6X6
natural state	T62.2X1	T62.2X2	T62.2X3	T62.2X4	—	—
Streptodornase	T45.3X1	T45.3X2	T45.3X3	T45.3X4	T45.3X5	T45.3X6
Streptoduocin	T36.5X1	T36.5X2	T36.5X3	T36.5X4	T36.5X5	T36.5X6
Streptokinase	T45.611	T45.612	T45.613	T45.614	T45.615	T45.616
Streptomycin (derivative)	T36.5X1	T36.5X2	T36.5X3	T36.5X4	T36.5X5	T36.5X6
Streptonivicin	T36.5X1	T36.5X2	T36.5X3	T36.5X4	T36.5X5	T36.5X6
Streptovarycin	T36.5X1	T36.5X2	T36.5X3	T36.5X4	T36.5X5	T36.5X6
Streptozocin	T45.1X1	T45.1X2	T45.1X3	T45.1X4	T45.1X5	T45.1X6
Streptozotocin	T45.1X1	T45.1X2	T45.1X3	T45.1X4	T45.1X5	T45.1X6
Stripper (paint) (solvent)	T52.8X1	T52.8X2	T52.8X3	T52.8X4	—	—
Strobane	T60.1X1	T60.1X2	T60.1X3	T60.1X4	—	—
Strofantina	T46.0X1	T46.0X2	T46.0X3	T46.0X4	T46.0X5	T46.0X6
Strophanthin (g) (k)	T46.0X1	T46.0X2	T46.0X3	T46.0X4	T46.0X5	T46.0X6
Strophanthus	T46.0X1	T46.0X2	T46.0X3	T46.0X4	T46.0X5	T46.0X6
Strophantin	T46.0X1	T46.0X2	T46.0X3	T46.0X4	T46.0X5	T46.0X6
Strophantin-g	T46.0X1	T46.0X2	T46.0X3	T46.0X4	T46.0X5	T46.0X6
Strychnine (nonmedicinal) (pesticide) (salts)	T65.1X1	T65.1X2	T65.1X3	T65.1X4	—	—
medicinal	T48.291	T48.292	T48.293	T48.294	T48.295	T48.296
Strychnos (ignatii) — see Strychnine						
Styramate	T42.8X1	T42.8X2	T42.8X3	T42.8X4	T42.8X5	T42.8X6
Styrene	T65.891	T65.892	T65.893	T65.894	—	—
Succinimide, antiepileptic or anticonvulsant	T42.2X1	T42.2X2	T42.2X3	T42.2X4	T42.2X5	T42.2X6
mercuric — see Mercury						
Succinylcholine	T48.1X1	T48.1X2	T48.1X3	T48.1X4	T48.1X5	T48.1X6
Succinylsulfathiazole	T37.0X1	T37.0X2	T37.0X3	T37.0X4	T37.0X5	T37.0X6
Sucralfate	T47.1X1	T47.1X2	T47.1X3	T47.1X4	T47.1X5	T47.1X6
Sucrose	T50.3X1	T50.3X2	T50.3X3	T50.3X4	T50.3X5	T50.3X6
Sufentanil	T40.4X1	T40.4X2	T40.4X3	T40.4X4	T40.4X5	T40.4X6
Sulbactam	T36.0X1	T36.0X2	T36.0X3	T36.0X4	T36.0X5	T36.0X6
Sulbenicillin	T36.0X1	T36.0X2	T36.0X3	T36.0X4	T36.0X5	T36.0X6
Sulbentine	T49.0X1	T49.0X2	T49.0X3	T49.0X4	T49.0X5	T49.0X6
Sulfacetamide	T49.0X1	T49.0X2	T49.0X3	T49.0X4	T49.0X5	T49.0X6
ophthalmic preparation	T49.5X1	T49.5X2	T49.5X3	T49.5X4	T49.5X5	T49.5X6
Sulfachlorpyridazine	T37.0X1	T37.0X2	T37.0X3	T37.0X4	T37.0X5	T37.0X6
Sulfacitine	T37.0X1	T37.0X2	T37.0X3	T37.0X4	T37.0X5	T37.0X6
Sulfadiasulfone sodium	T37.0X1	T37.0X2	T37.0X3	T37.0X4	T37.0X5	T37.0X6
Sulfadiazine	T37.0X1	T37.0X2	T37.0X3	T37.0X4	T37.0X5	T37.0X6
silver (topical)	T49.0X1	T49.0X2	T49.0X3	T49.0X4	T49.0X5	T49.0X6

	External Cause (T-Code)					
Substance	Poisoning, Accidental (Unintentional)	Poisoning, Intentional Self-Harm	Poisoning, Assault	Poisoning, Undetermined	Adverse Effect	Underdosing
Sulfadimethoxine	T37.0X1	T37.0X2	T37.0X3	T37.0X4	T37.0X5	T37.0X6
Sulfadimidine	T37.0X1	T37.0X2	T37.0X3	T37.0X4	T37.0X5	T37.0X6
Sulfadoxine	T37.0X1	T37.0X2	T37.0X3	T37.0X4	T37.0X5	T37.0X6
with pyrimethamine	T37.2X1	T37.2X2	T37.2X3	T37.2X4	T37.2X5	T37.2X6
Sulfaethidole	T37.0X1	T37.0X2	T37.0X3	T37.0X4	T37.0X5	T37.0X6
Sulfafurazole	T37.0X1	T37.0X2	T37.0X3	T37.0X4	T37.0X5	T37.0X6
Sulfaguanidine	T37.0X1	T37.0X2	T37.0X3	T37.0X4	T37.0X5	T37.0X6
Sulfalene	T37.0X1	T37.0X2	T37.0X3	T37.0X4	T37.0X5	T37.0X6
Sulfaloxate	T37.0X1	T37.0X2	T37.0X3	T37.0X4	T37.0X5	T37.0X6
Sulfaloxic acid	T37.0X1	T37.0X2	T37.0X3	T37.0X4	T37.0X5	T37.0X6
Sulfamazone	T39.2X1	T39.2X2	T39.2X3	T39.2X4	T39.2X5	T39.2X6
Sulfamerazine	T37.0X1	T37.0X2	T37.0X3	T37.0X4	T37.0X5	T37.0X6
Sulfameter	T37.0X1	T37.0X2	T37.0X3	T37.0X4	T37.0X5	T37.0X6
Sulfamethazine	T37.0X1	T37.0X2	T37.0X3	T37.0X4	T37.0X5	T37.0X6
Sulfamethizole	T37.0X1	T37.0X2	T37.0X3	T37.0X4	T37.0X5	T37.0X6
Sulfamethoxazole	T37.0X1	T37.0X2	T37.0X3	T37.0X4	T37.0X5	T37.0X6
with trimethoprim	T36.8X1	T36.8X2	T36.8X3	T36.8X4	T36.8X5	T36.8X6
Sulfamethoxydiazine	T37.0X1	T37.0X2	T37.0X3	T37.0X4	T37.0X5	T37.0X6
Sulfamethoxypyridazine	T37.0X1	T37.0X2	T37.0X3	T37.0X4	T37.0X5	T37.0X6
Sulfamethylthiazole	T37.0X1	T37.0X2	T37.0X3	T37.0X4	T37.0X5	T37.0X6
Sulfametoxydiazine	T37.0X1	T37.0X2	T37.0X3	T37.0X4	T37.0X5	T37.0X6
Sulfamidopyrine	T39.2X1	T39.2X2	T39.2X3	T39.2X4	T39.2X5	T39.2X6
Sulfamonomethoxine	T37.0X1	T37.0X2	T37.0X3	T37.0X4	T37.0X5	T37.0X6
Sulfamoxole	T37.0X1	T37.0X2	T37.0X3	T37.0X4	T37.0X5	T37.0X6
Sulfamylon	T49.0X1	T49.0X2	T49.0X3	T49.0X4	T49.0X5	T49.0X6
Sulfan blue (diagnostic dye)	T50.8X1	T50.8X2	T50.8X3	T50.8X4	T50.8X5	T50.8X6
Sulfanilamide	T37.0X1	T37.0X2	T37.0X3	T37.0X4	T37.0X5	T37.0X6
Sulfanilylguanidine	T37.0X1	T37.0X2	T37.0X3	T37.0X4	T37.0X5	T37.0X6
Sulfaperin	T37.0X1	T37.0X2	T37.0X3	T37.0X4	T37.0X5	T37.0X6
Sulfaphenazole	T37.0X1	T37.0X2	T37.0X3	T37.0X4	T37.0X5	T37.0X6
Sulfaphenylthiazole	T37.0X1	T37.0X2	T37.0X3	T37.0X4	T37.0X5	T37.0X6
Sulfaproxyline	T37.0X1	T37.0X2	T37.0X3	T37.0X4	T37.0X5	T37.0X6
Sulfapyridine	T37.0X1	T37.0X2	T37.0X3	T37.0X4	T37.0X5	T37.0X6
Sulfapyrimidine	T37.0X1	T37.0X2	T37.0X3	T37.0X4	T37.0X5	T37.0X6
Sulfarsphenamine	T37.8X1	T37.8X2	T37.8X3	T37.8X4	T37.8X5	T37.8X6
Sulfasalazine	T37.0X1	T37.0X2	T37.0X3	T37.0X4	T37.0X5	T37.0X6
Sulfasuxidine	T37.0X1	T37.0X2	T37.0X3	T37.0X4	T37.0X5	T37.0X6
Sulfasymazine	T37.0X1	T37.0X2	T37.0X3	T37.0X4	T37.0X5	T37.0X6
Sulfated amylopectin	T47.8X1	T47.8X2	T47.8X3	T47.8X4	T47.8X5	T47.8X6
Sulfathiazole	T37.0X1	T37.0X2	T37.0X3	T37.0X4	T37.0X5	T37.0X6
Sulfatostearate	T49.2X1	T49.2X2	T49.2X3	T49.2X4	T49.2X5	T49.2X6
Sulfinpyrazone	T50.4X1	T50.4X2	T50.4X3	T50.4X4	T50.4X5	T50.4X6

◄ New　◄▥ Revised　~~deleted~~ Deleted

Substance	Poisoning, Accidental (Unintentional)	Poisoning, Intentional Self-Harm	Poisoning, Assault	Poisoning, Undetermined	Adverse Effect	Underdosing
Sulfiram	T49.0X1	T49.0X2	T49.0X3	T49.0X4	T49.0X5	T49.0X6
Sulfisomidine	T37.0X1	T37.0X2	T37.0X3	T37.0X4	T37.0X5	T37.0X6
Sulfisoxazole	T37.0X1	T37.0X2	T37.0X3	T37.0X4	T37.0X5	T37.0X6
ophthalmic preparation	T49.5X1	T49.5X2	T49.5X3	T49.5X4	T49.5X5	T49.5X6
Sulfobromophthalein (sodium)	T50.8X1	T50.8X2	T50.8X3	T50.8X4	T50.8X5	T50.8X6
Sulfobromphthalein	T50.8X1	T50.8X2	T50.8X3	T50.8X4	T50.8X5	T50.8X6
Sulfogaiacol	T48.4X1	T48.4X2	T48.4X3	T48.4X4	T48.4X5	T48.4X6
Sulfomyxin	T36.8X1	T36.8X2	T36.8X3	T36.8X4	T36.8X5	T36.8X6
Sulfonal	T42.6X1	T42.6X2	T42.6X3	T42.6X4	T42.6X5	T42.6X6
Sulfonamide NEC	T37.0X1	T37.0X2	T37.0X3	T37.0X4	T37.0X5	T37.0X6
eye	T49.5X1	T49.5X2	T49.5X3	T49.5X4	T49.5X5	T49.5X6
Sulfonazide	T37.1X1	T37.1X2	T37.1X3	T37.1X4	T37.1X5	T37.1X6
Sulfones	T37.1X1	T37.1X2	T37.1X3	T37.1X4	T37.1X5	T37.1X6
Sulfonethylmethane	T42.6X1	T42.6X2	T42.6X3	T42.6X4	T42.6X5	T42.6X6
Sulfonmethane	T42.6X1	T42.6X2	T42.6X3	T42.6X4	T42.6X5	T42.6X6
Sulfonphthal, sulfonphthol	T50.8X1	T50.8X2	T50.8X3	T50.8X4	T50.8X5	T50.8X6
Sulfonylurea derivatives, oral	T38.3X1	T38.3X2	T38.3X3	T38.3X4	T38.3X5	T38.3X6
Sulforidazine	T43.3X1	T43.3X2	T43.3X3	T43.3X4	T43.3X5	T43.3X6
Sulfoxone	T37.1X1	T37.1X2	T37.1X3	T37.1X4	T37.1X5	T37.1X6
Sulfur, sulfurated, sulfuric, sulfurous, sulfuryl (compounds NEC) (medicinal)	T49.4X1	T49.4X2	T49.4X3	T49.4X4	T49.4X5	T49.4X6
acid	T54.2X1	T54.2X2	T54.2X3	T54.2X4	—	—
dioxide (gas)	T59.1X1	T59.1X2	T59.1X3	T59.1X4	—	—
ether — see Ether(s)						
hydrogen	T59.6X1	T59.6X2	T59.6X3	T59.6X4	—	—
medicinal (keratolytic) (ointment) NEC	T49.4X1	T49.4X2	T49.4X3	T49.4X4	T49.4X5	T49.4X6
ointment	T49.0X1	T49.0X2	T49.0X3	T49.0X4	T49.0X5	T49.0X6
pesticide (vapor)	T60.91	T60.92	T60.93	T60.94	—	—
vapor NEC	T59.891	T59.892	T59.893	T59.894	—	—
Sulfuric acid	T54.2X1	T54.2X2	T54.2X3	T54.2X4	—	—
Sulglicotide	T47.1X1	T47.1X2	T47.1X3	T47.1X4	T47.1X5	T47.1X6
Sulindac	T39.391	T39.392	T39.393	T39.394	T39.395	T39.396
Sulisatin	T47.2X1	T47.2X2	T47.2X3	T47.2X4	T47.2X5	T47.2X6
Sulisobenzone	T49.3X1	T49.3X2	T49.3X3	T49.3X4	T49.3X5	T49.3X6
Sulkowitch's reagent	T50.8X1	T50.8X2	T50.8X3	T50.8X4	T50.8X5	T50.8X6
Sulmetozine	T44.3X1	T44.3X2	T44.3X3	T44.3X4	T44.3X5	T44.3X6
Suloctidil	T46.7X1	T46.7X2	T46.7X3	T46.7X4	T46.7X5	T46.7X6
Sulph — see also Sulf-						
Sulphadiazine	T37.0X1	T37.0X2	T37.0X3	T37.0X4	T37.0X5	T37.0X6
Sulphadimethoxine	T37.0X1	T37.0X2	T37.0X3	T37.0X4	T37.0X5	T37.0X6
Sulphadimidine	T37.0X1	T37.0X2	T37.0X3	T37.0X4	T37.0X5	T37.0X6
Sulphadione	T37.1X1	T37.1X2	T37.1X3	T37.1X4	T37.1X5	T37.1X6
Sulphafurazole	T37.0X1	T37.0X2	T37.0X3	T37.0X4	T37.0X5	T37.0X6
Sulphamethizole	T37.0X1	T37.0X2	T37.0X3	T37.0X4	T37.0X5	T37.0X6
Sulphamethoxazole	T37.0X1	T37.0X2	T37.0X3	T37.0X4	T37.0X5	T37.0X6
Sulphan blue	T50.8X1	T50.8X2	T50.8X3	T50.8X4	T50.8X5	T50.8X6
Sulphaphenazole	T37.0X1	T37.0X2	T37.0X3	T37.0X4	T37.0X5	T37.0X6
Sulphapyridine	T37.0X1	T37.0X2	T37.0X3	T37.0X4	T37.0X5	T37.0X6
Sulphasalazine	T37.0X1	T37.0X2	T37.0X3	T37.0X4	T37.0X5	T37.0X6
Sulphinpyrazone	T50.4X1	T50.4X2	T50.4X3	T50.4X4	T50.4X5	T50.4X6
Sulpiride	T43.591	T43.592	T43.593	T43.594	T43.595	T43.596
Sulprostone	T48.0X1	T48.0X2	T48.0X3	T48.0X4	T48.0X5	T48.0X6
Sulpyrine	T39.2X1	T39.2X2	T39.2X3	T39.2X4	T39.2X5	T39.2X6
Sultamicillin	T36.0X1	T36.0X2	T36.0X3	T36.0X4	T36.0X5	T36.0X6
Sulthiame	T42.6X1	T42.6X2	T42.6X3	T42.6X4	T42.6X5	T42.6X6
Sultiame	T42.6X1	T42.6X2	T42.6X3	T42.6X4	T42.6X5	T42.6X6
Sultopride	T43.591	T43.592	T43.593	T43.594	T43.595	T43.596
Sumatriptan	T39.8X1	T39.8X2	T39.8X3	T39.8X4	T39.8X5	T39.8X6
Sunflower seed oil	T46.6X1	T46.6X2	T46.6X3	T46.6X4	T46.6X5	T46.6X6
Superinone	T48.4X1	T48.4X2	T48.4X3	T48.4X4	T48.4X5	T48.4X6
Suprofen	T39.311	T39.312	T39.313	T39.314	T39.315	T39.316
Suramin (sodium)	T37.4X1	T37.4X2	T37.4X3	T37.4X4	T37.4X5	T37.4X6
Surfacaine	T41.3X1	T41.3X2	T41.3X3	T41.3X4	T41.3X5	T41.3X6
Surital	T41.1X1	T41.1X2	T41.1X3	T41.1X4	T41.1X5	T41.1X6
Sutilains	T45.3X1	T45.3X2	T45.3X3	T45.3X4	T45.3X5	T45.3X6
Suxamethonium (chloride)	T48.1X1	T48.1X2	T48.1X3	T48.1X4	T48.1X5	T48.1X6
Suxethonium (chloride)	T48.1X1	T48.1X2	T48.1X3	T48.1X4	T48.1X5	T48.1X6
Suxibuzone	T39.2X1	T39.2X2	T39.2X3	T39.2X4	T39.2X5	T39.2X6
Sweet oil (birch)	T49.3X1	T49.3X2	T49.3X3	T49.3X4	T49.3X5	T49.3X6
Sweet niter spirit	T46.3X1	T46.3X2	T46.3X3	T46.3X4	T46.3X5	T46.3X6
Sweetener	T50.901	T50.902	T50.903	T50.904	T50.905	T50.906
Sym-dichloroethyl ether	T53.6X1	T53.6X2	T53.6X3	T53.6X4	—	—
Sympatholytic NEC	T44.8X1	T44.8X2	T44.8X3	T44.8X4	T44.8X5	T44.8X6
haloalkylamine	T44.8X1	T44.8X2	T44.8X3	T44.8X4	T44.8X5	T44.8X6
Sympathomimetic NEC	T44.901	T44.902	T44.903	T44.904	T44.905	T44.906
anti-common-cold	T48.5X1	T48.5X2	T48.5X3	T48.5X4	T48.5X5	T48.5X6
bronchodilator	T48.6X1	T48.6X2	T48.6X3	T48.6X4	T48.6X5	T48.6X6
specified NEC	T44.991	T44.992	T44.993	T44.994	T44.995	T44.996
Synagis	T50.B91	T50.B92	T50.B93	T50.B94	T50.B95	T50.B96
Synalar	T49.0X1	T49.0X2	T49.0X3	T49.0X4	T49.0X5	T49.0X6
Synthroid	T38.1X1	T38.1X2	T38.1X3	T38.1X4	T38.1X5	T38.1X6

◀ New   ◀▥ Revised   ~~deleted~~ Deleted

TABLE OF DRUGS AND CHEMICALS

Substance	Poisoning, Accidental (Unintentional)	Poisoning, Intentional Self-Harm	Poisoning, Assault	Poisoning, Undetermined	Adverse Effect	Underdosing
Syntocinon	T48.0X1	T48.0X2	T48.0X3	T48.0X4	T48.0X5	T48.0X6
Syrosingopine	T46.5X1	T46.5X2	T46.5X3	T46.5X4	T46.5X5	T46.5X6
Systemic drug	T45.91	T45.92	T45.93	T45.94	T45.95	T45.96
specified NEC	T45.8X1	T45.8X2	T45.8X3	T45.8X4	T45.8X5	T45.8X6
2,4,5-T	T60.3X1	T60.3X2	T60.3X3	T60.3X4	—	—

T

Substance	Poisoning, Accidental (Unintentional)	Poisoning, Intentional Self-Harm	Poisoning, Assault	Poisoning, Undetermined	Adverse Effect	Underdosing
Tablets — see also specified substance	T50.901	T50.902	T50.903	T50.904	T50.905	T50.906
Tace	T38.5X1	T38.5X2	T38.5X3	T38.5X4	T38.5X5	T38.5X6
Tacrine	T44.0X1	T44.0X2	T44.0X3	T44.0X4	T44.0X5	T44.0X6
Tadalafil	T46.7X1	T46.7X2	T46.7X3	T46.7X4	T46.7X5	T46.7X6
Talampicillin	T36.0X1	T36.0X2	T36.0X3	T36.0X4	T36.0X5	T36.0X6
Talbutal	T42.3X1	T42.3X2	T42.3X3	T42.3X4	T42.3X5	T42.3X6
Talc powder	T49.3X1	T49.3X2	T49.3X3	T49.3X4	T49.3X5	T49.3X6
Talcum	T49.3X1	T49.3X2	T49.3X3	T49.3X4	T49.3X5	T49.3X6
Taleranol	T38.6X1	T38.6X2	T38.6X3	T38.6X4	T38.6X5	T38.6X6
Tamoxifen	T38.6X1	T38.6X2	T38.6X3	T38.6X4	T38.6X5	T38.6X6
Tamsulosin	T44.6X1	T44.6X2	T44.6X3	T44.6X4	T44.6X5	T44.6X6
Tandearil, tanderil	T39.2X1	T39.2X2	T39.2X3	T39.2X4	T39.2X5	T39.2X6
Tannic acid	T49.2X1	T49.2X2	T49.2X3	T49.2X4	T49.2X5	T49.2X6
medicinal (astringent)	T49.2X1	T49.2X2	T49.2X3	T49.2X4	T49.2X5	T49.2X6
Tannin — see Tannic acid						
Tansy	T62.2X1	T62.2X2	T62.2X3	T62.2X4	—	—
TAO	T36.3X1	T36.3X2	T36.3X3	T36.3X4	T36.3X5	T36.3X6
Tapazole	T38.2X1	T38.2X2	T38.2X3	T38.2X4	T38.2X5	T38.2X6
Tar NEC	T52.0X1	T52.0X2	T52.0X3	T52.0X4	—	—
camphor	T60.1X1	T60.1X2	T60.1X3	T60.1X4	—	—
distillate	T49.1X1	T49.1X2	T49.1X3	T49.1X4	T49.1X5	T49.1X6
fumes	T59.891	T59.892	T59.893	T59.894	—	—
medicinal	T49.1X1	T49.1X2	T49.1X3	T49.1X4	T49.1X5	T49.1X6
ointment	T49.1X1	T49.1X2	T49.1X3	T49.1X4	T49.1X5	T49.1X6
Taractan	T43.591	T43.592	T43.593	T43.594	T43.595	T43.596
Tarantula (venomous)	T63.321	T63.322	T63.323	T63.324	—	—
Tartar emetic	T37.8X1	T37.8X2	T37.8X3	T37.8X4	T37.8X5	T37.8X6
Tartaric acid	T65.891	T65.892	T65.893	T65.894	—	—
Tartrated antimony (anti-infective)	T37.8X1	T37.8X2	T37.8X3	T37.8X4	T37.8X5	T37.8X6
Tartrate, laxative	T47.4X1	T47.4X2	T47.4X3	T47.4X4	T47.4X5	T47.4X6
Tauromustine	T45.1X1	T45.1X2	T45.1X3	T45.1X4	T45.1X5	T45.1X6
TCA — see Trichloroacetic acid						
TCDD	T53.7X1	T53.7X2	T53.7X3	T53.7X4	—	—
TDI (vapor)	T65.0X1	T65.0X2	T65.0X3	T65.0X4	—	—
Tear						
gas	T59.3X1	T59.3X2	T59.3X3	T59.3X4	—	—
solution	T49.5X1	T49.5X2	T49.5X3	T49.5X4	T49.5X5	T49.5X6
Teclothiazide	T50.2X1	T50.2X2	T50.2X3	T50.2X4	T50.2X5	T50.2X6
Teclozan	T37.3X1	T37.3X2	T37.3X3	T37.3X4	T37.3X5	T37.3X6
Tegafur	T45.1X1	T45.1X2	T45.1X3	T45.1X4	T45.1X5	T45.1X6
Tegretol	T42.1X1	T42.1X2	T42.1X3	T42.1X4	T42.1X5	T42.1X6
Teicoplanin	T36.8X1	T36.8X2	T36.8X3	T36.8X4	T36.8X5	T36.8X6
Telepaque	T50.8X1	T50.8X2	T50.8X3	T50.8X4	T50.8X5	T50.8X6
Tellurium	T56.891	T56.892	T56.893	T56.894	—	—
fumes	T56.891	T56.892	T56.893	T56.894	—	—
TEM	T45.1X1	T45.1X2	T45.1X3	T45.1X4	T45.1X5	T45.1X6
Temazepam	T42.4X1	T42.4X2	T42.4X3	T42.4X4	T42.4X5	T42.4X6
Temocillin	T36.0X1	T36.0X2	T36.0X3	T36.0X4	T36.0X5	T36.0X6
Tenamfetamine	T43.621	T43.622	T43.623	T43.624	T43.625	T43.626
Teniposide	T45.1X1	T45.1X2	T45.1X3	T45.1X4	T45.1X5	T45.1X6
Tenitramine	T46.3X1	T46.3X2	T46.3X3	T46.3X4	T46.3X5	T46.3X6
Tenoglicin	T48.4X1	T48.4X2	T48.4X3	T48.4X4	T48.4X5	T48.4X6
Tenonitrozole	T37.3X1	T37.3X2	T37.3X3	T37.3X4	T37.3X5	T37.3X6
Tenoxicam	T39.391	T39.392	T39.393	T39.394	T39.395	T39.396
TEPA	T45.1X1	T45.1X2	T45.1X3	T45.1X4	T45.1X5	T45.1X6
TEPP	T60.0X1	T60.0X2	T60.0X3	T60.0X4	—	—
Teprotide	T46.5X1	T46.5X2	T46.5X3	T46.5X4	T46.5X5	T46.5X6
Terazosin	T44.6X1	T44.6X2	T44.6X3	T44.6X4	T44.6X5	T44.6X6
Terbufos	T60.0X1	T60.0X2	T60.0X3	T60.0X4	—	—
Terbutaline	T48.6X1	T48.6X2	T48.6X3	T48.6X4	T48.6X5	T48.6X6
Terconazole	T49.0X1	T49.0X2	T49.0X3	T49.0X4	T49.0X5	T49.0X6
Terfenadine	T45.0X1	T45.0X2	T45.0X3	T45.0X4	T45.0X5	T45.0X6
Teriparatide (acetate)	T50.991	T50.992	T50.993	T50.994	T50.995	T50.996
Terizidone	T37.1X1	T37.1X2	T37.1X4	T37.1X4	T37.1X5	T37.1X6
Terlipressin	T38.891	T38.892	T38.893	T38.894	T38.895	T38.896
Terodiline	T46.3X1	T46.3X2	T46.3X3	T46.3X4	T46.3X5	T46.3X6
Teroxalene	T37.4X1	T37.4X2	T37.4X3	T37.4X4	T37.4X5	T37.4X6
Terpin(cis) hydrate	T48.4X1	T48.4X2	T48.4X3	T48.4X4	T48.4X5	T48.4X6
Terramycin	T36.4X1	T36.4X2	T36.4X3	T36.4X4	T36.4X5	T36.4X6
Tertatolol	T44.7X1	T44.7X2	T44.7X3	T44.7X4	T44.7X5	T44.7X6
Tessalon	T48.3X1	T48.3X2	T48.3X3	T48.3X4	T48.3X5	T48.3X6
Testolactone	T38.7X1	T38.7X2	T38.7X3	T38.7X4	T38.7X5	T38.7X6
Testosterone	T38.7X1	T38.7X2	T38.7X3	T38.7X4	T38.7X5	T38.7X6
Tetanus toxoid or vaccine	T50.A91	T50.A92	T50.A93	T50.A94	T50.A95	T50.A96
antitoxin	T50.Z11	T50.Z12	T50.Z13	T50.Z14	T50.Z15	T50.Z16
immune globulin (human)	T50.Z11	T50.Z12	T50.Z13	T50.Z14	T50.Z15	T50.Z16

Substance	External Cause (T-Code)					
	Poisoning, Accidental (Unintentional)	Poisoning, Intentional Self-Harm	Poisoning, Assault	Poisoning, Undetermined	Adverse Effect	Underdosing
Tetanus toxoid or vaccine *(Continued)*						
toxoid	T50.A91	T50.A92	T50.A93	T50.A94	T50.A95	T50.A96
with diphtheria toxoid	T50.A21	T50.A22	T50.A23	T50.A24	T50.A25	T50.A26
with pertussis	T50.A11	T50.A12	T50.A13	T50.A14	T50.A15	T50.A16
Tetrabenazine	T43.591	T43.592	T43.593	T43.594	T43.595	T43.596
Tetracaine	T41.3X1	T41.3X2	T41.3X3	T41.3X4	T41.3X5	T41.3X6
nerve block (peripheral) (plexus)	T41.3X1	T41.3X2	T41.3X3	T41.3X4	T41.3X5	T41.3X6
regional	T41.3X1	T41.3X2	T41.3X3	T41.3X4	T41.3X5	T41.3X6
spinal	T41.3X1	T41.3X2	T41.3X3	T41.3X4	T41.3X5	T41.3X6
Tetrachlorethylene — *see Tetrachloroethylene*						
Tetrachlormethiazide	T50.2X1	T50.2X2	T50.2X3	T50.2X4	T50.2X5	T50.2X6
2,3,7,8-Tetrachlorodibenzo-p-dioxin	T53.7X1	T53.7X2	T53.7X3	T53.7X4	—	—
Tetrachloroethane	T53.6X1	T53.6X2	T53.6X3	T53.6X4	—	—
vapor	T53.6X1	T53.6X2	T53.6X3	T53.6X4	—	—
paint or varnish	T53.6X1	T53.6X2	T53.6X3	T53.6X4	—	—
Tetrachloroethylene (liquid)	T53.3X1	T53.3X2	T53.3X3	T53.3X4	—	—
medicinal	T37.4X1	T37.4X2	T37.4X3	T37.4X4	T37.4X5	T37.4X6
vapor	T53.3X1	T53.3X2	T53.3X3	T53.3X4	—	—
Tetrachloromethane — *see Carbon tetrachloride*						
Tetracosactide	T38.811	T38.812	T38.813	T38.814	T38.815	T38.816
Tetracosactrin	T38.811	T38.812	T38.813	T38.814	T38.815	T38.816
Tetracycline	T36.4X1	T36.4X2	T36.4X3	T36.4X4	T36.4X5	T36.4X6
ophthalmic preparation	T49.5X1	T49.5X2	T49.5X3	T49.5X4	T49.5X5	T49.5X6
topical NEC	T49.0X1	T49.0X2	T49.0X3	T49.0X4	T49.0X5	T49.0X6
Tetradifon	T60.8X1	T60.8X2	T60.8X3	T60.8X4	—	—
Tetradotoxin	T61.771	T61.772	T61.773	T61.774		
Tetraethyl						
lead	T56.0X1	T56.0X2	T56.0X3	T56.0X4	—	—
pyrophosphate	T60.0X1	T60.0X2	T60.0X3	T60.0X4	—	—
Tetraethylammonium chloride	T44.2X1	T44.2X2	T44.2X3	T44.2X4	T44.2X5	T44.2X6
Tetraethylthiuram disulfide	T50.6X1	T50.6X2	T50.6X3	T50.6X4	T50.6X5	T50.6X6
Tetrahydroaminoacridine	T44.0X1	T44.0X2	T44.0X3	T44.0X4	T44.0X5	T44.0X6
Tetrahydrocannabinol	T40.7X1	T40.7X2	T40.7X3	T40.7X4	T40.7X5	T40.7X6
Tetrahydrofuran	T52.8X1	T52.8X2	T52.8X3	T52.8X4		
Tetrahydronaphthalene	T52.8X1	T52.8X2	T52.8X3	T52.8X4	—	—
Tetrahydrozoline	T49.5X1	T49.5X2	T49.5X3	T49.5X4	T49.5X5	T49.5X6
Tetralin	T52.8X1	T52.8X2	T52.8X3	T52.8X4	—	—
Tetramethrin	T60.2X1	T60.2X2	T60.2X3	T60.2X4	—	—

Substance	External Cause (T-Code)					
	Poisoning, Accidental (Unintentional)	Poisoning, Intentional Self-Harm	Poisoning, Assault	Poisoning, Undetermined	Adverse Effect	Underdosing
Tetramethylthiuram (disulfide) NEC	T60.3X1	T60.3X2	T60.3X3	T60.3X4	—	—
medicinal	T49.0X1	T49.0X2	T49.0X3	T49.0X4	T49.0X5	T49.0X6
Tetramisole	T37.4X1	T37.4X2	T37.4X3	T37.4X4	T37.4X5	T37.4X6
Tetranicotinoyl fructose	T46.7X1	T46.7X2	T46.7X3	T46.7X4	T46.7X5	T46.7X6
Tetronal	T42.6X1	T42.6X2	T42.6X3	T42.6X4	T42.6X5	T42.6X6
Tetrazepam	T42.4X1	T42.4X2	T42.4X3	T42.4X4	T42.4X5	T42.4X6
Tetryl	T65.3X1	T65.3X2	T65.3X3	T65.3X4	—	—
Tetrylammonium chloride	T44.2X1	T44.2X2	T44.2X3	T44.2X4	T44.2X5	T44.2X6
Tetryzoline	T49.5X1	T49.5X2	T49.5X3	T49.5X4	T49.5X5	T49.5X6
Thalidomide	T45.1X1	T45.1X2	T45.1X3	T45.1X4	T45.1X5	T45.1X6
Thallium (compounds) (dust) NEC	T56.811	T56.812	T56.813	T56.814	—	—
pesticide	T60.4X1	T60.4X2	T60.4X3	T60.4X4	—	—
THC	T40.7X1	T40.7X2	T40.7X3	T40.7X4	T40.7X5	T40.7X6
Thebacon	T48.3X1	T48.3X2	T48.3X3	T48.3X4	T48.3X5	T48.3X6
Thebaine	T40.2X1	T40.2X2	T40.2X3	T40.2X4	T40.2X5	T40.2X6
Thenoic acid	T49.6X1	T49.6X2	T49.6X3	T49.6X4	T49.6X5	T49.6X6
Thenyldiamine	T45.0X1	T45.0X2	T45.0X3	T45.0X4	T45.0X5	T45.0X6
Theobromine (calcium salicylate)	T48.6X1	T48.6X2	T48.6X3	T48.6X4	T48.6X5	T48.6X6
sodium salicylate	T48.6X1	T48.6X2	T48.6X3	T48.6X4	T48.6X5	T48.6X6
Theophyllamine	T48.6X1	T48.6X2	T48.6X3	T48.6X4	T48.6X5	T48.6X6
Theophylline	T48.6X1	T48.6X2	T48.6X3	T48.6X4	T48.6X5	T48.6X6
aminobenzoic acid	T48.6X1	T48.6X2	T48.6X3	T48.6X4	T48.6X5	T48.6X6
ethylenediamine	T48.6X1	T48.6X2	T48.6X3	T48.6X4	T48.6X5	T48.6X6
piperazine p-amino-benzoate	T48.6X1	T48.6X2	T48.6X3	T48.6X4	T48.6X5	T48.6X6
Thiabendazole	T37.4X1	T37.4X2	T37.4X3	T37.4X4	T37.4X5	T37.4X6
Thialbarbital	T41.1X1	T41.1X2	T41.1X3	T41.1X4	T41.1X5	T41.1X6
Thiamazole	T38.2X1	T38.2X2	T38.2X3	T38.2X4	T38.2X5	T38.2X6
Thiambutosine	T37.1X1	T37.1X2	T37.1X3	T37.1X4	T37.1X5	T37.1X6
Thiamine	T45.2X1	T45.2X2	T45.2X3	T45.2X4	T45.2X5	T45.2X6
Thiamphenicol	T36.2X1	T36.2X2	T36.2X3	T36.2X4	T36.2X5	T36.2X6
Thiamylal	T41.1X1	T41.1X2	T41.1X3	T41.1X4	T41.1X5	T41.1X6
sodium	T41.1X1	T41.1X2	T41.1X3	T41.1X4	T41.1X5	T41.1X6
Thiazesim	T43.291	T43.292	T43.293	T43.294	T43.295	T43.296
Thiazides (diuretics)	T50.2X1	T50.2X2	T50.2X3	T50.2X4	T50.2X5	T50.2X6
Thiazinamium metilsulfate	T43.3X1	T43.3X2	T43.3X3	T43.3X4	T43.3X5	T43.3X6
Thiethylperazine	T43.3X1	T43.3X2	T43.3X3	T43.3X4	T43.3X5	T43.3X6
Thimerosal	T49.0X1	T49.0X2	T49.0X3	T49.0X4	T49.0X5	T49.0X6
ophthalmic preparation	T49.5X1	T49.5X2	T49.5X3	T49.5X4	T49.5X5	T49.5X6
Thioacetazone	T37.1X1	T37.1X2	T37.1X3	T37.1X4	T37.1X5	T37.1X6
with isoniazid	T37.1X1	T37.1X2	T37.1X3	T37.1X4	T37.1X5	T37.1X6
Thiobarbital sodium	T41.1X1	T41.1X2	T41.1X3	T41.1X4	T41.1X5	T41.1X6

◀ New ⟵ Revised ~~deleted~~ Deleted

Substance	External Cause (T-Code)					
	Poisoning, Accidental (Unintentional)	Poisoning, Intentional Self-Harm	Poisoning, Assault	Poisoning, Undetermined	Adverse Effect	Underdosing
Thiobarbiturate anesthetic	T41.1X1	T41.1X2	T41.1X3	T41.1X4	T41.1X5	T41.1X6
Thiobismol	T37.8X1	T37.8X2	T37.8X3	T37.8X4	T37.8X5	T37.8X6
Thiobutabarbital sodium	T41.1X1	T41.1X2	T41.1X3	T41.1X4	T41.1X5	T41.1X6
Thiocarbamate (insecticide)	T60.0X1	T60.0X2	T60.0X3	T60.0X4	—	—
Thiocarbamide	T38.2X1	T38.2X2	T38.2X3	T38.2X4	T38.2X5	T38.2X6
Thiocarbarsone	T37.8X1	T37.8X2	T37.8X3	T37.8X4	T37.8X5	T37.8X6
Thiocarlide	T37.1X1	T37.1X2	T37.1X3	T37.1X4	T37.1X5	T37.1X6
Thioctamide	T50.991	T50.992	T50.993	T50.994	T50.995	T50.996
Thioctic acid	T50.991	T50.992	T50.993	T50.994	T50.995	T50.996
Thiofos	T60.0X1	T60.0X2	T60.0X3	T60.0X4	—	—
Thioglycolate	T49.4X1	T49.4X2	T49.4X3	T49.4X4	T49.4X5	T49.4X6
Thioglycolic acid	T65.891	T65.892	T65.893	T65.894		
Thioguanine	T45.1X1	T45.1X2	T45.1X3	T45.1X4	T45.1X5	T45.1X6
Thiomercaptomerin	T50.2X1	T50.2X2	T50.2X3	T50.2X4	T50.2X5	T50.2X6
Thiomerin	T50.2X1	T50.2X2	T50.2X3	T50.2X4	T50.2X5	T50.2X6
Thiomersal	T49.0X1	T49.0X2	T49.0X3	T49.0X4	T49.0X5	T49.0X6
Thionazin	T60.0X1	T60.0X2	T60.0X3	T60.0X4	—	—
Thiopental (sodium)	T41.1X1	T41.1X2	T41.1X3	T41.1X4	T41.1X5	T41.1X6
Thiopentone (sodium)	T41.1X1	T41.1X2	T41.1X3	T41.1X4	T41.1X5	T41.1X6
Thiopropazate	T43.3X1	T43.3X2	T43.3X3	T43.3X4	T43.3X5	T43.3X6
Thioproperazine	T43.3X1	T43.3X2	T43.3X3	T43.3X4	T43.3X5	T43.3X6
Thioridazine	T43.3X1	T43.3X2	T43.3X3	T43.3X4	T43.3X5	T43.3X6
Thiosinamine	T49.3X1	T49.3X2	T49.3X3	T49.3X4	T49.3X5	T49.3X6
Thiotepa	T45.1X1	T45.1X2	T45.1X3	T45.1X4	T45.1X5	T45.1X6
Thiothixene	T43.4X1	T43.4X2	T43.4X3	T43.4X4	T43.4X5	T43.4X6
Thiouracil (benzyl) (methyl) (propyl)	T38.2X1	T38.2X2	T38.2X3	T38.2X4	T38.2X5	T38.2X6
Thiourea	T38.2X1	T38.2X2	T38.2X3	T38.2X4	T38.2X5	T38.2X6
Thiphenamil	T44.3X1	T44.3X2	T44.3X3	T44.3X4	T44.3X5	T44.3X6
Thiram	T60.3X1	T60.3X2	T60.3X3	T60.3X4	—	—
medicinal	T49.2X1	T49.2X2	T49.2X3	T49.2X4	T49.2X5	T49.2X6
Thonzylamine (systemic)	T45.0X1	T45.0X2	T45.0X3	T45.0X4	T45.0X5	T45.0X6
mucosal decongestant	T48.5X1	T48.5X2	T48.5X3	T48.5X4	T48.5X5	T48.5X6
Thorazine	T43.3X1	T43.3X2	T43.3X3	T43.3X4	T43.3X5	T43.3X6
Thorium dioxide suspension	T50.8X1	T50.8X2	T50.8X3	T50.8X4	T50.8X5	T50.8X6
Thornapple	T62.2X1	T62.2X2	T62.2X3	T62.2X4	—	—
Throat drug NEC	T49.6X1	T49.6X2	T49.6X3	T49.6X4	T49.6X5	T49.6X6
Thrombin	T45.7X1	T45.7X2	T45.7X3	T45.7X4	T45.7X5	T45.7X6
Thrombolysin	T45.611	T45.612	T45.613	T45.614	T45.615	T45.616
Thromboplastin	T45.7X1	T45.7X2	T45.7X3	T45.7X4	T45.7X5	T45.7X6
Thurfyl nicotinate	T46.7X1	T46.7X2	T46.7X3	T46.7X4	T46.7X5	T46.7X6
Thymol	T49.0X1	T49.0X2	T49.0X3	T49.0X4	T49.0X5	T49.0X6

Substance	External Cause (T-Code)					
	Poisoning, Accidental (Unintentional)	Poisoning, Intentional Self-Harm	Poisoning, Assault	Poisoning, Undetermined	Adverse Effect	Underdosing
Thymopentin	T37.5X1	T37.5X2	T37.5X3	T37.5X4	T37.5X5	T37.5X6
Thymoxamine	T46.7X1	T46.7X2	T46.7X3	T46.7X4	T46.7X5	T46.7X6
Thymus extract	T38.891	T38.892	T38.893	T38.894	T38.895	T38.896
Thyreotrophic hormone	T38.811	T38.812	T38.813	T38.814	T38.815	T38.816
Thyroglobulin	T38.1X1	T38.1X2	T38.1X3	T38.1X4	T38.1X5	T38.1X6
Thyroid (hormone)	T38.1X1	T38.1X2	T38.1X3	T38.1X4	T38.1X5	T38.1X6
Thyrolar	T38.1X1	T38.1X2	T38.1X3	T38.1X4	T38.1X5	T38.1X6
Thyrotrophin	T38.811	T38.812	T38.813	T38.814	T38.815	T38.816
Thyrotropic hormone	T38.811	T38.812	T38.813	T38.814	T38.815	T38.816
Thyroxine	T38.1X1	T38.1X2	T38.1X3	T38.1X4	T38.1X5	T38.1X6
Tiabendazole	T37.4X1	T37.4X2	T37.4X3	T37.4X4	T37.4X5	T37.4X6
Tiamizide	T50.2X1	T50.2X2	T50.2X3	T50.2X4	T50.2X5	T50.2X6
Tianeptine	T43.291	T43.292	T43.293	T43.294	T43.295	T43.296
Tiapamil	T46.1X1	T46.1X2	T46.1X3	T46.1X4	T46.1X5	T46.1X6
Tiapride	T43.591	T43.592	T43.593	T43.594	T43.595	T43.596
Tiaprofenic acid	T39.311	T39.312	T39.313	T39.314	T39.315	T39.316
Tiaramide	T39.8X1	T39.8X2	T39.8X3	T39.8X4	T39.8X5	T39.8X6
Ticarcillin	T36.0X1	T36.0X2	T36.0X3	T36.0X4	T36.0X5	T36.0X6
Ticlatone	T49.0X1	T49.0X2	T49.0X3	T49.0X4	T49.0X5	T49.0X6
Ticlopidine	T45.521	T45.522	T45.523	T45.524	T45.525	T45.526
Ticrynafen	T50.1X1	T50.1X2	T50.1X3	T50.1X4	T50.1X5	T50.1X6
Tidiacic	T50.991	T50.992	T50.993	T50.994	T50.995	T50.996
Tiemonium	T44.3X1	T44.3X2	T44.3X3	T44.3X4	T44.3X5	T44.3X6
iodide	T44.3X1	T44.3X2	T44.3X3	T44.3X4	T44.3X5	T44.3X6
Tienilic acid	T50.1X1	T50.1X2	T50.1X3	T50.1X4	T50.1X5	T50.1X6
Tifenamil	T44.3X1	T44.3X2	T44.3X3	T44.3X4	T44.3X5	T44.3X6
Tigan	T45.0X1	T45.0X2	T45.0X3	T45.0X4	T45.0X5	T45.0X6
Tigloidine	T44.3X1	T44.3X2	T44.3X3	T44.3X4	T44.3X5	T44.3X6
Tilactase	T47.5X1	T47.5X2	T47.5X3	T47.5X4	T47.5X5	T47.5X6
Tiletamine	T41.291	T41.292	T41.293	T41.294	T41.295	T41.296
Tilidine	T40.4X1	T40.4X2	T40.4X3	T40.4X4	—	—
Timepidium bromide	T44.3X1	T44.3X2	T44.3X3	T44.3X4	T44.3X5	T44.3X6
Timiperone	T43.4X1	T43.4X2	T43.4X3	T43.4X4	T43.4X5	T43.4X6
Timolol	T44.7X1	T44.7X2	T44.7X3	T44.7X4	T44.7X5	T44.7X6
Tin (chloride) (dust) (oxide) NEC	T56.6X1	T56.6X2	T56.6X3	T56.6X4	—	—
anti-infectives	T37.8X1	T37.8X2	T37.8X3	T37.8X4	T37.8X5	T37.8X6
Tincture, iodine — see Iodine						
Tindal	T43.3X1	T43.3X2	T43.3X3	T43.3X4	T43.3X5	T43.3X6
Tinidazole	T37.3X1	T37.3X2	T37.3X3	T37.3X4	T37.3X5	T37.3X6
Tinoridine	T39.8X1	T39.8X2	T39.8X3	T39.8X4	T39.8X5	T39.8X6
Tiocarlide	T37.1X1	T37.1X2	T37.1X3	T37.1X4	T37.1X5	T37.1X6
Tioclomarol	T45.511	T45.512	T45.513	T45.514	T45.515	T45.516

◀ New ◀━ Revised ~~deleted~~ Deleted

Substance	Poisoning, Accidental (Unintentional)	Poisoning, Intentional Self-Harm	Poisoning, Assault	Poisoning, Undetermined	Adverse Effect	Underdosing
Tioconazole	T49.0X1	T49.0X2	T49.0X3	T49.0X4	T49.0X5	T49.0X6
Tioguanine	T45.1X1	T45.1X2	T45.1X3	T45.1X4	T45.1X5	T45.1X6
Tiopronin	T50.991	T50.992	T50.993	T50.994	T50.995	T50.996
Tiotixene	T43.4X1	T43.4X2	T43.4X3	T43.4X4	T43.4X5	T43.4X6
Tioxolone	T49.4X1	T49.4X2	T49.4X3	T49.4X4	T49.4X5	T49.4X6
Tipepidine	T48.3X1	T48.3X2	T48.3X3	T48.3X4	T48.3X5	T48.3X6
Tiquizium bromide	T44.3X1	T44.3X2	T44.3X3	T44.3X4	T44.3X5	T44.3X6
Tiratricol	T38.1X1	T38.1X2	T38.1X3	T38.1X4	T38.1X5	T38.1X6
Tisopurine	T50.4X1	T50.4X2	T50.4X3	T50.4X4	T50.4X5	T50.4X6
Titanium (compounds) (vapor)	T56.891	T56.892	T56.893	T56.894	—	—
dioxide	T49.3X1	T49.3X2	T49.3X3	T49.3X4	T49.3X5	T49.3X6
ointment	T49.3X1	T49.3X2	T49.3X3	T49.3X4	T49.3X5	T49.3X6
oxide	T49.3X1	T49.3X2	T49.3X3	T49.3X4	T49.3X5	T49.3X6
tetrachloride	T56.891	T56.892	T56.893	T56.894	—	—
Titanocene	T56.891	T56.892	T56.893	T56.894	—	—
Titroid	T38.1X1	T38.1X2	T38.1X3	T38.1X4	T38.1X5	T38.1X6
Tizanidine	T42.8X1	T42.8X2	T42.8X3	T42.8X4	T42.8X5	T42.8X6
TMTD	T60.3X1	T60.3X2	T60.3X3	T60.3X4	—	—
TNT (fumes)	T65.3X1	T65.3X2	T65.3X3	T65.3X4	—	—
Toadstool	T62.0X1	T62.0X2	T62.0X3	T62.0X4	—	—
Tobacco NEC	T65.291	T65.292	T65.293	T65.294	—	—
cigarettes	T65.221	T65.222	T65.223	T65.224	—	—
Indian	T62.2X1	T62.2X2	T62.2X3	T62.2X4	—	—
smoke, second-hand	T65.221	T65.222	T65.223	T65.224	—	—
Tobramycin	T36.5X1	T36.5X2	T36.5X3	T36.5X4	T36.5X5	T36.5X6
Tocainide	T46.2X1	T46.2X2	T46.2X3	T46.2X4	T46.2X5	T46.2X6
Tocoferol	T45.2X1	T45.2X2	T45.2X3	T45.2X4	T45.2X5	T45.2X6
Tocopherol	T45.2X1	T45.2X2	T45.2X3	T45.2X4	T45.2X5	T45.2X6
acetate	T45.2X1	T45.2X2	T45.2X3	T45.2X4	T45.2X5	T45.2X6
Tocosamine	T48.0X1	T48.0X2	T48.0X3	T48.0X4	T48.0X5	T48.0X6
Todralazine	T46.5X1	T46.5X2	T46.5X3	T46.5X4	T46.5X5	T46.5X6
Tofisopam	T42.4X1	T42.4X2	T42.4X3	T42.4X4	T42.4X5	T42.4X6
Tofranil	T43.011	T43.012	T43.013	T43.014	T43.015	T43.016
Toilet deodorizer	T65.891	T65.892	T65.893	T65.894	—	—
Tolamolol	T44.7X1	T44.7X2	T44.7X3	T44.7X4	T44.7X5	T44.7X6
Tolazamide	T38.3X1	T38.3X2	T38.3X3	T38.3X4	T38.3X5	T38.3X6
Tolazoline	T46.7X1	T46.7X2	T46.7X3	T46.7X4	T46.7X5	T46.7X6
Tolbutamide (sodium)	T38.3X1	T38.3X2	T38.3X3	T38.3X4	T38.3X5	T38.3X6
Tolciclate	T49.0X1	T49.0X2	T49.0X3	T49.0X4	T49.0X5	T49.0X6
Tolmetin	T39.391	T39.392	T39.393	T39.394	T39.395	T39.396
Tolnaftate	T49.0X1	T49.0X2	T49.0X3	T49.0X4	T49.0X5	T49.0X6
Tolonidine	T46.5X1	T46.5X2	T46.5X3	T46.5X4	T46.5X5	T46.5X6

Substance	Poisoning, Accidental (Unintentional)	Poisoning, Intentional Self-Harm	Poisoning, Assault	Poisoning, Undetermined	Adverse Effect	Underdosing
Toloxatone	T42.6X1	T42.6X2	T42.6X3	T42.6X4	T42.6X5	T42.6X6
Tolperisone	T44.3X1	T44.3X2	T44.3X3	T44.3X4	T44.3X5	T44.3X6
Tolserol	T42.8X1	T42.8X2	T42.8X3	T42.8X4	T42.8X5	T42.8X6
Toluene (liquid)	T52.2X1	T52.2X2	T52.2X3	T52.2X4	—	—
diisocyanate	T65.0X1	T65.0X2	T65.0X3	T65.0X4	—	—
Toluidine	T65.891	T65.892	T65.893	T65.894	—	—
vapor	T59.891	T59.892	T59.893	T59.894	—	—
Toluol (liquid)	T52.2X1	T52.2X2	T52.2X3	T52.2X4	—	—
vapor	T52.2X1	T52.2X2	T52.2X3	T52.2X4	—	—
Toluylenediamine	T65.3X1	T65.3X2	T65.3X3	T65.3X4	—	—
Tolylene-2,4-diisocyanate	T65.0X1	T65.0X2	T65.0X3	T65.0X4	—	—
Tonic NEC	T50.901	T50.902	T50.903	T50.904	T50.905	T50.906
Topical action drug NEC	T49.91	T49.92	T49.93	T49.94	T49.95	T49.96
ear, nose or throat	T49.6X1	T49.6X2	T49.6X3	T49.6X4	T49.6X5	T49.6X6
eye	T49.5X1	T49.5X2	T49.5X3	T49.5X4	T49.5X5	T49.5X6
skin	T49.91	T49.92	T49.93	T49.94	T49.95	T49.96
specified NEC	T49.8X1	T49.8X2	T49.8X3	T49.8X4	T49.8X5	T49.8X6
Toquizine	T44.3X1	T44.3X2	T44.3X3	T44.3X4	T44.3X5	T44.3X6
Toremifene	T38.6X1	T38.6X2	T38.6X3	T38.6X4	T38.6X5	T38.6X6
Tosylchloramide sodium	T49.8X1	T49.8X2	T49.8X3	T49.8X4	T49.8X5	T49.8X6
Toxaphene (dust) (spray)	T60.1X1	T60.1X2	T60.1X3	T60.1X4	—	—
Toxin, diphtheria (Schick Test)	T50.8X1	T50.8X2	T50.8X3	T50.8X4	T50.8X5	T50.8X6
Toxoid						
combined	T50.A21	T50.A22	T50.A23	T50.A24	T50.A25	T50.A26
diphtheria	T50.A91	T50.A92	T50.A93	T50.A94	T50.A95	T50.A96
tetanus	T50.A91	T50.A92	T50.A93	T50.A94	T50.A95	T50.A96
Trace element NEC	T45.8X1	T45.8X2	T45.8X3	T45.8X4	T45.8X5	T45.8X6
Tractor fuel NEC	T52.0X1	T52.0X2	T52.0X3	T52.0X4	—	—
Tragacanth	T50.991	T50.992	T50.993	T50.994	T50.995	T50.996
Tramadol	T40.4X1	T40.4X2	T40.4X3	T40.4X4	T40.4X5	T40.4X6
Tramazoline	T48.5X1	T48.5X2	T48.5X3	T48.5X4	T48.5X5	T48.5X6
Tranexamic acid	T45.621	T45.622	T45.623	T45.624	T45.625	T45.626
Tranilast	T45.0X1	T45.0X2	T45.0X3	T45.0X4	T45.0X5	T45.0X6
Tranquilizer NEC	T43.501	T43.502	T43.503	T43.504	T43.505	T43.506
with hypnotic or sedative	T42.6X1	T42.6X2	T42.6X3	T42.6X4	T42.6X5	T42.6X6
benzodiazepine NEC	T42.4X1	T42.4X2	T42.4X3	T42.4X4	T42.4X5	T42.4X6
butyrophenone NEC	T43.4X1	T43.4X2	T43.4X3	T43.4X4	T43.4X5	T43.4X6
carbamate	T43.591	T43.592	T43.593	T43.594	T43.595	T43.596
dimethylamine	T43.3X1	T43.3X2	T43.3X3	T43.3X4	T43.3X5	T43.3X6
ethylamine	T43.3X1	T43.3X2	T43.3X3	T43.3X4	T43.3X5	T43.3X6
hydroxyzine	T43.591	T43.592	T43.593	T43.594	T43.595	T43.596
major NEC	T43.501	T43.502	T43.503	T43.504	T43.505	T43.506

◀ New ◀ Revised ~~deleted~~ Deleted

Substance	Poisoning, Accidental (Unintentional)	Poisoning, Intentional Self-Harm	Poisoning, Assault	Poisoning, Undetermined	Adverse Effect	Underdosing
Tranquilizer NEC *(Continued)*						
penothiazine NEC	T43.3X1	T43.3X2	T43.3X3	T43.3X4	T43.3X5	T43.3X6
phenothiazine-based	T43.3X1	T43.3X2	T43.3X3	T43.3X4	T43.3X5	T43.3X6
piperazine NEC	T43.3X1	T43.3X2	T43.3X3	T43.3X4	T43.3X5	T43.3X6
piperidine	T43.3X1	T43.3X2	T43.3X3	T43.3X4	T43.3X5	T43.3X6
propylamine	T43.3X1	T43.3X2	T43.3X3	T43.3X4	T43.3X5	T43.3X6
specified NEC	T43.591	T43.592	T43.593	T43.594	T43.595	T43.596
thioxanthene NEC	T43.591	T43.592	T43.593	T43.594	T43.595	T43.596
Tranxene	T42.4X1	T42.4X2	T42.4X3	T42.4X4	T42.4X5	T42.4X6
Tranylcypromine	T43.1X1	T43.1X2	T43.1X3	T43.1X4	T43.1X5	T43.1X6
Trapidil	T46.3X1	T46.3X2	T46.3X3	T46.3X4	T46.3X5	T46.3X6
Trasentine	T44.3X1	T44.3X2	T44.3X3	T44.3X4	T44.3X5	T44.3X6
Travert	T50.3X1	T50.3X2	T50.3X3	T50.3X4	T50.3X5	T50.3X6
Trazodone	T43.211	T43.212	T43.213	T43.214	T43.215	T43.216
Trecator	T37.1X1	T37.1X2	T37.1X3	T37.1X4	T37.1X5	T37.1X6
Treosulfan	T45.1X1	T45.1X2	T45.1X3	T45.1X4	T45.1X5	T45.1X6
Tretamine	T45.1X1	T45.1X2	T45.1X3	T45.1X4	T45.1X5	T45.1X6
Tretinoin	T49.0X1	T49.0X2	T49.0X3	T49.0X4	T49.0X5	T49.0X6
Tretoquinol	T48.6X1	T48.6X2	T48.6X3	T48.6X4	T48.6X5	T48.6X6
Triacetin	T49.0X1	T49.0X2	T49.0X3	T49.0X4	T49.0X5	T49.0X6
Triacetoxyanthracene	T49.4X1	T49.4X2	T49.4X3	T49.4X4	T49.4X5	T49.4X6
Triacetyloleandomycin	T36.3X1	T36.3X2	T36.3X3	T36.3X4	T36.3X5	T36.3X6
Triamcinolone	T49.0X1	T49.0X2	T49.0X3	T49.0X4	T49.0X5	T49.0X6
ENT agent	T49.6X1	T49.6X2	T49.6X3	T49.6X4	T49.6X5	T49.6X6
hexacetonide	T49.0X1	T49.0X2	T49.0X3	T49.0X4	T49.0X5	T49.0X6
ophthalmic preparation	T49.5X1	T49.5X2	T49.5X3	T49.5X4	T49.5X5	T49.5X6
topical NEC	T49.0X1	T49.0X2	T49.0X3	T49.0X4	T49.0X5	T49.0X6
Triampyzine	T44.3X1	T44.3X2	T44.3X3	T44.3X4	T44.3X5	T44.3X6
Triamterene	T50.2X1	T50.2X2	T50.2X3	T50.2X4	T50.2X5	T50.2X6
Triazine (herbicide)	T60.3X1	T60.3X2	T60.3X3	T60.3X4	—	—
Triaziquone	T45.1X1	T45.1X2	T45.1X3	T45.1X4	T45.1X5	T45.1X6
Triazolam	T42.4X1	T42.4X2	T42.4X3	T42.4X4	T42.4X5	T42.4X6
Triazole (herbicide)	T60.3X1	T60.3X2	T60.3X3	T60.3X4	—	—
Tribenoside	T46.991	T46.992	T46.993	T46.994	T46.995	T46.996
Tribromacetaldehyde	T42.6X1	T42.6X2	T42.6X3	T42.6X4	T42.6X5	T42.6X6
Tribromoethanol, rectal	T41.291	T41.292	T41.293	T41.294	T41.295	T41.296
Tribromomethane	T42.6X1	T42.6X2	T42.6X3	T42.6X4	T42.6X5	T42.6X6
Trichlorethane	T53.2X1	T53.2X2	T53.2X3	T53.2X4	—	—
Trichlorethylene	T53.2X1	T53.2X2	T53.2X3	T53.2X4	—	—
Trichlorfon	T60.0X1	T60.0X2	T60.0X3	T60.0X4	—	—
Trichlormethiazide	T50.2X1	T50.2X2	T50.2X3	T50.2X4	T50.2X5	T50.2X6
Trichlormethine	T45.1X1	T45.1X2	T45.1X3	T45.1X4	T45.1X5	T45.1X6

Substance	Poisoning, Accidental (Unintentional)	Poisoning, Intentional Self-Harm	Poisoning, Assault	Poisoning, Undetermined	Adverse Effect	Underdosing
Trichloroacetic acid, Trichloracetic acid	T54.2X1	T54.2X2	T54.2X3	T54.2X4	—	—
medicinal	T49.4X1	T49.4X2	T49.4X3	T49.4X4	T49.4X5	T49.4X6
Trichloroethane	T53.2X1	T53.2X2	T53.2X3	T53.2X4	—	—
Trichloroethanol	T42.6X1	T42.6X2	T42.6X3	T42.6X4	T42.6X5	T42.6X6
Trichloroethylene (liquid) (vapor)	T53.2X1	T53.2X2	T53.2X3	T53.2X4	—	—
anesthetic (gas)	T41.0X1	T41.0X2	T41.0X3	T41.0X4	T41.0X5	T41.0X6
vapor NEC	T53.2X1	T53.2X2	T53.2X3	T53.2X4	—	—
Trichloroethyl phosphate	T42.6X1	T42.6X2	T42.6X3	T42.6X4	T42.6X5	T42.6X6
Trichlorofluoromethane NEC	T53.5X1	T53.5X2	T53.5X3	T53.5X4	—	—
Trichloronate	T60.0X1	T60.0X2	T60.0X3	T60.0X4	—	—
2,4,5-Trichlorophen-oxyacetic acid	T60.3X1	T60.3X2	T60.3X3	T60.3X4	—	—
Trichloropropane	T53.6X1	T53.6X2	T53.6X3	T53.6X4	—	—
Trichlorotriethylamine	T45.1X1	T45.1X2	T45.1X3	T45.1X4	T45.1X5	T45.1X6
Trichomonacides NEC	T37.3X1	T37.3X2	T37.3X3	T37.3X4	T37.3X5	T37.3X6
Trichomycin	T36.7X1	T36.7X2	T36.7X3	T36.7X4	T36.7X5	T36.7X6
Triclobisonium chloride	T49.0X1	T49.0X2	T49.0X3	T49.0X4	T49.0X5	T49.0X6
Triclocarban	T49.0X1	T49.0X2	T49.0X3	T49.0X4	T49.0X5	T49.0X6
Triclofos	T42.6X1	T42.6X2	T42.6X3	T42.6X4	T42.6X5	T42.6X6
Triclosan	T49.0X1	T49.0X2	T49.0X3	T49.0X4	T49.0X5	T49.0X6
Tricresyl phosphate	T65.891	T65.892	T65.893	T65.894	—	—
solvent	T52.91	T52.92	T52.93	T52.94	—	—
Tricyclamol chloride	T44.3X1	T44.3X2	T44.3X3	T44.3X4	T44.3X5	T44.3X6
Tridesilon	T49.0X1	T49.0X2	T49.0X3	T49.0X4	T49.0X5	T49.0X6
Tridihexethyl iodide	T44.3X1	T44.3X2	T44.3X3	T44.3X4	T44.3X5	T44.3X6
Tridione	T42.2X1	T42.2X2	T42.2X3	T42.2X4	T42.2X5	T42.2X6
Trientine	T45.8X1	T45.8X2	T45.8X3	T45.8X4	T45.8X5	T45.8X6
Triethanolamine NEC	T54.3X1	T54.3X2	T54.3X3	T54.3X4	—	—
detergent	T54.3X1	T54.3X2	T54.3X3	T54.3X4	—	—
trinitrate (biphosphate)	T46.3X1	T46.3X2	T46.3X3	T46.3X4	T46.3X5	T46.3X6
Triethanomelamine	T45.1X1	T45.1X2	T45.1X3	T45.1X4	T45.1X5	T45.1X6
Triethylenemelamine	T45.1X1	T45.1X2	T45.1X3	T45.1X4	T45.1X5	T45.1X6
Triethylenephosphoramide	T45.1X1	T45.1X2	T45.1X3	T45.1X4	T45.1X5	T45.1X6
Triethylenethiophosphoramide	T45.1X1	T45.1X2	T45.1X3	T45.1X4	T45.1X5	T45.1X6
Trifluoperazine	T43.3X1	T43.3X2	T43.3X3	T43.3X4	T43.3X5	T43.3X6
Trifluoroethyl vinyl ether	T41.0X1	T41.0X2	T41.0X3	T41.0X4	T41.0X5	T41.0X6
Trifluperidol	T43.4X1	T43.4X2	T43.4X3	T43.4X4	T43.4X5	T43.4X6
Triflupromazine	T43.3X1	T43.3X2	T43.3X3	T43.3X4	T43.3X5	T43.3X6
Trifluridine	T37.5X1	T37.5X2	T37.5X3	T37.5X4	T37.5X5	T37.5X6
Triflusal	T45.521	T45.522	T45.523	T45.524	T45.525	T45.526
Trihexyphenidyl	T44.3X1	T44.3X2	T44.3X3	T44.3X4	T44.3X5	T44.3X6
Triiodothyronine	T38.1X1	T38.1X2	T38.1X3	T38.1X4	T38.1X5	T38.1X6

◀ New   ◀═ Revised   ~~deleted~~ Deleted

	External Cause (T-Code)					
Substance	Poisoning, Accidental (Unintentional)	Poisoning, Intentional Self-Harm	Poisoning, Assault	Poisoning, Undetermined	Adverse Effect	Underdosing
Trilene	T41.0X1	T41.0X2	T41.0X3	T41.0X4	T41.0X5	T41.0X6
Trilostane	T38.991	T38.992	T38.993	T38.994	T38.995	T38.996
Trimebutine	T44.3X1	T44.3X2	T44.3X3	T44.3X4	T44.3X5	T44.3X6
Trimecaine	T41.3X1	T41.3X2	T41.3X3	T41.3X4	T41.3X5	T41.3X6
Trimeprazine (tartrate)	T44.3X1	T44.3X2	T44.3X3	T44.3X4	T44.3X5	T44.3X6
Trimetaphan camsilate	T44.2X1	T44.2X2	T44.2X3	T44.2X4	T44.2X5	T44.2X6
Trimetazidine	T46.7X1	T46.7X2	T46.7X3	T46.7X4	T46.7X5	T46.7X6
Trimethadione	T42.2X1	T42.2X2	T42.2X3	T42.2X4	T42.2X5	T42.2X6
Trimethaphan	T44.2X1	T44.2X2	T44.2X3	T44.2X4	T44.2X5	T44.2X6
Trimethidinium	T44.2X1	T44.2X2	T44.2X3	T44.2X4	T44.2X5	T44.2X6
Trimethobenzamide	T45.0X1	T45.0X2	T45.0X3	T45.0X4	T45.0X5	T45.0X6
Trimethoprim	T37.8X1	T37.8X2	T37.8X3	T37.8X4	T37.8X5	T37.8X6
with sulfamethoxazole	T36.8X1	T36.8X2	T36.8X3	T36.8X4	T36.8X5	T36.8X6
Trimethylcarbinol	T51.3X1	T51.3X2	T51.3X3	T51.3X4	—	—
Trimethylpsoralen	T49.3X1	T49.3X2	T49.3X3	T49.3X4	T49.3X5	T49.3X6
Trimeton	T45.0X1	T45.0X2	T45.0X3	T45.0X4	T45.0X5	T45.0X6
Trimetrexate	T45.1X1	T45.1X2	T45.1X3	T45.1X4	T45.1X5	T45.1X6
Trimipramine	T43.011	T43.012	T43.013	T43.014	T43.015	T43.016
Trimustine	T45.1X1	T45.1X2	T45.1X3	T45.1X4	T45.1X5	T45.1X6
Trinitrine	T46.3X1	T46.3X2	T46.3X3	T46.3X4	T46.3X5	T46.3X6
Trinitrobenzol	T65.3X1	T65.3X2	T65.3X3	T65.3X4	—	—
Trinitrophenol	T65.3X1	T65.3X2	T65.3X3	T65.3X4	—	—
Trinitrotoluene (fumes)	T65.3X1	T65.3X2	T65.3X3	T65.3X4	—	—
Trional	T42.6X1	T42.6X2	T42.6X3	T42.6X4	T42.6X5	T42.6X6
Triorthocresyl phosphate	T65.891	T65.892	T65.893	T65.894	—	—
Trioxide of arsenic	T57.0X1	T57.0X2	T57.0X3	T57.0X4		
Trioxysalen	T49.4X1	T49.4X2	T49.4X3	T49.4X4	T49.4X5	T49.4X6
Tripamide	T50.2X1	T50.2X2	T50.2X3	T50.2X4	T50.2X5	T50.2X6
Triparanol	T46.6X1	T46.6X2	T46.6X3	T46.6X4	T46.6X5	T46.6X6
Tripelennamine	T45.0X1	T45.0X2	T45.0X3	T45.0X4	T45.0X5	T45.0X6
Triperiden	T44.3X1	T44.3X2	T44.3X3	T44.3X4	T44.3X5	T44.3X6
Triperidol	T43.4X1	T43.4X2	T43.4X3	T43.4X4	T43.4X5	T43.4X6
Triphenylphosphate	T65.891	T65.892	T65.893	T65.894	—	—
Triple						
bromides	T42.6X1	T42.6X2	T42.6X3	T42.6X4	T42.6X5	T42.6X6
carbonate	T47.1X1	T47.1X2	T47.1X3	T47.1X4	T47.1X5	T47.1X6
vaccine						
DPT	T50.A11	T50.A12	T50.A13	T50.A14	T50.A15	T50.A16
including pertussis	T50.A11	T50.A12	T50.A13	T50.A14	T50.A15	T50.A16
MMR	T50.B91	T50.B92	—	—	—	—
Triprolidine	T45.0X1	T45.0X2	T45.0X3	T45.0X4	T45.0X5	T45.0X6
Trisodium hydrogen edetate	T50.6X1	T50.6X2	T50.6X3	T50.6X4	T50.6X5	T50.6X6

	External Cause (T-Code)					
Substance	Poisoning, Accidental (Unintentional)	Poisoning, Intentional Self-Harm	Poisoning, Assault	Poisoning, Undetermined	Adverse Effect	Underdosing
Trisoralen	T49.3X1	T49.3X2	T49.3X3	T49.3X4	T49.3X5	T49.3X6
Trisulfapyrimidines	T37.0X1	T37.0X2	T37.0X3	T37.0X4	T37.0X5	T37.0X6
Trithiozine	T44.3X1	T44.3X2	T44.3X3	T44.3X4	T44.3X5	T44.3X6
Tritiozine	T44.3X1	T44.3X2	T44.3X3	T44.3X4	T44.3X5	T44.3X6
Tritoqualine	T45.0X1	T45.0X2	T45.0X3	T45.0X4	T45.0X5	T45.0X6
Trofosfamide	T45.1X1	T45.1X2	T45.1X3	T45.1X4	T45.1X5	T45.1X6
Troleandomycin	T36.3X1	T36.3X2	T36.3X3	T36.3X4	T36.3X5	T36.3X6
Trolnitrate (phosphate)	T46.3X1	T46.3X2	T46.3X3	T46.3X4	T46.3X5	T46.3X6
Tromantadine	T37.5X1	T37.5X2	T37.5X3	T37.5X4	T37.5X5	T37.5X6
Trometamol	T50.2X1	T50.2X2	T50.2X3	T50.2X4	T50.2X5	T50.2X6
Tromethamine	T50.2X1	T50.2X2	T50.2X3	T50.2X4	T50.2X5	T50.2X6
Tronothane	T41.3X1	T41.3X2	T41.3X3	T41.3X4	T41.3X5	T41.3X6
Tropacine	T44.3X1	T44.3X2	T44.3X3	T44.3X4	T44.3X5	T44.3X6
Tropatepine	T44.3X1	T44.3X2	T44.3X3	T44.3X4	T44.3X5	T44.3X6
Tropicamide	T44.3X1	T44.3X2	T44.3X3	T44.3X4	T44.3X5	T44.3X6
Trospium chloride	T44.3X1	T44.3X2	T44.3X3	T44.3X4	T44.3X5	T44.3X6
Troxerutin	T46.991	T46.992	T46.993	T46.994	T46.995	T46.996
Troxidone	T42.2X1	T42.2X2	T42.2X3	T42.2X4	T42.2X5	T42.2X6
Tryparsamide	T37.3X1	T37.3X2	T37.3X3	T37.3X4	T37.3X5	T37.3X6
Trypsin	T45.3X1	T45.3X2	T45.3X3	T45.3X4	T45.3X5	T45.3X6
Tryptizol	T43.011	T43.012	T43.013	T43.014	T43.015	T43.016
TSH	T38.811	T38.812	T38.813	T38.814	T38.815	T38.816
Tuaminoheptane	T48.5X1	T48.5X2	T48.5X3	T48.5X4	T48.5X5	T48.5X6
Tuberculin, purified protein derivative (PPD)	T50.8X1	T50.8X2	T50.8X3	T50.8X4	T50.8X5	T50.8X6
Tubocurare	T48.1X1	T48.1X2	T48.1X3	T48.1X4	T48.1X5	T48.1X6
Tubocurarine (chloride)	T48.1X1	T48.1X2	T48.1X3	T48.1X4	T48.1X5	T48.1X6
Tulobuterol	T48.6X1	T48.6X2	T48.6X3	T48.6X4	T48.6X5	T48.6X6
Turpentine (spirits of)	T52.8X1	T52.8X2	T52.8X3	T52.8X4	—	—
vapor	T52.8X1	T52.8X2	T52.8X3	T52.8X4	—	—
Tybamate	T43.591	T43.592	T43.593	T43.594	T43.595	T43.596
Tyloxapol	T48.4X1	T48.4X2	T48.4X3	T48.4X4	T48.4X5	T48.4X6
Tymazoline	T48.5X1	T48.5X2	T48.5X3	T48.5X4	T48.5X5	T48.5X6
Typhoid-paratyphoid vaccine	T50.A91	T50.A92	T50.A93	T50.A94	T50.A95	T50.A96
Typhus vaccine	T50.A91	T50.A92	T50.A93	T50.A94	T50.A95	T50.A96
Tyropanoate	T50.8X1	T50.8X2	T50.8X3	T50.8X4	T50.8X5	T50.8X6
Tyrothricin	T49.6X1	T49.6X2	T49.6X3	T49.6X4	T49.6X5	T49.6X6
ENT agent	T49.6X1	T49.6X2	T49.6X3	T49.6X4	T49.6X5	T49.6X6
ophthalmic preparation	T49.5X1	T49.5X2	T49.5X3	T49.5X4	T49.5X5	T49.5X6
U						
Ufenamate	T39.391	T39.392	T39.393	T39.394	T39.395	T39.396
Ultraviolet light protectant	T49.3X1	T49.3X2	T49.3X3	T49.3X4	T49.3X5	T49.3X6

◀ New ◀▪▪ Revised ~~deleted~~ Deleted

Substance	Poisoning, Accidental (Unintentional)	Poisoning, Intentional Self-Harm	Poisoning, Assault	Poisoning, Undetermined	Adverse Effect	Underdosing
Undecenoic acid	T49.0X1	T49.0X2	T49.0X3	T49.0X4	T49.0X5	T49.0X6
Undecoylium	T49.0X1	T49.0X2	T49.0X3	T49.0X4	T49.0X5	T49.0X6
Undecylenic acid (derivatives)	T49.0X1	T49.0X2	T49.0X3	T49.0X4	T49.0X5	T49.0X6
Unna's boot	T49.3X1	T49.3X2	T49.3X3	T49.3X4	T49.3X5	T49.3X6
Unsaturated fatty acid	T46.6X1	T46.6X2	T46.6X3	T46.6X4	T46.6X5	T46.6X6
Uracil mustard	T45.1X1	T45.1X2	T45.1X3	T45.1X4	T45.1X5	T45.1X6
Uramustine	T45.1X1	T45.1X2	T45.1X3	T45.1X4	T45.1X5	T45.1X6
Urapidil	T46.5X1	T46.5X2	T46.5X3	T46.5X4	T46.5X5	T46.5X6
Urari	T48.1X1	T48.1X2	T48.1X3	T48.1X4	T48.1X5	T48.1X6
Urate oxidase	T50.4X1	T50.4X2	T50.4X3	T50.4X4	T50.4X5	T50.4X6
Urea	T47.3X1	T47.3X2	T47.3X3	T47.3X4	T47.3X5	T47.3X6
peroxide	T49.0X1	T49.0X2	T49.0X3	T49.0X4	T49.0X5	T49.0X6
stibamine	T37.4X1	T37.4X2	T37.4X3	T37.4X4	T37.4X5	T37.4X6
topical	T49.8X1	T49.8X2	T49.8X3	T49.8X4	T49.8X5	T49.8X6
Urethane	T45.1X1	T45.1X2	T45.1X3	T45.1X4	T45.1X5	T45.1X6
Urginea (maritima) (scilla) — see Squill						
Uric acid metabolism drug NEC	T50.4X1	T50.4X2	T50.4X3	T50.4X4	T50.4X5	T50.4X6
Uricosuric agent	T50.4X1	T50.4X2	T50.4X3	T50.4X4	T50.4X5	T50.4X6
Urinary anti-infective	T37.8X1	T37.8X2	T37.8X3	T37.8X4	T37.8X5	T37.8X6
Urofollitropin	T38.811	T38.812	T38.813	T38.814	T38.815	T38.816
Urokinase	T45.611	T45.612	T45.613	T45.614	T45.615	T45.616
Urokon	T50.8X1	T50.8X2	T50.8X3	T50.8X4	T50.8X5	T50.8X6
Ursodeoxycholic acid	T50.991	T50.992	T50.993	T50.994	T50.995	T50.996
Ursodiol	T50.991	T50.992	T50.993	T50.994	T50.995	T50.996
Urtica	T62.2X1	T62.2X2	T62.2X3	T62.2X4	—	—
Utility gas — see Gas, utility						
V						
Vaccine NEC	T50.Z91	T50.Z92	T50.Z93	T50.Z94	T50.Z95	T50.Z96
antineoplastic	T50.Z91	T50.Z92	T50.Z93	T50.Z94	T50.Z95	T50.Z96
bacterial NEC	T50.A91	T50.A92	T50.A93	T50.A94	T50.A95	T50.A96
with						
other bacterial component	T50.A91	T50.A92	T50.A93	T50.A94	T50.A95	T50.A96
pertussis component	T50.A91	T50.A92	T50.A93	T50.A94	T50.A95	T50.A96
viral-rickettsial component	T50.A91	T50.A92	T50.A93	T50.A94	T50.A95	T50.A96
mixed NEC	T50.A91	T50.A92	T50.A93	T50.A94	T50.A95	T50.A96
BCG	T50.A91	T50.A92	T50.A93	T50.A94	T50.A95	T50.A96
cholera	T50.A91	T50.A92	T50.A93	T50.A94	T50.A95	T50.A96
diphtheria	T50.A91	T50.A92	T50.A93	T50.A94	T50.A95	T50.A96
with tetanus	T50.A21	T50.A22	T50.A23	T50.A24	T50.A25	T50.A26
and pertussis	T50.A11	T50.A12	T50.A13	T50.A14	T50.A15	T50.A16

Substance	Poisoning, Accidental (Unintentional)	Poisoning, Intentional Self-Harm	Poisoning, Assault	Poisoning, Undetermined	Adverse Effect	Underdosing
Vaccine NEC *(Continued)*						
influenza	T50.B91	T50.B92	T50.B93	T50.B94	T50.B95	T50.B96
measles	T50.B91	T50.B92	T50.B93	T50.B94	T50.B95	T50.B96
with mumps and rubella	T50.B91	T50.B92	T50.B93	T50.B94	T50.B95	T50.B96
meningococcal	T50.A91	T50.A92	T50.A93	T50.A94	T50.A95	T50.A96
mumps	T50.B91	T50.B92	T50.B93	T50.B94	T50.B95	T50.B96
paratyphoid	T50.A91	T50.A92	T50.A93	T50.A94	T50.A95	T50.A96
pertussis	T50.A11	T50.A12	T50.A13	T50.A14	T50.A15	T50.A16
with diphtheria	T50.A11	T50.A12	T50.A13	T50.A14	T50.A15	T50.A16
and tetanus	T50.A11	T50.A12	T50.A13	T50.A14	T50.A15	T50.A16
plague	T50.A91	T50.A92	T50.A93	T50.A94	T50.A95	T50.A96
poliomyelitis	T50.B91	T50.B92	T50.B93	T50.B94	T50.B95	T50.B96
poliovirus	T50.B91	T50.B92	T50.B93	T50.B94	T50.B95	T50.B96
rabies	T50.B91	T50.B92	T50.B93	T50.B94	T50.B95	T50.B96
respiratory syncytial virus	T50.B91	T50.B92	T50.B93	T50.B94	T50.B95	T50.B96
rickettsial NEC	T50.A91	T50.A92	T50.A93	T50.A94	T50.A95	T50.A96
with						
bacterial component	T50.A21	T50.A22	T50.A23	T50.A24	T50.A25	T50.A26
Rocky Mountain spotted fever	T50.A91	T50.A92	T50.A93	T50.A94	T50.A95	T50.A96
rubella	T50.B91	T50.B92	T50.B93	T50.B94	T50.B95	T50.B96
sabin oral	T50.B91	T50.B92	T50.B93	T50.B94	T50.B95	T50.B96
smallpox	T50.B11	T50.B12	T50.B13	T50.B14	T50.B15	T50.B16
TAB	T50.A91	T50.A92	T50.A93	T50.A94	T50.A95	T50.A96
tetanus	T50.A91	T50.A92	T50.A93	T50.A94	T50.A95	T50.A96
typhoid	T50.A91	T50.A92	T50.A93	T50.A94	T50.A95	T50.A96
typhus	T50.A91	T50.A92	T50.A93	T50.A94	T50.A95	T50.A96
viral NEC	T50.B91	T50.B92	T50.B93	T50.B94	T50.B95	T50.B96
yellow fever	T50.B91	T50.B92	T50.B93	T50.B94	T50.B95	T50.B96
Vaccinia immune globulin	T50.Z11	T50.Z12	T50.Z13	T50.Z14	T50.Z15	T50.Z16
Vaginal contraceptives	T49.8X1	T49.8X2	T49.8X3	T49.8X4	T49.8X5	T49.8X6
Valerian						
root	T42.6X1	T42.6X2	T42.6X3	T42.6X4	T42.6X5	T42.6X6
tincture	T42.6X1	T42.6X2	T42.6X3	T42.6X4	T42.6X5	T42.6X6
Valethamate bromide	T44.3X1	T44.3X2	T44.3X3	T44.3X4	T44.3X5	T44.3X6
Valisone	T49.0X1	T49.0X2	T49.0X3	T49.0X4	T49.0X5	T49.0X6
Valium	T42.4X1	T42.4X2	T42.4X3	T42.4X4	T42.4X5	T42.4X6
Valmid	T42.6X1	T42.6X2	T42.6X3	T42.6X4	T42.6X5	T42.6X6
Valnoctamide	T42.6X1	T42.6X2	T42.6X3	T42.6X4	T42.6X5	T42.6X6
Valproate (sodium)	T42.6X1	T42.6X2	T42.6X3	T42.6X4	T42.6X5	T42.6X6
Valproic acid	T42.6X1	T42.6X2	T42.6X3	T42.6X4	T42.6X5	T42.6X6
Valpromide	T42.6X1	T42.6X2	T42.6X3	T42.6X4	T42.6X5	T42.6X6
Vanadium	T56.891	T56.892	T56.893	T56.894	—	—

◀ New ◀▌▌ Revised ~~deleted~~ Deleted

TABLE OF DRUGS AND CHEMICALS

Substance	Poisoning, Accidental (Unintentional)	Poisoning, Intentional Self-Harm	Poisoning, Assault	Poisoning, Undetermined	Adverse Effect	Underdosing
Vancomycin	T36.8X1	T36.8X2	T36.8X3	T36.8X4	T36.8X5	T36.8X6
Vapor — *see also Gas*	T59.91	T59.92	T59.93	T59.94	—	—
kiln (carbon monoxide)	T58.8X1	T58.8X2	T58.8X3	T58.8X4	—	—
lead — *see lead*						
specified source NEC	T59.891	T59.892	T59.893	T59.894	—	—
Vardenafil	T46.7X1	T46.7X2	T46.7X3	T46.7X4	T46.7X5	T46.7X6
Varicose reduction drug	T46.8X1	T46.8X2	T46.8X3	T46.8X4	T46.8X5	T46.8X6
Varnish	T65.4X1	T65.4X2	T65.4X3	T65.4X4		
cleaner	T52.91	T52.92	T52.93	T52.94	—	—
Vaseline	T49.3X1	T49.3X2	T49.3X3	T49.3X4	T49.3X5	T49.3X6
Vasodilan	T46.7X1	T46.7X2	T46.7X3	T46.7X4	T46.7X5	T46.7X6
Vasodilator						
coronary NEC	T46.3X1	T46.3X2	T46.3X3	T46.3X4	T46.3X5	T46.3X6
peripheral NEC	T46.7X1	T46.7X2	T46.7X3	T46.7X4	T46.7X5	T46.7X6
Vasopressin	T38.891	T38.892	T38.893	T38.894	T38.895	T38.896
Vasopressor drugs	T38.891	T38.892	T38.893	T38.894	T38.895	T38.896
Vecuronium bromide	T48.1X1	T48.1X2	T48.1X3	T48.1X4	T48.1X5	T48.1X6
Vegetable extract, astringent	T49.2X1	T49.2X2	T49.2X3	T49.2X4	T49.2X5	T49.2X6
Venlafaxine	T43.211	T43.212	T43.213	T43.214	T43.215	T43.216
Venom, venomous (bite) (sting)	T63.91	T63.92	T63.93	T63.94	—	—
amphibian NEC	T63.831	T63.832	T63.833	T63.834	—	—
animal NEC	T63.891	T63.892	T63.893	T63.894	—	—
ant	T63.421	T63.422	T63.423	T63.424	—	—
arthropod NEC	T63.481	T63.482	T63.483	T63.484	—	—
bee	T63.441	T63.442	T63.443	T63.444	—	—
centipede	T63.411	T63.412	T63.413	T63.414	—	—
fish	T63.591	T63.592	T63.593	T63.594	—	—
frog	T63.811	T63.812	T63.813	T63.814	—	—
hornet	T63.451	T63.452	T63.453	T63.454	—	—
insect NEC	T63.481	T63.482	T63.483	T63.484	—	—
lizard	T63.121	T63.122	T63.123	T63.124	—	—
marine						
animals	T63.691	T63.692	T63.693	T63.694	—	—
bluebottle	T63.611	T63.612	T63.613	T63.614	—	—
jellyfish NEC	T63.621	T63.622	T63.623	T63.624	—	—
Portugese Man-o-war	T63.611	T63.612	T63.613	T63.614	—	—
sea anemone	T63.631	T63.632	T63.633	T63.634	—	—
specified NEC	T63.691	T63.692	T63.693	T63.694	—	—
fish	T63.591	T63.592	T63.593	T63.594	—	—
plants	T63.711	T63.712	T63.713	T63.714	—	—
sting ray	T63.511	T63.512	T63.513	T63.514	—	—

Substance	Poisoning, Accidental (Unintentional)	Poisoning, Intentional Self-Harm	Poisoning, Assault	Poisoning, Undetermined	Adverse Effect	Underdosing
Venom, venomous *(Continued)*						
millipede (tropical)	T63.411	T63.412	T63.413	T63.414	—	—
plant NEC	T63.791	T63.792	T63.793	T63.794	—	—
marine	T63.711	T63.712	T63.713	T63.714	—	—
reptile	T63.191	T63.192	T63.193	T63.194	—	—
gila monster	T63.111	T63.112	T63.113	T63.114	—	—
lizard NEC	T63.121	T63.122	T63.123	T63.124	—	—
scorpion	T63.2X1	T63.2X2	T63.2X3	T63.2X4	—	—
snake	T63.001	T63.002	T63.003	T63.004	—	—
African NEC	T63.081	T63.082	T63.083	T63.084	—	—
American (North) (South) NEC	T63.061	T63.062	T63.063	T63.064	—	—
Asian	T63.081	T63.082	T63.083	T63.084	—	—
Australian	T63.071	T63.072	T63.073	T63.074	—	—
cobra	T63.041	T63.042	T63.043	T63.044	—	—
coral snake	T63.021	T63.022	T63.023	T63.024	—	—
rattlesnake	T63.011	T63.012	T63.013	T63.014	—	—
specified NEC	T63.091	T63.092	T63.093	T63.094	—	—
taipan	T63.031	T63.032	T63.033	T63.034	—	—
specified NEC	T63.891	T63.892	T63.893	T63.894	—	—
spider	T63.301	T63.302	T63.303	T63.304	—	—
black widow	T63.311	T63.312	T63.313	T63.314	—	—
brown recluse	T63.331	T63.332	T63.333	T63.334	—	—
specified NEC	T63.391	T63.392	T63.393	T63.394	—	—
tarantula	T63.321	T63.322	T63.323	T63.324	—	—
sting ray	T63.511	T63.512	T63.513	T63.514	—	—
toad	T63.821	T63.822	T63.823	T63.824	—	—
wasp	T63.461	T63.462	T63.463	T63.464	—	—
Venous sclerosing drug NEC	T46.8X1	T46.8X2	T46.8X3	T46.8X4	T46.8X5	T46.8X6
Ventolin — *see Albuterol*						
Verapamil	T46.1X1	T46.1X2	T46.1X3	T46.1X4	T46.1X5	T46.1X6
Veramon	T42.3X1	T42.3X2	T42.3X3	T42.3X4	T42.3X5	T42.3X6
Veratrine	T46.5X1	T46.5X2	T46.5X3	T46.5X4	T46.5X5	T46.5X6
Veratrum						
album	T62.2X1	T62.2X2	T62.2X3	T62.2X4	—	—
alkaloids	T46.5X1	T46.5X2	T46.5X3	T46.5X4	T46.5X5	T46.5X6
viride	T62.2X1	T62.2X2	T62.2X3	T62.2X4	—	—
Verdigris	T60.3X1	T60.3X2	T60.3X3	T60.3X4	—	—
Veronal	T42.3X1	T42.3X2	T42.3X3	T42.3X4	T42.3X5	T42.3X6
Veroxil	T37.4X1	T37.4X2	T37.4X3	T37.4X4	T37.4X5	T37.4X6
Versenate	T50.6X1	T50.6X2	T50.6X3	T50.6X4	T50.6X5	T50.6X6

◀ New ◀‖ Revised ~~deleted~~ Deleted

Substance	Poisoning, Accidental (Unintentional)	Poisoning, Intentional Self-Harm	Poisoning, Assault	Poisoning, Undetermined	Adverse Effect	Underdosing
Versidyne	T39.8X1	T39.8X2	T39.8X3	T39.8X4	T39.8X5	T39.8X6
Vetrabutine	T48.0X1	T48.0X2	T48.0X3	T48.0X4	T48.0X5	T48.0X6
Vidarabine	T37.5X1	T37.5X2	T37.5X3	T37.5X4	T37.5X5	T37.5X6
Vienna						
green	T57.0X1	T57.0X2	T57.0X3	T57.0X4	—	—
insecticide	T60.2X1	T60.2X2	T60.2X3	T60.2X4	—	—
red	T57.0X1	T57.0X2	T57.0X3	T57.0X4	—	—
pharmaceutical dye	T50.991	T50.992	T50.993	T50.994	T50.995	T50.996
Vigabatrin	T42.6X1	T42.6X2	T42.6X3	T42.6X4	T42.6X5	T42.6X6
Viloxazine	T43.291	T43.292	T43.293	T43.294	T43.295	T43.296
Viminol	T39.8X1	T39.8X2	T39.8X3	T39.8X4	T39.8X5	T39.8X6
Vinbarbital, vinbarbitone	T42.3X1	T42.3X2	T42.3X3	T42.3X4	T42.3X5	T42.3X6
Vinblastine	T45.1X1	T45.1X2	T45.1X3	T45.1X4	T45.1X5	T45.1X6
Vinburnine	T46.7X1	T46.7X2	T46.7X3	T46.7X4	T46.7X5	T46.7X6
Vincamine	T45.1X1	T45.1X2	T45.1X3	T45.1X4	T45.1X5	T45.1X6
Vincristine	T45.1X1	T45.1X2	T45.1X3	T45.1X4	T45.1X5	T45.1X6
Vindesine	T45.1X1	T45.1X2	T45.1X3	T45.1X4	T45.1X5	T45.1X6
Vinesthene, vinethene	T41.0X1	T41.0X2	T41.0X3	T41.0X4	T41.0X5	T41.0X6
Vinorelbine tartrate	T45.1X1	T45.1X2	T45.1X3	T45.1X4	T45.1X5	T45.1X6
Vinpocetine	T46.7X1	T46.7X2	T46.7X3	T46.7X4	T46.7X5	T46.7X6
Vinyl						
acetate	T65.891	T65.892	T65.893	T65.894	—	—
bital	T42.3X1	T42.3X2	T42.3X3	T42.3X4	T42.3X5	T42.3X6
bromide	T65.891	T65.892	T65.893	T65.894	—	—
chloride	T59.891	T59.892	T59.893	T59.894	—	—
ether	T41.0X1	T41.0X2	T41.0X3	T41.0X4	T41.0X5	T41.0X6
Vinylbital	T42.3X1	T42.3X2	T42.3X3	T42.3X4	T42.3X5	T42.3X6
Vinylidene chloride	T65.891	T65.892	T65.893	T65.894	—	—
Vioform	T37.8X1	T37.8X2	T37.8X3	T37.8X4	T37.8X5	T37.8X6
topical	T49.0X1	T49.0X2	T49.0X3	T49.0X4	T49.0X5	T49.0X6
Viomycin	T36.8X1	T36.8X2	T36.8X3	T36.8X4	T36.8X5	T36.8X6
Viosterol	T45.2X1	T45.2X2	T45.2X3	T45.2X4	T45.2X5	T45.2X6
Viper (venom)	T63.091	T63.092	T63.093	T63.094	—	—
Viprynium	T37.4X1	T37.4X2	T37.4X3	T37.4X4	T37.4X5	T37.4X6
Viquidil	T46.7X1	T46.7X2	T46.7X3	T46.7X4	T46.7X5	T46.7X6
Viral vaccine NEC	T50.B91	T50.B92	T50.B93	T50.B94	T50.B95	T50.B96
Virginiamycin	T36.8X1	T36.8X2	T36.8X3	T36.8X4	T36.8X5	T36.8X6
Virugon	T37.5X1	T37.5X2	T37.5X3	T37.5X4	T37.5X5	T37.5X6
Viscous agent	T50.901	T50.902	T50.903	T50.904	T50.905	T50.906
Visine	T49.5X1	T49.5X2	T49.5X3	T49.5X4	T49.5X5	T49.5X6
Visnadine	T46.3X1	T46.3X2	T46.3X3	T46.3X4	T46.3X5	T46.3X6

Substance	Poisoning, Accidental (Unintentional)	Poisoning, Intentional Self-Harm	Poisoning, Assault	Poisoning, Undetermined	Adverse Effect	Underdosing
Vitamin NEC	T45.2X1	T45.2X2	T45.2X3	T45.2X4	T45.2X5	T45.2X6
A	T45.2X1	T45.2X2	T45.2X3	T45.2X4	T45.2X5	T45.2X6
B NEC	T45.2X1	T45.2X2	T45.2X3	T45.2X4	T45.2X5	T45.2X6
nicotinic acid	T46.7X1	T46.7X2	T46.7X3	T46.7X4	T46.7X5	T46.7X6
B1	T45.2X1	T45.2X2	T45.2X3	T45.2X4	T45.2X5	T45.2X6
B2	T45.2X1	T45.2X2	T45.2X3	T45.2X4	T45.2X5	T45.2X6
B6	T45.2X1	T45.2X2	T45.2X3	T45.2X4	T45.2X5	T45.2X6
B12	T45.2X1	T45.2X2	T45.2X3	T45.2X4	T45.2X5	T45.2X6
B15	T45.2X1	T45.2X2	T45.2X3	T45.2X4	T45.2X5	T45.2X6
C	T45.2X1	T45.2X2	T45.2X3	T45.2X4	T45.2X5	T45.2X6
D	T45.2X1	T45.2X2	T45.2X3	T45.2X4	T45.2X5	T45.2X6
D2	T45.2X1	T45.2X2	T45.2X3	T45.2X4	T45.2X5	T45.2X6
D3	T45.2X1	T45.2X2	T45.2X3	T45.2X4	T45.2X5	T45.2X6
E	T45.2X1	T45.2X2	T45.2X3	T45.2X4	T45.2X5	T45.2X6
E acetate	T45.2X1	T45.2X2	T45.2X3	T45.2X4	T45.2X5	T45.2X6
hematopoietic	T45.8X1	T45.8X2	T45.8X3	T45.8X4	T45.8X5	T45.8X6
K NEC	T45.7X1	T45.7X2	T45.7X3	T45.7X4	T45.7X5	T45.7X6
K1	T45.7X1	T45.7X2	T45.7X3	T45.7X4	T45.7X5	T45.7X6
K2	T45.7X1	T45.7X2	T45.7X3	T45.7X4	T45.7X5	T45.7X6
PP	T45.2X1	T45.2X2	T45.2X3	T45.2X4	T45.2X5	T45.2X6
ulceroprotectant	T47.1X1	T47.1X2	T47.1X3	T47.1X4	T47.1X5	T47.1X6
Vleminckx's solution	T49.4X1	T49.4X2	T49.4X3	T49.4X4	T49.4X5	T49.4X6
Voltaren — see Diclofenac sodium						
W						
Warfarin	T45.511	T45.512	T45.513	T45.514	T45.515	T45.516
rodenticide	T60.4X1	T60.4X2	T60.4X3	T60.4X4	—	—
sodium	T60.4X1	T60.4X2	T60.4X3	T60.4X4	—	—
Wasp (sting)	T63.461	T63.462	T63.463	T63.464	—	—
Water						
balance drug	T50.3X1	T50.3X2	T50.3X3	T50.3X4	T50.3X5	T50.3X6
distilled	T50.3X1	T50.3X2	T50.3X3	T50.3X4	T50.3X5	T50.3X6
gas — see Gas, water						
incomplete combustion of — see Carbon, monoxide, fuel, utility						
hemlock	T62.2X1	T62.2X2	T62.2X3	T62.2X4	—	—
moccasin (venom)	T63.061	T63.062	T63.063	T63.064	—	—
purified	T50.3X1	T50.3X2	T50.3X3	T50.3X4	T50.3X5	T50.3X6
Wax (paraffin) (petroleum)	T52.0X1	T52.0X2	T52.0X3	T52.0X4	—	—
automobile	T65.891	T65.892	T65.893	T65.894	—	—
floor	T52.0X1	T52.0X2	T52.0X3	T52.0X4	—	—

TABLE OF DRUGS AND CHEMICALS

◄ New ◄Ⅲ Revised ~~deleted~~ Deleted

Substance	Poisoning, Accidental (Unintentional)	Poisoning, Intentional Self-Harm	Poisoning, Assault	Poisoning, Undetermined	Adverse Effect	Underdosing
Weed killers NEC	T60.3X1	T60.3X2	T60.3X3	T60.3X4	—	—
Welldorm	T42.6X1	T42.6X2	T42.6X3	T42.6X4	T42.6X5	T42.6X6
White						
arsenic	T57.0X1	T57.0X2	T57.0X3	T57.0X4	—	—
hellebore	T62.2X1	T62.2X2	T62.2X3	T62.2X4	—	—
lotion (keratolytic)	T49.4X1	T49.4X2	T49.4X3	T49.4X4	T49.4X5	T49.4X6
spirit	T52.0X1	T52.0X2	T52.0X3	T52.0X4	—	—
Whitewash	T65.891	T65.892	T65.893	T65.894	—	—
Whole blood (human)	T45.8X1	T45.8X2	T45.8X3	T45.8X4	T45.8X5	T45.8X6
Wild						
black cherry	T62.2X1	T62.2X2	T62.2X3	T62.2X4	—	—
poisonous plants NEC	T62.2X1	T62.2X2	T62.2X3	T62.2X4	—	—
Window cleaning fluid	T65.891	T65.892	T65.893	T65.894	—	—
Wintergreen (oil)	T49.3X1	T49.3X2	T49.3X3	T49.3X4	T49.3X5	T49.3X6
Wisterine	T62.2X1	T62.2X2	T62.2X3	T62.2X4	—	—
Witch hazel	T49.2X1	T49.2X2	T49.2X3	T49.2X4	T49.2X5	T49.2X6
Wood alcohol or spirit	T51.1X1	T51.1X2	T51.1X3	T51.1X4	—	—
Wool fat (hydrous)	T49.3X1	T49.3X2	T49.3X3	T49.3X4	T49.3X5	T49.3X6
Woorali	T48.1X1	T48.1X2	T48.1X3	T48.1X4	T48.1X5	T48.1X6
Wormseed, American	T37.4X1	T37.4X2	T37.4X3	T37.4X4	T37.4X5	T37.4X6
X						
Xamoterol	T44.5X1	T44.5X2	T44.5X3	T44.5X4	T44.5X5	T44.5X6
Xanthine diuretics	T50.2X1	T50.2X2	T50.2X3	T50.2X4	T50.2X5	T50.2X6
Xanthinol nicotinate	T46.7X1	T46.7X2	T46.7X3	T46.7X4	T46.7X5	T46.7X6
Xanthotoxin	T49.3X1	T49.3X2	T49.3X3	T49.3X4	T49.3X5	T49.3X6
Xantinol nicotinate	T46.7X1	T46.7X2	T46.7X3	T46.7X4	T46.7X5	T46.7X6
Xantocillin	T36.0X1	T36.0X2	T36.0X3	T36.0X4	T36.0X5	T36.0X6
Xenon (127Xe) (133Xe)	T50.8X1	T50.8X2	T50.8X3	T50.8X4	T50.8X5	T50.8X6
Xenysalate	T49.4X1	T49.4X2	T49.4X3	T49.4X4	T49.4X5	T49.4X6
Xibornol	T37.8X1	T37.8X2	T37.8X3	T37.8X4	T37.8X5	T37.8X6
Xigris	T45.511	T45.512	T45.513	T45.514	T45.515	T45.516
Xipamide	T50.2X1	T50.2X2	T50.2X3	T50.2X4	T50.2X5	T50.2X6
Xylene (vapor)	T52.2X1	T52.2X2	T52.2X3	T52.2X4	—	—
Xylocaine (infiltration) (topical)	T41.3X1	T41.3X2	T41.3X3	T41.3X4	T41.3X5	T41.3X6
nerve block (peripheral) (plexus)	T41.3X1	T41.3X2	T41.3X3	T41.3X4	T41.3X5	T41.3X6
spinal	T41.3X1	T41.3X2	T41.3X3	T41.3X4	T41.3X5	T41.3X6
Xylol (vapor)	T52.2X1	T52.2X2	T52.2X3	T52.2X4	—	—
Xylometazoline	T48.5X1	T48.5X2	T48.5X3	T48.5X4	T48.5X5	T48.5X6

Substance	Poisoning, Accidental (Unintentional)	Poisoning, Intentional Self-Harm	Poisoning, Assault	Poisoning, Undetermined	Adverse Effect	Underdosing
Y						
Yeast	T45.2X1	T45.2X2	T45.2X3	T45.2X4	T45.2X5	T45.2X6
dried	T45.2X1	T45.2X2	T45.2X3	T45.2X4	T45.2X5	T45.2X6
Yellow						
fever vaccine	T50.B91	T50.B92	T50.B93	T50.B94	T50.B95	T50.B96
jasmine	T62.2X1	T62.2X2	T62.2X3	T62.2X4	—	—
phenolphthalein	T47.2X1	T47.2X2	T47.2X3	T47.2X4	T47.2X5	T47.2X6
Yew	T62.2X1	T62.2X2	T62.2X3	T62.2X4	—	—
Yohimbic acid	T40.991	T40.992	T40.993	T40.994	T40.995	T40.996
Z						
Zactane	T39.8X1	T39.8X2	T39.8X3	T39.8X4	T39.8X5	T39.8X6
Zalcitabine	T37.5X1	T37.5X2	T37.5X3	T37.5X4	T37.5X5	T37.5X6
Zaroxolyn	T50.2X1	T50.2X2	T50.2X3	T50.2X4	T50.2X5	T50.2X6
Zephiran (topical)	T49.0X1	T49.0X2	T49.0X3	T49.0X4	T49.0X5	T49.0X6
ophthalmic preparation	T49.5X1	T49.5X2	T49.5X3	T49.5X4	T49.5X5	T49.5X6
Zeranol	T38.7X1	T38.7X2	T38.7X3	T38.7X4	T38.7X5	T38.7X6
Zerone	T51.1X1	T51.1X2	T51.1X3	T51.1X4	—	—
Zidovudine	T37.5X1	T37.5X2	T37.5X3	T37.5X4	T37.5X5	T37.5X6
Zimeldine	T43.221	T43.222	T43.223	T43.224	T43.225	T43.226
Zinc (compounds) (fumes) (vapor) NEC	T56.5X1	T56.5X2	T56.5X3	T56.5X4	—	—
anti-infectives	T49.0X1	T49.0X2	T49.0X3	T49.0X4	T49.0X5	T49.0X6
antivaricose	T46.8X1	T46.8X2	T46.8X3	T46.8X4	T46.8X5	T46.8X6
bacitracin	T49.0X1	T49.0X2	T49.0X3	T49.0X4	T49.0X5	T49.0X6
chloride (mouthwash)	T49.6X1	T49.6X2	T49.6X3	T49.6X4	T49.6X5	T49.6X6
chromate	T56.5X1	T56.5X2	T56.5X3	T56.5X4	—	—
gelatin	T49.3X1	T49.3X2	T49.3X3	T49.3X4	T49.3X5	T49.3X6
oxide	T49.3X1	T49.3X2	T49.3X3	T49.3X4	T49.3X5	T49.3X6
plaster	T49.3X1	T49.3X2	T49.3X3	T49.3X4	T49.3X5	T49.3X6
peroxide	T49.0X1	T49.0X2	T49.0X3	T49.0X4	T49.0X5	T49.0X6
pesticides	T56.5X1	T56.5X2	T56.5X3	T56.5X4	—	—
phosphide	T60.4X1	T60.4X2	T60.4X3	T60.4X4	—	—
pyrithionate	T49.4X1	T49.4X2	T49.4X3	T49.4X4	T49.4X5	T49.4X6
stearate	T49.3X1	T49.3X2	T49.3X3	T49.3X4	T49.3X5	T49.3X6
sulfate	T49.5X1	T49.5X2	T49.5X3	T49.5X4	T49.5X5	T49.5X6
ENT agent	T49.6X1	T49.6X2	T49.6X3	T49.6X4	T49.6X5	T49.6X6
ophthalmic solution	T49.5X1	T49.5X2	T49.5X3	T49.5X4	T49.5X5	T49.5X6
topical NEC	T49.0X1	T49.0X2	T49.0X3	T49.0X4	T49.0X5	T49.0X6
undecylenate	T49.0X1	T49.0X2	T49.0X3	T49.0X4	T49.0X5	T49.0X6

◄ New ◄▦ Revised ~~deleted~~ Deleted

Substance	External Cause (T-Code)					
	Poisoning, Accidental (Unintentional)	Poisoning, Intentional Self-Harm	Poisoning, Assault	Poisoning, Undetermined	Adverse Effect	Underdosing
Zineb	T60.0X1	T60.0X2	T60.0X3	T60.0X4	—	—
Zinostatin	T45.1X1	T45.1X2	T45.1X3	T45.1X4	T45.1X5	T45.1X6
Zipeprol	T48.3X1	T48.3X2	T48.3X3	T48.3X4	T48.3X5	T48.3X6
Zofenopril	T46.4X1	T46.4X2	T46.4X3	T46.4X4	T46.4X5	T46.4X6
Zolpidem	T42.6X1	T42.6X2	T42.6X3	T42.6X4	T42.6X5	T42.6X6
Zomepirac	T39.391	T39.392	T39.393	T39.394	T39.395	T39.396
Zopiclone	T42.6X1	T42.6X2	T42.6X3	T42.6X4	T42.6X5	T42.6X6

Substance	External Cause (T-Code)					
	Poisoning, Accidental (Unintentional)	Poisoning, Intentional Self-Harm	Poisoning, Assault	Poisoning, Undetermined	Adverse Effect	Underdosing
Zorubicin	T45.1X1	T45.1X2	T45.1X3	T45.1X4	T45.1X5	T45.1X6
Zotepine	T43.591	T43.592	T43.593	T43.594	T43.595	T43.596
Zovant	T45.511	T45.512	T45.513	T45.514	T45.515	T45.516
Zoxazolamine	T42.8X1	T42.8X2	T42.8X3	T42.8X4	T42.8X5	T42.8X6
Zuclopenthixol	T43.4X1	T43.4X2	T43.4X3	T43.4X4	T43.4X5	T43.4X6
Zygadenus (venenosus)	T62.2X1	T62.2X2	T62.2X3	T62.2X4	—	—
Zyprexa	T43.591	T43.592	T43.593	T43.594	T43.595	T43.596

◀ New ◀▥ Revised ~~deleted~~ Deleted

TABLE OF DRUGS AND CHEMICALS

External Cause
of Injuries Index

A

Abandonment (causing exposure to weather conditions) (with intent to injure or kill) NEC X58

Abuse (adult) (child) (mental) (physical) (sexual) X58

Accident (to) X58
aircraft (in transit) (powered) —see also Accident, transport, aircraft
due to, caused by cataclysm —see Forces of nature, by type
animal-drawn vehicle —see Accident, transport, animal-drawn vehicle occupant
animal-rider —see Accident, transport, animal-rider
automobile —see Accident, transport, car occupant
bare foot water skiier V94.4
boat, boating —see also Accident, watercraft
striking swimmer
powered V94.11
unpowered V94.12
bus —see Accident, transport, bus occupant
cable car, not on rails V98.0
on rails —see Accident, transport, streetcar occupant
car —see Accident, transport, car occupant
caused by, due to
animal NEC W64
chain hoist W24.0
cold (excessive) —see Exposure, cold
corrosive liquid, substance —see Table of Drugs and Chemicals ◀▥
cutting or piercing instrument —see Contact, with, by type of instrument
drive belt W24.0
electric
current —see Exposure, electric current
motor —see also Contact, with, by type of machine W31.3
current (of) W86.8
environmental factor NEC X58
explosive material —see Explosion
fire, flames —see Exposure, fire
firearm missile —see Discharge, firearm by type
heat (excessive) —see Heat
hot —see Contact, with, hot
ignition —see Ignition
lifting device W24.0
lightning —see subcategory T75.0
causing fire —see Exposure, fire
machine, machinery —see Contact, with, by type of machine
natural factor NEC X58
pulley (block) W24.0
radiation —see Radiation
steam X13.1
inhalation X13.0
pipe X16
thunderbolt —see subcategory T75.0
causing fire —see Exposure, fire
transmission device W24.1
coach —see Accident, transport, bus occupant
coal car —see Accident, transport, industrial vehicle occupant
diving —see also Fall, into, water
with
drowning or submersion —see Drowning
forklift —see Accident, transport, industrial vehicle occupant
heavy transport vehicle NOS —see Accident, transport, truck occupant
ice yacht V98.2

Accident (Continued)
in
medical, surgical procedure
as, or due to misadventure —see Misadventure
causing an abnormal reaction or later complication without mention of misadventure —see also Complication of or following, by type of procedure Y84.9
land yacht V98.1
late effect of —see W00-X58 with 7th character S
logging car —see Accident, transport, industrial vehicle occupant
machine, machinery —see also Contact, with, by type of machine
on board watercraft V93.69
explosion —see Explosion, in, watercraft
fire —see Burn, on board watercraft
powered craft V93.63
ferry boat V93.61
fishing boat V93.62
jetskis V93.63
liner V93.61
merchant ship V93.60
passenger ship V93.61
sailboat V93.64
mine tram —see Accident, transport, industrial vehicle occupant
mobility scooter (motorized) —see Accident, transport, pedestrian, conveyance, specified type NEC
motor scooter —see Accident, transport, motorcyclist
motor vehicle NOS (traffic) —see also Accident, transport V89.2
nontraffic V89.0
three-wheeled NOS —see Accident, transport, three-wheeled motor vehicle occupant
motorcycle NOS —see Accident, transport, motorcyclist
nonmotor vehicle NOS (nontraffic) —see also Accident, transport V89.1
traffic NOS V89.3
nontraffic (victim's mode of transport NOS) V88.9
collision (between) V88.7
bus and truck V88.5
car and:
bus V88.3
pickup V88.2
three-wheeled motor vehicle V88.0
train V88.6
truck V88.4
two-wheeled motor vehicle V88.0
van V88.2
specified vehicle NEC and:
three-wheeled motor vehicle V88.1
two-wheeled motor vehicle V88.1
known mode of transport —see Accident, transport, by type of vehicle
noncollision V88.8
on board watercraft V93.89
powered craft V93.83
ferry boat V93.81
fishing boat V93.82
jetskis V93.83
liner V93.81
merchant ship V93.80
passenger ship V93.81
unpowered craft V93.88
canoe V93.85
inflatable V93.86
in tow
recreational V94.31
specified NEC V94.32
kayak V93.85

Accident (Continued)
on board watercraft (Continued)
unpowered craft (Continued)
sailboat V93.84
surf-board V93.88
water skis V93.87
windsurfer V93.88
parachutist V97.29
entangled in object V97.21
injured on landing V97.22
pedal cycle —see Accident, transport, pedal cyclist
pedestrian (on foot)
with
another pedestrian W51
with fall W03
due to ice or snow W00.0
on pedestrian conveyance NEC V00.09
roller skater (in-line) V00.01
skate boarder V00.02
transport vehicle —see Accident, transport
on pedestrian conveyance —see Accident, transport, pedestrian, conveyance
pick-up truck or van —see Accident, transport, pickup truck occupant
quarry truck —see Accident, transport, industrial vehicle occupant
railway vehicle (any) (in motion) —see Accident, transport, railway vehicle occupant
due to cataclysm —see Forces of nature, by type
scooter (non-motorized) —see Accident, transport, pedestrian, conveyance, scooter
sequelae of —see W00-X58 with 7th character S
skateboard —see Accident, transport, pedestrian, conveyance, skateboard
ski (ing) —see Accident, transport, pedestrian, conveyance
lift V98.3
specified cause NEC X58
streetcar —see Accident, transport, streetcar occupant
traffic (victim's mode of transport NOS) V87.9
collision (between) V87.7
bus and truck V87.5
car and:
bus V87.3
pickup V87.2
three-wheeled motor vehicle V87.0
train V87.6
truck V87.4
two-wheeled motor vehicle V87.0
van V87.2
specified vehicle NEC and:
three-wheeled motor vehicle V87.1
two-wheeled motor vehicle V87.1
known mode of transport —see Accident, transport, by type of vehicle
noncollision V87.8
transport (involving injury to) V99
18 wheeler —see Accident, transport, truck occupant
agricultural vehicle occupant (nontraffic) V84.9
driver V84.5
hanger-on V84.7
passenger V84.6
traffic V84.3
driver V84.0
hanger-on V84.2
passenger V84.1
while boarding or alighting V84.4

Accident *(Continued)*
  transport *(Continued)*
    bus occupant *(Continued)*
      driver *(Continued)*
        collision *(Continued)*
          motor vehicle NOS (traffic) V79.40
            nontraffic V79.00
            specified type NEC (traffic)
              V79.49
              nontraffic V79.09
          pedal cycle (traffic) V71.5
            nontraffic V71.0
          pickup truck (traffic) V73.5
            nontraffic V73.0
          railway vehicle (traffic) V75.5
            nontraffic V75.0
          specified vehicle NEC (traffic)
            V76.5
            nontraffic V76.0
          stationary object (traffic) V77.5
            nontraffic V77.0
          streetcar (traffic) V76.5
            nontraffic V76.0
          three wheeled motor vehicle
            (traffic) V72.5
            nontraffic V72.0
          truck (traffic) V74.5
            nontraffic V74.0
          two wheeled motor vehicle (traffic)
            V72.5
            nontraffic V72.0
          van (traffic) V73.5
            nontraffic V73.0
        noncollision accident (traffic) V78.5
          nontraffic V78.0
      hanger-on
        collision (with)
          animal (traffic) V70.7
            being ridden (traffic) V76.7
              nontraffic V76.2
            nontraffic V70.2
          animal-drawn vehicle (traffic) V76.7
            nontraffic V76.2
          bus (traffic) V74.7
            nontraffic V74.2
          car (traffic) V73.7
            nontraffic V73.2
          pedal cycle (traffic) V71.7
            nontraffic V71.2
          pickup truck (traffic) V73.7
            nontraffic V73.2
          railway vehicle (traffic) V75.7
            nontraffic V75.2
          specified vehicle NEC (traffic) V76.7
            nontraffic V76.2
          stationary object (traffic) V77.7
            nontraffic V77.2
          streetcar (traffic) V76.7
            nontraffic V76.2
          three wheeled motor vehicle
            (traffic) V72.7
            nontraffic V72.2
          truck (traffic) V74.7
            nontraffic V74.2
          two wheeled motor vehicle (traffic)
            V72.7
            nontraffic V72.2
          van (traffic) V73.7
            nontraffic V73.2
        noncollision accident (traffic) V78.7
          nontraffic V78.2
      noncollision accident (traffic) V78.9
        nontraffic V78.3
        while boarding or alighting V78.4
      nontraffic V79.3
      passenger
        collision (with)
          animal (traffic) V70.6
            being ridden (traffic) V76.6
              nontraffic V76.1
            nontraffic V70.1

Accident *(Continued)*
  transport *(Continued)*
    bus occupant *(Continued)*
      passenger *(Continued)*
        collision *(Continued)*
          animal-drawn vehicle (traffic) V76.6
            nontraffic V76.1
          bus (traffic) V74.6
            nontraffic V74.1
          car (traffic) V73.6
            nontraffic V73.1
          motor vehicle NOS (traffic) V79.50
            nontraffic V79.10
            specified type NEC (traffic)
              V79.59
              nontraffic V79.19
          pedal cycle (traffic) V71.6
            nontraffic V71.1
          pickup truck (traffic) V73.6
            nontraffic V73.1
          railway vehicle (traffic) V75.6
            nontraffic V75.1
          specified vehicle NEC (traffic) V76.6
            nontraffic V76.1
          stationary object (traffic) V77.6
            nontraffic V77.1
          streetcar (traffic) V76.6
            nontraffic V76.1
          three wheeled motor vehicle
            (traffic) V72.6
            nontraffic V72.1
          truck (traffic) V74.6
            nontraffic V74.1
          two wheeled motor vehicle (traffic)
            V72.6
            nontraffic V72.1
          van (traffic) V73.6
            nontraffic V73.1
        noncollision accident (traffic) V78.6
          nontraffic V78.1
      specified type NEC V79.88
      military vehicle V79.81
  cable car, not on rails V98.0
    on rails —*see* Accident, transport,
      streetcar occupant
  car occupant V49.9
    ambulance occupant —*see* Accident,
      transport, ambulance occupant
    collision (with)
      animal (traffic) V40.9
        being ridden (traffic) V46.9
          nontraffic V46.3
          while boarding or alighting
            V46.4
        nontraffic V40.3
        while boarding or alighting V40.4
      animal-drawn vehicle (traffic) V46.9
        nontraffic V46.3
        while boarding or alighting V46.4
      bus (traffic) V44.9
        nontraffic V44.3
        while boarding or alighting V44.4
      car (traffic) V43.92
        nontraffic V43.32
        while boarding or alighting V43.42
      motor vehicle NOS (traffic) V49.60
        nontraffic V49.20
        specified type NEC (traffic) V49.69
          nontraffic V49.29
      pedal cycle (traffic) V41.9
        nontraffic V41.3
        while boarding or alighting V41.4
      pickup truck (traffic) V43.93
        nontraffic V43.33
        while boarding or alighting V43.43
      railway vehicle (traffic) V45.9
        nontraffic V45.3
        while boarding or alighting V45.4
      specified vehicle NEC (traffic) V46.9
        nontraffic V46.3
        while boarding or alighting V46.4

Accident *(Continued)*
  transport *(Continued)*
    car occupant *(Continued)*
      collision *(Continued)*
        sport utility vehicle (traffic) V43.91
          nontraffic V43.31
          while boarding or alighting V43.41
        stationary object (traffic) V47.92
          nontraffic V47.32
          while boarding or alighting V47.4
        streetcar (traffic) V46.9
          nontraffic V46.3
          while boarding or alighting V46.4
        three wheeled motor vehicle (traffic)
          V42.9
          nontraffic V42.3
          while boarding or alighting V42.4
        truck (traffic) V44.9
          nontraffic V44.3
          while boarding or alighting V44.4
        two wheeled motor vehicle (traffic)
          V42.9
          nontraffic V42.3
          while boarding or alighting V42.4
        van (traffic) V43.94
          nontraffic V43.34
          while boarding or alighting V43.44
      driver
        collision (with)
          animal (traffic) V40.5
            being ridden (traffic) V46.5
              nontraffic V46.0
            nontraffic V40.0
          animal-drawn vehicle (traffic) V46.5
            nontraffic V46.0
          bus (traffic) V44.5
            nontraffic V44.0
          car (traffic) V43.52
            nontraffic V43.02
          motor vehicle NOS (traffic) V49.40
            nontraffic V49.00
            specified type NEC (traffic)
              V49.49
              nontraffic V49.09
          pedal cycle (traffic) V41.5
            nontraffic V41.0
          pickup truck (traffic) V43.53
            nontraffic V43.03
          railway vehicle (traffic) V45.5
            nontraffic V45.0
          specified vehicle NEC (traffic) V46.5
            nontraffic V46.0
          sport utility vehicle (traffic) V43.51
            nontraffic V43.01
          stationary object (traffic) V47.52
            nontraffic V47.02
          streetcar (traffic) V46.5
            nontraffic V46.0
          three wheeled motor vehicle
            (traffic) V42.5
            nontraffic V42.0
          truck (traffic) V44.5
            nontraffic V44.0
          two wheeled motor vehicle (traffic)
            V42.5
            nontraffic V42.0
          van (traffic) V43.54
            nontraffic V43.04
        noncollision accident (traffic) V48.5
          nontraffic V48.0
      hanger-on
        collision (with)
          animal (traffic) V40.7
            being ridden (traffic) V46.7
              nontraffic V46.2
            nontraffic V40.2
          animal-drawn vehicle (traffic)
            V46.7
            nontraffic V46.2
          bus (traffic) V44.7
            nontraffic V44.2

Accident (Continued)
  transport (Continued)
    car occupant (Continued)
      hanger-on (Continued)
        collision (Continued)
          car (traffic) V43.72
            nontraffic V43.22
          pedal cycle (traffic) V41.7
            nontraffic V41.2
          pickup truck (traffic) V43.73
            nontraffic V43.23
          railway vehicle (traffic) V45.7
            nontraffic V45.2
          specified vehicle NEC (traffic) V46.7
            nontraffic V46.2
          sport utility vehicle (traffic) V43.71
            nontraffic V43.21
          stationary object (traffic) V47.7
            nontraffic V47.2
          streetcar (traffic) V46.7
            nontraffic V46.2
          three wheeled motor vehicle
            (traffic) V42.7
            nontraffic V42.2
          truck (traffic) V44.7
            nontraffic V44.2
          two wheeled motor vehicle (traffic)
            V42.7
            nontraffic V42.2
          van (traffic) V43.74
            nontraffic V43.24
        noncollision accident (traffic) V48.7
          nontraffic V48.2
      noncollision accident (traffic) V48.9
        nontraffic V48.3
        while boarding or alighting V48.4
      nontraffic V49.3
      passenger
        collision (with)
          animal (traffic) V40.6
            being ridden (traffic) V46.6
              nontraffic V46.1
            nontraffic V40.1
          animal-drawn vehicle (traffic) V46.6
            nontraffic V46.1
          bus (traffic) V44.6
            nontraffic V44.1
          car (traffic) V43.62
            nontraffic V43.12
          motor vehicle NOS (traffic) V49.50
            nontraffic V49.10
            specified type NEC (traffic) V49.59
              nontraffic V49.19
          pedal cycle (traffic) V41.6
            nontraffic V41.1
          pickup truck (traffic) V43.63
            nontraffic V43.13
          railway vehicle (traffic) V45.6
            nontraffic V45.1
          specified vehicle NEC (traffic) V46.6
            nontraffic V46.1
          sport utility vehicle (traffic) V43.61
            nontraffic V43.11
          stationary object (traffic) V47.62
            nontraffic V47.12
          streetcar (traffic) V46.6
            nontraffic V46.1
          three wheeled motor vehicle
            (traffic) V42.6
            nontraffic V42.1
          truck (traffic) V44.6
            nontraffic V44.1
          two wheeled motor vehicle (traffic)
            V42.6
            nontraffic V42.1
          van (traffic) V43.64
            nontraffic V43.14
        noncollision accident (traffic) V48.6
          nontraffic V48.1
      specified type NEC V49.88
      military vehicle V49.81

Accident (Continued)
  transport (Continued)
    coal car —see Accident, transport,
      industrial vehicle occupant
    construction vehicle occupant (nontraffic)
      V85.9
      driver V85.5
      hanger-on V85.7
      passenger V85.6
      traffic V85.3
        driver V85.0
        hanger-on V85.2
        passenger V85.1
      while boarding or alighting V85.4
    dirt bike rider —see Accident, transport,
      all-terrain vehicle occupant
    due to cataclysm —see Forces of nature,
      by type
    dune buggy occupant (nontraffic) V86.93
      driver V86.53
      hanger-on V86.73
      passenger V86.63
      traffic V86.33
        driver V86.03
        hanger-on V86.23
        passenger V86.13
      while boarding or alighting V86.43
    forklift —see Accident, transport, industrial
      vehicle occupant
    go cart —see Accident, transport, all-terrain
      vehicle occupant
    golf cart —see Accident, transport, all-
      terrain vehicle occupant
    heavy transport vehicle occupant —see
      Accident, transport, truck occupant
    ice yacht V98.2
    industrial vehicle occupant (nontraffic)
      V83.9
      driver V83.5
      hanger-on V83.7
      passenger V83.6
      traffic V83.3
        driver V83.0
        hanger-on V83.2
        passenger V83.1
      while boarding or alighting V83.4
    interurban electric car —see Accident,
      transport, streetcar
    land yacht V98.1
    logging car —see Accident, transport,
      industrial vehicle occupant
    military vehicle occupant (traffic) V86.34
      driver V86.04
      hanger-on V86.24
      nontraffic V86.94
        driver V86.54
        hanger-on V86.74
        passenger V86.64
      passenger V86.14
      while boarding or alighting V86.44
    mine tram —see Accident, transport,
      industrial vehicle occupant
    motor vehicle NEC occupant (traffic)
      V89.2 ◀▥
      ~~driver V86.09~~
      ~~hanger-on V86.29~~
      ~~nontraffic V86.99~~
        ~~driver V86.59~~
        ~~hanger-on V86.79~~
        ~~passenger V86.69~~
      ~~passenger V86.19~~
      ~~while boarding or alighting V86.49~~
    motorcoach —see Accident, transport, bus
      occupant
    motorcyclist V29.9
      collision (with)
        animal (traffic) V20.9
          being ridden (traffic) V26.9
            nontraffic V26.2
            while boarding or alighting V26.3
          nontraffic V20.2
          while boarding or alighting V20.3

Accident (Continued)
  transport (Continued)
    motorcyclist (Continued)
      collision (Continued)
        animal-drawn vehicle (traffic) V26.9
          nontraffic V26.2
          while boarding or alighting V26.3
        bus (traffic) V24.9
          nontraffic V24.2
          while boarding or alighting V24.3
        car (traffic) V23.9
          nontraffic V23.2
          while boarding or alighting V23.3
        motor vehicle NOS (traffic) V29.60
          nontraffic V29.20
          specified type NEC (traffic) V29.69
            nontraffic V29.29
        pedal cycle (traffic) V21.9
          nontraffic V21.2
          while boarding or alighting V21.3
        pickup truck (traffic) V23.9
          nontraffic V23.2
          while boarding or alighting V23.3
        railway vehicle (traffic) V25.9
          nontraffic V25.2
          while boarding or alighting V25.3
        specified vehicle NEC (traffic) V26.9
          nontraffic V26.2
          while boarding or alighting V26.3
        stationary object (traffic) V27.9
          nontraffic V27.2
          while boarding or alighting V27.3
        streetcar (traffic) V26.9
          nontraffic V26.2
          while boarding or alighting V26.3
        three wheeled motor vehicle (traffic)
          V22.9
          nontraffic V22.2
          while boarding or alighting V22.3
        truck (traffic) V24.9
          nontraffic V24.2
          while boarding or alighting V24.3
        two wheeled motor vehicle (traffic)
          V22.9
          nontraffic V22.2
          while boarding or alighting V22.3
        van (traffic) V23.9
          nontraffic V23.2
          while boarding or alighting V23.3
      driver
        collision (with)
          animal (traffic) V20.4
            being ridden (traffic) V26.4
              nontraffic V26.0
            nontraffic V20.0
          animal-drawn vehicle (traffic) V26.4
            nontraffic V26.0
          bus (traffic) V24.4
            nontraffic V24.0
          car (traffic) V23.4
            nontraffic V23.0
          motor vehicle NOS (traffic) V29.40
            nontraffic V29.00
            specified type NEC (traffic)
              V29.49
              nontraffic V29.09
          pedal cycle (traffic) V21.4
            nontraffic V21.0
          pickup truck (traffic) V23.4
            nontraffic V23.0
          railway vehicle (traffic) V25.4
            nontraffic V25.0
          specified vehicle NEC (traffic) V26.4
            nontraffic V26.0
          stationary object (traffic) V27.4
            nontraffic V27.0
          streetcar (traffic) V26.4
            nontraffic V26.0
          three wheeled motor vehicle
            (traffic) V22.4
            nontraffic V22.0

Accident *(Continued)*
　transport *(Continued)*
　　motorcyclist *(Continued)*
　　　driver *(Continued)*
　　　　collision *(Continued)*
　　　　　truck (traffic) V24.4
　　　　　　nontraffic V24.0
　　　　　two wheeled motor vehicle (traffic)
　　　　　　V22.4
　　　　　　nontraffic V22.0
　　　　　van (traffic) V23.4
　　　　　　nontraffic V23.0
　　　　noncollision accident (traffic) V28.4
　　　　　nontraffic V28.0
　　　　noncollision accident (traffic) V28.9
　　　　　nontraffic V28.2
　　　　while boarding or alighting V28.3
　　　　nontraffic V29.3
　　　passenger
　　　　collision (with)
　　　　　animal (traffic) V20.5
　　　　　　being ridden (traffic) V26.5
　　　　　　　nontraffic V26.1
　　　　　　nontraffic V20.1
　　　　　animal-drawn vehicle (traffic)
　　　　　　V26.5
　　　　　　nontraffic V26.1
　　　　　bus (traffic) V24.5
　　　　　　nontraffic V24.1
　　　　　car (traffic) V23.5
　　　　　　nontraffic V23.1
　　　　　motor vehicle NOS (traffic) V29.50
　　　　　　nontraffic V29.10
　　　　　　specified type NEC (traffic)
　　　　　　　V29.59
　　　　　　　nontraffic V29.19
　　　　　pedal cycle (traffic) V21.5
　　　　　　nontraffic V21.1
　　　　　pickup truck (traffic) V23.5
　　　　　　nontraffic V23.1
　　　　　railway vehicle (traffic) V25.5
　　　　　　nontraffic V25.1
　　　　　specified vehicle NEC (traffic)
　　　　　　V26.5
　　　　　　nontraffic V26.1
　　　　　stationary object (traffic) V27.5
　　　　　　nontraffic V27.1
　　　　　streetcar (traffic) V26.5
　　　　　　nontraffic V26.1
　　　　　three wheeled motor vehicle
　　　　　　(traffic) V22.5
　　　　　　nontraffic V22.1
　　　　　truck (traffic) V24.5
　　　　　　nontraffic V24.1
　　　　　two wheeled motor vehicle (traffic)
　　　　　　V22.5
　　　　　　nontraffic V22.1
　　　　　van (traffic) V23.5
　　　　　　nontraffic V23.1
　　　　noncollision accident (traffic) V28.5
　　　　　nontraffic V28.1
　　　specified type NEC V29.88
　　　military vehicle V29.81
　　occupant (of)
　　　aircraft (powered) V95.9
　　　　fixed wing
　　　　　commercial —*see* Accident,
　　　　　　transport, aircraft, occupant,
　　　　　　powered, fixed wing,
　　　　　　commercial
　　　　　private —*see* Accident, transport,
　　　　　　aircraft, occupant, powered,
　　　　　　fixed wing, private
　　　　nonpowered V96.9
　　　　specified NEC V95.8
　　　airport battery-powered vehicle —*see*
　　　　Accident, transport, industrial
　　　　vehicle occupant
　　　all-terrain vehicle (ATV) —*see* Accident,
　　　　transport, all-terrain vehicle
　　　　occupant

Accident *(Continued)*
　transport *(Continued)*
　　occupant *(Continued)*
　　　animal-drawn vehicle —*see* Accident,
　　　　transport, animal-drawn vehicle
　　　　occupant
　　　automobile —*see* Accident, transport, car
　　　　occupant
　　　balloon V96.00
　　　battery-powered vehicle —*see* Accident,
　　　　transport, industrial vehicle
　　　　occupant
　　　bicycle —*see* Accident, transport, pedal
　　　　cyclist
　　　　motorized —*see* Accident, transport,
　　　　　motorcycle rider
　　　boat NEC —*see* Accident, transport, watercraft
　　　bulldozer —*see* Accident, transport,
　　　　construction vehicle occupant
　　　bus —*see* Accident, transport, bus
　　　　occupant
　　　cable car (on rails) —*see also* Accident,
　　　　transport, streetcar occupant
　　　　not on rails V98.0
　　　car —*see also* Accident, transport, car
　　　　occupant
　　　　cable (on rails) —*see also* Accident,
　　　　　transport, streetcar occupant
　　　　not on rails V98.0
　　　coach —*see* Accident, transport, bus
　　　　occupant
　　　coal-car —*see* Accident, transport,
　　　　industrial vehicle occupant
　　　digger —*see* Accident, transport,
　　　　construction vehicle occupant
　　　dump truck —*see* Accident, transport,
　　　　construction vehicle occupant
　　　earth-leveler —*see* Accident, transport,
　　　　construction vehicle occupant
　　　farm machinery (self-propelled) —*see*
　　　　Accident, transport, agricultural
　　　　vehicle occupant
　　　forklift —*see* Accident, transport,
　　　　industrial vehicle occupant
　　　glider (unpowered) V96.20
　　　　hang V96.10
　　　　powered (microlight) (ultralight) —*see*
　　　　　Accident, transport, aircraft,
　　　　　occupant, powered, glider
　　　glider (unpowered) NEC V96.20
　　　hang-glider V96.10
　　　harvester —*see* Accident, transport,
　　　　agricultural vehicle occupant
　　　heavy (transport) vehicle —*see* Accident,
　　　　transport, truck occupant
　　　helicopter —*see* Accident, transport,
　　　　aircraft, occupant, helicopter
　　　ice-yacht V98.2
　　　kite (carrying person) V96.8
　　　land-yacht V98.1
　　　logging car —*see* Accident, transport,
　　　　industrial vehicle occupant
　　　mechanical shovel —*see* Accident,
　　　　transport, construction vehicle
　　　　occupant
　　　microlight —*see* Accident, transport,
　　　　aircraft, occupant, powered, glider
　　　minibus —*see* Accident, transport,
　　　　pickup truck occupant ◄░░░
　　　minivan —*see* Accident, transport,
　　　　pickup truck occupant ◄░░░
　　　moped —*see* Accident, transport,
　　　　motorcycle
　　　motor scooter —*see* Accident, transport,
　　　　motorcycle
　　　motorcycle (with sidecar) —*see* Accident,
　　　　transport, motorcycle
　　　pedal cycle —*see also* Accident,
　　　　transport, pedal cyclist
　　　pick-up (truck) —*see* Accident, transport,
　　　　pickup truck occupant

Accident *(Continued)*
　transport *(Continued)*
　　occupant *(Continued)*
　　　railway (train) (vehicle) (subterranean)
　　　　(elevated) —*see* Accident, transport,
　　　　railway vehicle occupant
　　　rickshaw —*see* Accident, transport,
　　　　pedal cycle
　　　　pedal driven —*see* Accident, transport,
　　　　　pedal cyclist
　　　road-roller —*see* Accident, transport,
　　　　construction vehicle occupant
　　　ship NOS V94.9
　　　ski-lift (chair) (gondola) V98.3
　　　snowmobile —*see* Accident, transport,
　　　　snowmobile occupant
　　　spacecraft, spaceship —*see* Accident,
　　　　transport, aircraft, occupant,
　　　　spacecraft
　　　sport utility vehicle —*see* Accident,
　　　　transport, pickup truck occupant ◄░░░
　　　streetcar (interurban) (operating on
　　　　public street or highway) —*see*
　　　　Accident, transport, streetcar
　　　　occupant
　　　SUV —*see* Accident, transport, pickup
　　　　truck occupant ◄░░░
　　　téléférique V98.0
　　　three-wheeled vehicle (motorized) —*see
　　　　also* Accident, transport, three-
　　　　wheeled motor vehicle occupant
　　　　nonmotorized —*see* Accident,
　　　　　transport, pedal cycle
　　　tractor (farm) (and trailer) —*see*
　　　　Accident, transport, agricultural
　　　　vehicle occupant
　　　train —*see* Accident, transport, railway
　　　　vehicle occupant
　　　tram —*see* Accident, transport, streetcar
　　　　occupant
　　　　in mine or quarry —*see* Accident,
　　　　　transport, industrial vehicle
　　　　　occupant
　　　tricycle —*see* Accident, transport, pedal
　　　　cycle
　　　　motorized —*see* Accident, transport,
　　　　　three-wheeled motor vehicle
　　　trolley —*see* Accident, transport,
　　　　streetcar occupant
　　　　in mine or quarry —*see* Accident,
　　　　　transport, industrial vehicle
　　　　　occupant
　　　tub, in mine or quarry —*see* Accident,
　　　　transport, industrial vehicle
　　　　occupant
　　　ultralight —*see* Accident, transport,
　　　　aircraft, occupant, powered, glider
　　　van —*see* Accident, transport, van
　　　　occupant
　　　vehicle NEC V89.9
　　　　heavy transport —*see* Accident,
　　　　　transport, truck occupant
　　　　motor (traffic) NEC V89.2
　　　　　nontraffic NEC V89.0
　　　watercraft NOS V94.9
　　　　causing drowning —*see* Drowning,
　　　　　resulting from accident to boat ◄
　　parachutist V97.29
　　　after accident to aircraft —*see* Accident,
　　　　transport, aircraft
　　　entangled in object V97.21
　　　injured on landing V97.22
　　pedal cyclist V19.9
　　　collision (with)
　　　　animal (traffic) V10.9
　　　　　being ridden (traffic) V16.9
　　　　　　nontraffic V16.2
　　　　　　while boarding or alighting
　　　　　　　V16.3
　　　　　nontraffic V10.2
　　　　　while boarding or alighting V10.3

◄ New　　◄░░░ Revised　　~~deleted~~ Deleted

Accident (Continued)
transport (Continued)
pedal cyclist (Continued)
collision (Continued)
animal-drawn vehicle (traffic) V16.9
nontraffic V16.2
while boarding or alighting V16.3
bus (traffic) V14.9
nontraffic V14.2
while boarding or alighting V14.3
car (traffic) V13.9
nontraffic V13.2
while boarding or alighting V13.3
motor vehicle NOS (traffic) V19.60
nontraffic V19.20
specified type NEC (traffic) V19.69
nontraffic V19.29
pedal cycle (traffic) V11.9
nontraffic V11.2
while boarding or alighting V11.3
pickup truck (traffic) V13.9
nontraffic V13.2
while boarding or alighting V13.3
railway vehicle (traffic) V15.9
nontraffic V15.2
while boarding or alighting V15.3
specified vehicle NEC (traffic) V16.9
nontraffic V16.2
while boarding or alighting V16.3
stationary object (traffic) V17.9
nontraffic V17.2
while boarding or alighting V17.3
streetcar (traffic) V16.9
nontraffic V16.2
while boarding or alighting V16.3
three wheeled motor vehicle (traffic)
V12.9
nontraffic V12.2
while boarding or alighting V12.3
truck (traffic) V14.9
nontraffic V14.2
while boarding or alighting V14.3
two wheeled motor vehicle (traffic)
V12.9
nontraffic V12.2
while boarding or alighting V12.3
van (traffic) V13.9
nontraffic V13.2
while boarding or alighting V13.3
driver
collision (with)
animal (traffic) V10.4
being ridden (traffic) V16.4
nontraffic V16.0
nontraffic V10.0
animal-drawn vehicle (traffic) V16.4
nontraffic V16.0
bus (traffic) V14.4
nontraffic V14.0
car (traffic) V13.4
nontraffic V13.0
motor vehicle NOS (traffic) V19.40
nontraffic V19.00
specified type NEC (traffic)
V19.49
nontraffic V19.09
pedal cycle (traffic) V11.4
nontraffic V11.0
pickup truck (traffic) V13.4
nontraffic V13.0
railway vehicle (traffic) V15.4
nontraffic V15.0
specified vehicle NEC (traffic) V16.4
nontraffic V16.0
stationary object (traffic) V17.4
nontraffic V17.0
streetcar (traffic) V16.4
nontraffic V16.0
three wheeled motor vehicle
(traffic) V12.4
nontraffic V12.0

Accident (Continued)
transport (Continued)
pedal cyclist (Continued)
driver (Continued)
collision (Continued)
truck (traffic) V14.4
nontraffic V14.0
two wheeled motor vehicle (traffic)
V12.4
nontraffic V12.0
van (traffic) V13.4
nontraffic V13.0
noncollision accident (traffic) V18.4
nontraffic V18.0
noncollision accident (traffic) V18.9
nontraffic V18.2
while boarding or alighting V18.3
nontraffic V19.3
passenger
collision (with)
animal (traffic) V10.5
being ridden (traffic) V16.5
nontraffic V16.1
nontraffic V10.1
animal-drawn vehicle (traffic) V16.5
nontraffic V16.1
bus (traffic) V14.5
nontraffic V14.1
car (traffic) V13.5
nontraffic V13.1
motor vehicle NOS (traffic) V19.50
nontraffic V19.10
specified type NEC (traffic)
V19.59
nontraffic V19.19
pedal cycle (traffic) V11.5
nontraffic V11.1
pickup truck (traffic) V13.5
nontraffic V13.1
railway vehicle (traffic) V15.5
nontraffic V15.1
specified vehicle NEC (traffic) V16.5
nontraffic V16.1
stationary object (traffic) V17.5
nontraffic V17.1
streetcar (traffic) V16.5
nontraffic V16.1
three wheeled motor vehicle
(traffic) V12.5
nontraffic V12.1
truck (traffic) V14.5
nontraffic V14.1
two wheeled motor vehicle (traffic)
V12.5
nontraffic V12.1
van (traffic) V13.5
nontraffic V13.1
noncollision accident (traffic) V18.5
nontraffic V18.1
specified type NEC V19.88
military vehicle V19.81
pedestrian
conveyance (occupant) V09.9
babystroller V00.828
collision (with) V09.9
animal being ridden or animal
drawn vehicle V06.99
nontraffic V06.09
traffic V06.19
bus or heavy transport V04.99
nontraffic V04.09
traffic V04.19
car V03.99
nontraffic V03.09
traffic V03.19
pedal cycle V01.99
nontraffic V01.09
traffic V01.19
pick-up truck or van V03.99
nontraffic V03.09
traffic V03.19

Accident (Continued)
transport (Continued)
pedestrian (Continued)
conveyance (Continued)
babystroller (Continued)
collision (Continued)
railway (train) (vehicle) V05.99
nontraffic V05.09
traffic V05.19
stationary object V00.822
streetcar V06.99
nontraffic V06.09
traffic V06.19
two- or three-wheeled motor
vehicle V02.99
nontraffic V02.09
traffic V02.19
vehicle V09.9
animal-drawn V06.99
nontraffic V06.09
traffic V06.19
motor
nontraffic V09.00
traffic V09.20
fall V00.821
nontraffic V09.1
involving motor vehicle NEC
V09.00
traffic V09.3
involving motor vehicle NEC
V09.20
flat-bottomed NEC V00.388
collision (with) V09.9
animal being ridden or animal
drawn vehicle V06.99
nontraffic V06.09
traffic V06.19
bus or heavy transport V04.99
nontraffic V04.09
traffic V04.19
car V03.99
nontraffic V03.09
traffic V03.19
pedal cycle V01.99
nontraffic V01.09
traffic V01.19
pick-up truck or van V03.99
nontraffic V03.09
traffic V03.19
railway (train) (vehicle) V05.99
nontraffic V05.09
traffic V05.19
stationary object V00.382
streetcar V06.99
nontraffic V06.09
traffic V06.19
two-or three-wheeled motor
vehicle V02.99
nontraffic V02.09
traffic V02.19
vehicle V09.9
animal-drawn V06.99
nontraffic V06.09
traffic V06.19
motor
nontraffic V09.00
traffic V09.20
fall V00.381
nontraffic V09.1
involving motor vehicle NEC
V09.00
snow
board —see Accident, transport,
pedestrian, conveyance,
snow board
ski —see Accident, transport,
pedestrian, conveyance, skis
(snow)
traffic V09.3
involving motor vehicle NEC
V09.20

Accident (Continued)
  transport (Continued)
    pedestrian (Continued)
      conveyance (Continued)
        gliding type NEC V00.288
          collision (with) V09.9
            animal being ridden or animal drawn vehicle V06.99
              nontraffic V06.09
              traffic V06.19
            bus or heavy transport V04.99
              nontraffic V04.09
              traffic V04.19
            car V03.99
              nontraffic V03.09
              traffic V03.19
            pedal cycle V01.99
              nontraffic V01.09
              traffic V01.19
            pick-up truck or van V03.99
              nontraffic V03.09
              traffic V03.19
            railway (train) (vehicle) V05.99
              nontraffic V05.09
              traffic V05.19
            stationary object V00.282
            streetcar V06.99
              nontraffic V06.09
              traffic V06.19
            two- or three-wheeled motor vehicle V02.99
              nontraffic V02.09
              traffic V02.19
            vehicle V09.9
              animal-drawn V06.99
                nontraffic V06.09
                traffic V06.19
              motor
                nontraffic V09.00
                traffic V09.20
          fall V00.281
        heelies —see Accident, transport, pedestrian, conveyance, heelies
        ice skate —see Accident, transport, pedestrian, conveyance, ice skate
        nontraffic V09.1
          involving motor vehicle NEC V09.00
        sled —see Accident, transport, pedestrian, conveyance, sled
        traffic V09.3
          involving motor vehicle NEC V09.20
          wheelies —see Accident, transport, pedestrian, conveyance, heelies
        heelies V00.158
          colliding with stationary object V00.152
          fall V00.151
        ice skates V00.218
          collision (with) V09.9
            animal being ridden or animal drawn vehicle V06.99
              nontraffic V06.09
              traffic V06.19
            bus or heavy transport V04.99
              nontraffic V04.09
              traffic V04.19
            car V03.99
              nontraffic V03.09
              traffic V03.19
            pedal cycle V01.99
              nontraffic V01.09
              traffic V01.19
            pick-up truck or van V03.99
              nontraffic V03.09
              traffic V03.19

Accident (Continued)
  transport (Continued)
    pedestrian (Continued)
      conveyance (Continued)
        ice skates (Continued)
          collision (Continued)
            railway (train) (vehicle) V05.99
              nontraffic V05.09
              traffic V05.19
            stationary object V00.212
            streetcar V06.99
              nontraffic V06.09
              traffic V06.19
            two- or three-wheeled motor vehicle V02.99
              nontraffic V02.09
              traffic V02.19
            vehicle V09.9
              animal-drawn V06.99
                nontraffic V06.09
                traffic V06.19
              motor
                nontraffic V09.00
                traffic V09.20
          fall V00.211
          nontraffic V09.1
            involving motor vehicle NEC V09.00
          traffic V09.3
            involving motor vehicle NEC V09.20
        motorized mobility scooter V00.838
          collision with stationary object V00.832
          fall from V00.831
        nontraffic V09.1
          involving motor vehicle V09.00
            military V09.01
            specified type NEC V09.09
        roller skates (non in-line) V00.128
          collision (with) V09.9
            animal being ridden or animal drawn vehicle V06.91
              nontraffic V06.01
              traffic V06.11
            bus or heavy transport V04.91
              nontraffic V04.01
              traffic V04.11
            car V03.91
              nontraffic V03.01
              traffic V03.11
            pedal cycle V01.91
              nontraffic V01.01
              traffic V01.11
            pick-up truck or van V03.91
              nontraffic V03.01
              traffic V03.11
            railway (train) (vehicle) V05.91
              nontraffic V05.01
              traffic V05.11
            stationary object V00.122
            streetcar V06.91
              nontraffic V06.01
              traffic V06.11
            two- or three-wheeled motor vehicle V02.91
              nontraffic V02.01
              traffic V02.11
            vehicle V09.9
              animal-drawn V06.91
                nontraffic V06.01
                traffic V06.11
              motor
                nontraffic V09.00
                traffic V09.20
          fall V00.121

Accident (Continued)
  transport (Continued)
    pedestrian (Continued)
      conveyance (Continued)
        roller skates (Continued)
          in-line V00.118
            collision —see also Accident, transport, pedestrian, conveyance occupant, roller skates, collision
              with stationary object V00.112
            fall V00.111
            nontraffic V09.1
              involving motor vehicle NEC V09.00
            traffic V09.3
              involving motor vehicle NEC V09.20
        rolling shoes V00.158
          colliding with stationary object V00.152
          fall V00.151
        rolling type NEC V00.188
          collision (with) V09.9
            animal being ridden or animal drawn vehicle V06.99
              nontraffic V06.09
              traffic V06.19
            bus or heavy transport V04.99
              nontraffic V04.09
              traffic V04.19
            car V03.99
              nontraffic V03.09
              traffic V03.19
            pedal cycle V01.99
              nontraffic V01.09
              traffic V01.19
            pick-up truck or van V03.99
              nontraffic V03.09
              traffic V03.19
            railway (train) (vehicle) V05.99
              nontraffic V05.09
              traffic V05.19
            stationary object V00.182
            streetcar V06.99
              nontraffic V06.09
              traffic V06.19
            two- or three-wheeled motor vehicle V02.99
              nontraffic V02.09
              traffic V02.19
            vehicle V09.9
              animal-drawn V06.99
                nontraffic V06.09
                traffic V06.19
              motor
                nontraffic V09.00
                traffic V09.20
          fall V00.181
        in-line roller skate —see Accident, transport, pedestrian, conveyance, roller skate, in-line
        nontraffic V09.1
          involving motor vehicle NEC V09.00
        roller skate —see Accident, transport, pedestrian, conveyance, roller skate
        scooter (non-motorized) — see Accident, transport, pedestrian, conveyance, scooter
        skateboard —see Accident, transport, pedestrian, conveyance, skateboard
        traffic V09.3
          involving motor vehicle NEC V09.20

◀ New   ◀▥ Revised   ~~deleted~~ Deleted

Accident (Continued)
transport (Continued)
pedestrian (Continued)
conveyance (Continued)
scooter (non-motorized) V00.148
collision (with) V09.9
animal being ridden or animal
drawn vehicle V06.99
nontraffic V06.09
traffic V06.19
bus or heavy transport
V04.99
nontraffic V04.09
traffic V04.19
car V03.99
nontraffic V03.09
traffic V03.19
pedal cycle V01.99
nontraffic V01.09
traffic V01.19
pick-up truck or van V03.99
nontraffic V03.09
traffic V03.19
railway (train) (vehicle)
V05.99
nontraffic V05.09
traffic V05.19
stationary object V00.142
streetcar V06.99
nontraffic V06.09
traffic V06.19
two- or three-wheeled motor
vehicle V02.99
nontraffic V02.09
traffic V02.19
vehicle V09.9
animal-drawn V06.99
nontraffic V06.09
traffic V06.19
motor
nontraffic V09.00
traffic V09.20
fall V00.141
nontraffic V09.1
involving motor vehicle NEC
V09.00
traffic V09.3
involving motor vehicle NEC
V09.20
skate board V00.138
collision (with) V09.9
animal being ridden or
animal drawn vehicle
V06.92
nontraffic V06.02
traffic V06.12
bus or heavy transport
V04.92
nontraffic V04.02
traffic V04.12
car V03.92
nontraffic V03.02
traffic V03.12
pedal cycle V01.92
nontraffic V01.02
traffic V01.12
pick-up truck or van V03.92
nontraffic V03.02
traffic V03.12
railway (train) (vehicle)
V05.92
nontraffic V05.02
traffic V05.12
stationary object V00.132
streetcar V06.92
nontraffic V06.02
traffic V06.12
two- or three-wheeled motor
vehicle V02.92
nontraffic V02.02
traffic V02.12

Accident (Continued)
transport (Continued)
pedestrian (Continued)
conveyance (Continued)
skate board (Continued)
collision (Continued)
vehicle V09.9
animal-drawn V06.92
nontraffic V06.02
traffic V06.12
motor
nontraffic V09.00
traffic V09.20
fall V00.131
nontraffic V09.1
involving motor vehicle NEC
V09.00
traffic V09.3
involving motor vehicle NEC
V09.20
skis (snow) V00.328
collision (with) V09.9
animal being ridden or animal
drawn vehicle V06.99
nontraffic V06.09
traffic V06.19
bus or heavy transport V04.99
nontraffic V04.09
traffic V04.19
car V03.99
nontraffic V03.09
traffic V03.19
pedal cycle V01.99
nontraffic V01.09
traffic V01.19
pick-up truck or van V03.99
nontraffic V03.09
traffic V03.19
railway (train) (vehicle) V05.99
nontraffic V05.09
traffic V05.19
stationary object V00.322
streetcar V06.99
nontraffic V06.09
traffic V06.19
two- or three-wheeled motor
vehicle V02.99
nontraffic V02.09
traffic V02.19
vehicle V09.9
animal-drawn V06.99
nontraffic V06.09
traffic V06.19
motor
nontraffic V09.00
traffic V09.20
fall V00.321
nontraffic V09.1
involving motor vehicle NEC
V09.00
traffic V09.3
involving motor vehicle NEC
V09.20
sled V00.228
collision (with) V09.9
animal being ridden or animal
drawn vehicle V06.99
nontraffic V06.09
traffic V06.19
bus or heavy transport V04.99
nontraffic V04.09
traffic V04.19
car V03.99
nontraffic V03.09
traffic V03.19
pedal cycle V01.99
nontraffic V01.09
traffic V01.19
pick-up truck or van V03.99
nontraffic V03.09
traffic V03.19

Accident (Continued)
transport (Continued)
pedestrian (Continued)
conveyance (Continued)
sled (Continued)
collision (Continued)
railway (train) (vehicle)
V05.99
nontraffic V05.09
traffic V05.19
stationary object V00.222
streetcar V06.99
nontraffic V06.09
traffic V06.19
two- or three-wheeled motor
vehicle V02.99
nontraffic V02.09
traffic V02.19
vehicle V09.9
animal-drawn V06.99
nontraffic V06.09
traffic V06.19
motor
nontraffic V09.00
traffic V09.20
fall V00.221
nontraffic V09.1
involving motor vehicle NEC
V09.00
traffic V09.3
involving motor vehicle NEC
V09.20
snow board V00.318
collision (with) V09.9
animal being ridden or animal
drawn vehicle V06.99
nontraffic V06.09
traffic V06.19
bus or heavy transport V04.99
nontraffic V04.09
traffic V04.19
car V03.99
nontraffic V03.09
traffic V03.19
pedal cycle V01.99
nontraffic V01.09
traffic V01.19
pick-up truck or van V03.99
nontraffic V03.09
traffic V03.19
railway (train) (vehicle) V05.99
nontraffic V05.09
traffic V05.19
stationary object V00.312
streetcar V06.99
nontraffic V06.09
traffic V06.19
two- or three-wheeled motor
vehicle V02.99
nontraffic V02.09
traffic V02.19
vehicle V09.9
animal-drawn V06.99
nontraffic V06.09
traffic V06.19
motor
nontraffic V09.00
traffic V09.20
fall V00.311
nontraffic V09.1
involving motor vehicle NEC
V09.00
traffic V09.3
involving motor vehicle NEC
V09.20
specified type NEC V00.898
collision (with) V09.9
animal being ridden or animal
drawn vehicle V06.99
nontraffic V06.09
traffic V06.19

◀ New   ◀◀◀ Revised   ~~deleted~~ Deleted

Accident *(Continued)*
  transport *(Continued)*
    pickup truck occupant *(Continued)*
      driver *(Continued)*
        collision *(Continued)*
          animal-drawn vehicle (traffic) V56.5
            nontraffic V56.0
          bus (traffic) V54.5
            nontraffic V54.0
          car (traffic) V53.5
            nontraffic V53.0
          motor vehicle NOS (traffic) V59.40
            nontraffic V59.00
            specified type NEC (traffic) V59.49
              nontraffic V59.09
          pedal cycle (traffic) V51.5
            nontraffic V51.0
          pickup truck (traffic) V53.5
            nontraffic V53.0
          railway vehicle (traffic) V55.5
            nontraffic V55.0
          specified vehicle NEC (traffic) V56.5
            nontraffic V56.0
          stationary object (traffic) V57.5
            nontraffic V57.0
          streetcar (traffic) V56.5
            nontraffic V56.0
          three wheeled motor vehicle (traffic) V52.5
            nontraffic V52.0
          truck (traffic) V54.5
            nontraffic V54.0
          two wheeled motor vehicle (traffic) V52.5
            nontraffic V52.0
          van (traffic) V53.5
            nontraffic V53.0
        noncollision accident (traffic) V58.5
          nontraffic V58.0
      hanger-on
        collision (with)
          animal (traffic) V50.7
            being ridden (traffic) V56.7
              nontraffic V56.2
            nontraffic V50.2
          animal-drawn vehicle (traffic) V56.7
            nontraffic V56.2
          bus (traffic) V54.7
            nontraffic V54.2
          car (traffic) V53.7
            nontraffic V53.2
          pedal cycle (traffic) V51.7
            nontraffic V51.2
          pickup truck (traffic) V53.7
            nontraffic V53.2
          railway vehicle (traffic) V55.7
            nontraffic V55.2
          specified vehicle NEC (traffic) V56.7
            nontraffic V56.2
          stationary object (traffic) V57.7
            nontraffic V57.2
          streetcar (traffic) V56.7
            nontraffic V56.2
          three wheeled motor vehicle (traffic) V52.7
            nontraffic V52.2
          truck (traffic) V54.7
            nontraffic V54.2
          two wheeled motor vehicle (traffic) V52.7
            nontraffic V52.2
          van (traffic) V53.7
            nontraffic V53.2
        noncollision accident (traffic) V58.7
          nontraffic V58.2
        noncollision accident (traffic) V58.9
          nontraffic V58.3
          while boarding or alighting V58.4
        nontraffic V59.3

Accident *(Continued)*
  transport *(Continued)*
    pickup truck occupant *(Continued)*
      passenger
        collision (with)
          animal (traffic) V50.6
            being ridden (traffic) V56.6
              nontraffic V56.1
            nontraffic V50.1
          animal-drawn vehicle (traffic) V56.6
            nontraffic V56.1
          bus (traffic) V54.6
            nontraffic V54.1
          car (traffic) V53.6
            nontraffic V53.1
          motor vehicle NOS (traffic) V59.50
            nontraffic V59.10
            specified type NEC (traffic) V59.59
              nontraffic V59.19
          pedal cycle (traffic) V51.6
            nontraffic V51.1
          pickup truck (traffic) V53.6
            nontraffic V53.1
          railway vehicle (traffic) V55.6
            nontraffic V55.1
          specified vehicle NEC (traffic) V56.6
            nontraffic V56.1
          stationary object (traffic) V57.6
            nontraffic V57.1
          streetcar (traffic) V56.6
            nontraffic V56.1
          three wheeled motor vehicle (traffic) V52.6
            nontraffic V52.1
          truck (traffic) V54.6
            nontraffic V54.1
          two wheeled motor vehicle (traffic) V52.6
            nontraffic V52.1
          van (traffic) V53.6
            nontraffic V53.1
        noncollision accident (traffic) V58.6
          nontraffic V58.1
      specified type NEC V59.88
      military vehicle V59.81
    quarry truck —*see* Accident, transport, industrial vehicle occupant
    race car —*see* Accident, transport, motor vehicle NEC occupant
    railway vehicle occupant V81.9
      collision (with) V81.3
        motor vehicle (non-military) (traffic) V81.1
          military V81.83
          nontraffic V81.0
        rolling stock V81.2
        specified object NEC V81.3
      during derailment V81.7
        with antecedent collision —*see* Accident, transport, railway vehicle occupant, collision ◄
      explosion V81.81
      fall (in railway vehicle) V81.5
        during derailment V81.7
          with antecedent collision —*see* Accident, transport, railway vehicle occupant, collision ◄
        from railway vehicle V81.6
          during derailment V81.7
            with antecedent collision —*see* Accident, transport, railway vehicle occupant, collision ◄
        while boarding or alighting V81.4
      fire V81.81
      object falling onto train V81.82
      specified type NEC V81.89
      while boarding or alighting V81.4
    ski lift V98.3

Accident *(Continued)*
  transport *(Continued)*
    snowmobile occupant (nontraffic) V86.92
      driver V86.52
      hanger-on V86.72
      passenger V86.62
      traffic V86.32
        driver V86.02
        hanger-on V86.22
        passenger V86.12
      while boarding or alighting V86.42
    specified NEC V98.8
    sport utility vehicle occupant —*see also* Accident, transport, pickup truck occupant ◄▥
      ~~collision (with)~~
        ~~stationary object (traffic) V47.91~~
          ~~nontraffic V47.31~~
      ~~driver~~
        ~~collision (with)~~
          ~~stationary object (traffic) V47.51~~
            ~~nontraffic V47.01~~
      ~~passenger~~
        ~~collision (with)~~
          ~~stationary object (traffic) V47.61~~
            ~~nontraffic V47.11~~
    streetcar occupant V82.9
      collision (with) V82.3
        motor vehicle (traffic) V82.1
          nontraffic V82.0
        rolling stock V82.2
      during derailment V82.7
        with antecedent collision —*see* Accident, transport, streetcar occupant, collision ◄
      fall (in streetcar) V82.5
        during derailment V82.7
          with antecedent collision —*see* Accident, transport, streetcar occupant, collision ◄
        from streetcar V82.6
          during derailment V82.7
            with antecedent collision —*see* Accident, transport, streetcar occupant, collision ◄
          while boarding or alighting V82.4
        while boarding or alighting V82.4
      specified type NEC V82.8
      while boarding or alighting V82.4
    three-wheeled motor vehicle occupant V39.9
      collision (with)
        animal (traffic) V30.9
          being ridden (traffic) V36.9
            nontraffic V36.3
            while boarding or alighting V36.4
          nontraffic V30.3
            while boarding or alighting V30.4
        animal-drawn vehicle (traffic) V36.9
          nontraffic V36.3
          while boarding or alighting V36.4
        bus (traffic) V34.9
          nontraffic V34.3
          while boarding or alighting V34.4
        car (traffic) V33.9
          nontraffic V33.3
          while boarding or alighting V33.4
        motor vehicle NOS (traffic) V39.60
          nontraffic V39.20
          specified type NEC (traffic) V39.69
            nontraffic V39.29
        pedal cycle (traffic) V31.9
          nontraffic V31.3
          while boarding or alighting V31.4
        pickup truck (traffic) V33.9
          nontraffic V33.3
          while boarding or alighting V33.4
        railway vehicle (traffic) V35.9
          nontraffic V35.3
          while boarding or alighting V35.4

Accident (Continued)
  transport (Continued)
    three-wheeled motor vehicle occupant
      (Continued)
      collision (Continued)
        specified vehicle NEC (traffic) V36.9
          nontraffic V36.3
          while boarding or alighting V36.4
        stationary object (traffic) V37.9
          nontraffic V37.3
          while boarding or alighting V37.4
        streetcar (traffic) V36.9
          nontraffic V36.3
          while boarding or alighting V36.4
        three wheeled motor vehicle (traffic)
          V32.9
          nontraffic V32.3
          while boarding or alighting V32.4
        truck (traffic) V34.9
          nontraffic V34.3
          while boarding or alighting V34.4
        two wheeled motor vehicle (traffic)
          V32.9
          nontraffic V32.3
          while boarding or alighting V32.4
        van (traffic) V33.9
          nontraffic V33.3
          while boarding or alighting V33.4
      driver
        collision (with)
          animal (traffic) V30.5
            being ridden (traffic) V36.5
              nontraffic V36.0
            nontraffic V30.0
          animal-drawn vehicle (traffic) V36.5
            nontraffic V36.0
          bus (traffic) V34.5
            nontraffic V34.0
          car (traffic) V33.5
            nontraffic V33.0
          motor vehicle NOS (traffic) V39.40
            nontraffic V39.00
            specified type NEC (traffic)
              V39.49
              nontraffic V39.09
          pedal cycle (traffic) V31.5
            nontraffic V31.0
          pickup truck (traffic) V33.5
            nontraffic V33.0
          railway vehicle (traffic) V35.5
            nontraffic V35.0
          specified vehicle NEC (traffic) V36.5
            nontraffic V36.0
          stationary object (traffic) V37.5
            nontraffic V37.0
          streetcar (traffic) V36.5
            nontraffic V36.0
          three wheeled motor vehicle
            (traffic) V32.5
            nontraffic V32.0
          truck (traffic) V34.5
            nontraffic V34.0
          two wheeled motor vehicle (traffic)
            V32.5
            nontraffic V32.0
          van (traffic) V33.5
            nontraffic V33.0
        noncollision accident (traffic) V38.5
          nontraffic V38.0
      hanger-on
        collision (with)
          animal (traffic) V30.7
            being ridden (traffic) V36.7
              nontraffic V36.2
            nontraffic V30.2
          animal-drawn vehicle (traffic) V36.7
            nontraffic V36.2
          bus (traffic) V34.7
            nontraffic V34.2
          car (traffic) V33.7
            nontraffic V33.2

Accident (Continued)
  transport (Continued)
    three-wheeled motor vehicle occupant
      (Continued)
      hanger-on (Continued)
        collision (Continued)
          pedal cycle (traffic) V31.7
            nontraffic V31.2
          pickup truck (traffic) V33.7
            nontraffic V33.2
          railway vehicle (traffic) V35.7
            nontraffic V35.2
          specified vehicle NEC (traffic) V36.7
            nontraffic V36.2
          stationary object (traffic) V37.7
            nontraffic V37.2
          streetcar (traffic) V36.7
            nontraffic V36.2
          three wheeled motor vehicle
            (traffic) V32.7
            nontraffic V32.2
          truck (traffic) V34.7
            nontraffic V34.2
          two wheeled motor vehicle (traffic)
            V32.7
            nontraffic V32.2
          van (traffic) V33.7
            nontraffic V33.2
        noncollision accident (traffic) V38.7
          nontraffic V38.2
      noncollision accident (traffic) V38.9
        nontraffic V38.3
        while boarding or alighting V38.4
      nontraffic V39.3
      passenger
        collision (with)
          animal (traffic) V30.6
            being ridden (traffic) V36.6
              nontraffic V36.1
            nontraffic V30.1
          animal-drawn vehicle (traffic) V36.6
            nontraffic V36.1
          bus (traffic) V34.6
            nontraffic V34.1
          car (traffic) V33.6
            nontraffic V33.1
          motor vehicle NOS (traffic) V39.50
            nontraffic V39.10
            specified type NEC (traffic)
              V39.59
              nontraffic V39.19
          pedal cycle (traffic) V31.6
            nontraffic V31.1
          pickup truck (traffic) V33.6
            nontraffic V33.1
          railway vehicle (traffic) V35.6
            nontraffic V35.1
          specified vehicle NEC (traffic)
            V36.6
            nontraffic V36.1
          stationary object (traffic) V37.6
            nontraffic V37.1
          streetcar (traffic) V36.6
            nontraffic V36.1
          three wheeled motor vehicle
            (traffic) V32.6
            nontraffic V32.1
          truck (traffic) V34.6
            nontraffic V34.1
          two wheeled motor vehicle (traffic)
            V32.6
            nontraffic V32.1
          van (traffic) V33.6
            nontraffic V33.1
        noncollision accident (traffic) V38.6
          nontraffic V38.1
      specified type NEC V39.89
      military vehicle V39.81
      tractor (farm) (and trailer) —see Accident,
        transport, agricultural vehicle
        occupant

Accident (Continued)
  transport (Continued)
    tram —see Accident, transport, streetcar
      in mine or quarry —see Accident,
        transport, industrial vehicle
        occupant
    trolley —see Accident, transport, streetcar
      in mine or quarry —see Accident,
        transport, industrial vehicle
        occupant
    truck (heavy) occupant V69.9
      collision (with)
        animal (traffic) V60.9
          being ridden (traffic) V66.9
            nontraffic V66.3
              while boarding or alighting V66.4
          nontraffic V60.3
          while boarding or alighting V60.4
        animal-drawn vehicle (traffic) V66.9
          nontraffic V66.3
          while boarding or alighting V66.4
        bus (traffic) V64.9
          nontraffic V64.3
          while boarding or alighting V64.4
        car (traffic) V63.9
          nontraffic V63.3
          while boarding or alighting V63.4
        motor vehicle NOS (traffic) V69.60
          nontraffic V69.20
          specified type NEC (traffic) V69.69
            nontraffic V69.29
        pedal cycle (traffic) V61.9
          nontraffic V61.3
          while boarding or alighting V61.4
        pickup truck (traffic) V63.9
          nontraffic V63.3
          while boarding or alighting V63.4
        railway vehicle (traffic) V65.9
          nontraffic V65.3
          while boarding or alighting V65.4
        specified vehicle NEC (traffic) V66.9
          nontraffic V66.3
          while boarding or alighting V66.4
        stationary object (traffic) V67.9
          nontraffic V67.3
          while boarding or alighting V67.4
        streetcar (traffic) V66.9
          nontraffic V66.3
          while boarding or alighting V66.4
        three wheeled motor vehicle (traffic)
          V62.9
          nontraffic V62.3
          while boarding or alighting V62.4
        truck (traffic) V64.9
          nontraffic V64.3
          while boarding or alighting V64.4
        two wheeled motor vehicle (traffic)
          V62.9
          nontraffic V62.3
          while boarding or alighting V62.4
        van (traffic) V63.9
          nontraffic V63.3
          while boarding or alighting V63.4
      driver
        collision (with)
          animal (traffic) V60.5
            being ridden (traffic) V66.5
              nontraffic V66.0
            nontraffic V60.0
          animal-drawn vehicle (traffic)
            V66.5
            nontraffic V66.0
          bus (traffic) V64.5
            nontraffic V64.0
          car (traffic) V63.5
            nontraffic V63.0
          motor vehicle NOS (traffic) V69.40
            nontraffic V69.00
            specified type NEC (traffic)
              V69.49
              nontraffic V69.09

◀ New   ◀⃪ Revised   ~~deleted~~ Deleted

Accident (*Continued*)
  transport (*Continued*)
    truck occupant (*Continued*)
      driver (*Continued*)
        collision (*Continued*)
          pedal cycle (traffic) V61.5
            nontraffic V61.0
          pickup truck (traffic) V63.5
            nontraffic V63.0
          railway vehicle (traffic) V65.5
            nontraffic V65.0
          specified vehicle NEC (traffic) V66.5
            nontraffic V66.0
          stationary object (traffic) V67.5
            nontraffic V67.0
          streetcar (traffic) V66.5
            nontraffic V66.0
          three wheeled motor vehicle
            (traffic) V62.5
            nontraffic V62.0
          truck (traffic) V64.5
            nontraffic V64.0
          two wheeled motor vehicle (traffic)
            V62.5
            nontraffic V62.0
          van (traffic) V63.5
            nontraffic V63.0
        noncollision accident (traffic) V68.5
          nontraffic V68.0
      dump —*see* Accident, transport,
        construction vehicle occupant
      hanger-on
        collision (with)
          animal (traffic) V60.7
            being ridden (traffic) V66.7
              nontraffic V66.2
            nontraffic V60.2
          animal-drawn vehicle (traffic) V66.7
            nontraffic V66.2
          bus (traffic) V64.7
            nontraffic V64.2
          car (traffic) V63.7
            nontraffic V63.2
          pedal cycle (traffic) V61.7
            nontraffic V61.2
          pickup truck (traffic) V63.7
            nontraffic V63.2
          railway vehicle (traffic) V65.7
            nontraffic V65.2
          specified vehicle NEC (traffic) V66.7
            nontraffic V66.2
          stationary object (traffic) V67.7
            nontraffic V67.2
          streetcar (traffic) V66.7
            nontraffic V66.2
          three wheeled motor vehicle
            (traffic) V62.7
            nontraffic V62.2
          truck (traffic) V64.7
            nontraffic V64.2
          two wheeled motor vehicle (traffic)
            V62.7
            nontraffic V62.2
          van (traffic) V63.7
            nontraffic V63.2
        noncollision accident (traffic) V68.7
          nontraffic V68.2
        noncollision accident (traffic) V68.9
        nontraffic V68.3
        while boarding or alighting V68.4
      nontraffic V69.3
      passenger
        collision (with)
          animal (traffic) V60.6
            being ridden (traffic) V66.6
              nontraffic V66.1
            nontraffic V60.1
          animal-drawn vehicle (traffic) V66.6
            nontraffic V66.1
          bus (traffic) V64.6
            nontraffic V64.1

Accident (*Continued*)
  transport (*Continued*)
    truck occupant (*Continued*)
      passenger (*Continued*)
        collision (*Continued*)
          car (traffic) V63.6
            nontraffic V63.1
          motor vehicle NOS (traffic) V69.50
            nontraffic V69.10
            specified type NEC (traffic)
              V69.59
              nontraffic V69.19
          pedal cycle (traffic) V61.6
            nontraffic V61.1
          pickup truck (traffic) V63.6
            nontraffic V63.1
          railway vehicle (traffic) V65.6
            nontraffic V65.1
          specified vehicle NEC (traffic)
            V66.6
            nontraffic V66.1
          stationary object (traffic) V67.6
            nontraffic V67.1
          streetcar (traffic) V66.6
            nontraffic V66.1
          three wheeled motor vehicle
            (traffic) V62.6
            nontraffic V62.1
          truck (traffic) V64.6
            nontraffic V64.1
          two wheeled motor vehicle (traffic)
            V62.6
            nontraffic V62.1
          van (traffic) V63.6
            nontraffic V63.1
        noncollision accident (traffic) V68.6
          nontraffic V68.1
      pickup —*see* Accident, transport, pickup
        truck occupant
      specified type NEC V69.88
      military vehicle V69.81
    van occupant V59.9
      collision (with)
        animal (traffic) V50.9
          being ridden (traffic) V56.9
            nontraffic V56.3
            while boarding or alighting
              V56.4
          nontraffic V50.3
          while boarding or alighting V50.4
         animal-drawn vehicle (traffic) V56.9
          nontraffic V56.3
          while boarding or alighting V56.4
        bus (traffic) V54.9
          nontraffic V54.3
          while boarding or alighting V54.4
        car (traffic) V53.9
          nontraffic V53.3
          while boarding or alighting V53.4
        motor vehicle NOS (traffic) V59.60
          nontraffic V59.20
          specified type NEC (traffic) V59.69
            nontraffic V59.29
        pedal cycle (traffic) V51.9
          nontraffic V51.3
          while boarding or alighting V51.4
        pickup truck (traffic) V53.9
          nontraffic V53.3
          while boarding or alighting V53.4
        railway vehicle (traffic) V55.9
          nontraffic V55.3
          while boarding or alighting V55.4
        specified vehicle NEC (traffic) V56.9
          nontraffic V56.3
          while boarding or alighting V56.4
        stationary object (traffic) V57.9
          nontraffic V57.3
          while boarding or alighting V57.4
        streetcar (traffic) V56.9
          nontraffic V56.3
          while boarding or alighting V56.4

Accident (*Continued*)
  transport (*Continued*)
    van occupant (*Continued*)
      collision (*Continued*)
        three wheeled motor vehicle (traffic)
          V52.9
          nontraffic V52.3
          while boarding or alighting V52.4
        truck (traffic) V54.9
          nontraffic V54.3
          while boarding or alighting V54.4
        two wheeled motor vehicle (traffic)
          V52.9
          nontraffic V52.3
          while boarding or alighting V52.4
        van (traffic) V53.9
          nontraffic V53.3
          while boarding or alighting V53.4
      driver
        collision (with)
          animal (traffic) V50.5
            being ridden (traffic) V56.5
              nontraffic V56.0
            nontraffic V50.0
          animal-drawn vehicle (traffic) V56.5
            nontraffic V56.0
          bus (traffic) V54.5
            nontraffic V54.0
          car (traffic) V53.5
            nontraffic V53.0
          motor vehicle NOS (traffic) V59.40
            nontraffic V59.00
            specified type NEC (traffic)
              V59.49
              nontraffic V59.09
          pedal cycle (traffic) V51.5
            nontraffic V51.0
          pickup truck (traffic) V53.5
            nontraffic V53.0
          railway vehicle (traffic) V55.5
            nontraffic V55.0
          specified vehicle NEC (traffic) V56.5
            nontraffic V56.0
          stationary object (traffic) V57.5
            nontraffic V57.0
          streetcar (traffic) V56.5
            nontraffic V56.0
          three wheeled motor vehicle
            (traffic) V52.5
            nontraffic V52.0
          truck (traffic) V54.5
            nontraffic V54.0
          two wheeled motor vehicle (traffic)
            V52.5
            nontraffic V52.0
          van (traffic) V53.5
            nontraffic V53.0
        noncollision accident (traffic) V58.5
          nontraffic V58.0
      hanger-on
        collision (with)
          animal (traffic) V50.7
            being ridden (traffic) V56.7
              nontraffic V56.2
            nontraffic V50.2
          animal-drawn vehicle (traffic) V56.7
            nontraffic V56.2
          bus (traffic) V54.7
            nontraffic V54.2
          car (traffic) V53.7
            nontraffic V53.2
          pedal cycle (traffic) V51.7
            nontraffic V51.2
          pickup truck (traffic) V53.7
            nontraffic V53.2
          railway vehicle (traffic) V55.7
            nontraffic V55.2
          specified vehicle NEC (traffic) V56.7
            nontraffic V56.2
          stationary object (traffic) V57.7
            nontraffic V57.2

Activity *(Continued)*
  digging
    dirt Y93.H1
  dirt digging Y93.H1
  dishwashing Y93.G1
  diving (platform) (springboard) Y93.12
    underwater Y93.15
  dodge ball Y93.6A
  downhill skiing Y93.23
  drum playing Y93.J2
  dumbbells Y93.B3
  electronic
    devices NEC Y93.C9
      hand held interactive Y93.C2
    game playing (using) (with)
      interactive device Y93.C2
      keyboard or other stationary device
        Y93.C1
  elliptical machine Y93.A1
  exercise (s)
    machines ((primarily) for)
      cardiorespiratory conditioning Y93.A1
      muscle strengthening Y93.B1
    muscle strengthening (non-machine) NEC
      Y93.B9
  external motion NEC Y93.I9
    rollercoaster Y93.I1
  fainting game Y93.85 ◄
  field hockey Y93.65
  figure skating (pairs) (singles) Y93.21
  flag football Y93.62
  floor mopping and cleaning Y93.E5
  food preparation and clean up Y93.G1
  football (American) NOS Y93.61
    flag Y93.62
    tackle Y93.61
    touch Y93.62
  four square Y93.6A
  free weights Y93.B3
  frisbee (ultimate) Y93.74
  furniture
    building Y93.D3
    finishing Y93.D3
    repair Y93.D3
  game playing (electronic)
    using interactive device Y93.C2
    using keyboard or other stationary device
      Y93.C1
  gardening Y93.H2
  golf Y93.53
  grass drills Y93.A6
  grilling and smoking food Y93.G2
  grooming and shearing an animal Y93.K3
  guerilla drills Y93.A6
  gymnastics (rhythmic) Y93.43
  hand held interactive electronic device Y93.C2
  handball Y93.73
  handcrafts NEC Y93.D9
  hang gliding Y93.35
  hiking (on level or elevated terrain) Y93.01
  hockey (ice) Y93.22
    field Y93.65
  horseback riding Y93.52
  household (interior) maintenance NEC Y93.E9
  ice NEC Y93.29
    dancing Y93.21
    hockey Y93.22
    skating Y93.21
  inline roller skating Y93.51
  ironing Y93.E4
  judo Y93.75
  jumping (off) NEC Y93.39
    BASE (Building, Antenna, Span, Earth)
      Y93.33
    bungee Y93.34
    jacks Y93.A2
    rope Y93.56
  jumping jacks Y93.A2
  jumping rope Y93.56
  karate Y93.75

Activity *(Continued)*
  kayaking (in calm and turbulent water) Y93.16
  keyboarding (computer) Y93.C1
  kickball Y93.6A
  knitting Y93.D1
  lacrosse Y93.65
  land maintenance NEC Y93.H9
  landscaping Y93.H2
  laundry Y93.E2
  machines (exercise)
    primarily for cardiorespiratory
      conditioning Y93.A1
    primarily for muscle strengthening Y93.B1
  maintenance
    exterior building NEC Y93.H9
    household (interior) NEC Y93.E9
    land Y93.H9
    property Y93.H9
  marching (on level or elevated terrain) Y93.01
  martial arts Y93.75
  microwave oven Y93.G3
  milking an animal Y93.K2
  mopping (floor) Y93.E5
  mountain climbing Y93.31
  muscle strengthening
    exercises (non-machine) NEC Y93.B9
    machines Y93.B1
  musical keyboard (electronic) playing Y93.J1
  nordic skiing Y93.24
  obstacle course Y93.A5
  oven (microwave) Y93.G3
  packing up and unpacking in moving to a
    new residence Y93.E6
  parasailing Y93.19
  pass out game Y93.85 ◄
  percussion instrument playing NEC Y93.J2
  personal
    bathing and showering Y93.E1
    hygiene NEC Y93.E8
    showering Y93.E1
  physical games generally associated with
    school recess, summer camp and
    children Y93.6A
  physical training NEC Y93.A9
  piano playing Y93.J1
  pilates Y93.B4
  platform diving Y93.12
  playing musical instrument
    brass instrument Y93.J4
    drum Y93.J2
    musical keyboard (electronic) Y93.J1
    percussion instrument NEC Y93.J2
    piano Y93.J1
    string instrument Y93.J3
    winds instrument Y93.J4
  property maintenance
    exterior NEC Y93.H9
    interior NEC Y93.E9
  pruning (garden and lawn) Y93.H2
  pull-ups Y93.B2
  push-ups Y93.B2
  racquetball Y93.73
  rafting (in calm and turbulent water) Y93.16
  raking (leaves) Y93.H1
  rappelling Y93.32
  refereeing a sports activity Y93.81
  residential relocation Y93.E6
  rhythmic gymnastics Y93.43
  rhythmic movement NEC Y93.49
  riding
    horseback Y93.52
    rollercoaster Y93.I1
  rock climbing Y93.31
  roller skating (inline) Y93.51
  rollercoaster riding Y93.I1
  rough housing and horseplay Y93.83
  rowing (in calm and turbulent water)
    Y93.16
  rugby Y93.63
  SCUBA diving Y93.15
  sewing Y93.D2

Activity *(Continued)*
  shoveling Y93.H1
    dirt Y93.H1
    snow Y93.H1
  showering (personal) Y93.E1
  sit-ups Y93.B2
  skateboarding Y93.51
  skating (ice) Y93.21
    roller Y93.51
  skiing (alpine) (downhill) Y93.23
    cross country Y93.24
    nordic Y93.24
    water Y93.17
  sledding (snow) Y93.23
  sleeping (sleep) Y93.84
  smoking and grilling food Y93.G2
  snorkeling Y93.15
  snow NEC Y93.29
    boarding Y93.23
    shoveling Y93.H1
    sledding Y93.23
    tubing Y93.23
  soccer Y93.66
  softball Y93.64
  specified NEC Y93.89
  spectator at an event Y93.82
  sports NEC Y93.79
    sports played as a team or group NEC
      Y93.69
    sports played individually NEC Y93.59
  springboard diving Y93.12
  squash Y93.73
  stationary bike Y93.A1
  step (stepping) exercise (class) Y93.A3
  stepper machine Y93.A1
  stove Y93.G3
  string instrument playing Y93.J3
  surfing Y93.18
    wind Y93.18
  swimming Y93.11
  tackle football Y93.61
  tap dancing Y93.41
  tennis Y93.73
  tobogganing Y93.23
  touch football Y93.62
  track and field events (non-running) Y93.57
    running Y93.02
  trampoline Y93.44
  treadmill Y93.A1
  trimming shrubs Y93.H2
  tubing (in calm and turbulent water) Y93.16
    snow Y93.23
  ultimate frisbee Y93.74
  underwater diving Y93.15
  unpacking in moving to a new residence
    Y93.E6
  use of stove, oven and microwave oven Y93.
    G3
  vacuuming Y93.E3
  volleyball (beach) (court) Y93.68
  wake boarding Y93.17
  walking (on level or elevated terrain) Y93.01
    an animal Y93.K1
  walking an animal Y93.K1
  wall climbing Y93.31
  warm up and cool down exercises Y93.A2
  water NEC Y93.19
    aerobics Y93.14
    craft NEC Y93.19
    exercise Y93.14
    polo Y93.13
    skiing Y93.17
    sliding Y93.18
    survival training and testing Y93.19
  weeding (garden and lawn) Y93.H2
  wind instrument playing Y93.J4
  windsurfing Y93.18
  wrestling Y93.72
  yoga Y93.42
Adverse effect of drugs —*see* Table of Drugs
  and Chemicals

Aerosinusitis —*see* Air, pressure
After-effect, late —*see* Sequelae
Air
  blast in war operations —*see* War operations,
    air blast
  pressure
    change, rapid
      during
        ascent W94.29
          while (in) (surfacing from)
            aircraft W94.23
            deep water diving W94.21
            underground W94.22
        descent W94.39
          in
            aircraft W94.31
            water W94.32
    high, prolonged W94.0
    low, prolonged W94.12
      due to residence or long visit at high
        altitude W94.11
Alpine sickness W94.11
Altitude sickness W94.11
Anaphylactic shock, anaphylaxis —*see* Table of
  Drugs and Chemicals ◀▥
Andes disease W94.11
Arachnidism, arachnoidism X58
Arson (with intent to injure or kill) X97
Asphyxia, asphyxiation
  by
    food (bone) (seed) —*see* categories T17
      and T18
    gas —*see also* Table of Drugs and
      Chemicals ◀▥
      legal
        execution —*see* Legal, intervention,
          gas
        intervention —*see* Legal, intervention,
          gas
  from
    fire —*see also* Exposure, fire
      in war operations —*see* War operations,
        fire
    ignition —*see* Ignition
    vomitus T17.81
  in war operations —*see* War operations,
    restriction of airway
Aspiration
  food (any type) (into respiratory tract) (with
    asphyxia, obstruction respiratory tract,
    suffocation) —*see* categories T17 and T18
  foreign body —*see* Foreign body, aspiration
  vomitus (with asphyxia, obstruction
    respiratory tract, suffocation) T17.81
Assassination (attempt) —*see* Assault
Assault (homicidal) (by) (in) Y09
  arson X97
  bite (of human being) Y04.1
  bodily force Y04.8
    bite Y04.1
    bumping into Y04.2
    sexual —*see* subcategories T74.0, T76.0
    unarmed fight Y04.0

Assault *(Continued)*
  bomb X96.9
    antipersonnel X96.0
    fertilizer X96.3
    gasoline X96.1
    letter X96.2
    petrol X96.1
    pipe X96.3
    specified NEC X96.8
  brawl (hand) (fists) (foot) (unarmed) Y04.0
  burning, burns (by fire) NEC X97
    acid Y08.89
    caustic, corrosive substance Y08.89
    chemical from swallowing caustic,
      corrosive substance —*see* Table of
        Drugs and Chemicals ◀▥
    cigarette(s) X97
    hot object X98.9
      fluid NEC X98.2
      household appliance X98.3
      specified NEC X98.8
      steam X98.0
      tap water X98.1
      vapors X98.0
    scalding —*see* Assault, burning
    steam X98.0
    vitriol Y08.89
  caustic, corrosive substance (gas) Y08.89
  crashing of
    aircraft Y08.81
    motor vehicle Y03.8
      pushed in front of Y02.0
      run over Y03.0
      specified NEC Y03.8
  cutting or piercing instrument X99.9
    dagger X99.2
    glass X99.0
    knife X99.1
    specified NEC X99.8
    sword X99.2
  dagger X99.2
  drowning (in) X92.9
    bathtub X92.0
    natural water X92.3
    specified NEC X92.8
    swimming pool X92.1
      following fall X92.2
  dynamite X96.8
  explosive (s) (material) X96.9
  fight (hand) (fists) (foot) (unarmed) Y04.0
    with weapon —*see* Assault, by type of
      weapon
  fire X97
  firearm X95.9
    airgun X95.01
    handgun X93
    hunting rifle X94.1
    larger X94.9
      specified NEC X94.8
    machine gun X94.2
    shotgun X94.0
    specified NEC X95.8

Assault *(Continued)*
  from high place Y01
  gunshot (wound) NEC —*see* Assault, firearm,
    by type
  incendiary device X97
  injury Y09
    to child due to criminal abortion attempt
      NEC Y08.89
  knife X99.1
  late effect of —*see* X92-Y08 with 7th character
    S
  placing before moving object NEC Y02.8
    motor vehicle Y02.0
  poisoning —*see* categories T36-T65 with 7th
    character S
  puncture, any part of body —*see* Assault,
    cutting or piercing instrument
  pushing
    before moving object NEC Y02.8
      motor vehicle Y02.0
      subway train Y02.1
      train Y02.1
  rape T74.2-
  scalding —*see* Assault, burning
  sequelae of —*see* X92-Y08 with 7th character
    S
  sexual (by bodily force) T74.2-
  shooting —*see* Assault, firearm
  specified means NEC Y08.89
  stab, any part of body —*see* Assault, cutting
    or piercing instrument
  steam X98.0
  striking against
    other person Y04.2
    sports equipment Y08.09
      baseball bat Y08.02
      hockey stick Y08.01
  struck by
    sports equipment Y08.09
      baseball bat Y08.02
      hockey stick Y08.01
  submersion —*see* Assault, drowning
  violence Y09
  weapon Y09
    blunt Y00
    cutting or piercing —*see* Assault, cutting or
      piercing instrument
    firearm —*see* Assault, firearm
  wound Y09
    cutting —*see* Assault, cutting or piercing
      instrument
    gunshot —*see* Assault, firearm
    knife X99.1
    piercing —*see* Assault, cutting or piercing
      instrument
    puncture —*see* Assault, cutting or piercing
      instrument
    stab —*see* Assault, cutting or piercing
      instrument
Attack by mammals NEC W55.89
Avalanche —*see* Landslide ◀
Aviator's disease —*see* Air, pressure

B

Barotitis, barodontalgia, barosinusitis, barotrauma (otitic) (sinus) —*see* Air, pressure
Battered (baby) (child) (person) (syndrome) X58
Bayonet wound W26.1
  in
    legal intervention —*see* Legal, intervention, sharp object, bayonet
    war operations —*see* War operations, combat
  stated as undetermined whether accidental or intentional Y28.8
  suicide (attempt) X78.2
Bean in nose —*see* categories T17 and T18
Bed set on fire NEC —*see* Exposure, fire, uncontrolled, building, bed
Beheading (by guillotine)
  homicide X99.9
  legal execution —*see* Legal, intervention
Bending, injury in (prolonged) (static) X50.1 ◀▥
Bends —*see* Air, pressure, change
Bite, bitten by
  alligator W58.01
  arthropod (nonvenomous) NEC W57
  bull W55.21
  cat W55.01
  cow W55.21
  crocodile W58.11
  dog W54.0
  goat W55.31
  hoof stock NEC W55.31
  horse W55.11
  human being (accidentally) W50.3
    with intent to injure or kill Y04.1
    as, or caused by, a crowd or human stampede (with fall) W52
    assault Y04.1
    homicide (attempt) Y04.1
    in
      fight Y04.1
  insect (nonvenomous) W57
  lizard (nonvenomous) W59.01
  mammal NEC W55.81
    marine W56.31 ◀
  marine animal (nonvenomous) W56.81
  millipede W57
  moray eel W56.51
  mouse W53.01
  person (s) (accidentally) W50.3
    with intent to injure or kill Y04.1
    as, or caused by, a crowd or human stampede (with fall) W52
    assault Y04.1
    homicide (attempt) Y04.1
    in
      fight Y04.1
  pig W55.41
  raccoon W55.51
  rat W53.11
  reptile W59.81
    lizard W59.01
    snake W59.11
    turtle W59.21
      terrestrial W59.81
  rodent W53.81
    mouse W53.01
    rat W53.11
    specified NEC W53.81
    squirrel W53.21
  shark W56.41
  sheep W55.31
  snake (nonvenomous) W59.11
  spider (nonvenomous) W57
  squirrel W53.21
Blast (air) in war operations —*see* War operations, blast
Blizzard X37.2

Blood alcohol level Y90.9
  20-39mg/100ml Y90.1
  40-59mg/100ml Y90.2
  60-79mg/100ml Y90.3
  80-99mg/100ml Y90.4
  100-119mg/100ml Y90.5
  120-199mg/100ml Y90.6
  200-239mg/100ml Y90.7
  less than 20mg/100ml Y90.0
  presence in blood, level not specified Y90.9
Blow X58
  by law-enforcing agent, police (on duty) —*see* Legal, intervention, manhandling
    blunt object —*see* Legal, intervention, blunt object
Blowing up —*see* Explosion
Brawl (hand) (fists) (foot) Y04.0
Breakage (accidental) (part of)
  ladder (causing fall) W11
  scaffolding (causing fall) W12
Broken
  glass, contact with —*see* Contact, with, glass
  power line (causing electric shock) W85
Bumping against, into (accidentally)
  object NEC W22.8
    with fall —*see* Fall, due to, bumping against, object
    caused by crowd or human stampede (with fall) W52
    sports equipment W21.9
  person (s) W51
    with fall W03
      due to ice or snow W00.0
    assault Y04.2
    caused by, a crowd or human stampede (with fall) W52
    homicide (attempt) Y04.2
  sports equipment W21.9
Burn, burned, burning (accidental) (by) (from) (on)
  acid NEC —*see* Table of Drugs and Chemicals ◀▥
  bed linen —*see* Exposure, fire, uncontrolled, in building, bed
  blowtorch X08.8
    with ignition of clothing NEC X06.2
      nightwear X05
  bonfire, campfire (controlled) —*see also* Exposure, fire, controlled, not in building
    uncontrolled —*see* Exposure, fire, uncontrolled, not in building
  candle X08.8
    with ignition of clothing NEC X06.2
      nightwear X05
  caustic liquid, substance (external) (internal) NEC —*see* Table of Drugs and Chemicals ◀▥
  chemical (external) (internal) —*see also* Table of Drugs and Chemicals ◀▥
    in war operations —*see* War operations, fire
  cigar (s) or cigarette (s) X08.8
    with ignition of clothing NEC X06.2
      nightwear X05
  clothes, clothing NEC (from controlled fire) X06.2
    with conflagration —*see* Exposure, fire, uncontrolled, building
      not in building or structure —*see* Exposure, fire, uncontrolled, not in building
  cooker (hot) X15.8
    stated as undetermined whether accidental or intentional Y27.3
    suicide (attempt) X77.3
  electric blanket X16
  engine (hot) X17
  fire, flames —*see* Exposure, fire
  flare, Very pistol —*see* Discharge, firearm NEC

Burn, burned, burning (Continued)
  heat
    from appliance (electrical) (household) X15.8
      cooker X15.8
      hotplate X15.2
      kettle X15.8
      light bulb X15.8
      saucepan X15.3
      skillet X15.3
      stated as undetermined whether accidental or intentional Y27.3
      stove X15.0
      suicide (attempt) X77.3
      toaster X15.1
    in local application or packing during medical or surgical procedure Y63.5
  heating
    appliance, radiator or pipe X16
  homicide (attempt) —*see* Assault, burning
  hot
    air X14.1
    cooker X15.8
    drink X10.0
    engine X17
    fat X10.2
    fluid NEC X12
    food X10.1
    gases X14.1
    heating appliance X16
    household appliance NEC X15.8
    kettle X15.8
    liquid NEC X12
    machinery X17
    metal (molten) (liquid) NEC X18
    object (not producing fire or flames) NEC X19
    oil (cooking) X10.2
    pipe (s) X16
    radiator X16
    saucepan (glass) (metal) X15.3
    stove (kitchen) X15.0
    substance NEC X19
      caustic or corrosive NEC —*see* Table of Drugs and Chemicals ◀▥
    toaster X15.1
    tool X17
    vapor X13.1
    water (tap) —*see* Contact, with, hot, tap water
  hotplate X15.2
    suicide (attempt) X77.3
  ignition —*see* Ignition
  in war operations —*see* War operations, fire
  inflicted by other person X97
    by hot objects, hot vapor, and steam —*see* Assault, burning, hot object
  internal, from swallowed caustic, corrosive liquid, substance —*see* Table of Drugs and Chemicals ◀▥
  iron (hot) X15.8
    stated as undetermined whether accidental or intentional Y27.3
    suicide (attempt) X77.3
  kettle (hot) X15.8
    stated as undetermined whether accidental or intentional Y27.3
    suicide (attempt) X77.3
  lamp (flame) X08.8
    with ignition of clothing NEC X06.2
      nightwear X05
  lighter (cigar) (cigarette) X08.8
    with ignition of clothing NEC X06.2
      nightwear X05
  lightning —*see* subcategory T75.0
    causing fire —*see* Exposure, fire
  liquid (boiling) (hot) NEC X12
    stated as undetermined whether accidental or intentional Y27.2
    suicide (attempt) X77.2

Burn, burned, burning *(Continued)*
  local application of externally applied
      substance in medical or surgical care
      Y63.5
  machinery (hot) X17
  matches X08.8
      with ignition of clothing NEC X06.2
          nightwear X05
  mattress —*see* Exposure, fire, uncontrolled,
      building, bed
  medicament, externally applied Y63.5
  metal (hot) (liquid) (molten) NEC X18
  nightwear (nightclothes, nightdress, gown,
      pajamas, robe) X05
  object (hot) NEC X19
  on board watercraft
      due to
          accident to watercraft V91.09
              powered craft V91.03
                  ferry boat V91.01
                  fishing boat V91.02
                  jetskis V91.03
                  liner V91.01
                  merchant ship V91.00
                  passenger ship V91.01
              unpowered craft V91.08
                  canoe V91.05
                  inflatable V91.06
                  kayak V91.05
                  sailboat V91.04
                  surf-board V91.08
                  water skis V91.07
                  windsurfer V91.08
          fire on board V93.09
              ferry boat V93.01
              fishing boat V93.02
              jetskis V93.03
              liner V93.01
              merchant ship V93.00
              passenger ship V93.01
              powered craft NEC V93.03
              sailboat V93.04

Burn, burned, burning *(Continued)*
  on board watercraft *(Continued)*
      due to *(Continued)*
          specified heat source NEC on board
              V93.19
              ferry boat V93.11
              fishing boat V93.12
              jetskis V93.13
              liner V93.11
              merchant ship V93.10
              passenger ship V93.11
              powered craft V93.13
              sailboat V93.14
  pipe (hot) X16
      smoking X08.8
          with ignition of clothing NEC X06.2
              nightwear X05
  powder —*see* Powder burn
  radiator (hot) X16
  saucepan (hot) (glass) (metal) X15.3
      stated as undetermined whether
          accidental or intentional
          Y27.3
      suicide (attempt) X77.3
  self-inflicted X76
      stated as undetermined whether
          accidental or intentional
          Y26
  stated as undetermined whether
      accidental or intentional Y27.0
  steam X13.1
      pipe X16
          stated as undetermined whether
              accidental or intentional
              Y27.8
      stated as undetermined whether
          accidental or intentional Y27.0
      suicide (attempt) X77.0
  stove (hot) (kitchen) X15.0
      stated as undetermined whether
          accidental or intentional Y27.3
      suicide (attempt) X77.3

Burn, burned, burning *(Continued)*
  substance (hot) NEC X19
      boiling X12
          stated as undetermined whether
              accidental or intentional Y27.2
          suicide (attempt) X77.2
      molten (metal) X18
  suicide (attempt) NEC X76
      hot
          household appliance X77.3
          object X77.9
      stated as undetermined whether accidental or
          intentional Y27.0
  therapeutic misadventure
      heat in local application or packing during
          medical or surgical procedure Y63.5
      overdose of radiation Y63.2
  toaster (hot) X15.1
      stated as undetermined whether accidental
          or intentional Y27.3
      suicide (attempt) X77.3
  tool (hot) X17
  torch, welding X08.8
      with ignition of clothing NEC X06.2
          nightwear X05
  trash fire (controlled) —*see* Exposure, fire,
      controlled, not in building
      uncontrolled —*see* Exposure, fire,
          uncontrolled, not in building
  vapor (hot) X13.1
      stated as undetermined whether accidental
          or intentional Y27.0
      suicide (attempt) X77.0
  Very pistol —*see* Discharge, firearm NEC
Butted by animal W55.82
  bull W55.22
  cow W55.22
  goat W55.32
  horse W55.12
  pig W55.42
  sheep W55.32

◄ New   ◄▥ Revised   ~~deleted~~ Deleted

C

Caisson disease —*see* Air, pressure, change
Campfire (exposure to) (controlled) —*see also* Exposure, fire, controlled, not in building
uncontrolled —*see* Exposure, fire, uncontrolled, not in building
Capital punishment (any means) —*see* Legal, intervention
Car sickness T75.3
Casualty (not due to war) NEC X58
war —*see* War operations
Cat
bite W55.Ø1
scratch W55.Ø3
Cataclysm, cataclysmic (any injury) NEC —*see* Forces of nature
Catching fire —*see* Exposure, fire
Caught
between
folding object W23.Ø
objects (moving) (stationary and moving) W23.Ø
and machinery —*see* Contact, with, by type of machine
stationary W23.1
sliding door and door frame W23.Ø
by, in
machinery (moving parts of) —*see* Contact, with, by type of machine
washing-machine wringer W23.Ø
under packing crate (due to losing grip) W23.1
Cave-in caused by cataclysmic earth surface movement or eruption —*see* Landslide
Change(s) in air pressure —*see* Air, pressure, change
Choked, choking (on) (any object except food or vomitus)
food (bone) (seed) —*see* categories T17 and T18
vomitus T17.81-
Civil insurrection —*see* War operations
Cloudburst (any injury) X37.8
Cold, exposure to (accidental) (excessive) (extreme) (natural) (place) NEC —*see* Exposure, cold
Collapse
building W2Ø.1
burning (uncontrolled fire) XØØ.2
dam or man-made structure (causing earth movement) X36.Ø
machinery —*see* Contact, with, by type of machine
structure W2Ø.1
burning (uncontrolled fire) XØØ.2
Collision (accidental) NEC —*see also* Accident, transport V89.9
pedestrian W51
with fall WØ3
due to ice or snow WØØ.Ø
involving pedestrian conveyance —*see* Accident, transport, pedestrian, conveyance
and
crowd or human stampede (with fall) W52
object W22.8
with fall —*see* Fall, due to, bumping against, object
person (s) —*see* Collision, pedestrian
transport vehicle NEC V89.9
and
avalanche, fallen or not moving —*see* Accident, transport
falling or moving —*see* Landslide ◀
landslide, fallen or not moving —*see* Accident, transport
falling or moving —*see* Landslide

Collision NEC (*Continued*)
transport vehicle NEC (*Continued*)
due to cataclysm —*see* Forces of nature, by type
intentional, purposeful suicide (attempt) —*see* Suicide, collision
Combustion, spontaneous —*see* Ignition
Complication (delayed) of or following (medical or surgical procedure) Y84.9
with misadventure —*see* Misadventure
amputation of limb (s) Y83.5
anastomosis (arteriovenous) (blood vessel) (gastrojejunal) (tendon) (natural or artificial material) Y83.2
aspiration (of fluid) Y84.4
tissue Y84.8
biopsy Y84.8
blood
sampling Y84.7
transfusion
procedure Y84.8
bypass Y83.2
catheterization (urinary) Y84.6
cardiac Y84.Ø
colostomy Y83.3
cystostomy Y83.3
dialysis (kidney) Y84.1
drug —*see* Table of Drugs and Chemicals ◀⃘
due to misadventure —*see* Misadventure
duodenostomy Y83.3
electroshock therapy Y84.3
external stoma, creation of Y83.3
formation of external stoma Y83.3
gastrostomy Y83.3
graft Y83.2
hypothermia (medically-induced) Y84.8
implant, implantation (of)
artificial
internal device (cardiac pacemaker) (electrodes in brain) (heart valve prosthesis) (orthopedic) Y83.1
material or tissue (for anastomosis or bypass) Y83.2
with creation of external stoma Y83.3
natural tissues (for anastomosis or bypass) Y83.2
with creation of external stoma Y83.3
infusion
procedure Y84.8
injection —*see* Table of Drugs and Chemicals ◀⃘
procedure Y84.8
insertion of gastric or duodenal sound Y84.5
insulin-shock therapy Y84.3
paracentesis (abdominal) (thoracic) (aspirative) Y84.4
procedures other than surgical operation —*see* Complication of or following, by type of procedure
radiological procedure or therapy Y84.2
removal of organ (partial) (total) NEC Y83.6
sampling
blood Y84.7
fluid NEC Y84.4
tissue Y84.8
shock therapy Y84.3
surgical operation NEC —*see also* Complication of or following, by type of operation Y83.9
reconstructive NEC Y83.4
with
anastomosis, bypass or graft Y83.2
formation of external stoma Y83.3
specified NEC Y83.8
transfusion —*see also* Table of Drugs and Chemicals ◀⃘
procedure Y84.8
transplant, transplantation (heart) (kidney) (liver) (whole organ, any) Y83.Ø
partial organ Y83.4
ureterostomy Y83.3

Complication of or following (*Continued*)
vaccination —*see also* Table of Drugs and Chemicals ◀⃘
procedure Y84.8
Compression
divers' squeeze —*see* Air, pressure, change
trachea by
food (lodged in esophagus) —*see* categories T17 and T18
vomitus (lodged in esophagus) T17.81-
Conflagration —*see* Exposure, fire, uncontrolled
Constriction (external)
hair W49.Ø1
jewelry W49.Ø4
ring W49.Ø4
rubber band W49.Ø3
specified item NEC W49.Ø9
string W49.Ø2
thread W49.Ø2
Contact (accidental)
with
abrasive wheel (metalworking) W31.1
alligator W58.Ø9
bite W58.Ø1
crushing W58.Ø3
strike W58.Ø2
amphibian W62.9
frog W62.Ø
toad W62.1
animal (nonvenomous) NEC W64
marine W56.89
bite W56.81
dolphin —*see* Contact, with, dolphin
fish NEC —*see* Contact, with, fish
mammal —*see* Contact, with, mammal, marine
orca —*see* Contact, with, orca
sea lion —*see* Contact, with, sea lion
shark —*see* Contact, with, shark
strike W56.82
animate mechanical force NEC W64
arrow W21.89
not thrown, projected or falling W45.8
arthropods (nonvenomous) W57
axe W27.Ø
band-saw (industrial) W31.2
bayonet —*see* Bayonet wound
bee (s) X58
bench-saw (industrial) W31.2
bird W61.99
bite W61.91
chicken —*see* Contact, with, chicken
duck —*see* Contact, with, duck
goose —*see* Contact, with, goose
macaw —*see* Contact, with, macaw
parrot —*see* Contact, with, parrot
psittacine —*see* Contact, with, psittacine
strike W61.92
turkey —*see* Contact, with, turkey
blender W29.Ø
boiling water X12
stated as undetermined whether accidental or intentional Y27.2
suicide (attempt) X77.2
bore, earth-drilling or mining (land) (seabed) W31.Ø
buffalo —*see* Contact, with, hoof stock NEC
bull W55.29
bite W55.21
gored W55.22
strike W55.22
bumper cars W31.81
camel —*see* Contact, with, hoof stock NEC
can
lid W26.8 ◀⃘
opener W27.4
powered W29.Ø
cat W55.Ø9
bite W55.Ø1
scratch W55.Ø3
caterpillar (venomous) X58

Contact *(Continued)*
  with *(Continued)*
    centipede (venomous) X58
    chain
      hoist W24.0
        agricultural operations W30.89
      saw W29.3
    chicken W61.39
      peck W61.33
      strike W61.32
    chisel W27.0
    circular saw W31.2
    cobra X58
    combine (harvester) W30.0
    conveyer belt W24.1
    cooker (hot) X15.8
      stated as undetermined whether
        accidental or intentional Y27.3
      suicide (attempt) X77.3
    coral X58
    cotton gin W31.82
    cow W55.29
      bite W55.21
      strike W55.22
    crane W24.0
      agricultural operations W30.89
    crocodile W58.19
      bite W58.11
      crushing W58.13
      strike W58.12
    dagger W26.1
      stated as undetermined whether
        accidental or intentional Y28.2
      suicide (attempt) X78.2
    dairy equipment W31.82
    dart W21.89
      not thrown, projected or falling W45.8
    deer —*see* Contact, with, hoof stock
      NEC
    derrick W24.0
      agricultural operations W30.89
        hay W30.2
    dog W54.8
      bite W54.0
      strike W54.1
    dolphin W56.09
      bite W56.01
      strike W56.02
    donkey —*see* Contact, with, hoof stock
      NEC
    drill (powered) W29.8
      earth (land) (seabed) W31.0
      nonpowered W27.8
    drive belt W24.0
      agricultural operations W30.89
    dry ice —*see* Exposure, cold, man-made
    dryer (clothes) (powered) (spin) W29.2
    duck W61.69
      bite W61.61
      strike W61.62
    earth(-)
      drilling machine (industrial) W31.0
      scraping machine in stationary use
        W31.83
    edge of stiff paper W26.2 ◀▥
    electric
      beater W29.0
      blanket X16
      fan W29.2
        commercial W31.82
      knife W29.1
      mixer W29.0
    elevator (building) W24.0
      agricultural operations W30.89
        grain W30.3
    engine (s), hot NEC X17
    excavating machine W31.0
    farm machine W30.9
    feces —*see* Contact, with, by type of
      animal
    fer de lance X58

Contact *(Continued)*
  with *(Continued)*
    fish W56.59
      bite W56.51
      shark —*see* Contact, with, shark
      strike W56.52
    flying horses W31.81
    forging (metalworking) machine
      W31.1
    fork W27.4
    forklift (truck) W24.0
      agricultural operations W30.89
    frog W62.0
    garden
      cultivator (powered) W29.3
        riding W30.89
      fork W27.1
    gas turbine W31.3
    Gila monster X58
    giraffe —*see* Contact, with, hoof stock
      NEC
    glass (sharp) (broken) W25
      with subsequent fall W18.02
      assault X99.0
      due to fall —*see* Fall, by type
      stated as undetermined whether
        accidental or intentional Y28. 0
      suicide (attempt) X78.0
    goat W55.39
      bite W55.31
      strike W55.32
    goose W61.59
      bite W61.51
      strike W61.52
    hand
      saw W27.0
      tool (not powered) NEC W27.8
        powered W29.8
    harvester W30.0
    hay-derrick W30.2
    heat NEC X19
      from appliance (electrical)
        (household) —*see* Contact, with,
        hot, household appliance
      heating appliance X16
    heating
      appliance (hot) X16
      pad (electric) X16
    hedge-trimmer (powered) W29.3
    hoe W27.1
    hoist (chain) (shaft) NEC W24.0
      agricultural W30.89
    hoof stock NEC W55.39
      bite W55.31
      strike W55.32
    hornet (s) X58
    horse W55.19
      bite W55.11
      strike W55.12
    hot
      air X14.1
        inhalation X14.0
      cooker X15.8
      drinks X10.0
      engine X17
      fats X10.2
      fluids NEC X12
        assault X98.2
        suicide (attempt) X77.2
        undetermined whether accidental or
          intentional Y27.2
      food X10.1
      gases X14.1
        inhalation X14.0
      heating appliance X16
      household appliance X15.8
        assault X98.3
        cooker X15.8
        hotplate X15.2
        kettle X15.8
        light bulb X15.8

Contact *(Continued)*
  with *(Continued)*
    hot *(Continued)*
      household appliance *(Continued)*
        object NEC X19
          assault X98.8
          stated as undetermined whether
            accidental or intentional Y27.9
          suicide (attempt) X77.8
        saucepan X15.3
        skillet X15.3
        stated as undetermined whether
          accidental or intentional Y27.3
        stove X15.0
        suicide (attempt) X77.3
        toaster X15.1
      kettle X15.8
      light bulb X15.8
      liquid NEC —*see also* Burn X12 ◀▥
        drinks X10.0
        stated as undetermined whether
          accidental or intentional Y27.2
        suicide (attempt) X77.2
        tap water X11.8
          stated as undetermined whether
            accidental or intentional Y27.1
          suicide (attempt) X77.1
      machinery X17
      metal (molten) (liquid) NEC X18
      object (not producing fire or flames)
        NEC X19
      oil (cooking) X10.2
      pipe X16
      plate X15.2
      radiator X16
      saucepan (glass) (metal) X15.3
      skillet X15.3
      stove (kitchen) X15.0
      substance NEC X19
      tap-water X11.8
        assault X98.1
        heated on stove X12
          stated as undetermined whether
            accidental or intentional Y27.2
          suicide (attempt) X77.2
        in bathtub X11.0
        running X11.1
        stated as undetermined whether
          accidental or intentional Y27.1
        suicide (attempt) X77.1
      toaster X15.1
      tool X17
      vapors X13.1
        inhalation X13.0
      water (tap) X11.8
        boiling X12
          stated as undetermined whether
            accidental or intentional Y27.2
          suicide (attempt) X77.2
        heated on stove X12
          stated as undetermined whether
            accidental or intentional Y27.2
          suicide (attempt) X77.2
        in bathtub X11.0
        running X11.1
        stated as undetermined whether
          accidental or intentional Y27.1
        suicide (attempt) X77.1
    hotplate X15.2
    ice-pick W27.4
    insect (nonvenomous) NEC W57
    kettle (hot) X15.8
    knife W26.0
      assault X99.1
      electric W29.1
      stated as undetermined whether
        accidental or intentional Y28.1
      suicide (attempt) X78.1
    lathe (metalworking) W31.1
      turnings W45.8
      woodworking W31.2

◀ New   ◀▥ Revised   ~~deleted~~ Deleted

Contact *(Continued)*
  with *(Continued)*
    lawnmower (powered) (ridden) W28
      causing electrocution W86.8
        suicide (attempt) X83.1
      unpowered W27.1
    lift, lifting (devices) W24.0
      agricultural operations W30.89
      shaft W24.0
    liquefied gas —*see* Exposure, cold,
      man-made
    liquid air, hydrogen, nitrogen —*see*
      Exposure, cold, man-made
    lizard (nonvenomous) W59.09
      bite W59.01
      strike W59.02
    llama —*see* Contact, with, hoof stock NEC
    macaw W61.19
      bite W61.11
      strike W61.12
    machine, machinery W31.9
      abrasive wheel W31.1
      agricultural including animal-powered
        W30.9
        combine harvester W30.0
        grain storage elevator W30.3
        hay derrick W30.2
        power take-off device W30.1
        reaper W30.0
        specified NEC W30.89
        thresher W30.0
        transport vehicle, stationary W30.81
      band saw W31.2
      bench saw W31.2
      circular saw W31.2
      commercial NEC W31.82
      drilling, metal (industrial) W31.1
      earth-drilling W31.0
      earthmoving or scraping W31.89
      excavating W31.89
      forging machine W31.1
      gas turbine W31.3
      hot X17
      internal combustion engine W31.3
      land drill W31.0
      lathe W31.1
      lifting (devices) W24.0
      metal drill W31.1
      metalworking (industrial) W31.1
      milling, metal W31.1
      mining W31.0
      molding W31.2
      overhead plane W31.2
      power press, metal W31.1
      prime mover W31.3
      printing W31.89
      radial saw W31.2
      recreational W31.81
      roller-coaster W31.81
      rolling mill, metal W31.1
      sander W31.2
      seabed drill W31.0
      shaft
        hoist W31.0
        lift W31.0
      specified NEC W31.89
      spinning W31.89
      steam engine W31.3
      transmission W24.1
      undercutter W31.0
      water driven turbine W31.3
      weaving W31.89
      woodworking or forming (industrial)
        W31.2
    mammal (feces) (urine) W55.89
      bull —*see* Contact, with, bull
      cat —*see* Contact, with, cat
      cow —*see* Contact, with, cow
      goat —*see* Contact, with, goat
      hoof stock —*see* Contact, with, hoof
        stock

Contact *(Continued)*
  with *(Continued)*
    mammal *(Continued)*
      horse —*see* Contact, with, horse
      marine W56.39
        dolphin —*see* Contact, with, dolphin
        orca —*see* Contact, with, orca
        sea lion —*see* Contact, with, sea lion
        specified NEC W56.39
          bite W56.31
          strike W56.32
      pig —*see* Contact, with, pig
      raccoon —*see* Contact, with, raccoon
      rodent —*see* Contact, with, rodent
      sheep —*see* Contact, with, sheep
      specified NEC W55.89
        bite W55.81
        strike W55.82
    marine
      animal W56.89
        bite W56.81
        dolphin —*see* Contact, with, dolphin
        fish NEC —*see* Contact, with, fish
        mammal —*see* Contact, with,
          mammal, marine
        orca —*see* Contact, with, orca
        sea lion —*see* Contact, with, sea lion
        shark —*see* Contact, with, shark
        strike W56.82
    meat
      grinder (domestic) W29.0
        industrial W31.82
        nonpowered W27.4
      slicer (domestic) W29.0
        industrial W31.82
    merry go round W31.81
    metal, (hot) (liquid) (molten) NEC X18
    millipede W57
    nail W45.0
      gun W29.4
    needle (sewing) W27.3
      hypodermic W46.0
        contaminated W46.1
    object (blunt) NEC
      hot NEC X19
      legal intervention —*see* Legal,
        intervention, blunt object
      sharp NEC W45.8
        inflicted by other person NEC W45.8
          stated as
            intentional homicide (attempt) —
              see Assault, cutting or
              piercing instrument
        legal intervention —*see* Legal,
          intervention, sharp object
        self-inflicted X78.9
    orca W56.29
      bite W56.21
      strike W56.22
    overhead plane W31.2
    paper (as sharp object) W26.2 ◀▥
    paper-cutter W27.5
    parrot W61.09
      bite W61.01
      strike W61.02
    pig W55.49
      bite W55.41
      strike W55.42
    pipe, hot X16
    pitchfork W27.1
    plane (metal) (wood) W27.0
      overhead W31.2
    plant thorns, spines, sharp leaves or other
      mechanisms W60
    powered
      garden cultivator W29.3
      household appliance, implement, or
        machine W29.8
      saw (industrial) W31.2
        hand W29.8
    printing machine W31.89

Contact *(Continued)*
  with *(Continued)*
    psittacine bird W61.29
      bite W61.21
      macaw —*see* Contact, with, macaw ◀▥
      parrot —*see* Contact, with, parrot
      strike W61.22
    pulley (block) (transmission) W24.0
      agricultural operations W30.89
    raccoon W55.59
      bite W55.51
      strike W55.52
    radial-saw (industrial) W31.2
    radiator (hot) X16
    rake W27.1
    rattlesnake X58
    reaper W30.0
    reptile W59.89
      lizard —*see* Contact, with, lizard
      snake —*see* Contact, with, snake
      specified NEC W59.89
        bite W59.81
        crushing W59.83
        strike W59.82
      turtle —*see* Contact, with, turtle
    rivet gun (powered) W29.4
    road scraper —*see* Accident, transport,
      construction vehicle
    rodent (feces) (urine) W53.89
      bite W53.81
      mouse W53.09
        bite W53.01
      rat W53.19
        bite W53.11
      specified NEC W53.89
        bite W53.81
      squirrel W53.29
        bite W53.21
    roller coaster W31.81
    rope NEC W24.0
      agricultural operations W30.89
    saliva —*see* Contact, with, by type of
      animal
    sander W29.8
      industrial W31.2
    saucepan (hot) (glass) (metal) X15.3
    saw W27.0
      band (industrial) W31.2
      bench (industrial) W31.2
      chain W29.3
      hand W27.0
    sawing machine, metal W31.1
    scissors W27.2
    scorpion X58
    screwdriver W27.0
      powered W29.8
    sea
      anemone, cucumber or urchin (spine)
        X58
      lion W56.19
        bite W56.11
        strike W56.12
    serpent —*see* Contact, with, snake, by type
    sewing-machine (electric) (powered) W29.2
      not powered W27.8
    shaft (hoist) (lift) (transmission) NEC W24.0
      agricultural W30.89
    shark W56.49
      bite W56.41
      strike W56.42
    sharp object(s) W26.9 ◀
      specified NEC W26.8 ◀
    shears (hand) W27.2
      powered (industrial) W31.1
        domestic W29.2
    sheep W55.39
      bite W55.31
      strike W55.32
    shovel W27.8
      steam —*see* Accident, transport,
        construction vehicle

Contact *(Continued)*
  with *(Continued)*
    snake (nonvenomous) W59.19
      bite W59.11
      crushing W59.13
      strike W59.12
    spade W27.1
    spider (venomous) X58
    spin-drier W29.2
    spinning machine W31.89
    splinter W45.8
    sports equipment W21.9
    staple gun (powered) W29.8
    steam X13.1
      engine W31.3
      inhalation X13.0
      pipe X16
      shovel W31.89
    stove (hot) (kitchen) X15.0
    substance, hot NEC X19
      molten (metal) X18
    sword W26.1
      assault X99.2
      stated as undetermined whether
        accidental or intentional
        Y28.2
      suicide (attempt) X78.2
    tarantula X58
    thresher W30.0
    tin can lid W26.8 ◀▥
    toad W62.1
    toaster (hot) X15.1
    tool W27.8
      hand (not powered) W27.8
        auger W27.0
        axe W27.0
        can opener W27.4
        chisel W27.0
        fork W27.4
        garden W27.1
        handsaw W27.0
        hoe W27.1
        ice-pick W27.4
        kitchen utensil W27.4
        manual
          lawn mower W27.1
          sewing machine W27.8
        meat grinder W27.4
        needle (sewing) W27.3
          hypodermic W46.0
            contaminated W46.1
        paper cutter W27.5
        pitchfork W27.1
        rake W27.1
        scissors W27.2
        screwdriver W27.0
        specified NEC W27.8
        workbench W27.0
      hot X17
      powered W29.8
        blender W29.0
          commercial W31.82
        can opener W29.0
          commercial W31.82
        chainsaw W29.3
        clothes dryer W29.2
          commercial W31.82
        dishwasher W29.2
          commercial W31.82
        edger W29.3
        electric fan W29.2
          commercial W31.82
        electric knife W29.1
        food processor W29.0
          commercial W31.82
        garbage disposal W29.0
          commercial W31.82

Contact *(Continued)*
  with *(Continued)*
    tool *(Continued)*
      powered *(Continued)*
        garden tool W29.3
        hedge trimmer W29.3
        ice maker W29.0
          commercial W31.82
        kitchen appliance W29.0
          commercial W31.82
        lawn mower W28
        meat grinder W29.0
          commercial W31.82
        mixer W29.0
          commercial W31.82
        rototiller W29.3
        sewing machine W29.2
          commercial W31.82
        washing machine W29.2
          commercial W31.82
      transmission device (belt, cable, chain,
        gear, pinion, shaft) W24.1
        agricultural operations W30.89
      turbine (gas) (water-driven) W31.3
      turkey W61.49
        peck W61.43
        strike W61.42
      turtle (nonvenomous) W59.29
        bite W59.21
        strike W59.22
        terrestrial W59.89
          bite W59.81
          crushing W59.83
          strike W59.82
      under-cutter W31.0
      urine —*see* Contact, with, by type of animal
      vehicle
        agricultural use (transport) —*see*
          Accident, transport, agricultural
          vehicle
          not on public highway W30.81
        industrial use (transport) —*see*
          Accident, transport, industrial
          vehicle
          not on public highway W31.83
        off-road use (transport) —*see* Accident,
          transport, all-terrain or off-road
          vehicle
          not on public highway W31.83
        special construction use (transport) —*see*
          Accident, transport, construction
          vehicle
          not on public highway W31.83
      venomous
        animal X58
        arthropods X58
        lizard X58
        marine animal NEC X58
        marine plant NEC X58
        millipedes (tropical) X58
        plant (s) X58
        snake X58
        spider X58
      viper X58
      washing-machine (powered) W29.2
      wasp X58
      weaving-machine W31.89
      winch W24.0
        agricultural operations W30.89
      wire NEC W24.0
        agricultural operations W30.89
      wood slivers W45.8
      yellow jacket X58
      zebra —*see* Contact, with, hoof stock NEC
    pressure X50.9 ◀
    stress X50.9 ◀
Coup de soleil X32

Crash
  aircraft (in transit) (powered) V95.9
    balloon V96.01
    fixed wing NEC (private) V95.21
      commercial V95.31
    glider V96.21
      hang V96.11
      powered V95.11
    helicopter V95.01
    in war operations —*see* War operations,
      destruction of aircraft
    microlight V95.11
    nonpowered V96.9
      specified NEC V96.8
    powered NEC V95.8
    stated as
      homicide (attempt) Y08.81
      suicide (attempt) X83.0
    ultralight V95.11
  spacecraft V95.41
  transport vehicle NEC —*see also* Accident,
    transport V89.9
    homicide (attempt) Y03.8
    motor NEC (traffic) V89.2
      homicide (attempt) Y03.8
      suicide (attempt) —*see* Suicide, collision
Cruelty (mental) (physical) (sexual) X58
Crushed (accidentally) X58
  between objects (moving) (stationary and
    moving) W23.0
    stationary W23.1
  by
    alligator W58.03
    avalanche NEC —*see* Landslide ◀
    cave-in W20.0
      caused by cataclysmic earth surface
        movement —*see* Landslide ◀
    crocodile W58.13
    crowd or human stampede W52
    falling
      aircraft V97.39
        in war operations —*see* War
          operations, destruction of aircraft
      earth, material W20.0
        caused by cataclysmic earth surface
          movement —*see* Landslide
      object NEC W20.8
    landslide NEC —*see* Landslide ◀
    lizard (nonvenomous) W59.09
    machinery —*see* Contact, with, by type of
      machine
    reptile NEC W59.89
    snake (nonvenomous) W59.13
  in
    machinery —*see* Contact, with, by type of
      machine
Cut, cutting (any part of body) (accidental) —
    see also Contact, with, by object or machine
  during medical or surgical treatment as
    misadventure —*see* Index to Diseases
    and Injuries, Complications ◀▥
  homicide (attempt) —*see* Assault, cutting or
    piercing instrument
  inflicted by other person —*see* Assault,
    cutting or piercing instrument
  legal
    execution —*see* Legal, intervention
    intervention —*see* Legal, intervention,
      sharp object
  machine NEC —*see also* Contact, with, by
    type of machine W31.9
  self-inflicted —*see* Suicide, cutting or piercing
    instrument
  suicide (attempt) —*see* Suicide, cutting or
    piercing instrument
Cyclone (any injury) X37.1

◀ New   ◀▥ Revised   ~~deleted~~ Deleted

D

Decapitation (accidental circumstances)
  NEC X58
  homicide X99.9
  legal execution —*see* Legal, intervention
Dehydration from lack of water X58
Deprivation X58
Derailment (accidental)
  railway (rolling stock) (train) (vehicle)
    (without antecedent collision) V81.7
    with antecedent collision —*see* Accident,
      transport, railway vehicle occupant
  streetcar (without antecedent collision)
    V82.7
    with antecedent collision —*see* Accident,
      transport, streetcar occupant
Descent
  parachute (voluntary) (without accident to
    aircraft) V97.29
  due to accident to aircraft —*see* Accident,
    transport, aircraft
Desertion X58
Destitution X58
Disability, late effect or sequela of injury —*see*
  Sequelae
Discharge (accidental)
  airgun W34.010
    assault X95.01
    homicide (attempt) X95.01
    stated as undetermined whether accidental
      or intentional Y24.0
    suicide (attempt) X74.01
  BB gun —*see* Discharge, airgun
  firearm (accidental) W34.00
    assault X95.9
    handgun (pistol) (revolver) W32.0
      assault X93
      homicide (attempt) X93
      legal intervention —*see* Legal,
        intervention, firearm, handgun
      stated as undetermined whether
        accidental or intentional Y22
      suicide (attempt) X72
    homicide (attempt) X95.9
    hunting rifle W33.02
      assault X94.1
      homicide (attempt) X94.1
      legal intervention
        injuring
          bystander Y35.032
          law enforcement personnel
            Y35.031
          suspect Y35.033
      stated as undetermined whether
        accidental or intentional Y23.1
      suicide (attempt) X73.1
    larger W33.00
      assault X94.9
      homicide (attempt) X94.9
      hunting rifle —*see* Discharge, firearm,
        hunting rifle
      legal intervention —*see* Legal,
        intervention, firearm by type of
        firearm
      machine gun —*see* Discharge, firearm,
        machine gun
      shotgun —*see* Discharge, firearm,
        shotgun
      specified NEC W33.09
        assault X94.8
        homicide (attempt) X94.8
        legal intervention
          injuring
            bystander Y35.092
            law enforcement personnel
              Y35.091
            suspect Y35.093
        stated as undetermined whether
          accidental or intentional Y23.8
        suicide (attempt) X73.8

Discharge (*Continued*)
  firearm (*Continued*)
    larger (*Continued*)
      stated as undetermined whether
        accidental or intentional Y23.9
      suicide (attempt) X73.9
    legal intervention
      injuring
        bystander Y35.002
        law enforcement personnel Y35.001
        suspect Y35.03
      using rubber bullet
        injuring
          bystander Y35.042
          law enforcement personnel
            Y35.041
          suspect Y35.043
    machine gun W33.03
      assault X94.2
      homicide (attempt) X94.2
      legal intervention —*see* Legal,
        intervention, firearm, machine gun
      stated as undetermined whether
        accidental or intentional Y23.3
      suicide (attempt) X73.2
    pellet gun —*see* Discharge, airgun
    shotgun W33.01
      assault X94.0
      homicide (attempt) X94.0
      legal intervention —*see* Legal,
        intervention, firearm, specified NEC
      stated as undetermined whether
        accidental or intentional Y23.0
      suicide (attempt) X73.0
    specified NEC W34.09
      assault X95.8
      homicide (attempt) X95.8
      legal intervention —*see* Legal,
        intervention, firearm, specified NEC
      stated as undetermined whether
        accidental or intentional Y24.8
      suicide (attempt) X74.8
    stated as undetermined whether accidental
      or intentional Y24.9
    suicide (attempt) X74.9
    Very pistol W34.09
      assault X95.8
      homicide (attempt) X95.8
      stated as undetermined whether
        accidental or intentional Y24.8
      suicide (attempt) X74.8
  firework (s) W39
    stated as undetermined whether accidental
      or intentional Y25
  gas-operated gun NEC W34.018
    airgun —*see* Discharge, airgun
    assault X95.09
    homicide (attempt) X95.09
    paintball gun —*see* Discharge, paintball
      gun
    stated as undetermined whether accidental
      or intentional Y24.8
    suicide (attempt) X74.09
  gun NEC —*see also* Discharge, firearm NEC
    air —*see* Discharge, airgun
    BB —*see* Discharge, airgun
    for single hand use —*see* Discharge,
      firearm, handgun
    hand —*see* Discharge, firearm, handgun
    machine —*see* Discharge, firearm, machine
      gun
    other specified —*see* Discharge, firearm
      NEC
    paintball —*see* Discharge, paintball gun
    pellet —*see* Discharge, airgun
  handgun —*see* Discharge, firearm, handgun
  machine gun —*see* Discharge, firearm,
    machine gun
  paintball gun W34.011
    assault X95.02
    homicide (attempt) X95.02

Discharge (*Continued*)
  paintball gun (*Continued*)
    stated as undetermined whether accidental
      or intentional Y24.8
    suicide (attempt) X74.02
  pistol —*see* Discharge, firearm, handgun
    flare —*see* Discharge, firearm, Very pistol
    pellet —*see* Discharge, airgun
    Very —*see* Discharge, firearm, Very pistol
  revolver —*see* Discharge, firearm, handgun
  rifle (hunting) —*see* Discharge, firearm,
    hunting rifle
  shotgun —*see* Discharge, firearm, shotgun
  spring-operated gun NEC W34.018
    assault X95.09
    homicide (attempt) X95.09
    stated as undetermined whether accidental
      or intentional Y24.8
    suicide (attempt) X74.09
Disease
  Andes W94.11
  aviator's —*see* Air, pressure
  range W94.11
Diver's disease, palsy, paralysis, squeeze —*see*
  Air, pressure
Diving (into water) —*see* Accident, diving
Dog bite W54.0
Dragged by transport vehicle NEC —*see also*
  Accident, transport V09.9
Drinking poison (accidental) —*see* Table of
  Drugs and Chemicals ◀▥
Dropped (accidentally) while being carried or
  supported by other person W04
Drowning (accidental) W74
  assault X92.9
  due to
    accident (to)
      machinery —*see* Contact, with, by type
        of machine
      watercraft V90.89
        burning V90.29
          powered V90.23
            fishing boat V90.22
            jetskis V90.23
            merchant ship V90.20
            passenger ship V90.21
          unpowered V90.28
            canoe V90.25
            inflatable V90.26
            kayak V90.25
            sailboat V90.24
            water skis V90.27
        crushed V90.39
          powered V90.33
            fishing boat V90.32
            jetskis V90.33
            merchant ship V90.30
            passenger ship V90.31
          unpowered V90.38
            canoe V90.35
            inflatable V90.36
            kayak V90.35
            sailboat V90.34
            water skis V90.37
        overturning V90.09
          powered V90.03
            fishing boat V90.02
            jetskis V90.03
            merchant ship V90.00
            passenger ship V90.01
          unpowered V90.08
            canoe V90.05
            inflatable V90.06
            kayak V90.05
            sailboat V90.04
        sinking V90.19
          powered V90.13
            fishing boat V90.12
            jetskis V90.13
            merchant ship V90.10
            passenger ship V90.11

Drowning (Continued)
  due to (Continued)
    accident (Continued)
      watercraft (Continued)
        sinking (Continued)
          unpowered V90.18
            canoe V90.15
            inflatable V90.16
            kayak V90.15
            sailboat V90.14
          specified type NEC V90.89
          powered V90.83
            fishing boat V90.82
            jetskis V90.83
            merchant ship V90.80
            passenger ship V90.81
          unpowered V90.88
            canoe V90.85
            inflatable V90.86
            kayak V90.85
            sailboat V90.84
            water skis V90.87
    avalanche —see Landslide ◀
    cataclysmic
      earth surface movement NEC —see
        Forces of nature, earth movement ◀
      storm —see Forces of nature, cataclysmic
        storm ◀
    cloudburst X37.8
    cyclone X37.1
    fall overboard (from) V92.09
      powered craft V92.03
        ferry boat V92.01
        fishing boat V92.02
        jetskis V92.03
        liner V92.01
        merchant ship V92.00
        passenger ship V92.01
      resulting from
        accident to watercraft —see Drowning,
          due to, accident to, watercraft
        being washed overboard (from)
          V92.29
          powered craft V92.23
            ferry boat V92.21
            fishing boat V92.22
            jetskis V92.23
            liner V92.21
            merchant ship V92.20
            passenger ship V92.21
          unpowered craft V92.28
            canoe V92.25
            inflatable V92.26
            kayak V92.25
            sailboat V92.24
            surf-board V92.28
            water skis V92.27
            windsurfer V92.28
        motion of watercraft V92.19
          powered craft V92.13
            ferry boat V92.11
            fishing boat V92.12
            jetskis V92.13
            liner V92.11
            merchant ship V92.10
            passenger ship V92.11
          unpowered craft
            canoe V92.15
            inflatable V92.16
            kayak V92.15
            sailboat V92.14
      unpowered craft V92.08
        canoe V92.05
        inflatable V92.06
        kayak V92.05

Drowning (Continued)
  due to (Continued)
    fall overboard (Continued)
      unpowered craft (Continued)
        sailboat V92.04
        surf-board V92.08
        water skis V92.07
        windsurfer V92.08
    hurricane X37.0
    jumping into water from watercraft
      (involved in accident) —see also
      Drowning, due to, accident to,
      watercraft
      without accident to or on watercraft
        W16.711
    tidal wave NEC —see Forces of nature,
      tidal wave ◀
    torrential rain X37.8
  following
    fall
      into
        bathtub W16.211
        bucket W16.221
        fountain —see Drowning, following,
          fall, into, water, specified NEC
        quarry —see Drowning, following,
          fall, into, water, specified NEC
        reservoir —see Drowning, following,
          fall, into, water, specified NEC
        swimming-pool W16.011
          stated as undetermined whether
            accidental or intentional
            Y21.3
          striking
            bottom W16.021
            wall W16.031
          suicide (attempt) X71.2
        water NOS W16.41
          natural (lake) (open sea) (river)
            (stream) (pond) W16.111
            striking
              bottom W16.121
              side W16.131
          specified NEC W16.311
            striking
              bottom W16.321
              wall W16.331
      overboard NEC —see Drowning, due to,
        fall overboard
    jump or dive
      from boat W16.711
        striking bottom W16.721
      into
        fountain —see Drowning, following,
          jump or dive, into, water,
          specified NEC
        quarry —see Drowning, following,
          jump or dive, into, water,
          specified NEC
        reservoir —see Drowning, following,
          jump or dive, into, water,
          specified NEC
        swimming-pool W16.511
          striking
            bottom W16.521
            wall W16.531
          suicide (attempt) X71.2
        water NOS W16.91
          natural (lake) (open sea) (river)
            (stream) (pond) W16.611
          specified NEC W16.811
            striking
             bottom W16.821
             wall W16.831
          striking bottom W16.621

Drowning (Continued)
  homicide (attempt) X92.9
  in
    bathtub (accidental) W65
      assault X92.0
      following fall W16.211
        stated as undetermined whether
          accidental or intentional
          Y21.1
      stated as undetermined whether
        accidental or intentional Y21.0
      suicide (attempt) X71.0
    lake —see Drowning, in, natural water
    natural water (lake) (open sea) (river)
      (stream) (pond) W69
      assault X92.3
      following
        dive or jump W16.611
          striking bottom W16.621
        fall W16.111
          striking
            bottom W16.121
            side W16.131
      stated as undetermined whether
        accidental or intentional Y21.4
      suicide (attempt) X71.3
    quarry —see Drowning, in, specified place
      NEC
    quenching tank —see Drowning, in,
      specified place NEC
    reservoir —see Drowning, in, specified
      place NEC
    river —see Drowning, in, natural water
    sea —see Drowning, in, natural water
    specified place NEC W73
      assault X92.8
      following
        dive or jump W16.811
          striking
            bottom W16.821
            wall W16.831
        fall W16.311
          striking
            bottom W16.321
            wall W16.331
      stated as undetermined whether
        accidental or intentional Y21.8
      suicide (attempt) X71.8
    stream —see Drowning, in, natural water
    swimming-pool W67
      assault X92.1
        following fall X92.2
      following
        dive or jump W16.511
          striking
            bottom W16.521
            wall W16.531
        fall W16.011
          striking
            bottom W16.021
            wall W16.031
      stated as undetermined whether
        accidental or intentional Y21.2
        following fall Y21.3
      suicide (attempt) X71.1
        following fall X71.2
  war operations —see War operations,
    restriction of airway
  resulting from accident to watercraft —see
    Drowning, due to, accident, watercraft
  self-inflicted X71.9
  stated as undetermined whether accidental or
    intentional Y21.9
  suicide (attempt) X71.9

E

Earth (surface) movement NEC —*see* Forces of
   nature, earth movement ⬅▬▬▬
Earth falling (on) W20.0
   caused by cataclysmic earth surface
      movement or eruption —*see* Landslide ◀
Earthquake (any injury) X34
Effect (s) (adverse) of
   air pressure (any) —*see* Air, pressure
   cold, excessive (exposure to) —*see* Exposure,
      cold
   heat (excessive) —*see* Heat
   hot place (weather) —*see* Heat ⬅▬▬▬
   insolation X30
   late —*see* Sequelae
   motion —*see* Motion
   nuclear explosion or weapon in war
      operations —*see* War operations, nuclear
      weapon
   radiation —*see* Radiation
   travel —*see* Travel
Electric shock (accidental) (by) (in) —*see*
   Exposure, electric current
Electrocution (accidental) —*see* Exposure,
   electric current
Endotracheal tube wrongly placed during
   anesthetic procedure Y65.3
Entanglement
   in
      bed linen, causing suffocation —*see*
         category T71
      wheel of pedal cycle V19.88
Entry of foreign body or material —*see* Foreign
   body
Environmental pollution related condition —
   see Z57
Execution, legal (any method) —*see* Legal,
   intervention
Exhaustion
   cold —*see* Exposure, cold
   due to excessive exertion —*see also*
      Overexertion X50.9 ⬅▬▬▬
   heat —*see* Heat
Explosion (accidental) (of) (with secondary fire)
   W40.9
   acetylene W40.1
   aerosol can W36.1
   air tank (compressed) (in machinery) W36.2
   aircraft (in transit) (powered) NEC V95.9
      balloon V96.05
      fixed wing NEC (private) V95.25
         commercial V95.35
      glider V96.25
         hang V96.15
         powered V95.15
      helicopter V95.05
      in war operations —*see* War operations,
         destruction of aircraft
      microlight V95.15
      nonpowered V96.9
         specified NEC V96.8
      powered NEC V95.8
      stated as
         homicide (attempt) Y03.8
         suicide (attempt) X83.0
      ultralight V95.15
   anesthetic gas in operating room W40.1
   antipersonnel bomb W40.8
      assault X96.0
      homicide (attempt) X96.0
      suicide (attempt) X75
   assault X96.9
   bicycle tire W37.0
   blasting (cap) (materials) W40.0
   boiler (machinery), not on transport vehicle
      W35
      on watercraft —*see* Explosion, in,
         watercraft
   butane W40.1
   caused by other person X96.9
   coal gas W40.1

Explosion *(Continued)*
   detonator W40.0
   dump (munitions) W40.8
   dynamite W40.0
      in
         assault X96.8
         homicide (attempt) X96.8
         legal intervention
            injuring
               bystander Y35.112
               law enforcement personnel Y35.111
               suspect Y35.113
         suicide (attempt) X75
   explosive (material) W40.9
      gas W40.1
      in blasting operation W40.0
      specified NEC W40.8
         in
            assault X96.8
            homicide (attempt) X96.8
            legal intervention
               injuring
                  bystander Y35.192
                  law enforcement personnel
                    Y35.191
                  suspect Y35.193
            suicide (attempt) X75
   factory (munitions) W40.8
   fertilizer bomb W40.8
      assault X96.3
      homicide (attempt) X96.3
      suicide (attempt) X75
   fire-damp W40.1
   firearm (parts) NEC W34.19
      airgun W34.110
      BB gun W34.110
      gas, air or spring-operated gun NEC
         W34.118
      handgun W32.1
      hunting rifle W33.12
      larger firearm W33.10
         specified NEC W33.19
      machine gun W33.13
      paintball gun W34.111
      pellet gun W34.110
      shotgun W33.11
      Very pistol [flare] W34.19
   fireworks W39
   gas (coal) (explosive) W40.1
      cylinder W36.9
         aerosol can W36.1
         air tank W36.2
         pressurized W36.3
         specified NEC W36.8
   gasoline (fumes) (tank) not in moving motor
      vehicle W40.1
      bomb W40.8
         assault X96.1
         homicide (attempt) X96.1
         suicide (attempt) X75
      in motor vehicle —*see* Accident, transport,
         by type of vehicle
   grain store W40.8
   grenade W40.8
      in
         assault X96.8
         homicide (attempt) X96.8
         legal intervention
            injuring
               bystander Y35.192
               law enforcement personnel
                 Y35.191
               suspect Y35.193
         suicide (attempt) X75
   handgun (parts) —*see* Explosion, firearm,
      handgun (parts)
   homicide (attempt) X96.9
      antipersonnel bomb —*see* Explosion,
         antipersonnel bomb
      fertilizer bomb —*see* Explosion, fertilizer
         bomb

Explosion *(Continued)*
   homicide *(Continued)*
      gasoline bomb —*see* Explosion, gasoline
         bomb
      letter bomb —*see* Explosion, letter bomb
      pipe bomb —*see* Explosion, pipe bomb
      specified NEC X96.8
   hose, pressurized W37.8
   hot water heater, tank (in machinery) W35
      on watercraft —*see* Explosion, in,
         watercraft
   in, on
      dump W40.8
      factory W40.8
      mine (of explosive gases) NEC W40.1
      watercraft V93.59
         powered craft V93.53
            ferry boat V93.51
            fishing boat V93.52
            jetskis V93.53
            liner V93.51
            merchant ship V93.50
            passenger ship V93.51
            sailboat V93.54
   letter bomb W40.8
      assault X96.2
      homicide (attempt) X96.2
      suicide (attempt) X75
   machinery —*see also* Contact, with, by type
      of machine
      on board watercraft —*see* Explosion, in,
         watercraft
      pressure vessel —*see* Explosion, by type
         of vessel
   methane W40.1
   mine W40.1
   missile NEC W40.8
   mortar bomb W40.8
      in
         assault X96.8
         homicide (attempt) X96.8
         legal intervention
            injuring
               bystander Y35.192
               law enforcement personnel
                 Y35.191
               suspect Y35.193
         suicide (attempt) X75
   munitions (dump) (factory) W40.8
   pipe, pressurized W37.8
      bomb W40.8
         assault X96.4
         homicide (attempt) X96.4
         suicide (attempt) X75
   pressure, pressurized
      cooker W38
      gas tank (in machinery) W36.3
      hose W37.8
      pipe W37.8
      specified device NEC W38
      tire W37.8
         bicycle W37.0
      vessel (in machinery) W38
   propane W40.1
   self-inflicted X75
   shell (artillery) NEC W40.8
      during war operations —*see* War
         operations, explosion
      in
         legal intervention
            injuring
               bystander Y35.122
               law enforcement personnel Y35.121
               suspect Y35.123
      war —*see* War operations, explosion
   spacecraft V95.45
   stated as undetermined whether accidental or
      intentional Y25
   steam or water lines (in machinery) W37.8
   stove W40.9
   suicide (attempt) X75

Explosion *(Continued)*
 tire, pressurized W37.8
  bicycle W37.0
 undetermined whether accidental or
  intentional Y25
 vehicle tire NEC W37.8
  bicycle W37.0
 war operations —*see* War operations,
  explosion
Exposure *(to)* X58
 air pressure change —*see* Air, pressure
 cold (accidental) (excessive) (extreme)
  (natural) (place) X31
  assault Y08.89
  due to
   man-made conditions W93.8
    dry ice (contact) W93.01
     inhalation W93.02
    liquid air (contact) (hydrogen)
     (nitrogen) W93.11
     inhalation W93.12
    refrigeration unit (deep freeze)
     W93.2
   suicide (attempt) X83.2
   weather (conditions) X31
  homicide (attempt) Y08.89
  self-inflicted X83.2
 due to abandonment or neglect X58
 electric current W86.8
  appliance (faulty) W86.8
   domestic W86.0
  caused by other person Y08.89
  conductor (faulty) W86.1
  control apparatus (faulty) W86.1
  electric power generating plant,
   distribution station W86.1
  electroshock gun —*see* Exposure, electric
   current, taser
  high-voltage cable W85
  homicide (attempt) Y08.89
  legal execution —*see* Legal, intervention,
   specified means NEC
  lightning —*see* subcategory T75.0
  live rail W86.8
  misadventure in medical or surgical
   procedure in electroshock therapy
   Y63.4
  motor (electric) (faulty) W86.8
   domestic W86.0
  self-inflicted X83.1
  specified NEC W86.8
   domestic W86.0
  stun gun —*see* Exposure, electric current,
   taser
  suicide (attempt) X83.1
  taser W86.8
   assault Y08.89
   legal intervention —*see* category Y35
   self-harm (intentional) X83.8
   undetermined intent Y33
  third rail W86.8
  transformer (faulty) W86.1
  transmission lines W85
 environmental tobacco smoke X58
 excessive
  cold —*see* Exposure, cold
  heat (natural) NEC X30
   man-made W92
 factor (s) NOS X58
  environmental NEC X58
   man-made NEC W99
   natural NEC —*see* Forces of nature ◄
  specified NEC X58
 fire, flames (accidental) X08.8
  assault X97
  campfire —*see* Exposure, fire, controlled,
   not in building
  controlled (in)
   with ignition (of) clothing —*see also*
    Ignition, clothes X06.2
    nightwear X05

Exposure *(Continued)*
 fire, flames *(Continued)*
  controlled *(Continued)*
   bonfire —*see* Exposure, fire, controlled,
    not in building
   brazier (in building or structure) —*see
    also* Exposure, fire, controlled,
    building
    not in building or structure —*see*
     Exposure, fire, controlled, not in
     building
   building or structure X02.0
    with
     fall from building X02.3
     from building X02.5
     injury due to building collapse
      X02.2
     smoke inhalation X02.1
    hit by object from building X02.4
    specified mode of injury NEC X02.8
   fireplace, furnace or stove —*see*
    Exposure, fire, controlled, building
   not in building or structure X03.0
    with
     fall X03.3
     smoke inhalation X03.1
    hit by object X03.4
    specified mode of injury NEC X03.8
   trash —*see* Exposure, fire, controlled, not
    in building
  fireplace —*see* Exposure, fire, controlled,
   building
  fittings or furniture (in building or
   structure) (uncontrolled) —*see*
   Exposure, fire, uncontrolled, building
  forest (uncontrolled) —*see* Exposure, fire,
   uncontrolled, not in building
  grass (uncontrolled) —*see* Exposure, fire,
   uncontrolled, not in building
  hay (uncontrolled) —*see* Exposure, fire,
   uncontrolled, not in building
  homicide (attempt) X97
  ignition of highly flammable material X04
  in, of, on, starting in
   machinery —*see* Contact, with, by type
    of machine
   motor vehicle (in motion) —*see also*
    Accident, transport, occupant by
    type of vehicle V87.8
    with collision —*see* Collision
   railway rolling stock, train, vehicle
    V81.81
    with collision —*see* Accident,
     transport, railway vehicle
     occupant
   street car (in motion) V82.8
    with collision —*see* Accident,
     transport, streetcar occupant
   transport vehicle NEC —*see also*
    Accident, transport
    with collision —*see* Collision
   war operations —*see also* War operations,
    fire
    from nuclear explosion —*see* War
     operations, nuclear weapons
   watercraft (in transit) (not in transit)
    V91.09
    localized —*see* Burn, on board
     watercraft, due to, fire on board
    powered craft V91.03
     ferry boat V91.01
     fishing boat V91.02
     jet skis V91.03
     liner V91.01
     merchant ship V91.00
     passenger ship V91.01
    unpowered craft V91.08
     canoe V91.05
     inflatable V91.06
     kayak V91.05
     sailboat V91.04

Exposure *(Continued)*
 fire, flames *(Continued)*
  in, of, on, starting in *(Continued)*
   watercraft *(Continued)*
    unpowered craft *(Continued)*
     surf-board V91.08
     waterskis V91.07
     windsurfer V91.08
  lumber (uncontrolled) —*see* Exposure, fire,
   uncontrolled, not in building
  mine (uncontrolled) —*see* Exposure, fire,
   uncontrolled, not in building
  prairie (uncontrolled) —*see* Exposure, fire,
   uncontrolled, not in building
  resulting from
   explosion —*see* Explosion
   lightning X08.8
  self-inflicted X76
  specified NEC X08.8
  started by other person X97
  stated as undetermined whether accidental
   or intentional Y26
  stove —*see* Exposure, fire, controlled,
   building
  suicide (attempt) X76
  tunnel (uncontrolled) —*see* Exposure, fire,
   uncontrolled, not in building
  uncontrolled
   in building or structure X00.0
    with
     fall from building X00.3
     injury due to building collapse
      X00.2
     jump from building X00.5
     smoke inhalation X00.1
    bed X08.00
     due to
      cigarette X08.01
      specified material NEC X08.09
    furniture NEC X08.20
     due to
      cigarette X08.21
      specified material NEC X08.29
    hit by object from building X00.4
    sofa X08.10
     due to
      cigarette X08.11
      specified material NEC
       X08.19
    specified mode of injury NEC
     X00.8
   not in building or structure (any)
    X01.0
    with
     fall X01.3
     smoke inhalation X01.1
    hit by object X01.4
    specified mode of injury NEC
     X01.8
  undetermined whether accidental or
   intentional Y26
 forces of nature NEC —*see* Forces of nature ◄
 G-forces (abnormal) W49.9
 gravitational forces (abnormal) W49.9
 heat (natural) NEC —*see* Heat
 high-pressure jet (hydraulic) (pneumatic)
  W49.9
 hydraulic jet W49.9
 inanimate mechanical force W49.9
 jet, high-pressure (hydraulic) (pneumatic)
  W49.9
 lightning —*see* subcategory T75.0
  causing fire —*see* Exposure, fire
 mechanical forces NEC W49.9
  animate NEC W64
  inanimate NEC W49.9
 noise W42.9
  supersonic W42.0
 noxious substance —*see* Table of Drugs and
  Chemicals ◄▥
 pneumatic jet W49.9

◄ New   ◄▥ Revised   ~~deleted~~ Deleted

Exposure *(Continued)*
prolonged in deep-freeze unit or refrigerator W93.2
radiation —*see* Radiation
smoke —*see also* Exposure, fire
tobacco, second hand Z77.22
specified factors NEC X58
sunlight X32
man-made (sun lamp) W89.8
tanning bed W89.1
supersonic waves W42.Ø
transmission line (s), electric W85
vibration W49.9

Exposure *(Continued)*
waves
infrasound W49.9
sound W42.9
supersonic W42.Ø
weather NEC —*see* Forces of nature ◄
External cause status Y99.9
child assisting in compensated work for family Y99.8
civilian activity done for financial or other compensation Y99.Ø
civilian activity done for income or pay Y99.Ø

External cause status *(Continued)*
family member assisting in compensated work for other family member Y99.8
hobby not done for income Y99.8
leisure activity Y99.8
military activity Y99.1
off-duty activity of military personnel Y99.8
recreation or sport not for income or while a student Y99.8
specified NEC Y99.8
student activity Y99.8
volunteer activity Y99.2

E

F

Factors, supplemental
alcohol
blood level
less than 20mg/100ml Y90.0
presence in blood, level not specified
Y90.9
20-39mg/100ml Y90.1
40-59mg/100ml Y90.2
60-79mg/100ml Y90.3
80-99mg/100ml Y90.4
100-119mg/100ml Y90.5
120-199mg/100ml Y90.6
200-239mg/100ml Y90.7
240mg/100ml or more Y90.8
presence in blood, but level not specified
Y90.9
environmental-pollution-related condition —
see Z57
nosocomial condition Y95
work-related condition Y99.0
Failure
in suture or ligature during surgical
procedure Y65.2
mechanical, of instrument or apparatus
(any) (during any medical or surgical
procedure) Y65.8
sterile precautions (during medical and
surgical care) —see Misadventure,
failure, sterile precautions, by type of
procedure
to
introduce tube or instrument Y65.4
endotracheal tube during anesthesia Y65.3
make curve (transport vehicle) NEC —see
Accident, transport
remove tube or instrument Y65.4
Fall, falling (accidental) W19
building W20.1
burning (uncontrolled fire) X00.3
down
embankment W17.81
escalator W10.0
hill W17.81
ladder W11
ramp W10.2
stairs, steps W10.9
due to
bumping against
object W18.00
sharp glass W18.02
specified NEC W18.09
sports equipment W18.01
person W03
due to ice or snow W00.0
on pedestrian conveyance —see
Accident, transport, pedestrian,
conveyance
collision with another person W03
due to ice or snow W00.0
involving pedestrian conveyance —see
Accident, transport, pedestrian,
conveyance
grocery cart tipping over W17.82
ice or snow W00.9
from one level to another W00.2
on stairs or steps W00.1
involving pedestrian conveyance —see
Accident, transport, pedestrian,
conveyance
on same level W00.0
slipping (on moving sidewalk) W01.0
with subsequent striking against object
W01.10
furniture W01.190
sharp object W01.119
glass W01.110
power tool or machine W01.111
specified NEC W01.118
specified NEC W01.198

Fall, falling (Continued)
due to (Continued)
striking against
object W18.00
sharp glass W18.02
specified NEC W18.09
sports equipment W18.01
person W03
due to ice or snow W00.0
on pedestrian conveyance —see
Accident, transport, pedestrian,
conveyance
earth (with asphyxia or suffocation (by
pressure)) —see Earth, falling
from, off, out of
aircraft NEC (with accident to aircraft
NEC) V97.0
while boarding or alighting V97.1
balcony W13.0
bed W06
boat, ship, watercraft NEC (with
drowning or submersion) —
see Drowning, due to, fall
overboard
with hitting bottom or object V94.0
bridge W13.1
building W13.9
burning (uncontrolled fire) X00.3
cavity W17.2
chair W07
cherry picker W17.89
cliff W15
dock W17.4
embankment W17.81
escalator W10.0
flagpole W13.8
furniture NEC W08
grocery cart W17.82
haystack W17.89
high place NEC W17.89
stated as undetermined whether
accidental or intentional Y30
hole W17.2
incline W10.2
ladder W11
lifting device W17.89
machine, machinery —see also Contact,
with, by type of machine
not in operation W17.89
manhole W17.1
mobile elevated work platform [MEWP]
W17.89
motorized mobility scooter W05.2
one level to another NEC W17.89
intentional, purposeful, suicide
(attempt) X80
stated as undetermined whether
accidental or intentional Y30
pit W17.2
playground equipment W09.8
jungle gym W09.2
slide W09.0
swing W09.1
quarry W17.89
railing W13.9
ramp W10.2
roof W13.2
scaffolding W12
scooter (nonmotorized) W05.1
motorized mobility W05.2
sky lift W17.89
stairs, steps W10.9
curb W10.1
due to ice or snow W00.1
escalator W10.0
incline W10.2
ramp W10.2
sidewalk curb W10.1
specified NEC W10.8
stepladder W11
storm drain W17.1

Fall, falling (Continued)
from, off, out of (Continued)
streetcar NEC V82.6
with antecedent collision —see
Accident, transport, streetcar
occupant
while boarding or alighting V82.4
structure NEC W13.8
burning (uncontrolled fire) X00.3
table W08
toilet W18.11
with subsequent striking against object
W18.12
train NEC V81.6
during derailment (without antecedent
collision) V81.7
with antecedent collision —see
Accident, transport, railway
vehicle occupant
while boarding or alighting V81.4
transport vehicle after collision —see
Accident, transport, by type of
vehicle, collision
tree W14
vehicle (in motion) NEC —see also
Accident, transport V89.9
motor NEC —see also Accident,
transport, occupant, by type of
vehicle V87.8
stationary W17.89
while boarding or alighting —see
Accident, transport, by type of
vehicle, while boarding or
alighting ◄
viaduct W13.8
wall W13.8
watercraft —see also Drowning, due to, fall
overboard
with hitting bottom or object V94.0
well W17.0
wheelchair, non-moving W05.0
powered —see Accident, transport,
pedestrian, conveyance occupant,
specified type NEC
window W13.4
in, on
aircraft NEC V97.0
with accident to aircraft V97.0
while boarding or alighting
V97.1
bathtub (empty) W18.2
filled W16.212
causing drowning W16.211
escalator W10.0
incline W10.2
ladder W11
machine, machinery —see Contact, with,
by type of machine
object, edged, pointed or sharp (with
cut) —see Fall, by type
playground equipment W09.8
jungle gym W09.2
slide W09.0
swing W09.1
ramp W10.2
scaffolding W12
shower W18.2
causing drowning W16.211
staircase, stairs, steps W10.9
curb W10.1
due to ice or snow W00.1
escalator W10.0
incline W10.2
specified NEC W10.8
streetcar (without antecedent collision)
V82.5
with antecedent collision —see
Accident, transport, streetcar
occupant
while boarding or alighting
V82.4

◄ New   ◄||||| Revised   ~~deleted~~ Deleted

Forces of nature *(Continued)*
  radiation (natural) X39.Ø8
    radon X39.Ø1
  radon X39.Ø1
  specified force NEC X39.8
  storm surge X37.Ø
  structure collapse causing
    earth movement
    X36.Ø
  sunlight X32
  tidal wave X37.41
    due to
      earthquake X37.41
      landslide X37.43
      storm X37.42
      volcanic eruption X37.41
  tornado X37.1

Forces of nature *(Continued)*
  tsunami X37.41
  twister X37.1
  typhoon X37.Ø
  volcanic eruption X35
Foreign body ◀
  aspiration - *see* Index to Diseases and
    Injuries, Foreign body, respitory
    tract ◀
  embedded in skin W45 ◀
  entering through skin W45.8 ◀
    can lid W26.2 ◀
    nail W45.Ø ◀
    paper W26.2 ◀
    specified NEC 45.8 ◀
    splinter W45.8 ◀

Forest fire (exposure to) —*see* Exposure, fire,
  uncontrolled, not in building
Found injured X58
  from exposure (to) —*see* Exposure
  on
    highway, road(way), street V89.9
    railway right of way V81.9
Fracture (circumstances unknown or
  unspecified) X58
  due to specified cause NEC X58
Freezing —*see* Exposure, cold
Frostbite X31
  due to man-made conditions —*see* Exposure,
    cold, man-made
Frozen —*see* Exposure, cold

G

Gored by bull W55.22
Gunshot wound W34.ØØ

H

Hailstones, injured by X39.8
Hanged herself or himself —*see* Hanging,
  self-inflicted
Hanging (accidental) —*see also* category T71
  legal execution —*see* Legal, intervention,
    specified means NEC
Heat (effects of) (excessive) X30
  due to
    man-made conditions W92
      on board watercraft V93.29
        fishing boat V93.22
        merchant ship V93.2Ø
        passenger ship V93.21
        sailboat V93.24
        specified powered craft NEC V93.23
  weather (conditions) X30

Heat *(Continued)*
  from
    electric heating apparatus causing
      burning X16
    nuclear explosion in war operations —
      see War operations, nuclear
      weapons
    inappropriate in local application or
      packing in medical or surgical
      procedure Y63.5
Hemorrhage
  delayed following medical or surgical
    treatment without mention of
    misadventure —*see* Index to Diseases
    and Injuries, Complication(s) ◀⃛
  during medical or surgical treatment as
    misadventure —*see* Index to Diseases
    and Injuries, Complication(s) ◀⃛

High
  altitude (effects) —*see* Air, pressure, low
  level of radioactivity, effects —*see* Radiation
  pressure (effects) —*see* Air, pressure, high
  temperature, effects —*see* Heat
Hit, hitting (accidental) by —*see* Struck by
Hitting against —*see* Striking against
Homicide (attempt) (justifiable) —*see* Assault
Hot
  place, effects —*see also* Heat
  weather, effects X30
House fire (uncontrolled) —*see* Exposure, fire,
  uncontrolled, building
Humidity, causing problem X39.8
Hunger X58
Hurricane (any injury) X37.Ø
Hypobarism, hypobaropathy —*see* Air,
  pressure, low

◀ New   ◀⃛ Revised   ~~deleted~~ Deleted

I

Ictus
  caloris —*see also* Heat
  solaris X30
Ignition (accidental) —*see also* Exposure, fire
    X08.8
  anesthetic gas in operating room W40.1
  apparel X06.2
    from highly flammable material X04
    nightwear X05
  bed linen (sheets) (spreads) (pillows)
      (mattress) —*see* Exposure, fire,
      uncontrolled, building, bed
  benzine X04
  clothes, clothing NEC (from controlled fire)
      X06.2
    from
        highly flammable material X04
  ether X04
    in operating room W40.1
  explosive material —*see* Explosion
  gasoline X04
  jewelry (plastic) (any) X06.0
  kerosene X04
  material
    explosive —*see* Explosion
    highly flammable with secondary
        explosion X04
  nightwear X05
  paraffin X04
  petrol X04
Immersion (accidental) —*see also* Drowning
  hand or foot due to cold (excessive) X31
Implantation of quills of porcupine
    W55.89
Inanition (from) (hunger) X58
  thirst X58.8
Inappropriate operation performed
  correct operation on wrong side or body
      part (wrong side) (wrong site)
      Y65.53
  operation intended for another patient done
      on wrong patient Y65.52
  wrong operation performed on correct
      patient Y65.51
Inattention after, at birth (homicidal intent)
    (infanticidal intent) X58
Incident, adverse
  device
    anesthesiology Y70.8
      accessory Y70.2
      diagnostic Y70.0
      miscellaneous Y70.8
      monitoring Y70.0
      prosthetic Y70.2
      rehabilitative Y70.1
      surgical Y70.3
      therapeutic Y70.1
    cardiovascular Y71.8
      accessory Y71.2
      diagnostic Y71.0
      miscellaneous Y71.8
      monitoring Y71.0
      prosthetic Y71.2
      rehabilitative Y71.1
      surgical Y71.3
      therapeutic Y71.1
    gastroenterology Y73.8
      accessory Y73.2
      diagnostic Y73.0
      miscellaneous Y73.8
      monitoring Y73.0
      prosthetic Y73.2
      rehabilitative Y73.1
      surgical Y73.3
      therapeutic Y73.1
    general
      hospital Y74.8
        accessory Y74.2
        diagnostic Y74.0

Incident, adverse *(Continued)*
  device *(Continued)*
    general *(Continued)*
      hospital *(Continued)*
        miscellaneous Y74.8
        monitoring Y74.0
        prosthetic Y74.2
        rehabilitative Y74.1
        surgical Y74.3
        therapeutic Y74.1
      surgical Y81.8
        accessory Y81.2
        diagnostic Y81.0
        miscellaneous Y81.8
        monitoring Y81.0
        prosthetic Y81.2
        rehabilitative Y81.1
        surgical Y81.3
        therapeutic Y81.1
    gynecological Y76.8
      accessory Y76.2
      diagnostic Y76.0
      miscellaneous Y76.8
      monitoring Y76.0
      prosthetic Y76.2
      rehabilitative Y76.1
      surgical Y76.3
      therapeutic Y76.1
    medical Y82.9
      specified type NEC Y82.8
    neurological Y75.8
      accessory Y75.2
      diagnostic Y75.0
      miscellaneous Y75.8
      monitoring Y75.0
      prosthetic Y75.2
      rehabilitative Y75.1
      surgical Y75.3
      therapeutic Y75.1
    obstetrical Y76.8
      accessory Y76.2
      diagnostic Y76.0
      miscellaneous Y76.8
      monitoring Y76.0
      prosthetic Y76.2
      rehabilitative Y76.1
      surgical Y76.3
      therapeutic Y76.1
    ophthalmic Y77.8
      accessory Y77.2
      diagnostic Y77.0
      miscellaneous Y77.8
      monitoring Y77.0
      prosthetic Y77.2
      rehabilitative Y77.1
      surgical Y77.3
      therapeutic Y77.1
    orthopedic Y79.8
      accessory Y79.2
      diagnostic Y79.0
      miscellaneous Y79.8
      monitoring Y79.0
      prosthetic Y79.2
      rehabilitative Y79.1
      surgical Y79.3
      therapeutic Y79.1
    otorhinolaryngological Y72.8
      accessory Y72.2
      diagnostic Y72.0
      miscellaneous Y72.8
      monitoring Y72.0
      prosthetic Y72.2
      rehabilitative Y72.1
      surgical Y72.3
      therapeutic Y72.1
    personal use Y74.8
      accessory Y74.2
      diagnostic Y74.0
      miscellaneous Y74.8
      monitoring Y74.0
      prosthetic Y74.2

Incident, adverse *(Continued)*
  device *(Continued)*
    personal use *(Continued)*
      rehabilitative Y74.1
      surgical Y74.3
      therapeutic Y74.1
    physical medicine Y80.8
      accessory Y80.2
      diagnostic Y80.0
      miscellaneous Y80.8
      monitoring Y80.0
      prosthetic Y80.2
      rehabilitative Y80.1
      surgical Y80.3
      therapeutic Y80.1
    plastic surgical Y81.8
      accessory Y81.2
      diagnostic Y81.0
      miscellaneous Y81.8
      monitoring Y81.0
      prosthetic Y81.2
      rehabilitative Y81.1
      surgical Y81.3
      therapeutic Y81.1
    radiological Y78.8
      accessory Y78.2
      diagnostic Y78.0
      miscellaneous Y78.8
      monitoring Y78.0
      prosthetic Y78.2
      rehabilitative Y78.1
      surgical Y78.3
      therapeutic Y78.1
    urology Y73.8
      accessory Y73.2
      diagnostic Y73.0
      miscellaneous Y73.8
      monitoring Y73.0
      prosthetic Y73.2
      rehabilitative Y73.1
      surgical Y73.3
      therapeutic Y73.1
Incineration (accidental) —*see* Exposure, fire
Infanticide —*see* Assault
Infrasound waves (causing injury) W49.9
Ingestion
  foreign body (causing injury) (with
      obstruction) —*see* Foreign body,
      alimentary canal
  poisonous
    plant (s) X58
    substance NEC —*see* Table of Drugs and
        Chemicals ◀▥
Inhalation
  excessively cold substance, man-made —*see*
      Exposure, cold, man-made
  food (any type) (into respiratory tract) (with
      asphyxia, obstruction respiratory tract,
      suffocation) —*see* categories T17 and T18
  foreign body —*see* Foreign body, aspiration
  gastric contents (with asphyxia, obstruction
      respiratory passage, suffocation) T17.81-
  hot air or gases X14.0
  liquid air, hydrogen, nitrogen W93.12
    suicide (attempt) X83.2
  steam X13.0
    assault X98.0
    stated as undetermined whether accidental
        or intentional Y27.0
    suicide (attempt) X77.0
  toxic gas —*see* Table of Drugs and
      Chemicals ◀▥
  vomitus (with asphyxia, obstruction
      respiratory passage, suffocation)T17.81-
Injury, injured (accidental(ly)) NOS X58
  by, caused by, from
    assault —*see* Assault
    law-enforcing agent, police, in course
        of legal intervention —*see* Legal
        intervention
    suicide (attempt) X83.8

Injury, injured NOS (Continued)
 due to, in
  civil insurrection —see War
   operations
  fight —see also Assault, fight
   Y04.0
  war operations —see War
   operations
 homicide —see also Assault Y09
 inflicted (by)
  in course of arrest (attempted), suppression
   of disturbance, maintenance of order,
   by law-enforcing agents —see Legal
   intervention

Injury, injured NOS (Continued)
 inflicted (Continued)
  other person
   stated as
    accidental X58
    intentional, homicide (attempt) —see
     Assault
    undetermined whether accidental or
     intentional Y33
  purposely (inflicted) by other person (s) —see
   Assault
  self-inflicted X83.8
   stated as accidental X58
  specified cause NEC X58

Injury, injured NOS (Continued)
 undetermined whether accidental or
  intentional Y33
Insolation, effects X30
Insufficient nourishment X58
Interruption of respiration (by)
 food (lodged in esophagus) —see categories
  T17 and T18
 vomitus (lodged in esophagus) T17.81-
Intervention, legal —see Legal intervention
Intoxication
 drug —see Table of Drugs and Chemicals ◀▥
 poison —see Table of Drugs and
  Chemicals ◀▥

J

Jammed (accidentally)
 between objects (moving) (stationary and
  moving) W23.0
 stationary W23.1
Jumped, jumping
 before moving object NEC X81.8
  motor vehicle X81.0
  subway train X81.1
  train X81.1
  undetermined whether accidental or
   intentional Y31
 from
  boat (into water) voluntarily,
   without accident (to or on boat)
   W16.712
   with
    accident to or on boat —see Accident,
     watercraft
    drowning or submersion W16.711
     suicide (attempt) X71.3

Jumped, jumping (Continued)
 from (Continued)
  boat voluntarily, without accident
   (Continued)
   striking bottom W16.722
    causing drowning W16.721
  building —see also Jumped, from,
   high place W13.9
   burning (uncontrolled fire)
    X00.5
  high place NEC W17.89
   suicide (attempt) X80
   undetermined whether accidental or
    intentional Y30
  structure —see also Jumped, from, high
   place W13.9
   burning (uncontrolled fire)
    X00.5
 into water W16.92
  causing drowning W16.91
  from, off watercraft —see Jumped, from,
   boat

Jumped, jumping (Continued)
 into water (Continued)
  in
   natural body W16.612
    causing drowning W16.611
    striking bottom W16.622
     causing drowning W16.621
   specified place NEC W16.812
    causing drowning W16.811
    striking
     bottom W16.822
      causing drowning W16.821
     wall W16.832
      causing drowning W16.831
   swimming pool W16.512
    causing drowning W16.511
    striking
     bottom W16.522
      causing drowning W16.521
     wall W16.532
      causing drowning W16.531
  suicide (attempt) X71.3

K

Kicked by
 animal NEC W55.82
 person (s) (accidentally) W50.1
  with intent to injure or kill Y04.0
  as, or caused by, a crowd or human
   stampede (with fall) W52
  assault Y04.0
  homicide (attempt) Y04.0
  in
   fight Y04.0
   legal intervention
    injuring
     bystander Y35.812
     law enforcement personnel Y35.811
     suspect Y35.813
~~Kicking against~~
~~object W22.8~~
 ~~sports equipment W21.9~~
 ~~stationary W22.09~~
  ~~sports equipment W21.89~~
~~person —see Striking against, person~~
~~sports equipment W21.9~~

Kicking ◀
 against ◀
  object W22.8 ◀
   sports equipment W21.9 ◀
   stationary W22.09 ◀
    sports equipment W21.89 ◀
  person —see Striking against, person ◀
  sports equipment W21.9 ◀
  carpet stretcher with knee X50.3 ◀
Killed, killing (accidentally) NOS —see also
 Injury X58
 in
  action —see War operations
  brawl, fight (hand) (fists) (foot) Y04.0
   by weapon —see also Assault
    cutting, piercing —see Assault, cutting
     or piercing instrument
    firearm —see Discharge, firearm, by
     type, homicide

Killed, killing NOS (Continued)
 self
  stated as
   accident NOS X58
   suicide —see Suicide
   undetermined whether accidental or
    intentional Y33
Kneeling (prolonged) (static) X50.1 ◀
Knocked down (accidentally) (by) NOS X58
 animal (not being ridden) NEC —see also
  Struck by, by type of animal
 crowd or human stampede W52
 person W51
  in brawl, fight Y04.0
 transport vehicle NEC —see also Accident,
  transport V09.9

◀ New ◀▥ Revised ~~deleted~~ Deleted

L

Laceration NEC —*see* Injury
Lack of
 care (helpless person) (infant) (newborn) X58
 food except as result of abandonment or
  neglect X58
  due to abandonment or neglect X58
 water except as result of transport accident X58
  due to transport accident —*see* Accident,
   transport, by type ◄
 helpless person, infant, newborn X58
Landslide (falling on transport vehicle) X36.1
 caused by collapse of man-made structure
  X36.0
Late effect —*see* Sequelae
Legal
 execution (any method) —*see* Legal,
  intervention
 intervention (by)
  baton —*see* Legal, intervention, blunt
   object, baton
  bayonet —*see* Legal, intervention, sharp
   object, bayonet
  blow —*see* Legal, intervention,
   manhandling
  blunt object
   baton
    injuring
     bystander Y35.312
     law enforcement personnel Y35.311
     suspect Y35.313
   injuring
    bystander Y35.302
    law enforcement personnel Y35.301
    suspect Y35.303
   specified NEC
    injuring
     bystander Y35.392
     law enforcement personnel Y35.391
     suspect Y35.393
   stave
    injuring
     bystander Y35.392
     law enforcement personnel Y35.391
     suspect Y35.393
  bomb —*see* Legal, intervention, explosive
  cutting or piercing instrument —*see* Legal,
   intervention, sharp object
  dynamite —*see* Legal, intervention,
   explosive, dynamite
  explosive (s)
   dynamite
    injuring
     bystander Y35.112
     law enforcement personnel Y35.111
     suspect Y35.113
   grenade
    injuring
     bystander Y35.192
     law enforcement personnel Y35.191
     suspect Y35.193
   injuring
    bystander Y35.102
    law enforcement personnel Y35.101
    suspect Y35.103

Legal *(Continued)*
 intervention *(Continued)*
  explosive *(Continued)*
   mortar bomb
    injuring
     bystander Y35.192
     law enforcement personnel
      Y35.191
     suspect Y35.193
   shell
    injuring
     bystander Y35.122
     law enforcement personnel Y35.121
     suspect Y35.123
   specified NEC
    injuring
     bystander Y35.192
     law enforcement personnel Y35.191
     suspect Y35.193
  firearm (s) (discharge)
   handgun
    injuring
     bystander Y35.022
     law enforcement personnel Y35.021
     suspect Y35.023
   injuring
    bystander Y35.002
    law enforcement personnel Y35.001
    suspect Y35.003
   machine gun
    injuring
     bystander Y35.012
     law enforcement personnel Y35.011
     suspect Y35.013
   rifle pellet
    injuring
     bystander Y35.032
     law enforcement personnel Y35.031
     suspect Y35.033
   rubber bullet
    injuring
     bystander Y35.042
     law enforcement personnel Y35.041
     suspect Y35.043
   shotgun —*see* Legal, intervention,
    firearm, specified NEC
   specified NEC
    injuring
     bystander Y35.092
     law enforcement personnel Y35.091
     suspect Y35.093
  gas (asphyxiation) (poisoning)
   injuring
    bystander Y35.202
    law enforcement personnel Y35.201
    suspect Y35.203
   specified NEC
    injuring
     bystander Y35.292
     law enforcement personnel Y35.291
     suspect Y35.293
   tear gas
    injuring
     bystander Y35.212
     law enforcement personnel Y35.211
     suspect Y35.213

Legal *(Continued)*
 intervention *(Continued)*
  grenade —*see* Legal, intervention,
   explosive, grenade
  injuring
   bystander Y35.92
   law enforcement personnel Y35.91
   suspect Y35.93
  late effect (of) —*see* with 7th character S
   Y35
  manhandling
   injuring
    bystander Y35.812
    law enforcement personnel Y35.811
    suspect Y35.813
  sequelae (of) —*see* with 7th character S
   Y35
  sharp objects
   bayonet
    injuring
     bystander Y35.412
     law enforcement personnel
      Y35.411
     suspect Y35.413
   injuring
    bystander Y35.402
    law enforcement personnel Y35.401
    suspect Y35.403
   specified NEC
    injuring
     bystander Y35.492
     law enforcement personnel Y35.491
     suspect Y35.493
  specified means NEC
   injuring
    bystander Y35.892
    law enforcement personnel Y35.891
    suspect Y35.893
  stabbing —*see* Legal, intervention, sharp
   object
  stave —*see* Legal, intervention, blunt
   object, stave
  tear gas —*see* Legal, intervention, gas, tear
   gas
  truncheon —*see* Legal, intervention, blunt
   object, stave
Lifting —*see also* Overexertion ◄
 heavy objects X50.0 ◄
 weights X50.0 ◄
Lightning (shock) (stroke) (struck by) —*see*
  subcategory T75.0
 causing fire —*see* Exposure, fire
Loss of control (transport vehicle) NEC —*see*
  Accident, transport
Lost at sea NOS —*see* Drowning, due to, fall
  overboard
Low
 pressure (effects) —*see* Air, pressure, low
 temperature (effects) —*see* Exposure, cold
Lying before train, vehicle or other moving
  object X81.8
 subway train X81.1
 train X81.1
 undetermined whether accidental or
  intentional Y31
Lynching —*see* Assault

M

Malfunction (mechanism or component) (of)
 firearm
  airgun W34.10
  BB gun W34.110
  gas, air or spring-operated gun NEC
   W34.118
  handgun W32.1
  hunting rifle W33.12
  larger firearm W33.10
   specified NEC W33.19
  machine gun W33.13
  paintball gun W34.111
  pellet gun W34.110
  shotgun W33.11
  specified NEC W34.19
  Very pistol [flare] W34.19
 handgun —see Malfunction, firearm,
  handgun
Maltreatment —see Perpetrator
Mangled (accidentally) NOS X58
Manhandling (in brawl, fight) Y04.0
 legal intervention —see Legal, intervention,
  manhandling
Manslaughter (nonaccidental) —see Assault
Mauled by animal NEC W55.89
Medical procedure, complication of
  (delayed or as an abnormal reaction
  without mention of misadventure) —see
  Complication of or following, by specified
  type of procedure
 due to or as a result of misadventure —see
  Misadventure
Melting (due to fire) —see also Exposure, fire
 apparel NEC X06.3
 clothes, clothing NEC X06.3
  nightwear X05
 fittings or furniture (burning building)
  (uncontrolled fire) X00.8
 nightwear X05
 plastic jewelry X06.1
Mental cruelty X58
Military operations (injuries to military and
  civilians occuring during peacetime on
  military property and during routine
  military exercises and operations) (by)
  (from) (involving) Y37.90-
 air blast Y37.20-
 aircraft
  destruction —see Military operations,
   destruction of aircraft
  airway restriction —see Military operations,
   restriction of airways
  asphyxiation —see Military operations,
   restriction of airways
 biological weapons Y37.6X-
 blast Y37.20-
 blast fragments Y37.20-
 blast wave Y37.20-
 blast wind Y37.20-
 bomb Y37.20-
  dirty Y37.50-
  gasoline Y37.31-
  incendiary Y37.31-
  petrol Y37.31-
 bullet Y37.43-
  incendiary Y37.32-
  rubber Y37.41-
 chemical weapons Y37.7X-
 combat
  hand to hand (unarmed) combat
   Y37.44-
  using blunt or piercing object Y37.45-
 conflagration —see Military operations, fire
 conventional warfare NEC Y37.49-
 depth-charge Y37.01-
 destruction of aircraft Y37.10-
  due to
   air to air missile Y37.11-
   collision with other aircraft Y37.12-

Military operations (Continued)
 destruction of aircraft (Continued)
  due to (Continued)
   detonation (accidental) of onboard
    munitions and explosives Y37.14-
   enemy fire or explosives Y37.11-
   explosive placed on aircraft Y37.11-
   onboard fire Y37.13-
   rocket propelled grenade [RPG] Y37.11-
   small arms fire Y37.11-
   surface to air missile Y37.11-
  specified NEC Y37.19-
 detonation (accidental) of
  onboard marine weapons Y37.05-
  own munitions or munitions launch device
   Y37.24-
 dirty bomb Y37.50-
 explosion (of) Y37.20-
  aerial bomb Y37.21-
  bomb NOS —see also Military operations,
   bomb (s) Y37.20-
  fragments Y37.20-
  grenade Y37.29-
  guided missile Y37.22-
  improvised explosive device [IED] (person-
   borne) (roadside) (vehicle-borne)
   Y37.23-
  land mine Y37.29-
  marine mine (at sea) (in harbor) Y37.02-
  marine weapon Y37.00-
   specified NEC Y37.09-
  own munitions or munitions launch device
   (accidental) Y37.24-
  sea-based artillery shell Y37.03-
  specified NEC Y37.29-
  torpedo Y37.04-
 fire Y37.30-
  specified NEC Y37.39-
 firearms
  discharge Y37.43-
  pellets Y37.42-
 flamethrower Y37.33-
 fragments (from) (of)
  improvised explosive device [IED] (person-
   borne) (roadside) (vehicle-borne)
   Y37.26-
  munitions Y37.25-
  specified NEC Y37.29-
  weapons Y37.27-
 friendly fire Y37.92-
 hand to hand (unarmed) combat Y37.44-
 hot substances —see Military operations, fire
 incendiary bullet Y37.32-
 nuclear weapon (effects of) Y37.50-
  acute radiation exposure Y37.54-
  blast pressure Y37.51-
  direct blast Y37.51-
  direct heat Y37.53-
  fallout exposure Y37.54-
  fireball Y37.53-
  indirect blast (struck or crushed by blast
   debris) (being thrown by blast)
   Y37.52-
  ionizing radiation (immediate exposure)
   Y37.54-
  nuclear radiation Y37.54-
  radiation
   ionizing (immediate exposure) Y37.54-
   nuclear Y37.54-
   thermal Y37.53-
  secondary effects Y37.54-
  specified NEC Y37.59-
  thermal radiation Y37.53-
 restriction of air (airway)
  intentional Y37.46-
  unintentional Y37.47-
 rubber bullets Y37.41-
 shrapnel NOS Y37.29-
 suffocation —see Military operations,
  restriction of airways
 unconventional warfare NEC Y37.7X-

Military operations (Continued)
 underwater blast NOS Y37.00-
 warfare
  conventional NEC Y37.49-
  unconventional NEC Y37.7X-
 weapon of mass destruction [WMD] Y37.91-
 weapons
  biological weapons Y37.6X-
  chemical Y37.7X-
  nuclear (effects of) Y37.50-
   acute radiation exposure Y37.54-
   blast pressure Y37.51-
   direct blast Y37.51-
   direct heat Y37.53-
   fallout exposure Y37.54-
   fireball Y37.53-
   ~~indirect blast (struck or crushed by blast~~
    ~~debris) (being thrown by blast)~~
    ~~Y37.52-~~
   radiation
    ionizing (immediate exposure) Y37.54-
    nuclear Y37.54-
    thermal Y37.53-
   secondary effects Y37.54-
   specified NEC Y37.59-
  of mass destruction [WMD] Y37.91-
**Misadventure (s) to patient (s) during surgical
 or medical care** Y69
 contaminated medical or biological substance
  (blood, drug, fluid) Y64.9
  administered (by) NEC Y64.9
   immunization Y64.1
   infusion Y64.0
   injection Y64.1
   specified means NEC Y64.8
   transfusion Y64.0
   vaccination Y64.1
 excessive amount of blood or other fluid
  during transfusion or infusion Y63.0
 failure
  in dosage Y63.9
   electroshock therapy Y63.4
   inappropriate temperature (too hot or
    too cold) in local application and
    packing Y63.5
   infusion
    excessive amount of fluid Y63.0
    incorrect dilution of fluid Y63.1
   insulin-shock therapy Y63.4
   nonadministration of necessary drug or
    biological substance Y63.6 ◄▥
   overdose —see Table of Drugs and
    Chemicals ◄▥
   radiation, in therapy Y63.2
   radiation
    overdose Y63.2
   specified procedure NEC Y63.8
   transfusion
    excessive amount of blood Y63.0
  mechanical, of instrument or apparatus
   (any) (during any procedure) Y65.8
  sterile precautions (during procedure)
   Y62.9
   aspiration of fluid or tissue (by puncture
    or catheterization, except heart)
    Y62.6
   biopsy (except needle aspiration) Y62.8
    needle (aspirating) Y62.6
   blood sampling Y62.6
   catheterization Y62.6
    heart Y62.5
   dialysis (kidney) Y62.2
   endoscopic examination Y62.4
   enema Y62.8
   immunization Y62.3
   infusion Y62.1
   injection Y62.3
   needle biopsy Y62.6
   paracentesis (abdominal) (thoracic)
    Y62.6
   perfusion Y62.2

◄ New   ◄▥ Revised   ~~deleted~~ Deleted

Misadventure (s) to patient (s) during surgical
  or medical care (*Continued*)
  failure (*Continued*)
    sterile precautions (*Continued*)
      puncture (lumbar) Y62.6
      removal of catheter or packing
        Y62.8
      specified procedure NEC Y62.8
      surgical operation Y62.0
      transfusion Y62.1
      vaccination Y62.3
    suture or ligature during surgical
      procedure Y65.2
    to introduce or to remove tube or
      instrument —*see* Failure, to ◀
  hemorrhage —*see* Index to Diseases and
    Injuries, Complication(s) ◀▥
  inadvertent exposure of patient to radiation
    Y63.3
  inappropriate
    operation performed —*see*
      Inappropriate operation
      performed
    temperature (too hot or too cold) in
      local application or packing
      Y63.5

Misadventure (s) to patient (s) during surgical
  or medical care (*Continued*)
  infusion —*see also* Misadventure, by type,
    infusion Y69
    excessive amount of fluid Y63.0
    incorrect dilution of fluid Y63.1
    wrong fluid Y65.1
  mismatched blood in transfusion Y65.0
  nonadministration of necessary drug or
    biological substance Y63.6 ◀▥
  overdose —*see* Table of Drugs and
    Chemicals ◀▥
  radiation (in therapy) Y63.2
  perforation —*see* Index to Diseases and
    Injuries, Complication(s) ◀▥
  performance of inappropriate operation —*see*
    Inappropriate operation performed
  puncture —*see* Index to Diseases and Injuries,
    Complication(s) ◀▥
  specified type NEC Y65.8
    failure
      suture or ligature during surgical
        operation Y65.2
      to introduce or to remove tube or
        instrument —*see* Failure, to ◀
    infusion of wrong fluid Y65.1

Misadventure (s) to patient (s) during surgical
  or medical care (*Continued*)
  specified type NEC (*Continued*)
    performance of inappropriate operation —
      see Inappropriate operation performed
    transfusion of mismatched blood Y65.0
    wrong
      fluid in infusion Y65.1
      placement of endotracheal tube during
        anesthetic procedure Y65.3
    transfusion —*see* Misadventure, by type,
      transfusion
      excessive amount of blood Y63.0
      mismatched blood Y65.0
    wrong
      drug given in error —*see* Table of Drugs
        and Chemicals ◀▥
      fluid in infusion Y65.1
      placement of endotracheal tube during
        anesthetic procedure Y65.3
Mismatched blood in transfusion Y65.0
Motion sickness T75.3
Mountain sickness W94.11
Mudslide (of cataclysmic nature) —*see*
  Landslide
Murder (attempt) —*see* Assault

N

Nail ◀
  contact with W45.0 ◀
    gun W29.4 ◀
  embedded in skin W45.0 ◀
  ~~Nail, contact with W45.0~~
    ~~gun W29.4~~

Neglect (criminal) (homicidal intent) X58
Noise (causing injury) (pollution) W42.9
  supersonic W42.0
Nonadministration (of)
  drug or biological substance (necessary)
    Y63.6 ◀▥
  surgical and medical care Y66
Nosocomial condition Y95

O

Object
  falling
    from, in, on, hitting
      machinery —*see* Contact, with, by type
        of machine
  set in motion by
    accidental explosion or rupture of pressure
      vessel W38
    firearm —*see* Discharge, firearm, by type
    machine (ry) —*see* Contact, with, by type
      of machine
Overdose (drug) —*see* Table of Drugs and
  Chemicals ◀▥
  radiation Y63.2

Overexertion X50.9 ◀▥
  from ◀
    prolonged static or awkward postures
      X50.1 ◀
    repetitive movements X50.3 ◀
    specified strenuous movements or postures
      NEC X50.9 ◀
    strenuous movement or load X50.0 ◀
Overexposure (accidental) (to)
  cold —*see also* Exposure, cold X31
    due to man-made conditions —*see*
      Exposure, cold, man-made
  heat —*see also* Heat X30
  radiation —*see* Radiation
  radioactivity W88.0
  sun (sunburn) X32

Overexposure (*Continued*)
  weather NEC —*see* Forces of nature ◀
  wind NEC —*see* Forces of nature ◀
Overheated —*see* Heat
Overturning (accidental)
  machinery —*see* Contact, with, by type of
    machine
  transport vehicle NEC —*see also* Accident,
    transport V89.9
  watercraft (causing drowning,
    submersion) —*see also* Drowning, due to,
    accident to, watercraft, overturning
    causing injury except drowning or
      submersion —*see* Accident, watercraft,
      causing, injury NEC ◀

P

Parachute descent (voluntary) (without accident to aircraft) V97.29
  due to accident to aircraft —*see* Accident, transport, aircraft
Pecked by bird W61.99
Perforation during medical or surgical treatment as misadventure —*see* Index to Diseases and Injuries, Complication(s) ◀▥
Perpetrator, perpetration, of assault, maltreatment and neglect (by) Y07.9
  boyfriend Y07.03
  brother Y07.410
    stepbrother Y07.435
  coach Y07.53
  cousin
    female Y07.491
    male Y07.490
  daycare provider Y07.519
    at-home
      adult care Y07.512
      childcare Y07.510
    care center
      adult care Y07.513
      childcare Y07.511
  family member NEC Y07.499
  father Y07.11
    adoptive Y07.13
    foster Y07.420
    stepfather Y07.430
  foster father Y07.420
  foster mother Y07.421
  girl friend Y07.04
  healthcare provider Y07.529
    mental health Y07.521
    specified NEC Y07.528
  husband Y07.01
  instructor Y07.53
  mother Y07.12
    adoptive Y07.14
    foster Y07.421
    stepmother Y07.433
  nonfamily member Y07.50
    specified NEC Y07.59
  nurse Y07.528
  occupational therapist Y07.528
  partner of parent
    female Y07.434
    male Y07.432
  physical therapist Y07.528
  sister Y07.411
  speech therapist Y07.528
  stepbrother Y07.435
  stepfather Y07.430
  stepmother Y07.433
  stepsister Y07.436
  teacher Y07.53
  wife Y07.02
Piercing —*see* Contact, with, by type of object or machine
Pinched
  between objects (moving) (stationary and moving) W23.0
    stationary W23.1
Pinned under machine (ry) —*see* Contact, with, by type of machine
Place of occurrence Y92.9
  abandoned house Y92.89
  airplane Y92.813
  airport Y92.520
  ambulatory health services establishment NEC Y92.538
  ambulatory surgery center Y92.530
  amusement park Y92.831
  apartment (co-op) —*see* Place of occurrence, residence, apartment
  assembly hall Y92.29
  bank Y92.510
  barn Y92.71
  baseball field Y92.320

Place of occurrence (*Continued*)
  basketball court Y92.310
  beach Y92.832
  boarding house —*see* Place of occurrence, residence, boarding house
  boat Y92.814
  bowling alley Y92.39
  bridge Y92.89
  building under construction Y92.61
  bus Y92.811
    station Y92.521
  cafe Y92.511
  campsite Y92.833
  campus —*see* Place of occurrence, school
  canal Y92.89
  car Y92.810
  casino Y92.59
  children's home —*see* Place of occurrence, residence, institutional, orphanage
  church Y92.22
  cinema Y92.26
  clubhouse Y92.29
  coal pit Y92.64
  college (community) Y92.214
  condominium —*see* Place of occurrence, residence, apartment
  construction area —*see* Place of occurrence, industrial and construction area
  convalescent home —*see* Place of occurrence, residence, institutional, nursing home
  court-house Y92.240
  cricket ground Y92.328
  cultural building Y92.258
    art gallery Y92.250
    museum Y92.251
    music hall Y92.252
    opera house Y92.253
    specified NEC Y92.258
    theater Y92.254
  dancehall Y92.252
  day nursery Y92.210
  dentist office Y92.531
  derelict house Y92.89
  desert Y92.820
  dock NOS Y92.89
  dockyard Y92.62
  doctor's office Y92.531
  dormitory —*see* Place of occurrence, residence, institutional, school dormitory
  dry dock Y92.62
  factory (building) (premises) Y92.63
  farm (land under cultivation) (outbuildings) Y92.79
    barn Y92.71
    chicken coop Y92.72
    field Y92.73
    hen house Y92.72
    house —*see* Place of occurrence, residence, house
    orchard Y92.74
    specified NEC Y92.79
  football field Y92.321
  forest Y92.821
  freeway Y92.411
  gallery Y92.250
  garage (commercial) Y92.59
    boarding house Y92.044
    military base Y92.135
    mobile home Y92.025
    nursing home Y92.124
    orphanage Y92.114
    private house Y92.015
    reform school Y92.155
  gas station Y92.524
  gasworks Y92.69
  golf course Y92.39
  gravel pit Y92.64
  grocery Y92.512
  gymnasium Y92.39
  handball court Y92.318
  harbor Y92.89

Place of occurrence (*Continued*)
  harness racing course Y92.39
  healthcare provider office Y92.531
  highway (interstate) Y92.411
  hill Y92.828
  hockey rink Y92.330
  home —*see* Place of occurrence, residence
  hospice —*see* Place of occurrence, residence, institutional, nursing home
  hospital Y92.239
    cafeteria Y92.233
    corridor Y92.232
    operating room Y92.234
    patient
      bathroom Y92.231
      room Y92.230
    specified NEC Y92.238
  hotel Y92.59
  house —*see also* Place of occurrence, residence
    abandoned Y92.89
    under construction Y92.61
  industrial and construction area (yard) Y92.69
    building under construction Y92.61
    dock Y92.62
    dry dock Y92.62
    factory Y92.63
    gasworks Y92.69
    mine Y92.64
    oil rig Y92.65
    pit Y92.64
    power station Y92.69
    shipyard Y92.62
    specified NEC Y92.69
    tunnel under construction Y92.69
    workshop Y92.69
  kindergarten Y92.211
  lacrosse field Y92.328
  lake Y92.828
  library Y92.241
  mall Y92.59
  market Y92.512
  marsh Y92.828
  military
    base —*see* Place of occurrence, residence, institutional, military base
    training ground Y92.84
  mine Y92.64
  mosque Y92.22
  motel Y92.59
  motorway (interstate) Y92.411
  mountain Y92.828
  movie-house Y92.26
  museum Y92.251
  music-hall Y92.252
  not applicable Y92.9
  nuclear power station Y92.69
  nursing home —*see* Place of occurrence, residence, institutional, nursing home
  office building Y92.59
  offshore installation Y92.65
  oil rig Y92.65
  old people's home —*see* Place of occurrence, residence, institutional, specified NEC
  opera-house Y92.253
  orphanage —*see* Place of occurrence, residence, institutional, orphanage
  outpatient surgery center Y92.530
  park (public) Y92.830
    amusement Y92.831
  parking garage Y92.89
    lot Y92.481
  pavement Y92.480
  physician office Y92.531
  polo field Y92.328
  pond Y92.828
  post office Y92.242
  power station Y92.69
  prairie Y92.828
  prison —*see* Place of occurrence, residence, institutional, prison

Place of occurrence *(Continued)*
  swimming pool *(Continued)*
    private *(Continued)*
      prison Y92.146
      reform school Y92.156
      single family residence
        Y92.016
  synagogue Y92.22
  television station Y92.59
  tennis court Y92.312
  theater Y92.254
  trade area Y92.59
    bank Y92.510
    cafe Y92.511
    casino Y92.59
    garage Y92.59
    hotel Y92.59
    market Y92.512
    office building Y92.59
    radio station Y92.59
    restaurant Y92.511
    shop Y92.513
    shopping mall Y92.59
    store Y92.512
    supermarket Y92.512
    television station Y92.59
    warehouse Y92.59
  trailer park, residential —*see* Place of
    occurrence, residence, mobile
    home
  trailer site NOS Y92.89
  train Y92.815
    station Y92.522
  truck Y92.812
  tunnel under construction Y92. 69
  university Y92.214
  urgent (health) care center Y92.532
  vehicle (transport) Y92.818
    airplane Y92.813
    boat Y92.814
    bus Y92.811
    car Y92.810
    specified NEC Y92.818
    subway car Y92.816
    train Y92.815
    truck Y92.812
  warehouse Y92.59
  water reservoir Y92.89
  wilderness area Y92.828
    desert Y92.820
    forest Y92.821
    marsh Y92.828
    mountain Y92.828
    prairie Y92.828
    specified NEC Y92.828
    swamp Y92.828
  workshop Y92.69
  yard, private Y92.096
    boarding house Y92.046
    mobile home Y92.027
    single family house Y92.017

Place of occurrence *(Continued)*
  youth center Y92.29
  zoo (zoological garden) Y92.834
Plumbism —*see* Table of Drugs and Chemicals,
  lead ◀
Poisoning (accidental) (by) —*see also* Table of
  Drugs and Chemicals ◀
  by plant, thorns, spines, sharp leaves or other
    mechanisms NEC X58
  carbon monoxide
    generated by
      motor vehicle —*see* Accident, transport
      watercraft (in transit) (not in transit)
        V93.89
        ferry boat V93.81
        fishing boat V93.82
        jet skis V93.83
        liner V93.81
        merchant ship V93.80
        passenger ship V93.81
        powered craft NEC V93.83
  caused by injection of poisons into skin by
    plant thorns, spines, sharp leaves X58
    marine or sea plants (venomous) X58
  exhaust gas
    generated by
      motor vehicle —*see* Accident, transport
      watercraft (in transit) (not in transit)
        V93.89
        ferry boat V93.81
        fishing boat V93.82
        jet skis V93.83
        liner V93.81
        merchant ship V93.80
        passenger ship V93.81
        powered craft NEC V93.83
  fumes or smoke due to
    explosion —*see also* Explosion W40.9
    fire —*see* Exposure, fire
    ignition —*see* Ignition
  gas
    in legal intervention —*see* Legal,
      intervention, gas
    legal execution —*see* Legal, intervention,
      gas
  in war operations —*see* War operations
  legal
    execution —*see* Legal, intervention, gas
    intervention
      by gas —*see* Legal, intervention, gas
      other specified means —*see* Legal,
        intervention, specified means
        NEC
Powder burn (by) (from)
  airgun W34.110
  BB gun W34.110
  firearm NEC W34.19
  gas, air or spring-operated gun NEC
    W34.118
  handgun W32.1
  hunting rifle W33.12

Powder burn *(Continued)*
  larger firearm W33.10
    specified NEC W33.19
  machine gun W33.13
  paintball gun W34.111
  pellet gun W34.110
  shotgun W33.11
  Very pistol [flare] W34.19
Premature cessation (of) surgical and medical
  care Y66
Privation (food) (water) X58
Procedure (operation)
  correct, on wrong side or body part (wrong
    side) (wrong site) Y65.53
  intended for another patient done on wrong
    patient Y65.52
  performed on patient not scheduled for
    surgery Y65.52
  performed on wrong patient Y65.52
  wrong, performed on correct patient Y65.51
Prolonged
  sitting in transport vehicle —*see* Travel, by
    type of vehicle
  stay in
    high altitude as cause of anoxia,
      barodontalgia, barotitis or hypoxia
      W94.11
    weightless environment X52
Pulling, excessive —*see also* Overexertion
  X50.9 ◀
Puncture, puncturing —*see also* Contact, with,
  by type of object or machine
  by
    plant thorns, spines, sharp leaves or other
      mechanisms NEC W60
  during medical or surgical treatment as
    misadventure —*see* Index to Diseases
    and Injuries, Complication(s) ◀
Pushed, pushing (accidental) (injury in) ◀
  by other person (s) (accidental) W51
    with fall W03
      due to ice or snow W00.0
    as, or caused by, a crowd or human
      stampede (with fall) W52
    before moving object NEC Y02.8
      motor vehicle Y02.0
      subway train Y02.1
      train Y02.1
    from
      high place NEC
        in accidental circumstances W17.89
        stated as
          intentional, homicide (attempt) Y01
          undetermined whether accidental
            or intentional Y30
      transport vehicle NEC —*see also*
        Accident, transport V89.9
        stated as
          intentional, homicide (attempt)
            Y08.89
      overexertion X50.9 ◀

R

Radiation (exposure to)
arc lamps W89.0
atomic power plant (malfunction) NEC
  W88.1
complication of or abnormal reaction to
  medical radiotherapy Y84.2
electromagnetic, ionizing W88.0
gamma rays W88.1
in
  war operations (from or following
    nuclear explosion) —see also War
    operations
inadvertent exposure of patient (receiving
  test or therapy) Y63.3
infrared (heaters and lamps) W90.1
  excessive heat from W92
ionized, ionizing (particles, artificially
  accelerated)
  radioisotopes W88.1
  specified NEC W88.8
  x-rays W88.0
isotopes, radioactive —see Radiation,
  radioactive isotopes
laser (s) W90.2
  in war operations —see War operations
  misadventure in medical care Y63.2
light sources (man-made visible and
  ultraviolet) W89.9
  natural X32
  specified NEC W89.8
  tanning bed W89.1
  welding light W89.0
man-made visible light W89.9
  specified NEC W89.8
  tanning bed W89.1
  welding light W89.0
microwave W90.8
misadventure in medical or surgical
  procedure Y63.2

Radiation (Continued)
natural NEC X39.08
  radon X39.01
overdose (in medical or surgical procedure)
  Y63.2
radar W90.0
radioactive isotopes (any) W88.1
  atomic power plant malfunction W88.1
  misadventure in medical or surgical
    treatment Y63.2
radiofrequency W90.0
radium NEC W88.1
sun X32
ultraviolet (light) (man-made) W89.9
  natural X32
  specified NEC W89.8
  tanning bed W89.1
  welding light W89.0
welding arc, torch, or light W89.0
  excessive heat from W92
x-rays (hard) (soft) W88.0
Range disease W94.11
Rape (attempted) T74.2-
Rat bite W53.11
Reaching (prolonged) (static) X50.1 ◀
Reaction, abnormal to medical procedure —see
  also Complication of or following, by type
  of procedure Y84.9
with misadventure —see Misadventure
biologicals —see Table of Drugs and
  Chemicals ◀▥
drugs —see Table of Drugs and Chemicals ◀▥
vaccine —see Table of Drugs and
  Chemicals ◀▥
Recoil
airgun W34.110
BB gun W34.110
firearm NEC W34.19
gas, air or spring-operated gun NEC W34.118

Recoil (Continued)
handgun W32.1
hunting rifle W33.12
larger firearm W33.10
  specified NEC W33.19
machine gun W33.13
paintball gun W34.111
pellet W34.110
shotgun W33.11
Very pistol [flare] W34.19
Reduction in
atmospheric pressure —see Air, pressure,
  change
Rock falling on or hitting (accidentally)
  (person) W20.8
in cave-in W20.0
Run over (accidentally) (by)
animal (not being ridden) NEC W55.89
machinery —see Contact, with, by specified
  type of machine
transport vehicle NEC —see also Accident,
  transport V09.9
  intentional homicide (attempt) Y03.0
  motor NEC V09.20
    intentional homicide (attempt) Y03.0
Running
before moving object X81.8
  motor vehicle X81.0
Running off, away
animal (being ridden) —see also Accident,
  transport V80.918
  not being ridden W55.89
animal-drawn vehicle NEC —see also
  Accident, transport V80.928
highway, road(way), street
  transport vehicle NEC —see also Accident,
    transport V89.9
Rupture pressurized devices —see Explosion,
  by type of device

S

Saturnism —*see* Table of Drugs and Chemicals, lead ◄▥

Scald, scalding (accidental) (by) (from) (in) X19
  air (hot) X14.1
  gases (hot) X14.1
  homicide (attempt) —*see* Assault, burning, hot object
  inflicted by other person
    stated as intentional, homicide (attempt) —
      see Assault, burning, hot object
  liquid (boiling) (hot) NEC X12
    stated as undetermined whether accidental or intentional Y27.2
    suicide (attempt) X77.2
  local application of externally applied substance in medical or surgical care Y63.5
  metal (molten) (liquid) (hot) NEC X18
  self-inflicted X77.9
  stated as undetermined whether accidental or intentional Y27.8
  steam X13.1
    assault X98.0
    stated as undetermined whether accidental or intentional Y27.0
    suicide (attempt) X77.0
  suicide (attempt) X77.9
  vapor (hot) X13.1
    assault X98.0
    stated as undetermined whether accidental or intentional Y27.0
    suicide (attempt) X77.0
Scratched by
  cat W55.03
  person (s) (accidentally) W50.4
    with intent to injure or kill Y04.0
    as, or caused by, a crowd or human stampede (with fall) W52
    assault Y04.0
    homicide (attempt) Y04.0
    in
      fight Y04.0
      legal intervention
        injuring
          bystander Y35.892
          law enforcement personnel Y35.891
          suspect Y35.893
Seasickness T75.3
Self-harm NEC —*see also* External cause by type, undetermined whether accidental or intentional
  intentional —*see* Suicide
  poisoning NEC —*see* Table of drugs and biologicals, accident
Self-inflicted (injury) NEC —*see also* External cause by type, undetermined whether accidental or intentional
  intentional —*see* Suicide
  poisoning NEC —*see* Table of drugs and biologicals, accident
Sequelae (of)
  accident NEC —*see* W00-X58 with 7th character S
  assault (homicidal) (any means) —*see* X92-Y08 with 7th character S
  homicide, attempt (any means) —*see* X92-Y08 with 7th character S
  injury undetermined whether accidentally or purposely inflicted —*see* Y21-Y33 with 7th character S
  intentional self-harm (classifiable to X71-X83) —*see* X71-X83 with 7th character S
  legal intervention (*see* with 7th character S Y35)
  motor vehicle accident —*see* V00-V99 with 7th character S
  suicide, attempt (any means) —*see* X71-X83 with 7th character S

Sequelae (*Continued*)
  transport accident —*see* V00-V99 with 7th character S
  war operations —*see* War operations
Shock
  electric —*see* Exposure, electric current
  from electric appliance (any) (faulty) W86.8
    domestic W86.0
    suicide (attempt) X83.1
Shooting, shot (accidental (ly)) —*see also* Discharge, firearm, by type
  herself or himself —*see* Discharge, firearm by type, self-inflicted
  homicide (attempt) —*see* Discharge, firearm by type, homicide
  in war operations —*see* War operations
  inflicted by other person —*see* Discharge, firearm by type, homicide
    accidental —*see* Discharge, firearm, by type of firearm
  legal
    execution —*see* Legal, intervention, firearm
    intervention —*see* Legal, intervention, firearm
  self-inflicted —*see* Discharge, firearm by type, suicide
    accidental —*see* Discharge, firearm, by type of firearm
  suicide (attempt) —*see* Discharge, firearm by type, suicide
Shoving (accidentally) by other person —*see* Pushed, by other person ◄▥
Sickness
  alpine W94.11
  motion —*see* Motion
  mountain W94.11
Sinking (accidental)
  watercraft (causing drowning, submersion) —*see also* Drowning, due to, accident to, watercraft, sinking
    causing injury except drowning or submersion —*see* Accident, watercraft, causing, injury NEC ◄
Siriasis X32
Sitting (prolonged) (static) X50.1 ◄
Slashed wrists —*see* Cut, self-inflicted
Slipping (accidental) (on same level) (with fall) W01.0
  without fall W18.40
    due to
      specified NEC W18.49
      stepping from one level to another W18.43
      stepping into hole or opening W18.42
      stepping on object W18.41
  on
    ice W00.0
      with skates —*see* Accident, transport, pedestrian, conveyance
    mud W01.0
    oil W01.0
    snow W00.0
      with skis —*see* Accident, transport, pedestrian, conveyance
    surface (slippery) (wet) NEC W01.0
Sliver, wood, contact with W45.8
Smoldering (due to fire) —*see* Exposure, fire
Sodomy (attempted) by force T74.2-
Sound waves (causing injury) W42.9
  supersonic W42.0
Splinter, contact with W45.8
Stab, stabbing —*see* Cut ◄
Standing (prolonged) (static) X50.1 ◄
Starvation X58
Status of external cause Y99.9
  child assisting in compensated work for family Y99.8
  civilian activity done for financial or other compensation Y99.0
  civilian activity done for income or pay Y99.0

Status of external cause (*Continued*)
  family member assisting in compensated work for other family member Y99.8
  hobby not done for income Y99.8
  leisure activity Y99.8
  military activity Y99.1
  off-duty activity of military personnel Y99.8
  recreation or sport not for income or while a student Y99.8
  specified NEC Y99.8
  student activity Y99.8
  volunteer activity Y99.2
Stepped on
  by
    animal (not being ridden) NEC W55.89
    crowd or human stampede W52
    person W50.0
Stepping on
  object W22.8
    with fall W18.31
      sports equipment W21.9
    stationary W22.09
      sports equipment W21.89
  person W51
    by crowd or human stampede W52
  sports equipment W21.9
Sting
  arthropod, nonvenomous W57
  insect, nonvenomous W57
Storm (cataclysmic) —*see* Forces of nature, cataclysmic storm ◄▥
Straining, excessive —*see also* Overexertion X50.9 ◄▥
Strangling —*see* Strangulation
Strangulation (accidental) —*see* category T71
Strenuous movements —*see also* Overexertion X50.9 ◄▥
Striking against
  airbag (automobile) W22.10
    driver side W22.11
    front passenger side W22.12
    specified NEC W22.19
  bottom when
    diving or jumping into water (in) W16.822
      causing drowning W16.821
      from boat W16.722
        causing drowning W16.721
      natural body W16.622
        causing drowning W16.821
      swimming pool W16.522
        causing drowning W16.521
    falling into water (in) W16.322
      causing drowning W16.321
      fountain —*see* Striking against, bottom when, falling into water, specified NEC
      natural body W16.122
        causing drowning W16.121
      reservoir —*see* Striking against, bottom when, falling into water, specified NEC
      specified NEC W16.322
        causing drowning W16.321
      swimming pool W16.022
        causing drowning W16.021
  diving board (swimming-pool) W21.4
  object W22.8
    with
      drowning or submersion —*see* Drowning
      fall —*see* Fall, due to, bumping against, object
    caused by crowd or human stampede (with fall) W52
    furniture W22.03
    lamppost W22.02
    sports equipment W21.9
    stationary W22.09
      sports equipment W21.89
    wall W22.01

◄ New   ◄▥ Revised   ~~deleted~~ Deleted

Struck by *(Continued)*
  sports equipment *(Continued)*
    ball *(Continued)*
      soft ball W21.07
      specified NEC W21.09
      volleyball W21.06
    bat or racquet
      baseball bat W21.11
        assault Y08.02
      golf club W21.13
        assault Y08.09
      specified NEC W21.19
      tennis racquet W21.12
        assault Y08.09
    cleats (shoe) W21.31
    foot wear NEC W21.39
    football helmet W21.81
    hockey (ice)
      field
        puck W21.221
        stick W21.211
      puck W21.220
      stick W21.210
        assault Y08.01
    skate blades W21.32
    specified NEC W21.89
      assault Y08.09
  thunderbolt —*see* subcategory
    T75.0
    causing fire —*see* Exposure, fire
  transport vehicle NEC —*see also* Accident,
    transport V09.9
    intentional, homicide (attempt) Y03.0
    motor NEC —*see also* Accident, transport
      V09.20
      homicide Y03.0
  vehicle (transport) NEC —*see* Accident,
    transport, by type of vehicle
    stationary (falling from jack,
      hydraulic lift, ramp)
      W20.8
Stumbling
  without fall W18.40
    due to
      specified NEC W18.49
      stepping from one level to another
        W18.43
      stepping into hole or opening W18.42
      stepping on object W18.41
  over
    animal NEC W01.0
      with fall W18.09
    carpet, rug or (small) object W22.8
      with fall W18.09
    person W51
      with fall W03
        due to ice or snow W00.0

Submersion (accidental) —*see* Drowning
Suffocation (accidental) (by external means) (by
    pressure) (mechanical) —*see also* category
    T71
  due to, by
    avalanche —*see* Landslide
    explosion —*see* Explosion
    fire —*see* Exposure, fire
    food, any type (aspiration) (ingestion)
      (inhalation) —*see* categories T17 and
      T18
    ignition —*see* Ignition
    landslide —*see* Landslide
    machine (ry) —*see* Contact, with, by type
      of machine
    vomitus (aspiration) (inhalation)
      T17.81-
  in
    burning building X00.8
Suicide, suicidal (attempted) (by) X83.8
  blunt object X79
  burning, burns X76
    hot object X77.9
      fluid NEC X77.2
      household appliance X77.3
      specified NEC X77.8
      steam X77.0
      tap water X77.1
      vapors X77.0
  caustic substance —*see* Table of Drugs and
    Chemicals ◀▥
  cold, extreme X83.2
  collision of motor vehicle with
    motor vehicle X82.0
    specified NEC X82.8
    train X82.1
    tree X82.2
  crashing of aircraft X83.0
  cut (any part of body) X78.9
  cutting or piercing instrument X78.9
    dagger X78.2
    glass X78.0
    knife X78.1
    specified NEC X78.8
    sword X78.2
  drowning (in) X71.9
    bathtub X71.0
    natural water X71.3
    specified NEC X71.8
    swimming pool X71.1
      following fall X71.2
  electrocution X83.1
  explosive (s) (material) X75
  fire, flames X76
  firearm X74.9
    airgun X74.01
    handgun X72

Suicide, suicidal *(Continued)*
  firearm *(Continued)*
    hunting rifle X73.1
    larger X73.9
      specified NEC X73.8
    machine gun X73.2
    shotgun X73.0
    specified NEC X74.8
  hanging X83.8
  hot object —*see* Suicide, burning, hot object
  jumping
    before moving object X81.8
      motor vehicle X81.0
      subway train X81.1
      train X81.1
    from high place X80
  late effect of attempt —*see* X71-X83 with 7th
    character S
  lying before moving object, train, vehicle X81.8
  poisoning —*see* Table of Drugs and
    Chemicals ◀▥
  puncture (any part of body) —*see* Suicide,
    cutting or piercing instrument
  scald —*see* Suicide, burning, hot object
  sequelae of attempt —*see* X71-X83 with 7th
    character S
  sharp object (any) —*see* Suicide, cutting or
    piercing instrument
  shooting —*see* Suicide, firearm
  specified means NEC X83.8
  stab (any part of body) —*see* Suicide, cutting
    or piercing instrument
  steam, hot vapors X77.0
  strangulation X83.8
  submersion —*see* Suicide, drowning
  suffocation X83.8
  wound NEC X83.8
Sunstroke X32
Supersonic waves (causing injury) W42.0
Surgical procedure, complication of (delayed
    or as an abnormal reaction without
    mention of misadventure) —*see also*
    Complication of or following, by type of
    procedure
  due to or as a result of misadventure —*see*
    Misadventure
Swallowed, swallowing
  foreign body —*see* Foreign body, alimentary
    canal
  poison —*see* Table of Drugs and Chemicals
  substance
    caustic or corrosive —*see* Table of Drugs
      and Chemicals
    poisonous —*see* Table of Drugs and
      Chemicals

◀ New   ◀▥ Revised   ~~deleted~~ Deleted

T

Tackle in sport W03
Terrorism (involving) Y38.80
  biological weapons Y38.6X-
  chemical weapons Y38.7X-
  conflagration Y38.3X-
  drowning and submersion Y38.89- ◀
  explosion Y38.2X-
    destruction of aircraft Y38.1X-
    marine weapons Y38.0X-
  fire Y38.3X-
  firearms Y38.4X-
  hot substances Y38.3X- ◀▥
  lasers Y38.89- ◀
  nuclear weapons Y38.5X-
  piercing or stabbing instruments
    Y38.89- ◀
  secondary effects Y38.9X- ◀
  specified method NEC Y38.89- ◀▥
  suicide bomber Y38.81- ◀
Thirst X58
Threat to breathing
  aspiration —see Aspiration
  due to cave-in, falling earth or substance
    NEC —see category T71
Thrown (accidentally)
  against part (any) of or object in transport
    vehicle (in motion) NEC —see also
    Accident, transport

Thrown (Continued)
  from
    high place, homicide (attempt) Y01
    machinery —see Contact, with, by type of
      machine
    transport vehicle NEC —see also Accident,
      transport V89.9
  off —see Thrown, from
Thunderbolt —see subcategory T75.0
  causing fire —see Exposure, fire
Tidal wave (any injury) NEC —see Forces of
  nature, tidal wave ◀▥
Took
  overdose (drug) —see Table of Drugs and
    Chemicals ◀▥
  poison —see Table of Drugs and
    Chemicals ◀▥
Tornado (any injury) X37.1
Torrential rain (any injury) X37.8
Torture X58
Trampled by animal NEC W55.89
Trapped (accidentally)
  between objects (moving) (stationary and
    moving) —see Caught
  by part (any) of
    motorcycle V29.88
    pedal cycle V19.88
    transport vehicle NEC —see also Accident,
      transport V89.9
Travel (effects) (sickness) T75.3

Tree falling on or hitting (accidentally)
  (person) W20.8
Tripping
  without fall W18.40
    due to
      specified NEC W18.49
      stepping from one level to another
        W18.43
      stepping into hole or opening
        W18.42
      stepping on object W18.41
    over
      animal W01.0
        with fall W01.0
      carpet, rug or (small) object W22.8
        with fall W18.09
      person W51
        with fall W03
          due to ice or snow W00.0
Twisted by person (s) (accidentally) W50.2
  with intent to injure or kill Y04.0
  as, or caused by, a crowd or human stampede
    (with fall) W52
  assault Y04.0
  homicide (attempt) Y04.0
  in
    fight Y04.0
    legal intervention —see Legal, intervention,
      manhandling
Twisting (prolonged) (static) X50.1 ◀

U

Underdosing of necessary drugs, medicaments
  or biological substances Y63.6 ◀▥
Undetermined intent (contact)
  (exposure)
  automobile collision Y32
  blunt object Y29
  drowning (submersion) (in) Y21.9
    bathtub Y21.0
      after fall Y21.1
    natural water (lake) (ocean) (pond) (river)
      (stream) Y21.4
    specified place NEC Y21.8
    swimming pool Y21.2
      after fall Y21.3
  explosive material Y25
  fall, jump or push from high place Y30
  falling, lying or running before moving object
    Y31
  fire Y26

Undetermined intent (Continued)
  firearm discharge Y24.9
    airgun (BB) (pellet) Y24.0
    handgun (pistol) (revolver)
      Y22
    hunting rifle Y23.1
    larger Y23.9
      hunting rifle Y23.1
      machine gun Y23.3
      military Y23.2
      shotgun Y23.0
      specified type NEC Y23.8
    machine gun Y23.3
    military Y23.2
    shotgun Y23.0
    specified type NEC Y24.8
    Very pistol Y24.8
  hot object Y27.9
    fluid NEC Y27.2
    household appliance Y27.3
    specified object NEC Y27.8

Undetermined intent (Continued)
  hot object (Continued)
    steam Y27.0
    tap water Y27.1
    vapor Y27.0
  jump, fall or push from high place Y30
  lying, falling or running before moving object
    Y31
  motor vehicle crash Y32
  push, fall or jump from high place Y30
  running, falling or lying before moving object
    Y31
  sharp object Y28.9
    dagger Y28.2
    glass Y28.0
    knife Y28.1
    specified object NEC Y28.8
    sword Y28.2
  smoke Y26
  specified event NEC Y33
Use of hand as hammer X50.3 ◀

V

Vibration (causing injury) W49.9
Victim (of)
  avalanche —see Landslide ◀
  earth movements NEC —see Forces of nature,
    earth movement ◀
  earthquake X34

Victim (Continued)
  flood —see Flood ◀
  landslide —see Landslide ◀
  lightning —see subcategory T75.0
    causing fire —see Exposure, fire
  storm (cataclysmic) NEC —see Forces of
    nature, cataclysmic storm ◀
  volcanic eruption X35

Volcanic eruption (any injury) X35
Vomitus, gastric contents in air passages
  (with asphyxia, obstruction or
  suffocation) T17.81-

T, U, & V

W

Walked into stationary object (any) W22.09
  furniture W22.03
  lamppost W22.02
  wall W22.01
War operations (injuries to military personnel
    and civilians during war, civil insurrection
    and peacekeeping missions) (by) (from)
    (involving) Y36.90-
  after cessation of hostilities Y36.89-
    explosion (of)
      bomb placed during war operations
        Y36.82-
      mine placed during war operations
        Y36.81-
    specified NEC Y36.88-
  air blast Y36.20-
  aircraft
    destruction —*see* War operations,
      destruction of aircraft
  airway restriction —*see* War operations,
    restriction of airways
  asphyxiation —*see* War operations, restriction
    of airways
  biological weapons Y36.6X-
  blast Y36.20-
  blast fragments Y36.20-
  blast wave Y36.20-
  blast wind Y36.20-
  bomb Y36.20-
    dirty Y36.50-
    gasoline Y36.31-
    incendiary Y36.31-
    petrol Y36.31-
  bullet Y36.43-
    incendiary Y36.32-
    rubber Y36.41-
  chemical weapons Y36.7X-
  combat
    hand to hand (unarmed) combat Y36.44-
    using blunt or piercing object Y36.45-
  conflagration —*see* War operations, fire
  conventional warfare NEC Y36.49-
  depth-charge Y36.01-
  destruction of aircraft Y36.10-
    due to
      air to air missile Y36.11-
      collision with other aircraft Y36.12-
      detonation (accidental) of onboard
        munitions and explosives Y36.14-
      enemy fire or explosives Y36.11-
      explosive placed on aircraft Y36.11-
      onboard fire Y36.13-
      rocket propelled grenade [RPG] Y36.11-
      small arms fire Y36.11-
      surface to air missile Y36.11-
    specified NEC Y36.19-
  detonation (accidental) of
    onboard marine weapons Y36.05-
    own munitions or munitions launch device
      Y36.24-

War operations (*Continued*)
  dirty bomb Y36.50-
  explosion (of) Y36.20-
    aerial bomb Y36.21-
    after cessation of hostilities
      bomb placed during war operations
        Y36.82-
      mine placed during war operations
        Y36.81-
    bomb NOS —*see also* War operations,
      bomb (s) Y36.20-
    fragments Y36.20-
    grenade Y36.29-
    guided missile Y36.22-
    improvised explosive device [IED]
      (person-borne) (roadside)
      (vehicle-borne) Y36.23-
    land mine Y36.29-
    marine mine (at sea) (in harbor)
      Y36.02-
    marine weapon Y36.00-
      specified NEC Y36.09-
    own munitions or munitions launch
      device (accidental) Y36.24-
    sea-based artillery shell Y36.03-
    specified NEC Y36.29-
    torpedo Y36.04-
  fire Y36.30-
    specified NEC Y36.39-
  firearms
    discharge Y36.43-
    pellets Y36.42-
  flamethrower Y36.33-
  fragments (from) (of)
    improvised explosive device [IED]
      (person-borne) (roadside)
      (vehicle-borne) Y36.26-
    munitions Y36.25-
    specified NEC Y36.29-
    weapons Y36.27-
  friendly fire Y36.92
  hand to hand (unarmed) combat
    Y36.44-
  hot substances —*see* War operations,
    fire
  incendiary bullet Y36.32-
  nuclear weapon (effects of) Y36.50-
    acute radiation exposure Y36.54-
    blast pressure Y36.51-
    direct blast Y36.51-
    direct heat Y36.53-
    fallout exposure Y36.54-
    fireball Y36.53-
    indirect blast (struck or crushed by blast
      debris) (being thrown by blast)
      Y36.52-
    ionizing radiation (immediate exposure)
      Y36.54-
    nuclear radiation Y36.54-
    radiation
      ionizing (immediate exposure)
        Y36.54-

War operations (*Continued*)
  nuclear weapon (*Continued*)
    radiation (*Continued*)
      nuclear Y36.54-
      thermal Y36.53-
    secondary effects Y36.54-
    specified NEC Y36.59-
    thermal radiation Y36.53-
  restriction of air (airway)
    intentional Y36.46-
    unintentional Y36.47-
  rubber bullets Y36.41-
  shrapnel NOS Y36.29-
  suffocation —*see* War operations, restriction
    of airways
  unconventional warfare NEC Y36.7X-
  underwater blast NOS Y36.00-
  warfare
    conventional NEC Y36.49-
    unconventional NEC Y36.7X-
  weapon of mass destruction [WMD] Y36.91
  weapons
    biological weapons Y36.6X-
    chemical Y36.7X-
    nuclear (effects of) Y36.50-
      acute radiation exposure Y36.54-
      blast pressure Y36.51-
      direct blast Y36.51-
      direct heat Y36.53-
      fallout exposure Y36.54-
      fireball Y36.53-
      ~~indirect blast (struck or crushed by blast~~
        ~~debris) (being thrown by blast)~~
        ~~Y36.52-~~
      radiation
        ionizing (immediate exposure) Y36.54-
        nuclear Y36.54-
        thermal Y36.53-
      secondary effects Y36.54-
      specified NEC Y36.59-
    of mass destruction [WMD] Y36.91-
Washed
  away by flood —*see* Flood
  off road by storm (transport vehicle) —*see*
    Forces of nature, cataclysmic storm
Weather exposure NEC —*see* Forces of nature
Weightlessness (causing injury) (effects of) (in
  spacecraft, real or simulated) X52
Work related condition Y99.0
Wound (accidental) NEC —*see also* Injury X58
  battle —*see also* War operations Y36.90
  gunshot —*see* Discharge, firearm by type
Wreck transport vehicle NEC —*see also*
  Accident, transport V89.9
Wrong
  device implanted into correct surgical site
    Y65.51
  fluid in infusion Y65.1
  patient, procedure performed on Y65.52
  procedure (operation) on correct patient
    Y65.51

◀ New   ⬅ Revised   ~~deleted~~ Deleted

ICD-10-CM Tabular List
of Diseases and Injuries

CHAPTER 1

CERTAIN INFECTIOUS AND PARASITIC DISEASES (A00-B99)

OGCR Chapter-Specific Coding Guidelines

1. **Chapter 1: Certain Infectious and Parasitic Diseases (A00-B99)**

   a. **Human Immunodeficiency Virus (HIV) Infections**

      1) **Code only confirmed cases**

      Code only confirmed cases of HIV infection/illness. This is an exception to the hospital inpatient guideline Section II, H.

      In this context, "confirmation" does not require documentation of positive serology or culture for HIV; the provider's diagnostic statement that the patient is HIV positive, or has an HIV-related illness is sufficient.

      2) **Selection and sequencing of HIV codes**

         (a) **Patient admitted for HIV-related condition**

         If a patient is admitted for an HIV-related condition, the principal diagnosis should be B20, Human immunodeficiency virus [HIV] disease followed by additional diagnosis codes for all reported HIV-related conditions.

         (b) **Patient with HIV disease admitted for unrelated condition**

         If a patient with HIV disease is admitted for an unrelated condition (such as a traumatic injury), the code for the unrelated condition (e.g., the nature of injury code) should be the principal diagnosis. Other diagnoses would be B20 followed by additional diagnosis codes for all reported HIV-related conditions.

         (c) **Whether the patient is newly diagnosed**

         Whether the patient is newly diagnosed or has had previous admissions/encounters for HIV conditions is irrelevant to the sequencing decision.

         (d) **Asymptomatic human immunodeficiency virus**

         Z21, Asymptomatic human immunodeficiency virus [HIV] infection status, is to be applied when the patient without any documentation of symptoms is listed as being "HIV positive," "known HIV," "HIV test positive," or similar terminology. Do not use this code if the term "AIDS" is used or if the patient is treated for any HIV-related illness or is described as having any condition(s) resulting from his/her HIV positive status; use B20 in these cases.

         (e) **Patients with inconclusive HIV serology**

         Patients with inconclusive HIV serology, but no definitive diagnosis or manifestations of the illness, may be assigned code R75, Inconclusive laboratory evidence of human immunodeficiency virus [HIV].

         (f) **Previously diagnosed HIV-related illness**

         Patients with any known prior diagnosis of an HIV-related illness should be coded to B20. Once a patient has developed an HIV-related illness, the patient should always be assigned code B20 on every subsequent admission/encounter. Patients previously diagnosed with any HIV illness (B20) should never be assigned to R75 or Z21, Asymptomatic human immunodeficiency virus [HIV] infection status.

         (g) **HIV Infection in Pregnancy, Childbirth and the Puerperium**

         During pregnancy, childbirth or the puerperium, a patient admitted (or presenting for a health care encounter) because of an HIV-related illness should receive a principal diagnosis code of O98.7-, Human immunodeficiency [HIV] disease complicating pregnancy, childbirth and the puerperium, followed by B20 and the code(s) for the HIV-related illness(es). Codes from Chapter 15 always take sequencing priority.

         Patients with asymptomatic HIV infection status admitted (or presenting for a health care encounter) during pregnancy, childbirth, or the puerperium should receive codes of O98.7- and Z21.

         (h) **Encounters for testing for HIV**

         If a patient is being seen to determine his/her HIV status, use code Z11.4, Encounter for screening for human immunodeficiency virus [HIV]. Use additional codes for any associated high risk behavior.

         If a patient with signs or symptoms is being seen for HIV testing, code the signs and symptoms. An additional counseling code Z71.7, Human immunodeficiency virus [HIV] counseling, may be used if counseling is provided during the encounter for the test.

         When a patient returns to be informed of his/her HIV test results and the test result is negative, use code Z71.7, Human immunodeficiency virus [HIV] counseling.

         If the results are positive, see previous guidelines and assign codes as appropriate.

   b. **Infectious agents as the cause of diseases classified to other chapters**

   Certain infections are classified in chapters other than Chapter 1 and no organism is identified as part of the infection code. In these instances, it is necessary to use an additional code from Chapter 1 to identify the organism. A code from category B95, Streptococcus, Staphylococcus, and Enterococcus as the cause of diseases classified to other chapters, B96, Other bacterial agents as the cause of diseases classified to other chapters, or B97, Viral agents as the cause of diseases classified to other chapters, is to be used as an additional code to identify the organism. An instructional note will be found at the infection code advising that an additional organism code is required.

   c. **Infections resistant to antibiotics**

   Many bacterial infections are resistant to current antibiotics. It is necessary to identify all infections documented as antibiotic resistant. Assign a code from category Z16, Resistance to antimicrobial drugs, following the infection code only if the infection code does not identify drug resistance.

   d. **Sepsis, Severe Sepsis, and Septic Shock**

      1) **Coding of Sepsis and Severe Sepsis**

         (a) **Sepsis**

         For a diagnosis of sepsis, assign the appropriate code for the underlying systemic infection. If the type of infection or causal organism is not further specified, assign code A41.9, Sepsis, unspecified organism.

         A code from subcategory R65.2, Severe sepsis, should not be assigned unless severe sepsis or an associated acute organ dysfunction is documented.

            (i) Negative or inconclusive blood cultures and sepsis
            Negative or inconclusive blood cultures do not preclude a diagnosis of sepsis in patients with clinical evidence of the condition, however, the provider should be queried.

            (ii) Urosepsis
            The term urosepsis is a nonspecific term. It is not to be considered synonymous with sepsis. It has no default code in the Alphabetic Index. Should a provider use this term, he/she must be queried for clarification.

            (iii) Sepsis with organ dysfunction
            If a patient has sepsis and associated acute organ dysfunction or multiple organ dysfunction (MOD), follow the instructions for coding severe sepsis.

            (iv) Acute organ dysfunction that is not clearly associated with the sepsis
            If a patient has sepsis and an acute organ dysfunction, but the medical record documentation indicates that the acute organ dysfunction is related to a medical condition other than the sepsis, do not assign a code from subcategory R65.2, Severe sepsis. An acute organ dysfunction must be associated with the sepsis in order to assign the severe sepsis code. If the documentation is not clear as to whether an acute organ dysfunction is related to the sepsis or another medical condition, query the provider.

         (b) **Severe sepsis**

         The coding of severe sepsis requires a minimum of 2 codes: first a code for the underlying systemic infection, followed by a code from subcategory R65.2, Severe sepsis. If the causal organism is not documented, assign code A41.9, Sepsis, unspecified organism, for the infection. Additional code(s) for the associated acute organ dysfunction are also required.

         Due to the complex nature of severe sepsis, some cases may require querying the provider prior to assignment of the codes.

◀ New ◀ Revised ~~deleted~~ Deleted | Excludes 1 | Excludes 2 | Includes | Use additional | Code first | Code also | Unspecified |

OGCR Official Guidelines   X Assign placeholder X   ● Use Additional Character(s)   ▶ Manifestation Code   **Coding Clinic**

2) Septic shock

(a) Septic shock generally refers to circulatory failure associated with severe sepsis, and therefore, it represents a type of acute organ dysfunction.

For all cases of septic shock, the code for the systemic infection should be sequenced first, followed by code R65.21, Severe sepsis with septic shock or code T81.12, Postprocedural septic shock. Any additional codes for the other acute organ dysfunctions should also be assigned. As noted in the sequencing instructions in the Tabular List, the code for septic shock cannot be assigned as a principal diagnosis.

3) Sequencing of severe sepsis

If severe sepsis is present on admission, and meets the definition of principal diagnosis, the underlying systemic infection should be assigned as principal diagnosis followed by the appropriate code from subcategory R65.2 as required by the sequencing rules in the Tabular List. A code from subcategory R65.2 can never be assigned as a principal diagnosis.

When severe sepsis develops during an encounter (it was not present on admission) the underlying systemic infection and the appropriate code from subcategory R65.2 should be assigned as secondary diagnoses.

Severe sepsis may be present on admission but the diagnosis may not be confirmed until sometime after admission. If the documentation is not clear whether severe sepsis was present on admission, the provider should be queried.

4) Sepsis and severe sepsis with a localized infection

If the reason for admission is both sepsis or severe sepsis and a localized infection, such as pneumonia or cellulitis, a code(s) for the underlying systemic infection should be assigned first and the code for the localized infection should be assigned as a secondary diagnosis. If the patient has severe sepsis, a code from subcategory R65.2 should also be assigned as a secondary diagnosis. If the patient is admitted with a localized infection, such as pneumonia, and sepsis/severe sepsis doesn't develop until after admission, the localized infection should be assigned first, followed by the appropriate sepsis/severe sepsis codes.

5) Sepsis due to a postprocedural infection

(a) Documentation of causal relationship

As with all postprocedural complications, code assignment is based on the provider's documentation of the relationship between the infection and the procedure.

(b) Sepsis due to a postprocedural infection

For such cases, the postprocedural infection code, such as, T80.2, Infections following infusion, transfusion, and therapeutic injection, T81.4, Infection following a procedure, T88.0, Infection following immunization, or O86.0, Infection of obstetric surgical wound, should be coded first, followed by the code for the specific infection. If the patient has severe sepsis the appropriate code from subcategory R65.2 should also be assigned with the additional code(s) for any acute organ dysfunction.

(c) Postprocedural infection and postprocedural septic shock

In cases where a postprocedural infection has occurred and has resulted in severe sepsis the code for the precipitating complication such as code T81.4, Infection following a procedure, or O86.0, Infection of obstetrical surgical wound should be coded first followed by code R65.20, Severe sepsis without septic shock. A Code for the systemic infection should also be assigned.

If a postprocedural infection has resulted in postprocedural septic shock, the code for the precipitating complication such as code T81.4, Infection following a procedure, or O86.0, Infection of obstetrical surgical wound should be coded first followed by code T81.12-, Postprocedural septic shock. A code for the systemic infection should also be assigned.

6) Sepsis and severe sepsis associated with a noninfectious process (condition)

In some cases a noninfectious process (condition), such as trauma, may lead to an infection which can result in sepsis or severe sepsis. If sepsis or severe sepsis is documented as associated with a noninfectious condition, such as a burn or serious injury, and this condition meets the definition for principal diagnosis, the code for the noninfectious condition should be sequenced first, followed by the code for the resulting infection. If severe sepsis is present, a code from subcategory R65.2 should also be assigned with any associated organ dysfunction(s) codes. It is not necessary to assign a code from subcategory R65.1, Systemic inflammatory response syndrome (SIRS) of non-infectious origin, for these cases.

If the infection meets the definition of principal diagnosis it should be sequenced before the non-infectious condition. When both the associated non-infectious condition and the infection meet the definition of principal diagnosis either may be assigned as principal diagnosis.

Only one code from category R65, Symptoms and signs specifically associated with systemic inflammation and infection, should be assigned. Therefore, when a non-infectious condition leads to an infection resulting in severe sepsis, assign the appropriate code from subcategory R65.2, Severe sepsis. Do not additionally assign a code from subcategory R65.1, Systemic inflammatory response syndrome (SIRS) of non-infectious origin.

See Section I.C.18. SIRS due to non-infectious process

7) Sepsis and septic shock complicating abortion, pregnancy, childbirth, and the puerperium

See Section I.C.15. Sepsis and septic shock complicating abortion, pregnancy, childbirth and the puerperium

8) Newborn sepsis

See Section I.C.16. f. Bacterial sepsis of Newborn

e. Methicillin Resistant Staphylococcus aureus (MRSA) Conditions

1) Selection and sequencing of MRSA codes

(a) Combination codes for MRSA infection

When a patient is diagnosed with an infection that is due to methicillin resistant *Staphylococcus aureus* (MRSA), and that infection has a combination code that includes the causal organism (e.g., sepsis, pneumonia) assign the appropriate combination code for the condition (e.g., code A41.02, Sepsis due to Methicillin resistant Staphylococcus aureus or code J15.212, Pneumonia due to Methicillin resistant Staphylococcus aureus). Do not assign code B95.62, Methicillin resistant Staphylococcus aureus infection as the cause of diseases classified elsewhere, as an additional code because the combination code includes the type of infection and the MRSA organism. Do not assign a code from subcategory Z16.11, Resistance to penicillins, as an additional diagnosis.

See Section C.1. for instructions on coding and sequencing of sepsis and severe sepsis.

(b) Other codes for MRSA infection

When there is documentation of a current infection (e.g., wound infection, stitch abscess, urinary tract infection) due to MRSA, and that infection does not have a combination code that includes the causal organism, assign the appropriate code to identify the condition along with code B95.62, Methicillin resistant Staphylococcus aureus infection as the cause of diseases classified elsewhere for the MRSA infection. Do not assign a code from subcategory Z16.11, Resistance to penicillins.

(c) Methicillin susceptible Staphylococcus aureus (MSSA) and MRSA colonization

The condition or state of being colonized or carrying MSSA or MRSA is called colonization or carriage, while an individual person is described as being colonized or being a carrier. Colonization means that MSSA or MSRA is present on or in the body without necessarily causing illness. A positive MRSA colonization test might be documented by the provider as "MRSA screen positive" or "MRSA nasal swab positive".

Assign code Z22.322, Carrier or suspected carrier of Methicillin resistant Staphylococcus aureus, for patients documented as having MRSA colonization. Assign code Z22.321, Carrier or suspected carrier of Methicillin susceptible Staphylococcus aureus, for patient documented as having MSSA colonization. Colonization is not necessarily indicative of a disease process or as the cause of a specific condition the patient may have unless documented as such by the provider.

(d) MRSA colonization and infection

If a patient is documented as having both MRSA colonization and infection during a hospital admission, code Z22.322, Carrier or suspected carrier of Methicillin resistant Staphylococcus aureus, and a code for the MRSA infection may both be assigned.

f. Zika virus infections

1) Code only confirmed cases

Code only a confirmed diagnosis of Zika virus (A92.5, Zika virus disease) as documented by the provider. This is an exception to the hospital inpatient guideline Section II, H.

In this context, "confirmation" does not require documentation of the type of test performed; the physician's diagnostic statement that the condition is confirmed is sufficient. This code should be assigned regardless of the stated mode of transmission.

If the provider documents "suspected", "possible" or "probable" Zika, do not assign code A92.5. Assign a code(s) explaining the reason for encounter (such as fever, rash, or joint pain) or Z20.828, Contact with and (suspected) exposure to other viral communicable diseases.

CHAPTER 1

CERTAIN INFECTIOUS AND PARASITIC DISEASES (A00-B99)

Includes   diseases generally recognized as communicable or transmissible

Use additional code to identify resistance to antimicrobial drugs (Z16.-)

Excludes1   certain localized infections - see body system-related chapters

Excludes2   carrier or suspected carrier of infectious disease (Z22.-)

infectious and parasitic diseases complicating pregnancy, childbirth and the puerperium (O98.-)

infectious and parasitic diseases specific to the perinatal period (P35-P39)

influenza and other acute respiratory infections (J00-J22)

This chapter contains the following blocks:

A00-A09	Intestinal infectious diseases
A15-A19	Tuberculosis
A20-A28	Certain zoonotic bacterial diseases
A30-A49	Other bacterial diseases
A50-A64	Infections with a predominantly sexual mode of transmission
A65-A69	Other spirochetal diseases
A70-A74	Other diseases caused by chlamydiae
A75-A79	Rickettsioses
A80-A89	Viral and prion infections of the central nervous system
A90-A99	Arthropod-borne viral fevers and viral hemorrhagic fevers
B00-B09	Viral infections characterized by skin and mucous membrane lesions
B10	Other human herpesviruses
B15-B19	Viral hepatitis
B20	Human immunodeficiency virus [HIV] disease
B25-B34	Other viral diseases
B35-B49	Mycoses
B50-B64	Protozoal diseases
B65-B83	Helminthiases
B85-B89	Pediculosis, acariasis and other infestations
B90-B94	Sequelae of infectious and parasitic diseases
B95-B97	Bacterial and viral infectious agents
B99	Other infectious diseases

INTESTINAL INFECTIOUS DISEASES (A00-A09)

● **A00**   **Cholera**
A serious, often deadly, infectious disease of the small intestine

    A00.0   **Cholera due to Vibrio cholerae 01, biovar cholerae**
Classical cholera

    A00.1   **Cholera due to Vibrio cholerae 01, biovar eltor**
Cholera eltor

    A00.9   **Cholera, unspecified**

● **A01**   **Typhoid and paratyphoid fevers**
Caused by Salmonella typhi and Salmonella paratyphi A, B, and C bacteria

    ● **A01.0**   **Typhoid fever**
Infection due to Salmonella typhi

       A01.00   **Typhoid fever, unspecified**

       A01.01   **Typhoid meningitis**

       A01.02   **Typhoid fever with heart involvement**
Typhoid endocarditis
Typhoid myocarditis

       A01.03   **Typhoid pneumonia**

       A01.04   **Typhoid arthritis**

       A01.05   **Typhoid osteomyelitis**

       A01.09   **Typhoid fever with other complications**

    A01.1   **Paratyphoid fever A**

    A01.2   **Paratyphoid fever B**

    A01.3   **Paratyphoid fever C**

    A01.4   **Paratyphoid fever, unspecified**
Infection due to Salmonella paratyphi NOS

● **A02**   **Other salmonella infections**

    Includes   infection or foodborne intoxication due to any Salmonella species other than S. typhi and S. paratyphi

    A02.0   **Salmonella enteritis**
Salmonellosis

    A02.1   **Salmonella sepsis**

    ● **A02.2**   **Localized salmonella infections**

       A02.20   **Localized salmonella infection, unspecified**
Specified in the documentation as localized, but unspecified as to type

       A02.21   **Salmonella meningitis**
Specified as localized in the meninges

       A02.22   **Salmonella pneumonia**
Specified as localized in the lungs

       A02.23   **Salmonella arthritis**
Specified as localized in the joints

       A02.24   **Salmonella osteomyelitis**
Specified as localized in bone

       A02.25   **Salmonella pyelonephritis**
Salmonella tubulo-interstitial nephropathy

       A02.29   **Salmonella with other localized infection**
Specified as localized (because it is still under localized heading) but does not assign into any of the above codes

    A02.8   **Other specified salmonella infections**
Any specified salmonella infection which does NOT assign into any of the above codes (not specified as localized)

    A02.9   **Salmonella infection, unspecified**
Unspecified in the documentation as to specific type of salmonella

● **A03**   **Shigellosis**
An infectious disease caused by bacteria (Shigella)

    A03.0   **Shigellosis due to Shigella dysenteriae**
Group A shigellosis [Shiga-Kruse dysentery]

    A03.1   **Shigellosis due to Shigella flexneri**
Group B shigellosis

    A03.2   **Shigellosis due to Shigella boydii**
Group C shigellosis

    A03.3   **Shigellosis due to Shigella sonnei**
Group D shigellosis

    A03.8   **Other shigellosis**

    A03.9   **Shigellosis, unspecified**
Bacillary dysentery NOS

Item 1–1   **Salmonella** is a bacterium that lives in the intestines of fowl and mammals and can spread to humans through improper food preparation and cooking. Salmonellosis is an infection with the bacterium. Symptoms include diarrhea, fever, and abdominal cramps 12 to 72 hours after infection. The illness usually lasts 4 to 7 days, and most persons recover without treatment. The diarrhea may be so severe that the patient needs to be hospitalized. Patients with immunocompromised systems in chronic, ill health are more likely to have the infection invade their bloodstream with life-threatening results. For example, patients with sickle cell disease are more prone to salmonella osteomyelitis than others.

◀ New   ◀▥ Revised   ~~deleted~~ Deleted   Excludes 1   Excludes 2   Includes   Use additional   Code first   Code also   Unspecified

OGCR Official Guidelines   X Assign placeholder X   ● Use Additional Character(s)   ▷ Manifestation Code   **Coding Clinic**

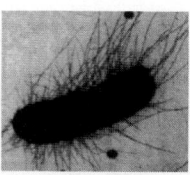

Figure 1-1 Electron micrograph of escherichia coli (E. coli) expressing P fimbriae. (From Mandell, Bennett, & Dolin: Principles and Practice of Infectious Diseases, ed 7, Churchill Livingstone, An Imprint of Elsevier, 2009)

Item 1–2 *Escherichia coli [E. coli]* is a gram-negative bacterium found in the intestinal tracts of humans and animals and is usually nonpathogenic. Pathogenic strains can cause diarrhea or pyogenic (pus-producing) infections. Can be a threat to food safety.

● **A04   Other bacterial intestinal infections**

> **Excludes1**   bacterial foodborne intoxications, NEC (A05.-)
> tuberculous enteritis (A18.32)

A04.0   Enteropathogenic Escherichia coli infection
Pertaining to or producing intestinal disease

A04.1   Enterotoxigenic Escherichia coli infection
Producing or containing intestinal toxin

A04.2   Enteroinvasive Escherichia coli infection
Capable of penetrating and spreading through intestinal mucosal epithelium

A04.3   Enterohemorrhagic Escherichia coli infection
Causing bloody diarrhea, resulting from microorganisms

A04.4   Other intestinal Escherichia coli infections
Escherichia coli enteritis NOS

A04.5   Campylobacter enteritis
Spiral shaped bacterium

A04.6   Enteritis due to Yersinia enterocolitica

> **Excludes1**   extraintestinal yersiniosis (A28.2)

Transmitted by infected food /water and person-to-person contact, affecting intestinal tract

A04.7   Enterocolitis due to Clostridium difficile
Foodborne intoxication by Clostridium difficile
Pseudomembraneous colitis
Marked by fibrinous deposit (false membrane) with enmeshed necrotic cells

A04.8   Other specified bacterial intestinal infections

A04.9   Bacterial intestinal infection, unspecified
Bacterial enteritis NOS

● **A05   Other bacterial foodborne intoxications, not elsewhere classified**

> **Excludes1**   Clostridium difficile foodborne intoxication and infection (A04.7)
> Escherichia coli infection (A04.0-A04.4)
> listeriosis (A32.-)
> salmonella foodborne intoxication and infection (A02.-)
> toxic effect of noxious foodstuffs (T61-T62)

A05.0   Foodborne staphylococcal intoxication

A05.1   Botulism food poisoning
Botulism NOS
Classical foodborne intoxication due to Clostridium botulinum

> **Excludes1**   infant botulism (A48.51)
> wound botulism (A48.52)

A05.2   Foodborne Clostridium perfringens [Clostridium welchii] intoxication
Type A causes gas gangrene and necrotizing colitis; major cause of food poisoning in humans
Enteritis necroticans
Pig-bel

A05.3   Foodborne Vibrio parahaemolyticus intoxication
Organism that survives only in high salt environment (halophilic), major cause of gastroenteritis due to consumption of raw or improperly cooked fish/seafood

A05.4   Foodborne Bacillus cereus intoxication
Spore-forming species commonly found in soil, causes food poisoning from formation of intestinal toxins in contaminated foods

A05.5   Foodborne Vibrio vulnificus intoxication
Species that survives in high salt environment (halophilic) with infection by eating raw seafood causes septicemia and cellulitis

A05.8   Other specified bacterial foodborne intoxications

A05.9   Bacterial foodborne intoxication, unspecified

● **A06   Amebiasis**
An intestinal illness caused by the microscopic parasite Entamoeba histolytica

> **Includes**   infection due to Entamoeba histolytica
> **Excludes1**   other protozoal intestinal diseases (A07.-)
> **Excludes2**   acanthamebiasis (B60.1-)
> Naegleriasis (B60.2)

A06.0   Acute amebic dysentery
Acute amebiasis
Intestinal amebiasis NOS

A06.1   Chronic intestinal amebiasis

A06.2   Amebic nondysenteric colitis
Pertaining to single cell microorganism

A06.3   Ameboma of intestine
Tumorlike mass produced by localized inflammation often in intestine
Ameboma NOS

A06.4   Amebic liver abscess
Hepatic amebiasis

A06.5   Amebic lung abscess
Amebic abscess of lung (and liver)

A06.6   Amebic brain abscess
Amebic abscess of brain (and liver) (and lung)

A06.7   Cutaneous amebiasis

● **A06.8   Amebic infection of other sites**

A06.81   Amebic cystitis

A06.82   Other amebic genitourinary infections
Amebic balanitis
Amebic vesiculitis
Amebic vulvovaginitis

A06.89   Other amebic infections
Amebic appendicitis
Amebic splenic abscess

A06.9   Amebiasis, unspecified

● **A07   Other protozoal intestinal diseases**

A07.0   Balantidiasis
Balantidial dysentery
Infection by protozoa that may cause diarrhea and dysentery, with ulceration of colonic mucous membranes

A07.1   Giardiasis [lambliasis]
Common infection in small intestine spread by contaminated food, water, or direct person-to-person contact

A07.2   Cryptosporidiosis
Human infection with protozoa usually seen as self-limited diarrhea in those who work with cattle

A07.3   Isosporiasis
Human intestinal disease caused by protozoa
Infection due to Isospora belli and Isospora hominis
Intestinal coccidiosis
Isosporosis

A07.4   Cyclosporiasis
Infection by protozoa with most common species infecting humans being C cayetanensis

CHAPTER 1 (A00-B99)

A07.8 Other specified protozoal intestinal diseases
Intestinal microsporidiosis
Intestinal trichomoniasis
Sarcocystosis
Sarcosporidiosis

A07.9 Protozoal intestinal disease, unspecified
Flagellate diarrhea
Protozoal colitis
Protozoal diarrhea
Protozoal dysentery

● **A08 Viral and other specified intestinal infections**
Excludes1   influenza with involvement of gastrointestinal tract (J09.X3, J10.2, J11.2)

A08.0 Rotaviral enteritis
● **A08.1 Acute gastroenteropathy due to Norwalk agent and other small round viruses**
A08.11 Acute gastroenteropathy due to Norwalk agent
Acute gastroenteropathy due to Norovirus
Acute gastroenteropathy due to Norwalk-like agent
A08.19 Acute gastroenteropathy due to other small round viruses
Acute gastroenteropathy due to small round virus [SRV] NOS

A08.2 Adenoviral enteritis
● **A08.3 Other viral enteritis**
A08.31 Calicivirus enteritis
A08.32 Astrovirus enteritis
A08.39 Other viral enteritis
Coxsackie virus enteritis
Echovirus enteritis
Enterovirus enteritis NEC
Torovirus enteritis

A08.4 Viral intestinal infection, unspecified
Viral enteritis NOS
Viral gastroenteritis NOS
Viral gastroenteropathy NOS

A08.8 Other specified intestinal infections

A09 Infectious gastroenteritis and colitis, unspecified
Infectious colitis NOS
Infectious enteritis NOS
Infectious gastroenteritis NOS
Excludes1   colitis NOS (K52.9)
diarrhea NOS (R19.7)
enteritis NOS (K52.9)
gastroenteritis NOS (K52.9)
noninfective gastroenteritis and colitis, unspecified (K52.9)

TUBERCULOSIS (A15-A19)

Includes   infections due to Mycobacterium tuberculosis and Mycobacterium bovis
Excludes1   congenital tuberculosis (P37.0)
nonspecific reaction to test for tuberculosis without active tuberculosis (R76.1-)
pneumoconiosis associated with tuberculosis, any type in A15 (J65)
positive PPD (R76.11)
positive tuberculin skin test without active tuberculosis (R76.11)
sequelae of tuberculosis (B90.-)
silicotuberculosis (J65)

● **A15 Respiratory tuberculosis**
A15.0 Tuberculosis of lung
Tuberculous bronchiectasis
Chronic dilatation of bronchi
Tuberculous fibrosis of lung
Tuberculous pneumonia
Tuberculous pneumothorax

Figure 1-2   Far advanced bilateral pulmonary tuberculosis before and after 8 months of treatment with streptomycin, PAS, and isoniazid. (From Hinshaw HC, Garland LH: Diseases of the Chest, ed 4, Philadelphia, WB Saunders, 1980)

Item 1-3 Tuberculosis is a common and deadly infectious disease caused by the *Mycobacterium tuberculosis* organism. The first tuberculosis infection is called the **primary infection** and most commonly attacks the lungs but can affect the central nervous system, lymphatic system, circulatory system, genitourinary system, bones, joints, and even the skin. A **Ghon** lesion is the **initial lesion.** A **secondary lesion** occurs when the tubercle bacilli are carried to other areas.

Item 1-4 Although it primarily affects the lungs, the bacteria ***Mycobacterium tuberculosis*** can travel from the pulmonary circulation to virtually any organ in the body, much as a cancer metastasizes to a secondary site. If the immune system becomes compromised by age or disease, what would otherwise be a self-limiting primary tuberculosis in the lungs will develop in other organs. These are known as extrapulmonary sites.

A15.4 Tuberculosis of intrathoracic lymph nodes
Tuberculosis of hilar lymph nodes
Tuberculosis of mediastinal lymph nodes
Tuberculosis of tracheobronchial lymph nodes
Excludes1   tuberculosis specified as primary (A15.7)
A15.5 Tuberculosis of larynx, trachea and bronchus
Tuberculosis of bronchus
Tuberculosis of glottis
Tuberculosis of larynx
Tuberculosis of trachea
A15.6 Tuberculous pleurisy
Tuberculosis of pleura
Tuberculous empyema
Excludes1   primary respiratory tuberculosis (A15.7)
A15.7 Primary respiratory tuberculosis
A15.8 Other respiratory tuberculosis
Mediastinal tuberculosis
Nasopharyngeal tuberculosis
Tuberculosis of nose
Tuberculosis of sinus [any nasal]
A15.9 Respiratory tuberculosis unspecified

● **A17 Tuberculosis of nervous system**
A17.0 Tuberculous meningitis
Tuberculosis of meninges (cerebral) (spinal)
Tuberculous leptomeningitis
Excludes1   tuberculous meningoencephalitis (A17.82)
A17.1 Meningeal tuberculoma
Tuberculoma of meninges (cerebral) (spinal)
Excludes2   tuberculoma of brain and spinal cord (A17.81)

◀ New   ◀ Revised   ~~deleted~~ Deleted   Excludes 1   Excludes 2   Includes   Use additional   Code first   Code also   Unspecified
OGCR Official Guidelines   X Assign placeholder X   ● Use Additional Character(s)   ▷ Manifestation Code   **Coding Clinic**
638

● A17.8 **Other tuberculosis of nervous system**
    A17.81 **Tuberculoma of brain and spinal cord**
        Tuberculous abscess of brain and spinal cord
    A17.82 **Tuberculous meningoencephalitis**
        Inflammation of brain and meninges; AKA
            cerebromeningitis and encephalomeningitis
        Tuberculous myelitis
    A17.83 **Tuberculous neuritis**
        Tuberculous mononeuropathy
    A17.89 **Other tuberculosis of nervous system**
        Tuberculous polyneuropathy
  A17.9 **Tuberculosis of nervous system, unspecified**

● **A18** **Tuberculosis of other organs**
  ● **A18.0** **Tuberculosis of bones and joints**
    A18.01 **Tuberculosis of spine**
        Pott's disease or curvature of spine
        Tuberculous arthritis
        Tuberculous osteomyelitis of spine
        Tuberculous spondylitis
    A18.02 **Tuberculous arthritis of other joints**
        Tuberculosis of hip (joint)
        Tuberculosis of knee (joint)
    A18.03 **Tuberculosis of other bones**
        Tuberculous mastoiditis
        Tuberculous osteomyelitis
    A18.09 **Other musculoskeletal tuberculosis**
        Tuberculous myositis
        Tuberculous synovitis
        Tuberculous tenosynovitis
  ● **A18.1** **Tuberculosis of genitourinary system**
    A18.10 **Tuberculosis of genitourinary system, unspecified**
    A18.11 **Tuberculosis of kidney and ureter**
    A18.12 **Tuberculosis of bladder**
    A18.13 **Tuberculosis of other urinary organs**
        Tuberculous urethritis
    A18.14 **Tuberculosis of prostate** ♂   **A**
    A18.15 **Tuberculosis of other male genital organs** ♂
    A18.16 **Tuberculosis of cervix** ♀
    A18.17 **Tuberculous female pelvic inflammatory disease** ♀
        Tuberculous endometritis
        Tuberculous oophoritis and salpingitis
            Oophoritis = inflammation of ovary
            Salpingitis = inflammation of fallopian tube
    A18.18 **Tuberculosis of other female genital organs** ♀
        Tuberculous ulceration of vulva
  ● **A18.2** **Tuberculous peripheral lymphadenopathy**
    Tuberculous adenitis
    Excludes2 tuberculosis of bronchial and mediastinal
            lymph nodes (A15.4)
            tuberculosis of mesenteric and
              retroperitoneal lymph nodes
              (A18.39)
            tuberculous tracheobronchial adenopathy
              (A15.4)
  ● **A18.3** **Tuberculosis of intestines, peritoneum and mesenteric glands**
    A18.31 **Tuberculous peritonitis**
        Tuberculous ascites
    A18.32 **Tuberculous enteritis**
        Tuberculosis of anus and rectum
        Tuberculosis of intestine (large) (small)
    A18.39 **Retroperitoneal tuberculosis**
        Tuberculosis of mesenteric glands
        Tuberculosis of retroperitoneal (lymph glands)

● **A18.4** **Tuberculosis of skin and subcutaneous tissue**
    Erythema induratum, tuberculous
    Lupus excedens
    Lupus vulgaris NOS
    Lupus vulgaris of eyelid
      Cutaneous tuberculosis characterized by reddish brown
        plaque on skin surrounded by papules and nodules
    Scrofuloderma
      Type of cutaneous tuberculosis, with direct extension of
        tuberculosis into skin from underlying structures;
        AKA tuberculosis colliquativa
    Tuberculosis of external ear
    Excludes2 lupus erythematosus (L93.-)
            lupus NOS (M32.9)
            systemic (M32.-)
● **A18.5** **Tuberculosis of eye**
    Excludes2 lupus vulgaris of eyelid (A18.4)
    A18.50 **Tuberculosis of eye, unspecified**
    A18.51 **Tuberculous episcleritis**
        Inflammation of episclera and adjacent tissues
    A18.52 **Tuberculous keratitis**
        Tuberculous interstitial keratitis
        Tuberculous keratoconjunctivitis (interstitial)
            (phlyctenular)
        Inflammation of cornea and conjunctiva
    A18.53 **Tuberculous chorioretinitis**
        Inflammation of choroid and retina;
            retinochoroiditis
    A18.54 **Tuberculous iridocyclitis**
        Inflammation of iris and ciliary body
    A18.59 **Other tuberculosis of eye**
        Tuberculous conjunctivitis
  A18.6 **Tuberculosis of (inner) (middle) ear**
    Tuberculous otitis media
    Excludes2 tuberculosis of external ear (A18.4)
            tuberculous mastoiditis (A18.03)
  A18.7 **Tuberculosis of adrenal glands**
    Tuberculous Addison's disease
● **A18.8** **Tuberculosis of other specified organs**
    A18.81 **Tuberculosis of thyroid gland**
    A18.82 **Tuberculosis of other endocrine glands**
        Tuberculosis of pituitary gland
        Tuberculosis of thymus gland
    A18.83 **Tuberculosis of digestive tract organs, not elsewhere classified**
      Excludes1 tuberculosis of intestine (A18.32)
    A18.84 **Tuberculosis of heart**
        Tuberculous cardiomyopathy
        Tuberculous endocarditis
        Tuberculous myocarditis
        Tuberculous pericarditis
    A18.85 **Tuberculosis of spleen**
    A18.89 **Tuberculosis of other sites**
        Tuberculosis of muscle
        Tuberculous cerebral arteritis

● **A19** **Miliary tuberculosis**
    Includes   disseminated tuberculosis
             generalized tuberculosis
             tuberculous polyserositis
  A19.0 **Acute miliary tuberculosis of a single specified site**
  A19.1 **Acute miliary tuberculosis of multiple sites**
  A19.2 **Acute miliary tuberculosis, unspecified**
  A19.8 **Other miliary tuberculosis**
  A19.9 **Miliary tuberculosis, unspecified**

Item 1-5 Miliary tuberculosis can be a life-threatening condition. If a tuberculous lesion enters a blood vessel, immense dissemination of tuberculous organisms can occur if the immune system is weak. High-risk populations—children under 4 years of age, the elderly, or the immunocompromised—are particularly prone to this type of infection. The lesions will have a millet seedlike appearance on chest x-ray. Bronchial washings and biopsy may aid in diagnosis.

CHAPTER 1 (A00-B99)

CERTAIN ZOONOTIC BACTERIAL DISEASES (A20-A28)

● **A20　Plague**
　　Infectious disease caused by a Yersinia pestis bacterium, transmitted by a rodent flea bite or handling of infected animal
　　Includes　infection due to Yersinia pestis

　　A20.0　Bubonic plague

　　A20.1　Cellulocutaneous plague
　　　　Skin and subcutaneous tissue plague

　　A20.2　Pneumonic plague

　　A20.3　Plague meningitis

　　A20.7　Septicemic plague

　　A20.8　Other forms of plague
　　　　Abortive plague
　　　　Asymptomatic plague
　　　　Pestis minor
　　　　　Systemic bacterial disease

　　A20.9　Plague, unspecified

● **A21　Tularemia**
　　Caused by Francisella tularensis bacterium found in rodents, rabbits, and hares and transmitted to humans by contact with infected animal tissues or by ticks, biting flies, or mosquitoes
　　Includes　deer-fly fever
　　　　　　　　infection due to Francisella tularensis
　　　　　　　　rabbit fever

　　A21.0　Ulceroglandular tularemia
　　　　Most common form of tularemia in humans is painful, swollen, erythematous papule at point of inoculation that ruptures to form shallow ulcer

　　A21.1　Oculoglandular tularemia
　　　　Primary site of entry is conjunctival sac, results in granulomatous corneal lesions
　　　　Ophthalmic tularemia

　　A21.2　Pulmonary tularemia

　　A21.3　Gastrointestinal tularemia
　　　　Abdominal tularemia

　　A21.7　Generalized tularemia

　　A21.8　Other forms of tularemia

　　A21.9　Tularemia, unspecified

● **A22　Anthrax**
　　An acute infectious disease caused by the spore-forming Bacillus anthracis; occurs in humans exposed to infected animals or tissue from infected animals
　　Includes　infection due to Bacillus anthracis

　　A22.0　Cutaneous anthrax
　　　　Malignant carbuncle
　　　　Malignant pustule

　　A22.1　Pulmonary anthrax
　　　　Inhalation anthrax
　　　　Ragpicker's disease
　　　　Woolsorter's disease

　　A22.2　Gastrointestinal anthrax

　　A22.7　Anthrax sepsis
　　　　Infectious bacterial disease

　　A22.8　Other forms of anthrax
　　　　Anthrax meningitis

　　A22.9　Anthrax, unspecified

Item 1-6　Brucellosis: An infectious disease caused by the bacterium Brucella. Humans are infected by contact with contaminated animals or animal products. In humans brucellosis symptoms that are similar to the flu include fever, sweats, headaches, back pains, and physical weakness. Severe infections of the central nervous system or lining of the heart may occur. Brucellosis can also cause chronic symptoms that include recurrent fevers, joint pain, and fatigue.

● **A23　Brucellosis**
　　Includes　Malta fever
　　　　　　　　Mediterranean fever
　　　　　　　　undulant fever

　　A23.0　Brucellosis due to Brucella melitensis
　　　　Resulting in flu-like symptoms that may lead to chronic symptoms that include recurrent fevers, joint pain, and fatigue

　　A23.1　Brucellosis due to Brucella abortus
　　　　Most common cause of brucellosis in humans; AKA Bang bacillus

　　A23.2　Brucellosis due to Brucella suis
　　　　Species found primarily in pigs, rabbits, and reindeer

　　A23.3　Brucellosis due to Brucella canis
　　　　Species that causes respiratory tract infection in humans

　　A23.8　Other brucellosis

　　A23.9　Brucellosis, unspecified

● **A24　Glanders and melioidosis**
　　Infection, usually of rodents, which spreads to other animals and humans, caused by Burkholderia pseudomallei through break in skin contaminated with infested soil or water

　　A24.0　Glanders
　　　　Infection due to Pseudomonas mallei
　　　　Malleus

　　A24.1　Acute and fulminating melioidosis
　　　　Melioidosis pneumonia
　　　　Melioidosis sepsis

　　A24.2　Subacute and chronic melioidosis

　　A24.3　Other melioidosis

　　A24.9　Melioidosis, unspecified
　　　　Infection due to Pseudomonas pseudomallei NOS
　　　　Whitmore's disease

● **A25　Rat-bite fevers**
　　RBF, infectious disease caused by Streptobacillus moniliformis or Spirillum minus.

　　A25.0　Spirillosis
　　　　Any disease condition caused by spirilla
　　　　Sodoku

　　A25.1　Streptobacillosis
　　　　Acute, febrile human illness caused by bacteria transmitted by rats in most cases, passed from rodent to human via rodent's urine or mucous secretions; AKA rat fever
　　　　Epidemic arthritic erythema
　　　　Haverhill fever
　　　　Streptobacillary rat-bite fever

　　A25.9　Rat-bite fever, unspecified

● **A26　Erysipeloid**
　　Infection with Erysipelothrix rhusiopathiae, occurring often as occupational disease resulting from handling infected fish, shellfish, meat, or poultry

　　A26.0　Cutaneous erysipeloid
　　　　Erythema migrans

　　A26.7　Erysipelothrix sepsis

　　A26.8　Other forms of erysipeloid

　　A26.9　Erysipeloid, unspecified

◀ New　　◀▥ Revised　　d̶e̶l̶e̶t̶e̶d̶ Deleted　　Excludes 1　　Excludes 2　　Includes　　Use additional　　Code first　　Code also　　Unspecified

OGCR Official Guidelines　　X Assign placeholder X　　● Use Additional Character(s)　　▶ Manifestation Code　　**Coding Clinic**

- **A27　Leptospirosis**
  Occurs most commonly in the tropics
  - **A27.0　Leptospirosis icterohemorrhagica**
    Leptospiral or spirochetal jaundice (hemorrhagic)
    Weil's disease
  - **A27.8　Other forms of leptospirosis**
    - **A27.81　Aseptic meningitis in leptospirosis**
    - **A27.89　Other forms of leptospirosis**
  - **A27.9　Leptospirosis, unspecified**

- **A28　Other zoonotic bacterial diseases, not elsewhere classified**
  - **A28.0　Pasteurellosis**
    Infection of humans or other animals by species of Pasteurella
  - **A28.1　Cat-scratch disease**
    Cat-scratch fever
  - **A28.2　Extraintestinal yersiniosis**
    Infection from Yersinia enterocolitica; AKA enteric yersiniosis, intestinal yersiniosis, Yersinia enteritis
    - **Excludes1**　enteritis due to Yersinia enterocolitica (A04.6)
      plague (A20.-)
  - **A28.8　Other specified zoonotic bacterial diseases, not elsewhere classified**
  - **A28.9　Zoonotic bacterial disease, unspecified**

OTHER BACTERIAL DISEASES (A30-A49)

- **A30　Leprosy [Hansen's disease]**
  Chronic infectious disease attacking the skin, peripheral nerves, and mucous membranes
  - **Includes**　infection due to Mycobacterium leprae
  - **Excludes1**　sequelae of leprosy (B92)
  - **A30.0　Indeterminate leprosy**
    I leprosy
  - **A30.1　Tuberculoid leprosy**
    TT leprosy
  - **A30.2　Borderline tuberculoid leprosy**
    BT leprosy
  - **A30.3　Borderline leprosy**
    BB leprosy
  - **A30.4　Borderline lepromatous leprosy**
    BL leprosy
  - **A30.5　Lepromatous leprosy**
    LL leprosy
  - **A30.8　Other forms of leprosy**
  - **A30.9　Leprosy, unspecified**

- **A31　Infection due to other mycobacteria**
  - **Excludes2**　leprosy (A30.-)
    tuberculosis (A15-A19)
  - **A31.0　Pulmonary mycobacterial infection**
    Infection due to Mycobacterium avium
    Infection due to Mycobacterium intracellulare [Battey bacillus]
    Infection due to Mycobacterium kansasii
  - **A31.1　Cutaneous mycobacterial infection**
    Buruli ulcer
    Infection due to Mycobacterium marinum
    Infection due to Mycobacterium ulcerans
  - **A31.2　Disseminated mycobacterium avium-intracellulare complex (DMAC)**
    MAC sepsis
  - **A31.8　Other mycobacterial infections**
  - **A31.9　Mycobacterial infection, unspecified**
    Atypical mycobacterial infection NOS
    Mycobacteriosis NOS

- **A32　Listeriosis**
  Infection caused by Listeria monocytogenes
  - **Includes**　listerial foodborne infection
  - **Excludes1**　neonatal (disseminated) listeriosis (P37.2)
  - **A32.0　Cutaneous listeriosis**
  - **A32.1　Listerial meningitis and meningoencephalitis**
    - **A32.11　Listerial meningitis**
    - **A32.12　Listerial meningoencephalitis**
  - **A32.7　Listerial sepsis**
  - **A32.8　Other forms of listeriosis**
    - **A32.81　Oculoglandular listeriosis**
      Primary infection site is conjunctival sac, which if untreated may result in perforation of cornea and optic atrophy
    - **A32.82　Listerial endocarditis**
      Exudative and proliferative inflammatory condition of endocardium caused by listeria bacteria
    - **A32.89　Other forms of listeriosis**
      Listerial cerebral arteritis
  - **A32.9　Listeriosis, unspecified**

- **A33　Tetanus neonatorum**　　　　　　　　　　　　　　　N
  Neonate = newborn

- **A34　Obstetrical tetanus ♀**　　　　　　　　　　　　　M

- **A35　Other tetanus**
  Tetanus NOS
  - **Excludes1**　tetanus neonatorum (A33)
    obstetrical tetanus (A34)

- **A36　Diphtheria**
  - **A36.0　Pharyngeal diphtheria**
    Diphtheritic membranous angina
    Tonsillar diphtheria
  - **A36.1　Nasopharyngeal diphtheria**
  - **A36.2　Laryngeal diphtheria**
    Diphtheritic laryngotracheitis
  - **A36.3　Cutaneous diphtheria**
    - **Excludes2**　erythrasma (L08.1)
  - **A36.8　Other diphtheria**
    - **A36.81　Diphtheritic cardiomyopathy**
      Diphtheritic myocarditis
    - **A36.82　Diphtheritic radiculomyelitis**
    - **A36.83　Diphtheritic polyneuritis**
    - **A36.84　Diphtheritic tubulo-interstitial nephropathy**
    - **A36.85　Diphtheritic cystitis**
    - **A36.86　Diphtheritic conjunctivitis**
    - **A36.89　Other diphtheritic complications**
      Diphtheritic peritonitis
  - **A36.9　Diphtheria, unspecified**

Item 1-7 Diptheria: A highly contagious bacterial disease that results in the formation of an adherent membrane in the throat that may lead to suffocation. In its most poisonous form, it attacks the heart and lungs. It is spread by direct physical contact or breathing the aerosolized secretions of infected individuals. The exact location is specified in the codes.

CHAPTER 1 (A00-B99)

● A37   Whooping cough
         Pertussis is a highly contagious disease caused by the bacterium
         Bordetella pertussis and results in a whooping sounding cough.
    ● A37.0   Whooping cough due to Bordetella pertussis
         A37.00   Whooping cough due to Bordetella pertussis
                  without pneumonia
         A37.01   Whooping cough due to Bordetella pertussis
                  with pneumonia
    ● A37.1   Whooping cough due to Bordetella parapertussis
         A37.10   Whooping cough due to Bordetella
                  parapertussis without pneumonia
         A37.11   Whooping cough due to Bordetella
                  parapertussis with pneumonia
    ● A37.8   Whooping cough due to other Bordetella species
         A37.80   Whooping cough due to other Bordetella
                  species without pneumonia
         A37.81   Whooping cough due to other Bordetella
                  species with pneumonia
    ● A37.9   Whooping cough, unspecified species
         A37.90   Whooping cough, unspecified species without
                  pneumonia
         A37.91   Whooping cough, unspecified species with
                  pneumonia

● A38   Scarlet fever
         Most commonly caused by the bacteria Streptococcus pneumoniae and
         Neisseria meningitides
         Includes   scarlatina
         Excludes2   streptococcal sore throat (J02.0)

    A38.0   Scarlet fever with otitis media
    A38.1   Scarlet fever with myocarditis
    A38.8   Scarlet fever with other complications
    A38.9   Scarlet fever, uncomplicated
            Scarlet fever, NOS

● A39   Meningococcal infection
         Most commonly caused by the bacteria Streptococcus pneumoniae and
         Neisseria meningitides
    A39.0   Meningococcal meningitis
    A39.1   Waterhouse-Friderichsen syndrome
            Fulminating complication of meningococcemia
            Meningococcal hemorrhagic adrenalitis
            Meningococcic adrenal syndrome
    A39.2   Acute meningococcemia
    A39.3   Chronic meningococcemia
    A39.4   Meningococcemia, unspecified
    ● A39.5   Meningococcal heart disease
         A39.50   Meningococcal carditis, unspecified
         A39.51   Meningococcal endocarditis
         A39.52   Meningococcal myocarditis
         A39.53   Meningococcal pericarditis
    ● A39.8   Other meningococcal infections
         A39.81   Meningococcal encephalitis
         A39.82   Meningococcal retrobulbar neuritis
                  Optic neuritis in portion of optic nerve posterior to
                  eyeball; AKA postocular optic neuritis
         A39.83   Meningococcal arthritis
         A39.84   Postmeningococcal arthritis
         A39.89   Other meningococcal infections
                  Meningococcal conjunctivitis
    A39.9   Meningococcal infection, unspecified
            Meningococcal disease NOS

● A40   Streptococcal sepsis
         Code first
            postprocedural streptococcal sepsis (T81.4-) ◀▥
            streptococcal sepsis during labor (O75.3)
            streptococcal sepsis following abortion or ectopic or molar
               pregnancy (O03-O07, O08.0)
            streptococcal sepsis following immunization (T88.0)
            streptococcal sepsis following infusion, transfusion or
               therapeutic injection (T80.2-)
         Excludes1   neonatal (P36.0-P36.1)
                           puerperal sepsis (O85)
                           sepsis due to Streptococcus, group D (A41.81)
    A40.0   Sepsis due to streptococcus, group A
    A40.1   Sepsis due to streptococcus, group B
    A40.3   Sepsis due to Streptococcus pneumoniae
            Pneumococcal sepsis
    A40.8   Other streptococcal sepsis
    A40.9   Streptococcal sepsis, unspecified

● A41   Other sepsis
         Code first
            postprocedural sepsis (T81.4-) ◀▥
            sepsis during labor (O75.3)
            sepsis following abortion, ectopic or molar pregnancy
               (O03-O07, O08.0)
            sepsis following immunization (T88.0)
            sepsis following infusion, transfusion or therapeutic injection
               (T80.2-)
         Excludes1   bacteremia NOS (R78.81)
                           neonatal (P36.-)
                           puerperal sepsis (O85)
                           sepsis NOS (A41.9)
                           streptococcal sepsis (A40.-)
         Excludes2   sepsis (due to) (in) actinomycotic (A42.7)
                           sepsis (due to) (in) anthrax (A22.7)
                           sepsis (due to) (in) candidal (B37.7)
                           sepsis (due to) (in) Erysipelothrix (A26.7)
                           sepsis (due to) (in) extraintestinal yersiniosis
                              (A28.2)
                           sepsis (due to) (in) gonococcal (A54.86)
                           sepsis (due to) (in) herpesviral (B00.7)
                           sepsis (due to) (in) listerial (A32.7)
                           sepsis (due to) (in) melioidosis (A24.1)
                           sepsis (due to) (in) meningococcal (A39.2-A39.4)
                           sepsis (due to) (in) plague (A20.7)
                           sepsis (due to) (in) tularemia (A21.7)
                           toxic shock syndrome (A48.3)
         Coding Clinic: 2016, Q1, P39
    ● A41.0   Sepsis due to Staphylococcus aureus
         A41.01   Sepsis due to Methicillin susceptible
                  Staphylococcus aureus
                  MSSA sepsis
                  Staphylococcus aureus sepsis NOS
         A41.02   Sepsis due to Methicillin resistant
                  Staphylococcus aureus
    A41.1   Sepsis due to other specified staphylococcus
            Coagulase negative staphylococcus sepsis
    A41.2   Sepsis due to unspecified staphylococcus
    A41.3   Sepsis due to Hemophilus influenzae
    A41.4   Sepsis due to anaerobes
         Excludes1   gas gangrene (A48.0)
    ● A41.5   Sepsis due to other Gram-negative organisms
         A41.50   Gram-negative sepsis, unspecified
                  Gram-negative sepsis NOS
         A41.51   Sepsis due to Escherichia coli [E. coli]
         A41.52   Sepsis due to Pseudomonas
                  Pseudomonas aeroginosa
         A41.53   Sepsis due to Serratia
         A41.59   Other Gram-negative sepsis

- A41.8   Other specified sepsis
  - A41.81   Sepsis due to Enterococcus
  - A41.89   Other specified sepsis
  - A41.9   Sepsis, unspecified organism
    - Septicemia NOS
- A42   Actinomycosis
  - Excludes1   actinomycetoma (B47.1)
  - A42.0   Pulmonary actinomycosis
  - A42.1   Abdominal actinomycosis
  - A42.2   Cervicofacial actinomycosis
  - A42.7   Actinomycotic sepsis
  - A42.8   Other forms of actinomycosis
    - A42.81   Actinomycotic meningitis
    - A42.82   Actinomycotic encephalitis
    - A42.89   Other forms of actinomycosis
  - A42.9   Actinomycosis, unspecified
- A43   Nocardiosis
  - A43.0   Pulmonary nocardiosis
  - A43.1   Cutaneous nocardiosis
  - A43.8   Other forms of nocardiosis
  - A43.9   Nocardiosis, unspecified
- A44   Bartonellosis
  - A44.0   Systemic bartonellosis
    - Oroya fever
  - A44.1   Cutaneous and mucocutaneous bartonellosis
    - Verruga peruana
  - A44.8   Other forms of bartonellosis
  - A44.9   Bartonellosis, unspecified
- A46   Erysipelas
  - Excludes1   postpartum or puerperal erysipelas (O86.89)
- A48   Other bacterial diseases, not elsewhere classified
  - Excludes1   actinomycetoma (B47.1)
  - A48.0   Gas gangrene
    - Clostridial cellulitis
    - Clostridial myonecrosis
  - A48.1   Legionnaires' disease
  - A48.2   Nonpneumonic Legionnaires' disease [Pontiac fever]
  - A48.3   Toxic shock syndrome
    - Use additional code to identify the organism (B95, B96)
    - Excludes1   endotoxic shock NOS (R57.8)
      - sepsis NOS (A41.9)
  - A48.4   Brazilian purpuric fever
    - Systemic Hemophilus aegyptius infection
  - A48.5   Other specified botulism
    - Non-foodborne intoxication due to toxins of Clostridium botulinum [C. botulinum]
    - Excludes1   food poisoning due to toxins of Clostridium botulinum (A05.1)
    - A48.51   Infant botulism   P
    - A48.52   Wound botulism
      - Non-foodborne botulism NOS
      - Use additional code for associated wound
  - A48.8   Other specified bacterial diseases

- A49   Bacterial infection of unspecified site
  - Excludes1   bacterial agents as the cause of diseases classified elsewhere (B95-B96)
    - chlamydial infection NOS (A74.9)
    - meningococcal infection NOS (A39.9)
    - rickettsial infection NOS (A79.9)
    - spirochetal infection NOS (A69.9)
  - A49.0   Staphylococcal infection, unspecified site
    - A49.01   Methicillin susceptible Staphylococcus aureus infection, unspecified site
      - Methicillin susceptible Staphylococcus aureus (MSSA) infection
      - Staphylococcus aureus infection NOS
    - A49.02   Methicillin resistant Staphylococcus aureus infection, unspecified site
      - Methicillin resistant Staphylococcus aureus (MRSA) infection
  - A49.1   Streptococcal infection, unspecified site
  - A49.2   Hemophilus influenzae infection, unspecified site
    - *Any of seven bacterium of genus Haemophilus*
  - A49.3   Mycoplasma infection, unspecified site
    - *Bacterium of class Mollicutes, unusual group of bacteria distinguished by absence of cell wall*
  - A49.8   Other bacterial infections of unspecified site
  - A49.9   Bacterial infection, unspecified
    - Excludes1   bacteremia NOS (R78.81)

INFECTIONS WITH A PREDOMINANTLY SEXUAL MODE OF TRANSMISSION (A50-A64)

- Excludes1   human immunodeficiency virus [HIV] disease (B20)
  - nonspecific and nongonococcal urethritis (N34.1)
  - Reiter's disease (M02.3-)

- A50   Congenital syphilis
  - A50.0   Early congenital syphilis, symptomatic
    - Any congenital syphilitic condition specified as early or manifest less than two years after birth
    - A50.01   Early congenital syphilitic oculopathy
    - A50.02   Early congenital syphilitic osteochondropathy
    - A50.03   Early congenital syphilitic pharyngitis
      - Early congenital syphilitic laryngitis
    - A50.04   Early congenital syphilitic pneumonia
    - A50.05   Early congenital syphilitic rhinitis
    - A50.06   Early cutaneous congenital syphilis
    - A50.07   Early mucocutaneous congenital syphilis
    - A50.08   Early visceral congenital syphilis
    - A50.09   Other early congenital syphilis, symptomatic

Figure 1-3   Chancre of primary syphilis. (From Mandell, Bennett, & Dolin: Principles and Practice of Infectious Diseases, ed 7, Churchill Livingstone, An Imprint of Elsevier, 2009)

Item 1-9   Syphilis, also known as lues, is the most serious of the venereal diseases caused by *Treponema pallidum*. The **primary** stage is characterized by an ulceration known as **chancre,** which usually appears on the genitals but can also develop on the anus, lips, tonsils, breasts, or fingers. Syphilis is easy to cure in its early stages. A single intramuscular injection of penicillin will usually cure a person who has had syphilis for less than a year.

The **secondary** stage is characterized by a rash that can affect any area of the body. **Latent** syphilis is divided into **early,** which is diagnosed within two years of infection, and **late,** which is diagnosed two years or more after infection. Additional doses of penicillin or another antibiotic are needed to treat someone who has had syphilis for longer than a year. For those allergic to penicillin, there are other antibiotic treatments. **Congenital** syphilis is also labeled **early** or **late** based on the time of diagnosis.

Item 1-8   Gas gangrene is a necrotizing subcutaneous infection that will cause tissue death. Patients with poor circulation (e.g., diabetes, peripheral nephropathy) will have low oxygen content in their tissues (hypoxia), which allows the Clostridium bacteria to flourish. Gas gangrene often occurs at the site of a surgical wound or trauma. Onset is sudden and dramatic. Treatment can include debridement, amputation, and/or hyperbaric oxygen treatments.

A50.1 **Early congenital syphilis, latent**
Congenital syphilis without clinical manifestations, with positive serological reaction and negative spinal fluid test, less than two years after birth

A50.2 **Early congenital syphilis, unspecified**
Congenital syphilis NOS less than two years after birth

● **A50.3** **Late congenital syphilitic oculopathy**

  | Excludes1 | Hutchinson's triad (A50.53)

  A50.30 **Late congenital syphilitic oculopathy, unspecified**

  A50.31 **Late congenital syphilitic interstitial keratitis**

  A50.32 **Late congenital syphilitic chorioretinitis**

  A50.39 **Other late congenital syphilitic oculopathy**

● **A50.4** **Late congenital neurosyphilis [juvenile neurosyphilis]**
Use additional code to identify any associated mental disorder

  | Excludes1 | Hutchinson's triad (A50.53)

  A50.40 **Late congenital neurosyphilis, unspecified**
Juvenile neurosyphilis NOS

  A50.41 **Late congenital syphilitic meningitis**

  A50.42 **Late congenital syphilitic encephalitis**

  A50.43 **Late congenital syphilitic polyneuropathy**

  A50.44 **Late congenital syphilitic optic nerve atrophy**

  A50.45 **Juvenile general paresis**
Dementia paralytica juvenilis
Juvenile tabetoparetic neurosyphilis

  A50.49 **Other late congenital neurosyphilis**
Juvenile tabes dorsalis

● **A50.5** **Other late congenital syphilis, symptomatic**
Any congenital syphilitic condition specified as late or manifest two years or more after birth

  A50.51 **Clutton's joints**

  A50.52 **Hutchinson's teeth**

  A50.53 **Hutchinson's triad**

  A50.54 **Late congenital cardiovascular syphilis**

  A50.55 **Late congenital syphilitic arthropathy**

  A50.56 **Late congenital syphilitic osteochondropathy**

  A50.57 **Syphilitic saddle nose**

  A50.59 **Other late congenital syphilis, symptomatic**

A50.6 **Late congenital syphilis, latent**
Congenital syphilis without clinical manifestations, with positive serological reaction and negative spinal fluid test, two years or more after birth.

A50.7 **Late congenital syphilis, unspecified**
Congenital syphilis NOS two years or more after birth.

A50.9 **Congenital syphilis, unspecified**

● **A51** **Early syphilis**

  A51.0 **Primary genital syphilis**
Syphilitic chancre NOS

  A51.1 **Primary anal syphilis**

  A51.2 **Primary syphilis of other sites**

● **A51.3** **Secondary syphilis of skin and mucous membranes**

  A51.31 **Condyloma latum**

  A51.32 **Syphilitic alopecia**

  A51.39 **Other secondary syphilis of skin**
Syphilitic leukoderma
Syphilitic mucous patch

    | Excludes1 | late syphilitic leukoderma (A52.79)

● **A51.4** **Other secondary syphilis**

  A51.41 **Secondary syphilitic meningitis**

  A51.42 **Secondary syphilitic female pelvic disease** ♀

  A51.43 **Secondary syphilitic oculopathy**
Secondary syphilitic chorioretinitis
Secondary syphilitic iridocyclitis, iritis
Secondary syphilitic uveitis

  A51.44 **Secondary syphilitic nephritis**

  A51.45 **Secondary syphilitic hepatitis**

  A51.46 **Secondary syphilitic osteopathy**

  A51.49 **Other secondary syphilitic conditions**
Secondary syphilitic lymphadenopathy
Secondary syphilitic myositis

A51.5 **Early syphilis, latent**
Syphilis (acquired) without clinical manifestations, with positive serological reaction and negative spinal fluid test, less than two years after infection.

A51.9 **Early syphilis, unspecified**

● **A52** **Late syphilis**

● **A52.0** **Cardiovascular and cerebrovascular syphilis**

  A52.00 **Cardiovascular syphilis, unspecified**

  A52.01 **Syphilitic aneurysm of aorta**

  A52.02 **Syphilitic aortitis**

  A52.03 **Syphilitic endocarditis**
Syphilitic aortic valve incompetence or stenosis
Syphilitic mitral valve stenosis
Syphilitic pulmonary valve regurgitation

  A52.04 **Syphilitic cerebral arteritis**

  A52.05 **Other cerebrovascular syphilis**
Syphilitic cerebral aneurysm (ruptured) (non-ruptured)
Syphilitic cerebral thrombosis

  A52.06 **Other syphilitic heart involvement**
Syphilitic coronary artery disease
Syphilitic myocarditis
Syphilitic pericarditis

  A52.09 **Other cardiovascular syphilis**

● **A52.1** **Symptomatic neurosyphilis**

  A52.10 **Symptomatic neurosyphilis, unspecified**

  A52.11 **Tabes dorsalis**
Cognitive decline with progressive degeneration of posterior columns, roots, and ganglia of spinal cord, occur 15-20 years after initial infection of syphilis; AKA Duchenne disease
Locomotor ataxia (progressive)
Tabetic neurosyphilis

  A52.12 **Other cerebrospinal syphilis**

  A52.13 **Late syphilitic meningitis**

  A52.14 **Late syphilitic encephalitis**

  A52.15 **Late syphilitic neuropathy**
Late syphilitic acoustic neuritis
Late syphilitic optic (nerve) atrophy
Late syphilitic polyneuropathy
Late syphilitic retrobulbar neuritis

  A52.16 **Charcôt's arthropathy (tabetic)**
Progressive musculoskeletal condition characterized by joint dislocation, fractures, and deformities, results in progressive destruction of bone and soft tissue of weight-bearing joints

  A52.17 **General paresis**
Chronic meningoencephalitis results in loss of cortical function, or progressive dementia and generalized paralysis, occurring 10-20 years after initial infection of syphilis; AKA Bayle disease, dementia paralytica, paralytic dementiaparetic neurosyphilis, syphilitic meningoencephalitis
Dementia paralytica

  A52.19 **Other symptomatic neurosyphilis**
Syphilitic parkinsonism

◀ New   ◀▦ Revised   ~~deleted~~ Deleted | Excludes 1 | | Excludes 2 | | Includes | | Use additional | | Code first | | Code also | | Unspecified |

644   OGCR Official Guidelines   X Assign placeholder X   ● Use Additional Character(s)   ▶ Manifestation Code   **Coding Clinic**

CHAPTER 1 (A00-B99)

A52.2   **Asymptomatic neurosyphilis**

A52.3   **Neurosyphilis,** unspecified
  Gumma (syphilitic)
  Destructive lesions of syphilis
  Syphilis (late)
  Syphiloma

● **A52.7**   **Other symptomatic late syphilis**

     A52.71   **Late syphilitic oculopathy**
  Late syphilitic chorioretinitis
  Late syphilitic episcleritis

     A52.72   **Syphilis of lung and bronchus**

     A52.73   **Symptomatic late syphilis of other respiratory organs**

     A52.74   **Syphilis of liver and other viscera**
  Late syphilitic peritonitis

     A52.75   **Syphilis of kidney and ureter**
  Syphilitic glomerular disease

     A52.76   **Other genitourinary symptomatic late syphilis**
  Late syphilitic female pelvic inflammatory disease

     A52.77   **Syphilis of bone and joint**

     A52.78   **Syphilis of other musculoskeletal tissue**
  Late syphilitic bursitis
  Syphilis [stage unspecified] of bursa
  Syphilis [stage unspecified] of muscle
  Syphilis [stage unspecified] of synovium
  Syphilis [stage unspecified] of tendon

     A52.79   **Other symptomatic late syphilis**
  Late syphilitic leukoderma
  Syphilis of adrenal gland
  Syphilis of pituitary gland
  Syphilis of thyroid gland
  Syphilitic splenomegaly
     Excludes1   syphilitic leukoderma (secondary) (A51.39)

A52.8   **Late syphilis, latent**
  Syphilis (acquired) without clinical manifestations, with positive serological reaction and negative spinal fluid test, two years or more after infection

A52.9   **Late syphilis,** unspecified

● **A53**   **Other and unspecified syphilis**

A53.0   **Latent syphilis,** unspecified **as early or late**
  Latent syphilis NOS
  Positive serological reaction for syphilis

A53.9   **Syphilis,** unspecified
  Infection due to Treponema pallidum NOS
  Syphilis (acquired) NOS
     Excludes1   syphilis NOS under two years of age (A50.2)

● **A54**   **Gonococcal infection**

● **A54.0**   **Gonococcal infection of lower genitourinary tract without periurethral or accessory gland abscess**
     Excludes1   gonococcal infection with genitourinary gland abscess (A54.1)
                     gonococcal infection with periurethral abscess (A54.1)

     A54.00   **Gonococcal infection of lower genitourinary tract,** unspecified

     A54.01   **Gonococcal cystitis and urethritis,** unspecified

     A54.02   **Gonococcal vulvovaginitis,** unspecified ♀

     A54.03   **Gonococcal cervicitis,** unspecified ♀

     A54.09   **Other gonococcal infection of lower genitourinary tract**

A54.1   **Gonococcal infection of lower genitourinary tract with periurethral and accessory gland abscess**
  Gonococcal Bartholin's gland abscess

Item 1-10 An STD (sexually transmitted disease) caused by **Neisseria gonorrhoeae** that flourishes in the warm, moist areas of the reproductive tract. Untreated gonorrhea spreads to other parts of the body, causing inflammation of the testes or prostate or pelvic inflammatory disease (PID).

● **A54.2**   **Gonococcal pelviperitonitis and other gonococcal genitourinary infection**

     A54.21   **Gonococcal infection of kidney and ureter**

     A54.22   **Gonococcal prostatitis** ♂

     A54.23   **Gonococcal infection of other male genital organs** ♂
  Gonococcal epididymitis
  Gonococcal orchitis

     A54.24   **Gonococcal female pelvic inflammatory disease** ♀
  Gonococcal pelviperitonitis
     Excludes1   gonococcal peritonitis (A54.85)

     A54.29   **Other gonococcal genitourinary infections**

● **A54.3**   **Gonococcal infection of eye**

     A54.30   **Gonococcal infection of eye,** unspecified

     A54.31   **Gonococcal conjunctivitis**
  Form of bacterial conjunctivitis contracted by newborns during delivery; AKA neonatal conjunctivitis
  Ophthalmia neonatorum due to gonococcus

     A54.32   **Gonococcal iridocyclitis**
  Inflammation of iris and of ciliary body due to gonococcal infection

     A54.33   **Gonococcal keratitis**
  Inflammation of cornea due to gonococcal infection; AKA keratoconjunctivitis, keratopathy

     A54.39   **Other gonococcal eye infection**
  Gonococcal endophthalmia

● **A54.4**   **Gonococcal infection of musculoskeletal system**

     A54.40   **Gonococcal infection of musculoskeletal system,** unspecified

     A54.41   **Gonococcal spondylopathy**
  Disorder of vertebrae due to gonococcal infection; AKA rachiopathy

     A54.42   **Gonococcal arthritis**
     Excludes2   gonococcal infection of spine (A54.41)

     A54.43   **Gonococcal osteomyelitis**
     Excludes2   gonococcal infection of spine (A54.41)

     A54.49   **Gonococcal infection of other musculoskeletal tissue**
  Gonococcal bursitis
  Gonococcal myositis
  Gonococcal synovitis
  Gonococcal tenosynovitis

A54.5   **Gonococcal pharyngitis**

A54.6   **Gonococcal infection of anus and rectum**

● **A54.8**   **Other gonococcal infections**

     A54.81   **Gonococcal meningitis**

     A54.82   **Gonococcal brain abscess**

     A54.83   **Gonococcal heart infection**
  Gonococcal endocarditis
  Gonococcal myocarditis
  Gonococcal pericarditis

     A54.84   **Gonococcal pneumonia**

     A54.85   **Gonococcal peritonitis**
     Excludes1   gonococcal pelviperitonitis (A54.24)

     A54.86   **Gonococcal sepsis**

     A54.89   **Other gonococcal infections**
  Gonococcal keratoderma
  Gonococcal lymphadenitis

A54.9   **Gonococcal infection,** unspecified

CHAPTER 1 (A00-B99)

A55   Chlamydial lymphogranuloma (venereum)
     Climatic or tropical bubo
     Durand-Nicolas-Favre disease
     Esthiomene
     Lymphogranuloma inguinale

● **A56   Other sexually transmitted chlamydial diseases**

     Includes   sexually transmitted diseases due to Chlamydia trachomatis

     Excludes1   neonatal chlamydial conjunctivitis (P39.1)
                    neonatal chlamydial pneumonia (P23.1)

     Excludes2   chlamydial lymphogranuloma (A55)
                    conditions classified to A74.-

   ● **A56.0   Chlamydial infection of lower genitourinary tract**

       A56.00   Chlamydial infection of lower genitourinary tract, unspecified

       A56.01   Chlamydial cystitis and urethritis

       A56.02   Chlamydial vulvovaginitis ♀

       A56.09   Other chlamydial infection of lower genitourinary tract
                    Chlamydial cervicitis

   ● **A56.1   Chlamydial infection of pelviperitoneum and other genitourinary organs**

       A56.11   Chlamydial female pelvic inflammatory disease ♀

       A56.19   Other chlamydial genitourinary infection
                    Chlamydial epididymitis
                    Chlamydial orchitis

     A56.2   Chlamydial infection of genitourinary tract, unspecified

     A56.3   Chlamydial infection of anus and rectum

     A56.4   Chlamydial infection of pharynx

     A56.8   Sexually transmitted chlamydial infection of other sites

A57   Chancroid
     Ulcus molle
     Sexually transmitted infection caused by bacteria, Haemophilus ducreyi

A58   Granuloma inguinale
     Chronic, progressive, ulcerative granulomatous disease
     Donovanosis

● **A59   Trichomoniasis**

     Excludes2   intestinal trichomoniasis (A07.8)

     A common STD caused by a parasite, Trichomonas vaginalis

   ● **A59.0   Urogenital trichomoniasis**

       A59.00   Urogenital trichomoniasis, unspecified
                    Fluor (vaginalis) due to Trichomonas
                    Leukorrhea (vaginalis) due to Trichomonas

       A59.01   Trichomonal vulvovaginitis ♀

       A59.02   Trichomonal prostatitis ♂

       A59.03   Trichomonal cystitis and urethritis

       A59.09   Other urogenital trichomoniasis
                    Common sexually transmitted disease (STD) caused by single-celled protozoan parasite; AKA trich
                    Trichomonas cervicitis

     A59.8   Trichomoniasis of other sites

     A59.9   Trichomoniasis, unspecified

● **A60   Anogenital herpesviral [herpes simplex] infections**

   ● **A60.0   Herpesviral infection of genitalia and urogenital tract**

       A60.00   Herpesviral infection of urogenital system, unspecified

       A60.01   Herpesviral infection of penis ♂

       A60.02   Herpesviral infection of other male genital organs ♂

       A60.03   Herpesviral cervicitis ♀

       A60.04   Herpesviral vulvovaginitis ♀
                    Herpesviral [herpes simplex] ulceration
                    Herpesviral [herpes simplex] vaginitis
                    Herpesviral [herpes simplex] vulvitis

       A60.09   Herpesviral infection of other urogenital tract

     A60.1   Herpesviral infection of perianal skin and rectum

     A60.9   Anogenital herpesviral infection, unspecified

● **A63   Other predominantly sexually transmitted diseases, not elsewhere classified**

     Excludes2   molluscum contagiosum (B08.1)
                    papilloma of cervix (D26.0)

     A63.0   Anogenital (venereal) warts
                  Anogenital warts due to (human) papillomavirus [HPV]
                  Condyloma acuminatum

     A63.8   Other specified predominantly sexually transmitted diseases

A64   Unspecified sexually transmitted disease

OTHER SPIROCHETAL DISEASES (A65-A69)

     Excludes2   leptospirosis (A27.-)
                    syphilis (A50-A53)

A65   Nonvenereal syphilis
     Bejel
     Endemic syphilis
     Njovera

● **A66   Yaws**
     Endemic, infectious, tropical disease caused by spirochete, spread by direct contact; AKA frambesia, framboesia, frambesia tropica

     Includes   bouba
                    frambesia (tropica)
                    pian

     A66.0   Initial lesions of yaws
                  Chancre of yaws
                  Frambesia, initial or primary
                  Initial frambesial ulcer
                  Mother yaw

     A66.1   Multiple papillomata and wet crab yaws
                  Frambesioma
                  Pianoma
                  Plantar or palmar papilloma of yaws

     A66.2   Other early skin lesions of yaws
                  Cutaneous yaws, less than five years after infection
                  Early yaws (cutaneous)(macular)(maculopapular) (micropapular)(papular)
                  Frambeside of early yaws

     A66.3   Hyperkeratosis of yaws
                  Hypertrophy of stratum corneum of skin in which there are small, hard, verrucous scales
                  Ghoul hand
                  Hyperkeratosis, palmar or plantar (early) (late) due to yaws
                  Worm-eaten soles

     A66.4   Gummata and ulcers of yaws
                  Small, rubbery granuloma with necrotic center and inflamed characteristic of advanced stage of syphilis; AKA syphiloma
                  Gummatous frambeside
                  Nodular late yaws (ulcerated)

     A66.5   Gangosa
                  Manifestation of yaws that develops in the soft palate and spreads eroding bone, cartilage, and soft tissue
                  Rhinopharyngitis mutilans

     A66.6   Bone and joint lesions of yaws
                  Yaws ganglion
                  Yaws goundou
                  Yaws gumma, bone
                  Yaws gummatous osteitis or periostitis
                  Yaws hydrarthrosis
                  Yaws osteitis
                  Yaws periostitis (hypertrophic)

◀ New   ⇐ Revised   ~~deleted~~ Deleted   Excludes 1   Excludes 2   Includes   Use additional   Code first   Code also   Unspecified

646   OGCR Official Guidelines   X Assign placeholder X   ● Use Additional Character(s)   ▶ Manifestation Code   **Coding Clinic**

A66.7   Other manifestations of yaws
Juxta-articular nodules of yaws
Mucosal yaws

A66.8   Latent yaws
Yaws without clinical manifestations, with positive serology

A66.9   Yaws, unspecified

● **A67   Pinta [carate]**
Group of nonvenereal diseases caused by Treponema species

A67.0   Primary lesions of pinta
Chancre (primary) of pinta
Papule (primary) of pinta

A67.1   Intermediate lesions of pinta
Erythematous plaques of pinta
Hyperchromic lesions of pinta
Hyperkeratosis of pinta
Pintids

A67.2   Late lesions of pinta
Achromic skin lesions of pinta
Cicatricial skin lesions of pinta
Dyschromic skin lesions of pinta

A67.3   Mixed lesions of pinta
Achromic with hyperchromic skin lesions of pinta [carate]

A67.9   Pinta, unspecified

● **A68   Relapsing fevers**
Includes   recurrent fever
Excludes2   Lyme disease (A69.2-)

A68.0   Louse-borne relapsing fever
Relapsing fever due to Borrelia recurrentis

A68.1   Tick-borne relapsing fever
Relapsing fever due to any Borrelia species other than Borrelia recurrentis

A68.9   Relapsing fever, unspecified

● **A69   Other spirochetal infections**

A69.0   Necrotizing ulcerative stomatitis
Cancrum oris
Fusospirochetal gangrene
Noma
Stomatitis gangrenosa

A69.1   Other Vincent's infections
Fusospirochetal pharyngitis
Necrotizing ulcerative (acute) gingivitis
Necrotizing ulcerative (acute) gingivostomatitis
Spirochetal stomatitis
Trench mouth
Vincent's angina
Vincent's gingivitis

● **A69.2   Lyme disease**
Erythema chronicum migrans due to Borrelia burgdorferi

A69.20   Lyme disease, unspecified

A69.21   Meningitis due to Lyme disease

A69.22   Other neurologic disorders in Lyme disease
Cranial neuritis
Meningoencephalitis
Polyneuropathy

A69.23   Arthritis due to Lyme disease

A69.29   Other conditions associated with Lyme disease
Myopericarditis due to Lyme disease

A69.8   Other specified spirochetal infections

A69.9   Spirochetal infection, unspecified

Item 1-11   Cancrum oris, also known as **noma** or **gangrenous stomatitis,** begins as an ulcer of the gingiva and results in a progressive gangrenous process.

OTHER DISEASES CAUSED BY CHLAMYDIAE (A70-A74)

Excludes1   sexually transmitted chlamydial diseases (A55-A56)

A70   Chlamydia psittaci infections
Ornithosis
Parrot fever
Psittacosis

● **A71   Trachoma**
Excludes1   sequelae of trachoma (B94.0)

A71.0   Initial stage of trachoma
Trachoma dubium

A71.1   Active stage of trachoma
Granular conjunctivitis (trachomatous)
Trachomatous follicular conjunctivitis
Trachomatous pannus

A71.9   Trachoma, unspecified

● **A74   Other diseases caused by chlamydiae**
Excludes1   neonatal chlamydial conjunctivitis (P39.1)
neonatal chlamydial pneumonia (P23.1)
Reiter's disease (M02.3-)
sexually transmitted chlamydial diseases (A55-A56)

Excludes2   chlamydial pneumonia (J16.0)

A74.0   Chlamydial conjunctivitis
Paratrachoma

● **A74.8   Other chlamydial diseases**
A74.81   Chlamydial peritonitis
A74.89   Other chlamydial diseases

A74.9   Chlamydial infection, unspecified
Chlamydiosis NOS

RICKETTSIOSES (A75-A79)

● **A75   Typhus fever**
Excludes1   rickettsiosis due to Ehrlichia sennetsu (A79.81)

A75.0   Epidemic louse-borne typhus fever due to Rickettsia prowazekii
Organisms transmitted between humans via louse
Classical typhus (fever)
Epidemic (louse-borne) typhus

A75.1   Recrudescent typhus [Brill's disease]
Brill-Zinsser disease

A75.2   Typhus fever due to Rickettsia typhi
Murine (flea-borne) typhus

A75.3   Typhus fever due to Rickettsia tsutsugamushi
Scrub (mite-borne) typhus
Tsutsugamushi fever

A75.9   Typhus fever, unspecified
Typhus (fever) NOS

Item 1-12   Rickettsioses are diseases spread from ticks, lice, fleas, or mites to humans.

Typhus is spread to humans chiefly by the fleas of rats.

Endemic identifies a disease as being present in low numbers of humans at all times, whereas **epidemic** identifies a disease as being present in high numbers of humans at a specific time. Morbidity (death) is higher in epidemic diseases.

Brill's disease, also known as **Brill-Zinsser disease,** is spread from human to human by body lice and also from the lice of flying squirrels. **Scrub typhus** is spread in the same ways as Brill's disease.

Malaria is spread to humans by mosquitoes.

CHAPTER 1 (A00-B99)

- A77   Spotted fever [tick-borne rickettsioses]
  - A77.0   **Spotted fever due to Rickettsia rickettsii**
    - Rocky Mountain spotted fever
    - Sao Paulo fever
  - A77.1   **Spotted fever due to Rickettsia conorii**
    - African tick typhus
    - Boutonneuse fever
    - India tick typhus
    - Kenya tick typhus
    - Marseilles fever
    - Mediterranean tick fever
  - A77.2   **Spotted fever due to Rickettsia siberica**
    - North Asian tick fever
    - Siberian tick typhus
  - A77.3   **Spotted fever due to Rickettsia australis**
    - Queensland tick typhus
  - A77.4   **Ehrlichiosis**
    - *Type of tick-borne fever caused by bacteria infection*
    - **Excludes1**   Rickettsiosis due to Ehrlichia sennetsu (A79.81)
    - A77.40   **Ehrlichiosis, unspecified**
    - A77.41   **Ehrlichiosis chafeensis [E. chafeensis]**
    - A77.49   **Other ehrlichiosis**
  - A77.8   **Other spotted fevers**
  - A77.9   **Spotted fever, unspecified**
    - Tick-borne typhus NOS

- A78   Q fever
  - Infection due to Coxiella burnetii
  - Nine Mile fever
  - Quadrilateral fever

- A79   Other rickettsioses
  - A79.0   **Trench fever**
    - Quintan fever
    - Wolhynian fever
  - A79.1   **Rickettsialpox due to Rickettsia akari**
    - Kew Garden fever
    - Vesicular rickettsiosis
  - A79.8   **Other specified rickettsioses**
    - A79.81   **Rickettsiosis due to Ehrlichia sennetsu**
    - A79.89   **Other specified rickettsioses**
  - A79.9   **Rickettsiosis, unspecified**
    - Rickettsial infection NOS

VIRAL AND PRION INFECTIONS OF THE CENTRAL NERVOUS SYSTEM (A80-A89)

- **Excludes1**   postpolio syndrome (G14)
  - sequelae of poliomyelitis (B91)
  - sequelae of viral encephalitis (B94.1)

- A80   Acute poliomyelitis
  - A80.0   **Acute paralytic poliomyelitis, vaccine-associated**
  - A80.1   **Acute paralytic poliomyelitis, wild virus, imported**
  - A80.2   **Acute paralytic poliomyelitis, wild virus, indigenous**
  - A80.3   **Acute paralytic poliomyelitis, other and unspecified**
    - A80.30   **Acute paralytic poliomyelitis, unspecified**
    - A80.39   **Other acute paralytic poliomyelitis**
  - A80.4   **Acute nonparalytic poliomyelitis**
  - A80.9   **Acute poliomyelitis, unspecified**

- A81   Atypical virus infections of central nervous system
  - **Includes**   diseases of the central nervous system caused by prions
  - Use additional code to identify:
    - dementia with behavioral disturbance (F02.81)
    - dementia without behavioral disturbance (F02.80)
  - A81.0   Creutzfeldt-Jakob disease
    - A81.00   **Creutzfeldt-Jakob disease, unspecified**
      - Jakob-Creutzfeldt disease, unspecified
    - A81.01   **Variant Creutzfeldt-Jakob disease**
      - vCJD
    - A81.09   **Other Creutzfeldt-Jakob disease**
      - CJD
      - Familial Creutzfeldt-Jakob disease
      - Iatrogenic Creutzfeldt-Jakob disease
      - Sporadic Creutzfeldt-Jakob disease
      - Subacute spongiform encephalopathy (with dementia)
  - A81.1   **Subacute sclerosing panencephalitis**
    - *Type of viral encephalitis that causes parenchymatous lesions in gray and white matter of brain*
    - Dawson's inclusion body encephalitis
    - Van Bogaert's sclerosing leukoencephalopathy
  - A81.2   **Progressive multifocal leukoencephalopathy**
    - *Group of diseases affecting white matter of brain*
    - Multifocal leukoencephalopathy NOS
  - A81.8   Other atypical virus infections of central nervous system
    - A81.81   **Kuru**
    - A81.82   **Gerstmann-Sträussler-Scheinker syndrome**
      - GSS syndrome
    - A81.83   **Fatal familial insomnia**
      - FFI
    - A81.89   **Other atypical virus infections of central nervous system**
  - A81.9   **Atypical virus infection of central nervous system, unspecified**
    - Prion diseases of the central nervous system NOS

- A82   Rabies
  - *Viral disease affecting the central nervous system and transmitted from infected mammals to man.*
  - A82.0   **Sylvatic rabies**
  - A82.1   **Urban rabies**
  - A82.9   **Rabies, unspecified**

- A83   Mosquito-borne viral encephalitis
  - *Inflammation of the brain caused most commonly by Herpes Simplex virus.*
  - **Includes**   mosquito-borne viral meningoencephalitis
  - **Excludes2**   Venezuelan equine encephalitis (A92.2)
    - West Nile fever (A92.3-)
    - West Nile virus (A92.3-)
  - A83.0   **Japanese encephalitis**
  - A83.1   **Western equine encephalitis**
  - A83.2   **Eastern equine encephalitis**
  - A83.3   **St. Louis encephalitis**
  - A83.4   **Australian encephalitis**
    - Kunjin virus disease
  - A83.5   **California encephalitis**
    - California meningoencephalitis
    - La Crosse encephalitis
  - A83.6   **Rocio virus disease**
    - *Mosquito-borne virus*
  - A83.8   **Other mosquito-borne viral encephalitis**
  - A83.9   **Mosquito-borne viral encephalitis, unspecified**

Item 1-13 Acute Poliomyelitis: Also called infantile paralysis and is caused by the poliovirus, which enters the body orally and infects the intestinal wall and then enters the blood stream and central nervous system, causing muscle weakness and paralysis. This disease has been nearly eradicated with the polio vaccine.

◀ New   ◀▥ Revised   ~~deleted~~ Deleted | Excludes 1 | | Excludes 2 | | Includes | | Use additional | | Code first | | Code also | | Unspecified |

OGCR Official Guidelines   X Assign placeholder X   ● Use Additional Character(s)   ▶ Manifestation Code   **Coding Clinic**

Item 1-14 **Encephalitis** is an inflammation of the brain most often caused by a virus but may also be caused by a bacteria and most commonly transmitted by a mosquito. **Myelitis** is an inflammation of the spinal cord that may disrupt CNS function. Untreated myelitis may rapidly lead to permanent damage to the spinal cord. **Encephalomyelitis** is a general term for an inflammation of the brain and spinal cord.

● **A84   Tick-borne viral encephalitis**

>   **Includes**   tick-borne viral meningoencephalitis

> **A84.0   Far Eastern tick-borne encephalitis [Russian spring-summer encephalitis]**

> **A84.1   Central European tick-borne encephalitis**

> **A84.8   Other tick-borne viral encephalitis**
> > Louping ill
> > Powassan virus disease

> **A84.9   Tick-borne viral encephalitis, unspecified**

● **A85   Other viral encephalitis, not elsewhere classified**

>   **Includes**   specified viral encephalomyelitis NEC
> > specified viral meningoencephalitis NEC

>   **Excludes1**   benign myalgic encephalomyelitis (G93.3)
> > encephalitis due to cytomegalovirus (B25.8)
> > encephalitis due to herpesvirus NEC (B10.0-)
> > encephalitis due to herpesvirus [herpes simplex] (B00.4)
> > encephalitis due to measles virus (B05.0)
> > encephalitis due to mumps virus (B26.2)
> > encephalitis due to poliomyelitis virus (A80.-)
> > encephalitis due to zoster (B02.0)
> > lymphocytic choriomeningitis (A87.2)

> **A85.0   Enteroviral encephalitis**
> > Enteroviral encephalomyelitis

> **A85.1   Adenoviral encephalitis**
> > Adenoviral meningoencephalitis

> **A85.2   Arthropod-borne viral encephalitis, unspecified**
> >   **Excludes1**   West nile virus with encephalitis (A92.31)

> **A85.8   Other specified viral encephalitis**
> > Encephalitis lethargica
> > Von Economo-Cruchet disease

● **A86   Unspecified viral encephalitis**
> Viral encephalomyelitis NOS
> Viral meningoencephalitis NOS

● **A87   Viral meningitis**

>   **Excludes1**   meningitis due to herpesvirus [herpes simplex] (B00.3)
> > meningitis due to measles virus (B05.1)
> > meningitis due to mumps virus (B26.1)
> > meningitis due to poliomyelitis virus (A80.-)
> > meningitis due to zoster (B02.1)

> **A87.0   Enteroviral meningitis**
> > *Group of common viruses responsible for the majority of viral meningitis*
> > Coxsackievirus meningitis
> > Echovirus meningitis

> **A87.1   Adenoviral meningitis**

> **A87.2   Lymphocytic choriomeningitis**
> > Lymphocytic meningoencephalitis

> **A87.8   Other viral meningitis**

> **A87.9   Viral meningitis, unspecified**

● **A88   Other viral infections of central nervous system, not elsewhere classified**

>   **Excludes1**   viral encephalitis NOS (A86)
> > viral meningitis NOS (A87.9)

> **A88.0   Enteroviral exanthematous fever [Boston exanthem]**
> > *Infectious skin eruption*

> **A88.1   Epidemic vertigo**

> **A88.8   Other specified viral infections of central nervous system**

● **A89   Unspecified viral infection of central nervous system**

ARTHROPOD-BORNE VIRAL FEVERS AND VIRAL HEMORRHAGIC FEVERS (A90-A99)

A90   Dengue fever [classical dengue]
> *Acute, self-limited disease, characterized by fever, prostration, severe muscle pains, headache, rash, lymphadenopathy, and leukopenia, caused by dengue virus; AKA breakbone, dandy*

>   **Excludes1**   dengue hemorrhagic fever (A91)

A91   Dengue hemorrhagic fever
> *Serious follow-up to regular dengue, with symptoms of hemorrhage*

● **A92   Other mosquito-borne viral fevers**

>   **Excludes1**   Ross River disease (B33.1)

> **A92.0   Chikungunya virus disease**
> > *Transmitted by mosquitoes*
> > Chikungunya (hemorrhagic) fever

> **A92.1   O'nyong-nyong fever**
> > *Acute, nonfatal febrile disease transmitted by mosquitoes, which clinically resembles dengue and chikungunya*

> **A92.2   Venezuelan equine fever**
> > Venezuelan equine encephalitis
> > Venezuelan equine encephalomyelitis virus disease

● **A92.3   West Nile virus infection**
> > West Nile fever

> > **A92.30   West Nile virus infection, unspecified**
> > > West Nile fever NOS
> > > West Nile fever without complications
> > > West Nile virus NOS

> > **A92.31   West Nile virus infection with encephalitis**
> > > West Nile encephalitis
> > > West Nile encephalomyelitis

> > **A92.32   West Nile virus infection with other neurologic manifestation**
> > > Use additional code to specify the neurologic manifestation

> > **A92.39   West Nile virus infection with other complications**
> > > Use additional code to specify the other conditions

> **A92.4   Rift Valley fever**

> **A92.5   Zika virus disease** ◄
> > Zika virus fever ◄
> > Zika virus infection ◄
> > Zika NOS ◄

> **A92.8   Other specified mosquito-borne viral fevers**

> **A92.9   Mosquito-borne viral fever, unspecified**

OGCR   Section I. C.1.f.

Certain Infectious and Parasitic Diseases (A00-B99)

Zika virus infections

Code only confirmed cases

Code only a confirmed diagnosis of Zika virus (A92.5, Zika virus disease) as documented by the provider. This is an exception to the hospital inpatient guideline Section II, H.

In this context, "confirmation" does not require documentation of the type of test performed; the physician's diagnostic statement that the condition is confirmed is sufficient. This code should be assigned regardless of the stated mode of transmission.

If the provider documents "suspected", "possible" or "probable" Zika, do not assign code A92.5. Assign a code(s) explaining the reason for encounter (such as fever, rash, or joint pain) or Z20.828, Contact with and (suspected) exposure to other viral communicable diseases.

CHAPTER 1 (A00-B99)

● A93   **Other arthropod-borne viral fevers, not elsewhere classified**

    A93.0   **Oropouche virus disease**
       Tropical viral infection
       Oropouche fever

    A93.1   **Sandfly fever**
       Pappataci fever
       Phlebotomus fever

    A93.2   **Colorado tick fever**

    A93.8   **Other specified arthropod-borne viral fevers**
       Piry virus disease
       Vesicular stomatitis virus disease [Indiana fever]

  A94   `Unspecified` **arthropod-borne viral fever**
       Arboviral fever NOS
       Arbovirus infection NOS

● A95   **Yellow fever**
     Acute infectious disease transmitted by mosquitoes

    A95.0   **Sylvatic yellow fever**
       Jungle yellow fever

    A95.1   **Urban yellow fever**

    A95.9   **Yellow fever,** `unspecified`

● A96   **Arenaviral hemorrhagic fever**
     Virus that causes various hemorrhagic fevers

    A96.0   **Junin hemorrhagic fever**
       Argentinian hemorrhagic fever

    A96.1   **Machupo hemorrhagic fever**
       Transmitted by contact with infected rodents
       Bolivian hemorrhagic fever

    A96.2   **Lassa fever**
       Acute type of hemorrhagic fever caused by contact with
       disease carrying mouse or person

    A96.8   **Other arenaviral hemorrhagic fevers**

    A96.9   **Arenaviral hemorrhagic fever,** `unspecified`

● A98   **Other viral hemorrhagic fevers, not elsewhere classified**
     `Excludes1`   chikungunya hemorrhagic fever (A92.0)
               dengue hemorrhagic fever (A91)

    A98.0   **Crimean-Congo hemorrhagic fever**
       Virus transmitted by ticks and contact with blood, secretions,
       or fluids from infected humans or animals
       Central Asian hemorrhagic fever

    A98.1   **Omsk hemorrhagic fever**
       Transmitted to humans by bites of infected ticks or contact
       with infected muskrats

    A98.2   **Kyasanur Forest disease**
       Transmitted via infected monkeys, voles, ticks

    A98.3   **Marburg virus disease**
       Rare, acute, often fatal type of hemorrhagic fever

    A98.4   **Ebola virus disease**

    A98.5   **Hemorrhagic fever with renal syndrome**
       Epidemic hemorrhagic fever
       Korean hemorrhagic fever
       Russian hemorrhagic fever
       Hantaan virus disease
       Hantavirus disease with renal manifestations
       Nephropathia epidemica
       Songo fever
      `Excludes1`   hantavirus (cardio)-pulmonary syndrome
                 (B33.4)

    A98.8   **Other specified viral hemorrhagic fevers**

  A99   `Unspecified` **viral hemorrhagic fever**

Figure 1-4   Primary herpes simplex in and around the mouth. The infection is usually acquired from siblings or parents and is readily transmitted to other direct contacts. (From Forbes, Jackson: Colour Atlas and Text of Clinical Medicine, International Edition, Mosby, 2002)

Item 1–15   **Herpes** is a viral disease for which there is no cure. There are two types of the herpes simplex virus: **Type I** causes **cold sores** or **fever blisters,** and **Type II** causes **genital herpes.** The virus can be spread from a sore on the lips to the genitals or from the genitals to the lips.

VIRAL INFECTIONS CHARACTERIZED BY SKIN AND MUCOUS MEMBRANE LESIONS (B00-B09)

● B00   **Herpesviral [herpes simplex] infections**
     `Excludes1`   congenital herpesviral infections (P35.2)
     `Excludes2`   anogenital herpesviral infection (A60.-)
               gammaherpesviral mononucleosis (B27.0-)
               herpangina (B08.5)

    B00.0   **Eczema herpeticum**
       Cutaneous eruption caused by herpes simplex virus (HSV)
         type 1, HSV-2, coxsackievirus A16, or vaccinia virus
       Kaposi's varicelliform eruption

    B00.1   **Herpesviral vesicular dermatitis**
       Vesicle formation; characteristics include formation of blisters
         and scabs on feet and legs
       Herpes simplex facialis
       Herpes simplex labialis
       Herpes simplex otitis externa
       Vesicular dermatitis of ear
       Vesicular dermatitis of lip

    B00.2   **Herpesviral gingivostomatitis and pharyngotonsillitis**
       Inflammation involving both gingivae and oral mucosa
       Herpesviral pharyngitis
       Inflammation of pharynx and tonsils; AKA
         tonsillopharyngitis

    B00.3   **Herpesviral meningitis**

    B00.4   **Herpesviral encephalitis**
       Herpesviral meningoencephalitis
       Simian B disease
      `Excludes1`   herpesviral encephalitis due to herpesvirus 6
                 and 7 (B10.01, B10.09)
                 non-simplex herpesviral encephalitis
                 (B10.0-)

● B00.5   **Herpesviral ocular disease**
    B00.50   **Herpesviral ocular disease,** `unspecified`

    B00.51   **Herpesviral iridocyclitis**
       Herpesviral iritis
       Herpesviral uveitis, anterior

    B00.52   **Herpesviral keratitis**
       Herpesviral keratoconjunctivitis

    B00.53   **Herpesviral conjunctivitis**

    B00.59   **Other herpesviral disease of eye**
       Herpesviral dermatitis of eyelid

    B00.7   **Disseminated herpesviral disease**
       Herpesviral sepsis

● B00.8   **Other forms of herpesviral infections**
    B00.81   **Herpesviral hepatitis**

    B00.82   **Herpes simplex myelitis**

    B00.89   **Other herpesviral infection**
       Herpesviral whitlow

    B00.9   **Herpesviral infection,** `unspecified`
       Herpes simplex infection NOS

◀ New   ◀━ Revised   ~~deleted~~ Deleted   `Excludes 1`   `Excludes 2`   `Includes`   `Use additional`   `Code first`   `Code also`   `Unspecified`

650   **OGCR** Official Guidelines   X Assign placeholder X   ● Use Additional Character(s)   ▶ Manifestation Code   **Coding Clinic**

Item 1-16 Zoster: Also known as *shingles* and is caused by the same virus as chickenpox. After exposure, the virus lies dormant in nerve tissue and is activated by factors including aging, stress, suppression of the immune system, and certain medication. It begins as a unilateral rash that leads to blisters and sores on the skin. It may involve the nerve pathways of the eye, forehead, nose, and eyelids and may be very painful with long-term systemic effects.

● **B01** **Varicella [chickenpox]**
  Very contagious disease caused by the varicella zoster virus that
  results in an itchy outbreak of skin blisters (varicella). The same
  virus causes shingles (zoster).
  B01.0 **Varicella meningitis**
● **B01.1** **Varicella encephalitis, myelitis and encephalomyelitis**
    Postchickenpox encephalitis, myelitis and
     encephalomyelitis
    B01.11 Varicella encephalitis and encephalomyelitis
      Postchickenpox encephalitis and
       encephalomyelitis
    B01.12 Varicella myelitis
      Postchickenpox myelitis
  B01.2 **Varicella pneumonia**
● **B01.8** **Varicella with other complications**
    B01.81 **Varicella keratitis**
    B01.89 **Other varicella complications**
  B01.9 **Varicella without complication**
    Varicella NOS

● **B02** **Zoster [herpes zoster]**
  | **Includes** | shingles |
        zona
  B02.0 **Zoster encephalitis**
    Zoster meningoencephalitis
  B02.1 **Zoster meningitis**
● **B02.2** **Zoster with other nervous system involvement**
    B02.21 **Postherpetic geniculate ganglionitis**
    B02.22 **Postherpetic trigeminal neuralgia**
    B02.23 **Postherpetic polyneuropathy**
    B02.24 **Postherpetic myelitis**
      Herpes zoster myelitis
    B02.29 **Other postherpetic nervous system involvement**
      Postherpetic radiculopathy
● **B02.3** **Zoster ocular disease**
    B02.30 **Zoster ocular disease, unspecified**
    B02.31 **Zoster conjunctivitis**
    B02.32 **Zoster iridocyclitis**
    B02.33 **Zoster keratitis**
      Herpes zoster keratoconjunctivitis
    B02.34 **Zoster scleritis**
    B02.39 **Other herpes zoster eye disease**
      Zoster blepharitis
  B02.7 **Disseminated zoster**
  B02.8 **Zoster with other complications**
    Herpes zoster otitis externa
  B02.9 **Zoster without complications**
    Zoster NOS

B03 **Smallpox**
  Note: In 1980 the 33rd World Health Assembly declared
   that smallpox had been eradicated. The classification is
   maintained for surveillance purposes.

B04 **Monkeypox**
  Disease occurring in captive monkeys and other mammals that may
   be transmitted to humans, clinically similar to smallpox

● **B05** **Measles**
  | **Includes** | morbilli |
  | **Excludes1** | subacute sclerosing panencephalitis (A81.1) |
  B05.0 **Measles complicated by encephalitis**
    Postmeasles encephalitis
  B05.1 **Measles complicated by meningitis**
    Postmeasles meningitis
  B05.2 **Measles complicated by pneumonia**
    Postmeasles pneumonia
  B05.3 **Measles complicated by otitis media**
    Postmeasles otitis media
  B05.4 **Measles with intestinal complications**
● **B05.8** **Measles with other complications**
    B05.81 **Measles keratitis and keratoconjunctivitis**
    B05.89 **Other measles complications**
  B05.9 **Measles without complication**
    Measles NOS

● **B06** **Rubella [German measles]**
  | **Excludes1** | congenital rubella (P35.0) |
● **B06.0** **Rubella with neurological complications**
    B06.00 **Rubella with neurological complication, unspecified**
    B06.01 **Rubella encephalitis**
      Rubella meningoencephalitis
    B06.02 **Rubella meningitis**
    B06.09 **Other neurological complications of rubella**
● **B06.8** **Rubella with other complications**
    B06.81 **Rubella pneumonia**
    B06.82 **Rubella arthritis**
    B06.89 **Other rubella complications**
  B06.9 **Rubella without complication**
    Rubella NOS

● **B07** **Viral warts**
  | **Includes** | verruca simplex |
        verruca vulgaris
        viral warts due to human papillomavirus
  | **Excludes2** | anogenital (venereal) warts (A63.0) |
        papilloma of bladder (D41.4)
        papilloma of cervix (D26.0)
        papilloma larynx (D14.1)
  B07.0 **Plantar wart**
    Verruca plantaris
  B07.8 **Other viral warts**
    Common wart
    Flat wart
    Verruca plana
  B07.9 **Viral wart, unspecified**

CHAPTER 1 (A00–B99)

Figure 1-5 Photograph of eyelids with marginal blepharitis. (From Mandell, Bennett, & Dolin: Principles and Practice of Infectious Diseases, ed 7, Churchill Livingstone, An Imprint of Elsevier, 2009)

Item 1-17 Blepharitis is a common condition in which the eyelid is swollen and yellow scaling and conjunctivitis develop. Usually the hair on the scalp and brow is involved.

CHAPTER 1 (A00–B99)

● **B08** **Other viral infections characterized by skin and mucous membrane lesions, not elsewhere classified**

> Excludes1   vesicular stomatitis virus disease (A93.8)

● **B08.0** **Other orthopoxvirus infections**

> Excludes2   monkeypox (B04)

● **B08.01** **Cowpox and vaccinia not from vaccine**

B08.010 **Cowpox**

B08.011 **Vaccinia not from vaccine**

> Excludes1   vaccinia (from vaccination) (generalized) (T88.1)

B08.02 **Orf virus disease**
Contagious pustular dermatitis
Ecthyma contagiosum

B08.03 **Pseudocowpox [milker's node]**

B08.04 **Paravaccinia, unspecified**

B08.09 **Other orthopoxvirus infections**
Orthopoxvirus infection NOS

B08.1 **Molluscum contagiosum**
Various skin diseases characterized by soft, rounded, cutaneous lesions

● **B08.2** **Exanthema subitum [sixth disease] Roseola infantum**
Acute, short-lived high fever in infants and young children followed by a rash mainly on the trunk, caused by human herpesvirus 6

B08.20 **Exanthema subitum [sixth disease], unspecified Roseola infantum, unspecified**   P

B08.21 **Exanthema subitum [sixth disease] due to human herpesvirus 6 Roseola infantum due to human herpesvirus 6**   P
Virus results in sudden rash; infection results in lifelong persistence

B08.22 **Exanthema subitum [sixth disease] due to human herpesvirus 7 Roseola infantum due to human herpesvirus 7**   P

B08.3 **Erythema infectiosum [fifth disease]**
Moderately contagious, epidemic disease in children caused by B19 virus; onset of rash that begins as redness of cheeks, later there is rash on trunk and limbs; when this fades, there may be central clearing that leaves lacelike pattern

B08.4 **Enteroviral vesicular stomatitis with exanthem**
Hand, foot and mouth disease
Check your documentation—this code is HAND, foot, and mouth disease. Code B08.8 is foot and mouth disease.

B08.5 **Enteroviral vesicular pharyngitis**
Herpangina

● **B08.6** **Parapoxvirus infections**

B08.60 **Parapoxvirus infection, unspecified**

B08.61 **Bovine stomatitis**

B08.62 **Sealpox**

B08.69 **Other parapoxvirus infections**

● **B08.7** **Yatapoxvirus infections**

B08.70 **Yatapoxvirus infection, unspecified**

B08.71 **Tanapox virus disease**

B08.72 **Yaba pox virus disease**
Yaba monkey tumor disease

B08.79 **Other yatapoxvirus infections**

B08.8 **Other specified viral infections characterized by skin and mucous membrane lesions**
Enteroviral lymphonodular pharyngitis
Foot-and-mouth disease
Check your documentation. Code B08.4 is for HAND, foot, and mouth disease.
Poxvirus NEC

B09 **Unspecified viral infection characterized by skin and mucous membrane lesions**
Viral enanthema NOS
Viral exanthema NOS

OTHER HUMAN HERPESVIRUSES (B10)

● **B10** **Other human herpesviruses**

> Excludes2   cytomegalovirus (B25.9)
> Epstein-Barr virus (B27.0-)
> herpes NOS (B00.9)
> herpes simplex (B00.-)
> herpes zoster (B02.-)
> human herpesvirus NOS (B00.-)
> human herpesvirus 1 and 2 (B00.-)
> human herpesvirus 3 (B01.-, B02.-)
> human herpesvirus 4 (B27.0-)
> human herpesvirus 5 (B25.-)
> varicella (B01.-)
> zoster (B02.-)

● **B10.0** **Other human herpesvirus encephalitis**

> Excludes2   herpes encephalitis NOS (B00.4)
> herpes simplex encephalitis (B00.4)
> human herpesvirus encephalitis (B00.4)
> simian B herpes virus encephalitis (B00.4)

B10.01 **Human herpesvirus 6 encephalitis**
Sudden rash or roseola

B10.09 **Other human herpesvirus encephalitis**
Human herpesvirus 7 encephalitis
Virus closely related to human herpesvirus 6, but not known to cause any disease

● **B10.8** **Other human herpesvirus infection**

B10.81 **Human herpesvirus 6 infection**
Causative agent of exanthema subitum that results in sudden rash

B10.82 **Human herpesvirus 7 infection**
Closely related to human herpesvirus 6, but not known cause any disease

B10.89 **Other human herpesvirus infection**
Human herpesvirus 8 infection
May be the cause of Kaposi sarcoma, a malignant tumor
Kaposi's sarcoma-associated herpesvirus infection

VIRAL HEPATITIS (B15-B19)

> Excludes1   sequelae of viral hepatitis (B94.2)
> Excludes2   cytomegaloviral hepatitis (B25.1)
> herpesviral [herpes simplex] hepatitis (B00.81)

● **B15** **Acute hepatitis A**

B15.0 **Hepatitis A with hepatic coma**

B15.9 **Hepatitis A without hepatic coma**
Hepatitis A (acute) (viral) NOS

● **B17** **Other acute viral hepatitis**

B17.0 **Acute delta-(super) infection of hepatitis B carrier**

● **B17.1** **Acute hepatitis C**

B17.10 **Acute hepatitis C without hepatic coma**
Acute hepatitis C NOS

B17.11 **Acute hepatitis C with hepatic coma**

B17.2 **Acute hepatitis E**

B17.8 **Other specified acute viral hepatitis**
Hepatitis non-A non-B (acute) (viral) NEC

B17.9 **Acute viral hepatitis, unspecified**
Acute hepatitis NOS
Acute infectious hepatitis NOS ◄

◄ New   ◄━ Revised   ~~deleted~~ Deleted   Excludes 1   Excludes 2   Includes   Use additional   Code first   Code also   Unspecified

OGCR Official Guidelines   X Assign placeholder X   ● Use Additional Character(s)   ▷ Manifestation Code   **Coding Clinic**

Figure 1-6 Hepatitis B viral infection. **A.** Liver parenchyma showing hepatocytes with diffuse granular cytoplasm, so-called ground glass hepatocytes (H&E). **B.** Immunoperoxidase stains from the same case, showing cytoplasmic inclusions of viral particles. (From Kumar: Robbins and Cotran: Pathologic Basis of Disease, ed 8, Saunders, An Imprint of Elsevier, 2009)

Item 1–18 **Hepatitis A (HAV)** was formerly called epidemic, infectious, short-incubation, or acute catarrhal jaundice hepatitis. The primary transmission mode is the oral–fecal route. **Hepatitis B (HBV)** was formerly called long-incubation period, serum, or homologous serum hepatitis. Transmission modes are through blood from infected persons and from body fluids of infected mother to neonate. **Hepatitis C (HCV),** caused by the hepatitis C virus, is primarily transfusion associated. **Hepatitis D (HDV),** also called delta hepatitis, is caused by the hepatitis D virus in patients formerly or currently infected with hepatitis B. **Hepatitis E (HEV)** is also called enterically transmitted non-A, non-B hepatitis. The primary transmission mode is the oral–fecal route, usually through contaminated water.

● **B18** **Chronic viral hepatitis**
     Includes   Carrier of viral hepatitis ◀
  B18.0 **Chronic viral hepatitis B with delta-agent**
  B18.1 **Chronic viral hepatitis B without delta-agent**
          Carrier of viral hepatitis B ◀
          Chronic (viral) hepatitis B
  B18.2 **Chronic viral hepatitis C**
          Carrier of viral hepatitis C ◀
  B18.8 **Other chronic viral hepatitis**
          Carrier of other viral hepatitis ◀
  B18.9 **Chronic viral hepatitis, unspecified**
          Carrier of unspecified viral hepatitis ◀

● **B19** **Unspecified viral hepatitis**
  B19.0 **Unspecified viral hepatitis with hepatic coma**
  ● **B19.1** **Unspecified viral hepatitis B**
     B19.10 **Unspecified viral hepatitis B without hepatic coma**
               Unspecified viral hepatitis B NOS
     B19.11 **Unspecified viral hepatitis B with hepatic coma**
  ● **B19.2** **Unspecified viral hepatitis C**
     B19.20 **Unspecified viral hepatitis C without hepatic coma**
               Viral hepatitis C NOS
     B19.21 **Unspecified viral hepatitis C with hepatic coma**
  B19.9 **Unspecified viral hepatitis without hepatic coma**
          Viral hepatitis NOS

Figure 1-7 Kaposi's sarcoma. There are large confluent hyperpigmented patch-stage lesions with lymphedema. (From Cohen & Powderly: Infectious Diseases, ed 3, Mosby, An Imprint of Elsevier, 2010)

Item 1–19 **AIDS** (acquired immune deficiency syndrome) is caused by **HIV** (human immunodeficiency virus). HIV affects certain white blood cells (T-4 lymphocytes) and destroys the ability of the cells to fight infections, making patients susceptible to a host of infectious diseases (e.g., **Pneumocystis carinii pneumonia (PCP), Kaposi's sarcoma,** and **lymphoma**). **AIDS-related complex (ARC)** is an early stage of AIDS in which tests for HIV are positive but the symptoms are mild.

OGCR Section I. C.1.a
   Certain Infectious and Parasitic Diseases (A00-B99)
   a. Human Immunodeficiency Virus (HIV) Infections
      1) Code only confirmed cases
         Code only confirmed cases of HIV infection illness. This is an exception to the hospital inpatient guideline Section II, H.
         In this context, "confirmation" does not require documentation of positive serology or culture for HIV; the provider's diagnostic statement that the patient is HIV positive, or has an HIV-related illness is sufficient.

HUMAN IMMUNODEFICIENCY VIRUS [HIV] DISEASE (B20)

B20 **Human immunodeficiency virus [HIV] disease**
     Includes   acquired immune deficiency syndrome [AIDS]
                    AIDS-related complex [ARC]
                    HIV infection, symptomatic
     Code first Human immunodeficiency virus [HIV] disease complicating pregnancy, childbirth and the puerperium, if applicable (O98.7-)
     Use additional code(s) to identify all manifestations of HIV infection
     Excludes1   asymptomatic human immunodeficiency virus [HIV] infection status (Z21)
                    exposure to HIV virus (Z20.6)
                    inconclusive serologic evidence of HIV (R75)

OTHER VIRAL DISEASES (B25-B34)

● **B25** **Cytomegaloviral disease**
     AKA: HCMV or Human Herpesvirus 5 (HHV-5)
     Excludes1   congenital cytomegalovirus infection (P35.1)
                    cytomegaloviral mononucleosis (B27.1-)
  B25.0 **Cytomegaloviral pneumonitis**
  B25.1 **Cytomegaloviral hepatitis**
  B25.2 **Cytomegaloviral pancreatitis**
  B25.8 **Other cytomegaloviral diseases**
          Cytomegaloviral encephalitis
  B25.9 **Cytomegaloviral disease, unspecified**

● **B26** **Mumps**
     Includes   epidemic parotitis
                    infectious parotitis
     Acute, contagious, viral disease
  B26.0 **Mumps orchitis** ♂
  B26.1 **Mumps meningitis**
  B26.2 **Mumps encephalitis**
  B26.3 **Mumps pancreatitis**
  ● **B26.8** **Mumps with other complications**
     B26.81 **Mumps hepatitis**
     B26.82 **Mumps myocarditis**
     B26.83 **Mumps nephritis**
     B26.84 **Mumps polyneuropathy**
     B26.85 **Mumps arthritis**
     B26.89 **Other mumps complications**
  B26.9 **Mumps without complication**
          Mumps NOS
          Mumps parotitis NOS

CHAPTER 1 (A00-B99)

CHAPTER 1 (A00-B99)

● **B27　Infectious mononucleosis**

> | Includes | glandular fever |
> | --- | --- |
> | | monocytic angina |
> | | Pfeiffer's disease |

● **B27.0　Gammaherpesviral mononucleosis**
　　　　AKA: Pfeiffer's disease, infective mononucleosis
　　　　Mononucleosis due to Epstein-Barr virus

　　B27.00　Gammaherpesviral mononucleosis without complication
　　　　　Infective mononucleosis

　　B27.01　Gammaherpesviral mononucleosis with polyneuropathy

　　B27.02　Gammaherpesviral mononucleosis with meningitis

　　B27.09　Gammaherpesviral mononucleosis with other complications
　　　　　Hepatomegaly in gammaherpesviral mononucleosis

● **B27.1　Cytomegaloviral mononucleosis**
　　　　Infectious disease resembling infectious mononucleosis

　　B27.10　Cytomegaloviral mononucleosis without complications

　　B27.11　Cytomegaloviral mononucleosis with polyneuropathy

　　B27.12　Cytomegaloviral mononucleosis with meningitis

　　B27.19　Cytomegaloviral mononucleosis with other complication
　　　　　Hepatomegaly in cytomegaloviral mononucleosis

● **B27.8　Other infectious mononucleosis**

　　B27.80　Other infectious mononucleosis without complication

　　B27.81　Other infectious mononucleosis with polyneuropathy

　　B27.82　Other infectious mononucleosis with meningitis

　　B27.89　Other infectious mononucleosis with other complication
　　　　　Hepatomegaly in other infectious mononucleosis

● **B27.9　Infectious mononucleosis, unspecified**

　　B27.90　Infectious mononucleosis, unspecified without complication

　　B27.91　Infectious mononucleosis, unspecified with polyneuropathy

　　B27.92　Infectious mononucleosis, unspecified with meningitis

　　B27.99　Infectious mononucleosis, unspecified with other complication
　　　　　Hepatomegaly in unspecified infectious mononucleosis

● **B30　Viral conjunctivitis**

> | Excludes1 | herpesviral [herpes simplex] ocular disease (B00.5) |
> | --- | --- |
> | | ocular zoster (B02.3) |

B30.0　Keratoconjunctivitis due to adenovirus
　　　Epidemic keratoconjunctivitis
　　　Shipyard eye

B30.1　Conjunctivitis due to adenovirus
　　　Acute adenoviral follicular conjunctivitis
　　　Swimming-pool conjunctivitis

B30.2　Viral pharyngoconjunctivitis

B30.3　Acute epidemic hemorrhagic conjunctivitis (enteroviral)
　　　Conjunctivitis due to coxsackievirus 24
　　　Conjunctivitis due to enterovirus 70
　　　Hemorrhagic conjunctivitis (acute)(epidemic)

B30.8　Other viral conjunctivitis
　　　Newcastle conjunctivitis

B30.9　Viral conjunctivitis, unspecified

● **B33　Other viral diseases, not elsewhere classified**

B33.0　Epidemic myalgia
　　　Acute infectious disease, caused by group A coxsackie viruses or other enteroviruses with symptoms that include sudden pain in chest or upper abdomen with fever
　　　Bornholm disease

B33.1　Ross River disease
　　　Epidemic polyarthritis and exanthema
　　　Ross River fever

● **B33.2　Viral carditis**
　　　Coxsackie (virus) carditis

　　B33.20　Viral carditis, unspecified

　　B33.21　Viral endocarditis

　　B33.22　Viral myocarditis

　　B33.23　Viral pericarditis

　　B33.24　Viral cardiomyopathy

B33.3　Retrovirus infections, not elsewhere classified
　　　Retrovirus infection NOS

B33.4　Hantavirus (cardio)-pulmonary syndrome [HPS] [HCPS]
　　　Hantavirus disease with pulmonary manifestations
　　　Sin nombre virus disease

> Use additional code to identify any associated acute kidney failure (N17.9)

> | Excludes1 | hantavirus disease with renal manifestations (A98.5) |
> | --- | --- |
> | | hemorrhagic fever with renal manifestations (A98.5) |

B33.8　Other specified viral diseases

> | Excludes1 | anogenital human papillomavirus infection (A63.0) |
> | --- | --- |
> | | viral warts due to human papillomavirus infection (B07) |

● **B34　Viral infection of unspecified site**

> | Excludes1 | anogenital human papillomavirus infection (A63.0) |
> | --- | --- |
> | | cytomegaloviral disease NOS (B25.9) |
> | | herpesvirus [herpes simplex] infection NOS (B00.9) |
> | | retrovirus infection NOS (B33.3) |
> | | viral agents as the cause of diseases classified elsewhere (B97.-) |
> | | viral warts due to human papillomavirus infection (B07) |

B34.0　Adenovirus infection, unspecified

B34.1　Enterovirus infection, unspecified
　　　Intestinal tract infection
　　　Coxsackievirus infection NOS
　　　Echovirus infection NOS

B34.2　Coronavirus infection, unspecified

> | Excludes1 | pneumonia due to SARS-associated coronavirus (J12.81) |
> | --- | --- |

B34.3　Parvovirus infection, unspecified

B34.4　Papovavirus infection, unspecified

B34.8　Other viral infections of unspecified site

B34.9　Viral infection, unspecified
　　　Viremia NOS

◀ New　　◀▥ Revised　　deleted Deleted　　Excludes 1　　Excludes 2　　Includes　　Use additional　　Code first　　Code also　　Unspecified

OGCR Official Guidelines　　X Assign placeholder X　　● Use Additional Character(s)　　▸ Manifestation Code　　**Coding Clinic**

MYCOSES (B35-B49)

Excludes2   hypersensitivity pneumonitis due to organic dust (J67.-)
mycosis fungoides (C84.0-)

● **B35**   **Dermatophytosis**
AKA tinea or ringworm

    Includes   favus
infections due to species of Epidermophyton, Micro-sporum and Trichophyton
tinea, any type except those in B36.-

B35.0   **Tinea barbae and tinea capitis**
Beard ringworm
Kerion
Scalp ringworm
Sycosis, mycotic

B35.1   **Tinea unguium**
White patches or pits on surface or edges of nails, followed by infection under nail plate
Dermatophytic onychia
Dermatophytosis of nail
Onychomycosis
Ringworm of nails

B35.2   **Tinea manuum**
Tinea of hands
Dermatophytosis of hand
Hand ringworm

B35.3   **Tinea pedis**
Tinea affecting feet
Athlete's foot
Dermatophytosis of foot
Foot ringworm

B35.4   **Tinea corporis**
Infecting skin areas other than hands
Ringworm of the body

B35.5   **Tinea imbricata**
Chronic tropical tinea corporis; AKA Oriental ringworm, tinea inguinalis, tinea cruris
Tokelau

B35.6   **Tinea cruris**
In groin or perineal area, spreading to adjacent regions; AKA jock itch, eczema marginatum, ringworm of groin, or t inguinalis
Dhobi itch
Groin ringworm
Jock itch

B35.8   **Other dermatophytoses**
Disseminated dermatophytosis
Granulomatous dermatophytosis

B35.9   **Dermatophytosis, unspecified**
Ringworm NOS

● **B36**   **Other superficial mycoses**

B36.0   **Pityriasis versicolor**
Common, chronic, symptomless disorder that includes macular patches of various sizes and shapes; AKA liver spots
Tinea flava
Tinea versicolor

B36.1   **Tinea nigra**
Minor fungal infection, with dark lesions, usually on skin of hands
Keratomycosis nigricans palmaris
Microsporosis nigra
Pityriasis nigra

B36.2   **White piedra**
White to light brown nodules on hair of beard, axilla, or groin; AKA trichosporosis
Tinea blanca

B36.3   **Black piedra**
Characterized by small black or brown nodules on shafts of scalp hair

B36.8   **Other specified superficial mycoses**

B36.9   **Superficial mycosis, unspecified**

Figure 1-8   Oral candidiasis (thrush). *(Courtesy of Stephen Raffanti, MD, MPH.)* (From Mandell, Bennett, & Dolin: Principles and Practice of Infectious Diseases, ed 7, Churchill Livingstone, An Imprint of Elsevier, 2009)

Item 1–20 Candidiasis, also called oidiomycosis or moniliasis, is a fungal infection. It most often appears on moist cutaneous areas of the body but can also be responsible for a variety of systemic infections such as endocarditis, meningitis, arthritis, and myositis. Antifungal medications cure most yeast infections.

● **B37**   **Candidiasis**

    Includes   candidosis
moniliasis

    Excludes1   neonatal candidiasis (P37.5)

B37.0   **Candidal stomatitis**
Oral thrush

B37.1   **Pulmonary candidiasis**
Candidal bronchitis
Candidal pneumonia

B37.2   **Candidiasis of skin and nail**
Candidal onychia
Candidal paronychia

    Excludes2   diaper dermatitis (L22)

B37.3   **Candidiasis of vulva and vagina ♀**
Candidal vulvovaginitis
Monilial vulvovaginitis
Vaginal thrush

● **B37.4**   **Candidiasis of other urogenital sites**

     B37.41   **Candidal cystitis and urethritis**

     B37.42   **Candidal balanitis**
Male condition only

     B37.49   **Other urogenital candidiasis**
Candidal pyelonephritis

B37.5   **Candidal meningitis**

B37.6   **Candidal endocarditis**

B37.7   **Candidal sepsis**
Disseminated candidiasis systemic candidiasis

● **B37.8**   **Candidiasis of other sites**

     B37.81   **Candidal esophagitis**

     B37.82   **Candidal enteritis**
Candidal proctitis

     B37.83   **Candidal cheilitis**
Inflammation affecting lip

     B37.84   **Candidal otitis externa**
Inflammation of external auditory canal

     B37.89   **Other sites of candidiasis**
Infection manifested by invasive candidiasis
Candidal osteomyelitis

B37.9   **Candidiasis, unspecified**
Thrush NOS

● **B38**   **Coccidioidomycosis**
Fungal disease; AKA coccidioidosis, coccidioidal granuloma, Posadas, or Posadas-Wernicke disease

B38.0   **Acute pulmonary coccidioidomycosis**

B38.1   **Chronic pulmonary coccidioidomycosis**

B38.2   **Pulmonary coccidioidomycosis, unspecified**

B38.3   **Cutaneous coccidioidomycosis**

B38.4   **Coccidioidomycosis meningitis**

B38.7   **Disseminated coccidioidomycosis**
Generalized coccidioidomycosis

● **B38.8**   **Other forms of coccidioidomycosis**

     B38.81   **Prostatic coccidioidomycosis ♂**

     B38.89   **Other forms of coccidioidomycosis**

B38.9   **Coccidioidomycosis, unspecified**

CHAPTER 1 (A00-B99)

Item 1-21 Bird and bat droppings that fall into the soil give rise to a fungus that can spread airborne spores. When inhaled into the lungs, these spores divide and multiply into lesions. Histoplasmosis capsulatum takes three forms: primary (lodged in the lungs only), chronic (resembles TB), and disseminated (infection has moved to other organs). This is an opportunistic infection in immunosuppressed patients.

● **B39　Histoplasmosis**
Infection resulting from inhalation or ingestion of spores; AKA Darling disease

　　Code first associated AIDS (B20)
　　Use additional code for any associated manifestations, such as:
　　　　endocarditis (I39)
　　　　meningitis (G02)
　　　　pericarditis (I32)
　　　　retinitits (H32)

　B39.0　Acute pulmonary histoplasmosis capsulati
　B39.1　Chronic pulmonary histoplasmosis capsulati
　B39.2　Pulmonary histoplasmosis capsulati, unspecified
　B39.3　Disseminated histoplasmosis capsulati
　　　　Generalized histoplasmosis capsulati
　B39.4　Histoplasmosis capsulati, unspecified
　　　　American histoplasmosis
　B39.5　Histoplasmosis duboisii
　　　　African histoplasmosis
　B39.9　Histoplasmosis, unspecified

● **B40　Blastomycosis**
Rare and potentially fatal infection caused by inhaling fungus found in moist soil in temperate climates.

　　Excludes1　Brazilian blastomycosis (B41.-)
　　　　　　　keloidal blastomycosis (B48.0)

　B40.0　Acute pulmonary blastomycosis
　B40.1　Chronic pulmonary blastomycosis
　B40.2　Pulmonary blastomycosis, unspecified
　B40.3　Cutaneous blastomycosis
　B40.7　Disseminated blastomycosis
　　　　Generalized blastomycosis
　● **B40.8　Other forms of blastomycosis**
　　　B40.81　Blastomycotic meningoencephalitis
　　　　　　Meningomyelitis due to blastomycosis
　　　B40.89　Other forms of blastomycosis
　B40.9　Blastomycosis, unspecified

● **B41　Paracoccidioidomycosis**
Fungal infection usually chronic that begins in lungs, spreads to mucocutaneous areas which may extend to skin, tonsils, gastrointestinal lymphatics, liver, and spleen; AKA Almeida or Lutz-Splendore-Almeida disease, Brazilian or South American blastomycosis, or paracoccidioidal granuloma

　　Includes　Brazilian blastomycosis
　　　　　　Lutz' disease

　B41.0　Pulmonary paracoccidioidomycosis
　B41.7　Disseminated paracoccidioidomycosis
　　　　Generalized paracoccidioidomycosis
　B41.8　Other forms of paracoccidioidomycosis
　B41.9　Paracoccidioidomycosis, unspecified

● **B42　Sporotrichosis**
Chronic fungal infection with nodular lesions

　B42.0　Pulmonary sporotrichosis
　B42.1　Lymphocutaneous sporotrichosis
　B42.7　Disseminated sporotrichosis
　　　　Generalized sporotrichosis
　● **B42.8　Other forms of sporotrichosis**
　　　B42.81　Cerebral sporotrichosis
　　　　　　Meningitis due to sporotrichosis
　　　B42.82　Sporotrichosis arthritis
　　　B42.89　Other forms of sporotrichosis
　B42.9　Sporotrichosis, unspecified

● **B43　Chromomycosis and pheomycotic abscess**
Chronic fungal infection of skin, initiated at site of puncture affecting lower limb or foot (mossy foot)

　B43.0　Cutaneous chromomycosis
　　　　Dermatitis verrucosa
　B43.1　Pheomycotic brain abscess
　　　　Cerebral chromomycosis
　B43.2　Subcutaneous pheomycotic abscess and cyst
　B43.8　Other forms of chromomycosis
　B43.9　Chromomycosis, unspecified

● **B44　Aspergillosis**
Infection marked by inflammatory lesions in skin, ear, orbit, nasal sinuses, lungs, and occasionally bones and meninges

　　Includes　aspergilloma

　B44.0　Invasive pulmonary aspergillosis
　B44.1　Other pulmonary aspergillosis
　B44.2　Tonsillar aspergillosis
　B44.7　Disseminated aspergillosis
　　　　Generalized aspergillosis
　● **B44.8　Other forms of aspergillosis**
　　　B44.81　Allergic bronchopulmonary aspergillosis
　　　B44.89　Other forms of aspergillosis
　B44.9　Aspergillosis, unspecified

● **B45　Cryptococcosis**
Infection in the immunocompromised and fatal if left untreated; AKA torulosis, Buschke, or Busse-Buschke disease

　B45.0　Pulmonary cryptococcosis
　B45.1　Cerebral cryptococcosis
　　　　Cryptococcal meningitis
　　　　Cryptococcosis meningocerebralis
　B45.2　Cutaneous cryptococcosis
　B45.3　Osseous cryptococcosis
　B45.7　Disseminated cryptococcosis
　　　　Generalized cryptococcosis
　B45.8　Other forms of cryptococcosis
　B45.9　Cryptococcosis, unspecified

● **B46　Zygomycosis**
Fungal infections including subcutaneous lesions and infection of sinuses, brain, or lungs

　B46.0　Pulmonary mucormycosis
　　　　Fungal infection affecting lung
　B46.1　Rhinocerebral mucormycosis
　B46.2　Gastrointestinal mucormycosis
　B46.3　Cutaneous mucormycosis
　　　　Subcutaneous mucormycosis
　B46.4　Disseminated mucormycosis
　　　　Generalized mucormycosis
　B46.5　Mucormycosis, unspecified
　B46.8　Other zygomycoses
　　　　Entomophthoromycosis
　B46.9　Zygomycosis, unspecified
　　　　Phycomycosis NOS

● **B47　Mycetoma**
Slow progressive, destructive fungal infection of cutaneous and subcutaneous tissues, fascia, and bone, primarily seen in foot (Madura foot) or leg

　B47.0　Eumycetoma
　　　　Madura foot, mycotic Maduromycosis
　B47.1　Actinomycetoma
　B47.9　Mycetoma, unspecified
　　　　Madura foot NOS

CHAPTER 1 (A00-B99)

◀ New　◀▥ Revised　~~deleted~~ Deleted　Excludes 1　Excludes 2　Includes　Use additional　Code first　Code also　Unspecified
OGCR Official Guidelines　X Assign placeholder X　● Use Additional Character(s)　▌ Manifestation Code　**Coding Clinic**

● **B48** **Other mycoses, not elsewhere classified**

    B48.0 **Lobomycosis**
         Infection with symptoms of red, smooth, hard cutaneous
            nodules resembling keloids
         Keloidal blastomycosis
         Lobo's disease

    B48.1 **Rhinosporidiosis**
         Chronic, localized granulomatous fungal infection, affecting
            mucocutaneous tissues, usually of nose characterized by
            polyps, papillomas, and wartlike lesions

    B48.2 **Allescheriasis**
         Fungal infection
         Infection due to Pseudallescheria boydii
         Excludes1 eumycetoma (B47.0)

    B48.3 **Geotrichosis**
         Fungal infection usually of bronchi, lungs, mouth, or
            intestinal tract
         Geotrichum stomatitis

    B48.4 **Penicillosis**
         Fungal infection

    B48.8 **Other specified mycoses**
         Adiaspiromycosis
         Infection of tissue and organs by Alternaria
         Infection of tissue and organs by Drechslera
         Infection of tissue and organs by Fusarium
         Infection of tissue and organs by saprophytic fungi
            NEC

B49 **Unspecified mycosis**
      Fungemia NOS

PROTOZOAL DISEASES (B50-B64)

    Excludes1 amebiasis (A06.-)
           other protozoal intestinal diseases (A07.-)

● **B50** **Plasmodium falciparum malaria**
    Severe form of malaria that can be fatal
    Includes mixed infections of Plasmodium falciparum with
           any other Plasmodium species

    B50.0 **Plasmodium falciparum malaria with cerebral**
         complications
         Cerebral malaria NOS

    B50.8 **Other severe and complicated Plasmodium falciparum**
         malaria
         Severe or complicated Plasmodium falciparum malaria
            NOS

    B50.9 **Plasmodium falciparum malaria, unspecified**

● **B51** **Plasmodium vivax malaria**
    Includes mixed infections of Plasmodium vivax with other
           Plasmodium species, except Plasmodium
           falciparum
    Excludes1 plasmodium vivav with Plasmodium falciparum
           (B50.-)

    B51.0 **Plasmodium vivax malaria with rupture of spleen**
    B51.8 **Plasmodium vivax malaria with other complications**
    B51.9 **Plasmodium vivax malaria without complication**
         Plasmodium vivax malaria NOS

● **B52** **Plasmodium malariae malaria**
    Causes fever that recurs at approximately three-day intervals (quartan
      fever), longer than two-day (tertian) intervals of other malarial
      parasites
    Includes mixed infections of Plasmodium malariae
           with other Plasmodium species, except
           Plasmodium falciparum and Plasmodium
           vivax
    Excludes1 plasmodium falciparum (B50.-)
           plasmodium vivax (B51.-)

    B52.0 **Plasmodium malariae malaria with nephropathy**
    B52.8 **Plasmodium malariae malaria with other complications**
    B52.9 **Plasmodium malariae malaria without complication**
         Plasmodium malariae malaria NOS

● **B53** **Other specified malaria**
    B53.0 **Plasmodium ovale malaria**
         Least diagnosed type of malaria spread by female mosquitoes
            of rare species
         Excludes1 plasmodium ovale with Plasmodium
              falciparum (B50.-)
              plasmodium ovale with Plasmodium
                malariae (B52.-)
              plasmodium ovale with Plasmodium
                vivax (B51.-)

    B53.1 **Malaria due to simian plasmodia**
         Malaria-like disease (parasite infection)
         Excludes1 malaria due to simian plasmodia with
              Plasmodium falciparum (B50.-)
              malaria due to simian plasmodia with
                Plasmodium malariae (B52.-)
              malaria due to simian plasmodia with
                Plasmodium ovale (B53.0)
              malaria due to simian plasmodia with
                Plasmodium vivax (B51.-)

    B53.8 **Other malaria, not elsewhere classified**

  B54 **Unspecified malaria**

● **B55** **Leishmaniasis**
    Protozoal infection
    B55.0 **Visceral leishmaniasis**
         Kala-azar
         Post-kala-azar dermal leishmaniasis

    B55.1 **Cutaneous leishmaniasis**
    B55.2 **Mucocutaneous leishmaniasis**
    B55.9 **Leishmaniasis, unspecified**

● **B56** **African trypanosomiasis**
    Human African trypanosomiasis (HAT) is transmitted by fly bites
    B56.0 **Gambiense trypanosomiasis**
         Infection due to Trypanosoma brucei gambiense
         West African sleeping sickness

    B56.1 **Rhodesiense trypanosomiasis**
         East African sleeping sickness
         Infection due to Trypanosoma brucei rhodesiense

    B56.9 **African trypanosomiasis, unspecified**
         Sleeping sickness NOS

● **B57** **Chagas' disease**
    Tropical parasitic disease
    Includes American trypanosomiasis
           infection due to Trypanosoma cruzi

    B57.0 **Acute Chagas' disease with heart involvement**
         Acute Chagas' disease with myocarditis

    B57.1 **Acute Chagas' disease without heart involvement**
         Acute Chagas' disease NOS

    B57.2 **Chagas' disease (chronic) with heart involvement**
         American trypanosomiasis NOS
         Chagas' disease (chronic) NOS
         Chagas' disease (chronic) with myocarditis
         Trypanosomiasis NOS

● **B57.3** **Chagas' disease (chronic) with digestive system**
      involvement
        B57.30 **Chagas' disease with digestive system**
            involvement, unspecified
        B57.31 **Megaesophagus in Chagas' disease**
        B57.32 **Megacolon in Chagas' disease**
        B57.39 **Other digestive system involvement in Chagas'**
            disease

● **B57.4** **Chagas' disease (chronic) with nervous system**
      involvement
        B57.40 **Chagas' disease with nervous system**
            involvement, unspecified
        B57.41 **Meningitis in Chagas' disease**
        B57.42 **Meningoencephalitis in Chagas' disease**
        B57.49 **Other nervous system involvement in Chagas'**
            disease

    B57.5 **Chagas' disease (chronic) with other organ involvement**

Item 1–22 Toxoplasmosis is caused by the protozoa **Toxoplasma gondii,** of which the house cat can be a host. Human infection occurs when contact is made with materials containing the pathogen, such as feces, contaminated soil, or ingestion of infected lamb, goat, or pork. Of the infected, very few have symptoms because a healthy person's immune system keeps the parasite from causing illness. When the immune system is compromised, symptoms may occur. Clinical symptoms include flu-like symptoms, but the disease progresses to include the eyes and the brain in babies.

● **B58** **Toxoplasmosis**
    Infection by protozoon transmitted in cysts in feces of cats
    Includes   infection due to Toxoplasma gondii
    Excludes1   congenital toxoplasmosis (P37.1)
  ● **B58.0** **Toxoplasma oculopathy**
     B58.00   **Toxoplasma oculopathy,** unspecified
     B58.01   **Toxoplasma chorioretinitis**
     B58.09   **Other toxoplasma oculopathy**
          Toxoplasma uveitis
   B58.1   **Toxoplasma hepatitis**
   B58.2   **Toxoplasma meningoencephalitis**
   B58.3   **Pulmonary toxoplasmosis**
  ● **B58.8** **Toxoplasmosis with other organ involvement**
     B58.81   **Toxoplasma myocarditis**
     B58.82   **Toxoplasma myositis**
     B58.83   **Toxoplasma tubulo-interstitial nephropathy**
          Toxoplasma pyelonephritis
     B58.89   **Toxoplasmosis with other organ involvement**
   B58.9   **Toxoplasmosis,** unspecified

  B59   **Pneumocystosis**
    Caused by fungus
    Pneumonia due to Pneumocystis carinii
    Pneumonia due to Pneumocystis jiroveci

● **B60** **Other protozoal diseases, not elsewhere classified**
    Excludes1   cryptosporidiosis (A07.2)
          intestinal microsporidiosis (A07.8)
          isosporiasis (A07.3)
   B60.0   **Babesiosis**
     Tickborne disease caused by microscopic organisms
     Piroplasmosis
  ● **B60.1** **Acanthamebiasis**
     B60.10   **Acanthamebiasis,** unspecified
     B60.11   **Meningoencephalitis due to Acanthamoeba (culbertsoni)**
     B60.12   **Conjunctivitis due to Acanthamoeba**
     B60.13   **Keratoconjunctivitis due to Acanthamoeba**
     B60.19   **Other acanthamebic disease**
   B60.2   **Naegleriasis**
     Infection with microscopic organisms
     Primary amebic meningoencephalitis
   B60.8   **Other specified protozoal diseases**
     Microsporidiosis

  B64   Unspecified **protozoal disease**

HELMINTHIASES (B65-B83)

Diseases or infestations caused by parasitic worms

● **B65** **Schistosomiasis [bilharziasis]**
    Infection with flukes (flat parasitic worms)
    Includes   snail fever
   B65.0   **Schistosomiasis due to Schistosoma haematobium [urinary schistosomiasis]**
   B65.1   **Schistosomiasis due to Schistosoma mansoni [intestinal schistosomiasis]**

   B65.2   **Schistosomiasis due to Schistosoma japonicum**
     Asiatic schistosomiasis
   B65.3   **Cercarial dermatitis**
     Swimmer's itch
   B65.8   **Other schistosomiasis**
     Infection due to Schistosoma intercalatum
     Infection due to Schistosoma mattheei
     Infection due to Schistosoma mekongi
   B65.9   **Schistosomiasis,** unspecified
● **B66** **Other fluke infections**
    Trematode (parasitic worms)
   B66.0   **Opisthorchiasis**
     Infection due to cat liver fluke
     Infection due to Opisthorchis (felineus)(viverrini)
   B66.1   **Clonorchiasis**
     Chinese liver fluke disease
     Infection due to Clonorchis sinensis
     Oriental liver fluke disease
   B66.2   **Dicroceliasis**
     Liver fluke
     Infection due to Dicrocoelium dendriticum
     Lancet fluke infection
   B66.3   **Fascioliasis**
     Infection due to Fasciola gigantica
     Infection due to Fasciola hepatica
     Infection due to Fasciola indica
     Sheep liver fluke disease
   B66.4   **Paragonimiasis**
     Infection due to Paragonimus species
     Lung fluke disease
     Pulmonary distomiasis
   B66.5   **Fasciolopsiasis**
     Largest intestinal fluke in humans
     Infection due to Fasciolopsis buski
     Intestinal distomiasis
   B66.8   **Other specified fluke infections**
     Echinostomiasis
     Heterophyiasis
     Metagonimiasis
     Nanophyetiasis
     Watsoniasis
   B66.9   **Fluke infection,** unspecified
● **B67** **Echinococcosis**
    Larval forms of tapeworms usually of liver or lungs
    Includes   hydatidosis
   B67.0   **Echinococcus granulosus infection of liver**
   B67.1   **Echinococcus granulosus infection of lung**
   B67.2   **Echinococcus granulosus infection of bone**
  ● **B67.3** **Echinococcus granulosus infection, other and multiple sites**
     B67.31   **Echinococcus granulosus infection, thyroid gland**
     B67.32   **Echinococcus granulosus infection, multiple sites**
     B67.39   **Echinococcus granulosus infection, other sites**
   B67.4   **Echinococcus granulosus infection,** unspecified
     Dog tapeworm (infection)
   B67.5   **Echinococcus multilocularis infection of liver**

Item 1-23 Echinococcosis: Also known as hydatid disease; is caused by Echinococcus granulosus, E. multilocularis, and E. vogeli tapeworms; and is contracted from infected food. Found in southern South America, the Mediterranean, the Middle East, central Asia, and Africa and uncommon in the United States but has been reported in California, New Mexico, Arizona and Utah. The disease is treated with medication over a long course as it is resistive.

◀ New   ◀‖‖ Revised   deleted Deleted   Excludes 1   Excludes 2   Includes   Use additional   Code first   Code also   Unspecified

658   OGCR Official Guidelines   X Assign placeholder X   ● Use Additional Character(s)   ▌ Manifestation Code   **Coding Clinic**

● **B67.6** **Echinococcus multilocularis infection, other and multiple sites**

     B67.61 **Echinococcus multilocularis infection, multiple sites**

     B67.69 **Echinococcus multilocularis infection, other sites**

   B67.7 **Echinococcus multilocularis infection, unspecified**

   B67.8 **Echinococcosis, unspecified, of liver**

● **B67.9** **Echinococcosis, other and unspecified**

     B67.90 **Echinococcosis, unspecified**
       Echinococcosis NOS

     B67.99 **Other echinococcosis**

● **B68** **Taeniasis**
   Intestinal tapeworm (cestode) infection from raw or undercooked meat of infected animal

     Excludes1   cysticercosis (B69.-)

   B68.0 **Taenia solium taeniasis**
     Pork tapeworm (infection)

   B68.1 **Taenia saginata taeniasis**
     Beef tapeworm (infection)
     Infection due to adult tapeworm Taenia saginata

   B68.9 **Taeniasis, unspecified**

● **B69** **Cysticercosis**
   Systemic illness caused by the larvae of pork tapeworm

     Includes   cysticerciasis infection due to larval form of Taenia solium

   B69.0 **Cysticercosis of central nervous system**

   B69.1 **Cysticercosis of eye**

● **B69.8** **Cysticercosis of other sites**

     B69.81 **Myositis in cysticercosis**

     B69.89 **Cysticercosis of other sites**

   B69.9 **Cysticercosis, unspecified**

● **B70** **Diphyllobothriasis and sparganosis**
   Infection with tapeworms seen most often from inadequately cooked fish

   B70.0 **Diphyllobothriasis**
     Diphyllobothrium (adult) (latum) (pacificum) infection
     Fish tapeworm (infection)

     Excludes2   larval diphyllobothriasis (B70.1)

   B70.1 **Sparganosis**
     Infection with migrating tapeworm larvae, which invade subcutaneous tissues, causing inflammation and fibrosis that resembles cellulitis
     Infection due to Sparganum (mansoni) (proliferum)
     Infection due to Spirometra larva
     Larval diphyllobothriasis
     Spirometrosis

● **B71** **Other cestode infections**

   B71.0 **Hymenolepiasis**
     Intestinal infestation with tapeworms
     Dwarf tapeworm infection
     Rat tapeworm (infection)

   B71.1 **Dipylidiasis**
     Infection with tapeworm common to dogs and cats and seen in children having close contact with infected pets

   B71.8 **Other specified cestode infections**
     Infection by the larval stage of a tapeworm, usually through fruit or vegetables
     Coenurosis

   B71.9 **Cestode infection, unspecified**
     Tapeworm (infection) NOS

   B72 **Dracunculiasis**
   Infection with roundworms

     Includes   guinea worm infection
       infection due to Dracunculus medinensis

● **B73** **Onchocerciasis**
   Infection with parasitic worm

     Includes   onchocerca volvulus infection
       onchocercosis
       river blindness

● **B73.0** **Onchocerciasis with eye disease**

     B73.00 **Onchocerciasis with eye involvement, unspecified**

     B73.01 **Onchocerciasis with endophthalmitis**

     B73.02 **Onchocerciasis with glaucoma**

     B73.09 **Onchocerciasis with other eye involvement**
       Infestation of eyelid due to onchocerciasis

   B73.1 **Onchocerciasis without eye disease**

● **B74** **Filariasis**
   Infestation with slender threadlike worms

     Excludes2   onchocerciasis (B73)
       tropical (pulmonary) eosinophilia NOS (J82)

   B74.0 **Filariasis due to Wuchereria bancrofti**
     Bancroftian elephantiasis
     Bancroftian filariasis

   B74.1 **Filariasis due to Brugia malayi**

   B74.2 **Filariasis due to Brugia timori**

   B74.3 **Loiasis**
     Infection with round worms growing in subcutaneous connective tissue
     Calabar swelling
     Eyeworm disease of Africa
     Loa loa infection

   B74.4 **Mansonelliasis**
     Infection with filarial parasite
     Infection due to Mansonella ozzardi
     Infection due to Mansonella perstans
     Infection due to Mansonella streptocerca

   B74.8 **Other filariases**
     Dirofilariasis

   B74.9 **Filariasis, unspecified**

   B75 **Trichinellosis**
   Infestation with parasitic roundworms ingested in undercooked contaminated meat

     Includes   infection due to Trichinella species trichiniasis

● **B76** **Hookworm diseases**
   Occurs in hot, humid parts of world where larvae are soil borne, enter digestive tract through skin of feet/legs or in contaminated food/water; AKA ground itch

     Includes   uncinariasis

   B76.0 **Ancylostomiasis**
     Infection due to Ancylostoma species

   B76.1 **Necatoriasis**
     Infection due to Necator americanus

   B76.8 **Other hookworm diseases**

   B76.9 **Hookworm disease, unspecified**
     Cutaneous larva migrans NOS

● **B77** **Ascariasis**
   Infection by roundworm in small intestine

     Includes   ascaridiasis
       roundworm infection

   B77.0 **Ascariasis with intestinal complications**

● **B77.8** **Ascariasis with other complications**

     B77.81 **Ascariasis pneumonia**

     B77.89 **Ascariasis with other complications**

   B77.9 **Ascariasis, unspecified**

CHAPTER 1 (A00-B99)

● **B78**   **Strongyloidiasis**
Infection with adult female roundworms
> **Excludes1**   trichostrongyliasis (B81.2)

   B78.0   **Intestinal strongyloidiasis**
   B78.1   **Cutaneous strongyloidiasis**
   B78.7   **Disseminated strongyloidiasis**
   B78.9   **Strongyloidiasis, unspecified**

   B79   **Trichuriasis**
Intestinal infection with roundworms
> **Includes**   trichocephaliasis
>   whipworm (disease)(infection)

   B80   **Enterobiasis**
Intestinal infection with pinworms
> **Includes**   oxyuriasis
>   pinworm infection
>   threadworm infection

● **B81**   **Other intestinal helminthiases, not elsewhere classified**
Diseases or infestations caused by parasitic worms
> **Excludes1**   angiostrongyliasis due to Parastrongylus
>   cantonensis (B83.2)

   B81.0   **Anisakiasis**
Roundworm infection via contaminated undercooked infected fish or marine mammals
Infection due to Anisakis larva

   B81.1   **Intestinal capillariasis**
Infestation with of parasites (nematodes)
Capillariasis NOS
Infection due to Capillaria philippinensis
> **Excludes2**   hepatic capillariasis (B83.8)

   B81.2   **Trichostrongyliasis**
   B81.3   **Intestinal angiostrongyliasis**
Angiostrongyliasis due to Parastrongylus costaricensis

   B81.4   **Mixed intestinal helminthiases**
Infection due to intestinal helminths classified to more than one of the categories B65.0-B81.3 and B81.8
Mixed helminthiasis NOS

   B81.8   **Other specified intestinal helminthiases**
Infection due to Oesophagostomum species [esophagostomiasis]
Infection due to Ternidens diminutus [ternidensiasis]

● **B82**   **Unspecified intestinal parasitism**
   B82.0   **Intestinal helminthiasis, unspecified**
Infected with worms
   B82.9   **Intestinal parasitism, unspecified**

● **B83**   **Other helminthiases**
Caused by parasitic worms
> **Excludes1**   capillariasis NOS (B81.1)
> **Excludes2**   intestinal capillariasis (B81.1)

   B83.0   **Visceral larva migrans**
Prolonged migration of nematode larvae
Toxocariasis

   B83.1   **Gnathostomiasis**
Infection with nematode occurring from ingested undercooked fish contaminated with larvae; larvae migrate to subcutaneous tissue or deeper tissues, results are abscesses
Wandering swelling

   B83.2   **Angiostrongyliasis due to Parastrongylus cantonensis**
Nematode infection caused by eating contaminated raw snails, slugs, or paratenic hosts such as prawns or crabs; larval worms migrate to central nervous system resulting in eosinophilic meningitis
Eosinophilic meningoencephalitis due to Parastrongylus cantonensis
> **Excludes2**   intestinal angiostrongyliasis (B81.3)

   B83.3   **Syngamiasis**
Infestation with gapeworm from turkey, pheasant, guinea fowl, goose, and wild birds
Syngamosis

   B83.4   **Internal hirudiniasis**
Infestation by leeches
> **Excludes2**   external hirudiniasis (B88.3)

   B83.8   **Other specified helminthiases**
Parasitic worm infestation
Acanthocephaliasis
Gongylonemiasis
Hepatic capillariasis
Metastrongyliasis
Thelaziasis

   B83.9   **Helminthiasis, unspecified**
Worms NOS
> **Excludes1**   intestinal helminthiasis NOS (B82.0)

PEDICULOSIS, ACARIASIS AND OTHER INFESTATIONS (B85-B89)

● **B85**   **Pediculosis and phthiriasis**
Infestation of lice
   B85.0   **Pediculosis due to Pediculus humanus capitis**
Head-louse infestation

   B85.1   **Pediculosis due to Pediculus humanus corporis**
Body-louse infestation

   B85.2   **Pediculosis, unspecified**
   B85.3   **Phthiriasis**
Crab or pubic lice
Infestation by crab-louse
Infestation by Phthirus pubis

   B85.4   **Mixed pediculosis and phthiriasis**
Infestation classifiable to more than one of the categories B85.0-B85.3

   B86   **Scabies**
Sarcoptic itch
Contagious dermatitis caused by mites

● **B87**   **Myiasis**
Infestation by fly maggots
> **Includes**   infestation by larva of flies

   B87.0   **Cutaneous myiasis**
Creeping myiasis

   B87.1   **Wound myiasis**
Traumatic myiasis

   B87.2   **Ocular myiasis**
   B87.3   **Nasopharyngeal myiasis**
Laryngeal myiasis

   B87.4   **Aural myiasis**
● **B87.8**   **Myiasis of other sites**
     B87.81   **Genitourinary myiasis**
     B87.82   **Intestinal myiasis**
     B87.89   **Myiasis of other sites**

   B87.9   **Myiasis, unspecified**

◀ New   ◀━ Revised   ~~deleted~~ Deleted   Excludes 1   Excludes 2   Includes   Use additional   Code first   Code also   Unspecified

OGCR Official Guidelines   X Assign placeholder X   ● Use Additional Character(s)   ▶ Manifestation Code   **Coding Clinic**

660

● **B88   Other infestations**

   B88.0   Other acariasis
      Acarine dermatitis
      Dermatitis due to Demodex species
      Dermatitis due to Dermanyssus gallinae
      Dermatitis due to Liponyssoides sanguineus
      Trombiculosis
      Excludes2   scabies (B86)

   B88.1   Tungiasis [sandflea infestation]
      Inflammatory skin disease caused by infestation of fleas

   B88.2   Other arthropod infestations
      Scarabiasis

   B88.3   External hirudiniasis
      Leech infestation NOS
      Excludes2   internal hirudiniasis (B83.4)

   B88.8   Other specified infestations
      Infection of topical fresh water fish parasite
      Ichthyoparasitism due to Vandellia cirrhosa
      Linguatulosis
      Porocephaliasis

   B88.9   Infestation, unspecified
      Infestation (skin) NOS
      Infestation by mites NOS
      Skin parasites NOS

B89   Unspecified parasitic disease

SEQUELAE OF INFECTIOUS AND PARASITIC DISEASES (B90-B94)

Note: Categories B90-B94 are to be used to indicate conditions in categories A00-B89 as the cause of sequelae, which are themselves classified elsewhere. The 'sequelae' include conditions specified as such; they also include residuals of diseases classifiable to the above categories if there is evidence that the disease itself is no longer present. Codes from these categories are not to be used for chronic infections. Code chronic current infections to active infectious disease as appropriate.

Code first condition resulting from (sequela) the infectious or parasitic disease

● **B90   Sequelae of tuberculosis**
    Condition resulting from tuberculosis

   B90.0   Sequelae of central nervous system tuberculosis

   B90.1   Sequelae of genitourinary tuberculosis

   B90.2   Sequelae of tuberculosis of bones and joints

   B90.8   Sequelae of tuberculosis of other organs
      Excludes2   sequelae of respiratory tuberculosis (B90.9)

   B90.9   Sequelae of respiratory and unspecified tuberculosis
      Sequelae of tuberculosis NOS

B91   Sequelae of poliomyelitis
      Excludes1   postpolio syndrome (G14)

B92   Sequelae of leprosy

● **B94   Sequelae of other and unspecified infectious and parasitic diseases**

   B94.0   Sequelae of trachoma

   B94.1   Sequelae of viral encephalitis

   B94.2   Sequelae of viral hepatitis

   B94.8   Sequelae of other specified infectious and parasitic diseases

   B94.9   Sequelae of unspecified infectious and parasitic disease

OGCR Section I.C.1.b

> Certain infectious and parasitic diseases
> Infectious agents as the cause of diseases classified to other chapters
> Certain infections are classified in chapters other than Chapter 1 and no organism is identified as part of the infection code. In these instances, it is necessary to use an additional code from Chapter 1 to identify the organism. A code from category B95, Streptococcus, Staphylococcus, and Enterococcus as the cause of diseases classified to other chapters, B96, Other bacterial agents as the cause of diseases classified to other chapters, or B97, Viral agents as the cause of diseases classified to other chapters, is to be used as an additional code to identify the organism. An instructional note will be found at the infection code advising that an additional organism code is required.

BACTERIAL AND VIRAL INFECTIOUS AGENTS (B95-B97)

Note: These categories are provided for use as supplementary or additional codes to identify the infectious agent(s) in diseases classified elsewhere.
Code the disease first, then the bacterium. Do not report codes from B95-B97 for sepsis.

● **B95   Streptococcus, Staphylococcus, and Enterococcus as the cause of diseases classified elsewhere**

   B95.0   Streptococcus, group A, as the cause of diseases classified elsewhere

   B95.1   Streptococcus, group B, as the cause of diseases classified elsewhere

   B95.2   Enterococcus as the cause of diseases classified elsewhere

   B95.3   Streptococcus pneumoniae as the cause of diseases classified elsewhere

   B95.4   Other streptococcus as the cause of diseases classified elsewhere

   B95.5   Unspecified streptococcus as the cause of diseases classified elsewhere

   ● **B95.6   Staphylococcus aureus as the cause of diseases classified elsewhere**

     B95.61   Methicillin susceptible Staphylococcus aureus infection as the cause of diseases classified elsewhere
       Methicillin susceptible Staphylococcus aureus (MSSA) infection as the cause of diseases classified elsewhere
       Staphylococcus aureus infection NOS as the cause of diseases classified elsewhere

     B95.62   Methicillin resistant Staphylococcus aureus infection as the cause of diseases classified elsewhere
       Methicillin resistant staphylococcus aureus (MRSA) infection as the cause of diseases classified elsewhere
       Coding Clinic: 2016, Q1, P13

   B95.7   Other staphylococcus as the cause of diseases classified elsewhere

   B95.8   Unspecified staphylococcus as the cause of diseases classified elsewhere

● **B96   Other bacterial agents as the cause of diseases classified elsewhere**

   B96.0   Mycoplasma pneumoniae [M. pneumoniae] as the cause of diseases classified elsewhere
      Pleuro-pneumonia-like-organism [PPLO]

   B96.1   Klebsiella pneumoniae [K. pneumoniae] as the cause of diseases classified elsewhere

CHAPTER 1 (A00-B99)

● **B96.2** **Escherichia coli [E. coli] as the cause of diseases classified elsewhere**

     B96.20 Unspecified Escherichia coli [E. coli] as the cause of diseases classified elsewhere

         Escherichia coli [E. coli] NOS

     B96.21 **Shiga toxin-producing Escherichia coli [E. coli] (STEC) O157 as the cause of diseases classified elsewhere**

         E. coli O157:H- (nonmotile) with confirmation of Shiga toxin

         E. coli O157 with confirmation of Shiga toxin when H antigen is unknown, or is not H7

         O157:H7 Escherichia coli [E.coli] with or without confirmation of Shiga toxin-production

         Shiga toxin-producing Escherichia coli [E.coli] O157:H7 with or without confirmation of Shiga toxin-production

         STEC O157:H7 with or without confirmation of Shiga toxin-production

     B96.22 **Other specified Shiga toxin-producing Escherichia coli [E. coli] (STEC) as the cause of diseases classified elsewhere**

         Non-O157 Shiga toxin-producing Escherichia coli [E.coli]

         Non-O157 Shiga toxin-producing Escherichia coli [E.coli] with known O group

     B96.23 Unspecified Shiga toxin-producing Escherichia coli [E. coli] (STEC) as the cause of diseases classified elsewhere

         Shiga toxin-producing Escherichia coli [E. coli] with unspecified O group

         STEC NOS

     B96.29 **Other Escherichia coli [E. coli] as the cause of diseases classified elsewhere**

         Non-Shiga toxin-producing E. coli

   B96.3 **Hemophilus influenzae [H. influenzae] as the cause of diseases classified elsewhere**

   B96.4 **Proteus (mirabilis) (morganii) as the cause of diseases classified elsewhere**

   B96.5 **Pseudomonas (aeruginosa) (mallei) (pseudomallei) as the cause of diseases classified elsewhere**

     Coding Clinic: 2015, Q1, P18

   B96.6 **Bacteroides fragilis [B. fragilis] as the cause of diseases classified elsewhere**

   B96.7 **Clostridium perfringens [C. perfringens] as the cause of diseases classified elsewhere**

● **B96.8** **Other specified bacterial agents as the cause of diseases classified elsewhere**

     B96.81 **Helicobacter pylori [H. pylori] as the cause of diseases classified elsewhere**

     B96.82 **Vibrio vulnificus as the cause of diseases classified elsewhere**

     B96.89 **Other specified bacterial agents as the cause of diseases classified elsewhere**

● **B97** **Viral agents as the cause of diseases classified elsewhere**

   B97.0 **Adenovirus as the cause of diseases classified elsewhere**

● **B97.1** **Enterovirus as the cause of diseases classified elsewhere**

     B97.10 Unspecified enterovirus as the cause of diseases classified elsewhere

     B97.11 **Coxsackievirus as the cause of diseases classified elsewhere**

     B97.12 **Echovirus as the cause of diseases classified elsewhere**

     B97.19 **Other enterovirus as the cause of diseases classified elsewhere**

● **B97.2** **Coronavirus as the cause of diseases classified elsewhere**

     B97.21 **SARS-associated coronavirus as the cause of diseases classified elsewhere**

         Excludes1   pneumonia due to SARS-associated coronavirus (J12.81)

     B97.29 **Other coronavirus as the cause of diseases classified elsewhere**

● **B97.3** **Retrovirus as the cause of diseases classified elsewhere**

     Excludes1   human immunodeficiency virus [HIV] disease (B20)

     B97.30 Unspecified retrovirus as the cause of diseases classified elsewhere

     B97.31 **Lentivirus as the cause of diseases classified elsewhere**

     B97.32 **Oncovirus as the cause of diseases classified elsewhere**

     B97.33 **Human T-cell lymphotrophic virus, type I [HTLV-I] as the cause of diseases classified elsewhere**

     B97.34 **Human T-cell lymphotrophic virus, type II [HTLV-II] as the cause of diseases classified elsewhere**

Item 1–24   **Retrovirus** develops by copying its RNA, genetic materials, into the DNA, which then produces new virus particles. It is from the Retroviridae virus family. **Human T-cell lymphotropic virus, Type I (HTLV-I)** is also called human T-cell leukemia virus, Type I, and is a retrovirus thought to cause T-cell leukemia/lymphoma. **Human T-cell lymphotropic virus, Type II (HTLV-II),** is also called human T-cell leukemia virus, Type II, and is a retrovirus associated with hematologic disorders.

     HIV-2 is one of the serotypes of HIV and is usually confined to West Africa, whereas HIV-**1** is found worldwide.

     B97.35 **Human immunodeficiency virus, type 2 [HIV 2] as the cause of diseases classified elsewhere**

     B97.39 **Other retrovirus as the cause of diseases classified elsewhere**

   B97.4 **Respiratory syncytial virus as the cause of diseases classified elsewhere**

   B97.5 **Reovirus as the cause of diseases classified elsewhere**

   B97.6 **Parvovirus as the cause of diseases classified elsewhere**

   B97.7 **Papillomavirus as the cause of diseases classified elsewhere**

● **B97.8** **Other viral agents as the cause of diseases classified elsewhere**

     B97.81 **Human metapneumovirus as the cause of diseases classified elsewhere**

     B97.89 **Other viral agents as the cause of diseases classified elsewhere**

OTHER INFECTIOUS DISEASES (B99)

● **B99** **Other and unspecified infectious diseases**

   B99.8 **Other infectious disease**

   B99.9 Unspecified infectious disease

◀ New   ⬅ Revised   ~~deleted~~ Deleted   Excludes 1   Excludes 2   Includes   Use additional   Code first   Code also   Unspecified

OGCR Official Guidelines   **X** Assign placeholder X   ● Use Additional Character(s)   ▶ Manifestation Code   **Coding Clinic**

CHAPTER 2

NEOPLASMS (C00-D49)

OGCR Chapter-Specific Coding Guidelines

2. **Chapter 2: Neoplasms (C00-D49)**
   General guidelines
   Chapter 2 of the ICD-10-CM contains the codes for most benign and all malignant neoplasms. Certain benign neoplasms, such as prostatic adenomas, may be found in the specific body system chapters. To properly code a neoplasm it is necessary to determine from the record if the neoplasm is benign, in-situ, malignant, or of uncertain histologic behavior. If malignant, any secondary (metastatic) sites should also be determined.

   Primary malignant neoplasms overlapping site boundaries
   A primary malignant neoplasm that overlaps two or more contiguous (next to each other) sites should be classified to the subcategory/code .8 ('overlapping lesion'), unless the combination is specifically indexed elsewhere. For multiple neoplasms of the same site that are not contiguous such as tumors in different quadrants of the same breast, codes for each site should be assigned.

   Malignant neoplasm of ectopic tissue
   Malignant neoplasms of ectopic tissue are to be coded to the site of origin mentioned, e.g., ectopic pancreatic malignant neoplasms involving the stomach are coded to pancreas, unspecified (C25.9).

   The neoplasm table in the Alphabetic Index should be referenced first. However, if the histological term is documented, that term should be referenced first, rather than going immediately to the Neoplasm Table, in order to determine which column in the Neoplasm Table is appropriate. For example, if the documentation indicates "adenoma," refer to the term in the Alphabetic Index to review the entries under this term and the instructional note to "see also neoplasm, by site, benign." The table provides the proper code based on the type of neoplasm and the site. It is important to select the proper column in the table that corresponds to the type of neoplasm. The Tabular List should then be referenced to verify that the correct code has been selected from the table and that a more specific site code does not exist.

   See Section I.C.21. Factors influencing health status and contact with health services, Status, for information regarding Z15.0, codes for genetic susceptibility to cancer.

   a. **Treatment directed at the malignancy**
   If the treatment is directed at the malignancy, designate the malignancy as the principal diagnosis.

   The only exception to this guideline is if a patient admission/encounter is solely for the administration of chemotherapy, immunotherapy or radiation therapy, assign the appropriate Z51.— code as the first-listed or principal diagnosis, and the diagnosis or problem for which the service is being performed as a secondary diagnosis.

   b. **Treatment of secondary site**
   When a patient is admitted because of a primary neoplasm with metastasis and treatment is directed toward the secondary site only, the secondary neoplasm is designated as the principal diagnosis even though the primary malignancy is still present.

   c. **Coding and sequencing of complications**
   Coding and sequencing of complications associated with the malignancies or with the therapy thereof are subject to the following guidelines:

   1) **Anemia associated with malignancy**
   When admission/encounter is for management of an anemia associated with the malignancy, and the treatment is only for anemia, the appropriate code for the malignancy is sequenced as the principal or first-listed diagnosis followed by the appropriate code for the anemia (such as code D63.0, Anemia in neoplastic disease).

   2) **Anemia associated with chemotherapy, immunotherapy and radiation therapy**
   When the admission/encounter is for management of an anemia associated with an adverse effect of the administration of chemotherapy or immunotherapy and the only treatment is for the anemia, the anemia code is sequenced first followed by the appropriate codes for the neoplasm and the adverse effect

(T45.1X5, Adverse effect of antineoplastic and immunosuppressive drugs).

When the admission/encounter is for management of an anemia associated with an adverse effect of radiotherapy, the anemia code should be sequenced first, followed by the appropriate neoplasm code and code Y84.2, Radiological procedure and radiotherapy as the cause of abnormal reaction of the patient, or of later complication, without mention of misadventure at the time of the procedure.

   3) **Management of dehydration due to the malignancy**
   When the admission/encounter is for management of dehydration due to the malignancy and only the dehydration is being treated (intravenous rehydration), the dehydration is sequenced first, followed by the code(s) for the malignancy.

   4) **Treatment of a complication resulting from a surgical procedure**
   When the admission/encounter is for treatment of a complication resulting from a surgical procedure, designate the complication as the principal or first-listed diagnosis if treatment is directed at resolving the complication.

   d. **Primary malignancy previously excised**
   When a primary malignancy has been previously excised or eradicated from its site and there is no further treatment directed to that site and there is no evidence of any existing primary malignancy, a code from category Z85, Personal history of malignant neoplasm, should be used to indicate the former site of the malignancy. Any mention of extension, invasion, or metastasis to another site is coded as a secondary malignant neoplasm to that site. The secondary site may be the principal or first-listed with the Z85 code used as a secondary code.

   e. **Admissions/Encounters involving chemotherapy, immunotherapy and radiation therapy**

   1) **Episode of care involves surgical removal of neoplasm**
   When an episode of care involves the surgical removal of a neoplasm, primary or secondary site, followed by adjunct chemotherapy or radiation treatment during the same episode of care, the code for the neoplasm should be assigned as principal or first-listed diagnosis.

   2) **Patient admission/encounter solely for administration of chemotherapy, immunotherapy and radiation therapy**
   If a patient admission/encounter is solely for the administration of chemotherapy, immunotherapy or radiation therapy assign code Z51.0, Encounter for antineoplastic radiation therapy, or Z51.11, Encounter for antineoplastic chemotherapy, or Z51.12, Encounter for antineoplastic immunotherapy as the first-listed or principal diagnosis. If a patient receives more than one of these therapies during the same admission more than one of these codes may be assigned, in any sequence.

   The malignancy for which the therapy is being administered should be assigned as a secondary diagnosis.

   3) **Patient admitted for radiation therapy, chemotherapy or immunotherapy and develops complications**
   When a patient is admitted for the purpose of radiotherapy, immunotherapy or chemotherapy and develops complications such as uncontrolled nausea and vomiting or dehydration, the principal or first-listed diagnosis is Z51.0, Encounter for antineoplastic radiation therapy, or Z51.11, Encounter for antineoplastic chemotherapy, or Z51.12, Encounter for antineoplastic immunotherapy followed by any codes for the complications.

   f. **Admission/encounter to determine extent of malignancy**
   When the reason for admission/encounter is to determine the extent of the malignancy, or for a procedure such as paracentesis or thoracentesis, the primary malignancy or appropriate metastatic site is designated as the principal or first-listed diagnosis, even though chemotherapy or radiotherapy is administered.

   g. **Symptoms, signs, and abnormal findings listed in Chapter 18 associated with neoplasms**
   Symptoms, signs, and ill-defined conditions listed in Chapter 18 characteristic of, or associated with, an existing primary or secondary site malignancy cannot be used to replace the malignancy as principal or first-listed diagnosis, regardless of the number of admissions or encounters for treatment and care of the neoplasm.

See section I.C.21. Factors influencing health status and contact with health services, Encounter for prophylactic organ removal.

h. Admission/encounter for pain control/management
See Section I.C.6. for information on coding admission/encounter for pain control/management.

i. Malignancy in two or more noncontiguous sites
A patient may have more than one malignant tumor in the same organ. These tumors may represent different primaries or metastatic disease, depending on the site. Should the documentation be unclear, the provider should be queried as to the status of each tumor so that the correct codes can be assigned.

j. Disseminated malignant neoplasm, unspecified
Code C80.0, Disseminated malignant neoplasm, unspecified, is for use only in those cases where the patient has advanced metastatic disease and no known primary or secondary sites are specified. It should not be used in place of assigning codes for the primary site and all known secondary sites.

k. Malignant neoplasm without specification of site
Code C80.1, Malignant (primary) neoplasm, unspecified, equates to Cancer, unspecified. This code should only be used when no determination can be made as to the primary site of a malignancy. This code should rarely be used in the inpatient setting.

l. Sequencing of neoplasm codes
1) Encounter for treatment of primary malignancy
If the reason for the encounter is for treatment of a primary malignancy, assign the malignancy as the principal/first-listed diagnosis. The primary site is to be sequenced first, followed by any metastatic sites.

2) Encounter for treatment of secondary malignancy
When an encounter is for a primary malignancy with metastasis and treatment is directed toward the metastatic (secondary) site(s) only, the metastatic site(s) is designated as the principal/first-listed diagnosis. The primary malignancy is coded as an additional code.

3) Malignant neoplasm in a pregnant patient
When a pregnant woman has a malignant neoplasm, a code from subcategory O9A.1-, Malignant neoplasm complicating pregnancy, childbirth, and the puerperium, should be sequenced first, followed by the appropriate code from Chapter 2 to indicate the type of neoplasm.

4) Encounter for complication associated with a neoplasm
When an encounter is for management of a complication associated with a neoplasm, such as dehydration, and the treatment is only for the complication, the complication is coded first, followed by the appropriate code(s) for the neoplasm.

The exception to this guideline is anemia. When the admission/encounter is for management of an anemia associated with the malignancy, and the treatment is only for anemia, the appropriate code for the malignancy is sequenced as the principal or first-listed diagnosis followed by code D63.0, Anemia in neoplastic disease.

5) Complication from surgical procedure for treatment of a neoplasm
When an encounter is for treatment of a complication resulting from a surgical procedure performed for the treatment of the neoplasm, designate the complication as the principal/first-listed diagnosis. See guideline regarding the coding of a current malignancy versus personal history to determine if the code for the neoplasm should also be assigned.

6) Pathologic fracture due to a neoplasm
When an encounter is for a pathological fracture due to a neoplasm, and the focus of treatment is the fracture, a code from subcategory M84.5, Pathological fracture in neoplastic disease, should be sequenced first, followed by the code for the neoplasm.

If the focus of treatment is the neoplasm with an associated pathological fracture, the neoplasm code should be sequenced first, followed by a code from M84.5 for the pathological fracture.

m. Current malignancy versus personal history of malignancy
When a primary malignancy has been excised but further treatment, such as an additional surgery for the malignancy, radiation therapy or chemotherapy is directed to that site, the primary malignancy code should be used until treatment is completed.

When a primary malignancy has been previously excised or eradicated from its site, there is no further treatment (of the malignancy) directed to that site, and there is no evidence of any existing primary malignancy, a code from category Z85, Personal history of malignant neoplasm, should be used to indicate the former site of the malignancy.
See Section I.C.21. Factors influencing health status and contact with health services, History (of)

n. Leukemia, Multiple Myeloma, and Malignant Plasma Cell Neoplasms in remission versus personal history
The categories for leukemia, and category C90, Multiple myeloma and malignant plasma cell neoplasms, have codes indicating whether or not the leukemia has achieved remission. There are also codes Z85.6, Personal history of leukemia, and Z85.79, Personal history of other malignant neoplasms of lymphoid, hematopoietic and related tissues. If the documentation is unclear, as to whether the leukemia has achieved remission, the provider should be queried.
See Section I.C.21. Factors influencing health status and contact with health services, History (of)

o. Aftercare following surgery for neoplasm
See Section I.C.21. Factors influencing health status and contact with health services, Aftercare

p. Follow-up care for completed treatment of a malignancy
See Section I.C.21. Factors influencing health status and contact with health services, Follow-up

q. Prophylactic organ removal for prevention of malignancy
See Section I.C. 21, Factors influencing health status and contact with health services, Prophylactic organ removal

r. Malignant neoplasm associated with transplanted organ
A malignant neoplasm of a transplanted organ should be coded as a transplant complication. Assign first the appropriate code from category T86.-, Complications of transplanted organs and tissue, followed by code C80.2, Malignant neoplasm associated with transplanted organ. Use an additional code for the specific malignancy.

Item 2–1 Neoplasm: Neo = new, plasm = growth, development, formation. This new growth (mass, tumor) can be malignant or benign, which is confirmed by the pathology report. Do not assign a code to a neoplasm until you review the pathology report. Certain CPT codes will specify benign or malignant lesion, so be certain the diagnosis code supports the procedure code.

CHAPTER 2

NEOPLASMS (C00-D49)

This chapter contains the following blocks:

C00-C14	Malignant neoplasms of lip, oral cavity and pharynx
C15-C26	Malignant neoplasms of digestive organs
C30-C39	Malignant neoplasms of respiratory and intrathoracic organs
C40-C41	Malignant neoplasms of bone and articular cartilage
C43-C44	Melanoma and other malignant neoplasms of skin
C45-C49	Malignant neoplasms of mesothelial and soft tissue
C50	Malignant neoplasms of breast
C51-C58	Malignant neoplasms of female genital organs
C60-C63	Malignant neoplasms of male genital organs
C64-C68	Malignant neoplasms of urinary tract
C69-C72	Malignant neoplasms of eye, brain and other parts of central nervous system
C73-C75	Malignant neoplasms of thyroid and other endocrine glands
C7A	Malignant neuroendocrine tumors
C7B	Secondary neuroendocrine tumors
C76-C80	Malignant neoplasms of ill-defined, other secondary and unspecified sites
C81-C96	Malignant neoplasms of lymphoid, hematopoietic and related tissue
D00-D09	In situ neoplasms
D10-D36	Benign neoplasms, except benign neuroendocrine tumors
D3A	Benign neuroendocrine tumors
D37-D48	Neoplasms of uncertain behavior, polycythemia vera and myelodysplastic syndromes
D49	Neoplasms of unspecified behavior

Notes: Functional activity

All neoplasms are classified in this chapter, whether they are functionally active or not. An additional code from Chapter 4 may be used, to identify functional activity associated with any neoplasm.

Morphology [Histology]

Chapter 2 classifies neoplasms primarily by site (topography), with broad groupings for behavior, malignant, in situ, benign, etc. The Table of Neoplasms should be used to identify the correct topography code. In a few cases, such as for malignant melanoma and certain neuroendocrine tumors, the morphology (histologic type) is included in the category and codes.

Primary malignant neoplasms overlapping site boundaries

A primary malignant neoplasm that overlaps two or more contiguous (next to each other) sites should be classified to the subcategory/code .8 ('overlapping lesion'), unless the combination is specifically indexed elsewhere. For multiple neoplasms of the same site that are not contiguous, such as tumors in different quadrants of the same breast, codes for each site should be assigned.

Malignant neoplasm of ectopic tissue

Malignant neoplasms of ectopic tissue are to be coded to the site mentioned, e.g., ectopic pancreatic malignant neoplasms are coded to pancreas, unspecified (C25.9).

MALIGNANT NEOPLASMS (C00-C96)

MALIGNANT NEOPLASMS, STATED OR PRESUMED TO BE PRIMARY (OF SPECIFIED SITES), AND CERTAIN SPECIFIED HISTOLOGIES, EXCEPT NEUROENDOCRINE, AND OF LYMPHOID, HEMATOPOIETIC AND RELATED TISSUE (C00-C75)

MALIGNANT NEOPLASMS OF LIP, ORAL CAVITY AND PHARYNX (C00-C14)

● **C00**   **Malignant neoplasm of lip**

Use additional code to identify:
alcohol abuse and dependence (F10.-)
history of tobacco dependence (Z87.891) ◄━━━
tobacco dependence (F17.-)
tobacco use (Z72.0)

Excludes1   malignant melanoma of lip (C43.0)
Merkel cell carcinoma of lip (C4A.0)
other and unspecified malignant neoplasm of skin of lip (C44.0-)

C00.0   **Malignant neoplasm of external upper lip**
Malignant neoplasm of lipstick area of upper lip
Malignant neoplasm of upper lip NOS
Malignant neoplasm of vermilion border of upper lip

C00.1   **Malignant neoplasm of external lower lip**
Malignant neoplasm of lower lip NOS
Malignant neoplasm of lipstick area of lower lip
Malignant neoplasm of vermilion border of lower lip

C00.2   **Malignant neoplasm of external lip, unspecified**
Malignant neoplasm of vermilion border of lip NOS

C00.3   **Malignant neoplasm of upper lip, inner aspect**
Malignant neoplasm of buccal aspect of upper lip
Malignant neoplasm of frenulum of upper lip
Malignant neoplasm of mucosa of upper lip
Malignant neoplasm of oral aspect of upper lip

C00.4   **Malignant neoplasm of lower lip, inner aspect**
Malignant neoplasm of buccal aspect of lower lip
Malignant neoplasm of frenulum of lower lip
Malignant neoplasm of mucosa of lower lip
Malignant neoplasm of oral aspect of lower lip

C00.5   **Malignant neoplasm of lip, unspecified, inner aspect**
Malignant neoplasm of buccal aspect of lip, unspecified
Malignant neoplasm of frenulum of lip, unspecified
Malignant neoplasm of mucosa of lip, unspecified
Malignant neoplasm of oral aspect of lip, unspecified

C00.6   **Malignant neoplasm of commissure of lip, unspecified**
Commissure: Site of union of corresponding parts

C00.8   **Malignant neoplasm of overlapping sites of lip**

C00.9   **Malignant neoplasm of lip, unspecified**

Transitional or vermilion surfaces

A Lips are connected to the gums by frenulum

Hard palate
Soft palate
Vestibule
Uvula
Tonsil
Dorsal surface (anterior two-thirds of tongue)

B

Ventral surface

Lingual frenum

C

Figure 2-1 Anatomical structures of the mouth and lips. **A.** Transitional or vermilion borders. Lips are connected to the gums by frenulum. **B.** Dorsal surface. **C.** Ventral surface.

C01   Malignant neoplasm of base of tongue
　　Malignant neoplasm of dorsal surface of base of tongue
　　Malignant neoplasm of fixed part of tongue NOS
　　Malignant neoplasm of posterior third of tongue
　　Use additional code to identify:
　　　alcohol abuse and dependence (F10.-)
　　　history of tobacco dependence (Z87.891) ◀▥
　　　tobacco dependence (F17.-)
　　　tobacco use (Z72.0)

● **C02   Malignant neoplasm of other and unspecified parts of tongue**
　　Use additional code to identify:
　　　alcohol abuse and dependence (F10.-)
　　　history of tobacco dependence (Z87.891) ◀▥
　　　tobacco dependence (F17.-)
　　　tobacco use (Z72.0)
　　C02.0   Malignant neoplasm of dorsal surface of tongue
　　　　Malignant neoplasm of anterior two-thirds of tongue, dorsal surface
　　　　Excludes2   malignant neoplasm of dorsal surface of base of tongue (C01)
　　C02.1   Malignant neoplasm of border of tongue
　　　　Malignant neoplasm of tip of tongue
　　C02.2   Malignant neoplasm of ventral surface of tongue
　　　　Malignant neoplasm of anterior two-thirds of tongue, ventral surface
　　　　Malignant neoplasm of frenulum linguae
　　C02.3   Malignant neoplasm of anterior two-thirds of tongue, part unspecified
　　　　Malignant neoplasm of middle third of tongue NOS
　　　　Malignant neoplasm of mobile part of tongue NOS
　　C02.4   Malignant neoplasm of lingual tonsil
　　　　Lingual tonsil: Aggregation of lymph follicles at root of tongue
　　　　Excludes2   malignant neoplasm of tonsil NOS (C09.9)
　　C02.8   Malignant neoplasm of overlapping sites of tongue
　　　　Malignant neoplasm of two or more contiguous sites of tongue
　　C02.9   Malignant neoplasm of tongue, unspecified

● **C03   Malignant neoplasm of gum**
　　Includes   malignant neoplasm of alveolar (ridge) mucosa
　　　　　　　malignant neoplasm of gingiva
　　Use additional code to identify:
　　　alcohol abuse and dependence (F10.-)
　　　history of tobacco dependence (Z87.891) ◀▥
　　　tobacco dependence (F17.-)
　　　tobacco use (Z72.0)
　　Excludes2   malignant odontogenic neoplasms (C41.0-C41.1)
　　C03.0   Malignant neoplasm of upper gum
　　C03.1   Malignant neoplasm of lower gum
　　C03.9   Malignant neoplasm of gum, unspecified

● **C04   Malignant neoplasm of floor of mouth**
　　Use additional code to identify:
　　　alcohol abuse and dependence (F10.-)
　　　history of tobacco dependence (Z87.891) ◀▥
　　　tobacco dependence (F17.-)
　　　tobacco use (Z72.0)
　　C04.0   Malignant neoplasm of anterior floor of mouth
　　　　Malignant neoplasm of anterior to the premolar-canine junction
　　C04.1   Malignant neoplasm of lateral floor of mouth
　　C04.8   Malignant neoplasm of overlapping sites of floor of mouth
　　C04.9   Malignant neoplasm of floor of mouth, unspecified

● **C05   Malignant neoplasm of palate**
　　Use additional code to identify:
　　　alcohol abuse and dependence (F10.-)
　　　history of tobacco dependence (Z87.891) ◀▥
　　　tobacco dependence (F17.-)
　　　tobacco use (Z72.0)
　　Excludes1   Kaposi's sarcoma of palate (C46.2)
　　C05.0   Malignant neoplasm of hard palate
　　C05.1   Malignant neoplasm of soft palate
　　　　Excludes2   malignant neoplasm of nasopharyngeal surface of soft palate (C11.3)
　　C05.2   Malignant neoplasm of uvula
　　C05.8   Malignant neoplasm of overlapping sites of palate
　　C05.9   Malignant neoplasm of palate, unspecified
　　　　Malignant neoplasm of roof of mouth

● **C06   Malignant neoplasm of other and unspecified parts of mouth**
　　Use additional code to identify:
　　　alcohol abuse and dependence (F10.-)
　　　history of tobacco dependence (Z87.891) ◀▥
　　　tobacco dependence (F17.-)
　　　tobacco use (Z72.0)
　　C06.0   Malignant neoplasm of cheek mucosa
　　　　Malignant neoplasm of buccal mucosa NOS
　　　　Malignant neoplasm of internal cheek
　　C06.1   Malignant neoplasm of vestibule of mouth
　　　　Malignant neoplasm of buccal sulcus (upper) (lower)
　　　　Malignant neoplasm of labial sulcus (upper) (lower)
　　C06.2   Malignant neoplasm of retromolar area
　● **C06.8   Malignant neoplasm of overlapping sites of other and unspecified parts of mouth**
　　　　C06.80   Malignant neoplasm of overlapping sites of unspecified parts of mouth
　　　　C06.89   Malignant neoplasm of overlapping sites of other parts of mouth 'book leaf' neoplasm [ventral surface of tongue and floor of mouth]
　　C06.9   Malignant neoplasm of mouth, unspecified
　　　　Malignant neoplasm of minor salivary gland, unspecified site
　　　　Malignant neoplasm of oral cavity NOS

CHAPTER 2 (C00-D49)

Parotid
gland
Sublingual
gland
Submandibular
gland

Figure 2-2 Major salivary glands.

C07　Malignant neoplasm of parotid gland
Use additional code to identify:
alcohol abuse and dependence (F10.-)
exposure to environmental tobacco smoke (Z77.22)
exposure to tobacco smoke in the perinatal period (P96.81)
history of tobacco dependence (Z87.891) ◀▥
occupational exposure to environmental tobacco smoke
(Z57.31)
tobacco dependence (F17.-)
tobacco use (Z72.0)

● C08　Malignant neoplasm of other and unspecified major salivary glands
Includes　　malignant neoplasm of salivary ducts
Use additional code to identify:
alcohol abuse and dependence (F10.-)
exposure to environmental tobacco smoke (Z77.22)
exposure to tobacco smoke in the perinatal period (P96.81)
history of tobacco dependence (Z87.891) ◀▥
occupational exposure to environmental tobacco smoke
(Z57.31)
tobacco dependence (F17.-)
tobacco use (Z72.0)
Excludes1　　malignant neoplasms of specified minor salivary
glands which are classified according to their
anatomical location
Excludes2　　malignant neoplasms of minor salivary glands
NOS (C06.9)
malignant neoplasm of parotid gland (C07)

C08.0　Malignant neoplasm of submandibular gland
Malignant neoplasm of submaxillary gland

C08.1　Malignant neoplasm of sublingual gland

C08.9　Malignant neoplasm of major salivary gland, unspecified
Malignant neoplasm of salivary gland (major) NOS

★ **(See Plate 61 on page 73.)**

● C09　Malignant neoplasm of tonsil
Use additional code to identify:
alcohol abuse and dependence (F10.-)
exposure to environmental tobacco smoke (Z77.22)
exposure to tobacco smoke in the perinatal period (P96.81)
history of tobacco dependence (Z87.891) ◀▥
occupational exposure to environmental tobacco smoke
(Z57.31)
tobacco dependence (F17.-)
tobacco use (Z72.0)
Excludes2　　malignant neoplasm of lingual tonsil (C02.4)
malignant neoplasm of pharyngeal tonsil (C11.1)

C09.0　Malignant neoplasm of tonsillar fossa
Surface of palatine (two masses of lymphatic tissue on sides of throat) tonsils

C09.1　Malignant neoplasm of tonsillar pillar (anterior) (posterior)
Extension from palatine (two masses of lymphatic tissue on sides of throat) tonsils

C09.8　Malignant neoplasm of overlapping sites of tonsil

C09.9　Malignant neoplasm of tonsil, unspecified
Malignant neoplasm of tonsil NOS
Malignant neoplasm of faucial tonsils
Malignant neoplasm of palatine tonsils

● C10　Malignant neoplasm of oropharynx
Area of throat at back of mouth
Use additional code to identify:
alcohol abuse and dependence (F10.-)
exposure to environmental tobacco smoke (Z77.22)
exposure to tobacco smoke in the perinatal period (P96.81)
history of tobacco dependence (Z87.891) ◀▥
occupational exposure to environmental tobacco smoke
(Z57.31)
tobacco dependence (F17.-)
tobacco use (Z72.0)
Excludes2　　malignant neoplasm of tonsil (C09.-)

C10.0　Malignant neoplasm of vallecula
Vallecula, depression or furrow

C10.1　Malignant neoplasm of anterior surface of epiglottis
Malignant neoplasm of epiglottis, free border [margin]
Malignant neoplasm of glossoepiglottic fold(s)
Excludes2　　malignant neoplasm of epiglottis
(suprahyoid portion) NOS (C32.1)

C10.2　Malignant neoplasm of lateral wall of oropharynx

C10.3　Malignant neoplasm of posterior wall of oropharynx

C10.4　Malignant neoplasm of branchial cleft
Congenital slitlike openings formed between branchial arches pharyngeal groove
Malignant neoplasm of branchial cyst [site of neoplasm]

C10.8　Malignant neoplasm of overlapping sites of oropharynx
Malignant neoplasm of junctional region of oropharynx

C10.9　Malignant neoplasm of oropharynx, unspecified

● C11　Malignant neoplasm of nasopharynx
Use additional code to identify:
exposure to environmental tobacco smoke (Z77.22)
exposure to tobacco smoke in the perinatal period (P96.81)
history of tobacco dependence (Z87.891) ◀▥
occupational exposure to environmental tobacco smoke
(Z57.31)
tobacco dependence (F17.-)
tobacco use (Z72.0)

C11.0　Malignant neoplasm of superior wall of nasopharynx
Part of pharynx that lies above soft palate
Malignant neoplasm of roof of nasopharynx

C11.1　Malignant neoplasm of posterior wall of nasopharynx
Malignant neoplasm of adenoid
Malignant neoplasm of pharyngeal tonsil

C11.2　Malignant neoplasm of lateral wall of nasopharynx
Malignant neoplasm of fossa of Rosenmüller
Malignant neoplasm of opening of auditory tube
Malignant neoplasm of pharyngeal recess

C11.3　Malignant neoplasm of anterior wall of nasopharynx
Malignant neoplasm of floor of nasopharynx
Malignant neoplasm of nasopharyngeal (anterior)
(posterior) surface of soft palate
Malignant neoplasm of posterior margin of nasal
choana
Malignant neoplasm of posterior margin of nasal
septum

C11.8　Malignant neoplasm of overlapping sites of nasopharynx

C11.9　Malignant neoplasm of nasopharynx, unspecified
Malignant neoplasm of nasopharyngeal wall NOS

C12　Malignant neoplasm of pyriform sinus
Malignant neoplasm of pyriform fossa
Use additional code to identify:
exposure to environmental tobacco smoke (Z77.22)
exposure to tobacco smoke in the perinatal period (P96.81)
history of tobacco dependence (Z87.891) ◀▥
occupational exposure to environmental tobacco smoke
(Z57.31)
tobacco dependence (F17.-)
tobacco use (Z72.0)

CHAPTER 2 (C00-D49)

● **C13**   **Malignant neoplasm of hypopharynx**

Use additional code to identify:
exposure to environmental tobacco smoke (Z77.22)
exposure to tobacco smoke in the perinatal period (P96.81)
history of tobacco dependence (Z87.891) ◀▦▦
occupational exposure to environmental tobacco smoke (Z57.31)
tobacco dependence (F17.-)
tobacco use (Z72.0)

Excludes2   malignant neoplasm of pyriform sinus (C12)

C13.0   **Malignant neoplasm of postcricoid region**
Behind the cricoid cartilage of neck

C13.1   **Malignant neoplasm of aryepiglottic fold, hypopharyngeal aspect**
Arytenoepiglottic fold, triangular opening between side of epiglottis and apex of arytenoid cartilage
Malignant neoplasm of aryepiglottic fold, marginal zone
Malignant neoplasm of aryepiglottic fold NOS
Malignant neoplasm of interarytenoid fold, marginal zone
Malignant neoplasm of interarytenoid fold NOS

Excludes2   malignant neoplasm of aryepiglottic fold or interarytenoid fold, laryngeal aspect (C32.1)

C13.2   **Malignant neoplasm of posterior wall of hypopharynx**

C13.8   **Malignant neoplasm of overlapping sites of hypopharynx**

C13.9   **Malignant neoplasm of hypopharynx, unspecified**
Malignant neoplasm of hypopharyngeal wall NOS

● **C14**   **Malignant neoplasm of other and ill-defined sites in the lip, oral cavity and pharynx**

Use additional code to identify:
alcohol abuse and dependence (F10.-)
exposure to environmental tobacco smoke (Z77.22)
exposure to tobacco smoke in the perinatal period (P96.81)
history of tobacco dependence (Z87.891) ◀▦▦
occupational exposure to environmental tobacco smoke (Z57.31)
tobacco dependence (F17.-)
tobacco use (Z72.0)

Excludes1   malignant neoplasm of oral cavity NOS (C06.9)

C14.0   **Malignant neoplasm of pharynx, unspecified**

C14.2   **Malignant neoplasm of Waldeyer's ring**

C14.8   **Malignant neoplasm of overlapping sites of lip, oral cavity and pharynx**
Primary malignant neoplasm of two or more contiguous sites of lip, oral cavity and pharynx

Excludes1   'book leaf' neoplasm [ventral surface of tongue and floor of mouth] (C06.89)

MALIGNANT NEOPLASM OF DIGESTIVE ORGANS (C15-C26)

Excludes1   Kaposi's sarcoma of gastrointestinal sites (C46.4)

Excludes2   gastrointestinal stromal tumors (C49.A-) ◀

● **C15**   **Malignant neoplasms of esophagus**

Use additional code to identify:
alcohol abuse and dependence (F10.-)

C15.3   **Malignant neoplasm of upper third of esophagus**

C15.4   **Malignant neoplasm of middle third of esophagus**

C15.5   **Malignant neoplasm of lower third of esophagus**

Excludes1   malignant neoplasm of cardio-esophageal junction (C16.0)

C15.8   **Malignant neoplasm of overlapping sites of esophagus**

C15.9   **Malignant neoplasm of esophagus, unspecified**

● **C16**   **Malignant neoplasm of stomach**

Use additional code to identify:
alcohol abuse and dependence (F10.-)

Excludes2   malignant carcinoid tumor of the stomach (C7A.092)

C16.0   **Malignant neoplasm of cardia**
Malignant neoplasm of cardiac orifice
Malignant neoplasm of cardio-esophageal junction
Malignant neoplasm of esophagus and stomach
Malignant neoplasm of gastro-esophageal junction

C16.1   **Malignant neoplasm of fundus of stomach**

C16.2   **Malignant neoplasm of body of stomach**

C16.3   **Malignant neoplasm of pyloric antrum**
Malignant neoplasm of gastric antrum

C16.4   **Malignant neoplasm of pylorus**
Malignant neoplasm of prepylorus
Malignant neoplasm of pyloric canal

C16.5   **Malignant neoplasm of lesser curvature of stomach, unspecified**
Malignant neoplasm of lesser curvature of stomach, not classifiable to C16.1-C16.4

C16.6   **Malignant neoplasm of greater curvature of stomach, unspecified**
Malignant neoplasm of greater curvature of stomach, not classifiable to C16.0-C16.4

C16.8   **Malignant neoplasm of overlapping sites of stomach**

C16.9   **Malignant neoplasm of stomach, unspecified**
Gastric cancer NOS

Figure 2-3   The esophagus is the muscular tube that connects the pharynx and the stomach. The 10 inch (25 cm) long esophagus is divided into three parts: **cervical, thoracic,** and **abdominal.**

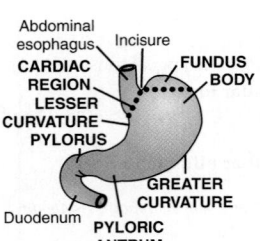

Figure 2-4   Parts of the stomach.

Item 2-2   The esophagus opens into the stomach through the **cardiac orifice,** also called the **cardioesophageal junction.** The **cardia** is adjacent to the cardiac orifice. The stomach widens into the **greater** and **lesser curvatures.** The **pyloric antrum** precedes the **pylorus,** which opens to the duodenum.

◀ New   ▥▥ Revised   ~~deleted~~ Deleted   Excludes 1   Excludes 2   Includes   Use additional   Code first   Code also   Unspecified

668   **OGCR** Official Guidelines   X Assign placeholder X   ● Use Additional Character(s)   ▶ Manifestation Code   **Coding Clinic**

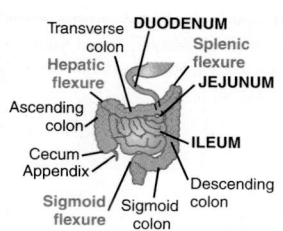

Figure 2-5   Small intestine and colon.

● **C17   Malignant neoplasm of small intestine**

> **Excludes1**   malignant carcinoid tumor of the small intestine (C7A.Ø1)

C17.Ø   Malignant neoplasm of duodenum
> *First or proximal portion of small intestine, extending from pylorus to jejunum*

C17.1   Malignant neoplasm of jejunum
> *Second section of small intestine, extending from duodenum to ileum*

C17.2   Malignant neoplasm of ileum
> *Distal and longest portion of small intestine, extending from jejunum to cecum*

> **Excludes1**   malignant neoplasm of ileocecal valve (C18.Ø)

C17.3   Meckel's diverticulum, malignant
> *Appendage of ileum*

> **Excludes1**   Meckel's diverticulum, congenital (Q43.Ø)

C17.8   Malignant neoplasm of overlapping sites of small intestine

C17.9   Malignant neoplasm of small intestine, unspecified

● **C18   Malignant neoplasm of colon**

> **Excludes1**   malignant carcinoid tumors of the colon (C7A.Ø2)

C18.Ø   Malignant neoplasm of cecum
> *First section of large intestine*
> Malignant neoplasm of ileocecal valve

C18.1   Malignant neoplasm of appendix
> *Blind ended tube connected to the cecum; AKA vermiform appendix*

C18.2   Malignant neoplasm of ascending colon
> *Ascending colon is between cecum and right colic flexure*

C18.3   Malignant neoplasm of hepatic flexure
> *A flexure is a bending in a structure or organ. Note the three flexures illustrated in Figure 2–5.*

C18.4   Malignant neoplasm of transverse colon
> *Portion of colon that runs transversely across upper part of abdomen, between right and left colic flexures*

C18.5   Malignant neoplasm of splenic flexure
> *Bend at junction of transverse and descending colon*

C18.6   Malignant neoplasm of descending colon
> *Portion between left colic flexure and sigmoid colon at pelvic brim; AKA iliac colon*

C18.7   Malignant neoplasm of sigmoid colon
> *S-shaped part of colon extending from pelvic brim to third segment of sacrum*
> Malignant neoplasm of sigmoid (flexure)

> **Excludes1**   malignant neoplasm of rectosigmoid junction (C19)

C18.8   Malignant neoplasm of overlapping sites of colon

C18.9   Malignant neoplasm of colon, unspecified
> Malignant neoplasm of large intestine NOS

C19   Malignant neoplasm of rectosigmoid junction
> Malignant neoplasm of colon with rectum
> Malignant neoplasm of rectosigmoid (colon)

> **Excludes1**   malignant carcinoid tumors of the colon (C7A.Ø2-)

C20   Malignant neoplasm of rectum
> Malignant neoplasm of rectal ampulla

> **Excludes1**   malignant carcinoid tumor of the rectum (C7A.Ø26)

● **C21   Malignant neoplasm of anus and anal canal**

> **Excludes2**   malignant carcinoid tumors of the colon (C7A.Ø2-)
> malignant melanoma of anal margin (C43.51)
> malignant melanoma of anal skin (C43.51)
> malignant melanoma of perianal skin (C43.51)
> other and unspecified malignant neoplasm of anal margin (C44.5ØØ, C44.51Ø, C44.52Ø, C44.59Ø)
> other and unspecified malignant neoplasm of anal skin (C44.5ØØ, C44.51Ø, C44.52Ø, C44.59Ø)
> other and unspecified malignant neoplasm of perianal skin (C44.5ØØ, C44.51Ø, C44.52Ø, C44.59Ø)

C21.Ø   Malignant neoplasm of anus, unspecified

C21.1   Malignant neoplasm of anal canal
> *Terminal part of large intestine*
> Malignant neoplasm of anal sphincter

C21.2   Malignant neoplasm of cloacogenic zone

C21.8   Malignant neoplasm of overlapping sites of rectum, anus and anal canal
> Malignant neoplasm of anorectal junction
> Malignant neoplasm of anorectum
> Primary malignant neoplasm of two or more contiguous sites of rectum, anus and anal canal

● **C22   Malignant neoplasm of liver and intrahepatic bile ducts**
> *Intrahepatic: Within liver*

> Use additional code to identify:
> alcohol abuse and dependence (F1Ø.-)
> hepatitis B (B16.-, B18.Ø-B18.1) hepatitis C (B17.1-, B18.2)

> **Excludes1**   malignant neoplasm of biliary tract NOS (C24.9)
> secondary malignant neoplasm of liver and intrahepatic bile duct (C78.7)

C22.Ø   Liver cell carcinoma
> Hepatocellular carcinoma
> Hepatoma

C22.1   Intrahepatic bile duct carcinoma
> Cholangiocarcinoma
> *Adenocarcinoma (cancer that originates in glandular tissue) arising from epithelium of intrahepatic bile ducts*

> **Excludes1**   malignant neoplasm of hepatic duct (C24.Ø)

C22.2   Hepatoblastoma
> *Malignant intrahepatic tumor*

C22.3   Angiosarcoma of liver
> Kupffer cell sarcoma

C22.4   Other sarcomas of liver

C22.7   Other specified carcinomas of liver

C22.8   Malignant neoplasm of liver, primary, unspecified as to type

C22.9   Malignant neoplasm of liver, not specified as primary or secondary

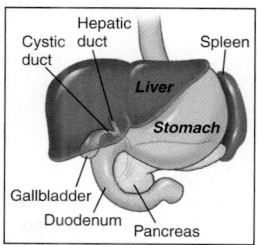

Figure 2-6   Diagram of liver, gallbladder, hepatic duct, pancreas, and spleen. (From Thibodeau and Patton: Anatomy and Physiology, ed 7, Mosby, 2010)

CHAPTER 2 (C00–D49)

C23   **Malignant neoplasm of gallbladder**

● **C24**   **Malignant neoplasm of other and unspecified parts of biliary tract**

     Excludes1   malignant neoplasm of intrahepatic bile duct (C22.1)

     C24.0   **Malignant neoplasm of extrahepatic bile duct**
         Extrahepatic = outside the liver
         Malignant neoplasm of biliary duct or passage NOS
         Malignant neoplasm of common bile duct
         Malignant neoplasm of cystic duct
         Malignant neoplasm of hepatic duct

     C24.1   **Malignant neoplasm of ampulla of Vater**
         Union of pancreatic duct and common bile duct

     C24.8   **Malignant neoplasm of overlapping sites of biliary tract**
         Malignant neoplasm involving both intrahepatic and extrahepatic bile ducts
         Primary malignant neoplasm of two or more contiguous sites of biliary tract

     C24.9   **Malignant neoplasm of biliary tract, unspecified**

● **C25**   **Malignant neoplasm of pancreas**
     Check documentation for specific site.
     Code also exocrine pancreatic insufficiency (K86.81) ◄
     Use additional code to identify:
         alcohol abuse and dependence (F10.-)

     C25.0   **Malignant neoplasm of head of pancreas**

     C25.1   **Malignant neoplasm of body of pancreas**

     C25.2   **Malignant neoplasm of tail of pancreas**

     C25.3   **Malignant neoplasm of pancreatic duct**

     C25.4   **Malignant neoplasm of endocrine pancreas**
         Malignant neoplasm of islets of Langerhans
         That part of the pancreas that acts as endocrine gland and consists of islets of Langerhans
         Use additional code to identify any functional activity.

     C25.7   **Malignant neoplasm of other parts of pancreas**
         Malignant neoplasm of neck of pancreas

     C25.8   **Malignant neoplasm of overlapping sites of pancreas**

     C25.9   **Malignant neoplasm of pancreas, unspecified**

● **C26**   **Malignant neoplasm of other and ill-defined digestive organs**

     Excludes1   malignant neoplasm of peritoneum and retroperitoneum (C48.-)

     C26.0   **Malignant neoplasm of intestinal tract, part unspecified**
         Malignant neoplasm of intestine NOS

     C26.1   **Malignant neoplasm of spleen**

         Excludes1   Hodgkin lymphoma (C81.-)
                  non-Hodgkin lymphoma (C82-C85)

     C26.9   **Malignant neoplasm of ill-defined sites within the digestive system**
         Malignant neoplasm of alimentary canal or tract NOS
         Malignant neoplasm of gastrointestinal tract NOS

         Excludes1   malignant neoplasm of abdominal NOS (C76.2)
                  malignant neoplasm of intra-abdominal NOS (C76.2)

Figure 2-7   Paranasal sinuses. (From Buck CJ: Step-by-Step Medical Coding, ed 2016, St. Louis, Elsevier, 2016)

MALIGNANT NEOPLASMS OF RESPIRATORY AND INTRATHORACIC ORGANS (C30-C39)

     Includes   malignant neoplasm of middle ear
     Excludes1   mesothelioma (C45.-)

● **C30**   **Malignant neoplasm of nasal cavity and middle ear**

     C30.0   **Malignant neoplasm of nasal cavity**
         Malignant neoplasm of cartilage of nose
         Malignant neoplasm of nasal concha
         Malignant neoplasm of internal nose
         Malignant neoplasm of septum of nose
         Malignant neoplasm of vestibule of nose
         Anterior part of nasal cavity

         Excludes1   malignant neoplasm of nasal bone (C41.0)
                  malignant neoplasm of nose NOS (C76.0)
                  malignant neoplasm of olfactory bulb (C72.2-)
                  malignant neoplasm of posterior margin of nasal septum and choana (C11.3)
                  malignant melanoma of skin of nose (C43.31)
                  malignant neoplasm of turbinates (C41.0)
                  other and unspecified malignant neoplasm of skin of nose C44.301, C44.311, C44.321, C44.391)

     C30.1   **Malignant neoplasm of middle ear**
         Malignant neoplasm of antrum tympanicum
         Boney cavity or chamber
         Malignant neoplasm of auditory tube
         Malignant neoplasm of eustachian tube
         Malignant neoplasm of inner ear
         Malignant neoplasm of mastoid air cells
         Malignant neoplasm of tympanic cavity

         Excludes1   malignant neoplasm of auricular canal (external) (C43.2-, C44.2-)
                  malignant neoplasm of bone of ear (meatus) (C41.0)
                  malignant neoplasm of cartilage of ear (C49.0)
                  malignant melanoma of skin of (external) ear (C43.2-)
                  other and unspecified malignant neoplasm of skin of (external) ear (C44.2-)

● **C31**   **Malignant neoplasm of accessory sinuses**
     Paired sinuses in bones of face

     C31.0   **Malignant neoplasm of maxillary sinus**
         Malignant neoplasm of antrum (Highmore) (maxillary)

     C31.1   **Malignant neoplasm of ethmoidal sinus**

     C31.2   **Malignant neoplasm of frontal sinus**

     C31.3   **Malignant neoplasm of sphenoid sinus**

     C31.8   **Malignant neoplasm of overlapping sites of accessory sinuses**

     C31.9   **Malignant neoplasm of accessory sinus, unspecified**

Item 2–3   **Islets** of Langerhans (endocrine producing cells comprising 1% to 2% of the pancreatic mass) make and secrete hormones that regulate the body's production of insulin, glucagon, and stomach acid. Breakdown of the insulin-producing cells can cause diabetes mellitus. Islet cell tumors can be benign or malignant and include glucagonomas, insulinomas, gastrinomas, and neuroendocrine tumor. The neoplasm table must be consulted for the correct neoplasm code.

◄ New   ⬸ Revised   ~~deleted~~ Deleted   Excludes 1   Excludes 2   Includes   Use additional   Code first   Code also   Unspecified

● **C32   Malignant neoplasm of larynx**
     Use additional code to identify:
          alcohol abuse and dependence (F10.-)
          exposure to environmental tobacco smoke (Z77.22)
          exposure to tobacco smoke in the perinatal period (P96.81)
          history of tobacco dependence (Z87.891) ◀▥
          occupational exposure to environmental tobacco smoke
               (Z57.31)
          tobacco dependence (F17.-)
          tobacco use (Z72.0)

   C32.0   Malignant neoplasm of glottis
          *Vocal apparatus of larynx, consisting of true vocal cords
               (plicae vocales) and opening between them (rima
               glottidis)*
          Malignant neoplasm of intrinsic larynx
          Malignant neoplasm of laryngeal commissure (anterior)
               (posterior)
          Malignant neoplasm of vocal cord (true) NOS
               True *vocal cords ("lower vocal folds") produce vocalization
                    when air from the lungs passes between them. Check
                    your documentation. Code C32.1 is for malignant
                    neoplasm of the **false** vocal cords.*

   C32.1   Malignant neoplasm of supraglottis
          Area of pharynx above glottis
          Malignant neoplasm of aryepiglottic fold or
               interarytenoid fold, laryngeal aspect
          Malignant neoplasm of epiglottis (suprahyoid portion)
               NOS
          Malignant neoplasm of extrinsic larynx
          Malignant neoplasm of false vocal cord
               False *vocal cords ("upper vocal folds") are not involved in
                    vocalization. Check your documentation. Code C32.0 is
                    for true vocal cords.*
          Malignant neoplasm of posterior (laryngeal) surface of
               epiglottis
          Malignant neoplasm of ventricular bands
               Excludes2   malignant neoplasm of anterior surface of
                                   epiglottis (C10.1)
                              malignant neoplasm of aryepiglottic
                                   fold or interarytenoid fold,
                                   hypopharyngeal aspect (C13.1)
                              malignant neoplasm of aryepiglottic fold
                                   or interarytenoid fold, marginal zone
                                   (C13.1)
                              malignant neoplasm of aryepiglottic fold
                                   or interarytenoid fold NOS (C13.1)

   C32.2   Malignant neoplasm of subglottis
          *Lowest part of larynx from just below vocal cords down to top
               of trachea*

   C32.3   Malignant neoplasm of laryngeal cartilage
          *Cartilages of larynx, including cricoid, thyroid, and
               epiglottic, and two each of arytenoid, corniculate, and
               cuneiform*

   C32.8   Malignant neoplasm of overlapping sites of larynx

   C32.9   Malignant neoplasm of larynx, unspecified

C33   Malignant neoplasm of trachea
     Use additional code to identify:
          exposure to environmental tobacco smoke (Z77.22)
          exposure to tobacco smoke in the perinatal period (P96.81)
          history of tobacco dependence (Z87.891) ◀▥
          occupational exposure to environmental tobacco smoke
               (Z57.31)
          tobacco dependence (F17.-)
          tobacco use (Z72.0)

● **C34   Malignant neoplasm of bronchus and lung**
     Use additional code to identify:
          exposure to environmental tobacco smoke (Z77.22)
          exposure to tobacco smoke in the perinatal period (P96.81)
          history of tobacco dependence (Z87.891) ◀▥
          occupational exposure to environmental tobacco smoke
               (Z57.31)
          tobacco dependence (F17.-)
          tobacco use (Z72.0)
          Excludes1   Kaposi's sarcoma of lung (C46.5-)
                        malignant carcinoid tumor of the bronchus and
                             lung (C7A.090)

● **C34.0   Malignant neoplasm of main bronchus**
          Malignant neoplasm of carina
               Ridgelike structure
          Malignant neoplasm of hilus (of lung)
               Anatomic depression or pit

     **C34.00   Malignant neoplasm of unspecified main
                  bronchus**
     C34.01   Malignant neoplasm of right main bronchus
     C34.02   Malignant neoplasm of left main bronchus

● **C34.1   Malignant neoplasm of upper lobe, bronchus or lung**
     **C34.10   Malignant neoplasm of unspecified bronchus
                  or lung**
     **C34.11   Malignant neoplasm of upper lobe, right
                  bronchus or lung**
     **C34.12   Malignant neoplasm of upper lobe, left
                  bronchus or lung**

   C34.2   Malignant neoplasm of middle lobe, bronchus or lung

● **C34.3   Malignant neoplasm of lower lobe, bronchus or lung**
     **C34.30   Malignant neoplasm of lower lobe, unspecified
                  bronchus or lung**
     **C34.31   Malignant neoplasm of lower lobe, right
                  bronchus or lung**
     **C34.32   Malignant neoplasm of lower lobe, left
                  bronchus or lung**

● **C34.8   Malignant neoplasm of overlapping sites of bronchus
            and lung**
     **C34.80   Malignant neoplasm of overlapping sites
                  of unspecified bronchus and lung**
     **C34.81   Malignant neoplasm of overlapping sites of
                  right bronchus and lung**
     **C34.82   Malignant neoplasm of overlapping sites of left
                  bronchus and lung**

● **C34.9   Malignant neoplasm of unspecified part of bronchus or
            lung**
     **C34.90   Malignant neoplasm of unspecified part of
                  unspecified bronchus or lung**
                  Lung cancer NOS
     **C34.91   Malignant neoplasm of unspecified part of
                  right bronchus or lung**
     **C34.92   Malignant neoplasm of unspecified part of left
                  bronchus or lung**

C37   Malignant neoplasm of thymus
     Excludes1   malignant carcinoid tumor of the thymus
                     (C7A.091)

● **C38**   **Malignant neoplasm of heart, mediastinum and pleura**
    Excludes1   mesothelioma (C45.-)

    C38.0   **Malignant neoplasm of heart**
         Malignant neoplasm of pericardium
         Excludes1   malignant neoplasm of great vessels
                          (C49.3)

    C38.1   **Malignant neoplasm of anterior mediastinum**
    C38.2   **Malignant neoplasm of posterior mediastinum**
    C38.3   **Malignant neoplasm of mediastinum, part unspecified**
    C38.4   **Malignant neoplasm of pleura**
    C38.8   **Malignant neoplasm of overlapping sites of heart, mediastinum and pleura**
         Pleura are comprised of serous membrane that lines the thoracic cavity (parietal) and covers the lungs (visceral).

● **C39**   **Malignant neoplasm of other and ill-defined sites in the respiratory system and intrathoracic organs**
         Intrathoracic: within thorax/chest
         Use additional code to identify:
             exposure to environmental tobacco smoke (Z77.22)
             exposure to tobacco smoke in the perinatal period (P96.81)
             history of tobacco dependence (Z87.891) ◀▥▥
             occupational exposure to environmental tobacco smoke
                 (Z57.31)
             tobacco dependence (F17.-)
             tobacco use (Z72.0)
         Excludes1   intrathoracic malignant neoplasm NOS (C76.1)
                          thoracic malignant neoplasm NOS (C76.1)

    C39.0   **Malignant neoplasm of upper respiratory tract, part unspecified**
    C39.9   **Malignant neoplasm of lower respiratory tract, part unspecified**
         Malignant neoplasm of respiratory tract NOS

MALIGNANT NEOPLASMS OF BONE AND ARTICULAR CARTILAGE (C40-C41)

    Includes   malignant neoplasm of cartilage (articular) (joint)
                    malignant neoplasm of periosteum
    Excludes1   malignant neoplasm of bone marrow NOS (C96.9)
                    malignant neoplasm of synovia (C49.-)

● **C40**   **Malignant neoplasm of bone and articular cartilage of limbs**
         Use additional code to identify major osseous defect, if
             applicable (M89.7-)

    ● **C40.0**   **Malignant neoplasm of scapula and long bones of upper limb**
        C40.00   **Malignant neoplasm of scapula and long bones of unspecified upper limb**
        C40.01   **Malignant neoplasm of scapula and long bones of right upper limb**
        C40.02   **Malignant neoplasm of scapula and long bones of left upper limb**

    ● **C40.1**   **Malignant neoplasm of short bones of upper limb**
        C40.10   **Malignant neoplasm of short bones of unspecified upper limb**
        C40.11   **Malignant neoplasm of short bones of right upper limb**
        C40.12   **Malignant neoplasm of short bones of left upper limb**

    ● **C40.2**   **Malignant neoplasm of long bones of lower limb**
        C40.20   **Malignant neoplasm of long bones of unspecified lower limb**
        C40.21   **Malignant neoplasm of long bones of right lower limb**
        C40.22   **Malignant neoplasm of long bones of left lower limb**

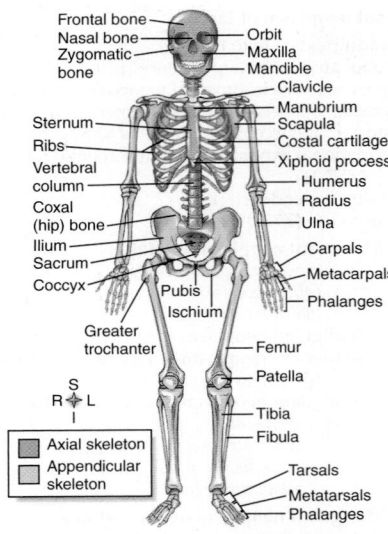

Figure 2-8   Diagram of skeleton of trunk and limbs with bones labeled. (From Thibodeau and Patton: Anatomy and Physiology, ed 7, Mosby, 2010)

    ● **C40.3**   **Malignant neoplasm of short bones of lower limb**
        C40.30   **Malignant neoplasm of short bones of unspecified lower limb**
        C40.31   **Malignant neoplasm of short bones of right lower limb**
        C40.32   **Malignant neoplasm of short bones of left lower limb**

    ● **C40.8**   **Malignant neoplasm of overlapping sites of bone and articular cartilage of limb**
        C40.80   **Malignant neoplasm of overlapping sites of bone and articular cartilage of unspecified limb**
        C40.81   **Malignant neoplasm of overlapping sites of bone and articular cartilage of right limb**
        C40.82   **Malignant neoplasm of overlapping sites of bone and articular cartilage of left limb**

    ● **C40.9**   **Malignant neoplasm of unspecified bones and articular cartilage of limb**
        C40.90   **Malignant neoplasm of unspecified bones and articular cartilage of unspecified limb**
        C40.91   **Malignant neoplasm of unspecified bones and articular cartilage of right limb**
        C40.92   **Malignant neoplasm of unspecified bones and articular cartilage of left limb**

● **C41**   **Malignant neoplasm of bone and articular cartilage of other and unspecified sites**
    Excludes1   malignant neoplasm of bones of limbs (C40.-)
                    malignant neoplasm of cartilage of ear (C49.0)
                    malignant neoplasm of cartilage of eyelid (C49.0)
                    malignant neoplasm of cartilage of larynx (C32.3)
                    malignant neoplasm of cartilage of limbs (C40.-)
                    malignant neoplasm of cartilage of nose (C30.0)

    C41.0   **Malignant neoplasm of bones of skull and face**
         Malignant neoplasm of maxilla (superior)
         Malignant neoplasm of orbital bone
         Excludes2   carcinoma, any type except intraosseous
                          or odontogenic of:
                              maxillary sinus (C31.0)
                              upper jaw (C03.0)
                          malignant neoplasm of jaw bone (lower)
                              (C41.1)

◀ New   ◀▥▥ Revised   ~~deleted~~ Deleted   Excludes 1   Excludes 2   Includes   Use additional   Code first   Code also   Unspecified

672   OGCR Official Guidelines   X Assign placeholder X   ● Use Additional Character(s)   ▌ Manifestation Code   **Coding Clinic**

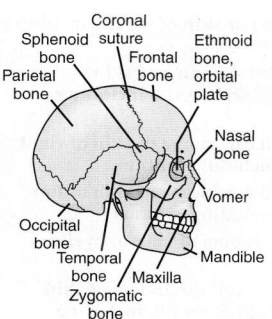

Figure 2-9 Bones of the skull.

Figure 2-10 Malignant melanoma of skin. (From Goldman: Cecil Textbook of Medicine, ed 22, Saunders, 2004)

Item 2–4 Malignant melanoma is a serious form of skin cancer that affects the melanocytes (pigment-forming cells) and is caused by ultraviolet (UV) rays from the sun that damage skin. It is most commonly seen in the 4Ø- to 6Ø-year-olds with fair skin, blue or green eyes, and red or blond hair who sunburn easily.

Melanoma can spread very rapidly and is the most deadly form of skin cancer. It is less common than other types of skin cancer. The rate of melanoma is increasing and currently is the leading cause of death from skin disease.

C41.1 Malignant neoplasm of mandible
        Malignant neoplasm of inferior maxilla
        Malignant neoplasm of lower jaw bone
    Excludes2 carcinoma, any type except intraosseous or odontogenic of:
                jaw NOS (CØ3.9)
                lower (CØ3.1)
                malignant neoplasm of upper jaw bone (C41.Ø)

C41.2 Malignant neoplasm of vertebral column
    Excludes1 malignant neoplasm of sacrum and coccyx (C41.4)

C41.3 Malignant neoplasm of ribs, sternum and clavicle

C41.4 Malignant neoplasm of pelvic bones, sacrum and coccyx

C41.9 Malignant neoplasm of bone and articular cartilage, unspecified

---

MELANOMA AND OTHER MALIGNANT NEOPLASMS OF SKIN (C43-C44)

● **C43 Malignant melanoma of skin**
    Excludes1 melanoma in situ (DØ3.-)
    Excludes2 malignant melanoma of skin of genital organs (C51-C52, C6Ø.-, C63.-)
                Merkel cell carcinoma (C4A.-)
                sites other than skin-code to malignant neoplasm of the site

C43.Ø Malignant melanoma of lip
    Excludes1 malignant neoplasm of vermilion border of lip (CØØ.Ø-CØØ.2)

● **C43.1 Malignant melanoma of eyelid, including canthus**
    Canthus: Either corner of eye where upper and lower eyelids meet
    C43.1Ø Malignant melanoma of unspecified eyelid, including canthus
    C43.11 Malignant melanoma of right eyelid, including canthus
    C43.12 Malignant melanoma of left eyelid, including canthus

● **C43.2 Malignant melanoma of ear and external auricular canal**
    C43.2Ø Malignant melanoma of unspecified ear and external auricular canal
    C43.21 Malignant melanoma of right ear and external auricular canal
    C43.22 Malignant melanoma of left ear and external auricular canal

● **C43.3 Malignant melanoma of other and unspecified parts of face**
    C43.3Ø Malignant melanoma of unspecified part of face
    C43.31 Malignant melanoma of nose
    C43.39 Malignant melanoma of other parts of face

C43.4 Malignant melanoma of scalp and neck

● **C43.5 Malignant melanoma of trunk**
    Excludes2 malignant neoplasm of anus NOS (C21.Ø)
                malignant neoplasm of scrotum (C63.2)
    C43.51 Malignant melanoma of anal skin
            Malignant melanoma of anal margin
            Malignant melanoma of perianal skin
    C43.52 Malignant melanoma of skin of breast
    C43.59 Malignant melanoma of other part of trunk

● **C43.6 Malignant melanoma of upper limb, including shoulder**
    C43.6Ø Malignant melanoma of upper limb, including shoulder, unspecified side
    C43.61 Malignant melanoma of right upper limb, including shoulder
    C43.62 Malignant melanoma of left upper limb, including shoulder

● **C43.7 Malignant melanoma of lower limb, including hip**
    C43.7Ø Malignant melanoma of unspecified lower limb, including hip
    C43.71 Malignant melanoma of right lower limb, including hip
    C43.72 Malignant melanoma of left lower limb, including hip

C43.8 Malignant melanoma of overlapping sites of skin

C43.9 Malignant melanoma of skin, unspecified
        Malignant melanoma of unspecified site of skin
        Melanoma (malignant) NOS

● **C4A Merkel cell carcinoma**
    C4A.Ø Merkel cell carcinoma of lip
        Excludes1 malignant neoplasm of vermilion border of lip (CØØ.Ø-CØØ.2)

● **C4A.1 Merkel cell carcinoma of eyelid, including canthus**
    C4A.1Ø Merkel cell carcinoma of unspecified eyelid, including canthus
    C4A.11 Merkel cell carcinoma of right eyelid, including canthus
    C4A.12 Merkel cell carcinoma of left eyelid, including canthus

● **C4A.2 Merkel cell carcinoma of ear and external auricular canal**
    C4A.2Ø Merkel cell carcinoma of unspecified ear and external auricular canal
    C4A.21 Merkel cell carcinoma of right ear and external auricular canal
    C4A.22 Merkel cell carcinoma of left ear and external auricular canal

CHAPTER 2 (CØØ-D49)

● **C4A.3 Merkel cell carcinoma of other and unspecified parts of face**

    C4A.30 Merkel cell carcinoma of unspecified part of face

    C4A.31 Merkel cell carcinoma of nose

    C4A.39 Merkel cell carcinoma of other parts of face

● **C4A.4 Merkel cell carcinoma of scalp and neck**

● **C4A.5 Merkel cell carcinoma of trunk**

    Excludes2   malignant neoplasm of anus NOS (C21.0)
                         malignant neoplasm of scrotum (C63.2)

    C4A.51 Merkel cell carcinoma of anal skin
            Merkel cell carcinoma of anal margin
            Merkel cell carcinoma of perianal skin

    C4A.52 Merkel cell carcinoma of skin of breast

    C4A.59 Merkel cell carcinoma of other part of trunk

● **C4A.6 Merkel cell carcinoma of upper limb, including shoulder**

    C4A.60 Merkel cell carcinoma of unspecified upper limb, including shoulder

    C4A.61 Merkel cell carcinoma of right upper limb, including shoulder

    C4A.62 Merkel cell carcinoma of left upper limb, including shoulder

● **C4A.7 Merkel cell carcinoma of lower limb, including hip**

    C4A.70 Merkel cell carcinoma of unspecified lower limb, including hip

    C4A.71 Merkel cell carcinoma of right lower limb, including hip

    C4A.72 Merkel cell carcinoma of left lower limb, including hip

  C4A.8 Merkel cell carcinoma of overlapping sites

  C4A.9 Merkel cell carcinoma, unspecified
         Merkel cell carcinoma of unspecified site
         Merkel cell carcinoma NOS

● **C44 Other and unspecified malignant neoplasm of skin**

    Includes   malignant neoplasm of sebaceous glands
                  malignant neoplasm of sweat glands

    Excludes1   Kaposi's sarcoma of skin (C46.0)
                  malignant melanoma of skin (C43.-)
                  malignant neoplasm of skin of genital organs
                     (C51-C52, C60.-, C63.2)
                  Merkel cell carcinoma (C4A.-)

● **C44.0 Other and unspecified malignant neoplasm of skin of lip**

    Excludes1   malignant neoplasm of lip (C00.-)

    C44.00 Unspecified malignant neoplasm of skin of lip

    C44.01 Basal cell carcinoma of skin of lip

    C44.02 Squamous cell carcinoma of skin of lip

    C44.09 Other specified malignant neoplasm of skin of lip

● **C44.1 Other and unspecified malignant neoplasm of skin of eyelid, including canthus**

    Excludes1   connective tissue of eyelid (C49.0)

  ● **C44.10 Unspecified malignant neoplasm of skin of eyelid, including canthus**

    C44.101 Unspecified malignant neoplasm of skin of unspecified eyelid, including canthus

    C44.102 Unspecified malignant neoplasm of skin of right eyelid, including canthus

    C44.109 Unspecified malignant neoplasm of skin of left eyelid, including canthus

● **C44.11 Basal cell carcinoma of skin of eyelid, including canthus**

    C44.111 Basal cell carcinoma of skin of unspecified eyelid, including canthus

    C44.112 Basal cell carcinoma of skin of right eyelid, including canthus

    C44.119 Basal cell carcinoma of skin of left eyelid, including canthus

● **C44.12 Squamous cell carcinoma of skin of eyelid, including canthus**

    C44.121 Squamous cell carcinoma of skin of unspecified eyelid, including canthus

    C44.122 Squamous cell carcinoma of skin of right eyelid, including canthus

    C44.129 Squamous cell carcinoma of skin of left eyelid, including canthus

● **C44.19 Other specified malignant neoplasm of skin of eyelid, including canthus**

    C44.191 Other specified malignant neoplasm of skin of unspecified eyelid, including canthus

    C44.192 Other specified malignant neoplasm of skin of right eyelid, including canthus

    C44.199 Other specified malignant neoplasm of skin of left eyelid, including canthus

● **C44.2 Other and unspecified malignant neoplasm of skin of ear and external auricular canal**

    Excludes1   connective tissue of ear (C49.0)

  ● **C44.20 Unspecified malignant neoplasm of skin of ear and external auricular canal**

    C44.201 Unspecified malignant neoplasm of skin of unspecified ear and external auricular canal

    C44.202 Unspecified malignant neoplasm of skin of right ear and external auricular canal

    C44.209 Unspecified malignant neoplasm of skin of left ear and external auricular canal

  ● **C44.21 Basal cell carcinoma of skin of ear and external auricular canal**

    C44.211 Basal cell carcinoma of skin of unspecified ear and external auricular canal

    C44.212 Basal cell carcinoma of skin of right ear and external auricular canal

    C44.219 Basal cell carcinoma of skin of left ear and external auricular canal

  ● **C44.22 Squamous cell carcinoma of skin of ear and external auricular canal**

    C44.221 Squamous cell carcinoma of skin of unspecified ear and external auricular canal

    C44.222 Squamous cell carcinoma of skin of right ear and external auricular canal

    C44.229 Squamous cell carcinoma of skin of left ear and external auricular canal

  ● **C44.29 Other specified malignant neoplasm of skin of ear and external auricular canal**

    C44.291 Other specified malignant neoplasm of skin of unspecified ear and external auricular canal

    C44.292 Other specified malignant neoplasm of skin of right ear and external auricular canal

    C44.299 Other specified malignant neoplasm of skin of left ear and external auricular canal

◀ New   ◀ Revised   ~~deleted~~ Deleted   Excludes 1   Excludes 2   Includes   Use additional   Code first   Code also   Unspecified

674   **OGCR** Official Guidelines   X Assign placeholder X   ● Use Additional Character(s)   ▶ Manifestation Code   **Coding Clinic**

- ● C44.3   **Other and unspecified malignant neoplasm of skin of other and unspecified parts of face**
  - ● C44.30   Unspecified malignant neoplasm of skin of other and unspecified parts of face
    - C44.300   Unspecified malignant neoplasm of skin of unspecified part of face
    - C44.301   Unspecified malignant neoplasm of skin of nose
    - C44.309   Unspecified malignant neoplasm of skin of other parts of face
  - ● C44.31   Basal cell carcinoma of skin of other and unspecified parts of face
    - C44.310   Basal cell carcinoma of skin of unspecified parts of face
    - C44.311   Basal cell carcinoma of skin of nose
    - C44.319   Basal cell carcinoma of skin of other parts of face
  - ● C44.32   Squamous cell carcinoma of skin of other and unspecified parts of face
    - C44.320   Squamous cell carcinoma of skin of unspecified parts of face
    - C44.321   Squamous cell carcinoma of skin of nose
    - C44.329   Squamous cell carcinoma of skin of other parts of face
  - ● C44.39   Other specified malignant neoplasm of skin of other and unspecified parts of face
    - C44.390   Other specified malignant neoplasm of skin of unspecified parts of face
    - C44.391   Other specified malignant neoplasm of skin of nose
    - C44.399   Other specified malignant neoplasm of skin of other parts of face
- ● C44.4   **Other and unspecified malignant neoplasm of skin of scalp and neck**
  - C44.40   Unspecified malignant neoplasm of skin of scalp and neck
  - C44.41   Basal cell carcinoma of skin of scalp and neck
  - C44.42   Squamous cell carcinoma of skin of scalp and neck
  - C44.49   Other specified malignant neoplasm of skin of scalp and neck
- ● C44.5   **Other and unspecified malignant neoplasm of skin of trunk**

  > **Excludes1**   anus NOS (C21.0)
  >   scrotum (C63.2)

  - ● C44.50   Unspecified malignant neoplasm of skin of trunk
    - C44.500   Unspecified malignant neoplasm of anal skin
      Unspecified malignant neoplasm of anal margin
      Unspecified malignant neoplasm of perianal skin
    - C44.501   Unspecified malignant neoplasm of skin of breast
    - C44.509   Unspecified malignant neoplasm of skin of other part of trunk
  - ● C44.51   Basal cell carcinoma of skin of trunk
    - C44.510   Basal cell carcinoma of anal skin
      Basal cell carcinoma of anal margin
      Basal cell carcinoma of perianal skin
    - C44.511   Basal cell carcinoma of skin of breast
    - C44.519   Basal cell carcinoma of skin of other part of trunk

- ● C44.52   Squamous cell carcinoma of skin of trunk
  - C44.520   Squamous cell carcinoma of anal skin
    Squamous cell carcinoma of anal margin
    Squamous cell carcinoma of perianal skin
  - C44.521   Squamous cell carcinoma of skin of breast
  - C44.529   Squamous cell carcinoma of skin of other part of trunk
- ● C44.59   Other specified malignant neoplasm of skin of trunk
  - C44.590   Other specified malignant neoplasm of anal skin
    Other specified malignant neoplasm of anal margin
    Other specified malignant neoplasm of perianal skin
  - C44.591   Other specified malignant neoplasm of skin of breast
  - C44.599   Other specified malignant neoplasm of skin of other part of trunk
- ● C44.6   **Other and unspecified malignant neoplasm of skin of upper limb, including shoulder**
  - ● C44.60   Unspecified malignant neoplasm of skin of upper limb, including shoulder
    - C44.601   Unspecified malignant neoplasm of skin of unspecified upper limb, including shoulder
    - C44.602   Unspecified malignant neoplasm of skin of right upper limb, including shoulder
    - C44.609   Unspecified malignant neoplasm of skin of left upper limb, including shoulder
  - ● C44.61   Basal cell carcinoma of skin of upper limb, including shoulder
    - C44.611   Basal cell carcinoma of skin of unspecified upper limb, including shoulder
    - C44.612   Basal cell carcinoma of skin of right upper limb, including shoulder
    - C44.619   Basal cell carcinoma of skin of left upper limb, including shoulder
  - ● C44.62   Squamous cell carcinoma of skin of upper limb, including shoulder
    - C44.621   Squamous cell carcinoma of skin of unspecified upper limb, including shoulder
    - C44.622   Squamous cell carcinoma of skin of right upper limb, including shoulder
    - C44.629   Squamous cell carcinoma of skin of left upper limb, including shoulder
  - ● C44.69   Other specified malignant neoplasm of skin of upper limb, including shoulder
    - C44.691   Other specified malignant neoplasm of skin of unspecified upper limb, including shoulder
    - C44.692   Other specified malignant neoplasm of skin of right upper limb, including shoulder
    - C44.699   Other specified malignant neoplasm of skin of left upper limb, including shoulder

CHAPTER 2 (C00-D49)

CHAPTER 2 (C00-D49)

●C44.7   **Other and unspecified malignant neoplasm of skin of lower limb, including hip**
     ●C44.70   **Unspecified malignant neoplasm of skin of lower limb, including hip**
         C44.701   Unspecified malignant neoplasm of skin of unspecified lower limb, including hip
         C44.702   Unspecified malignant neoplasm of skin of right lower limb, including hip
         C44.709   Unspecified malignant neoplasm of skin of left lower limb, including hip
     ●C44.71   **Basal cell carcinoma of skin of lower limb, including hip**
         C44.711   Basal cell carcinoma of skin of unspecified lower limb, including hip
         C44.712   Basal cell carcinoma of skin of right lower limb, including hip
         C44.719   Basal cell carcinoma of skin of left lower limb, including hip
     ●C44.72   **Squamous cell carcinoma of skin of lower limb, including hip**
         C44.721   Squamous cell carcinoma of skin of unspecified lower limb, including hip
         C44.722   Squamous cell carcinoma of skin of right lower limb, including hip
         C44.729   Squamous cell carcinoma of skin of left lower limb, including hip
     ●C44.79   **Other specified malignant neoplasm of skin of lower limb, including hip**
         C44.791   Other specified malignant neoplasm of skin of unspecified lower limb, including hip
         C44.792   Other specified malignant neoplasm of skin of right lower limb, including hip
         C44.799   Other specified malignant neoplasm of skin of left lower limb, including hip
●C44.8   **Other and unspecified malignant neoplasm of overlapping sites of skin**
     C44.80   Unspecified malignant neoplasm of overlapping sites of skin
     C44.81   Basal cell carcinoma of overlapping sites of skin
     C44.82   Squamous cell carcinoma of overlapping sites of skin
     C44.89   Other specified malignant neoplasm of overlapping sites of skin
●C44.9   **Other and unspecified malignant neoplasm of skin, unspecified**
     C44.90   Unspecified malignant neoplasm of skin, unspecified
         Malignant neoplasm of unspecified site of skin
     C44.91   Basal cell carcinoma of skin, unspecified
     C44.92   Squamous cell carcinoma of skin, unspecified
     C44.99   Other specified malignant neoplasm of skin, unspecified

---

MALIGNANT NEOPLASMS OF MESOTHELIAL AND SOFT TISSUE (C45-C49)

●C45   **Mesothelioma**
   Malignant cells develop in protective lining that covers internal organs (mesothelium) caused by exposure to asbestos
     C45.0   **Mesothelioma of pleura**
         Excludes1   other malignant neoplasm of pleura (C38.4)
     C45.1   **Mesothelioma of peritoneum**
         Mesothelioma of cul-de-sac
         Mesothelioma of mesentery
         Mesothelioma of mesocolon
         Mesothelioma of omentum
         Mesothelioma of peritoneum (parietal) (pelvic)
         Excludes1   other malignant neoplasm of soft tissue of peritoneum (C48.-)

Figure 2-11 Kaposi's sarcoma. There are large confluent hyperpigmented patch-stage lesions with lymphedema. (From Cohen & Powderly: Infectious Diseases, ed 3, Mosby, An Imprint of Elsevier, 2010)

Item 2–5   Kaposi's sarcoma is a cancer that causes patches of abnormal tissue to grow under the skin; in the lining of the mouth, nose, and throat; or in other organs, often beginning and spreading to other organs. Patients who have had organ transplants or patients with AIDS are at high risk for this malignancy.

     C45.2   **Mesothelioma of pericardium**
         Excludes1   other malignant neoplasm of pericardium (C38.0)
     C45.7   **Mesothelioma of other sites**
     C45.9   **Mesothelioma, unspecified**
●C46   **Kaposi's sarcoma**
   Code first any human immunodeficiency virus [HIV] disease (B20)
     C46.0   **Kaposi's sarcoma of skin**
     C46.1   **Kaposi's sarcoma of soft tissue**
         Kaposi's sarcoma of blood vessel
         Kaposi's sarcoma of connective tissue
         Kaposi's sarcoma of fascia
         Kaposi's sarcoma of ligament
         Kaposi's sarcoma of lymphatic(s) NEC
         Kaposi's sarcoma of muscle
         Excludes2   Kaposi's sarcoma of lymph glands and nodes (C46.3)
     C46.2   **Kaposi's sarcoma of palate**
     C46.3   **Kaposi's sarcoma of lymph nodes**
     C46.4   **Kaposi's sarcoma of gastrointestinal sites**
     ●C46.5   **Kaposi's sarcoma of lung**
         C46.50   Kaposi's sarcoma of unspecified lung
         C46.51   Kaposi's sarcoma of right lung
         C46.52   Kaposi's sarcoma of left lung
     C46.7   **Kaposi's sarcoma of other sites**
     ●C46.9   **Kaposi's sarcoma, unspecified**
         Kaposi's sarcoma of unspecified site
●C47   **Malignant neoplasm of peripheral nerves and autonomic nervous system**
     Includes   malignant neoplasm of sympathetic and parasympathetic nerves and ganglia
     Excludes1   Kaposi's sarcoma of soft tissue (C46.1)
     C47.0   **Malignant neoplasm of peripheral nerves of head, face and neck**
         Excludes1   malignant neoplasm of peripheral nerves of orbit (C69.6-)
     ●C47.1   **Malignant neoplasm of peripheral nerves of upper limb, including shoulder**
         C47.10   Malignant neoplasm of peripheral nerves of unspecified upper limb, including shoulder
         C47.11   Malignant neoplasm of peripheral nerves of right upper limb, including shoulder
         C47.12   Malignant neoplasm of peripheral nerves of left upper limb, including shoulder
     ●C47.2   **Malignant neoplasm of peripheral nerves of lower limb, including hip**
         C47.20   Malignant neoplasm of peripheral nerves of unspecified lower limb, including hip
         C47.21   Malignant neoplasm of peripheral nerves of right lower limb, including hip
         C47.22   Malignant neoplasm of peripheral nerves of left lower limb, including hip

◀ New   ◀▥ Revised   ~~deleted~~ Deleted   Excludes 1   Excludes 2   Includes   Use additional   Code first   Code also   Unspecified

676   **OGCR** Official Guidelines   X Assign placeholder X   ● Use Additional Character(s)   ▌ Manifestation Code   **Coding Clinic**

C47.3   **Malignant neoplasm of peripheral nerves of thorax**

C47.4   **Malignant neoplasm of peripheral nerves of abdomen**

C47.5   **Malignant neoplasm of peripheral nerves of pelvis**

C47.6   **Malignant neoplasm of peripheral nerves of trunk, unspecified**
Malignant neoplasm of peripheral nerves of unspecified part of trunk

C47.8   **Malignant neoplasm of overlapping sites of peripheral nerves and autonomic nervous system**

C47.9   **Malignant neoplasm of peripheral nerves and autonomic nervous system, unspecified**
Malignant neoplasm of unspecified site of peripheral nerves and autonomic nervous system

● **C48**   **Malignant neoplasm of retroperitoneum and peritoneum**

    Excludes1   Kaposi's sarcoma of connective tissue (C46.1)
mesothelioma (C45.-)

C48.0   **Malignant neoplasm of retroperitoneum**
Behind/outside of peritoneum

C48.1   **Malignant neoplasm of specified parts of peritoneum**
Serous membrane lining abdominopelvic walls and covering viscera
Malignant neoplasm of cul-de-sac
Malignant neoplasm of mesentery
Malignant neoplasm of mesocolon
Malignant neoplasm of omentum
Malignant neoplasm of parietal peritoneum
Malignant neoplasm of pelvic peritoneum

C48.2   **Malignant neoplasm of peritoneum, unspecified**

C48.8   **Malignant neoplasm of overlapping sites of retroperitoneum and peritoneum**

● **C49**   **Malignant neoplasm of other connective and soft tissue**

    Includes   malignant neoplasm of blood vessel
malignant neoplasm of bursa
malignant neoplasm of cartilage
malignant neoplasm of fascia
malignant neoplasm of fat
malignant neoplasm of ligament, except uterine
malignant neoplasm of lymphatic vessel
malignant neoplasm of muscle
malignant neoplasm of synovia
malignant neoplasm of tendon (sheath)

    Excludes1   malignant neoplasm of cartilage (of):
articular (C40-C41)
larynx (C32.3)
nose (C30.0)
malignant neoplasm of connective tissue of breast (C50.-)

    Excludes2   Kaposi's sarcoma of soft tissue (C46.1)
malignant neoplasm of heart (C38.0)
malignant neoplasm of peripheral nerves and autonomic nervous system (C47.-)
malignant neoplasm of peritoneum (C48.2)
malignant neoplasm of retroperitoneum (C48.0)
malignant neoplasm of uterine ligament (C57.3)
mesothelioma (C45.-)

C49.0   **Malignant neoplasm of connective and soft tissue of head, face and neck**
Malignant neoplasm of connective tissue of ear
Malignant neoplasm of connective tissue of eyelid
    Excludes1   connective tissue of orbit (C69.6-)

● C49.1   **Malignant neoplasm of connective and soft tissue of upper limb, including shoulder**

C49.10   **Malignant neoplasm of connective and soft tissue of unspecified upper limb, including shoulder**

C49.11   **Malignant neoplasm of connective and soft tissue of right upper limb, including shoulder**

C49.12   **Malignant neoplasm of connective and soft tissue of left upper limb, including shoulder**

● C49.2   **Malignant neoplasm of connective and soft tissue of lower limb, including hip**

C49.20   **Malignant neoplasm of connective and soft tissue of unspecified lower limb, including hip**

C49.21   **Malignant neoplasm of connective and soft tissue of right lower limb, including hip**

C49.22   **Malignant neoplasm of connective and soft tissue of left lower limb, including hip**

C49.3   **Malignant neoplasm of connective and soft tissue of thorax**
Malignant neoplasm of axilla
Malignant neoplasm of diaphragm
Malignant neoplasm of great vessels
    Excludes1   malignant neoplasm of breast (C50.-)
malignant neoplasm of heart (C38.0)
malignant neoplasm of mediastinum (C38.1-C38.3)
malignant neoplasm of thymus (C37)
    Coding Clinic: 2015, Q3, P19

C49.4   **Malignant neoplasm of connective and soft tissue of abdomen**
Malignant neoplasm of abdominal wall
Malignant neoplasm of hypochondrium

C49.5   **Malignant neoplasm of connective and soft tissue of pelvis**
Malignant neoplasm of buttock
Malignant neoplasm of groin
Malignant neoplasm of perineum

C49.6   **Malignant neoplasm of connective and soft tissue of trunk, unspecified**
Malignant neoplasm of back NOS

C49.8   **Malignant neoplasm of overlapping sites of connective and soft tissue**
Primary malignant neoplasm of two or more contiguous sites of connective and soft tissue

C49.9   **Malignant neoplasm of connective and soft tissue, unspecified**

● C49.A   **Gastrointestinal stromal tumor** ◀

C49.A0   **Gastrointestinal stromal tumor, unspecified site** ◀

C49.A1   **Gastrointestinal stromal tumor of esophagus** ◀

C49.A2   **Gastrointestinal stromal tumor of stomach** ◀

C49.A3   **Gastrointestinal stromal tumor of small intestine** ◀

C49.A4   **Gastrointestinal stromal tumor of large intestine** ◀

C49.A5   **Gastrointestinal stromal tumor of rectum** ◀

C49.A9   **Gastrointestinal stromal tumor of other sites** ◀

MALIGNANT NEOPLASMS OF BREAST (C50)

● C50   **Malignant neoplasm of breast**

    Includes   connective tissue of breast
Paget's disease of breast
Paget's disease of nipple
Intraductal carcinoma of breast characterized by eczema-like inflammatory skin changes
Use additional code to identify estrogen receptor status (Z17.0, Z17.1)
    Excludes1   skin of breast (C44.501, C44.511, C44.521, C44.591)

● C50.0   **Malignant neoplasm of nipple and areola**

● C50.01   **Malignant neoplasm of nipple and areola, female**

C50.011   **Malignant neoplasm of nipple and areola, right female breast** ♀

C50.012   **Malignant neoplasm of nipple and areola, left female breast** ♀

C50.019   **Malignant neoplasm of nipple and areola, unspecified female breast** ♀

CHAPTER 2 (C00-D49)

● C50.02　Malignant neoplasm of nipple and areola, male

　　C50.021　Malignant neoplasm of nipple and areola, right male breast ♂

　　C50.022　Malignant neoplasm of nipple and areola, left male breast ♂

　　C50.029　Malignant neoplasm of nipple and areola, unspecified male breast ♂

● C50.1　Malignant neoplasm of central portion of breast

　● C50.11　Malignant neoplasm of central portion of breast, female

　　C50.111　Malignant neoplasm of central portion of right female breast ♀

　　C50.112　Malignant neoplasm of central portion of left female breast ♀

　　C50.119　Malignant neoplasm of central portion of unspecified female breast ♀

　● C50.12　Malignant neoplasm of central portion of breast, male

　　C50.121　Malignant neoplasm of central portion of right male breast ♂

　　C50.122　Malignant neoplasm of central portion of left male breast ♂

　　C50.129　Malignant neoplasm of central portion of unspecified male breast ♂

● C50.2　Malignant neoplasm of upper-inner quadrant of breast

　● C50.21　Malignant neoplasm of upper-inner quadrant of breast, female

　　C50.211　Malignant neoplasm of upper-inner quadrant of right female breast ♀

　　C50.212　Malignant neoplasm of upper-inner quadrant of left female breast ♀

　　C50.219　Malignant neoplasm of upper-inner quadrant of unspecified female breast ♀

　● C50.22　Malignant neoplasm of upper-inner quadrant of breast, male

　　C50.221　Malignant neoplasm of upper-inner quadrant of right male breast ♂

　　C50.222　Malignant neoplasm of upper-inner quadrant of left male breast ♂

　　C50.229　Malignant neoplasm of upper-inner quadrant of unspecified male breast ♂

● C50.3　Malignant neoplasm of lower-inner quadrant of breast

　● C50.31　Malignant neoplasm of lower-inner quadrant of breast, female

　　C50.311　Malignant neoplasm of lower-inner quadrant of right female breast ♀

　　C50.312　Malignant neoplasm of lower-inner quadrant of left female breast ♀

　　C50.319　Malignant neoplasm of lower-inner quadrant of unspecified female breast ♀

Figure 2-12　Female breast quadrants and axillary tail.

● C50.32　Malignant neoplasm of lower-inner quadrant of breast, male

　　C50.321　Malignant neoplasm of lower-inner quadrant of right male breast ♂

　　C50.322　Malignant neoplasm of lower-inner quadrant of left male breast ♂

　　C50.329　Malignant neoplasm of lower-inner quadrant of unspecified male breast ♂

● C50.4　Malignant neoplasm of upper-outer quadrant of breast

　● C50.41　Malignant neoplasm of upper-outer quadrant of breast, female

　　C50.411　Malignant neoplasm of upper-outer quadrant of right female breast ♀

　　C50.412　Malignant neoplasm of upper-outer quadrant of left female breast ♀

　　C50.419　Malignant neoplasm of upper-outer quadrant of unspecified female breast ♀

　● C50.42　Malignant neoplasm of upper-outer quadrant of breast, male

　　C50.421　Malignant neoplasm of upper-outer quadrant of right male breast ♂

　　C50.422　Malignant neoplasm of upper-outer quadrant of left male breast ♂

　　C50.429　Malignant neoplasm of upper-outer quadrant of unspecified male breast ♂

● C50.5　Malignant neoplasm of lower-outer quadrant of breast

　● C50.51　Malignant neoplasm of lower-outer quadrant of breast, female

　　C50.511　Malignant neoplasm of lower-outer quadrant of right female breast ♀

　　C50.512　Malignant neoplasm of lower-outer quadrant of left female breast ♀

　　C50.519　Malignant neoplasm of lower-outer quadrant of unspecified female breast ♀

　● C50.52　Malignant neoplasm of lower-outer quadrant of breast, male

　　C50.521　Malignant neoplasm of lower-outer quadrant of right male breast ♂

　　C50.522　Malignant neoplasm of lower-outer quadrant of left male breast ♂

　　C50.529　Malignant neoplasm of lower-outer quadrant of unspecified male breast ♂

● C50.6　Malignant neoplasm of axillary tail of breast

　● C50.61　Malignant neoplasm of axillary tail of breast, female

　　C50.611　Malignant neoplasm of axillary tail of right female breast ♀

　　C50.612　Malignant neoplasm of axillary tail of left female breast ♀

　　C50.619　Malignant neoplasm of axillary tail of unspecified female breast ♀

　● C50.62　Malignant neoplasm of axillary tail of breast, male

　　C50.621　Malignant neoplasm of axillary tail of right male breast ♂

　　C50.622　Malignant neoplasm of axillary tail of left male breast ♂

　　C50.629　Malignant neoplasm of axillary tail of unspecified male breast ♂

● C50.8　Malignant neoplasm of overlapping sites of breast

　● C50.81　Malignant neoplasm of overlapping sites of breast, female

　　C50.811　Malignant neoplasm of overlapping sites of right female breast ♀

　　C50.812　Malignant neoplasm of overlapping sites of left female breast ♀

　　C50.819　Malignant neoplasm of overlapping sites of unspecified female breast ♀

◀ New　⬅ Revised　~~deleted~~ Deleted　Excludes 1　Excludes 2　Includes　Use additional　Code first　Code also　Unspecified

OGCR Official Guidelines　X Assign placeholder X　● Use Additional Character(s)　▶ Manifestation Code　**Coding Clinic**

● **C50.82**   Malignant neoplasm of overlapping sites of breast, male
  C50.821   Malignant neoplasm of overlapping sites of right male breast ♂
  C50.822   Malignant neoplasm of overlapping sites of left male breast ♂
  C50.829   Malignant neoplasm of overlapping sites of unspecified male breast ♂
● **C50.9**   Malignant neoplasm of breast of unspecified site
  ● **C50.91**   Malignant neoplasm of breast of unspecified site, female
    C50.911   Malignant neoplasm of unspecified site of right female breast ♀
    C50.912   Malignant neoplasm of unspecified site of left female breast ♀
    C50.919   Malignant neoplasm of unspecified site of unspecified female breast ♀
  ● **C50.92**   Malignant neoplasm of breast of unspecified site, male
    C50.921   Malignant neoplasm of unspecified site of right male breast ♂
    C50.922   Malignant neoplasm of unspecified site of left male breast ♂
    C50.929   Malignant neoplasm of unspecified site of unspecified male breast ♂

MALIGNANT NEOPLASMS OF FEMALE GENITAL ORGANS (C51-C58)

Includes   malignant neoplasm of skin of female genital organs

● **C51**   Malignant neoplasm of vulva
  Excludes1   carcinoma in situ of vulva (D07.1)
  C51.0   Malignant neoplasm of labium majus ♀
    Outer folds of skin external female genitalia
    Malignant neoplasm of Bartholin's [greater vestibular] gland
  C51.1   Malignant neoplasm of labium minus ♀
    Two inner folds surrounding vulva in female genitalia
  C51.2   Malignant neoplasm of clitoris ♀
  C51.8   Malignant neoplasm of overlapping sites of vulva ♀
  C51.9   Malignant neoplasm of vulva, unspecified ♀
    Malignant neoplasm of external female genitalia NOS
    Malignant neoplasm of pudendum

C52   Malignant neoplasm of vagina ♀
  Excludes1   carcinoma in situ of vagina (D07.2)

● **C53**   Malignant neoplasm of cervix uteri
  Excludes1   carcinoma in situ of cervix uteri (D06.-)
  C53.0   Malignant neoplasm of endocervix ♀
    Inside the cervix
  C53.1   Malignant neoplasm of exocervix ♀
    Outside the cervix
  C53.8   Malignant neoplasm of overlapping sites of cervix uteri ♀
  C53.9   Malignant neoplasm of cervix uteri, unspecified ♀

● **C54**   Malignant neoplasm of corpus uteri
  C54.0   Malignant neoplasm of isthmus uteri ♀
    Constricted part of uterus between cervix and body
    Malignant neoplasm of lower uterine segment
  C54.1   Malignant neoplasm of endometrium ♀
    Lining of uterus
  C54.2   Malignant neoplasm of myometrium ♀
    Middle layer of uterine wall consisting of smooth muscle supporting stromal and vascular tissue
  C54.3   Malignant neoplasm of fundus uteri ♀
    Top rounded portion of uterus
  C54.8   Malignant neoplasm of overlapping sites of corpus uteri ♀
    Main body of uterus
  C54.9   Malignant neoplasm of corpus uteri, unspecified ♀

C55   Malignant neoplasm of uterus, part unspecified ♀

● **C56**   Malignant neoplasm of ovary
    Use additional code to identify any functional activity
  C56.1   Malignant neoplasm of right ovary ♀
  C56.2   Malignant neoplasm of left ovary ♀
  C56.9   Malignant neoplasm of unspecified ovary ♀

● **C57**   Malignant neoplasm of other and unspecified female genital organs
  ● **C57.0**   Malignant neoplasm of fallopian tube
    Malignant neoplasm of oviduct
    Malignant neoplasm of uterine tube
    C57.00   Malignant neoplasm of unspecified fallopian tube ♀
    C57.01   Malignant neoplasm of right fallopian tube ♀
    C57.02   Malignant neoplasm of left fallopian tube ♀
  ● **C57.1**   Malignant neoplasm of broad ligament
    C57.10   Malignant neoplasm of unspecified broad ligament ♀
    C57.11   Malignant neoplasm of right broad ligament ♀
    C57.12   Malignant neoplasm of left broad ligament ♀
  ● **C57.2**   Malignant neoplasm of round ligament
    C57.20   Malignant neoplasm of unspecified round ligament ♀
    C57.21   Malignant neoplasm of right round ligament ♀
    C57.22   Malignant neoplasm of left round ligament ♀
  C57.3   Malignant neoplasm of parametrium ♀
    Malignant neoplasm of uterine ligament NOS
  C57.4   Malignant neoplasm of uterine adnexa, unspecified ♀
  C57.7   Malignant neoplasm of other specified female genital organs ♀
    Malignant neoplasm of wolffian body or duct
  C57.8   Malignant neoplasm of overlapping sites of female genital organs ♀
    Primary malignant neoplasm of two or more contiguous sites of the female genital organs whose point of origin cannot be determined
    Primary tubo-ovarian malignant neoplasm whose point of origin cannot be determined
    Primary utero-ovarian malignant neoplasm whose point of origin cannot be determined
  C57.9   Malignant neoplasm of female genital organ, unspecified ♀
    Malignant neoplasm of female genitourinary tract NOS

Figure 2-13   Cervix uteri.

CHAPTER 2 (C00-D49)

CHAPTER 2 (C00-D49)

C58   Malignant neoplasm of placenta ♀   **M**

    Includes   choriocarcinoma NOS
               chorionepithelioma NOS

    Excludes1   chorioadenoma (destruens) (D39.2)
               hydatidiform mole NOS (O01.9)
               invasive hydatidiform mole (D39.2)
               male choriocarcinoma NOS (C62.9-)
               malignant hydatidiform mole (D39.2)

MALIGNANT NEOPLASMS OF MALE GENITAL ORGANS (C60-C63)

    Includes   malignant neoplasm of skin of male genital organs

C60   Malignant neoplasm of penis
    C60.0   Malignant neoplasm of prepuce ♂
          Malignant neoplasm of foreskin
    C60.1   Malignant neoplasm of glans penis ♂
    C60.2   Malignant neoplasm of body of penis ♂
          Malignant neoplasm of corpus cavernosum
    C60.8   Malignant neoplasm of overlapping sites of penis ♂
    C60.9   Malignant neoplasm of penis, unspecified ♂
          Malignant neoplasm of skin of penis NOS

C61   Malignant neoplasm of prostate ♂
    Use additional code to identify: ◄
    hormone sensitivity status (Z19.1-Z19.2) ◄
    rising PSA following treatment for malignant neoplasm of prostate (R97.21) ◄
    Excludes1   malignant neoplasm of seminal vesicle (C63.7)

C62   Malignant neoplasm of testis
    Use additional code to identify any functional activity.
    C62.0   Malignant neoplasm of undescended testis
          Malignant neoplasm of ectopic testis
          Malignant neoplasm of retained testis
       C62.00   Malignant neoplasm of unspecified undescended testis ♂
       C62.01   Malignant neoplasm of undescended right testis ♂
       C62.02   Malignant neoplasm of undescended left testis ♂
    C62.1   Malignant neoplasm of descended testis
          Malignant neoplasm of scrotal testis
       C62.10   Malignant neoplasm of unspecified descended testis, unspecified side ♂
       C62.11   Malignant neoplasm of descended right testis ♂
       C62.12   Malignant neoplasm of descended left testis ♂
    C62.9   Malignant neoplasm of testis, unspecified whether descended or undescended
       C62.90   Malignant neoplasm of unspecified testis, unspecified whether descended or undescended ♂
          Malignant neoplasm of testis NOS
       C62.91   Malignant neoplasm of right testis, unspecified whether descended or undescended ♂
       C62.92   Malignant neoplasm of left testis, unspecified whether descended or undescended ♂

C63   Malignant neoplasm of other and unspecified male genital organs
    C63.0   Malignant neoplasm of epididymis
       C63.00   Malignant neoplasm of unspecified epididymis ♂
       C63.01   Malignant neoplasm of right epididymis ♂
       C63.02   Malignant neoplasm of left epididymis ♂
    C63.1   Malignant neoplasm of spermatic cord
       C63.10   Malignant neoplasm of unspecified spermatic cord ♂
       C63.11   Malignant neoplasm of right spermatic cord ♂
       C63.12   Malignant neoplasm of left spermatic cord ♂
    C63.2   Malignant neoplasm of scrotum ♂
          Malignant neoplasm of skin of scrotum
    C63.7   Malignant neoplasm of other specified male genital organs ♂
          Malignant neoplasm of seminal vesicle
          Malignant neoplasm of tunica vaginalis
    C63.8   Malignant neoplasm of overlapping sites of male genital organs ♂
          Primary malignant neoplasm of two or more contiguous sites of male genital organs whose point of origin cannot be determined
    C63.9   Malignant neoplasm of male genital organ, unspecified ♂
          Malignant neoplasm of male genitourinary tract NOS

MALIGNANT NEOPLASMS OF URINARY TRACT (C64-C68)

C64   Malignant neoplasm of kidney, except renal pelvis
    Excludes1   malignant carcinoid tumor of the kidney (C7A.093)
          malignant neoplasm of renal calyces (C65.-)
          malignant neoplasm of renal pelvis (C65.-)
    C64.1   Malignant neoplasm of right kidney, except renal pelvis
    C64.2   Malignant neoplasm of left kidney, except renal pelvis
    C64.9   Malignant neoplasm of unspecified kidney, except renal pelvis

C65   Malignant neoplasm of renal pelvis
    Includes   malignant neoplasm of pelviureteric junction
          malignant neoplasm of renal calyces
    C65.1   Malignant neoplasm of right renal pelvis
    C65.2   Malignant neoplasm of left renal pelvis
    C65.9   Malignant neoplasm of unspecified renal pelvis

C66   Malignant neoplasm of ureter
    Excludes1   malignant neoplasm of ureteric orifice of bladder (C67.6)
    C66.1   Malignant neoplasm of right ureter
    C66.2   Malignant neoplasm of left ureter
    C66.9   Malignant neoplasm of unspecified ureter

C67   Malignant neoplasm of bladder
    C67.0   Malignant neoplasm of trigone of bladder
          Triangular area formed by three openings in the floor of urinary bladder
    C67.1   Malignant neoplasm of dome of bladder
          Vaulted roof
    C67.2   Malignant neoplasm of lateral wall of bladder
          Side walls
    C67.3   Malignant neoplasm of anterior wall of bladder
          Front wall
    C67.4   Malignant neoplasm of posterior wall of bladder
          Back wall
    C67.5   Malignant neoplasm of bladder neck
          Joining of bladder and urethra
          Malignant neoplasm of internal urethral orifice
    C67.6   Malignant neoplasm of ureteric orifice
          Opening from bladder to ureters

Figure 2-14 Penis and other male genital organs.

◄ New   ◄ Revised   ~~deleted~~ Deleted   Excludes 1   Excludes 2   Includes   Use additional   Code first   Code also   Unspecified
OGCR Official Guidelines   X Assign placeholder X   ● Use Additional Character(s)   ▶ Manifestation Code   **Coding Clinic**

C67.7   **Malignant neoplasm of urachus**
Embryonic canal that connects the urinary bladder with the structure that forms the umbilical cord (allantois)

C67.8   **Malignant neoplasm of overlapping sites of bladder**

C67.9   **Malignant neoplasm of bladder, unspecified**
Coding Clinic: 2016, Q1, P19

● **C68**   **Malignant neoplasm of other and unspecified urinary organs**
Excludes1   malignant neoplasm of female genitourinary tract NOS (C57.9)
malignant neoplasm of male genitourinary tract NOS (C63.9)

C68.0   **Malignant neoplasm of urethra**
Excludes1   malignant neoplasm of urethral orifice of bladder (C67.5)

C68.1   **Malignant neoplasm of paraurethral glands**
Group of glands of female urethra drained by paraurethral ducts; AKA Skene glands, female prostate

C68.8   **Malignant neoplasm of overlapping sites of urinary organs**
Primary malignant neoplasm of two or more contiguous sites of urinary organs whose point of origin cannot be determined

C68.9   **Malignant neoplasm of urinary organ, unspecified**
Malignant neoplasm of urinary system NOS

MALIGNANT NEOPLASMS OF EYE, BRAIN AND OTHER PARTS OF CENTRAL NERVOUS SYSTEM (C69-C72)

● **C69**   **Malignant neoplasm of eye and adnexa**
Excludes1   malignant neoplasm of connective tissue of eyelid (C49.0)
malignant neoplasm of eyelid (skin) (C43.1-, C44.1-)
malignant neoplasm of optic nerve (C72.3-)

● **C69.0**   **Malignant neoplasm of conjunctiva**
C69.00   **Malignant neoplasm of unspecified conjunctiva**
C69.01   **Malignant neoplasm of right conjunctiva**
C69.02   **Malignant neoplasm of left conjunctiva**

● **C69.1**   **Malignant neoplasm of cornea**
C69.10   **Malignant neoplasm of unspecified cornea**
C69.11   **Malignant neoplasm of right cornea**
C69.12   **Malignant neoplasm of left cornea**

● **C69.2**   **Malignant neoplasm of retina**
Excludes1   dark area on retina (D49.81)
neoplasm of unspecified behavior of retina and choroid (D49.81)
retinal freckle (D49.81)
C69.20   **Malignant neoplasm of unspecified retina**
C69.21   **Malignant neoplasm of right retina**
C69.22   **Malignant neoplasm of left retina**

● **C69.3**   **Malignant neoplasm of choroid**
C69.30   **Malignant neoplasm of unspecified choroid**
C69.31   **Malignant neoplasm of right choroid**
C69.32   **Malignant neoplasm of left choroid**

● **C69.4**   **Malignant neoplasm of ciliary body**
C69.40   **Malignant neoplasm of unspecified ciliary body**
C69.41   **Malignant neoplasm of right ciliary body**
C69.42   **Malignant neoplasm of left ciliary body**

● **C69.5**   **Malignant neoplasm of lacrimal gland and duct**
Malignant neoplasm of lacrimal sac
Malignant neoplasm of nasolacrimal duct
C69.50   **Malignant neoplasm of unspecified lacrimal gland and duct**
C69.51   **Malignant neoplasm of right lacrimal gland and duct**
C69.52   **Malignant neoplasm of left lacrimal gland and duct**

Figure 2-15   The brain.

● **C69.6**   **Malignant neoplasm of orbit**
Malignant neoplasm of connective tissue of orbit
Malignant neoplasm of extraocular muscle
Malignant neoplasm of peripheral nerves of orbit
Malignant neoplasm of retrobulbar tissue
Malignant neoplasm of retro-ocular tissue
Excludes1   malignant neoplasm of orbital bone (C41.0)
C69.60   **Malignant neoplasm of unspecified orbit**
C69.61   **Malignant neoplasm of right orbit**
C69.62   **Malignant neoplasm of left orbit**

● **C69.8**   **Malignant neoplasm of overlapping sites of eye and adnexa**
C69.80   **Malignant neoplasm of overlapping sites of unspecified eye and adnexa**
C69.81   **Malignant neoplasm of overlapping sites of right eye and adnexa**
C69.82   **Malignant neoplasm of overlapping sites of left eye and adnexa**

● **C69.9**   **Malignant neoplasm of unspecified site of eye**
Malignant neoplasm of eyeball
C69.90   **Malignant neoplasm of unspecified site of unspecified eye**
C69.91   **Malignant neoplasm of unspecified site of right eye**
C69.92   **Malignant neoplasm of unspecified site of left eye**

● **C70**   **Malignant neoplasm of meninges**
C70.0   **Malignant neoplasm of cerebral meninges**
C70.1   **Malignant neoplasm of spinal meninges**
C70.9   **Malignant neoplasm of meninges, unspecified**

● **C71**   **Malignant neoplasm of brain**
Excludes1   malignant neoplasm of cranial nerves (C72.2-C72.5)
retrobulbar malignant neoplasm (C69.6-)
C71.0   **Malignant neoplasm of cerebrum, except lobes and ventricles**
Malignant neoplasm of supratentorial NOS
C71.1   **Malignant neoplasm of frontal lobe**
C71.2   **Malignant neoplasm of temporal lobe**
C71.3   **Malignant neoplasm of parietal lobe**
C71.4   **Malignant neoplasm of occipital lobe**
C71.5   **Malignant neoplasm of cerebral ventricle**
Excludes1   malignant neoplasm of fourth cerebral ventricle (C71.7)
C71.6   **Malignant neoplasm of cerebellum**
C71.7   **Malignant neoplasm of brain stem**
Malignant neoplasm of fourth cerebral ventricle
Infratentorial malignant neoplasm NOS
C71.8   **Malignant neoplasm of overlapping sites of brain**
C71.9   **Malignant neoplasm of brain, unspecified**

CHAPTER 2 (C00-D49)

● **C72**   **Malignant neoplasm of spinal cord, cranial nerves and other parts of central nervous system**

> **Excludes1**   malignant neoplasm of meninges (C70.-)
> malignant neoplasm of peripheral nerves and autonomic nervous system (C47.-)

   C72.0   **Malignant neoplasm of spinal cord**

   C72.1   **Malignant neoplasm of cauda equina**
> *Lower end of spinal column*

● **C72.2**   **Malignant neoplasm of olfactory nerve**
> Malignant neoplasm of olfactory bulb

     C72.20   Malignant neoplasm of unspecified olfactory nerve

     C72.21   Malignant neoplasm of right olfactory nerve

     C72.22   Malignant neoplasm of left olfactory nerve

● **C72.3**   **Malignant neoplasm of optic nerve**

     C72.30   Malignant neoplasm of unspecified optic nerve

     C72.31   Malignant neoplasm of right optic nerve

     C72.32   Malignant neoplasm of left optic nerve

● **C72.4**   **Malignant neoplasm of acoustic nerve**

     C72.40   Malignant neoplasm of unspecified acoustic nerve

     C72.41   Malignant neoplasm of right acoustic nerve

     C72.42   Malignant neoplasm of left acoustic nerve

● **C72.5**   **Malignant neoplasm of other and unspecified cranial nerves**

     C72.50   Malignant neoplasm of unspecified cranial nerve
> Malignant neoplasm of cranial nerve NOS

     C72.59   Malignant neoplasm of other cranial nerves

   C72.9   **Malignant neoplasm of central nervous system, unspecified**
> Malignant neoplasm of unspecified site of central nervous system
> Malignant neoplasm of nervous system NOS

MALIGNANT NEOPLASMS OF THYROID AND OTHER ENDOCRINE GLANDS (C73-C75)

   C73   **Malignant neoplasm of thyroid gland**
> Use additional code to identify any functional activity

● **C74**   **Malignant neoplasm of adrenal gland**

● **C74.0**   **Malignant neoplasm of cortex of adrenal gland**

     C74.00   Malignant neoplasm of cortex of unspecified adrenal gland

     C74.01   Malignant neoplasm of cortex of right adrenal gland

     C74.02   Malignant neoplasm of cortex of left adrenal gland

● **C74.1**   **Malignant neoplasm of medulla of adrenal gland**
> *Pair of glands situated on top of or above each kidney ("suprarenal")*

     C74.10   Malignant neoplasm of medulla of unspecified adrenal gland

     C74.11   Malignant neoplasm of medulla of right adrenal gland

     C74.12   Malignant neoplasm of medulla of left adrenal gland

● **C74.9**   **Malignant neoplasm of unspecified part of adrenal gland**

     C74.90   Malignant neoplasm of unspecified part of unspecified adrenal gland

     C74.91   Malignant neoplasm of unspecified part of right adrenal gland

     C74.92   Malignant neoplasm of unspecified part of left adrenal gland

● **C75**   **Malignant neoplasm of other endocrine glands and related structures**

> **Excludes1**   malignant carcinoid tumors (C7A.0-)
> malignant neoplasm of adrenal gland (C74.-)
> malignant neoplasm of endocrine pancreas (C25.4)
> malignant neoplasm of islets of Langerhans (C25.4)
> malignant neoplasm of ovary (C56.-)
> malignant neoplasm of testis (C62.-)
> malignant neoplasm of thymus (C37)
> malignant neoplasm of thyroid gland (C73)
> malignant neuroendocrine tumors (C7A.-)

   C75.0   **Malignant neoplasm of parathyroid gland**

   C75.1   **Malignant neoplasm of pituitary gland**

   C75.2   **Malignant neoplasm of craniopharyngeal duct**

   C75.3   **Malignant neoplasm of pineal gland**

   C75.4   **Malignant neoplasm of carotid body**

   C75.5   **Malignant neoplasm of aortic body and other paraganglia**

   C75.8   **Malignant neoplasm with pluriglandular involvement, unspecified**

   C75.9   **Malignant neoplasm of endocrine gland, unspecified**

MALIGNANT NEUROENDOCRINE TUMORS (C7A)

● **C7A**   **Malignant neuroendocrine tumors**
> Code also any associated multiple endocrine neoplasia [MEN] syndromes (E31.2-)
> Use additional code to identify any associated endocrine syndrome, such as:
> carcinoid syndrome (E34.0)

> **Excludes2**   malignant pancreatic islet cell tumors (C25.4)
> Merkel cell carcinoma (C4A.-)

● **C7A.0**   **Malignant carcinoid tumors**

     C7A.00   Malignant carcinoid tumor of unspecified site

● **C7A.01**   **Malignant carcinoid tumors of the small intestine**

     C7A.010   Malignant carcinoid tumor of the duodenum

     C7A.011   Malignant carcinoid tumor of the jejunum

     C7A.012   Malignant carcinoid tumor of the ileum

     C7A.019   Malignant carcinoid tumor of the small intestine, unspecified portion

● **C7A.02**   **Malignant carcinoid tumors of the appendix, large intestine, and rectum**

     C7A.020   Malignant carcinoid tumor of the appendix

     C7A.021   Malignant carcinoid tumor of the cecum

     C7A.022   Malignant carcinoid tumor of the ascending colon

     C7A.023   Malignant carcinoid tumor of the transverse colon

     C7A.024   Malignant carcinoid tumor of the descending colon

     C7A.025   Malignant carcinoid tumor of the sigmoid colon

     C7A.026   Malignant carcinoid tumor of the rectum

     C7A.029   Malignant carcinoid tumor of the large intestine, unspecified portion
> Malignant carcinoid tumor of the colon NOS

◀ New   ◀ Revised   ~~deleted~~ Deleted   Excludes 1   Excludes 2   Includes   Use additional   Code first   Code also   Unspecified

682   **OGCR** Official Guidelines   X Assign placeholder X   ● Use Additional Character(s)   ▶ Manifestation Code   **Coding Clinic**

● **C7A.09   Malignant carcinoid tumors of other sites**

     C7A.090   Malignant carcinoid tumor of the bronchus and lung

     C7A.091   Malignant carcinoid tumor of the thymus

     C7A.092   Malignant carcinoid tumor of the stomach

     C7A.093   Malignant carcinoid tumor of the kidney

     C7A.094   Malignant carcinoid tumor of the foregut, unspecified ◀▥

     C7A.095   Malignant carcinoid tumor of the midgut, unspecified ◀▥

     C7A.096   Malignant carcinoid tumor of the hindgut, unspecified ◀▥

     C7A.098   Malignant carcinoid tumors of other sites

C7A.1   Malignant poorly differentiated neuroendocrine tumors

     Malignant poorly differentiated neuroendocrine tumor NOS

     Malignant poorly differentiated neuroendocrine carcinoma, any site

     High grade neuroendocrine carcinoma, any site

C7A.8   Other malignant neuroendocrine tumors

     Secondary neuroendocrine tumors (C7B)

SECONDARY NEUROENDOCRINE TUMORS (C7B)

● **C7B   Secondary neuroendocrine tumors**

     Use additional code to identify any functional activity

● **C7B.0   Secondary carcinoid tumors**

     C7B.00   Secondary carcinoid tumors, unspecified site

     C7B.01   Secondary carcinoid tumors of distant lymph nodes

     C7B.02   Secondary carcinoid tumors of liver

     C7B.03   Secondary carcinoid tumors of bone

     C7B.04   Secondary carcinoid tumors of peritoneum
         Mesentary metastasis of carcinoid tumor

     C7B.09   Secondary carcinoid tumors of other sites

C7B.1   Secondary Merkel cell carcinoma

     Merkel cell carcinoma nodal presentation

     Merkel cell carcinoma visceral metastatic presentation

C7B.8   Other secondary neuroendocrine tumors

MALIGNANT NEOPLASMS OF ILL-DEFINED, OTHER SECONDARY AND UNSPECIFIED SITES (C76-C80)

● **C76   Malignant neoplasm of other and ill-defined sites**

     Excludes1   malignant neoplasm of female genitourinary tract NOS (C57.9)

             malignant neoplasm of male genitourinary tract NOS (C63.9)

             malignant neoplasm of lymphoid, hematopoietic and related tissue (C81-C96)

             malignant neoplasm of skin (C44.-)

             malignant neoplasm of unspecified site NOS (C80.1)

C76.0   Malignant neoplasm of head, face and neck

     Malignant neoplasm of cheek NOS

     Malignant neoplasm of nose NOS

C76.1   Malignant neoplasm of thorax

     Intrathoracic malignant neoplasm NOS

     Malignant neoplasm of axilla NOS

     Thoracic malignant neoplasm NOS

C76.2   Malignant neoplasm of abdomen

C76.3   Malignant neoplasm of pelvis

     Malignant neoplasm of groin NOS

     Malignant neoplasm of sites overlapping systems within the pelvis

     Rectovaginal (septum) malignant neoplasm
         Between rectum and vagina

     Rectovesical (septum) malignant neoplasm
         Between rectum and urinary bladder; AKA vesicorectal

● **C76.4   Malignant neoplasm of upper limb**

     C76.40   Malignant neoplasm of unspecified upper limb

     C76.41   Malignant neoplasm of right upper limb

     C76.42   Malignant neoplasm of left upper limb

● **C76.5   Malignant neoplasm of lower limb**

     C76.50   Malignant neoplasm of unspecified lower limb

     C76.51   Malignant neoplasm of right lower limb

     C76.52   Malignant neoplasm of left lower limb

C76.8   Malignant neoplasm of other specified ill-defined sites

     Malignant neoplasm of overlapping ill-defined sites

● **C77   Secondary and unspecified malignant neoplasm of lymph nodes**

     Excludes1   malignant neoplasm of lymph nodes, specified as primary (C81-C86, C88, C96.-)

             mesentary metastasis of carcinoid tumor (C7B.04)

             secondary carcinoid tumors of distant lymph nodes (C7B.01)

C77.0   Secondary and unspecified malignant neoplasm of lymph nodes of head, face and neck

     Secondary and unspecified malignant neoplasm of supraclavicular lymph nodes

C77.1   Secondary and unspecified malignant neoplasm of intrathoracic lymph nodes

C77.2   Secondary and unspecified malignant neoplasm of intra-abdominal lymph nodes

C77.3   Secondary and unspecified malignant neoplasm of axilla and upper limb lymph nodes

     Secondary and unspecified malignant neoplasm of pectoral lymph nodes

C77.4   Secondary and unspecified malignant neoplasm of inguinal and lower limb lymph nodes

C77.5   Secondary and unspecified malignant neoplasm of intrapelvic lymph nodes

C77.8   Secondary and unspecified malignant neoplasm of lymph nodes of multiple regions

C77.9   Secondary and unspecified malignant neoplasm of lymph node, unspecified

● **C78   Secondary malignant neoplasm of respiratory and digestive organs**

     Excludes1   secondary carcinoid tumors of liver (C7B.02)

             secondary carcinoid tumors of peritoneum (C7B.04)

     Excludes2   lymph node metastases (C77.0) ◀

● **C78.0   Secondary malignant neoplasm of lung**

     C78.00   Secondary malignant neoplasm of unspecified lung

     C78.01   Secondary malignant neoplasm of right lung

     C78.02   Secondary malignant neoplasm of left lung

C78.1   Secondary malignant neoplasm of mediastinum
     Thoracic cavity between pleural cavities

C78.2   Secondary malignant neoplasm of pleura
     Serous membrane covering lungs and lining thoracic cavity

● **C78.3   Secondary malignant neoplasm of other and unspecified respiratory organs**

     C78.30   Secondary malignant neoplasm of unspecified respiratory organ

     C78.39   Secondary malignant neoplasm of other respiratory organs

CHAPTER 2 (C00-D49)

Item 2–6 The adrenal glands are a pair of glands situated on top of or above each kidney ("suprarenal") and chiefly responsible for regulating the stress response through the synthesis of corticosteroids and catecholamines, including cortisol and adrenaline.

C78.4 **Secondary malignant neoplasm of small intestine**

C78.5 **Secondary malignant neoplasm of large intestine and rectum**

C78.6 **Secondary malignant neoplasm of retroperitoneum and peritoneum**

C78.7 **Secondary malignant neoplasm of liver and intrahepatic bile duct**

● C78.8 **Secondary malignant neoplasm of other and unspecified digestive organs**

     C78.80 **Secondary malignant neoplasm of** `unspecified` **digestive organ**

     C78.89 **Secondary malignant neoplasm of other digestive organs**

         Code also exocrine pancreatic insufficiency (K86.81) ◀

● C79 **Secondary malignant neoplasm of other and unspecified sites**

     `Excludes1` secondary carcinoid tumors (C7B.-)
                  secondary neuroendocrine tumors (C7B.-)

     `Excludes2` lymph node metastases (C77.0) ◀

● C79.0 **Secondary malignant neoplasm of kidney and renal pelvis**

     C79.00 **Secondary malignant neoplasm of** `unspecified` **kidney and renal pelvis**

     C79.01 **Secondary malignant neoplasm of right kidney and renal pelvis**

     C79.02 **Secondary malignant neoplasm of left kidney and renal pelvis**

● C79.1 **Secondary malignant neoplasm of bladder and other and unspecified urinary organs**

     C79.10 **Secondary malignant neoplasm of** `unspecified` **urinary organs**

     C79.11 **Secondary malignant neoplasm of bladder**

     C79.19 **Secondary malignant neoplasm of other urinary organs**

C79.2 **Secondary malignant neoplasm of skin**

     `Excludes1` secondary Merkel cell carcinoma (C7B.1)

● C79.3 **Secondary malignant neoplasm of brain and cerebral meninges**

     C79.31 **Secondary malignant neoplasm of brain**

     C79.32 **Secondary malignant neoplasm of cerebral meninges**

● C79.4 **Secondary malignant neoplasm of other and unspecified parts of nervous system**

     C79.40 **Secondary malignant neoplasm of** `unspecified` **part of nervous system**

     C79.49 **Secondary malignant neoplasm of other parts of nervous system**

● C79.5 **Secondary malignant neoplasm of bone and bone marrow**

     `Excludes1` secondary carcinoid tumors of bone (C7B.03)

     C79.51 **Secondary malignant neoplasm of bone**

     C79.52 **Secondary malignant neoplasm of bone marrow**

● C79.6 **Secondary malignant neoplasm of ovary**

     C79.60 **Secondary malignant neoplasm of** `unspecified` **ovary** ♀

     C79.61 **Secondary malignant neoplasm of right ovary** ♀

     C79.62 **Secondary malignant neoplasm of left ovary** ♀

● C79.7 **Secondary malignant neoplasm of adrenal gland**

     C79.70 **Secondary malignant neoplasm of** `unspecified` **adrenal gland**

     C79.71 **Secondary malignant neoplasm of right adrenal gland**

     C79.72 **Secondary malignant neoplasm of left adrenal gland**

● C79.8 **Secondary malignant neoplasm of other specified sites**

     C79.81 **Secondary malignant neoplasm of breast**

     C79.82 **Secondary malignant neoplasm of genital organs**

     C79.89 **Secondary malignant neoplasm of other specified sites**

● C79.9 **Secondary malignant neoplasm of** `unspecified` **site**

     Metastatic cancer NOS
     Metastatic disease NOS

     `Excludes1` carcinomatosis NOS (C80.0)
              generalized cancer NOS (C80.0)
              malignant (primary) neoplasm of unspecified site (C80.1)

OGCR Section I.C.2.j and k

Disseminated malignant neoplasm, unspecified

j. Code C80.0, Disseminated malignant neoplasm, unspecified, is for use only in those cases where the patient has advanced metastatic disease and no known primary or secondary sites are specified. It should not be used in place of assigning codes for the primary site and all known secondary sites.

Malignant neoplasm without specification of site

k. Code C80.1, Malignant (primary) neoplasm, unspecified, equates to Cancer, unspecified. This code should only be used when no determination can be made as to the primary site of a malignancy. This code should rarely be used in the inpatient setting.

● C80 **Malignant neoplasm without specification of site**

     `Excludes1` malignant carcinoid tumor of unspecified site (C7A.00)
              malignant neoplasm of specified multiple sites- code to each site

C80.0 **Disseminated malignant neoplasm,** `unspecified`

     Carcinomatosis NOS
     Generalized cancer, unspecified site (primary) (secondary)
     Generalized malignancy, unspecified site (primary) (secondary)

C80.1 **Malignant (primary) neoplasm,** `unspecified`

     Cancer NOS
     Cancer unspecified site (primary)
     Carcinoma unspecified site (primary)
     Malignancy unspecified site (primary)

     `Excludes1` secondary malignant neoplasm of unspecified site (C79.9)

C80.2 **Malignant neoplasm associated with transplanted organ**

     Code first complication of transplanted organ (T86.-)

     Use additional code to identify the specific malignancy

◀ New   ⫷ Revised   ~~deleted~~ Deleted   Excludes 1   Excludes 2   Includes   Use additional   Code first   Code also   Unspecified

684   OGCR Official Guidelines   X Assign placeholder X   ● Use Additional Character(s)   ▶ Manifestation Code   **Coding Clinic**

★**(See Plate 315 on page 49.)**

MALIGNANT NEOPLASMS OF LYMPHOID, HEMATOPOIETIC AND RELATED TISSUE (C81-C96)

Excludes2   Kaposi's sarcoma of lymph nodes (C46.3)
secondary and unspecified neoplasm of lymph nodes (C77.-)
secondary neoplasm of bone marrow (C79.52)
secondary neoplasm of spleen (C78.89)

● **C81**   **Hodgkin lymphoma**
Form of malignant lymphoma with four types, nodular sclerosis, mixed cellularity, lymphocyte depleted, and lymphocyte predominant

     Excludes1   personal history of Hodgkin lymphoma (Z85.71)

● **C81.0**   **Nodular lymphocyte predominant Hodgkin lymphoma**
Least aggressive, least common, typically no symptoms
Lymphocytic-histiocytic predominance Hodgkin's disease

     C81.00   Nodular lymphocyte predominant Hodgkin lymphoma, unspecified site

     C81.01   Nodular lymphocyte predominant Hodgkin lymphoma, lymph nodes of head, face, and neck

     C81.02   Nodular lymphocyte predominant Hodgkin lymphoma, intrathoracic lymph nodes

     C81.03   Nodular lymphocyte predominant Hodgkin lymphoma, intra-abdominal lymph nodes

     C81.04   Nodular lymphocyte predominant Hodgkin lymphoma, lymph nodes of axilla and upper limb

     C81.05   Nodular lymphocyte predominant Hodgkin lymphoma, lymph nodes of inguinal region and lower limb

     C81.06   Nodular lymphocyte predominant Hodgkin lymphoma, intrapelvic lymph nodes

     C81.07   Nodular lymphocyte predominant Hodgkin lymphoma, spleen

     C81.08   Nodular lymphocyte predominant Hodgkin lymphoma, lymph nodes of multiple sites

     C81.09   Nodular lymphocyte predominant Hodgkin lymphoma, extranodal and solid organ sites

● **C81.1**   **Nodular sclerosis Hodgkin lymphoma** ◀▥
Nodular sclerosis classical Hodgkin lymphoma ◀
Moderately aggressive; most common in young adults

     C81.10   Nodular sclerosis Hodgkin lymphoma, unspecified site ◀▥

     C81.11   Nodular sclerosis Hodgkin lymphoma, lymph nodes of head, face, and neck ◀▥

     C81.12   Nodular sclerosis Hodgkin lymphoma, intrathoracic lymph nodes ◀▥

     C81.13   Nodular sclerosis Hodgkin lymphoma, intra-abdominal lymph nodes ◀▥

     C81.14   Nodular sclerosis Hodgkin lymphoma, lymph nodes of axilla and upper limb ◀▥

     C81.15   Nodular sclerosis Hodgkin lymphoma, lymph nodes of inguinal region and lower limb ◀▥

     C81.16   Nodular sclerosis Hodgkin lymphoma, intrapelvic lymph nodes ◀▥

     C81.17   Nodular sclerosis Hodgkin lymphoma, spleen ◀▥

     C81.18   Nodular sclerosis Hodgkin lymphoma, lymph nodes of multiple sites ◀▥

     C81.19   Nodular sclerosis Hodgkin lymphoma, extranodal and solid organ sites ◀▥

● **C81.2**   **Mixed cellularity Hodgkin lymphoma** ◀▥
Mixed cellularity classical Hodgkin lymphoma ◀
A type of Hodgkin's that is moderately aggressive with mixed cell types

     C81.20   Mixed cellularity Hodgkin lymphoma, unspecified site ◀▥

     C81.21   Mixed cellularity Hodgkin lymphoma, lymph nodes of head, face, and neck ◀▥

     C81.22   Mixed cellularity Hodgkin lymphoma, intrathoracic lymph nodes ◀▥

     C81.23   Mixed cellularity Hodgkin lymphoma, intra-abdominal lymph nodes ◀▥

     C81.24   Mixed cellularity Hodgkin lymphoma, lymph nodes of axilla and upper limb ◀▥

     C81.25   Mixed cellularity Hodgkin lymphoma, lymph nodes of inguinal region and lower limb ◀▥

     C81.26   Mixed cellularity Hodgkin lymphoma, intrapelvic lymph nodes ◀▥

     C81.27   Mixed cellularity Hodgkin lymphoma, spleen ◀▥

     C81.28   Mixed cellularity Hodgkin lymphoma, lymph nodes of multiple sites ◀▥

     C81.29   Mixed cellularity Hodgkin lymphoma, extranodal and solid organ sites ◀▥

● **C81.3**   **Lymphocyte depleted Hodgkin lymphoma** ◀▥
Lymphocyte depleted classical Hodgkin lymphoma ◀
Most aggressive type with poor prognosis

     C81.30   Lymphocyte depleted Hodgkin lymphoma, unspecified site ◀▥

     C81.31   Lymphocyte depleted Hodgkin lymphoma, lymph nodes of head, face, and neck ◀▥

     C81.32   Lymphocyte depleted Hodgkin lymphoma, intrathoracic lymph nodes ◀▥

     C81.33   Lymphocyte depleted Hodgkin lymphoma, intra-abdominal lymph nodes ◀▥

     C81.34   Lymphocyte depleted Hodgkin lymphoma, lymph nodes of axilla and upper limb ◀▥

     C81.35   Lymphocyte depleted Hodgkin lymphoma, lymph nodes of inguinal region and lower limb ◀▥

     C81.36   Lymphocyte depleted Hodgkin lymphoma, intrapelvic lymph nodes ◀▥

     C81.37   Lymphocyte depleted Hodgkin lymphoma, spleen ◀▥

     C81.38   Lymphocyte depleted Hodgkin lymphoma, lymph nodes of multiple sites ◀▥

     C81.39   Lymphocyte depleted Hodgkin lymphoma, extranodal and solid organ sites ◀▥

● **C81.4**   **Lymphocyte-rich Hodgkin lymphoma** ◀▥
Lymphocyte-rich classical Hodgkin lymphoma ◀

     Excludes1   nodular lymphocyte predominant Hodgkin lymphoma (C81.0-)

     C81.40   Lymphocyte-rich Hodgkin lymphoma, unspecified site ◀▥

     C81.41   Lymphocyte-rich Hodgkin lymphoma, lymph nodes of head, face, and neck ◀▥

     C81.42   Lymphocyte-rich Hodgkin lymphoma, intrathoracic lymph nodes ◀▥

     C81.43   Lymphocyte-rich Hodgkin lymphoma, intra-abdominal lymph nodes ◀▥

     C81.44   Lymphocyte-rich Hodgkin lymphoma, lymph nodes of axilla and upper limb ◀▥

     C81.45   Lymphocyte-rich Hodgkin lymphoma, lymph nodes of inguinal region and lower limb ◀▥

     C81.46   Lymphocyte-rich Hodgkin lymphoma, intrapelvic lymph nodes ◀▥

     C81.47   Lymphocyte-rich Hodgkin lymphoma, spleen ◀▥

     C81.48   Lymphocyte-rich Hodgkin lymphoma, lymph nodes of multiple sites ◀▥

     C81.49   Lymphocyte-rich Hodgkin lymphoma, extranodal and solid organ sites ◀▥

CHAPTER 2 (C00-D49)

- **C81.7 Other Hodgkin lymphoma**
    Classical Hodgkin lymphoma NOS
    Other classical Hodgkin lymphoma
    - C81.70 Other Hodgkin lymphoma, unspecified site
    - C81.71 Other Hodgkin lymphoma, lymph nodes of head, face, and neck
    - C81.72 Other Hodgkin lymphoma, intrathoracic lymph nodes
    - C81.73 Other Hodgkin lymphoma, intra-abdominal lymph nodes
    - C81.74 Other Hodgkin lymphoma, lymph nodes of axilla and upper limb
    - C81.75 Other Hodgkin lymphoma, lymph nodes of inguinal region and lower limb
    - C81.76 Other Hodgkin lymphoma, intrapelvic lymph nodes
    - C81.77 Other Hodgkin lymphoma, spleen
    - C81.78 Other Hodgkin lymphoma, lymph nodes of multiple sites
    - C81.79 Other Hodgkin lymphoma, extranodal and solid organ sites
- **C81.9 Hodgkin lymphoma, unspecified**
    - C81.90 Hodgkin lymphoma, unspecified, unspecified site
    - C81.91 Hodgkin lymphoma, unspecified, lymph nodes of head, face, and neck
    - C81.92 Hodgkin lymphoma, unspecified, intrathoracic lymph nodes
    - C81.93 Hodgkin lymphoma, unspecified, intra-abdominal lymph nodes
    - C81.94 Hodgkin lymphoma, unspecified, lymph nodes of axilla and upper limb
    - C81.95 Hodgkin lymphoma, unspecified, lymph nodes of inguinal region and lower limb
    - C81.96 Hodgkin lymphoma, unspecified, intrapelvic lymph nodes
    - C81.97 Hodgkin lymphoma, unspecified, spleen
    - C81.98 Hodgkin lymphoma, unspecified, lymph nodes of multiple sites
    - C81.99 Hodgkin lymphoma, unspecified, extranodal and solid organ sites
- **C82 Follicular lymphoma**
    Group of malignant lymphomas
    Includes follicular lymphoma with or without diffuse areas
    Excludes1 mature T/NK-cell lymphomas (C84.-)
    personal history of non-Hodgkin lymphoma (Z85.72)
    - **C82.0 Follicular lymphoma grade I**
        - C82.00 Follicular lymphoma grade I, unspecified site
        - C82.01 Follicular lymphoma grade I, lymph nodes of head, face, and neck
        - C82.02 Follicular lymphoma grade I, intrathoracic lymph nodes
        - C82.03 Follicular lymphoma grade I, intra-abdominal lymph nodes
        - C82.04 Follicular lymphoma grade I, lymph nodes of axilla and upper limb
        - C82.05 Follicular lymphoma grade I, lymph nodes of inguinal region and lower limb
        - C82.06 Follicular lymphoma grade I, intrapelvic lymph nodes
        - C82.07 Follicular lymphoma grade I, spleen
        - C82.08 Follicular lymphoma grade I, lymph nodes of multiple sites
        - C82.09 Follicular lymphoma grade I, extranodal and solid organ sites

- **C82.1 Follicular lymphoma grade II**
    - C82.10 Follicular lymphoma grade II, unspecified site
    - C82.11 Follicular lymphoma grade II, lymph nodes of head, face, and neck
    - C82.12 Follicular lymphoma grade II, intrathoracic lymph nodes
    - C82.13 Follicular lymphoma grade II, intra-abdominal lymph nodes
    - C82.14 Follicular lymphoma grade II, lymph nodes of axilla and upper limb
    - C82.15 Follicular lymphoma grade II, lymph nodes of inguinal region and lower limb
    - C82.16 Follicular lymphoma grade II, intrapelvic lymph nodes
    - C82.17 Follicular lymphoma grade II, spleen
    - C82.18 Follicular lymphoma grade II, lymph nodes of multiple sites
    - C82.19 Follicular lymphoma grade II, extranodal and solid organ sites
- **C82.2 Follicular lymphoma grade III, unspecified**
    - C82.20 Follicular lymphoma grade III, unspecified, unspecified site
    - C82.21 Follicular lymphoma grade III, unspecified, lymph nodes of head, face, and neck
    - C82.22 Follicular lymphoma grade III, unspecified, intrathoracic lymph nodes
    - C82.23 Follicular lymphoma grade III, unspecified, intra-abdominal lymph nodes
    - C82.24 Follicular lymphoma grade III, unspecified, lymph nodes of axilla and upper limb
    - C82.25 Follicular lymphoma grade III, unspecified, lymph nodes of inguinal region and lower limb
    - C82.26 Follicular lymphoma grade III, unspecified, intrapelvic lymph nodes
    - C82.27 Follicular lymphoma grade III, unspecified, spleen
    - C82.28 Follicular lymphoma grade III, unspecified, lymph nodes of multiple sites
    - C82.29 Follicular lymphoma grade III, unspecified, extranodal and solid organ sites
- **C82.3 Follicular lymphoma grade IIIa**
    - C82.30 Follicular lymphoma grade IIIa, unspecified site
    - C82.31 Follicular lymphoma grade IIIa, lymph nodes of head, face, and neck
    - C82.32 Follicular lymphoma grade IIIa, intrathoracic lymph nodes
    - C82.33 Follicular lymphoma grade IIIa, intra-abdominal lymph nodes
    - C82.34 Follicular lymphoma grade IIIa, lymph nodes of axilla and upper limb
    - C82.35 Follicular lymphoma grade IIIa, lymph nodes of inguinal region and lower limb
    - C82.36 Follicular lymphoma grade IIIa, intrapelvic lymph nodes
    - C82.37 Follicular lymphoma grade IIIa, spleen
    - C82.38 Follicular lymphoma grade IIIa, lymph nodes of multiple sites
    - C82.39 Follicular lymphoma grade IIIa, extranodal and solid organ sites

◀ New   ◀▥ Revised   deleted Deleted   Excludes 1   Excludes 2   Includes   Use additional   Code first   Code also   Unspecified
OGCR Official Guidelines   X Assign placeholder X   ● Use Additional Character(s)   ▶ Manifestation Code   **Coding Clinic**

● **C82.4**   Follicular lymphoma grade IIIb

     C82.40   Follicular lymphoma grade IIIb, unspecified site

     C82.41   Follicular lymphoma grade IIIb, lymph nodes of head, face, and neck

     C82.42   Follicular lymphoma grade IIIb, intrathoracic lymph nodes

     C82.43   Follicular lymphoma grade IIIb, intra-abdominal lymph nodes

     C82.44   Follicular lymphoma grade IIIb, lymph nodes of axilla and upper limb

     C82.45   Follicular lymphoma grade IIIb, lymph nodes of inguinal region and lower limb

     C82.46   Follicular lymphoma grade IIIb, intrapelvic lymph nodes

     C82.47   Follicular lymphoma grade IIIb, spleen

     C82.48   Follicular lymphoma grade IIIb, lymph nodes of multiple sites

     C82.49   Follicular lymphoma grade IIIb, extranodal and solid organ sites

● **C82.5**   Diffuse follicle center lymphoma

     C82.50   Diffuse follicle center lymphoma, unspecified site

     C82.51   Diffuse follicle center lymphoma, lymph nodes of head, face, and neck

     C82.52   Diffuse follicle center lymphoma, intrathoracic lymph nodes

     C82.53   Diffuse follicle center lymphoma, intra-abdominal lymph nodes

     C82.54   Diffuse follicle center lymphoma, lymph nodes of axilla and upper limb

     C82.55   Diffuse follicle center lymphoma, lymph nodes of inguinal region and lower limb

     C82.56   Diffuse follicle center lymphoma, intrapelvic lymph nodes

     C82.57   Diffuse follicle center lymphoma, spleen

     C82.58   Diffuse follicle center lymphoma, lymph nodes of multiple sites

     C82.59   Diffuse follicle center lymphoma, extranodal and solid organ sites

● **C82.6**   Cutaneous follicle center lymphoma

     C82.60   Cutaneous follicle center lymphoma, unspecified site

     C82.61   Cutaneous follicle center lymphoma, lymph nodes of head, face, and neck

     C82.62   Cutaneous follicle center lymphoma, intrathoracic lymph nodes

     C82.63   Cutaneous follicle center lymphoma, intra-abdominal lymph nodes

     C82.64   Cutaneous follicle center lymphoma, lymph nodes of axilla and upper limb

     C82.65   Cutaneous follicle center lymphoma, lymph nodes of inguinal region and lower limb

     C82.66   Cutaneous follicle center lymphoma, intrapelvic lymph nodes

     C82.67   Cutaneous follicle center lymphoma, spleen

     C82.68   Cutaneous follicle center lymphoma, lymph nodes of multiple sites

     C82.69   Cutaneous follicle center lymphoma, extranodal and solid organ sites

● **C82.8**   Other types of follicular lymphoma

     C82.80   Other types of follicular lymphoma, unspecified site

     C82.81   Other types of follicular lymphoma, lymph nodes of head, face, and neck

     C82.82   Other types of follicular lymphoma, intrathoracic lymph nodes

     C82.83   Other types of follicular lymphoma, intra-abdominal lymph nodes

     C82.84   Other types of follicular lymphoma, lymph nodes of axilla and upper limb

     C82.85   Other types of follicular lymphoma, lymph nodes of inguinal region and lower limb

     C82.86   Other types of follicular lymphoma, intrapelvic lymph nodes

     C82.87   Other types of follicular lymphoma, spleen

     C82.88   Other types of follicular lymphoma, lymph nodes of multiple sites

     C82.89   Other types of follicular lymphoma, extranodal and solid organ sites

● **C82.9**   Follicular lymphoma, unspecified

     C82.90   Follicular lymphoma, unspecified, unspecified site

     C82.91   Follicular lymphoma, unspecified, lymph nodes of head, face, and neck

     C82.92   Follicular lymphoma, unspecified, intrathoracic lymph nodes

     C82.93   Follicular lymphoma, unspecified, intra-abdominal lymph nodes

     C82.94   Follicular lymphoma, unspecified, lymph nodes of axilla and upper limb

     C82.95   Follicular lymphoma, unspecified, lymph nodes of inguinal region and lower limb

     C82.96   Follicular lymphoma, unspecified, intrapelvic lymph nodes

     C82.97   Follicular lymphoma, unspecified, spleen

     C82.98   Follicular lymphoma, unspecified, lymph nodes of multiple sites

     C82.99   Follicular lymphoma, unspecified, extranodal and solid organ sites

● **C83**   Non-follicular lymphoma

     Excludes1   personal history of non-Hodgkin lymphoma (Z85.72)

  ● **C83.0**   Small cell B-cell lymphoma

     Lymphoplasmacytic lymphoma
     Nodal marginal zone lymphoma
     Non-leukemic variant of B-CLL
     Splenic marginal zone lymphoma

     Excludes1   chronic lymphocytic leukemia (C91.1)
                      mature T/NK-cell lymphomas (C84.-)
                      Waldenström macroglobulinemia (C88.0)

     C83.00   Small cell B-cell lymphoma, unspecified site

     C83.01   Small cell B-cell lymphoma, lymph nodes of head, face, and neck

     C83.02   Small cell B-cell lymphoma, intrathoracic lymph nodes

     C83.03   Small cell B-cell lymphoma, intra-abdominal lymph nodes

     C83.04   Small cell B-cell lymphoma, lymph nodes of axilla and upper limb

     C83.05   Small cell B-cell lymphoma, lymph nodes of inguinal region and lower limb

     C83.06   Small cell B-cell lymphoma, intrapelvic lymph nodes

     C83.07   Small cell B-cell lymphoma, spleen

     C83.08   Small cell B-cell lymphoma, lymph nodes of multiple sites

     C83.09   Small cell B-cell lymphoma, extranodal and solid organ sites

CHAPTER 2 (C00-D49)

● **C83.1**   **Mantle cell lymphoma**
       Centrocytic lymphoma
       Malignant lymphomatous polyposis

   C83.10   Mantle cell lymphoma, `unspecified` site

   C83.11   Mantle cell lymphoma, lymph nodes of head, face, and neck

   C83.12   Mantle cell lymphoma, intrathoracic lymph nodes

   C83.13   Mantle cell lymphoma, intra-abdominal lymph nodes

   C83.14   Mantle cell lymphoma, lymph nodes of axilla and upper limb

   C83.15   Mantle cell lymphoma, lymph nodes of inguinal region and lower limb

   C83.16   Mantle cell lymphoma, intrapelvic lymph nodes

   C83.17   Mantle cell lymphoma, spleen

   C83.18   Mantle cell lymphoma, lymph nodes of multiple sites

   C83.19   Mantle cell lymphoma, extranodal and solid organ sites

● **C83.3**   **Diffuse large B-cell lymphoma**
       Anaplastic diffuse large B-cell lymphoma
       CD30-positive diffuse large B-cell lymphoma
       Centroblastic diffuse large B-cell lymphoma
       Diffuse large B-cell lymphoma, subtype not specified
       Immunoblastic diffuse large B-cell lymphoma
       Plasmablastic diffuse large B-cell lymphoma
       Diffuse large B-cell lymphoma, subtype not specified
       T-cell rich diffuse large B-cell lymphoma

     Excludes1   mediastinal (thymic) large B-cell lymphoma (C85.2-)
                  mature T/NK-cell lymphomas (C84.-)

   C83.30   Diffuse large B-cell lymphoma, `unspecified` site

   C83.31   Diffuse large B-cell lymphoma, lymph nodes of head, face, and neck

   C83.32   Diffuse large B-cell lymphoma, intrathoracic lymph nodes

   C83.33   Diffuse large B-cell lymphoma, intra-abdominal lymph nodes

   C83.34   Diffuse large B-cell lymphoma, lymph nodes of axilla and upper limb

   C83.35   Diffuse large B-cell lymphoma, lymph nodes of inguinal region and lower limb

   C83.36   Diffuse large B-cell lymphoma, intrapelvic lymph nodes

   C83.37   Diffuse large B-cell lymphoma, spleen

   C83.38   Diffuse large B-cell lymphoma, lymph nodes of multiple sites

   C83.39   Diffuse large B-cell lymphoma, extranodal and solid organ sites

● **C83.5**   **Lymphoblastic (diffuse) lymphoma**
       Highly malignant type of non-Hodgkin lymphoma with diffuse infiltration
       B-precursor lymphoma
       Lymphoblastic B-cell lymphoma
       Lymphoblastic lymphoma NOS
       Lymphoblastic T-cell lymphoma
       T-precursor lymphoma

   C83.50   Lymphoblastic (diffuse) lymphoma, `unspecified` site

   C83.51   Lymphoblastic (diffuse) lymphoma, lymph nodes of head, face, and neck

   C83.52   Lymphoblastic (diffuse) lymphoma, intrathoracic lymph nodes

   C83.53   Lymphoblastic (diffuse) lymphoma, intra-abdominal lymph nodes

   C83.54   Lymphoblastic (diffuse) lymphoma, lymph nodes of axilla and upper limb

   C83.55   Lymphoblastic (diffuse) lymphoma, lymph nodes of inguinal region and lower limb

   C83.56   Lymphoblastic (diffuse) lymphoma, intrapelvic lymph nodes

   C83.57   Lymphoblastic (diffuse) lymphoma, spleen

   C83.58   Lymphoblastic (diffuse) lymphoma, lymph nodes of multiple sites

   C83.59   Lymphoblastic (diffuse) lymphoma, extranodal and solid organ sites

● **C83.7**   **Burkitt lymphoma**
       Form of small cell lymphoma
       Atypical Burkitt lymphoma
       Burkitt-like lymphoma

     Excludes1   mature B-cell leukemia Burkitt type (C91.A-)

   C83.70   Burkitt lymphoma, `unspecified` site

   C83.71   Burkitt lymphoma, lymph nodes of head, face, and neck

   C83.72   Burkitt lymphoma, intrathoracic lymph nodes

   C83.73   Burkitt lymphoma, intra-abdominal lymph nodes

   C83.74   Burkitt lymphoma, lymph nodes of axilla and upper limb

   C83.75   Burkitt lymphoma, lymph nodes of inguinal region and lower limb

   C83.76   Burkitt lymphoma, intrapelvic lymph nodes

   C83.77   Burkitt lymphoma, spleen

   C83.78   Burkitt lymphoma, lymph nodes of multiple sites

   C83.79   Burkitt lymphoma, extranodal and solid organ sites

● **C83.8**   **Other non-follicular lymphoma**
       Intravascular large B-cell lymphoma
       Lymphoid granulomatosis
       Primary effusion B-cell lymphoma

     Excludes1   mediastinal (thymic) large B-cell lymphoma (C85.2-)
                  T-cell rich B-cell lymphoma (C83.3-)

   C83.80   Other non-follicular lymphoma, `unspecified` site

   C83.81   Other non-follicular lymphoma, lymph nodes of head, face, and neck

   C83.82   Other non-follicular lymphoma, intrathoracic lymph nodes

   C83.83   Other non-follicular lymphoma, intra-abdominal lymph nodes

   C83.84   Other non-follicular lymphoma, lymph nodes of axilla and upper limb

   C83.85   Other non-follicular lymphoma, lymph nodes of inguinal region and lower limb

   C83.86   Other non-follicular lymphoma, intrapelvic lymph nodes

   C83.87   Other non-follicular lymphoma, spleen

   C83.88   Other non-follicular lymphoma, lymph nodes of multiple sites

   C83.89   Other non-follicular lymphoma, extranodal and solid organ sites

◀ New   ⬅ Revised   ~~deleted~~ Deleted   Excludes 1   Excludes 2   Includes   Use additional   Code first   Code also   Unspecified

OGCR Official Guidelines   X Assign placeholder X   ● Use Additional Character(s)   ▶ Manifestation Code   **Coding Clinic**

● C83.9   Non-follicular (diffuse) lymphoma, unspecified

　C83.90   Non-follicular (diffuse) lymphoma, unspecified, unspecified site

　C83.91   Non-follicular (diffuse) lymphoma, unspecified, lymph nodes of head, face, and neck

　C83.92   Non-follicular (diffuse) lymphoma, unspecified, intrathoracic lymph nodes

　C83.93   Non-follicular (diffuse) lymphoma, unspecified, intra-abdominal lymph nodes

　C83.94   Non-follicular (diffuse) lymphoma, unspecified, lymph nodes of axilla and upper limb

　C83.95   Non-follicular (diffuse) lymphoma, unspecified, lymph nodes of inguinal region and lower limb

　C83.96   Non-follicular (diffuse) lymphoma, unspecified, intrapelvic lymph nodes

　C83.97   Non-follicular (diffuse) lymphoma, unspecified, spleen

　C83.98   Non-follicular (diffuse) lymphoma, unspecified, lymph nodes of multiple sites

　C83.99   Non-follicular (diffuse) lymphoma, unspecified, extranodal and solid organ sites

● C84   Mature T/NK-cell lymphomas

　Excludes1   personal history of non-Hodgkin lymphoma (Z85.72)

● C84.0   Mycosis fungoides
　Chronic or rapidly progressive form of cutaneous T-cell lymphoma; AKA granuloma fungoides

　Excludes1   peripheral T-cell lymphoma, not classified (C84.4-)

　C84.00   Mycosis fungoides, unspecified site

　C84.01   Mycosis fungoides, lymph nodes of head, face, and neck

　C84.02   Mycosis fungoides, intrathoracic lymph nodes

　C84.03   Mycosis fungoides, intra-abdominal lymph nodes

　C84.04   Mycosis fungoides, lymph nodes of axilla and upper limb

　C84.05   Mycosis fungoides, lymph nodes of inguinal region and lower limb

　C84.06   Mycosis fungoides, intrapelvic lymph nodes

　C84.07   Mycosis fungoides, spleen

　C84.08   Mycosis fungoides, lymph nodes of multiple sites

　C84.09   Mycosis fungoides, extranodal and solid organ sites

● C84.1   Sézary disease
　Type of cutaneous lymphoma affecting T-cells

　C84.10   Sézary disease, unspecified site

　C84.11   Sézary disease, lymph nodes of head, face, and neck

　C84.12   Sézary disease, intrathoracic lymph nodes

　C84.13   Sézary disease, intra-abdominal lymph nodes

　C84.14   Sézary disease, lymph nodes of axilla and upper limb

　C84.15   Sézary disease, lymph nodes of inguinal region and lower limb

　C84.16   Sézary disease, intrapelvic lymph nodes

　C84.17   Sézary disease, spleen

　C84.18   Sézary disease, lymph nodes of multiple sites

　C84.19   Sézary disease, extranodal and solid organ sites

Item 2–7 Lymphosarcoma, also known as malignant lymphoma, is a cancer of the lymph system exhibiting abnormal cells encompassing an entire lymph node creating a diffuse pattern without any definite organization. Diffuse pattern lymphoma has a more unfavorable survival outlook than those with a follicular or nodular pattern. Reticulosarcoma is the most common aggressive form of non-Hodgkin's lymphoma.

● C84.4   Peripheral T-cell lymphoma, not classified
　Diverse group of blood carcinomas originating from T-cells, requiring aggressive chemotherapy
　Lennert's lymphoma
　Lymphoepithelioid lymphoma
　Mature T-cell lymphoma, not elsewhere classified

　C84.40   Peripheral T-cell lymphoma, not classified, unspecified site

　C84.41   Peripheral T-cell lymphoma, not classified, lymph nodes of head, face, and neck

　C84.42   Peripheral T-cell lymphoma, not classified, intrathoracic lymph nodes

　C84.43   Peripheral T-cell lymphoma, not classified, intra-abdominal lymph nodes

　C84.44   Peripheral T-cell lymphoma, not classified, lymph nodes of axilla and upper limb

　C84.45   Peripheral T-cell lymphoma, not classified, lymph nodes of inguinal region and lower limb

　C84.46   Peripheral T-cell lymphoma, not classified, intrapelvic lymph nodes

　C84.47   Peripheral T-cell lymphoma, not classified, spleen

　C84.48   Peripheral T-cell lymphoma, not classified, lymph nodes of multiple sites

　C84.49   Peripheral T-cell lymphoma, not classified, extranodal and solid organ sites

● C84.6   Anaplastic large cell lymphoma, ALK-positive
　Anaplastic large cell lymphoma, CD30-positive

　C84.60   Anaplastic large cell lymphoma, ALK-positive, unspecified site

　C84.61   Anaplastic large cell lymphoma, ALK-positive, lymph nodes of head, face, and neck

　C84.62   Anaplastic large cell lymphoma, ALK-positive, intrathoracic lymph nodes

　C84.63   Anaplastic large cell lymphoma, ALK-positive, intra-abdominal lymph nodes

　C84.64   Anaplastic large cell lymphoma, ALK-positive, lymph nodes of axilla and upper limb

　C84.65   Anaplastic large cell lymphoma, ALK-positive, lymph nodes of inguinal region and lower limb

　C84.66   Anaplastic large cell lymphoma, ALK-positive, intrapelvic lymph nodes

　C84.67   Anaplastic large cell lymphoma, ALK-positive, spleen

　C84.68   Anaplastic large cell lymphoma, ALK-positive, lymph nodes of multiple sites

　C84.69   Anaplastic large cell lymphoma, ALK-positive, extranodal and solid organ sites

● C84.7   Anaplastic large cell lymphoma, ALK-negative

　Excludes1   primary cutaneous CD30-positive T-cell proliferations (C86.6-)

　C84.70   Anaplastic large cell lymphoma, ALK-negative, unspecified site

　C84.71   Anaplastic large cell lymphoma, ALK-negative, lymph nodes of head, face, and neck

　C84.72   Anaplastic large cell lymphoma, ALK-negative, intrathoracic lymph nodes

　C84.73   Anaplastic large cell lymphoma, ALK-negative, intra-abdominal lymph nodes

　C84.74   Anaplastic large cell lymphoma, ALK-negative, lymph nodes of axilla and upper limb

　C84.75   Anaplastic large cell lymphoma, ALK-negative, lymph nodes of inguinal region and lower limb

　C84.76   Anaplastic large cell lymphoma, ALK-negative, intrapelvic lymph nodes

　C84.77   Anaplastic large cell lymphoma, ALK-negative, spleen

　C84.78   Anaplastic large cell lymphoma, ALK-negative, lymph nodes of multiple sites

　C84.79   Anaplastic large cell lymphoma, ALK-negative, extranodal and solid organ sites

CHAPTER 2 (C00-D49)

● **C84.A** **Cutaneous T-cell lymphoma, unspecified**

 C84.A0 **Cutaneous T-cell lymphoma, unspecified, unspecified site**

 C84.A1 **Cutaneous T-cell lymphoma, unspecified lymph nodes of head, face, and neck**

 C84.A2 **Cutaneous T-cell lymphoma, unspecified, intrathoracic lymph nodes**

 C84.A3 **Cutaneous T-cell lymphoma, unspecified, intra-abdominal lymph nodes**

 C84.A4 **Cutaneous T-cell lymphoma, unspecified, lymph nodes of axilla and upper limb**

 C84.A5 **Cutaneous T-cell lymphoma, unspecified, lymph nodes of inguinal region and lower limb**

 C84.A6 **Cutaneous T-cell lymphoma, unspecified, intrapelvic lymph nodes**

 C84.A7 **Cutaneous T-cell lymphoma, unspecified, spleen**

 C84.A8 **Cutaneous T-cell lymphoma, unspecified, lymph nodes of multiple sites**

 C84.A9 **Cutaneous T-cell lymphoma, unspecified, extranodal and solid organ sites**

● **C84.Z** **Other mature T/NK-cell lymphomas**

 Note: If T-cell lineage or involvement is mentioned in conjunction with a specific lymphoma, code to the more specific description.

 Excludes1 angioimmunoblastic T-cell lymphoma (C86.5)
     blastic NK-cell lymphoma (C86.4)
     enteropathy-type T-cell lymphoma (C86.2)
     extranodal NK-cell lymphoma, nasal type (C86.0)
     hepatosplenic T-cell lymphoma (C86.1)
     primary cutaneous CD30-positive T-cell proliferations (C86.6)
     subcutaneous panniculitis-like T-cell lymphoma (C86.3)
     T-cell leukemia (C91.1-)

 C84.Z0 **Other mature T/NK-cell lymphomas, unspecified site**

 C84.Z1 **Other mature T/NK-cell lymphomas, lymph nodes of head, face, and neck**

 C84.Z2 **Other mature T/NK-cell lymphomas, intrathoracic lymph nodes**

 C84.Z3 **Other mature T/NK-cell lymphomas, intra-abdominal lymph nodes**

 C84.Z4 **Other mature T/NK-cell lymphomas, lymph nodes of axilla and upper limb**

 C84.Z5 **Other mature T/NK-cell lymphomas, lymph nodes of inguinal region and lower limb**

 C84.Z6 **Other mature T/NK-cell lymphomas, intrapelvic lymph nodes**

 C84.Z7 **Other mature T/NK-cell lymphomas, spleen**

 C84.Z8 **Other mature T/NK-cell lymphomas, lymph nodes of multiple sites**

 C84.Z9 **Other mature T/NK-cell lymphomas, extranodal and solid organ sites**

● **C84.9** **Mature T/NK-cell lymphomas, unspecified**
 NK/T cell lymphoma NOS

 Excludes1 mature T-cell lymphoma, not elsewhere classified (C84.4-)

 C84.90 **Mature T/NK-cell lymphomas, unspecified, unspecified site**

 C84.91 **Mature T/NK-cell lymphomas, unspecified, lymph nodes of head, face, and neck**

 C84.92 **Mature T/NK-cell lymphomas, unspecified, intrathoracic lymph nodes**

 C84.93 **Mature T/NK-cell lymphomas, unspecified, intra-abdominal lymph nodes**

 C84.94 **Mature T/NK-cell lymphomas, unspecified, lymph nodes of axilla and upper limb**

 C84.95 **Mature T/NK-cell lymphomas, unspecified, lymph nodes of inguinal region and lower limb**

 C84.96 **Mature T/NK-cell lymphomas, unspecified, intrapelvic lymph nodes**

 C84.97 **Mature T/NK-cell lymphomas, unspecified, spleen**

 C84.98 **Mature T/NK-cell lymphomas, unspecified, lymph nodes of multiple sites**

 C84.99 **Mature T/NK-cell lymphomas, unspecified, extranodal and solid organ sites**

● **C85** **Other specified and unspecified types of non-Hodgkin lymphoma**

 Excludes1 other specified types of T/NK-cell lymphoma (C86.-)
     personal history of non-Hodgkin lymphoma (Z85.72)

● **C85.1** **Unspecified B-cell lymphoma**

 Note: If B-cell lineage or involvement is mentioned in conjunction with a specific lymphoma, code to the more specific description.

 C85.10 **Unspecified B-cell lymphoma, unspecified site**

 C85.11 **Unspecified B-cell lymphoma, lymph nodes of head, face, and neck**

 C85.12 **Unspecified B-cell lymphoma, intrathoracic lymph nodes**

 C85.13 **Unspecified B-cell lymphoma, intra-abdominal lymph nodes**

 C85.14 **Unspecified B-cell lymphoma, lymph nodes of axilla and upper limb**

 C85.15 **Unspecified B-cell lymphoma, lymph nodes of inguinal region and lower limb**

 C85.16 **Unspecified B-cell lymphoma, intrapelvic lymph nodes**

 C85.17 **Unspecified B-cell lymphoma, spleen**

 C85.18 **Unspecified B-cell lymphoma, lymph nodes of multiple sites**

 C85.19 **Unspecified B-cell lymphoma, extranodal and solid organ sites**

● **C85.2** **Mediastinal (thymic) large B-cell lymphoma**

 C85.20 **Mediastinal (thymic) large B-cell lymphoma, unspecified site**

 C85.21 **Mediastinal (thymic) large B-cell lymphoma, lymph nodes of head, face, and neck**

 C85.22 **Mediastinal (thymic) large B-cell lymphoma, intrathoracic lymph nodes**

 C85.23 **Mediastinal (thymic) large B-cell lymphoma, intra-abdominal lymph nodes**

 C85.24 **Mediastinal (thymic) large B-cell lymphoma, lymph nodes of axilla and upper limb**

 C85.25 **Mediastinal (thymic) large B-cell lymphoma, lymph nodes of inguinal region and lower limb**

 C85.26 **Mediastinal (thymic) large B-cell lymphoma, intrapelvic lymph nodes**

 C85.27 **Mediastinal (thymic) large B-cell lymphoma, spleen**

 C85.28 **Mediastinal (thymic) large B-cell lymphoma, lymph nodes of multiple sites**

 C85.29 **Mediastinal (thymic) large B-cell lymphoma, extranodal and solid organ sites**

◀ New ◀┅ Revised ~~deleted~~ Deleted Excludes 1 Excludes 2 Includes Use additional Code first Code also Unspecified

OGCR Official Guidelines X Assign placeholder X ● Use Additional Character(s) ▶ Manifestation Code **Coding Clinic**

●C85.8   **Other specified types of non-Hodgkin lymphoma**
- C85.80   Other specified types of non-Hodgkin lymphoma, unspecified site
- C85.81   Other specified types of non-Hodgkin lymphoma, lymph nodes of head, face, and neck
- C85.82   Other specified types of non-Hodgkin lymphoma, intrathoracic lymph nodes
- C85.83   Other specified types of non-Hodgkin lymphoma, intra-abdominal lymph nodes
- C85.84   Other specified types of non-Hodgkin lymphoma, lymph nodes of axilla and upper limb
- C85.85   Other specified types of non-Hodgkin lymphoma, lymph nodes of inguinal region and lower limb
- C85.86   Other specified types of non-Hodgkin lymphoma, intrapelvic lymph nodes
- C85.87   Other specified types of non-Hodgkin lymphoma, spleen
- C85.88   Other specified types of non-Hodgkin lymphoma, lymph nodes of multiple sites
- C85.89   Other specified types of non-Hodgkin lymphoma, extranodal and solid organ sites

●C85.9   **Non-Hodgkin lymphoma, unspecified**
Lymphoma NOS
Malignant lymphoma NOS
Non-Hodgkin lymphoma NOS
- C85.90   Non-Hodgkin lymphoma, unspecified, unspecified site
- C85.91   Non-Hodgkin lymphoma, unspecified, lymph nodes of head, face, and neck
- C85.92   Non-Hodgkin lymphoma, unspecified, intrathoracic lymph nodes
- C85.93   Non-Hodgkin lymphoma, unspecified, intra-abdominal lymph nodes
- C85.94   Non-Hodgkin lymphoma, unspecified, lymph nodes of axilla and upper limb
- C85.95   Non-Hodgkin lymphoma, unspecified, lymph nodes of inguinal region and lower limb
- C85.96   Non-Hodgkin lymphoma, unspecified, intrapelvic lymph nodes
- C85.97   Non-Hodgkin lymphoma, unspecified, spleen
- C85.98   Non-Hodgkin lymphoma, unspecified, lymph nodes of multiple sites
- C85.99   Non-Hodgkin lymphoma, unspecified, extranodal and solid organ sites

●C86   **Other specified types of T/NK-cell lymphoma**
> **Excludes1**   anaplastic large cell lymphoma, ALK negative (C84.7-)
> anaplastic large cell lymphoma, ALK positive (C84.6-)
> mature T/NK-cell lymphomas (C84.-)
> other specified types of non-Hodgkin lymphoma (C85.8-)

C86.0   **Extranodal NK/T-cell lymphoma, nasal type**

C86.1   **Hepatosplenic T-cell lymphoma**
Alpha-beta and gamma delta types

C86.2   **Enteropathy-type (intestinal) T-cell lymphoma**
Enteropathy associated T-cell lymphoma

C86.3   **Subcutaneous panniculitis-like T-cell lymphoma**

C86.4   **Blastic NK-cell lymphoma**

C86.5   **Angioimmunoblastic T-cell lymphoma**
Angioimmunoblastic lymphadenopathy with dysproteinemia (AILD)

C86.6   **Primary cutaneous CD30-positive T-cell proliferations**
Lymphomatoid papulosis
Primary cutaneous anaplastic large cell lymphoma
Primary cutaneous CD30-positive large T-cell lymphoma

●C88   **Malignant immunoproliferative diseases and certain other B-cell lymphomas**
Diseases involving immune system
> **Excludes1**   B-cell lymphoma, unspecified (C85.1-)
> personal history of other malignant neoplasms of lymphoid, hematopoietic and related tissues (Z85.79)

C88.0   **Waldenström's macroglobulinemia**
Lymphoplasmacytic lymphoma with IgM-production
Macroglobulinemia (idiopathic) (primary)
> **Excludes1**   small cell B-cell lymphoma (C83.0)

C88.2   **Heavy chain disease**
Franklin disease
Gamma heavy chain disease
Mu heavy chain disease

C88.3   **Immunoproliferative small intestinal disease**
Alpha heavy chain disease
Mediterranean lymphoma

C88.4   **Extranodal marginal zone B-cell lymphoma of mucosa-associated lymphoid tissue [MALT-lymphoma]**
Lymphoma of skin-associated lymphoid tissue [SALT-lymphoma]
Lymphoma of bronchial-associated lymphoid tissue [BALT-lymphoma]
> **Excludes1**   high malignant (diffuse large B-cell) lymphoma (C83.3-)

C88.8   **Other malignant immunoproliferative diseases**

C88.9   **Malignant immunoproliferative disease, unspecified**
Immunoproliferative disease NOS

●C90   **Multiple myeloma and malignant plasma cell neoplasms**
> **Excludes1**   personal history of other malignant neoplasms of lymphoid, hematopoietic and related tissues (Z85.79)

●C90.0   **Multiple myeloma**
Kahler's disease
Medullary plasmacytoma
Myelomatosis
Plasma cell myeloma
> **Excludes1**   solitary myeloma (C90.3-)
> solitary plasmacytoma (C90.3-)
- C90.00   Multiple myeloma not having achieved remission
  Multiple myeloma with failed remission
  Multiple myeloma NOS
- C90.01   Multiple myeloma in remission
- C90.02   Multiple myeloma in relapse

●C90.1   **Plasma cell leukemia**
Rare type of acute leukemia
Plasmacytic leukemia
- C90.10   Plasma cell leukemia not having achieved remission
  Plasma cell leukemia with failed remission
  Plasma cell leukemia NOS
- C90.11   Plasma cell leukemia in remission
- C90.12   Plasma cell leukemia in relapse

●C90.2   **Extramedullary plasmacytoma**
Malignant monoclonal plasma cell tumor growing in soft tissue; AKA plasma cell dyscrasias
- C90.20   Extramedullary plasmacytoma not having achieved remission
  Extramedullary plasmacytoma with failed remission
  Extramedullary plasmacytoma NOS
- C90.21   Extramedullary plasmacytoma in remission
- C90.22   Extramedullary plasmacytoma in relapse

Item 2–8 Multiple myeloma is a cancer of a plasma cell (a type of white blood cell) and is an incurable but treatable disease. Immunoproliferative neoplasm is a term for diseases (mostly cancers) in which the immune system cells proliferate.

CHAPTER 2 (C00-D49)

- **C90.3   Solitary plasmacytoma**
  - Localized malignant plasma cell tumor NOS
  - Plasmacytoma NOS
  - Solitary myeloma
  - **C90.30   Solitary plasmacytoma not having achieved remission**
    - Solitary plasmacytoma with failed remission
    - Solitary plasmacytoma NOS
  - **C90.31   Solitary plasmacytoma in remission**
  - **C90.32   Solitary plasmacytoma in relapse**

- **C91   Lymphoid leukemia**
  - *Type of leukemia affecting circulating cells of lymphoid origin*
  - **Excludes1**   personal history of leukemia (Z85.6)
  - **C91.0   Acute lymphoblastic leukemia [ALL]**
    - **Note:** Code C91.0 should only be used for T-cell and B-cell precursor leukemia
    - **C91.00   Acute lymphoblastic leukemia not having achieved remission**
      - Acute lymphoblastic leukemia with failed remission
      - Acute lymphoblastic leukemia NOS
    - **C91.01   Acute lymphoblastic leukemia, in remission**
    - **C91.02   Acute lymphoblastic leukemia, in relapse**
  - **C91.1   Chronic lymphocytic leukemia of B-cell type**
    - Lymphoplasmacytic leukemia
    - Richter syndrome
    - **Excludes1**   lymphoplasmacytic lymphoma (C83.0-)
    - **C91.10   Chronic lymphocytic leukemia of B-cell type not having achieved remission**
      - Chronic lymphocytic leukemia of B-cell type with failed remission
      - Chronic lymphocytic leukemia of B-cell type NOS
    - **C91.11   Chronic lymphocytic leukemia of B-cell type in remission**
    - **C91.12   Chronic lymphocytic leukemia of B-cell type in relapse**
  - **C91.3   Prolymphocytic leukemia of B-cell type**
    - *Chronic leukemia with symptoms of large number of circulating lymphocytes*
    - **C91.30   Prolymphocytic leukemia of B-cell type not having achieved remission**
      - Prolymphocytic leukemia of B-cell type with failed remission
      - Prolymphocytic leukemia of B-cell type NOS
    - **C91.31   Prolymphocytic leukemia of B-cell type, in remission**
    - **C91.32   Prolymphocytic leukemia of B-cell type, in relapse**
  - **C91.4   Hairy cell leukemia**
    - *Chronic leukemia with splenomegaly and excessive number of abnormal large mononuclear cells covered by hairlike villi*
    - Leukemic reticuloendotheliosis
    - **C91.40   Hairy cell leukemia not having achieved remission**
      - Hairy cell leukemia with failed remission
      - Hairy cell leukemia NOS
    - **C91.41   Hairy cell leukemia, in remission**
    - **C91.42   Hairy cell leukemia, in relapse**

- **C91.5   Adult T-cell lymphoma/leukemia (HTLV-1-associated)**
  - Acute variant of adult T-cell lymphoma/leukemia (HTLV-1-associated)
  - Chronic variant of adult T-cell lymphoma/leukemia (HTLV-1-associated)
  - Lymphomatoid variant of adult T-cell lymphoma/leukemia (HTLV-1-associated)
  - Smouldering variant of adult T-cell lymphoma/leukemia (HTLV-1-associated)
  - **C91.50   Adult T-cell lymphoma/leukemia (HTLV-1-associated) not having achieved remission**   A
    - Adult T-cell lymphoma/leukemia (HTLV-1-associated) with failed remission
    - Adult T-cell lymphoma/leukemia (HTLV-1-associated) NOS
  - **C91.51   Adult T-cell lymphoma/leukemia (HTLV-1-associated), in remission**   A
  - **C91.52   Adult T-cell lymphoma/leukemia (HTLV-1-associated), in relapse**   A
- **C91.6   Prolymphocytic leukemia of T-cell type**
  - **C91.60   Prolymphocytic leukemia of T-cell type not having achieved remission**
    - Prolymphocytic leukemia of T-cell type with failed remission
    - Prolymphocytic leukemia of T-cell type NOS
  - **C91.61   Prolymphocytic leukemia of T-cell type, in remission**
  - **C91.62   Prolymphocytic leukemia of T-cell type, in relapse**
- **C91.A   Mature B-cell leukemia Burkitt-type**
  - **Excludes1**   Burkitt lymphoma (C83.7-)
  - **C91.A0   Mature B-cell leukemia Burkitt-type not having achieved remission**
    - Mature B-cell leukemia Burkitt-type with failed remission
    - Mature B-cell leukemia Burkitt-type NOS
  - **C91.A1   Mature B-cell leukemia Burkitt-type, in remission**
  - **C91.A2   Mature B-cell leukemia Burkitt-type, in relapse**
- **C91.Z   Other lymphoid leukemia**
  - T-cell large granular lymphocytic leukemia (associated with rheumatoid arthritis)
  - **C91.Z0   Other lymphoid leukemia not having achieved remission**
    - Other lymphoid leukemia with failed remission
    - Other lymphoid leukemia NOS
  - **C91.Z1   Other lymphoid leukemia, in remission**
  - **C91.Z2   Other lymphoid leukemia, in relapse**
- **C91.9   Lymphoid leukemia, unspecified**
  - **C91.90   Lymphoid leukemia, unspecified not having achieved remission**
    - Lymphoid leukemia with failed remission
    - Lymphoid leukemia NOS
  - **C91.91   Lymphoid leukemia, unspecified, in remission**
  - **C91.92   Lymphoid leukemia, unspecified, in relapse**

Item 2-9 Leukemia is a cancer (acute or chronic) of the blood-forming tissues of the bone marrow. Blood cells all start out as stem cells. They mature and become red cells, white cells, or platelets. There are three main types of leukocytes (white cells that fight infection): monocytes, lymphocytes, and granulocytes. **Acute monocytic leukemia** (AML) affects monocytes. **Acute lymphoid leukemia** (ALL) affects lymphocytes, and **acute myeloid leukemia** (AML) affects cells that typically develop into white blood cells (not lymphocytes), though it may develop in other blood cells.

- **C92   Myeloid leukemia**
  - **Includes**   granulocytic leukemia
  - myelogenous leukemia
  - **Excludes1**   personal history of leukemia (Z85.6)
  - **C92.0   Acute myeloblastic leukemia**
    - Acute myeloblastic leukemia, minimal differentiation
    - Acute myeloblastic leukemia (with maturation)
    - Acute myeloblastic leukemia 1/ETO
    - Acute myeloblastic leukemia MØ
    - Acute myeloblastic leukemia M1
    - Acute myeloblastic leukemia M2
    - Acute myeloblastic leukemia with t(8;21)
    - Acute myeloblastic leukemia (without a FAB classification) NOS
    - Refractory anemia with excess blasts in transformation [RAEB T]
      - **Excludes1**   acute exacerbation of chronic myeloid leukemia (C92.1Ø)
      - refractory anemia with excess of blasts not in transformation (D46.2-)
    - **C92.00   Acute myeloblastic leukemia, not having achieved remission**
      - Acute myeloblastic leukemia with failed remission
      - Acute myeloblastic leukemia NOS
    - **C92.Ø1   Acute myeloblastic leukemia, in remission**
    - **C92.Ø2   Acute myeloblastic leukemia, in relapse**
  - **C92.1   Chronic myeloid leukemia, BCR/ABL-positive**
    - Chronic myelogenous leukemia, Philadelphia chromosome (Ph1) positive
    - Chronic myelogenous leukemia, t(9;22) (q34;q11)
    - Chronic myelogenous leukemia with crisis of blast cells
      - **Excludes1**   atypical chronic myeloid leukemia BCR/ABL-negative (C92.2-)
      - chronic myelomonocytic leukemia (C93.1-)
      - chronic myeloproliferative disease (D47.1)
    - **C92.1Ø   Chronic myeloid leukemia, BCR/ABL-positive, not having achieved remission**
      - Chronic myeloid leukemia, BCR/ABL-positive with failed remission
      - Chronic myeloid leukemia, BCR/ABL-positive NOS
    - **C92.11   Chronic myeloid leukemia, BCR/ABL-positive, in remission**
    - **C92.12   Chronic myeloid leukemia, BCR/ABL-positive, in relapse**
  - **C92.2   Atypical chronic myeloid leukemia, BCR/ABL-negative**
    - **C92.2Ø   Atypical chronic myeloid leukemia, BCR/ABL-negative, not having achieved remission**
      - Atypical chronic myeloid leukemia, BCR/ABL-negative with failed remission
      - Atypical chronic myeloid leukemia, BCR/ABL-negative NOS
    - **C92.21   Atypical chronic myeloid leukemia, BCR/ABL-negative, in remission**
    - **C92.22   Atypical chronic myeloid leukemia, BCR/ABL-negative, in relapse**
  - **C92.3   Myeloid sarcoma**
    - A malignant tumor of immature myeloid cells
    - Chloroma
    - Granulocytic sarcoma
    - **C92.3Ø   Myeloid sarcoma, not having achieved remission**
      - Myeloid sarcoma with failed remission
      - Myeloid sarcoma NOS
    - **C92.31   Myeloid sarcoma, in remission**
    - **C92.32   Myeloid sarcoma, in relapse**
  - **C92.4   Acute promyelocytic leukemia**
    - AML M3
    - AML Me with t(15;17) and variants
    - **C92.4Ø   Acute promyelocytic leukemia, not having achieved remission**
      - Acute promyelocytic leukemia with failed remission
      - Acute promyelocytic leukemia NOS
    - **C92.41   Acute promyelocytic leukemia, in remission**
    - **C92.42   Acute promyelocytic leukemia, in relapse**
  - **C92.5   Acute myelomonocytic leukemia**
    - AML M4
    - AML M4 Eo with inv(16) or t(16;16)
    - **C92.5Ø   Acute myelomonocytic leukemia, not having achieved remission**
      - Acute myelomonocytic leukemia with failed remission
      - Acute myelomonocytic leukemia NOS
    - **C92.51   Acute myelomonocytic leukemia, in remission**
    - **C92.52   Acute myelomonocytic leukemia, in relapse**
  - **C92.6   Acute myeloid leukemia with 11q23-abnormality**
    - Acute myeloid leukemia with variation of MLL-gene
    - **C92.6Ø   Acute myeloid leukemia with 11q23-abnormality not having achieved remission**
      - Acute myeloid leukemia with 11q23-abnormality with failed remission
      - Acute myeloid leukemia with 11q23-abnormality NOS
    - **C92.61   Acute myeloid leukemia with 11q23-abnormality in remission**
    - **C92.62   Acute myeloid leukemia with 11q23-abnormality in relapse**
  - **C92.A   Acute myeloid leukemia with multilineage dysplasia**
    - Acute myeloid leukemia with dysplasia of remaining hematopoesis and/or myelodysplastic disease in its history
    - **C92.AØ   Acute myeloid leukemia with multilineage dysplasia, not having achieved remission**
      - Acute myeloid leukemia with multilineage dysplasia with failed remission
      - Acute myeloid leukemia with multilineage dysplasia NOS
    - **C92.A1   Acute myeloid leukemia with multilineage dysplasia, in remission**
    - **C92.A2   Acute myeloid leukemia with multilineage dysplasia, in relapse**
  - **C92.Z   Other myeloid leukemia**
    - **C92.ZØ   Other myeloid leukemia not having achieved remission**
      - Myeloid leukemia NEC with failed remission
      - Myeloid leukemia NEC
    - **C92.Z1   Other myeloid leukemia, in remission**
    - **C92.Z2   Other myeloid leukemia, in relapse**
  - **C92.9   Myeloid leukemia, unspecified**
    - **C92.9Ø   Myeloid leukemia, unspecified, not having achieved remission**
      - Myeloid leukemia, unspecified with failed remission
      - Myeloid leukemia, unspecified NOS
    - **C92.91   Myeloid leukemia, unspecified in remission**
    - **C92.92   Myeloid leukemia, unspecified in relapse**

● **C93**   **Monocytic leukemia**
- **Includes**   monocytoid leukemia
- **Excludes1**   personal history of leukemia (Z85.6)

● **C93.0**   **Acute monoblastic/monocytic leukemia**
- AML M5
- AML M5a
- AML M5b

- **C93.00**   **Acute monoblastic/monocytic leukemia, not having achieved remission**
  - Acute monoblastic/monocytic leukemia with failed remission
  - Acute monoblastic/monocytic leukemia NOS
- **C93.01**   **Acute monoblastic/monocytic leukemia, in remission**
- **C93.02**   **Acute monoblastic/monocytic leukemia, in relapse**

● **C93.1**   **Chronic myelomonocytic leukemia**
- Chronic monocytic leukemia
- CMML-1
- CMML-2
- CMML with eosinophilia

- **C93.10**   **Chronic myelomonocytic leukemia not having achieved remission**
  - Chronic myelomonocytic leukemia with failed remission
  - Chronic myelomonocytic leukemia NOS
- **C93.11**   **Chronic myelomonocytic leukemia, in remission**
- **C93.12**   **Chronic myelomonocytic leukemia, in relapse**

● **C93.3**   **Juvenile myelomonocytic leukemia**
- **C93.30**   **Juvenile myelomonocytic leukemia, not having achieved remission**   P
  - Juvenile myelomonocytic leukemia with failed remission
  - Juvenile myelomonocytic leukemia NOS
- **C93.31**   **Juvenile myelomonocytic leukemia, in remission**   P
- **C93.32**   **Juvenile myelomonocytic leukemia, in relapse** P

● **C93.Z**   **Other monocytic leukemia**
- **C93.Z0**   **Other monocytic leukemia, not having achieved remission**
  - Other monocytic leukemia NOS
- **C93.Z1**   **Other monocytic leukemia, in remission**
- **C93.Z2**   **Other monocytic leukemia, in relapse**

● **C93.9**   **Monocytic leukemia, unspecified**
- **C93.90**   **Monocytic leukemia, unspecified, not having achieved remission**
  - Monocytic leukemia, unspecified with failed remission
  - Monocytic leukemia, unspecified NOS
- **C93.91**   **Monocytic leukemia, unspecified in remission**
- **C93.92**   **Monocytic leukemia, unspecified in relapse**

● **C94**   **Other leukemias of specified cell type**
- **Excludes1**   leukemic reticuloendotheliosis (C91.4-)
  - myelodysplastic syndromes (D46.-)
  - personal history of leukemia (Z85.6)
  - plasma cell leukemia (C90.1-)

● **C94.0**   **Acute erythroid leukemia**
- Acute myeloid leukemia M6(a)(b)
- Erythroleukemia

- **C94.00**   **Acute erythroid leukemia, not having achieved remission**
  - Acute erythroid leukemia with failed remission
  - Acute erythroid leukemia NOS
- **C94.01**   **Acute erythroid leukemia, in remission**
- **C94.02**   **Acute erythroid leukemia, in relapse**

● **C94.2**   **Acute megakaryoblastic leukemia**
- Acute myeloid leukemia M7
- Acute megakaryocytic leukemia

- **C94.20**   **Acute megakaryoblastic leukemia not having achieved remission**
  - Acute megakaryoblastic leukemia with failed remission ◄▥
  - Acute megakaryoblastic leukemia NOS
- **C94.21**   **Acute megakaryoblastic leukemia, in remission**
- **C94.22**   **Acute megakaryoblastic leukemia, in relapse**

● **C94.3**   **Mast cell leukemia**
- **C94.30**   **Mast cell leukemia not having achieved remission**
  - Mast cell leukemia with failed remission
  - Mast cell leukemia NOS
- **C94.31**   **Mast cell leukemia, in remission**
- **C94.32**   **Mast cell leukemia, in relapse**

● **C94.4**   **Acute panmyelosis with myelofibrosis**
- Acute myelofibrosis
- **Excludes1**   myelofibrosis NOS (D75.81)
  - secondary myelofibrosis NOS (D75.81)

- **C94.40**   **Acute panmyelosis with myelofibrosis not having achieved remission**
  - Acute myelofibrosis NOS
  - Acute panmyelosis with myelofibrosis with failed remission
  - Acute panmyelosis NOS
- **C94.41**   **Acute panmyelosis with myelofibrosis, in remission**
- **C94.42**   **Acute panmyelosis with myelofibrosis, in relapse**

- **C94.6**   **Myelodysplastic disease, not classified**
  - Myeloproliferative disease, not classified

● **C94.8**   **Other specified leukemias**
- Aggressive NK-cell leukemia
- Acute basophilic leukemia

- **C94.80**   **Other specified leukemias not having achieved remission**
  - Other specified leukemia with failed remission
  - Other specified leukemias NOS
- **C94.81**   **Other specified leukemias, in remission**
- **C94.82**   **Other specified leukemias, in relapse**

● **C95**   **Leukemia of unspecified cell type**
- **Excludes1**   personal history of leukemia (Z85.6)

● **C95.0**   **Acute leukemia of unspecified cell type**
- Acute bilineal leukemia
- Acute mixed lineage leukemia
- Biphenotypic acute leukemia
- Stem cell leukemia of unclear lineage
- **Excludes1**   acute exacerbation of unspecified chronic leukemia (C95.10)

- **C95.00**   **Acute leukemia of unspecified cell type not having achieved remission**
  - Acute leukemia of unspecified cell type with failed remission
  - Acute leukemia NOS
- **C95.01**   **Acute leukemia of unspecified cell type, in remission**
- **C95.02**   **Acute leukemia of unspecified cell type, in relapse**

● **C95.1**   **Chronic leukemia of unspecified cell type**
- **C95.10**   **Chronic leukemia of unspecified cell type not having achieved remission**
  - Chronic leukemia of unspecified cell type with failed remission
  - Chronic leukemia NOS
- **C95.11**   **Chronic leukemia of unspecified cell type, in remission**
- **C95.12**   **Chronic leukemia of unspecified cell type, in relapse**

◄ New   ◄▥ Revised   ~~deleted~~ Deleted   Excludes 1   Excludes 2   Includes   Use additional   Code first   Code also   Unspecified

694   OGCR Official Guidelines   X Assign placeholder X   ● Use Additional Character(s)   ▶ Manifestation Code   **Coding Clinic**

● C95.9 **Leukemia, unspecified**

    C95.90   **Leukemia, unspecified not having achieved remission**
          Leukemia, unspecified with failed remission
          Leukemia NOS

    C95.91   **Leukemia, unspecified, in remission**

    C95.92   **Leukemia, unspecified, in relapse**

● C96 **Other and unspecified malignant neoplasms of lymphoid, hematopoietic and related tissue**

    Excludes1   personal history of other malignant neoplasms of lymphoid, hematopoietic and related tissues (Z85.79)

    C96.0 **Multifocal and multisystemic (disseminated) Langerhans-cell histiocytosis**
        Histiocytosis X, multisystemic
        Letterer-Siwe disease

        Excludes1   adult pulmonary Langerhans cell histiocytosis (J84.82)
                multifocal and unisystemic Langerhans-cell histiocytosis (C96.5)
                unifocal Langerhans-cell histiocytosis (C96.6)

    C96.2 **Malignant mast cell tumor**
        Aggressive systemic mastocytosis
        Mast cell sarcoma

        Excludes1   indolent mastocytosis (D47.0)
                mast cell leukemia (C94.30)
                mastocytosis (congenital) (cutaneous) (Q82.2)

    C96.4 **Sarcoma of dendritic cells (accessory cells)**
        Follicular dendritic cell sarcoma
        Interdigitating dendritic cell sarcoma
        Langerhans cell sarcoma

    C96.5 **Multifocal and unisystemic Langerhans-cell histiocytosis**
        Hand-Schüller-Christian disease
        Histiocytosis X, multifocal

        Excludes1   multifocal and multisystemic (disseminated) Langerhans-cell histiocytosis (C96.0)
                unifocal Langerhans-cell histiocytosis (C96.6)

    C96.6 **Unifocal Langerhans-cell histiocytosis**
        Eosinophilic granuloma
        Histiocytosis X, unifocal
        Histiocytosis X NOS
        Langerhans-cell histiocytosis NOS

        Excludes1   multifocal and multisysemic (disseminated) Langerhans-cell histiocytosis (C96.0)
                multifocal and unisystemic Langerhans-cell histiocytosis (C96.5)

    C96.A **Histiocytic sarcoma**
        Malignant histiocytosis

    C96.Z **Other specified malignant neoplasms of lymphoid, hematopoietic and related tissue**

    C96.9 **Malignant neoplasm of lymphoid, hematopoietic and related tissue, unspecified**

    In situ is carcinoma involving cells in localized tissues that has not spread to nearby tissues

---

IN SITU NEOPLASMS (D00-D09)

    Includes   Bowen's disease
               erythroplasia
               grade III intraepithelial neoplasia
               Queyrat's erythroplasia

● D00 **Carcinoma in situ of oral cavity, esophagus and stomach**

    Excludes1   melanoma in situ (D03.-)

  ● D00.0 **Carcinoma in situ of lip, oral cavity and pharynx**
        Use additional code to identify:
        exposure to environmental tobacco smoke (Z77.22)
        exposure to tobacco smoke in the perinatal period (P96.81)
        history of tobacco dependence (Z87.891) ◀▦
        occupational exposure to environmental tobacco smoke (Z57.31)
        tobacco dependence (F17.-)
        tobacco use (Z72.0)

        Excludes1   carcinoma in situ of aryepiglottic fold or interarytenoid fold, laryngeal aspect (D02.0)
                carcinoma in situ of epiglottis NOS (D02.0)
                carcinoma in situ of epiglottis suprahyoid portion (D02.0)
                carcinoma in situ of skin of lip (D03.0, D04.0)

      D00.00   **Carcinoma in situ of oral cavity, unspecified site**

      D00.01   **Carcinoma in situ of labial mucosa and vermilion border**

      D00.02   **Carcinoma in situ of buccal mucosa**

      D00.03   **Carcinoma in situ of gingiva and edentulous alveolar ridge**

      D00.04   **Carcinoma in situ of soft palate**

      D00.05   **Carcinoma in situ of hard palate**

      D00.06   **Carcinoma in situ of floor of mouth**

      D00.07   **Carcinoma in situ of tongue**

      D00.08   **Carcinoma in situ of pharynx**
          Carcinoma in situ of aryepiglottic fold NOS
          Carcinoma in situ of hypopharyngeal aspect of aryepiglottic fold
          Carcinoma in situ of marginal zone of aryepiglottic fold

    D00.1 **Carcinoma in situ of esophagus**

    D00.2 **Carcinoma in situ of stomach**

● D01 **Carcinoma in situ of other and unspecified digestive organs**

    Excludes1   melanoma in situ (D03.-)

    D01.0 **Carcinoma in situ of colon**

        Excludes1   carcinoma in situ of rectosigmoid junction (D01.1)

    D01.1 **Carcinoma in situ of rectosigmoid junction**

    D01.2 **Carcinoma in situ of rectum**

    D01.3 **Carcinoma in situ of anus and anal canal**
        Anal intraepithelial neoplasia III [AIN III] ◀
        Severe dysplasia of anus ◀

        Excludes1   anal intraepithelial neoplasia I and II [AIN I and AIN II] (K62.82) ◀
                carcinoma in situ of anal margin (D04.5)
                carcinoma in situ of anal skin (D04.5)
                carcinoma in situ of perianal skin (D04.5)

  ● D01.4 **Carcinoma in situ of other and unspecified parts of intestine**

        Excludes1   carcinoma in situ of ampulla of Vater (D01.5)

      D01.40   **Carcinoma in situ of unspecified part of intestine**

      D01.49   **Carcinoma in situ of other parts of intestine**

D01.5 Carcinoma in situ of liver, gallbladder and bile ducts
Carcinoma in situ of ampulla of Vater

D01.7 Carcinoma in situ of other specified digestive organs
Carcinoma in situ of pancreas

D01.9 Carcinoma in situ of digestive organ, unspecified

● **D02 Carcinoma in situ of middle ear and respiratory system**
Use additional code to identify:
exposure to environmental tobacco smoke (Z77.22)
exposure to tobacco smoke in the perinatal period (P96.81)
history of tobacco dependence (Z87.891) ◄▥
occupational exposure to environmental tobacco smoke (Z57.31)
tobacco dependence (F17.-)
tobacco use (Z72.0)
Excludes1   melanoma in situ (D03.-)

D02.0 Carcinoma in situ of larynx
Carcinoma in situ of aryepiglottic fold or interarytenoid fold, laryngeal aspect
Carcinoma in situ of epiglottis (suprahyoid portion)
Excludes1   carcinoma in situ of aryepiglottic fold or interarytenoid fold NOS (D00.08)
carcinoma in situ of hypopharyngeal aspect (D00.08)
carcinoma in situ of marginal zone (D00.08)

D02.1 Carcinoma in situ of trachea

● **D02.2 Carcinoma in situ of bronchus and lung**
D02.20 Carcinoma in situ of unspecified bronchus and lung
D02.21 Carcinoma in situ of right bronchus and lung
D02.22 Carcinoma in situ of left bronchus and lung

D02.3 Carcinoma in situ of other parts of respiratory system
Carcinoma in situ of accessory sinuses
Carcinoma in situ of middle ear
Carcinoma in situ of nasal cavities
Excludes1   carcinoma in situ of ear (external) (skin) (D04.2-)
carcinoma in situ of nose NOS (D09.8)
carcinoma in situ of skin of nose (D04.3)

D02.4 Carcinoma in situ of respiratory system, unspecified

● **D03 Melanoma in situ**
D03.0 Melanoma in situ of lip

● **D03.1 Melanoma in situ of eyelid, including canthus**
D03.10 Melanoma in situ of unspecified eyelid, including canthus
D03.11 Melanoma in situ of right eyelid, including canthus
D03.12 Melanoma in situ of left eyelid, including canthus

● **D03.2 Melanoma in situ of ear and external auricular canal**
D03.20 Melanoma in situ of unspecified ear and external auricular canal
D03.21 Melanoma in situ of right ear and external auricular canal
D03.22 Melanoma in situ of left ear and external auricular canal

● **D03.3 Melanoma in situ of other and unspecified parts of face**
D03.30 Melanoma in situ of unspecified part of face
D03.39 Melanoma in situ of other parts of face

D03.4 Melanoma in situ of scalp and neck

● **D03.5 Melanoma in situ of trunk**
D03.51 Melanoma in situ of anal skin
Melanoma in situ of anal margin
Melanoma in situ of perianal skin
D03.52 Melanoma in situ of breast (skin) (soft tissue)
D03.59 Melanoma in situ of other part of trunk

● **D03.6 Melanoma in situ of upper limb, including shoulder**
D03.60 Melanoma in situ of unspecified upper limb, including shoulder
D03.61 Melanoma in situ of right upper limb, including shoulder
D03.62 Melanoma in situ of left upper limb, including shoulder

● **D03.7 Melanoma in situ of lower limb, including hip**
D03.70 Melanoma in situ of unspecified lower limb, including hip ◄▥
D03.71 Melanoma in situ of right lower limb, including hip
D03.72 Melanoma in situ of left lower limb, including hip

D03.8 Melanoma in situ of other sites
Melanoma in situ of scrotum
Excludes1   carcinoma in situ of scrotum (D07.61)

D03.9 Melanoma in situ, unspecified

● **D04 Carcinoma in situ of skin**
Excludes1   erythroplasia of Queyrat (penis) NOS (D07.4)
melanoma in situ (D03.-)

D04.0 Carcinoma in situ of skin of lip
Excludes1   carcinoma in situ of vermilion border of lip (D00.01)

● **D04.1 Carcinoma in situ of skin of eyelid, including canthus**
D04.10 Carcinoma in situ of skin of unspecified eyelid, including canthus
D04.11 Carcinoma in situ of skin of right eyelid, including canthus
D04.12 Carcinoma in situ of skin of left eyelid, including canthus

● **D04.2 Carcinoma in situ of skin of ear and external auricular canal**
D04.20 Carcinoma in situ of skin of unspecified ear and external auricular canal
D04.21 Carcinoma in situ of skin of right ear and external auricular canal
D04.22 Carcinoma in situ of skin of left ear and external auricular canal

● **D04.3 Carcinoma in situ of skin of other and unspecified parts of face**
D04.30 Carcinoma in situ of skin of unspecified part of face
D04.39 Carcinoma in situ of skin of other parts of face

D04.4 Carcinoma in situ of skin of scalp and neck

D04.5 Carcinoma in situ of skin of trunk
Carcinoma in situ of anal margin
Carcinoma in situ of anal skin
Carcinoma in situ of perianal skin
Carcinoma in situ of skin of breast
Excludes1   carcinoma in situ of anus NOS (D01.3)
carcinoma in situ of scrotum (D07.61)
carcinoma in situ of skin of genital organs (D07.-)

● **D04.6 Carcinoma in situ of skin of upper limb, including shoulder**
D04.60 Carcinoma in situ of skin of unspecified upper limb, including shoulder
D04.61 Carcinoma in situ of skin of right upper limb, including shoulder
D04.62 Carcinoma in situ of skin of left upper limb, including shoulder

● **D04.7 Carcinoma in situ of skin of lower limb, including hip**
   D04.70 Carcinoma in situ of skin of unspecified lower limb, including hip
   D04.71 Carcinoma in situ of skin of right lower limb, including hip
   D04.72 Carcinoma in situ of skin of left lower limb, including hip
D04.8 Carcinoma in situ of skin of other sites
D04.9 Carcinoma in situ of skin, unspecified

● **D05 Carcinoma in situ of breast**
   Excludes1 carcinoma in situ of skin of breast (D04.5)
   melanoma in situ of breast (skin) (D03.5)
   Paget's disease of breast or nipple (C50.-)
● **D05.0 Lobular carcinoma in situ of breast**
   D05.00 Lobular carcinoma in situ of unspecified breast
   D05.01 Lobular carcinoma in situ of right breast
   D05.02 Lobular carcinoma in situ of left breast
● **D05.1 Intraductal carcinoma in situ of breast**
   D05.10 Intraductal carcinoma in situ of unspecified breast
   D05.11 Intraductal carcinoma in situ of right breast
   D05.12 Intraductal carcinoma in situ of left breast
● **D05.8 Other specified type of carcinoma in situ of breast**
   D05.80 Other specified type of carcinoma in situ of unspecified breast
   D05.81 Other specified type of carcinoma in situ of right breast
   D05.82 Other specified type of carcinoma in situ of left breast
● **D05.9 Unspecified type of carcinoma in situ of breast**
   D05.90 Unspecified type of carcinoma in situ of unspecified breast
   D05.91 Unspecified type of carcinoma in situ of right breast
   D05.92 Unspecified type of carcinoma in situ of left breast

● **D06 Carcinoma in situ of cervix uteri**
   Includes cervical adenocarcinoma in situ
   cervical intraepithelial glandular neoplasia
   cervical intraepithelial neoplasia III [CIN III]
   severe dysplasia of cervix uteri
   Excludes1 cervical intraepithelial neoplasia II [CIN II] (N87.1)
   cytologic evidence of malignancy of cervix without histologic confirmation (R87.614)
   high grade squamous intraepithelial lesion (HGSIL) of cervix (R87.613)
   melanoma in situ of cervix (D03.5)
   moderate cervical dysplasia (N87.1)
   D06.0 Carcinoma in situ of endocervix ♀
   D06.1 Carcinoma in situ of exocervix ♀
   D06.7 Carcinoma in situ of other parts of cervix ♀
   D06.9 Carcinoma in situ of cervix, unspecified ♀

● **D07 Carcinoma in situ of other and unspecified genital organs**
   Excludes1 melanoma in situ of trunk (D03.5)
   D07.0 Carcinoma in situ of endometrium ♀
   D07.1 Carcinoma in situ of vulva ♀
   Severe dysplasia of vulva
   Vulvar intraepithelial neoplasia III [VIN III]
   Excludes1 moderate dysplasia of vulva (N90.1)
   vulvar intraepithelial neoplasia II [VIN II] (N90.1)
   D07.2 Carcinoma in situ of vagina ♀
   Severe dysplasia of vagina
   Vaginal intraepithelial neoplasia III [VIN III]
   Excludes1 moderate dysplasia of vagina (N89.1)
   vaginal intraepithelial neoplasia II [VIN II] (N89.1)

● **D07.3 Carcinoma in situ of other and unspecified female genital organs**
   D07.30 Carcinoma in situ of unspecified female genital organs ♀
   D07.39 Carcinoma in situ of other female genital organs ♀
D07.4 Carcinoma in situ of penis ♂
   Erythroplasia of Queyrat NOS
D07.5 Carcinoma in situ of prostate ♂
   Prostatic intraepithelial neoplasia III (PIN III)
   Severe dysplasia of prostate
   Excludes1 dysplasia (mild) (moderate) of prostate (N42.3-) ◀
   prostatic intraepithelial neoplasia II [PIN II] (N42.3-) ◀
● **D07.6 Carcinoma in situ of other and unspecified male genital organs**
   D07.60 Carcinoma in situ of unspecified male genital organs ♂
   D07.61 Carcinoma in situ of scrotum ♂
   D07.69 Carcinoma in situ of other male genital organs ♂

● **D09 Carcinoma in situ of other and unspecified sites**
   Excludes1 melanoma in situ (D03.-)
D09.0 Carcinoma in situ of bladder
● **D09.1 Carcinoma in situ of other and unspecified urinary organs**
   D09.10 Carcinoma in situ of unspecified urinary organ
   D09.19 Carcinoma in situ of other urinary organs
● **D09.2 Carcinoma in situ of eye**
   Excludes1 carcinoma in situ of skin of eyelid (D04.1-)
   D09.20 Carcinoma in situ of unspecified eye
   D09.21 Carcinoma in situ of right eye
   D09.22 Carcinoma in situ of left eye
D09.3 Carcinoma in situ of thyroid and other endocrine glands
   Excludes1 carcinoma in situ of endocrine pancreas (D01.7)
   carcinoma in situ of ovary (D07.39)
   carcinoma in situ of testis (D07.69)
D09.8 Carcinoma in situ of other specified sites
D09.9 Carcinoma in situ, unspecified

BENIGN NEOPLASMS, EXCEPT BENIGN NEUROENDOCRINE TUMORS (D10-D36)

● **D10 Benign neoplasm of mouth and pharynx**
   D10.0 Benign neoplasm of lip
   Benign neoplasm of lip (frenulum) (inner aspect) (mucosa) (vermilion border)
   Excludes1 benign neoplasm of skin of lip (D22.0, D23.0)
   D10.1 Benign neoplasm of tongue
   Benign neoplasm of lingual tonsil
   D10.2 Benign neoplasm of floor of mouth
● **D10.3 Benign neoplasm of other and unspecified parts of mouth ◀**
   D10.30 Benign neoplasm of unspecified part of mouth
   D10.39 Benign neoplasm of other parts of mouth
   Benign neoplasm of minor salivary gland NOS
   Excludes1 benign odontogenic neoplasms (D16.4-D16.5)
   benign neoplasm of mucosa of lip (D10.0)
   benign neoplasm of nasopharyngeal surface of soft palate (D10.6)

CHAPTER 2 (C00-D49)

Figure 2-16 The esophagus is the muscular tube that connects the pharynx and the stomach. The 10 inch (25 cm) long esophagus is divided into three parts: **cervical, thoracic,** and **abdominal.**

D10.4   Benign neoplasm of tonsil
Benign neoplasm of tonsil (faucial) (palatine)

> **Excludes1**   benign neoplasm of lingual tonsil (D10.1)
> benign neoplasm of pharyngeal tonsil (D10.6)
> benign neoplasm of tonsillar fossa (D10.5)
> benign neoplasm of tonsillar pillars (D10.5)

D10.5   Benign neoplasm of other parts of oropharynx
Division of pharynx lying between soft palate and upper edge of epiglottis
Benign neoplasm of epiglottis, anterior aspect
Benign neoplasm of tonsillar fossa
Benign neoplasm of tonsillar pillars
Benign neoplasm of vallecula

> **Excludes1**   benign neoplasm of epiglottis NOS (D14.1)
> benign neoplasm of epiglottis, suprahyoid portion (D14.1)

D10.6   Benign neoplasm of nasopharynx
Segment of pharynx that lies above soft palate
Benign neoplasm of pharyngeal tonsil
Benign neoplasm of posterior margin of septum and choanae

D10.7   Benign neoplasm of hypopharynx
Segment of pharynx that lies below upper edge of epiglottis and opens into larynx and esophagus

D10.9   Benign neoplasm of pharynx, unspecified

● **D11   Benign neoplasm of major salivary glands**

> **Excludes1**   benign neoplasms of specified minor salivary glands which are classified according to their anatomical location
> benign neoplasms of minor salivary glands NOS (D10.39)

D11.0   Benign neoplasm of parotid gland

D11.7   Benign neoplasm of other major salivary glands
Benign neoplasm of sublingual salivary gland
Benign neoplasm of submandibular salivary gland

D11.9   Benign neoplasm of major salivary gland, unspecified

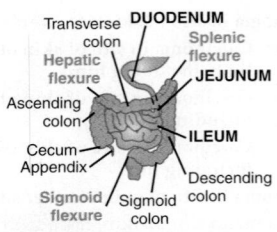

Figure 2-17 Small intestine and colon.

● **D12   Benign neoplasm of colon, rectum, anus and anal canal**

> **Excludes1**   benign carcinoid tumors of the large intestine, and rectum (D3A.02-)

Coding Clinic: 2015, Q2, P14

D12.0   Benign neoplasm of cecum
Benign neoplasm of ileocecal valve

D12.1   Benign neoplasm of appendix

> **Excludes1**   benign carcinoid tumor of the appendix (D3A.020)

D12.2   Benign neoplasm of ascending colon

D12.3   Benign neoplasm of transverse colon
Benign neoplasm of hepatic flexure
Benign neoplasm of splenic flexure
Flexure is a bending in a structure or organ. Note the three flexures illustrated in Figure 2–17. Hepatic = liver, sigmoid = colon, splenic = spleen.

D12.4   Benign neoplasm of descending colon
Coding Clinic: 2015, Q2, P14

D12.5   Benign neoplasm of sigmoid colon

D12.6   Benign neoplasm of colon, unspecified
Adenomatosis of colon
Benign neoplasm of large intestine NOS
Polyposis (hereditary) of colon

> **Excludes1**   inflammatory polyp of colon (K51.4-)
> polyp of colon NOS (K63.5)

D12.7   Benign neoplasm of rectosigmoid junction
Angle where sigmoid colon becomes rectum

D12.8   Benign neoplasm of rectum

> **Excludes1**   benign carcinoid tumor of the rectum (D3A.026)

D12.9   Benign neoplasm of anus and anal canal
Benign neoplasm of anus NOS

> **Excludes1**   benign neoplasm of anal margin (D22.5, D23.5)
> benign neoplasm of anal skin (D22.5, D23.5)
> benign neoplasm of perianal skin (D22.5, D23.5)

● **D13   Benign neoplasm of other and ill-defined parts of digestive system**

> **Excludes1**   benign stromal tumors of digestive system (D21.4)

D13.0   Benign neoplasm of esophagus

D13.1   Benign neoplasm of stomach

> **Excludes1**   benign carcinoid tumor of the stomach (D3A.092)

D13.2   Benign neoplasm of duodenum

> **Excludes1**   benign carcinoid tumor of the duodenum (D3A.010)

◀ New   ◀▬ Revised   ~~deleted~~ Deleted   Excludes 1   Excludes 2   Includes   Use additional   Code first   Code also   Unspecified

OGCR Official Guidelines   X Assign placeholder X   ● Use Additional Character(s)   ▶ Manifestation Code   **Coding Clinic**

698

● **D13.3** **Benign neoplasm of other and unspecified parts of small intestine**

> **Excludes1**   benign carcinoid tumors of the small intestine (D3A.Ø1-)
> benign neoplasm of ileocecal valve (D12.Ø)

     D13.3Ø **Benign neoplasm of unspecified part of small intestine**

     D13.39 **Benign neoplasm of other parts of small intestine**

D13.4 **Benign neoplasm of liver**
Benign neoplasm of intrahepatic bile ducts

D13.5 **Benign neoplasm of extrahepatic bile ducts**
Extensions of common hepatic bile duct (tube that collects bile from liver)

D13.6 **Benign neoplasm of pancreas**

> **Excludes1**   benign neoplasm of endocrine pancreas (D13.7)

D13.7 **Benign neoplasm of endocrine pancreas**
Pancreatic islets: Cells scattered throughout pancreas
Islet cell tumor
Benign neoplasm of islets of Langerhans
Use additional code to identify any functional activity.

D13.9 **Benign neoplasm of ill-defined sites within the digestive system**
Benign neoplasm of digestive system NOS
Benign neoplasm of intestine NOS
Benign neoplasm of spleen

● **D14** **Benign neoplasm of middle ear and respiratory system**

     D14.Ø **Benign neoplasm of middle ear, nasal cavity and accessory sinuses**
Benign neoplasm of cartilage of nose

> **Excludes1**   benign neoplasm of auricular canal (external) (D22.2-, D23.2-)
> benign neoplasm of bone of ear (D16.4)
> benign neoplasm of bone of nose (D16.4)
> benign neoplasm of cartilage of ear (D21.Ø)
> benign neoplasm of ear (external) (skin) (D22.2-, D23.2-)
> benign neoplasm of nose NOS (D36.7)
> benign neoplasm of skin of nose (D22.39, D23.39)
> benign neoplasm of olfactory bulb (D33.3)
> benign neoplasm of posterior margin of septum and choanae (D1Ø.6)
> polyp of accessory sinus (J33.8)
> polyp of ear (middle) (H74.4)
> polyp of nasal (cavity) (J33.-)

     D14.1 **Benign neoplasm of larynx**
Adenomatous polyp of larynx
Benign neoplasm of epiglottis (suprahyoid portion)
Horseshoe shaped bone in anterior midline of neck between chin and thyroid cartilage

> **Excludes1**   benign neoplasm of epiglottis, anterior aspect (D1Ø.5)
> polyp (nonadenomatous) of vocal cord or larynx (J38.1)

     D14.2 **Benign neoplasm of trachea**

● **D14.3** **Benign neoplasm of bronchus and lung**

> **Excludes1**   benign carcinoid tumor of the bronchus and lung (D3A.Ø9Ø)

     D14.3Ø **Benign neoplasm of unspecified bronchus and lung**

     D14.31 **Benign neoplasm of right bronchus and lung**

     D14.32 **Benign neoplasm of left bronchus and lung**

     D14.4 **Benign neoplasm of respiratory system, unspecified**

● **D15** **Benign neoplasm of other and unspecified intrathoracic organs**

> **Excludes1**   benign neoplasm of mesothelial tissue (D19.-)

     D15.Ø **Benign neoplasm of thymus**

> **Excludes1**   benign carcinoid tumor of the thymus (D3A.Ø91)

     D15.1 **Benign neoplasm of heart**

> **Excludes1**   benign neoplasm of great vessels (D21.3)

     D15.2 **Benign neoplasm of mediastinum**

     D15.7 **Benign neoplasm of other specified intrathoracic organs**

     D15.9 **Benign neoplasm of intrathoracic organ, unspecified**

● **D16** **Benign neoplasm of bone and articular cartilage**

> **Excludes1**   benign neoplasm of connective tissue of ear (D21.Ø)
> benign neoplasm of connective tissue of eyelid (D21.Ø)
> benign neoplasm of connective tissue of larynx (D14.1)
> benign neoplasm of connective tissue of nose (D14.Ø)
> benign neoplasm of synovia (D21.-)

● **D16.Ø** **Benign neoplasm of scapula and long bones of upper limb**

     D16.ØØ **Benign neoplasm of scapula and long bones of unspecified upper limb**

     D16.Ø1 **Benign neoplasm of scapula and long bones of right upper limb**

     D16.Ø2 **Benign neoplasm of scapula and long bones of left upper limb**

● **D16.1** **Benign neoplasm of short bones of upper limb**

     D16.1Ø **Benign neoplasm of short bones of unspecified upper limb**

     D16.11 **Benign neoplasm of short bones of right upper limb**

     D16.12 **Benign neoplasm of short bones of left upper limb**

● **D16.2** **Benign neoplasm of long bones of lower limb**

     D16.2Ø **Benign neoplasm of long bones of unspecified lower limb**

     D16.21 **Benign neoplasm of long bones of right lower limb**

     D16.22 **Benign neoplasm of long bones of left lower limb**

● **D16.3** **Benign neoplasm of short bones of lower limb**

     D16.3Ø **Benign neoplasm of short bones of unspecified lower limb**

     D16.31 **Benign neoplasm of short bones of right lower limb**

     D16.32 **Benign neoplasm of short bones of left lower limb**

     D16.4 **Benign neoplasm of bones of skull and face**
Benign neoplasm of maxilla (superior)
Benign neoplasm of orbital bone
Cavity or socket of skull in which eye and its appendages are located
Keratocyst of maxilla
Keratocystic odontogenic tumor of maxilla

> **Excludes2**   benign neoplasm of lower jaw bone (D16.5) ◄

     D16.5 **Benign neoplasm of lower jaw bone**
Keratocyst of mandible
Keratocystic odontogenic tumor of mandible

     D16.6 **Benign neoplasm of vertebral column**

> **Excludes1**   benign neoplasm of sacrum and coccyx (D16.8)

     D16.7 **Benign neoplasm of ribs, sternum and clavicle**

     D16.8 **Benign neoplasm of pelvic bones, sacrum and coccyx**

     D16.9 **Benign neoplasm of bone and articular cartilage, unspecified**

CHAPTER 2 (CØØ-D49)

● **D17** **Benign lipomatous neoplasm**
Slow-growing benign tumors (rubbery masses) of mature fat cells enclosed in a thin fibrous capsule

    D17.0 **Benign lipomatous neoplasm of skin and subcutaneous tissue of head, face and neck**

    D17.1 **Benign lipomatous neoplasm of skin and subcutaneous tissue of trunk**

●   **D17.2** **Benign lipomatous neoplasm of skin and subcutaneous tissue of limb**

        D17.20 **Benign lipomatous neoplasm of skin and subcutaneous tissue of** `unspecified` **limb**

        D17.21 **Benign lipomatous neoplasm of skin and subcutaneous tissue of right arm**

        D17.22 **Benign lipomatous neoplasm of skin and subcutaneous tissue of left arm**

        D17.23 **Benign lipomatous neoplasm of skin and subcutaneous tissue of right leg**

        D17.24 **Benign lipomatous neoplasm of skin and subcutaneous tissue of left leg**

●   **D17.3** **Benign lipomatous neoplasm of skin and subcutaneous tissue of other and unspecified sites**

        D17.30 **Benign lipomatous neoplasm of skin and subcutaneous tissue of** `unspecified` **sites**

        D17.39 **Benign lipomatous neoplasm of skin and subcutaneous tissue of other sites**

    D17.4 **Benign lipomatous neoplasm of intrathoracic organs**

    D17.5 **Benign lipomatous neoplasm of intra-abdominal organs**

        `Excludes1` benign lipomatous neoplasm of peritoneum and retroperitoneum (D17.79)

    D17.6 **Benign lipomatous neoplasm of spermatic cord ♂**

●   **D17.7** **Benign lipomatous neoplasm of other sites**

        D17.71 **Benign lipomatous neoplasm of kidney**

        D17.72 **Benign lipomatous neoplasm of other genitourinary organ**

        D17.79 **Benign lipomatous neoplasm of other sites**
            Benign lipomatous neoplasm of peritoneum
            Benign lipomatous neoplasm of retroperitoneum

    D17.9 **Benign lipomatous neoplasm,** `unspecified`
        Lipoma NOS

● **D18** **Hemangioma and lymphangioma, any site**

    `Excludes1` benign neoplasm of glomus jugulare (D35.6)
        blue or pigmented nevus (D22.-)
        nevus NOS (D22.-)
        vascular nevus (Q82.5)

●   **D18.0** **Hemangioma**
Common type of vascular malformation
        Angioma NOS
        Cavernous nevus

        D18.00 **Hemangioma** `unspecified` **site**

        D18.01 **Hemangioma of skin and subcutaneous tissue**

        D18.02 **Hemangioma of intracranial structures**

        D18.03 **Hemangioma of intra-abdominal structures**

        D18.09 **Hemangioma of other sites**

    D18.1 **Lymphangioma, any site**

Item 2–10 **Hemangiomas** are abnormally dense collections of dilated capillaries that occur on the skin or in internal organs. Hemangiomas are both deep and superficial and undergo a rapid growth phase when the size increases rapidly, followed by a rest phase, in which the tumor changes very little, followed by an involutional phase in which the tumor begins to and can disappear altogether. **Lymphangiomas** or cystic hygroma are benign collections of overgrown lymph vessels and, although rare, may occur anywhere but most commonly on the head and neck of children and infants. Visceral organs, lungs, and gastrointestinal tract may also be involved.

● **D19** **Benign neoplasm of mesothelial tissue**
Mesothelial tissue is the membrane lining several body cavities

    D19.0 **Benign neoplasm of mesothelial tissue of pleura**

    D19.1 **Benign neoplasm of mesothelial tissue of peritoneum**

    D19.7 **Benign neoplasm of mesothelial tissue of other sites**

    D19.9 **Benign neoplasm of mesothelial tissue,** `unspecified`
        Benign mesothelioma NOS

● **D20** **Benign neoplasm of soft tissue of retroperitoneum and peritoneum**

    `Excludes1` benign lipomatous neoplasm of peritoneum and retroperitoneum (D17.79)
        benign neoplasm of mesothelial tissue (D19.-)

    D20.0 **Benign neoplasm of soft tissue of retroperitoneum**

    D20.1 **Benign neoplasm of soft tissue of peritoneum**

● **D21** **Other benign neoplasms of connective and other soft tissue**

    `Includes` benign neoplasm of blood vessel
        benign neoplasm of bursa
        benign neoplasm of cartilage
        benign neoplasm of fascia
        benign neoplasm of fat
        benign neoplasm of ligament, except uterine
        benign neoplasm of lymphatic channel
        benign neoplasm of muscle
        benign neoplasm of synovia
        benign neoplasm of tendon (sheath)
        benign stromal tumors

    `Excludes1` benign neoplasm of articular cartilage (D16.-)
        benign neoplasm of cartilage of larynx (D14.1)
        benign neoplasm of cartilage of nose (D14.0)
        benign neoplasm of connective tissue of breast (D24.-)
        benign neoplasm of peripheral nerves and autonomic nervous system (D36.1-)
        benign neoplasm of peritoneum (D20.1)
        benign neoplasm of retroperitoneum (D20.0)
        benign neoplasm of uterine ligament, any (D28.2)
        benign neoplasm of vascular tissue (D18.-)
        hemangioma (D18.0-)
        lipomatous neoplasm (D17.-)
        lymphangioma (D18.1)
        uterine leiomyoma (D25.-)

    D21.0 **Benign neoplasm of connective and other soft tissue of head, face and neck**
        Benign neoplasm of connective tissue of ear
        Benign neoplasm of connective tissue of eyelid

        `Excludes1` benign neoplasm of connective tissue of orbit (D31.6-)

●   **D21.1** **Benign neoplasm of connective and other soft tissue of upper limb, including shoulder**

        D21.10 **Benign neoplasm of connective and other soft tissue of** `unspecified` **upper limb, including shoulder**

        D21.11 **Benign neoplasm of connective and other soft tissue of right upper limb, including shoulder**

        D21.12 **Benign neoplasm of connective and other soft tissue of left upper limb, including shoulder**

Figure 2-18 Hemangioma of skin and subcutaneous tissue. (From Yanoff: Ophthalmology, ed 3, Mosby, Inc., 2008)

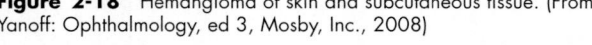

◄ New   ◄ Revised   ~~deleted~~ Deleted   Excludes 1   Excludes 2   Includes   Use additional   Code first   Code also   Unspecified
OGCR Official Guidelines   X Assign placeholder X   ● Use Additional Character(s)   ▶ Manifestation Code   **Coding Clinic**

● **D21.2** **Benign neoplasm of connective and other soft tissue of lower limb, including hip**
     D21.20 Benign neoplasm of connective and other soft tissue of unspecified lower limb, including hip
     D21.21 Benign neoplasm of connective and other soft tissue of right lower limb, including hip
     D21.22 Benign neoplasm of connective and other soft tissue of left lower limb, including hip
   D21.3 **Benign neoplasm of connective and other soft tissue of thorax**
     Benign neoplasm of axilla
     Benign neoplasm of diaphragm
     Benign neoplasm of great vessels
     Excludes1 benign neoplasm of heart (D15.1)
         benign neoplasm of mediastinum (D15.2)
         benign neoplasm of thymus (D15.0)
   D21.4 **Benign neoplasm of connective and other soft tissue of abdomen Benign stromal tumors of abdomen**
   D21.5 **Benign neoplasm of connective and other soft tissue of pelvis**
     Excludes1 benign neoplasm of any uterine ligament (D28.2)
         uterine leiomyoma (D25.-)
   D21.6 **Benign neoplasm of connective and other soft tissue of trunk, unspecified**
     Benign neoplasm of back NOS
   D21.9 **Benign neoplasm of connective and other soft tissue, unspecified**

● **D22** **Melanocytic nevi**
     Includes atypical nevus
         blue hairy pigmented nevus
         nevus NOS
   D22.0 **Melanocytic nevi of lip**
     Skin lesions composed of nests of nevus cells with macules/papules
● **D22.1** **Melanocytic nevi of eyelid, including canthus**
     D22.10 Melanocytic nevi of unspecified eyelid, including canthus
     D22.11 Melanocytic nevi of right eyelid, including canthus
     D22.12 Melanocytic nevi of left eyelid, including canthus
● **D22.2** **Melanocytic nevi of ear and external auricular canal**
     D22.20 Melanocytic nevi of unspecified ear and external auricular canal
     D22.21 Melanocytic nevi of right ear and external auricular canal
     D22.22 Melanocytic nevi of left ear and external auricular canal
● **D22.3** **Melanocytic nevi of other and unspecified parts of face**
     D22.30 Melanocytic nevi of unspecified part of face
     D22.39 Melanocytic nevi of other parts of face
   D22.4 **Melanocytic nevi of scalp and neck**
   D22.5 **Melanocytic nevi of trunk**
     Melanocytic nevi of anal margin
     Melanocytic nevi of anal skin
     Melanocytic nevi of perianal skin
     Melanocytic nevi of skin of breast
● **D22.6** **Melanocytic nevi of upper limb, including shoulder**
     D22.60 Melanocytic nevi of unspecified upper limb, including shoulder
     D22.61 Melanocytic nevi of right upper limb, including shoulder
     D22.62 Melanocytic nevi of left upper limb, including shoulder

● **D22.7** **Melanocytic nevi of lower limb, including hip**
     D22.70 Melanocytic nevi of unspecified lower limb, including hip
     D22.71 Melanocytic nevi of right lower limb, including hip
     D22.72 Melanocytic nevi of left lower limb, including hip
   D22.9 **Melanocytic nevi, unspecified**

● **D23** **Other benign neoplasms of skin**
     Includes benign neoplasm of hair follicles
         benign neoplasm of sebaceous glands
         benign neoplasm of sweat glands
     Excludes1 benign lipomatous neoplasms of skin (D17.0-D17.3)
         melanocytic nevi (D22.-)
   D23.0 **Other benign neoplasm of skin of lip**
     Excludes1 benign neoplasm of vermilion border of lip (D10.0)
● **D23.1** **Other benign neoplasm of skin of eyelid, including canthus**
     D23.10 Other benign neoplasm of skin unspecified of eyelid, including canthus
     D23.11 Other benign neoplasm of skin of right eyelid, including canthus
     D23.12 Other benign neoplasm of skin of left eyelid, including canthus
● **D23.2** **Other benign neoplasm of skin of ear and external auricular canal**
     D23.20 Other benign neoplasm of skin of unspecified ear and external auricular canal
     D23.21 Other benign neoplasm of skin of right ear and external auricular canal
     D23.22 Other benign neoplasm of skin of left ear and external auricular canal
● **D23.3** **Other benign neoplasm of skin of other and unspecified parts of face**
     D23.30 Other benign neoplasm of skin of unspecified part of face
     D23.39 Other benign neoplasm of skin of other parts of face
   D23.4 **Other benign neoplasm of skin of scalp and neck**
   D23.5 **Other benign neoplasm of skin of trunk**
     Other benign neoplasm of anal margin
     Other benign neoplasm of anal skin
     Other benign neoplasm of perianal skin
     Other benign neoplasm of skin of breast
     Excludes1 benign neoplasm of anus NOS (D12.9)
● **D23.6** **Other benign neoplasm of skin of upper limb, including shoulder**
     D23.60 Other benign neoplasm of skin of unspecified upper limb, including shoulder
     D23.61 Other benign neoplasm of skin of right upper limb, including shoulder
     D23.62 Other benign neoplasm of skin of left upper limb, including shoulder
● **D23.7** **Other benign neoplasm of skin of lower limb, including hip**
     D23.70 Other benign neoplasm of skin of unspecified lower limb, including hip
     D23.71 Other benign neoplasm of skin of right lower limb, including hip
     D23.72 Other benign neoplasm of skin of left lower limb, including hip
   D23.9 **Other benign neoplasm of skin, unspecified**

CHAPTER 2 (C00-D49)

● **D24 Benign neoplasm of breast**
   Includes benign neoplasm of connective tissue of breast
         benign neoplasm of soft parts of breast
         fibroadenoma of breast
   Excludes2 adenofibrosis of breast (N60.2)
         benign cyst of breast (N60.-)
         benign mammary dysplasia (N60.-)
         benign neoplasm of skin of breast (D22.5, D23.5)
         fibrocystic disease of breast (N60.-)
   D24.1 Benign neoplasm of right breast
   D24.2 Benign neoplasm of left breast
   D24.9 Benign neoplasm of unspecified breast

● **D25 Leiomyoma of uterus**
   Benign tumors or nodules of the uterine wall
   Includes uterine fibroid
         uterine fibromyoma
         uterine myoma
   D25.0 Submucous leiomyoma of uterus ♀
   D25.1 Intramural leiomyoma of uterus ♀
         Interstitial leiomyoma of uterus
   D25.2 Subserosal leiomyoma of uterus ♀
         Subperitoneal leiomyoma of uterus
   D25.9 Leiomyoma of uterus, unspecified ♀

● **D26 Other benign neoplasms of uterus**
   D26.0 Other benign neoplasm of cervix uteri ♀
   D26.1 Other benign neoplasm of corpus uteri ♀
   D26.7 Other benign neoplasm of other parts of uterus ♀
   D26.9 Other benign neoplasm of uterus, unspecified ♀

● **D27 Benign neoplasm of ovary**
   Use additional code to identify any functional activity.
   Excludes2 corpus albicans cyst (N83.2-) ◀
         corpus luteum cyst (N83.1-) ◀
         endometrial cyst (N80.1)
         follicular (atretic) cyst (N83.0-) ◀
         graafian follicle cyst (N83.0-) ◀
         ovarian cyst NEC (N83.2-) ◀
         ovarian retention cyst (N83.2-) ◀
   D27.0 Benign neoplasm of right ovary ♀
   D27.1 Benign neoplasm of left ovary ♀
   D27.9 Benign neoplasm of unspecified ovary ♀

● **D28 Benign neoplasm of other and unspecified female genital organs**
   Includes adenomatous polyp
         benign neoplasm of skin of female genital organs
         benign teratoma
   Excludes1 epoophoron cyst (Q50.5)
         fimbrial cyst (Q50.4)
         Gartner's duct cyst (Q52.4)
         parovarian cyst (Q50.5)
   D28.0 Benign neoplasm of vulva ♀
   D28.1 Benign neoplasm of vagina ♀
   D28.2 Benign neoplasm of uterine tubes and ligaments ♀
         Benign neoplasm of fallopian tube
         Benign neoplasm of uterine ligament (broad) (round)
   D28.7 Benign neoplasm of other specified female genital organs ♀
   D28.9 Benign neoplasm of female genital organ, unspecified ♀

● **D29 Benign neoplasm of male genital organs**
   Includes benign neoplasm of skin of male genital organs
   D29.0 Benign neoplasm of penis ♂
   D29.1 Benign neoplasm of prostate ♂
        Excludes1 enlarged prostate (N40.-)
   ● **D29.2** Benign neoplasm of testis
         Use additional code to identify any functional activity.
        D29.20 Benign neoplasm of unspecified testis ♂
        D29.21 Benign neoplasm of right testis ♂
        D29.22 Benign neoplasm of left testis ♂
   ● **D29.3** Benign neoplasm of epididymis
        D29.30 Benign neoplasm of unspecified epididymis ♂
        D29.31 Benign neoplasm of right epididymis ♂
        D29.32 Benign neoplasm of left epididymis ♂
   D29.4 Benign neoplasm of scrotum ♂
         Benign neoplasm of skin of scrotum
   D29.8 Benign neoplasm of other specified male genital organs ♂
         Benign neoplasm of seminal vesicle
         Benign neoplasm of spermatic cord
         Benign neoplasm of tunica vaginalis
   D29.9 Benign neoplasm of male genital organ, unspecified ♂

● **D30 Benign neoplasm of urinary organs**
   ● **D30.0** Benign neoplasm of kidney
        Excludes1 benign carcinoid tumor of the kidney (D3A.093)
         benign neoplasm of renal calyces (D30.1-)
         benign neoplasm of renal pelvis (D30.1-)
        D30.00 Benign neoplasm of unspecified kidney
        D30.01 Benign neoplasm of right kidney
        D30.02 Benign neoplasm of left kidney
   ● **D30.1** Benign neoplasm of renal pelvis
        D30.10 Benign neoplasm of unspecified renal pelvis
        D30.11 Benign neoplasm of right renal pelvis
        D30.12 Benign neoplasm of left renal pelvis
   ● **D30.2** Benign neoplasm of ureter
        Excludes1 benign neoplasm of ureteric orifice of bladder (D30.3)
        D30.20 Benign neoplasm of unspecified ureter
        D30.21 Benign neoplasm of right ureter
        D30.22 Benign neoplasm of left ureter
   D30.3 Benign neoplasm of bladder
         Benign neoplasm of ureteric orifice of bladder
         Benign neoplasm of urethral orifice of bladder
   D30.4 Benign neoplasm of urethra
        Excludes1 benign neoplasm of urethral orifice of bladder (D30.3)
   D30.8 Benign neoplasm of other specified urinary organs
         Benign neoplasm of paraurethral glands
   D30.9 Benign neoplasm of urinary organ, unspecified
         Benign neoplasm of urinary system NOS

● **D31 Benign neoplasm of eye and adnexa**
   Excludes1 benign neoplasm of connective tissue of eyelid (D21.0)
         benign neoplasm of optic nerve (D33.3)
         benign neoplasm of skin of eyelid (D22.1-, D23.1-)
   ● **D31.0** Benign neoplasm of conjunctiva
        D31.00 Benign neoplasm of unspecified conjunctiva
        D31.01 Benign neoplasm of right conjunctiva
        D31.02 Benign neoplasm of left conjunctiva
   ● **D31.1** Benign neoplasm of cornea
        D31.10 Benign neoplasm of unspecified cornea
        D31.11 Benign neoplasm of right cornea
        D31.12 Benign neoplasm of left cornea

Item 2–11 Teratoma: terat = monster, oma = mass, tumor. Alternate terms: dermoid cyst of the ovary, ovarian teratoma. Teratomas are neoplasms and arise from germ cells (ovaries in female and testes in male) and can be benign or malignant. Teratomas have been known to contain hair, nails, and teeth, giving them a bizarre ("monster") appearance.

● **D31.2**   **Benign neoplasm of retina**
> **Excludes1**   dark area on retina (D49.81)
> hemangioma of retina (D49.81)
> neoplasm of unspecified behavior of
> retina and choroid (D49.81)
> retinal freckle (D49.81)

    D31.20   Benign neoplasm of unspecified retina
    D31.21   Benign neoplasm of right retina
    D31.22   Benign neoplasm of left retina

● **D31.3**   **Benign neoplasm of choroid**
    D31.30   Benign neoplasm of unspecified choroid
    D31.31   Benign neoplasm of right choroid
    D31.32   Benign neoplasm of left choroid

● **D31.4**   **Benign neoplasm of ciliary body**
    D31.40   Benign neoplasm of unspecified ciliary body
    D31.41   Benign neoplasm of right ciliary body
    D31.42   Benign neoplasm of left ciliary body

● **D31.5**   **Benign neoplasm of lacrimal gland and duct**
> Benign neoplasm of lacrimal sac
> Benign neoplasm of nasolacrimal duct

    D31.50   Benign neoplasm of unspecified lacrimal gland and duct
    D31.51   Benign neoplasm of right lacrimal gland and duct
    D31.52   Benign neoplasm of left lacrimal gland and duct

● **D31.6**   **Benign neoplasm of unspecified site of orbit**
> Benign neoplasm of connective tissue of orbit
> Benign neoplasm of extraocular muscle
> Benign neoplasm of peripheral nerves of orbit
> Benign neoplasm of retrobulbar tissue
> Benign neoplasm of retro-ocular tissue

> **Excludes1**   benign neoplasm of orbital bone (D16.4)

    D31.60   Benign neoplasm of unspecified site of unspecified orbit
    D31.61   Benign neoplasm of unspecified site of right orbit
    D31.62   Benign neoplasm of unspecified site of left orbit

● **D31.9**   **Benign neoplasm of unspecified part of eye**
> Benign neoplasm of eyeball

    D31.90   Benign neoplasm of unspecified part of unspecified eye
    D31.91   Benign neoplasm of unspecified part of right eye
    D31.92   Benign neoplasm of unspecified part of left eye

● **D32**   **Benign neoplasm of meninges**
    D32.0   **Benign neoplasm of cerebral meninges**
    D32.1   **Benign neoplasm of spinal meninges**
    D32.9   **Benign neoplasm of meninges, unspecified**
> Meningioma NOS

● **D33**   **Benign neoplasm of brain and other parts of central nervous system**
> **Excludes1**   angioma (D18.0-)
> benign neoplasm of meninges (D32.-)
> benign neoplasm of peripheral nerves and
> autonomic nervous system (D36.1-)
> hemangioma (D18.0-)
> neurofibromatosis (Q85.0-)
> retro-ocular benign neoplasm (D31.6-)

    D33.0   **Benign neoplasm of brain, supratentorial**
> Benign neoplasm of cerebral ventricle
> Benign neoplasm of cerebrum
> Benign neoplasm of frontal lobe
> Benign neoplasm of occipital lobe
> Benign neoplasm of parietal lobe
> Benign neoplasm of temporal lobe

> **Excludes1**   benign neoplasm of fourth ventricle (D33.1)

    D33.1   **Benign neoplasm of brain, infratentorial**
> Benign neoplasm of brain stem
> Benign neoplasm of cerebellum
> Benign neoplasm of fourth ventricle

    D33.2   **Benign neoplasm of brain, unspecified**
    D33.3   **Benign neoplasm of cranial nerves**
> Benign neoplasm of olfactory bulb

    D33.4   **Benign neoplasm of spinal cord**
    D33.7   **Benign neoplasm of other specified parts of central nervous system**
    D33.9   **Benign neoplasm of central nervous system, unspecified**
> Benign neoplasm of nervous system (central) NOS

● **D34**   **Benign neoplasm of thyroid gland**
> Use additional code to identify any functional activity.

● **D35**   **Benign neoplasm of other and unspecified endocrine glands**
> Use additional code to identify any functional activity.

> **Excludes1**   benign neoplasm of endocrine pancreas (D13.7)
> benign neoplasm of ovary (D27.-)
> benign neoplasm of testis (D29.2.-)
> benign neoplasm of thymus (D15.0)

● **D35.0**   **Benign neoplasm of adrenal gland**
    D35.00   Benign neoplasm of unspecified adrenal gland
    D35.01   Benign neoplasm of right adrenal gland
    D35.02   Benign neoplasm of left adrenal gland

    D35.1   **Benign neoplasm of parathyroid gland**
    D35.2   **Benign neoplasm of pituitary gland**
    D35.3   **Benign neoplasm of craniopharyngeal duct**
    D35.4   **Benign neoplasm of pineal gland**
    D35.5   **Benign neoplasm of carotid body**
    D35.6   **Benign neoplasm of aortic body and other paraganglia**
> Benign tumor of glomus jugulare

    D35.7   **Benign neoplasm of other specified endocrine glands**
    D35.9   **Benign neoplasm of endocrine gland, unspecified**
> Benign neoplasm of unspecified endocrine gland

● **D36**   **Benign neoplasm of other and unspecified sites**
    D36.0   **Benign neoplasm of lymph nodes**
> **Excludes1**   lymphangioma (D18.1)

● **D36.1**   **Benign neoplasm of peripheral nerves and autonomic nervous system**
> **Excludes1**   benign neoplasm of peripheral nerves of
> orbit (D31.6-)
> neurofibromatosis (Q85.0-)

    D36.10   Benign neoplasm of peripheral nerves and autonomic nervous system, unspecified
    D36.11   Benign neoplasm of peripheral nerves and autonomic nervous system of face, head, and neck
    D36.12   Benign neoplasm of peripheral nerves and autonomic nervous system, upper limb, including shoulder
    D36.13   Benign neoplasm of peripheral nerves and autonomic nervous system of lower limb, including hip
    D36.14   Benign neoplasm of peripheral nerves and autonomic nervous system of thorax
    D36.15   Benign neoplasm of peripheral nerves and autonomic nervous system of abdomen
    D36.16   Benign neoplasm of peripheral nerves and autonomic nervous system of pelvis
    D36.17   Benign neoplasm of peripheral nerves and autonomic nervous system of trunk, unspecified

    D36.7   **Benign neoplasm of other specified sites**
> Benign neoplasm of nose NOS

    D36.9   **Benign neoplasm, unspecified site**

BENIGN NEUROENDOCRINE TUMORS (D3A)

● **D3A** **Benign neuroendocrine tumors**

Code also any associated multiple endocrine neoplasia [MEN] syndromes (E31.2-)

Use additional code to identify any associated endocrine syndrome, such as:
carcinoid syndrome (E34.0)

Excludes2   benign pancreatic islet cell tumors (D13.7)

● **D3A.0** **Benign carcinoid tumors**

     D3A.00 **Benign carcinoid tumor of unspecified site**
         Carcinoid tumor NOS

     ● **D3A.01** **Benign carcinoid tumors of the small intestine**

         D3A.010 **Benign carcinoid tumor of the duodenum**

         D3A.011 **Benign carcinoid tumor of the jejunum**

         D3A.012 **Benign carcinoid tumor of the ileum**

         D3A.019 **Benign carcinoid tumor of the small intestine, unspecified portion**

     ● **D3A.02** **Benign carcinoid tumors of the appendix, large intestine, and rectum**

         D3A.020 **Benign carcinoid tumor of the appendix**

         D3A.021 **Benign carcinoid tumor of the cecum**

         D3A.022 **Benign carcinoid tumor of the ascending colon**

         D3A.023 **Benign carcinoid tumor of the transverse colon**

         D3A.024 **Benign carcinoid tumor of the descending colon**

         D3A.025 **Benign carcinoid tumor of the sigmoid colon**

         D3A.026 **Benign carcinoid tumor of the rectum**

         D3A.029 **Benign carcinoid tumor of the large intestine, unspecified portion**
             Benign carcinoid tumor of the colon NOS

     ● **D3A.09** **Benign carcinoid tumors of other sites**

         D3A.090 **Benign carcinoid tumor of the bronchus and lung**

         D3A.091 **Benign carcinoid tumor of the thymus**

         D3A.092 **Benign carcinoid tumor of the stomach**

         D3A.093 **Benign carcinoid tumor of the kidney**

         D3A.094 **Benign carcinoid tumor of the foregut, unspecified** ◀▥

         D3A.095 **Benign carcinoid tumor of the midgut, unspecified** ◀▥

         D3A.096 **Benign carcinoid tumor of the hindgut, unspecified** ◀▥

         D3A.098 **Benign carcinoid tumors of other sites**

     D3A.8 **Other benign neuroendocrine tumors**
         Neuroendocrine tumor NOS

NEOPLASMS OF UNCERTAIN BEHAVIOR, POLYCYTHEMIA VERA AND MYELODYSPLASTIC SYNDROMES (D37-D48)

Note: Categories D37-D44, and D48 classify by site neoplasms of uncertain behavior, i.e., histologic confirmation whether the neoplasm is malignant or benign cannot be made.

     Excludes1   neoplasms of unspecified behavior (D49.-)

● **D37** **Neoplasm of uncertain behavior of oral cavity and digestive organs**

     Excludes1   stromal tumors of uncertain behavior of digestive system (D48.1)

   ● **D37.0** **Neoplasm of uncertain behavior of lip, oral cavity and pharynx**

     Excludes1   neoplasm of uncertain behavior of aryepiglottic fold or interarytenoid fold, laryngeal aspect (D38.0)
                neoplasm of uncertain behavior of epiglottis NOS (D38.0)
                neoplasm of uncertain behavior of skin of lip (D48.5)
                neoplasm of uncertain behavior of suprahyoid portion of epiglottis (D38.0)

     D37.01 **Neoplasm of uncertain behavior of lip**
         Neoplasm of uncertain behavior of vermilion border of lip

     D37.02 **Neoplasm of uncertain behavior of tongue**

   ● **D37.03** **Neoplasm of uncertain behavior of the major salivary glands**

         D37.030 **Neoplasm of uncertain behavior of the parotid salivary glands**

         D37.031 **Neoplasm of uncertain behavior of the sublingual salivary glands**

         D37.032 **Neoplasm of uncertain behavior of the submandibular salivary glands**

         D37.039 **Neoplasm of uncertain behavior of the major salivary glands, unspecified**

     D37.04 **Neoplasm of uncertain behavior of the minor salivary glands**
         Neoplasm of uncertain behavior of submucosal salivary glands of lip
         Neoplasm of uncertain behavior of submucosal salivary glands of cheek
         Neoplasm of uncertain behavior of submucosal salivary glands of hard palate
         Neoplasm of uncertain behavior of submucosal salivary glands of soft palate

     D37.05 **Neoplasm of uncertain behavior of pharynx**
         Neoplasm of uncertain behavior of aryepiglottic fold of pharynx NOS
         Neoplasm of uncertain behavior of hypopharyngeal aspect of aryepiglottic fold of pharynx
         Neoplasm of uncertain behavior of marginal zone of aryepiglottic fold of pharynx

     D37.09 **Neoplasm of uncertain behavior of other specified sites of the oral cavity**

Figure 2-19   Major salivary glands.

Parotid gland
Sublingual gland
Submandibular gland

◀ New   ◀▥ Revised   ~~deleted~~ Deleted   Excludes 1   Excludes 2   Includes   Use additional   Code first   Code also   Unspecified

OGCR Official Guidelines   X Assign placeholder X   ● Use Additional Character(s)   ▌ Manifestation Code   **Coding Clinic**

D37.1   **Neoplasm of uncertain behavior of stomach**

D37.2   **Neoplasm of uncertain behavior of small intestine**

D37.3   **Neoplasm of uncertain behavior of appendix**

D37.4   **Neoplasm of uncertain behavior of colon**

D37.5   **Neoplasm of uncertain behavior of rectum**
      Neoplasm of uncertain behavior of rectosigmoid junction
      Rectosigmoid junction: Angle where sigmoid colon becomes rectum

D37.6   **Neoplasm of uncertain behavior of liver, gallbladder and bile ducts**
      Neoplasm of uncertain behavior of ampulla of Vater
      Ampulla of Vater: Enlarged segment of ducts from liver and pancreas at entry point to small intestine

D37.8   **Neoplasm of uncertain behavior of other specified digestive organs**
      Neoplasm of uncertain behavior of anal canal
      Neoplasm of uncertain behavior of anal sphincter
      Neoplasm of uncertain behavior of anus NOS
      Neoplasm of uncertain behavior of esophagus
      Neoplasm of uncertain behavior of intestine NOS
      Neoplasm of uncertain behavior of pancreas

      Excludes1   neoplasm of uncertain behavior of anal margin (D48.5)
              neoplasm of uncertain behavior of anal skin (D48.5)
              neoplasm of uncertain behavior of perianal skin (D48.5)

D37.9   **Neoplasm of uncertain behavior of digestive organ, unspecified**

● D38   **Neoplasm of uncertain behavior of middle ear and respiratory and intrathoracic organs**
      Excludes1   neoplasm of uncertain behavior of heart (D48.7)

D38.0   **Neoplasm of uncertain behavior of larynx**
      Neoplasm of uncertain behavior of aryepiglottic fold or interarytenoid fold, laryngeal aspect
      Neoplasm of uncertain behavior of epiglottis (suprahyoid portion)

      Excludes1   neoplasm of uncertain behavior of aryepiglottic fold or interarytenoid fold NOS (D37.05)
              neoplasm of uncertain behavior of hypopharyngeal aspect of aryepiglottic fold (D37.05)
              neoplasm of uncertain behavior of marginal zone of aryepiglottic fold (D37.05)

D38.1   **Neoplasm of uncertain behavior of trachea, bronchus and lung**

D38.2   **Neoplasm of uncertain behavior of pleura**

D38.3   **Neoplasm of uncertain behavior of mediastinum**

D38.4   **Neoplasm of uncertain behavior of thymus**

D38.5   **Neoplasm of uncertain behavior of other respiratory organs**
      Neoplasm of uncertain behavior of accessory sinuses
      Neoplasm of uncertain behavior of cartilage of nose
      Neoplasm of uncertain behavior of middle ear
      Neoplasm of uncertain behavior of nasal cavities

      Excludes1   neoplasm of uncertain behavior of ear (external) (skin) (D48.5)
              neoplasm of uncertain behavior of nose NOS (D48.7)
              neoplasm of uncertain behavior of skin of nose (D48.5)

D38.6   **Neoplasm of uncertain behavior of respiratory organ, unspecified**

● D39   **Neoplasm of uncertain behavior of female genital organs**

D39.0   **Neoplasm of uncertain behavior of uterus** ♀

● D39.1   **Neoplasm of uncertain behavior of ovary**
      Use additional code to identify any functional activity.

      D39.10   **Neoplasm of uncertain behavior of unspecified ovary** ♀

      D39.11   **Neoplasm of uncertain behavior of right ovary** ♀

      D39.12   **Neoplasm of uncertain behavior of left ovary** ♀

D39.2   **Neoplasm of uncertain behavior of placenta** ♀   M
      Chorioadenoma destruens
      Invasive hydatidiform mole
      Malignant hydatidiform mole

      Excludes1   hydatidiform mole NOS (O01.9)

D39.8   **Neoplasm of uncertain behavior of other specified female genital organs** ♀
      Neoplasm of uncertain behavior of skin of female genital organs

D39.9   **Neoplasm of uncertain behavior of female genital organ, unspecified** ♀

● D40   **Neoplasm of uncertain behavior of male genital organs**

D40.0   **Neoplasm of uncertain behavior of prostate** ♂

● D40.1   **Neoplasm of uncertain behavior of testis**

      D40.10   **Neoplasm of uncertain behavior of unspecified testis** ♂

      D40.11   **Neoplasm of uncertain behavior of right testis** ♂

      D40.12   **Neoplasm of uncertain behavior of left testis** ♂

D40.8   **Neoplasm of uncertain behavior of other specified male genital organs** ♂
      Neoplasm of uncertain behavior of skin of male genital organs

D40.9   **Neoplasm of uncertain behavior of male genital organ, unspecified** ♂

● D41   **Neoplasm of uncertain behavior of urinary organs**

● D41.0   **Neoplasm of uncertain behavior of kidney**
      Excludes1   neoplasm of uncertain behavior of renal pelvis (D41.1-)

      D41.00   **Neoplasm of uncertain behavior of unspecified kidney**

      D41.01   **Neoplasm of uncertain behavior of right kidney**

      D41.02   **Neoplasm of uncertain behavior of left kidney**

● D41.1   **Neoplasm of uncertain behavior of renal pelvis**

      D41.10   **Neoplasm of uncertain behavior of unspecified renal pelvis**

      D41.11   **Neoplasm of uncertain behavior of right renal pelvis**

      D41.12   **Neoplasm of uncertain behavior of left renal pelvis**

● D41.2   **Neoplasm of uncertain behavior of ureter**

      D41.20   **Neoplasm of uncertain behavior of unspecified ureter**

      D41.21   **Neoplasm of uncertain behavior of right ureter**

      D41.22   **Neoplasm of uncertain behavior of left ureter**

D41.3   **Neoplasm of uncertain behavior of urethra**

D41.4   **Neoplasm of uncertain behavior of bladder**

D41.8   **Neoplasm of uncertain behavior of other specified urinary organs**

D41.9   **Neoplasm of uncertain behavior of unspecified urinary organ**

CHAPTER 2 (C00-D49)

CHAPTER 2 (C00-D49)

● **D42   Neoplasm of uncertain behavior of meninges**

     D42.0   Neoplasm of uncertain behavior of cerebral meninges

     D42.1   Neoplasm of uncertain behavior of spinal meninges

     D42.9   Neoplasm of uncertain behavior of meninges, unspecified

● **D43   Neoplasm of uncertain behavior of brain and central nervous system**

     Excludes1   neoplasm of uncertain behavior of peripheral nerves and autonomic nervous system (D48.2)

     D43.0   Neoplasm of uncertain behavior of brain, supratentorial
        Superior to tentorium of cerebellum
        Neoplasm of uncertain behavior of cerebral ventricle
        Neoplasm of uncertain behavior of cerebrum
        Neoplasm of uncertain behavior of frontal lobe
        Neoplasm of uncertain behavior of occipital lobe
        Neoplasm of uncertain behavior of parietal lobe
        Neoplasm of uncertain behavior of temporal lobe

        Excludes1   neoplasm of uncertain behavior of fourth ventricle (D43.1)

     D43.1   Neoplasm of uncertain behavior of brain, infratentorial
        Beneath the tentorium of cerebellum
        Neoplasm of uncertain behavior of brain stem
        Neoplasm of uncertain behavior of cerebellum
        Neoplasm of uncertain behavior of fourth ventricle

     D43.2   Neoplasm of uncertain behavior of brain, unspecified

     D43.3   Neoplasm of uncertain behavior of cranial nerves

     D43.4   Neoplasm of uncertain behavior of spinal cord

     D43.8   Neoplasm of uncertain behavior of other specified parts of central nervous system

     D43.9   Neoplasm of uncertain behavior of central nervous system, unspecified
        Neoplasm of uncertain behavior of nervous system (central) NOS

● **D44   Neoplasm of uncertain behavior of endocrine glands**

     Excludes1   multiple endocrine adenomatosis (E31.2-)
        multiple endocrine neoplasia (E31.2-)
        neoplasm of uncertain behavior of endocrine pancreas (D37.8)
        neoplasm of uncertain behavior of ovary (D39.1-)
        neoplasm of uncertain behavior of testis (D40.1-)
        neoplasm of uncertain behavior of thymus (D38.4)

     D44.0   Neoplasm of uncertain behavior of thyroid gland

●   **D44.1   Neoplasm of uncertain behavior of adrenal gland**
        Use additional code to identify any functional activity.

        D44.10   Neoplasm of uncertain behavior of unspecified adrenal gland

        D44.11   Neoplasm of uncertain behavior of right adrenal gland

        D44.12   Neoplasm of uncertain behavior of left adrenal gland

     D44.2   Neoplasm of uncertain behavior of parathyroid gland

     D44.3   Neoplasm of uncertain behavior of pituitary gland
        Use additional code to identify any functional activity.

     D44.4   Neoplasm of uncertain behavior of craniopharyngeal duct

     D44.5   Neoplasm of uncertain behavior of pineal gland

     D44.6   Neoplasm of uncertain behavior of carotid body

     D44.7   Neoplasm of uncertain behavior of aortic body and other paraganglia

     D44.9   Neoplasm of uncertain behavior of unspecified endocrine gland

● **D45   Polycythemia vera**

     Excludes1   familial polycythemia (D75.0)
        secondary polycythemia (D75.1)
     Primary polycythemia. Secondary polycythemia is D75.1. Check your documentation. Polycythemia is caused by too many red blood cells, which increase the thickness of blood (viscosity). This can cause engorgement of the spleen (splenomegaly) with extra RBCs and potential clot formation.

● **D46   Myelodysplastic syndromes**

     Use additional code for adverse effect, if applicable, to identify drug (T36-T50 with fifth or sixth character 5)

     Excludes2   drug-induced aplastic anemia (D61.1)

     D46.0   Refractory anemia without ring sideroblasts, so stated
        Refractory anemia without sideroblasts, without excess of blasts

     D46.1   Refractory anemia with ring sideroblasts RARS

●   **D46.2   Refractory anemia with excess of blasts [RAEB]** ◀▥
        Form of myelodysplasia with increased immature white blood cells (blasts) in bone marrow

        D46.20   Refractory anemia with excess of blasts, unspecified RAEB NOS

        D46.21   Refractory anemia with excess of blasts 1 RAEB 1
           Bone marrow disease which results in insufficient RBCs (anemia) in which level of blasts is less than 10%

        D46.22   Refractory anemia with excess of blasts 2 RAEB 2
           Bone marrow disease manifested by insufficient numbers of RBCs (anemia) with level of blasts 10-20%

     D46.A   Refractory cytopenia with multilineage dysplasia

     D46.B   Refractory cytopenia with multilineage dysplasia and ring sideroblasts
        RCMD RS

     D46.C   Myelodysplastic syndrome with isolated del(5q) chromosomal abnormality
        Myelodysplastic syndrome with 5q deletion
        5q minus syndrome NOS

     D46.4   Refractory anemia, unspecified

     D46.Z   Other myelodysplastic syndromes
        Excludes1   chronic myelomonocytic leukemia (C93.1-)

     D46.9   Myelodysplastic syndrome, unspecified
        Myelodysplasia NOS

● **D47   Other neoplasms of uncertain behavior of lymphoid, hematopoietic and related tissue**

     D47.0   Histiocytic and mast cell tumors of uncertain behavior
        Indolent systemic mastocytosis
        Mast cell tumor NOS
        Mastocytoma NOS

        Excludes1   malignant mast cell tumor (C96.2)
           mastocytosis (congenital) (cutaneous) (Q82.2)

     D47.1   Chronic myeloproliferative disease
        Chronic neutrophilic leukemia
        Myeloproliferative disease, unspecified

        Excludes1   atypical chronic myeloid leukemia BCR/ABL-negative (C92.2-)
           chronic myeloid leukemia BCR/ABL-positive (C92.1-)
           myelofibrosis NOS (D75.81)
           myelophthisic anemia (D61.82)
           myelophthisis (D61.82)
           secondary myelofibrosis NOS (D75.81)

     D47.2   Monoclonal gammopathy
        Monoclonal gammopathy of undetermined significance [MGUS]

     D47.3   Essential (hemorrhagic) thrombocythemia
        Essential thrombocytosis
        Idiopathic hemorrhagic thrombocythemia

D47.4   Osteomyelofibrosis
Chronic idiopathic myelofibrosis
Myelofibrosis (idiopathic) (with myeloid metaplasia)
Myelosclerosis (megakaryocytic) with myeloid
    metaplasia
Secondary myelofibrosis in myeloproliferative disease
> **Excludes1**   acute myelofibrosis (C94.4-)

● **D47.Z   Other specified neoplasms of uncertain behavior of lymphoid, hematopoietic and related tissue**

    D47.Z1   Post-transplant lymphoproliferative disorder (PTLD)
> *Code first* complications of transplanted organs and tissue (T86.-)

    D47.Z2   Castleman disease ◄
> Code also if applicable human herpesvirus 8 infection (B10.89) ◄
> **Excludes2**   Kaposi's sarcoma (C46-) ◄

    D47.Z9   Other specified neoplasms of uncertain behavior of lymphoid, hematopoietic and related tissue
Histiocytic tumors of uncertain behavior

D47.9   Neoplasm of uncertain behavior of lymphoid, hematopoietic and related tissue, unspecified
Lymphoproliferative disease NOS

● **D48   Neoplasm of uncertain behavior of other and unspecified sites**
> **Excludes1**   neurofibromatosis (nonmalignant) (Q85.0-)

D48.0   Neoplasm of uncertain behavior of bone and articular cartilage
> **Excludes1**   neoplasm of uncertain behavior of cartilage of ear (D48.1)
> neoplasm of uncertain behavior of cartilage of larynx (D38.0)
> neoplasm of uncertain behavior of cartilage of nose (D38.5)
> neoplasm of uncertain behavior of connective tissue of eyelid (D48.1)
> neoplasm of uncertain behavior of synovia (D48.1)

D48.1   Neoplasm of uncertain behavior of connective and other soft tissue
Neoplasm of uncertain behavior of connective tissue of ear
Neoplasm of uncertain behavior of connective tissue of eyelid
Stromal tumors of uncertain behavior of digestive system
> **Excludes1**   neoplasm of uncertain behavior of articular cartilage (D48.0)
> neoplasm of uncertain behavior of cartilage of larynx (D38.0)
> neoplasm of uncertain behavior of cartilage of nose (D38.5)
> neoplasm of uncertain behavior of connective tissue of breast (D48.6-)

D48.2   Neoplasm of uncertain behavior of peripheral nerves and autonomic nervous system
> **Excludes1**   neoplasm of uncertain behavior of peripheral nerves of orbit (D48.7)

D48.3   Neoplasm of uncertain behavior of retroperitoneum

D48.4   Neoplasm of uncertain behavior of peritoneum

D48.5   Neoplasm of uncertain behavior of skin
Neoplasm of uncertain behavior of anal margin
Neoplasm of uncertain behavior of anal skin
Neoplasm of uncertain behavior of perianal skin
Neoplasm of uncertain behavior of skin of breast
> **Excludes1**   neoplasm of uncertain behavior of anus NOS (D37.8)
> neoplasm of uncertain behavior of skin of genital organs (D39.8, D40.8)
> neoplasm of uncertain behavior of vermilion border of lip (D37.0)

● **D48.6   Neoplasm of uncertain behavior of breast**
Neoplasm of uncertain behavior of connective tissue of breast
Cystosarcoma phyllodes
> **Excludes1**   neoplasm of uncertain behavior of skin of breast (D48.5)

    D48.60   Neoplasm of uncertain behavior of unspecified breast

    D48.61   Neoplasm of uncertain behavior of right breast

    D48.62   Neoplasm of uncertain behavior of left breast

D48.7   Neoplasm of uncertain behavior of other specified sites
Neoplasm of uncertain behavior of eye
Neoplasm of uncertain behavior of heart
Neoplasm of uncertain behavior of peripheral nerves of orbit
> **Excludes1**   neoplasm of uncertain behavior of connective tissue (D48.1)
> neoplasm of uncertain behavior of skin of eyelid (D48.5)

D48.9   Neoplasm of uncertain behavior, unspecified

● **D49   Neoplasms of unspecified behavior**
> **Note:** Category D49 classifies by site neoplasms of unspecified morphology and behavior. The term 'mass,' unless otherwise stated, is not to be regarded as a neoplastic growth.
> **Includes**   'growth' NOS
> neoplasm NOS
> new growth NOS
> tumor NOS
> **Excludes1**   neoplasms of uncertain behavior (D37-D44, D48)

D49.0   Neoplasm of unspecified behavior of digestive system
> **Excludes1**   neoplasm of unspecified behavior of margin of anus (D49.2)
> neoplasm of unspecified behavior of perianal skin (D49.2)
> neoplasm of unspecified behavior of skin of anus (D49.2)

D49.1   Neoplasm of unspecified behavior of respiratory system

D49.2   Neoplasm of unspecified behavior of bone, soft tissue, and skin
> **Excludes1**   neoplasm of unspecified behavior of anal canal (D49.0)
> neoplasm of unspecified behavior of anus NOS (D49.0)
> neoplasm of unspecified behavior of bone marrow (D49.89)
> neoplasm of unspecified behavior of cartilage of larynx (D49.1)
> neoplasm of unspecified behavior of cartilage of nose (D49.1)
> neoplasm of unspecified behavior of connective tissue of breast (D49.3)
> neoplasm of unspecified behavior of skin of genital organs (D49.59) ◄▥
> neoplasm of unspecified behavior of vermilion border of lip (D49.0)

D49.3   Neoplasm of unspecified behavior of breast
> **Excludes1**   neoplasm of unspecified behavior of skin of breast (D49.2)

D49.4   Neoplasm of unspecified behavior of bladder

● D49.5　Neoplasm of unspecified behavior of other genitourinary organs
　● D49.51　Neoplasm of unspecified behavior of kidney ◀
　　D49.511　Neoplasm of unspecified behavior of right kidney ◀
　　D49.512　Neoplasm of unspecified behavior of left kidney ◀
　　D49.519　Neoplasm of unspecified behavior of unspecified kidney ◀
　　D49.59　Neoplasm of unspecified behavior of other genitourinary organ ◀

D49.6　Neoplasm of unspecified behavior of brain
　Excludes1　neoplasm of unspecified behavior of cerebral meninges (D49.7)
　　neoplasm of unspecified behavior of cranial nerves (D49.7)

D49.7　Neoplasm of unspecified behavior of endocrine glands and other parts of nervous system
　Excludes1　neoplasm of unspecified behavior of peripheral, sympathetic, and parasympathetic nerves and ganglia (D49.2)

● D49.8　Neoplasm of unspecified behavior of other specified sites
　Excludes1　neoplasm of unspecified behavior of eyelid (skin) (D49.2)
　　neoplasm of unspecified behavior of eyelid cartilage (D49.2)
　　neoplasm of unspecified behavior of great vessels (D49.2)
　　neoplasm of unspecified behavior of optic nerve (D49.7)

D49.81　Neoplasm of unspecified behavior of retina and choroid
　Dark area on retina
　Retinal freckle

D49.89　Neoplasm of unspecified behavior of other specified sites

D49.9　Neoplasm of unspecified behavior of unspecified site

CHAPTER 3

DISEASES OF THE BLOOD AND BLOOD-FORMING ORGANS AND CERTAIN DISORDERS INVOLVING THE IMMUNE MECHANISM (D50-D89)

Excludes2   autoimmune disease (systemic) NOS (M35.9)
certain conditions originating in the perinatal period (P00-P96)
complications of pregnancy, childbirth and the puerperium (O00-O9A)
congenital malformations, deformations and chromosomal abnormalities (Q00-Q99)
endocrine, nutritional and metabolic diseases (E00-E88)
human immunodeficiency virus [HIV] disease (B20)
injury, poisoning and certain other consequences of external causes (S00-T88)
neoplasms (C00-D49)
symptoms, signs and abnormal clinical and laboratory findings, not elsewhere classified (R00-R94)

This chapter contains the following blocks:

D50-D53	Nutritional anemias
D55-D59	Hemolytic anemias
D60-D64	Aplastic and other anemias and other bone marrow failure syndromes
D65-D69	Coagulation defects, purpura and other hemorrhagic conditions
D70-D77	Other disorders of blood and blood-forming organs
D78	Intraoperative and postprocedural complications of the spleen
D80-D89	Certain disorders involving the immune mechanism

NUTRITIONAL ANEMIAS (D50-D53)

● **D50**   **Iron deficiency anemia**
A disease characterized by a decrease in the number of red cells (hemoglobin) in the blood.

    Includes   asiderotic anemia
hypochromic anemia

   D50.0   **Iron deficiency anemia secondary to blood loss (chronic)**
Posthemorrhagic anemia (chronic)

     Excludes1   acute posthemorrhagic anemia (D62)
congenital anemia from fetal blood loss (P61.3)

   D50.1   **Sideropenic dysphagia**
Web-like growth of membranes in throat that makes swallowing difficult
Kelly-Paterson syndrome
Plummer-Vinson syndrome

   D50.8   **Other iron deficiency anemias**
Iron deficiency anemia due to inadequate dietary iron intake

   D50.9   **Iron deficiency anemia, unspecified**

● **D51**   **Vitamin B12 deficiency anemia**

    Excludes1   vitamin B12 deficiency (E53.8)

   D51.0   **Vitamin B12 deficiency anemia due to intrinsic factor deficiency**
Addison anemia
Biermer anemia
Pernicious (congenital) anemia
Congenital intrinsic factor deficiency

   D51.1   **Vitamin B12 deficiency anemia due to selective vitamin B12 malabsorption with proteinuria**
Imerslund (Gräsbeck) syndrome
Megaloblastic hereditary anemia

   D51.2   **Transcobalamin II deficiency**

   D51.3   **Other dietary vitamin B12 deficiency anemia**
Vegan anemia

   D51.8   **Other vitamin B12 deficiency anemias**

   D51.9   **Vitamin B12 deficiency anemia, unspecified**

● **D52**   **Folate deficiency anemia**

    Excludes1   folate deficiency without anemia (E53.8)

   D52.0   **Dietary folate deficiency anemia**
Nutritional megaloblastic anemia

   D52.1   **Drug-induced folate deficiency anemia**
Use additional code for adverse effect, if applicable, to identify drug (T36-T50 with fifth or sixth character 5)

   D52.8   **Other folate deficiency anemias**

   D52.9   **Folate deficiency anemia, unspecified**
Folic acid deficiency anemia NOS

● **D53**   **Other nutritional anemias**

    Includes   megaloblastic anemia unresponsive to vitamin B12 or folate therapy

   D53.0   **Protein deficiency anemia**
Amino-acid deficiency anemia
Orotaciduric anemia

     Excludes1   Lesch-Nyhan syndrome (E79.1)

   D53.1   **Other megaloblastic anemias, not elsewhere classified**
Megaloblastic anemia NOS

     Excludes1   Di Guglielmo's disease (C94.0)

   D53.2   **Scorbutic anemia**
Anemia resulting from deficiency of ascorbic acid (vitamin C)

     Excludes1   scurvy (E54)

   D53.8   **Other specified nutritional anemias**
Anemia associated with deficiency of copper
Anemia associated with deficiency of molybdenum
Anemia associated with deficiency of zinc

     Excludes1   nutritional deficiencies without anemia, such as:
copper deficiency NOS (E61.0)
molybdenum deficiency NOS (E61.5)
zinc deficiency NOS (E60)

   D53.9   **Nutritional anemia, unspecified**
Simple chronic anemia

     Excludes1   anemia NOS (D64.9)

CHAPTER 3 (D50-D89)

HEMOLYTIC ANEMIAS (D55-D59)

● **D55   Anemia due to enzyme disorders**

> **Excludes1**   drug-induced enzyme deficiency anemia (D59.2)

D55.0   Anemia due to glucose-6-phosphate dehydrogenase [G6PD] deficiency
Favism
G6PD deficiency anemia

D55.1   Anemia due to other disorders of glutathione metabolism
Anemia (due to) enzyme deficiencies, except G6PD, related to the hexose monophosphate [HMP] shunt pathway
Anemia (due to) hemolytic nonspherocytic (hereditary), type I

D55.2   Anemia due to disorders of glycolytic enzymes
Hemolytic nonspherocytic (hereditary) anemia, type II
Hexokinase deficiency anemia
Pyruvate kinase [PK] deficiency anemia
Triose-phosphate isomerase deficiency anemia

> **Excludes1**   disorders of glycolysis not associated with anemia (E74.8)

D55.3   Anemia due to disorders of nucleotide metabolism

D55.8   Other anemias due to enzyme disorders

D55.9   Anemia due to enzyme disorder, unspecified

● **D56   Thalassemia**

> *Hereditary disorders characterized by low production of hemoglobin or excessive destruction of red blood cells*

> **Excludes1**   sickle-cell thalassemia (D57.4-)

D56.0   Alpha thalassemia
Alpha thalassemia major
Hemoglobin H Constant Spring
Hemoglobin H disease
Hydrops fetalis due to alpha thalassemia
Severe alpha thalassemia
Triple gene defect alpha thalassemia

> Use additional code, if applicable, for hydrops fetalis due to alpha thalassemia (P56.99)

> **Excludes1**   alpha thalassemia trait or minor (D56.3)
> asymptomatic alpha thalassemia (D56.3)
> hydrops fetalis due to isoimmunization (P56.0)
> hydrops fetalis not due to immune hemolysis (P83.2)

D56.1   Beta thalassemia
Beta thalassemia major
Cooley's anemia
Homozygous beta thalassemia
Severe beta thalassemia
Thalassemia intermedia
Thalassemia major

> **Excludes1**   beta thalassemia minor (D56.3)
> beta thalassemia trait (D56.3)
> delta-beta thalassemia (D56.2)
> hemoglobin E-beta thalassemia (D56.5)
> sickle-cell beta thalassemia (D57.4-)

D56.2   Delta-beta thalassemia
Homozygous delta-beta thalassemia

> **Excludes1**   delta-beta thalassemia minor (D56.3)
> delta-beta thalassemia trait (D56.3)

D56.3   Thalassemia minor
> *Genetic disorders that have in common defective production of hemoglobin*
Alpha thalassemia minor
Alpha thalassemia silent carrier
Alpha thalassemia trait
Beta thalassemia minor
Beta thalassemia trait
Delta-beta thalassemia minor
Delta-beta thalassemia trait
Thalassemia trait NOS

> **Excludes1**   alpha thalassemia (D56.0)
> beta thalassemia (D56.1)
> delta-beta thalassemia (D56.2)
> hemoglobin E-beta thalassemia (D56.5)
> sickle-cell trait (D57.3)

D56.4   Hereditary persistence of fetal hemoglobin [HPFH]
> *Persistent production of hemoglobin*

D56.5   Hemoglobin E-beta thalassemia

> **Excludes1**   beta thalassemia (D56.1)
> beta thalassemia minor (D56.3)
> beta thalassemia trait (D56.3)
> delta-beta thalassemia (D56.2)
> delta-beta thalassemia trait (D56.3)
> hemoglobin E disease (D58.2)
> other hemoglobinopathies (D58.2)
> sickle-cell beta thalassemia (D57.4-)

D56.8   Other thalassemias
Dominant thalassemia
Hemoglobin C thalassemia
Mixed thalassemia
Thalassemia with other hemoglobinopathy

> **Excludes1**   hemoglobin C disease (D58.2)
> hemoglobin E disease (D58.2)
> other hemoglobinopathies (D58.2)
> sickle cell anemia (D57.-)
> sickle-cell thalassemia (D57.4)

D56.9   Thalassemia, unspecified
Mediterranean anemia (with other hemoglobinopathy)

● **D57   Sickle-cell disorders**
> *Inherited disease in which red blood cells, normally disc-shaped, become crescent shaped*

> Use additional code for any associated fever (R50.81)

> **Excludes1**   other hemoglobinopathies (D58.-)

● **D57.0   Hb-SS disease with crisis**
Sickle-cell disease NOS with crisis
Hb-SS disease with vasoocclusive pain

D57.00   Hb-SS disease with crisis, unspecified

D57.01   Hb-SS disease with acute chest syndrome

D57.02   Hb-SS disease with splenic sequestration

D57.1   Sickle-cell disease without crisis Hb-SS disease without crisis
Sickle-cell anemia NOS
Sickle-cell disease NOS
Sickle-cell disorder NOS

● **D57.2   Sickle-cell/Hb-C disease**
Hb-SC disease
Hb-S/Hb-C disease

D57.20   Sickle-cell/Hb-C disease without crisis

● **D57.21   Sickle-cell/Hb-C disease with crisis**

D57.211   Sickle-cell/Hb-C disease with acute chest syndrome

D57.212   Sickle-cell/Hb-C disease with splenic sequestration

D57.219   Sickle-cell/Hb-C disease with crisis, unspecified
Sickle-cell/Hb-C disease with crisis NOS

◀ New   ◀◀ Revised   ~~deleted~~ Deleted   Excludes 1   Excludes 2   Includes   Use additional   Code first   Code also   Unspecified

OGCR Official Guidelines   X Assign placeholder X   ● Use Additional Character(s)   ▶ Manifestation Code   **Coding Clinic**

D57.3   Sickle-cell trait
Hb-S trait
Heterozygous hemoglobin S

D57.4   Sickle-cell thalassemia
Sickle-cell beta thalassemia
Thalassemia Hb-S disease

    D57.40   Sickle-cell thalassemia without crisis
Microdrepanocytosis
Sickle-cell thalassemia NOS

    D57.41   Sickle-cell thalassemia with crisis
Sickle-cell "crisis" is precipitated when abnormally crescent-shaped red blood cells form clots and interrupt blood flow to major organs, causing severe pain and organ damage.
Sickle-cell thalassemia with vasoocclusive pain

       D57.411   Sickle-cell thalassemia with acute chest syndrome

       D57.412   Sickle-cell thalassemia with splenic sequestration

       D57.419   Sickle-cell thalassemia with crisis, unspecified
Sickle-cell thalassemia with crisis NOS

D57.8   Other sickle-cell disorders
Hb-SD disease
Hb-SE disease

    D57.80   Other sickle-cell disorders without crisis

    D57.81   Other sickle-cell disorders with crisis

       D57.811   Other sickle-cell disorders with acute chest syndrome

       D57.812   Other sickle-cell disorders with splenic sequestration

       D57.819   Other sickle-cell disorders with crisis, unspecified
Other sickle-cell disorders with crisis NOS

D58   Other hereditary hemolytic anemias
Genetic condition in which bone marrow is unable to compensate for premature destruction of red blood cells
    Excludes1   hemolytic anemia of the newborn (P55.-)

D58.0   Hereditary spherocytosis
Presence of spherocytes (spherically shaped red blood cells)
Acholuric (familial) jaundice
Congenital (spherocytic) hemolytic icterus
Minkowski-Chauffard syndrome

D58.1   Hereditary elliptocytosis
Presence of large numbers of elliptocytes in blood
Elliptocytosis (congenital)
Ovalocytosis (congenital) (hereditary)

D58.2   Other hemoglobinopathies
Abnormal hemoglobin NOS
Congenital Heinz body anemia
Hb-C disease
Hb-D disease
Hb-E disease
Hemoglobinopathy NOS
Unstable hemoglobin hemolytic disease
    Excludes1   familial polycythemia (D75.0)
Hb-M disease (D74.0)
hemoglobin E-beta thalassemia (D56.5)
hereditary persistence of fetal hemoglobin [HPFH] (D56.4)
high-altitude polycythemia (D75.1)
methemoglobinemia (D74.-)
other hemoglobinopathies with thalassemia (D56.8)

D58.8   Other specified hereditary hemolytic anemias
Stomatocytosis

D58.9   Hereditary hemolytic anemia, unspecified

D59   Acquired hemolytic anemia

    D59.0   Drug-induced autoimmune hemolytic anemia
Use additional code for adverse effect, if applicable, to identify drug (T36-T50 with fifth or sixth character 5)

    D59.1   Other autoimmune hemolytic anemias
Autoimmune hemolytic disease (cold type) (warm type)
Chronic cold hemagglutinin disease
Cold agglutinin disease
Cold agglutinin hemoglobinuria
Cold type (secondary) (symptomatic) hemolytic anemia
Warm type (secondary) (symptomatic) hemolytic anemia
    Excludes1   Evans syndrome (D69.41)
hemolytic disease of newborn (P55.-)
paroxysmal cold hemoglobinuria (D59.6)

    D59.2   Drug-induced nonautoimmune hemolytic anemia
Drug-induced enzyme deficiency anemia
Use additional code for adverse effect, if applicable, to identify drug (T36-T50 with fifth or sixth character 5)

    D59.3   Hemolytic-uremic syndrome
Use additional code to identify associated:
    E. coli infection (B96.2-)
    Pneumococcal pneumonia (J13)
    Shigella dysenteriae (A03.9)

    D59.4   Other nonautoimmune hemolytic anemias
Mechanical hemolytic anemia
Microangiopathic hemolytic anemia
Toxic hemolytic anemia

    D59.5   Paroxysmal nocturnal hemoglobinuria [Marchiafava-Micheli]
    Excludes1   hemoglobinuria NOS (R82.3)

    D59.6   Hemoglobinuria due to hemolysis from other external causes
Hemoglobinuria from exertion
March hemoglobinuria
Paroxysmal cold hemoglobinuria
Use additional code (Chapter 20) to identify external cause
    Excludes1   hemoglobinuria NOS (R82.3)

    D59.8   Other acquired hemolytic anemias

    D59.9   Acquired hemolytic anemia, unspecified
Idiopathic hemolytic anemia, chronic

APLASTIC AND OTHER ANEMIAS AND OTHER BONE MARROW FAILURE SYNDROMES (D60-D64)

D60   Acquired pure red cell aplasia [erythroblastopenia]
Deficiency of erythroblasts
    Includes   red cell aplasia (acquired) (adult) (with thymoma)
    Excludes1   congenital red cell aplasia (D61.01)

    D60.0   Chronic acquired pure red cell aplasia
Lack of development of blood cell

    D60.1   Transient acquired pure red cell aplasia

    D60.8   Other acquired pure red cell aplasias

    D60.9   Acquired pure red cell aplasia, unspecified

D61   Other aplastic anemias and other bone marrow failure syndromes
    Excludes1   neutropenia (D70.-)

    D61.0   Constitutional aplastic anemia
Condition where bone marrow is unable to produce blood cells

       D61.01   Constitutional (pure) red blood cell aplasia
Blackfan-Diamond syndrome
Congenital (pure) red cell aplasia
Familial hypoplastic anemia
Primary (pure) red cell aplasia
Red cell (pure) aplasia of infants
    Excludes1   acquired red cell aplasia (D60.9)

       D61.09   Other constitutional aplastic anemia
Fanconi's anemia
Pancytopenia with malformations

D61.1　Drug-induced aplastic anemia
> Use additional code for adverse effect, if applicable, to identify drug (T36-T50 with fifth or sixth character 5)

D61.2　Aplastic anemia due to other external agents
> *Code first*, if applicable, toxic effects of substances chiefly nonmedicinal as to source (T51-T65)

D61.3　Idiopathic aplastic anemia

● **D61.8　Other specified aplastic anemias and other bone marrow failure syndromes**

　● **D61.81　Pancytopenia**
> *Marked deficiency of all the blood elements: Red blood cells (erythrocytes), white blood cells (leukocytes), and platelets (thrombocytes). Check laboratory results.*

> **Excludes1** pancytopenia (due to) (with) aplastic anemia (D61.9)
> pancytopenia (due to) (with) bone marrow infiltration (D61.82)
> pancytopenia (due to) (with) congenital (pure) red cell aplasia (D61.01)
> pancytopenia (due to) (with) hairy cell leukemia (C91.4-)
> pancytopenia (due to) (with) human immunodeficiency virus disease (B20.-)
> pancytopenia (due to) (with) leukoerythroblastic anemia (D61.82)
> pancytopenia (due to) (with) myeloproliferative disease (D47.1)

> **Excludes2** pancytopenia (due to) (with) myelodysplastic syndromes (D46.-) ◀

　　D61.810　Antineoplastic chemotherapy induced pancytopenia
> **Excludes2** aplastic anemia due to antineoplastic chemotherapy (D61.1)

　　D61.811　Other drug-induced pancytopenia
> **Excludes2** aplastic anemia due to drugs (D61.1)

　　D61.818　Other pancytopenia

　D61.82　Myelophthisis
> Leukoerythroblastic anemia
> Myelophthisic anemia
> Panmyelophthisis

> Code also the underlying disorder, such as:
> malignant neoplasm of breast (C50.-)
> tuberculosis (A15.-)

> **Excludes1** idiopathic myelofibrosis (D47.1)
> myelofibrosis NOS (D75.81)
> myelofibrosis with myeloid metaplasia (D47.4)
> primary myelofibrosis (D47.1)
> secondary myelofibrosis (D75.81)

　D61.89　Other specified aplastic anemias and other bone marrow failure syndromes

D61.9　Aplastic anemia, unspecified
> Hypoplastic anemia NOS
> Medullary hypoplasia

D62　Acute posthemorrhagic anemia
> **Excludes1** anemia due to chronic blood loss (D50.0)
> blood loss anemia NOS (D50.0)
> congenital anemia from fetal blood loss (P61.3)

● **D63　Anemia in chronic diseases classified elsewhere**

▷ **D63.0　*Anemia in neoplastic disease***
> *Code first* neoplasm (C00-D49)
> **Excludes1** anemia due to antineoplastic chemotherapy (D64.81)
> aplastic anemia due to antineoplastic chemotherapy (D61.1)

> **OGCR** Section I.C.2.e.2.

> 2) Anemia associated with chemotherapy, immunotherapy and radiation therapy
> When the admission/encounter is for management of an anemia associated with an adverse effect of the administration of chemotherapy or immunotherapy and the only treatment is for the anemia, the anemia code is sequenced first followed by the appropriate codes for the neoplasm and the adverse effect (T45.1X5, Adverse effect of antineoplastic and immunosuppressive drugs).

▷ **D63.1　*Anemia in chronic kidney disease***
> Erythropoietin resistant anemia (EPO resistant anemia)
> *Code first* underlying chronic kidney disease (CKD) (N18.-)

▷ **D63.8　*Anemia in other chronic diseases classified elsewhere***
> *Code first* underlying disease, such as:
> diphyllobothriasis (B70.0)
> hookworm disease (B76.0-B76.9)
> hypothyroidism (E00.0-E03.9)
> malaria (B50.0-B54)
> symptomatic late syphilis (A52.79)
> tuberculosis (A18.89)

● **D64　Other anemias**
> **Excludes1** refractory anemia (D46.-)
> refractory anemia with excess blasts in transformation [RAEB T] (C92.0-)

D64.0　Hereditary sideroblastic anemia
> *Abnormal production RBCs (erythrocytes)*
> Sex-linked hypochromic sideroblastic anemia

▷ **D64.1　*Secondary sideroblastic anemia due to disease***
> *Code first* underlying disease

D64.2　Secondary sideroblastic anemia due to drugs and toxins
> *Code first* poisoning due to drug or toxin, if applicable (T36-T65 with fifth or sixth character 1-4 or 6)
> Use additional code for adverse effect, if applicable, to identify drug (T36-T50 with fifth or sixth character 5)

D64.3　Other sideroblastic anemias
> Sideroblastic anemia NOS
> Pyridoxine-responsive sideroblastic anemia NEC

D64.4　Congenital dyserythropoietic anemia
> *Any of several rare hereditary anemias, mostly types of macrocytic anemia*
> Dyshematopoietic anemia (congenital)
> **Excludes1** Blackfan-Diamond syndrome (D61.01)
> Di Guglielmo's disease (C94.0)

● **D64.8　Other specified anemias**

　D64.81　Anemia due to antineoplastic chemotherapy
> Antineoplastic chemotherapy induced anemia
> **Excludes1** aplastic anemia due to antineoplastic chemotherapy (D61.1)
> **Excludes2** anemia in neoplastic disease (D63.0) ◀

　D64.89　Other specified anemias
> Infantile pseudoleukemia

D64.9　Anemia, unspecified

◀ New　◀━ Revised　~~deleted~~ Deleted　Excludes 1　Excludes 2　Includes　Use additional　Code first　Code also　Unspecified

712　　**OGCR** Official Guidelines　X Assign placeholder X　● Use Additional Character(s)　▷ Manifestation Code　**Coding Clinic**

CHAPTER 3 (D50-D89)

COAGULATION DEFECTS, PURPURA AND OTHER HEMORRHAGIC CONDITIONS (D65-D69)

D65   Disseminated intravascular coagulation [defibrination syndrome]
Blood clots form and consume all coagulation proteins and platelets and disrupt normal coagulation, resulting in abnormal bleeding
Afibrinogenemia, acquired
Consumption coagulopathy
Diffuse or disseminated intravascular coagulation [DIC]
Fibrinolytic hemorrhage, acquired
Fibrinolytic purpura
Purpura fulminans

> **Excludes1**   disseminated intravascular coagulation (complicating):
> abortion or ectopic or molar pregnancy (O00-O07, O08.1)
> in newborn (P60)
> pregnancy, childbirth and the puerperium (O45.0, O46.0, O67.0, O72.3)

D66   Hereditary factor VIII deficiency
Inherited coagulation disorder carried by females but most often affecting males
Classical hemophilia
Deficiency factor VIII (with functional defect)
Hemophilia NOS
Hemophilia A

> **Excludes1**   factor VIII deficiency with vascular defect (D68.0)

D67   Hereditary factor IX deficiency
Christmas disease
Factor IX deficiency (with functional defect)
Hemophilia B
Plasma thromboplastin component [PTC] deficiency

● **D68   Other coagulation defects**

> **Excludes1**   abnormal coagulation profile (R79.1)
> coagulation defects complicating abortion or ectopic or molar pregnancy (O00-O07, O08.1)
> coagulation defects complicating pregnancy, childbirth and the puerperium (O45.0, O46.0, O67.0, O72.3)

Coding Clinic: 2016, Q1, P14

D68.0   Von Willebrand's disease
Congenital bleeding disorder
Angiohemophilia
Factor VIII deficiency with vascular defect
Vascular hemophilia

> **Excludes1**   capillary fragility (hereditary) (D69.8)
> factor VIII deficiency NOS (D66)
> factor VIII deficiency with functional defect (D66)

D68.1   Hereditary factor XI deficiency
Deficiency of blood coagulation resulting in systemic blood-clotting defect
Hemophilia C
Plasma thromboplastin antecedent [PTA] deficiency
Rosenthal's disease

D68.2   Hereditary deficiency of other clotting factors
Blood clotting disorders caused by hereditary deficiencies of one or more clotting factors
AC globulin deficiency
Congenital afibrinogenemia
Deficiency of factor I [fibrinogen]
Deficiency of factor II [prothrombin]
Deficiency of factor V [labile]
Deficiency of factor VII [stable]
Deficiency of factor X [Stuart-Prower]
Deficiency of factor XII [Hageman]
Deficiency of factor XIII [fibrin stabilizing]
Dysfibrinogenemia (congenital)
Hypoproconvertinemia
Owren's disease
Proaccelerin deficiency

● **D68.3   Hemorrhagic disorder due to circulating anticoagulants**
Blood clotting disorders caused by anticoagulants (warfarin and heparin)

● **D68.31   Hemorrhagic disorder due to intrinsic circulating anticoagulants, antibodies, or inhibitors**

D68.311   Acquired hemophilia
Autoimmune hemophilia
Autoimmune inhibitors to clotting factors
Secondary hemophilia

D68.312   Antiphospholipid antibody with hemorrhagic disorder
Lupus anticoagulant (LAC) with hemorrhagic disorder
Systemic lupus erythematosus [SLE] inhibitor with hemorrhagic disorder

> **Excludes1**   antiphospholipid antibody, finding without diagnosis (R76.0)
> antiphospholipid antibody syndrome (D68.61)
> antiphospholipid antibody with hypercoagulable state (D68.61)
> lupus anticoagulant (LAC) finding without diagnosis (R76.0)
> lupus anticoagulant (LAC) with hypercoagulable state (D68.62)
> systemic lupus erythematosus [SLE] inhibitor finding without diagnosis (R76.0)
> systemic lupus erythematosus [SLE] inhibitor with hypercoagulable state (D68.62)

D68.318   Other hemorrhagic disorder due to intrinsic circulating anticoagulants, antibodies, or inhibitors
Antithromboplastinemia
Antithromboplastinogenemia
Hemorrhagic disorder due to intrinsic increase in antithrombin
Hemorrhagic disorder due to intrinsic increase in anti-VIIIa
Hemorrhagic disorder due to intrinsic increase in anti-IXa
Hemorrhagic disorder due to intrinsic increase in anti-XIa

D68.32   Hemorrhagic disorder due to extrinsic circulating anticoagulants
Drug-induced hemorrhagic disorder
Hemorrhagic disorder due to increase in anti-IIa
Hemorrhagic disorder due to increase in anti-Xa
Hyperheparinemia

> Use additional code for adverse effect, if applicable, to identify drug (T45.515, T45.525)

Coding Clinic: 2016, Q1, P14-15

CHAPTER 3 (D50-D89)

D68.4   Acquired coagulation factor deficiency
Deficiency of coagulation factor due to liver disease
Deficiency of coagulation factor due to vitamin K
deficiency
> **Excludes1**   vitamin K deficiency of newborn (P53)

● **D68.5   Primary thrombophilia**
AKA idiopathic thrombocytopenia, may be acquired or congenital and is a common cause of coagulation disorders.
Primary hypercoagulable states
> **Excludes1**   antiphospholipid syndrome (D68.61)
> lupus anticoagulant (D68.62)
> secondary activated protein C resistance
> (D68.69)
> secondary antiphospholipid antibody
> syndrome (D68.69)
> secondary lupus anticoagulant with
> hypercoagulable state (D68.69)
> secondary systemic lupus erythematosus
> [SLE] inhibitor with hypercoagulable
> state (D68.69)
> systemic lupus erythematosus [SLE]
> inhibitor finding without diagnosis
> (R76.0)
> systemic lupus erythematosus [SLE]
> inhibitor with hemorrhagic disorder
> (D68.312)
> thrombotic thrombocytopenic purpura
> (M31.1)

   D68.51   Activated protein C resistance
      Factor V Leiden mutation

   D68.52   Prothrombin gene mutation

   D68.59   Other primary thrombophilia
      Antithrombin III deficiency
      Hypercoagulable state NOS
      Primary hypercoagulable state NEC
      Primary thrombophilia NEC
      Protein C deficiency
      Protein S deficiency
      Thrombophilia NOS

● **D68.6   Other thrombophilia**
Other hypercoagulable states
> **Excludes1**   diffuse or disseminated intravascular
> coagulation [DIC] (D65)
> heparin induced thrombocytopenia (HIT)
> (D75.82)
> hyperhomocysteinemia (E72.11)

   D68.61   Antiphospholipid syndrome
      Anticardiolipin syndrome
      Antiphospholipid antibody syndrome
> **Excludes1**   anti-phospholipid antibody,
> finding without diagnosis
> (R76.0)
> anti-phospholipid antibody
> with hemorrhagic disorder
> (D68.312)
> lupus anticoagulant syndrome
> (D68.62)

   D68.62   Lupus anticoagulant syndrome
      Lupus anticoagulant
      Presence of systemic lupus erythematosus
      [SLE] inhibitor
> **Excludes1**   anticardiolipin syndrome
> (D68.61)
> antiphospholipid syndrome
> (D68.61)
> lupus anticoagulant (LAC)
> finding without diagnosis
> (R76.0) ◀
> lupus anticoagulant (LAC)
> with hemorrhagic disorder
> (D68.312)

   D68.69   Other thrombophilia
      Hypercoagulable states NEC
      Secondary hypercoagulable state NOS

D68.8   Other specified coagulation defects
> **Excludes1**   hemorrhagic disease of newborn (P53)

D68.9   Coagulation defect, unspecified

● **D69   Purpura and other hemorrhagic conditions**
Group of conditions characterized by small hemorrhages in skin, mucous membranes, or serosal surfaces
> **Excludes1**   benign hypergammaglobulinemic purpura
> (D89.0)
> cryoglobulinemic purpura (D89.1)
> essential (hemorrhagic) thrombocythemia (D47.3)
> hemorrhagic thrombocythemia (D47.3)
> purpura fulminans (D65)
> thrombotic thrombocytopenic purpura (M31.1)
> Waldenström hypergammaglobulinemic purpura
> (D89.0)

D69.0   Allergic purpura
Allergic vasculitis
Nonthrombocytopenic hemorrhagic purpura
Nonthrombocytopenic idiopathic purpura
Purpura anaphylactoid
Purpura Henoch(-Schönlein)
Purpura rheumatica
Vascular purpura
> **Excludes1**   thrombocytopenic hemorrhagic purpura
> (D69.3)

D69.1   Qualitative platelet defects
Bernard-Soulier [giant platelet] syndrome
Glanzmann's disease
Grey platelet syndrome
Thromboasthenia (hemorrhagic) (hereditary)
Thrombocytopathy
> **Excludes1**   von Willebrand's disease (D68.0)

D69.2   Other nonthrombocytopenic purpura
Purpura NOS
Purpura simplex
Senile purpura

D69.3   Immune thrombocytopenic purpura
Hemorrhagic (thrombocytopenic) purpura
Idiopathic thrombocytopenic purpura
Tidal platelet dysgenesis

● **D69.4   Other primary thrombocytopenia**
> **Excludes1**   transient neonatal thrombocytopenia
> (P61.0)
> Wiskott-Aldrich syndrome (D82.0)

   D69.41   Evans syndrome
      Acquired hemolytic anemia and thrombocytopenia

   D69.42   Congenital and hereditary thrombocytopenia purpura
      Congenital thrombocytopenia
      Hereditary thrombocytopenia
      Code first congenital or hereditary disorder, such as:
      thrombocytopenia with absent radius (TAR syndrome) (Q87.2)

   D69.49   Other primary thrombocytopenia
      Megakaryocytic hypoplasia
      Primary thrombocytopenia NOS

● **D69.5   Secondary thrombocytopenia**
Acquired reduction of number of platelets required for blood clotting
> **Excludes1**   heparin induced thrombocytopenia (HIT)
> (D75.82)
> transient thrombocytopenia of newborn
> (P61.0)

   D69.51   Posttransfusion purpura
      Posttransfusion purpura from whole blood
      (fresh) or blood products PTP

   D69.59   Other secondary thrombocytopenia

D69.6   Thrombocytopenia, unspecified

D69.8   Other specified hemorrhagic conditions
Capillary fragility (hereditary)
Vascular pseudohemophilia

D69.9   Hemorrhagic condition, unspecified

OTHER DISORDERS OF BLOOD AND BLOOD-FORMING ORGANS (D70-D77)

● **D70 Neutropenia**
Decrease in number of neutrophils (type of white blood cell)
> **Includes**   agranulocytosis
>   decreased absolute neurophile count (ANC)

Use additional code for any associated:
fever (R50.81)
mucositis (J34.81, K12.3-, K92.81, N76.81)
> **Excludes1**   neutropenic splenomegaly (D73.81)
>   transient neonatal neutropenia (P61.5)

D70.0 Congenital agranulocytosis
Reduced numbers of neutrophils (type of white blood cell)
Congenital neutropenia
Infantile genetic agranulocytosis
Kostmann's disease

D70.1 Agranulocytosis secondary to cancer chemotherapy
Decreased numbers of granulocytes (type of white blood cell)
Code also *underlying neoplasm*
Use additional code for adverse effect, if applicable, to identify drug (T45.1X5)

D70.2 Other drug-induced agranulocytosis
Use additional code for adverse effect, if applicable, to identify drug (T36-T50 with fifth or sixth character 5)

D70.3 Neutropenia due to infection

D70.4 Cyclic neutropenia
Chronic neutropenia (low number of type of white blood cell)
Cyclic hematopoiesis
Periodic neutropenia

D70.8 Other neutropenia

D70.9 Neutropenia, unspecified

D71 Functional disorders of polymorphonuclear neutrophils
Polymorphonuclear: varying shapes of nucleus; AKA PMNs
Cell membrane receptor complex [CR3] defect
Chronic (childhood) granulomatous disease
Congenital dysphagocytosis
Progressive septic granulomatosis

● **D72 Other disorders of white blood cells**
> **Excludes1**   basophilia (D72.824)
>   immunity disorders (D80-D89)
>   neutropenia (D70)
>   preleukemia (syndrome) (D46.9)

D72.0 Genetic anomalies of leukocytes
Alder (granulation) (granulocyte) anomaly
Alder syndrome
Hereditary leukocytic hypersegmentation
Hereditary leukocytic hyposegmentation
Hereditary leukomelanopathy
May-Hegglin (granulation) (granulocyte) anomaly
May-Hegglin syndrome
Pelger-Huët (granulation) (granulocyte) anomaly
Pelger-Huët syndrome
> **Excludes1**   Chédiak (-Steinbrinck)-Higashi syndrome (E70.330)

D72.1 Eosinophilia
Formation and accumulation of high number of white cells in blood/tissue
Allergic eosinophilia
Hereditary eosinophilia
> **Excludes1**   Löffler's syndrome (J82)
>   pulmonary eosinophilia (J82)

● **D72.8 Other specified disorders of white blood cells**
> **Excludes1**   leukemia (C91-C95)

  ● **D72.81 Decreased white blood cell count**
> **Excludes1**   neutropenia (D70.-)

    D72.810 Lymphocytopenia
Decreased lymphocytes
Reduction in number of lympho cytes in blood

D72.818 Other decreased white blood cell count
Basophilic leukopenia
Eosinophilic leukopenia
Monocytopenia
Other decreased leukocytes
Plasmacytopenia

D72.819 Decreased white blood cell count, unspecified
Decreased leukocytes, unspecified
Leukocytopenia, unspecified
Leukopenia
> **Excludes1**   malignant leukopenia (D70.9)

● **D72.82 Elevated white blood cell count**
> **Excludes1**   eosinophilia (D72.1)

D72.820 Lymphocytosis (symptomatic)
Elevated lymphocytes
Excess of normal lymphocytes

D72.821 Monocytosis (symptomatic)
> **Excludes1**   infectious mononucleosis (B27.-)

D72.822 Plasmacytosis
Presence of excess plasma cells

D72.823 Leukemoid reaction
Basophilic leukemoid reaction
Leukemoid reaction NOS
Lymphocytic leukemoid reaction
Monocytic leukemoid reaction
Myelocytic leukemoid reaction
Neutrophilic leukemoid reaction

D72.824 Basophilia
Increase of basophils in blood

D72.825 Bandemia
Bandemia without diagnosis of specific infection
Excess number of band cells (immature white blood cells) released by bone marrow
> **Excludes1**   confirmed infection -code to infection
>   leukemia (C91.-, C92.-, C93.-, C94.-, C95.-)

D72.828 Other elevated white blood cell count

D72.829 Elevated white blood cell count, unspecified
Elevated leukocytes, unspecified
Leukocytosis, unspecified

D72.89 Other specified disorders of white blood cells
Abnormality of white blood cells NEC

D72.9 Disorder of white blood cells, unspecified
Abnormal leukocyte differential NOS

● **D73 Diseases of spleen**

D73.0 Hyposplenism
Diminished functioning of spleen
Atrophy of spleen
> **Excludes1**   asplenia (congenital) (Q89.01)
>   postsurgical absence of spleen (Z90.81)

D73.1 Hypersplenism
Accelerated function of spleen
> **Excludes1**   neutropenic splenomegaly (D73.81)
>   primary splenic neutropenia (D73.81)
>   splenitis, splenomegaly in late syphilis (A52.79)
>   splenitis, splenomegaly in tuberculosis (A18.85)
>   splenomegaly NOS (R16.1)
>   splenomegaly congenital (Q89.0)

CHAPTER 3 (D50-D89)

D73.2   Chronic congestive splenomegaly
Enlargement of spleen

D73.3   Abscess of spleen

D73.4   Cyst of spleen

D73.5   Infarction of spleen
Splenic rupture, nontraumatic
Torsion of spleen

> **Excludes1**   rupture of spleen due to Plasmodium vivax malaria (B51.0)
> traumatic rupture of spleen (S36.03-)

● **D73.8   Other diseases of spleen**

     D73.81   Neutropenic splenomegaly
Werner-Schultz disease
Enlarged spleen responding to inadequate number of neutrophils

     D73.89   Other diseases of spleen
Fibrosis of spleen NOS
Perisplenitis
Splenitis NOS

D73.9   Disease of spleen, unspecified

● **D74   Methemoglobinemia**
Excessive methemoglobin (form of hemoglobin)

     D74.0   Congenital methemoglobinemia
Congenital NADH-methemoglobin reductase deficiency
Hemoglobin-M [Hb-M] disease
Methemoglobinemia, hereditary

     D74.8   Other methemoglobinemias
Acquired methemoglobinemia (with sulfhemoglobinemia)
Toxic methemoglobinemia

     D74.9   Methemoglobinemia, unspecified

● **D75   Other and unspecified diseases of blood and blood-forming organs**

> **Excludes2**   acute lymphadenitis (L04.-)
> chronic lymphadenitis (I88.1)
> enlarged lymph nodes (R59.-)
> hypergammaglobulinemia NOS (D89.2)
> lymphadenitis NOS (I88.9)
> mesenteric lymphadenitis (acute) (chronic) (I88.0)

     D75.0   Familial erythrocytosis
Genetic mutation of gene that results in increased circulating RBCs
Benign polycythemia
Familial polycythemia

> **Excludes1**   hereditary ovalocytosis (D58.1)

     D75.1   Secondary polycythemia
Increase in total red cell mass
Acquired polycythemia
Emotional polycythemia
Erythrocytosis NOS
Hypoxemic polycythemia
Nephrogenous polycythemia
Polycythemia due to erythropoietin
Polycythemia due to fall in plasma volume
Polycythemia due to high altitude
Polycythemia due to stress
Polycythemia NOS
Relative polycythemia

> **Excludes1**   polycythemia neonatorum (P61.1)
> polycythemia vera (D45)

● **D75.8   Other specified diseases of blood and blood-forming organs**

     ▌ **D75.81   *Myelofibrosis***
Replacing bone marrow by fibrous tissue
Myelofibrosis NOS
Secondary myelofibrosis NOS

> *Code first* the underlying disorder, such as:
> malignant neoplasm of breast (C50.-)

> Use additional code, if applicable, for associated therapy-related myelodysplastic syndrome (D46.-)

> Use additional code for adverse effect, if applicable, to identify drug (T45.1X5)

> **Excludes1**   acute myelofibrosis (C94.4-)
> idiopathic myelofibrosis (D47.1)
> leukoerythroblastic anemia (D61.82)
> myelofibrosis with myeloid metaplasia (D47.4)
> myelophthisic anemia (D61.82)
> myelophthisis (D61.82)
> primary myelofibrosis (D47.1)

     D75.82   Heparin induced thrombocytopenia (HIT)

     D75.89   Other specified diseases of blood and blood-forming organs

D75.9   Disease of blood and blood-forming organs, unspecified

● **D76   Other specified diseases with participation of lymphoreticular and reticulohistiocytic tissue**

> **Excludes1**   (Abt-) Letterer-Siwe disease (C96.0)
> eosinophilic granuloma (C96.6)
> Hand-Schüller-Christian disease (C96.5)
> histiocytic medullary reticulosis (C96.9) ◄
> histiocytic sarcoma (C96.A)
> histiocytosis X, multifocal (C96.5)
> histiocytosis X, unifocal (C96.6)
> Langerhans-cell histiocytosis, multifocal (C96.5)
> Langerhans-cell histiocytosis NOS (C96.6)
> Langerhans-cell histiocytosis, unifocal (C96.6)
> leukemic reticuloendotheliosis (C91.4-) ◄
> lipomelanotic reticulosis (I89.8) ◄
> malignant histiocytosis (C96.A)
> malignant reticulosis (C86.0) ◄
> nonlipid reticuloendotheliosis (C96.0) ◄

     D76.1   Hemophagocytic lymphohistiocytosis
Familial hemophagocytic reticulosis
Histiocytoses of mononuclear phagocytes

     D76.2   Hemophagocytic syndrome, infection-associated
Use additional code to identify infectious agent or disease.

     D76.3   Other histiocytosis syndromes
Reticulohistiocytoma (giant-cell)
Sinus histiocytosis with massive lymphadenopathy
Xanthogranuloma

▌ **D77   *Other disorders of blood and blood-forming organs in diseases classified elsewhere***

> *Code first* underlying disease, such as:
> amyloidosis (E85.-)
> congenital early syphilis (A50.0)
> echinococcosis (B67.0-B67.9)
> malaria (B50.0-B54)
> schistosomiasis [bilharziasis] (B65.0-B65.9)
> vitamin C deficiency (E54)

> **Excludes1**   rupture of spleen due to Plasmodium vivax malaria (B51.0)
> splenitis, splenomegaly in late syphilis (A52.79)
> splenitis, splenomegaly in tuberculosis (A18.85)

◄ New   ◀▬ Revised   ~~deleted~~ Deleted   Excludes 1   Excludes 2   Includes   Use additional   Code first   Code also   Unspecified

716   **OGCR** Official Guidelines   X Assign placeholder X   ● Use Additional Character(s)   ▌ Manifestation Code   **Coding Clinic**

INTRAOPERATIVE AND POSTPROCEDURAL COMPLICATIONS OF THE SPLEEN (D78)

● **D78** Intraoperative and postprocedural complications of the spleen

● **D78.0** Intraoperative hemorrhage and hematoma of the spleen complicating a procedure

> **Excludes1** intraoperative hemorrhage and hematoma of the spleen due to accidental puncture or laceration during a procedure (D78.1-)

D78.01 Intraoperative hemorrhage and hematoma of the spleen complicating a procedure on the spleen

D78.02 Intraoperative hemorrhage and hematoma of the spleen complicating other procedure

● **D78.1** Accidental puncture and laceration of the spleen during a procedure

D78.11 Accidental puncture and laceration of the spleen during a procedure on the spleen

D78.12 Accidental puncture and laceration of the spleen during other procedure

● **D78.2** Postprocedural hemorrhage of the spleen following a procedure ◀▥

D78.21 Postprocedural hemorrhage of the spleen following a procedure on the spleen ◀▥

D78.22 Postprocedural hemorrhage of the spleen following other procedure ◀▥

● **D78.3** Postprocedural hematoma and seroma of the spleen following a procedure ◀

D78.31 Postprocedural hematoma of the spleen following a procedure on the spleen ◀

D78.32 Postprocedural hematoma of the spleen following other procedure ◀

D78.33 Postprocedural seroma of the spleen following a procedure on the spleen ◀

D78.34 Postprocedural seroma of the spleen following other procedure ◀

● **D78.8** Other intraoperative and postprocedural complications of the spleen

> Use additional code, if applicable, to further specify disorder

D78.81 Other intraoperative complications of the spleen

D78.89 Other postprocedural complications of the spleen

CERTAIN DISORDERS INVOLVING THE IMMUNE MECHANISM (D80-D89)

> **Includes** defects in the complement system
> immunodeficiency disorders, except human immunodeficiency virus [HIV] disease
> sarcoidosis

> **Excludes1** autoimmune disease (systemic) NOS (M35.9)
> functional disorders of polymorphonuclear neutrophils (D71)
> human immunodeficiency virus [HIV] disease (B20)

● **D80** Immunodeficiency with predominantly antibody defects

D80.0 Hereditary hypogammaglobulinemia
Autosomal recessive agammaglobulinemia (Swiss type)
X-linked agammaglobulinemia [Bruton] (with growth hormone deficiency)

D80.1 Nonfamilial hypogammaglobulinemia
Abnormally low levels of all classes of immunoglobulins
Agammaglobulinemia with immunoglobulin-bearing B-lymphocytes
Common variable agammaglobulinemia [CVAgamma]
Hypogammaglobulinemia NOS

D80.2 Selective deficiency of immunoglobulin A [IgA]

D80.3 Selective deficiency of immunoglobulin G [IgG] subclasses

D80.4 Selective deficiency of immunoglobulin M [IgM]

D80.5 Immunodeficiency with increased immunoglobulin M [IgM]

D80.6 Antibody deficiency with near-normal immunoglobulins or with hyperimmunoglobulinemia
Abnormally high levels of immunoglobulins in serum

D80.7 Transient hypogammaglobulinemia of infancy

D80.8 Other immunodeficiencies with predominantly antibody defects
Kappa light chain deficiency

D80.9 Immunodeficiency with predominantly antibody defects, unspecified

● **D81** Combined immunodeficiencies

> **Excludes1** autosomal recessive agammaglobulinemia (Swiss type) (D80.0)

D81.0 Severe combined immunodeficiency [SCID] with reticular dysgenesis

D81.1 Severe combined immunodeficiency [SCID] with low T- and B-cell numbers

D81.2 Severe combined immunodeficiency [SCID] with low or normal B-cell numbers

D81.3 Adenosine deaminase [ADA] deficiency

D81.4 Nezelof's syndrome

D81.5 Purine nucleoside phosphorylase [PNP] deficiency

D81.6 Major histocompatibility complex class I deficiency
Bare lymphocyte syndrome

D81.7 Major histocompatibility complex class II deficiency

● **D81.8** Other combined immunodeficiencies

● **D81.81** Biotin-dependent carboxylase deficiency
Multiple carboxylase deficiency

> **Excludes1** biotin-dependent carboxylase deficiency due to dietary deficiency of biotin (E53.8)

D81.810 Biotinidase deficiency

D81.818 Other biotin-dependent carboxylase deficiency
Holocarboxylase synthetase deficiency
Other multiple carboxylase deficiency

D81.819 Biotin-dependent carboxylase deficiency, unspecified
Multiple carboxylase deficiency, unspecified

D81.89 Other combined immunodeficiencies

D81.9 Combined immunodeficiency, unspecified
Severe combined immunodeficiency disorder [SCID] NOS

● **D82** Immunodeficiency associated with other major defects

> **Excludes1** ataxia telangiectasia [Louis-Bar] (G11.3)

D82.0 Wiskott-Aldrich syndrome
X-linked immunodeficiency
Immunodeficiency with thrombocytopenia and eczema

D82.1 Di George's syndrome
Congenital disorder with defective development of third and fourth pharyngeal pouches
Pharyngeal pouch syndrome
Thymic alymphoplasia
Thymic aplasia or hypoplasia with immunodeficiency

D82.2 Immunodeficiency with short-limbed stature

D82.3 Immunodeficiency following hereditary defective response to Epstein-Barr virus
X-linked lymphoproliferative disease

D82.4 Hyperimmunoglobulin E [IgE] syndrome
Suspected genetic defect that produces high levels of antibody immunoglobulin (IgE) that causes skin and lung infections and eczema

D82.8 Immunodeficiency associated with other specified major defects

D82.9 Immunodeficiency associated with major defect, unspecified

CHAPTER 3 (D50-D89)

Item 3-1 Sarcoidosis: A symptom of an inflammation producing tiny lumps of cells (granulomas) in various organs, most commonly the lungs and lymph nodes, that affect organ function. Cause is unknown occurring primarily in 20- to 40-year-olds, African-American, especially women, and those of Asian, German, Irish, Scandinavian, and Puerto Rican heritage.

● **D83** **Common variable immunodeficiency**
   D83.0 **Common variable immunodeficiency with predominant abnormalities of B-cell numbers and function**
   D83.1 **Common variable immunodeficiency with predominant immunoregulatory T-cell disorders**
   D83.2 **Common variable immunodeficiency with autoantibodies to B- or T-cells**
   D83.8 **Other common variable immunodeficiencies**
   D83.9 **Common variable immunodeficiency, unspecified**

● **D84** **Other immunodeficiencies**
   D84.0 **Lymphocyte function antigen-1 [LFA-1] defect**
   D84.1 **Defects in the complement system**
      C1 esterase inhibitor [C1-INH] deficiency
   D84.8 **Other specified immunodeficiencies**
   D84.9 **Immunodeficiency, unspecified**

● **D86** **Sarcoidosis**
   D86.0 **Sarcoidosis of lung**
   D86.1 **Sarcoidosis of lymph nodes**
   D86.2 **Sarcoidosis of lung with sarcoidosis of lymph nodes**
   D86.3 **Sarcoidosis of skin**
   ● **D86.8** **Sarcoidosis of other sites**
      D86.81 **Sarcoid meningitis**
      D86.82 **Multiple cranial nerve palsies in sarcoidosis**
      D86.83 **Sarcoid iridocyclitis**
         Rare large tumor with irregular surface of iris
      D86.84 **Sarcoid pyelonephritis**
         Systemic disease of unknown etiology characterized by chronic granulomatous inflammation with tissue destruction of pelvis kidney
         Tubulo-interstitial nephropathy in sarcoidosis
      D86.85 **Sarcoid myocarditis**
      D86.86 **Sarcoid arthropathy**
         Polyarthritis in sarcoidosis
      D86.87 **Sarcoid myositis**
         Granumloma of muscle
      D86.89 **Sarcoidosis of other sites**
         Hepatic granuloma
         Uveoparotid fever [Heerfordt]
   D86.9 **Sarcoidosis, unspecified**

● **D89** **Other disorders involving the immune mechanism, not elsewhere classified**
   Excludes1 hyperglobulinemia NOS (R77.1)
      monoclonal gammopathy (of undetermined significance) (D47.2)
   Excludes2 transplant failure and rejection (T86.-)
   D89.0 **Polyclonal hypergammaglobulinemia**
      Benign hypergammaglobulinemic purpura
      Polyclonal gammopathy NOS
   D89.1 **Cryoglobulinemia**
      Cryoglobulin (proteins) in blood that precipitate temperatures below 98.6° F; usually symptomatic of underlying disease
      Cryoglobulinemic purpura
      Cryoglobulinemic vasculitis
      Essential cryoglobulinemia
      Idiopathic cryoglobulinemia
      Mixed cryoglobulinemia
      Primary cryoglobulinemia
      Secondary cryoglobulinemia

   D89.2 **Hypergammaglobulinemia, unspecified**
   D89.3 **Immune reconstitution syndrome**
      Immune reconstitution inflammatory syndrome [IRIS]
      Use additional code for adverse effect, if applicable, to identify drug (T36-T50 with fifth or sixth character 5)
● **D89.4** **Mast cell activation syndrome and related disorders** ◄
      Excludes1 aggressive systemic mastocytosis (C96.2) ◄
         cutaneous mastocytosis (Q82.2) ◄
         indolent systemic mastocytosis (D47.0) ◄
         malignant mastocytoma (C96.2) ◄
         mast cell leukemia (C94.3-) ◄
         mastocytoma (D47.0) ◄
         systemic mastocytosis associated with a clonal hematologic non-mast cell lineage disease (SM-AHNMD) (D47.0) ◄
      D89.40 **Mast cell activation, unspecified** ◄
         Mast cell activation disorder, unspecified ◄
         Mast cell activation syndrome, NOS ◄
      D89.41 **Monoclonal mast cell activation syndrome** ◄
      D89.42 **Idiopathic mast cell activation syndrome** ◄
      D89.43 **Secondary mast cell activation** ◄
         Secondary mast cell activation syndrome ◄
         Code also underlying etiology, if known ◄
      D89.49 **Other mast cell activation disorder** ◄
         Other mast cell activation syndrome ◄
● **D89.8** **Other specified disorders involving the immune mechanism, not elsewhere classified**
   ● **D89.81** **Graft-versus-host disease**
         Code first underlying cause, such as:
            complications of transplanted organs and tissue (T86.-)
            complications of blood transfusion (T80.89)
         Use additional code to identify associated manifestations, such as:
            desquamative dermatitis (L30.8)
            diarrhea (R19.7)
            elevated bilirubin (R17)
            hair loss (L65.9)
      D89.810 **Acute graft-versus-host disease**
      D89.811 **Chronic graft-versus-host disease**
      D89.812 **Acute on chronic graft-versus-host disease**
      D89.813 **Graft-versus-host disease, unspecified**
   D89.82 **Autoimmune lymphoproliferative syndrome [ALPS]**
   D89.89 **Other specified disorders involving the immune mechanism, not elsewhere classified**
      Excludes1 human immunodeficiency virus disease (B20)
   D89.9 **Disorder involving the immune mechanism, unspecified**
      Immune disease NOS
      Coding Clinic: 2015, Q3, P22

◄ New   ◄═ Revised   ~~deleted~~ Deleted   Excludes 1   Excludes 2   Includes   Use additional   Code first   Code also   Unspecified
OGCR Official Guidelines   X Assign placeholder X   ● Use Additional Character(s)   ▶ Manifestation Code   **Coding Clinic**

CHAPTER 4

ENDOCRINE, NUTRITIONAL AND METABOLIC DISEASES (E00-E89)

OGCR Chapter-Specific Coding Guidelines

4. **Chapter 4: Endocrine, Nutritional, and Metabolic Diseases (E00-E89)**

   a. **Diabetes mellitus**
   The diabetes mellitus codes are combination codes that include the type of diabetes mellitus, the body system affected, and the complications affecting that body system. As many codes within a particular category as are necessary to describe all of the complications of the disease may be used. They should be sequenced based on the reason for a particular encounter. Assign as many codes from categories E08 – E13 as needed to identify all of the associated conditions that the patient has.

   1) **Type of diabetes**
   The age of a patient is not the sole determining factor, though most type 1 diabetics develop the condition before reaching puberty. For this reason type 1 diabetes mellitus is also referred to as juvenile diabetes.

   2) **Type of diabetes mellitus not documented**
   If the type of diabetes mellitus is not documented in the medical record the default is E11.-, Type 2 diabetes mellitus.

   3) **Diabetes mellitus and the use of insulin oral hypoglycemics**
   If the documentation in a medical record does not indicate the type of diabetes but does indicate that the patient uses insulin, code E11, Type 2 diabetes mellitus, should be assigned. Code Z79.4, Long-term (current) use of insulin **or Z79.84, Long term (current) use of oral hypoglycemic drugs,** should also be assigned to indicate that the patient uses insulin **or hypoglycemic drugs**. Code Z79.4 should not be assigned if insulin is given temporarily to bring a type 2 patient's blood sugar under control during an encounter.

   4) **Diabetes mellitus in pregnancy and gestational diabetes**
   See Section I.C.15. Diabetes mellitus in pregnancy.
   See Section I.C.15. Gestational (pregnancy induced) diabetes

   5) **Complications due to insulin pump malfunction**
      (a) **Underdose of insulin due to insulin pump failure**
   An underdose of insulin due to an insulin pump failure should be assigned to a code from subcategory T85.6, Mechanical complication of other specified internal and external prosthetic devices, implants and grafts, that specifies the type of pump malfunction, as the principal or first-listed code, followed by code T38.3X6-, Underdosing of insulin and oral hypoglycemic [antidiabetic] drugs. Additional codes for the type of diabetes mellitus and any associated complications due to the underdosing should also be assigned.

      (b) **Overdose of insulin due to insulin pump failure**
   The principal or first-listed code for an encounter due to an insulin pump malfunction resulting in an overdose of insulin, should also be T85.6-, Mechanical complication of other specified internal and external prosthetic devices, implants and grafts, followed by code T38.3X1-, Poisoning by insulin and oral hypoglycemic [antidiabetic] drugs, accidental (unintentional).

   6) **Secondary diabetes mellitus**
   Codes under categories E08, Diabetes mellitus due to underlying condition, E09, Drug or chemical induced diabetes mellitus and E13, Other specified diabetes mellitus, identify complications/manifestations associated with secondary diabetes mellitus. Secondary diabetes is always caused by another condition or event (e.g., cystic fibrosis, malignant neoplasm of pancreas, pancreatectomy, adverse effect of drug, or poisoning).

      (a) **Secondary diabetes mellitus and the use of insulin or hypoglycemic drugs**
   For patients who routinely use insulin **or hypoglycemic drugs,** code Z79.4, Long-term (current) use of insulin **or Z79.84, Long term (current) use of oral hypoglycemic drugs,** should also be assigned. Code Z79.4 should not be assigned if insulin is given temporarily to bring a patient's blood sugar under control during an encounter.

      (b) **Assigning and sequencing secondary diabetes codes and its causes**
   The sequencing of the secondary diabetes codes in relationship to codes for the cause of the diabetes is based on the Tabular List instructions for categories E08, E09 and E13.

         (i) **Secondary diabetes mellitus due to pancreatectomy** For postpancreatectomy diabetes mellitus (lack of insulin due to the surgical removal of all or part of the pancreas), assign code E89.1, Postprocedural hypoinsulinemia. Assign a code from category E13 and a code from subcategory Z90.41-, Acquired absence of pancreas, as additional codes.

         (ii) **Secondary diabetes due to drugs** Secondary diabetes may be caused by an adverse effect of correctly administered medications, poisoning or sequela of poisoning.
   See section I.C.19.e for coding of adverse effects and poisoning, and section I.C.20 for external cause code reporting.

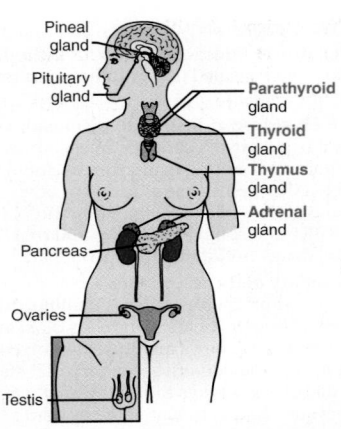

Figure 4-1 The endocrine system. (From Buck CJ: Step-by-Step Medical Coding, ed 2016, St. Louis, Elsevier, 2016)

CHAPTER 4

ENDOCRINE, NUTRITIONAL AND METABOLIC DISEASES (E00-E89)

All neoplasms, whether functionally active or not, are classified in Chapter 2. Appropriate codes in this chapter (i.e., E05.8, E07.0, E16-E31, E34.-) may be used as additional codes to indicate either functional activity by neoplasms and ectopic endocrine tissue or hyperfunction and hypofunction of endocrine glands associated with neoplasms and other conditions classified elsewhere.

Excludes1 transitory endocrine and metabolic disorders specific to newborn (P70-P74)

This chapter contains the following blocks:

E00-E07	Disorders of thyroid gland
E08-E13	Diabetes mellitus
E15-E16	Other disorders of glucose regulation and pancreatic internal secretion
E20-E35	Disorders of other endocrine glands
E36	Intraoperative complications of endocrine system
E40-E46	Malnutrition
E50-E64	Other nutritional deficiencies
E65-E68	Overweight, obesity and other hyperalimentation
E70-E88	Metabolic disorders
E89	Postprocedural endocrine and metabolic complications and disorders, not elsewhere classified

DISORDERS OF THYROID GLAND (E00-E07)

● **E00** **Congenital iodine-deficiency syndrome**

Use additional code (F70-F79) to identify associated intellectual disabilities.

Excludes1 subclinical iodine-deficiency hypothyroidism (E02)

E00.0 **Congenital iodine-deficiency syndrome, neurological type**
Endemic cretinism, neurological type

E00.1 **Congenital iodine-deficiency syndrome, myxedematous type**
Dry, waxy type of swelling (nonpitting edema) with abnormal deposits of mucin in skin (mucinosis) and other tissues
Endemic hypothyroid cretinism
Endemic cretinism, myxedematous type

E00.2 **Congenital iodine-deficiency syndrome, mixed type**
Endemic cretinism, mixed type

E00.9 **Congenital iodine-deficiency syndrome, unspecified**
Congenital iodine-deficiency hypothyroidism NOS
Endemic cretinism NOS

Figure 4-2 **Goiter** is an enlargement of the thyroid gland.

Item 4–1 **Simple** goiter indicates no nodules are present. The most common type of goiter is a **diffuse colloidal**, also called a **nontoxic** or **endemic** goiter.

● **E01** **Iodine-deficiency related thyroid disorders and allied conditions**

Excludes1 congenital iodine-deficiency syndrome (E00.-)
subclinical iodine-deficiency hypothyroidism (E02)

E01.0 **Iodine-deficiency related diffuse (endemic) goiter**
Thyroid gland is enlarged

E01.1 **Iodine-deficiency related multinodular (endemic) goiter**
Iodine-deficiency related nodular goiter

E01.2 **Iodine-deficiency related (endemic) goiter, unspecified**
Endemic goiter NOS

E01.8 **Other iodine-deficiency related thyroid disorders and allied conditions**
Acquired iodine-deficiency hypothyroidism NOS

E02 **Subclinical iodine-deficiency hypothyroidism**

● **E03** **Other hypothyroidism**

Excludes1 iodine-deficiency related hypothyroidism (E00-E02)
postprocedural hypothyroidism (E89.0)

E03.0 **Congenital hypothyroidism with diffuse goiter**
Congenital parenchymatous goiter (nontoxic)
Congenital goiter (nontoxic) NOS

Excludes1 transitory congenital goiter with normal function (P72.0)

E03.1 **Congenital hypothyroidism without goiter**
Aplasia of thyroid (with myxedema)
Congenital atrophy of thyroid
Congenital hypothyroidism NOS

E03.2 **Hypothyroidism due to medicaments and other exogenous substances**
Code first poisoning due to drug or toxin, if applicable (T36-T65 with fifth or sixth character 1-4 or 6)
Use additional code for adverse effect, if applicable, to identify drug (T36-T50 with fifth or sixth character 5)

E03.3 **Postinfectious hypothyroidism**

E03.4 **Atrophy of thyroid (acquired)**

Excludes1 congenital atrophy of thyroid (E03.1)

E03.5 **Myxedema coma**
Often fatal complication of long-term hypothyroidism

E03.8 **Other specified hypothyroidism**

E03.9 **Hypothyroidism, unspecified**
Myxedema NOS

Item 4–2 **Hypothyroidism** is a condition in which there are insufficient levels of thyroxine. **Cretinism** is congenital hypothyroidism, which can result in mental and physical retardation.

Figure 4-3 Typical appearance of patients with moderately severe primary hypothyroidism or myxedema. (From Larsen: Williams Textbook of Endocrinology, ed 10, Saunders, An Imprint of Elsevier, 2003)

● **E04 Other nontoxic goiter**

> **Excludes1** congenital goiter (NOS) (diffuse)
> (parenchymatous) (E03.0)
> iodine-deficiency related goiter (E00-E02)

E04.0 **Nontoxic diffuse goiter**
Thyroid gland is enlarged
Diffuse (colloid) nontoxic goiter
Simple nontoxic goiter

E04.1 **Nontoxic single thyroid nodule**
Colloid nodule (cystic) (thyroid)
Nontoxic uninodular goiter
Thyroid (cystic) nodule NOS

E04.2 **Nontoxic multinodular goiter**
Enlarged thyroid gland with multiple nodules
Cystic goiter NOS
Multinodular (cystic) goiter NOS

E04.8 **Other specified nontoxic goiter**

E04.9 **Nontoxic goiter, unspecified**
Goiter NOS
Nodular goiter (nontoxic) NOS

● **E05 Thyrotoxicosis [hyperthyroidism]**
Enlarged thyroid gland with multiple nodules

> **Excludes1** chronic thyroiditis with transient thyrotoxicosis
> (E06.2)
> neonatal thyrotoxicosis (P72.1)

● E05.0 **Thyrotoxicosis with diffuse goiter**
Exophthalmic or toxic goiter NOS
Graves' disease
Toxic diffuse goiter

E05.00 **Thyrotoxicosis with diffuse goiter without thyrotoxic crisis or storm**

E05.01 **Thyrotoxicosis with diffuse goiter with thyrotoxic crisis or storm**

● E05.1 **Thyrotoxicosis with toxic single thyroid nodule**
Thyrotoxicosis with toxic uninodular goiter

E05.10 **Thyrotoxicosis with toxic single thyroid nodule without thyrotoxic crisis or storm**

E05.11 **Thyrotoxicosis with toxic single thyroid nodule with thyrotoxic crisis or storm**

● E05.2 **Thyrotoxicosis with toxic multinodular goiter**
Toxic nodular goiter NOS

E05.20 **Thyrotoxicosis with toxic multinodular goiter without thyrotoxic crisis or storm**

E05.21 **Thyrotoxicosis with toxic multinodular goiter with thyrotoxic crisis or storm**

● E05.3 **Thyrotoxicosis from ectopic thyroid tissue**

E05.30 **Thyrotoxicosis from ectopic thyroid tissue without thyrotoxic crisis or storm**

E05.31 **Thyrotoxicosis from ectopic thyroid tissue with thyrotoxic crisis or storm**

● E05.4 **Thyrotoxicosis factitia**

E05.40 **Thyrotoxicosis factitia without thyrotoxic crisis or storm**

E05.41 **Thyrotoxicosis factitia with thyrotoxic crisis or storm**

● E05.8 **Other thyrotoxicosis**
Overproduction of thyroid-stimulating hormone

E05.80 **Other thyrotoxicosis without thyrotoxic crisis or storm**

E05.81 **Other thyrotoxicosis with thyrotoxic crisis or storm**

● E05.9 **Thyrotoxicosis, unspecified**
Hyperthyroidism NOS

E05.90 **Thyrotoxicosis, unspecified without thyrotoxic crisis or storm**

E05.91 **Thyrotoxicosis, unspecified with thyrotoxic crisis or storm**

● **E06 Thyroiditis**
An inflammation of the thyroid gland which results in an inability to convert iodine into thyroid hormone

> **Excludes1** postpartum thyroiditis (O90.5)

E06.0 **Acute thyroiditis**
Abscess of thyroid
Pyogenic thyroiditis
Suppurative thyroiditis
Use additional code (B95-B97) to identify infectious agent.

E06.1 **Subacute thyroiditis**
Inflammation of thyroid gland following viral upper respiratory infection
de Quervain thyroiditis
Giant-cell thyroiditis
Granulomatous thyroiditis
Nonsuppurative thyroiditis
Viral thyroiditis

> **Excludes1** autoimmune thyroiditis (E06.3)

E06.2 **Chronic thyroiditis with transient thyrotoxicosis**
Chronic inflammation of thyroid gland with intermittent overproduction of thyroid hormone

> **Excludes1** autoimmune thyroiditis (E06.3)

E06.3 **Autoimmune thyroiditis**
Hashimoto's thyroiditis
Hashitoxicosis (transient)
Lymphadenoid goiter
Lymphocytic thyroiditis
Struma lymphomatosa

E06.4 **Drug-induced thyroiditis**
Use additional code for adverse effect, if applicable, to identify drug (T36-T50 with fifth or sixth character 5)

E06.5 **Other chronic thyroiditis**
Chronic fibrous thyroiditis
Chronic thyroiditis NOS
Ligneous thyroiditis
Riedel thyroiditis

E06.9 **Thyroiditis, unspecified**

● **E07 Other disorders of thyroid**

E07.0 **Hypersecretion of calcitonin**
C-cell hyperplasia of thyroid
Hypersecretion of thyrocalcitonin

E07.1 **Dyshormogenetic goiter**
Group of several types of goiter resulting from enzyme defects in hormone synthesis
Familial dyshormogenetic goiter
Pendred's syndrome

> **Excludes1** transitory congenital goiter with normal function (P72.0)

Figure 4-4 Graves' disease. In Graves' disease, exophthalmos often looks more pronounced than it actually is because of the extreme lid retraction that may occur. This patient, for instance, had minimal proptosis of the left eye but marked lid retraction.

(Courtesy Dr. HG Scheie. From Yanoff M, Fine BS: Ocular Pathology, ed 6, St. Louis, Mosby, 2008)

Item 4–3 Thyrotoxicosis is a condition caused by excessive amounts of the thyroid hormone thyroxine production or hyperthyroidism. **Graves' disease is associated with hyperthyroidism** (known as **Basedow's disease** in Europe).

● **E07.8**   **Other specified disorders of thyroid**

    E07.81   **Sick-euthyroid syndrome**
          Euthyroid sick-syndrome

    E07.89   **Other specified disorders of thyroid**
          Abnormality of thyroid-binding globulin
          Hemorrhage of thyroid
          Infarction of thyroid

   E07.9   **Disorder of thyroid, unspecified**

OGCR Section I.C.4.a

Diabetes mellitus

The diabetes mellitus codes are combination codes that include the type of diabetes mellitus, body system affected, and the complications affecting that body system. As many codes within a particular category as are necessary to describe all of the complications of the disease may be used. They should be sequenced based on the reason for a particular visit. Assign as many codes from categories E08–E13 as needed to identify all of the associated conditions that the patient has.

DIABETES MELLITUS (E08-E13)

A metabolic disease that results in persistent hyperglycemia.

● **E08**   **Diabetes mellitus due to underlying condition**
    Code first the underlying condition, such as:
      congenital rubella (P35.0)
      Cushing's syndrome (E24.-)
      cystic fibrosis (E84.-)
      malignant neoplasm (C00-C96)
      malnutrition (E40-E46)
      pancreatitis and other diseases of the pancreas (K85-K86.-)
    Use additional code to identify control using:
      insulin (Z79.4)
      oral antidiabetic drugs (Z79.84)
      oral hypoglycemic drugs (Z79.84)
    Excludes1   drug or chemical induced diabetes mellitus (E09.-)
          gestational diabetes (O24.4-)
          neonatal diabetes mellitus (P70.2)
          postpancreatectomy diabetes mellitus (E13.-)
          postprocedural diabetes mellitus (E13.-)
          secondary diabetes mellitus NEC (E13.-)
          type 1 diabetes mellitus (E10.-)
          type 2 diabetes mellitus (E11.-)

● **E08.0**   **Diabetes mellitus due to underlying condition with hyperosmolarity**

   E08.00   *Diabetes mellitus due to underlying condition with hyperosmolarity without nonketotic hyperglycemic-hyperosmolar coma (NKHHC)*

   E08.01   *Diabetes mellitus due to underlying condition with hyperosmolarity with coma*

● **E08.1**   **Diabetes mellitus due to underlying condition with ketoacidosis**

   E08.10   *Diabetes mellitus due to underlying condition with ketoacidosis without coma*

   E08.11   *Diabetes mellitus due to underlying condition with ketoacidosis with coma*

● **E08.2**   **Diabetes mellitus due to underlying condition with kidney complications**

   E08.21   *Diabetes mellitus due to underlying condition with diabetic nephropathy*
      Diabetes mellitus due to underlying condition with intercapillary glomerulosclerosis
      Diabetes mellitus due to underlying condition with intracapillary glomerulonephrosis
      Diabetes mellitus due to underlying condition with Kimmelstiel-Wilson disease

   E08.22   *Diabetes mellitus due to underlying condition with diabetic chronic kidney disease*
      Use additional code to identify stage of chronic kidney disease (N18.1-N18.6)

   E08.29   *Diabetes mellitus due to underlying condition with other diabetic kidney complication*
      Renal tubular degeneration in diabetes mellitus due to underlying condition

● **E08.3**   **Diabetes mellitus due to underlying condition with ophthalmic complications**
    Changes in blood vessels of retina in which blood vessels swell and leak fluid into retinal surface.

● **E08.31**   **Diabetes mellitus due to underlying condition with unspecified diabetic retinopathy**

   E08.311   *Diabetes mellitus due to underlying condition with unspecified diabetic retinopathy with macular edema*

   E08.319   *Diabetes mellitus due to underlying condition with unspecified diabetic retinopathy without macular edema*

● **E08.32**   **Diabetes mellitus due to underlying condition with mild nonproliferative diabetic retinopathy**
    Diabetes mellitus due to underlying condition with nonproliferative diabetic retinopathy NOS

    One of the following 7th characters is to be assigned to codes in subcategory E08.32 to designate laterality of the disease:

    1   right eye
    2   left eye
    3   bilateral
    9   unspecified eye

   E08.321   *Diabetes mellitus due to underlying condition with mild nonproliferative diabetic retinopathy with macular edema*

   E08.329   *Diabetes mellitus due to underlying condition with mild nonproliferative diabetic retinopathy without macular edema*

● **E08.33**   **Diabetes mellitus due to underlying condition with moderate nonproliferative diabetic retinopathy**

    One of the following 7th characters is to be assigned to codes in subcategory E08.33 to designate laterality of the disease:

    1   right eye
    2   left eye
    3   bilateral
    9   unspecified eye

   E08.331   *Diabetes mellitus due to underlying condition with moderate nonproliferative diabetic retinopathy with macular edema*

   E08.339   *Diabetes mellitus due to underlying condition with moderate nonproliferative diabetic retinopathy without macular edema*

● **E08.34**   **Diabetes mellitus due to underlying condition with severe nonproliferative diabetic retinopathy**

    One of the following 7th characters is to be assigned to codes in subcategory E08.34 to designate laterality of the disease:

    1   right eye
    2   left eye
    3   bilateral
    9   unspecified eye

   E08.341   *Diabetes mellitus due to underlying condition with severe nonproliferative diabetic retinopathy with macular edema*

   E08.349   *Diabetes mellitus due to underlying condition with severe nonproliferative diabetic retinopathy without macular edema*

◄ New   ◄▥ Revised   ~~deleted~~ Deleted   Excludes 1   Excludes 2   Includes   Use additional   Code first   Code also   Unspecified

OGCR Official Guidelines   X Assign placeholder X   ● Use Additional Character(s)   ▣ Manifestation Code   **Coding Clinic**

● **E08.35**   **Diabetes mellitus due to underlying condition with proliferative diabetic retinopathy**

One of the following 7th characters is to be assigned to codes in subcategory E08.35 to designate laterality of the disease: ◄

1	right eye ◄
2	left eye ◄
3	bilateral ◄
9	unspecified eye ◄

   ● ▶ *E08.351*   *Diabetes mellitus due to underlying condition with proliferative diabetic retinopathy with macular edema*

   ● ▶ *E08.352*   *Diabetes mellitus due to underlying condition with proliferative diabetic retinopathy with traction retinal detachment involving the macula* ◄

   ● ▶ *E08.353*   *Diabetes mellitus due to underlying condition with proliferative diabetic retinopathy with traction retinal detachment not involving the macula* ◄

   ● ▶ *E08.354*   *Diabetes mellitus due to underlying condition with proliferative diabetic retinopathy with combined traction retinal detachment and rhegmatogenous retinal detachment* ◄

   ● ▶ *E08.355*   *Diabetes mellitus due to underlying condition with stable proliferative diabetic retinopathy* ◄

   ● ▶ *E08.359*   *Diabetes mellitus due to underlying condition with proliferative diabetic retinopathy without macular edema*

  ▶ *E08.36*   *Diabetes mellitus due to underlying condition with diabetic cataract*

X ● ▶ *E08.37*   *Diabetes mellitus due to underlying condition with diabetic macular edema, resolved following treatment* ◄

One of the following 7th characters is to be assigned to code E08.37 to designate laterality of the disease: ◄

1	right eye ◄
2	left eye ◄
3	bilateral ◄
9	unspecified eye ◄

  ▶ *E08.39*   *Diabetes mellitus due to underlying condition with other diabetic ophthalmic complication*

    Use additional code to identify manifestation, such as:
      diabetic glaucoma (H40-H42)

● **E08.4**   **Diabetes mellitus due to underlying condition with neurological complications**

  ▶ *E08.40*   *Diabetes mellitus due to underlying condition with diabetic neuropathy, unspecified*

  ▶ *E08.41*   *Diabetes mellitus due to underlying condition with diabetic mononeuropathy*

  ▶ *E08.42*   *Diabetes mellitus due to underlying condition with diabetic polyneuropathy*
    Diabetes mellitus due to underlying condition with diabetic neuralgia

  ▶ *E08.43*   *Diabetes mellitus due to underlying condition with diabetic autonomic (poly)neuropathy*
    Diabetes mellitus due to underlying condition with diabetic gastroparesis

  ▶ *E08.44*   *Diabetes mellitus due to underlying condition with diabetic amyotrophy*

  ▶ *E08.49*   *Diabetes mellitus due to underlying condition with other diabetic neurological complication*

● **E08.5**   **Diabetes mellitus due to underlying condition with circulatory complications**

  ▶ *E08.51*   *Diabetes mellitus due to underlying condition with diabetic peripheral angiopathy without gangrene*

  ▶ *E08.52*   *Diabetes mellitus due to underlying condition with diabetic peripheral angiopathy with gangrene*
    Diabetes mellitus due to underlying condition with diabetic gangrene

  ▶ *E08.59*   *Diabetes mellitus due to underlying condition with other circulatory complications*

● **E08.6**   **Diabetes mellitus due to underlying condition with other specified complications**

  ● **E08.61**   **Diabetes mellitus due to underlying condition with diabetic arthropathy**

   ▶ *E08.610*   *Diabetes mellitus due to underlying condition with diabetic neuropathic arthropathy*
     Diabetes mellitus due to underlying condition with Charcôt's joints

   ▶ *E08.618*   *Diabetes mellitus due to underlying condition with other diabetic arthropathy*

  ● **E08.62**   **Diabetes mellitus due to underlying condition with skin complications**

   ▶ *E08.620*   *Diabetes mellitus due to underlying condition with diabetic dermatitis*
     Diabetes mellitus due to underlying condition with diabetic necrobiosis lipoidica

   ▶ *E08.621*   *Diabetes mellitus due to underlying condition with foot ulcer*
     Use additional code to identify site of ulcer (L97.4-, L97.5-)

   ▶ *E08.622*   *Diabetes mellitus due to underlying condition with other skin ulcer*
     Use additional code to identify site of ulcer (L97.1-L97.9, L98.41-L98.49)

   ▶ *E08.628*   *Diabetes mellitus due to underlying condition with other skin complications*

  ● **E08.63**   **Diabetes mellitus due to underlying condition with oral complications**

   ▶ *E08.630*   *Diabetes mellitus due to underlying condition with periodontal disease*

   ▶ *E08.638*   *Diabetes mellitus due to underlying condition with other oral complications*

  ● **E08.64**   **Diabetes mellitus due to underlying condition with hypoglycemia**

   ▶ *E08.641*   *Diabetes mellitus due to underlying condition with hypoglycemia with coma*

   ▶ *E08.649*   *Diabetes mellitus due to underlying condition with hypoglycemia without coma*

  ▶ *E08.65*   *Diabetes mellitus due to underlying condition with hyperglycemia*

  ▶ *E08.69*   *Diabetes mellitus due to underlying condition with other specified complication*
    Use additional code to identify complication

▶ *E08.8*   *Diabetes mellitus due to underlying condition with unspecified complications*

▶ *E08.9*   *Diabetes mellitus due to underlying condition without complications*

CHAPTER 4 (E00-E90)

● **E09   Drug or chemical induced diabetes mellitus**

Code first poisoning due to drug or toxin, if applicable (T36-T65 with fifth or sixth character 1-4 or 6)

Use additional code for adverse effect, if applicable, to identify drug (T36-T50 with fifth or sixth character 5)

Use additional code to identify control using: ◀━━
    insulin (Z79.4) ◀
    oral antidiabetic drugs (Z79.84) ◀
    oral hypoglycemic drugs (Z79.84) ◀

Excludes1   diabetes mellitus due to underlying condition (E08.-)
        gestational diabetes (O24.4-)
        neonatal diabetes mellitus (P70.2)
        postpancreatectomy diabetes mellitus (E13.-)
        postprocedural diabetes mellitus (E13.-)
        secondary diabetes mellitus NEC (E13.-)
        type 1 diabetes mellitus (E10.-)
        type 2 diabetes mellitus (E11.-)

● **E09.0   Drug or chemical induced diabetes mellitus with hyperosmolarity**

    E09.00   **Drug or chemical induced diabetes mellitus with hyperosmolarity without nonketotic hyperglycemic-hyperosmolar coma (NKHHC)**

    E09.01   **Drug or chemical induced diabetes mellitus with hyperosmolarity with coma**

● **E09.1   Drug or chemical induced diabetes mellitus with ketoacidosis**

    E09.10   **Drug or chemical induced diabetes mellitus with ketoacidosis without coma**

    E09.11   **Drug or chemical induced diabetes mellitus with ketoacidosis with coma**

● **E09.2   Drug or chemical induced diabetes mellitus with kidney complications**

    E09.21   **Drug or chemical induced diabetes mellitus with diabetic nephropathy**
        Drug or chemical induced diabetes mellitus with intercapillary glomerulosclerosis
        Drug or chemical induced diabetes mellitus with intracapillary glomerulonephrosis
        Drug or chemical induced diabetes mellitus with Kimmelstiel-Wilson disease

    E09.22   **Drug or chemical induced diabetes mellitus with diabetic chronic kidney disease**
        Use additional code to identify stage of chronic kidney disease (N18.1-N18.6)

    E09.29   **Drug or chemical induced diabetes mellitus with other diabetic kidney complication**
        Drug or chemical induced diabetes mellitus with renal tubular degeneration

● **E09.3   Drug or chemical induced diabetes mellitus with ophthalmic complications**

  ● **E09.31**   **Drug or chemical induced diabetes mellitus with unspecified diabetic retinopathy**

        E09.311   **Drug or chemical induced diabetes mellitus with unspecified diabetic retinopathy with macular edema**

        E09.319   **Drug or chemical induced diabetes mellitus with unspecified diabetic retinopathy without macular edema**

● **E09.32**   **Drug or chemical induced diabetes mellitus with mild nonproliferative diabetic retinopathy**
        Drug or chemical induced diabetes mellitus with nonproliferative diabetic retinopathy NOS

        One of the following 7th characters is to be assigned to codes in subcategory E09.32 to designate laterality of the disease: ◀

1	right eye ◀
2	left eye ◀
3	bilateral ◀
9	unspecified eye ◀

  ● **E09.321**   **Drug or chemical induced diabetes mellitus with mild nonproliferative diabetic retinopathy with macular edema**

  ● **E09.329**   **Drug or chemical induced diabetes mellitus with mild nonproliferative diabetic retinopathy without macular edema**

● **E09.33**   **Drug or chemical induced diabetes mellitus with moderate nonproliferative diabetic retinopathy**

        One of the following 7th characters is to be assigned to codes in subcategory E09.33 to designate laterality of the disease: ◀

1	right eye ◀
2	left eye ◀
3	bilateral ◀
9	unspecified eye ◀

  ● **E09.331**   **Drug or chemical induced diabetes mellitus with moderate nonproliferative diabetic retinopathy with macular edema**

  ● **E09.339**   **Drug or chemical induced diabetes mellitus with moderate nonproliferative diabetic retinopathy without macular edema**

● **E09.34**   **Drug or chemical induced diabetes mellitus with severe nonproliferative diabetic retinopathy**

        One of the following 7th characters is to be assigned to codes in subcategory E09.34 to designate laterality of the disease: ◀

1	right eye ◀
2	left eye ◀
3	bilateral ◀
9	unspecified eye ◀

  ● **E09.341**   **Drug or chemical induced diabetes mellitus with severe nonproliferative diabetic retinopathy with macular edema**

  ● **E09.349**   **Drug or chemical induced diabetes mellitus with severe nonproliferative diabetic retinopathy without macular edema**

● **E09.35**   **Drug or chemical induced diabetes mellitus with proliferative diabetic retinopathy**

One of the following 7th characters is to be assigned to codes in subcategory E09.35 to designate laterality of the disease: ◄

1	right eye ◄
2	left eye ◄
3	bilateral ◄
9	unspecified eye ◄

● **E09.351**   Drug or chemical induced diabetes mellitus with proliferative diabetic retinopathy with macular edema

● **E09.352**   Drug or chemical induced diabetes mellitus with proliferative diabetic retinopathy with traction retinal detachment involving the macula ◄

● **E09.353**   Drug or chemical induced diabetes mellitus with proliferative diabetic retinopathy with traction retinal detachment not involving the macula ◄

● **E09.354**   Drug or chemical induced diabetes mellitus with proliferative diabetic retinopathy with combined traction retinal detachment and rhegmatogenous retinal detachment ◄

● **E09.355**   Drug or chemical induced diabetes mellitus with stable proliferative diabetic retinopathy ◄

● **E09.359**   Drug or chemical induced diabetes mellitus with proliferative diabetic retinopathy without macular edema

E09.36   **Drug or chemical induced diabetes mellitus with diabetic cataract**

X ● **E09.37**   **Drug or chemical induced diabetes mellitus with diabetic macular edema, resolved following treatment** ◄

One of the following 7th characters is to be assigned to code E09.37 to designate laterality of the disease: ◄

1	right eye ◄
2	left eye ◄
3	bilateral ◄
9	unspecified eye ◄

E09.39   **Drug or chemical induced diabetes mellitus with other diabetic ophthalmic complication**

Use additional code to identify manifestation, such as:
    diabetic glaucoma (H40-H42)

● **E09.4**   **Drug or chemical induced diabetes mellitus with neurological complications**

E09.40   **Drug or chemical induced diabetes mellitus with neurological complications with diabetic neuropathy, unspecified**

E09.41   **Drug or chemical induced diabetes mellitus with neurological complications with diabetic mononeuropathy**

E09.42   **Drug or chemical induced diabetes mellitus with neurological complications with diabetic polyneuropathy**
Drug or chemical induced diabetes mellitus with diabetic neuralgia

E09.43   **Drug or chemical induced diabetes mellitus with neurological complications with diabetic autonomic (poly)neuropathy**
Drug or chemical induced diabetes mellitus with diabetic gastroparesis

E09.44   **Drug or chemical induced diabetes mellitus with neurological complications with diabetic amyotrophy**

E09.49   **Drug or chemical induced diabetes mellitus with neurological complications with other diabetic neurological complication**

● **E09.5**   **Drug or chemical induced diabetes mellitus with circulatory complications**

E09.51   **Drug or chemical induced diabetes mellitus with diabetic peripheral angiopathy without gangrene**

E09.52   **Drug or chemical induced diabetes mellitus with diabetic peripheral angiopathy with gangrene**
Drug or chemical induced diabetes mellitus with diabetic gangrene

E09.59   **Drug or chemical induced diabetes mellitus with other circulatory complications**

● **E09.6**   **Drug or chemical induced diabetes mellitus with other specified complications**

● **E09.61**   **Drug or chemical induced diabetes mellitus with diabetic arthropathy**

E09.610   Drug or chemical induced diabetes mellitus with diabetic neuropathic arthropathy
Drug or chemical induced diabetes mellitus with Charcôt's joints
Progressive degeneration of weight-bearing joint

E09.618   Drug or chemical induced diabetes mellitus with other diabetic arthropathy

● **E09.62**   **Drug or chemical induced diabetes mellitus with skin complications**

E09.620   Drug or chemical induced diabetes mellitus with diabetic dermatitis
Drug or chemical induced diabetes mellitus with diabetic necrobiosis lipoidica
Necrotizing skin condition

E09.621   Drug or chemical induced diabetes mellitus with foot ulcer
Use additional code to identify site of ulcer (L97.4-, L97.5-)

E09.622   Drug or chemical induced diabetes mellitus with other skin ulcer
Use additional code to identify site of ulcer (L97.1-L97.9, L98.41-L98.49)

E09.628   Drug or chemical induced diabetes mellitus with other skin complications

● **E09.63**   **Drug or chemical induced diabetes mellitus with oral complications**

E09.630   Drug or chemical induced diabetes mellitus with periodontal disease

E09.638   Drug or chemical induced diabetes mellitus with other oral complications

● **E09.64**   **Drug or chemical induced diabetes mellitus with hypoglycemia**

E09.641   Drug or chemical induced diabetes mellitus with hypoglycemia with coma

E09.649   Drug or chemical induced diabetes mellitus with hypoglycemia without coma

E09.65   **Drug or chemical induced diabetes mellitus with hyperglycemia**

E09.69   **Drug or chemical induced diabetes mellitus with other specified complication**
Use additional code to identify complication

E09.8   **Drug or chemical induced diabetes mellitus with unspecified complications**

E09.9   **Drug or chemical induced diabetes mellitus without complications**

CHAPTER 4 (E00-E90)

● E10　　Type 1 diabetes mellitus

Includes　　brittle diabetes (mellitus)
　　　　　　diabetes (mellitus) due to autoimmune process
　　　　　　diabetes (mellitus) due to immune mediated
　　　　　　　　pancreatic islet beta-cell destruction
　　　　　　idiopathic diabetes (mellitus)
　　　　　　juvenile onset diabetes (mellitus)
　　　　　　ketosis-prone diabetes (mellitus)

Excludes1　　diabetes mellitus due to underlying condition
　　　　　　　　(E08.-)
　　　　　　drug or chemical induced diabetes mellitus (E09.-)
　　　　　　gestational diabetes (O24.4-)
　　　　　　hyperglycemia NOS (R73.9)
　　　　　　neonatal diabetes mellitus (P70.2)
　　　　　　postpancreatectomy diabetes mellitus (E13.-)
　　　　　　postprocedural diabetes mellitus (E13.-)
　　　　　　secondary diabetes mellitus NEC (E13.-)
　　　　　　type 2 diabetes mellitus (E11.-)

● E10.1　　**Type 1 diabetes mellitus with ketoacidosis**
　　　　　Acidosis accompanied by accumulation of ketone bodies
　　　　　(ketosis) in body tissues and fluids

　　　E10.10　　**Type 1 diabetes mellitus with ketoacidosis**
　　　　　　　without coma
　　　　　　　Coding Clinic: 2013, Q3, P20

　　　E10.11　　**Type 1 diabetes mellitus with ketoacidosis with**
　　　　　　　coma

● E10.2　　**Type 1 diabetes mellitus with kidney complications**
　　　E10.21　　**Type 1 diabetes mellitus with diabetic**
　　　　　　　nephropathy
　　　　　　　Type 1 diabetes mellitus with intercapillary
　　　　　　　　glomerulosclerosis
　　　　　　　Type 1 diabetes mellitus with intracapillary
　　　　　　　　glomerulonephrosis
　　　　　　　Type 1 diabetes mellitus with Kimmelstiel-
　　　　　　　　Wilson disease

　　　E10.22　　**Type 1 diabetes mellitus with diabetic chronic**
　　　　　　　kidney disease
　　　　　　　　Use additional code to identify stage of chronic
　　　　　　　　　kidney disease (N18.1-N18.6)

　　　E10.29　　**Type 1 diabetes mellitus with other diabetic**
　　　　　　　kidney complication
　　　　　　　Type 1 diabetes mellitus with renal tubular
　　　　　　　　degeneration
　　　　　　　Coding Clinic: 2016, Q1, P13

● E10.3　　**Type 1 diabetes mellitus with ophthalmic complications**
　● E10.31　　**Type 1 diabetes mellitus with unspecified**
　　　　　　　diabetic retinopathy
　　　　　E10.311　　**Type 1 diabetes mellitus**
　　　　　　　　with unspecified diabetic retinopathy
　　　　　　　　with macular edema
　　　　　E10.319　　**Type 1 diabetes mellitus**
　　　　　　　　with unspecified diabetic retinopathy
　　　　　　　　without macular edema
　● E10.32　　**Type 1 diabetes mellitus with mild**
　　　　　　　nonproliferative diabetic retinopathy
　　　　　　　Type 1 diabetes mellitus with nonproliferative
　　　　　　　　diabetic retinopathy NOS

　　　　　　　One of the following 7th characters is to be
　　　　　　　　assigned to codes in subcategory E10.32 to
　　　　　　　　designate laterality of the disease: ◄

1	right eye ◄
2	left eye ◄
3	bilateral ◄
9	unspecified eye ◄

　　　　　● E10.321　　**Type 1 diabetes mellitus with mild**
　　　　　　　　nonproliferative diabetic retinopathy
　　　　　　　　with macular edema
　　　　　● E10.329　　**Type 1 diabetes mellitus with mild**
　　　　　　　　nonproliferative diabetic retinopathy
　　　　　　　　without macular edema

● E10.33　　**Type 1 diabetes mellitus with moderate**
　　　　　　nonproliferative diabetic retinopathy
　　　　　　One of the following 7th characters is to be
　　　　　　　assigned to codes in subcategory E10.33 to
　　　　　　　designate laterality of the disease: ◄

1	right eye ◄
2	left eye ◄
3	bilateral ◄
9	unspecified eye ◄

　● E10.331　　**Type 1 diabetes mellitus with**
　　　　　　　moderate nonproliferative diabetic
　　　　　　　retinopathy with macular edema
　● E10.339　　**Type 1 diabetes mellitus with**
　　　　　　　moderate nonproliferative diabetic
　　　　　　　retinopathy without macular edema

● E10.34　　**Type 1 diabetes mellitus with severe**
　　　　　　nonproliferative diabetic retinopathy
　　　　　　One of the following 7th characters is to be
　　　　　　　assigned to codes in subcategory E10.34 to
　　　　　　　designate laterality of the disease: ◄

1	right eye ◄
2	left eye ◄
3	bilateral ◄
9	unspecified eye ◄

　● E10.341　　**Type 1 diabetes mellitus with severe**
　　　　　　　nonproliferative diabetic retinopathy
　　　　　　　with macular edema
　● E10.349　　**Type 1 diabetes mellitus with severe**
　　　　　　　nonproliferative diabetic retinopathy
　　　　　　　without macular edema

● E10.35　　**Type 1 diabetes mellitus with proliferative**
　　　　　　diabetic retinopathy
　　　　　　One of the following 7th characters is to be
　　　　　　　assigned to codes in subcategory E10.35 to
　　　　　　　designate laterality of the disease: ◄

1	right eye ◄
2	left eye ◄
3	bilateral ◄
9	unspecified eye ◄

　● E10.351　　**Type 1 diabetes mellitus with**
　　　　　　　proliferative diabetic retinopathy
　　　　　　　with macular edema
　● E10.352　　**Type 1 diabetes mellitus with**
　　　　　　　proliferative diabetic retinopathy
　　　　　　　with traction retinal detachment
　　　　　　　involving the macula ◄
　● E10.353　　**Type 1 diabetes mellitus with**
　　　　　　　proliferative diabetic retinopathy
　　　　　　　with traction retinal detachment not
　　　　　　　involving the macula ◄
　● E10.354　　**Type 1 diabetes mellitus with**
　　　　　　　proliferative diabetic retinopathy
　　　　　　　with combined traction retinal
　　　　　　　detachment and rhegmatogenous
　　　　　　　retinal detachment ◄
　● E10.355　　**Type 1 diabetes mellitus with stable**
　　　　　　　proliferative diabetic retinopathy ◄
　● E10.359　　**Type 1 diabetes mellitus with**
　　　　　　　proliferative diabetic retinopathy
　　　　　　　without macular edema

◄ New　　◄■ Revised　　d̶e̶l̶e̶t̶e̶d̶ Deleted　　Excludes 1　　Excludes 2　　Includes　　Use additional　　Code first　　Code also　　Unspecified

OGCR Official Guidelines　　X Assign placeholder X　　● Use Additional Character(s)　　▶ Manifestation Code　　**Coding Clinic**

E10.36   Type 1 diabetes mellitus with diabetic cataract

X ● E10.37   Type 1 diabetes mellitus with diabetic macular edema, resolved following treatment ◄

> One of the following 7th characters is to be assigned to code E10.37 to designate laterality of the disease: ◄

> | | |
> |---|---|
> | 1 | right eye ◄ |
> | 2 | left eye ◄ |
> | 3 | bilateral ◄ |
> | 9 | unspecified eye ◄ |

E10.39   Type 1 diabetes mellitus with other diabetic ophthalmic complication
> Use additional code to identify manifestation, such as:
> diabetic glaucoma (H40-H42)

● E10.4   Type 1 diabetes mellitus with neurological complications

E10.40   Type 1 diabetes mellitus with diabetic neuropathy, unspecified

E10.41   Type 1 diabetes mellitus with diabetic mononeuropathy

E10.42   Type 1 diabetes mellitus with diabetic polyneuropathy
> Type 1 diabetes mellitus with diabetic neuralgia

E10.43   Type 1 diabetes mellitus with diabetic autonomic (poly)neuropathy
> Type 1 diabetes mellitus with diabetic gastroparesis

E10.44   Type 1 diabetes mellitus with diabetic amyotrophy

E10.49   Type 1 diabetes mellitus with other diabetic neurological complication

● E10.5   Type 1 diabetes mellitus with circulatory complications

E10.51   Type 1 diabetes mellitus with diabetic peripheral angiopathy without gangrene

E10.52   Type 1 diabetes mellitus with diabetic peripheral angiopathy with gangrene
> Type 1 diabetes mellitus with diabetic gangrene

E10.59   Type 1 diabetes mellitus with other circulatory complications

● E10.6   Type 1 diabetes mellitus with other specified complications

● E10.61   Type 1 diabetes mellitus with diabetic arthropathy

E10.610   Type 1 diabetes mellitus with diabetic neuropathic arthropathy
> Type 1 diabetes mellitus with Charcôt's joints

E10.618   Type 1 diabetes mellitus with other diabetic arthropathy

● E10.62   Type 1 diabetes mellitus with skin complications

E10.620   Type 1 diabetes mellitus with diabetic dermatitis
> Type 1 diabetes mellitus with diabetic necrobiosis lipoidica

E10.621   Type 1 diabetes mellitus with foot ulcer
> Use additional code to identify site of ulcer (L97.4-, L97.5-)

E10.622   Type 1 diabetes mellitus with other skin ulcer
> Use additional code to identify site of ulcer (L97.1-L97.9, L98.41-L98.49)

E10.628   Type 1 diabetes mellitus with other skin complications

● E10.63   Type 1 diabetes mellitus with oral complications

E10.630   Type 1 diabetes mellitus with periodontal disease

E10.638   Type 1 diabetes mellitus with other oral complications

● E10.64   Type 1 diabetes mellitus with hypoglycemia

E10.641   Type 1 diabetes mellitus with hypoglycemia with coma

E10.649   Type 1 diabetes mellitus with hypoglycemia without coma
> **Coding Clinic: 2016, Q1, P13**

E10.65   Type 1 diabetes mellitus with hyperglycemia
> **Coding Clinic: 2013, Q3, P20**

E10.69   Type 1 diabetes mellitus with other specified complication
> Use additional code to identify complication
> *Use this code with E10.65 to report hyperosmolarity in a Type 1 patient*

E10.8   Type 1 diabetes mellitus with unspecified complications

E10.9   Type 1 diabetes mellitus without complications

● E11   Type 2 diabetes mellitus
> **Includes**   diabetes (mellitus) due to insulin secretory defect
> diabetes NOS
> insulin resistant diabetes (mellitus)

> Use additional code to identify control using: ◄
> insulin (Z79.4) ◄
> oral antidiabetic drugs (Z79.84) ◄
> oral hypoglycemic drugs (Z79.84) ◄

> **Excludes1**   diabetes mellitus due to underlying condition (E08.-)
> drug or chemical induced diabetes mellitus (E09.-)
> gestational diabetes (O24.4-)
> neonatal diabetes mellitus (P70.2)
> postpancreatectomy diabetes mellitus (E13.-)
> postprocedural diabetes mellitus (E13.-)
> secondary diabetes mellitus NEC (E13.-)
> type 1 diabetes mellitus (E10.-)
> **Coding Clinic: 2016, Q2, P10**

● E11.0   Type 2 diabetes mellitus with hyperosmolarity

E11.00   Type 2 diabetes mellitus with hyperosmolarity without nonketotic hyperglycemic-hyperosmolar coma (NKHHC)

E11.01   Type 2 diabetes mellitus with hyperosmolarity with coma

● E11.2   Type 2 diabetes mellitus with kidney complications

E11.21   Type 2 diabetes mellitus with diabetic nephropathy
> Type 2 diabetes mellitus with intercapillary glomerulosclerosis
> Type 2 diabetes mellitus with intracapillary glomerulonephrosis
> Type 2 diabetes mellitus with Kimmelstiel-Wilson disease

E11.22   Type 2 diabetes mellitus with diabetic chronic kidney disease
> Use additional code to identify stage of chronic kidney disease (N18.1-N18.6)
> **Coding Clinic: 2016, Q2, P36, Q1, P13**

E11.29   Type 2 diabetes mellitus with other diabetic kidney complication
> Type 2 diabetes mellitus with renal tubular degeneration

CHAPTER 4 (E00-E90)

● **E11.3**   **Type 2 diabetes mellitus with ophthalmic complications**

   ● **E11.31**   **Type 2 diabetes mellitus with unspecified diabetic retinopathy**

       E11.311   **Type 2 diabetes mellitus with unspecified diabetic retinopathy with macular edema**

       E11.319   **Type 2 diabetes mellitus with unspecified diabetic retinopathy without macular edema**
          Coding Clinic: 2013, Q3, P20

   ● **E11.32**   **Type 2 diabetes mellitus with mild nonproliferative diabetic retinopathy**

       Type 2 diabetes mellitus with nonproliferative diabetic retinopathy NOS

       One of the following 7th characters is to be assigned to codes in subcategory E11.32 to designate laterality of the disease: ◀

         1   right eye ◀
         2   left eye ◀
         3   bilateral ◀
         9   unspecified eye ◀

     ● **E11.321**   **Type 2 diabetes mellitus with mild nonproliferative diabetic retinopathy with macular edema**

     ● **E11.329**   **Type 2 diabetes mellitus with mild nonproliferative diabetic retinopathy without macular edema**

   ● **E11.33**   **Type 2 diabetes mellitus with moderate nonproliferative diabetic retinopathy**

       One of the following 7th characters is to be assigned to codes in subcategory E11.33 to designate laterality of the disease: ◀

         1   right eye ◀
         2   left eye ◀
         3   bilateral ◀
         9   unspecified eye ◀

     ● **E11.331**   **Type 2 diabetes mellitus with moderate nonproliferative diabetic retinopathy with macular edema**

     ● **E11.339**   **Type 2 diabetes mellitus with moderate nonproliferative diabetic retinopathy without macular edema**

   ● **E11.34**   **Type 2 diabetes mellitus with severe nonproliferative diabetic retinopathy**

       One of the following 7th characters is to be assigned to codes in subcategory E11.34 to designate laterality of the disease: ◀

         1   right eye ◀
         2   left eye ◀
         3   bilateral ◀
         9   unspecified eye ◀

     ● **E11.341**   **Type 2 diabetes mellitus with severe nonproliferative diabetic retinopathy with macular edema**

     ● **E11.349**   **Type 2 diabetes mellitus with severe nonproliferative diabetic retinopathy without macular edema**

   ● **E11.35**   **Type 2 diabetes mellitus with proliferative diabetic retinopathy**

       One of the following 7th characters is to be assigned to codes in subcategory E11.35 to designate laterality of the disease: ◀

         1   right eye ◀
         2   left eye ◀
         3   bilateral ◀
         9   unspecified eye ◀

     ● **E11.351**   **Type 2 diabetes mellitus with proliferative diabetic retinopathy with macular edema**

     ● **E11.352**   **Type 2 diabetes mellitus with proliferative diabetic retinopathy with traction retinal detachment involving the macula ◀**

     ● **E11.353**   **Type 2 diabetes mellitus with proliferative diabetic retinopathy with traction retinal detachment not involving the macula ◀**

     ● **E11.354**   **Type 2 diabetes mellitus with proliferative diabetic retinopathy with combined traction retinal detachment and rhegmatogenous retinal detachment ◀**

     ● **E11.355**   **Type 2 diabetes mellitus with stable proliferative diabetic retinopathy ◀**

     ● **E11.359**   **Type 2 diabetes mellitus with proliferative diabetic retinopathy without macular edema**

   E11.36   **Type 2 diabetes mellitus with diabetic cataract**
       Coding Clinic: 2016, Q2, P36

X ● **E11.37**   **Type 2 diabetes mellitus with diabetic macular edema, resolved following treatment ◀**

       One of the following 7th characters is to be assigned to code E11.37 to designate laterality of the disease: ◀

         1   right eye ◀
         2   left eye ◀
         3   bilateral ◀
         9   unspecified eye ◀

   E11.39   **Type 2 diabetes mellitus with other diabetic ophthalmic complication**

       Use additional code to identify manifestation, such as:
         diabetic glaucoma (H40-H42)

● **E11.4**   **Type 2 diabetes mellitus with neurological complications**

   E11.40   **Type 2 diabetes mellitus with diabetic neuropathy, unspecified**

   E11.41   **Type 2 diabetes mellitus with diabetic mononeuropathy**

   E11.42   **Type 2 diabetes mellitus with diabetic polyneuropathy**
       Type 2 diabetes mellitus with diabetic neuralgia
       Coding Clinic: 2016, Q1, P13

   E11.43   **Type 2 diabetes mellitus with diabetic autonomic (poly)neuropathy**
       Type 2 diabetes mellitus with diabetic gastroparesis
       Coding Clinic: 2016, Q2, P36

   E11.44   **Type 2 diabetes mellitus with diabetic amyotrophy**
       Coding Clinic: 2016, Q2, P36

   E11.49   **Type 2 diabetes mellitus with other diabetic neurological complication**

◀ New   ◀▥ Revised   ~~deleted~~ Deleted   Excludes 1   Excludes 2   Includes   Use additional   Code first   Code also   Unspecified

OGCR Official Guidelines   X Assign placeholder X   ● Use Additional Character(s)   ▶ Manifestation Code   **Coding Clinic**

● **E11.5 Type 2 diabetes mellitus with circulatory complications**

    E11.51 Type 2 diabetes mellitus with diabetic peripheral angiopathy without gangrene

    E11.52 Type 2 diabetes mellitus with diabetic peripheral angiopathy with gangrene
        Type 2 diabetes mellitus with diabetic gangrene

    E11.59 Type 2 diabetes mellitus with other circulatory complications

● **E11.6 Type 2 diabetes mellitus with other specified complications**

  ● **E11.61 Type 2 diabetes mellitus with diabetic arthropathy**

    E11.610 Type 2 diabetes mellitus with diabetic neuropathic arthropathy
        Type 2 diabetes mellitus with Charcôt's joints
        Coding Clinic: 2016, Q2, P36

    E11.618 Type 2 diabetes mellitus with other diabetic arthropathy
        Coding Clinic: 2016, Q2, P36

  ● **E11.62 Type 2 diabetes mellitus with skin complications**

    E11.620 Type 2 diabetes mellitus with diabetic dermatitis
        Type 2 diabetes mellitus with diabetic necrobiosis lipoidica

    E11.621 Type 2 diabetes mellitus with foot ulcer
        Use additional code to identify site of ulcer (L97.4-, L97.5-)
        Coding Clinic: 2016, Q1, P12

    E11.622 Type 2 diabetes mellitus with other skin ulcer
        Use additional code to identify site of ulcer (L97.1-L97.9, L98.41-L98.49)

    E11.628 Type 2 diabetes mellitus with other skin complications

  ● **E11.63 Type 2 diabetes mellitus with oral complications**

    E11.630 Type 2 diabetes mellitus with periodontal disease

    E11.638 Type 2 diabetes mellitus with other oral complications

  ● **E11.64 Type 2 diabetes mellitus with hypoglycemia**

    E11.641 Type 2 diabetes mellitus with hypoglycemia with coma

    E11.649 Type 2 diabetes mellitus with hypoglycemia without coma
        Coding Clinic: 2015, Q3, P21

    E11.65 Type 2 diabetes mellitus with hyperglycemia
        Coding Clinic: 2013, Q3, P20

    E11.69 Type 2 diabetes mellitus with other specified complication
        Use additional code to identify complication
        Use this code with E11.65 to report DKA in a Type 2 patient

E11.8 Type 2 diabetes mellitus with unspecified complications

E11.9 Type 2 diabetes mellitus without complications
  Coding Clinic: 2016, Q2, P36

● **E13 Other specified diabetes mellitus**

  Includes   diabetes mellitus due to genetic defects of beta-cell function
        diabetes mellitus due to genetic defects in insulin action
        postpancreatectomy diabetes mellitus
        postprocedural diabetes mellitus
        secondary diabetes mellitus NEC

Use additional code to identify control using: ◀━
  insulin (Z79.4) ◀
  oral antidiabetic drugs (Z79.84) ◀
  oral hypoglycemic drugs (Z79.84) ◀

  Excludes1   diabetes (mellitus) due to autoimmune process (E10.-)
        diabetes (mellitus) due to immune mediated pancreatic islet beta-cell destruction (E10.-)
        diabetes mellitus due to underlying condition (E08.-)
        drug or chemical induced diabetes mellitus (E09.-)
        gestational diabetes (O24.4-)
        neonatal diabetes mellitus (P70.2)
        type 1 diabetes mellitus (E10.-) ◀
        type 2 diabetes mellitus (E11.-)

● **E13.0 Other specified diabetes mellitus with hyperosmolarity**

    E13.00 Other specified diabetes mellitus with hyperosmolarity without nonketotic hyperglycemic-hyperosmolar coma (NKHHC)

    E13.01 Other specified diabetes mellitus with hyperosmolarity with coma

● **E13.1 Other specified diabetes mellitus with ketoacidosis**

    E13.10 Other specified diabetes mellitus with ketoacidosis without coma
        Coding Clinic: 2016, Q2, P10; 2013, Q1, P26

    E13.11 Other specified diabetes mellitus with ketoacidosis with coma

● **E13.2 Other specified diabetes mellitus with kidney complications**

    E13.21 Other specified diabetes mellitus with diabetic nephropathy
        Other specified diabetes mellitus with intercapillary glomerulosclerosis
        Other specified diabetes mellitus with intracapillary glomerulonephrosis
        Other specified diabetes mellitus with Kimmelstiel-Wilson disease

    E13.22 Other specified diabetes mellitus with diabetic chronic kidney disease
        Use additional code to identify stage of chronic kidney disease (N18.1-N18.6)

    E13.29 Other specified diabetes mellitus with other diabetic kidney complication
        Other specified diabetes mellitus with renal tubular degeneration

● **E13.3 Other specified diabetes mellitus with ophthalmic complications**

  ● **E13.31 Other specified diabetes mellitus with unspecified diabetic retinopathy**

    E13.311 Other specified diabetes mellitus with unspecified diabetic retinopathy with macular edema

    E13.319 Other specified diabetes mellitus with unspecified diabetic retinopathy without macular edema

● **E13.32** **Other specified diabetes mellitus with mild nonproliferative diabetic retinopathy**
Other specified diabetes mellitus with nonproliferative diabetic retinopathy NOS

One of the following 7th characters is to be assigned to codes in subcategory E13.32 to designate laterality of the disease: ◄

> 1　right eye ◄
> 2　left eye ◄
> 3　bilateral ◄
> 9　unspecified eye ◄

● **E13.321** **Other specified diabetes mellitus with mild nonproliferative diabetic retinopathy with macular edema**

● **E13.329** **Other specified diabetes mellitus with mild nonproliferative diabetic retinopathy without macular edema**

● **E13.33** **Other specified diabetes mellitus with moderate nonproliferative diabetic retinopathy**

One of the following 7th characters is to be assigned to codes in subcategory E13.33 to designate laterality of the disease: ◄

> 1　right eye ◄
> 2　left eye ◄
> 3　bilateral ◄
> 9　unspecified eye ◄

● **E13.331** **Other specified diabetes mellitus with moderate nonproliferative diabetic retinopathy with macular edema**

● **E13.339** **Other specified diabetes mellitus with moderate nonproliferative diabetic retinopathy without macular edema**

● **E13.34** **Other specified diabetes mellitus with severe nonproliferative diabetic retinopathy**

One of the following 7th characters is to be assigned to codes in subcategory E13.34 to designate laterality of the disease: ◄

> 1　right eye ◄
> 2　left eye ◄
> 3　bilateral ◄
> 9　unspecified eye ◄

● **E13.341** **Other specified diabetes mellitus with severe nonproliferative diabetic retinopathy with macular edema**

● **E13.349** **Other specified diabetes mellitus with severe nonproliferative diabetic retinopathy without macular edema**

● **E13.35** **Other specified diabetes mellitus with proliferative diabetic retinopathy**

One of the following 7th characters is to be assigned to codes in subcategory E13.35 to designate laterality of the disease: ◄

> 1　right eye ◄
> 2　left eye ◄
> 3　bilateral ◄
> 9　unspecified eye ◄

● **E13.351** **Other specified diabetes mellitus with proliferative diabetic retinopathy with macular edema**

● **E13.352** **Other specified diabetes mellitus with proliferative diabetic retinopathy with traction retinal detachment involving the macula** ◄

● **E13.353** **Other specified diabetes mellitus with proliferative diabetic retinopathy with traction retinal detachment not involving the macula** ◄

● **E13.354** **Other specified diabetes mellitus with proliferative diabetic retinopathy with combined traction retinal detachment and rhegmatogenous retinal detachment** ◄

● **E13.355** **Other specified diabetes mellitus with stable proliferative diabetic retinopathy** ◄

● **E13.359** **Other specified diabetes mellitus with proliferative diabetic retinopathy without macular edema**

E13.36 **Other specified diabetes mellitus with diabetic cataract**

X ● **E13.37** **Other specified diabetes mellitus with diabetic macular edema, resolved following treatment**

One of the following 7th characters is to be assigned to code E13.37 to designate laterality of the disease: ◄

> 1　right eye ◄
> 2　left eye ◄
> 3　bilateral ◄
> 9　unspecified eye ◄

E13.39 **Other specified diabetes mellitus with other diabetic ophthalmic complication**
Use additional code to identify manifestation, such as:
diabetic glaucoma (H40-H42)

● **E13.4** **Other specified diabetes mellitus with neurological complications**

E13.40 **Other specified diabetes mellitus with diabetic neuropathy, unspecified**

E13.41 **Other specified diabetes mellitus with diabetic mononeuropathy**

E13.42 **Other specified diabetes mellitus with diabetic polyneuropathy**
Other specified diabetes mellitus with diabetic neuralgia

E13.43 **Other specified diabetes mellitus with diabetic autonomic (poly)neuropathy**
Other specified diabetes mellitus with diabetic gastroparesis

E13.44 **Other specified diabetes mellitus with diabetic amyotrophy**

E13.49 **Other specified diabetes mellitus with other diabetic neurological complication**

● **E13.5** **Other specified diabetes mellitus with circulatory complications**

E13.51 **Other specified diabetes mellitus with diabetic peripheral angiopathy without gangrene**

E13.52 **Other specified diabetes mellitus with diabetic peripheral angiopathy with gangrene**
Other specified diabetes mellitus with diabetic gangrene

E13.59 **Other specified diabetes mellitus with other circulatory complications**

● **E13.6** **Other specified diabetes mellitus with other specified complications**

● **E13.61** **Other specified diabetes mellitus with diabetic arthropathy**

E13.610 **Other specified diabetes mellitus with diabetic neuropathic arthropathy**
Other specified diabetes mellitus with Charcôt's joints

E13.618 **Other specified diabetes mellitus with other diabetic arthropathy**

◄ New　◄▥ Revised　~~deleted~~ Deleted　Excludes 1　Excludes 2　Includes　Use additional　Code first　Code also　Unspecified
OGCR Official Guidelines　X Assign placeholder X　● Use Additional Character(s)　▶ Manifestation Code　Coding Clinic

● E13.62   **Other specified diabetes mellitus with skin complications**

　　E13.620   **Other specified diabetes mellitus with diabetic dermatitis**
　　　　　Other specified diabetes mellitus with diabetic necrobiosis lipoidica

　　E13.621   **Other specified diabetes mellitus with foot ulcer**
　　　　　Use additional code to identify site of ulcer (L97.4-, L97.5-)

　　E13.622   **Other specified diabetes mellitus with other skin ulcer**
　　　　　Use additional code to identify site of ulcer (L97.1-L97.9, L98.41-L98.49)

　　E13.628   **Other specified diabetes mellitus with other skin complications**

● E13.63   **Other specified diabetes mellitus with oral complications**

　　E13.630   **Other specified diabetes mellitus with periodontal disease**

　　E13.638   **Other specified diabetes mellitus with other oral complications**

● E13.64   **Other specified diabetes mellitus with hypoglycemia**

　　E13.641   **Other specified diabetes mellitus with hypoglycemia with coma**

　　E13.649   **Other specified diabetes mellitus with hypoglycemia without coma**

　E13.65   **Other specified diabetes mellitus with hyperglycemia**

　E13.69   **Other specified diabetes mellitus with other specified complication**
　　　　Use additional code to identify complication

E13.8   **Other specified diabetes mellitus with unspecified complications**

E13.9   **Other specified diabetes mellitus without complications**

OTHER DISORDERS OF GLUCOSE REGULATION AND PANCREATIC INTERNAL SECRETION (E15-E16)

E15   **Nondiabetic hypoglycemic coma**
　　Includes   drug-induced insulin coma in nondiabetic
　　　　hyperinsulinism with hypoglycemic coma
　　　　hypoglycemic coma NOS

● E16   **Other disorders of pancreatic internal secretion**

　E16.0   **Drug-induced hypoglycemia without coma**
　　Excludes1   diabetes with hypoglycemia without coma (E09.692) ◀
　　Use additional code for adverse effect, if applicable, to identify drug (T36-T50 with fifth or sixth character 5)

　E16.1   **Other hypoglycemia**
　　Functional hyperinsulinism
　　Functional nonhyperinsulinemic hypoglycemia
　　Hyperinsulinism NOS
　　Hyperplasia of pancreatic islet beta cells NOS
　　Excludes1   diabetes with hypoglycemia (E08.649, E10.649, E11.649, E13.649) ◀
　　　　hypoglycemia in infant of diabetic mother (P70.1)
　　　　neonatal hypoglycemia (P70.4)

　E16.2   **Hypoglycemia, unspecified**
　　Excludes1   diabetes with hypoglycemia (E08.649, E10.649, E11.649, E13.649) ◀

　E16.3   **Increased secretion of glucagon**
　　Hyperplasia of pancreatic endocrine cells with glucagon excess

　E16.4   **Increased secretion of gastrin**
　　Hypergastrinemia
　　Hyperplasia of pancreatic endocrine cells with gastrin excess
　　Zollinger-Ellison syndrome

　E16.8   **Other specified disorders of pancreatic internal secretion**
　　Increased secretion from endocrine pancreas of growth hormone-releasing hormone
　　Increased secretion from endocrine pancreas of pancreatic polypeptide
　　Increased secretion from endocrine pancreas of somatostatin
　　Increased secretion from endocrine pancreas of vasoactive-intestinal polypeptide

　E16.9   **Disorder of pancreatic internal secretion, unspecified**
　　Islet-cell hyperplasia NOS
　　Pancreatic endocrine cell hyperplasia NOS

DISORDERS OF OTHER ENDOCRINE GLANDS (E20-E35)

Excludes1   galactorrhea (N64.3)
　　　　gynecomastia (N62)

● E20   **Hypoparathyroidism**
　　Greatly reduced function of parathyroid glands; AKA parathyroid insufficiency
　　Excludes1   Di George's syndrome (D82.1)
　　　　postprocedural hypoparathyroidism (E89.2)
　　　　tetany NOS (R29.0)
　　　　transitory neonatal hypoparathyroidism (P71.4)

　E20.0   **Idiopathic hypoparathyroidism**
　　Rare condition, unknown cause; short dwarf-like with round face

　E20.1   **Pseudohypoparathyroidism**
　　Hereditary condition resembling hypoparathyroidism, but caused by inability to respond to parathyroid hormone

　E20.8   **Other hypoparathyroidism**

　E20.9   **Hypoparathyroidism, unspecified**
　　Parathyroid tetany

● E21   **Hyperparathyroidism and other disorders of parathyroid gland**
　　Excludes1   adult osteomalacia (M83.-)
　　　　ectopic hyperparathyroidism (E34.2)
　　　　familial hypocalciuric hypercalcemia (E83.52)
　　　　hungry bone syndrome (E83.81)
　　　　infantile and juvenile osteomalacia (E55.0)

　E21.0   **Primary hyperparathyroidism**
　　Hyperplasia of parathyroid
　　Osteitis fibrosa cystica generalisata [von Recklinghausen's disease of bone]

　E21.1   **Secondary hyperparathyroidism, not elsewhere classified**
　　Excludes1   secondary hyperparathyroidism of renal origin (N25.81)

　E21.2   **Other hyperparathyroidism**
　　Tertiary hyperparathyroidism
　　Excludes1   familial hypocalciuric hypercalcemia (E83.52)

　E21.3   **Hyperparathyroidism, unspecified**

　E21.4   **Other specified disorders of parathyroid gland**

　E21.5   **Disorder of parathyroid gland, unspecified**

Item 4–4   Hyperparathyroidism is an overactive parathyroid gland that secretes excessive parathormone, causing increased levels of circulating calcium. This results in a loss of calcium in the bone (osteoporosis).

Hypoparathyroidism is an underactive parathyroid gland that results in decreased levels of circulating calcium. The primary manifestation is **tetany,** a continuous muscle spasm.

Figure 4-5   Tetany caused by hypoparathyroidism.

CHAPTER 4 (E00-E90)

Item 4–5 **Hyperadrenalism** is overactivity of the adrenal cortex, which secretes corticosteroid hormones. Excessive glucocorticoid hormone results in hyperglycemia **(Cushing's syndrome),** and excessive aldosterone results in **Conn's syndrome. Adrenogenital syndrome** is the result of excessive secretion of androgens, male hormones, which stimulates premature sexual development. **Hypoadrenalism, Addison's disease,** is a condition in which the adrenal glands atrophy.

Figure 4-6 Centripetal and generalized obesity and dorsal kyphosis in a 30-year-old woman with Cushing's disease. (From Larsen: Williams Textbook of Endocrinology, ed 10, Saunders, An Imprint of Elsevier, 2003)

● **E22 Hyperfunction of pituitary gland**
    Excludes1 Cushing's syndrome (E24.-)
         Nelson's syndrome (E24.1)
         overproduction of ACTH not associated with Cushing's disease (E27.0)
         overproduction of pituitary ACTH (E24.0)
         overproduction of thyroid-stimulating hormone (E05.8-)

   E22.0 Acromegaly and pituitary gigantism
     Chronic disease caused by hypersecretion of growth hormone
     Overproduction of growth hormone
     Excludes1 constitutional gigantism (E34.4)
         constitutional tall stature (E34.4)
         increased secretion from endocrine pancreas of growth hormone-releasing hormone (E16.8)

   E22.1 Hyperprolactinemia
     Increased levels of prolactin
     Use additional code for adverse effect, if applicable, to identify drug (T36-T50 with fifth or sixth character 5)

   E22.2 Syndrome of inappropriate secretion of antidiuretic hormone

   E22.8 Other hyperfunction of pituitary gland
     Central precocious puberty

   E22.9 Hyperfunction of pituitary gland, unspecified

● **E23 Hypofunction and other disorders of the pituitary gland**
    Includes the listed conditions whether the disorder is in the pituitary or the hypothalamus
    Excludes1 postprocedural hypopituitarism (E89.3)

   E23.0 Hypopituitarism
     Fertile eunuch syndrome
     Hypogonadotropic hypogonadism
     Idiopathic growth hormone deficiency
     Isolated deficiency of gonadotropin
     Isolated deficiency of growth hormone
     Isolated deficiency of pituitary hormone
     Kallmann's syndrome
     Lorain-Levi short stature
     Necrosis of pituitary gland (postpartum)
     Panhypopituitarism
     Pituitary cachexia
     Pituitary insufficiency NOS
     Pituitary short stature
     Sheehan's syndrome
     Simmonds' disease

   E23.1 Drug-induced hypopituitarism
     Use additional code for adverse effect, if applicable, to identify drug (T36-T50 with fifth or sixth character 5)

   E23.2 Diabetes insipidus
     Excludes1 nephrogenic diabetes insipidus (N25.1)

   E23.3 Hypothalamic dysfunction, not elsewhere classified
     Excludes1 Prader-Willi syndrome (Q87.1)
         Russell-Silver syndrome (Q87.1)

   E23.6 Other disorders of pituitary gland
     Abscess of pituitary
     Adiposogenital dystrophy

   E23.7 Disorder of pituitary gland, unspecified

● **E24 Cushing's syndrome**
    Excludes1 congenital adrenal hyperplasia (E25.0)

   E24.0 Pituitary-dependent Cushing's disease
     Overproduction of pituitary ACTH
     Pituitary-dependent hypercorticalism

   E24.1 Nelson's syndrome

   E24.2 Drug-induced Cushing's syndrome
     Use additional code for adverse effect, if applicable, to identify drug (T36-T50 with fifth or sixth character 5)

   E24.3 Ectopic ACTH syndrome

   E24.4 Alcohol-induced pseudo-Cushing's syndrome

   E24.8 Other Cushing's syndrome

   E24.9 Cushing's syndrome, unspecified

● **E25 Adrenogenital disorders**
    Disorder of production of steroid hormone in adrenal gland
    Includes adrenogenital syndromes, virilizing or feminizing, whether acquired or due to adrenal hyperplasia consequent on inborn enzyme defects in hormone synthesis
        female adrenal pseudohermaphroditism
        female heterosexual precocious pseudopuberty
        male isosexual precocious pseudopuberty
        male macrogenitosomia praecox
        male sexual precocity with adrenal hyperplasia
        male virilization (female)
    Excludes1 indeterminate sex and pseudohermaphroditism (Q56)
        chromosomal abnormalities (Q90-Q99)

   E25.0 Congenital adrenogenital disorders associated with enzyme deficiency
     Congenital adrenal hyperplasia
     21-Hydroxylase deficiency
     Salt-losing congenital adrenal hyperplasia

   E25.8 Other adrenogenital disorders
     Idiopathic adrenogenital disorder
     Use additional code for adverse effect, if applicable, to identify drug (T36-T50 with fifth or sixth character 5)

   E25.9 Adrenogenital disorder, unspecified
     Adrenogenital syndrome NOS

● **E26 Hyperaldosteronism**
    Abnormality of electrolyte metabolism caused by excessive secretion of aldosterone

  ● **E26.0 Primary hyperaldosteronism**
    E26.01 Conn's syndrome
       Code also adrenal adenoma (D35.0-)

    E26.02 Glucocorticoid-remediable aldosteronism
       Familial aldosteronism type I

    E26.09 Other primary hyperaldosteronism
       Primary aldosteronism due to adrenal hyperplasia (bilateral)

◄ New   ◄◄◄ Revised   ~~deleted~~ Deleted   Excludes 1   Excludes 2   Includes   Use additional   Code first   Code also   Unspecified
OGCR Official Guidelines   X Assign placeholder X   ● Use Additional Character(s)   ▶ Manifestation Code   **Coding Clinic**

E26.1   **Secondary hyperaldosteronism**

● E26.8   **Other hyperaldosteronism**

     E26.81   **Bartter's syndrome**

     E26.89   **Other hyperaldosteronism**

E26.9   **Hyperaldosteronism, unspecified**
     Aldosteronism NOS
     Hyperaldosteronism NOS

● **E27**   **Other disorders of adrenal gland**

E27.0   **Other adrenocortical overactivity**
     Overproduction of ACTH, not associated with
        Cushing's disease
     Premature adrenarche

     Excludes1   Cushing's syndrome (E24.-)

E27.1   **Primary adrenocortical insufficiency**
     Addison's disease
     Autoimmune adrenalitis

     Excludes1   Addison only phenotype
                 adrenoleukodystrophy (E71.528)
              amyloidosis (E85.-)
              tuberculous Addison's disease (A18.7)
              Waterhouse-Friderichsen syndrome
                 (A39.1)

E27.2   **Addisonian crisis**
     Acute onset of adrenocortical insufficiency
     Adrenal crisis
     Adrenocortical crisis

E27.3   **Drug-induced adrenocortical insufficiency**
     Use additional code for adverse effect, if applicable,
        to identify drug (T36-T50 with fifth or sixth
        character 5)

● E27.4   **Other and unspecified adrenocortical insufficiency**

     Excludes1   adrenoleukodystrophy [Addison-
                 Schilder] (E71.528)
              Waterhouse-Friderichsen syndrome
                 (A39.1)

     E27.40   **Unspecified adrenocortical insufficiency**
          Adrenocortical insufficiency NOS
          Hypoaldosteronism

     E27.49   **Other adrenocortical insufficiency**
          Adrenal hemorrhage
          Adrenal infarction

E27.5   **Adrenomedullary hyperfunction**
     Adrenomedullary hyperplasia
     Catecholamine hypersecretion

E27.8   **Other specified disorders of adrenal gland**
     Abnormality of cortisol-binding globulin

E27.9   **Disorder of adrenal gland, unspecified**

● **E28**   **Ovarian dysfunction**

     Excludes1   isolated gonadotropin deficiency (E23.0)
                 postprocedural ovarian failure (E89.4-)

E28.0   **Estrogen excess** ♀
     Use additional code for adverse effect, if applicable,
        to identify drug (T36-T50 with fifth or sixth
        character 5)

E28.1   **Androgen excess** ♀
     Hypersecretion of ovarian androgens
     Use additional code for adverse effect, if applicable,
        to identify drug (T36-T50 with fifth or sixth
        character 5)

E28.2   **Polycystic ovarian syndrome** ♀
     Sclerocystic ovary syndrome
     Stein-Leventhal syndrome

● E28.3   **Primary ovarian failure**

     Excludes1   pure gonadal dysgenesis (Q99.1)
                 Turner's syndrome (Q96.-)

   ● E28.31   **Premature menopause**

     E28.310   **Symptomatic premature**
           menopause ♀   A
            Symptoms such as flushing,
               sleeplessness, headache, lack of
               concentration, associated with
               premature menopause

     E28.319   **Asymptomatic premature menopause**
           ♀   A
            Premature menopause NOS

     E28.39   **Other primary ovarian failure** ♀
          Decreased estrogen
          Resistant ovary syndrome

E28.8   **Other ovarian dysfunction** ♀
     Ovarian hyperfunction NOS

     Excludes1   postprocedural ovarian failure (E89.4-)

E28.9   **Ovarian dysfunction, unspecified** ♀

● **E29**   **Testicular dysfunction**

     Excludes1   androgen insensitivity syndrome (E34.5-)
                 azoospermia or oligospermia NOS (N46.0-N46.1)
              isolated gonadotropin deficiency (E23.0)
              Klinefelter's syndrome (Q98.0-Q98.1, Q98.4) ◀

E29.0   **Testicular hyperfunction** ♂
     Hypersecretion of testicular hormones

E29.1   **Testicular hypofunction** ♂
     Defective biosynthesis of testicular androgen NOS
     5-delta-Reductase deficiency (with male
        pseudohermaphroditism)
     Testicular hypogonadism NOS

     Use additional code for adverse effect, if applicable,
        to identify drug (T36-T50 with fifth or sixth
        character 5)

     Excludes1   postprocedural testicular hypofunction
                 (E89.5)

E29.8   **Other testicular dysfunction** ♂

E29.9   **Testicular dysfunction, unspecified** ♂

● **E30**   **Disorders of puberty, not elsewhere classified**

E30.0   **Delayed puberty**
     Constitutional delay of puberty
     Delayed sexual development

E30.1   **Precocious puberty**   P
     Sexual maturation at earlier age than normal, or before age
        8 in girls and 9 in boys, usually hormonal; AKA sexual
        precocity or pubertas praecox
     Precocious menstruation

     Excludes1   Albright (-McCune) (-Sternberg)
                 syndrome (Q78.1)
              central precocious puberty (E22.8)
              congenital adrenal hyperplasia (E25.0)
              female heterosexual precocious
                 pseudopuberty (E25.-)
              male isosexual precocious pseudopuberty
                 (E25.-)

E30.8   **Other disorders of puberty**   P
     Premature thelarche

E30.9   **Disorder of puberty, unspecified**

● **E31**   **Polyglandular dysfunction**

     Excludes1   ataxia telangiectasia [Louis-Bar] (G11.3)
                 dystrophia myotonica [Steinert] (G71.11)
                 pseudohypoparathyroidism (E20.1)

   E31.0   **Autoimmune polyglandular failure**
         Schmidt's syndrome

   E31.1   **Polyglandular hyperfunction**

       Excludes1   multiple endocrine adenomatosis (E31.2-)
                  multiple endocrine neoplasia (E31.2-)

●   **E31.2**   **Multiple endocrine neoplasia [MEN] syndromes**
         Adenomatous hyperplasia and malignant tumors in endocrine glands
         Multiple endocrine adenomatosis
         Code also any associated malignancies and other conditions associated with the syndromes

     E31.20   **Multiple endocrine neoplasia [MEN] syndrome, unspecified**
            Multiple endocrine adenomatosis NOS
            Multiple endocrine neoplasia [MEN] syndrome NOS

     E31.21   **Multiple endocrine neoplasia [MEN] type I**
            Wermer's syndrome

     E31.22   **Multiple endocrine neoplasia [MEN] type IIA**
            Sipple's syndrome

     E31.23   **Multiple endocrine neoplasia [MEN] type IIB**

   E31.8   **Other polyglandular dysfunction**

   E31.9   **Polyglandular dysfunction, unspecified**

● **E32**   **Diseases of thymus**

     Excludes1   aplasia or hypoplasia of thymus with immunodeficiency (D82.1)
                 myasthenia gravis (G70.0)

   E32.0   **Persistent hyperplasia of thymus**
         Hypertrophy of thymus

   E32.1   **Abscess of thymus**

   E32.8   **Other diseases of thymus**

       Excludes1   aplasia or hypoplasia with immunodeficiency (D82.1)
                  thymoma (D15.0)

   E32.9   **Disease of thymus, unspecified**

● **E34**   **Other endocrine disorders**

     Excludes1   pseudohypoparathyroidism (E20.1)

   E34.0   **Carcinoid syndrome**
         Note: May be used as an additional code to identify functional activity associated with a carcinoid tumor.

   E34.1   **Other hypersecretion of intestinal hormones**

   E34.2   **Ectopic hormone secretion, not elsewhere classified**

       Excludes1   ectopic ACTH syndrome (E24.3)

   E34.3   **Short stature due to endocrine disorder**
         Constitutional short stature
         Laron-type short stature

       Excludes1   achondroplastic short stature (Q77.4)
                  hypochondroplastic short stature (Q77.4)
                  nutritional short stature (E45)
                  pituitary short stature (E23.0)
                  progeria (E34.8)
                  renal short stature (N25.0)
                  Russell-Silver syndrome (Q87.1)
                  short-limbed stature with immunodeficiency (D82.2)
                  short stature in specific dysmorphic syndromes - code to syndrome - see Alphabetical Index
                  short stature NOS (R62.52)

   E34.4   **Constitutional tall stature**
         Constitutional gigantism

●   **E34.5**   **Androgen insensitivity syndrome**

     E34.50   **Androgen insensitivity syndrome, unspecified**
            Androgen insensitivity NOS

     E34.51   **Complete androgen insensitivity syndrome**
            Complete androgen insensitivity
            de Quervain syndrome
            Goldberg-Maxwell syndrome

     E34.52   **Partial androgen insensitivity syndrome**
            Partial androgen insensitivity
            Reifenstein syndrome

   E34.8   **Other specified endocrine disorders**
         Pineal gland dysfunction
         Progeria

       Excludes2   pseudohypoparathyroidism (E20.1)

   E34.9   **Endocrine disorder, unspecified**
         Endocrine disturbance NOS
         Hormone disturbance NOS

▷ **E35**   *Disorders of endocrine glands in diseases classified elsewhere*

     Code first underlying disease, such as:
         late congenital syphilis of thymus gland [Dubois disease] (A50.5)

     Use additional code, if applicable, to identify:
         sequelae of tuberculosis of other organs (B90.8)

     Excludes1   Echinococcus granulosus infection of thyroid gland (B67.3)
                 meningococcal hemorrhagic adrenalitis (A39.1)
                 syphilis of endocrine gland (A52.79)
                 tuberculosis of adrenal gland, except calcification (A18.7)
                 tuberculosis of endocrine gland NEC (A18.82)
                 tuberculosis of thyroid gland (A18.81)
                 Waterhouse-Friderichsen syndrome (A39.1)

INTRAOPERATIVE COMPLICATIONS OF ENDOCRINE SYSTEM (E36)

● **E36**   **Intraoperative complications of endocrine system**

     Excludes2   postprocedural endocrine and metabolic complications and disorders, not elsewhere classified (E89.-)

●   **E36.0**   **Intraoperative hemorrhage and hematoma of an endocrine system organ or structure complicating a procedure**

       Excludes1   intraoperative hemorrhage and hematoma of an endocrine system organ or structure due to accidental puncture or laceration during a procedure (E36.1-)

     E36.01   **Intraoperative hemorrhage and hematoma of an endocrine system organ or structure complicating an endocrine system procedure**

     E36.02   **Intraoperative hemorrhage and hematoma of an endocrine system organ or structure complicating other procedure**

●   **E36.1**   **Accidental puncture and laceration of an endocrine system organ or structure during a procedure**

     E36.11   **Accidental puncture and laceration of an endocrine system organ or structure during an endocrine system procedure**

     E36.12   **Accidental puncture and laceration of an endocrine system organ or structure during other procedure**

     E36.8   **Other intraoperative complications of endocrine system**
            Use additional code, if applicable, to further specify disorder

◀ New   ◀ Revised   ~~deleted~~ Deleted   Excludes 1   Excludes 2   Includes   Use additional   Code first   Code also   Unspecified

734   **OGCR** Official Guidelines   X Assign placeholder X   ● Use Additional Character(s)   ▷ Manifestation Code   **Coding Clinic**

MALNUTRITION (E40-E46)

Excludes1   intestinal malabsorption (K90.-)
sequelae of protein-calorie malnutrition (E64.0)

Excludes2   nutritional anemias (D50-D53)
starvation (T73.0)

E40   Kwashiorkor
Malnutrition produced by severe protein deficiency
Severe malnutrition with nutritional edema with
dyspigmentation of skin and hair
    Excludes1   marasmic kwashiorkor (E42)

E41   Nutritional marasmus
Severe malnutrition with marasmus
    Excludes1   marasmic kwashiorkor (E42)

E42   Marasmic kwashiorkor
Severe protein malnutrition
Intermediate form severe protein-calorie malnutrition
Severe protein-calorie malnutrition with signs of both
kwashiorkor and marasmus

E43   Unspecified severe protein-calorie malnutrition
Starvation edema

● E44   Protein-calorie malnutrition of moderate and mild degree
   E44.0   Moderate protein-calorie malnutrition
   E44.1   Mild protein-calorie malnutrition

E45   Retarded development following protein-calorie malnutrition
Nutritional short stature
Nutritional stunting
Physical retardation due to malnutrition

E46   Unspecified protein-calorie malnutrition
Malnutrition NOS
Protein-calorie imbalance NOS
    Excludes1   nutritional deficiency NOS (E63.9)

OTHER NUTRITIONAL DEFICIENCIES (E50-E64)

Excludes2   nutritional anemias (D50-D53)

● E50   Vitamin A deficiency
    Excludes1   sequelae of vitamin A deficiency (E64.1)
   E50.0   Vitamin A deficiency with conjunctival xerosis
   E50.1   Vitamin A deficiency with Bitot's spot and conjunctival xerosis
      Bitot's spot in the young child
   E50.2   Vitamin A deficiency with corneal xerosis
   E50.3   Vitamin A deficiency with corneal ulceration and xerosis
   E50.4   Vitamin A deficiency with keratomalacia
      Eye disorder that results in dry cornea caused by vitamin A deficiency
   E50.5   Vitamin A deficiency with night blindness
   E50.6   Vitamin A deficiency with xerophthalmic scars of cornea
      Abnormal dryness and thickening of conjunctiva and cornea due to vitamin A deficiency

   E50.7   Other ocular manifestations of vitamin A deficiency
      Xerophthalmia NOS
   E50.8   Other manifestations of vitamin A deficiency
      Follicular keratosis
      Xeroderma
   E50.9   Vitamin A deficiency, unspecified
      Hypovitaminosis A NOS

● E51   Thiamine deficiency
    Excludes1   sequelae of thiamine deficiency (E64.8)
 ● E51.1   Beriberi
     E51.11   Dry beriberi
        Thiamine deficiency with nervous system manifestation most often caused by excessive alcohol consumption
        Beriberi NOS
        Beriberi with polyneuropathy
     E51.12   Wet beriberi
        Thiamine deficiency with cardiovascular manifestation most often caused by excessive alcohol consumption
        Beriberi with cardiovascular manifestations
        Cardiovascular beriberi
        Shoshin disease

   E51.2   Wernicke's encephalopathy
      Acute disease of brain due to thiamine deficiency most often associated with excessive alcohol consumption

   E51.8   Other manifestations of thiamine deficiency
   E51.9   Thiamine deficiency, unspecified

E52   Niacin deficiency [pellagra]
Niacin (-tryptophan) deficiency
Nicotinamide deficiency
Pellagra (alcoholic)
    Excludes1   sequelae of niacin deficiency (E64.8)

● E53   Deficiency of other B group vitamins
    Excludes1   sequelae of vitamin B deficiency (E64.8)
   E53.0   Riboflavin deficiency
      Ariboflavinosis
      Vitamin B2 deficiency
   E53.1   Pyridoxine deficiency
      Vitamin B6 deficiency
      Excludes1   pyridoxine-responsive sideroblastic anemia (D64.3)
   E53.8   Deficiency of other specified B group vitamins
      Biotin deficiency
      Cyanocobalamin deficiency
      Folate deficiency
      Folic acid deficiency
      Pantothenic acid deficiency
      Vitamin B12 deficiency
      Excludes1   folate deficiency anemia (D52.-)
          vitamin B12 deficiency anemia (D51.-)
   E53.9   Vitamin B deficiency, unspecified

Item 4–6   Bitot's spots are the result of a buildup of keratin debris found on the superficial surface the conjunctiva; oval, triangular, or irregular in shape; and a sign of vitamin A deficiency and associated with night blindness. The disease may progress to **keratomalacia,** which can result in eventual prolapse of the iris and loss of the lens.

Figure 4-7   Bitot's spot on the conjunctiva.

Figure 4-8   The sharply demarcated, characteristic scaling dermatitis of pellagra. (From Kumar: Robbins and Cotran: Pathologic Basis of Disease, ed 8, Saunders, An Imprint of Elsevier, 2009)

Item 4–7   Pellagra is associated with a deficiency of niacin and its precursor, **tryptophan.** Characteristics of the condition include diarrhea, dermatitis on exposed skin surfaces, dementia, and death. It is prevalent in developing countries where nutrition is inadequate. **Beriberi** is associated with thiamine deficiency.

CHAPTER 4 (E00-E90)

● **E54** **Ascorbic acid deficiency**
Deficiency of vitamin C
Scurvy
> **Excludes1**   scorbutic anemia (D53.2)
> sequelae of vitamin C deficiency (E64.2)

● **E55** **Vitamin D deficiency**
> **Excludes1**   adult osteomalacia (M83.-)
> osteoporosis (M80.-)
> sequelae of rickets (E64.3)

E55.0 **Rickets, active**
Infantile osteomalacia
Juvenile osteomalacia
Softening of bone
> **Excludes1**   celiac rickets (K90.0)
> Crohn's rickets (K50.-)
> hereditary vitamin D-dependent rickets
> (E83.32)
> inactive rickets (E64.3)
> renal rickets (N25.0)
> sequelae of rickets (E64.3)
> vitamin D-resistant rickets (E83.31)

E55.9 **Vitamin D deficiency, unspecified**
Avitaminosis D

● **E56** **Other vitamin deficiencies**
> **Excludes1**   sequelae of other vitamin deficiencies (E64.8)

E56.0 **Deficiency of vitamin E**
E56.1 **Deficiency of vitamin K**
> **Excludes1**   deficiency of coagulation factor due to
> vitamin K deficiency (D68.4)
> vitamin K deficiency of newborn (P53)

E56.8 **Deficiency of other vitamins**
E56.9 **Vitamin deficiency, unspecified**

E58 **Dietary calcium deficiency**
> **Excludes1**   disorders of calcium metabolism (E83.5-)
> sequelae of calcium deficiency (E64.8)

E59 **Dietary selenium deficiency**
Keshan disease
> **Excludes1**   sequelae of selenium deficiency (E64.8)

E60 **Dietary zinc deficiency**

● **E61** **Deficiency of other nutrient elements**
Use additional code for adverse effect, if applicable, to identify
drug (T36-T50 with fifth or sixth character 5)
> **Excludes1**   disorders of mineral metabolism (E83.-)
> iodine deficiency related thyroid disorders
> (E00-E02)
> sequelae of malnutrition and other nutritional
> deficiencies (E64.-)

E61.0 **Copper deficiency**
E61.1 **Iron deficiency**
> **Excludes1**   iron deficiency anemia (D50.-)

E61.2 **Magnesium deficiency**
E61.3 **Manganese deficiency**
E61.4 **Chromium deficiency**
E61.5 **Molybdenum deficiency**
E61.6 **Vanadium deficiency**
E61.7 **Deficiency of multiple nutrient elements**
E61.8 **Deficiency of other specified nutrient elements**
E61.9 **Deficiency of nutrient element, unspecified**

● **E63** **Other nutritional deficiencies**
> **Excludes1**   dehydration (E86.0)
> failure to thrive, adult (R62.7)
> failure to thrive, child (R62.51)
> feeding problems in newborn (P92.-)
> sequelae of malnutrition and other nutritional
> deficiencies (E64.-)

E63.0 **Essential fatty acid [EFA] deficiency**
E63.1 **Imbalance of constituents of food intake**
E63.8 **Other specified nutritional deficiencies**
E63.9 **Nutritional deficiency, unspecified**

● **E64** **Sequelae of malnutrition and other nutritional deficiencies**
Pathological condition resulting from disease, injury, or other trauma
Note: This category is to be used to indicate conditions in
categories E43, E44, E46, E50-E63 as the cause of sequelae,
which are themselves classified elsewhere. The 'sequelae'
include conditions specified as such; they also include the
late effects of diseases classifiable to the above categories if
the disease itself is no longer present
*Code first condition resulting from (sequela) of malnutrition and
other nutritional deficiencies*

E64.0 **Sequelae of protein-calorie malnutrition**
> **Excludes2**   retarded development following protein-
> calorie malnutrition (E45)

E64.1 **Sequelae of vitamin A deficiency**
E64.2 **Sequelae of vitamin C deficiency**
E64.3 **Sequelae of rickets**
E64.8 **Sequelae of other nutritional deficiencies**
E64.9 **Sequelae of unspecified nutritional deficiency**

OVERWEIGHT, OBESITY AND OTHER HYPERALIMENTATION (E65-E68)

E65 **Localized adiposity**
Fat pad

● **E66** **Overweight and obesity**
*Code first obesity complicating pregnancy, childbirth and the
puerperium, if applicable (O99.21-)*
Use additional code to identify body mass index (BMI), if
known (Z68.-)
> **Excludes1**   adiposogenital dystrophy (E23.6)
> lipomatosis NOS (E88.2)
> lipomatosis dolorosa [Dercum] (E88.2)
> Prader-Willi syndrome (Q87.1)

● **E66.0** **Obesity due to excess calories**
E66.01 **Morbid (severe) obesity due to excess calories**
> **Excludes1**   morbid (severe) obesity with
> alveolar hypoventilation
> (E66.2)

E66.09 **Other obesity due to excess calories**
E66.1 **Drug-induced obesity**
Use additional code for adverse effect, if applicable,
to identify drug (T36-T50 with fifth or sixth
character 5)

E66.2 **Morbid (severe) obesity with alveolar hypoventilation**
*Uncommon condition of unknown cause leading to
inadequate ventilation in lungs, even though lungs and
airways are normal*
Obesity hypoventilation syndrome (OHS) ◀
Pickwickian syndrome

E66.3 **Overweight**
E66.8 **Other obesity**
E66.9 **Obesity, unspecified**
Obesity NOS

◀ New   ◀═ Revised   ~~deleted~~ Deleted   Excludes 1   Excludes 2   Includes   Use additional   Code first   Code also   Unspecified
OGCR Official Guidelines   X Assign placeholder X   ● Use Additional Character(s)   ▶ Manifestation Code   **Coding Clinic**

● **E67 Other hyperalimentation**
Ingestion of more than optimal amount of nutrients

Excludes1 hyperalimentation NOS (R63.2)
sequelae of hyperalimentation (E68)

E67.0 Hypervitaminosis A

E67.1 Hypercarotinemia

E67.2 Megavitamin-B6 syndrome

E67.3 Hypervitaminosis D

E67.8 Other specified hyperalimentation

E68 Sequelae of hyperalimentation
Code first condition resulting from (sequela) of hyperalimentation

METABOLIC DISORDERS (E70-E88)

Excludes1 androgen insensitivity syndrome (E34.5-)
congenital adrenal hyperplasia (E25.0)
Ehlers-Danlos syndrome (Q79.6)
hemolytic anemias attributable to enzyme
   disorders (D55.-)
Marfan's syndrome (Q87.4)
5-alpha-reductase deficiency (E29.1)

● **E70 Disorders of aromatic amino-acid metabolism**

E70.0 Classical phenylketonuria
Inherited disorder that increases to harmful levels amino acid phenylalanine

E70.1 Other hyperphenylalaninemias

● **E70.2 Disorders of tyrosine metabolism**

Excludes1 transitory tyrosinemia of newborn (P74.5)

E70.20 Disorder of tyrosine metabolism, unspecified
Tyrosine: Nonessential amino acid occurring in most proteins

E70.21 Tyrosinemia
Congenital amino acid metabolism
Hypertyrosinemia

E70.29 Other disorders of tyrosine metabolism
Alkaptonuria
Ochronosis

● **E70.3 Albinism**
Congenital condition of reduced or absent pigment in eyes, skin, and hair

E70.30 Albinism, unspecified

● **E70.31 Ocular albinism**

E70.310 X-linked ocular albinism

E70.311 Autosomal recessive ocular albinism

E70.318 Other ocular albinism

E70.319 Ocular albinism, unspecified

● **E70.32 Oculocutaneous albinism**
Partial or total lack of melanin pigment in eyes

Excludes1 Chediak-Higashi syndrome
   (E70.330)
Hermansky-Pudlak syndrome
   (E70.331)

E70.320 Tyrosinase negative oculocutaneous albinism
Albinism I
Oculocutaneous albinism ty-neg

E70.321 Tyrosinase positive oculocutaneous albinism
Albinism II
Oculocutaneous albinism ty-pos

E70.328 Other oculocutaneous albinism
Cross syndrome

E70.329 Oculocutaneous albinism, unspecified

● **E70.33 Albinism with hematologic abnormality**

E70.330 Chediak-Higashi syndrome

E70.331 Hermansky-Pudlak syndrome

E70.338 Other albinism with hematologic abnormality

E70.339 Albinism with hematologic abnormality, unspecified

E70.39 Other specified albinism
Piebaldism

● **E70.4 Disorders of histidine metabolism**

E70.40 Disorders of histidine metabolism, unspecified

E70.41 Histidinemia

E70.49 Other disorders of histidine metabolism

E70.5 Disorders of tryptophan metabolism

E70.8 Other disorders of aromatic amino-acid metabolism

E70.9 Disorder of aromatic amino-acid metabolism, unspecified

● **E71 Disorders of branched-chain amino-acid metabolism and fatty-acid metabolism**

E71.0 Maple-syrup-urine disease
Due to defect in amino acid catabolism, causing severe ketoacidosis with smell of maple syrup in urine and on body

● **E71.1 Other disorders of branched-chain amino-acid metabolism**

● **E71.11 Branched-chain organic acidurias**

E71.110 Isovaleric acidemia

E71.111 3-methylglutaconic aciduria

E71.118 Other branched-chain organic acidurias

● **E71.12 Disorders of propionate metabolism**

E71.120 Methylmalonic acidemia

E71.121 Propionic acidemia

E71.128 Other disorders of propionate metabolism

E71.19 Other disorders of branched-chain amino-acid metabolism
Hyperleucine-isoleucinemia
Hypervalinemia

E71.2 Disorder of branched-chain amino-acid metabolism, unspecified

● **E71.3 Disorders of fatty-acid metabolism**

Excludes1 peroxisomal disorders (E71.5)
Refsum's disease (G60.1)
Schilder's disease (G37.0)

Excludes2 carnitine deficiency due to inborn error of
   metabolism (E71.42)

E71.30 Disorder of fatty-acid metabolism, unspecified

● **E71.31 Disorders of fatty-acid oxidation**

E71.310 Long chain/very long chain acyl CoA dehydrogenase deficiency
LCAD
VLCAD

E71.311 Medium chain acyl CoA dehydrogenase deficiency
MCAD

E71.312 Short chain acyl CoA dehydrogenase deficiency
SCAD

E71.313 Glutaric aciduria type II
Glutaric aciduria type II A
Glutaric aciduria type II B
Glutaric aciduria type II C

Excludes1 glutaric aciduria (type
   1) NOS (E72.3)

E71.314 Muscle carnitine palmitoyltransferase deficiency

E71.318 Other disorders of fatty-acid oxidation

E71.32 Disorders of ketone metabolism

E71.39 Other disorders of fatty-acid metabolism

CHAPTER 4 (E00-E90)

● **E71.4   Disorders of carnitine metabolism**

> **Excludes1**   muscle carnitine palmitoyltransferase
> deficiency (E71.314)

E71.40   Disorder of carnitine metabolism, unspecified

E71.41   Primary carnitine deficiency

E71.42   Carnitine deficiency due to inborn errors of metabolism

> Code also associated inborn error or
> metabolism

E71.43   Iatrogenic carnitine deficiency

> *Iatrogenic: Outcomes from activity of physicians*
> Carnitine deficiency due to hemodialysis
> Carnitine deficiency due to Valproic acid
> therapy

● **E71.44   Other secondary carnitine deficiency**

E71.440   Ruvalcaba-Myhre-Smith syndrome

E71.448   Other secondary carnitine deficiency

● **E71.5   Peroxisomal disorders**

> *Class of conditions which lead to disorders of lipid metabolism*

> **Excludes1**   Schilder's disease (G37.0)

E71.50   Peroxisomal disorder, unspecified

● **E71.51   Disorders of peroxisome biogenesis**

> Group 1 peroxisomal disorders

> **Excludes1**   Refsum's disease (G60.1)

E71.510   Zellweger syndrome

E71.511   Neonatal adrenoleukodystrophy

> **Excludes1**   X-linked adrenoleuko-
> dystrophy
> (E71.42-)

E71.518   Other disorders of peroxisome biogenesis

● **E71.52   X-linked adrenoleukodystrophy**

E71.520   Childhood cerebral X-linked adrenoleukodystrophy

E71.521   Adolescent X-linked adrenoleukodystrophy

E71.522   Adrenomyeloneuropathy

E71.528   Other X-linked adrenoleukodystrophy

> Addison only phenotype
> adrenoleukodystrophy
> Addison-Schilder
> adrenoleukodystrophy

E71.529   X-linked adrenoleukodystrophy, unspecified type

E71.53   Other group 2 peroxisomal disorders

● **E71.54   Other peroxisomal disorders**

E71.540   Rhizomelic chondrodysplasia punctata

> *Rare, severe, inherited disorder with limb shortening, bone and cartilage abnormalities, abnormal facial appearance, severe mental retardation, psychomotor retardation, and cataracts*

> **Excludes1**   chondrodysplasia
> punctata NOS
> (Q77.3)

E71.541   Zellweger-like syndrome

E71.542   Other group 3 peroxisomal disorders

E71.548   Other peroxisomal disorders

● **E72   Other disorders of amino-acid metabolism**

> **Excludes1**   disorders of:
> aromatic amino-acid metabolism (E70.-)
> branched-chain amino-acid metabolism
> (E71.0-E71.2)
> fatty-acid metabolism (E71.3)
> purine and pyrimidine metabolism (E79.-)
> gout (M1A.-, M10.-)

● **E72.0   Disorders of amino-acid transport**

> **Excludes1**   disorders of tryptophan metabolism
> (E70.5)

E72.00   Disorders of amino-acid transport, unspecified

E72.01   Cystinuria

> *Hereditary aminoaciduria due to impairment of renal transport with predominant symptom of urinary cystine calculi*

E72.02   Hartnup's disease

> *Inborn error of metabolism*

E72.03   Lowe's syndrome

> *X-linked disorder with rickets, hydrophthalmia, congenital glaucoma, cataracts, mental retardation, and renal tubule dysfunction*

> Use additional code for associated glaucoma
> (H42)

E72.04   Cystinosis

> *Genetic disease with excessive depostits of amino acid cystine in cells*
> Fanconi (-de Toni) (-Debré) syndrome with
> cystinosis

> **Excludes1**   Fanconi (-de Toni) (-Debré)
> syndrome without
> cystinosis (E72.09)

E72.09   Other disorders of amino-acid transport

> Fanconi (-de Toni) (-Debré) syndrome,
> unspecified

● **E72.1   Disorders of sulfur-bearing amino-acid metabolism**

> **Excludes1**   cystinosis (E72.04)
> cystinuria (E72.01)
> transcobalamin II deficiency (D51.2)

E72.10   Disorders of sulfur-bearing amino-acid metabolism, unspecified

E72.11   Homocystinuria

> Cystathionine synthase deficiency

E72.12   Methylenetetrahydrofolate reductase deficiency

E72.19   Other disorders of sulfur-bearing amino-acid metabolism

> Cystathioninuria
> Methioninemia
> Sulfite oxidase deficiency

● **E72.2   Disorders of urea cycle metabolism**

> **Excludes1**   disorders of ornithine metabolism (E72.4)

E72.20   Disorder of urea cycle metabolism, unspecified

> Hyperammonemia
> *Elevated levels of ammonia*

> **Excludes1**   hyperammonemia-
> hyperornithinemia-
> homocitrullinemia
> syndrome E72.4
> transient hyperammonemia of
> newborn (P74.6)

E72.21   Argininemia

> *Disorder in which deficiency of enzyme arginase causes build up of arginine and ammonia in blood*

E72.22   Arginosuccinic aciduria

> *Gene disorder of urea cycle resulting accumulation of ammonia*

E72.23   Citrullinemia

> *Urea cycle disorder that causes ammonia and other toxic substances to accumulate in blood*

E72.29   Other disorders of urea cycle metabolism

◀ New   ◀ Revised   ~~deleted~~ Deleted   Excludes 1   Excludes 2   Includes   Use additional   Code first   Code also   Unspecified

738   OGCR Official Guidelines   X Assign placeholder X   ● Use Additional Character(s)   ▶ Manifestation Code   **Coding Clinic**

E72.3　**Disorders of lysine and hydroxylysine metabolism**
　　　　Glutaric aciduria NOS
　　　　Glutaric aciduria (type I)
　　　　Hydroxylysinemia
　　　　Hyperlysinemia
　　　　Excludes1　glutaric aciduria type II (E71.313)
　　　　　　　　　Refsum's disease (G60.1)
　　　　　　　　　Zellweger syndrome (E71.510)

E72.4　**Disorders of ornithine metabolism**
　　　　Hyperammonemia-Hyperornithinemia-
　　　　　　Homocitrullinemia syndrome
　　　　Ornithinemia (types I, II)
　　　　Ornithine transcarbamylase deficiency
　　　　Excludes1　hereditary choroidal dystrophy (H31.2-)

● E72.5　**Disorders of glycine metabolism**
　　　E72.50　**Disorder of glycine metabolism, unspecified**
　　　E72.51　**Non-ketotic hyperglycinemia**
　　　E72.52　**Trimethylaminuria**
　　　E72.53　**Hyperoxaluria**
　　　　　　　Oxalosis
　　　　　　　Oxaluria
　　　E72.59　**Other disorders of glycine metabolism**
　　　　　　　D-glycericacidemia
　　　　　　　Hyperhydroxyprolinemia
　　　　　　　Hyperprolinemia (types I, II)
　　　　　　　Sarcosinemia

E72.8　**Other specified disorders of amino-acid metabolism**
　　　　Disorders of beta-amino-acid metabolism
　　　　Disorders of gamma-glutamyl cycle

E72.9　**Disorder of amino-acid metabolism, unspecified**

● E73　**Lactose intolerance**
　　Intolerance for lactose, due to inherited deficiency of lactase activity in intestinal mucosa
　　E73.0　**Congenital lactase deficiency**
　　E73.1　**Secondary lactase deficiency**
　　E73.8　**Other lactose intolerance**
　　E73.9　**Lactose intolerance, unspecified**

● E74　**Other disorders of carbohydrate metabolism**
　　　Excludes1　diabetes mellitus (E08-E13)
　　　　　　　hypoglycemia NOS (E16.2)
　　　　　　　increased secretion of glucagon (E16.3)
　　　　　　　mucopolysaccharidosis (E76.0-E76.3)

● E74.0　**Glycogen storage disease**
　　　E74.00　**Glycogen storage disease, unspecified**
　　　E74.01　**von Gierke's disease**
　　　　　　　Type I glycogen storage disease
　　　E74.02　**Pompe disease**
　　　　　　　Cardiac glycogenosis
　　　　　　　Type II glycogen storage disease
　　　E74.03　**Cori disease**
　　　　　　　Forbes' disease
　　　　　　　Type III glycogen storage disease
　　　E74.04　**McArdle disease**
　　　　　　　Type V glycogen storage disease
　　　E74.09　**Other glycogen storage disease**
　　　　　　　Andersen disease
　　　　　　　Hers disease
　　　　　　　Tauri disease
　　　　　　　Glycogen storage disease, types 0, IV, VI-XI
　　　　　　　Liver phosphorylase deficiency
　　　　　　　Muscle phosphofructokinase deficiency

● E74.1　**Disorders of fructose metabolism**
　　　Excludes1　muscle phosphofructokinase deficiency (E74.09)
　　　E74.10　**Disorder of fructose metabolism, unspecified**
　　　E74.11　**Essential fructosuria**
　　　　　　　Fructokinase deficiency
　　　E74.12　**Hereditary fructose intolerance**
　　　　　　　Fructosemia
　　　E74.19　**Other disorders of fructose metabolism**
　　　　　　　Fructose-1, 6-diphosphatase deficiency

● E74.2　**Disorders of galactose metabolism**
　　　E74.20　**Disorders of galactose metabolism, unspecified**
　　　E74.21　**Galactosemia**
　　　　　　　Genetic disorders resulting from defective simple sugar (galactose) metabolism
　　　E74.29　**Other disorders of galactose metabolism**
　　　　　　　Galactokinase deficiency

● E74.3　**Other disorders of intestinal carbohydrate absorption**
　　　Excludes2　lactose intolerance (E73.-)
　　　E74.31　**Sucrase-isomaltase deficiency**
　　　　　　　Deficiency in metabolism in intestinal mucosa results in malabsorption of sucrose and starch
　　　E74.39　**Other disorders of intestinal carbohydrate absorption**
　　　　　　　Disorder of intestinal carbohydrate absorption NOS
　　　　　　　Glucose-galactose malabsorption
　　　　　　　Sucrase deficiency

E74.4　**Disorders of pyruvate metabolism and gluconeogenesis**
　　　　Deficiency of phosphoenolpyruvate carboxykinase
　　　　Deficiency of pyruvate carboxylase
　　　　Deficiency of pyruvate dehydrogenase
　　　Excludes1　disorders of pyruvate metabolism and gluconeogenesis with anemia (D55.-)
　　　　　　　Leigh's syndrome (G31.82)

E74.8　**Other specified disorders of carbohydrate metabolism**
　　　　Essential pentosuria
　　　　Renal glycosuria

E74.9　**Disorder of carbohydrate metabolism, unspecified**

● E75　**Disorders of sphingolipid metabolism and other lipid storage disorders**
　　　Excludes1　mucolipidosis, types I-III (E77.0-E77.1)
　　　　　　　Refsum's disease (G60.1)

● E75.0　**GM2 gangliosidosis**
　　　Rare metabolic disorder that causes destruction of nerve cells of brain and spinal cord
　　　E75.00　**GM2 gangliosidosis, unspecified**
　　　E75.01　**Sandhoff disease**
　　　E75.02　**Tay-Sachs disease**
　　　E75.09　**Other GM2 gangliosidosis**
　　　　　　　Adult GM2 gangliosidosis
　　　　　　　Juvenile GM2 gangliosidosis

● E75.1　**Other and unspecified gangliosidosis**
　　　E75.10　**Unspecified gangliosidosis**
　　　　　　　Gangliosidosis NOS
　　　E75.11　**Mucolipidosis IV**
　　　　　　　Disorder with symptoms of psychomotor retardation and severe visual impairment
　　　E75.19　**Other gangliosidosis**
　　　　　　　GM1 gangliosidosis
　　　　　　　GM3 gangliosidosis

CHAPTER 4 (E00-E90)

Item 4–8 Leukodystrophy is characterized by degeneration and/or failure of the myelin formation of the central nervous system and sometimes of the peripheral nervous system. The disease is inherited and progressive.

- ● **E75.2 Other sphingolipidosis**
  - *Lysosomal (a particle in a cytoplasm cell that contains digestive enzymes) storage diseases with symptoms of abnormal storage of amino acids*
    - Excludes1   adrenoleukodystrophy [Addison-Schilder] (E71.528)
  - **E75.21 Fabry (-Anderson) disease**
  - **E75.22 Gaucher disease**
  - **E75.23 Krabbe disease**
  - ● **E75.24 Niemann-Pick disease**
    - **E75.240 Niemann-Pick disease type A**
    - **E75.241 Niemann-Pick disease type B**
    - **E75.242 Niemann-Pick disease type C**
    - **E75.243 Niemann-Pick disease type D**
    - **E75.248 Other Niemann-Pick disease**
    - **E75.249 Niemann-Pick disease, unspecified**
  - **E75.25 Metachromatic leukodystrophy**
  - **E75.29 Other sphingolipidosis**
    - Farber's syndrome
    - Sulfatase deficiency
    - Sulfatide lipidosis
- **E75.3 Sphingolipidosis, unspecified**
- **E75.4 Neuronal ceroid lipofuscinosis**
  - Batten disease
  - Bielschowsky-Jansky disease
  - Kufs disease
  - Spielmeyer-Vogt disease
- **E75.5 Other lipid storage disorders**
  - Cerebrotendinous cholesterosis [van Bogaert-Scherer-Epstein]
  - Wolman's disease
- **E75.6 Lipid storage disorder, unspecified**
- ● **E76 Disorders of glycosaminoglycan metabolism**
  - ● **E76.0 Mucopolysaccharidosis, type I**
    - *Inborn metabolic disorder of enzymes that break down carbohydrates*
    - **E76.01 Hurler's syndrome**
    - **E76.02 Hurler-Scheie syndrome**
    - **E76.03 Scheie's syndrome**
  - **E76.1 Mucopolysaccharidosis, type II**
    - *Inborn metabolic disorder of enzymes that break down carbohydrates occurs in 2-4 year old males*
    - Hunter's syndrome
  - ● **E76.2 Other mucopolysaccharidoses**
    - ● **E76.21 Morquio mucopolysaccharidoses**
      - **E76.210 Morquio A mucopolysaccharidoses**
        - Classic Morquio syndrome
        - Morquio syndrome A
        - Mucopolysaccharidosis, type IVA
      - **E76.211 Morquio B mucopolysaccharidoses**
        - Morquio-like mucopolysaccharidoses
        - Morquio-like syndrome
        - Morquio syndrome B
        - Mucopolysaccharidosis, type IVB
      - **E76.219 Morquio mucopolysaccharidoses, unspecified**
        - Morquio syndrome
        - Mucopolysaccharidosis, type IV

- **E76.22 Sanfilippo mucopolysaccharidoses**
  - Mucopolysaccharidosis, type III (A) (B) (C) (D)
  - Sanfilippo A syndrome
  - Sanfilippo B syndrome
  - Sanfilippo C syndrome
  - Sanfilippo D syndrome
- **E76.29 Other mucopolysaccharidoses**
  - beta-Glucuronidase deficiency
  - Maroteaux-Lamy (mild) (severe) syndrome
  - Mucopolysaccharidosis, types VI, VII
- **E76.3 Mucopolysaccharidosis, unspecified**
- **E76.8 Other disorders of glucosaminoglycan metabolism**
- **E76.9 Glucosaminoglycan metabolism disorder, unspecified**
- ● **E77 Disorders of glycoprotein metabolism**
  - **E77.0 Defects in post-translational modification of lysosomal enzymes**
    - Mucolipidosis II [I-cell disease]
    - Mucolipidosis III [pseudo-Hurler polydystrophy]
  - **E77.1 Defects in glycoprotein degradation**
    - Aspartylglucosaminuria
    - Fucosidosis
    - Mannosidosis
    - Sialidosis [mucolipidosis I]
  - **E77.8 Other disorders of glycoprotein metabolism**
  - **E77.9 Disorder of glycoprotein metabolism, unspecified**
- ● **E78 Disorders of lipoprotein metabolism and other lipidemias**
  - Excludes1   sphingolipidosis (E75.0-E75.3)
  - ● **E78.0 Pure hypercholesterolemia**
    - ~~Familial hypercholesterolemia~~
    - ~~Hyperlipidemia, Group A~~
    - **E78.00 Pure hypercholesterolemia, unspecified ◀**
      - Fredrickson's hyperlipoproteinemia, type IIa ◀
      - Hyperbetalipoproteinemia ◀
      - Low-density-lipoprotein-type [LDL] hyperlipoproteinemia ◀
    - **E78.01 Familial hypercholesterolemia ◀**
  - **E78.1 Pure hyperglyceridemia**
    - Elevated fasting triglycerides
    - Endogenous hyperglyceridemia
    - Fredrickson's hyperlipoproteinemia, type IV
    - Hyperlipidemia, group B
    - Hyperprebetalipoproteinemia
    - Very-low-density-lipoprotein-type [VLDL] hyperlipoproteinemia
  - **E78.2 Mixed hyperlipidemia**
    - Broad- or floating-betalipoproteinemia
    - Combined hyperlipidemia NOS
    - Elevated cholesterol with elevated triglycerides NEC
    - Fredrickson's hyperlipoproteinemia, type IIb or III
    - Hyperbetalipoproteinemia with prebetalipoproteinemia
    - Hypercholesteremia with endogenous hyperglyceridemia
    - Hyperlipidemia, group C
    - Tubo-eruptive xanthoma
    - Xanthoma tuberosum
    - Excludes1   cerebrotendinous cholesterosis [van Bogaert-Scherer-Epstein] (E75.5)
      - familial combined hyperlipidemia (E78.4)
  - **E78.3 Hyperchylomicronemia**
    - Chylomicron retention disease
    - Fredrickson's hyperlipoproteinemia, type I or V
    - Hyperlipidemia, group D
    - Mixed hyperglyceridemia
  - **E78.4 Other hyperlipidemia**
    - Familial combined hyperlipidemia

E78.5 Hyperlipidemia, unspecified

E78.6 Lipoprotein deficiency
    Abetalipoproteinemia
    Depressed HDL cholesterol
    High-density lipoprotein deficiency
    Hypoalphalipoproteinemia
    Hypobetalipoproteinemia (familial)
    Lecithin cholesterol acyltransferase deficiency
    Tangier disease

● **E78.7 Disorders of bile acid and cholesterol metabolism**
    Excludes1   Niemann-Pick disease type C (E75.242)

    E78.70 Disorder of bile acid and cholesterol metabolism, unspecified

    E78.71 Barth syndrome

    E78.72 Smith-Lemli-Opitz syndrome

    E78.79 Other disorders of bile acid and cholesterol metabolism

● **E78.8 Other disorders of lipoprotein metabolism**

    E78.81 Lipoid dermatoarthritis

    E78.89 Other lipoprotein metabolism disorders

E78.9 Disorder of lipoprotein metabolism, unspecified

● **E79 Disorders of purine and pyrimidine metabolism**
    Purines, along with pyrimidines, signal RNA and DNA production
    Excludes1   Ataxia-telangiectasia (Q87.1)
        Bloom's syndrome (Q82.8)
        Cockayne's syndrome (Q87.1)
        calculus of kidney (N20.0)
        combined immunodeficiency disorders (D81.-)
        Fanconi's anemia (D61.09)
        gout (M1A.-, M10.-)
        orotaciduric anemia (D53.0)
        progeria (E34.8)
        Werner's syndrome (E34.8)
        xeroderma pigmentosum (Q82.1)

E79.0 Hyperuricemia without signs of inflammatory arthritis and tophaceous disease
    Asymptomatic hyperuricemia

E79.1 Lesch-Nyhan syndrome
    HGPRT deficiency

E79.2 Myoadenylate deaminase deficiency

E79.8 Other disorders of purine and pyrimidine metabolism
    Hereditary xanthinuria

E79.9 Disorder of purine and pyrimidine metabolism, unspecified

● **E80 Disorders of porphyrin and bilirubin metabolism**
    Group of chemical compounds in RBC's that combine with iron to form heme
    Includes   defects of catalase and peroxidase

E80.0 Hereditary erythropoietic porphyria
    Congenital erythropoietic porphyria
    Erythropoietic protoporphyria

E80.1 Porphyria cutanea tarda

● **E80.2 Other and unspecified porphyria**

    E80.20 Unspecified porphyria
        Porphyria NOS

    E80.21 Acute intermittent (hepatic) porphyria

    E80.29 Other porphyria
        Hereditary coproporphyria

E80.3 Defects of catalase and peroxidase
    Acatalasia [Takahara]

E80.4 Gilbert syndrome

E80.5 Crigler-Najjar syndrome

E80.6 Other disorders of bilirubin metabolism
    Dubin-Johnson syndrome
    Rotor's syndrome

E80.7 Disorder of bilirubin metabolism, unspecified

● **E83 Disorders of mineral metabolism**
    Excludes1   dietary mineral deficiency (E58-E61)
        parathyroid disorders (E20-E21)
        vitamin D deficiency (E55.-)

● **E83.0 Disorders of copper metabolism**

    E83.00 Disorder of copper metabolism, unspecified

    E83.01 Wilson's disease
        Code also associated Kayser Fleischer ring (H18.04-)

    E83.09 Other disorders of copper metabolism
        Menkes' (kinky hair) (steely hair) disease

● **E83.1 Disorders of iron metabolism**
    Excludes1   iron deficiency anemia (D50.-)
        sideroblastic anemia (D64.0-D64.3)

    E83.10 Disorder of iron metabolism, unspecified

●   **E83.11 Hemochromatosis**

        E83.110 Hereditary hemochromatosis
            Bronzed diabetes
            Pigmentary cirrhosis (of liver)
            Primary (hereditary) hemochromatosis

        E83.111 Hemochromatosis due to repeated red blood cell transfusions
            Iron overload due to repeated red blood cell transfusions
            Transfusion (red blood cell) associated hemochromatosis

        E83.118 Other hemochromatosis

        E83.119 Hemochromatosis, unspecified

    E83.19 Other disorders of iron metabolism
        Use additional code, if applicable, for idiopathic pulmonary hemosiderosis (J84.03)

E83.2 Disorders of zinc metabolism
    Acrodermatitis enteropathica

● **E83.3 Disorders of phosphorus metabolism and phosphatases**
    Excludes1   adult osteomalacia (M83.-)
        osteoporosis (M80.-)

    E83.30 Disorder of phosphorus metabolism, unspecified

    E83.31 Familial hypophosphatemia
        Vitamin D-resistant osteomalacia
        Vitamin D-resistant rickets
        Excludes1   vitamin D-deficiency rickets (E55.0)

    E83.32 Hereditary vitamin D-dependent rickets (type 1) (type 2)
        25-hydroxyvitamin D 1-alpha-hydroxylase deficiency
        Pseudovitamin D deficiency
        Vitamin D receptor defect

    E83.39 Other disorders of phosphorus metabolism
        Acid phosphatase deficiency
        Hypophosphatasia

● **E83.4 Disorders of magnesium metabolism**

    E83.40 Disorders of magnesium metabolism, unspecified

    E83.41 Hypermagnesemia

    E83.42 Hypomagnesemia

    E83.49 Other disorders of magnesium metabolism

● **E83.5 Disorders of calcium metabolism**
    Excludes1   chondrocalcinosis (M11.1-M11.2)
        hungry bone syndrome (E83.81)
        hyperparathyroidism (E21.0-E21.3)

    E83.50 Unspecified disorder of calcium metabolism

    E83.51 Hypocalcemia

    E83.52 Hypercalcemia
        Familial hypocalciuric hypercalcemia

    E83.59 Other disorders of calcium metabolism
        Idiopathic hypercalciuria

CHAPTER 4 (E00-E90)

● E83.8   **Other disorders of mineral metabolism**
    E83.81   **Hungry bone syndrome**
    E83.89   **Other disorders of mineral metabolism**
  E83.9   **Disorder of mineral metabolism, unspecified**

● E84   **Cystic fibrosis**
    Includes   mucoviscidosis

    Code also exocrine pancreatic insufficiency (K86.81) ◀

  E84.0   **Cystic fibrosis with pulmonary manifestations**
    Use additional code to identify any infectious organism present, such as:
    Pseudomonas (B96.5)

● E84.1   **Cystic fibrosis with intestinal manifestations**
    E84.11   **Meconium ileus in cystic fibrosis**   N
        Excludes1   meconium ileus not due to cystic fibrosis (P76.0)
    E84.19   **Cystic fibrosis with other intestinal manifestations**
        Distal intestinal obstruction syndrome

  E84.8   **Cystic fibrosis with other manifestations**
  E84.9   **Cystic fibrosis, unspecified**

● E85   **Amyloidosis**
    A disorder resulting from the abnormal deposition of a particular protein (amyloid) into tissues of the body

    Excludes1   Alzheimer's disease (G30.0-)

  E85.0   **Non-neuropathic heredofamilial amyloidosis**
    ~~Familial Mediterranean fever~~
    Hereditary amyloid nephropathy

  E85.1   **Neuropathic heredofamilial amyloidosis**
    Amyloid polyneuropathy (Portuguese)
    Coding Clinic: 2012, Q4, P100

  E85.2   **Heredofamilial amyloidosis, unspecified**
  E85.3   **Secondary systemic amyloidosis**
    Hemodialysis-associated amyloidosis

  E85.4   **Organ-limited amyloidosis**
    Localized amyloidosis

  E85.8   **Other amyloidosis**
  E85.9   **Amyloidosis, unspecified**

● E86   **Volume depletion**
    Excludes1   dehydration of newborn (P74.1)
        hypovolemic shock NOS (R57.1)
        postprocedural hypovolemic shock (T81.19)
        traumatic hypovolemic shock (T79.4)

    Use additional code(s) for any associated disorders of electrolyte and acid-base balance (E87.-) ◀

  E86.0   **Dehydration**
    Excessive loss of body water

  E86.1   **Hypovolemia**
    Diminished volume of circulating blood
    Depletion of volume of plasma

  E86.9   **Volume depletion, unspecified**

● E87   **Other disorders of fluid, electrolyte and acid-base balance**
    Excludes1   diabetes insipidus (E23.2)
        electrolyte imbalance associated with hyperemesis gravidarum (O21.1)
        electrolyte imbalance following ectopic or molar pregnancy (O08.5)
        familial periodic paralysis (G72.3)

  E87.0   **Hyperosmolality and hypernatremia**
    Sodium [Na] excess
    Sodium [Na] overload

  E87.1   **Hypo-osmolality and hyponatremia**
    Sodium [Na] deficiency
    Excludes1   syndrome of inappropriate secretion of antidiuretic hormone (E22.2)

  E87.2   **Acidosis**
    Acidosis NOS
    Lactic acidosis
    Metabolic acidosis
    Respiratory acidosis
    Excludes1   diabetic acidosis - see categories E08-E10, E13 with ketoacidosis

  E87.3   **Alkalosis**
    Alkalosis NOS
    Metabolic alkalosis
    Respiratory alkalosis

  E87.4   **Mixed disorder of acid-base balance**
  E87.5   **Hyperkalemia**
    Potassium [K] excess
    Potassium [K] overload

  E87.6   **Hypokalemia**
    Potassium [K] deficiency

● E87.7   **Fluid overload**
    Excludes1   edema NOS (R60.9)
        fluid retention (R60.9)
    E87.70   **Fluid overload, unspecified**
    E87.71   **Transfusion associated circulatory overload**
        Fluid overload due to transfusion (blood) (blood components) TACO
    E87.79   **Other fluid overload**

  E87.8   **Other disorders of electrolyte and fluid balance, not elsewhere classified**
    Electrolyte imbalance NOS
    Hyperchloremia
    Hypochloremia

● E88   **Other and unspecified metabolic disorders**
    Use additional codes for associated conditions
    Excludes1   histiocytosis X (chronic) (C96.6)

● E88.0   **Disorders of plasma-protein metabolism, not elsewhere classified**
    Excludes1   disorder of lipoprotein metabolism (E78.-)
        monoclonal gammopathy (of undetermined significance) (D47.2)
        polyclonal hypergammaglobulinemia (D89.0)
        Waldenström macroglobulinemia (C88.0)
    E88.01   **Alpha-1-antitrypsin deficiency AAT deficiency**
    E88.09   **Other disorders of plasma-protein metabolism, not elsewhere classified**
        Bisalbuminemia

  E88.1   **Lipodystrophy, not elsewhere classified**
    Defective fat metabolism resulting in absence of subcutaneous fat
    Lipodystrophy NOS
    Excludes1   Whipple's disease (K90.81)

  E88.2   **Lipomatosis, not elsewhere classified**
    Abnormal tumorlike accumulations of fat in tissue
    Lipomatosis NOS
    Lipomatosis (Check) dolorosa [Dercum]

Item 4–9 Circulating fluid volume is regulated by the amount of water and sodium ingested, excreted by the kidneys into the urine, and lost through the gastrointestinal tract, lungs, and skin. To maintain blood volume within a normal range, the kidneys regulate the amount of water and sodium lost into the urine. Too much (**fluid overload**) or too little fluid volume (**volume depletion**) will affect blood pressure. Severe cases of vomiting, diarrhea, bleeding, and burns (fluid loss through exposed burn surface area) can contribute to fluid loss. Internal body environment must maintain a precise balance (homeostasis) between too much fluid and too little fluid. This complex balancing mechanism is critical to good health.

◀ New   ◀▥ Revised   ~~deleted~~ Deleted   Excludes 1   Excludes 2   Includes   Use additional   Code first   Code also   Unspecified
OGCR Official Guidelines   X Assign placeholder X   ● Use Additional Character(s)   ▶ Manifestation Code   **Coding Clinic**

E88.3   **Tumor lysis syndrome**
> Tumor lysis syndrome (spontaneous)
> Tumor lysis syndrome following antineoplastic drug chemotherapy
>
> Use additional code for adverse effect, if applicable, to identify drug (T45.1X5)

● **E88.4**   **Mitochondrial metabolism disorders**
> *Congenital disorder of metabolism*
>
> | Excludes1 | disorders of pyruvate metabolism (E74.4) |
> |---|---|
> | | Kearns-Sayre syndrome (H49.81) |
> | | Leber's disease (H47.22) |
> | | Leigh's encephalopathy (G31.82) |
> | | Mitochondrial myopathy, NEC (G71.3) |
> | | Reye's syndrome (G93.7) |

     E88.40   **Mitochondrial metabolism disorder, unspecified**

     E88.41   **MELAS syndrome**
> Mitochondrial myopathy, encephalopathy, lactic acidosis and stroke-like episodes

     E88.42   **MERRF syndrome**
> Myoclonic epilepsy associated with ragged-red fibers
>
> Code also progressive myoclonic epilepsy (G40.3-) ◄▥

     E88.49   **Other mitochondrial metabolism disorders**

● **E88.8**   **Other specified metabolic disorders**

     E88.81   **Metabolic syndrome**
> Dysmetabolic syndrome X
>
> Use additional codes for associated manifestations, such as:
> obesity (E66.-)

     E88.89   **Other specified metabolic disorders**
> Launois-Bensaude adenolipomatosis
>
> | Excludes1 | adult pulmonary Langerhans cell histiocytosis (J84.82) |
> |---|---|

E88.9   **Metabolic disorder, unspecified**

POSTPROCEDURAL ENDOCRINE AND METABOLIC COMPLICATIONS AND DISORDERS, NOT ELSEWHERE CLASSIFIED (E89)

● **E89**   **Postprocedural endocrine and metabolic complications and disorders, not elsewhere classified**
> | Excludes2 | intraoperative complications of endocrine system organ or structure (E36.0-, E36.1-, E36.8) |
> |---|---|

E89.0   **Postprocedural hypothyroidism**
> Postirradiation hypothyroidism
> Postsurgical hypothyroidism

E89.1   **Postprocedural hypoinsulinemia**
> Postpancreatectomy hyperglycemia
> Postsurgical hypoinsulinemia
>
> Use additional code, if applicable, to identify:
> acquired absence of pancreas (Z90.41-)
> diabetes mellitus (postpancreatectomy) (postprocedural) (E13.-)
> insulin use (Z79.4)
>
> | Excludes1 | transient postprocedural hyperglycemia (R73.9) |
> |---|---|
> | | transient postprocedural hypoglycemia (E16.2) |

E89.2   **Postprocedural hypoparathyroidism**
> Parathyroprival tetany

E89.3   **Postprocedural hypopituitarism**
> Postirradiation hypopituitarism

● **E89.4**   **Postprocedural ovarian failure**

     E89.40   **Asymptomatic postprocedural ovarian failure** ♀
> Postprocedural ovarian failure NOS

     E89.41   **Symptomatic postprocedural ovarian failure** ♀
> Symptoms such as flushing, sleeplessness, headache, lack of concentration, associated with postprocedural menopause

E89.5   **Postprocedural testicular hypofunction** ♂

E89.6   **Postprocedural adrenocortical (-medullary) hypofunction**

● **E89.8**   **Other postprocedural endocrine and metabolic complications and disorders**

     ● **E89.81**   **Postprocedural hemorrhage of an endocrine system organ or structure following a procedure** ◄▥

         E89.810   **Postprocedural hemorrhage of an endocrine system organ or structure following an endocrine system procedure** ◄▥

         E89.811   **Postprocedural hemorrhage of an endocrine system organ or structure following other procedure** ◄▥

     ● **E89.82**   **Postprocedural hematoma and seroma of an endocrine system organ or structure** ◄

         E89.820   **Postprocedural hematoma of an endocrine system organ or structure following an endocrine system procedure** ◄

         E89.821   **Postprocedural hematoma of an endocrine system organ or structure following other procedure** ◄

         E89.822   **Postprocedural seroma of an endocrine system organ or structure following an endocrine system procedure** ◄

         E89.823   **Postprocedural seroma of an endocrine system organ or structure following other procedure** ◄

     E89.89   **Other postprocedural endocrine and metabolic complications and disorders**
> Use additional code, if applicable, to further specify disorder

CHAPTER 5

MENTAL, BEHAVIORAL AND NEURODEVELOPMENTAL DISORDERS (F01-F99)

OGCR Chapter-Specific Coding Guidelines

5. Chapter 5: Mental, Behavioral and Neurodevelopmental disorders (F01 – F99)

a. **Pain disorders related to psychological factors**

Assign code F45.41, for pain that is exclusively related to psychological disorders. As indicated by the Excludes 1 note under category G89, a code from category G89 should not be assigned with code F45.41

Code F45.42, Pain disorders with related psychological factors, should be used with a code from category G89, Pain, not elsewhere classified, if there is documentation of a psychological component for a patient with acute or chronic pain.

See Section I.C.6. Pain

c. **Mental and behavioral disorders due to psychoactive substance use**

1) **In Remission**

Selection of codes for "in remission" for categories F10-F19, Mental and behavioral disorders due to psychoactive substance use (categories F10-F19 with -.21) requires the provider's clinical judgment. The appropriate codes for "in remission" are assigned only on the basis of provider documentation (as defined in the Official Guidelines for Coding and Reporting).

2) **Psychoactive Substance Use, Abuse And Dependence**

When the provider documentation refers to use, abuse and dependence of the same substance (e.g. alcohol, opioid, cannabis, etc.), only one code should be assigned to identify the pattern of use based on the following hierarchy:

- If both use and abuse are documented, assign only the code for abuse
- If both abuse and dependence are documented, assign only the code for dependence
- If use, abuse and dependence are all documented, assign only the code for dependence
- If both use and dependence are documented, assign only the code for dependence.

3) **Psychoactive Substance Use**

As with all other diagnoses, the codes for psychoactive substance use (F10.9-, F11.9-, F12.9-, F13.9-, F14.9-, F15.9-, F16.9-) should only be assigned based on provider documentation and when they meet the definition of a reportable diagnosis (see Section III, Reporting Additional Diagnoses). The codes are to be used only when the psychoactive substance use is associated with a mental or behavioral disorder, and such a relationship is documented by the provider.

CHAPTER 5

MENTAL, BEHAVIORAL AND NEURODEVELOPMENTAL DISORDERS (F01-F99)

Includes disorders of psychological development

Excludes2 symptoms, signs and abnormal clinical laboratory findings, not elsewhere classified (R00-R99)

This chapter contains the following blocks:

F01-F09	Mental disorders due to known physiological conditions
F10-F19	Mental and behavioral disorders due to psychoactive substance use
F20-F29	Schizophrenia, schizotypal, delusional, and other non-mood psychotic disorders
F30-F39	Mood [affective] disorders
F40-F48	Anxiety, dissociative, stress-related, somatoform and other nonpsychotic mental disorders
F50-F59	Behavioral syndromes associated with physiological disturbances and physical factors
F60-F69	Disorders of adult personality and behavior
F70-F79	Intellectual disabilities
F80-F89	Pervasive and specific developmental disorders
F90-F98	Behavioral and emotional disorders with onset usually occurring in childhood and adolescence
F99	Unspecified mental disorder

MENTAL DISORDERS DUE TO KNOWN PHYSIOLOGICAL CONDITIONS (F01-F09)

This block comprises a range of mental disorders grouped together on the basis of their having in common a demonstrable etiology in cerebral disease, brain injury, or other insult leading to cerebral dysfunction. The dysfunction may be primary, as in diseases, injuries, and insults that affect the brain directly and selectively; or secondary, as in systemic diseases and disorders that attack the brain only as one of the multiple organs or systems of the body that are involved.

● **F01 Vascular dementia**

Vascular dementia as a result of infarction of the brain due to vascular disease, including hypertensive cerebrovascular disease.

Includes arteriosclerotic dementia

Code first the underlying physiological condition or sequelae of cerebrovascular disease.

● **F01.5 Vascular dementia**

F01.50 Vascular dementia without behavioral disturbance A

Major neurocognitive disorder without behavioral disturbance ◀

F01.51 Vascular dementia with behavioral disturbance A

Major neurocognitive disorder due to vascular disease, with behavioral disturbance ◀
Major neurocognitive disorder with aggressive behavior ◀
Major neurocognitive disorder with combative behavior ◀
Major neurocognitive disorder with violent behavior ◀
Vascular dementia with aggressive behavior
Vascular dementia with combative behavior
Vascular dementia with violent behavior

Use additional code, if applicable, to identify wandering in vascular dementia (Z91.83)

◀ New   ◀ Revised   ~~deleted~~ Deleted   Excludes 1   Excludes 2   Includes   Use additional   Code first   Code also   Unspecified

OGCR Official Guidelines   X Assign placeholder X   ● Use Additional Character(s)   ▶ Manifestation Code   **Coding Clinic**

● **F02**   **Dementia in other diseases classified elsewhere**

> *Code first* the underlying physiological condition, such as:
> Alzheimer's (G30.-)
> cerebral lipidosis (E75.4)
> Creutzfeldt-Jakob disease (A81.0-)
> dementia with Lewy bodies (G31.83)
> dementia with Parkinsonism (G31.83) ◄
> epilepsy and recurrent seizures (G40.-)
> frontotemporal dementia (G31.09)
> hepatolenticular degeneration (E83.0)
> human immunodeficiency virus [HIV] disease (B20)
> Huntington's disease (G10) ◄
> hypercalcemia (E83.52)
> hypothyroidism, acquired (E00-E03.-)
> intoxications (T36-T65)
> Jakob-Creutzfeldt disease (A81.0-)
> multiple sclerosis (G35)
> neurosyphilis (A52.17)
> niacin deficiency [pellagra] (E52)
> Parkinson's disease (G20)
> Pick's disease (G31.01)
> polyarteritis nodosa (M30.0)
> prion disease (A81.9) ◄
> systemic lupus erythematosus (M32.-)
> traumatic brain injury (S06.-) ◄
> trypanosomiasis (B56.-, B57.-)
> vitamin B deficiency (E53.8)

>   **Includes**   Major neurocognitive disorder in other diseases classified elsewhere ◄

>   **Excludes2**   dementia in alcohol and psychoactive substance disorders (F10-F19, with .17, .27, .97)
>   vascular dementia (F01.5-)

● **F02.8**   **Dementia in other diseases classified elsewhere**

> ▸ *F02.80*   *Dementia in other diseases classified elsewhere without behavioral disturbance*
>   Dementia in other diseases classified elsewhere NOS
>   Major neurocognitive disorder in other diseases classified elsewhere ◄
>   **Coding Clinic: 2016, Q2, P6**

> ▸ *F02.81*   *Dementia in other diseases classified elsewhere with behavioral disturbance*
>   Dementia in other diseases classified elsewhere with aggressive behavior
>   Dementia in other diseases classified elsewhere with combative behavior
>   Dementia in other diseases classified elsewhere with violent behavior
>   Major neurocognitive disorder in other diseases classified elsewhere with aggressive behavior ◄
>   Major neurocognitive disorder in other diseases classified elsewhere with combative behavior ◄
>   Major neurocognitive disorder in other diseases classified elsewhere with violent behavior ◄
>   Use additional code, if applicable, to identify wandering in dementia in conditions classified elsewhere (Z91.83)

Item 5-1 Psychosis was a term formerly applied to any mental disorder but is now restricted to disturbances of a great magnitude in which there is a personality disintegration and loss of contact with reality.

● **F03**   **Unspecified dementia**

> Presenile dementia NOS
> Presenile psychosis NOS
> Primary degenerative dementia NOS
> Senile dementia NOS
> Senile dementia depressed or paranoid type
> Senile psychosis NOS

>   **Excludes1**   senility NOS (R41.81)

>   **Excludes2**   mild memory disturbance due to known physiological condition (F06.8)
>   senile dementia with delirium or acute confusional state (F05)

● **F03.9**   **Unspecified dementia**

> **F03.90**   **Unspecified dementia without behavioral disturbance**   A
>   Dementia NOS
>   **Coding Clinic: 2012, Q4, P92**

> **F03.91**   **Unspecified dementia with behavioral disturbance**   A
>   Unspecified dementia with aggressive behavior
>   Unspecified dementia with combative behavior
>   Unspecified dementia with violent behavior
>   Use additional code, if applicable, to identify wandering in unspecified dementia (Z91.83)

F04   **Amnestic disorder due to known physiological condition**

> Korsakov's psychosis or syndrome, nonalcoholic

> *Code first* the underlying physiological condition

>   **Excludes1**   amnesia NOS (R41.3)
>   anterograde amnesia (R41.1)
>   dissociative amnesia (F44.0)
>   retrograde amnesia (R41.2)

>   **Excludes2**   alcohol-induced or unspecified Korsakov's syndrome (F10.26, F10.96)
>   Korsakov's syndrome induced by other psychoactive substances (F13.26, F13.96, F19.16, F19.26, F19.96)

F05   **Delirium due to known physiological condition**

> Acute or subacute brain syndrome
> Acute or subacute confusional state (nonalcoholic)
> Acute or subacute infective psychosis
> Acute or subacute organic reaction
> Acute or subacute psycho-organic syndrome
> Delirium of mixed etiology
> Delirium superimposed on dementia
> Sundowning

> *Code first* the underlying physiological condition

>   **Excludes1**   delirium NOS (R41.0)

>   **Excludes2**   delirium tremens alcohol-induced or unspecified (F10.231, F10.921)

CHAPTER 5 (F01-F99)

● **F06**   **Other mental disorders due to known physiological condition**

     Includes   mental disorders due to endocrine disorder
                       mental disorders due to exogenous hormone
                       mental disorders due to exogenous toxic
                           substance
                       mental disorders due to primary cerebral disease
                       mental disorders due to somatic illness
                       mental disorders due to systemic disease
                         affecting the brain

     Code first the underlying physiological condition

     Excludes1   unspecified dementia (F03)

     Excludes2   delirium due to known physiological condition
                       (F05)
                   dementia as classified in F01-F02
                   other mental disorders associated with alcohol
                       and other psychoactive substances (F10-F19)

   F06.0   **Psychotic disorder with hallucinations due to known physiological condition**
         Organic hallucinatory state (nonalcoholic)

     Excludes2   hallucinations and perceptual disturbance
                       induced by alcohol and other
                       psychoactive substances (F10-F19
                       with .151, .251, .951)
                       schizophrenia (F20.-)

   F06.1   **Catatonic disorder due to known physiological condition**
         Catatonia associated with another mental disorder ◀
         Catatonia NOS ◀

     Excludes1   catatonic stupor (R40.1)
                       stupor NOS (R40.1)

     Excludes2   catatonic schizophrenia (F20.2)
                       dissociative stupor (F44.2)

   F06.2   **Psychotic disorder with delusions due to known physiological condition**
         Paranoid and paranoid-hallucinatory organic states
         Schizophrenia-like psychosis in epilepsy

     Excludes2   alcohol and drug-induced psychotic
                       disorder (F10-F19 with .150, .250,
                       .950)
                   brief psychotic disorder (F23)
                   delusional disorder (F22)
                   schizophrenia (F20.-)

● **F06.3**   **Mood disorder due to known physiological condition**

     Excludes2   mood disorders due to alcohol and other
                       psychoactive
                       substances (F10-F19 with .14, .24, .94)
                   mood disorders, not due to known
                       physiological condition or
                       unspecified (F30-F39)

     F06.30   **Mood disorder due to known physiological condition, unspecified**

     F06.31   **Mood disorder due to known physiological condition with depressive features**

     F06.32   **Mood disorder due to known physiological condition with major depressive-like episode**

     F06.33   **Mood disorder due to known physiological condition with manic features**

     F06.34   **Mood disorder due to known physiological condition with mixed features**

   F06.4   **Anxiety disorder due to known physiological condition**

     Excludes2   anxiety disorders due to alcohol and
                       other psychoactive substances
                       (F10-F19 with .180, .280, .980)
                   anxiety disorders, not due to known
                       physiological condition or
                       unspecified (F40.-, F41.-)

   F06.8   **Other specified mental disorders due to known physiological condition**
         Epileptic psychosis NOS
         Organic dissociative disorder
         Organic emotionally labile [asthenic] disorder

● **F07**   **Personality and behavioral disorders due to known physiological condition**

     Code first the underlying physiological condition

   F07.0   **Personality change due to known physiological condition**
         Frontal lobe syndrome
         Limbic epilepsy personality syndrome
         Lobotomy syndrome
         Organic personality disorder
         Organic pseudopsychopathic personality
         Organic pseudoretarded personality
         Postleucotomy syndrome

     Code first underlying physiological condition

     Excludes1   mild cognitive impairment (G31.84)
                       postconcussional syndrome (F07.81)
                       postencephalitic syndrome (F07.89)
                       signs and symptoms involving emotional
                         state (R45.-)

     Excludes2   specific personality disorder (F60.-)

● **F07.8**   **Other personality and behavioral disorders due to known physiological condition**

     F07.81   **Postconcussional syndrome**
         Postcontusional syndrome (encephalopathy)
         Post-traumatic brain syndrome, nonpsychotic

         Use additional code to identify associated
                 post-traumatic headache, if applicable
                 (G44.3-)

         Excludes1   current concussion (brain)
                         (S06.0-)
                       postencephalitic syndrome
                       (F07.89)

     F07.89   **Other personality and behavioral disorders due to known physiological condition**
         Postencephalitic syndrome
         Damage to temporal brain lobes with memory
         loss and abnormal behavior
         Right hemispheric organic affective disorder

   F07.9   **Unspecified personality and behavioral disorder due to known physiological condition**
         Organic psychosyndrome
         Due to exposure to organic solvents

   F09   **Unspecified mental disorder due to known physiological condition**
         Mental disorder NOS due to known physiological condition
         Organic brain syndrome NOS
         Organic mental disorder NOS
         Organic psychosis NOS
         Symptomatic psychosis NOS

     Code first the underlying physiological condition

     Excludes1   psychosis NOS (F29)

MENTAL AND BEHAVIORAL DISORDERS DUE TO PSYCHOACTIVE SUBSTANCE USE (F10-F19)

● **F10**   **Alcohol related disorders**
     Use additional code for blood alcohol level, if applicable (Y90.-)

● **F10.1**   **Alcohol abuse**

     Excludes1   alcohol dependence (F10.2-)
                       alcohol use, unspecified (F10.9-)

     F10.10   **Alcohol abuse, uncomplicated**
         Alcohol use disorder, mild ◀

●   **F10.12**   **Alcohol abuse with intoxication**

         F10.120   **Alcohol abuse with intoxication, uncomplicated**

         F10.121   **Alcohol abuse with intoxication, delirium**

         F10.129   **Alcohol abuse with intoxication, unspecified**

◀ New   ◀▥ Revised   ~~deleted~~ Deleted   Excludes 1   Excludes 2   Includes   Use additional   Code first   Code also   Unspecified

OGCR Official Guidelines   X Assign placeholder X   ● Use Additional Character(s)   ▶ Manifestation Code   **Coding Clinic**

F10.14 **Alcohol abuse with alcohol-induced mood disorder**
  Alcohol use disorder, mild, with alcohol-induced bipolar or related disorder ◄
  Alcohol use disorder, mild, with alcohol-induced depressive disorder ◄

● F10.15 **Alcohol abuse with alcohol-induced psychotic disorder**
  F10.150 **Alcohol abuse with alcohol-induced psychotic disorder with delusions**
  F10.151 **Alcohol abuse with alcohol-induced psychotic disorder with hallucinations**
  F10.159 **Alcohol abuse with alcohol-induced psychotic disorder, unspecified**

● F10.18 **Alcohol abuse with other alcohol-induced disorders**
  F10.180 **Alcohol abuse with alcohol-induced anxiety disorder**
  F10.181 **Alcohol abuse with alcohol-induced sexual dysfunction**
  F10.182 **Alcohol abuse with alcohol-induced sleep disorder**
  F10.188 **Alcohol abuse with other alcohol-induced disorder**

F10.19 **Alcohol abuse with unspecified alcohol-induced disorder**

● F10.2 **Alcohol dependence**
  Excludes1   alcohol abuse (F10.1-)
     alcohol use, unspecified (F10.9-)
  Excludes2   toxic effect of alcohol (T51.0-)

F10.20 **Alcohol dependence, uncomplicated**
  Alcohol use disorder, moderate ◄
  Alcohol use disorder, severe ◄

F10.21 **Alcohol dependence, in remission**

● F10.22 **Alcohol dependence with intoxication**
  Acute drunkenness (in alcoholism)
  Excludes2   alcohol dependence with withdrawal (F10.23-) ◄
  F10.220 **Alcohol dependence with intoxication, uncomplicated**
  F10.221 **Alcohol dependence with intoxication delirium**
  F10.229 **Alcohol dependence with intoxication, unspecified**

● F10.23 **Alcohol dependence with withdrawal**
  Excludes2   alcohol dependence with intoxication (F10.22-) ◄
  F10.230 **Alcohol dependence with withdrawal, uncomplicated**
  F10.231 **Alcohol dependence with withdrawal delirium**
  F10.232 **Alcohol dependence with withdrawal with perceptual disturbance**
  F10.239 **Alcohol dependence with withdrawal, unspecified**
  Coding Clinic: 2015, Q2, P15

F10.24 **Alcohol dependence with alcohol-induced mood disorder**
  Alcohol use disorder, moderate, with alcohol-induced bipolar or related disorder ◄
  Alcohol use disorder, moderate, with alcohol-induced depressive disorder ◄
  Alcohol use disorder, severe, with alcohol-induced bipolar or related disorder ◄
  Alcohol use disorder, severe, with alcohol-induced depressive disorder ◄

● F10.25 **Alcohol dependence with alcohol-induced psychotic disorder**
  F10.250 **Alcohol dependence with alcohol-induced psychotic disorder with delusions**
  F10.251 **Alcohol dependence with alcohol-induced psychotic disorder with hallucinations**
  F10.259 **Alcohol dependence with alcohol-induced psychotic disorder, unspecified**

F10.26 **Alcohol dependence with alcohol-induced persisting amnestic disorder**
  Alcohol use disorder, moderate, with alcohol-induced major neurocognitive disorder, amnestic-confabulatory type ◄
  Alcohol use disorder, severe, with alcohol-induced major neurocognitive disorder, amnestic-confabulatory type ◄

F10.27 **Alcohol dependence with alcohol-induced persisting dementia**
  Alcohol use disorder, moderate, with alcohol-induced major neurocognitive disorder, nonamnestic-confabulatory type ◄
  Alcohol use disorder, severe, with alcohol-induced major neurocognitive disorder, nonamnestic-confabulatory type ◄

● F10.28 **Alcohol dependence with other alcohol-induced disorders**
  F10.280 **Alcohol dependence with alcohol-induced anxiety disorder**
  F10.281 **Alcohol dependence with alcohol-induced sexual dysfunction**
  F10.282 **Alcohol dependence with alcohol-induced sleep disorder**
  F10.288 **Alcohol dependence with other alcohol-induced disorder**
    Alcohol use disorder, moderate, with alcohol-induced mild neurocognitive disorder ◄
    Alcohol use disorder, severe, with alcohol-induced mild neurocognitive disorder ◄

F10.29 **Alcohol dependence with unspecified alcohol-induced disorder**

● F10.9 **Alcohol use, unspecified**
  Excludes1   alcohol abuse (F10.1-)
     alcohol dependence (F10.2-)

● F10.92 **Alcohol use, unspecified with intoxication**
  F10.920 **Alcohol use, unspecified with intoxication, uncomplicated**
  F10.921 **Alcohol use, unspecified with intoxication delirium**
  F10.929 **Alcohol use, unspecified with intoxication, unspecified**

F10.94 **Alcohol use, unspecified with alcohol-induced mood disorder**
  Alcohol-induced bipolar or related disorder, without use disorder ◄
  Alcohol-induced depressive disorder, without use disorder ◄

CHAPTER 5 (F01-F99)

● **F10.95** **Alcohol use, unspecified with alcohol-induced psychotic disorder**

    F10.950 Alcohol use, unspecified with alcohol-induced psychotic disorder with delusions

    F10.951 Alcohol use, unspecified with alcohol-induced psychotic disorder with hallucinations

    F10.959 Alcohol use, unspecified with alcohol-induced psychotic disorder, unspecified
        Alcohol-induced psychotic disorder without use disorder ◄

  F10.96 Alcohol use, unspecified with alcohol-induced persisting amnestic disorder
    Alcohol-induced major neurocognitive disorder, amnestic-confabulatory type, without use disorder ◄

  F10.97 Alcohol use, unspecified with alcohol-induced persisting dementia
    Alcohol-induced major neurocognitive disorder, nonamnestic-confabulatory type, without use disorder ◄

● **F10.98** **Alcohol use, unspecified with other alcohol-induced disorders**

    F10.980 Alcohol use, unspecified with alcohol-induced anxiety disorder
        Alcohol-induced anxiety disorder, without use disorder ◄

    F10.981 Alcohol use, unspecified with alcohol-induced sexual dysfunction
        Alcohol-induced sexual dysfunction, without use disorder ◄

    F10.982 Alcohol use, unspecified with alcohol-induced sleep disorder
        Alcohol-induced sleep disorder, without use disorder ◄

    F10.988 Alcohol use, unspecified with other alcohol-induced disorder
        Alcohol-induced mild neurocognitive disorder, without use disorder ◄

  F10.99 Alcohol use, unspecified with unspecified alcohol-induced disorder

● **F11** **Opioid related disorders**

● **F11.1** **Opioid abuse**

    Excludes1 opioid dependence (F11.2-)
        opioid use, unspecified (F11.9-)

  F11.10 Opioid abuse, uncomplicated
    Opioid use disorder, mild ◄

● **F11.12** **Opioid abuse with intoxication**

    F11.120 Opioid abuse with intoxication, uncomplicated

    F11.121 Opioid abuse with intoxication delirium

    F11.122 Opioid abuse with intoxication with perceptual disturbance

    F11.129 Opioid abuse with intoxication, unspecified

  F11.14 Opioid abuse with opioid-induced mood disorder
    Opioid use disorder, mild, with opioid-induced depressive disorder ◄

● **F11.15** **Opioid abuse with opioid-induced psychotic disorder**

    F11.150 Opioid abuse with opioid-induced psychotic disorder with delusions

    F11.151 Opioid abuse with opioid-induced psychotic disorder with hallucinations

    F11.159 Opioid abuse with opioid-induced psychotic disorder, unspecified

● **F11.18** **Opioid abuse with other opioid-induced disorder**

    F11.181 Opioid abuse with opioid-induced sexual dysfunction

    F11.182 Opioid abuse with opioid-induced sleep disorder

    F11.188 Opioid abuse with other opioid-induced disorder

  F11.19 Opioid abuse with unspecified opioid-induced disorder

● **F11.2** **Opioid dependence**

    Excludes1 opioid abuse (F11.1-)
        opioid use, unspecified (F11.9-)

    Excludes2 opioid poisoning (T40.0--T40.2-)

  F11.20 Opioid dependence, uncomplicated
    Opioid use disorder, moderate ◄
    Opioid use disorder, severe ◄

  F11.21 Opioid dependence, in remission

● **F11.22** **Opioid dependence with intoxication**

    Excludes1 opioid dependence with withdrawal (F11.23)

    F11.220 Opioid dependence with intoxication, uncomplicated

    F11.221 Opioid dependence with intoxication delirium

    F11.222 Opioid dependence with intoxication with perceptual disturbance

    F11.229 Opioid dependence with intoxication, unspecified

  F11.23 Opioid dependence with withdrawal
    Excludes1 opioid dependence with intoxication (F11.22-)

  F11.24 Opioid dependence with opioid-induced mood disorder
    Opioid use disorder, moderate, with opioid-induced depressive disorder ◄

● **F11.25** **Opioid dependence with opioid-induced psychotic disorder**

    F11.250 Opioid dependence with opioid-induced psychotic disorder with delusions

    F11.251 Opioid dependence with opioid-induced psychotic disorder with hallucinations

    F11.259 Opioid dependence with opioid-induced psychotic disorder, unspecified

● **F11.28** **Opioid dependence with other opioid-induced disorder**

    F11.281 Opioid dependence with opioid-induced sexual dysfunction

    F11.282 Opioid dependence with opioid-induced sleep disorder

    F11.288 Opioid dependence with other opioid-induced disorder

  F11.29 Opioid dependence with unspecified opioid-induced disorder

◄ New   ◄▥ Revised   ~~deleted~~ Deleted   Excludes 1   Excludes 2   Includes   Use additional   Code first   Code also   Unspecified

OGCR Official Guidelines   X Assign placeholder X   ● Use Additional Character(s)   ▶ Manifestation Code   **Coding Clinic**

● F11.9　Opioid use, unspecified
　　　Excludes1　opioid abuse (F11.1-)
　　　　　　　　　opioid dependence (F11.2-)
　　F11.90　Opioid use, unspecified, uncomplicated
● F11.92　Opioid use, unspecified with intoxication
　　　Excludes1　opioid use, unspecified with
　　　　　　　　　withdrawal (F11.93)
　　　F11.920　Opioid use, unspecified with
　　　　　　　　intoxication, uncomplicated
　　　F11.921　Opioid use, unspecified with
　　　　　　　　intoxication delirium
　　　　　　　　　Opioid-induced delirium ◄
　　　F11.922　Opioid use, unspecified with
　　　　　　　　intoxication with perceptual
　　　　　　　　disturbance
　　　F11.929　Opioid use, unspecified with
　　　　　　　　intoxication, unspecified
　　F11.93　Opioid use, unspecified with withdrawal
　　　　Excludes1　opioid use, unspecified with
　　　　　　　　　intoxication (F11.92-)
　　F11.94　Opioid use, unspecified with opioid-induced
　　　　　　mood disorder
　　　　　　Opioid-induced depressive disorder, without
　　　　　　　use disorder ◄
● F11.95　Opioid use, unspecified with opioid-induced
　　　　　　psychotic disorder
　　　F11.950　Opioid use, unspecified with opioid-
　　　　　　　　induced psychotic disorder with
　　　　　　　　delusions
　　　F11.951　Opioid use, unspecified with opioid-
　　　　　　　　induced psychotic disorder with
　　　　　　　　hallucinations
　　　F11.959　Opioid use, unspecified with
　　　　　　　　opioid-induced psychotic disorder,
　　　　　　　　unspecified
● F11.98　Opioid use, unspecified with other specified
　　　　　　opioid-induced disorder
　　　F11.981　Opioid use, unspecified with opioid-
　　　　　　　　induced sexual dysfunction
　　　　　　　　　Opioid-induced sexual dysfunction,
　　　　　　　　　　without use disorder ◄
　　　F11.982　Opioid use, unspecified with opioid-
　　　　　　　　induced sleep disorder
　　　　　　　　　Opioid-induced sleep disorder,
　　　　　　　　　　without use disorder ◄
　　　F11.988　Opioid use, unspecified with other
　　　　　　　　opioid-induced disorder
　　　　　　　　　Opioid-induced anxiety disorder,
　　　　　　　　　　without use disorder ◄
　　F11.99　Opioid use, unspecified with unspecified
　　　　　　opioid-induced disorder

● F12　Cannabis related disorders
　　　Includes　marijuana
● F12.1　Cannabis abuse
　　　Excludes1　cannabis dependence (F12.2-)
　　　　　　　　　cannabis use, unspecified (F12.9-)
　　F12.10　Cannabis abuse, uncomplicated
　　　　　　Cannabis use disorder, mild ◄
● F12.12　Cannabis abuse with intoxication
　　　F12.120　Cannabis abuse with intoxication,
　　　　　　　　uncomplicated
　　　F12.121　Cannabis abuse with intoxication
　　　　　　　　delirium
　　　F12.122　Cannabis abuse with intoxication
　　　　　　　　with perceptual disturbance
　　　F12.129　Cannabis abuse with
　　　　　　　　intoxication, unspecified

● F12.15　Cannabis abuse with psychotic disorder
　　　F12.150　Cannabis abuse with psychotic
　　　　　　　　disorder with delusions
　　　F12.151　Cannabis abuse with psychotic
　　　　　　　　disorder with hallucinations
　　　F12.159　Cannabis abuse with psychotic
　　　　　　　　disorder, unspecified
● F12.18　Cannabis abuse with other cannabis-induced
　　　　　　disorder
　　　F12.180　Cannabis abuse with cannabis-
　　　　　　　　induced anxiety disorder
　　　F12.188　Cannabis abuse with other cannabis-
　　　　　　　　induced disorder
　　　　　　　　　Cannabis use disorder, mild, with
　　　　　　　　　　cannabis-induced sleep
　　　　　　　　　　disorder ◄
　　F12.19　Cannabis abuse with unspecified cannabis-
　　　　　　induced disorder
● F12.2　Cannabis dependence
　　　Excludes1　cannabis abuse (F12.1-)
　　　　　　　　　cannabis use, unspecified (F12.9-)
　　　Excludes2　cannabis poisoning (T40.7-)
　　F12.20　Cannabis dependence, uncomplicated
　　　　　　Cannabis use disorder, moderate ◄
　　　　　　Cannabis use disorder, severe ◄
　　F12.21　Cannabis dependence, in remission
● F12.22　Cannabis dependence with intoxication
　　　F12.220　Cannabis dependence with
　　　　　　　　intoxication, uncomplicated
　　　F12.221　Cannabis dependence with
　　　　　　　　intoxication delirium
　　　F12.222　Cannabis dependence with
　　　　　　　　intoxication with perceptual
　　　　　　　　disturbance
　　　F12.229　Cannabis dependence with
　　　　　　　　intoxication, unspecified
● F12.25　Cannabis dependence with psychotic disorder
　　　F12.250　Cannabis dependence with psychotic
　　　　　　　　disorder with delusions
　　　F12.251　Cannabis dependence with psychotic
　　　　　　　　disorder with hallucinations
　　　F12.259　Cannabis dependence with psychotic
　　　　　　　　disorder, unspecified
● F12.28　Cannabis dependence with other cannabis-
　　　　　　induced disorder
　　　F12.280　Cannabis dependence with cannabis-
　　　　　　　　induced anxiety disorder
　　　F12.288　Cannabis dependence with other
　　　　　　　　cannabis-induced disorder
　　　　　　　　　Cannabis use disorder, moderate,
　　　　　　　　　　with cannabis-induced sleep
　　　　　　　　　　disorder ◄
　　　　　　　　　Cannabis use disorder, severe, with
　　　　　　　　　　cannabis-induced sleep
　　　　　　　　　　disorder ◄
　　　　　　　　　Cannabis withdrawal ◄
　　F12.29　Cannabis dependence with unspecified
　　　　　　cannabis-induced disorder
● F12.9　Cannabis use, unspecified
　　　Excludes1　cannabis abuse (F12.1-)
　　　　　　　　　cannabis dependence (F12.2-)
　　F12.90　Cannabis use, unspecified, uncomplicated
● F12.92　Cannabis use, unspecified with intoxication
　　　F12.920　Cannabis use, unspecified with
　　　　　　　　intoxication, uncomplicated
　　　F12.921　Cannabis use, unspecified with
　　　　　　　　intoxication delirium
　　　F12.922　Cannabis use, unspecified with
　　　　　　　　intoxication with perceptual
　　　　　　　　disturbance
　　　F12.929　Cannabis use, unspecified with
　　　　　　　　intoxication, unspecified

CHAPTER 5 (F01-F99)

CHAPTER 5 (F01-F99)

● **F12.95**   **Cannabis use, unspecified with psychotic disorder**

     F12.950   **Cannabis use, unspecified with psychotic disorder with delusions**

     F12.951   **Cannabis use, unspecified with psychotic disorder with hallucinations**

     F12.959   **Cannabis use, unspecified with psychotic disorder, unspecified**
         Cannabis-induced psychotic disorder, without use disorder ◀

● **F12.98**   **Cannabis use, unspecified with other cannabis-induced disorder**

     F12.980   **Cannabis use, unspecified with anxiety disorder**
         Cannabis-induced anxiety disorder, without use disorder ◀

     F12.988   **Cannabis use, unspecified with other cannabis-induced disorder**
         Cannabis-induced sleep disorder, without use disorder ◀

     F12.99   **Cannabis use, unspecified with unspecified cannabis-induced disorder**

● **F13**   **Sedative, hypnotic, or anxiolytic related disorders**

   ● **F13.1**   **Sedative, hypnotic or anxiolytic-related abuse**

     Excludes1   sedative, hypnotic or anxiolytic-related dependence (F13.2-)
         sedative, hypnotic, or anxiolytic use, unspecified (F13.9-)

     F13.10   **Sedative, hypnotic or anxiolytic abuse, uncomplicated**
         Sedative, hypnotic, or anxiolytic use disorder, mild ◀

   ● **F13.12**   **Sedative, hypnotic or anxiolytic abuse with intoxication**

     F13.120   **Sedative, hypnotic or anxiolytic abuse with intoxication, uncomplicated**

     F13.121   **Sedative, hypnotic or anxiolytic abuse with intoxication delirium**

     F13.129   **Sedative, hypnotic or anxiolytic abuse with intoxication, unspecified**

     F13.14   **Sedative, hypnotic or anxiolytic abuse with sedative, hypnotic or anxiolytic-induced mood disorder**
         Sedative, hypnotic, or anxiolytic use disorder, mild, with sedative, hypnotic, or anxiolytic-induced bipolar or related disorder ◀
         Sedative, hypnotic, or anxiolytic use disorder, mild, with sedative, hypnotic, or anxiolytic-induced depressive disorder ◀

   ● **F13.15**   **Sedative, hypnotic or anxiolytic abuse with sedative, hypnotic or anxiolytic-induced psychotic disorder**

     F13.150   **Sedative, hypnotic or anxiolytic abuse with sedative, hypnotic or anxiolytic-induced psychotic disorder with delusions**

     F13.151   **Sedative, hypnotic or anxiolytic abuse with sedative, hypnotic or anxiolytic-induced psychotic disorder with hallucinations**

     F13.159   **Sedative, hypnotic or anxiolytic abuse with sedative, hypnotic or anxiolytic-induced psychotic disorder, unspecified**

   ● **F13.18**   **Sedative, hypnotic or anxiolytic abuse with other sedative, hypnotic or anxiolytic-induced disorders**

     F13.180   **Sedative, hypnotic or anxiolytic abuse with sedative, hypnotic or anxiolytic-induced anxiety disorder**

     F13.181   **Sedative, hypnotic or anxiolytic abuse with sedative, hypnotic or anxiolytic-induced sexual dysfunction**

     F13.182   **Sedative, hypnotic or anxiolytic abuse with sedative, hypnotic or anxiolytic-induced sleep disorder**

     F13.188   **Sedative, hypnotic or anxiolytic abuse with other sedative, hypnotic or anxiolytic-induced disorder**

     F13.19   **Sedative, hypnotic or anxiolytic abuse with unspecified sedative, hypnotic or anxiolytic-induced disorder**

   ● **F13.2**   **Sedative, hypnotic or anxiolytic-related dependence**

     Excludes1   sedative, hypnotic or anxiolytic-related abuse (F13.1-)
         sedative, hypnotic, or anxiolytic use, unspecified (F13.9-)

     Excludes2   sedative, hypnotic, or anxiolytic poisoning (T42.-)

     F13.20   **Sedative, hypnotic or anxiolytic dependence, uncomplicated**

     F13.21   **Sedative, hypnotic or anxiolytic dependence, in remission**

   ● **F13.22**   **Sedative, hypnotic or anxiolytic dependence with intoxication**

     Excludes1   sedative, hypnotic or anxiolytic dependence with withdrawal (F13.23-)

     F13.220   **Sedative, hypnotic or anxiolytic dependence with intoxication, uncomplicated**

     F13.221   **Sedative, hypnotic or anxiolytic dependence with intoxication delirium**

     F13.229   **Sedative, hypnotic or anxiolytic dependence with intoxication, unspecified**

   ● **F13.23**   **Sedative, hypnotic or anxiolytic dependence with withdrawal**
         Sedative, hypnotic, or anxiolytic use disorder, moderate ◀
         Sedative, hypnotic, or anxiolytic use disorder, severe ◀

     Excludes1   sedative, hypnotic or anxiolytic dependence with intoxication (F13.22-)

     F13.230   **Sedative, hypnotic or anxiolytic dependence with withdrawal, uncomplicated**

     F13.231   **Sedative, hypnotic or anxiolytic dependence with withdrawal delirium**

     F13.232   **Sedative, hypnotic or anxiolytic dependence with withdrawal with perceptual disturbance**
         Sedative, hypnotic, or anxiolytic withdrawal with perceptual disturbances ◀

     F13.239   **Sedative, hypnotic or anxiolytic dependence with withdrawal, unspecified**
         Sedative, hypnotic, or anxiolytic withdrawal without perceptual disturbances ◀

F13.24   **Sedative, hypnotic or anxiolytic dependence with sedative, hypnotic or anxiolytic-induced mood disorder**

> Sedative, hypnotic, or anxiolytic use disorder, moderate, with sedative, hypnotic, or anxiolytic-induced bipolar or related disorder ◄
>
> Sedative, hypnotic, or anxiolytic use disorder, moderate, with sedative, hypnotic, or anxiolytic-induced depressive disorder ◄
>
> Sedative, hypnotic, or anxiolytic use disorder, severe, with sedative, hypnotic, or anxiolytic-induced bipolar or related disorder ◄
>
> Sedative, hypnotic, or anxiolytic use disorder, severe, with sedative, hypnotic, or anxiolytic-induced depressive disorder ◄

● **F13.25**   **Sedative, hypnotic or anxiolytic dependence with sedative, hypnotic or anxiolytic-induced psychotic disorder**

     F13.250   **Sedative, hypnotic or anxiolytic dependence with sedative, hypnotic or anxiolytic-induced psychotic disorder with delusions**

     F13.251   **Sedative, hypnotic or anxiolytic dependence with sedative, hypnotic or anxiolytic-induced psychotic disorder with hallucinations**

     F13.259   **Sedative, hypnotic or anxiolytic dependence with sedative, hypnotic or anxiolytic-induced psychotic disorder, unspecified**

F13.26   **Sedative, hypnotic or anxiolytic dependence with sedative, hypnotic or anxiolytic-induced persisting amnestic disorder**

F13.27   **Sedative, hypnotic or anxiolytic dependence with sedative, hypnotic or anxiolytic-induced persisting dementia**

> Sedative, hypnotic, or anxiolytic use disorder, moderate, with sedative, hypnotic, or anxiolytic-induced major neurocognitive disorder ◄
>
> Sedative, hypnotic, or anxiolytic use disorder, severe, with sedative, hypnotic, or anxiolytic-induced major neurocognitive disorder ◄

● **F13.28**   **Sedative, hypnotic or anxiolytic dependence with other sedative, hypnotic or anxiolytic-induced disorders**

     F13.280   **Sedative, hypnotic or anxiolytic dependence with sedative, hypnotic or anxiolytic-induced anxiety disorder**

     F13.281   **Sedative, hypnotic or anxiolytic dependence with sedative, hypnotic or anxiolytic-induced sexual dysfunction**

     F13.282   **Sedative, hypnotic or anxiolytic dependence with sedative, hypnotic or anxiolytic-induced sleep disorder**

     F13.288   **Sedative, hypnotic or anxiolytic dependence with other sedative, hypnotic or anxiolytic-induced disorder**

> Sedative, hypnotic, or anxiolytic use disorder, moderate, with sedative, hypnotic, or anxiolytic-induced mild neurocognitive disorder ◄
>
> Sedative, hypnotic, or anxiolytic use disorder, severe, with sedative, hypnotic, or anxiolytic-induced mild neurocognitive disorder ◄

F13.29   **Sedative, hypnotic or anxiolytic dependence with unspecified sedative, hypnotic or anxiolytic-induced disorder**

● **F13.9**   **Sedative, hypnotic or anxiolytic-related use, unspecified**

> **Excludes1**   sedative, hypnotic or anxiolytic-related abuse (F13.1-)
> sedative, hypnotic or anxiolytic-related dependence (F13.2-)

F13.90   **Sedative, hypnotic, or anxiolytic use, unspecified, uncomplicated**

● **F13.92**   **Sedative, hypnotic or anxiolytic use, unspecified with intoxication**

> **Excludes1**   sedative, hypnotic or anxiolytic use, unspecified with withdrawal (F13.93-)

     F13.920   **Sedative, hypnotic or anxiolytic use, unspecified with intoxication, uncomplicated**

     F13.921   **Sedative, hypnotic or anxiolytic use, unspecified with intoxication delirium**

> Sedative, hypnotic, or anxiolytic-induced delirium ◄

     F13.929   **Sedative, hypnotic or anxiolytic use, unspecified with intoxication, unspecified**

● **F13.93**   **Sedative, hypnotic or anxiolytic use, unspecified with withdrawal**

> **Excludes1**   sedative, hypnotic or anxiolytic use, unspecified with intoxication (F13.92-)

     F13.930   **Sedative, hypnotic or anxiolytic use, unspecified with withdrawal, uncomplicated**

     F13.931   **Sedative, hypnotic or anxiolytic use, unspecified with withdrawal delirium**

     F13.932   **Sedative, hypnotic or anxiolytic use, unspecified with withdrawal with perceptual disturbances**

     F13.939   **Sedative, hypnotic or anxiolytic use, unspecified with withdrawal, unspecified**

F13.94   **Sedative, hypnotic or anxiolytic use, unspecified with sedative, hypnotic or anxiolytic-induced mood disorder**

> Sedative, hypnotic, or anxiolytic-induced bipolar or related disorder, without use disorder ◄
>
> Sedative, hypnotic, or anxiolytic-induced depressive disorder, without use disorder ◄

● **F13.95**   **Sedative, hypnotic or anxiolytic use, unspecified with sedative, hypnotic or anxiolytic-induced psychotic disorder**

     F13.950   **Sedative, hypnotic or anxiolytic use, unspecified with sedative, hypnotic or anxiolytic-induced psychotic disorder with delusions**

     F13.951   **Sedative, hypnotic or anxiolytic use, unspecified with sedative, hypnotic or anxiolytic-induced psychotic disorder with hallucinations**

     F13.959   **Sedative, hypnotic or anxiolytic use, unspecified with sedative, hypnotic or anxiolytic-induced psychotic disorder, unspecified**

> Sedative, hypnotic, or anxiolytic-induced psychotic disorder, without use disorder ◄

F13.96   Sedative, hypnotic or anxiolytic use, unspecified with sedative, hypnotic or anxiolytic-induced persisting amnestic disorder

F13.97   Sedative, hypnotic or anxiolytic use, unspecified with sedative, hypnotic or anxiolytic-induced persisting dementia
> Sedative, hypnotic, or anxiolytic-induced major neurocognitive disorder, without use disorder ◄

● F13.98   Sedative, hypnotic or anxiolytic use, unspecified with other sedative, hypnotic or anxiolytic-induced disorders

     F13.980   Sedative, hypnotic or anxiolytic use, unspecified with sedative, hypnotic or anxiolytic-induced anxiety disorder
> Sedative, hypnotic, or anxiolytic-induced anxiety disorder, without use disorder ◄

     F13.981   Sedative, hypnotic or anxiolytic use, unspecified with sedative, hypnotic or anxiolytic-induced sexual dysfunction
> Sedative, hypnotic, or anxiolytic-induced sexual dysfunction disorder, without use disorder ◄

     F13.982   Sedative, hypnotic or anxiolytic use, unspecified with sedative, hypnotic or anxiolytic-induced sleep disorder
> Sedative, hypnotic, or anxiolytic-induced sleep disorder, without use disorder ◄

     F13.988   Sedative, hypnotic or anxiolytic use, unspecified with other sedative, hypnotic or anxiolytic-induced disorder
> Sedative, hypnotic, or anxiolytic-induced mild neurocognitive disorder ◄

F13.99   Sedative, hypnotic or anxiolytic use, unspecified with unspecified sedative, hypnotic or anxiolytic-induced disorder

● F14   Cocaine related disorders
> **Excludes2**   other stimulant-related disorders (F15.-)

● F14.1   Cocaine abuse
> **Excludes1**   cocaine dependence (F14.2-)
>   cocaine use, unspecified (F14.9-)

     F14.10   Cocaine abuse, uncomplicated
> Cocaine use disorder, mild ◄

  ● F14.12   Cocaine abuse with intoxication

     F14.120   Cocaine abuse with intoxication, uncomplicated

     F14.121   Cocaine abuse with intoxication with delirium

     F14.122   Cocaine abuse with intoxication with perceptual disturbance

     F14.129   Cocaine abuse with intoxication, unspecified

     F14.14   Cocaine abuse with cocaine-induced mood disorder
> Cocaine use disorder, mild, with cocaine-induced bipolar or related disorder ◄
> Cocaine use disorder, mild, with cocaine-induced depressive disorder ◄

  ● F14.15   Cocaine abuse with cocaine-induced psychotic disorder

     F14.150   Cocaine abuse with cocaine-induced psychotic disorder with delusions

     F14.151   Cocaine abuse with cocaine-induced psychotic disorder with hallucinations

     F14.159   Cocaine abuse with cocaine-induced psychotic disorder, unspecified

  ● F14.18   Cocaine abuse with other cocaine-induced disorder

     F14.180   Cocaine abuse with cocaine-induced anxiety disorder

     F14.181   Cocaine abuse with cocaine-induced sexual dysfunction

     F14.182   Cocaine abuse with cocaine-induced sleep disorder

     F14.188   Cocaine abuse with other cocaine-induced disorder
> Cocaine use disorder, mild, with cocaine-induced obsessive-compulsive or related disorder ◄

     F14.19   Cocaine abuse with unspecified cocaine-induced disorder

● F14.2   Cocaine dependence
> **Excludes1**   cocaine abuse (F14.1-)
>   cocaine use, unspecified (F14.9-)
> **Excludes2**   cocaine poisoning (T40.5-)

     F14.20   Cocaine dependence, uncomplicated
> Cocaine use disorder, moderate ◄
> Cocaine use disorder, severe ◄

     F14.21   Cocaine dependence, in remission

  ● F14.22   Cocaine dependence with intoxication
> **Excludes1**   cocaine dependence with withdrawal (F14.23)

     F14.220   Cocaine dependence with intoxication, uncomplicated

     F14.221   Cocaine dependence with intoxication delirium

     F14.222   Cocaine dependence with intoxication with perceptual disturbance

     F14.229   Cocaine dependence with intoxication, unspecified

     F14.23   Cocaine dependence with withdrawal
> **Excludes1**   cocaine dependence with intoxication (F14.22-)

     F14.24   Cocaine dependence with cocaine-induced mood disorder
> Cocaine use disorder, moderate, with cocaine-induced bipolar or related disorder ◄
> Cocaine use disorder, moderate, with cocaine-induced depressive disorder ◄
> Cocaine use disorder, severe, with cocaine-induced bipolar or related disorder ◄
> Cocaine use disorder, severe, with cocaine-induced depressive disorder ◄

  ● F14.25   Cocaine dependence with cocaine-induced psychotic disorder

     F14.250   Cocaine dependence with cocaine-induced psychotic disorder with delusions

     F14.251   Cocaine dependence with cocaine-induced psychotic disorder with hallucinations

     F14.259   Cocaine dependence with cocaine-induced psychotic disorder, unspecified

◄ New   ◄▪▪ Revised   ~~deleted~~ Deleted   Excludes 1   Excludes 2   Includes   Use additional   Code first   Code also   Unspecified

752   OGCR Official Guidelines   X Assign placeholder X   ● Use Additional Character(s)   ▶ Manifestation Code   **Coding Clinic**

● **F14.28**   **Cocaine dependence with other cocaine-induced disorder**

    F14.280   **Cocaine dependence with cocaine-induced anxiety disorder**

    F14.281   **Cocaine dependence with cocaine-induced sexual dysfunction**

    F14.282   **Cocaine dependence with cocaine-induced sleep disorder**

    F14.288   **Cocaine dependence with other cocaine-induced disorder**
       Cocaine use disorder, moderate, with cocaine-induced obsessive-compulsive or related disorder ◄
       Cocaine use disorder, severe, with cocaine-induced obsessive-compulsive or related disorder ◄

   F14.29   **Cocaine dependence with unspecified cocaine-induced disorder**

● **F14.9**   **Cocaine use, unspecified**

    Excludes1   cocaine abuse (F14.1-)
             cocaine dependence (F14.2-)

   F14.90   **Cocaine use, unspecified, uncomplicated**

● **F14.92**   **Cocaine use, unspecified with intoxication**

    F14.920   **Cocaine use, unspecified with intoxication, uncomplicated**

    F14.921   **Cocaine use, unspecified with intoxication delirium**

    F14.922   **Cocaine use, unspecified with intoxication with perceptual disturbance**

    F14.929   **Cocaine use, unspecified with intoxication, unspecified**

   F14.94   **Cocaine use, unspecified with cocaine-induced mood disorder**
       Cocaine-induced bipolar or related disorder, without use disorder ◄
       Cocaine-induced depressive disorder, without use disorder ◄

● **F14.95**   **Cocaine use, unspecified with cocaine-induced psychotic disorder**

    F14.950   **Cocaine use, unspecified with cocaine-induced psychotic disorder with delusions**

    F14.951   **Cocaine use, unspecified with cocaine-induced psychotic disorder with hallucinations**

    F14.959   **Cocaine use, unspecified with cocaine-induced psychotic disorder, unspecified**
       Cocaine-induced psychotic disorder, without use disorder ◄

● **F14.98**   **Cocaine use, unspecified with other specified cocaine-induced disorder**

    F14.980   **Cocaine use, unspecified with cocaine-induced anxiety disorder**
       Cocaine-induced anxiety disorder, without use disorder ◄

    F14.981   **Cocaine use, unspecified with cocaine-induced sexual dysfunction**
       Cocaine-induced sexual dysfunction, without use disorder ◄

    F14.982   **Cocaine use, unspecified with cocaine-induced sleep disorder**
       Cocaine-induced sleep disorder, without use disorder ◄

    F14.988   **Cocaine use, unspecified with other cocaine-induced disorder**
       Cocaine-induced obsessive-compulsive or related disorder ◄

   F14.99   **Cocaine use, unspecified with unspecified cocaine-induced disorder**

● **F15**   **Other stimulant related disorders**

    Includes   amphetamine-related disorders
            caffeine

    Excludes2   cocaine-related disorders (F14.-)

● **F15.1**   **Other stimulant abuse**

    Excludes1   other stimulant dependence (F15.2-)
            other stimulant use, unspecified (F15.9-)

    F15.10   **Other stimulant abuse, uncomplicated**
       Amphetamine type substance use disorder, mild ◄
       Other or unspecified stimulant use disorder, mild ◄

● **F15.12**   **Other stimulant abuse with intoxication**

    F15.120   **Other stimulant abuse with intoxication, uncomplicated**

    F15.121   **Other stimulant abuse with intoxication delirium**

    F15.122   **Other stimulant abuse with intoxication with perceptual disturbance**
       Amphetamine or other stimulant use disorder, mild, with amphetamine or other stimulant intoxication, with perceptual disturbances ◄

    F15.129   **Other stimulant abuse with intoxication, unspecified**
       Amphetamine or other stimulant use disorder, mild, with amphetamine or other stimulant intoxication, without perceptual disturbances ◄

   F15.14   **Other stimulant abuse with stimulant-induced mood disorder**
       Amphetamine or other stimulant use disorder, mild, with amphetamine or other stimulant-induced bipolar or related disorder ◄
       Amphetamine or other stimulant use disorder, mild, with amphetamine or other stimulant-induced depressive disorder ◄

● **F15.15**   **Other stimulant abuse with stimulant-induced psychotic disorder**

    F15.150   **Other stimulant abuse with stimulant-induced psychotic disorder with delusions**

    F15.151   **Other stimulant abuse with stimulant-induced psychotic disorder with hallucinations**

    F15.159   **Other stimulant abuse with stimulant-induced psychotic disorder, unspecified**

● **F15.18**   **Other stimulant abuse with other stimulant-induced disorder**

    F15.180   **Other stimulant abuse with stimulant-induced anxiety disorder**

    F15.181   **Other stimulant abuse with stimulant-induced sexual dysfunction**

    F15.182   **Other stimulant abuse with stimulant-induced sleep disorder**

    F15.188   **Other stimulant abuse with other stimulant-induced disorder**
       Amphetamine or other stimulant use disorder, mild, with amphetamine or other stimulant-induced obsessive-compulsive or related disorder ◄

   F15.19   **Other stimulant abuse with unspecified stimulant-induced disorder**

CHAPTER 5 (F01-F99)

● F15.2　Other stimulant dependence
　　Excludes1　other stimulant abuse (F15.1-)
　　　　　　　　other stimulant use, unspecified (F15.9-)

F15.20　Other stimulant dependence, uncomplicated
　　　　Amphetamine type substance use disorder, moderate ◄
　　　　Amphetamine type substance use disorder, severe ◄
　　　　Other or unspecified stimulant use disorder, moderate ◄
　　　　Other or unspecified stimulant use disorder, severe ◄

F15.21　Other stimulant dependence, in remission

● F15.22　Other stimulant dependence with intoxication
　　Excludes1　other stimulant dependence with withdrawal (F15.23)

F15.220　Other stimulant dependence with intoxication, uncomplicated

F15.221　Other stimulant dependence with intoxication delirium

F15.222　Other stimulant dependence with intoxication with perceptual disturbance
　　　　Amphetamine or other stimulant use disorder, moderate, with amphetamine or other stimulant intoxication, with perceptual disturbances ◄
　　　　Amphetamine or other stimulant use disorder, severe, with amphetamine or other stimulant intoxication, with perceptual disturbances ◄

F15.229　Other stimulant dependence with intoxication, unspecified
　　　　Amphetamine or other stimulant use disorder, moderate, with amphetamine or other stimulant intoxication, without perceptual disturbances ◄
　　　　Amphetamine or other stimulant use disorder, severe, with amphetamine or other stimulant intoxication, without perceptual disturbances ◄

F15.23　Other stimulant dependence with withdrawal
　　　　Amphetamine or other stimulant withdrawal ◄
　　Excludes1　other stimulant dependence with intoxication (F15.22-)

F15.24　Other stimulant dependence with stimulant-induced mood disorder
　　　　Amphetamine or other stimulant use disorder, moderate, with amphetamine or other stimulant-induced bipolar or related disorder ◄
　　　　Amphetamine or other stimulant use disorder, moderate, with amphetamine or other stimulant-induced depressive disorder ◄
　　　　Amphetamine or other stimulant use disorder, severe, with amphetamine or other stimulant-induced bipolar or related disorder ◄
　　　　Amphetamine or other stimulant use disorder, severe, with amphetamine or other stimulant-induced depressive disorder ◄

F15.25　Other stimulant dependence with stimulant-induced psychotic disorder
　F15.250　Other stimulant dependence with stimulant-induced psychotic disorder with delusions
　F15.251　Other stimulant dependence with stimulant-induced psychotic disorder with hallucinations
　F15.259　Other stimulant dependence with stimulant-induced psychotic disorder, unspecified

● F15.28　Other stimulant dependence with other stimulant-induced disorder
　F15.280　Other stimulant dependence with stimulant-induced anxiety disorder
　F15.281　Other stimulant dependence with stimulant-induced sexual dysfunction
　F15.282　Other stimulant dependence with stimulant-induced sleep disorder
　F15.288　Other stimulant dependence with other stimulant-induced disorder
　　　　Amphetamine or other stimulant use disorder, moderate, with amphetamine or other stimulant-induced obsessive-compulsive or related disorder ◄
　　　　Amphetamine or other stimulant use disorder, severe, with amphetamine or other stimulant-induced obsessive-compulsive or related disorder ◄

F15.29　Other stimulant dependence with unspecified stimulant-induced disorder

● F15.9　Other stimulant use, unspecified
　　Excludes1　other stimulant abuse (F15.1-)
　　　　　　　　other stimulant dependence (F15.2-)

F15.90　Other stimulant use, unspecified, uncomplicated

● F15.92　Other stimulant use, unspecified with intoxication
　　Excludes1　other stimulant use, unspecified with withdrawal (F15.93)

　F15.920　Other stimulant use, unspecified with intoxication, uncomplicated
　F15.921　Other stimulant use, unspecified with intoxication delirium
　　　　Amphetamine or other stimulant-induced delirium ◄
　F15.922　Other stimulant use, unspecified with intoxication with perceptual disturbance
　F15.929　Other stimulant use, unspecified with intoxication, unspecified
　　　　Caffeine intoxication ◄

F15.93　Other stimulant use, unspecified with withdrawal
　　　　Caffeine withdrawal ◄
　　Excludes1　other stimulant use, unspecified with intoxication (F15.92-)

F15.94　Other stimulant use, unspecified with stimulant-induced mood disorder
　　　　Amphetamine or other stimulant-induced bipolar or related disorder, without use disorder ◄
　　　　Amphetamine or other stimulant-induced depressive disorder, without use disorder ◄

◄ New　◄▪ Revised　d̶e̶l̶e̶t̶e̶d̶ Deleted　Excludes 1　Excludes 2　Includes　Use additional　Code first　Code also　Unspecified
OGCR Official Guidelines　X Assign placeholder X　● Use Additional Character(s)　▷ Manifestation Code　Coding Clinic

● **F15.95**   **Other stimulant use, unspecified with stimulant-induced psychotic disorder**

    F15.950   **Other stimulant use, unspecified with stimulant-induced psychotic disorder with delusions**

    F15.951   **Other stimulant use, unspecified with stimulant-induced psychotic disorder with hallucinations**

    F15.959   **Other stimulant use, unspecified with stimulant-induced psychotic disorder, unspecified**
        Amphetamine or other stimulant-induced psychotic disorder, without use disorder ◄

● **F15.98**   **Other stimulant use, unspecified with other stimulant-induced disorder**

    F15.980   **Other stimulant use, unspecified with stimulant-induced anxiety disorder**
        Amphetamine or other stimulant-induced anxiety disorder, without use disorder ◄
        Caffeine-induced anxiety disorder, without use disorder ◄

    F15.981   **Other stimulant use, unspecified with stimulant-induced sexual dysfunction**
        Amphetamine or other stimulant-induced sexual dysfunction, without use disorder ◄

    F15.982   **Other stimulant use, unspecified with stimulant-induced sleep disorder**
        Amphetamine or other stimulant-induced sleep disorder, without use disorder ◄
        Caffeine-induced sleep disorder, without use disorder ◄

    F15.988   **Other stimulant use, unspecified with other stimulant-induced disorder**
        Amphetamine or other stimulant-induced obsessive-compulsive or related disorder, without use disorder ◄

    F15.99   **Other stimulant use, unspecified with unspecified stimulant-induced disorder**

● **F16**   **Hallucinogen related disorders**

    Includes   ecstasy
                PCP
                phencyclidine

● **F16.1**   **Hallucinogen abuse**

    Excludes1   hallucinogen dependence (F16.2-)
               hallucinogen use, unspecified (F16.9-)

    F16.10   **Hallucinogen abuse, uncomplicated**
        Other hallucinogen use disorder, mild ◄
        Phencyclidine use disorder, mild ◄

●   **F16.12**   **Hallucinogen abuse with intoxication**

    F16.120   **Hallucinogen abuse with intoxication, uncomplicated**

    F16.121   **Hallucinogen abuse with intoxication with delirium**

    F16.122   **Hallucinogen abuse with intoxication with perceptual disturbance**

    F16.129   **Hallucinogen abuse with intoxication, unspecified**

    F16.14   **Hallucinogen abuse with hallucinogen-induced mood disorder**
        Other hallucinogen use disorder, mild, with other hallucinogen-induced bipolar or related disorder ◄
        Other hallucinogen use disorder, mild, with other hallucinogen-induced depressive disorder ◄
        Phencyclidine use disorder, mild, with phencyclidine-induced bipolar or related disorder ◄
        Phencyclidine use disorder, mild, with phencyclidine-induced depressive disorder ◄

● **F16.15**   **Hallucinogen abuse with hallucinogen-induced psychotic disorder**

    F16.150   **Hallucinogen abuse with hallucinogen-induced psychotic disorder with delusions**

    F16.151   **Hallucinogen abuse with hallucinogen-induced psychotic disorder with hallucinations**

    F16.159   **Hallucinogen abuse with hallucinogen-induced psychotic disorder, unspecified**

● **F16.18**   **Hallucinogen abuse with other hallucinogen-induced disorder**

    F16.180   **Hallucinogen abuse with hallucinogen-induced anxiety disorder**

    F16.183   **Hallucinogen abuse with hallucinogen persisting perception disorder (flashbacks)**

    F16.188   **Hallucinogen abuse with other hallucinogen-induced disorder**

    F16.19   **Hallucinogen abuse with unspecified hallucinogen-induced disorder**

● **F16.2**   **Hallucinogen dependence**

    Excludes1   hallucinogen abuse (F16.1-)
              hallucinogen use, unspecified (F16.9-)

    F16.20   **Hallucinogen dependence, uncomplicated**
        Other hallucinogen use disorder, moderate ◄
        Other hallucinogen use disorder, severe ◄
        Phencyclidine use disorder, moderate ◄
        Phencyclidine use disorder, severe ◄

    F16.21   **Hallucinogen dependence, in remission**

● **F16.22**   **Hallucinogen dependence with intoxication**

    F16.220   **Hallucinogen dependence with intoxication, uncomplicated**

    F16.221   **Hallucinogen dependence with intoxication with delirium**

    F16.229   **Hallucinogen dependence with intoxication, unspecified**

    F16.24   **Hallucinogen dependence with hallucinogen-induced mood disorder**
        Other hallucinogen use disorder, moderate, with other hallucinogen-induced bipolar or related disorder ◄
        Other hallucinogen use disorder, moderate, with other hallucinogen-induced depressive disorder ◄
        Other hallucinogen use disorder, severe, with other hallucinogen-induced bipolar or related disorder ◄
        Other hallucinogen use disorder, severe, with other hallucinogen-induced depressive disorder ◄
        Phencyclidine use disorder, moderate, with phencyclidine-induced bipolar or related disorder ◄
        Phencyclidine use disorder, moderate, with phencyclidine-induced depressive disorder ◄
        Phencyclidine use disorder, severe, with phencyclidine-induced bipolar or related disorder ◄
        Phencyclidine use disorder, severe, with phencyclidine-induced depressive disorder ◄

CHAPTER 5 (F01-F99)

CHAPTER 5 (F01-F99)

- **F16.25**   Hallucinogen dependence with hallucinogen-induced psychotic disorder
  - F16.250   Hallucinogen dependence with hallucinogen-induced psychotic disorder with delusions
  - F16.251   Hallucinogen dependence with hallucinogen-induced psychotic disorder with hallucinations
  - F16.259   Hallucinogen dependence with hallucinogen-induced psychotic disorder, unspecified
- **F16.28**   Hallucinogen dependence with other hallucinogen-induced disorder
  - F16.280   Hallucinogen dependence with hallucinogen-induced anxiety disorder
  - F16.283   Hallucinogen dependence with hallucinogen persisting perception disorder (flashbacks)
  - F16.288   Hallucinogen dependence with other hallucinogen-induced disorder
- F16.29   Hallucinogen dependence with unspecified hallucinogen-induced disorder
- **F16.9**   Hallucinogen use, unspecified
  - **Excludes1**   hallucinogen abuse (F16.1-)
    hallucinogen dependence (F16.2-)
  - F16.90   Hallucinogen use, unspecified, uncomplicated
- **F16.92**   Hallucinogen use, unspecified with intoxication
  - F16.920   Hallucinogen use, unspecified with intoxication, uncomplicated
  - F16.921   Hallucinogen use, unspecified with intoxication with delirium
    Other hallucinogen intoxication delirium ◀
  - F16.929   Hallucinogen use, unspecified with intoxication, unspecified
  - F16.94   Hallucinogen use, unspecified with hallucinogen-induced mood disorder
    Other hallucinogen-induced bipolar or related disorder, without use disorder ◀
    Other hallucinogen-induced depressive disorder, without use disorder ◀
    Phencyclidine-induced bipolar or related disorder, without use disorder ◀
    Phencyclidine-induced depressive disorder, without use disorder ◀
- **F16.95**   Hallucinogen use, unspecified with hallucinogen-induced psychotic disorder
  - F16.950   Hallucinogen use, unspecified with hallucinogen-induced psychotic disorder with delusions
  - F16.951   Hallucinogen use, unspecified with hallucinogen-induced psychotic disorder with hallucinations
  - F16.959   Hallucinogen use, unspecified with hallucinogen-induced psychotic disorder, unspecified
    Other hallucinogen-induced psychotic disorder, without use disorder ◀
    Phencyclidine-induced psychotic disorder, without use disorder ◀
- **F16.98**   Hallucinogen use, unspecified with other specified hallucinogen-induced disorder
  - F16.980   Hallucinogen use, unspecified with hallucinogen-induced anxiety disorder
    Other hallucinogen-induced anxiety disorder, without use disorder ◀
    Phencyclidine-induced anxiety disorder, without use disorder ◀

-    F16.983   Hallucinogen use, unspecified with hallucinogen persisting perception disorder (flashbacks)
-    F16.988   Hallucinogen use, unspecified with other hallucinogen-induced disorder
- F16.99   Hallucinogen use, unspecified with unspecified hallucinogen-induced disorder
- **F17**   **Nicotine dependence**
  - **Excludes1**   history of tobacco dependence (Z87.891)
    tobacco use NOS (Z72.0)
  - **Excludes2**   tobacco use (smoking) during pregnancy, childbirth and the puerperium (O99.33-)
    toxic effect of nicotine (T65.2-)
- **F17.2**   Nicotine dependence
  - **F17.20**   Nicotine dependence, unspecified
    - F17.200   Nicotine dependence, unspecified, uncomplicated
      Tobacco use disorder, mild ◀
      Tobacco use disorder, moderate ◀
      Tobacco use disorder, severe ◀
      Coding Clinic: 2016, Q1, P37
    - F17.201   Nicotine dependence, unspecified, in remission
    - F17.203   Nicotine dependence unspecified, with withdrawal
      Tobacco withdrawal ◀
    - F17.208   Nicotine dependence, unspecified, with other nicotine-induced disorders
    - F17.209   Nicotine dependence, unspecified, with unspecified nicotine-induced disorders
  - **F17.21**   Nicotine dependence, cigarettes
    - F17.210   Nicotine dependence, cigarettes, uncomplicated
    - F17.211   Nicotine dependence, cigarettes, in remission
    - F17.213   Nicotine dependence, cigarettes, with withdrawal
    - F17.218   Nicotine dependence, cigarettes, with other nicotine-induced disorders
    - F17.219   Nicotine dependence, cigarettes, with unspecified nicotine-induced disorders
  - **F17.22**   Nicotine dependence, chewing tobacco
    - F17.220   Nicotine dependence, chewing tobacco, uncomplicated
    - F17.221   Nicotine dependence, chewing tobacco, in remission
    - F17.223   Nicotine dependence, chewing tobacco, with withdrawal
    - F17.228   Nicotine dependence, chewing tobacco, with other nicotine-induced disorders
    - F17.229   Nicotine dependence, chewing tobacco, with unspecified nicotine-induced disorders
  - **F17.29**   Nicotine dependence, other tobacco product
    - F17.290   Nicotine dependence, other tobacco product, uncomplicated
    - F17.291   Nicotine dependence, other tobacco product, in remission
    - F17.293   Nicotine dependence, other tobacco product, with withdrawal
    - F17.298   Nicotine dependence, other tobacco product, with other nicotine-induced disorders
    - F17.299   Nicotine dependence, other tobacco product, with unspecified nicotine-induced disorders

◀ New   ◀▥ Revised   ~~deleted~~ Deleted   Excludes 1   Excludes 2   Includes   Use additional   Code first   Code also   Unspecified

756

OGCR Official Guidelines   X Assign placeholder X   ● Use Additional Character(s)   ▶ Manifestation Code   **Coding Clinic**

● **F18**   **Inhalant related disorders**
    Includes   volatile solvents

● **F18.1**   **Inhalant abuse**
    Excludes1   inhalant dependence (F18.2-)
               inhalant use, unspecified (F18.9-)

   F18.10   **Inhalant abuse, uncomplicated**
           Inhalant use disorder, mild ◀

● **F18.12**   **Inhalant abuse with intoxication**
     F18.120   **Inhalant abuse with intoxication, uncomplicated**
     F18.121   **Inhalant abuse with intoxication delirium**
     F18.129   **Inhalant abuse with intoxication, unspecified**

   F18.14   **Inhalant abuse with inhalant-induced mood disorder**
           Inhalant use disorder, mild, with inhalant-induced depressive disorder ◀

● **F18.15**   **Inhalant abuse with inhalant-induced psychotic disorder**
     F18.150   **Inhalant abuse with inhalant-induced psychotic disorder with delusions**
     F18.151   **Inhalant abuse with inhalant-induced psychotic disorder with hallucinations**
     F18.159   **Inhalant abuse with inhalant-induced psychotic disorder, unspecified**

   F18.17   **Inhalant abuse with inhalant-induced dementia**
           Inhalant use disorder, mild, with inhalant-induced major neurocognitive disorder ◀

● **F18.18**   **Inhalant abuse with other inhalant-induced disorders**
     F18.180   **Inhalant abuse with inhalant-induced anxiety disorder**
     F18.188   **Inhalant abuse with other inhalant-induced disorder**
               Inhalant use disorder, mild, with inhalant-induced mild neurocognitive disorder ◀

   F18.19   **Inhalant abuse with unspecified inhalant-induced disorder**

● **F18.2**   **Inhalant dependence**
    Excludes1   inhalant abuse (F18.1-)
               inhalant use, unspecified (F18.9-)

   F18.20   **Inhalant dependence, uncomplicated**
           Inhalant use disorder, moderate ◀
           Inhalant use disorder, severe ◀

   F18.21   **Inhalant dependence, in remission**

● **F18.22**   **Inhalant dependence with intoxication**
     F18.220   **Inhalant dependence with intoxication, uncomplicated**
     F18.221   **Inhalant dependence with intoxication delirium**
     F18.229   **Inhalant dependence with intoxication, unspecified**

   F18.24   **Inhalant dependence with inhalant-induced mood disorder**
           Inhalant use disorder, moderate, with inhalant-induced depressive disorder ◀
           Inhalant use disorder, severe, with inhalant-induced depressive disorder ◀

● **F18.25**   **Inhalant dependence with inhalant-induced psychotic disorder**
     F18.250   **Inhalant dependence with inhalant-induced psychotic disorder with delusions**
     F18.251   **Inhalant dependence with inhalant-induced psychotic disorder with hallucinations**
     F18.259   **Inhalant dependence with inhalant-induced psychotic disorder, unspecified**

   F18.27   **Inhalant dependence with inhalant-induced dementia**
           Inhalant use disorder, moderate, with inhalant-induced major neurocognitive disorder ◀
           Inhalant use disorder, severe, with inhalant-induced major neurocognitive disorder ◀

● **F18.28**   **Inhalant dependence with other inhalant-induced disorders**
     F18.280   **Inhalant dependence with inhalant-induced anxiety disorder**
     F18.288   **Inhalant dependence with other inhalant-induced disorder**
               Inhalant use disorder, moderate, with inhalant-induced mild neurocognitive disorder ◀
               Inhalant use disorder, severe, with inhalant-induced mild neurocognitive disorder ◀

   F18.29   **Inhalant dependence with unspecified inhalant-induced disorder**

● **F18.9**   **Inhalant use, unspecified**
    Excludes1   inhalant abuse (F18.1-)
               inhalant dependence (F18.2-)

   F18.90   **Inhalant use, unspecified, uncomplicated**

● **F18.92**   **Inhalant use, unspecified with intoxication**
     F18.920   **Inhalant use, unspecified with intoxication, uncomplicated**
     F18.921   **Inhalant use, unspecified with intoxication with delirium**
     F18.929   **Inhalant use, unspecified with intoxication, unspecified**

   F18.94   **Inhalant use, unspecified with inhalant-induced mood disorder**
           Inhalant-induced depressive disorder ◀

● **F18.95**   **Inhalant use, unspecified with inhalant-induced psychotic disorder**
     F18.950   **Inhalant use, unspecified with inhalant-induced psychotic disorder with delusions**
     F18.951   **Inhalant use, unspecified with inhalant-induced psychotic disorder with hallucinations**
     F18.959   **Inhalant use, unspecified with inhalant-induced psychotic disorder, unspecified**

   F18.97   **Inhalant use, unspecified with inhalant-induced persisting dementia**
           Inhalant-induced major neurocognitive disorder ◀

● **F18.98**   **Inhalant use, unspecified with other inhalant-induced disorders**
     F18.980   **Inhalant use, unspecified with inhalant-induced anxiety disorder**
     F18.988   **Inhalant use, unspecified with other inhalant-induced disorder**
               Inhalant-induced mild neurocognitive disorder ◀

   F18.99   **Inhalant use, unspecified with unspecified inhalant-induced disorder**

CHAPTER 5 (F01-F99)

CHAPTER 5 (F01-F99)

● **F19** **Other psychoactive substance related disorders**
    Includes   polysubstance drug use (indiscriminate drug use)

● **F19.1** **Other psychoactive substance abuse**
    Excludes1   other psychoactive substance dependence (F19.2-)
           other psychoactive substance use, unspecified (F19.9-)

     F19.10 **Other psychoactive substance abuse, uncomplicated**
         Other (or unknown) substance use disorder, mild ◄

● **F19.12** **Other psychoactive substance abuse with intoxication**
        F19.120 **Other psychoactive substance abuse with intoxication, uncomplicated**
        F19.121 **Other psychoactive substance abuse with intoxication delirium**
        F19.122 **Other psychoactive substance abuse with intoxication with perceptual disturbances**
        F19.129 **Other psychoactive substance abuse with intoxication, unspecified**

     F19.14 **Other psychoactive substance abuse with psychoactive substance-induced mood disorder**
         Other (or unknown) substance use disorder, mild, with other (or unknown) substance-induced bipolar or related disorder ◄
         Other (or unknown) substance use disorder, mild, with other (or unknown) substance-induced depressive disorder ◄

● **F19.15** **Other psychoactive substance abuse with psychoactive substance-induced psychotic disorder**
        F19.150 **Other psychoactive substance abuse with psychoactive substance-induced psychotic disorder with delusions**
        F19.151 **Other psychoactive substance abuse with psychoactive substance-induced psychotic disorder with hallucinations**
        F19.159 **Other psychoactive substance abuse with psychoactive substance-induced psychotic disorder, unspecified**

     F19.16 **Other psychoactive substance abuse with psychoactive substance-induced persisting amnestic disorder**

     F19.17 **Other psychoactive substance abuse with psychoactive substance-induced persisting dementia**
         Other (or unknown) substance use disorder, mild, with other (or unknown) substance-induced major neurocognitive disorder ◄

● **F19.18** **Other psychoactive substance abuse with other psychoactive substance-induced disorders**
        F19.180 **Other psychoactive substance abuse with psychoactive substance-induced anxiety disorder**
        F19.181 **Other psychoactive substance abuse with psychoactive substance-induced sexual dysfunction**
        F19.182 **Other psychoactive substance abuse with psychoactive substance-induced sleep disorder**
        F19.188 **Other psychoactive substance abuse with other psychoactive substance-induced disorder**
          Other (or unknown) substance use disorder, mild, with other (or unknown) substance-induced mild neurocognitive disorder ◄
          Other (or unknown) substance use disorder, mild, with other (or unknown) substance-induced obsessive-compulsive or related disorder ◄

     F19.19 **Other psychoactive substance abuse with unspecified psychoactive substance-induced disorder**

● **F19.2** **Other psychoactive substance dependence**
    Excludes1   other psychoactive substance abuse (F19.1-)
           other psychoactive substance use, unspecified (F19.9-)

     F19.20 **Other psychoactive substance dependence, uncomplicated**
         Other (or unknown) substance use disorder, moderate ◄
         Other (or unknown) substance use disorder, severe ◄

     F19.21 **Other psychoactive substance dependence, in remission**

● **F19.22** **Other psychoactive substance dependence with intoxication**
    Excludes1   other psychoactive substance dependence with withdrawal (F19.23-)

        F19.220 **Other psychoactive substance dependence with intoxication, uncomplicated**
        F19.221 **Other psychoactive substance dependence with intoxication delirium**
        F19.222 **Other psychoactive substance dependence with intoxication with perceptual disturbance**
        F19.229 **Other psychoactive substance dependence with intoxication, unspecified**

● **F19.23** **Other psychoactive substance dependence with withdrawal**
    Excludes1   other psychoactive substance dependence with intoxication (F19.22-)

        F19.230 **Other psychoactive substance dependence with withdrawal, uncomplicated**
        F19.231 **Other psychoactive substance dependence with withdrawal delirium**

◄ New   ◄▥ Revised   ~~deleted~~ Deleted   Excludes 1   Excludes 2   Includes   Use additional   Code first   Code also   Unspecified
OGCR Official Guidelines   X Assign placeholder X   ● Use Additional Character(s)   ▌ Manifestation Code   **Coding Clinic**

F19.232   Other psychoactive substance dependence with withdrawal with perceptual disturbance

F19.239   Other psychoactive substance dependence with withdrawal, unspecified

F19.24   Other psychoactive substance dependence with psychoactive substance-induced mood disorder

Other (or unknown) substance use disorder, moderate, with other (or unknown) substance-induced bipolar or related disorder ◀

Other (or unknown) substance use disorder, moderate, with other (or unknown) substance-induced depressive disorder ◀

Other (or unknown) substance use disorder, severe, with other (or unknown) substance-induced bipolar or related disorder ◀

Other (or unknown) substance use disorder, severe, with other (or unknown) substance-induced depressive disorder ◀

● **F19.25   Other psychoactive substance dependence with psychoactive substance-induced psychotic disorder**

F19.250   Other psychoactive substance dependence with psychoactive substance-induced psychotic disorder with delusions

F19.251   Other psychoactive substance dependence with psychoactive substance-induced psychotic disorder with hallucinations

F19.259   Other psychoactive substance dependence with psychoactive substance-induced psychotic disorder, unspecified

F19.26   Other psychoactive substance dependence with psychoactive substance-induced persisting amnestic disorder

F19.27   Other psychoactive substance dependence with psychoactive substance-induced persisting dementia

Other (or unknown) substance use disorder, moderate, with other (or unknown) substance-induced major neurocognitive disorder ◀

Other (or unknown) substance use disorder, severe, with other (or unknown) substance-induced major neurocognitive disorder ◀

● **F19.28   Other psychoactive substance dependence with other psychoactive substance-induced disorders**

F19.280   Other psychoactive substance dependence with psychoactive substance-induced anxiety disorder

F19.281   Other psychoactive substance dependence with psychoactive substance-induced sexual dysfunction

F19.282   Other psychoactive substance dependence with psychoactive substance-induced sleep disorder

F19.288   Other psychoactive substance dependence with other psychoactive substance-induced disorder

Other (or unknown) substance use disorder, moderate, with other (or unknown) substance-induced mild neurocognitive disorder ◀

Other (or unknown) substance use disorder, severe, with other (or unknown) substance-induced mild neurocognitive disorder ◀

Other (or unknown) substance use disorder, moderate, with other (or unknown) substance-induced obsessive-compulsive or related disorder ◀

Other (or unknown) substance use disorder, severe, with other (or unknown) substance-induced obsessive-compulsive or related disorder ◀

F19.29   Other psychoactive substance dependence with unspecified psychoactive substance-induced disorder

● **F19.9   Other psychoactive substance use, unspecified**

     Excludes1   other psychoactive substance abuse (F19.1-)
                 other psychoactive substance dependence (F19.2-)

F19.90   Other psychoactive substance use, unspecified, uncomplicated

● **F19.92   Other psychoactive substance use, unspecified with intoxication**

     Excludes1   other psychoactive substance use, unspecified with withdrawal (F19.93)

F19.920   Other psychoactive substance use, unspecified with intoxication, uncomplicated

F19.921   Other psychoactive substance use, unspecified with intoxication with delirium

       Other (or unknown) substance-induced delirium ◀

F19.922   Other psychoactive substance use, unspecified with intoxication with perceptual disturbance

F19.929   Other psychoactive substance use, unspecified with intoxication, unspecified

● **F19.93   Other psychoactive substance use, unspecified with withdrawal**

     Excludes1   other psychoactive substance use, unspecified with intoxication (F19.92-)

F19.930   Other psychoactive substance use, unspecified with withdrawal, uncomplicated

F19.931   Other psychoactive substance use, unspecified with withdrawal delirium

F19.932   Other psychoactive substance use, unspecified with withdrawal with perceptual disturbance

F19.939   Other psychoactive substance use, unspecified with withdrawal, unspecified

CHAPTER 5 (F01-F99)

CHAPTER 5 (FØ1-F99)

F19.94   Other psychoactive substance use, unspecified with psychoactive substance-induced mood disorder
> Other (or unknown) substance-induced bipolar or related disorder, without use disorder ◀
> Other (or unknown) substance-induced depressive disorder, without use disorder ◀

● **F19.95**   Other psychoactive substance use, unspecified with psychoactive substance-induced psychotic disorder

     F19.950   Other psychoactive substance use, unspecified with psychoactive substance-induced psychotic disorder with delusions

     F19.951   Other psychoactive substance use, unspecified with psychoactive substance-induced psychotic disorder with hallucinations

     F19.959   Other psychoactive substance use, unspecified with psychoactive substance-induced psychotic disorder, unspecified
> Other or unknown substance-induced psychotic disorder, without use disorder ◀

F19.96   Other psychoactive substance use, unspecified with psychoactive substance-induced persisting amnestic disorder

F19.97   Other psychoactive substance use, unspecified with psychoactive substance-induced persisting dementia
> Other (or unknown) substance-induced major neurocognitive disorder, without use disorder ◀

● **F19.98**   Other psychoactive substance use, unspecified with other psychoactive substance-induced disorders

     F19.980   Other psychoactive substance use, unspecified with psychoactive substance-induced anxiety disorder
> Other (or unknown) substance-induced anxiety disorder, without use disorder ◀

     F19.981   Other psychoactive substance use, unspecified with psychoactive substance-induced sexual dysfunction
> Other (or unknown) substance-induced sexual dysfunction, without use disorder ◀

     F19.982   Other psychoactive substance use, unspecified with psychoactive substance-induced sleep disorder
> Other (or unknown) substance-induced sleep disorder, without use disorder ◀

     F19.988   Other psychoactive substance use, unspecified with other psychoactive substance-induced disorder
> Other (or unknown) substance-induced mild neurocognitive disorder, without use disorder ◀
> Other (or unknown) substance-induced obsessive-compulsive or related disorder, without use disorder ◀

F19.99   Other psychoactive substance use, unspecified with unspecified psychoactive substance-induced disorder

---

SCHIZOPHRENIA, SCHIZOTYPAL, DELUSIONAL, AND OTHER NON-MOOD PSYCHOTIC DISORDERS (F2Ø-F29)

● **F2Ø**   **Schizophrenia**
Personality disorders characterized by multiple mental and behavioral irregularities (may exhibit disorganized thinking, delusions, and auditory hallucinations)

> **Excludes1**   brief psychotic disorder (F23)
> cyclic schizophrenia (F25.Ø)
> mood [affective] disorders with psychotic symptoms (F3Ø.2, F31.2, F31.5, F31.64, F32.3, F33.3)
> schizoaffective disorder (F25.-)
> schizophrenic reaction NOS (F23)

> **Excludes2**   schizophrenic reaction in:
> alcoholism (F1Ø.15-, F1Ø.25-, F1Ø.95-)
> brain disease (FØ6.2)
> epilepsy (FØ6.2)
> psychoactive drug use (F11-F19 with .15, .25, .95)
> schizotypal disorder (F21)

F2Ø.Ø   **Paranoid schizophrenia**
> Paraphrenic schizophrenia
> **Excludes1**   involutional paranoid state (F22)
> paranoia (F22)

F2Ø.1   **Disorganized schizophrenia**
> Hebephrenic schizophrenia
> Hebephrenia

F2Ø.2   **Catatonic schizophrenia**
> Schizophrenic catalepsy
> Schizophrenic catatonia
> Schizophrenic flexibilitas cerea
> **Excludes1**   catatonic stupor (R4Ø.1)

F2Ø.3   **Undifferentiated schizophrenia**
> Atypical schizophrenia
> **Excludes1**   acute schizophrenia-like psychotic disorder (F23)
> **Excludes2**   post-schizophrenic depression (F32.89) ◀▥

F2Ø.5   **Residual schizophrenia**
> Restzustand (schizophrenic)
> Schizophrenic residual state

● **F2Ø.8**   **Other schizophrenia**

     F2Ø.81   **Schizophreniform disorder**
> Schizophreniform psychosis NOS

     F2Ø.89   **Other schizophrenia**
> Cenesthopathic schizophrenia
> Simple schizophrenia

F2Ø.9   **Schizophrenia, unspecified**

F21   **Schizotypal disorder**
Personality disorder characterized by need for social isolation, odd behavior and thinking, and often unconventional beliefs
> Borderline schizophrenia
> Latent schizophrenia
> Latent schizophrenic reaction
> Prepsychotic schizophrenia
> Prodromal schizophrenia
> Pseudoneurotic schizophrenia
> Pseudopsychopathic schizophrenia
> Schizotypal personality disorder
> **Excludes2**   Asperger's syndrome (F84.5)
> schizoid personality disorder (F6Ø.1)

◀ New   ◀▥ Revised   ~~deleted~~ Deleted   Excludes 1   Excludes 2   Includes   Use additional   Code first   Code also   Unspecified

OGCR Official Guidelines   X Assign placeholder X   ● Use Additional Character(s)   ▶ Manifestation Code   **Coding Clinic**

F22　Delusional disorders
Delusional dysmorphophobia
Involutional paranoid state
Paranoia
Paranoia querulans
Paranoid psychosis
Paranoid state
Paraphrenia (late)
Sensitiver Beziehungswahn

> **Excludes1**　mood [affective] disorders with psychotic
> symptoms (F30.2, F31.2, F31.5, F31.64, F32.3,
> F33.3)
> paranoid schizophrenia (F20.0)
>
> **Excludes2**　paranoid personality disorder (F60.0)
> paranoid psychosis, psychogenic (F23)
> paranoid reaction (F23)

F23　Brief psychotic disorder
Paranoid reaction
Psychogenic paranoid psychosis

> **Excludes2**　mood [affective] disorders with psychotic
> symptoms (F30.2, F31.2, F31.5, F31.64, F32.3,
> F33.3)

F24　Shared psychotic disorder
Folie à deux
Induced paranoid disorder
Induced psychotic disorder

● **F25　Schizoaffective disorders**
*Mental disorder exhibiting major depressive episode, manic episode,
or mixed episode occurs with symptoms of schizophrenia, and
mood disorder*

> **Excludes1**　mood [affective] disorders with psychotic
> symptoms (F30.2, F31.2, F31.5, F31.64, F32.3,
> F33.3)
> schizophrenia (F20.-)

　F25.0　Schizoaffective disorder, bipolar type
Cyclic schizophrenia
Schizoaffective disorder, manic type
Schizoaffective disorder, mixed type
Schizoaffective psychosis, bipolar type
Schizophreniform psychosis, manic type

　F25.1　Schizoaffective disorder, depressive type
Schizoaffective psychosis, depressive type
Schizophreniform psychosis, depressive type

　F25.8　Other schizoaffective disorders

　F25.9　Schizoaffective disorder, unspecified
Schizoaffective psychosis NOS

**F28　Other psychotic disorder not due to a substance or known
physiological condition**
Chronic hallucinatory psychosis

**F29　Unspecified psychosis not due to a substance or known
physiological condition**
Psychosis NOS

> **Excludes1**　mental disorder NOS (F99)
> unspecified mental disorder due to known
> physiological condition (F09)

MOOD [AFFECTIVE] DISORDERS (F30-F39)

● **F30　Manic episode**
Elevated, expansive, or irritable mood

> **Includes**　bipolar disorder, single manic episode
> mixed affective episode
>
> **Excludes1**　bipolar disorder (F31.-)
> major depressive disorder, single episode (F32.-)
> major depressive disorder, recurrent (F33.-)

● **F30.1　Manic episode without psychotic symptoms**

　**F30.10　Manic episode without psychotic
symptoms, unspecified**

　**F30.11　Manic episode without psychotic symptoms,
mild**

　**F30.12　Manic episode without psychotic symptoms,
moderate**

　**F30.13　Manic episode, severe, without psychotic
symptoms**

F30.2　Manic episode, severe with psychotic symptoms
Manic stupor
Mania with mood-congruent psychotic symptoms
Mania with mood-incongruent psychotic symptoms

F30.3　Manic episode in partial remission

F30.4　Manic episode in full remission

F30.8　Other manic episodes
Abnormality of mood resembling mania but less intense
Hypomania

F30.9　Manic episode, unspecified
Mania NOS

● **F31　Bipolar disorder**
Mood disorders with history of manic, mixed, or hypomanic episodes

> **Includes**　manic-depressive illness
> manic-depressive psychosis
> manic-depressive reaction
>
> **Excludes1**　bipolar disorder, single manic episode (F30.-)
> major depressive disorder, single episode (F32.-)
> major depressive disorder, recurrent (F33.-)
>
> **Excludes2**　cyclothymia (F34.0)

F31.0　Bipolar disorder, current episode hypomanic

● **F31.1　Bipolar disorder, current episode manic without
psychotic features**

　**F31.10　Bipolar disorder, current episode manic without
psychotic features, unspecified**

　**F31.11　Bipolar disorder, current episode manic without
psychotic features, mild**

　**F31.12　Bipolar disorder, current episode manic without
psychotic features, moderate**

　**F31.13　Bipolar disorder, current episode manic without
psychotic features, severe**

**F31.2　Bipolar disorder, current episode manic severe with
psychotic features**
Bipolar disorder, current episode manic with mood-
congruent psychotic symptoms
Bipolar disorder, current episode manic with mood-
incongruent psychotic symptoms

● **F31.3　Bipolar disorder, current episode depressed, mild or
moderate severity**

　**F31.30　Bipolar disorder, current episode depressed,
mild or moderate severity, unspecified**

　**F31.31　Bipolar disorder, current episode depressed,
mild**

　**F31.32　Bipolar disorder, current episode depressed,
moderate**

**F31.4　Bipolar disorder, current episode depressed, severe,
without psychotic features**

**F31.5　Bipolar disorder, current episode depressed, severe, with
psychotic features**
Bipolar disorder, current episode depressed with mood-
incongruent psychotic symptoms
Bipolar disorder, current episode depressed with mood-
congruent psychotic symptoms

● **F31.6　Bipolar disorder, current episode mixed**

　**F31.60　Bipolar disorder, current episode
mixed, unspecified**

　F31.61　Bipolar disorder, current episode mixed, mild

　**F31.62　Bipolar disorder, current episode mixed,
moderate**

　**F31.63　Bipolar disorder, current episode mixed, severe,
without psychotic features**

　**F31.64　Bipolar disorder, current episode mixed, severe,
with psychotic features**
Bipolar disorder, current episode mixed with
mood-congruent psychotic symptoms
Bipolar disorder, current episode mixed with
mood-incongruent psychotic symptoms

CHAPTER 5 (F01-F99)

● **F31.7**   **Bipolar disorder, currently in remission**

     F31.70   Bipolar disorder, currently in remission, most recent episode unspecified

     F31.71   Bipolar disorder, in partial remission, most recent episode hypomanic

     F31.72   Bipolar disorder, in full remission, most recent episode hypomanic

     F31.73   Bipolar disorder, in partial remission, most recent episode manic

     F31.74   Bipolar disorder, in full remission, most recent episode manic

     F31.75   Bipolar disorder, in partial remission, most recent episode depressed

     F31.76   Bipolar disorder, in full remission, most recent episode depressed

     F31.77   Bipolar disorder, in partial remission, most recent episode mixed

     F31.78   Bipolar disorder, in full remission, most recent episode mixed

● **F31.8**   **Other bipolar disorders**

     F31.81   **Bipolar II disorder**

     F31.89   **Other bipolar disorder**
           Recurrent manic episodes NOS

   F31.9   **Bipolar disorder, unspecified**

● **F32**   **Major depressive disorder, single episode**

   Includes   single episode of agitated depression
           single episode of depressive reaction
           single episode of major depression
           single episode of psychogenic depression
           single episode of reactive depression
           single episode of vital depression

   Excludes1   bipolar disorder (F31.-)
           manic episode (F30.-)
           recurrent depressive disorder (F33.-)

   Excludes2   adjustment disorder (F43.2)

   F32.0   **Major depressive disorder, single episode, mild**

   F32.1   **Major depressive disorder, single episode, moderate**

   F32.2   **Major depressive disorder, single episode, severe without psychotic features**

   F32.3   **Major depressive disorder, single episode, severe with psychotic features**
         Single episode of major depression with mood-congruent psychotic symptoms
         Single episode of major depression with mood-incongruent psychotic symptoms
         Single episode of major depression with psychotic symptoms
         Single episode of psychogenic depressive psychosis
         Single episode of psychotic depression
         Single episode of reactive depressive psychosis

   F32.4   **Major depressive disorder, single episode, in partial remission**

   F32.5   **Major depressive disorder, single episode, in full remission**

● **F32.8**   **Other depressive episodes**

     F32.81   **Premenstrual dysphoric disorder** ♀ ◀

         Excludes1   premenstrual tension syndrome (N94.3) ◀

     F32.89   **Other specified depressive episodes** ◀
         Atypical depression ◀
         Post-schizophrenic depression ◀
         Single episode of 'masked' depression NOS ◀

   F32.9   **Major depressive disorder, single episode, unspecified**
       Depression NOS
       Depressive disorder NOS
       Major depression NOS

Figure 5-1   PET scan of depressed individual's brain before and after recovery. (From Fortinash KM: Psychiatric Mental Health Nursing, ed 4, St. Louis, Mosby, 2008)

● **F33**   **Major depressive disorder, recurrent**

   Includes   recurrent episodes of depressive reaction
           recurrent episodes of endogenous depression
           recurrent episodes of major depression
           recurrent episodes of psychogenic depression
           recurrent episodes of reactive depression
           recurrent episodes of seasonal depressive disorder
           recurrent episodes of vital depression

   Excludes1   bipolar disorder (F31.-)
           manic episode (F30.-)

   F33.0   **Major depressive disorder, recurrent, mild**

   F33.1   **Major depressive disorder, recurrent, moderate**

   F33.2   **Major depressive disorder, recurrent severe without psychotic features**

   F33.3   **Major depressive disorder, recurrent, severe with psychotic symptoms**
         Endogenous depression with psychotic symptoms
         Recurrent severe episodes of major depression with mood-congruent psychotic symptoms
         Recurrent severe episodes of major depression with mood-incongruent psychotic symptoms
         Recurrent severe episodes of major depression with psychotic symptoms
         Recurrent severe episodes of psychogenic depressive psychosis
         Recurrent severe episodes of psychotic depression
         Recurrent severe episodes of reactive depressive psychosis

● **F33.4**   **Major depressive disorder, recurrent, in remission**

     F33.40   **Major depressive disorder, recurrent, in remission, unspecified**

     F33.41   **Major depressive disorder, recurrent, in partial remission**

     F33.42   **Major depressive disorder, recurrent, in full remission**

   F33.8   **Other recurrent depressive disorders**
       Recurrent brief depressive episodes

   F33.9   **Major depressive disorder, recurrent, unspecified**
       Monopolar depression NOS

◀ New   ◀▥ Revised   ~~deleted~~ Deleted   Excludes 1   Excludes 2   Includes   Use additional   Code first   Code also   Unspecified

762   **OGCR** Official Guidelines   X Assign placeholder X   ● Use Additional Character(s)   ▶ Manifestation Code   **Coding Clinic**

● **F34** **Persistent mood [affective] disorders**

    F34.0 **Cyclothymic disorder**
        Affective personality disorder
        Cycloid personality
        Cyclothymia
        Cyclothymic personality

    F34.1 **Dysthymic disorder**
        Depressive neurosis
        Depressive personality disorder
        Dysthymia
        Neurotic depression
        Persistent anxiety depression
        Persistent depressive disorder ◄

        Excludes2   anxiety depression (mild or not persistent) (F41.8)

    F34.8 **Other persistent mood [affective] disorders**
        F34.81 **Disruptive mood dysregulation disorder** ◄
        F34.89 **Other specified persistent mood disorders** ◄
    F34.9 **Persistent mood [affective] disorder, unspecified**

F39 **Unspecified mood [affective] disorder**
    Affective psychosis NOS

ANXIETY, DISSOCIATIVE, STRESS-RELATED, SOMATOFORM AND OTHER NONPSYCHOTIC MENTAL DISORDERS (F40-F48)

● **F40** **Phobic anxiety disorders**
    Irrational fear with avoidance of the feared subject, activity, or situation even though the individual knows that the reaction is excessive

● **F40.0** **Agoraphobia**
    Intense, irrational fear of open spaces

    F40.00 **Agoraphobia, unspecified**

    F40.01 **Agoraphobia with panic disorder**
        Panic disorder with agoraphobia

        Excludes1   panic disorder without agoraphobia (F41.0)

    F40.02 **Agoraphobia without panic disorder**

● **F40.1** **Social phobias**
    Anthropophobia
    Social anxiety disorder of childhood
    Social neurosis

    F40.10 **Social phobia, unspecified**
    F40.11 **Social phobia, generalized**

● **F40.2** **Specific (isolated) phobias**
        Excludes2   dysmorphophobia (nondelusional) (F45.22)
                  nosophobia (F45.22)

  ● **F40.21** **Animal type phobia**
        F40.210 **Arachnophobia**
            Fear of spiders
        F40.218 **Other animal type phobia**

  ● **F40.22** **Natural environment type phobia**
        F40.220 **Fear of thunderstorms**
        F40.228 **Other natural environment type phobia**

  ● **F40.23** **Blood, injection, injury type phobia**
        F40.230 **Fear of blood**
        F40.231 **Fear of injections and transfusions**
        F40.232 **Fear of other medical care**
        F40.233 **Fear of injury**

  ● **F40.24** **Situational type phobia**
        F40.240 **Claustrophobia**
            Fear of closed spaces
        F40.241 **Acrophobia**
            Fear of heights
        F40.242 **Fear of bridges**
        F40.243 **Fear of flying**
        F40.248 **Other situational type phobia**

  ● **F40.29** **Other specified phobia**
        F40.290 **Androphobia**
            Fear of men
        F40.291 **Gynephobia**
            Fear of women
        F40.298 **Other specified phobia**

    F40.8 **Other phobic anxiety disorders**
        Phobic anxiety disorder of childhood

    F40.9 **Phobic anxiety disorder, unspecified**
        Phobia NOS
        Phobic state NOS

● **F41** **Other anxiety disorders**
        Excludes2   anxiety in:
                acute stress reaction (F43.0)
                transient adjustment reaction (F43.2)
                neurasthenia (F48.8)
                psychophysiologic disorders (F45.-)
                separation anxiety (F93.0)

    F41.0 **Panic disorder [episodic paroxysmal anxiety] without agoraphobia**
        Panic attack
        Panic state

        Excludes1   panic disorder with agoraphobia (F40.01)

    F41.1 **Generalized anxiety disorder**
        Anxiety neurosis
        Anxiety reaction
        Anxiety state
        Overanxious disorder

        Excludes2   neurasthenia (F48.8)

    F41.3 **Other mixed anxiety disorders**

    F41.8 **Other specified anxiety disorders**
        Anxiety depression (mild or not persistent)
        Anxiety hysteria
        Mixed anxiety and depressive disorder

    F41.9 **Anxiety disorder, unspecified**
        Anxiety NOS

● **F42** **Obsessive-compulsive disorder**
    Anxiety disorder with recurrent obsessions or compulsions
        Excludes2   obsessive-compulsive personality (disorder) (F60.5)
                obsessive-compulsive symptoms occurring in depression (F32-F33)
                obsessive-compulsive symptoms occurring in schizophrenia (F20.-)

    F42.2 **Mixed obsessional thoughts and acts** ◄
    F42.3 **Hoarding disorder** ◄
    F42.4 **Excoriation (skin-picking) disorder** ◄
        Excludes1   factitial dermatitis (L98.1) ◄
                other specified behavioral and emotional disorders with onset usually occurring in early childhood and adolescence (F98.8) ◄

    F42.8 **Other obsessive-compulsive disorder** ◄
        Anancastic neurosis ◄
        Obsessive-compulsive neurosis ◄

    F42.9 **Obsessive-compulsive disorder, unspecified** ◄

● **F43** **Reaction to severe stress and adjustment disorders**

    F43.0 **Acute stress reaction**
        Acute crisis reaction
        Acute reaction to stress
        Combat and operational stress reaction
        Combat fatigue
        Crisis state
        Psychic shock

  ● **F43.1** **Post-traumatic stress disorder (PTSD)**
        Traumatic neurosis
        F43.10 **Post-traumatic stress disorder, unspecified**
        F43.11 **Post-traumatic stress disorder, acute**
        F43.12 **Post-traumatic stress disorder, chronic**

● **F43.2 Adjustment disorders**
    Culture shock
    Grief reaction
    Hospitalism in children
    Excludes2   separation anxiety disorder of childhood
        (F93.0)

    F43.20 Adjustment disorder, unspecified

    F43.21 Adjustment disorder with depressed mood

    F43.22 Adjustment disorder with anxiety

    F43.23 Adjustment disorder with mixed anxiety and depressed mood

    F43.24 Adjustment disorder with disturbance of conduct

    F43.25 Adjustment disorder with mixed disturbance of emotions and conduct

    F43.29 Adjustment disorder with other symptoms

F43.8 Other reactions to severe stress
    Other specified trauma and stressor-related disorder ◄

F43.9 Reaction to severe stress, unspecified
    Trauma and stressor-related disorder, NOS ◄

● **F44 Dissociative and conversion disorders**
    Includes   conversion hysteria
         conversion reaction
         hysteria
         hysterical psychosis
    Excludes2   malingering [conscious simulation] (Z76.5)

F44.0 Dissociative amnesia
    Sudden loss of memory for personal information
    Excludes1   amnesia NOS (R41.3)
         anterograde amnesia (R41.1)
         dissociative amnesia with dissociative
          fugue (F44.1) ◄
         retrograde amnesia (R41.2)
    Excludes2   alcohol-or other psychoactive substance-
          induced amnestic disorder (F10, F13,
          F19 with .26, .96)
         amnestic disorder due to known
          physiological condition (F04)
         postictal amnesia in epilepsy (G40.-)

F44.1 Dissociative fugue
    Characterized by episode of sudden, unexpected travel with amnesia for past and partial to total confusion about identity or assumption of new identity
    Dissociative amnesia with dissociative fugue ◄
    Excludes2   postictal fugue in epilepsy (G40.-)

F44.2 Dissociative stupor
    Profound diminution or absence of voluntary movement and responsiveness to external stimuli
    Excludes1   catatonic stupor (R40.1)
         stupor NOS (R40.1)
    Excludes2   catatonic disorder due to known
          physiological condition (F06.1)
         depressive stupor (F32, F33)
         manic stupor (F30, F31)

F44.4 Conversion disorder with motor symptom or deficit
    Dissociative motor disorders
    Psychogenic aphonia
    Psychogenic dysphonia

F44.5 Conversion disorder with seizures or convulsions
    Dissociative convulsions

F44.6 Conversion disorder with sensory symptom or deficit
    Dissociative anesthesia and sensory loss
    Psychogenic deafness

F44.7 Conversion disorder with mixed symptom presentation

● **F44.8 Other dissociative and conversion disorders**
    F44.81 Dissociative identity disorder
         Multiple personality disorder

    F44.89 Other dissociative and conversion disorders
         Ganser's syndrome
         Psychogenic confusion
         Psychogenic twilight state
         Trance and possession disorders

F44.9 Dissociative and conversion disorder, unspecified
    Dissociative disorder NOS

OGCR Section I.C.5.a

Pain disorders related to psychological factors

Assign code F45.41, for pain that is exclusively psychological. Code F45.41, Pain disorder exclusively related to psychological factors, should be used following the appropriate code from category G89, Pain, not elsewhere classified, if there is documentation of a psychological component for a patient with acute or chronic pain.
See Section I.C.6. Pain

● **F45 Somatoform disorders**
    Mental disorders characterized by symptoms suggesting general medical condition
    Excludes2   dissociative and conversion disorders (F44.-)
         factitious disorders (F68.1-)
         hair-plucking (F63.3)
         lalling (F80.0)
         lisping (F80.0)
         malingering [conscious simulation] (Z76.5)
         nail-biting (F98.8)
         psychological or behavioral factors associated
          with disorders or diseases classified
          elsewhere (F54)
         sexual dysfunction, not due to a substance or
          known physiological condition (F52.-)
         thumb-sucking (F98.8)
         tic disorders (in childhood and adolescence) (F95.-)
         Tourette's syndrome (F95.2)
         trichotillomania (F63.3)

F45.0 Somatization disorder
    Briquet's disorder
    Multiple psychosomatic disorder

F45.1 Undifferentiated somatoform disorder
    Somatic symptom disorder ◄
    Undifferentiated psychosomatic disorder

● **F45.2 Hypochondriacal disorders**
    Persistent, unrealistic preoccupation with possibility of having serious disease
    Excludes2   delusional dysmorphophobia (F22)
         fixed delusions about bodily functions or
          shape (F22)

    F45.20 Hypochondriacal disorder, unspecified

    F45.21 Hypochondriasis
         Hypochondriacal neurosis
         Illness anxiety disorder ◄

    F45.22 Body dysmorphic disorder
         Dysmorphophobia (nondelusional)
         Nosophobia

    F45.29 Other hypochondriacal disorders

● **F45.4 Pain disorders related to psychological factors**
    Excludes1   pain NOS (R52)

    F45.41 Pain disorder exclusively related to psychological factors
         Somatoform pain disorder (persistent)

    F45.42 Pain disorder with related psychological factors
         Code also associated acute or chronic pain
          (G89.-)

F45.8   **Other somatoform disorders**
Psychogenic dysmenorrhea
Psychogenic dysphagia, including 'globus hystericus'
Psychogenic pruritus
Psychogenic torticollis
Somatoform autonomic dysfunction
Teeth grinding
> **Excludes1**   sleep related teeth grinding (G47.63)

F45.9   **Somatoform disorder, unspecified**
Psychosomatic disorder NOS

● **F48**   **Other nonpsychotic mental disorders**

F48.1   **Depersonalization-derealization syndrome**

F48.2   **Pseudobulbar affect**
Involuntary emotional expression disorder
Code first underlying cause, if known, such as:
    amyotrophic lateral sclerosis (G12.21)
    multiple sclerosis (G35)
    sequelae of cerebrovascular disease (I69.-)
    sequelae of traumatic intracranial injury (S06.-)

F48.8   **Other specified nonpsychotic mental disorders**
Dhat syndrome
Neurasthenia
Occupational neurosis, including writer's cramp
Psychasthenia
Psychasthenic neurosis
Psychogenic syncope

F48.9   **Nonpsychotic mental disorder, unspecified**
Neurosis NOS

BEHAVIORAL SYNDROMES ASSOCIATED WITH PHYSIOLOGICAL DISTURBANCES AND PHYSICAL FACTORS (F50-F59)

● **F50**   **Eating disorders**
> **Excludes1**   anorexia NOS (R63.0)
>   feeding difficulties (R63.3)
>   polyphagia (R63.2)
> **Excludes2**   feeding disorder in infancy or childhood (F98.2-)

● **F50.0**   **Anorexia nervosa**
> **Excludes1**   loss of appetite (R63.0)
>   psychogenic loss of appetite (F50.89) ◀──

   F50.00   **Anorexia nervosa, unspecified**

   F50.01   **Anorexia nervosa, restricting type**

   F50.02   **Anorexia nervosa, binge eating/purging type**
> **Excludes1**   bulimia nervosa (F50.2)

F50.2   **Bulimia nervosa**
Bulimia NOS
Hyperorexia nervosa
> **Excludes1**   anorexia nervosa, binge eating/purging type (F50.02)

● **F50.8**   **Other eating disorders**
> **Excludes2**   pica of infancy and childhood (F98.3)

   F50.81   **Binge eating disorder** ◀

   F50.89   **Other specified eating disorder** ◀
     Pica in adults ◀
     Psychogenic loss of appetite ◀

F50.9   **Eating disorder, unspecified**
Atypical anorexia nervosa
Atypical bulimia nervosa

● **F51**   **Sleep disorders not due to a substance or known physiological condition**
> **Excludes2**   organic sleep disorders (G47.-)

● **F51.0**   **Insomnia not due to a substance or known physiological condition**
> **Excludes2**   alcohol related insomnia (F10.182, F10.282, F10.982)
>   drug-related insomnia (F11.182, F11.282, F11.982, F13.182, F13.282, F13.982, F14.182, F14.282, F14.982, F15.182, F15.282, F15.982, F19.182, F19.282, F19.982)
>   insomnia NOS (G47.0-)
>   insomnia due to known physiological condition (G47.0-)
>   organic insomnia (G47.0-)
>   sleep deprivation (Z72.820)

   F51.01   **Primary insomnia**
     Idiopathic insomnia

   F51.02   **Adjustment insomnia**

   F51.03   **Paradoxical insomnia**

   F51.04   **Psychophysiologic insomnia**

   F51.05   **Insomnia due to other mental disorder**
     Code also associated mental disorder

   F51.09   **Other insomnia not due to a substance or known physiological condition**

● **F51.1**   **Hypersomnia not due to a substance or known physiological condition**
Hypersomnia: Excessive sleeping/sleepiness
> **Excludes2**   alcohol related hypersomnia (F10.182, F10.282, F10.982)
>   drug-related hypersomnia (F11.182, F11.282, F11.982, F13.182, F13.282, F13.982, F14.182, F14.282, F14.982, F15.182, F15.282, F15.982, F19.182, F19.282, F19.982)
>   hypersomnia NOS (G47.10)
>   hypersomnia due to known physiological condition (G47.10)
>   idiopathic hypersomnia (G47.11, G47.12)
>   narcolepsy (G47.4-)

   F51.11   **Primary hypersomnia**

   F51.12   **Insufficient sleep syndrome**
> **Excludes1**   sleep deprivation (Z72.820)

   F51.13   **Hypersomnia due to other mental disorder**
     Code also associated mental disorder

   F51.19   **Other hypersomnia not due to a substance or known physiological condition**

F51.3   **Sleepwalking [somnambulism]**

F51.4   **Sleep terrors [night terrors]**

F51.5   **Nightmare disorder**
Dream anxiety disorder

F51.8   **Other sleep disorders not due to a substance or known physiological condition**

F51.9   **Sleep disorder not due to a substance or known physiological condition, unspecified**
Emotional sleep disorder NOS

CHAPTER 5 (F01-F99)

CHAPTER 5 (F01-F99)

● **F52** **Sexual dysfunction not due to a substance or known physiological condition**
> **Excludes2**   Dhat syndrome (F48.8)

F52.0 **Hypoactive sexual desire disorder**
Total loss of feeling of sexual pleasure
Lack or loss of sexual desire
Sexual anhedonia ◄
> **Excludes1**   decreased libido (R68.82)

F52.1 **Sexual aversion disorder**
Sexual aversion and lack of sexual enjoyment

● **F52.2** **Sexual arousal disorders**
Failure of genital response

    F52.21 **Male erectile disorder** ♂
    Psychogenic impotence
>   **Excludes1**   impotence of organic origin (N52.-)
>   impotence NOS (N52.-)

    F52.22 **Female sexual arousal disorder** ♀
    ~~Frigidity~~

● **F52.3** **Orgasmic disorder**
Inhibited orgasm
Psychogenic anorgasmy

    F52.31 **Female orgasmic disorder** ♀

    F52.32 **Male orgasmic disorder** ♂
    Delayed ejaculation ◄

F52.4 **Premature ejaculation** ♂

F52.5 **Vaginismus not due to a substance or known physiological condition** ♀
Psychogenic vaginismus
> **Excludes2**   vaginismus (due to a known physiological condition) (N94.2)

F52.6 **Dyspareunia not due to a substance or known physiological condition** ♀
Dyspareunia: Difficult or painful sexual intercourse
Genito-pelvic pain penetration disorder ◄
Psychogenic dyspareunia
> **Excludes2**   dyspareunia (due to a known physiological condition) (N94.1-) ◄▦

F52.8 **Other sexual dysfunction not due to a substance or known physiological condition**
Excessive sexual drive
Nymphomania
Satyriasis

F52.9 **Unspecified sexual dysfunction not due to a substance or known physiological condition**
Sexual dysfunction NOS

F53 **Puerperal psychosis** ♀   **M**
Postpartum depression
Acute mental illness with sudden onset following childbirth with symptoms of affective psychosis, disorientation, and confusion are prevalent
> **Excludes1**   mood disorders with psychotic features (F30.2, F31.2, F31.5, F31.64, F32.3, F33.3)
>   postpartum dysphoria (O90.6)
>   psychosis in schizophrenia, schizotypal, delusional, and other psychotic disorders (F20-F29)

▶ **F54** *Psychological and behavioral factors associated with disorders or diseases classified elsewhere*
Psychological factors affecting physical conditions
Code first the associated physical disorder, such as:
asthma (J45.-)
dermatitis (L23-L25)
gastric ulcer (K25.-)
mucous colitis (K58.-)
ulcerative colitis (K51.-)
urticaria (L50.-)
> **Excludes2**   tension-type headache (G44.2)

● **F55** **Abuse of non-psychoactive substances**
> **Excludes2**   abuse of psychoactive substances (F10-F19)

F55.0 **Abuse of antacids**

F55.1 **Abuse of herbal or folk remedies**

F55.2 **Abuse of laxatives**

F55.3 **Abuse of steroids or hormones**

F55.4 **Abuse of vitamins**

F55.8 **Abuse of other non-psychoactive substances**

F59 **Unspecified behavioral syndromes associated with physiological disturbances and physical factors**
Psychogenic physiological dysfunction NOS

DISORDERS OF ADULT PERSONALITY AND BEHAVIOR (F60-F69)

● **F60** **Specific personality disorders**
Long-term patterns of thoughts and behaviors causing serious problems with relationships and work.

F60.0 **Paranoid personality disorder**
Hostile, devious, and combative response to disappointments
Expansive paranoid personality (disorder)
Fanatic personality (disorder)
Querulant personality (disorder)
Paranoid personality (disorder)
Sensitive paranoid personality (disorder)
> **Excludes2**   paranoia (F22)
>   paranoia querulans (F22)
>   paranoid psychosis (F22)
>   paranoid schizophrenia (F20.0)
>   paranoid state (F22)

F60.1 **Schizoid personality disorder**
Detachment from social relationships with minimal emotional experiences and expressions
> **Excludes2**   Asperger's syndrome (F84.5)
>   delusional disorder (F22)
>   schizoid disorder of childhood (F84.5)
>   schizophrenia (F20.-)
>   schizotypal disorder (F21)

F60.2 **Antisocial personality disorder**
Continuous and chronic antisocial behavior
Amoral personality (disorder)
Asocial personality (disorder)
Dissocial personality disorder
Psychopathic personality (disorder)
Sociopathic personality (disorder)
> **Excludes1**   conduct disorders (F91.-)
> **Excludes2**   borderline personality disorder (F60.3)

F60.3 **Borderline personality disorder**
Instability of mood, self-image or sense of self, and interpersonal relationships
Aggressive personality (disorder)
Emotionally unstable personality disorder
Explosive personality (disorder)
> **Excludes2**   antisocial personality disorder (F60.2)

F60.4 **Histrionic personality disorder**
Personality disorder with excessive emotional and attention-seeking behavior
Hysterical personality (disorder)
Psychoinfantile personality (disorder)

F60.5 **Obsessive-compulsive personality disorder**
Anankastic personality (disorder)
Compulsive personality (disorder)
Obsessional personality (disorder)
> **Excludes2**   obsessive-compulsive disorder (F42-) ◄▦

F60.6 **Avoidant personality disorder**
Anxious personality disorder

F60.7 **Dependent personality disorder**
Asthenic personality (disorder)
Inadequate personality (disorder)
Passive personality (disorder)

◄ New   ◄▦ Revised   ~~deleted~~ Deleted   Excludes 1   Excludes 2   Includes   Use additional   Code first   Code also   Unspecified

766   OGCR Official Guidelines   X Assign placeholder X   ● Use Additional Character(s)   ▶ Manifestation Code   **Coding Clinic**

- **F60.8** **Other specific personality disorders**
  - **F60.81** **Narcissistic personality disorder**
    Vanity, conceit, egotism or indifference to plight of others
  - **F60.89** **Other specific personality disorders**
    Eccentric personality disorder
    'Haltlose' type personality disorder
    Immature personality disorder
    Passive-aggressive personality disorder
    Psychoneurotic personality disorder
    Self-defeating personality disorder
  - **F60.9** **Personality disorder, unspecified**
    Character disorder NOS
    Character neurosis NOS
    Pathological personality NOS
- **F63** **Impulse disorders**
  - **Excludes2** habitual excessive use of alcohol or psychoactive substances (F10-F19)
    impulse disorders involving sexual behavior (F65.-)
  - **F63.0** **Pathological gambling**
    Compulsive gambling
    - **Excludes1** gambling and betting NOS (Z72.6)
    - **Excludes2** excessive gambling by manic patients (F30, F31)
      gambling in antisocial personality disorder (F60.2)
  - **F63.1** **Pyromania**
    Pathological fire-setting
    - **Excludes2** fire-setting (by) (in):
      adult with antisocial personality disorder (F60.2)
      alcohol or psychoactive substance intoxication (F10-F19)
      conduct disorders (F91.-)
      mental disorders due to known physiological condition (F01-F09)
      schizophrenia (F20.-)
  - **F63.2** **Kleptomania**
    Pathological stealing
    - **Excludes1** shoplifting as the reason for observation for suspected mental disorder (Z03.8)
    - **Excludes2** depressive disorder with stealing (F31-F33)
      stealing due to underlying mental condition-code to mental condition
      stealing in mental disorders due to known physiological condition (F01-F09)
  - **F63.3** **Trichotillomania**
    Hair plucking
    - **Excludes2** other stereotyped movement disorder (F98.4)
- **F63.8** **Other impulse disorders**
  - **F63.81** **Intermittent explosive disorder**
  - **F63.89** **Other impulse disorders**
  - **F63.9** **Impulse disorder, unspecified**
    Impulse control disorder NOS
- **F64** **Gender identity disorders**
  - **F64.0** **Transsexualism** ◀
    Gender identity disorder in adolescence and adulthood ◀
    Gender dysphoria in adolescents and adults ◀
  - **F64.1** **Dual role transvestism** ◀
    Use additional code to identify sex reassignment status (Z87.890)
    - **Excludes1** gender identity disorder in childhood (F64.2)
    - **Excludes2** fetishistic transvestism (F65.1)

- **F64.2** **Gender identity disorder of childhood**   P
  Gender dysphoria in children ◀
  - **Excludes1** gender identity disorder in adolescence and adulthood (F64.0) ◀
  - **Excludes2** sexual maturation disorder (F66)
- **F64.8** **Other gender identity disorders**
- **F64.9** **Gender identity disorder, unspecified**
  Gender-role disorder NOS
- **F65** **Paraphilias**
  - **F65.0** **Fetishism**
    Intense sexual urges and arousing fantasies using inanimate objects
  - **F65.1** **Transvestic fetishism**
    Intense sexual urges, arousal, or orgasm associated with fantasized/actual cross-dressing
    Fetishistic transvestism
  - **F65.2** **Exhibitionism**
  - **F65.3** **Voyeurism**
    Sexual urges or arousal involving real or fantasized observation of unsuspecting people who are naked, disrobing, or engaging in sexual activity
  - **F65.4** **Pedophilia**
- **F65.5** **Sadomasochism**
  - **F65.50** **Sadomasochism, unspecified**
  - **F65.51** **Sexual masochism**
  - **F65.52** **Sexual sadism**
- **F65.8** **Other paraphilias**
  - **F65.81** **Frotteurism**
    Sexual arousal or orgasm is achieved by rubbing up against another person (or fantasies of), in crowded place with unsuspecting victim
  - **F65.89** **Other paraphilias**
    Necrophilia
  - **F65.9** **Paraphilia, unspecified**
    Sexual deviation NOS
- **F66** **Other sexual disorders**
  Sexual maturation disorder
  Sexual relationship disorder
- **F68** **Other disorders of adult personality and behavior**
  - **F68.1** **Factitious disorder**
    Compensation neurosis
    Elaboration of physical symptoms for psychological reasons
    Hospital hopper syndrome
    Münchhausen's syndrome
    Peregrinating patient
    - **Excludes2** factitial dermatitis (L98.1)
      person feigning illness (with obvious motivation) (Z76.5)
    - **F68.10** **Factitious disorder, unspecified**
    - **F68.11** **Factitious disorder with predominantly psychological signs and symptoms**
    - **F68.12** **Factitious disorder with predominantly physical signs and symptoms**
    - **F68.13** **Factitious disorder with combined psychological and physical signs and symptoms**
  - **F68.8** **Other specified disorders of adult personality and behavior**
- **F69** **Unspecified disorder of adult personality and behavior**   A

CHAPTER 5 (F01-F99)

INTELLECTUAL DISABILITIES (F70-F79)

Code first any associated physical or developmental disorders

> **Excludes1**   borderline intellectual functioning, IQ above 70 to 84 (R41.83)

F70   **Mild intellectual disabilities**
IQ level 50-55 to approximately 70
Mild mental subnormality

F71   **Moderate intellectual disabilities**
IQ level 35-40 to 50-55
Moderate mental subnormality

F72   **Severe intellectual disabilities**
IQ 20-25 to 35-40
Severe mental subnormality

F73   **Profound intellectual disabilities**
IQ level below 20-25
Profound mental subnormality

F78   **Other intellectual disabilities**

F79   **Unspecified intellectual disabilities**
Mental deficiency NOS
Mental subnormality NOS

PERVASIVE AND SPECIFIC DEVELOPMENTAL DISORDERS (F80-F89)

● **F80**   **Specific developmental disorders of speech and language**

    F80.0   **Phonological disorder**
Communication disorder of unknown cause, characterized by failure to use age-appropriate sounds
Dyslalia
Functional speech articulation disorder
Lalling
Lisping
Phonological developmental disorder
Speech articulation developmental disorder
Speech-sound disorder ◀

> **Excludes1**   speech articulation impairment due to aphasia NOS (R47.01)
> speech articulation impairment due to apraxia (R48.2)

> **Excludes2**   speech articulation impairment due to hearing loss (F80.4)
> speech articulation impairment due to intellectual disabilities (F70-F79)
> speech articulation impairment with expressive language developmental disorder (F80.1)
> speech articulation impairment with mixed receptive expressive language developmental disorder (F80.2)

    F80.1   **Expressive language disorder**
Developmental dysphasia or aphasia, expressive type

> **Excludes1**   mixed receptive-expressive language disorder (F80.2)
> dysphasia and aphasia NOS (R47.-)

> **Excludes2**   acquired aphasia with epilepsy [Landau-Kleffner] (G40.80-)
> intellectual disabilities (F70-F79)
> pervasive developmental disorders (F84.-)
> selective mutism (F94.0)

    F80.2   **Mixed receptive-expressive language disorder**
Developmental dysphasia or aphasia, receptive type
Developmental Wernicke's aphasia

> **Excludes1**   central auditory processing disorder (H93.25)
> dysphasia or aphasia NOS (R47.-)
> expressive language disorder (F80.1)
> expressive type dysphasia or aphasia (F80.1)
> word deafness (H93.25)

> **Excludes2**   acquired aphasia with epilepsy [Landau-Kleffner] (G40.80-)
> intellectual disabilities (F70-F79)
> pervasive developmental disorders (F84.-)
> selective mutism (F94.0)

    F80.4   **Speech and language development delay due to hearing loss**
Code also type of hearing loss (H90.-, H91.-)

● **F80.8**   **Other developmental disorders of speech or language**

    F80.81   **Childhood onset fluency disorder**
Cluttering NOS
Stuttering NOS

> **Excludes1**   adult onset fluency disorder (F98.5)
> fluency disorder in conditions classified elsewhere (R47.82)
> fluency disorder (stuttering) following cerebrovascular disease (I69. with final characters -23)

    F80.82   **Social pragmatic communication disorder** ◀

> **Excludes1**   Asperger's syndrome (F84.5) ◀
> autistic disorder (F84.0) ◀

    F80.89   **Other developmental disorders of speech and language**

    F80.9   **Developmental disorder of speech and language, unspecified**
Communication disorder NOS
Language disorder NOS

● **F81**   **Specific developmental disorders of scholastic skills**

    F81.0   **Specific reading disorder**
'Backward reading'
Developmental dyslexia
Specific reading retardation

> **Excludes1**   alexia NOS (R48.0)
> dyslexia NOS (R48.0)

    F81.2   **Mathematics disorder**
Developmental acalculia
Developmental arithmetical disorder
Developmental Gerstmann's syndrome

> **Excludes1**   acalculia NOS (R48.8)

> **Excludes2**   arithmetical difficulties associated with a reading disorder (F81.0)
> arithmetical difficulties associated with a spelling disorder (F81.81)
> arithmetical difficulties due to inadequate teaching (Z55.8)

● **F81.8**   **Other developmental disorders of scholastic skills**

    F81.81   **Disorder of written expression**
Specific spelling disorder

    F81.89   **Other developmental disorders of scholastic skills**

    F81.9   **Developmental disorder of scholastic skills, unspecified**
Knowledge acquisition disability NOS
Learning disability NOS
Learning disorder NOS

◀ New   ◀▥ Revised   ~~deleted~~ Deleted   Excludes 1   Excludes 2   Includes   Use additional   Code first   Code also   Unspecified

OGCR Official Guidelines   X Assign placeholder X   ● Use Additional Character(s)   ▶ Manifestation Code   **Coding Clinic**

F82   Specific developmental disorder of motor function
    Clumsy child syndrome
    Developmental coordination disorder
    Developmental dyspraxia

> **Excludes1**   abnormalities of gait and mobility (R26.-)
>   lack of coordination (R27.-)

> **Excludes2**   lack of coordination secondary to intellectual
>   disabilities (F70-F79)

● **F84   Pervasive developmental disorders**
    Use additional code to identify any associated medical
    condition and intellectual disabilities.

    F84.0   Autistic disorder
       Autism spectrum disorder ◄
       Infantile autism
       Infantile psychosis
       Kanner's syndrome

> **Excludes1**   Asperger's syndrome (F84.5)

    F84.2   Rett's syndrome
       Neurodevelopmental disorder

> **Excludes1**   Asperger's syndrome (F84.5)
>   Autistic disorder (F84.0)
>   other childhood disintegrative disorder
>   (F84.3)

    F84.3   Other childhood disintegrative disorder   P
       Dementia infantilis
       At least two years of normal development followed by
       *   significant loss of language abilities, social skills,*
       *   bowel/bladder control, motor skills*
       Disintegrative psychosis
       Heller's syndrome
       At least two years of normal development followed by
       *   significant loss of language abilities, social skills,*
       *   bowel/bladder control, motor skills*
       Symbiotic psychosis
       Abnormal relationship to mothering figure, characterized
       *   by intense separation anxiety, severe regression,*
       *   giving up of useful speech, and autism*
       Use additional code to identify any associated
       neurological condition.

> **Excludes1**   Asperger's syndrome (F84.5)
>   Autistic disorder (F84.0)
>   Rett's syndrome (F84.2)

    F84.5   Asperger's syndrome
       Developmental disorder
       Asperger's disorder
       Autistic psychopathy
       Schizoid disorder of childhood

    F84.8   Other pervasive developmental disorders
       Overactive disorder associated with intellectual
          disabilities and stereotyped movements

    F84.9   Pervasive developmental disorder, unspecified
       Atypical autism

F88   Other disorders of psychological development
    Developmental agnosia
    Global developmental delay ◄
    Other specified neurodevelopmental disorder ◄

F89   Unspecified disorder of psychological development
    Developmental disorder NOS
    Neurodevelopmental disorder NOS ◄

BEHAVIORAL AND EMOTIONAL DISORDERS WITH ONSET USUALLY OCCURRING IN CHILDHOOD AND ADOLESCENCE (F90-F98)

Note: Codes within categories F90-F98 may be used regardless
of the age of a patient. These disorders generally have onset
within the childhood or adolescent years, but may continue
throughout life or not be diagnosed until adulthood.

● **F90   Attention-deficit hyperactivity disorders**
    Attention deficit disorder with hyperactivity=ADHD

> **Includes**   attention deficit disorder with hyperactivity
>   attention deficit syndrome with hyperactivity

> **Excludes2**   anxiety disorders (F40.-, F41.-)
>   mood [affective] disorders (F30-F39)
>   pervasive developmental disorders (F84.-)
>   schizophrenia (F20.-)

    F90.0   Attention-deficit hyperactivity disorder, predominantly inattentive type
    F90.1   Attention-deficit hyperactivity disorder, predominantly hyperactive type
    F90.2   Attention-deficit hyperactivity disorder, combined type
    F90.8   Attention-deficit hyperactivity disorder, other type
    F90.9   Attention-deficit hyperactivity disorder, unspecified type
       Attention-deficit hyperactivity disorder of childhood or
          adolescence NOS
       Attention-deficit hyperactivity disorder NOS

● **F91   Conduct disorders**
    Childhood/adolescence disruptive behavior disorder

> **Excludes1**   antisocial behavior (Z72.81-)
>   antisocial personality disorder (F60.2)

> **Excludes2**   conduct problems associated with attention-
>   deficit hyperactivity disorder (F90.-)
>   mood [affective] disorders (F30-F39)
>   pervasive developmental disorders (F84.-)
>   schizophrenia (F20.-)

    F91.0   Conduct disorder confined to family context
    F91.1   Conduct disorder, childhood-onset type
       Unsocialized conduct disorder
       Conduct disorder, solitary aggressive type
       Unsocialized aggressive disorder
    F91.2   Conduct disorder, adolescent-onset type
       Socialized conduct disorder
       Conduct disorder, group type
    F91.3   Oppositional defiant disorder
    F91.8   Other conduct disorders
       Other specified conduct disorder ◄
       Other specified disruptive disorder ◄
    F91.9   Conduct disorder, unspecified
       Behavioral disorder NOS
       Conduct disorder NOS
       Disruptive behavior disorder NOS
       Disruptive disorder NOS ◄

● **F93   Emotional disorders with onset specific to childhood**
    F93.0   Separation anxiety disorder of childhood

> **Excludes2**   mood [affective] disorders (F30-F39)
>   nonpsychotic mental disorders (F40-F48)
>   phobic anxiety disorder of childhood
>   (F40.8)
>   social phobia (F40.1)

    F93.8   Other childhood emotional disorders
       Identity disorder

> **Excludes2**   gender identity disorder of childhood
>   (F64.2)

    F93.9   Childhood emotional disorder, unspecified

CHAPTER 5 (F01-F99)

● **F94**   **Disorders of social functioning with onset specific to childhood and adolescence**

     F94.0   **Selective mutism**
          Elective mutism
          Excludes2   pervasive developmental disorders (F84.-)
                           schizophrenia (F20.-)
                           specific developmental disorders of speech and language (F80.-)
                           transient mutism as part of separation anxiety in young children (F93.0)

     F94.1   **Reactive attachment disorder of childhood**
          Use additional code to identify any associated failure to thrive or growth retardation
          Excludes1   disinhibited attachment disorder of childhood (F94.2)
                           normal variation in pattern of selective attachment
          Excludes2   Asperger's syndrome (F84.5)
                           maltreatment syndromes (T74.-)
                           sexual or physical abuse in childhood, resulting in psychosocial problems (Z62.81-)

     F94.2   **Disinhibited attachment disorder of childhood**
          Affectionless psychopathy
          Institutional syndrome
          Excludes1   reactive attachment disorder of childhood (F94.1)
          Excludes2   Asperger's syndrome (F84.5)
                           attention-deficit hyperactivity disorders (F90.-)
                           hospitalism in children (F43.2-)

     F94.8   **Other childhood disorders of social functioning**

     F94.9   **Childhood disorder of social functioning, unspecified**

● **F95**   **Tic disorder**
          Involuntary twitch

     F95.0   **Transient tic disorder**
          Provisional tic disorder ◀

     F95.1   **Chronic motor or vocal tic disorder**

     F95.2   **Tourette's disorder**
          Combined vocal and multiple motor tic disorder [de la Tourette]
          Tourette's syndrome

     F95.8   **Other tic disorders**

     F95.9   **Tic disorder, unspecified**
          Tic NOS

● **F98**   **Other behavioral and emotional disorders with onset usually occurring in childhood and adolescence**
          Excludes2   breath-holding spells (R06.89)
                           gender identity disorder of childhood (F64.2)
                           Kleine-Levin syndrome (G47.13)
                           obsessive-compulsive disorder (F42-) ◀▥
                           sleep disorders not due to a substance or known physiological condition (F51.-)

     F98.0   **Enuresis not due to a substance or known physiological condition**
          Enuresis: Urinary incontinence
          Enuresis (primary) (secondary) of nonorganic origin
          Functional enuresis
          Psychogenic enuresis
          Urinary incontinence of nonorganic origin
          Excludes1   enuresis NOS (R32)

     F98.1   **Encopresis not due to a substance or known physiological condition**
          Encopresis: Fecal incontinence
          Functional encopresis
          Incontinence of feces of nonorganic origin
          Psychogenic encopresis
          Use additional code to identify the cause of any coexisting constipation.
          Excludes1   encopresis NOS (R15.-)

● **F98.2**   **Other feeding disorders of infancy and childhood**
          Excludes1   feeding difficulties (R63.3)
          Excludes2   anorexia nervosa and other eating disorders (F50.-)
                           feeding problems of newborn (P92.-)
                           pica of infancy or childhood (F98.3)

     F98.21   **Rumination disorder of infancy**

     F98.29   **Other feeding disorders of infancy and early childhood**

     F98.3   **Pica of infancy and childhood**
          Craving and eating substances such as paint, clay, or dirt to replace a nutritional deficit in the body.

     F98.4   **Stereotyped movement disorders**
          Stereotype/habit disorder
          Excludes1   abnormal involuntary movements (R25.-)
          Excludes2   compulsions in obsessive-compulsive disorder (F42-) ◀▥
                           hair plucking (F63.3)
                           movement disorders of organic origin (G20-G25)
                           nail-biting (F98.8)
                           nose-picking (F98.8)
                           stereotypies that are part of a broader psychiatric condition (F01-F95)
                           thumb-sucking (F98.8)
                           tic disorders (F95.-)
                           trichotillomania (F63.3)

     F98.5   **Adult onset fluency disorder**
          Excludes1   childhood onset fluency disorder (F80.81)
                           dysphasia (R47.02)
                           fluency disorder in conditions classified elsewhere (R47.82)
                           fluency disorder (stuttering) following cerebrovascular disease (I69. with final characters -23)
                           tic disorders (F95.-)

     F98.8   **Other specified behavioral and emotional disorders with onset usually occurring in childhood and adolescence**
          Excessive masturbation
          Nail-biting
          Nose-picking
          Thumb-sucking

     F98.9   **Unspecified behavioral and emotional disorders with onset usually occurring in childhood and adolescence**

UNSPECIFIED MENTAL DISORDER (F99)

F99   **Mental disorder, not otherwise specified**
          Mental illness NOS
          Excludes1   unspecified mental disorder due to known physiological condition (F09)

Item 5–2 Enuresis: Bed wetting by children at night. Causes can be either psychological or medical (diabetes, urinary tract infections, or abnormalities). **Encopresis:** Overflow incontinence of bowels sometimes resulting from chronic constipation or fecal impaction. Check the documentation for additional diagnoses.

◀ New   ◀▥ Revised   ~~deleted~~ Deleted   Excludes 1   Excludes 2   Includes   Use additional   Code first   Code also   Unspecified

OGCR Official Guidelines   X Assign placeholder X   ● Use Additional Character(s)   ▐ Manifestation Code   **Coding Clinic**

CHAPTER 6

DISEASES OF THE NERVOUS SYSTEM
(G00-G99)

OGCR Chapter-Specific Coding Guidelines

6. **Chapter 6: Diseases of the Nervous System (G00-G99)**

   a. **Dominant/nondominant side**

   Codes from category G81, Hemiplegia and hemiparesis, and subcategories, G83.1, Monoplegia of lower limb, G83.2, Monoplegia of upper limb, and G83.3, Monoplegia, unspecified, identify whether the dominant or nondominant side is affected. Should the affected side be documented, but not specified as dominant or nondominant, and the classification system does not indicate a default, code selection is as follows:

   - For ambidextrous patients, the default should be dominant.
   - If the left side is affected, the default is non-dominant.
   - If the right side is affected, the default is dominant.

   b. **Pain - Category G89**

   1) **General coding information**

   Codes in category G89, Pain, not elsewhere classified, may be used in conjunction with codes from other categories and chapters to provide more detail about acute or chronic pain and neoplasm-related pain, unless otherwise indicated below.

   If the pain is not specified as acute or chronic, post-thoracotomy, postprocedural, or neoplasm-related, do not assign codes from category G89.

   A code from category G89 should not be assigned if the underlying (definitive) diagnosis is known, unless the reason for the encounter is pain control/management and not management of the underlying condition.

   When an admission or encounter is for a procedure aimed at treating the underlying condition (e.g., spinal fusion, kyphoplasty), a code for the underlying condition (e.g., vertebral fracture, spinal stenosis) should be assigned as the principal diagnosis. No code from category G89 should be assigned.

   (a) **Category G89 Codes as Principal or First-Listed Diagnosis**

   Category G89 codes are acceptable as principal diagnosis or the first-listed code:

   - When pain control or pain management is the reason for the admission/encounter (e.g., a patient with displaced intervertebral disc, nerve impingement and severe back pain presents for injection of steroid into the spinal canal). The underlying cause of the pain should be reported as an additional diagnosis, if known.
   - When a patient is admitted for the insertion of a neurostimulator for pain control, assign the appropriate pain code as the principal or first-listed diagnosis. When an admission or encounter is for a procedure aimed at treating the underlying condition and a neurostimulator is inserted for pain control during the same admission/encounter, a code for the underlying condition should be assigned as the principal diagnosis and the appropriate pain code should be assigned as a secondary diagnosis.

   (b) **Use of Category G89 Codes in Conjunction with Site Specific Pain Codes**

   (i) **Assigning Category G89 and Site-Specific Pain Codes**

   Codes from category G89 may be used in conjunction with codes that identify the site of pain (including codes from chapter 18) if the category G89 code provides additional information. For example, if the code describes the site of the pain, but does not fully describe whether the pain is acute or chronic, then both codes should be assigned.

   (ii) **Sequencing of Category G89 Codes with Site-Specific Pain Codes**

   The sequencing of category G89 codes with site-specific pain codes (including chapter 18 codes), is dependent on the circumstances of the encounter/admission as follows:

   - If the encounter is for pain control or pain management, assign the code from category G89 followed by the code identifying the specific site of pain (e.g., encounter for pain management for acute neck pain from trauma is assigned code G89.11, Acute pain due to trauma, followed by code M54.2, Cervicalgia, to identify the site of pain).
   - If the encounter is for any other reason except pain control or pain management, and a related definitive diagnosis has not been established (confirmed) by the provider, assign the code for the specific site of pain first, followed by the appropriate code from category G89.

   2) **Pain due to devices, implants and grafts**
   See Section I.C.19. Pain due to medical devices

   3) **Postoperative Pain**

   The provider's documentation should be used to guide the coding of postoperative pain, as well as Section III. Reporting Additional Diagnoses and Section IV. Diagnostic Coding and Reporting in the Outpatient Setting.

   The default for post-thoracotomy and other postoperative pain not specified as acute or chronic is the code for the acute form.

   Routine or expected postoperative pain immediately after surgery should not be coded.

   (a) **Postoperative pain not associated with specific postoperative complication**

   Postoperative pain not associated with a specific postoperative complication is assigned to the appropriate postoperative pain code in category G89.

   (b) **Postoperative pain associated with specific postoperative complication**

   Postoperative pain associated with a specific postoperative complication (such as painful wire sutures) is assigned to the appropriate code(s) found in Chapter 19, Injury, poisoning, and certain other consequences of external causes. If appropriate, use additional code(s) from category G89 to identify acute or chronic pain (G89.18 or G89.28).

   4) **Chronic pain**

   Chronic pain is classified to subcategory G89.2. There is no time frame defining when pain becomes chronic pain. The provider's documentation should be used to guide use of these codes.

   5) **Neoplasm Related Pain**

   Code G89.3 is assigned to pain documented as being related, associated or due to cancer, primary or secondary malignancy, or tumor. This code is assigned regardless of whether the pain is acute or chronic.

   This code may be assigned as the principal or first-listed code when the stated reason for the admission/encounter is documented as pain control/pain management. The underlying neoplasm should be reported as an additional diagnosis.

   When the reason for the admission/encounter is management of the neoplasm and the pain associated with the neoplasm is also documented, code G89.3 may be assigned as an additional diagnosis. It is not necessary to assign an additional code for the site of the pain.

   See Section I.C.2 for instructions on the sequencing of neoplasms for all other stated reasons for the admission/encounter (except for pain control/pain management).

   6) **Chronic pain syndrome**

   Central pain syndrome (G89.0) and chronic pain syndrome (G89.4) are different than the term "chronic pain," and therefore codes should only be used when the provider has specifically documented this condition.

   See Section I.C.5. Pain disorders related to psychological factors

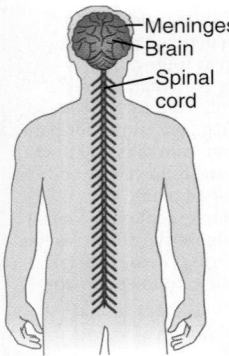

—Meninges
—Brain
—Spinal cord

Figure 6-1 The brain and spinal cord make up the central nervous system.

Item 6–1 The two major classifications of the nervous system are the peripheral nervous system and the central nervous system (CNS). The central nervous system is comprised of the brain and the spinal cord. The peripheral nervous system is comprised of the parasympathetic and sympathetic systems. **Encephalitis** is the swelling of the brain. **Meningitis** is swelling of the covering of the brain, the meninges. Types and causes of brain infections are:

Type	Cause
purulent	bacterial
aseptic/abacterial	viral
chronic meningitis	mycobacterial and fungal

CHAPTER 6

DISEASES OF THE NERVOUS SYSTEM (G00-G99)

Excludes2   certain conditions originating in the perinatal period (P04-P96)
certain infectious and parasitic diseases (A00-B99)
complications of pregnancy, childbirth and the puerperium (O00-O9A)
congenital malformations, deformations, and chromosomal abnormalities (Q00-Q99)
endocrine, nutritional and metabolic diseases (E00-E88)
injury, poisoning and certain other consequences of external causes (S00-T88)
neoplasms (C00-D49)
symptoms, signs and abnormal clinical and laboratory findings, not elsewhere classified (R00-R94)

This chapter contains the following blocks:

G00-G09	Inflammatory diseases of the central nervous system
G10-G14	Systemic atrophies primarily affecting the central nervous system
G20-G26	Extrapyramidal and movement disorders
G30-G32	Other degenerative diseases of the nervous system
G35-G37	Demyelinating diseases of the central nervous system
G40-G47	Episodic and paroxysmal disorders
G50-G59	Nerve, nerve root and plexus disorders
G60-G65	Polyneuropathies and other disorders of the peripheral nervous system
G70-G73	Diseases of myoneural junction and muscle
G80-G83	Cerebral palsy and other paralytic syndromes
G89-G99	Other disorders of the nervous system

INFLAMMATORY DISEASES OF THE CENTRAL NERVOUS SYSTEM (G00-G09)

● **G00   Bacterial meningitis, not elsewhere classified**
An infection of the cerebrospinal fluid surrounding the spinal cord and brain.

Includes   bacterial arachnoiditis
bacterial leptomeningitis
bacterial meningitis
bacterial pachymeningitis

Excludes1   bacterial:
meningoencephalitis (G04.2)
meningomyelitis (G04.2)

G00.0   Hemophilus meningitis
Meningitis due to Hemophilus influenzae

G00.1   Pneumococcal meningitis
Meningitis due to Streptococcal pneumoniae ◄

G00.2   Streptococcal meningitis
Use additional code to further identify organism (B95.0-B95.5)

G00.3   Staphylococcal meningitis
Use additional code to further identify organism (B95.61-B95.8)

G00.8   Other bacterial meningitis
Meningitis due to Escherichia coli
Meningitis due to Friedländer bacillus
Meningitis due to Klebsiella
Use additional code to further identify organism (B96.-)

G00.9   Bacterial meningitis, unspecified
Meningitis due to gram-negative bacteria, unspecified
Purulent meningitis NOS
Pyogenic meningitis NOS
Suppurative meningitis NOS

▶ **G01   Meningitis in bacterial diseases classified elsewhere**
Code first underlying disease
Excludes1   meningitis (in):
gonococcal (A54.81)
leptospirosis (A27.81)
listeriosis (A32.11)
Lyme disease (A69.21)
meningococcal (A39.0)
neurosyphilis (A52.13)
tuberculosis (A17.0)
meningoencephalitis and meningomyelitis in bacterial diseases classified elsewhere (G05)

▶ **G02   Meningitis in other infectious and parasitic diseases classified elsewhere**
Code first underlying disease, such as:
African trypanosomiasis (B56.-)
poliovirus infection (A80.-)
Excludes1   candidal meningitis (B37.5)
coccidioidomycosis meningitis (B38.4)
cryptococcal meningitis (B45.1)
herpesviral [herpes simplex] meningitis (B00.3)
infectious mononucleosis complicated by meningitis (B27.- with fourth character 2)
measles complicated by meningitis (B05.1)
meningoencephalitis and meningomyelitis in other infectious and parasitic diseases classified elsewhere (G05)
mumps meningitis (B26.1)
rubella meningitis (B06.02)
varicella [chickenpox] meningitis (B01.0)
zoster meningitis (B02.1)

◄ New   ◀═ Revised   ~~deleted~~ Deleted   Excludes 1   Excludes 2   Includes   Use additional   Code first   Code also   Unspecified
OGCR Official Guidelines   X Assign placeholder X   ● Use Additional Character(s)   ▶ Manifestation Code   **Coding Clinic**

● **G03 Meningitis due to other and unspecified causes**

Includes arachnoiditis NOS
leptomeningitis NOS
meningitis NOS
pachymeningitis NOS

Excludes1 meningoencephalitis (G04.-)
meningomyelitis (G04.-)

G03.0 Nonpyogenic meningitis
Aseptic meningitis
Nonbacterial meningitis

G03.1 Chronic meningitis

G03.2 Benign recurrent meningitis [Mollaret]

G03.8 Meningitis due to other specified causes

G03.9 Meningitis, unspecified
Arachnoiditis (spinal) NOS

● **G04 Encephalitis, myelitis and encephalomyelitis**

Includes acute ascending myelitis
meningoencephalitis
meningomyelitis

Excludes1 encephalopathy NOS (G93.40)
other noninfectious acute disseminated
encephalomyelitis (noninfectious ADEM)
(G04.81)

Excludes2 acute transverse myelitis (G37.3-)
alcoholic encephalopathy (G31.2)
benign myalgic encephalomyelitis (G93.3)
multiple sclerosis (G35)
subacute necrotizing myelitis (G37.4)
toxic encephalitis (G92)
toxic encephalopathy (G92)

● **G04.0 Acute disseminated encephalitis and encephalomyelitis (ADEM)**

Excludes1 acute necrotizing hemorrhagic
encephalopathy (G04.3-)

G04.00 Acute disseminated encephalitis and encephalomyelitis, unspecified

▷ **G04.01** *Postinfectious acute disseminated encephalitis and encephalomyelitis (postinfectious ADEM)*

Excludes1 post chickenpox encephalitis
(B01.1)
post measles encephalitis (B05.0)
post measles myelitis (B05.1)

G04.02 Postimmunization acute disseminated encephalitis, myelitis and encephalomyelitis
Encephalitis, post immunization
Encephalomyelitis, post immunization
Use additional code to identify the vaccine
(T50.A-, T50.B-, T50.Z-)

G04.1 Tropical spastic paraplegia

G04.2 Bacterial meningoencephalitis and meningomyelitis, not elsewhere classified

● **G04.3 Acute necrotizing hemorrhagic encephalopathy**
Sudden and severe CNS disease with pathology of hemorrhages and necrosis of white matter

Excludes1 acute disseminated encephalitis and
encephalomyelitis (G04.0-)

G04.30 Acute necrotizing hemorrhagic encephalopathy, unspecified

G04.31 Postinfectious acute necrotizing hemorrhagic encephalopathy

G04.32 Postimmunization acute necrotizing hemorrhagic encephalopathy
Use additional code to identify vaccine
(T50.A-, T50.B-, T50.Z-)

G04.39 Other acute necrotizing hemorrhagic encephalopathy
Code also underlying etiology, if applicable

● **G04.8 Other encephalitis, myelitis and encephalomyelitis**
Code also any associated seizure (G40.-, R56.9)

G04.81 Other encephalitis and encephalomyelitis
Noninfectious acute disseminated
encephalomyelitis (noninfectious ADEM)

G04.89 Other myelitis

● **G04.9 Encephalitis, myelitis and encephalomyelitis, unspecified**

G04.90 Encephalitis and encephalomyelitis, unspecified
Ventriculitis (cerebral) NOS

G04.91 Myelitis, unspecified

● **G05 Encephalitis, myelitis and encephalomyelitis in diseases classified elsewhere**
Code first underlying disease, such as:
human immunodeficiency virus [HIV] disease (B20)
poliovirus (A80.-)
suppurative otitis media (H66.01-H66.4)
trichinellosis (B75)

Excludes1 adenoviral encephalitis, myelitis and
encephalomyelitis (A85.1)
congenital toxoplasmosis encephalitis, myelitis
and encephalomyelitis (P37.1)
cytomegaloviral encephalitis, myelitis and
encephalomyelitis (B25.8)
encephalitis, myelitis and encephalomyelitis (in)
measles (B05.0)
encephalitis, myelitis and encephalomyelitis (in)
systemic lupus erythematosus (M32.19)
enteroviral encephalitis, myelitis and
encephalomyelitis (A85.0)
herpesviral [herpes simplex] encephalitis,
myelitis and encephalomyelitis (B00.4)
listerial encephalitis, myelitis and
encephalomyelitis (A32.12)
meningococcal encephalitis, myelitis and
encephalomyelitis (A39.81)
mumps encephalitis, myelitis and
encephalomyelitis (B26.2)
postchickenpox encephalitis, myelitis and
encephalomyelitis (B01.1-)
rubella encephalitis, myelitis and
encephalomyelitis (B06.01)
toxoplasmosis encephalitis, myelitis and
encephalomyelitis (B58.2)
zoster encephalitis, myelitis and
encephalomyelitis (B02.0)

▷ **G05.3** *Encephalitis and encephalomyelitis in diseases classified elsewhere*
Meningoencephalitis in diseases classified elsewhere

▷ **G05.4** *Myelitis in diseases classified elsewhere*
Meningomyelitis in diseases classified elsewhere

● **G06 Intracranial and intraspinal abscess and granuloma**
An accumulation of pus in either the brain or spinal cord
Use additional code (B95-B97) to identify infectious agent.

G06.0 Intracranial abscess and granuloma
Brain [any part] abscess (embolic)
Cerebellar abscess (embolic)
Cerebral abscess (embolic)
Intracranial epidural abscess or granuloma
Intracranial extradural abscess or granuloma
Intracranial subdural abscess or granuloma
Otogenic abscess (embolic)

Excludes1 tuberculous intracranial abscess and
granuloma (A17.81)

G06.1 Intraspinal abscess and granuloma
Abscess (embolic) of spinal cord [any part]
Intraspinal epidural abscess or granuloma
Intraspinal extradural abscess or granuloma
Intraspinal subdural abscess or granuloma

Excludes1 tuberculous intraspinal abscess and
granuloma (A17.81)

G06.2 Extradural and subdural abscess, unspecified

G07 *Intracranial and intraspinal abscess and granuloma in diseases classified elsewhere*

> *Code first* underlying disease, such as:
> schistosomiasis granuloma of brain (B65.-)
>
> **Excludes1** abscess of brain:
> amebic (A06.6)
> chromomycotic (B43.1)
> gonococcal (A54.82)
> tuberculous (A17.81)
> tuberculoma of meninges (A17.1)

G08 **Intracranial and intraspinal phlebitis and thrombophlebitis**

> Septic embolism of intracranial or intraspinal venous sinuses and veins
> Septic endophlebitis of intracranial or intraspinal venous sinuses and veins
> Septic phlebitis of intracranial or intraspinal venous sinuses and veins
> Septic thrombophlebitis of intracranial or intraspinal venous sinuses and veins
> Septic thrombosis of intracranial or intraspinal venous sinuses and veins
>
> **Excludes1** intracranial phlebitis and thrombophlebitis complicating:
> abortion, ectopic or molar pregnancy (O00-O07, O08.7)
> pregnancy, childbirth and the puerperium (O22.5, O87.3)
> nonpyogenic intracranial phlebitis and thrombophlebitis (I67.6)
>
> **Excludes2** intracranial phlebitis and thrombophlebitis complicating nonpyogenic intraspinal phlebitis and thrombophlebitis (G95.1)

G09 **Sequelae of inflammatory diseases of central nervous system**

> **Note:** Category G09 is to be used to indicate conditions whose primary classification is to G00-G08 as the cause of sequelae, themselves classifiable elsewhere. The 'sequelae' include conditions specified as residuals.
>
> *Code first* condition resulting from (sequela) of inflammatory diseases of central nervous system

SYSTEMIC ATROPHIES PRIMARILY AFFECTING THE CENTRAL NERVOUS SYSTEM (G10-G14)

G10 **Huntington's disease**

> *Genetic disease with degeneration of cells of the nervous system, including brain*
> Huntington's chorea
> Huntington's dementia

● **G11** **Hereditary ataxia**

> *Genetic neurological disorder affecting coordination*
>
> **Excludes2** cerebral palsy (G80.-)
> hereditary and idiopathic neuropathy (G60.-)
> metabolic disorders (E70-E88)

G11.0 **Congenital nonprogressive ataxia**

G11.1 **Early-onset cerebellar ataxia**
> Early-onset cerebellar ataxia with essential tremor
> Early-onset cerebellar ataxia with myoclonus [Hunt's ataxia]
> Early-onset cerebellar ataxia with retained tendon reflexes
> Friedreich's ataxia (autosomal recessive)
> X-linked recessive spinocerebellar ataxia

G11.2 **Late-onset cerebellar ataxia**   A

G11.3 **Cerebellar ataxia with defective DNA repair**
> Ataxia telangiectasia [Louis-Bar]
>
> **Excludes2** Cockayne's syndrome (Q87.1)
> other disorders of purine and pyrimidine metabolism (E79.-)
> xeroderma pigmentosum (Q82.1)

G11.4 **Hereditary spastic paraplegia**

G11.8 **Other hereditary ataxias**

G11.9 **Hereditary ataxia, unspecified**
> Hereditary cerebellar ataxia NOS
> Hereditary cerebellar degeneration
> Hereditary cerebellar disease
> Hereditary cerebellar syndrome

● **G12** **Spinal muscular atrophy and related syndromes**

G12.0 **Infantile spinal muscular atrophy, type I [Werdnig-Hoffman]**

G12.1 **Other inherited spinal muscular atrophy**
> Adult form spinal muscular atrophy
> Childhood form, type II spinal muscular atrophy
> Distal spinal muscular atrophy
> Juvenile form, type III spinal muscular atrophy [Kugelberg-Welander]
> Progressive bulbar palsy of childhood [Fazio-Londe]
> Scapuloperoneal form spinal muscular atrophy

● **G12.2** **Motor neuron disease**
> *Progressive disease of motor neurons that carry impulses to muscles to move*

G12.20 **Motor neuron disease, unspecified**

G12.21 **Amyotrophic lateral sclerosis**   A
> *Lou Gehrig's disease (ALS)*
> Progressive spinal muscle atrophy

G12.22 **Progressive bulbar palsy**

G12.29 **Other motor neuron disease**
> Familial motor neuron disease
> Primary lateral sclerosis

G12.8 **Other spinal muscular atrophies and related syndromes**

G12.9 **Spinal muscular atrophy, unspecified**

● **G13** **Systemic atrophies primarily affecting central nervous system in diseases classified elsewhere**

▶ **G13.0** *Paraneoplastic neuromyopathy and neuropathy*
> Carcinomatous neuromyopathy
> Sensorial paraneoplastic neuropathy [Denny Brown]
> *Code first* underlying neoplasm (C00-D49)

▶ **G13.1** *Other systemic atrophy primarily affecting central nervous system in neoplastic disease*
> Paraneoplastic limbic encephalopathy
> *Code first* underlying neoplasm (C00-D49)

▶ **G13.2** *Systemic atrophy primarily affecting the central nervous system in myxedema*
> *Code first* underlying disease, such as:
> hypothyroidism (E03.-)
> myxedematous congenital iodine deficiency (E00.1)

▶ **G13.8** *Systemic atrophy primarily affecting central nervous system in other diseases classified elsewhere*
> *Code first* underlying disease

G14 **Postpolio syndrome**
> **Includes** Postpolio myelitic syndrome
> **Excludes1** sequelae of poliomyelitis (B91)

EXTRAPYRAMIDAL AND MOVEMENT DISORDERS (G20-G26)

G20 **Parkinson's disease**
> *Progressive disease of the nervous system that affects muscle coordination*
> Hemiparkinsonism
> Idiopathic Parkinsonism or Parkinson's disease
> Paralysis agitans
> Parkinsonism or Parkinson's disease NOS
> Primary Parkinsonism or Parkinson's disease
>
> **Excludes1** dementia with Parkinsonism (G31.83)
>
> **Coding Clinic: 2016, Q2, P7**

Item 6–2 Huntington's chorea is an inherited degenerative disorder of the central nervous system and is characterized by ceaseless, jerky movements and progressive cognitive and behavioral deterioration.

New ◀ Revised ◀▥ ~~deleted~~ Deleted   Excludes 1   Excludes 2   Includes   Use additional   Code first   Code also   Unspecified
OGCR Official Guidelines   X Assign placeholder X   ● Use Additional Character(s)   ▶ Manifestation Code   **Coding Clinic**

● **G21 Secondary parkinsonism**
Symptoms of Parkinson's caused by medicines, illness, or other nervous system disorder
Excludes1 dementia with Parkinsonism (G31.83)
Huntington's disease (G10)
Shy-Drager syndrome (G90.3)
syphilitic Parkinsonism (A52.19)

G21.0 Malignant neuroleptic syndrome
Use additional code for adverse effect, if applicable, to identify drug (T43.3X5, T43.4X5, T43.505, T43.595)
Excludes1 neuroleptic induced parkinsonism (G21.11)

● **G21.1 Other drug-induced secondary parkinsonism**
G21.11 Neuroleptic induced parkinsonism
Use additional code for adverse effect, if applicable, to identify drug (T43.3X5, T43.4X5, T43.505, T43.595)
Excludes1 malignant neuroleptic syndrome (G21.0)

G21.19 Other drug induced secondary parkinsonism
Use additional code for adverse effect, if applicable, to identify drug (T36-T50 with fifth or sixth character 5)

G21.2 Secondary parkinsonism due to other external agents
Code first (T51-T65) to identify external agent

G21.3 Postencephalitic parkinsonism

G21.4 Vascular parkinsonism

G21.8 Other secondary parkinsonism

G21.9 Secondary parkinsonism, unspecified

● **G23 Other degenerative diseases of basal ganglia**
Excludes2 multi-system degeneration of the autonomic nervous system (G90.3)

G23.0 Hallervorden-Spatz disease
Pigmentary pallidal degeneration

G23.1 Progressive supranuclear ophthalmoplegia [Steele-Richardson-Olszewski]
Progressive supranuclear palsy

G23.2 Striatonigral degeneration

G23.8 Other specified degenerative diseases of basal ganglia
Calcification of basal ganglia

G23.9 Degenerative disease of basal ganglia, unspecified

● **G24 Dystonia**
Involuntary movements
Includes dyskinesia
Excludes2 athetoid cerebral palsy (G80.3)

● **G24.0 Drug induced dystonia**
Use additional code for adverse effect, if applicable, to identify drug (T36-T50 with fifth or sixth character 5)

G24.01 Drug induced subacute dyskinesia
Drug induced blepharospasm
Drug induced orofacial dyskinesia
Neuroleptic induced tardive dyskinesia
Tardive dyskinesia

G24.02 Drug induced acute dystonia
Acute dystonic reaction to drugs
Neuroleptic induced acute dystonia

G24.09 Other drug induced dystonia

G24.1 Genetic torsion dystonia
Dystonia deformans progressiva
Dystonia musculorum deformans
Familial torsion dystonia
Idiopathic familial dystonia
Idiopathic (torsion) dystonia NOS
(Schwalbe-) Ziehen-Oppenheim disease

G24.2 Idiopathic nonfamilial dystonia

G24.3 Spasmodic torticollis
Head tilts toward one side and chin is elevated and turned toward opposite side (wry neck)
Excludes1 congenital torticollis (Q68.0)
hysterical torticollis (F44.4)
ocular torticollis (R29.891)
psychogenic torticollis (F45.8)
torticollis NOS (M43.6)
traumatic recurrent torticollis (S13.4)

G24.4 Idiopathic orofacial dystonia
Orofacial dyskinesia
Excludes1 drug induced orofacial dyskinesia (G24.01)

G24.5 Blepharospasm
Tonic spasm of orbicularis oculi muscle, producing closure of eyelids
Excludes1 drug induced blepharospasm (G24.01)

G24.8 Other dystonia
Acquired torsion dystonia NOS

G24.9 Dystonia, unspecified
Dyskinesia NOS

● **G25 Other extrapyramidal and movement disorders**
Extrapyramidal: Other than pyramidal tracts
Excludes2 sleep related movement disorders (G47.6-)

G25.0 Essential tremor
Familial tremor
Excludes1 tremor NOS (R25.1)

G25.1 Drug-induced tremor
Use additional code for adverse effect, if applicable, to identify drug (T36-T50 with fifth or sixth character 5)

G25.2 Other specified forms of tremor
Intention tremor

G25.3 Myoclonus
Shocklike contractions muscle(s)
Drug-induced myoclonus
Palatal myoclonus
Use additional code for adverse effect, if applicable, to identify drug (T36-T50 with fifth or sixth character 5)
Excludes1 facial myokymia (G51.4)
myoclonic epilepsy (G40.-)

G25.4 Drug-induced chorea
Use additional code for adverse effect, if applicable, to identify drug (T36-T50 with fifth or sixth character 5)

G25.5 Other chorea
Continual, involuntary, jerky, movements
Chorea NOS
Excludes1 chorea NOS with heart involvement (I02.0)
Huntington's chorea (G10)
rheumatic chorea (I02.-)
Sydenham's chorea (I02.-)

● **G25.6 Drug induced tics and other tics of organic origin**
G25.61 Drug induced tics
Use additional code for adverse effect, if applicable, to identify drug (T36-T50 with fifth or sixth character 5)

G25.69 Other tics of organic origin
Excludes1 habit spasm (F95.9)
tic NOS (F95.9)
Tourette's syndrome (F95.2)

● G25.7 Other and unspecified drug induced movement disorders

> Use additional code for adverse effect, if applicable, to identify drug (T36-T50 with fifth or sixth character 5)

> **G25.70 Drug induced movement disorder, unspecified**

> **G25.71 Drug induced akathisia**
> > Drug induced acathisia
> > Neuroleptic induced acute akathisia

> **G25.79 Other drug induced movement disorders**

● G25.8 Other specified extrapyramidal and movement disorders

> **G25.81 Restless legs syndrome**

> **G25.82 Stiff-man syndrome**

> **G25.83 Benign shuddering attacks**

> **G25.89 Other specified extrapyramidal and movement disorders**

G25.9 Extrapyramidal and movement disorder, unspecified

▌ G26 Extrapyramidal and movement disorders in diseases classified elsewhere

> *Code first* underlying disease

OTHER DEGENERATIVE DISEASES OF THE NERVOUS SYSTEM (G30-G32)

● G30 Alzheimer's disease

> *Progressive central neurodegenerative disorder*

> **Includes**   Alzheimer's dementia senile and presenile forms

> Use additional code to identify:
> > delirium, if applicable (F05)
> > dementia with behavioral disturbance (F02.81)
> > dementia without behavioral disturbance (F02.80)

> **Excludes1**   senile degeneration of brain NEC (G31.1)
> > senile dementia NOS (F03)
> > senility NOS (R41.81)

> **G30.0 Alzheimer's disease with early onset**

> **G30.1 Alzheimer's disease with late onset**   A

> **G30.8 Other Alzheimer's disease**

> **G30.9 Alzheimer's disease, unspecified**
> > Coding Clinic: 2016, Q2, P6; 2012, Q4, P95

● G31 Other degenerative diseases of nervous system, not elsewhere classified

> Use additional code to identify:
> > dementia with behavioral disturbance (F02.81)
> > dementia without behavioral disturbance (F02.80)

> **Excludes2**   Reye's syndrome (G93.7)

● G31.0 Frontotemporal dementia

> **G31.01 Pick's disease**
> > Primary progressive aphasia
> > Progressive isolated aphasia

> **G31.09 Other frontotemporal dementia**
> > Frontal dementia

> **G31.1 Senile degeneration of brain, not elsewhere classified**

> > **Excludes1**   Alzheimer's disease (G30.-)
> > > senility NOS (R41.81)

> **G31.2 Degeneration of nervous system due to alcohol**
> > Alcoholic cerebellar ataxia
> > Alcoholic cerebellar degeneration
> > Alcoholic cerebral degeneration
> > Alcoholic encephalopathy
> > Dysfunction of the autonomic nervous system due to alcohol
> > *Code also* associated alcoholism (F10.-)

● G31.8 Other specified degenerative diseases of nervous system

> **G31.81 Alpers' disease**
> > *Rare neuronal degeneration of cerebral cortex disease of young children*
> > Grey-matter degeneration

> **G31.82 Leigh's disease**
> > *Rare neurometabolic disorder that affects central nervous system*
> > Subacute necrotizing encephalopathy

G31.83 Dementia with Lewy bodies
> *Closely allied to Parkinson's Disease*
> Dementia with Parkinsonism
> Lewy body dementia
> Lewy body disease

G31.84 Mild cognitive impairment, so stated

> **Excludes1**   age related cognitive decline (R41.81)
> > altered mental status (R41.82)
> > cerebral degeneration (G31.9)
> > change in mental status (R41.82)
> > cognitive deficits following (sequelae of) cerebral hemorrhage or infarction (I69.01-, I69.11-, I69.21-, I69.31-, I69.81-, I69.91-) ◀▥
> > cognitive impairment due to intracranial or head injury (S06.-)
> > dementia (F01.-, F02.-, F03)
> > mild memory disturbance (F06.8)
> > neurologic neglect syndrome (R41.4)
> > personality change, nonpsychotic (F68.8)

G31.85 Corticobasal degeneration

G31.89 Other specified degenerative diseases of nervous system

G31.9 Degenerative disease of nervous system, unspecified

● G32 Other degenerative disorders of nervous system in diseases classified elsewhere

▌ G32.0 Subacute combined degeneration of spinal cord in diseases classified elsewhere
> Dana-Putnam syndrome
> Sclerosis of spinal cord (combined) (dorsolateral) (posterolateral)

> *Code first* underlying disease, such as:
> > anemia (D51.9)
> > dietary (D51.3)
> > pernicious (D51.0)
> > vitamin B12 deficiency (E53.8)

> **Excludes1**   syphilitic combined degeneration of spinal cord (A52.11)

● G32.8 Other specified degenerative disorders of nervous system in diseases classified elsewhere

> *Code first* underlying disease, such as:
> > amyloidosis cerebral degeneration (E85.-)
> > cerebral degeneration (due to) hypothyroidism (E00.0-E03.9)
> > cerebral degeneration (due to) neoplasm (C00-D49)
> > cerebral degeneration (due to) vitamin B deficiency, except thiamine (E52-E53.-)

> **Excludes1**   superior hemorrhagic polioencephalitis [Wernicke's encephalopathy] (E51.2)

▌ G32.81 Cerebellar ataxia in diseases classified elsewhere

> *Code first* underlying disease, such as:
> > celiac disease (with gluten ataxia) (K90.0)
> > cerebellar ataxia (in) neoplastic disease (paraneoplastic cerebellar degeneration) (C00-D49)
> > non-celiac gluten ataxia (M35.9)

> **Excludes1**   systemic atrophy primarily affecting the central nervous system in alcoholic cerebellar ataxia (G31.2)
> > systemic atrophy primarily affecting the central nervous system in myxedema (G13.2)

▌ G32.89 Other specified degenerative disorders of nervous system in diseases classified elsewhere
> Degenerative encephalopathy in diseases classified elsewhere

---

◀ New   ◀▥ Revised   ~~deleted~~ Deleted   Excludes 1   Excludes 2   Includes   Use additional   Code first   Code also   Unspecified

776   OGCR Official Guidelines   X Assign placeholder X   ● Use Additional Character(s)   ▌ Manifestation Code   **Coding Clinic**

DEMYELINATING DISEASES OF THE CENTRAL NERVOUS SYSTEM (G35-G37)

G35   Multiple sclerosis
     Destruction of central nervous system; four types: relapsing
     remitting, secondary progressive, primary progressive, and
     progressive relapsing
     Disseminated multiple sclerosis
     Generalized multiple sclerosis
     Multiple sclerosis NOS
     Multiple sclerosis of brain stem
     Multiple sclerosis of cord

● **G36   Other acute disseminated demyelination**
     Excludes1   postinfectious encephalitis and encephalomyelitis
                   NOS (G04.01)

     G36.0   Neuromyelitis optica [Devic]
         Inflammatory disorder in which immune system attacks optic
           nerves and spinal cord producing inflammation of optic
           nerve (optic neuritis) and spinal cord (myelitis)
         Demyelination in optic neuritis
         Excludes1   optic neuritis NOS (H46)

     **G36.1   Acute and subacute hemorrhagic leukoencephalitis
              [Hurst]**
     G36.8   Other specified acute disseminated demyelination
     G36.9   Acute disseminated demyelination, unspecified

● **G37   Other demyelinating diseases of central nervous system**
     Destruction of central nervous system

     G37.0   Diffuse sclerosis of central nervous system
         Periaxial encephalitis
         Schilder's disease
         Excludes1   X linked adrenoleukodystrophy (E71.52-)

     G37.1   Central demyelination of corpus callosum
     G37.2   Central pontine myelinolysis
     **G37.3   Acute transverse myelitis in demyelinating disease of
              central nervous system**
         Acute transverse myelitis NOS
         Acute transverse myelopathy
         Excludes1   multiple sclerosis (G35)
                        neuromyelitis optica [Devic] (G36.0)

     G37.4   Subacute necrotizing myelitis of central nervous system
     G37.5   Concentric sclerosis [Baló] of central nervous system
     **G37.8   Other specified demyelinating diseases of central
              nervous system**
     **G37.9   Demyelinating disease of central nervous
              system, unspecified**

EPISODIC AND PAROXYSMAL DISORDERS (G40-G47)

● **G40   Epilepsy and recurrent seizures**
     Note: The following terms are to be considered equivalent
         to intractable: pharmacoresistant (pharmacologically
         resistant), treatment resistant, refractory (medically) and
         poorly controlled
     Excludes1   conversion disorder with seizures (F44.5)
                   convulsions NOS (R56.9)
                   post traumatic seizures (R56.1)
                   seizure (convulsive) NOS (R56.9)
                   seizure of newborn (P90)
     Excludes2   hippocampal sclerosis (G93.81) ◄
                   mesial temporal sclerosis (G93.81) ◄
                   temporal sclerosis (G93.81) ◄
                   Todd's paralysis (G83.84) ◄

● **G40.0   Localization-related (focal) (partial) idiopathic epilepsy
         and epileptic syndromes with seizures of localized onset**
     Benign childhood epilepsy with centrotemporal EEG
         spikes
     Childhood epilepsy with occipital EEG paroxysms
     Excludes1   adult onset localization-related epilepsy
                   (G40.1-, G40.2-)

● **G40.00   Localization-related (focal) (partial) idiopathic
           epilepsy and epileptic syndromes with seizures
           of localized onset, not intractable**
         Localization-related (focal) (partial) idiopathic
           epilepsy and epileptic syndromes with
           seizures of localized onset without
           intractability

         **G40.001   Localization-related (focal) (partial)
                 idiopathic epilepsy and epileptic
                 syndromes with seizures of localized
                 onset, not intractable, with status
                 epilepticus**

         **G40.009   Localization-related (focal) (partial)
                 idiopathic epilepsy and epileptic
                 syndromes with seizures of localized
                 onset, not intractable, without status
                 epilepticus**
                 Localization-related (focal) (partial)
                   idiopathic epilepsy and
                   epileptic syndromes with
                   seizures of localized onset NOS

● **G40.01   Localization-related (focal) (partial) idiopathic
           epilepsy and epileptic syndromes with seizures of
           localized onset, intractable**

         **G40.011   Localization-related (focal) (partial)
                 idiopathic epilepsy and epileptic
                 syndromes with seizures of localized
                 onset, intractable, with status
                 epilepticus**

         **G40.019   Localization-related (focal) (partial)
                 idiopathic epilepsy and epileptic
                 syndromes with seizures of localized
                 onset, intractable, without status
                 epilepticus**

Item 6-3   Multiple sclerosis (MS) is a nervous system disease affecting the brain and spinal cord by damaging the myelin sheath surrounding and protecting nerve cells. The damage slows down/blocks messages between the brain and body. Symptoms are: visual disturbances, muscle weakness, coordination and balance issues, numbness, prickling, thinking and memory problems. The cause is unknown, though it is thought that it may be an autoimmune disease. It affects women more than men, between 20 and 40 years of age. MS can be mild, but it may cause the loss of ability to write, walk, and speak. There is no cure, but medication may slow or control symptoms.

● **G40.1   Localization-related (focal) (partial) symptomatic epilepsy and epileptic syndromes with simple partial seizures**
> Attacks without alteration of consciousness
> Epilepsia partialis continua [Kozhevnikof]
> Simple partial seizures developing into secondarily generalized seizures

● **G40.10   Localization-related (focal) (partial) symptomatic epilepsy and epileptic syndromes with simple partial seizures, not intractable**
> Localization-related (focal) (partial) symptomatic epilepsy and epileptic syndromes with simple partial seizures without intractability

  G40.101   Localization-related (focal) (partial) symptomatic epilepsy and epileptic syndromes with simple partial seizures, not intractable, with status epilepticus

  G40.109   Localization-related (focal) (partial) symptomatic epilepsy and epileptic syndromes with simple partial seizures, not intractable, without status epilepticus
> Localization-related (focal) (partial) symptomatic epilepsy and epileptic syndromes with simple partial seizures NOS

● **G40.11   Localization-related (focal) (partial) symptomatic epilepsy and epileptic syndromes with simple partial seizures, intractable**

  G40.111   Localization-related (focal) (partial) symptomatic epilepsy and epileptic syndromes with simple partial seizures, intractable, with status epilepticus

  G40.119   Localization-related (focal) (partial) symptomatic epilepsy and epileptic syndromes with simple partial seizures, intractable, without status epilepticus

● **G40.2   Localization-related (focal) (partial) symptomatic epilepsy and epileptic syndromes with complex partial seizures**
> Attacks with alteration of consciousness, often with automatisms
> Complex partial seizures developing into secondarily generalized seizures

● **G40.20   Localization-related (focal) (partial) symptomatic epilepsy and epileptic syndromes with complex partial seizures, not intractable**
> Localization-related (focal) (partial) symptomatic epilepsy and epileptic syndromes with complex partial seizures without intractability

  G40.201   Localization-related (focal) (partial) symptomatic epilepsy and epileptic syndromes with complex partial seizures, not intractable, with status epilepticus

  G40.209   Localization-related (focal) (partial) symptomatic epilepsy and epileptic syndromes with complex partial seizures, not intractable, without status epilepticus
> Localization-related (focal) (partial) symptomatic epilepsy and epileptic syndromes with complex partial seizures NOS

● **G40.21   Localization-related (focal) (partial) symptomatic epilepsy and epileptic syndromes with complex partial seizures, intractable**

  G40.211   Localization-related (focal) (partial) symptomatic epilepsy and epileptic syndromes with complex partial seizures, intractable, with status epilepticus

  G40.219   Localization-related (focal) (partial) symptomatic epilepsy and epileptic syndromes with complex partial seizures, intractable, without status epilepticus

● **G40.3   Generalized idiopathic epilepsy and epileptic syndromes**
> Code also MERRF syndrome, if applicable (E88.42)

● **G40.30   Generalized idiopathic epilepsy and epileptic syndromes, not intractable**
> Generalized idiopathic epilepsy and epileptic syndromes without intractability

  G40.301   Generalized idiopathic epilepsy and epileptic syndromes, not intractable, with status epilepticus

  G40.309   Generalized idiopathic epilepsy and epileptic syndromes, not intractable, without status epilepticus
> Generalized idiopathic epilepsy and epileptic syndromes NOS

● **G40.31   Generalized idiopathic epilepsy and epileptic syndromes, intractable**

  G40.311   Generalized idiopathic epilepsy and epileptic syndromes, intractable, with status epilepticus

  G40.319   Generalized idiopathic epilepsy and epileptic syndromes, intractable, without status epilepticus

● **G40.A   Absence epileptic syndrome**
> Childhood absence epilepsy [pyknolepsy]
> Juvenile absence epilepsy
> Absence epileptic syndrome, NOS

● **G40.A0   Absence epileptic syndrome, not intractable**

  G40.A01   Absence epileptic syndrome, not intractable, with status epilepticus

  G40.A09   Absence epileptic syndrome, not intractable, without status epilepticus

● **G40.A1   Absence epileptic syndrome, intractable**

  G40.A11   Absence epileptic syndrome, intractable, with status epilepticus

  G40.A19   Absence epileptic syndrome, intractable, without status epilepticus

● **G40.B   Juvenile myoclonic epilepsy [impulsive petit mal]**

● **G40.B0   Juvenile myoclonic epilepsy, not intractable**

  G40.B01   Juvenile myoclonic epilepsy, not intractable, with status epilepticus

  G40.B09   Juvenile myoclonic epilepsy, not intractable, without status epilepticus

● **G40.B1   Juvenile myoclonic epilepsy, intractable**

  G40.B11   Juvenile myoclonic epilepsy, intractable, with status epilepticus

  G40.B19   Juvenile myoclonic epilepsy, intractable, without status epilepticus

◀ New   ◀▥ Revised   ~~deleted~~ Deleted   Excludes 1   Excludes 2   Includes   Use additional   Code first   Code also   Unspecified

OGCR Official Guidelines   X Assign placeholder X   ● Use Additional Character(s)   ▶ Manifestation Code   **Coding Clinic**

● **G40.4   Other generalized epilepsy and epileptic syndromes**
    Epilepsy with grand mal seizures on awakening
    Epilepsy with myoclonic absences
    Epilepsy with myoclonic-astatic seizures
    Grand mal seizure NOS
    Nonspecific atonic epileptic seizures
    Nonspecific clonic epileptic seizures
    Nonspecific myoclonic epileptic seizures
    Nonspecific tonic epileptic seizures
    Nonspecific tonic-clonic epileptic seizures
    Symptomatic early myoclonic encephalopathy

  ● **G40.40   Other generalized epilepsy and epileptic syndromes, not intractable**
      Other generalized epilepsy and epileptic syndromes without intractability
      Other generalized epilepsy and epileptic syndromes NOS

    G40.401   Other generalized epilepsy and epileptic syndromes, not intractable, with status epilepticus

    G40.409   Other generalized epilepsy and epileptic syndromes, not intractable, without status epilepticus

  ● **G40.41   Other generalized epilepsy and epileptic syndromes, intractable**

    G40.411   Other generalized epilepsy and epileptic syndromes, intractable, with status epilepticus

    G40.419   Other generalized epilepsy and epileptic syndromes, intractable, without status epilepticus

● **G40.5   Epileptic seizures related to external causes**
    Epileptic seizures related to alcohol
    Epileptic seizures related to drugs
    Epileptic seizures related to hormonal changes
    Epileptic seizures related to sleep deprivation
    Epileptic seizures related to stress

    `Code also`, if applicable, associated epilepsy and recurrent seizures (G40.-)

    `Use additional` code for adverse effect, if applicable, to identify drug (T36-T50 with fifth or sixth character 5)

  ● **G40.50   Epileptic seizures related to external causes, not intractable**

    G40.501   Epileptic seizures related to external causes, not intractable, with status epilepticus

    G40.509   Epileptic seizures related to external causes, not intractable, without status epilepticus
      Epileptic seizures related to external causes, NOS

● **G40.8   Other epilepsy and recurrent seizures**
    Epilepsies and epileptic syndromes undetermined as to whether they are focal or generalized
    Landau-Kleffner syndrome

  ● **G40.80   Other epilepsy**

    G40.801   Other epilepsy, not intractable, with status epilepticus
      Other epilepsy without intractability with status epilepticus

    G40.802   Other epilepsy, not intractable, without status epilepticus
      Other epilepsy NOS
      Other epilepsy without intractability without status epilepticus

    G40.803   Other epilepsy, intractable, with status epilepticus

    G40.804   Other epilepsy, intractable, without status epilepticus

  ● **G40.81   Lennox-Gastaut syndrome**

    G40.811   Lennox-Gastaut syndrome, not intractable, with status epilepticus

    G40.812   Lennox-Gastaut syndrome, not intractable, without status epilepticus

    G40.813   Lennox-Gastaut syndrome, intractable, with status epilepticus

    G40.814   Lennox-Gastaut syndrome, intractable, without status epilepticus

  ● **G40.82   Epileptic spasms**
    Infantile spasms
    Salaam attacks
    West's syndrome

    G40.821   Epileptic spasms, not intractable, with status epilepticus

    G40.822   Epileptic spasms, not intractable, without status epilepticus

    G40.823   Epileptic spasms, intractable, with status epilepticus

    G40.824   Epileptic spasms, intractable, without status epilepticus

  G40.89   Other seizures
    `Excludes1`   post traumatic seizures (R56.1)
      recurrent seizures NOS (G40.909)
      seizure NOS (R56.9)

● **G40.9   Epilepsy, unspecified**

  ● **G40.90   Epilepsy, unspecified, not intractable**
    Epilepsy, unspecified, without intractability

    G40.901   Epilepsy, unspecified, not intractable, with status epilepticus

    G40.909   Epilepsy, unspecified, not intractable, without status epilepticus
      Epilepsy NOS
      Epileptic convulsions NOS
      Epileptic fits NOS
      Epileptic seizures NOS
      Recurrent seizures NOS
      Seizure disorder NOS

  ● **G40.91   Epilepsy, unspecified, intractable**
    Intractable seizure disorder NOS

    G40.911   Epilepsy, unspecified, intractable, with status epilepticus

    G40.919   Epilepsy, unspecified, intractable, without status epilepticus

● **G43   Migraine**
    Note: The following terms are to be considered equivalent to intractable: pharmacoresistant (pharmacologically resistant), treatment resistant, refractory (medically) and poorly controlled

    `Use additional` code for adverse effect, if applicable, to identify drug (T36-T50 with fifth or sixth character 5)

    `Excludes1`   headache NOS (R51)
      lower half migraine (G44.00)

    `Excludes2`   headache syndromes (G44.-)

● **G43.0   Migraine without aura**
    Neurological disorder, generally recurring headaches without early symptom (aura)
    Common migraine

    `Excludes1`   chronic migraine without aura (G43.7-)

  ● **G43.00   Migraine without aura, not intractable**
    Neurological disorder, generally recurring headaches without early symptom (aura); resistant to cure, relief, or control
    Migraine without aura without mention of refractory migraine

    G43.001   Migraine without aura, not intractable, with status migrainosus

    G43.009   Migraine without aura, not intractable, without status migrainosus
      Migraine without aura NOS

CHAPTER 6 (G00-G99)

Item 6–4   Migraine headache is described as an intense pulsing or throbbing pain in one area of the head. It can be accompanied by extreme sensitivity to light (photophobic) and sound and is three times more common in women than in men. Symptoms include nausea and vomiting. Research indicates migraine headaches are caused by inherited abnormalities in genes that control the activities of certain cell populations in the brain.

● **G43.01**   **Migraine without aura, intractable**
      Intractable migraine: Not easily cured or managed; relentless pain from a migraine
      Migraine without aura with refractory migraine

      G43.011   **Migraine without aura, intractable, with status migrainosus**

      G43.019   **Migraine without aura, intractable, without status migrainosus**

● **G43.1**   **Migraine with aura**
      Basilar migraine
      Classical migraine
      Migraine equivalents
      Migraine preceded or accompanied by transient focal neurological phenomena
      Migraine triggered seizures
      Migraine with acute-onset aura
      Migraine with aura without headache (migraine equivalents)
      Migraine with prolonged aura
      Migraine with typical aura
      Retinal migraine
      Code also any associated seizure (G40.-, R56.9)
      Excludes1   persistent migraine aura (G43.5-, G43.6-)

● **G43.10**   **Migraine with aura, not intractable**
      Migraine with aura without mention of refractory migraine

      G43.101   **Migraine with aura, not intractable, with status migrainosus**

      G43.109   **Migraine with aura, not intractable, without status migrainosus**
            Migraine with aura NOS

● **G43.11**   **Migraine with aura, intractable**
      Migraine with aura with refractory migraine

      G43.111   **Migraine with aura, intractable, with status migrainosus**

      G43.119   **Migraine with aura, intractable, without status migrainosus**

● **G43.4**   **Hemiplegic migraine**
      Inherited migraine disorder causing temporary paralysis of one side of body followed by severe headache and nausea
      Familial migraine
      Sporadic migraine

● **G43.40**   **Hemiplegic migraine, not intractable**
      Hemiplegic migraine without refractory migraine

      G43.401   **Hemiplegic migraine, not intractable, with status migrainosus**

      G43.409   **Hemiplegic migraine, not intractable, without status migrainosus**
            Hemiplegic migraine NOS

● **G43.41**   **Hemiplegic migraine, intractable**
      Hemiplegic migraine with refractory migraine

      G43.411   **Hemiplegic migraine, intractable, with status migrainosus**

      G43.419   **Hemiplegic migraine, intractable, without status migrainosus**

● **G43.5**   **Persistent migraine aura without cerebral infarction**
● **G43.50**   **Persistent migraine aura without cerebral infarction, not intractable**
      Persistent migraine aura without cerebral infarction, without refractory migraine

      G43.501   **Persistent migraine aura without cerebral infarction, not intractable, with status migrainosus**

      G43.509   **Persistent migraine aura without cerebral infarction, not intractable, without status migrainosus**
            Persistent migraine aura NOS

● **G43.51**   **Persistent migraine aura without cerebral infarction, intractable**
      Persistent migraine aura without cerebral infarction, with refractory migraine

      G43.511   **Persistent migraine aura without cerebral infarction, intractable, with status migrainosus**

      G43.519   **Persistent migraine aura without cerebral infarction, intractable, without status migrainosus**

● **G43.6**   **Persistent migraine aura with cerebral infarction**
      Visual, motor, or psychic disturbances, paresthesias, and related neurologic abnormalities accompanying migraine
      Code also the type of cerebral infarction (I63.-)

● **G43.60**   **Persistent migraine aura with cerebral infarction, not intractable**
      Persistent migraine aura with cerebral infarction, without refractory migraine

      G43.601   **Persistent migraine aura with cerebral infarction, not intractable, with status migrainosus**

      G43.609   **Persistent migraine aura with cerebral infarction, not intractable, without status migrainosus**

● **G43.61**   **Persistent migraine aura with cerebral infarction, intractable**
      Persistent migraine aura with cerebral infarction, with refractory migraine

      G43.611   **Persistent migraine aura with cerebral infarction, intractable, with status migrainosus**

      G43.619   **Persistent migraine aura with cerebral infarction, intractable, without status migrainosus**

● **G43.7**   **Chronic migraine without aura**
      Transformed migraine
      Excludes1   migraine without aura (G43.0-)

● **G43.70**   **Chronic migraine without aura, not intractable**
      Chronic migraine without aura, without refractory migraine

      G43.701   **Chronic migraine without aura, not intractable, with status migrainosus**

      G43.709   **Chronic migraine without aura, not intractable, without status migrainosus**
            Chronic migraine without aura NOS

● **G43.71**   **Chronic migraine without aura, intractable**
      Chronic migraine without aura, with refractory migraine

      G43.711   **Chronic migraine without aura, intractable, with status migrainosus**

      G43.719   **Chronic migraine without aura, intractable, without status migrainosus**

◄ New   ◄ Revised   ~~deleted~~ Deleted   Excludes 1   Excludes 2   Includes   Use additional   Code first   Code also   Unspecified

OGCR Official Guidelines   X Assign placeholder X   ● Use Additional Character(s)   ▷ Manifestation Code   **Coding Clinic**

● **G43.A Cyclical vomiting**
   G43.AØ Cyclical vomiting, not intractable
        Cyclical vomiting, without refractory migraine
   G43.A1 Cyclical vomiting, intractable
        Cyclical vomiting, with refractory migraine
● **G43.B Ophthalmoplegic migraine**
   G43.BØ Ophthalmoplegic migraine, not intractable
        Ophthalmoplegic migraine, without refractory
        migraine
   G43.B1 Ophthalmoplegic migraine, intractable
        Ophthalmoplegic migraine, with refractory
        migraine
● **G43.C Periodic headache syndromes in child or adult**
   **G43.CØ Periodic headache syndromes in child or adult,
        not intractable**
        Periodic headache syndromes in child or adult,
        without refractory migraine
   **G43.C1 Periodic headache syndromes in child or adult,
        intractable**
        Periodic headache syndromes in child or adult,
        with refractory migraine
● **G43.D Abdominal migraine**
   G43.DØ Abdominal migraine, not intractable
        Abdominal migraine, without refractory
        migraine
   G43.D1 Abdominal migraine, intractable
        Abdominal migraine, with refractory migraine
● **G43.8 Other migraine**
   ● **G43.8Ø Other migraine, not intractable**
        Other migraine, without refractory migraine
        **G43.8Ø1 Other migraine, not intractable, with
            status migrainosus**
        **G43.8Ø9 Other migraine, not intractable,
            without status migrainosus**
   ● **G43.81 Other migraine, intractable**
        Other migraine, with refractory migraine
        **G43.811 Other migraine, intractable, with
            status migrainosus**
        **G43.819 Other migraine, intractable, without
            status migrainosus**
   ● **G43.82 Menstrual migraine, not intractable**
        Menstrual headache, not intractable
        Menstrual migraine, without refractory
        migraine
        Menstrually related migraine, not intractable
        Pre-menstrual headache, not intractable
        Pre-menstrual migraine, not intractable
        Pure menstrual migraine, not intractable
        Code also associated premenstrual tension
        syndrome (N94.3)
        **G43.821 Menstrual migraine, not intractable,
            with status migrainosus ♀**
        **G43.829 Menstrual migraine, not intractable,
            without status migrainosus ♀**
            Menstrual migraine NOS
   ● **G43.83 Menstrual migraine, intractable**
        Menstrual headache, intractable
        Menstrual migraine, with refractory migraine
        Menstrually related migraine, intractable
        Pre-menstrual headache, intractable
        Pre-menstrual migraine, intractable
        Pure menstrual migraine, intractable
        Code also associated premenstrual tension
        syndrome (N94.3)
        **G43.831 Menstrual migraine, intractable, with
            status migrainosus ♀**
        **G43.839 Menstrual migraine, intractable,
            without status migrainosus ♀**

● **G43.9 Migraine, unspecified**
   ● **G43.9Ø Migraine, unspecified, not intractable**
        Migraine, unspecified, without refractory
        migraine
        **G43.9Ø1 Migraine, unspecified, not intractable,
            with status migrainosus**
            Status migrainosus NOS
        **G43.9Ø9 Migraine, unspecified, not intractable,
            without status migrainosus**
            Migraine NOS
   ● **G43.91 Migraine, unspecified, intractable**
        Migraine, unspecified, with refractory
        migraine
        **G43.911 Migraine, unspecified, intractable,
            with status migrainosus**
        **G43.919 Migraine, unspecified, intractable,
            without status migrainosus**
● **G44 Other headache syndromes**
   Excludes1 headache NOS (R51)
   Excludes2 atypical facial pain (G5Ø.1)
        headache due to lumbar puncture (G97.1)
        migraines (G43.-)
        trigeminal neuralgia (G5Ø.Ø)
   ● **G44.Ø Cluster headaches and other trigeminal autonomic
        cephalgias (TAC)**
      ● **G44.ØØ Cluster headache syndrome, unspecified**
            Ciliary neuralgia
            Cluster headache NOS
            Histamine cephalgia
            Lower half migraine
            Migrainous neuralgia
            **G44.ØØ1 Cluster headache
                syndrome, unspecified, intractable**
            **G44.ØØ9 Cluster headache
                syndrome, unspecified, not intractable**
                Cluster headache syndrome NOS
      ● **G44.Ø1 Episodic cluster headache**
            G44.Ø11 Episodic cluster headache, intractable
            **G44.Ø19 Episodic cluster headache, not
                intractable**
                Episodic cluster headache NOS
      ● **G44.Ø2 Chronic cluster headache**
            G44.Ø21 Chronic cluster headache, intractable
            **G44.Ø29 Chronic cluster headache, not
                intractable**
                Chronic cluster headache NOS
      ● **G44.Ø3 Episodic paroxysmal hemicrania**
            Paroxysmal hemicrania NOS
            **G44.Ø31 Episodic paroxysmal hemicrania,
                intractable**
            **G44.Ø39 Episodic paroxysmal hemicrania, not
                intractable**
                Episodic paroxysmal hemicrania
                NOS
      ● **G44.Ø4 Chronic paroxysmal hemicrania**
            Unilateral headache
            **G44.Ø41 Chronic paroxysmal hemicrania,
                intractable**
            **G44.Ø49 Chronic paroxysmal hemicrania, not
                intractable**
                Chronic paroxysmal hemicrania
                NOS

CHAPTER 6 (G00-G99)

● **G44.05** **Short lasting unilateral neuralgiform headache with conjunctival injection and tearing (SUNCT)**

    G44.051 **Short lasting unilateral neuralgiform headache with conjunctival injection and tearing (SUNCT), intractable**

    G44.059 **Short lasting unilateral neuralgiform headache with conjunctival injection and tearing (SUNCT), not intractable**
        Short lasting unilateral neuralgiform headache with conjunctival injection and tearing (SUNCT) NOS

● **G44.09** **Other trigeminal autonomic cephalgias (TAC)**
    Cluster headaches

    G44.091 **Other trigeminal autonomic cephalgias (TAC), intractable**

    G44.099 **Other trigeminal autonomic cephalgias (TAC), not intractable**

G44.1 **Vascular headache, not elsewhere classified**

    Excludes2   cluster headache (G44.0)
        complicated headache syndromes (G44.5-)
        drug-induced headache (G44.4-)
        migraine (G43.-)
        other specified headache syndromes (G44.8-)
        post-traumatic headache (G44.3-)
        tension-type headache (G44.2-)

● **G44.2** **Tension-type headache**

  ● **G44.20** **Tension-type headache, unspecified**

    G44.201 **Tension-type headache, unspecified, intractable**

    G44.209 **Tension-type headache, unspecified, not intractable**
        Tension headache NOS

  ● **G44.21** **Episodic tension-type headache**

    G44.211 **Episodic tension-type headache, intractable**

    G44.219 **Episodic tension-type headache, not intractable**
        Episodic tension-type headache NOS

  ● **G44.22** **Chronic tension-type headache**

    G44.221 **Chronic tension-type headache, intractable**

    G44.229 **Chronic tension-type headache, not intractable**
        Chronic tension-type headache NOS

● **G44.3** **Post-traumatic headache**

  ● **G44.30** **Post-traumatic headache, unspecified**

    G44.301 **Post-traumatic headache, unspecified, intractable**

    G44.309 **Post-traumatic headache, unspecified, not intractable**
        Post-traumatic headache NOS

  ● **G44.31** **Acute post-traumatic headache**

    G44.311 **Acute post-traumatic headache, intractable**

    G44.319 **Acute post-traumatic headache, not intractable**
        Acute post-traumatic headache NOS

  ● **G44.32** **Chronic post-traumatic headache**

    G44.321 **Chronic post-traumatic headache, intractable**

    G44.329 **Chronic post-traumatic headache, not intractable**
        Chronic post-traumatic headache NOS

● **G44.4** **Drug-induced headache, not elsewhere classified**
    Medication overuse headache

    Use additional code for adverse effect, if applicable, to identify drug (T36-T50 with fifth or sixth character 5)

    G44.40 **Drug-induced headache, not elsewhere classified, not intractable**

    G44.41 **Drug-induced headache, not elsewhere classified, intractable**

● **G44.5** **Complicated headache syndromes**

    G44.51 **Hemicrania continua**
        Persistent unilateral headache

    G44.52 **New daily persistent headache (NDPH)**

    G44.53 **Primary thunderclap headache**

    G44.59 **Other complicated headache syndrome**

● **G44.8** **Other specified headache syndromes**

    G44.81 **Hypnic headache**
        Benign primary headaches

    G44.82 **Headache associated with sexual activity**
        Orgasmic headache
        Preorgasmic headache

    G44.83 **Primary cough headache**

    G44.84 **Primary exertional headache**

    G44.85 **Primary stabbing headache**

    G44.89 **Other headache syndrome**

● **G45** **Transient cerebral ischemic attacks and related syndromes**

    Excludes1 neonatal cerebral ischemia (P91.0)
        transient retinal artery occlusion (H34.0-)

  G45.0 **Vertebro-basilar artery syndrome**

  G45.1 **Carotid artery syndrome (hemispheric)**

  G45.2 **Multiple and bilateral precerebral artery syndromes**

  G45.3 **Amaurosis fugax**
    Transient visual loss in one eye

  G45.4 **Transient global amnesia**
    Episode of short-term memory loss, nonrecurrent, lasting few hours

    Excludes1 amnesia NOS (R41.3)

  G45.8 **Other transient cerebral ischemic attacks and related syndromes**

  G45.9 **Transient cerebral ischemic attack, unspecified**
    Spasm of cerebral artery
    TIA
    Transient cerebral ischemia NOS

● **G46** **Vascular syndromes of brain in cerebrovascular diseases**
    Code first underlying cerebrovascular disease (I60-I69)

  G46.0 **Middle cerebral artery syndrome**

  G46.1 **Anterior cerebral artery syndrome**

  G46.2 **Posterior cerebral artery syndrome**

  G46.3 **Brain stem stroke syndrome**
    Benedikt syndrome
    Claude syndrome
    Foville syndrome
    Millard-Gubler syndrome
    Wallenberg syndrome
    Weber syndrome

  G46.4 **Cerebellar stroke syndrome**

  G46.5 **Pure motor lacunar syndrome**
    Occlusion of single deep penetrating artery

  G46.6 **Pure sensory lacunar syndrome**

  G46.7 **Other lacunar syndromes**

  G46.8 **Other vascular syndromes of brain in cerebrovascular diseases**

◄ New   ◄▦ Revised   ~~deleted~~ Deleted   Excludes 1   Excludes 2   Includes   Use additional   Code first   Code also   Unspecified

OGCR Official Guidelines   **X** Assign placeholder X   ● Use Additional Character(s)   ▶ Manifestation Code   **Coding Clinic**

● **G47   Sleep disorders**

     Excludes2   nightmares (F51.5)
                    nonorganic sleep disorders (F51.-)
                    sleep terrors (F51.4)
                    sleepwalking (F51.3)

● **G47.0   Insomnia**

     Excludes2   alcohol related insomnia (F10.182, F10.282, F10.982)
                    drug-related insomnia (F11.182, F11.282, F11.982, F13.182, F13.282, F13.982, F14.182, F14.282, F14.982, F15.182, F15.282, F15.982, F19.182, F19.282, F19.982)
                    idiopathic insomnia (F51.01)
                    insomnia due to a mental disorder (F51.05)
                    insomnia not due to a substance or known physiological condition (F51.0-)
                    nonorganic insomnia (F51.0-)
                    primary insomnia (F51.01)
                    sleep apnea (G47.3-)

     G47.00   Insomnia, unspecified
                Insomnia NOS

     G47.01   Insomnia due to medical condition
                Code also associated medical condition

     G47.09   Other insomnia

● **G47.1   Hypersomnia**

     Excludes2   alcohol-related hypersomnia (F10.182, F10.282, F10.982)
                    drug-related hypersomnia (F11.182, F11.282, F11.982, F13.182, F13.282, F13.982, F14.182, F14.282, F14.982, F15.182, F15.282, F15.982, F19.182, F19.282, F19.982)
                    hypersomnia due to a mental disorder (F51.13)
                    hypersomnia not due to a substance or known physiological condition (F51.1-)
                    primary hypersomnia (F51.11)
                    sleep apnea (G47.3-)

     G47.10   Hypersomnia, unspecified
                Hypersomnia NOS

     G47.11   Idiopathic hypersomnia with long sleep time
                Idiopathic hypersomnia NOS

     G47.12   Idiopathic hypersomnia without long sleep time

     G47.13   Recurrent hypersomnia
                Kleine-Levin syndrome
                Menstrual related hypersomnia

     G47.14   Hypersomnia due to medical condition
                Code also associated medical condition

     G47.19   Other hypersomnia

● **G47.2   Circadian rhythm sleep disorders**
           Disorders of the sleep wake schedule
           Inversion of nyctohemeral rhythm
           Inversion of sleep rhythm

     G47.20   Circadian rhythm sleep disorder, unspecified type
                Sleep wake schedule disorder NOS

     G47.21   Circadian rhythm sleep disorder, delayed sleep phase type
                Delayed sleep phase syndrome

     G47.22   Circadian rhythm sleep disorder, advanced sleep phase type

     G47.23   Circadian rhythm sleep disorder, irregular sleep wake type
                Irregular sleep-wake pattern

     G47.24   Circadian rhythm sleep disorder, free running type

     G47.25   Circadian rhythm sleep disorder, jet lag type

     G47.26   Circadian rhythm sleep disorder, shift work type

▶ **G47.27   *Circadian rhythm sleep disorder in conditions classified elsewhere***
                Code first underlying condition

     G47.29   Other circadian rhythm sleep disorder

● **G47.3   Sleep apnea**
           Characterized by episodes in which breathing stops during sleep
           Code also any associated underlying condition

     Excludes1   apnea NOS (R06.81)
                    Cheyne-Stokes breathing (R06.3)
                    pickwickian syndrome (E66.2)
                    sleep apnea of newborn (P28.3)

     G47.30   Sleep apnea, unspecified
                Sleep apnea NOS

     G47.31   Primary central sleep apnea

     G47.32   High altitude periodic breathing

     G47.33   Obstructive sleep apnea (adult) (pediatric)
          Excludes1   obstructive sleep apnea of newborn (P28.3)

     G47.34   Idiopathic sleep related nonobstructive alveolar hypoventilation
                Sleep related hypoxia

     G47.35   Congenital central alveolar hypoventilation syndrome

▶ **G47.36   *Sleep related hypoventilation in conditions classified elsewhere***
                Sleep related hypoxemia in conditions classified elsewhere
                Code first underlying condition

▶ **G47.37   *Central sleep apnea in conditions classified elsewhere***
                Code first underlying condition

     G47.39   Other sleep apnea

● **G47.4   Narcolepsy and cataplexy**
           *Cataplexy is a disorder evidenced by seizures including minor slacking of the facial muscles to complete collapse and often affects people who have **narcolepsy**, a disorder in which there is great difficulty remaining awake during the daytime.*

     ● **G47.41   Narcolepsy**

         G47.411   Narcolepsy with cataplexy

         G47.419   Narcolepsy without cataplexy
                    Narcolepsy NOS

     ● **G47.42   Narcolepsy in conditions classified elsewhere**
                Code first underlying condition

         ▶ **G47.421   *Narcolepsy in conditions classified elsewhere with cataplexy***

         ▶ **G47.429   *Narcolepsy in conditions classified elsewhere without cataplexy***

● **G47.5   Parasomnia**

     Excludes1   alcohol induced parasomnia (F10.182, F10.282, F10.982)
                    drug induced parasomnia (F11.182, F11.282, F11.982, F13.182, F13.282, F13.982, F14.182, F14.282, F14.982, F15.182, F15.282, F15.982, F19.182, F19.282, F19.982)
                    parasomnia not due to a substance or known physiological condition (F51.8)

     G47.50   Parasomnia, unspecified
                Parasomnia NOS

     G47.51   Confusional arousals

     G47.52   REM sleep behavior disorder

     G47.53   Recurrent isolated sleep paralysis

▶ **G47.54   *Parasomnia in conditions classified elsewhere***
                Code first underlying condition

     G47.59   Other parasomnia

CHAPTER 6 (G00-G99)

CHAPTER 6 (G00-G99)

● G47.6   **Sleep related movement disorders**
> **Excludes2**   restless legs syndrome (G25.81)

    G47.61   **Periodic limb movement disorder**
> Periodic limb movement disorder

    G47.62   **Sleep related leg cramps**

    G47.63   **Sleep related bruxism**
> **Excludes1**   psychogenic bruxism (F45.8)

    G47.69   **Other sleep related movement disorders**

   G47.8   **Other sleep disorders**

   G47.9   **Sleep disorder, unspecified**
> Sleep disorder NOS

★**(See Plate 118 on page 54.)**

NERVE, NERVE ROOT AND PLEXUS DISORDERS (G50-G59)

> **Excludes1**   current traumatic nerve, nerve root and plexus disorders - see Injury, nerve by body region
> neuralgia NOS (M79.2)
> neuritis NOS (M79.2)
> peripheral neuritis in pregnancy (O26.82-)
> radiculitis NOS (M54.1-)

● G50   **Disorders of trigeminal nerve**
> **Includes**   disorders of 5th cranial nerve

   G50.0   **Trigeminal neuralgia**
> Syndrome of paroxysmal facial pain
> Tic douloureux

   G50.1   **Atypical facial pain**

   G50.8   **Other disorders of trigeminal nerve**

   G50.9   **Disorder of trigeminal nerve, unspecified**

● G51   **Facial nerve disorders**
> **Includes**   disorders of 7th cranial nerve

   G51.0   **Bell's palsy**
> Facial palsy

   G51.1   **Geniculate ganglionitis**
> *Rare disorder with symptoms of severe pain deep in ear, spreading to ear canal, outer ear, mastoid or eye regions*
> **Excludes1**   postherpetic geniculate ganglionitis (B02.21)

   G51.2   **Melkersson's syndrome**
> Melkersson-Rosenthal syndrome

   G51.3   **Clonic hemifacial spasm**

   G51.4   **Facial myokymia**
> *Involuntary facial muscle movement*

   G51.8   **Other disorders of facial nerve**

   G51.9   **Disorder of facial nerve, unspecified**

● G52   **Disorders of other cranial nerves**
> **Excludes2**   disorders of acoustic [8th] nerve (H93.3)
> disorders of optic [2nd] nerve (H46, H47.0)
> paralytic strabismus due to nerve palsy (H49.0-H49.2)

   G52.0   **Disorders of olfactory nerve**
> Disorders of 1st cranial nerve

   G52.1   **Disorders of glossopharyngeal nerve**
> Disorder of 9th cranial nerve
> Glossopharyngeal neuralgia

   G52.2   **Disorders of vagus nerve**
> Disorders of pneumogastric [10th] nerve

   G52.3   **Disorders of hypoglossal nerve**
> Disorders of 12th cranial nerve

Item 6-5   **Trigeminal neuralgia,** tic douloureux, is a pain syndrome diagnosed from the patient's history alone. The condition is characterized by pain and a brief facial spasm or tic. Pain is unilateral and follows the sensory distribution of cranial nerve V, typically radiating to the maxillary (V2) or mandibular (V3) area.

Item 6-6   The most common facial nerve disorder is **Bell's Palsy,** which occurs suddenly and results in facial drooping unilaterally. This disorder is the result of a reaction to a virus that causes the facial nerve in the ear to swell resulting in pressure in the bony canal.

   G52.7   **Disorders of multiple cranial nerves**
> Polyneuritis cranialis

   G52.8   **Disorders of other specified cranial nerves**

   G52.9   **Cranial nerve disorder, unspecified**

▌ G53   *Cranial nerve disorders in diseases classified elsewhere*
> *Code first* underlying disease, such as:
> neoplasm (C00-D49)
> **Excludes1**   multiple cranial nerve palsy in sarcoidosis (D86.82)
> multiple cranial nerve palsy in syphilis (A52.15)
> postherpetic geniculate ganglionitis (B02.21)
> postherpetic trigeminal neuralgia (B02.22)

● G54   **Nerve root and plexus disorders**
> *Raiculopathy (nerve root disorder) caused by pressure on nerve root, most common cause is herniation of intervertebral disk. Plexus disorders (plexopathies) are due to compression or injury.*
> **Excludes1**   current traumatic nerve root and plexus disorders - see nerve injury by body region
> intervertebral disc disorders (M50-M51)
> neuralgia or neuritis NOS (M79.2)
> neuritis or radiculitis brachial NOS (M54.13)
> neuritis or radiculitis lumbar NOS (M54.16)
> neuritis or radiculitis lumbosacral NOS (M54.17)
> neuritis or radiculitis thoracic NOS (M54.14)
> radiculitis NOS (M54.10)
> radiculopathy NOS (M54.10)
> spondylosis (M47.-)

   G54.0   **Brachial plexus disorders**
> Thoracic outlet syndrome

   G54.1   **Lumbosacral plexus disorders**

   G54.2   **Cervical root disorders, not elsewhere classified**

   G54.3   **Thoracic root disorders, not elsewhere classified**

   G54.4   **Lumbosacral root disorders, not elsewhere classified**

   G54.5   **Neuralgic amyotrophy**
> Parsonage-Aldren-Turner syndrome
> Shoulder-girdle neuritis
> **Excludes1**   neuralgic amyotrophy in diabetes mellitus (E08-E13 with .44)

   G54.6   **Phantom limb syndrome with pain**
> *Sensations (cramping, itching) in a limb that no longer exists*

   G54.7   **Phantom limb syndrome without pain**
> Phantom limb syndrome NOS

   G54.8   **Other nerve root and plexus disorders**

   G54.9   **Nerve root and plexus disorder, unspecified**

▌ G55   *Nerve root and plexus compressions in diseases classified elsewhere*
> *Code first* underlying disease, such as:
> neoplasm (C00-D49)
> **Excludes1**   nerve root compression (due to) (in) ankylosing spondylitis (M45.-)
> nerve root compression (due to) (in)dorsopathies (M53.-, M54.-)
> nerve root compression (due to) (in)intervertebral disc disorders (M50.1.-, M51.1.-)
> nerve root compression (due to) (in) spondylopathies (M46.-, M48.-)

★**(See Plates 472 and 473 on pages 56 and 57.)**

● G56   **Mononeuropathies of upper limb**
> **Excludes1**   current traumatic nerve disorder - see nerve injury by body region

   ● **G56.0**   **Carpal tunnel syndrome**

     G56.00   **Carpal tunnel syndrome, unspecified upper limb**

     G56.01   **Carpal tunnel syndrome, right upper limb**

     G56.02   **Carpal tunnel syndrome, left upper limb**

     G56.03   **Carpal tunnel syndrome, bilateral upper limbs** ◀

◀ New   ⇐ Revised   ~~deleted~~ Deleted   Excludes 1   Excludes 2   Includes   Use additional   Code first   Code also   Unspecified

OGCR Official Guidelines   X Assign placeholder X   ● Use Additional Character(s)   ▌ Manifestation Code   **Coding Clinic**

● **G56.1**   **Other lesions of median nerve**
     G56.10   Other lesions of median nerve, unspecified side
     G56.11   Other lesions of median nerve, right upper limb
     G56.12   Other lesions of median nerve, left upper limb
     G56.13   Other lesions of median nerve, bilateral upper limbs ◄

● **G56.2**   **Lesion of ulnar nerve**
     Tardy ulnar nerve palsy
     G56.20   Lesion of ulnar nerve, unspecified upper limb
     G56.21   Lesion of ulnar nerve, right upper limb
     G56.22   Lesion of ulnar nerve, left upper limb
     G56.23   Lesion of ulnar nerve, bilateral upper limbs ◄

● **G56.3**   **Lesion of radial nerve**
     G56.30   Lesion of radial nerve, unspecified upper limb
     G56.31   Lesion of radial nerve, right upper limb
     G56.32   Lesion of radial nerve, left upper limb
     G56.33   Lesion of radial nerve, bilateral upper limbs ◄

● **G56.4**   **Causalgia of upper limb**
     Intense burning pain and sensitivity to slight touch
     Complex regional pain syndrome II of upper limb

     Excludes1   complex regional pain syndrome I of lower limb (G90.52-)
                complex regional pain syndrome I of upper limb (G90.51-)
                complex regional pain syndrome II of lower limb (G57.7-)
                reflex sympathetic dystrophy of lower limb (G90.52-)
                reflex sympathetic dystrophy (G90.51-)

     G56.40   Causalgia of unspecified upper limb
     G56.41   Causalgia of right upper limb
     G56.42   Causalgia of left upper limb
     G56.43   Causalgia of bilateral upper limbs ◄

● **G56.8**   **Other specified mononeuropathies of upper limb**
     Disease of a single nerve
     Interdigital neuroma of upper limb
     G56.80   Other specified mononeuropathies of unspecified upper limb
     G56.81   Other specified mononeuropathies of right upper limb
     G56.82   Other specified mononeuropathies of left upper limb
     G56.83   Other specified mononeuropathies of bilateral upper limbs ◄

● **G56.9**   **Unspecified mononeuropathy of upper limb**
     Disease of a single nerve
     G56.90   Unspecified mononeuropathy of unspecified upper limb
     G56.91   Unspecified mononeuropathy of right upper limb
     G56.92   Unspecified mononeuropathy of left upper limb
     G56.93   Unspecified mononeuropathy of bilateral upper limbs ◄

● **G57**   **Mononeuropathies of lower limb**
     Excludes1   current traumatic nerve disorder - see nerve injury by body region

★ **(See Plates 544 and 545 on pages 58 and 59.)**

   ● **G57.0**   **Lesion of sciatic nerve**
     Excludes1   sciatica NOS (M54.3-)
     Excludes2   sciatica attributed to intervertebral disc disorder (M51.1.-)
     G57.00   Lesion of sciatic nerve, unspecified lower limb
     G57.01   Lesion of sciatic nerve, right lower limb
     G57.02   Lesion of sciatic nerve, left lower limb
     G57.03   Lesion of sciatic nerve, bilateral lower limbs ◄

● **G57.1**   **Meralgia paresthetica**
     Numbness or pain in outer thigh caused by injury to nerve
     Lateral cutaneous nerve of thigh syndrome
     G57.10   Meralgia paresthetica, unspecified lower limb
     G57.11   Meralgia paresthetica, right lower limb
     G57.12   Meralgia paresthetica, left lower limb
     G57.13   Meralgia paresthetica, bilateral lower limbs ◄

● **G57.2**   **Lesion of femoral nerve**
     G57.20   Lesion of femoral nerve, unspecified lower limb
     G57.21   Lesion of femoral nerve, right lower limb
     G57.22   Lesion of femoral nerve, left lower limb
     G57.23   Lesion of femoral nerve, bilateral lower limbs ◄

● **G57.3**   **Lesion of lateral popliteal nerve**
     Peroneal nerve palsy
     G57.30   Lesion of lateral popliteal nerve, unspecified lower limb
     G57.31   Lesion of lateral popliteal nerve, right lower limb
     G57.32   Lesion of lateral popliteal nerve, left lower limb
     G57.33   Lesion of lateral popliteal nerve, bilateral lower limbs ◄

● **G57.4**   **Lesion of medial popliteal nerve**
     G57.40   Lesion of medial popliteal nerve, unspecified lower limb
     G57.41   Lesion of medial popliteal nerve, right lower limb
     G57.42   Lesion of medial popliteal nerve, left lower limb
     G57.43   Lesion of medial popliteal nerve, bilateral lower limbs ◄

● **G57.5**   **Tarsal tunnel syndrome**
     G57.50   Tarsal tunnel syndrome, unspecified lower limb
     G57.51   Tarsal tunnel syndrome, right lower limb
     G57.52   Tarsal tunnel syndrome, left lower limb
     G57.53   Tarsal tunnel syndrome, bilateral lower limbs ◄

● **G57.6**   **Lesion of plantar nerve**
     Morton's metatarsalgia
     G57.60   Lesion of plantar nerve, unspecified lower limb
     G57.61   Lesion of plantar nerve, right lower limb
     G57.62   Lesion of plantar nerve, left lower limb
     G57.63   Lesion of plantar nerve, bilateral lower limbs ◄

● **G57.7**   **Causalgia of lower limb**
     Complex regional pain syndrome II of lower limb

     Excludes1   complex regional pain syndrome I of lower limb (G90.52-)
                complex regional pain syndrome I of upper limb (G90.51-)
                complex regional pain syndrome II of upper limb (G56.4-)
                reflex sympathetic dystrophy of lower limb (G90.52-)
                reflex sympathetic dystrophy of upper limb (G90.51-)

     G57.70   Causalgia of unspecified lower limb
     G57.71   Causalgia of right lower limb
     G57.72   Causalgia of left lower limb
     G57.73   Causalgia of bilateral lower limbs ◄

● **G57.8**   **Other specified mononeuropathies of lower limb**
     Interdigital neuroma of lower limb
     G57.80   Other specified mononeuropathies of unspecified lower limb
     G57.81   Other specified mononeuropathies of right lower limb
     G57.82   Other specified mononeuropathies of left lower limb
     G57.83   Other specified mononeuropathies of bilateral lower limbs ◄

CHAPTER 6 (G00-G99)

● G57.9   Unspecified mononeuropathy of lower limb
  G57.90   Unspecified mononeuropathy of unspecified lower limb
  G57.91   Unspecified mononeuropathy of right lower limb
  G57.92   Unspecified mononeuropathy of left lower limb
  G57.93   Unspecified mononeuropathy of bilateral lower limbs ◀

● G58   Other mononeuropathies
  G58.0   Intercostal neuropathy
  G58.7   Mononeuritis multiplex
  G58.8   Other specified mononeuropathies
  G58.9   Mononeuropathy, unspecified

▶ G59   *Mononeuropathy in diseases classified elsewhere*
        Code first underlying disease
        Excludes1   diabetic mononeuropathy (E08-E13 with .41)
                        syphilitic nerve paralysis (A52.19)
                        syphilitic neuritis (A52.15)
                        tuberculous mononeuropathy (A17.83)

POLYNEUROPATHIES AND OTHER DISORDERS OF THE PERIPHERAL NERVOUS SYSTEM (G60-G65)

        Excludes1   neuralgia NOS (M79.2)
                        neuritis NOS (M79.2)
                        peripheral neuritis in pregnancy (O26.82-)
                        radiculitis NOS (M54.10)

● G60   Hereditary and idiopathic neuropathy
  G60.0   **Hereditary motor and sensory neuropathy**
          Charcot-Marie-Tooth disease
          Déjerine-Sottas disease
          Hereditary motor and sensory neuropathy, types I-IV
          Hypertrophic neuropathy of infancy
          Peroneal muscular atrophy (axonal type) (hypertrophic type)
          Roussy-Lévy syndrome
  G60.1   **Refsum's disease**
          Genetic disorder affecting fatty acid metabolism
          Infantile Refsum disease
  G60.2   **Neuropathy in association with hereditary ataxia**

Item 6-7   The **peripheral nervous system** consists of 31 pairs of spinal nerves, 12 pairs of cranial nerves, and the autonomic nerves, which are divided into the parasympathetic and sympathetic nerves. The cranial nerves are: olfactory (I), optic (II), oculomotor (III), trochlear (IV), trigeminal (V), abducens (VI), facial (VII), vestibulocochlear (VIII), glossopharyngeal (IX), vagus (X), accessory (XI), and hypoglossal (XII).

  G60.3   **Idiopathic progressive neuropathy**
  G60.8   **Other hereditary and idiopathic neuropathies**
          Dominantly inherited sensory neuropathy
          Morvan's disease
          Nelaton's syndrome
          Recessively inherited sensory neuropathy
  G60.9   **Hereditary and idiopathic neuropathy, unspecified**

● G61   Inflammatory polyneuropathy
  G61.0   **Guillain-Barré syndrome**
          Autoimmune disease affecting peripheral nervous system
          Acute (post-)infective polyneuritis
          Miller Fisher Syndrome
  G61.1   **Serum neuropathy**
          Use additional code for adverse effect, if applicable, to identify serum (T50.-)
● G61.8   **Other inflammatory polyneuropathies**
  G61.81   Chronic inflammatory demyelinating polyneuritis
  G61.82   Multifocal motor neuropathy ◀
           MMN ◀
  G61.89   Other inflammatory polyneuropathies
  G61.9   Inflammatory polyneuropathy, unspecified

● G62   Other and unspecified polyneuropathies
  G62.0   **Drug-induced polyneuropathy**
          Use additional code for adverse effect, if applicable, to identify drug (T36-T50 with fifth or sixth character 5)
  G62.1   **Alcoholic polyneuropathy**
          Malfunction of many peripheral nerves throughout the body
  G62.2   **Polyneuropathy due to other toxic agents**
          Code first (T51-T65) to identify toxic agent

SYMPATHETIC	PARASYMPATHETIC
Pupils dilated	Pupils constricted
Salivation inhibited	Salivation stimulated
Increased respiration	Decreased respiration
Bronchial passages dilated	Bronchial passages constricted
Increased heart rate	Decreased heart rate
Increased secretion by sweat glands	
Hair follicles raised; goose bumps	
Secretion of adrenal hormones	
Digestion inhibited	Digestion stimulated
Bladder muscles relaxed (filling)	Bladder muscles contracted (emptying)

Figure 6-2   Actions of parasympathetic and sympathetic nerves. (From Chabner: The Language of Medicine, ed 9, St. Louis, Saunders, 2011)

◀ New   ◀▥ Revised   ~~deleted~~ Deleted   Excludes 1   Excludes 2   Includes   Use additional   Code first   Code also   Unspecified

786   OGCR Official Guidelines   X Assign placeholder X   ● Use Additional Character(s)   ▶ Manifestation Code   **Coding Clinic**

● G62.8   Other specified polyneuropathies
　　　 G62.81   Critical illness polyneuropathy
　　　　　 Acute motor neuropathy
　　　 G62.82   Radiation-induced polyneuropathy
　　　　　 Use additional external cause code (W88-W90, X39.0-) to identify cause
　　　 G62.89   Other specified polyneuropathies
　　　　　 Coding Clinic: 2016, Q2, P11
　 G62.9   Polyneuropathy, unspecified
　　　 Neuropathy NOS

▷ G63   *Polyneuropathy in diseases classified elsewhere*
　　 Code first underlying disease, such as:
　　　 amyloidosis (E85.-)
　　　 endocrine disease, except diabetes (E00-E07, E15-E16, E20-E34)
　　　 metabolic diseases (E70-E88)
　　　 neoplasm (C00-D49)
　　　 nutritional deficiency (E40-E64)
　　 Excludes1   polyneuropathy (in):
　　　　　 diabetes mellitus (E08-E13 with .42)
　　　　　 diphtheria (A36.83)
　　　　　 infectious mononucleosis (B27.0-B27.9 with 1)
　　　　　 Lyme disease (A69.22)
　　　　　 mumps (B26.84)
　　　　　 postherpetic (B02.23)
　　　　　 rheumatoid arthritis (M05.33)
　　　　　 scleroderma (M34.83)
　　　　　 systemic lupus erythematosus (M32.19)
　　 Coding Clinic: 2012, Q4, P100

G64   Other disorders of peripheral nervous system
　　　 Disorder of peripheral nervous system NOS

● G65   Sequelae of inflammatory and toxic polyneuropathies
　　 Code first condition resulting from (sequela) of inflammatory and toxic polyneuropathies
　　 G65.0   Sequelae of Guillain-Barré syndrome
　　 G65.1   Sequelae of other inflammatory polyneuropathy
　　 G65.2   Sequelae of toxic polyneuropathy

DISEASES OF MYONEURAL JUNCTION AND MUSCLE (G70-G73)

● G70   Myasthenia gravis and other myoneural disorders
　　 Excludes1   botulism (A05.1, A48.51-A48.52)
　　　　　 transient neonatal myasthenia gravis (P94.0)
　 ● G70.0   Myasthenia gravis
　　　 Acquired and results in fatigable muscle weakness exacerbated by activity and improved with rest
　　　 G70.00   Myasthenia gravis without (acute) exacerbation
　　　　　 Myasthenia gravis NOS
　　　 G70.01   Myasthenia gravis with (acute) exacerbation
　　　　　 Myasthenia gravis in crisis
　　 G70.1   Toxic myoneural disorders
　　　 Dysfunction at junction of muscle and motor nerve (myoneural junction)
　　　 Code first (T51-T65) to identify toxic agent
　　 G70.2   Congenital and developmental myasthenia
　 ● G70.8   Other specified myoneural disorders
　　　 G70.80   Lambert-Eaton syndrome, unspecified
　　　　　 Lambert-Eaton syndrome NOS
　　 ▷ G70.81   *Lambert-Eaton syndrome in disease classified elsewhere*
　　　　　 Code first underlying disease
　　　　　 Excludes1   Lambert-Eaton syndrome in neoplastic disease (G73.1)
　　　 G70.89   Other specified myoneural disorders
　　 G70.9   Myoneural disorder, unspecified

Item 6-8   Muscular dystrophies (MD) are a group of rare inherited muscle diseases. Voluntary muscles become progressively weaker. In the late stages of MD, fat and connective tissue replace muscle fibers. In some types of muscular dystrophy, heart muscles, other involuntary muscles, and other organs are affected. **Myopathies** is a general term for neuromuscular diseases in which the muscle fibers dysfunction for any one of many reasons, resulting in muscular weakness.

● G71   Primary disorders of muscles
　　 Excludes2   arthrogryposis multiplex congenita (Q74.3)
　　　　　 metabolic disorders (E70-E88)
　　　　　 myositis (M60.-)
　　 G71.0   Muscular dystrophy
　　　 Autosomal recessive, childhood type, muscular dystrophy resembling Duchenne or Becker muscular dystrophy
　　　 Benign [Becker] muscular dystrophy
　　　 Benign scapuloperoneal muscular dystrophy with early contractures [Emery-Dreifuss]
　　　 Congenital muscular dystrophy NOS
　　　 Congenital muscular dystrophy with specific morphological abnormalities of the muscle fiber
　　　 Distal muscular dystrophy
　　　 Facioscapulohumeral muscular dystrophy
　　　 Limb-girdle muscular dystrophy
　　　 Ocular muscular dystrophy
　　　 Oculopharyngeal muscular dystrophy
　　　 Scapuloperoneal muscular dystrophy
　　　 Severe [Duchenne] muscular dystrophy
　 ● G71.1   Myotonic disorders
　　　 Inherited disorder that affects muscles tone
　　　 G71.11   Myotonic muscular dystrophy
　　　　　 Dystrophia myotonica [Steinert]
　　　　　 Myotonia atrophica
　　　　　 Myotonic dystrophy
　　　　　 Proximal myotonic myopathy (PROMM)
　　　　　 Steinert disease
　　　 G71.12   Myotonia congenita
　　　　　 Acetazolamide responsive myotonia congenita
　　　　　 Dominant myotonia congenita [Thomsen disease]
　　　　　 Myotonia levior
　　　　　 Recessive myotonia congenita [Becker disease]
　　　 G71.13   Myotonic chondrodystrophy
　　　　　 Chondrodystrophic myotonia
　　　　　 Congenital myotonic chondrodystrophy
　　　　　 Schwartz-Jampel disease
　　　 G71.14   Drug induced myotonia
　　　　　 Use additional code for adverse effect, if applicable, to identify drug (T36-T50 with fifth or sixth character 5)
　　　 G71.19   Other specified myotonic disorders
　　　　　 Myotonia fluctuans
　　　　　 Myotonia permanens
　　　　　 Neuromyotonia [Isaacs]
　　　　　 Paramyotonia congenita (of von Eulenburg)
　　　　　 Pseudomyotonia
　　　　　 Symptomatic myotonia
　　 G71.2   Congenital myopathies
　　　 Central core disease
　　　 Fiber-type disproportion
　　　 Minicore disease
　　　 Multicore disease
　　　 Myotubular (centronuclear) myopathy
　　　 Nemaline myopathy
　　　 Excludes1   arthrogryposis multiplex congenita (Q74.3)

CHAPTER 6 (G00-G99)

G71.3 Mitochondrial myopathy, not elsewhere classified
Myopathies associated with increased number of enlarged, often abnormal, mitochondria in muscle fibers

> **Excludes1**   Kearns-Sayre syndrome (H49.81)
> Leber's disease (H47.21)
> Leigh's encephalopathy (G31.82)
> mitochondrial metabolism disorders (E88.4.-)
> Reye's syndrome (G93.7)

G71.8 Other primary disorders of muscles

G71.9 Primary disorder of muscle, unspecified
Hereditary myopathy NOS

● G72 Other and unspecified myopathies

> **Excludes1**   arthrogryposis multiplex congenita (Q74.3)
> dermatopolymyositis (M33.-)
> ischemic infarction of muscle (M62.2-)
> myositis (M60.-)
> polymyositis (M33.2-)

G72.0 Drug-induced myopathy
Use additional code for adverse effect, if applicable, to identify drug (T36-T50 with fifth or sixth character 5)

G72.1 Alcoholic myopathy
Use additional code to identify alcoholism (F10.-)

G72.2 Myopathy due to other toxic agents
Code first (T51-T65) to identify toxic agent

G72.3 Periodic paralysis
Familial periodic paralysis
Hyperkalemic periodic paralysis (familial)
Hypokalemic periodic paralysis (familial)
Myotonic periodic paralysis (familial)
Normokalemic paralysis (familial)
Potassium sensitive periodic paralysis

> **Excludes1**   paramyotonia congenita (of von Eulenburg) (G71.19)

● G72.4 Inflammatory and immune myopathies, not elsewhere classified

> **G72.41 Inclusion body myositis [IBM]**
> **G72.49 Other inflammatory and immune myopathies, not elsewhere classified**
> Inflammatory myopathy NOS

● G72.8 Other specified myopathies

> **G72.81 Critical illness myopathy**
> Acute necrotizing myopathy
> Acute quadriplegic myopathy
> Intensive care (ICU) myopathy
> Myopathy of critical illness
> **G72.89 Other specified myopathies**

G72.9 Myopathy, unspecified

● G73 Disorders of myoneural junction and muscle in diseases classified elsewhere

> **▷ G73.1 Lambert-Eaton syndrome in neoplastic disease**
> *Rare autoimmune disorder affecting calcium channels of nerve-muscle (neuromuscular) junction*
> *Code first underlying neoplasm (C00-D49)*
>
> > **Excludes1**   Lambert-Eaton syndrome not associated with neoplasm (G70.80-G70.81)
>
> **▷ G73.3 Myasthenic syndromes in other diseases classified elsewhere**
> *Code first underlying disease, such as:*
> neoplasm (C00-D49)
> thyrotoxicosis (E05.-)

▷ G73.7 Myopathy in diseases classified elsewhere
Code first underlying disease, such as:
hyperparathyroidism (E21.0, E21.3)
hypoparathyroidism (E20.-)
glycogen storage disease (E74.0)
lipid storage disorders (E75.-)

> **Excludes1**   myopathy in:
> rheumatoid arthritis (M05.32)
> sarcoidosis (D86.87)
> scleroderma (M34.82)
> sicca syndrome [Sjögren] (M35.03)
> systemic lupus erythematosus (M32.19)

CEREBRAL PALSY AND OTHER PARALYTIC SYNDROMES (G80-G83)

● G80 Cerebral palsy

> **Excludes1**   hereditary spastic paraplegia (G11.4)

G80.0 Spastic quadriplegic cerebral palsy
Congenital spastic paralysis (cerebral)

G80.1 Spastic diplegic cerebral palsy
Spastic cerebral palsy NOS

G80.2 Spastic hemiplegic cerebral palsy

G80.3 Athetoid cerebral palsy
Result of damage to cerebellum or basal ganglia responsible for processing neuromuscular signals
Double athetosis (syndrome)
Dyskinetic cerebral palsy
Dystonic cerebral palsy
Vogt disease

G80.4 Ataxic cerebral palsy
Poor muscle tone and coordination

G80.8 Other cerebral palsy
Mixed cerebral palsy syndromes

G80.9 Cerebral palsy, unspecified
Cerebral palsy NOS

OGCR Section I.C.6.a.

Dominant/nondominant side

Codes from category G81, Hemiplegia and hemiparesis, and subcategories, G83.1, Monoplegia of lower limb, G83.2, Monoplegia of upper limb, and G83.3, Monoplegia, unspecified, identify whether the dominant and nondominant side is affected. Should the affected side be documented, but not specified as dominant or nondominant, and the classification system does not indicate a default, code selection is as follows:

- For ambidextrous patients, the default should be dominant.
- If the left side is affected, the default is non-dominant.
- If the right side is affected, the default is dominant.

● G81 Hemiplegia and hemiparesis

> **Note:** This category is to be used only when hemiplegia (complete)(incomplete) is reported without further specification, or is stated to be old or longstanding but of unspecified cause. The category is also for use in multiple coding to identify these types of hemiplegia resulting from any cause.

> **Excludes1**   congenital cerebral palsy (G80.-)
> hemiplegia and hemiparesis due to sequela of cerebrovascular disease (I69.05-, I69.15-, I69.25-, I69.35-, I69.85-, I69.95-)

Coding Clinic: 2012, Q4, P106

● G81.0 Flaccid hemiplegia
Paralysis of half of body with loss of tone of muscles of paralyzed part and absence of tendon reflexes

> **G81.00 Flaccid hemiplegia affecting unspecified side**
> **G81.01 Flaccid hemiplegia affecting right dominant side**
> **G81.02 Flaccid hemiplegia affecting left dominant side**
> **G81.03 Flaccid hemiplegia affecting right nondominant side**
> **G81.04 Flaccid hemiplegia affecting left nondominant side**

Item 6–9 Hemiplegia is complete paralysis of one side of the body— arm, leg, and trunk. **Hemiparesis** is a generalized weakness or incomplete paralysis of one side of the body. If most activities (eating, writing) are performed with the right hand, the right is the dominant side, and the left is the nondominant side. **Quadriplegia,** also called tetraplegia, is the complete paralysis of all four limbs. **Quadriparesis** is the incomplete paralysis of all four limbs. Nerve damage in C1–C4 is associated with lower limb paralysis, and C5–C7 damage is associated with upper limb paralysis. **Diplegia** is the paralysis of the upper limbs. **Monoplegia** is the complete paralysis of one limb.

● **G81.1 Spastic hemiplegia**
     Paralysis of half of body with spasticity of muscles of paralyzed part and increased tendon reflexes
     G81.10 Spastic hemiplegia affecting `unspecified` **side**
     G81.11 Spastic hemiplegia affecting right dominant side
     G81.12 Spastic hemiplegia affecting left dominant side
     G81.13 Spastic hemiplegia affecting right nondominant side
     G81.14 Spastic hemiplegia affecting left nondominant side

● **G81.9 Hemiplegia, unspecified**
     G81.90 Hemiplegia, `unspecified` **affecting unspecified side**
     G81.91 Hemiplegia, `unspecified` **affecting right dominant side**
     G81.92 Hemiplegia, `unspecified` **affecting left dominant side**
     G81.93 Hemiplegia, `unspecified` **affecting right nondominant side**
     G81.94 Hemiplegia, `unspecified` **affecting left nondominant side**
     Coding Clinic: 2015, Q1, P26

● **G82 Paraplegia (paraparesis) and quadriplegia (quadriparesis)**
     Note: This category is to be used only when the listed conditions are reported without further specification, or are stated to be old or longstanding but of unspecified cause. The category is also for use in multiple coding to identify these conditions resulting from any cause.
     `Excludes1` congenital cerebral palsy (G80.-)
              functional quadriplegia (R53.2)
              hysterical paralysis (F44.4)

● **G82.2 Paraplegia**
     Paralysis of both lower limbs NOS
     Paraparesis (lower) NOS
     Paraplegia (lower) NOS
     G82.20 Paraplegia, `unspecified`
     G82.21 Paraplegia, complete
     G82.22 Paraplegia, incomplete

● **G82.5 Quadriplegia**
     Paralysis of all limbs; AKA tetraplegia
     G82.50 Quadriplegia, `unspecified`
     G82.51 Quadriplegia, C1-C4 complete
     G82.52 Quadriplegia, C1-C4 incomplete
     G82.53 Quadriplegia, C5-C7 complete
     G82.54 Quadriplegia, C5-C7 incomplete

● **G83 Other paralytic syndromes**
     Note: This category is to be used only when the listed conditions are reported without further specification, or are stated to be old or longstanding but of unspecified cause. The category is also for use in multiple coding to identify these conditions resulting from any cause.
     `Includes` paralysis (complete) (incomplete), except as in G80-G82

G83.0 Diplegia of upper limbs
     Paralysis affecting limbs on both sides; AKA bilateral paralysis
     Diplegia (upper)
     Paralysis of both upper limbs

● **G83.1 Monoplegia of lower limb**
     Paralysis of limb on one side
     Paralysis of lower limb
     `Excludes1` monoplegia of lower limbs due to sequela of cerebrovascular disease (I69.04-, I69.14-, I69.24-, I69.34-, I69.84-, I69.94-)
     Coding Clinic: 2012, Q4, P106
     G83.10 Monoplegia of lower limb affecting `unspecified` **side**
     G83.11 Monoplegia of lower limb affecting right dominant side
     G83.12 Monoplegia of lower limb affecting left dominant side
     G83.13 Monoplegia of lower limb affecting right nondominant side
     G83.14 Monoplegia of lower limb affecting left nondominant side

● **G83.2 Monoplegia of upper limb**
     Paralysis of upper limb
     `Excludes1` monoplegia of upper limbs due to sequela of cerebrovascular disease (I69.03-, I69.13-, I69.23-, I69.33-, I69.83-, I69.93-)
     Coding Clinic: 2012, Q4, P106
     G83.20 Monoplegia of upper limb affecting `unspecified` **side**
     G83.21 Monoplegia of upper limb affecting right dominant side
     G83.22 Monoplegia of upper limb affecting left dominant side
     G83.23 Monoplegia of upper limb affecting right nondominant side
     G83.24 Monoplegia of upper limb affecting left nondominant side

● **G83.3 Monoplegia, unspecified**
     Coding Clinic: 2012, Q4, P106
     G83.30 Monoplegia, `unspecified` **affecting unspecified side**
     G83.31 Monoplegia, `unspecified` **affecting right dominant side**
     G83.32 Monoplegia, `unspecified` **affecting left dominant side**
     G83.33 Monoplegia, `unspecified` **affecting right nondominant side**
     G83.34 Monoplegia, `unspecified` **affecting left nondominant side**

G83.4 Cauda equina syndrome
     Aching pain due to compression of spinal nerve roots
     Neurogenic bladder due to cauda equina syndrome
     `Excludes1` cord bladder NOS (G95.89)
              neurogenic bladder NOS (N31.9)

G83.5 Locked-in state

● **G83.8 Other specified paralytic syndromes**
     `Excludes1` paralytic syndromes due to current spinal cord injury-code to spinal cord injury (S14, S24, S34)
     G83.81 Brown-Séquard syndrome
     G83.82 Anterior cord syndrome
     G83.83 Posterior cord syndrome
     G83.84 Todd's paralysis (postepileptic)
     G83.89 Other specified paralytic syndromes

G83.9 Paralytic syndrome, `unspecified`

CHAPTER 6 (G00-G99)

OTHER DISORDERS OF THE NERVOUS SYSTEM (G89-G99)

● **G89**   **Pain, not elsewhere classified**

Code also related psychological factors associated with pain (F45.42)

     Excludes1   generalized pain NOS (R52)
                  pain disorders exclusively related to psychological factors (F45.41)
                  pain NOS (R52)

     Excludes2   atypical face pain (G50.1)
                  headache syndromes (G44.-)
                  localized pain, unspecified type - code to pain by site, such as:
                      abdomen pain (R10.-)
                      back pain (M54.9)
                      breast pain (N64.4)
                      chest pain (R07.1-R07.9)
                      ear pain (H92.0-)
                      eye pain (H57.1)
                      headache (R51)
                      joint pain (M25.5-)
                      limb pain (M79.6-)
                      lumbar region pain (M54.5)
                      painful urination (R30.9)
                      pelvic and perineal pain (R10.2)
                      shoulder pain (M25.51-)
                      spine pain (M54.-)
                      throat pain (R07.0)
                      tongue pain (K14.6)
                      tooth pain (K08.8)
                  renal colic (N23)
                  migraines (G43.-)
                  myalgia (M79.1)
                  pain from prosthetic devices, implants, and grafts (T82.84, T83.84, T84.84, T85.84-) ◀▥
                  phantom limb syndrome with pain (G54.6)
                  vulvar vestibulitis (N94.810)
                  vulvodynia (N94.81-)

     G89.0   **Central pain syndrome**
              Neurological condition causing intractable pain resulting from damage to CNS
              Déjérine-Roussy syndrome
              Myelopathic pain syndrome
              Thalamic pain syndrome (hyperesthetic)

● **G89.1**   **Acute pain, not elsewhere classified**

     G89.11   **Acute pain due to trauma**

     G89.12   **Acute post-thoracotomy pain**
              Post-thoracotomy pain NOS

     G89.18   **Other acute postprocedural pain**
              Postoperative pain NOS
              Postprocedural pain NOS

● **G89.2**   **Chronic pain, not elsewhere classified**

     Excludes1   causalgia, lower limb (G57.7-)
                  causalgia, upper limb (G56.4-)
                  central pain syndrome (G89.0)
                  chronic pain syndrome (G89.4)
                  complex regional pain syndrome II, lower limb (G57.7-)
                  complex regional pain syndrome II, upper limb (G56.4-)
                  neoplasm related chronic pain (G89.3)
                  reflex sympathetic dystrophy (G90.5-)

     G89.21   **Chronic pain due to trauma**

     G89.22   **Chronic post-thoracotomy pain**

     G89.28   **Other chronic postprocedural pain**
              Other chronic postoperative pain

     G89.29   **Other chronic pain**

     G89.3   **Neoplasm related pain (acute) (chronic)**
              Cancer associated pain
              Pain due to malignancy (primary) (secondary)
              Tumor associated pain

     G89.4   **Chronic pain syndrome**
              Chronic pain associated with significant psychosocial dysfunction

● **G90**   **Disorders of autonomic nervous system**

     Excludes1   dysfunction of the autonomic nervous system due to alcohol (G31.2)

● **G90.0**   **Idiopathic peripheral autonomic neuropathy**

     G90.01   **Carotid sinus syncope**
              Carotid sinus syndrome

     G90.09   **Other idiopathic peripheral autonomic neuropathy**
              Idiopathic peripheral autonomic neuropathy NOS

     G90.1   **Familial dysautonomia [Riley-Day]**
              Inherited disorder that affects nerve function

     G90.2   **Horner's syndrome**
              Due to damage of the sympathetic nervous system
              Bernard(-Horner) syndrome
              Cervical sympathetic dystrophy or paralysis

     G90.3   **Multi-system degeneration of the autonomic nervous system**
              Neurogenic orthostatic hypotension [Shy-Drager]
         Excludes1   orthostatic hypotension NOS (I95.1)

     G90.4   **Autonomic dysreflexia**
              Syndrome resulting from lesions of spinal cord
              Use additional code to identify the cause, such as:
                  fecal impaction (K56.41)
                  pressure ulcer (pressure area) (L89.-)
                  urinary tract infection (N39.0)

● **G90.5**   **Complex regional pain syndrome I (CRPS I)**
              Reflex sympathetic dystrophy
         Excludes1   causalgia of lower limb (G57.7-)
                          causalgia of upper limb (G56.4-)
                          complex regional pain syndrome II of lower limb (G57.7-)
                          complex regional pain syndrome II of upper limb (G56.4-)

     G90.50   **Complex regional pain syndrome I, unspecified**

● **G90.51**   **Complex regional pain syndrome I of upper limb**

     G90.511   **Complex regional pain syndrome I of right upper limb**

     G90.512   **Complex regional pain syndrome I of left upper limb**

     G90.513   **Complex regional pain syndrome I of upper limb, bilateral**

     G90.519   **Complex regional pain syndrome I of unspecified upper limb**

● **G90.52**   **Complex regional pain syndrome I of lower limb**

     G90.521   **Complex regional pain syndrome I of right lower limb**

     G90.522   **Complex regional pain syndrome I of left lower limb**

     G90.523   **Complex regional pain syndrome I of lower limb, bilateral**

     G90.529   **Complex regional pain syndrome I of unspecified lower limb**

     G90.59   **Complex regional pain syndrome I of other specified site**

     G90.8   **Other disorders of autonomic nervous system**

     G90.9   **Disorder of the autonomic nervous system, unspecified**

◀ New   ◀▥ Revised   ~~deleted~~ Deleted   Excludes 1   Excludes 2   Includes   Use additional   Code first   Code also   Unspecified

OGCR Official Guidelines   X Assign placeholder X   ● Use Additional Character(s)   ▸ Manifestation Code   **Coding Clinic**

● **G91**   **Hydrocephalus**
Dilatation of cerebral ventricles, accompanied by accumulation of cerebrospinal fluid
> **Includes**   acquired hydrocephalus
> **Excludes1**   Arnold-Chiari syndrome with hydrocephalus (Q07.-)
> congenital hydrocephalus (Q03.-)
> spina bifida with hydrocephalus (Q05.-)

   G91.0   **Communicating hydrocephalus**
     Secondary normal pressure hydrocephalus

   G91.1   **Obstructive hydrocephalus**

   G91.2   **(Idiopathic) normal pressure hydrocephalus**
     Normal pressure hydrocephalus NOS

   G91.3   **Post-traumatic hydrocephalus, unspecified**

▶ **G91.4**   *Hydrocephalus in diseases classified elsewhere*
> *Code first underlying condition, such as:*
> congenital syphilis (A50.4-)
> neoplasm (C00-D49)
> **Excludes1**   hydrocephalus due to congenital toxoplasmosis (P37.1)

   G91.8   **Other hydrocephalus**

   G91.9   **Hydrocephalus, unspecified**

● **G92**   **Toxic encephalopathy**
Disorder or disease of brain caused by chemicals
Toxic encephalitis
Toxic metabolic encephalopathy
Code first (T51-T65) to identify toxic agent

● **G93**   **Other disorders of brain**

   G93.0   **Cerebral cysts**
     Arachnoid cyst
     Porencephalic cyst, acquired
> **Excludes1**   acquired periventricular cysts of newborn (P91.1)
> congenital cerebral cysts (Q04.6)

   G93.1   **Anoxic brain damage, not elsewhere classified**
     Permanent brain damage by lack of oxygen perfusion through brain tissues.
> **Excludes1**   cerebral anoxia due to anesthesia during labor and delivery (O74.3)
> cerebral anoxia due to anesthesia during the puerperium (O89.2)
> neonatal anoxia (P84)

   G93.2   **Benign intracranial hypertension**
> **Excludes1**   hypertensive encephalopathy (I67.4)

   G93.3   **Postviral fatigue syndrome**
     Benign myalgic encephalomyelitis
> **Excludes1**   chronic fatigue syndrome NOS (R53.82)

● **G93.4**   **Other and unspecified encephalopathy**
> **Excludes1**   alcoholic encephalopathy (G31.2)
> encephalopathy in diseases classified elsewhere (G94)
> hypertensive encephalopathy (I67.4)
> toxic (metabolic) encephalopathy (G92)

   G93.40   **Encephalopathy, unspecified**

   G93.41   **Metabolic encephalopathy**
     Septic encephalopathy
     Coding Clinic: 2015, Q3, P21

   G93.49   **Other encephalopathy**
     Encephalopathy NEC

   G93.5   **Compression of brain**
     Arnold-Chiari type 1 compression of brain
     Compression of brain (stem)
     Herniation of brain (stem)
> **Excludes1**   diffuse traumatic compression of brain (S06.2-)
> focal traumatic compression of brain (S06.3-)

   G93.6   **Cerebral edema**
> **Excludes1**   cerebral edema due to birth injury (P11.0)
> traumatic cerebral edema (S06.1-)

   G93.7   **Reye's syndrome**   P
     Life-threatening neurological condition, usually follows viral illness
     Code first (T39.0-), if salicylates-induced

● **G93.8**   **Other specified disorders of brain**

   G93.81   **Temporal sclerosis**
     Hippocampal sclerosis
     Mesial temporal sclerosis

   G93.82   **Brain death**

   G93.89   **Other specified disorders of brain**
     Postradiation encephalopathy

   G93.9   **Disorder of brain, unspecified**

▶ **G94**   *Other disorders of brain in diseases classified elsewhere*
     Code first underlying disease
> **Excludes1**   encephalopathy in congenital syphilis (A50.49)
> encephalopathy in influenza (J09.X9, J10.81, J11.81)
> encephalopathy in syphilis (A52.19)
> hydrocephalus in diseases classified elsewhere (G91.4)

● **G95**   **Other and unspecified diseases of spinal cord**
> **Excludes2**   myelitis (G04.-)

   G95.0   **Syringomyelia and syringobulbia**

● **G95.1**   **Vascular myelopathies**
> **Excludes2**   intraspinal phlebitis and thrombophlebitis, except non-pyogenic (G08)

   G95.11   **Acute infarction of spinal cord (embolic) (nonembolic)**
     Anoxia of spinal cord
     Arterial thrombosis of spinal cord

   G95.19   **Other vascular myelopathies**
     Edema of spinal cord
     Hematomyelia
     Nonpyogenic intraspinal phlebitis and thrombophlebitis
     Subacute necrotic myelopathy

● **G95.2**   **Other and unspecified cord compression**

   G95.20   **Unspecified cord compression**

   G95.29   **Other cord compression**

● **G95.8**   **Other specified diseases of spinal cord**
> **Excludes1**   neurogenic bladder NOS (N31.9)
> neurogenic bladder due to cauda equina syndrome (G83.4)
> neuromuscular dysfunction of bladder without spinal cord lesion (N31.-)

   G95.81   **Conus medullaris syndrome**
     Damage to gray matter and/or nerve roots in lower end of spinal cord

   G95.89   **Other specified diseases of spinal cord**
     Cord bladder NOS
     Drug-induced myelopathy
     Radiation-induced myelopathy
> **Excludes1**   myelopathy NOS (G95.9)

   G95.9   **Disease of spinal cord, unspecified**
     Myelopathy NOS

CHAPTER 6 (G00-G99)

● **G96** **Other disorders of central nervous system**

    G96.0 **Cerebrospinal fluid leak**

         Excludes1 cerebrospinal fluid leak from spinal puncture (G97.0)

  ● **G96.1** **Disorders of meninges, not elsewhere classified**

      G96.11 **Dural tear**

           Excludes1 accidental puncture or laceration of dura during a procedure (G97.41)

      G96.12 **Meningeal adhesions (cerebral) (spinal)**

      G96.19 **Other disorders of meninges, not elsewhere classified**

    G96.8 **Other specified disorders of central nervous system**

    G96.9 **Disorder of central nervous system, unspecified**

● **G97** **Intraoperative and postprocedural complications and disorders of nervous system, not elsewhere classified**

        Excludes2 intraoperative and postprocedural cerebrovascular infarction (I97.81-, I97.82-)

    G97.0 **Cerebrospinal fluid leak from spinal puncture**

    G97.1 **Other reaction to spinal and lumbar puncture**
        Headache due to lumbar puncture

    G97.2 **Intracranial hypotension following ventricular shunting**

  ● **G97.3** **Intraoperative hemorrhage and hematoma of a nervous system organ or structure complicating a procedure**

         Excludes1 intraoperative hemorrhage and hematoma of a nervous system organ or structure due to accidental puncture and laceration during a procedure (G97.4-)

      G97.31 **Intraoperative hemorrhage and hematoma of a nervous system organ or structure complicating a nervous system procedure**

      G97.32 **Intraoperative hemorrhage and hematoma of a nervous system organ or structure complicating other procedure**

  ● **G97.4** **Accidental puncture and laceration of a nervous system organ or structure during a procedure**

      G97.41 **Accidental puncture or laceration of dura during a procedure**
          Incidental (inadvertent) durotomy

      G97.48 **Accidental puncture and laceration of other nervous system organ or structure during a nervous system procedure**

      G97.49 **Accidental puncture and laceration of other nervous system organ or structure during other procedure**

  ● **G97.5** **Postprocedural hemorrhage of a nervous system organ or structure following a procedure** ◀⃫

      G97.51 **Postprocedural hemorrhage of a nervous system organ or structure following a nervous system procedure** ◀⃫

      G97.52 **Postprocedural hemorrhage of a nervous system organ or structure following other procedure** ◀⃫

● **G97.6** **Postprocedural hematoma and seroma of a nervous system organ or structure following a procedure** ◀

      G97.61 **Postprocedural hematoma of a nervous system organ or structure following a nervous system procedure** ◀

      G97.62 **Postprocedural hematoma of a nervous system organ or structure following other procedure** ◀

      G97.63 **Postprocedural seroma of a nervous system organ or structure following a nervous system procedure** ◀

      G97.64 **Postprocedural seroma of a nervous system organ or structure following other procedure** ◀

● **G97.8** **Other intraoperative and postprocedural complications and disorders of nervous system**

      Use additional code to further specify disorder

      G97.81 **Other intraoperative complications of nervous system**

      G97.82 **Other postprocedural complications and disorders of nervous system**

● **G98** **Other disorders of nervous system not elsewhere classified**

      Includes nervous system disorder NOS

    G98.0 **Neurogenic arthritis, not elsewhere classified**
        Nonsyphilitic neurogenic arthropathy NEC
        Nonsyphilitic neurogenic spondylopathy NEC

         Excludes1 spondylopathy (in):
            syringomyelia and syringobulbia (G95.0)

             tabes dorsalis (A52.11)

    G98.8 **Other disorders of nervous system**
        Nervous system disorder NOS

● **G99** **Other disorders of nervous system in diseases classified elsewhere**

  ▌ *G99.0* *Autonomic neuropathy in diseases classified elsewhere*

      Code first *underlying disease, such as:*
        amyloidosis (E85.-)
        gout (M1A.-, M10.-)
        hyperthyroidism (E05.-)

         Excludes1 diabetic autonomic neuropathy (E08-E13 with .43)

  ▌ *G99.2* *Myelopathy in diseases classified elsewhere*

      Code first *underlying disease, such as:*
        neoplasm (C00-D49)

         Excludes1 myelopathy in:
            intervertebral disease (M50.0-, M51.0-)

             spondylosis (M47.0-, M47.1-)

  ▌ *G99.8* *Other specified disorders of nervous system in diseases classified elsewhere*

      Code first *underlying disorder, such as:*
        amyloidosis (E85.-)
        avitaminosis (E56.9)

         Excludes1 nervous system involvement in:
            cysticercosis (B69.0)
            rubella (B06.0-)
            syphilis (A52.1-)

◀ New   ◀⃫ Revised   ~~deleted~~ Deleted   Excludes 1   Excludes 2   Includes   Use additional   Code first   Code also   Unspecified

792   **OGCR** Official Guidelines   X Assign placeholder X   ● Use Additional Character(s)   ▌ Manifestation Code   **Coding Clinic**

CHAPTER 7

DISEASES OF THE EYE AND ADNEXA (H00-H59)

OGCR Chapter-Specific Coding Guidelines

7. Chapter 7: Diseases of the Eye and Adnexa (H00-H59)

a. Glaucoma

1) **Assigning Glaucoma Codes**

Assign as many codes from category H40, Glaucoma, as needed to identify the type of glaucoma, the affected eye, and the glaucoma stage.

2) **Bilateral glaucoma with same type and stage**

When a patient has bilateral glaucoma and both eyes are documented as being the same type and stage, and there is a code for bilateral glaucoma, report only the code for the type of glaucoma, bilateral, with the seventh character for the stage.

When a patient has bilateral glaucoma and both eyes are documented as being the same type and stage, and the classification does not provide a code for bilateral glaucoma (i.e. subcategories H40.10, H40.11 and H40.20) report only one code for the type of glaucoma with the appropriate seventh character for the stage.

3) **Bilateral glaucoma stage with different types or stages**

When a patient has bilateral glaucoma and each eye is documented as having a different type or stage, and the classification distinguishes laterality, assign the appropriate code for each eye rather than the code for bilateral glaucoma.

When a patient has bilateral glaucoma and each eye is documented as having a different type, and the classification does not distinguish laterality (i.e. subcategories H40.10, H40.11 and H40.20), assign one code for each type of glaucoma with the appropriate seventh character for the stage.

When a patient has bilateral glaucoma and each eye is documented as having the same type, but different stage, and the classification does not distinguish laterality (i.e. subcategories H40.10, H40.11 and H40.20), assign a code for the type of glaucoma for each eye with the seventh character for the specific glaucoma stage documented for each eye.

4) **Patient admitted with glaucoma and stage evolves during the admission**

If a patient is admitted with glaucoma and the stage progresses during the admission, assign the code for highest stage documented.

5) **Indeterminate stage glaucoma**

Assignment of the seventh character "4" for "indeterminate stage" should be based on the clinical documentation. The seventh character "4" is used for glaucomas whose stage cannot be clinically determined. This seventh character should not be confused with the seventh character "0", unspecified, which should be assigned when there is no documentation regarding the stage of the glaucoma.

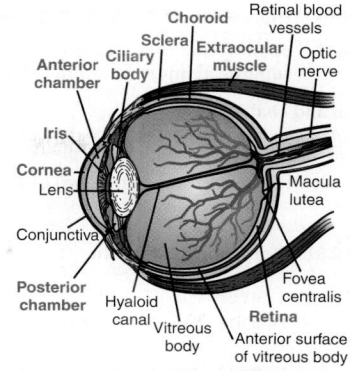

Figure 7-1 Eye and ocular adnexa. (From Buck CJ: Step-by-Step Medical Coding, ed 2016, St. Louis, Elsevier, 2016)

★ **(See Plate 87 on page 63.)**

CHAPTER 7

DISEASES OF THE EYE AND ADNEXA (H00-H59)

Note: Use an external cause code following the code for the eye condition, if applicable, to identify the cause of the eye condition

Excludes2   certain conditions originating in the perinatal period (P04-P96)

certain infectious and parasitic diseases (A00-B99)

complications of pregnancy, childbirth and the puerperium (O00-O9A)

congenital malformations, deformations, and chromosomal abnormalities (Q00-Q99)

diabetes mellitus related eye conditions (E09.3-, E10.3-, E11.3-, E13.3-)

endocrine, nutritional and metabolic diseases (E00-E88)

injury (trauma) of eye and orbit (S05.-)

injury, poisoning and certain other consequences of external causes (S00-T88)

neoplasms (C00-D49)

symptoms, signs and abnormal clinical and laboratory findings, not elsewhere classified (R00-R94)

syphilis related eye disorders (A50.01, A50.3-, A51.43, A52.71)

This chapter contains the following blocks:

H00-H05	Disorders of eyelid, lacrimal system and orbit
H10-H11	Disorders of conjunctiva
H15-H22	Disorders of sclera, cornea, iris and ciliary body
H25-H28	Disorders of lens
H30-H36	Disorders of choroid and retina
H40-H42	Glaucoma
H43-H44	Disorders of vitreous body and globe
H46-H47	Disorders of optic nerve and visual pathways
H49-H52	Disorders of ocular muscles, binocular movement, accommodation and refraction
H53-H54	Visual disturbances and blindness
H55-H57	Other disorders of eye and adnexa
H59	Intraoperative and postprocedural complications and disorders of eye and adnexa, not elsewhere classified

DISORDERS OF EYELID, LACRIMAL SYSTEM AND ORBIT (H00-H05)

Excludes2   open wound of eyelid (S01.1-)
              superficial injury of eyelid (S00.1-, S00.2-)

● **H00   Hordeolum and chalazion**
     Hordeolum: inflammatory staphylococcal infection of sebaceous
     glands of eyelids; AKA stye. Chalazion: eyelid mass

● **H00.0   Hordeolum (externum) (internum) of eyelid**
     Bacterial infection (staphylococcus) of the sebaceous gland of
     the eyelid (stye)

   ● **H00.01   Hordeolum externum**
              Hordeolum NOS
              Stye
       H00.011   Hordeolum externum right upper eyelid
       H00.012   Hordeolum externum right lower eyelid
       H00.013   Hordeolum externum right eye, unspecified eyelid
       H00.014   Hordeolum externum left upper eyelid
       H00.015   Hordeolum externum left lower eyelid
       H00.016   Hordeolum externum left eye, unspecified eyelid
       H00.019   Hordeolum externum unspecified eye, unspecified eyelid

   ● **H00.02   Hordeolum internum**
              Infection of meibomian gland
       H00.021   Hordeolum internum right upper eyelid
       H00.022   Hordeolum internum right lower eyelid
       H00.023   Hordeolum internum right eye, unspecified eyelid
       H00.024   Hordeolum internum left upper eyelid
       H00.025   Hordeolum internum left lower eyelid
       H00.026   Hordeolum internum left eye, unspecified eyelid
       H00.029   Hordeolum internum unspecified eye, unspecified eyelid

   ● **H00.03   Abscess of eyelid**
              Furuncle of eyelid
       H00.031   Abscess of right upper eyelid
       H00.032   Abscess of right lower eyelid
       H00.033   Abscess of eyelid right eye, unspecified eyelid
       H00.034   Abscess of left upper eyelid
       H00.035   Abscess of left lower eyelid
       H00.036   Abscess of eyelid left eye, unspecified eyelid
       H00.039   Abscess of eyelid unspecified eye, unspecified eyelid

● **H00.1   Chalazion**
     Often caused by accumulation of meibomian gland secretions
     resulting from a blockage of duct.
     Meibomian (gland) cyst
     Excludes2   infected meibomian gland (H00.02-)
   H00.11   Chalazion right upper eyelid
   H00.12   Chalazion right lower eyelid
   H00.13   Chalazion right eye, unspecified eyelid
   H00.14   Chalazion left upper eyelid
   H00.15   Chalazion left lower eyelid
   H00.16   Chalazion left eye, unspecified eyelid
   H00.19   Chalazion unspecified eye, unspecified eyelid

● **H01   Other inflammation of eyelid**

   ● **H01.0   Blepharitis**
       Inflammation of eyelids
       Excludes1   blepharoconjunctivitis (H10.5-)

   ● **H01.00   Unspecified blepharitis**
       H01.001   Unspecified blepharitis right upper eyelid
       H01.002   Unspecified blepharitis right lower eyelid
       H01.003   Unspecified blepharitis right eye, unspecified eyelid
       H01.004   Unspecified blepharitis left upper eyelid
       H01.005   Unspecified blepharitis left lower eyelid
       H01.006   Unspecified blepharitis left eye, unspecified eyelid
       H01.009   Unspecified blepharitis unspecified eye, unspecified eyelid

   ● **H01.01   Ulcerative blepharitis**
       H01.011   Ulcerative blepharitis right upper eyelid
       H01.012   Ulcerative blepharitis right lower eyelid
       H01.013   Ulcerative blepharitis right eye, unspecified eyelid
       H01.014   Ulcerative blepharitis left upper eyelid
       H01.015   Ulcerative blepharitis left lower eyelid
       H01.016   Ulcerative blepharitis left eye, unspecified eyelid
       H01.019   Ulcerative blepharitis unspecified eye, unspecified eyelid

   ● **H01.02   Squamous blepharitis**
       H01.021   Squamous blepharitis right upper eyelid
       H01.022   Squamous blepharitis right lower eyelid
       H01.023   Squamous blepharitis right eye, unspecified eyelid
       H01.024   Squamous blepharitis left upper eyelid
       H01.025   Squamous blepharitis left lower eyelid
       H01.026   Squamous blepharitis left eye, unspecified eyelid
       H01.029   Squamous blepharitis unspecified eye, unspecified eyelid

   ● **H01.1   Noninfectious dermatoses of eyelid**

   ● **H01.11   Allergic dermatitis of eyelid**
       Contact dermatitis of eyelid
       H01.111   Allergic dermatitis of right upper eyelid
       H01.112   Allergic dermatitis of right lower eyelid
       H01.113   Allergic dermatitis of right eye, unspecified eyelid
       H01.114   Allergic dermatitis of left upper eyelid
       H01.115   Allergic dermatitis of left lower eyelid
       H01.116   Allergic dermatitis of left eye, unspecified eyelid
       H01.119   Allergic dermatitis of unspecified eye, unspecified eyelid

◀ New   ◀⋯ Revised   ~~deleted~~ Deleted   Excludes 1   Excludes 2   Includes   Use additional   Code first   Code also   Unspecified
OGCR Official Guidelines   X Assign placeholder X   ● Use Additional Character(s)   ▷ Manifestation Code   **Coding Clinic**

● **H01.12   Discoid lupus erythematosus of eyelid**

 H01.121 Discoid lupus erythematosus of right upper eyelid

 H01.122 Discoid lupus erythematosus of right lower eyelid

 H01.123 Discoid lupus erythematosus of right eye, <mark>unspecified</mark> eyelid

 H01.124 Discoid lupus erythematosus of left upper eyelid

 H01.125 Discoid lupus erythematosus of left lower eyelid

 H01.126 Discoid lupus erythematosus of left eye, <mark>unspecified</mark> eyelid

 H01.129 Discoid lupus erythematosus of unspecified eye, <mark>unspecified</mark> eyelid

● **H01.13   Eczematous dermatitis of eyelid**

 H01.131 Eczematous dermatitis of right upper eyelid

 H01.132 Eczematous dermatitis of right lower eyelid

 H01.133 Eczematous dermatitis of right eye, <mark>unspecified</mark> eyelid

 H01.134 Eczematous dermatitis of left upper eyelid

 H01.135 Eczematous dermatitis of left lower eyelid

 H01.136 Eczematous dermatitis of left eye, <mark>unspecified</mark> eyelid

 H01.139 Eczematous dermatitis of <mark>unspecified</mark> eye, unspecified eyelid

● **H01.14   Xeroderma of eyelid**
 Abnormally dry

 H01.141 Xeroderma of right upper eyelid

 H01.142 Xeroderma of right lower eyelid

 H01.143 Xeroderma of right eye, <mark>unspecified</mark> eyelid

 H01.144 Xeroderma of left upper eyelid

 H01.145 Xeroderma of left lower eyelid

 H01.146 Xeroderma of left eye, <mark>unspecified</mark> eyelid

 H01.149 Xeroderma of unspecified eye, <mark>unspecified</mark> eyelid

H01.8 Other specified inflammations of eyelid

H01.9 <mark>Unspecified</mark> inflammation of eyelid
 Inflammation of eyelid NOS

● **H02   Other disorders of eyelid**
 Turning inward (inversion) of eyelid margin and ingrowing eyelashes

 Excludes1 congenital malformations of eyelid (Q10.0-Q10.3)

● **H02.0   Entropion and trichiasis of eyelid**

● **H02.00   Unspecified entropion of eyelid**

 H02.001 <mark>Unspecified</mark> entropion of right upper eyelid

 H02.002 <mark>Unspecified</mark> entropion of right lower eyelid

 H02.003 <mark>Unspecified</mark> entropion of right eye, unspecified eyelid

 H02.004 <mark>Unspecified</mark> entropion of left upper eyelid

 H02.005 <mark>Unspecified</mark> entropion of left lower eyelid

 H02.006 <mark>Unspecified</mark> entropion of left eye, unspecified eyelid

 H02.009 <mark>Unspecified</mark> entropion of unspecified eye, unspecified eyelid

● **H02.01   Cicatricial entropion of eyelid**
 Scar

 H02.011 Cicatricial entropion of right upper eyelid

 H02.012 Cicatricial entropion of right lower eyelid

 H02.013 Cicatricial entropion of right eye, <mark>unspecified</mark> eyelid

 H02.014 Cicatricial entropion of left upper eyelid

 H02.015 Cicatricial entropion of left lower eyelid

 H02.016 Cicatricial entropion of left eye, <mark>unspecified</mark> eyelid

 H02.019 Cicatricial entropion of <mark>unspecified</mark> eye, unspecified eyelid

● **H02.02   Mechanical entropion of eyelid**
 Turning inward (inversion) of eyelid margin due to lack of support

 H02.021 Mechanical entropion of right upper eyelid

 H02.022 Mechanical entropion of right lower eyelid

 H02.023 Mechanical entropion of right eye, <mark>unspecified</mark> eyelid

 H02.024 Mechanical entropion of left upper eyelid

 H02.025 Mechanical entropion of left lower eyelid

 H02.026 Mechanical entropion of left eye, <mark>unspecified</mark> eyelid

 H02.029 Mechanical entropion of <mark>unspecified</mark> eye, unspecified eyelid

● **H02.03   Senile entropion of eyelid**
 Turning inward (inversion) of eyelid margin due to aging

 H02.031 Senile entropion of right upper eyelid A

 H02.032 Senile entropion of right lower eyelid A

 H02.033 Senile entropion of right eye, <mark>unspecified</mark> eyelid A

 H02.034 Senile entropion of left upper eyelid A

 H02.035 Senile entropion of left lower eyelid A

 H02.036 Senile entropion of left eye, <mark>unspecified</mark> eyelid A

 H02.039 Senile entropion of unspecified eye, <mark>unspecified</mark> eyelid A

● **H02.04   Spastic entropion of eyelid**
 Turning inward (inversion) of eyelid margin caused by spasm of muscle

 H02.041 Spastic entropion of right upper eyelid

 H02.042 Spastic entropion of right lower eyelid

 H02.043 Spastic entropion of right eye, <mark>unspecified</mark> eyelid

 H02.044 Spastic entropion of left upper eyelid

 H02.045 Spastic entropion of left lower eyelid

 H02.046 Spastic entropion of left eye, <mark>unspecified</mark> eyelid

 H02.049 Spastic entropion of unspecified eye, <mark>unspecified</mark> eyelid

Figure 7-2 Right lower eyelid entropion. Note the inward rotation of the tarsal plate about the horizontal axis and the resultant contact between the mucocutaneous junction and ocular surface. (From Yanoff: Ophthalmology, ed 3, Mosby, Inc., 2008)

CHAPTER 7 (H00-H59)

CHAPTER 7 (H00-H59)

● H02.05   **Trichiasis without entropian**
Ingrowing hairs of eyelashes

    H02.051   **Trichiasis without entropian right upper eyelid**

    H02.052   **Trichiasis without entropian right lower eyelid**

    H02.053   **Trichiasis without entropian right eye, unspecified eyelid**

    H02.054   **Trichiasis without entropian left upper eyelid**

    H02.055   **Trichiasis without entropian left lower eyelid**

    H02.056   **Trichiasis without entropian left eye, unspecified eyelid**

    H02.059   **Trichiasis without entropian unspecified eye, unspecified eyelid**

● H02.1   **Ectropion of eyelid**
Eversion (pulling away) of eyelid

 ● H02.10   **Unspecified ectropion of eyelid**

    H02.101   **Unspecified ectropion of right upper eyelid**

    H02.102   **Unspecified ectropion of right lower eyelid**

    H02.103   **Unspecified ectropion of right eye, unspecified eyelid**

    H02.104   **Unspecified ectropion of left upper eyelid**

    H02.105   **Unspecified ectropion of left lower eyelid**

    H02.106   **Unspecified ectropion of left eye, unspecified eyelid**

    H02.109   **Unspecified ectropion of unspecified eye, unspecified eyelid**

 ● H02.11   **Cicatricial ectropion of eyelid**
Pulling of eyelid down and away from eye due to scar or tightening

    H02.111   **Cicatricial ectropion of right upper eyelid**

    H02.112   **Cicatricial ectropion of right lower eyelid**

    H02.113   **Cicatricial ectropion of right eye, unspecified eyelid**

    H02.114   **Cicatricial ectropion of left upper eyelid**

    H02.115   **Cicatricial ectropion of left lower eyelid**

    H02.116   **Cicatricial ectropion of left eye, unspecified eyelid**

    H02.119   **Cicatricial ectropion of unspecified eye, unspecified eyelid**

 ● H02.12   **Mechanical ectropion of eyelid**
Eversion (pulling away) of eyelid due to lack of support

    H02.121   **Mechanical ectropion of right upper eyelid**

    H02.122   **Mechanical ectropion of right lower eyelid**

    H02.123   **Mechanical ectropion of right eye, unspecified eyelid**

    H02.124   **Mechanical ectropion of left upper eyelid**

    H02.125   **Mechanical ectropion of left lower eyelid**

    H02.126   **Mechanical ectropion of left eye, unspecified eyelid**

    H02.129   **Mechanical ectropion of unspecified eye, unspecified eyelid**

● H02.13   **Senile ectropion of eyelid**
Eversion (pulling away) of eyelid due to age

    H02.131   **Senile ectropion of right upper eyelid**   A

    H02.132   **Senile ectropion of right lower eyelid**   A

    H02.133   **Senile ectropion of right eye, unspecified eyelid**   A

    H02.134   **Senile ectropion of left upper eyelid**   A

    H02.135   **Senile ectropion of left lower eyelid**   A

    H02.136   **Senile ectropion of left eye, unspecified eyelid**   A

    H02.139   **Senile ectropion of unspecified eye, unspecified eyelid**   A

● H02.14   **Spastic ectropion of eyelid**
Eversion (pulling away) of eyelid due to tonic muscle spasm

    H02.141   **Spastic ectropion of right upper eyelid**

    H02.142   **Spastic ectropion of right lower eyelid**

    H02.143   **Spastic ectropion of right eye, unspecified eyelid**

    H02.144   **Spastic ectropion of left upper eyelid**

    H02.145   **Spastic ectropion of left lower eyelid**

    H02.146   **Spastic ectropion of left eye, unspecified eyelid**

    H02.149   **Spastic ectropion of unspecified eye, unspecified eyelid**

● H02.2   **Lagophthalmos**
Condition in which eye cannot completely close

 ● H02.20   **Unspecified lagophthalmos**

    H02.201   **Unspecified lagophthalmos right upper eyelid**

    H02.202   **Unspecified lagophthalmos right lower eyelid**

    H02.203   **Unspecified lagophthalmos right eye, unspecified eyelid**

    H02.204   **Unspecified lagophthalmos left upper eyelid**

    H02.205   **Unspecified lagophthalmos left lower eyelid**

    H02.206   **Unspecified lagophthalmos left eye, unspecified eyelid**

    H02.209   **Unspecified lagophthalmos unspecified eye, unspecified eyelid**

 ● H02.21   **Cicatricial lagophthalmos**
Upper or lower eyelid does not close due to scar or tightening

    H02.211   **Cicatricial lagophthalmos right upper eyelid**

    H02.212   **Cicatricial lagophthalmos right lower eyelid**

    H02.213   **Cicatricial lagophthalmos right eye, unspecified eyelid**

    H02.214   **Cicatricial lagophthalmos left upper eyelid**

    H02.215   **Cicatricial lagophthalmos left lower eyelid**

    H02.216   **Cicatricial lagophthalmos left eye, unspecified eyelid**

    H02.219   **Cicatricial lagophthalmos unspecified eye, unspecified eyelid**

● **H02.22   Mechanical lagophthalmos**
Inability to close lids due to structural disorder

    H02.221   Mechanical lagophthalmos right upper eyelid
    H02.222   Mechanical lagophthalmos right lower eyelid
    H02.223   Mechanical lagophthalmos right eye, unspecified eyelid
    H02.224   Mechanical lagophthalmos left upper eyelid
    H02.225   Mechanical lagophthalmos left lower eyelid
    H02.226   Mechanical lagophthalmos left eye, unspecified eyelid
    H02.229   Mechanical lagophthalmos unspecified eye, unspecified eyelid

● **H02.23   Paralytic lagophthalmos**
Eyelids do not close due to paralysis

    H02.231   Paralytic lagophthalmos right upper eyelid
    H02.232   Paralytic lagophthalmos right lower eyelid
    H02.233   Paralytic lagophthalmos right eye, unspecified eyelid
    H02.234   Paralytic lagophthalmos left upper eyelid
    H02.235   Paralytic lagophthalmos left lower eyelid
    H02.236   Paralytic lagophthalmos left eye, unspecified eyelid
    H02.239   Paralytic lagophthalmos unspecified eye, unspecified eyelid

★ **(See Plate 81, middle, on page 65.)**

● **H02.3   Blepharochalasis**
Relaxation of skin of eyelid, due to atrophy of intercellular tissue
Pseudoptosis

    H02.30   Blepharochalasis unspecified eye, unspecified eyelid
    H02.31   Blepharochalasis right upper eyelid
    H02.32   Blepharochalasis right lower eyelid
    H02.33   Blepharochalasis right eye, unspecified eyelid
    H02.34   Blepharochalasis left upper eyelid
    H02.35   Blepharochalasis left lower eyelid
    H02.36   Blepharochalasis left eye, unspecified eyelid

● **H02.4   Ptosis of eyelid**
Falling forward, drooping, sagging of eyelid

  ● **H02.40   Unspecified ptosis of eyelid**
    H02.401   Unspecified ptosis of right eyelid
    H02.402   Unspecified ptosis of left eyelid
    H02.403   Unspecified ptosis of bilateral eyelids
    H02.409   Unspecified ptosis of unspecified eyelid

  ● **H02.41   Mechanical ptosis of eyelid**
    H02.411   Mechanical ptosis of right eyelid
    H02.412   Mechanical ptosis of left eyelid
    H02.413   Mechanical ptosis of bilateral eyelids
    H02.419   Mechanical ptosis of unspecified eyelid

● **H02.42   Myogenic ptosis of eyelid**
    H02.421   Myogenic ptosis of right eyelid
    H02.422   Myogenic ptosis of left eyelid
    H02.423   Myogenic ptosis of bilateral eyelids
    H02.429   Myogenic ptosis of unspecified eyelid

● **H02.43   Paralytic ptosis of eyelid**
Neurogenic ptosis of eyelid
    H02.431   Paralytic ptosis of right eyelid
    H02.432   Paralytic ptosis of left eyelid
    H02.433   Paralytic ptosis of bilateral eyelids
    H02.439   Paralytic ptosis unspecified eyelid

● **H02.5   Other disorders affecting eyelid function**
    Excludes2   blepharospasm (G24.5)
                organic tic (G25.69)
                psychogenic tic (F95.-)

  ● **H02.51   Abnormal innervation syndrome**
    H02.511   Abnormal innervation syndrome right upper eyelid
    H02.512   Abnormal innervation syndrome right lower eyelid
    H02.513   Abnormal innervation syndrome right eye, unspecified eyelid
    H02.514   Abnormal innervation syndrome left upper eyelid
    H02.515   Abnormal innervation syndrome left lower eyelid
    H02.516   Abnormal innervation syndrome left eye, unspecified eyelid
    H02.519   Abnormal innervation syndrome unspecified eye, unspecified eyelid

  ● **H02.52   Blepharophimosis**
Drooping of eyelid with reduced lid size
Ankyloblepharon
    H02.521   Blepharophimosis right upper eyelid
    H02.522   Blepharophimosis right lower eyelid
    H02.523   Blepharophimosis right eye, unspecified eyelid
    H02.524   Blepharophimosis left upper eyelid
    H02.525   Blepharophimosis left lower eyelid
    H02.526   Blepharophimosis left eye, unspecified eyelid
    H02.529   Blepharophimosis unspecified eye, unspecified lid

  ● **H02.53   Eyelid retraction**
Eyelid lag
    H02.531   Eyelid retraction right upper eyelid
    H02.532   Eyelid retraction right lower eyelid
    H02.533   Eyelid retraction right eye, unspecified eyelid
    H02.534   Eyelid retraction left upper eyelid
    H02.535   Eyelid retraction left lower eyelid
    H02.536   Eyelid retraction left eye, unspecified eyelid
    H02.539   Eyelid retraction unspecified eye, unspecified lid

    H02.59   Other disorders affecting eyelid function
Deficient blink reflex
Sensory disorders

Figure 7-3   Ptosis of eyelid. (From Yanoff: Ophthalmology, ed 3, Mosby, Inc., 2008)

Item 7-1   Ptosis of eyelid is drooping of the upper eyelid over the pupil when the eyes are fully opened resulting from nerve or muscle damage, which may require surgical correction.

● **H02.6 Xanthelasma of eyelid**
  Yellow-to-orange patches or pimples clustered together on eyelid

H02.60 Xanthelasma of unspecified eye, unspecified eyelid

H02.61 Xanthelasma of right upper eyelid

H02.62 Xanthelasma of right lower eyelid

H02.63 Xanthelasma of right eye, unspecified eyelid

H02.64 Xanthelasma of left upper eyelid

H02.65 Xanthelasma of left lower eyelid

H02.66 Xanthelasma of left eye, unspecified eyelid

● **H02.7 Other and unspecified degenerative disorders of eyelid and periocular area**

H02.70 Unspecified degenerative disorders of eyelid and periocular area

● **H02.71 Chloasma of eyelid and periocular area**
  Dyspigmentation of eyelid
  Hyperpigmentation of eyelid

H02.711 Chloasma of right upper eyelid and periocular area

H02.712 Chloasma of right lower eyelid and periocular area

H02.713 Chloasma of right eye, unspecified eyelid and periocular area

H02.714 Chloasma of left upper eyelid and periocular area

H02.715 Chloasma of left lower eyelid and periocular area

H02.716 Chloasma of left eye, unspecified eyelid and periocular area

H02.719 Chloasma of unspecified eye, unspecified eyelid and periocular area

● **H02.72 Madarosis of eyelid and periocular area**
  Loss of eyelashes and/or eyebrows
  Hypotrichosis of eyelid

H02.721 Madarosis of right upper eyelid and periocular area

H02.722 Madarosis of right lower eyelid and periocular area

H02.723 Madarosis of right eye, unspecified eyelid and periocular area

H02.724 Madarosis of left upper eyelid and periocular area

H02.725 Madarosis of left lower eyelid and periocular area

H02.726 Madarosis of left eye, unspecified eyelid and periocular area

H02.729 Madarosis of unspecified eye, unspecified eyelid and periocular area

● **H02.73 Vitiligo of eyelid and periocular area**
  Skin pigmentation disease characterized by white patches
  Hypopigmentation of eyelid

H02.731 Vitiligo of right upper eyelid and periocular area

H02.732 Vitiligo of right lower eyelid and periocular area

H02.733 Vitiligo of right eye, unspecified eyelid and periocular area

H02.734 Vitiligo of left upper eyelid and periocular area

H02.735 Vitiligo of left lower eyelid and periocular area

H02.736 Vitiligo of left eye, unspecified eyelid and periocular area

H02.739 Vitiligo of unspecified eye, unspecified eyelid and periocular area

H02.79 Other degenerative disorders of eyelid and periocular area

● **H02.8 Other specified disorders of eyelid**

● **H02.81 Retained foreign body in eyelid**
  Use additional code to identify the type of retained foreign body (Z18.-)

  Excludes1   laceration of eyelid with foreign body (S01.12-)
  retained intraocular foreign body (H44.6-, H44.7-)
  superficial foreign body of eyelid and periocular area (S00.25-)

H02.811 Retained foreign body in right upper eyelid

H02.812 Retained foreign body in right lower eyelid

H02.813 Retained foreign body in right eye, unspecified eyelid

H02.814 Retained foreign body in left upper eyelid

H02.815 Retained foreign body in left lower eyelid

H02.816 Retained foreign body in left eye, unspecified eyelid

H02.819 Retained foreign body in unspecified eye, unspecified eyelid

● **H02.82 Cysts of eyelid**
  Sebaceous cyst of eyelid

H02.821 Cysts of right upper eyelid

H02.822 Cysts of right lower eyelid

H02.823 Cysts of right eye, unspecified eyelid

H02.824 Cysts of left upper eyelid

H02.825 Cysts of left lower eyelid

H02.826 Cysts of left eye, unspecified eyelid

H02.829 Cysts of unspecified eye, unspecified eyelid

● **H02.83 Dermatochalasis of eyelid**
  Skin is inelastic and hangs loosely in folds

H02.831 Dermatochalasis of right upper eyelid

H02.832 Dermatochalasis of right lower eyelid

H02.833 Dermatochalasis of right eye, unspecified eyelid

H02.834 Dermatochalasis of left upper eyelid

H02.835 Dermatochalasis of left lower eyelid

H02.836 Dermatochalasis of left eye, unspecified eyelid

H02.839 Dermatochalasis of unspecified eye, unspecified eyelid

● **H02.84 Edema of eyelid**
  Hyperemia of eyelid

H02.841 Edema of right upper eyelid

H02.842 Edema of right lower eyelid

H02.843 Edema of right eye, unspecified eyelid

H02.844 Edema of left upper eyelid

H02.845 Edema of left lower eyelid

H02.846 Edema of left eye, unspecified eyelid

H02.849 Edema of unspecified eye, unspecified eyelid

● **H02.85 Elephantiasis of eyelid**
  Massive secondary lymphedema with hypertrophy of skin and subcutaneous tissues (pachyderma)

H02.851 Elephantiasis of right upper eyelid

H02.852 Elephantiasis of right lower eyelid

H02.853 Elephantiasis of right eye, unspecified eyelid

H02.854 Elephantiasis of left upper eyelid

H02.855 Elephantiasis of left lower eyelid

CHAPTER 7 (H00-H59)

◀ New   ◀‖ Revised   ~~deleted~~ Deleted   Excludes 1   Excludes 2   Includes   Use additional   Code first   Code also   Unspecified

OGCR Official Guidelines   X Assign placeholder X   ● Use Additional Character(s)   ▷ Manifestation Code   **Coding Clinic**

H02.856 Elephantiasis of left eye, unspecified eyelid

H02.859 Elephantiasis of unspecified eye, unspecified eyelid

● H02.86 Hypertrichosis of eyelid
Excessive growth of hair

H02.861 Hypertrichosis of right upper eyelid

H02.862 Hypertrichosis of right lower eyelid

H02.863 Hypertrichosis of right eye, unspecified eyelid

H02.864 Hypertrichosis of left upper eyelid

H02.865 Hypertrichosis of left lower eyelid

H02.866 Hypertrichosis of left eye, unspecified eyelid

H02.869 Hypertrichosis of unspecified eye, unspecified eyelid

● H02.87 Vascular anomalies of eyelid

H02.871 Vascular anomalies of right upper eyelid

H02.872 Vascular anomalies of right lower eyelid

H02.873 Vascular anomalies of right eye, unspecified eyelid

H02.874 Vascular anomalies of left upper eyelid

H02.875 Vascular anomalies of left lower eyelid

H02.876 Vascular anomalies of left eye, unspecified eyelid

H02.879 Vascular anomalies of unspecified eye, unspecified eyelid

H02.89 Other specified disorders of eyelid
Hemorrhage of eyelid

H02.9 Unspecified disorder of eyelid
Disorder of eyelid NOS

● H04 Disorders of lacrimal system
   Excludes1 congenital malformations of lacrimal system (Q10.4-Q10.6)

● H04.0 Dacryoadenitis
Inflammation of lacrimal gland

● H04.00 Unspecified dacryoadenitis

H04.001 Unspecified dacryoadenitis, right lacrimal gland

H04.002 Unspecified dacryoadenitis, left lacrimal gland

H04.003 Unspecified dacryoadenitis, bilateral lacrimal glands

H04.009 Unspecified dacryoadenitis, unspecified lacrimal gland

● H04.01 Acute dacryoadenitis

H04.011 Acute dacryoadenitis, right lacrimal gland

H04.012 Acute dacryoadenitis, left lacrimal gland

H04.013 Acute dacryoadenitis, bilateral lacrimal glands

H04.019 Acute dacryoadenitis, unspecified lacrimal gland

● H04.02 Chronic dacryoadenitis

H04.021 Chronic dacryoadenitis, right lacrimal gland

H04.022 Chronic dacryoadenitis, left lacrimal gland

H04.023 Chronic dacryoadenitis, bilateral lacrimal gland

H04.029 Chronic dacryoadenitis, unspecified lacrimal gland

● H04.03 Chronic enlargement of lacrimal gland

H04.031 Chronic enlargement of right lacrimal gland

H04.032 Chronic enlargement of left lacrimal gland

H04.033 Chronic enlargement of bilateral lacrimal glands

H04.039 Chronic enlargement of unspecified lacrimal gland

● H04.1 Other disorders of lacrimal gland

● H04.11 Dacryops
Watery eye or distention of lacrimal duct due to fluid

H04.111 Dacryops of right lacrimal gland

H04.112 Dacryops of left lacrimal gland

H04.113 Dacryops of bilateral lacrimal glands

H04.119 Dacryops of unspecified lacrimal gland

● H04.12 Dry eye syndrome
Tear film insufficiency, NOS

H04.121 Dry eye syndrome of right lacrimal gland

H04.122 Dry eye syndrome of left lacrimal gland

H04.123 Dry eye syndrome of bilateral lacrimal glands

H04.129 Dry eye syndrome of unspecified lacrimal gland

● H04.13 Lacrimal cyst
Lacrimal cystic degeneration

H04.131 Lacrimal cyst right lacrimal gland

H04.132 Lacrimal cyst left lacrimal gland

H04.133 Lacrimal cyst bilateral lacrimal glands

H04.139 Lacrimal cyst unspecified lacrimal gland

● H04.14 Primary lacrimal gland atrophy

H04.141 Primary lacrimal gland atrophy, right lacrimal gland

H04.142 Primary lacrimal gland atrophy, left lacrimal gland

H04.143 Primary lacrimal gland atrophy, bilateral lacrimal glands

H04.149 Primary lacrimal gland atrophy, unspecified lacrimal gland

● H04.15 Secondary lacrimal gland atrophy

H04.151 Secondary lacrimal gland atrophy, right lacrimal gland

H04.152 Secondary lacrimal gland atrophy, left lacrimal gland

H04.153 Secondary lacrimal gland atrophy, bilateral lacrimal glands

H04.159 Secondary lacrimal gland atrophy, unspecified lacrimal gland

● H04.16 Lacrimal gland dislocation

H04.161 Lacrimal gland dislocation, right lacrimal gland

H04.162 Lacrimal gland dislocation, left lacrimal gland

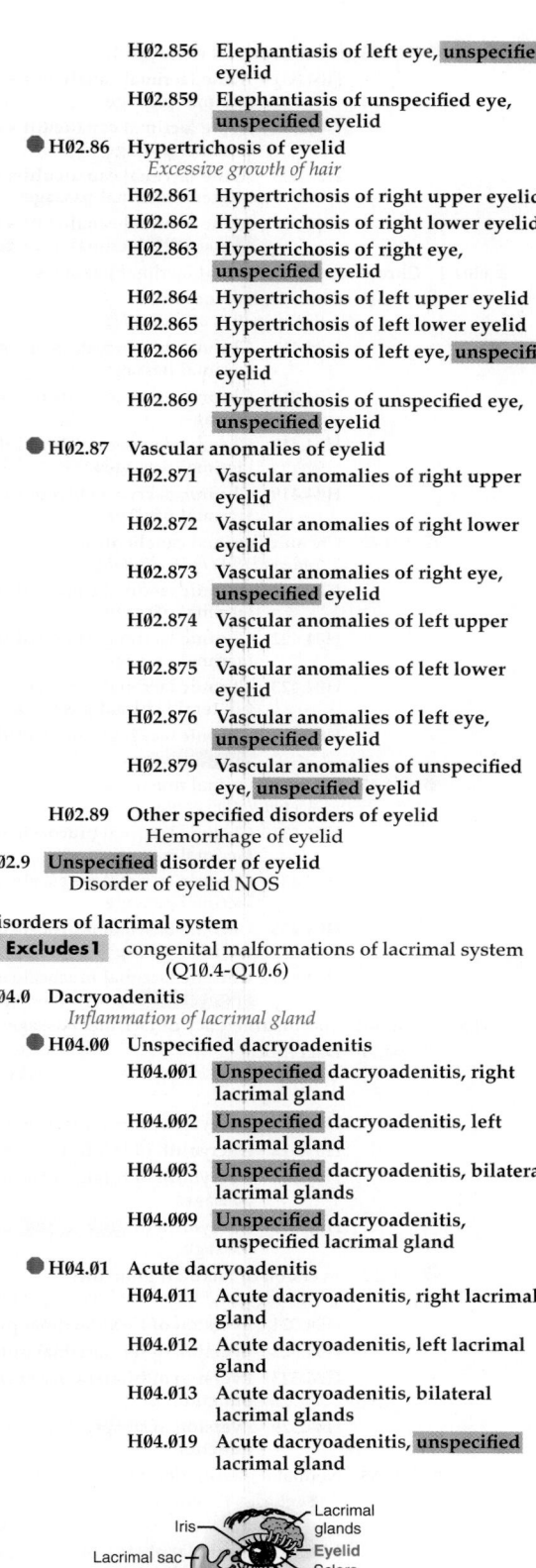

Figure 7-4 Lacrimal apparatus. (From Buck CJ: Step-by-Step Medical Coding, 2016, St. Louis, Elsevier, 2016)

★ **(See Plate 82 on page 67.)**

CHAPTER 7 (H00-H59)

H04.163 Lacrimal gland dislocation, bilateral lacrimal glands
H04.169 Lacrimal gland dislocation, **unspecified** lacrimal gland
H04.19 Other specified disorders of lacrimal gland
● H04.2 Epiphora
Overflow of tears due to stricture of lacrimal passages; AKA lacrimation
● H04.20 Unspecified epiphora
H04.201 **Unspecified** epiphora, right lacrimal gland
H04.202 **Unspecified** epiphora, left lacrimal gland
H04.203 **Unspecified** epiphora, bilateral lacrimal glands
H04.209 **Unspecified** epiphora, unspecified lacrimal gland
● H04.21 Epiphora due to excess lacrimation
H04.211 Epiphora due to excess lacrimation, right lacrimal gland
H04.212 Epiphora due to excess lacrimation, left lacrimal gland
H04.213 Epiphora due to excess lacrimation, bilateral lacrimal glands
H04.219 Epiphora due to excess lacrimation, **unspecified** lacrimal gland
● H04.22 Epiphora due to insufficient drainage
H04.221 Epiphora due to insufficient drainage, right lacrimal gland
H04.222 Epiphora due to insufficient drainage, left lacrimal gland
H04.223 Epiphora due to insufficient drainage, bilateral lacrimal glands
H04.229 Epiphora due to insufficient drainage, **unspecified** lacrimal gland
● H04.3 Acute and unspecified inflammation of lacrimal passages
Excludes1 neonatal dacryocystitis (P39.1)
● H04.30 Unspecified dacryocystitis
H04.301 **Unspecified** dacryocystitis of right lacrimal passage
H04.302 **Unspecified** dacryocystitis of left lacrimal passage
H04.303 **Unspecified** dacryocystitis of bilateral lacrimal passages
H04.309 **Unspecified** dacryocystitis of unspecified lacrimal passage
● H04.31 Phlegmonous dacryocystitis
Cellulitis of lacrimal sac
H04.311 Phlegmonous dacryocystitis of right lacrimal passage
H04.312 Phlegmonous dacryocystitis of left lacrimal passage
H04.313 Phlegmonous dacryocystitis of bilateral lacrimal passages
H04.319 Phlegmonous dacryocystitis of **unspecified** lacrimal passage
● H04.32 Acute dacryocystitis
Acute dacryopericystitis
H04.321 Acute dacryocystitis of right lacrimal passage
H04.322 Acute dacryocystitis of left lacrimal passage
H04.323 Acute dacryocystitis of bilateral lacrimal passages
H04.329 Acute dacryocystitis of **unspecified** lacrimal passage

● H04.33 Acute lacrimal canaliculitis
H04.331 Acute lacrimal canaliculitis of right lacrimal passage
H04.332 Acute lacrimal canaliculitis of left lacrimal passage
H04.333 Acute lacrimal canaliculitis of bilateral lacrimal passages
H04.339 Acute lacrimal canaliculitis of **unspecified** lacrimal passage
● H04.4 Chronic inflammation of lacrimal passages
● H04.41 Chronic dacryocystitis
Inflammation of lacrimal sac
H04.411 Chronic dacryocystitis of right lacrimal passage
H04.412 Chronic dacryocystitis of left lacrimal passage
H04.413 Chronic dacryocystitis of bilateral lacrimal passages
H04.419 Chronic dacryocystitis of **unspecified** lacrimal passage
● H04.42 Chronic lacrimal canaliculitis
Inflammation of lacrimal ducts
H04.421 Chronic lacrimal canaliculitis of right lacrimal passage
H04.422 Chronic lacrimal canaliculitis of left lacrimal passage
H04.423 Chronic lacrimal canaliculitis of bilateral lacrimal passages
H04.429 Chronic lacrimal canaliculitis of **unspecified** lacrimal passage
● H04.43 Chronic lacrimal mucocele
Accumulation of mucous secretion
H04.431 Chronic lacrimal mucocele of right lacrimal passage
H04.432 Chronic lacrimal mucocele of left lacrimal passage
H04.433 Chronic lacrimal mucocele of bilateral lacrimal passages
H04.439 Chronic lacrimal mucocele of **unspecified** lacrimal passage
● H04.5 Stenosis and insufficiency of lacrimal passages
● H04.51 Dacryolith
Concretion in lacrimal sac/duct; AKA lacrimal calculus
H04.511 Dacryolith of right lacrimal passage
H04.512 Dacryolith of left lacrimal passage
H04.513 Dacryolith of bilateral lacrimal passages
H04.519 Dacryolith of **unspecified** lacrimal passage
● H04.52 Eversion of lacrimal punctum
Turning out of lacrimal drainage opening
H04.521 Eversion of right lacrimal punctum
H04.522 Eversion of left lacrimal punctum
H04.523 Eversion of bilateral lacrimal punctum
H04.529 Eversion of **unspecified** lacrimal punctum
● H04.53 Neonatal obstruction of nasolacrimal duct
Excludes1 congenital stenosis and stricture of lacrimal duct (Q10.5)
H04.531 Neonatal obstruction of right nasolacrimal duct   N
H04.532 Neonatal obstruction of left nasolacrimal duct   N
H04.533 Neonatal obstruction of bilateral nasolacrimal duct   N
H04.539 Neonatal obstruction of **unspecified** nasolacrimal duct   N

◀ New ◀▦ Revised ~~deleted~~ Deleted | Excludes 1 | Excludes 2 | Includes | Use additional | Code first | Code also | Unspecified
OGCR Official Guidelines X Assign placeholder X ● Use Additional Character(s) ▌ Manifestation Code **Coding Clinic**

- **H04.54**　Stenosis of lacrimal canaliculi
  - H04.541　Stenosis of right lacrimal canaliculi
  - H04.542　Stenosis of left lacrimal canaliculi
  - H04.543　Stenosis of bilateral lacrimal canaliculi
  - H04.549　Stenosis of unspecified lacrimal canaliculi
- **H04.55**　Acquired stenosis of nasolacrimal duct
  - H04.551　Acquired stenosis of right nasolacrimal duct
  - H04.552　Acquired stenosis of left nasolacrimal duct
  - H04.553　Acquired stenosis of bilateral nasolacrimal duct
  - H04.559　Acquired stenosis of unspecified nasolacrimal duct
- **H04.56**　Stenosis of lacrimal punctum
  - H04.561　Stenosis of right lacrimal punctum
  - H04.562　Stenosis of left lacrimal punctum
  - H04.563　Stenosis of bilateral lacrimal punctum
  - H04.569　Stenosis of unspecified lacrimal punctum
- **H04.57**　Stenosis of lacrimal sac
  - H04.571　Stenosis of right lacrimal sac
  - H04.572　Stenosis of left lacrimal sac
  - H04.573　Stenosis of bilateral lacrimal sac
  - H04.579　Stenosis of unspecified lacrimal sac
- **H04.6**　Other changes of lacrimal passages
  - **H04.61**　Lacrimal fistula
    - H04.611　Lacrimal fistula right lacrimal passage
    - H04.612　Lacrimal fistula left lacrimal passage
    - H04.613　Lacrimal fistula bilateral lacrimal passages
    - H04.619　Lacrimal fistula unspecified lacrimal passage
  - H04.69　Other changes of lacrimal passages
- **H04.8**　Other disorders of lacrimal system
  - **H04.81**　Granuloma of lacrimal passages
    - *Inflammatory response due to infectious or noninfectious agents*
    - H04.811　Granuloma of right lacrimal passage
    - H04.812　Granuloma of left lacrimal passage
    - H04.813　Granuloma of bilateral lacrimal passages
    - H04.819　Granuloma of unspecified lacrimal passage
  - H04.89　Other disorders of lacrimal system
- **H04.9**　Disorder of lacrimal system, unspecified

- **H05**　**Disorders of orbit**
  - **Excludes1**　congenital malformation of orbit (Q10.7)
  - **H05.0**　Acute inflammation of orbit
    - H05.00　Unspecified acute inflammation of orbit
    - **H05.01**　Cellulitis of orbit
      - *Infection of soft tissue of orbit*
      - Abscess of orbit
      - H05.011　Cellulitis of right orbit
      - H05.012　Cellulitis of left orbit
      - H05.013　Cellulitis of bilateral orbits
      - H05.019　Cellulitis of unspecified orbit

- **H05.02**　Osteomyelitis of orbit
  - *Infection of boney orbit of eye*
  - H05.021　Osteomyelitis of right orbit
  - H05.022　Osteomyelitis of left orbit
  - H05.023　Osteomyelitis of bilateral orbits
  - H05.029　Osteomyelitis of unspecified orbit
- **H05.03**　Periostitis of orbit
  - *Inflammation of periosteum (membrane covering bone surface)*
  - H05.031　Periostitis of right orbit
  - H05.032　Periostitis of left orbit
  - H05.033　Periostitis of bilateral orbits
  - H05.039　Periostitis of unspecified orbit
- **H05.04**　Tenonitis of orbit
  - *Inflammation of tenon capsule (space enclosing fascia of Tenon between eyeball and fat of orbit)*
  - H05.041　Tenonitis of right orbit
  - H05.042　Tenonitis of left orbit
  - H05.043　Tenonitis of bilateral orbits
  - H05.049　Tenonitis of unspecified orbit
- **H05.1**　Chronic inflammatory disorders of orbit
  - H05.10　Unspecified chronic inflammatory disorders of orbit
  - **H05.11**　Granuloma of orbit
    - Pseudotumor (inflammatory) of orbit
    - H05.111　Granuloma of right orbit
    - H05.112　Granuloma of left orbit
    - H05.113　Granuloma of bilateral orbits
    - H05.119　Granuloma of unspecified orbit
  - **H05.12**　Orbital myositis
    - *Inflammation of extraocular muscles of orbit*
    - H05.121　Orbital myositis, right orbit
    - H05.122　Orbital myositis, left orbit
    - H05.123　Orbital myositis, bilateral
    - H05.129　Orbital myositis, unspecified orbit
- **H05.2**　Exophthalmic conditions
  - *Bulging eyes*
  - H05.20　Unspecified exophthalmos
  - **H05.21**　Displacement (lateral) of globe
    - H05.211　Displacement (lateral) of globe, right eye
    - H05.212　Displacement (lateral) of globe, left eye
    - H05.213　Displacement (lateral) of globe, bilateral
    - H05.219　Displacement (lateral) of globe, unspecified eye
  - **H05.22**　Edema of orbit
    - Orbital congestion
    - H05.221　Edema of right orbit
    - H05.222　Edema of left orbit
    - H05.223　Edema of bilateral orbit
    - H05.229　Edema of unspecified orbit
  - **H05.23**　Hemorrhage of orbit
    - H05.231　Hemorrhage of right orbit
    - H05.232　Hemorrhage of left orbit
    - H05.233　Hemorrhage of bilateral orbit
    - H05.239　Hemorrhage of unspecified orbit

CHAPTER 7 (H00-H59)

Figure 7-5   Exophthalmos. (From Stein: The Ophthalmic Assistant: Fundamentals and Clinical Practice, ed 6, London, Mosby, 1994)

● H05.24   Constant exophthalmos
Constant bulging eyes, often symptom of Graves disease
    H05.241   Constant exophthalmos, right eye
    H05.242   Constant exophthalmos, left eye
    H05.243   Constant exophthalmos, bilateral
    H05.249   Constant exophthalmos, unspecified eye

● H05.25   Intermittent exophthalmos
Intermittent bulging eye occurring with bending forward or sharp turning of head
    H05.251   Intermittent exophthalmos, right eye
    H05.252   Intermittent exophthalmos, left eye
    H05.253   Intermittent exophthalmos, bilateral
    H05.259   Intermittent exophthalmos, unspecified eye

● H05.26   Pulsating exophthalmos
Bulging eyes with pulsation and bruit, often due to aneurysm pushing eye forward
    H05.261   Pulsating exophthalmos, right eye
    H05.262   Pulsating exophthalmos, left eye
    H05.263   Pulsating exophthalmos, bilateral
    H05.269   Pulsating exophthalmos, unspecified eye

● H05.3   Deformity of orbit
    Excludes1   congenital deformity of orbit (Q10.7)
                    hypertelorism (Q75.2)
    H05.30   Unspecified deformity of orbit
● H05.31   Atrophy of orbit
    H05.311   Atrophy of right orbit
    H05.312   Atrophy of left orbit
    H05.313   Atrophy of bilateral orbit
    H05.319   Atrophy of unspecified orbit
● H05.32   Deformity of orbit due to bone disease
    Code also associated bone disease
    H05.321   Deformity of right orbit due to bone disease
    H05.322   Deformity of left orbit due to bone disease
    H05.323   Deformity of bilateral orbits due to bone disease
    H05.329   Deformity of unspecified orbit due to bone disease
● H05.33   Deformity of orbit due to trauma or surgery
    H05.331   Deformity of right orbit due to trauma or surgery
    H05.332   Deformity of left orbit due to trauma or surgery
    H05.333   Deformity of bilateral orbits due to trauma or surgery
    H05.339   Deformity of unspecified orbit due to trauma or surgery

● H05.34   Enlargement of orbit
    H05.341   Enlargement of right orbit
    H05.342   Enlargement of left orbit
    H05.343   Enlargement of bilateral orbits
    H05.349   Enlargement of unspecified orbit
● H05.35   Exostosis of orbit
    H05.351   Exostosis of right orbit
    H05.352   Exostosis of left orbit
    H05.353   Exostosis of bilateral orbits
    H05.359   Exostosis of unspecified orbit

● H05.4   Enophthalmos
Recessed eyeball into orbit
● H05.40   Unspecified enophthalmos
    H05.401   Unspecified enophthalmos, right eye
    H05.402   Unspecified enophthalmos, left eye
    H05.403   Unspecified enophthalmos, bilateral
    H05.409   Unspecified enophthalmos, unspecified eye
● H05.41   Enophthalmos due to atrophy of orbital tissue
    H05.411   Enophthalmos due to atrophy of orbital tissue, right eye
    H05.412   Enophthalmos due to atrophy of orbital tissue, left eye
    H05.413   Enophthalmos due to atrophy of orbital tissue, bilateral
    H05.419   Enophthalmos due to atrophy of orbital tissue, unspecified eye
● H05.42   Enophthalmos due to trauma or surgery
    H05.421   Enophthalmos due to trauma or surgery, right eye
    H05.422   Enophthalmos due to trauma or surgery, left eye
    H05.423   Enophthalmos due to trauma or surgery, bilateral
    H05.429   Enophthalmos due to trauma or surgery, unspecified eye
● H05.5   Retained (old) foreign body following penetrating wound of orbit
    Retrobulbar foreign body
    Use additional code to identify the type of retained foreign body (Z18.-)
    Excludes1   current penetrating wound of orbit (S05.4-)
    Excludes2   retained foreign body of eyelid (H02.81-)
                    retained intraocular foreign body (H44.6-, H44.7-)
    H05.50   Retained (old) foreign body following penetrating wound of unspecified orbit
    H05.51   Retained (old) foreign body following penetrating wound of right orbit
    H05.52   Retained (old) foreign body following penetrating wound of left orbit
    H05.53   Retained (old) foreign body following penetrating wound of bilateral orbits
● H05.8   Other disorders of orbit
● H05.81   Cyst of orbit
    Encephalocele of orbit
    H05.811   Cyst of right orbit
    H05.812   Cyst of left orbit
    H05.813   Cyst of bilateral orbits
    H05.819   Cyst of unspecified orbit

◀ New   ◀▥ Revised   ~~deleted~~ Deleted   Excludes 1   Excludes 2   Includes   Use additional   Code first   Code also   Unspecified
OGCR Official Guidelines   X Assign placeholder X   ● Use Additional Character(s)   ▶ Manifestation Code   **Coding Clinic**

● H05.82   **Myopathy of extraocular muscles**
     Weakness of muscles of eye

     H05.821   **Myopathy of extraocular muscles, right orbit**

     H05.822   **Myopathy of extraocular muscles, left orbit**

     H05.823   **Myopathy of extraocular muscles, bilateral**

     H05.829   **Myopathy of extraocular muscles, unspecified orbit**

   H05.89   **Other disorders of orbit**

H05.9   **Unspecified disorder of orbit**

DISORDERS OF CONJUNCTIVA (H10-H11)

★ **(See Plate 81, upper, on page 66.)**

● H10   **Conjunctivitis**
     Inflammation of membrane of the inside of the eyelid or on surface of eye (conjunctiva)

     Excludes1   keratoconjunctivitis (H16.2-)

● H10.0   **Mucopurulent conjunctivitis**

   ● H10.01   **Acute follicular conjunctivitis**

     H10.011   **Acute follicular conjunctivitis, right eye**

     H10.012   **Acute follicular conjunctivitis, left eye**

     H10.013   **Acute follicular conjunctivitis, bilateral**

     H10.019   **Acute follicular conjunctivitis, unspecified eye**

   ● H10.02   **Other mucopurulent conjunctivitis**

     H10.021   **Other mucopurulent conjunctivitis, right eye**

     H10.022   **Other mucopurulent conjunctivitis, left eye**

     H10.023   **Other mucopurulent conjunctivitis, bilateral**

     H10.029   **Other mucopurulent conjunctivitis, unspecified eye**

● H10.1   **Acute atopic conjunctivitis**
     Acute papillary conjunctivitis

   H10.10   **Acute atopic conjunctivitis, unspecified eye**

   H10.11   **Acute atopic conjunctivitis, right eye**

   H10.12   **Acute atopic conjunctivitis, left eye**

   H10.13   **Acute atopic conjunctivitis, bilateral**

● H10.2   **Other acute conjunctivitis**

   ● H10.21   **Acute toxic conjunctivitis**
     Acute chemical conjunctivitis

     Code first (T51-T65) *to identify chemical and intent*

     Excludes1   burn and corrosion of eye and adnexa (T26.-)

     H10.211   **Acute toxic conjunctivitis, right eye**

     H10.212   **Acute toxic conjunctivitis, left eye**

     H10.213   **Acute toxic conjunctivitis, bilateral**

     H10.219   **Acute toxic conjunctivitis, unspecified eye**

   ● H10.22   **Pseudomembranous conjunctivitis**

     H10.221   **Pseudomembranous conjunctivitis, right eye**

     H10.222   **Pseudomembranous conjunctivitis, left eye**

     H10.223   **Pseudomembranous conjunctivitis, bilateral**

     H10.229   **Pseudomembranous conjunctivitis, unspecified eye**

● H10.23   **Serous conjunctivitis, except viral**

     Excludes1   viral conjunctivitis (B30.-)

     H10.231   **Serous conjunctivitis, except viral, right eye**

     H10.232   **Serous conjunctivitis, except viral, left eye**

     H10.233   **Serous conjunctivitis, except viral, bilateral**

     H10.239   **Serous conjunctivitis, except viral, unspecified eye**

● H10.3   **Unspecified acute conjunctivitis**

     Excludes1   ophthalmia neonatorum NOS (P39.1)

   H10.30   **Unspecified acute conjunctivitis, unspecified eye**

   H10.31   **Unspecified acute conjunctivitis, right eye**

   H10.32   **Unspecified acute conjunctivitis, left eye**

   H10.33   **Unspecified acute conjunctivitis, bilateral**

● H10.4   **Chronic conjunctivitis**

   ● H10.40   **Unspecified chronic conjunctivitis**

     H10.401   **Unspecified chronic conjunctivitis, right eye**

     H10.402   **Unspecified chronic conjunctivitis, left eye**

     H10.403   **Unspecified chronic conjunctivitis, bilateral**

     H10.409   **Unspecified chronic conjunctivitis, unspecified eye**

   ● H10.41   **Chronic giant papillary conjunctivitis**
     Inflammation of membrane of the inside of the eyelid or on surface of eye often associated with contact lens wear

     H10.411   **Chronic giant papillary conjunctivitis, right eye**

     H10.412   **Chronic giant papillary conjunctivitis, left eye**

     H10.413   **Chronic giant papillary conjunctivitis, bilateral**

     H10.419   **Chronic giant papillary conjunctivitis, unspecified eye**

   ● H10.42   **Simple chronic conjunctivitis**

     H10.421   **Simple chronic conjunctivitis, right eye**

     H10.422   **Simple chronic conjunctivitis, left eye**

     H10.423   **Simple chronic conjunctivitis, bilateral**

     H10.429   **Simple chronic conjunctivitis, unspecified eye**

   ● H10.43   **Chronic follicular conjunctivitis**
     Inflammation of membrane of the inside of the eyelid or on surface of eye due to topical medications or infection

     H10.431   **Chronic follicular conjunctivitis, right eye**

     H10.432   **Chronic follicular conjunctivitis, left eye**

     H10.433   **Chronic follicular conjunctivitis, bilateral**

     H10.439   **Chronic follicular conjunctivitis, unspecified eye**

   H10.44   **Vernal conjunctivitis**
     Affecting children, especially boys in which there are flattened papules with thick, gelatinous exudate on conjunctivae on inside of upper lid

     Excludes1   vernal keratoconjunctivitis with limbar and corneal involvement (H16.26-)

   H10.45   **Other chronic allergic conjunctivitis**

CHAPTER 7 (H00-H59)

● **H10.5 Blepharoconjunctivitis**
Inflammation of eyelids and conjunctiva

  ● **H10.50 Unspecified blepharoconjunctivitis**

    H10.501 Unspecified blepharoconjunctivitis, right eye

    H10.502 Unspecified blepharoconjunctivitis, left eye

    H10.503 Unspecified blepharoconjunctivitis, bilateral

    H10.509 Unspecified blepharoconjunctivitis, unspecified eye

  ● **H10.51 Ligneous conjunctivitis**

    H10.511 Ligneous conjunctivitis, right eye

    H10.512 Ligneous conjunctivitis, left eye

    H10.513 Ligneous conjunctivitis, bilateral

    H10.519 Ligneous conjunctivitis, unspecified eye

  ● **H10.52 Angular blepharoconjunctivitis**

    H10.521 Angular blepharoconjunctivitis, right eye

    H10.522 Angular blepharoconjunctivitis, left eye

    H10.523 Angular blepharoconjunctivitis, bilateral

    H10.529 Angular blepharoconjunctivitis, unspecified eye

  ● **H10.53 Contact blepharoconjunctivitis**

    H10.531 Contact blepharoconjunctivitis, right eye

    H10.532 Contact blepharoconjunctivitis, left eye

    H10.533 Contact blepharoconjunctivitis, bilateral

    H10.539 Contact blepharoconjunctivitis, unspecified eye

  ● **H10.8 Other conjunctivitis**

  ● **H10.81 Pingueculitis**
Inflammation of a yellow, raised thickening on the white of the eye associated with chronic dry eyes

    Excludes1 pinguecula (H11.15-)

    H10.811 Pingueculitis, right eye

    H10.812 Pingueculitis, left eye

    H10.813 Pingueculitis, bilateral

    H10.819 Pingueculitis, unspecified eye

    H10.89 Other conjunctivitis

    H10.9 Unspecified conjunctivitis

● **H11 Other disorders of conjunctiva**

  Excludes1 keratoconjunctivitis (H16.2-)

  ● **H11.0 Pterygium of eye**

    Excludes1 pseudopterygium (H11.81-)

  ● **H11.00 Unspecified pterygium of eye**

    H11.001 Unspecified pterygium of right eye

    H11.002 Unspecified pterygium of left eye

    H11.003 Unspecified pterygium of eye, bilateral

    H11.009 Unspecified pterygium of unspecified eye

  ● **H11.01 Amyloid pterygium**

    H11.011 Amyloid pterygium of right eye

    H11.012 Amyloid pterygium of left eye

    H11.013 Amyloid pterygium of eye, bilateral

    H11.019 Amyloid pterygium of unspecified eye

Figure 7-6 Double pterygium. Note both nasal and temporal pterygia in a 57-year-old farmer. (From Yanoff: Ophthalmology, ed 3, Mosby, Inc., 2008)

Item 7–2 **Pterygium** is Greek for batlike. The condition is characterized by a membrane that extends from the limbus to the center of the cornea and resembles a wing.

  ● **H11.02 Central pterygium of eye**

    H11.021 Central pterygium of right eye

    H11.022 Central pterygium of left eye

    H11.023 Central pterygium of eye, bilateral

    H11.029 Central pterygium of unspecified eye

  ● **H11.03 Double pterygium of eye**

    H11.031 Double pterygium of right eye

    H11.032 Double pterygium of left eye

    H11.033 Double pterygium of eye, bilateral

    H11.039 Double pterygium of unspecified eye

  ● **H11.04 Peripheral pterygium of eye, stationary**

    H11.041 Peripheral pterygium, stationary, right eye

    H11.042 Peripheral pterygium, stationary, left eye

    H11.043 Peripheral pterygium, stationary, bilateral

    H11.049 Peripheral pterygium, stationary, unspecified eye

  ● **H11.05 Peripheral pterygium of eye, progressive**

    H11.051 Peripheral pterygium, progressive, right eye

    H11.052 Peripheral pterygium, progressive, left eye

    H11.053 Peripheral pterygium, progressive, bilateral

    H11.059 Peripheral pterygium, progressive, unspecified eye

  ● **H11.06 Recurrent pterygium of eye**

    H11.061 Recurrent pterygium of right eye

    H11.062 Recurrent pterygium of left eye

    H11.063 Recurrent pterygium of eye, bilateral

    H11.069 Recurrent pterygium of unspecified eye

  ● **H11.1 Conjunctival degenerations and deposits**

    Excludes2 pseudopterygium (H11.81)

    H11.10 Unspecified conjunctival degenerations

  ● **H11.11 Conjunctival deposits**

    H11.111 Conjunctival deposits, right eye

    H11.112 Conjunctival deposits, left eye

    H11.113 Conjunctival deposits, bilateral

    H11.119 Conjunctival deposits, unspecified eye

  ● **H11.12 Conjunctival concretions**
White to yellow nodules within or beneath conjunctiva

    H11.121 Conjunctival concretions, right eye

    H11.122 Conjunctival concretions, left eye

    H11.123 Conjunctival concretions, bilateral

    H11.129 Conjunctival concretions, unspecified eye

  ● **H11.13 Conjunctival pigmentations**
Conjunctival argyrosis [argyria]

    H11.131 Conjunctival pigmentations, right eye

    H11.132 Conjunctival pigmentations, left eye

    H11.133 Conjunctival pigmentations, bilateral

    H11.139 Conjunctival pigmentations, unspecified eye

◀ New   ◀▥ Revised   ~~deleted~~ Deleted   Excludes 1   Excludes 2   Includes   Use additional   Code first   Code also   Unspecified

OGCR Official Guidelines   X Assign placeholder X   ● Use Additional Character(s)   ▶ Manifestation Code   **Coding Clinic**

● **H11.14**   Conjunctival xerosis, unspecified
>   **Excludes1**   xerosis of conjunctiva due to
>   vitamin A deficiency (E50.0,
>   E50.1)

    H11.141   Conjunctival xerosis, unspecified, right eye

    H11.142   Conjunctival xerosis, unspecified, left eye

    H11.143   Conjunctival xerosis, unspecified, bilateral

    H11.149   Conjunctival xerosis, unspecified, unspecified eye

● **H11.15**   Pinguecula
>   *Yellowish spot near sclerocorneal junction, usually*
>   *on nasal side; associated with aging*
>   **Excludes1**   pingueculitis (H10.81-)

    H11.151   Pinguecula, right eye

    H11.152   Pinguecula, left eye

    H11.153   Pinguecula, bilateral

    H11.159   Pinguecula, unspecified eye

● **H11.2**   Conjunctival scars

  ● **H11.21**   Conjunctival adhesions and strands (localized)

    H11.211   Conjunctival adhesions and strands (localized), right eye

    H11.212   Conjunctival adhesions and strands (localized), left eye

    H11.213   Conjunctival adhesions and strands (localized), bilateral

    H11.219   Conjunctival adhesions and strands (localized), unspecified eye

  ● **H11.22**   Conjunctival granuloma

    H11.221   Conjunctival granuloma, right eye

    H11.222   Conjunctival granuloma, left eye

    H11.223   Conjunctival granuloma, bilateral

    H11.229   Conjunctival granuloma, unspecified

  ● **H11.23**   Symblepharon
>   *Adhesion between tarsal conjunctiva and bulbar*
>   *conjunctiva*

    H11.231   Symblepharon, right eye

    H11.232   Symblepharon, left eye

    H11.233   Symblepharon, bilateral

    H11.239   Symblepharon, unspecified eye

  ● **H11.24**   Scarring of conjunctiva

    H11.241   Scarring of conjunctiva, right eye

    H11.242   Scarring of conjunctiva, left eye

    H11.243   Scarring of conjunctiva, bilateral

    H11.249   Scarring of conjunctiva, unspecified eye

● **H11.3**   Conjunctival hemorrhage
>   Subconjunctival hemorrhage

    H11.30   Conjunctival hemorrhage, unspecified eye

    H11.31   Conjunctival hemorrhage, right eye

    H11.32   Conjunctival hemorrhage, left eye

    H11.33   Conjunctival hemorrhage, bilateral

● **H11.4**   Other conjunctival vascular disorders and cysts

  ● **H11.41**   Vascular abnormalities of conjunctiva
>   Conjunctival aneurysm

    H11.411   Vascular abnormalities of conjunctiva, right eye

    H11.412   Vascular abnormalities of conjunctiva, left eye

    H11.413   Vascular abnormalities of conjunctiva, bilateral

    H11.419   Vascular abnormalities of conjunctiva, unspecified eye

● **H11.42**   Conjunctival edema

    H11.421   Conjunctival edema, right eye

    H11.422   Conjunctival edema, left eye

    H11.423   Conjunctival edema, bilateral

    H11.429   Conjunctival edema, unspecified eye

● **H11.43**   Conjunctival hyperemia

    H11.431   Conjunctival hyperemia, right eye

    H11.432   Conjunctival hyperemia, left eye

    H11.433   Conjunctival hyperemia, bilateral

    H11.439   Conjunctival hyperemia, unspecified eye

● **H11.44**   Conjunctival cysts

    H11.441   Conjunctival cysts, right eye

    H11.442   Conjunctival cysts, left eye

    H11.443   Conjunctival cysts, bilateral

    H11.449   Conjunctival cysts, unspecified eye

● **H11.8**   Other specified disorders of conjunctiva

  ● **H11.81**   Pseudopterygium of conjunctiva
>   *Conjunctival scar attached to cornea*

    H11.811   Pseudopterygium of conjunctiva, right eye

    H11.812   Pseudopterygium of conjunctiva, left eye

    H11.813   Pseudopterygium of conjunctiva, bilateral

    H11.819   Pseudopterygium of conjunctiva, unspecified eye

  ● **H11.82**   Conjunctivochalasis
>   *Conjunctiva bulges over eyelid margin or covers*
>   *lower punctum*

    H11.821   Conjunctivochalasis, right eye

    H11.822   Conjunctivochalasis, left eye

    H11.823   Conjunctivochalasis, bilateral

    H11.829   Conjunctivochalasis, unspecified eye

    H11.89   Other specified disorders of conjunctiva

  H11.9   Unspecified disorder of conjunctiva

DISORDERS OF SCLERA, CORNEA, IRIS AND CILIARY BODY (H15-H22)

● **H15**   Disorders of sclera

  ● **H15.0**   Scleritis
>   *Inflammation of the white (sclera and episclera) of the eye.*

    ● **H15.00**   Unspecified scleritis

      H15.001   Unspecified scleritis, right eye

      H15.002   Unspecified scleritis, left eye

      H15.003   Unspecified scleritis, bilateral

      H15.009   Unspecified scleritis, unspecified eye

    ● **H15.01**   Anterior scleritis

      H15.011   Anterior scleritis, right eye

      H15.012   Anterior scleritis, left eye

      H15.013   Anterior scleritis, bilateral

      H15.019   Anterior scleritis, unspecified eye

    ● **H15.02**   Brawny scleritis
>   *Swelling around the cornea that is gelantinous in*
>   *appearance*

      H15.021   Brawny scleritis, right eye

      H15.022   Brawny scleritis, left eye

      H15.023   Brawny scleritis, bilateral

      H15.029   Brawny scleritis, unspecified eye

    ● **H15.03**   Posterior scleritis
>   Sclerotenonitis

      H15.031   Posterior scleritis, right eye

      H15.032   Posterior scleritis, left eye

      H15.033   Posterior scleritis, bilateral

      H15.039   Posterior scleritis, unspecified eye

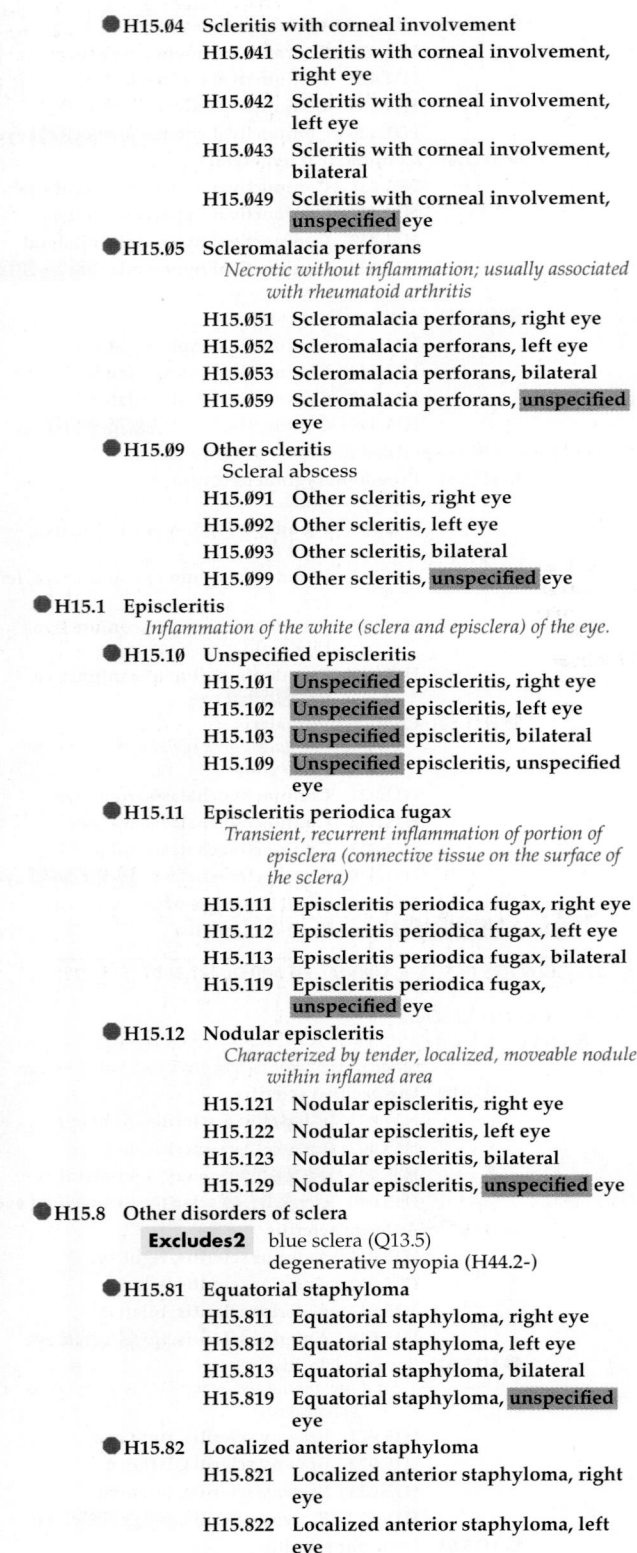

● H15.04   Scleritis with corneal involvement
    H15.041   Scleritis with corneal involvement, right eye
    H15.042   Scleritis with corneal involvement, left eye
    H15.043   Scleritis with corneal involvement, bilateral
    H15.049   Scleritis with corneal involvement, unspecified eye

● H15.05   Scleromalacia perforans
    Necrotic without inflammation; usually associated with rheumatoid arthritis
    H15.051   Scleromalacia perforans, right eye
    H15.052   Scleromalacia perforans, left eye
    H15.053   Scleromalacia perforans, bilateral
    H15.059   Scleromalacia perforans, unspecified eye

● H15.09   Other scleritis
    Scleral abscess
    H15.091   Other scleritis, right eye
    H15.092   Other scleritis, left eye
    H15.093   Other scleritis, bilateral
    H15.099   Other scleritis, unspecified eye

● H15.1   Episcleritis
    Inflammation of the white (sclera and episclera) of the eye.

● H15.10   Unspecified episcleritis
    H15.101   Unspecified episcleritis, right eye
    H15.102   Unspecified episcleritis, left eye
    H15.103   Unspecified episcleritis, bilateral
    H15.109   Unspecified episcleritis, unspecified eye

● H15.11   Episcleritis periodica fugax
    Transient, recurrent inflammation of portion of episclera (connective tissue on the surface of the sclera)
    H15.111   Episcleritis periodica fugax, right eye
    H15.112   Episcleritis periodica fugax, left eye
    H15.113   Episcleritis periodica fugax, bilateral
    H15.119   Episcleritis periodica fugax, unspecified eye

● H15.12   Nodular episcleritis
    Characterized by tender, localized, moveable nodule within inflamed area
    H15.121   Nodular episcleritis, right eye
    H15.122   Nodular episcleritis, left eye
    H15.123   Nodular episcleritis, bilateral
    H15.129   Nodular episcleritis, unspecified eye

● H15.8   Other disorders of sclera
    Excludes2   blue sclera (Q13.5)
                  degenerative myopia (H44.2-)

● H15.81   Equatorial staphyloma
    H15.811   Equatorial staphyloma, right eye
    H15.812   Equatorial staphyloma, left eye
    H15.813   Equatorial staphyloma, bilateral
    H15.819   Equatorial staphyloma, unspecified eye

● H15.82   Localized anterior staphyloma
    H15.821   Localized anterior staphyloma, right eye
    H15.822   Localized anterior staphyloma, left eye
    H15.823   Localized anterior staphyloma, bilateral
    H15.829   Localized anterior staphyloma, unspecified eye

● H15.83   Staphyloma posticum
    H15.831   Staphyloma posticum, right eye
    H15.832   Staphyloma posticum, left eye
    H15.833   Staphyloma posticum, bilateral
    H15.839   Staphyloma posticum, unspecified eye

● H15.84   Scleral ectasia
    H15.841   Scleral ectasia, right eye
    H15.842   Scleral ectasia, left eye
    H15.843   Scleral ectasia, bilateral
    H15.849   Scleral ectasia, unspecified eye

● H15.85   Ring staphyloma
    H15.851   Ring staphyloma, right eye
    H15.852   Ring staphyloma, left eye
    H15.853   Ring staphyloma, bilateral
    H15.859   Ring staphyloma, unspecified eye

    H15.89   Other disorders of sclera
  H15.9   Unspecified disorder of sclera

● H16   Keratitis
  ● H16.0   Corneal ulcer
   ● H16.00   Unspecified corneal ulcer
    H16.001   Unspecified corneal ulcer, right eye
    H16.002   Unspecified corneal ulcer, left eye
    H16.003   Unspecified corneal ulcer, bilateral
    H16.009   Unspecified corneal ulcer, unspecified eye

   ● H16.01   Central corneal ulcer
    H16.011   Central corneal ulcer, right eye
    H16.012   Central corneal ulcer, left eye
    H16.013   Central corneal ulcer, bilateral
    H16.019   Central corneal ulcer, unspecified eye

   ● H16.02   Ring corneal ulcer
    H16.021   Ring corneal ulcer, right eye
    H16.022   Ring corneal ulcer, left eye
    H16.023   Ring corneal ulcer, bilateral
    H16.029   Ring corneal ulcer, unspecified eye

   ● H16.03   Corneal ulcer with hypopyon
    H16.031   Corneal ulcer with hypopyon, right eye
    H16.032   Corneal ulcer with hypopyon, left eye
    H16.033   Corneal ulcer with hypopyon, bilateral
    H16.039   Corneal ulcer with hypopyon, unspecified eye

Marginal (catarrhal) ulcer   Ring ulcer   Central corneal ulcer   Rosacea ulcer   Mooren's (rodent) ulcer

Figure 7-7   Corneal ulcers: marginal, ring, central corneal, rosacea, and Mooren's.

Item 7-3   An infected ulcer is usually called a **serpiginous** or **hypopyon** ulcer which is a pus sac in the anterior chamber of the eye. **Marginal** ulcers are usually asymptomatic, not primary, and are often superficial and simple. More severe marginal ulcers spread to form a ring ulcer. **Ring** ulcers can extend around the entire corneal periphery. **Central corneal** ulcers develop when there is an abrasion to the epithelium and an infection develops in the eroded area. The **pyocyaneal** ulcer is the most serious corneal infection, which, if left untreated, can lead to loss of the eye.

◀ New   ◀ Revised   ~~deleted~~ Deleted   Excludes 1   Excludes 2   Includes   Use additional   Code first   Code also   Unspecified
OGCR Official Guidelines   X Assign placeholder X   ● Use Additional Character(s)   ▶ Manifestation Code   **Coding Clinic**

● **H16.04**   **Marginal corneal ulcer**
     H16.041   Marginal corneal ulcer, right eye
     H16.042   Marginal corneal ulcer, left eye
     H16.043   Marginal corneal ulcer, bilateral
     H16.049   Marginal corneal ulcer, unspecified eye

● **H16.05**   **Mooren's corneal ulcer**
     H16.051   Mooren's corneal ulcer, right eye
     H16.052   Mooren's corneal ulcer, left eye
     H16.053   Mooren's corneal ulcer, bilateral
     H16.059   Mooren's corneal ulcer, unspecified eye

● **H16.06**   **Mycotic corneal ulcer**
     H16.061   Mycotic corneal ulcer, right eye
     H16.062   Mycotic corneal ulcer, left eye
     H16.063   Mycotic corneal ulcer, bilateral
     H16.069   Mycotic corneal ulcer, unspecified eye

● **H16.07**   **Perforated corneal ulcer**
     H16.071   Perforated corneal ulcer, right eye
     H16.072   Perforated corneal ulcer, left eye
     H16.073   Perforated corneal ulcer, bilateral
     H16.079   Perforated corneal ulcer, unspecified eye

● **H16.1**   **Other and unspecified superficial keratitis without conjunctivitis**

   ● **H16.10**   Unspecified superficial keratitis
     H16.101   Unspecified superficial keratitis, right eye
     H16.102   Unspecified superficial keratitis, left eye
     H16.103   Unspecified superficial keratitis, bilateral
     H16.109   Unspecified superficial keratitis, unspecified eye

   ● **H16.11**   Macular keratitis
     Areolar keratitis
     Nummular keratitis
     Stellate keratitis
     Striate keratitis
     H16.111   Macular keratitis, right eye
     H16.112   Macular keratitis, left eye
     H16.113   Macular keratitis, bilateral
     H16.119   Macular keratitis, unspecified eye

   ● **H16.12**   Filamentary keratitis
     H16.121   Filamentary keratitis, right eye
     H16.122   Filamentary keratitis, left eye
     H16.123   Filamentary keratitis, bilateral
     H16.129   Filamentary keratitis, unspecified eye

   ● **H16.13**   Photokeratitis
     Snow blindness
     Welders' keratitis
     H16.131   Photokeratitis, right eye
     H16.132   Photokeratitis, left eye
     H16.133   Photokeratitis, bilateral
     H16.139   Photokeratitis, unspecified eye

   ● **H16.14**   Punctate keratitis
     H16.141   Punctate keratitis, right eye
     H16.142   Punctate keratitis, left eye
     H16.143   Punctate keratitis, bilateral
     H16.149   Punctate keratitis, unspecified eye

● **H16.2**   **Keratoconjunctivitis**

   ● **H16.20**   Unspecified keratoconjunctivitis
     Superficial keratitis with conjunctivitis NOS
     H16.201   Unspecified keratoconjunctivitis, right eye
     H16.202   Unspecified keratoconjunctivitis, left eye
     H16.203   Unspecified keratoconjunctivitis, bilateral
     H16.209   Unspecified keratoconjunctivitis, unspecified eye

   ● **H16.21**   Exposure keratoconjunctivitis
     H16.211   Exposure keratoconjunctivitis, right eye
     H16.212   Exposure keratoconjunctivitis, left eye
     H16.213   Exposure keratoconjunctivitis, bilateral
     H16.219   Exposure keratoconjunctivitis, unspecified eye

   ● **H16.22**   Keratoconjunctivitis sicca, not specified as Sjögren's

     Excludes1   Sjogren's syndrome (M35.01)

     H16.221   Keratoconjunctivitis sicca, not specified as Sjögren's, right eye
     H16.222   Keratoconjunctivitis sicca, not specified as Sjögren's, left eye
     H16.223   Keratoconjunctivitis sicca, not specified as Sjögren's, bilateral
     H16.229   Keratoconjunctivitis sicca, not specified as Sjögren's, unspecified eye

   ● **H16.23**   Neurotrophic keratoconjunctivitis
     H16.231   Neurotrophic keratoconjunctivitis, right eye
     H16.232   Neurotrophic keratoconjunctivitis, left eye
     H16.233   Neurotrophic keratoconjunctivitis, bilateral
     H16.239   Neurotrophic keratoconjunctivitis, unspecified eye

   ● **H16.24**   Ophthalmia nodosa
     H16.241   Ophthalmia nodosa, right eye
     H16.242   Ophthalmia nodosa, left eye
     H16.243   Ophthalmia nodosa, bilateral
     H16.249   Ophthalmia nodosa, unspecified eye

   ● **H16.25**   Phlyctenular keratoconjunctivitis
     H16.251   Phlyctenular keratoconjunctivitis, right eye
     H16.252   Phlyctenular keratoconjunctivitis, left eye
     H16.253   Phlyctenular keratoconjunctivitis, bilateral
     H16.259   Phlyctenular keratoconjunctivitis, unspecified eye

   ● **H16.26**   Vernal keratoconjunctivitis, with limbar and corneal involvement

     Excludes1   vernal conjunctivitis without limbar and corneal involvement (H10.44)

     H16.261   Vernal keratoconjunctivitis, with limbar and corneal involvement, right eye
     H16.262   Vernal keratoconjunctivitis, with limbar and corneal involvement, left eye

CHAPTER 7 (H00-H59)

H16.263   Vernal keratoconjunctivitis, with limbar and corneal involvement, bilateral

H16.269   Vernal keratoconjunctivitis, with limbar and corneal involvement, unspecified eye

● H16.29   Other keratoconjunctivitis

H16.291   Other keratoconjunctivitis, right eye

H16.292   Other keratoconjunctivitis, left eye

H16.293   Other keratoconjunctivitis, bilateral

H16.299   Other keratoconjunctivitis, unspecified eye

● H16.3   Interstitial and deep keratitis

● H16.30   Unspecified interstitial keratitis

H16.301   Unspecified interstitial keratitis, right eye

H16.302   Unspecified interstitial keratitis, left eye

H16.303   Unspecified interstitial keratitis, bilateral

H16.309   Unspecified interstitial keratitis, unspecified eye

● H16.31   Corneal abscess

H16.311   Corneal abscess, right eye

H16.312   Corneal abscess, left eye

H16.313   Corneal abscess, bilateral

H16.319   Corneal abscess, unspecified eye

● H16.32   Diffuse interstitial keratitis
          Cogan's syndrome

H16.321   Diffuse interstitial keratitis, right eye

H16.322   Diffuse interstitial keratitis, left eye

H16.323   Diffuse interstitial keratitis, bilateral

H16.329   Diffuse interstitial keratitis, unspecified eye

● H16.33   Sclerosing keratitis

H16.331   Sclerosing keratitis, right eye

H16.332   Sclerosing keratitis, left eye

H16.333   Sclerosing keratitis, bilateral

H16.339   Sclerosing keratitis, unspecified eye

● H16.39   Other interstitial and deep keratitis

H16.391   Other interstitial and deep keratitis, right eye

H16.392   Other interstitial and deep keratitis, left eye

H16.393   Other interstitial and deep keratitis, bilateral

H16.399   Other interstitial and deep keratitis, unspecified eye

● H16.4   Corneal neovascularization

● H16.40   Unspecified corneal neovascularization

H16.401   Unspecified corneal neovascularization, right eye

H16.402   Unspecified corneal neovascularization, left eye

H16.403   Unspecified corneal neovascularization, bilateral

H16.409   Unspecified corneal neovascularization, unspecified eye

● H16.41   Ghost vessels (corneal)

H16.411   Ghost vessels (corneal), right eye

H16.412   Ghost vessels (corneal), left eye

H16.413   Ghost vessels (corneal), bilateral

H16.419   Ghost vessels (corneal), unspecified eye

● H16.42   Pannus (corneal)

H16.421   Pannus (corneal), right eye

H16.422   Pannus (corneal), left eye

H16.423   Pannus (corneal), bilateral

H16.429   Pannus (corneal), unspecified eye

● H16.43   Localized vascularization of cornea

H16.431   Localized vascularization of cornea, right eye

H16.432   Localized vascularization of cornea, left eye

H16.433   Localized vascularization of cornea, bilateral

H16.439   Localized vascularization of cornea, unspecified eye

● H16.44   Deep vascularization of cornea

H16.441   Deep vascularization of cornea, right eye

H16.442   Deep vascularization of cornea, left eye

H16.443   Deep vascularization of cornea, bilateral

H16.449   Deep vascularization of cornea, unspecified eye

H16.8   Other keratitis

H16.9   Unspecified keratitis

● H17   Corneal scars and opacities

● H17.0   Adherent leukoma

H17.00   Adherent leukoma, unspecified eye

H17.01   Adherent leukoma, right eye

H17.02   Adherent leukoma, left eye

H17.03   Adherent leukoma, bilateral

● H17.1   Central corneal opacity

H17.10   Central corneal opacity, unspecified eye

H17.11   Central corneal opacity, right eye

H17.12   Central corneal opacity, left eye

H17.13   Central corneal opacity, bilateral

● H17.8   Other corneal scars and opacities

● H17.81   Minor opacity of cornea
          Corneal nebula

H17.811   Minor opacity of cornea, right eye

H17.812   Minor opacity of cornea, left eye

H17.813   Minor opacity of cornea, bilateral

H17.819   Minor opacity of cornea, unspecified eye

● H17.82   Peripheral opacity of cornea

H17.821   Peripheral opacity of cornea, right eye

H17.822   Peripheral opacity of cornea, left eye

H17.823   Peripheral opacity of cornea, bilateral

H17.829   Peripheral opacity of cornea, unspecified eye

H17.89   Other corneal scars and opacities

H17.9   Unspecified corneal scar and opacity

● H18   Other disorders of cornea

● H18.0   Corneal pigmentations and deposits

● H18.00   Unspecified corneal deposit

H18.001   Unspecified corneal deposit, right eye

H18.002   Unspecified corneal deposit, left eye

H18.003   Unspecified corneal deposit, bilateral

H18.009   Unspecified corneal deposit, unspecified eye

● H18.01   Anterior corneal pigmentations
          Staehli's line

H18.011   Anterior corneal pigmentations, right eye

H18.012   Anterior corneal pigmentations, left eye

◀ New   ◀┅ Revised   ~~deleted~~ Deleted   Excludes 1   Excludes 2   Includes   Use additional   Code first   Code also   Unspecified

OGCR Official Guidelines   X Assign placeholder X   ● Use Additional Character(s)   ▶ Manifestation Code   Coding Clinic

H18.013   Anterior corneal pigmentations, bilateral

H18.019   Anterior corneal pigmentations, unspecified eye

● H18.02   Argentous corneal deposits

H18.021   Argentous corneal deposits, right eye

H18.022   Argentous corneal deposits, left eye

H18.023   Argentous corneal deposits, bilateral

H18.029   Argentous corneal deposits, unspecified eye

● H18.03   Corneal deposits in metabolic disorders

     Code also associated metabolic disorder

H18.031   Corneal deposits in metabolic disorders, right eye

H18.032   Corneal deposits in metabolic disorders, left eye

H18.033   Corneal deposits in metabolic disorders, bilateral

H18.039   Corneal deposits in metabolic disorders, unspecified eye

● H18.04   Kayser-Fleischer ring

     Code also associated Wilson's disease (E83.01)

H18.041   Kayser-Fleischer ring, right eye

H18.042   Kayser-Fleischer ring, left eye

H18.043   Kayser-Fleischer ring, bilateral

H18.049   Kayser-Fleischer ring, unspecified eye

● H18.05   Posterior corneal pigmentations

     Krukenberg's spindle

H18.051   Posterior corneal pigmentations, right eye

H18.052   Posterior corneal pigmentations, left eye

H18.053   Posterior corneal pigmentations, bilateral

H18.059   Posterior corneal pigmentations, unspecified eye

● H18.06   Stromal corneal pigmentations

     Hematocornea

H18.061   Stromal corneal pigmentations, right eye

H18.062   Stromal corneal pigmentations, left eye

H18.063   Stromal corneal pigmentations, bilateral

H18.069   Stromal corneal pigmentations, unspecified eye

● H18.1   Bullous keratopathy

H18.10   Bullous keratopathy, unspecified eye

H18.11   Bullous keratopathy, right eye

H18.12   Bullous keratopathy, left eye

H18.13   Bullous keratopathy, bilateral

● H18.2   Other and unspecified corneal edema

H18.20   Unspecified corneal edema

● H18.21   Corneal edema secondary to contact lens

     Excludes2   other corneal disorders due to contact lens (H18.82-)

H18.211   Corneal edema secondary to contact lens, right eye

H18.212   Corneal edema secondary to contact lens, left eye

H18.213   Corneal edema secondary to contact lens, bilateral

H18.219   Corneal edema secondary to contact lens, unspecified eye

● H18.22   Idiopathic corneal edema

H18.221   Idiopathic corneal edema, right eye

H18.222   Idiopathic corneal edema, left eye

H18.223   Idiopathic corneal edema, bilateral

H18.229   Idiopathic corneal edema, unspecified eye

● H18.23   Secondary corneal edema

H18.231   Secondary corneal edema, right eye

H18.232   Secondary corneal edema, left eye

H18.233   Secondary corneal edema, bilateral

H18.239   Secondary corneal edema, unspecified eye

● H18.3   Changes of corneal membranes

H18.30   Unspecified corneal membrane change

● H18.31   Folds and rupture in Bowman's membrane

H18.311   Folds and rupture in Bowman's membrane, right eye

H18.312   Folds and rupture in Bowman's membrane, left eye

H18.313   Folds and rupture in Bowman's membrane, bilateral

H18.319   Folds and rupture in Bowman's membrane, unspecified eye

● H18.32   Folds in Descemet's membrane

H18.321   Folds in Descemet's membrane, right eye

H18.322   Folds in Descemet's membrane, left eye

H18.323   Folds in Descemet's membrane, bilateral

H18.329   Folds in Descemet's membrane, unspecified eye

● H18.33   Rupture in Descemet's membrane

H18.331   Rupture in Descemet's membrane, right eye

H18.332   Rupture in Descemet's membrane, left eye

H18.333   Rupture in Descemet's membrane, bilateral

H18.339   Rupture in Descemet's membrane, unspecified eye

● H18.4   Corneal degeneration

     Excludes1   Mooren's ulcer (H16.0-)
            recurrent erosion of cornea (H18.83-)

H18.40   Unspecified corneal degeneration

● H18.41   Arcus senilis

     Senile corneal changes

H18.411   Arcus senilis, right eye

H18.412   Arcus senilis, left eye

H18.413   Arcus senilis, bilateral

H18.419   Arcus senilis, unspecified eye

● H18.42   Band keratopathy

H18.421   Band keratopathy, right eye

H18.422   Band keratopathy, left eye

H18.423   Band keratopathy, bilateral

H18.429   Band keratopathy, unspecified eye

H18.43   Other calcerous corneal degeneration

● H18.44   Keratomalacia

     Excludes1   keratomalacia due to vitamin A deficiency (E50.4)

H18.441   Keratomalacia, right eye

H18.442   Keratomalacia, left eye

H18.443   Keratomalacia, bilateral

H18.449   Keratomalacia, unspecified eye

CHAPTER 7 (H00-H59)

● H18.45   Nodular corneal degeneration
     H18.451   Nodular corneal degeneration, right eye
     H18.452   Nodular corneal degeneration, left eye
     H18.453   Nodular corneal degeneration, bilateral
     H18.459   Nodular corneal degeneration, unspecified eye

● H18.46   Peripheral corneal degeneration
     H18.461   Peripheral corneal degeneration, right eye
     H18.462   Peripheral corneal degeneration, left eye
     H18.463   Peripheral corneal degeneration, bilateral
     H18.469   Peripheral corneal degeneration, unspecified eye

     H18.49   Other corneal degeneration

● H18.5   Hereditary corneal dystrophies
     H18.50   Unspecified hereditary corneal dystrophies
     H18.51   Endothelial corneal dystrophy
         Fuchs' dystrophy
     H18.52   Epithelial (juvenile) corneal dystrophy
     H18.53   Granular corneal dystrophy
     H18.54   Lattice corneal dystrophy
     H18.55   Macular corneal dystrophy
     H18.59   Other hereditary corneal dystrophies

● H18.6   Keratoconus
   ● H18.60   Keratoconus, unspecified
     H18.601   Keratoconus, unspecified, right eye
     H18.602   Keratoconus, unspecified, left eye
     H18.603   Keratoconus, unspecified, bilateral
     H18.609   Keratoconus, unspecified, unspecified eye

   ● H18.61   Keratoconus, stable
     H18.611   Keratoconus, stable, right eye
     H18.612   Keratoconus, stable, left eye
     H18.613   Keratoconus, stable, bilateral
     H18.619   Keratoconus, stable, unspecified eye

   ● H18.62   Keratoconus, unstable
         Acute hydrops
     H18.621   Keratoconus, unstable, right eye
     H18.622   Keratoconus, unstable, left eye
     H18.623   Keratoconus, unstable, bilateral
     H18.629   Keratoconus, unstable, unspecified eye

● H18.7   Other and unspecified corneal deformities
     Excludes1   congenital malformations of cornea (Q13.3-Q13.4)
     H18.70   Unspecified corneal deformity
   ● H18.71   Corneal ectasia
     H18.711   Corneal ectasia, right eye
     H18.712   Corneal ectasia, left eye
     H18.713   Corneal ectasia, bilateral
     H18.719   Corneal ectasia, unspecified eye

   ● H18.72   Corneal staphyloma
     H18.721   Corneal staphyloma, right eye
     H18.722   Corneal staphyloma, left eye
     H18.723   Corneal staphyloma, bilateral
     H18.729   Corneal staphyloma, unspecified eye

   ● H18.73   Descemetocele
     H18.731   Descemetocele, right eye
     H18.732   Descemetocele, left eye
     H18.733   Descemetocele, bilateral
     H18.739   Descemetocele, unspecified eye

   ● H18.79   Other corneal deformities
     H18.791   Other corneal deformities, right eye
     H18.792   Other corneal deformities, left eye
     H18.793   Other corneal deformities, bilateral
     H18.799   Other corneal deformities, unspecified eye

● H18.8   Other specified disorders of cornea
   ● H18.81   Anesthesia and hypoesthesia of cornea
     H18.811   Anesthesia and hypoesthesia of cornea, right eye
     H18.812   Anesthesia and hypoesthesia of cornea, left eye
     H18.813   Anesthesia and hypoesthesia of cornea, bilateral
     H18.819   Anesthesia and hypoesthesia of cornea, unspecified eye

   ● H18.82   Corneal disorder due to contact lens
     Excludes2   corneal edema due to contact lens (H18.21-)
     H18.821   Corneal disorder due to contact lens, right eye
     H18.822   Corneal disorder due to contact lens, left eye
     H18.823   Corneal disorder due to contact lens, bilateral
     H18.829   Corneal disorder due to contact lens, unspecified eye

   ● H18.83   Recurrent erosion of cornea
     H18.831   Recurrent erosion of cornea, right eye
     H18.832   Recurrent erosion of cornea, left eye
     H18.833   Recurrent erosion of cornea, bilateral
     H18.839   Recurrent erosion of cornea, unspecified eye

   ● H18.89   Other specified disorders of cornea
     H18.891   Other specified disorders of cornea, right eye
     H18.892   Other specified disorders of cornea, left eye
     H18.893   Other specified disorders of cornea, bilateral
     H18.899   Other specified disorders of cornea, unspecified eye

H18.9   Unspecified disorder of cornea

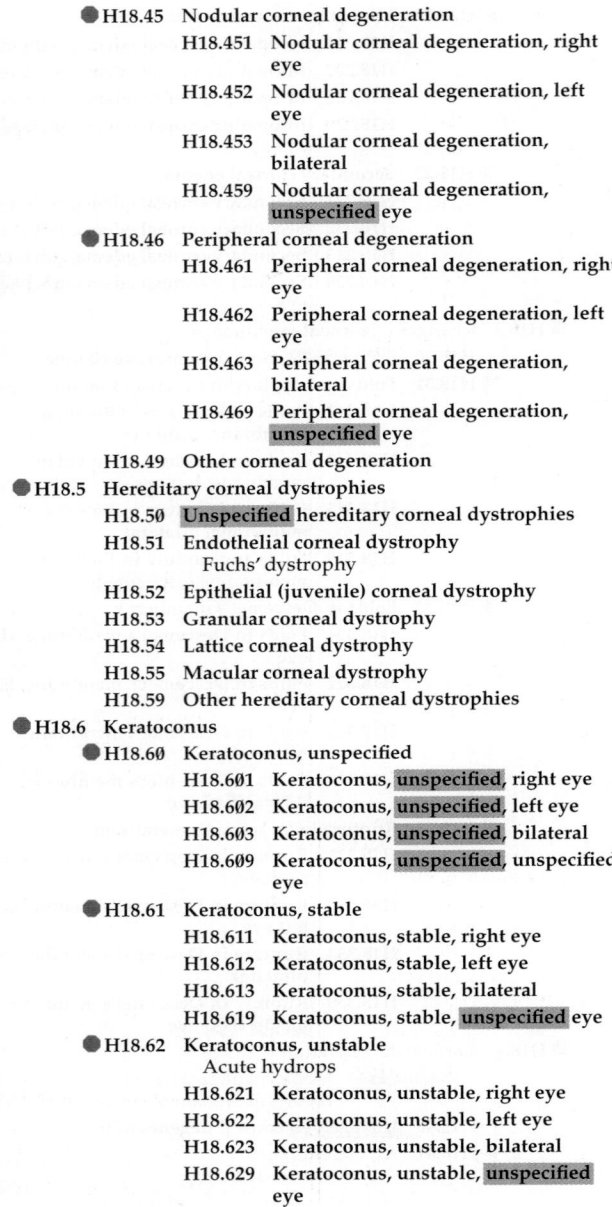

Figure 7-8   Lateral view of the displacement of the cone apex in keratoconus. (From Yanoff: Ophthalmology, ed 3, Mosby, Inc., 2008)

Item 7–4   Keratoconus results in corneal degeneration that begins in childhood, gradually changes the cornea from a round to cone shape, decreasing visual acuity. Treatment includes contact lenses. In severe cases the need for corneal transplant may be the treatment of choice; however, newer technologies may use high frequency radio energy to shrink the edges of the cornea, pulling the central area back to a more normal shape. It can help delay or avoid the need for a corneal transplantation.

◀ New   ◀▥ Revised   ~~deleted~~ Deleted   Excludes 1   Excludes 2   Includes   Use additional   Code first   Code also   Unspecified

810   OGCR Official Guidelines   X Assign placeholder X   ● Use Additional Character(s)   ▶ Manifestation Code   **Coding Clinic**

● **H20** **Iridocyclitis**
   ● **H20.0** **Acute and subacute iridocyclitis**
        Acute anterior uveitis
        Acute cyclitis
        Acute iritis
        Subacute anterior uveitis
        Subacute cyclitis
        Subacute iritis

        Excludes1 iridocyclitis, iritis, uveitis (due to) (in) diabetes mellitus (E08-E13 with .39)
                iridocyclitis, iritis, uveitis (due to) (in) diphtheria (A36.89)
                iridocyclitis, iritis, uveitis (due to) (in) gonococcal (A54.32)
                iridocyclitis, iritis, uveitis (due to) (in) herpes (simplex) (B00.51)
                iridocyclitis, iritis, uveitis (due to) (in) herpes zoster (B02.32)
                iridocyclitis, iritis, uveitis (due to) (in) late congenital syphilis (A50.39)
                iridocyclitis, iritis, uveitis (due to) (in) late syphilis (A52.71)
                iridocyclitis, iritis, uveitis (due to) (in) sarcoidosis (D86.83)
                iridocyclitis, iritis, uveitis (due to) (in) syphilis (A51.43)
                iridocyclitis, iritis, uveitis (due to) (in) toxoplasmosis (B58.09)
                iridocyclitis, iritis, uveitis (due to) (in) tuberculosis (A18.54)

      H20.00 Unspecified acute and subacute iridocyclitis
    ● **H20.01** Primary iridocyclitis
        H20.011 Primary iridocyclitis, right eye
        H20.012 Primary iridocyclitis, left eye
        H20.013 Primary iridocyclitis, bilateral
        H20.019 Primary iridocyclitis, unspecified eye
    ● **H20.02** Recurrent acute iridocyclitis
        H20.021 Recurrent acute iridocyclitis, right eye
        H20.022 Recurrent acute iridocyclitis, left eye
        H20.023 Recurrent acute iridocyclitis, bilateral
        H20.029 Recurrent acute iridocyclitis, unspecified eye
    ● **H20.03** Secondary infectious iridocyclitis
        H20.031 Secondary infectious iridocyclitis, right eye
        H20.032 Secondary infectious iridocyclitis, left eye
        H20.033 Secondary infectious iridocyclitis, bilateral
        H20.039 Secondary infectious iridocyclitis, unspecified eye
    ● **H20.04** Secondary noninfectious iridocyclitis
        H20.041 Secondary noninfectious iridocyclitis, right eye
        H20.042 Secondary noninfectious iridocyclitis, left eye
        H20.043 Secondary noninfectious iridocyclitis, bilateral
        H20.049 Secondary noninfectious iridocyclitis, unspecified eye
    ● **H20.05** Hypopyon
        H20.051 Hypopyon, right eye
        H20.052 Hypopyon, left eye
        H20.053 Hypopyon, bilateral
        H20.059 Hypopyon, unspecified eye

   ● **H20.1** **Chronic iridocyclitis**
        Use additional code for any associated cataract (H26.21-)
        Excludes2 posterior cyclitis (H30.2-)
        H20.10 Chronic iridocyclitis, unspecified eye
        H20.11 Chronic iridocyclitis, right eye
        H20.12 Chronic iridocyclitis, left eye
        H20.13 Chronic iridocyclitis, bilateral
   ● **H20.2** **Lens-induced iridocyclitis**
        H20.20 Lens-induced iridocyclitis, unspecified eye
        H20.21 Lens-induced iridocyclitis, right eye
        H20.22 Lens-induced iridocyclitis, left eye
        H20.23 Lens-induced iridocyclitis, bilateral
   ● **H20.8** **Other iridocyclitis**
        Excludes2 glaucomatocyclitis crises (H40.4-)
                posterior cyclitis (H30.2-)
                sympathetic uveitis (H44.13-)
    ● **H20.81** Fuchs' heterochromic cyclitis
        H20.811 Fuchs' heterochromic cyclitis, right eye
        H20.812 Fuchs' heterochromic cyclitis, left eye
        H20.813 Fuchs' heterochromic cyclitis, bilateral
        H20.819 Fuchs' heterochromic cyclitis, unspecified eye
    ● **H20.82** Vogt-Koyanagi syndrome
        H20.821 Vogt-Koyanagi syndrome, right eye
        H20.822 Vogt-Koyanagi syndrome, left eye
        H20.823 Vogt-Koyanagi syndrome, bilateral
        H20.829 Vogt-Koyanagi syndrome, unspecified eye
   ● **H20.9** Unspecified iridocyclitis
        Uveitis NOS

● **H21** **Other disorders of iris and ciliary body**
        Excludes2 sympathetic uveitis (H44.1-)
   ● **H21.0** **Hyphema**
        Excludes1 traumatic hyphema (S05.1-)
        H21.00 Hyphema, unspecified eye
        H21.01 Hyphema, right eye
        H21.02 Hyphema, left eye
        H21.03 Hyphema, bilateral
   ● **H21.1** **Other vascular disorders of iris and ciliary body**
        Neovascularization of iris or ciliary body
        Rubeosis iridis
        Rubeosis of iris
    ● **H21.1X** Other vascular disorders of iris and ciliary body
        H21.1X1 Other vascular disorders of iris and ciliary body, right eye
        H21.1X2 Other vascular disorders of iris and ciliary body, left eye
        H21.1X3 Other vascular disorders of iris and ciliary body, bilateral
        H21.1X9 Other vascular disorders of iris and ciliary body, unspecified eye
   ● **H21.2** **Degeneration of iris and ciliary body**
    ● **H21.21** Degeneration of chamber angle
        H21.211 Degeneration of chamber angle, right eye
        H21.212 Degeneration of chamber angle, left eye
        H21.213 Degeneration of chamber angle, bilateral
        H21.219 Degeneration of chamber angle, unspecified eye

CHAPTER 7 (H00-H59)

● **H21.22 Degeneration of ciliary body**
    H21.221 Degeneration of ciliary body, right eye
    H21.222 Degeneration of ciliary body, left eye
    H21.223 Degeneration of ciliary body, bilateral
    H21.229 Degeneration of ciliary body, unspecified eye

● **H21.23 Degeneration of iris (pigmentary)**
        Translucency of iris
    H21.231 Degeneration of iris (pigmentary), right eye
    H21.232 Degeneration of iris (pigmentary), left eye
    H21.233 Degeneration of iris (pigmentary), bilateral
    H21.239 Degeneration of iris (pigmentary), unspecified eye

● **H21.24 Degeneration of pupillary margin**
    H21.241 Degeneration of pupillary margin, right eye
    H21.242 Degeneration of pupillary margin, left eye
    H21.243 Degeneration of pupillary margin, bilateral
    H21.249 Degeneration of pupillary margin, unspecified eye

● **H21.25 Iridoschisis**
    H21.251 Iridoschisis, right eye
    H21.252 Iridoschisis, left eye
    H21.253 Iridoschisis, bilateral
    H21.259 Iridoschisis, unspecified eye

● **H21.26 Iris atrophy (essential) (progressive)**
    H21.261 Iris atrophy (essential) (progressive), right eye
    H21.262 Iris atrophy (essential) (progressive), left eye
    H21.263 Iris atrophy (essential) (progressive), bilateral
    H21.269 Iris atrophy (essential) (progressive), unspecified eye

● **H21.27 Miotic pupillary cyst**
    H21.271 Miotic pupillary cyst, right eye
    H21.272 Miotic pupillary cyst, left eye
    H21.273 Miotic pupillary cyst, bilateral
    H21.279 Miotic pupillary cyst, unspecified eye
    H21.29 Other iris atrophy

● **H21.3 Cyst of iris, ciliary body and anterior chamber**
        Excludes2 miotic pupillary cyst (H21.27-)

● **H21.30 Idiopathic cysts of iris, ciliary body or anterior chamber**
        Cyst of iris, ciliary body or anterior chamber NOS
    H21.301 Idiopathic cysts of iris, ciliary body or anterior chamber, right eye
    H21.302 Idiopathic cysts of iris, ciliary body or anterior chamber, left eye
    H21.303 Idiopathic cysts of iris, ciliary body or anterior chamber, bilateral
    H21.309 Idiopathic cysts of iris, ciliary body or anterior chamber, unspecified eye

● **H21.31 Exudative cysts of iris or anterior chamber**
    H21.311 Exudative cysts of iris or anterior chamber, right eye
    H21.312 Exudative cysts of iris or anterior chamber, left eye
    H21.313 Exudative cysts of iris or anterior chamber, bilateral
    H21.319 Exudative cysts of iris or anterior chamber, unspecified eye

● **H21.32 Implantation cysts of iris, ciliary body or anterior chamber**
    H21.321 Implantation cysts of iris, ciliary body or anterior chamber, right eye
    H21.322 Implantation cysts of iris, ciliary body or anterior chamber, left eye
    H21.323 Implantation cysts of iris, ciliary body or anterior chamber, bilateral
    H21.329 Implantation cysts of iris, ciliary body or anterior chamber, unspecified eye

● **H21.33 Parasitic cyst of iris, ciliary body or anterior chamber**
    H21.331 Parasitic cyst of iris, ciliary body or anterior chamber, right eye
    H21.332 Parasitic cyst of iris, ciliary body or anterior chamber, left eye
    H21.333 Parasitic cyst of iris, ciliary body or anterior chamber, bilateral
    H21.339 Parasitic cyst of iris, ciliary body or anterior chamber, unspecified eye

● **H21.34 Primary cyst of pars plana**
    H21.341 Primary cyst of pars plana, right eye
    H21.342 Primary cyst of pars plana, left eye
    H21.343 Primary cyst of pars plana, bilateral
    H21.349 Primary cyst of pars plana, unspecified eye

● **H21.35 Exudative cyst of pars plana**
    H21.351 Exudative cyst of pars plana, right eye
    H21.352 Exudative cyst of pars plana, left eye
    H21.353 Exudative cyst of pars plana, bilateral
    H21.359 Exudative cyst of pars plana, unspecified eye

● **H21.4 Pupillary membranes**
        Iris bombé
        Pupillary occlusion
        Pupillary seclusion
        Excludes1 congenital pupillary membranes (Q13.8)
    H21.40 Pupillary membranes, unspecified eye
    H21.41 Pupillary membranes, right eye
    H21.42 Pupillary membranes, left eye
    H21.43 Pupillary membranes, bilateral

● **H21.5 Other and unspecified adhesions and disruptions of iris and ciliary body**
        Excludes1 corectopia (Q13.2)

● **H21.50 Unspecified adhesions of iris**
        Synechia (iris) NOS
    H21.501 Unspecified adhesions of iris, right eye
    H21.502 Unspecified adhesions of iris, left eye
    H21.503 Unspecified adhesions of iris, bilateral
    H21.509 Unspecified adhesions of iris and ciliary body, unspecified eye

● **H21.51 Anterior synechiae (iris)**
    H21.511 Anterior synechiae (iris), right eye
    H21.512 Anterior synechiae (iris), left eye
    H21.513 Anterior synechiae (iris), bilateral
    H21.519 Anterior synechiae (iris), unspecified eye

● **H21.52 Goniosynechiae**
    H21.521 Goniosynechiae, right eye
    H21.522 Goniosynechiae, left eye
    H21.523 Goniosynechiae, bilateral
    H21.529 Goniosynechiae, unspecified eye

● **H21.53 Iridodialysis**
  H21.531 Iridodialysis, right eye
  H21.532 Iridodialysis, left eye
  H21.533 Iridodialysis, bilateral
  H21.539 Iridodialysis, unspecified eye
● **H21.54 Posterior synechiae (iris)**
  H21.541 Posterior synechiae (iris), right eye
  H21.542 Posterior synechiae (iris), left eye
  H21.543 Posterior synechiae (iris), bilateral
  H21.549 Posterior synechiae (iris), unspecified eye
● **H21.55 Recession of chamber angle**
  H21.551 Recession of chamber angle, right eye
  H21.552 Recession of chamber angle, left eye
  H21.553 Recession of chamber angle, bilateral
  H21.559 Recession of chamber angle, unspecified eye
● **H21.56 Pupillary abnormalities**
    Deformed pupil
    Ectopic pupil
    Rupture of sphincter, pupil
    Excludes1 congenital deformity of pupil (Q13.2-)
  H21.561 Pupillary abnormality, right eye
  H21.562 Pupillary abnormality, left eye
  H21.563 Pupillary abnormality, bilateral
  H21.569 Pupillary abnormality, unspecified eye
● **H21.8 Other specified disorders of iris and ciliary body**
  H21.81 Floppy iris syndrome
    Intraoperative floppy iris syndrome (IFIS)
    Use additional code for adverse effect, if applicable, to identify drug (T36-T50 with fifth or sixth character 5)
  H21.82 Plateau iris syndrome (post-iridectomy) (postprocedural)
  H21.89 Other specified disorders of iris and ciliary body
● **H21.9 Unspecified disorder of iris and ciliary body**

▶ *H22 Disorders of iris and ciliary body in diseases classified elsewhere*
    Code first underlying disease, such as:
      gout (M1A.-, M10.-)
      leprosy (A30.-)
      parasitic disease (B89)

DISORDERS OF LENS (H25-H28)

● **H25 Age-related cataract**
    Senile cataract
    Excludes2 capsular glaucoma with pseudoexfoliation of lens (H40.1-)
● **H25.0 Age-related incipient cataract**
  ● **H25.01 Cortical age-related cataract**
    H25.011 Cortical age-related cataract, right eye A
    H25.012 Cortical age-related cataract, left eye A
    H25.013 Cortical age-related cataract, bilateral A
    H25.019 Cortical age-related cataract, unspecified eye A
  ● **H25.03 Anterior subcapsular polar age-related cataract**
    H25.031 Anterior subcapsular polar age-related cataract, right eye A
    H25.032 Anterior subcapsular polar age-related cataract, left eye A
    H25.033 Anterior subcapsular polar age-related cataract, bilateral A
    H25.039 Anterior subcapsular polar age-related cataract, unspecified eye A

Figure 7-9 Age-related cataract. Nuclear sclerosis and cortical lens opacities are present. (From Yanoff: Ophthalmology, ed 3, Mosby, Inc., 2008)

Item 7–5 Senile cataracts are linked to the aging process. The most common area for the formation of a cataract is the cortical area of the lens. **Polar cataracts** can be either anterior or posterior. **Anterior polar cataracts** are more common and are small, white, capsular cataracts located on the anterior portion of the lens. **Total cataracts,** also called **complete** or **mature,** cause an opacity of all fibers of the lens. **Hypermature** describes a mature cataract with a swollen, milky cortex that covers the entire lens. **Immature,** also called **incipient,** cataracts have a clear cortex and are only slightly opaque. Treatment for all cataracts is the removal of the lens.

  ● **H25.04 Posterior subcapsular polar age-related cataract**
    H25.041 Posterior subcapsular polar age-related cataract, right eye A
    H25.042 Posterior subcapsular polar age-related cataract, left eye A
    H25.043 Posterior subcapsular polar age-related cataract, bilateral A
    H25.049 Posterior subcapsular polar age-related cataract, unspecified eye A
  ● **H25.09 Other age-related incipient cataract**
    Coronary age-related cataract
    Punctate age-related cataract
    Water clefts
    H25.091 Other age-related incipient cataract, right eye A
    H25.092 Other age-related incipient cataract, left eye A
    H25.093 Other age-related incipient cataract, bilateral A
    H25.099 Other age-related incipient cataract, unspecified eye A
● **H25.1 Age-related nuclear cataract**
    Cataracta brunescens
    Nuclear sclerosis cataract
  H25.10 Age-related nuclear cataract, unspecified eye A
  H25.11 Age-related nuclear cataract, right eye A
  H25.12 Age-related nuclear cataract, left eye A
    Coding Clinic: 2016, Q1, P33
  H25.13 Age-related nuclear cataract, bilateral A
    Coding Clinic: 2016, Q1, P32
● **H25.2 Age-related cataract, morgagnian type**
    Age-related hypermature cataract
  H25.20 Age-related cataract, morgagnian type, unspecified eye A
  H25.21 Age-related cataract, morgagnian type, right eye A
  H25.22 Age-related cataract, morgagnian type, left eye A
  H25.23 Age-related cataract, morgagnian type, bilateral A
● **H25.8 Other age-related cataract**
  ● **H25.81 Combined forms of age-related cataract**
    H25.811 Combined forms of age-related cataract, right eye A
    H25.812 Combined forms of age-related cataract, left eye A
    H25.813 Combined forms of age-related cataract, bilateral A
    H25.819 Combined forms of age-related cataract, unspecified eye A
  H25.89 Other age-related cataract A
● **H25.9 Unspecified age-related cataract** A

CHAPTER 7 (H00-H59)

CHAPTER 7 (H00-H59)

● H26   Other cataract

  Excludes1   congenital cataract (Q12.0)

  ● H26.0   Infantile and juvenile cataract

    ● H26.00   Unspecified infantile and juvenile cataract

      H26.001   Unspecified infantile and juvenile cataract, right eye   P

      H26.002   Unspecified infantile and juvenile cataract, left eye   P

      H26.003   Unspecified infantile and juvenile cataract, bilateral   P

      H26.009   Unspecified infantile and juvenile cataract, unspecified eye   P

    ● H26.01   Infantile and juvenile cortical, lamellar, or zonular cataract

      H26.011   Infantile and juvenile cortical, lamellar, or zonular cataract, right eye   P

      H26.012   Infantile and juvenile cortical, lamellar, or zonular cataract, left eye   P

      H26.013   Infantile and juvenile cortical, lamellar, or zonular cataract, bilateral   P

      H26.019   Infantile and juvenile cortical, lamellar, or zonular cataract, unspecified eye   P

    ● H26.03   Infantile and juvenile nuclear cataract

      H26.031   Infantile and juvenile nuclear cataract, right eye   P

      H26.032   Infantile and juvenile nuclear cataract, left eye   P

      H26.033   Infantile and juvenile nuclear cataract, bilateral   P

      H26.039   Infantile and juvenile nuclear cataract, unspecified eye   P

    ● H26.04   Anterior subcapsular polar infantile and juvenile cataract

      H26.041   Anterior subcapsular polar infantile and juvenile cataract, right eye   P

      H26.042   Anterior subcapsular polar infantile and juvenile cataract, left eye   P

      H26.043   Anterior subcapsular polar infantile and juvenile cataract, bilateral   P

      H26.049   Anterior subcapsular polar infantile and juvenile cataract, unspecified eye   P

    ● H26.05   Posterior subcapsular polar infantile and juvenile cataract

      H26.051   Posterior subcapsular polar infantile and juvenile cataract, right eye   P

      H26.052   Posterior subcapsular polar infantile and juvenile cataract, left eye   P

      H26.053   Posterior subcapsular polar infantile and juvenile cataract, bilateral   P

      H26.059   Posterior subcapsular polar infantile and juvenile cataract, unspecified eye   P

    ● H26.06   Combined forms of infantile and juvenile cataract

      H26.061   Combined forms of infantile and juvenile cataract, right eye   P

      H26.062   Combined forms of infantile and juvenile cataract, left eye   P

      H26.063   Combined forms of infantile and juvenile cataract bilateral   P

      H26.069   Combined forms of infantile and juvenile cataract, unspecified eye   P

    H26.09   Other infantile and juvenile cataract   P

  ● H26.1   Traumatic cataract

    Use additional code (Chapter 20) to identify external cause

    ● H26.10   Unspecified traumatic cataract

      H26.101   Unspecified traumatic cataract, right eye

      H26.102   Unspecified traumatic cataract, left eye

      H26.103   Unspecified traumatic cataract, bilateral

      H26.109   Unspecified traumatic cataract, unspecified eye

    ● H26.11   Localized traumatic opacities

      H26.111   Localized traumatic opacities, right eye

      H26.112   Localized traumatic opacities, left eye

      H26.113   Localized traumatic opacities, bilateral

      H26.119   Localized traumatic opacities, unspecified eye

    ● H26.12   Partially resolved traumatic cataract

      H26.121   Partially resolved traumatic cataract, right eye

      H26.122   Partially resolved traumatic cataract, left eye

      H26.123   Partially resolved traumatic cataract, bilateral

      H26.129   Partially resolved traumatic cataract, unspecified eye

    ● H26.13   Total traumatic cataract

      H26.131   Total traumatic cataract, right eye

      H26.132   Total traumatic cataract, left eye

      H26.133   Total traumatic cataract, bilateral

      H26.139   Total traumatic cataract, unspecified eye

  ● H26.2   Complicated cataract

    H26.20   Unspecified complicated cataract

      Cataracta complicata NOS

    ● H26.21   Cataract with neovascularization

      Code also associated condition, such as: chronic iridocyclitis (H20.1-)

      H26.211   Cataract with neovascularization, right eye

      H26.212   Cataract with neovascularization, left eye

      H26.213   Cataract with neovascularization, bilateral

      H26.219   Cataract with neovascularization, unspecified eye

    ● H26.22   Cataract secondary to ocular disorders (degenerative) (inflammatory)

      Code also associated ocular disorder

      H26.221   Cataract secondary to ocular disorders (degenerative) (inflammatory), right eye

      H26.222   Cataract secondary to ocular disorders (degenerative) (inflammatory), left eye

      H26.223   Cataract secondary to ocular disorders (degenerative) (inflammatory), bilateral

      H26.229   Cataract secondary to ocular disorders (degenerative) (inflammatory), unspecified eye

    ● H26.23   Glaucomatous flecks (subcapsular)

      Code first underlying glaucoma (H40-H42)

      H26.231   Glaucomatous flecks (subcapsular), right eye

      H26.232   Glaucomatous flecks (subcapsular), left eye

◀ New   ◀≡ Revised   ~~deleted~~ Deleted   Excludes 1   Excludes 2   Includes   Use additional   Code first   Code also   Unspecified

OGCR Official Guidelines   X Assign placeholder X   ● Use Additional Character(s)   ▶ Manifestation Code   **Coding Clinic**

        H26.233   Glaucomatous flecks (subcapsular), bilateral

        H26.239   Glaucomatous flecks (subcapsular), unspecified eye

● **H26.3**   Drug-induced cataract
    Toxic cataract

    Use additional code for adverse effect, if applicable, to identify drug (T36-T50 with fifth or sixth character 5)

    H26.30   Drug-induced cataract, unspecified eye

    H26.31   Drug-induced cataract, right eye

    H26.32   Drug-induced cataract, left eye

    H26.33   Drug-induced cataract, bilateral

● **H26.4**   Secondary cataract

    H26.40   Unspecified secondary cataract

    ● H26.41   Soemmering's ring

        H26.411   Soemmering's ring, right eye

        H26.412   Soemmering's ring, left eye

        H26.413   Soemmering's ring, bilateral

        H26.419   Soemmering's ring, unspecified eye

    ● H26.49   Other secondary cataract

        H26.491   Other secondary cataract, right eye

        H26.492   Other secondary cataract, left eye

        H26.493   Other secondary cataract, bilateral

        H26.499   Other secondary cataract, unspecified eye

H26.8   Other specified cataract

H26.9   Unspecified cataract

● **H27**   Other disorders of lens

    Excludes1   congenital lens malformations (Q12.-)

        mechanical complications of intraocular lens implant (T85.2)

        pseudophakia (Z96.1)

● **H27.0**   Aphakia

    Acquired absence of lens

    Acquired aphakia

    Aphakia due to trauma

    Excludes1   cataract extraction status (Z98.4-)

        congenital absence of lens (Q12.3)

        congenital aphakia (Q12.3)

    H27.00   Aphakia, unspecified eye

    H27.01   Aphakia, right eye

    H27.02   Aphakia, left eye

    H27.03   Aphakia, bilateral

● **H27.1**   Dislocation of lens

    H27.10   Unspecified dislocation of lens

    ● H27.11   Subluxation of lens

        H27.111   Subluxation of lens, right eye

        H27.112   Subluxation of lens, left eye

        H27.113   Subluxation of lens, bilateral

        H27.119   Subluxation of lens, unspecified eye

    ● H27.12   Anterior dislocation of lens

        H27.121   Anterior dislocation of lens, right eye

        H27.122   Anterior dislocation of lens, left eye

        H27.123   Anterior dislocation of lens, bilateral

        H27.129   Anterior dislocation of lens, unspecified eye

    ● H27.13   Posterior dislocation of lens

        H27.131   Posterior dislocation of lens, right eye

        H27.132   Posterior dislocation of lens, left eye

        H27.133   Posterior dislocation of lens, bilateral

        H27.139   Posterior dislocation of lens, unspecified eye

H27.8   Other specified disorders of lens

H27.9   Unspecified disorder of lens

▶ **H28**   *Cataract in diseases classified elsewhere*

    Code first underlying disease, such as:

    hypoparathyroidism (E20.-)

    myotonia (G71.1-)

    myxedema (E03.-)

    protein-calorie malnutrition (E40-E46)

    Excludes1   cataract in diabetes mellitus (E08.36, E09.36, E10.36, E11.36, E13.36)

DISORDERS OF CHOROID AND RETINA (H30-H36)

★ **(See Plate 90 on page 64.)**

● **H30**   Chorioretinal inflammation

    ● **H30.0**   Focal chorioretinal inflammation

        Focal chorioretinitis

        Focal choroiditis

        Focal retinitis

        Focal retinochoroiditis

        ● H30.00   Unspecified focal chorioretinal inflammation

            Focal chorioretinitis NOS

            Focal choroiditis NOS

            Focal retinitis NOS

            Focal retinochoroiditis NOS

            H30.001   Unspecified focal chorioretinal inflammation, right eye

            H30.002   Unspecified focal chorioretinal inflammation, left eye

            H30.003   Unspecified focal chorioretinal inflammation, bilateral

            H30.009   Unspecified focal chorioretinal inflammation, unspecified eye

        ● H30.01   Focal chorioretinal inflammation, juxtapapillary

            H30.011   Focal chorioretinal inflammation, juxtapapillary, right eye

            H30.012   Focal chorioretinal inflammation, juxtapapillary, left eye

            H30.013   Focal chorioretinal inflammation, juxtapapillary, bilateral

            H30.019   Focal chorioretinal inflammation, juxtapapillary, unspecified eye

        ● H30.02   Focal chorioretinal inflammation of posterior pole

            H30.021   Focal chorioretinal inflammation of posterior pole, right eye

            H30.022   Focal chorioretinal inflammation of posterior pole, left eye

            H30.023   Focal chorioretinal inflammation of posterior pole, bilateral

            H30.029   Focal chorioretinal inflammation of posterior pole, unspecified eye

        ● H30.03   Focal chorioretinal inflammation, peripheral

            H30.031   Focal chorioretinal inflammation, peripheral, right eye

            H30.032   Focal chorioretinal inflammation, peripheral, left eye

            H30.033   Focal chorioretinal inflammation, peripheral, bilateral

            H30.039   Focal chorioretinal inflammation, peripheral, unspecified eye

        ● H30.04   Focal chorioretinal inflammation, macular or paramacular

            H30.041   Focal chorioretinal inflammation, macular or paramacular, right eye

            H30.042   Focal chorioretinal inflammation, macular or paramacular, left eye

            H30.043   Focal chorioretinal inflammation, macular or paramacular, bilateral

            H30.049   Focal chorioretinal inflammation, macular or paramacular, unspecified eye

● **H30.1**   **Disseminated chorioretinal inflammation**
      Disseminated chorioretinitis
      Disseminated choroiditis
      Disseminated retinitis
      Disseminated retinochoroiditis

      Excludes2   exudative retinopathy (H35.02-)

  ● **H30.10**   **Unspecified disseminated chorioretinal inflammation**
        Disseminated chorioretinitis NOS
        Disseminated choroiditis NOS
        Disseminated retinitis NOS
        Disseminated retinochoroiditis NOS

     H30.101   Unspecified disseminated chorioretinal inflammation, right eye

     H30.102   Unspecified disseminated chorioretinal inflammation, left eye

     H30.103   Unspecified disseminated chorioretinal inflammation, bilateral

     H30.109   Unspecified disseminated chorioretinal inflammation, unspecified eye

  ● **H30.11**   **Disseminated chorioretinal inflammation of posterior pole**

     H30.111   Disseminated chorioretinal inflammation of posterior pole, right eye

     H30.112   Disseminated chorioretinal inflammation of posterior pole, left eye

     H30.113   Disseminated chorioretinal inflammation of posterior pole, bilateral

     H30.119   Disseminated chorioretinal inflammation of posterior pole, unspecified eye

  ● **H30.12**   **Disseminated chorioretinal inflammation, peripheral**

     H30.121   Disseminated chorioretinal inflammation, peripheral right eye

     H30.122   Disseminated chorioretinal inflammation, peripheral, left eye

     H30.123   Disseminated chorioretinal inflammation, peripheral, bilateral

     H30.129   Disseminated chorioretinal inflammation, peripheral, unspecified eye

  ● **H30.13**   **Disseminated chorioretinal inflammation, generalized**

     H30.131   Disseminated chorioretinal inflammation, generalized, right eye

     H30.132   Disseminated chorioretinal inflammation, generalized, left eye

     H30.133   Disseminated chorioretinal inflammation, generalized, bilateral

     H30.139   Disseminated chorioretinal inflammation, generalized, unspecified eye

  ● **H30.14**   **Acute posterior multifocal placoid pigment epitheliopathy**

     H30.141   Acute posterior multifocal placoid pigment epitheliopathy, right eye

     H30.142   Acute posterior multifocal placoid pigment epitheliopathy, left eye

     H30.143   Acute posterior multifocal placoid pigment epitheliopathy, bilateral

     H30.149   Acute posterior multifocal placoid pigment epitheliopathy, unspecified eye

● **H30.2**   **Posterior cyclitis**
      Pars planitis

  H30.20   Posterior cyclitis, unspecified eye

  H30.21   Posterior cyclitis, right eye

  H30.22   Posterior cyclitis, left eye

  H30.23   Posterior cyclitis, bilateral

● **H30.8**   **Other chorioretinal inflammations**

  ● **H30.81**   **Harada's disease**

     H30.811   Harada's disease, right eye

     H30.812   Harada's disease, left eye

     H30.813   Harada's disease, bilateral

     H30.819   Harada's disease, unspecified eye

  ● **H30.89**   **Other chorioretinal inflammations**

     H30.891   Other chorioretinal inflammations, right eye

     H30.892   Other chorioretinal inflammations, left eye

     H30.893   Other chorioretinal inflammations, bilateral

     H30.899   Other chorioretinal inflammations, unspecified eye

● **H30.9**   **Unspecified chorioretinal inflammation**
      Chorioretinitis NOS
      Choroiditis NOS
      Neuroretinitis NOS
      Retinitis NOS
      Retinochoroiditis NOS

  H30.90   Unspecified chorioretinal inflammation, unspecified eye

  H30.91   Unspecified chorioretinal inflammation, right eye

  H30.92   Unspecified chorioretinal inflammation, left eye

  H30.93   Unspecified chorioretinal inflammation, bilateral

● **H31**   **Other disorders of choroid**

  ● **H31.0**   **Chorioretinal scars**

      Excludes2   postsurgical chorioretinal scars (H59.81-)

  ● **H31.00**   **Unspecified chorioretinal scars**

     H31.001   Unspecified chorioretinal scars, right eye

     H31.002   Unspecified chorioretinal scars, left eye

     H31.003   Unspecified chorioretinal scars, bilateral

     H31.009   Unspecified chorioretinal scars, unspecified eye

  ● **H31.01**   **Macula scars of posterior pole (postinflammatory) (post-traumatic)**

      Excludes1   postprocedural chorioretinal scar (H59.81-)

     H31.011   Macula scars of posterior pole (postinflammatory) (post-traumatic), right eye

     H31.012   Macula scars of posterior pole (postinflammatory) (post-traumatic), left eye

     H31.013   Macula scars of posterior pole (postinflammatory) (post-traumatic), bilateral

     H31.019   Macula scars of posterior pole (postinflammatory) (post-traumatic), unspecified eye

◀ New   ◀ Revised   ~~deleted~~ Deleted   Excludes 1   Excludes 2   Includes   Use additional   Code first   Code also   Unspecified

OGCR Official Guidelines   X Assign placeholder X   ● Use Additional Character(s)   ◗ Manifestation Code   **Coding Clinic**

● H31.02   Solar retinopathy
     H31.021   Solar retinopathy, right eye
     H31.022   Solar retinopathy, left eye
     H31.023   Solar retinopathy, bilateral
     H31.029   Solar retinopathy, unspecified eye

● H31.09   Other chorioretinal scars
     H31.091   Other chorioretinal scars, right eye
     H31.092   Other chorioretinal scars, left eye
     H31.093   Other chorioretinal scars, bilateral
     H31.099   Other chorioretinal scars, unspecified eye

● H31.1   Choroidal degeneration
     Excludes2   angioid streaks of macula (H35.33)

  ● H31.10   Unspecified choroidal degeneration
      Choroidal sclerosis NOS
     H31.101   Choroidal degeneration, unspecified, right eye
     H31.102   Choroidal degeneration, unspecified, left eye
     H31.103   Choroidal degeneration, unspecified, bilateral
     H31.109   Choroidal degeneration, unspecified, unspecified eye

  ● H31.11   Age-related choroidal atrophy
     H31.111   Age-related choroidal atrophy, right eye   A
     H31.112   Age-related choroidal atrophy, left eye   A
     H31.113   Age-related choroidal atrophy, bilateral   A
     H31.119   Age-related choroidal atrophy, unspecified eye   A

  ● H31.12   Diffuse secondary atrophy of choroid
     H31.121   Diffuse secondary atrophy of choroid, right eye
     H31.122   Diffuse secondary atrophy of choroid, left eye
     H31.123   Diffuse secondary atrophy of choroid, bilateral
     H31.129   Diffuse secondary atrophy of choroid, unspecified eye

● H31.2   Hereditary choroidal dystrophy
     Excludes2   hyperornithinemia (E72.4)
                 ornithinemia (E72.4)
     H31.20   Hereditary choroidal dystrophy, unspecified
     H31.21   Choroideremia
     H31.22   Choroidal dystrophy (central areolar) (generalized) (peripapillary)
     H31.23   Gyrate atrophy, choroid
     H31.29   Other hereditary choroidal dystrophy

● H31.3   Choroidal hemorrhage and rupture
  ● H31.30   Unspecified choroidal hemorrhage
     H31.301   Unspecified choroidal hemorrhage, right eye
     H31.302   Unspecified choroidal hemorrhage, left eye
     H31.303   Unspecified choroidal hemorrhage, bilateral
     H31.309   Unspecified choroidal hemorrhage, unspecified eye

  ● H31.31   Expulsive choroidal hemorrhage
     H31.311   Expulsive choroidal hemorrhage, right eye
     H31.312   Expulsive choroidal hemorrhage, left eye
     H31.313   Expulsive choroidal hemorrhage, bilateral
     H31.319   Expulsive choroidal hemorrhage, unspecified eye

  ● H31.32   Choroidal rupture
     H31.321   Choroidal rupture, right eye
     H31.322   Choroidal rupture, left eye
     H31.323   Choroidal rupture, bilateral
     H31.329   Choroidal rupture, unspecified eye

● H31.4   Choroidal detachment
  ● H31.40   Unspecified choroidal detachment
     H31.401   Unspecified choroidal detachment, right eye
     H31.402   Unspecified choroidal detachment, left eye
     H31.403   Unspecified choroidal detachment, bilateral
     H31.409   Unspecified choroidal detachment, unspecified eye

  ● H31.41   Hemorrhagic choroidal detachment
     H31.411   Hemorrhagic choroidal detachment, right eye
     H31.412   Hemorrhagic choroidal detachment, left eye
     H31.413   Hemorrhagic choroidal detachment, bilateral
     H31.419   Hemorrhagic choroidal detachment, unspecified eye

  ● H31.42   Serous choroidal detachment
     H31.421   Serous choroidal detachment, right eye
     H31.422   Serous choroidal detachment, left eye
     H31.423   Serous choroidal detachment, bilateral
     H31.429   Serous choroidal detachment, unspecified eye

   H31.8   Other specified disorders of choroid
   H31.9   Unspecified disorder of choroid

▶ *H32*   *Chorioretinal disorders in diseases classified elsewhere*
     Code first underlying disease, such as:
       congenital toxoplasmosis (P37.1)
       histoplasmosis (B39.-)
       leprosy (A30.-)
     Excludes1   chorioretinitis (in):
           toxoplasmosis (acquired) (B58.01)
           tuberculosis (A18.53)

● H33   Retinal detachments and breaks
     Excludes1   detachment of retinal pigment epithelium (H35.72-, H35.73-)

  ● H33.0   Retinal detachment with retinal break
      Rhegmatogenous retinal detachment
     Excludes1   serous retinal detachment (without retinal break) (H33.2-)

    ● H33.00   Unspecified retinal detachment with retinal break
       H33.001   Unspecified retinal detachment with retinal break, right eye
       H33.002   Unspecified retinal detachment with retinal break, left eye
       H33.003   Unspecified retinal detachment with retinal break, bilateral
       H33.009   Unspecified retinal detachment with retinal break, unspecified eye

CHAPTER 7 (H00-H59)

NON-RHEGMATOGENOUS
RETINAL DETACHMENT

- Vitreous
- Retina
- Protein-rich fluid in sub-retinal space
- Retinal pigment epithelium

VITREOUS DETACHMENT

- Vitreous
- Posterior hyaloid
- Internal limiting membrane

RHEGMATOGENOUS
RETINAL DETACHMENT

- Blood
- Vitreous
- Posterior hyaloid
- Retina
- Retinal tear
- Liquified vitreous
- Retinal pigment epithelium

Figure 7-10 Retinal detachment. (From Kumar: Robbins and Cotran: Pathologic Basis of Disease, ed 7, Saunders, 2005)

Item 7-6 Retinal detachments and defects are conditions of the eye in which the retina separates from the underlying tissue. Initial detachment may be localized, requiring rapid treatment (medical emergency) to avoid the entire retina from detaching which leads to vision loss and blindness.

- ● H33.01   **Retinal detachment with single break**
  - H33.011   **Retinal detachment with single break, right eye**
  - H33.012   **Retinal detachment with single break, left eye**
  - H33.013   **Retinal detachment with single break, bilateral**
  - H33.019   **Retinal detachment with single break, unspecified eye**
- ● H33.02   **Retinal detachment with multiple breaks**
  - H33.021   **Retinal detachment with multiple breaks, right eye**
  - H33.022   **Retinal detachment with multiple breaks, left eye**
  - H33.023   **Retinal detachment with multiple breaks, bilateral**
  - H33.029   **Retinal detachment with multiple breaks, unspecified eye**
- ● H33.03   **Retinal detachment with giant retinal tear**
  - H33.031   **Retinal detachment with giant retinal tear, right eye**
  - H33.032   **Retinal detachment with giant retinal tear, left eye**
  - H33.033   **Retinal detachment with giant retinal tear, bilateral**
  - H33.039   **Retinal detachment with giant retinal tear, unspecified eye**

- ● H33.04   **Retinal detachment with retinal dialysis**
  - H33.041   **Retinal detachment with retinal dialysis, right eye**
  - H33.042   **Retinal detachment with retinal dialysis, left eye**
  - H33.043   **Retinal detachment with retinal dialysis, bilateral**
  - H33.049   **Retinal detachment with retinal dialysis, unspecified eye**
- ● H33.05   **Total retinal detachment**
  - H33.051   **Total retinal detachment, right eye**
  - H33.052   **Total retinal detachment, left eye**
  - H33.053   **Total retinal detachment, bilateral**
  - H33.059   **Total retinal detachment, unspecified eye**
- ● H33.1   **Retinoschisis and retinal cysts**
  - **Excludes1**   congenital retinoschisis (Q14.1)
    microcystoid degeneration of retina (H35.42-)
  - ● H33.10   **Unspecified retinoschisis**
    - H33.101   **Unspecified retinoschisis, right eye**
    - H33.102   **Unspecified retinoschisis, left eye**
    - H33.103   **Unspecified retinoschisis, bilateral**
    - H33.109   **Unspecified retinoschisis, unspecified eye**
  - ● H33.11   **Cyst of ora serrata**
    - H33.111   **Cyst of ora serrata, right eye**
    - H33.112   **Cyst of ora serrata, left eye**
    - H33.113   **Cyst of ora serrata, bilateral**
    - H33.119   **Cyst of ora serrata, unspecified eye**
  - ● H33.12   **Parasitic cyst of retina**
    - H33.121   **Parasitic cyst of retina, right eye**
    - H33.122   **Parasitic cyst of retina, left eye**
    - H33.123   **Parasitic cyst of retina, bilateral**
    - H33.129   **Parasitic cyst of retina, unspecified eye**
  - ● H33.19   **Other retinoschisis and retinal cysts**
    Pseudocyst of retina
    - H33.191   **Other retinoschisis and retinal cysts, right eye**
    - H33.192   **Other retinoschisis and retinal cysts, left eye**
    - H33.193   **Other retinoschisis and retinal cysts, bilateral**
    - H33.199   **Other retinoschisis and retinal cysts, unspecified eye**
- ● H33.2   **Serous retinal detachment**
  Retinal detachment NOS
  Retinal detachment without retinal break
  - **Excludes1**   central serous chorioretinopathy (H35.71-)
  - H33.20   **Serous retinal detachment, unspecified eye**
  - H33.21   **Serous retinal detachment, right eye**
  - H33.22   **Serous retinal detachment, left eye**
  - H33.23   **Serous retinal detachment, bilateral**
- ● H33.3   **Retinal breaks without detachment**
  - **Excludes1**   chorioretinal scars after surgery for detachment (H59.81-)
    peripheral retinal degeneration without break (H35.4-)
  - ● H33.30   **Unspecified retinal break**
    - H33.301   **Unspecified retinal break, right eye**
    - H33.302   **Unspecified retinal break, left eye**
    - H33.303   **Unspecified retinal break, bilateral**
    - H33.309   **Unspecified retinal break, unspecified eye**

- **H33.31**   **Horseshoe tear of retina without detachment**
  Operculum of retina without detachment
  - **H33.311**   **Horseshoe tear of retina without detachment, right eye**
  - **H33.312**   **Horseshoe tear of retina without detachment, left eye**
  - **H33.313**   **Horseshoe tear of retina without detachment, bilateral**
  - **H33.319**   **Horseshoe tear of retina without detachment, unspecified eye**
- **H33.32**   **Round hole of retina without detachment**
  - **H33.321**   **Round hole, right eye**
  - **H33.322**   **Round hole, left eye**
  - **H33.323**   **Round hole, bilateral**
  - **H33.329**   **Round hole, unspecified eye**
- **H33.33**   **Multiple defects of retina without detachment**
  - **H33.331**   **Multiple defects of retina without detachment, right eye**
  - **H33.332**   **Multiple defects of retina without detachment, left eye**
  - **H33.333**   **Multiple defects of retina without detachment, bilateral**
  - **H33.339**   **Multiple defects of retina without detachment, unspecified eye**
- **H33.4**   **Traction detachment of retina**
  Proliferative vitreo-retinopathy with retinal detachment
  - **H33.40**   **Traction detachment of retina, unspecified eye**
  - **H33.41**   **Traction detachment of retina, right eye**
  - **H33.42**   **Traction detachment of retina, left eye**
  - **H33.43**   **Traction detachment of retina, bilateral**
- **H33.8**   **Other retinal detachments**
- **H34**   **Retinal vascular occlusions**
  Blockage in vessel of the retina
  Excludes1   amaurosis fugax (G45.3)
  - **H34.0**   **Transient retinal artery occlusion**
    - **H34.00**   **Transient retinal artery occlusion, unspecified eye**
    - **H34.01**   **Transient retinal artery occlusion, right eye**
    - **H34.02**   **Transient retinal artery occlusion, left eye**
    - **H34.03**   **Transient retinal artery occlusion, bilateral**
  - **H34.1**   **Central retinal artery occlusion**
    - **H34.10**   **Central retinal artery occlusion, unspecified eye**
    - **H34.11**   **Central retinal artery occlusion, right eye**
    - **H34.12**   **Central retinal artery occlusion, left eye**
    - **H34.13**   **Central retinal artery occlusion, bilateral**
  - **H34.2**   **Other retinal artery occlusions**
    - **H34.21**   **Partial retinal artery occlusion**
      Hollenhorst's plaque
      Retinal microembolism
      - **H34.211**   **Partial retinal artery occlusion, right eye**
      - **H34.212**   **Partial retinal artery occlusion, left eye**
      - **H34.213**   **Partial retinal artery occlusion, bilateral**
      - **H34.219**   **Partial retinal artery occlusion, unspecified eye**
    - **H34.23**   **Retinal artery branch occlusion**
      - **H34.231**   **Retinal artery branch occlusion, right eye**
      - **H34.232**   **Retinal artery branch occlusion, left eye**
      - **H34.233**   **Retinal artery branch occlusion, bilateral**
      - **H34.239**   **Retinal artery branch occlusion, unspecified eye**

- **H34.8**   **Other retinal vascular occlusions**
  - **H34.81**   **Central retinal vein occlusion**
    One of the following 7th characters is to be assigned to codes in subcategory H34.81 to designate the severity of the occlusion: ◄

Ø	with macular edema ◄
1	with retinal neovascularization ◄
2	stable ◄
	Old central retinal vein occlusion ◄

    - **H34.811**   **Central retinal vein occlusion, right eye**
    - **H34.812**   **Central retinal vein occlusion, left eye**
    - **H34.813**   **Central retinal vein occlusion, bilateral**
    - **H34.819**   **Central retinal vein occlusion, unspecified eye**
  - **H34.82**   **Venous engorgement**
    Incipient retinal vein occlusion
    Partial retinal vein occlusion
    - **H34.821**   **Venous engorgement, right eye**
    - **H34.822**   **Venous engorgement, left eye**
    - **H34.823**   **Venous engorgement, bilateral**
    - **H34.829**   **Venous engorgement, unspecified eye**
  - **H34.83**   **Tributary (branch) retinal vein occlusion**
    One of the following 7th characters is to be assigned to codes in subcategory H34.83 to designate the severity of the occlusion: ◄

Ø	with macular edema ◄
1	with retinal neovascularization ◄
2	stable ◄
	Old tributary (branch) retinal vein occlusion ◄

    - **H34.831**   **Tributary (branch) retinal vein occlusion, right eye**
    - **H34.832**   **Tributary (branch) retinal vein occlusion, left eye**
    - **H34.833**   **Tributary (branch) retinal vein occlusion, bilateral**
    - **H34.839**   **Tributary (branch) retinal vein occlusion, unspecified eye**
  - **H34.9**   **Unspecified retinal vascular occlusion**
- **H35**   **Other retinal disorders**
  Excludes2   diabetic retinal disorders (E08.311-E08.359, E09.311-E09.359, E10.311-E10.359, E11.311-E11.359, E13.311-E13.359)
  - **H35.0**   **Background retinopathy and retinal vascular changes**
    Code also any associated hypertension (I10.-)
    OGCR Section I. C.9.a.5.

    Hypertensive Retinopathy
    Subcategory H35.0, Background retinopathy and retinal vascular changes, should be used with a code from category I10–I15, Hypertensive disease to include the systemic hypertension. The sequencing is based on the reason for the encounter.

    - **H35.00**   **Unspecified background retinopathy**
    - **H35.01**   **Changes in retinal vascular appearance**
      Retinal vascular sheathing
      - **H35.011**   **Changes in retinal vascular appearance, right eye**
      - **H35.012**   **Changes in retinal vascular appearance, left eye**
      - **H35.013**   **Changes in retinal vascular appearance, bilateral**
      - **H35.019**   **Changes in retinal vascular appearance, unspecified eye**

CHAPTER 7 (H00-H59)

● H35.02 **Exudative retinopathy**
  Coats retinopathy
  H35.021 Exudative retinopathy, right eye
  H35.022 Exudative retinopathy, left eye
  H35.023 Exudative retinopathy, bilateral
  H35.029 Exudative retinopathy, unspecified eye
● H35.03 **Hypertensive retinopathy**
  H35.031 Hypertensive retinopathy, right eye
  H35.032 Hypertensive retinopathy, left eye
  H35.033 Hypertensive retinopathy, bilateral
  H35.039 Hypertensive retinopathy, unspecified eye
● H35.04 **Retinal micro-aneurysms, unspecified**
  H35.041 Retinal micro-aneurysms, unspecified, right eye
  H35.042 Retinal micro-aneurysms, unspecified, left eye
  H35.043 Retinal micro-aneurysms, unspecified, bilateral
  H35.049 Retinal micro-aneurysms, unspecified, unspecified eye
● H35.05 **Retinal neovascularization, unspecified**
  H35.051 Retinal neovascularization, unspecified, right eye
  H35.052 Retinal neovascularization, unspecified, left eye
  H35.053 Retinal neovascularization, unspecified, bilateral
  H35.059 Retinal neovascularization, unspecified, unspecified eye
● H35.06 **Retinal vasculitis**
  Eales disease
  Retinal perivasculitis
  H35.061 Retinal vasculitis, right eye
  H35.062 Retinal vasculitis, left eye
  H35.063 Retinal vasculitis, bilateral
  H35.069 Retinal vasculitis, unspecified eye
● H35.07 **Retinal telangiectasis**
  H35.071 Retinal telangiectasis, right eye
  H35.072 Retinal telangiectasis, left eye
  H35.073 Retinal telangiectasis, bilateral
  H35.079 Retinal telangiectasis, unspecified eye
  H35.09 **Other intraretinal microvascular abnormalities**
  Retinal varices
● H35.1 **Retinopathy of prematurity**
● H35.10 **Retinopathy of prematurity, unspecified**
  Retinopathy of prematurity NOS
  H35.101 Retinopathy of prematurity, unspecified, right eye
  H35.102 Retinopathy of prematurity, unspecified, left eye
  H35.103 Retinopathy of prematurity, unspecified, bilateral
  H35.109 Retinopathy of prematurity, unspecified, unspecified eye
● H35.11 **Retinopathy of prematurity, stage 0**
  H35.111 Retinopathy of prematurity, stage 0, right eye
  H35.112 Retinopathy of prematurity, stage 0, left eye
  H35.113 Retinopathy of prematurity, stage 0, bilateral
  H35.119 Retinopathy of prematurity, stage 0, unspecified eye

● H35.12 **Retinopathy of prematurity, stage 1**
  H35.121 Retinopathy of prematurity, stage 1, right eye
  H35.122 Retinopathy of prematurity, stage 1, left eye
  H35.123 Retinopathy of prematurity, stage 1, bilateral
  H35.129 Retinopathy of prematurity, stage 1, unspecified eye
● H35.13 **Retinopathy of prematurity, stage 2**
  H35.131 Retinopathy of prematurity, stage 2, right eye
  H35.132 Retinopathy of prematurity, stage 2, left eye
  H35.133 Retinopathy of prematurity, stage 2, bilateral
  H35.139 Retinopathy of prematurity, stage 2, unspecified eye
● H35.14 **Retinopathy of prematurity, stage 3**
  H35.141 Retinopathy of prematurity, stage 3, right eye
  H35.142 Retinopathy of prematurity, stage 3, left eye
  H35.143 Retinopathy of prematurity, stage 3, bilateral
  H35.149 Retinopathy of prematurity, stage 3, unspecified eye
● H35.15 **Retinopathy of prematurity, stage 4**
  H35.151 Retinopathy of prematurity, stage 4, right eye
  H35.152 Retinopathy of prematurity, stage 4, left eye
  H35.153 Retinopathy of prematurity, stage 4, bilateral
  H35.159 Retinopathy of prematurity, stage 4, unspecified eye
● H35.16 **Retinopathy of prematurity, stage 5**
  H35.161 Retinopathy of prematurity, stage 5, right eye
  H35.162 Retinopathy of prematurity, stage 5, left eye
  H35.163 Retinopathy of prematurity, stage 5, bilateral
  H35.169 Retinopathy of prematurity, stage 5, unspecified eye
● H35.17 **Retrolental fibroplasia**
  H35.171 Retrolental fibroplasia, right eye
  H35.172 Retrolental fibroplasia, left eye
  H35.173 Retrolental fibroplasia, bilateral
  H35.179 Retrolental fibroplasia, unspecified eye
● H35.2 **Other non-diabetic proliferative retinopathy**
  Proliferative vitreo-retinopathy
  Excludes1 proliferative vitreo-retinopathy with retinal detachment (H33.4-)
  H35.20 Other non-diabetic proliferative retinopathy, unspecified eye
  H35.21 Other non-diabetic proliferative retinopathy, right eye
  H35.22 Other non-diabetic proliferative retinopathy, left eye
  H35.23 Other non-diabetic proliferative retinopathy, bilateral

◄ New   ◄■ Revised   ~~deleted~~ Deleted   Excludes 1   Excludes 2   Includes   Use additional   Code first   Code also   Unspecified

OGCR Official Guidelines   X Assign placeholder X   ● Use Additional Character(s)   ▶ Manifestation Code   **Coding Clinic**

Item 7–7 Macular degeneration is typically age-related, chronic, and is evidenced by deterioration of the macula (the part of the retina that provides for central field vision), resulting in blurred vision or a blind spot in the center of visual field while not affecting peripheral vision.

● H35.3   **Degeneration of macula and posterior pole**

    H35.30   Unspecified macular degeneration   A
          Age-related macular degeneration

● H35.31   **Nonexudative age-related macular degeneration**
       Atrophic age-related macular degeneration
       Dry age-related macular degeneration ◄
       One of the following 7th characters is to be assigned to codes in subcategory H35.31 to designate the stage of the disease: ◄

> | | |
> |---|---|
> | Ø | stage unspecified ◄ |
> | 1 | early dry stage ◄ |
> | 2 | intermediate dry stage ◄ |
> | 3 | advanced atrophic without subfoveal involvement ◄ |
> | | advanced dry stage ◄ |
> | 4 | advanced atrophic with subfoveal involvement ◄ |

   ● H35.311   Nonexudative age-related macular degeneration, right eye ◄   A
   ● H35.312   Nonexudative age-related macular degeneration, left eye ◄   A
   ● H35.313   Nonexudative age-related macular degeneration, bilateral ◄   A
   ● H35.319   Nonexudative age-related macular degeneration, unspecified eye ◄   A

● H35.32   **Exudative age-related macular degeneration**
       Wet age-related macular degeneration ◄
       One of the following 7th characters is to be assigned to codes in subcategory H35.32 to designate the stage of the disease: ◄

> | | |
> |---|---|
> | Ø | stage unspecified ◄ |
> | 1 | with active choroidal neovascularization ◄ |
> | 2 | with inactive choroidal neovascularization ◄ |
> | | with involuted or regressed neovascularization ◄ |
> | 3 | with inactive scar ◄ |

   ● H35.321   Exudative age-related macular degeneration, right eye ◄   A
   ● H35.322   Exudative age-related macular degeneration, left eye ◄   A
   ● H35.323   Exudative age-related macular degeneration, bilateral ◄   A
   ● H35.329   Exudative age-related macular degeneration, unspecified eye ◄   A

    H35.33   Angioid streaks of macula

● H35.34   **Macular cyst, hole, or pseudohole**
    H35.341   Macular cyst, hole, or pseudohole, right eye
    H35.342   Macular cyst, hole, or pseudohole, left eye
    H35.343   Macular cyst, hole, or pseudohole, bilateral
    H35.349   Macular cyst, hole, or pseudohole, unspecified eye

● H35.35   **Cystoid macular degeneration**
     Excludes1   cystoid macular edema following cataract surgery (H59.Ø3-)
    H35.351   Cystoid macular degeneration, right eye
    H35.352   Cystoid macular degeneration, left eye
    H35.353   Cystoid macular degeneration, bilateral
    H35.359   Cystoid macular degeneration, unspecified eye

● H35.36   **Drusen (degenerative) of macula**
    H35.361   Drusen (degenerative) of macula, right eye
    H35.362   Drusen (degenerative) of macula, left eye
    H35.363   Drusen (degenerative) of macula, bilateral
    H35.369   Drusen (degenerative) of macula, unspecified eye

● H35.37   **Puckering of macula**
    H35.371   Puckering of macula, right eye
    H35.372   Puckering of macula, left eye
    H35.373   Puckering of macula, bilateral
    H35.379   Puckering of macula, unspecified eye

● H35.38   **Toxic maculopathy**
     Code first poisoning due to drug or toxin, if applicable (T36-T65 with fifth or sixth character 1-4 or 6)
     Use additional code for adverse effect, if applicable, to identify drug (T36-T5Ø with fifth or sixth character 5)
    H35.381   Toxic maculopathy, right eye
    H35.382   Toxic maculopathy, left eye
    H35.383   Toxic maculopathy, bilateral
    H35.389   Toxic maculopathy, unspecified eye

● H35.4   **Peripheral retinal degeneration**
     Excludes1   hereditary retinal degeneration (dystrophy) (H35.5-)
          peripheral retinal degeneration with retinal break (H33.3-)
    H35.4Ø   Unspecified peripheral retinal degeneration

● H35.41   **Lattice degeneration of retina**
       Palisade degeneration of retina
    H35.411   Lattice degeneration of retina, right eye
    H35.412   Lattice degeneration of retina, left eye
    H35.413   Lattice degeneration of retina, bilateral
    H35.419   Lattice degeneration of retina, unspecified eye

● H35.42   **Microcystoid degeneration of retina**
    H35.421   Microcystoid degeneration of retina, right eye
    H35.422   Microcystoid degeneration of retina, left eye
    H35.423   Microcystoid degeneration of retina, bilateral
    H35.429   Microcystoid degeneration of retina, unspecified eye

CHAPTER 7 (HØØ-H59)

● H35.43   Paving stone degeneration of retina
- H35.431   Paving stone degeneration of retina, right eye
- H35.432   Paving stone degeneration of retina, left eye
- H35.433   Paving stone degeneration of retina, bilateral
- H35.439   Paving stone degeneration of retina, unspecified eye

● H35.44   Age-related reticular degeneration of retina
- H35.441   Age-related reticular degeneration of retina, right eye   A
- H35.442   Age-related reticular degeneration of retina, left eye   A
- H35.443   Age-related reticular degeneration of retina, bilateral   A
- H35.449   Age-related reticular degeneration of retina, unspecified eye   A

● H35.45   Secondary pigmentary degeneration
- H35.451   Secondary pigmentary degeneration, right eye
- H35.452   Secondary pigmentary degeneration, left eye
- H35.453   Secondary pigmentary degeneration, bilateral
- H35.459   Secondary pigmentary degeneration, unspecified eye

● H35.46   Secondary vitreoretinal degeneration
- H35.461   Secondary vitreoretinal degeneration, right eye
- H35.462   Secondary vitreoretinal degeneration, left eye
- H35.463   Secondary vitreoretinal degeneration, bilateral
- H35.469   Secondary vitreoretinal degeneration, unspecified eye

● H35.5   Hereditary retinal dystrophy

> **Excludes1**   dystrophies primarily involving Bruch's membrane (H31.1-)

- H35.50   Unspecified hereditary retinal dystrophy
- H35.51   Vitreoretinal dystrophy
- H35.52   Pigmentary retinal dystrophy
  - Albipunctate retinal dystrophy
  - Retinitis pigmentosa
  - Tapetoretinal dystrophy
- H35.53   Other dystrophies primarily involving the sensory retina
  - Stargardt's disease
- H35.54   Dystrophies primarily involving the retinal pigment epithelium
  - Vitelliform retinal dystrophy

● H35.6   Retinal hemorrhage
- H35.60   Retinal hemorrhage, unspecified eye
- H35.61   Retinal hemorrhage, right eye
- H35.62   Retinal hemorrhage, left eye
- H35.63   Retinal hemorrhage, bilateral

● H35.7   Separation of retinal layers

> **Excludes1**   retinal detachment (serous) (H33.2-)
> rhegmatogenous retinal detachment (H33.0-)

- H35.70   Unspecified separation of retinal layers

● H35.71   Central serous chorioretinopathy
- H35.711   Central serous chorioretinopathy, right eye
- H35.712   Central serous chorioretinopathy, left eye
- H35.713   Central serous chorioretinopathy, bilateral
- H35.719   Central serous chorioretinopathy, unspecified eye

● H35.72   Serous detachment of retinal pigment epithelium
- H35.721   Serous detachment of retinal pigment epithelium, right eye
- H35.722   Serous detachment of retinal pigment epithelium, left eye
- H35.723   Serous detachment of retinal pigment epithelium, bilateral
- H35.729   Serous detachment of retinal pigment epithelium, unspecified eye

● H35.73   Hemorrhagic detachment of retinal pigment epithelium
- H35.731   Hemorrhagic detachment of retinal pigment epithelium, right eye
- H35.732   Hemorrhagic detachment of retinal pigment epithelium, left eye
- H35.733   Hemorrhagic detachment of retinal pigment epithelium, bilateral
- H35.739   Hemorrhagic detachment of retinal pigment epithelium, unspecified eye

● H35.8   Other specified retinal disorders

> **Excludes2**   retinal hemorrhage (H35.6-)

- H35.81   Retinal edema
  - Retinal cotton wool spots
- H35.82   Retinal ischemia
- H35.89   Other specified retinal disorders

H35.9   Unspecified retinal disorder

▷ *H36*   *Retinal disorders in diseases classified elsewhere*

> *Code first* underlying disease, such as:
> lipid storage disorders (E75.-)
> sickle-cell disorders (D57.-)

> **Excludes1**   arteriosclerotic retinopathy (H35.0-)
> diabetic retinopathy (E08.3-, E09.3-, E10.3-, E11.3-, E13.3-)

GLAUCOMA (H40-H42)

● H40   Glaucoma

> *Intraocular pressure (IOP) that is too high results from too much aqueous humor and because of excess production or inadequate drainage, optic nerve damage and vision loss may occur.*

> **Excludes1**   absolute glaucoma (H44.51-)
> congenital glaucoma (Q15.0)
> traumatic glaucoma due to birth injury (P15.3)

● H40.0   Glaucoma suspect

● H40.00   Preglaucoma, unspecified
- H40.001   Preglaucoma, unspecified, right eye
- H40.002   Preglaucoma, unspecified, left eye
- H40.003   Preglaucoma, unspecified, bilateral
- H40.009   Preglaucoma, unspecified, unspecified eye

● H40.01   Open angle with borderline findings, low risk
  - Open angle, low risk
- H40.011   Open angle with borderline findings, low risk, right eye
- H40.012   Open angle with borderline findings, low risk, left eye
- H40.013   Open angle with borderline findings, low risk, bilateral
- H40.019   Open angle with borderline findings, low risk, unspecified eye

● H40.02   Open angle with borderline findings, high risk
     Open angle, high risk

     H40.021   Open angle with borderline findings, high risk, right eye

     H40.022   Open angle with borderline findings, high risk, left eye

     H40.023   Open angle with borderline findings, high risk, bilateral

     H40.029   Open angle with borderline findings, high risk, unspecified eye

● H40.03   Anatomical narrow angle
     Primary angle closure suspect

     H40.031   Anatomical narrow angle, right eye

     H40.032   Anatomical narrow angle, left eye

     H40.033   Anatomical narrow angle, bilateral

     H40.039   Anatomical narrow angle, unspecified eye

● H40.04   Steroid responder

     H40.041   Steroid responder, right eye

     H40.042   Steroid responder, left eye

     H40.043   Steroid responder, bilateral

     H40.049   Steroid responder, unspecified eye

● H40.05   Ocular hypertension

     H40.051   Ocular hypertension, right eye

     H40.052   Ocular hypertension, left eye

     H40.053   Ocular hypertension, bilateral

     H40.059   Ocular hypertension, unspecified eye

● H40.06   Primary angle closure without glaucoma damage

     H40.061   Primary angle closure without glaucoma damage, right eye

     H40.062   Primary angle closure without glaucoma damage, left eye

     H40.063   Primary angle closure without glaucoma damage, bilateral

     H40.069   Primary angle closure without glaucoma damage, unspecified eye

● H40.1   Open-angle glaucoma

X ● H40.10   Unspecified open-angle glaucoma

     One of the following 7th characters is to be assigned to code H40.10 to designate the stage of glaucoma

0	stage unspecified
1	mild stage
2	moderate stage
3	severe stage
4	indeterminate stage

● H40.11   Primary open-angle glaucoma
     Chronic simple glaucoma

     One of the following 7th characters is to be assigned to each code in subcategory H40.11 to designate the stage of glaucoma ◀▥

0	stage unspecified
1	mild stage
2	moderate stage
3	severe stage
4	indeterminate stage

     ● H40.111   Primary open-angle glaucoma, right eye ◀

     ● H40.112   Primary open-angle glaucoma, left eye ◀

     ● H40.113   Primary open-angle glaucoma, bilateral ◀

     ● H40.119   Primary open-angle glaucoma, unspecified eye ◀

● H40.12   Low-tension glaucoma

     One of the following 7th characters is to be assigned to each code in subcategory H40.12 to designate the stage of glaucoma

0	stage unspecified
1	mild stage
2	moderate stage
3	severe stage
4	indeterminate stage

     ● H40.121   Low-tension glaucoma, right eye

     ● H40.122   Low-tension glaucoma, left eye

     ● H40.123   Low-tension glaucoma, bilateral

     ● H40.129   Low-tension glaucoma, unspecified eye

● H40.13   Pigmentary glaucoma

     One of the following 7th characters is to be assigned to each code in subcategory H40.13 to designate the stage of glaucoma

0	stage unspecified
1	mild stage
2	moderate stage
3	severe stage
4	indeterminate stage

     ● H40.131   Pigmentary glaucoma, right eye

     ● H40.132   Pigmentary glaucoma, left eye

     ● H40.133   Pigmentary glaucoma, bilateral

     ● H40.139   Pigmentary glaucoma, unspecified eye

● H40.14   Capsular glaucoma with pseudoexfoliation of lens

     One of the following 7th characters is to be assigned to each code in subcategory H40.14 to designate the stage of glaucoma

0	stage unspecified
1	mild stage
2	moderate stage
3	severe stage
4	indeterminate stage

     ● H40.141   Capsular glaucoma with pseudoexfoliation of lens, right eye

     ● H40.142   Capsular glaucoma with pseudoexfoliation of lens, left eye

     ● H40.143   Capsular glaucoma with pseudoexfoliation of lens, bilateral

     ● H40.149   Capsular glaucoma with pseudoexfoliation of lens, unspecified eye

● H40.15   Residual stage of open-angle glaucoma

     H40.151   Residual stage of open-angle glaucoma, right eye

     H40.152   Residual stage of open-angle glaucoma, left eye

     H40.153   Residual stage of open-angle glaucoma, bilateral

     H40.159   Residual stage of open-angle glaucoma, unspecified eye

CHAPTER 7 (H00-H59)

● H40.2   Primary angle-closure glaucoma

     Excludes1   aqueous misdirection (H40.83-)
                        malignant glaucoma (H40.83-)

X ● H40.20   Unspecified primary angle-closure glaucoma

     One of the following 7th characters is to be assigned to code H40.20 to designate the stage of glaucoma

0	stage unspecified
1	mild stage
2	moderate stage
3	severe stage
4	indeterminate stage

● H40.21   Acute angle-closure glaucoma

     Acute angle-closure glaucoma attack
     Acute angle-closure glaucoma crisis

     H40.211   Acute angle-closure glaucoma, right eye

     H40.212   Acute angle-closure glaucoma, left eye

     H40.213   Acute angle-closure glaucoma, bilateral

     H40.219   Acute angle-closure glaucoma, unspecified eye

● H40.22   Chronic angle-closure glaucoma

     Chronic primary angle closure glaucoma

     One of the following 7th characters is to be assigned to each code in subcategory H40.22 to designate the stage of glaucoma

0	stage unspecified
1	mild stage
2	moderate stage
3	severe stage
4	indeterminate stage

     ● H40.221   Chronic angle-closure glaucoma, right eye

     ● H40.222   Chronic angle-closure glaucoma, left eye

     ● H40.223   Chronic angle-closure glaucoma, bilateral

     ● H40.229   Chronic angle-closure glaucoma, unspecified eye

● H40.23   Intermittent angle-closure glaucoma

     H40.231   Intermittent angle-closure glaucoma, right eye

     H40.232   Intermittent angle-closure glaucoma, left eye

     H40.233   Intermittent angle-closure glaucoma, bilateral

     H40.239   Intermittent angle-closure glaucoma, unspecified eye

● H40.24   Residual stage of angle-closure glaucoma

     H40.241   Residual stage of angle-closure glaucoma, right eye

     H40.242   Residual stage of angle-closure glaucoma, left eye

     H40.243   Residual stage of angle-closure glaucoma, bilateral

     H40.249   Residual stage of angle-closure glaucoma, unspecified eye

● H40.3   Glaucoma secondary to eye trauma

     Code also underlying condition

     One of the following 7th characters is to be assigned to each code in subcategory H40.3 to designate the stage of glaucoma

0	stage unspecified
1	mild stage
2	moderate stage
3	severe stage
4	indeterminate stage

X ● H40.30   Glaucoma secondary to eye trauma, unspecified eye

X ● H40.31   Glaucoma secondary to eye trauma, right eye

X ● H40.32   Glaucoma secondary to eye trauma, left eye

X ● H40.33   Glaucoma secondary to eye trauma, bilateral

● H40.4   Glaucoma secondary to eye inflammation

     Code also underlying condition

     One of the following 7th characters is to be assigned to each code in subcategory H40.4 to designate the stage of glaucoma

0	stage unspecified
1	mild stage
2	moderate stage
3	severe stage
4	indeterminate stage

X ● H40.40   Glaucoma secondary to eye inflammation, unspecified eye

X ● H40.41   Glaucoma secondary to eye inflammation, right eye

X ● H40.42   Glaucoma secondary to eye inflammation, left eye

X ● H40.43   Glaucoma secondary to eye inflammation, bilateral

● H40.5   Glaucoma secondary to other eye disorders

     Code also underlying eye disorder

     One of the following 7th characters is to be assigned to each code in subcategory H40.5 to designate the stage of glaucoma

0	stage unspecified
1	mild stage
2	moderate stage
3	severe stage
4	indeterminate stage

X ● H40.50   Glaucoma secondary to other eye disorders, unspecified eye

X ● H40.51   Glaucoma secondary to other eye disorders, right eye

X ● H40.52   Glaucoma secondary to other eye disorders, left eye

X ● H40.53   Glaucoma secondary to other eye disorders, bilateral

◀ New   ◀▥ Revised   ~~deleted~~ Deleted   Excludes 1   Excludes 2   Includes   Use additional   Code first   Code also   Unspecified

OGCR Official Guidelines   X Assign placeholder X   ● Use Additional Character(s)   ▶ Manifestation Code   **Coding Clinic**

● **H40.6**   **Glaucoma secondary to drugs**

Use additional code for adverse effect, if applicable, to identify drug (T36-T50 with fifth or sixth character 5)

One of the following 7th characters is to be assigned to each code in subcategory H40.6 to designate the stage of glaucoma

Ø	stage unspecified
1	mild stage
2	moderate stage
3	severe stage
4	indeterminate stage

X● **H40.60**   Glaucoma secondary to drugs, unspecified eye
X● **H40.61**   Glaucoma secondary to drugs, right eye
X● **H40.62**   Glaucoma secondary to drugs, left eye
X● **H40.63**   Glaucoma secondary to drugs, bilateral

● **H40.8**   **Other glaucoma**

  ● **H40.81**   Glaucoma with increased episcleral venous pressure

     H40.811   Glaucoma with increased episcleral venous pressure, right eye

     H40.812   Glaucoma with increased episcleral venous pressure, left eye

     H40.813   Glaucoma with increased episcleral venous pressure, bilateral

     H40.819   Glaucoma with increased episcleral venous pressure, unspecified eye

  ● **H40.82**   Hypersecretion glaucoma

     H40.821   Hypersecretion glaucoma, right eye
     H40.822   Hypersecretion glaucoma, left eye
     H40.823   Hypersecretion glaucoma, bilateral
     H40.829   Hypersecretion glaucoma, unspecified eye

  ● **H40.83**   Aqueous misdirection
     Malignant glaucoma

     H40.831   Aqueous misdirection, right eye
     H40.832   Aqueous misdirection, left eye
     H40.833   Aqueous misdirection, bilateral
     H40.839   Aqueous misdirection, unspecified eye

     H40.89   Other specified glaucoma

  H40.9   Unspecified glaucoma

▶ *H42*   *Glaucoma in diseases classified elsewhere*

     Code first underlying condition, such as:
       amyloidosis (E85.-)
       aniridia (Q13.1)
       Lowe's syndrome (E72.03)
       Reiger's anomaly (Q13.81)
       specified metabolic disorder (E70-E88)

     Excludes1   glaucoma (in) onchocerciasis (B73.02) ◀▥
              glaucoma (in) syphilis (A52.71) ◀▥
              glaucoma (in) tuberculous (A18.59) ◀▥

     Excludes2   glaucoma (in) diabetes mellitus (E08.39, E09.39, E10.39, E11.39, E13.39) ◀

DISORDERS OF VITREOUS BODY AND GLOBE (H43-H44)

● **H43**   **Disorders of vitreous body**

  ● **H43.0**   **Vitreous prolapse**

     Excludes1   vitreous syndrome following cataract surgery (H59.0-)
                  traumatic vitreous prolapse (S05.2-)

     H43.00   Vitreous prolapse, unspecified eye
     H43.01   Vitreous prolapse, right eye
     H43.02   Vitreous prolapse, left eye
     H43.03   Vitreous prolapse, bilateral

  ● **H43.1**   **Vitreous hemorrhage**

     H43.10   Vitreous hemorrhage, unspecified eye
     H43.11   Vitreous hemorrhage, right eye
     H43.12   Vitreous hemorrhage, left eye
     H43.13   Vitreous hemorrhage, bilateral

  ● **H43.2**   **Crystalline deposits in vitreous body**

     H43.20   Crystalline deposits in vitreous body, unspecified eye
     H43.21   Crystalline deposits in vitreous body, right eye
     H43.22   Crystalline deposits in vitreous body, left eye
     H43.23   Crystalline deposits in vitreous body, bilateral

  ● **H43.3**   **Other vitreous opacities**

    ● **H43.31**   Vitreous membranes and strands

       H43.311   Vitreous membranes and strands, right eye
       H43.312   Vitreous membranes and strands, left eye
       H43.313   Vitreous membranes and strands, bilateral
       H43.319   Vitreous membranes and strands, unspecified eye

    ● **H43.39**   Other vitreous opacities
       Vitreous floaters
       Small clumps of cells that float in the vitreous of the eye, appearing as black specks or dots in the field of vision and common in the aging eye.

       H43.391   Other vitreous opacities, right eye
       H43.392   Other vitreous opacities, left eye
       H43.393   Other vitreous opacities, bilateral
       H43.399   Other vitreous opacities, unspecified eye

  ● **H43.8**   **Other disorders of vitreous body**

     Excludes1   proliferative vitreo-retinopathy with retinal detachment (H33.4)

     Excludes2   vitreous abscess (H44.02-)

    ● **H43.81**   Vitreous degeneration
       Vitreous detachment

       H43.811   Vitreous degeneration, right eye
       H43.812   Vitreous degeneration, left eye
       H43.813   Vitreous degeneration, bilateral
       H43.819   Vitreous degeneration, unspecified eye

    ● **H43.82**   Vitreomacular adhesion
       Vitreomacular traction

       H43.821   Vitreomacular adhesion, right eye   A
       H43.822   Vitreomacular adhesion, left eye   A
       H43.823   Vitreomacular adhesion, bilateral   A
       H43.829   Vitreomacular adhesion, unspecified eye   A

     H43.89   Other disorders of vitreous body

  H43.9   Unspecified disorder of vitreous body

● H44 Disorders of globe
    Includes disorders affecting multiple structures of eye
 ● H44.0 Purulent endophthalmitis
    Use additional code to identify organism
    Excludes1 bleb associated endophthalmitis (H59.4-)
  ● H44.00 Unspecified purulent endophthalmitis
    H44.001 Unspecified purulent endophthalmitis, right eye
    H44.002 Unspecified purulent endophthalmitis, left eye
    H44.003 Unspecified purulent endophthalmitis, bilateral
    H44.009 Unspecified purulent endophthalmitis, unspecified eye
  ● H44.01 Panophthalmitis (acute)
    H44.011 Panophthalmitis (acute), right eye
    H44.012 Panophthalmitis (acute), left eye
    H44.013 Panophthalmitis (acute), bilateral
    H44.019 Panophthalmitis (acute), unspecified eye
  ● H44.02 Vitreous abscess (chronic)
    H44.021 Vitreous abscess (chronic), right eye
    H44.022 Vitreous abscess (chronic), left eye
    H44.023 Vitreous abscess (chronic), bilateral
    H44.029 Vitreous abscess (chronic), unspecified eye
 ● H44.1 Other endophthalmitis
    Excludes1 bleb associated endophthalmitis (H59.4-)
    Excludes2 ophthalmia nodosa (H16.2-)
  ● H44.11 Panuveitis
    H44.111 Panuveitis, right eye
    H44.112 Panuveitis, left eye
    H44.113 Panuveitis, bilateral
    H44.119 Panuveitis, unspecified eye
  ● H44.12 Parasitic endophthalmitis, unspecified
    H44.121 Parasitic endophthalmitis, unspecified, right eye
    H44.122 Parasitic endophthalmitis, unspecified, left eye
    H44.123 Parasitic endophthalmitis, unspecified, bilateral
    H44.129 Parasitic endophthalmitis, unspecified, unspecified eye
  ● H44.13 Sympathetic uveitis
    H44.131 Sympathetic uveitis, right eye
    H44.132 Sympathetic uveitis, left eye
    H44.133 Sympathetic uveitis, bilateral
    H44.139 Sympathetic uveitis, unspecified eye
    H44.19 Other endophthalmitis
 ● H44.2 Degenerative myopia
    Malignant myopia
    H44.20 Degenerative myopia, unspecified eye
    H44.21 Degenerative myopia, right eye
    H44.22 Degenerative myopia, left eye
    H44.23 Degenerative myopia, bilateral
 ● H44.3 Other and unspecified degenerative disorders of globe
    H44.30 Unspecified degenerative disorder of globe
  ● H44.31 Chalcosis
    H44.311 Chalcosis, right eye
    H44.312 Chalcosis, left eye
    H44.313 Chalcosis, bilateral
    H44.319 Chalcosis, unspecified eye

  ● H44.32 Siderosis of eye
    H44.321 Siderosis of eye, right eye
    H44.322 Siderosis of eye, left eye
    H44.323 Siderosis of eye, bilateral
    H44.329 Siderosis of eye, unspecified eye
  ● H44.39 Other degenerative disorders of globe
    H44.391 Other degenerative disorders of globe, right eye
    H44.392 Other degenerative disorders of globe, left eye
    H44.393 Other degenerative disorders of globe, bilateral
    H44.399 Other degenerative disorders of globe, unspecified eye
 ● H44.4 Hypotony of eye
    H44.40 Unspecified hypotony of eye
  ● H44.41 Flat anterior chamber hypotony of eye
    H44.411 Flat anterior chamber hypotony of right eye
    H44.412 Flat anterior chamber hypotony of left eye
    H44.413 Flat anterior chamber hypotony of eye, bilateral
    H44.419 Flat anterior chamber hypotony of unspecified eye
  ● H44.42 Hypotony of eye due to ocular fistula
    H44.421 Hypotony of right eye due to ocular fistula
    H44.422 Hypotony of left eye due to ocular fistula
    H44.423 Hypotony of eye due to ocular fistula, bilateral
    H44.429 Hypotony of unspecified eye due to ocular fistula
  ● H44.43 Hypotony of eye due to other ocular disorders
    H44.431 Hypotony of eye due to other ocular disorders, right eye
    H44.432 Hypotony of eye due to other ocular disorders, left eye
    H44.433 Hypotony of eye due to other ocular disorders, bilateral
    H44.439 Hypotony of eye due to other ocular disorders, unspecified eye
  ● H44.44 Primary hypotony of eye
    H44.441 Primary hypotony of right eye
    H44.442 Primary hypotony of left eye
    H44.443 Primary hypotony of eye, bilateral
    H44.449 Primary hypotony of unspecified eye
 ● H44.5 Degenerated conditions of globe
    H44.50 Unspecified degenerated conditions of globe
  ● H44.51 Absolute glaucoma
    H44.511 Absolute glaucoma, right eye
    H44.512 Absolute glaucoma, left eye
    H44.513 Absolute glaucoma, bilateral
    H44.519 Absolute glaucoma, unspecified eye
  ● H44.52 Atrophy of globe
    Phthisis bulbi
    H44.521 Atrophy of globe, right eye
    H44.522 Atrophy of globe, left eye
    H44.523 Atrophy of globe, bilateral
    H44.529 Atrophy of globe, unspecified eye
  ● H44.53 Leucocoria
    H44.531 Leucocoria, right eye
    H44.532 Leucocoria, left eye
    H44.533 Leucocoria, bilateral
    H44.539 Leucocoria, unspecified eye

◀ New   ◀▥ Revised   deleted Deleted   Excludes 1   Excludes 2   Includes   Use additional   Code first   Code also   Unspecified
    OGCR Official Guidelines   X Assign placeholder X   ● Use Additional Character(s)   ▶ Manifestation Code   **Coding Clinic**

● **H44.6**   Retained (old) intraocular foreign body, magnetic

Use additional code to identify magnetic foreign body (Z18.11)

Excludes1   current intraocular foreign body (S05.-)

Excludes2   retained foreign body in eyelid (H02.81-)
retained (old) foreign body following penetrating wound of orbit (H05.5-)
retained (old) intraocular foreign body, nonmagnetic (H44.7-)

● **H44.60**   Unspecified retained (old) intraocular foreign body, magnetic

H44.601   Unspecified retained (old) intraocular foreign body, magnetic, right eye

H44.602   Unspecified retained (old) intraocular foreign body, magnetic, left eye

H44.603   Unspecified retained (old) intraocular foreign body, magnetic, bilateral

H44.609   Unspecified retained (old) intraocular foreign body, magnetic, unspecified eye

● **H44.61**   Retained (old) magnetic foreign body in anterior chamber

H44.611   Retained (old) magnetic foreign body in anterior chamber, right eye

H44.612   Retained (old) magnetic foreign body in anterior chamber, left eye

H44.613   Retained (old) magnetic foreign body in anterior chamber, bilateral

H44.619   Retained (old) magnetic foreign body in anterior chamber, unspecified eye

● **H44.62**   Retained (old) magnetic foreign body in iris or ciliary body

H44.621   Retained (old) magnetic foreign body in iris or ciliary body, right eye

H44.622   Retained (old) magnetic foreign body in iris or ciliary body, left eye

H44.623   Retained (old) magnetic foreign body in iris or ciliary body, bilateral

H44.629   Retained (old) magnetic foreign body in iris or ciliary body, unspecified eye

● **H44.63**   Retained (old) magnetic foreign body in lens

H44.631   Retained (old) magnetic foreign body in lens, right eye

H44.632   Retained (old) magnetic foreign body in lens, left eye

H44.633   Retained (old) magnetic foreign body in lens, bilateral

H44.639   Retained (old) magnetic foreign body in lens, unspecified eye

● **H44.64**   Retained (old) magnetic foreign body in posterior wall of globe

H44.641   Retained (old) magnetic foreign body in posterior wall of globe, right eye

H44.642   Retained (old) magnetic foreign body in posterior wall of globe, left eye

H44.643   Retained (old) magnetic foreign body in posterior wall of globe, bilateral

H44.649   Retained (old) magnetic foreign body in posterior wall of globe, unspecified eye

● **H44.65**   Retained (old) magnetic foreign body in vitreous body

H44.651   Retained (old) magnetic foreign body in vitreous body, right eye

H44.652   Retained (old) magnetic foreign body in vitreous body, left eye

H44.653   Retained (old) magnetic foreign body in vitreous body, bilateral

H44.659   Retained (old) magnetic foreign body in vitreous body, unspecified eye

● **H44.69**   Retained (old) intraocular foreign body, magnetic, in other or multiple sites

H44.691   Retained (old) intraocular foreign body, magnetic, in other or multiple sites, right eye

H44.692   Retained (old) intraocular foreign body, magnetic, in other or multiple sites, left eye

H44.693   Retained (old) intraocular foreign body, magnetic, in other or multiple sites, bilateral

H44.699   Retained (old) intraocular foreign body, magnetic, in other or multiple sites, unspecified eye

● **H44.7**   Retained (old) intraocular foreign body, nonmagnetic

Use additional code to identify nonmagnetic foreign body (Z18.01-Z18.10, Z18.12, Z18.2-Z18.9)

Excludes1   current intraocular foreign body (S05.-)

Excludes2   retained foreign body in eyelid (H02.81-)
retained (old) foreign body following penetrating wound of orbit (H05.5-)
retained (old) intraocular foreign body, magnetic (H44.6-)

● **H44.70**   Unspecified retained (old) intraocular foreign body, nonmagnetic

H44.701   Unspecified retained (old) intraocular foreign body, nonmagnetic, right eye

H44.702   Unspecified retained (old) intraocular foreign body, nonmagnetic, left eye

H44.703   Unspecified retained (old) intraocular foreign body, nonmagnetic, bilateral

H44.709   Unspecified retained (old) intraocular foreign body, nonmagnetic, unspecified eye
Retained (old) intraocular foreign body NOS

● **H44.71**   Retained (nonmagnetic) (old) foreign body in anterior chamber

H44.711   Retained (nonmagnetic) (old) foreign body in anterior chamber, right eye

H44.712   Retained (nonmagnetic) (old) foreign body in anterior chamber, left eye

H44.713   Retained (nonmagnetic) (old) foreign body in anterior chamber, bilateral

H44.719   Retained (nonmagnetic) (old) foreign body in anterior chamber, unspecified eye

● **H44.72**   Retained (nonmagnetic) (old) foreign body in iris or ciliary body

H44.721   Retained (nonmagnetic) (old) foreign body in iris or ciliary body, right eye

H44.722   Retained (nonmagnetic) (old) foreign body in iris or ciliary body, left eye

H44.723   Retained (nonmagnetic) (old) foreign body in iris or ciliary body, bilateral

H44.729   Retained (nonmagnetic) (old) foreign body in iris or ciliary body, unspecified eye

CHAPTER 7 (H00-H59)

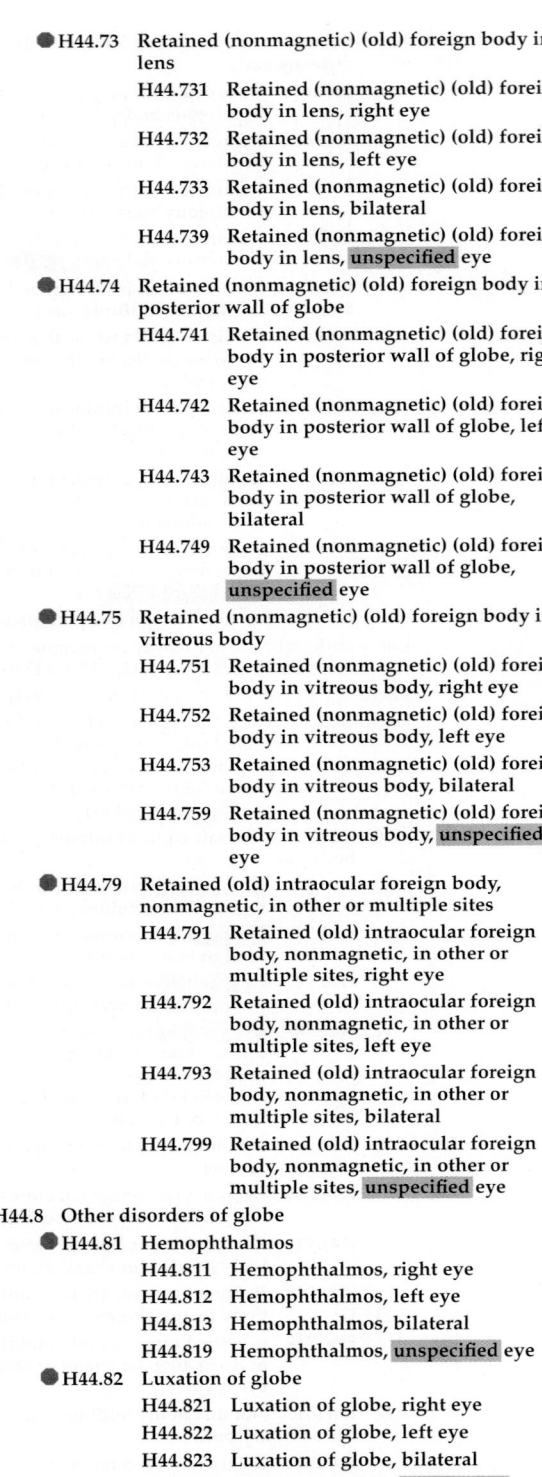

- H44.73 Retained (nonmagnetic) (old) foreign body in lens
  - H44.731 Retained (nonmagnetic) (old) foreign body in lens, right eye
  - H44.732 Retained (nonmagnetic) (old) foreign body in lens, left eye
  - H44.733 Retained (nonmagnetic) (old) foreign body in lens, bilateral
  - H44.739 Retained (nonmagnetic) (old) foreign body in lens, unspecified eye
- H44.74 Retained (nonmagnetic) (old) foreign body in posterior wall of globe
  - H44.741 Retained (nonmagnetic) (old) foreign body in posterior wall of globe, right eye
  - H44.742 Retained (nonmagnetic) (old) foreign body in posterior wall of globe, left eye
  - H44.743 Retained (nonmagnetic) (old) foreign body in posterior wall of globe, bilateral
  - H44.749 Retained (nonmagnetic) (old) foreign body in posterior wall of globe, unspecified eye
- H44.75 Retained (nonmagnetic) (old) foreign body in vitreous body
  - H44.751 Retained (nonmagnetic) (old) foreign body in vitreous body, right eye
  - H44.752 Retained (nonmagnetic) (old) foreign body in vitreous body, left eye
  - H44.753 Retained (nonmagnetic) (old) foreign body in vitreous body, bilateral
  - H44.759 Retained (nonmagnetic) (old) foreign body in vitreous body, unspecified eye
- H44.79 Retained (old) intraocular foreign body, nonmagnetic, in other or multiple sites
  - H44.791 Retained (old) intraocular foreign body, nonmagnetic, in other or multiple sites, right eye
  - H44.792 Retained (old) intraocular foreign body, nonmagnetic, in other or multiple sites, left eye
  - H44.793 Retained (old) intraocular foreign body, nonmagnetic, in other or multiple sites, bilateral
  - H44.799 Retained (old) intraocular foreign body, nonmagnetic, in other or multiple sites, unspecified eye
- H44.8 Other disorders of globe
  - H44.81 Hemophthalmos
    - H44.811 Hemophthalmos, right eye
    - H44.812 Hemophthalmos, left eye
    - H44.813 Hemophthalmos, bilateral
    - H44.819 Hemophthalmos, unspecified eye
  - H44.82 Luxation of globe
    - H44.821 Luxation of globe, right eye
    - H44.822 Luxation of globe, left eye
    - H44.823 Luxation of globe, bilateral
    - H44.829 Luxation of globe, unspecified eye
  - H44.89 Other disorders of globe
- H44.9 Unspecified disorder of globe

★ (See Plate 86 on page 55.)

DISORDERS OF OPTIC NERVE AND VISUAL PATHWAYS (H46-H47)

- H46 Optic neuritis
  - Excludes2   ischemic optic neuropathy (H47.01-)
           neuromyelitis optica [Devic] (G36.0)
  - H46.0 Optic papillitis
    - H46.00 Optic papillitis, unspecified eye
    - H46.01 Optic papillitis, right eye
    - H46.02 Optic papillitis, left eye
    - H46.03 Optic papillitis, bilateral
  - H46.1 Retrobulbar neuritis
    Retrobulbar neuritis NOS
    - Excludes1   syphilitic retrobulbar neuritis (A52.15)
    - H46.10 Retrobulbar neuritis, unspecified eye
    - H46.11 Retrobulbar neuritis, right eye
    - H46.12 Retrobulbar neuritis, left eye
    - H46.13 Retrobulbar neuritis, bilateral
  - H46.2 Nutritional optic neuropathy
  - H46.3 Toxic optic neuropathy
    Code first (T51-T65) to identify cause
  - H46.8 Other optic neuritis
  - H46.9 Unspecified optic neuritis
- H47 Other disorders of optic [2nd] nerve and visual pathways
  - H47.0 Disorders of optic nerve, not elsewhere classified
    - H47.01 Ischemic optic neuropathy
      - H47.011 Ischemic optic neuropathy, right eye
      - H47.012 Ischemic optic neuropathy, left eye
      - H47.013 Ischemic optic neuropathy, bilateral
      - H47.019 Ischemic optic neuropathy, unspecified eye
    - H47.02 Hemorrhage in optic nerve sheath
      - H47.021 Hemorrhage in optic nerve sheath, right eye
      - H47.022 Hemorrhage in optic nerve sheath, left eye
      - H47.023 Hemorrhage in optic nerve sheath, bilateral
      - H47.029 Hemorrhage in optic nerve sheath, unspecified eye
    - H47.03 Optic nerve hypoplasia
      - H47.031 Optic nerve hypoplasia, right eye
      - H47.032 Optic nerve hypoplasia, left eye
      - H47.033 Optic nerve hypoplasia, bilateral
      - H47.039 Optic nerve hypoplasia, unspecified eye
    - H47.09 Other disorders of optic nerve, not elsewhere classified
      Compression of optic nerve
      - H47.091 Other disorders of optic nerve, not elsewhere classified, right eye
      - H47.092 Other disorders of optic nerve, not elsewhere classified, left eye
      - H47.093 Other disorders of optic nerve, not elsewhere classified, bilateral
      - H47.099 Other disorders of optic nerve, not elsewhere classified, unspecified eye

◀ New   ◀ Revised   ~~deleted~~ Deleted   Excludes 1   Excludes 2   Includes   Use additional   Code first   Code also   Unspecified
OGCR Official Guidelines   X Assign placeholder X   ● Use Additional Character(s)   ▶ Manifestation Code   **Coding Clinic**

Figure 7-11   Papilledema. (From Behrma: Nelson Textbook of Pediatrics, ed 17, Saunders, 2004)

Item 7–8   Papilledema is swelling of the optic disc caused by increased intracranial pressure. It is most often bilateral and occurs quickly (hours) or over weeks of time. It is a common symptom of a brain tumor. The term should not be used to describe optic disc swelling with underlying infectious, infiltrative, or inflammatory etiologies.

● H47.1   **Papilledema**
- H47.10   Unspecified papilledema
- H47.11   Papilledema associated with increased intracranial pressure
- H47.12   Papilledema associated with decreased ocular pressure
- H47.13   Papilledema associated with retinal disorder
- ● H47.14   Foster-Kennedy syndrome
  - H47.141   Foster-Kennedy syndrome, right eye
  - H47.142   Foster-Kennedy syndrome, left eye
  - H47.143   Foster-Kennedy syndrome, bilateral
  - H47.149   Foster-Kennedy syndrome, unspecified eye

● H47.2   **Optic atrophy**
- H47.20   Unspecified optic atrophy
- ● H47.21   Primary optic atrophy
  - H47.211   Primary optic atrophy, right eye
  - H47.212   Primary optic atrophy, left eye
  - H47.213   Primary optic atrophy, bilateral
  - H47.219   Primary optic atrophy, unspecified eye
- H47.22   Hereditary optic atrophy
  - Leber's optic atrophy
- ● H47.23   Glaucomatous optic atrophy
  - H47.231   Glaucomatous optic atrophy, right eye
  - H47.232   Glaucomatous optic atrophy, left eye
  - H47.233   Glaucomatous optic atrophy, bilateral
  - H47.239   Glaucomatous optic atrophy, unspecified eye
- ● H47.29   Other optic atrophy
  - Temporal pallor of optic disc
  - H47.291   Other optic atrophy, right eye
  - H47.292   Other optic atrophy, left eye
  - H47.293   Other optic atrophy, bilateral
  - H47.299   Other optic atrophy, unspecified eye

● H47.3   **Other disorders of optic disc**
- ● H47.31   Coloboma of optic disc
  - H47.311   Coloboma of optic disc, right eye
  - H47.312   Coloboma of optic disc, left eye
  - H47.313   Coloboma of optic disc, bilateral
  - H47.319   Coloboma of optic disc, unspecified eye
- ● H47.32   Drusen of optic disc
  - H47.321   Drusen of optic disc, right eye
  - H47.322   Drusen of optic disc, left eye
  - H47.323   Drusen of optic disc, bilateral
  - H47.329   Drusen of optic disc, unspecified eye
- ● H47.33   Pseudopapilledema of optic disc
  - H47.331   Pseudopapilledema of optic disc, right eye
  - H47.332   Pseudopapilledema of optic disc, left eye
  - H47.333   Pseudopapilledema of optic disc, bilateral
  - H47.339   Pseudopapilledema of optic disc, unspecified eye
- ● H47.39   Other disorders of optic disc
  - H47.391   Other disorders of optic disc, right eye
  - H47.392   Other disorders of optic disc, left eye
  - H47.393   Other disorders of optic disc, bilateral
  - H47.399   Other disorders of optic disc, unspecified eye

● H47.4   **Disorders of optic chiasm**
- Code also underlying condition
- H47.41   Disorders of optic chiasm in (due to) inflammatory disorders
- H47.42   Disorders of optic chiasm in (due to) neoplasm
- H47.43   Disorders of optic chiasm in (due to) vascular disorders
- H47.49   Disorders of optic chiasm in (due to) other disorders

● H47.5   **Disorders of other visual pathways**
- Disorders of optic tracts, geniculate nuclei and optic radiations
- Code also underlying condition
- ● H47.51   Disorders of visual pathways in (due to) inflammatory disorders
  - H47.511   Disorders of visual pathways in (due to) inflammatory disorders, right side
  - H47.512   Disorders of visual pathways in (due to) inflammatory disorders, left side
  - H47.519   Disorders of visual pathways in (due to) inflammatory disorders, unspecified side
- ● H47.52   Disorders of visual pathways in (due to) neoplasm
  - H47.521   Disorders of visual pathways in (due to) neoplasm, right side
  - H47.522   Disorders of visual pathways in (due to) neoplasm, left side
  - H47.529   Disorders of visual pathways in (due to) neoplasm, unspecified side
- ● H47.53   Disorders of visual pathways in (due to) vascular disorders
  - H47.531   Disorders of visual pathways in (due to) vascular disorders, right side
  - H47.532   Disorders of visual pathways in (due to) vascular disorders, left side
  - H47.539   Disorders of visual pathways in (due to) vascular disorders, unspecified side

CHAPTER 7 (H00-H59)

CHAPTER 7 (H00–H59)

● H47.6   Disorders of visual cortex
     Code also underlying condition
     Excludes1   injury to visual cortex S04.04

    ● H47.61   Cortical blindness
        H47.611   Cortical blindness, right side of brain
        H47.612   Cortical blindness, left side of brain
        H47.619   Cortical blindness, unspecified side of brain

    ● H47.62   Disorders of visual cortex in (due to) inflammatory disorders
        H47.621   Disorders of visual cortex in (due to) inflammatory disorders, right side of brain
        H47.622   Disorders of visual cortex in (due to) inflammatory disorders, left side of brain
        H47.629   Disorders of visual cortex in (due to) inflammatory disorders, unspecified side of brain

    ● H47.63   Disorders of visual cortex in (due to) neoplasm
        H47.631   Disorders of visual cortex in (due to) neoplasm, right side of brain
        H47.632   Disorders of visual cortex in (due to) neoplasm, left side of brain
        H47.639   Disorders of visual cortex in (due to) neoplasm, unspecified side of brain

    ● H47.64   Disorders of visual cortex in (due to) vascular disorders
        H47.641   Disorders of visual cortex in (due to) vascular disorders, right side of brain
        H47.642   Disorders of visual cortex in (due to) vascular disorders, left side of brain
        H47.649   Disorders of visual cortex in (due to) vascular disorders, unspecified side of brain

  H47.9   Unspecified disorder of visual pathways

DISORDERS OF OCULAR MUSCLES, BINOCULAR MOVEMENT, ACCOMMODATION AND REFRACTION (H49-H52)

    Excludes2   nystagmus and other irregular eye movements (H55)

● H49   Paralytic strabismus
    Excludes2   internal ophthalmoplegia (H52.51-)
                   internuclear ophthalmoplegia (H51.2-)
                   progressive supranuclear ophthalmoplegia (G23.1)

    ● H49.0   Third [oculomotor] nerve palsy
        H49.00   Third [oculomotor] nerve palsy, unspecified eye
        H49.01   Third [oculomotor] nerve palsy, right eye
        H49.02   Third [oculomotor] nerve palsy, left eye
        H49.03   Third [oculomotor] nerve palsy, bilateral

Item 7–9 Strabismus or esotropia (crossed eyes) is a condition of the extraocular eye muscles, resulting in an inability of the eyes to focus and also affects depth perception.

A

B

Figure 7-12 **A.** Image of strabismus. **B.** Exotropia. (**A** from Yanoff: Ophthalmology, ed 3, Mosby, Inc., 2008. **B** from Rakel: Textbook of Family Practice, ed 7, Saunders, 2007)

    ● H49.1   Fourth [trochlear] nerve palsy
        H49.10   Fourth [trochlear] nerve palsy, unspecified eye
        H49.11   Fourth [trochlear] nerve palsy, right eye
        H49.12   Fourth [trochlear] nerve palsy, left eye
        H49.13   Fourth [trochlear] nerve palsy, bilateral

    ● H49.2   Sixth [abducent] nerve palsy
        H49.20   Sixth [abducent] nerve palsy, unspecified eye
        H49.21   Sixth [abducent] nerve palsy, right eye
        H49.22   Sixth [abducent] nerve palsy, left eye
        H49.23   Sixth [abducent] nerve palsy, bilateral

    ● H49.3   Total (external) ophthalmoplegia
        H49.30   Total (external) ophthalmoplegia, unspecified eye
        H49.31   Total (external) ophthalmoplegia, right eye
        H49.32   Total (external) ophthalmoplegia, left eye
        H49.33   Total (external) ophthalmoplegia, bilateral

    ● H49.4   Progressive external ophthalmoplegia
        Excludes1   Kearns-Sayre syndrome (H49.81-)
        H49.40   Progressive external ophthalmoplegia, unspecified eye
        H49.41   Progressive external ophthalmoplegia, right eye
        H49.42   Progressive external ophthalmoplegia, left eye
        H49.43   Progressive external ophthalmoplegia, bilateral

    ● H49.8   Other paralytic strabismus
      ● H49.81   Kearns-Sayre syndrome
           Progressive external ophthalmoplegia with pigmentary retinopathy
           Use additional code for other manifestation, such as:
               heart block (I45.9)
        H49.811   Kearns-Sayre syndrome, right eye
        H49.812   Kearns-Sayre syndrome, left eye
        H49.813   Kearns-Sayre syndrome, bilateral
        H49.819   Kearns-Sayre syndrome, unspecified eye

      ● H49.88   Other paralytic strabismus
           External ophthalmoplegia NOS
        H49.881   Other paralytic strabismus, right eye
        H49.882   Other paralytic strabismus, left eye
        H49.883   Other paralytic strabismus, bilateral
        H49.889   Other paralytic strabismus, unspecified eye

  H49.9   Unspecified paralytic strabismus

● H50   Other strabismus
    ● H50.0   Esotropia
        Convergent concomitant strabismus
        Excludes1   intermittent esotropia (H50.31-, H50.32)
       H50.00   Unspecified esotropia
      ● H50.01   Monocular esotropia
        H50.011   Monocular esotropia, right eye
        H50.012   Monocular esotropia, left eye
      ● H50.02   Monocular esotropia with A pattern
        H50.021   Monocular esotropia with A pattern, right eye
        H50.022   Monocular esotropia with A pattern, left eye
      ● H50.03   Monocular esotropia with V pattern
        H50.031   Monocular esotropia with V pattern, right eye
        H50.032   Monocular esotropia with V pattern, left eye

- **H50.04** Monocular esotropia with other noncomitancies
  - **H50.041** Monocular esotropia with other noncomitancies, right eye
  - **H50.042** Monocular esotropia with other noncomitancies, left eye
- **H50.05** Alternating esotropia
- **H50.06** Alternating esotropia with A pattern
- **H50.07** Alternating esotropia with V pattern
- **H50.08** Alternating esotropia with other noncomitancies
- **H50.1** Exotropia
  - *Misalignment in which one eye deviates outward (away from nose) while the other fixates normally*
  - Divergent concomitant strabismus
  - **Excludes1**   intermittent exotropia (H50.33-, H50.34)
  - **H50.10** Unspecified exotropia
  - **H50.11** Monocular exotropia
    - **H50.111** Monocular exotropia, right eye
    - **H50.112** Monocular exotropia, left eye
  - **H50.12** Monocular exotropia with A pattern
    - **H50.121** Monocular exotropia with A pattern, right eye
    - **H50.122** Monocular exotropia with A pattern, left eye
  - **H50.13** Monocular exotropia with V pattern
    - **H50.131** Monocular exotropia with V pattern, right eye
    - **H50.132** Monocular exotropia with V pattern, left eye
  - **H50.14** Monocular exotropia with other noncomitancies
    - **H50.141** Monocular exotropia with other noncomitancies, right eye
    - **H50.142** Monocular exotropia with other noncomitancies, left eye
  - **H50.15** Alternating exotropia
  - **H50.16** Alternating exotropia with A pattern
  - **H50.17** Alternating exotropia with V pattern
  - **H50.18** Alternating exotropia with other noncomitancies
- **H50.2** Vertical strabismus
  - Hypertropia
  - **H50.21** Vertical strabismus, right eye
  - **H50.22** Vertical strabismus, left eye
- **H50.3** Intermittent heterotropia
  - *Displacement of an organ or part of an organ from its normal position*
  - **H50.30** Unspecified intermittent heterotropia
  - **H50.31** Intermittent monocular esotropia
    - **H50.311** Intermittent monocular esotropia, right eye
    - **H50.312** Intermittent monocular esotropia, left eye
  - **H50.32** Intermittent alternating esotropia
  - **H50.33** Intermittent monocular exotropia
    - **H50.331** Intermittent monocular exotropia, right eye
    - **H50.332** Intermittent monocular exotropia, left eye
  - **H50.34** Intermittent alternating exotropia

- **H50.4** Other and unspecified heterotropia
  - **H50.40** Unspecified heterotropia
  - **H50.41** Cyclotropia
    - **H50.411** Cyclotropia, right eye
    - **H50.412** Cyclotropia, left eye
  - **H50.42** Monofixation syndrome
  - **H50.43** Accommodative component in esotropia
- **H50.5** Heterophoria
  - *One or both eyes wander away from the position where both eyes are looking together in the same direction*
  - **H50.50** Unspecified heterophoria
  - **H50.51** Esophoria
    - *Eye deviates inward (toward the nose)*
  - **H50.52** Exophoria
    - *Eye deviates outward (toward the ear)*
  - **H50.53** Vertical heterophoria
  - **H50.54** Cyclophoria
  - **H50.55** Alternating heterophoria
- **H50.6** Mechanical strabismus
  - **H50.60** Mechanical strabismus, unspecified
  - **H50.61** Brown's sheath syndrome
    - **H50.611** Brown's sheath syndrome, right eye
    - **H50.612** Brown's sheath syndrome, left eye
  - **H50.69** Other mechanical strabismus
    - Strabismus due to adhesions
    - Traumatic limitation of duction of eye muscle
- **H50.8** Other specified strabismus
  - **H50.81** Duane's syndrome
    - **H50.811** Duane's syndrome, right eye
    - **H50.812** Duane's syndrome, left eye
  - **H50.89** Other specified strabismus
- **H50.9** Unspecified strabismus

- **H51** Other disorders of binocular movement
  - **H51.0** Palsy (spasm) of conjugate gaze
  - **H51.1** Convergence insufficiency and excess
    - **H51.11** Convergence insufficiency
    - **H51.12** Convergence excess
  - **H51.2** Internuclear ophthalmoplegia
    - **H51.20** Internuclear ophthalmoplegia, unspecified eye
    - **H51.21** Internuclear ophthalmoplegia, right eye
    - **H51.22** Internuclear ophthalmoplegia, left eye
    - **H51.23** Internuclear ophthalmoplegia, bilateral
  - **H51.8** Other specified disorders of binocular movement
  - **H51.9** Unspecified disorder of binocular movement

- **H52** Disorders of refraction and accommodation
  - **H52.0** Hypermetropia
    - **H52.00** Hypermetropia, unspecified eye
    - **H52.01** Hypermetropia, right eye
    - **H52.02** Hypermetropia, left eye
    - **H52.03** Hypermetropia, bilateral
  - **H52.1** Myopia
    - **Excludes1**   degenerative myopia (H44.2-)
    - **H52.10** Myopia, unspecified eye
    - **H52.11** Myopia, right eye
    - **H52.12** Myopia, left eye
    - **H52.13** Myopia, bilateral

CHAPTER 7 (H00–H59)

Item 7–10 Disorders of refraction: **Hypermetropia,** or farsightedness, means focus at a distance is adequate but not on close objects. **Myopia** is near-sightedness or short-sightedness and means the focus on nearby objects is clear but distant objects appear blurred. **Astigmatism** is warping of the curvature of the cornea so light rays entering do not meet a single focal point, resulting in a distorted image. **Anisometropia** is unequal refractive power in which one eye may be myopic (near-sighted) and the other hyperopic (far-sighted). **Presbyopia** is the loss of focus on near objects, which occurs with age because the lens loses elasticity.

- H52.2 Astigmatism
  - H52.20 Unspecified astigmatism
    - H52.201 Unspecified astigmatism, right eye
    - H52.202 Unspecified astigmatism, left eye
    - H52.203 Unspecified astigmatism, bilateral
    - H52.209 Unspecified astigmatism, unspecified eye
  - H52.21 Irregular astigmatism
    - H52.211 Irregular astigmatism, right eye
    - H52.212 Irregular astigmatism, left eye
    - H52.213 Irregular astigmatism, bilateral
    - H52.219 Irregular astigmatism, unspecified eye
  - H52.22 Regular astigmatism
    - H52.221 Regular astigmatism, right eye
    - H52.222 Regular astigmatism, left eye
    - H52.223 Regular astigmatism, bilateral
    - H52.229 Regular astigmatism, unspecified eye
- H52.3 Anisometropia and aniseikonia
  - H52.31 Anisometropia
  - H52.32 Aniseikonia
- H52.4 Presbyopia
- H52.5 Disorders of accommodation
  - H52.51 Internal ophthalmoplegia (complete) (total)
    - H52.511 Internal ophthalmoplegia (complete) (total), right eye
    - H52.512 Internal ophthalmoplegia (complete) (total), left eye
    - H52.513 Internal ophthalmoplegia (complete) (total), bilateral
    - H52.519 Internal ophthalmoplegia (complete) (total), unspecified eye
  - H52.52 Paresis of accommodation
    - H52.521 Paresis of accommodation, right eye
    - H52.522 Paresis of accommodation, left eye
    - H52.523 Paresis of accommodation, bilateral
    - H52.529 Paresis of accommodation, unspecified eye
  - H52.53 Spasm of accommodation
    - H52.531 Spasm of accommodation, right eye
    - H52.532 Spasm of accommodation, left eye
    - H52.533 Spasm of accommodation, bilateral
    - H52.539 Spasm of accommodation, unspecified eye
- H52.6 Other disorders of refraction
- H52.7 Unspecified disorder of refraction

VISUAL DISTURBANCES AND BLINDNESS (H53-H54)

- H53 Visual disturbances
  - H53.0 Amblyopia ex anopsia
    - Excludes1 amblyopia due to vitamin A deficiency (E50.5)
    - H53.00 Unspecified amblyopia
      - H53.001 Unspecified amblyopia, right eye
      - H53.002 Unspecified amblyopia, left eye
      - H53.003 Unspecified amblyopia, bilateral
      - H53.009 Unspecified amblyopia, unspecified eye
    - H53.01 Deprivation amblyopia
      - H53.011 Deprivation amblyopia, right eye
      - H53.012 Deprivation amblyopia, left eye
      - H53.013 Deprivation amblyopia, bilateral
      - H53.019 Deprivation amblyopia, unspecified eye
    - H53.02 Refractive amblyopia
      - H53.021 Refractive amblyopia, right eye
      - H53.022 Refractive amblyopia, left eye
      - H53.023 Refractive amblyopia, bilateral
      - H53.029 Refractive amblyopia, unspecified eye
    - H53.03 Strabismic amblyopia
      - Excludes1 strabismus (H50.-)
      - H53.031 Strabismic amblyopia, right eye
      - H53.032 Strabismic amblyopia, left eye
      - H53.033 Strabismic amblyopia, bilateral
      - H53.039 Strabismic amblyopia, unspecified eye
    - H53.04 Amblyopia suspect ◄
      - H53.041 Amblyopia suspect, right eye ◄
      - H53.042 Amblyopia suspect, left eye ◄
      - H53.043 Amblyopia suspect, bilateral ◄
      - H53.049 Amblyopia suspect, unspecified eye ◄
  - H53.1 Subjective visual disturbances
    - Excludes1 subjective visual disturbances due to vitamin A deficiency (E50.5)
      visual hallucinations (R44.1)
    - H53.10 Unspecified subjective visual disturbances
    - H53.11 Day blindness
      Hemeralopia
    - H53.12 Transient visual loss
      Scintillating scotoma
      - Excludes1 amaurosis fugax (G45.3-)
        transient retinal artery occlusion (H34.0-)
      - H53.121 Transient visual loss, right eye
      - H53.122 Transient visual loss, left eye
      - H53.123 Transient visual loss, bilateral
      - H53.129 Transient visual loss, unspecified eye
    - H53.13 Sudden visual loss
      - H53.131 Sudden visual loss, right eye
      - H53.132 Sudden visual loss, left eye
      - H53.133 Sudden visual loss, bilateral
      - H53.139 Sudden visual loss, unspecified eye

◄ New ◄= Revised ~~deleted~~ Deleted | Excludes 1 | Excludes 2 | Includes | Use additional | Code first | Code also | Unspecified |
OGCR Official Guidelines X Assign placeholder X ● Use Additional Character(s) ▶ Manifestation Code **Coding Clinic**

- **H53.14** Visual discomfort
  Asthenopia
  Photophobia
  - **H53.141** Visual discomfort, right eye
  - **H53.142** Visual discomfort, left eye
  - **H53.143** Visual discomfort, bilateral
  - **H53.149** Visual discomfort, unspecified
- **H53.15** Visual distortions of shape and size
  Metamorphopsia
- **H53.16** Psychophysical visual disturbances
- **H53.19** Other subjective visual disturbances
  Visual halos
- **H53.2** Diplopia
  Double vision
- **H53.3** Other and unspecified disorders of binocular vision
  - **H53.30** Unspecified disorder of binocular vision
  - **H53.31** Abnormal retinal correspondence
  - **H53.32** Fusion with defective stereopsis
  - **H53.33** Simultaneous visual perception without fusion
  - **H53.34** Suppression of binocular vision
- **H53.4** Visual field defects
  - **H53.40** Unspecified visual field defects
  - **H53.41** Scotoma involving central area
    Central scotoma
    - **H53.411** Scotoma involving central area, right eye
    - **H53.412** Scotoma involving central area, left eye
    - **H53.413** Scotoma involving central area, bilateral
    - **H53.419** Scotoma involving central area, unspecified eye
  - **H53.42** Scotoma of blind spot area
    Enlarged blind spot
    - **H53.421** Scotoma of blind spot area, right eye
    - **H53.422** Scotoma of blind spot area, left eye
    - **H53.423** Scotoma of blind spot area, bilateral
    - **H53.429** Scotoma of blind spot area, unspecified eye
  - **H53.43** Sector or arcuate defects
    Arcuate scotoma
    Bjerrum scotoma
    - **H53.431** Sector or arcuate defects, right eye
    - **H53.432** Sector or arcuate defects, left eye
    - **H53.433** Sector or arcuate defects, bilateral
    - **H53.439** Sector or arcuate defects, unspecified eye
  - **H53.45** Other localized visual field defect
    Peripheral visual field defect
    Ring scotoma NOS
    Scotoma NOS
    - **H53.451** Other localized visual field defect, right eye
    - **H53.452** Other localized visual field defect, left eye
    - **H53.453** Other localized visual field defect, bilateral
    - **H53.459** Other localized visual field defect, unspecified eye
- **H53.46** Homonymous bilateral field defects
  Homonymous hemianopia
  Homonymous hemianopsia
  Quadrant anopia
  Quadrant anopsia
  - **H53.461** Homonymous bilateral field defects, right side
  - **H53.462** Homonymous bilateral field defects, left side
  - **H53.469** Homonymous bilateral field defects, unspecified side
    Homonymous bilateral field defects NOS
- **H53.47** Heteronymous bilateral field defects
  Heteronymous hemianop(s)ia
- **H53.48** Generalized contraction of visual field
  - **H53.481** Generalized contraction of visual field, right eye
  - **H53.482** Generalized contraction of visual field, left eye
  - **H53.483** Generalized contraction of visual field, bilateral
  - **H53.489** Generalized contraction of visual field, unspecified eye
- **H53.5** Color vision deficiencies
  Color blindness
  Excludes2 day blindness (H53.11)
  - **H53.50** Unspecified color vision deficiencies
    Color blindness NOS
  - **H53.51** Achromatopsia
  - **H53.52** Acquired color vision deficiency
  - **H53.53** Deuteranomaly
    Deuteranopia
  - **H53.54** Protanomaly
    Protanopia
  - **H53.55** Tritanomaly
    Tritanopia
  - **H53.59** Other color vision deficiencies
- **H53.6** Night blindness
  Excludes1 night blindness due to vitamin A deficiency (E50.5)
  - **H53.60** Unspecified night blindness
  - **H53.61** Abnormal dark adaptation curve
  - **H53.62** Acquired night blindness
  - **H53.63** Congenital night blindness
  - **H53.69** Other night blindness
- **H53.7** Vision sensitivity deficiencies
  - **H53.71** Glare sensitivity
  - **H53.72** Impaired contrast sensitivity
- **H53.8** Other visual disturbances
- **H53.9** Unspecified visual disturbance

CHAPTER 7 (H00-H59)

● **H54 Blindness and low vision**
   Note: For definition of visual impairment categories see table below.
   Code first any associated underlying cause of the blindness
   Excludes1   amaurosis fugax (G45.3)
  H54.0 Blindness, both eyes
    Visual impairment categories 3, 4, 5 in both eyes.
● **H54.1 Blindness, one eye, low vision other eye**
    Visual impairment categories 3, 4, 5 in one eye, with categories 1 or 2 in the other eye.
    H54.10 Blindness, one eye, low vision other eye, **unspecified** eyes
    H54.11 Blindness, right eye, low vision left eye
    H54.12 Blindness, left eye, low vision right eye
  H54.2 Low vision, both eyes
    Visual impairment categories 1 or 2 in both eyes.
  H54.3 Unqualified visual loss, both eyes
    Visual impairment category 9 in both eyes.
● **H54.4 Blindness, one eye**
    Visual impairment categories 3, 4, 5 in one eye [normal vision in other eye]
    H54.40 Blindness, one eye, **unspecified** eye
    H54.41 Blindness, right eye, normal vision left eye
    H54.42 Blindness, left eye, normal vision right eye
● **H54.5 Low vision, one eye**
    Visual impairment categories 1 or 2 in one eye [normal vision in other eye].
    H54.50 Low vision, one eye, **unspecified** eye
    H54.51 Low vision, right eye, normal vision left eye
    H54.52 Low vision, left eye, normal vision right eye
● **H54.6 Unqualified visual loss, one eye**
    Visual impairment category 9 in one eye [normal vision in other eye].
    H54.60 Unqualified visual loss, one eye, **unspecified**
    H54.61 Unqualified visual loss, right eye, normal vision left eye
    H54.62 Unqualified visual loss, left eye, normal vision right eye
  H54.7 Unspecified visual loss
    Visual impairment category 9 NOS
  H54.8 Legal blindness, as defined in USA
    Blindness NOS according to USA definition
    Excludes1 legal blindness with specification of impairment level (H54.0-H54.7)
    Note: The table below gives a classification of severity of visual impairment recommended by a WHO Study Group on the Prevention of Blindness, Geneva, 6-10 November 1972.
    The term 'low vision' in category H54 comprises categories 1 and 2 of the table, the term 'blindness' categories 3, 4 and 5, and the term 'unqualified visual loss' category 9.
    If the extent of the visual field is taken into account, patients with a field no greater than 10 but greater than 5 around central fixation should be placed in category 3 and patients with a field no greater than 5 around central fixation should be placed in category 4, even if the central acuity is not impaired.

(Document 508 compliance requires all cells in the following table to be filled.)

Category of visual impairment	Visual acuity with best possible correction	
	Maximum less than:	**Minimum equal to or better than:**
—	6/18	6/60
3/10 (0.3)	1/10 (0.1)	—
20/70	20/200	—
—	6/60	3/60
1/10 (0.1)	1/20 (0.05)	—
20/200	20/400	—
—	3/60	1/60 (finger counting at one meter)
1/20 (0.05)	1/50 (0.02)	—
20/400	5/300 (20/1200)	—
—	1/60 (finger counting at one meter)	Light perception
1/50 (0.02)	—	—
5/300	—	—
—	No light perception	
—	Undetermined or unspecified	

OTHER DISORDERS OF EYE AND ADNEXA (H55-H57)

● **H55 Nystagmus and other irregular eye movements**
  ● **H55.0 Nystagmus**
    Rapid, involuntary movements of the eyes in the horizontal or vertical direction
    H55.00 **Unspecified** nystagmus
    H55.01 Congenital nystagmus
    H55.02 Latent nystagmus
    H55.03 Visual deprivation nystagmus
    H55.04 Dissociated nystagmus
    H55.09 Other forms of nystagmus
  ● **H55.8 Other irregular eye movements**
    H55.81 Saccadic eye movements
    H55.89 Other irregular eye movements

● **H57 Other disorders of eye and adnexa**
  ● **H57.0 Anomalies of pupillary function**
    H57.00 **Unspecified** anomaly of pupillary function
    H57.01 Argyll Robertson pupil, atypical
      Excludes1 syphilitic Argyll Robertson pupil (A52.19)
    H57.02 Anisocoria
    H57.03 Miosis
    H57.04 Mydriasis
  ● **H57.05** Tonic pupil
    H57.051 Tonic pupil, right eye
    H57.052 Tonic pupil, left eye
    H57.053 Tonic pupil, bilateral
    H57.059 Tonic pupil, **unspecified** eye
    H57.09 Other anomalies of pupillary function
  ● **H57.1 Ocular pain**
    H57.10 Ocular pain, **unspecified** eye
    H57.11 Ocular pain, right eye
    H57.12 Ocular pain, left eye
    H57.13 Ocular pain, bilateral
  H57.8 Other specified disorders of eye and adnexa
  H57.9 Unspecified disorder of eye and adnexa

◀ New   ◀▦ Revised   ~~deleted~~ Deleted   Excludes 1   Excludes 2   Includes   Use additional   Code first   Code also   Unspecified
OGCR Official Guidelines   X Assign placeholder X   ● Use Additional Character(s)   ▶ Manifestation Code   **Coding Clinic**

INTRAOPERATIVE AND POSTPROCEDURAL COMPLICATIONS AND DISORDERS OF EYE AND ADNEXA, NOT ELSEWHERE CLASSIFIED (H59)

● **H59　Intraoperative and postprocedural complications and disorders of eye and adnexa, not elsewhere classified**

> **Excludes1**　mechanical complication of intraocular lens (T85.2)
> mechanical complication of other ocular prosthetic devices, implants and grafts (T85.3)
> pseudophakia (Z96.1)
> secondary cataracts (H26.4-)

● **H59.0　Disorders of the eye following cataract surgery**

　● **H59.01　Keratopathy (bullous aphakic) following cataract surgery**
　　　Vitreal corneal syndrome
　　　Vitreous (touch) syndrome

　　　H59.011　Keratopathy (bullous aphakic) following cataract surgery, right eye

　　　H59.012　Keratopathy (bullous aphakic) following cataract surgery, left eye

　　　H59.013　Keratopathy (bullous aphakic) following cataract surgery, bilateral

　　　H59.019　Keratopathy (bullous aphakic) following cataract surgery, unspecified eye

　● **H59.02　Cataract (lens) fragments in eye following cataract surgery**

　　　H59.021　Cataract (lens) fragments in eye following cataract surgery, right eye

　　　H59.022　Cataract (lens) fragments in eye following cataract surgery, left eye

　　　H59.023　Cataract (lens) fragments in eye following cataract surgery, bilateral

　　　H59.029　Cataract (lens) fragments in eye following cataract surgery, unspecified eye

　● **H59.03　Cystoid macular edema following cataract surgery**

　　　H59.031　Cystoid macular edema following cataract surgery, right eye

　　　H59.032　Cystoid macular edema following cataract surgery, left eye

　　　H59.033　Cystoid macular edema following cataract surgery, bilateral

　　　H59.039　Cystoid macular edema following cataract surgery, unspecified eye

　● **H59.09　Other disorders of the eye following cataract surgery**

　　　H59.091　Other disorders of the right eye following cataract surgery

　　　H59.092　Other disorders of the left eye following cataract surgery

　　　H59.093　Other disorders of the eye following cataract surgery, bilateral

　　　H59.099　Other disorders of unspecified eye following cataract surgery

● **H59.1　Intraoperative hemorrhage and hematoma of eye and adnexa complicating a procedure**

> **Excludes1**　intraoperative hemorrhage and hematoma of eye and adnexa due to accidental puncture or laceration during a procedure (H59.2-)

　● **H59.11　Intraoperative hemorrhage and hematoma of eye and adnexa complicating an ophthalmic procedure**

　　　H59.111　Intraoperative hemorrhage and hematoma of right eye and adnexa complicating an ophthalmic procedure

　　　H59.112　Intraoperative hemorrhage and hematoma of left eye and adnexa complicating an ophthalmic procedure

　　　H59.113　Intraoperative hemorrhage and hematoma of eye and adnexa complicating an ophthalmic procedure, bilateral

　　　H59.119　Intraoperative hemorrhage and hematoma of unspecified eye and adnexa complicating an ophthalmic procedure

　● **H59.12　Intraoperative hemorrhage and hematoma of eye and adnexa complicating other procedure**

　　　H59.121　Intraoperative hemorrhage and hematoma of right eye and adnexa complicating other procedure

　　　H59.122　Intraoperative hemorrhage and hematoma of left eye and adnexa complicating other procedure

　　　H59.123　Intraoperative hemorrhage and hematoma of eye and adnexa complicating other procedure, bilateral

　　　H59.129　Intraoperative hemorrhage and hematoma of unspecified eye and adnexa complicating other procedure

● **H59.2　Accidental puncture and laceration of eye and adnexa during a procedure**

　● **H59.21　Accidental puncture and laceration of eye and adnexa during an ophthalmic procedure**

　　　H59.211　Accidental puncture and laceration of right eye and adnexa during an ophthalmic procedure

　　　H59.212　Accidental puncture and laceration of left eye and adnexa during an ophthalmic procedure

　　　H59.213　Accidental puncture and laceration of eye and adnexa during an ophthalmic procedure, bilateral

　　　H59.219　Accidental puncture and laceration of unspecified eye and adnexa during an ophthalmic procedure

　● **H59.22　Accidental puncture and laceration of eye and adnexa during other procedure**

　　　H59.221　Accidental puncture and laceration of right eye and adnexa during other procedure

　　　H59.222　Accidental puncture and laceration of left eye and adnexa during other procedure

　　　H59.223　Accidental puncture and laceration of eye and adnexa during other procedure, bilateral

　　　H59.229　Accidental puncture and laceration of unspecified eye and adnexa during other procedure

CHAPTER 7 (H00-H59)

- H59.3   Postprocedural hemorrhage, hematoma, and seroma of eye and adnexa following other procedure ◀═
  - H59.31   Postprocedural hemorrhage of eye and adnexa following an ophthalmic procedure ◀═
    - H59.311   Postprocedural hemorrhage of right eye and adnexa following an ophthalmic procedure ◀═
    - H59.312   Postprocedural hemorrhage of left eye and adnexa following an ophthalmic procedure ◀═
    - H59.313   Postprocedural hemorrhage of eye and adnexa following an ophthalmic procedure, bilateral ◀═
    - H59.319   Postprocedural hemorrhage of unspecified eye and adnexa following an ophthalmic procedure ◀═
  - H59.32   Postprocedural hemorrhage of eye and adnexa following other procedure ◀═
    - H59.321   Postprocedural hemorrhage of right eye and adnexa following other procedure ◀═
    - H59.322   Postprocedural hemorrhage of left eye and adnexa following other procedure ◀═
    - H59.323   Postprocedural hemorrhage of eye and adnexa following other procedure, bilateral ◀═
    - H59.329   Postprocedural hemorrhage of unspecified eye and adnexa following other procedure ◀═
  - H59.33   Postprocedural hematoma of eye and adnexa following an ophthalmic procedure ◀
    - H59.331   Postprocedural hematoma of right eye and adnexa following an ophthalmic procedure ◀
    - H59.332   Postprocedural hematoma of left eye and adnexa following an ophthalmic procedure ◀
    - H59.333   Postprocedural hematoma of eye and adnexa following an ophthalmic procedure, bilateral ◀
    - H59.339   Postprocedural hematoma of unspecified eye and adnexa following an ophthalmic procedure ◀
  - H59.34   Postprocedural hematoma of eye and adnexa following other procedure ◀
    - H59.341   Postprocedural hematoma of right eye and adnexa following other procedure ◀
    - H59.342   Postprocedural hematoma of left eye and adnexa following other procedure ◀
    - H59.343   Postprocedural hematoma of eye and adnexa following other procedure, bilateral ◀
    - H59.349   Postprocedural hematoma of unspecified eye and adnexa following other procedure ◀

- H59.35   Postprocedural seroma of eye and adnexa following an ophthalmic procedure ◀
  - H59.351   Postprocedural seroma of right eye and adnexa following an ophthalmic procedure ◀
  - H59.352   Postprocedural seroma of left eye and adnexa following an ophthalmic procedure ◀
  - H59.353   Postprocedural seroma of eye and adnexa following an ophthalmic procedure, bilateral ◀
  - H59.359   Postprocedural seroma of unspecified eye and adnexa following an ophthalmic procedure ◀
- H59.36   Postprocedural seroma of eye and adnexa following other procedure ◀
  - H59.361   Postprocedural seroma of right eye and adnexa following other procedure ◀
  - H59.362   Postprocedural seroma of left eye and adnexa following other procedure ◀
  - H59.363   Postprocedural seroma of eye and adnexa following other procedure, bilateral ◀
  - H59.369   Postprocedural seroma of unspecified eye and adnexa following other procedure ◀
- H59.4   Inflammation (infection) of postprocedural bleb
  Postprocedural blebitis
  > **Excludes1**   filtering (vitreous) bleb after glaucoma surgery status (Z98.83)
  - H59.40   Inflammation (infection) of postprocedural bleb, unspecified
  - H59.41   Inflammation (infection) of postprocedural bleb, stage 1
  - H59.42   Inflammation (infection) of postprocedural bleb, stage 2
  - H59.43   Inflammation (infection) of postprocedural bleb, stage 3
    Bleb endophthalmitis
- H59.8   Other intraoperative and postprocedural complications and disorders of eye and adnexa, not elsewhere classified
  - H59.81   Chorioretinal scars after surgery for detachment
    - H59.811   Chorioretinal scars after surgery for detachment, right eye
    - H59.812   Chorioretinal scars after surgery for detachment, left eye
    - H59.813   Chorioretinal scars after surgery for detachment, bilateral
    - H59.819   Chorioretinal scars after surgery for detachment, unspecified eye
  - H59.88   Other intraoperative complications of eye and adnexa, not elsewhere classified
  - H59.89   Other postprocedural complications and disorders of eye and adnexa, not elsewhere classified

◀ New   ◀═ Revised   deleted Deleted   Excludes 1   Excludes 2   Includes   Use additional   Code first   Code also   Unspecified

836   OGCR Official Guidelines   X Assign placeholder X   ● Use Additional Character(s)   ▶ Manifestation Code   **Coding Clinic**

CHAPTER 8

DISEASES OF THE EAR AND MASTOID PROCESS (H60-H95)

OGCR Chapter-Specific Coding Guidelines

> 8. Chapter 8: Diseases of the Ear and Mastoid Process (H60-H95)
> Reserved for future guideline expansion

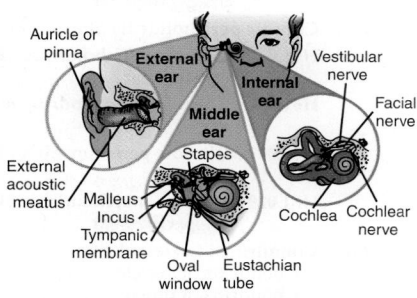

Figure 8-1 Auditory system. (From Buck CJ: Step-by-Step Medical Coding, ed 2016, St. Louis, Elsevier, 2016)

★ **(See Plate 92 on page 68.)**

CHAPTER 8

DISEASES OF THE EAR AND MASTOID PROCESS (H60-H95)

Note: Use an external cause code following the code for the ear condition, if applicable, to identify the cause of the ear condition

Excludes2 certain conditions originating in the perinatal period (P04-P96)
certain infectious and parasitic diseases (A00-B99)
complications of pregnancy, childbirth and the puerperium (O00-O9A)
congenital malformations, deformations and chromosomal abnormalities (Q00-Q99)
endocrine, nutritional and metabolic diseases (E00-E88)
injury, poisoning and certain other consequences of external causes (S00-T88)
neoplasms (C00-D49)
symptoms, signs and abnormal clinical and laboratory findings, not elsewhere classified (R00-R94)

This chapter contains the following blocks:

H60-H62	Diseases of external ear
H65-H75	Diseases of middle ear and mastoid
H80-H83	Diseases of inner ear
H90-H94	Other disorders of ear
H95	Intraoperative and postprocedural complications and disorders of ear and mastoid process, not elsewhere classified

DISEASES OF EXTERNAL EAR (H60-H62)

● **H60**   **Otitis externa**

  ● **H60.0**   **Abscess of external ear**
        Boil of external ear
        Carbuncle of auricle or external auditory canal
        Furuncle of external ear
        H60.00   Abscess of external ear, unspecified ear
        H60.01   Abscess of right external ear
        H60.02   Abscess of left external ear
        H60.03   Abscess of external ear, bilateral

● **H60.1**   **Cellulitis of external ear**
        Cellulitis of auricle
        Cellulitis of external auditory canal
        H60.10   Cellulitis of external ear, unspecified ear
        H60.11   Cellulitis of right external ear
        H60.12   Cellulitis of left external ear
        H60.13   Cellulitis of external ear, bilateral

● **H60.2**   **Malignant otitis externa**
        H60.20   Malignant otitis externa, unspecified ear
        H60.21   Malignant otitis externa, right ear
        H60.22   Malignant otitis externa, left ear
        H60.23   Malignant otitis externa, bilateral

● **H60.3**   **Other infective otitis externa**
  ● **H60.31**   **Diffuse otitis externa**
        H60.311   Diffuse otitis externa, right ear
        H60.312   Diffuse otitis externa, left ear
        H60.313   Diffuse otitis externa, bilateral
        H60.319   Diffuse otitis externa, unspecified ear
  ● **H60.32**   **Hemorrhagic otitis externa**
        H60.321   Hemorrhagic otitis externa, right ear
        H60.322   Hemorrhagic otitis externa, left ear
        H60.323   Hemorrhagic otitis externa, bilateral
        H60.329   Hemorrhagic otitis externa, unspecified ear
  ● **H60.33**   **Swimmer's ear**
        H60.331   Swimmer's ear, right ear
        H60.332   Swimmer's ear, left ear
        H60.333   Swimmer's ear, bilateral
        H60.339   Swimmer's ear, unspecified ear
  ● **H60.39**   **Other infective otitis externa**
        H60.391   Other infective otitis externa, right ear
        H60.392   Other infective otitis externa, left ear
        H60.393   Other infective otitis externa, bilateral
        H60.399   Other infective otitis externa, unspecified ear

● **H60.4**   **Cholesteatoma of external ear**
        Keratosis obturans of external ear (canal)
        Excludes2   cholesteatoma of middle ear (H71.-)
            recurrent cholesteatoma of postmastoidectomy cavity (H95.0-)
        H60.40   Cholesteatoma of external ear, unspecified ear
        H60.41   Cholesteatoma of right external ear
        H60.42   Cholesteatoma of left external ear
        H60.43   Cholesteatoma of external ear, bilateral

● **H60.5**   **Acute noninfective otitis externa**
  ● **H60.50**   **Unspecified acute noninfective otitis externa**
        Acute otitis externa NOS
        H60.501   Unspecified acute noninfective otitis externa, right ear
        H60.502   Unspecified acute noninfective otitis externa, left ear
        H60.503   Unspecified acute noninfective otitis externa, bilateral
        H60.509   Unspecified acute noninfective otitis externa, unspecified ear
  ● **H60.51**   **Acute actinic otitis externa**
        H60.511   Acute actinic otitis externa, right ear
        H60.512   Acute actinic otitis externa, left ear
        H60.513   Acute actinic otitis externa, bilateral
        H60.519   Acute actinic otitis externa, unspecified ear

● H60.52 Acute chemical otitis externa
  H60.521 Acute chemical otitis externa, right ear
  H60.522 Acute chemical otitis externa, left ear
  H60.523 Acute chemical otitis externa, bilateral
  H60.529 Acute chemical otitis externa, unspecified ear

● H60.53 Acute contact otitis externa
  H60.531 Acute contact otitis externa, right ear
  H60.532 Acute contact otitis externa, left ear
  H60.533 Acute contact otitis externa, bilateral
  H60.539 Acute contact otitis externa, unspecified ear

● H60.54 Acute eczematoid otitis externa
  H60.541 Acute eczematoid otitis externa, right ear
  H60.542 Acute eczematoid otitis externa, left ear
  H60.543 Acute eczematoid otitis externa, bilateral
  H60.549 Acute eczematoid otitis externa, unspecified ear

● H60.55 Acute reactive otitis externa
  H60.551 Acute reactive otitis externa, right ear
  H60.552 Acute reactive otitis externa, left ear
  H60.553 Acute reactive otitis externa, bilateral
  H60.559 Acute reactive otitis externa, unspecified ear

● H60.59 Other noninfective acute otitis externa
  H60.591 Other noninfective acute otitis externa, right ear
  H60.592 Other noninfective acute otitis externa, left ear
  H60.593 Other noninfective acute otitis externa, bilateral
  H60.599 Other noninfective acute otitis externa, unspecified ear

● H60.6 Unspecified chronic otitis externa
  H60.60 Unspecified chronic otitis externa, unspecified ear
  H60.61 Unspecified chronic otitis externa, right ear
  H60.62 Unspecified chronic otitis externa, left ear
  H60.63 Unspecified chronic otitis externa, bilateral

● H60.8 Other otitis externa
  ● H60.8X Other otitis externa
    H60.8X1 Other otitis externa, right ear
    H60.8X2 Other otitis externa, left ear
    H60.8X3 Other otitis externa, bilateral
    H60.8X9 Other otitis externa, unspecified ear

● H60.9 Unspecified otitis externa
  H60.90 Unspecified otitis externa, unspecified ear
  H60.91 Unspecified otitis externa, right ear
  H60.92 Unspecified otitis externa, left ear
  H60.93 Unspecified otitis externa, bilateral

● H61 Other disorders of external ear
  ● H61.0 Chondritis and perichondritis of external ear
    Chondrodermatitis nodularis chronica helicis
    Perichondritis of auricle
    Perichondritis of pinna
    ● H61.00 Unspecified perichondritis of external ear
      H61.001 Unspecified perichondritis of right external ear
      H61.002 Unspecified perichondritis of left external ear
      H61.003 Unspecified perichondritis of external ear, bilateral
      H61.009 Unspecified perichondritis of external ear, unspecified ear

● H61.01 Acute perichondritis of external ear
  H61.011 Acute perichondritis of right external ear
  H61.012 Acute perichondritis of left external ear
  H61.013 Acute perichondritis of external ear, bilateral
  H61.019 Acute perichondritis of external ear, unspecified ear

● H61.02 Chronic perichondritis of external ear
  H61.021 Chronic perichondritis of right external ear
  H61.022 Chronic perichondritis of left external ear
  H61.023 Chronic perichondritis of external ear, bilateral
  H61.029 Chronic perichondritis of external ear, unspecified ear

● H61.03 Chondritis of external ear
  Chondritis of auricle
  Chondritis of pinna
  H61.031 Chondritis of right external ear
  H61.032 Chondritis of left external ear
    Coding Clinic: 2015, Q1, P18
  H61.033 Chondritis of external ear, bilateral
  H61.039 Chondritis of external ear, unspecified ear

● H61.1 Noninfective disorders of pinna
  Excludes2 cauliflower ear (M95.1-)
                 gouty tophi of ear (M1A.-)
  ● H61.10 Unspecified noninfective disorders of pinna
    Disorder of pinna NOS
    H61.101 Unspecified noninfective disorders of pinna, right ear
    H61.102 Unspecified noninfective disorders of pinna, left ear
    H61.103 Unspecified noninfective disorders of pinna, bilateral
    H61.109 Unspecified noninfective disorders of pinna, unspecified ear

● H61.11 Acquired deformity of pinna
  Acquired deformity of auricle
  Excludes2 cauliflower ear (M95.1-)
  H61.111 Acquired deformity of pinna, right ear
  H61.112 Acquired deformity of pinna, left ear
  H61.113 Acquired deformity of pinna, bilateral
  H61.119 Acquired deformity of pinna, unspecified ear

● H61.12 Hematoma of pinna
  Hematoma of auricle
  H61.121 Hematoma of pinna, right ear
  H61.122 Hematoma of pinna, left ear
  H61.123 Hematoma of pinna, bilateral
  H61.129 Hematoma of pinna, unspecified ear

● H61.19 Other noninfective disorders of pinna
  H61.191 Noninfective disorders of pinna, right ear
  H61.192 Noninfective disorders of pinna, left ear
  H61.193 Noninfective disorders of pinna, bilateral
  H61.199 Noninfective disorders of pinna, unspecified ear

◀ New   ◀▪▪ Revised   ~~deleted~~ Deleted   Excludes 1   Excludes 2   Includes   Use additional   Code first   Code also   Unspecified
OGCR Official Guidelines   X Assign placeholder X   ● Use Additional Character(s)   ▶ Manifestation Code   Coding Clinic

- **H61.2 Impacted cerumen**
  Wax in ear
  - H61.2Ø   Impacted cerumen, unspecified ear
  - H61.21   Impacted cerumen, right ear
  - H61.22   Impacted cerumen, left ear
  - H61.23   Impacted cerumen, bilateral
- **H61.3 Acquired stenosis of external ear canal**
  Collapse of external ear canal

Excludes1	postprocedural stenosis of external ear canal (H95.81-)

  - **H61.3Ø   Acquired stenosis of external ear canal, unspecified**
    - H61.3Ø1   Acquired stenosis of right external ear canal, unspecified
    - H61.3Ø2   Acquired stenosis of left external ear canal, unspecified
    - H61.3Ø3   Acquired stenosis of external ear canal, unspecified, bilateral
    - H61.3Ø9   Acquired stenosis of external ear canal, unspecified, unspecified ear
  - **H61.31   Acquired stenosis of external ear canal secondary to trauma**
    - H61.311   Acquired stenosis of right external ear canal secondary to trauma
    - H61.312   Acquired stenosis of left external ear canal secondary to trauma
    - H61.313   Acquired stenosis of external ear canal secondary to trauma, bilateral
    - H61.319   Acquired stenosis of external ear canal secondary to trauma, unspecified ear
  - **H61.32   Acquired stenosis of external ear canal secondary to inflammation and infection**
    - H61.321   Acquired stenosis of right external ear canal secondary to inflammation and infection
    - H61.322   Acquired stenosis of left external ear canal secondary to inflammation and infection
    - H61.323   Acquired stenosis of external ear canal secondary to inflammation and infection, bilateral
    - H61.329   Acquired stenosis of external ear canal secondary to inflammation and infection, unspecified ear
  - **H61.39   Other acquired stenosis of external ear canal**
    - H61.391   Other acquired stenosis of right external ear canal
    - H61.392   Other acquired stenosis of left external ear canal
    - H61.393   Other acquired stenosis of external ear canal, bilateral
    - H61.399   Other acquired stenosis of external ear canal, unspecified ear
- **H61.8 Other specified disorders of external ear**
  - **H61.81   Exostosis of external canal**
    - H61.811   Exostosis of right external canal
    - H61.812   Exostosis of left external canal
    - H61.813   Exostosis of external canal, bilateral
    - H61.819   Exostosis of external canal, unspecified ear
  - **H61.89   Other specified disorders of external ear**
    - H61.891   Other specified disorders of right external ear
    - H61.892   Other specified disorders of left external ear
    - H61.893   Other specified disorders of external ear, bilateral
    - H61.899   Other specified disorders of external ear, unspecified ear

- **H61.9 Disorder of external ear, unspecified**
  - H61.9Ø   Disorder of external ear, unspecified, unspecified ear
  - H61.91   Disorder of right external ear, unspecified
  - H61.92   Disorder of left external ear, unspecified
  - H61.93   Disorder of external ear, unspecified, bilateral
- **H62 Disorders of external ear in diseases classified elsewhere**
  - **H62.4 Otitis externa in other diseases classified elsewhere**
    Code first underlying disease, such as:
    erysipelas (A46)
    impetigo (LØ1.Ø)

Excludes1	otitis externa (in): candidiasis (B37.84) herpes viral [herpes simplex] (BØØ.1) herpes zoster (BØ2.8)

    - *H62.4Ø   Otitis externa in other diseases classified elsewhere, unspecified ear*
    - *H62.41   Otitis externa in other diseases classified elsewhere, right ear*
    - *H62.42   Otitis externa in other diseases classified elsewhere, left ear*
    - *H62.43   Otitis externa in other diseases classified elsewhere, bilateral*
  - **H62.8 Other disorders of external ear in diseases classified elsewhere**
    Code first underlying disease, such as:
    gout (M1A.-, M1Ø.-)
    - **H62.8X   Other disorders of external ear in diseases classified elsewhere**
      - *H62.8X1   Other disorders of right external ear in diseases classified elsewhere*
      - *H62.8X2   Other disorders of left external ear in diseases classified elsewhere*
      - *H62.8X3   Other disorders of external ear in diseases classified elsewhere, bilateral*
      - *H62.8X9   Other disorders of external ear in diseases classified elsewhere, unspecified ear*

DISEASES OF MIDDLE EAR AND MASTOID (H65-H75)

★ **(See Plate 94 on page 69.)**

- **H65 Nonsuppurative otitis media**
  Bacterial or viral infection or inflammation of the middle ear; may result in fluid accumulation with pain and temporary hearing loss.

Includes	nonsuppurative otitis media with myringitis

  Use additional code for any associated perforated tympanic membrane (H72.-)
  Use additional code to identify:
  exposure to environmental tobacco smoke (Z77.22)
  exposure to tobacco smoke in the perinatal period (P96.81)
  history of tobacco dependence (Z87.891) ◀▥
  occupational exposure to environmental tobacco smoke (Z57.31)
  tobacco dependence (F17.-)
  tobacco use (Z72.Ø)
  - **H65.Ø Acute serous otitis media**
    Acute and subacute secretory otitis
    - H65.ØØ   Acute serous otitis media, unspecified ear
    - H65.Ø1   Acute serous otitis media, right ear
    - H65.Ø2   Acute serous otitis media, left ear
    - H65.Ø3   Acute serous otitis media, bilateral
    - H65.Ø4   Acute serous otitis media, recurrent, right ear
    - H65.Ø5   Acute serous otitis media, recurrent, left ear
    - H65.Ø6   Acute serous otitis media, recurrent, bilateral
    - H65.Ø7   Acute serous otitis media, recurrent, unspecified ear

● **H65.1 Other acute nonsuppurative otitis media**

   Excludes1 otitic barotrauma (T70.0)
                  otitis media (acute) NOS (H66.9)

● **H65.11 Acute and subacute allergic otitis media (mucoid) (sanguinous) (serous)**

   H65.111 Acute and subacute allergic otitis media (mucoid) (sanguinous) (serous), right ear

   H65.112 Acute and subacute allergic otitis media (mucoid) (sanguinous) (serous), left ear

   H65.113 Acute and subacute allergic otitis media (mucoid) (sanguinous) (serous), bilateral

   H65.114 Acute and subacute allergic otitis media (mucoid) (sanguinous) (serous), recurrent, right ear

   H65.115 Acute and subacute allergic otitis media (mucoid) (sanguinous) (serous), recurrent, left ear

   H65.116 Acute and subacute allergic otitis media (mucoid) (sanguinous) (serous), recurrent, bilateral

   H65.117 Acute and subacute allergic otitis media (mucoid) (sanguinous) (serous), recurrent, unspecified ear

   H65.119 Acute and subacute allergic otitis media (mucoid) (sanguinous) (serous), unspecified ear

● **H65.19 Other acute nonsuppurative otitis media**

   Acute and subacute mucoid otitis media
   Acute and subacute nonsuppurative otitis media NOS
   Acute and subacute sanguinous otitis media
   Acute and subacute seromucinous otitis media

   H65.191 Other acute nonsuppurative otitis media, right ear

   H65.192 Other acute nonsuppurative otitis media, left ear

   H65.193 Other acute nonsuppurative otitis media, bilateral

   H65.194 Other acute nonsuppurative otitis media, recurrent, right ear

   H65.195 Other acute nonsuppurative otitis media, recurrent, left ear

   H65.196 Other acute nonsuppurative otitis media, recurrent, bilateral

   H65.197 Other acute nonsuppurative otitis media recurrent, unspecified ear

   H65.199 Other acute nonsuppurative otitis media, unspecified ear

● **H65.2 Chronic serous otitis media**

   Chronic tubotympanal catarrh

   H65.20 Chronic serous otitis media, unspecified ear

   H65.21 Chronic serous otitis media, right ear

   H65.22 Chronic serous otitis media, left ear

   H65.23 Chronic serous otitis media, bilateral

● **H65.3 Chronic mucoid otitis media**

   Chronic mucinous otitis media
   Chronic secretory otitis media
   Chronic transudative otitis media
   Glue ear

   Excludes1 adhesive middle ear disease (H74.1)

   H65.30 Chronic mucoid otitis media, unspecified ear

   H65.31 Chronic mucoid otitis media, right ear

   H65.32 Chronic mucoid otitis media, left ear

   H65.33 Chronic mucoid otitis media, bilateral

● **H65.4 Other chronic nonsuppurative otitis media**

● **H65.41 Chronic allergic otitis media**

   H65.411 Chronic allergic otitis media, right ear

   H65.412 Chronic allergic otitis media, left ear

   H65.413 Chronic allergic otitis media, bilateral

   H65.419 Chronic allergic otitis media, unspecified ear

● **H65.49 Other chronic nonsuppurative otitis media**

   Chronic exudative otitis media
   Chronic nonsuppurative otitis media NOS
   Chronic otitis media with effusion (nonpurulent)
   Chronic seromucinous otitis media

   H65.491 Other chronic nonsuppurative otitis media, right ear

   H65.492 Other chronic nonsuppurative otitis media, left ear

   H65.493 Other chronic nonsuppurative otitis media, bilateral

   H65.499 Other chronic nonsuppurative otitis media, unspecified ear

● **H65.9 Unspecified nonsuppurative otitis media**

   Allergic otitis media NOS
   Catarrhal otitis media NOS
   Exudative otitis media NOS
   Mucoid otitis media NOS
   Otitis media with effusion (nonpurulent) NOS
   Secretory otitis media NOS
   Seromucinous otitis media NOS
   Serous otitis media NOS
   Transudative otitis media NOS

   H65.90 Unspecified nonsuppurative otitis media, unspecified ear

   H65.91 Unspecified nonsuppurative otitis media, right ear

   H65.92 Unspecified nonsuppurative otitis media, left ear

   H65.93 Unspecified nonsuppurative otitis media, bilateral

● **H66 Suppurative and unspecified otitis media**

   Suppurative: Discharging pus

   Includes suppurative and unspecified otitis media with myringitis

   Use additional code to identify:
   exposure to environmental tobacco smoke (Z77.22)
   exposure to tobacco smoke in the perinatal period (P96.81)
   history of tobacco dependence (Z87.891) ◄▥▥
   occupational exposure to environmental tobacco smoke (Z57.31)
   tobacco dependence (F17.-)
   tobacco use (Z72.0)

● **H66.0 Acute suppurative otitis media**

● **H66.00 Acute suppurative otitis media without spontaneous rupture of ear drum**

   H66.001 Acute suppurative otitis media without spontaneous rupture of ear drum, right ear
            Coding Clinic: 2016, Q1, P34

   H66.002 Acute suppurative otitis media without spontaneous rupture of ear drum, left ear

   H66.003 Acute suppurative otitis media without spontaneous rupture of ear drum, bilateral

   H66.004 Acute suppurative otitis media without spontaneous rupture of ear drum, recurrent, right ear

   H66.005 Acute suppurative otitis media without spontaneous rupture of ear drum, recurrent, left ear

   H66.006 Acute suppurative otitis media without spontaneous rupture of ear drum, recurrent, bilateral

◄ New   ◄▥▥ Revised   ~~deleted~~ Deleted   Excludes 1   Excludes 2   Includes   Use additional   Code first   Code also   Unspecified

OGCR Official Guidelines   X Assign placeholder X   ● Use Additional Character(s)   ▶ Manifestation Code   **Coding Clinic**

H66.007   Acute suppurative otitis media without spontaneous rupture of ear drum, recurrent, unspecified ear

H66.009   Acute suppurative otitis media without spontaneous rupture of ear drum, unspecified ear

● H66.01   Acute suppurative otitis media with spontaneous rupture of ear drum

H66.011   Acute suppurative otitis media with spontaneous rupture of ear drum, right ear

H66.012   Acute suppurative otitis media with spontaneous rupture of ear drum, left ear

H66.013   Acute suppurative otitis media with spontaneous rupture of ear drum, bilateral

H66.014   Acute suppurative otitis media with spontaneous rupture of ear drum, recurrent, right ear

H66.015   Acute suppurative otitis media with spontaneous rupture of ear drum, recurrent, left ear

H66.016   Acute suppurative otitis media with spontaneous rupture of ear drum, recurrent, bilateral

H66.017   Acute suppurative otitis media with spontaneous rupture of ear drum, recurrent, unspecified ear

H66.019   Acute suppurative otitis media with spontaneous rupture of ear drum, unspecified ear

● H66.1   Chronic tubotympanic suppurative otitis media

Benign chronic suppurative otitis media

Chronic tubotympanic disease

Use additional code for any associated perforated tympanic membrane (H72.-)

H66.10   Chronic tubotympanic suppurative otitis media, unspecified

H66.11   Chronic tubotympanic suppurative otitis media, right ear

H66.12   Chronic tubotympanic suppurative otitis media, left ear

H66.13   Chronic tubotympanic suppurative otitis media, bilateral

● H66.2   Chronic atticoantral suppurative otitis media

Chronic atticoantral disease

Use additional code for any associated perforated tympanic membrane (H72.-)

H66.20   Chronic atticoantral suppurative otitis media, unspecified ear

H66.21   Chronic atticoantral suppurative otitis media, right ear

H66.22   Chronic atticoantral suppurative otitis media, left ear

H66.23   Chronic atticoantral suppurative otitis media, bilateral

● H66.3   Other chronic suppurative otitis media

Chronic suppurative otitis media NOS

Use additional code for any associated perforated tympanic membrane (H72.-)

Excludes1   tuberculous otitis media (A18.6)

● H66.3X   Other chronic suppurative otitis media

H66.3X1   Other chronic suppurative otitis media, right ear

H66.3X2   Other chronic suppurative otitis media, left ear

H66.3X3   Other chronic suppurative otitis media, bilateral

H66.3X9   Other chronic suppurative otitis media, unspecified ear

● H66.4   Suppurative otitis media, unspecified

Purulent otitis media NOS

Use additional code for any associated perforated tympanic membrane (H72.-)

H66.40   Suppurative otitis media, unspecified, unspecified ear

H66.41   Suppurative otitis media, unspecified, right ear

H66.42   Suppurative otitis media, unspecified, left ear

H66.43   Suppurative otitis media, unspecified, bilateral

● H66.9   Otitis media, unspecified

Otitis media NOS

Acute otitis media NOS

Chronic otitis media NOS

Use additional code for any associated perforated tympanic membrane (H72.-)

H66.90   Otitis media, unspecified, unspecified ear

H66.91   Otitis media, unspecified, right ear

H66.92   Otitis media, unspecified, left ear

H66.93   Otitis media, unspecified, bilateral

● H67   Otitis media in diseases classified elsewhere

Code first underlying disease, such as:
viral disease NEC (B00-B34)

Use additional code for any associated perforated tympanic membrane (H72.-)

Excludes1   otitis media in:
influenza (J09.X9, J10.83, J11.83)
measles (B05.3)
scarlet fever (A38.0)
tuberculosis (A18.6)

▸ *H67.1   Otitis media in diseases classified elsewhere, right ear*

▸ *H67.2   Otitis media in diseases classified elsewhere, left ear*

▸ *H67.3   Otitis media in diseases classified elsewhere, bilateral*

▸ *H67.9   Otitis media in diseases classified elsewhere, unspecified ear*

● H68   Eustachian salpingitis and obstruction

● H68.0   Eustachian salpingitis

● H68.00   Unspecified Eustachian salpingitis

H68.001   Unspecified Eustachian salpingitis, right ear

H68.002   Unspecified Eustachian salpingitis, left ear

H68.003   Unspecified Eustachian salpingitis, bilateral

H68.009   Unspecified Eustachian salpingitis, unspecified ear

● H68.01   Acute Eustachian salpingitis

H68.011   Acute Eustachian salpingitis, right ear

H68.012   Acute Eustachian salpingitis, left ear

H68.013   Acute Eustachian salpingitis, bilateral

H68.019   Acute Eustachian salpingitis, unspecified ear

● H68.02   Chronic Eustachian salpingitis

H68.021   Chronic Eustachian salpingitis, right ear

H68.022   Chronic Eustachian salpingitis, left ear

H68.023   Chronic Eustachian salpingitis, bilateral

H68.029   Chronic Eustachian salpingitis, unspecified ear

CHAPTER 8 (H60-H95)

- **H68.1** **Obstruction of Eustachian tube**
  Stenosis of Eustachian tube
  Stricture of Eustachian tube
  - **H68.10** **Unspecified obstruction of Eustachian tube**
    - H68.101 Unspecified obstruction of Eustachian tube, right ear
    - H68.102 Unspecified obstruction of Eustachian tube, left ear
    - H68.103 Unspecified obstruction of Eustachian tube, bilateral
    - H68.109 Unspecified obstruction of Eustachian tube, unspecified ear
  - **H68.11** **Osseous obstruction of Eustachian tube**
    - H68.111 Osseous obstruction of Eustachian tube, right ear
    - H68.112 Osseous obstruction of Eustachian tube, left ear
    - H68.113 Osseous obstruction of Eustachian tube, bilateral
    - H68.119 Osseous obstruction of Eustachian tube, unspecified ear
  - **H68.12** **Intrinsic cartilagenous obstruction of Eustachian tube**
    - H68.121 Intrinsic cartilagenous obstruction of Eustachian tube, right ear
    - H68.122 Intrinsic cartilagenous obstruction of Eustachian tube, left ear
    - H68.123 Intrinsic cartilagenous obstruction of Eustachian tube, bilateral
    - H68.129 Intrinsic cartilagenous obstruction of Eustachian tube, unspecified ear
  - **H68.13** **Extrinsic cartilagenous obstruction of Eustachian tube**
    Compression of Eustachian tube
    - H68.131 Extrinsic cartilagenous obstruction of Eustachian tube, right ear
    - H68.132 Extrinsic cartilagenous obstruction of Eustachian tube, left ear
    - H68.133 Extrinsic cartilagenous obstruction of Eustachian tube, bilateral
    - H68.139 Extrinsic cartilagenous obstruction of Eustachian tube, unspecified ear
- **H69** **Other and unspecified disorders of Eustachian tube**
  - **H69.0** **Patulous Eustachian tube**
    - H69.00 Patulous Eustachian tube, unspecified ear
    - H69.01 Patulous Eustachian tube, right ear
    - H69.02 Patulous Eustachian tube, left ear
    - H69.03 Patulous Eustachian tube, bilateral
  - **H69.8** **Other specified disorders of Eustachian tube**
    - H69.80 Other specified disorders of Eustachian tube, unspecified ear
    - H69.81 Other specified disorders of Eustachian tube, right ear
    - H69.82 Other specified disorders of Eustachian tube, left ear
    - H69.83 Other specified disorders of Eustachian tube, bilateral
  - **H69.9** **Unspecified Eustachian tube disorder**
    - H69.90 Unspecified Eustachian tube disorder, unspecified ear
    - H69.91 Unspecified Eustachian tube disorder, right ear
    - H69.92 Unspecified Eustachian tube disorder, left ear
    - H69.93 Unspecified Eustachian tube disorder, bilateral

- **H70** **Mastoiditis and related conditions**
  - **H70.0** **Acute mastoiditis**
    Abscess of mastoid
    Empyema of mastoid
    - **H70.00** **Acute mastoiditis without complications**
      - H70.001 Acute mastoiditis without complications, right ear
      - H70.002 Acute mastoiditis without complications, left ear
      - H70.003 Acute mastoiditis without complications, bilateral
      - H70.009 Acute mastoiditis without complications, unspecified ear
    - **H70.01** **Subperiosteal abscess of mastoid**
      - H70.011 Subperiosteal abscess of mastoid, right ear
      - H70.012 Subperiosteal abscess of mastoid, left ear
      - H70.013 Subperiosteal abscess of mastoid, bilateral
      - H70.019 Subperiosteal abscess of mastoid, unspecified ear
    - **H70.09** **Acute mastoiditis with other complications**
      - H70.091 Acute mastoiditis with other complications, right ear
      - H70.092 Acute mastoiditis with other complications, left ear
      - H70.093 Acute mastoiditis with other complications, bilateral
      - H70.099 Acute mastoiditis with other complications, unspecified ear
  - **H70.1** **Chronic mastoiditis**
    Caries of mastoid
    Fistula of mastoid
    Excludes1   tuberculous mastoiditis (A18.03)
    - H70.10 Chronic mastoiditis, unspecified ear
    - H70.11 Chronic mastoiditis, right ear
    - H70.12 Chronic mastoiditis, left ear
    - H70.13 Chronic mastoiditis, bilateral
  - **H70.2** **Petrositis**
    Inflammation of petrous bone
    - **H70.20** **Unspecified petrositis**
      - H70.201 Unspecified petrositis, right ear
      - H70.202 Unspecified petrositis, left ear
      - H70.203 Unspecified petrositis, bilateral
      - H70.209 Unspecified petrositis, unspecified ear
    - **H70.21** **Acute petrositis**
      - H70.211 Acute petrositis, right ear
      - H70.212 Acute petrositis, left ear
      - H70.213 Acute petrositis, bilateral
      - H70.219 Acute petrositis, unspecified ear
    - **H70.22** **Chronic petrositis**
      - H70.221 Chronic petrositis, right ear
      - H70.222 Chronic petrositis, left ear
      - H70.223 Chronic petrositis, bilateral
      - H70.229 Chronic petrositis, unspecified ear

◀ New   ◀▪▪▪ Revised   deleted Deleted   Excludes 1   Excludes 2   Includes   Use additional   Code first   Code also   Unspecified

OGCR Official Guidelines   X Assign placeholder X   ● Use Additional Character(s)   ▶ Manifestation Code   **Coding Clinic**

842

Item 8–1   **Mastoiditis** is an infection of the portion of the temporal bone of the skull that is behind the ear (mastoid process) caused by an untreated otitis media, leading to an infection of the surrounding structures which may include the brain.

● **H70.8**   **Other mastoiditis and related conditions**
    Excludes1   preauricular sinus and cyst (Q18.1)
                  sinus, fistula, and cyst of branchial cleft (Q18.0)
   ● **H70.81**   Postauricular fistula
       H70.811   Postauricular fistula, right ear
       H70.812   Postauricular fistula, left ear
       H70.813   Postauricular fistula, bilateral
       H70.819   Postauricular fistula, unspecified ear
   ● **H70.89**   Other mastoiditis and related conditions
       H70.891   Other mastoiditis and related conditions, right ear
       H70.892   Other mastoiditis and related conditions, left ear
       H70.893   Other mastoiditis and related conditions, bilateral
       H70.899   Other mastoiditis and related conditions, unspecified ear

● **H70.9**   **Unspecified mastoiditis**
     H70.90   Unspecified mastoiditis, unspecified ear
     H70.91   Unspecified mastoiditis, right ear
     H70.92   Unspecified mastoiditis, left ear
     H70.93   Unspecified mastoiditis, bilateral

● **H71**   **Cholesteatoma of middle ear**
    Excludes2   cholesteatoma of external ear (H60.4-)
                  recurrent cholesteatoma of postmastoidectomy cavity (H95.0-)
   ● **H71.0**   Cholesteatoma of attic
       H71.00   Cholesteatoma of attic, unspecified ear
       H71.01   Cholesteatoma of attic, right ear
       H71.02   Cholesteatoma of attic, left ear
       H71.03   Cholesteatoma of attic, bilateral
   ● **H71.1**   Cholesteatoma of tympanum
       H71.10   Cholesteatoma of tympanum, unspecified ear
       H71.11   Cholesteatoma of tympanum, right ear
       H71.12   Cholesteatoma of tympanum, left ear
       H71.13   Cholesteatoma of tympanum, bilateral
   ● **H71.2**   Cholesteatoma of mastoid
       H71.20   Cholesteatoma of mastoid, unspecified ear
       H71.21   Cholesteatoma of mastoid, right ear
       H71.22   Cholesteatoma of mastoid, left ear
       H71.23   Cholesteatoma of mastoid, bilateral
   ● **H71.3**   Diffuse cholesteatosis
       H71.30   Diffuse cholesteatosis, unspecified ear
       H71.31   Diffuse cholesteatosis, right ear
       H71.32   Diffuse cholesteatosis, left ear
       H71.33   Diffuse cholesteatosis, bilateral
   ● **H71.9**   Unspecified cholesteatoma
       H71.90   Unspecified cholesteatoma, unspecified ear
       H71.91   Unspecified cholesteatoma, right ear
       H71.92   Unspecified cholesteatoma, left ear
       H71.93   Unspecified cholesteatoma, bilateral

★**(See Plate 93 on page 69.)**

● **H72**   **Perforation of tympanic membrane**
     Hole or rupture in ear drum
    Includes   persistent post-traumatic perforation of ear drum
              postinflammatory perforation of ear drum
    Code first any associated otitis media (H65.-, H66.1-, H66.2-, H66.3-, H66.4-, H66.9-, H67.-)
    Excludes1   acute suppurative otitis media with rupture of the tympanic membrane (H66.01-)
                  traumatic rupture of ear drum (S09.2-)
   ● **H72.0**   Central perforation of tympanic membrane
       H72.00   Central perforation of tympanic membrane, unspecified ear
       H72.01   Central perforation of tympanic membrane, right ear
       H72.02   Central perforation of tympanic membrane, left ear
       H72.03   Central perforation of tympanic membrane, bilateral
   ● **H72.1**   Attic perforation of tympanic membrane
       Perforation of pars flaccida
       H72.10   Attic perforation of tympanic membrane, unspecified ear
       H72.11   Attic perforation of tympanic membrane, right ear
       H72.12   Attic perforation of tympanic membrane, left ear
       H72.13   Attic perforation of tympanic membrane, bilateral
   ● **H72.2**   Other marginal perforations of tympanic membrane
    ● **H72.2X**   Other marginal perforations of tympanic membrane
       H72.2X1   Other marginal perforations of tympanic membrane, right ear
       H72.2X2   Other marginal perforations of tympanic membrane, left ear
       H72.2X3   Other marginal perforations of tympanic membrane, bilateral
       H72.2X9   Other marginal perforations of tympanic membrane, unspecified ear
   ● **H72.8**   Other perforations of tympanic membrane
    ● **H72.81**   Multiple perforations of tympanic membrane
       H72.811   Multiple perforations of tympanic membrane, right ear
       H72.812   Multiple perforations of tympanic membrane, left ear
       H72.813   Multiple perforations of tympanic membrane, bilateral
       H72.819   Multiple perforations of tympanic membrane, unspecified ear
    ● **H72.82**   Total perforations of tympanic membrane
       H72.821   Total perforations of tympanic membrane, right ear
       H72.822   Total perforations of tympanic membrane, left ear
       H72.823   Total perforations of tympanic membrane, bilateral
       H72.829   Total perforations of tympanic membrane, unspecified ear
   ● **H72.9**   Unspecified perforation of tympanic membrane
       H72.90   Unspecified perforation of tympanic membrane, unspecified ear
       H72.91   Unspecified perforation of tympanic membrane, right ear
       H72.92   Unspecified perforation of tympanic membrane, left ear
       H72.93   Unspecified perforation of tympanic membrane, bilateral

CHAPTER 8 (H60-H95)

● **H73   Other disorders of tympanic membrane**
   ● **H73.0   Acute myringitis**
      Excludes1   acute myringitis with otitis media (H65, H66)
     ● **H73.00   Unspecified acute myringitis**
        Acute tympanitis NOS
        H73.001   Acute myringitis, right ear
        H73.002   Acute myringitis, left ear
        H73.003   Acute myringitis, bilateral
        H73.009   Acute myringitis, unspecified ear
     ● **H73.01   Bullous myringitis**
        H73.011   Bullous myringitis, right ear
        H73.012   Bullous myringitis, left ear
        H73.013   Bullous myringitis, bilateral
        H73.019   Bullous myringitis, unspecified ear
     ● **H73.09   Other acute myringitis**
        H73.091   Other acute myringitis, right ear
        H73.092   Other acute myringitis, left ear
        H73.093   Other acute myringitis, bilateral
        H73.099   Other acute myringitis, unspecified ear
   ● **H73.1   Chronic myringitis**
      Chronic tympanitis
      Excludes1   chronic myringitis with otitis media (H65, H66)
     H73.10   Chronic myringitis, unspecified ear
     H73.11   Chronic myringitis, right ear
     H73.12   Chronic myringitis, left ear
     H73.13   Chronic myringitis, bilateral
   ● **H73.2   Unspecified myringitis**
     H73.20   Unspecified myringitis, unspecified ear
     H73.21   Unspecified myringitis, right ear
     H73.22   Unspecified myringitis, left ear
     H73.23   Unspecified myringitis, bilateral
   ● **H73.8   Other specified disorders of tympanic membrane**
     ● **H73.81   Atrophic flaccid tympanic membrane**
        H73.811   Atrophic flaccid tympanic membrane, right ear
        H73.812   Atrophic flaccid tympanic membrane, left ear
        H73.813   Atrophic flaccid tympanic membrane, bilateral
        H73.819   Atrophic flaccid tympanic membrane, unspecified ear
     ● **H73.82   Atrophic nonflaccid tympanic membrane**
        H73.821   Atrophic nonflaccid tympanic membrane, right ear
        H73.822   Atrophic nonflaccid tympanic membrane, left ear
        H73.823   Atrophic nonflaccid tympanic membrane, bilateral
        H73.829   Atrophic nonflaccid tympanic membrane, unspecified ear
     ● **H73.89   Other specified disorders of tympanic membrane**
        H73.891   Other specified disorders of tympanic membrane, right ear
        H73.892   Other specified disorders of tympanic membrane, left ear
        H73.893   Other specified disorders of tympanic membrane, bilateral
        H73.899   Other specified disorders of tympanic membrane, unspecified ear

   ● **H73.9   Unspecified disorder of tympanic membrane**
     H73.90   Unspecified disorder of tympanic membrane, unspecified ear
     H73.91   Unspecified disorder of tympanic membrane, right ear
     H73.92   Unspecified disorder of tympanic membrane, left ear
     H73.93   Unspecified disorder of tympanic membrane, bilateral
● **H74   Other disorders of middle ear mastoid**
      Excludes2   mastoiditis (H70.-)
   ● **H74.0   Tympanosclerosis**
     H74.01   Tympanosclerosis, right ear
     H74.02   Tympanosclerosis, left ear
     H74.03   Tympanosclerosis, bilateral
     H74.09   Tympanosclerosis, unspecified ear
   ● **H74.1   Adhesive middle ear disease**
      Adhesive otitis
      Excludes1   glue ear (H65.3-)
     H74.11   Adhesive right middle ear disease
     H74.12   Adhesive left middle ear disease
     H74.13   Adhesive middle ear disease, bilateral
     H74.19   Adhesive middle ear disease, unspecified ear
   ● **H74.2   Discontinuity and dislocation of ear ossicles**
     H74.20   Discontinuity and dislocation of ear ossicles, unspecified ear
     H74.21   Discontinuity and dislocation of right ear ossicles
     H74.22   Discontinuity and dislocation of left ear ossicles
     H74.23   Discontinuity and dislocation of ear ossicles, bilateral
   ● **H74.3   Other acquired abnormalities of ear ossicles**
     ● **H74.31   Ankylosis of ear ossicles**
        H74.311   Ankylosis of ear ossicles, right ear
        H74.312   Ankylosis of ear ossicles, left ear
        H74.313   Ankylosis of ear ossicles, bilateral
        H74.319   Ankylosis of ear ossicles, unspecified ear
     ● **H74.32   Partial loss of ear ossicles**
        H74.321   Partial loss of ear ossicles, right ear
        H74.322   Partial loss of ear ossicles, left ear
        H74.323   Partial loss of ear ossicles, bilateral
        H74.329   Partial loss of ear ossicles, unspecified ear
     ● **H74.39   Other acquired abnormalities of ear ossicles**
        H74.391   Other acquired abnormalities of right ear ossicles
        H74.392   Other acquired abnormalities of left ear ossicles
        H74.393   Other acquired abnormalities of ear ossicles, bilateral
        H74.399   Other acquired abnormalities of ear ossicles, unspecified ear
   ● **H74.4   Polyp of middle ear**
     H74.40   Polyp of middle ear, unspecified ear
     H74.41   Polyp of right middle ear
     H74.42   Polyp of left middle ear
     H74.43   Polyp of middle ear, bilateral

◀ New   ◀◀◀ Revised   deleted Deleted   Excludes 1   Excludes 2   Includes   Use additional   Code first   Code also   Unspecified

844   OGCR Official Guidelines   X Assign placeholder X   ● Use Additional Character(s)   ▶ Manifestation Code   **Coding Clinic**

● **H74.8** Other specified disorders of middle ear and mastoid

  ● **H74.8X** Other specified disorders of middle ear and mastoid

     H74.8X1 Other specified disorders of right middle ear and mastoid

     H74.8X2 Other specified disorders of left middle ear and mastoid

     H74.8X3 Other specified disorders of middle ear and mastoid, bilateral

     H74.8X9 Other specified disorders of middle ear and mastoid, unspecified ear

  ● **H74.9** Unspecified disorder of middle ear and mastoid

     H74.90 Unspecified disorder of middle ear and mastoid, unspecified ear

     H74.91 Unspecified disorder of right middle ear and mastoid

     H74.92 Unspecified disorder of left middle ear and mastoid

     H74.93 Unspecified disorder of middle ear and mastoid, bilateral

● **H75** Other disorders of middle ear and mastoid in diseases classified elsewhere

     Code first underlying disease

  ● **H75.0** Mastoiditis in infectious and parasitic diseases classified elsewhere

     Excludes1   mastoiditis (in):
                syphilis (A52.77)
                tuberculosis (A18.03)

     ▹ *H75.00   Mastoiditis in infectious and parasitic diseases classified elsewhere, unspecified ear*

     ▹ *H75.01   Mastoiditis in infectious and parasitic diseases classified elsewhere, right ear*

     ▹ *H75.02   Mastoiditis in infectious and parasitic diseases classified elsewhere, left ear*

     ▹ *H75.03   Mastoiditis in infectious and parasitic diseases classified elsewhere, bilateral*

  ● **H75.8** Other specified disorders of middle ear and mastoid in diseases classified elsewhere

     ▹ *H75.80   Other specified disorders of middle ear and mastoid in diseases classified elsewhere, unspecified ear*

     ▹ *H75.81   Other specified disorders of right middle ear and mastoid in diseases classified elsewhere*

     ▹ *H75.82   Other specified disorders of left middle ear and mastoid in diseases classified elsewhere*

     ▹ *H75.83   Other specified disorders of middle ear and mastoid in diseases classified elsewhere, bilateral*

DISEASES OF INNER EAR (H80-H83)

★ **(See Plate 95 on page 69.)**

● **H80** Otosclerosis

     Inherited middle ear spongelike bone growth causing hearing loss

     Includes   Otospongiosis

  ● **H80.0** Otosclerosis involving oval window, nonobliterative

     H80.00 Otosclerosis involving oval window, nonobliterative, unspecified ear

     H80.01 Otosclerosis involving oval window, nonobliterative, right ear

     H80.02 Otosclerosis involving oval window, nonobliterative, left ear

     H80.03 Otosclerosis involving oval window, nonobliterative, bilateral

  ● **H80.1** Otosclerosis involving oval window, obliterative

     H80.10 Otosclerosis involving oval window, obliterative, unspecified ear

     H80.11 Otosclerosis involving oval window, obliterative, right ear

     H80.12 Otosclerosis involving oval window, obliterative, left ear

     H80.13 Otosclerosis involving oval window, obliterative, bilateral

  ● **H80.2** Cochlear otosclerosis

     Otosclerosis involving otic capsule
     Otosclerosis involving round window

     H80.20 Cochlear otosclerosis, unspecified ear

     H80.21 Cochlear otosclerosis, right ear

     H80.22 Cochlear otosclerosis, left ear

     H80.23 Cochlear otosclerosis, bilateral

  ● **H80.8** Other otosclerosis

     H80.80 Other otosclerosis, unspecified ear

     H80.81 Other otosclerosis, right ear

     H80.82 Other otosclerosis, left ear

     H80.83 Other otosclerosis, bilateral

  ● **H80.9** Unspecified otosclerosis

     H80.90 Unspecified otosclerosis, unspecified ear

     H80.91 Unspecified otosclerosis, right ear

     H80.92 Unspecified otosclerosis, left ear

     H80.93 Unspecified otosclerosis, bilateral

● **H81** Disorders of vestibular function

     Excludes1   epidemic vertigo (A88.1)
                vertigo NOS (R42)

  ● **H81.0** Ménière's disease

     Vestibular disorder that produces recurring symptoms including severe and intermittent hearing loss including the feeling of ear pressure or pain

     Labyrinthine hydrops
     Ménière's syndrome or vertigo

     H81.01 Ménière's disease, right ear

     H81.02 Ménière's disease, left ear

     H81.03 Ménière's disease, bilateral

     H81.09 Ménière's disease, unspecified ear

  ● **H81.1** Benign paroxysmal vertigo

     H81.10 Benign paroxysmal vertigo, unspecified ear

     H81.11 Benign paroxysmal vertigo, right ear

     H81.12 Benign paroxysmal vertigo, left ear

     H81.13 Benign paroxysmal vertigo, bilateral

  ● **H81.2** Vestibular neuronitis

     H81.20 Vestibular neuronitis, unspecified ear

     H81.21 Vestibular neuronitis, right ear

     H81.22 Vestibular neuronitis, left ear

     H81.23 Vestibular neuronitis, bilateral

  ● **H81.3** Other peripheral vertigo

    ● **H81.31** Aural vertigo

       H81.311 Aural vertigo, right ear

       H81.312 Aural vertigo, left ear

       H81.313 Aural vertigo, bilateral

       H81.319 Aural vertigo, unspecified ear

    ● **H81.39** Other peripheral vertigo

       Lermoyez' syndrome
       Otogenic vertigo
       Peripheral vertigo NOS

       H81.391 Other peripheral vertigo, right ear

       H81.392 Other peripheral vertigo, left ear

       H81.393 Other peripheral vertigo, bilateral

       H81.399 Other peripheral vertigo, unspecified ear

CHAPTER 8 (H60-H95)

- H81.4   **Vertigo of central origin**
  Central positional nystagmus
  - H81.41   **Vertigo of central origin, right ear**
  - H81.42   **Vertigo of central origin, left ear**
  - H81.43   **Vertigo of central origin, bilateral**
  - H81.49   **Vertigo of central origin, unspecified ear**
- H81.8   **Other disorders of vestibular function**
  - H81.8X   **Other disorders of vestibular function**
    - H81.8X1   **Other disorders of vestibular function, right ear**
    - H81.8X2   **Other disorders of vestibular function, left ear**
    - H81.8X3   **Other disorders of vestibular function, bilateral**
    - H81.8X9   **Other disorders of vestibular function, unspecified ear**
- H81.9   **Unspecified disorder of vestibular function**
  Vertiginous syndrome NOS
  - H81.90   **Unspecified disorder of vestibular function, unspecified ear**
  - H81.91   **Unspecified disorder of vestibular function, right ear**
  - H81.92   **Unspecified disorder of vestibular function, left ear**
  - H81.93   **Unspecified disorder of vestibular function, bilateral**
- H82   **Vertiginous syndromes in diseases classified elsewhere**
  Code first underlying disease
  Excludes1   epidemic vertigo (A88.1)
  - H82.1   *Vertiginous syndromes in diseases classified elsewhere, right ear*
  - H82.2   *Vertiginous syndromes in diseases classified elsewhere, left ear*
  - H82.3   *Vertiginous syndromes in diseases classified elsewhere, bilateral*
  - H82.9   *Vertiginous syndromes in diseases classified elsewhere, unspecified ear*
- H83   **Other diseases of inner ear**
  - H83.0   **Labyrinthitis**
    Balance disorder that follows URI or head injury
    - H83.01   **Labyrinthitis, right ear**
    - H83.02   **Labyrinthitis, left ear**
    - H83.03   **Labyrinthitis, bilateral**
    - H83.09   **Labyrinthitis, unspecified ear**
  - H83.1   **Labyrinthine fistula**
    - H83.11   **Labyrinthine fistula, right ear**
    - H83.12   **Labyrinthine fistula, left ear**
    - H83.13   **Labyrinthine fistula, bilateral**
    - H83.19   **Labyrinthine fistula, unspecified ear**
  - H83.2   **Labyrinthine dysfunction**
    Labyrinthine hypersensitivity
    Labyrinthine hypofunction
    Labyrinthine loss of function
    - H83.2X   **Labyrinthine dysfunction**
      - H83.2X1   **Labyrinthine dysfunction, right ear**
      - H83.2X2   **Labyrinthine dysfunction, left ear**
      - H83.2X3   **Labyrinthine dysfunction, bilateral**
      - H83.2X9   **Labyrinthine dysfunction, unspecified ear**

- H83.3   **Noise effects on inner ear**
  Acoustic trauma of inner ear
  Noise-induced hearing loss of inner ear
  - H83.3X   **Noise effects on inner ear**
    - H83.3X1   **Noise effects on right inner ear**
    - H83.3X2   **Noise effects on left inner ear**
    - H83.3X3   **Noise effects on inner ear, bilateral**
    - H83.3X9   **Noise effects on inner ear, unspecified ear**
- H83.8   **Other specified diseases of inner ear**
  - H83.8X   **Other specified diseases of inner ear**
    - H83.8X1   **Other specified diseases of right inner ear**
    - H83.8X2   **Other specified diseases of left inner ear**
    - H83.8X3   **Other specified diseases of inner ear, bilateral**
    - H83.8X9   **Other specified diseases of inner ear, unspecified ear**
- H83.9   **Unspecified disease of inner ear**
  - H83.90   **Unspecified disease of inner ear, unspecified ear**
  - H83.91   **Unspecified disease of right inner ear**
  - H83.92   **Unspecified disease of left inner ear**
  - H83.93   **Unspecified disease of inner ear, bilateral**

OTHER DISORDERS OF EAR (H90-H94)

- H90   **Conductive and sensorineural hearing loss**
  Excludes1   deaf nonspeaking NEC (H91.3)
  deafness NOS (H91.9-)
  hearing loss NOS (H91.9-)
  noise-induced hearing loss (H83.3-)
  ototoxic hearing loss (H91.0-)
  sudden (idiopathic) hearing loss (H91.2-)
  - H90.0   **Conductive hearing loss, bilateral**
  - H90.1   **Conductive hearing loss, unilateral with unrestricted hearing on the contralateral side**
    - H90.11   **Conductive hearing loss, unilateral, right ear, with unrestricted hearing on the contralateral side**
    - H90.12   **Conductive hearing loss, unilateral, left ear, with unrestricted hearing on the contralateral side**
  - H90.2   **Conductive hearing loss, unspecified**
    Conductive deafness NOS
  - H90.3   **Sensorineural hearing loss, bilateral**
  - H90.4   **Sensorineural hearing loss, unilateral with unrestricted hearing on the contralateral side**
    - H90.41   **Sensorineural hearing loss, unilateral, right ear, with unrestricted hearing on the contralateral side**
    - H90.42   **Sensorineural hearing loss, unilateral, left ear, with unrestricted hearing on the contralateral side**
  - H90.5   **Unspecified sensorineural hearing loss**
    Central hearing loss NOS
    Congenital deafness NOS
    Neural hearing loss NOS
    Perceptive hearing loss NOS
    Sensorineural deafness NOS
    Sensory hearing loss NOS
    Excludes1   abnormal auditory perception (H93.2-)
    psychogenic deafness (F44.6)
  - H90.6   **Mixed conductive and sensorineural hearing loss, bilateral**
    Coding Clinic: 2015, Q2, P7

◀ New   ◀▥ Revised   ~~deleted~~ Deleted   Excludes 1   Excludes 2   Includes   Use additional   Code first   Code also   Unspecified
OGCR Official Guidelines   X Assign placeholder X   ● Use Additional Character(s)   ▶ Manifestation Code   **Coding Clinic**

● H90.7 Mixed conductive and sensorineural hearing loss, unilateral with unrestricted hearing on the contralateral side
  H90.71 Mixed conductive and sensorineural hearing loss, unilateral, right ear, with unrestricted hearing on the contralateral side
  H90.72 Mixed conductive and sensorineural hearing loss, unilateral, left ear, with unrestricted hearing on the contralateral side
H90.8 Mixed conductive and sensorineural hearing loss, unspecified
● H90.A Conductive and sensorineural hearing loss with restricted hearing on the contralateral side ◄
  ● H90.A1 Conductive hearing loss, unilateral, with restricted hearing on the contralateral side ◄
    H90.A11 Conductive hearing loss, unilateral, right ear with restricted hearing on the contralateral side ◄
    H90.A12 Conductive hearing loss, unilateral, left ear with restricted hearing on the contralateral side ◄
  ● H90.A2 Sensorineural hearing loss, unilateral, with restricted hearing on the contralateral side ◄
    H90.A21 Sensorineural hearing loss, unilateral, right ear, with restricted hearing on the contralateral side ◄
    H90.A22 Sensorineural hearing loss, unilateral, left ear, with restricted hearing on the contralateral side ◄
  ● H90.A3 Mixed conductive and sensorineural hearing loss, unilateral with restricted hearing on the contralateral side ◄
    H90.A31 Mixed conductive and sensorineural hearing loss, unilateral, right ear with restricted hearing on the contralateral side ◄
    H90.A32 Mixed conductive and sensorineural hearing loss, unilateral, left ear with restricted hearing on the contralateral side ◄

● H91 Other and unspecified hearing loss
  Excludes1 abnormal auditory perception (H93.2-)
    hearing loss as classified in H90.-
    impacted cerumen (H61.2-)
    noise-induced hearing loss (H83.3-)
    psychogenic deafness (F44.6)
    transient ischemic deafness (H93.01-)
  ● H91.0 Ototoxic hearing loss
    Code first poisoning due to drug or toxin, if applicable (T36-T65 with fifth or sixth character 1-4 or 6)
    Use additional code for adverse effect, if applicable, to identify drug (T36-T50 with fifth or sixth character 5)
    H91.01 Ototoxic hearing loss, right ear
    H91.02 Ototoxic hearing loss, left ear
    H91.03 Ototoxic hearing loss, bilateral
    H91.09 Ototoxic hearing loss, unspecified ear
  ● H91.1 Presbycusis
    Presbyacusia
    H91.10 Presbycusis, unspecified ear
    H91.11 Presbycusis, right ear
    H91.12 Presbycusis, left ear
    H91.13 Presbycusis, bilateral

● H91.2 Sudden idiopathic hearing loss
    Sudden hearing loss NOS
    H91.20 Sudden idiopathic hearing loss, unspecified ear
    H91.21 Sudden idiopathic hearing loss, right ear
    H91.22 Sudden idiopathic hearing loss, left ear
    H91.23 Sudden idiopathic hearing loss, bilateral
  H91.3 Deaf nonspeaking, not elsewhere classified
● H91.8 Other specified hearing loss
  ● H91.8X Other specified hearing loss
    H91.8X1 Other specified hearing loss, right ear
    H91.8X2 Other specified hearing loss, left ear
    H91.8X3 Other specified hearing loss, bilateral
    H91.8X9 Other specified hearing loss, unspecified ear
● H91.9 Unspecified hearing loss
    Deafness NOS
    High frequency deafness
    Low frequency deafness
    H91.90 Unspecified hearing loss, unspecified ear
    H91.91 Unspecified hearing loss, right ear
    H91.92 Unspecified hearing loss, left ear
    H91.93 Unspecified hearing loss, bilateral

● H92 Otalgia and effusion of ear
  ● H92.0 Otalgia
    H92.01 Otalgia, right ear
    H92.02 Otalgia, left ear
    H92.03 Otalgia, bilateral
    H92.09 Otalgia, unspecified ear
  ● H92.1 Otorrhea
    Excludes1 leakage of cerebrospinal fluid through ear (G96.0)
    H92.10 Otorrhea, unspecified ear
    H92.11 Otorrhea, right ear
    H92.12 Otorrhea, left ear
    H92.13 Otorrhea, bilateral
  ● H92.2 Otorrhagia
    Excludes1 traumatic otorrhagia - code to injury
    H92.20 Otorrhagia, unspecified ear
    H92.21 Otorrhagia, right ear
    H92.22 Otorrhagia, left ear
    H92.23 Otorrhagia, bilateral

● H93 Other disorders of ear, not elsewhere classified
  ● H93.0 Degenerative and vascular disorders of ear
    Excludes1 presbycusis (H91.1)
    ● H93.01 Transient ischemic deafness
      H93.011 Transient ischemic deafness, right ear
      H93.012 Transient ischemic deafness, left ear
      H93.013 Transient ischemic deafness, bilateral
      H93.019 Transient ischemic deafness, unspecified ear
    ● H93.09 Unspecified degenerative and vascular disorders of ear
      H93.091 Unspecified degenerative and vascular disorders of right ear
      H93.092 Unspecified degenerative and vascular disorders of left ear
      H93.093 Unspecified degenerative and vascular disorders of ear, bilateral
      H93.099 Unspecified degenerative and vascular disorders of unspecified ear

CHAPTER 8 (H60-H95)

● **H93.1**   **Tinnitus**
> *Perception of sound (ringing, buzzing, humming, whistling tunes, or singing)*

    H93.11   **Tinnitus, right ear**

    H93.12   **Tinnitus, left ear**

    H93.13   **Tinnitus, bilateral**

    H93.19   **Tinnitus, unspecified ear**

● **H93.A**   **Pulsatile tinnitus** ◀

    H93.A1   **Pulsatile tinnitus, right ear** ◀

    H93.A2   **Pulsatile tinnitus, left ear** ◀

    H93.A3   **Pulsatile tinnitus, bilateral** ◀

    H93.A9   **Pulsatile tinnitus, unspecified ear** ◀

● **H93.2**   **Other abnormal auditory perceptions**

    Excludes2   auditory hallucinations (R44.0)

   ● H93.21   **Auditory recruitment**

     H93.211   **Auditory recruitment, right ear**

     H93.212   **Auditory recruitment, left ear**

     H93.213   **Auditory recruitment, bilateral**

     H93.219   **Auditory recruitment, unspecified ear**

   ● H93.22   **Diplacusis**

     H93.221   **Diplacusis, right ear**

     H93.222   **Diplacusis, left ear**

     H93.223   **Diplacusis, bilateral**

     H93.229   **Diplacusis, unspecified ear**

   ● H93.23   **Hyperacusis**

     H93.231   **Hyperacusis, right ear**

     H93.232   **Hyperacusis, left ear**

     H93.233   **Hyperacusis, bilateral**

     H93.239   **Hyperacusis, unspecified ear**

   ● H93.24   **Temporary auditory threshold shift**

     H93.241   **Temporary auditory threshold shift, right ear**

     H93.242   **Temporary auditory threshold shift, left ear**

     H93.243   **Temporary auditory threshold shift, bilateral**

     H93.249   **Temporary auditory threshold shift, unspecified ear**

    H93.25   **Central auditory processing disorder**
> Congenital auditory imperception
> Word deafness

     Excludes1   mixed receptive-expressive language disorder (F80.2)

   ● H93.29   **Other abnormal auditory perceptions**

     H93.291   **Other abnormal auditory perceptions, right ear**

     H93.292   **Other abnormal auditory perceptions, left ear**

     H93.293   **Other abnormal auditory perceptions, bilateral**

     H93.299   **Other abnormal auditory perceptions, unspecified ear**

● **H93.3**   **Disorders of acoustic nerve**
> Disorder of 8th cranial nerve

    Excludes1   acoustic neuroma (D33.3)
> syphilitic acoustic neuritis (A52.15)

   ● H93.3X   **Disorders of acoustic nerve**

     H93.3X1   **Disorders of right acoustic nerve**

     H93.3X2   **Disorders of left acoustic nerve**

     H93.3X3   **Disorders of bilateral acoustic nerves**

     H93.3X9   **Disorders of unspecified acoustic nerve**

● **H93.8**   **Other specified disorders of ear**

   ● H93.8X   **Other specified disorders of ear**

     H93.8X1   **Other specified disorders of right ear**

     H93.8X2   **Other specified disorders of left ear**

     H93.8X3   **Other specified disorders of ear, bilateral**

     H93.8X9   **Other specified disorders of ear, unspecified ear**

● **H93.9**   **Unspecified disorder of ear**

    H93.90   **Unspecified disorder of ear, unspecified ear**

    H93.91   **Unspecified disorder of right ear**

    H93.92   **Unspecified disorder of left ear**

    H93.93   **Unspecified disorder of ear, bilateral**

● **H94**   **Other disorders of ear in diseases classified elsewhere**

   ● H94.0   **Acoustic neuritis in infectious and parasitic diseases classified elsewhere**
> *Code first* underlying disease, such as:
> parasitic disease (B65-B89)

    Excludes1   acoustic neuritis (in):
> herpes zoster (B02.29)
> syphilis (A52.15)

    ▌*H94.00*   *Acoustic neuritis in infectious and parasitic diseases classified elsewhere, unspecified ear*

    ▌*H94.01*   *Acoustic neuritis in infectious and parasitic diseases classified elsewhere, right ear*

    ▌*H94.02*   *Acoustic neuritis in infectious and parasitic diseases classified elsewhere, left ear*

    ▌*H94.03*   *Acoustic neuritis in infectious and parasitic diseases classified elsewhere, bilateral*

   ● H94.8   **Other specified disorders of ear in diseases classified elsewhere**
> *Code first* underlying disease, such as:
> congenital syphilis (A50.0)

    Excludes1   aural myiasis (B87.4)
> syphilitic labyrinthitis (A52.79)

    ▌*H94.80*   *Other specified disorders of ear in diseases classified elsewhere, unspecified ear*

    ▌*H94.81*   *Other specified disorders of right ear in diseases classified elsewhere*

    ▌*H94.82*   *Other specified disorders of left ear in diseases classified elsewhere*

    ▌*H94.83*   *Other specified disorders of ear in diseases classified elsewhere, bilateral*

● **H95**   **Intraoperative and postprocedural complications and disorders of ear and mastoid process, not elsewhere classified**

   ● H95.0   **Recurrent cholesteatoma of postmastoidectomy cavity**

    H95.00   **Recurrent cholesteatoma of postmastoidectomy cavity, unspecified ear**

    H95.01   **Recurrent cholesteatoma of postmastoidectomy cavity, right ear**

    H95.02   **Recurrent cholesteatoma of postmastoidectomy cavity, left ear**

    H95.03   **Recurrent cholesteatoma of postmastoidectomy cavity, bilateral ears**

◀ New   ◀▥ Revised   ~~deleted~~ Deleted   Excludes 1   Excludes 2   Includes   Use additional   Code first   Code also   Unspecified

848   **OGCR** Official Guidelines   X Assign placeholder X   ● Use Additional Character(s)   ▌ Manifestation Code   **Coding Clinic**

● H95.1   **Other disorders of ear and mastoid process following mastoidectomy**

  ● H95.11   Chronic inflammation of postmastoidectomy cavity

     H95.111   Chronic inflammation of postmastoidectomy cavity, right ear

     H95.112   Chronic inflammation of postmastoidectomy cavity, left ear

     H95.113   Chronic inflammation of postmastoidectomy cavity, bilateral ears

     H95.119   Chronic inflammation of postmastoidectomy cavity, unspecified ear

  ● H95.12   Granulation of postmastoidectomy cavity

     H95.121   Granulation of postmastoidectomy cavity, right ear

     H95.122   Granulation of postmastoidectomy cavity, left ear

     H95.123   Granulation of postmastoidectomy cavity, bilateral ears

     H95.129   Granulation of postmastoidectomy cavity, unspecified ear

  ● H95.13   Mucosal cyst of postmastoidectomy cavity

     H95.131   Mucosal cyst of postmastoidectomy cavity, right ear

     H95.132   Mucosal cyst of postmastoidectomy cavity, left ear

     H95.133   Mucosal cyst of postmastoidectomy cavity, bilateral ears

     H95.139   Mucosal cyst of postmastoidectomy cavity, unspecified ear

  ● H95.19   Other disorders following mastoidectomy

     H95.191   Other disorders following mastoidectomy, right ear

     H95.192   Other disorders following mastoidectomy, left ear

     H95.193   Other disorders following mastoidectomy, bilateral ears

     H95.199   Other disorders following mastoidectomy, unspecified ear

● H95.2   **Intraoperative hemorrhage and hematoma of ear and mastoid process complicating a procedure**

     Excludes1   intraoperative hemorrhage and hematoma of ear and mastoid process due to accidental puncture or laceration during a procedure (H95.3-)

     H95.21   Intraoperative hemorrhage and hematoma of ear and mastoid process complicating a procedure on the ear and mastoid process

     H95.22   Intraoperative hemorrhage and hematoma of ear and mastoid process complicating other procedure

● H95.3   **Accidental puncture and laceration of ear and mastoid process during a procedure**

     H95.31   Accidental puncture and laceration of the ear and mastoid process during a procedure on the ear and mastoid process

     H95.32   Accidental puncture and laceration of the ear and mastoid process during other procedure

● H95.4   **Postprocedural hemorrhage of ear and mastoid process following a procedure** ◀▥

     H95.41   Postprocedural hemorrhage of ear and mastoid process following a procedure on the ear and mastoid process ◀▥

     H95.42   Postprocedural hemorrhage of ear and mastoid process following other procedure ◀▥

● H95.5   **Postprocedural hematoma and seroma of ear and mastoid process following a procedure** ◀

     H95.51   Postprocedural hematoma of ear and mastoid process following a procedure on the ear and mastoid process ◀

     H95.52   Postprocedural hematoma of ear and mastoid process following other procedure ◀

     H95.53   Postprocedural seroma of ear and mastoid process following a procedure on the ear and mastoid process ◀

     H95.54   Postprocedural seroma of ear and mastoid process following other procedure ◀

● H95.8   **Other intraoperative and postprocedural complications and disorders of the ear and mastoid process, not elsewhere classified**

     Excludes2   postprocedural complications and disorders following mastoidectomy (H95.0-, H95.1-)

  ● H95.81   Postprocedural stenosis of external ear canal

     H95.811   Postprocedural stenosis of right external ear canal

     H95.812   Postprocedural stenosis of left external ear canal

     H95.813   Postprocedural stenosis of external ear canal, bilateral

     H95.819   Postprocedural stenosis of unspecified external ear canal

     H95.88   Other intraoperative complications and disorders of the ear and mastoid process, not elsewhere classified

       Use additional code, if applicable, to further specify disorder

     H95.89   Other postprocedural complications and disorders of the ear and mastoid process, not elsewhere classified

       Use additional code, if applicable, to further specify disorder

CHAPTER 8 (H60-H95)

CHAPTER 9   DISEASES OF THE CIRCULATORY SYSTEM (I00-I99)

OGCR Chapter-Specific Coding Guidelines

9. **Chapter 9: Diseases of the Circulatory System (I00-I99)**

a. **Hypertension**
The classification presumes a causal relationship between hypertension and heart involvement and between hypertension and kidney involvement, as the two conditions are linked by the term "with" in the Alphabetic Index. These conditions should be coded as related even in the absence of provider documentation explicitly linking them, unless the documentation clearly states the conditions are unrelated.

For hypertension and conditions not specifically linked by relational terms such as "with," "associated with" or "due to" in the classification, provider documentation must link the conditions in order to code them as related.

1) **Hypertension with Heart Disease**
Hypertension with heart conditions classified to I50.- or I51.4-I51.9, are assigned to, a code from category I11, Hypertensive heart disease. Use an additional code from category I50, Heart failure, to identify the type of heart failure in those patients with heart failure.

The same heart conditions (I50.-, I51.4-I51.9) with hypertension, are coded separately **if the provider has specifically documented a different cause.** Sequence according to the circumstances of the admission/encounter.

2) **Hypertensive Chronic Kidney Disease**
Assign codes from category I12, Hypertensive chronic kidney disease, when both hypertension and a condition classifiable to category N18, Chronic kidney disease (CKD), are present. **CKD should not be coded as hypertensive if the physician has specifically documented a different cause.**

The appropriate code from category N18 should be used as a secondary code with a code from category I12 to identify the stage of chronic kidney disease.
See Section I.C.14. Chronic kidney disease.
If a patient has hypertensive chronic kidney disease and acute renal failure, an additional code for the acute renal failure is required.

3) **Hypertensive Heart and Chronic Kidney Disease**
Assign codes from combination category I13, Hypertensive heart and chronic kidney disease, when **there is hypertension with both heart and kidney involvement.** If heart failure is present, assign an additional code from category I50 to identify the type of heart failure.

The appropriate code from category N18, Chronic kidney disease, should be used as a secondary code with a code from category I13 to identify the stage of chronic kidney disease.
See Section I.C.14. Chronic kidney disease.
The codes in category I13, Hypertensive heart and chronic kidney disease, are combination codes that include hypertension, heart disease and chronic kidney disease. The Includes note at I13 specifies that the conditions included at I11 and I12 are included together in I13. If a patient has hypertension, heart disease and chronic kidney disease then a code from I13 should be used, not individual codes for hypertension, heart disease and chronic kidney disease, or codes from I11 or I12.

For patients with both acute renal failure and chronic kidney disease an additional code for acute renal failure is required.

4) **Hypertensive Cerebrovascular Disease**
For hypertensive cerebrovascular disease, first assign the appropriate code from categories I60-I69, followed by the appropriate hypertension code.

5) **Hypertensive Retinopathy**
Subcategory H35.0, Background retinopathy and retinal vascular changes, should be used with a code from category I10 – I15, Hypertensive disease to include the systemic hypertension. The sequencing is based on the reason for the encounter.

6) **Hypertension, Secondary**
Secondary hypertension is due to an underlying condition. Two codes are required: one to identify the underlying etiology and one from category I15 to identify the hypertension. Sequencing of codes is determined by the reason for admission/encounter.

7) **Hypertension, Transient**
Assign code R03.0, Elevated blood pressure reading without diagnosis of hypertension, unless patient has an established diagnosis of hypertension. Assign code O13.-, Gestational [pregnancy-induced] hypertension without significant proteinuria, or O14.-, Pre-eclampsia, for transient hypertension of pregnancy.

8) **Hypertension, Controlled**
This diagnostic statement usually refers to an existing state of hypertension under control by therapy. Assign the appropriate code from categories I10-I15, Hypertensive diseases.

9) **Hypertension, Uncontrolled**
Uncontrolled hypertension may refer to untreated hypertension or hypertension not responding to current therapeutic regimen. In either case, assign the appropriate code from categories I10-I15, Hypertensive diseases.

10) **Hypertensive Crisis**
Assign a code from category I16, Hypertensive crisis, for documented hypertensive urgency, hypertensive emergency or unspecified hypertensive crisis. Code also any identified hypertensive disease (I10-I15). The sequencing is based on the reason for the encounter.

b. **Atherosclerotic Coronary Artery Disease and Angina**
ICD-10-CM has combination codes for atherosclerotic heart disease with angina pectoris. The subcategories for these codes are I25.11, Atherosclerotic heart disease of native coronary artery with angina pectoris and I25.7, Atherosclerosis of coronary artery bypass graft(s) and coronary artery of transplanted heart with angina pectoris.

When using one of these combination codes it is not necessary to use an additional code for angina pectoris. A causal relationship can be assumed in a patient with both atherosclerosis and angina pectoris, unless the documentation indicates the angina is due to something other than the atherosclerosis.

If a patient with coronary artery disease is admitted due to an acute myocardial infarction (AMI), the AMI should be sequenced before the coronary artery disease.
See Section I.C.9. Acute myocardial infarction (AMI)

c. **Intraoperative and Postprocedural Cerebrovascular Accident**
Medical record documentation should clearly specify the cause-and-effect relationship between the medical intervention and the cerebrovascular accident in order to assign a code for intraoperative or postprocedural cerebrovascular accident.

Proper code assignment depends on whether it was an infarction or hemorrhage and whether it occurred intraoperatively or postoperatively. If it was a cerebral hemorrhage, code assignment depends on the type of procedure performed.

d. **Sequelae of Cerebrovascular Disease**

1) **Category I69, Sequelae of Cerebrovascular disease**
Category I69 is used to indicate conditions classifiable to categories I60-I67 as the causes of sequela (neurologic deficits), themselves classified elsewhere. These "late effects" include neurologic deficits that persist after initial onset of conditions classifiable to categories I60-I67. The neurologic deficits caused by cerebrovascular disease may be present from the onset or may arise at any time after the onset of the condition classifiable to categories I60-I67.

Codes from category I69, Sequelae of cerebrovascular disease, that specify hemiplegia, hemiparesis and monoplegia identify whether the dominant or nondominant side is affected. Should the affected side be documented, but not specified as dominant or nondominant, and the classification system does not indicate a default, code selection is as follows:
- For ambidextrous patients, the default should be dominant.
- If the left side is affected, the default is non-dominant.
- If the right side is affected, the default is dominant.

2) Codes from category I69 with codes from I60-I67
Codes from category I69 may be assigned on a health care record with codes from I60-I67, if the patient has a current cerebrovascular disease and deficits from an old cerebrovascular disease.

3) Codes from category I69 and Personal history of transient ischemic attack (TIA) and cerebral infarction (Z86.73)
Codes from category I69 should not be assigned if the patient does not have neurologic deficits.
See Section I.C.21. 4. History (of) for use of personal history codes

e. **Acute myocardial infarction (AMI)**

1) ST elevation myocardial infarction (STEMI) and non ST elevation myocardial infarction (NSTEMI)
The ICD-10-CM codes for acute myocardial infarction (AMI) identify the site, such as anterolateral wall or true posterior wall. Subcategories I21.0-I21.2 and code I21.3 are used for ST elevation myocardial infarction (STEMI). Code I21.4, Non-ST elevation (NSTEMI) myocardial infarction, is used for non ST elevation myocardial infarction (NSTEMI) and nontransmural MIs.

If NSTEMI evolves to STEMI, assign the STEMI code. If STEMI converts to NSTEMI due to thrombolytic therapy, it is still coded as STEMI.

For encounters occurring while the myocardial infarction is equal to, or less than, four weeks old, including transfers to another acute setting or a postacute setting, and the myocardial infarction **meets the definition for "other diagnoses" (see Section III, Reporting Additional Diagnoses)**, codes from category I21 may continue to be reported. For encounters after the 4 week time frame and the patient is still receiving care related to the myocardial infarction, the appropriate aftercare code should be assigned, rather than a code from category I21. For old or healed myocardial infarctions not requiring further care, code I25.2, Old myocardial infarction, may be assigned.

2) Acute myocardial infarction, unspecified
Code I21.3, ST elevation (STEMI) myocardial infarction of unspecified site, is the default for unspecified acute myocardial infarction. If only STEMI or transmural MI without the site is documented, assign code I21.3.

3) AMI documented as nontransmural or subendocardial but site provided
If an AMI is documented as nontransmural or subendocardial, but the site is provided, it is still coded as a subendocardial AMI.
See Section I.C.21.3 for information on coding status post administration of tPA in a different facility within the last 24 hours.

4) Subsequent acute myocardial infarction
A code from category I22, Subsequent ST elevation (STEMI) and non ST elevation (NSTEMI) myocardial infarction, is to be used when a patient who has suffered an AMI has a new AMI within the 4 week time frame of the initial AMI. A code from category I22 must be used in conjunction with a code from category I21. The sequencing of the I22 and I21 codes depends on the circumstances of the encounter.

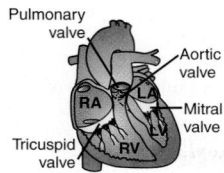

Figure 9-1 Cardiovascular valves.

Item 9-1 Rheumatic fever is the inflammation of the valve(s) of the heart, usually the mitral or aortic, which leads to valve damage. Rheumatic heart inflammations are usually **pericarditis** (sac surrounding heart), **endocarditis** (heart cavity), or **myocarditis** (heart muscle).

CHAPTER 9   DISEASES OF THE CIRCULATORY SYSTEM (I00-I99)

Excludes2   certain conditions originating in the perinatal period (P04-P96)
certain infectious and parasitic diseases (A00-B99)
complications of pregnancy, childbirth and the puerperium (O00-O9A)
congenital malformations, deformations, and chromosomal abnormalities (Q00-Q99)
endocrine, nutritional and metabolic diseases (E00-E88)
injury, poisoning and certain other consequences of external causes (S00-T88)
neoplasms (C00-D49)
symptoms, signs and abnormal clinical and laboratory findings, not elsewhere classified (R00-R94)
systemic connective tissue disorders (M30-M36)
transient cerebral ischemic attacks and related syndromes (G45.-)

This chapter contains the following blocks:

I00-I02	Acute rheumatic fever
I05-I09	Chronic rheumatic heart diseases
I10-I16	Hypertensive diseases ◄
I20-I25	Ischemic heart diseases
I26-I28	Pulmonary heart disease and diseases of pulmonary circulation
I30-I52	Other forms of heart disease
I60-I69	Cerebrovascular diseases
I70-I79	Diseases of arteries, arterioles and capillaries
I80-I89	Diseases of veins, lymphatic vessels and lymph nodes, not elsewhere classified
I95-I99	Other and unspecified disorders of the circulatory system

ACUTE RHEUMATIC FEVER (I00-I02)

I00   Rheumatic fever without heart involvement
Includes   arthritis, rheumatic, acute or subacute
Excludes1   rheumatic fever with heart involvement (I01.0-I01.9)

● **I01   Rheumatic fever with heart involvement**
Excludes1   chronic diseases of rheumatic origin (I05-I09) unless rheumatic fever is also present or there is evidence of reactivation or activity of the rheumatic process.

I01.0   Acute rheumatic pericarditis
Any condition in I00 with pericarditis
Rheumatic pericarditis (acute)
Excludes1   acute pericarditis not specified as rheumatic (I30.-)

I01.1   Acute rheumatic endocarditis
Any condition in I00 with endocarditis or valvulitis
Acute rheumatic valvulitis

Item 9-2 Rheumatic chorea, also called Sydenham's, juvenile, minor, simple, or St. Vitus' dance, is a major symptom of rheumatic fever and is characterized by ceaseless, involuntary, jerky, purposeless movements.

CHAPTER 9 (I00-I99)

I01.2   **Acute rheumatic myocarditis**
Any condition in I00 with myocarditis

I01.8   **Other acute rheumatic heart disease**
Any condition in I00 with other or multiple types of heart involvement
Acute rheumatic pancarditis

I01.9   **Acute rheumatic heart disease, unspecified**
Any condition in I00 with unspecified type of heart involvement
Rheumatic carditis, acute
Rheumatic heart disease, active or acute

● **I02**   **Rheumatic chorea**

   Includes   Sydenham's chorea

   Excludes1   chorea NOS (G25.5)
     Huntington's chorea (G10)

I02.0   **Rheumatic chorea with heart involvement**
Chorea NOS with heart involvement
Rheumatic chorea with heart involvement of any type classifiable under I01.-

I02.9   **Rheumatic chorea without heart involvement**
Rheumatic chorea NOS

CHRONIC RHEUMATIC HEART DISEASES (I05-I09)

● **I05**   **Rheumatic mitral valve diseases**

   Includes   conditions classifiable to both I05.0 and I05.2-I05.9, whether specified as rheumatic or not

   Excludes1   mitral valve disease specified as nonrheumatic (I34.-)
     mitral valve disease with aortic and/or tricuspid valve involvement (I08.-)

I05.0   **Rheumatic mitral stenosis**
Mitral (valve) obstruction (rheumatic)

I05.1   **Rheumatic mitral insufficiency**
Rheumatic mitral incompetence
Rheumatic mitral regurgitation

   Excludes1   mitral insufficiency not specified as rheumatic (I34.0)

I05.2   **Rheumatic mitral stenosis with insufficiency**
Rheumatic mitral stenosis with incompetence or regurgitation

I05.8   **Other rheumatic mitral valve diseases**
Rheumatic mitral (valve) failure

I05.9   **Rheumatic mitral valve disease, unspecified**
Rheumatic mitral (valve) disorder (chronic) NOS

● **I06**   **Rheumatic aortic valve diseases**

   Excludes1   aortic valve disease not specified as rheumatic (I35.-)
     aortic valve disease with mitral and/or tricuspid valve involvement (I08.-)

I06.0   **Rheumatic aortic stenosis**
Rheumatic aortic (valve) obstruction

I06.1   **Rheumatic aortic insufficiency**
Rheumatic aortic incompetence
Rheumatic aortic regurgitation

I06.8   **Other rheumatic aortic valve diseases**

I06.9   **Rheumatic aortic valve disease, unspecified**
Rheumatic aortic (valve) disease NOS

★ **(See Plate 244 on page 78.)**

I06.2   **Rheumatic aortic stenosis with insufficiency**
Rheumatic aortic stenosis with incompetence or regurgitation

Item 9–3 Mitral stenosis is the narrowing of the mitral valve separating the left atrium from the left ventricle. **Mitral insufficiency** is the improper closure of the mitral valve which may lead to enlargement (hypertrophy) of the left atrium.

Item 9–4 Aortic stenosis is the narrowing of the aortic valve located between the left ventricle and the aorta. **Aortic insufficiency** is the improper closure of the aortic valve which may lead to enlargement (hypertrophy) of the left ventricle.

● **I07**   **Rheumatic tricuspid valve diseases**

   Includes   rheumatic tricuspid valve diseases specified as rheumatic or unspecified

   Excludes1   tricuspid valve disease specified as nonrheumatic (I36.-)
     tricuspid valve disease with aortic and/or mitral valve involvement (I08.-)

I07.0   **Rheumatic tricuspid stenosis**
Tricuspid (valve) stenosis (rheumatic)

I07.1   **Rheumatic tricuspid insufficiency**
Tricuspid (valve) insufficiency (rheumatic)

I07.2   **Rheumatic tricuspid stenosis and insufficiency**

I07.8   **Other rheumatic tricuspid valve diseases**

I07.9   **Rheumatic tricuspid valve disease, unspecified**
Rheumatic tricuspid valve disorder NOS

● **I08**   **Multiple valve diseases**

   Includes   multiple valve diseases specified as rheumatic or unspecified

   Excludes1   endocarditis, valve unspecified (I38)
     multiple valve disease specified a nonrheumatic (I34.-, I35.-, I36.-, I37.-, I38.-, Q22.-, Q23.-, Q24.8-)
     rheumatic valve disease NOS (I09.1)

I08.0   **Rheumatic disorders of both mitral and aortic valves**
Involvement of both mitral and aortic valves specified as rheumatic or unspecified

I08.1   **Rheumatic disorders of both mitral and tricuspid valves**

I08.2   **Rheumatic disorders of both aortic and tricuspid valves**

I08.3   **Combined rheumatic disorders of mitral, aortic and tricuspid valves**

I08.8   **Other rheumatic multiple valve diseases**

I08.9   **Rheumatic multiple valve disease, unspecified**

● **I09**   **Other rheumatic heart diseases**

I09.0   **Rheumatic myocarditis**

   Excludes1   myocarditis not specified as rheumatic (I51.4)

I09.1   **Rheumatic diseases of endocardium, valve unspecified**
Rheumatic endocarditis (chronic)
Rheumatic valvulitis (chronic)

   Excludes1   endocarditis, valve unspecified (I38)

I09.2   **Chronic rheumatic pericarditis**
Adherent pericardium, rheumatic
Chronic rheumatic mediastinopericarditis
Chronic rheumatic myopericarditis

   Excludes1   chronic pericarditis not specified as rheumatic (I31.-)

● **I09.8**   **Other specified rheumatic heart diseases**

I09.81   **Rheumatic heart failure**
Use additional code to identify type of heart failure (I50.-)

I09.89   **Other specified rheumatic heart diseases**
Rheumatic disease of pulmonary valve

I09.9   **Rheumatic heart disease, unspecified**
Rheumatic carditis

   Excludes1   rheumatoid carditis (M05.31)

◀ New   ◀▦ Revised   ~~deleted~~ Deleted   Excludes 1   Excludes 2   Includes   Use additional   Code first   Code also   Unspecified

OGCR Official Guidelines   X Assign placeholder X   ● Use Additional Character(s)   ▶ Manifestation Code   **Coding Clinic**

Item 9–5 Hypertension is caused by high arterial blood pressure in the arteries. **Essential, primary,** or **idiopathic** hypertension occurs without identifiable organic cause. **Secondary** hypertension is that which has an organic cause. **Malignant** hypertension is severely elevated blood pressure. **Benign** hypertension is mildly elevated blood pressure.

HYPERTENSIVE DISEASES (I10-I16) ◄▦

Use additional code to identify:
- exposure to environmental tobacco smoke (Z77.22)
- history of tobacco dependence (Z87.891) ◄▦
- occupational exposure to environmental tobacco smoke (Z57.31)
- tobacco dependence (F17.-)
- tobacco use (Z72.0)

| Excludes1 | neonatal hypertension (P29.2) |
| | primary pulmonary hypertension (I27.0) |

| Excludes2 | hypertensive disease complicating pregnancy, childbirth and the puerperium (O10-O11, O13-O16) ◄ |

I10   Essential (primary) hypertension

| Includes | high blood pressure |
| | hypertension (arterial) (benign) (essential) (malignant) (primary) (systemic) |

| Excludes1 | hypertensive disease complicating pregnancy, childbirth and the puerperium (O10-O11, O13-O16) |

| Excludes2 | essential (primary) hypertension involving vessels of brain (I60-I69) |
| | essential (primary) hypertension involving vessels of eye (H35.0-) |

● **I11   Hypertensive heart disease**

| Includes | any condition in I51.4-I51.9 due to hypertension |

I11.0   Hypertensive heart disease with heart failure
Hypertensive heart failure

Use additional code to identify type of heart failure (I50.-)

I11.9   Hypertensive heart disease without heart failure
Hypertensive heart disease NOS

OGCR Section I.C.9.a.2

Hypertensive Chronic Kidney Disease

Assign codes from category I12, Hypertensive chronic kidney disease, when both hypertension and a condition classifiable to category N18, Chronic kidney disease (CKD), are present. **CKD should not be coded as hypertensive if the physician has specifically documented a different cause.**

The appropriate code from category N18 should be used as a secondary code with a code from category I12 to identify the stage of chronic kidney disease.

See Section I.C.14. Chronic kidney disease.

If a patient has hypertensive chronic kidney disease and acute renal failure, an additional code for the acute renal failure is required.

● **I12   Hypertensive chronic kidney disease**

Includes	any condition in N18 and N26 - due to hypertension
	arteriosclerosis of kidney
	arteriosclerotic nephritis (chronic) (interstitial)
	hypertensive nephropathy
	nephrosclerosis

Excludes1	hypertension due to kidney disease (I15.0, I15.1)
	renovascular hypertension (I15.0)
	secondary hypertension (I15.-)

| Excludes2 | acute kidney failure (N17.-) |

I12.0   Hypertensive chronic kidney disease with stage 5 chronic kidney disease or end stage renal disease

Use additional code to identify the stage of chronic kidney disease (N18.5, N18.6)

I12.9   Hypertensive chronic kidney disease with stage 1 through stage 4 chronic kidney disease, or unspecified chronic kidney disease
Hypertensive chronic kidney disease NOS
Hypertensive renal disease NOS

Use additional code to identify the stage of chronic kidney disease (N18.1-N18.4, N18.9)

OGCR Section I.c.9.a.3

Hypertensive Heart and Chronic Kidney Disease

Assign codes from combination category I13, Hypertensive heart and chronic kidney disease, when **there is hypertension with both heart and kidney involvement.** If heart failure is present, assign an additional code from category I50 to identify the type of heart failure.

The appropriate code from category N18, Chronic kidney disease, should be used as a secondary code with a code from category I13 to identify the stage of chronic kidney disease.

See Section I.C.14. Chronic kidney disease.

The codes in category I13, Hypertensive heart and chronic kidney disease, are combination codes that include hypertension, heart disease and chronic kidney disease. The Includes note at I13 specifies that the conditions included at I11 and I12 are included together in I13. If a patient has hypertension, heart disease and chronic kidney disease then a code from I13 should be used, not individual codes for hypertension, heart disease and chronic kidney disease, or codes from I11 or I12.

For patients with both acute renal failure and chronic kidney disease an additional code for acute renal failure is required.

● **I13   Hypertensive heart and chronic kidney disease**

Includes	any condition in I11.- with any condition in I12.-
	cardiorenal disease
	cardiovascular renal disease

I13.0   Hypertensive heart and chronic kidney disease with heart failure and stage 1 through stage 4 chronic kidney disease, or unspecified chronic kidney disease

Use additional code to identify type of heart failure (I50.-)

Use additional code to identify stage of chronic kidney disease (N18.1-N18.4, N18.9)

● **I13.1   Hypertensive heart and chronic kidney disease without heart failure**

I13.10   Hypertensive heart and chronic kidney disease without heart failure, with stage 1 through stage 4 chronic kidney disease, or unspecified chronic kidney disease
Hypertensive heart disease and hypertensive chronic kidney disease NOS

Use additional code to identify the stage of chronic kidney disease (N18.1-N18.4, N18.9)

I13.11   Hypertensive heart and chronic kidney disease without heart failure, with stage 5 chronic kidney disease, or end stage renal disease

Use additional code to identify the stage of chronic kidney disease (N18.5, N18.6)

I13.2   Hypertensive heart and chronic kidney disease with heart failure and with stage 5 chronic kidney disease, or end stage renal disease

Use additional code to identify type of heart failure (I50.-)

Use additional code to identify the stage of chronic kidney disease (N18.5, N18.6)

CHAPTER 9 (I00-I99)

Hypertension, Secondary

Secondary hypertension is due to an underlying condition. Two codes are required: one to identify the underlying etiology and one from category I15 to identify the hypertension. Sequencing of codes is determined by the reason for admission/encounter.

● I15   **Secondary hypertension**
    Code also underlying condition
    Excludes1   postprocedural hypertension (I97.3)
    Excludes2   secondary hypertension involving vessels of brain (I60-I69)
           secondary hypertension involving vessels of eye (H35.0-)
   I15.0   **Renovascular hypertension**
   I15.1   **Hypertension secondary to other renal disorders**
   I15.2   **Hypertension secondary to endocrine disorders**
   I15.8   **Other secondary hypertension**
   I15.9   **Secondary hypertension, unspecified**

● I16   **Hypertensive crisis** ◄
    Code also any identified hypertensive disease (I10-I15) ◄
   I16.0   **Hypertensive urgency** ◄
   I16.1   **Hypertensive emergency** ◄
   I16.9   **Hypertensive crisis, unspecified** ◄

ISCHEMIC HEART DISEASES (I20-I25)

Use additional code to identify presence of hypertension (I10-I16) ◄▥

● I20   **Angina pectoris**
Chest pain/discomfort due to lack of oxygen to the heart muscle. Principal symptom of myocardial infarction.
Use additional code to identify:
    exposure to environmental tobacco smoke (Z77.22)
    history of tobacco dependence (Z87.891) ◄▥
    occupational exposure to environmental tobacco smoke (Z57.31)
    tobacco dependence (F17.-)
    tobacco use (Z72.0)
   Excludes1   angina pectoris with atherosclerotic heart disease of native coronary arteries (I25.1-)
          atherosclerosis of coronary artery bypass graft(s) and coronary artery of transplanted heart with angina pectoris (I25.7-)
          postinfarction angina (I23.7)
   I20.0   **Unstable angina**
     Accelerated angina
     Crescendo angina
     De novo effort angina
     Intermediate coronary syndrome
     Preinfarction syndrome
     Worsening effort angina
   I20.1   **Angina pectoris with documented spasm**
     Angiospastic angina
     Prinzmetal angina
     Spasm-induced angina
     Variant angina

   I20.8   **Other forms of angina pectoris**
     Angina equivalent
     Angina of effort
     Coronary slow flow syndrome
     Stable angina ◄
     Stenocardia
     Use additional code(s) for symptoms associated with angina equivalent
   I20.9   **Angina pectoris, unspecified**
     Angina NOS
     Anginal syndrome
     Cardiac angina
     Ischemic chest pain

● I21   **ST elevation (STEMI) and non-ST elevation (NSTEMI) myocardial infarction**
   Includes   cardiac infarction
         coronary (artery) embolism
         coronary (artery) occlusion
         coronary (artery) rupture
         coronary (artery) thrombosis
         infarction of heart, myocardium, or ventricle
         myocardial infarction specified as acute or with a stated duration of 4 weeks (28 days) or less from onset
   Use additional code, if applicable, to identify:
    exposure to environmental tobacco smoke (Z77.22)
    history of tobacco dependence (Z87.891) ◄▥
    occupational exposure to environmental tobacco smoke (Z57.31)
    status post administration of tPA (rtPA) in a different facility within the last 24 hours prior to admission to current facility (Z92.82)
    tobacco dependence (F17.-)
    tobacco use (Z72.0)
   Excludes2   old myocardial infarction (I25.2)
         postmyocardial infarction syndrome (I24.1)
         subsequent myocardial infarction (I22.-)
   Coding Clinic: 2013, Q1, P25-26; 2012, Q4, P103
● I21.0   **ST elevation (STEMI) myocardial infarction of anterior wall**
    Coding Clinic: 2013, Q1, P26
   I21.01   **ST elevation (STEMI) myocardial infarction involving left main coronary artery**
   I21.02   **ST elevation (STEMI) myocardial infarction involving left anterior descending coronary artery**
     ST elevation (STEMI) myocardial infarction involving diagonal coronary artery
     Coding Clinic: 2013, Q1, P26
   I21.09   **ST elevation (STEMI) myocardial infarction involving other coronary artery of anterior wall**
     Acute transmural myocardial infarction of anterior wall
     Anteroapical transmural (Q wave) infarction (acute)
     Anterolateral transmural (Q wave) infarction (acute)
     Anteroseptal transmural (Q wave) infarction (acute)
     Transmural (Q wave) infarction (acute) (of) anterior (wall) NOS
     Coding Clinic: 2012, Q4, P102, 104

◄ New   ◄▥ Revised   ~~deleted~~ Deleted   Excludes 1   Excludes 2   Includes   Use additional   Code first   Code also   Unspecified
OGCR Official Guidelines   X Assign placeholder X   ● Use Additional Character(s)   ▶ Manifestation Code   **Coding Clinic**

● **I21.1**   **ST elevation (STEMI) myocardial infarction of inferior wall**
Coding Clinic: 2013, Q1, P26

    I21.11   **ST elevation (STEMI) myocardial infarction involving right coronary artery**
          Inferoposterior transmural (Q wave) infarction (acute)

    I21.19   **ST elevation (STEMI) myocardial infarction involving other coronary artery of inferior wall**
          Acute transmural myocardial infarction of inferior wall
          Inferolateral transmural (Q wave) infarction (acute)
          Transmural (Q wave) infarction (acute) (of) diaphragmatic wall
          Transmural (Q wave) infarction (acute) (of) inferior (wall) NOS

       Excludes2   ST elevation (STEMI) myocardial infarction involving left circumflex coronary artery (I21.21)

        Coding Clinic: 2012, Q4, P97

● **I21.2**   **ST elevation (STEMI) myocardial infarction of other sites**
Coding Clinic: 2013, Q1, P26

    I21.21   **ST elevation (STEMI) myocardial infarction involving left circumflex coronary artery**
          ST elevation (STEMI) myocardial infarction involving oblique marginal coronary artery

    I21.29   **ST elevation (STEMI) myocardial infarction involving other sites**
          Acute transmural myocardial infarction of other sites
          Apical-lateral transmural (Q wave) infarction (acute)
          Basal-lateral transmural (Q wave) infarction (acute)
          High lateral transmural (Q wave) infarction (acute)
          Lateral (wall) NOS transmural (Q wave) infarction (acute)
          Posterior (true) transmural (Q wave) infarction (acute)
          Posterobasal transmural (Q wave) infarction (acute)
          Posterolateral transmural (Q wave) infarction (acute)
          Posteroseptal transmural (Q wave) infarction (acute)
          Septal transmural (Q wave) infarction (acute) NOS

OGCR Section I.c.9.e.2

Acute myocardial infarction, unspecified

Code I21.3, ST elevation (STEMI) myocardial infarction of unspecified site, is the default for unspecified acute myocardial infarction. If only STEMI or transmural MI without the site is documented, assign I21.3.

I21.3   **ST elevation (STEMI) myocardial infarction of unspecified site**
       Acute transmural myocardial infarction of unspecified site
       Myocardial infarction (acute) NOS
       Transmural (Q wave) myocardial infarction NOS
       Coding Clinic: 2013, Q1, P26

I21.4   **Non-ST elevation (NSTEMI) myocardial infarction**
       Acute subendocardial myocardial infarction
       Non-Q wave myocardial infarction NOS
       Nontransmural myocardial infarction NOS
       Coding Clinic: 2015, Q2, P16; 2013, Q1, P26

● **I22**   **Subsequent ST elevation (STEMI) and non-ST elevation (NSTEMI) myocardial infarction**

    Includes   acute myocardial infarction occurring within four weeks (28 days) of a previous acute myocardial infarction, regardless of site
          cardiac infarction
          coronary (artery) embolism
          coronary (artery) occlusion
          coronary (artery) rupture
          coronary (artery) thrombosis
          infarction of heart, myocardium, or ventricle
          recurrent myocardial infarction
          reinfarction of myocardium
          rupture of heart, myocardium, or ventricle

Use additional code, if applicable, to identify:
    exposure to environmental tobacco smoke (Z77.22)
    history of tobacco dependence (Z87.891) ◀▥
    occupational exposure to environmental tobacco smoke (Z57.31)
    status post administration of tPA (rtPA) in a different facility within the last 24 hours prior to admission to current facility (Z92.82)
    tobacco dependence (F17.-)
    tobacco use (Z72.0)
Coding Clinic: 2013, Q1, P25; 2012, Q4, P103

I22.0   **Subsequent ST elevation (STEMI) myocardial infarction of anterior wall**
       Subsequent acute transmural myocardial infarction of anterior wall
       Subsequent transmural (Q wave) infarction (acute)(of) anterior (wall) NOS
       Subsequent anteroapical transmural (Q wave) infarction (acute)
       Subsequent anterolateral transmural (Q wave) infarction (acute)
       Subsequent anteroseptal transmural (Q wave) infarction (acute)

I22.1   **Subsequent ST elevation (STEMI) myocardial infarction of inferior wall**
       Subsequent acute transmural myocardial infarction of inferior wall
       Subsequent transmural (Q wave) infarction (acute)(of) diaphragmatic wall
       Subsequent transmural (Q wave) infarction (acute)(of) inferior (wall) NOS
       Subsequent inferolateral transmural (Q wave) infarction (acute)
       Subsequent inferoposterior transmural (Q wave) infarction (acute)
       Coding Clinic: 2012, Q4, P97, 102, 104

I22.2   **Subsequent non-ST elevation (NSTEMI) myocardial infarction**
       Subsequent acute subendocardial myocardial infarction
       Subsequent non-Q wave myocardial infarction NOS
       Subsequent nontransmural myocardial infarction NOS

I22.8   **Subsequent ST elevation (STEMI) myocardial infarction of other sites**
       Subsequent acute transmural myocardial infarction of other sites
       Subsequent apical-lateral transmural (Q wave) myocardial infarction (acute)
       Subsequent basal-lateral transmural (Q wave) myocardial infarction (acute)
       Subsequent high lateral transmural (Q wave) myocardial infarction (acute)
       Subsequent transmural (Q wave) myocardial infarction (acute)(of) lateral (wall) NOS
       Subsequent posterior (true) transmural (Q wave) myocardial infarction (acute)
       Subsequent posterobasal transmural (Q wave) myocardial infarction (acute)
       Subsequent posterolateral transmural (Q wave) myocardial infarction (acute)
       Subsequent posteroseptal transmural (Q wave) myocardial infarction (acute)
       Subsequent septal NOS transmural (Q wave) myocardial infarction (acute)

CHAPTER 9 (I00-I99)

I22.9 **Subsequent ST elevation (STEMI) myocardial infarction of unspecified site**
Subsequent acute myocardial infarction of unspecified site
Subsequent myocardial infarction (acute) NOS

● **I23** **Certain current complications following ST elevation (STEMI) and non-ST elevation (NSTEMI) myocardial infarction (within the 28 day period)**

I23.0 **Hemopericardium as current complication following acute myocardial infarction** A
> Excludes1   hemopericardium not specified as current complication following acute myocardial infarction (I31.2)

I23.1 **Atrial septal defect as current complication following acute myocardial infarction** A
> Excludes1   acquired atrial septal defect not specified as current complication following acute myocardial infarction (I51.0)

I23.2 **Ventricular septal defect as current complication following acute myocardial infarction** A
> Excludes1   acquired ventricular septal defect not specified as current complication following acute myocardial infarction (I51.0)

I23.3 **Rupture of cardiac wall without hemopericardium as current complication following acute myocardial infarction** A

I23.4 **Rupture of chordae tendineae as current complication following acute myocardial infarction**
> Excludes1   rupture of chordae tendineae not specified as current complication following acute myocardial infarction (I51.1)

I23.5 **Rupture of papillary muscle as current complication following acute myocardial infarction**
> Excludes1   rupture of papillary muscle not specified as current complication following acute myocardial infarction (I51.2)

I23.6 **Thrombosis of atrium, auricular appendage, and ventricle as current complications following acute myocardial infarction** A
> Excludes1   thrombosis of atrium, auricular appendage, and ventricle not specified as current complication following acute myocardial infarction (I51.3)

I23.7 **Postinfarction angina** A
Coding Clinic: 2015, Q2, P16-17

I23.8 **Other current complications following acute myocardial infarction** A

● **I24** **Other acute ischemic heart diseases**
> Excludes1   angina pectoris (I20.-)
> transient myocardial ischemia in newborn (P29.4)

I24.0 **Acute coronary thrombosis not resulting in myocardial infarction**
Acute coronary (artery) (vein) embolism not resulting in myocardial infarction
Acute coronary (artery) (vein) occlusion not resulting in myocardial infarction
Acute coronary (artery) (vein) thromboembolism not resulting in myocardial infarction
> Excludes1   atherosclerotic heart disease (I25.1-)
Coding Clinic: 2013, Q1, P24

I24.1 **Dressler's syndrome**
Postmyocardial infarction syndrome
> Excludes1   postinfarction angina (I23.7)

I24.8 **Other forms of acute ischemic heart disease**

I24.9 **Acute ischemic heart disease, unspecified**
> Excludes1   ischemic heart disease (chronic) NOS (I25.9)

● **I25** **Chronic ischemic heart disease**
Use additional code to identify:
chronic total occlusion of coronary artery (I25.82)
exposure to environmental tobacco smoke (Z77.22)
history of tobacco dependence (Z87.891) ◀▥
occupational exposure to environmental tobacco smoke (Z57.31)
tobacco dependence (F17.-)
tobacco use (Z72.0)

★ **(See Plates 218 and 219 on pages 74 and 75.)**

● **I25.1** **Atherosclerotic heart disease of native coronary artery**
Disease in which fatty deposits form on the walls of arteries
Atherosclerotic cardiovascular disease
Coronary (artery) atheroma
Coronary (artery) atherosclerosis
Coronary (artery) disease
Coronary (artery) sclerosis
Use additional code, if applicable, to identify:
coronary atherosclerosis due to calcified coronary lesion (I25.84)
coronary atherosclerosis due to lipid rich plaque (I25.83)
> Excludes2   atheroembolism (I75.-)
> atherosclerosis of coronary artery bypass graft(s) and transplanted heart (I25.7-)

I25.10 **Atherosclerotic heart disease of native coronary artery without angina pectoris** A
Atherosclerotic heart disease NOS
Coding Clinic: 2015, Q2, P17; 2012, Q4, P92

OGCR See Section I.9.b.

> Atherosclerotic Coronary Artery Disease and Angina
> ICD-10-CM has combination codes for atherosclerotic heart disease with angina pectoris. The subcategories for these codes are I25.11, Atherosclerotic heart disease of native coronary artery with angina pectoris and I25.7, Atherosclerosis of coronary artery bypass graft(s) and coronary artery of transplanted heart with angina pectoris.
>
> When using one of these combination codes it is not necessary to use an additional code for angina pectoris. A causal relationship can be assumed in a patient with both atherosclerosis and angina pectoris, unless the documentation indicates the angina is due to something other than the atherosclerosis.
>
> If a patient with coronary artery disease is admitted due to an acute myocardial infarction (AMI), the AMI should be sequenced before the coronary artery disease.
> *See Section I.C.9. Acute myocardial infarction (AMI)*

● **I25.11** **Atherosclerotic heart disease of native coronary artery with angina pectoris**

I25.110 **Atherosclerotic heart disease of native coronary artery with unstable angina pectoris** A
> Excludes1   unstable angina without atherosclerotic heart disease (I20.0)

I25.111 **Atherosclerotic heart disease of native coronary artery with angina pectoris with documented spasm** A
> Excludes1   angina pectoris with documented spasm without atherosclerotic heart disease (I20.1)

Item 9–6   Classification is based on the location of the atherosclerosis. **"Of native coronary artery"** indicates the atherosclerosis is within an original heart artery. **"Of autologous vein bypass graft"** indicates that the atherosclerosis is within a vein graft that was taken from within the patient. **"Of nonautologous biological bypass graft"** indicates the atherosclerosis is within a vessel grafted from other than the patient. **"Of artery bypass graft"** indicates the atherosclerosis is within an artery that was grafted from within the patient.

Figure 9-2   Atherosclerotic plaque.

Atherosclerotic plaque (atheromas)

I25.118   Atherosclerotic heart disease of native coronary artery with other forms of angina pectoris   A
   Excludes1   other forms of angina pectoris without atherosclerotic heart disease (I20.8)
    Coding Clinic: 2015, Q2, P16-17

I25.119   Atherosclerotic heart disease of native coronary artery with unspecified angina pectoris   A
   Atherosclerotic heart disease with angina NOS
   Atherosclerotic heart disease with ischemic chest pain
   Excludes1   unspecified angina pectoris without atherosclerotic heart disease (I20.9)

I25.2   Old myocardial infarction
   Healed myocardial infarction
   Past myocardial infarction diagnosed by ECG or other investigation, but currently presenting no symptoms

I25.3   Aneurysm of heart
   Mural aneurysm
   Ventricular aneurysm

● **I25.4   Coronary artery aneurysm and dissection**
   I25.41   Coronary artery aneurysm
     Coronary arteriovenous fistula, acquired
     Excludes1   congenital coronary (artery) aneurysm (Q24.5)
   I25.42   Coronary artery dissection

I25.5   Ischemic cardiomyopathy
   Excludes2   coronary atherosclerosis (I25.1-, I25.7-)

I25.6   Silent myocardial ischemia

● **I25.7   Atherosclerosis of coronary artery bypass graft(s) and coronary artery of transplanted heart with angina pectoris**
   Use additional code, if applicable, to identify:
     coronary atherosclerosis due to calcified coronary lesion (I25.84)
     coronary atherosclerosis due to lipid rich plaque (I25.83)
   Excludes1   atherosclerosis of bypass graft(s) of transplanted heart without angina pectoris (I25.812)
     atherosclerosis of coronary artery bypass graft(s) without angina pectoris (I25.810)
     atherosclerosis of native coronary artery of transplanted heart without angina pectoris (I25.811)
     embolism or thrombus of coronary artery bypass graft(s) (T82.8-)

● **I25.70   Atherosclerosis of coronary artery bypass graft(s), unspecified, with angina pectoris**
   I25.700   Atherosclerosis of coronary artery bypass graft(s), unspecified, with unstable angina pectoris   A
     Excludes1   unstable angina pectoris without atherosclerosis of coronary artery bypass graft (I20.0)
   I25.701   Atherosclerosis of coronary artery bypass graft(s), unspecified, with angina pectoris with documented spasm   A
     Excludes1   angina pectoris with documented spasm without atherosclerosis of coronary artery bypass graft (I20.1)
   I25.708   Atherosclerosis of coronary artery bypass graft(s), unspecified, with other forms of angina pectoris   A
     Excludes1   other forms of angina pectoris without atherosclerosis of coronary artery bypass graft (I20.8)
   I25.709   Atherosclerosis of coronary artery bypass graft(s), unspecified, with unspecified angina pectoris   A
     Excludes1   unspecified angina pectoris without atherosclerosis of coronary artery bypass graft (I20.9)

CHAPTER 9 (I00-I99)

●I25.71 **Atherosclerosis of autologous vein coronary artery bypass graft(s) with angina pectoris**

    I25.710 **Atherosclerosis of autologous vein coronary artery bypass graft(s) with unstable angina pectoris** A

        Excludes1 unstable angina without atherosclerosis of autologous vein coronary artery bypass graft(s) (I20.0)

    I25.711 **Atherosclerosis of autologous vein coronary artery bypass graft(s) with angina pectoris with documented spasm** A

        Excludes1 angina pectoris with documented spasm without atherosclerosis of autologous vein coronary artery bypass graft(s) (I20.1)

    I25.718 **Atherosclerosis of autologous vein coronary artery bypass graft(s) with other forms of angina pectoris** A

        Excludes1 other forms of angina pectoris without atherosclerosis of autologous vein coronary artery bypass graft(s) (I20.8)

    I25.719 **Atherosclerosis of autologous vein coronary artery bypass graft(s) with unspecified angina pectoris** A

        Excludes1 unspecified angina pectoris without atherosclerosis of autologous vein coronary artery bypass graft(s) (I20.9)

●I25.72 **Atherosclerosis of autologous artery coronary artery bypass graft(s) with angina pectoris**
    Atherosclerosis of internal mammary artery graft with angina pectoris

    I25.720 **Atherosclerosis of autologous artery coronary artery bypass graft(s) with unstable angina pectoris** A

        Excludes1 unstable angina without atherosclerosis of autologous artery coronary artery bypass graft(s) (I20.0)

    I25.721 **Atherosclerosis of autologous artery coronary artery bypass graft(s) with angina pectoris with documented spasm** A

        Excludes1 angina pectoris with documented spasm without atherosclerosis of autologous artery coronary artery bypass graft(s) (I20.1)

    I25.728 **Atherosclerosis of autologous artery coronary artery bypass graft(s) with other forms of angina pectoris** A

        Excludes1 other forms of angina pectoris without atherosclerosis of autologous artery coronary artery bypass graft(s) (I20.8)

    I25.729 **Atherosclerosis of autologous artery coronary artery bypass graft(s) with unspecified angina pectoris** A

        Excludes1 unspecified angina pectoris without atherosclerosis of autologous artery coronary artery bypass graft(s) (I20.9)

●I25.73 **Atherosclerosis of nonautologous biological coronary artery bypass graft(s) with angina pectoris**

    I25.730 **Atherosclerosis of nonautologous biological coronary artery bypass graft(s) with unstable angina pectoris** A

        Excludes1 unstable angina without atherosclerosis of nonautologous biological coronary artery bypass graft(s) (I20.0)

    I25.731 **Atherosclerosis of nonautologous biological coronary artery bypass graft(s) with angina pectoris with documented spasm** A

        Excludes1 angina pectoris with documented spasm without atherosclerosis of nonautologous biological coronary artery bypass graft(s) (I20.1)

    I25.738 **Atherosclerosis of nonautologous biological coronary artery bypass graft(s) with other forms of angina pectoris** A

        Excludes1 other forms of angina pectoris without atherosclerosis of nonautologous biological coronary artery bypass graft(s) (I20.8)

    I25.739 **Atherosclerosis of nonautologous biological coronary artery bypass graft(s) with unspecified angina pectoris** A

        Excludes1 unspecified angina pectoris without atherosclerosis of nonautologous biological coronary artery bypass graft(s) (I20.9)

◀ New ◀▦ Revised ~~deleted~~ Deleted Excludes 1 Excludes 2 Includes Use additional Code first Code also Unspecified
OGCR Official Guidelines X Assign placeholder X ● Use Additional Character(s) ▶ Manifestation Code **Coding Clinic**

● **I25.75** **Atherosclerosis of native coronary artery of transplanted heart with angina pectoris**

> **Excludes1**   atherosclerosis of native coronary artery of transplanted heart without angina pectoris (I25.811)

I25.750 **Atherosclerosis of native coronary artery of transplanted heart with unstable angina**

I25.751 **Atherosclerosis of native coronary artery of transplanted heart with angina pectoris with documented spasm**

I25.758 **Atherosclerosis of native coronary artery of transplanted heart with other forms of angina pectoris**

I25.759 **Atherosclerosis of native coronary artery of transplanted heart with** unspecified **angina pectoris**

● **I25.76** **Atherosclerosis of bypass graft of coronary artery of transplanted heart with angina pectoris**

> **Excludes1**   atherosclerosis of bypass graft of coronary artery of transplanted heart without angina pectoris (I25.812)

I25.760 **Atherosclerosis of bypass graft of coronary artery of transplanted heart with unstable angina**   A

I25.761 **Atherosclerosis of bypass graft of coronary artery of transplanted heart with angina pectoris with documented spasm**   A

I25.768 **Atherosclerosis of bypass graft of coronary artery of transplanted heart with other forms of angina pectoris**   A

I25.769 **Atherosclerosis of bypass graft of coronary artery of transplanted heart with** unspecified **angina pectoris**   A

● **I25.79** **Atherosclerosis of other coronary artery bypass graft(s) with angina pectoris**   A

I25.790 **Atherosclerosis of other coronary artery bypass graft(s) with unstable angina pectoris**

> **Excludes1**   unstable angina without atherosclerosis of other coronary artery bypass graft(s) (I20.0)

I25.791 **Atherosclerosis of other coronary artery bypass graft(s) with angina pectoris with documented spasm**   A

> **Excludes1**   angina pectoris with documented spasm without atherosclerosis of other coronary artery bypass graft(s) (I20.1)

I25.798 **Atherosclerosis of other coronary artery bypass graft(s) with other forms of angina pectoris**   A

> **Excludes1**   other forms of angina pectoris without atherosclerosis of other coronary artery bypass graft(s) (I20.8)

I25.799 **Atherosclerosis of other coronary artery bypass graft(s) with** unspecified **angina pectoris**   A

> **Excludes1**   unspecified angina pectoris without atherosclerosis of other coronary artery bypass graft(s) (I20.9)

● **I25.8** **Other forms of chronic ischemic heart disease**

● **I25.81** **Atherosclerosis of other coronary vessels without angina pectoris**

> Use additional code, if applicable, to identify:
> coronary atherosclerosis due to calcified coronary lesion (I25.84)
> coronary atherosclerosis due to lipid rich plaque (I25.83)

> **Excludes1**   atherosclerotic heart disease of native coronary artery without angina pectoris (I25.10)

I25.810 **Atherosclerosis of coronary artery bypass graft(s) without angina pectoris**   A

> Atherosclerosis of coronary artery bypass graft NOS

> **Excludes1**   atherosclerosis of coronary bypass graft(s) with angina pectoris (I25.70- -I25.73-, I25.79-)

I25.811 **Atherosclerosis of native coronary artery of transplanted heart without angina pectoris**

> Atherosclerosis of native coronary artery of transplanted heart NOS

> **Excludes1**   atherosclerosis of native coronary artery of transplanted heart with angina pectoris (I25.75-)

I25.812 **Atherosclerosis of bypass graft of coronary artery of transplanted heart without angina pectoris**   A

> Atherosclerosis of bypass graft of transplanted heart NOS

> **Excludes1**   atherosclerosis of bypass graft of transplanted heart with angina pectoris (I25.76)

I25.82 **Chronic total occlusion of coronary artery**

> Complete occlusion of coronary artery
> Total occlusion of coronary artery

> *Code first coronary atherosclerosis (I25.1-, I25.7-, I25.81-)*

> **Excludes1**   acute coronary occulsion with myocardial infarction (I21.-, I22.-)
> acute coronary occulsion without myocardial infarction (I24.0)

I25.83 **Coronary atherosclerosis due to lipid rich plaque**   A

> *Code first coronary atherosclerosis (I25.1-, I25.7-, I25.81-)*

CHAPTER 9 (I00-I99)

CHAPTER 9 (I00-I99)

I25.84   **Coronary atherosclerosis due to calcified coronary lesion**
Coronary atherosclerosis due to severely calcified coronary lesion

Code first coronary atherosclerosis (I25.1-, I25.7-, I25.81-)

I25.89   **Other forms of chronic ischemic heart disease**

I25.9   **Chronic ischemic heart disease, unspecified**
Ischemic heart disease (chronic) NOS

PULMONARY HEART DISEASE AND DISEASES OF PULMONARY CIRCULATION (I26-I28)

● **I26**   **Pulmonary embolism**

Includes   pulmonary (acute)(artery)(vein) infarction
pulmonary (acute)(artery)(vein) thromboembolism
pulmonary (acute)(artery)(vein) thrombosis

Excludes2   chronic pulmonary embolism (I27.82)
personal history of pulmonary embolism (Z86.711)
pulmonary embolism due to trauma (T79.0, T79.1)
pulmonary embolism due to complications of surgical and medical care (T80.0, T81.7-, T82.8-)
pulmonary embolism complicating abortion, ectopic or molar pregnancy (O00-O07, O08.2)
pulmonary embolism complicating pregnancy, childbirth and the puerperium (O88.-)
septic (non-pulmonary) arterial embolism (I76)

● **I26.0**   **Pulmonary embolism with acute cor pulmonale**

I26.01   **Septic pulmonary embolism with acute cor pulmonale**

Code first underlying infection

I26.02   **Saddle embolus of pulmonary artery with acute cor pulmonale**

I26.09   **Other pulmonary embolism with acute cor pulmonale**
Acute cor pulmonale NOS

I26.9   **Pulmonary embolism without acute cor pulmonale**

I26.90   **Septic pulmonary embolism without acute cor pulmonale**

Code first underlying infection

I26.92   **Saddle embolus of pulmonary artery without acute cor pulmonale**

I26.99   **Other pulmonary embolism without acute cor pulmonale**
Acute pulmonary embolism NOS
Pulmonary embolism NOS

● **I27**   **Other pulmonary heart diseases**

I27.0   **Primary pulmonary hypertension**

Excludes1   pulmonary hypertension NOS (I27.2)
secondary pulmonary hypertension (I27.2)

I27.1   **Kyphoscoliotic heart disease**

I27.2   **Other secondary pulmonary hypertension**
Pulmonary hypertension NOS

Code also associated underlying condition
Coding Clinic: 2016, Q2, P8

● **I27.8**   **Other specified pulmonary heart diseases**

I27.81   **Cor pulmonale (chronic)**
Cor pulmonale NOS

Excludes1   acute cor pulmonale (I26.0-)

I27.82   **Chronic pulmonary embolism**

Use additional code, if applicable, for associated long-term (current) use of anticoagulants (Z79.01)

Excludes1   personal history of pulmonary embolism (Z86.711)

I27.89   **Other specified pulmonary heart diseases**
Eisenmenger's complex
Eisenmenger's syndrome

Excludes1   Eisenmenger's defect (Q21.8)

I27.9   **Pulmonary heart disease, unspecified**
Chronic cardiopulmonary disease

● **I28**   **Other diseases of pulmonary vessels**

I28.0   **Arteriovenous fistula of pulmonary vessels**

Excludes1   congenital arteriovenous fistula (Q25.72)

I28.1   **Aneurysm of pulmonary artery**

Excludes1   congenital aneurysm (Q25.79)
congenital arteriovenous aneurysm (Q25.72)

I28.8   **Other diseases of pulmonary vessels**
Pulmonary arteritis
Pulmonary endarteritis
Rupture of pulmonary vessels
Stenosis of pulmonary vessels
Stricture of pulmonary vessels

I28.9   **Disease of pulmonary vessels, unspecified**

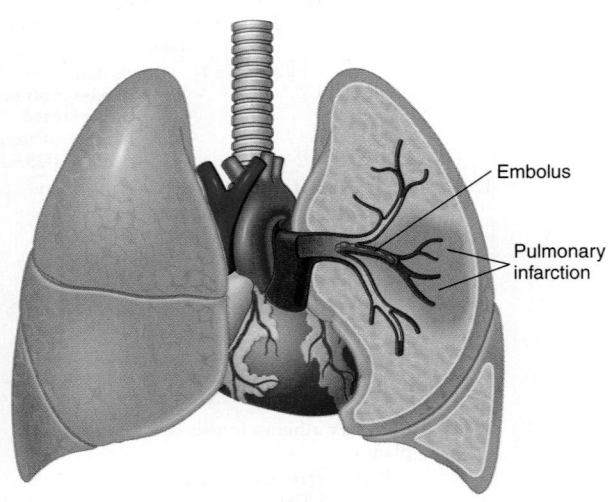

Embolus

Pulmonary infarction

Figure 9-3   Pulmonary Embolism. (From Chabner: The Language of Medicine, ed 8, St. Louis, Saunders, 2007)

Item 9–7   Pulmonary heart disease or **cor pulmonale** is right ventricle hypertrophy or RVH as a result of a respiratory disorder increasing back flow pressure to the right ventricle. Left untreated, cor pulmonale leads to right-heart failure and death.

◀ New   ◀ Revised   ~~deleted~~ Deleted   Excludes 1   Excludes 2   Includes   Use additional   Code first   Code also   Unspecified

OTHER FORMS OF HEART DISEASE (I30-I52)

● **I30 Acute pericarditis**

Inflammation of pericardium (sac surrounding the heart) caused by an infection

Includes	acute mediastinopericarditis
	acute myopericarditis
	acute pericardial effusion
	acute pleuropericarditis
	acute pneumopericarditis

Excludes1	Dressler's syndrome (I24.1)
	rheumatic pericarditis (acute) (I01.0)

I30.0 Acute nonspecific idiopathic pericarditis

I30.1 Infective pericarditis

Pneumococcal pericarditis
Pneumopyopericardium
Purulent pericarditis
Pyopericarditis
Pyopericardium
Pyopneumopericardium
Staphylococcal pericarditis
Streptococcal pericarditis
Suppurative pericarditis
Viral pericarditis

Use additional code (B95-B97) to identify infectious agent

I30.8 Other forms of acute pericarditis

I30.9 Acute pericarditis, unspecified

● **I31 Other diseases of pericardium**

Excludes1	diseases of pericardium specified as rheumatic (I09.2)
	postcardiotomy syndrome (I97.0)
	traumatic injury to pericardium (S26.-)

I31.0 Chronic adhesive pericarditis

Accretio cordis
Adherent pericardium
Adhesive mediastinopericarditis

I31.1 Chronic constrictive pericarditis

Concretio cordis
Pericardial calcification

I31.2 Hemopericardium, not elsewhere classified

Excludes1	hemopericardium as current complication following acute myocardial infarction (I23.0)

I31.3 Pericardial effusion (noninflammatory)

Chylopericardium

Excludes1	acute pericardial effusion (I30.9)

I31.4 Cardiac tamponade

Code first underlying cause

I31.8 Other specified diseases of pericardium

Epicardial plaques
Focal pericardial adhesions

I31.9 Disease of pericardium, unspecified

Pericarditis (chronic) NOS

▷ **I32 *Pericarditis in diseases classified elsewhere***

Code first underlying disease

Excludes1	pericarditis (in):
	coxsackie (virus) (B33.23)
	gonococcal (A54.83)
	meningococcal (A39.53)
	rheumatoid (arthritis) (M05.31)
	syphilitic (A52.06)
	systemic lupus erythematosus (M32.12)
	tuberculosis (A18.84)

● **I33 Acute and subacute endocarditis**

Inflammation/infection of lining of heart, affecting heart valves including replacement valves and is usually caused by a bacterial infection

Excludes1	acute rheumatic endocarditis (I01.1)
	endocarditis NOS (I38)

I33.0 Acute and subacute infective endocarditis

Bacterial endocarditis (acute) (subacute)
Infective endocarditis (acute) (subacute) NOS
Endocarditis lenta (acute) (subacute)
Malignant endocarditis (acute) (subacute)
Purulent endocarditis (acute) (subacute)
Septic endocarditis (acute) (subacute)
Ulcerative endocarditis (acute) (subacute)
Vegetative endocarditis (acute) (subacute)

Use additional code (B95-B97) to identify infectious agent

I33.9 Acute and subacute endocarditis, unspecified

Acute endocarditis NOS
Acute myoendocarditis NOS
Acute periendocarditis NOS
Subacute endocarditis NOS
Subacute myoendocarditis NOS
Subacute periendocarditis NOS

● **I34 Nonrheumatic mitral valve disorders**

Excludes1	mitral valve disease (I05.9)
	mitral valve failure (I05.8)
	mitral valve stenosis (I05.0)
	mitral valve disorder of unspecified cause with diseases of aortic and/or tricuspid valve(s) (I08.-)
	mitral valve disorder of unspecified cause with mitral stenosis or obstruction (I05.0)
	mitral valve disorder specified as congenital (Q23.2, Q23.3)
	mitral valve disorder specified as rheumatic (I05.-)

I34.0 Nonrheumatic mitral (valve) insufficiency

Nonrheumatic mitral (valve) incompetence NOS
Nonrheumatic mitral (valve) regurgitation NOS

I34.1 Nonrheumatic mitral (valve) prolapse

Floppy nonrheumatic mitral valve syndrome

Excludes1	Marfan's syndrome (Q87.4-)

I34.2 Nonrheumatic mitral (valve) stenosis

I34.8 Other nonrheumatic mitral valve disorders

I34.9 Nonrheumatic mitral valve disorder, unspecified

● **I35 Nonrheumatic aortic valve disorders**

Excludes1	aortic valve disorder of unspecified cause but with diseases of mitral and/or tricuspid valve(s) (I08.-)
	aortic valve disorder specified as congenital (Q23.0, Q23.1)
	aortic valve disorder specified as rheumatic (I06.-)
	hypertrophic subaortic stenosis (I42.1)

I35.0 Nonrheumatic aortic (valve) stenosis

I35.1 Nonrheumatic aortic (valve) insufficiency

Nonrheumatic aortic (valve) incompetence NOS
Nonrheumatic aortic (valve) regurgitation NOS

I35.2 Nonrheumatic aortic (valve) stenosis with insufficiency

I35.8 Other nonrheumatic aortic valve disorders

I35.9 Nonrheumatic aortic valve disorder, unspecified

CHAPTER 9 (I00-I99)

● **I36　Nonrheumatic tricuspid valve disorders**
　　Excludes1　tricuspid valve disorders of unspecified cause (I07.-)
　　　　　　　tricuspid valve disorders specified as congenital (Q22.4, Q22.8, Q22.9)
　　　　　　　tricuspid valve disorders specified as rheumatic (I07.-)
　　　　　　　tricuspid valve disorders with aortic and/or mitral valve involvement (I08.-)
　　I36.0　Nonrheumatic tricuspid (valve) stenosis
　　I36.1　Nonrheumatic tricuspid (valve) insufficiency
　　　　　Nonrheumatic tricuspid (valve) incompetence
　　　　　Nonrheumatic tricuspid (valve) regurgitation
　　I36.2　Nonrheumatic tricuspid (valve) stenosis with insufficiency
　　I36.8　Other nonrheumatic tricuspid valve disorders
　　I36.9　Nonrheumatic tricuspid valve disorder, unspecified

● **I37　Nonrheumatic pulmonary valve disorders**
　　Excludes1　pulmonary valve disorder specified as congenital (Q22.1, Q22.2, Q22.3)
　　　　　　　pulmonary valve disorder specified as rheumatic (I09.89)
　　I37.0　Nonrheumatic pulmonary valve stenosis
　　I37.1　Nonrheumatic pulmonary valve insufficiency
　　　　　Nonrheumatic pulmonary valve incompetence
　　　　　Nonrheumatic pulmonary valve regurgitation
　　I37.2　Nonrheumatic pulmonary valve stenosis with insufficiency
　　I37.8　Other nonrheumatic pulmonary valve disorders
　　I37.9　Nonrheumatic pulmonary valve disorder, unspecified

I38　Endocarditis, valve unspecified
　　Includes　endocarditis (chronic) NOS
　　　　　　valvular incompetence NOS
　　　　　　valvular insufficiency NOS
　　　　　　valvular regurgitation NOS
　　　　　　valvular stenosis NOS
　　　　　　valvulitis (chronic) NOS
　　Excludes1　congenital insufficiency of cardiac valve NOS (Q24.8)
　　　　　　　congenital stenosis of cardiac valve NOS (Q24.8)
　　　　　　　endocardial fibroelastosis (I42.4)
　　　　　　　endocarditis specified as rheumatic (I09.1)

▶ **I39　*Endocarditis and heart valve disorders in diseases classified elsewhere***
　　Code first underlying disease, such as:
　　　　Q fever (A78)
　　Excludes1　endocardial involvement in:
　　　　　　　candidiasis (B37.6)
　　　　　　　gonococcal infection (A54.83)
　　　　　　　Libman-Sacks disease (M32.11)
　　　　　　　listerosis (A32.82)
　　　　　　　meningococcal infection (A39.51)
　　　　　　　rheumatoid arthritis (M05.31)
　　　　　　　syphilis (A52.03)
　　　　　　　tuberculosis (A18.84)
　　　　　　　typhoid fever (A01.02)

● **I40　Acute myocarditis**
　　Inflammation of heart muscle due to infection (viral/bacterial)
　　Includes　subacute myocarditis
　　Excludes1　acute rheumatic myocarditis (I01.2)
　　I40.0　Infective myocarditis
　　　　　Septic myocarditis
　　　　　Use additional code (B95-B97) to identify infectious agent
　　I40.1　Isolated myocarditis
　　　　　Fiedler's myocarditis
　　　　　Giant cell myocarditis
　　　　　Idiopathic myocarditis
　　I40.8　Other acute myocarditis
　　I40.9　Acute myocarditis, unspecified

▶ **I41　*Myocarditis in diseases classified elsewhere***
　　Code first underlying disease, such as:
　　　　typhus (A75.0-A75.9)
　　Excludes1　myocarditis (in):
　　　　　　　Chagas' disease (chronic) (B57.2)
　　　　　　　acute (B57.0)
　　　　　　　coxsackie (virus) infection (B33.22)
　　　　　　　diphtheritic (A36.81)
　　　　　　　gonococcal (A54.83)
　　　　　　　influenzal (J09.X9, J10.82, J11.82)
　　　　　　　meningococcal (A39.52)
　　　　　　　mumps (B26.82)
　　　　　　　rheumatoid arthritis (M05.31)
　　　　　　　sarcoid (D86.85)
　　　　　　　syphilis (A52.06)
　　　　　　　toxoplasmosis (B58.81)
　　　　　　　tuberculous (A18.84)

● **I42　Cardiomyopathy**
　　Disease of the heart muscle resulting in an abnormally enlarged, weakened, thickened, and/or stiffened muscles
　　Includes　myocardiopathy
　　Code first pre-existing cardiomyopathy complicating pregnancy and puerperium (O99.4)
　　Excludes2　ischemic cardiomyopathy (I25.5) ◀
　　　　　　　peripartum cardiomyopathy (O90.3) ◀
　　　　　　　ventricular hypertrophy (I51.7)
　　I42.0　Dilated cardiomyopathy
　　　　　Congestive cardiomyopathy
　　I42.1　Obstructive hypertrophic cardiomyopathy
　　　　　Hypertrophic subaortic stenosis (idiopathic)
　　I42.2　Other hypertrophic cardiomyopathy
　　　　　Nonobstructive hypertrophic cardiomyopathy
　　I42.3　Endomyocardial (eosinophilic) disease
　　　　　Endomyocardial (tropical) fibrosis
　　　　　Löffler's endocarditis
　　I42.4　Endocardial fibroelastosis
　　　　　Congenital cardiomyopathy
　　　　　Elastomyofibrosis
　　I42.5　Other restrictive cardiomyopathy
　　　　　Constrictive cardiomyopathy NOS
　　I42.6　Alcoholic cardiomyopathy
　　　　　Code also presence of alcoholism (F10.-)
　　I42.7　Cardiomyopathy due to drug and external agent
　　　　　Code first poisoning due to drug or toxin, if applicable (T36-T65 with fifth or sixth character 1-4 or 6)
　　　　　Use additional code for adverse effect, if applicable, to identify drug (T36-T50 with fifth or sixth character 5)
　　I42.8　Other cardiomyopathies
　　I42.9　Cardiomyopathy, unspecified
　　　　　Cardiomyopathy (primary) (secondary) NOS

▶ **I43　*Cardiomyopathy in diseases classified elsewhere***
　　Code first underlying disease, such as:
　　　　amyloidosis (E85.-)
　　　　glycogen storage disease (E74.0)
　　　　gout (M10.0-)
　　　　thyrotoxicosis (E05.0-E05.9-)
　　Excludes1　cardiomyopathy (in):
　　　　　　　coxsackie (virus) (B33.24)
　　　　　　　diphtheria (A36.81)
　　　　　　　sarcoidosis (D86.85)
　　　　　　　tuberculosis (A18.84)

◀ New　◀◀ Revised　~~deleted~~ Deleted　Excludes 1　Excludes 2　Includes　Use additional　Code first　Code also　Unspecified

 OGCR Official Guidelines　X Assign placeholder X　● Use Additional Character(s)　▶ Manifestation Code　**Coding Clinic**

● **I44 Atrioventricular and left bundle-branch block**

Conduction problem resulting in arrhythmias/dysrhythmias due to a lack of electrical impulses being transmitted normally through the heart

I44.0 Atrioventricular block, first degree

I44.1 Atrioventricular block, second degree
Atrioventricular block, type I and II
Möbitz block, type I and II
Second degree block, type I and II
Wenckebach's block

I44.2 Atrioventricular block, complete
Complete heart block NOS
Third degree block

● **I44.3 Other and unspecified atrioventricular block**
Atrioventricular block NOS

　　I44.30 Unspecified atrioventricular block

　　I44.39 Other atrioventricular block

I44.4 Left anterior fascicular block

I44.5 Left posterior fascicular block

● **I44.6 Other and unspecified fascicular block**

　　I44.60 Unspecified fascicular block
　　　　Left bundle-branch hemiblock NOS

　　I44.69 Other fascicular block

I44.7 Left bundle-branch block, unspecified

● **I45 Other conduction disorders**

I45.0 Right fascicular block

● **I45.1 Other and unspecified right bundle-branch block**

　　I45.10 Unspecified right bundle-branch block
　　　　Right bundle-branch block NOS

　　I45.19 Other right bundle-branch block

I45.2 Bifascicular block

I45.3 Trifascicular block

I45.4 Nonspecific intraventricular block
Bundle-branch block NOS

I45.5 Other specified heart block
Sinoatrial block
Sinoauricular block

　　Excludes1 heart block NOS (I45.9)

I45.6 Pre-excitation syndrome
Accelerated atrioventricular conduction
Accessory atrioventricular conduction
Anomalous atrioventricular excitation
Lown-Ganong-Levine syndrome
Pre-excitation atrioventricular conduction
Wolff-Parkinson-White syndrome

● **I45.8 Other specified conduction disorders**

　　I45.81 Long QT syndrome

　　I45.89 Other specified conduction disorders
　　　　Atrioventricular [AV] dissociation
　　　　Interference dissociation
　　　　Isorhythmic dissociation
　　　　Nonparoxysmal AV nodal tachycardia
　　　　Coding Clinic: 2013, Q2, P32

I45.9 Conduction disorder, unspecified
Heart block NOS
Stokes-Adams syndrome

● **I46 Cardiac arrest**

　　Excludes1 cardiogenic shock (R57.0)

I46.2 Cardiac arrest due to underlying cardiac condition
Code first underlying cardiac condition

I46.8 Cardiac arrest due to other underlying condition
Code first underlying condition

I46.9 Cardiac arrest, cause unspecified

● **I47 Paroxysmal tachycardia**

Code first tachycardia complicating:
abortion or ectopic or molar pregnancy (O00-O07, O08.8)
obstetric surgery and procedures (O75.4)

　　Excludes1 tachycardia NOS (R00.0)
　　　　sinoauricular tachycardia NOS (R00.0)
　　　　sinus [sinusal] tachycardia NOS (R00.0)

I47.0 Re-entry ventricular arrhythmia

I47.1 Supraventricular tachycardia
Atrial (paroxysmal) tachycardia
Atrioventricular [AV] (paroxysmal) tachycardia
Atrioventricular re-entrant (nodal) tachycardia
[AVNRT] [AVRT]
Junctional (paroxysmal) tachycardia
Nodal (paroxysmal) tachycardia

I47.2 Ventricular tachycardia
Coding Clinic: 2013, Q3, P23

I47.9 Paroxysmal tachycardia, unspecified
Bouveret (-Hoffman) syndrome

● **I48 Atrial fibrillation and flutter**

Most common abnormal heart rhythm (arrhythmia) presenting as irregular, rapid beating (tachycardia) of the heart's upper chamber.

I48.0 Paroxysmal atrial fibrillation

I48.1 Persistent atrial fibrillation
Rapid contractions of the upper heart chamber

I48.2 Chronic atrial fibrillation
Permanent atrial fibrillation

I48.3 Typical atrial flutter
Type I atrial flutter

I48.4 Atypical atrial flutter
Type II atrial flutter

● **I48.9 Unspecified atrial fibrillation and atrial flutter**

　　I48.91 Unspecified atrial fibrillation

　　I48.92 Unspecified atrial flutter

● **I49 Other cardiac arrhythmias**

Code first cardiac arrhythmia complicating:
abortion or ectopic or molar pregnancy (O00-O07, O08.8)
obstetric surgery and procedures (O75.4)

　　Excludes1 bradycardia NOS (R00.1)
　　　　neonatal dysrhythmia (P29.1-)
　　　　sinoatrial bradycardia (R00.1)
　　　　sinus bradycardia (R00.1)
　　　　vagal bradycardia (R00.1)

● **I49.0 Ventricular fibrillation and flutter**

　　I49.01 Ventricular fibrillation

　　I49.02 Ventricular flutter

I49.1 Atrial premature depolarization
Atrial premature beats

I49.2 Junctional premature depolarization

I49.3 Ventricular premature depolarization

● **I49.4 Other and unspecified premature depolarization**

　　I49.40 Unspecified premature depolarization
　　　　Premature beats NOS

　　I49.49 Other premature depolarization
　　　　Ectopic beats
　　　　Extrasystoles
　　　　Extrasystolic arrhythmias
　　　　Premature contractions

I49.5 Sick sinus syndrome
Tachycardia-bradycardia syndrome

I49.8 Other specified cardiac arrhythmias
Coronary sinus rhythm disorder
Ectopic rhythm disorder
Nodal rhythm disorder

● **I49.9 Cardiac arrhythmia, unspecified**
Arrhythmia (cardiac) NOS

CHAPTER 9 (I00-I99)

● **I50**   **Heart failure**
Code first heart failure complicating abortion or ectopic or molar
    pregnancy (O00-O07, O08.8)
    heart failure due to hypertension (I11.0)
    heart failure due to hypertension with chronic kidney disease
      (I13.-)
    heart failure following surgery (I97.13-)
    obstetric surgery and procedures (O75.4)
    rheumatic heart failure (I09.81)

    Excludes1   neonatal cardiac failure (P29.0)

    Excludes2   cardiac arrest (I46.-) ◀

    Coding Clinic: 2016, Q1, P38; 2015, Q2, P15

I50.1   **Left ventricular failure**
    Cardiac asthma
    Edema of lung with heart disease NOS
    Edema of lung with heart failure
    Left heart failure
    Pulmonary edema with heart disease NOS
    Pulmonary edema with heart failure

      Excludes1   edema of lung without heart disease or
         heart failure (J81.-)
         pulmonary edema without heart disease
         or failure (J81.-)

● **I50.2**   **Systolic (congestive) heart failure**

      Excludes1   combined systolic (congestive) and
         diastolic (congestive) heart failure
         (I50.4-)

   I50.20   **Unspecified systolic (congestive) heart failure**

   I50.21   **Acute systolic (congestive) heart failure**
      Presenting a short and relatively severe episode

   I50.22   **Chronic systolic (congestive) heart failure**
      Long-lasting, presenting over time

   I50.23   **Acute on chronic systolic (congestive) heart
      failure**
      *Combination code. What was a chronic condition
        now has an acute exacerbation (to make more
        severe).*
      Coding Clinic: 2013, Q2, P33

● **I50.3**   **Diastolic (congestive) heart failure**

      Excludes1   combined systolic (congestive) and
         diastolic (congestive) heart failure
         (I50.4-)

   I50.30   **Unspecified diastolic (congestive) heart failure**

   I50.31   **Acute diastolic (congestive) heart failure**

   I50.32   **Chronic diastolic (congestive) heart failure**

   I50.33   **Acute on chronic diastolic (congestive) heart
      failure**

● **I50.4**   **Combined systolic (congestive) and diastolic
(congestive) heart failure**

   I50.40   **Unspecified combined systolic (congestive) and
      diastolic (congestive) heart failure**

   I50.41   **Acute combined systolic (congestive) and
      diastolic (congestive) heart failure**

   I50.42   **Chronic combined systolic (congestive) and
      diastolic (congestive) heart failure**

   I50.43   **Acute on chronic combined systolic (congestive)
      and diastolic (congestive) heart failure**

I50.9   **Heart failure, unspecified**
    Biventricular (heart) failure NOS
    Cardiac, heart or myocardial failure NOS
    Congestive heart disease
    Congestive heart failure NOS
    Right ventricular failure (secondary to left heart failure)

      Excludes2   fluid overload (E87.70) ◀
    Coding Clinic: 2015, Q2, P15; 2012, Q4, P92

● **I51**   **Complications and ill-defined descriptions of heart disease**

    Excludes1   any condition in I51.4-I51.9 due to hypertension
        (I11.-)
        any condition in I51.4-I51.9 due to hypertension
        and chronic kidney disease (I13.-)
        heart disease specified as rheumatic (I00-I09)

I51.0   **Cardiac septal defect, acquired**   A
    Acquired septal atrial defect (old)
    Acquired septal auricular defect (old)
    Acquired septal ventricular defect (old)

      Excludes1   cardiac septal defect as current
         complication following acute
         myocardial infarction (I23.1, I23.2)

I51.1   **Rupture of chordae tendineae, not elsewhere classified**

      Excludes1   rupture of chordae tendineae as current
         complication following acute
         myocardial infarction (I23.4)

I51.2   **Rupture of papillary muscle, not elsewhere classified**

      Excludes1   rupture of papillary muscle as current
         complication following acute
         myocardial infarction (I23.5)

I51.3   **Intracardiac thrombosis, not elsewhere classified**
    Apical thrombosis (old)
    Atrial thrombosis (old)
    Auricular thrombosis (old)
    Mural thrombosis (old)
    Ventricular thrombosis (old)

      Excludes1   intracardiac thrombosis as current
         complication following acute
         myocardial infarction (I23.6)
    Coding Clinic: 2013, Q1, P24

I51.4   **Myocarditis, unspecified**
    Chronic (interstitial) myocarditis
    Myocardial fibrosis
    Myocarditis NOS

      Excludes1   acute or subacute myocarditis (I40.-)

I51.5   **Myocardial degeneration**
    Fatty degeneration of heart or myocardium
    Myocardial disease
    Senile degeneration of heart or myocardium

I51.7   **Cardiomegaly**
    Cardiac dilatation
    Cardiac hypertrophy
    Ventricular dilatation

● **I51.8**   **Other ill-defined heart diseases**

   I51.81   **Takotsubo syndrome**
      Reversible left ventricular dysfunction
        following sudden emotional stress
      Stress induced cardiomyopathy
      Takotsubo cardiomyopathy
      Transient left ventricular apical ballooning
        syndrome

   I51.89   **Other ill-defined heart diseases**
      Carditis (acute)(chronic)
      Pancarditis (acute)(chronic)

I51.9   **Heart disease, unspecified**

▷ **I52**   *Other heart disorders in diseases classified elsewhere*
    Code first underlying disease, such as:
    congenital syphilis (A50.5)
    mucopolysaccharidosis (E76.3)
    schistosomiasis (B65.0-B65.9)

    Excludes1   heart disease (in):
        gonococcal infection (A54.83)
        meningococcal infection (A39.50)
        rheumatoid arthritis (M05.31)
        syphilis (A52.06)

Item 9–8 Congestive heart failure (CHF) is a condition in which the
left ventricle of the heart cannot pump enough blood to the body. The blood
flow from the heart slows or returns to the heart from the venous system back
flow resulting in congestion (fluid accumulation) particularly in the abdomen.
Most commonly, fluid collects in the lungs and results in shortness of breath,
especially when in a reclining position.

Sidebar: CHAPTER 9 (I00-I99)

◀ New   ⬅ Revised   ~~deleted~~ Deleted   Excludes 1   Excludes 2   Includes   Use additional   Code first   Code also   Unspecified

OGCR Official Guidelines   X Assign placeholder X   ● Use Additional Character(s)   ▷ Manifestation Code   **Coding Clinic**

CEREBROVASCULAR DISEASES (I6Ø-I69)

Use additional code to identify presence of:
   alcohol abuse and dependence (F10.-)
   exposure to environmental tobacco smoke (Z77.22)
   history of tobacco dependence (Z87.891) ◄▥
   hypertension (I10-I15)
   occupational exposure to environmental tobacco smoke
     (Z57.31)
   tobacco dependence (F17.-)
   tobacco use (Z72.0)

> **Excludes1**   transient cerebral ischemic attacks and related
>   syndromes (G45.-)
>   traumatic intracranial hemorrhage (S06.-)

Coding Clinic: 2Ø15, Q4, P4Ø

● **I6Ø**   **Nontraumatic subarachnoid hemorrhage**
> **Includes**   ruptured cerebral aneurysm
> **Excludes1**   syphilitic ruptured cerebral aneurysm (A52.Ø5)
> **Excludes2**   sequelae of subarachnoid hemorrhage (I69.0-) ◄

● **I6Ø.Ø**   **Nontraumatic subarachnoid hemorrhage from carotid siphon and bifurcation**

   I6Ø.ØØ   **Nontraumatic subarachnoid hemorrhage from unspecified carotid siphon and bifurcation**

   I6Ø.Ø1   **Nontraumatic subarachnoid hemorrhage from right carotid siphon and bifurcation**

   I6Ø.Ø2   **Nontraumatic subarachnoid hemorrhage from left carotid siphon and bifurcation**

● **I6Ø.1**   **Nontraumatic subarachnoid hemorrhage from middle cerebral artery**

   I6Ø.1Ø   **Nontraumatic subarachnoid hemorrhage from unspecified middle cerebral artery**

   I6Ø.11   **Nontraumatic subarachnoid hemorrhage from right middle cerebral artery**

   I6Ø.12   **Nontraumatic subarachnoid hemorrhage from left middle cerebral artery**

I6Ø.2   **Nontraumatic subarachnoid hemorrhage from anterior communicating artery**

   ~~I6Ø.2Ø~~   ~~Nontraumatic subarachnoid hemorrhage from unspecified anterior communicating artery~~

   ~~I6Ø.21~~   ~~Nontraumatic subarachnoid hemorrhage from right anterior communicating artery~~

   ~~I6Ø.22~~   ~~Nontraumatic subarachnoid hemorrhage from left anterior communicating artery~~

● **I6Ø.3**   **Nontraumatic subarachnoid hemorrhage from posterior communicating artery**

   I6Ø.3Ø   **Nontraumatic subarachnoid hemorrhage from unspecified posterior communicating artery**

   I6Ø.31   **Nontraumatic subarachnoid hemorrhage from right posterior communicating artery**

   I6Ø.32   **Nontraumatic subarachnoid hemorrhage from left posterior communicating artery**

I6Ø.4   **Nontraumatic subarachnoid hemorrhage from basilar artery**

● **I6Ø.5**   **Nontraumatic subarachnoid hemorrhage from vertebral artery**

   I6Ø.5Ø   **Nontraumatic subarachnoid hemorrhage from unspecified vertebral artery**

   I6Ø.51   **Nontraumatic subarachnoid hemorrhage from right vertebral artery**

   I6Ø.52   **Nontraumatic subarachnoid hemorrhage from left vertebral artery**

I6Ø.6   **Nontraumatic subarachnoid hemorrhage from other intracranial arteries**

I6Ø.7   **Nontraumatic subarachnoid hemorrhage from unspecified intracranial artery**
   Ruptured (congenital) berry aneurysm
   Ruptured (congenital) cerebral aneurysm
   Subarachnoid hemorrhage (nontraumatic) from cerebral artery NOS
   Subarachnoid hemorrhage (nontraumatic) from communicating artery NOS

> **Excludes1**   berry aneurysm, nonruptured (I67.1)

I6Ø.8   **Other nontraumatic subarachnoid hemorrhage**
   Meningeal hemorrhage
   Rupture of cerebral arteriovenous malformation

I6Ø.9   **Nontraumatic subarachnoid hemorrhage, unspecified**

● **I61**   **Nontraumatic intracerebral hemorrhage**
> **Excludes2**   sequelae of intracerebral hemorrhage (I69.1-) ◄

I61.Ø   **Nontraumatic intracerebral hemorrhage in hemisphere, subcortical**
   Deep intracerebral hemorrhage (nontraumatic)

I61.1   **Nontraumatic intracerebral hemorrhage in hemisphere, cortical**
   Cerebral lobe hemorrhage (nontraumatic)
   Superficial intracerebral hemorrhage (nontraumatic)

I61.2   **Nontraumatic intracerebral hemorrhage in hemisphere, unspecified**

I61.3   **Nontraumatic intracerebral hemorrhage in brain stem**

I61.4   **Nontraumatic intracerebral hemorrhage in cerebellum**

I61.5   **Nontraumatic intracerebral hemorrhage, intraventricular**

I61.6   **Nontraumatic intracerebral hemorrhage, multiple localized**

I61.8   **Other nontraumatic intracerebral hemorrhage**

I61.9   **Nontraumatic intracerebral hemorrhage, unspecified**

● **I62**   **Other and unspecified nontraumatic intracranial hemorrhage**
> **Excludes2**   sequelae of intracranial hemorrhage (I69.2) ◄

● **I62.Ø**   **Nontraumatic subdural hemorrhage**

   I62.ØØ   **Nontraumatic subdural hemorrhage, unspecified**

   I62.Ø1   **Nontraumatic acute subdural hemorrhage**

   I62.Ø2   **Nontraumatic subacute subdural hemorrhage**

   I62.Ø3   **Nontraumatic chronic subdural hemorrhage**

I62.1   **Nontraumatic extradural hemorrhage**
   Nontraumatic epidural hemorrhage

I62.9   **Nontraumatic intracranial hemorrhage, unspecified**

★ **(See Plate 141 on page 76.)**

● **I63**   **Cerebral infarction**
> **Includes**   occlusion and stenosis of cerebral and precerebral arteries, resulting in cerebral infarction

Use additional code, if applicable, to identify status post administration of tPA (rtPA) in a different facility within the last 24 hours prior to admission to current facility (Z92.82)

Use additional code, if known, to indicate National Institutes of Health Stroke Scale (NIHSS) score (R29.7-) ◄

> **Excludes2**   sequelae of cerebral infarction (I69.3-) ◄

● **I63.Ø**   **Cerebral infarction due to thrombosis of precerebral arteries**

   I63.ØØ   **Cerebral infarction due to thrombosis of unspecified precerebral artery**

   ● **I63.Ø1**   **Cerebral infarction due to thrombosis of vertebral artery**

      I63.Ø11   **Cerebral infarction due to thrombosis of right vertebral artery**

      I63.Ø12   **Cerebral infarction due to thrombosis of left vertebral artery**

      I63.Ø13   **Cerebral infarction due to thrombosis of bilateral vertebral arteries** ◄

      I63.Ø19   **Cerebral infarction due to thrombosis of unspecified vertebral artery**

Cerebral
embolus

Cerebral
hemorrhage

Cerebral
thrombosis

Figure 9-4 Events causing a stroke. (From Shiland: Mastering Healthcare Terminology, ed 1, St. Louis, Mosby, 2003)

I63.02   Cerebral infarction due to thrombosis of basilar artery

● I63.03   Cerebral infarction due to thrombosis of carotid artery
  I63.031   Cerebral infarction due to thrombosis of right carotid artery
  I63.032   Cerebral infarction due to thrombosis of left carotid artery
  I63.033   Cerebral infarction due to thrombosis of bilateral carotid arteries ◀
  I63.039   Cerebral infarction due to thrombosis of unspecified carotid artery

I63.09   Cerebral infarction due to thrombosis of other precerebral artery

● I63.1   Cerebral infarction due to embolism of precerebral arteries
  I63.10   Cerebral infarction due to embolism of unspecified precerebral artery

● I63.11   Cerebral infarction due to embolism of vertebral artery
  I63.111   Cerebral infarction due to embolism of right vertebral artery
  I63.112   Cerebral infarction due to embolism of left vertebral artery
  I63.113   Cerebral infarction due to embolism of bilateral vertebral arteries ◀
  I63.119   Cerebral infarction due to embolism of unspecified vertebral artery

I63.12   Cerebral infarction due to embolism of basilar artery

● I63.13   Cerebral infarction due to embolism of carotid artery
  I63.131   Cerebral infarction due to embolism of right carotid artery
  I63.132   Cerebral infarction due to embolism of left carotid artery
  I63.133   Cerebral infarction due to embolism of bilateral carotid arteries ◀
  I63.139   Cerebral infarction due to embolism of unspecified carotid artery

I63.19   Cerebral infarction due to embolism of other precerebral artery

● I63.2   Cerebral infarction due to unspecified occlusion or stenosis of precerebral arteries
  I63.20   Cerebral infarction due to unspecified occlusion or stenosis of unspecified precerebral arteries

● I63.21   Cerebral infarction due to unspecified occlusion or stenosis of vertebral arteries
  I63.211   Cerebral infarction due to unspecified occlusion or stenosis of right vertebral arteries
  I63.212   Cerebral infarction due to unspecified occlusion or stenosis of left vertebral arteries
  I63.213   Cerebral infarction due to unspecified occlusion or stenosis of bilateral vertebral arteries ◀
  I63.219   Cerebral infarction due to unspecified occlusion or stenosis of unspecified vertebral arteries

I63.22   Cerebral infarction due to unspecified occlusion or stenosis of basilar arteries

● I63.23   Cerebral infarction due to unspecified occlusion or stenosis of carotid arteries
  I63.231   Cerebral infarction due to unspecified occlusion or stenosis of right carotid arteries
  I63.232   Cerebral infarction due to unspecified occlusion or stenosis of left carotid arteries
  I63.233   Cerebral infarction due to unspecified occlusion or stenosis of bilateral carotid arteries ◀
  I63.239   Cerebral infarction due to unspecified occlusion or stenosis of unspecified carotid arteries

I63.29   Cerebral infarction due to unspecified occlusion or stenosis of other precerebral arteries

● I63.3   Cerebral infarction due to thrombosis of cerebral arteries
  I63.30   Cerebral infarction due to thrombosis of unspecified cerebral artery

● I63.31   Cerebral infarction due to thrombosis of middle cerebral artery
  I63.311   Cerebral infarction due to thrombosis of right middle cerebral artery
  I63.312   Cerebral infarction due to thrombosis of left middle cerebral artery
  I63.313   Cerebral infarction due to thrombosis of bilateral middle cerebral arteries ◀
  I63.319   Cerebral infarction due to thrombosis of unspecified middle cerebral artery

● I63.32   Cerebral infarction due to thrombosis of anterior cerebral artery
  I63.321   Cerebral infarction due to thrombosis of right anterior cerebral artery
  I63.322   Cerebral infarction due to thrombosis of left anterior cerebral artery
  I63.323   Cerebral infarction due to thrombosis of bilateral anterior arteries ◀
  I63.329   Cerebral infarction due to thrombosis of unspecified anterior cerebral artery

● I63.33   Cerebral infarction due to thrombosis of posterior cerebral artery
  I63.331   Cerebral infarction due to thrombosis of right posterior cerebral artery
  I63.332   Cerebral infarction due to thrombosis of left posterior cerebral artery
  I63.333   Cerebral infarction to thrombosis of bilateral posterior arteries ◀
  I63.339   Cerebral infarction due to thrombosis of unspecified posterior cerebral artery

◀ New   ◀━ Revised   ̶d̶e̶l̶e̶t̶e̶d̶ Deleted   Excludes 1   Excludes 2   Includes   Use additional   Code first   Code also   Unspecified

866   OGCR Official Guidelines   X Assign placeholder X   ● Use Additional Character(s)   ▶ Manifestation Code   **Coding Clinic**

● **I63.34** Cerebral infarction due to thrombosis of cerebellar artery

    I63.341 Cerebral infarction due to thrombosis of right cerebellar artery

    I63.342 Cerebral infarction due to thrombosis of left cerebellar artery

    I63.343 Cerebral infarction to thrombosis of bilateral cerebellar arteries ◀

    I63.349 Cerebral infarction due to thrombosis of unspecified cerebellar artery

  I63.39 Cerebral infarction due to thrombosis of other cerebral artery

● **I63.4** Cerebral infarction due to embolism of cerebral arteries

  I63.40 Cerebral infarction due to embolism of unspecified cerebral artery

● **I63.41** Cerebral infarction due to embolism of middle cerebral artery

    I63.411 Cerebral infarction due to embolism of right middle cerebral artery

    I63.412 Cerebral infarction due to embolism of left middle cerebral artery

    I63.413 Cerebral infarction due to embolism of bilateral middle cerebral arteries ◀

    I63.419 Cerebral infarction due to embolism of unspecified middle cerebral artery

● **I63.42** Cerebral infarction due to embolism of anterior cerebral artery

    I63.421 Cerebral infarction due to embolism of right anterior cerebral artery

    I63.422 Cerebral infarction due to embolism of left anterior cerebral artery

    I63.423 Cerebral infarction due to embolism of bilateral anterior cerebral arteries ◀

    I63.429 Cerebral infarction due to embolism of unspecified anterior cerebral artery

● **I63.43** Cerebral infarction due to embolism of posterior cerebral artery

    I63.431 Cerebral infarction due to embolism of right posterior cerebral artery

    I63.432 Cerebral infarction due to embolism of left posterior cerebral artery

    I63.433 Cerebral infarction due to embolism of bilateral posterior cerebral arteries ◀

    I63.439 Cerebral infarction due to embolism of unspecified posterior cerebral artery

● **I63.44** Cerebral infarction due to embolism of cerebellar artery

    I63.441 Cerebral infarction due to embolism of right cerebellar artery

    I63.442 Cerebral infarction due to embolism of left cerebellar artery

    I63.443 Cerebral infarction due to embolism of bilateral cerebellar arteries ◀

    I63.449 Cerebral infarction due to embolism of unspecified cerebellar artery

  I63.49 Cerebral infarction due to embolism of other cerebral artery

● **I63.5** Cerebral infarction due to unspecified occlusion or stenosis of cerebral arteries

  I63.50 Cerebral infarction due to unspecified occlusion or stenosis of unspecified cerebral artery

● **I63.51** Cerebral infarction due to unspecified occlusion or stenosis of middle cerebral artery

    I63.511 Cerebral infarction due to unspecified occlusion or stenosis of right middle cerebral artery

    I63.512 Cerebral infarction due to unspecified occlusion or stenosis of left middle cerebral artery

    I63.513 Cerebral infarction due to unspecified occlusion or stenosis of bilateral middle arteries ◀

    I63.519 Cerebral infarction due to unspecified occlusion or stenosis of unspecified middle cerebral artery

● **I63.52** Cerebral infarction due to unspecified occlusion or stenosis of anterior cerebral artery

    I63.521 Cerebral infarction due to unspecified occlusion or stenosis of right anterior cerebral artery

    I63.522 Cerebral infarction due to unspecified occlusion or stenosis of left anterior cerebral artery

    I63.523 Cerebral infarction due to unspecified occlusion or stenosis of bilateral anterior arteries ◀

    I63.529 Cerebral infarction due to unspecified occlusion or stenosis of unspecified anterior cerebral artery

● **I63.53** Cerebral infarction due to unspecified occlusion or stenosis of posterior cerebral artery

    I63.531 Cerebral infarction due to unspecified occlusion or stenosis of right posterior cerebral artery

    I63.532 Cerebral infarction due to unspecified occlusion or stenosis of left posterior cerebral artery

    I63.533 Cerebral infarction due to unspecified occlusion or stenosis of bilateral posterior arteries ◀

    I63.539 Cerebral infarction due to unspecified occlusion or stenosis of unspecified posterior cerebral artery

● **I63.54** Cerebral infarction due to unspecified occlusion or stenosis of cerebellar artery

    I63.541 Cerebral infarction due to unspecified occlusion or stenosis of right cerebellar artery

    I63.542 Cerebral infarction due to unspecified occlusion or stenosis of left cerebellar artery

    I63.543 Cerebral infarction due to unspecified occlusion or stenosis of bilateral cerebellar arteries ◀

    I63.549 Cerebral infarction due to unspecified occlusion or stenosis of unspecified cerebellar artery

  I63.59 Cerebral infarction due to unspecified occlusion or stenosis of other cerebral artery

I63.6 Cerebral infarction due to cerebral venous thrombosis, nonpyogenic

I63.8 Other cerebral infarction

I63.9 Cerebral infarction, unspecified
    Stroke NOS
    Coding Clinic: 2015, Q1, P26

CHAPTER 9 (I00–I99)

● **I65** **Occlusion and stenosis of precerebral arteries, not resulting in cerebral infarction**

    Includes   embolism of precerebral artery
            narrowing of precerebral artery
            obstruction (complete) (partial) of precerebral artery
            thrombosis of precerebral artery

    Excludes1   insufficiency, NOS, of precerebral artery (G45.-)
            insufficiency of precerebral arteries causing cerebral infarction (I63.0-I63.2)

● **I65.0** **Occlusion and stenosis of vertebral artery**
    I65.01 Occlusion and stenosis of right vertebral artery
    I65.02 Occlusion and stenosis of left vertebral artery
    I65.03 Occlusion and stenosis of bilateral vertebral arteries
    I65.09 Occlusion and stenosis of unspecified vertebral artery

I65.1 **Occlusion and stenosis of basilar artery**

● **I65.2** **Occlusion and stenosis of carotid artery**
    I65.21 Occlusion and stenosis of right carotid artery
    I65.22 Occlusion and stenosis of left carotid artery
    I65.23 Occlusion and stenosis of bilateral carotid arteries
    I65.29 Occlusion and stenosis of unspecified carotid artery

I65.8 **Occlusion and stenosis of other precerebral arteries**

I65.9 **Occlusion and stenosis of unspecified precerebral artery**
    Occlusion and stenosis of precerebral artery NOS

● **I66** **Occlusion and stenosis of cerebral arteries, not resulting in cerebral infarction**

    Includes   embolism of cerebral artery
            narrowing of cerebral artery
            obstruction (complete) (partial) of cerebral artery
            thrombosis of cerebral artery

    Excludes1   occlusion and stenosis of cerebral artery causing cerebral infarction (I63.3-I63.5)

● **I66.0** **Occlusion and stenosis of middle cerebral artery**
    I66.01 Occlusion and stenosis of right middle cerebral artery
    I66.02 Occlusion and stenosis of left middle cerebral artery
    I66.03 Occlusion and stenosis of bilateral middle cerebral arteries
    I66.09 Occlusion and stenosis of unspecified middle cerebral artery

● **I66.1** **Occlusion and stenosis of anterior cerebral artery**
    I66.11 Occlusion and stenosis of right anterior cerebral artery
    I66.12 Occlusion and stenosis of left anterior cerebral artery
    I66.13 Occlusion and stenosis of bilateral anterior cerebral arteries
    I66.19 Occlusion and stenosis of unspecified anterior cerebral artery

● **I66.2** **Occlusion and stenosis of posterior cerebral artery**
    I66.21 Occlusion and stenosis of right posterior cerebral artery
    I66.22 Occlusion and stenosis of left posterior cerebral artery
    I66.23 Occlusion and stenosis of bilateral posterior cerebral arteries
    I66.29 Occlusion and stenosis of unspecified posterior cerebral artery

I66.3 **Occlusion and stenosis of cerebellar arteries**

I66.8 **Occlusion and stenosis of other cerebral arteries**
    Occlusion and stenosis of perforating arteries

I66.9 **Occlusion and stenosis of unspecified cerebral artery**

● **I67** **Other cerebrovascular diseases**

    Excludes2   sequelae of the listed conditions (I69.8) ◄

I67.0 **Dissection of cerebral arteries, nonruptured**
    Excludes1   ruptured cerebral arteries (I60.7)

I67.1 **Cerebral aneurysm, nonruptured**
    Cerebral aneurysm NOS
    Cerebral arteriovenous fistula, acquired
    Internal carotid artery aneurysm, intracranial portion
    Internal carotid artery aneurysm, NOS
    Excludes1   congenital cerebral aneurysm, nonruptured (Q28.-)
            ruptured cerebral aneurysm (I60.7)

I67.2 **Cerebral atherosclerosis**
    Atheroma of cerebral and precerebral arteries

I67.3 **Progressive vascular leukoencephalopathy**
    Binswanger's disease

I67.4 **Hypertensive encephalopathy**

I67.5 **Moyamoya disease**

I67.6 **Nonpyogenic thrombosis of intracranial venous system**
    Nonpyogenic thrombosis of cerebral vein
    Nonpyogenic thrombosis of intracranial venous sinus
    Excludes1   nonpyogenic thrombosis of intracranial venous system causing infarction (I63.6)

I67.7 **Cerebral arteritis, not elsewhere classified**
    Granulomatous angiitis of the nervous system
    Excludes1   allergic granulomatous angiitis (M30.1)

● **I67.8** **Other specified cerebrovascular diseases**
    I67.81 **Acute cerebrovascular insufficiency**
         Acute cerebrovascular insufficiency unspecified as to location or reversibility
    I67.82 **Cerebral ischemia**
         Chronic cerebral ischemia
    I67.83 **Posterior reversible encephalopathy syndrome**
         PRES
    ● **I67.84** **Cerebral vasospasm and vasoconstriction**
        I67.841 **Reversible cerebrovascular vasoconstriction syndrome**
             Call-Fleming syndrome
             Code first underlying condition, if applicable, such as eclampsia (O15.00-O15.9)
        I67.848 **Other cerebrovascular vasospasm and vasoconstriction**
    I67.89 **Other cerebrovascular disease**

I67.9 **Cerebrovascular disease, unspecified**

● **I68** **Cerebrovascular disorders in diseases classified elsewhere**

▌ *I68.0* *Cerebral amyloid angiopathy*
    Code first underlying amyloidosis (E85.-)

▌ *I68.2* *Cerebral arteritis in other diseases classified elsewhere*
    Code first underlying disease
    Excludes1   cerebral arteritis (in):
            listerosis (A32.89)
            systemic lupus erythematosus (M32.19)
            syphilis (A52.04)
            tuberculosis (A18.89)

▌ *I68.8* *Other cerebrovascular disorders in diseases classified elsewhere*
    Code first underlying disease
    Excludes1   syphilitic cerebral aneurysm (A52.05)

◄ New   ◄▌ Revised   ~~deleted~~ Deleted   Excludes 1   Excludes 2   Includes   Use additional   Code first   Code also   Unspecified
OGCR Official Guidelines   X Assign placeholder X   ● Use Additional Character(s)   ▌ Manifestation Code   **Coding Clinic**

OGCR Section I.c.9.d.

Sequelae of Cerebrovascular Disease

1) Category I69, Sequelae of Cerebrovascular disease

Category I69 is used to indicate conditions classifiable to categories I60-I67 as the causes of sequela (neurologic deficits), themselves classified elsewhere. These "late effects" include neurologic deficits that persist after initial onset of conditions classifiable to categories I60-I67. The neurologic deficits caused by cerebrovascular disease may be present from the onset of may arise at any time after the onset of the condition classifiable to categories I60-I67.

Codes from category I69, Sequelae of cerebrovascular disease, that specify hemiplegia, hemiparesis and monoplegia identify whether the dominant or nondominant side is affected. Should the affected side be documented, but not specified as dominant or nondominant, and the classification system does not indicate a default, code selection is as follows:

For ambidextrous patients, the default should be dominant.

If the left side is affected, the default is non-dominant.

If the right side is affected, the default is dominant.

2) Codes from category I69 with codes from I60-I67

Codes from category I69 may be assigned on a health care record with codes from I60-I67, if the patient has a current cerebrovascular disease and deficits from an old cerebrovascular disease.

● **I69**   **Sequelae of cerebrovascular disease**

     Note: Category I69 is to be used to indicate conditions in I60-I67 as the cause of sequelae. The 'sequelae' include conditions specified as such or as residuals which may occur at any time after the onset of the causal condition.

     Excludes1   personal history of cerebral infarction without residual deficit (Z86.73)

            personal history of prolonged reversible ischemic neurologic deficit (PRIND) (Z86.73)

            personal history of reversible ischemic neurolgcial deficit (RIND) (Z86.73)

            sequelae of traumatic intracranial injury (S06.-)

            transient ischemic attack (TIA) (G45.9)

     Coding Clinic: 2015, Q4, P40; 2012, Q4, P107

● **I69.Ø**   **Sequelae of nontraumatic subarachnoid hemorrhage**

     I69.ØØ   **Unspecified sequelae of nontraumatic subarachnoid hemorrhage**

     ● **I69.Ø1**   **Cognitive deficits following nontraumatic subarachnoid hemorrhage**

         I69.Ø1Ø   **Attention and concentration deficit following nontraumatic subarachnoid hemorrhage** ◄

         I69.Ø11   **Memory deficit following nontraumatic subarachnoid hemorrhage** ◄

         I69.Ø12   **Visuospatial deficit and spatial neglect following nontraumatic subarachnoid hemorrhage** ◄

         I69.Ø13   **Psychomotor deficit following nontraumatic subarachnoid hemorrhage** ◄

         I69.Ø14   **Frontal lobe and executive function deficit following nontraumatic subarachnoid hemorrhage** ◄

         I69.Ø15   **Cognitive social or emotional deficit following nontraumatic subarachnoid hemorrhage** ◄

         I69.Ø18   **Other symptoms and signs involving cognitive functions following nontraumatic subarachnoid hemorrhage** ◄

         I69.Ø19   **Unspecified symptoms and signs involving cognitive functions following nontraumatic subarachnoid hemorrhage** ◄

● **I69.Ø2**   **Speech and language deficits following nontraumatic subarachnoid hemorrhage**

     I69.Ø2Ø   **Aphasia following nontraumatic subarachnoid hemorrhage**

     I69.Ø21   **Dysphasia following nontraumatic subarachnoid hemorrhage**

     I69.Ø22   **Dysarthria following nontraumatic subarachnoid hemorrhage**

     I69.Ø23   **Fluency disorder following nontraumatic subarachnoid hemorrhage**

         Stuttering following nontraumatic subarachnoid hemorrhage

     I69.Ø28   **Other speech and language deficits following nontraumatic subarachnoid hemorrhage**

● **I69.Ø3**   **Monoplegia of upper limb following nontraumatic subarachnoid hemorrhage**

     I69.Ø31   **Monoplegia of upper limb following nontraumatic subarachnoid hemorrhage affecting right dominant side**

     I69.Ø32   **Monoplegia of upper limb following nontraumatic subarachnoid hemorrhage affecting left dominant side**

     I69.Ø33   **Monoplegia of upper limb following nontraumatic subarachnoid hemorrhage affecting right non-dominant side**

     I69.Ø34   **Monoplegia of upper limb following nontraumatic subarachnoid hemorrhage affecting left non-dominant side**

     I69.Ø39   **Monoplegia of upper limb following nontraumatic subarachnoid hemorrhage affecting unspecified side**

● **I69.Ø4**   **Monoplegia of lower limb following nontraumatic subarachnoid hemorrhage**

     I69.Ø41   **Monoplegia of lower limb following nontraumatic subarachnoid hemorrhage affecting right dominant side**

     I69.Ø42   **Monoplegia of lower limb following nontraumatic subarachnoid hemorrhage affecting left dominant side**

     I69.Ø43   **Monoplegia of lower limb following nontraumatic subarachnoid hemorrhage affecting right non-dominant side**

     I69.Ø44   **Monoplegia of lower limb following nontraumatic subarachnoid hemorrhage affecting left non-dominant side**

     I69.Ø49   **Monoplegia of lower limb following nontraumatic subarachnoid hemorrhage affecting unspecified side**

● I69.05   Hemiplegia and hemiparesis following
            nontraumatic subarachnoid hemorrhage
            I69.051   Hemiplegia and hemiparesis
                       following nontraumatic subarachnoid
                       hemorrhage affecting right dominant
                       side
            I69.052   Hemiplegia and hemiparesis
                       following nontraumatic subarachnoid
                       hemorrhage affecting left dominant
                       side
            I69.053   Hemiplegia and hemiparesis
                       following nontraumatic subarachnoid
                       hemorrhage affecting right non-
                       dominant side
            I69.054   Hemiplegia and hemiparesis
                       following nontraumatic subarachnoid
                       hemorrhage affecting left non-
                       dominant side
            I69.059   Hemiplegia and hemiparesis
                       following nontraumatic subarachnoid
                       hemorrhage affecting unspecified side

● I69.06   Other paralytic syndrome following
            nontraumatic subarachnoid hemorrhage
            Use additional code to identify type of
              paralytic syndrome, such as:
              locked-in state (G83.5)
              quadriplegia (G82.5-)

            Excludes1   hemiplegia/hemiparesis
                         following nontraumatic
                         subarachnoid hemorrhage
                         (I69.05-)
                         monoplegia of lower limb
                         following nontraumatic
                         subarachnoid hemorrhage
                         (I69.04-)
                         monoplegia of upper limb
                         following nontraumatic
                         subarachnoid hemorrhage
                         (I69.03-)

            I69.061   Other paralytic syndrome following
                       nontraumatic subarachnoid
                       hemorrhage affecting right dominant
                       side
            I69.062   Other paralytic syndrome following
                       nontraumatic subarachnoid
                       hemorrhage affecting left dominant
                       side
            I69.063   Other paralytic syndrome following
                       nontraumatic subarachnoid
                       hemorrhage affecting right non-
                       dominant side
            I69.064   Other paralytic syndrome following
                       nontraumatic subarachnoid
                       hemorrhage affecting left non-
                       dominant side
            I69.065   Other paralytic syndrome following
                       nontraumatic subarachnoid
                       hemorrhage, bilateral
            I69.069   Other paralytic syndrome following
                       nontraumatic subarachnoid
                       hemorrhage affecting unspecified side

● I69.09   Other sequelae of nontraumatic subarachnoid
            hemorrhage
            I69.090   Apraxia following nontraumatic
                       subarachnoid hemorrhage
            I69.091   Dysphagia following nontraumatic
                       subarachnoid hemorrhage
                       Use additional code to identify the
                         type of dysphagia, if known
                         (R13.1-)
            I69.092   Facial weakness following
                       nontraumatic subarachnoid
                       hemorrhage
                       Facial droop following nontraumatic
                         subarachnoid hemorrhage
            I69.093   Ataxia following nontraumatic
                       subarachnoid hemorrhage
            I69.098   Other sequelae following
                       nontraumatic subarachnoid
                       hemorrhage
                       Alterations of sensation following
                         nontraumatic subarachnoid
                         hemorrhage
                       Disturbance of vision following
                         nontraumatic subarachnoid
                         hemorrhage
                       Use additional code to identify the
                         sequelae

● I69.1   Sequelae of nontraumatic intracerebral hemorrhage
            I69.10   Unspecified sequelae of nontraumatic
                       intracerebral hemorrhage
● I69.11   Cognitive deficits following nontraumatic
            intracerebral hemorrhage
            I69.110   Attention and concentration deficit
                       following nontraumatic intracerebral
                       hemorrhage ◄
            I69.111   Memory deficit following
                       nontraumatic intracerebral
                       hemorrhage ◄
            I69.112   Visuospatial deficit and spatial
                       neglect following nontraumatic
                       intracerebral hemorrhage ◄
            I69.113   Psychomotor deficit following
                       nontraumatic intracerebral
                       hemorrhage ◄
            I69.114   Frontal lobe and executive function
                       deficit following nontraumatic
                       intracerebral hemorrhage ◄
            I69.115   Cognitive social or emotional deficit
                       following nontraumatic intracerebral
                       hemorrhage ◄
            I69.118   Other symptoms and signs involving
                       cognitive functions following
                       nontraumatic intracerebral
                       hemorrhage ◄
            I69.119   Unspecified symptoms and signs
                       involving cognitive functions
                       following nontraumatic intracerebral
                       hemorrhage ◄
● I69.12   Speech and language deficits following
            nontraumatic intracerebral hemorrhage
            I69.120   Aphasia following nontraumatic
                       intracerebral hemorrhage
            I69.121   Dysphasia following nontraumatic
                       intracerebral hemorrhage
            I69.122   Dysarthria following nontraumatic
                       intracerebral hemorrhage
            I69.123   Fluency disorder following
                       nontraumatic intracerebral
                       hemorrhage
                       Stuttering following nontraumatic
                         intracerebral hemorrhage ◄▥
            I69.128   Other speech and language deficits
                       following nontraumatic intracerebral
                       hemorrhage

CHAPTER 9 (I00-I99)

● **I69.13** **Monoplegia of upper limb following nontraumatic intracerebral hemorrhage**

    I69.131 **Monoplegia of upper limb following nontraumatic intracerebral hemorrhage affecting right dominant side**

    I69.132 **Monoplegia of upper limb following nontraumatic intracerebral hemorrhage affecting left dominant side**

    I69.133 **Monoplegia of upper limb following nontraumatic intracerebral hemorrhage affecting right non-dominant side**

    I69.134 **Monoplegia of upper limb following nontraumatic intracerebral hemorrhage affecting left non-dominant side**

    I69.139 **Monoplegia of upper limb following nontraumatic intracerebral hemorrhage affecting unspecified side**

● **I69.14** **Monoplegia of lower limb following nontraumatic intracerebral hemorrhage**

    I69.141 **Monoplegia of lower limb following nontraumatic intracerebral hemorrhage affecting right dominant side**

    I69.142 **Monoplegia of lower limb following nontraumatic intracerebral hemorrhage affecting left dominant side**

    I69.143 **Monoplegia of lower limb following nontraumatic intracerebral hemorrhage affecting right non-dominant side**

    I69.144 **Monoplegia of lower limb following nontraumatic intracerebral hemorrhage affecting left non-dominant side**

    I69.149 **Monoplegia of lower limb following nontraumatic intracerebral hemorrhage affecting unspecified side**

● **I69.15** **Hemiplegia and hemiparesis following nontraumatic intracerebral hemorrhage**

    I69.151 **Hemiplegia and hemiparesis following nontraumatic intracerebral hemorrhage affecting right dominant side**

    I69.152 **Hemiplegia and hemiparesis following nontraumatic intracerebral hemorrhage affecting left dominant side**

    I69.153 **Hemiplegia and hemiparesis following nontraumatic intracerebral hemorrhage affecting right non-dominant side**

    I69.154 **Hemiplegia and hemiparesis following nontraumatic intracerebral hemorrhage affecting left non-dominant side**

    I69.159 **Hemiplegia and hemiparesis following nontraumatic intracerebral hemorrhage affecting unspecified side**

● **I69.16** **Other paralytic syndrome following nontraumatic intracerebral hemorrhage**

    Use additional code to identify type of paralytic syndrome, such as:
    locked-in state (G83.5)
    quadriplegia (G82.5-)

    Excludes1 hemiplegia/hemiparesis following nontraumatic intracerebral hemorrhage (I69.15-)
        monoplegia of lower limb following nontraumatic intracerebral hemorrhage (I69.14-)
        monoplegia of upper limb following nontraumatic intracerebral hemorrhage (I69.13-)

    I69.161 **Other paralytic syndrome following nontraumatic intracerebral hemorrhage affecting right dominant side**

    I69.162 **Other paralytic syndrome following nontraumatic intracerebral hemorrhage affecting left dominant side**

    I69.163 **Other paralytic syndrome following nontraumatic intracerebral hemorrhage affecting right non-dominant side**

    I69.164 **Other paralytic syndrome following nontraumatic intracerebral hemorrhage affecting left non-dominant side**

    I69.165 **Other paralytic syndrome following nontraumatic intracerebral hemorrhage, bilateral**

    I69.169 **Other paralytic syndrome following nontraumatic intracerebral hemorrhage affecting unspecified side**

● **I69.19** **Other sequelae of nontraumatic intracerebral hemorrhage**

    I69.190 **Apraxia following nontraumatic intracerebral hemorrhage**

    I69.191 **Dysphagia following nontraumatic intracerebral hemorrhage**

        Use additional code to identify the type of dysphagia, if known (R13.1-)

    I69.192 **Facial weakness following nontraumatic intracerebral hemorrhage**

        Facial droop following nontraumatic intracerebral hemorrhage

    I69.193 **Ataxia following nontraumatic intracerebral hemorrhage**

    I69.198 **Other sequelae of nontraumatic intracerebral hemorrhage**

        Alteration of sensations following nontraumatic intracerebral hemorrhage
        Disturbance of vision following nontraumatic intracerebral hemorrhage

        Use additional code to identify the sequelae

CHAPTER 9 (I00-I99)

● **I69.2**   **Sequelae of other nontraumatic intracranial hemorrhage**

    I69.20   Unspecified sequelae of other nontraumatic intracranial hemorrhage

●   **I69.21**   **Cognitive deficits following other nontraumatic intracranial hemorrhage**

       I69.210   Attention and concentration deficit following other nontraumatic intracranial hemorrhage ◀

       I69.211   Memory deficit following other nontraumatic intracranial hemorrhage ◀

       I69.212   Visuospatial deficit and spatial neglect following other nontraumatic intracranial hemorrhage ◀

       I69.213   Psychomotor deficit following other nontraumatic intracranial hemorrhage ◀

       I69.214   Frontal lobe and executive function deficit following other nontraumatic intracranial hemorrhage ◀

       I69.215   Cognitive social or emotional deficit following other nontraumatic intracranial hemorrhage ◀

       I69.218   Other symptoms and signs involving cognitive functions following other nontraumatic intracranial hemorrhage ◀

       I69.219   Unspecified symptoms and signs involving cognitive functions following other nontraumatic intracranial hemorrhage ◀

●   **I69.22**   **Speech and language deficits following other nontraumatic intracranial hemorrhage**

       I69.220   Aphasia following other nontraumatic intracranial hemorrhage

       I69.221   Dysphasia following other nontraumatic intracranial hemorrhage

       I69.222   Dysarthria following other nontraumatic intracranial hemorrhage

       I69.223   Fluency disorder following other nontraumatic intracranial hemorrhage

         Stuttering following other nontraumatic intracranial hemorrhage ◀▥

       I69.228   Other speech and language deficits following other nontraumatic intracranial hemorrhage

●   **I69.23**   **Monoplegia of upper limb following other nontraumatic intracranial hemorrhage**

       I69.231   Monoplegia of upper limb following other nontraumatic intracranial hemorrhage affecting right dominant side

       I69.232   Monoplegia of upper limb following other nontraumatic intracranial hemorrhage affecting left dominant side

       I69.233   Monoplegia of upper limb following other nontraumatic intracranial hemorrhage affecting right non-dominant side

       I69.234   Monoplegia of upper limb following other nontraumatic intracranial hemorrhage affecting left non-dominant side

       I69.239   Monoplegia of upper limb following other nontraumatic intracranial hemorrhage affecting unspecified side

●   **I69.24**   **Monoplegia of lower limb following other nontraumatic intracranial hemorrhage**

       I69.241   Monoplegia of lower limb following other nontraumatic intracranial hemorrhage affecting right dominant side

       I69.242   Monoplegia of lower limb following other nontraumatic intracranial hemorrhage affecting left dominant side

       I69.243   Monoplegia of lower limb following other nontraumatic intracranial hemorrhage affecting right non-dominant side

       I69.244   Monoplegia of lower limb following other nontraumatic intracranial hemorrhage affecting left non-dominant side

       I69.249   Monoplegia of lower limb following other nontraumatic intracranial hemorrhage affecting unspecified side

●   **I69.25**   **Hemiplegia and hemiparesis following other nontraumatic intracranial hemorrhage**

       I69.251   Hemiplegia and hemiparesis following other nontraumatic intracranial hemorrhage affecting right dominant side

       I69.252   Hemiplegia and hemiparesis following other nontraumatic intracranial hemorrhage affecting left dominant side

       I69.253   Hemiplegia and hemiparesis following other nontraumatic intracranial hemorrhage affecting right non-dominant side

       I69.254   Hemiplegia and hemiparesis following other nontraumatic intracranial hemorrhage affecting left non-dominant side

       I69.259   Hemiplegia and hemiparesis following other nontraumatic intracranial hemorrhage affecting unspecified side

●   **I69.26**   **Other paralytic syndrome following other nontraumatic intracranial hemorrhage**

      Use additional code to identify type of paralytic syndrome, such as:
        locked-in state (G83.5)
        quadriplegia (G82.5-)

      Excludes1   hemiplegia/hemiparesis following other nontraumatic intracranial hemorrhage (I69.25-)
         monoplegia of lower limb following other nontraumatic intracranial hemorrhage (I69.24-)
         monoplegia of upper limb following other nontraumatic intracranial hemorrhage (I69.23-)

       I69.261   Other paralytic syndrome following other nontraumatic intracranial hemorrhage affecting right dominant side

       I69.262   Other paralytic syndrome following other nontraumatic intracranial hemorrhage affecting left dominant side

---

I69.263   Other paralytic syndrome following other nontraumatic intracranial hemorrhage affecting right non-dominant side

I69.264   Other paralytic syndrome following other nontraumatic intracranial hemorrhage affecting left non-dominant side

I69.265   Other paralytic syndrome following other nontraumatic intracranial hemorrhage, bilateral

I69.269   Other paralytic syndrome following other nontraumatic intracranial hemorrhage affecting unspecified side

● I69.29   Other sequelae of other nontraumatic intracranial hemorrhage

I69.290   Apraxia following other nontraumatic intracranial hemorrhage

I69.291   Dysphagia following other nontraumatic intracranial hemorrhage

      Use additional code to identify the type of dysphagia, if known (R13.1-)

I69.292   Facial weakness following other nontraumatic intracranial hemorrhage

      Facial droop following other nontraumatic intracranial hemorrhage

I69.293   Ataxia following other nontraumatic intracranial hemorrhage

I69.298   Other sequelae of other nontraumatic intracranial hemorrhage

      Alteration of sensation following other nontraumatic intracranial hemorrhage

      Disturbance of vision following other nontraumatic intracranial hemorrhage

      Use additional code to identify the sequelae

● I69.3   Sequelae of cerebral infarction

      Sequelae of stroke NOS

      Coding Clinic: 2012, Q4, P92, 95

I69.30   Unspecified sequelae of cerebral infarction

● I69.31   Cognitive deficits following cerebral infarction

I69.310   Attention and concentration deficit following cerebral infarction ◄

I69.311   Memory deficit following cerebral infarction ◄

I69.312   Visuospatial deficit and spatial neglect following cerebral infarction ◄

I69.313   Psychomotor deficit following cerebral infarction ◄

I69.314   Frontal lobe and executive function deficit following cerebral infarction ◄

I69.315   Cognitive social or emotional deficit following cerebral infarction ◄

I69.318   Other symptoms and signs involving cognitive functions following cerebral infarction ◄

I69.319   Unspecified symptoms and signs involving cognitive functions following cerebral infarction ◄

● I69.32   Speech and language deficits following cerebral infarction

I69.320   Aphasia following cerebral infarction

I69.321   Dysphasia following cerebral infarction

      Coding Clinic: 2012, Q4, P91

I69.322   Dysarthria following cerebral infarction

I69.323   Fluency disorder following cerebral infarction

      Stuttering following cerebral infarction ◄

I69.328   Other speech and language deficits following cerebral infarction

● I69.33   Monoplegia of upper limb following cerebral infarction

I69.331   Monoplegia of upper limb following cerebral infarction affecting right dominant side

I69.332   Monoplegia of upper limb following cerebral infarction affecting left dominant side

I69.333   Monoplegia of upper limb following cerebral infarction affecting right non-dominant side

I69.334   Monoplegia of upper limb following cerebral infarction affecting left non-dominant side

I69.339   Monoplegia of upper limb following cerebral infarction affecting unspecified side

● I69.34   Monoplegia of lower limb following cerebral infarction

I69.341   Monoplegia of lower limb following cerebral infarction affecting right dominant side

I69.342   Monoplegia of lower limb following cerebral infarction affecting left dominant side

I69.343   Monoplegia of lower limb following cerebral infarction affecting right non-dominant side

I69.344   Monoplegia of lower limb following cerebral infarction affecting left non-dominant side

I69.349   Monoplegia of lower limb following cerebral infarction affecting unspecified side

● I69.35   Hemiplegia and hemiparesis following cerebral infarction

I69.351   Hemiplegia and hemiparesis following cerebral infarction affecting right dominant side

      Coding Clinic: 2015, Q1, P25

I69.352   Hemiplegia and hemiparesis following cerebral infarction affecting left dominant side

I69.353   Hemiplegia and hemiparesis following cerebral infarction affecting right non-dominant side

I69.354   Hemiplegia and hemiparesis following cerebral infarction affecting left non-dominant side

      Coding Clinic: 2012, Q4, P91

I69.359   Hemiplegia and hemiparesis following cerebral infarction affecting unspecified side

CHAPTER 9 (I00-I99)

● **I69.36 Other paralytic syndrome following cerebral infarction**

    Use additional code to identify type of paralytic syndrome, such as:
        locked-in state (G83.5)
        quadriplegia (G82.5-)

    Excludes1 hemiplegia/hemiparesis following cerebral infarction (I69.35-)
          monoplegia of lower limb following cerebral infarction (I69.34-)
          monoplegia of upper limb following cerebral infarction (I69.33-)

    I69.361   **Other paralytic syndrome following cerebral infarction affecting right dominant side**

    I69.362   **Other paralytic syndrome following cerebral infarction affecting left dominant side**

    I69.363   **Other paralytic syndrome following cerebral infarction affecting right non-dominant side**

    I69.364   **Other paralytic syndrome following cerebral infarction affecting left non-dominant side**

    I69.365   **Other paralytic syndrome following cerebral infarction, bilateral**

    I69.369   **Other paralytic syndrome following cerebral infarction affecting unspecified side**

● **I69.39 Other sequelae of cerebral infarction**

    I69.390   **Apraxia following cerebral infarction**

    I69.391   **Dysphagia following cerebral infarction**

        Use additional code to identify the type of dysphagia, if known (R13.1-)

    I69.392   **Facial weakness following cerebral infarction**
        Facial droop following cerebral infarction

    I69.393   **Ataxia following cerebral infarction**

    I69.398   **Other sequelae of cerebral infarction**
        Alteration of sensation following cerebral infarction
        Disturbance of vision following cerebral infarction
        Use additional code to identify the sequelae

● **I69.8 Sequelae of other cerebrovascular diseases**

    Excludes1 sequelae of traumatic intracranial injury (S06.-)

  I69.80   **Unspecified sequelae of other cerebrovascular disease**

● I69.81 **Cognitive deficits following other cerebrovascular disease**

    I69.810   **Attention and concentration deficit following other cerebrovascular disease** ◄

    I69.811   **Memory deficit following other cerebrovascular disease** ◄

    I69.812   **Visuospatial deficit and spatial neglect following other cerebrovascular disease** ◄

    I69.813   **Psychomotor deficit following other cerebrovascular disease** ◄

    I69.814   **Frontal lobe and executive function deficit following other cerebrovascular disease** ◄

    I69.815   **Cognitive social or emotional deficit following other cerebrovascular disease** ◄

    I69.818   **Other symptoms and signs involving cognitive functions following other cerebrovascular disease** ◄

    I69.819   **Unspecified symptoms and signs involving cognitive functions following other cerebrovascular disease** ◄

● **I69.82 Speech and language deficits following other cerebrovascular disease**

    I69.820   **Aphasia following other cerebrovascular disease**

    I69.821   **Dysphasia following other cerebrovascular disease**

    I69.822   **Dysarthria following other cerebrovascular disease**

    I69.823   **Fluency disorder following other cerebrovascular disease**
        Stuttering following other cerebrovascular disease ◄▪▪▪

    I69.828   **Other speech and language deficits following other cerebrovascular disease**

● **I69.83 Monoplegia of upper limb following other cerebrovascular disease**

    I69.831   **Monoplegia of upper limb following other cerebrovascular disease affecting right dominant side**

    I69.832   **Monoplegia of upper limb following other cerebrovascular disease affecting left dominant side**

    I69.833   **Monoplegia of upper limb following other cerebrovascular disease affecting right non-dominant side**

    I69.834   **Monoplegia of upper limb following other cerebrovascular disease affecting left non-dominant side**

    I69.839   **Monoplegia of upper limb following other cerebrovascular disease affecting unspecified side**

● **I69.84 Monoplegia of lower limb following other cerebrovascular disease**

    I69.841   **Monoplegia of lower limb following other cerebrovascular disease affecting right dominant side**

    I69.842   **Monoplegia of lower limb following other cerebrovascular disease affecting left dominant side**

    I69.843   **Monoplegia of lower limb following other cerebrovascular disease affecting right non-dominant side**

    I69.844   **Monoplegia of lower limb following other cerebrovascular disease affecting left non-dominant side**

    I69.849   **Monoplegia of lower limb following other cerebrovascular disease affecting unspecified side**

● **I69.85 Hemiplegia and hemiparesis following other cerebrovascular disease**

    I69.851   **Hemiplegia and hemiparesis following other cerebrovascular disease affecting right dominant side**

    I69.852   **Hemiplegia and hemiparesis following other cerebrovascular disease affecting left dominant side**

    I69.853   **Hemiplegia and hemiparesis following other cerebrovascular disease affecting right non-dominant side**

I69.854   Hemiplegia and hemiparesis following other cerebrovascular disease affecting left non-dominant side

I69.859   Hemiplegia and hemiparesis following other cerebrovascular disease affecting unspecified side

● **I69.86**   Other paralytic syndrome following other cerebrovascular disease

Use additional code to identify type of paralytic syndrome, such as:
locked-in state (G83.5)
quadriplegia (G82.5-)

Excludes1   hemiplegia/hemiparesis following other cerebrovascular disease (I69.85-)
monoplegia of lower limb following other cerebrovascular disease (I69.84-)
monoplegia of upper limb following other cerebrovascular disease (I69.83-)

I69.861   Other paralytic syndrome following other cerebrovascular disease affecting right dominant side

I69.862   Other paralytic syndrome following other cerebrovascular disease affecting left dominant side

I69.863   Other paralytic syndrome following other cerebrovascular disease affecting right non-dominant side

I69.864   Other paralytic syndrome following other cerebrovascular disease affecting left non-dominant side

I69.865   Other paralytic syndrome following other cerebrovascular disease, bilateral

I69.869   Other paralytic syndrome following other cerebrovascular disease affecting unspecified side

● **I69.89**   Other sequelae of other cerebrovascular disease

I69.890   Apraxia following other cerebrovascular disease

I69.891   Dysphagia following other cerebrovascular disease

Use additional code to identify the type of dysphagia, if known (R13.1-)

I69.892   Facial weakness following other cerebrovascular disease
Facial droop following other cerebrovascular disease

I69.893   Ataxia following other cerebrovascular disease

I69.898   Other sequelae of other cerebrovascular disease
Alteration of sensation following other cerebrovascular disease
Disturbance of vision following other cerebrovascular disease

Use additional code to identify the sequelae

● **I69.9**   Sequelae of unspecified cerebrovascular diseases

Excludes1   sequelae of stroke (I69.3)
sequelae of traumatic intracranial injury (S06.-)

I69.90   Unspecified sequelae of unspecified cerebrovascular disease

● **I69.91**   Cognitive deficits following unspecified cerebrovascular disease

I69.910   Attention and concentration deficit following unspecified cerebrovascular disease ◄

I69.911   Memory deficit following unspecified cerebrovascular disease ◄

I69.912   Visuospatial deficit and spatial neglect following unspecified cerebrovascular disease ◄

I69.913   Psychomotor deficit following unspecified cerebrovascular disease ◄

I69.914   Frontal lobe and executive function deficit following unspecified cerebrovascular disease ◄

I69.915   Cognitive social or emotional deficit following unspecified cerebrovascular disease ◄

I69.918   Other symptoms and signs involving cognitive functions following unspecified cerebrovascular disease ◄

I69.919   Unspecified symptoms and signs involving cognitive functions following unspecified cerebrovascular disease ◄

● **I69.92**   Speech and language deficits following unspecified cerebrovascular disease

I69.920   Aphasia following unspecified cerebrovascular disease

I69.921   Dysphasia following unspecified cerebrovascular disease

I69.922   Dysarthria following unspecified cerebrovascular disease

I69.923   Fluency disorder following unspecified cerebrovascular disease
Stuttering following unspecified cerebrovascular disease ◄||||

I69.928   Other speech and language deficits following unspecified cerebrovascular disease

● **I69.93**   Monoplegia of upper limb following unspecified cerebrovascular disease

I69.931   Monoplegia of upper limb following unspecified cerebrovascular disease affecting right dominant side

I69.932   Monoplegia of upper limb following unspecified cerebrovascular disease affecting left dominant side

I69.933   Monoplegia of upper limb following unspecified cerebrovascular disease affecting right non-dominant side

I69.934   Monoplegia of upper limb following unspecified cerebrovascular disease affecting left non-dominant side

I69.939   Monoplegia of upper limb following unspecified cerebrovascular disease affecting unspecified side

● **I69.94** **Monoplegia of lower limb following unspecified cerebrovascular disease**

    I69.941 **Monoplegia of lower limb following unspecified cerebrovascular disease affecting right dominant side**

    I69.942 **Monoplegia of lower limb following unspecified cerebrovascular disease affecting left dominant side**

    I69.943 **Monoplegia of lower limb following unspecified cerebrovascular disease affecting right non-dominant side**

    I69.944 **Monoplegia of lower limb following unspecified cerebrovascular disease affecting left non-dominant side**

    I69.949 **Monoplegia of lower limb following unspecified cerebrovascular disease affecting unspecified side**

● **I69.95** **Hemiplegia and hemiparesis following unspecified cerebrovascular disease**

    I69.951 **Hemiplegia and hemiparesis following unspecified cerebrovascular disease affecting right dominant side**

    I69.952 **Hemiplegia and hemiparesis following unspecified cerebrovascular disease affecting left dominant side**

    I69.953 **Hemiplegia and hemiparesis following unspecified cerebrovascular disease affecting right non-dominant side**

    I69.954 **Hemiplegia and hemiparesis following unspecified cerebrovascular disease affecting left non-dominant side**

    I69.959 **Hemiplegia and hemiparesis following unspecified cerebrovascular disease affecting unspecified side**

● **I69.96** **Other paralytic syndrome following unspecified cerebrovascular disease**

    Use additional code to identify type of paralytic syndrome, such as:
    locked-in state (G83.5)
    quadriplegia (G82.5-)

    Excludes1 hemiplegia/hemiparesis following unspecified cerebrovascular disease (I69.95-)
    monoplegia of lower limb following unspecified cerebrovascular disease (I69.94-)
    monoplegia of upper limb following unspecified cerebrovascular disease (I69.93-)

    I69.961 **Other paralytic syndrome following unspecified cerebrovascular disease affecting right dominant side**

    I69.962 **Other paralytic syndrome following unspecified cerebrovascular disease affecting left dominant side**

    I69.963 **Other paralytic syndrome following unspecified cerebrovascular disease affecting right non-dominant side**

    I69.964 **Other paralytic syndrome following unspecified cerebrovascular disease affecting left non-dominant side**

    I69.965 **Other paralytic syndrome following unspecified cerebrovascular disease, bilateral**

    I69.969 **Other paralytic syndrome following unspecified cerebrovascular disease affecting unspecified side**

● **I69.99** **Other sequelae of unspecified cerebrovascular disease**

    I69.990 **Apraxia following unspecified cerebrovascular disease**

    I69.991 **Dysphagia following unspecified cerebrovascular disease**

    Use additional code to identify the type of dysphagia, if known (R13.1-)

    I69.992 **Facial weakness following unspecified cerebrovascular disease**
    Facial droop following unspecified cerebrovascular disease

    I69.993 **Ataxia following unspecified cerebrovascular disease**

    I69.998 **Other sequelae following unspecified cerebrovascular disease**
    Alteration in sensation following unspecified cerebrovascular disease
    Disturbance of vision following unspecified cerebrovascular disease

    Use additional code to identify the sequelae

DISEASES OF ARTERIES, ARTERIOLES AND CAPILLARIES (I70-I79)

● **I70** **Atherosclerosis**

    Includes arteriolosclerosis
    arterial degeneration
    arteriosclerosis
    arteriosclerotic vascular disease
    arteriovascular degeneration
    atheroma
    endarteritis deformans or obliterans
    senile arteritis
    senile endarteritis
    vascular degeneration

    Use additional code to identify:
    exposure to environmental tobacco smoke (Z77.22)
    history of tobacco dependence (Z87.891)
    occupational exposure to environmental tobacco smoke (Z57.31)
    tobacco dependence (F17.-)
    tobacco use (Z72.0)

    Excludes2 arteriosclerotic cardiovascular disease (I25.1-)
    arteriosclerotic heart disease (I25.1-)
    atheroembolism (I75.-)
    cerebral atherosclerosis (I67.2)
    coronary atherosclerosis (I25.1-)
    mesenteric atherosclerosis (K55.1)
    precerebral atherosclerosis (I67.2)
    primary pulmonary atherosclerosis (I27.0)

I70.0 **Atherosclerosis of aorta**

I70.1 **Atherosclerosis of renal artery**
    Goldblatt's kidney

    Excludes2 atherosclerosis of renal arterioles (I12.-)

◀ New ◀ Revised ~~deleted~~ Deleted | Excludes 1 | Excludes 2 | Includes | Use additional | Code first | Code also | Unspecified
OGCR Official Guidelines X Assign placeholder X ● Use Additional Character(s) ▶ Manifestation Code **Coding Clinic**

★**(See Plates 500, 501, and 502 on pages 60 – 62.)**

● **I70.2 Atherosclerosis of native arteries of the extremities**
Mönckeberg's (medial) sclerosis
Use additional code, if applicable, to identify chronic total occlusion of artery of extremity (I70.92)

Excludes2   atherosclerosis of bypass graft of extremities (I70.30-I70.79)

● **I70.20 Unspecified atherosclerosis of native arteries of extremities**

I70.201 Unspecified atherosclerosis of native arteries of extremities, right leg   A

I70.202 Unspecified atherosclerosis of native arteries of extremities, left leg   A

I70.203 Unspecified atherosclerosis of native arteries of extremities, bilateral legs   A

I70.208 Unspecified atherosclerosis of native arteries of extremities, other extremity   A

I70.209 Unspecified atherosclerosis of native arteries of extremities, unspecified extremity   A

● **I70.21 Atherosclerosis of native arteries of extremities with intermittent claudication**

I70.211 Atherosclerosis of native arteries of extremities with intermittent claudication, right leg   A

I70.212 Atherosclerosis of native arteries of extremities with intermittent claudication, left leg   A

I70.213 Atherosclerosis of native arteries of extremities with intermittent claudication, bilateral legs   A

I70.218 Atherosclerosis of native arteries of extremities with intermittent claudication, other extremity   A

I70.219 Atherosclerosis of native arteries of extremities with intermittent claudication, unspecified extremity   A

● **I70.22 Atherosclerosis of native arteries of extremities with rest pain**

Includes   any condition classifiable to I70.21-

I70.221 Atherosclerosis of native arteries of extremities with rest pain, right leg   A

I70.222 Atherosclerosis of native arteries of extremities with rest pain, left leg   A

I70.223 Atherosclerosis of native arteries of extremities with rest pain, bilateral legs   A

I70.228 Atherosclerosis of native arteries of extremities with rest pain, other extremity   A

I70.229 Atherosclerosis of native arteries of extremities with rest pain, unspecified extremity   A

● **I70.23 Atherosclerosis of native arteries of right leg with ulceration**

Includes   any condition classifiable to I70.211 and I70.221

Use additional code to identify severity of ulcer (L97.-)

I70.231 Atherosclerosis of native arteries of right leg with ulceration of thigh   A

I70.232 Atherosclerosis of native arteries of right leg with ulceration of calf   A

I70.233 Atherosclerosis of native arteries of right leg with ulceration of ankle   A

I70.234 Atherosclerosis of native arteries of right leg with ulceration of heel and midfoot   A
Atherosclerosis of native arteries of right leg with ulceration of plantar surface of midfoot

I70.235 Atherosclerosis of native arteries of right leg with ulceration of other part of foot   A
Atherosclerosis of native arteries of right leg extremities with ulceration of toe

I70.238 Atherosclerosis of native arteries of right leg with ulceration of other part of lower right leg   A

I70.239 Atherosclerosis of native arteries of right leg with ulceration of unspecified site   A

● **I70.24 Atherosclerosis of native arteries of left leg with ulceration**

Includes   any condition classifiable to I70.212 and I70.222

Use additional code to identify severity of ulcer (L97.-)

I70.241 Atherosclerosis of native arteries of left leg with ulceration of thigh   A

I70.242 Atherosclerosis of native arteries of left leg with ulceration of calf   A

I70.243 Atherosclerosis of native arteries of left leg with ulceration of ankle   A

I70.244 Atherosclerosis of native arteries of left leg with ulceration of heel and midfoot   A
Atherosclerosis of native arteries of left leg with ulceration of plantar surface of midfoot

I70.245 Atherosclerosis of native arteries of left leg with ulceration of other part of foot   A
Atherosclerosis of native arteries of left leg extremities with ulceration of toe

I70.248 Atherosclerosis of native arteries of left leg with ulceration of other part of lower left leg   A

I70.249 Atherosclerosis of native arteries of left leg with ulceration of unspecified site   A

I70.25 Atherosclerosis of native arteries of other extremities with ulceration   A

Includes   any condition classifiable to I70.218 and I70.228

Use additional code to identify the severity of the ulcer (L98.49-)

CHAPTER 9 (I00-I99)

● **I70.26** **Atherosclerosis of native arteries of extremities with gangrene**

     Includes   any condition classifiable to I70.21-, I70.22-, I70.23-, I70.24-, and I70.25-

     Use additional code to identify the severity of any ulcer (L97.-, L98.49-), if applicable

     I70.261   Atherosclerosis of native arteries of extremities with gangrene, right leg   A

     I70.262   Atherosclerosis of native arteries of extremities with gangrene, left leg   A

     I70.263   Atherosclerosis of native arteries of extremities with gangrene, bilateral legs   A

     I70.268   Atherosclerosis of native arteries of extremities with gangrene, other extremity   A

     I70.269   Atherosclerosis of native arteries of extremities with gangrene, **unspecified** extremity   A

● **I70.29** **Other atherosclerosis of native arteries of extremities**

     I70.291   Other atherosclerosis of native arteries of extremities, right leg   A

     I70.292   Other atherosclerosis of native arteries of extremities, left leg   A

     I70.293   Other atherosclerosis of native arteries of extremities, bilateral legs   A

     I70.298   Other atherosclerosis of native arteries of extremities, other extremity   A

     I70.299   Other atherosclerosis of native arteries of extremities, **unspecified** extremity   A

● **I70.3** **Atherosclerosis of unspecified type of bypass graft(s) of the extremities**

     Use additional code, if applicable, to identify chronic total occlusion of artery of extremity (I70.92)

     Excludes1   embolism or thrombus of bypass graft(s) of extremities (T82.8-)

● **I70.30** **Unspecified atherosclerosis of unspecified type of bypass graft(s) of the extremities**

     70.301   **Unspecified** atherosclerosis of unspecified type of bypass graft(s) of the extremities, right leg   A

     I70.302   **Unspecified** atherosclerosis of unspecified type of bypass graft(s) of the extremities, left leg   A

     I70.303   **Unspecified** atherosclerosis of unspecified type of bypass graft(s) of the extremities, bilateral legs   A

     I70.308   **Unspecified** atherosclerosis of unspecified type of bypass graft(s) of the extremities, other extremity   A

     I70.309   **Unspecified** atherosclerosis of unspecified type of bypass graft(s) of the extremities, unspecified extremity   A

● **I70.31** **Atherosclerosis of unspecified type of bypass graft(s) of the extremities with intermittent claudication**

     I70.311   Atherosclerosis of **unspecified** type of bypass graft(s) of the extremities with intermittent claudication, right leg   A

     I70.312   Atherosclerosis of **unspecified** type of bypass graft(s) of the extremities with intermittent claudication, left leg   A

     I70.313   Atherosclerosis of **unspecified** type of bypass graft(s) of the extremities with intermittent claudication, bilateral legs   A

     I70.318   Atherosclerosis of **unspecified** type of bypass graft(s) of the extremities with intermittent claudication, other extremity   A

     I70.319   Atherosclerosis of **unspecified** type of bypass graft(s) of the extremities with intermittent claudication, unspecified extremity   A

● **I70.32** **Atherosclerosis of unspecified type of bypass graft(s) of the extremities with rest pain**

     Includes   any condition classifiable to I70.31-

     I70.321   Atherosclerosis of **unspecified** type of bypass graft(s) of the extremities with rest pain, right leg   A

     I70.322   Atherosclerosis of **unspecified** type of bypass graft(s) of the extremities with rest pain, left leg   A

     I70.323   Atherosclerosis of **unspecified** type of bypass graft(s) of the extremities with rest pain, bilateral legs   A

     I70.328   Atherosclerosis of **unspecified** type of bypass graft(s) of the extremities with rest pain, other extremity   A

     I70.329   Atherosclerosis of **unspecified** type of bypass graft(s) of the extremities with rest pain, unspecified extremity   A

● **I70.33** **Atherosclerosis of unspecified type of bypass graft(s) of the right leg with ulceration**

     Includes   any condition classifiable to I70.311 and I70.321

     Use additional code to identify severity of ulcer (L97.-)

     I70.331   Atherosclerosis of **unspecified** type of bypass graft(s) of the right leg with ulceration of thigh   A

     I70.332   Atherosclerosis of **unspecified** type of bypass graft(s) of the right leg with ulceration of calf   A

     I70.333   Atherosclerosis of **unspecified** type of bypass graft(s) of the right leg with ulceration of ankle   A

     I70.334   Atherosclerosis of **unspecified** type of bypass graft(s) of the right leg with ulceration of heel and midfoot   A

       Atherosclerosis of unspecified type of bypass graft(s) of right leg with ulceration of plantar surface of midfoot

     I70.335   Atherosclerosis of **unspecified** type of bypass graft(s) of the right leg with ulceration of other part of foot   A

       Atherosclerosis of unspecified type of bypass graft(s) of the right leg with ulceration of toe

     I70.338   Atherosclerosis of **unspecified** type of bypass graft(s) of the right leg with ulceration of other part of lower leg   A

     I70.339   Atherosclerosis of **unspecified** type of bypass graft(s) of the right leg with ulceration of unspecified site   A

◀ New   ◀▥ Revised   ~~deleted~~ Deleted   Excludes 1   Excludes 2   Includes   Use additional   Code first   Code also   Unspecified

OGCR Official Guidelines   X Assign placeholder X   ● Use Additional Character(s)   ▶ Manifestation Code   **Coding Clinic**

● **I70.34** **Atherosclerosis of unspecified type of bypass graft(s) of the left leg with ulceration**

> **Includes**   any condition classifiable to I70.312 and I70.322

> Use additional code to identify severity of ulcer (L97.-)

I70.341 Atherosclerosis of unspecified type of bypass graft(s) of the left leg with ulceration of thigh   A

I70.342 Atherosclerosis of unspecified type of bypass graft(s) of the left leg with ulceration of calf   A

I70.343 Atherosclerosis of unspecified type of bypass graft(s) of the left leg with ulceration of ankle   A

I70.344 Atherosclerosis of unspecified type of bypass graft(s) of the left leg with ulceration of heel and midfoot   A
> Atherosclerosis of unspecified type of bypass graft(s) of left leg with ulceration of plantar surface of midfoot

I70.345 Atherosclerosis of unspecified type of bypass graft(s) of the left leg with ulceration of other part of foot   A
> Atherosclerosis of unspecified type of bypass graft(s) of the left leg with ulceration of toe

I70.348 Atherosclerosis of unspecified type of bypass graft(s) of the left leg with ulceration of other part of lower leg   A

I70.349 Atherosclerosis of unspecified type of bypass graft(s) of the left leg with ulceration of unspecified site   A

I70.35 Atherosclerosis of unspecified type of bypass graft(s) of other extremity with ulceration   A
> **Includes**   any condition classifiable to I70.318 and I70.328
> Use additional code to identify severity of ulcer (L98.49-)

● **I70.36** **Atherosclerosis of unspecified type of bypass graft(s) of the extremities with gangrene**
> **Includes**   any condition classifiable to I70.31-, I70.32-, I70.33-, I70.34-, I70.35
> Use additional code to identify the severity of any ulcer (L97.-, L98.49-), if applicable

I70.361 Atherosclerosis of unspecified type of bypass graft(s) of the extremities with gangrene, right leg   A

I70.362 Atherosclerosis of unspecified type of bypass graft(s) of the extremities with gangrene, left leg   A

I70.363 Atherosclerosis of unspecified type of bypass graft(s) of the extremities with gangrene, bilateral legs   A

I70.368 Atherosclerosis of unspecified type of bypass graft(s) of the extremities with gangrene, other extremity   A

I70.369 Atherosclerosis of unspecified type of bypass graft(s) of the extremities with gangrene, unspecified extremity   A

● **I70.39** Other atherosclerosis of unspecified type of bypass graft(s) of the extremities

I70.391 Other atherosclerosis of unspecified type of bypass graft(s) of the extremities, right leg   A

I70.392 Other atherosclerosis of unspecified type of bypass graft(s) of the extremities, left leg   A

I70.393 Other atherosclerosis of unspecified type of bypass graft(s) of the extremities, bilateral legs   A

I70.398 Other atherosclerosis of unspecified type of bypass graft(s) of the extremities, other extremity   A

I70.399 Other atherosclerosis of unspecified type of bypass graft(s) of the extremities, unspecified extremity   A

● **I70.4** **Atherosclerosis of autologous vein bypass graft(s) of the extremities**
> Use additional code, if applicable, to identify chronic total occlusion of artery of extremity (I70.92)

● **I70.40** Unspecified atherosclerosis of autologous vein bypass graft(s) of the extremities

I70.401 Unspecified atherosclerosis of autologous vein bypass graft(s) of the extremities, right leg   A

I70.402 Unspecified atherosclerosis of autologous vein bypass graft(s) of the extremities, left leg   A

I70.403 Unspecified atherosclerosis of autologous vein bypass graft(s) of the extremities, bilateral legs   A

I70.408 Unspecified atherosclerosis of autologous vein bypass graft(s) of the extremities, other extremity   A

I70.409 Unspecified atherosclerosis of autologous vein bypass graft(s) of the extremities, unspecified extremity   A

● **I70.41** Atherosclerosis of autologous vein bypass graft(s) of the extremities with intermittent claudication

I70.411 Atherosclerosis of autologous vein bypass graft(s) of the extremities with intermittent claudication, right leg   A

I70.412 Atherosclerosis of autologous vein bypass graft(s) of the extremities with intermittent claudication, left leg   A

I70.413 Atherosclerosis of autologous vein bypass graft(s) of the extremities with intermittent claudication, bilateral legs   A

I70.418 Atherosclerosis of autologous vein bypass graft(s) of the extremities with intermittent claudication, other extremity   A

I70.419 Atherosclerosis of autologous vein bypass graft(s) of the extremities with intermittent claudication, unspecified extremity   A

● **I70.42** Atherosclerosis of autologous vein bypass graft(s) of the extremities with rest pain
> **Includes**   any condition classifiable to I70.41-

I70.421 Atherosclerosis of autologous vein bypass graft(s) of the extremities with rest pain, right leg   A

I70.422 Atherosclerosis of autologous vein bypass graft(s) of the extremities with rest pain, left leg   A

I70.423 Atherosclerosis of autologous vein bypass graft(s) of the extremities with rest pain, bilateral legs   A

I70.428 Atherosclerosis of autologous vein bypass graft(s) of the extremities with rest pain, other extremity   A

I70.429 Atherosclerosis of autologous vein bypass graft(s) of the extremities with rest pain, unspecified extremity   A

CHAPTER 9 (I00-I99)

● **I70.43** **Atherosclerosis of autologous vein bypass graft(s) of the right leg with ulceration**
>> **Includes**   any condition classifiable to I70.411 and I70.421
>> Use additional code to identify severity of ulcer (L97.-)

>> **I70.431** Atherosclerosis of autologous vein bypass graft(s) of the right leg with ulceration of thigh   A
>> **I70.432** Atherosclerosis of autologous vein bypass graft(s) of the right leg with ulceration of calf   A
>> **I70.433** Atherosclerosis of autologous vein bypass graft(s) of the right leg with ulceration of ankle   A
>> **I70.434** Atherosclerosis of autologous vein bypass graft(s) of the right leg with ulceration of heel and midfoot   A
>>> Atherosclerosis of autologous vein bypass graft(s) of right leg with ulceration of plantar surface of midfoot
>> **I70.435** Atherosclerosis of autologous vein bypass graft(s) of the right leg with ulceration of other part of foot   A
>>> Atherosclerosis of autologous vein bypass graft(s) of right leg with ulceration of toe
>> **I70.438** Atherosclerosis of autologous vein bypass graft(s) of the right leg with ulceration of other part of lower leg   A
>> **I70.439** Atherosclerosis of autologous vein bypass graft(s) of the right leg with ulceration of unspecified site   A

● **I70.44** **Atherosclerosis of autologous vein bypass graft(s) of the left leg with ulceration**
>> **Includes**   any condition classifiable to I70.412 and I70.422
>> Use additional code to identify severity of ulcer (L97.-)

>> **I70.441** Atherosclerosis of autologous vein bypass graft(s) of the left leg with ulceration of thigh   A
>> **I70.442** Atherosclerosis of autologous vein bypass graft(s) of the left leg with ulceration of calf   A
>> **I70.443** Atherosclerosis of autologous vein bypass graft(s) of the left leg with ulceration of ankle   A
>> **I70.444** Atherosclerosis of autologous vein bypass graft(s) of the left leg with ulceration of heel and midfoot   A
>>> Atherosclerosis of autologous vein bypass graft(s) of left leg with ulceration of plantar surface of midfoot
>> **I70.445** Atherosclerosis of autologous vein bypass graft(s) of the left leg with ulceration of other part of foot   A
>>> Atherosclerosis of autologous vein bypass graft(s) of left leg with ulceration of toe
>> **I70.448** Atherosclerosis of autologous vein bypass graft(s) of the left leg with ulceration of other part of lower leg   A
>> **I70.449** Atherosclerosis of autologous vein bypass graft(s) of the left leg with ulceration of unspecified site   A

I70.45 **Atherosclerosis of autologous vein bypass graft(s) of other extremity with ulceration**   A
>> **Includes**   any condition classifiable to I70.418, I70.428, and I70.438
>> Use additional code to identify severity of ulcer (L98.49-)

● **I70.46** **Atherosclerosis of autologous vein bypass graft(s) of the extremities with gangrene**
>> **Includes**   any condition classifiable to I70.41-, I70.42-, and I70.43-, I70.44-, I70.45
>> Use additional code to identify the severity of any ulcer (L97.-, L98.49-), if applicable

>> **I70.461** Atherosclerosis of autologous vein bypass graft(s) of the extremities with gangrene, right leg   A
>> **I70.462** Atherosclerosis of autologous vein bypass graft(s) of the extremities with gangrene, left leg   A
>> **I70.463** Atherosclerosis of autologous vein bypass graft(s) of the extremities with gangrene, bilateral legs   A
>> **I70.468** Atherosclerosis of autologous vein bypass graft(s) of the extremities with gangrene, other extremity   A
>> **I70.469** Atherosclerosis of autologous vein bypass graft(s) of the extremities with gangrene, unspecified extremity   A

● **I70.49** **Other atherosclerosis of autologous vein bypass graft(s) of the extremities**
>> **I70.491** Other atherosclerosis of autologous vein bypass graft(s) of the extremities, right leg   A
>> **I70.492** Other atherosclerosis of autologous vein bypass graft(s) of the extremities, left leg   A
>> **I70.493** Other atherosclerosis of autologous vein bypass graft(s) of the extremities, bilateral legs   A
>> **I70.498** Other atherosclerosis of autologous vein bypass graft(s) of the extremities, other extremity   A
>> **I70.499** Other atherosclerosis of autologous vein bypass graft(s) of the extremities, unspecified extremity   A

● **I70.5** **Atherosclerosis of nonautologous biological bypass graft(s) of the extremities**
>> Use additional code, if applicable, to identify chronic total occlusion of artery of extremity (I70.92)

● **I70.50** **Unspecified atherosclerosis of nonautologous biological bypass graft(s) of the extremities**
>> **I70.501** Unspecified atherosclerosis of nonautologous biological bypass graft(s) of the extremities, right leg   A
>> **I70.502** Unspecified atherosclerosis of nonautologous biological bypass graft(s) of the extremities, left leg   A
>> **I70.503** Unspecified atherosclerosis of nonautologous biological bypass graft(s) of the extremities, bilateral legs   A
>> **I70.508** Unspecified atherosclerosis of nonautologous biological bypass graft(s) of the extremities, other extremity   A
>> **I70.509** Unspecified atherosclerosis of nonautologous biological bypass graft(s) of the extremities, unspecified extremity

● **I70.51**   **Atherosclerosis of nonautologous biological bypass graft(s) of the extremities intermittent claudication**

    I70.511   Atherosclerosis of nonautologous biological bypass graft(s) of the extremities with intermittent claudication, right leg   **A**

    I70.512   Atherosclerosis of nonautologous biological bypass graft(s) of the extremities with intermittent claudication, left leg   **A**

    I70.513   Atherosclerosis of nonautologous biological bypass graft(s) of the extremities with intermittent claudication, bilateral legs   **A**

    I70.518   Atherosclerosis of nonautologous biological bypass graft(s) of the extremities with intermittent claudication, other extremity   **A**

    I70.519   Atherosclerosis of nonautologous biological bypass graft(s) of the extremities with intermittent claudication, unspecified extremity   **A**

● **I70.52**   **Atherosclerosis of nonautologous biological bypass graft(s) of the extremities with rest pain**

    Includes   any condition classifiable to I70.51-

    I70.521   Atherosclerosis of nonautologous biological bypass graft(s) of the extremities with rest pain, right leg   **A**

    I70.522   Atherosclerosis of nonautologous biological bypass graft(s) of the extremities with rest pain, left leg   **A**

    I70.523   Atherosclerosis of nonautologous biological bypass graft(s) of the extremities with rest pain, bilateral legs   **A**

    I70.528   Atherosclerosis of nonautologous biological bypass graft(s) of the extremities with rest pain, other extremity   **A**

    I70.529   Atherosclerosis of nonautologous biological bypass graft(s) of the extremities with rest pain, unspecified extremity   **A**

● **I70.53**   **Atherosclerosis of nonautologous biological bypass graft(s) of the right leg with ulceration**

    Includes   any condition classifiable to I70.511 and I70.521

    Use additional code to identify severity of ulcer (L97.-)

    I70.531   Atherosclerosis of nonautologous biological bypass graft(s) of the right leg with ulceration of thigh   **A**

    I70.532   Atherosclerosis of nonautologous biological bypass graft(s) of the right leg with ulceration of calf   **A**

    I70.533   Atherosclerosis of nonautologous biological bypass graft(s) of the right leg with ulceration of ankle   **A**

    I70.534   Atherosclerosis of nonautologous biological bypass graft(s) of the right leg with ulceration of heel and midfoot   **A**

        Atherosclerosis of nonautologous biological bypass graft(s) of right leg with ulceration of plantar surface of midfoot

    I70.535   Atherosclerosis of nonautologous biological bypass graft(s) of the right leg with ulceration of other part of foot   **A**

        Atherosclerosis of nonautologous biological bypass graft(s) of the right leg with ulceration of toe

    I70.538   Atherosclerosis of nonautologous biological bypass graft(s) of the right leg with ulceration of other part of lower leg   **A**

    I70.539   Atherosclerosis of nonautologous biological bypass graft(s) of the right leg with ulceration of unspecified site   **A**

● **I70.54**   **Atherosclerosis of nonautologous biological bypass graft(s) of the left leg with ulceration**

    Includes   any condition classifiable to I70.512 and I70.522

    Use additional code to identify severity of ulcer (L97.-)

    I70.541   Atherosclerosis of nonautologous biological bypass graft(s) of the left leg with ulceration of thigh   **A**

    I70.542   Atherosclerosis of nonautologous biological bypass graft(s) of the left leg with ulceration of calf   **A**

    I70.543   Atherosclerosis of nonautologous biological bypass graft(s) of the left leg with ulceration of ankle   **A**

    I70.544   Atherosclerosis of nonautologous biological bypass graft(s) of the left leg with ulceration of heel and midfoot   **A**

        Atherosclerosis of nonautologous biological bypass graft(s) of left leg with ulceration of plantar surface of midfoot

    I70.545   Atherosclerosis of nonautologous biological bypass graft(s) of the left leg with ulceration of other part of foot   **A**

        Atherosclerosis of nonautologous biological bypass graft(s) of the left leg with ulceration of toe

    I70.548   Atherosclerosis of nonautologous biological bypass graft(s) of the left leg with ulceration of other part of lower leg   **A**

    I70.549   Atherosclerosis of nonautologous biological bypass graft(s) of the left leg with ulceration of unspecified site   **A**

I70.55   Atherosclerosis of nonautologous biological bypass graft(s) of other extremity with ulceration   **A**

    Includes   any condition classifiable to I70.518, I70.528, and I70.538

    Use additional code to identify severity of ulcer (L98.49)

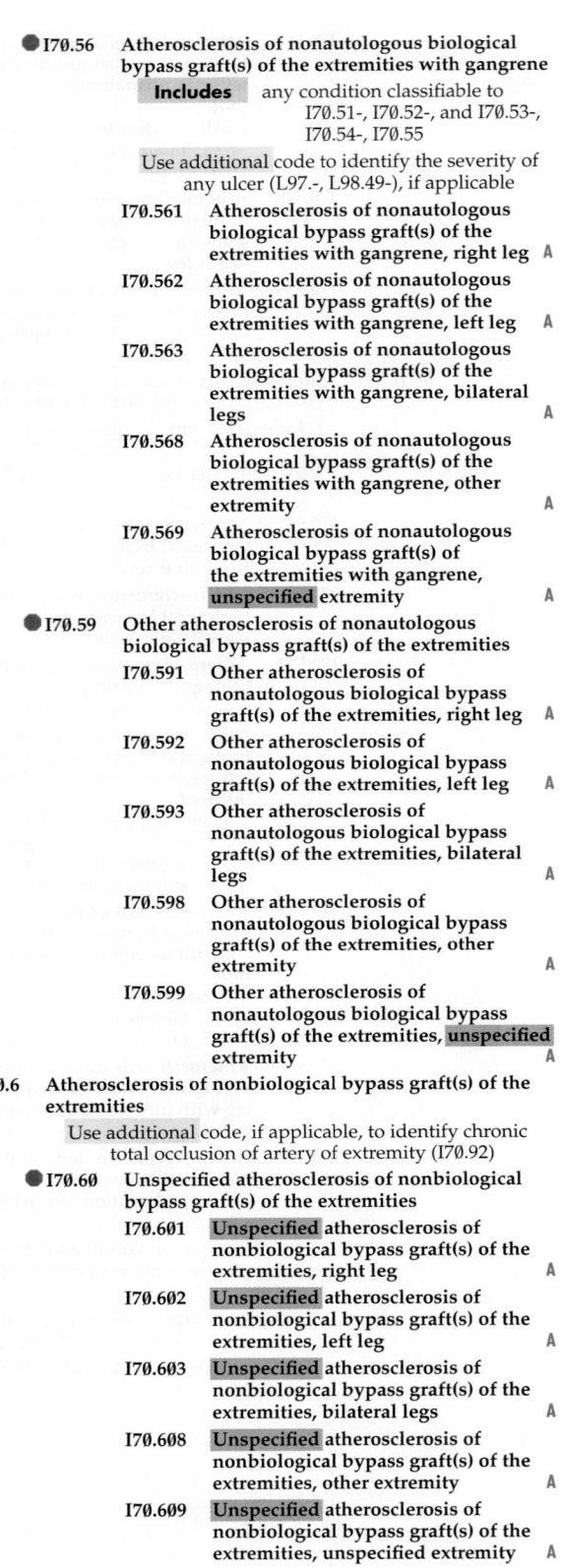

● I70.56 **Atherosclerosis of nonautologous biological bypass graft(s) of the extremities with gangrene**

> **Includes** any condition classifiable to I70.51-, I70.52-, and I70.53-, I70.54-, I70.55

Use additional code to identify the severity of any ulcer (L97.-, L98.49-), if applicable

I70.561 Atherosclerosis of nonautologous biological bypass graft(s) of the extremities with gangrene, right leg   A

I70.562 Atherosclerosis of nonautologous biological bypass graft(s) of the extremities with gangrene, left leg   A

I70.563 Atherosclerosis of nonautologous biological bypass graft(s) of the extremities with gangrene, bilateral legs   A

I70.568 Atherosclerosis of nonautologous biological bypass graft(s) of the extremities with gangrene, other extremity   A

I70.569 Atherosclerosis of nonautologous biological bypass graft(s) of the extremities with gangrene, unspecified extremity   A

● I70.59 **Other atherosclerosis of nonautologous biological bypass graft(s) of the extremities**

I70.591 Other atherosclerosis of nonautologous biological bypass graft(s) of the extremities, right leg   A

I70.592 Other atherosclerosis of nonautologous biological bypass graft(s) of the extremities, left leg   A

I70.593 Other atherosclerosis of nonautologous biological bypass graft(s) of the extremities, bilateral legs   A

I70.598 Other atherosclerosis of nonautologous biological bypass graft(s) of the extremities, other extremity   A

I70.599 Other atherosclerosis of nonautologous biological bypass graft(s) of the extremities, unspecified extremity   A

● I70.6 **Atherosclerosis of nonbiological bypass graft(s) of the extremities**

> Use additional code, if applicable, to identify chronic total occlusion of artery of extremity (I70.92)

● I70.60 **Unspecified atherosclerosis of nonbiological bypass graft(s) of the extremities**

I70.601 Unspecified atherosclerosis of nonbiological bypass graft(s) of the extremities, right leg   A

I70.602 Unspecified atherosclerosis of nonbiological bypass graft(s) of the extremities, left leg   A

I70.603 Unspecified atherosclerosis of nonbiological bypass graft(s) of the extremities, bilateral legs   A

I70.608 Unspecified atherosclerosis of nonbiological bypass graft(s) of the extremities, other extremity   A

I70.609 Unspecified atherosclerosis of nonbiological bypass graft(s) of the extremities, unspecified extremity   A

● I70.61 **Atherosclerosis of nonbiological bypass graft(s) of the extremities with intermittent claudication**

I70.611 Atherosclerosis of nonbiological bypass graft(s) of the extremities with intermittent claudication, right leg   A

I70.612 Atherosclerosis of nonbiological bypass graft(s) of the extremities with intermittent claudication, left leg   A

I70.613 Atherosclerosis of nonbiological bypass graft(s) of the extremities with intermittent claudication, bilateral legs   A

I70.618 Atherosclerosis of nonbiological bypass graft(s) of the extremities with intermittent claudication, other extremity   A

I70.619 Atherosclerosis of nonbiological bypass graft(s) of the extremities with intermittent claudication, unspecified extremity   A

● I70.62 **Atherosclerosis of nonbiological bypass graft(s) of the extremities with rest pain**

> **Includes** any condition classifiable to I70.61-

I70.621 Atherosclerosis of nonbiological bypass graft(s) of the extremities with rest pain, right leg   A

I70.622 Atherosclerosis of nonbiological bypass graft(s) of the extremities with rest pain, left leg   A

I70.623 Atherosclerosis of nonbiological bypass graft(s) of the extremities with rest pain, bilateral legs   A

I70.628 Atherosclerosis of nonbiological bypass graft(s) of the extremities with rest pain, other extremity   A

I70.629 Atherosclerosis of nonbiological bypass graft(s) of the extremities with rest pain, unspecified extremity   A

● I70.63 **Atherosclerosis of nonbiological bypass graft(s) of the right leg with ulceration**

> **Includes** any condition classifiable to I70.611 and I70.621

Use additional code to identify severity of ulcer (L97.-)

I70.631 Atherosclerosis of nonbiological bypass graft(s) of the right leg with ulceration of thigh   A

I70.632 Atherosclerosis of nonbiological bypass graft(s) of the right leg with ulceration of calf   A

I70.633 Atherosclerosis of nonbiological bypass graft(s) of the right leg with ulceration of ankle   A

I70.634 Atherosclerosis of nonbiological bypass graft(s) of the right leg with ulceration of heel and midfoot
Atherosclerosis of nonbiological bypass graft(s) of right leg with ulceration of plantar surface of midfoot

I70.635 Atherosclerosis of nonbiological bypass graft(s) of the right leg with ulceration of other part of foot   A
Atherosclerosis of nonbiological bypass graft(s) of the right leg with ulceration of toe

I70.638 Atherosclerosis of nonbiological bypass graft(s) of the right leg with ulceration of other part of lower leg   A

I70.639 Atherosclerosis of nonbiological bypass graft(s) of the right leg with ulceration of unspecified site   A

◀ New   ◀ Revised   deleted Deleted   Excludes 1   Excludes 2   Includes   Use additional   Code first   Code also   Unspecified

882   OGCR Official Guidelines   X Assign placeholder X   ● Use Additional Character(s)   ▶ Manifestation Code   **Coding Clinic**

● **I70.64**   **Atherosclerosis of nonbiological bypass graft(s) of the left leg with ulceration**

     Includes   any condition classifiable to I70.612 and I70.622

     Use additional code to identify severity of ulcer (L97.-)

   I70.641   Atherosclerosis of nonbiological bypass graft(s) of the left leg with ulceration of thigh   A

   I70.642   Atherosclerosis of nonbiological bypass graft(s) of the left leg with ulceration of calf   A

   I70.643   Atherosclerosis of nonbiological bypass graft(s) of the left leg with ulceration of ankle   A

   I70.644   Atherosclerosis of nonbiological bypass graft(s) of the left leg with ulceration of heel and midfoot   A
     Atherosclerosis of nonbiological bypass graft(s) of left leg with ulceration of plantar surface of midfoot

   I70.645   Atherosclerosis of nonbiological bypass graft(s) of the left leg with ulceration of other part of foot   A
     Atherosclerosis of nonbiological bypass graft(s) of the left leg with ulceration of toe

   I70.648   Atherosclerosis of nonbiological bypass graft(s) of the left leg with ulceration of other part of lower leg   A

   I70.649   Atherosclerosis of nonbiological bypass graft(s) of the left leg with ulceration of unspecified site   A

  I70.65   **Atherosclerosis of nonbiological bypass graft(s) of other extremity with ulceration**   A

     Includes   any condition classifiable to I70.618 and I70.628

     Use additional code to identify severity of ulcer (L98.49-)

● **I70.66**   **Atherosclerosis of nonbiological bypass graft(s) of the extremities with gangrene**

     Includes   any condition classifiable to I70.61-, I70.62-, I70.63-, I70.64-, I70.65

     Use additional code to identify the severity of any ulcer (L97.-, L98.49-), if applicable

   I70.661   Atherosclerosis of nonbiological bypass graft(s) of the extremities with gangrene, right leg   A

   I70.662   Atherosclerosis of nonbiological bypass graft(s) of the extremities with gangrene, left leg   A

   I70.663   Atherosclerosis of nonbiological bypass graft(s) of the extremities with gangrene, bilateral legs   A

   I70.668   Atherosclerosis of nonbiological bypass graft(s) of the extremities with gangrene, other extremity   A

   I70.669   Atherosclerosis of nonbiological bypass graft(s) of the extremities with gangrene, unspecified extremity   A

● **I70.69**   **Other atherosclerosis of nonbiological bypass graft(s) of the extremities**

   I70.691   Other atherosclerosis of nonbiological bypass graft(s) of the extremities, right leg   A

   I70.692   Other atherosclerosis of nonbiological bypass graft(s) of the extremities, left leg   A

   I70.693   Other atherosclerosis of nonbiological bypass graft(s) of the extremities, bilateral legs   A

   I70.698   Other atherosclerosis of nonbiological bypass graft(s) of the extremities, other extremity   A

   I70.699   Other atherosclerosis of nonbiological bypass graft(s) of the extremities, unspecified extremity   A

● **I70.7**   **Atherosclerosis of other type of bypass graft(s) of the extremities**

     Use additional code, if applicable, to identify chronic total occlusion of artery of extremity (I70.92)

● **I70.70**   **Unspecified atherosclerosis of other type of bypass graft(s) of the extremities**

   I70.701   Unspecified atherosclerosis of other type of bypass graft(s) of the extremities, right leg   A

   I70.702   Unspecified atherosclerosis of other type of bypass graft(s) of the extremities, left leg   A

   I70.703   Unspecified atherosclerosis of other type of bypass graft(s) of the extremities, bilateral legs   A

   I70.708   Unspecified atherosclerosis of other type of bypass graft(s) of the extremities, other extremity   A

   I70.709   Unspecified atherosclerosis of other type of bypass graft(s) of the extremities, unspecified extremity   A

● **I70.71**   **Atherosclerosis of other type of bypass graft(s) of the extremities with intermittent claudication**

   I70.711   Atherosclerosis of other type of bypass graft(s) of the extremities with intermittent claudication, right leg   A

   I70.712   Atherosclerosis of other type of bypass graft(s) of the extremities with intermittent claudication, left leg   A

   I70.713   Atherosclerosis of other type of bypass graft(s) of the extremities with intermittent claudication, bilateral legs   A

   I70.718   Atherosclerosis of other type of bypass graft(s) of the extremities with intermittent claudication, other extremity   A

   I70.719   Atherosclerosis of other type of bypass graft(s) of the extremities with intermittent claudication, unspecified extremity   A

● **I70.72**   **Atherosclerosis of other type of bypass graft(s) of the extremities with rest pain**

     Includes   any condition classifiable to I70.71-

   I70.721   Atherosclerosis of other type of bypass graft(s) of the extremities with rest pain, right leg   A

   I70.722   Atherosclerosis of other type of bypass graft(s) of the extremities with rest pain, left leg   A

   I70.723   Atherosclerosis of other type of bypass graft(s) of the extremities with rest pain, bilateral legs   A

   I70.728   Atherosclerosis of other type of bypass graft(s) of the extremities with rest pain, other extremity   A

   I70.729   Atherosclerosis of other type of bypass graft(s) of the extremities with rest pain, unspecified extremity   A

CHAPTER 9 (I00-I99)

● **I70.73   Atherosclerosis of other type of bypass graft(s) of the right leg with ulceration**

> **Includes**   any condition classifiable to I70.711 and I70.721

> Use additional code to identify severity of ulcer (L97.-)

I70.731   Atherosclerosis of other type of bypass graft(s) of the right leg with ulceration of thigh   A

I70.732   Atherosclerosis of other type of bypass graft(s) of the right leg with ulceration of calf   A

I70.733   Atherosclerosis of other type of bypass graft(s) of the right leg with ulceration of ankle   A

I70.734   Atherosclerosis of other type of bypass graft(s) of the right leg with ulceration of heel and midfoot   A
> Atherosclerosis of other type of bypass graft(s) of right leg with ulceration of plantar surface of midfoot

I70.735   Atherosclerosis of other type of bypass graft(s) of the right leg with ulceration of other part of foot   A
> Atherosclerosis of other type of bypass graft(s) of right leg with ulceration of toe

I70.738   Atherosclerosis of other type of bypass graft(s) of the right leg with ulceration of other part of lower leg   A

I70.739   Atherosclerosis of other type of bypass graft(s) of the right leg with ulceration of unspecified site   A

● **I70.74   Atherosclerosis of other type of bypass graft(s) of the left leg with ulceration**

> **Includes**   any condition classifiable to I70.712 and I70.722

> Use additional code to identify severity of ulcer (L97.-)

I70.741   Atherosclerosis of other type of bypass graft(s) of the left leg with ulceration of thigh   A

I70.742   Atherosclerosis of other type of bypass graft(s) of the left leg with ulceration of calf   A

I70.743   Atherosclerosis of other type of bypass graft(s) of the left leg with ulceration of ankle   A

I70.744   Atherosclerosis of other type of bypass graft(s) of the left leg with ulceration of heel and midfoot   A
> Atherosclerosis of other type of bypass graft(s) of left leg with ulceration of plantar surface of midfoot

I70.745   Atherosclerosis of other type of bypass graft(s) of the left leg with ulceration of other part of foot   A
> Atherosclerosis of other type of bypass graft(s) of left leg with ulceration of toe

I70.748   Atherosclerosis of other type of bypass graft(s) of the left leg with ulceration of other part of lower leg   A

I70.749   Atherosclerosis of other type of bypass graft(s) of the left leg with ulceration of unspecified site   A

I70.75   Atherosclerosis of other type of bypass graft(s) of other extremity with ulceration   A

> **Includes**   any condition classifiable to I70.718 and I70.728

> Use additional code to identify severity of ulcer (L98.49)

● **I70.76   Atherosclerosis of other type of bypass graft(s) of the extremities with gangrene**

> **Includes**   any condition classifiable to I70.71-, I70.72-, I70.73-, I70.74-, I70.75

> Use additional code to identify the severity of any ulcer (L97.-, L98.49-), if applicable

I70.761   Atherosclerosis of other type of bypass graft(s) of the extremities with gangrene, right leg   A

I70.762   Atherosclerosis of other type of bypass graft(s) of the extremities with gangrene, left leg   A

I70.763   Atherosclerosis of other type of bypass graft(s) of the extremities with gangrene, bilateral legs   A

I70.768   Atherosclerosis of other type of bypass graft(s) of the extremities with gangrene, other extremity   A

I70.769   Atherosclerosis of other type of bypass graft(s) of the extremities with gangrene, unspecified extremity   A

● **I70.79   Other atherosclerosis of other type of bypass graft(s) of the extremities**

I70.791   Other atherosclerosis of other type of bypass graft(s) of the extremities, right leg   A

I70.792   Other atherosclerosis of other type of bypass graft(s) of the extremities, left leg   A

I70.793   Other atherosclerosis of other type of bypass graft(s) of the extremities, bilateral legs   A

I70.798   Other atherosclerosis of other type of bypass graft(s) of the extremities, other extremity   A

I70.799   Other atherosclerosis of other type of bypass graft(s) of the extremities, unspecified extremity   A

I70.8   Atherosclerosis of other arteries   A

● **I70.9   Other and unspecified atherosclerosis**

I70.90   Unspecified atherosclerosis   A

I70.91   Generalized atherosclerosis   A

I70.92   Chronic total occlusion of artery of the extremities   A
> Complete occlusion of artery of the extremities
> Total occlusion of artery of the extremities
> *Code first* atherosclerosis of arteries of the extremities (I70.2-, I70.3-, I70.4-, I70.5-, I70.6-, I70.7-)

● **I71**   **Aortic aneurysm and dissection**
     Excludes1   aortic ectasia (I77.81-)
                    syphilitic aortic aneurysm (A52.01)
                    traumatic aortic aneurysm (S25.09, S35.09)

   ● **I71.0**   **Dissection of aorta**
       I71.00   **Dissection of unspecified site of aorta**
       I71.01   **Dissection of thoracic aorta**
       I71.02   **Dissection of abdominal aorta**
       I71.03   **Dissection of thoracoabdominal aorta**

     I71.1   **Thoracic aortic aneurysm, ruptured**
     I71.2   **Thoracic aortic aneurysm, without rupture**
     I71.3   **Abdominal aortic aneurysm, ruptured**
     I71.4   **Abdominal aortic aneurysm, without rupture**
     I71.5   **Thoracoabdominal aortic aneurysm, ruptured**
     I71.6   **Thoracoabdominal aortic aneurysm, without rupture**
     I71.8   **Aortic aneurysm of unspecified site, ruptured**
          Rupture of aorta NOS
     I71.9   **Aortic aneurysm of unspecified site, without rupture**
          Aneurysm of aorta
          Dilatation of aorta
          Hyaline necrosis of aorta

● **I72**   **Other aneurysm**
     Includes   aneurysm (cirsoid) (false) (ruptured)
     Excludes2   acquired aneurysm (I77.0)
                   aneurysm (of) aorta (I71.-)
                   aneurysm (of) arteriovenous NOS (Q27.3-)
                   carotid artery dissection (I77.71)
                   cerebral (nonruptured) aneurysm (I67.1)
                   coronary aneurysm (I25.4)
                   coronary artery dissection (I25.42)
                   dissection of artery NEC (I77.79)
                   dissection of precerebral artery, congenital
                       (nonruptured) (Q28.1) ◄
                   heart aneurysm (I25.3)
                   iliac artery dissection (I77.72)
                   pulmonary artery aneurysm (I28.1)
                   renal artery dissection (I77.73)
                   retinal aneurysm (H35.0)
                   ruptured cerebral aneurysm (I60.7)
                   varicose aneurysm (I77.0)
                   vertebral artery dissection (I77.74)

     I72.0   **Aneurysm of carotid artery**
          Aneurysm of common carotid artery
          Aneurysm of external carotid artery
          Aneurysm of internal carotid artery, extracranial
             portion
       Excludes1   aneurysm of internal carotid artery,
                      intracranial portion (I67.1)
                    aneurysm of internal carotid artery NOS
                      (I67.1)
     I72.1   **Aneurysm of artery of upper extremity**
     I72.2   **Aneurysm of renal artery**
     I72.3   **Aneurysm of iliac artery**
     I72.4   **Aneurysm of artery of lower extremity**
     I72.5   **Aneurysm of other precerebral arteries** ◄
          Aneurysm of basilar artery (trunk) ◄
       Excludes2   aneurysm of carotid artery (I72.0) ◄
                    aneurysm of vertebral artery (I72.6) ◄
                    dissection of carotid artery (I77.71) ◄
                    dissection of other precerebral arteries
                      (I77.75) ◄
                    dissection of vertebral artery (I77.74) ◄
     I72.6   **Aneurysm of vertebral artery** ◄
       Excludes2   dissection of vertebral artery (I77.74) ◄
     I72.8   **Aneurysm of other specified arteries**
     I72.9   **Aneurysm of unspecified site**

Figure 9-5   Raynaud's syndrome. (From Hallett: Comprehensive Vascular and Endovascular Surgery, ed 2, Philadelphia, Mosby Ltd., 2010)

● **I73**   **Other peripheral vascular diseases**
     Excludes2   chilblains (T69.1)
                   frostbite (T33-T34)
                   immersion hand or foot (T69.0-)
                   spasm of cerebral artery (G45.9)

   ● **I73.0**   **Raynaud's syndrome**
          Diminishing oxygen supply to fingers, toes, nose, and ears
              when exposed to temperature changes or stress
          Raynaud's disease
          Raynaud's phenomenon (secondary)
       I73.00   **Raynaud's syndrome without gangrene**
       I73.01   **Raynaud's syndrome with gangrene**
     I73.1   **Thromboangiitis obliterans [Buerger's disease]**
          Inflammatory occlusive disease resulting in poor circulation
             to the legs, feet, and sometimes the hands due to
             progressive inflammatory narrowing and eventually
             obliteration of the small arteries
   ● **I73.8**   **Other specified peripheral vascular diseases**
       Excludes1   diabetic (peripheral) angiopathy
                    (E08-E13 with .51-.52)
       I73.81   **Erythromelalgia**
       I73.89   **Other specified peripheral vascular diseases**
             Acrocyanosis
             Erythrocyanosis
             Simple acroparesthesia [Schultze's type]
             Vasomotor acroparesthesia [Nothnagel's type]
     I73.9   **Peripheral vascular disease, unspecified**
          Intermittent claudication
          Peripheral angiopathy NOS
          Spasm of artery
       Excludes1   atherosclerosis of the extremities
                    (I70.2--I70.7-)

● **I74   Arterial embolism and thrombosis**

Includes   embolic infarction
embolic occlusion
thrombotic infarction
thrombotic occlusion

Code first embolism and thrombosis complicating abortion or ectopic or molar pregnancy (O00-O07, O08.2)
embolism and thrombosis complicating pregnancy, childbirth and the puerperium (O88.-)

Excludes2   atheroembolism (I75.-)
basilar embolism and thrombosis (I63.0-I63.2, I65.1)
carotid embolism and thrombosis (I63.0-I63.2, I65.2)
cerebral embolism and thrombosis (I63.3-I63.5, I66.-)
coronary embolism and thrombosis (I21-I25)
mesenteric embolism and thrombosis (K55.0-) ◀▥
ophthalmic embolism and thrombosis (H34.-)
precerebral embolism and thrombosis NOS (I63.0-I63.2, I65.9)
pulmonary embolism and thrombosis (I26.-)
renal embolism and thrombosis (N28.0)
retinal embolism and thrombosis (H34.-)
septic embolism and thrombosis (I76)
vertebral embolism and thrombosis (I63.0-I63.2, I65.0)

● **I74.0   Embolism and thrombosis of abdominal aorta**

I74.01   **Saddle embolus of abdominal aorta**

I74.09   **Other arterial embolism and thrombosis of abdominal aorta**
Aortic bifurcation syndrome
Aortoiliac obstruction
Leriche's syndrome

● **I74.1   Embolism and thrombosis of other and unspecified parts of aorta**

I74.10   **Embolism and thrombosis of unspecified parts of aorta**

I74.11   **Embolism and thrombosis of thoracic aorta**

I74.19   **Embolism and thrombosis of other parts of aorta**

I74.2   **Embolism and thrombosis of arteries of the upper extremities**

I74.3   **Embolism and thrombosis of arteries of the lower extremities**

I74.4   **Embolism and thrombosis of arteries of extremities, unspecified**
Peripheral arterial embolism NOS

I74.5   **Embolism and thrombosis of iliac artery**

I74.8   **Embolism and thrombosis of other arteries**

I74.9   **Embolism and thrombosis of unspecified artery**

● **I75   Atheroembolism**

Includes   atherothrombotic microembolism
cholesterol embolism

● **I75.0   Atheroembolism of extremities**

● **I75.01   Atheroembolism of upper extremity**

I75.011   **Atheroembolism of right upper extremity**

I75.012   **Atheroembolism of left upper extremity**

I75.013   **Atheroembolism of bilateral upper extremities**

I75.019   **Atheroembolism of unspecified upper extremity**

● **I75.02   Atheroembolism of lower extremity**

I75.021   **Atheroembolism of right lower extremity**

I75.022   **Atheroembolism of left lower extremity**

I75.023   **Atheroembolism of bilateral lower extremities**

I75.029   **Atheroembolism of unspecified lower extremity**

● **I75.8   Atheroembolism of other sites**

I75.81   **Atheroembolism of kidney**
Use additional code for any associated acute kidney failure and chronic kidney disease (N17.-, N18.-)

I75.89   **Atheroembolism of other site**

I76   **Septic arterial embolism**
Code first underlying infection, such as:
infective endocarditis (I33.0)
lung abscess (J85.-)
Use additional code to identify the site of the embolism (I74.-)
Excludes2   septic pulmonary embolism (I26.01, I26.90)

● **I77   Other disorders of arteries and arterioles**

Excludes2   collagen (vascular) diseases (M30-M36)
hypersensitivity angiitis (M31.0)
pulmonary artery (I28.-)

I77.0   **Arteriovenous fistula, acquired**
Aneurysmal varix
Arteriovenous aneurysm, acquired
Excludes1   arteriovenous aneurysm NOS (Q27.3-)
presence of arteriovenous shunt (fistula) for dialysis (Z99.2)
traumatic - see injury of blood vessel by body region
Excludes2   cerebral (I67.1)
coronary (I25.4)

I77.1   **Stricture of artery**
Narrowing of artery

I77.2   **Rupture of artery**
Erosion of artery
Fistula of artery
Ulcer of artery
Excludes1   traumatic rupture of artery - see injury of blood vessel by body region

Item 9-9   An **embolus** is a mass of undissolved matter present in the blood that is transported by the blood current. A **thrombus** is a blood clot that occludes or shuts off a vessel. When a thrombus is dislodged, it becomes an embolus.

Embolus

Figure 9-6   An arterial embolus.

◀ New   ◀▥ Revised   ~~deleted~~ Deleted   Excludes 1   Excludes 2   Includes   Use additional   Code first   Code also   Unspecified

OGCR Official Guidelines   X Assign placeholder X   ● Use Additional Character(s)   ▶ Manifestation Code   **Coding Clinic**

I77.3   **Arterial fibromuscular dysplasia**
Fibromuscular hyperplasia (of) carotid artery
Fibromuscular hyperplasia (of) renal artery

I77.4   **Celiac artery compression syndrome**

I77.5   **Necrosis of artery**

I77.6   **Arteritis, unspecified**
Aortitis NOS
Endarteritis NOS
   Excludes1   arteritis or endarteritis:
aortic arch (M31.4)
cerebral NEC (I67.7)
coronary (I25.89)
deformans (I70.-)
giant cell (M31.5., M31.6)
obliterans (I70.-)
senile (I70.-)

I77.7   **Other arterial dissection**
   Excludes2   dissection of aorta (I71.0-)
dissection of coronary artery (I25.42)

   I77.70   **Dissection of unspecified artery** ◀

   I77.71   **Dissection of carotid artery**

   I77.72   **Dissection of iliac artery**

   I77.73   **Dissection of renal artery**

   I77.74   **Dissection of vertebral artery**
     Excludes2   aneurysm of vertebral artery (I72.6) ◀

   I77.75   **Dissection of other precerebral arteries** ◀
Dissection of basilar artery (trunk) ◀
     Excludes2   aneurysm of carotid artery (I72.0) ◀
aneurysm of other precerebral arteries (I72.5) ◀
aneurysm of vertebral artery (I72.6) ◀
dissection of carotid artery (I77.71) ◀
dissection of vertebral artery (I77.74) ◀

   I77.76   **Dissection of artery of upper extremity** ◀

   I77.77   **Dissection of artery of lower extremity** ◀

   I77.79   **Dissection of other specified artery** ◀⫿

I77.8   **Other specified disorders of arteries and arterioles**

   I77.81   **Aortic ectasia**
Ectasis aorta
     Excludes1   aortic aneurysm and dissection (I71.0-)

     I77.810   **Thoracic aortic ectasia**
     I77.811   **Abdominal aortic ectasia**
     I77.812   **Thoracoabdominal aortic ectasia**
     I77.819   **Aortic ectasia, unspecified site**

   I77.89   **Other specified disorders of arteries and arterioles**

I77.9   **Disorder of arteries and arterioles, unspecified**

I78   **Diseases of capillaries**

I78.0   **Hereditary hemorrhagic telangiectasia**
Rendu-Osler-Weber disease

I78.1   **Nevus, non-neoplastic**
Araneus nevus   Spider nevus
Senile nevus   Stellar nevus
   Excludes1   nevus NOS (D22.-)
vascular NOS (Q82.5)
   Excludes2   blue nevus (D22.-)
flammeus nevus (Q82.5)
hairy nevus (D22.-)
melanocytic nevus (D22.-)
pigmented nevus (D22.-)
portwine nevus (Q82.5)
sanguineous nevus (Q82.5)
strawberry nevus (Q82.5)
verrucous nevus (Q82.5)

I78.8   **Other diseases of capillaries**

I78.9   **Disease of capillaries, unspecified**

I79   **Disorders of arteries, arterioles and capillaries in diseases classified elsewhere**

   I79.0   *Aneurysm of aorta in diseases classified elsewhere*
Code first underlying disease
   Excludes1   syphilitic aneurysm (A52.01)

   I79.1   *Aortitis in diseases classified elsewhere*
Code first underlying disease
   Excludes1   syphilitic aortitis (A52.02)

   I79.8   *Other disorders of arteries, arterioles and capillaries in diseases classified elsewhere*
Code first underlying disease, such as:
amyloidosis (E85.-)
   Excludes1   diabetic (peripheral) angiopathy (E08-E13 with .51-.52)
syphilitic endarteritis (A52.09)
tuberculous endarteritis (A18.89)

DISEASES OF VEINS, LYMPHATIC VESSELS AND LYMPH NODES, NOT ELSEWHERE CLASSIFIED (I80-I89)

I80   **Phlebitis and thrombophlebitis**
Inflammation of a vein with infiltration of walls (phlebitis).
   Includes   endophlebitis
inflammation, vein
periphlebitis
suppurative phlebitis
Code first phlebitis and thrombophlebitis complicating abortion, ectopic or molar pregnancy (O00-O07, O08.7)
phlebitis and thrombophlebitis complicating pregnancy, childbirth and the puerperium (O22.-, O87.-)
   Excludes1   venous embolism and thrombosis of lower extremities (I82.4-, I82.5-, I82.81-)

I80.0   **Phlebitis and thrombophlebitis of superficial vessels of lower extremities**
Phlebitis and thrombophlebitis of femoropopliteal vein

   I80.00   **Phlebitis and thrombophlebitis of superficial vessels of unspecified lower extremity**

   I80.01   **Phlebitis and thrombophlebitis of superficial vessels of right lower extremity**

   I80.02   **Phlebitis and thrombophlebitis of superficial vessels of left lower extremity**

   I80.03   **Phlebitis and thrombophlebitis of superficial vessels of lower extremities, bilateral**

● **I80.1**   **Phlebitis and thrombophlebitis of femoral vein**

    I80.10   Phlebitis and thrombophlebitis of unspecified femoral vein

    I80.11   Phlebitis and thrombophlebitis of right femoral vein

    I80.12   Phlebitis and thrombophlebitis of left femoral vein

    I80.13   Phlebitis and thrombophlebitis of femoral vein, bilateral

● **I80.2**   **Phlebitis and thrombophlebitis of other and unspecified deep vessels of lower extremities**

    ● **I80.20**   Phlebitis and thrombophlebitis of unspecified deep vessels of lower extremities

      I80.201   Phlebitis and thrombophlebitis of unspecified deep vessels of right lower extremity

      I80.202   Phlebitis and thrombophlebitis of unspecified deep vessels of left lower extremity

      I80.203   Phlebitis and thrombophlebitis of unspecified deep vessels of lower extremities, bilateral

      I80.209   Phlebitis and thrombophlebitis of unspecified deep vessels of unspecified lower extremity

    ● **I80.21**   Phlebitis and thrombophlebitis of iliac vein

      I80.211   Phlebitis and thrombophlebitis of right iliac vein

      I80.212   Phlebitis and thrombophlebitis of left iliac vein

      I80.213   Phlebitis and thrombophlebitis of iliac vein, bilateral

      I80.219   Phlebitis and thrombophlebitis of unspecified iliac vein

    ● **I80.22**   Phlebitis and thrombophlebitis of popliteal vein

      I80.221   Phlebitis and thrombophlebitis of right popliteal vein

      I80.222   Phlebitis and thrombophlebitis of left popliteal vein

      I80.223   Phlebitis and thrombophlebitis of popliteal vein, bilateral

      I80.229   Phlebitis and thrombophlebitis of unspecified popliteal vein

    ● **I80.23**   Phlebitis and thrombophlebitis of tibial vein

      I80.231   Phlebitis and thrombophlebitis of right tibial vein

      I80.232   Phlebitis and thrombophlebitis of left tibial vein

      I80.233   Phlebitis and thrombophlebitis of tibial vein, bilateral

      I80.239   Phlebitis and thrombophlebitis of unspecified tibial vein

    ● **I80.29**   Phlebitis and thrombophlebitis of other deep vessels of lower extremities

      I80.291   Phlebitis and thrombophlebitis of other deep vessels of right lower extremity

      I80.292   Phlebitis and thrombophlebitis of other deep vessels of left lower extremity

      I80.293   Phlebitis and thrombophlebitis of other deep vessels of lower extremity, bilateral

      I80.299   Phlebitis and thrombophlebitis of other deep vessels of unspecified lower extremity

   I80.3   Phlebitis and thrombophlebitis of lower extremities, unspecified

   I80.8   Phlebitis and thrombophlebitis of other sites

   I80.9   Phlebitis and thrombophlebitis of unspecified site

   I81   **Portal vein thrombosis**

     Portal (vein) obstruction

     Excludes2   hepatic vein thrombosis (I82.0)
               phlebitis of portal vein (K75.1)

● **I82**   **Other venous embolism and thrombosis**

     Code first venous embolism and thrombosis complicating:
      abortion, ectopic or molar pregnancy (O00-O07, O08.7)
      pregnancy, childbirth and the puerperium (O22.-, O87.-)

     Excludes2   venous embolism and thrombosis (of):
               cerebral (I63.6, I67.6)
               coronary (I21-I25)
               intracranial and intraspinal, septic or NOS (G08)
               intracranial, nonpyogenic (I67.6)
               intraspinal, nonpyogenic (G95.1)
               mesenteric (K55.0-) ◀▥
               portal (I81)
               pulmonary (I26.-)

   I82.0   **Budd-Chiari syndrome**
      Hepatic vein thrombosis

   I82.1   **Thrombophlebitis migrans**
      "White leg" is the other term to describe a migrating thrombus.

● **I82.2**   **Embolism and thrombosis of vena cava and other thoracic veins**

    ● **I82.21**   Embolism and thrombosis of superior vena cava

      I82.210   **Acute embolism and thrombosis of superior vena cava**
         Embolism and thrombosis of superior vena cava NOS

      I82.211   **Chronic embolism and thrombosis of superior vena cava**

    ● **I82.22**   Embolism and thrombosis of inferior vena cava

      I82.220   **Acute embolism and thrombosis of inferior vena cava**
         Embolism and thrombosis of inferior vena cava NOS

      I82.221   **Chronic embolism and thrombosis of inferior vena cava**

    ● **I82.29**   Embolism and thrombosis of other thoracic veins
      Embolism and thrombosis of brachiocephalic (innominate) vein

      I82.290   **Acute embolism and thrombosis of other thoracic veins**

      I82.291   **Chronic embolism and thrombosis of other thoracic veins**

   I82.3   **Embolism and thrombosis of renal vein**

● **I82.4**   **Acute embolism and thrombosis of deep veins of lower extremity**

    I82.40   **Acute embolism and thrombosis of unspecified deep veins of lower extremity**
      Deep vein thrombosis NOS
      DVT NOS

      Excludes1   acute embolism and thrombosis of unspecified deep veins of distal lower extremity (I82.4Z-)
           acute embolism and thrombosis of unspecified deep veins of proximal lower extremity (I82.4Y-)

      I82.401   **Acute embolism and thrombosis of unspecified deep veins of right lower extremity**

      I82.402   **Acute embolism and thrombosis of unspecified deep veins of left lower extremity**

      I82.403   **Acute embolism and thrombosis of unspecified deep veins of lower extremity, bilateral**

      I82.409   **Acute embolism and thrombosis of unspecified deep veins of unspecified lower extremity**

◀ New   ◀▥ Revised   ~~deleted~~ Deleted   Excludes 1   Excludes 2   Includes   Use additional   Code first   Code also   Unspecified

888   OGCR Official Guidelines   X Assign placeholder X   ● Use Additional Character(s)   ▷ Manifestation Code   **Coding Clinic**

● **I82.41**   Acute embolism and thrombosis of femoral vein

     I82.411   Acute embolism and thrombosis of right femoral vein

     I82.412   Acute embolism and thrombosis of left femoral vein

     I82.413   Acute embolism and thrombosis of femoral vein, bilateral

     I82.419   Acute embolism and thrombosis of unspecified femoral vein

● **I82.42**   Acute embolism and thrombosis of iliac vein

     I82.421   Acute embolism and thrombosis of right iliac vein

     I82.422   Acute embolism and thrombosis of left iliac vein

     I82.423   Acute embolism and thrombosis of iliac vein, bilateral

     I82.429   Acute embolism and thrombosis of unspecified iliac vein

● **I82.43**   Acute embolism and thrombosis of popliteal vein

     I82.431   Acute embolism and thrombosis of right popliteal vein

     I82.432   Acute embolism and thrombosis of left popliteal vein

     I82.433   Acute embolism and thrombosis of popliteal vein, bilateral

     I82.439   Acute embolism and thrombosis of unspecified popliteal vein

● **I82.44**   Acute embolism and thrombosis of tibial vein

     I82.441   Acute embolism and thrombosis of right tibial vein

     I82.442   Acute embolism and thrombosis of left tibial vein

     I82.443   Acute embolism and thrombosis of tibial vein, bilateral

     I82.449   Acute embolism and thrombosis of unspecified tibial vein

● **I82.49**   Acute embolism and thrombosis of other specified deep vein of lower extremity

     I82.491   Acute embolism and thrombosis of other specified deep vein of right lower extremity

     I82.492   Acute embolism and thrombosis of other specified deep vein of left lower extremity

     I82.493   Acute embolism and thrombosis of other specified deep vein of lower extremity, bilateral

     I82.499   Acute embolism and thrombosis of other specified deep vein of unspecified lower extremity

● **I82.4Y**   Acute embolism and thrombosis of unspecified deep veins of proximal lower extremity

     Acute embolism and thrombosis of deep vein of thigh NOS

     Acute embolism and thrombosis of deep vein of upper leg NOS

     I82.4Y1   Acute embolism and thrombosis of unspecified deep veins of right proximal lower extremity

     I82.4Y2   Acute embolism and thrombosis of unspecified deep veins of left proximal lower extremity

     I82.4Y3   Acute embolism and thrombosis of unspecified deep veins of proximal lower extremity, bilateral

     I82.4Y9   Acute embolism and thrombosis of unspecified deep veins of unspecified proximal lower extremity

● **I82.4Z**   Acute embolism and thrombosis of unspecified deep veins of distal lower extremity

     Acute embolism and thrombosis of deep vein of calf NOS

     Acute embolism and thrombosis of deep vein of lower leg NOS

     I82.4Z1   Acute embolism and thrombosis of unspecified deep veins of right distal lower extremity

     I82.4Z2   Acute embolism and thrombosis of unspecified deep veins of left distal lower extremity

     I82.4Z3   Acute embolism and thrombosis of unspecified deep veins of distal lower extremity, bilateral

     I82.4Z9   Acute embolism and thrombosis of unspecified deep veins of unspecified distal lower extremity

● **I82.5**   Chronic embolism and thrombosis of deep veins of lower extremity

     Use additional code, if applicable, for associated long-term (current) use of anticoagulants (Z79.01)

     Excludes1   personal history of venous embolism and thrombosis (Z86.718)

   ● **I82.50**   Chronic embolism and thrombosis of unspecified deep veins of lower extremity

     Excludes1   chronic embolism and thrombosis of unspecified deep veins of distal lower extremity (I82.5Z-)

                 chronic embolism and thrombosis of unspecified deep veins of proximal lower extremity (I82.5Y-)

     I82.501   Chronic embolism and thrombosis of unspecified deep veins of right lower extremity

     I82.502   Chronic embolism and thrombosis of unspecified deep veins of left lower extremity

     I82.503   Chronic embolism and thrombosis of unspecified deep veins of lower extremity, bilateral

     I82.509   Chronic embolism and thrombosis of unspecified deep veins of unspecified lower extremity

   ● **I82.51**   Chronic embolism and thrombosis of femoral vein

     I82.511   Chronic embolism and thrombosis of right femoral vein

     I82.512   Chronic embolism and thrombosis of left femoral vein

     I82.513   Chronic embolism and thrombosis of femoral vein, bilateral

     I82.519   Chronic embolism and thrombosis of unspecified femoral vein

   ● **I82.52**   Chronic embolism and thrombosis of iliac vein

     I82.521   Chronic embolism and thrombosis of right iliac vein

     I82.522   Chronic embolism and thrombosis of left iliac vein

     I82.523   Chronic embolism and thrombosis of iliac vein, bilateral

     I82.529   Chronic embolism and thrombosis of unspecified iliac vein

CHAPTER 9 (I00-I99)

Item 9–10 Varicose/Varicosities (varix = singular, varices = plural): Enlarged, engorged, tortuous, twisted vascular vessels (veins, arteries, lymphatics). As such, the condition can present in various parts of the body, although the most familiar locations are the lower extremities. A common complication of varices is thrombophlebitis. Varicosities of the anus and rectum are called hemorrhoids.

Figure 9-7 Varicose veins of the legs. (From Goldman: Cecil Medicine, ed 23, Saunders, 2008)

- **I82.53 Chronic embolism and thrombosis of popliteal vein**
  - I82.531 Chronic embolism and thrombosis of right popliteal vein
  - I82.532 Chronic embolism and thrombosis of left popliteal vein
  - I82.533 Chronic embolism and thrombosis of popliteal vein, bilateral
  - I82.539 Chronic embolism and thrombosis of unspecified popliteal vein
- **I82.54 Chronic embolism and thrombosis of tibial vein**
  - I82.541 Chronic embolism and thrombosis of right tibial vein
  - I82.542 Chronic embolism and thrombosis of left tibial vein
  - I82.543 Chronic embolism and thrombosis of tibial vein, bilateral
  - I82.549 Chronic embolism and thrombosis of unspecified tibial vein
- **I82.59 Chronic embolism and thrombosis of other specified deep vein of lower extremity**
  - I82.591 Chronic embolism and thrombosis of other specified deep vein of right lower extremity
  - I82.592 Chronic embolism and thrombosis of other specified deep vein of left lower extremity
  - I82.593 Chronic embolism and thrombosis of other specified deep vein of lower extremity, bilateral
  - I82.599 Chronic embolism and thrombosis of other specified deep vein of unspecified lower extremity
- **I82.5Y Chronic embolism and thrombosis of unspecified deep veins of proximal lower extremity**
  Chronic embolism and thrombosis of deep veins of thigh NOS
  Chronic embolism and thrombosis of deep veins of upper leg NOS
  - I82.5Y1 Chronic embolism and thrombosis of unspecified deep veins of right proximal lower extremity
  - I82.5Y2 Chronic embolism and thrombosis of unspecified deep veins of left proximal lower extremity
  - I82.5Y3 Chronic embolism and thrombosis of unspecified deep veins of proximal lower extremity, bilateral
  - I82.5Y9 Chronic embolism and thrombosis of unspecified deep veins of unspecified proximal lower extremity

- **I82.5Z Chronic embolism and thrombosis of unspecified deep veins of distal lower extremity**
  Chronic embolism and thrombosis of deep veins of calf NOS
  Chronic embolism and thrombosis of deep veins of lower leg NOS
  - I82.5Z1 Chronic embolism and thrombosis of unspecified deep veins of right distal lower extremity
  - I82.5Z2 Chronic embolism and thrombosis of unspecified deep veins of left distal lower extremity
  - I82.5Z3 Chronic embolism and thrombosis of unspecified deep veins of distal lower extremity, bilateral
  - I82.5Z9 Chronic embolism and thrombosis of unspecified deep veins of unspecified distal lower extremity
- **I82.6 Acute embolism and thrombosis of veins of upper extremity**
  - **I82.60 Acute embolism and thrombosis of unspecified veins of upper extremity**
    - I82.601 Acute embolism and thrombosis of unspecified veins of right upper extremity
    - I82.602 Acute embolism and thrombosis of unspecified veins of left upper extremity
    - I82.603 Acute embolism and thrombosis of unspecified veins of upper extremity, bilateral
    - I82.609 Acute embolism and thrombosis of unspecified veins of unspecified upper extremity
  - **I82.61 Acute embolism and thrombosis of superficial veins of upper extremity**
    Acute embolism and thrombosis of antecubital vein
    Acute embolism and thrombosis of basilic vein
    Acute embolism and thrombosis of cephalic vein
    - I82.611 Acute embolism and thrombosis of superficial veins of right upper extremity
    - I82.612 Acute embolism and thrombosis of superficial veins of left upper extremity
    - I82.613 Acute embolism and thrombosis of superficial veins of upper extremity, bilateral
    - I82.619 Acute embolism and thrombosis of superficial veins of unspecified upper extremity
  - **I82.62 Acute embolism and thrombosis of deep veins of upper extremity**
    Acute embolism and thrombosis of brachial vein
    Acute embolism and thrombosis of radial vein
    Acute embolism and thrombosis of ulnar vein
    - I82.621 Acute embolism and thrombosis of deep veins of right upper extremity
    - I82.622 Acute embolism and thrombosis of deep veins of left upper extremity
    - I82.623 Acute embolism and thrombosis of deep veins of upper extremity, bilateral
    - I82.629 Acute embolism and thrombosis of deep veins of unspecified upper extremity

◀ New   ◀▦ Revised   ~~deleted~~ Deleted   Excludes 1   Excludes 2   Includes   Use additional   Code first   Code also   Unspecified

890   **OGCR** Official Guidelines   X Assign placeholder X   ● Use Additional Character(s)   ▶ Manifestation Code   **Coding Clinic**

● **I82.7**   **Chronic embolism and thrombosis of veins of upper extremity**

> Use additional code, if applicable, for associated long-term (current) use of anticoagulants (Z79.01)
>
> **Excludes1**   personal history of venous embolism and thrombosis (Z86.718)

  ● **I82.70**   **Chronic embolism and thrombosis of unspecified veins of upper extremity**

     I82.701   Chronic embolism and thrombosis of unspecified veins of right upper extremity

     I82.702   Chronic embolism and thrombosis of unspecified veins of left upper extremity

     I82.703   Chronic embolism and thrombosis of unspecified veins of upper extremity, bilateral

     I82.709   Chronic embolism and thrombosis of unspecified veins of unspecified upper extremity

  ● **I82.71**   **Chronic embolism and thrombosis of superficial veins of upper extremity**

> Chronic embolism and thrombosis of antecubital vein
> Chronic embolism and thrombosis of basilic vein
> Chronic embolism and thrombosis of cephalic vein

     I82.711   Chronic embolism and thrombosis of superficial veins of right upper extremity

     I82.712   Chronic embolism and thrombosis of superficial veins of left upper extremity

     I82.713   Chronic embolism and thrombosis of superficial veins of upper extremity, bilateral

     I82.719   Chronic embolism and thrombosis of superficial veins of unspecified upper extremity

  ● **I82.72**   **Chronic embolism and thrombosis of deep veins of upper extremity**

> Chronic embolism and thrombosis of brachial vein
> Chronic embolism and thrombosis of radial vein
> Chronic embolism and thrombosis of ulnar vein

     I82.721   Chronic embolism and thrombosis of deep veins of right upper extremity

     I82.722   Chronic embolism and thrombosis of deep veins of left upper extremity

     I82.723   Chronic embolism and thrombosis of deep veins of upper extremity, bilateral

     I82.729   Chronic embolism and thrombosis of deep veins of unspecified upper extremity

● **I82.A**   **Embolism and thrombosis of axillary vein**

  ● **I82.A1**   **Acute embolism and thrombosis of axillary vein**

     I82.A11   Acute embolism and thrombosis of right axillary vein

     I82.A12   Acute embolism and thrombosis of left axillary vein

     I82.A13   Acute embolism and thrombosis of axillary vein, bilateral

     I82.A19   Acute embolism and thrombosis of unspecified axillary vein

  ● **I82.A2**   **Chronic embolism and thrombosis of axillary vein**

     I82.A21   Chronic embolism and thrombosis of right axillary vein

     I82.A22   Chronic embolism and thrombosis of left axillary vein

     I82.A23   Chronic embolism and thrombosis of axillary vein, bilateral

     I82.A29   Chronic embolism and thrombosis of unspecified axillary vein

● **I82.B**   **Embolism and thrombosis of subclavian vein**

  ● **I82.B1**   **Acute embolism and thrombosis of subclavian vein**

     I82.B11   Acute embolism and thrombosis of right subclavian vein

     I82.B12   Acute embolism and thrombosis of left subclavian vein

     I82.B13   Acute embolism and thrombosis of subclavian vein, bilateral

     I82.B19   Acute embolism and thrombosis of unspecified subclavian vein

  ● **I82.B2**   **Chronic embolism and thrombosis of subclavian vein**

     I82.B21   Chronic embolism and thrombosis of right subclavian vein

     I82.B22   Chronic embolism and thrombosis of left subclavian vein

     I82.B23   Chronic embolism and thrombosis of subclavian vein, bilateral

     I82.B29   Chronic embolism and thrombosis of unspecified subclavian vein

● **I82.C**   **Embolism and thrombosis of internal jugular vein**

  ● **I82.C1**   **Acute embolism and thrombosis of internal jugular vein**

     I82.C11   Acute embolism and thrombosis of right internal jugular vein

     I82.C12   Acute embolism and thrombosis of left internal jugular vein

     I82.C13   Acute embolism and thrombosis of internal jugular vein, bilateral

     I82.C19   Acute embolism and thrombosis of unspecified internal jugular vein

  ● **I82.C2**   **Chronic embolism and thrombosis of internal jugular vein**

     I82.C21   Chronic embolism and thrombosis of right internal jugular vein

     I82.C22   Chronic embolism and thrombosis of left internal jugular vein

     I82.C23   Chronic embolism and thrombosis of internal jugular vein, bilateral

     I82.C29   Chronic embolism and thrombosis of unspecified internal jugular vein

● **I82.8**   **Embolism and thrombosis of other specified veins**

> Use additional code, if applicable, for associated long-term (current) use of anticoagulants (Z79.01)

  ● **I82.81**   **Embolism and thrombosis of superficial veins of lower extremities**

> Embolism and thrombosis of saphenous vein (greater) (lesser)

     I82.811   Embolism and thrombosis of superficial veins of right lower extremities

     I82.812   Embolism and thrombosis of superficial veins of left lower extremities

     I82.813   Embolism and thrombosis of superficial veins of lower extremities, bilateral

     I82.819   Embolism and thrombosis of superficial veins of unspecified lower extremities

CHAPTER 9 (I00-I99)

● **I82.89**   **Embolism and thrombosis of other specified veins**

     I82.890   **Acute embolism and thrombosis of other specified veins**

     I82.891   **Chronic embolism and thrombosis of other specified veins**

● **I82.9**   **Embolism and thrombosis of unspecified vein**

     I82.90   **Acute embolism and thrombosis of** `unspecified` **vein**

         Embolism of vein NOS

         Thrombosis (vein) NOS

     I82.91   **Chronic embolism and thrombosis of** `unspecified` **vein**

● **I83**   **Varicose veins of lower extremities**

     `Excludes1`   varicose veins complicating pregnancy (O22.0-)

               varicose veins complicating the puerperium (O87.4)

● **I83.0**   **Varicose veins of lower extremities with ulcer**

     Use additional code to identify severity of ulcer (L97.-)

  ● **I83.00**   **Varicose veins of unspecified lower extremity with ulcer**

     I83.001   **Varicose veins of** `unspecified` **lower extremity with ulcer of thigh**   A

     I83.002   **Varicose veins of** `unspecified` **lower extremity with ulcer of calf**   A

     I83.003   **Varicose veins of** `unspecified` **lower extremity with ulcer of ankle**   A

     I83.004   **Varicose veins of** `unspecified` **lower extremity with ulcer of heel and midfoot**   A

         Varicose veins of unspecified lower extremity with ulcer of plantar surface of midfoot

     I83.005   **Varicose veins of** `unspecified` **lower extremity with ulcer other part of foot**   A

         Varicose veins of unspecified lower extremity with ulcer of toe

     I83.008   **Varicose veins of** `unspecified` **lower extremity with ulcer other part of lower leg**   A

     I83.009   **Varicose veins of** `unspecified` **lower extremity with ulcer of unspecified site**   A

  ● **I83.01**   **Varicose veins of right lower extremity with ulcer**

     I83.011   **Varicose veins of right lower extremity with ulcer of thigh**   A

     I83.012   **Varicose veins of right lower extremity with ulcer of calf**   A

     I83.013   **Varicose veins of right lower extremity with ulcer of ankle**   A

     I83.014   **Varicose veins of right lower extremity with ulcer of heel and midfoot**   A

         Varicose veins of right lower extremity with ulcer of plantar surface of midfoot

     I83.015   **Varicose veins of right lower extremity with ulcer other part of foot**   A

         Varicose veins of right lower extremity with ulcer of toe

     I83.018   **Varicose veins of right lower extremity with ulcer other part of lower leg**   A

     I83.019   **Varicose veins of right lower extremity with ulcer of** `unspecified` **site**   A

● **I83.02**   **Varicose veins of left lower extremity with ulcer**

     I83.021   **Varicose veins of left lower extremity with ulcer of thigh**   A

     I83.022   **Varicose veins of left lower extremity with ulcer of calf**   A

     I83.023   **Varicose veins of left lower extremity with ulcer of ankle**   A

     I83.024   **Varicose veins of left lower extremity with ulcer of heel and midfoot**   A

         Varicose veins of left lower extremity with ulcer of plantar surface of midfoot

     I83.025   **Varicose veins of left lower extremity with ulcer other part of foot**   A

         Varicose veins of left lower extremity with ulcer of toe

     I83.028   **Varicose veins of left lower extremity with ulcer other part of lower leg**   A

     I83.029   **Varicose veins of left lower extremity with ulcer of** `unspecified` **site**   A

● **I83.1**   **Varicose veins of lower extremities with inflammation**

     ~~Stasis dermatitis~~

     I83.10   **Varicose veins of** `unspecified` **lower extremity with inflammation**   A

     I83.11   **Varicose veins of right lower extremity with inflammation**   A

     I83.12   **Varicose veins of left lower extremity with inflammation**   A

● **I83.2**   **Varicose veins of lower extremities with both ulcer and inflammation**

     Use additional code to identify severity of ulcer (L97.-)

  ● **I83.20**   **Varicose veins of unspecified lower extremity with both ulcer and inflammation**

     I83.201   **Varicose veins of** `unspecified` **lower extremity with both ulcer of thigh and inflammation**   A

     I83.202   **Varicose veins of** `unspecified` **lower extremity with both ulcer of calf and inflammation**   A

     I83.203   **Varicose veins of** `unspecified` **lower extremity with both ulcer of ankle and inflammation**   A

     I83.204   **Varicose veins of** `unspecified` **lower extremity with both ulcer of heel and midfoot and inflammation**   A

         Varicose veins of unspecified lower extremity with both ulcer of plantar surface of midfoot and inflammation

     I83.205   **Varicose veins of** `unspecified` **lower extremity with both ulcer other part of foot and inflammation**   A

         Varicose veins of unspecified lower extremity with both ulcer of toe and inflammation

     I83.208   **Varicose veins of** `unspecified` **lower extremity with both ulcer of other part of lower extremity and inflammation**   A

     I83.209   **Varicose veins of** `unspecified` **lower extremity with both ulcer of unspecified site and inflammation**   A

◄ New   ⬅ Revised   ~~deleted~~ Deleted   `Excludes 1`   Excludes 2   Includes   Use additional   Code first   Code also   `Unspecified`

OGCR Official Guidelines   X Assign placeholder X   ● Use Additional Character(s)   ▶ Manifestation Code   **Coding Clinic**

● **I83.21** **Varicose veins of right lower extremity with both ulcer and inflammation**
- **I83.211** **Varicose veins of right lower extremity with both ulcer of thigh and inflammation**   A
- **I83.212** **Varicose veins of right lower extremity with both ulcer of calf and inflammation**   A
- **I83.213** **Varicose veins of right lower extremity with both ulcer of ankle and inflammation**   A
- **I83.214** **Varicose veins of right lower extremity with both ulcer of heel and midfoot and inflammation**   A
  Varicose veins of right lower extremity with both ulcer of plantar surface of midfoot and inflammation
- **I83.215** **Varicose veins of right lower extremity with both ulcer other part of foot and inflammation**   A
  Varicose veins of right lower extremity with both ulcer of toe and inflammation
- **I83.218** **Varicose veins of right lower extremity with both ulcer of other part of lower extremity and inflammation**   A
- **I83.219** **Varicose veins of right lower extremity with both ulcer of unspecified site and inflammation**   A

● **I83.22** **Varicose veins of left lower extremity with both ulcer and inflammation**
- **I83.221** **Varicose veins of left lower extremity with both ulcer of thigh and inflammation**   A
- **I83.222** **Varicose veins of left lower extremity with both ulcer of calf and inflammation**   A
- **I83.223** **Varicose veins of left lower extremity with both ulcer of ankle and inflammation**   A
- **I83.224** **Varicose veins of left lower extremity with both ulcer of heel and midfoot and inflammation**   A
  Varicose veins of left lower extremity with both ulcer of plantar surface of midfoot and inflammation
- **I83.225** **Varicose veins of left lower extremity with both ulcer other part of foot and inflammation**   A
  Varicose veins of left lower extremity with both ulcer of toe and inflammation
- **I83.228** **Varicose veins of left lower extremity with both ulcer of other part of lower extremity and inflammation**   A
- **I83.229** **Varicose veins of left lower extremity with both ulcer of unspecified site and inflammation**   A

● **I83.8** **Varicose veins of lower extremities with other complications**
● **I83.81** **Varicose veins of lower extremities with pain**
- **I83.811** **Varicose veins of right lower extremities with pain**   A
- **I83.812** **Varicose veins of left lower extremities with pain**   A
- **I83.813** **Varicose veins of bilateral lower extremities with pain**   A
- **I83.819** **Varicose veins of unspecified lower extremities with pain**   A

● **I83.89** **Varicose veins of lower extremities with other complications**
  Varicose veins of lower extremities with edema
  Varicose veins of lower extremities with swelling
- **I83.891** **Varicose veins of right lower extremities with other complications** A
- **I83.892** **Varicose veins of left lower extremities with other complications** A
- **I83.893** **Varicose veins of bilateral lower extremities with other complications** A
- **I83.899** **Varicose veins of unspecified lower extremities with other complications** A

● **I83.9** **Asymptomatic varicose veins of lower extremities**
  Phlebectasia of lower extremities
  Varicose veins of lower extremities
  Varix of lower extremities
- **I83.90** **Asymptomatic varicose veins of unspecified lower extremity**   A
  Varicose veins NOS
- **I83.91** **Asymptomatic varicose veins of right lower extremity**   A
- **I83.92** **Asymptomatic varicose veins of left lower extremity**   A
- **I83.93** **Asymptomatic varicose veins of bilateral lower extremities**   A

● **I85** **Esophageal varices**
  Use additional code to identify:
  alcohol abuse and dependence (F10.-)
● **I85.0** **Esophageal varices**
  Idiopathic esophageal varices
  Primary esophageal varices
- **I85.00** **Esophageal varices without bleeding**
  Esophageal varices NOS
- **I85.01** **Esophageal varices with bleeding**
● **I85.1** **Secondary esophageal varices**
  Esophageal varices secondary to alcoholic liver disease
  Esophageal varices secondary to cirrhosis of liver
  Esophageal varices secondary to schistosomiasis
  Esophageal varices secondary to toxic liver disease
  Code first underlying disease
- **I85.10** **Secondary esophageal varices without bleeding**
- **I85.11** **Secondary esophageal varices with bleeding**

● **I86** **Varicose veins of other sites**
  Excludes1   varicose veins of unspecified site (I83.9-)
  Excludes2   retinal varices (H35.0-)
- **I86.0** **Sublingual varices**
- **I86.1** **Scrotal varices** ♂
  Varicocele
- **I86.2** **Pelvic varices**
- **I86.3** **Vulval varices** ♀
  Excludes1   vulval varices complicating childbirth and the puerperium (O87.8)
  vulval varices complicating pregnancy (O22.1-)
- **I86.4** **Gastric varices**
- **I86.8** **Varicose veins of other specified sites**   A
  Varicose ulcer of nasal septum

CHAPTER 9 (I00–I99)

● **I87**   **Other disorders of veins**
  ● **I87.0**   **Postthrombotic syndrome**
     Chronic venous hypertension due to deep vein thrombosis
     Postphlebitic syndrome
     Excludes1   chronic venous hypertension without deep vein thrombosis (I87.3-)
    ● **I87.00**   **Postthrombotic syndrome without complications**
      Asymptomatic Postthrombotic syndrome
      I87.001   Postthrombotic syndrome without complications of right lower extremity
      I87.002   Postthrombotic syndrome without complications of left lower extremity
      I87.003   Postthrombotic syndrome without complications of bilateral lower extremity
      I87.009   Postthrombotic syndrome without complications of unspecified extremity
       Postthrombotic syndrome NOS
    ● **I87.01**   **Postthrombotic syndrome with ulcer**
      Use additional code to specify site and severity of ulcer (L97.-)
      I87.011   Postthrombotic syndrome with ulcer of right lower extremity
      I87.012   Postthrombotic syndrome with ulcer of left lower extremity
      I87.013   Postthrombotic syndrome with ulcer of bilateral lower extremity
      I87.019   Postthrombotic syndrome with ulcer of unspecified lower extremity
    ● **I87.02**   **Postthrombotic syndrome with inflammation**
      I87.021   Postthrombotic syndrome with inflammation of right lower extremity
      I87.022   Postthrombotic syndrome with inflammation of left lower extremity
      I87.023   Postthrombotic syndrome with inflammation of bilateral lower extremity
      I87.029   Postthrombotic syndrome with inflammation of unspecified lower extremity
    ● **I87.03**   **Postthrombotic syndrome with ulcer and inflammation**
      Use additional code to specify site and severity of ulcer (L97.-)
      I87.031   Postthrombotic syndrome with ulcer and inflammation of right lower extremity
      I87.032   Postthrombotic syndrome with ulcer and inflammation of left lower extremity
      I87.033   Postthrombotic syndrome with ulcer and inflammation of bilateral lower extremity
      I87.039   Postthrombotic syndrome with ulcer and inflammation of unspecified lower extremity

    ● **I87.09**   **Postthrombotic syndrome with other complications**
      I87.091   Postthrombotic syndrome with other complications of right lower extremity
      I87.092   Postthrombotic syndrome with other complications of left lower extremity
      I87.093   Postthrombotic syndrome with other complications of bilateral lower extremity
      I87.099   Postthrombotic syndrome with other complications of unspecified lower extremity
  I87.1   **Compression of vein**
     Stricture of vein
     Vena cava syndrome (inferior) (superior)
     Excludes2   compression of pulmonary vein (I28.8)
  I87.2   **Venous insufficiency (chronic) (peripheral)**
     Stasis dermatitis ◀
     Excludes1   stasis dermatitis with varicose veins of lower extremities (I83.1-, I83.2-) ◀
  ● **I87.3**   **Chronic venous hypertension (idiopathic)**
     Stasis edema
     Excludes1   chronic venous hypertension due to deep vein thrombosis (I87.0-)
      varicose veins of lower extremities (I83.-)
    ● **I87.30**   **Chronic venous hypertension (idiopathic) without complications**
      Asymptomatic chronic venous hypertension (idiopathic)
      I87.301   Chronic venous hypertension (idiopathic) without complications of right lower extremity
      I87.302   Chronic venous hypertension (idiopathic) without complications of left lower extremity
      I87.303   Chronic venous hypertension (idiopathic) without complications of bilateral lower extremity
      I87.309   Chronic venous hypertension (idiopathic) without complications of unspecified lower extremity
       Chronic venous hypertension NOS
    ● **I87.31**   **Chronic venous hypertension (idiopathic) with ulcer**
      Use additional code to specify site and severity of ulcer (L97.-)
      I87.311   Chronic venous hypertension (idiopathic) with ulcer of right lower extremity
      I87.312   Chronic venous hypertension (idiopathic) with ulcer of left lower extremity
      I87.313   Chronic venous hypertension (idiopathic) with ulcer of bilateral lower extremity
      I87.319   Chronic venous hypertension (idiopathic) with ulcer of unspecified lower extremity

● **I87.32**   **Chronic venous hypertension (idiopathic) with inflammation**
    I87.321   Chronic venous hypertension (idiopathic) with inflammation of right lower extremity
    I87.322   Chronic venous hypertension (idiopathic) with inflammation of left lower extremity
    I87.323   Chronic venous hypertension (idiopathic) with inflammation of bilateral lower extremity
    I87.329   Chronic venous hypertension (idiopathic) with inflammation of unspecified lower extremity

● **I87.33**   **Chronic venous hypertension (idiopathic) with ulcer and inflammation**
    Use additional code to specify site and severity of ulcer (L97.-)
    I87.331   Chronic venous hypertension (idiopathic) with ulcer and inflammation of right lower extremity
    I87.332   Chronic venous hypertension (idiopathic) with ulcer and inflammation of left lower extremity
    I87.333   Chronic venous hypertension (idiopathic) with ulcer and inflammation of bilateral lower extremity
    I87.339   Chronic venous hypertension (idiopathic) with ulcer and inflammation of unspecified lower extremity

● **I87.39**   **Chronic venous hypertension (idiopathic) with other complications**
    I87.391   Chronic venous hypertension (idiopathic) with other complications of right lower extremity
    I87.392   Chronic venous hypertension (idiopathic) with other complications of left lower extremity
    I87.393   Chronic venous hypertension (idiopathic) with other complications of bilateral lower extremity
    I87.399   Chronic venous hypertension (idiopathic) with other complications of unspecified lower extremity

I87.8   **Other specified disorders of veins**
    Phlebosclerosis
    Venofibrosis

I87.9   **Disorder of vein, unspecified**

● **I88**   **Nonspecific lymphadenitis**
    Excludes1 acute lymphadenitis, except mesenteric (L04.-)
        enlarged lymph nodes NOS (R59.-)
        human immunodeficiency virus [HIV] disease resulting in generalized lymphadenopathy (B20)

I88.0   **Nonspecific mesenteric lymphadenitis**
    Mesenteric lymphadenitis (acute)(chronic)

I88.1   **Chronic lymphadenitis, except mesenteric**
    Adenitis
    Lymphadenitis

I88.8   **Other nonspecific lymphadenitis**

I88.9   **Nonspecific lymphadenitis, unspecified**
    Lymphadenitis NOS

● **I89**   **Other noninfective disorders of lymphatic vessels and lymph nodes**
    Excludes1 chylocele, tunica vaginalis (nonfilarial) NOS (N50.89) ◄▥
        enlarged lymph nodes NOS (R59.-)
        filarial chylocele (B74.-)
        hereditary lymphedema (Q82.0)

I89.0   **Lymphedema, not elsewhere classified**
    Elephantiasis (nonfilarial) NOS
    Lymphangiectasis
    Obliteration, lymphatic vessel
    Praecox lymphedema
    Secondary lymphedema
    Excludes1 postmastectomy lymphedema (I97.2)

I89.1   **Lymphangitis**
    Chronic lymphangitis
    Lymphangitis NOS
    Subacute lymphangitis
    Excludes1 acute lymphangitis (L03.-)

I89.8   **Other specified noninfective disorders of lymphatic vessels and lymph nodes**
    Chylocele (nonfilarial)
    Chylous ascites
    Chylous cyst
    Lipomelanotic reticulosis
    Lymph node or vessel fistula
    Lymph node or vessel infarction
    Lymph node or vessel rupture

I89.9   **Noninfective disorder of lymphatic vessels and lymph nodes, unspecified**
    Disease of lymphatic vessels NOS

OTHER AND UNSPECIFIED DISORDERS OF THE CIRCULATORY SYSTEM (I95-I99)

● **I95**   **Hypotension**
    Subnormal arterial blood pressure
    Excludes1 cardiovascular collapse (R57.9)
        maternal hypotension syndrome (O26.5-)
        nonspecific low blood pressure reading NOS (R03.1)

I95.0   **Idiopathic hypotension**

I95.1   **Orthostatic hypotension**
    Hypotension, postural
    Moving from a sitting or reclining position to a standing position precipitates a sudden drop in blood pressure (hypotension).
    Excludes1 neurogenic orthostatic hypotension [Shy-Drager] (G90.3)
        orthostatic hypotension due to drugs (I95.2)

I95.2   **Hypotension due to drugs**
    Orthostatic hypotension due to drugs
    Use additional code for adverse effect, if applicable, to identify drug (T36-T50 with fifth or sixth character 5)

I95.3   **Hypotension of hemodialysis**
    Intra-dialytic hypotension

● **I95.8**   **Other hypotension**
    I95.81   Postprocedural hypotension
    I95.89   Other hypotension
        Chronic hypotension

I95.9   **Hypotension, unspecified**

I96   Gangrene, not elsewhere classified
   Gangrenous cellulitis
   Excludes1   gangrene in atherosclerosis of native arteries of
                  the extremities (I70.26)
                  gangrene of certain specified sites - *see*
                  Alphabetical Index
                  gangrene in diabetes mellitus
                  (E08-E13 with .52) ◀▥
                  gangrene in hernia (K40.1, K40.4, K41.1, K41.4,
                  K42.1, K43.1-, K44.1, K45.1, K46.1)
                  gangrene in other peripheral vascular diseases
                  (I73.-)
                  gas gangrene (A48.0)
                  pyoderma gangrenosum (L88)
   Coding Clinic: 2013, Q2, P35

● **I97   Intraoperative and postprocedural complications and disorders
         of circulatory system, not elsewhere classified**
   Excludes2   postprocedural shock (T81.1-)
   I97.0   Postcardiotomy syndrome
● **I97.1   Other postprocedural cardiac functional disturbances**
   Excludes2   acute pulmonary insufficiency following
                  thoracic surgery (J95.1)
                  intraoperative cardiac functional
                  disturbances (I97.7-)
   ● **I97.11   Postprocedural cardiac insufficiency**
      **I97.110   Postprocedural cardiac insufficiency
                  following cardiac surgery**
      **I97.111   Postprocedural cardiac insufficiency
                  following other surgery**
   ● **I97.12   Postprocedural cardiac arrest**
      **I97.120   Postprocedural cardiac arrest
                  following cardiac surgery**
      **I97.121   Postprocedural cardiac arrest
                  following other surgery**
   ● **I97.13   Postprocedural heart failure**
         Use additional code to identify the heart
         failure (I50.-)
      **I97.130   Postprocedural heart failure
                  following cardiac surgery**
      **I97.131   Postprocedural heart failure
                  following other surgery**
   ● **I97.19   Other postprocedural cardiac functional
               disturbances**
         Use additional code, if applicable, to further
         specify disorder
      **I97.190   Other postprocedural cardiac
                  functional disturbances following
                  cardiac surgery**
      **I97.191   Other postprocedural cardiac
                  functional disturbances following
                  other surgery**
   I97.2   Postmastectomy lymphedema syndrome   A
         Elephantiasis due to mastectomy
         Obliteration of lymphatic vessels
   I97.3   Postprocedural hypertension

● **I97.4   Intraoperative hemorrhage and hematoma of a
         circulatory system organ or structure complicating a
         procedure**
   Excludes1   intraoperative hemorrhage and
                  hematoma of a circulatory system
                  organ or structure due to accidental
                  puncture and laceration during a
                  procedure (I97.5-)
   Excludes2   intraoperative cerebrovascular
                  hemorrhage complicating a
                  procedure (G97.3-)
   ● **I97.41   Intraoperative hemorrhage and hematoma
               of a circulatory system organ or structure
               complicating a circulatory system procedure**
      **I97.410   Intraoperative hemorrhage and
                  hematoma of a circulatory system
                  organ or structure complicating a
                  cardiac catheterization**
      **I97.411   Intraoperative hemorrhage and
                  hematoma of a circulatory system
                  organ or structure complicating a
                  cardiac bypass**
      **I97.418   Intraoperative hemorrhage and
                  hematoma of a circulatory system
                  organ or structure complicating other
                  circulatory system procedure**
   **I97.42   Intraoperative hemorrhage and hematoma
               of a circulatory system organ or structure
               complicating other procedure**
● **I97.5   Accidental puncture and laceration of a circulatory
         system organ or structure during a procedure**
   Excludes2   accidental puncture and laceration of
                  brain during a procedure (G97.4-)
   **I97.51   Accidental puncture and laceration of a
               circulatory system organ or structure during a
               circulatory system procedure**
   **I97.52   Accidental puncture and laceration of a
               circulatory system organ or structure during
               other procedure**
● **I97.6   Postprocedural hemorrhage, hematoma and seroma of a
         circulatory system organ or structure following a
         procedure** ◀▥
   Excludes2   postprocedural cerebrovascular
                  hemorrhage complicating a
                  procedure (G97.5-)
   ● **I97.61   Postprocedural hemorrhage of a circulatory
               system organ or structure following a
               circulatory system procedure** ◀▥
      **I97.610   Postprocedural hemorrhage of a
                  circulatory system organ or structure
                  following a cardiac catheterization** ◀▥
      **I97.611   Postprocedural hemorrhage of a
                  circulatory system organ or structure
                  following cardiac bypass** ◀▥
      **I97.618   Postprocedural hemorrhage of a
                  circulatory system organ or structure
                  following other circulatory system
                  procedure** ◀▥

● **I97.62** **Postprocedural hemorrhage, hematoma and seroma of a circulatory system organ or structure following other procedure** ◀▥

     I97.620 **Postprocedural hemorrhage of a circulatory system organ or structure following other procedure** ◀

     I97.621 **Postprocedural hematoma of a circulatory system organ or structure following other procedure** ◀

     I97.622 **Postprocedural seroma of a circulatory system organ or structure following other procedure** ◀

● **I97.63** **Postprocedural hematoma of a circulatory system organ or structure following a circulatory system procedure** ◀

     I97.630 **Postprocedural hematoma of a circulatory system organ or structure following a cardiac catheterization** ◀

     I97.631 **Postprocedural hematoma of a circulatory system organ or structure following cardiac bypass** ◀

     I97.638 **Postprocedural hematoma of a circulatory system organ or structure following other circulatory system procedure** ◀

● **I97.64** **Postprocedural seroma of a circulatory system organ or structure following a circulatory system procedure** ◀

     I97.640 **Postprocedural seroma of a circulatory system organ or structure following a cardiac catheterization** ◀

     I97.641 **Postprocedural seroma of a circulatory system organ or structure following cardiac bypass** ◀

     I97.648 **Postprocedural seroma of a circulatory system organ or structure following other circulatory system procedure** ◀

● **I97.7** **Intraoperative cardiac functional disturbances**

     Excludes2   acute pulmonary insufficiency following thoracic surgery (J95.1)
         postprocedural cardiac functional disturbances (I97.1-)

   ● **I97.71** **Intraoperative cardiac arrest**

     I97.710 **Intraoperative cardiac arrest during cardiac surgery**

     I97.711 **Intraoperative cardiac arrest during other surgery**

   ● **I97.79** **Other intraoperative cardiac functional disturbances**

     Use additional code, if applicable, to further specify disorder

     I97.790 **Other intraoperative cardiac functional disturbances during cardiac surgery**

     I97.791 **Other intraoperative cardiac functional disturbances during other surgery**

● **I97.8** **Other intraoperative and postprocedural complications and disorders of the circulatory system, not elsewhere classified**

     Use additional code, if applicable, to further specify disorder

   ● **I97.81** **Intraoperative cerebrovascular infarction**

     I97.810 **Intraoperative cerebrovascular infarction during cardiac surgery**

     I97.811 **Intraoperative cerebrovascular infarction during other surgery**

   ● **I97.82** **Postprocedural cerebrovascular infarction**

     I97.820 **Postprocedural cerebrovascular infarction following cardiac surgery** ◀▥

     I97.821 **Postprocedural cerebrovascular infarction following other surgery** ◀▥

     I97.88 **Other intraoperative complications of the circulatory system, not elsewhere classified**

     I97.89 **Other postprocedural complications and disorders of the circulatory system, not elsewhere classified**

● **I99** **Other and unspecified disorders of circulatory system**

     I99.8 **Other disorder of circulatory system**

     I99.9 Unspecified **disorder of circulatory system**

CHAPTER 9 (I00-I99)

CHAPTER 10

DISEASES OF THE RESPIRATORY SYSTEM (J00-J99)

OGCR Chapter-Specific Coding Guidelines

10. Chapter 10: Diseases of the Respiratory System (J00-J99)

a. Chronic Obstructive Pulmonary Disease [COPD] and Asthma

1) Acute exacerbation of chronic obstructive bronchitis and asthma

The codes in categories J44 and J45 distinguish between uncomplicated cases and those in acute exacerbation. An acute exacerbation is a worsening or a decompensation of a chronic condition. An acute exacerbation is not equivalent to an infection superimposed on a chronic condition, though an exacerbation may be triggered by an infection.

b. Acute Respiratory Failure

1) Acute respiratory failure as principal diagnosis

A code from subcategory J96.0, Acute respiratory failure, or subcategory J96.2, Acute and chronic respiratory failure, may be assigned as a principal diagnosis when it is the condition established after study to be chiefly responsible for occasioning the admission to the hospital, and the selection is supported by the Alphabetic Index and Tabular List. However, chapter-specific coding guidelines (such as obstetrics, poisoning, HIV, newborn) that provide sequencing direction take precedence.

2) Acute respiratory failure as secondary diagnosis

Respiratory failure may be listed as a secondary diagnosis if it occurs after admission, or if it is present on admission, but does not meet the definition of principal diagnosis.

3) Sequencing of acute respiratory failure and another acute condition

When a patient is admitted with respiratory failure and another acute condition, (e.g., myocardial infarction, cerebrovascular accident, aspiration pneumonia), the principal diagnosis will not be the same in every situation. This applies whether the other acute condition is a respiratory or nonrespiratory condition. Selection of the principal diagnosis will be dependent on the circumstances of admission. If both the respiratory failure and the other acute condition are equally responsible for occasioning the admission to the hospital, and there are no chapter-specific sequencing rules, the guideline regarding two or more diagnoses that equally meet the definition for principal diagnosis *(Section II, C.)* may be applied in these situations.

If the documentation is not clear as to whether acute respiratory failure and another condition are equally responsible for occasioning the admission, query the provider for clarification.

c. Influenza due to certain identified influenza viruses

Code only confirmed cases of influenza due to certain identified influenza viruses (category J09), and due to other identified influenza virus (category J10). This is an exception to the hospital inpatient guideline Section II, H. (Uncertain Diagnosis).

In this context, "confirmation" does not require documentation of positive laboratory testing specific for avian or other novel influenza A or other identified influenza virus. However, coding should be based on the provider's diagnostic statement that the patient has avian influenza, or other novel influenza A, for category J09, or has another particular identified strain of influenza, such as H1N1 or H3N2, but not identified as novel or variant, for category J10.

If the provider records "suspected" or "possible" or "probable" avian influenza, or novel influenza, or other identified influenza, then the appropriate influenza code from category J11, Influenza due to unidentified influenza virus, should be assigned. A code from category J09, Influenza due to certain identified influenza viruses, should not be assigned nor should a code from category J10, Influenza due to other identified influenza virus.

d. Ventilator associated Pneumonia

1) Documentation of Ventilator associated Pneumonia

As with all procedural or postprocedural complications, code assignment is based on the provider's documentation of the relationship between the condition and the procedure.

Code J95.851, Ventilator associated pneumonia, should be assigned only when the provider has documented ventilator associated pneumonia (VAP). An additional code to identify the organism (e.g., Pseudomonas aeruginosa, code B96.5) should also be assigned. Do not assign an additional code from categories J12-J18 to identify the type of pneumonia.

Code J95.851 should not be assigned for cases where the patient has pneumonia and is on a mechanical ventilator and the provider has not specifically stated that the pneumonia is ventilator-associated pneumonia. If the documentation is unclear as to whether the patient has a pneumonia that is a complication attributable to the mechanical ventilator, query the provider.

2) Ventilator associated Pneumonia Develops after Admission

A patient may be admitted with one type of pneumonia (e.g., code J13, Pneumonia due to Streptococcus pneumonia) and subsequently develop VAP. In this instance, the principal diagnosis would be the appropriate code from categories J12-J18 for the pneumonia diagnosed at the time of admission. Code J95.851, Ventilator associated pneumonia, would be assigned as an additional diagnosis when the provider has also documented the presence of ventilator associated pneumonia.

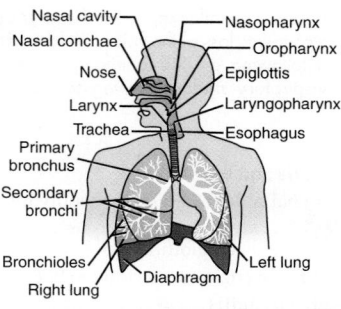

Figure 10-1 Respiratory system. (From Buck CJ: Step-by-Step Medical Coding, ed 2016, St. Louis, Elsevier, 2016)

Figure 10-2 Paranasal sinuses. (From Buck CJ: Step-by-Step Medical Coding, ed 2016, St. Louis, Elsevier, 2016)

Item 10–1 Pharyngitis is painful inflammation of the pharynx (sore throat). Ninety percent of the infections are caused by a virus with the remaining being bacterial and rarely a fungus (candidiasis). Other irritants such as pollutants, chemicals, or smoke may cause similar symptoms.

CHAPTER 10

DISEASES OF THE RESPIRATORY SYSTEM (J00-J99)

Note: When a respiratory condition is described as occurring in more than one site and is not specifically indexed, it should be classified to the lower anatomic site (e.g., tracheobronchitis to bronchitis in J40).

Use additional code, where applicable, to identify:
   exposure to environmental tobacco smoke (Z77.22)
   exposure to tobacco smoke in the perinatal period (P96.81)
   history of tobacco dependence (Z87.891) ◀▥
   occupational exposure to environmental tobacco smoke (Z57.31)
   tobacco dependence (F17.-)
   tobacco use (Z72.0)

Excludes2   certain conditions originating in the perinatal period (P04-P96)
   certain infectious and parasitic diseases (A00-B99)
   complications of pregnancy, childbirth and the puerperium (O00-O99A)
   congenital malformations, deformations and chromosomal abnormalities (Q00-Q99)
   endocrine, nutritional and metabolic diseases (E00-E88)
   injury, poisoning and certain other consequences of external causes (S00-T88)
   neoplasms (C00-D49)
   smoke inhalation (T59.81-)
   symptoms, signs and abnormal clinical and laboratory findings, not elsewhere classified (R00-R94)

This chapter contains the following blocks:

J00-J06	Acute upper respiratory infections
J09-J18	Influenza and pneumonia
J20-J22	Other acute lower respiratory infections
J30-J39	Other diseases of upper respiratory tract
J40-J47	Chronic lower respiratory diseases
J60-J70	Lung diseases due to external agents
J80-J84	Other respiratory diseases principally affecting the interstitium
J85-J86	Suppurative and necrotic conditions of the lower respiratory tract
J90-J94	Other diseases of the pleura
J95	Intraoperative and postprocedural complications and disorders of respiratory system, not elsewhere classified
J96-J99	Other diseases of the respiratory system

ACUTE UPPER RESPIRATORY INFECTIONS (J00-J06)

Excludes1   chronic obstructive pulmonary disease with acute lower respiratory infection (J44.0)
   influenza virus with other respiratory manifestations (J09.X2, J10.1, J11.1)

J00   Acute nasopharyngitis [common cold]
   Acute rhinitis
   Coryza (acute)
   Infective nasopharyngitis NOS
   Infective rhinitis
   Nasal catarrh, acute
   Nasopharyngitis NOS

Excludes1   acute pharyngitis (J02.-)
   acute sore throat NOS (J02.9)
   pharyngitis NOS (J02.9)
   rhinitis NOS (J31.0)
   sore throat NOS (J02.9)

Excludes2   allergic rhinitis (J30.1-J30.9)
   chronic pharyngitis (J31.2)
   chronic rhinitis (J31.0)
   chronic sore throat (J31.2)
   nasopharyngitis, chronic (J31.1)
   vasomotor rhinitis (J30.0)

★ **(See Plate 49 on page 72.)**

● **J01   Acute sinusitis**
   Includes   acute abscess of sinus
      acute empyema of sinus
      acute infection of sinus
      acute inflammation of sinus
      acute suppuration of sinus
   Use additional code (B95-B97) to identify infectious agent.
   Excludes1   sinusitis NOS (J32.9)
   Excludes2   chronic sinusitis (J32.0-J32.8)

● **J01.0   Acute maxillary sinusitis**
   Acute antritis
   J01.00   Acute maxillary sinusitis, **unspecified**
   J01.01   Acute recurrent maxillary sinusitis

● **J01.1   Acute frontal sinusitis**
   J01.10   Acute frontal sinusitis, **unspecified**
   J01.11   Acute recurrent frontal sinusitis

● **J01.2   Acute ethmoidal sinusitis**
   J01.20   Acute ethmoidal sinusitis, **unspecified**
   J01.21   Acute recurrent ethmoidal sinusitis

● **J01.3   Acute sphenoidal sinusitis**
   J01.30   Acute sphenoidal sinusitis, **unspecified**
   J01.31   Acute recurrent sphenoidal sinusitis

● **J01.4   Acute pansinusitis**
   J01.40   Acute pansinusitis, **unspecified**
   J01.41   Acute recurrent pansinusitis

● **J01.8**   **Other acute sinusitis**

    J01.80   **Other acute sinusitis**
         Acute sinusitis involving more than one sinus but not pansinusitis

    J01.81   **Other acute recurrent sinusitis**
         Acute recurrent sinusitis involving more than one sinus but not pansinusitis

● **J01.9**   **Acute sinusitis, unspecified**

    J01.90   **Acute sinusitis, unspecified**

    J01.91   **Acute recurrent sinusitis, unspecified**

● **J02**   **Acute pharyngitis**

    Includes   acute sore throat

    Excludes1   acute laryngopharyngitis (J06.0)
         peritonsillar abscess (J36)
         pharyngeal abscess (J39.1)
         retropharyngeal abscess (J39.0)

    Excludes2   chronic pharyngitis (J31.2)

    J02.0   **Streptococcal pharyngitis**
         Septic pharyngitis
         Streptococcal sore throat

       Excludes2   scarlet fever (A38.-)

    J02.8   **Acute pharyngitis due to other specified organisms**
         Use additional code (B95-B97) to identify infectious agent

       Excludes1   pharyngitis due to coxsackie virus (B08.5)
         pharyngitis due to gonococcus (A54.5)
         acute pharyngitis due to herpes [simplex] virus (B00.2)
         acute pharyngitis due to infectious mononucleosis (B27.-)
         enteroviral vesicular pharyngitis (B08.5)

    J02.9   **Acute pharyngitis, unspecified**
         Gangrenous pharyngitis (acute)
         Infective pharyngitis (acute) NOS
         Pharyngitis (acute) NOS
         Sore throat (acute) NOS
         Suppurative pharyngitis (acute)
         Ulcerative pharyngitis (acute)

● **J03**   **Acute tonsillitis**
    Inflammation of pharyngeal tonsils caused by virus or bacteria

    Excludes1   acute sore throat (J02.-)
         hypertrophy of tonsils (J35.1)
         peritonsillar abscess (J36)
         sore throat NOS (J02.9)
         streptococcal sore throat (J02.0)

    Excludes2   chronic tonsillitis (J35.0)

● **J03.0**   **Streptococcal tonsillitis**

    J03.00   **Acute streptococcal tonsillitis, unspecified**

    J03.01   **Acute recurrent streptococcal tonsillitis**

● **J03.8**   **Acute tonsillitis due to other specified organisms**
         Use additional code (B95-B97) to identify infectious agent.

       Excludes1   diphtheritic tonsillitis (A36.0)
         herpesviral pharyngotonsillitis (B00.2)
         streptococcal tonsillitis (J03.0)
         tuberculous tonsillitis (A15.8)
         Vincent's tonsillitis (A69.1)

    J03.80   **Acute tonsillitis due to other specified organisms**

    J03.81   **Acute recurrent tonsillitis due to other specified organisms**

● **J03.9**   **Acute tonsillitis, unspecified**
         Follicular tonsillitis (acute)
         Gangrenous tonsillitis (acute)
         Infective tonsillitis (acute)
         Tonsillitis (acute) NOS
         Ulcerative tonsillitis (acute)

    J03.90   **Acute tonsillitis, unspecified**

    J03.91   **Acute recurrent tonsillitis, unspecified**

Item 10–2   **Laryngitis** is an inflammation of the larynx (voice box) resulting in hoarse voice or the complete loss of the voice. **Tracheitis** is an inflammation of the trachea (often following a URI) commonly caused by *staphylococcus aureus* resulting in inspiratory stridor (crowing sound on inspiration) and a croup like cough.

● **J04**   **Acute laryngitis and tracheitis**
         Use additional code (B95-B97) to identify infectious agent.

    Excludes1   acute obstructive laryngitis [croup] and epiglottitis (J05.-)

    Excludes2   laryngismus (stridulus) (J38.5)

    J04.0   **Acute laryngitis**
         Edematous laryngitis (acute)
         Laryngitis (acute) NOS
         Subglottic laryngitis (acute)
         Suppurative laryngitis (acute)
         Ulcerative laryngitis (acute)

       Excludes1   acute obstructive laryngitis (J05.0)
       Excludes2   chronic laryngitis (J37.0)

● **J04.1**   **Acute tracheitis**
         Acute viral tracheitis
         Catarrhal tracheitis (acute)
         Tracheitis (acute) NOS

       Excludes2   chronic tracheitis (J42)

    J04.10   **Acute tracheitis without obstruction**

    J04.11   **Acute tracheitis with obstruction**

    J04.2   **Acute laryngotracheitis**
         Laryngotracheitis NOS
         Tracheitis (acute) with laryngitis (acute)

       Excludes1   acute obstructive laryngotracheitis (J05.0)
       Excludes2   chronic laryngotracheitis (J37.1)

● **J04.3**   **Supraglottitis, unspecified**

    J04.30   **Supraglottitis, unspecified, without obstruction**

    J04.31   **Supraglottitis, unspecified, with obstruction**

● **J05**   **Acute obstructive laryngitis [croup] and epiglottitis**
         Use additional code (B95-B97) to identify infectious agent.

    J05.0   **Acute obstructive laryngitis [croup]**
         Obstructive laryngitis (acute) NOS
         Obstructive laryngotracheitis NOS

    J05.1   **Acute epiglottitis**

       Excludes2   epiglottitis, chronic (J37.0)

    J05.10   **Acute epiglottitis without obstruction**
         Epiglottitis NOS

    J05.11   **Acute epiglottitis with obstruction**

● **J06**   **Acute upper respiratory infections of multiple and unspecified sites**

    Excludes1   acute respiratory infection NOS (J22)
         streptococcal pharyngitis (J02.0)

    J06.0   **Acute laryngopharyngitis**

    J06.9   **Acute upper respiratory infection, unspecified**
         Upper respiratory disease, acute
         Upper respiratory infection NOS

◀ New   ⬅ Revised   ~~deleted~~ Deleted   Excludes 1   Excludes 2   Includes   Use additional   Code first   Code also   Unspecified

OGCR Official Guidelines   X Assign placeholder X   ● Use Additional Character(s)   ▶ Manifestation Code   **Coding Clinic**

INFLUENZA AND PNEUMONIA (J09-J18)

 Excludes2 allergic or eosinophilic pneumonia (J82)
     aspiration pneumonia NOS (J69.0)
     meconium pneumonia (P24.01)
     neonatal aspiration pneumonia (P24.-)
     pneumonia due to solids and liquids (J69.-)
     congenital pneumonia (P23.9)
     lipid pneumonia (J69.1)
     rheumatic pneumonia (I00)
     ventilator associated pneumonia (J95.851)

● **J09** **Influenza due to certain identified influenza viruses**

  Excludes1 influenza due to other influenza viruses (J10.-)
     influenza due to unidentified influenza virus (J11.-)
     seasonal influenza due to other identified influenza virus (J10.-)
     seasonal influenza due to unidentified influenza virus (J11.-)

● **J09.X** **Influenza due to identified novel influenza A virus**
   Avian influenza
   Bird influenza
   Influenza A/H5N1
   Influenza of other animal origin, not bird or swine
   Swine influenza virus (viruses that normally cause infections in pigs)

 J09.X1 **Influenza due to identified novel influenza A virus with pneumonia**
   Code also , if applicable, associated:
    lung abscess (J85.1)
    other specified type of pneumonia

 J09.X2 **Influenza due to identified novel influenza A virus with other respiratory manifestations**
   Influenza due to identified novel influenza A virus NOS
   Influenza due to identified novel influenza A virus with laryngitis
   Influenza due to identified novel influenza A virus with pharyngitis
   Influenza due to identified novel influenza A virus with upper respiratory symptoms
   Use additional code, if applicable, for associated:
    pleural effusion (J91.8)
    sinusitis (J01.-)

 J09.X3 **Influenza due to identified novel influenza A virus with gastrointestinal manifestations**
   Influenza due to identified novel influenza A virus gastroenteritis
   Excludes1 'intestinal flu' [viral gastroenteritis] (A08.-)

 J09.X9 **Influenza due to identified novel influenza A virus with other manifestations**
   Influenza due to identified novel influenza A virus with encephalopathy
   Influenza due to identified novel influenza A virus with myocarditis
   Influenza due to identified novel influenza A virus with otitis media
   Use additional code to identify manifestation

● **J10** **Influenza due to other identified influenza virus**

  Excludes1 influenza due to avian influenza virus (J09.X-)
     influenza due to swine flu (J09.X-)
     influenza due to unidentified influenza virus (J11.-)

● **J10.0** **Influenza due to other identified influenza virus with pneumonia**
   Code also associated lung abscess, if applicable (J85.1)

 J10.00 **Influenza due to other identified influenza virus with unspecified type of pneumonia**

 J10.01 **Influenza due to other identified influenza virus with the same other identified influenza virus pneumonia**

 J10.08 **Influenza due to other identified influenza virus with other specified pneumonia**
   Code also other specified type of pneumonia

 J10.1 **Influenza due to other identified influenza virus with other respiratory manifestations**
   Influenza due to other identified influenza virus NOS
   Influenza due to other identified influenza virus with laryngitis
   Influenza due to other identified influenza virus with pharyngitis
   Influenza due to other identified influenza virus with upper respiratory symptoms
   Use additional code for associated pleural effusion, if applicable (J91.8)
   Use additional code for associated sinusitis, if applicable (J01.-)

 J10.2 **Influenza due to other identified influenza virus with gastrointestinal manifestations**
   Influenza due to other identified influenza virus gastroenteritis
   Excludes1 'intestinal flu' [viral gastroenteritis] (A08.-)

● **J10.8** **Influenza due to other identified influenza virus with other manifestations**

 J10.81 **Influenza due to other identified influenza virus with encephalopathy**

 J10.82 **Influenza due to other identified influenza virus with myocarditis**

 J10.83 **Influenza due to other identified influenza virus with otitis media**
   Use additional code for any associated perforated tympanic membrane (H72.-)

 J10.89 **Influenza due to other identified influenza virus with other manifestations**
   Use additional codes to identify the manifestations

● **J11** **Influenza due to unidentified influenza virus**

● **J11.0** **Influenza due to unidentified influenza virus with pneumonia**
   Code also associated lung abscess, if applicable (J85.1)

 J11.00 **Influenza due to unidentified influenza virus with unspecified type of pneumonia**
   Influenza with pneumonia NOS

 J11.08 **Influenza due to unidentified influenza virus with specified pneumonia**
   Code also other specified type of pneumonia

 J11.1 **Influenza due to unidentified influenza virus with other respiratory manifestations**
   Influenza NOS
   Influenzal laryngitis NOS
   Influenzal pharyngitis NOS
   Influenza with upper respiratory symptoms NOS
   Use additional code for associated pleural effusion, if applicable (J91.8)
   Use additional code for associated sinusitis, if applicable (J01.-)

CHAPTER 10 (J00-J99)

CHAPTER 10 (J00–J99)

J11.2   **Influenza due to unidentified influenza virus with gastrointestinal manifestations**
       Influenza gastroenteritis NOS
       Excludes1   'intestinal flu' [viral gastroenteritis] (A08.-)

● **J11.8**   **Influenza due to unidentified influenza virus with other manifestations**

     J11.81   **Influenza due to unidentified influenza virus with encephalopathy**
          Influenzal encephalopathy NOS

     J11.82   **Influenza due to unidentified influenza virus with myocarditis**
          Influenzal myocarditis NOS

     J11.83   **Influenza due to unidentified influenza virus with otitis media**
          Influenzal otitis media NOS
          Use additional code for any associated perforated tympanic membrane (H72.-)

     J11.89   **Influenza due to unidentified influenza virus with other manifestations**
          Use additional codes to identify the manifestations

● **J12**   **Viral pneumonia, not elsewhere classified**
       Includes   bronchopneumonia due to viruses other than influenza viruses
       Code first associated influenza, if applicable (J09.X1, J10.0-, J11.0-)
       Code also associated abscess, if applicable (J85.1)
       Excludes1   aspiration pneumonia due to anesthesia during labor and delivery (O74.0)
                   aspiration pneumonia due to anesthesia during pregnancy (O29)
                   aspiration pneumonia due to anesthesia during puerperium (O89.0)
                   aspiration pneumonia due to solids and liquids (J69.-)
                   aspiration pneumonia NOS (J69.0)
                   congenital pneumonia (P23.0)
                   congenital rubella pneumonitis (P35.0)
                   interstitial pneumonia NOS (J84.9)
                   lipid pneumonia (J69.1)
                   neonatal aspiration pneumonia (P24.-)

     J12.0   **Adenoviral pneumonia**

     J12.1   **Respiratory syncytial virus pneumonia**

     J12.2   **Parainfluenza virus pneumonia**

     J12.3   **Human metapneumovirus pneumonia**

●   **J12.8**   **Other viral pneumonia**

       J12.81   **Pneumonia due to SARS-associated coronavirus**
           Severe acute respiratory syndrome NOS

       J12.89   **Other viral pneumonia**

     J12.9   **Viral pneumonia, unspecified**

J13   **Pneumonia due to Streptococcus pneumoniae**
       Bronchopneumonia due to S. pneumoniae
       Code first associated influenza, if applicable (J09.X1, J10.0-, J11.0-)
       Code also associated abscess, if applicable (J85.1)
       Excludes1   congenital pneumonia due to S. pneumoniae (P23.6)
                   lobar pneumonia, unspecified organism (J18.1)
                   pneumonia due to other streptococci (J15.3-J15.4)

Item 10–3   Pneumonia is an infection of the lungs, caused by a variety of microorganisms, including viruses, most commonly the Streptococcus pneumoniae (pneumococcus) bacteria, fungi, and parasites. Pneumonia occurs when the immune system is weakened, often by a URI or influenza.

J14   **Pneumonia due to Hemophilus influenzae**
       Bronchopneumonia due to H. influenzae
       Code first associated influenza, if applicable (J09.X1, J10.0-, J11.0-)
       Code also associated abscess, if applicable (J85.1)
       Excludes1   congenital pneumonia due to H. influenzae (P23.6)

● **J15**   **Bacterial pneumonia, not elsewhere classified**
       Includes   bronchopneumonia due to bacteria other than S. pneumoniae and H. influenzae
       Code first associated influenza, if applicable (J09.X1, J10.0-, J11.0-)
       Code also associated abscess, if applicable (J85.1)
       Excludes1   chlamydial pneumonia (J16.0)
                   congenital pneumonia (P23.-)
                   Legionnaires' disease (A48.1)
                   spirochetal pneumonia (A69.8)

     J15.0   **Pneumonia due to Klebsiella pneumoniae**

     J15.1   **Pneumonia due to Pseudomonas**

●   **J15.2**   **Pneumonia due to staphylococcus**

       J15.20   **Pneumonia due to staphylococcus, unspecified**

●   **J15.21**   **Pneumonia due to staphylococcus aureus**

         J15.211   **Pneumonia due to Methicillin susceptible Staphylococcus aureus**
            MSSA pneumonia
            Pneumonia due to Staphylococcus aureus NOS

         J15.212   **Pneumonia due to Methicillin resistant Staphylococcus aureus**

       J15.29   **Pneumonia due to other staphylococcus**

     J15.3   **Pneumonia due to streptococcus, group B**

     J15.4   **Pneumonia due to other streptococci**
       Excludes1   pneumonia due to streptococcus, group B (J15.3)
                   pneumonia due to Streptococcus pneumoniae (J13)

     J15.5   **Pneumonia due to Escherichia coli**

     J15.6   **Pneumonia due to other aerobic Gram-negative bacteria**
       Pneumonia due to Serratia marcescens

     J15.7   **Pneumonia due to Mycoplasma pneumoniae**

     J15.8   **Pneumonia due to other specified bacteria**

     J15.9   **Unspecified bacterial pneumonia**
       Pneumonia due to gram-positive bacteria

● **J16**   **Pneumonia due to other infectious organisms, not elsewhere classified**
       Code first associated influenza, if applicable (J09.X1, J10.0-, J11.0-)
       Code also associated abscess, if applicable (J85.1)
       Excludes1   congenital pneumonia (P23.-)
                   ornithosis (A70)
                   pneumocystosis (B59)
                   pneumonia NOS (J18.9)

     J16.0   **Chlamydial pneumonia**

     J16.8   **Pneumonia due to other specified infectious organisms**

◄ New   ◄◄ Revised   ~~deleted~~ Deleted   Excludes 1   Excludes 2   Includes   Use additional   Code first   Code also   Unspecified

OGCR Official Guidelines   X Assign placeholder X   ● Use Additional Character(s)   ▶ Manifestation Code   **Coding Clinic**

▶ J17   *Pneumonia in diseases classified elsewhere*

    Code first underlying disease, such as:
      Q fever (A78)
      rheumatic fever (I00)
      schistosomiasis (B65.0-B65.9)

    Excludes1   candidial pneumonia (B37.1)
         chlamydial pneumonia (J16.0)
         gonorrheal pneumonia (A54.84)
         histoplasmosis pneumonia (B39.0-B39.2)
         measles pneumonia (B05.2)
         nocardiosis pneumonia (A43.0)
         pneumocystosis (B59)
         pneumonia due to Pneumocystis carinii (B59)
         pneumonia due to Pneumocystis jiroveci (B59)
         pneumonia in actinomycosis (A42.0)
         pneumonia in anthrax (A22.1)
         pneumonia in ascariasis (B77.81)
         pneumonia in aspergillosis (B44.0-B44.1)
         pneumonia in coccidioidomycosis (B38.0-B38.2)
         pneumonia in cytomegalovirus disease (B25.0)
         pneumonia in toxoplasmosis (B58.3)
         rubella pneumonia (B06.81)
         salmonella pneumonia (A02.22)
         spirochetal infection NEC with pneumonia (A69.8)
         tularemia pneumonia (A21.2)
         typhoid fever with pneumonia (A01.03)
         varicella pneumonia (B01.2)
         whooping cough with pneumonia (A37 with fifth-character 1)

● J18   **Pneumonia, unspecified organism**

    Code first associated influenza, if applicable (J09.X1, J10.0-, J11.0-)

    Excludes1   abscess of lung with pneumonia (J85.1)
         aspiration pneumonia due to anesthesia during labor and delivery (O74.0)
         aspiration pneumonia due to anesthesia during pregnancy (O29)
         aspiration pneumonia due to anesthesia during puerperium (O89.0)
         aspiration pneumonia due to solids and liquids (J69.-)
         aspiration pneumonia NOS (J69.0)
         congenital pneumonia (P23.0)
         drug-induced interstitial lung disorder (J70.2-J70.4)
         interstitial pneumonia NOS (J84.9)
         lipid pneumonia (J69.1)
         neonatal aspiration pneumonia (P24.-)
         pneumonitis due to external agents (J67-J70)
         pneumonitis due to fumes and vapors (J68.0)
         usual interstitial pneumonia (J84.17)

J18.0   **Bronchopneumonia, unspecified organism**

    Excludes1   hypostatic bronchopneumonia (J18.2)
         lipid pneumonia (J69.1)

    Excludes2   acute bronchiolitis (J21.-)
         chronic bronchiolitis (J44.9)

J18.1   **Lobar pneumonia, unspecified organism**

J18.2   **Hypostatic pneumonia, unspecified organism**
     Hypostatic bronchopneumonia
     Passive pneumonia

J18.8   **Other pneumonia, unspecified organism**

J18.9   **Pneumonia, unspecified organism**
     Coding Clinic: 2012, Q4, P94

OTHER ACUTE LOWER RESPIRATORY INFECTIONS (J20-J22)

    Excludes2   chronic obstructive pulmonary disease with acute lower respiratory infection (J44.0)

● J20   **Acute bronchitis**
     Inflammation/irritation of the bronchial tubes lasting 2-3 weeks, most commonly caused by a virus

    Includes   acute and subacute bronchitis (with) bronchospasm
         acute and subacute bronchitis (with) tracheitis
         acute and subacute bronchitis (with) tracheobronchitis, acute
         acute and subacute fibrinous bronchitis
         acute and subacute membranous bronchitis
         acute and subacute purulent bronchitis
         acute and subacute septic bronchitis

    Excludes1   bronchitis NOS (J40)
         tracheobronchitis NOS (J40)

    Excludes2   acute bronchitis with bronchiectasis (J47.0)
         acute bronchitis with chronic obstructive asthma (J44.0)
         acute bronchitis with chronic obstructive pulmonary disease (J44.0)
         allergic bronchitis NOS (J45.909-)
         bronchitis due to chemicals, fumes and vapors (J68.0)
         chronic bronchitis NOS (J42)
         chronic mucopurulent bronchitis (J41.1)
         chronic obstructive bronchitis (J44.-)
         chronic obstructive tracheobronchitis (J44.-)
         chronic simple bronchitis (J41.0)
         chronic tracheobronchitis (J42)

J20.0   **Acute bronchitis due to Mycoplasma pneumoniae**

J20.1   **Acute bronchitis due to Hemophilus influenzae**

J20.2   **Acute bronchitis due to streptococcus**

J20.3   **Acute bronchitis due to coxsackievirus**

J20.4   **Acute bronchitis due to parainfluenza virus**

J20.5   **Acute bronchitis due to respiratory syncytial virus**

J20.6   **Acute bronchitis due to rhinovirus**

J20.7   **Acute bronchitis due to echovirus**

J20.8   **Acute bronchitis due to other specified organisms**

J20.9   **Acute bronchitis, unspecified**

● J21   **Acute bronchiolitis**
     Bronchiolitis obliterans with organizing pneumonia (BOOP) inflammation of bronchioles and surrounding tissue in lung

    Includes   acute bronchiolitis with bronchospasm

    Excludes2   respiratory bronchiolitis interstitial lung disease (J84.115)

J21.0   **Acute bronchiolitis due to respiratory syncytial virus**

J21.1   **Acute bronchiolitis due to human metapneumovirus**

J21.8   **Acute bronchiolitis due to other specified organisms**

J21.9   **Acute bronchiolitis, unspecified**
     Bronchiolitis (acute)

    Excludes1   chronic bronchiolitis (J44.-)

J22   **Unspecified acute lower respiratory infection**
     Acute (lower) respiratory (tract) infection NOS

    Excludes1   upper respiratory infection (acute) (J06.9)

CHAPTER 10 (J00-J99)

CHAPTER 10 (J00-J99)

OTHER DISEASES OF UPPER RESPIRATORY TRACT (J30-J39)

● **J30**   **Vasomotor and allergic rhinitis**

> **Includes**   spasmodic rhinorrhea
>
> **Excludes1**   allergic rhinitis with asthma (bronchial) (J45.909)
> rhinitis NOS (J31.0)

  J30.0   **Vasomotor rhinitis**

  J30.1   **Allergic rhinitis due to pollen**
> Allergy NOS due to pollen
> Hay fever
> Pollinosis

  J30.2   **Other seasonal allergic rhinitis**

  J30.5   **Allergic rhinitis due to food**

● **J30.8**   **Other allergic rhinitis**

      J30.81   **Allergic rhinitis due to animal (cat) (dog) hair and dander**

      J30.89   **Other allergic rhinitis**
>   Perennial allergic rhinitis

  J30.9   **Allergic rhinitis, unspecified**

● **J31**   **Chronic rhinitis, nasopharyngitis and pharyngitis**

> Use additional code to identify:
> exposure to environmental tobacco smoke (Z77.22)
> exposure to tobacco smoke in the perinatal period (P96.81)
> history of tobacco dependence (Z87.891) ◀▥
> occupational exposure to environmental tobacco smoke (Z57.31)
> tobacco dependence (F17.-)
> tobacco use (Z72.0)

  J31.0   **Chronic rhinitis**
> Atrophic rhinitis (chronic)
> Granulomatous rhinitis (chronic)
> Hypertrophic rhinitis (chronic)
> Obstructive rhinitis (chronic)
> Ozena
> Purulent rhinitis (chronic)
> Rhinitis (chronic) NOS
> Ulcerative rhinitis (chronic)
>
> **Excludes1**   allergic rhinitis (J30.1-J30.9)
>   vasomotor rhinitis (J30.0)

  J31.1   **Chronic nasopharyngitis**
> **Excludes2**   acute nasopharyngitis (J00)

  J31.2   **Chronic pharyngitis**
> Chronic sore throat
> Atrophic pharyngitis (chronic)
> Granular pharyngitis (chronic)
> Hypertrophic pharyngitis (chronic)
>
> **Excludes2**   acute pharyngitis (J02.9)

● **J32**   **Chronic sinusitis**

> **Includes**   sinus abscess
>   sinus empyema
>   sinus infection
>   sinus suppuration

> Use additional code to identify:
> exposure to environmental tobacco smoke (Z77.22)
> exposure to tobacco smoke in the perinatal period (P96.81)
> history of tobacco dependence (Z87.891) ◀▥
> infectious agent (B95-B97)
> occupational exposure to environmental tobacco smoke (Z57.31)
> tobacco dependence (F17.-)
> tobacco use (Z72.0)
>
> **Excludes2**   acute sinusitis (J01.-)

  J32.0   **Chronic maxillary sinusitis**
> Antritis (chronic)
> Maxillary sinusitis NOS

  J32.1   **Chronic frontal sinusitis**
> Frontal sinusitis NOS

Item 10–4 Nasal polyps are an abnormal growth of tissue (tumor) projecting from a mucous membrane and attached to the surface by a narrow elongated stalk (pedunculated). Nasal polyps usually originate in the ethmoid sinus but also may occur in the maxillary sinus. Symptoms are nasal block, sinusitis, anosmia, and secondary infections.

  J32.2   **Chronic ethmoidal sinusitis**
> Ethmoidal sinusitis NOS
>
> **Excludes1**   Woakes' ethmoiditis (J33.1)

  J32.3   **Chronic sphenoidal sinusitis**
> Sphenoidal sinusitis NOS

  J32.4   **Chronic pansinusitis**
> Pansinusitis NOS

  J32.8   **Other chronic sinusitis**
> Sinusitis (chronic) involving more than one sinus but not pansinusitis

  J32.9   **Chronic sinusitis, unspecified**
> Sinusitis (chronic) NOS

● **J33**   **Nasal polyp**

> Use additional code to identify:
> exposure to environmental tobacco smoke (Z77.22)
> exposure to tobacco smoke in the perinatal period (P96.81)
> history of tobacco dependence (Z87.891) ◀▥
> occupational exposure to environmental tobacco smoke (Z57.31)
> tobacco dependence (F17.-)
> tobacco use (Z72.0)
>
> **Excludes1**   adenomatous polyps (D14.0)

  J33.0   **Polyp of nasal cavity**
> Choanal polyp
> Nasopharyngeal polyp

  J33.1   **Polypoid sinus degeneration**
> Woakes' syndrome or ethmoiditis

  J33.8   **Other polyp of sinus**
> Accessory polyp of sinus
> Ethmoidal polyp of sinus
> Maxillary polyp of sinus
> Sphenoidal polyp of sinus

  J33.9   **Nasal polyp, unspecified**

● **J34**   **Other and unspecified disorders of nose and nasal sinuses**
> **Excludes2**   varicose ulcer of nasal septum (I86.8)

  J34.0   **Abscess, furuncle and carbuncle of nose**
> Cellulitis of nose
> Necrosis of nose
> Ulceration of nose

  J34.1   **Cyst and mucocele of nose and nasal sinus**

  J34.2   **Deviated nasal septum**
> Deflection or deviation of septum (nasal) (acquired)
>
> **Excludes1**   congenital deviated nasal septum (Q67.4)

  J34.3   **Hypertrophy of nasal turbinates**

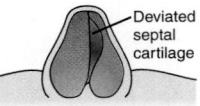

Deviated septal cartilage

Figure 10-3   Deviated nasal septum.

Item 10–5 A **deviated nasal septum** is the displacement of the septal cartilage that separates the nares. This displacement causes obstructed air flow through the nasal passages. A child can be born with this displacement (congenital), or the condition may be acquired through trauma, such as a sports injury. Symptoms include nasal block, sinusitis, and related secondary infections. Septoplasty is surgical repair of this condition.

◀ New	◀▥ Revised	~~deleted~~ Deleted	Excludes 1	Excludes 2	Includes	Use additional	Code first	Code also	Unspecified

OGCR Official Guidelines   **X** Assign placeholder X   ● Use Additional Character(s)   ▶ Manifestation Code   **Coding Clinic**

● **J34.8   Other specified disorders of nose and nasal sinuses**

J34.81   Nasal mucositis (ulcerative)

Code also type of associated therapy, such as:
antineoplastic and immunosuppressive
drugs (T45.1X-)
radiological procedure and radiotherapy
(Y84.2)

Excludes2   gastrointestinal mucositis
(ulcerative) (K92.81)
mucositis (ulcerative) of vagina
and vulva (N76.81)
oral mucositis (ulcerative)
(K12.3-)

**J34.89   Other specified disorders of nose and nasal
sinuses**
Perforation of nasal septum NOS
Rhinolith

J34.9   Unspecified disorder of nose and nasal sinuses

● **J35   Chronic diseases of tonsils and adenoids**
Use additional code to identify:
exposure to environmental tobacco smoke (Z77.22)
exposure to tobacco smoke in the perinatal period (P96.81)
history of tobacco dependence (Z87.891) ◀▬▬
occupational exposure to environmental tobacco smoke
(Z57.31)
tobacco dependence (F17.-)
tobacco use (Z72.0)

● **J35.0   Chronic tonsillitis and adenoiditis**
Excludes2   acute tonsillitis (J03.-)

J35.01   Chronic tonsillitis

J35.02   Chronic adenoiditis

J35.03   Chronic tonsillitis and adenoiditis

J35.1   Hypertrophy of tonsils
Enlargement of tonsils
Excludes1   hypertrophy of tonsils with tonsillitis
(J35.0-)

J35.2   Hypertrophy of adenoids
Enlargement of adenoids
Excludes1   hypertrophy of adenoids with adenoiditis
(J35.0-)

J35.3   Hypertrophy of tonsils with hypertrophy of adenoids
Excludes1   hypertrophy of tonsils and adenoids with
tonsillitis and adenoiditis (J35.03)

J35.8   Other chronic diseases of tonsils and adenoids
Adenoid vegetations
Amygdalolith
Calculus, tonsil
Cicatrix of tonsil (and adenoid)
Tonsillar tag
Ulcer of tonsil

J35.9   Chronic disease of tonsils and adenoids, unspecified
Disease (chronic) of tonsils and adenoids NOS

J36   Peritonsillar abscess
Includes   abscess of tonsil
peritonsillar cellulitis
quinsy
Use additional code (B95-B97) to identify infectious agent.
Excludes1   acute tonsillitis (J03.-)
chronic tonsillitis (J35.0)
retropharyngeal abscess (J39.0)
tonsillitis NOS (J03.9-)

● **J37   Chronic laryngitis and laryngotracheitis**
Use additional code to identify:
exposure to environmental tobacco smoke (Z77.22)
exposure to tobacco smoke in the perinatal period (P96.81)
history of tobacco dependence (Z87.891) ◀▬▬
infectious agent (B95-B97)
occupational exposure to environmental tobacco smoke
(Z57.31)
tobacco dependence (F17.-)
tobacco use (Z72.0)

J37.0   Chronic laryngitis
Catarrhal laryngitis
Hypertrophic laryngitis
Sicca laryngitis
Excludes2   acute laryngitis (J04.0)
obstructive (acute) laryngitis (J05.0)

J37.1   Chronic laryngotracheitis
Laryngitis, chronic, with tracheitis (chronic)
Tracheitis, chronic, with laryngitis
Excludes1   chronic tracheitis (J42)
Excludes2   acute laryngotracheitis (J04.2)
acute tracheitis (J04.1)

● **J38   Diseases of vocal cords and larynx, not elsewhere classified**
Use additional code to identify:
exposure to environmental tobacco smoke (Z77.22)
exposure to tobacco smoke in the perinatal period (P96.81)
history of tobacco dependence (Z87.891) ◀▬▬
occupational exposure to environmental tobacco smoke
(Z57.31)
tobacco dependence (F17.-)
tobacco use (Z72.0)
Excludes1   congenital laryngeal stridor (P28.89)
obstructive laryngitis (acute) (J05.0)
postprocedural subglottic stenosis (J95.5)
stridor (R06.1)
ulcerative laryngitis (J04.0)

● **J38.0   Paralysis of vocal cords and larynx**
Laryngoplegia
Paralysis of glottis

J38.00   Paralysis of vocal cords and larynx, unspecified

J38.01   Paralysis of vocal cords and larynx, unilateral

J38.02   Paralysis of vocal cords and larynx, bilateral

J38.1   Polyp of vocal cord and larynx
Excludes1   adenomatous polyps (D14.1)

J38.2   Nodules of vocal cords
Chorditis (fibrinous)(nodosa)(tuberosa)
Singer's nodes
Teacher's nodes

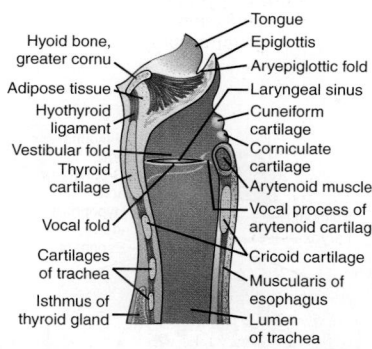

Figure 10-4   Coronal section of the larynx.

Item 10–6   The **larynx** extends from the tongue to the trachea and is divided into an upper and lower portion separated by folds. The framework of the larynx is cartilage composed of the single cricoid, thyroid, and epiglottic cartilages, and the paired arytenoid, cuneiform, and corniculate cartilages.

J38.3 Other diseases of vocal cords
Abscess of vocal cords
Cellulitis of vocal cords
Granuloma of vocal cords
Leukokeratosis of vocal cords
Leukoplakia of vocal cords

J38.4 Edema of larynx
Edema (of) glottis
Subglottic edema
Supraglottic edema
> Excludes1   acute obstructive laryngitis [croup] (J05.0)
> edematous laryngitis (J04.0)

J38.5 Laryngeal spasm
Laryngismus (stridulus)

J38.6 Stenosis of larynx

J38.7 Other diseases of larynx
Abscess of larynx
Cellulitis of larynx
Disease of larynx NOS
Necrosis of larynx
Pachyderma of larynx
Perichondritis of larynx
Ulcer of larynx

● J39 Other diseases of upper respiratory tract
> Excludes1   acute respiratory infection NOS (J22)
> acute upper respiratory infection (J06.9)
> upper respiratory inflammation due to chemicals, gases, fumes or vapors (J68.2)

J39.0 Retropharyngeal and parapharyngeal abscess
Peripharyngeal abscess
> Excludes1   peritonsillar abscess (J36)

J39.1 Other abscess of pharynx
Cellulitis of pharynx
Nasopharyngeal abscess

J39.2 Other diseases of pharynx
Cyst of pharynx
Edema of pharynx
> Excludes2   chronic pharyngitis (J31.2)
> ulcerative pharyngitis (J02.9)

J39.3 Upper respiratory tract hypersensitivity reaction, site unspecified
> Excludes1   hypersensitivity reaction of upper respiratory tract, such as:
> extrinsic allergic alveolitis (J67.9)
> pneumoconiosis (J60-J67.9)

J39.8 Other specified diseases of upper respiratory tract

J39.9 Disease of upper respiratory tract, unspecified

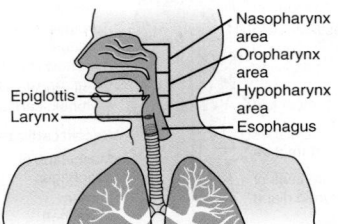
Figure 10-5 The pharynx.

Item 10-7 The **pharynx** is the passage for both food and air between the mouth and the esophagus and is divided into three areas: nasopharynx, oropharynx, and hypopharynx. The hypopharynx branches into the esophagus and the voice box.

Item 10-8 Chronic bronchitis is usually defined as being present in any patient who has persistent cough with sputum production for at least three months in at least two consecutive years. **Simple chronic bronchitis** is marked by a productive cough but no pathological airflow obstruction. **Chronic obstructive pulmonary disease (COPD)** is a group of conditions—bronchitis, emphysema, asthma, bronchiectasis, allergic alveolitis—marked by dyspnea. **Catarrhal** bronchitis is an acute form of bronchitis marked by profuse mucus and pus production (**mucopurulent** discharge). **Croupous** bronchitis, also known as pseudomembranous, fibrinous, plastic, exudative, or membranous, is marked by a violent cough and dyspnea.

CHRONIC LOWER RESPIRATORY DISEASES (J40-J47)
> Excludes1   bronchitis due to chemicals, gases, fumes and vapors (J68.0)
> Excludes2   cystic fibrosis (E84.-)

J40 Bronchitis, not specified as acute or chronic
Bronchitis NOS
Catarrhal bronchitis
Bronchitis with tracheitis NOS
Tracheobronchitis NOS
Use additional code to identify:
exposure to environmental tobacco smoke (Z77.22)
exposure to tobacco smoke in the perinatal period (P96.81)
history of tobacco dependence (Z87.891)
occupational exposure to environmental tobacco smoke (Z57.31)
tobacco dependence (F17.-)
tobacco use (Z72.0)
> Excludes1   acute bronchitis (J20.-)
> allergic bronchitis NOS (J45.909-)
> asthmatic bronchitis NOS (J45.9-)
> bronchitis due to chemicals, gases, fumes and vapors (J68.0)

● J41 Simple and mucopurulent chronic bronchitis
Use additional code to identify:
exposure to environmental tobacco smoke (Z77.22)
exposure to tobacco smoke in the perinatal period (P96.81)
history of tobacco dependence (Z87.891)
occupational exposure to environmental tobacco smoke (Z57.31)
tobacco dependence (F17.-)
tobacco use (Z72.0)
> Excludes1   chronic bronchitis NOS (J42)
> chronic obstructive bronchitis (J44.-)

J41.0 Simple chronic bronchitis
J41.1 Mucopurulent chronic bronchitis
J41.8 Mixed simple and mucopurulent chronic bronchitis

J42 Unspecified chronic bronchitis
Chronic bronchitis NOS
Chronic tracheitis
Chronic tracheobronchitis
Use additional code to identify:
exposure to environmental tobacco smoke (Z77.22)
exposure to tobacco smoke in the perinatal period (P96.81)
history of tobacco dependence (Z87.891)
occupational exposure to environmental tobacco smoke (Z57.31)
tobacco dependence (F17.-)
tobacco use (Z72.0)
> Excludes1   chronic asthmatic bronchitis (J44.-)
> chronic bronchitis with airways obstruction (J44.-)
> chronic emphysematous bronchitis (J44.-)
> chronic obstructive pulmonary disease NOS (J44.9)
> simple and mucopurulent chronic bronchitis (J41.-)

● **J43   Emphysema**
    Use additional code to identify:
        exposure to environmental tobacco smoke (Z77.22)
        history of tobacco dependence (Z87.891) ◀▥
        occupational exposure to environmental tobacco smoke
          (Z57.31)
        tobacco dependence (F17.-)
        tobacco use (Z72.0)

    | Excludes1 | compensatory emphysema (J98.3) |

            emphysema due to inhalation of chemicals, gases,
                fumes or vapors (J68.4)
            emphysema with chronic (obstructive) bronchitis
                (J44.-)
            emphysematous (obstructive) bronchitis (J44.-)
            interstitial emphysema (J98.2)
            mediastinal emphysema (J98.2)
            neonatal interstitial emphysema (P25.0)
            surgical (subcutaneous) emphysema (T81.82)
            traumatic subcutaneous emphysema (T79.7)

    **J43.0   Unilateral pulmonary emphysema [MacLeod's
         syndrome]**
         Swyer-James syndrome
         Unilateral emphysema
         Unilateral hyperlucent lung
         Unilateral pulmonary artery functional hypoplasia
         Unilateral transparency of lung

    J43.1   Panlobular emphysema
         Panacinar emphysema

    J43.2   Centrilobular emphysema

    J43.8   Other emphysema

    J43.9   Emphysema, unspecified
         Bullous emphysema (lung)(pulmonary)
         Emphysema (lung)(pulmonary) NOS
         Emphysematous bleb
         Vesicular emphysema (lung)(pulmonary)

● **J44   Other chronic obstructive pulmonary disease**

    | Includes | asthma with chronic obstructive pulmonary |

               disease
            chronic asthmatic (obstructive) bronchitis
            chronic bronchitis with airways obstruction
            chronic bronchitis with emphysema
            chronic emphysematous bronchitis
            chronic obstructive asthma
            chronic obstructive bronchitis
            chronic obstructive tracheobronchitis

    Code also type of asthma, if applicable (J45.-)
    Use additional code to identify:
        exposure to environmental tobacco smoke (Z77.22)
        history of tobacco dependence (Z87.891) ◀▥
        occupational exposure to environmental tobacco smoke
          (Z57.31)
        tobacco dependence (F17.-)
        tobacco use (Z72.0)

    | Excludes1 | bronchiectasis (J47.-) |

            chronic bronchitis NOS (J42)
            chronic simple and mucopurulent bronchitis (J41.-)
            chronic tracheitis (J42)
            chronic tracheobronchitis (J42)
            emphysema without chronic bronchitis (J43.-)

    | Excludes2 | lung diseases due to external agents (J60-J70) ◀ |

    **J44.0   Chronic obstructive pulmonary disease with acute lower
         respiratory infection**
         Use additional code to identify the infection

    **J44.1   Chronic obstructive pulmonary disease with (acute)
         exacerbation**
         Decompensated COPD
         Decompensated COPD with (acute) exacerbation

        | Excludes2 | chronic obstructive pulmonary disease |

                [COPD] with acute bronchitis (J44.0)
        Coding Clinic: 2016, Q1, P36

    J44.9   Chronic obstructive pulmonary disease, unspecified
         Chronic obstructive airway disease NOS
         Chronic obstructive lung disease NOS
         Coding Clinic: 2016, Q1, P37

    Normal alveoli   Walls of
                              alveoli enlarge
                              and fuse into
                              large air spaces
                Emphysema

Figure 10-6   Emphysema. (From Shiland, BJ: Medical Terminology &
Anatomy for ICD-10 Coding, ed 2, Mosby, 2015)

● **J45   Asthma**
        Allergic (predominantly) asthma
        Allergic bronchitis NOS
        Allergic rhinitis with asthma
        Atopic asthma
        Extrinsic allergic asthma
        Hay fever with asthma
        Idiosyncratic asthma
        Intrinsic nonallergic asthma
        Nonallergic asthma
    Use additional code to identify:
        exposure to environmental tobacco smoke (Z77.22)
        exposure to tobacco smoke in the perinatal period (P96.81)
        history of tobacco dependence (Z87.891) ◀▥
        occupational exposure to environmental tobacco smoke
          (Z57.31)
        tobacco dependence (F17.-)
        tobacco use (Z72.0)

    | Excludes1 | detergent asthma (J69.8) |

            eosinophilic asthma (J82)
            lung diseases due to external agents (J60-J70)
            miner's asthma (J60)
            wheezing NOS (R06.2)
            wood asthma (J67.8)

    | Excludes2 | asthma with chronic obstructive pulmonary |

                disease (J44.9)
            chronic asthmatic (obstructive) bronchitis (J44.9)
            chronic obstructive asthma (J44.9)

●   **J45.2   Mild intermittent asthma**

      J45.20   Mild intermittent asthma, uncomplicated
          Mild intermittent asthma NOS

      **J45.21   Mild intermittent asthma with (acute)
          exacerbation**

      **J45.22   Mild intermittent asthma with status
          asthmaticus**

●   **J45.3   Mild persistent asthma**

      J45.30   Mild persistent asthma, uncomplicated
          Mild persistent asthma NOS

      **J45.31   Mild persistent asthma with (acute)
          exacerbation**
          Coding Clinic: 2016, Q1, P35

      J45.32   Mild persistent asthma with status asthmaticus

●   **J45.4   Moderate persistent asthma**

      J45.40   Moderate persistent asthma, uncomplicated
          Moderate persistent asthma NOS

      **J45.41   Moderate persistent asthma with (acute)
          exacerbation**

      **J45.42   Moderate persistent asthma with status
          asthmaticus**

●   **J45.5   Severe persistent asthma**

      J45.50   Severe persistent asthma, uncomplicated
          Severe persistent asthma NOS

      **J45.51   Severe persistent asthma with (acute)
          exacerbation**

      **J45.52   Severe persistent asthma with status
          asthmaticus**

Item 10–9 **Asthma** is a bronchial condition marked by airway obstruction, hyper-responsiveness, and inflammation. **Extrinsic** asthma, also known as allergic asthma, is characterized by the same symptoms that occur with exposure to allergens and is divided into the following types: **atopic, occupational, and allergic bronchopulmonary aspergillosis. Intrinsic** asthma occurs in patients who have no history of allergy or sensitivities to allergens and is divided into the following types: **nonreaginic and pharmacologic. Status asthmaticus** is the most severe form of asthma attack and can last for days or weeks.

Figure 10-8 Progressive massive fibrosis superimposed on coal workers' pneumoconiosis. The large, blackened scars are located principally in the upper lobe. (From Cotran R, Kumar V, Collins T: Robbins Pathologic Basis of Disease, ed 8, Philadelphia, WB Saunders, 2009. Courtesy of Dr. Warner Laquer, Dr. Jerome Kleinerman, and the National Institute of Occupational Safety and Health, Morgantown, WV)

Figure 10-7 Factors causing expiratory obstruction in asthma. **A.** Cross section of a bronchiole occluded by muscle spasm, swollen mucosa, and mucus. **B.** Longitudinal section of an obstructed bronchiole. **C.** Cross-section of a clear bronchiole. (From Shiland: Mastering Healthcare Terminology, ed 1, St. Louis, Mosby, 2003)

● J45.9   **Other and unspecified asthma**
  ● J45.90   **Unspecified asthma**
    Asthmatic bronchitis NOS
    Childhood asthma NOS
    Late onset asthma
    J45.901   **Unspecified** asthma with (acute) exacerbation
    J45.902   **Unspecified** asthma with status asthmaticus
    J45.909   **Unspecified** asthma, uncomplicated
      Asthma NOS
  ● J45.99   **Other asthma**
    J45.990   **Exercise induced bronchospasm**
    J45.991   **Cough variant asthma**
    J45.998   **Other asthma**

● J47   **Bronchiectasis**
  Includes   bronchiolectasis
  Use additional code to identify:
    exposure to environmental tobacco smoke (Z77.22)
    exposure to tobacco smoke in the perinatal period (P96.81)
    history of tobacco dependence (Z87.891) ◀━
    occupational exposure to environmental tobacco smoke (Z57.31)
    tobacco dependence (F17.-)
    tobacco use (Z72.0)
  Excludes1   congenital bronchiectasis (Q33.4)
      tuberculous bronchiectasis (current disease) (A15.0)
  J47.0   **Bronchiectasis with acute lower respiratory infection**
    Bronchiectasis with acute bronchitis
    Use additional code to identify the infection ◀
  J47.1   **Bronchiectasis with (acute) exacerbation**
  J47.9   **Bronchiectasis, uncomplicated**
    Bronchiectasis NOS

Item 10–10 **Pneumoconiosis** refers to a lung condition resulting from exposure to inorganic or organic airborne particles, such as coal dust or moldy hay, as well as chemical fumes and vapors, such as insecticides. In this condition, the lungs retain the airborne particles.

LUNG DISEASES DUE TO EXTERNAL AGENTS (J60-J70)

  Excludes2   asthma (J45.-)
    malignant neoplasm of bronchus and lung (C34.-)

J60   **Coalworker's pneumoconiosis**   A
  Anthracosilicosis
  Anthracosis
  Black lung disease
  Coalworker's lung
  Excludes1   coalworker pneumoconiosis with tuberculosis, any type in A15 (J65)

J61   **Pneumoconiosis due to asbestos and other mineral fibers**   A
  Asbestosis
  Excludes1   pleural plaque with asbestosis (J92.0)
    pneumoconiosis with tuberculosis, any type in A15 (J65)

● J62   **Pneumoconiosis due to dust containing silica**
  Includes   silicotic fibrosis (massive) of lung
  Excludes1   pneumoconiosis with tuberculosis, any type in A15 (J65)
  J62.0   **Pneumoconiosis due to talc dust**
  J62.8   **Pneumoconiosis due to other dust containing silica**
    Silicosis NOS

● J63   **Pneumoconiosis due to other inorganic dusts**
  Excludes1   pneumoconiosis with tuberculosis, any type in A15 (J65)
  J63.0   **Aluminosis (of lung)**
  J63.1   **Bauxite fibrosis (of lung)**
  J63.2   **Berylliosis**
  J63.3   **Graphite fibrosis (of lung)**
  J63.4   **Siderosis**
  J63.5   **Stannosis**
  J63.6   **Pneumoconiosis due to other specified inorganic dusts**

J64   **Unspecified pneumoconiosis**
  Excludes1   pneumonoconiosis with tuberculosis, any type in A15 (J65)

J65   **Pneumoconiosis associated with tuberculosis**
  Any condition in J60-J64 with tuberculosis, any type in A15
  Silicotuberculosis

● J66   **Airway disease due to specific organic dust**
  Excludes2   allergic alveolitis (J67.-)
    asbestosis (J61)
    bagassosis (J67.1)
    farmer's lung (J67.0)
    hypersensitivity pneumonitis due to organic dust (J67.-)
    reactive airways dysfunction syndrome (J68.3)
  J66.0   **Byssinosis**
    Airway disease due to cotton dust
  J66.1   **Flax-dressers' disease**
  J66.2   **Cannabinosis**
  J66.8   **Airway disease due to other specific organic dusts**

◀ New   ◀━ Revised   ̶d̶e̶l̶e̶t̶e̶d̶ Deleted   Excludes 1   Excludes 2   Includes   Use additional   Code first   Code also   Unspecified

908
  OGCR Official Guidelines   X Assign placeholder X   ● Use Additional Character(s)   ▸ Manifestation Code   **Coding Clinic**

● **J67　Hypersensitivity pneumonitis due to organic dust**

> **Includes**　allergic alveolitis and pneumonitis due to inhaled organic dust and particles of fungal, actinomycetic or other origin
>
> **Excludes1**　pneumonitis due to inhalation of chemicals, gases, fumes or vapors (J68.0)

J67.0　**Farmer's lung**
Harvester's lung
Haymaker's lung
Moldy hay disease

J67.1　**Bagassosis**
Bagasse disease
Bagasse pneumonitis

J67.2　**Bird fancier's lung**
Budgerigar fancier's disease or lung
Pigeon fancier's disease or lung

J67.3　**Suberosis**
Corkhandler's disease or lung
Corkworker's disease or lung

J67.4　**Maltworker's lung**
Alveolitis due to Aspergillus clavatus

J67.5　**Mushroom-worker's lung**

J67.6　**Maple-bark-stripper's lung**
Alveolitis due to Cryptostroma corticale
Cryptostromosis

J67.7　**Air conditioner and humidifier lung**
Allergic alveolitis due to fungal, thermophilic actinomycetes and other organisms growing in ventilation [air conditioning] systems

J67.8　**Hypersensitivity pneumonitis due to other organic dusts**
Cheese-washer's lung
Coffee-worker's lung
Fish-meal worker's lung
Furrier's lung
Sequoiosis

J67.9　**Hypersensitivity pneumonitis due to unspecified organic dust**
Allergic alveolitis (extrinsic) NOS
Hypersensitivity pneumonitis NOS

● **J68　Respiratory conditions due to inhalation of chemicals, gases, fumes and vapors**

> *Code first (T51-T65) to identify cause*
> Use additional code to identify associated respiratory conditions, such as:
> acute respiratory failure (J96.0-)

J68.0　**Bronchitis and pneumonitis due to chemicals, gases, fumes and vapors**
Chemical bronchitis (acute)

J68.1　**Pulmonary edema due to chemicals, gases, fumes and vapors**
Chemical pulmonary edema (acute) (chronic)
> **Excludes1**　pulmonary edema (acute) (chronic) NOS (J81.-)

J68.2　**Upper respiratory inflammation due to chemicals, gases, fumes and vapors, not elsewhere classified**

J68.3　**Other acute and subacute respiratory conditions due to chemicals, gases, fumes and vapors**
Reactive airways dysfunction syndrome

J68.4　**Chronic respiratory conditions due to chemicals, gases, fumes and vapors**
Emphysema (diffuse) (chronic) due to inhalation of chemicals, gases, fumes and vapors
Obliterative bronchiolitis (chronic) (subacute) due to inhalation of chemicals, gases, fumes and vapors
Pulmonary fibrosis (chronic) due to inhalation of chemicals, gases, fumes and vapors
> **Excludes1**　chronic pulmonary edema due to chemicals, gases, fumes and vapors (J68.1)

J68.8　**Other respiratory conditions due to chemicals, gases, fumes and vapors**

J68.9　**Unspecified respiratory condition due to chemicals, gases, fumes and vapors**

● **J69　Pneumonitis due to solids and liquids**

> **Excludes1**　neonatal aspiration syndromes (P24.-)
> postprocedural pneumonitis (J95.4)

J69.0　**Pneumonitis due to inhalation of food and vomit**
Aspiration pneumonia NOS
Aspiration pneumonia (due to) food (regurgitated)
Aspiration pneumonia (due to) gastric secretions
Aspiration pneumonia (due to) milk
Aspiration pneumonia (due to) vomit
Code also any associated foreign body in respiratory tract (T17.-)
> **Excludes1**　chemical pneumonitis due to anesthesia (J95.4)
> obstetric aspiration pneumonitis (O74.0)

J69.1　**Pneumonitis due to inhalation of oils and essences**
Exogenous lipoid pneumonia
Lipid pneumonia NOS
Code first (T51-T65) to identify substance
> **Excludes1**　endogenous lipoid pneumonia (J84.89)

J69.8　**Pneumonitis due to inhalation of other solids and liquids**
Pneumonitis due to aspiration of blood
Pneumonitis due to aspiration of detergent
Code first (T51-T65) to identify substance

● **J70　Respiratory conditions due to other external agents**

J70.0　**Acute pulmonary manifestations due to radiation**
Radiation pneumonitis
Use additional code (W88-W90, X39.0-) to identify the external cause

J70.1　**Chronic and other pulmonary manifestations due to radiation**
Fibrosis of lung following radiation
Use additional code (W88-W90, X39.0-) to identify the external cause

J70.2　**Acute drug-induced interstitial lung disorders**
Use additional code for adverse effect, if applicable, to identify drug (T36-T50 with fifth or sixth character 5)
> **Excludes1**　interstitial pneumonia NOS (J84.9)
> lymphoid interstitial pneumonia (J84.2)

J70.3　**Chronic drug-induced interstitial lung disorders**
Use additional code for adverse effect, if applicable, to identify drug (T36-T50 with fifth or sixth character 5)
> **Excludes1**　interstitial pneumonia NOS (J84.9)
> lymphoid interstitial pneumonia (J84.2)

J70.4　**Drug-induced interstitial lung disorders, unspecified**
Use additional code for adverse effect, if applicable, to identify drug (T36-T50 with fifth or sixth character 5)
> **Excludes1**　interstitial pneumonia NOS (J84.9)
> lymphoid interstitial pneumonia (J84.2)

J70.5　**Respiratory conditions due to smoke inhalation**
Smoke inhalation NOS
> **Excludes1**　smoke inhalation due to chemicals, gases, fumes and vapors (J68.9)

J70.8　**Respiratory conditions due to other specified external agents**
Code first (T51-T65) to identify the external agent

J70.9　**Respiratory conditions due to unspecified external agent**
Code first (T51-T65) to identify the external agent

CHAPTER 10 (J00-J99)

Figure 10-9 Bullous emphysema with large subpleural bullae *(upper left)*. (From Kumar: Robbins and Cotran: Pathologic Basis of Disease, ed 8, Saunders, An Imprint of Elsevier, 2009)

CHAPTER 10 (J00-J99)

OTHER RESPIRATORY DISEASES PRINCIPALLY AFFECTING THE INTERSTITIUM (J80-J84)

J80   **Acute respiratory distress syndrome**
Acute respiratory distress syndrome in adult or child
Adult hyaline membrane disease
> **Excludes1**   respiratory distress syndrome in newborn (perinatal) (P22.0)

● **J81**   **Pulmonary edema**
Use additional code to identify:
    exposure to environmental tobacco smoke (Z77.22)
    history of tobacco dependence (Z87.891) ◀▦
    occupational exposure to environmental tobacco smoke (Z57.31)
    tobacco dependence (F17.-)
    tobacco use (Z72.0)
> **Excludes1**   chemical (acute) pulmonary edema (J68.1)
>   hypostatic pneumonia (J18.2)
>   passive pneumonia (J18.2)
>   pulmonary edema due to external agents (J60-J70)
>   pulmonary edema with heart disease NOS (I50.1)
>   pulmonary edema with heart failure (I50.1)

     J81.0   **Acute pulmonary edema**
              Acute edema of lung

     J81.1   **Chronic pulmonary edema**
              Pulmonary congestion (chronic) (passive)
              Pulmonary edema NOS

J82   **Pulmonary eosinophilia, not elsewhere classified**
Allergic pneumonia
Eosinophilic asthma
Eosinophilic pneumonia
Löffler's pneumonia
Tropical (pulmonary) eosinophilia NOS
> **Excludes1**   pulmonary eosinophilia due to aspergillosis (B44.-)
>   pulmonary eosinophilia due to drugs (J70.2-J70.4)
>   pulmonary eosinophilia due to specified parasitic infection (B50-B83)
>   pulmonary eosinophilia due to systemic connective tissue disorders (M30-M36)
>   pulmonary infiltrate NOS (R91.8)

● **J84**   **Other interstitial pulmonary diseases**
> **Excludes1**   drug-induced interstitial lung disorders (J70.2-J70.4)
>   interstitial emphysema (J98.2)
>   lung diseases due to external agents (J60-J70)

   ● **J84.0**   **Alveolar and parieto-alveolar conditions**
       J84.01   **Alveolar proteinosis**
       J84.02   **Pulmonary alveolar microlithiasis**
     ▷ **J84.03**   *Idiopathic pulmonary hemosiderosis*
                Essential brown induration of lung
                Code first underlying disease, such as:
                  disorders of iron metabolism (E83.1-)
>   **Excludes1**   acute idiopathic pulmonary hemorrhage in infants [AIPHI] (R04.81)
       J84.09   **Other alveolar and parieto-alveolar conditions**

● **J84.1**   **Other interstitial pulmonary diseases with fibrosis**
> **Excludes1**   pulmonary fibrosis (chronic) due to inhalation of chemicals, gases, fumes or vapors (J68.4)
>   pulmonary fibrosis (chronic) following radiation (J70.1)

     J84.10   **Pulmonary fibrosis, unspecified**
              Capillary fibrosis of lung
              Cirrhosis of lung (chronic) NOS
              Fibrosis of lung (atrophic) (chronic) (confluent) (massive) (perialveolar) (peribronchial) NOS
              Induration of lung (chronic) NOS
              Postinflammatory pulmonary fibrosis

   ● **J84.11**   **Idiopathic interstitial pneumonia**
> **Excludes1**   lymphoid interstitial pneumonia (J84.2)
>   pneumocystis pneumonia (B59)

       J84.111   **Idiopathic interstitial pneumonia, not otherwise specified**
       J84.112   **Idiopathic pulmonary fibrosis**
              Cryptogenic fibrosing alveolitis
              Idiopathic fibrosing alveolitis
       J84.113   **Idiopathic non-specific interstitial pneumonitis**
>   **Excludes1**   non-specific interstitial pneumonia NOS, or due to known underlying cause (J84.89)
       J84.114   **Acute interstitial pneumonitis**
              Hamman-Rich syndrome
>   **Excludes1**   pneumocystis pneumonia (B59)
       J84.115   **Respiratory bronchiolitis interstitial lung disease**
       J84.116   **Cryptogenic organizing pneumonia**
>   **Excludes1**   organizing pneumonia NOS, or due to known underlying cause (J84.89)
       J84.117   **Desquamative interstitial pneumonia**

    ▷ **J84.17**   *Other interstitial pulmonary diseases with fibrosis in diseases classified elsewhere*
            Interstitial pneumonia (nonspecific) (usual) due to collagen vascular disease
            Interstitial pneumonia (nonspecific) (usual) in diseases classified elsewhere
            Organizing pneumonia due to collagen vascular disease
            Organizing pneumonia in diseases classified elsewhere
            Code first underlying disease, such as:
               progressive systemic sclerosis (M34.0)
               rheumatoid arthritis (M05.00-M06.9)
               systemic lupus erythematosis (M32.0-M32.9)

   J84.2   **Lymphoid interstitial pneumonia**
          Lymphoid interstitial pneumonitis

● **J84.8**   **Other specified interstitial pulmonary diseases**
> **Excludes1**   exogenous lipoid pneumonia (J69.1)
>   unspecified lipoid pneumonia (J69.1)

     J84.81   **Lymphangioleiomyomatosis ♀**
              Lymphangiomyomatosis
     J84.82   **Adult pulmonary Langerhans cell histiocytosis**
              Adult PLCH
     J84.83   **Surfactant mutations of the lung**

A

● **J84.84**   **Other interstitial lung diseases of childhood**

     J84.841   **Neuroendocrine cell hyperplasia of infancy**

     J84.842   **Pulmonary interstitial glycogenosis**

     J84.843   **Alveolar capillary dysplasia with vein misalignment**

     J84.848   **Other interstitial lung diseases of childhood**

   J84.89   **Other specified interstitial pulmonary diseases**

       Endogenous lipoid pneumonia
       Interstitial pneumonitis
       Non-specific interstitial pneumonitis NOS
       ~~Organizing pneumonia due to known underlying cause~~
       Organizing pneumonia NOS

       Code first, if applicable:
       poisoning due to drug or toxin (T51-T65 with fifth or sixth character to indicate intent), for toxic pneumonopathy underlying cause of pneumonopathy, if known

       Use additional code, for adverse effect, to identify drug (T36-T50 with fifth or sixth character 5), if drug-induced

       Excludes1   cryptogenic organizing pneumonia (J84.116)
            idiopathic non-specific interstitial pneumonitis (J84.113)
            lipoid pneumonia, exogenous or unspecified (J69.1)
            lymphoid interstitial pneumonia (J84.2)

   J84.9   **Interstitial pulmonary disease, unspecified**
       Interstitial pneumonia NOS

SUPPURATIVE AND NECROTIC CONDITIONS OF THE LOWER RESPIRATORY TRACT (J85-J86)

● **J85**   **Abscess of lung and mediastinum**
       Use additional code (B95-B97) to identify infectious agent.

   J85.0   **Gangrene and necrosis of lung**

   J85.1   **Abscess of lung with pneumonia**
       Code also the type of pneumonia

   J85.2   **Abscess of lung without pneumonia**
       Abscess of lung NOS

   J85.3   **Abscess of mediastinum**

● **J86**   **Pyothorax**
       Use additional code (B95-B97) to identify infectious agent.

       Excludes1   abscess of lung (J85.-)
            pyothorax due to tuberculosis (A15.6)

   J86.0   **Pyothorax with fistula**
       Bronchocutaneous fistula
       Bronchopleural fistula
       Hepatopleural fistula
       Mediastinal fistula
       Pleural fistula
       Thoracic fistula
       Any condition classifiable to J86.9 with fistula

   J86.9   **Pyothorax without fistula**
       Abscess of pleura
       Abscess of thorax
       Empyema (chest) (lung) (pleura)
       Fibrinopurulent pleurisy
       Purulent pleurisy
       Pyopneumothorax
       Septic pleurisy
       Seropurulent pleurisy
       Suppurative pleurisy

OTHER DISEASES OF THE PLEURA (J90-J94)

   J90   **Pleural effusion, not elsewhere classified**
       Encysted pleurisy
       Pleural effusion NOS
       Pleurisy with effusion (exudative) (serous)

       Excludes1   chylous (pleural) effusion (J94.0)
            malignant pleural effusion (J91.0))
            pleurisy NOS (R09.1)
            tuberculous pleural effusion (A15.6)
       Coding Clinic: 2015, Q2, P16

● **J91**   **Pleural effusion in conditions classified elsewhere**
       Excludes2   pleural effusion in heart failure (I50.-)
            pleural effusion in systemic lupus erythematosus (M32.13)

   J91.0   *Malignant pleural effusion*
       Code first underlying neoplasm

   J91.8   *Pleural effusion in other conditions classified elsewhere*
       Code first underlying disease, such as:
       filariasis (B74.0-B74.9)
       influenza (J09.X2, J10.1, J11.1)
       Coding Clinic: 2015, Q2, P16

● **J92**   **Pleural plaque**
       Includes   pleural thickening

   J92.0   **Pleural plaque with presence of asbestos**

   J92.9   **Pleural plaque without asbestos**
       Pleural plaque NOS

● **J93**   **Pneumothorax and air leak**
       Collapsed lung

       Excludes1   congenital or perinatal pneumothorax (P25.1)
            postprocedural air leak (J95.812)
            postprocedural pneumothorax (J95.811)
            traumatic pneumothorax (S27.0)
            tuberculous (current disease) pneumothorax (A15.-)
            pyopneumothorax (J86.-)

   J93.0   **Spontaneous tension pneumothorax**
       Tension pneumothorax (most serious type) occurs when air (positive pressure) collects in the pleural space

● **J93.1**   **Other spontaneous pneumothorax**

     J93.11   **Primary spontaneous pneumothorax**

     J93.12   **Secondary spontaneous pneumothorax**

       Code first underlying condition, such as:
       catamenial pneumothorax due to endometriosis (N80.8)
       cystic fibrosis (E84.-)
       eosinophilic pneumonia (J82)
       lymphangioleiomyomatosis (J84.81)
       malignant neoplasm of bronchus and lung (C34.-)
       Marfan's syndrome (Q87.4)
       pneumonia due to Pneumocystis carinii (B59)
       secondary malignant neoplasm of lung (C78.0-)
       spontaneous rupture of the esophagus (K22.3)

● **J93.8**   **Other pneumothorax and air leak**

     J93.81   **Chronic pneumothorax**

     J93.82   **Other air leak**
       Persistent air leak

     J93.83   **Other pneumothorax**
       Acute pneumothorax
       Spontaneous pneumothorax NOS

   J93.9   **Pneumothorax, unspecified**
       Pneumothorax NOS

Item 10–11   **Empyema** is a condition in which pus accumulates in a body cavity. Empyema **with fistula** occurs when the pus passes from one cavity to another organ or structure.

CHAPTER 10 (J00-J99)

● **J94   Other pleural conditions**
     Excludes1   pleurisy NOS (R09.1)
                   traumatic hemopneumothorax (S27.2)
                   traumatic hemothorax (S27.1)
                   tuberculous pleural conditions (current disease)
                      (A15.-)

     J94.0   Chylous effusion
            Chyliform effusion

     J94.1   Fibrothorax

     J94.2   Hemothorax
            Hemopneumothorax

     J94.8   Other specified pleural conditions
            Hydropneumothorax
            Hydrothorax

     J94.9   Pleural condition, unspecified

INTRAOPERATIVE AND POSTPROCEDURAL COMPLICATIONS AND DISORDERS OF RESPIRATORY SYSTEM, NOT ELSEWHERE CLASSIFIED (J95)

● **J95   Intraoperative and postprocedural complications and disorders of respiratory system, not elsewhere classified**
     Excludes2   aspiration pneumonia (J69.-)
                   emphysema (subcutaneous) resulting from a
                      procedure (T81.82)
                   hypostatic pneumonia (J18.2)
                   pulmonary manifestations due to radiation
                      (J70.0- J70.1)

● **J95.0   Tracheostomy complications**
       J95.00   Unspecified tracheostomy complication
       J95.01   Hemorrhage from tracheostomy stoma
       J95.02   Infection of tracheostomy stoma
               Use additional code to identify type of
                   infection, such as:
                   cellulitis of neck (L03.8)
                   sepsis (A40, A41.-)
       J95.03   Malfunction of tracheostomy stoma
               Mechanical complication of tracheostomy
                   stoma
               Obstruction of tracheostomy airway
               Tracheal stenosis due to tracheostomy
       J95.04   Tracheo-esophageal fistula following tracheostomy
       J95.09   Other tracheostomy complication

     J95.1   Acute pulmonary insufficiency following thoracic surgery
         Excludes2   functional disturbances following cardiac
                      surgery (I97.0, I97.1-)

     J95.2   Acute pulmonary insufficiency following nonthoracic surgery
         Excludes2   functional disturbances following cardiac
                      surgery (I97.0, I97.1-)

     J95.3   Chronic pulmonary insufficiency following surgery
         Excludes2   functional disturbances following cardiac
                      surgery (I97.0, I97.1-)

     J95.4   Chemical pneumonitis due to anesthesia
            Mendelson's syndrome
            Postprocedural aspiration pneumonia
            Use additional code for adverse effect, if applicable, to
               identify drug (T41.- with fifth or sixth character 5)
         Excludes1   aspiration pneumonitis due to anesthesia
                      complicating labor and delivery
                      (O74.0)
                   aspiration pneumonitis due to anesthesia
                      complicating pregnancy (O29)
                   aspiration pneumonitis due to anesthesia
                      complicating the puerperium
                      (O89.01)

     J95.5   Postprocedural subglottic stenosis

● **J95.6   Intraoperative hemorrhage and hematoma of a respiratory system organ or structure complicating a procedure**
         Excludes1   intraoperative hemorrhage and
                      hematoma of a respiratory system
                      organ or structure due to accidental
                      puncture and laceration during
                      procedure (J95.7-)

     J95.61   Intraoperative hemorrhage and hematoma of a respiratory system organ or structure complicating a respiratory system procedure

     J95.62   Intraoperative hemorrhage and hematoma of a respiratory system organ or structure complicating other procedure

● **J95.7   Accidental puncture and laceration of a respiratory system organ or structure during a procedure**
         Excludes2   postprocedural pneumothorax (J95.811)

     J95.71   Accidental puncture and laceration of a respiratory system organ or structure during a respiratory system procedure

     J95.72   Accidental puncture and laceration of a respiratory system organ or structure during other procedure

● **J95.8   Other intraoperative and postprocedural complications and disorders of respiratory system, not elsewhere classified**

● **J95.81   Postprocedural pneumothorax and air leak**
       J95.811   Postprocedural pneumothorax
       J95.812   Postprocedural air leak

● **J95.82   Postprocedural respiratory failure**
         Excludes1   Respiratory failure in other
                      conditions (J96.-)
       J95.821   Acute postprocedural respiratory failure
              Postprocedural respiratory failure NOS
       J95.822   Acute and chronic postprocedural respiratory failure

● **J95.83   Postprocedural hemorrhage of a respiratory system organ or structure following a procedure** ◀▥
       J95.830   Postprocedural hemorrhage of a respiratory system organ or structure following a respiratory system procedure ◀▥
       J95.831   Postprocedural hemorrhage of a respiratory system organ or structure following other procedure ◀▥

     J95.84   Transfusion-related acute lung injury (TRALI)

● **J95.85   Complication of respirator [ventilator]**
       J95.850   Mechanical complication of respirator
           Excludes1   encounter for
                      respirator
                      [ventilator]
                      dependence
                      during power
                      failure (Z99.12)
       J95.851   Ventilator associated pneumonia
              Ventilator associated pneumonitis
              Use additional code to identify the
                   organism, if known (B95.-,
                   B96.-, B97.-)
           Excludes1   ventilator lung in
                      newborn (P27.8)
       J95.859   Other complication of respirator [ventilator]

◀ New   ◀▥ Revised   ~~deleted~~ Deleted   Excludes 1   Excludes 2   Includes   Use additional   Code first   Code also   Unspecified
OGCR Official Guidelines   X Assign placeholder X   ● Use Additional Character(s)   ▶ Manifestation Code   **Coding Clinic**

● J95.86   Postprocedural hematoma and seroma of a respiratory system organ or structure following a procedure ◄

    J95.860   Postprocedural hematoma of a respiratory system organ or structure following a respiratory system procedure ◄

    J95.861   Postprocedural hematoma of a respiratory system organ or structure following other procedure ◄

    J95.862   Postprocedural seroma of a respiratory system organ or structure following a respiratory system procedure ◄

    J95.863   Postprocedural seroma of a respiratory system organ or structure following other procedure ◄

J95.88   Other intraoperative complications of respiratory system, not elsewhere classified

J95.89   Other postprocedural complications and disorders of respiratory system, not elsewhere classified

    Use additional code to identify disorder, such as:
       aspiration pneumonia (J69.-)
       bacterial or viral pneumonia (J12-J18)

    Excludes2   acute pulmonary insufficiency following thoracic surgery (J95.1)
               postprocedural subglottic stenosis (J95.5)

OTHER DISEASES OF THE RESPIRATORY SYSTEM (J96-J99)

● J96   Respiratory failure, not elsewhere classified

    Excludes1   acute respiratory distress syndrome (J80)
              cardiorespiratory failure (R09.2)
              newborn respiratory distress syndrome (P22.0)
              postprocedural respiratory failure (J95.82-)
              respiratory arrest (R09.2)
              respiratory arrest of newborn (P28.81)
              respiratory failure of newborn (P28.5)

● J96.0   Acute respiratory failure

    J96.00   Acute respiratory failure, unspecified whether with hypoxia or hypercapnia

    J96.01   Acute respiratory failure with hypoxia

    J96.02   Acute respiratory failure with hypercapnia

● J96.1   Chronic respiratory failure

    J96.10   Chronic respiratory failure, unspecified whether with hypoxia or hypercapnia
           Coding Clinic: 2016, Q1, P38; 2015, Q1, P21

    J96.11   Chronic respiratory failure with hypoxia

    J96.12   Chronic respiratory failure with hypercapnia

● J96.2   Acute and chronic respiratory failure
    Acute on chronic respiratory failure

    J96.20   Acute and chronic respiratory failure, unspecified whether with hypoxia or hypercapnia

    J96.21   Acute and chronic respiratory failure with hypoxia

    J96.22   Acute and chronic respiratory failure with hypercapnia

● J96.9   Respiratory failure, unspecified

    J96.90   Respiratory failure, unspecified, unspecified whether with hypoxia or hypercapnia

    J96.91   Respiratory failure, unspecified with hypoxia

    J96.92   Respiratory failure, unspecified with hypercapnia

● J98   Other respiratory disorders

    Use additional code to identify:
       exposure to environmental tobacco smoke (Z77.22)
       exposure to tobacco smoke in the perinatal period (P96.81)
       history of tobacco dependence (Z87.891) ◄▥
       occupational exposure to environmental tobacco smoke (Z57.31)
       tobacco dependence (F17.-)
       tobacco use (Z72.0)

    Excludes1   newborn apnea (P28.4)
              newborn sleep apnea (P28.3)

    Excludes2   apnea NOS (R06.81)
              sleep apnea (G47.3-)

● J98.0   Diseases of bronchus, not elsewhere classified

    J98.01   Acute bronchospasm

       Excludes1   acute bronchiolitis with bronchospasm (J21.-)
                acute bronchitis with bronchospasm (J20.-)
                asthma (J45.-)
                exercise induced bronchospasm (J45.990)

    J98.09   Other diseases of bronchus, not elsewhere classified
           Broncholithiasis
           Calcification of bronchus
           Stenosis of bronchus
           Tracheobronchial collapse
           Tracheobronchial dyskinesia
           Ulcer of bronchus

● J98.1   Pulmonary collapse

    Excludes1   therapeutic collapse of lung status (Z98.3)

    J98.11   Atelectasis

       Excludes1   newborn atelectasis
                tuberculous atelectasis (current disease) (A15)

    J98.19   Other pulmonary collapse

J98.2   Interstitial emphysema
    Mediastinal emphysema

    Excludes1   emphysema NOS (J43.9)
              emphysema in newborn (P25.0)
              surgical emphysema (subcutaneous) (T81.82)
              traumatic subcutaneous emphysema (T79.7)

J98.3   Compensatory emphysema

J98.4   Other disorders of lung
    Calcification of lung
    Cystic lung disease (acquired)
    Lung disease NOS
    Pulmolithiasis

    Excludes1   acute interstitial pneumonitis (J84.114)
              pulmonary insufficiency following surgery (J95.1-J95.2)

CHAPTER 10 (J00-J99)

● **J98.5** **Diseases of mediastinum, not elsewhere classified**

     Excludes2   abscess of mediastinum (J85.3)

     J98.51   **Mediastinitis** ◀

         Code first underlying condition, if applicable, such as postoperative mediastinitis (T81.-) ◀

     J98.59   **Other diseases of mediastinum, not elsewhere classified** ◀

         Fibrosis of mediastinum ◀

         Hernia of mediastinum ◀

         Retraction of mediastinum ◀

J98.6 **Disorders of diaphragm**

     Diaphragmatitis

     Paralysis of diaphragm

     Relaxation of diaphragm

     Excludes1   congenital malformation of diaphragm NEC (Q79.1)

               congenital diaphragmatic hernia (Q79.0)

     Excludes2   diaphragmatic hernia (K44.-)

J98.8 **Other specified respiratory disorders**

J98.9 **Respiratory disorder, unspecified**

     Respiratory disease (chronic) NOS

▌ *J99*   *Respiratory disorders in diseases classified elsewhere*

     Code first underlying disease, such as:

         amyloidosis (E85.-)

         ankylosing spondylitis (M45)

         congenital syphilis (A50.5)

         cryoglobulinemia (D89.1)

         early congenital syphilis (A50.0)

         schistosomiasis (B65.0-B65.9)

     Excludes1   respiratory disorders in:

         amebiasis (A06.5)

         blastomycosis (B40.0-B40.2)

         candidiasis (B37.1)

         coccidioidomycosis (B38.0-B38.2)

         cystic fibrosis with pulmonary manifestations (E84.0)

         dermatomyositis (M33.01, M33.11)

         histoplasmosis (B39.0-B39.2)

         late syphilis (A52.72, A52.73)

         polymyositis (M33.21)

         sicca syndrome (M35.02)

         systemic lupus erythematosus (M32.13)

         systemic sclerosis (M34.81)

         Wegener's granulomatosis (M31.30-M31.31)

CHAPTER 11

DISEASES OF THE DIGESTIVE SYSTEM (K00-K95)

OGCR Chapter-Specific Coding Guidelines

> 11. **Chapter 11: Diseases of the Digestive System (K00-K95)**
> Reserved for future guideline expansion

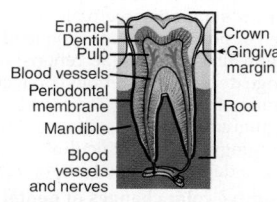

Figure 11-1 Anatomy of a tooth.

Item 11–1 **Anodontia** is the congenital absence of teeth. **Hypodontia** is partial anodontia. **Oligodontia** is the congenital absence of some teeth, whereas **supernumerary** is having more teeth than the normal number. **Mesiodens** are small extra teeth that often appear in pairs, although single small teeth are not uncommon.

CHAPTER 11

DISEASES OF THE DIGESTIVE SYSTEM (K00-K95)

Excludes2   certain conditions originating in the perinatal period (P04-P96)
certain infectious and parasitic diseases (A00-B99)
complications of pregnancy, childbirth and the puerperium (O00-O9A)
congenital malformations, deformations and chromosomal abnormalities (Q00-Q99)
endocrine, nutritional and metabolic diseases (E00-E88)
injury, poisoning and certain other consequences of external causes (S00-T88)
neoplasms (C00-D49)
symptoms, signs and abnormal clinical and laboratory findings, not elsewhere classified (R00-R94)

This chapter contains the following blocks:

K00-K14	Diseases of oral cavity and salivary glands
K20-K31	Diseases of esophagus, stomach and duodenum
K35-K38	Diseases of appendix
K40-K46	Hernia
K50-K52	Noninfective enteritis and colitis
K55-K64	Other diseases of intestines
K65-K68	Diseases of peritoneum and retroperitoneum
K70-K77	Diseases of liver
K80-K87	Disorders of gallbladder, biliary tract and pancreas
K90-K95	Other diseases of the digestive system

DISEASES OF ORAL CAVITY AND SALIVARY GLANDS (K00-K14)

● **K00**   **Disorders of tooth development and eruption**
    Excludes2   embedded and impacted teeth (K01.-)
    K00.0   **Anodontia**
       Hypodontia
       Oligodontia
       Excludes1   acquired absence of teeth (K08.1-)
    K00.1   **Supernumerary teeth**
       Distomolar
       Fourth molar
       Mesiodens
       Paramolar
       Supplementary teeth
       Excludes2   supernumerary roots (K00.2)

K00.2   **Abnormalities of size and form of teeth**
    Concrescence of teeth
    Fusion of teeth
    Gemination of teeth
    Dens evaginatus
    Dens in dente
    Dens invaginatus
    Enamel pearls
    Macrodontia
    Microdontia
    Peg-shaped [conical] teeth
    Supernumerary roots
    Taurodontism
    Tuberculum paramolare
    Excludes1   abnormalities of teeth due to congenital syphilis (A50.5)
          tuberculum Carabelli, which is regarded as a normal variation and should not be coded

K00.3   **Mottled teeth**
    Dental fluorosis
    Mottling of enamel
    Nonfluoride enamel opacities
    Excludes2   deposits [accretions] on teeth (K03.6)

K00.4   **Disturbances in tooth formation**
    Aplasia and hypoplasia of cementum
    Dilaceration of tooth
    Enamel hypoplasia (neonatal) (postnatal) (prenatal)
    Regional odontodysplasia
    Turner's tooth
    Excludes1   Hutchinson's teeth and mulberry molars in congenital syphilis (A50.5)
    Excludes2   mottled teeth (K00.3)

K00.5   **Hereditary disturbances in tooth structure, not elsewhere classified**
    Amelogenesis imperfecta
    Dentinogenesis imperfecta
    Odontogenesis imperfecta
    Dentinal dysplasia
    Shell teeth

K00.6   **Disturbances in tooth eruption**
    Dentia praecox
    Natal tooth
    Neonatal tooth
    Premature eruption of tooth
    Premature shedding of primary [deciduous] tooth
    Prenatal teeth
    Retained [persistent] primary tooth
    Excludes2   embedded and impacted teeth (K01.-)

K00.7   **Teething syndrome**

K00.8   **Other disorders of tooth development**
    Color changes during tooth formation
    Intrinsic staining of teeth NOS
    Excludes2   posteruptive color changes (K03.7)

K00.9   **Disorder of tooth development, unspecified**
    Disorder of odontogenesis NOS

● **K01**   **Embedded and impacted teeth**
    Excludes1   abnormal position of fully erupted teeth (M26.3-)
    K01.0   **Embedded teeth**
    K01.1   **Impacted teeth**

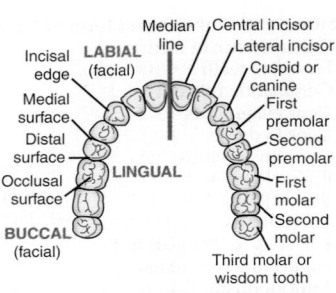

Figure 11-2 The permanent teeth within the dental arch.

Item 11–2 Each dental arch (jaw) normally contains 16 teeth. Tooth decay or **dental caries** is a disease of the enamel, dentin, and cementum of the tooth and can result in a cavity.

● **K02   Dental caries**
  Includes   caries of dentine ◀
            dental cavities
            early childhood caries ◀
            pre-eruptive caries ◀
            recurrent caries (dentino enamel junction)
              (enamel) (to the pulp) ◀
            tooth decay

   K02.3   Arrested dental caries
            Arrested coronal and root caries

● **K02.5   Dental caries on pit and fissure surface**
            Dental caries on chewing surface of tooth

   K02.51   Dental caries on pit and fissure surface limited to enamel
            White spot lesions [initial caries] on pit and fissure surface of tooth

   K02.52   Dental caries on pit and fissure surface penetrating into dentin
            Primary dental caries, cervical origin ◀

   K02.53   Dental caries on pit and fissure surface penetrating into pulp

● **K02.6   Dental caries on smooth surface**

   K02.61   Dental caries on smooth surface limited to enamel
            White spot lesions [initial caries] on smooth surface of tooth

   K02.62   Dental caries on smooth surface penetrating into dentin

   K02.63   Dental caries on smooth surface penetrating into pulp

   K02.7   Dental root caries
   K02.9   Dental caries, unspecified

● **K03   Other diseases of hard tissues of teeth**
  Excludes2   bruxism (F45.8)
            dental caries (K02.-)
            teeth-grinding NOS (F45.8)

   K03.0   Excessive attrition of teeth
            Approximal wear of teeth
            Occlusal wear of teeth

   K03.1   Abrasion of teeth
            Dentifrice abrasion of teeth
            Habitual abrasion of teeth
            Occupational abrasion of teeth
            Ritual abrasion of teeth
            Traditional abrasion of teeth
            Wedge defect NOS

   K03.2   Erosion of teeth
            Erosion of teeth due to diet
            Erosion of teeth due to drugs and medicaments
            Erosion of teeth due to persistent vomiting
            Erosion of teeth NOS
            Idiopathic erosion of teeth
            Occupational erosion of teeth

   K03.3   Pathological resorption of teeth
            Internal granuloma of pulp
            Resorption of teeth (external)

   K03.4   Hypercementosis
            Cementation hyperplasia

   K03.5   Ankylosis of teeth

   K03.6   Deposits [accretions] on teeth
            Betel deposits [accretions] on teeth
            Black deposits [accretions] on teeth
            Extrinsic staining of teeth NOS
            Green deposits [accretions] on teeth
            Materia alba deposits [accretions] on teeth
            Orange deposits [accretions] on teeth
            Staining of teeth NOS
            Subgingival dental calculus
            Supragingival dental calculus
            Tobacco deposits [accretions] on teeth

   K03.7   Posteruptive color changes of dental hard tissues
            Excludes2   deposits [accretions] on teeth (K03.6)

● **K03.8   Other specified diseases of hard tissues of teeth**

   K03.81   Cracked tooth
            Excludes1   asymptomatic craze lines in enamel - omit code
                      broken or fractured tooth due to trauma (S02.5)

   K03.89   Other specified diseases of hard tissues of teeth
   K03.9   Disease of hard tissues of teeth, unspecified

● **K04   Diseases of pulp and periapical tissues**
● **K04.0   Pulpitis**
            Acute pulpitis
            Chronic (hyperplastic) (ulcerative) pulpitis

   K04.01   Reversible pulpitis ◀
   K04.02   Irreversible pulpitis ◀

   K04.1   Necrosis of pulp
            Pulpal gangrene

   K04.2   Pulp degeneration
            Denticles
            Pulpal calcifications
            Pulpal stones

   K04.3   Abnormal hard tissue formation in pulp
            Secondary or irregular dentine

   K04.4   Acute apical periodontitis of pulpal origin
            Acute apical periodontitis NOS
            Excludes1   acute periodontitis (K05.2-)

   K04.5   Chronic apical periodontitis
            Apical or periapical granuloma
            Apical periodontitis NOS
            Excludes1   chronic periodontitis (K05.3-)

   K04.6   Periapical abscess with sinus
            Dental abscess with sinus
            Dentoalveolar abscess with sinus

   K04.7   Periapical abscess without sinus
            Dental abscess without sinus
            Dentoalveolar abscess without sinus
            Periapical abscess without sinus

   K04.8   Radicular cyst
            Apical (periodontal) cyst
            Periapical cyst
            Residual radicular cyst
            Excludes2   lateral periodontal cyst (K09.0)

● **K04.9   Other and unspecified diseases of pulp and periapical tissues**

   K04.90   Unspecified diseases of pulp and periapical tissues

   K04.99   Other diseases of pulp and periapical tissues

◀ New   ◀┅ Revised   ~~deleted~~ Deleted   Excludes 1   Excludes 2   Includes   Use additional   Code first   Code also   Unspecified
OGCR Official Guidelines   X Assign placeholder X   ● Use Additional Character(s)   ▌ Manifestation Code   **Coding Clinic**

Item 11–3 **Acute gingivitis,** also known as orilitis or ulitis, is the short-term, severe inflammation of the gums (gingiva) caused by bacteria. **Chronic gingivitis** is persistent inflammation of the gums. When the gingivitis moves into the periodontium it is called periodontitis, also known as paradentitis.

● **K05 Gingivitis and periodontal diseases**
      Use additional code to identify:
        alcohol abuse and dependence (F10.-)
        exposure to environmental tobacco smoke (Z77.22)
        exposure to tobacco smoke in the perinatal period (P96.81)
        history of tobacco dependence (Z87.891) ◀▥
        occupational exposure to environmental tobacco smoke (Z57.31)
        tobacco dependence (F17.-)
        tobacco use (Z72.0)

● **K05.0 Acute gingivitis**
      Excludes1 acute necrotizing ulcerative gingivitis (A69.1)
                  herpesviral [herpes simplex] gingivostomatitis (B00.2)

      K05.00 Acute gingivitis, plaque induced
           Acute gingivitis NOS
           Plaque induced gingival disease ◀

      K05.01 Acute gingivitis, non-plaque induced

● **K05.1 Chronic gingivitis**
      Desquamative gingivitis (chronic)
      Gingivitis (chronic) NOS
      Hyperplastic gingivitis (chronic)
      Pregnancy associated gingivitis ◀
      Simple marginal gingivitis (chronic)
      Ulcerative gingivitis (chronic)
      Code first, if applicable, diseases of the digestive system complicating pregnancy (O99.61-) ◀

      K05.10 Chronic gingivitis, plaque induced
           Chronic gingivitis NOS
           Gingivitis NOS

      K05.11 Chronic gingivitis, non-plaque induced

● **K05.2 Aggressive periodontitis**
      Acute pericoronitis
      Excludes1 acute apical periodontitis (K04.4)
                  periapical abscess (K04.7)
                  periapical abscess with sinus (K04.6)

      K05.20 Aggressive periodontitis, unspecified
●   **K05.21 Aggressive periodontitis, localized**
           Periodontal abscess

           K05.211 Aggressive periodontitis, localized, slight ◀
           K05.212 Aggressive periodontitis, localized, moderate ◀
           K05.213 Aggressive periodontitis, localized, severe ◀
           K05.219 Aggressive periodontitis, localized, unspecified severity ◀

●   **K05.22 Aggressive periodontitis, generalized**
           K05.221 Aggressive periodontitis, generalized, slight ◀
           K05.222 Aggressive periodontitis, generalized, moderate ◀
           K05.223 Aggressive periodontitis, generalized, severe ◀
           K05.229 Aggressive periodontitis, generalized, unspecified severity ◀

● **K05.3 Chronic periodontitis**
      Chronic pericoronitis
      Complex periodontitis
      Periodontitis NOS
      Simplex periodontitis
      Excludes1 chronic apical periodontitis (K04.5)

      K05.30 Chronic periodontitis, unspecified
●   **K05.31 Chronic periodontitis, localized**
           K05.311 Chronic periodontitis, localized, slight ◀
           K05.312 Chronic periodontitis, localized, moderate ◀
           K05.313 Chronic periodontitis, localized, severe ◀
           K05.319 Chronic periodontitis, localized, unspecified severity ◀

●   **K05.32 Chronic periodontitis, generalized**
           K05.321 Chronic periodontitis, generalized, slight ◀
           K05.322 Chronic periodontitis, generalized, moderate ◀
           K05.323 Chronic periodontitis, generalized, severe ◀
           K05.329 Chronic periodontitis, generalized, unspecified severity ◀

  K05.4 Periodontosis
      Juvenile periodontosis

  K05.5 Other periodontal diseases
      Combined periodontic-endodontic lesion ◀
      Narrow gingival width (of periodontal soft tissue) ◀
      Excludes2 leukoplakia of gingiva (K13.21)

  K05.6 Periodontal disease, unspecified

● **K06 Other disorders of gingiva and edentulous alveolar ridge**
      Excludes2 acute gingivitis (K05.0)
                  atrophy of edentulous alveolar ridge (K08.2)
                  chronic gingivitis (K05.1)
                  gingivitis NOS (K05.1)

  K06.0 Gingival recession
      Gingival recession (generalized) (localized) (postinfective) (postprocedural)

  K06.1 Gingival enlargement
      Gingival fibromatosis

  K06.2 Gingival and edentulous alveolar ridge lesions associated with trauma
      Irritative hyperplasia of edentulous ridge [denture hyperplasia]
      Use additional code (Chapter 20) to identify external cause or denture status (Z97.2)

  K06.3 Horizontal alveolar bone loss ◀

  K06.8 Other specified disorders of gingiva and edentulous alveolar ridge
      Fibrous epulis
      Flabby alveolar ridge
      Giant cell epulis
      Peripheral giant cell granuloma of gingiva
      Pyogenic granuloma of gingiva
      Vertical ridge deficiency ◀
      Excludes2 gingival cyst (K09.0)

  K06.9 Disorder of gingiva and edentulous alveolar ridge, unspecified

CHAPTER 11 (K00-K95)

● **K08** **Other disorders of teeth and supporting structures**

    Excludes2 dentofacial anomalies [including malocclusion] (M26.-)

               disorders of jaw (M27.-)

  K08.0 **Exfoliation of teeth due to systemic causes**

      Code also underlying systemic condition

● **K08.1** **Complete loss of teeth**

      Acquired loss of teeth, complete

    Excludes1 congenital absence of teeth (K00.0)

            exfoliation of teeth due to systemic causes (K08.0)

            partial loss of teeth (K08.4-)

●   **K08.10** **Complete loss of teeth, unspecified cause**

      K08.101 Complete loss of teeth, unspecified cause, class I

      K08.102 Complete loss of teeth, unspecified cause, class II

      K08.103 Complete loss of teeth, unspecified cause, class III

      K08.104 Complete loss of teeth, unspecified cause, class IV

      K08.109 Complete loss of teeth, unspecified cause, unspecified class

            Edentulism NOS

●   **K08.11** **Complete loss of teeth due to trauma**

      K08.111 Complete loss of teeth due to trauma, class I

      K08.112 Complete loss of teeth due to trauma, class II

      K08.113 Complete loss of teeth due to trauma, class III

      K08.114 Complete loss of teeth due to trauma, class IV

      K08.119 Complete loss of teeth due to trauma, unspecified class

●   **K08.12** **Complete loss of teeth due to periodontal diseases**

      K08.121 Complete loss of teeth due to periodontal diseases, class I

      K08.122 Complete loss of teeth due to periodontal diseases, class II

      K08.123 Complete loss of teeth due to periodontal diseases, class III

      K08.124 Complete loss of teeth due to periodontal diseases, class IV

      K08.129 Complete loss of teeth due to periodontal diseases, unspecified class

●   **K08.13** **Complete loss of teeth due to caries**

      K08.131 Complete loss of teeth due to caries, class I

      K08.132 Complete loss of teeth due to caries, class II

      K08.133 Complete loss of teeth due to caries, class III

      K08.134 Complete loss of teeth due to caries, class IV

      K08.139 Complete loss of teeth due to caries, unspecified class

●   **K08.19** **Complete loss of teeth due to other specified cause**

      K08.191 Complete loss of teeth due to other specified cause, class I

      K08.192 Complete loss of teeth due to other specified cause, class II

      K08.193 Complete loss of teeth due to other specified cause, class III

      K08.194 Complete loss of teeth due to other specified cause, class IV

      K08.199 Complete loss of teeth due to other specified cause, unspecified class

● **K08.2** **Atrophy of edentulous alveolar ridge**

    K08.20 **Unspecified atrophy of edentulous alveolar ridge**

      Atrophy of the mandible NOS

      Atrophy of the maxilla NOS

    K08.21 **Minimal atrophy of the mandible**

      Minimal atrophy of the edentulous mandible

    K08.22 **Moderate atrophy of the mandible**

      Moderate atrophy of the edentulous mandible

    K08.23 **Severe atrophy of the mandible**

      Severe atrophy of the edentulous mandible

    K08.24 **Minimal atrophy of maxilla**

      Minimal atrophy of the edentulous maxilla

    K08.25 **Moderate atrophy of the maxilla**

      Moderate atrophy of the edentulous maxilla

    K08.26 **Severe atrophy of the maxilla**

      Severe atrophy of the edentulous maxilla

  K08.3 **Retained dental root**

● **K08.4** **Partial loss of teeth**

      Acquired loss of teeth, partial

    Excludes1 complete loss of teeth (K08.1-)

            congenital absence of teeth (K00.0)

    Excludes2 exfoliation of teeth due to systemic causes (K08.0)

●   **K08.40** **Partial loss of teeth, unspecified cause**

      K08.401 Partial loss of teeth, unspecified cause, class I

      K08.402 Partial loss of teeth, unspecified cause, class II

      K08.403 Partial loss of teeth, unspecified cause, class III

      K08.404 Partial loss of teeth, unspecified cause, class IV

      K08.409 Partial loss of teeth, unspecified cause, unspecified class

            Tooth extraction status NOS

●   **K08.41** **Partial loss of teeth due to trauma**

      K08.411 Partial loss of teeth due to trauma, class I

      K08.412 Partial loss of teeth due to trauma, class II

      K08.413 Partial loss of teeth due to trauma, class III

      K08.414 Partial loss of teeth due to trauma, class IV

      K08.419 Partial loss of teeth due to trauma, unspecified class

●   **K08.42** **Partial loss of teeth due to periodontal diseases**

      K08.421 Partial loss of teeth due to periodontal diseases, class I

      K08.422 Partial loss of teeth due to periodontal diseases, class II

      K08.423 Partial loss of teeth due to periodontal diseases, class III

      K08.424 Partial loss of teeth due to periodontal diseases, class IV

      K08.429 Partial loss of teeth due to periodontal diseases, unspecified class

●   **K08.43** **Partial loss of teeth due to caries**

      K08.431 Partial loss of teeth due to caries, class I

      K08.432 Partial loss of teeth due to caries, class II

      K08.433 Partial loss of teeth due to caries, class III

      K08.434 Partial loss of teeth due to caries, class IV

      K08.439 Partial loss of teeth due to caries, unspecified class

◄ New   ◄▬ Revised   ~~deleted~~ Deleted   Excludes 1   Excludes 2   Includes   Use additional   Code first   Code also   Unspecified

OGCR Official Guidelines   X Assign placeholder X   ● Use Additional Character(s)   ▶ Manifestation Code   **Coding Clinic**

● **K08.49   Partial loss of teeth due to other specified cause**
     K08.491   Partial loss of teeth due to other specified cause, class I
     K08.492   Partial loss of teeth due to other specified cause, class II
     K08.493   Partial loss of teeth due to other specified cause, class III
     K08.494   Partial loss of teeth due to other specified cause, class IV
     K08.499   Partial loss of teeth due to other specified cause, unspecified class

● **K08.5   Unsatisfactory restoration of tooth**
     Defective bridge, crown, filling
     Defective dental restoration
     Excludes1   dental restoration status (Z98.811)
     Excludes2   endosseous dental implant failure (M27.6-)
          unsatisfactory endodontic treatment (M27.5-)
     K08.50   Unsatisfactory restoration of tooth, unspecified
          Defective dental restoration NOS
     K08.51   Open restoration margins of tooth
          Dental restoration failure of marginal integrity
          Open margin on tooth restoration
          Poor gingival margin to tooth restoration
     K08.52   Unrepairable overhanging of dental restorative materials
          Overhanging of tooth restoration
●   **K08.53   Fractured dental restorative material**
          Excludes1   cracked tooth (K03.81)
             traumatic fracture of tooth (S02.5)
          K08.530   Fractured dental restorative material without loss of material
          K08.531   Fractured dental restorative material with loss of material
          K08.539   Fractured dental restorative material, unspecified
     K08.54   Contour of existing restoration of tooth biologically incompatible with oral health
          Dental restoration failure of periodontal anatomical integrity
          Unacceptable contours of existing restoration of tooth
          Unacceptable morphology of existing restoration of tooth
     K08.55   Allergy to existing dental restorative material
          Use additional code to identify the specific type of allergy
     K08.56   Poor aesthetic of existing restoration of tooth
          Dental restoration aesthetically inadequate or displeasing
     K08.59   Other unsatisfactory restoration of tooth
          Other defective dental restoration
● **K08.8   Other specified disorders of teeth and supporting structures**
     K08.81   Primary occlusal trauma ◄
     K08.82   Secondary occlusal trauma ◄
     K08.89   Other specified disorders of teeth and supporting structures ◄
          Enlargement of alveolar ridge NOS ◄
          Insufficient anatomic crown height ◄
          Insufficient clinical crown length ◄
          Irregular alveolar process ◄
          Toothache NOS ◄
K08.9   Disorder of teeth and supporting structures, unspecified

● **K09   Cysts of oral region, not elsewhere classified**
     Includes   lesions showing histological features both of aneurysmal cyst and of another fibro-osseous lesion
     Excludes2   cysts of jaw (M27.0-, M27.4-)
          radicular cyst (K04.8)
     K09.0   Developmental odontogenic cysts
          Dentigerous cyst
          Eruption cyst
          Follicular cyst
          Gingival cyst
          Lateral periodontal cyst
          Primordial cyst
          Excludes2   keratocysts (D16.4, D16.5)
             odontogenic keratocystic tumors (D16.4, D16.5)
     K09.1   Developmental (nonodontogenic) cysts of oral region
          Cyst (of) incisive canal
          Cyst (of) palatine of papilla
          Globulomaxillary cyst
          Median palatal cyst
          Nasoalveolar cyst
          Nasolabial cyst
          Nasopalatine duct cyst
     K09.8   Other cysts of oral region, not elsewhere classified
          Dermoid cyst
          Epidermoid cyst
          Lymphoepithelial cyst
          Epstein's pearl
     K09.9   Cyst of oral region, unspecified

★ **(See Plate 61 on page 73.)**

● **K11   Diseases of salivary glands**
     Use additional code to identify:
          alcohol abuse and dependence (F10.-)
          exposure to environmental tobacco smoke (Z77.22)
          exposure to tobacco smoke in the perinatal period (P96.81)
          history of tobacco dependence (Z87.891) ◄▥
          occupational exposure to environmental tobacco smoke (Z57.31)
          tobacco dependence (F17.-)
          tobacco use (Z72.0)
     K11.0   Atrophy of salivary gland
     K11.1   Hypertrophy of salivary gland
●   **K11.2   Sialoadenitis**
          Parotitis
     Excludes1   epidemic parotitis (B26.-)
          mumps (B26.-)
          uveoparotid fever [Heerfordt] (D86.89)
     K11.20   Sialoadenitis, unspecified
     K11.21   Acute sialoadenitis
          Excludes1   acute recurrent sialoadenitis (K11.22)
     K11.22   Acute recurrent sialoadenitis
     K11.23   Chronic sialoadenitis

Item 11–4   Atrophy is wasting away of a tissue or organ, whereas **hypertrophy** is overdevelopment or enlargement of a tissue or organ. **Sialoadenitis** is salivary gland inflammation. **Parotitis** is the inflammation of the parotid gland. In the epidemic form, parotitis is also known as mumps. **Sialolithiasis** is the formation of calculus within a salivary gland. **Mucocele** is a polyp composed of mucus.

Figure 11-3   Major salivary glands.

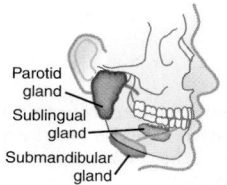

Parotid gland
Sublingual gland
Submandibular gland

CHAPTER 11 (K00-K95)

K11.3 **Abscess of salivary gland**

K11.4 **Fistula of salivary gland**

> **Excludes1** congenital fistula of salivary gland (Q38.4)

K11.5 **Sialolithiasis**
Calculus of salivary gland or duct
Stone of salivary gland or duct

K11.6 **Mucocele of salivary gland**
Mucous extravasation cyst of salivary gland
Mucous retention cyst of salivary gland
Ranula

K11.7 **Disturbances of salivary secretion**
Hypoptyalism
Ptyalism
Xerostomia

> **Excludes2** dry mouth NOS (R68.2)

K11.8 **Other diseases of salivary glands**
Benign lymphoepithelial lesion of salivary gland
Mikulicz' disease
Necrotizing sialometaplasia
Sialectasia
Stenosis of salivary duct
Stricture of salivary duct

> **Excludes1** sicca syndrome [Sjögren] (M35.0-)

K11.9 **Disease of salivary gland, unspecified**
Sialoadenopathy NOS

● **K12** **Stomatitis and related lesions**
Use additional code to identify:
alcohol abuse and dependence (F10.-)
exposure to environmental tobacco smoke (Z77.22)
exposure to tobacco smoke in the perinatal period (P96.81)
history of tobacco dependence (Z87.891) ◄▥
occupational exposure to environmental tobacco smoke (Z57.31)
tobacco dependence (F17.-)
tobacco use (Z72.0)

> **Excludes1** cancrum oris (A69.0)
> cheilitis (K13.0)
> gangrenous stomatitis (A69.0)
> herpesviral [herpes simplex] gingivostomatitis (B00.2)
> noma (A69.0)

K12.0 **Recurrent oral aphthae**
Aphthous stomatitis (major) (minor)
Bednar's aphthae
Periadenitis mucosa necrotica recurrens
Recurrent aphthous ulcer
Stomatitis herpetiformis

K12.1 **Other forms of stomatitis**
Stomatitis NOS
Denture stomatitis
Ulcerative stomatitis
Vesicular stomatitis

> **Excludes1** acute necrotizing ulcerative stomatitis (A69.1)
> Vincent's stomatitis (A69.1)

K12.2 **Cellulitis and abscess of mouth**
Cellulitis of mouth (floor)
Submandibular abscess

> **Excludes2** abscess of salivary gland (K11.3)
> abscess of tongue (K14.0)
> periapical abscess (K04.6-K04.7)
> periodontal abscess (K05.21)
> peritonsillar abscess (J36)

● **K12.3** **Oral mucositis (ulcerative)**
Mucositis (oral) (oropharyneal)

> **Excludes2** gastrointestinal mucositis (ulcerative) (K92.81)
> mucositis (ulcerative) of vagina and vulva (N76.81)
> nasal mucositis (ulcerative) (J34.81)

K12.30 **Oral mucositis (ulcerative), unspecified**

K12.31 **Oral mucositis (ulcerative) due to antineoplastic therapy**

> Use additional code for adverse effect, if applicable, to identify antineoplastic and immunosuppressive drugs (T45.1X5)
>
> Use additional code for other antineoplastic therapy, such as:
> radiological procedure and radiotherapy (Y84.2)

K12.32 **Oral mucositis (ulcerative) due to other drugs**

> Use additional code for adverse effect, if applicable, to identify drug (T36-T50 with fifth or sixth character 5)

K12.33 **Oral mucositis (ulcerative) due to radiation**

> Use additional external cause code (W88-W90, X39.0-) to identify cause

K12.39 **Other oral mucositis (ulcerative)**
Viral oral mucositis (ulcerative)

● **K13** **Other diseases of lip and oral mucosa**

> **Includes** epithelial disturbances of tongue

Use additional code to identify:
alcohol abuse and dependence (F10.-)
exposure to environmental tobacco smoke (Z77.22)
exposure to tobacco smoke in the perinatal period (P96.81)
history of tobacco dependence (Z87.891) ◄▥
occupational exposure to environmental tobacco smoke (Z57.31)
tobacco dependence (F17.-)
tobacco use (Z72.0)

> **Excludes2** certain disorders of gingiva and edentulous alveolar ridge (K05-K06)
> cysts of oral region (K09.-)
> diseases of tongue (K14.-)
> stomatitis and related lesions (K12.-)

K13.0 **Diseases of lips**
Abscess of lips
Angular cheilitis
Cellulitis of lips
Cheilitis NOS
Cheilodynia
Cheilosis
Exfoliative cheilitis
Fistula of lips
Glandular cheilitis
Hypertrophy of lips
Perlèche NEC

> **Excludes1** ariboflavinosis (E53.0)
> cheilitis due to radiation-related disorders (L55-L59)
> congenital fistula of lips (Q38.0)
> congenital hypertrophy of lips (Q18.6)
> Perlèche due to candidiasis (B37.83)
> Perlèche due to riboflavin deficiency (E53.0)

K13.1 **Cheek and lip biting**

Item 11–5 **Stomatitis** is the inflammation of the oral mucosa. **Mucositis** is the inflammation of the mucous membranes lining the digestive tract from the mouth to the anus. It is a common side effect of chemotherapy and of radiotherapy that involves any part of the digestive tract.

Figure 11-4   Oral leukoplakia and associated squamous carcinoma. (From Feldman: Sleisenger & Fordtran's Gastrointestinal and Liver Disease, ed 8, Saunders, An Imprint of Elsevier, 2006)

● **K13.2**   **Leukoplakia and other disturbances of oral epithelium, including tongue**

> **Excludes1**   carcinoma in situ of oral epithelium (D00.0-)
> hairy leukoplakia (K13.3)

    K13.21   **Leukoplakia of oral mucosa, including tongue**
Considered precancerous and evidenced by thickened white patches of epithelium on mucous membranes
Leukokeratosis of oral mucosa
Leukoplakia of gingiva, lips, tongue

> **Excludes1**   hairy leukoplakia (K13.3)
> leukokeratosis nicotina palati (K13.24)

    K13.22   **Minimal keratinized residual ridge mucosa**
Minimal keratinization of alveolar ridge mucosa

    K13.23   **Excessive keratinized residual ridge mucosa**
Excessive keratinization of alveolar ridge mucosa

    K13.24   **Leukokeratosis nicotina palati**
Smoker's palate

    K13.29   **Other disturbances of oral epithelium, including tongue**
Erythroplakia of mouth or tongue
Focal epithelial hyperplasia of mouth or tongue
Leukoedema of mouth or tongue
Other oral epithelium disturbances

K13.3   **Hairy leukoplakia**

K13.4   **Granuloma and granuloma-like lesions of oral mucosa**
Eosinophilic granuloma
Granuloma pyogenicum
Verrucous xanthoma

K13.5   **Oral submucous fibrosis**
Submucous fibrosis of tongue

K13.6   **Irritative hyperplasia of oral mucosa**

> **Excludes2**   irritative hyperplasia of edentulous ridge [denture hyperplasia] (K06.2)

● **K13.7**   **Other and unspecified lesions of oral mucosa**

    K13.70   **Unspecified lesions of oral mucosa**

    K13.79   **Other lesions of oral mucosa**
Focal oral mucinosis

★ **(See Plate 58 on page 71.)**

● **K14**   **Diseases of tongue**
Use additional code to identify:
alcohol abuse and dependence (F10.-)
exposure to environmental tobacco smoke (Z77.22)
history of tobacco dependence (Z87.891) ◀━
occupational exposure to environmental tobacco smoke (Z57.31)
tobacco dependence (F17.-)
tobacco use (Z72.0)

> **Excludes2**   erythroplakia (K13.29)
> focal epithelial hyperplasia (K13.29)
> leukedema of tongue (K13.29)
> leukoplakia of tongue (K13.21)
> hairy leukoplakia (K13.3)
> macroglossia (congenital) (Q38.2)
> submucous fibrosis of tongue (K13.5)

    K14.0   **Glossitis**
Abscess of tongue
Ulceration (traumatic) of tongue

> **Excludes1**   atrophic glossitis (K14.4)

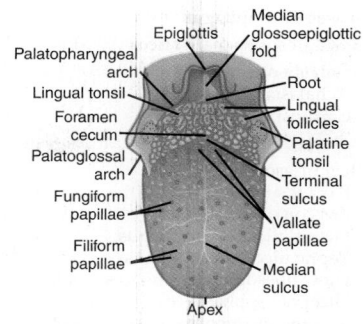

Figure 11-5   Structure of the tongue.

    K14.1   **Geographic tongue**
Benign migratory glossitis
Glossitis areata exfoliativa

    K14.2   **Median rhomboid glossitis**

    K14.3   **Hypertrophy of tongue papillae**
Black hairy tongue
Coated tongue
Hypertrophy of foliate papillae
Lingua villosa nigra

    K14.4   **Atrophy of tongue papillae**
Atrophic glossitis

    K14.5   **Plicated tongue**
Fissured tongue   Scrotal tongue
Furrowed tongue

> **Excludes1**   fissured tongue, congenital (Q38.3)

    K14.6   **Glossodynia**
Glossopyrosis   Painful tongue

    K14.8   **Other diseases of tongue**
Atrophy of tongue   Glossocele
Crenated tongue   Glossoptosis
Enlargement of tongue   Hypertrophy of tongue

    K14.9   **Disease of tongue, unspecified**
Glossopathy NOS

DISEASES OF ESOPHAGUS, STOMACH AND DUODENUM (K20-K31)

> **Excludes2**   hiatus hernia (K44.-)

● **K20**   **Esophagitis**
Use additional code to identify:
alcohol abuse and dependence (F10.-)

> **Excludes1**   erosion of esophagus (K22.1-)
> esophagitis with gastro-esophageal reflux disease (K21.0)
> reflux esophagitis (K21.0)
> ulcerative esophagitis (K22.1-)

> **Excludes2**   eosinophilic gastritis or gastroenteritis (K52.81)

    K20.0   **Eosinophilic esophagitis**

    K20.8   **Other esophagitis**
Abscess of esophagus

    K20.9   **Esophagitis, unspecified**
Esophagitis NOS

● **K21**   **Gastro-esophageal reflux disease**

> **Excludes1**   newborn esophageal reflux (P78.83)

    K21.0   **Gastro-esophageal reflux disease with esophagitis**
Reflux esophagitis

    K21.9   **Gastro-esophageal reflux disease without esophagitis**
Esophageal reflux NOS
Coding Clinic: 2016, Q1, P18

● **K22　Other diseases of esophagus**
　　Excludes2　esophageal varices (I85.-)
　　K22.0　Achalasia of cardia
　　　　Achalasia NOS
　　　　Cardiospasm
　　　　Excludes1　congenital cardiospasm (Q39.5)
● **K22.1　Ulcer of esophagus**
　　　　Barrett's ulcer
　　　　Erosion of esophagus
　　　　Fungal ulcer of esophagus
　　　　Peptic ulcer of esophagus
　　　　Ulcer of esophagus due to ingestion of chemicals
　　　　Ulcer of esophagus due to ingestion of drugs and
　　　　　medicaments
　　　　Ulcerative esophagitis
　　　　Code first poisoning due to drug or toxin, if applicable
　　　　　(T36-T65 with fifth or sixth character 1-4 or 6)
　　　　Use additional code for adverse effect, if applicable,
　　　　　to identify drug (T36-T50 with fifth or sixth
　　　　　character 5)
　　　　Excludes1　Barrett's esophagus (K22.87-)
　　K22.10　Ulcer of esophagus without bleeding
　　　　　Ulcer of esophagus NOS
　　K22.11　Ulcer of esophagus with bleeding
　　　　　Excludes2　bleeding esophageal varices
　　　　　　　　　　　　(I85.01, I85.11)
　　K22.2　Esophageal obstruction
　　　　Compression of esophagus
　　　　Constriction of esophagus
　　　　Stenosis of esophagus
　　　　Stricture of esophagus
　　　　Excludes1　congenital stenosis or stricture of
　　　　　　　　　　　esophagus (Q39.3)
　　K22.3　Perforation of esophagus
　　　　Rupture of esophagus
　　　　Excludes1　traumatic perforation of (thoracic)
　　　　　　　　　　　esophagus (S27.8-)
　　K22.4　Dyskinesia of esophagus
　　　　Difficulty in moving
　　　　Corkscrew esophagus
　　　　Diffuse esophageal spasm
　　　　Spasm of esophagus
　　　　Excludes1　cardiospasm (K22.0)
　　K22.5　Diverticulum of esophagus, acquired
　　　　Esophageal pouch, acquired
　　　　Excludes1　diverticulum of esophagus (congenital)
　　　　　　　　　　　(Q39.6)

Item 11-6　Esophageal reflux is the return flow of the contents of the stomach to the esophagus and is referred to as GERD and/or "heartburn." **Gastroesophageal reflux** is the return flow of the contents of the stomach and duodenum to the esophagus. **Esophageal leukoplakia** are white areas on the mucous membrane of the esophagus for which no specific cause can be identified.

Item 11-7　Achalasia is a condition in which the smooth muscle fibers of the esophagus do not relax. Most frequently, this condition occurs at the esophagogastric sphincter. **Cardiospasm,** also known as **megaesophagus,** is achalasia of the thoracic esophagus.

　　K22.6　Gastro-esophageal laceration-hemorrhage syndrome
　　　　Mallory-Weiss syndrome
● **K22.7　Barrett's esophagus**
　　　　Barrett's disease
　　　　Barrett's syndrome
　　　　Excludes1　Barrett's ulcer (K22.1)
　　　　　　　　　　　malignant neoplasm of esophagus
　　　　　　　　　　　　(C15.-)
　　K22.70　Barrett's esophagus without dysplasia
　　　　　Barrett's esophagus NOS
● **K22.71　Barrett's esophagus with dysplasia**
　　　　**K22.710　Barrett's esophagus with low grade
　　　　　　　　　dysplasia**
　　　　**K22.711　Barrett's esophagus with high grade
　　　　　　　　　dysplasia**
　　　　**K22.719　Barrett's esophagus with dysplasia,
　　　　　　　　　unspecified**
　　K22.8　Other specified diseases of esophagus
　　　　Hemorrhage of esophagus NOS
　　　　Excludes2　esophageal varices (I85.-)
　　　　　　　　　　　Paterson-Kelly syndrome (D50.1)
　　K22.9　Disease of esophagus, unspecified

▷ **K23　*Disorders of esophagus in diseases classified elsewhere***
　　　　Code first underlying disease, such as:
　　　　　congenital syphilis (A50.5)
　　　　Excludes1　late syphilis (A52.79)
　　　　　　　　　　　megaesophagus due to Chagas' disease (B57.31)
　　　　　　　　　　　tuberculosis (A18.83)

● **K25　Gastric ulcer**
　　　　Includes　erosion (acute) of stomach
　　　　　　　　　　pylorus ulcer (peptic)
　　　　　　　　　　stomach ulcer (peptic)
　　　　Use additional code to identify:
　　　　　alcohol abuse and dependence (F10.-)
　　　　Excludes1　acute gastritis (K29.0-)
　　　　　　　　　　　peptic ulcer NOS (K27.-)
　　K25.0　Acute gastric ulcer with hemorrhage
　　K25.1　Acute gastric ulcer with perforation
　　**K25.2　Acute gastric ulcer with both hemorrhage and
　　　　　　perforation**
　　K25.3　Acute gastric ulcer without hemorrhage or perforation
　　K25.4　Chronic or unspecified gastric ulcer with hemorrhage
　　K25.5　Chronic or unspecified gastric ulcer with perforation
　　**K25.6　Chronic or unspecified gastric ulcer with both
　　　　　　hemorrhage and perforation**
　　K25.7　Chronic gastric ulcer without hemorrhage or perforation
　　**K25.9　Gastric ulcer, unspecified as acute or chronic, without
　　　　　　hemorrhage or perforation**

Figure 11-6　The esophagus is the muscular tube that connects the pharynx and the stomach. The 10 inch (25 cm) long esophagus is divided into three parts: **cervical, thoracic,** and **abdominal.**

CERVICAL ESOPHAGUS
Left subclavian artery
First rib
Arch of aorta
Diaphragm
THORACIC ESOPHAGUS
ABDOMINAL ESOPHAGUS
Stomach

◀ New　　◀▦ Revised　　~~deleted~~ Deleted　　Excludes 1　　Excludes 2　　Includes　　Use additional　　Code first　　Code also　　Unspecified
　　OGCR Official Guidelines　　X Assign placeholder X　　● Use Additional Character(s)　　▷ Manifestation Code　　**Coding Clinic**

CHAPTER 11 (K00-K95)

Figure 11-7 A. Ulcer. **B.** Perforated ulcer. **C.** Laparoscopic view of a perforated duodenal ulcer *(arrow)* with fibrinous exudate on the adjacent peritoneum. (**C** from Feldman: Sleisenger & Fordtran's Gastrointestinal and Liver Disease, ed 8, Saunders, An Imprint of Elsevier, 2006)

Item 11-8   Gastric ulcers are lesions of the stomach that result in the death of the tissue and a defect of the surface. **Perforated ulcers** are those in which the lesion penetrates the gastric wall, leaving a hole. **Peptic ulcers** are lesions of the stomach or the duodenum. **Peptic** refers to the gastric juice, pepsin.

● **K26   Duodenal ulcer**
  Includes   erosion (acute) of duodenum
               duodenum ulcer (peptic)
               postpyloric ulcer (peptic)
  Use additional code to identify:
    alcohol abuse and dependence (F10.-)
  Excludes1   peptic ulcer NOS (K27.-)
  K26.0   Acute duodenal ulcer with hemorrhage
  K26.1   Acute duodenal ulcer with perforation
  K26.2   Acute duodenal ulcer with both hemorrhage and perforation
  K26.3   Acute duodenal ulcer without hemorrhage or perforation
  K26.4   Chronic or unspecified duodenal ulcer with hemorrhage
               Coding Clinic: 2016, Q1, P14
  K26.5   Chronic or unspecified duodenal ulcer with perforation
  K26.6   Chronic or unspecified duodenal ulcer with both hemorrhage and perforation
  K26.7   Chronic duodenal ulcer without hemorrhage or perforation
  K26.9   Duodenal ulcer, unspecified as acute or chronic, without hemorrhage or perforation

● **K27   Peptic ulcer, site unspecified**
  Includes   gastroduodenal ulcer NOS
               peptic ulcer NOS
  Use additional code to identify:
    alcohol abuse and dependence (F10.-)
  Excludes1   peptic ulcer of newborn (P78.82)
  K27.0   Acute peptic ulcer, site unspecified, with hemorrhage
  K27.1   Acute peptic ulcer, site unspecified, with perforation
  K27.2   Acute peptic ulcer, site unspecified, with both hemorrhage and perforation
  K27.3   Acute peptic ulcer, site unspecified, without hemorrhage or perforation
  K27.4   Chronic or unspecified peptic ulcer, site unspecified, with hemorrhage
  K27.5   Chronic or unspecified peptic ulcer, site unspecified, with perforation
  K27.6   Chronic or unspecified peptic ulcer, site unspecified, with both hemorrhage and perforation
  K27.7   Chronic peptic ulcer, site unspecified, without hemorrhage or perforation
  K27.9   Peptic ulcer, site unspecified, unspecified as acute or chronic, without hemorrhage or perforation

● **K28   Gastrojejunal ulcer**
  Includes   anastomotic ulcer (peptic) or erosion
               gastrocolic ulcer (peptic) or erosion
               gastrointestinal ulcer (peptic) or erosion
               gastrojejunal ulcer (peptic) or erosion
               jejunal ulcer (peptic) or erosion
               marginal ulcer (peptic) or erosion
               stomal ulcer (peptic) or erosion
  Use additional code to identify:
    alcohol abuse and dependence (F10.-)
  Excludes1   primary ulcer of small intestine (K63.3)
  K28.0   Acute gastrojejunal ulcer with hemorrhage
  K28.1   Acute gastrojejunal ulcer with perforation
  K28.2   Acute gastrojejunal ulcer with both hemorrhage and perforation
  K28.3   Acute gastrojejunal ulcer without hemorrhage or perforation
  K28.4   Chronic or unspecified gastrojejunal ulcer with hemorrhage
  K28.5   Chronic or unspecified gastrojejunal ulcer with perforation
  K28.6   Chronic or unspecified gastrojejunal ulcer with both hemorrhage and perforation
  K28.7   Chronic gastrojejunal ulcer without hemorrhage or perforation
  K28.9   Gastrojejunal ulcer, unspecified as acute or chronic, without hemorrhage or perforation

● **K29   Gastritis and duodenitis**
  Excludes1   eosinophilic gastritis or gastroenteritis (K52.81)
               Zollinger-Ellison syndrome (E16.4)
  ● **K29.0   Acute gastritis**
    Use additional code to identify:
      alcohol abuse and dependence (F10.-)
    Excludes1   erosion (acute) of stomach (K25.-)
    K29.00   Acute gastritis without bleeding
    K29.01   Acute gastritis with bleeding
  ● **K29.2   Alcoholic gastritis**
    Use additional code to identify:
      alcohol abuse and dependence (F10.-)
    K29.20   Alcoholic gastritis without bleeding
    K29.21   Alcoholic gastritis with bleeding
  ● **K29.3   Chronic superficial gastritis**
    K29.30   Chronic superficial gastritis without bleeding
    K29.31   Chronic superficial gastritis with bleeding
  ● **K29.4   Chronic atrophic gastritis**
      Gastric atrophy
    K29.40   Chronic atrophic gastritis without bleeding
    K29.41   Chronic atrophic gastritis with bleeding
  ● **K29.5   Unspecified chronic gastritis**
      Chronic antral gastritis
      Chronic fundal gastritis
    K29.50   Unspecified chronic gastritis without bleeding
    K29.51   Unspecified chronic gastritis with bleeding
  ● **K29.6   Other gastritis**
      Giant hypertrophic gastritis
      Granulomatous gastritis
      Ménétrier's disease
    K29.60   Other gastritis without bleeding
    K29.61   Other gastritis with bleeding

Item 11-9   Gastritis is a severe inflammation of the stomach. **Atrophic gastritis** is a chronic inflammation of the stomach that results in destruction of the cells of the mucosa of the stomach. Duodenitis is an inflammation of the duodenum, the first section of the small intestine.

CHAPTER 11 (K00-K95)

● **K29.7 Gastritis, unspecified**
    K29.70 Gastritis, unspecified, without bleeding
    K29.71 Gastritis, unspecified, with bleeding
● **K29.8 Duodenitis**
    K29.80 Duodenitis without bleeding
    K29.81 Duodenitis with bleeding
● **K29.9 Gastroduodenitis, unspecified**
    K29.90 Gastroduodenitis, unspecified, without bleeding
    K29.91 Gastroduodenitis, unspecified, with bleeding

K30 Functional dyspepsia
    Indigestion
    Excludes1 dyspepsia NOS (R10.13)
          heartburn (R12)
          nervous dyspepsia (F45.8)
          neurotic dyspepsia (F45.8)
          psychogenic dyspepsia (F45.8)

● **K31 Other diseases of stomach and duodenum**
    Includes   functional disorders of stomach
    Excludes2 diabetic gastroparesis (E08.43, E09.43, E10.43, E11.43, E13.43)
          diverticulum of duodenum (K57.00-K57.13)
    K31.0 Acute dilatation of stomach
        Acute distention of stomach
    K31.1 Adult hypertrophic pyloric stenosis   A
        Pyloric stenosis NOS
        Excludes1 congenital or infantile pyloric stenosis (Q40.0)
    K31.2 Hourglass stricture and stenosis of stomach
        Excludes1 congenital hourglass stomach (Q40.2)
           hourglass contraction of stomach (K31.89)
    K31.3 Pylorospasm, not elsewhere classified
        Excludes1 congenital or infantile pylorospasm (Q40.0)
           neurotic pylorospasm (F45.8)
           psychogenic pylorospasm (F45.8)
    K31.4 Gastric diverticulum
        Excludes1 congenital diverticulum of stomach (Q40.2)
    K31.5 Obstruction of duodenum
        Constriction of duodenum
        Duodenal ileus (chronic)
        Stenosis of duodenum
          Narrowing
        Stricture of duodenum
          Narrowing
        Volvulus of duodenum
          Twisting/knotting
        Excludes1 congenital stenosis of duodenum (Q41.0)
    K31.6 Fistula of stomach and duodenum
        Gastrocolic fistula
        Gastrojejunocolic fistula
    K31.7 Polyp of stomach and duodenum
        Excludes1 adenomatous polyp of stomach (D13.1)
● **K31.8 Other specified diseases of stomach and duodenum**
    ● **K31.81 Angiodysplasia of stomach and duodenum**
        K31.811 Angiodysplasia of stomach and duodenum with bleeding
        K31.819 Angiodysplasia of stomach and duodenum without bleeding
             Angiodysplasia of stomach and duodenum NOS

K31.82 Dieulafoy lesion (hemorrhagic) of stomach and duodenum
    Excludes2 Dieulafoy lesion of intestine (K63.81)
K31.83 Achlorhydria
K31.84 Gastroparesis
    Gastroparalysis
    Code first underlying disease, if known, such as:
      anorexia nervosa (F50.0-)
      diabetes mellitus (E08.43, E09.43, E10.43, E11.43, E13.43)
      scleroderma (M34.-)
K31.89 Other diseases of stomach and duodenum
K31.9 Disease of stomach and duodenum, unspecified

DISEASES OF APPENDIX (K35-K38)

● **K35 Acute appendicitis**
    K35.2 Acute appendicitis with generalized peritonitis
        Appendicitis (acute) with generalized (diffuse) peritonitis following rupture or perforation of appendix
        Perforated appendix NOS
        Ruptured appendix NOS
    K35.3 Acute appendicitis with localized peritonitis
        Acute appendicitis with or without perforation or rupture with peritonitis NOS ◀
        Acute appendicitis with or without perforation or rupture with localized peritonitis
        Acute appendicitis with peritoneal abscess
    ● **K35.8 Other and unspecified acute appendicitis**
        K35.80 Unspecified acute appendicitis
            Acute appendicitis NOS
            Acute appendicitis without (localized) (generalized) peritonitis
        K35.89 Other acute appendicitis

K36 Other appendicitis
    Chronic appendicitis
    Recurrent appendicitis

K37 Unspecified appendicitis
    Excludes1 -unspecified appendicitis with peritonitis (K35.2-K35.3)

● **K38 Other diseases of appendix**
    K38.0 Hyperplasia of appendix
    K38.1 Appendicular concretions
        Fecalith of appendix
        Stercolith of appendix
    K38.2 Diverticulum of appendix
    K38.3 Fistula of appendix
    K38.8 Other specified diseases of appendix
        Intussusception of appendix
    K38.9 Disease of appendix, unspecified

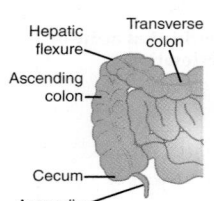

Figure 11-8 Acute appendicitis is the inflammation of the appendix, usually associated with obstruction. Most often this is a disease of adolescents and young adults.

Hepatic flexure — Transverse colon — Ascending colon — Cecum — Appendix

Item 11-10 Achlorhydria, also known as gastric anacidity, is the absence of gastric acid.

◀ New   ◀ Revised   ~~deleted~~ Deleted   Excludes 1   Excludes 2   Includes   Use additional   Code first   Code also   Unspecified
OGCR Official Guidelines   X Assign placeholder X   ● Use Additional Character(s)   ▶ Manifestation Code   **Coding Clinic**

Item 11–11 **Hernias** of the groin are the most common type, accounting for 80 percent of all hernias. There are two major types of inguinal hernias: indirect (oblique) affecting men only and direct. **Indirect inguinal hernias** result when the intestines emerge through the abdominal wall in an indirect fashion through the inguinal canal. **Direct inguinal hernias** penetrate through the abdominal wall in a direct fashion. **Femoral hernias** occur at the femoral ring where the femoral vessels enter the thigh and is most common in women. An abdominal wall hernia is also called a ventral or epigastric hernia and occurs in both sexes. Classification is based on location of the hernia and whether there is obstruction or gangrene.

Ventral, epigastric, or incisional hernia occurs on the abdominal surface caused by musculature weakness or a tear at a previous surgical site and is evidenced by a bulge that changes in size, becoming larger with exertion. An **incarcerated** hernia is one in which the intestines become trapped in the hernia. A **strangulated** hernia is one in which the blood supply to the intestines is lost. Hiatal hernia occurs when a loop of the stomach protrudes upward through the small opening in the diaphragm through which the esophagus passes, leaving the abdominal cavity and entering the chest. It occurs in both sexes.

Figure 11-9 Inguinal hernias are those that are located in the inguinal or iliac areas of the abdomen.

HERNIA (K40-K46)

Note: Hernia with both gangrene and obstruction is classified to hernia with gangrene.

Includes   acquired hernia
congenital [except diaphragmatic or hiatus] hernia
recurrent hernia

● **K40 Inguinal hernia**

Includes   bubonocele
direct inguinal hernia
double inguinal hernia
indirect inguinal hernia
inguinal hernia NOS
oblique inguinal hernia
scrotal hernia

● **K40.0 Bilateral inguinal hernia, with obstruction, without gangrene**
Inguinal hernia (bilateral) causing obstruction without gangrene
Incarcerated inguinal hernia (bilateral) without gangrene
Irreducible inguinal hernia (bilateral) without gangrene
Strangulated inguinal hernia (bilateral) without gangrene

K40.00 Bilateral inguinal hernia, with obstruction, without gangrene, not specified as recurrent
Bilateral inguinal hernia, with obstruction, without gangrene NOS

K40.01 Bilateral inguinal hernia, with obstruction, without gangrene, recurrent

● **K40.1 Bilateral inguinal hernia, with gangrene**

K40.10 Bilateral inguinal hernia, with gangrene, not specified as recurrent
Bilateral inguinal hernia, with gangrene NOS

K40.11 Bilateral inguinal hernia, with gangrene, recurrent

● **K40.2 Bilateral inguinal hernia, without obstruction or gangrene**

K40.20 Bilateral inguinal hernia, without obstruction or gangrene, not specified as recurrent
Bilateral inguinal hernia NOS

K40.21 Bilateral inguinal hernia, without obstruction or gangrene, recurrent

● **K40.3 Unilateral inguinal hernia, with obstruction, without gangrene**
Inguinal hernia (unilateral) causing obstruction without gangrene
Incarcerated inguinal hernia (unilateral) without gangrene
Irreducible inguinal hernia (unilateral) without gangrene
Strangulated inguinal hernia (unilateral) without gangrene

K40.30 Unilateral inguinal hernia, with obstruction, without gangrene, not specified as recurrent
Inguinal hernia, with obstruction NOS
Unilateral inguinal hernia, with obstruction, without gangrene NOS

K40.31 Unilateral inguinal hernia, with obstruction, without gangrene, recurrent

● **K40.4 Unilateral inguinal hernia, with gangrene**

K40.40 Unilateral inguinal hernia, with gangrene, not specified as recurrent
Inguinal hernia with gangrene NOS
Unilateral inguinal hernia with gangrene NOS

K40.41 Unilateral inguinal hernia, with gangrene, recurrent

● **K40.9 Unilateral inguinal hernia, without obstruction or gangrene**

K40.90 Unilateral inguinal hernia, without obstruction or gangrene, not specified as recurrent
Inguinal hernia NOS
Unilateral inguinal hernia NOS

K40.91 Unilateral inguinal hernia, without obstruction or gangrene, recurrent

● **K41 Femoral hernia**

● **K41.0 Bilateral femoral hernia, with obstruction, without gangrene**
Femoral hernia (bilateral) causing obstruction, without gangrene
Incarcerated femoral hernia (bilateral), without gangrene
Irreducible femoral hernia (bilateral), without gangrene
Strangulated femoral hernia (bilateral), without gangrene

K41.00 Bilateral femoral hernia, with obstruction, without gangrene, not specified as recurrent
Bilateral femoral hernia, with obstruction, without gangrene NOS

K41.01 Bilateral femoral hernia, with obstruction, without gangrene, recurrent

● **K41.1 Bilateral femoral hernia, with gangrene**

K41.10 Bilateral femoral hernia, with gangrene, not specified as recurrent
Bilateral femoral hernia, with gangrene NOS

K41.11 Bilateral femoral hernia, with gangrene, recurrent

● **K41.2 Bilateral femoral hernia, without obstruction or gangrene**

K41.20 Bilateral femoral hernia, without obstruction or gangrene, not specified as recurrent
Bilateral femoral hernia NOS

K41.21 Bilateral femoral hernia, without obstruction or gangrene, recurrent

CHAPTER 11 (K00-K95)

● **K41.3**   **Unilateral femoral hernia, with obstruction, without gangrene**
     Femoral hernia (unilateral) causing obstruction, without gangrene
     Incarcerated femoral hernia (unilateral), without gangrene
     Irreducible femoral hernia (unilateral), without gangrene
     Strangulated femoral hernia (unilateral), without gangrene

    K41.30   **Unilateral femoral hernia, with obstruction, without gangrene, not specified as recurrent**
       Femoral hernia, with obstruction NOS
       Unilateral femoral hernia, with obstruction NOS

    K41.31   **Unilateral femoral hernia, with obstruction, without gangrene, recurrent**

● **K41.4**   **Unilateral femoral hernia, with gangrene**

    K41.40   **Unilateral femoral hernia, with gangrene, not specified as recurrent**
       Femoral hernia, with gangrene NOS
       Unilateral femoral hernia, with gangrene NOS

    K41.41   **Unilateral femoral hernia, with gangrene, recurrent**

● **K41.9**   **Unilateral femoral hernia, without obstruction or gangrene**

    K41.90   **Unilateral femoral hernia, without obstruction or gangrene, not specified as recurrent**
       Femoral hernia NOS
       Unilateral femoral hernia NOS

    K41.91   **Unilateral femoral hernia, without obstruction or gangrene, recurrent**

● **K42**   **Umbilical hernia**
    Includes   paraumbilical hernia
    Excludes1   omphalocele (Q79.2)

    K42.0   **Umbilical hernia with obstruction, without gangrene**
       Umbilical hernia causing obstruction, without gangrene
       Incarcerated umbilical hernia, without gangrene
       Irreducible umbilical hernia, without gangrene
       Strangulated umbilical hernia, without gangrene

    K42.1   **Umbilical hernia with gangrene**
       Gangrenous umbilical hernia

    K42.9   **Umbilical hernia without obstruction or gangrene**
       Umbilical hernia NOS

● **K43**   **Ventral hernia**

    K43.0   **Incisional hernia with obstruction, without gangrene**
       Incisional hernia causing obstruction, without gangrene
       Incarcerated incisional hernia, without gangrene
       Irreducible incisional hernia, without gangrene
       Strangulated incisional hernia, without gangrene

    K43.1   **Incisional hernia with gangrene**
       Gangrenous incisional hernia

    K43.2   **Incisional hernia without obstruction or gangrene**
       Incisional hernia NOS

    K43.3   **Parastomal hernia with obstruction, without gangrene**
       Incarcerated parastomal hernia, without gangrene
       Irreducible parastomal hernia, without gangrene
       Parastomal hernia causing obstruction, without gangrene
       Strangulated parastomal hernia, without gangrene

    K43.4   **Parastomal hernia with gangrene**
       Gangrenous parastomal hernia

    K43.5   **Parastomal hernia without obstruction or gangrene**
       Parastomal hernia NOS

    K43.6   **Other and unspecified ventral hernia with obstruction, without gangrene**
       Epigastric hernia causing obstruction, without gangrene
       Hypogastric hernia causing obstruction, without gangrene
       Incarcerated epigastric hernia without gangrene
       Incarcerated hypogastric hernia without gangrene
       Incarcerated midline hernia without gangrene
       Incarcerated spigelian hernia without gangrene
       Incarcerated subxiphoid hernia without gangrene
       Irreducible epigastric hernia without gangrene
       Irreducible hypogastric hernia without gangrene
       Irreducible midline hernia without gangrene
       Irreducible spigelian hernia without gangrene
       Irreducible subxiphoid hernia without gangrene
       Midline hernia causing obstruction, without gangrene
       Spigelian hernia causing obstruction, without gangrene
       Strangulated epigastric hernia without gangrene
       Strangulated hypogastric hernia without gangrene
       Strangulated midline hernia without gangrene
       Strangulated spigelian hernia without gangrene
       Strangulated subxiphoid hernia without gangrene
       Subxiphoid hernia causing obstruction, without gangrene

    K43.7   **Other and unspecified ventral hernia with gangrene**
       Any condition listed under K43.6 specified as gangrenous

    K43.9   **Ventral hernia without obstruction or gangrene**
       Epigastric hernia
       Ventral hernia NOS

● **K44**   **Diaphragmatic hernia**
    Includes   hiatus hernia (esophageal) (sliding)
             paraesophageal hernia
    Excludes1   congenital diaphragmatic hernia (Q79.0)
              congenital hiatus hernia (Q40.1)

    K44.0   **Diaphragmatic hernia with obstruction, without gangrene**
       Diaphragmatic hernia causing obstruction
       Incarcerated diaphragmatic hernia
       Irreducible diaphragmatic hernia
       Strangulated diaphragmatic hernia

    K44.1   **Diaphragmatic hernia with gangrene**
       Gangrenous diaphragmatic hernia

    K44.9   **Diaphragmatic hernia without obstruction or gangrene**
       Diaphragmatic hernia NOS

● **K45**   **Other abdominal hernia**
    Includes   abdominal hernia, specified site NEC
             lumbar hernia
             obturator hernia
             pudendal hernia
             retroperitoneal hernia
             sciatic hernia

    K45.0   **Other specified abdominal hernia with obstruction, without gangrene**
       Other specified abdominal hernia causing obstruction
       Other specified incarcerated abdominal hernia
       Other specified irreducible abdominal hernia
       Other specified strangulated abdominal hernia

    K45.1   **Other specified abdominal hernia with gangrene**
       Any condition listed under K45 specified as gangrenous

    K45.8   **Other specified abdominal hernia without obstruction or gangrene**

▷ New   ◁▥ Revised   ~~deleted~~ Deleted   Excludes 1   Excludes 2   Includes   Use additional   Code first   Code also   Unspecified

926   OGCR Official Guidelines   X Assign placeholder X   ● Use Additional Character(s)   ▷ Manifestation Code   **Coding Clinic**

● **K46**   **Unspecified abdominal hernia**

     Includes   enterocele
                      epiplocele
                      hernia NOS
                      interstitial hernia
                      intestinal hernia
                      intra-abdominal hernia

     Excludes1   vaginal enterocele (N81.5)

   K46.0   **Unspecified abdominal hernia with obstruction, without gangrene**
         Unspecified abdominal hernia causing obstruction
         Unspecified incarcerated abdominal hernia
         Unspecified irreducible abdominal hernia
         Unspecified strangulated abdominal hernia

   K46.1   **Unspecified abdominal hernia with gangrene**
         Any condition listed under K46 specified as gangrenous

   K46.9   **Unspecified abdominal hernia without obstruction or gangrene**
         Abdominal hernia NOS

★ **(See Plate 284 on page 77.)**

NONINFECTIVE ENTERITIS AND COLITIS (K50-K52)

     Includes   noninfective inflammatory bowel disease
     Excludes1   irritable bowel syndrome (K58.-)
                   megacolon (K59.3-) ◀

● **K50**   **Crohn's disease [regional enteritis]**

     Includes   granulomatous enteritis

     Use additional code to identify manifestations, such as:
       pyoderma gangrenosum (L88)

     Excludes1   ulcerative colitis (K51.-)

●   **K50.0**   **Crohn's disease of small intestine**
         Crohn's disease [regional enteritis] of duodenum
         Crohn's disease [regional enteritis] of ileum
         Crohn's disease [regional enteritis] of jejunum
         Regional ileitis
         Terminal ileitis

       Excludes1   Crohn's disease of both small and large intestine (K50.8-)

     K50.00   Crohn's disease of small intestine without complications

●   **K50.01**   Crohn's disease of small intestine with complications
       K50.011   Crohn's disease of small intestine with rectal bleeding
       K50.012   Crohn's disease of small intestine with intestinal obstruction
       K50.013   Crohn's disease of small intestine with fistula
       K50.014   Crohn's disease of small intestine with abscess
           Coding Clinic: 2012, Q4, P104
       K50.018   Crohn's disease of small intestine with other complication
       K50.019   Crohn's disease of small intestine with unspecified complications

Item 11–12 Crohn's disease, also known as **regional enteritis,** is a chronic inflammatory disease of the intestines. Classification is based on location in the small (duodenum, ileum, jejunum) or large (cecum, colon, rectum, anal canal) intestine.

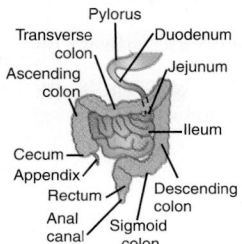

Figure 11-10   Small and large intestines.

● **K50.1**   **Crohn's disease of large intestine**
         Crohn's disease [regional enteritis] of colon
         Crohn's disease [regional enteritis] of large bowel
         Crohn's disease [regional enteritis] of rectum
         Granulomatous colitis
         Regional colitis

       Excludes1   Crohn's disease of both small and large intestine (K50.8)

   K50.10   Crohn's disease of large intestine without complications

●   **K50.11**   Crohn's disease of large intestine with complications
       K50.111   Crohn's disease of large intestine with rectal bleeding
       K50.112   Crohn's disease of large intestine with intestinal obstruction
       K50.113   Crohn's disease of large intestine with fistula
       K50.114   Crohn's disease of large intestine with abscess
           Coding Clinic: 2012, Q4, P104
       K50.118   Crohn's disease of large intestine with other complication
       K50.119   Crohn's disease of large intestine with unspecified complications

● **K50.8**   **Crohn's disease of both small and large intestine**
   K50.80   Crohn's disease of both small and large intestine without complications

●   **K50.81**   Crohn's disease of both small and large intestine with complications
       K50.811   Crohn's disease of both small and large intestine with rectal bleeding
       K50.812   Crohn's disease of both small and large intestine with intestinal obstruction
       K50.813   Crohn's disease of both small and large intestine with fistula
       K50.814   Crohn's disease of both small and large intestine with abscess
           Coding Clinic: 2012, Q4, P104
       K50.818   Crohn's disease of both small and large intestine with other complication
       K50.819   Crohn's disease of both small and large intestine with unspecified complications

● **K50.9**   **Crohn's disease, unspecified**
   K50.90   Crohn's disease, unspecified, without complications
         Crohn's disease NOS
         Regional enteritis NOS

●   **K50.91**   Crohn's disease, unspecified, with complications
       K50.911   Crohn's disease, unspecified, with rectal bleeding
       K50.912   Crohn's disease, unspecified, with intestinal obstruction
       K50.913   Crohn's disease, unspecified, with fistula
       K50.914   Crohn's disease, unspecified, with abscess
           Coding Clinic: 2012, Q4, P104
       K50.918   Crohn's disease, unspecified, with other complication
       K50.919   Crohn's disease, unspecified, with unspecified complications

Item 11-13 Ulcerative colitis attacks the colonic mucosa and forms abscesses. The disease involves the intestines. Classification is based on the location:
- Enterocolitis: large and small intestine
- Ileocolitis: ileum and colon
- Proctitis: rectum
- Proctosigmoiditis: sigmoid colon and rectum

● **K51 Ulcerative colitis**
  Use additional code to identify manifestations, such as: pyoderma gangrenosum (L88)
  Excludes1 Crohn's disease [regional enteritis] (K50.-)

  ● **K51.0 Ulcerative (chronic) pancolitis**
    Backwash ileitis
    K51.00 Ulcerative (chronic) pancolitis without complications
      Ulcerative (chronic) pancolitis NOS
    ● **K51.01 Ulcerative (chronic) pancolitis with complications**
      K51.011 Ulcerative (chronic) pancolitis with rectal bleeding
      K51.012 Ulcerative (chronic) pancolitis with intestinal obstruction
      K51.013 Ulcerative (chronic) pancolitis with fistula
      K51.014 Ulcerative (chronic) pancolitis with abscess
      K51.018 Ulcerative (chronic) pancolitis with other complication
      K51.019 Ulcerative (chronic) pancolitis with unspecified complications

  ● **K51.2 Ulcerative (chronic) proctitis**
    K51.20 Ulcerative (chronic) proctitis without complications
      Ulcerative (chronic) proctitis NOS
    ● **K51.21 Ulcerative (chronic) proctitis with complications**
      K51.211 Ulcerative (chronic) proctitis with rectal bleeding
      K51.212 Ulcerative (chronic) proctitis with intestinal obstruction
      K51.213 Ulcerative (chronic) proctitis with fistula
      K51.214 Ulcerative (chronic) proctitis with abscess
      K51.218 Ulcerative (chronic) proctitis with other complication
      K51.219 Ulcerative (chronic) proctitis with unspecified complications

  ● **K51.3 Ulcerative (chronic) rectosigmoiditis**
    K51.30 Ulcerative (chronic) rectosigmoiditis without complications
      Ulcerative (chronic) rectosigmoiditis NOS
    ● **K51.31 Ulcerative (chronic) rectosigmoiditis with complications**
      K51.311 Ulcerative (chronic) rectosigmoiditis with rectal bleeding
      K51.312 Ulcerative (chronic) rectosigmoiditis with intestinal obstruction
      K51.313 Ulcerative (chronic) rectosigmoiditis with fistula
      K51.314 Ulcerative (chronic) rectosigmoiditis with abscess
      K51.318 Ulcerative (chronic) rectosigmoiditis with other complication
      K51.319 Ulcerative (chronic) rectosigmoiditis with unspecified complications

● **K51.4 Inflammatory polyps of colon**
  Excludes1 adenomatous polyp of colon (D12.6)
           polyposis of colon (D12.6)
           polyps of colon NOS (K63.5)
  K51.40 Inflammatory polyps of colon without complications
    Inflammatory polyps of colon NOS
  ● **K51.41 Inflammatory polyps of colon with complications**
    K51.411 Inflammatory polyps of colon with rectal bleeding
    K51.412 Inflammatory polyps of colon with intestinal obstruction
    K51.413 Inflammatory polyps of colon with fistula
    K51.414 Inflammatory polyps of colon with abscess
    K51.418 Inflammatory polyps of colon with other complication
    K51.419 Inflammatory polyps of colon with unspecified complications

● **K51.5 Left sided colitis**
  Left hemicolitis
  K51.50 Left sided colitis without complications
    Left sided colitis NOS
  ● **K51.51 Left sided colitis with complications**
    K51.511 Left sided colitis with rectal bleeding
    K51.512 Left sided colitis with intestinal obstruction
    K51.513 Left sided colitis with fistula
    K51.514 Left sided colitis with abscess
    K51.518 Left sided colitis with other complication
    K51.519 Left sided colitis with unspecified complications

● **K51.8 Other ulcerative colitis**
  K51.80 Other ulcerative colitis without complications
  ● **K51.81 Other ulcerative colitis with complications**
    K51.811 Other ulcerative colitis with rectal bleeding
    K51.812 Other ulcerative colitis with intestinal obstruction
    K51.813 Other ulcerative colitis with fistula
    K51.814 Other ulcerative colitis with abscess
    K51.818 Other ulcerative colitis with other complication
    K51.819 Other ulcerative colitis with unspecified complications

● **K51.9 Ulcerative colitis, unspecified**
  K51.90 Ulcerative colitis, unspecified, without complications
  ● **K51.91 Ulcerative colitis, unspecified, with complications**
    K51.911 Ulcerative colitis, unspecified with rectal bleeding
    K51.912 Ulcerative colitis, unspecified with intestinal obstruction
    K51.913 Ulcerative colitis, unspecified with fistula
    K51.914 Ulcerative colitis, unspecified with abscess
    K51.918 Ulcerative colitis, unspecified with other complication
    K51.919 Ulcerative colitis, unspecified with unspecified complications

◀ New   ◀ Revised   deleted Deleted   Excludes 1   Excludes 2   Includes   Use additional   Code first   Code also   Unspecified

928   OGCR Official Guidelines   X Assign placeholder X   ● Use Additional Character(s)   ▶ Manifestation Code   **Coding Clinic**

● **K52   Other and unspecified noninfective gastroenteritis and colitis**
   K52.0   Gastroenteritis and colitis due to radiation
   K52.1   Toxic gastroenteritis and colitis
     Drug-induced gastroenteritis and colitis
     Code first (T51-T65) *to identify toxic agent*
     Use additional code for adverse effect, if applicable, to identify drug (T36-T50 with fifth or sixth character 5)
● **K52.2   Allergic and dietetic gastroenteritis and colitis**
     Food hypersensitivity gastroenteritis or colitis
     Use additional code to identify type of food allergy (Z91.01-, Z91.02-)
     Excludes2   allergic eosinophilic colitis (K52.82) ◄
               allergic eosinophilic esophagitis (K20.0)
               allergic eosinophilic gastritis (K52.81) ◄
               allergic eosinophilic gastroenteritis (K52.81) ◄
               food protein-induced proctocolitis (K52.82) ◄
     K52.21   Food protein-induced enterocolitis syndrome ◄
         Use additional code for hypovolemic shock, if present (R57.1) ◄
     K52.22   Food protein-induced enteropathy ◄
     K52.29   Other allergic and dietetic gastroenteritis and colitis ◄
         Food hypersensitivity gastroenteritis or colitis ◄
         Immediate gastrointestinal hypersensitivity ◄
   K52.3   Indeterminate colitis ◄
     Colonic inflammatory bowel disease unclassified (IBDU) ◄
     Excludes1   unspecified colitis (K52.9) ◄
● **K52.8   Other specified noninfective gastroenteritis and colitis**
     K52.81   Eosinophilic gastritis or gastroenteritis
         Eosinophilic enteritis
         Excludes2   eosinophilic esophagitis (K20.0) ◄
     K52.82   Eosinophilic colitis
         Allergic proctocolitis ◄
         Food-induced eosinophilic proctocolitis ◄
         Food protein-induced proctocolitis ◄
         Milk protein-induced proctocolitis ◄
     ● **K52.83   Microscopic colitis** ◄
         K52.831   Collagenous colitis ◄
         K52.832   Lymphocytic colitis ◄
         K52.838   Other microscopic colitis ◄
         K52.839   Microscopic colitis, unspecified ◄
     K52.89   Other specified noninfective gastroenteritis and colitis
   K52.9   Noninfective gastroenteritis and colitis, unspecified
     Colitis NOS   Ileitis NOS
     Enteritis NOS   Jejunitis NOS
     Gastroenteritis NOS   Sigmoiditis NOS
     Excludes1   diarrhea NOS (R19.7)
               functional diarrhea (K59.1)
               infectious gastroenteritis and colitis NOS (A09)
               neonatal diarrhea (noninfective) (P78.3)
               psychogenic diarrhea (F45.8)

OTHER DISEASES OF INTESTINES (K55-K64)

● **K55   Vascular disorders of intestine**
   Excludes1   necrotizing enterocolitis of newborn (P77.-)
● **K55.0   Acute vascular disorders of intestine**
     Infarction of appendices epiploicae
     Mesenteric (artery) (vein) embolism
     Mesenteric (artery) (vein) infarction
     Mesenteric (artery) (vein) thrombosis
     ● **K55.01   Acute (reversible) ischemia of small intestine** ◄
         K55.011   Focal (segmental) acute (reversible) ischemia of small intestine ◄
         K55.012   Diffuse acute (reversible) ischemia of small intestine ◄
         K55.019   Acute (reversible) ischemia of small intestine, extent unspecified ◄
     ● **K55.02   Acute infarction of small intestine** ◄
         Gangrene of small intestine ◄
         Necrosis of small intestine ◄
         K55.021   Focal (segmental) acute infarction of small intestine ◄
         K55.022   Diffuse acute infarction of small intestine ◄
         K55.029   Acute infarction of small intestine, extent unspecified ◄
     ● **K55.03   Acute (reversible) ischemia of large intestine** ◄
         Acute fulminant ischemic colitis ◄
         Subacute ischemic colitis ◄
         K55.031   Focal (segmental) acute (reversible) ischemia of large intestine ◄
         K55.032   Diffuse acute (reversible) ischemia of large intestine ◄
         K55.039   Acute (reversible) ischemia of large intestine, extent unspecified ◄
     ● **K55.04   Acute infarction of large intestine** ◄
         Gangrene of large intestine ◄
         Necrosis of large intestine ◄
         K55.041   Focal (segmental) acute infarction of large intestine ◄
         K55.042   Diffuse acute infarction of large intestine ◄
         K55.049   Acute infarction of large intestine, extent unspecified ◄
     ● **K55.05   Acute (reversible) ischemia of intestine, part unspecified** ◄
         K55.051   Focal (segmental) acute (reversible) ischemia of intestine, part unspecified ◄
         K55.052   Diffuse acute (reversible) ischemia of intestine, part unspecified ◄
         K55.059   Acute (reversible) ischemia of intestine, part and extent unspecified ◄
     ● **K55.06   Acute infarction of intestine, part unspecified** ◄
         Acute intestinal infarction ◄
         Gangrene of intestine ◄
         Necrosis of intestine ◄
         K55.061   Focal (segmental) acute infarction of intestine, part unspecified ◄
         K55.062   Diffuse acute infarction of intestine, part unspecified ◄
         K55.069   Acute infarction of intestine, part and extent unspecified ◄
   K55.1   Chronic vascular disorders of intestine
     Chronic ischemic colitis
     Chronic ischemic enteritis
     Chronic ischemic enterocolitis
     Ischemic stricture of intestine
     Mesenteric atherosclerosis
     Mesenteric vascular insufficiency

CHAPTER 11 (K00-K95)

CHAPTER 11 (K00-K95)

● **K55.2**   **Angiodysplasia of colon**
    K55.20   **Angiodysplasia of colon without hemorrhage**
    K55.21   **Angiodysplasia of colon with hemorrhage**
● **K55.3**   **Necrotizing enterocolitis** ◀
    Excludes1   necrotizing enterocolitis of newborn (P77.-) ◀
    Excludes2   necrotizing enterocolitis due to Clostridium difficile (A04.7) ◀
    K55.30   **Necrotizing enterocolitis, unspecified** ◀
      Necrotizing enterocolitis, NOS ◀
    K55.31   **Stage 1 necrotizing enterocolitis** ◀
      Necrotizing enterocolitis without pneumatosis, without perforation ◀
    K55.32   **Stage 2 necrotizing enterocolitis** ◀
      Necrotizing enterocolitis with pneumatosis, without perforation ◀
    K55.33   **Stage 3 necrotizing enterocolitis** ◀
      Necrotizing enterocolitis with perforation ◀
      Necrotizing enterocolitis with pneumatosis and perforation ◀
    K55.8   **Other vascular disorders of intestine**
    K55.9   **Vascular disorder of intestine, unspecified**
      Ischemic colitis
      Ischemic enteritis
      Ischemic enterocolitis

● **K56**   **Paralytic ileus and intestinal obstruction without hernia**
    Excludes1   congenital stricture or stenosis of intestine (Q41-Q42)
      cystic fibrosis with meconium ileus (E84.11)
      ischemic stricture of intestine (K55.1)
      meconium ileus NOS (P76.0)
      neonatal intestinal obstructions classifiable to P76.-
      obstruction of duodenum (K31.5)
      postprocedural intestinal obstruction (K91.3)
      stenosis of anus or rectum (K62.4)
      intestinal obstruction with hernia (K40-K46)
    K56.0   **Paralytic ileus**
      Paralysis of bowel
      Paralysis of colon
      Paralysis of intestine
      Excludes1   gallstone ileus (K56.3)
       ileus NOS (K56.7)
       obstructive ileus NOS (K56.69)
    K56.1   **Intussusception**
      Intussusception or invagination of bowel
      Intussusception or invagination of colon
      Intussusception or invagination of intestine
      Intussusception or invagination of rectum
      Excludes2   intussusception of appendix (K38.8)

SIMPLE TYPES   DOUBLE TYPES
Cecum and appendix
Ileum
Ileocecal valve   Ileum   Ileocecal valve
ILEOCOLIC
ILEOCECAL

Figure 11-11   Types of intussusception.

Item 11-14   **Intussusception** is the prolapse (telescoping) of a part of the intestine into another adjacent part of the intestine. Intussusception may be enteric (ileoileal, jejunoileal, jejunojejunal), colic (colocolic), or intracolic (ileocecal, ileocolic).

Item 11-15   **Volvulus** is the twisting of a segment of the intestine, resulting in obstruction. Paralytic ileus is paralysis of the intestine. It need not be a complete paralysis, but it must prohibit the passage of food through the intestine and lead to intestinal blockage. It is a common aftermath of some types of surgery.

    K56.2   **Volvulus**
      Strangulation of colon or intestine
      Torsion of colon or intestine
      Twist of colon or intestine
      Excludes1   volvulus of duodenum (K31.5)
    K56.3   **Gallstone ileus**
      Obstruction of intestine by gallstone
●   **K56.4**   **Other impaction of intestine**
    K56.41   **Fecal impaction**
      Excludes1   constipation (K59.0-)
       incomplete defecation (R15.0)
    K56.49   **Other impaction of intestine**
    K56.5   **Intestinal adhesions [bands] with obstruction (postprocedural) (postinfection)**
      Abdominal hernia due to adhesions with obstruction
      Peritoneal adhesions [bands] with intestinal obstruction (postprocedural) (postinfection)
●   **K56.6**   **Other and unspecified intestinal obstruction**
    K56.60   **Unspecified intestinal obstruction Intestinal obstruction NOS**
      Excludes1   intestinal obstruction due to specified condition-code to condition
    K56.69   **Other intestinal obstruction**
      Enterostenosis NOS
      Obstructive ileus NOS
      Occlusion of colon or intestine NOS
      Stenosis of colon or intestine NOS
      Stricture of colon or intestine NOS
      Excludes1   intestinal obstruction due to specified condition-code to condition
    K56.7   **Ileus, unspecified**
      Excludes1   obstructive ileus (K56.69)

● **K57**   **Diverticular disease of intestine**
    Excludes1   congenital diverticulum of intestine (Q43.8)
      Meckel's diverticulum (Q43.0)
    Excludes2   diverticulum of appendix (K38.2)
●   **K57.0**   **Diverticulitis of small intestine with perforation and abscess**
      Diverticulitis of small intestine with peritonitis
      Excludes1   diverticulitis of both small and large intestine with perforation and abscess (K57.4-)
    K57.00   **Diverticulitis of small intestine with perforation and abscess without bleeding**
    K57.01   **Diverticulitis of small intestine with perforation and abscess with bleeding**
●   **K57.1**   **Diverticular disease of small intestine without perforation or abscess**
      Excludes1   diverticular disease of both small and large intestine without perforation or abscess (K57.5-)
    K57.10   **Diverticulosis of small intestine without perforation or abscess without bleeding**
      Diverticular disease of small intestine NOS
    K57.11   **Diverticulosis of small intestine without perforation or abscess with bleeding**
    K57.12   **Diverticulitis of small intestine without perforation or abscess without bleeding**
    K57.13   **Diverticulitis of small intestine without perforation or abscess with bleeding**

◀ New   ◀▥ Revised   ~~deleted~~ Deleted   Excludes 1   Excludes 2   Includes   Use additional   Code first   Code also   Unspecified
OGCR Official Guidelines   X Assign placeholder X   ● Use Additional Character(s)   ▷ Manifestation Code   Coding Clinic
930

● **K57.2** **Diverticulitis of large intestine with perforation and abscess**
Diverticulitis of colon with peritonitis
> **Excludes1** diverticulitis of both small and large intestine with perforation and abscess (K57.4-)

     K57.20 **Diverticulitis of large intestine with perforation and abscess without bleeding**

     K57.21 **Diverticulitis of large intestine with perforation and abscess with bleeding**

● **K57.3** **Diverticular disease of large intestine without perforation or abscess**
> **Excludes1** diverticular disease of both small and large intestine without perforation or abscess (K57.5-)

     K57.30 **Diverticulosis of large intestine without perforation or abscess without bleeding**
Diverticular disease of colon NOS

     K57.31 **Diverticulosis of large intestine without perforation or abscess with bleeding**

     K57.32 **Diverticulitis of large intestine without perforation or abscess without bleeding**

     K57.33 **Diverticulitis of large intestine without perforation or abscess with bleeding**

● **K57.4** **Diverticulitis of both small and large intestine with perforation and abscess**
Diverticulitis of both small and large intestine with peritonitis

     K57.40 **Diverticulitis of both small and large intestine with perforation and abscess without bleeding**

     K57.41 **Diverticulitis of both small and large intestine with perforation and abscess with bleeding**

● **K57.5** **Diverticular disease of both small and large intestine without perforation or abscess**

     K57.50 **Diverticulosis of both small and large intestine without perforation or abscess without bleeding**
Diverticular disease of both small and large intestine NOS

     K57.51 **Diverticulosis of both small and large intestine without perforation or abscess with bleeding**

     K57.52 **Diverticulitis of both small and large intestine without perforation or abscess without bleeding**

     K57.53 **Diverticulitis of both small and large intestine without perforation or abscess with bleeding**

Figure 11-12 Diverticulosis. (From Shiland: Mastering Healthcare Terminology, ed 4, St. Louis, Mosby, 2012)

Item 11-16 **Diverticula** of the intestines are acquired herniations of the mucosa. Diverticulum (singular): Pocket or pouch that bulges outward through a weak spot (herniation) in the colon. Diverticula (plural). **Diverticulosis** is the condition of having diverticula. **Diverticulitis** is inflammation of these pouches or herniations. Classification is based on location (small intestine or colon) and whether it occurs with or without hemorrhage.

● **K57.8** **Diverticulitis of intestine, part unspecified, with perforation and abscess**
Diverticulitis of intestine NOS with peritonitis

     K57.80 **Diverticulitis of intestine, part unspecified, with perforation and abscess without bleeding**

     K57.81 **Diverticulitis of intestine, part unspecified, with perforation and abscess with bleeding**

● **K57.9** **Diverticular disease of intestine, part unspecified, without perforation or abscess**

     K57.90 **Diverticulosis of intestine, part unspecified, without perforation or abscess without bleeding**
Diverticular disease of intestine NOS

     K57.91 **Diverticulosis of intestine, part unspecified, without perforation or abscess with bleeding**

     K57.92 **Diverticulitis of intestine, part unspecified, without perforation or abscess without bleeding**

     K57.93 **Diverticulitis of intestine, part unspecified, without perforation or abscess with bleeding**

● **K58** **Irritable bowel syndrome**
> **Includes** irritable colon
> spastic colon

     K58.0 **Irritable bowel syndrome with diarrhea**

     K58.1 **Irritable bowel syndrome with constipation** ◄

     K58.2 **Mixed irritable bowel syndrome** ◄

     K58.8 **Other irritable bowel syndrome** ◄

     K58.9 **Irritable bowel syndrome without diarrhea**
Irritable bowel syndrome NOS

● **K59** **Other functional intestinal disorders**
> **Excludes1** change in bowel habit NOS (R19.4)
> intestinal malabsorption (K90.-)
> psychogenic intestinal disorders (F45.8)
> **Excludes2** functional disorders of stomach (K31.-)

● **K59.0** **Constipation**
Use additional code for adverse effect, if applicable, to identify drug (T36-T50 with fifth or sixth character 5) ◄
> **Excludes1** fecal impaction (K56.41)
> incomplete defecation (R15.0)

     K59.00 **Constipation, unspecified**

     K59.01 **Slow transit constipation**

     K59.02 **Outlet dysfunction constipation**

     K59.03 **Drug induced constipation** ◄
Use additional code for adverse effect, if applicable, to identify drug (T36-T50 with fifth or sixth character 5) ◄

     K59.04 **Chronic idiopathic constipation** ◄
Functional constipation ◄

     K59.09 **Other constipation**
Chronic constipation ◄

     K59.1 **Functional diarrhea**
> **Excludes1** diarrhea NOS (R19.7)
> irritable bowel syndrome with diarrhea (K58.0)

     K59.2 **Neurogenic bowel, not elsewhere classified**

● **K59.3** **Megacolon, not elsewhere classified**
Dilatation of colon
Code first, if applicable (T51-T65) to identify toxic agent ◄
> **Excludes1** congenital megacolon (aganglionic) (Q43.1)
> megacolon (due to) (in) Chagas' disease (B57.32)
> megacolon (due to) (in) Clostridium difficile (A04.7)
> megacolon (due to) (in) Hirschsprung's disease (Q43.1)

     K59.31 **Toxic megacolon** ◄

     K59.39 **Other megacolon** ◄
Megacolon NOS ◄

CHAPTER 11 (K00-K95)

Item 11–17 A **fissure** is a groove in the surface, whereas a **fistula** is an abnormal passage. An **abscess** is an accumulation of pus in a tissue cavity resulting from a bacterial or parasitic infection.

K59.4 Anal spasm
Proctalgia fugax

K59.8 Other specified functional intestinal disorders
Atony of colon Pseudo-obstruction (acute) (chronic) of intestine

K59.9 Functional intestinal disorder, unspecified

● **K60 Fissure and fistula of anal and rectal regions**
> Excludes1   fissure and fistula of anal and rectal regions with abscess or cellulitis (K61.-)
> Excludes2   anal sphincter tear (healed) (nontraumatic) (old) (K62.81)

K60.0 Acute anal fissure
K60.1 Chronic anal fissure
K60.2 Anal fissure, unspecified
K60.3 Anal fistula
K60.4 Rectal fistula
Fistula of rectum to skin
> Excludes1   rectovaginal fistula (N82.3)
> vesicorectal fistula (N32.1)

K60.5 Anorectal fistula

● **K61 Abscess of anal and rectal regions**
> Includes   abscess of anal and rectal regions
> cellulitis of anal and rectal regions

K61.0 Anal abscess
Perianal abscess
> Excludes1   intrasphincteric abscess (K61.4)

K61.1 Rectal abscess
Perirectal abscess
> Excludes1   ischiorectal abscess (K61.3)
> Coding Clinic: 2012, Q4, P104

K61.2 Anorectal abscess
K61.3 Ischiorectal abscess
Abscess of ischiorectal fossa

K61.4 Intrasphincteric abscess

● **K62 Other diseases of anus and rectum**
> Includes   anal canal
> Excludes2   colostomy and enterostomy malfunction (K94.0-, K91.4-)
> fecal incontinence (R15.-)
> hemorrhoids (K64.-)

K62.0 Anal polyp
K62.1 Rectal polyp
> Excludes1   adenomatous polyp (D12.8)

K62.2 Anal prolapse
Prolapse of anal canal

K62.3 Rectal prolapse
Prolapse of rectal mucosa

K62.4 Stenosis of anus and rectum
Stricture of anus (sphincter)

K62.5 Hemorrhage of anus and rectum
> Excludes1   gastrointestinal bleeding NOS (K92.2)
> melena (K92.1)
> neonatal rectal hemorrhage (P54.2)

K62.6 Ulcer of anus and rectum
Solitary ulcer of anus and rectum
Stercoral ulcer of anus and rectum
> Excludes1   fissure and fistula of anus and rectum (K60.-)
> ulcerative colitis (K51.-)

K62.7 Radiation proctitis
Use additional code to identify the type of radiation (W90.-)

● **K62.8 Other specified diseases of anus and rectum**
> Excludes2   ulcerative proctitis (K51.2)

K62.81 Anal sphincter tear (healed) (nontraumatic) (old)
Tear of anus, nontraumatic
Use additional code for any associated fecal incontinence (R15.-)
> Excludes2   anal fissure (K60.-)
> anal sphincter tear (healed) (old) complicating delivery (O34.7-)
> traumatic tear of anal sphincter (S31.831)

K62.82 Dysplasia of anus
Anal intraepithelial neoplasia I and II (AIN I and II) (histologically confirmed)
Dysplasia of anus NOS
Mild and moderate dysplasia of anus (histologically confirmed)
> Excludes1   abnormal results from anal cytologic examination without histologic confirmation (R85.61-)
> anal intraepithelial neoplasia III (D01.3)
> carcinoma in situ of anus (D01.3)
> HGSIL of anus (R85.613)
> severe dysplasia of anus (D01.3)

K62.89 Other specified diseases of anus and rectum
Proctitis NOS
Use additional code for any associated fecal incontinence (R15.-)

K62.9 Disease of anus and rectum, unspecified

● **K63 Other diseases of intestine**
K63.0 Abscess of intestine
> Excludes1   abscess of intestine with Crohn's disease (K50.014, K50.114, K50.814, K50.914)
> abscess of intestine with diverticular disease (K57.0, K57.2, K57.4, K57.8)
> abscess of intestine with ulcerative colitis (K51.014, K51.214, K51.314, K51.414, K51.514, K51.814, K51.914)
> Excludes2   abscess of anal and rectal regions (K61.-)
> abscess of appendix (K35.3)

K63.1 Perforation of intestine (nontraumatic)
Perforation (nontraumatic) of rectum
> Excludes1   perforation (nontraumatic) of duodenum (K26.-)
> perforation (nontraumatic) of intestine with diverticular disease (K57.0, K57.2, K57.4, K57.8)
> Excludes2   perforation (nontraumatic) of appendix (K35.2, K35.3)

K63.2 Fistula of intestine
> Excludes1   fistula of duodenum (K31.6)
> fistula of intestine with Crohn's disease (K50.013, K50.113, K50.813, K50.913)
> fistula of intestine with ulcerative colitis (K51.013, K51.213, K51.313, K51.413, K51.513, K51.813, K51.913)
> Excludes2   fistula of anal and rectal regions (K60.-)
> fistula of appendix (K38.3)
> intestinal-genital fistula, female (N82.2-N82.4)
> vesicointestinal fistula (N32.1)

K63.3   **Ulcer of intestine**
Primary ulcer of small intestine

> **Excludes1**   duodenal ulcer (K26.-)
> gastrointestinal ulcer (K28.-)
> gastrojejunal ulcer (K28.-)
> jejunal ulcer (K28.-)
> peptic ulcer, site unspecified (K27.-)
> ulcer of intestine with perforation (K63.1)
> ulcer of anus or rectum (K62.6)
> ulcerative colitis (K51.-)

K63.4   **Enteroptosis**

K63.5   **Polyp of colon**

> **Excludes1**   adenomatous polyp of colon (D12.6)
> inflammatory polyp of colon (K51.4-)
> polyposis of colon (D12.6)

Coding Clinic: 2015, Q2, P14

● **K63.8**   **Other specified diseases of intestine**

     K63.81   **Dieulafoy lesion of intestine**

> **Excludes2**   Dieulafoy lesion of stomach and duodenum (K31.82)

     K63.89   **Other specified diseases of intestine**
Coding Clinic: 2013, Q2, P31

K63.9   **Disease of intestine, unspecified**

● **K64**   **Hemorrhoids and perianal venous thrombosis**

> **Includes**   piles
> **Excludes1**   hemorrhoids complicating childbirth and the puerperium (O87.2)
> hemorrhoids complicating pregnancy (O22.4)

K64.0   **First degree hemorrhoids**
Grade/stage I hemorrhoids
Hemorrhoids (bleeding) without prolapse outside of anal canal

K64.1   **Second degree hemorrhoids**
Grade/stage II hemorrhoids
Hemorrhoids (bleeding) that prolapse with straining, but retract spontaneously

K64.2   **Third degree hemorrhoids**
Grade/stage III hemorrhoids
Hemorrhoids (bleeding) that prolapse with straining and require manual replacement back inside anal canal

K64.3   **Fourth degree hemorrhoids**
Grade/stage IV hemorrhoids
Hemorrhoids (bleeding) with prolapsed tissue that cannot be manually replaced

K64.4   **Residual hemorrhoidal skin tags**
External hemorrhoids, NOS
Skin tags of anus

K64.5   **Perianal venous thrombosis**
External hemorrhoids with thrombosis
Perianal hematoma
Thrombosed hemorrhoids NOS

K64.8   **Other hemorrhoids**
Internal hemorrhoids, without mention of degree
Prolapsed hemorrhoids, degree not specified

K64.9   **Unspecified hemorrhoids**
Hemorrhoids (bleeding) NOS
Hemorrhoids (bleeding) without mention of degree

Item 11-18   **Peritonitis** is an inflammation of the lining (peritoneum) of the abdominal cavity and surface of the intestines.

DISEASES OF PERITONEUM AND RETROPERITONEUM (K65-K68)

● **K65**   **Peritonitis**

Use additional code (B95-B97), to identify infectious agent

> **Excludes1**   acute appendicitis with generalized peritonitis (K35.2)
> aseptic peritonitis (T81.6)
> benign paroxysmal peritonitis (E85.0)
> chemical peritonitis (T81.6)
> diverticulitis of both small and large intestine with peritonitis (K57.4-)
> diverticulitis of colon with peritonitis (K57.2-)
> diverticulitis of intestine, NOS, with peritonitis (K57.8-)
> diverticulitis of small intestine with peritonitis (K57.0-)
> gonococcal peritonitis (A54.85)
> neonatal peritonitis (P78.0-P78.1)
> pelvic peritonitis, female (N73.3-N73.5)
> periodic familial peritonitis (E85.0)
> peritonitis due to talc or other foreign substance (T81.6)
> peritonitis in chlamydia (A74.81)
> peritonitis in diphtheria (A36.89)
> peritonitis in syphilis (late) (A52.74)
> peritonitis in tuberculosis (A18.31)
> peritonitis with or following abortion or ectopic or molar pregnancy (O00-O07, O08.0)
> peritonitis with or following appendicitis (K35.-)
> peritonitis with or following diverticular disease of intestine (K57.-)
> puerperal peritonitis (O85)
> retroperitoneal infections (K68.-)

K65.0   **Generalized (acute) peritonitis**
Pelvic peritonitis (acute), male
Subphrenic peritonitis (acute)
Suppurative peritonitis (acute)

K65.1   **Peritoneal abscess**
Abdominopelvic abscess
Abscess (of) omentum
Abscess (of) peritoneum
Mesenteric abscess
Retrocecal abscess
Subdiaphragmatic abscess
Subhepatic abscess
Subphrenic abscess

K65.2   **Spontaneous bacterial peritonitis**

> **Excludes1**   bacterial peritonitis NOS (K65.9)

K65.3   **Choleperitonitis**
Peritonitis due to bile

K65.4   **Sclerosing mesenteritis**
Fat necrosis of peritoneum
(Idiopathic) sclerosing mesenteric fibrosis
Mesenteric lipodystrophy
Mesenteric panniculitis
Retractile mesenteritis

K65.8   **Other peritonitis**
Chronic proliferative peritonitis
Peritonitis due to urine

K65.9   **Peritonitis, unspecified**
Bacterial peritonitis NOS
Coding Clinic: 2013, Q2, P31

CHAPTER 11 (K00-K95)

Item 11-19 Retroperitoneal infections occur between the posterior parietal peritoneum and posterior abdominal wall where the kidneys, adrenal glands, ureters, duodenum, ascending colon, descending colon, pancreas, and the large vessels and nerves are located.

● **K66**   **Other disorders of peritoneum**
> **Excludes2**   ascites (R18.-)
> peritoneal effusion (chronic) (R18.8)

> **K66.0**   **Peritoneal adhesions (postprocedural) (postinfection)**
> Adhesions (of) abdominal (wall)
> Adhesions (of) diaphragm
> Adhesions (of) intestine
> Adhesions (of) male pelvis
> Adhesions (of) omentum
> Adhesions (of) stomach
> Adhesive bands
> Mesenteric adhesions
>> **Excludes1**   female pelvic adhesions [bands] (N73.6)
>> peritoneal adhesions with intestinal obstruction (K56.5)

> **K66.1**   **Hemoperitoneum**
>> **Excludes1**   traumatic hemoperitoneum (S36.8-)

> **K66.8**   **Other specified disorders of peritoneum**

> **K66.9**   **Disorder of peritoneum, unspecified**

▶ **K67**   *Disorders of peritoneum in infectious diseases classified elsewhere*
> *Code first underlying disease, such as:*
> congenital syphilis (A50.0)
> helminthiasis (B65.0-B83.9)
>> **Excludes1**   peritonitis in chlamydia (A74.81)
>> peritonitis in diphtheria (A36.89)
>> peritonitis in gonococcal (A54.85)
>> peritonitis in syphilis (late) (A52.74)
>> peritonitis in tuberculosis (A18.31)

● **K68**   **Disorders of retroperitoneum**
> ● **K68.1**   **Retroperitoneal abscess**
>> **K68.11**   **Postprocedural retroperitoneal abscess**
>> **K68.12**   **Psoas muscle abscess**
>> **K68.19**   **Other retroperitoneal abscess**
> **K68.9**   **Other disorders of retroperitoneum**

DISEASES OF LIVER (K70-K77)

> **Excludes1**   jaundice NOS (R17)
> **Excludes2**   hemochromatosis (E83.11-)
> Reye's syndrome (G93.7)
> viral hepatitis (B15-B19)
> Wilson's disease (E83.0)

● **K70**   **Alcoholic liver disease**
> Use additional code to identify:
> alcohol abuse and dependence (F10.-)

> **K70.0**   **Alcoholic fatty liver**   A
> ● **K70.1**   **Alcoholic hepatitis**
>> **K70.10**   **Alcoholic hepatitis without ascites**   A
>> **K70.11**   **Alcoholic hepatitis with ascites**   A
> **K70.2**   **Alcoholic fibrosis and sclerosis of liver**   A
> ● **K70.3**   **Alcoholic cirrhosis of liver**
> Alcoholic cirrhosis NOS
>> **K70.30**   **Alcoholic cirrhosis of liver without ascites**   A
>> **K70.31**   **Alcoholic cirrhosis of liver with ascites**   A

> ● **K70.4**   **Alcoholic hepatic failure**
> Acute alcoholic hepatic failure
> Alcoholic hepatic failure NOS
> Chronic alcoholic hepatic failure
> Subacute alcoholic hepatic failure
>> **K70.40**   **Alcoholic hepatic failure without coma**   A
>> **K70.41**   **Alcoholic hepatic failure with coma**   A
> **K70.9**   **Alcoholic liver disease, unspecified**   A

● **K71**   **Toxic liver disease**
> **Includes**   drug-induced idiosyncratic (unpredictable) liver disease
> drug-induced toxic (predictable) liver disease
> *Code first poisoning due to drug or toxin, if applicable (T36-T65 with fifth or sixth character 1-4 or 6)*
> Use additional code for adverse effect, if applicable, to identify drug (T36-T50 with fifth or sixth character 5)
>> **Excludes2**   alcoholic liver disease (K70.-)
>> Budd-Chiari syndrome (I82.0)

> **K71.0**   **Toxic liver disease with cholestasis**
> Cholestasis with hepatocyte injury
> 'Pure' cholestasis

> ● **K71.1**   **Toxic liver disease with hepatic necrosis**
> Hepatic failure (acute) (chronic) due to drugs
>> **K71.10**   **Toxic liver disease with hepatic necrosis, without coma**
>> **K71.11**   **Toxic liver disease with hepatic necrosis, with coma**

> **K71.2**   **Toxic liver disease with acute hepatitis**
> **K71.3**   **Toxic liver disease with chronic persistent hepatitis**
> **K71.4**   **Toxic liver disease with chronic lobular hepatitis**
> ● **K71.5**   **Toxic liver disease with chronic active hepatitis**
> Toxic liver disease with lupoid hepatitis
>> **K71.50**   **Toxic liver disease with chronic active hepatitis without ascites**
>> **K71.51**   **Toxic liver disease with chronic active hepatitis with ascites**

> **K71.6**   **Toxic liver disease with hepatitis, not elsewhere classified**
> **K71.7**   **Toxic liver disease with fibrosis and cirrhosis of liver**
> **K71.8**   **Toxic liver disease with other disorders of liver**
> Toxic liver disease with focal nodular hyperplasia
> Toxic liver disease with hepatic granulomas
> Toxic liver disease with peliosis hepatis
> Toxic liver disease with veno-occlusive disease of liver
> **K71.9**   **Toxic liver disease, unspecified**

Item 11-20 Cirrhosis is the progressive fibrosis of the liver resulting in loss of liver function. The main causes of cirrhosis of the liver are alcohol abuse, chronic hepatitis (inflammation of the liver), biliary disease, and excessive amounts of iron. **Alcoholic cirrhosis of the liver** is also called portal, Laënnec's, or fatty nutritional cirrhosis.

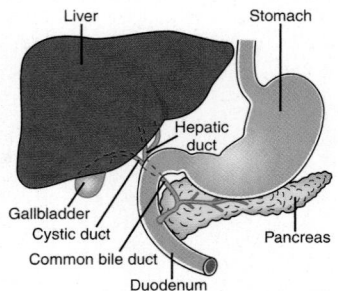

Figure 11-13   Liver and bile ducts.

◀ New   ◀ Revised   ~~deleted~~ Deleted   Excludes 1   Excludes 2   Includes   Use additional   Code first   Code also   Unspecified

OGCR Official Guidelines   X Assign placeholder X   ▶ Use Additional Character(s)   ▶ Manifestation Code   **Coding Clinic**

● **K72   Hepatic failure, not elsewhere classified**

Includes	~~acute hepatitis NEC, with hepatic failure~~
	fulminant hepatitis NEC, with hepatic failure
	hepatic encephalopathy NOS
	liver (cell) necrosis with hepatic failure
	malignant hepatitis NEC, with hepatic failure
	yellow liver atrophy or dystrophy
Excludes1	alcoholic hepatic failure (K70.4)
	hepatic failure with toxic liver disease (K71.1-)
	icterus of newborn (P55-P59)
	postprocedural hepatic failure (K91.82)
Excludes2	hepatic failure complicating abortion or ectopic or molar pregnancy (O00-O07, O08.8)
	hepatic failure complicating pregnancy, childbirth and the puerperium (O26.6-)
	viral hepatitis with hepatic coma (B15-B19) ◄

● **K72.0   Acute and subacute hepatic failure**
Acute non-viral hepatitis NOS ◄
Coding Clinic: 2015, Q2, P17

　　K72.00   Acute and subacute hepatic failure without coma
　　　　Coding Clinic: 2015, Q2, P17

　　K72.01   Acute and subacute hepatic failure with coma

● **K72.1   Chronic hepatic failure**

　　K72.10   Chronic hepatic failure without coma

　　K72.11   Chronic hepatic failure with coma

● **K72.9   Hepatic failure, unspecified**

　　K72.90   Hepatic failure, unspecified without coma

　　K72.91   Hepatic failure, unspecified with coma
　　　　Hepatic coma NOS
　　　　Coding Clinic: 2016, Q2, P35

● **K73   Chronic hepatitis, not elsewhere classified**

Excludes1	alcoholic hepatitis (chronic) (K70.1-)
	drug-induced hepatitis (chronic) (K71.-)
	granulomatous hepatitis (chronic) NEC (K75.3)
	reactive, nonspecific hepatitis (chronic) (K75.2)
	viral hepatitis (chronic) (B15-B19)

K73.0   Chronic persistent hepatitis, not elsewhere classified

K73.1   Chronic lobular hepatitis, not elsewhere classified

K73.2   Chronic active hepatitis, not elsewhere classified

K73.8   Other chronic hepatitis, not elsewhere classified

K73.9   Chronic hepatitis, unspecified

● **K74   Fibrosis and cirrhosis of liver**
Code also, if applicable, viral hepatitis (acute) (chronic) (B15-B19)

Excludes1	alcoholic cirrhosis (of liver) (K70.3)
	alcoholic fibrosis of liver (K70.2)
	cardiac sclerosis of liver (K76.1)
	cirrhosis (of liver) with toxic liver disease (K71.7)
	congenital cirrhosis (of liver) (P78.81)
	pigmentary cirrhosis (of liver) (E83.110)

K74.0   Hepatic fibrosis

K74.1   Hepatic sclerosis

K74.2   Hepatic fibrosis with hepatic sclerosis

K74.3   Primary biliary cirrhosis
Chronic nonsuppurative destructive cholangitis

K74.4   Secondary biliary cirrhosis

K74.5   Biliary cirrhosis, unspecified

● **K74.6   Other and unspecified cirrhosis of liver**

　　K74.60   Unspecified cirrhosis of liver
　　　　Cirrhosis (of liver) NOS

　　K74.69   Other cirrhosis of liver
　　　　Cryptogenic cirrhosis (of liver)
　　　　Macronodular cirrhosis (of liver)
　　　　Micronodular cirrhosis (of liver)
　　　　Mixed type cirrhosis (of liver)
　　　　Portal cirrhosis (of liver)
　　　　Postnecrotic cirrhosis (of liver)

● **K75   Other inflammatory liver diseases**

Excludes2	toxic liver disease (K71.-)

K75.0   Abscess of liver
Cholangitic hepatic abscess
Hematogenic hepatic abscess
Hepatic abscess NOS
Lymphogenic hepatic abscess
Pylephlebitic hepatic abscess

Excludes1	amebic liver abscess (A06.4)
	cholangitis without liver abscess (K83.0)
	pylephlebitis without liver abscess (K75.1)
Excludes2	acute or subacute hepatitis NOS (B17.9) ◄
	acute or subacute non-viral hepatitis (K72.0) ◄
	chronic hepatitis NEC (K73.8) ◄

K75.1   Phlebitis of portal vein
Pylephlebitis

Excludes1	pylephlebitic liver abscess (K75.0)

K75.2   Nonspecific reactive hepatitis

Excludes1	acute or subacute hepatitis (K72.0-)
	chronic hepatitis NEC (K73.-)
	viral hepatitis (B15-B19)

K75.3   Granulomatous hepatitis, not elsewhere classified

Excludes1	acute or subacute hepatitis (K72.0-)
	chronic hepatitis NEC (K73.-)
	viral hepatitis (B15-B19)

K75.4   Autoimmune hepatitis
Lupoid hepatitis NEC

● **K75.8   Other specified inflammatory liver diseases**

　　K75.81   Nonalcoholic steatohepatitis (NASH)

　　K75.89   Other specified inflammatory liver diseases

K75.9   Inflammatory liver disease, unspecified
Hepatitis NOS

Excludes1	acute or subacute hepatitis (K72.0-)
	chronic hepatitis NEC (K73.-)
	viral hepatitis (B15-B19)

Coding Clinic: 2015, Q2, P17

● **K76   Other diseases of liver**

Excludes2	alcoholic liver disease (K70.-)
	amyloid degeneration of liver (E85.-)
	cystic disease of liver (congenital) (Q44.6)
	hepatic vein thrombosis (I82.0)
	hepatomegaly NOS (R16.0)
	pigmentary cirrhosis (of liver) (E83.110)
	portal vein thrombosis (I81)
	toxic liver disease (K71.-)

K76.0   Fatty (change of) liver, not elsewhere classified
Nonalcoholic fatty liver disease (NAFLD)

Excludes1	nonalcoholic steatohepatitis (NASH) (K75.81)

K76.1   Chronic passive congestion of liver
Cardiac cirrhosis
Cardiac sclerosis

K76.2   Central hemorrhagic necrosis of liver

Excludes1	liver necrosis with hepatic failure (K72.-)

K76.3   Infarction of liver

K76.4   Peliosis hepatis
Hepatic angiomatosis

K76.5   Hepatic veno-occlusive disease

Excludes1	Budd-Chiari syndrome (I82.0)

K76.6   Portal hypertension
Use additional code for any associated complications, such as:
portal hypertensive gastropathy (K31.89)

K76.7   Hepatorenal syndrome

Excludes1	hepatorenal syndrome following labor and delivery (O90.4)
	postprocedural hepatorenal syndrome (K91.83) ◄

CHAPTER 11 (K00-K95)

CHAPTER 11 (K00-K95)

● K76.8 **Other specified diseases of liver**

  K76.81 **Hepatopulmonary syndrome**
      Code first underlying liver disease, such as:
          alcoholic cirrhosis of liver (K70.3-)
          cirrhosis of liver without mention of alcohol
              (K74.6-)

  K76.89 **Other specified diseases of liver**
          Cyst (simple) of liver
          Focal nodular hyperplasia of liver
          Hepatoptosis

  K76.9 **Liver disease, unspecified**

▶ K77 *Liver disorders in diseases classified elsewhere*
      Code first underlying disease, such as:
          amyloidosis (E85.-)
          congenital syphilis (A50.0, A50.5)
          congenital toxoplasmosis (P37.1)
          schistosomiasis (B65.0-B65.9)
      Excludes1 alcoholic hepatitis (K70.1-)
                  alcoholic liver disease (K70.-)
                  cytomegaloviral hepatitis (B25.1)
                  herpesviral [herpes simplex] hepatitis (B00.81)
                  infectious mononucleosis with liver disease
                      (B27.0-B27.9 with .9)
                  mumps hepatitis (B26.81)
                  sarcoidosis with liver disease (D86.89)
                  secondary syphilis with liver disease (A51.45)
                  syphilis (late) with liver disease (A52.74)
                  toxoplasmosis (acquired) hepatitis (B58.1)
                  tuberculosis with liver disease (A18.83)

DISORDERS OF GALLBLADDER, BILIARY TRACT AND PANCREAS (K80–K87)

● K80 **Cholelithiasis**
      Presence or formation of gallstones
      Excludes1 retained cholelithiasis following cholecystectomy
                  (K91.86)

● K80.0 **Calculus of gallbladder with acute cholecystitis**
      Any condition listed in K80.2 with acute cholecystitis
      *Check documentation for acute/chronic gallbladder/common
      bile duct either with or without obstruction.*

  K80.00 **Calculus of gallbladder with acute cholecystitis
          without obstruction**

  K80.01 **Calculus of gallbladder with acute cholecystitis
          with obstruction**

● K80.1 **Calculus of gallbladder with other cholecystitis**

  K80.10 **Calculus of gallbladder with chronic
          cholecystitis without obstruction**
          Cholelithiasis with cholecystitis NOS

  K80.11 **Calculus of gallbladder with chronic
          cholecystitis with obstruction**

  K80.12 **Calculus of gallbladder with acute and chronic
          cholecystitis without obstruction**

  K80.13 **Calculus of gallbladder with acute and chronic
          cholecystitis with obstruction**

  K80.18 **Calculus of gallbladder with other cholecystitis
          without obstruction**

  K80.19 **Calculus of gallbladder with other cholecystitis
          with obstruction**

● K80.2 **Calculus of gallbladder without cholecystitis**
          Cholecystolithiasis without cholecystitis
          Cholelithiasis (without cholecystitis)
          Colic (recurrent) of gallbladder (without cholecystitis)
          Gallstone (impacted) of cystic duct (without
              cholecystitis)
          Gallstone (impacted) of gallbladder (without
              cholecystitis)

  K80.20 **Calculus of gallbladder without cholecystitis
          without obstruction**

  K80.21 **Calculus of gallbladder without cholecystitis
          with obstruction**

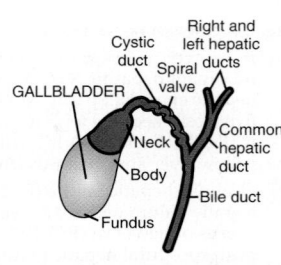

Figure 11-14 *Gallbladder and bile ducts.*

● K80.3 **Calculus of bile duct with cholangitis**
      Any condition listed in K80.5 with cholangitis

  K80.30 **Calculus of bile duct with cholangitis,
          unspecified, without obstruction**

  K80.31 **Calculus of bile duct with cholangitis,
          unspecified, with obstruction**

  K80.32 **Calculus of bile duct with acute cholangitis
          without obstruction**

  K80.33 **Calculus of bile duct with acute cholangitis
          with obstruction**

  K80.34 **Calculus of bile duct with chronic cholangitis
          without obstruction**

  K80.35 **Calculus of bile duct with chronic cholangitis
          with obstruction**

  K80.36 **Calculus of bile duct with acute and chronic
          cholangitis without obstruction**

  K80.37 **Calculus of bile duct with acute and chronic
          cholangitis with obstruction**

● K80.4 **Calculus of bile duct with cholecystitis**
      Any condition listed in K80.5 with cholecystitis (with
          cholangitis)

  K80.40 **Calculus of bile duct with cholecystitis,
          unspecified, without obstruction**

  K80.41 **Calculus of bile duct with cholecystitis,
          unspecified, with obstruction**

  K80.42 **Calculus of bile duct with acute cholecystitis
          without obstruction**

  K80.43 **Calculus of bile duct with acute cholecystitis
          with obstruction**

  K80.44 **Calculus of bile duct with chronic cholecystitis
          without obstruction**

  K80.45 **Calculus of bile duct with chronic cholecystitis
          with obstruction**

  K80.46 **Calculus of bile duct with acute and chronic
          cholecystitis without obstruction**

  K80.47 **Calculus of bile duct with acute and chronic
          cholecystitis with obstruction**

● K80.5 **Calculus of bile duct without cholangitis or cholecystitis**
          Choledocholithiasis (without cholangitis or
              cholecystitis)
          Gallstone (impacted) of bile duct NOS (without
              cholangitis or cholecystitis)
          Gallstone (impacted) of common duct (without
              cholangitis or cholecystitis)
          Gallstone (impacted) of hepatic duct (without
              cholangitis or cholecystitis)
          Hepatic cholelithiasis (without cholangitis or
              cholecystitis)
          Hepatic colic (recurrent) (without cholangitis or
              cholecystitis)

  K80.50 **Calculus of bile duct without cholangitis or
          cholecystitis without obstruction**

  K80.51 **Calculus of bile duct without cholangitis or
          cholecystitis with obstruction**

● **K80.6   Calculus of gallbladder and bile duct with cholecystitis**

    K80.60   Calculus of gallbladder and bile duct with cholecystitis, unspecified, without obstruction

    K80.61   Calculus of gallbladder and bile duct with cholecystitis, unspecified, with obstruction

    K80.62   Calculus of gallbladder and bile duct with acute cholecystitis without obstruction

    K80.63   Calculus of gallbladder and bile duct with acute cholecystitis with obstruction

    K80.64   Calculus of gallbladder and bile duct with chronic cholecystitis without obstruction

    K80.65   Calculus of gallbladder and bile duct with chronic cholecystitis with obstruction

    K80.66   Calculus of gallbladder and bile duct with acute and chronic cholecystitis without obstruction

    K80.67   Calculus of gallbladder and bile duct with acute and chronic cholecystitis with obstruction

● **K80.7   Calculus of gallbladder and bile duct without cholecystitis**

    K80.70   Calculus of gallbladder and bile duct without cholecystitis without obstruction

    K80.71   Calculus of gallbladder and bile duct without cholecystitis with obstruction

● **K80.8   Other cholelithiasis**

    K80.80   Other cholelithiasis without obstruction

    K80.81   Other cholelithiasis with obstruction

● **K81   Cholecystitis**

    Chronic or acute inflammation of the gallbladder

    Excludes1   cholecystitis with cholelithiasis (K80.-)

   K81.0   Acute cholecystitis

     Abscess of gallbladder

     Angiocholecystitis

     Emphysematous (acute) cholecystitis

     Empyema of gallbladder

     Gangrene of gallbladder

     Gangrenous cholecystitis

     Suppurative cholecystitis

   K81.1   Chronic cholecystitis

   K81.2   Acute cholecystitis with chronic cholecystitis

   K81.9   Cholecystitis, unspecified

● **K82   Other diseases of gallbladder**

    Excludes1   nonvisualization of gallbladder (R93.2)

               postcholecystectomy syndrome (K91.5)

   K82.0   Obstruction of gallbladder

     Occlusion of cystic duct or gallbladder without cholelithiasis

     Stenosis of cystic duct or gallbladder without cholelithiasis

     Stricture of cystic duct or gallbladder without cholelithiasis

     Excludes1   obstruction of gallbladder with cholelithiasis (K80.-)

   K82.1   Hydrops of gallbladder

     Mucocele of gallbladder

   K82.2   Perforation of gallbladder

     Rupture of cystic duct or gallbladder

   K82.3   Fistula of gallbladder

     Cholecystocolic fistula

     Cholecystoduodenal fistula

   K82.4   Cholesterolosis of gallbladder

     Strawberry gallbladder

     Excludes1   cholesterolosis of gallbladder with cholecystitis (K81.-)

                 cholesterolosis of gallbladder with cholelithiasis (K80.-)

● **K82.8   Other specified diseases of gallbladder**

     Adhesions of cystic duct or gallbladder

     Atrophy of cystic duct or gallbladder

     Cyst of cystic duct or gallbladder

     Dyskinesia of cystic duct or gallbladder

     Hypertrophy of cystic duct or gallbladder

     Nonfunctioning of cystic duct or gallbladder

     Ulcer of cystic duct or gallbladder

   K82.9   Disease of gallbladder, unspecified

● **K83   Other diseases of biliary tract**

    Excludes1   postcholecystectomy syndrome (K91.5)

    Excludes2   conditions involving the gallbladder (K81-K82)

                 conditions involving the cystic duct (K81-K82)

   K83.0   Cholangitis

     Ascending cholangitis   Sclerosing cholangitis

     Cholangitis NOS   Secondary cholangitis

     Primary cholangitis   Stenosing cholangitis

     Recurrent cholangitis   Suppurative cholangitis

     Excludes1   cholangitic liver abscess (K75.0)

                 cholangitis with choledocholithiasis (K80.3-, K80.4-)

                 chronic nonsuppurative destructive cholangitis (K74.3)

   K83.1   Obstruction of bile duct

     Occlusion of bile duct without cholelithiasis

     Stenosis of bile duct without cholelithiasis

     Stricture of bile duct without cholelithiasis

     Excludes1   congenital obstruction of bile duct (Q44.3)

                 obstruction of bile duct with cholelithiasis (K80.-)

     Coding Clinic: 2016, Q1, P18

   K83.2   Perforation of bile duct

     Rupture of bile duct

   K83.3   Fistula of bile duct

     Choledochoduodenal fistula

   K83.4   Spasm of sphincter of Oddi

   K83.5   Biliary cyst

   K83.8   Other specified diseases of biliary tract

     Adhesions of biliary tract

     Atrophy of biliary tract

     Hypertrophy of biliary tract

     Ulcer of biliary tract

   K83.9   Disease of biliary tract, unspecified

● **K85   Acute pancreatitis**

    Inflammatory process in which pancreatic enzymes autodigest the gland

    Includes   ~~abscess of pancreas~~

                 ~~acute necrosis of pancreas~~

                 acute (recurrent) pancreatitis

                 ~~gangrene of (gangrenous) pancreas~~

                 ~~hemorrhagic pancreatitis~~

                 ~~infective necrosis of pancreas~~

                 subacute pancreatitis

                 ~~suppurative pancreatitis~~

● **K85.0   Idiopathic acute pancreatitis**

    K85.00   Idiopathic acute pancreatitis without necrosis or infection ◄

    K85.01   Idiopathic acute pancreatitis with uninfected necrosis ◄

    K85.02   Idiopathic acute pancreatitis with infected necrosis ◄

● **K85.1   Biliary acute pancreatitis**

     Gallstone pancreatitis

    K85.10   Biliary acute pancreatitis without necrosis or infection ◄

    K85.11   Biliary acute pancreatitis with uninfected necrosis ◄

    K85.12   Biliary acute pancreatitis with infected necrosis ◄

CHAPTER 11 (K00-K95)

CHAPTER 11 (K00-K95)

● **K85.2** **Alcohol induced acute pancreatitis**

    Excludes2   alcohol induced chronic pancreatitis (K86.0)

  K85.20   **Alcohol induced acute pancreatitis without necrosis or infection** ◀

  K85.21   **Alcohol induced acute pancreatitis with uninfected necrosis** ◀

  K85.22   **Alcohol induced acute pancreatitis with infected necrosis** ◀

● **K85.3** **Drug induced acute pancreatitis**

    Use additional code for adverse effect, if applicable, to identify drug (T36-T50 with fifth or sixth character 5)

    Use additional code to identify drug abuse and dependence (F11.-F17.-)

  K85.30   **Drug induced acute pancreatitis without necrosis or infection** ◀

  K85.31   **Drug induced acute pancreatitis with uninfected necrosis** ◀

  K85.32   **Drug induced acute pancreatitis with infected necrosis** ◀

● **K85.8** **Other acute pancreatitis**

  K85.80   **Other acute pancreatitis without necrosis or infection** ◀

  K85.81   **Other acute pancreatitis with uninfected necrosis** ◀

  K85.82   **Other acute pancreatitis with infected necrosis** ◀

● **K85.9** **Acute pancreatitis, unspecified**

    Pancreatitis NOS

  K85.90   **Acute pancreatitis without necrosis or infection, unspecified** ◀

  K85.91   **Acute pancreatitis with uninfected necrosis, unspecified** ◀

  K85.92   **Acute pancreatitis with infected necrosis, unspecified** ◀

● **K86** **Other diseases of pancreas**

    Excludes2   fibrocystic disease of pancreas (E84.-)
islet cell tumor (of pancreas) (D13.7)
pancreatic steatorrhea (K90.3)

  K86.0   **Alcohol-induced chronic pancreatitis**

    Use additional code to identify:
alcohol abuse and dependence (F10.-)

    Code also exocrine pancreatic insufficiency (K86.81) ◀

    Excludes2   alcohol induced acute pancreatitis (K85.2-) ◀

  K86.1   **Other chronic pancreatitis**

    Chronic pancreatitis NOS
Infectious chronic pancreatitis
Recurrent chronic pancreatitis
Relapsing chronic pancreatitis

    Code also exocrine pancreatic insufficiency (K86.81) ◀

  K86.2   **Cyst of pancreas**

  K86.3   **Pseudocyst of pancreas**

● **K86.8**   **Other specified diseases of pancreas**

  K86.81   **Exocrine pancreatic insufficiency** ◀

  K86.89   **Other specified diseases of pancreas** ◀

    Aseptic pancreatic necrosis, unrelated to acute pancreatitis ◀
Atrophy of pancreas ◀
Calculus of pancreas ◀
Cirrhosis of pancreas ◀
Fibrosis of pancreas ◀
Pancreatic fat necrosis, unrelated to acute pancreatitis ◀
Pancreatic infantilism ◀
Pancreatic necrosis NOS, unrelated to acute pancreatitis ◀

  K86.9   **Disease of pancreas, unspecified**

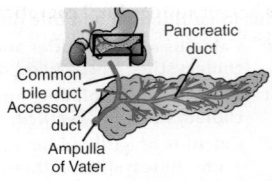

Figure 11-15   Pancreatic ductal system.

▶ **K87** *Disorders of gallbladder, biliary tract and pancreas in diseases classified elsewhere*

    Code first underlying disease

    Excludes1   cytomegaloviral pancreatitis (B25.2)
mumps pancreatitis (B26.3)
syphilitic gallbladder (A52.74)
syphilitic pancreas (A52.74)
tuberculosis of gallbladder (A18.83)
tuberculosis of pancreas (A18.83)

OTHER DISEASES OF THE DIGESTIVE SYSTEM (K90-K95)

● **K90** **Intestinal malabsorption**

    Excludes1   intestinal malabsorption following gastrointestinal surgery (K91.2)

  K90.0   **Celiac disease**

    Celiac disease with steatorrhea ◀
Gluten-sensitive enteropathy
~~Idiopathic steatorrhea~~
Nontropical sprue

    Use additional code for associated disorders including:
dermatitis herpetiformis (L13.0)
gluten ataxia (G32.81)

    Code also exocrine pancreatic insufficiency (K86.81) ◀

  K90.1   **Tropical sprue**

    Sprue NOS
Tropical steatorrhea

  K90.2   **Blind loop syndrome, not elsewhere classified**

    Blind loop syndrome NOS

    Excludes1   congenital blind loop syndrome (Q43.8)
postsurgical blind loop syndrome (K91.2)

  K90.3   **Pancreatic steatorrhea**

● **K90.4**   **Other malabsorption due to intolerance** ◀▥

    Excludes2   gluten-sensitive enteropathy (K90.0)
lactose intolerance (E73.-)

  K90.41   **Non-celiac gluten sensitivity** ◀

    Gluten sensitivity NOS ◀
Non-celiac gluten sensitive enteropathy ◀

  K90.49   **Malabsorption due to intolerance, not elsewhere classified** ◀

    Malabsorption due to intolerance to carbohydrate ◀
Malabsorption due to intolerance to fat ◀
Malabsorption due to intolerance to protein ◀
Malabsorption due to intolerance to starch ◀

● **K90.8**   **Other intestinal malabsorption**

  K90.81   **Whipple's disease**

  K90.89   **Other intestinal malabsorption**

  K90.9   **Intestinal malabsorption, unspecified**

◀ New   ◀▥ Revised   ~~deleted~~ Deleted   Excludes 1   Excludes 2   Includes   Use additional   Code first   Code also   Unspecified

OGCR Official Guidelines   X Assign placeholder X   ● Use Additional Character(s)   ▶ Manifestation Code   **Coding Clinic**

● **K91 Intraoperative and postprocedural complications and disorders of digestive system, not elsewhere classified**

    Excludes2   complications of artificial opening of digestive system (K94.-)
               complications of bariatric procedures (K95.-)
               gastrojejunal ulcer (K28.-)
               postprocedural (radiation) retroperitoneal abscess (K68.11)
               radiation colitis (K52.0)
               radiation gastroenteritis (K52.0)
               radiation proctitis (K62.7)

K91.0 Vomiting following gastrointestinal surgery

K91.1 Postgastric surgery syndromes
    Dumping syndrome
    Postgastrectomy syndrome
    Postvagotomy syndrome

K91.2 Postsurgical malabsorption, not elsewhere classified
    Postsurgical blind loop syndrome

    Excludes1   malabsorption osteomalacia in adults (M83.2)
               malabsorption osteoporosis, postsurgical (M80.8-, M81.8)

K91.3 Postprocedural intestinal obstruction

K91.5 Postcholecystectomy syndrome

● **K91.6 Intraoperative hemorrhage and hematoma of a digestive system organ or structure complicating a procedure**

    Excludes1   intraoperative hemorrhage and hematoma of a digestive system organ or structure due to accidental puncture and laceration during a procedure (K91.7-)

    K91.61 Intraoperative hemorrhage and hematoma of a digestive system organ or structure complicating a digestive system procedure ◀▥

    K91.62 Intraoperative hemorrhage and hematoma of a digestive system organ or structure complicating other procedure

● **K91.7 Accidental puncture and laceration of a digestive system organ or structure during a procedure**

    K91.71 Accidental puncture and laceration of a digestive system organ or structure during a digestive system procedure

    K91.72 Accidental puncture and laceration of a digestive system organ or structure during other procedure

● **K91.8 Other intraoperative and postprocedural complications and disorders of digestive system**

    K91.81 Other intraoperative complications of digestive system

    K91.82 Postprocedural hepatic failure

    K91.83 Postprocedural hepatorenal syndrome

    ● **K91.84 Postprocedural hemorrhage of a digestive system organ or structure following a procedure** ◀▥

        K91.840 Postprocedural hemorrhage of a digestive system organ or structure following a digestive system procedure ◀▥
           Coding Clinic: 2016, Q1, P15

        K91.841 Postprocedural hemorrhage of a digestive system organ or structure following other procedure ◀▥

    ● **K91.85 Complications of intestinal pouch**

        K91.850 Pouchitis
            Inflammation of internal ileoanal pouch

        K91.858 Other complications of intestinal pouch

    K91.86 Retained cholelithiasis following cholecystectomy

● **K91.87 Postprocedural hematoma and seroma of a digestive system organ or structure following a procedure** ◀

    K91.870 Postprocedural hematoma of a digestive system organ or structure following a digestive system procedure ◀

    K91.871 Postprocedural hematoma of a digestive system organ or structure following other procedure ◀

    K91.872 Postprocedural seroma of a digestive system organ or structure following a digestive system procedure ◀

    K91.873 Postprocedural seroma of a digestive system organ or structure following other procedure ◀

  K91.89 Other postprocedural complications and disorders of digestive system

    Use additional code, if applicable, to further specify disorder

    Excludes2   postprocedural retroperitoneal abscess (K68.11)

● **K92 Other diseases of digestive system**

    Excludes1   neonatal gastrointestinal hemorrhage (P54.0-P54.3)

K92.0 Hematemesis

K92.1 Melena

    Excludes1   occult blood in feces (R19.5)

K92.2 Gastrointestinal hemorrhage, unspecified
    Gastric hemorrhage NOS
    Intestinal hemorrhage NOS

    Excludes1   acute hemorrhagic gastritis (K29.01)
               hemorrhage of anus and rectum (K62.5)
               angiodysplasia of stomach with hemorrhage (K31.811)
               diverticular disease with hemorrhage (K57.-)
               gastritis and duodenitis with hemorrhage (K29.-)
               peptic ulcer with hemorrhage (K25-K28)

● **K92.8 Other specified diseases of the digestive system**

    K92.81 Gastrointestinal mucositis (ulcerative)

        Code also type of associated therapy, such as:
        antineoplastic and immunosuppressive drugs (T45.1X-)
        radiological procedure and radiotherapy (Y84.2)

        Excludes2   mucositis (ulcerative) of vagina and vulva (N76.81)
                 nasal mucositis (ulcerative) (J34.81)
                 oral mucositis (ulcerative) (K12.3-)

    K92.89 Other specified diseases of the digestive system

K92.9 Disease of digestive system, unspecified

● **K94 Complications of artificial openings of the digestive system**

● **K94.0 Colostomy complications**

    K94.00 Colostomy complication, unspecified

    K94.01 Colostomy hemorrhage

    K94.02 Colostomy infection

        Use additional code to specify type of infection, such as:
        cellulitis of abdominal wall (L03.311)
        sepsis (A40.-, A41.-)

    K94.03 Colostomy malfunction
        Mechanical complication of colostomy

    K94.09 Other complications of colostomy

CHAPTER 11 (K00-K95)

● **K94.1   Enterostomy complications**
     K94.10   Enterostomy complication, unspecified
     K94.11   Enterostomy hemorrhage
     K94.12   Enterostomy infection
         Use additional code to specify type of infection, such as:
            cellulitis of abdominal wall (L03.311)
            sepsis (A40.-, A41.-)
     K94.13   Enterostomy malfunction
         Mechanical complication of enterostomy
     K94.19   Other complications of enterostomy
● **K94.2   Gastrostomy complications**
     K94.20   Gastrostomy complication, unspecified
     K94.21   Gastrostomy hemorrhage
     K94.22   Gastrostomy infection
         Use additional code to specify type of infection, such as:
            cellulitis of abdominal wall (L03.311)
            sepsis (A40.-, A41.-)
     K94.23   Gastrostomy malfunction
         Mechanical complication of gastrostomy
     K94.29   Other complications of gastrostomy
● **K94.3   Esophagostomy complications**
     K94.30   Esophagostomy complications, unspecified
     K94.31   Esophagostomy hemorrhage
     K94.32   Esophagostomy infection
         Use additional code to identify the infection
     K94.33   Esophagostomy malfunction
         Mechanical complication of esophagostomy
     K94.39   Other complications of esophagostomy

● **K95   Complications of bariatric procedures**
   ● **K95.0   Complications of gastric band procedure**
     K95.01   Infection due to gastric band procedure
         Use additional code to specify type of infection or organism, such as:
            bacterial and viral infectious agents (B95.-, B96.-)
            cellulitis of abdominal wall (L03.311)
            sepsis (A40.-, A41.-)
     K95.09   Other complications of gastric band procedure
         Use additional code, if applicable, to further specify complication
   ● **K95.8   Complications of other bariatric procedure**
     Excludes1   complications of gastric band surgery (K95.0-)
     K95.81   Infection due to other bariatric procedure
         Use additional code to specify type of infection or organism, such as:
            bacterial and viral infectious agents (B95.-, B96.-)
            cellulitis of abdominal wall (L03.311)
            sepsis (A40.-, A41.-)
     K95.89   Other complications of other bariatric procedure
         Use additional code, if applicable, to further specify complication

CHAPTER 12

DISEASES OF THE SKIN AND SUBCUTANEOUS TISSUE (L00-L99)

OGCR Chapter-Specific Coding Guidelines

12. **Chapter 12: Diseases of the Skin and Subcutaneous Tissue (L00-L99)**

   a. **Pressure ulcer stage codes**

   1) **Pressure ulcer stages**
   Codes from category L89, Pressure ulcer, identify the site of the pressure ulcer as well as the stage of the ulcer.
   The ICD-10-CM classifies pressure ulcer stages based on severity, which is designated by stages 1-4, unspecified stage and unstageable.
   Assign as many codes from category L89 as needed to identify all the pressure ulcers the patient has, if applicable.

   2) **Unstageable pressure ulcers**
   Assignment of the code for unstageable pressure ulcer (L89.--0) should be based on the clinical documentation. These codes are used for pressure ulcers whose stage cannot be clinically determined (e.g., the ulcer is covered by eschar or has been treated with a skin or muscle graft) and pressure ulcers that are documented as deep tissue injury but not documented as due to trauma. This code should not be confused with the codes for unspecified stage (L89.--9). When there is no documentation regarding the stage of the pressure ulcer, assign the appropriate code for unspecified stage (L89.--9).

   3) **Documented pressure ulcer stage**
   Assignment of the pressure ulcer stage code should be guided by clinical documentation of the stage or documentation of the terms found in the Alphabetic Index. For clinical terms describing the stage that are not found in the Alphabetic Index, and there is no documentation of the stage, the provider should be queried.

   4) **Patients admitted with pressure ulcers documented as healed**
   No code is assigned if the documentation states that the pressure ulcer is completely healed.

   5) **Patients admitted with pressure ulcers documented as healing**
   Pressure ulcers described as healing should be assigned the appropriate pressure ulcer stage code based on the documentation in the medical record. If the documentation does not provide information about the stage of the healing pressure ulcer, assign the appropriate code for unspecified stage.
   If the documentation is unclear as to whether the patient has a current (new) pressure ulcer or if the patient is being treated for a healing pressure ulcer, query the provider.
   For ulcers that were present on admission but healed at the time of discharge, assign the code for the site and stage of the pressure ulcer at the time of admission.

   6) **Patient admitted with pressure ulcer evolving into another stage during the admission**
   If a patient is admitted with a pressure ulcer at one stage and it progresses to a higher stage, **two separate codes should be assigned: one code for the site and stage of the ulcer on admission and a second code for the same ulcer site and the highest stage reported during the stay.**

Figure 12-1 Furuncle, also known as a boil, is a staphylococcal infection. The organism enters the body through a hair follicle and so furuncles usually appear in hairy areas of the body. A cluster of furuncles is known as a carbuncle and involves infection into the deep subcutaneous fascia. These usually appear on the back and neck. (**B** from Habif: Clinical Dermatology, ed 5, Mosby, 2009)

CHAPTER 12

DISEASES OF THE SKIN AND SUBCUTANEOUS TISSUE (L00-L99)

Excludes2 certain conditions originating in the perinatal period (P04-P96)
certain infectious and parasitic diseases (A00-B99)
complications of pregnancy, childbirth and the puerperium (O00-O9A)
congenital malformations, deformations, and chromosomal abnormalities (Q00-Q99)
endocrine, nutritional and metabolic diseases (E00-E88)
lipomelanotic reticulosis (I89.8)
neoplasms (C00-D49)
symptoms, signs and abnormal clinical and laboratory findings, not elsewhere classified (R00-R94)
systemic connective tissue disorders (M30-M36)
viral warts (B07.-)

This chapter contains the following blocks:

L00-L08	Infections of the skin and subcutaneous tissue
L10-L14	Bullous disorders
L20-L30	Dermatitis and eczema
L40-L45	Papulosquamous disorders
L49-L54	Urticaria and erythema
L55-L59	Radiation-related disorders of the skin and subcutaneous tissue
L60-L75	Disorders of skin appendages
L76	Intraoperative and postprocedural complications of skin and subcutaneous tissue
L80-L99	Other disorders of the skin and subcutaneous tissue

INFECTIONS OF THE SKIN AND SUBCUTANEOUS TISSUE (L00-L08)

Use additional code (B95-B97) to identify infectious agent.

Excludes2   hordeolum (H00.0)
infective dermatitis (L30.3)
local infections of skin classified in Chapter 1
lupus panniculitis (L93.2)
panniculitis NOS (M79.3)
panniculitis of neck and back (M54.0-)
Perlèche NOS (K13.0)
Perlèche due to candidiasis (B37.0)
Perlèche due to riboflavin deficiency (E53.0)
pyogenic granuloma (L98.0)
relapsing panniculitis [Weber-Christian] (M35.6)
viral warts (B07.-)
zoster (B02.-)

L00   **Staphylococcal scalded skin syndrome**
Ritter's disease

Use additional code to identify percentage of skin exfoliation
(L49.-)

Excludes1   bullous impetigo (L01.03)
pemphigus neonatorum (L01.03)
toxic epidermal necrolysis [Lyell] (L51.2)

● **L01**   **Impetigo**
Contagious skin infection caused by a streptococcus or staphylococcus aureus, common skin infections among children

Excludes1   impetigo herpetiformis (L40.1)

● **L01.0**   **Impetigo**
Impetigo contagiosa
Impetigo vulgaris

     L01.00   **Impetigo, unspecified**
Impetigo NOS

     L01.01   **Non-bullous impetigo**

     L01.02   **Bockhart's impetigo**
Impetigo follicularis
Perifolliculitis NOS
Superficial pustular perifolliculitis

     L01.03   **Bullous impetigo**
Impetigo neonatorum
Pemphigus neonatorum
Neonate = newborn

     L01.09   **Other impetigo**
Ulcerative impetigo

   L01.1   **Impetiginization of other dermatoses**

● **L02**   **Cutaneous abscess, furuncle and carbuncle**
Use additional code to identify organism (B95-B96)

Excludes2   abscess of anus and rectal regions (K61.-)
abscess of female genital organs (external) (N76.4)
abscess of male genital organs (external) (N48.2, N49.-)

● **L02.0**   **Cutaneous abscess, furuncle and carbuncle of face**

     Excludes2   abscess of ear, external (H60.0)
abscess of eyelid (H00.0)
abscess of head [any part, except face] (L02.8)
abscess of lacrimal gland (H04.0)
abscess of lacrimal passages (H04.3)
abscess of mouth (K12.2)
abscess of nose (J34.0)
abscess of orbit (H05.0)
submandibular abscess (K12.2)

     L02.01   **Cutaneous abscess of face**

     L02.02   **Furuncle of face**
Boil of face
Folliculitis of face

     L02.03   **Carbuncle of face**

● **L02.1**   **Cutaneous abscess, furuncle and carbuncle of neck**

     L02.11   **Cutaneous abscess of neck**

     L02.12   **Furuncle of neck**
Boil of neck
Folliculitis of neck

     L02.13   **Carbuncle of neck**

● **L02.2**   **Cutaneous abscess, furuncle and carbuncle of trunk**

     Excludes1   non-newborn omphalitis (L08.82)
omphalitis of newborn (P38.-)

     Excludes2   abscess of breast (N61.1) ◄━
abscess of buttocks (L02.3)
abscess of female external genital organs (N76.4)
abscess of male external genital organs (N48.2, N49.-)
abscess of hip (L02.4)

     ● **L02.21**   **Cutaneous abscess of trunk**

         L02.211   **Cutaneous abscess of abdominal wall**

         L02.212   **Cutaneous abscess of back [any part, except buttock]**

         L02.213   **Cutaneous abscess of chest wall**

         L02.214   **Cutaneous abscess of groin**

         L02.215   **Cutaneous abscess of perineum**

         L02.216   **Cutaneous abscess of umbilicus**

         L02.219   **Cutaneous abscess of trunk, unspecified**

     ● **L02.22**   **Furuncle of trunk**
Boil of trunk
Folliculitis of trunk

         L02.221   **Furuncle of abdominal wall**

         L02.222   **Furuncle of back [any part, except buttock]**

         L02.223   **Furuncle of chest wall**

         L02.224   **Furuncle of groin**

         L02.225   **Furuncle of perineum**

         L02.226   **Furuncle of umbilicus**

         L02.229   **Furuncle of trunk, unspecified**

     ● **L02.23**   **Carbuncle of trunk**

         L02.231   **Carbuncle of abdominal wall**

         L02.232   **Carbuncle of back [any part, except buttock]**

         L02.233   **Carbuncle of chest wall**

         L02.234   **Carbuncle of groin**

         L02.235   **Carbuncle of perineum**

         L02.236   **Carbuncle of umbilicus**

         L02.239   **Carbuncle of trunk, unspecified**

● **L02.3**   **Cutaneous abscess, furuncle and carbuncle of buttock**

     Excludes1   pilonidal cyst with abscess (L05.01)

     L02.31   **Cutaneous abscess of buttock**
Cutaneous abscess of gluteal region

     L02.32   **Furuncle of buttock**
Boil of buttock
Folliculitis of buttock
Furuncle of gluteal region

     L02.33   **Carbuncle of buttock**
Carbuncle of gluteal region

◄ New   ◄━ Revised   ~~deleted~~ Deleted   Excludes 1   Excludes 2   Includes   Use additional   Code first   Code also   Unspecified
OGCR Official Guidelines   X Assign placeholder X   ● Use Additional Character(s)   ▌ Manifestation Code   **Coding Clinic**

● **L02.4**   **Cutaneous abscess, furuncle and carbuncle of limb**
     Excludes2   Cutaneous abscess, furuncle and carbuncle of groin (L02.214, L02.224, L02.234)
           Cutaneous abscess, furuncle and carbuncle of hand (L02.5-)
           Cutaneous abscess, furuncle and carbuncle of foot (L02.6-)
    ● **L02.41**   **Cutaneous abscess of limb**
        L02.411   **Cutaneous abscess of right axilla**
        L02.412   **Cutaneous abscess of left axilla**
        L02.413   **Cutaneous abscess of right upper limb**
        L02.414   **Cutaneous abscess of left upper limb**
        L02.415   **Cutaneous abscess of right lower limb**
        L02.416   **Cutaneous abscess of left lower limb**
        L02.419   **Cutaneous abscess of limb, unspecified**
    ● **L02.42**   **Furuncle of limb**
        Boil of limb
        Folliculitis of limb
        L02.421   **Furuncle of right axilla**
        L02.422   **Furuncle of left axilla**
        L02.423   **Furuncle of right upper limb**
        L02.424   **Furuncle of left upper limb**
        L02.425   **Furuncle of right lower limb**
        L02.426   **Furuncle of left lower limb**
        L02.429   **Furuncle of limb, unspecified**
    ● **L02.43**   **Carbuncle of limb**
        L02.431   **Carbuncle of right axilla**
        L02.432   **Carbuncle of left axilla**
        L02.433   **Carbuncle of right upper limb**
        L02.434   **Carbuncle of left upper limb**
        L02.435   **Carbuncle of right lower limb**
        L02.436   **Carbuncle of left lower limb**
        L02.439   **Carbuncle of limb, unspecified**
● **L02.5**   **Cutaneous abscess, furuncle and carbuncle of hand**
    ● **L02.51**   **Cutaneous abscess of hand**
        L02.511   **Cutaneous abscess of right hand**
        L02.512   **Cutaneous abscess of left hand**
        L02.519   **Cutaneous abscess of unspecified hand**
    ● **L02.52**   **Furuncle hand**
        Boil of hand
        Folliculitis of hand
        L02.521   **Furuncle right hand**
        L02.522   **Furuncle left hand**
        L02.529   **Furuncle unspecified hand**
    ● **L02.53**   **Carbuncle of hand**
        L02.531   **Carbuncle of right hand**
        L02.532   **Carbuncle of left hand**
        L02.539   **Carbuncle of unspecified hand**
● **L02.6**   **Cutaneous abscess, furuncle and carbuncle of foot**
    ● **L02.61**   **Cutaneous abscess of foot**
        L02.611   **Cutaneous abscess of right foot**
        L02.612   **Cutaneous abscess of left foot**
        L02.619   **Cutaneous abscess of unspecified foot**
    ● **L02.62**   **Furuncle of foot**
        Boil of foot
        Folliculitis of foot
        L02.621   **Furuncle of right foot**
        L02.622   **Furuncle of left foot**
        L02.629   **Furuncle of unspecified foot**

    ● **L02.63**   **Carbuncle of foot**
        L02.631   **Carbuncle of right foot**
        L02.632   **Carbuncle of left foot**
        L02.639   **Carbuncle of unspecified foot**
● **L02.8**   **Cutaneous abscess, furuncle and carbuncle of other sites**
    ● **L02.81**   **Cutaneous abscess of other sites**
        L02.811   **Cutaneous abscess of head [any part, except face]**
        L02.818   **Cutaneous abscess of other sites**
    ● **L02.82**   **Furuncle of other sites**
        Boil of other sites
        Folliculitis of other sites
        L02.821   **Furuncle of head [any part, except face]**
        L02.828   **Furuncle of other sites**
    ● **L02.83**   **Carbuncle of other sites**
        L02.831   **Carbuncle of head [any part, except face]**
        L02.838   **Carbuncle of other sites**
● **L02.9**   **Cutaneous abscess, furuncle and carbuncle, unspecified**
    L02.91   **Cutaneous abscess, unspecified**
    L02.92   **Furuncle, unspecified**
        Boil NOS
        Furunculosis NOS
    L02.93   **Carbuncle, unspecified**
● **L03**   **Cellulitis and acute lymphangitis**
     Excludes2   cellulitis of anal and rectal region (K61.-)
           cellulitis of external auditory canal (H60.1)
           cellulitis of eyelid (H00.0)
           cellulitis of female external genital organs (N76.4)
           cellulitis of lacrimal apparatus (H04.3)
           cellulitis of male external genital organs (N48.2, N49.-)
           cellulitis of mouth (K12.2)
           cellulitis of nose (J34.0)
           eosinophilic cellulitis [Wells] (L98.3)
           febrile neutrophilic dermatosis [Sweet] (L98.2)
           lymphangitis (chronic) (subacute) (I89.1)
● **L03.0**   **Cellulitis and acute lymphangitis of finger and toe**
       Infection of nail
       Onychia
       Paronychia
       Perionychia
    ● **L03.01**   **Cellulitis of finger**
        Felon
        Whitlow
        Excludes1   herpetic whitlow (B00.89)
        L03.011   **Cellulitis of right finger**
        L03.012   **Cellulitis of left finger**
        L03.019   **Cellulitis of unspecified finger**
    ● **L03.02**   **Acute lymphangitis of finger**
        Hangnail with lymphangitis of finger
        L03.021   **Acute lymphangitis of right finger**
        L03.022   **Acute lymphangitis of left finger**
        L03.029   **Acute lymphangitis of unspecified finger**
    ● **L03.03**   **Cellulitis of toe**
        L03.031   **Cellulitis of right toe**
        L03.032   **Cellulitis of left toe**
        L03.039   **Cellulitis of unspecified toe**
    ● **L03.04**   **Acute lymphangitis of toe**
        Hangnail with lymphangitis of toe
        L03.041   **Acute lymphangitis of right toe**
        L03.042   **Acute lymphangitis of left toe**
        L03.049   **Acute lymphangitis of unspecified toe**

Item 12-1   **Onychia** is an inflammation of the tissue surrounding the nail with pus accumulation and loss of the nail, resulting from microscopic pathogens entering through small wounds. **Paronychia** is a nail disease also known as felon or whitlow and is a bacterial or fungal infection.

CHAPTER 12 (L00–L99)

● **L03.1**   **Cellulitis and acute lymphangitis of other parts of limb**
  ● **L03.11**   **Cellulitis of other parts of limb**
     Excludes2   cellulitis of fingers (L03.01-)
                        cellulitis of toes (L03.03-)
                        groin (L03.314)
     L03.111   **Cellulitis of right axilla**
     L03.112   **Cellulitis of left axilla**
     L03.113   **Cellulitis of right upper limb**
     L03.114   **Cellulitis of left upper limb**
     L03.115   **Cellulitis of right lower limb**
     L03.116   **Cellulitis of left lower limb**
     L03.119   **Cellulitis of** unspecified **part of limb**
  ● **L03.12**   **Acute lymphangitis of other parts of limb**
     Excludes2   acute lymphangitis of fingers (L03.2-)
                        acute lymphangitis of toes (L03.04-)
                        acute lymphangitis of groin (L03.324)
     L03.121   **Acute lymphangitis of right axilla**
     L03.122   **Acute lymphangitis of left axilla**
     L03.123   **Acute lymphangitis of right upper limb**
     L03.124   **Acute lymphangitis of left upper limb**
     L03.125   **Acute lymphangitis of right lower limb**
     L03.126   **Acute lymphangitis of left lower limb**
     L03.129   **Acute lymphangitis of** unspecified **part of limb**
● **L03.2**   **Cellulitis and acute lymphangitis of face and neck**
  ● **L03.21**   **Cellulitis and acute lymphangitis of face**
     L03.211   **Cellulitis of face**
         Excludes2   abscess of orbit (H05.01-) ◀
                      cellulitis of ear (H60.1-)
                      cellulitis of eyelid (H00.0-)
                      cellulitis of head (L03.81)
                      cellulitis of lacrimal apparatus (H04.3)
                      cellulitis of lip (K13.0)
                      cellulitis of mouth (K12.2)
                      cellulitis of nose (internal) (J34.0)
                      cellulitis of orbit (H05.01-) ◀
                      cellulitis of scalp (L03.81)
     L03.212   **Acute lymphangitis of face**
     L03.213   **Periorbital cellulitis** ◀
            Preseptal cellulitis ◀
  ● **L03.22**   **Cellulitis and acute lymphangitis of neck**
     L03.221   **Cellulitis of neck**
     L03.222   **Acute lymphangitis of neck**

Item 12-2   **Cellulitis** is an acute spreading bacterial infection below the surface of the skin characterized by redness (erythema), warmth, swelling, pain, fever, chills, and enlarged lymph nodes ("swollen glands").

● **L03.3**   **Cellulitis and acute lymphangitis of trunk**
  ● **L03.31**   **Cellulitis of trunk**
     Excludes2   cellulitis of anal and rectal regions (K61.-)
                      cellulitis of breast NOS (N61.0) ◀
                      cellulitis of female external genital organs (N76.4)
                      cellulitis of male external genital organs (N48.2, N49.-)
                      omphalitis of newborn (P38.-)
                      puerperal cellulitis of breast (O91.2)
     L03.311   **Cellulitis of abdominal wall**
         Excludes2   cellulitis of umbilicus (L03.316)
                      cellulitis of groin (L03.314)
     L03.312   **Cellulitis of back [any part except buttock]**
     L03.313   **Cellulitis of chest wall**
     L03.314   **Cellulitis of groin**
     L03.315   **Cellulitis of perineum**
     L03.316   **Cellulitis of umbilicus**
     L03.317   **Cellulitis of buttock**
     L03.319   **Cellulitis of trunk,** unspecified
  ● **L03.32**   **Acute lymphangitis of trunk**
     L03.321   **Acute lymphangitis of abdominal wall**
     L03.322   **Acute lymphangitis of back [any part except buttock]**
     L03.323   **Acute lymphangitis of chest wall**
     L03.324   **Acute lymphangitis of groin**
     L03.325   **Acute lymphangitis of perineum**
     L03.326   **Acute lymphangitis of umbilicus**
     L03.327   **Acute lymphangitis of buttock**
     L03.329   **Acute lymphangitis of trunk,** unspecified
● **L03.8**   **Cellulitis and acute lymphangitis of other sites**
  ● **L03.81**   **Cellulitis of other sites**
     L03.811   **Cellulitis of head [any part, except face]**
         Cellulitis of scalp
         Excludes2   cellulitis of face (L03.211)
     L03.818   **Cellulitis of other sites**
  ● **L03.89**   **Acute lymphangitis of other sites**
     L03.891   **Acute lymphangitis of head [any part, except face]**
     L03.898   **Acute lymphangitis of other sites**
● **L03.9**   **Cellulitis and acute lymphangitis, unspecified**
     L03.90   **Cellulitis,** unspecified
     L03.91   **Acute lymphangitis,** unspecified
         Excludes1   lymphangitis NOS (I89.1)

◀ New   ◀≡ Revised   ~~deleted~~ Deleted   Excludes 1   Excludes 2   Includes   Use additional   Code first   Code also   Unspecified
OGCR Official Guidelines   X Assign placeholder X   ● Use Additional Character(s)   ▌ Manifestation Code   **Coding Clinic**

Item 12–3   **Abscess** is a localized collection of pus in tissues or organs and is a sign of infection resulting in swelling and inflammation.

Item 12–4   **Pilonidal cyst,** also called a coccygeal cyst, is the result of a disorder called pilonidal disease. The cyst usually contains hair and pus.

● **L04**   **Acute lymphadenitis**
> *Short-term inflammation of lymph nodes which can be regionalized to involve a given area of the lymph system or systemic involving much of the body*

    Includes   abscess (acute) of lymph nodes, except mesenteric
                 acute lymphadenitis, except mesenteric

    Excludes1   chronic or subacute lymphadenitis, except mesenteric (I88.1)
                 enlarged lymph nodes (R59.-)
                 human immunodeficiency virus [HIV] disease resulting in generalized lymphadenopathy (B20)
                 lymphadenitis NOS (I88.9)
                 nonspecific mesenteric lymphadenitis (I88.0)

    L04.0   **Acute lymphadenitis of face, head and neck**
    L04.1   **Acute lymphadenitis of trunk**
    L04.2   **Acute lymphadenitis of upper limb**
            Acute lymphadenitis of axilla
            Acute lymphadenitis of shoulder
    L04.3   **Acute lymphadenitis of lower limb**
            Acute lymphadenitis of hip
          Excludes2   acute lymphadenitis of groin (L04.1)
    L04.8   **Acute lymphadenitis of other sites**
    L04.9   **Acute lymphadenitis, unspecified**

● **L05**   **Pilonidal cyst and sinus**
  ● **L05.0**   **Pilonidal cyst and sinus with abscess**
        L05.01   **Pilonidal cyst with abscess**
                Pilonidal abscess
                Pilonidal dimple with abscess
                Postanal dimple with abscess
             Excludes2   congenital sacral dimple (Q82.6) ◄
                          parasacral dimple (Q82.6) ◄
        L05.02   **Pilonidal sinus with abscess**
                Coccygeal fistula with abscess
                Coccygeal sinus with abscess
                Pilonidal fistula with abscess
  ● **L05.9**   **Pilonidal cyst and sinus without abscess**
        L05.91   **Pilonidal cyst without abscess**
                Pilonidal dimple
                Postanal dimple
                Pilonidal cyst NOS
             Excludes2   congenital sacral dimple (Q82.6) ◄
                          parasacral dimple (Q82.6) ◄
        L05.92   **Pilonidal sinus without abscess**
                Coccygeal fistula
                Coccygeal sinus without abscess
                Pilonidal fistula

● **L08**   **Other local infections of skin and subcutaneous tissue**
    L08.0   **Pyoderma**
            Dermatitis gangrenosa
            Purulent dermatitis
             Septic dermatitis
            Suppurative dermatitis
         Excludes1   pyoderma gangrenosum (L88)
                     pyoderma vegetans (L08.81)
    L08.1   **Erythrasma**

    ● **L08.8**   **Other specified local infections of the skin and subcutaneous tissue**
        L08.81   **Pyoderma vegetans**
             Excludes1   pyoderma gangrenosum (L88)
                        pyoderma NOS (L08.0)
        L08.82   **Omphalitis not of newborn**
             Excludes1   omphalitis of newborn (P38.-)
        L08.89   **Other specified local infections of the skin and subcutaneous tissue**
    L08.9   **Local infection of the skin and subcutaneous tissue, unspecified**

BULLOUS DISORDERS (L10-L14)

    Excludes1   benign familial pemphigus [Hailey-Hailey] (Q82.8)
                 staphylococcal scalded skin syndrome (L00)
                 toxic epidermal necrolysis [Lyell] (L51.2)

● **L10**   **Pemphigus**
    Excludes1   pemphigus neonatorum (L01.03)
    L10.0   **Pemphigus vulgaris**
    L10.1   **Pemphigus vegetans**
    L10.2   **Pemphigus foliaceous**
    L10.3   **Brazilian pemphigus [fogo selvagem]**
    L10.4   **Pemphigus erythematosus**
            Senear-Usher syndrome
    L10.5   **Drug-induced pemphigus**
            Use additional code for adverse effect, if applicable, to identify drug (T36-T50 with fifth or sixth character 5)
    ● **L10.8**   **Other pemphigus**
        L10.81   **Paraneoplastic pemphigus**
        L10.89   **Other pemphigus**
    L10.9   **Pemphigus, unspecified**

● **L11**   **Other acantholytic disorders**
    L11.0   **Acquired keratosis follicularis**
          Excludes1   keratosis follicularis (congenital) [Darier-White] (Q82.8)
    L11.1   **Transient acantholytic dermatosis [Grover]**
    L11.8   **Other specified acantholytic disorders**
    L11.9   **Acantholytic disorder, unspecified**

● **L12**   **Pemphigoid**
    Excludes1   herpes gestationis (O26.4-)
                 impetigo herpetiformis (L40.1)
    L12.0   **Bullous pemphigoid**
    L12.1   **Cicatricial pemphigoid**
            Benign mucous membrane pemphigoid
    L12.2   **Chronic bullous disease of childhood**   P
            Juvenile dermatitis herpetiformis
    ● **L12.3**   **Acquired epidermolysis bullosa**
          Excludes1   epidermolysis bullosa (congenital) (Q81.-)
        L12.30   **Acquired epidermolysis bullosa, unspecified**
        L12.31   **Epidermolysis bullosa due to drug**
             Use additional code for adverse effect, if applicable, to identify drug (T36-T50 with fifth or sixth character 5)
        L12.35   **Other acquired epidermolysis bullosa**
    L12.8   **Other pemphigoid**
    L12.9   **Pemphigoid, unspecified**

Figure 12-2   Impetigo. A thick, honey-yellow adherent crust covers the entire eroded surface. (From Habif: Clinical Dermatology, ed 4, Mosby, Inc., 2004)

CHAPTER 12 (L00-L99)

● **L13   Other bullous disorders**

  L13.0   Dermatitis herpetiformis
       Duhring's disease
       Hydroa herpetiformis
       Excludes1   juvenile dermatitis herpetiformis (L12.2)
                    senile dermatitis herpetiformis (L12.0)

  L13.1   Subcorneal pustular dermatitis
       Sneddon-Wilkinson disease

  L13.8   Other specified bullous disorders

  L13.9   Bullous disorder, unspecified

▸ *L14   Bullous disorders in diseases classified elsewhere*
       Code first underlying disease

DERMATITIS AND ECZEMA (L20-L30)

  Note: In this block the terms dermatitis and eczema are used
  synonymously and interchangeably.
       Excludes2   chronic (childhood) granulomatous disease (D71)
                    dermatitis gangrenosa (L08.0)
                    dermatitis herpetiformis (L13.0)
                    dry skin dermatitis (L85.3)
                    factitial dermatitis (L98.1)
                    perioral dermatitis (L71.0)
                    radiation-related disorders of the skin and
                        subcutaneous tissue (L55-L59)
                    stasis dermatitis (I87.2) ◀▥▥

● **L20   Atopic dermatitis**

  L20.0   Besnier's prurigo

● **L20.8   Other atopic dermatitis**
       Excludes2   circumscribed neurodermatitis (L28.0)

       L20.81   Atopic neurodermatitis
                 Diffuse neurodermatitis

       L20.82   Flexural eczema

       L20.83   Infantile (acute) (chronic) eczema   P

       L20.84   Intrinsic (allergic) eczema

       L20.89   Other atopic dermatitis

  L20.9   Atopic dermatitis, unspecified

● **L21   Seborrheic dermatitis**
       Excludes2   infective dermatitis (L30.3)
                    seborrheic keratosis (L82.-)

  L21.0   Seborrhea capitis   P
       Cradle cap

  L21.1   Seborrheic infantile dermatitis   P

  L21.8   Other seborrheic dermatitis

  L21.9   Seborrheic dermatitis, unspecified
       Seborrhea NOS

Item 12–5 Dermatitis herpetiformis, also known as Duhring's
disease, is a systemic disease characterized by small blisters (3 to 5 mm) and
occasionally large bullae (> 5 mm).

Figure 12-3 Dermatitis herpetiformis. (From Arnold HL, Odom RB,
James WD: Andrews' Diseases of the Skin, Clinical Dermatology, ed 8,
Philadelphia, WB Saunders, 1990)

Item 12–6 Seborrheic dermatitis is characterized by greasy, scaly, red
patches and is associated with oily skin and scalp.

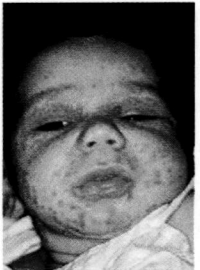

Figure 12-4 Seborrheic dermatitis. (From
Cohen BA: Atlas of Pediatric Dermatology,
St. Louis, Mosby, 1993)

Item 12–7 Atopic dermatitis, also known as atopic eczema, infantile
eczema, disseminated neuro dermatitis, flexural eczema, and *prurigo
diathesique* (Besnier), is characterized by intense itching and is often hereditary.

Figure 12-5 Atopic dermatitis. (From
Moschella SL, Hurley HJ: Dermatology, ed 3,
Philadelphia, WB Saunders, 1993)

  L22   Diaper dermatitis
       Diaper erythema
       Diaper rash
       Psoriasiform diaper rash

● **L23   Allergic contact dermatitis**
       Excludes1   allergy NOS (T78.40)
                    contact dermatitis NOS (L25.9)
                    dermatitis NOS (L30.9)
       Excludes2   dermatitis due to substances taken internally
                        (L27.-)
                    dermatitis of eyelid (H01.1-)
                    diaper dermatitis (L22)
                    eczema of external ear (H60.5-)
                    irritant contact dermatitis (L24.-)
                    perioral dermatitis (L71.0)
                    radiation-related disorders of the skin and
                        subcutaneous tissue (L55-L59)

  L23.0   Allergic contact dermatitis due to metals
       Allergic contact dermatitis due to chromium
       Allergic contact dermatitis due to nickel

  L23.1   Allergic contact dermatitis due to adhesives

  L23.2   Allergic contact dermatitis due to cosmetics

  **L23.3   Allergic contact dermatitis due to drugs in contact with
       skin**
       Use additional code for adverse effect, if applicable,
           to identify drug (T36-T50 with fifth or sixth
           character 5)
       Excludes2   dermatitis due to ingested drugs and
                        medicaments (L27.0-L27.1)

  L23.4   Allergic contact dermatitis due to dyes

  **L23.5   Allergic contact dermatitis due to other chemical
       products**
       Allergic contact dermatitis due to cement
       Allergic contact dermatitis due to insecticide
       Allergic contact dermatitis due to plastic
       Allergic contact dermatitis due to rubber

L23.6   Allergic contact dermatitis due to food in contact with the skin
>   **Excludes2**   dermatitis due to ingested food (L27.2)

L23.7   Allergic contact dermatitis due to plants, except food
>   **Excludes2**   allergy NOS due to pollen (J30.1)

● **L23.8   Allergic contact dermatitis due to other agents**
>   **L23.81   Allergic contact dermatitis due to animal (cat) (dog) dander**
>   Allergic contact dermatitis due to animal (cat) (dog) hair
>
>   **L23.89   Allergic contact dermatitis due to other agents**

L23.9   Allergic contact dermatitis, unspecified cause
> Allergic contact eczema NOS

● **L24   Irritant contact dermatitis**
>   **Excludes1**   allergy NOS (T78.40)
>   contact dermatitis NOS (L25.9)
>   dermatitis NOS (L30.9)
>
>   **Excludes2**   allergic contact dermatitis (L23.-)
>   dermatitis due to substances taken internally (L27.-)
>   dermatitis of eyelid (H01.1-)
>   diaper dermatitis (L22)
>   eczema of external ear (H60.5-)
>   perioral dermatitis (L71.0)
>   radiation-related disorders of the skin and subcutaneous tissue (L55-L59)

L24.0   Irritant contact dermatitis due to detergents

L24.1   Irritant contact dermatitis due to oils and greases

L24.2   Irritant contact dermatitis due to solvents
> Irritant contact dermatitis due to chlorocompound
> Irritant contact dermatitis due to cyclohexane
> Irritant contact dermatitis due to ester
> Irritant contact dermatitis due to glycol
> Irritant contact dermatitis due to hydrocarbon
> Irritant contact dermatitis due to ketone

L24.3   Irritant contact dermatitis due to cosmetics

L24.4   Irritant contact dermatitis due to drugs in contact with skin
>   Use additional code for adverse effect, if applicable, to identify drug (T36-T50 with fifth or sixth character 5)

L24.5   Irritant contact dermatitis due to other chemical products
> Irritant contact dermatitis due to cement
> Irritant contact dermatitis due to insecticide
> Irritant contact dermatitis due to plastic
> Irritant contact dermatitis due to rubber

L24.6   Irritant contact dermatitis due to food in contact with skin
>   **Excludes2**   dermatitis due to ingested food (L27.2)

L24.7   Irritant contact dermatitis due to plants, except food
>   **Excludes2**   allergy NOS to pollen (J30.1)

● **L24.8   Irritant contact dermatitis due to other agents**
>   **L24.81   Irritant contact dermatitis due to metals**
>   Irritant contact dermatitis due to chromium
>   Irritant contact dermatitis due to nickel
>
>   **L24.89   Irritant contact dermatitis due to other agents**
>   Irritant contact dermatitis due to dyes

L24.9   Irritant contact dermatitis, unspecified cause
> Irritant contact eczema NOS

● **L25   Unspecified contact dermatitis**
>   **Excludes1**   allergic contact dermatitis (L23.-)
>   allergy NOS (T78.40)
>   dermatitis NOS (L30.9)
>   irritant contact dermatitis (L24.-)
>
>   **Excludes2**   dermatitis due to ingested substances (L27.-)
>   dermatitis of eyelid (H01.1-)
>   eczema of external ear (H60.5-)
>   perioral dermatitis (L71.0)
>   radiation-related disorders of the skin and subcutaneous tissue (L55-L59)

L25.0   Unspecified contact dermatitis due to cosmetics

L25.1   Unspecified contact dermatitis due to drugs in contact with skin
>   Use additional code for adverse effect, if applicable, to identify drug (T36-T50 with fifth or sixth character 5)
>   **Excludes2**   dermatitis due to ingested drugs and medicaments (L27.0-L27.1)

L25.2   Unspecified contact dermatitis due to dyes

L25.3   Unspecified contact dermatitis due to other chemical products
> Unspecified contact dermatitis due to cement
> Unspecified contact dermatitis due to insecticide

L25.4   Unspecified contact dermatitis due to food in contact with skin
>   **Excludes2**   dermatitis due to ingested food (L27.2)

L25.5   Unspecified contact dermatitis due to plants, except food
>   **Excludes1**   nettle rash (L50.9)
>   **Excludes2**   allergy NOS due to pollen (J30.1)

L25.8   Unspecified contact dermatitis due to other agents

L25.9   Unspecified contact dermatitis, unspecified cause
> Contact dermatitis (occupational) NOS
> Contact eczema (occupational) NOS

L26   Exfoliative dermatitis
> Hebra's pityriasis
>   **Excludes1**   Ritter's disease (L00)

● **L27   Dermatitis due to substances taken internally**
>   **Excludes1**   allergy NOS (T78.40)
>   **Excludes2**   adverse food reaction, except dermatitis (T78.0-T78.1)
>   contact dermatitis (L23-L25)
>   drug photoallergic response (L56.1)
>   drug phototoxic response (L56.0)
>   urticaria (L50.-)

L27.0   Generalized skin eruption due to drugs and medicaments taken internally
>   Use additional code for adverse effect, if applicable, to identify drug (T36-T50 with fifth or sixth character 5)

L27.1   Localized skin eruption due to drugs and medicaments taken internally
>   Use additional code for adverse effect, if applicable, to identify drug (T36-T50 with fifth or sixth character 5)

L27.2   Dermatitis due to ingested food
>   **Excludes2**   dermatitis due to food in contact with skin (L23.6, L24.6, L25.4)

L27.8   Dermatitis due to other substances taken internally

L27.9   Dermatitis due to unspecified substance taken internally

CHAPTER 12 (L00-L99)

● L28 Lichen simplex chronicus and prurigo
    L28.0 Lichen simplex chronicus
        Circumscribed neurodermatitis
        Lichen NOS
    L28.1 Prurigo nodularis
    L28.2 Other prurigo
        Prurigo NOS   Prurigo mitis
        Prurigo Hebra   Urticaria papulosa

● L29 Pruritus
    Excludes1 neurotic excoriation (L98.1)
           psychogenic pruritus (F45.8)
    L29.0 Pruritus ani
    L29.1 Pruritus scroti ♂
    L29.2 Pruritus vulvae ♀
    L29.3 Anogenital pruritus, **unspecified**
    L29.8 Other pruritus
    L29.9 Pruritus, **unspecified**
        Itch NOS

● L30 Other and unspecified dermatitis
    Excludes2 contact dermatitis (L23-L25)
           dry skin dermatitis (L85.3)
           small plaque parapsoriasis (L41.3)
           stasis dermatitis (I87.2) ◀▥
    L30.0 Nummular dermatitis
    L30.1 Dyshidrosis [pompholyx]
    L30.2 Cutaneous autosensitization
        Candidid [levurid]   Eczematid
        Dermatophytid
    L30.3 Infective dermatitis
        Infectious eczematoid dermatitis
    L30.4 Erythema intertrigo
    L30.5 Pityriasis alba
    L30.8 Other specified dermatitis
    L30.9 Dermatitis, **unspecified**
        Eczema NOS

PAPULOSQUAMOUS DISORDERS (L40-L45)

● L40 Psoriasis
    L40.0 Psoriasis vulgaris
        Nummular psoriasis   Plaque psoriasis
    L40.1 Generalized pustular psoriasis
        Impetigo herpetiformis
        Von Zumbusch's disease
    L40.2 Acrodermatitis continua
    L40.3 Pustulosis palmaris et plantaris
    L40.4 Guttate psoriasis
   ● L40.5 Arthropathic psoriasis
        L40.50 Arthropathic psoriasis, **unspecified**
        L40.51 Distal interphalangeal psoriatic arthropathy
        L40.52 Psoriatic arthritis mutilans
        L40.53 Psoriatic spondylitis
        L40.54 Psoriatic juvenile arthropathy
        L40.59 Other psoriatic arthropathy
    L40.8 Other psoriasis
        Flexural psoriasis
    L40.9 Psoriasis, **unspecified**

● L41 Parapsoriasis
    Excludes1 poikiloderma vasculare atrophicans (L94.5)
    L41.0 Pityriasis lichenoides et varioliformis acuta
        Mucha-Habermann disease
    L41.1 Pityriasis lichenoides chronica
    L41.3 Small plaque parapsoriasis
    L41.4 Large plaque parapsoriasis
    L41.5 Retiform parapsoriasis
    L41.8 Other parapsoriasis
    L41.9 Parapsoriasis, **unspecified**

  L42 Pityriasis rosea

● L43 Lichen planus
    Excludes1 lichen planopilaris (L66.1)
    L43.0 Hypertrophic lichen planus
    L43.1 Bullous lichen planus
    L43.2 Lichenoid drug reaction
        Use additional code for adverse effect, if applicable, to identify drug (T36-T50 with fifth or sixth character 5)
    L43.3 Subacute (active) lichen planus
        Lichen planus tropicus
    L43.8 Other lichen planus
    L43.9 Lichen planus, **unspecified**

● L44 Other papulosquamous disorders
    L44.0 Pityriasis rubra pilaris
    L44.1 Lichen nitidus
    L44.2 Lichen striatus
    L44.3 Lichen ruber moniliformis
    L44.4 Infantile papular acrodermatitis [Gianotti-Crosti]   P
    L44.8 Other specified papulosquamous disorders
    L44.9 Papulosquamous disorder, **unspecified**

▌ L45 *Papulosquamous disorders in diseases classified elsewhere*
    Code first underlying disease

URTICARIA AND ERYTHEMA (L49-L54)

    Excludes1 Lyme disease (A69.2-)
           rosacea (L71.-)

● L49 Exfoliation due to erythematous conditions according to extent of body surface involved
    Code first erythematous condition causing exfoliation, such as:
        Ritter's disease (L00)
        (Staphylococcal) scalded skin syndrome (L00)
        Stevens-Johnson syndrome (L51.1)
        Stevens-Johnson syndrome-toxic epidermal necrolysis overlap syndrome (L51.3)
        Toxic epidermal necrolysis (L51.2)
    L49.0 Exfoliation due to erythematous condition involving less than 10 percent of body surface
        Exfoliation due to erythematous condition NOS
    L49.1 Exfoliation due to erythematous condition involving 10-19 percent of body surface
    L49.2 Exfoliation due to erythematous condition involving 20-29 percent of body surface
    L49.3 Exfoliation due to erythematous condition involving 30-39 percent of body surface
    L49.4 Exfoliation due to erythematous condition involving 40-49 percent of body surface
    L49.5 Exfoliation due to erythematous condition involving 50-59 percent of body surface

Item 12–8 Psoriasis is a chronic, recurrent inflammatory skin disease characterized by small patches covered with thick silvery scales. **Parapsoriasis** is a treatment-resistant erythroderma. **Pityriasis rosea** is characterized by a herald patch that is a single large lesion and that usually appears on the trunk and is followed by scattered, smaller lesions.

CHAPTER 12 (L00-L99)

◀ New   ◀▥ Revised   ~~deleted~~ Deleted   Excludes 1   Excludes 2   Includes   Use additional   Code first   Code also   Unspecified
OGCR Official Guidelines   X Assign placeholder X   ● Use Additional Character(s)   ▌ Manifestation Code   **Coding Clinic**

Figure 12-6 Erythematous plaques with silvery scales in a patient with psoriasis. (From Goldman: Cecil Textbook of Medicine, ed 22, Saunders, 2004)

L49.6   **Exfoliation due to erythematous condition involving 60-69 percent of body surface**

L49.7   **Exfoliation due to erythematous condition involving 70-79 percent of body surface**

L49.8   **Exfoliation due to erythematous condition involving 80-89 percent of body surface**

L49.9   **Exfoliation due to erythematous condition involving 90 or more percent of body surface**

● **L50   Urticaria**

> **Excludes1**   allergic contact dermatitis (L23.-)
> angioneurotic edema (T78.3)
> giant urticaria (T78.3)
> hereditary angio-edema (D84.1)
> Quincke's edema (T78.3)
> serum urticaria (T80.6-)
> solar urticaria (L56.3)
> urticaria neonatorum (P83.8)
> urticaria papulosa (L28.2)
> urticaria pigmentosa (Q82.2)

L50.0   **Allergic urticaria**

L50.1   **Idiopathic urticaria**

L50.2   **Urticaria due to cold and heat**

> **Excludes2**   familial cold urticaria (M04.2) ◄

L50.3   **Dermatographic urticaria**

L50.4   **Vibratory urticaria**

L50.5   **Cholinergic urticaria**

L50.6   **Contact urticaria**

L50.8   **Other urticaria**
> Chronic urticaria
> Recurrent periodic urticaria

L50.9   **Urticaria, unspecified**

Figure 12-7 Urticaria (hives). *(Courtesy of David Effron, MD.)* (From Marx: Rosen's Emergency Medicine: Concepts and Clinical Practice, ed 6, Mosby, Inc., 2006)

Item 12–9   Urticaria is a vascular reaction in which wheals surrounded by a red halo appear and cause severe itching. The causes of urticaria or hives are extensive and varied (e.g., food, heat, cold, drugs, stress, infections).

● **L51   Erythema multiforme**

> Use additional code for adverse effect, if applicable, to identify drug (T36-T50 with fifth or sixth character 5)

> Use additional code to identify associated manifestations, such as:
> arthropathy associated with dermatological disorders (M14.8-)
> conjunctival edema (H11.42)
> conjunctivitis (H10.22-)
> corneal scars and opacities (H17.-)
> corneal ulcer (H16.0-)
> edema of eyelid (H02.84)
> inflammation of eyelid (H01.8)
> keratoconjunctivitis sicca (H16.22-)
> mechanical lagophthalmos (H02.22-)
> stomatitis (K12.-)
> symblepharon (H11.23-)

> Use additional code to identify percentage of skin exfoliation (L49.-)

> **Excludes1**   staphylococcal scalded skin syndrome (L00)
> Ritter's disease (L00)

L51.0   **Nonbullous erythema multiforme**

L51.1   **Stevens-Johnson syndrome**

L51.2   **Toxic epidermal necrolysis [Lyell]**

L51.3   **Stevens-Johnson syndrome-toxic epidermal necrolysis overlap syndrome**
> SJS-TEN overlap syndrome

L51.8   **Other erythema multiforme**

L51.9   **Erythema multiforme, unspecified**
> Erythema iris
> Erythema multiforme major NOS
> Erythema multiforme minor NOS
> Herpes iris

● **L52   Erythema nodosum**

> **Excludes1**   tuberculous erythema nodosum (A18.4)

● **L53   Other erythematous conditions**

> **Excludes1**   erythema ab igne (L59.0)
> erythema due to external agents in contact with skin (L23-L25)
> erythema intertrigo (L30.4)

L53.0   **Toxic erythema**
> *Code first* poisoning due to drug or toxin, if applicable (T36-T65 with fifth or sixth character 1-4 or 6)

> Use additional code for adverse effect, if applicable, to identify drug (T36-T50 with fifth or sixth character 5)

> **Excludes1**   neonatal erythema toxicum (P83.1)

L53.1   **Erythema annulare centrifugum**

L53.2   **Erythema marginatum**

L53.3   **Other chronic figurate erythema**

L53.8   **Other specified erythematous conditions**

L53.9   **Erythematous condition, unspecified**
> Erythema NOS
> Erythroderma NOS

◗ **L54   *Erythema in diseases classified elsewhere***
> *Code first* underlying disease

RADIATION-RELATED DISORDERS OF THE SKIN AND SUBCUTANEOUS TISSUE (L55-L59)

● **L55   Sunburn**

L55.0   **Sunburn of first degree**

L55.1   **Sunburn of second degree**

L55.2   **Sunburn of third degree**

L55.9   **Sunburn, unspecified**

CHAPTER 12 (L00-L99)

● **L56** **Other acute skin changes due to ultraviolet radiation**
Use additional code to identify the source of the ultraviolet radiation (W89, X32)

    L56.0 **Drug phototoxic response**
Use additional code for adverse effect, if applicable, to identify drug (T36-T50 with fifth or sixth character 5)

    L56.1 **Drug photoallergic response**
Use additional code for adverse effect, if applicable, to identify drug (T36-T50 with fifth or sixth character 5)

    L56.2 **Photocontact dermatitis [berloque dermatitis]**

    L56.3 **Solar urticaria**

    L56.4 **Polymorphous light eruption**

    L56.5 **Disseminated superficial actinic porokeratosis (DSAP)**

    L56.8 **Other specified acute skin changes due to ultraviolet radiation**

    L56.9 **Acute skin change due to ultraviolet radiation, unspecified**

● **L57** **Skin changes due to chronic exposure to nonionizing radiation**
Use additional code to identify the source of the ultraviolet radiation (W89, X32)

    L57.0 **Actinic keratosis**
Keratosis NOS   Solar keratosis
Senile keratosis

    L57.1 **Actinic reticuloid**

    L57.2 **Cutis rhomboidalis nuchae**

    L57.3 **Poikiloderma of Civatte**

    L57.4 **Cutis laxa senilis**
Elastosis senilis

    L57.5 **Actinic granuloma**

    L57.8 **Other skin changes due to chronic exposure to nonionizing radiation**
Farmer's skin   Solar dermatitis
Sailor's skin

    L57.9 **Skin changes due to chronic exposure to nonionizing radiation, unspecified**

● **L58** **Radiodermatitis**
Use additional code to identify the source of the radiation (W88, W90)

    L58.0 **Acute radiodermatitis**

    L58.1 **Chronic radiodermatitis**

    L58.9 **Radiodermatitis, unspecified**

● **L59** **Other disorders of skin and subcutaneous tissue related to radiation**

    L59.0 **Erythema ab igne [dermatitis ab igne]**

    L59.8 **Other specified disorders of the skin and subcutaneous tissue related to radiation**

    L59.9 **Disorder of the skin and subcutaneous tissue related to radiation, unspecified**

DISORDERS OF SKIN APPENDAGES (L60-L75)

Excludes1   congenital malformations of integument (Q84.-)

● **L60** **Nail disorders**

    Excludes2   clubbing of nails (R68.3)
onychia and paronychia (L03.0-)

    L60.0 **Ingrowing nail**

    L60.1 **Onycholysis**

    L60.2 **Onychogryphosis**

    L60.3 **Nail dystrophy**

    L60.4 **Beau's lines**

    L60.5 **Yellow nail syndrome**

    L60.8 **Other nail disorders**

    L60.9 **Nail disorder, unspecified**

▶ *L62* *Nail disorders in diseases classified elsewhere*
Code first underlying disease, such as:
pachydermoperiostosis (M89.4-)

Item 12–10 **Alopecia** is lack of hair and takes many forms. The most common is male pattern alopecia, also known as **androgenetic alopecia.** **Telogen effluvium** is early and excessive loss of hair resulting from a trauma to the hair follicle (fever, drugs, surgery, etc.).

Figure 12-8 Male pattern alopecia.

● **L63** **Alopecia areata**

    L63.0 **Alopecia (capitis) totalis**

    L63.1 **Alopecia universalis**

    L63.2 **Ophiasis**

    L63.8 **Other alopecia areata**

    L63.9 **Alopecia areata, unspecified**

● **L64** **Androgenic alopecia**

    Includes   male-pattern baldness

    L64.0 **Drug-induced androgenic alopecia**
Use additional code for adverse effect, if applicable, to identify drug (T36-T50 with fifth or sixth character 5)

    L64.8 **Other androgenic alopecia**

    L64.9 **Androgenic alopecia, unspecified**

● **L65** **Other nonscarring hair loss**
Use additional code for adverse effect, if applicable, to identify drug (T36-T50 with fifth or sixth character 5)

    Excludes1   trichotillomania (F63.3)

    L65.0 **Telogen effluvium**

    L65.1 **Anagen effluvium**

    L65.2 **Alopecia mucinosa**

    L65.8 **Other specified nonscarring hair loss**

    L65.9 **Nonscarring hair loss, unspecified**
Alopecia NOS

● **L66** **Cicatricial alopecia [scarring hair loss]**

    L66.0 **Pseudopelade**

    L66.1 **Lichen planopilaris**
Follicular lichen planus

    L66.2 **Folliculitis decalvans**

    L66.3 **Perifolliculitis capitis abscedens**

    L66.4 **Folliculitis ulerythematosa reticulata**

    L66.8 **Other cicatricial alopecia**
Coding Clinic: 2015, Q1, P19

    L66.9 **Cicatricial alopecia, unspecified**

● **L67** **Hair color and hair shaft abnormalities**

    Excludes1   monilethrix (Q84.1)
pili annulati (Q84.1)
telogen effluvium (L65.0)

    L67.0 **Trichorrhexis nodosa**

    L67.1 **Variations in hair color**
Canities
Greyness, hair (premature)
Heterochromia of hair
Poliosis circumscripta, acquired
Poliosis NOS

    L67.8 **Other hair color and hair shaft abnormalities**
Fragilitas crinium

    L67.9 **Hair color and hair shaft abnormality, unspecified**

● **L68**   **Hypertrichosis**
     Includes   excess hair
     Excludes1   congenital hypertrichosis (Q84.2)
                   persistent lanugo (Q84.2)

     L68.0   **Hirsutism**
           Excessive growth of hair
     L68.1   **Acquired hypertrichosis lanuginosa**
     L68.2   **Localized hypertrichosis**
     L68.3   **Polytrichia**
     L68.8   **Other hypertrichosis**
     L68.9   **Hypertrichosis, unspecified**

● **L70**   **Acne**
     Excludes2   acne keloid (L73.0)
     L70.0   **Acne vulgaris**
     L70.1   **Acne conglobata**
     L70.2   **Acne varioliformis**
           Acne necrotica miliaris
     L70.3   **Acne tropica**
     L70.4   **Infantile acne**   P
     L70.5   **Acné excoriée** ◀▥
           Acné excoriée des jeunes filles ◀
           Picker's acne
     L70.8   **Other acne**
     L70.9   **Acne, unspecified**

● **L71**   **Rosacea**
     Use additional code for adverse effect, if applicable, to identify drug (T36-T50 with fifth or sixth character 5)
     L71.0   **Perioral dermatitis**
     L71.1   **Rhinophyma**
     L71.8   **Other rosacea**
     L71.9   **Rosacea, unspecified**

● **L72**   **Follicular cysts of skin and subcutaneous tissue**
     L72.0   **Epidermal cyst**
   ● L72.1   **Pilar and trichodermal cyst**
         L72.11   **Pilar cyst**
         L72.12   **Trichodermal cyst**
                Trichilemmal (proliferating) cyst
     L72.3   **Sebaceous cyst**
         Excludes2   pilar cyst (L72.11)
                      trichilemmal (proliferating) cyst (L72.12)
     L72.2   **Steatocystoma multiplex**
     L72.8   **Other follicular cysts of the skin and subcutaneous tissue**
     L72.9   **Follicular cyst of the skin and subcutaneous tissue, unspecified**

● **L73**   **Other follicular disorders**
     L73.0   **Acne keloid**
     L73.1   **Pseudofolliculitis barbae**
     L73.2   **Hidradenitis suppurativa**
     L73.8   **Other specified follicular disorders**
           Sycosis barbae
     L73.9   **Follicular disorder, unspecified**

● **L74**   **Eccrine sweat disorders**
     Excludes2   generalized hyperhidrosis (R61)
     L74.0   **Miliaria rubra**
     L74.1   **Miliaria crystallina**
     L74.2   **Miliaria profunda**
           Miliaria tropicalis
     L74.3   **Miliaria, unspecified**
     L74.4   **Anhidrosis**
           Hypohidrosis

● L74.5   **Focal hyperhidrosis**
   ● L74.51   **Primary focal hyperhidrosis**
         L74.510   **Primary focal hyperhidrosis, axilla**
         L74.511   **Primary focal hyperhidrosis, face**
         L74.512   **Primary focal hyperhidrosis, palms**
         L74.513   **Primary focal hyperhidrosis, soles**
         L74.519   **Primary focal hyperhidrosis, unspecified**
     L74.52   **Secondary focal hyperhidrosis**
           Frey's syndrome
     L74.8   **Other eccrine sweat disorders**
     L74.9   **Eccrine sweat disorder, unspecified**
           Sweat gland disorder NOS

● **L75**   **Apocrine sweat disorders**
     Excludes1   dyshidrosis (L30.1)
                     hidradenitis suppurativa (L73.2)
     L75.0   **Bromhidrosis**
     L75.1   **Chromhidrosis**
     L75.2   **Apocrine miliaria**
           Fox-Fordyce disease
     L75.8   **Other apocrine sweat disorders**
     L75.9   **Apocrine sweat disorder, unspecified**
           Intraoperative and postprocedural complications of skin and subcutaneous tissue (L76)

INTRAOPERATIVE AND POSTPROCEDURAL COMPLICATIONS OF SKIN AND SUBCUTANEOUS TISSUE (L76)

● **L76**   **Intraoperative and postprocedural complications of skin and subcutaneous tissue**
   ● L76.0   **Intraoperative hemorrhage and hematoma of skin and subcutaneous tissue complicating a procedure**
         Excludes1   intraoperative hemorrhage and hematoma of skin and subcutaneous tissue due to accidental puncture and laceration during a procedure (L76.1-)
         L76.01   **Intraoperative hemorrhage and hematoma of skin and subcutaneous tissue complicating a dermatologic procedure**
         L76.02   **Intraoperative hemorrhage and hematoma of skin and subcutaneous tissue complicating other procedure**
   ● L76.1   **Accidental puncture and laceration of skin and subcutaneous tissue during a procedure**
         L76.11   **Accidental puncture and laceration of skin and subcutaneous tissue during a dermatologic procedure**
         L76.12   **Accidental puncture and laceration of skin and subcutaneous tissue during other procedure**
   ● L76.2   **Postprocedural hemorrhage of skin and subcutaneous tissue following a procedure** ◀▥
         L76.21   **Postprocedural hemorrhage of skin and subcutaneous tissue following a dermatologic procedure** ◀▥
         L76.22   **Postprocedural hemorrhage of skin and subcutaneous tissue following other procedure** ◀▥
   ● L76.3   **Postprocedural hematoma and seroma of skin and subcutaneous tissue following a procedure** ◀
         L76.31   **Postprocedural hematoma of skin and subcutaneous tissue following a dermatologic procedure** ◀
         L76.32   **Postprocedural hematoma of skin and subcutaneous tissue following other procedure** ◀
         L76.33   **Postprocedural seroma of skin and subcutaneous tissue following a dermatologic procedure** ◀
         L76.34   **Postprocedural seroma of skin and subcutaneous tissue following other procedure** ◀

● **L76.8** **Other intraoperative and postprocedural complications of skin and subcutaneous tissue**
> Use additional code, if applicable, to further specify disorder

     L76.81 **Other intraoperative complications of skin and subcutaneous tissue**

     L76.82 **Other postprocedural complications of skin and subcutaneous tissue**

OTHER DISORDERS OF THE SKIN AND SUBCUTANEOUS TISSUE (L80-L99)

L80 **Vitiligo**
> **Excludes2**   vitiligo of eyelids (H02.73-)
> vitiligo of vulva (N90.89)

● **L81** **Other disorders of pigmentation**
> **Excludes1**   birthmark NOS (Q82.5)
> Peutz-Jeghers syndrome (Q85.8)
>
> **Excludes2**   nevus - see Alphabetical Index

     L81.0 **Postinflammatory hyperpigmentation**

     L81.1 **Chloasma**

     L81.2 **Freckles**

     L81.3 **Café au lait spots**

     L81.4 **Other melanin hyperpigmentation**
> Lentigo

     L81.5 **Leukoderma, not elsewhere classified**

     L81.6 **Other disorders of diminished melanin formation**

     L81.7 **Pigmented purpuric dermatosis**
> Angioma serpiginosum

     L81.8 **Other specified disorders of pigmentation**
> Iron pigmentation
> Tattoo pigmentation

     L81.9 **Disorder of pigmentation, unspecified**

● **L82** **Seborrheic keratosis**
> **Includes**   basal cell papilloma ◀
> dermatosis papulosa nigra
> Leser-Trélat disease
>
> **Excludes2**   seborrheic dermatitis (L21.-)

     L82.0 **Inflamed seborrheic keratosis**

     L82.1 **Other seborrheic keratosis**
> Seborrheic keratosis NOS

L83 **Acanthosis nigricans**
> Confluent and reticulated papillomatosis

L84 **Corns and callosities**
> Callus
> Clavus

● **L85** **Other epidermal thickening**
> **Excludes2**   hypertrophic disorders of the skin (L91.-)

     L85.0 **Acquired ichthyosis**
> > **Excludes1**   congenital ichthyosis (Q80.-)

     L85.1 **Acquired keratosis [keratoderma] palmaris et plantaris**
> > **Excludes1**   inherited keratosis palmaris et plantaris (Q82.8)

     L85.2 **Keratosis punctata (palmaris et plantaris)**

     L85.3 **Xerosis cutis**
> Dry skin dermatitis

     L85.8 **Other specified epidermal thickening**
> Cutaneous horn

     L85.9 **Epidermal thickening, unspecified**

▌ *L86* *Keratoderma in diseases classified elsewhere*
> *Firm horny papules that have a cobblestone appearance.*
>
> *Code first underlying disease, such as:*
> Reiter's disease (M02.3-)
>
> **Excludes1**   gonococcal keratoderma (A54.89)
> gonococcal keratosis (A54.89)
> keratoderma due to vitamin A deficiency (E50.8)
> keratosis due to vitamin A deficiency (E50.8)
> xeroderma due to vitamin A deficiency (E50.8)

● **L87** **Transepidermal elimination disorders**
> **Excludes1**   granuloma annulare (perforating) (L92.0)

     L87.0 **Keratosis follicularis et parafollicularis in cutem penetrans**
> Kyrle disease
> Hyperkeratosis follicularis penetrans

     L87.1 **Reactive perforating collagenosis**

     L87.2 **Elastosis perforans serpiginosa**

     L87.8 **Other transepidermal elimination disorders**

     L87.9 **Transepidermal elimination disorder, unspecified**

L88 **Pyoderma gangrenosum**
> Phagedenic pyoderma
>
> **Excludes1**   dermatitis gangrenosa (L08.0)

OGCR Section I.B.14.

> General Coding Guidelines
>
> Documentation for BMI, *Depth of* Non-pressure ulcers, Pressure Ulcer Stages, **Coma Scale, and** *NIH Stroke Scale*
>
> For the Body Mass Index (BMI), depth of non-pressure chronic ulcers, pressure ulcer stage, **coma scale, and NIH stroke scale (NIHSS) codes,** code assignment may be based on medical record documentation from clinicians who are not the patient's provider (i.e., physician or other qualified healthcare practitioner legally accountable for establishing the patient's diagnosis), since this information is typically documented by other clinicians involved in the care of the patient (e.g., a dietitian often documents the BMI, a nurse often documents the pressure ulcer stages, **and an emergency medical technician often documents the coma scale**). However, the associated diagnosis (such as overweight, obesity, **acute stroke,** or pressure ulcer) must be documented by the patient's provider. If there is conflicting medical record documentation, either from the same clinician or different clinicians, the patient's attending provider should be queried for clarification. The BMI, **coma scale, and NHSS** codes should only be reported as secondary diagnoses.

● **L89** **Pressure ulcer**
> **Includes**   bed sore   pressure area
> decubitus ulcer   pressure sore
> plaster ulcer
>
> *Code first any associated gangrene (I96)*
>
> **Excludes2**   decubitus (trophic) ulcer of cervix (uteri) (N86)
> diabetic ulcers (E08.621, E08.622, E09.621, E09.622, E10.621, E10.622, E11.621, E11.622, E13.621, E13.622)
> non-pressure chronic ulcer of skin (L97.-)
> skin infections (L00-L08)
> varicose ulcer (I83.0, I83.2)

     ● **L89.0** **Pressure ulcer of elbow**

       ● **L89.00** **Pressure ulcer of unspecified elbow**

         L89.000 **Pressure ulcer of unspecified elbow, unstageable**

         L89.001 **Pressure ulcer of unspecified elbow, stage 1**
> Healing pressure ulcer of unspecified elbow, stage 1
> Pressure pre-ulcer skin changes limited to persistent focal edema, unspecified elbow

         L89.002 **Pressure ulcer of unspecified elbow, stage 2**
> Healing pressure ulcer of unspecified elbow, stage 2
> Pressure ulcer with abrasion, blister, partial thickness skin loss involving epidermis and/or dermis, unspecified elbow

         L89.003 **Pressure ulcer of unspecified elbow, stage 3**
> Healing pressure ulcer of unspecified elbow, stage 3
> Pressure ulcer with full thickness skin loss involving damage or necrosis of subcutaneous tissue, unspecified elbow

◀ New   ◀◀ Revised   deleted Deleted   Excludes 1   Excludes 2   Includes   Use additional   Code first   Code also   Unspecified

952   OGCR Official Guidelines   X Assign placeholder X   ● Use Additional Character(s)   ▌ Manifestation Code   **Coding Clinic**

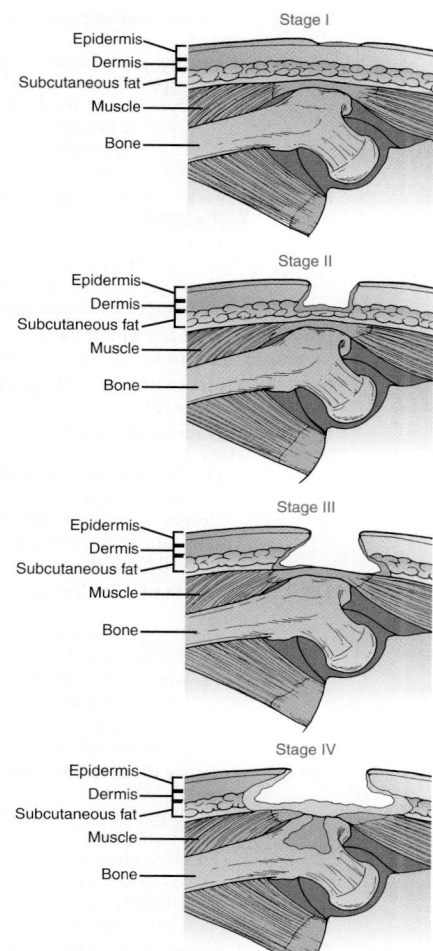

Figure 12-9   Stage I, II, III, and IV of pressure ulcers.

L89.004   **Pressure ulcer of unspecified elbow,
            stage 4**
            Healing pressure ulcer of
                unspecified elbow, stage 4
            Pressure ulcer with necrosis of soft
                tissues through to underlying
                muscle, tendon, or bone,
                unspecified elbow

L89.009   **Pressure ulcer of unspecified elbow,
            unspecified stage**
            Healing pressure ulcer of elbow
                NOS
            Healing pressure ulcer of
                unspecified elbow, unspecified
                stage

● L89.01   **Pressure ulcer of right elbow**

L89.010   **Pressure ulcer of right elbow,
            unstageable**

L89.011   **Pressure ulcer of right elbow, stage 1**
            Healing pressure ulcer of right
                elbow, stage 1
            Pressure pre-ulcer skin changes
                limited to persistent focal
                edema, right elbow

L89.012   **Pressure ulcer of right elbow, stage 2**
            Healing pressure ulcer of right
                elbow, stage 2
            Pressure ulcer with abrasion, blister,
                partial thickness skin loss
                involving epidermis and/or
                dermis, right elbow

L89.013   **Pressure ulcer of right elbow, stage 3**
            Healing pressure ulcer of right
                elbow, stage 3
            Pressure ulcer with full thickness
                skin loss involving damage or
                necrosis of subcutaneous tissue,
                right elbow

L89.014   **Pressure ulcer of right elbow, stage 4**
            Healing pressure ulcer of right
                elbow, stage 4
            Pressure ulcer with necrosis of soft
                tissues through to underlying
                muscle, tendon, or bone, right
                elbow

L89.019   **Pressure ulcer of right elbow,
            unspecified stage**
            Healing pressure right of elbow
                NOS
            Healing pressure ulcer of
                unspecified elbow, unspecified
                stage

● L89.02   **Pressure ulcer of left elbow**

L89.020   **Pressure ulcer of left elbow,
            unstageable**

L89.021   **Pressure ulcer of left elbow, stage 1**
            Healing pressure ulcer of left elbow,
                stage 1
            Pressure pre-ulcer skin changes
                limited to persistent focal
                edema, left elbow

L89.022   **Pressure ulcer of left elbow, stage 2**
            Healing pressure ulcer of left elbow,
                stage 2
            Pressure ulcer with abrasion, blister,
                partial thickness skin loss
                involving epidermis and/or
                dermis, left elbow

L89.023   **Pressure ulcer of left elbow, stage 3**
            Healing pressure ulcer of left elbow,
                stage 3
            Pressure ulcer with full thickness
                skin loss involving damage or
                necrosis of subcutaneous tissue,
                left elbow

L89.024   **Pressure ulcer of left elbow, stage 4**
            Healing pressure ulcer of left elbow,
                stage 4
            Pressure ulcer with necrosis of soft
                tissues through to underlying
                muscle, tendon, or bone, left
                elbow

L89.029   **Pressure ulcer of left elbow,
            unspecified stage**
            Healing pressure ulcer of left of
                elbow NOS
            Healing pressure ulcer of
                unspecified elbow, unspecified
                stage

CHAPTER 12 (L00-L99)

● **L89.1   Pressure ulcer of back**

  ● **L89.10   Pressure ulcer of unspecified part of back**

    L89.100   Pressure ulcer of unspecified part of back, unstageable

    L89.101   Pressure ulcer of unspecified part of back, stage 1
      Healing pressure ulcer of unspecified part of back, stage 1
      Pressure pre-ulcer skin changes limited to persistent focal edema, unspecified part of back

    L89.102   Pressure ulcer of unspecified part of back, stage 2
      Healing pressure ulcer of unspecified part of back, stage 2
      Pressure ulcer with abrasion, blister, partial thickness skin loss involving epidermis and/or dermis, unspecified part of back

    L89.103   Pressure ulcer of unspecified part of back, stage 3
      Healing pressure ulcer of unspecified part of back, stage 3
      Pressure ulcer with full thickness skin loss involving damage or necrosis of subcutaneous tissue, unspecified part of back

    L89.104   Pressure ulcer of unspecified part of back, stage 4
      Healing pressure ulcer of unspecified part of back, stage 4
      Pressure ulcer with necrosis of soft tissues through to underlying muscle, tendon, or bone, unspecified part of back

    L89.109   Pressure ulcer of unspecified part of back, unspecified stage
      Healing pressure ulcer of unspecified part of back NOS
      Healing pressure ulcer of unspecified part of back, unspecified stage

  ● **L89.11   Pressure ulcer of right upper back**
    Pressure ulcer of right shoulder blade

    L89.110   Pressure ulcer of right upper back, unstageable

    L89.111   Pressure ulcer of right upper back, stage 1
      Healing pressure ulcer of right upper back, stage 1
      Pressure pre-ulcer skin changes limited to persistent focal edema, right upper back

    L89.112   Pressure ulcer of right upper back, stage 2
      Healing pressure ulcer of right upper back, stage 2
      Pressure ulcer with abrasion, blister, partial thickness skin loss involving epidermis and/or dermis, right upper back

    L89.113   Pressure ulcer of right upper back, stage 3
      Healing pressure ulcer of right upper back, stage 3
      Pressure ulcer with full thickness skin loss involving damage or necrosis of subcutaneous tissue, right upper back

    L89.114   Pressure ulcer of right upper back, stage 4
      Healing pressure ulcer of right upper back, stage 4
      Pressure ulcer with necrosis of soft tissues through to underlying muscle, tendon, or bone, right upper back

    L89.119   Pressure ulcer of right upper back, unspecified stage
      Healing pressure ulcer of right upper back NOS
      Healing pressure ulcer of right upper back, unspecified stage

  ● **L89.12   Pressure ulcer of left upper back**
    Pressure ulcer of left shoulder blade

    L89.120   Pressure ulcer of left upper back, unstageable

    L89.121   Pressure ulcer of left upper back, stage 1
      Healing pressure ulcer of left upper back, stage 1
      Pressure pre-ulcer skin changes limited to persistent focal edema, left upper back

    L89.122   Pressure ulcer of left upper back, stage 2
      Healing pressure ulcer of left upper back, stage 2
      Pressure ulcer with abrasion, blister, partial thickness skin loss involving epidermis and/or dermis, left upper back

    L89.123   Pressure ulcer of left upper back, stage 3
      Healing pressure ulcer of left upper back, stage 3
      Pressure ulcer with full thickness skin loss involving damage or necrosis of subcutaneous tissue, left upper back

    L89.124   Pressure ulcer of left upper back, stage 4
      Healing pressure ulcer of left upper back, stage 4
      Pressure ulcer with necrosis of soft tissues through to underlying muscle, tendon, or bone, left upper back

    L89.129   Pressure ulcer of left upper back, unspecified stage
      Healing pressure ulcer of left upper back NOS
      Healing pressure ulcer of left upper back, unspecified stage

  ● **L89.13   Pressure ulcer of right lower back**

    L89.130   Pressure ulcer of right lower back, unstageable

    L89.131   Pressure ulcer of right lower back, stage 1
      Healing pressure ulcer of right lower back, stage 1
      Pressure pre-ulcer skin changes limited to persistent focal edema, right lower back

    L89.132   Pressure ulcer of right lower back, stage 2
      Healing pressure ulcer of right lower back, stage 2
      Pressure ulcer with abrasion, blister, partial thickness skin loss involving epidermis and/or dermis, right lower back

◄ New   ◄◄◄ Revised   ~~deleted~~ Deleted   Excludes 1   Excludes 2   Includes   Use additional   Code first   Code also   Unspecified
OGCR Official Guidelines   X Assign placeholder X   ● Use Additional Character(s)   ▶ Manifestation Code   **Coding Clinic**

L89.133   **Pressure ulcer of right lower back, stage 3**
     Healing pressure ulcer of right lower back, stage 3
     Pressure ulcer with full thickness skin loss involving damage or necrosis of subcutaneous tissue, right lower back

L89.134   **Pressure ulcer of right lower back, stage 4**
     Healing pressure ulcer of right lower back, stage 4
     Pressure ulcer with necrosis of soft tissues through to underlying muscle, tendon, or bone, right lower back

L89.139   **Pressure ulcer of right lower back, unspecified stage**
     Healing pressure ulcer of right lower back NOS
     Healing pressure ulcer of right lower back, unspecified stage

● **L89.14**   **Pressure ulcer of left lower back**

L89.140   **Pressure ulcer of left lower back, unstageable**

L89.141   **Pressure ulcer of left lower back, stage 1**
     Healing pressure ulcer of left lower back, stage 1
     Pressure pre-ulcer skin changes limited to persistent focal edema, left lower back

L89.142   **Pressure ulcer of left lower back, stage 2**
     Healing pressure ulcer of left lower back, stage 2
     Pressure ulcer with abrasion, blister, partial thickness skin loss involving epidermis and/or dermis, left lower back

L89.143   **Pressure ulcer of left lower back, stage 3**
     Healing pressure ulcer of left lower back, stage 3
     Pressure ulcer with full thickness skin loss involving damage or necrosis of subcutaneous tissue, left lower back

L89.144   **Pressure ulcer of left lower back, stage 4**
     Healing pressure ulcer of left lower back, stage 4
     Pressure ulcer with necrosis of soft tissues through to underlying muscle, tendon, or bone, left lower back

L89.149   **Pressure ulcer of left lower back, unspecified stage**
     Healing pressure ulcer of left lower back NOS
     Healing pressure ulcer of left lower back, unspecified stage

● **L89.15**   **Pressure ulcer of sacral region**
     Pressure ulcer of coccyx
     Pressure ulcer of tailbone

L89.150   **Pressure ulcer of sacral region, unstageable**

L89.151   **Pressure ulcer of sacral region, stage 1**
     Healing pressure ulcer of sacral region, stage 1
     Pressure pre-ulcer skin changes limited to persistent focal edema, sacral region

L89.152   **Pressure ulcer of sacral region, stage 2**
     Healing pressure ulcer of sacral region, stage 2
     Pressure ulcer with abrasion, blister, partial thickness skin loss involving epidermis and/or dermis, sacral region

L89.153   **Pressure ulcer of sacral region, stage 3**
     Healing pressure ulcer of sacral region, stage 3
     Pressure ulcer with full thickness skin loss involving damage or necrosis of subcutaneous tissue, sacral region

L89.154   **Pressure ulcer of sacral region, stage 4**
     Healing pressure ulcer of sacral region, stage 4
     Pressure ulcer with necrosis of soft tissues through to underlying muscle, tendon, or bone, sacral region

L89.159   **Pressure ulcer of sacral region, unspecified stage**
     Healing pressure ulcer of sacral region NOS
     Healing pressure ulcer of sacral region, unspecified stage

● **L89.2**   **Pressure ulcer of hip**

● **L89.20**   **Pressure ulcer of unspecified hip**

L89.200   **Pressure ulcer of unspecified hip, unstageable**

L89.201   **Pressure ulcer of unspecified hip, stage 1**
     Healing pressure ulcer of unspecified hip back, stage 1
     Pressure pre-ulcer skin changes limited to persistent focal edema, unspecified hip

L89.202   **Pressure ulcer of unspecified hip, stage 2**
     Healing pressure ulcer of unspecified hip, stage 2
     Pressure ulcer with abrasion, blister, partial thickness skin loss involving epidermis and/or dermis, unspecified hip

L89.203   **Pressure ulcer of unspecified hip, stage 3**
     Healing pressure ulcer of unspecified hip, stage 3
     Pressure ulcer with full thickness skin loss involving damage or necrosis of subcutaneous tissue, unspecified hip

L89.204   **Pressure ulcer of unspecified hip, stage 4**
     Healing pressure ulcer of unspecified hip, stage 4
     Pressure ulcer with necrosis of soft tissues through to underlying muscle, tendon, or bone, unspecified hip

L89.209   **Pressure ulcer of unspecified hip, unspecified stage**
     Healing pressure ulcer of unspecified hip NOS
     Healing pressure ulcer of unspecified hip, unspecified stage

CHAPTER 12 (L00-L99)

● **L89.21   Pressure ulcer of right hip**

L89.210   Pressure ulcer of right hip, unstageable

L89.211   Pressure ulcer of right hip, stage 1
Healing pressure ulcer of right hip back, stage 1
Pressure pre-ulcer skin changes limited to persistent focal edema, right hip

L89.212   Pressure ulcer of right hip, stage 2
Healing pressure ulcer of right hip, stage 2
Pressure ulcer with abrasion, blister, partial thickness skin loss involving epidermis and/or dermis, right hip

L89.213   Pressure ulcer of right hip, stage 3
Healing pressure ulcer of right hip, stage 3
Pressure ulcer with full thickness skin loss involving damage or necrosis of subcutaneous tissue, right hip

L89.214   Pressure ulcer of right hip, stage 4
Healing pressure ulcer of right hip, stage 4
Pressure ulcer with necrosis of soft tissues through to underlying muscle, tendon, or bone, right hip

L89.219   Pressure ulcer of right hip, unspecified stage
Healing pressure ulcer of right hip NOS
Healing pressure ulcer of right hip, unspecified stage

● **L89.22   Pressure ulcer of left hip**

L89.220   Pressure ulcer of left hip, unstageable

L89.221   Pressure ulcer of left hip, stage 1
Healing pressure ulcer of left hip back, stage 1
Pressure pre-ulcer skin changes limited to persistent focal edema, left hip

L89.222   Pressure ulcer of left hip, stage 2
Healing pressure ulcer of left hip, stage 2
Pressure ulcer with abrasion, blister, partial thickness skin loss involving epidermis and/or dermis, left hip

L89.223   Pressure ulcer of left hip, stage 3
Healing pressure ulcer of left hip, stage 3
Pressure ulcer with full thickness skin loss involving damage or necrosis of subcutaneous tissue, left hip

L89.224   Pressure ulcer of left hip, stage 4
Healing pressure ulcer of left hip, stage 4
Pressure ulcer with necrosis of soft tissues through to underlying muscle, tendon, or bone, left hip

L89.229   Pressure ulcer of left hip, unspecified stage
Healing pressure ulcer of left hip NOS
Healing pressure ulcer of left hip, unspecified stage

● **L89.3   Pressure ulcer of buttock**

● **L89.30   Pressure ulcer of unspecified buttock**

L89.300   Pressure ulcer of unspecified buttock, unstageable

L89.301   Pressure ulcer of unspecified buttock, stage 1
Healing pressure ulcer of unspecified buttock, stage 1
Pressure pre-ulcer skin changes limited to persistent focal edema, unspecified buttock

L89.302   Pressure ulcer of unspecified buttock, stage 2
Healing pressure ulcer of unspecified buttock, stage 2
Pressure ulcer with abrasion, blister, partial thickness skin loss involving epidermis and/or dermis, unspecified buttock

L89.303   Pressure ulcer of unspecified buttock, stage 3
Healing pressure ulcer of unspecified buttock, stage 3
Pressure ulcer with full thickness skin loss involving damage or necrosis of subcutaneous tissue, unspecified buttock

L89.304   Pressure ulcer of unspecified buttock, stage 4
Healing pressure ulcer of unspecified buttock, stage 4
Pressure ulcer with necrosis of soft tissues through to underlying muscle, tendon, or bone, unspecified buttock

L89.309   Pressure ulcer of unspecified buttock, unspecified stage
Healing pressure ulcer of unspecified buttock NOS
Healing pressure ulcer of unspecified buttock, unspecified stage

● **L89.31   Pressure ulcer of right buttock**

L89.310   Pressure ulcer of right buttock, unstageable

L89.311   Pressure ulcer of right buttock, stage 1
Healing pressure ulcer of right buttock, stage 1
Pressure pre-ulcer skin changes limited to persistent focal edema, right buttock

L89.312   Pressure ulcer of right buttock, stage 2
Healing pressure ulcer of right buttock, stage 2
Pressure ulcer with abrasion, blister, partial thickness skin loss involving epidermis and/or dermis, right buttock

L89.313   Pressure ulcer of right buttock, stage 3
Healing pressure ulcer of right buttock, stage 3
Pressure ulcer with full thickness skin loss involving damage or necrosis of subcutaneous tissue, right buttock

◀ New   ◀▥ Revised   deleted Deleted   Excludes 1   Excludes 2   Includes   Use additional   Code first   Code also   Unspecified

OGCR Official Guidelines   X Assign placeholder X   ● Use Additional Character(s)   ▶ Manifestation Code   **Coding Clinic**

L89.314   Pressure ulcer of right buttock, stage 4
    Healing pressure ulcer of right buttock, stage 4
    Pressure ulcer with necrosis of soft tissues through to underlying muscle, tendon, or bone, right buttock

L89.319   Pressure ulcer of right buttock, unspecified stage
    Healing pressure ulcer of right buttock NOS
    Healing pressure ulcer of right buttock, unspecified stage

● **L89.32**   Pressure ulcer of left buttock

L89.320   Pressure ulcer of left buttock, unstageable

L89.321   Pressure ulcer of left buttock, stage 1
    Healing pressure ulcer of left buttock, stage 1
    Pressure pre-ulcer skin changes limited to persistent focal edema, left buttock

L89.322   Pressure ulcer of left buttock, stage 2
    Healing pressure ulcer of left buttock, stage 2
    Pressure ulcer with abrasion, blister, partial thickness skin loss involving epidermis and/or dermis, left buttock

L89.323   Pressure ulcer of left buttock, stage 3
    Healing pressure ulcer of left buttock, stage 3
    Pressure ulcer with full thickness skin loss involving damage or necrosis of subcutaneous tissue, left buttock

L89.324   Pressure ulcer of left buttock, stage 4
    Healing pressure ulcer of left buttock, stage 4
    Pressure ulcer with necrosis of soft tissues through to underlying muscle, tendon, or bone, left buttock

L89.329   Pressure ulcer of left buttock, unspecified stage
    Healing pressure ulcer of left buttock NOS
    Healing pressure ulcer of left buttock, unspecified stage

● **L89.4**   Pressure ulcer of contiguous site of back, buttock and hip

L89.40   Pressure ulcer of contiguous site of back, buttock and hip, unspecified stage
    Healing pressure ulcer of contiguous site of back, buttock and hip NOS
    Healing pressure ulcer of contiguous site of back, buttock and hip, unspecified stage

L89.41   Pressure ulcer of contiguous site of back, buttock and hip, stage 1
    Healing pressure ulcer of contiguous site of back, buttock and hip, stage 1
    Pressure pre-ulcer skin changes limited to persistent focal edema, contiguous site of back, buttock and hip

L89.42   Pressure ulcer of contiguous site of back, buttock and hip, stage 2
    Healing pressure ulcer of contiguous site of back, buttock and hip, stage 2
    Pressure ulcer with abrasion, blister, partial thickness skin loss involving epidermis and/or dermis, contiguous site of back, buttock and hip

L89.43   Pressure ulcer of contiguous site of back, buttock and hip, stage 3
    Healing pressure ulcer of contiguous site of back, buttock and hip, stage 3
    Pressure ulcer with full thickness skin loss involving damage or necrosis of subcutaneous tissue, contiguous site of back, buttock and hip

L89.44   Pressure ulcer of contiguous site of back, buttock and hip, stage 4
    Healing pressure ulcer of contiguous site of back, buttock and hip, stage 4
    Pressure ulcer with necrosis of soft tissues through to underlying muscle, tendon, or bone, contiguous site of back, buttock and hip

L89.45   Pressure ulcer of contiguous site of back, buttock and hip, unstageable

● **L89.5**   Pressure ulcer of ankle

● **L89.50**   Pressure ulcer of unspecified ankle

L89.500   Pressure ulcer of unspecified ankle, unstageable

L89.501   Pressure ulcer of unspecified ankle, stage 1
    Healing pressure ulcer of unspecified ankle, stage 1
    Pressure pre-ulcer skin changes limited to persistent focal edema, unspecified ankle

L89.502   Pressure ulcer of unspecified ankle, stage 2
    Healing pressure ulcer of unspecified ankle, stage 2
    Pressure ulcer with abrasion, blister, partial thickness skin loss involving epidermis and/or dermis, unspecified ankle

L89.503   Pressure ulcer of unspecified ankle, stage 3
    Healing pressure ulcer of unspecified ankle, stage 3
    Pressure ulcer with full thickness skin loss involving damage or necrosis of subcutaneous tissue, unspecified ankle

L89.504   Pressure ulcer of unspecified ankle, stage 4
    Healing pressure ulcer of unspecified ankle, stage 4
    Pressure ulcer with necrosis of soft tissues through to underlying muscle, tendon, or bone, unspecified ankle

L89.509   Pressure ulcer of unspecified ankle, unspecified stage
    Healing pressure ulcer of unspecified ankle NOS
    Healing pressure ulcer of unspecified ankle, unspecified stage

CHAPTER 12 (L00-L99)

CHAPTER 12 (L00–L99)

● **L89.51**   **Pressure ulcer of right ankle**

    L89.510   **Pressure ulcer of right ankle, unstageable**

    L89.511   **Pressure ulcer of right ankle, stage 1**
       Healing pressure ulcer of right ankle, stage 1
       Pressure pre-ulcer skin changes limited to persistent focal edema, right ankle

    L89.512   **Pressure ulcer of right ankle, stage 2**
       Healing pressure ulcer of right ankle, stage 2
       Pressure ulcer with abrasion, blister, partial thickness skin loss involving epidermis and/or dermis, right ankle

    L89.513   **Pressure ulcer of right ankle, stage 3**
       Healing pressure ulcer of right ankle, stage 3
       Pressure ulcer with full thickness skin loss involving damage or necrosis of subcutaneous tissue, right ankle

    L89.514   **Pressure ulcer of right ankle, stage 4**
       Healing pressure ulcer of right ankle, stage 4
       Pressure ulcer with necrosis of soft tissues through to underlying muscle, tendon, or bone, right ankle

    L89.519   **Pressure ulcer of right ankle, unspecified stage**
       Healing pressure ulcer of right ankle NOS
       Healing pressure ulcer of right ankle, unspecified stage

● **L89.52**   **Pressure ulcer of left ankle**

    L89.520   **Pressure ulcer of left ankle, unstageable**

    L89.521   **Pressure ulcer of left ankle, stage 1**
       Healing pressure ulcer of left ankle, stage 1
       Pressure pre-ulcer skin changes limited to persistent focal edema, left ankle ◀▥

    L89.522   **Pressure ulcer of left ankle, stage 2**
       Healing pressure ulcer of left ankle, stage 2
       Pressure ulcer with abrasion, blister, partial thickness skin loss involving epidermis and/or dermis, left ankle

    L89.523   **Pressure ulcer of left ankle, stage 3**
       Healing pressure ulcer of left ankle, stage 3
       Pressure ulcer with full thickness skin loss involving damage or necrosis of subcutaneous tissue, left ankle

    L89.524   **Pressure ulcer of left ankle, stage 4**
       Healing pressure ulcer of left ankle, stage 4
       Pressure ulcer with necrosis of soft tissues through to underlying muscle, tendon, or bone, left ankle

    L89.529   **Pressure ulcer of left ankle, unspecified stage**
       Healing pressure ulcer of left ankle NOS
       Healing pressure ulcer of left ankle, unspecified stage

● **L89.6**   **Pressure ulcer of heel**

  ● **L89.60**   **Pressure ulcer of unspecified heel**

    L89.600   **Pressure ulcer of unspecified heel, unstageable**

    L89.601   **Pressure ulcer of unspecified heel, stage 1**
       Healing pressure ulcer of unspecified heel, stage 1
       Pressure pre-ulcer skin changes limited to persistent focal edema, unspecified heel

    L89.602   **Pressure ulcer of unspecified heel, stage 2**
       Healing pressure ulcer of unspecified heel, stage 2
       Pressure ulcer with abrasion, blister, partial thickness skin loss involving epidermis and/or dermis, unspecified heel

    L89.603   **Pressure ulcer of unspecified heel, stage 3**
       Healing pressure ulcer of unspecified heel, stage 3
       Pressure ulcer with full thickness skin loss involving damage or necrosis of subcutaneous tissue, unspecified heel

    L89.604   **Pressure ulcer of unspecified heel, stage 4**
       Healing pressure ulcer of unspecified heel, stage 4
       Pressure ulcer with necrosis of soft tissues through to underlying muscle, tendon, or bone, unspecified heel

    L89.609   **Pressure ulcer of unspecified heel, unspecified stage**
       Healing pressure ulcer of unspecified heel NOS
       Healing pressure ulcer of unspecified heel, unspecified stage

  ● **L89.61**   **Pressure ulcer of right heel**

    L89.610   **Pressure ulcer of right heel, unstageable**

    L89.611   **Pressure ulcer of right heel, stage 1**
       Healing pressure ulcer of right heel, stage 1
       Pressure pre-ulcer skin changes limited to persistent focal edema, right heel

    L89.612   **Pressure ulcer of right heel, stage 2**
       Healing pressure ulcer of right heel, stage 2
       Pressure ulcer with abrasion, blister, partial thickness skin loss involving epidermis and/or dermis, right heel

    L89.613   **Pressure ulcer of right heel, stage 3**
       Healing pressure ulcer of right heel, stage 3
       Pressure ulcer with full thickness skin loss involving damage or necrosis of subcutaneous tissue, right heel

    L89.614   **Pressure ulcer of right heel, stage 4**
       Healing pressure ulcer of right heel, stage 4
       Pressure ulcer with necrosis of soft tissues through to underlying muscle, tendon, or bone, right heel

    L89.619   **Pressure ulcer of right heel, unspecified stage**
       Healing pressure ulcer of right heel NOS
       Healing pressure ulcer of unspecified heel, right stage

◀ New   ◀▥ Revised   ~~deleted~~ Deleted   Excludes 1   Excludes 2   Includes   Use additional   Code first   Code also   Unspecified

OGCR Official Guidelines   X Assign placeholder X   ● Use Additional Character(s)   ▶ Manifestation Code   **Coding Clinic**

● **L89.62**   **Pressure ulcer of left heel**

     L89.620   **Pressure ulcer of left heel, unstageable**

     L89.621   **Pressure ulcer of left heel, stage 1**
         Healing pressure ulcer of left heel, stage 1
         Pressure pre-ulcer skin changes limited to persistent focal edema, left heel

     L89.622   **Pressure ulcer of left heel, stage 2**
         Healing pressure ulcer of left heel, stage 2
         Pressure ulcer with abrasion, blister, partial thickness skin loss involving epidermis and/or dermis, left heel

     L89.623   **Pressure ulcer of left heel, stage 3**
         Healing pressure ulcer of left heel, stage 3
         Pressure ulcer with full thickness skin loss involving damage or necrosis of subcutaneous tissue, left heel

     L89.624   **Pressure ulcer of left heel, stage 4**
         Healing pressure ulcer of left heel, stage 4
         Pressure ulcer with necrosis of soft tissues through to underlying muscle, tendon, or bone, left heel

     L89.629   **Pressure ulcer of left heel, unspecified stage**
         Healing pressure ulcer of left heel NOS
         Healing pressure ulcer of left heel, unspecified stage

● **L89.8**   **Pressure ulcer of other site**

   ● **L89.81**   **Pressure ulcer of head**
         Pressure ulcer of face

     L89.810   **Pressure ulcer of head, unstageable**

     L89.811   **Pressure ulcer of head, stage 1**
         Healing pressure ulcer of head, stage 1
         Pressure pre-ulcer skin changes limited to persistent focal edema, head

     L89.812   **Pressure ulcer of head, stage 2**
         Healing pressure ulcer of head, stage 2
         Pressure ulcer with abrasion, blister, partial thickness skin loss involving epidermis and/or dermis, head

     L89.813   **Pressure ulcer of head, stage 3**
         Healing pressure ulcer of head, stage 3
         Pressure ulcer with full thickness skin loss involving damage or necrosis of subcutaneous tissue, head

     L89.814   **Pressure ulcer of head, stage 4**
         Healing pressure ulcer of head, stage 4
         Pressure ulcer with necrosis of soft tissues through to underlying muscle, tendon, or bone, head

     L89.819   **Pressure ulcer of head, unspecified stage**
         Healing pressure ulcer of head NOS
         Healing pressure ulcer of head, unspecified stage

● **L89.89**   **Pressure ulcer of other site**

     L89.890   **Pressure ulcer of other site, unstageable**

     L89.891   **Pressure ulcer of other site, stage 1**
         Healing pressure ulcer of other site, stage 1
         Pressure pre-ulcer skin changes limited to persistent focal edema, other site

     L89.892   **Pressure ulcer of other site, stage 2**
         Healing pressure ulcer of other site, stage 2
         Pressure ulcer with abrasion, blister, partial thickness skin loss involving epidermis and/or dermis, other site

     L89.893   **Pressure ulcer of other site, stage 3**
         Healing pressure ulcer of other site, stage 3
         Pressure ulcer with full thickness skin loss involving damage or necrosis of subcutaneous tissue, other site

     L89.894   **Pressure ulcer of other site, stage 4**
         Healing pressure ulcer of other site, stage 4
         Pressure ulcer with necrosis of soft tissues through to underlying muscle, tendon, or bone, other site

     L89.899   **Pressure ulcer of other site, unspecified stage**
         Healing pressure ulcer of other site NOS
         Healing pressure ulcer of other site, unspecified stage

● **L89.9**   **Pressure ulcer of unspecified site**

     L89.90   **Pressure ulcer of unspecified site, unspecified stage**
         Healing pressure ulcer of unspecified site NOS
         Healing pressure ulcer of unspecified site, unspecified stage

     L89.91   **Pressure ulcer of unspecified site, stage 1**
         Healing pressure ulcer of unspecified site, stage 1
         Pressure pre-ulcer skin changes limited to persistent focal edema, unspecified site

     L89.92   **Pressure ulcer of unspecified site, stage 2**
         Healing pressure ulcer of unspecified site, stage 2
         Pressure ulcer with abrasion, blister, partial thickness skin loss involving epidermis and/or dermis, unspecified site

     L89.93   **Pressure ulcer of unspecified site, stage 3**
         Healing pressure ulcer of unspecified site, stage 3
         Pressure ulcer with full thickness skin loss involving damage or necrosis of subcutaneous tissue, unspecified site

     L89.94   **Pressure ulcer of unspecified site, stage 4**
         Healing pressure ulcer of unspecified site, stage 4
         Pressure ulcer with necrosis of soft tissues through to underlying muscle, tendon, or bone, unspecified site

     L89.95   **Pressure ulcer of unspecified site, unstageable**

CHAPTER 12 (L00-L99)

CHAPTER 12 (L00-L99)

● **L90 Atrophic disorders of skin**

L90.0 Lichen sclerosus et atrophicus

> **Excludes2** lichen sclerosus of external female genital organs (N90.4)
> lichen sclerosus of external male genital organs (N48.0)

L90.1 Anetoderma of Schweninger-Buzzi

L90.2 Anetoderma of Jadassohn-Pellizzari

L90.3 Atrophoderma of Pasini and Pierini

L90.4 Acrodermatitis chronica atrophicans

L90.5 Scar conditions and fibrosis of skin
> Adherent scar (skin)
> Cicatrix
> Disfigurement of skin due to scar
> Fibrosis of skin NOS
> Scar NOS

> **Excludes2** hypertrophic scar (L91.0)
> keloid scar (L91.0)
> Coding Clinic: 2016, Q2, P5; 2015, Q1, P19

L90.6 Striae atrophicae

L90.8 Other atrophic disorders of skin

L90.9 Atrophic disorder of skin, unspecified

● **L91 Hypertrophic disorders of skin**

L91.0 Keloid scar
> Hypertrophic scar
> Keloid

> **Excludes2** acne keloid (L73.0)
> scar NOS (L90.5)

L91.8 Other hypertrophic disorders of the skin

L91.9 Hypertrophic disorder of the skin, unspecified

● **L92 Granulomatous disorders of skin and subcutaneous tissue**

> **Excludes2** actinic granuloma (L57.5)

L92.0 Granuloma annulare
> Perforating granuloma annulare

L92.1 Necrobiosis lipoidica, not elsewhere classified

> **Excludes1** necrobiosis lipoidica associated with diabetes mellitus (E08-E13 with .620)

L92.2 Granuloma faciale [eosinophilic granuloma of skin]

L92.3 Foreign body granuloma of the skin and subcutaneous tissue

> Use additional code to identify the type of retained foreign body (Z18.-)

L92.8 Other granulomatous disorders of the skin and subcutaneous tissue

L92.9 Granulomatous disorder of the skin and subcutaneous tissue, unspecified

● **L93 Lupus erythematosus**

> Use additional code for adverse effect, if applicable, to identify drug (T36-T50 with fifth or sixth character 5)

> **Excludes1** lupus exedens (A18.4)
> lupus vulgaris (A18.4)
> scleroderma (M34.-)
> systemic lupus erythematosus (M32.-)

L93.0 Discoid lupus erythematosus
> Lupus erythematosus NOS

L93.1 Subacute cutaneous lupus erythematosus

L93.2 Other local lupus erythematosus
> Lupus erythematosus profundus
> Lupus panniculitis

● **L94 Other localized connective tissue disorders**

> **Excludes1** systemic connective tissue disorders (M30-M36)

L94.0 Localized scleroderma [morphea]
> Circumscribed scleroderma

L94.1 Linear scleroderma
> En coup de sabre lesion

L94.2 Calcinosis cutis

L94.3 Sclerodactyly

L94.4 Gottron's papules

L94.5 Poikiloderma vasculare atrophicans

L94.6 Ainhum

L94.8 Other specified localized connective tissue disorders

L94.9 Localized connective tissue disorder, unspecified

● **L95 Vasculitis limited to skin, not elsewhere classified**

> **Excludes1** angioma serpiginosum (L81.7)
> Henoch(-Schönlein) purpura (D69.0)
> hypersensitivity angiitis (M31.0)
> lupus panniculitis (L93.2)
> panniculitis NOS (M79.3)
> panniculitis of neck and back (M54.0-)
> polyarteritis nodosa (M30.0)
> relapsing panniculitis (M35.6)
> rheumatoid vasculitis (M05.2)
> serum sickness (T80.6-)
> urticaria (L50.-)
> Wegener's granulomatosis (M31.3-)

L95.0 Livedoid vasculitis
> Atrophie blanche (en plaque)

L95.1 Erythema elevatum diutinum

L95.8 Other vasculitis limited to the skin

L95.9 Vasculitis limited to the skin, unspecified

● **L97 Non-pressure chronic ulcer of lower limb, not elsewhere classified**

> **Includes** chronic ulcer of skin of lower limb NOS
> non-healing ulcer of skin
> non-infected sinus of skin
> trophic ulcer NOS
> tropical ulcer NOS
> ulcer of skin of lower limb NOS

> *Code first any associated underlying condition, such as:*
> any associated gangrene (I96)
> atherosclerosis of the lower extremities (I70.23-, I70.24-, I70.33-, I70.34-, I70.43-, I70.44-, I70.53-, I70.54-, I70.63-, I70.64-, I70.73-, I70.74-)
> chronic venous hypertension (I87.31-, I87.33-)
> diabetic ulcers (E08.621, E08.622, E09.621, E09.622, E10.621, E10.622, E11.621, E11.622, E13.621, E13.622)
> postphlebitic syndrome (I87.01-, I87.03-)
> postthrombotic syndrome (I87.01-, I87.03-)
> varicose ulcer (I83.0-, I83.2-)

> **Excludes2** pressure ulcer (pressure area) (L89.-)
> skin infections (L00-L08)
> specific infections classified to A00-B99

● **L97.1 Non-pressure chronic ulcer of thigh**

● **L97.10 Non-pressure chronic ulcer of unspecified thigh**

L97.101 Non-pressure chronic ulcer of unspecified thigh limited to breakdown of skin

L97.102 Non-pressure chronic ulcer of unspecified thigh with fat layer exposed

L97.103 Non-pressure chronic ulcer of unspecified thigh with necrosis of muscle

L97.104 Non-pressure chronic ulcer of unspecified thigh with necrosis of bone

L97.109 Non-pressure chronic ulcer of unspecified thigh with unspecified severity

Item 12–11 Scleroderma means hard skin. It is a group of diseases that causes abnormal growth of connective tissues that support the skin and organs. There are two types: localized scleroderma affecting the skin and systemic scleroderma affecting blood vessels and internal organs and the skin.

◀ New   ◀ Revised   ~~deleted~~ Deleted   Excludes 1   Excludes 2   Includes   Use additional   Code first   Code also   Unspecified

OGCR Official Guidelines   X Assign placeholder X   ● Use Additional Character(s)   ▶ Manifestation Code   **Coding Clinic**

● L97.11   Non-pressure chronic ulcer of right thigh

     L97.111   Non-pressure chronic ulcer of right thigh limited to breakdown of skin

     L97.112   Non-pressure chronic ulcer of right thigh with fat layer exposed

     L97.113   Non-pressure chronic ulcer of right thigh with necrosis of muscle

     L97.114   Non-pressure chronic ulcer of right thigh with necrosis of bone

     L97.119   Non-pressure chronic ulcer of right thigh with unspecified severity

● L97.12   Non-pressure chronic ulcer of left thigh

     L97.121   Non-pressure chronic ulcer of left thigh limited to breakdown of skin

     L97.122   Non-pressure chronic ulcer of left thigh with fat layer exposed

     L97.123   Non-pressure chronic ulcer of left thigh with necrosis of muscle

     L97.124   Non-pressure chronic ulcer of left thigh with necrosis of bone

     L97.129   Non-pressure chronic ulcer of left thigh with unspecified severity

● L97.2   Non-pressure chronic ulcer of calf

 ● L97.20   Non-pressure chronic ulcer of unspecified calf

     L97.201   Non-pressure chronic ulcer of unspecified calf limited to breakdown of skin

     L97.202   Non-pressure chronic ulcer of unspecified calf with fat layer exposed

     L97.203   Non-pressure chronic ulcer of unspecified calf with necrosis of muscle

     L97.204   Non-pressure chronic ulcer of unspecified calf with necrosis of bone

     L97.209   Non-pressure chronic ulcer of unspecified calf with unspecified severity

 ● L97.21   Non-pressure chronic ulcer of right calf

     L97.211   Non-pressure chronic ulcer of right calf limited to breakdown of skin

     L97.212   Non-pressure chronic ulcer of right calf with fat layer exposed

     L97.213   Non-pressure chronic ulcer of right calf with necrosis of muscle

     L97.214   Non-pressure chronic ulcer of right calf with necrosis of bone

     L97.219   Non-pressure chronic ulcer of right calf with unspecified severity

 ● L97.22   Non-pressure chronic ulcer of left calf

     L97.221   Non-pressure chronic ulcer of left calf limited to breakdown of skin

     L97.222   Non-pressure chronic ulcer of left calf with fat layer exposed

     L97.223   Non-pressure chronic ulcer of left calf with necrosis of muscle

     L97.224   Non-pressure chronic ulcer of left calf with necrosis of bone

     L97.229   Non-pressure chronic ulcer of left calf with unspecified severity

● L97.3   Non-pressure chronic ulcer of ankle

 ● L97.30   Non-pressure chronic ulcer of unspecified ankle

     L97.301   Non-pressure chronic ulcer of unspecified ankle limited to breakdown of skin

     L97.302   Non-pressure chronic ulcer of unspecified ankle with fat layer exposed

     L97.303   Non-pressure chronic ulcer of unspecified ankle with necrosis of muscle

     L97.304   Non-pressure chronic ulcer of unspecified ankle with necrosis of bone

     L97.309   Non-pressure chronic ulcer of unspecified ankle with unspecified severity

● L97.31   Non-pressure chronic ulcer of right ankle

     L97.311   Non-pressure chronic ulcer of right ankle limited to breakdown of skin

     L97.312   Non-pressure chronic ulcer of right ankle with fat layer exposed

     L97.313   Non-pressure chronic ulcer of right ankle with necrosis of muscle

     L97.314   Non-pressure chronic ulcer of right ankle with necrosis of bone

     L97.319   Non-pressure chronic ulcer of right ankle with unspecified severity

● L97.32   Non-pressure chronic ulcer of left ankle

     L97.321   Non-pressure chronic ulcer of left ankle limited to breakdown of skin

     L97.322   Non-pressure chronic ulcer of left ankle with fat layer exposed

     L97.323   Non-pressure chronic ulcer of left ankle with necrosis of muscle

     L97.324   Non-pressure chronic ulcer of left ankle with necrosis of bone

     L97.329   Non-pressure chronic ulcer of left ankle with unspecified severity

● L97.4   Non-pressure chronic ulcer of heel and midfoot

     Non-pressure chronic ulcer of plantar surface of midfoot

 ● L97.40   Non-pressure chronic ulcer of unspecified heel and midfoot

     L97.401   Non-pressure chronic ulcer of unspecified heel and midfoot limited to breakdown of skin

     L97.402   Non-pressure chronic ulcer of unspecified heel and midfoot with fat layer exposed

     L97.403   Non-pressure chronic ulcer of unspecified heel and midfoot with necrosis of muscle

     L97.404   Non-pressure chronic ulcer of unspecified heel and midfoot with necrosis of bone

     L97.409   Non-pressure chronic ulcer of unspecified heel and midfoot with unspecified severity

 ● L97.41   Non-pressure chronic ulcer of right heel and midfoot

     L97.411   Non-pressure chronic ulcer of right heel and midfoot limited to breakdown of skin

     L97.412   Non-pressure chronic ulcer of right heel and midfoot with fat layer exposed

     L97.413   Non-pressure chronic ulcer of right heel and midfoot with necrosis of muscle

     L97.414   Non-pressure chronic ulcer of right heel and midfoot with necrosis of bone

     L97.419   Non-pressure chronic ulcer of right heel and midfoot with unspecified severity

● **L97.42** Non-pressure chronic ulcer of left heel and midfoot

    L97.421 Non-pressure chronic ulcer of left heel and midfoot limited to breakdown of skin
        Coding Clinic: 2016, Q1, P13

    L97.422 Non-pressure chronic ulcer of left heel and midfoot with fat layer exposed

    L97.423 Non-pressure chronic ulcer of left heel and midfoot with necrosis of muscle

    L97.424 Non-pressure chronic ulcer of left heel and midfoot with necrosis of bone

    L97.429 Non-pressure chronic ulcer of left heel and midfoot with unspecified severity

● **L97.5** Non-pressure chronic ulcer of other part of foot
    Non-pressure chronic ulcer of toe

  ● **L97.50** Non-pressure chronic ulcer of other part of unspecified foot

    L97.501 Non-pressure chronic ulcer of other part of unspecified foot limited to breakdown of skin

    L97.502 Non-pressure chronic ulcer of other part of unspecified foot with fat layer exposed

    L97.503 Non-pressure chronic ulcer of other part of unspecified foot with necrosis of muscle

    L97.504 Non-pressure chronic ulcer of other part of unspecified foot with necrosis of bone

    L97.509 Non-pressure chronic ulcer of other part of unspecified foot with unspecified severity

  ● **L97.51** Non-pressure chronic ulcer of other part of right foot

    L97.511 Non-pressure chronic ulcer of other part of right foot limited to breakdown of skin

    L97.512 Non-pressure chronic ulcer of other part of right foot with fat layer exposed

    L97.513 Non-pressure chronic ulcer of other part of right foot with necrosis of muscle

    L97.514 Non-pressure chronic ulcer of other part of right foot with necrosis of bone

    L97.519 Non-pressure chronic ulcer of other part of right foot with unspecified severity

  ● **L97.52** Non-pressure chronic ulcer of other part of left foot

    L97.521 Non-pressure chronic ulcer of other part of left foot limited to breakdown of skin

    L97.522 Non-pressure chronic ulcer of other part of left foot with fat layer exposed

    L97.523 Non-pressure chronic ulcer of other part of left foot with necrosis of muscle

    L97.524 Non-pressure chronic ulcer of other part of left foot with necrosis of bone

    L97.529 Non-pressure chronic ulcer of other part of left foot with unspecified severity

● **L97.8** Non-pressure chronic ulcer of other part of lower leg

  ● **L97.80** Non-pressure chronic ulcer of other part of unspecified lower leg

    L97.801 Non-pressure chronic ulcer of other part of unspecified lower leg limited to breakdown of skin

    L97.802 Non-pressure chronic ulcer of other part of unspecified lower leg with fat layer exposed

    L97.803 Non-pressure chronic ulcer of other part of unspecified lower leg with necrosis of muscle

    L97.804 Non-pressure chronic ulcer of other part of unspecified lower leg with necrosis of bone

    L97.809 Non-pressure chronic ulcer of other part of unspecified lower leg with unspecified severity

  ● **L97.81** Non-pressure chronic ulcer of other part of right lower leg

    L97.811 Non-pressure chronic ulcer of other part of right lower leg limited to breakdown of skin

    L97.812 Non-pressure chronic ulcer of other part of right lower leg with fat layer exposed

    L97.813 Non-pressure chronic ulcer of other part of right lower leg with necrosis of muscle

    L97.814 Non-pressure chronic ulcer of other part of right lower leg with necrosis of bone

    L97.819 Non-pressure chronic ulcer of other part of right lower leg with unspecified severity

  ● **L97.82** Non-pressure chronic ulcer of other part of left lower leg

    L97.821 Non-pressure chronic ulcer of other part of left lower leg limited to breakdown of skin

    L97.822 Non-pressure chronic ulcer of other part of left lower leg with fat layer exposed

    L97.823 Non-pressure chronic ulcer of other part of left lower leg with necrosis of muscle

    L97.824 Non-pressure chronic ulcer of other part of left lower leg with necrosis of bone

    L97.829 Non-pressure chronic ulcer of other part of left lower leg with unspecified severity

● **L97.9** Non-pressure chronic ulcer of unspecified part of lower leg

  ● **L97.90** Non-pressure chronic ulcer of unspecified part of unspecified lower leg

    L97.901 Non-pressure chronic ulcer of unspecified part of unspecified lower leg limited to breakdown of skin

    L97.902 Non-pressure chronic ulcer of unspecified part of unspecified lower leg with fat layer exposed

    L97.903 Non-pressure chronic ulcer of unspecified part of unspecified lower leg with necrosis of muscle

    L97.904 Non-pressure chronic ulcer of unspecified part of unspecified lower leg with necrosis of bone

    L97.909 Non-pressure chronic ulcer of unspecified part of unspecified lower leg with unspecified severity

◀ New   ◀━ Revised   ~~deleted~~ Deleted   Excludes 1   Excludes 2   Includes   Use additional   Code first   Code also   Unspecified

962   OGCR Official Guidelines   X Assign placeholder X   ● Use Additional Character(s)   ▷ Manifestation Code   **Coding Clinic**

CHAPTER 12 (L00-L99)

● **L97.91**   **Non-pressure chronic ulcer of unspecified part of right lower leg**

    L97.911   Non-pressure chronic ulcer of unspecified part of right lower leg limited to breakdown of skin

    L97.912   Non-pressure chronic ulcer of unspecified part of right lower leg with fat layer exposed

    L97.913   Non-pressure chronic ulcer of unspecified part of right lower leg with necrosis of muscle

    L97.914   Non-pressure chronic ulcer of unspecified part of right lower leg with necrosis of bone

    L97.919   Non-pressure chronic ulcer of unspecified part of right lower leg with unspecified severity

● **L97.92**   **Non-pressure chronic ulcer of unspecified part of left lower leg**

    L97.921   Non-pressure chronic ulcer of unspecified part of left lower leg limited to breakdown of skin

    L97.922   Non-pressure chronic ulcer of unspecified part of left lower leg with fat layer exposed

    L97.923   Non-pressure chronic ulcer of unspecified part of left lower leg with necrosis of muscle

    L97.924   Non-pressure chronic ulcer of unspecified part of left lower leg with necrosis of bone

    L97.929   Non-pressure chronic ulcer of unspecified part of left lower leg with unspecified severity

● **L98**   **Other disorders of skin and subcutaneous tissue, not elsewhere classified**

   L98.0   **Pyogenic granuloma**

     Excludes2   pyogenic granuloma of gingiva (K06.8)
         pyogenic granuloma of maxillary alveolar ridge (K04.5)
         pyogenic granuloma of oral mucosa (K13.4)

   L98.1   **Factitial dermatitis**
     Neurotic excoriation

     Excludes1   Excoriation (skin-picking) disorder (F42.4) ◄

   L98.2   **Febrile neutrophilic dermatosis [Sweet]**

   L98.3   **Eosinophilic cellulitis [Wells]**

● **L98.4**   **Non-pressure chronic ulcer of skin, not elsewhere classified**
     Chronic ulcer of skin NOS
     Tropical ulcer NOS
     Ulcer of skin NOS

     Excludes2   pressure ulcer (pressure area) (L89.-)
         gangrene (I96)
         skin infections (L00-L08)
         specific infections classified to A00-B99
         ulcer of lower limb NEC (L97.-)
         varicose ulcer (I83.0-I82.2)

● **L98.41**   **Non-pressure chronic ulcer of buttock**

    L98.411   Non-pressure chronic ulcer of buttock limited to breakdown of skin

    L98.412   Non-pressure chronic ulcer of buttock with fat layer exposed

    L98.413   Non-pressure chronic ulcer of buttock with necrosis of muscle

    L98.414   Non-pressure chronic ulcer of buttock with necrosis of bone

    L98.419   Non-pressure chronic ulcer of buttock with unspecified severity

● **L98.42**   **Non-pressure chronic ulcer of back**

    L98.421   Non-pressure chronic ulcer of back limited to breakdown of skin

    L98.422   Non-pressure chronic ulcer of back with fat layer exposed

    L98.423   Non-pressure chronic ulcer of back with necrosis of muscle

    L98.424   Non-pressure chronic ulcer of back with necrosis of bone

    L98.429   Non-pressure chronic ulcer of back with unspecified severity

● **L98.49**   **Non-pressure chronic ulcer of skin of other sites**
     Non-pressure chronic ulcer of skin NOS

    L98.491   Non-pressure chronic ulcer of skin of other sites limited to breakdown of skin

    L98.492   Non-pressure chronic ulcer of skin of other sites with fat layer exposed

    L98.493   Non-pressure chronic ulcer of skin of other sites with necrosis of muscle

    L98.494   Non-pressure chronic ulcer of skin of other sites with necrosis of bone

    L98.499   Non-pressure chronic ulcer of skin of other sites with unspecified severity

   L98.5   **Mucinosis of the skin**
     Focal mucinosis
     Lichen myxedematosus
     Reticular erythematous mucinosis

     Excludes1   focal oral mucinosis (K13.79)
         myxedema (E03.9)

   L98.6   **Other infiltrative disorders of the skin and subcutaneous tissue**

     Excludes1   hyalinosis cutis et mucosae (E78.89)

   L98.7   **Excessive and redundant skin and subcutaneous tissue** ◄
     Loose or sagging skin following bariatric surgery weight loss ◄
     Loose or sagging skin following dietary weight loss ◄
     Loose or sagging skin, NOS ◄

     Excludes2   acquired excess or redundant skin of eyelid (H02.3-) ◄
         congenital excess or redundant skin of eyelid (Q10.3) ◄
         skin changes due to chronic exposure to nonionizing radiation (L57.-) ◄

   L98.8   **Other specified disorders of the skin and subcutaneous tissue**
     Coding Clinic: 2013, Q2, P32

   L98.9   **Disorder of the skin and subcutaneous tissue, unspecified**

▶ *L99*   *Other disorders of skin and subcutaneous tissue in diseases classified elsewhere*

     Code first underlying disease, such as:
     amyloidosis (E85.-)

     Excludes1   skin disorders in diabetes (E08-E13 with .62)
         skin disorders in gonorrhea (A54.89)
         skin disorders in syphilis (A51.31, A52.79)

CHAPTER 12 (L00-L99)

CHAPTER 13

DISEASES OF THE MUSCULOSKELETAL SYSTEM AND CONNECTIVE TISSUE (M00-M99)

OGCR Chapter-Specific Coding Guidelines

13. **Chapter 13: Diseases of the Musculoskeletal System and Connective Tissue (M00-M99)**

a. Site and laterality

Most of the codes within Chapter 13 have site and laterality designations. The site represents the bone, joint or the muscle involved. For some conditions where more than one bone, joint or muscle is usually involved, such as osteoarthritis, there is a "multiple sites" code available. For categories where no multiple site code is provided and more than one bone, joint or muscle is involved, multiple codes should be used to indicate the different sites involved.

1) Bone versus joint

For certain conditions, the bone may be affected at the upper or lower end, (e.g., avascular necrosis of bone, M87, Osteoporosis, M80, M81). Though the portion of the bone affected may be at the joint, the site designation will be the bone, not the joint.

b. Acute traumatic versus chronic or recurrent musculoskeletal conditions

Many musculoskeletal conditions are a result of previous injury or trauma to a site, or are recurrent conditions. Bone, joint or muscle conditions that are the result of a healed injury are usually found in chapter 13. Recurrent bone, joint or muscle conditions are also usually found in chapter 13. Any current, acute injury should be coded to the appropriate injury code from chapter 19. Chronic or recurrent conditions should generally be coded with a code from chapter 13. If it is difficult to determine from the documentation in the record which code is best to describe a condition, query the provider.

c. Coding of Pathologic Fractures

7th character A is for use as long as the patient is receiving active treatment for the fracture. While the patient may be seen by a new or different provider over the course of treatment for a pathological fracture, assignment of the 7th character is based on whether the patient is undergoing active treatment and not whether the provider is seeing the patient for the first time.

7th character, D is to be used for encounters after the patient has completed active treatment. The other 7th characters, listed under each subcategory in the Tabular List, are to be used for subsequent encounters for **routine care of fractures during the healing and recovery phase as well as** treatment of problems associated with the healing, such as malunions, nonunions, and sequelae.

Care for complications of surgical treatment for fracture repairs during the healing or recovery phase should be coded with the appropriate complication codes.

See Section I.C.19. Coding of traumatic fractures.

d. Osteoporosis

Osteoporosis is a systemic condition, meaning that all bones of the musculoskeletal system are affected. Therefore, site is not a component of the codes under category M81, Osteoporosis without current pathological fracture. The site codes under category M80, Osteoporosis with current pathological fracture, identify the site of the fracture, not the osteoporosis.

1) Osteoporosis without pathological fracture

Category M81, Osteoporosis without current pathological fracture, is for use for patients with osteoporosis who do not currently have a pathologic fracture due to the osteoporosis, even if they have had a fracture in the past. For patients with a history of osteoporosis fractures, status code Z87.310, Personal history of (healed) osteoporosis fracture, should follow the code from M81.

2) Osteoporosis with current pathological fracture

Category M80, Osteoporosis with current pathological fracture, is for patients who have a current pathologic fracture at the time of an encounter. The codes under M80 identify the site of the fracture. A code from category M80, not a traumatic fracture code, should be used for any patient with known osteoporosis who suffers a fracture, even if the patient had a minor fall or trauma, if that fall or trauma would not usually break a normal, healthy bone.

CHAPTER 13

DISEASES OF THE MUSCULOSKELETAL SYSTEM AND CONNECTIVE TISSUE (M00-M99)

Note: Use an external cause code following the code for the musculoskeletal condition, if applicable, to identify the cause of the musculoskeletal condition

Excludes2 arthropathic psoriasis (L40.5-)
certain conditions originating in the perinatal period (P04-P96)
certain infectious and parasitic diseases (A00-B99)
compartment syndrome (traumatic) (T79.A-)
complications of pregnancy, childbirth and the puerperium (O00-O9A)
congenital malformations, deformations, and chromosomal abnormalities (Q00-Q99)
endocrine, nutritional and metabolic diseases (E00-E88)
injury, poisoning and certain other consequences of external causes (S00-T88)
neoplasms (C00-D49)
symptoms, signs and abnormal clinical and laboratory findings, not elsewhere classified (R00-R94)

This chapter contains the following blocks:

M00-M02	Infectious arthropathies
M04	Autoinflammatory syndromes ◀
M05-M14	Inflammatory polyarthropathies
M15-M19	Osteoarthritis
M20-M25	Other joint disorders
M26-M27	Dentofacial anomalies [including malocclusion] and other disorders of jaw
M30-M36	Systemic connective tissue disorders
M40-M43	Deforming dorsopathies
M45-M49	Spondylopathies
M50-M54	Other dorsopathies
M60-M63	Disorders of muscles
M65-M67	Disorders of synovium and tendon
M70-M79	Other soft tissue disorders
M80-M85	Disorders of bone density and structure
M86-M90	Other osteopathies
M91-M94	Chondropathies
M95	Other disorders of the musculoskeletal system and connective tissue
M96	Intraoperative and postprocedural complications and disorders of musculoskeletal system, not elsewhere classified
M97	Periprosthetic fracture around internal prosthetic joint ◀
M99	Biomechanical lesions, not elsewhere classified

ARTHROPATHIES (M00-M25)

Includes Disorders affecting predominantly peripheral (limb) joints

INFECTIOUS ARTHROPATHIES (M00-M02)

Note: This block comprises arthropathies due to microbiological agents.

Distinction is made between the following types of etiological relationship:

a) direct infection of joint, where organisms invade synovial tissue and microbial antigen is present in the joint;

b) indirect infection, which may be of two types: a reactive arthropathy, where microbial infection of the body is established but neither organisms nor antigens can be identified in the joint, and a postinfective arthropathy, where microbial antigen is present but recovery of an organism is inconstant and evidence of local multiplication is lacking.

◀ New   ◀▥ Revised   ~~deleted~~ Deleted   Excludes 1   Excludes 2   Includes   Use additional   Code first   Code also   Unspecified

OGCR Official Guidelines   X Assign placeholder X   ● Use Additional Character(s)   ▶ Manifestation Code   **Coding Clinic**

● **M00** **Pyogenic arthritis**

  ● **M00.0** **Staphylococcal arthritis and polyarthritis**

    Use additional code (B95.61-B95.8) to identify bacterial agent

      Excludes2   infection and inflammatory reaction due to internal joint prosthesis (T84.5-)

    M00.00 Staphylococcal arthritis, unspecified joint

   ● **M00.01** Staphylococcal arthritis, shoulder

      M00.011 Staphylococcal arthritis, right shoulder

      M00.012 Staphylococcal arthritis, left shoulder

      M00.019 Staphylococcal arthritis, unspecified shoulder

   ● **M00.02** Staphylococcal arthritis, elbow

      M00.021 Staphylococcal arthritis, right elbow

      M00.022 Staphylococcal arthritis, left elbow

      M00.029 Staphylococcal arthritis, unspecified elbow

   ● **M00.03** Staphylococcal arthritis, wrist

      Staphylococcal arthritis of carpal bones

      M00.031 Staphylococcal arthritis, right wrist

      M00.032 Staphylococcal arthritis, left wrist

      M00.039 Staphylococcal arthritis, unspecified wrist

   ● **M00.04** Staphylococcal arthritis, hand

      Staphylococcal arthritis of metacarpus and phalanges

      M00.041 Staphylococcal arthritis, right hand

      M00.042 Staphylococcal arthritis, left hand

      M00.049 Staphylococcal arthritis, unspecified hand

   ● **M00.05** Staphylococcal arthritis, hip

      M00.051 Staphylococcal arthritis, right hip

      M00.052 Staphylococcal arthritis, left hip

      M00.059 Staphylococcal arthritis, unspecified hip

   ● **M00.06** Staphylococcal arthritis, knee

      M00.061 Staphylococcal arthritis, right knee

      M00.062 Staphylococcal arthritis, left knee

      M00.069 Staphylococcal arthritis, unspecified knee

   ● **M00.07** Staphylococcal arthritis, ankle and foot

      Staphylococcal arthritis, tarsus, metatarsus and phalanges

      M00.071 Staphylococcal arthritis, right ankle and foot

      M00.072 Staphylococcal arthritis, left ankle and foot

      M00.079 Staphylococcal arthritis, unspecified ankle and foot

    M00.08 Staphylococcal arthritis, vertebrae

    M00.09 Staphylococcal polyarthritis

  ● **M00.1** Pneumococcal arthritis and polyarthritis

    M00.10 Pneumococcal arthritis, unspecified joint

   ● **M00.11** Pneumococcal arthritis, shoulder

      M00.111 Pneumococcal arthritis, right shoulder

      M00.112 Pneumococcal arthritis, left shoulder

      M00.119 Pneumococcal arthritis, unspecified shoulder

   ● **M00.12** Pneumococcal arthritis, elbow

      M00.121 Pneumococcal arthritis, right elbow

      M00.122 Pneumococcal arthritis, left elbow

      M00.129 Pneumococcal arthritis, unspecified elbow

   ● **M00.13** Pneumococcal arthritis, wrist

      Pneumococcal arthritis of carpal bones

      M00.131 Pneumococcal arthritis, right wrist

      M00.132 Pneumococcal arthritis, left wrist

      M00.139 Pneumococcal arthritis, unspecified wrist

   ● **M00.14** Pneumococcal arthritis, hand

      Pneumococcal arthritis of metacarpus and phalanges

      M00.141 Pneumococcal arthritis, right hand

      M00.142 Pneumococcal arthritis, left hand

      M00.149 Pneumococcal arthritis, unspecified hand

   ● **M00.15** Pneumococcal arthritis, hip

      M00.151 Pneumococcal arthritis, right hip

      M00.152 Pneumococcal arthritis, left hip

      M00.159 Pneumococcal arthritis, unspecified hip

   ● **M00.16** Pneumococcal arthritis, knee

      M00.161 Pneumococcal arthritis, right knee

      M00.162 Pneumococcal arthritis, left knee

      M00.169 Pneumococcal arthritis, unspecified knee

   ● **M00.17** Pneumococcal arthritis, ankle and foot

      Pneumococcal arthritis, tarsus, metatarsus and phalanges

      M00.171 Pneumococcal arthritis, right ankle and foot

      M00.172 Pneumococcal arthritis, left ankle and foot

      M00.179 Pneumococcal arthritis, unspecified ankle and foot

    M00.18 Pneumococcal arthritis, vertebrae

    M00.19 Pneumococcal polyarthritis

  ● **M00.2** Other streptococcal arthritis and polyarthritis

    Use additional code (B95.0-B95.2, B95.4-B95.5) to identify bacterial agent

    M00.20 Other streptococcal arthritis, unspecified joint

   ● **M00.21** Other streptococcal arthritis, shoulder

      M00.211 Other streptococcal arthritis, right shoulder

      M00.212 Other streptococcal arthritis, left shoulder

      M00.219 Other streptococcal arthritis, unspecified shoulder

   ● **M00.22** Other streptococcal arthritis, elbow

      M00.221 Other streptococcal arthritis, right elbow

      M00.222 Other streptococcal arthritis, left elbow

      M00.229 Other streptococcal arthritis, unspecified elbow

   ● **M00.23** Other streptococcal arthritis, wrist

      Other streptococcal arthritis of carpal bones

      M00.231 Other streptococcal arthritis, right wrist

      M00.232 Other streptococcal arthritis, left wrist

      M00.239 Other streptococcal arthritis, unspecified wrist

   ● **M00.24** Other streptococcal arthritis, hand

      Other streptococcal arthritis metacarpus and phalanges

      M00.241 Other streptococcal arthritis, right hand

      M00.242 Other streptococcal arthritis, left hand

      M00.249 Other streptococcal arthritis, unspecified hand

CHAPTER 13 (M00-M99)

- M00.25 Other streptococcal arthritis, hip
  - M00.251 Other streptococcal arthritis, right hip
  - M00.252 Other streptococcal arthritis, left hip
  - M00.259 Other streptococcal arthritis, unspecified hip
- M00.26 Other streptococcal arthritis, knee
  - M00.261 Other streptococcal arthritis, right knee
  - M00.262 Other streptococcal arthritis, left knee
  - M00.269 Other streptococcal arthritis, unspecified knee
- M00.27 Other streptococcal arthritis, ankle and foot
  - Other streptococcal arthritis, tarsus, metatarsus and phalanges
  - M00.271 Other streptococcal arthritis, right ankle and foot
  - M00.272 Other streptococcal arthritis, left ankle and foot
  - M00.279 Other streptococcal arthritis, unspecified ankle and foot
  - M00.28 Other streptococcal arthritis, vertebrae
  - M00.29 Other streptococcal polyarthritis
- M00.8 Arthritis and polyarthritis due to other bacteria
  - Use additional code (B96) to identify bacteria
  - M00.80 Arthritis due to other bacteria, unspecified joint
- M00.81 Arthritis due to other bacteria, shoulder
  - M00.811 Arthritis due to other bacteria, right shoulder
  - M00.812 Arthritis due to other bacteria, left shoulder
  - M00.819 Arthritis due to other bacteria, unspecified shoulder
- M00.82 Arthritis due to other bacteria, elbow
  - M00.821 Arthritis due to other bacteria, right elbow
  - M00.822 Arthritis due to other bacteria, left elbow
  - M00.829 Arthritis due to other bacteria, unspecified elbow
- M00.83 Arthritis due to other bacteria, wrist
  - Arthritis due to other bacteria, carpal bones
  - M00.831 Arthritis due to other bacteria, right wrist
  - M00.832 Arthritis due to other bacteria, left wrist
  - M00.839 Arthritis due to other bacteria, unspecified wrist
- M00.84 Arthritis due to other bacteria, hand
  - Arthritis due to other bacteria, metacarpus and phalanges
  - M00.841 Arthritis due to other bacteria, right hand
  - M00.842 Arthritis due to other bacteria, left hand
  - M00.849 Arthritis due to other bacteria, unspecified hand
- M00.85 Arthritis due to other bacteria, hip
  - M00.851 Arthritis due to other bacteria, right hip
  - M00.852 Arthritis due to other bacteria, left hip
  - M00.859 Arthritis due to other bacteria, unspecified hip

- M00.86 Arthritis due to other bacteria, knee
  - M00.861 Arthritis due to other bacteria, right knee
  - M00.862 Arthritis due to other bacteria, left knee
  - M00.869 Arthritis due to other bacteria, unspecified knee
- M00.87 Arthritis due to other bacteria, ankle and foot
  - Arthritis due to other bacteria, tarsus, metatarsus, and phalanges
  - M00.871 Arthritis due to other bacteria, right ankle and foot
  - M00.872 Arthritis due to other bacteria, left ankle and foot
  - M00.879 Arthritis due to other bacteria, unspecified ankle and foot
  - M00.88 Arthritis due to other bacteria, vertebrae
  - M00.89 Polyarthritis due to other bacteria
- M00.9 Pyogenic arthritis, unspecified
  - Infective arthritis NOS
- M01 Direct infections of joint in infectious and parasitic diseases classified elsewhere

  Code first underlying disease, such as:
  - leprosy [Hansen's disease] (A30.-)
  - mycoses (B35-B49)
  - O'nyong-nyong fever (A92.1)
  - paratyphoid fever (A01.1-A01.4)

  Excludes1 arthropathy in Lyme disease (A69.23)
  - gonococcal arthritis (A54.42)
  - meningococcal arthritis (A39.83)
  - mumps arthritis (B26.85)
  - postinfective arthropathy (M02.-)
  - postmeningococcal arthritis (A39.84)
  - reactive arthritis (M02.3)
  - rubella arthritis (B06.82)
  - sarcoidosis arthritis (D86.86)
  - typhoid fever arthritis (A01.04)
  - tuberculosis arthritis (A18.01-A18.02)

- M01.X Direct infection of joint in infectious and parasitic diseases classified elsewhere
  - *M01.X0 Direct infection of unspecified joint in infectious and parasitic diseases classified elsewhere*
  - M01.X1 Direct infection of shoulder joint in infectious and parasitic diseases classified elsewhere
    - *M01.X11 Direct infection of right shoulder in infectious and parasitic diseases classified elsewhere*
    - *M01.X12 Direct infection of left shoulder in infectious and parasitic diseases classified elsewhere*
    - *M01.X19 Direct infection of unspecified shoulder in infectious and parasitic diseases classified elsewhere*
  - M01.X2 Direct infection of elbow in infectious and parasitic diseases classified elsewhere
    - *M01.X21 Direct infection of right elbow in infectious and parasitic diseases classified elsewhere*
    - *M01.X22 Direct infection of left elbow in infectious and parasitic diseases classified elsewhere*
    - *M01.X29 Direct infection of unspecified elbow in infectious and parasitic diseases classified elsewhere*

New   Revised   deleted Deleted   Excludes 1   Excludes 2   Includes   Use additional   Code first   Code also   Unspecified
OGCR Official Guidelines   X Assign placeholder X   Use Additional Character(s)   Manifestation Code   Coding Clinic

● **M01.X3** **Direct infection of wrist in infectious and parasitic diseases classified elsewhere**
Direct infection of carpal bones in infectious and parasitic diseases classified elsewhere

▷ *M01.X31* *Direct infection of right wrist in infectious and parasitic diseases classified elsewhere*

▷ *M01.X32* *Direct infection of left wrist in infectious and parasitic diseases classified elsewhere*

▷ *M01.X39* *Direct infection of unspecified wrist in infectious and parasitic diseases classified elsewhere*

● **M01.X4** **Direct infection of hand in infectious and parasitic diseases classified elsewhere**
Direct infection of metacarpus and phalanges in infectious and parasitic diseases classified elsewhere

▷ *M01.X41* *Direct infection of right hand in infectious and parasitic diseases classified elsewhere*

▷ *M01.X42* *Direct infection of left hand in infectious and parasitic diseases classified elsewhere*

▷ *M01.X49* *Direct infection of unspecified hand in infectious and parasitic diseases classified elsewhere*

● **M01.X5** **Direct infection of hip in infectious and parasitic diseases classified elsewhere**

▷ *M01.X51* *Direct infection of right hip in infectious and parasitic diseases classified elsewhere*

▷ *M01.X52* *Direct infection of left hip in infectious and parasitic diseases classified elsewhere*

▷ *M01.X59* *Direct infection of unspecified hip in infectious and parasitic diseases classified elsewhere*

● **M01.X6** **Direct infection of knee in infectious and parasitic diseases classified elsewhere**

▷ *M01.X61* *Direct infection of right knee in infectious and parasitic diseases classified elsewhere*

▷ *M01.X62* *Direct infection of left knee in infectious and parasitic diseases classified elsewhere*

▷ *M01.X69* *Direct infection of unspecified knee in infectious and parasitic diseases classified elsewhere*

● **M01.X7** **Direct infection of ankle and foot in infectious and parasitic diseases classified elsewhere**
Direct infection of tarsus, metatarsus and phalanges in infectious and parasitic diseases classified elsewhere

▷ *M01.X71* *Direct infection of right ankle and foot in infectious and parasitic diseases classified elsewhere*

▷ *M01.X72* *Direct infection of left ankle and foot in infectious and parasitic diseases classified elsewhere*

▷ *M01.X79* *Direct infection of unspecified ankle and foot in infectious and parasitic diseases classified elsewhere*

▷ *M01.X8* *Direct infection of vertebrae in infectious and parasitic diseases classified elsewhere*

▷ *M01.X9* *Direct infection of multiple joints in infectious and parasitic diseases classified elsewhere*

● **M02** **Postinfective and reactive arthropathies**
Code first underlying disease, such as:
   congenital syphilis [Clutton's joints] (A50.5)
   enteritis due to Yersinia enterocolitica (A04.6)
   infective endocarditis (I33.0)
   viral hepatitis (B15-B19)

Excludes1   Behçet's disease (M35.2)
   direct infections of joint in infectious and parasitic diseases classified elsewhere (M01.-)
   postmeningococcal arthritis (A39.84)
   mumps arthritis (B26.85)
   rubella arthritis (B06.82)
   syphilis arthritis (late) (A52.77)
   rheumatic fever (I00)
   tabetic arthropathy [Charcôt's] (A52.16)

● **M02.0** **Arthropathy following intestinal bypass**

M02.00 **Arthropathy following intestinal bypass, unspecified site**

● **M02.01** **Arthropathy following intestinal bypass, shoulder**

M02.011 **Arthropathy following intestinal bypass, right shoulder**

M02.012 **Arthropathy following intestinal bypass, left shoulder**

M02.019 **Arthropathy following intestinal bypass, unspecified shoulder**

● **M02.02** **Arthropathy following intestinal bypass, elbow**

M02.021 **Arthropathy following intestinal bypass, right elbow**

M02.022 **Arthropathy following intestinal bypass, left elbow**

M02.029 **Arthropathy following intestinal bypass, unspecified elbow**

● **M02.03** **Arthropathy following intestinal bypass, wrist**
Arthropathy following intestinal bypass, carpal bones

M02.031 **Arthropathy following intestinal bypass, right wrist**

M02.032 **Arthropathy following intestinal bypass, left wrist**

M02.039 **Arthropathy following intestinal bypass, unspecified wrist**

● **M02.04** **Arthropathy following intestinal bypass, hand**
Arthropathy following intestinal bypass, metacarpals and phalanges

M02.041 **Arthropathy following intestinal bypass, right hand**

M02.042 **Arthropathy following intestinal bypass, left hand**

M02.049 **Arthropathy following intestinal bypass, unspecified hand**

● **M02.05** **Arthropathy following intestinal bypass, hip**

M02.051 **Arthropathy following intestinal bypass, right hip**

M02.052 **Arthropathy following intestinal bypass, left hip**

M02.059 **Arthropathy following intestinal bypass, unspecified hip**

● **M02.06** **Arthropathy following intestinal bypass, knee**

M02.061 **Arthropathy following intestinal bypass, right knee**

M02.062 **Arthropathy following intestinal bypass, left knee**

M02.069 **Arthropathy following intestinal bypass, unspecified knee**

● **M02.07**   **Arthropathy following intestinal bypass, ankle and foot**
Arthropathy following intestinal bypass, tarsus, metatarsus and phalanges

     M02.071   Arthropathy following intestinal bypass, right ankle and foot

     M02.072   Arthropathy following intestinal bypass, left ankle and foot

     M02.079   Arthropathy following intestinal bypass, unspecified ankle and foot

   M02.08   Arthropathy following intestinal bypass, vertebrae

   M02.09   Arthropathy following intestinal bypass, multiple sites

● **M02.1**   Postdysenteric arthropathy

   M02.10   Postdysenteric arthropathy, unspecified site

● **M02.11**   Postdysenteric arthropathy, shoulder

     M02.111   Postdysenteric arthropathy, right shoulder

     M02.112   Postdysenteric arthropathy, left shoulder

     M02.119   Postdysenteric arthropathy, unspecified shoulder

● **M02.12**   Postdysenteric arthropathy, elbow

     M02.121   Postdysenteric arthropathy, right elbow

     M02.122   Postdysenteric arthropathy, left elbow

     M02.129   Postdysenteric arthropathy, unspecified elbow

● **M02.13**   Postdysenteric arthropathy, wrist
Postdysenteric arthropathy, carpal bones

     M02.131   Postdysenteric arthropathy, right wrist

     M02.132   Postdysenteric arthropathy, left wrist

     M02.139   Postdysenteric arthropathy, unspecified wrist

● **M02.14**   Postdysenteric arthropathy, hand
Postdysenteric arthropathy, metacarpus and phalanges

     M02.141   Postdysenteric arthropathy, right hand

     M02.142   Postdysenteric arthropathy, left hand

     M02.149   Postdysenteric arthropathy, unspecified hand

● **M02.15**   Postdysenteric arthropathy, hip

     M02.151   Postdysenteric arthropathy, right hip

     M02.152   Postdysenteric arthropathy, left hip

     M02.159   Postdysenteric arthropathy, unspecified hip

● **M02.16**   Postdysenteric arthropathy, knee

     M02.161   Postdysenteric arthropathy, right knee

     M02.162   Postdysenteric arthropathy, left knee

     M02.169   Postdysenteric arthropathy, unspecified knee

● **M02.17**   Postdysenteric arthropathy, ankle and foot
Postdysenteric arthropathy, tarsus, metatarsus and phalanges

     M02.171   Postdysenteric arthropathy, right ankle and foot

     M02.172   Postdysenteric arthropathy, left ankle and foot

     M02.179   Postdysenteric arthropathy, unspecified ankle and foot

   M02.18   Postdysenteric arthropathy, vertebrae

   M02.19   Postdysenteric arthropathy, multiple sites

● **M02.2**   Postimmunization arthropathy

   M02.20   Postimmunization arthropathy, unspecified site

● **M02.21**   Postimmunization arthropathy, shoulder

     M02.211   Postimmunization arthropathy, right shoulder

     M02.212   Postimmunization arthropathy, left shoulder

     M02.219   Postimmunization arthropathy, unspecified shoulder

● **M02.22**   Postimmunization arthropathy, elbow

     M02.221   Postimmunization arthropathy, right elbow

     M02.222   Postimmunization arthropathy, left elbow

     M02.229   Postimmunization arthropathy, unspecified elbow

● **M02.23**   Postimmunization arthropathy, wrist
Postimmunization arthropathy, carpal bones

     M02.231   Postimmunization arthropathy, right wrist

     M02.232   Postimmunization arthropathy, left wrist

     M02.239   Postimmunization arthropathy, unspecified wrist

● **M02.24**   Postimmunization arthropathy, hand
Postimmunization arthropathy, metacarpus and phalanges

     M02.241   Postimmunization arthropathy, right hand

     M02.242   Postimmunization arthropathy, left hand

     M02.249   Postimmunization arthropathy, unspecified hand

● **M02.25**   Postimmunization arthropathy, hip

     M02.251   Postimmunization arthropathy, right hip

     M02.252   Postimmunization arthropathy, left hip

     M02.259   Postimmunization arthropathy, unspecified hip

● **M02.26**   Postimmunization arthropathy, knee

     M02.261   Postimmunization arthropathy, right knee

     M02.262   Postimmunization arthropathy, left knee

     M02.269   Postimmunization arthropathy, unspecified knee

● **M02.27**   Postimmunization arthropathy, ankle and foot
Postimmunization arthropathy, tarsus, metatarsus and phalanges

     M02.271   Postimmunization arthropathy, right ankle and foot

     M02.272   Postimmunization arthropathy, left ankle and foot

     M02.279   Postimmunization arthropathy, unspecified ankle and foot

   M02.28   Postimmunization arthropathy, vertebrae

   M02.29   Postimmunization arthropathy, multiple sites

● **M02.3**   Reiter's disease
Reactive arthritis

   M02.30   Reiter's disease, unspecified site

● **M02.31**   Reiter's disease, shoulder

     M02.311   Reiter's disease, right shoulder

     M02.312   Reiter's disease, left shoulder

     M02.319   Reiter's disease, unspecified shoulder

● **M02.32 Reiter's disease, elbow**
     M02.321 Reiter's disease, right elbow
     M02.322 Reiter's disease, left elbow
     M02.329 Reiter's disease, unspecified elbow
● **M02.33 Reiter's disease, wrist**
     Reiter's disease, carpal bones
     M02.331 Reiter's disease, right wrist
     M02.332 Reiter's disease, left wrist
     M02.339 Reiter's disease, unspecified wrist
● **M02.34 Reiter's disease, hand**
     Reiter's disease, metacarpus and phalanges
     M02.341 Reiter's disease, right hand
     M02.342 Reiter's disease, left hand
     M02.349 Reiter's disease, unspecified hand
● **M02.35 Reiter's disease, hip**
     M02.351 Reiter's disease, right hip
     M02.352 Reiter's disease, left hip
     M02.359 Reiter's disease, unspecified hip
● **M02.36 Reiter's disease, knee**
     M02.361 Reiter's disease, right knee
     M02.362 Reiter's disease, left knee
     M02.369 Reiter's disease, unspecified knee
● **M02.37 Reiter's disease, ankle and foot**
     Reiter's disease, tarsus, metatarsus and phalanges
     M02.371 Reiter's disease, right ankle and foot
     M02.372 Reiter's disease, left ankle and foot
     M02.379 Reiter's disease, unspecified ankle and foot
     M02.38 Reiter's disease, vertebrae
     M02.39 Reiter's disease, multiple sites
● **M02.8 Other reactive arthropathies**
    ▌ *M02.80 Other reactive arthropathies, unspecified site*
● **M02.81 Other reactive arthropathies, shoulder**
    ▌ *M02.811 Other reactive arthropathies, right shoulder*
    ▌ *M02.812 Other reactive arthropathies, left shoulder*
    ▌ *M02.819 Other reactive arthropathies, unspecified shoulder*
● **M02.82 Other reactive arthropathies, elbow**
    ▌ *M02.821 Other reactive arthropathies, right elbow*
    ▌ *M02.822 Other reactive arthropathies, left elbow*
    ▌ *M02.829 Other reactive arthropathies, unspecified elbow*
● **M02.83 Other reactive arthropathies, wrist**
     Other reactive arthropathies, carpal bones
    ▌ *M02.831 Other reactive arthropathies, right wrist*
    ▌ *M02.832 Other reactive arthropathies, left wrist*
    ▌ *M02.839 Other reactive arthropathies, unspecified wrist*
● **M02.84 Other reactive arthropathies, hand**
     Other reactive arthropathies, metacarpus and phalanges
    ▌ *M02.841 Other reactive arthropathies, right hand*
    ▌ *M02.842 Other reactive arthropathies, left hand*
    ▌ *M02.849 Other reactive arthropathies, unspecified hand*

● **M02.85 Other reactive arthropathies, hip**
    ▌ *M02.851 Other reactive arthropathies, right hip*
    ▌ *M02.852 Other reactive arthropathies, left hip*
    ▌ *M02.859 Other reactive arthropathies, unspecified hip*
● **M02.86 Other reactive arthropathies, knee**
    ▌ *M02.861 Other reactive arthropathies, right knee*
    ▌ *M02.862 Other reactive arthropathies, left knee*
    ▌ *M02.869 Other reactive arthropathies, unspecified knee*
● **M02.87 Other reactive arthropathies, ankle and foot**
     Other reactive arthropathies, tarsus, metatarsus and phalanges
    ▌ *M02.871 Other reactive arthropathies, right ankle and foot*
    ▌ *M02.872 Other reactive arthropathies, left ankle and foot*
    ▌ *M02.879 Other reactive arthropathies, unspecified ankle and foot*
    ▌ *M02.88 Other reactive arthropathies, vertebrae*
    ▌ *M02.89 Other reactive arthropathies, multiple sites*
    ▌ *M02.9 Reactive arthropathy, unspecified*

AUTOINFLAMMATORY SYNDROMES (M04) ◄

● **M04 Autoinflammatory syndromes** ◄
    Excludes2   Crohn's disease (K50.-) ◄
    M04.1 Periodic fever syndromes ◄
     Familial Mediterranean fever ◄
     Hyperimmunoglobin D syndrome ◄
     Mevalonate kinase deficiency ◄
     Tumor necrosis factor receptor associated periodic syndrome [TRAPS] ◄
    M04.2 Cryopyrin-associated periodic syndromes ◄
     Chronic infantile neurological, cutaneous and articular syndrome [CINCA] ◄
     Familial cold autoinflammatory syndrome ◄
     Familial cold urticaria ◄
     Muckle-Wells syndrome ◄
     Neonatal onset multisystemic inflammatory disorder [NOMID] ◄
    M04.8 Other autoinflammatory syndromes ◄
     Blau syndrome ◄
     Deficiency of interleukin 1 receptor antagonist [DIRA] ◄
     Majeed syndrome ◄
     Periodic fever, aphthous stomatitis, pharyngitis, and adenopathy syndrome [PFAPA] ◄
     Pyogenic arthritis, pyoderma gangrenosum, and acne syndrome [PAPA] ◄
    M04.9 Autoinflammatory syndrome, unspecified ◄

INFLAMMATORY POLYARTHROPATHIES (M05-M14)

● **M05 Rheumatoid arthritis with rheumatoid factor**
    Excludes1   rheumatic fever (I00)
     juvenile rheumatoid arthritis (M08.-)
     rheumatoid arthritis of spine (M45.-)
● **M05.0 Felty's syndrome**
     Rheumatoid arthritis with splenoadenomegaly and leukopenia
     M05.00 Felty's syndrome, unspecified site
● **M05.01 Felty's syndrome, shoulder**
     M05.011 Felty's syndrome, right shoulder
     M05.012 Felty's syndrome, left shoulder
     M05.019 Felty's syndrome, unspecified shoulder

Item 13-1   Rheumatoid arthritis (RA) is a chronic systemic inflammatory autoimmune disease of undetermined etiology involving primarily the synovial membranes and articular structures of multiple joints. It can also affect other organs, including the eyes, blood vessels, heart, and lungs. The disease is often progressive. In late stages, deformity, ankylosis, and other **inflammatory polyarthropathies** develop.

● M05.02   Felty's syndrome, elbow
     M05.021   Felty's syndrome, right elbow
     M05.022   Felty's syndrome, left elbow
     M05.029   Felty's syndrome, unspecified elbow

● M05.03   Felty's syndrome, wrist
     Felty's syndrome, carpal bones
     M05.031   Felty's syndrome, right wrist
     M05.032   Felty's syndrome, left wrist
     M05.039   Felty's syndrome, unspecified wrist

● M05.04   Felty's syndrome, hand
     Felty's syndrome, metacarpus and phalanges
     M05.041   Felty's syndrome, right hand
     M05.042   Felty's syndrome, left hand
     M05.049   Felty's syndrome, unspecified hand

● M05.05   Felty's syndrome, hip
     M05.051   Felty's syndrome, right hip
     M05.052   Felty's syndrome, left hip
     M05.059   Felty's syndrome, unspecified hip

● M05.06   Felty's syndrome, knee
     M05.061   Felty's syndrome, right knee
     M05.062   Felty's syndrome, left knee
     M05.069   Felty's syndrome, unspecified knee

● M05.07   Felty's syndrome, ankle and foot
     Felty's syndrome, tarsus, metatarsus and phalanges
     M05.071   Felty's syndrome, right ankle and foot
     M05.072   Felty's syndrome, left ankle and foot
     M05.079   Felty's syndrome, unspecified ankle and foot

     M05.09   Felty's syndrome, multiple sites

● M05.1   Rheumatoid lung disease with rheumatoid arthritis
     M05.10   Rheumatoid lung disease with rheumatoid arthritis of unspecified site

● M05.11   Rheumatoid lung disease with rheumatoid arthritis of shoulder
     M05.111   Rheumatoid lung disease with rheumatoid arthritis of right shoulder
     M05.112   Rheumatoid lung disease with rheumatoid arthritis of left shoulder
     M05.119   Rheumatoid lung disease with rheumatoid arthritis of unspecified shoulder

● M05.12   Rheumatoid lung disease with rheumatoid arthritis of elbow
     M05.121   Rheumatoid lung disease with rheumatoid arthritis of right elbow
     M05.122   Rheumatoid lung disease with rheumatoid arthritis of left elbow
     M05.129   Rheumatoid lung disease with rheumatoid arthritis of unspecified elbow

● M05.13   Rheumatoid lung disease with rheumatoid arthritis of wrist
     Rheumatoid lung disease with rheumatoid arthritis, carpal bones
     M05.131   Rheumatoid lung disease with rheumatoid arthritis of right wrist
     M05.132   Rheumatoid lung disease with rheumatoid arthritis of left wrist
     M05.139   Rheumatoid lung disease with rheumatoid arthritis of unspecified wrist

● M05.14   Rheumatoid lung disease with rheumatoid arthritis of hand
     Rheumatoid lung disease with rheumatoid arthritis, metacarpus and phalanges
     M05.141   Rheumatoid lung disease with rheumatoid arthritis of right hand
     M05.142   Rheumatoid lung disease with rheumatoid arthritis of left hand
     M05.149   Rheumatoid lung disease with rheumatoid arthritis of unspecified hand

● M05.15   Rheumatoid lung disease with rheumatoid arthritis of hip
     M05.151   Rheumatoid lung disease with rheumatoid arthritis of right hip
     M05.152   Rheumatoid lung disease with rheumatoid arthritis of left hip
     M05.159   Rheumatoid lung disease with rheumatoid arthritis of unspecified hip

● M05.16   Rheumatoid lung disease with rheumatoid arthritis of knee
     M05.161   Rheumatoid lung disease with rheumatoid arthritis of right knee
     M05.162   Rheumatoid lung disease with rheumatoid arthritis of left knee
     M05.169   Rheumatoid lung disease with rheumatoid arthritis of unspecified knee

● M05.17   Rheumatoid lung disease with rheumatoid arthritis of ankle and foot
     Rheumatoid lung disease with rheumatoid arthritis, tarsus, metatarsus and phalanges
     M05.171   Rheumatoid lung disease with rheumatoid arthritis of right ankle and foot
     M05.172   Rheumatoid lung disease with rheumatoid arthritis of left ankle and foot
     M05.179   Rheumatoid lung disease with rheumatoid arthritis of unspecified ankle and foot

     M05.19   Rheumatoid lung disease with rheumatoid arthritis of multiple sites

● M05.2   Rheumatoid vasculitis with rheumatoid arthritis
     M05.20   Rheumatoid vasculitis with rheumatoid arthritis of unspecified site

● M05.21   Rheumatoid vasculitis with rheumatoid arthritis of shoulder
     M05.211   Rheumatoid vasculitis with rheumatoid arthritis of right shoulder
     M05.212   Rheumatoid vasculitis with rheumatoid arthritis of left shoulder
     M05.219   Rheumatoid vasculitis with rheumatoid arthritis of unspecified shoulder

● M05.22   Rheumatoid vasculitis with rheumatoid arthritis of elbow
     M05.221   Rheumatoid vasculitis with rheumatoid arthritis of right elbow
     M05.222   Rheumatoid vasculitis with rheumatoid arthritis of left elbow
     M05.229   Rheumatoid vasculitis with rheumatoid arthritis of unspecified elbow

◀ New   ◀ Revised   deleted Deleted   Excludes 1   Excludes 2   Includes   Use additional   Code first   Code also   Unspecified
OGCR Official Guidelines   X Assign placeholder X   ● Use Additional Character(s)   ▶ Manifestation Code   **Coding Clinic**

● **M05.23**   **Rheumatoid vasculitis with rheumatoid arthritis of wrist**
> Rheumatoid vasculitis with rheumatoid arthritis, carpal bones

    M05.231   Rheumatoid vasculitis with rheumatoid arthritis of right wrist

    M05.232   Rheumatoid vasculitis with rheumatoid arthritis of left wrist

    M05.239   Rheumatoid vasculitis with rheumatoid arthritis of unspecified wrist

● **M05.24**   **Rheumatoid vasculitis with rheumatoid arthritis of hand**
> Rheumatoid vasculitis with rheumatoid arthritis, metacarpus and phalanges

    M05.241   Rheumatoid vasculitis with rheumatoid arthritis of right hand

    M05.242   Rheumatoid vasculitis with rheumatoid arthritis of left hand

    M05.249   Rheumatoid vasculitis with rheumatoid arthritis of unspecified hand

● **M05.25**   **Rheumatoid vasculitis with rheumatoid arthritis of hip**

    M05.251   Rheumatoid vasculitis with rheumatoid arthritis of right hip

    M05.252   Rheumatoid vasculitis with rheumatoid arthritis of left hip

    M05.259   Rheumatoid vasculitis with rheumatoid arthritis of unspecified hip

● **M05.26**   **Rheumatoid vasculitis with rheumatoid arthritis of knee**

    M05.261   Rheumatoid vasculitis with rheumatoid arthritis of right knee

    M05.262   Rheumatoid vasculitis with rheumatoid arthritis of left knee

    M05.269   Rheumatoid vasculitis with rheumatoid arthritis of unspecified knee

● **M05.27**   **Rheumatoid vasculitis with rheumatoid arthritis of ankle and foot**
> Rheumatoid vasculitis with rheumatoid arthritis, tarsus, metatarsus and phalanges

    M05.271   Rheumatoid vasculitis with rheumatoid arthritis of right ankle and foot

    M05.272   Rheumatoid vasculitis with rheumatoid arthritis of left ankle and foot

    M05.279   Rheumatoid vasculitis with rheumatoid arthritis of unspecified ankle and foot

   M05.29   **Rheumatoid vasculitis with rheumatoid arthritis of multiple sites**

● **M05.3**   **Rheumatoid heart disease with rheumatoid arthritis**
> Rheumatoid carditis
> Rheumatoid endocarditis
> Rheumatoid myocarditis
> Rheumatoid pericarditis

   M05.30   **Rheumatoid heart disease with rheumatoid arthritis of unspecified site**

● **M05.31**   **Rheumatoid heart disease with rheumatoid arthritis of shoulder**

    M05.311   Rheumatoid heart disease with rheumatoid arthritis of right shoulder

    M05.312   Rheumatoid heart disease with rheumatoid arthritis of left shoulder

    M05.319   Rheumatoid heart disease with rheumatoid arthritis of unspecified shoulder

● **M05.32**   **Rheumatoid heart disease with rheumatoid arthritis of elbow**

    M05.321   Rheumatoid heart disease with rheumatoid arthritis of right elbow

    M05.322   Rheumatoid heart disease with rheumatoid arthritis of left elbow

    M05.329   Rheumatoid heart disease with rheumatoid arthritis of unspecified elbow

● **M05.33**   **Rheumatoid heart disease with rheumatoid arthritis of wrist**
> Rheumatoid heart disease with rheumatoid arthritis, carpal bones

    M05.331   Rheumatoid heart disease with rheumatoid arthritis of right wrist

    M05.332   Rheumatoid heart disease with rheumatoid arthritis of left wrist

    M05.339   Rheumatoid heart disease with rheumatoid arthritis of unspecified wrist

● **M05.34**   **Rheumatoid heart disease with rheumatoid arthritis of hand**
> Rheumatoid heart disease with rheumatoid arthritis, metacarpus and phalanges

    M05.341   Rheumatoid heart disease with rheumatoid arthritis of right hand

    M05.342   Rheumatoid heart disease with rheumatoid arthritis of left hand

    M05.349   Rheumatoid heart disease with rheumatoid arthritis of unspecified hand

● **M05.35**   **Rheumatoid heart disease with rheumatoid arthritis of hip**

    M05.351   Rheumatoid heart disease with rheumatoid arthritis of right hip

    M05.352   Rheumatoid heart disease with rheumatoid arthritis of left hip

    M05.359   Rheumatoid heart disease with rheumatoid arthritis of unspecified hip

● **M05.36**   **Rheumatoid heart disease with rheumatoid arthritis of knee**

    M05.361   Rheumatoid heart disease with rheumatoid arthritis of right knee

    M05.362   Rheumatoid heart disease with rheumatoid arthritis of left knee

    M05.369   Rheumatoid heart disease with rheumatoid arthritis of unspecified knee

● **M05.37**   **Rheumatoid heart disease with rheumatoid arthritis of ankle and foot**
> Rheumatoid heart disease with rheumatoid arthritis, tarsus, metatarsus and phalanges

    M05.371   Rheumatoid heart disease with rheumatoid arthritis of right ankle and foot

    M05.372   Rheumatoid heart disease with rheumatoid arthritis of left ankle and foot

    M05.379   Rheumatoid heart disease with rheumatoid arthritis of unspecified ankle and foot

   M05.39   **Rheumatoid heart disease with rheumatoid arthritis of multiple sites**

CHAPTER 13 (M00-M99)

● **M05.4 Rheumatoid myopathy with rheumatoid arthritis**

  M05.40 Rheumatoid myopathy with rheumatoid arthritis of unspecified site

● **M05.41** Rheumatoid myopathy with rheumatoid arthritis of shoulder

    M05.411 Rheumatoid myopathy with rheumatoid arthritis of right shoulder

    M05.412 Rheumatoid myopathy with rheumatoid arthritis of left shoulder

    M05.419 Rheumatoid myopathy with rheumatoid arthritis of unspecified shoulder

● **M05.42** Rheumatoid myopathy with rheumatoid arthritis of elbow

    M05.421 Rheumatoid myopathy with rheumatoid arthritis of right elbow

    M05.422 Rheumatoid myopathy with rheumatoid arthritis of left elbow

    M05.429 Rheumatoid myopathy with rheumatoid arthritis of unspecified elbow

● **M05.43** Rheumatoid myopathy with rheumatoid arthritis of wrist
     Rheumatoid myopathy with rheumatoid arthritis, carpal bones

    M05.431 Rheumatoid myopathy with rheumatoid arthritis of right wrist

    M05.432 Rheumatoid myopathy with rheumatoid arthritis of left wrist

    M05.439 Rheumatoid myopathy with rheumatoid arthritis of unspecified wrist

● **M05.44** Rheumatoid myopathy with rheumatoid arthritis of hand
     Rheumatoid myopathy with rheumatoid arthritis, metacarpus and phalanges

    M05.441 Rheumatoid myopathy with rheumatoid arthritis of right hand

    M05.442 Rheumatoid myopathy with rheumatoid arthritis of left hand

    M05.449 Rheumatoid myopathy with rheumatoid arthritis of unspecified hand

● **M05.45** Rheumatoid myopathy with rheumatoid arthritis of hip

    M05.451 Rheumatoid myopathy with rheumatoid arthritis of right hip

    M05.452 Rheumatoid myopathy with rheumatoid arthritis of left hip

    M05.459 Rheumatoid myopathy with rheumatoid arthritis of unspecified hip

● **M05.46** Rheumatoid myopathy with rheumatoid arthritis of knee

    M05.461 Rheumatoid myopathy with rheumatoid arthritis of right knee

    M05.462 Rheumatoid myopathy with rheumatoid arthritis of left knee

    M05.469 Rheumatoid myopathy with rheumatoid arthritis of unspecified knee

● **M05.47** Rheumatoid myopathy with rheumatoid arthritis of ankle and foot
     Rheumatoid myopathy with rheumatoid arthritis, tarsus, metatarsus and phalanges

    M05.471 Rheumatoid myopathy with rheumatoid arthritis of right ankle and foot

    M05.472 Rheumatoid myopathy with rheumatoid arthritis of left ankle and foot

    M05.479 Rheumatoid myopathy with rheumatoid arthritis of unspecified ankle and foot

  M05.49 Rheumatoid myopathy with rheumatoid arthritis of multiple sites

● **M05.5 Rheumatoid polyneuropathy with rheumatoid arthritis**

  M05.50 Rheumatoid polyneuropathy with rheumatoid arthritis of unspecified site

● **M05.51** Rheumatoid polyneuropathy with rheumatoid arthritis of shoulder

    M05.511 Rheumatoid polyneuropathy with rheumatoid arthritis of right shoulder

    M05.512 Rheumatoid polyneuropathy with rheumatoid arthritis of left shoulder

    M05.519 Rheumatoid polyneuropathy with rheumatoid arthritis of unspecified shoulder

● **M05.52** Rheumatoid polyneuropathy with rheumatoid arthritis of elbow

    M05.521 Rheumatoid polyneuropathy with rheumatoid arthritis of right elbow

    M05.522 Rheumatoid polyneuropathy with rheumatoid arthritis of left elbow

    M05.529 Rheumatoid polyneuropathy with rheumatoid arthritis of unspecified elbow

● **M05.53** Rheumatoid polyneuropathy with rheumatoid arthritis of wrist
     Rheumatoid polyneuropathy with rheumatoid arthritis, carpal bones

    M05.531 Rheumatoid polyneuropathy with rheumatoid arthritis of right wrist

    M05.532 Rheumatoid polyneuropathy with rheumatoid arthritis of left wrist

    M05.539 Rheumatoid polyneuropathy with rheumatoid arthritis of unspecified wrist

● **M05.54** Rheumatoid polyneuropathy with rheumatoid arthritis of hand
     Rheumatoid polyneuropathy with rheumatoid arthritis, metacarpus and phalanges

    M05.541 Rheumatoid polyneuropathy with rheumatoid arthritis of right hand

    M05.542 Rheumatoid polyneuropathy with rheumatoid arthritis of left hand

    M05.549 Rheumatoid polyneuropathy with rheumatoid arthritis of unspecified hand

● **M05.55** Rheumatoid polyneuropathy with rheumatoid arthritis of hip

    M05.551 Rheumatoid polyneuropathy with rheumatoid arthritis of right hip

    M05.552 Rheumatoid polyneuropathy with rheumatoid arthritis of left hip

    M05.559 Rheumatoid polyneuropathy with rheumatoid arthritis of unspecified hip

◀ New   ◀Ⅲ Revised   ~~deleted~~ Deleted   Excludes 1   Excludes 2   Includes   Use additional   Code first   Code also   Unspecified

OGCR Official Guidelines   X Assign placeholder X   ● Use Additional Character(s)   ▶ Manifestation Code   **Coding Clinic**

● M05.56   Rheumatoid polyneuropathy with rheumatoid arthritis of knee

    M05.561   Rheumatoid polyneuropathy with rheumatoid arthritis of right knee

    M05.562   Rheumatoid polyneuropathy with rheumatoid arthritis of left knee

    M05.569   Rheumatoid polyneuropathy with rheumatoid arthritis of unspecified knee

● M05.57   Rheumatoid polyneuropathy with rheumatoid arthritis of ankle and foot

    Rheumatoid polyneuropathy with rheumatoid arthritis, tarsus, metatarsus and phalanges

    M05.571   Rheumatoid polyneuropathy with rheumatoid arthritis of right ankle and foot

    M05.572   Rheumatoid polyneuropathy with rheumatoid arthritis of left ankle and foot

    M05.579   Rheumatoid polyneuropathy with rheumatoid arthritis of unspecified ankle and foot

    M05.59   Rheumatoid polyneuropathy with rheumatoid arthritis of multiple sites

● M05.6   Rheumatoid arthritis with involvement of other organs and systems

    M05.60   Rheumatoid arthritis of unspecified site with involvement of other organs and systems

● M05.61   Rheumatoid arthritis of shoulder with involvement of other organs and systems

    M05.611   Rheumatoid arthritis of right shoulder with involvement of other organs and systems

    M05.612   Rheumatoid arthritis of left shoulder with involvement of other organs and systems

    M05.619   Rheumatoid arthritis of unspecified shoulder with involvement of other organs and systems

● M05.62   Rheumatoid arthritis of elbow with involvement of other organs and systems

    M05.621   Rheumatoid arthritis of right elbow with involvement of other organs and systems

    M05.622   Rheumatoid arthritis of left elbow with involvement of other organs and systems

    M05.629   Rheumatoid arthritis of unspecified elbow with involvement of other organs and systems

● M05.63   Rheumatoid arthritis of wrist with involvement of other organs and systems

    Rheumatoid arthritis of carpal bones with involvement of other organs and systems

    M05.631   Rheumatoid arthritis of right wrist with involvement of other organs and systems

    M05.632   Rheumatoid arthritis of left wrist with involvement of other organs and systems

    M05.639   Rheumatoid arthritis of unspecified wrist with involvement of other organs and systems

● M05.64   Rheumatoid arthritis of hand with involvement of other organs and systems

    Rheumatoid arthritis of metacarpus and phalanges with involvement of other organs and systems

    M05.641   Rheumatoid arthritis of right hand with involvement of other organs and systems

    M05.642   Rheumatoid arthritis of left hand with involvement of other organs and systems

    M05.649   Rheumatoid arthritis of unspecified hand with involvement of other organs and systems

● M05.65   Rheumatoid arthritis of hip with involvement of other organs and systems

    M05.651   Rheumatoid arthritis of right hip with involvement of other organs and systems

    M05.652   Rheumatoid arthritis of left hip with involvement of other organs and systems

    M05.659   Rheumatoid arthritis of unspecified hip with involvement of other organs and systems

● M05.66   Rheumatoid arthritis of knee with involvement of other organs and systems

    M05.661   Rheumatoid arthritis of right knee with involvement of other organs and systems

    M05.662   Rheumatoid arthritis of left knee with involvement of other organs and systems

    M05.669   Rheumatoid arthritis of unspecified knee with involvement of other organs and systems

● M05.67   Rheumatoid arthritis of ankle and foot with involvement of other organs and systems

    Rheumatoid arthritis of tarsus, metatarsus and phalanges with involvement of other organs and systems

    M05.671   Rheumatoid arthritis of right ankle and foot with involvement of other organs and systems

    M05.672   Rheumatoid arthritis of left ankle and foot with involvement of other organs and systems

    M05.679   Rheumatoid arthritis of unspecified ankle and foot with involvement of other organs and systems

    M05.69   Rheumatoid arthritis of multiple sites with involvement of other organs and systems

● M05.7   Rheumatoid arthritis with rheumatoid factor without organ or systems involvement

    M05.70   Rheumatoid arthritis with rheumatoid factor of unspecified site without organ or systems involvement

● M05.71   Rheumatoid arthritis with rheumatoid factor of shoulder without organ or systems involvement

    M05.711   Rheumatoid arthritis with rheumatoid factor of right shoulder without organ or systems involvement

    M05.712   Rheumatoid arthritis with rheumatoid factor of left shoulder without organ or systems involvement

    M05.719   Rheumatoid arthritis with rheumatoid factor of unspecified shoulder without organ or systems involvement

CHAPTER 13 (M00-M99)

● **M05.72** Rheumatoid arthritis with rheumatoid factor of elbow without organ or systems involvement

    M05.721 Rheumatoid arthritis with rheumatoid factor of right elbow without organ or systems involvement

    M05.722 Rheumatoid arthritis with rheumatoid factor of left elbow without organ or systems involvement

    M05.729 Rheumatoid arthritis with rheumatoid factor of unspecified elbow without organ or systems involvement

● **M05.73** Rheumatoid arthritis with rheumatoid factor of wrist without organ or systems involvement

    M05.731 Rheumatoid arthritis with rheumatoid factor of right wrist without organ or systems involvement

    M05.732 Rheumatoid arthritis with rheumatoid factor of left wrist without organ or systems involvement

    M05.739 Rheumatoid arthritis with rheumatoid factor of unspecified wrist without organ or systems involvement

● **M05.74** Rheumatoid arthritis with rheumatoid factor of hand without organ or systems involvement

    M05.741 Rheumatoid arthritis with rheumatoid factor of right hand without organ or systems involvement

    M05.742 Rheumatoid arthritis with rheumatoid factor of left hand without organ or systems involvement

    M05.749 Rheumatoid arthritis with rheumatoid factor of unspecified hand without organ or systems involvement

● **M05.75** Rheumatoid arthritis with rheumatoid factor of hip without organ or systems involvement

    M05.751 Rheumatoid arthritis with rheumatoid factor of right hip without organ or systems involvement

    M05.752 Rheumatoid arthritis with rheumatoid factor of left hip without organ or systems involvement

    M05.759 Rheumatoid arthritis with rheumatoid factor of unspecified hip without organ or systems involvement

● **M05.76** Rheumatoid arthritis with rheumatoid factor of knee without organ or systems involvement

    M05.761 Rheumatoid arthritis with rheumatoid factor of right knee without organ or systems involvement

    M05.762 Rheumatoid arthritis with rheumatoid factor of left knee without organ or systems involvement

    M05.769 Rheumatoid arthritis with rheumatoid factor of unspecified knee without organ or systems involvement

● **M05.77** Rheumatoid arthritis with rheumatoid factor of ankle and foot without organ or systems involvement

    M05.771 Rheumatoid arthritis with rheumatoid factor of right ankle and foot without organ or systems involvement

    M05.772 Rheumatoid arthritis with rheumatoid factor of left ankle and foot without organ or systems involvement

    M05.779 Rheumatoid arthritis with rheumatoid factor of unspecified ankle and foot without organ or systems involvement

    M05.79 Rheumatoid arthritis with rheumatoid factor of multiple sites without organ or systems involvement

● **M05.8** Other rheumatoid arthritis with rheumatoid factor

    M05.80 Other rheumatoid arthritis with rheumatoid factor of unspecified site

●   **M05.81** Other rheumatoid arthritis with rheumatoid factor of shoulder

    M05.811 Other rheumatoid arthritis with rheumatoid factor of right shoulder

    M05.812 Other rheumatoid arthritis with rheumatoid factor of left shoulder

    M05.819 Other rheumatoid arthritis with rheumatoid factor of unspecified shoulder

●   **M05.82** Other rheumatoid arthritis with rheumatoid factor of elbow

    M05.821 Other rheumatoid arthritis with rheumatoid factor of right elbow

    M05.822 Other rheumatoid arthritis with rheumatoid factor of left elbow

    M05.829 Other rheumatoid arthritis with rheumatoid factor of unspecified elbow

●   **M05.83** Other rheumatoid arthritis with rheumatoid factor of wrist

    M05.831 Other rheumatoid arthritis with rheumatoid factor of right wrist

    M05.832 Other rheumatoid arthritis with rheumatoid factor of left wrist

    M05.839 Other rheumatoid arthritis with rheumatoid factor of unspecified wrist

●   **M05.84** Other rheumatoid arthritis with rheumatoid factor of hand

    M05.841 Other rheumatoid arthritis with rheumatoid factor of right hand

    M05.842 Other rheumatoid arthritis with rheumatoid factor of left hand

    M05.849 Other rheumatoid arthritis with rheumatoid factor of unspecified hand

●   **M05.85** Other rheumatoid arthritis with rheumatoid factor of hip

    M05.851 Other rheumatoid arthritis with rheumatoid factor of right hip

    M05.852 Other rheumatoid arthritis with rheumatoid factor of left hip

    M05.859 Other rheumatoid arthritis with rheumatoid factor of unspecified hip

● **M05.86**   Other rheumatoid arthritis with rheumatoid factor of knee

     M05.861   Other rheumatoid arthritis with rheumatoid factor of right knee

     M05.862   Other rheumatoid arthritis with rheumatoid factor of left knee

     M05.869   Other rheumatoid arthritis with rheumatoid factor of unspecified knee

● **M05.87**   Other rheumatoid arthritis with rheumatoid factor of ankle and foot

     M05.871   Other rheumatoid arthritis with rheumatoid factor of right ankle and foot

     M05.872   Other rheumatoid arthritis with rheumatoid factor of left ankle and foot

     M05.879   Other rheumatoid arthritis with rheumatoid factor of unspecified ankle and foot

   M05.89   Other rheumatoid arthritis with rheumatoid factor of multiple sites

M05.9   Rheumatoid arthritis with rheumatoid factor, unspecified

● **M06**   Other rheumatoid arthritis

   ● **M06.0**   Rheumatoid arthritis without rheumatoid factor

     M06.00   Rheumatoid arthritis without rheumatoid factor, unspecified site

     ● M06.01   Rheumatoid arthritis without rheumatoid factor, shoulder

       M06.011   Rheumatoid arthritis without rheumatoid factor, right shoulder

       M06.012   Rheumatoid arthritis without rheumatoid factor, left shoulder

       M06.019   Rheumatoid arthritis without rheumatoid factor, unspecified shoulder

     ● M06.02   Rheumatoid arthritis without rheumatoid factor, elbow

       M06.021   Rheumatoid arthritis without rheumatoid factor, right elbow

       M06.022   Rheumatoid arthritis without rheumatoid factor, left elbow

       M06.029   Rheumatoid arthritis without rheumatoid factor, unspecified elbow

     ● M06.03   Rheumatoid arthritis without rheumatoid factor, wrist

       M06.031   Rheumatoid arthritis without rheumatoid factor, right wrist

       M06.032   Rheumatoid arthritis without rheumatoid factor, left wrist

       M06.039   Rheumatoid arthritis without rheumatoid factor, unspecified wrist

     ● M06.04   Rheumatoid arthritis without rheumatoid factor, hand

       M06.041   Rheumatoid arthritis without rheumatoid factor, right hand

       M06.042   Rheumatoid arthritis without rheumatoid factor, left hand

       M06.049   Rheumatoid arthritis without rheumatoid factor, unspecified hand

     ● M06.05   Rheumatoid arthritis without rheumatoid factor, hip

       M06.051   Rheumatoid arthritis without rheumatoid factor, right hip

       M06.052   Rheumatoid arthritis without rheumatoid factor, left hip

       M06.059   Rheumatoid arthritis without rheumatoid factor, unspecified hip

● **M06.06**   Rheumatoid arthritis without rheumatoid factor, knee

     M06.061   Rheumatoid arthritis without rheumatoid factor, right knee

     M06.062   Rheumatoid arthritis without rheumatoid factor, left knee

     M06.069   Rheumatoid arthritis without rheumatoid factor, unspecified knee

● **M06.07**   Rheumatoid arthritis without rheumatoid factor, ankle and foot

     M06.071   Rheumatoid arthritis without rheumatoid factor, right ankle and foot

     M06.072   Rheumatoid arthritis without rheumatoid factor, left ankle and foot

     M06.079   Rheumatoid arthritis without rheumatoid factor, unspecified ankle and foot

   M06.08   Rheumatoid arthritis without rheumatoid factor, vertebrae

   M06.09   Rheumatoid arthritis without rheumatoid factor, multiple sites

M06.1   Adult-onset Still's disease   A

     Excludes1   Still's disease NOS (M08.2-)

● M06.2   Rheumatoid bursitis

   M06.20   Rheumatoid bursitis, unspecified site

   ● M06.21   Rheumatoid bursitis, shoulder

     M06.211   Rheumatoid bursitis, right shoulder

     M06.212   Rheumatoid bursitis, left shoulder

     M06.219   Rheumatoid bursitis, unspecified shoulder

   ● M06.22   Rheumatoid bursitis, elbow

     M06.221   Rheumatoid bursitis, right elbow

     M06.222   Rheumatoid bursitis, left elbow

     M06.229   Rheumatoid bursitis, unspecified elbow

   ● M06.23   Rheumatoid bursitis, wrist

     M06.231   Rheumatoid bursitis, right wrist

     M06.232   Rheumatoid bursitis, left wrist

     M06.239   Rheumatoid bursitis, unspecified wrist

   ● M06.24   Rheumatoid bursitis, hand

     M06.241   Rheumatoid bursitis, right hand

     M06.242   Rheumatoid bursitis, left hand

     M06.249   Rheumatoid bursitis, unspecified hand

   ● M06.25   Rheumatoid bursitis, hip

     M06.251   Rheumatoid bursitis, right hip

     M06.252   Rheumatoid bursitis, left hip

     M06.259   Rheumatoid bursitis, unspecified hip

   ● M06.26   Rheumatoid bursitis, knee

     M06.261   Rheumatoid bursitis, right knee

     M06.262   Rheumatoid bursitis, left knee

     M06.269   Rheumatoid bursitis, unspecified knee

   ● M06.27   Rheumatoid bursitis, ankle and foot

     M06.271   Rheumatoid bursitis, right ankle and foot

     M06.272   Rheumatoid bursitis, left ankle and foot

     M06.279   Rheumatoid bursitis, unspecified ankle and foot

   M06.28   Rheumatoid bursitis, vertebrae

   M06.29   Rheumatoid bursitis, multiple sites

CHAPTER 13 (M00-M99)

● M06.3   **Rheumatoid nodule**
    M06.30   Rheumatoid nodule, unspecified site
● M06.31   Rheumatoid nodule, shoulder
       M06.311   Rheumatoid nodule, right shoulder
       M06.312   Rheumatoid nodule, left shoulder
       M06.319   Rheumatoid nodule, unspecified shoulder
● M06.32   Rheumatoid nodule, elbow
       M06.321   Rheumatoid nodule, right elbow
       M06.322   Rheumatoid nodule, left elbow
       M06.329   Rheumatoid nodule, unspecified elbow
● M06.33   Rheumatoid nodule, wrist
       M06.331   Rheumatoid nodule, right wrist
       M06.332   Rheumatoid nodule, left wrist
       M06.339   Rheumatoid nodule, unspecified wrist
● M06.34   Rheumatoid nodule, hand
       M06.341   Rheumatoid nodule, right hand
       M06.342   Rheumatoid nodule, left hand
       M06.349   Rheumatoid nodule, unspecified hand
● M06.35   Rheumatoid nodule, hip
       M06.351   Rheumatoid nodule, right hip
       M06.352   Rheumatoid nodule, left hip
       M06.359   Rheumatoid nodule, unspecified hip
● M06.36   Rheumatoid nodule, knee
       M06.361   Rheumatoid nodule, right knee
       M06.362   Rheumatoid nodule, left knee
       M06.369   Rheumatoid nodule, unspecified knee
● M06.37   Rheumatoid nodule, ankle and foot
       M06.371   Rheumatoid nodule, right ankle and foot
       M06.372   Rheumatoid nodule, left ankle and foot
       M06.379   Rheumatoid nodule, unspecified ankle and foot
    M06.38   Rheumatoid nodule, vertebrae
    M06.39   Rheumatoid nodule, multiple sites
  M06.4   **Inflammatory polyarthropathy**
      Excludes1   polyarthritis NOS (M13.0)
● M06.8   **Other specified rheumatoid arthritis**
    M06.80   Other specified rheumatoid arthritis, unspecified site
● M06.81   Other specified rheumatoid arthritis, shoulder
       M06.811   Other specified rheumatoid arthritis, right shoulder
       M06.812   Other specified rheumatoid arthritis, left shoulder
       M06.819   Other specified rheumatoid arthritis, unspecified shoulder
● M06.82   Other specified rheumatoid arthritis, elbow
       M06.821   Other specified rheumatoid arthritis, right elbow
       M06.822   Other specified rheumatoid arthritis, left elbow
       M06.829   Other specified rheumatoid arthritis, unspecified elbow
● M06.83   Other specified rheumatoid arthritis, wrist
       M06.831   Other specified rheumatoid arthritis, right wrist
       M06.832   Other specified rheumatoid arthritis, left wrist
       M06.839   Other specified rheumatoid arthritis, unspecified wrist

● M06.84   Other specified rheumatoid arthritis, hand
       M06.841   Other specified rheumatoid arthritis, right hand
       M06.842   Other specified rheumatoid arthritis, left hand
       M06.849   Other specified rheumatoid arthritis, unspecified hand
● M06.85   Other specified rheumatoid arthritis, hip
       M06.851   Other specified rheumatoid arthritis, right hip
       M06.852   Other specified rheumatoid arthritis, left hip
       M06.859   Other specified rheumatoid arthritis, unspecified hip
● M06.86   Other specified rheumatoid arthritis, knee
       M06.861   Other specified rheumatoid arthritis, right knee
       M06.862   Other specified rheumatoid arthritis, left knee
       M06.869   Other specified rheumatoid arthritis, unspecified knee
● M06.87   Other specified rheumatoid arthritis, ankle and foot
       M06.871   Other specified rheumatoid arthritis, right ankle and foot
       M06.872   Other specified rheumatoid arthritis, left ankle and foot
       M06.879   Other specified rheumatoid arthritis, unspecified ankle and foot
    M06.88   Other specified rheumatoid arthritis, vertebrae
    M06.89   Other specified rheumatoid arthritis, multiple sites
  M06.9   **Rheumatoid arthritis, unspecified**

● M07   **Enteropathic arthropathies**
    Code also associated enteropathy, such as:
      regional enteritis [Crohn's disease] (K50.-)
      ulcerative colitis (K51.-)
      Excludes1   psoriatic arthropathies (L40.5-)
● M07.6   **Enteropathic arthropathies**
    M07.60   Enteropathic arthropathies, unspecified site
● M07.61   Enteropathic arthropathies, shoulder
       M07.611   Enteropathic arthropathies, right shoulder
       M07.612   Enteropathic arthropathies, left shoulder
       M07.619   Enteropathic arthropathies, unspecified shoulder
● M07.62   Enteropathic arthropathies, elbow
       M07.621   Enteropathic arthropathies, right elbow
       M07.622   Enteropathic arthropathies, left elbow
       M07.629   Enteropathic arthropathies, unspecified elbow
● M07.63   Enteropathic arthropathies, wrist
       M07.631   Enteropathic arthropathies, right wrist
       M07.632   Enteropathic arthropathies, left wrist
       M07.639   Enteropathic arthropathies, unspecified wrist
● M07.64   Enteropathic arthropathies, hand
       M07.641   Enteropathic arthropathies, right hand
       M07.642   Enteropathic arthropathies, left hand
       M07.649   Enteropathic arthropathies, unspecified hand

◄ New   ⬅ Revised   ~~deleted~~ Deleted   Excludes 1   Excludes 2   Includes   Use additional   Code first   Code also   Unspecified

OGCR Official Guidelines   X Assign placeholder X   ● Use Additional Character(s)   ▶ Manifestation Code   **Coding Clinic**

976

● M07.65   Enteropathic arthropathies, hip
     M07.651   Enteropathic arthropathies, right hip
     M07.652   Enteropathic arthropathies, left hip
     M07.659   Enteropathic arthropathies, unspecified hip

● M07.66   Enteropathic arthropathies, knee
     M07.661   Enteropathic arthropathies, right knee
     M07.662   Enteropathic arthropathies, left knee
     M07.669   Enteropathic arthropathies, unspecified knee

● M07.67   Enteropathic arthropathies, ankle and foot
     M07.671   Enteropathic arthropathies, right ankle and foot
     M07.672   Enteropathic arthropathies, left ankle and foot
     M07.679   Enteropathic arthropathies, unspecified ankle and foot

   M07.68   Enteropathic arthropathies, vertebrae

   M07.69   Enteropathic arthropathies, multiple sites

● **M08   Juvenile arthritis**
     Code also any associated underlying condition, such as:
       regional enteritis [Crohn's disease] (K50.-)
       ulcerative colitis (K51.-)
     Excludes1   arthropathy in Whipple's disease (M14.8)
               Felty's syndrome (M05.0)
               juvenile dermatomyositis (M33.0-)
               psoriatic juvenile arthropathy (L40.54)

● M08.0   Unspecified juvenile rheumatoid arthritis
     Juvenile rheumatoid arthritis with or without rheumatoid factor
     M08.00   Unspecified juvenile rheumatoid arthritis of unspecified site
   ● M08.01   Unspecified juvenile rheumatoid arthritis, shoulder
     M08.011   Unspecified juvenile rheumatoid arthritis, right shoulder
     M08.012   Unspecified juvenile rheumatoid arthritis, left shoulder
     M08.019   Unspecified juvenile rheumatoid arthritis, unspecified shoulder
   ● M08.02   Unspecified juvenile rheumatoid arthritis of elbow
     M08.021   Unspecified juvenile rheumatoid arthritis, right elbow
     M08.022   Unspecified juvenile rheumatoid arthritis, left elbow
     M08.029   Unspecified juvenile rheumatoid arthritis, unspecified elbow
   ● M08.03   Unspecified juvenile rheumatoid arthritis, wrist
     M08.031   Unspecified juvenile rheumatoid arthritis, right wrist
     M08.032   Unspecified juvenile rheumatoid arthritis, left wrist
     M08.039   Unspecified juvenile rheumatoid arthritis, unspecified wrist
   ● M08.04   Unspecified juvenile rheumatoid arthritis, hand
     M08.041   Unspecified juvenile rheumatoid arthritis, right hand
     M08.042   Unspecified juvenile rheumatoid arthritis, left hand
     M08.049   Unspecified juvenile rheumatoid arthritis, unspecified hand
   ● M08.05   Unspecified juvenile rheumatoid arthritis, hip
     M08.051   Unspecified juvenile rheumatoid arthritis, right hip
     M08.052   Unspecified juvenile rheumatoid arthritis, left hip
     M08.059   Unspecified juvenile rheumatoid arthritis, unspecified hip

● M08.06   Unspecified juvenile rheumatoid arthritis, knee
     M08.061   Unspecified juvenile rheumatoid arthritis, right knee
     M08.062   Unspecified juvenile rheumatoid arthritis, left knee
     M08.069   Unspecified juvenile rheumatoid arthritis, unspecified knee
   ● M08.07   Unspecified juvenile rheumatoid arthritis, ankle and foot
     M08.071   Unspecified juvenile rheumatoid arthritis, right ankle and foot
     M08.072   Unspecified juvenile rheumatoid arthritis, left ankle and foot
     M08.079   Unspecified juvenile rheumatoid arthritis, unspecified ankle and foot
   M08.08   Unspecified juvenile rheumatoid arthritis, vertebrae
   M08.09   Unspecified juvenile rheumatoid arthritis, multiple sites

M08.1   Juvenile ankylosing spondylitis
     Excludes1   ankylosing spondylitis in adults (M45.0-)

● M08.2   Juvenile rheumatoid arthritis with systemic onset
     Still's disease NOS
     Excludes1   adult-onset Still's disease (M06.1-)
     M08.20   Juvenile rheumatoid arthritis with systemic onset, unspecified site
   ● M08.21   Juvenile rheumatoid arthritis with systemic onset, shoulder
     M08.211   Juvenile rheumatoid arthritis with systemic onset, right shoulder
     M08.212   Juvenile rheumatoid arthritis with systemic onset, left shoulder
     M08.219   Juvenile rheumatoid arthritis with systemic onset, unspecified shoulder
   ● M08.22   Juvenile rheumatoid arthritis with systemic onset, elbow
     M08.221   Juvenile rheumatoid arthritis with systemic onset, right elbow
     M08.222   Juvenile rheumatoid arthritis with systemic onset, left elbow
     M08.229   Juvenile rheumatoid arthritis with systemic onset, unspecified elbow
   ● M08.23   Juvenile rheumatoid arthritis with systemic onset, wrist
     M08.231   Juvenile rheumatoid arthritis with systemic onset, right wrist
     M08.232   Juvenile rheumatoid arthritis with systemic onset, left wrist
     M08.239   Juvenile rheumatoid arthritis with systemic onset, unspecified wrist
   ● M08.24   Juvenile rheumatoid arthritis with systemic onset, hand
     M08.241   Juvenile rheumatoid arthritis with systemic onset, right hand
     M08.242   Juvenile rheumatoid arthritis with systemic onset, left hand
     M08.249   Juvenile rheumatoid arthritis with systemic onset, unspecified hand
   ● M08.25   Juvenile rheumatoid arthritis with systemic onset, hip
     M08.251   Juvenile rheumatoid arthritis with systemic onset, right hip
     M08.252   Juvenile rheumatoid arthritis with systemic onset, left hip
     M08.259   Juvenile rheumatoid arthritis with systemic onset, unspecified hip

CHAPTER 13 (M00-M99)

● **M08.26** Juvenile rheumatoid arthritis with systemic onset, knee

　　M08.261　Juvenile rheumatoid arthritis with systemic onset, right knee

　　M08.262　Juvenile rheumatoid arthritis with systemic onset, left knee

　　M08.269　Juvenile rheumatoid arthritis with systemic onset, unspecified knee

● **M08.27** Juvenile rheumatoid arthritis with systemic onset, ankle and foot

　　M08.271　Juvenile rheumatoid arthritis with systemic onset, right ankle and foot

　　M08.272　Juvenile rheumatoid arthritis with systemic onset, left ankle and foot

　　M08.279　Juvenile rheumatoid arthritis with systemic onset, unspecified ankle and foot

　M08.28　Juvenile rheumatoid arthritis with systemic onset, vertebrae

　M08.29　Juvenile rheumatoid arthritis with systemic onset, multiple sites

M08.3　Juvenile rheumatoid polyarthritis (seronegative)

● M08.4　Pauciarticular juvenile rheumatoid arthritis

　M08.40　Pauciarticular juvenile rheumatoid arthritis, unspecified site

● M08.41　Pauciarticular juvenile rheumatoid arthritis, shoulder

　　M08.411　Pauciarticular juvenile rheumatoid arthritis, right shoulder

　　M08.412　Pauciarticular juvenile rheumatoid arthritis, left shoulder

　　M08.419　Pauciarticular juvenile rheumatoid arthritis, unspecified shoulder

● M08.42　Pauciarticular juvenile rheumatoid arthritis, elbow

　　M08.421　Pauciarticular juvenile rheumatoid arthritis, right elbow

　　M08.422　Pauciarticular juvenile rheumatoid arthritis, left elbow

　　M08.429　Pauciarticular juvenile rheumatoid arthritis, unspecified elbow

● M08.43　Pauciarticular juvenile rheumatoid arthritis, wrist

　　M08.431　Pauciarticular juvenile rheumatoid arthritis, right wrist

　　M08.432　Pauciarticular juvenile rheumatoid arthritis, left wrist

　　M08.439　Pauciarticular juvenile rheumatoid arthritis, unspecified wrist

● M08.44　Pauciarticular juvenile rheumatoid arthritis, hand

　　M08.441　Pauciarticular juvenile rheumatoid arthritis, right hand

　　M08.442　Pauciarticular juvenile rheumatoid arthritis, left hand

　　M08.449　Pauciarticular juvenile rheumatoid arthritis, unspecified hand

● M08.45　Pauciarticular juvenile rheumatoid arthritis, hip

　　M08.451　Pauciarticular juvenile rheumatoid arthritis, right hip

　　M08.452　Pauciarticular juvenile rheumatoid arthritis, left hip

　　M08.459　Pauciarticular juvenile rheumatoid arthritis, unspecified hip

● M08.46　Pauciarticular juvenile rheumatoid arthritis, knee

　　M08.461　Pauciarticular juvenile rheumatoid arthritis, right knee

　　M08.462　Pauciarticular juvenile rheumatoid arthritis, left knee

　　M08.469　Pauciarticular juvenile rheumatoid arthritis, unspecified knee

● M08.47　Pauciarticular juvenile rheumatoid arthritis, ankle and foot

　　M08.471　Pauciarticular juvenile rheumatoid arthritis, right ankle and foot

　　M08.472　Pauciarticular juvenile rheumatoid arthritis, left ankle and foot

　　M08.479　Pauciarticular juvenile rheumatoid arthritis, unspecified ankle and foot

　M08.48　Pauciarticular juvenile rheumatoid arthritis, vertebrae

● M08.8　Other juvenile arthritis

　M08.80　Other juvenile arthritis, unspecified site

● M08.81　Other juvenile arthritis, shoulder

　　M08.811　Other juvenile arthritis, right shoulder

　　M08.812　Other juvenile arthritis, left shoulder

　　M08.819　Other juvenile arthritis, unspecified shoulder

● M08.82　Other juvenile arthritis, elbow

　　M08.821　Other juvenile arthritis, right elbow

　　M08.822　Other juvenile arthritis, left elbow

　　M08.829　Other juvenile arthritis, unspecified elbow

● M08.83　Other juvenile arthritis, wrist

　　M08.831　Other juvenile arthritis, right wrist

　　M08.832　Other juvenile arthritis, left wrist

　　M08.839　Other juvenile arthritis, unspecified wrist

● M08.84　Other juvenile arthritis, hand

　　M08.841　Other juvenile arthritis, right hand

　　M08.842　Other juvenile arthritis, left hand

　　M08.849　Other juvenile arthritis, unspecified hand

● M08.85　Other juvenile arthritis, hip

　　M08.851　Other juvenile arthritis, right hip

　　M08.852　Other juvenile arthritis, left hip

　　M08.859　Other juvenile arthritis, unspecified hip

● M08.86　Other juvenile arthritis, knee

　　M08.861　Other juvenile arthritis, right knee

　　M08.862　Other juvenile arthritis, left knee

　　M08.869　Other juvenile arthritis, unspecified knee

● M08.87　Other juvenile arthritis, ankle and foot

　　M08.871　Other juvenile arthritis, right ankle and foot

　　M08.872　Other juvenile arthritis, left ankle and foot

　　M08.879　Other juvenile arthritis, unspecified ankle and foot

　M08.88　Other juvenile arthritis, other specified site
　　　　　Other juvenile arthritis, vertebrae

　M08.89　Other juvenile arthritis, multiple sites

◀ New　◀▦ Revised　deleted Deleted　Excludes 1　Excludes 2　Includes　Use additional　Code first　Code also　Unspecified

OGCR Official Guidelines　X Assign placeholder X　● Use Additional Character(s)　▌ Manifestation Code　**Coding Clinic**

● **M08.9 Juvenile arthritis, unspecified**

     Excludes1   juvenile rheumatoid arthritis, unspecified (M08.0-)

     M08.90   Juvenile arthritis, unspecified, unspecified site

● **M08.91**   Juvenile arthritis, unspecified, shoulder

      M08.911   Juvenile arthritis, unspecified, right shoulder

      M08.912   Juvenile arthritis, unspecified, left shoulder

      M08.919   Juvenile arthritis, unspecified, unspecified shoulder

● **M08.92**   Juvenile arthritis, unspecified, elbow

      M08.921   Juvenile arthritis, unspecified, right elbow

      M08.922   Juvenile arthritis, unspecified, left elbow

      M08.929   Juvenile arthritis, unspecified, unspecified elbow

● **M08.93**   Juvenile arthritis, unspecified, wrist

      M08.931   Juvenile arthritis, unspecified, right wrist

      M08.932   Juvenile arthritis, unspecified, left wrist

      M08.939   Juvenile arthritis, unspecified, unspecified wrist

● **M08.94**   Juvenile arthritis, unspecified, hand

      M08.941   Juvenile arthritis, unspecified, right hand

      M08.942   Juvenile arthritis, unspecified, left hand

      M08.949   Juvenile arthritis, unspecified, unspecified hand

● **M08.95**   Juvenile arthritis, unspecified, hip

      M08.951   Juvenile arthritis, unspecified, right hip

      M08.952   Juvenile arthritis, unspecified, left hip

      M08.959   Juvenile arthritis, unspecified, unspecified hip

● **M08.96**   Juvenile arthritis, unspecified, knee

      M08.961   Juvenile arthritis, unspecified, right knee

      M08.962   Juvenile arthritis, unspecified, left knee

      M08.969   Juvenile arthritis, unspecified, unspecified knee

● **M08.97**   Juvenile arthritis, unspecified, ankle and foot

      M08.971   Juvenile arthritis, unspecified, right ankle and foot

      M08.972   Juvenile arthritis, unspecified, left ankle and foot

      M08.979   Juvenile arthritis, unspecified, unspecified ankle and foot

     M08.98   Juvenile arthritis, unspecified, vertebrae

     M08.99   Juvenile arthritis, unspecified, multiple sites

● **M1A Chronic gout**

     Use additional code to identify:

       Autonomic neuropathy in diseases classified elsewhere (G99.0)

       Calculus of urinary tract in diseases classified elsewhere (N22)

       Cardiomyopathy in diseases classified elsewhere (I43)

       Disorders of external ear in diseases classified elsewhere (H61.1-, H62.8-)

       Disorders of iris and ciliary body in diseases classified elsewhere (H22)

       Glomerular disorders in diseases classified elsewhere (N08)

     Excludes1   gout NOS (M10.-)

     Excludes2   acute gout (M10.-) ◄

     The appropriate 7th character is to be added to each code from category M1A

>   Ø   without tophus (tophi)
>   1   with tophus (tophi)

● **M1A.Ø Idiopathic chronic gout**

       Chronic gouty bursitis

       Primary chronic gout

X ● **M1A.00**   Idiopathic chronic gout, unspecified site

● **M1A.01**   Idiopathic chronic gout, shoulder

      ● **M1A.011**   Idiopathic chronic gout, right shoulder

      ● **M1A.012**   Idiopathic chronic gout, left shoulder

      ● **M1A.019**   Idiopathic chronic gout, unspecified shoulder

● **M1A.02**   Idiopathic chronic gout, elbow

      ● **M1A.021**   Idiopathic chronic gout, right elbow

      ● **M1A.022**   Idiopathic chronic gout, left elbow

      ● **M1A.029**   Idiopathic chronic gout, unspecified elbow

● **M1A.03**   Idiopathic chronic gout, wrist

      ● **M1A.031**   Idiopathic chronic gout, right wrist

      ● **M1A.032**   Idiopathic chronic gout, left wrist

      ● **M1A.039**   Idiopathic chronic gout, unspecified wrist

● **M1A.04**   Idiopathic chronic gout, hand

      ● **M1A.041**   Idiopathic chronic gout, right hand

      ● **M1A.042**   Idiopathic chronic gout, left hand

      ● **M1A.049**   Idiopathic chronic gout, unspecified hand

● **M1A.05**   Idiopathic chronic gout, hip

      ● **M1A.051**   Idiopathic chronic gout, right hip

      ● **M1A.052**   Idiopathic chronic gout, left hip

      ● **M1A.059**   Idiopathic chronic gout, unspecified hip

● **M1A.06**   Idiopathic chronic gout, knee

      ● **M1A.061**   Idiopathic chronic gout, right knee

      ● **M1A.062**   Idiopathic chronic gout, left knee

      ● **M1A.069**   Idiopathic chronic gout, unspecified knee

● **M1A.07**   Idiopathic chronic gout, ankle and foot

      ● **M1A.071**   Idiopathic chronic gout, right ankle and foot

      ● **M1A.072**   Idiopathic chronic gout, left ankle and foot

      ● **M1A.079**   Idiopathic chronic gout, unspecified ankle and foot

X ● **M1A.08**   Idiopathic chronic gout, vertebrae

X ● **M1A.09**   Idiopathic chronic gout, multiple sites

CHAPTER 13 (M00-M99)

● **M1A.1** Lead-induced chronic gout
> *Code first* toxic effects of lead and its compounds (T56.0-)

X ● **M1A.10** Lead-induced chronic gout, ==unspecified== site
● **M1A.11** Lead-induced chronic gout, shoulder
  ● **M1A.111** Lead-induced chronic gout, right shoulder
  ● **M1A.112** Lead-induced chronic gout, left shoulder
  ● **M1A.119** Lead-induced chronic gout, ==unspecified== shoulder
● **M1A.12** Lead-induced chronic gout, elbow
  ● **M1A.121** Lead-induced chronic gout, right elbow
  ● **M1A.122** Lead-induced chronic gout, left elbow
  ● **M1A.129** Lead-induced chronic gout, ==unspecified== elbow
● **M1A.13** Lead-induced chronic gout, wrist
  ● **M1A.131** Lead-induced chronic gout, right wrist
  ● **M1A.132** Lead-induced chronic gout, left wrist
  ● **M1A.139** Lead-induced chronic gout, ==unspecified== wrist
● **M1A.14** Lead-induced chronic gout, hand
  ● **M1A.141** Lead-induced chronic gout, right hand
  ● **M1A.142** Lead-induced chronic gout, left hand
  ● **M1A.149** Lead-induced chronic gout, ==unspecified== hand
● **M1A.15** Lead-induced chronic gout, hip
  ● **M1A.151** Lead-induced chronic gout, right hip
  ● **M1A.152** Lead-induced chronic gout, left hip
  ● **M1A.159** Lead-induced chronic gout, ==unspecified== hip
● **M1A.16** Lead-induced chronic gout, knee
  ● **M1A.161** Lead-induced chronic gout, right knee
  ● **M1A.162** Lead-induced chronic gout, left knee
  ● **M1A.169** Lead-induced chronic gout, ==unspecified== knee
● **M1A.17** Lead-induced chronic gout, ankle and foot
  ● **M1A.171** Lead-induced chronic gout, right ankle and foot
  ● **M1A.172** Lead-induced chronic gout, left ankle and foot
  ● **M1A.179** Lead-induced chronic gout, ==unspecified== ankle and foot
X ● **M1A.18** Lead-induced chronic gout, vertebrae
X ● **M1A.19** Lead-induced chronic gout, multiple sites
● **M1A.2** Drug-induced chronic gout
> *Use additional* code for adverse effect, if applicable, to identify drug (T36-T50 with fifth or sixth character 5)

X ● **M1A.20** Drug-induced chronic gout, ==unspecified== site
● **M1A.21** Drug-induced chronic gout, shoulder
  ● **M1A.211** Drug-induced chronic gout, right shoulder
  ● **M1A.212** Drug-induced chronic gout, left shoulder
  ● **M1A.219** Drug-induced chronic gout, ==unspecified== shoulder
● **M1A.22** Drug-induced chronic gout, elbow
  ● **M1A.221** Drug-induced chronic gout, right elbow
  ● **M1A.222** Drug-induced chronic gout, left elbow
  ● **M1A.229** Drug-induced chronic gout, ==unspecified== elbow

● **M1A.23** Drug-induced chronic gout, wrist
  ● **M1A.231** Drug-induced chronic gout, right wrist
  ● **M1A.232** Drug-induced chronic gout, left wrist
  ● **M1A.239** Drug-induced chronic gout, ==unspecified== wrist
● **M1A.24** Drug-induced chronic gout, hand
  ● **M1A.241** Drug-induced chronic gout, right hand
  ● **M1A.242** Drug-induced chronic gout, left hand
  ● **M1A.249** Drug-induced chronic gout, ==unspecified== hand
● **M1A.25** Drug-induced chronic gout, hip
  ● **M1A.251** Drug-induced chronic gout, right hip
  ● **M1A.252** Drug-induced chronic gout, left hip
  ● **M1A.259** Drug-induced chronic gout, ==unspecified== hip
● **M1A.26** Drug-induced chronic gout, knee
  ● **M1A.261** Drug-induced chronic gout, right knee
  ● **M1A.262** Drug-induced chronic gout, left knee
  ● **M1A.269** Drug-induced chronic gout, ==unspecified== knee
● **M1A.27** Drug-induced chronic gout, ankle and foot
  ● **M1A.271** Drug-induced chronic gout, right ankle and foot
  ● **M1A.272** Drug-induced chronic gout, left ankle and foot
  ● **M1A.279** Drug-induced chronic gout, ==unspecified== ankle and foot
X ● **M1A.28** Drug-induced chronic gout, vertebrae
X ● **M1A.29** Drug-induced chronic gout, multiple sites
● **M1A.3** Chronic gout due to renal impairment
> *Code first* associated renal disease

X ● **M1A.30** Chronic gout due to renal impairment, ==unspecified== site
● **M1A.31** Chronic gout due to renal impairment, shoulder
  ● **M1A.311** Chronic gout due to renal impairment, right shoulder
  ● **M1A.312** Chronic gout due to renal impairment, left shoulder
  ● **M1A.319** Chronic gout due to renal impairment, ==unspecified== shoulder
● **M1A.32** Chronic gout due to renal impairment, elbow
  ● **M1A.321** Chronic gout due to renal impairment, right elbow
  ● **M1A.322** Chronic gout due to renal impairment, left elbow
  ● **M1A.329** Chronic gout due to renal impairment, ==unspecified== elbow
● **M1A.33** Chronic gout due to renal impairment, wrist
  ● **M1A.331** Chronic gout due to renal impairment, right wrist
  ● **M1A.332** Chronic gout due to renal impairment, left wrist
  ● **M1A.339** Chronic gout due to renal impairment, ==unspecified== wrist
● **M1A.34** Chronic gout due to renal impairment, hand
  ● **M1A.341** Chronic gout due to renal impairment, right hand
  ● **M1A.342** Chronic gout due to renal impairment, left hand
  ● **M1A.349** Chronic gout due to renal impairment, ==unspecified== hand

◀ New   ◀◀◀ Revised   ~~deleted~~ Deleted   Excludes 1   Excludes 2   Includes   Use additional   Code first   Code also   Unspecified

980   OGCR Official Guidelines   X Assign placeholder X   ● Use Additional Character(s)   ▶ Manifestation Code   **Coding Clinic**

- M1A.35 Chronic gout due to renal impairment, hip
  - M1A.351 Chronic gout due to renal impairment, right hip
  - M1A.352 Chronic gout due to renal impairment, left hip
  - M1A.359 Chronic gout due to renal impairment, unspecified hip
- M1A.36 Chronic gout due to renal impairment, knee
  - M1A.361 Chronic gout due to renal impairment, right knee
  - M1A.362 Chronic gout due to renal impairment, left knee
  - M1A.369 Chronic gout due to renal impairment, unspecified knee
- M1A.37 Chronic gout due to renal impairment, ankle and foot
  - M1A.371 Chronic gout due to renal impairment, right ankle and foot
  - M1A.372 Chronic gout due to renal impairment, left ankle and foot
  - M1A.379 Chronic gout due to renal impairment, unspecified ankle and foot
- X M1A.38 Chronic gout due to renal impairment, vertebrae
- X M1A.39 Chronic gout due to renal impairment, multiple sites
- M1A.4 Other secondary chronic gout
  - *Code first* associated condition
  - X M1A.40 Other secondary chronic gout, unspecified site
  - M1A.41 Other secondary chronic gout, shoulder
    - M1A.411 Other secondary chronic gout, right shoulder
    - M1A.412 Other secondary chronic gout, left shoulder
    - M1A.419 Other secondary chronic gout, unspecified shoulder
  - M1A.42 Other secondary chronic gout, elbow
    - M1A.421 Other secondary chronic gout, right elbow
    - M1A.422 Other secondary chronic gout, left elbow
    - M1A.429 Other secondary chronic gout, unspecified elbow
  - M1A.43 Other secondary chronic gout, wrist
    - M1A.431 Other secondary chronic gout, right wrist
    - M1A.432 Other secondary chronic gout, left wrist
    - M1A.439 Other secondary chronic gout, unspecified wrist
  - M1A.44 Other secondary chronic gout, hand
    - M1A.441 Other secondary chronic gout, right hand
    - M1A.442 Other secondary chronic gout, left hand
    - M1A.449 Other secondary chronic gout, unspecified hand
  - M1A.45 Other secondary chronic gout, hip
    - M1A.451 Other secondary chronic gout, right hip
    - M1A.452 Other secondary chronic gout, left hip
    - M1A.459 Other secondary chronic gout, unspecified hip

- M1A.46 Other secondary chronic gout, knee
  - M1A.461 Other secondary chronic gout, right knee
  - M1A.462 Other secondary chronic gout, left knee
  - M1A.469 Other secondary chronic gout, unspecified knee
- M1A.47 Other secondary chronic gout, ankle and foot
  - M1A.471 Other secondary chronic gout, right ankle and foot
  - M1A.472 Other secondary chronic gout, left ankle and foot
  - M1A.479 Other secondary chronic gout, unspecified ankle and foot
- X M1A.48 Other secondary chronic gout, vertebrae
- X M1A.49 Other secondary chronic gout, multiple sites
- X M1A.9 Chronic gout, unspecified

- M10 **Gout**
  - *Accumulation of uric acid that results in swollen, red, hot, painful, stiff joints*
  - Acute gout
  - Gout attack
  - Gout flare
  - Podagra
  - Use additional code to identify:
    - Autonomic neuropathy in diseases classified elsewhere (G99.0)
    - Calculus of urinary tract in diseases classified elsewhere (N22)
    - Cardiomyopathy in diseases classified elsewhere (I43)
    - Disorders of external ear in diseases classified elsewhere (H61.1-, H62.8-)
    - Disorders of iris and ciliary body in diseases classified elsewhere (H22)
    - Glomerular disorders in diseases classified elsewhere (N08)
  - **Excludes2** chronic gout (M1A.-) ◄
  - M10.0 **Idiopathic gout**
    - Gouty bursitis
    - Primary gout
    - M10.00 Idiopathic gout, unspecified site
    - M10.01 Idiopathic gout, shoulder
      - M10.011 Idiopathic gout, right shoulder
      - M10.012 Idiopathic gout, left shoulder
      - M10.019 Idiopathic gout, unspecified shoulder
    - M10.02 Idiopathic gout, elbow
      - M10.021 Idiopathic gout, right elbow
      - M10.022 Idiopathic gout, left elbow
      - M10.029 Idiopathic gout, unspecified elbow
    - M10.03 Idiopathic gout, wrist
      - M10.031 Idiopathic gout, right wrist
      - M10.032 Idiopathic gout, left wrist
      - M10.039 Idiopathic gout, unspecified wrist
    - M10.04 Idiopathic gout, hand
      - M10.041 Idiopathic gout, right hand
      - M10.042 Idiopathic gout, left hand
      - M10.049 Idiopathic gout, unspecified hand
    - M10.05 Idiopathic gout, hip
      - M10.051 Idiopathic gout, right hip
      - M10.052 Idiopathic gout, left hip
      - M10.059 Idiopathic gout, unspecified hip
    - M10.06 Idiopathic gout, knee
      - M10.061 Idiopathic gout, right knee
      - M10.062 Idiopathic gout, left knee
      - M10.069 Idiopathic gout, unspecified knee

● M10.07   Idiopathic gout, ankle and foot
     M10.071   Idiopathic gout, right ankle and foot
     M10.072   Idiopathic gout, left ankle and foot
     M10.079   Idiopathic gout, unspecified ankle and foot
   M10.08   Idiopathic gout, vertebrae
   M10.09   Idiopathic gout, multiple sites

● M10.1   Lead-induced gout
     Code first toxic effects of lead and its compounds (T56.0-)
   M10.10   Lead-induced gout, unspecified site
● M10.11   Lead-induced gout, shoulder
     M10.111   Lead-induced gout, right shoulder
     M10.112   Lead-induced gout, left shoulder
     M10.119   Lead-induced gout, unspecified shoulder
● M10.12   Lead-induced gout, elbow
     M10.121   Lead-induced gout, right elbow
     M10.122   Lead-induced gout, left elbow
     M10.129   Lead-induced gout, unspecified elbow
● M10.13   Lead-induced gout, wrist
     M10.131   Lead-induced gout, right wrist
     M10.132   Lead-induced gout, left wrist
     M10.139   Lead-induced gout, unspecified wrist
● M10.14   Lead-induced gout, hand
     M10.141   Lead-induced gout, right hand
     M10.142   Lead-induced gout, left hand
     M10.149   Lead-induced gout, unspecified hand
● M10.15   Lead-induced gout, hip
     M10.151   Lead-induced gout, right hip
     M10.152   Lead-induced gout, left hip
     M10.159   Lead-induced gout, unspecified hip
● M10.16   Lead-induced gout, knee
     M10.161   Lead-induced gout, right knee
     M10.162   Lead-induced gout, left knee
     M10.169   Lead-induced gout, unspecified knee
● M10.17   Lead-induced gout, ankle and foot
     M10.171   Lead-induced gout, right ankle and foot
     M10.172   Lead-induced gout, left ankle and foot
     M10.179   Lead-induced gout, unspecified ankle and foot
   M10.18   Lead-induced gout, vertebrae
   M10.19   Lead-induced gout, multiple sites

● M10.2   Drug-induced gout
     Use additional code for adverse effect, if applicable, to identify drug (T36-T50 with fifth or sixth character 5)
   M10.20   Drug-induced gout, unspecified site
● M10.21   Drug-induced gout, shoulder
     M10.211   Drug-induced gout, right shoulder
     M10.212   Drug-induced gout, left shoulder
     M10.219   Drug-induced gout, unspecified shoulder
● M10.22   Drug-induced gout, elbow
     M10.221   Drug-induced gout, right elbow
     M10.222   Drug-induced gout, left elbow
     M10.229   Drug-induced gout, unspecified elbow
● M10.23   Drug-induced gout, wrist
     M10.231   Drug-induced gout, right wrist
     M10.232   Drug-induced gout, left wrist
     M10.239   Drug-induced gout, unspecified wrist

● M10.24   Drug-induced gout, hand
     M10.241   Drug-induced gout, right hand
     M10.242   Drug-induced gout, left hand
     M10.249   Drug-induced gout, unspecified hand
● M10.25   Drug-induced gout, hip
     M10.251   Drug-induced gout, right hip
     M10.252   Drug-induced gout, left hip
     M10.259   Drug-induced gout, unspecified hip
● M10.26   Drug-induced gout, knee
     M10.261   Drug-induced gout, right knee
     M10.262   Drug-induced gout, left knee
     M10.269   Drug-induced gout, unspecified knee
● M10.27   Drug-induced gout, ankle and foot
     M10.271   Drug-induced gout, right ankle and foot
     M10.272   Drug-induced gout, left ankle and foot
     M10.279   Drug-induced gout, unspecified ankle and foot
   M10.28   Drug-induced gout, vertebrae
   M10.29   Drug-induced gout, multiple sites

● M10.3   Gout due to renal impairment
     Code also associated renal disease
   M10.30   Gout due to renal impairment, unspecified site
● M10.31   Gout due to renal impairment, shoulder
     M10.311   Gout due to renal impairment, right shoulder
     M10.312   Gout due to renal impairment, left shoulder
     M10.319   Gout due to renal impairment, unspecified shoulder
● M10.32   Gout due to renal impairment, elbow
     M10.321   Gout due to renal impairment, right elbow
     M10.322   Gout due to renal impairment, left elbow
     M10.329   Gout due to renal impairment, unspecified elbow
● M10.33   Gout due to renal impairment, wrist
     M10.331   Gout due to renal impairment, right wrist
     M10.332   Gout due to renal impairment, left wrist
     M10.339   Gout due to renal impairment, unspecified wrist
● M10.34   Gout due to renal impairment, hand
     M10.341   Gout due to renal impairment, right hand
     M10.342   Gout due to renal impairment, left hand
     M10.349   Gout due to renal impairment, unspecified hand
● M10.35   Gout due to renal impairment, hip
     M10.351   Gout due to renal impairment, right hip
     M10.352   Gout due to renal impairment, left hip
     M10.359   Gout due to renal impairment, unspecified hip
● M10.36   Gout due to renal impairment, knee
     M10.361   Gout due to renal impairment, right knee
     M10.362   Gout due to renal impairment, left knee
     M10.369   Gout due to renal impairment, unspecified knee

● **M10.37**   Gout due to renal impairment, ankle and foot

     M10.371   Gout due to renal impairment, right ankle and foot

     M10.372   Gout due to renal impairment, left ankle and foot

     M10.379   Gout due to renal impairment, unspecified ankle and foot

     M10.38   Gout due to renal impairment, vertebrae

     M10.39   Gout due to renal impairment, multiple sites

● **M10.4**   Other secondary gout

     Code first associated condition

     M10.40   Other secondary gout, unspecified site

● **M10.41**   Other secondary gout, shoulder

     M10.411   Other secondary gout, right shoulder

     M10.412   Other secondary gout, left shoulder

     M10.419   Other secondary gout, unspecified shoulder

● **M10.42**   Other secondary gout, elbow

     M10.421   Other secondary gout, right elbow

     M10.422   Other secondary gout, left elbow

     M10.429   Other secondary gout, unspecified elbow

● **M10.43**   Other secondary gout, wrist

     M10.431   Other secondary gout, right wrist

     M10.432   Other secondary gout, left wrist

     M10.439   Other secondary gout, unspecified wrist

● **M10.44**   Other secondary gout, hand

     M10.441   Other secondary gout, right hand

     M10.442   Other secondary gout, left hand

     M10.449   Other secondary gout, unspecified hand

● **M10.45**   Other secondary gout, hip

     M10.451   Other secondary gout, right hip

     M10.452   Other secondary gout, left hip

     M10.459   Other secondary gout, unspecified hip

● **M10.46**   Other secondary gout, knee

     M10.461   Other secondary gout, right knee

     M10.462   Other secondary gout, left knee

     M10.469   Other secondary gout, unspecified knee

● **M10.47**   Other secondary gout, ankle and foot

     M10.471   Other secondary gout, right ankle and foot

     M10.472   Other secondary gout, left ankle and foot

     M10.479   Other secondary gout, unspecified ankle and foot

     M10.48   Other secondary gout, vertebrae

     M10.49   Other secondary gout, multiple sites

● **M10.9**   Gout, unspecified

     Gout NOS

● **M11**   Other crystal arthropathies

● **M11.0**   Hydroxyapatite deposition disease

     M11.00   Hydroxyapatite deposition disease, unspecified site

● **M11.01**   Hydroxyapatite deposition disease, shoulder

     M11.011   Hydroxyapatite deposition disease, right shoulder

     M11.012   Hydroxyapatite deposition disease, left shoulder

     M11.019   Hydroxyapatite deposition disease, unspecified shoulder

● **M11.02**   Hydroxyapatite deposition disease, elbow

     M11.021   Hydroxyapatite deposition disease, right elbow

     M11.022   Hydroxyapatite deposition disease, left elbow

     M11.029   Hydroxyapatite deposition disease, unspecified elbow

● **M11.03**   Hydroxyapatite deposition disease, wrist

     M11.031   Hydroxyapatite deposition disease, right wrist

     M11.032   Hydroxyapatite deposition disease, left wrist

     M11.039   Hydroxyapatite deposition disease, unspecified wrist

● **M11.04**   Hydroxyapatite deposition disease, hand

     M11.041   Hydroxyapatite deposition disease, right hand

     M11.042   Hydroxyapatite deposition disease, left hand

     M11.049   Hydroxyapatite deposition disease, unspecified hand

● **M11.05**   Hydroxyapatite deposition disease, hip

     M11.051   Hydroxyapatite deposition disease, right hip

     M11.052   Hydroxyapatite deposition disease, left hip

     M11.059   Hydroxyapatite deposition disease, unspecified hip

● **M11.06**   Hydroxyapatite deposition disease, knee

     M11.061   Hydroxyapatite deposition disease, right knee

     M11.062   Hydroxyapatite deposition disease, left knee

     M11.069   Hydroxyapatite deposition disease, unspecified knee

● **M11.07**   Hydroxyapatite deposition disease, ankle and foot

     M11.071   Hydroxyapatite deposition disease, right ankle and foot

     M11.072   Hydroxyapatite deposition disease, left ankle and foot

     M11.079   Hydroxyapatite deposition disease, unspecified ankle and foot

     M11.08   Hydroxyapatite deposition disease, vertebrae

     M11.09   Hydroxyapatite deposition disease, multiple sites

● **M11.1**   Familial chondrocalcinosis

     M11.10   Familial chondrocalcinosis, unspecified site

● **M11.11**   Familial chondrocalcinosis, shoulder

     M11.111   Familial chondrocalcinosis, right shoulder

     M11.112   Familial chondrocalcinosis, left shoulder

     M11.119   Familial chondrocalcinosis, unspecified shoulder

● **M11.12**   Familial chondrocalcinosis, elbow

     M11.121   Familial chondrocalcinosis, right elbow

     M11.122   Familial chondrocalcinosis, left elbow

     M11.129   Familial chondrocalcinosis, unspecified elbow

● **M11.13**   Familial chondrocalcinosis, wrist

     M11.131   Familial chondrocalcinosis, right wrist

     M11.132   Familial chondrocalcinosis, left wrist

     M11.139   Familial chondrocalcinosis, unspecified wrist

CHAPTER 13 (M00-M99)

● M11.14   Familial chondrocalcinosis, hand
     M11.141   Familial chondrocalcinosis, right hand
     M11.142   Familial chondrocalcinosis, left hand
     M11.149   Familial chondrocalcinosis, unspecified hand

● M11.15   Familial chondrocalcinosis, hip
     M11.151   Familial chondrocalcinosis, right hip
     M11.152   Familial chondrocalcinosis, left hip
     M11.159   Familial chondrocalcinosis, unspecified hip

● M11.16   Familial chondrocalcinosis, knee
     M11.161   Familial chondrocalcinosis, right knee
     M11.162   Familial chondrocalcinosis, left knee
     M11.169   Familial chondrocalcinosis, unspecified knee

● M11.17   Familial chondrocalcinosis, ankle and foot
     M11.171   Familial chondrocalcinosis, right ankle and foot
     M11.172   Familial chondrocalcinosis, left ankle and foot
     M11.179   Familial chondrocalcinosis, unspecified ankle and foot

     M11.18   Familial chondrocalcinosis, vertebrae
     M11.19   Familial chondrocalcinosis, multiple sites

● M11.2   Other chondrocalcinosis
     Chondrocalcinosis NOS
     M11.20   Other chondrocalcinosis, unspecified site

● M11.21   Other chondrocalcinosis, shoulder
     M11.211   Other chondrocalcinosis, right shoulder
     M11.212   Other chondrocalcinosis, left shoulder
     M11.219   Other chondrocalcinosis, unspecified shoulder

● M11.22   Other chondrocalcinosis, elbow
     M11.221   Other chondrocalcinosis, right elbow
     M11.222   Other chondrocalcinosis, left elbow
     M11.229   Other chondrocalcinosis, unspecified elbow

● M11.23   Other chondrocalcinosis, wrist
     M11.231   Other chondrocalcinosis, right wrist
     M11.232   Other chondrocalcinosis, left wrist
     M11.239   Other chondrocalcinosis, unspecified wrist

● M11.24   Other chondrocalcinosis, hand
     M11.241   Other chondrocalcinosis, right hand
     M11.242   Other chondrocalcinosis, left hand
     M11.249   Other chondrocalcinosis, unspecified hand

● M11.25   Other chondrocalcinosis, hip
     M11.251   Other chondrocalcinosis, right hip
     M11.252   Other chondrocalcinosis, left hip
     M11.259   Other chondrocalcinosis, unspecified hip

● M11.26   Other chondrocalcinosis, knee
     M11.261   Other chondrocalcinosis, right knee
     M11.262   Other chondrocalcinosis, left knee
     M11.269   Other chondrocalcinosis, unspecified knee

● M11.27   Other chondrocalcinosis, ankle and foot
     M11.271   Other chondrocalcinosis, right ankle and foot
     M11.272   Other chondrocalcinosis, left ankle and foot
     M11.279   Other chondrocalcinosis, unspecified ankle and foot

     M11.28   Other chondrocalcinosis, vertebrae
     M11.29   Other chondrocalcinosis, multiple sites

● M11.8   Other specified crystal arthropathies
     M11.80   Other specified crystal arthropathies, unspecified site

● M11.81   Other specified crystal arthropathies, shoulder
     M11.811   Other specified crystal arthropathies, right shoulder
     M11.812   Other specified crystal arthropathies, left shoulder
     M11.819   Other specified crystal arthropathies, unspecified shoulder

● M11.82   Other specified crystal arthropathies, elbow
     M11.821   Other specified crystal arthropathies, right elbow
     M11.822   Other specified crystal arthropathies, left elbow
     M11.829   Other specified crystal arthropathies, unspecified elbow

● M11.83   Other specified crystal arthropathies, wrist
     M11.831   Other specified crystal arthropathies, right wrist
     M11.832   Other specified crystal arthropathies, left wrist
     M11.839   Other specified crystal arthropathies, unspecified wrist

● M11.84   Other specified crystal arthropathies, hand
     M11.841   Other specified crystal arthropathies, right hand
     M11.842   Other specified crystal arthropathies, left hand
     M11.849   Other specified crystal arthropathies, unspecified hand

● M11.85   Other specified crystal arthropathies, hip
     M11.851   Other specified crystal arthropathies, right hip
     M11.852   Other specified crystal arthropathies, left hip
     M11.859   Other specified crystal arthropathies, unspecified hip

● M11.86   Other specified crystal arthropathies, knee
     M11.861   Other specified crystal arthropathies, right knee
     M11.862   Other specified crystal arthropathies, left knee
     M11.869   Other specified crystal arthropathies, unspecified knee

● M11.87   Other specified crystal arthropathies, ankle and foot
     M11.871   Other specified crystal arthropathies, right ankle and foot
     M11.872   Other specified crystal arthropathies, left ankle and foot
     M11.879   Other specified crystal arthropathies, unspecified ankle and foot

     M11.88   Other specified crystal arthropathies, vertebrae
     M11.89   Other specified crystal arthropathies, multiple sites

M11.9   Crystal arthropathy, unspecified

◀ New   ◀ Revised   ~~deleted~~ Deleted   Excludes 1   Excludes 2   Includes   Use additional   Code first   Code also   Unspecified
OGCR Official Guidelines   X Assign placeholder X   ● Use Additional Character(s)   ▶ Manifestation Code   Coding Clinic

● **M12 Other and unspecified arthropathy**

> **Excludes1**   arthrosis (M15-M19)
> cricoarytenoid arthropathy (J38.7)

● **M12.0 Chronic postrheumatic arthropathy [Jaccoud]**

    M12.00 Chronic postrheumatic arthropathy [Jaccoud], unspecified site

●   **M12.01** Chronic postrheumatic arthropathy [Jaccoud], shoulder

      M12.011 Chronic postrheumatic arthropathy [Jaccoud], right shoulder

      M12.012 Chronic postrheumatic arthropathy [Jaccoud], left shoulder

      M12.019 Chronic postrheumatic arthropathy [Jaccoud], unspecified shoulder

●   **M12.02** Chronic postrheumatic arthropathy [Jaccoud], elbow

      M12.021 Chronic postrheumatic arthropathy [Jaccoud], right elbow

      M12.022 Chronic postrheumatic arthropathy [Jaccoud], left elbow

      M12.029 Chronic postrheumatic arthropathy [Jaccoud], unspecified elbow

●   **M12.03** Chronic postrheumatic arthropathy [Jaccoud], wrist

      M12.031 Chronic postrheumatic arthropathy [Jaccoud], right wrist

      M12.032 Chronic postrheumatic arthropathy [Jaccoud], left wrist

      M12.039 Chronic postrheumatic arthropathy [Jaccoud], unspecified wrist

●   **M12.04** Chronic postrheumatic arthropathy [Jaccoud], hand

      M12.041 Chronic postrheumatic arthropathy [Jaccoud], right hand

      M12.042 Chronic postrheumatic arthropathy [Jaccoud], left hand

      M12.049 Chronic postrheumatic arthropathy [Jaccoud], unspecified hand

●   **M12.05** Chronic postrheumatic arthropathy [Jaccoud], hip

      M12.051 Chronic postrheumatic arthropathy [Jaccoud], right hip

      M12.052 Chronic postrheumatic arthropathy [Jaccoud], left hip

      M12.059 Chronic postrheumatic arthropathy [Jaccoud], unspecified hip

●   **M12.06** Chronic postrheumatic arthropathy [Jaccoud], knee

      M12.061 Chronic postrheumatic arthropathy [Jaccoud], right knee

      M12.062 Chronic postrheumatic arthropathy [Jaccoud], left knee

      M12.069 Chronic postrheumatic arthropathy [Jaccoud], unspecified knee

●   **M12.07** Chronic postrheumatic arthropathy [Jaccoud], ankle and foot

      M12.071 Chronic postrheumatic arthropathy [Jaccoud], right ankle and foot

      M12.072 Chronic postrheumatic arthropathy [Jaccoud], left ankle and foot

      M12.079 Chronic postrheumatic arthropathy [Jaccoud], unspecified ankle and foot

    M12.08 Chronic postrheumatic arthropathy [Jaccoud], other specified site

> Chronic postrheumatic arthropathy [Jaccoud], vertebrae

    M12.09 Chronic postrheumatic arthropathy [Jaccoud], multiple sites

● **M12.1 Kaschin-Beck disease**

> Osteochondroarthrosis deformans endemica

    M12.10 Kaschin-Beck disease, unspecified site

●   **M12.11** Kaschin-Beck disease, shoulder

      M12.111 Kaschin-Beck disease, right shoulder

      M12.112 Kaschin-Beck disease, left shoulder

      M12.119 Kaschin-Beck disease, unspecified shoulder

●   **M12.12** Kaschin-Beck disease, elbow

      M12.121 Kaschin-Beck disease, right elbow

      M12.122 Kaschin-Beck disease, left elbow

      M12.129 Kaschin-Beck disease, unspecified elbow

●   **M12.13** Kaschin-Beck disease, wrist

      M12.131 Kaschin-Beck disease, right wrist

      M12.132 Kaschin-Beck disease, left wrist

      M12.139 Kaschin-Beck disease, unspecified wrist

●   **M12.14** Kaschin-Beck disease, hand

      M12.141 Kaschin-Beck disease, right hand

      M12.142 Kaschin-Beck disease, left hand

      M12.149 Kaschin-Beck disease, unspecified hand

●   **M12.15** Kaschin-Beck disease, hip

      M12.151 Kaschin-Beck disease, right hip

      M12.152 Kaschin-Beck disease, left hip

      M12.159 Kaschin-Beck disease, unspecified hip

●   **M12.16** Kaschin-Beck disease, knee

      M12.161 Kaschin-Beck disease, right knee

      M12.162 Kaschin-Beck disease, left knee

      M12.169 Kaschin-Beck disease, unspecified knee

●   **M12.17** Kaschin-Beck disease, ankle and foot

      M12.171 Kaschin-Beck disease, right ankle and foot

      M12.172 Kaschin-Beck disease, left ankle and foot

      M12.179 Kaschin-Beck disease, unspecified ankle and foot

    M12.18 Kaschin-Beck disease, vertebrae

    M12.19 Kaschin-Beck disease, multiple sites

● **M12.2 Villonodular synovitis (pigmented)**

    M12.20 Villonodular synovitis (pigmented), unspecified site

●   **M12.21** Villonodular synovitis (pigmented), shoulder

      M12.211 Villonodular synovitis (pigmented), right shoulder

      M12.212 Villonodular synovitis (pigmented), left shoulder

      M12.219 Villonodular synovitis (pigmented), unspecified shoulder

●   **M12.22** Villonodular synovitis (pigmented), elbow

      M12.221 Villonodular synovitis (pigmented), right elbow

      M12.222 Villonodular synovitis (pigmented), left elbow

      M12.229 Villonodular synovitis (pigmented), unspecified elbow

●   **M12.23** Villonodular synovitis (pigmented), wrist

      M12.231 Villonodular synovitis (pigmented), right wrist

      M12.232 Villonodular synovitis (pigmented), left wrist

      M12.239 Villonodular synovitis (pigmented), unspecified wrist

CHAPTER 13 (M00-M99)

● M12.24 Villonodular synovitis (pigmented), hand
    M12.241 Villonodular synovitis (pigmented), right hand
    M12.242 Villonodular synovitis (pigmented), left hand
    M12.249 Villonodular synovitis (pigmented), unspecified hand

● M12.25 Villonodular synovitis (pigmented), hip
    M12.251 Villonodular synovitis (pigmented), right hip
    M12.252 Villonodular synovitis (pigmented), left hip
    M12.259 Villonodular synovitis (pigmented), unspecified hip

● M12.26 Villonodular synovitis (pigmented), knee
    M12.261 Villonodular synovitis (pigmented), right knee
    M12.262 Villonodular synovitis (pigmented), left knee
    M12.269 Villonodular synovitis (pigmented), unspecified knee

● M12.27 Villonodular synovitis (pigmented), ankle and foot
    M12.271 Villonodular synovitis (pigmented), right ankle and foot
    M12.272 Villonodular synovitis (pigmented), left ankle and foot
    M12.279 Villonodular synovitis (pigmented), unspecified ankle and foot

  M12.28 Villonodular synovitis (pigmented), other specified site
    Villonodular synovitis (pigmented), vertebrae

  M12.29 Villonodular synovitis (pigmented), multiple sites

● M12.3 Palindromic rheumatism
  M12.30 Palindromic rheumatism, unspecified site

● M12.31 Palindromic rheumatism, shoulder
    M12.311 Palindromic rheumatism, right shoulder
    M12.312 Palindromic rheumatism, left shoulder
    M12.319 Palindromic rheumatism, unspecified shoulder

● M12.32 Palindromic rheumatism, elbow
    M12.321 Palindromic rheumatism, right elbow
    M12.322 Palindromic rheumatism, left elbow
    M12.329 Palindromic rheumatism, unspecified elbow

● M12.33 Palindromic rheumatism, wrist
    M12.331 Palindromic rheumatism, right wrist
    M12.332 Palindromic rheumatism, left wrist
    M12.339 Palindromic rheumatism, unspecified wrist

● M12.34 Palindromic rheumatism, hand
    M12.341 Palindromic rheumatism, right hand
    M12.342 Palindromic rheumatism, left hand
    M12.349 Palindromic rheumatism, unspecified hand

● M12.35 Palindromic rheumatism, hip
    M12.351 Palindromic rheumatism, right hip
    M12.352 Palindromic rheumatism, left hip
    M12.359 Palindromic rheumatism, unspecified hip

● M12.36 Palindromic rheumatism, knee
    M12.361 Palindromic rheumatism, right knee
    M12.362 Palindromic rheumatism, left knee
    M12.369 Palindromic rheumatism, unspecified knee

● M12.37 Palindromic rheumatism, ankle and foot
    M12.371 Palindromic rheumatism, right ankle and foot
    M12.372 Palindromic rheumatism, left ankle and foot
    M12.379 Palindromic rheumatism, unspecified ankle and foot

  M12.38 Palindromic rheumatism, other specified site
    Palindromic rheumatism, vertebrae

  M12.39 Palindromic rheumatism, multiple sites

● M12.4 Intermittent hydrarthrosis
  M12.40 Intermittent hydrarthrosis, unspecified site

● M12.41 Intermittent hydrarthrosis, shoulder
    M12.411 Intermittent hydrarthrosis, right shoulder
    M12.412 Intermittent hydrarthrosis, left shoulder
    M12.419 Intermittent hydrarthrosis, unspecified shoulder

● M12.42 Intermittent hydrarthrosis, elbow
    M12.421 Intermittent hydrarthrosis, right elbow
    M12.422 Intermittent hydrarthrosis, left elbow
    M12.429 Intermittent hydrarthrosis, unspecified elbow

● M12.43 Intermittent hydrarthrosis, wrist
    M12.431 Intermittent hydrarthrosis, right wrist
    M12.432 Intermittent hydrarthrosis, left wrist
    M12.439 Intermittent hydrarthrosis, unspecified wrist

● M12.44 Intermittent hydrarthrosis, hand
    M12.441 Intermittent hydrarthrosis, right hand
    M12.442 Intermittent hydrarthrosis, left hand
    M12.449 Intermittent hydrarthrosis, unspecified hand

● M12.45 Intermittent hydrarthrosis, hip
    M12.451 Intermittent hydrarthrosis, right hip
    M12.452 Intermittent hydrarthrosis, left hip
    M12.459 Intermittent hydrarthrosis, unspecified hip

● M12.46 Intermittent hydrarthrosis, knee
    M12.461 Intermittent hydrarthrosis, right knee
    M12.462 Intermittent hydrarthrosis, left knee
    M12.469 Intermittent hydrarthrosis, unspecified knee

● M12.47 Intermittent hydrarthrosis, ankle and foot
    M12.471 Intermittent hydrarthrosis, right ankle and foot
    M12.472 Intermittent hydrarthrosis, left ankle and foot
    M12.479 Intermittent hydrarthrosis, unspecified ankle and foot

  M12.48 Intermittent hydrarthrosis, other site
  M12.49 Intermittent hydrarthrosis, multiple sites

◀ New   ◀◀ Revised   ~~deleted~~ Deleted   Excludes 1   Excludes 2   Includes   Use additional   Code first   Code also   Unspecified

OGCR Official Guidelines   X Assign placeholder X   ● Use Additional Character(s)   ▶ Manifestation Code   **Coding Clinic**

● **M12.5 Traumatic arthropathy**
     Excludes1   current injury-see Alphabetic Index
              post-traumatic osteoarthritis of first
                carpometacarpal joint (M18.2-M18.3)
              post-traumatic osteoarthritis of hip
                (M16.4-M16.5)
              post-traumatic osteoarthritis of knee
                (M17.2-M17.3)
              post-traumatic osteoarthritis NOS
                (M19.1-)
              post-traumatic osteoarthritis of other
                single joints (M19.1-)

     M12.50   Traumatic arthropathy, unspecified site
●   **M12.51**   Traumatic arthropathy, shoulder
        M12.511   Traumatic arthropathy, right shoulder
        M12.512   Traumatic arthropathy, left shoulder
        M12.519   Traumatic arthropathy, unspecified shoulder
●   **M12.52**   Traumatic arthropathy, elbow
        M12.521   Traumatic arthropathy, right elbow
        M12.522   Traumatic arthropathy, left elbow
        M12.529   Traumatic arthropathy, unspecified elbow
●   **M12.53**   Traumatic arthropathy, wrist
        M12.531   Traumatic arthropathy, right wrist
        M12.532   Traumatic arthropathy, left wrist
        M12.539   Traumatic arthropathy, unspecified wrist
●   **M12.54**   Traumatic arthropathy, hand
        M12.541   Traumatic arthropathy, right hand
        M12.542   Traumatic arthropathy, left hand
        M12.549   Traumatic arthropathy, unspecified hand
●   **M12.55**   Traumatic arthropathy, hip
        M12.551   Traumatic arthropathy, right hip
        M12.552   Traumatic arthropathy, left hip
           Coding Clinic: 2015, Q1, P17
        M12.559   Traumatic arthropathy, unspecified hip
●   **M12.56**   Traumatic arthropathy, knee
        M12.561   Traumatic arthropathy, right knee
        M12.562   Traumatic arthropathy, left knee
        M12.569   Traumatic arthropathy, unspecified knee
●   **M12.57**   Traumatic arthropathy, ankle and foot
        M12.571   Traumatic arthropathy, right ankle and foot
        M12.572   Traumatic arthropathy, left ankle and foot
        M12.579   Traumatic arthropathy, unspecified ankle and foot
     M12.58   Traumatic arthropathy, other specified site
           Traumatic arthropathy, vertebrae
     M12.59   Traumatic arthropathy, multiple sites
● **M12.8 Other specific arthropathies, not elsewhere classified**
          Transient arthropathy
     M12.80   Other specific arthropathies, not elsewhere classified, unspecified site
●   **M12.81**   Other specific arthropathies, not elsewhere classified, shoulder
        M12.811   Other specific arthropathies, not elsewhere classified, right shoulder
        M12.812   Other specific arthropathies, not elsewhere classified, left shoulder
        M12.819   Other specific arthropathies, not elsewhere classified, unspecified shoulder

●   **M12.82**   Other specific arthropathies, not elsewhere classified, elbow
        M12.821   Other specific arthropathies, not elsewhere classified, right elbow
        M12.822   Other specific arthropathies, not elsewhere classified, left elbow
        M12.829   Other specific arthropathies, not elsewhere classified, unspecified elbow
●   **M12.83**   Other specific arthropathies, not elsewhere classified, wrist
        M12.831   Other specific arthropathies, not elsewhere classified, right wrist
        M12.832   Other specific arthropathies, not elsewhere classified, left wrist
        M12.839   Other specific arthropathies, not elsewhere classified, unspecified wrist
●   **M12.84**   Other specific arthropathies, not elsewhere classified, hand
        M12.841   Other specific arthropathies, not elsewhere classified, right hand
        M12.842   Other specific arthropathies, not elsewhere classified, left hand
        M12.849   Other specific arthropathies, not elsewhere classified, unspecified hand
●   **M12.85**   Other specific arthropathies, not elsewhere classified, hip
        M12.851   Other specific arthropathies, not elsewhere classified, right hip
        M12.852   Other specific arthropathies, not elsewhere classified, left hip
        M12.859   Other specific arthropathies, not elsewhere classified, unspecified hip
●   **M12.86**   Other specific arthropathies, not elsewhere classified, knee
        M12.861   Other specific arthropathies, not elsewhere classified, right knee
        M12.862   Other specific arthropathies, not elsewhere classified, left knee
        M12.869   Other specific arthropathies, not elsewhere classified, unspecified knee
●   **M12.87**   Other specific arthropathies, not elsewhere classified, ankle and foot
        M12.871   Other specific arthropathies, not elsewhere classified, right ankle and foot
        M12.872   Other specific arthropathies, not elsewhere classified, left ankle and foot
        M12.879   Other specific arthropathies, not elsewhere classified, unspecified ankle and foot
     M12.88   Other specific arthropathies, not elsewhere classified, other specified site
          Other specific arthropathies, not elsewhere classified, vertebrae
     M12.89   Other specific arthropathies, not elsewhere classified, multiple sites
M12.9 Arthropathy, unspecified

● **M13 Other arthritis**

     Excludes1   arthrosis (M15-M19)
                   osteoarthritis (M15-M19)

    M13.0   Polyarthritis, unspecified

●   M13.1   Monoarthritis, not elsewhere classified

      M13.10   Monoarthritis, not elsewhere classified, unspecified site

   ● M13.11   Monoarthritis, not elsewhere classified, shoulder

       M13.111   Monoarthritis, not elsewhere classified, right shoulder

       M13.112   Monoarthritis, not elsewhere classified, left shoulder

       M13.119   Monoarthritis, not elsewhere classified, unspecified shoulder

   ● M13.12   Monoarthritis, not elsewhere classified, elbow

       M13.121   Monoarthritis, not elsewhere classified, right elbow

       M13.122   Monoarthritis, not elsewhere classified, left elbow

       M13.129   Monoarthritis, not elsewhere classified, unspecified elbow

   ● M13.13   Monoarthritis, not elsewhere classified, wrist

       M13.131   Monoarthritis, not elsewhere classified, right wrist

       M13.132   Monoarthritis, not elsewhere classified, left wrist

       M13.139   Monoarthritis, not elsewhere classified, unspecified wrist

   ● M13.14   Monoarthritis, not elsewhere classified, hand

       M13.141   Monoarthritis, not elsewhere classified, right hand

       M13.142   Monoarthritis, not elsewhere classified, left hand

       M13.149   Monoarthritis, not elsewhere classified, unspecified hand

   ● M13.15   Monoarthritis, not elsewhere classified, hip

       M13.151   Monoarthritis, not elsewhere classified, right hip

       M13.152   Monoarthritis, not elsewhere classified, left hip

       M13.159   Monoarthritis, not elsewhere classified, unspecified hip

   ● M13.16   Monoarthritis, not elsewhere classified, knee

       M13.161   Monoarthritis, not elsewhere classified, right knee

       M13.162   Monoarthritis, not elsewhere classified, left knee

       M13.169   Monoarthritis, not elsewhere classified, unspecified knee

   ● M13.17   Monoarthritis, not elsewhere classified, ankle and foot

       M13.171   Monoarthritis, not elsewhere classified, right ankle and foot

       M13.172   Monoarthritis, not elsewhere classified, left ankle and foot

       M13.179   Monoarthritis, not elsewhere classified, unspecified ankle and foot

●   M13.8   Other specified arthritis

      Allergic arthritis

      Excludes1   osteoarthritis (M15-M19)

      M13.80   Other specified arthritis, unspecified site

   ● M13.81   Other specified arthritis, shoulder

       M13.811   Other specified arthritis, right shoulder

       M13.812   Other specified arthritis, left shoulder

       M13.819   Other specified arthritis, unspecified shoulder

● M13.82   Other specified arthritis, elbow

       M13.821   Other specified arthritis, right elbow

       M13.822   Other specified arthritis, left elbow

       M13.829   Other specified arthritis, unspecified elbow

● M13.83   Other specified arthritis, wrist

       M13.831   Other specified arthritis, right wrist

       M13.832   Other specified arthritis, left wrist

       M13.839   Other specified arthritis, unspecified wrist

● M13.84   Other specified arthritis, hand

       M13.841   Other specified arthritis, right hand

       M13.842   Other specified arthritis, left hand

       M13.849   Other specified arthritis, unspecified hand

● M13.85   Other specified arthritis, hip

       M13.851   Other specified arthritis, right hip

       M13.852   Other specified arthritis, left hip

       M13.859   Other specified arthritis, unspecified hip

● M13.86   Other specified arthritis, knee

       M13.861   Other specified arthritis, right knee

       M13.862   Other specified arthritis, left knee

       M13.869   Other specified arthritis, unspecified knee

● M13.87   Other specified arthritis, ankle and foot

       M13.871   Other specified arthritis, right ankle and foot

       M13.872   Other specified arthritis, left ankle and foot

       M13.879   Other specified arthritis, unspecified ankle and foot

    M13.88   Other specified arthritis, other site

    M13.89   Other specified arthritis, multiple sites

● **M14 Arthropathies in other diseases classified elsewhere**

     Excludes1   arthropathy in:
                 diabetes mellitus (E08-E13 with .61-)
                 hematological disorders (M36.2-M36.3)
                 hypersensitivity reactions (M36.4)
                 neoplastic disease (M36.1)
                 neurosyphillis (A52.16)
                 sarcoidosis (D86.86)
             enteropathic arthropathies (M07.0-)
             juvenile psoriatic arthropathy (L40.54)
             lipoid dermatoarthritis (E78.81)

●   M14.6   Charcôt's joint

      Neuropathic arthropathy

      Excludes1   Charcôt's joint in diabetes mellitus (E08-E13 with .610)
                      Charcôt's joint in tabes dorsalis (A52.16)

      M14.60   Charcôt's joint, unspecified site

   ● M14.61   Charcôt's joint, shoulder

       M14.611   Charcôt's joint, right shoulder

       M14.612   Charcôt's joint, left shoulder

       M14.619   Charcôt's joint, unspecified shoulder

   ● M14.62   Charcôt's joint, elbow

       M14.621   Charcôt's joint, right elbow

       M14.622   Charcôt's joint, left elbow

       M14.629   Charcôt's joint, unspecified elbow

   ● M14.63   Charcôt's joint, wrist

       M14.631   Charcôt's joint, right wrist

       M14.632   Charcôt's joint, left wrist

       M14.639   Charcôt's joint, unspecified wrist

◀ New   ◀▥ Revised   ~~deleted~~ Deleted   Excludes 1   Excludes 2   Includes   Use additional   Code first   Code also   Unspecified

OGCR Official Guidelines   X Assign placeholder X   ● Use Additional Character(s)   ▶ Manifestation Code   **Coding Clinic**

● M14.64 Charcôt's joint, hand
    M14.641 Charcôt's joint, right hand
    M14.642 Charcôt's joint, left hand
    M14.649 Charcôt's joint, unspecified hand
● M14.65 Charcôt's joint, hip
    M14.651 Charcôt's joint, right hip
    M14.652 Charcôt's joint, left hip
    M14.659 Charcôt's joint, unspecified hip
● M14.66 Charcôt's joint, knee
    M14.661 Charcôt's joint, right knee
    M14.662 Charcôt's joint, left knee
    M14.669 Charcôt's joint, unspecified knee
● M14.67 Charcôt's joint, ankle and foot
    M14.671 Charcôt's joint, right ankle and foot
    M14.672 Charcôt's joint, left ankle and foot
    M14.679 Charcôt's joint, unspecified ankle and foot
    M14.68 Charcôt's joint, vertebrae
    M14.69 Charcôt's joint, multiple sites
● M14.8 Arthropathies in other specified diseases classified elsewhere

    Code first underlying disease, such as:
      amyloidosis (E85.-)
      erythema multiforme (L51.-)
      erythema nodosum (L52)
      hemochromatosis (E83.11-)
      hyperparathyroidism (E21.-)
      hypothyroidism (E00-E03)
      sickle-cell disorders (D57.-)
      thyrotoxicosis [hyperthyroidism] (E05.-)
      Whipple's disease (K90.81)

  ▷ *M14.80 Arthropathies in other specified diseases classified elsewhere, unspecified site*
● M14.81 Arthropathies in other specified diseases classified elsewhere, shoulder
  ▷ *M14.811 Arthropathies in other specified diseases classified elsewhere, right shoulder*
  ▷ *M14.812 Arthropathies in other specified diseases classified elsewhere, left shoulder*
  ▷ *M14.819 Arthropathies in other specified diseases classified elsewhere, unspecified shoulder*
● M14.82 Arthropathies in other specified diseases classified elsewhere, elbow
  ▷ *M14.821 Arthropathies in other specified diseases classified elsewhere, right elbow*
  ▷ *M14.822 Arthropathies in other specified diseases classified elsewhere, left elbow*
  ▷ *M14.829 Arthropathies in other specified diseases classified elsewhere, unspecified elbow*
● M14.83 Arthropathies in other specified diseases classified elsewhere, wrist
  ▷ *M14.831 Arthropathies in other specified diseases classified elsewhere, right wrist*
  ▷ *M14.832 Arthropathies in other specified diseases classified elsewhere, left wrist*
  ▷ *M14.839 Arthropathies in other specified diseases classified elsewhere, unspecified wrist*

● M14.84 Arthropathies in other specified diseases classified elsewhere, hand
  ▷ *M14.841 Arthropathies in other specified diseases classified elsewhere, right hand*
  ▷ *M14.842 Arthropathies in other specified diseases classified elsewhere, left hand*
  ▷ *M14.849 Arthropathies in other specified diseases classified elsewhere, unspecified hand*
● M14.85 Arthropathies in other specified diseases classified elsewhere, hip
  ▷ *M14.851 Arthropathies in other specified diseases classified elsewhere, right hip*
  ▷ *M14.852 Arthropathies in other specified diseases classified elsewhere, left hip*
  ▷ *M14.859 Arthropathies in other specified diseases classified elsewhere, unspecified hip*
● M14.86 Arthropathies in other specified diseases classified elsewhere, knee
  ▷ *M14.861 Arthropathies in other specified diseases classified elsewhere, right knee*
  ▷ *M14.862 Arthropathies in other specified diseases classified elsewhere, left knee*
  ▷ *M14.869 Arthropathies in other specified diseases classified elsewhere, unspecified knee*
● M14.87 Arthropathies in other specified diseases classified elsewhere, ankle and foot
  ▷ *M14.871 Arthropathies in other specified diseases classified elsewhere, right ankle and foot*
  ▷ *M14.872 Arthropathies in other specified diseases classified elsewhere, left ankle and foot*
  ▷ *M14.879 Arthropathies in other specified diseases classified elsewhere, unspecified ankle and foot*
  ▷ *M14.88 Arthropathies in other specified diseases classified elsewhere, vertebrae*
  ▷ *M14.89 Arthropathies in other specified diseases classified elsewhere, multiple sites*

OSTEOARTHRITIS (M15-M19)

Osteoarthritis is the most common degenerative joint disease and form of arthritis that breaks down the cartilage causing pain, swelling, and reduced motion in the joints.

  Excludes2 osteoarthritis of spine (M47.-)

● M15 Polyosteoarthritis
  Includes arthritis of multiple sites
  Excludes1 bilateral involvement of single joint (M16-M19)
  M15.0 Primary generalized (osteo)arthritis
  M15.1 Heberden's nodes (with arthropathy)
    Interphalangeal distal osteoarthritis
  M15.2 Bouchard's nodes (with arthropathy)
    Juxtaphalangeal distal osteoarthritis
  M15.3 Secondary multiple arthritis
    Post-traumatic polyosteoarthritis
  M15.4 Erosive (osteo)arthritis
  M15.8 Other polyosteoarthritis
  M15.9 Polyosteoarthritis, unspecified
    Generalized osteoarthritis NOS

● M16 Osteoarthritis of hip
    M16.0 Bilateral primary osteoarthritis of hip
  ● M16.1 Unilateral primary osteoarthritis of hip
        Primary osteoarthritis of hip NOS
      M16.10 Unilateral primary osteoarthritis, unspecified hip
      M16.11 Unilateral primary osteoarthritis, right hip
      M16.12 Unilateral primary osteoarthritis, left hip
    M16.2 Bilateral osteoarthritis resulting from hip dysplasia
  ● M16.3 Unilateral osteoarthritis resulting from hip dysplasia
        Dysplastic osteoarthritis of hip NOS
      M16.30 Unilateral osteoarthritis resulting from hip dysplasia, unspecified hip
      M16.31 Unilateral osteoarthritis resulting from hip dysplasia, right hip
      M16.32 Unilateral osteoarthritis resulting from hip dysplasia, left hip
    M16.4 Bilateral post-traumatic osteoarthritis of hip
  ● M16.5 Unilateral post-traumatic osteoarthritis of hip
        Post-traumatic osteoarthritis of hip NOS
      M16.50 Unilateral post-traumatic osteoarthritis, unspecified hip
      M16.51 Unilateral post-traumatic osteoarthritis, right hip
      M16.52 Unilateral post-traumatic osteoarthritis, left hip
    M16.6 Other bilateral secondary osteoarthritis of hip
    M16.7 Other unilateral secondary osteoarthritis of hip
        Secondary osteoarthritis of hip NOS
    M16.9 Osteoarthritis of hip, unspecified

● M17 Osteoarthritis of knee
    M17.0 Bilateral primary osteoarthritis of knee
  ● M17.1 Unilateral primary osteoarthritis of knee
        Primary osteoarthritis of knee NOS
      M17.10 Unilateral primary osteoarthritis, unspecified knee
      M17.11 Unilateral primary osteoarthritis, right knee
      M17.12 Unilateral primary osteoarthritis, left knee
    M17.2 Bilateral post-traumatic osteoarthritis of knee
  ● M17.3 Unilateral post-traumatic osteoarthritis of knee
        Post-traumatic osteoarthritis of knee NOS
      M17.30 Unilateral post-traumatic osteoarthritis, unspecified knee
      M17.31 Unilateral post-traumatic osteoarthritis, right knee
      M17.32 Unilateral post-traumatic osteoarthritis, left knee
    M17.4 Other bilateral secondary osteoarthritis of knee
    M17.5 Other unilateral secondary osteoarthritis of knee
        Secondary osteoarthritis of knee NOS
    M17.9 Osteoarthritis of knee, unspecified

● M18 Osteoarthritis of first carpometacarpal joint
    M18.0 Bilateral primary osteoarthritis of first carpometacarpal joints
  ● M18.1 Unilateral primary osteoarthritis of first carpometacarpal joint
        Primary osteoarthritis of first carpometacarpal joint NOS
      M18.10 Unilateral primary osteoarthritis of first carpometacarpal joint, unspecified hand
      M18.11 Unilateral primary osteoarthritis of first carpometacarpal joint, right hand
      M18.12 Unilateral primary osteoarthritis of first carpometacarpal joint, left hand

    M18.2 Bilateral post-traumatic osteoarthritis of first carpometacarpal joints
  ● M18.3 Unilateral post-traumatic osteoarthritis of first carpometacarpal joint
        Post-traumatic osteoarthritis of first carpometacarpal joint NOS
      M18.30 Unilateral post-traumatic osteoarthritis of first carpometacarpal joint, unspecified hand
      M18.31 Unilateral post-traumatic osteoarthritis of first carpometacarpal joint, right hand
      M18.32 Unilateral post-traumatic osteoarthritis of first carpometacarpal joint, left hand
    M18.4 Other bilateral secondary osteoarthritis of first carpometacarpal joints
  ● M18.5 Other unilateral secondary osteoarthritis of first carpometacarpal joint
        Secondary osteoarthritis of first carpometacarpal joint NOS
      M18.50 Other unilateral secondary osteoarthritis of first carpometacarpal joint, unspecified hand
      M18.51 Other unilateral secondary osteoarthritis of first carpometacarpal joint, right hand
      M18.52 Other unilateral secondary osteoarthritis of first carpometacarpal joint, left hand
    M18.9 Osteoarthritis of first carpometacarpal joint, unspecified

● M19 Other and unspecified osteoarthritis
    Excludes1 polyarthritis (M15.-)
    Excludes2 arthrosis of spine (M47.-)
              hallux rigidus (M20.2)
              osteoarthritis of spine (M47.-)
  ● M19.0 Primary osteoarthritis of other joints
    ● M19.01 Primary osteoarthritis, shoulder
        M19.011 Primary osteoarthritis, right shoulder
        M19.012 Primary osteoarthritis, left shoulder
        M19.019 Primary osteoarthritis, unspecified shoulder
    ● M19.02 Primary osteoarthritis, elbow
        M19.021 Primary osteoarthritis, right elbow
        M19.022 Primary osteoarthritis, left elbow
        M19.029 Primary osteoarthritis, unspecified elbow
    ● M19.03 Primary osteoarthritis, wrist
        M19.031 Primary osteoarthritis, right wrist
        M19.032 Primary osteoarthritis, left wrist
        M19.039 Primary osteoarthritis, unspecified wrist
    ● M19.04 Primary osteoarthritis, hand
        Excludes2 primary osteoarthritis of first carpometacarpal joint (M18.0-, M18.1-)
        M19.041 Primary osteoarthritis, right hand
        M19.042 Primary osteoarthritis, left hand
        M19.049 Primary osteoarthritis, unspecified hand
    ● M19.07 Primary osteoarthritis ankle and foot
        M19.071 Primary osteoarthritis, right ankle and foot
        M19.072 Primary osteoarthritis, left ankle and foot
        M19.079 Primary osteoarthritis, unspecified ankle and foot

● M19.1   Post-traumatic osteoarthritis of other joints
   ● M19.11   Post-traumatic osteoarthritis, shoulder
     M19.111   Post-traumatic osteoarthritis, right shoulder
     M19.112   Post-traumatic osteoarthritis, left shoulder
     M19.119   Post-traumatic osteoarthritis, unspecified shoulder
   ● M19.12   Post-traumatic osteoarthritis, elbow
     M19.121   Post-traumatic osteoarthritis, right elbow
     M19.122   Post-traumatic osteoarthritis, left elbow
     M19.129   Post-traumatic osteoarthritis, unspecified elbow
   ● M19.13   Post-traumatic osteoarthritis, wrist
     M19.131   Post-traumatic osteoarthritis, right wrist
     M19.132   Post-traumatic osteoarthritis, left wrist
     M19.139   Post-traumatic osteoarthritis, unspecified wrist
   ● M19.14   Post-traumatic osteoarthritis, hand
     Excludes2   post-traumatic osteoarthritis of first carpometacarpal joint (M18.2-, M18.3-)
     M19.141   Post-traumatic osteoarthritis, right hand
     M19.142   Post-traumatic osteoarthritis, left hand
     M19.149   Post-traumatic osteoarthritis, unspecified hand
   ● M19.17   Post-traumatic osteoarthritis, ankle and foot
     M19.171   Post-traumatic osteoarthritis, right ankle and foot
     M19.172   Post-traumatic osteoarthritis, left ankle and foot
     M19.179   Post-traumatic osteoarthritis, unspecified ankle and foot
● M19.2   Secondary osteoarthritis of other joints
   ● M19.21   Secondary osteoarthritis, shoulder
     M19.211   Secondary osteoarthritis, right shoulder
     M19.212   Secondary osteoarthritis, left shoulder
     M19.219   Secondary osteoarthritis, unspecified shoulder
   ● M19.22   Secondary osteoarthritis, elbow
     M19.221   Secondary osteoarthritis, right elbow
     M19.222   Secondary osteoarthritis, left elbow
     M19.229   Secondary osteoarthritis, unspecified elbow
   ● M19.23   Secondary osteoarthritis, wrist
     M19.231   Secondary osteoarthritis, right wrist
     M19.232   Secondary osteoarthritis, left wrist
     M19.239   Secondary osteoarthritis, unspecified wrist
   ● M19.24   Secondary osteoarthritis, hand
     M19.241   Secondary osteoarthritis, right hand
     M19.242   Secondary osteoarthritis, left hand
     M19.249   Secondary osteoarthritis, unspecified hand

   ● M19.27   Secondary osteoarthritis, ankle and foot
     M19.271   Secondary osteoarthritis, right ankle and foot
     M19.272   Secondary osteoarthritis, left ankle and foot
     M19.279   Secondary osteoarthritis, unspecified ankle and foot
● M19.9   Osteoarthritis, unspecified site
   M19.90   Unspecified osteoarthritis, unspecified site
     Arthrosis NOS
     Arthritis NOS
     Osteoarthritis NOS
   M19.91   Primary osteoarthritis, unspecified site
     Primary osteoarthritis NOS
   M19.92   Post-traumatic osteoarthritis, unspecified site
     Post-traumatic osteoarthritis NOS
   M19.93   Secondary osteoarthritis, unspecified site
     Secondary osteoarthritis NOS

OTHER JOINT DISORDERS (M20-M25)

Excludes2   joints of the spine (M40-M54)

● M20   Acquired deformities of fingers and toes
   Excludes1   acquired absence of fingers and toes (Z89.-)
     congenital absence of fingers and toes (Q71.3-, Q72.3-)
     congenital deformities and malformations of fingers and toes (Q66.-, Q68-Q70, Q74.-)
   ● M20.0   Deformity of finger(s)
     Excludes1   clubbing of fingers (R68.3)
       palmar fascial fibromatosis [Dupuytren] (M72.0)
       trigger finger (M65.3)
     ● M20.00   Unspecified deformity of finger(s)
       M20.001   Unspecified deformity of right finger(s)
       M20.002   Unspecified deformity of left finger(s)
       M20.009   Unspecified deformity of unspecified finger(s)
     ● M20.01   Mallet finger
       M20.011   Mallet finger of right finger(s)
       M20.012   Mallet finger of left finger(s)
       M20.019   Mallet finger of unspecified finger(s)
     ● M20.02   Boutonnière deformity
       M20.021   Boutonnière deformity of right finger(s)
       M20.022   Boutonnière deformity of left finger(s)
       M20.029   Boutonnière deformity of unspecified finger(s)
     ● M20.03   Swan-neck deformity
       M20.031   Swan-neck deformity of right finger(s)
       M20.032   Swan-neck deformity of left finger(s)
       M20.039   Swan-neck deformity of unspecified finger(s)
     ● M20.09   Other deformity of finger(s)
       M20.091   Other deformity of right finger(s)
       M20.092   Other deformity of left finger(s)
       M20.099   Other deformity of finger(s), unspecified finger(s)

Figure 13-1   Hallux valgus or bunion.

Item 13–2   Hallux valgus or bunion is a sometimes painful structural deformity caused by an inflammation of the bursal sac at the base of the metatarsophalangeal joint (big toe). **Hallus varus** is a deviation of the great toe to the inner side of the foot or away from the next toe.

- **M20.1   Hallux valgus (acquired)**
  - **Excludes2**   bunion (M21.6-) ◀
  - M20.10   Hallux valgus (acquired), unspecified foot
  - M20.11   Hallux valgus (acquired), right foot
  - M20.12   Hallux valgus (acquired), left foot
- **M20.2   Hallux rigidus**
  - M20.20   Hallux rigidus, unspecified foot
  - M20.21   Hallux rigidus, right foot
  - M20.22   Hallux rigidus, left foot
- **M20.3   Hallux varus (acquired)**
  - M20.30   Hallux varus (acquired), unspecified foot
  - M20.31   Hallux varus (acquired), right foot
  - M20.32   Hallux varus (acquired), left foot
- **M20.4   Other hammer toe(s) (acquired)**
  - M20.40   Other hammer toe(s) (acquired), unspecified foot
  - M20.41   Other hammer toe(s) (acquired), right foot
  - M20.42   Other hammer toe(s) (acquired), left foot
- **M20.5   Other deformities of toe(s) (acquired)**
  - **M20.5X   Other deformities of toe(s) (acquired)**
    - M20.5X1   Other deformities of toe(s) (acquired), right foot
    - M20.5X2   Other deformities of toe(s) (acquired), left foot
    - M20.5X9   Other deformities of toe(s) (acquired), unspecified foot
- **M20.6   Acquired deformities of toe(s), unspecified**
  - M20.60   Acquired deformities of toe(s), unspecified, unspecified foot
  - M20.61   Acquired deformities of toe(s), unspecified, right foot
  - M20.62   Acquired deformities of toe(s), unspecified, left foot

Item 13–3   Cubitus valgus is a deformity of the elbow resulting in an increased carrying angle in which the arm extends at the side and the palm faces forward, which results in the forearm and hand extended at a greater than 15 degrees.

Item 13–4   Cubitus varus is a deformity of the elbow resulting in the arm extended at the side and the palm facing forward so that the forearm and hand are held at less than 5 degrees, decreasing the carrying angle.

- **M21   Other acquired deformities of limbs**
  - **Excludes1**   acquired absence of limb (Z89.-)
    - congenital absence of limbs (Q71-Q73)
    - congenital deformities and malformations of limbs (Q65-Q66, Q68-Q74)
  - **Excludes2**   acquired deformities of fingers or toes (M20.-)
    - coxa plana (M91.2)
  - **M21.0   Valgus deformity, not elsewhere classified**
    - **Excludes1**   metatarsus valgus (Q66.6)
      - talipes calcaneovalgus (Q66.4)
    - M21.00   Valgus deformity, not elsewhere classified, unspecified site
    - **M21.02   Valgus deformity, not elsewhere classified, elbow**
      - Cubitus valgus
      - M21.021   Valgus deformity, not elsewhere classified, right elbow
      - M21.022   Valgus deformity, not elsewhere classified, left elbow
      - M21.029   Valgus deformity, not elsewhere classified, unspecified elbow
    - **M21.05   Valgus deformity, not elsewhere classified, hip**
      - M21.051   Valgus deformity, not elsewhere classified, right hip
      - M21.052   Valgus deformity, not elsewhere classified, left hip
      - M21.059   Valgus deformity, not elsewhere classified, unspecified hip
    - **M21.06   Valgus deformity, not elsewhere classified, knee**
      - Genu valgum
      - Knock knee
      - M21.061   Valgus deformity, not elsewhere classified, right knee
      - M21.062   Valgus deformity, not elsewhere classified, left knee
      - M21.069   Valgus deformity, not elsewhere classified, unspecified knee
    - **M21.07   Valgus deformity, not elsewhere classified, ankle**
      - M21.071   Valgus deformity, not elsewhere classified, right ankle
      - M21.072   Valgus deformity, not elsewhere classified, left ankle
      - M21.079   Valgus deformity, not elsewhere classified, unspecified ankle
  - **M21.1   Varus deformity, not elsewhere classified**
    - **Excludes1**   metatarsus varus (Q66.22) ◀
      - tibia vara (M92.5)
    - M21.10   Varus deformity, not elsewhere classified, unspecified site
    - **M21.12   Varus deformity, not elsewhere classified, elbow**
      - Cubitus varus, elbow
      - M21.121   Varus deformity, not elsewhere classified, right elbow
      - M21.122   Varus deformity, not elsewhere classified, left elbow
      - M21.129   Varus deformity, not elsewhere classified, unspecified elbow

◀ New   ◀ Revised   ~~deleted~~ Deleted   Excludes 1   Excludes 2   Includes   Use additional   Code first   Code also   Unspecified

OGCR Official Guidelines   X Assign placeholder X   ● Use Additional Character(s)   ▶ Manifestation Code   **Coding Clinic**

● **M21.15**   Varus deformity, not elsewhere classified, hip
    M21.151   Varus deformity, not elsewhere classified, right hip
    M21.152   Varus deformity, not elsewhere classified, left hip
    M21.159   Varus deformity, not elsewhere classified, unspecified

● **M21.16**   Varus deformity, not elsewhere classified, knee
    Bow leg
    Genu varum
    M21.161   Varus deformity, not elsewhere classified, right knee
    M21.162   Varus deformity, not elsewhere classified, left knee
    M21.169   Varus deformity, not elsewhere classified, unspecified knee

● **M21.17**   Varus deformity, not elsewhere classified, ankle
    M21.171   Varus deformity, not elsewhere classified, right ankle
    M21.172   Varus deformity, not elsewhere classified, left ankle
    M21.179   Varus deformity, not elsewhere classified, unspecified ankle

● **M21.2**   Flexion deformity
    M21.20   Flexion deformity, unspecified site
● **M21.21**   Flexion deformity, shoulder
    M21.211   Flexion deformity, right shoulder
    M21.212   Flexion deformity, left shoulder
    M21.219   Flexion deformity, unspecified shoulder
● **M21.22**   Flexion deformity, elbow
    M21.221   Flexion deformity, right elbow
    M21.222   Flexion deformity, left elbow
    M21.229   Flexion deformity, unspecified elbow
● **M21.23**   Flexion deformity, wrist
    M21.231   Flexion deformity, right wrist
    M21.232   Flexion deformity, left wrist
    M21.239   Flexion deformity, unspecified wrist
● **M21.24**   Flexion deformity, finger joints
    M21.241   Flexion deformity, right finger joints
    M21.242   Flexion deformity, left finger joints
    M21.249   Flexion deformity, unspecified finger joints
● **M21.25**   Flexion deformity, hip
    M21.251   Flexion deformity, right hip
    M21.252   Flexion deformity, left hip
    M21.259   Flexion deformity, unspecified hip
● **M21.26**   Flexion deformity, knee
    M21.261   Flexion deformity, right knee
    M21.262   Flexion deformity, left knee
    M21.269   Flexion deformity, unspecified knee
● **M21.27**   Flexion deformity, ankle and toes
    M21.271   Flexion deformity, right ankle and toes
    M21.272   Flexion deformity, left ankle and toes
    M21.279   Flexion deformity, unspecified ankle and toes

● **M21.3**   Wrist or foot drop (acquired)
● **M21.33**   Wrist drop (acquired)
    M21.331   Wrist drop, right wrist
    M21.332   Wrist drop, left wrist
    M21.339   Wrist drop, unspecified wrist
● **M21.37**   Foot drop (acquired)
    M21.371   Foot drop, right foot
    M21.372   Foot drop, left foot
    M21.379   Foot drop, unspecified foot

● **M21.4**   Flat foot [pes planus] (acquired)
    Excludes1   congenital pes planus (Q66.5-)
    M21.40   Flat foot [pes planus] (acquired), unspecified foot
    M21.41   Flat foot [pes planus] (acquired), right foot
    M21.42   Flat foot [pes planus] (acquired), left foot

● **M21.5**   Acquired clawhand, clubhand, clawfoot and clubfoot
    Excludes1   clubfoot, not specified as acquired (Q66.89)
● **M21.51**   Acquired clawhand
    M21.511   Acquired clawhand, right hand
    M21.512   Acquired clawhand, left hand
    M21.519   Acquired clawhand, unspecified hand
● **M21.52**   Acquired clubhand
    M21.521   Acquired clubhand, right hand
    M21.522   Acquired clubhand, left hand
    M21.529   Acquired clubhand, unspecified hand
● **M21.53**   Acquired clawfoot
    M21.531   Acquired clawfoot, right foot
    M21.532   Acquired clawfoot, left foot
    M21.539   Acquired clawfoot, unspecified foot
● **M21.54**   Acquired clubfoot
    M21.541   Acquired clubfoot, right foot
    M21.542   Acquired clubfoot, left foot
    M21.549   Acquired clubfoot, unspecified foot

● **M21.6**   Other acquired deformities of foot
    Excludes2   deformities of toe (acquired) (M20.1-M20.6-) ◀▥
● **M21.61**   Bunion ◀
    M21.611   Bunion of right foot ◀
    M21.612   Bunion of left foot ◀
    M21.619   Bunion of unspecified foot ◀
● **M21.62**   Bunionette ◀
    M21.621   Bunionette of right foot ◀
    M21.622   Bunionette of left foot ◀
    M21.629   Bunionette of unspecified foot ◀
● **M21.6X**   Other acquired deformities of foot
    M21.6X1   Other acquired deformities of right foot
    M21.6X2   Other acquired deformities of left foot
    M21.6X9   Other acquired deformities of unspecified foot

● **M21.7**   Unequal limb length (acquired)
    Note: The site used should correspond to the shorter limb.
    M21.70   Unequal limb length (acquired), unspecified site
● **M21.72**   Unequal limb length (acquired), humerus
    M21.721   Unequal limb length (acquired), right humerus
    M21.722   Unequal limb length (acquired), left humerus
    M21.729   Unequal limb length (acquired), unspecified humerus
● **M21.73**   Unequal limb length (acquired), ulna and radius
    M21.731   Unequal limb length (acquired), right ulna
    M21.732   Unequal limb length (acquired), left ulna
    M21.733   Unequal limb length (acquired), right radius
    M21.734   Unequal limb length (acquired), left radius
    M21.739   Unequal limb length (acquired), unspecified ulna and radius

CHAPTER 13 (M00-M99)

M21.75 **Unequal limb length (acquired), femur**
  M21.751 Unequal limb length (acquired), right femur
  M21.752 Unequal limb length (acquired), left femur
  M21.759 Unequal limb length (acquired), unspecified femur

M21.76 **Unequal limb length (acquired), tibia and fibula**
  M21.761 Unequal limb length (acquired), right tibia
  M21.762 Unequal limb length (acquired), left tibia
  M21.763 Unequal limb length (acquired), right fibula
  M21.764 Unequal limb length (acquired), left fibula
  M21.769 Unequal limb length (acquired), unspecified tibia and fibula

M21.8 **Other specified acquired deformities of limbs**
  Excludes2 coxa plana (M91.2)
  M21.80 Other specified acquired deformities of unspecified limb
  M21.82 Other specified acquired deformities of upper arm
    M21.821 Other specified acquired deformities of right upper arm
    M21.822 Other specified acquired deformities of left upper arm
    M21.829 Other specified acquired deformities of unspecified upper arm
  M21.83 Other specified acquired deformities of forearm
    M21.831 Other specified acquired deformities of right forearm
    M21.832 Other specified acquired deformities of left forearm
    M21.839 Other specified acquired deformities of unspecified forearm
  M21.85 Other specified acquired deformities of thigh
    M21.851 Other specified acquired deformities of right thigh
    M21.852 Other specified acquired deformities of left thigh
    M21.859 Other specified acquired deformities of unspecified thigh
  M21.86 Other specified acquired deformities of lower leg
    M21.861 Other specified acquired deformities of right lower leg
    M21.862 Other specified acquired deformities of left lower leg
    M21.869 Other specified acquired deformities of unspecified lower leg

M21.9 **Unspecified acquired deformity of limb and hand**
  M21.90 Unspecified acquired deformity of unspecified limb
  M21.92 Unspecified acquired deformity of upper arm
    M21.921 Unspecified acquired deformity of right upper arm
    M21.922 Unspecified acquired deformity of left upper arm
    M21.929 Unspecified acquired deformity of unspecified upper arm
  M21.93 Unspecified acquired deformity of forearm
    M21.931 Unspecified acquired deformity of right forearm
    M21.932 Unspecified acquired deformity of left forearm
    M21.939 Unspecified acquired deformity of unspecified forearm

M21.94 **Unspecified acquired deformity of hand**
  M21.941 Unspecified acquired deformity of hand, right hand
  M21.942 Unspecified acquired deformity of hand, left hand
  M21.949 Unspecified acquired deformity of hand, unspecified hand

M21.95 **Unspecified acquired deformity of thigh**
  M21.951 Unspecified acquired deformity of right thigh
  M21.952 Unspecified acquired deformity of left thigh
  M21.959 Unspecified acquired deformity of unspecified thigh

M21.96 **Unspecified acquired deformity of lower leg**
  M21.961 Unspecified acquired deformity of right lower leg
  M21.962 Unspecified acquired deformity of left lower leg
  M21.969 Unspecified acquired deformity of unspecified lower leg

M22 Disorder of patella
  Excludes1 traumatic dislocation of patella (S83.0-)
  M22.0 **Recurrent dislocation of patella**
    M22.00 Recurrent dislocation of patella, unspecified knee
    M22.01 Recurrent dislocation of patella, right knee
    M22.02 Recurrent dislocation of patella, left knee
  M22.1 **Recurrent subluxation of patella**
    Incomplete dislocation of patella
    M22.10 Recurrent subluxation of patella, unspecified knee
    M22.11 Recurrent subluxation of patella, right knee
    M22.12 Recurrent subluxation of patella, left knee
  M22.2 **Patellofemoral disorders**
    M22.2X Patellofemoral disorders
      M22.2X1 Patellofemoral disorders, right knee
      M22.2X2 Patellofemoral disorders, left knee
      M22.2X9 Patellofemoral disorders, unspecified knee
  M22.3 **Other derangements of patella**
    M22.3X Other derangements of patella
      M22.3X1 Other derangements of patella, right knee
      M22.3X2 Other derangements of patella, left knee
      M22.3X9 Other derangements of patella, unspecified knee
  M22.4 **Chondromalacia patellae**
    M22.40 Chondromalacia patellae, unspecified knee
    M22.41 Chondromalacia patellae, right knee
    M22.42 Chondromalacia patellae, left knee
  M22.8 **Other disorders of patella**
    M22.8X Other disorders of patella
      M22.8X1 Other disorders of patella, right knee
      M22.8X2 Other disorders of patella, left knee
      M22.8X9 Other disorders of patella, unspecified knee
  M22.9 **Unspecified disorder of patella**
    M22.90 Unspecified disorder of patella, unspecified knee
    M22.91 Unspecified disorder of patella, right knee
    M22.92 Unspecified disorder of patella, left knee

◀ New   ◀█ Revised   ~~deleted~~ Deleted   Excludes 1   Excludes 2   Includes   Use additional   Code first   Code also   Unspecified
OGCR Official Guidelines   X Assign placeholder X   ▶ Use Additional Character(s)   ▶ Manifestation Code   **Coding Clinic**

● **M23　Internal derangement of knee**

> **Excludes1**　ankylosis (M24.66)
> current injury - see injury of knee and lower leg (S80-S89)
> deformity of knee (M21.-)
> osteochondritis dissecans (M93.2)
> recurrent dislocation or subluxation of joints (M24.4)
> recurrent dislocation or subluxation of patella (M22.0-M22.1)

● **M23.0　Cystic meniscus**

　● **M23.00　Cystic meniscus, unspecified meniscus**
　　　Cystic meniscus, unspecified lateral meniscus
　　　Cystic meniscus, unspecified medial meniscus

　　M23.000　Cystic meniscus, unspecified lateral meniscus, right knee
　　M23.001　Cystic meniscus, unspecified lateral meniscus, left knee
　　M23.002　Cystic meniscus, unspecified lateral meniscus, unspecified knee
　　M23.003　Cystic meniscus, unspecified medial meniscus, right knee
　　M23.004　Cystic meniscus, unspecified medial meniscus, left knee
　　M23.005　Cystic meniscus, unspecified medial meniscus, unspecified knee
　　M23.006　Cystic meniscus, unspecified meniscus, right knee
　　M23.007　Cystic meniscus, unspecified meniscus, left knee
　　M23.009　Cystic meniscus, unspecified meniscus, unspecified knee

　● **M23.01　Cystic meniscus, anterior horn of medial meniscus**
　　M23.011　Cystic meniscus, anterior horn of medial meniscus, right knee
　　M23.012　Cystic meniscus, anterior horn of medial meniscus, left knee
　　M23.019　Cystic meniscus, anterior horn of medial meniscus, unspecified knee

　● **M23.02　Cystic meniscus, posterior horn of medial meniscus**
　　M23.021　Cystic meniscus, posterior horn of medial meniscus, right knee
　　M23.022　Cystic meniscus, posterior horn of medial meniscus, left knee
　　M23.029　Cystic meniscus, posterior horn of medial meniscus, unspecified knee

　● **M23.03　Cystic meniscus, other medial meniscus**
　　M23.031　Cystic meniscus, other medial meniscus, right knee
　　M23.032　Cystic meniscus, other medial meniscus, left knee
　　M23.039　Cystic meniscus, other medial meniscus, unspecified knee

　● **M23.04　Cystic meniscus, anterior horn of lateral meniscus**
　　M23.041　Cystic meniscus, anterior horn of lateral meniscus, right knee
　　M23.042　Cystic meniscus, anterior horn of lateral meniscus, left knee
　　M23.049　Cystic meniscus, anterior horn of lateral meniscus, unspecified knee

　● **M23.05　Cystic meniscus, posterior horn of lateral meniscus**
　　M23.051　Cystic meniscus, posterior horn of lateral meniscus, right knee
　　M23.052　Cystic meniscus, posterior horn of lateral meniscus, left knee
　　M23.059　Cystic meniscus, posterior horn of lateral meniscus, unspecified knee

● **M23.06　Cystic meniscus, other lateral meniscus**
　　M23.061　Cystic meniscus, other lateral meniscus, right knee
　　M23.062　Cystic meniscus, other lateral meniscus, left knee
　　M23.069　Cystic meniscus, other lateral meniscus, unspecified knee

★ **(See Plate 509 on page 79.)**

● **M23.2　Derangement of meniscus due to old tear or injury**
　　Old bucket-handle tear

　● **M23.20　Derangement of unspecified meniscus due to old tear or injury**
　　　Derangement of unspecified lateral meniscus due to old tear or injury
　　　Derangement of unspecified medial meniscus due to old tear or injury

　　M23.200　Derangement of unspecified lateral meniscus due to old tear or injury, right knee
　　M23.201　Derangement of unspecified lateral meniscus due to old tear or injury, left knee
　　M23.202　Derangement of unspecified lateral meniscus due to old tear or injury, unspecified knee
　　M23.203　Derangement of unspecified medial meniscus due to old tear or injury, right knee
　　M23.204　Derangement of unspecified medial meniscus due to old tear or injury, left knee
　　M23.205　Derangement of unspecified medial meniscus due to old tear or injury, unspecified knee
　　M23.206　Derangement of unspecified meniscus due to old tear or injury, right knee
　　M23.207　Derangement of unspecified meniscus due to old tear or injury, left knee
　　M23.209　Derangement of unspecified meniscus due to old tear or injury, unspecified knee

　● **M23.21　Derangement of anterior horn of medial meniscus due to old tear or injury**
　　M23.211　Derangement of anterior horn of medial meniscus due to old tear or injury, right knee
　　M23.212　Derangement of anterior horn of medial meniscus due to old tear or injury, left knee
　　M23.219　Derangement of anterior horn of medial meniscus due to old tear or injury, unspecified knee

　● **M23.22　Derangement of posterior horn of medial meniscus due to old tear or injury**
　　M23.221　Derangement of posterior horn of medial meniscus due to old tear or injury, right knee
　　M23.222　Derangement of posterior horn of medial meniscus due to old tear or injury, left knee
　　M23.229　Derangement of posterior horn of medial meniscus due to old tear or injury, unspecified knee

CHAPTER 13 (M00-M99)

● M23.23 Derangement of other medial meniscus due to old tear or injury

    M23.231 Derangement of other medial meniscus due to old tear or injury, right knee

    M23.232 Derangement of other medial meniscus due to old tear or injury, left knee

    M23.239 Derangement of other medial meniscus due to old tear or injury, unspecified knee

● M23.24 Derangement of anterior horn of lateral meniscus due to old tear or injury

    M23.241 Derangement of anterior horn of lateral meniscus due to old tear or injury, right knee

    M23.242 Derangement of anterior horn of lateral meniscus due to old tear or injury, left knee

    M23.249 Derangement of anterior horn of lateral meniscus due to old tear or injury, unspecified knee

● M23.25 Derangement of posterior horn of lateral meniscus due to old tear or injury

    M23.251 Derangement of posterior horn of lateral meniscus due to old tear or injury, right knee

    M23.252 Derangement of posterior horn of lateral meniscus due to old tear or injury, left knee

    M23.259 Derangement of posterior horn of lateral meniscus due to old tear or injury, unspecified knee

● M23.26 Derangement of other lateral meniscus due to old tear or injury

    M23.261 Derangement of other lateral meniscus due to old tear or injury, right knee

    M23.262 Derangement of other lateral meniscus due to old tear or injury, left knee

    M23.269 Derangement of other lateral meniscus due to old tear or injury, unspecified knee

● M23.3 Other meniscus derangements
    Degenerate meniscus
    Detached meniscus
    Retained meniscus

● M23.30 Other meniscus derangements, unspecified meniscus
    Other meniscus derangements, unspecified lateral meniscus
    Other meniscus derangements, unspecified medial meniscus

    M23.300 Other meniscus derangements, unspecified lateral meniscus, right knee

    M23.301 Other meniscus derangements, unspecified lateral meniscus, left knee

    M23.302 Other meniscus derangements, unspecified lateral meniscus, unspecified knee

    M23.303 Other meniscus derangements, unspecified medial meniscus, right knee

    M23.304 Other meniscus derangements, unspecified medial meniscus, left knee

    M23.305 Other meniscus derangements, unspecified medial meniscus, unspecified knee

    M23.306 Other meniscus derangements, unspecified meniscus, right knee

    M23.307 Other meniscus derangements, unspecified meniscus, left knee

    M23.309 Other meniscus derangements, unspecified meniscus, unspecified knee

● M23.31 Other meniscus derangements, anterior horn of medial meniscus

    M23.311 Other meniscus derangements, anterior horn of medial meniscus, right knee

    M23.312 Other meniscus derangements, anterior horn of medial meniscus, left knee

    M23.319 Other meniscus derangements, anterior horn of medial meniscus, unspecified knee

● M23.32 Other meniscus derangements, posterior horn of medial meniscus

    M23.321 Other meniscus derangements, posterior horn of medial meniscus, right knee

    M23.322 Other meniscus derangements, posterior horn of medial meniscus, left knee

    M23.329 Other meniscus derangements, posterior horn of medial meniscus, unspecified knee

● M23.33 Other meniscus derangements, other medial meniscus

    M23.331 Other meniscus derangements, other medial meniscus, right knee

    M23.332 Other meniscus derangements, other medial meniscus, left knee

    M23.339 Other meniscus derangements, other medial meniscus, unspecified knee

● M23.34 Other meniscus derangements, anterior horn of lateral meniscus

    M23.341 Other meniscus derangements, anterior horn of lateral meniscus, right knee

    M23.342 Other meniscus derangements, anterior horn of lateral meniscus, left knee

    M23.349 Other meniscus derangements, anterior horn of lateral meniscus, unspecified knee

● M23.35 Other meniscus derangements, posterior horn of lateral meniscus

    M23.351 Other meniscus derangements, posterior horn of lateral meniscus, right knee

    M23.352 Other meniscus derangements, posterior horn of lateral meniscus, left knee

    M23.359 Other meniscus derangements, posterior horn of lateral meniscus, unspecified knee

● M23.36 Other meniscus derangements, other lateral meniscus

    M23.361 Other meniscus derangements, other lateral meniscus, right knee

    M23.362 Other meniscus derangements, other lateral meniscus, left knee

    M23.369 Other meniscus derangements, other lateral meniscus, unspecified knee

◀ New   ◀━━ Revised   deleted Deleted   Excludes 1   Excludes 2   Includes   Use additional   Code first   Code also   Unspecified

OGCR Official Guidelines   X Assign placeholder X   ● Use Additional Character(s)   ▶ Manifestation Code   Coding Clinic

● M23.4   Loose body in knee
    M23.4Ø   Loose body in knee, unspecified knee
    M23.41   Loose body in knee, right knee
    M23.42   Loose body in knee, left knee

● M23.5   Chronic instability of knee
    M23.5Ø   Chronic instability of knee, unspecified knee
    M23.51   Chronic instability of knee, right knee
    M23.52   Chronic instability of knee, left knee

● M23.6   Other spontaneous disruption of ligament(s) of knee
   ● M23.6Ø   Other spontaneous disruption of unspecified ligament of knee
      M23.6Ø1   Other spontaneous disruption of unspecified ligament of right knee
      M23.6Ø2   Other spontaneous disruption of unspecified ligament of left knee
      M23.6Ø9   Other spontaneous disruption of unspecified ligament of unspecified knee
   ● M23.61   Other spontaneous disruption of anterior cruciate ligament of knee
      M23.611   Other spontaneous disruption of anterior cruciate ligament of right knee
      M23.612   Other spontaneous disruption of anterior cruciate ligament of left knee
      M23.619   Other spontaneous disruption of anterior cruciate ligament of unspecified knee
   ● M23.62   Other spontaneous disruption of posterior cruciate ligament of knee
      M23.621   Other spontaneous disruption of posterior cruciate ligament of right knee
      M23.622   Other spontaneous disruption of posterior cruciate ligament of left knee
      M23.629   Other spontaneous disruption of posterior cruciate ligament of unspecified knee
   ● M23.63   Other spontaneous disruption of medial collateral ligament of knee
      M23.631   Other spontaneous disruption of medial collateral ligament of right knee
      M23.632   Other spontaneous disruption of medial collateral ligament of left knee
      M23.639   Other spontaneous disruption of medial collateral ligament of unspecified knee
   ● M23.64   Other spontaneous disruption of lateral collateral ligament of knee
      M23.641   Other spontaneous disruption of lateral collateral ligament of right knee
      M23.642   Other spontaneous disruption of lateral collateral ligament of left knee
      M23.649   Other spontaneous disruption of lateral collateral ligament of unspecified knee

   ● M23.67   Other spontaneous disruption of capsular ligament of knee
      M23.671   Other spontaneous disruption of capsular ligament of right knee
      M23.672   Other spontaneous disruption of capsular ligament of left knee
      M23.679   Other spontaneous disruption of capsular ligament of unspecified knee

● M23.8   Other internal derangements of knee
    Laxity of ligament of knee
    Snapping knee
   ● M23.8X   Other internal derangements of knee
      M23.8X1   Other internal derangements of right knee
      M23.8X2   Other internal derangements of left knee
      M23.8X9   Other internal derangements of unspecified knee

● M23.9   Unspecified internal derangement of knee
    M23.9Ø   Unspecified internal derangement of unspecified knee
    M23.91   Unspecified internal derangement of right knee
    M23.92   Unspecified internal derangement of left knee

● M24   Other specific joint derangements
    Excludes1   current injury - see injury of joint by body region
    Excludes2   ganglion (M67.4)
              snapping knee (M23.8-)
              temporomandibular joint disorders (M26.6-)
   ● M24.Ø   Loose body in joint
      Excludes2   loose body in knee (M23.4)
     M24.ØØ   Loose body in unspecified joint
    ● M24.Ø1   Loose body in shoulder
      M24.Ø11   Loose body in right shoulder
      M24.Ø12   Loose body in left shoulder
      M24.Ø19   Loose body in unspecified shoulder
    ● M24.Ø2   Loose body in elbow
      M24.Ø21   Loose body in right elbow
      M24.Ø22   Loose body in left elbow
      M24.Ø29   Loose body in unspecified elbow
    ● M24.Ø3   Loose body in wrist
      M24.Ø31   Loose body in right wrist
      M24.Ø32   Loose body in left wrist
      M24.Ø39   Loose body in unspecified wrist
    ● M24.Ø4   Loose body in finger joints
      M24.Ø41   Loose body in right finger joint(s)
      M24.Ø42   Loose body in left finger joint(s)
      M24.Ø49   Loose body in unspecified finger joint(s)
    ● M24.Ø5   Loose body in hip
      M24.Ø51   Loose body in right hip
      M24.Ø52   Loose body in left hip
      M24.Ø59   Loose body in unspecified hip
    ● M24.Ø7   Loose body in ankle and toe joints
      M24.Ø71   Loose body in right ankle
      M24.Ø72   Loose body in left ankle
      M24.Ø73   Loose body in unspecified ankle
      M24.Ø74   Loose body in right toe joint(s)
      M24.Ø75   Loose body in left toe joint(s)
      M24.Ø76   Loose body in unspecified toe joints
    M24.Ø8   Loose body, other site

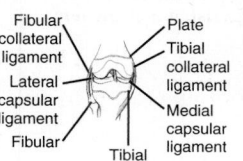

Figure 13-2   Collateral and cruciate ligament of knee. (From DeLee: DeLee and Drez's Orthopaedic Sports Medicine, ed 3, Saunders, 2009)

CHAPTER 13 (MØØ–M99)

● M24.1   Other articular cartilage disorders
    Excludes2   chondrocalcinosis (M11.1, M11.2-)
                  internal derangement of knee (M23.-)
                  metastatic calcification (E83.5)
                  ochronosis (E70.2)
   M24.10   Other articular cartilage disorders, unspecified site
● M24.11   Other articular cartilage disorders, shoulder
    M24.111   Other articular cartilage disorders, right shoulder
    M24.112   Other articular cartilage disorders, left shoulder
    M24.119   Other articular cartilage disorders, unspecified shoulder
● M24.12   Other articular cartilage disorders, elbow
    M24.121   Other articular cartilage disorders, right elbow
    M24.122   Other articular cartilage disorders, left elbow
    M24.129   Other articular cartilage disorders, unspecified elbow
● M24.13   Other articular cartilage disorders, wrist
    M24.131   Other articular cartilage disorders, right wrist
    M24.132   Other articular cartilage disorders, left wrist
    M24.139   Other articular cartilage disorders, unspecified wrist
● M24.14   Other articular cartilage disorders, hand
    M24.141   Other articular cartilage disorders, right hand
    M24.142   Other articular cartilage disorders, left hand
    M24.149   Other articular cartilage disorders, unspecified hand
● M24.15   Other articular cartilage disorders, hip
    M24.151   Other articular cartilage disorders, right hip
    M24.152   Other articular cartilage disorders, left hip
    M24.159   Other articular cartilage disorders, unspecified hip
● M24.17   Other articular cartilage disorders, ankle and foot
    M24.171   Other articular cartilage disorders, right ankle
    M24.172   Other articular cartilage disorders, left ankle
    M24.173   Other articular cartilage disorders, unspecified ankle
    M24.174   Other articular cartilage disorders, right foot
    M24.175   Other articular cartilage disorders, left foot
    M24.176   Other articular cartilage disorders, unspecified foot
● M24.2   Disorder of ligament
   Instability secondary to old ligament injury
   Ligamentous laxity NOS
    Excludes1   familial ligamentous laxity (M35.7)
    Excludes2   internal derangement of knee (M23.5-M23.89)
   M24.20   Disorder of ligament, unspecified site
● M24.21   Disorder of ligament, shoulder
    M24.211   Disorder of ligament, right shoulder
    M24.212   Disorder of ligament, left shoulder
    M24.219   Disorder of ligament, unspecified shoulder

● M24.22   Disorder of ligament, elbow
    M24.221   Disorder of ligament, right elbow
    M24.222   Disorder of ligament, left elbow
    M24.229   Disorder of ligament, unspecified elbow
● M24.23   Disorder of ligament, wrist
    M24.231   Disorder of ligament, right wrist
    M24.232   Disorder of ligament, left wrist
    M24.239   Disorder of ligament, unspecified wrist
● M24.24   Disorder of ligament, hand
    M24.241   Disorder of ligament, right hand
    M24.242   Disorder of ligament, left hand
    M24.249   Disorder of ligament, unspecified hand
● M24.25   Disorder of ligament, hip
    M24.251   Disorder of ligament, right hip
    M24.252   Disorder of ligament, left hip
    M24.259   Disorder of ligament, unspecified hip
● M24.27   Disorder of ligament, ankle and foot
    M24.271   Disorder of ligament, right ankle
    M24.272   Disorder of ligament, left ankle
    M24.273   Disorder of ligament, unspecified ankle
    M24.274   Disorder of ligament, right foot
    M24.275   Disorder of ligament, left foot
    M24.276   Disorder of ligament, unspecified foot
   M24.28   Disorder of ligament, vertebrae
● M24.3   Pathological dislocation of joint, not elsewhere classified
    Excludes1   congenital dislocation or displacement of joint - see congenital malformations and deformations of the musculoskeletal system (Q65-Q79)
              current injury - see injury of joints and ligaments by body region
              recurrent dislocation of joint (M24.4-)
   M24.30   Pathological dislocation of unspecified joint, not elsewhere classified
● M24.31   Pathological dislocation of shoulder, not elsewhere classified
    M24.311   Pathological dislocation of right shoulder, not elsewhere classified
    M24.312   Pathological dislocation of left shoulder, not elsewhere classified
    M24.319   Pathological dislocation of unspecified shoulder, not elsewhere classified
● M24.32   Pathological dislocation of elbow, not elsewhere classified
    M24.321   Pathological dislocation of right elbow, not elsewhere classified
    M24.322   Pathological dislocation of left elbow, not elsewhere classified
    M24.329   Pathological dislocation of unspecified elbow, not elsewhere classified
● M24.33   Pathological dislocation of wrist, not elsewhere classified
    M24.331   Pathological dislocation of right wrist, not elsewhere classified
    M24.332   Pathological dislocation of left wrist, not elsewhere classified
    M24.339   Pathological dislocation of unspecified wrist, not elsewhere classified

◀ New   ◀▥ Revised   ~~deleted~~ Deleted   Excludes 1   Excludes 2   Includes   Use additional   Code first   Code also   Unspecified
OGCR Official Guidelines   X Assign placeholder X   ● Use Additional Character(s)   ▶ Manifestation Code   **Coding Clinic**

● **M24.34** Pathological dislocation of hand, not elsewhere classified

    M24.341 Pathological dislocation of right hand, not elsewhere classified

    M24.342 Pathological dislocation of left hand, not elsewhere classified

    M24.349 Pathological dislocation of unspecified hand, not elsewhere classified

● **M24.35** Pathological dislocation of hip, not elsewhere classified

    M24.351 Pathological dislocation of right hip, not elsewhere classified

    M24.352 Pathological dislocation of left hip, not elsewhere classified

    M24.359 Pathological dislocation of unspecified hip, not elsewhere classified

● **M24.36** Pathological dislocation of knee, not elsewhere classified

    M24.361 Pathological dislocation of right knee, not elsewhere classified

    M24.362 Pathological dislocation of left knee, not elsewhere classified

    M24.369 Pathological dislocation of unspecified knee, not elsewhere classified

● **M24.37** Pathological dislocation of ankle and foot, not elsewhere classified

    M24.371 Pathological dislocation of right ankle, not elsewhere classified

    M24.372 Pathological dislocation of left ankle, not elsewhere classified

    M24.373 Pathological dislocation of unspecified ankle, not elsewhere classified

    M24.374 Pathological dislocation of right foot, not elsewhere classified

    M24.375 Pathological dislocation of left foot, not elsewhere classified

    M24.376 Pathological dislocation of unspecified foot, not elsewhere classified

● **M24.4** Recurrent dislocation of joint

    Recurrent subluxation of joint

    Excludes2   recurrent dislocation of patella (M22.0-M22.1)

               recurrent vertebral dislocation (M43.3-, M43.4, M43.5-)

    M24.40 Recurrent dislocation, unspecified joint

● **M24.41** Recurrent dislocation, shoulder

    M24.411 Recurrent dislocation, right shoulder

    M24.412 Recurrent dislocation, left shoulder

    M24.419 Recurrent dislocation, unspecified shoulder

● **M24.42** Recurrent dislocation, elbow

    M24.421 Recurrent dislocation, right elbow

    M24.422 Recurrent dislocation, left elbow

    M24.429 Recurrent dislocation, unspecified elbow

● **M24.43** Recurrent dislocation, wrist

    M24.431 Recurrent dislocation, right wrist

    M24.432 Recurrent dislocation, left wrist

    M24.439 Recurrent dislocation, unspecified wrist

● **M24.44** Recurrent dislocation, hand and finger(s)

    M24.441 Recurrent dislocation, right hand

    M24.442 Recurrent dislocation, left hand

    M24.443 Recurrent dislocation, unspecified hand

    M24.444 Recurrent dislocation, right finger

    M24.445 Recurrent dislocation, left finger

    M24.446 Recurrent dislocation, unspecified finger

● **M24.45** Recurrent dislocation, hip

    M24.451 Recurrent dislocation, right hip

    M24.452 Recurrent dislocation, left hip

    M24.459 Recurrent dislocation, unspecified hip

● **M24.46** Recurrent dislocation, knee

    M24.461 Recurrent dislocation, right knee

    M24.462 Recurrent dislocation, left knee

    M24.469 Recurrent dislocation, unspecified knee

● **M24.47** Recurrent dislocation, ankle, foot and toes

    M24.471 Recurrent dislocation, right ankle

    M24.472 Recurrent dislocation, left ankle

    M24.473 Recurrent dislocation, unspecified ankle

    M24.474 Recurrent dislocation, right foot

    M24.475 Recurrent dislocation, left foot

    M24.476 Recurrent dislocation, unspecified foot

    M24.477 Recurrent dislocation, right toe(s)

    M24.478 Recurrent dislocation, left toe(s)

    M24.479 Recurrent dislocation, unspecified toe(s)

● **M24.5** Contracture of joint

    Excludes1   contracture of muscle without contracture of joint (M62.4-)

               contracture of tendon (sheath) without contracture of joint (M62.4-)

               Dupuytren's contracture (M72.0)

    Excludes2   acquired deformities of limbs (M20-M21)

    M24.50 Contracture, unspecified joint

● **M24.51** Contracture, shoulder

    M24.511 Contracture, right shoulder

    M24.512 Contracture, left shoulder

    M24.519 Contracture, unspecified shoulder

● **M24.52** Contracture, elbow

    M24.521 Contracture, right elbow

    M24.522 Contracture, left elbow

    M24.529 Contracture, unspecified elbow

● **M24.53** Contracture, wrist

    M24.531 Contracture, right wrist

    M24.532 Contracture, left wrist

    M24.539 Contracture, unspecified wrist

● **M24.54** Contracture, hand

    M24.541 Contracture, right hand

    M24.542 Contracture, left hand

    M24.549 Contracture, unspecified hand

● **M24.55** Contracture, hip

    M24.551 Contracture, right hip
           Coding Clinic: 2016, Q2, P6

    M24.552 Contracture, left hip
           Coding Clinic: 2016, Q2, P6

    M24.559 Contracture, unspecified hip

CHAPTER 13 (M00-M99)

● M24.56 Contracture, knee
    M24.561 Contracture, right knee
          Coding Clinic: 2016, Q2, P6
    M24.562 Contracture, left knee
          Coding Clinic: 2016, Q2, P6
    M24.569 Contracture, unspecified knee

● M24.57 Contracture, ankle and foot
    M24.571 Contracture, right ankle
    M24.572 Contracture, left ankle
    M24.573 Contracture, unspecified ankle
    M24.574 Contracture, right foot
    M24.575 Contracture, left foot
    M24.576 Contracture, unspecified foot

● M24.6 Ankylosis of joint
    Excludes1   stiffness of joint without ankylosis
               (M25.6-)
    Excludes2   spine (M43.2-)
    M24.60 Ankylosis, unspecified joint

● M24.61 Ankylosis, shoulder
    M24.611 Ankylosis, right shoulder
    M24.612 Ankylosis, left shoulder
    M24.619 Ankylosis, unspecified shoulder

● M24.62 Ankylosis, elbow
    M24.621 Ankylosis, right elbow
    M24.622 Ankylosis, left elbow
    M24.629 Ankylosis, unspecified elbow

● M24.63 Ankylosis, wrist
    M24.631 Ankylosis, right wrist
    M24.632 Ankylosis, left wrist
    M24.639 Ankylosis, unspecified wrist

● M24.64 Ankylosis, hand
    M24.641 Ankylosis, right hand
    M24.642 Ankylosis, left hand
    M24.649 Ankylosis, unspecified hand

● M24.65 Ankylosis, hip
    M24.651 Ankylosis, right hip
    M24.652 Ankylosis, left hip
    M24.659 Ankylosis, unspecified hip

● M24.66 Ankylosis, knee
    M24.661 Ankylosis, right knee
    M24.662 Ankylosis, left knee
    M24.669 Ankylosis, unspecified knee

● M24.67 Ankylosis, ankle and foot
    M24.671 Ankylosis, right ankle
    M24.672 Ankylosis, left ankle
    M24.673 Ankylosis, unspecified ankle
    M24.674 Ankylosis, right foot
    M24.675 Ankylosis, left foot
    M24.676 Ankylosis, unspecified foot

  M24.7 Protrusio acetabuli
● M24.8 Other specific joint derangements, not elsewhere classified
    Excludes2   iliotibial band syndrome (M76.3)
    M24.80 Other specific joint derangements of unspecified joint, not elsewhere classified

● M24.81 Other specific joint derangements of shoulder, not elsewhere classified
    M24.811 Other specific joint derangements of right shoulder, not elsewhere classified
    M24.812 Other specific joint derangements of left shoulder, not elsewhere classified
    M24.819 Other specific joint derangements of unspecified shoulder, not elsewhere classified

● M24.82 Other specific joint derangements of elbow, not elsewhere classified
    M24.821 Other specific joint derangements of right elbow, not elsewhere classified
    M24.822 Other specific joint derangements of left elbow, not elsewhere classified
    M24.829 Other specific joint derangements of unspecified elbow, not elsewhere classified

● M24.83 Other specific joint derangements of wrist, not elsewhere classified
    M24.831 Other specific joint derangements of right wrist, not elsewhere classified
    M24.832 Other specific joint derangements of left wrist, not elsewhere classified
    M24.839 Other specific joint derangements of unspecified wrist, not elsewhere classified

● M24.84 Other specific joint derangements of hand, not elsewhere classified
    M24.841 Other specific joint derangements of right hand, not elsewhere classified
    M24.842 Other specific joint derangements of left hand, not elsewhere classified
    M24.849 Other specific joint derangements of unspecified hand, not elsewhere classified

● M24.85 Other specific joint derangements of hip, not elsewhere classified
    Irritable hip
    M24.851 Other specific joint derangements of right hip, not elsewhere classified
    M24.852 Other specific joint derangements of left hip, not elsewhere classified
    M24.859 Other specific joint derangements of unspecified hip, not elsewhere classified

● M24.87 Other specific joint derangements of ankle and foot, not elsewhere classified
    M24.871 Other specific joint derangements of right ankle, not elsewhere classified
    M24.872 Other specific joint derangements of left ankle, not elsewhere classified
    M24.873 Other specific joint derangements of unspecified ankle, not elsewhere classified
    M24.874 Other specific joint derangements of right foot, not elsewhere classified
    M24.875 Other specific joint derangements left foot, not elsewhere classified
    M24.876 Other specific joint derangements of unspecified foot, not elsewhere classified

  M24.9 Joint derangement, unspecified

CHAPTER 13 (M00-M99)

Item 13–5 Ankylosis or arthrokleisis is a consolidation of a joint due to disease, injury, or surgical procedure. Spondylosis is the degeneration of the vertebral processes and formation of osteophytes and commonly occurs with age. **Spondylitis** or ankylosing spondylitis is a type of arthritis that affects the spine or backbone causing back pain and stiffness.

◄ New   ◄▥ Revised   ~~deleted~~ Deleted   Excludes 1   Excludes 2   Includes   Use additional   Code first   Code also   Unspecified

OGCR Official Guidelines   X Assign placeholder X   ● Use Additional Character(s)   ▶ Manifestation Code   **Coding Clinic**

● **M25   Other joint disorder, not elsewhere classified**

    Excludes2   abnormality of gait and mobility (R26.-)
                      acquired deformities of limb (M20-M21)
                      calcification of bursa (M71.4-)
                      calcification of shoulder (joint) (M75.3)
                      calcification of tendon (M65.2-)
                      difficulty in walking (R26.2)
                      temporomandibular joint disorder (M26.6-)

● **M25.0   Hemarthrosis**

    Excludes1   current injury - see injury of joint by body
                      region
                      hemophilic arthropathy (M36.2)

     M25.00   Hemarthrosis, unspecified joint

  ● M25.01   Hemarthrosis, shoulder

       M25.011   Hemarthrosis, right shoulder

       M25.012   Hemarthrosis, left shoulder

       M25.019   Hemarthrosis, unspecified shoulder

  ● M25.02   Hemarthrosis, elbow

       M25.021   Hemarthrosis, right elbow

       M25.022   Hemarthrosis, left elbow

       M25.029   Hemarthrosis, unspecified elbow

  ● M25.03   Hemarthrosis, wrist

       M25.031   Hemarthrosis, right wrist

       M25.032   Hemarthrosis, left wrist

       M25.039   Hemarthrosis, unspecified wrist

  ● M25.04   Hemarthrosis, hand

       M25.041   Hemarthrosis, right hand

       M25.042   Hemarthrosis, left hand

       M25.049   Hemarthrosis, unspecified hand

  ● M25.05   Hemarthrosis, hip

       M25.051   Hemarthrosis, right hip

       M25.052   Hemarthrosis, left hip

       M25.059   Hemarthrosis, unspecified hip

  ● M25.06   Hemarthrosis, knee

       M25.061   Hemarthrosis, right knee

       M25.062   Hemarthrosis, left knee

       M25.069   Hemarthrosis, unspecified knee

  ● M25.07   Hemarthrosis, ankle and foot

       M25.071   Hemarthrosis, right ankle

       M25.072   Hemarthrosis, left ankle

       M25.073   Hemarthrosis, unspecified ankle

       M25.074   Hemarthrosis, right foot

       M25.075   Hemarthrosis, left foot

       M25.076   Hemarthrosis, unspecified foot

     M25.08   Hemarthrosis, other specified site
              Hemarthrosis, vertebrae

● **M25.1   Fistula of joint**

     M25.10   Fistula, unspecified joint

  ● M25.11   Fistula, shoulder

       M25.111   Fistula, right shoulder

       M25.112   Fistula, left shoulder

       M25.119   Fistula, unspecified shoulder

  ● M25.12   Fistula, elbow

       M25.121   Fistula, right elbow

       M25.122   Fistula, left elbow

       M25.129   Fistula, unspecified elbow

  ● M25.13   Fistula, wrist

       M25.131   Fistula, right wrist

       M25.132   Fistula, left wrist

       M25.139   Fistula, unspecified wrist

  ● M25.14   Fistula, hand

       M25.141   Fistula, right hand

       M25.142   Fistula, left hand

       M25.149   Fistula, unspecified hand

  ● M25.15   Fistula, hip

       M25.151   Fistula, right hip

       M25.152   Fistula, left hip

       M25.159   Fistula, unspecified hip

  ● M25.16   Fistula, knee

       M25.161   Fistula, right knee

       M25.162   Fistula, left knee

       M25.169   Fistula, unspecified knee

  ● M25.17   Fistula, ankle and foot

       M25.171   Fistula, right ankle

       M25.172   Fistula, left ankle

       M25.173   Fistula, unspecified ankle

       M25.174   Fistula, right foot

       M25.175   Fistula, left foot

       M25.176   Fistula, unspecified foot

     M25.18   Fistula, other specified site
              Fistula, vertebrae

● **M25.2   Flail joint**

     M25.20   Flail joint, unspecified joint

  ● M25.21   Flail joint, shoulder

       M25.211   Flail joint, right shoulder

       M25.212   Flail joint, left shoulder

       M25.219   Flail joint, unspecified shoulder

  ● M25.22   Flail joint, elbow

       M25.221   Flail joint, right elbow

       M25.222   Flail joint, left elbow

       M25.229   Flail joint, unspecified elbow

  ● M25.23   Flail joint, wrist

       M25.231   Flail joint, right wrist

       M25.232   Flail joint, left wrist

       M25.239   Flail joint, unspecified wrist

  ● M25.24   Flail joint, hand

       M25.241   Flail joint, right hand

       M25.242   Flail joint, left hand

       M25.249   Flail joint, unspecified hand

  ● M25.25   Flail joint, hip

       M25.251   Flail joint, right hip

       M25.252   Flail joint, left hip

       M25.259   Flail joint, unspecified hip

  ● M25.26   Flail joint, knee

       M25.261   Flail joint, right knee

       M25.262   Flail joint, left knee

       M25.269   Flail joint, unspecified knee

  ● M25.27   Flail joint, ankle and foot

       M25.271   Flail joint, right ankle and foot

       M25.272   Flail joint, left ankle and foot

       M25.279   Flail joint, unspecified ankle and foot

     M25.28   Flail joint, other site

● **M25.3   Other instability of joint**

     Excludes1   instability of joint secondary to old
                      ligament injury (M24.2-)
                  instability of joint secondary to removal
                      of joint prosthesis (M96.8-)

     Excludes2   spinal instabilities (M53.2-)

     M25.30   Other instability, unspecified joint

  ● M25.31   Other instability, shoulder

       M25.311   Other instability, right shoulder

       M25.312   Other instability, left shoulder

       M25.319   Other instability, unspecified
                   shoulder

  ● M25.32   Other instability, elbow

       M25.321   Other instability, right elbow

       M25.322   Other instability, left elbow

       M25.329   Other instability, unspecified elbow

CHAPTER 13 (MØØ-M99)

● M25.33 Other instability, wrist
   M25.331 Other instability, right wrist
   M25.332 Other instability, left wrist
   M25.339 Other instability, unspecified wrist
● M25.34 Other instability, hand
   M25.341 Other instability, right hand
   M25.342 Other instability, left hand
   M25.349 Other instability, unspecified hand
● M25.35 Other instability, hip
   M25.351 Other instability, right hip
   M25.352 Other instability, left hip
   M25.359 Other instability, unspecified hip
● M25.36 Other instability, knee
   M25.361 Other instability, right knee
   M25.362 Other instability, left knee
   M25.369 Other instability, unspecified knee
● M25.37 Other instability, ankle and foot
   M25.371 Other instability, right ankle
   M25.372 Other instability, left ankle
   M25.373 Other instability, unspecified ankle
   M25.374 Other instability, right foot
   M25.375 Other instability, left foot
   M25.376 Other instability, unspecified foot
● M25.4 Effusion of joint
   Excludes1 hydrarthrosis in yaws (A66.6)
      intermittent hydrarthrosis (M12.4-)
      other infective (teno)synovitis (M65.1-)
   M25.40 Effusion, unspecified joint
● M25.41 Effusion, shoulder
   M25.411 Effusion, right shoulder
   M25.412 Effusion, left shoulder
   M25.419 Effusion, unspecified shoulder
● M25.42 Effusion, elbow
   M25.421 Effusion, right elbow
   M25.422 Effusion, left elbow
   M25.429 Effusion, unspecified elbow
● M25.43 Effusion, wrist
   M25.431 Effusion, right wrist
   M25.432 Effusion, left wrist
   M25.439 Effusion, unspecified wrist
● M25.44 Effusion, hand
   M25.441 Effusion, right hand
   M25.442 Effusion, left hand
   M25.449 Effusion, unspecified hand
● M25.45 Effusion, hip
   M25.451 Effusion, right hip
   M25.452 Effusion, left hip
   M25.459 Effusion, unspecified hip
● M25.46 Effusion, knee
   M25.461 Effusion, right knee
   M25.462 Effusion, left knee
   M25.469 Effusion, unspecified knee
● M25.47 Effusion, ankle and foot
   M25.471 Effusion, right ankle
   M25.472 Effusion, left ankle
   M25.473 Effusion, unspecified ankle
   M25.474 Effusion, right foot
   M25.475 Effusion, left foot
   M25.476 Effusion, unspecified foot
   M25.48 Effusion, other site

● M25.5 Pain in joint
   Excludes2 pain in hand (M79.64-)
      pain in fingers (M79.64-)
      pain in foot (M79.67-)
      pain in limb (M79.6-)
      pain in toes (M79.67-)
   M25.50 Pain in unspecified joint
● M25.51 Pain in shoulder
   M25.511 Pain in right shoulder
   M25.512 Pain in left shoulder
   M25.519 Pain in unspecified shoulder
● M25.52 Pain in elbow
   M25.521 Pain in right elbow
   M25.522 Pain in left elbow
   M25.529 Pain in unspecified elbow
● M25.53 Pain in wrist
   M25.531 Pain in right wrist
   M25.532 Pain in left wrist
   M25.539 Pain in unspecified wrist
● M25.54 Pain in joints of hand ◄
   M25.541 Pain in joints of right hand ◄
   M25.542 Pain in joints of left hand ◄
   M25.549 Pain in joints of unspecified hand ◄
      Pain in joints of hand NOS ◄
● M25.55 Pain in hip
   M25.551 Pain in right hip
   M25.552 Pain in left hip
   M25.559 Pain in unspecified hip
● M25.56 Pain in knee
   M25.561 Pain in right knee
   M25.562 Pain in left knee
   M25.569 Pain in unspecified knee
● M25.57 Pain in ankle and joints of foot
   M25.571 Pain in right ankle and joints of right foot
   M25.572 Pain in left ankle and joints of left foot
   M25.579 Pain in unspecified ankle and joints of unspecified foot
● M25.6 Stiffness of joint, not elsewhere classified
   Excludes1 ankylosis of joint (M24.6-)
      contracture of joint (M24.5-)
   M25.60 Stiffness of unspecified joint, not elsewhere classified
● M25.61 Stiffness of shoulder, not elsewhere classified
   M25.611 Stiffness of right shoulder, not elsewhere classified
   M25.612 Stiffness of left shoulder, not elsewhere classified
   M25.619 Stiffness of unspecified shoulder, not elsewhere classified
● M25.62 Stiffness of elbow, not elsewhere classified
   M25.621 Stiffness of right elbow, not elsewhere classified
   M25.622 Stiffness of left elbow, not elsewhere classified
   M25.629 Stiffness of unspecified elbow, not elsewhere classified
● M25.63 Stiffness of wrist, not elsewhere classified
   M25.631 Stiffness of right wrist, not elsewhere classified
   M25.632 Stiffness of left wrist, not elsewhere classified
   M25.639 Stiffness of unspecified wrist, not elsewhere classified

◄ New   ◀ Revised   ~~deleted~~ Deleted   Excludes 1   Excludes 2   Includes   Use additional   Code first   Code also   Unspecified
OGCR Official Guidelines   X Assign placeholder X   ● Use Additional Character(s)   ▶ Manifestation Code   **Coding Clinic**

● M25.64 Stiffness of hand, not elsewhere classified
    M25.641 Stiffness of right hand, not elsewhere classified
    M25.642 Stiffness of left hand, not elsewhere classified
    M25.649 Stiffness of unspecified hand, not elsewhere classified
● M25.65 Stiffness of hip, not elsewhere classified
    M25.651 Stiffness of right hip, not elsewhere classified
    M25.652 Stiffness of left hip, not elsewhere classified
    M25.659 Stiffness of unspecified hip, not elsewhere classified
● M25.66 Stiffness of knee, not elsewhere classified
    M25.661 Stiffness of right knee, not elsewhere classified
    M25.662 Stiffness of left knee, not elsewhere classified
    M25.669 Stiffness of unspecified knee, not elsewhere classified
● M25.67 Stiffness of ankle and foot, not elsewhere classified
    M25.671 Stiffness of right ankle, not elsewhere classified
    M25.672 Stiffness of left ankle, not elsewhere classified
    M25.673 Stiffness of unspecified ankle, not elsewhere classified
    M25.674 Stiffness of right foot, not elsewhere classified
    M25.675 Stiffness of left foot, not elsewhere classified
    M25.676 Stiffness of unspecified foot, not elsewhere classified
● M25.7 Osteophyte
    M25.70 Osteophyte, unspecified joint
● M25.71 Osteophyte, shoulder
    M25.711 Osteophyte, right shoulder
    M25.712 Osteophyte, left shoulder
    M25.719 Osteophyte, unspecified shoulder
● M25.72 Osteophyte, elbow
    M25.721 Osteophyte, right elbow
    M25.722 Osteophyte, left elbow
    M25.729 Osteophyte, unspecified elbow
● M25.73 Osteophyte, wrist
    M25.731 Osteophyte, right wrist
    M25.732 Osteophyte, left wrist
    M25.739 Osteophyte, unspecified wrist
● M25.74 Osteophyte, hand
    M25.741 Osteophyte, right hand
    M25.742 Osteophyte, left hand
    M25.749 Osteophyte, unspecified hand
● M25.75 Osteophyte, hip
    M25.751 Osteophyte, right hip
    M25.752 Osteophyte, left hip
    M25.759 Osteophyte, unspecified hip
● M25.76 Osteophyte, knee
    M25.761 Osteophyte, right knee
    M25.762 Osteophyte, left knee
    M25.769 Osteophyte, unspecified knee

● M25.77 Osteophyte, ankle and foot
    M25.771 Osteophyte, right ankle
    M25.772 Osteophyte, left ankle
    M25.773 Osteophyte, unspecified ankle
    M25.774 Osteophyte, right foot
    M25.775 Osteophyte, left foot
    M25.776 Osteophyte, unspecified foot
    M25.78 Osteophyte, vertebrae
● M25.8 Other specified joint disorders
    M25.80 Other specified joint disorders, unspecified joint
● M25.81 Other specified joint disorders, shoulder
    M25.811 Other specified joint disorders, right shoulder
    M25.812 Other specified joint disorders, left shoulder
    M25.819 Other specified joint disorders, unspecified shoulder
● M25.82 Other specified joint disorders, elbow
    M25.821 Other specified joint disorders, right elbow
    M25.822 Other specified joint disorders, left elbow
    M25.829 Other specified joint disorders, unspecified elbow
● M25.83 Other specified joint disorders, wrist
    M25.831 Other specified joint disorders, right wrist
    M25.832 Other specified joint disorders, left wrist
    M25.839 Other specified joint disorders, unspecified wrist
● M25.84 Other specified joint disorders, hand
    M25.841 Other specified joint disorders, right hand
    M25.842 Other specified joint disorders, left hand
    M25.849 Other specified joint disorders, unspecified hand
● M25.85 Other specified joint disorders, hip
    M25.851 Other specified joint disorders, right hip
    M25.852 Other specified joint disorders, left hip
    M25.859 Other specified joint disorders, unspecified hip
● M25.86 Other specified joint disorders, knee
    M25.861 Other specified joint disorders, right knee
    M25.862 Other specified joint disorders, left knee
    M25.869 Other specified joint disorders, unspecified knee
● M25.87 Other specified joint disorders, ankle and foot
    M25.871 Other specified joint disorders, right ankle and foot
    M25.872 Other specified joint disorders, left ankle and foot
    M25.879 Other specified joint disorders, unspecified ankle and foot
  M25.9 Joint disorder, unspecified

CHAPTER 13 (M00-M99)

Figure 13-3   Dentofacial malocclusion.

Item 13–6 Hyperplasia is a condition of overdevelopment, whereas **hypoplasia** is a condition of underdevelopment. **Macrogenia** is overdevelopment of the chin, whereas **microgenia** is underdevelopment of the chin.

DENTOFACIAL ANOMALIES [INCLUDING MALOCCLUSION] AND OTHER DISORDERS OF JAW (M26-M27)

> Excludes1   hemifacial atrophy or hypertrophy (Q67.4)
> unilateral condylar hyperplasia or hypoplasia (M27.8)

● **M26   Dentofacial anomalies [including malocclusion]**

  ● **M26.0   Major anomalies of jaw size**

> Excludes1   acromegaly (E22.0)
> Robin's syndrome (Q87.0)

    M26.00   Unspecified anomaly of jaw size

    M26.01   Maxillary hyperplasia

    M26.02   Maxillary hypoplasia

    M26.03   Mandibular hyperplasia

    M26.04   Mandibular hypoplasia

    M26.05   Macrogenia

    M26.06   Microgenia

    M26.07   Excessive tuberosity of jaw
         Entire maxillary tuberosity

    M26.09   Other specified anomalies of jaw size

  ● **M26.1   Anomalies of jaw-cranial base relationship**

    M26.10   Unspecified anomaly of jaw-cranial base relationship

    M26.11   Maxillary asymmetry

    M26.12   Other jaw asymmetry

    M26.19   Other specified anomalies of jaw-cranial base relationship

  ● **M26.2   Anomalies of dental arch relationship**

    M26.20   Unspecified anomaly of dental arch relationship

    ● M26.21   Malocclusion, Angle's class

         M26.211   Malocclusion, Angle's class I
             Neutro-occlusion

         M26.212   Malocclusion, Angle's class II
             Disto-occlusion Division I
             Disto-occlusion Division II

         M26.213   Malocclusion, Angle's class III
             Mesio-occlusion

         M26.219   Malocclusion, Angle's class, unspecified

    ● M26.22   Open occlusal relationship

         M26.220   Open anterior occlusal relationship
             Anterior openbite

         M26.221   Open posterior occlusal relationship
             Posterior openbite

    M26.23   Excessive horizontal overlap
         Excessive horizontal overjet

    M26.24   Reverse articulation
         Crossbite (anterior) (posterior)

    M26.25   Anomalies of interarch distance

    M26.29   Other anomalies of dental arch relationship
         Midline deviation of dental arch
         Overbite (excessive) deep
         Overbite (excessive) horizontal
         Overbite (excessive) vertical
         Posterior lingual occlusion of mandibular teeth

● **M26.3   Anomalies of tooth position of fully erupted tooth or teeth**

> Excludes2   embedded and impacted teeth (K01.-)

    M26.30   Unspecified anomaly of tooth position of fully erupted tooth or teeth
         Abnormal spacing of fully erupted tooth or teeth NOS
         Displacement of fully erupted tooth or teeth NOS
         Transposition of fully erupted tooth or teeth NOS

    M26.31   Crowding of fully erupted teeth

    M26.32   Excessive spacing of fully erupted teeth
         Diastema of fully erupted tooth or teeth NOS

    M26.33   Horizontal displacement of fully erupted tooth or teeth
         Tipped tooth or teeth
         Tipping of fully erupted tooth

    M26.34   Vertical displacement of fully erupted tooth or teeth
         Extruded tooth
         Infraeruption of tooth or teeth
         Supraeruption of tooth or teeth

    M26.35   Rotation of fully erupted tooth or teeth

    M26.36   Insufficient interocclusal distance of fully erupted teeth (ridge)
         Lack of adequate intermaxillary vertical dimension of fully erupted teeth

    M26.37   Excessive interocclusal distance of fully erupted teeth
         Excessive intermaxillary vertical dimension of fully erupted teeth
         Loss of occlusal vertical dimension of fully erupted teeth

    M26.39   Other anomalies of tooth position of fully erupted tooth or teeth

  M26.4   Malocclusion, unspecified

● **M26.5   Dentofacial functional abnormalities**

> Excludes1   bruxism (F45.8)
> teeth-grinding NOS (F45.8)

    M26.50   Dentofacial functional abnormalities, unspecified

    M26.51   Abnormal jaw closure

    M26.52   Limited mandibular range of motion

    M26.53   Deviation in opening and closing of the mandible

    M26.54   Insufficient anterior guidance
         Insufficient anterior occlusal guidance

    M26.55   Centric occlusion maximum intercuspation discrepancy

> Excludes1   centric occlusion NOS (M26.59)

    M26.56   Non-working side interference
         Balancing side interference

    M26.57   Lack of posterior occlusal support

    M26.59   Other dentofacial functional abnormalities
         Centric occlusion (of teeth) NOS
         Malocclusion due to abnormal swallowing
         Malocclusion due to mouth breathing
         Malocclusion due to tongue, lip or finger habits

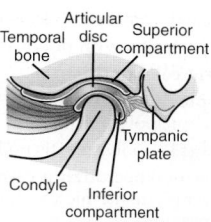

Figure 13-4   Temporomandibular joint.

Item 13–7   Dysfunction of the temporomandibular joint is termed **temporomandibular joint (TMJ) syndrome** and is characterized by pain and tenderness/spasm of the muscles of mastication, joint noise, and in the later stages, limited mandibular movement.

● M26.6   **Temporomandibular joint disorders**
> **Excludes2**   current temporomandibular joint dislocation (S03.0)
> current temporomandibular joint sprain (S03.4)

  ● M26.60   **Temporomandibular joint disorder, unspecified**

    M26.601   Right temporomandibular joint disorder, unspecified ◄

    M26.602   Left temporomandibular joint disorder, unspecified ◄

    M26.603   Bilateral temporomandibular joint disorder, unspecified ◄

    M26.609   Unspecified temporomandibular joint disorder, unspecified side ◄
        Temporomandibular joint disorder NOS ◄

  ● M26.61   **Adhesions and ankylosis of temporomandibular joint**

    M26.611   Adhesions and ankylosis of right temporomandibular joint ◄

    M26.612   Adhesions and ankylosis of left temporomandibular joint ◄

    M26.613   Adhesions and ankylosis of bilateral temporomandibular joint ◄

    M26.619   Adhesions and ankylosis of temporomandibular joint, unspecified side ◄

  ● M26.62   **Arthralgia of temporomandibular joint**

    M26.621   Arthralgia of right temporomandibular joint ◄

    M26.622   Arthralgia of left temporomandibular joint ◄

    M26.623   Arthralgia of bilateral temporomandibular joint ◄

    M26.629   Arthralgia of temporomandibular joint, unspecified side ◄

  ● M26.63   **Articular disc disorder of temporomandibular joint**

    M26.631   Articular disc disorder of right temporomandibular joint ◄

    M26.632   Articular disc disorder of left temporomandibular joint ◄

    M26.633   Articular disc disorder of bilateral temporomandibular joint ◄

    M26.639   Articular disc disorder of temporomandibular joint, unspecified side ◄

    M26.69   Other specified disorders of temporomandibular joint

● M26.7   **Dental alveolar anomalies**

    M26.70   Unspecified alveolar anomaly

    M26.71   Alveolar maxillary hyperplasia

    M26.72   Alveolar mandibular hyperplasia

    M26.73   Alveolar maxillary hypoplasia

    M26.74   Alveolar mandibular hypoplasia

    M26.79   Other specified alveolar anomalies

● M26.8   **Other dentofacial anomalies**

    M26.81   Anterior soft tissue impingement
        Anterior soft tissue impingement on teeth

    M26.82   Posterior soft tissue impingement
        Posterior soft tissue impingement on teeth

    M26.89   Other dentofacial anomalies

  M26.9   Dentofacial anomaly, unspecified

● M27   **Other diseases of jaws**

  M27.0   **Developmental disorders of jaws**
     Latent bone cyst of jaw
     Stafne's cyst
     Torus mandibularis
     Torus palatinus

  M27.1   **Giant cell granuloma, central**
     Giant cell granuloma NOS
> **Excludes1**   peripheral giant cell granuloma (K06.8)

  M27.2   **Inflammatory conditions of jaws**
     Osteitis of jaw(s)
     Osteomyelitis (neonatal) jaw(s)
     Osteoradionecrosis jaw(s)
     Periostitis jaw(s)
     Sequestrum of jaw bone
     Use additional code (W88-W90, X39.0) to identify radiation, if radiation-induced
> **Excludes2**   osteonecrosis of jaw due to drug (M87.180)

  M27.3   **Alveolitis of jaws**
     Alveolar osteitis
     Dry socket

● M27.4   **Other and unspecified cysts of jaw**
> **Excludes1**   cysts of oral region (K09.-)
> latent bone cyst of jaw (M27.0)
> Stafne's cyst (M27.0)

    M27.40   Unspecified cyst of jaw
        Cyst of jaw NOS

    M27.49   Other cysts of jaw
        Aneurysmal cyst of jaw
        Hemorrhagic cyst of jaw
        Traumatic cyst of jaw

● M27.5   **Periradicular pathology associated with previous endodontic treatment**

    M27.51   Perforation of root canal space due to endodontic treatment

    M27.52   Endodontic overfill

    M27.53   Endodontic underfill

    M27.59   Other periradicular pathology associated with previous endodontic treatment

● M27.6   **Endosseous dental implant failure**

    M27.61   Osseointegration failure of dental implant
        Hemorrhagic complications of dental implant placement
        Iatrogenic osseointegration failure of dental implant
        Osseointegration failure of dental implant due to complications of systemic disease
        Osseointegration failure of dental implant due to poor bone quality
        Pre-integration failure of dental implant NOS
        Pre-osseointegration failure of dental implant

CHAPTER 13 (M00-M99)

M27.62 Post-osseointegration biological failure of dental implant
Failure of dental implant due to lack of attached gingiva
Failure of dental implant due to occlusal trauma (caused by poor prosthetic design)
Failure of dental implant due to parafunctional habits
Failure of dental implant due to periodontal infection (peri–implantitis)
Failure of dental implant due to poor oral hygiene
Iatrogenic post-osseointegration failure of dental implant
Post-osseointegration failure of dental implant due to complications of systemic disease

M27.63 Post-osseointegration mechanical failure of dental implant
Failure of dental prosthesis causing loss of dental implant
Fracture of dental implant
Excludes2 cracked tooth (K03.81)
fractured dental restorative material with loss of material (K08.531)
fractured dental restorative material without loss of material (K08.530)
fractured tooth (S02.5)

M27.69 Other endosseous dental implant failure
Dental implant failure NOS

M27.8 Other specified diseases of jaws
Cherubism
Exostosis
Fibrous dysplasia
Unilateral condylar hyperplasia
Unilateral condylar hypoplasia
Excludes1 jaw pain (R68.84)

M27.9 Disease of jaws, unspecified

SYSTEMIC CONNECTIVE TISSUE DISORDERS (M30-M36)

Includes autoimmune disease NOS
collagen (vascular) disease NOS
systemic autoimmune disease
systemic collagen (vascular) disease

Excludes1 autoimmune disease, single organ or single cell-type - code to relevant condition category

● **M30 Polyarteritis nodosa and related conditions**
Excludes1 microscopic polyarteritis (M31.7)

M30.0 Polyarteritis nodosa

M30.1 Polyarteritis with lung involvement [Churg-Strauss]
Allergic granulomatous angiitis

M30.2 Juvenile polyarteritis

M30.3 Mucocutaneous lymph node syndrome [Kawasaki]

M30.8 Other conditions related to polyarteritis nodosa
Polyangiitis overlap syndrome

● **M31 Other necrotizing vasculopathies**
M31.0 Hypersensitivity angiitis
Goodpasture's syndrome

M31.1 Thrombotic microangiopathy
Thrombotic thrombocytopenic purpura

M31.2 Lethal midline granuloma

● **M31.3 Wegener's granulomatosis**
Necrotizing respiratory granulomatosis

M31.30 Wegener's granulomatosis without renal involvement
Wegener's granulomatosis NOS

M31.31 Wegener's granulomatosis with renal involvement

M31.4 Aortic arch syndrome [Takayasu]

M31.5 Giant cell arteritis with polymyalgia rheumatica

M31.6 Other giant cell arteritis

M31.7 Microscopic polyangiitis
Microscopic polyarteritis
Excludes1 polyarteritis nodosa (M30.0)

M31.8 Other specified necrotizing vasculopathies
Hypocomplementemic vasculitis
Septic vasculitis

M31.9 Necrotizing vasculopathy, unspecified

● **M32 Systemic lupus erythematosus (SLE)**
Autoimmune inflammatory connective tissue disease of unknown cause that occurs most often in women
Excludes1 lupus erythematosus (discoid) (NOS) (L93.0)

M32.0 Drug-induced systemic lupus erythematosus
Use additional code for adverse effect, if applicable, to identify drug (T36-T50 with fifth or sixth character 5)

● **M32.1 Systemic lupus erythematosus with organ or system involvement**
M32.10 Systemic lupus erythematosus, organ or system involvement unspecified

M32.11 Endocarditis in systemic lupus erythematosus
Libman-Sacks disease

M32.12 Pericarditis in systemic lupus erythematosus
Lupus pericarditis

M32.13 Lung involvement in systemic lupus erythematosus
Pleural effusion due to systemic lupus erythematosus

M32.14 Glomerular disease in systemic lupus erythematosus
Lupus renal disease NOS

M32.15 Tubulo-interstitial nephropathy in systemic lupus erythematosus

M32.19 Other organ or system involvement in systemic lupus erythematosus

M32.8 Other forms of systemic lupus erythematosus

M32.9 Systemic lupus erythematosus, unspecified
SLE NOS
Systemic lupus erythematosus NOS
Systemic lupus erythematosus without organ involvement

● **M33 Dermatopolymyositis**
● **M33.0 Juvenile dermatopolymyositis**
M33.00 Juvenile dermatopolymyositis, organ involvement unspecified

M33.01 Juvenile dermatopolymyositis with respiratory involvement

M33.02 Juvenile dermatopolymyositis with myopathy

M33.09 Juvenile dermatopolymyositis with other organ involvement

● **M33.1 Other dermatopolymyositis**
M33.10 Other dermatopolymyositis, organ involvement unspecified

M33.11 Other dermatopolymyositis with respiratory involvement

M33.12 Other dermatopolymyositis with myopathy

M33.19 Other dermatopolymyositis with other organ involvement

● **M33.2 Polymyositis**
M33.20 Polymyositis, organ involvement unspecified

M33.21 Polymyositis with respiratory involvement

M33.22 Polymyositis with myopathy

M33.29 Polymyositis with other organ involvement

Item 13–8 Polymyalgia rheumatica is a syndrome characterized by aching and morning stiffness and is related to aging and hereditary predisposition.

◀ New   ⇇ Revised   ~~deleted~~ Deleted   Excludes 1   Excludes 2   Includes   Use additional   Code first   Code also   Unspecified
OGCR Official Guidelines   X Assign placeholder X   ● Use Additional Character(s)   ▶ Manifestation Code   **Coding Clinic**

● **M33.9**   **Dermatopolymyositis, unspecified**

    M33.90   **Dermatopolymyositis, unspecified, organ involvement unspecified**

    M33.91   **Dermatopolymyositis, unspecified with respiratory involvement**

    M33.92   **Dermatopolymyositis, unspecified with myopathy**

    M33.99   **Dermatopolymyositis, unspecified with other organ involvement**

● **M34**   **Systemic sclerosis [scleroderma]**

    Excludes1   circumscribed scleroderma (L94.0)
            neonatal scleroderma (P83.8)

    M34.0   **Progressive systemic sclerosis**

    M34.1   **CR(E)ST syndrome**
         Combination of calcinosis, Raynaud's phenomenon, esophageal dysfunction, sclerodactyly, telangiectasia

    M34.2   **Systemic sclerosis induced by drug and chemical**
         Code first poisoning due to drug or toxin, if applicable (T36-T65 with fifth or sixth character 1-4 or 6)
         Use additional code for adverse effect, if applicable, to identify drug (T36-T50 with fifth or sixth character 5)

● **M34.8**   **Other forms of systemic sclerosis**

    M34.81   **Systemic sclerosis with lung involvement**

    M34.82   **Systemic sclerosis with myopathy**

    M34.83   **Systemic sclerosis with polyneuropathy**

    M34.89   **Other systemic sclerosis**

    M34.9   **Systemic sclerosis, unspecified**

● **M35**   **Other systemic involvement of connective tissue**

    Excludes1   reactive perforating collagenosis (L87.1)

● **M35.0**   **Sicca syndrome [Sjögren]**

    M35.00   **Sicca syndrome, unspecified**

    M35.01   **Sicca syndrome with keratoconjunctivitis**

    M35.02   **Sicca syndrome with lung involvement**

    M35.03   **Sicca syndrome with myopathy**

    M35.04   **Sicca syndrome with tubulo-interstitial nephropathy**
         Renal tubular acidosis in sicca syndrome

    M35.09   **Sicca syndrome with other organ involvement**

    M35.1   **Other overlap syndromes**
         Mixed connective tissue disease

         Excludes1   polyangiitis overlap syndrome (M30.8)

    M35.2   **Behçet's disease**

    M35.3   **Polymyalgia rheumatica**

         Excludes1   polymyalgia rheumatica with giant cell arteritis (M31.5)

    M35.4   **Diffuse (eosinophilic) fasciitis**

    M35.5   **Multifocal fibrosclerosis**

    M35.6   **Relapsing panniculitis [Weber-Christian]**

         Excludes1   lupus panniculitis (L93.2)
                   panniculitis NOS (M79.3-)

    M35.7   **Hypermobility syndrome**
         Familial ligamentous laxity

         Excludes1   Ehlers-Danlos syndrome (Q79.6)
                   ligamentous laxity, NOS (M24.2-)

    M35.8   **Other specified systemic involvement of connective tissue**

    M35.9   **Systemic involvement of connective tissue, unspecified**
         Autoimmune disease (systemic) NOS
         Collagen (vascular) disease NOS

● **M36**   **Systemic disorders of connective tissue in diseases classified elsewhere**

    Excludes2   arthropathies in diseases classified elsewhere (M14.-)

▷ **M36.0**   *Dermato(poly)myositis in neoplastic disease*
         Code first underlying neoplasm (C00-D49)

▷ **M36.1**   *Arthropathy in neoplastic disease*
         Code first underlying neoplasm, such as:
           leukemia (C91-C95)
           malignant histiocytosis (C96.A)
           multiple myeloma (C90.0)

▷ **M36.2**   *Hemophilic arthropathy*
         Hemarthrosis in hemophilic arthropathy

         Code first underlying disease, such as:
           factor VIII deficiency (D66)
           with vascular defect (D68.0)
           factor IX deficiency (D67)
           hemophilia (classical) (D66)
           hemophilia B (D67)
           hemophilia C (D68.1)

▷ **M36.3**   *Arthropathy in other blood disorders*

▷ **M36.4**   *Arthropathy in hypersensitivity reactions classified elsewhere*
         Code first underlying disease, such as:
           Henoch (-Schönlein) purpura (D69.0)
           serum sickness (T80.6-)

▷ **M36.8**   *Systemic disorders of connective tissue in other diseases classified elsewhere*
         Code first underlying disease, such as:
           alkaptonuria (E70.2)
           hypogammaglobulinemia (D80.-)
           ochronosis (E70.2)

DORSOPATHIES (M40-M54)

DEFORMING DORSOPATHIES (M40-M43)

● **M40**   **Kyphosis and lordosis**

    Excludes1   congenital kyphosis and lordosis (Q76.4)
            kyphoscoliosis (M41.-)
            postprocedural kyphosis and lordosis (M96.-)

● **M40.0**   **Postural kyphosis**

         Excludes1   osteochondrosis of spine (M42.-)

    M40.00   **Postural kyphosis, site unspecified**

    M40.03   **Postural kyphosis, cervicothoracic region**

    M40.04   **Postural kyphosis, thoracic region**

    M40.05   **Postural kyphosis, thoracolumbar region**

● **M40.1**   **Other secondary kyphosis**

    M40.10   **Other secondary kyphosis, site unspecified**

    M40.12   **Other secondary kyphosis, cervical region**

    M40.13   **Other secondary kyphosis, cervicothoracic region**

    M40.14   **Other secondary kyphosis, thoracic region**

    M40.15   **Other secondary kyphosis, thoracolumbar region**

● **M40.2**   **Other and unspecified kyphosis**

    ● **M40.20**   **Unspecified kyphosis**

         M40.202   **Unspecified kyphosis, cervical region**

         M40.203   **Unspecified kyphosis, cervicothoracic region**

         M40.204   **Unspecified kyphosis, thoracic region**

         M40.205   **Unspecified kyphosis, thoracolumbar region**

         M40.209   **Unspecified kyphosis, site unspecified**

CHAPTER 13 (M00-M99)

CHAPTER 13 (M00-M99)

M40.29   ICD-10-CM   M41.27

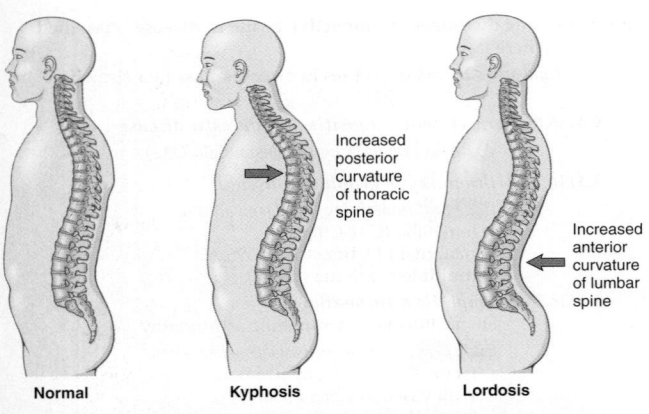

Figure 13-5 Kyphosis, Lordosis, Scoliosis. (From Chabner: The Language of Medicine, ed 8, St. Louis, Saunders, 2007)

Item 13–9 Kyphosis is an abnormal curvature of the spine. **Senile kyphosis** is a result of disc degeneration causing ossification (turning to bone). **Adolescent** or **juvenile** kyphosis is also known as **Scheuermann's disease,** a condition in which the discs of the lower thoracic spine herniate, causing the disc space to narrow and the spine to tilt forward. This condition is attributed to poor posture. Lordosis or swayback is an abnormal curvature of the spine resulting in an inward curve of the lumbar spine just above the buttocks. Scoliosis causes a sideways curve to the spine. The curves are S- or C-shaped, and it is most commonly acquired in late childhood and early teen years, when growth is fast.

- **M40.29 Other kyphosis**
  - M40.292 Other kyphosis, cervical region
  - M40.293 Other kyphosis, cervicothoracic region
  - M40.294 Other kyphosis, thoracic region
  - M40.295 Other kyphosis, thoracolumbar region
  - M40.299 Other kyphosis, site unspecified
- **M40.3 Flatback syndrome**
  - M40.30 Flatback syndrome, site unspecified
  - M40.35 Flatback syndrome, thoracolumbar region
  - M40.36 Flatback syndrome, lumbar region
  - M40.37 Flatback syndrome, lumbosacral region
- **M40.4 Postural lordosis**
  - *Abnormal increase in the normal curvature of the lumbar spine (sway back)*
  - Acquired lordosis
  - M40.40 Postural lordosis, site unspecified
  - M40.45 Postural lordosis, thoracolumbar region
  - M40.46 Postural lordosis, lumbar region
  - M40.47 Postural lordosis, lumbosacral region
- **M40.5 Lordosis, unspecified**
  - M40.50 Lordosis, unspecified, site unspecified
  - M40.55 Lordosis, unspecified, thoracolumbar region
  - M40.56 Lordosis, unspecified, lumbar region
  - M40.57 Lordosis, unspecified, lumbosacral region

- **M41 Scoliosis**
  - **Includes** kyphoscoliosis
  - **Excludes1** congenital scoliosis NOS (Q67.5)
    congenital scoliosis due to bony malformation (Q76.3)
    postural congenital scoliosis (Q67.5)
    kyphoscoliotic heart disease (I27.1)
    postprocedural scoliosis (M96.-)
- **M41.0 Infantile idiopathic scoliosis**
  - M41.00 Infantile idiopathic scoliosis, site unspecified
  - M41.02 Infantile idiopathic scoliosis, cervical region
  - M41.03 Infantile idiopathic scoliosis, cervicothoracic region
  - M41.04 Infantile idiopathic scoliosis, thoracic region
  - M41.05 Infantile idiopathic scoliosis, thoracolumbar region
  - M41.06 Infantile idiopathic scoliosis, lumbar region
  - M41.07 Infantile idiopathic scoliosis, lumbosacral region
  - M41.08 Infantile idiopathic scoliosis, sacral and sacrococcygeal region
- **M41.1 Juvenile and adolescent idiopathic scoliosis**
  - **M41.11 Juvenile idiopathic scoliosis**
    - M41.112 Juvenile idiopathic scoliosis, cervical region
    - M41.113 Juvenile idiopathic scoliosis, cervicothoracic region
    - M41.114 Juvenile idiopathic scoliosis, thoracic region
    - M41.115 Juvenile idiopathic scoliosis, thoracolumbar region
    - M41.116 Juvenile idiopathic scoliosis, lumbar region
    - M41.117 Juvenile idiopathic scoliosis, lumbosacral region
    - M41.119 Juvenile idiopathic scoliosis, site unspecified
  - **M41.12 Adolescent scoliosis**
    - M41.122 Adolescent idiopathic scoliosis, cervical region
    - M41.123 Adolescent idiopathic scoliosis, cervicothoracic region
    - M41.124 Adolescent idiopathic scoliosis, thoracic region
    - M41.125 Adolescent idiopathic scoliosis, thoracolumbar region
    - M41.126 Adolescent idiopathic scoliosis, lumbar region
    - M41.127 Adolescent idiopathic scoliosis, lumbosacral region
    - M41.129 Adolescent idiopathic scoliosis, site unspecified
- **M41.2 Other idiopathic scoliosis**
  - M41.20 Other idiopathic scoliosis, site unspecified
  - M41.22 Other idiopathic scoliosis, cervical region
  - M41.23 Other idiopathic scoliosis, cervicothoracic region
  - M41.24 Other idiopathic scoliosis, thoracic region
  - M41.25 Other idiopathic scoliosis, thoracolumbar region
  - M41.26 Other idiopathic scoliosis, lumbar region
  - M41.27 Other idiopathic scoliosis, lumbosacral region

◄ New ◄■ Revised ~~deleted~~ Deleted | Excludes 1 | Excludes 2 | Includes | Use additional | Code first | Code also | Unspecified

OGCR Official Guidelines   X Assign placeholder X   ● Use Additional Character(s)   ▶ Manifestation Code   **Coding Clinic**

1008

● **M41.3   Thoracogenic scoliosis**
     M41.30   Thoracogenic scoliosis, site unspecified
     M41.34   Thoracogenic scoliosis, thoracic region
     M41.35   Thoracogenic scoliosis, thoracolumbar region

● **M41.4   Neuromuscular scoliosis**
     Scoliosis secondary to cerebral palsy, Friedreich's ataxia, poliomyelitis and other neuromuscular disorders
     Code also underlying condition
     M41.40   Neuromuscular scoliosis, site unspecified
     M41.41   Neuromuscular scoliosis, occipito-atlanto-axial region
     M41.42   Neuromuscular scoliosis, cervical region
     M41.43   Neuromuscular scoliosis, cervicothoracic region
     M41.44   Neuromuscular scoliosis, thoracic region
     M41.45   Neuromuscular scoliosis, thoracolumbar region
     M41.46   Neuromuscular scoliosis, lumbar region
     M41.47   Neuromuscular scoliosis, lumbosacral region

● **M41.5   Other secondary scoliosis**
     M41.50   Other secondary scoliosis, site unspecified
     M41.52   Other secondary scoliosis, cervical region
     M41.53   Other secondary scoliosis, cervicothoracic region
     M41.54   Other secondary scoliosis, thoracic region
     M41.55   Other secondary scoliosis, thoracolumbar region
     M41.56   Other secondary scoliosis, lumbar region
     M41.57   Other secondary scoliosis, lumbosacral region

● **M41.8   Other forms of scoliosis**
     M41.80   Other forms of scoliosis, site unspecified
     M41.82   Other forms of scoliosis, cervical region
     M41.83   Other forms of scoliosis, cervicothoracic region
     M41.84   Other forms of scoliosis, thoracic region
     M41.85   Other forms of scoliosis, thoracolumbar region
     M41.86   Other forms of scoliosis, lumbar region
     M41.87   Other forms of scoliosis, lumbosacral region

     M41.9   Scoliosis, unspecified

● **M42   Spinal osteochondrosis**
● **M42.0   Juvenile osteochondrosis of spine**
     Calvé's disease
     Scheuermann's disease
     Excludes1   postural kyphosis (M40.0)
     M42.00   Juvenile osteochondrosis of spine, site unspecified
     M42.01   Juvenile osteochondrosis of spine, occipito-atlanto-axial region
     M42.02   Juvenile osteochondrosis of spine, cervical region
     M42.03   Juvenile osteochondrosis of spine, cervicothoracic region
     M42.04   Juvenile osteochondrosis of spine, thoracic region
     M42.05   Juvenile osteochondrosis of spine, thoracolumbar region
     M42.06   Juvenile osteochondrosis of spine, lumbar region
     M42.07   Juvenile osteochondrosis of spine, lumbosacral region
     M42.08   Juvenile osteochondrosis of spine, sacral and sacrococcygeal region
     M42.09   Juvenile osteochondrosis of spine, multiple sites in spine

● **M42.1   Adult osteochondrosis of spine**
     M42.10   Adult osteochondrosis of spine, site unspecified   A
     M42.11   Adult osteochondrosis of spine, occipitoatlanto-axial region   A
     M42.12   Adult osteochondrosis of spine, cervical region   A
     M42.13   Adult osteochondrosis of spine, cervicothoracic region   A
     M42.14   Adult osteochondrosis of spine, thoracic region   A
     M42.15   Adult osteochondrosis of spine, thoracolumbar region   A
     M42.16   Adult osteochondrosis of spine, lumbar region   A
     M42.17   Adult osteochondrosis of spine, lumbosacral region   A
     M42.18   Adult osteochondrosis of spine, sacral and sacrococcygeal region   A
     M42.19   Adult osteochondrosis of spine, multiple sites in spine   A

     M42.9   Spinal osteochondrosis, unspecified

● **M43   Other deforming dorsopathies**
     Excludes1   congenital spondylolysis and spondylolisthesis (Q76.2)
         hemivertebra (Q76.3-Q76.4)
         Klippel-Feil syndrome (Q76.1)
         lumbarization and sacralization (Q76.4)
         platyspondylisis (Q76.4)
         spina bifida occulta (Q76.0)
         spinal curvature in osteoporosis (M80.-)
         spinal curvature in Paget's disease of bone [osteitis deformans] (M88.-)

● **M43.0   Spondylolysis**
     Excludes1   congenital spondylolysis (Q76.2)
         spondylolisthesis (M43.1)
     M43.00   Spondylolysis, site unspecified
     M43.01   Spondylolysis, occipito-atlanto-axial region
     M43.02   Spondylolysis, cervical region
     M43.03   Spondylolysis, cervicothoracic region
     M43.04   Spondylolysis, thoracic region
     M43.05   Spondylolysis, thoracolumbar region
     M43.06   Spondylolysis, lumbar region
     M43.07   Spondylolysis, lumbosacral region
     M43.08   Spondylolysis, sacral and sacrococcygeal region
     M43.09   Spondylolysis, multiple sites in spine

● **M43.1   Spondylolisthesis**
     Excludes1   acute traumatic of lumbosacral region (S33.1)
         acute traumatic of sites other than lumbosacral - code to Fracture, vertebra, by region
         congenital spondylolisthesis (Q76.2)
     M43.10   Spondylolisthesis, site unspecified
     M43.11   Spondylolisthesis, occipito-atlanto-axial region
     M43.12   Spondylolisthesis, cervical region
     M43.13   Spondylolisthesis, cervicothoracic region
     M43.14   Spondylolisthesis, thoracic region
     M43.15   Spondylolisthesis, thoracolumbar region
     M43.16   Spondylolisthesis, lumbar region
     M43.17   Spondylolisthesis, lumbosacral region
     M43.18   Spondylolisthesis, sacral and sacrococcygeal region
     M43.19   Spondylolisthesis, multiple sites in spine

Item 13-10 Spondylolisthesis is a condition caused by the slipping forward of one disc over another.

CHAPTER 13 (M00-M99)

● **M43.2 Fusion of spine**
Ankylosis of spinal joint

> **Excludes1**   ankylosing spondylitis (M45.0-)
> congenital fusion of spine (Q76.4)

> **Excludes2**   arthrodesis status (Z98.1)
> pseudoarthrosis after fusion or arthrodesis (M96.0)

M43.20 Fusion of spine, site unspecified
M43.21 Fusion of spine, occipito-atlanto-axial region
M43.22 Fusion of spine, cervical region
M43.23 Fusion of spine, cervicothoracic region
M43.24 Fusion of spine, thoracic region
M43.25 Fusion of spine, thoracolumbar region
M43.26 Fusion of spine, lumbar region
M43.27 Fusion of spine, lumbosacral region
M43.28 Fusion of spine, sacral and sacrococcygeal region

M43.3 Recurrent atlantoaxial dislocation with myelopathy
M43.4 Other recurrent atlantoaxial dislocation

● **M43.5 Other recurrent vertebral dislocation**

> **Excludes1**   biomechanical lesions NEC (M99.-)

● **M43.5X Other recurrent vertebral dislocation**

M43.5X2 Other recurrent vertebral dislocation, cervical region
M43.5X3 Other recurrent vertebral dislocation, cervicothoracic region
M43.5X4 Other recurrent vertebral dislocation, thoracic region
M43.5X5 Other recurrent vertebral dislocation, thoracolumbar region
M43.5X6 Other recurrent vertebral dislocation, lumbar region
M43.5X7 Other recurrent vertebral dislocation, lumbosacral region
M43.5X8 Other recurrent vertebral dislocation, sacral and sacrococcygeal region
M43.5X9 Other recurrent vertebral dislocation, site unspecified

M43.6 Torticollis

> **Excludes1**   congenital (sternomastoid) torticollis (Q68.0)
> current injury - see Injury, of spine, by body region ocular torticollis (R29.891)
> psychogenic torticollis (F45.8)
> spasmodic torticollis (G24.3)
> torticollis due to birth injury (P15.2)

● **M43.8 Other specified deforming dorsopathies**

> **Excludes2**   kyphosis and lordosis (M40.-)
> scoliosis (M41.-)

● **M43.8X Other specified deforming dorsopathies**

M43.8X1 Other specified deforming dorsopathies, occipito-atlanto-axial region
M43.8X2 Other specified deforming dorsopathies, cervical region
M43.8X3 Other specified deforming dorsopathies, cervicothoracic region
M43.8X4 Other specified deforming dorsopathies, thoracic region
M43.8X5 Other specified deforming dorsopathies, thoracolumbar region
M43.8X6 Other specified deforming dorsopathies, lumbar region
M43.8X7 Other specified deforming dorsopathies, lumbosacral region
M43.8X8 Other specified deforming dorsopathies, sacral and sacrococcygeal region
M43.8X9 Other specified deforming dorsopathies, site unspecified

M43.9 Deforming dorsopathy, unspecified
Curvature of spine NOS

SPONDYLOPATHIES (M45-M49)

● **M45 Ankylosing spondylitis**
Rheumatoid arthritis of spine

> **Excludes1**   arthropathy in Reiter's disease (M02.3-)
> juvenile (ankylosing) spondylitis (M08.1)

> **Excludes2**   Behçet's disease (M35.2)

M45.0 Ankylosing spondylitis of multiple sites in spine
M45.1 Ankylosing spondylitis of occipito-atlanto-axial region
M45.2 Ankylosing spondylitis of cervical region
M45.3 Ankylosing spondylitis of cervicothoracic region
M45.4 Ankylosing spondylitis of thoracic region
M45.5 Ankylosing spondylitis of thoracolumbar region
M45.6 Ankylosing spondylitis lumbar region
M45.7 Ankylosing spondylitis of lumbosacral region
M45.8 Ankylosing spondylitis sacral and sacrococcygeal region
M45.9 Ankylosing spondylitis of unspecified sites in spine

● **M46 Other inflammatory spondylopathies**
● **M46.0 Spinal enthesopathy**
Disorder of ligamentous or muscular attachments of spine

M46.00 Spinal enthesopathy, site unspecified
M46.01 Spinal enthesopathy, occipito-atlanto-axial region
M46.02 Spinal enthesopathy, cervical region
M46.03 Spinal enthesopathy, cervicothoracic region
M46.04 Spinal enthesopathy, thoracic region
M46.05 Spinal enthesopathy, thoracolumbar region
M46.06 Spinal enthesopathy, lumbar region
M46.07 Spinal enthesopathy, lumbosacral region
M46.08 Spinal enthesopathy, sacral and sacrococcygeal region
M46.09 Spinal enthesopathy, multiple sites in spine

M46.1 Sacroiliitis, not elsewhere classified
● **M46.2 Osteomyelitis of vertebra**

M46.20 Osteomyelitis of vertebra, site unspecified
M46.21 Osteomyelitis of vertebra, occipito-atlanto-axial region
M46.22 Osteomyelitis of vertebra, cervical region
M46.23 Osteomyelitis of vertebra, cervicothoracic region
M46.24 Osteomyelitis of vertebra, thoracic region
M46.25 Osteomyelitis of vertebra, thoracolumbar region
M46.26 Osteomyelitis of vertebra, lumbar region
M46.27 Osteomyelitis of vertebra, lumbosacral region
M46.28 Osteomyelitis of vertebra, sacral and sacrococcygeal region

● **M46.3 Infection of intervertebral disc (pyogenic)**
      Use additional code (B95-B97) to identify infectious
      agent
   M46.30 Infection of intervertebral disc (pyogenic), site
              unspecified
   M46.31 Infection of intervertebral disc (pyogenic),
              occipito-atlanto-axial region
   M46.32 Infection of intervertebral disc (pyogenic),
              cervical region
   M46.33 Infection of intervertebral disc (pyogenic),
              cervicothoracic region
   M46.34 Infection of intervertebral disc (pyogenic),
              thoracic region
   M46.35 Infection of intervertebral disc (pyogenic),
              thoracolumbar region
   M46.36 Infection of intervertebral disc (pyogenic),
              lumbar region
   M46.37 Infection of intervertebral disc (pyogenic),
              lumbosacral region
   M46.38 Infection of intervertebral disc (pyogenic),
              sacral and sacrococcygeal region
   M46.39 Infection of intervertebral disc (pyogenic),
              multiple sites in spine
● **M46.4 Discitis, unspecified**
   M46.40 Discitis, unspecified, site unspecified
   M46.41 Discitis, unspecified, occipito-atlanto-axial
              region
   M46.42 Discitis, unspecified, cervical region
   M46.43 Discitis, unspecified, cervicothoracic region
   M46.44 Discitis, unspecified, thoracic region
   M46.45 Discitis, unspecified, thoracolumbar region
   M46.46 Discitis, unspecified, lumbar region
   M46.47 Discitis, unspecified, lumbosacral region
   M46.48 Discitis, unspecified, sacral and sacrococcygeal
              region
   M46.49 Discitis, unspecified, multiple sites in spine
● **M46.5 Other infective spondylopathies**
   M46.50 Other infective spondylopathies, site
              unspecified
   M46.51 Other infective spondylopathies,
              occipitoatlanto-axial region
   M46.52 Other infective spondylopathies, cervical
              region
   M46.53 Other infective spondylopathies,
              cervicothoracic region
   M46.54 Other infective spondylopathies, thoracic
              region
   M46.55 Other infective spondylopathies,
              thoracolumbar region
   M46.56 Other infective spondylopathies, lumbar region
   M46.57 Other infective spondylopathies, lumbosacral
              region
   M46.58 Other infective spondylopathies, sacral and
              sacrococcygeal region
   M46.59 Other infective spondylopathies, multiple sites
              in spine
● **M46.8 Other specified inflammatory spondylopathies**
   M46.80 Other specified inflammatory spondylopathies,
              site unspecified
   M46.81 Other specified inflammatory spondylopathies,
              occipito-atlanto-axial region
   M46.82 Other specified inflammatory spondylopathies,
              cervical region

   M46.83 Other specified inflammatory spondylopathies,
              cervicothoracic region
   M46.84 Other specified inflammatory spondylopathies,
              thoracic region
   M46.85 Other specified inflammatory spondylopathies,
              thoracolumbar region
   M46.86 Other specified inflammatory spondylopathies,
              lumbar region
   M46.87 Other specified inflammatory spondylopathies,
              lumbosacral region
   M46.88 Other specified inflammatory spondylopathies,
              sacral and sacrococcygeal region
   M46.89 Other specified inflammatory spondylopathies,
              multiple sites in spine
● **M46.9 Unspecified inflammatory spondylopathy**
   M46.90 Unspecified inflammatory spondylopathy, site
              unspecified
   M46.91 Unspecified inflammatory spondylopathy,
              occipito-atlanto-axial region
   M46.92 Unspecified inflammatory spondylopathy,
              cervical region
   M46.93 Unspecified inflammatory spondylopathy,
              cervicothoracic region
   M46.94 Unspecified inflammatory spondylopathy,
              thoracic region
   M46.95 Unspecified inflammatory spondylopathy,
              thoracolumbar region
   M46.96 Unspecified inflammatory spondylopathy,
              lumbar region
   M46.97 Unspecified inflammatory spondylopathy,
              lumbosacral region
   M46.98 Unspecified inflammatory spondylopathy,
              sacral and sacrococcygeal region
   M46.99 Unspecified inflammatory spondylopathy,
              multiple sites in spine
● **M47 Spondylosis**
      Includes   arthrosis or osteoarthritis of spine
                    degeneration of facet joints
   ● **M47.0 Anterior spinal and vertebral artery compression
            syndromes**
      ● **M47.01 Anterior spinal artery compression syndromes**
         M47.011 Anterior spinal artery compression
                    syndromes, occipito-atlanto-axial
                    region
         M47.012 Anterior spinal artery compression
                    syndromes, cervical region
         M47.013 Anterior spinal artery compression
                    syndromes, cervicothoracic region
         M47.014 Anterior spinal artery compression
                    syndromes, thoracic region
         M47.015 Anterior spinal artery compression
                    syndromes, thoracolumbar region
         M47.016 Anterior spinal artery compression
                    syndromes, lumbar region
         M47.019 Anterior spinal artery compression
                    syndromes, site unspecified
      ● **M47.02 Vertebral artery compression syndromes**
         M47.021 Vertebral artery compression
                    syndromes, occipito-atlanto-axial
                    region
         M47.022 Vertebral artery compression
                    syndromes, cervical region
         M47.029 Vertebral artery compression
                    syndromes, site unspecified

CHAPTER 13 (M00-M99)

CHAPTER 13 (M00-M99)

● **M47.1**   **Other spondylosis with myelopathy**
Spondylogenic compression of spinal cord
> **Excludes1**   vertebral subluxation (M43.3-M43.59)

     M47.10   Other spondylosis with myelopathy, site unspecified

     M47.11   Other spondylosis with myelopathy, occipito-atlanto-axial region

     M47.12   Other spondylosis with myelopathy, cervical region

     M47.13   Other spondylosis with myelopathy, cervicothoracic region

     M47.14   Other spondylosis with myelopathy, thoracic region

     M47.15   Other spondylosis with myelopathy, thoracolumbar region

     M47.16   Other spondylosis with myelopathy, lumbar region

● **M47.2**   **Other spondylosis with radiculopathy**

     M47.20   Other spondylosis with radiculopathy, site unspecified

     M47.21   Other spondylosis with radiculopathy, occipito-atlanto-axial region

     M47.22   Other spondylosis with radiculopathy, cervical region

     M47.23   Other spondylosis with radiculopathy, cervicothoracic region

     M47.24   Other spondylosis with radiculopathy, thoracic region

     M47.25   Other spondylosis with radiculopathy, thoracolumbar region

     M47.26   Other spondylosis with radiculopathy, lumbar region

     M47.27   Other spondylosis with radiculopathy, lumbosacral region

     M47.28   Other spondylosis with radiculopathy, sacral and sacrococcygeal region

● **M47.8**   **Other spondylosis**

 ● M47.81   Spondylosis without myelopathy or radiculopathy

     M47.811   Spondylosis without myelopathy or radiculopathy, occipito-atlanto-axial region

     M47.812   Spondylosis without myelopathy or radiculopathy, cervical region

     M47.813   Spondylosis without myelopathy or radiculopathy, cervicothoracic region

     M47.814   Spondylosis without myelopathy or radiculopathy, thoracic region

     M47.815   Spondylosis without myelopathy or radiculopathy, thoracolumbar region

     M47.816   Spondylosis without myelopathy or radiculopathy, lumbar region

     M47.817   Spondylosis without myelopathy or radiculopathy, lumbosacral region

     M47.818   Spondylosis without myelopathy or radiculopathy, sacral and sacrococcygeal region

     M47.819   Spondylosis without myelopathy or radiculopathy, site unspecified

 ● M47.89   Other spondylosis

     M47.891   Other spondylosis, occipito-atlanto-axial region

     M47.892   Other spondylosis, cervical region

     M47.893   Other spondylosis, cervicothoracic region

     M47.894   Other spondylosis, thoracic region

     M47.895   Other spondylosis, thoracolumbar region

     M47.896   Other spondylosis, lumbar region

     M47.897   Other spondylosis, lumbosacral region

     M47.898   Other spondylosis, sacral and sacrococcygeal region

     M47.899   Other spondylosis, site unspecified

   M47.9   **Spondylosis, unspecified**

● **M48**   **Other spondylopathies**

 ● **M48.0**   **Spinal stenosis**
Caudal stenosis

     M48.00   Spinal stenosis, site unspecified

     M48.01   Spinal stenosis, occipito-atlanto-axial region

     M48.02   Spinal stenosis, cervical region

     M48.03   Spinal stenosis, cervicothoracic region

     M48.04   Spinal stenosis, thoracic region

     M48.05   Spinal stenosis, thoracolumbar region

     M48.06   Spinal stenosis, lumbar region

     M48.07   Spinal stenosis, lumbosacral region

     M48.08   Spinal stenosis, sacral and sacrococcygeal region

 ● **M48.1**   **Ankylosing hyperostosis [Forestier]**
Diffuse idiopathic skeletal hyperostosis [DISH]

     M48.10   Ankylosing hyperostosis [Forestier], site unspecified

     M48.11   Ankylosing hyperostosis [Forestier], occipito-atlanto-axial region

     M48.12   Ankylosing hyperostosis [Forestier], cervical region

     M48.13   Ankylosing hyperostosis [Forestier], cervicothoracic region

     M48.14   Ankylosing hyperostosis [Forestier], thoracic region

     M48.15   Ankylosing hyperostosis [Forestier], thoracolumbar region

     M48.16   Ankylosing hyperostosis [Forestier], lumbar region

     M48.17   Ankylosing hyperostosis [Forestier], lumbosacral region

     M48.18   Ankylosing hyperostosis [Forestier], sacral and sacrococcygeal region

     M48.19   Ankylosing hyperostosis [Forestier], multiple sites in spine

 ● **M48.2**   **Kissing spine**

     M48.20   Kissing spine, site unspecified

     M48.21   Kissing spine, occipito-atlanto-axial region

     M48.22   Kissing spine, cervical region

     M48.23   Kissing spine, cervicothoracic region

     M48.24   Kissing spine, thoracic region

     M48.25   Kissing spine, thoracolumbar region

     M48.26   Kissing spine, lumbar region

     M48.27   Kissing spine, lumbosacral region

 ● **M48.3**   **Traumatic spondylopathy**

     M48.30   Traumatic spondylopathy, site unspecified

     M48.31   Traumatic spondylopathy, occipito-atlanto-axial region

     M48.32   Traumatic spondylopathy, cervical region

     M48.33   Traumatic spondylopathy, cervicothoracic region

     M48.34   Traumatic spondylopathy, thoracic region

     M48.35   Traumatic spondylopathy, thoracolumbar region

     M48.36   Traumatic spondylopathy, lumbar region

     M48.37   Traumatic spondylopathy, lumbosacral region

     M48.38   Traumatic spondylopathy, sacral and sacrococcygeal region

◀ New   ◀▥ Revised   ~~deleted~~ Deleted   Excludes 1   Excludes 2   Includes   Use additional   Code first   Code also   Unspecified

1012   OGCR Official Guidelines   X Assign placeholder X   ▷ Use Additional Character(s)   ▷ Manifestation Code   **Coding Clinic**

● **M48.4   Fatigue fracture of vertebra**
Stress fracture of vertebra

> **Excludes1**   pathological fracture NOS (M84.4-)
> pathological fracture of vertebra due to
> neoplasm (M84.58)
> pathological fracture of vertebra due to
> other diagnosis (M84.68)
> pathological fracture of vertebra due to
> osteoporosis (M80.-)
> traumatic fracture of vertebrae
> (S12.0-S12.3-, S22.0-, S32.0-)

The appropriate 7th character is to be added to each
code from subcategory M48.4:

> A   initial encounter for fracture
> D   subsequent encounter for fracture with routine
> healing
> G   subsequent encounter for fracture with
> delayed healing
> S   sequela of fracture

X● **M48.40**   Fatigue fracture of vertebra, site unspecified
X● **M48.41**   Fatigue fracture of vertebra, occipitoatlanto-
axial region
X● **M48.42**   Fatigue fracture of vertebra, cervical region
X● **M48.43**   Fatigue fracture of vertebra, cervicothoracic
region
X● **M48.44**   Fatigue fracture of vertebra, thoracic region
X● **M48.45**   Fatigue fracture of vertebra, thoracolumbar
region
X● **M48.46**   Fatigue fracture of vertebra, lumbar region
X● **M48.47**   Fatigue fracture of vertebra, lumbosacral region
X● **M48.48**   Fatigue fracture of vertebra, sacral and
sacrococcygeal region

● **M48.5   Collapsed vertebra, not elsewhere classified**
Collapsed vertebra NOS
Compression fracture of vertebra NOS ◄
Wedging of vertebra NOS

> **Excludes1**   current injury - see Injury of spine, by
> body region
> fatigue fracture of vertebra (M48.4)
> pathological fracture of vertebra due to
> neoplasm (M84.58)
> pathological fracture of vertebra due to
> other diagnosis (M84.68)
> pathological fracture of vertebra due to
> osteoporosis (M80.-)
> pathological fracture NOS (M84.4-)
> stress fracture of vertebra (M48.4-)
> traumatic fracture of vertebra (S12.-, S22.-,
> S32.-)

The appropriate 7th character is to be added to each
code from subcategory M48.5:

> A   initial encounter for fracture
> D   subsequent encounter for fracture with routine
> healing
> G   subsequent encounter for fracture with
> delayed healing
> S   sequela of fracture

X● **M48.50**   Collapsed vertebra, not elsewhere classified,
site unspecified
X● **M48.51**   Collapsed vertebra, not elsewhere classified,
occipito-atlanto-axial region
X● **M48.52**   Collapsed vertebra, not elsewhere classified,
cervical region
X● **M48.53**   Collapsed vertebra, not elsewhere classified,
cervicothoracic region
X● **M48.54**   Collapsed vertebra, not elsewhere classified,
thoracic region

X● **M48.55**   Collapsed vertebra, not elsewhere classified,
thoracolumbar region
X● **M48.56**   Collapsed vertebra, not elsewhere classified,
lumbar region
X● **M48.57**   Collapsed vertebra, not elsewhere classified,
lumbosacral region
X● **M48.58**   Collapsed vertebra, not elsewhere classified,
sacral and sacrococcygeal region

● **M48.8   Other specified spondylopathies**
Ossification of posterior longitudinal ligament

● **M48.8X   Other specified spondylopathies**

**M48.8X1   Other specified spondylopathies,
occipito-atlanto-axial region**
**M48.8X2   Other specified spondylopathies,
cervical region**
**M48.8X3   Other specified spondylopathies,
cervicothoracic region**
**M48.8X4   Other specified spondylopathies,
thoracic region**
**M48.8X5   Other specified spondylopathies,
thoracolumbar region**
**M48.8X6   Other specified spondylopathies,
lumbar region**
**M48.8X7   Other specified spondylopathies,
lumbosacral region**
**M48.8X8   Other specified spondylopathies,
sacral and sacrococcygeal region**
**M48.8X9   Other specified spondylopathies, site
unspecified**

M48.9   Spondylopathy, unspecified

● **M49   Spondylopathies in diseases classified elsewhere**

> **Includes**   curvature of spine in diseases classified elsewhere
> deformity of spine in diseases classified
> elsewhere
> kyphosis in diseases classified elsewhere
> scoliosis in diseases classified elsewhere
> spondylopathy in diseases classified elsewhere

Code first underlying disease, such as:
brucellosis (A23.-)
Charcot-Marie-Tooth disease (G60.0)
enterobacterial infections (A01-A04)
osteitis fibrosa cystica (E21.0)

> **Excludes1**   curvature of spine in tuberculosis [Pott's]
> (A18.01)
> enteropathic arthropathies (M07.-)
> gonococcal spondylitis (A54.41)
> neuropathic [tabes dorsalis] spondylitis (A52.11)
> neuropathic spondylopathy in syringomyelia
> (G95.0)
> neuropathic spondylopathy in tabes dorsalis
> (A52.11)
> nonsyphilitic neuropathic spondylopathy NEC
> (G98.0)
> spondylitis in syphilis (acquired) (A52.77)
> tuberculous spondylitis (A18.01)
> typhoid fever spondylitis (A01.05)

● **M49.8   Spondylopathy in diseases classified elsewhere**

▷ *M49.80   Spondylopathy in diseases classified elsewhere,
site unspecified*
▷ *M49.81   Spondylopathy in diseases classified elsewhere,
occipito-atlanto-axial region*
▷ *M49.82   Spondylopathy in diseases classified elsewhere,
cervical region*
▷ *M49.83   Spondylopathy in diseases classified elsewhere,
cervicothoracic region*
▷ *M49.84   Spondylopathy in diseases classified elsewhere,
thoracic region*
▷ *M49.85   Spondylopathy in diseases classified elsewhere,
thoracolumbar region*

CHAPTER 13 (M00-M99)

▸ *M49.86*   *Spondylopathy in diseases classified elsewhere, lumbar region*

▸ *M49.87*   *Spondylopathy in diseases classified elsewhere, lumbosacral region*

▸ *M49.88*   *Spondylopathy in diseases classified elsewhere, sacral and sacrococcygeal region*

▸ *M49.89*   *Spondylopathy in diseases classified elsewhere, multiple sites in spine*

OTHER DORSOPATHIES (M50-M54)

Excludes1   current injury - see injury of spine by body region
discitis NOS (M46.4-)

● **M50** **Cervical disc disorders**
  Note: Code to the most superior level of disorder.
  Includes   cervicothoracic disc disorders with cervicalgia
             cervicothoracic disc disorders
  Coding Clinic: 2016, Q1, P17

● **M50.0** **Cervical disc disorder with myelopathy**

  M50.00   **Cervical disc disorder with myelopathy, unspecified cervical region**

  M50.01   **Cervical disc disorder with myelopathy, high cervical region**
          C2-C3 disc disorder with myelopathy
          C3-C4 disc disorder with myelopathy
          Coding Clinic: 2016, Q1, P17

● **M50.02**   **Cervical disc disorder with myelopathy, mid-cervical region**

    M50.020   **Cervical disc disorder with myelopathy, mid-cervical region, unspecified level** ◀

    M50.021   **Cervical disc disorder at C4-C5 level with myelopathy** ◀
            C4-C5 disc disorder with myelopathy ◀

    M50.022   **Cervical disc disorder at C5-C6 level with myelopathy** ◀
            C5-C6 disc disorder with myelopathy ◀

    M50.023   **Cervical disc disorder at C6-C7 level with myelopathy** ◀
            C6-C7 disc disorder with myelopathy ◀

  M50.03   **Cervical disc disorder with myelopathy, cervicothoracic region**
          C7-T1 disc disorder with myelopathy

● **M50.1** **Cervical disc disorder with radiculopathy**
  Excludes2   brachial radiculitis NOS (M54.13)

  M50.10   **Cervical disc disorder with radiculopathy, unspecified cervical region**

  M50.11   **Cervical disc disorder with radiculopathy, high cervical region**
          C2-C3 disc disorder with radiculopathy
          C3 radiculopathy due to disc disorder
          C3-C4 disc disorder with radiculopathy
          C4 radiculopathy due to disc disorder

● **M50.12**   **Cervical disc disorder with radiculopathy, mid-cervical region**

    M50.120   **Mid-cervical disc disorder, unspecified** ◀

    M50.121   **Cervical disc disorder at C4-C5 level with radiculopathy** ◀
            C4-C5 disc disorder with radiculopathy ◀
            C5 radiculopathy due to disc disorder ◀

    M50.122   **Cervical disc disorder at C5-C6 level with radiculopathy** ◀
            C5-C6 disc disorder with radiculopathy ◀
            C6 radiculopathy due to disc disorder ◀

    M50.123   **Cervical disc disorder at C6-C7 level with radiculopathy** ◀
            C6-C7 disc disorder with radiculopathy ◀
            C7 radiculopathy due to disc disorder ◀

  M50.13   **Cervical disc disorder with radiculopathy, cervicothoracic region**
          C7-T1 disc disorder with radiculopathy
          C8 radiculopathy due to disc disorder

● **M50.2** **Other cervical disc displacement**

  M50.20   **Other cervical disc displacement, unspecified cervical region**

  M50.21   **Other cervical disc displacement, high cervical region**
          Other C2-C3 cervical disc displacement
          Other C3-C4 cervical disc displacement

● **M50.22**   **Other cervical disc displacement, mid-cervical region**

    M50.220   **Other cervical disc displacement, mid-cervical region, unspecified level** ◀

    M50.221   **Other cervical disc displacement at C4-C5 level** ◀
            Other C4-C5 cervical disc displacement ◀

    M50.222   **Other cervical disc displacement at C5-C6 level** ◀
            Other C5-C6 cervical disc displacement ◀

    M50.223   **Other cervical disc displacement at C6-C7 level** ◀
            Other C6-C7 cervical disc displacement ◀

  M50.23   **Other cervical disc displacement, cervicothoracic region**
          Other C7-T1 cervical disc displacement

● **M50.3** **Other cervical disc degeneration**

  M50.30   **Other cervical disc degeneration, unspecified cervical region**

  M50.31   **Other cervical disc degeneration, high cervical region**
          Other C2-C3 cervical disc degeneration
          Other C3-C4 cervical disc degeneration

● **M50.32**   **Other cervical disc degeneration, mid-cervical region**

    M50.320   **Other cervical disc degeneration, mid-cervical region, unspecified level** ◀

    M50.321   **Other cervical disc degeneration at C4-C5 level** ◀
            Other C4-C5 cervical disc degeneration ◀

    M50.322   **Other cervical disc degeneration at C5-C6 level** ◀
            Other C5-C6 cervical disc degeneration ◀

    M50.323   **Other cervical disc degeneration at C6-C7 level** ◀
            Other C6-C7 cervical disc degeneration ◀

  M50.33   **Other cervical disc degeneration, cervicothoracic region**
          Other C7-T1 cervical disc degeneration

● **M50.8** **Other cervical disc disorders**

  M50.80   **Other cervical disc disorders, unspecified cervical region**

  M50.81   **Other cervical disc disorders, high cervical region**
          Other C2-C3 cervical disc disorders
          Other C3-C4 cervical disc disorders

◀ New   ◀▥ Revised   ~~deleted~~ Deleted   Excludes 1   Excludes 2   Includes   Use additional   Code first   Code also   Unspecified

OGCR Official Guidelines   X Assign placeholder X   ● Use Additional Character(s)   ▸ Manifestation Code   **Coding Clinic**

● **M50.82** **Other cervical disc disorders, mid-cervical region**
     M50.820 **Other cervical disc disorders, mid-cervical region, unspecified level** ◄
     M50.821 **Other cervical disc disorders at C4-C5 level** ◄
        Other C4-C5 cervical disc disorders ◄
     M50.822 **Other cervical disc disorders at C5-C6 level** ◄
        Other C5-C6 cervical disc disorders ◄
     M50.823 **Other cervical disc disorders at C6-C7 level** ◄
        Other C6-C7 cervical disc disorders ◄
   M50.83 **Other cervical disc disorders, cervicothoracic region**
     Other C7-T1 cervical disc disorders

● **M50.9** **Cervical disc disorder, unspecified**
   M50.90 **Cervical disc disorder, unspecified, unspecified cervical region**
   M50.91 **Cervical disc disorder, unspecified, high cervical region**
     C2-C3 cervical disc disorder, unspecified
     C3-C4 cervical disc disorder, unspecified
● **M50.92** **Cervical disc disorder, unspecified, mid-cervical region**
     M50.920 **Unspecified cervical disc disorder, mid-cervical region, unspecified level** ◄
     M50.921 **Unspecified cervical disc disorder at C4-C5 level** ◄
        Unspecified C4-C5 cervical disc disorder ◄
     M50.922 **Unspecified cervical disc disorder at C5-C6 level** ◄
        Unspecified C5-C6 cervical disc disorder ◄
     M50.923 **Unspecified cervical disc disorder at C6-C7 level** ◄
        Unspecified C6-C7 cervical disc disorder ◄
   M50.93 **Cervical disc disorder, unspecified, cervicothoracic region**
     C7-T1 cervical disc disorder, unspecified

● **M51** **Thoracic, thoracolumbar, and lumbosacral intervertebral disc disorders**
   Excludes2   cervical and cervicothoracic disc disorders (M50.-)
             sacral and sacrococcygeal disorders (M53.3)

● **M51.0** **Thoracic, thoracolumbar and lumbosacral intervertebral disc disorders with myelopathy**
   M51.04 **Intervertebral disc disorders with myelopathy, thoracic region**
   M51.05 **Intervertebral disc disorders with myelopathy, thoracolumbar region**
   M51.06 **Intervertebral disc disorders with myelopathy, lumbar region**

● **M51.1** **Thoracic, thoracolumbar and lumbosacral intervertebral disc disorders with radiculopathy**
   Sciatica due to intervertebral disc disorder
   Excludes1   lumbar radiculitis NOS (M54.16)
             sciatica NOS (M54.3)
   M51.14 **Intervertebral disc disorders with radiculopathy, thoracic region**
   M51.15 **Intervertebral disc disorders with radiculopathy, thoracolumbar region**

   M51.16 **Intervertebral disc disorders with radiculopathy, lumbar region**
   M51.17 **Intervertebral disc disorders with radiculopathy, lumbosacral region**

● **M51.2** **Other thoracic, thoracolumbar and lumbosacral intervertebral disc displacement**
   Lumbago due to displacement of intervertebral disc
   M51.24 **Other intervertebral disc displacement, thoracic region**
   M51.25 **Other intervertebral disc displacement, thoracolumbar region**
   M51.26 **Other intervertebral disc displacement, lumbar region**
   M51.27 **Other intervertebral disc displacement, lumbosacral region**

● **M51.3** **Other thoracic, thoracolumbar and lumbosacral intervertebral disc degeneration**
   Coding Clinic: 2013, Q3, P22
   M51.34 **Other intervertebral disc degeneration, thoracic region**
   M51.35 **Other intervertebral disc degeneration, thoracolumbar region**
   M51.36 **Other intervertebral disc degeneration, lumbar region**
   M51.37 **Other intervertebral disc degeneration, lumbosacral region**

● **M51.4** **Schmorl's nodes**
   M51.44 **Schmorl's nodes, thoracic region**
   M51.45 **Schmorl's nodes, thoracolumbar region**
   M51.46 **Schmorl's nodes, lumbar region**
   M51.47 **Schmorl's nodes, lumbosacral region**

● **M51.8** **Other thoracic, thoracolumbar and lumbosacral intervertebral disc disorders**
   M51.84 **Other intervertebral disc disorders, thoracic region**
   M51.85 **Other intervertebral disc disorders, thoracolumbar region**
   M51.86 **Other intervertebral disc disorders, lumbar region**
   M51.87 **Other intervertebral disc disorders, lumbosacral region**

● **M51.9** **Unspecified thoracic, thoracolumbar and lumbosacral intervertebral disc disorder**

● **M53** **Other and unspecified dorsopathies, not elsewhere classified**
   M53.0 **Cervicocranial syndrome**
     Posterior cervical sympathetic syndrome
   M53.1 **Cervicobrachial syndrome**
     Excludes2   cervical disc disorder (M50.-)
               thoracic outlet syndrome (G54.0)

● **M53.2** **Spinal instabilities**
   ● **M53.2X** **Spinal instabilities**
     M53.2X1 **Spinal instabilities, occipito-atlanto-axial region**
     M53.2X2 **Spinal instabilities, cervical region**
     M53.2X3 **Spinal instabilities, cervicothoracic region**
     M53.2X4 **Spinal instabilities, thoracic region**
     M53.2X5 **Spinal instabilities, thoracolumbar region**
     M53.2X6 **Spinal instabilities, lumbar region**
     M53.2X7 **Spinal instabilities, lumbosacral region**
     M53.2X8 **Spinal instabilities, sacral and sacrococcygeal region**
     M53.2X9 **Spinal instabilities, site unspecified**

CHAPTER 13 (M00-M99)

CHAPTER 13 (M00-M99)

M53.3 Sacrococcygeal disorders, not elsewhere classified
    Coccygodynia
● M53.8 Other specified dorsopathies
  M53.80 Other specified dorsopathies, site unspecified
  M53.81 Other specified dorsopathies, occipito-atlanto-axial region
  M53.82 Other specified dorsopathies, cervical region
  M53.83 Other specified dorsopathies, cervicothoracic region
  M53.84 Other specified dorsopathies, thoracic region
  M53.85 Other specified dorsopathies, thoracolumbar region
  M53.86 Other specified dorsopathies, lumbar region
  M53.87 Other specified dorsopathies, lumbosacral region
  M53.88 Other specified dorsopathies, sacral and sacrococcygeal region
M53.9 Dorsopathy, unspecified

● M54 Dorsalgia
  Excludes1 psychogenic dorsalgia (F45.41)
● M54.0 Panniculitis affecting regions of neck and back
  Excludes1 lupus panniculitis (L93.2)
    panniculitis NOS (M79.3)
    relapsing [Weber-Christian] panniculitis (M35.6)
  M54.00 Panniculitis affecting regions of neck and back, site unspecified
  M54.01 Panniculitis affecting regions of neck and back, occipito-atlanto-axial region
  M54.02 Panniculitis affecting regions of neck and back, cervical region
  M54.03 Panniculitis affecting regions of neck and back, cervicothoracic region
  M54.04 Panniculitis affecting regions of neck and back, thoracic region
  M54.05 Panniculitis affecting regions of neck and back, thoracolumbar region
  M54.06 Panniculitis affecting regions of neck and back, lumbar region
  M54.07 Panniculitis affecting regions of neck and back, lumbosacral region
  M54.08 Panniculitis affecting regions of neck and back, sacral and sacrococcygeal region
  M54.09 Panniculitis affecting regions, neck and back, multiple sites in spine
● M54.1 Radiculopathy
  Brachial neuritis or radiculitis NOS
  Lumbar neuritis or radiculitis NOS
  Lumbosacral neuritis or radiculitis NOS
  Thoracic neuritis or radiculitis NOS
  Radiculitis NOS
  Excludes1 neuralgia and neuritis NOS (M79.2)
    radiculopathy with cervical disc disorder (M50.1)
    radiculopathy with lumbar and other intervertebral disc disorder (M51.1-)
    radiculopathy with spondylosis (M47.2-)
  M54.10 Radiculopathy, site unspecified
  M54.11 Radiculopathy, occipito-atlanto-axial region
  M54.12 Radiculopathy, cervical region
  M54.13 Radiculopathy, cervicothoracic region
  M54.14 Radiculopathy, thoracic region
  M54.15 Radiculopathy, thoracolumbar region
  M54.16 Radiculopathy, lumbar region
  M54.17 Radiculopathy, lumbosacral region
  M54.18 Radiculopathy, sacral and sacrococcygeal region

M54.2 Cervicalgia
  Excludes1 cervicalgia due to intervertebral cervical disc disorder (M50.-)
● M54.3 Sciatica
  Excludes1 lesion of sciatic nerve (G57.0)
    sciatica due to intervertebral disc disorder (M51.1-)
    sciatica with lumbago (M54.4-)
  M54.30 Sciatica, unspecified side
  M54.31 Sciatica, right side
  M54.32 Sciatica, left side
● M54.4 Lumbago with sciatica
  Excludes1 lumbago with sciatica due to intervertebral disc disorder (M51.1-)
  M54.40 Lumbago with sciatica, unspecified side
  M54.41 Lumbago with sciatica, right side
  M54.42 Lumbago with sciatica, left side
    Coding Clinic: 2016, Q2, P7
M54.5 Low back pain
  Loin pain
  Lumbago NOS
  Excludes1 low back strain (S39.012)
    lumbago due to intervertebral disc displacement (M51.2-)
    lumbago with sciatica (M54.4-)
M54.6 Pain in thoracic spine
  Excludes1 pain in thoracic spine due to intervertebral disc disorder (M51.)
● M54.8 Other dorsalgia
  Excludes1 dorsalgia in thoracic region (M54.6)
    low back pain (M54.5)
  M54.81 Occipital neuralgia
  M54.89 Other dorsalgia
M54.9 Dorsalgia, unspecified
  Backache NOS
  Back pain NOS

SOFT TISSUE DISORDERS (M60-M79)

DISORDERS OF MUSCLES (M60-M63)

Excludes1 dermatopolymyositis (M33.-)
  muscular dystrophies and myopathies (G71-G72)
  myopathy in amyloidosis (E85.-)
  myopathy in polyarteritis nodosa (M30.0)
  myopathy in rheumatoid arthritis (M05.32)
  myopathy in scleroderma (M34.-)
  myopathy in Sjögren's syndrome (M35.03)
  myopathy in systemic lupus erythematosus (M32.-)

● M60 Myositis
  Excludes2 inclusion body myositis [IBM] (G72.41)
● M60.0 Infective myositis
  Tropical pyomyositis
  Use additional code (B95-B97) to identify infectious agent
  ● M60.00 Infective myositis, unspecified site
    M60.000 Infective myositis, unspecified right arm
      Infective myositis, right upper limb NOS
    M60.001 Infective myositis, unspecified left arm
      Infective myositis, left upper limb NOS
    M60.002 Infective myositis, unspecified arm
      Infective myositis, upper limb NOS

◀ New ◀ Revised ~~deleted~~ Deleted Excludes 1 Excludes 2 Includes Use additional Code first Code also Unspecified
OGCR Official Guidelines X Assign placeholder X ● Use Additional Character(s) ▶ Manifestation Code **Coding Clinic**

M60.003　Infective myositis, unspecified right leg
　　　　Infective myositis, right lower limb NOS
M60.004　Infective myositis, unspecified left leg
　　　　Infective myositis, left lower limb NOS
M60.005　Infective myositis, unspecified leg
　　　　Infective myositis, lower limb NOS
M60.009　Infective myositis, unspecified site
● M60.01　Infective myositis, shoulder
M60.011　Infective myositis, right shoulder
M60.012　Infective myositis, left shoulder
M60.019　Infective myositis, unspecified shoulder
● M60.02　Infective myositis, upper arm
M60.021　Infective myositis, right upper arm
M60.022　Infective myositis, left upper arm
M60.029　Infective myositis, unspecified upper arm
● M60.03　Infective myositis, forearm
M60.031　Infective myositis, right forearm
M60.032　Infective myositis, left forearm
M60.039　Infective myositis, unspecified forearm
● M60.04　Infective myositis, hand and fingers
M60.041　Infective myositis, right hand
M60.042　Infective myositis, left hand
M60.043　Infective myositis, unspecified hand
M60.044　Infective myositis, right finger(s)
M60.045　Infective myositis, left finger(s)
M60.046　Infective myositis, unspecified finger(s)
● M60.05　Infective myositis, thigh
M60.051　Infective myositis, right thigh
M60.052　Infective myositis, left thigh
M60.059　Infective myositis, unspecified thigh
● M60.06　Infective myositis, lower leg
M60.061　Infective myositis, right lower leg
M60.062　Infective myositis, left lower leg
M60.069　Infective myositis, unspecified lower leg
● M60.07　Infective myositis, ankle, foot and toes
M60.070　Infective myositis, right ankle
M60.071　Infective myositis, left ankle
M60.072　Infective myositis, unspecified ankle
M60.073　Infective myositis, right foot
M60.074　Infective myositis, left foot
M60.075　Infective myositis, unspecified foot
M60.076　Infective myositis, right toe(s)
M60.077　Infective myositis, left toe(s)
M60.078　Infective myositis, unspecified toe(s)
M60.08　Infective myositis, other site
M60.09　Infective myositis, multiple sites
● M60.1　Interstitial myositis
M60.10　Interstitial myositis of unspecified site
● M60.11　Interstitial myositis, shoulder
M60.111　Interstitial myositis, right shoulder
M60.112　Interstitial myositis, left shoulder
M60.119　Interstitial myositis, unspecified shoulder

● M60.12　Interstitial myositis, upper arm
M60.121　Interstitial myositis, right upper arm
M60.122　Interstitial myositis, left upper arm
M60.129　Interstitial myositis, unspecified upper arm
● M60.13　Interstitial myositis, forearm
M60.131　Interstitial myositis, right forearm
M60.132　Interstitial myositis, left forearm
M60.139　Interstitial myositis, unspecified forearm
● M60.14　Interstitial myositis, hand
M60.141　Interstitial myositis, right hand
M60.142　Interstitial myositis, left hand
M60.149　Interstitial myositis, unspecified hand
● M60.15　Interstitial myositis, thigh
M60.151　Interstitial myositis, right thigh
M60.152　Interstitial myositis, left thigh
M60.159　Interstitial myositis, unspecified thigh
● M60.16　Interstitial myositis, lower leg
M60.161　Interstitial myositis, right lower leg
M60.162　Interstitial myositis, left lower leg
M60.169　Interstitial myositis, unspecified lower leg
● M60.17　Interstitial myositis, ankle and foot
M60.171　Interstitial myositis, right ankle and foot
M60.172　Interstitial myositis, left ankle and foot
M60.179　Interstitial myositis, unspecified ankle and foot
M60.18　Interstitial myositis, other site
M60.19　Interstitial myositis, multiple sites
● M60.2　Foreign body granuloma of soft tissue, not elsewhere classified
　　　Use additional code to identify the type of retained foreign body (Z18.-)
　　　Excludes1　foreign body granuloma of skin and subcutaneous tissue (L92.3)
M60.20　Foreign body granuloma of soft tissue, not elsewhere classified, unspecified site
● M60.21　Foreign body granuloma of soft tissue, not elsewhere classified, shoulder
M60.211　Foreign body granuloma of soft tissue, not elsewhere classified, right shoulder
M60.212　Foreign body granuloma of soft tissue, not elsewhere classified, left shoulder
M60.219　Foreign body granuloma of soft tissue, not elsewhere classified, unspecified shoulder
● M60.22　Foreign body granuloma of soft tissue, not elsewhere classified, upper arm
M60.221　Foreign body granuloma of soft tissue, not elsewhere classified, right upper arm
M60.222　Foreign body granuloma of soft tissue, not elsewhere classified, left upper arm
M60.229　Foreign body granuloma of soft tissue, not elsewhere classified, unspecified upper arm

● M60.23   Foreign body granuloma of soft tissue, not elsewhere classified, forearm

    M60.231   Foreign body granuloma of soft tissue, not elsewhere classified, right forearm

    M60.232   Foreign body granuloma of soft tissue, not elsewhere classified, left forearm

    M60.239   Foreign body granuloma of soft tissue, not elsewhere classified, unspecified forearm

● M60.24   Foreign body granuloma of soft tissue, not elsewhere classified, hand

    M60.241   Foreign body granuloma of soft tissue, not elsewhere classified, right hand

    M60.242   Foreign body granuloma of soft tissue, not elsewhere classified, left hand

    M60.249   Foreign body granuloma of soft tissue, not elsewhere classified, unspecified hand

● M60.25   Foreign body granuloma of soft tissue, not elsewhere classified, thigh

    M60.251   Foreign body granuloma of soft tissue, not elsewhere classified, right thigh

    M60.252   Foreign body granuloma of soft tissue, not elsewhere classified, left thigh

    M60.259   Foreign body granuloma of soft tissue, not elsewhere classified, unspecified thigh

● M60.26   Foreign body granuloma of soft tissue, not elsewhere classified, lower leg

    M60.261   Foreign body granuloma of soft tissue, not elsewhere classified, right lower leg

    M60.262   Foreign body granuloma of soft tissue, not elsewhere classified, left lower leg

    M60.269   Foreign body granuloma of soft tissue, not elsewhere classified, unspecified lower leg

● M60.27   Foreign body granuloma of soft tissue, not elsewhere classified, ankle and foot

    M60.271   Foreign body granuloma of soft tissue, not elsewhere classified, right ankle and foot

    M60.272   Foreign body granuloma of soft tissue, not elsewhere classified, left ankle and foot

    M60.279   Foreign body granuloma of soft tissue, not elsewhere classified, unspecified ankle and foot

    M60.28   Foreign body granuloma of soft tissue, not elsewhere classified, other site

● M60.8   Other myositis

    M60.80   Other myositis, unspecified site

● M60.81   Other myositis shoulder

    M60.811   Other myositis, right shoulder

    M60.812   Other myositis, left shoulder

    M60.819   Other myositis, unspecified shoulder

● M60.82   Other myositis, upper arm

    M60.821   Other myositis, right upper arm

    M60.822   Other myositis, left upper arm

    M60.829   Other myositis, unspecified upper arm

● M60.83   Other myositis, forearm

    M60.831   Other myositis, right forearm

    M60.832   Other myositis, left forearm

    M60.839   Other myositis, unspecified forearm

● M60.84   Other myositis, hand

    M60.841   Other myositis, right hand

    M60.842   Other myositis, left hand

    M60.849   Other myositis, unspecified hand

● M60.85   Other myositis, thigh

    M60.851   Other myositis, right thigh

    M60.852   Other myositis, left thigh

    M60.859   Other myositis, unspecified thigh

● M60.86   Other myositis, lower leg

    M60.861   Other myositis, right lower leg

    M60.862   Other myositis, left lower leg

    M60.869   Other myositis, unspecified lower leg

● M60.87   Other myositis, ankle and foot

    M60.871   Other myositis, right ankle and foot

    M60.872   Other myositis, left ankle and foot

    M60.879   Other myositis, unspecified ankle and foot

    M60.88   Other myositis, other site

    M60.89   Other myositis, multiple sites

   M60.9   Myositis, unspecified

● M61   Calcification and ossification of muscle

   ● M61.0   Myositis ossificans traumatica

    M61.00   Myositis ossificans traumatica, unspecified site

   ● M61.01   Myositis ossificans traumatica, shoulder

    M61.011   Myositis ossificans traumatica, right shoulder

    M61.012   Myositis ossificans traumatica, left shoulder

    M61.019   Myositis ossificans traumatica, unspecified shoulder

   ● M61.02   Myositis ossificans traumatica, upper arm

    M61.021   Myositis ossificans traumatica, right upper arm

    M61.022   Myositis ossificans traumatica, left upper arm

    M61.029   Myositis ossificans traumatica, unspecified upper arm

   ● M61.03   Myositis ossificans traumatica, forearm

    M61.031   Myositis ossificans traumatica, right forearm

    M61.032   Myositis ossificans traumatica, left forearm

    M61.039   Myositis ossificans traumatica, unspecified forearm

   ● M61.04   Myositis ossificans traumatica, hand

    M61.041   Myositis ossificans traumatica, right hand

    M61.042   Myositis ossificans traumatica, left hand

    M61.049   Myositis ossificans traumatica, unspecified hand

   ● M61.05   Myositis ossificans traumatica, thigh

    M61.051   Myositis ossificans traumatica, right thigh

    M61.052   Myositis ossificans traumatica, left thigh

    M61.059   Myositis ossificans traumatica, unspecified thigh

● **M61.06** Myositis ossificans traumatica, lower leg
     M61.061 Myositis ossificans traumatica, right lower leg
     M61.062 Myositis ossificans traumatica, left lower leg
     M61.069 Myositis ossificans traumatica, unspecified lower leg
● **M61.07** Myositis ossificans traumatica, ankle and foot
     M61.071 Myositis ossificans traumatica, right ankle and foot
     M61.072 Myositis ossificans traumatica, left ankle and foot
     M61.079 Myositis ossificans traumatica, unspecified ankle and foot
     M61.08 Myositis ossificans traumatica, other site
     M61.09 Myositis ossificans traumatica, multiple sites
● **M61.1** Myositis ossificans progressiva
     Fibrodysplasia ossificans progressiva
     M61.10 Myositis ossificans progressiva, unspecified site
● **M61.11** Myositis ossificans progressiva, shoulder
     M61.111 Myositis ossificans progressiva, right shoulder
     M61.112 Myositis ossificans progressiva, left shoulder
     M61.119 Myositis ossificans progressiva, unspecified shoulder
● **M61.12** Myositis ossificans progressiva, upper arm
     M61.121 Myositis ossificans progressiva, right upper arm
     M61.122 Myositis ossificans progressiva, left upper arm
     M61.129 Myositis ossificans progressiva, unspecified arm
● **M61.13** Myositis ossificans progressiva, forearm
     M61.131 Myositis ossificans progressiva, right forearm
     M61.132 Myositis ossificans progressiva, left forearm
     M61.139 Myositis ossificans progressiva, unspecified forearm
● **M61.14** Myositis ossificans progressiva, hand and finger(s)
     M61.141 Myositis ossificans progressiva, right hand
     M61.142 Myositis ossificans progressiva, left hand
     M61.143 Myositis ossificans progressiva, unspecified hand
     M61.144 Myositis ossificans progressiva, right finger(s)
     M61.145 Myositis ossificans progressiva, left finger(s)
     M61.146 Myositis ossificans progressiva, unspecified finger(s)
● **M61.15** Myositis ossificans progressiva, thigh
     M61.151 Myositis ossificans progressiva, right thigh
     M61.152 Myositis ossificans progressiva, left thigh
     M61.159 Myositis ossificans progressiva, unspecified thigh
● **M61.16** Myositis ossificans progressiva, lower leg
     M61.161 Myositis ossificans progressiva, right lower leg
     M61.162 Myositis ossificans progressiva, left lower leg
     M61.169 Myositis ossificans progressiva, unspecified lower leg

● **M61.17** Myositis ossificans progressiva, ankle, foot and toe(s)
     M61.171 Myositis ossificans progressiva, right ankle
     M61.172 Myositis ossificans progressiva, left ankle
     M61.173 Myositis ossificans progressiva, unspecified ankle
     M61.174 Myositis ossificans progressiva, right foot
     M61.175 Myositis ossificans progressiva, left foot
     M61.176 Myositis ossificans progressiva, unspecified foot
     M61.177 Myositis ossificans progressiva, right toe(s)
     M61.178 Myositis ossificans progressiva, left toe(s)
     M61.179 Myositis ossificans progressiva, unspecified toe(s)
     M61.18 Myositis ossificans progressiva, other site
     M61.19 Myositis ossificans progressiva, multiple sites
● **M61.2** Paralytic calcification and ossification of muscle
     Myositis ossificans associated with quadriplegia or paraplegia
     M61.20 Paralytic calcification and ossification of muscle, unspecified site
● **M61.21** Paralytic calcification and ossification of muscle, shoulder
     M61.211 Paralytic calcification and ossification of muscle, right shoulder
     M61.212 Paralytic calcification and ossification of muscle, left shoulder
     M61.219 Paralytic calcification and ossification of muscle, unspecified shoulder
● **M61.22** Paralytic calcification and ossification of muscle, upper arm
     M61.221 Paralytic calcification and ossification of muscle, right upper arm
     M61.222 Paralytic calcification and ossification of muscle, left upper arm
     M61.229 Paralytic calcification and ossification of muscle, unspecified upper arm
● **M61.23** Paralytic calcification and ossification of muscle, forearm
     M61.231 Paralytic calcification and ossification of muscle, right forearm
     M61.232 Paralytic calcification and ossification of muscle, left forearm
     M61.239 Paralytic calcification and ossification of muscle, unspecified forearm
● **M61.24** Paralytic calcification and ossification of muscle, hand
     M61.241 Paralytic calcification and ossification of muscle, right hand
     M61.242 Paralytic calcification and ossification of muscle, left hand
     M61.249 Paralytic calcification and ossification of muscle, unspecified hand
● **M61.25** Paralytic calcification and ossification of muscle, thigh
     M61.251 Paralytic calcification and ossification of muscle, right thigh
     M61.252 Paralytic calcification and ossification of muscle, left thigh
     M61.259 Paralytic calcification and ossification of muscle, unspecified thigh

CHAPTER 13 (M00-M99)

M61.26 Paralytic calcification and ossification of muscle, lower leg
- M61.261 Paralytic calcification and ossification of muscle, right lower leg
- M61.262 Paralytic calcification and ossification of muscle, left lower leg
- M61.269 Paralytic calcification and ossification of muscle, unspecified lower leg

M61.27 Paralytic calcification and ossification of muscle, ankle and foot
- M61.271 Paralytic calcification and ossification of muscle, right ankle and foot
- M61.272 Paralytic calcification and ossification of muscle, left ankle and foot
- M61.279 Paralytic calcification and ossification of muscle, unspecified ankle and foot

M61.28 Paralytic calcification and ossification of muscle, other site

M61.29 Paralytic calcification and ossification of muscle, multiple sites

M61.3 Calcification and ossification of muscles associated with burns
Myositis ossificans associated with burns

M61.30 Calcification and ossification of muscles associated with burns, unspecified site

M61.31 Calcification and ossification of muscles associated with burns, shoulder
- M61.311 Calcification and ossification of muscles associated with burns, right shoulder
- M61.312 Calcification and ossification of muscles associated with burns, left shoulder
- M61.319 Calcification and ossification of muscles associated with burns, unspecified shoulder

M61.32 Calcification and ossification of muscles associated with burns, upper arm
- M61.321 Calcification and ossification of muscles associated with burns, right upper arm
- M61.322 Calcification and ossification of muscles associated with burns, left upper arm
- M61.329 Calcification and ossification of muscles associated with burns, unspecified upper arm

M61.33 Calcification and ossification of muscles associated with burns, forearm
- M61.331 Calcification and ossification of muscles associated with burns, right forearm
- M61.332 Calcification and ossification of muscles associated with burns, left forearm
- M61.339 Calcification and ossification of muscles associated with burns, unspecified forearm

M61.34 Calcification and ossification of muscles associated with burns, hand
- M61.341 Calcification and ossification of muscles associated with burns, right hand
- M61.342 Calcification and ossification of muscles associated with burns, left hand
- M61.349 Calcification and ossification of muscles associated with burns, unspecified hand

M61.35 Calcification and ossification of muscles associated with burns, thigh
- M61.351 Calcification and ossification of muscles associated with burns, right thigh
- M61.352 Calcification and ossification of muscles associated with burns, left thigh
- M61.359 Calcification and ossification of muscles associated with burns, unspecified thigh

M61.36 Calcification and ossification of muscles associated with burns, lower leg
- M61.361 Calcification and ossification of muscles associated with burns, right lower leg
- M61.362 Calcification and ossification of muscles associated with burns, left lower leg
- M61.369 Calcification and ossification of muscles associated with burns, unspecified lower leg

M61.37 Calcification and ossification of muscles associated with burns, ankle and foot
- M61.371 Calcification and ossification of muscles associated with burns, right ankle and foot
- M61.372 Calcification and ossification of muscles associated with burns, left ankle and foot
- M61.379 Calcification and ossification of muscles associated with burns, unspecified ankle and foot

M61.38 Calcification and ossification of muscles associated with burns, other site

M61.39 Calcification and ossification of muscles associated with burns, multiple sites

M61.4 Other calcification of muscle
Excludes1: calcific tendinitis NOS (M65.2-)
calcific tendinitis of shoulder (M75.3)

M61.40 Other calcification of muscle, unspecified site

M61.41 Other calcification of muscle, shoulder
- M61.411 Other calcification of muscle, right shoulder
- M61.412 Other calcification of muscle, left shoulder
- M61.419 Other calcification of muscle, unspecified shoulder

M61.42 Other calcification of muscle, upper arm
- M61.421 Other calcification of muscle, right upper arm
- M61.422 Other calcification of muscle, left upper arm
- M61.429 Other calcification of muscle, unspecified upper arm

M61.43 Other calcification of muscle, forearm
- M61.431 Other calcification of muscle, right forearm
- M61.432 Other calcification of muscle, left forearm
- M61.439 Other calcification of muscle, unspecified forearm

M61.44 Other calcification of muscle, hand
- M61.441 Other calcification of muscle, right hand
- M61.442 Other calcification of muscle, left hand
- M61.449 Other calcification of muscle, unspecified hand

●M61.45   Other calcification of muscle, thigh
     M61.451   Other calcification of muscle, right thigh
     M61.452   Other calcification of muscle, left thigh
     M61.459   Other calcification of muscle, unspecified thigh

●M61.46   Other calcification of muscle, lower leg
     M61.461   Other calcification of muscle, right lower leg
     M61.462   Other calcification of muscle, left lower leg
     M61.469   Other calcification of muscle, unspecified lower leg

●M61.47   Other calcification of muscle, ankle and foot
     M61.471   Other calcification of muscle, right ankle and foot
     M61.472   Other calcification of muscle, left ankle and foot
     M61.479   Other calcification of muscle, unspecified ankle and foot

     M61.48   Other calcification of muscle, other site
     M61.49   Other calcification of muscle, multiple sites

●M61.5   Other ossification of muscle
     M61.50   Other ossification of muscle, unspecified site
●M61.51   Other ossification of muscle, shoulder
     M61.511   Other ossification of muscle, right shoulder
     M61.512   Other ossification of muscle, left shoulder
     M61.519   Other ossification of muscle, unspecified shoulder

●M61.52   Other ossification of muscle, upper arm
     M61.521   Other ossification of muscle, right upper arm
     M61.522   Other ossification of muscle, left upper arm
     M61.529   Other ossification of muscle, unspecified upper arm

●M61.53   Other ossification of muscle, forearm
     M61.531   Other ossification of muscle, right forearm
     M61.532   Other ossification of muscle, left forearm
     M61.539   Other ossification of muscle, unspecified forearm

●M61.54   Other ossification of muscle, hand
     M61.541   Other ossification of muscle, right hand
     M61.542   Other ossification of muscle, left hand
     M61.549   Other ossification of muscle, unspecified hand

●M61.55   Other ossification of muscle, thigh
     M61.551   Other ossification of muscle, right thigh
     M61.552   Other ossification of muscle, left thigh
     M61.559   Other ossification of muscle, unspecified thigh

●M61.56   Other ossification of muscle, lower leg
     M61.561   Other ossification of muscle, right lower leg
     M61.562   Other ossification of muscle, left lower leg
     M61.569   Other ossification of muscle, unspecified lower leg

●M61.57   Other ossification of muscle, ankle and foot
     M61.571   Other ossification of muscle, right ankle and foot
     M61.572   Other ossification of muscle, left ankle and foot
     M61.579   Other ossification of muscle, unspecified ankle and foot

     M61.58   Other ossification of muscle, other site
     M61.59   Other ossification of muscle, multiple sites

   M61.9   Calcification and ossification of muscle, unspecified

●M62   **Other disorders of muscle**
     Excludes1   alcoholic myopathy (G72.1)
              cramp and spasm (R25.2)
              drug-induced myopathy (G72.0)
              myalgia (M79.1)
              stiff-man syndrome (G25.82)
     Excludes2   nontraumatic hematoma of muscle (M79.81)

●M62.0   Separation of muscle (nontraumatic)
       Diastasis of muscle
     Excludes1   diastasis recti complicating pregnancy, labor and delivery (O71.8)
              traumatic separation of muscle - see strain of muscle by body region

     M62.00   Separation of muscle (nontraumatic), unspecified site
●M62.01   Separation of muscle (nontraumatic), shoulder
     M62.011   Separation of muscle (nontraumatic), right shoulder
     M62.012   Separation of muscle (nontraumatic), left shoulder
     M62.019   Separation of muscle (nontraumatic), unspecified shoulder

●M62.02   Separation of muscle (nontraumatic), upper arm
     M62.021   Separation of muscle (nontraumatic), right upper arm
     M62.022   Separation of muscle (nontraumatic), left upper arm
     M62.029   Separation of muscle (nontraumatic), unspecified upper arm

●M62.03   Separation of muscle (nontraumatic), forearm
     M62.031   Separation of muscle (nontraumatic), right forearm
     M62.032   Separation of muscle (nontraumatic), left forearm
     M62.039   Separation of muscle (nontraumatic), unspecified forearm

●M62.04   Separation of muscle (nontraumatic), hand
     M62.041   Separation of muscle (nontraumatic), right hand
     M62.042   Separation of muscle (nontraumatic), left hand
     M62.049   Separation of muscle (nontraumatic), unspecified hand

●M62.05   Separation of muscle (nontraumatic), thigh
     M62.051   Separation of muscle (nontraumatic), right thigh
     M62.052   Separation of muscle (nontraumatic), left thigh
     M62.059   Separation of muscle (nontraumatic), unspecified thigh

●M62.06   Separation of muscle (nontraumatic), lower leg
     M62.061   Separation of muscle (nontraumatic), right lower leg
     M62.062   Separation of muscle (nontraumatic), left lower leg
     M62.069   Separation of muscle (nontraumatic), unspecified lower leg

CHAPTER 13 (M00-M99)

● **M62.07** Separation of muscle (nontraumatic), ankle and foot
   M62.071 Separation of muscle (nontraumatic), right ankle and foot
   M62.072 Separation of muscle (nontraumatic), left ankle and foot
   M62.079 Separation of muscle (nontraumatic), unspecified ankle and foot
  M62.08 Separation of muscle (nontraumatic), other site
● **M62.1** Other rupture of muscle (nontraumatic)
  Excludes1 traumatic rupture of muscle - see strain of muscle by body region
  Excludes2 rupture of tendon (M66.-)
  M62.10 Other rupture of muscle (nontraumatic), unspecified site
● **M62.11** Other rupture of muscle (nontraumatic), shoulder
   M62.111 Other rupture of muscle (nontraumatic), right shoulder
   M62.112 Other rupture of muscle (nontraumatic), left shoulder
   M62.119 Other rupture of muscle (nontraumatic), unspecified shoulder
● **M62.12** Other rupture of muscle (nontraumatic), upper arm
   M62.121 Other rupture of muscle (nontraumatic), right upper arm
   M62.122 Other rupture of muscle (nontraumatic), left upper arm
   M62.129 Other rupture of muscle (nontraumatic), unspecified upper arm
● **M62.13** Other rupture of muscle (nontraumatic), forearm
   M62.131 Other rupture of muscle (nontraumatic), right forearm
   M62.132 Other rupture of muscle (nontraumatic), left forearm
   M62.139 Other rupture of muscle (nontraumatic), unspecified forearm
● **M62.14** Other rupture of muscle (nontraumatic), hand
   M62.141 Other rupture of muscle (nontraumatic), right hand
   M62.142 Other rupture of muscle (nontraumatic), left hand
   M62.149 Other rupture of muscle (nontraumatic), unspecified hand
● **M62.15** Other rupture of muscle (nontraumatic), thigh
   M62.151 Other rupture of muscle (nontraumatic), right thigh
   M62.152 Other rupture of muscle (nontraumatic), left thigh
   M62.159 Other rupture of muscle (nontraumatic), unspecified thigh
● **M62.16** Other rupture of muscle (nontraumatic), lower leg
   M62.161 Other rupture of muscle (nontraumatic), right lower leg
   M62.162 Other rupture of muscle (nontraumatic), left lower leg
   M62.169 Other rupture of muscle (nontraumatic), unspecified lower leg

● **M62.17** Other rupture of muscle (nontraumatic), ankle and foot
   M62.171 Other rupture of muscle (nontraumatic), right ankle and foot
   M62.172 Other rupture of muscle (nontraumatic), left ankle and foot
   M62.179 Other rupture of muscle (nontraumatic), unspecified ankle and foot
  M62.18 Other rupture of muscle (nontraumatic), other site
● **M62.2** Nontraumatic ischemic infarction of muscle
  Excludes1 compartment syndrome (traumatic) (T79.A-)
    nontraumatic compartment syndrome (M79.A-)
    traumatic ischemia of muscle (T79.6)
    rhabdomyolysis (M62.82)
    Volkmann's ischemic contracture (T79.6)
  M62.20 Nontraumatic ischemic infarction of muscle, unspecified site
● **M62.21** Nontraumatic ischemic infarction of muscle, shoulder
   M62.211 Nontraumatic ischemic infarction of muscle, right shoulder
   M62.212 Nontraumatic ischemic infarction of muscle, left shoulder
   M62.219 Nontraumatic ischemic infarction of muscle, unspecified shoulder
● **M62.22** Nontraumatic ischemic infarction of muscle, upper arm
   M62.221 Nontraumatic ischemic infarction of muscle, right upper arm
   M62.222 Nontraumatic ischemic infarction of muscle, left upper arm
   M62.229 Nontraumatic ischemic infarction of muscle, unspecified upper arm
● **M62.23** Nontraumatic ischemic infarction of muscle, forearm
   M62.231 Nontraumatic ischemic infarction of muscle, right forearm
   M62.232 Nontraumatic ischemic infarction of muscle, left forearm
   M62.239 Nontraumatic ischemic infarction of muscle, unspecified forearm
● **M62.24** Nontraumatic ischemic infarction of muscle, hand
   M62.241 Nontraumatic ischemic infarction of muscle, right hand
   M62.242 Nontraumatic ischemic infarction of muscle, left hand
   M62.249 Nontraumatic ischemic infarction of muscle, unspecified hand
● **M62.25** Nontraumatic ischemic infarction of muscle, thigh
   M62.251 Nontraumatic ischemic infarction of muscle, right thigh
   M62.252 Nontraumatic ischemic infarction of muscle, left thigh
   M62.259 Nontraumatic ischemic infarction of muscle, unspecified thigh

◄ New   ◀ Revised   ~~deleted~~ Deleted   Excludes 1   Excludes 2   Includes   Use additional   Code first   Code also   Unspecified
OGCR Official Guidelines   X Assign placeholder X   ● Use Additional Character(s)   ▶ Manifestation Code   **Coding Clinic**

● M62.26   Nontraumatic ischemic infarction of muscle, lower leg

     M62.261   Nontraumatic ischemic infarction of muscle, right lower leg

     M62.262   Nontraumatic ischemic infarction of muscle, left lower leg

     M62.269   Nontraumatic ischemic infarction of muscle, unspecified lower leg

● M62.27   Nontraumatic ischemic infarction of muscle, ankle and foot

     M62.271   Nontraumatic ischemic infarction of muscle, right ankle and foot

     M62.272   Nontraumatic ischemic infarction of muscle, left ankle and foot

     M62.279   Nontraumatic ischemic infarction of muscle, unspecified ankle and foot

     M62.28   Nontraumatic ischemic infarction of muscle, other site

M62.3   Immobility syndrome (paraplegic)

M62.4   Contracture of muscle

CONTRACTURE OF TENDON (SHEATH)

Excludes1   contracture of joint (M24.5-)

     M62.40   Contracture of muscle, unspecified site

● M62.41   Contracture of muscle, shoulder

     M62.411   Contracture of muscle, right shoulder

     M62.412   Contracture of muscle, left shoulder

     M62.419   Contracture of muscle, unspecified shoulder

● M62.42   Contracture of muscle, upper arm

     M62.421   Contracture of muscle, right upper arm

     M62.422   Contracture of muscle, left upper arm

     M62.429   Contracture of muscle, unspecified upper arm

● M62.43   Contracture of muscle, forearm

     M62.431   Contracture of muscle, right forearm

     M62.432   Contracture of muscle, left forearm

     M62.439   Contracture of muscle, unspecified forearm

● M62.44   Contracture of muscle, hand

     M62.441   Contracture of muscle, right hand

     M62.442   Contracture of muscle, left hand

     M62.449   Contracture of muscle, unspecified hand

● M62.45   Contracture of muscle, thigh

     M62.451   Contracture of muscle, right thigh

     M62.452   Contracture of muscle, left thigh

     M62.459   Contracture of muscle, unspecified thigh

● M62.46   Contracture of muscle, lower leg

     M62.461   Contracture of muscle, right lower leg

     M62.462   Contracture of muscle, left lower leg

     M62.469   Contracture of muscle, unspecified lower leg

● M62.47   Contracture of muscle, ankle and foot

     M62.471   Contracture of muscle, right ankle and foot

     M62.472   Contracture of muscle, left ankle and foot

     M62.479   Contracture of muscle, unspecified ankle and foot

     M62.48   Contracture of muscle, other site

     M62.49   Contracture of muscle, multiple sites

● M62.5   Muscle wasting and atrophy, not elsewhere classified

Disuse atrophy NEC

Excludes1   neuralgic amyotrophy (G54.5)

     progressive muscular atrophy (G12.29)

     sarcopenia (M62.84) ◄

Excludes2   pelvic muscle wasting (N81.84)

     M62.50   Muscle wasting and atrophy, not elsewhere classified, unspecified site

● M62.51   Muscle wasting and atrophy, not elsewhere classified, shoulder

     M62.511   Muscle wasting and atrophy, not elsewhere classified, right shoulder

     M62.512   Muscle wasting and atrophy, not elsewhere classified, left shoulder

     M62.519   Muscle wasting and atrophy, not elsewhere classified, unspecified shoulder

● M62.52   Muscle wasting and atrophy, not elsewhere classified, upper arm

     M62.521   Muscle wasting and atrophy, not elsewhere classified, right upper arm

     M62.522   Muscle wasting and atrophy, not elsewhere classified, left upper arm

     M62.529   Muscle wasting and atrophy, not elsewhere classified, unspecified upper arm

● M62.53   Muscle wasting and atrophy, not elsewhere classified, forearm

     M62.531   Muscle wasting and atrophy, not elsewhere classified, right forearm

     M62.532   Muscle wasting and atrophy, not elsewhere classified, left forearm

     M62.539   Muscle wasting and atrophy, not elsewhere classified, unspecified forearm

● M62.54   Muscle wasting and atrophy, not elsewhere classified, hand

     M62.541   Muscle wasting and atrophy, not elsewhere classified, right hand

     M62.542   Muscle wasting and atrophy, not elsewhere classified, left hand

     M62.549   Muscle wasting and atrophy, not elsewhere classified, unspecified hand

● M62.55   Muscle wasting and atrophy, not elsewhere classified, thigh

     M62.551   Muscle wasting and atrophy, not elsewhere classified, right thigh

     M62.552   Muscle wasting and atrophy, not elsewhere classified, left thigh

     M62.559   Muscle wasting and atrophy, not elsewhere classified, unspecified thigh

● M62.56   Muscle wasting and atrophy, not elsewhere classified, lower leg

     M62.561   Muscle wasting and atrophy, not elsewhere classified, right lower leg

     M62.562   Muscle wasting and atrophy, not elsewhere classified, left lower leg

     M62.569   Muscle wasting and atrophy, not elsewhere classified, unspecified lower leg

CHAPTER 13 (M00-M99)

● M62.57 Muscle wasting and atrophy, not elsewhere classified, ankle and foot

    M62.571 Muscle wasting and atrophy, not elsewhere classified, right ankle and foot

    M62.572 Muscle wasting and atrophy, not elsewhere classified, left ankle and foot

    M62.579 Muscle wasting and atrophy, not elsewhere classified, unspecified ankle and foot

    M62.58 Muscle wasting and atrophy, not elsewhere classified, other site

    M62.59 Muscle wasting and atrophy, not elsewhere classified, multiple sites

● M62.8 Other specified disorders of muscle

    Excludes2 nontraumatic hematoma of muscle (M79.81)

    M62.81 Muscle weakness (generalized)

      Excludes1 muscle weakness in sarcopenia (M62.84) ◀

    M62.82 Rhabdomyolysis

      Excludes1 traumatic rhabdomyolysis (T79.6)

● M62.83 Muscle spasm

    M62.830 Muscle spasm of back

    M62.831 Muscle spasm of calf
      Charley-horse

    M62.838 Other muscle spasm

    M62.84 Sarcopenia ◀
      Age-related sarcopenia ◀
      Code first underlying disease, if applicable, such as:
        disorders of myoneural junction and muscle disease in diseases classified elsewhere (G73.-) ◀
        other and unspecified myopathies (G72.-) ◀
        primary disorders of muscles (G71.-) ◀

    M62.89 Other specified disorders of muscle
      Muscle (sheath) hernia

    M62.9 Disorder of muscle, unspecified

● M63 Disorders of muscle in diseases classified elsewhere

    Code first underlying disease, such as:
      leprosy (A30.-)
      neoplasm (C49.-, C79.89, D21.-, D48.1)
      schistosomiasis (B65.-)
      trichinellosis (B75)

    Excludes1 myopathy in cysticercosis (B69.81)
      myopathy in endocrine diseases (G73.7)
      myopathy in metabolic diseases (G73.7)
      myopathy in sarcoidosis (D86.87)
      myopathy in secondary syphilis (A51.49)
      myopathy in syphilis (late) (A52.78)
      myopathy in toxoplasmosis (B58.82)
      myopathy in tuberculosis (A18.09)

● M63.8 Disorders of muscle in diseases classified elsewhere

    ▶M63.80 *Disorders of muscle in diseases classified elsewhere, unspecified site*

● M63.81 Disorders of muscle in diseases classified elsewhere, shoulder

    ▶M63.811 *Disorders of muscle in diseases classified elsewhere, right shoulder*

    ▶M63.812 *Disorders of muscle in diseases classified elsewhere, left shoulder*

    ▶M63.819 *Disorders of muscle in diseases classified elsewhere, unspecified shoulder*

● M63.82 Disorders of muscle in diseases classified elsewhere, upper arm

    ▶M63.821 *Disorders of muscle in diseases classified elsewhere, right upper arm*

    ▶M63.822 *Disorders of muscle in diseases classified elsewhere, left upper arm*

    ▶M63.829 *Disorders of muscle in diseases classified elsewhere, unspecified upper arm*

● M63.83 Disorders of muscle in diseases classified elsewhere, forearm

    ▶M63.831 *Disorders of muscle in diseases classified elsewhere, right forearm*

    ▶M63.832 *Disorders of muscle in diseases classified elsewhere, left forearm*

    ▶M63.839 *Disorders of muscle in diseases classified elsewhere, unspecified forearm*

● M63.84 Disorders of muscle in diseases classified elsewhere, hand

    ▶M63.841 *Disorders of muscle in diseases classified elsewhere, right hand*

    ▶M63.842 *Disorders of muscle in diseases classified elsewhere, left hand*

    ▶M63.849 *Disorders of muscle in diseases classified elsewhere, unspecified hand*

● M63.85 Disorders of muscle in diseases classified elsewhere, thigh

    ▶M63.851 *Disorders of muscle in diseases classified elsewhere, right thigh*

    ▶M63.852 *Disorders of muscle in diseases classified elsewhere, left thigh*

    ▶M63.859 *Disorders of muscle in diseases classified elsewhere, unspecified thigh*

● M63.86 Disorders of muscle in diseases classified elsewhere, lower leg

    ▶M63.861 *Disorders of muscle in diseases classified elsewhere, right lower leg*

    ▶M63.862 *Disorders of muscle in diseases classified elsewhere, left lower leg*

    ▶M63.869 *Disorders of muscle in diseases classified elsewhere, unspecified lower leg*

● M63.87 Disorders of muscle in diseases classified elsewhere, ankle and foot

    ▶M63.871 *Disorders of muscle in diseases classified elsewhere, right ankle and foot*

    ▶M63.872 *Disorders of muscle in diseases classified elsewhere, left ankle and foot*

    ▶M63.879 *Disorders of muscle in diseases classified elsewhere, unspecified ankle and foot*

    ▶M63.88 *Disorders of muscle in diseases classified elsewhere, other site*

    ▶M63.89 *Disorders of muscle in diseases classified elsewhere, multiple sites*

◀ New   ◀▥ Revised   deleted Deleted   Excludes 1   Excludes 2   Includes   Use additional   Code first   Code also   Unspecified
OGCR Official Guidelines   X Assign placeholder X   ● Use Additional Character(s)   ▶ Manifestation Code   **Coding Clinic**

Item 13-11 **Synovitis** is an inflammation of a synovial membrane resulting in pain on motion and is characterized by fluctuating swelling due to effusion in a synovial sac. **Tenosynovitis** is an inflammation of a tendon sheath and occurs most commonly in the wrists, hands, and feet. Bursitis is inflammation of a bursa (fluid filled sac) caused by repetitive use, trauma, infection, or systemic inflammatory disease. Bursae act as protectors and facilitate movement between bones and overlapping muscles (deep bursae) or between bones and tendons/skin (superficial bursae).

DISORDERS OF SYNOVIUM AND TENDON (M65-M67)

- M65 **Synovitis and tenosynovitis**
  - **Excludes1**   chronic crepitant synovitis of hand and wrist (M70.0-)
    - current injury - see injury of ligament or tendon by body region
    - soft tissue disorders related to use, overuse and pressure (M70.-)
  - M65.0 **Abscess of tendon sheath**
    - Use additional code (B95-B96) to identify bacterial agent
    - M65.00   Abscess of tendon sheath, unspecified site
    - M65.01   Abscess of tendon sheath, shoulder
      - M65.011   Abscess of tendon sheath, right shoulder
      - M65.012   Abscess of tendon sheath, left shoulder
      - M65.019   Abscess of tendon sheath, unspecified shoulder
    - M65.02   Abscess of tendon sheath, upper arm
      - M65.021   Abscess of tendon sheath, right upper arm
      - M65.022   Abscess of tendon sheath, left upper arm
      - M65.029   Abscess of tendon sheath, unspecified upper arm
    - M65.03   Abscess of tendon sheath, forearm
      - M65.031   Abscess of tendon sheath, right forearm
      - M65.032   Abscess of tendon sheath, left forearm
      - M65.039   Abscess of tendon sheath, unspecified forearm
    - M65.04   Abscess of tendon sheath, hand
      - M65.041   Abscess of tendon sheath, right hand
      - M65.042   Abscess of tendon sheath, left hand
      - M65.049   Abscess of tendon sheath, unspecified hand
    - M65.05   Abscess of tendon sheath, thigh
      - M65.051   Abscess of tendon sheath, right thigh
      - M65.052   Abscess of tendon sheath, left thigh
      - M65.059   Abscess of tendon sheath, unspecified thigh
    - M65.06   Abscess of tendon sheath, lower leg
      - M65.061   Abscess of tendon sheath, right lower leg
      - M65.062   Abscess of tendon sheath, left lower leg
      - M65.069   Abscess of tendon sheath, unspecified lower leg
    - M65.07   Abscess of tendon sheath, ankle and foot
      - M65.071   Abscess of tendon sheath, right ankle and foot
      - M65.072   Abscess of tendon sheath, left ankle and foot
      - M65.079   Abscess of tendon sheath, unspecified ankle and foot
    - M65.08   Abscess of tendon sheath, other site

- M65.1 **Other infective (teno)synovitis**
  - M65.10   Other infective (teno)synovitis, unspecified site
  - M65.11   Other infective (teno)synovitis, shoulder
    - M65.111   Other infective (teno)synovitis, right shoulder
    - M65.112   Other infective (teno)synovitis, left shoulder
    - M65.119   Other infective (teno)synovitis, unspecified shoulder
  - M65.12   Other infective (teno)synovitis, elbow
    - M65.121   Other infective (teno)synovitis, right elbow
    - M65.122   Other infective (teno)synovitis, left elbow
    - M65.129   Other infective (teno)synovitis, unspecified elbow
  - M65.13   Other infective (teno)synovitis, wrist
    - M65.131   Other infective (teno)synovitis, right wrist
    - M65.132   Other infective (teno)synovitis, left wrist
    - M65.139   Other infective (teno)synovitis, unspecified wrist
  - M65.14   Other infective (teno)synovitis, hand
    - M65.141   Other infective (teno)synovitis, right hand
    - M65.142   Other infective (teno)synovitis, left hand
    - M65.149   Other infective (teno)synovitis, unspecified hand
  - M65.15   Other infective (teno)synovitis, hip
    - M65.151   Other infective (teno)synovitis, right hip
    - M65.152   Other infective (teno)synovitis, left hip
    - M65.159   Other infective (teno)synovitis, unspecified hip
  - M65.16   Other infective (teno)synovitis, knee
    - M65.161   Other infective (teno)synovitis, right knee
    - M65.162   Other infective (teno)synovitis, left knee
    - M65.169   Other infective (teno)synovitis, unspecified knee
  - M65.17   Other infective (teno)synovitis, ankle and foot
    - M65.171   Other infective (teno)synovitis, right ankle and foot
    - M65.172   Other infective (teno)synovitis, left ankle and foot
    - M65.179   Other infective (teno)synovitis, unspecified ankle and foot
  - M65.18   Other infective (teno)synovitis, other site
  - M65.19   Other infective (teno)synovitis, multiple sites
- M65.2 **Calcific tendinitis**
  - **Excludes1**   tendinitis as classified in M75-M77
    - calcified tendinitis of shoulder (M75.3)
  - M65.20   Calcific tendinitis, unspecified site
  - M65.22   Calcific tendinitis, upper arm
    - M65.221   Calcific tendinitis, right upper arm
    - M65.222   Calcific tendinitis, left upper arm
    - M65.229   Calcific tendinitis, unspecified upper arm
  - M65.23   Calcific tendinitis, forearm
    - M65.231   Calcific tendinitis, right forearm
    - M65.232   Calcific tendinitis, left forearm
    - M65.239   Calcific tendinitis, unspecified forearm

● M65.24   Calcific tendinitis, hand
    M65.241   Calcific tendinitis, right hand
    M65.242   Calcific tendinitis, left hand
    M65.249   Calcific tendinitis, unspecified hand
● M65.25   Calcific tendinitis, thigh
    M65.251   Calcific tendinitis, right thigh
    M65.252   Calcific tendinitis, left thigh
    M65.259   Calcific tendinitis, unspecified thigh
● M65.26   Calcific tendinitis, lower leg
    M65.261   Calcific tendinitis, right lower leg
    M65.262   Calcific tendinitis, left lower leg
    M65.269   Calcific tendinitis, unspecified lower leg
● M65.27   Calcific tendinitis, ankle and foot
    M65.271   Calcific tendinitis, right ankle and foot
    M65.272   Calcific tendinitis, left ankle and foot
    M65.279   Calcific tendinitis, unspecified ankle and foot
  M65.28   Calcific tendinitis, other site
  M65.29   Calcific tendinitis, multiple sites
● M65.3   Trigger finger
    Nodular tendinous disease
  M65.30   Trigger finger, unspecified finger
● M65.31   Trigger thumb
    M65.311   Trigger thumb, right thumb
    M65.312   Trigger thumb, left thumb
    M65.319   Trigger thumb, unspecified thumb
● M65.32   Trigger finger, index finger
    M65.321   Trigger finger, right index finger
    M65.322   Trigger finger, left index finger
    M65.329   Trigger finger, unspecified index finger
● M65.33   Trigger finger, middle finger
    M65.331   Trigger finger, right middle finger
    M65.332   Trigger finger, left middle finger
    M65.339   Trigger finger, unspecified middle finger
● M65.34   Trigger finger, ring finger
    M65.341   Trigger finger, right ring finger
    M65.342   Trigger finger, left ring finger
    M65.349   Trigger finger, unspecified ring finger
● M65.35   Trigger finger, little finger
    M65.351   Trigger finger, right little finger
    M65.352   Trigger finger, left little finger
    M65.359   Trigger finger, unspecified little finger
  M65.4   Radial styloid tenosynovitis [de Quervain]
● M65.8   Other synovitis and tenosynovitis
  M65.80   Other synovitis and tenosynovitis, unspecified site
● M65.81   Other synovitis and tenosynovitis, shoulder
    M65.811   Other synovitis and tenosynovitis, right shoulder
    M65.812   Other synovitis and tenosynovitis, left shoulder
    M65.819   Other synovitis and tenosynovitis, unspecified shoulder
● M65.82   Other synovitis and tenosynovitis, upper arm
    M65.821   Other synovitis and tenosynovitis, right upper arm
    M65.822   Other synovitis and tenosynovitis, left upper arm
    M65.829   Other synovitis and tenosynovitis, unspecified upper arm

● M65.83   Other synovitis and tenosynovitis, forearm
    M65.831   Other synovitis and tenosynovitis, right forearm
    M65.832   Other synovitis and tenosynovitis, left forearm
    M65.839   Other synovitis and tenosynovitis, unspecified forearm
● M65.84   Other synovitis and tenosynovitis, hand
    M65.841   Other synovitis and tenosynovitis, right hand
    M65.842   Other synovitis and tenosynovitis, left hand
    M65.849   Other synovitis and tenosynovitis, unspecified hand
● M65.85   Other synovitis and tenosynovitis, thigh
    M65.851   Other synovitis and tenosynovitis, right thigh
    M65.852   Other synovitis and tenosynovitis, left thigh
    M65.859   Other synovitis and tenosynovitis, unspecified thigh
● M65.86   Other synovitis and tenosynovitis, lower leg
    M65.861   Other synovitis and tenosynovitis, right lower leg
    M65.862   Other synovitis and tenosynovitis, left lower leg
    M65.869   Other synovitis and tenosynovitis, unspecified lower leg
● M65.87   Other synovitis and tenosynovitis, ankle and foot
    M65.871   Other synovitis and tenosynovitis, right ankle and foot
    M65.872   Other synovitis and tenosynovitis, left ankle and foot
    M65.879   Other synovitis and tenosynovitis, unspecified ankle and foot
  M65.88   Other synovitis and tenosynovitis, other site
  M65.89   Other synovitis and tenosynovitis, multiple sites
  M65.9   Synovitis and tenosynovitis, unspecified
● M66   Spontaneous rupture of synovium and tendon
  Includes   rupture that occurs when a normal force is applied to tissues that are inferred to have less than normal strength
  Excludes2   rotator cuff syndrome (M75.1-)
    rupture where an abnormal force is applied to normal tissue - see injury of tendon by body region
  M66.0   Rupture of popliteal cyst
● M66.1   Rupture of synovium
    Rupture of synovial cyst
    Excludes2   rupture of popliteal cyst (M66.0)
  M66.10   Rupture of synovium, unspecified joint
● M66.11   Rupture of synovium, shoulder
    M66.111   Rupture of synovium, right shoulder
    M66.112   Rupture of synovium, left shoulder
    M66.119   Rupture of synovium, unspecified shoulder
● M66.12   Rupture of synovium, elbow
    M66.121   Rupture of synovium, right elbow
    M66.122   Rupture of synovium, left elbow
    M66.129   Rupture of synovium, unspecified elbow
● M66.13   Rupture of synovium, wrist
    M66.131   Rupture of synovium, right wrist
    M66.132   Rupture of synovium, left wrist
    M66.139   Rupture of synovium, unspecified wrist

◀ New   ◀▦ Revised   ~~deleted~~ Deleted   Excludes 1   Excludes 2   Includes   Use additional   Code first   Code also   Unspecified

1026   OGCR Official Guidelines   X Assign placeholder X   ● Use Additional Character(s)   ▶ Manifestation Code   **Coding Clinic**

● M66.14   Rupture of synovium, hand and fingers
    M66.141   Rupture of synovium, right hand
    M66.142   Rupture of synovium, left hand
    M66.143   Rupture of synovium, unspecified hand
    M66.144   Rupture of synovium, right finger(s)
    M66.145   Rupture of synovium, left finger(s)
    M66.146   Rupture of synovium, unspecified finger(s)
● M66.15   Rupture of synovium, hip
    M66.151   Rupture of synovium, right hip
    M66.152   Rupture of synovium, left hip
    M66.159   Rupture of synovium, unspecified hip
● M66.17   Rupture of synovium, ankle, foot and toes
    M66.171   Rupture of synovium, right ankle
    M66.172   Rupture of synovium, left ankle
    M66.173   Rupture of synovium, unspecified ankle
    M66.174   Rupture of synovium, right foot
    M66.175   Rupture of synovium, left foot
    M66.176   Rupture of synovium, unspecified foot
    M66.177   Rupture of synovium, right toe(s)
    M66.178   Rupture of synovium, left toe(s)
    M66.179   Rupture of synovium, unspecified toe(s)
    M66.18   Rupture of synovium, other site
● M66.2   Spontaneous rupture of extensor tendons
    M66.20   Spontaneous rupture of extensor tendons, unspecified site
● M66.21   Spontaneous rupture of extensor tendons, shoulder
    M66.211   Spontaneous rupture of extensor tendons, right shoulder
    M66.212   Spontaneous rupture of extensor tendons, left shoulder
    M66.219   Spontaneous rupture of extensor tendons, unspecified shoulder
● M66.22   Spontaneous rupture of extensor tendons, upper arm
    M66.221   Spontaneous rupture of extensor tendons, right upper arm
    M66.222   Spontaneous rupture of extensor tendons, left upper arm
    M66.229   Spontaneous rupture of extensor tendons, unspecified upper arm
● M66.23   Spontaneous rupture of extensor tendons, forearm
    M66.231   Spontaneous rupture of extensor tendons, right forearm
    M66.232   Spontaneous rupture of extensor tendons, left forearm
    M66.239   Spontaneous rupture of extensor tendons, unspecified forearm
● M66.24   Spontaneous rupture of extensor tendons, hand
    M66.241   Spontaneous rupture of extensor tendons, right hand
    M66.242   Spontaneous rupture of extensor tendons, left hand
    M66.249   Spontaneous rupture of extensor tendons, unspecified hand
● M66.25   Spontaneous rupture of extensor tendons, thigh
    M66.251   Spontaneous rupture of extensor tendons, right thigh
    M66.252   Spontaneous rupture of extensor tendons, left thigh
    M66.259   Spontaneous rupture of extensor tendons, unspecified thigh

● M66.26   Spontaneous rupture of extensor tendons, lower leg
    M66.261   Spontaneous rupture of extensor tendons, right lower leg
    M66.262   Spontaneous rupture of extensor tendons, left lower leg
    M66.269   Spontaneous rupture of extensor tendons, unspecified lower leg
● M66.27   Spontaneous rupture of extensor tendons, ankle and foot
    M66.271   Spontaneous rupture of extensor tendons, right ankle and foot
    M66.272   Spontaneous rupture of extensor tendons, left ankle and foot
    M66.279   Spontaneous rupture of extensor tendons, unspecified ankle and foot
    M66.28   Spontaneous rupture of extensor tendons, other site
    M66.29   Spontaneous rupture of extensor tendons, multiple sites
● M66.3   Spontaneous rupture of flexor tendons
    M66.30   Spontaneous rupture of flexor tendons, unspecified site
● M66.31   Spontaneous rupture of flexor tendons, shoulder
    M66.311   Spontaneous rupture of flexor tendons, right shoulder
    M66.312   Spontaneous rupture of flexor tendons, left shoulder
    M66.319   Spontaneous rupture of flexor tendons, unspecified shoulder
● M66.32   Spontaneous rupture of flexor tendons, upper arm
    M66.321   Spontaneous rupture of flexor tendons, right upper arm
    M66.322   Spontaneous rupture of flexor tendons, left upper arm
    M66.329   Spontaneous rupture of flexor tendons, unspecified upper arm
● M66.33   Spontaneous rupture of flexor tendons, forearm
    M66.331   Spontaneous rupture of flexor tendons, right forearm
    M66.332   Spontaneous rupture of flexor tendons, left forearm
    M66.339   Spontaneous rupture of flexor tendons, unspecified forearm
● M66.34   Spontaneous rupture of flexor tendons, hand
    M66.341   Spontaneous rupture of flexor tendons, right hand
    M66.342   Spontaneous rupture of flexor tendons, left hand
    M66.349   Spontaneous rupture of flexor tendons, unspecified hand
● M66.35   Spontaneous rupture of flexor tendons, thigh
    M66.351   Spontaneous rupture of flexor tendons, right thigh
    M66.352   Spontaneous rupture of flexor tendons, left thigh
    M66.359   Spontaneous rupture of flexor tendons, unspecified thigh
● M66.36   Spontaneous rupture of flexor tendons, lower leg
    M66.361   Spontaneous rupture of flexor tendons, right lower leg
    M66.362   Spontaneous rupture of flexor tendons, left lower leg
    M66.369   Spontaneous rupture of flexor tendons, unspecified lower leg

CHAPTER 13 (M00-M99)

● **M66.37** Spontaneous rupture of flexor tendons, ankle and foot
   M66.371 Spontaneous rupture of flexor tendons, right ankle and foot
   M66.372 Spontaneous rupture of flexor tendons, left ankle and foot
   M66.379 Spontaneous rupture of flexor tendons, unspecified ankle and foot
  M66.38 Spontaneous rupture of flexor tendons, other site
  M66.39 Spontaneous rupture of flexor tendons, multiple sites

● **M66.8** Spontaneous rupture of other tendons
  M66.80 Spontaneous rupture of other tendons, unspecified site
● **M66.81** Spontaneous rupture of other tendons, shoulder
   M66.811 Spontaneous rupture of other tendons, right shoulder
   M66.812 Spontaneous rupture of other tendons, left shoulder
   M66.819 Spontaneous rupture of other tendons, unspecified shoulder
● **M66.82** Spontaneous rupture of other tendons, upper arm
   M66.821 Spontaneous rupture of other tendons, right upper arm
   M66.822 Spontaneous rupture of other tendons, left upper arm
   M66.829 Spontaneous rupture of other tendons, unspecified upper arm
● **M66.83** Spontaneous rupture of other tendons, forearm
   M66.831 Spontaneous rupture of other tendons, right forearm
   M66.832 Spontaneous rupture of other tendons, left forearm
   M66.839 Spontaneous rupture of other tendons, unspecified forearm
● **M66.84** Spontaneous rupture of other tendons, hand
   M66.841 Spontaneous rupture of other tendons, right hand
   M66.842 Spontaneous rupture of other tendons, left hand
   M66.849 Spontaneous rupture of other tendons, unspecified hand
● **M66.85** Spontaneous rupture of other tendons, thigh
   M66.851 Spontaneous rupture of other tendons, right thigh
   M66.852 Spontaneous rupture of other tendons, left thigh
   M66.859 Spontaneous rupture of other tendons, unspecified thigh
● **M66.86** Spontaneous rupture of other tendons, lower leg
   M66.861 Spontaneous rupture of other tendons, right lower leg
   M66.862 Spontaneous rupture of other tendons, left lower leg
   M66.869 Spontaneous rupture of other tendons, unspecified lower leg

● **M66.87** Spontaneous rupture of other tendons, ankle and foot
   M66.871 Spontaneous rupture of other tendons, right ankle and foot
   M66.872 Spontaneous rupture of other tendons, left ankle and foot
   M66.879 Spontaneous rupture of other tendons, unspecified ankle and foot
  M66.88 Spontaneous rupture of other tendons, other
  M66.89 Spontaneous rupture of other tendons, multiple sites
M66.9 Spontaneous rupture of unspecified tendon
  Rupture at musculotendinous junction, nontraumatic

● **M67** Other disorders of synovium and tendon
  Excludes1 palmar fascial fibromatosis [Dupuytren] (M72.0)
    tendinitis NOS (M77.9-)
    xanthomatosis localized to tendons (E78.2)
● **M67.0** Short Achilles tendon (acquired)
  M67.00 Short Achilles tendon (acquired), unspecified ankle
  M67.01 Short Achilles tendon (acquired), right ankle
  M67.02 Short Achilles tendon (acquired), left ankle
● **M67.2** Synovial hypertrophy, not elsewhere classified
  Excludes1 villonodular synovitis (pigmented) (M12.2-)
  M67.20 Synovial hypertrophy, not elsewhere classified, unspecified site
● **M67.21** Synovial hypertrophy, not elsewhere classified, shoulder
   M67.211 Synovial hypertrophy, not elsewhere classified, right shoulder
   M67.212 Synovial hypertrophy, not elsewhere classified, left shoulder
   M67.219 Synovial hypertrophy, not elsewhere classified, unspecified shoulder
● **M67.22** Synovial hypertrophy, not elsewhere classified, upper arm
   M67.221 Synovial hypertrophy, not elsewhere classified, right upper arm
   M67.222 Synovial hypertrophy, not elsewhere classified, left upper arm
   M67.229 Synovial hypertrophy, not elsewhere classified, unspecified upper arm
● **M67.23** Synovial hypertrophy, not elsewhere classified, forearm
   M67.231 Synovial hypertrophy, not elsewhere classified, right forearm
   M67.232 Synovial hypertrophy, not elsewhere classified, left forearm
   M67.239 Synovial hypertrophy, not elsewhere classified, unspecified forearm
● **M67.24** Synovial hypertrophy, not elsewhere classified, hand
   M67.241 Synovial hypertrophy, not elsewhere classified, right hand
   M67.242 Synovial hypertrophy, not elsewhere classified, left hand
   M67.249 Synovial hypertrophy, not elsewhere classified, unspecified hand

● **M67.25** Synovial hypertrophy, not elsewhere classified, thigh

   M67.251 Synovial hypertrophy, not elsewhere classified, right thigh

   M67.252 Synovial hypertrophy, not elsewhere classified, left thigh

   M67.259 Synovial hypertrophy, not elsewhere classified, unspecified thigh

● **M67.26** Synovial hypertrophy, not elsewhere classified, lower leg

   M67.261 Synovial hypertrophy, not elsewhere classified, right lower leg

   M67.262 Synovial hypertrophy, not elsewhere classified, left lower leg

   M67.269 Synovial hypertrophy, not elsewhere classified, unspecified lower leg

● **M67.27** Synovial hypertrophy, not elsewhere classified, ankle and foot

   M67.271 Synovial hypertrophy, not elsewhere classified, right ankle and foot

   M67.272 Synovial hypertrophy, not elsewhere classified, left ankle and foot

   M67.279 Synovial hypertrophy, not elsewhere classified, unspecified ankle and foot

  M67.28 Synovial hypertrophy, not elsewhere classified, other site

  M67.29 Synovial hypertrophy, not elsewhere classified, multiple sites

● **M67.3** Transient synovitis

   Toxic synovitis

   Excludes1 palindromic rheumatism (M12.3-)

  M67.30 Transient synovitis, unspecified site

● **M67.31** Transient synovitis, shoulder

   M67.311 Transient synovitis, right shoulder

   M67.312 Transient synovitis, left shoulder

   M67.319 Transient synovitis, unspecified shoulder

● **M67.32** Transient synovitis, elbow

   M67.321 Transient synovitis, right elbow

   M67.322 Transient synovitis, left elbow

   M67.329 Transient synovitis, unspecified elbow

● **M67.33** Transient synovitis, wrist

   M67.331 Transient synovitis, right wrist

   M67.332 Transient synovitis, left wrist

   M67.339 Transient synovitis, unspecified wrist

● **M67.34** Transient synovitis, hand

   M67.341 Transient synovitis, right hand

   M67.342 Transient synovitis, left hand

   M67.349 Transient synovitis, unspecified hand

● **M67.35** Transient synovitis, hip

   M67.351 Transient synovitis, right hip

   M67.352 Transient synovitis, left hip

   M67.359 Transient synovitis, unspecified hip

● **M67.36** Transient synovitis, knee

   M67.361 Transient synovitis, right knee

   M67.362 Transient synovitis, left knee

   M67.369 Transient synovitis, unspecified knee

● **M67.37** Transient synovitis, ankle and foot

   M67.371 Transient synovitis, right ankle and foot

   M67.372 Transient synovitis, left ankle and foot

   M67.379 Transient synovitis, unspecified ankle and foot

  M67.38 Transient synovitis, other site

  M67.39 Transient synovitis, multiple sites

● **M67.4** Ganglion

   Ganglion of joint or tendon (sheath)

   Excludes1 ganglion in yaws (A66.6)

   Excludes2 cyst of bursa (M71.2-M71.3)

         cyst of synovium (M71.2-M71.3)

  M67.40 Ganglion, unspecified site

● **M67.41** Ganglion, shoulder

   M67.411 Ganglion, right shoulder

   M67.412 Ganglion, left shoulder

   M67.419 Ganglion, unspecified shoulder

● **M67.42** Ganglion, elbow

   M67.421 Ganglion, right elbow

   M67.422 Ganglion, left elbow

   M67.429 Ganglion, unspecified elbow

● **M67.43** Ganglion, wrist

   M67.431 Ganglion, right wrist

   M67.432 Ganglion, left wrist

   M67.439 Ganglion, unspecified wrist

● **M67.44** Ganglion, hand

   M67.441 Ganglion, right hand

   M67.442 Ganglion, left hand

   M67.449 Ganglion, unspecified hand

● **M67.45** Ganglion, hip

   M67.451 Ganglion, right hip

   M67.452 Ganglion, left hip

   M67.459 Ganglion, unspecified hip

● **M67.46** Ganglion, knee

   M67.461 Ganglion, right knee

   M67.462 Ganglion, left knee

   M67.469 Ganglion, unspecified knee

● **M67.47** Ganglion, ankle and foot

   M67.471 Ganglion, right ankle and foot

   M67.472 Ganglion, left ankle and foot

   M67.479 Ganglion, unspecified ankle and foot

  M67.48 Ganglion, other site

  M67.49 Ganglion, multiple sites

● **M67.5** Plica syndrome

   Plica knee

  M67.50 Plica syndrome, unspecified knee

  M67.51 Plica syndrome, right knee

  M67.52 Plica syndrome, left knee

● **M67.8** Other specified disorders of synovium and tendon

  M67.80 Other specified disorders of synovium and tendon, unspecified site

● **M67.81** Other specified disorders of synovium and tendon, shoulder

   M67.811 Other specified disorders of synovium, right shoulder

   M67.812 Other specified disorders of synovium, left shoulder

   M67.813 Other specified disorders of tendon, right shoulder

   M67.814 Other specified disorders of tendon, left shoulder

   M67.819 Other specified disorders of synovium and tendon, unspecified shoulder

CHAPTER 13 (M00-M99)

● M67.82 Other specified disorders of synovium and tendon, elbow
    M67.821 Other specified disorders of synovium, right elbow
    M67.822 Other specified disorders of synovium, left elbow
    M67.823 Other specified disorders of tendon, right elbow
    M67.824 Other specified disorders of tendon, left elbow
    M67.829 Other specified disorders of synovium and tendon, unspecified elbow

● M67.83 Other specified disorders of synovium and tendon, wrist
    M67.831 Other specified disorders of synovium, right wrist
    M67.832 Other specified disorders of synovium, left wrist
    M67.833 Other specified disorders of tendon, right wrist
    M67.834 Other specified disorders of tendon, left wrist
    M67.839 Other specified disorders of synovium and tendon, unspecified forearm

● M67.84 Other specified disorders of synovium and tendon, hand
    M67.841 Other specified disorders of synovium, right hand
    M67.842 Other specified disorders of synovium, left hand
    M67.843 Other specified disorders of tendon, right hand
    M67.844 Other specified disorders of tendon, left hand
    M67.849 Other specified disorders of synovium and tendon, unspecified hand

● M67.85 Other specified disorders of synovium and tendon, hip
    M67.851 Other specified disorders of synovium, right hip
    M67.852 Other specified disorders of synovium, left hip
    M67.853 Other specified disorders of tendon, right hip
    M67.854 Other specified disorders of tendon, left hip
    M67.859 Other specified disorders of synovium and tendon, unspecified hip

● M67.86 Other specified disorders of synovium and tendon, knee
    M67.861 Other specified disorders of synovium, right knee
    M67.862 Other specified disorders of synovium, left knee
    M67.863 Other specified disorders of tendon, right knee
    M67.864 Other specified disorders of tendon, left knee
    M67.869 Other specified disorders of synovium and tendon, unspecified knee

● M67.87 Other specified disorders of synovium and tendon, ankle and foot
    M67.871 Other specified disorders of synovium, right ankle and foot
    M67.872 Other specified disorders of synovium, left ankle and foot
    M67.873 Other specified disorders of tendon, right ankle and foot
    M67.874 Other specified disorders of tendon, left ankle and foot
    M67.879 Other specified disorders of synovium and tendon, unspecified ankle and foot

    M67.88 Other specified disorders of synovium and tendon, other site
    M67.89 Other specified disorders of synovium and tendon, multiple sites

● M67.9 Unspecified disorder of synovium and tendon
    M67.90 Unspecified disorder of synovium and tendon, unspecified site
● M67.91 Unspecified disorder of synovium and tendon, shoulder
    M67.911 Unspecified disorder of synovium and tendon, right shoulder
    M67.912 Unspecified disorder of synovium and tendon, left shoulder
    M67.919 Unspecified disorder of synovium and tendon, unspecified shoulder

● M67.92 Unspecified disorder of synovium and tendon, upper arm
    M67.921 Unspecified disorder of synovium and tendon, right upper arm
    M67.922 Unspecified disorder of synovium and tendon, left upper arm
    M67.929 Unspecified disorder of synovium and tendon, unspecified upper arm

● M67.93 Unspecified disorder of synovium and tendon, forearm
    M67.931 Unspecified disorder of synovium and tendon, right forearm
    M67.932 Unspecified disorder of synovium and tendon, left forearm
    M67.939 Unspecified disorder of synovium and tendon, unspecified forearm

● M67.94 Unspecified disorder of synovium and tendon, hand
    M67.941 Unspecified disorder of synovium and tendon, right hand
    M67.942 Unspecified disorder of synovium and tendon, left hand
    M67.949 Unspecified disorder of synovium and tendon, unspecified hand

● M67.95 Unspecified disorder of synovium and tendon, thigh
    M67.951 Unspecified disorder of synovium and tendon, right thigh
    M67.952 Unspecified disorder of synovium and tendon, left thigh
    M67.959 Unspecified disorder of synovium and tendon, unspecified thigh

● M67.96 Unspecified disorder of synovium and tendon, lower leg
    M67.961 Unspecified disorder of synovium and tendon, right lower leg
    M67.962 Unspecified disorder of synovium and tendon, left lower leg
    M67.969 Unspecified disorder of synovium and tendon, unspecified lower leg

◀ New   ◀▥ Revised   ~~deleted~~ Deleted   Excludes 1   Excludes 2   Includes   Use additional   Code first   Code also   Unspecified
OGCR Official Guidelines   X Assign placeholder X   ● Use Additional Character(s)   ▶ Manifestation Code   Coding Clinic

● M67.97   Unspecified disorder of synovium and tendon, ankle and foot
    M67.971   Unspecified disorder of synovium and tendon, right ankle and foot
    M67.972   Unspecified disorder of synovium and tendon, left ankle and foot
    M67.979   Unspecified disorder of synovium and tendon, unspecified ankle and foot
   M67.98   Unspecified disorder of synovium and tendon, other site
   M67.99   Unspecified disorder of synovium and tendon, multiple sites

OTHER SOFT TISSUE DISORDERS (M70-M79)

● M70   Soft tissue disorders related to use, overuse and pressure
    Includes   soft tissue disorders of occupational origin
    Use additional external cause code to identify activity causing disorder (Y93.-)
    Excludes1   bursitis NOS (M71.9-)
    Excludes2   bursitis of shoulder (M75.5)
                enthesopathies (M76-M77)
                pressure ulcer (pressure area) (L89.-)

● M70.0   Crepitant synovitis (acute) (chronic) of hand and wrist
   ● M70.03   Crepitant synovitis (acute) (chronic), wrist
     M70.031   Crepitant synovitis (acute) (chronic), right wrist
     M70.032   Crepitant synovitis (acute) (chronic), left wrist
     M70.039   Crepitant synovitis (acute) (chronic), unspecified wrist
   ● M70.04   Crepitant synovitis (acute) (chronic), hand
     M70.041   Crepitant synovitis (acute) (chronic), right hand
     M70.042   Crepitant synovitis (acute) (chronic), left hand
     M70.049   Crepitant synovitis (acute) (chronic), unspecified hand

● M70.1   Bursitis of hand
   M70.10   Bursitis, unspecified hand
   M70.11   Bursitis, right hand
   M70.12   Bursitis, left hand

● M70.2   Olecranon bursitis
   M70.20   Olecranon bursitis, unspecified elbow
   M70.21   Olecranon bursitis, right elbow
   M70.22   Olecranon bursitis, left elbow

● M70.3   Other bursitis of elbow
   M70.30   Other bursitis of elbow, unspecified elbow
   M70.31   Other bursitis of elbow, right elbow
   M70.32   Other bursitis of elbow, left elbow

● M70.4   Prepatellar bursitis
   M70.40   Prepatellar bursitis, unspecified knee
   M70.41   Prepatellar bursitis, right knee
   M70.42   Prepatellar bursitis, left knee

● M70.5   Other bursitis of knee
   M70.50   Other bursitis of knee, unspecified knee
   M70.51   Other bursitis of knee, right knee
   M70.52   Other bursitis of knee, left knee

● M70.6   Trochanteric bursitis
    Trochanteric tendinitis
   M70.60   Trochanteric bursitis, unspecified hip
   M70.61   Trochanteric bursitis, right hip
   M70.62   Trochanteric bursitis, left hip

● M70.7   Other bursitis of hip
    Ischial bursitis
   M70.70   Other bursitis of hip, unspecified hip
   M70.71   Other bursitis of hip, right hip
   M70.72   Other bursitis of hip, left hip

● M70.8   Other soft tissue disorders related to use, overuse and pressure
   M70.80   Other soft tissue disorders related to use, overuse and pressure of unspecified site
   ● M70.81   Other soft tissue disorders related to use, overuse and pressure of shoulder
     M70.811   Other soft tissue disorders related to use, overuse and pressure, right shoulder
     M70.812   Other soft tissue disorders related to use, overuse and pressure, left shoulder
     M70.819   Other soft tissue disorders related to use, overuse and pressure, unspecified shoulder
   ● M70.82   Other soft tissue disorders related to use, overuse and pressure of upper arm
     M70.821   Other soft tissue disorders related to use, overuse and pressure, right upper arm
     M70.822   Other soft tissue disorders related to use, overuse and pressure, left upper arm
     M70.829   Other soft tissue disorders related to use, overuse and pressure, unspecified upper arms
   ● M70.83   Other soft tissue disorders related to use, overuse and pressure of forearm
     M70.831   Other soft tissue disorders related to use, overuse and pressure, right forearm
     M70.832   Other soft tissue disorders related to use, overuse and pressure, left forearm
     M70.839   Other soft tissue disorders related to use, overuse and pressure, unspecified forearm
   ● M70.84   Other soft tissue disorders related to use, overuse and pressure of hand
     M70.841   Other soft tissue disorders related to use, overuse and pressure, right hand
     M70.842   Other soft tissue disorders related to use, overuse and pressure, left hand
     M70.849   Other soft tissue disorders related to use, overuse and pressure, unspecified hand
   ● M70.85   Other soft tissue disorders related to use, overuse and pressure of thigh
     M70.851   Other soft tissue disorders related to use, overuse and pressure, right thigh
     M70.852   Other soft tissue disorders related to use, overuse and pressure, left thigh
     M70.859   Other soft tissue disorders related to use, overuse and pressure, unspecified thigh
   ● M70.86   Other soft tissue disorders related to use, overuse and pressure lower leg
     M70.861   Other soft tissue disorders related to use, overuse and pressure, right lower leg
     M70.862   Other soft tissue disorders related to use, overuse and pressure, left lower leg
     M70.869   Other soft tissue disorders related to use, overuse and pressure, unspecified leg

● M70.87   Other soft tissue disorders related to use, overuse and pressure of ankle and foot
    M70.871   Other soft tissue disorders related to use, overuse and pressure, right ankle and foot
    M70.872   Other soft tissue disorders related to use, overuse and pressure, left ankle and foot
    M70.879   Other soft tissue disorders related to use, overuse and pressure, unspecified ankle and foot
   M70.88   Other soft tissue disorders related to use, overuse and pressure other site
   M70.89   Other soft tissue disorders related to use, overuse and pressure multiple sites
● M70.9   Unspecified soft tissue disorder related to use, overuse and pressure
   M70.90   Unspecified soft tissue disorder related to use, overuse and pressure of unspecified site
● M70.91   Unspecified soft tissue disorder related to use, overuse and pressure of shoulder
    M70.911   Unspecified soft tissue disorder related to use, overuse and pressure, right shoulder
    M70.912   Unspecified soft tissue disorder related to use, overuse and pressure, left shoulder
    M70.919   Unspecified soft tissue disorder related to use, overuse and pressure, unspecified shoulder
● M70.92   Unspecified soft tissue disorder related to use, overuse and pressure of upper arm
    M70.921   Unspecified soft tissue disorder related to use, overuse and pressure, right upper arm
    M70.922   Unspecified soft tissue disorder related to use, overuse and pressure, left upper arm
    M70.929   Unspecified soft tissue disorder related to use, overuse and pressure, unspecified upper arm
● M70.93   Unspecified soft tissue disorder related to use, overuse and pressure of forearm
    M70.931   Unspecified soft tissue disorder related to use, overuse and pressure, right forearm
    M70.932   Unspecified soft tissue disorder related to use, overuse and pressure, left forearm
    M70.939   Unspecified soft tissue disorder related to use, overuse and pressure, unspecified forearm
● M70.94   Unspecified soft tissue disorder related to use, overuse and pressure of hand
    M70.941   Unspecified soft tissue disorder related to use, overuse and pressure, right hand
    M70.942   Unspecified soft tissue disorder related to use, overuse and pressure, left hand
    M70.949   Unspecified soft tissue disorder related to use, overuse and pressure, unspecified hand

● M70.95   Unspecified soft tissue disorder related to use, overuse and pressure of thigh
    M70.951   Unspecified soft tissue disorder related to use, overuse and pressure, right thigh
    M70.952   Unspecified soft tissue disorder related to use, overuse and pressure, left thigh
    M70.959   Unspecified soft tissue disorder related to use, overuse and pressure, unspecified thigh
● M70.96   Unspecified soft tissue disorder related to use, overuse and pressure lower leg
    M70.961   Unspecified soft tissue disorder related to use, overuse and pressure, right lower leg
    M70.962   Unspecified soft tissue disorder related to use, overuse and pressure, left lower leg
    M70.969   Unspecified soft tissue disorder related to use, overuse and pressure, unspecified lower leg
● M70.97   Unspecified soft tissue disorder related to use, overuse and pressure of ankle and foot
    M70.971   Unspecified soft tissue disorder related to use, overuse and pressure, right ankle and foot
    M70.972   Unspecified soft tissue disorder related to use, overuse and pressure, left ankle and foot
    M70.979   Unspecified soft tissue disorder related to use, overuse and pressure, unspecified ankle and foot
   M70.98   Unspecified soft tissue disorder related to use, overuse and pressure other
   M70.99   Unspecified soft tissue disorder related to use, overuse and pressure multiple sites

● M71   Other bursopathies
   Excludes1   bunion (M20.1)
         bursitis related to use, overuse or pressure (M70.-)
         enthesopathies (M76-M77)
● M71.0   Abscess of bursa
    Use additional code (B95.-, B96.-) to identify causative organism
   M71.00   Abscess of bursa, unspecified site
● M71.01   Abscess of bursa, shoulder
    M71.011   Abscess of bursa, right shoulder
    M71.012   Abscess of bursa, left shoulder
    M71.019   Abscess of bursa, unspecified shoulder
● M71.02   Abscess of bursa, elbow
    M71.021   Abscess of bursa, right elbow
    M71.022   Abscess of bursa, left elbow
    M71.029   Abscess of bursa, unspecified elbow
● M71.03   Abscess of bursa, wrist
    M71.031   Abscess of bursa, right wrist
    M71.032   Abscess of bursa, left wrist
    M71.039   Abscess of bursa, unspecified wrist
● M71.04   Abscess of bursa, hand
    M71.041   Abscess of bursa, right hand
    M71.042   Abscess of bursa, left hand
    M71.049   Abscess of bursa, unspecified hand

● M71.05   Abscess of bursa, hip
     M71.051   Abscess of bursa, right hip
     M71.052   Abscess of bursa, left hip
     M71.059   Abscess of bursa, unspecified hip

● M71.06   Abscess of bursa, knee
     M71.061   Abscess of bursa, right knee
     M71.062   Abscess of bursa, left knee
     M71.069   Abscess of bursa, unspecified knee

● M71.07   Abscess of bursa, ankle and foot
     M71.071   Abscess of bursa, right ankle and foot
     M71.072   Abscess of bursa, left ankle and foot
     M71.079   Abscess of bursa, unspecified ankle and foot

     M71.08   Abscess of bursa, other site
     M71.09   Abscess of bursa, multiple sites

● M71.1   Other infective bursitis
     Use additional code (B95.-, B96.-) to identify causative organism
     M71.10   Other infective bursitis, unspecified site

● M71.11   Other infective bursitis, shoulder
     M71.111   Other infective bursitis, right shoulder
     M71.112   Other infective bursitis, left shoulder
     M71.119   Other infective bursitis, unspecified shoulder

● M71.12   Other infective bursitis, elbow
     M71.121   Other infective bursitis, right elbow
     M71.122   Other infective bursitis, left elbow
     M71.129   Other infective bursitis, unspecified elbow

● M71.13   Other infective bursitis, wrist
     M71.131   Other infective bursitis, right wrist
     M71.132   Other infective bursitis, left wrist
     M71.139   Other infective bursitis, unspecified wrist

● M71.14   Other infective bursitis, hand
     M71.141   Other infective bursitis, right hand
     M71.142   Other infective bursitis, left hand
     M71.149   Other infective bursitis, unspecified hand

● M71.15   Other infective bursitis, hip
     M71.151   Other infective bursitis, right hip
     M71.152   Other infective bursitis, left hip
     M71.159   Other infective bursitis, unspecified hip

● M71.16   Other infective bursitis, knee
     M71.161   Other infective bursitis, right knee
     M71.162   Other infective bursitis, left knee
     M71.169   Other infective bursitis, unspecified knee

● M71.17   Other infective bursitis, ankle and foot
     M71.171   Other infective bursitis, right ankle and foot
     M71.172   Other infective bursitis, left ankle and foot
     M71.179   Other infective bursitis, unspecified ankle and foot

     M71.18   Other infective bursitis, other site
     M71.19   Other infective bursitis, multiple sites

● M71.2   Synovial cyst of popliteal space [Baker]
     Popliteal space = popliteal cavity, popliteal fossa. Depression in the posterior aspect of the knee (behind the knee).
     Excludes1   synovial cyst of popliteal space with rupture (M66.0)
     M71.20   Synovial cyst of popliteal space [Baker], unspecified knee
     M71.21   Synovial cyst of popliteal space [Baker], right knee
     M71.22   Synovial cyst of popliteal space [Baker], left knee

● M71.3   Other bursal cyst
     Synovial cyst NOS
     Excludes1   synovial cyst with rupture (M66.1-)
     M71.30   Other bursal cyst, unspecified site

● M71.31   Other bursal cyst, shoulder
     M71.311   Other bursal cyst, right shoulder
     M71.312   Other bursal cyst, left shoulder
     M71.319   Other bursal cyst, unspecified shoulder

● M71.32   Other bursal cyst, elbow
     M71.321   Other bursal cyst, right elbow
     M71.322   Other bursal cyst, left elbow
     M71.329   Other bursal cyst, unspecified elbow

● M71.33   Other bursal cyst, wrist
     M71.331   Other bursal cyst, right wrist
     M71.332   Other bursal cyst, left wrist
     M71.339   Other bursal cyst, unspecified wrist

● M71.34   Other bursal cyst, hand
     M71.341   Other bursal cyst, right hand
     M71.342   Other bursal cyst, left hand
     M71.349   Other bursal cyst, unspecified hand

● M71.35   Other bursal cyst, hip
     M71.351   Other bursal cyst, right hip
     M71.352   Other bursal cyst, left hip
     M71.359   Other bursal cyst, unspecified hip

● M71.37   Other bursal cyst, ankle and foot
     M71.371   Other bursal cyst, right ankle and foot
     M71.372   Other bursal cyst, left ankle and foot
     M71.379   Other bursal cyst, unspecified ankle and foot

     M71.38   Other bursal cyst, other site
     M71.39   Other bursal cyst, multiple sites

● M71.4   Calcium deposit in bursa
     Excludes2   calcium deposit in bursa of shoulder (M75.3)
     M71.40   Calcium deposit in bursa, unspecified site

● M71.42   Calcium deposit in bursa, elbow
     M71.421   Calcium deposit in bursa, right elbow
     M71.422   Calcium deposit in bursa, left elbow
     M71.429   Calcium deposit in bursa, unspecified elbow

● M71.43   Calcium deposit in bursa, wrist
     M71.431   Calcium deposit in bursa, right wrist
     M71.432   Calcium deposit in bursa, left wrist
     M71.439   Calcium deposit in bursa, unspecified wrist

● M71.44   Calcium deposit in bursa, hand
     M71.441   Calcium deposit in bursa, right hand
     M71.442   Calcium deposit in bursa, left hand
     M71.449   Calcium deposit in bursa, unspecified hand

CHAPTER 13 (M00-M99)

● M71.45 Calcium deposit in bursa, hip
  M71.451 Calcium deposit in bursa, right hip
  M71.452 Calcium deposit in bursa, left hip
  M71.459 Calcium deposit in bursa, unspecified hip
● M71.46 Calcium deposit in bursa, knee
  M71.461 Calcium deposit in bursa, right knee
  M71.462 Calcium deposit in bursa, left knee
  M71.469 Calcium deposit in bursa, unspecified knee
● M71.47 Calcium deposit in bursa, ankle and foot
  M71.471 Calcium deposit in bursa, right ankle and foot
  M71.472 Calcium deposit in bursa, left ankle and foot
  M71.479 Calcium deposit in bursa, unspecified ankle and foot
 M71.48 Calcium deposit in bursa, other site
 M71.49 Calcium deposit in bursa, multiple sites
● M71.5 Other bursitis, not elsewhere classified
  Excludes1 bursitis NOS (M71.9-)
  Excludes2 bursitis of shoulder (M75.5)
    bursitis of tibial collateral [Pellegrini-Stieda] (M76.4-) ◀▥
 M71.50 Other bursitis, not elsewhere classified, unspecified site
● M71.52 Other bursitis, not elsewhere classified, elbow
  M71.521 Other bursitis, not elsewhere classified, right elbow
  M71.522 Other bursitis, not elsewhere classified, left elbow
  M71.529 Other bursitis, not elsewhere classified, unspecified elbow
● M71.53 Other bursitis, not elsewhere classified, wrist
  M71.531 Other bursitis, not elsewhere classified, right wrist
  M71.532 Other bursitis, not elsewhere classified, left wrist
  M71.539 Other bursitis, not elsewhere classified, unspecified wrist
● M71.54 Other bursitis, not elsewhere classified, hand
  M71.541 Other bursitis, not elsewhere classified, right hand
  M71.542 Other bursitis, not elsewhere classified, left hand
  M71.549 Other bursitis, not elsewhere classified, unspecified hand
● M71.55 Other bursitis, not elsewhere classified, hip
  M71.551 Other bursitis, not elsewhere classified, right hip
  M71.552 Other bursitis, not elsewhere classified, left hip
  M71.559 Other bursitis, not elsewhere classified, unspecified hip
● M71.56 Other bursitis, not elsewhere classified, knee
  M71.561 Other bursitis, not elsewhere classified, right knee
  M71.562 Other bursitis, not elsewhere classified, left knee
  M71.569 Other bursitis, not elsewhere classified, unspecified knee

● M71.57 Other bursitis, not elsewhere classified, ankle and foot
  M71.571 Other bursitis, not elsewhere classified, right ankle and foot
  M71.572 Other bursitis, not elsewhere classified, left ankle and foot
  M71.579 Other bursitis, not elsewhere classified, unspecified ankle and foot
 M71.58 Other bursitis, not elsewhere classified, other site
● M71.8 Other specified bursopathies
 M71.80 Other specified bursopathies, unspecified site
● M71.81 Other specified bursopathies, shoulder
  M71.811 Other specified bursopathies, right shoulder
  M71.812 Other specified bursopathies, left shoulder
  M71.819 Other specified bursopathies, unspecified shoulder
● M71.82 Other specified bursopathies, elbow
  M71.821 Other specified bursopathies, right elbow
  M71.822 Other specified bursopathies, left elbow
  M71.829 Other specified bursopathies, unspecified elbow
● M71.83 Other specified bursopathies, wrist
  M71.831 Other specified bursopathies, right wrist
  M71.832 Other specified bursopathies, left wrist
  M71.839 Other specified bursopathies, unspecified wrist
● M71.84 Other specified bursopathies, hand
  M71.841 Other specified bursopathies, right hand
  M71.842 Other specified bursopathies, left hand
  M71.849 Other specified bursopathies, unspecified hand
● M71.85 Other specified bursopathies, hip
  M71.851 Other specified bursopathies, right hip
  M71.852 Other specified bursopathies, left hip
  M71.859 Other specified bursopathies, unspecified hip
● M71.86 Other specified bursopathies, knee
  M71.861 Other specified bursopathies, right knee
  M71.862 Other specified bursopathies, left knee
  M71.869 Other specified bursopathies, unspecified knee
● M71.87 Other specified bursopathies, ankle and foot
  M71.871 Other specified bursopathies, right ankle and foot
  M71.872 Other specified bursopathies, left ankle and foot
  M71.879 Other specified bursopathies, unspecified ankle and foot
 M71.88 Other specified bursopathies, other site
 M71.89 Other specified bursopathies, multiple sites
M71.9 Bursopathy, unspecified
 Bursitis NOS

◀ New ◀▥ Revised ~~deleted~~ Deleted Excludes 1 Excludes 2 Includes Use additional Code first Code also Unspecified
OGCR Official Guidelines X Assign placeholder X ● Use Additional Character(s) ▶ Manifestation Code **Coding Clinic**

● **M72 Fibroblastic disorders**

    Excludes2   retroperitoneal fibromatosis (D48.3)

  M72.0 **Palmar fascial fibromatosis [Dupuytren]**   A

  M72.1 **Knuckle pads**

  M72.2 **Plantar fascial fibromatosis**
        Plantar fasciitis

  M72.4 **Pseudosarcomatous fibromatosis**
        Nodular fasciitis

  M72.6 **Necrotizing fasciitis**
        Use additional code (B95.-, B96.-) to identify causative organism

  M72.8 **Other fibroblastic disorders**
        Abscess of fascia
        Fasciitis NEC
        Other infective fasciitis
        Use additional code to (B95.-, B96.-) identify causative organism

        Excludes1   diffuse (eosinophilic) fasciitis (M35.4)
                   necrotizing fasciitis (M72.6)
                   nodular fasciitis (M72.4)
                   perirenal fasciitis NOS (N13.5)
                   perirenal fasciitis with infection (N13.6)
                   plantar fasciitis (M72.2)

  M72.9 **Fibroblastic disorder, unspecified**
        Fasciitis NOS
        Fibromatosis NOS

● **M75 Shoulder lesions**

    Excludes2   shoulder-hand syndrome (M89.0-)

  ● **M75.0 Adhesive capsulitis of shoulder**
        Frozen shoulder
        Periarthritis of shoulder

    M75.00 **Adhesive capsulitis of unspecified shoulder**

    M75.01 **Adhesive capsulitis of right shoulder**

    M75.02 **Adhesive capsulitis of left shoulder**
        Coding Clinic: 2015, Q2, P23

  ● **M75.1 Rotator cuff tear or rupture, not specified as traumatic**
        Rotator cuff syndrome
        Supraspinatus syndrome
        Supraspinatus tear or rupture, not specified as traumatic

        Excludes1   tear of rotator cuff, traumatic (S46.01-)

        Gradual onset due to repetitive stress to rotator cuff

    ● **M75.10 Unspecified rotator cuff tear or rupture, not specified as traumatic**

        M75.100 **Unspecified rotator cuff tear or rupture of unspecified shoulder, not specified as traumatic**

        M75.101 **Unspecified rotator cuff tear or rupture of right shoulder, not specified as traumatic**

        M75.102 **Unspecified rotator cuff tear or rupture of left shoulder, not specified as traumatic**

    ● **M75.11 Incomplete rotator cuff tear or rupture not specified as traumatic**

        M75.110 **Incomplete rotator cuff tear or rupture of unspecified shoulder, not specified as traumatic**

        M75.111 **Incomplete rotator cuff tear or rupture of right shoulder, not specified as traumatic**

        M75.112 **Incomplete rotator cuff tear or rupture of left shoulder, not specified as traumatic**

  ● **M75.12 Complete rotator cuff tear or rupture not specified as traumatic**

        M75.120 **Complete rotator cuff tear or rupture of unspecified shoulder, not specified as traumatic**

        M75.121 **Complete rotator cuff tear or rupture of right shoulder, not specified as traumatic**

        M75.122 **Complete rotator cuff tear or rupture of left shoulder, not specified as traumatic**

  ● **M75.2 Bicipital tendinitis**

    M75.20 **Bicipital tendinitis, unspecified shoulder**

    M75.21 **Bicipital tendinitis, right shoulder**

    M75.22 **Bicipital tendinitis, left shoulder**

  ● **M75.3 Calcific tendinitis of shoulder**
        Calcified bursa of shoulder

    M75.30 **Calcific tendinitis of unspecified shoulder**

    M75.31 **Calcific tendinitis of right shoulder**

    M75.32 **Calcific tendinitis of left shoulder**

  ● **M75.4 Impingement syndrome of shoulder**

    M75.40 **Impingement syndrome of unspecified shoulder**

    M75.41 **Impingement syndrome of right shoulder**

    M75.42 **Impingement syndrome of left shoulder**

  ● **M75.5 Bursitis of shoulder**

    M75.50 **Bursitis of unspecified shoulder**

    M75.51 **Bursitis of right shoulder**

    M75.52 **Bursitis of left shoulder**

  ● **M75.8 Other shoulder lesions**

    M75.80 **Other shoulder lesions, unspecified shoulder**

    M75.81 **Other shoulder lesions, right shoulder**

    M75.82 **Other shoulder lesions, left shoulder**

  ● **M75.9 Shoulder lesion, unspecified**

    M75.90 **Shoulder lesion, unspecified, unspecified shoulder**

    M75.91 **Shoulder lesion, unspecified, right shoulder**

    M75.92 **Shoulder lesion, unspecified, left shoulder**

● **M76 Enthesopathies, lower limb, excluding foot**

    Excludes2   bursitis due to use, overuse and pressure (M70.-)
                   enthesopathies of ankle and foot (M77.5-)

  ● **M76.0 Gluteal tendinitis**

    M76.00 **Gluteal tendinitis, unspecified hip**

    M76.01 **Gluteal tendinitis, right hip**

    M76.02 **Gluteal tendinitis, left hip**

  ● **M76.1 Psoas tendinitis**

    M76.10 **Psoas tendinitis, unspecified hip**

    M76.11 **Psoas tendinitis, right hip**

    M76.12 **Psoas tendinitis, left hip**

  ● **M76.2 Iliac crest spur**

    M76.20 **Iliac crest spur, unspecified hip**

    M76.21 **Iliac crest spur, right hip**

    M76.22 **Iliac crest spur, left hip**

  ● **M76.3 Iliotibial band syndrome**

    M76.30 **Iliotibial band syndrome, unspecified leg**

    M76.31 **Iliotibial band syndrome, right leg**

    M76.32 **Iliotibial band syndrome, left leg**

  ● **M76.4 Tibial collateral bursitis [Pellegrini-Stieda]**

    M76.40 **Tibial collateral bursitis [Pellegrini-Stieda], unspecified leg**

    M76.41 **Tibial collateral bursitis [Pellegrini-Stieda], right leg**

    M76.42 **Tibial collateral bursitis [Pellegrini-Stieda], left leg**

CHAPTER 13 (M00-M99)

● M76.5 Patellar tendinitis
  M76.50 Patellar tendinitis, unspecified knee
  M76.51 Patellar tendinitis, right knee
  M76.52 Patellar tendinitis, left knee
● M76.6 Achilles tendinitis
    Achilles bursitis
  M76.60 Achilles tendinitis, unspecified leg
  M76.61 Achilles tendinitis, right leg
  M76.62 Achilles tendinitis, left leg
● M76.7 Peroneal tendinitis
  M76.70 Peroneal tendinitis, unspecified leg
  M76.71 Peroneal tendinitis, right leg
  M76.72 Peroneal tendinitis, left leg
● M76.8 Other specified enthesopathies of lower limb, excluding foot
  ● M76.81 Anterior tibial syndrome
    M76.811 Anterior tibial syndrome, right leg
    M76.812 Anterior tibial syndrome, left leg
    M76.819 Anterior tibial syndrome, unspecified leg
  ● M76.82 Posterior tibial tendinitis
    M76.821 Posterior tibial tendinitis, right leg
    M76.822 Posterior tibial tendinitis, left leg
    M76.829 Posterior tibial tendinitis, unspecified leg
  ● M76.89 Other specified enthesopathies of lower limb, excluding foot
    M76.891 Other specified enthesopathies of right lower limb, excluding foot
    M76.892 Other specified enthesopathies of left lower limb, excluding foot
    M76.899 Other specified enthesopathies of unspecified lower limb, excluding foot
  M76.9 Unspecified enthesopathy, lower limb, excluding foot
● M77 Other enthesopathies
    Excludes1   bursitis NOS (M71.9-)
    Excludes2   bursitis due to use, overuse and pressure (M70.-)
                osteophyte (M25.7)
                spinal enthesopathy (M46.0-)
  ● M77.0 Medial epicondylitis
    M77.00 Medial epicondylitis, unspecified elbow
    M77.01 Medial epicondylitis, right elbow
    M77.02 Medial epicondylitis, left elbow
  ● M77.1 Lateral epicondylitis
      Tennis elbow
    M77.10 Lateral epicondylitis, unspecified elbow
    M77.11 Lateral epicondylitis, right elbow
    M77.12 Lateral epicondylitis, left elbow
  ● M77.2 Periarthritis of wrist
    M77.20 Periarthritis, unspecified wrist
    M77.21 Periarthritis, right wrist
    M77.22 Periarthritis, left wrist
  ● M77.3 Calcaneal spur
    M77.30 Calcaneal spur, unspecified foot
    M77.31 Calcaneal spur, right foot
    M77.32 Calcaneal spur, left foot
  ● M77.4 Metatarsalgia
      Excludes1   Morton's metatarsalgia (G57.6)
    M77.40 Metatarsalgia, unspecified foot
    M77.41 Metatarsalgia, right foot
    M77.42 Metatarsalgia, left foot

● M77.5 Other enthesopathy of foot
  M77.50 Other enthesopathy of unspecified foot
  M77.51 Other enthesopathy of right foot
  M77.52 Other enthesopathy of left foot
M77.8 Other enthesopathies, not elsewhere classified
M77.9 Enthesopathy, unspecified
    Bone spur NOS
    Capsulitis NOS
    Periarthritis NOS
    Tendinitis NOS
● M79 Other and unspecified soft tissue disorders, not elsewhere classified
    Excludes1   psychogenic rheumatism (F45.8)
                soft tissue pain, psychogenic (F45.41)
  M79.0 Rheumatism, unspecified
    Excludes1   fibromyalgia (M79.7)
                palindromic rheumatism (M12.3-)
  M79.1 Myalgia
      Myofascial pain syndrome
    Excludes1   fibromyalgia (M79.7)
                myositis (M60.-)
  M79.2 Neuralgia and neuritis, unspecified
    Excludes1   brachial radiculitis NOS (M54.1)
                lumbosacral radiculitis NOS (M54.1)
                mononeuropathies (G56-G58)
                radiculitis NOS (M54.1)
                sciatica (M54.3-M54.4)
  M79.3 Panniculitis, unspecified
    Excludes1   lupus panniculitis (L93.2)
                neck and back panniculitis (M54.0-)
                relapsing [Weber-Christian] panniculitis (M35.6)
  M79.4 Hypertrophy of (infrapatellar) fat pad
  M79.5 Residual foreign body in soft tissue
    Excludes1   foreign body granuloma of skin and subcutaneous tissue (L92.3)
                foreign body granuloma of soft tissue (M60.2-)
  ● M79.6 Pain in limb, hand, foot, fingers and toes
      Excludes2   pain in joint (M25.5-)
    ● M79.60 Pain in limb, unspecified
      M79.601 Pain in right arm
          Pain in right upper limb NOS
      M79.602 Pain in left arm
          Pain in left upper limb NOS
      M79.603 Pain in arm, unspecified
          Pain in upper limb NOS
      M79.604 Pain in right leg
          Pain in right lower limb NOS
      M79.605 Pain in left leg
          Pain in left lower limb NOS
      M79.606 Pain in leg, unspecified
          Pain in lower limb NOS
      M79.609 Pain in unspecified limb
          Pain in limb NOS
    ● M79.62 Pain in upper arm
          Pain in axillary region
      M79.621 Pain in right upper arm
      M79.622 Pain in left upper arm
      M79.629 Pain in unspecified upper arm
    ● M79.63 Pain in forearm
      M79.631 Pain in right forearm
      M79.632 Pain in left forearm
      M79.639 Pain in unspecified forearm

◀ New   ◀▥ Revised   d̶e̶l̶e̶t̶e̶d̶ Deleted   Excludes 1   Excludes 2   Includes   Use additional   Code first   Code also   Unspecified
OGCR Official Guidelines   X Assign placeholder X   ● Use Additional Character(s)   ▶ Manifestation Code   Coding Clinic

● M79.64   **Pain in hand and fingers**
    M79.641   **Pain in right hand**
    M79.642   **Pain in left hand**
    M79.643   **Pain in unspecified hand**
    M79.644   **Pain in right finger(s)**
    M79.645   **Pain in left finger(s)**
    M79.646   **Pain in unspecified finger(s)**
● M79.65   **Pain in thigh**
    M79.651   **Pain in right thigh**
    M79.652   **Pain in left thigh**
    M79.659   **Pain in unspecified thigh**
● M79.66   **Pain in lower leg**
    M79.661   **Pain in right lower leg**
    M79.662   **Pain in left lower leg**
    M79.669   **Pain in unspecified lower leg**
● M79.67   **Pain in foot and toes**
    M79.671   **Pain in right foot**
    M79.672   **Pain in left foot**
    M79.673   **Pain in unspecified foot**
    M79.674   **Pain in right toe(s)**
    M79.675   **Pain in left toe(s)**
    M79.676   **Pain in unspecified toe(s)**

M79.7   **Fibromyalgia**
    Fibromyositis
    Fibrositis
    Myofibrositis

● M79.A **Nontraumatic compartment syndrome**
    Code first, if applicable, associated postprocedural complication
    Excludes1   compartment syndrome NOS (T79.A-)
            fibromyalgia (M79.7) nontraumatic ischemic infarction of muscle (M62.2-)
            traumatic compartment syndrome (T79.A-)

● M79.A1 **Nontraumatic compartment syndrome of upper extremity**
    Nontraumatic compartment syndrome of shoulder, arm, forearm, wrist, hand, and fingers
    M79.A11   **Nontraumatic compartment syndrome of right upper extremity**
    M79.A12   **Nontraumatic compartment syndrome of left upper extremity**
    M79.A19   **Nontraumatic compartment syndrome of unspecified upper extremity**

● M79.A2 **Nontraumatic compartment syndrome of lower extremity**
    Nontraumatic compartment syndrome of hip, buttock, thigh, leg, foot, and toes
    M79.A21   **Nontraumatic compartment syndrome of right lower extremity**
    M79.A22   **Nontraumatic compartment syndrome of left lower extremity**
    M79.A29   **Nontraumatic compartment syndrome of unspecified lower extremity**

M79.A3   **Nontraumatic compartment syndrome of abdomen**
M79.A9   **Nontraumatic compartment syndrome of other sites**

● M79.8 **Other specified soft tissue disorders**
    M79.81   **Nontraumatic hematoma of soft tissue**
        Nontraumatic hematoma of muscle
        Nontraumatic seroma of muscle and soft tissue
    M79.89   **Other specified soft tissue disorders**
        Polyalgia

M79.9   **Soft tissue disorder, unspecified**

OGCR See Section I.C., Chapter 13.d.

Osteoporosis

Osteoporosis is a systemic condition, meaning that all bones of the musculoskeletal system are affected. Therefore, site is not a component of the codes under category M81, Osteoporosis without current pathological fracture. The site codes under category M80, Osteoporosis with current pathological fracture, identify the site of the fracture, not the osteoporosis.

1) Osteoporosis without pathological fracture

Category M81, Osteoporosis without current pathological fracture, is for use for patients with osteoporosis who do not currently have a pathologic fracture due to the osteoporosis, even if they have had a fracture in the past. For patients with a history of osteoporosis fractures, status code Z87.310, Personal history of (healed) osteoporosis fracture, should follow the code from M81.

2) Osteoporosis with current pathological fracture

Category M80, Osteoporosis with current pathological fracture, is for patients who have a current pathologic fracture at the time of an encounter. The codes under M80 identify the site of the fracture. A code from category M80, not a traumatic fracture code, should be used for any patient with known osteoporosis who suffers a fracture, even if the patient had a minor fall or trauma, if that fall or trauma would not usually break a normal, healthy bone.

OSTEOPATHIES AND CHONDROPATHIES (M80-M94)

DISORDERS OF BONE DENSITY AND STRUCTURE (M80-M85)

M80   **Osteoporosis with current pathological fracture**
    Excessive skeletal fragility (porous bone) resulting in bone fractures
    Includes   osteoporosis with current fragility fracture
    Use additional code to identify major osseous defect, if applicable (M89.7-)
    Excludes1   collapsed vertebra NOS (M48.5)
            pathological fracture NOS (M84.4)
            wedging of vertebra NOS (M48.5)
    Excludes2   personal history of (healed) osteoporosis fracture (Z87.310)
    The appropriate 7th character is to be added to each code from category M80:

A	initial encounter for fracture *All encounters involving diagnosis and treatment*
D	subsequent encounter for fracture with routine healing
G	subsequent encounter for fracture with delayed healing *Encounters for attention to casting or fixation devices, medication, and follow-up visits during the healing phase*
K	subsequent encounter for fracture with nonunion *Total failure of fracture healing*
P	subsequent encounter for fracture with malunion *Fracture ends do not heal together correctly.*
S	sequela

● M80.0 **Age-related osteoporosis with current pathological fracture**
    Involutional osteoporosis with current pathological fracture
    Osteoporosis NOS with current pathological fracture
    Postmenopausal osteoporosis with current pathological fracture
    Senile osteoporosis with current pathological fracture
  X ● M80.00   **Age-related osteoporosis with current pathological fracture, unspecified site**   A
    ● M80.01   **Age-related osteoporosis with current pathological fracture, shoulder**
      ● M80.011   **Age-related osteoporosis with current pathological fracture, right shoulder** A
      ● M80.012   **Age-related osteoporosis with current pathological fracture, left shoulder** A
      ● M80.019   **Age-related osteoporosis with current pathological fracture, unspecified shoulder** A

CHAPTER 13 (M00-M99)

● **M80.02**   **Age-related osteoporosis with current pathological fracture, humerus**
- ● **M80.021**   Age-related osteoporosis with current pathological fracture, right humerus   A
- ● **M80.022**   Age-related osteoporosis with current pathological fracture, left humerus   A
- ● **M80.029**   Age-related osteoporosis with current pathological fracture, unspecified humerus   A

● **M80.03**   **Age-related osteoporosis with current pathological fracture, forearm**
    Age-related osteoporosis with current pathological fracture of wrist
- ● **M80.031**   Age-related osteoporosis with current pathological fracture, right forearm   A
- ● **M80.032**   Age-related osteoporosis with current pathological fracture, left forearm   A
- ● **M80.039**   Age-related osteoporosis with current pathological fracture, unspecified forearm   A

● **M80.04**   **Age-related osteoporosis with current pathological fracture, hand**
- ● **M80.041**   Age-related osteoporosis with current pathological fracture, right hand   A
- ● **M80.042**   Age-related osteoporosis with current pathological fracture, left hand   A
- ● **M80.049**   Age-related osteoporosis with current pathological fracture, unspecified hand   A

● **M80.05**   **Age-related osteoporosis with current pathological fracture, femur**
    Age-related osteoporosis with current pathological fracture of hip
- ● **M80.051**   Age-related osteoporosis with current pathological fracture, right femur   A
- ● **M80.052**   Age-related osteoporosis with current pathological fracture, left femur   A
- ● **M80.059**   Age-related osteoporosis with current pathological fracture, unspecified femur   A

● **M80.06**   **Age-related osteoporosis with current pathological fracture, lower leg**
- ● **M80.061**   Age-related osteoporosis with current pathological fracture, right lower leg   A
- ● **M80.062**   Age-related osteoporosis with current pathological fracture, left lower leg   A
- ● **M80.069**   Age-related osteoporosis with current pathological fracture, unspecified lower leg   A

● **M80.07**   **Age-related osteoporosis with current pathological fracture, ankle and foot**
- ● **M80.071**   Age-related osteoporosis with current pathological fracture, right ankle and foot   A
- ● **M80.072**   Age-related osteoporosis with current pathological fracture, left ankle and foot   A
- ● **M80.079**   Age-related osteoporosis with current pathological fracture, unspecified ankle and foot   A

X ● **M80.08**   **Age-related osteoporosis with current pathological fracture, vertebra(e)**   A

● **M80.8**   **Other osteoporosis with current pathological fracture**
    Drug-induced osteoporosis with current pathological fracture
    Idiopathic osteoporosis with current pathological fracture
    Osteoporosis of disuse with current pathological fracture
    Postoophorectomy osteoporosis with current pathological fracture
    Postsurgical malabsorption osteoporosis with current pathological fracture
    Post-traumatic osteoporosis with current pathological fracture
    Use additional code for adverse effect, if applicable, to identify drug (T36-T50 with fifth or sixth character 5)

X ● **M80.80**   Other osteoporosis with current pathological fracture, unspecified site   A

● **M80.81**   **Other osteoporosis with pathological fracture, shoulder**
- ● **M80.811**   Other osteoporosis with current pathological fracture, right shoulder
- ● **M80.812**   Other osteoporosis with current pathological fracture, left shoulder
- ● **M80.819**   Other osteoporosis with current pathological fracture, unspecified shoulder

● **M80.82**   **Other osteoporosis with current pathological fracture, humerus**
- ● **M80.821**   Other osteoporosis with current pathological fracture, right humerus
- ● **M80.822**   Other osteoporosis with current pathological fracture, left humerus
- ● **M80.829**   Other osteoporosis with current pathological fracture, unspecified humerus

● **M80.83**   **Other osteoporosis with current pathological fracture, forearm**
    Other osteoporosis with current pathological fracture of wrist
- ● **M80.831**   Other osteoporosis with current pathological fracture, right forearm
- ● **M80.832**   Other osteoporosis with current pathological fracture, left forearm
- ● **M80.839**   Other osteoporosis with current pathological fracture, unspecified forearm

● **M80.84**   **Other osteoporosis with current pathological fracture, hand**
- ● **M80.841**   Other osteoporosis with current pathological fracture, right hand
- ● **M80.842**   Other osteoporosis with current pathological fracture, left hand
- ● **M80.849**   Other osteoporosis with current pathological fracture, unspecified hand

● **M80.85**   **Other osteoporosis with current pathological fracture, femur**
    Other osteoporosis with current pathological fracture of hip
- ● **M80.851**   Other osteoporosis with current pathological fracture, right femur
- ● **M80.852**   Other osteoporosis with current pathological fracture, left femur
- ● **M80.859**   Other osteoporosis with current pathological fracture, unspecified femur

◀ New   ◀▥ Revised   ~~deleted~~ Deleted   Excludes 1   Excludes 2   Includes   Use additional   Code first   Code also   Unspecified

1038   OGCR Official Guidelines   X Assign placeholder X   ● Use Additional Character(s)   ▶ Manifestation Code   **Coding Clinic**

● **M80.86**   Other osteoporosis with current pathological fracture, lower leg
  - ● **M80.861**   Other osteoporosis with current pathological fracture, right lower leg
  - ● **M80.862**   Other osteoporosis with current pathological fracture, left lower leg
  - ● **M80.869**   Other osteoporosis with current pathological fracture, unspecified lower leg

● **M80.87**   Other osteoporosis with current pathological fracture, ankle and foot
  - ● **M80.871**   Other osteoporosis with current pathological fracture, right ankle and foot
  - ● **M80.872**   Other osteoporosis with current pathological fracture, left ankle and foot
  - ● **M80.879**   Other osteoporosis with current pathological fracture, unspecified ankle and foot

X ● **M80.88**   Other osteoporosis with current pathological fracture, vertebra(e)

● **M81**   **Osteoporosis without current pathological fracture**
  Use additional code to identify:
  major osseous defect, if applicable (M89.7-)
  personal history of (healed) osteoporosis fracture, if applicable (Z87.310)

  Excludes1   osteoporosis with current pathological fracture (M80.-)
                Sudeck's atrophy (M89.0)

  M81.0   **Age-related osteoporosis without current pathological fracture**   A
  Involutional osteoporosis without current pathological fracture
  Osteoporosis NOS
  Postmenopausal osteoporosis without current pathological fracture
  Senile osteoporosis without current pathological fracture

  M81.6   **Localized osteoporosis [Lequesne]**
     Excludes1   Sudeck's atrophy (M89.0)

  M81.8   **Other osteoporosis without current pathological fracture**
  Drug-induced osteoporosis without current pathological fracture
  Idiopathic osteoporosis without current pathological fracture
  Osteoporosis of disuse without current pathological fracture
  Postoophorectomy osteoporosis without current pathological fracture
  Postsurgical malabsorption osteoporosis without current pathological fracture
  Post-traumatic osteoporosis without current pathological fracture
  Use additional code for adverse effect, if applicable, to identify drug (T36-T50 with fifth or sixth character 5)

● **M83**   **Adult osteomalacia**
  Excludes1   infantile and juvenile osteomalacia (E55.0)
                renal osteodystrophy (N25.0)
                rickets (active) (E55.0)
                rickets (active) sequelae (E64.3)
                vitamin D-resistant osteomalacia (E83.3)
                vitamin D-resistant rickets (active) (E83.3)

  M83.0   **Puerperal osteomalacia** ♀   M
  M83.1   **Senile osteomalacia**   A
  M83.2   **Adult osteomalacia due to malabsorption**   A
  Postsurgical malabsorption osteomalacia in adults
  M83.3   **Adult osteomalacia due to malnutrition**   A
  M83.4   **Aluminum bone disease**

M83.5   **Other drug-induced osteomalacia in adults**   A
Use additional code for adverse effect, if applicable, to identify drug (T36-T50 with fifth or sixth character 5)

M83.8   **Other adult osteomalacia**   A
M83.9   **Adult osteomalacia, unspecified**   A

● **M84**   **Disorder of continuity of bone**
  Excludes2   traumatic fracture of bone-see fracture, by site

  ● **M84.3**   **Stress fracture**
  Fatigue fracture
  March fracture
  Stress fracture NOS
  Stress reaction
  Use additional external cause code(s) to identify the cause of the stress fracture

  Excludes1   pathological fracture NOS (M84.4.-)
             pathological fracture due to osteoporosis (M80.-)
             traumatic fracture (S12.-, S22.-, S32.-, S42.-, S52.-, S62.-, S72.-, S82.-, S92.-)

  Excludes2   personal history of (healed) stress (fatigue) fracture (Z87.312)
             stress fracture of vertebra (M48.4-)

  The appropriate 7th character is to be added to each code from subcategory M84.3:

A	initial encounter for fracture
D	subsequent encounter for fracture with routine healing
G	subsequent encounter for fracture with delayed healing
K	subsequent encounter for fracture with nonunion
P	subsequent encounter for fracture with malunion
S	sequela

  X ● **M84.30**   Stress fracture, unspecified site
  ● **M84.31**   Stress fracture, shoulder
  - ● **M84.311**   Stress fracture, right shoulder
  - ● **M84.312**   Stress fracture, left shoulder
  - ● **M84.319**   Stress fracture, unspecified shoulder
  ● **M84.32**   Stress fracture, humerus
  - ● **M84.321**   Stress fracture, right humerus
  - ● **M84.322**   Stress fracture, left humerus
  - ● **M84.329**   Stress fracture, unspecified humerus
  ● **M84.33**   Stress fracture, ulna and radius
  - ● **M84.331**   Stress fracture, right ulna
  - ● **M84.332**   Stress fracture, left ulna
  - ● **M84.333**   Stress fracture, right radius
  - ● **M84.334**   Stress fracture, left radius
  - ● **M84.339**   Stress fracture, unspecified ulna and radius
  ● **M84.34**   Stress fracture, hand and fingers
  - ● **M84.341**   Stress fracture, right hand
  - ● **M84.342**   Stress fracture, left hand
  - ● **M84.343**   Stress fracture, unspecified hand
  - ● **M84.344**   Stress fracture, right finger(s)
  - ● **M84.345**   Stress fracture, left finger(s)
  - ● **M84.346**   Stress fracture, unspecified finger(s)
  ● **M84.35**   Stress fracture, pelvis and femur
        Stress fracture, hip
  - ● **M84.350**   Stress fracture, pelvis
  - ● **M84.351**   Stress fracture, right femur
  - ● **M84.352**   Stress fracture, left femur
  - ● **M84.353**   Stress fracture, unspecified femur
  - ● **M84.359**   Stress fracture, hip, unspecified

CHAPTER 13 (M00-M99)

● M84.36 Stress fracture, tibia and fibula
  ● M84.361 Stress fracture, right tibia
  ● M84.362 Stress fracture, left tibia
  ● M84.363 Stress fracture, right fibula
  ● M84.364 Stress fracture, left fibula
  ● M84.369 Stress fracture, unspecified tibia and fibula
● M84.37 Stress fracture, ankle, foot and toes
  ● M84.371 Stress fracture, right ankle
  ● M84.372 Stress fracture, left ankle
  ● M84.373 Stress fracture, unspecified ankle
  ● M84.374 Stress fracture, right foot
  ● M84.375 Stress fracture, left foot
  ● M84.376 Stress fracture, unspecified foot
  ● M84.377 Stress fracture, right toe(s)
  ● M84.378 Stress fracture, left toe(s)
  ● M84.379 Stress fracture, unspecified toe(s)
X ● M84.38 Stress fracture, other site

Excludes2   stress fracture of vertebra (M48.4-)

● M84.4 Pathological fracture, not elsewhere classified
  Chronic fracture
  Pathological fracture NOS

Excludes1   collapsed vertebra NEC (M48.5)
pathological fracture in neoplastic disease (M84.5-)
pathological fracture in osteoporosis (M80.-)
pathological fracture in other disease (M84.6-)
stress fracture (M84.3-)
traumatic fracture (S12.-, S22.-, S32.-, S42.-, S52.-, S62.-, S72.-, S82.-, S92.-)

Excludes2   personal history of (healed) pathological fracture (Z87.311)

The appropriate 7th character is to be added to each code from subcategory M84.4:

A	initial encounter for fracture
D	subsequent encounter for fracture with routine healing
G	subsequent encounter for fracture with delayed healing
K	subsequent encounter for fracture with nonunion
P	subsequent encounter for fracture with malunion
S	sequela

X ● M84.40 Pathological fracture, unspecified site
● M84.41 Pathological fracture, shoulder
  ● M84.411 Pathological fracture, right shoulder
  ● M84.412 Pathological fracture, left shoulder
  ● M84.419 Pathological fracture, unspecified shoulder

● M84.42 Pathological fracture, humerus
  ● M84.421 Pathological fracture, right humerus
  ● M84.422 Pathological fracture, left humerus
  ● M84.429 Pathological fracture, unspecified humerus
● M84.43 Pathological fracture, ulna and radius
  ● M84.431 Pathological fracture, right ulna
  ● M84.432 Pathological fracture, left ulna
  ● M84.433 Pathological fracture, right radius
  ● M84.434 Pathological fracture, left radius
  ● M84.439 Pathological fracture, unspecified ulna and radius
● M84.44 Pathological fracture, hand and fingers
  ● M84.441 Pathological fracture, right hand
  ● M84.442 Pathological fracture, left hand
  ● M84.443 Pathological fracture, unspecified hand
  ● M84.444 Pathological fracture, right finger(s)
  ● M84.445 Pathological fracture, left finger(s)
  ● M84.446 Pathological fracture, unspecified finger(s)
● M84.45 Pathological fracture, femur and pelvis
  ● M84.451 Pathological fracture, right femur
  ● M84.452 Pathological fracture, left femur
  ● M84.453 Pathological fracture, unspecified femur
  ● M84.454 Pathological fracture, pelvis
  ● M84.459 Pathological fracture, hip, unspecified
● M84.46 Pathological fracture, tibia and fibula
  ● M84.461 Pathological fracture, right tibia
  ● M84.462 Pathological fracture, left tibia
  ● M84.463 Pathological fracture, right fibula
  ● M84.464 Pathological fracture, left fibula
  ● M84.469 Pathological fracture, unspecified tibia and fibula
● M84.47 Pathological fracture, ankle, foot and toes
  ● M84.471 Pathological fracture, right ankle
  ● M84.472 Pathological fracture, left ankle
  ● M84.473 Pathological fracture, unspecified ankle
  ● M84.474 Pathological fracture, right foot
  ● M84.475 Pathological fracture, left foot
  ● M84.476 Pathological fracture, unspecified foot
  ● M84.477 Pathological fracture, right toe(s)
  ● M84.478 Pathological fracture, left toe(s)
  ● M84.479 Pathological fracture, unspecified toe(s)
X ● M84.48 Pathological fracture, other site

◄ New   ◄║║║ Revised   deleted Deleted   Excludes 1   Excludes 2   Includes   Use additional   Code first   Code also   Unspecified
OGCR Official Guidelines   X Assign placeholder X   ● Use Additional Character(s)   ▶ Manifestation Code   Coding Clinic

OGCR Section I.a, Chapter 13.C.

Coding of Pathologic Fractures

7th character A is for use as long as the patient is receiving active treatment for the fracture. While the patient may be seen by a new or different provider over the course of treatment for a pathological fracture, assignment of the 7th character is based on whether the patient is undergoing active treatment and not whether the provider is seeing the patient for the first time.3. 7th character, D is to be used for encounters after the patient has completed active treatment. The other 7th characters, listed under each subcategory in the Tabular List, are to be used for subsequent encounters for **routine care of fractures during the healing and recovery phase as well as** treatment of problems associated with the healing, such as malunions, nonunions, and sequelae.

Care for complications of surgical treatment for fracture repairs during the healing or recovery phase should be coded with the appropriate complication codes.

See Section I.C.19. Coding of traumatic fractures.

● **M84.5 Pathological fracture in neoplastic disease**

    Code also underlying neoplasm

    The appropriate 7th character is to be added to each code from subcategory M84.5:

A	initial encounter for fracture
D	subsequent encounter for fracture with routine healing
G	subsequent encounter for fracture with delayed healing
K	subsequent encounter for fracture with nonunion
P	subsequent encounter for fracture with malunion
S	sequela

X ● **M84.50 Pathological fracture in neoplastic disease, unspecified site**

● **M84.51 Pathological fracture in neoplastic disease, shoulder**

    ● **M84.511 Pathological fracture in neoplastic disease, right shoulder**

    ● **M84.512 Pathological fracture in neoplastic disease, left shoulder**

    ● **M84.519 Pathological fracture in neoplastic disease, unspecified shoulder**

● **M84.52 Pathological fracture in neoplastic disease, humerus**

    ● **M84.521 Pathological fracture in neoplastic disease, right humerus**

    ● **M84.522 Pathological fracture in neoplastic disease, left humerus**

    ● **M84.529 Pathological fracture in neoplastic disease, unspecified humerus**

● **M84.53 Pathological fracture in neoplastic disease, ulna and radius**

    ● **M84.531 Pathological fracture in neoplastic disease, right ulna**

    ● **M84.532 Pathological fracture in neoplastic disease, left ulna**

● **M84.533 Pathological fracture in neoplastic disease, right radius**

● **M84.534 Pathological fracture in neoplastic disease, left radius**

● **M84.539 Pathological fracture in neoplastic disease, unspecified ulna and radius**

● **M84.54 Pathological fracture in neoplastic disease, hand**

    ● **M84.541 Pathological fracture in neoplastic disease, right hand**

    ● **M84.542 Pathological fracture in neoplastic disease, left hand**

    ● **M84.549 Pathological fracture in neoplastic disease, unspecified hand**

● **M84.55 Pathological fracture in neoplastic disease, pelvis and femur**

    ● **M84.550 Pathological fracture in neoplastic disease, pelvis**

    ● **M84.551 Pathological fracture in neoplastic disease, right femur**

    ● **M84.552 Pathological fracture in neoplastic disease, left femur**

    ● **M84.553 Pathological fracture in neoplastic disease, unspecified femur**

    ● **M84.559 Pathological fracture in neoplastic disease, hip, unspecified**

● **M84.56 Pathological fracture in neoplastic disease, tibia and fibula**

    ● **M84.561 Pathological fracture in neoplastic disease, right tibia**

    ● **M84.562 Pathological fracture in neoplastic disease, left tibia**

    ● **M84.563 Pathological fracture in neoplastic disease, right fibula**

    ● **M84.564 Pathological fracture in neoplastic disease, left fibula**

    ● **M84.569 Pathological fracture in neoplastic disease, unspecified tibia and fibula**

● **M84.57 Pathological fracture in neoplastic disease, ankle and foot**

    ● **M84.571 Pathological fracture in neoplastic disease, right ankle**

    ● **M84.572 Pathological fracture in neoplastic disease, left ankle**

    ● **M84.573 Pathological fracture in neoplastic disease, unspecified ankle**

    ● **M84.574 Pathological fracture in neoplastic disease, right foot**

    ● **M84.575 Pathological fracture in neoplastic disease, left foot**

    ● **M84.576 Pathological fracture in neoplastic disease, unspecified foot**

X ● **M84.58 Pathological fracture in neoplastic disease, other specified site**

    Pathological fracture in neoplastic disease, vertebrae

CHAPTER 13 (M00-M99)

● **M84.6** **Pathological fracture in other disease**
  Code also underlying condition
  Excludes1 pathological fracture in osteoporosis
                 (M80.-)
  The appropriate 7th character is to be added to each
  code from subcategory M84.6:

A	initial encounter for fracture
D	subsequent encounter for fracture with routine healing
G	subsequent encounter for fracture with delayed healing
K	subsequent encounter for fracture with nonunion
P	subsequent encounter for fracture with malunion
S	sequela

  X ● **M84.60** **Pathological fracture in other disease, unspecified site**
  ● **M84.61** **Pathological fracture in other disease, shoulder**
      ● **M84.611** Pathological fracture in other disease, right shoulder
      ● **M84.612** Pathological fracture in other disease, left shoulder
      ● **M84.619** Pathological fracture in other disease, unspecified shoulder
  ● **M84.62** **Pathological fracture in other disease, humerus**
      ● **M84.621** Pathological fracture in other disease, right humerus
      ● **M84.622** Pathological fracture in other disease, left humerus
      ● **M84.629** Pathological fracture in other disease, unspecified humerus
  ● **M84.63** **Pathological fracture in other disease, ulna and radius**
      ● **M84.631** Pathological fracture in other disease, right ulna
      ● **M84.632** Pathological fracture in other disease, left ulna
      ● **M84.633** Pathological fracture in other disease, right radius
      ● **M84.634** Pathological fracture in other disease, left radius
      ● **M84.639** Pathological fracture in other disease, unspecified ulna and radius
  ● **M84.64** **Pathological fracture in other disease, hand**
      ● **M84.641** Pathological fracture in other disease, right hand
      ● **M84.642** Pathological fracture in other disease, left hand
      ● **M84.649** Pathological fracture in other disease, unspecified hand
  ● **M84.65** **Pathological fracture in other disease, pelvis and femur**
      ● **M84.650** Pathological fracture in other disease, pelvis
      ● **M84.651** Pathological fracture in other disease, right femur
      ● **M84.652** Pathological fracture in other disease, left femur
      ● **M84.653** Pathological fracture in other disease, unspecified femur
      ● **M84.659** Pathological fracture in other disease, hip, unspecified

● **M84.66** **Pathological fracture in other disease, tibia and fibula**
    ● **M84.661** Pathological fracture in other disease, right tibia
    ● **M84.662** Pathological fracture in other disease, left tibia
    ● **M84.663** Pathological fracture in other disease, right fibula
    ● **M84.664** Pathological fracture in other disease, left fibula
    ● **M84.669** Pathological fracture in other disease, unspecified tibia and fibula
● **M84.67** **Pathological fracture in other disease, ankle and foot**
    ● **M84.671** Pathological fracture in other disease, right ankle
    ● **M84.672** Pathological fracture in other disease, left ankle
    ● **M84.673** Pathological fracture in other disease, unspecified ankle
    ● **M84.674** Pathological fracture in other disease, right foot
    ● **M84.675** Pathological fracture in other disease, left foot
    ● **M84.676** Pathological fracture in other disease, unspecified foot
  X ● **M84.68** **Pathological fracture in other disease, other site**
● **M84.7** **Nontraumatic fracture, not elsewhere classified** ◀
  ● **M84.75** **Atypical femoral fracture** ◀
    The appropriate 7th character is to be added to
    each code from M84.75: ◀

A	initial encounter for fracture ◀
D	subsequent encounter for fracture with routine healing ◀
G	subsequent encounter for fracture with delayed healing ◀
K	subsequent encounter for fracture with nonunion ◀
P	subsequent encounter for fracture with malunion ◀
S	sequela ◀

    ● **M84.750** Atypical femoral fracture, unspecified ◀
    ● **M84.751** Incomplete atypical femoral fracture, right leg ◀
    ● **M84.752** Incomplete atypical femoral fracture, left leg ◀
    ● **M84.753** Incomplete atypical femoral fracture, unspecified leg ◀
    ● **M84.754** Complete transverse atypical femoral fracture, right leg ◀
    ● **M84.755** Complete transverse atypical femoral fracture, left leg ◀
    ● **M84.756** Complete transverse atypical femoral fracture, unspecified leg ◀
    ● **M84.757** Complete oblique atypical femoral fracture, right leg ◀
    ● **M84.758** Complete oblique atypical femoral fracture, left leg ◀
    ● **M84.759** Complete oblique atypical femoral fracture, unspecified leg ◀

◀ New   ◀▥ Revised   ~~deleted~~ Deleted   Excludes 1   Excludes 2   Includes   Use additional   Code first   Code also   Unspecified

OGCR Official Guidelines   X Assign placeholder X   ● Use Additional Character(s)   ▶ Manifestation Code   **Coding Clinic**

CHAPTER 13 (M00-M99)

● M84.8   Other disorders of continuity of bone

    M84.80   Other disorders of continuity of bone, unspecified site

   ● M84.81   Other disorders of continuity of bone, shoulder

       M84.811   Other disorders of continuity of bone, right shoulder

       M84.812   Other disorders of continuity of bone, left shoulder

       M84.819   Other disorders of continuity of bone, unspecified shoulder

   ● M84.82   Other disorders of continuity of bone, humerus

       M84.821   Other disorders of continuity of bone, right humerus

       M84.822   Other disorders of continuity of bone, left humerus

       M84.829   Other disorders of continuity of bone, unspecified humerus

   ● M84.83   Other disorders of continuity of bone, ulna and radius

       M84.831   Other disorders of continuity of bone, right ulna

       M84.832   Other disorders of continuity of bone, left ulna

       M84.833   Other disorders of continuity of bone, right radius

       M84.834   Other disorders of continuity of bone, left radius

       M84.839   Other disorders of continuity of bone, unspecified ulna and radius

   ● M84.84   Other disorders of continuity of bone, hand

       M84.841   Other disorders of continuity of bone, right hand

       M84.842   Other disorders of continuity of bone, left hand

       M84.849   Other disorders of continuity of bone, unspecified hand

   ● M84.85   Other disorders of continuity of bone, pelvic region and thigh

       M84.851   Other disorders of continuity of bone, right pelvic region and thigh

       M84.852   Other disorders of continuity of bone, left pelvic region and thigh

       M84.859   Other disorders of continuity of bone, unspecified pelvic region and thigh

   ● M84.86   Other disorders of continuity of bone, tibia and fibula

       M84.861   Other disorders of continuity of bone, right tibia

       M84.862   Other disorders of continuity of bone, left tibia

       M84.863   Other disorders of continuity of bone, right fibula

       M84.864   Other disorders of continuity of bone, left fibula

       M84.869   Other disorders of continuity of bone, unspecified tibia and fibula

   ● M84.87   Other disorders of continuity of bone, ankle and foot

       M84.871   Other disorders of continuity of bone, right ankle and foot

       M84.872   Other disorders of continuity of bone, left ankle and foot

       M84.879   Other disorders of continuity of bone, unspecified ankle and foot

     M84.88   Other disorders of continuity of bone, other site

  M84.9   Disorder of continuity of bone, unspecified

● M85   Other disorders of bone density and structure

    Excludes1   osteogenesis imperfecta (Q78.0)
               osteopetrosis (Q78.2)
               osteopoikilosis (Q78.8)
               polyostotic fibrous dysplasia (Q78.1)

  ● M85.0   Fibrous dysplasia (monostotic)

     Excludes2   fibrous dysplasia of jaw (M27.8)

     M85.00   Fibrous dysplasia (monostotic), unspecified site

   ● M85.01   Fibrous dysplasia (monostotic), shoulder

       M85.011   Fibrous dysplasia (monostotic), right shoulder

       M85.012   Fibrous dysplasia (monostotic), left shoulder

       M85.019   Fibrous dysplasia (monostotic), unspecified shoulder

   ● M85.02   Fibrous dysplasia (monostotic), upper arm

       M85.021   Fibrous dysplasia (monostotic), right upper arm

       M85.022   Fibrous dysplasia (monostotic), left upper arm

       M85.029   Fibrous dysplasia (monostotic), unspecified upper arm

   ● M85.03   Fibrous dysplasia (monostotic), forearm

       M85.031   Fibrous dysplasia (monostotic), right forearm

       M85.032   Fibrous dysplasia (monostotic), left forearm

       M85.039   Fibrous dysplasia (monostotic), unspecified forearm

   ● M85.04   Fibrous dysplasia (monostotic), hand

       M85.041   Fibrous dysplasia (monostotic), right hand

       M85.042   Fibrous dysplasia (monostotic), left hand

       M85.049   Fibrous dysplasia (monostotic), unspecified hand

   ● M85.05   Fibrous dysplasia (monostotic), thigh

       M85.051   Fibrous dysplasia (monostotic), right thigh

       M85.052   Fibrous dysplasia (monostotic), left thigh

       M85.059   Fibrous dysplasia (monostotic), unspecified thigh

   ● M85.06   Fibrous dysplasia (monostotic), lower leg

       M85.061   Fibrous dysplasia (monostotic), right lower leg

       M85.062   Fibrous dysplasia (monostotic), left lower leg

       M85.069   Fibrous dysplasia (monostotic), unspecified lower leg

   ● M85.07   Fibrous dysplasia (monostotic), ankle and foot

       M85.071   Fibrous dysplasia (monostotic), right ankle and foot

       M85.072   Fibrous dysplasia (monostotic), left ankle and foot

       M85.079   Fibrous dysplasia (monostotic), unspecified ankle and foot

     M85.08   Fibrous dysplasia (monostotic), other site

     M85.09   Fibrous dysplasia (monostotic), multiple sites

  ● M85.1   Skeletal fluorosis

     M85.10   Skeletal fluorosis, unspecified site

   ● M85.11   Skeletal fluorosis, shoulder

       M85.111   Skeletal fluorosis, right shoulder

       M85.112   Skeletal fluorosis, left shoulder

       M85.119   Skeletal fluorosis, unspecified shoulder

CHAPTER 13 (M00-M99)

- ● **M85.12** Skeletal fluorosis, upper arm
  - **M85.121** Skeletal fluorosis, right upper arm
  - **M85.122** Skeletal fluorosis, left upper arm
  - **M85.129** Skeletal fluorosis, unspecified upper arm
- ● **M85.13** Skeletal fluorosis, forearm
  - **M85.131** Skeletal fluorosis, right forearm
  - **M85.132** Skeletal fluorosis, left forearm
  - **M85.139** Skeletal fluorosis, unspecified forearm
- ● **M85.14** Skeletal fluorosis, hand
  - **M85.141** Skeletal fluorosis, right hand
  - **M85.142** Skeletal fluorosis, left hand
  - **M85.149** Skeletal fluorosis, unspecified hand
- ● **M85.15** Skeletal fluorosis, thigh
  - **M85.151** Skeletal fluorosis, right thigh
  - **M85.152** Skeletal fluorosis, left thigh
  - **M85.159** Skeletal fluorosis, unspecified thigh
- ● **M85.16** Skeletal fluorosis, lower leg
  - **M85.161** Skeletal fluorosis, right lower leg
  - **M85.162** Skeletal fluorosis, left lower leg
  - **M85.169** Skeletal fluorosis, unspecified lower leg
- ● **M85.17** Skeletal fluorosis, ankle and foot
  - **M85.171** Skeletal fluorosis, right ankle and foot
  - **M85.172** Skeletal fluorosis, left ankle and foot
  - **M85.179** Skeletal fluorosis, unspecified ankle and foot
- **M85.18** Skeletal fluorosis, other site
- **M85.19** Skeletal fluorosis, multiple sites
- **M85.2** Hyperostosis of skull
- ● **M85.3** Osteitis condensans
  - **M85.30** Osteitis condensans, unspecified site
- ● **M85.31** Osteitis condensans, shoulder
  - **M85.311** Osteitis condensans, right shoulder
  - **M85.312** Osteitis condensans, left shoulder
  - **M85.319** Osteitis condensans, unspecified shoulder
- ● **M85.32** Osteitis condensans, upper arm
  - **M85.321** Osteitis condensans, right upper arm
  - **M85.322** Osteitis condensans, left upper arm
  - **M85.329** Osteitis condensans, unspecified upper arm
- ● **M85.33** Osteitis condensans, forearm
  - **M85.331** Osteitis condensans, right forearm
  - **M85.332** Osteitis condensans, left forearm
  - **M85.339** Osteitis condensans, unspecified forearm
- ● **M85.34** Osteitis condensans, hand
  - **M85.341** Osteitis condensans, right hand
  - **M85.342** Osteitis condensans, left hand
  - **M85.349** Osteitis condensans, unspecified hand
- ● **M85.35** Osteitis condensans, thigh
  - **M85.351** Osteitis condensans, right thigh
  - **M85.352** Osteitis condensans, left thigh
  - **M85.359** Osteitis condensans, unspecified thigh
- ● **M85.36** Osteitis condensans, lower leg
  - **M85.361** Osteitis condensans, right lower leg
  - **M85.362** Osteitis condensans, left lower leg
  - **M85.369** Osteitis condensans, unspecified lower leg

- ● **M85.37** Osteitis condensans, ankle and foot
  - **M85.371** Osteitis condensans, right ankle and foot
  - **M85.372** Osteitis condensans, left ankle and foot
  - **M85.379** Osteitis condensans, unspecified ankle and foot
- **M85.38** Osteitis condensans, other site
- **M85.39** Osteitis condensans, multiple sites
- ● **M85.4** Solitary bone cyst
  - **Excludes2** solitary cyst of jaw (M27.4)
  - **M85.40** Solitary bone cyst, unspecified site
- ● **M85.41** Solitary bone cyst, shoulder
  - **M85.411** Solitary bone cyst, right shoulder
  - **M85.412** Solitary bone cyst, left shoulder
  - **M85.419** Solitary bone cyst, unspecified shoulder
- ● **M85.42** Solitary bone cyst, humerus
  - **M85.421** Solitary bone cyst, right humerus
  - **M85.422** Solitary bone cyst, left humerus
  - **M85.429** Solitary bone cyst, unspecified humerus
- ● **M85.43** Solitary bone cyst, ulna and radius
  - **M85.431** Solitary bone cyst, right ulna and radius
  - **M85.432** Solitary bone cyst, left ulna and radius
  - **M85.439** Solitary bone cyst, unspecified ulna and radius
- ● **M85.44** Solitary bone cyst, hand
  - **M85.441** Solitary bone cyst, right hand
  - **M85.442** Solitary bone cyst, left hand
  - **M85.449** Solitary bone cyst, unspecified hand
- ● **M85.45** Solitary bone cyst, pelvis
  - **M85.451** Solitary bone cyst, right pelvis
  - **M85.452** Solitary bone cyst, left pelvis
  - **M85.459** Solitary bone cyst, unspecified pelvis
- ● **M85.46** Solitary bone cyst, tibia and fibula
  - **M85.461** Solitary bone cyst, right tibia and fibula
  - **M85.462** Solitary bone cyst, left tibia and fibula
  - **M85.469** Solitary bone cyst, unspecified tibia and fibula
- ● **M85.47** Solitary bone cyst, ankle and foot
  - **M85.471** Solitary bone cyst, right ankle and foot
  - **M85.472** Solitary bone cyst, left ankle and foot
  - **M85.479** Solitary bone cyst, unspecified ankle and foot
- **M85.48** Solitary bone cyst, other site
- ● **M85.5** Aneurysmal bone cyst
  - **Excludes2** aneurysmal cyst of jaw (M27.4)
  - **M85.50** Aneurysmal bone cyst, unspecified site
- ● **M85.51** Aneurysmal bone cyst, shoulder
  - **M85.511** Aneurysmal bone cyst, right shoulder
  - **M85.512** Aneurysmal bone cyst, left shoulder
  - **M85.519** Aneurysmal bone cyst, unspecified shoulder
- ● **M85.52** Aneurysmal bone cyst, upper arm
  - **M85.521** Aneurysmal bone cyst, right upper arm
  - **M85.522** Aneurysmal bone cyst, left upper arm
  - **M85.529** Aneurysmal bone cyst, unspecified upper arm

1044

◀ New ◀▪▪ Revised ~~deleted~~ Deleted Excludes 1 Excludes 2 Includes Use additional Code first Code also Unspecified
OGCR Official Guidelines X Assign placeholder X ● Use Additional Character(s) ▶ Manifestation Code **Coding Clinic**

● M85.53   Aneurysmal bone cyst, forearm
     M85.531   Aneurysmal bone cyst, right forearm
     M85.532   Aneurysmal bone cyst, left forearm
     M85.539   Aneurysmal bone cyst, unspecified forearm
● M85.54   Aneurysmal bone cyst, hand
     M85.541   Aneurysmal bone cyst, right hand
     M85.542   Aneurysmal bone cyst, left hand
     M85.549   Aneurysmal bone cyst, unspecified hand
● M85.55   Aneurysmal bone cyst, thigh
     M85.551   Aneurysmal bone cyst, right thigh
     M85.552   Aneurysmal bone cyst, left thigh
     M85.559   Aneurysmal bone cyst, unspecified thigh
● M85.56   Aneurysmal bone cyst, lower leg
     M85.561   Aneurysmal bone cyst, right lower leg
     M85.562   Aneurysmal bone cyst, left lower leg
     M85.569   Aneurysmal bone cyst, unspecified lower leg
● M85.57   Aneurysmal bone cyst, ankle and foot
     M85.571   Aneurysmal bone cyst, right ankle and foot
     M85.572   Aneurysmal bone cyst, left ankle and foot
     M85.579   Aneurysmal bone cyst, unspecified ankle and foot
   M85.58   Aneurysmal bone cyst, other site
   M85.59   Aneurysmal bone cyst, multiple sites
● M85.6   **Other cyst of bone**
     Excludes1   cyst of jaw NEC (M27.4)
               osteitis fibrosa cystica generalisata [von Recklinghausen's disease of bone] (E21.0)
   M85.60   Other cyst of bone, unspecified site
● M85.61   Other cyst of bone, shoulder
     M85.611   Other cyst of bone, right shoulder
     M85.612   Other cyst of bone, left shoulder
     M85.619   Other cyst of bone, unspecified shoulder
● M85.62   Other cyst of bone, upper arm
     M85.621   Other cyst of bone, right upper arm
     M85.622   Other cyst of bone, left upper arm
     M85.629   Other cyst of bone, unspecified upper arm
● M85.63   Other cyst of bone, forearm
     M85.631   Other cyst of bone, right forearm
     M85.632   Other cyst of bone, left forearm
     M85.639   Other cyst of bone, unspecified forearm
● M85.64   Other cyst of bone, hand
     M85.641   Other cyst of bone, right hand
     M85.642   Other cyst of bone, left hand
     M85.649   Other cyst of bone, unspecified hand
● M85.65   Other cyst of bone, thigh
     M85.651   Other cyst of bone, right thigh
     M85.652   Other cyst of bone, left thigh
     M85.659   Other cyst of bone, unspecified thigh
● M85.66   Other cyst of bone, lower leg
     M85.661   Other cyst of bone, right lower leg
     M85.662   Other cyst of bone, left lower leg
     M85.669   Other cyst of bone, unspecified lower leg

● M85.67   Other cyst of bone, ankle and foot
     M85.671   Other cyst of bone, right ankle and foot
     M85.672   Other cyst of bone, left ankle and foot
     M85.679   Other cyst of bone, unspecified ankle and foot
   M85.68   Other cyst of bone, other site
   M85.69   Other cyst of bone, multiple sites
● M85.8   **Other specified disorders of bone density and structure**
     Hyperostosis of bones, except skull
     Osteosclerosis, acquired
     Excludes1   diffuse idiopathic skeletal hyperostosis [DISH] (M48.1)
               osteosclerosis congenita (Q77.4)
               osteosclerosis fragilitas (generalista) (Q78.2)
               osteosclerosis myelofibrosis (D75.81)
   M85.80   Other specified disorders of bone density and structure, unspecified site
● M85.81   Other specified disorders of bone density and structure, shoulder
     M85.811   Other specified disorders of bone density and structure, right shoulder
     M85.812   Other specified disorders of bone density and structure, left shoulder
     M85.819   Other specified disorders of bone density and structure, unspecified shoulder
● M85.82   Other specified disorders of bone density and structure, upper arm
     M85.821   Other specified disorders of bone density and structure, right upper arm
     M85.822   Other specified disorders of bone density and structure, left upper arm
     M85.829   Other specified disorders of bone density and structure, unspecified upper arm
● M85.83   Other specified disorders of bone density and structure, forearm
     M85.831   Other specified disorders of bone density and structure, right forearm
     M85.832   Other specified disorders of bone density and structure, left forearm
     M85.839   Other specified disorders of bone density and structure, unspecified forearm
● M85.84   Other specified disorders of bone density and structure, hand
     M85.841   Other specified disorders of bone density and structure, right hand
     M85.842   Other specified disorders of bone density and structure, left hand
     M85.849   Other specified disorders of bone density and structure, unspecified hand
● M85.85   Other specified disorders of bone density and structure, thigh
     M85.851   Other specified disorders of bone density and structure, right thigh
     M85.852   Other specified disorders of bone density and structure, left thigh
     M85.859   Other specified disorders of bone density and structure, unspecified thigh

CHAPTER 13 (M00-M99)

● **M85.86** Other specified disorders of bone density and structure, lower leg

  M85.861 Other specified disorders of bone density and structure, right lower leg

  M85.862 Other specified disorders of bone density and structure, left lower leg

  M85.869 Other specified disorders of bone density and structure, unspecified lower leg

● **M85.87** Other specified disorders of bone density and structure, ankle and foot

  M85.871 Other specified disorders of bone density and structure, right ankle and foot

  M85.872 Other specified disorders of bone density and structure, left ankle and foot

  M85.879 Other specified disorders of bone density and structure, unspecified ankle and foot

  M85.88 Other specified disorders of bone density and structure, other site

  M85.89 Other specified disorders of bone density and structure, multiple sites

 M85.9 Disorder of bone density and structure, unspecified

OTHER OSTEOPATHIES (M86-M90)

Excludes1   postprocedural osteopathies (M96.-)

● **M86 Osteomyelitis**

  Use additional code (B95-B97) to identify infectious agent

  Use additional code to identify major osseous defect, if applicable (M89.7-)

  Excludes1   osteomyelitis due to:
    echinococcus (B67.2)
    gonococcus (A54.43)
    salmonella (AØ2.24)

  Excludes2   ostemyelitis of:
    orbit (HØ5.0-)
    petrous bone (H70.2-)
    vertebra (M46.2-)

● **M86.Ø** Acute hematogenous osteomyelitis

  M86.ØØ Acute hematogenous osteomyelitis, unspecified site

● **M86.Ø1** Acute hematogenous osteomyelitis, shoulder

  M86.Ø11 Acute hematogenous osteomyelitis, right shoulder

  M86.Ø12 Acute hematogenous osteomyelitis, left shoulder

  M86.Ø19 Acute hematogenous osteomyelitis, unspecified shoulder

● **M86.Ø2** Acute hematogenous osteomyelitis, humerus

  M86.Ø21 Acute hematogenous osteomyelitis, right humerus

  M86.Ø22 Acute hematogenous osteomyelitis, left humerus

  M86.Ø29 Acute hematogenous osteomyelitis, unspecified humerus

● **M86.Ø3** Acute hematogenous osteomyelitis, radius and ulna

  M86.Ø31 Acute hematogenous osteomyelitis, right radius and ulna

  M86.Ø32 Acute hematogenous osteomyelitis, left radius and ulna

  M86.Ø39 Acute hematogenous osteomyelitis, unspecified radius and ulna

Figure 13-6 Osteomyelitis of the spine. A lateral view of the lower thoracic spine demonstrates destruction of the disk space *(arrow)* as well as destruction of the adjoining vertebral bodies. (From Mettler: Essentials of Radiology, ed 2, Saunders, An Imprint of Elsevier, 2005)

Item 13–12 Osteomyelitis is an inflammation of the bone. **Acute osteomyelitis** is a rapidly destructive, pus-producing infection capable of causing severe bone destruction. **Chronic osteomyelitis** can remain long after the initial acute episode has passed and may lead to a recurrence of the acute phase. **Brodie's abscess** is an encapsulated focal abscess that must be surgically drained. Periostitis is an inflammation of the periosteum, a dense membrane composed of fibrous connective tissue that closely wraps all bone, except those with articulating surfaces in joints, which are covered by synovial membranes.

● **M86.Ø4** Acute hematogenous osteomyelitis, hand

  M86.Ø41 Acute hematogenous osteomyelitis, right hand

  M86.Ø42 Acute hematogenous osteomyelitis, left hand

  M86.Ø49 Acute hematogenous osteomyelitis, unspecified hand

● **M86.Ø5** Acute hematogenous osteomyelitis, femur

  M86.Ø51 Acute hematogenous osteomyelitis, right femur

  M86.Ø52 Acute hematogenous osteomyelitis, left femur

  M86.Ø59 Acute hematogenous osteomyelitis, unspecified femur

● **M86.Ø6** Acute hematogenous osteomyelitis, tibia and fibula

  M86.Ø61 Acute hematogenous osteomyelitis, right tibia and fibula

  M86.Ø62 Acute hematogenous osteomyelitis, left tibia and fibula

  M86.Ø69 Acute hematogenous osteomyelitis, unspecified tibia and fibula

● **M86.Ø7** Acute hematogenous osteomyelitis, ankle and foot

  M86.Ø71 Acute hematogenous osteomyelitis, right ankle and foot

  M86.Ø72 Acute hematogenous osteomyelitis, left ankle and foot

  M86.Ø79 Acute hematogenous osteomyelitis, unspecified ankle and foot

  M86.Ø8 Acute hematogenous osteomyelitis, other sites

  M86.Ø9 Acute hematogenous osteomyelitis, multiple sites

● **M86.1** Other acute osteomyelitis

  M86.1Ø Other acute osteomyelitis, unspecified site

● **M86.11** Other acute osteomyelitis, shoulder

  M86.111 Other acute osteomyelitis, right shoulder

  M86.112 Other acute osteomyelitis, left shoulder

  M86.119 Other acute osteomyelitis, unspecified shoulder

●M86.12   Other acute osteomyelitis, humerus
     M86.121   Other acute osteomyelitis, right humerus
     M86.122   Other acute osteomyelitis, left humerus
     M86.129   Other acute osteomyelitis, unspecified humerus
●M86.13   Other acute osteomyelitis, radius and ulna
     M86.131   Other acute osteomyelitis, right radius and ulna
     M86.132   Other acute osteomyelitis, left radius and ulna
     M86.139   Other acute osteomyelitis, unspecified radius and ulna
●M86.14   Other acute osteomyelitis, hand
     M86.141   Other acute osteomyelitis, right hand
     M86.142   Other acute osteomyelitis, left hand
     M86.149   Other acute osteomyelitis, unspecified hand
●M86.15   Other acute osteomyelitis, femur
     M86.151   Other acute osteomyelitis, right femur
     M86.152   Other acute osteomyelitis, left femur
     M86.159   Other acute osteomyelitis, unspecified femur
●M86.16   Other acute osteomyelitis, tibia and fibula
     M86.161   Other acute osteomyelitis, right tibia and fibula
     M86.162   Other acute osteomyelitis, left tibia and fibula
     M86.169   Other acute osteomyelitis, unspecified tibia and fibula
●M86.17   Other acute osteomyelitis, ankle and foot
     M86.171   Other acute osteomyelitis, right ankle and foot
     M86.172   Other acute osteomyelitis, left ankle and foot
     M86.179   Other acute osteomyelitis, unspecified ankle and foot
     M86.18   Other acute osteomyelitis, other site
     M86.19   Other acute osteomyelitis, multiple sites
●M86.2   Subacute osteomyelitis
     M86.20   Subacute osteomyelitis, unspecified site
●M86.21   Subacute osteomyelitis, shoulder
     M86.211   Subacute osteomyelitis, right shoulder
     M86.212   Subacute osteomyelitis, left shoulder
     M86.219   Subacute osteomyelitis, unspecified shoulder
●M86.22   Subacute osteomyelitis, humerus
     M86.221   Subacute osteomyelitis, right humerus
     M86.222   Subacute osteomyelitis, left humerus
     M86.229   Subacute osteomyelitis, unspecified humerus
●M86.23   Subacute osteomyelitis, radius and ulna
     M86.231   Subacute osteomyelitis, right radius and ulna
     M86.232   Subacute osteomyelitis, left radius and ulna
     M86.239   Subacute osteomyelitis, unspecified radius and ulna
●M86.24   Subacute osteomyelitis, hand
     M86.241   Subacute osteomyelitis, right hand
     M86.242   Subacute osteomyelitis, left hand
     M86.249   Subacute osteomyelitis, unspecified hand

●M86.25   Subacute osteomyelitis, femur
     M86.251   Subacute osteomyelitis, right femur
     M86.252   Subacute osteomyelitis, left femur
     M86.259   Subacute osteomyelitis, unspecified femur
●M86.26   Subacute osteomyelitis, tibia and fibula
     M86.261   Subacute osteomyelitis, right tibia and fibula
     M86.262   Subacute osteomyelitis, left tibia and fibula
     M86.269   Subacute osteomyelitis, unspecified tibia and fibula
●M86.27   Subacute osteomyelitis, ankle and foot
     M86.271   Subacute osteomyelitis, right ankle and foot
     M86.272   Subacute osteomyelitis, left ankle and foot
     M86.279   Subacute osteomyelitis, unspecified ankle and foot
     M86.28   Subacute osteomyelitis, other site
     M86.29   Subacute osteomyelitis, multiple sites
●M86.3   Chronic multifocal osteomyelitis
     M86.30   Chronic multifocal osteomyelitis, unspecified site
●M86.31   Chronic multifocal osteomyelitis, shoulder
     M86.311   Chronic multifocal osteomyelitis, right shoulder
     M86.312   Chronic multifocal osteomyelitis, left shoulder
     M86.319   Chronic multifocal osteomyelitis, unspecified shoulder
●M86.32   Chronic multifocal osteomyelitis, humerus
     M86.321   Chronic multifocal osteomyelitis, right humerus
     M86.322   Chronic multifocal osteomyelitis, left humerus
     M86.329   Chronic multifocal osteomyelitis, unspecified humerus
●M86.33   Chronic multifocal osteomyelitis, radius and ulna
     M86.331   Chronic multifocal osteomyelitis, right radius and ulna
     M86.332   Chronic multifocal osteomyelitis, left radius and ulna
     M86.339   Chronic multifocal osteomyelitis, unspecified radius and ulna
●M86.34   Chronic multifocal osteomyelitis, hand
     M86.341   Chronic multifocal osteomyelitis, right hand
     M86.342   Chronic multifocal osteomyelitis, left hand
     M86.349   Chronic multifocal osteomyelitis, unspecified hand
●M86.35   Chronic multifocal osteomyelitis, femur
     M86.351   Chronic multifocal osteomyelitis, right femur
     M86.352   Chronic multifocal osteomyelitis, left femur
     M86.359   Chronic multifocal osteomyelitis, unspecified femur
●M86.36   Chronic multifocal osteomyelitis, tibia and fibula
     M86.361   Chronic multifocal osteomyelitis, right tibia and fibula
     M86.362   Chronic multifocal osteomyelitis, left tibia and fibula
     M86.369   Chronic multifocal osteomyelitis, unspecified tibia and fibula

CHAPTER 13 (M00-M99)

CHAPTER 13 (M00-M99)

● M86.37   Chronic multifocal osteomyelitis, ankle and foot

     M86.371   Chronic multifocal osteomyelitis, right ankle and foot

     M86.372   Chronic multifocal osteomyelitis, left ankle and foot

     M86.379   Chronic multifocal osteomyelitis, unspecified ankle and foot

   M86.38   Chronic multifocal osteomyelitis, other site

   M86.39   Chronic multifocal osteomyelitis, multiple sites

● M86.4   Chronic osteomyelitis with draining sinus

   M86.40   Chronic osteomyelitis with draining sinus, unspecified site

● M86.41   Chronic osteomyelitis with draining sinus, shoulder

     M86.411   Chronic osteomyelitis with draining sinus, right shoulder

     M86.412   Chronic osteomyelitis with draining sinus, left shoulder

     M86.419   Chronic osteomyelitis with draining sinus, unspecified shoulder

● M86.42   Chronic osteomyelitis with draining sinus, humerus

     M86.421   Chronic osteomyelitis with draining sinus, right humerus

     M86.422   Chronic osteomyelitis with draining sinus, left humerus

     M86.429   Chronic osteomyelitis with draining sinus, unspecified humerus

● M86.43   Chronic osteomyelitis with draining sinus, radius and ulna

     M86.431   Chronic osteomyelitis with draining sinus, right radius and ulna

     M86.432   Chronic osteomyelitis with draining sinus, left radius and ulna

     M86.439   Chronic osteomyelitis with draining sinus, unspecified radius and ulna

● M86.44   Chronic osteomyelitis with draining sinus, hand

     M86.441   Chronic osteomyelitis with draining sinus, right hand

     M86.442   Chronic osteomyelitis with draining sinus, left hand

     M86.449   Chronic osteomyelitis with draining sinus, unspecified hand

● M86.45   Chronic osteomyelitis with draining sinus, femur

     M86.451   Chronic osteomyelitis with draining sinus, right femur

     M86.452   Chronic osteomyelitis with draining sinus, left femur

     M86.459   Chronic osteomyelitis with draining sinus, unspecified femur

● M86.46   Chronic osteomyelitis with draining sinus, tibia and fibula

     M86.461   Chronic osteomyelitis with draining sinus, right tibia and fibula

     M86.462   Chronic osteomyelitis with draining sinus, left tibia and fibula

     M86.469   Chronic osteomyelitis with draining sinus, unspecified tibia and fibula

● M86.47   Chronic osteomyelitis with draining sinus, ankle and foot

     M86.471   Chronic osteomyelitis with draining sinus, right ankle and foot

     M86.472   Chronic osteomyelitis with draining sinus, left ankle and foot

     M86.479   Chronic osteomyelitis with draining sinus, unspecified ankle and foot

   M86.48   Chronic osteomyelitis with draining sinus, other site

   M86.49   Chronic osteomyelitis with draining sinus, multiple sites

● M86.5   Other chronic hematogenous osteomyelitis

   M86.50   Other chronic hematogenous osteomyelitis, unspecified site

● M86.51   Other chronic hematogenous osteomyelitis, shoulder

     M86.511   Other chronic hematogenous osteomyelitis, right shoulder

     M86.512   Other chronic hematogenous osteomyelitis, left shoulder

     M86.519   Other chronic hematogenous osteomyelitis, unspecified shoulder

● M86.52   Other chronic hematogenous osteomyelitis, humerus

     M86.521   Other chronic hematogenous osteomyelitis, right humerus

     M86.522   Other chronic hematogenous osteomyelitis, left humerus

     M86.529   Other chronic hematogenous osteomyelitis, unspecified humerus

● M86.53   Other chronic hematogenous osteomyelitis, radius and ulna

     M86.531   Other chronic hematogenous osteomyelitis, right radius and ulna

     M86.532   Other chronic hematogenous osteomyelitis, left radius and ulna

     M86.539   Other chronic hematogenous osteomyelitis, unspecified radius and ulna

● M86.54   Other chronic hematogenous osteomyelitis, hand

     M86.541   Other chronic hematogenous osteomyelitis, right hand

     M86.542   Other chronic hematogenous osteomyelitis, left hand

     M86.549   Other chronic hematogenous osteomyelitis, unspecified hand

● M86.55   Other chronic hematogenous osteomyelitis, femur

     M86.551   Other chronic hematogenous osteomyelitis, right femur

     M86.552   Other chronic hematogenous osteomyelitis, left femur

     M86.559   Other chronic hematogenous osteomyelitis, unspecified femur

● M86.56   Other chronic hematogenous osteomyelitis, tibia and fibula

     M86.561   Other chronic hematogenous osteomyelitis, right tibia and fibula

     M86.562   Other chronic hematogenous osteomyelitis, left tibia and fibula

     M86.569   Other chronic hematogenous osteomyelitis, unspecified tibia and fibula

● M86.57   Other chronic hematogenous osteomyelitis, ankle and foot

     M86.571   Other chronic hematogenous osteomyelitis, right ankle and foot

     M86.572   Other chronic hematogenous osteomyelitis, left ankle and foot

     M86.579   Other chronic hematogenous osteomyelitis, unspecified ankle and foot

   M86.58   Other chronic hematogenous osteomyelitis, other site

   M86.59   Other chronic hematogenous osteomyelitis, multiple sites

● **M86.6 Other chronic osteomyelitis**
    M86.60 Other chronic osteomyelitis, unspecified site
  ● M86.61 Other chronic osteomyelitis, shoulder
      M86.611 Other chronic osteomyelitis, right shoulder
      M86.612 Other chronic osteomyelitis, left shoulder
      M86.619 Other chronic osteomyelitis, unspecified shoulder
  ● M86.62 Other chronic osteomyelitis, humerus
      M86.621 Other chronic osteomyelitis, right humerus
      M86.622 Other chronic osteomyelitis, left humerus
      M86.629 Other chronic osteomyelitis, unspecified humerus
  ● M86.63 Other chronic osteomyelitis, radius and ulna
      M86.631 Other chronic osteomyelitis, right radius and ulna
      M86.632 Other chronic osteomyelitis, left radius and ulna
      M86.639 Other chronic osteomyelitis, unspecified radius and ulna
  ● M86.64 Other chronic osteomyelitis, hand
      M86.641 Other chronic osteomyelitis, right hand
      M86.642 Other chronic osteomyelitis, left hand
      M86.649 Other chronic osteomyelitis, unspecified hand
  ● M86.65 Other chronic osteomyelitis, thigh
      M86.651 Other chronic osteomyelitis, right thigh
      M86.652 Other chronic osteomyelitis, left thigh
      M86.659 Other chronic osteomyelitis, unspecified thigh
  ● M86.66 Other chronic osteomyelitis, tibia and fibula
      M86.661 Other chronic osteomyelitis, right tibia and fibula
      M86.662 Other chronic osteomyelitis, left tibia and fibula
      M86.669 Other chronic osteomyelitis, unspecified tibia and fibula
  ● M86.67 Other chronic osteomyelitis, ankle and foot
      M86.671 Other chronic osteomyelitis, right ankle and foot
         Coding Clinic: 2016, Q1, P13
      M86.672 Other chronic osteomyelitis, left ankle and foot
      M86.679 Other chronic osteomyelitis, unspecified ankle and foot
    M86.68 Other chronic osteomyelitis, other site
    M86.69 Other chronic osteomyelitis, multiple sites
● **M86.8 Other osteomyelitis**
    Brodie's abscess
  ● M86.8X Other osteomyelitis
      M86.8X0 Other osteomyelitis, multiple sites
      M86.8X1 Other osteomyelitis, shoulder
      M86.8X2 Other osteomyelitis, upper arm
      M86.8X3 Other osteomyelitis, forearm
      M86.8X4 Other osteomyelitis, hand
      M86.8X5 Other osteomyelitis, thigh
      M86.8X6 Other osteomyelitis, lower leg
      M86.8X7 Other osteomyelitis, ankle and foot
      M86.8X8 Other osteomyelitis, other site
      M86.8X9 Other osteomyelitis, unspecified sites
M86.9 Osteomyelitis, unspecified
    Infection of bone NOS
    Periostitis without osteomyelitis

● **M87 Osteonecrosis**
    Includes   avascular necrosis of bone
    Use additional code to identify major osseous defect, if applicable (M89.7-)
    Excludes1   juvenile osteonecrosis (M91-M92)
          osteochondropathies (M90-M93)
  ● **M87.0 Idiopathic aseptic necrosis of bone**
    M87.00 Idiopathic aseptic necrosis of unspecified bone
  ● M87.01 Idiopathic aseptic necrosis of shoulder
      Idiopathic aseptic necrosis of clavicle and scapula
      M87.011 Idiopathic aseptic necrosis of right shoulder
      M87.012 Idiopathic aseptic necrosis of left shoulder
      M87.019 Idiopathic aseptic necrosis of unspecified shoulder
  ● M87.02 Idiopathic aseptic necrosis of humerus
      M87.021 Idiopathic aseptic necrosis of right humerus
      M87.022 Idiopathic aseptic necrosis of left humerus
      M87.029 Idiopathic aseptic necrosis of unspecified humerus
  ● M87.03 Idiopathic aseptic necrosis of radius, ulna and carpus
      M87.031 Idiopathic aseptic necrosis of right radius
      M87.032 Idiopathic aseptic necrosis of left radius
      M87.033 Idiopathic aseptic necrosis of unspecified radius
      M87.034 Idiopathic aseptic necrosis of right ulna
      M87.035 Idiopathic aseptic necrosis of left ulna
      M87.036 Idiopathic aseptic necrosis of unspecified ulna
      M87.037 Idiopathic aseptic necrosis of right carpus
      M87.038 Idiopathic aseptic necrosis of left carpus
      M87.039 Idiopathic aseptic necrosis of unspecified carpus
  ● M87.04 Idiopathic aseptic necrosis of hand and fingers
      Idiopathic aseptic necrosis of metacarpals and phalanges of hands
      M87.041 Idiopathic aseptic necrosis of right hand
      M87.042 Idiopathic aseptic necrosis of left hand
      M87.043 Idiopathic aseptic necrosis of unspecified hand
      M87.044 Idiopathic aseptic necrosis of right finger(s)
      M87.045 Idiopathic aseptic necrosis of left finger(s)
      M87.046 Idiopathic aseptic necrosis of unspecified finger(s)
  ● M87.05 Idiopathic aseptic necrosis of pelvis and femur
      M87.050 Idiopathic aseptic necrosis of pelvis
      M87.051 Idiopathic aseptic necrosis of right femur
      M87.052 Idiopathic aseptic necrosis of left femur
      M87.059 Idiopathic aseptic necrosis of unspecified femur
         Idiopathic aseptic necrosis of hip NOS

CHAPTER 13 (M00-M99)

● M87.06 Idiopathic aseptic necrosis of tibia and fibula
  M87.061 Idiopathic aseptic necrosis of right tibia
  M87.062 Idiopathic aseptic necrosis of left tibia
  M87.063 Idiopathic aseptic necrosis of unspecified tibia
  M87.064 Idiopathic aseptic necrosis of right fibula
  M87.065 Idiopathic aseptic necrosis of left fibula
  M87.066 Idiopathic aseptic necrosis of unspecified fibula
● M87.07 Idiopathic aseptic necrosis of ankle, foot and toes
  Idiopathic aseptic necrosis of metatarsus, tarsus, and phalanges of toes
  M87.071 Idiopathic aseptic necrosis of right ankle
  M87.072 Idiopathic aseptic necrosis of left ankle
  M87.073 Idiopathic aseptic necrosis of unspecified ankle
  M87.074 Idiopathic aseptic necrosis of right foot
  M87.075 Idiopathic aseptic necrosis of left foot
  M87.076 Idiopathic aseptic necrosis of unspecified foot
  M87.077 Idiopathic aseptic necrosis of right toe(s)
  M87.078 Idiopathic aseptic necrosis of left toe(s)
  M87.079 Idiopathic aseptic necrosis of unspecified toe(s)
 M87.08 Idiopathic aseptic necrosis of bone, other site
 M87.09 Idiopathic aseptic necrosis of bone, multiple sites
● M87.1 Osteonecrosis due to drugs
  Use additional code for adverse effect, if applicable, to identify drug (T36-T50 with fifth or sixth character 5)
 M87.10 Osteonecrosis due to drugs, unspecified bone
● M87.11 Osteonecrosis due to drugs, shoulder
  M87.111 Osteonecrosis due to drugs, right shoulder
  M87.112 Osteonecrosis due to drugs, left shoulder
  M87.119 Osteonecrosis due to drugs, unspecified shoulder
● M87.12 Osteonecrosis due to drugs, humerus
  M87.121 Osteonecrosis due to drugs, right humerus
  M87.122 Osteonecrosis due to drugs, left humerus
  M87.129 Osteonecrosis due to drugs, unspecified humerus
● M87.13 Osteonecrosis due to drugs of radius, ulna and carpus
  M87.131 Osteonecrosis due to drugs of right radius
  M87.132 Osteonecrosis due to drugs of left radius
  M87.133 Osteonecrosis due to drugs of unspecified radius
  M87.134 Osteonecrosis due to drugs of right ulna
  M87.135 Osteonecrosis due to drugs of left ulna
  M87.136 Osteonecrosis due to drugs of unspecified ulna
  M87.137 Osteonecrosis due to drugs of right carpus
  M87.138 Osteonecrosis due to drugs of left carpus
  M87.139 Osteonecrosis due to drugs of unspecified carpus
● M87.14 Osteonecrosis due to drugs, hand and fingers
  M87.141 Osteonecrosis due to drugs, right hand
  M87.142 Osteonecrosis due to drugs, left hand
  M87.143 Osteonecrosis due to drugs, unspecified hand
  M87.144 Osteonecrosis due to drugs, right finger(s)
  M87.145 Osteonecrosis due to drugs, left finger(s)
  M87.146 Osteonecrosis due to drugs, unspecified finger(s)
● M87.15 Osteonecrosis due to drugs, pelvis and femur
  M87.150 Osteonecrosis due to drugs, pelvis
  M87.151 Osteonecrosis due to drugs, right femur
  M87.152 Osteonecrosis due to drugs, left femur
  M87.159 Osteonecrosis due to drugs, unspecified femur
● M87.16 Osteonecrosis due to drugs, tibia and fibula
  M87.161 Osteonecrosis due to drugs, right tibia
  M87.162 Osteonecrosis due to drugs, left tibia
  M87.163 Osteonecrosis due to drugs, unspecified tibia
  M87.164 Osteonecrosis due to drugs, right fibula
  M87.165 Osteonecrosis due to drugs, left fibula
  M87.166 Osteonecrosis due to drugs, unspecified fibula
● M87.17 Osteonecrosis due to drugs, ankle, foot and toes
  M87.171 Osteonecrosis due to drugs, right ankle
  M87.172 Osteonecrosis due to drugs, left ankle
  M87.173 Osteonecrosis due to drugs, unspecified ankle
  M87.174 Osteonecrosis due to drugs, right foot
  M87.175 Osteonecrosis due to drugs, left foot
  M87.176 Osteonecrosis due to drugs, unspecified foot
  M87.177 Osteonecrosis due to drugs, right toe(s)
  M87.178 Osteonecrosis due to drugs, left toe(s)
  M87.179 Osteonecrosis due to drugs, unspecified toe(s)
● M87.18 Osteonecrosis due to drugs, other site
  M87.180 Osteonecrosis due to drugs, jaw
  M87.188 Osteonecrosis due to drugs, other site
 M87.19 Osteonecrosis due to drugs, multiple sites
● M87.2 Osteonecrosis due to previous trauma
 M87.20 Osteonecrosis due to previous trauma, unspecified bone
● M87.21 Osteonecrosis due to previous trauma, shoulder
  M87.211 Osteonecrosis due to previous trauma, right shoulder
  M87.212 Osteonecrosis due to previous trauma, left shoulder
  M87.219 Osteonecrosis due to previous trauma, unspecified shoulder

CHAPTER 13 (M00-M99)

◀ New   ◀▪▪ Revised   ~~deleted~~ Deleted   Excludes 1   Excludes 2   Includes   Use additional   Code first   Code also   Unspecified
OGCR Official Guidelines   X Assign placeholder X   ● Use Additional Character(s)   ▶ Manifestation Code   **Coding Clinic**

- M87.22　Osteonecrosis due to previous trauma, humerus
  - M87.221　Osteonecrosis due to previous trauma, right humerus
  - M87.222　Osteonecrosis due to previous trauma, left humerus
  - M87.229　Osteonecrosis due to previous trauma, unspecified humerus
- M87.23　Osteonecrosis due to previous trauma of radius, ulna and carpus
  - M87.231　Osteonecrosis due to previous trauma of right radius
  - M87.232　Osteonecrosis due to previous trauma of left radius
  - M87.233　Osteonecrosis due to previous trauma of unspecified radius
  - M87.234　Osteonecrosis due to previous trauma of right ulna
  - M87.235　Osteonecrosis due to previous trauma of left ulna
  - M87.236　Osteonecrosis due to previous trauma of unspecified ulna
  - M87.237　Osteonecrosis due to previous trauma of right carpus
  - M87.238　Osteonecrosis due to previous trauma of left carpus
  - M87.239　Osteonecrosis due to previous trauma of unspecified carpus
- M87.24　Osteonecrosis due to previous trauma, hand and fingers
  - M87.241　Osteonecrosis due to previous trauma, right hand
  - M87.242　Osteonecrosis due to previous trauma, left hand
  - M87.243　Osteonecrosis due to previous trauma, unspecified hand
  - M87.244　Osteonecrosis due to previous trauma, right finger(s)
  - M87.245　Osteonecrosis due to previous trauma, left finger(s)
  - M87.246　Osteonecrosis due to previous trauma, unspecified finger(s)
- M87.25　Osteonecrosis due to previous trauma, pelvis and femur
  - M87.250　Osteonecrosis due to previous trauma, pelvis
  - M87.251　Osteonecrosis due to previous trauma, right femur
  - M87.252　Osteonecrosis due to previous trauma, left femur
  - M87.256　Osteonecrosis due to previous trauma, unspecified femur
- M87.26　Osteonecrosis due to previous trauma, tibia and fibula
  - M87.261　Osteonecrosis due to previous trauma, right tibia
  - M87.262　Osteonecrosis due to previous trauma, left tibia
  - M87.263　Osteonecrosis due to previous trauma, unspecified tibia
  - M87.264　Osteonecrosis due to previous trauma, right fibula
  - M87.265　Osteonecrosis due to previous trauma, left fibula
  - M87.266　Osteonecrosis due to previous trauma, unspecified fibula

- M87.27　Osteonecrosis due to previous trauma, ankle, foot and toes
  - M87.271　Osteonecrosis due to previous trauma, right ankle
  - M87.272　Osteonecrosis due to previous trauma, left ankle
  - M87.273　Osteonecrosis due to previous trauma, unspecified ankle
  - M87.274　Osteonecrosis due to previous trauma, right foot
  - M87.275　Osteonecrosis due to previous trauma, left foot
  - M87.276　Osteonecrosis due to previous trauma, unspecified foot
  - M87.277　Osteonecrosis due to previous trauma, right toe(s)
  - M87.278　Osteonecrosis due to previous trauma, left toe(s)
  - M87.279　Osteonecrosis due to previous trauma, unspecified toe(s)
- M87.28　Osteonecrosis due to previous trauma, other site
- M87.29　Osteonecrosis due to previous trauma, multiple sites
- M87.3　Other secondary osteonecrosis
  - M87.30　Other secondary osteonecrosis, unspecified bone
  - M87.31　Other secondary osteonecrosis, shoulder
    - M87.311　Other secondary osteonecrosis, right shoulder
    - M87.312　Other secondary osteonecrosis, left shoulder
    - M87.319　Other secondary osteonecrosis, unspecified shoulder
  - M87.32　Other secondary osteonecrosis, humerus
    - M87.321　Other secondary osteonecrosis, right humerus
    - M87.322　Other secondary osteonecrosis, left humerus
    - M87.329　Other secondary osteonecrosis, unspecified humerus
  - M87.33　Other secondary osteonecrosis of radius, ulna and carpus
    - M87.331　Other secondary osteonecrosis of right radius
    - M87.332　Other secondary osteonecrosis of left radius
    - M87.333　Other secondary osteonecrosis of unspecified radius
    - M87.334　Other secondary osteonecrosis of right ulna
    - M87.335　Other secondary osteonecrosis of left ulna
    - M87.336　Other secondary osteonecrosis of unspecified ulna
    - M87.337　Other secondary osteonecrosis of right carpus
    - M87.338　Other secondary osteonecrosis of left carpus
    - M87.339　Other secondary osteonecrosis of unspecified carpus

● M87.34   **Other secondary osteonecrosis, hand and fingers**
  M87.341   Other secondary osteonecrosis, right hand
  M87.342   Other secondary osteonecrosis, left hand
  M87.343   Other secondary osteonecrosis, unspecified hand
  M87.344   Other secondary osteonecrosis, right finger(s)
  M87.345   Other secondary osteonecrosis, left finger(s)
  M87.346   Other secondary osteonecrosis, unspecified finger(s)

● M87.35   **Other secondary osteonecrosis, pelvis and femur**
  M87.350   Other secondary osteonecrosis, pelvis
  M87.351   Other secondary osteonecrosis, right femur
  M87.352   Other secondary osteonecrosis, left femur
  M87.353   Other secondary osteonecrosis, unspecified femur

● M87.36   **Other secondary osteonecrosis, tibia and fibula**
  M87.361   Other secondary osteonecrosis, right tibia
  M87.362   Other secondary osteonecrosis, left tibia
  M87.363   Other secondary osteonecrosis, unspecified tibia
  M87.364   Other secondary osteonecrosis, right fibula
  M87.365   Other secondary osteonecrosis, left fibula
  M87.366   Other secondary osteonecrosis, unspecified fibula

● M87.37   **Other secondary osteonecrosis, ankle and foot**
  M87.371   Other secondary osteonecrosis, right ankle
  M87.372   Other secondary osteonecrosis, left ankle
  M87.373   Other secondary osteonecrosis, unspecified ankle
  M87.374   Other secondary osteonecrosis, right foot
  M87.375   Other secondary osteonecrosis, left foot
  M87.376   Other secondary osteonecrosis, unspecified foot
  M87.377   Other secondary osteonecrosis, right toe(s)
  M87.378   Other secondary osteonecrosis, left toe(s)
  M87.379   Other secondary osteonecrosis, unspecified toe(s)

  M87.38   Other secondary osteonecrosis, other site
  M87.39   Other secondary osteonecrosis, multiple sites

● M87.8   **Other osteonecrosis**
  M87.80   Other osteonecrosis, unspecified bone

● M87.81   **Other osteonecrosis, shoulder**
  M87.811   Other osteonecrosis, right shoulder
  M87.812   Other osteonecrosis, left shoulder
  M87.819   Other osteonecrosis, unspecified shoulder

● M87.82   **Other osteonecrosis, humerus**
  M87.821   Other osteonecrosis, right humerus
  M87.822   Other osteonecrosis, left humerus
  M87.829   Other osteonecrosis, unspecified humerus

● M87.83   **Other osteonecrosis of radius, ulna and carpus**
  M87.831   Other osteonecrosis of right radius
  M87.832   Other osteonecrosis of left radius
  M87.833   Other osteonecrosis of unspecified radius
  M87.834   Other osteonecrosis of right ulna
  M87.835   Other osteonecrosis of left ulna
  M87.836   Other osteonecrosis of unspecified ulna
  M87.837   Other osteonecrosis of right carpus
  M87.838   Other osteonecrosis of left carpus
  M87.839   Other osteonecrosis of unspecified carpus

● M87.84   **Other osteonecrosis, hand and fingers**
  M87.841   Other osteonecrosis, right hand
  M87.842   Other osteonecrosis, left hand
  M87.843   Other osteonecrosis, unspecified hand
  M87.844   Other osteonecrosis, right finger(s)
  M87.845   Other osteonecrosis, left finger(s)
  M87.849   Other osteonecrosis, unspecified finger(s)

● M87.85   **Other osteonecrosis, pelvis and femur**
  M87.850   Other osteonecrosis, pelvis
  M87.851   Other osteonecrosis, right femur
  M87.852   Other osteonecrosis, left femur
  M87.859   Other osteonecrosis, unspecified femur

● M87.86   **Other osteonecrosis, tibia and fibula**
  M87.861   Other osteonecrosis, right tibia
  M87.862   Other osteonecrosis, left tibia
  M87.863   Other osteonecrosis, unspecified tibia
  M87.864   Other osteonecrosis, right fibula
  M87.865   Other osteonecrosis, left fibula
  M87.869   Other osteonecrosis, unspecified fibula

● M87.87   **Other osteonecrosis, ankle, foot and toes**
  M87.871   Other osteonecrosis, right ankle
  M87.872   Other osteonecrosis, left ankle
  M87.873   Other osteonecrosis, unspecified ankle
  M87.874   Other osteonecrosis, right foot
  M87.875   Other osteonecrosis, left foot
  M87.876   Other osteonecrosis, unspecified foot
  M87.877   Other osteonecrosis, right toe(s)
  M87.878   Other osteonecrosis, left toe(s)
  M87.879   Other osteonecrosis, unspecified toe(s)

  M87.88   Other osteonecrosis, other site
  M87.89   Other osteonecrosis, multiple sites

M87.9   **Osteonecrosis, unspecified**
  Necrosis of bone NOS

◀ New   ◀▦ Revised   ~~deleted~~ Deleted   Excludes 1   Excludes 2   Includes   Use additional   Code first   Code also   Unspecified

OGCR Official Guidelines   X Assign placeholder X   ● Use Additional Character(s)   ▷ Manifestation Code   **Coding Clinic**

● **M88 Osteitis deformans [Paget's disease of bone]**
Chronic disorder that results in enlarged and deformed bones. The excessive breakdown and formation of bone tissue causes bones to weaken and results in bone pain, arthritis, deformities, and fractures.

Excludes1   osteitis deformans in neoplastic disease (M90.6)

M88.0 Osteitis deformans of skull

M88.1 Osteitis deformans of vertebrae

● **M88.8 Osteitis deformans of other bones**

   ● **M88.81 Osteitis deformans of shoulder**
      M88.811 Osteitis deformans of right shoulder
      M88.812 Osteitis deformans of left shoulder
      M88.819 Osteitis deformans of unspecified shoulder

   ● **M88.82 Osteitis deformans of upper arm**
      M88.821 Osteitis deformans of right upper arm
      M88.822 Osteitis deformans of left upper arm
      M88.829 Osteitis deformans of unspecified upper arm

   ● **M88.83 Osteitis deformans of forearm**
      M88.831 Osteitis deformans of right forearm
      M88.832 Osteitis deformans of left forearm
      M88.839 Osteitis deformans of unspecified forearm

   ● **M88.84 Osteitis deformans of hand**
      M88.841 Osteitis deformans of right hand
      M88.842 Osteitis deformans of left hand
      M88.849 Osteitis deformans of unspecified hand

   ● **M88.85 Osteitis deformans of thigh**
      M88.851 Osteitis deformans of right thigh
      M88.852 Osteitis deformans of left thigh
      M88.859 Osteitis deformans of unspecified thigh

   ● **M88.86 Osteitis deformans of lower leg**
      M88.861 Osteitis deformans of right lower leg
      M88.862 Osteitis deformans of left lower leg
      M88.869 Osteitis deformans of unspecified lower leg

   ● **M88.87 Osteitis deformans of ankle and foot**
      M88.871 Osteitis deformans of right ankle and foot
      M88.872 Osteitis deformans of left ankle and foot
      M88.879 Osteitis deformans of unspecified ankle and foot

   M88.88 Osteitis deformans of other bones
      Excludes2   osteitis deformans of skull (M88.0)
                   osteitis deformans of vertebrae (M88.1)

   M88.89 Osteitis deformans of multiple sites

M88.9 Osteitis deformans of unspecified bone

● **M89 Other disorders of bone**

  ● **M89.0 Algoneurodystrophy**
     Shoulder-hand syndrome
     Sudeck's atrophy

    Excludes1   causalgia, lower limb (G57.7-)
              causalgia, upper limb (G56.4-)
              complex regional pain syndrome II, lower limb (G57.7-)
              complex regional pain syndrome II, upper limb (G56.4-)
              reflex sympathetic dystrophy (G90.5-)

   M89.00 Algoneurodystrophy, unspecified site

   ● **M89.01 Algoneurodystrophy, shoulder**
      M89.011 Algoneurodystrophy, right shoulder
      M89.012 Algoneurodystrophy, left shoulder
      M89.019 Algoneurodystrophy, unspecified shoulder

   ● **M89.02 Algoneurodystrophy, upper arm**
      M89.021 Algoneurodystrophy, right upper arm
      M89.022 Algoneurodystrophy, left upper arm
      M89.029 Algoneurodystrophy, unspecified upper arm

   ● **M89.03 Algoneurodystrophy, forearm**
      M89.031 Algoneurodystrophy, right forearm
      M89.032 Algoneurodystrophy, left forearm
      M89.039 Algoneurodystrophy, unspecified forearm

   ● **M89.04 Algoneurodystrophy, hand**
      M89.041 Algoneurodystrophy, right hand
      M89.042 Algoneurodystrophy, left hand
      M89.049 Algoneurodystrophy, unspecified hand

   ● **M89.05 Algoneurodystrophy, thigh**
      M89.051 Algoneurodystrophy, right thigh
      M89.052 Algoneurodystrophy, left thigh
      M89.059 Algoneurodystrophy, unspecified thigh

   ● **M89.06 Algoneurodystrophy, lower leg**
      M89.061 Algoneurodystrophy, right lower leg
      M89.062 Algoneurodystrophy, left lower leg
      M89.069 Algoneurodystrophy, unspecified lower leg

   ● **M89.07 Algoneurodystrophy, ankle and foot**
      M89.071 Algoneurodystrophy, right ankle and foot
      M89.072 Algoneurodystrophy, left ankle and foot
      M89.079 Algoneurodystrophy, unspecified ankle and foot

   M89.08 Algoneurodystrophy, other site

   M89.09 Algoneurodystrophy, multiple sites

CHAPTER 13 (M00-M99)

● **M89.1　Physeal arrest**
　　　Arrest of growth plate
　　　Epiphyseal arrest
　　　Growth plate arrest

● **M89.12　Physeal arrest, humerus**

　　M89.121　Complete physeal arrest, right proximal humerus

　　M89.122　Complete physeal arrest, left proximal humerus

　　M89.123　Partial physeal arrest, right proximal humerus

　　M89.124　Partial physeal arrest, left proximal humerus

　　M89.125　Complete physeal arrest, right distal humerus

　　M89.126　Complete physeal arrest, left distal humerus

　　M89.127　Partial physeal arrest, right distal humerus

　　M89.128　Partial physeal arrest, left distal humerus

　　M89.129　Physeal arrest, humerus, unspecified

● **M89.13　Physeal arrest, forearm**

　　M89.131　Complete physeal arrest, right distal radius

　　M89.132　Complete physeal arrest, left distal radius

　　M89.133　Partial physeal arrest, right distal radius

　　M89.134　Partial physeal arrest, left distal radius

　　M89.138　Other physeal arrest of forearm

　　M89.139　Physeal arrest, forearm, unspecified

● **M89.15　Physeal arrest, femur**

　　M89.151　Complete physeal arrest, right proximal femur

　　M89.152　Complete physeal arrest, left proximal femur

　　M89.153　Partial physeal arrest, right proximal femur

　　M89.154　Partial physeal arrest, left proximal femur

　　M89.155　Complete physeal arrest, right distal femur

　　M89.156　Complete physeal arrest, left distal femur

　　M89.157　Partial physeal arrest, right distal femur

　　M89.158　Partial physeal arrest, left distal femur

　　M89.159　Physeal arrest, femur, unspecified

● **M89.16　Physeal arrest, lower leg**

　　M89.160　Complete physeal arrest, right proximal tibia

　　M89.161　Complete physeal arrest, left proximal tibia

　　M89.162　Partial physeal arrest, right proximal tibia

　　M89.163　Partial physeal arrest, left proximal tibia

　　M89.164　Complete physeal arrest, right distal tibia

　　M89.165　Complete physeal arrest, left distal tibia

　　M89.166　Partial physeal arrest, right distal tibia

　　M89.167　Partial physeal arrest, left distal tibia

　　M89.168　Other physeal arrest of lower leg

　　M89.169　Physeal arrest, lower leg, unspecified

　M89.18　Physeal arrest, other site

● **M89.2　Other disorders of bone development and growth**

　M89.20　Other disorders of bone development and growth, unspecified site

● **M89.21　Other disorders of bone development and growth, shoulder**

　　M89.211　Other disorders of bone development and growth, right shoulder

　　M89.212　Other disorders of bone development and growth, left shoulder

　　M89.219　Other disorders of bone development and growth, unspecified shoulder

● **M89.22　Other disorders of bone development and growth, humerus**

　　M89.221　Other disorders of bone development and growth, right humerus

　　M89.222　Other disorders of bone development and growth, left humerus

　　M89.229　Other disorders of bone development and growth, unspecified humerus

● **M89.23　Other disorders of bone development and growth, ulna and radius**

　　M89.231　Other disorders of bone development and growth, right ulna

　　M89.232　Other disorders of bone development and growth, left ulna

　　M89.233　Other disorders of bone development and growth, right radius

　　M89.234　Other disorders of bone development and growth, left radius

　　M89.239　Other disorders of bone development and growth, unspecified ulna and radius

● **M89.24　Other disorders of bone development and growth, hand**

　　M89.241　Other disorders of bone development and growth, right hand

　　M89.242　Other disorders of bone development and growth, left hand

　　M89.249　Other disorders of bone development and growth, unspecified hand

● **M89.25　Other disorders of bone development and growth, femur**

　　M89.251　Other disorders of bone development and growth, right femur

　　M89.252　Other disorders of bone development and growth, left femur

　　M89.259　Other disorders of bone development and growth, unspecified femur

● **M89.26　Other disorders of bone development and growth, tibia and fibula**

　　M89.261　Other disorders of bone development and growth, right tibia

　　M89.262　Other disorders of bone development and growth, left tibia

　　M89.263　Other disorders of bone development and growth, right fibula

　　M89.264　Other disorders of bone development and growth, left fibula

　　M89.269　Other disorders of bone development and growth, unspecified lower leg

● **M89.27　Other disorders of bone development and growth, ankle and foot**

　　M89.271　Other disorders of bone development and growth, right ankle and foot

　　M89.272　Other disorders of bone development and growth, left ankle and foot

　　M89.279　Other disorders of bone development and growth, unspecified ankle and foot

◀ New　　◀⋅⋅⋅ Revised　　deleted Deleted　　Excludes 1　　Excludes 2　　Includes　　Use additional　　Code first　　Code also　　Unspecified

OGCR Official Guidelines　　X Assign placeholder X　　● Use Additional Character(s)　　▷ Manifestation Code　　**Coding Clinic**

M89.28   Other disorders of bone development and growth, other site

M89.29   Other disorders of bone development and growth, multiple sites

● M89.3   Hypertrophy of bone

     M89.30   Hypertrophy of bone, unspecified site

   ● M89.31   Hypertrophy of bone, shoulder

       M89.311   Hypertrophy of bone, right shoulder

       M89.312   Hypertrophy of bone, left shoulder

       M89.319   Hypertrophy of bone, unspecified shoulder

   ● M89.32   Hypertrophy of bone, humerus

       M89.321   Hypertrophy of bone, right humerus

       M89.322   Hypertrophy of bone, left humerus

       M89.329   Hypertrophy of bone, unspecified humerus

   ● M89.33   Hypertrophy of bone, ulna and radius

       M89.331   Hypertrophy of bone, right ulna

       M89.332   Hypertrophy of bone, left ulna

       M89.333   Hypertrophy of bone, right radius

       M89.334   Hypertrophy of bone, left radius

       M89.339   Hypertrophy of bone, unspecified ulna and radius

   ● M89.34   Hypertrophy of bone, hand

       M89.341   Hypertrophy of bone, right hand

       M89.342   Hypertrophy of bone, left hand

       M89.349   Hypertrophy of bone, unspecified hand

   ● M89.35   Hypertrophy of bone, femur

       M89.351   Hypertrophy of bone, right femur

       M89.352   Hypertrophy of bone, left femur

       M89.359   Hypertrophy of bone, unspecified femur

   ● M89.36   Hypertrophy of bone, tibia and fibula

       M89.361   Hypertrophy of bone, right tibia

       M89.362   Hypertrophy of bone, left tibia

       M89.363   Hypertrophy of bone, right fibula

       M89.364   Hypertrophy of bone, left fibula

       M89.369   Hypertrophy of bone, unspecified tibia and fibula

   ● M89.37   Hypertrophy of bone, ankle and foot

       M89.371   Hypertrophy of bone, right ankle and foot

       M89.372   Hypertrophy of bone, left ankle and foot

       M89.379   Hypertrophy of bone, unspecified ankle and foot

     M89.38   Hypertrophy of bone, other site

     M89.39   Hypertrophy of bone, multiple sites

● M89.4   Other hypertrophic osteoarthropathy

     Marie-Bamberger disease

     Pachydermoperiostosis

     M89.40   Other hypertrophic osteoarthropathy, unspecified site

   ● M89.41   Other hypertrophic osteoarthropathy, shoulder

       M89.411   Other hypertrophic osteoarthropathy, right shoulder

       M89.412   Other hypertrophic osteoarthropathy, left shoulder

       M89.419   Other hypertrophic osteoarthropathy, unspecified shoulder

   ● M89.42   Other hypertrophic osteoarthropathy, upper arm

       M89.421   Other hypertrophic osteoarthropathy, right upper arm

       M89.422   Other hypertrophic osteoarthropathy, left upper arm

       M89.429   Other hypertrophic osteoarthropathy, unspecified upper arm

   ● M89.43   Other hypertrophic osteoarthropathy, forearm

       M89.431   Other hypertrophic osteoarthropathy, right forearm

       M89.432   Other hypertrophic osteoarthropathy, left forearm

       M89.439   Other hypertrophic osteoarthropathy, unspecified forearm

   ● M89.44   Other hypertrophic osteoarthropathy, hand

       M89.441   Other hypertrophic osteoarthropathy, right hand

       M89.442   Other hypertrophic osteoarthropathy, left hand

       M89.449   Other hypertrophic osteoarthropathy, unspecified hand

   ● M89.45   Other hypertrophic osteoarthropathy, thigh

       M89.451   Other hypertrophic osteoarthropathy, right thigh

       M89.452   Other hypertrophic osteoarthropathy, left thigh

       M89.459   Other hypertrophic osteoarthropathy, unspecified thigh

   ● M89.46   Other hypertrophic osteoarthropathy, lower leg

       M89.461   Other hypertrophic osteoarthropathy, right lower leg

       M89.462   Other hypertrophic osteoarthropathy, left lower leg

       M89.469   Other hypertrophic osteoarthropathy, unspecified lower leg

   ● M89.47   Other hypertrophic osteoarthropathy, ankle and foot

       M89.471   Other hypertrophic osteoarthropathy, right ankle and foot

       M89.472   Other hypertrophic osteoarthropathy, left ankle and foot

       M89.479   Other hypertrophic osteoarthropathy, unspecified ankle and foot

     M89.48   Other hypertrophic osteoarthropathy, other site

     M89.49   Other hypertrophic osteoarthropathy, multiple sites

● M89.5   Osteolysis

     Use additional code to identify major osseous defect, if applicable (M89.7-)

     Excludes2   periprosthetic osteolysis of internal prosthetic joint (T84.05-)

     M89.50   Osteolysis, unspecified site

   ● M89.51   Osteolysis, shoulder

       M89.511   Osteolysis, right shoulder

       M89.512   Osteolysis, left shoulder

       M89.519   Osteolysis, unspecified shoulder

   ● M89.52   Osteolysis, upper arm

       M89.521   Osteolysis, right upper arm

       M89.522   Osteolysis, left upper arm

       M89.529   Osteolysis, unspecified upper arm

   ● M89.53   Osteolysis, forearm

       M89.531   Osteolysis, right forearm

       M89.532   Osteolysis, left forearm

       M89.539   Osteolysis, unspecified forearm

CHAPTER 13 (M00-M99)

● **M89.54 Osteolysis, hand**
    M89.541 Osteolysis, right hand
    M89.542 Osteolysis, left hand
    M89.549 Osteolysis, unspecified hand
● **M89.55 Osteolysis, thigh**
    M89.551 Osteolysis, right thigh
    M89.552 Osteolysis, left thigh
    M89.559 Osteolysis, unspecified thigh
● **M89.56 Osteolysis, lower leg**
    M89.561 Osteolysis, right lower leg
    M89.562 Osteolysis, left lower leg
    M89.569 Osteolysis, unspecified lower leg
● **M89.57 Osteolysis, ankle and foot**
    M89.571 Osteolysis, right ankle and foot
    M89.572 Osteolysis, left ankle and foot
    M89.579 Osteolysis, unspecified ankle and foot
  M89.58 Osteolysis, other site
  M89.59 Osteolysis, multiple sites
● **M89.6 Osteopathy after poliomyelitis**
    Use additional code (B91) to identify previous poliomyelitis
    Excludes1 postpolio syndrome (G14)
  M89.60 Osteopathy after poliomyelitis, unspecified site
● **M89.61 Osteopathy after poliomyelitis, shoulder**
    M89.611 Osteopathy after poliomyelitis, right shoulder
    M89.612 Osteopathy after poliomyelitis, left shoulder
    M89.619 Osteopathy after poliomyelitis, unspecified shoulder
● **M89.62 Osteopathy after poliomyelitis, upper arm**
    M89.621 Osteopathy after poliomyelitis, right upper arm
    M89.622 Osteopathy after poliomyelitis, left upper arm
    M89.629 Osteopathy after poliomyelitis, unspecified upper arm
● **M89.63 Osteopathy after poliomyelitis, forearm**
    M89.631 Osteopathy after poliomyelitis, right forearm
    M89.632 Osteopathy after poliomyelitis, left forearm
    M89.639 Osteopathy after poliomyelitis, unspecified forearm
● **M89.64 Osteopathy after poliomyelitis, hand**
    M89.641 Osteopathy after poliomyelitis, right hand
    M89.642 Osteopathy after poliomyelitis, left hand
    M89.649 Osteopathy after poliomyelitis, unspecified hand
● **M89.65 Osteopathy after poliomyelitis, thigh**
    M89.651 Osteopathy after poliomyelitis, right thigh
    M89.652 Osteopathy after poliomyelitis, left thigh
    M89.659 Osteopathy after poliomyelitis, unspecified thigh
● **M89.66 Osteopathy after poliomyelitis, lower leg**
    M89.661 Osteopathy after poliomyelitis, right lower leg
    M89.662 Osteopathy after poliomyelitis, left lower leg
    M89.669 Osteopathy after poliomyelitis, unspecified lower leg

● **M89.67 Osteopathy after poliomyelitis, ankle and foot**
    M89.671 Osteopathy after poliomyelitis, right ankle and foot
    M89.672 Osteopathy after poliomyelitis, left ankle and foot
    M89.679 Osteopathy after poliomyelitis, unspecified ankle and foot
  M89.68 Osteopathy after poliomyelitis, other site
  M89.69 Osteopathy after poliomyelitis, multiple sites
● **M89.7 Major osseous defect**
    Code first underlying disease, if known, such as:
    aseptic necrosis of bone (M87.-)
    malignant neoplasm of bone (C40.-)
    osteolysis (M89.5)
    osteomyelitis (M86.-)
    osteonecrosis (M87.-)
    osteoporosis (M80.-, M81.-)
    periprosthetic osteolysis (T84.05-)
  M89.70 Major osseous defect, unspecified site
● **M89.71 Major osseous defect, shoulder region**
    Major osseous defect clavicle or scapula
    M89.711 Major osseous defect, right shoulder region
    M89.712 Major osseous defect, left shoulder region
    M89.719 Major osseous defect, unspecified shoulder region
● **M89.72 Major osseous defect, humerus**
    M89.721 Major osseous defect, right humerus
    M89.722 Major osseous defect, left humerus
    M89.729 Major osseous defect, unspecified humerus
● **M89.73 Major osseous defect, forearm**
    Major osseous defect of radius and ulna
    M89.731 Major osseous defect, right forearm
    M89.732 Major osseous defect, left forearm
    M89.739 Major osseous defect, unspecified forearm
● **M89.74 Major osseous defect, hand**
    Major osseous defect of carpus, fingers, metacarpus
    M89.741 Major osseous defect, right hand
    M89.742 Major osseous defect, left hand
    M89.749 Major osseous defect, unspecified hand
● **M89.75 Major osseous defect, pelvic region and thigh**
    Major osseous defect of femur and pelvis
    M89.751 Major osseous defect, right pelvic region and thigh
    M89.752 Major osseous defect, left pelvic region and thigh
    M89.759 Major osseous defect, unspecified pelvic region and thigh
● **M89.76 Major osseous defect, lower leg**
    Major osseous defect of fibula and tibia
    M89.761 Major osseous defect, right lower leg
    M89.762 Major osseous defect, left lower leg
    M89.769 Major osseous defect, unspecified lower leg
● **M89.77 Major osseous defect, ankle and foot**
    Major osseous defect of metatarsus, tarsus, toes
    M89.771 Major osseous defect, right ankle and foot
    M89.772 Major osseous defect, left ankle and foot
    M89.779 Major osseous defect, unspecified ankle and foot
  M89.78 Major osseous defect, other site
  M89.79 Major osseous defect, multiple sites

● **M89.8   Other specified disorders of bone**
     Infantile cortical hyperostoses
     Post-traumatic subperiosteal ossification
   ● **M89.8X   Other specified disorders of bone**
     M89.8X0   Other specified disorders of bone, multiple sites
     M89.8X1   Other specified disorders of bone, shoulder
     M89.8X2   Other specified disorders of bone, upper arm
     M89.8X3   Other specified disorders of bone, forearm
     M89.8X4   Other specified disorders of bone, hand
     M89.8X5   Other specified disorders of bone, thigh
     M89.8X6   Other specified disorders of bone, lower leg
     M89.8X7   Other specified disorders of bone, ankle and foot
     M89.8X8   Other specified disorders of bone, other site
     M89.8X9   Other specified disorders of bone, unspecified site

   M89.9   Disorder of bone, unspecified

● **M90   Osteopathies in diseases classified elsewhere**
   Excludes1   osteochondritis, osteomyelitis, and osteopathy (in):
     cryptococcosis (B45.3)
     diabetes mellitus (E08-E13 with .69-) ◀
     gonococcal (A54.43)
     neurogenic syphilis (A52.11)
     renal osteodystrophy (N25.0)
     salmonellosis (A02.24)
     secondary syphilis (A51.46)
     syphilis (late) (A52.77)

● **M90.5   Osteonecrosis in diseases classified elsewhere**
   Code first underlying disease, such as:
     caisson disease (T70.3)
     hemoglobinopathy (D50-D64)
   ▷ *M90.50   Osteonecrosis in diseases classified elsewhere, unspecified site*
   ● **M90.51   Osteonecrosis in diseases classified elsewhere, shoulder**
     ▷ *M90.511   Osteonecrosis in diseases classified elsewhere, right shoulder*
     ▷ *M90.512   Osteonecrosis in diseases classified elsewhere, left shoulder*
     ▷ *M90.519   Osteonecrosis in diseases classified elsewhere, unspecified shoulder*
   ● **M90.52   Osteonecrosis in diseases classified elsewhere, upper arm**
     ▷ *M90.521   Osteonecrosis in diseases classified elsewhere, right upper arm*
     ▷ *M90.522   Osteonecrosis in diseases classified elsewhere, left upper arm*
     ▷ *M90.529   Osteonecrosis in diseases classified elsewhere, unspecified upper arm*
   ● **M90.53   Osteonecrosis in diseases classified elsewhere, forearm**
     ▷ *M90.531   Osteonecrosis in diseases classified elsewhere, right forearm*
     ▷ *M90.532   Osteonecrosis in diseases classified elsewhere, left forearm*
     ▷ *M90.539   Osteonecrosis in diseases classified elsewhere, unspecified forearm*

● **M90.54   Osteonecrosis in diseases classified elsewhere, hand**
     ▷ *M90.541   Osteonecrosis in diseases classified elsewhere, right hand*
     ▷ *M90.542   Osteonecrosis in diseases classified elsewhere, left hand*
     ▷ *M90.549   Osteonecrosis in diseases classified elsewhere, unspecified hand*
● **M90.55   Osteonecrosis in diseases classified elsewhere, thigh**
     ▷ *M90.551   Osteonecrosis in diseases classified elsewhere, right thigh*
     ▷ *M90.552   Osteonecrosis in diseases classified elsewhere, left thigh*
     ▷ *M90.559   Osteonecrosis in diseases classified elsewhere, unspecified thigh*
● **M90.56   Osteonecrosis in diseases classified elsewhere, lower leg**
     ▷ *M90.561   Osteonecrosis in diseases classified elsewhere, right lower leg*
     ▷ *M90.562   Osteonecrosis in diseases classified elsewhere, left lower leg*
     ▷ *M90.569   Osteonecrosis in diseases classified elsewhere, unspecified lower leg*
● **M90.57   Osteonecrosis in diseases classified elsewhere, ankle and foot**
     ▷ *M90.571   Osteonecrosis in diseases classified elsewhere, right ankle and foot*
     ▷ *M90.572   Osteonecrosis in diseases classified elsewhere, left ankle and foot*
     ▷ *M90.579   Osteonecrosis in diseases classified elsewhere, unspecified ankle and foot*
   ▷ *M90.58   Osteonecrosis in diseases classified elsewhere, other site*
   ▷ *M90.59   Osteonecrosis in diseases classified elsewhere, multiple sites*

● **M90.6   Osteitis deformans in neoplastic diseases**
     Osteitis deformans in malignant neoplasm of bone
   Code first the neoplasm (C40.-, C41.-)
   Excludes1   osteitis deformans [Paget's disease of bone] (M88.-)
   ▷ *M90.60   Osteitis deformans in neoplastic diseases, unspecified site*
   ● **M90.61   Osteitis deformans in neoplastic diseases, shoulder**
     ▷ *M90.611   Osteitis deformans in neoplastic diseases, right shoulder*
     ▷ *M90.612   Osteitis deformans in neoplastic diseases, left shoulder*
     ▷ *M90.619   Osteitis deformans in neoplastic diseases, unspecified shoulder*
   ● **M90.62   Osteitis deformans in neoplastic diseases, upper arm**
     ▷ *M90.621   Osteitis deformans in neoplastic diseases, right upper arm*
     ▷ *M90.622   Osteitis deformans in neoplastic diseases, left upper arm*
     ▷ *M90.629   Osteitis deformans in neoplastic diseases, unspecified upper arm*
   ● **M90.63   Osteitis deformans in neoplastic diseases, forearm**
     ▷ *M90.631   Osteitis deformans in neoplastic diseases, right forearm*
     ▷ *M90.632   Osteitis deformans in neoplastic diseases, left forearm*
     ▷ *M90.639   Osteitis deformans in neoplastic diseases, unspecified forearm*

CHAPTER 13 (M00-M99)

● **M90.64** Osteitis deformans in neoplastic diseases, hand
  ▶ *M90.641 Osteitis deformans in neoplastic diseases, right hand*
  ▶ *M90.642 Osteitis deformans in neoplastic diseases, left hand*
  ▶ *M90.649 Osteitis deformans in neoplastic diseases, unspecified hand*
● **M90.65** Osteitis deformans in neoplastic diseases, thigh
  ▶ *M90.651 Osteitis deformans in neoplastic diseases, right thigh*
  ▶ *M90.652 Osteitis deformans in neoplastic diseases, left thigh*
  ▶ *M90.659 Osteitis deformans in neoplastic diseases, unspecified thigh*
● **M90.66** Osteitis deformans in neoplastic diseases, lower leg
  ▶ *M90.661 Osteitis deformans in neoplastic diseases, right lower leg*
  ▶ *M90.662 Osteitis deformans in neoplastic diseases, left lower leg*
  ▶ *M90.669 Osteitis deformans in neoplastic diseases, unspecified lower leg*
● **M90.67** Osteitis deformans in neoplastic diseases, ankle and foot
  ▶ *M90.671 Osteitis deformans in neoplastic diseases, right ankle and foot*
  ▶ *M90.672 Osteitis deformans in neoplastic diseases, left ankle and foot*
  ▶ *M90.679 Osteitis deformans in neoplastic diseases, unspecified ankle and foot*
  ▶ *M90.68 Osteitis deformans in neoplastic diseases, other site*
  ▶ *M90.69 Osteitis deformans in neoplastic diseases, multiple sites*
● **M90.8** Osteopathy in diseases classified elsewhere
    Code first underlying disease, such as:
      rickets (E55.0)
      vitamin-D-resistant rickets (E83.3)
  ▶ *M90.80 Osteopathy in diseases classified elsewhere, unspecified site*
● **M90.81** Osteopathy in diseases classified elsewhere, shoulder
  ▶ *M90.811 Osteopathy in diseases classified elsewhere, right shoulder*
  ▶ *M90.812 Osteopathy in diseases classified elsewhere, left shoulder*
  ▶ *M90.819 Osteopathy in diseases classified elsewhere, unspecified shoulder*
● **M90.82** Osteopathy in diseases classified elsewhere, upper arm
  ▶ *M90.821 Osteopathy in diseases classified elsewhere, right upper arm*
  ▶ *M90.822 Osteopathy in diseases classified elsewhere, left upper arm*
  ▶ *M90.829 Osteopathy in diseases classified elsewhere, unspecified upper arm*
● **M90.83** Osteopathy in diseases classified elsewhere, forearm
  ▶ *M90.831 Osteopathy in diseases classified elsewhere, right forearm*
  ▶ *M90.832 Osteopathy in diseases classified elsewhere, left forearm*
  ▶ *M90.839 Osteopathy in diseases classified elsewhere, unspecified forearm*

● **M90.84** Osteopathy in diseases classified elsewhere, hand
  ▶ *M90.841 Osteopathy in diseases classified elsewhere, right hand*
  ▶ *M90.842 Osteopathy in diseases classified elsewhere, left hand*
  ▶ *M90.849 Osteopathy in diseases classified elsewhere, unspecified hand*
● **M90.85** Osteopathy in diseases classified elsewhere, thigh
  ▶ *M90.851 Osteopathy in diseases classified elsewhere, right thigh*
  ▶ *M90.852 Osteopathy in diseases classified elsewhere, left thigh*
  ▶ *M90.859 Osteopathy in diseases classified elsewhere, unspecified thigh*
● **M90.86** Osteopathy in diseases classified elsewhere, lower leg
  ▶ *M90.861 Osteopathy in diseases classified elsewhere, right lower leg*
  ▶ *M90.862 Osteopathy in diseases classified elsewhere, left lower leg*
  ▶ *M90.869 Osteopathy in diseases classified elsewhere, unspecified lower leg*
● **M90.87** Osteopathy in diseases classified elsewhere, ankle and foot
  ▶ *M90.871 Osteopathy in diseases classified elsewhere, right ankle and foot*
  ▶ *M90.872 Osteopathy in diseases classified elsewhere, left ankle and foot*
  ▶ *M90.879 Osteopathy in diseases classified elsewhere, unspecified ankle and foot*
  ▶ *M90.88 Osteopathy in diseases classified elsewhere, other site*
  ▶ *M90.89 Osteopathy in diseases classified elsewhere, multiple sites*

CHONDROPATHIES (M91-M94)

Excludes1 postprocedural chondropathies (M96.-)

● M91 Juvenile osteochondrosis of hip and pelvis
    Excludes1 slipped upper femoral epiphysis (nontraumatic) (M93.0)
  M91.0 Juvenile osteochondrosis of pelvis
      Osteochondrosis (juvenile) of acetabulum
      Osteochondrosis (juvenile) of iliac crest [Buchanan]
      Osteochondrosis (juvenile) of ischiopubic synchondrosis [van Neck]
      Osteochondrosis (juvenile) of symphysis pubis [Pierson]
  ● **M91.1** Juvenile osteochondrosis of head of femur [Legg-Calvé-Perthes]
      M91.10 Juvenile osteochondrosis of head of femur [Legg-Calvé-Perthes], unspecified leg
      M91.11 Juvenile osteochondrosis of head of femur [Legg-Calvé-Perthes], right leg
      M91.12 Juvenile osteochondrosis of head of femur [Legg-Calvé-Perthes], left leg
  ● **M91.2** Coxa plana
      Hip deformity due to previous juvenile osteochondrosis
      M91.20 Coxa plana, unspecified hip
      M91.21 Coxa plana, right hip
      M91.22 Coxa plana, left hip
  ● **M91.3** Pseudocoxalgia
      M91.30 Pseudocoxalgia, unspecified hip
      M91.31 Pseudocoxalgia, right hip
      M91.32 Pseudocoxalgia, left hip

◀ New   ◀⚎ Revised   ~~deleted~~ Deleted   Excludes 1   Excludes 2   Includes   Use additional   Code first   Code also   Unspecified
OGCR Official Guidelines   X Assign placeholder X   ● Use Additional Character(s)   ▶ Manifestation Code   **Coding Clinic**

● **M91.4 Coxa magna**
  M91.40 Coxa magna, unspecified hip
  M91.41 Coxa magna, right hip
  M91.42 Coxa magna, left hip
● **M91.8 Other juvenile osteochondrosis of hip and pelvis**
  Juvenile osteochondrosis after reduction of congenital dislocation of hip
  M91.80 Other juvenile osteochondrosis of hip and pelvis, unspecified leg
  M91.81 Other juvenile osteochondrosis of hip and pelvis, right leg
  M91.82 Other juvenile osteochondrosis of hip and pelvis, left leg
● **M91.9 Juvenile osteochondrosis of hip and pelvis, unspecified**
  M91.90 Juvenile osteochondrosis of hip and pelvis, unspecified, unspecified leg
  M91.91 Juvenile osteochondrosis of hip and pelvis, unspecified, right leg
  M91.92 Juvenile osteochondrosis of hip and pelvis, unspecified, left leg
● **M92 Other juvenile osteochondrosis**
  ● **M92.0 Juvenile osteochondrosis of humerus**
    Osteochondrosis (juvenile) of capitulum of humerus [Panner]
    Osteochondrosis (juvenile) of head of humerus [Haas]
    M92.00 Juvenile osteochondrosis of humerus, unspecified arm
    M92.01 Juvenile osteochondrosis of humerus, right arm
    M92.02 Juvenile osteochondrosis of humerus, left arm
  ● **M92.1 Juvenile osteochondrosis of radius and ulna**
    Osteochondrosis (juvenile) of lower ulna [Burns]
    Osteochondrosis (juvenile) of radial head [Brailsford]
    M92.10 Juvenile osteochondrosis of radius and ulna, unspecified arm
    M92.11 Juvenile osteochondrosis of radius and ulna, right arm
    M92.12 Juvenile osteochondrosis of radius and ulna, left arm
  ● **M92.2 Juvenile osteochondrosis, hand**
    ● M92.20 Unspecified juvenile osteochondrosis, hand
      M92.201 Unspecified juvenile osteochondrosis, right hand
      M92.202 Unspecified juvenile osteochondrosis, left hand
      M92.209 Unspecified juvenile osteochondrosis, unspecified hand
    ● M92.21 Osteochondrosis (juvenile) of carpal lunate [Kienböck]
      M92.211 Osteochondrosis (juvenile) of carpal lunate [Kienböck], right hand
      M92.212 Osteochondrosis (juvenile) of carpal lunate [Kienböck], left hand
      M92.219 Osteochondrosis (juvenile) of carpal lunate [Kienböck], unspecified hand
    ● M92.22 Osteochondrosis (juvenile) of metacarpal heads [Mauclaire]
      M92.221 Osteochondrosis (juvenile) of metacarpal heads [Mauclaire], right hand
      M92.222 Osteochondrosis (juvenile) of metacarpal heads [Mauclaire], left hand
      M92.229 Osteochondrosis (juvenile) of metacarpal heads [Mauclaire], unspecified hand

● M92.29 Other juvenile osteochondrosis, hand
  M92.291 Other juvenile osteochondrosis, right hand
  M92.292 Other juvenile osteochondrosis, left hand
  M92.299 Other juvenile osteochondrosis, unspecified hand
● **M92.3 Other juvenile osteochondrosis, upper limb**
  M92.30 Other juvenile osteochondrosis, unspecified upper limb
  M92.31 Other juvenile osteochondrosis, right upper limb
  M92.32 Other juvenile osteochondrosis, left upper limb
● **M92.4 Juvenile osteochondrosis of patella**
  Osteochondrosis (juvenile) of primary patellar center [Köhler]
  Osteochondrosis (juvenile) of secondary patellar center [Sinding Larsen]
  M92.40 Juvenile osteochondrosis of patella, unspecified knee
  M92.41 Juvenile osteochondrosis of patella, right knee
  M92.42 Juvenile osteochondrosis of patella, left knee
● **M92.5 Juvenile osteochondrosis of tibia and fibula**
  Osteochondrosis (juvenile) of proximal tibia [Blount]
  Osteochondrosis (juvenile) of tibial tubercle [Osgood-Schlatter]
  Tibia vara
  M92.50 Juvenile osteochondrosis of tibia and fibula, unspecified leg
  M92.51 Juvenile osteochondrosis of tibia and fibula, right leg
  M92.52 Juvenile osteochondrosis of tibia and fibula, left leg
● **M92.6 Juvenile osteochondrosis of tarsus**
  Osteochondrosis (juvenile) of calcaneum [Sever]
  Osteochondrosis (juvenile) of os tibiale externum [Haglund]
  Osteochondrosis (juvenile) of talus [Diaz]
  Osteochondrosis (juvenile) of tarsal navicular [Köhler]
  M92.60 Juvenile osteochondrosis of tarsus, unspecified ankle
  M92.61 Juvenile osteochondrosis of tarsus, right ankle
  M92.62 Juvenile osteochondrosis of tarsus, left ankle
● **M92.7 Juvenile osteochondrosis of metatarsus**
  Osteochondrosis (juvenile) of fifth metatarsus [Iselin]
  Osteochondrosis (juvenile) of second metatarsus [Freiberg]
  M92.70 Juvenile osteochondrosis of metatarsus, unspecified foot
  M92.71 Juvenile osteochondrosis of metatarsus, right foot
  M92.72 Juvenile osteochondrosis of metatarsus, left foot
M92.8 Other specified juvenile osteochondrosis
  Calcaneal apophysitis
M92.9 Juvenile osteochondrosis, unspecified
  Juvenile apophysitis NOS
  Juvenile epiphysitis NOS
  Juvenile osteochondritis NOS
  Juvenile osteochondrosis NOS

CHAPTER 13 (M00-M99)

● **M93   Other osteochondropathies**
     Excludes2   osteochondrosis of spine (M42.-)

    ● **M93.0   Slipped upper femoral epiphysis (nontraumatic)**
        Use additional code for associated chondrolysis (M94.3)

      ● **M93.00   Unspecified slipped upper femoral epiphysis (nontraumatic)**
         M93.001   Unspecified slipped upper femoral epiphysis (nontraumatic), right hip
         M93.002   Unspecified slipped upper femoral epiphysis (nontraumatic), left hip
         M93.003   Unspecified slipped upper femoral epiphysis (nontraumatic), unspecified hip

      ● **M93.01   Acute slipped upper femoral epiphysis (nontraumatic)**
         M93.011   Acute slipped upper femoral epiphysis (nontraumatic), right hip
         M93.012   Acute slipped upper femoral epiphysis (nontraumatic), left hip
         M93.013   Acute slipped upper femoral epiphysis (nontraumatic), unspecified hip

      ● **M93.02   Chronic slipped upper femoral epiphysis (nontraumatic)**
         M93.021   Chronic slipped upper femoral epiphysis (nontraumatic), right hip
         M93.022   Chronic slipped upper femoral epiphysis (nontraumatic), left hip
         M93.023   Chronic slipped upper femoral epiphysis (nontraumatic), unspecified hip

      ● **M93.03   Acute on chronic slipped upper femoral epiphysis (nontraumatic)**
         M93.031   Acute on chronic slipped upper femoral epiphysis (nontraumatic), right hip
         M93.032   Acute on chronic slipped upper femoral epiphysis (nontraumatic), left hip
         M93.033   Acute on chronic slipped upper femoral epiphysis (nontraumatic), unspecified hip

    M93.1   Kienböck's disease of adults   A
        Adult osteochondrosis of carpal lunates

    ● **M93.2   Osteochondritis dissecans**
       M93.20   Osteochondritis dissecans of unspecified site
      ● M93.21   Osteochondritis dissecans of shoulder
         M93.211   Osteochondritis dissecans, right shoulder
         M93.212   Osteochondritis dissecans, left shoulder
         M93.219   Osteochondritis dissecans, unspecified shoulder
      ● M93.22   Osteochondritis dissecans of elbow
         M93.221   Osteochondritis dissecans, right elbow
         M93.222   Osteochondritis dissecans, left elbow
         M93.229   Osteochondritis dissecans, unspecified elbow
      ● M93.23   Osteochondritis dissecans of wrist
         M93.231   Osteochondritis dissecans, right wrist
         M93.232   Osteochondritis dissecans, left wrist
         M93.239   Osteochondritis dissecans, unspecified wrist

      ● M93.24   Osteochondritis dissecans of joints of hand
         M93.241   Osteochondritis dissecans, joints of right hand
         M93.242   Osteochondritis dissecans, joints of left hand
         M93.249   Osteochondritis dissecans, joints of unspecified hand
      ● M93.25   Osteochondritis dissecans of hip
         M93.251   Osteochondritis dissecans, right hip
         M93.252   Osteochondritis dissecans, left hip
         M93.259   Osteochondritis dissecans, unspecified hip
      ● M93.26   Osteochondritis dissecans knee
         M93.261   Osteochondritis dissecans, right knee
         M93.262   Osteochondritis dissecans, left knee
         M93.269   Osteochondritis dissecans, unspecified knee
      ● M93.27   Osteochondritis dissecans of ankle and joints of foot
         M93.271   Osteochondritis dissecans, right ankle and joints of right foot
         M93.272   Osteochondritis dissecans, left ankle and joints of left foot
         M93.279   Osteochondritis dissecans, unspecified ankle and joints of foot
       M93.28   Osteochondritis dissecans other site
       M93.29   Osteochondritis dissecans multiple sites

    ● **M93.8   Other specified osteochondropathies**
       M93.80   Other specified osteochondropathies of unspecified site
      ● M93.81   Other specified osteochondropathies of shoulder
         M93.811   Other specified osteochondropathies, right shoulder
         M93.812   Other specified osteochondropathies, left shoulder
         M93.819   Other specified osteochondropathies, unspecified shoulder
      ● M93.82   Other specified osteochondropathies of upper arm
         M93.821   Other specified osteochondropathies, right upper arm
         M93.822   Other specified osteochondropathies, left upper arm
         M93.829   Other specified osteochondropathies, unspecified upper arm
      ● M93.83   Other specified osteochondropathies of forearm
         M93.831   Other specified osteochondropathies, right forearm
         M93.832   Other specified osteochondropathies, left forearm
         M93.839   Other specified osteochondropathies, unspecified forearm
      ● M93.84   Other specified osteochondropathies of hand
         M93.841   Other specified osteochondropathies, right hand
         M93.842   Other specified osteochondropathies, left hand
         M93.849   Other specified osteochondropathies, unspecified hand
      ● M93.85   Other specified osteochondropathies of thigh
         M93.851   Other specified osteochondropathies, right thigh
         M93.852   Other specified osteochondropathies, left thigh
         M93.859   Other specified osteochondropathies, unspecified thigh

◀ New   ◀ⁱ Revised   ~~deleted~~ Deleted   Excludes 1   Excludes 2   Includes   Use additional   Code first   Code also   Unspecified
OGCR Official Guidelines   X Assign placeholder X   ● Use Additional Character(s)   ▶ Manifestation Code   **Coding Clinic**

● M93.86 Other specified osteochondropathies lower leg
 M93.861 Other specified osteochondropathies, right lower leg
 M93.862 Other specified osteochondropathies, left lower leg
 M93.869 Other specified osteochondropathies, unspecified lower leg
● M93.87 Other specified osteochondropathies of ankle and foot
 M93.871 Other specified osteochondropathies, right ankle and foot
 M93.872 Other specified osteochondropathies, left ankle and foot
 M93.879 Other specified osteochondropathies, unspecified ankle and foot
 M93.88 Other specified osteochondropathies other
 M93.89 Other specified osteochondropathies multiple sites
M93.9 Osteochondropathy, unspecified
 Apophysitis NOS
 Epiphysitis NOS
 Osteochondritis NOS
 Osteochondrosis NOS
 M93.90 Osteochondropathy, unspecified of unspecified site
● M93.91 Osteochondropathy, unspecified of shoulder
 M93.911 Osteochondropathy, unspecified, right shoulder
 M93.912 Osteochondropathy, unspecified, left shoulder
 M93.919 Osteochondropathy, unspecified, unspecified shoulder
● M93.92 Osteochondropathy, unspecified of upper arm
 M93.921 Osteochondropathy, unspecified, right upper arm
 M93.922 Osteochondropathy, unspecified, left upper arm
 M93.929 Osteochondropathy, unspecified, unspecified upper arm
● M93.93 Osteochondropathy, unspecified of forearm
 M93.931 Osteochondropathy, unspecified, right forearm
 M93.932 Osteochondropathy, unspecified, left forearm
 M93.939 Osteochondropathy, unspecified, unspecified forearm
● M93.94 Osteochondropathy, unspecified of hand
 M93.941 Osteochondropathy, unspecified, right hand
 M93.942 Osteochondropathy, unspecified, left hand
 M93.949 Osteochondropathy, unspecified, unspecified hand
● M93.95 Osteochondropathy, unspecified of thigh
 M93.951 Osteochondropathy, unspecified, right thigh
 M93.952 Osteochondropathy, unspecified, left thigh
 M93.959 Osteochondropathy, unspecified, unspecified thigh

● M93.96 Osteochondropathy, unspecified lower leg
 M93.961 Osteochondropathy, unspecified, right lower leg
 M93.962 Osteochondropathy, unspecified, left lower leg
 M93.969 Osteochondropathy, unspecified, unspecified lower leg
● M93.97 Osteochondropathy, unspecified of ankle and foot
 M93.971 Osteochondropathy, unspecified, right ankle and foot
 M93.972 Osteochondropathy, unspecified, left ankle and foot
 M93.979 Osteochondropathy, unspecified, unspecified ankle and foot
 M93.98 Osteochondropathy, unspecified other
 M93.99 Osteochondropathy, unspecified multiple sites
● M94 Other disorders of cartilage
 M94.0 Chondrocostal junction syndrome [Tietze]
 Costochondritis
 M94.1 Relapsing polychondritis
● M94.2 Chondromalacia
 Excludes1   chondromalacia patellae (M22.4)
 M94.20 Chondromalacia, unspecified site
● M94.21 Chondromalacia, shoulder
 M94.211 Chondromalacia, right shoulder
 M94.212 Chondromalacia, left shoulder
 M94.219 Chondromalacia, unspecified shoulder
● M94.22 Chondromalacia, elbow
 M94.221 Chondromalacia, right elbow
 M94.222 Chondromalacia, left elbow
 M94.229 Chondromalacia, unspecified elbow
● M94.23 Chondromalacia, wrist
 M94.231 Chondromalacia, right wrist
 M94.232 Chondromalacia, left wrist
 M94.239 Chondromalacia, unspecified wrist
● M94.24 Chondromalacia, joints of hand
 M94.241 Chondromalacia, joints of right hand
 M94.242 Chondromalacia, joints of left hand
 M94.249 Chondromalacia, joints of unspecified hand
● M94.25 Chondromalacia, hip
 M94.251 Chondromalacia, right hip
 M94.252 Chondromalacia, left hip
 M94.259 Chondromalacia, unspecified hip
● M94.26 Chondromalacia, knee
 M94.261 Chondromalacia, right knee
 M94.262 Chondromalacia, left knee
 M94.269 Chondromalacia, unspecified knee
● M94.27 Chondromalacia, ankle and joints of foot
 M94.271 Chondromalacia, right ankle and joints of right foot
 M94.272 Chondromalacia, left ankle and joints of left foot
 M94.279 Chondromalacia, unspecified ankle and joints of foot
 M94.28 Chondromalacia, other site
 M94.29 Chondromalacia, multiple sites

CHAPTER 13 (M00-M99)

● M94.3   Chondrolysis

Code first any associated slipped upper femoral epiphysis (nontraumatic) (M93.0-)

    ● M94.35   Chondrolysis, hip

       M94.351   Chondrolysis, right hip

       M94.352   Chondrolysis, left hip

       M94.359   Chondrolysis, unspecified hip

● M94.8   Other specified disorders of cartilage

    ● M94.8X   Other specified disorders of cartilage

       M94.8X0   Other specified disorders of cartilage, multiple sites

       M94.8X1   Other specified disorders of cartilage, shoulder

       M94.8X2   Other specified disorders of cartilage, upper arm

       M94.8X3   Other specified disorders of cartilage, forearm

       M94.8X4   Other specified disorders of cartilage, hand

       M94.8X5   Other specified disorders of cartilage, thigh

       M94.8X6   Other specified disorders of cartilage, lower leg

       M94.8X7   Other specified disorders of cartilage, ankle and foot

       M94.8X8   Other specified disorders of cartilage, other site

       M94.8X9   Other specified disorders of cartilage, unspecified sites

M94.9   Disorder of cartilage, unspecified

OTHER DISORDERS OF THE MUSCULOSKELETAL SYSTEM AND CONNECTIVE TISSUE (M95)

● M95   Other acquired deformities of musculoskeletal system and connective tissue

    Excludes2   acquired absence of limbs and organs (Z89-Z90)

acquired deformities of limbs (M20-M21)

congenital malformations and deformations of the musculoskeletal system (Q65-Q79)

deforming dorsopathies (M40-M43)

dentofacial anomalies [including malocclusion] (M26.-)

postprocedural musculoskeletal disorders (M96.-)

M95.0   Acquired deformity of nose

    Excludes2   deviated nasal septum (J34.2)

● M95.1   Cauliflower ear

    Excludes2   other acquired deformities of ear (H61.1)

    M95.10   Cauliflower ear, unspecified ear

    M95.11   Cauliflower ear, right ear

    M95.12   Cauliflower ear, left ear

M95.2   Other acquired deformity of head

M95.3   Acquired deformity of neck

M95.4   Acquired deformity of chest and rib

M95.5   Acquired deformity of pelvis

    Excludes1   maternal care for known or suspected disproportion (O33.-)

M95.8   Other specified acquired deformities of musculoskeletal system

M95.9   Acquired deformity of musculoskeletal system, unspecified

INTRAOPERATIVE AND POSTPROCEDURAL COMPLICATIONS AND DISORDERS OF MUSCULOSKELETAL SYSTEM, NOT ELSEWHERE CLASSIFIED (M96)

● M96   Intraoperative and postprocedural complications and disorders of musculoskeletal system, not elsewhere classified

    Excludes2   arthropathy following intestinal bypass (M02.0-)

complications of internal orthopedic prosthetic devices, implants and grafts (T84.-)

disorders associated with osteoporosis (M80)

periprosthetic fracture around internal prosthetic joint (M97.-) ◀

presence of functional implants and other devices (Z96-Z97)

M96.0   Pseudarthrosis after fusion or arthrodesis

M96.1   Postlaminectomy syndrome, not elsewhere classified

M96.2   Postradiation kyphosis

M96.3   Postlaminectomy kyphosis

M96.4   Postsurgical lordosis

M96.5   Postradiation scoliosis

● M96.6   Fracture of bone following insertion of orthopedic implant, joint prosthesis, or bone plate

Intraoperative fracture of bone during insertion of orthopedic implant, joint prosthesis, or bone plate

    Excludes2   complication of internal orthopedic devices, implants or grafts (T84.-)

    ● M96.62   Fracture of humerus following insertion of orthopedic implant, joint prosthesis, or bone plate

       M96.621   Fracture of humerus following insertion of orthopedic implant, joint prosthesis, or bone plate, right arm

       M96.622   Fracture of humerus following insertion of orthopedic implant, joint prosthesis, or bone plate, left arm

       M96.629   Fracture of humerus following insertion of orthopedic implant, joint prosthesis, or bone plate, unspecified arm

    ● M96.63   Fracture of radius or ulna following insertion of orthopedic implant, joint prosthesis, or bone plate

       M96.631   Fracture of radius or ulna following insertion of orthopedic implant, joint prosthesis, or bone plate, right arm

       M96.632   Fracture of radius or ulna following insertion of orthopedic implant, joint prosthesis, or bone plate, left arm

       M96.639   Fracture of radius or ulna following insertion of orthopedic implant, joint prosthesis, or bone plate, unspecified arm

    M96.65   Fracture of pelvis following insertion of orthopedic implant, joint prosthesis, or bone plate

    ● M96.66   Fracture of femur following insertion of orthopedic implant, joint prosthesis, or bone plate

       M96.661   Fracture of femur following insertion of orthopedic implant, joint prosthesis, or bone plate, right leg

       M96.662   Fracture of femur following insertion of orthopedic implant, joint prosthesis, or bone plate, left leg

       M96.669   Fracture of femur following insertion of orthopedic implant, joint prosthesis, or bone plate, unspecified leg

◀ New   ◀▥ Revised   ~~deleted~~ Deleted   Excludes 1   Excludes 2   Includes   Use additional   Code first   Code also   Unspecified

OGCR Official Guidelines   X Assign placeholder X   ● Use Additional Character(s)   ▎ Manifestation Code   **Coding Clinic**

1062

● **M96.67**   **Fracture of tibia or fibula following insertion of orthopedic implant, joint prosthesis, or bone plate**

     M96.671   Fracture of tibia or fibula following insertion of orthopedic implant, joint prosthesis, or bone plate, right leg

     M96.672   Fracture of tibia or fibula following insertion of orthopedic implant, joint prosthesis, or bone plate, left leg

     M96.679   Fracture of tibia or fibula following insertion of orthopedic implant, joint prosthesis, or bone plate, unspecified leg

     M96.69   Fracture of other bone following insertion of orthopedic implant, joint prosthesis, or bone plate

● **M96.8**   **Other intraoperative and postprocedural complications and disorders of musculoskeletal system, not elsewhere classified**

     ● **M96.81**   **Intraoperative hemorrhage and hematoma of a musculoskeletal structure complicating a procedure**

         Excludes1   intraoperative hemorrhage and hematoma of a musculoskeletal structure due to accidental puncture and laceration during a procedure (M96.82-)

         M96.810   Intraoperative hemorrhage and hematoma of a musculoskeletal structure complicating a musculoskeletal system procedure

         M96.811   Intraoperative hemorrhage and hematoma of a musculoskeletal structure complicating other procedure

     ● **M96.82**   **Accidental puncture and laceration of a musculoskeletal structure during a procedure**

         M96.820   Accidental puncture and laceration of a musculoskeletal structure during a musculoskeletal system procedure

         M96.821   Accidental puncture and laceration of a musculoskeletal structure during other procedure

     ● **M96.83**   **Postprocedural hemorrhage of a musculoskeletal structure following a procedure**

         M96.830   Postprocedural hemorrhage of a musculoskeletal structure following a musculoskeletal system procedure

         M96.831   Postprocedural hemorrhage of a musculoskeletal structure following other procedure

     ● **M96.84**   **Postprocedural hematoma and seroma of a musculoskeletal structure following a procedure**

         M96.840   Postprocedural hematoma of a musculoskeletal structure following a musculoskeletal system procedure

         M96.841   Postprocedural hematoma of a musculoskeletal structure following other procedure

         M96.842   Postprocedural seroma of a musculoskeletal structure following a musculoskeletal system procedure

         M96.843   Postprocedural seroma of a musculoskeletal structure following other procedure

     M96.89   **Other intraoperative and postprocedural complications and disorders of the musculoskeletal system**

         Instability of joint secondary to removal of joint prosthesis

         Use additional code, if applicable, to further specify disorder

PERIPROSTHETIC FRACTURE AROUND INTERNAL PROSTHETIC JOINT (M97) ◄

● **M97**   **Periprosthetic fracture around internal prosthetic joint** ◄

     Excludes2   fracture of bone following insertion of orthopedic implant, joint prosthesis or bone plate (M96.6-) ◄

         breakage (fracture) of prosthetic joint (T84.01-) ◄

     The appropriate 7th character is to be added to each code from category M97: ◄

> A   initial encounter ◄
> D   subsequent encounter ◄
> S   sequela ◄

● **M97.0**   **Periprosthetic fracture around internal prosthetic hip joint**

   X ● **M97.01**   Periprosthetic fracture around internal prosthetic right hip joint ◄

   X ● **M97.02**   Periprosthetic fracture around internal prosthetic left hip joint ◄

● **M97.1**   **Periprosthetic fracture around internal prosthetic knee joint** ◄

   X ● **M97.11**   Periprosthetic fracture around internal prosthetic right knee joint ◄

   X ● **M97.12**   Periprosthetic fracture around internal prosthetic left knee joint ◄

● **M97.2**   **Periprosthetic fracture around internal prosthetic ankle joint** ◄

   X ● **M97.21**   Periprosthetic fracture around internal prosthetic right ankle joint ◄

   X ● **M97.22**   Periprosthetic fracture around internal prosthetic left ankle joint ◄

● **M97.3**   **Periprosthetic fracture around internal prosthetic shoulder joint** ◄

   X ● **M97.31**   Periprosthetic fracture around internal prosthetic right shoulder joint ◄

   X ● **M97.32**   Periprosthetic fracture around internal prosthetic left shoulder joint ◄

● **M97.4**   **Periprosthetic fracture around internal prosthetic elbow joint** ◄

   X ● **M97.41**   Periprosthetic fracture around internal prosthetic right elbow joint ◄

   X ● **M97.42**   Periprosthetic fracture around internal prosthetic left elbow joint ◄

   X ● **M97.8**   **Periprosthetic fracture around other internal prosthetic joint** ◄

     Periprosthetic fracture around internal prosthetic finger joint ◄

     Periprosthetic fracture around internal prosthetic spinal joint ◄

     Periprosthetic fracture around internal prosthetic toe joint ◄

     Periprosthetic fracture around internal prosthetic wrist joint ◄

     Use additional code to identify the joint (Z96.6-) ◄

   X ● **M97.9**   **Periprosthetic fracture around unspecified internal prosthetic joint** ◄

BIOMECHANICAL LESIONS, NOT ELSEWHERE CLASSIFIED (M99)

● **M99 Biomechanical lesions, not elsewhere classified**

    Note: This category should not be used if the condition can be classified elsewhere.

  ● **M99.0 Segmental and somatic dysfunction**

    M99.00 Segmental and somatic dysfunction of head region

    M99.01 Segmental and somatic dysfunction of cervical region

    M99.02 Segmental and somatic dysfunction of thoracic region

    M99.03 Segmental and somatic dysfunction of lumbar region

    M99.04 Segmental and somatic dysfunction of sacral region

    M99.05 Segmental and somatic dysfunction of pelvic region

    M99.06 Segmental and somatic dysfunction of lower extremity

    M99.07 Segmental and somatic dysfunction of upper extremity

    M99.08 Segmental and somatic dysfunction of rib cage

    M99.09 Segmental and somatic dysfunction of abdomen and other regions

  ● **M99.1 Subluxation complex (vertebral)**

    M99.10 Subluxation complex (vertebral) of head region

    M99.11 Subluxation complex (vertebral) of cervical region

    M99.12 Subluxation complex (vertebral) of thoracic region

    M99.13 Subluxation complex (vertebral) of lumbar region

    M99.14 Subluxation complex (vertebral) of sacral region

    M99.15 Subluxation complex (vertebral) of pelvic region

    M99.16 Subluxation complex (vertebral) of lower extremity

    M99.17 Subluxation complex (vertebral) of upper extremity

    M99.18 Subluxation complex (vertebral) of rib cage

    M99.19 Subluxation complex (vertebral) of abdomen and other regions

  ● **M99.2 Subluxation stenosis of neural canal**

    M99.20 Subluxation stenosis of neural canal of head region

    M99.21 Subluxation stenosis of neural canal of cervical region

    M99.22 Subluxation stenosis of neural canal of thoracic region

    M99.23 Subluxation stenosis of neural canal of lumbar region

    M99.24 Subluxation stenosis of neural canal of sacral region

    M99.25 Subluxation stenosis of neural canal of pelvic region

    M99.26 Subluxation stenosis of neural canal of lower extremity

    M99.27 Subluxation stenosis of neural canal of upper extremity

    M99.28 Subluxation stenosis of neural canal of rib cage

    M99.29 Subluxation stenosis of neural canal of abdomen and other regions

  ● **M99.3 Osseous stenosis of neural canal**

    M99.30 Osseous stenosis of neural canal of head region

    M99.31 Osseous stenosis of neural canal of cervical region

    M99.32 Osseous stenosis of neural canal of thoracic region

    M99.33 Osseous stenosis of neural canal of lumbar region

    M99.34 Osseous stenosis of neural canal of sacral region

    M99.35 Osseous stenosis of neural canal of pelvic region

    M99.36 Osseous stenosis of neural canal of lower extremity

    M99.37 Osseous stenosis of neural canal of upper extremity

    M99.38 Osseous stenosis of neural canal of rib cage

    M99.39 Osseous stenosis of neural canal of abdomen and other regions

  ● **M99.4 Connective tissue stenosis of neural canal**

    M99.40 Connective tissue stenosis of neural canal of head region

    M99.41 Connective tissue stenosis of neural canal of cervical region

    M99.42 Connective tissue stenosis of neural canal of thoracic region

    M99.43 Connective tissue stenosis of neural canal of lumbar region

    M99.44 Connective tissue stenosis of neural canal of sacral region

    M99.45 Connective tissue stenosis of neural canal of pelvic region

    M99.46 Connective tissue stenosis of neural canal of lower extremity

    M99.47 Connective tissue stenosis of neural canal of upper extremity

    M99.48 Connective tissue stenosis of neural canal of rib cage

    M99.49 Connective tissue stenosis of neural canal of abdomen and other regions

  ● **M99.5 Intervertebral disc stenosis of neural canal**

    M99.50 Intervertebral disc stenosis of neural canal of head region

    M99.51 Intervertebral disc stenosis of neural canal of cervical region

    M99.52 Intervertebral disc stenosis of neural canal of thoracic region

    M99.53 Intervertebral disc stenosis of neural canal of lumbar region

    M99.54 Intervertebral disc stenosis of neural canal of sacral region

    M99.55 Intervertebral disc stenosis of neural canal of pelvic region

    M99.56 Intervertebral disc stenosis of neural canal of lower extremity

    M99.57 Intervertebral disc stenosis of neural canal of upper extremity

    M99.58 Intervertebral disc stenosis of neural canal of rib cage

    M99.59 Intervertebral disc stenosis of neural canal of abdomen and other regions

◀ New   ◀◀ Revised   ~~deleted~~ Deleted   Excludes 1   Excludes 2   Includes   Use additional   Code first   Code also   Unspecified
OGCR Official Guidelines   X Assign placeholder X   ● Use Additional Character(s)   ▶ Manifestation Code   **Coding Clinic**

● **M99.6 Osseous and subluxation stenosis of intervertebral foramina**

M99.60 Osseous and subluxation stenosis of intervertebral foramina of head region

M99.61 Osseous and subluxation stenosis of intervertebral foramina of cervical region

M99.62 Osseous and subluxation stenosis of intervertebral foramina of thoracic region

M99.63 Osseous and subluxation stenosis of intervertebral foramina of lumbar region

M99.64 Osseous and subluxation stenosis of intervertebral foramina of sacral region

M99.65 Osseous and subluxation stenosis of intervertebral foramina of pelvic region

M99.66 Osseous and subluxation stenosis of intervertebral foramina of lower extremity

M99.67 Osseous and subluxation stenosis of intervertebral foramina of upper extremity

M99.68 Osseous and subluxation stenosis of intervertebral foramina of rib cage

M99.69 Osseous and subluxation stenosis of intervertebral foramina of abdomen and other regions

● **M99.7 Connective tissue and disc stenosis of intervertebral foramina**

M99.70 Connective tissue and disc stenosis of intervertebral foramina of head region

M99.71 Connective tissue and disc stenosis of intervertebral foramina of cervical region

M99.72 Connective tissue and disc stenosis of intervertebral foramina of thoracic region

M99.73 Connective tissue and disc stenosis of intervertebral foramina of lumbar region

M99.74 Connective tissue and disc stenosis of intervertebral foramina of sacral region

M99.75 Connective tissue and disc stenosis of intervertebral foramina of pelvic region

M99.76 Connective tissue and disc stenosis of intervertebral foramina of lower extremity

M99.77 Connective tissue and disc stenosis of intervertebral foramina of upper extremity

M99.78 Connective tissue and disc stenosis of intervertebral foramina of rib cage

M99.79 Connective tissue and disc stenosis of intervertebral foramina of abdomen and other regions

● **M99.8 Other biomechanical lesions**

M99.80 Other biomechanical lesions of head region

M99.81 Other biomechanical lesions of cervical region

M99.82 Other biomechanical lesions of thoracic region

M99.83 Other biomechanical lesions of lumbar region

M99.84 Other biomechanical lesions of sacral region

M99.85 Other biomechanical lesions of pelvic region

M99.86 Other biomechanical lesions of lower extremity

M99.87 Other biomechanical lesions of upper extremity

M99.88 Other biomechanical lesions of rib cage

M99.89 Other biomechanical lesions of abdomen and other regions

M99.9 Biomechanical lesion, unspecified

CHAPTER 14

DISEASES OF THE GENITOURINARY SYSTEM (N00-N99)

14. **Chapter 14: Diseases of Genitourinary System (N00-N99)**
    a. **Chronic kidney disease**
        1) **Stages of chronic kidney disease (CKD)**
    The ICD-10-CM classifies CKD based on severity. The severity of CKD is designated by stages 1-5. Stage 2, code N18.2, equates to mild CKD; stage 3, code N18.3, equates to moderate CKD; and stage 4, code N18.4, equates to severe CKD. Code N18.6, End stage renal disease (ESRD), is assigned when the provider has documented end-stage-renal disease (ESRD).
    If both a stage of CKD and ESRD are documented, assign code N18.6 only.
        2) **Chronic kidney disease and kidney transplant status**
    Patients who have undergone kidney transplant may still have some form of chronic kidney disease CKD because the kidney transplant may not fully restore kidney function. Therefore, the presence of CKD alone does not constitute a transplant complication. Assign the appropriate N18 code for the patient's stage of CKD and code Z94.0, Kidney transplant status. If a transplant complication such as failure or rejection or other transplant complication is documented, see section I.C.19.g for information on coding complications of a kidney transplant. If the documentation is unclear as to whether the patient has a complication of the transplant, query the provider.
        3) **Chronic kidney disease with other conditions**
    Patients with CKD may also suffer from other serious conditions, most commonly diabetes mellitus and hypertension. The sequencing of the CKD code in relationship to codes for other contributing conditions is based on the conventions in the Tabular List.
    See I.C.9. Hypertensive chronic kidney disease.
    See I.C.19. Chronic kidney disease and kidney transplant complications.

Item 14–1 Nephritis (inflammation) or **nephropathy** (disease) **with lesion of proliferative glomerulonephritis** results from a streptococcal infection.
Nephritis (inflammation) or **nephropathy** (disease) **with lesion of membranous glomerulonephritis** is characterized by deposits along the epithelial side of the basement membrane.
Nephritis (inflammation) or **nephropathy** (disease) **with lesion of membranoproliferative glomerulonephritis** is characterized by alterations in the basement membranes of the kidney and the glomerular cells.
Nephritis (inflammation) or **nephropathy** (disease) **with lesion of rapidly progressive glomerulonephritis** is characterized by rapid and progressive decline in renal function.
Nephritis (inflammation) or **nephropathy** (disease) **with lesion of renal cortical necrosis** is characterized by death of the cortical tissues.
Nephritis (inflammation) or **nephropathy** (disease) **with lesion of renal medullary necrosis** is characterized by death of the tissues that collect urine.

Figure 14-1 Kidneys within the urinary system.

Item 14–2 Glomerulonephritis is nephritis accompanied by inflammation of the glomeruli of the kidney, resulting in the degeneration of the glomeruli and the nephrons.
Acute glomerulonephritis primarily affects children and young adults and is usually a result of a streptococcal infection.
Proliferative glomerulonephritis is the acute form of the disease resulting from a streptococcal infection.
Rapidly progressive glomerulonephritis, also known as **crescentic** or **malignant glomerulonephritis**, is the acute form of the disease, which leads quickly to rapid and progressive decline in renal function.

CHAPTER 14

DISEASES OF THE GENITOURINARY SYSTEM (N00-N99)

Excludes2 certain conditions originating in the perinatal period (P04-P96)
certain infectious and parasitic diseases (A00-B99)
complications of pregnancy, childbirth and the puerperium (O00-O9A)
congenital malformations, deformations and chromosomal abnormalities (Q00-Q99)
endocrine, nutritional and metabolic diseases (E00-E88)
injury, poisoning and certain other consequences of external causes (S00-T88)
neoplasms (C00-D49)
symptoms, signs and abnormal clinical and laboratory findings, not elsewhere classified (R00-R94)

This chapter contains the following blocks:

N00-N08	Glomerular diseases
N10-N16	Renal tubulo-interstitial diseases
N17-N19	Acute kidney failure and chronic kidney disease
N20-N23	Urolithiasis
N25-N29	Other disorders of kidney and ureter
N30-N39	Other diseases of the urinary system
N40-N53	Diseases of male genital organs
N60-N65	Disorders of breast
N70-N77	Inflammatory diseases of female pelvic organs
N80-N98	Noninflammatory disorders of female genital tract
N99	Intraoperative and postprocedural complications and disorders of genitourinary system, not elsewhere classified

GLOMERULAR DISEASES (N00-N08)

Code also any associated kidney failure (N17-N19)
Excludes1 hypertensive chronic kidney disease (I12.-)

● **N00 Acute nephritic syndrome**
   Includes acute glomerular disease
             acute glomerulonephritis
             acute nephritis
   Excludes1 acute tubulo-interstitial nephritis (N10)
             nephritic syndrome NOS (N05.-)

  N00.0 Acute nephritic syndrome with minor glomerular abnormality
     Acute nephritic syndrome with minimal change lesion

  N00.1 Acute nephritic syndrome with focal and segmental glomerular lesions
     Acute nephritic syndrome with focal and segmental hyalinosis
     Acute nephritic syndrome with focal and segmental sclerosis
     Acute nephritic syndrome with focal glomerulonephritis

◀ New   ⬸ Revised   ~~deleted~~ Deleted   Excludes 1   Excludes 2   Includes   Use additional   Code first   Code also   Unspecified
OGCR Official Guidelines   X Assign placeholder X   ● Use Additional Character(s)   ▶ Manifestation Code   **Coding Clinic**

N00.2   **Acute nephritic syndrome with diffuse membranous glomerulonephritis**

N00.3   **Acute nephritic syndrome with diffuse mesangial proliferative glomerulonephritis**

N00.4   **Acute nephritic syndrome with diffuse endocapillary proliferative glomerulonephritis**

N00.5   **Acute nephritic syndrome with diffuse mesangiocapillary glomerulonephritis**
> Acute nephritic syndrome with membranoproliferative glomerulonephritis, types 1 and 3, or NOS

N00.6   **Acute nephritic syndrome with dense deposit disease**
> Acute nephritic syndrome with membranoproliferative glomerulonephritis, type 2

N00.7   **Acute nephritic syndrome with diffuse crescentic glomerulonephritis**
> Acute nephritic syndrome with extracapillary glomerulonephritis

N00.8   **Acute nephritic syndrome with other morphologic changes**
> Acute nephritic syndrome with proliferative glomerulonephritis NOS

N00.9   **Acute nephritic syndrome with unspecified morphologic changes**

● **N01**   **Rapidly progressive nephritic syndrome**

> **Includes**   rapidly progressive glomerular disease
> rapidly progressive glomerulonephritis
> rapidly progressive nephritis

> **Excludes1**   nephritic syndrome NOS (N05.-)

N01.0   **Rapidly progressive nephritic syndrome with minor glomerular abnormality**
> Rapidly progressive nephritic syndrome with minimal change lesion

N01.1   **Rapidly progressive nephritic syndrome with focal and segmental glomerular lesions**
> Rapidly progressive nephritic syndrome with focal and segmental hyalinosis
> Rapidly progressive nephritic syndrome with focal and segmental sclerosis
> Rapidly progressive nephritic syndrome with focal glomerulonephritis

N01.2   **Rapidly progressive nephritic syndrome with diffuse membranous glomerulonephritis**

N01.3   **Rapidly progressive nephritic syndrome with diffuse mesangial proliferative glomerulonephritis**

N01.4   **Rapidly progressive nephritic syndrome with diffuse endocapillary proliferative glomerulonephritis**

N01.5   **Rapidly progressive nephritic syndrome with diffuse mesangiocapillary glomerulonephritis**
> Rapidly progressive nephritic syndrome with membranoproliferative glomerulonephritis, types 1 and 3, or NOS

N01.6   **Rapidly progressive nephritic syndrome with dense deposit disease**
> Rapidly progressive nephritic syndrome with membranoproliferative glomerulonephritis, type 2

N01.7   **Rapidly progressive nephritic syndrome with diffuse crescentic glomerulonephritis**
> Rapidly progressive nephritic syndrome with extracapillary glomerulonephritis

N01.8   **Rapidly progressive nephritic syndrome with other morphologic changes**
> Rapidly progressive nephritic syndrome with proliferative glomerulonephritis NOS

N01.9   **Rapidly progressive nephritic syndrome with unspecified morphologic changes**

● **N02**   **Recurrent and persistent hematuria**

> **Excludes1**   acute cystitis with hematuria (N30.01)
> hematuria NOS (R31.9)
> hematuria not associated with specified morphologic lesions (R31.-)

N02.0   **Recurrent and persistent hematuria with minor glomerular abnormality**
> Recurrent and persistent hematuria with minimal change lesion

N02.1   **Recurrent and persistent hematuria with focal and segmental glomerular lesions**
> Recurrent and persistent hematuria with focal and segmental hyalinosis
> Recurrent and persistent hematuria with focal and segmental sclerosis
> Recurrent and persistent hematuria with focal glomerulonephritis

N02.2   **Recurrent and persistent hematuria with diffuse membranous glomerulonephritis**

N02.3   **Recurrent and persistent hematuria with diffuse mesangial proliferative glomerulonephritis**

N02.4   **Recurrent and persistent hematuria with diffuse endocapillary proliferative glomerulonephritis**

N02.5   **Recurrent and persistent hematuria with diffuse mesangiocapillary glomerulonephritis**
> Recurrent and persistent hematuria with membranoproliferative glomerulonephritis, types 1 and 3, or NOS

N02.6   **Recurrent and persistent hematuria with dense deposit disease**
> Recurrent and persistent hematuria with membranoproliferative glomerulonephritis, type 2

N02.7   **Recurrent and persistent hematuria with diffuse crescentic glomerulonephritis**
> Recurrent and persistent hematuria with extracapillary glomerulonephritis

N02.8   **Recurrent and persistent hematuria with other morphologic changes**
> Recurrent and persistent hematuria with proliferative glomerulonephritis NOS

N02.9   **Recurrent and persistent hematuria with unspecified morphologic changes**

● **N03**   **Chronic nephritic syndrome**

> **Includes**   chronic glomerular disease
> chronic glomerulonephritis
> chronic nephritis

> **Excludes1**   chronic tubulo-interstitial nephritis (N11.-)
> diffuse sclerosing glomerulonephritis (N05.8-)
> nephritic syndrome NOS (N05.-)

N03.0   **Chronic nephritic syndrome with minor glomerular abnormality**
> Chronic nephritic syndrome with minimal change lesion

N03.1   **Chronic nephritic syndrome with focal and segmental glomerular lesions**
> Chronic nephritic syndrome with focal and segmental hyalinosis
> Chronic nephritic syndrome with focal and segmental sclerosis
> Chronic nephritic syndrome with focal glomerulonephritis

N03.2   **Chronic nephritic syndrome with diffuse membranous glomerulonephritis**

N03.3   **Chronic nephritic syndrome with diffuse mesangial proliferative glomerulonephritis**

N03.4   **Chronic nephritic syndrome with diffuse endocapillary proliferative glomerulonephritis**

N03.5   **Chronic nephritic syndrome with diffuse mesangiocapillary glomerulonephritis**
> Chronic nephritic syndrome with membranoproliferative glomerulonephritis, types 1 and 3, or NOS

CHAPTER 14 (N00-N99)

CHAPTER 14 (N00–N99)

Item 14–3 Chronic glomerulonephritis (GN) persists over a period of years, with remissions and exacerbation.

Chronic GN with lesion of proliferative glomerulonephritis results from a streptococcal infection.

Chronic GN with lesion of membranous glomerulonephritis, also known as membranous nephropathy, is characterized by deposits along the epithelial side of the basement membrane.

Chronic GN with lesion of membrano-proliferative glomerulonephritis (MPGN) is a group of disorders characterized by alterations in the basement membranes of the kidney and the glomerular cells.

Chronic GN with lesion of rapidly progressive glomerulonephritis is characterized by necrosis, endothelial proliferation, and mesangial proliferation. The condition is marked by rapid and progressive decline in renal function.

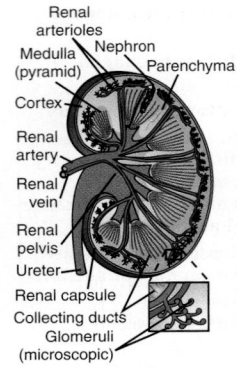

Figure 14-2 Kidney cross section.

Labels: Renal arterioles, Medulla (pyramid), Nephron, Parenchyma, Cortex, Renal artery, Renal vein, Renal pelvis, Ureter, Renal capsule, Collecting ducts, Glomeruli (microscopic)

N03.6   Chronic nephritic syndrome with dense deposit disease
　　　　　Chronic nephritic syndrome with membranoproliferative glomerulonephritis, type 2

N03.7   Chronic nephritic syndrome with diffuse crescentic glomerulonephritis
　　　　　Chronic nephritic syndrome with extracapillary glomerulonephritis

N03.8   Chronic nephritic syndrome with other morphologic changes
　　　　　Chronic nephritic syndrome with proliferative glomerulonephritis NOS

N03.9   Chronic nephritic syndrome with unspecified morphologic changes

● **N04   Nephrotic syndrome**
　　Includes　　congenital nephrotic syndrome
　　　　　　　　　lipoid nephrosis

N04.0   Nephrotic syndrome with minor glomerular abnormality
　　　　　Nephrotic syndrome with minimal change lesion

N04.1   Nephrotic syndrome with focal and segmental glomerular lesions
　　　　　Nephrotic syndrome with focal and segmental hyalinosis
　　　　　Nephrotic syndrome with focal and segmental sclerosis
　　　　　Nephrotic syndrome with focal glomerulonephritis

N04.2   Nephrotic syndrome with diffuse membranous glomerulonephritis

N04.3   Nephrotic syndrome with diffuse mesangial proliferative glomerulonephritis

N04.4   Nephrotic syndrome with diffuse endocapillary proliferative glomerulonephritis

N04.5   Nephrotic syndrome with diffuse mesangiocapillary glomerulonephritis
　　　　　Nephrotic syndrome with membranoproliferative glomerulonephritis, types 1 and 3, or NOS

N04.6   Nephrotic syndrome with dense deposit disease
　　　　　Nephrotic syndrome with membranoproliferative glomerulonephritis, type 2

N04.7   Nephrotic syndrome with diffuse crescentic glomerulonephritis
　　　　　Nephrotic syndrome with extracapillary glomerulonephritis

N04.8   Nephrotic syndrome with other morphologic changes
　　　　　Nephrotic syndrome with proliferative glomerulonephritis NOS

N04.9   Nephrotic syndrome with unspecified morphologic changes

Item 14–4 Nephrotic syndrome (NS) is marked by massive proteinuria (protein in the urine) and water retention. Patients with NS are particularly vulnerable to staphylococcal and pneumococcal infections. NS with lesion of proliferative glomerulonephritis results from a streptococcal infection. NS with lesion of membranous glomerulonephritis results in thickening of the capillary walls. NS with lesion of minimal change glomerulonephritis is usually a benign disorder that occurs mostly in children and requires electron microscopy (biopsy) to verify changes in the glomeruli.

● **N05   Unspecified nephritic syndrome**
　　Includes　　glomerular disease NOS
　　　　　　　　　glomerulonephritis NOS
　　　　　　　　　nephritis NOS
　　　　　　　　　nephropathy NOS and renal disease NOS with morphological lesion specified in .0-.8

　　Excludes1　nephropathy NOS with no stated morphological lesion (N28.9)
　　　　　　　　　renal disease NOS with no stated morphological lesion (N28.9)
　　　　　　　　　tubulo-interstitial nephritis NOS (N12)

N05.0   Unspecified nephritic syndrome with minor glomerular abnormality
　　　　　Unspecified nephritic syndrome with minimal change lesion

N05.1   Unspecified nephritic syndrome with focal and segmental glomerular lesions
　　　　　Unspecified nephritic syndrome with focal and segmental hyalinosis
　　　　　Unspecified nephritic syndrome with focal and segmental sclerosis
　　　　　Unspecified nephritic syndrome with focal glomerulonephritis

N05.2   Unspecified nephritic syndrome with diffuse membranous glomerulonephritis

N05.3   Unspecified nephritic syndrome with diffuse mesangial proliferative glomerulonephritis

N05.4   Unspecified nephritic syndrome with diffuse endocapillary proliferative glomerulonephritis

N05.5   Unspecified nephritic syndrome with diffuse mesangiocapillary glomerulonephritis
　　　　　Unspecified nephritic syndrome with membranoproliferative glomerulonephritis, types 1 and 3, or NOS

N05.6   Unspecified nephritic syndrome with dense deposit disease
　　　　　Unspecified nephritic syndrome with membranoproliferative glomerulonephritis, type 2

N05.7   Unspecified nephritic syndrome with diffuse crescentic glomerulonephritis
　　　　　Unspecified nephritic syndrome with extracapillary glomerulonephritis

N05.8   Unspecified nephritic syndrome with other morphologic changes
　　　　　Unspecified nephritic syndrome with proliferative glomerulonephritis NOS

N05.9   Unspecified nephritic syndrome with unspecified morphologic changes

◄ New　◄▬ Revised　~~deleted~~ Deleted　Excludes 1　Excludes 2　Includes　Use additional　Code first　Code also　Unspecified
OGCR Official Guidelines　X Assign placeholder X　● Use Additional Character(s)　▶ Manifestation Code　**Coding Clinic**

● **N06 Isolated proteinuria with specified morphological lesion**

    Excludes1   proteinuria not associated with specific morphologic lesions (R80.0)

N06.0 Isolated proteinuria with minor glomerular abnormality
Isolated proteinuria with minimal change lesion

N06.1 Isolated proteinuria with focal and segmental glomerular lesions
Isolated proteinuria with focal and segmental hyalinosis
Isolated proteinuria with focal and segmental sclerosis
Isolated proteinuria with focal glomerulonephritis

N06.2 Isolated proteinuria with diffuse membranous glomerulonephritis

N06.3 Isolated proteinuria with diffuse mesangial proliferative glomerulonephritis

N06.4 Isolated proteinuria with diffuse endocapillary proliferative glomerulonephritis

N06.5 Isolated proteinuria with diffuse mesangiocapillary glomerulonephritis
Isolated proteinuria with membranoproliferative glomerulonephritis, types 1 and 3, or NOS

N06.6 Isolated proteinuria with dense deposit disease
Isolated proteinuria with membranoproliferative glomerulonephritis, type 2

N06.7 Isolated proteinuria with diffuse crescentic glomerulonephritis
Isolated proteinuria with extracapillary glomerulonephritis

N06.8 Isolated proteinuria with other morphologic lesion
Isolated proteinuria with proliferative glomerulonephritis NOS

N06.9 Isolated proteinuria with unspecified morphologic lesion

● **N07 Hereditary nephropathy, not elsewhere classified**

    Excludes2   Alport's syndrome (Q87.81-)
hereditary amyloid nephropathy (E85.-)
nail patella syndrome (Q87.2)
non-neuropathic heredofamilial amyloidosis (E85.-)

N07.0 Hereditary nephropathy, not elsewhere classified with minor glomerular abnormality
Hereditary nephropathy, not elsewhere classified with minimal change lesion

N07.1 Hereditary nephropathy, not elsewhere classified with focal and segmental glomerular lesions
Hereditary nephropathy, not elsewhere classified with focal and segmental hyalinosis
Hereditary nephropathy, not elsewhere classified with focal and segmental sclerosis
Hereditary nephropathy, not elsewhere classified with focal glomerulonephritis

N07.2 Hereditary nephropathy, not elsewhere classified with diffuse membranous glomerulonephritis

N07.3 Hereditary nephropathy, not elsewhere classified with diffuse mesangial proliferative glomerulonephritis

N07.4 Hereditary nephropathy, not elsewhere classified with diffuse endocapillary proliferative glomerulonephritis

N07.5 Hereditary nephropathy, not elsewhere classified with diffuse mesangiocapillary glomerulonephritis
Hereditary nephropathy, not elsewhere classified with membranoproliferative glomerulonephritis, types 1 and 3, or NOS

N07.6 Hereditary nephropathy, not elsewhere classified with dense deposit disease
Hereditary nephropathy, not elsewhere classified with membranoproliferative glomerulonephritis, type 2

N07.7 Hereditary nephropathy, not elsewhere classified with diffuse crescentic glomerulonephritis
Hereditary nephropathy, not elsewhere classified with extracapillary glomerulonephritis

N07.8 Hereditary nephropathy, not elsewhere classified with other morphologic lesions
Hereditary nephropathy, not elsewhere classified with proliferative glomerulonephritis NOS

N07.9 Hereditary nephropathy, not elsewhere classified with unspecified morphologic lesions

▷ **N08 Glomerular disorders in diseases classified elsewhere**
Glomerulonephritis
Nephritis
Nephropathy
Code first underlying disease, such as:
amyloidosis (E85.-)
congenital syphilis (A50.5)
cryoglobulinemia (D89.1)
disseminated intravascular coagulation (D65)
gout (M1A.-, M10.-)
microscopic polyangiitis (M31.7)
multiple myeloma (C90.0-)
sepsis (A40.0-A41.9)
sickle-cell disease (D57.0-D57.8)

    Excludes1   glomerulonephritis, nephritis and nephropathy (in):
antiglomerular basement membrane disease (M31.0)
diabetes (E08-E13 with .21)
gonococcal (A54.21)
Goodpasture's syndrome (M31.0)
hemolytic-uremic syndrome (D59.3)
lupus (M32.14)
mumps (B26.83)
syphilis (A52.75)
systemic lupus erythematosus (M32.14)
Wegener's granulomatosis (M31.31)
pyelonephritis in diseases classified elsewhere (N16)
renal tubulo-interstitial disorders classified elsewhere (N16)

RENAL TUBULO-INTERSTITIAL DISEASES (N10-N16)

    Includes   pyelonephritis
    Excludes1   pyeloureteritis cystica (N28.85)

N10 Acute pyelonephritis ◀
Acute infectious interstitial nephritis
Acute pyelitis
Acute tubulo-interstitial nephritis ◀
Hemoglobin nephrosis
Myoglobin nephrosis
Use additional code (B95-B97), to identify infectious agent

● **N11 Chronic tubulo-interstitial nephritis**
    Includes   chronic infectious interstitial nephritis
chronic pyelitis
chronic pyelonephritis
Use additional code (B95-B97), to identify infectious agent

N11.0 Nonobstructive reflux-associated chronic pyelonephritis
Pyelonephritis (chronic) associated with (vesicoureteral) reflux
    Excludes1   vesicoureteral reflux NOS (N13.70)

N11.1 Chronic obstructive pyelonephritis
Pyelonephritis (chronic) associated with anomaly of pelviureteric junction
Pyelonephritis (chronic) associated with anomaly of pyeloureteric junction
Pyelonephritis (chronic) associated with crossing of vessel
Pyelonephritis (chronic) associated with kinking of ureter
Pyelonephritis (chronic) associated with obstruction of ureter
Pyelonephritis (chronic) associated with stricture of pelviureteric junction
Pyelonephritis (chronic) associated with stricture of ureter
    Excludes1   calculous pyelonephritis (N20.9)
obstructive uropathy (N13.-)

CHAPTER 14 (N00-N99)

Figure 14-3   Acute pyelonephritis. Cortical surface exhibits grayish white areas of inflammation and abscess formation. (From Kumar: Robbins and Cotran: Pathologic Basis of Disease, ed 8, Saunders, An Imprint of Elsevier, 2009)

Item 14–5 Pyelonephritis is an infection of the kidneys and ureters and may be chronic or acute in one or both kidneys.

N11.8   **Other chronic tubulo-interstitial nephritis**
    Nonobstructive chronic pyelonephritis NOS

N11.9   **Chronic tubulo-interstitial nephritis, unspecified**
    Chronic interstitial nephritis NOS
    Chronic pyelitis NOS
    Chronic pyelonephritis NOS

N12   **Tubulo-interstitial nephritis, not specified as acute or chronic**
    Interstitial nephritis NOS
    Pyelitis NOS
    Pyelonephritis NOS
    Excludes1   calculous pyelonephritis (N20.9)

● **N13**   **Obstructive and reflux uropathy**
    Excludes2   calculus of kidney and ureter without hydronephrosis (N20.-)
       congenital obstructive defects of renal pelvis and ureter (Q62.0-Q62.3)
       hydronephrosis with ureteropelvic junction obstruction (Q62.1)
       obstructive pyelonephritis (N11.1)

N13.0   **Hydronephrosis with ureteropelvic junction obstruction** ◀
    Hydronephrosis due to acquired occlusion of ureteropelvic junction ◀
    Excludes2   Hydronephrosis with ureteropelvic junction obstruction due to calculus (N13.2) ◀

N13.1   **Hydronephrosis with ureteral stricture, not elsewhere classified**
    Excludes1   hydronephrosis with ureteral stricture with infection (N13.6)

N13.2   **Hydronephrosis with renal and ureteral calculous obstruction**
    Excludes1   hydronephrosis with renal and ureteral calculous obstruction with infection (N13.6)

● **N13.3**   **Other and unspecified hydronephrosis**
    Excludes1   hydronephrosis with infection (N13.6)
   N13.30   **Unspecified hydronephrosis**
   N13.39   **Other hydronephrosis**

N13.4   **Hydroureter**
    Excludes1   congenital hydroureter (Q62.3-)
       hydroureter with infection (N13.6)
       vesicoureteral-reflux with hydroureter (N13.73-)

N13.5   **Crossing vessel and stricture of ureter without hydronephrosis**
    Kinking and stricture of ureter without hydronephrosis
    Excludes1   crossing vessel and stricture of ureter without hydronephrosis with infection (N13.6)

N13.6   **Pyonephrosis**
    Conditions in N13.0-N13.5 with infection ◀▥
    Obstructive uropathy with infection
    Use additional code (B95-B97), to identify infectious agent

● **N13.7**   **Vesicoureteral-reflux**
    Excludes1   reflux-associated pyelonephritis (N11.0)
   N13.70   **Vesicoureteral-reflux, unspecified**
      Occurs when urine flows from bladder back into ureters
      Vesicoureteral-reflux NOS
   N13.71   **Vesicoureteral-reflux without reflux nephropathy**
   ● **N13.72**   **Vesicoureteral-reflux with reflux nephropathy without hydroureter**
     N13.721   **Vesicoureteral-reflux with reflux nephropathy without hydroureter, unilateral**
     N13.722   **Vesicoureteral-reflux with reflux nephropathy without hydroureter, bilateral**
     N13.729   **Vesicoureteral-reflux with reflux nephropathy without hydroureter, unspecified**
   ● **N13.73**   **Vesicoureteral-reflux with reflux nephropathy with hydroureter**
     N13.731   **Vesicoureteral-reflux with reflux nephropathy with hydroureter, unilateral**
     N13.732   **Vesicoureteral-reflux with reflux nephropathy with hydroureter, bilateral**
     N13.739   **Vesicoureteral-reflux with reflux nephropathy with hydroureter, unspecified**

N13.8   **Other obstructive and reflux uropathy**
    Urinary tract obstruction due to specified cause
    Code first, if applicable, any causal condition first, such as: enlarged prostate (N40.1)

N13.9   **Obstructive and reflux uropathy, unspecified**
    Urinary tract obstruction NOS

● **N14**   **Drug- and heavy-metal-induced tubulo-interstitial and tubular conditions**
    Code first poisoning due to drug or toxin, if applicable (T36-T65 with fifth or sixth character 1-4 or 6)
    Use additional code for adverse effect, if applicable, to identify drug (T36-T50 with fifth or sixth character 5)

N14.0   **Analgesic nephropathy**
N14.1   **Nephropathy induced by other drugs, medicaments and biological substances**
N14.2   **Nephropathy induced by unspecified drug, medicament or biological substance**
N14.3   **Nephropathy induced by heavy metals**
N14.4   **Toxic nephropathy, not elsewhere classified**

● **N15**   **Other renal tubulo-interstitial diseases**
N15.0   **Balkan nephropathy**
    Balkan endemic nephropathy
N15.1   **Renal and perinephric abscess**
N15.8   **Other specified renal tubulo-interstitial diseases**
N15.9   **Renal tubulo-interstitial disease, unspecified**
    Infection of kidney NOS
    Excludes1   urinary tract infection NOS (N39.0)

Figure 14-4   Hydronephrosis of the kidney, with marked dilatation of pelvis and calyces and thinning of renal parenchyma. (From Kumar: Robbins and Cotran: Pathologic Basis of Disease, ed 8, Saunders, An Imprint of Elsevier, 2009)

◀ New   ◀▥ Revised   ~~deleted~~ Deleted   Excludes 1   Excludes 2   Includes   Use additional   Code first   Code also   Unspecified

OGCR Official Guidelines   X Assign placeholder X   ● Use Additional Character(s)   ▶ Manifestation Code   **Coding Clinic**

CHAPTER 14 (N00-N99)

▶ *N16*   *Renal tubulo-interstitial disorders in diseases classified elsewhere*
     Pyelonephritis
     Tubulo-interstitial nephritis
     Code first underlying disease, such as:
        brucellosis (A23.0-A23.9)
        cryoglobulinemia (D89.1)
        glycogen storage disease (E74.0)
        leukemia (C91-C95)
        lymphoma (C81.0-C85.9, C96.0-C96.9)
        multiple myeloma (C90.0-)
        sepsis (A40.0-A41.9)
        Wilson's disease (E83.0)

     Excludes1   diphtheritic pyelonephritis and tubulo-interstitial nephritis (A36.84)
         pyelonephritis and tubulo-interstitial nephritis in candidiasis (B37.49)
         pyelonephritis and tubulo-interstitial nephritis in cystinosis (E72.04)
         pyelonephritis and tubulo-interstitial nephritis in salmonella infection (A02.25)
         pyelonephritis and tubulo-interstitial nephritis in sarcoidosis (D86.84)
         pyelonephritis and tubulo-interstitial nephritis in sicca syndrome [Sjogren's] (M35.04)
         pyelonephritis and tubulo-interstitial nephritis in systemic lupus erythematosus (M32.15)
         pyelonephritis and tubulo-interstitial nephritis in toxoplasmosis (B58.83)
         renal tubular degeneration in diabetes (E08-E13 with .29)
         syphilitic pyelonephritis and tubulo-interstitial nephritis (A52.75)

ACUTE KIDNEY FAILURE AND CHRONIC KIDNEY DISEASE (N17-N19)

     Excludes2   congenital renal failure (P96.0)
         drug- and heavy-metal-induced tubulo-interstitial and tubular conditions (N14.-)
         extrarenal uremia (R39.2)
         hemolytic-uremic syndrome (D59.3)
         hepatorenal syndrome (K76.7)
         postpartum hepatorenal syndrome (O90.4)
         posttraumatic renal failure (T79.5)
         prerenal uremia (R39.2)
         renal failure complicating abortion or ectopic or molar pregnancy (O00-O07, O08.4)
         renal failure following labor and delivery (O90.4)
         renal failure postprocedural (N99.0)

● **N17**   **Acute kidney failure**
     Code also associated underlying condition
     Excludes1   posttraumatic renal failure (T79.5)

N17.0   **Acute kidney failure with tubular necrosis**
     Acute tubular necrosis
     Renal tubular necrosis
     Tubular necrosis NOS

N17.1   **Acute kidney failure with acute cortical necrosis**
     Acute cortical necrosis
     Cortical necrosis NOS
     Renal cortical necrosis

N17.2   **Acute kidney failure with medullary necrosis**
     Medullary [papillary] necrosis NOS
     Acute medullary [papillary] necrosis
     Renal medullary [papillary] necrosis

N17.8   **Other acute kidney failure**

N17.9   **Acute kidney failure, unspecified**
     Acute kidney injury (nontraumatic)
     Excludes2   traumatic kidney injury (S37.0-)

Item 14–6 Decreased blood flow is the usual cause of **acute renal failure** that offers a good prognosis for recovery.
     Chronic renal failure is usually the result of long-standing kidney disease and is a very serious condition that generally results in death.

● **N18**   **Chronic kidney disease (CKD)**
     Code first any associated:
        diabetic chronic kidney disease (E08.22, E09.22, E10.22, E11.22, E13.22)
        hypertensive chronic kidney disease (I12.-, I13.-)
     Use additional code to identify kidney transplant status, if applicable, (Z94.0)

N18.1   **Chronic kidney disease, stage 1**

N18.2   **Chronic kidney disease, stage 2 (mild)**

N18.3   **Chronic kidney disease, stage 3 (moderate)**

N18.4   **Chronic kidney disease, stage 4 (severe)**
     Coding Clinic: 2013, Q1, P24

N18.5   **Chronic kidney disease, stage 5**
     Excludes1   chronic kidney disease, stage 5 requiring chronic dialysis (N18.6)

N18.6   **End stage renal disease**
     Chronic kidney disease requiring chronic dialysis
     Use additional code to identify dialysis status (Z99.2)
     Coding Clinic: 2016, Q1, P13

N18.9   **Chronic kidney disease, unspecified**
     Chronic renal disease
     Chronic renal failure NOS
     Chronic renal insufficiency
     Chronic uremia

N19   **Unspecified kidney failure**
     Uremia NOS
     Excludes1   acute kidney failure (N17.-)
         chronic kidney disease (N18.-)
         chronic uremia (N18.9)
         extrarenal uremia (R39.2)
         prerenal uremia (R39.2)
         renal insufficiency (acute) (N28.9)
         uremia of newborn (P96.0)

UROLITHIASIS (N20-N23)

● **N20**   **Calculus of kidney and ureter**
     Calculous pyelonephritis
     Excludes1   nephrocalcinosis (E83.5)
         that with hydronephrosis (N13.2)

N20.0   **Calculus of kidney**
     Nephrolithiasis NOS   Staghorn calculus
     Renal calculus   Stone in kidney
     Renal stone

N20.1   **Calculus of ureter**
     Ureteric stone

N20.2   **Calculus of kidney with calculus of ureter**

N20.9   **Urinary calculus, unspecified**

● **N21**   **Calculus of lower urinary tract**
     Includes   calculus of lower urinary tract with cystitis and urethritis

N21.0   **Calculus in bladder**
     Calculus in diverticulum of bladder
     Urinary bladder stone
     Excludes2   staghorn calculus (N20.0)
     Coding Clinic: 2015, Q2, P9

N21.1   **Calculus in urethra**
     Excludes2   calculus of prostate (N42.0)

N21.8   **Other lower urinary tract calculus**

N21.9   **Calculus of lower urinary tract, unspecified**
     Excludes1   calculus of urinary tract NOS (N20.9)

CHAPTER 14 (N00-N99)

Figure 14-5   Multiple urinary calculi.

Multiple calculi

▶N22   *Calculus of urinary tract in diseases classified elsewhere*
     Code first underlying disease, such as:
       gout (M1A.-, M10.-)
       schistosomiasis (B65.0-B65.9)

N23   **Unspecified** renal colic

OTHER DISORDERS OF KIDNEY AND URETER (N25-N29)
    Excludes2   disorders of kidney and ureter with urolithiasis (N20-N23)

●N25   **Disorders resulting from impaired renal tubular function**
     Excludes1   metabolic disorders classifiable to E70-E88
    N25.0   **Renal osteodystrophy**
       Azotemic osteodystrophy
       Phosphate-losing tubular disorders
       Renal rickets
       Renal short stature
    N25.1   **Nephrogenic diabetes insipidus**
       Excludes1   diabetes insipidus NOS (E23.2)
  ●N25.8   **Other disorders resulting from impaired renal tubular function**
     N25.81   **Secondary hyperparathyroidism of renal origin**
       Excludes1   secondary hyperparathyroidism, non-renal (E21.1)
     N25.89   **Other disorders resulting from impaired renal tubular function**
       Hypokalemic nephropathy
       Lightwood-Albright syndrome
       Renal tubular acidosis NOS
    N25.9   **Disorder resulting from impaired renal tubular function, unspecified**

●N26   **Unspecified contracted kidney**
     Excludes1   contracted kidney due to hypertension (I12.-)
       diffuse sclerosing glomerulonephritis (N05.8.-)
       hypertensive nephrosclerosis (arteriolar) (arteriosclerotic) (I12.-)
       small kidney of unknown cause (N27.-)
    N26.1   **Atrophy of kidney (terminal)**
    N26.2   **Page kidney**
    N26.9   **Renal sclerosis, unspecified**

●N27   **Small kidney of unknown cause**
     Includes   oligonephronia
    N27.0   **Small kidney, unilateral**
    N27.1   **Small kidney, bilateral**
    N27.9   **Small kidney, unspecified**

●N28   **Other disorders of kidney and ureter, not elsewhere classified**
    N28.0   **Ischemia and infarction of kidney**
       Renal artery embolism
       Renal artery obstruction
       Renal artery occlusion
       Renal artery thrombosis
       Renal infarct
       Excludes1   atherosclerosis of renal artery (extrarenal part) (I70.1)
       congenital stenosis of renal artery (Q27.1)
       Goldblatt's kidney (I70.1)
    N28.1   **Cyst of kidney, acquired**
       Cyst (multiple)(solitary) of kidney, acquired
       Excludes1   cystic kidney disease (congenital) (Q61.-)

●N28.8   **Other specified disorders of kidney and ureter**
     Excludes1   hydroureter (N13.4)
       ureteric stricture with hydronephrosis (N13.1)
       ureteric stricture without hydronephrosis (N13.5)
    N28.81   **Hypertrophy of kidney**
    N28.82   **Megaloureter**
    N28.83   **Nephroptosis**
    N28.84   **Pyelitis cystica**
    N28.85   **Pyeloureteritis cystica**
    N28.86   **Ureteritis cystica**
    N28.89   **Other specified disorders of kidney and ureter**
    N28.9   **Disorder of kidney and ureter, unspecified**
       Nephropathy NOS
       Renal disease (acute) NOS
       Renal insufficiency (acute)
       Excludes1   chronic renal insufficiency (N18.9)
       unspecified nephritic syndrome (N05.-)
       Coding Clinic: 2016, Q1, P13

▶N29   *Other disorders of kidney and ureter in diseases classified elsewhere*
     Code first underlying disease, such as:
       amyloidosis (E85.-)
       nephrocalcinosis (E83.5)
       schistosomiasis (B65.0-B65.9)
     Excludes1   disorders of kidney and ureter in:
       cystinosis (E72.0)
       gonorrhea (A54.21)
       syphilis (A52.75)
       tuberculosis (A18.11)

OTHER DISEASES OF THE URINARY SYSTEM (N30-N39)
    Excludes1   urinary infection (complicating):
       abortion or ectopic or molar pregnancy (O00-O07, O08.8)
       pregnancy, childbirth and the puerperium (O23.-, O75.3, O86.2-)

●N30   **Cystitis**
     Infection of bladder and irritation in lower urinary tract
     Use additional code to identify infectious agent (B95-B97)
     Excludes1   prostatocystitis (N41.3)
  ●N30.0   **Acute cystitis**
       Excludes1   irradiation cystitis (N30.4-)
       trigonitis (N30.3-)
    N30.00   **Acute cystitis without hematuria**
    N30.01   **Acute cystitis with hematuria**
  ●N30.1   **Interstitial cystitis (chronic)**
     Ongoing infection of kidney glomeruli and tubules
    N30.10   **Interstitial cystitis (chronic) without hematuria**
    N30.11   **Interstitial cystitis (chronic) with hematuria**
  ●N30.2   **Other chronic cystitis**
    N30.20   **Other chronic cystitis without hematuria**
    N30.21   **Other chronic cystitis with hematuria**
  ●N30.3   **Trigonitis**
     Inflammation of triangular area of bladder (where the ureters and urethra come together)
     Urethrotrigonitis
    N30.30   **Trigonitis without hematuria**
    N30.31   **Trigonitis with hematuria**
  ●N30.4   **Irradiation cystitis**
    N30.40   **Irradiation cystitis without hematuria**
    N30.41   **Irradiation cystitis with hematuria**

◀ New   ◀▬ Revised   ~~deleted~~ Deleted   Excludes 1   Excludes 2   Includes   Use additional   Code first   Code also   Unspecified
OGCR Official Guidelines   X Assign placeholder X   ● Use Additional Character(s)   ▶ Manifestation Code   **Coding Clinic**

● **N30.8　Other cystitis**
　　　Abscess of bladder
　　N30.80　Other cystitis without hematuria
　　N30.81　Other cystitis with hematuria
● **N30.9　Cystitis, unspecified**
　　N30.90　Cystitis, unspecified without hematuria
　　N30.91　Cystitis, unspecified with hematuria

● **N31　Neuromuscular dysfunction of bladder, not elsewhere classified**
　　Use additional code to identify any associated urinary
　　incontinence (N39.3-N39.4-)
　　Excludes1　cord bladder NOS (G95.89)
　　　　　　　　neurogenic bladder due to cauda equina
　　　　　　　　　　syndrome (G83.4)
　　　　　　　　neuromuscular dysfunction due to spinal cord
　　　　　　　　　　lesion (G95.89)
　　N31.0　Uninhibited neuropathic bladder, not elsewhere classified
　　N31.1　Reflex neuropathic bladder, not elsewhere classified
　　N31.2　Flaccid neuropathic bladder, not elsewhere classified
　　　　Atonic (motor) (sensory) neuropathic bladder
　　　　Diminished tone of bladder muscle
　　　　Autonomous neuropathic bladder
　　　　Nonreflex neuropathic bladder
　　N31.8　Other neuromuscular dysfunction of bladder
　　N31.9　Neuromuscular dysfunction of bladder, unspecified
　　　　Neurogenic bladder dysfunction NOS

● **N32　Other disorders of bladder**
　　Excludes2　calculus of bladder (N21.0)
　　　　　　　　cystocele (N81.1-)
　　　　　　　　hernia or prolapse of bladder, female (N81.1-)
　　N32.0　Bladder-neck obstruction
　　　　Bladder-neck stenosis (acquired)
　　　　Excludes1　congenital bladder-neck obstruction
　　　　　　　　　　(Q64.3-)
　　N32.1　Vesicointestinal fistula
　　　　Vesicorectal fistula
　　N32.2　Vesical fistula, not elsewhere classified
　　　　Excludes1　fistula between bladder and female
　　　　　　　　　　genital tract (N82.0-N82.1)
　　N32.3　Diverticulum of bladder
　　　　Formation of sac from a herniation of wall of bladder
　　　　Excludes1　congenital diverticulum of bladder
　　　　　　　　　　(Q64.6)
　　　　　　　　　　diverticulitis of bladder (N30.8-)
● **N32.8　Other specified disorders of bladder**
　　N32.81　Overactive bladder
　　　　Detrusor muscle hyperactivity
　　　　Excludes1　frequent urination due to
　　　　　　　　　　specified bladder condition-
　　　　　　　　　　code to condition
　　N32.89　Other specified disorders of bladder
　　　　Bladder hemorrhage
　　　　Bladder hypertrophy
　　　　Calcified bladder
　　　　Contracted bladder
　　N32.9　Bladder disorder, unspecified

▷ *N33　Bladder disorders in diseases classified elsewhere*
　　Code first underlying disease, such as:
　　　schistosomiasis (B65.0-B65.9)
　　Excludes1　bladder disorder in syphilis (A52.76)
　　　　　　　　bladder disorder in tuberculosis (A18.12)
　　　　　　　　candidal cystitis (B37.41)
　　　　　　　　chlamydial cystitis(A56.01)
　　　　　　　　cystitis in gonorrhea (A54.01)
　　　　　　　　cystitis in neurogenic bladder (N31.-)
　　　　　　　　diphtheritic cystitis (A36.85)
　　　　　　　　syphilitic cystitis (A52.76)
　　　　　　　　trichomonal cystitis (A59.03)

● **N34　Urethritis and urethral syndrome**
　　Use additional code (B95-B97), to identify infectious agent
　　Excludes2　Reiter's disease (M02.3-)
　　　　　　　　urethritis in diseases with a predominantly sexual
　　　　　　　　　　mode of transmission (A50-A64)
　　　　　　　　urethrotrigonitis (N30.3-)
　　N34.0　Urethral abscess
　　　　Abscess (of) Cowper's gland
　　　　Abscess (of) Littré's gland
　　　　Abscess (of) urethral (gland)
　　　　Periurethral abscess
　　　　Excludes1　urethral caruncle (N36.2)
　　N34.1　Nonspecific urethritis
　　　　Nongonococcal urethritis
　　　　Nonvenereal urethritis
　　N34.2　Other urethritis
　　　　Inflammation of urethra
　　　　Meatitis, urethral
　　　　Postmenopausal urethritis
　　　　Ulcer of urethra (meatus)
　　　　Urethritis NOS
　　N34.3　Urethral syndrome, unspecified

● **N35　Urethral stricture**
　　Narrowing of lumen of urethra caused by scarring due to infection or injury
　　Excludes1　congenital urethral stricture (Q64.3-)
　　　　　　　　postprocedural urethral stricture (N99.1-)
● **N35.0　Post-traumatic urethral stricture**
　　　Urethral stricture due to injury
　　　Excludes1　postprocedural urethral stricture (N99.1-)
　● **N35.01　Post-traumatic urethral stricture, male**
　　　　N35.010　Post-traumatic urethral stricture, male, meatal ♂
　　　　N35.011　Post-traumatic bulbous urethral stricture
　　　　N35.012　Post-traumatic membranous urethral stricture
　　　　N35.013　Post-traumatic anterior urethral stricture
　　　　N35.014　Post-traumatic urethral stricture, male, unspecified ♂
　● **N35.02　Post-traumatic urethral stricture, female**
　　　　N35.021　Urethral stricture due to childbirth ♀
　　　　N35.028　Other post-traumatic urethral stricture, female ♀
● **N35.1　Postinfective urethral stricture, not elsewhere classified**
　　Excludes1　urethral stricture associated with
　　　　　　　　　　schistosomiasis (B65.-, N29)
　　　　　　　　gonococcal urethral stricture (A54.01)
　　　　　　　　syphilitic urethral stricture (A52.76)
　● **N35.11　Postinfective urethral stricture, not elsewhere classified, male**
　　　　N35.111　Postinfective urethral stricture, not elsewhere classified, male, meatal ♂
　　　　N35.112　Postinfective bulbous urethral stricture, not elsewhere classified
　　　　N35.113　Postinfective membranous urethral stricture, not elsewhere classified
　　　　N35.114　Postinfective anterior urethral stricture, not elsewhere classified
　　　　N35.119　Postinfective urethral stricture, not elsewhere classified, male, unspecified ♂
　　N35.12　Postinfective urethral stricture, not elsewhere classified, female ♀
　　N35.8　Other urethral stricture
　　　Excludes1　postprocedural urethral stricture (N99.1-)
　　N35.9　Urethral stricture, unspecified

CHAPTER 14 (N00-N99)

● N36 Other disorders of urethra

N36.0 Urethral fistula
Urethroperineal fistula
Urethrorectal fistula
Urinary fistula NOS
> **Excludes1** urethroscrotal fistula (N50.89) ◀▥
> urethrovaginal fistula (N82.1)
> urethrovesicovaginal fistula (N82.1)

N36.1 Urethral diverticulum

N36.2 Urethral caruncle

● N36.4 Urethral functional and muscular disorders
Use additional code to identify associated urinary stress incontinence (N39.3)

N36.41 Hypermobility of urethra

N36.42 Intrinsic sphincter deficiency (ISD)

N36.43 Combined hypermobility of urethra and intrinsic sphincter deficiency

N36.44 Muscular disorders of urethra
Bladder sphincter dyssynergy

N36.5 Urethral false passage

N36.8 Other specified disorders of urethra
> **Excludes1** congenital urethrocele (Q64.7) ◀
> female urethrocele (N81.0) ◀

N36.9 Urethral disorder, unspecified

▶ N37 *Urethral disorders in diseases classified elsewhere*
Code first underlying disease
> **Excludes1** urethritis (in):
> candidal infection (B37.41)
> chlamydial (A56.01)
> gonorrhea (A54.01)
> syphilis (A52.76)
> trichomonal infection (A59.03)
> tuberculosis (A18.13)

● N39 Other disorders of urinary system
> **Excludes2** hematuria NOS (R31.-)
> recurrent or persistent hematuria (N02.-)
> recurrent or persistent hematuria with specified morphological lesion (N02.-)
> proteinuria NOS (R80.-)

N39.0 Urinary tract infection, site not specified
Use additional code (B95-B97), to identify infectious agent
> **Excludes1** candidiasis of urinary tract (B37.4-)
> neonatal urinary tract infection (P39.3)
> urinary tract infection of specified site, such as:
> cystitis (N30.-)
> urethritis (N34.-)

Coding Clinic: 2012, Q4, P94

N39.3 Stress incontinence (female) (male)
Code also any associated overactive bladder (N32.81)
> **Excludes1** mixed incontinence (N39.46)

● N39.4 Other specified urinary incontinence
Code also any associated overactive bladder (N32.81)
> **Excludes1** enuresis NOS (R32)
> functional urinary incontinence (R39.81)
> urinary incontinence associated with cognitive impairment (R39.81)
> urinary incontinence NOS (R32)
> urinary incontinence of nonorganic origin (F98.0)

N39.41 Urge incontinence
> **Excludes1** mixed incontinence (N39.46)

N39.42 Incontinence without sensory awareness
Insensible (urinary) incontinence ◀

N39.43 Post-void dribbling

N39.44 Nocturnal enuresis

N39.45 Continuous leakage

N39.46 Mixed incontinence
Urge and stress incontinence

● N39.49 Other specified urinary incontinence

N39.490 Overflow incontinence

N39.491 Coital incontinence ◀

N39.492 Postural (urinary) incontinence ◀

N39.498 Other specified urinary incontinence
Reflex incontinence
Total incontinence

N39.8 Other specified disorders of urinary system

N39.9 Disorder of urinary system, unspecified

DISEASES OF MALE GENITAL ORGANS (N40-N53)

★ **(See Plate 387 on page 53.)**

● N40 Benign prostatic hyperplasia ◀▥
> **Includes** adenofibromatous hypertrophy of prostate
> benign hypertrophy of the prostate
> *Enlargement of prostate gland usually occurring with age and causing obstructed urine flow*
> benign prostatic hypertrophy
> BPH
> enlarged prostate ◀
> nodular prostate
> polyp of prostate

> **Excludes1** benign neoplasms of prostate (adenoma, benign) (fibroadenoma) (fibroma) (myoma) (D29.1)
> malignant neoplasm of prostate (C61)

N40.0 Benign prostatic hyperplasia without lower urinary tract symptoms ♂ ◀▥   A
Enlarged prostate without LUTS
Enlarged prostate NOS

N40.1 Benign prostatic hyperplasia with lower urinary tract symptoms ♂ ◀▥   A
Enlarged prostate with LUTS
Use additional code for associated symptoms, when specified:
incomplete bladder emptying (R39.14)
nocturia (R35.1)
straining on urination (R39.16)
urinary frequency (R35.0)
urinary hesitancy (R39.11)
urinary incontinence (N39.4-)
urinary obstruction (N13.8)
urinary retention (R33.8)
urinary urgency (R39.15)
weak urinary stream (R39.12)

N40.2 Nodular prostate without lower urinary tract symptoms ♂   A
Nodular prostate without LUTS

Figure 14-6 Benign prostatic hyperplasia. (From Shiland: Mastering Healthcare Terminology, ed 3, St. Louis, Mosby, 2010)

◀ New   ◀▥ Revised   ~~deleted~~ Deleted   Excludes 1   Excludes 2   Includes   Use additional   Code first   Code also   Unspecified

OGCR Official Guidelines   X Assign placeholder X   ● Use Additional Character(s)   ▶ Manifestation Code   **Coding Clinic**

N40.3   Nodular prostate with lower urinary tract symptoms ♂ A
     Use additional code for associated symptoms, when
       specified:
       incomplete bladder emptying (R39.14)
       nocturia (R35.1)
       straining on urination (R39.16)
       urinary frequency (R35.0)
       urinary hesitancy (R39.11)
       urinary incontinence (N39.4-)
       urinary obstruction (N13.8)
       urinary retention (R33.8)
       urinary urgency (R39.15)
       weak urinary stream (R39.12)

● **N41   Inflammatory diseases of prostate**
     Use additional code (B95-B97), to identify infectious agent
   N41.0   Acute prostatitis ♂   A
   N41.1   Chronic prostatitis ♂   A
   N41.2   Abscess of prostate ♂   A
   N41.3   Prostatocystitis ♂   A
   N41.4   Granulomatous prostatitis ♂   A
   N41.8   Other inflammatory diseases of prostate ♂   A
   N41.9   Inflammatory disease of prostate, unspecified ♂   A
       Prostatitis NOS

● **N42   Other and unspecified disorders of prostate**
   N42.0   Calculus of prostate ♂   A
       Prostatic stone
   N42.1   Congestion and hemorrhage of prostate ♂   A
     Excludes1   enlarged prostate (N40.-)
                hematuria (R31.-)
                hyperplasia of prostate (N40.-)
                inflammatory diseases of prostate (N41.-)
 ● **N42.3   Dysplasia of prostate**
     N42.30   Unspecified dysplasia of prostate ♂ ◀
     N42.31   Prostatic intraepithelial neoplasia ♂ ◀
         PIN ◀
         Prostatic intraepithelial neoplasia I (PIN I) ◀
         Prostatic intraepithelial neoplasia II (PIN II) ◀
       Excludes1   prostatic intraepithelial neoplasia
                III (PIN III) (D07.5) ◀
     **N42.32   Atypical small acinar proliferation of
             prostate** ♂ ◀
     N42.39   Other dysplasia of prostate ♂ ◀
 ● **N42.8   Other specified disorders of prostate**
     N42.81   Prostatodynia syndrome ♂   A
         Painful prostate syndrome
     N42.82   Prostatosis syndrome ♂   A
     N42.83   Cyst of prostate ♂   A
     N42.89   Other specified disorders of prostate ♂   A
   N42.9   Disorder of prostate, unspecified ♂   A

● **N43   Hydrocele and spermatocele**
     Includes   hydrocele of spermatic cord, testis or tunica
               vaginalis
     Excludes1   congenital hydrocele (P83.5)
   N43.0   Encysted hydrocele ♂
   N43.1   Infected hydrocele ♂
     Use additional code (B95-B97), to identify infectious
       agent
   N43.2   Other hydrocele ♂
   N43.3   Hydrocele, unspecified ♂

Item 14–7   Hydrocele is a sac of fluid accumulating in the testes membrane.

Figure 14-7   A. Hydrocele. **B.** Newborn with large right hydrocele. (**B** from Behrman: Nelson Textbook of Pediatrics, ed 18, Saunders, An Imprint of Elsevier, 2007)

 ● **N43.4   Spermatocele of epididymis**
     Spermatic cyst
     N43.40   Spermatocele of epididymis, unspecified ♂
     N43.41   Spermatocele of epididymis, single ♂
     N43.42   Spermatocele of epididymis, multiple ♂

● **N44   Noninflammatory disorders of testis**
 ● **N44.0   Torsion of testis**
     N44.00   Torsion of testis, unspecified ♂
     N44.01   Extravaginal torsion of spermatic cord ♂
     N44.02   Intravaginal torsion of spermatic cord ♂
         Torsion of spermatic cord NOS
     N44.03   Torsion of appendix testis ♂
     N44.04   Torsion of appendix epididymis ♂
   N44.1   Cyst of tunica albuginea testis ♂
   N44.2   Benign cyst of testis ♂
   N44.8   Other noninflammatory disorders of the testis ♂

● **N45   Orchitis and epididymitis**
     *Orchitis is inflammation of one or both of the testes as a result of
       mumps or other infection, trauma, or metastasis. Epididymitis
       is inflammation of the tubular structure that connects the testicle
       with the vas deferens.*
     Use additional code (B95-B97), to identify infectious agent
   N45.1   Epididymitis ♂
   N45.2   Orchitis ♂
   N45.3   Epididymo-orchitis ♂
   N45.4   Abscess of epididymis or testis ♂

● **N46   Male infertility**
     Excludes1   vasectomy status (Z98.52)
 ● **N46.0   Azoospermia**
     Absolute male infertility
     Male infertility due to germinal (cell) aplasia
     Male infertility due to spermatogenic arrest (complete)
     N46.01   Organic azoospermia ♂   A
         Azoospermia NOS
  ● **N46.02   Azoospermia due to extratesticular causes**
       Code also associated cause
       N46.021   Azoospermia due to drug therapy ♂   A
       N46.022   Azoospermia due to infection ♂   A
       **N46.023   Azoospermia due to obstruction of
            efferent ducts** ♂   A
       N46.024   Azoospermia due to radiation ♂   A
       **N46.025   Azoospermia due to systemic
            disease** ♂   A
       **N46.029   Azoospermia due to other
            extratesticular causes** ♂   A

Item 14-8 Male infertility is the inability of the female sex partner to conceive after one year of unprotected intercourse.
    Azoospermia is no sperm ejaculated and **oligospermia** is few sperm ejaculated—both resulting in infertility. Extratesticular causes such as injury, infections, radiation, and chemotherapy may also cause male infertility.

CHAPTER 14 (N00-N99)

● **N46.1 Oligospermia**
    Male infertility due to germinal cell desquamation
    Male infertility due to hypospermatogenesis
    Male infertility due to incomplete spermatogenic arrest
    N46.11 Organic oligospermia ♂   A
        Oligospermia NOS
  ● **N46.12 Oligospermia due to extratesticular causes** ♂
        Code also associated cause
        N46.121 Oligospermia due to drug therapy ♂   A
        N46.122 Oligospermia due to infection ♂   A
        N46.123 Oligospermia due to obstruction of efferent ducts ♂   A
        N46.124 Oligospermia due to radiation ♂   A
        N46.125 Oligospermia due to systemic disease ♂   A
        N46.129 Oligospermia due to other extratesticular causes ♂   A
  N46.8 Other male infertility ♂   A
  N46.9 Male infertility, `unspecified` ♂   A

● **N47 Disorders of prepuce**
  N47.0 Adherent prepuce, newborn ♂   N
  N47.1 Phimosis ♂
  N47.2 Paraphimosis ♂
  N47.3 Deficient foreskin ♂
  N47.4 Benign cyst of prepuce ♂
  N47.5 Adhesions of prepuce and glans penis ♂
  N47.6 Balanoposthitis ♂
    Use additional code (B95-B97), to identify infectious agent
    Excludes1 balanitis (N48.1)
  N47.7 Other inflammatory diseases of prepuce ♂
    Use additional code (B95-B97), to identify infectious agent
  N47.8 Other disorders of prepuce ♂

● **N48 Other disorders of penis**
  N48.0 Leukoplakia of penis ♂
    Balanitis xerotica obliterans
    Kraurosis of penis
    Lichen sclerosus of external male genital organs
    Excludes1 carcinoma in situ of penis (D07.4)
  N48.1 Balanitis ♂
    Use additional code (B95-B97), to identify infectious agent
    Excludes1 amebic balanitis (A06.8)
        balanitis xerotica obliterans (N48.0)
        candidal balanitis (B37.42)
        gonococcal balanitis (A54.23)
        herpesviral [herpes simplex] balanitis (A60.01)
● **N48.2 Other inflammatory disorders of penis**
    Use additional code (B95-B97), to identify infectious agent
    Excludes1 balanitis (N48.1)
        balanitis xerotica obliterans (N48.0)
        balanoposthitis (N47.6)
    N48.21 Abscess of corpus cavernosum and penis ♂
    N48.22 Cellulitis of corpus cavernosum and penis ♂
    N48.29 Other inflammatory disorders of penis ♂
● **N48.3 Priapism**
    Painful erection
    Code first underlying cause
    N48.30 Priapism, `unspecified` ♂
    N48.31 Priapism due to trauma ♂
  ▸ **N48.32 Priapism due to disease classified elsewhere** ♂
    N48.33 Priapism, drug-induced ♂
    N48.39 Other priapism ♂

N48.5 Ulcer of penis ♂
N48.6 Induration penis plastica ♂
    Peyronie's disease
    Plastic induration of penis
● **N48.8 Other specified disorders of penis** ♂
  N48.81 Thrombosis of superficial vein of penis ♂
  N48.82 Acquired torsion of penis ♂
    Acquired torsion of penis NOS
    Excludes1 congenital torsion of penis (Q55.63)
  N48.83 Acquired buried penis ♂
    Excludes1 congenital hidden penis (Q55.64)
  N48.89 Other specified disorders of penis ♂
N48.9 Disorder of penis, `unspecified` ♂

● **N49 Inflammatory disorders of male genital organs, not elsewhere classified**
  Use additional code (B95-B97), to identify infectious agent
  Excludes1 inflammation of penis (N48.1, N48.2-)
        orchitis and epididymitis (N45.-)
  N49.0 Inflammatory disorders of seminal vesicle ♂
    Vesiculitis NOS
  N49.1 Inflammatory disorders of spermatic cord, tunica vaginalis and vas deferens ♂
    Vasitis
  N49.2 Inflammatory disorders of scrotum ♂
  N49.3 Fournier gangrene ♂
  N49.8 Inflammatory disorders of other specified male genital organs ♂
    Inflammation of multiple sites in male genital organs
  N49.9 Inflammatory disorder of `unspecified` **male genital organ** ♂
    Abscess of unspecified male genital organ
    Boil of unspecified male genital organ
    Carbuncle of unspecified male genital organ
    Cellulitis of unspecified male genital organ

● **N50 Other and unspecified disorders of male genital organs**
  Excludes2 torsion of testis (N44.0-)
  N50.0 Atrophy of testis ♂
  N50.1 Vascular disorders of male genital organs ♂
    Hematocele, NOS, of male genital organs
    Hemorrhage of male genital organs
    Thrombosis of male genital organs
  N50.3 Cyst of epididymis ♂

Item 14–9 Seminal vesiculitis is an inflammation of the seminal vesicle. Spermatocele is a benign cystic accumulation of sperm arising from the head of the epididymis. Torsion of the testis is a medical emergency occurring most commonly in boys 7 to 12 years of age and results from a congenital abnormality of the covering of the testis allowing the testis to twist within its sac and cutting off the blood supply to the testis.

Figure 14-8 A. Torsion of testis. **B.** Torsion of the testis. (**B** from Kumar: Robbins and Cotran: Pathologic Basis of Disease, ed 8, Saunders, An Imprint of Elsevier, 2009)

◄ New   ⬅ Revised   ~~deleted~~ Deleted   Excludes 1   Excludes 2   Includes   Use additional   Code first   Code also   Unspecified
OGCR Official Guidelines   X Assign placeholder X   ● Use Additional Character(s)   ▸ Manifestation Code   **Coding Clinic**

● **N50.8**   **Other specified disorders of male genital organs**
   ● **N50.81**   Testicular pain ◀
     N50.811   Right testicular pain ♂ ◀
     N50.812   Left testicular pain ♂ ◀
     N50.819   Testicular pain, unspecified ♂ ◀
   N50.82   Scrotal pain ♂ ◀
   N50.89   Other specified disorders of the male genital organs ♂ ◀
     Atrophy of scrotum, seminal vesicle, spermatic cord, tunica vaginalis and vas deferens ◀
     Chylocele, tunica vaginalis (nonfilarial) NOS ◀
     Edema of scrotum, seminal vesicle, spermatic cord, tunica vaginalis and vas deferens ◀
     Hypertrophy of scrotum, seminal vesicle, spermatic cord, tunica vaginalis and vas deferens ◀
     Stricture of spermatic cord, tunica vaginalis, and vas deferens ◀
     Ulcer of scrotum, seminal vesicle, spermatic cord, testis, tunica vaginalis and vas deferens ◀
     Urethroscrotal fistula ◀
   N50.9   **Disorder of male genital organs, unspecified** ♂

▷ *N51*   *Disorders of male genital organs in diseases classified elsewhere* ♂
   Code first underlying disease, such as:
   filariasis (B74.0-B74.9)
   Excludes1   amebic balanitis (A06.8)
     candidal balanitis (B37.42)
     gonococcal balanitis (A54.23)
     gonococcal prostatitis (A54.22)
     herpesviral [herpes simplex] balanitis (A60.01)
     trichomonal prostatitis (A59.02)
     tuberculous prostatitis (A18.14)

● **N52**   **Male erectile dysfunction**
   Excludes1   psychogenic impotence (F52.21)
   ● **N52.0**   **Vasculogenic erectile dysfunction**
     N52.01   Erectile dysfunction due to arterial insufficiency ♂   A
     N52.02   Corporo-venous occlusive erectile dysfunction ♂   A
     N52.03   Combined arterial insufficiency and corporo-venous occlusive erectile dysfunction ♂   A
   ▷ *N52.1*   *Erectile dysfunction due to diseases classified elsewhere* ♂   A
     Code first underlying disease
   N52.2   **Drug-induced erectile dysfunction** ♂   A
   ● **N52.3**   **Postprocedural erectile dysfunction** ◀▥
     N52.31   Erectile dysfunction following radical prostatectomy ♂   A
     N52.32   Erectile dysfunction following radical cystectomy ♂   A
     N52.33   Erectile dysfunction following urethral surgery ♂   A
     N52.34   Erectile dysfunction following simple prostatectomy ♂   A
     N52.35   Erectile dysfunction following radiation therapy ♂ ◀   A
     N52.36   Erectile dysfunction following interstitial seed therapy ♂ ◀   A
     N52.37   Erectile dysfunction following prostate ablative therapy ♂ ◀   A
     Erectile dysfunction following cryotherapy ◀
     Erectile dysfunction following other prostate ablative therapies ◀
     Erectile dysfunction following ultrasound ablative therapies ◀
     N52.39   Other and unspecified postprocedural erectile dysfunction ♂ ◀▥   A

   N52.8   Other male erectile dysfunction ♂   A
   N52.9   Male erectile dysfunction, unspecified ♂   A
     Impotence NOS
● **N53**   **Other male sexual dysfunction**
   Excludes1   psychogenic sexual dysfunction (F52.-)
   ● **N53.1**   **Ejaculatory dysfunction**
     Excludes1   premature ejaculation (F52.4)
     N53.11   Retarded ejaculation ♂
     N53.12   Painful ejaculation ♂
     N53.13   Anejaculatory orgasm ♂
     N53.14   Retrograde ejaculation ♂
     N53.19   Other ejaculatory dysfunction ♂
     Ejaculatory dysfunction NOS
   N53.8   Other male sexual dysfunction ♂
   N53.9   Unspecified male sexual dysfunction ♂

DISORDERS OF BREAST (N60-N65)

   Excludes1   disorders of breast associated with childbirth (O91-O92)

● **N60**   **Benign mammary dysplasia**
   Benign lumpiness of breast
   Includes   fibrocystic mastopathy
   ● **N60.0**   **Solitary cyst of breast**
     Cyst of breast
     N60.01   Solitary cyst of right breast
     N60.02   Solitary cyst of left breast
     N60.09   Solitary cyst of unspecified breast
   ● **N60.1**   **Diffuse cystic mastopathy**
     Cystic breast
     Fibrocystic disease of breast
     Excludes1   diffuse cystic mastopathy with epithelial proliferation (N60.3-)
     N60.11   Diffuse cystic mastopathy of right breast   A
     N60.12   Diffuse cystic mastopathy of left breast   A
     N60.19   Diffuse cystic mastopathy of unspecified breast   A
   ● **N60.2**   **Fibroadenosis of breast**
     Adenofibrosis of breast
     Excludes2   fibroadenoma of breast (D24.-)
     N60.21   Fibroadenosis of right breast
     N60.22   Fibroadenosis of left breast
     N60.29   Fibroadenosis of unspecified breast
   ● **N60.3**   **Fibrosclerosis of breast**
     Cystic mastopathy with epithelial proliferation
     N60.31   Fibrosclerosis of right breast
     N60.32   Fibrosclerosis of left breast
     N60.39   Fibrosclerosis of unspecified breast
   ● **N60.4**   **Mammary duct ectasia**
     N60.41   Mammary duct ectasia of right breast
     N60.42   Mammary duct ectasia of left breast
     N60.49   Mammary duct ectasia of unspecified breast

Figure 14-9 Breast.

● N60.8   Other benign mammary dysplasias
   N60.81   Other benign mammary dysplasias of right breast
   N60.82   Other benign mammary dysplasias of left breast
   N60.89   Other benign mammary dysplasias of unspecified breast
● N60.9   Unspecified benign mammary dysplasia
   N60.91   Unspecified benign mammary dysplasia of right breast
   N60.92   Unspecified benign mammary dysplasia of left breast
   N60.99   Unspecified benign mammary dysplasia of unspecified breast

● N61   Inflammatory disorders of breast
   Excludes1   inflammatory carcinoma of breast (C50.9)
           inflammatory disorder of breast associated with childbirth (O91.-)
           neonatal infective mastitis (P39.0)
           thrombophlebitis of breast [Mondor's disease] (I80.8)
  N61.0   Mastitis without abscess ◀
      Infective mastitis (acute) (nonpuerperal) (subacute) ◀
      Mastitis (acute) (nonpuerperal) (subacute) NOS ◀
      Cellulitis (acute) (nonpuerperal) (subacute) of breast NOS ◀
      Cellulitis (acute) (nonpuerperal) (subacute) of nipple NOS ◀
  N61.1   Abscess of the breast and nipple ◀
      Abscess (acute) (chronic) (nonpuerperal) of areola ◀
      Abscess (acute) (chronic) (nonpuerperal) of breast ◀
      Carbuncle of breast ◀
      Mastitis with abscess ◀

N62   Hypertrophy of breast
      Gynecomastia
      Hypertrophy of breast NOS
      Massive pubertal hypertrophy of breast
   Excludes1   breast engorgement of newborn (P83.4)
           disproportion of reconstructed breast (N65.1)

N63   Unspecified lump in breast
      Nodule(s) NOS in breast

● N64   Other disorders of breast
   Excludes2   mechanical complication of breast prosthesis and implant (T85.4-)
  N64.0   Fissure and fistula of nipple
  N64.1   Fat necrosis of breast
      Fat necrosis (segmental) of breast
      Code first breast necrosis due to breast graft (T85.898) ◀▦
  N64.2   Atrophy of breast
  N64.3   Galactorrhea not associated with childbirth
      Excessive or spontaneous flow of milk
  N64.4   Mastodynia
● N64.5   Other signs and symptoms in breast
   Excludes2   abnormal findings on diagnostic imaging of breast (R92.-)
   N64.51   Induration of breast
   N64.52   Nipple discharge
      Excludes1   abnormal findings in nipple discharge (R89.-)
   N64.53   Retraction of nipple
   N64.59   Other signs and symptoms in breast

● N64.8   Other specified disorders of breast
   N64.81   Ptosis of breast   A
      Excludes1   ptosis of native breast in relation to reconstructed breast (N65.1)
   N64.82   Hypoplasia of breast   A
      Micromastia
      Excludes1   congenital absence of breast (Q83.0)
             hypoplasia of native breast in relation to reconstructed breast (N65.1)
   N64.89   Other specified disorders of breast
      Galactocele
      Subinvolution of breast (postlactational)
  N64.9   Disorder of breast, unspecified

● N65   Deformity and disproportion of reconstructed breast
  N65.0   Deformity of reconstructed breast   A
      Contour irregularity in reconstructed breast
      Excess tissue in reconstructed breast
      Misshapen reconstructed breast
  N65.1   Disproportion of reconstructed breast   A
      Breast asymmetry between native breast and reconstructed breast
      Disproportion between native breast and reconstructed breast

INFLAMMATORY DISEASES OF FEMALE PELVIC ORGANS (N70-N77)

   Excludes1   inflammatory diseases of female pelvic organs complicating:
      abortion or ectopic or molar pregnancy (O00-O07, O08.0)
      pregnancy, childbirth and the puerperium (O23.-, O75.3, O85, O86.-)

★ **(See Plate 360 on page 80.)**

● N70   Salpingitis and oophoritis
    Oophoritis = inflammation of ovary
    Salpingitis = inflammation of fallopian tube
   Includes   abscess (of) fallopian tube
      abscess (of) ovary
      pyosalpinx
      salpingo-oophoritis
      tubo-ovarian abscess
      tubo-ovarian inflammatory disease
   Use additional code (B95-B97), to identify infectious agent
   Excludes1   gonococcal infection (A54.24)
      tuberculous infection (A18.17)
● N70.0   Acute salpingitis and oophoritis
   N70.01   Acute salpingitis ♀
   N70.02   Acute oophoritis ♀
   N70.03   Acute salpingitis and oophoritis ♀
● N70.1   Chronic salpingitis and oophoritis
      Hydrosalpinx
   N70.11   Chronic salpingitis ♀
   N70.12   Chronic oophoritis ♀
   N70.13   Chronic salpingitis and oophoritis ♀
● N70.9   Salpingitis and oophoritis, unspecified
   N70.91   Salpingitis, unspecified ♀
   N70.92   Oophoritis, unspecified ♀
   N70.93   Salpingitis and oophoritis, unspecified ♀

A   Female Genital System   B   *The three parts of the vulva

Figure 14-10   A. Female genital system. **B.** External female genital system. (From Buck CJ: Step-by-Step Medical Coding, ed 2016, St. Louis, Elsevier, 2016)

Item 14–10 Salpingitis is an infection of one or both fallopian tubes. **Oophoritis** is an infection of one or both ovaries.

● **N71   Inflammatory disease of uterus, except cervix**
  Includes   endo (myo) metritis
                metritis
                myometritis
                pyometra
                uterine abscess
  Use additional code (B95-B97), to identify infectious agent
  Excludes1   hyperplastic endometritis (N85.0-)
                infection of uterus following delivery (O85, O86.-)
  N71.0   Acute inflammatory disease of uterus ♀
  N71.1   Chronic inflammatory disease of uterus ♀
  N71.9   Inflammatory disease of uterus, unspecified ♀

N72   Inflammatory disease of cervix uteri ♀
  Includes   cervicitis (with or without erosion or ectropion)
                endocervicitis (with or without erosion or ectropion)
                exocervicitis (with or without erosion or ectropion)
  Use additional code (B95-B97), to identify infectious agent
  Excludes1   erosion and ectropion of cervix without cervicitis (N86)

● **N73   Other female pelvic inflammatory diseases**
  Use additional code (B95-B97), to identify infectious agent
  N73.0   Acute parametritis and pelvic cellulitis ♀
            Abscess of broad ligament
            Abscess of parametrium
            Pelvic cellulitis, female
  N73.1   Chronic parametritis and pelvic cellulitis ♀
            Any condition in N73.0 specified as chronic
            Excludes1   tuberculous parametritis and pelvic cellultis (A18.17)
  N73.2   Unspecified parametritis and pelvic cellulitis ♀
            Any condition in N73.0 unspecified whether acute or chronic
  N73.3   Female acute pelvic peritonitis ♀
  N73.4   Female chronic pelvic peritonitis ♀
            Excludes1   tuberculous pelvic (female) peritonitis (A18.17)
  N73.5   Female pelvic peritonitis, unspecified ♀
  N73.6   Female pelvic peritoneal adhesions (postinfective) ♀
            Excludes2   postprocedural pelvic peritoneal adhesions (N99.4)
  N73.8   Other specified female pelvic inflammatory diseases ♀
  N73.9   Female pelvic inflammatory disease, unspecified ♀
            Female pelvic infection or inflammation NOS

▶ **N74   *Female pelvic inflammatory disorders in diseases classified elsewhere* ♀**
  Code first underlying disease
  Excludes1   chlamydial cervicitis (A56.02)
                chlamydial pelvic inflammatory disease (A56.11)
                gonococcal cervicitis (A54.03)
                gonococcal pelvic inflammatory disease (A54.24)
                herpesviral [herpes simplex] cervicitis (A60.03)
                herpesviral [herpes simplex] pelvic inflammatory disease (A60.09)
                syphilitic cervicitis (A52.76)
                syphilitic pelvic inflammatory disease (A52.76)
                trichomonal cervicitis (A59.09)
                tuberculous cervicitis (A18.16)
                tuberculous pelvic inflammatory disease (A18.17)

● **N75   Diseases of Bartholin's gland**
  N75.0   Cyst of Bartholin's gland ♀
            Cysts filled with liquid or semisolid material
  N75.1   Abscess of Bartholin's gland ♀
            Localized collection of pus
  N75.8   Other diseases of Bartholin's gland ♀
            Bartholinitis
  N75.9   Disease of Bartholin's gland, unspecified ♀

● **N76   Other inflammation of vagina and vulva**
  Use additional code (B95-B97), to identify infectious agent
  Excludes2   senile (atrophic) vaginitis (N95.2)
                vulvar vestibulitis (N94.810)
  N76.0   Acute vaginitis ♀
            Acute vulvovaginitis
            Vaginitis NOS
            Vulvovaginitis NOS
  N76.1   Subacute and chronic vaginitis ♀
            Chronic vulvovaginitis
            Subacute vulvovaginitis
  N76.2   Acute vulvitis ♀
            Vulvitis NOS
  N76.3   Subacute and chronic vulvitis ♀
  N76.4   Abscess of vulva ♀
            Furuncle of vulva
  N76.5   Ulceration of vagina ♀
  N76.6   Ulceration of vulva ♀
  ● **N76.8   Other specified inflammation of vagina and vulva**
            N76.81   Mucositis (ulcerative) of vagina and vulva ♀
                    Code also type of associated therapy, such as:
                        antineoplastic and immunosuppressive drugs (T45.1X-)
                        radiological procedure and radiotherapy (Y84.2)
                    Excludes2   gastrointestinal mucositis (ulcerative) (K92.81)
                                nasal mucositis (ulcerative) (J34.81)
                                oral mucositis (ulcerative) (K12.3-)
            N76.89   Other specified inflammation of vagina and vulva ♀

● **N77   Vulvovaginal ulceration and inflammation in diseases classified elsewhere**
  ▶ **N77.0   *Ulceration of vulva in diseases classified elsewhere* ♀**
            Code first underlying disease, such as:
                Behçet's disease (M35.2)
            Excludes1   ulceration of vulva in gonococcal infection (A54.02)
                        ulceration of vulva in herpesviral [herpes simplex] infection (A60.04)
                        ulceration of vulva in syphilis (A51.0)
                        ulceration of vulva in tuberculosis (A18.18)

CHAPTER 14 (N00-N99)

CHAPTER 14 (N00-N99)

> **N77.1   Vaginitis, vulvitis and vulvovaginitis in diseases classified elsewhere ♀**
>> Code first *underlying disease, such as:*
>> pinworm (B80)
>>> **Excludes1**   candidial vulvovaginitis (B37.3)
>>> chlamydial vulvovaginitis (A56.02)
>>> gonococcal vulvovaginitis (A54.02)
>>> herpesviral [herpes simplex]
>>>   vulvovaginitis (A60.04)
>>> trichomonal vulvovaginitis (A59.01)
>>> tuberculous vulvovaginitis (A18.18)
>>> vulvovaginitis in early syphilis (A51.0)
>>> vulvovaginitis in late syphilis (A52.76)

NONINFLAMMATORY DISORDERS OF FEMALE GENITAL TRACT (N80-N98)

- **N80   Endometriosis**
  - **N80.0   Endometriosis of uterus ♀**
    - Adenomyosis
    - **Excludes1**   stromal endometriosis (D39.0)
  - **N80.1   Endometriosis of ovary ♀**
  - **N80.2   Endometriosis of fallopian tube ♀**
  - **N80.3   Endometriosis of pelvic peritoneum ♀**
  - **N80.4   Endometriosis of rectovaginal septum and vagina ♀**
  - **N80.5   Endometriosis of intestine ♀**
  - **N80.6   Endometriosis in cutaneous scar ♀**
  - **N80.8   Other endometriosis ♀**
  - **N80.9   Endometriosis, unspecified ♀**

- **N81   Female genital prolapse**
  - **Excludes1**   genital prolapse complicating pregnancy, labor or delivery (O34.5-)
    - prolapse and hernia of ovary and fallopian tube (N83.4-) ◀▬
    - prolapse of vaginal vault after hysterectomy (N99.3)
  - **N81.0   Urethrocele ♀**
    - **Excludes1**   urethrocele with cystocele (N81.1-)
      - urethrocele with prolapse of uterus (N81.2-N81.4)
  - **N81.1   Cystocele**
    - Cystocele with urethrocele
    - Cystourethrocele
    - **Excludes1**   cystocele with prolapse of uterus (N81.2-N81.4)
    - **N81.10   Cystocele, unspecified ♀**
      - Prolapse of (anterior) vaginal wall NOS
    - **N81.11   Cystocele, midline ♀**
    - **N81.12   Cystocele, lateral ♀**
      - Paravaginal cystocele

Figure 14-12   Three stages of uterine prolapse. **A.** Uterus is prolapsed. **B.** Vagina and uterus are prolapsed (incomplete uterovaginal prolapse). **C.** Vagina and uterus are completely prolapsed and are exposed through the external genitalia (complete uterovaginal prolapse).

  - **N81.2   Incomplete uterovaginal prolapse ♀**
    - First degree uterine prolapse
    - Prolapse of cervix NOS
    - Second degree uterine prolapse
    - **Excludes1**   cervical stump prolaspe (N81.85)
  - **N81.3   Complete uterovaginal prolapse ♀**
    - Procidentia (uteri) NOS
    - Third degree uterine prolapse
  - **N81.4   Uterovaginal prolapse, unspecified ♀**
    - Prolapse of uterus NOS
  - **N81.5   Vaginal enterocele ♀**
    - **Excludes1**   enterocele with prolapse of uterus (N81.2-N81.4)
  - **N81.6   Rectocele ♀**
    - Prolapse of posterior vaginal wall
    - Use additional code for any associated fecal incontinence, if applicable (R15.-)
    - **Excludes2**   perineocele (N81.81)
      - rectal prolapse (K62.3)
      - rectocele with prolapse of uterus (N81.2-N81.4)
  - **N81.8   Other female genital prolapse**
    - **N81.81   Perineocele ♀**
    - **N81.82   Incompetence or weakening of pubocervical tissue ♀**
    - **N81.83   Incompetence or weakening of rectovaginal tissue ♀**
    - **N81.84   Pelvic muscle wasting ♀**
      - Disuse atrophy of pelvic muscles and anal sphincter
    - **N81.85   Cervical stump prolapse ♀**
    - **N81.89   Other female genital prolapse ♀**
      - Deficient perineum
      - Old laceration of muscles of pelvic floor
  - **N81.9   Female genital prolapse, unspecified ♀**

- **N82   Fistulae involving female genital tract**
  - **Excludes1**   vesicointestinal fistulae (N32.1)
  - **N82.0   Vesicovaginal fistula ♀**
  - **N82.1   Other female urinary-genital tract fistulae ♀**
    - Cervicovesical fistula
    - Ureterovaginal fistula
    - Urethrovaginal fistula
    - Uteroureteric fistula
    - Uterovesical fistula
  - **N82.2   Fistula of vagina to small intestine ♀**
  - **N82.3   Fistula of vagina to large intestine ♀**
    - Rectovaginal fistula
  - **N82.4   Other female intestinal-genital tract fistulae ♀**
    - Intestinouterine fistula
  - **N82.5   Female genital tract-skin fistulae ♀**
    - Uterus to abdominal wall fistula
    - Vaginoperineal fistula
  - **N82.8   Other female genital tract fistulae ♀**
  - **N82.9   Female genital tract fistula, unspecified ♀**

Item 14–11 Endometriosis is a condition for which no clear cause has been identified. Endometrial tissue is expelled from the uterus into the abdominal cavity and can implant onto a variety of organs. Classification is based on the site of implant of the endometrial tissue.

Figure 14-11   Sites of potential endometrial implants.

◀ New   ◀▬ Revised   ~~deleted~~ Deleted   Excludes 1   Excludes 2   Includes   Use additional   Code first   Code also   Unspecified
OGCR Official Guidelines   X Assign placeholder X   ● Use Additional Character(s)   ▶ Manifestation Code   **Coding Clinic**

● **N83**   **Noninflammatory disorders of ovary, fallopian tube and broad ligament**

     Excludes2   hydrosalpinx (N70.1-)

● **N83.0**   **Follicular cyst of ovary**
         Cyst of graafian follicle
         Hemorrhagic follicular cyst (of ovary)

     N83.00   Follicular cyst of ovary, unspecified side ♀ ◄

     N83.01   Follicular cyst of right ovary ♀ ◄

     N83.02   Follicular cyst of left ovary ♀ ◄

● **N83.1**   **Corpus luteum cyst**
         Hemorrhagic corpus luteum cyst

     N83.10   Corpus luteum cyst of ovary, unspecified side ♀ ◄

     N83.11   Corpus luteum cyst of right ovary ♀ ◄

     N83.12   Corpus luteum cyst of left ovary ♀ ◄

● **N83.2**   **Other and unspecified ovarian cysts**

     Excludes1   developmental ovarian cyst (Q50.1)
                     neoplastic ovarian cyst (D27.-)
                     polycystic ovarian syndrome (E28.2)
                     Stein-Leventhal syndrome (E28.2)

   ● **N83.20**   Unspecified ovarian cysts

       N83.201   Unspecified ovarian cyst, right side ♀ ◄

       N83.202   Unspecified ovarian cyst, left side ♀ ◄

       N83.209   Unspecified ovarian cyst, unspecified side ♀ ◄
                 Ovarian cyst, NOS ◄

   ● **N83.29**   Other ovarian cysts
         Retention cyst of ovary
         Simple cyst of ovary

       N83.291   Other ovarian cyst, right side ♀ ◄

       N83.292   Other ovarian cyst, left side ♀ ◄

       N83.299   Other ovarian cyst, unspecified side ♀ ◄

● **N83.3**   **Acquired atrophy of ovary and fallopian tube**

   ● **N83.31**   Acquired atrophy of ovary

       N83.311   Acquired atrophy of right ovary ♀ ◄

       N83.312   Acquired atrophy of left ovary ♀ ◄

       N83.319   Acquired atrophy of ovary, unspecified side ♀ ◄
                 Acquired atrophy of ovary, NOS ◄

   ● **N83.32**   Acquired atrophy of fallopian tube

       N83.321   Acquired atrophy of right fallopian tube ♀ ◄

       N83.322   Acquired atrophy of left fallopian tube ♀ ◄

       N83.329   Acquired atrophy of fallopian tube, unspecified side ♀ ◄
                 Acquired atrophy of fallopian tube, NOS ◄

   ● **N83.33**   Acquired atrophy of ovary and fallopian tube

       N83.331   Acquired atrophy of right ovary and fallopian tube ♀ ◄

       N83.332   Acquired atrophy of left ovary and fallopian tube ♀ ◄

       N83.339   Acquired atrophy of ovary and fallopian tube, unspecified side ♀ ◄
                 Acquired atrophy of ovary and fallopian tube, NOS ◄

● **N83.4**   **Prolapse and hernia of ovary and fallopian tube**

     N83.40   Prolapse and hernia of ovary and fallopian tube, unspecified side ♀ ◄
               Prolapse and hernia of ovary and fallopian tube, NOS ◄

     N83.41   Prolapse and hernia of right ovary and fallopian tube ♀ ◄

     N83.42   Prolapse and hernia of left ovary and fallopian tube ♀ ◄

● **N83.5**   **Torsion of ovary, ovarian pedicle and fallopian tube**
         Torsion of accessory tube

   ● **N83.51**   Torsion of ovary and ovarian pedicle

       N83.511   Torsion of right ovary and ovarian pedicle ♀ ◄

       N83.512   Torsion of left ovary and ovarian pedicle ♀ ◄

       N83.519   Torsion of ovary and ovarian pedicle, unspecified side ♀ ◄
                 Torsion of ovary and ovarian pedicle, NOS ◄

   ● **N83.52**   Torsion of fallopian tube
         Torsion of hydatid of Morgagni

       N83.521   Torsion of right fallopian tube ♀ ◄

       N83.522   Torsion of left fallopian tube ♀ ◄

       N83.529   Torsion of fallopian tube, unspecified side ♀ ◄
                 Torsion of fallopian tube, NOS ◄

     N83.53   Torsion of ovary, ovarian pedicle and fallopian tube ♀

● **N83.6**   **Hematosalpinx** ♀

     Excludes1   hematosalpinx (with) (in):
                     hematocolpos (N89.7)
                     hematometra (N85.7)
                     tubal pregnancy (O00.1-) ◄

● **N83.7**   **Hematoma of broad ligament** ♀

● **N83.8**   **Other noninflammatory disorders of ovary, fallopian tube and broad ligament** ♀
         Broad ligament laceration syndrome [Allen-Masters]

● **N83.9**   **Noninflammatory disorder of ovary, fallopian tube and broad ligament, unspecified** ♀

● **N84**   **Polyp of female genital tract**

     Excludes1   adenomatous polyp (D28.-)
                     placental polyp (O90.89)

N84.0   **Polyp of corpus uteri** ♀
         Polyp of endometrium
         Polyp of uterus NOS

     Excludes1   polypoid endometrial hyperplasia (N85.0-)

N84.1   **Polyp of cervix uteri** ♀
         Mucous polyp of cervix

N84.2   **Polyp of vagina** ♀

N84.3   **Polyp of vulva** ♀
         Polyp of labia

N84.8   **Polyp of other parts of female genital tract** ♀

N84.9   **Polyp of female genital tract, unspecified** ♀

● **N85**   **Other noninflammatory disorders of uterus, except cervix**

     Excludes1   endometriosis (N80.-)
                     inflammatory diseases of uterus (N71.-)
                     noninflammatory disorders of cervix, except malposition (N86-N88)
                     polyp of corpus uteri (N84.0)
                     uterine prolapse (N81.-)

● **N85.0**   **Endometrial hyperplasia**

     N85.00   Endometrial hyperplasia, unspecified ♀
               Hyperplasia (adenomatous) (cystic) (glandular) of endometrium
               Hyperplastic endometritis

     N85.01   Benign endometrial hyperplasia ♀
               Endometrial hyperplasia (complex) (simple) without atypia

     N85.02   Endometrial intraepithelial neoplasia [EIN] ♀
               Endometrial hyperplasia with atypia

       Excludes1   malignant neoplasm of endometrium (with endometrial intraepithelial neoplasia [EIN]) (C54.1)

N85.2   Hypertrophy of uterus ♀
Bulky or enlarged uterus
> **Excludes1**   puerperal hypertrophy of uterus (O90.89)

N85.3   Subinvolution of uterus ♀
> **Excludes1**   puerperal subinvolution of uterus (O90.89)

N85.4   Malposition of uterus ♀
Anteversion of uterus
Retroflexion of uterus
Retroversion of uterus
> **Excludes1**   malposition of uterus complicating pregnancy, labor or delivery (O34.5-, O65.5)

N85.5   Inversion of uterus ♀
> **Excludes1**   current obstetric trauma (O71.2)
> postpartum inversion of uterus (O71.2)

N85.6   Intrauterine synechiae ♀

N85.7   Hematometra ♀
Hematosalpinx with hematometra
> **Excludes1**   hematometra with hematocolpos (N89.7)

N85.8   Other specified noninflammatory disorders of uterus ♀
Atrophy of uterus, acquired
Fibrosis of uterus NOS

N85.9   Noninflammatory disorder of uterus, unspecified ♀
Disorder of uterus NOS

N86   Erosion and ectropion of cervix uteri ♀
Decubitus (trophic) ulcer of cervix
Eversion of cervix
> **Excludes1**   erosion and ectropion of cervix with cervicitis (N72)

● N87   Dysplasia of cervix uteri
> **Excludes1**   abnormal results from cervical cytologic examination without histologic confirmation (R87.61-)
> carcinoma in situ of cervix uteri (D06.-)
> cervical intraepithelial neoplasia III [CIN III] (D06.-)
> HGSIL of cervix (R87.613)
> severe dysplasia of cervix uteri (D06.-)

N87.0   Mild cervical dysplasia ♀
Cervical intraepithelial neoplasia I [CIN I]

N87.1   Moderate cervical dysplasia ♀
Cervical intraepithelial neoplasia II [CIN II]

N87.9   Dysplasia of cervix uteri, unspecified ♀
Anaplasia of cervix
Cervical atypism
Cervical dysplasia NOS

● N88   Other noninflammatory disorders of cervix uteri
> **Excludes2**   inflammatory disease of cervix (N72)
> polyp of cervix (N84.1)

N88.0   Leukoplakia of cervix uteri ♀

N88.1   Old laceration of cervix uteri ♀
Adhesions of cervix
> **Excludes1**   current obstetric trauma (O71.3)

N88.2   Stricture and stenosis of cervix uteri ♀
> **Excludes1**   stricture and stenosis of cervix uteri complicating labor (O65.5)

N88.3   Incompetence of cervix uteri ♀
Investigation and management of (suspected) cervical incompetence in a nonpregnant woman
> **Excludes1**   cervical incompetence complicating pregnancy (O34.3-)

N88.4   Hypertrophic elongation of cervix uteri ♀

N88.8   Other specified noninflammatory disorders of cervix uteri ♀
> **Excludes1**   current obstetric trauma (O71.3)

N88.9   Noninflammatory disorder of cervix uteri, unspecified ♀

● N89   Other noninflammatory disorders of vagina
> **Excludes1**   abnormal results from vaginal cytologic examination without histologic confirmation (R87.62-)
> carcinoma in situ of vagina (D07.2)
> HGSIL of vagina (R87.623)
> inflammation of vagina (N76.-)
> senile (atrophic) vaginitis (N95.2)
> severe dysplasia of vagina (D07.2)
> trichomonal leukorrhea (A59.00)
> vaginal intraepithelial neoplasia [VAIN], grade III (D07.2)

N89.0   Mild vaginal dysplasia ♀
Vaginal intraepithelial neoplasia [VAIN], grade I

N89.1   Moderate vaginal dysplasia ♀
Vaginal intraepithelial neoplasia [VAIN], grade II

N89.3   Dysplasia of vagina, unspecified ♀

N89.4   Leukoplakia of vagina ♀

N89.5   Stricture and atresia of vagina ♀
Vaginal adhesions   Vaginal stenosis
> **Excludes1**   congenital atresia or stricture (Q52.4)
> postprocedural adhesions of vagina (N99.2)

N89.6   Tight hymenal ring ♀
Rigid hymen   Tight introitus
> **Excludes1**   imperforate hymen (Q52.3)

N89.7   Hematocolpos ♀
Hematocolpos with hematometra or hematosalpinx

N89.8   Other specified noninflammatory disorders of vagina ♀
Leukorrhea NOS
Old vaginal laceration
Pessary ulcer of vagina
> **Excludes1**   current obstetric trauma (O70.-, O71.4, O71.7-O71.8)
> old laceration involving muscles of pelvic floor (N81.8)

N89.9   Noninflammatory disorder of vagina, unspecified ♀

● N90   Other noninflammatory disorders of vulva and perineum
> **Excludes1**   anogenital (venereal) warts (A63.0)
> carcinoma in situ of vulva (D07.1)
> condyloma acuminatum (A63.0)
> current obstetric trauma (O70.-, O71.7-O71.8)
> inflammation of vulva (N76.-)
> severe dysplasia of vulva (D07.1)
> vulvar intraepithelial neoplasm III [VIN III] (D07.1)

N90.0   Mild vulvar dysplasia ♀
Vulvar intraepithelial neoplasia [VIN], grade I

N90.1   Moderate vulvar dysplasia ♀
Vulvar intraepithelial neoplasia [VIN], grade II

N90.3   Dysplasia of vulva, unspecified ♀

N90.4   Leukoplakia of vulva ♀
Dystrophy of vulva
Kraurosis of vulva
Lichen sclerosus of external female genital organs

N90.5   Atrophy of vulva ♀
Stenosis of vulva

● N90.6   Hypertrophy of vulva
> **N90.60   Unspecified hypertrophy of vulva ♀ ◀**
> Unspecified hypertrophy of labia ◀
>
> **N90.61   Childhood asymmetric labium majus enlargement ♀ ◀**
> CALME ◀
>
> **N90.69   Other specified hypertrophy of vulva ♀ ◀**
> Other specified hypertrophy of labia ◀

N90.7   Vulvar cyst ♀

◀ New   ◀⁞ Revised   ~~deleted~~ Deleted   Excludes 1   Excludes 2   Includes   Use additional   Code first   Code also   Unspecified

1082   OGCR Official Guidelines   X Assign placeholder X   ● Use Additional Character(s)   ▶ Manifestation Code   **Coding Clinic**

● **N90.8**   **Other specified noninflammatory disorders of vulva and perineum**
  ● **N90.81**   **Female genital mutilation status**
     Female genital cutting status
      N90.810   **Female genital mutilation status, unspecified** ♀
        Female genital cutting status, unspecified
        Female genital mutilation status NOS
      N90.811   **Female genital mutilation Type I status** ♀
        Clitorectomy status
        Female genital cutting Type I status
      N90.812   **Female genital mutilation Type II status** ♀
        Clitorectomy with excision of labia minora status
        Female genital cutting Type II status
      N90.813   **Female genital mutilation Type III status** ♀
        Female genital cutting Type III status
        Infibulation status
      N90.818   **Other female genital mutilation status** ♀
        Female genital cutting Type IV status
        Female genital mutilation Type IV status
        Other female genital cutting status
     N90.89   **Other specified noninflammatory disorders of vulva and perineum** ♀
       Adhesions of vulva
       Hypertrophy of clitoris
   N90.9   **Noninflammatory disorder of vulva and perineum, unspecified** ♀

● **N91**   **Absent, scanty and rare menstruation**
   Excludes1   ovarian dysfunction (E28.-)
   N91.0   **Primary amenorrhea** ♀
   N91.1   **Secondary amenorrhea** ♀
   N91.2   **Amenorrhea, unspecified** ♀
   N91.3   **Primary oligomenorrhea** ♀
   N91.4   **Secondary oligomenorrhea** ♀
   N91.5   **Oligomenorrhea, unspecified** ♀
     Hypomenorrhea NOS

● **N92**   **Excessive, frequent and irregular menstruation**
   Excludes1   postmenopausal bleeding (N95.0)
       precocious puberty (menstruation) (E30.1)
   N92.0   **Excessive and frequent menstruation with regular cycle** ♀
     Heavy periods NOS   Polymenorrhea
     Menorrhagia NOS
   N92.1   **Excessive and frequent menstruation with irregular cycle** ♀
     Irregular intermenstrual bleeding
     Irregular, shortened intervals between menstrual bleeding
     Menometrorrhagia
     Metrorrhagia
   N92.2   **Excessive menstruation at puberty** ♀   P
     Excessive bleeding associated with onset of menstrual periods
     Pubertal menorrhagia
     Puberty bleeding
   N92.3   **Ovulation bleeding** ♀
     Regular intermenstrual bleeding

   N92.4   **Excessive bleeding in the premenopausal period** ♀
     Climacteric menorrhagia or metrorrhagia
     Menopausal menorrhagia or metrorrhagia
     Preclimacteric menorrhagia or metrorrhagia
     Premenopausal menorrhagia or metrorrhagia
   N92.5   **Other specified irregular menstruation** ♀
   N92.6   **Irregular menstruation, unspecified** ♀
     Irregular bleeding NOS
     Irregular periods NOS
     Excludes1   irregular menstruation with:
         lengthened intervals or scanty bleeding (N91.3-N91.5)
         shortened intervals or excessive bleeding (N92.1)

● **N93**   **Other abnormal uterine and vaginal bleeding**
   Excludes1   neonatal vaginal hemorrhage (P54.6)
       precocious puberty (menstruation) (E30.1)
       pseudomenses (P54.6)
   N93.0   **Postcoital and contact bleeding** ♀
   N93.1   **Pre-pubertal vaginal bleeding** ♀ ◀
   N93.8   **Other specified abnormal uterine and vaginal bleeding** ♀
     Dysfunctional or functional uterine or vaginal bleeding NOS
   N93.9   **Abnormal uterine and vaginal bleeding, unspecified** ♀

● **N94**   **Pain and other conditions associated with female genital organs and menstrual cycle**
   N94.0   **Mittelschmerz** ♀
     Ovulation pain
  ● **N94.1**   **Dyspareunia**
     Painful intercourse/coitus
     Excludes1   psychogenic dyspareunia (F52.6)
     N94.10   **Unspecified dyspareunia** ♀ ◀
     N94.11   **Superficial (introital) dyspareunia** ♀ ◀
     N94.12   **Deep dyspareunia** ♀ ◀
     N94.19   **Other specified dyspareunia** ♀ ◀
   N94.2   **Vaginismus** ♀
     Vagina tightness
     Excludes1   psychogenic vaginismus (F52.5)
   N94.3   **Premenstrual tension syndrome** ♀
     AKA: PMS
     Premenstrual dysphoric disorder
     Code also associated menstrual migraine (G43.82-, G43.83-)
     Excludes1   Premenstrual dysphoric disorder (F32.81) ◀
   N94.4   **Primary dysmenorrhea** ♀
     Lifelong painful menstruation
   N94.5   **Secondary dysmenorrhea** ♀
     Later onset of painful menstruation
   N94.6   **Dysmenorrhea, unspecified** ♀
     Excludes1   psychogenic dysmenorrhea (F45.8)
  ● **N94.8**   **Other specified conditions associated with female genital organs and menstrual cycle**
    ● **N94.81**   **Vulvodynia**
       N94.810   **Vulvar vestibulitis** ♀
       N94.818   **Other vulvodynia** ♀
       N94.819   **Vulvodynia, unspecified** ♀
         Vulvodynia NOS
     N94.89   **Other specified conditions associated with female genital organs and menstrual cycle** ♀
   N94.9   **Unspecified condition associated with female genital organs and menstrual cycle** ♀

CHAPTER 14 (N00-N99)

● **N95   Menopausal and other perimenopausal disorders**
Menopausal and other perimenopausal disorders due to
naturally occurring (age-related) menopause and
perimenopause

Excludes1   excessive bleeding in the premenopausal period
(N92.4)
menopausal and perimenopausal disorders due
to artificial or premature menopause (E89.4-,
E28.31-)
premature menopause (E28.31-)

Excludes2   postmenopausal osteoporosis (M81.0-)
postmenopausal osteoporosis with current
pathological fracture (M80.0-)
postmenopausal urethritis (N34.2)

N95.0   Postmenopausal bleeding ♀

N95.1   Menopausal and female climacteric states ♀
Symptoms such as flushing, sleeplessness, headache,
lack of concentration, associated with natural (age-
related) menopause

Use additional code for associated symptoms

Excludes1   asymptomatic menopausal state (Z78.0)
symptoms associated with artificial
menopause (E89.41)
symptoms associated with premature
menopause (E28.310)

N95.2   Postmenopausal atrophic vaginitis ♀
Senile (atrophic) vaginitis

**N95.8   Other specified menopausal and perimenopausal
disorders** ♀

N95.9   Unspecified menopausal and perimenopausal disorder ♀

N96   Recurrent pregnancy loss ♀
Investigation or care in a nonpregnant woman with history of
recurrent pregnancy loss

Excludes1   recurrent pregnancy loss with current pregnancy
(O26.2-)

● **N97   Female infertility**

Includes   inability to achieve a pregnancy
sterility, female NOS

Excludes1   female infertility associated with:
hypopituitarism (E23.0)
Stein-Leventhal syndrome (E28.2)

Excludes2   incompetence of cervix uteri (N88.3)

N97.0   Female infertility associated with anovulation ♀

N97.1   Female infertility of tubal origin ♀
Female infertility associated with congenital anomaly
of tube
Female infertility due to tubal block
Female infertility due to tubal occlusion
Female infertility due to tubal stenosis

N97.2   Female infertility of uterine origin ♀
Female infertility associated with congenital anomaly
of uterus
Female infertility due to nonimplantation of ovum

N97.8   Female infertility of other origin ♀

N97.9   Female infertility, unspecified ♀

● **N98   Complications associated with artificial fertilization**

N98.0   Infection associated with artificial insemination ♀

N98.1   Hyperstimulation of ovaries ♀
Hyperstimulation of ovaries NOS
Hyperstimulation of ovaries associated with induced
ovulation

**N98.2   Complications of attempted introduction of fertilized
ovum following in vitro fertilization** ♀

**N98.3   Complications of attempted introduction of embryo in
embryo transfer** ♀

**N98.8   Other complications associated with artificial
fertilization** ♀

**N98.9   Complication associated with artificial fertilization,
unspecified** ♀

**INTRAOPERATIVE AND POSTPROCEDURAL COMPLICATIONS AND DISORDERS
OF GENITOURINARY SYSTEM, NOT ELSEWHERE CLASSIFIED (N99)**

● **N99   Intraoperative and postprocedural complications and disorders
of genitourinary system, not elsewhere classified**

Excludes2   irradiation cystitis (N30.4-)
postoophorectomy osteoporosis with current
pathological fracture (M80.8-)
postoophorectomy osteoporosis without current
pathological fracture (M81.8)

N99.0   Postprocedural (acute) (chronic) kidney failure
Use additional code to type of kidney disease

● **N99.1   Postprocedural urethral stricture**
Postcatheterization urethral stricture

● **N99.11   Postprocedural urethral stricture, male**

**N99.110   Postprocedural urethral stricture,
male, meatal** ♂

**N99.111   Postprocedural bulbous urethral
stricture** ♂

**N99.112   Postprocedural membranous urethral
stricture** ♂

**N99.113   Postprocedural anterior bulbous
urethral stricture** ♂ ◀▥

**N99.114   Postprocedural urethral stricture,
male, unspecified** ♂

**N99.115   Postprocedural fossa navicularis
urethral stricture** ◀

N99.12   Postprocedural urethral stricture, female ♀

N99.2   Postprocedural adhesions of vagina ♀

N99.3   Prolapse of vaginal vault after hysterectomy ♀

N99.4   Postprocedural pelvic peritoneal adhesions

Excludes2   pelvic peritoneal adhesions NOS (N73.6)
postinfective pelvic peritoneal adhesions
(N73.6)

● **N99.5   Complications of stoma of urinary tract**

Excludes2   mechanical complication of urinary
catheter (T83.0-) ◀▥

● **N99.51   Complication of cystostomy**

N99.510   Cystostomy hemorrhage

N99.511   Cystostomy infection

N99.512   Cystostomy malfunction

N99.518   Other cystostomy complication

● **N99.52   Complication of incontinent external stoma of
urinary tract** ◀▥

**N99.520   Hemorrhage of incontinent external
stoma of urinary tract** ◀▥

**N99.521   Infection of incontinent external
stoma of urinary tract** ◀▥

**N99.522   Malfunction of incontinent external
stoma of urinary tract** ◀▥

**N99.523   Herniation of incontinent stoma of
urinary tract** ◀

**N99.524   Stenosis of incontinent stoma of
urinary tract** ◀

**N99.528   Other complication of incontinent
external stoma of urinary tract** ◀▥

◀ New   ◀▥ Revised   ~~deleted~~ Deleted   Excludes 1   Excludes 2   Includes   Use additional   Code first   Code also   Unspecified
OGCR Official Guidelines   X Assign placeholder X   ● Use Additional Character(s)   ▶ Manifestation Code   **Coding Clinic**

● **N99.53**   **Complication of continent stoma of urinary tract** ◀▥

     N99.530   Hemorrhage of continent stoma of urinary tract ◀▥

     N99.531   Infection of continent stoma of urinary tract ◀▥

     N99.532   Malfunction of continent stoma of urinary tract ◀▥

     N99.533   Herniation of continent stoma of urinary tract ◀

     N99.534   Stenosis of continent stoma of urinary tract ◀

     N99.538   Other complication of continent stoma of urinary tract ◀▥

● **N99.6**   **Intraoperative hemorrhage and hematoma of a genitourinary system organ or structure complicating a procedure**

     | **Excludes1** | intraoperative hemorrhage and hematoma of a genitourinary system organ or structure due to accidental puncture or laceration during a procedure (N99.7-) |

     N99.61   Intraoperative hemorrhage and hematoma of a genitourinary system organ or structure complicating a genitourinary system procedure

     N99.62   Intraoperative hemorrhage and hematoma of a genitourinary system organ or structure complicating other procedure

● **N99.7**   **Accidental puncture and laceration of a genitourinary system organ or structure during a procedure**

     N99.71   Accidental puncture and laceration of a genitourinary system organ or structure during a genitourinary system procedure

     N99.72   Accidental puncture and laceration of a genitourinary system organ or structure during other procedure

● **N99.8**   **Other intraoperative and postprocedural complications and disorders of genitourinary system**

     N99.81   Other intraoperative complications of genitourinary system

●   **N99.82**   Postprocedural hemorrhage of a genitourinary system organ or structure following a procedure ◀▥

     N99.820   Postprocedural hemorrhage of a genitourinary system organ or structure following a genitourinary system procedure ◀▥

     N99.821   Postprocedural hemorrhage of a genitourinary system organ or structure following other procedure ◀▥

     N99.83   Residual ovary syndrome ♀

●   **N99.84**   Postprocedural hematoma and seroma of a genitourinary system organ or structure following a procedure ◀

     N99.840   Postprocedural hematoma of a genitourinary system organ or structure following a genitourinary system procedure ◀

     N99.841   Postprocedural hematoma of a genitourinary system organ or structure following other procedure ◀

     N99.842   Postprocedural seroma of a genitourinary system organ or structure following a genitourinary system procedure ◀

     N99.843   Postprocedural seroma of a genitourinary system organ or structure following other procedure ◀

     N99.89   Other postprocedural complications and disorders of genitourinary system

CHAPTER 14 (N00-N99)

CHAPTER 15

PREGNANCY, CHILDBIRTH AND THE PUERPERIUM (O00-O9A)

OGCR Chapter-Specific Coding Guidelines

15. **Chapter 15: Pregnancy, Childbirth, and the Puerperium (O00-O9A)**

a. **General Rules for Obstetric Cases**

1) Codes from chapter 15 and sequencing priority
Obstetric cases require codes from chapter 15, codes in the range O00-O9A, Pregnancy, Childbirth, and the Puerperium. Chapter 15 codes have sequencing priority over codes from other chapters. Additional codes from other chapters may be used in conjunction with chapter 15 codes to further specify conditions. Should the provider document that the pregnancy is incidental to the encounter, then code Z33.1, Pregnant state, incidental, should be used in place of any chapter 15 codes. It is the provider's responsibility to state that the condition being treated is not affecting the pregnancy.

2) Chapter 15 codes used only on the maternal record
Chapter 15 codes are to be used only on the maternal record, never on the record of the newborn.

3) Final character for trimester
The majority of codes in Chapter 15 have a final character indicating the trimester of pregnancy. The timeframes for the trimesters are indicated at the beginning of the chapter. If trimester is not a component of a code it is because the condition always occurs in a specific trimester, or the concept of trimester of pregnancy is not applicable. Certain codes have characters for only certain trimesters because the condition does not occur in all trimesters, but it may occur in more than just one.

Assignment of the final character for trimester should be based on the provider's documentation of the trimester (or number of weeks) for the current admission/encounter. This applies to the assignment of trimester for pre-existing conditions as well as those that develop during or are due to the pregnancy. The provider's documentation of the number of weeks may be used to assign the appropriate code identifying the trimester.

Whenever delivery occurs during the current admission, and there is an "in childbirth" option for the obstetric complication being coded, the "in childbirth" code should be assigned.

4) Selection of trimester for inpatient admissions that encompass more than one trimester
In instances when a patient is admitted to a hospital for complications of pregnancy during one trimester and remains in the hospital into a subsequent trimester, the trimester character for the antepartum complication code should be assigned on the basis of the trimester when the complication developed, not the trimester of the discharge. If the condition developed prior to the current admission/encounter or represents a pre-existing condition, the trimester character for the trimester at the time of the admission/encounter should be assigned.

5) Unspecified trimester
Each category that includes codes for trimester has a code for "unspecified trimester." The "unspecified trimester" code should rarely be used, such as when the documentation in the record is insufficient to determine the trimester and it is not possible to obtain clarification.

6) 7th character for Fetus Identification
Where applicable, a 7th character is to be assigned for certain categories (O31, O32, O33.3 - O33.6, O35, O36, O40, O41, O60.1, O60.2, O64, and O69) to identify the fetus for which the complication code applies.

Assign 7th character "0":
- For single gestations
- When the documentation in the record is insufficient to determine the fetus affected and it is not possible to obtain clarification.
- When it is not possible to clinically determine which fetus is affected.

b. **Selection of OB Principal or First-listed Diagnosis**

1) Routine outpatient prenatal visits
For routine outpatient prenatal visits when no complications are present, a code from category Z34, Encounter for supervision of normal pregnancy, should be used as the first-listed diagnosis. These codes should not be used in conjunction with chapter 15 codes.

2) *Supervision of High-Risk Pregnancy*
Codes from category O09, Supervision of high-risk pregnancy, are intended for use only during the prenatal period. For complications during the labor or delivery episode as a result of a high-risk pregnancy, assign the applicable complication codes from Chapter 15. If there are no complications during the labor or delivery episode, assign code O80, Encounter for full-term uncomplicated delivery.

For routine prenatal outpatient visits for patients with high-risk pregnancies, a code from category O09, Supervision of high-risk pregnancy, should be used as the first-listed diagnosis. Secondary chapter 15 codes may be used in conjunction with these codes if appropriate.

3) Episodes when no delivery occurs
In episodes when no delivery occurs, the principal diagnosis should correspond to the principal complication of the pregnancy which necessitated the encounter. Should more than one complication exist, all of which are treated or monitored, any of the complications codes may be sequenced first.

4) When a delivery occurs
When an obstetric patient is admitted and delivers during that admission, the condition that prompted the admission should be sequenced as the principal diagnosis. If multiple conditions prompted the admission, sequence the one most related to the delivery as the principal diagnosis. A code for any complication of the delivery should be assigned as an additional diagnosis. In cases of cesarean delivery, if the patient was admitted with a condition that resulted in the performance of a cesarean procedure, that condition should be selected as the principal diagnosis. If the reason for the admission was unrelated to the condition resulting in the cesarean delivery, the condition related to the reason for the admission should be selected as the principal diagnosis.

5) Outcome of delivery
A code from category Z37, Outcome of delivery, should be included on every maternal record when a delivery has occurred. These codes are not to be used on subsequent records or on the newborn record.

c. **Pre-existing conditions versus conditions due to the pregnancy**
Certain categories in Chapter 15 distinguish between conditions of the mother that existed prior to pregnancy (pre-existing) and those that are a direct result of pregnancy. When assigning codes from Chapter 15, it is important to assess if a condition was pre-existing prior to pregnancy or developed during or due to the pregnancy in order to assign the correct code.

Categories that do not distinguish between pre-existing and pregnancy-related conditions may be used for either. It is acceptable to use codes specifically for the puerperium with codes complicating pregnancy and childbirth if a condition arises postpartum during the delivery encounter.

d. **Pre-existing hypertension in pregnancy**
Category O10, Pre-existing hypertension complicating pregnancy, childbirth and the puerperium, includes codes for hypertensive heart and hypertensive chronic kidney disease. When assigning one of the O10 codes that includes hypertensive heart disease or hypertensive chronic kidney disease, it is necessary to add a secondary code from the appropriate hypertension category to specify the type of heart failure or chronic kidney disease.
See Section I.C.9. Hypertension.

e. **Fetal Conditions Affecting the Management of the Mother**

1) Codes from categories O35 and O36
Codes from categories O35, Maternal care for known or suspected fetal abnormality and damage, and O36, Maternal care for other fetal problems, are assigned only when the fetal condition is actually responsible for modifying the management of the mother, i.e., by requiring diagnostic studies, additional observation, special care, or termination of pregnancy. The fact that the fetal condition exists does not justify assigning a code from this series to the mother's record.

2) In utero surgery
In cases when surgery is performed on the fetus, a diagnosis code from category O35, Maternal care for known or suspected fetal abnormality and damage, should be assigned identifying the fetal condition. Assign the appropriate procedure code for the procedure performed.

No code from Chapter 16, the perinatal codes, should be used on the mother's record to identify fetal conditions. Surgery performed in utero on a fetus is still to be coded as an obstetric encounter.

f. **HIV Infection in Pregnancy, Childbirth and the Puerperium**
During pregnancy, childbirth or the puerperium, a patient admitted because of an HIV-related illness should receive a principal diagnosis from subcategory O98.7-, Human immunodeficiency [HIV] disease complicating pregnancy, childbirth and the puerperium, followed by the code(s) for the HIV-related illness(es).

Patients with asymptomatic HIV infection status admitted during pregnancy, childbirth, or the puerperium should receive codes of O98.7- and Z21, Asymptomatic human immunodeficiency virus [HIV] infection status.

g. **Diabetes mellitus in pregnancy**
Diabetes mellitus is a significant complicating factor in pregnancy. Pregnant women who are diabetic should be assigned a code from category O24, Diabetes mellitus in pregnancy, childbirth, and the puerperium, first, followed by the appropriate diabetes code(s) (E08-E13) from Chapter 4.

h. Long term use of insulin and oral hypoglycemics
Code Z79.4, Long-term (current) use of insulin **or code Z79.84, Long-term (current) use of oral hypoglycemic drugs,** should also be assigned if the diabetes mellitus is being treated with insulin **or oral medications. If the patient is treated with both oral medications and insulin, only the code for insulin-controlled should be assigned.**

i. Gestational (pregnancy induced) diabetes
Gestational (pregnancy induced) diabetes can occur during the second and third trimester of pregnancy in women who were not diabetic prior to pregnancy. Gestational diabetes can cause complications in the pregnancy similar to those of pre-existing diabetes mellitus. It also puts the woman at greater risk of developing diabetes after the pregnancy. Codes for gestational diabetes are in subcategory O24.4, Gestational diabetes mellitus. No other code from category O24, Diabetes mellitus in pregnancy, childbirth, and the puerperium, should be used with a code from O24.4.

The codes under subcategory O24.4 include diet controlled, insulin controlled, **and controlled by oral hypoglycemic drugs.** If a patient with gestational diabetes is treated with both diet and insulin, only the code for insulin-controlled is required. **If a patient with gestational diabetes is treated with both diet and oral hypoglycemic medications, only the code for "controlled by oral hypoglycemic drugs" is required.** Code Z79.4, Long-term (current) use of insulin **or code Z79.84, Long-term (current) use of oral hypoglycemic drugs,** should not be assigned with codes from subcategory O24.4.

An abnormal glucose tolerance in pregnancy is assigned a code from subcategory O99.81, Abnormal glucose complicating pregnancy, childbirth, and the puerperium.

j. Sepsis and septic shock complicating abortion, pregnancy, childbirth and the puerperium
When assigning a chapter 15 code for sepsis complicating abortion, pregnancy, childbirth, and the puerperium, a code for the specific type of infection should be assigned as an additional diagnosis. If severe sepsis is present, a code from subcategory R65.2, Severe sepsis, and code(s) for associated organ dysfunction(s) should also be assigned as additional diagnoses.

k. Puerperal sepsis
Code O85, Puerperal sepsis, should be assigned with a secondary code to identify the causal organism (e.g., for a bacterial infection, assign a code from category B95-B96, Bacterial infections in conditions classified elsewhere). A code from category A40, Streptococcal sepsis, or A41, Other sepsis, should not be used for puerperal sepsis. If applicable, use additional codes to identify severe sepsis (R65.2-) and any associated acute organ dysfunction.

l. Alcohol and tobacco use during pregnancy, childbirth and the puerperium
1) Alcohol use during pregnancy, childbirth and the puerperium
Codes under subcategory O99.31, Alcohol use complicating pregnancy, childbirth, and the puerperium, should be assigned for any pregnancy case when a mother uses alcohol during the pregnancy or postpartum. A secondary code from category F10, Alcohol related disorders, should also be assigned to identify manifestations of the alcohol use.

2) Tobacco use during pregnancy, childbirth and the puerperium
Codes under subcategory O99.33, Smoking (tobacco) complicating pregnancy, childbirth, and the puerperium, should be assigned for any pregnancy case when a mother uses any type of tobacco product during the pregnancy or postpartum. A secondary code from category F17, Nicotine dependence, should also be assigned to identify the type of nicotine dependence.

m. Poisoning, toxic effects, adverse effects and underdosing in a pregnant patient
A code from subcategory O9A.2, Injury, poisoning and certain other consequences of external causes complicating pregnancy, childbirth, and the puerperium, should be sequenced first, followed by the appropriate injury, poisoning, toxic effect, adverse effect or underdosing code, and then the additional code(s) that specifies the condition caused by the poisoning, toxic effect, adverse effect or underdosing.
See Section I.C.19. Adverse effects, poisoning, underdosing and toxic effects.

n. Normal Delivery, Code O80
1) Encounter for full term uncomplicated delivery
Code O80 should be assigned when a woman is admitted for a full-term normal delivery and delivers a single, healthy infant without any complications antepartum, during the delivery, or postpartum during the delivery episode. Code O80 is always a principal diagnosis. It is not to be used if any other code from chapter 15 is

needed to describe a current complication of the antenatal, delivery, or perinatal period. Additional codes from other chapters may be used with code O80 if they are not related to or are in any way complicating the pregnancy.

2) Uncomplicated delivery with resolved antepartum complication
Code O80 may be used if the patient had a complication at some point during the pregnancy, but the complication is not present at the time of the admission for delivery.

3) Outcome of delivery for O80
Z37.0, Single live birth, is the only outcome of delivery code appropriate for use with O80.

o. The Peripartum and Postpartum Periods
1) Peripartum and Postpartum periods
The postpartum period begins immediately after delivery and continues for six weeks following delivery. The peripartum period is defined as the last month of pregnancy to five months postpartum.

2) Peripartum and postpartum complication
A postpartum complication is any complication occurring within the six-week period.

3) Pregnancy-related complications after 6 week period
Chapter 15 codes may also be used to describe pregnancy-related complications after the peripartum or postpartum period if the provider documents that a condition is pregnancy related.

4) Admission for routine postpartum care following delivery outside hospital
When the mother delivers outside the hospital prior to admission and is admitted for routine postpartum care and no complications are noted, code Z39.0, Encounter for care and examination of mother immediately after delivery, should be assigned as the principal diagnosis.

5) Pregnancy associated cardiomyopathy
Pregnancy associated cardiomyopathy, code O90.3, is unique in that it may be diagnosed in the third trimester of pregnancy but may continue to progress months after delivery. For this reason, it is referred to as peripartum cardiomyopathy. Code O90.3 is only for use when the cardiomyopathy develops as a result of pregnancy in a woman who did not have pre-existing heart disease.

p. Code O94, Sequelae of complication of pregnancy, childbirth, and the puerperium
1) Code O94
Code O94, Sequelae of complication of pregnancy, childbirth, and the puerperium, is for use in those cases when an initial complication of a pregnancy develops a sequelae requiring care or treatment at a future date.

2) After the initial postpartum period
This code may be used at any time after the initial postpartum period.

3) Sequencing of Code O94
This code, like all sequela codes, is to be sequenced following the code describing the sequelae of the complication.

q. *Termination of Pregnancy and Spontaneous abortions*
1) Abortion with Liveborn Fetus
When an attempted termination of pregnancy results in a liveborn fetus assign code Z33.2, Encounter for elective termination of pregnancy and a code from category Z37, Outcome of Delivery.

2) Retained Products of Conception following an abortion
Subsequent encounters for retained products of conception following a spontaneous abortion or elective termination of pregnancy are assigned the appropriate code from category O03, Spontaneous abortion, or codes O07.4, Failed attempted termination of pregnancy without complication and Z33.2, Encounter for elective termination of pregnancy. This advice is appropriate even when the patient was discharged previously with a discharge diagnosis of complete abortion.

3) Complications leading to abortion
Codes from Chapter 15 may be used as additional codes to identify any documented complications of the pregnancy in conjunction with codes in categories in O07 and O08.

r. Abuse in a pregnant patient
For suspected or confirmed cases of abuse of a pregnant patient, a code(s) from subcategories O9A.3, Physical abuse complicating pregnancy, childbirth, and the puerperium, O9A.4, Sexual abuse complicating pregnancy, childbirth, and the puerperium, and O9A.5, Psychological abuse complicating pregnancy, childbirth, and the puerperium, should be sequenced first, followed by the appropriate codes (if applicable) to identify any associated current injury due to physical abuse, sexual abuse, and the perpetrator of abuse.
See Section I.C.19. Adult and child abuse, neglect and other maltreatment.

CHAPTER 15 (O00-O9A)

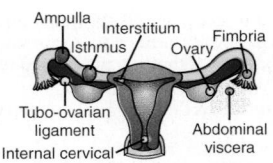

Figure 15-1 Implantation sites of ectopic pregnancy.

Item 15–1 Ectopic pregnancy most often occurs in the fallopian tube. Pregnancy outside the uterus may end in a lifethreatening rupture.

★**(See Plate 375 on page 52.)**

CHAPTER 15

PREGNANCY, CHILDBIRTH AND THE PUERPERIUM (O00-O9A)

Note: CODES FROM THIS CHAPTER ARE FOR USE ONLY ON MATERNAL RECORDS, NEVER ON NEWBORN RECORDS

Codes from this chapter are for use for conditions related to or aggravated by the pregnancy, childbirth, or by the puerperium (maternal causes or obstetric causes)

Trimesters are counted from the first day of the last menstrual period. They are defined as follows:

1st trimester - less than 14 weeks 0 days

2nd trimester - 14 weeks 0 days to less than 28 weeks 0 days

3rd trimester - 28 weeks 0 days until delivery

Use additional code from category Z3A, Weeks of gestation, to identify the specific week of the pregnancy, if known. ◀▥

Excludes1 supervision of normal pregnancy (Z34.-)

Excludes2 mental and behavioral disorders associated with the puerperium (F53)
obstetrical tetanus (A34)
postpartum necrosis of pituitary gland (E23.0)
puerperal osteomalacia (M83.0)

This chapter contains the following blocks:

O00-O08	Pregnancy with abortive outcome
O09	Supervision of high risk pregnancy
O10-O16	Edema, proteinuria and hypertensive disorders in pregnancy, childbirth and the puerperium
O20-O29	Other maternal disorders predominantly related to pregnancy
O30-O48	Maternal care related to the fetus and amniotic cavity and possible delivery problems
O60-O77	Complications of labor and delivery
O80, O82	Encounter for delivery
O85-O92	Complications predominantly related to the puerperium
O94-O9A	Other obstetric conditions, not elsewhere classified

PREGNANCY WITH ABORTIVE OUTCOME (O00-O08)

Excludes1 continuing pregnancy in multiple gestation after abortion of one fetus or more (O31.1-, O31.3-)

● **O00 Ectopic pregnancy**
  Includes ruptured ectopic pregnancy
  Use additional code from category O08 to identify any associated complication

● **O00.0 Abdominal pregnancy**
    Excludes1 maternal care for viable fetus in abdominal pregnancy (O36.7-)
    O00.00 **Abdominal pregnancy without intrauterine pregnancy** ♀ ◀   M
        Abdominal pregnancy NOS ◀
    O00.01 **Abdominal pregnancy with intrauterine pregnancy** ♀ ◀   M

Item 15–2 A **hydatidiform** mole is an overproduction of placental tissue. The tumor secretes a hormone, chorionic gonadotropic hormone (CGH), that indicates a positive pregnancy test. There is no viable fetus. More than 80% of hydatidiform moles are noncancerous.

● **O00.1 Tubal pregnancy**
    Fallopian pregnancy
    Rupture of (fallopian) tube due to pregnancy
    Tubal abortion
    O00.10 **Tubal pregnancy without intrauterine pregnancy** ♀ ◀   M
        Tubal pregnancy NOS ◀
    O00.11 **Tubal pregnancy with intrauterine pregnancy** ♀ ◀   M
● **O00.2 Ovarian pregnancy**
    O00.20 **Ovarian pregnancy without intrauterine pregnancy** ♀ ◀   M
        Ovarian pregnancy NOS ◀
    O00.21 **Ovarian pregnancy with intrauterine pregnancy** ♀ ◀   M
● **O00.8 Other ectopic pregnancy**
    Cervical pregnancy
    Cornual pregnancy
    Intraligamentous pregnancy
    Mural pregnancy
    O00.80 **Other ectopic pregnancy without intrauterine pregnancy** ♀ ◀   M
        Other ectopic pregnancy NOS ◀
    O00.81 **Other ectopic pregnancy with intrauterine pregnancy** ♀ ◀   M
● **O00.9 Ectopic pregnancy, unspecified**
    O00.90 **Unspecified ectopic pregnancy without intrauterine pregnancy** ♀ ◀   M
        Ectopic pregnancy NOS ◀
    O00.91 **Unspecified ectopic pregnancy with intrauterine pregnancy** ♀ ◀   M

● **O01 Hydatidiform mole**
  Use additional code from category O08 to identify any associated complication
  Excludes1 chorioadenoma (destruens) (D39.2)
    malignant hydatidiform mole (D39.2)
  O01.0 **Classical hydatidiform mole**   M
    Complete hydatidiform mole
  O01.1 **Incomplete and partial hydatidiform mole** ♀   M
  O01.9 **Hydatidiform mole, unspecified** ♀   M
    Trophoblastic disease NOS
    Vesicular mole NOS

● **O02 Other abnormal products of conception**
  Use additional code from category O08 to identify any associated complication
  Excludes1 papyraceous fetus (O31.0-)
  O02.0 **Blighted ovum and nonhydatidiform mole** ♀   M
    Carneous mole   Molar pregnancy NEC
    Fleshy mole   Pathological ovum
    Intrauterine mole NOS
  O02.1 **Missed abortion** ♀   M
    Early fetal death, before completion of 20 weeks of gestation, with retention of dead fetus
    Excludes1 failed induced abortion (O07.-)
      fetal death (intrauterine) (late) (O36.4)
      missed abortion with blighted ovum (O02.0)
      missed abortion with hydatidiform mole (O01.-)
      missed abortion with nonhydatidiform (O02.0)
      missed abortion with other abnormal products of conception (O02.8-)
      missed delivery (O36.4)
      stillbirth (P95)

◀ New   ◀▥ Revised   ~~deleted~~ Deleted   Excludes 1   Excludes 2   Includes   Use additional   Code first   Code also   Unspecified
OGCR Official Guidelines   X Assign placeholder X   ● Use Additional Character(s)   ▶ Manifestation Code   **Coding Clinic**

● **O02.8**   **Other specified abnormal products of conception**

     Excludes1   abnormal products of conception with blighted ovum (O02.0)

          abnormal products of conception with hydatidiform mole (O01.-)

          abnormal products of conception with nonhydatidiform mole (O02.0)

    O02.81   **Inappropriate change in quantitative human chorionic gonadotropin (hCG) in early pregnancy** ♀   M

       Biochemical pregnancy

       Chemical pregnancy

       Inappropriate level of quantitative human chorionic gonadotropin (hCG) for gestational age in early pregnancy

    O02.89   **Other abnormal products of conception** ♀   M

● **O02.9**   **Abnormal product of conception, unspecified** ♀   M

● **O03**   **Spontaneous abortion**

    Note: Incomplete abortion includes retained products of conception following spontaneous abortion.

     Includes   miscarriage

    O03.0   **Genital tract and pelvic infection following incomplete spontaneous abortion** ♀   M

       Endometritis following incomplete spontaneous abortion

       Oophoritis following incomplete spontaneous abortion

       Parametritis following incomplete spontaneous abortion

       Pelvic peritonitis following incomplete spontaneous abortion

       Salpingitis following incomplete spontaneous abortion

       Salpingo-oophoritis following incomplete spontaneous abortion

      Excludes1   sepsis following incomplete spontaneous abortion (O03.37)

          urinary tract infection following incomplete spontaneous abortion (O03.38)

    O03.1   **Delayed or excessive hemorrhage following incomplete spontaneous abortion** ♀   M

       Afibrinogenemia following incomplete spontaneous abortion

       Defibrination syndrome following incomplete spontaneous abortion

       Hemolysis following incomplete spontaneous abortion

       Intravascular coagulation following incomplete spontaneous abortion

    O03.2   **Embolism following incomplete spontaneous abortion** ♀   M

       Air embolism following incomplete spontaneous abortion

       Amniotic fluid embolism following incomplete spontaneous abortion

       Blood-clot embolism following incomplete spontaneous abortion

       Embolism NOS following incomplete spontaneous abortion

       Fat embolism following incomplete spontaneous abortion

       Pulmonary embolism following incomplete spontaneous abortion

       Pyemic embolism following incomplete spontaneous abortion

       Septic or septicopyemic embolism following incomplete spontaneous abortion

       Soap embolism following incomplete spontaneous abortion

● **O03.3**   **Other and unspecified complications following incomplete spontaneous abortion**

    O03.30   **Unspecified complication following incomplete spontaneous abortion** ♀   M

    O03.31   **Shock following incomplete spontaneous abortion** ♀   M

       Circulatory collapse following incomplete spontaneous abortion

       Shock (postprocedural) following incomplete spontaneous abortion

      Excludes1   shock due to infection following incomplete spontaneous abortion (O03.37)

    O03.32   **Renal failure following incomplete spontaneous abortion** ♀   M

       Kidney failure (acute) following incomplete spontaneous abortion

       Oliguria following incomplete spontaneous abortion

       Renal shutdown following incomplete spontaneous abortion

       Renal tubular necrosis following incomplete spontaneous abortion

       Uremia following incomplete spontaneous abortion

    O03.33   **Metabolic disorder following incomplete spontaneous abortion** ♀   M

    O03.34   **Damage to pelvic organs following incomplete spontaneous abortion** ♀   M

       Laceration, perforation, tear or chemical damage of bladder following incomplete spontaneous abortion

       Laceration, perforation, tear or chemical damage of bowel following incomplete spontaneous abortion

       Laceration, perforation, tear or chemical damage of broad ligament following incomplete spontaneous abortion

       Laceration, perforation, tear or chemical damage of cervix following incomplete spontaneous abortion

       Laceration, perforation, tear or chemical damage of periurethral tissue following incomplete spontaneous abortion

       Laceration, perforation, tear or chemical damage of uterus following incomplete spontaneous abortion

       Laceration, perforation, tear or chemical damage of vagina following incomplete spontaneous abortion

    O03.35   **Other venous complications following incomplete spontaneous abortion** ♀   M

    O03.36   **Cardiac arrest following incomplete spontaneous abortion** ♀   M

    O03.37   **Sepsis following incomplete spontaneous abortion** ♀   M

       Use additional code to identify infectious agent (B95-B97)

       Use additional code to identify severe sepsis, if applicable (R65.2-)

      Excludes1   septic or septicopyemic embolism following incomplete spontaneous abortion (O03.2)

    O03.38   **Urinary tract infection following incomplete spontaneous abortion** ♀   M

       Cystitis following incomplete spontaneous abortion

    O03.39   **Incomplete spontaneous abortion with other complications** ♀   M

CHAPTER 15 (O00-O9A)

O03.4 **Incomplete spontaneous abortion without complication** ♀ M

O03.5 **Genital tract and pelvic infection following complete or unspecified spontaneous abortion** ♀ M

Endometritis following complete or unspecified spontaneous abortion
Oophoritis following complete or unspecified spontaneous abortion
Parametritis following complete or unspecified spontaneous abortion
Pelvic peritonitis following complete or unspecified spontaneous abortion
Salpingitis following complete or unspecified spontaneous abortion
Salpingo-oophoritis following complete or unspecified spontaneous abortion

> **Excludes1** sepsis following complete or unspecified spontaneous abortion (O03.87)
> urinary tract infection following complete or unspecified spontaneous abortion (O03.88)

O03.6 **Delayed or excessive hemorrhage following complete or unspecified spontaneous abortion** ♀ M

Afibrinogenemia following complete or unspecified spontaneous abortion
Defibrination syndrome following complete or unspecified spontaneous abortion
Hemolysis following complete or unspecified spontaneous abortion
Intravascular coagulation following complete or unspecified spontaneous abortion

O03.7 **Embolism following complete or unspecified spontaneous abortion** ♀ M

Air embolism following complete or unspecified spontaneous abortion
Amniotic fluid embolism following complete or unspecified spontaneous abortion
Blood-clot embolism following complete or unspecified spontaneous abortion
Embolism NOS following complete or unspecified spontaneous abortion
Fat embolism following complete or unspecified spontaneous abortion
Pulmonary embolism following complete or unspecified spontaneous abortion
Pyemic embolism following complete or unspecified spontaneous abortion
Septic or septicopyemic embolism following complete or unspecified spontaneous abortion
Soap embolism following complete or unspecified spontaneous abortion

● O03.8 **Other and unspecified complications following complete or unspecified spontaneous abortion**

O03.80 **Unspecified complication following complete or unspecified spontaneous abortion** ♀ M

O03.81 **Shock following complete or unspecified spontaneous abortion** ♀ M

Circulatory collapse following complete or unspecified spontaneous abortion
Shock (postprocedural) following complete or unspecified spontaneous abortion

> **Excludes1** shock due to infection following complete or unspecified spontaneous abortion (O03.87)

O03.82 **Renal failure following complete or unspecified spontaneous abortion** ♀ M

Kidney failure (acute) following complete or unspecified spontaneous abortion
Oliguria following complete or unspecified spontaneous abortion
Renal shutdown following complete or unspecified spontaneous abortion
Renal tubular necrosis following complete or unspecified spontaneous abortion
Uremia following complete or unspecified spontaneous abortion

O03.83 **Metabolic disorder following complete or unspecified spontaneous abortion** ♀ M

O03.84 **Damage to pelvic organs following complete or unspecified spontaneous abortion** ♀ M

Laceration, perforation, tear or chemical damage of bladder following complete or unspecified spontaneous abortion
Laceration, perforation, tear or chemical damage of bowel following complete or unspecified spontaneous abortion
Laceration, perforation, tear or chemical damage of broad ligament following complete or unspecified spontaneous abortion
Laceration, perforation, tear or chemical damage of cervix following complete or unspecified spontaneous abortion
Laceration, perforation, tear or chemical damage of periurethral tissue following complete or unspecified spontaneous abortion
Laceration, perforation, tear or chemical damage of uterus following complete or unspecified spontaneous abortion
Laceration, perforation, tear or chemical damage of vagina following complete or unspecified spontaneous abortion

O03.85 **Other venous complications following complete or unspecified spontaneous abortion** ♀ M

O03.86 **Cardiac arrest following complete or unspecified spontaneous abortion** ♀ M

O03.87 **Sepsis following complete or unspecified spontaneous abortion** ♀ M

> Use additional code to identify infectious agent (B95-B97)
> Use additional code to identify severe sepsis, if applicable (R65.2-)
> **Excludes1** septic or septicopyemic embolism following complete or unspecified spontaneous abortion (O03.7)

O03.88 **Urinary tract infection following complete or unspecified spontaneous abortion** ♀ M

Cystitis following complete or unspecified spontaneous abortion

O03.89 **Complete or unspecified spontaneous abortion with other complications** ♀ M

O03.9 **Complete or unspecified spontaneous abortion without complication** ♀ M

Miscarriage NOS
Spontaneous abortion NOS

◀ New ◀⋯ Revised ~~deleted~~ Deleted Excludes 1 Excludes 2 Includes Use additional Code first Code also Unspecified
OGCR Official Guidelines X Assign placeholder X ● Use Additional Character(s) ▶ Manifestation Code **Coding Clinic**

● O04   **Complications following (induced) termination of pregnancy**

   Includes   complications following (induced) termination of pregnancy

   Excludes1   encounter for elective termination of pregnancy, uncomplicated (Z33.2)
   failed attempted termination of pregnancy (O07.-)

O04.5   **Genital tract and pelvic infection following (induced) termination of pregnancy ♀**   M
   Endometritis following (induced) termination of pregnancy
   Oophoritis following (induced) termination of pregnancy
   Parametritis following (induced) termination of pregnancy
   Pelvic peritonitis following (induced) termination of pregnancy
   Salpingitis following (induced) termination of pregnancy
   Salpingo-oophoritis following (induced) termination of pregnancy

   Excludes1   sepsis following (induced) termination of pregnancy (O04.87)
   urinary tract infection following (induced) termination of pregnancy (O04.88)

O04.6   **Delayed or excessive hemorrhage following (induced) termination of pregnancy ♀**   M
   Afibrinogenemia following (induced) termination of pregnancy
   Defibrination syndrome following (induced) termination of pregnancy
   Hemolysis following (induced) termination of pregnancy
   Intravascular coagulation following (induced) termination of pregnancy

O04.7   **Embolism following (induced) termination of pregnancy ♀**   M
   Air embolism following (induced) termination of pregnancy
   Amniotic fluid embolism following (induced) termination of pregnancy
   Blood-clot embolism following (induced) termination of pregnancy
   Embolism NOS following (induced) termination of pregnancy
   Fat embolism following (induced) termination of pregnancy
   Pulmonary embolism following (induced) termination of pregnancy
   Pyemic embolism following (induced) termination of pregnancy
   Septic or septicopyemic embolism following (induced) termination of pregnancy
   Soap embolism following (induced) termination of pregnancy

● O04.8   **(Induced) termination of pregnancy with other and unspecified complications**

   O04.80   **(Induced) termination of pregnancy with unspecified complications ♀**   M

   O04.81   **Shock following (induced) termination of pregnancy ♀**   M
   Circulatory collapse following (induced) termination of pregnancy
   Shock (postprocedural) following (induced) termination of pregnancy

   Excludes1   shock due to infection following (induced) termination of pregnancy (O04.87)

O04.82   **Renal failure following (induced) termination of pregnancy ♀**   M
   Kidney failure (acute) following (induced) termination of pregnancy
   Oliguria following (induced) termination of pregnancy
   Renal shutdown following (induced) termination of pregnancy
   Renal tubular necrosis following (induced) termination of pregnancy
   Uremia following (induced) termination of pregnancy

O04.83   **Metabolic disorder following (induced) termination of pregnancy ♀**   M

O04.84   **Damage to pelvic organs following (induced) termination of pregnancy ♀**   M
   Laceration, perforation, tear or chemical damage of bladder following (induced) termination of pregnancy
   Laceration, perforation, tear or chemical damage of bowel following (induced) termination of pregnancy
   Laceration, perforation, tear or chemical damage of broad ligament following (induced) termination of pregnancy
   Laceration, perforation, tear or chemical damage of cervix following (induced) termination of pregnancy
   Laceration, perforation, tear or chemical damage of periurethral tissue following (induced) termination of pregnancy
   Laceration, perforation, tear or chemical damage of uterus following (induced) termination of pregnancy
   Laceration, perforation, tear or chemical damage of vagina following (induced) termination of pregnancy

O04.85   **Other venous complications following (induced) termination of pregnancy ♀**   M

O04.86   **Cardiac arrest following (induced) termination of pregnancy ♀**   M

O04.87   **Sepsis following (induced) termination of pregnancy ♀**   M
   Use additional code to identify infectious agent (B95-B97)
   Use additional code to identify severe sepsis, if applicable (R65.2-)

   Excludes1   septic or septicopyemic embolism following (induced) termination of pregnancy (O04.7)

O04.88   **Urinary tract infection following (induced) termination of pregnancy ♀**   M
   Cystitis following (induced) termination of pregnancy

O04.89   **(Induced) termination of pregnancy with other complications ♀**   M

CHAPTER 15 (O00-O9A)

● **O07** **Failed attempted termination of pregnancy**

      Includes   failure of attempted induction of termination of pregnancy
                        incomplete elective abortion

      Excludes1   incomplete spontaneous abortion (O03.0-)

O07.0 **Genital tract and pelvic infection following failed attempted termination of pregnancy** ♀   M

    Endometritis following failed attempted termination of pregnancy
    Oophoritis following failed attempted termination of pregnancy
    Parametritis following failed attempted termination of pregnancy
    Pelvic peritonitis following failed attempted termination of pregnancy
    Salpingitis following failed attempted termination of pregnancy
    Salpingo-oophoritis following failed attempted termination of pregnancy

      Excludes1   sepsis following failed attempted termination of pregnancy (O07.37)
                     urinary tract infection following failed attempted termination of pregnancy (O07.38)

O07.1 **Delayed or excessive hemorrhage following failed attempted termination of pregnancy** ♀   M

    Afibrinogenemia following failed attempted termination of pregnancy
    Defibrination syndrome following failed attempted termination of pregnancy
    Hemolysis following failed attempted termination of pregnancy
    Intravascular coagulation following failed attempted termination of pregnancy

O07.2 **Embolism following failed attempted termination of pregnancy** ♀   M

    Air embolism following failed attempted termination of pregnancy
    Amniotic fluid embolism following failed attempted termination of pregnancy
    Blood-clot embolism following failed attempted termination of pregnancy
    Embolism NOS following failed attempted termination of pregnancy
    Fat embolism following failed attempted termination of pregnancy
    Pulmonary embolism following failed attempted termination of pregnancy
    Pyemic embolism following failed attempted termination of pregnancy
    Septic or septicopyemic embolism following failed attempted termination of pregnancy
    Soap embolism following failed attempted termination of pregnancy

● **O07.3** **Failed attempted termination of pregnancy with other and unspecified complications**

    O07.30 **Failed attempted termination of pregnancy with unspecified complications** ♀   M

    O07.31 **Shock following failed attempted termination of pregnancy** ♀   M

        Circulatory collapse following failed attempted termination of pregnancy
        Shock (postprocedural) following failed attempted termination of pregnancy

        Excludes1   shock due to infection following failed attempted termination of pregnancy (O07.37)

O07.32 **Renal failure following failed attempted termination of pregnancy** ♀   M

    Kidney failure (acute) following failed attempted termination of pregnancy
    Oliguria following failed attempted termination of pregnancy
    Renal shutdown following failed attempted termination of pregnancy
    Renal tubular necrosis following failed attempted termination of pregnancy
    Uremia following failed attempted termination of pregnancy

O07.33 **Metabolic disorder following failed attempted termination of pregnancy** ♀   M

O07.34 **Damage to pelvic organs following failed attempted termination of pregnancy** ♀   M

    Laceration, perforation, tear or chemical damage of bladder following failed attempted termination of pregnancy
    Laceration, perforation, tear or chemical damage of bowel following failed attempted termination of pregnancy
    Laceration, perforation, tear or chemical damage of broad ligament following failed attempted termination of pregnancy
    Laceration, perforation, tear or chemical damage of cervix following failed attempted termination of pregnancy
    Laceration, perforation, tear or chemical damage of periurethral tissue following failed attempted termination of pregnancy
    Laceration, perforation, tear or chemical damage of uterus following failed attempted termination of pregnancy
    Laceration, perforation, tear or chemical damage of vagina following failed attempted termination of pregnancy

O07.35 **Other venous complications following failed attempted termination of pregnancy** ♀   M

O07.36 **Cardiac arrest following failed attempted termination of pregnancy** ♀   M

O07.37 **Sepsis following failed attempted termination of pregnancy** ♀   M

    Use additional code (B95-B97), to identify infectious agent
    Use additional code (R65.2-) to identify severe sepsis, if applicable

    Excludes1   septic or septicopyemic embolism following failed attempted termination of pregnancy (O07.2)

O07.38 **Urinary tract infection following failed attempted termination of pregnancy** ♀   M

    Cystitis following failed attempted termination of pregnancy

O07.39 **Failed attempted termination of pregnancy with other complications** ♀   M

O07.4 **Failed attempted termination of pregnancy without complication** ♀   M

◄ New   ◄▥ Revised   ~~deleted~~ Deleted   Excludes 1   Excludes 2   Includes   Use additional   Code first   Code also   Unspecified

OGCR Official Guidelines   X Assign placeholder X   ● Use Additional Character(s)   ▶ Manifestation Code   **Coding Clinic**

● **O08   Complications following ectopic and molar pregnancy**
This category is for use with categories O00-O02 to identify any associated complications.

O08.0   Genital tract and pelvic infection following ectopic and molar pregnancy ♀   M
Endometritis following ectopic and molar pregnancy
Oophoritis following ectopic and molar pregnancy
Parametritis following ectopic and molar pregnancy
Pelvic peritonitis following ectopic and molar pregnancy
Salpingitis following ectopic and molar pregnancy
Salpingo-oophoritis following ectopic and molar pregnancy

Excludes1   sepsis following ectopic and molar pregnancy (O08.82)
urinary tract infection (O08.83)

O08.1   Delayed or excessive hemorrhage following ectopic and molar pregnancy ♀   M
Afibrinogenemia following ectopic and molar pregnancy
Defibrination syndrome following ectopic and molar pregnancy
Hemolysis following ectopic and molar pregnancy
Intravascular coagulation following ectopic and molar pregnancy

Excludes1   delayed or excessive hemorrhage due to incomplete abortion (O03.1)

O08.2   Embolism following ectopic and molar pregnancy ♀   M
Air embolism following ectopic and molar pregnancy
Amniotic fluid embolism following ectopic and molar pregnancy
Blood-clot embolism following ectopic and molar pregnancy
Embolism NOS following ectopic and molar pregnancy
Fat embolism following ectopic and molar pregnancy
Pulmonary embolism following ectopic and molar pregnancy
Pyemic embolism following ectopic and molar pregnancy
Septic or septicopyemic embolism following ectopic and molar pregnancy
Soap embolism following ectopic and molar pregnancy

O08.3   Shock following ectopic and molar pregnancy ♀   M
Circulatory collapse following ectopic and molar pregnancy
Shock (postprocedural) following ectopic and molar pregnancy

Excludes1   shock due to infection following ectopic and molar pregnancy (O08.82)

O08.4   Renal failure following ectopic and molar pregnancy ♀   M
Kidney failure (acute) following ectopic and molar pregnancy
Oliguria following ectopic and molar pregnancy
Renal shutdown following ectopic and molar pregnancy
Renal tubular necrosis following ectopic and molar pregnancy
Uremia following ectopic and molar pregnancy

O08.5   Metabolic disorders following an ectopic and molar pregnancy ♀   M

O08.6   Damage to pelvic organs and tissues following an ectopic and molar pregnancy ♀   M
Laceration, perforation, tear or chemical damage of bladder following an ectopic and molar pregnancy
Laceration, perforation, tear or chemical damage of bowel following an ectopic and molar pregnancy
Laceration, perforation, tear or chemical damage of broad ligament following an ectopic and molar pregnancy
Laceration, perforation, tear or chemical damage of cervix following an ectopic and molar pregnancy
Laceration, perforation, tear or chemical damage of periurethral tissue following an ectopic and molar pregnancy
Laceration, perforation, tear or chemical damage of uterus following an ectopic and molar pregnancy
Laceration, perforation, tear or chemical damage of vagina following an ectopic and molar pregnancy

O08.7   Other venous complications following an ectopic and molar pregnancy ♀

● **O08.8   Other complications following an ectopic and molar pregnancy**

O08.81   Cardiac arrest following an ectopic and molar pregnancy ♀   M

O08.82   Sepsis following ectopic and molar pregnancy ♀   M
Use additional code (B95-B97), to identify infectious agent
Use additional code (R65.2-) to identify severe sepsis, if applicable

Excludes1   septic or septicopyemic embolism following ectopic and molar pregnancy (O08.2)

O08.83   Urinary tract infection following an ectopic and molar pregnancy ♀   M
Cystitis following an ectopic and molar pregnancy

O08.89   Other complications following an ectopic and molar pregnancy ♀

O08.9   Unspecified complication following an ectopic and molar pregnancy ♀   M

SUPERVISION OF HIGH RISK PREGNANCY (O09)

● **O09   Supervision of high risk pregnancy**

● **O09.0   Supervision of pregnancy with history of infertility**

O09.00   Supervision of pregnancy with history of infertility, unspecified trimester ♀   M

O09.01   Supervision of pregnancy with history of infertility, first trimester ♀   M

O09.02   Supervision of pregnancy with history of infertility, second trimester ♀   M

O09.03   Supervision of pregnancy with history of infertility, third trimester ♀   M

● **O09.1   Supervision of pregnancy with history of ectopic pregnancy** ◀▥

O09.10   Supervision of pregnancy with history of ectopic pregnancy, unspecified trimester ♀ ◀▥ M

O09.11   Supervision of pregnancy with history of ectopic pregnancy, first trimester ♀ ◀▥ M

O09.12   Supervision of pregnancy with history of ectopic pregnancy, second trimester ♀ ◀▥ M

O09.13   Supervision of pregnancy with history of ectopic pregnancy, third trimester ♀ ◀▥ M

CHAPTER 15 (O00-O9A)

O09.A Supervision of pregnancy with history of molar pregnancy ◀

O09.A0 Supervision of pregnancy with history of molar pregnancy, unspecified trimester ♀ ◀   M

O09.A1 Supervision of pregnancy with history of molar pregnancy, first trimester ♀ ◀   M

O09.A2 Supervision of pregnancy with history of molar pregnancy, second trimester ♀ ◀   M

O09.A3 Supervision of pregnancy with history of molar pregnancy, third trimester ♀ ◀   M

O09.2 Supervision of pregnancy with other poor reproductive or obstetric history

  Excludes2 pregnancy care for patient with history of recurrent pregnancy loss (O26.2-)

O09.21 Supervision of pregnancy with history of pre-term labor

O09.211 Supervision of pregnancy with history of pre-term labor, first trimester ♀   M

O09.212 Supervision of pregnancy with history of pre-term labor, second trimester ♀ M

O09.213 Supervision of pregnancy with history of pre-term labor, third trimester ♀   M

O09.219 Supervision of pregnancy with history of pre-term labor, unspecified trimester ♀   M

O09.29 Supervision of pregnancy with other poor reproductive or obstetric history
Supervision of pregnancy with history of neonatal death
Supervision of pregnancy with history of stillbirth

O09.291 Supervision of pregnancy with other poor reproductive or obstetric history, first trimester ♀   M

O09.292 Supervision of pregnancy with other poor reproductive or obstetric history, second trimester ♀   M

O09.293 Supervision of pregnancy with other poor reproductive or obstetric history, third trimester ♀   M

O09.299 Supervision of pregnancy with other poor reproductive or obstetric history, unspecified trimester ♀   M

O09.3 Supervision of pregnancy with insufficient antenatal care
Supervision of concealed pregnancy
Supervision of hidden pregnancy

O09.30 Supervision of pregnancy with insufficient antenatal care, unspecified trimester ♀   M

O09.31 Supervision of pregnancy with insufficient antenatal care, first trimester ♀   M

O09.32 Supervision of pregnancy with insufficient antenatal care, second trimester ♀   M

O09.33 Supervision of pregnancy with insufficient antenatal care, third trimester ♀   M

O09.4 Supervision of pregnancy with grand multiparity

O09.40 Supervision of pregnancy with grand multiparity, unspecified trimester ♀   M

O09.41 Supervision of pregnancy with grand multiparity, first trimester ♀   M

O09.42 Supervision of pregnancy with grand multiparity, second trimester ♀   M

O09.43 Supervision of pregnancy with grand multiparity, third trimester ♀   M

O09.5 Supervision of elderly primigravida and multigravida
Pregnancy for a female 35 years and older at expected date of delivery

O09.51 Supervision of elderly primigravida

O09.511 Supervision of elderly primigravida, first trimester ♀   M

O09.512 Supervision of elderly primigravida, second trimester ♀   M

O09.513 Supervision of elderly primigravida, third trimester ♀   M

O09.519 Supervision of elderly primigravida, unspecified trimester ♀   M

O09.52 Supervision of elderly multigravida

O09.521 Supervision of elderly multigravida, first trimester ♀   M

O09.522 Supervision of elderly multigravida, second trimester ♀   M

O09.523 Supervision of elderly multigravida, third trimester ♀   M

O09.529 Supervision of elderly multigravida, unspecified trimester ♀   M

O09.6 Supervision of young primigravida and multigravida
Supervision of pregnancy for a female less than 16 years old at expected date of delivery

O09.61 Supervision of young primigravida

O09.611 Supervision of young primigravida, first trimester ♀   M

O09.612 Supervision of young primigravida, second trimester ♀   M

O09.613 Supervision of young primigravida, third trimester ♀   M

O09.619 Supervision of young primigravida, unspecified trimester ♀   M

O09.62 Supervision of young multigravida

O09.621 Supervision of young multigravida, first trimester ♀   M

O09.622 Supervision of young multigravida, second trimester ♀   M

O09.623 Supervision of young multigravida, third trimester ♀   M

O09.629 Supervision of young multigravida, unspecified trimester ♀   M

O09.7 Supervision of high risk pregnancy due to social problems

O09.70 Supervision of high risk pregnancy due to social problems, unspecified trimester ♀   M

O09.71 Supervision of high risk pregnancy due to social problems, first trimester ♀   M

O09.72 Supervision of high risk pregnancy due to social problems, second trimester ♀   M

O09.73 Supervision of high risk pregnancy due to social problems, third trimester ♀   M

O09.8 Supervision of other high risk pregnancies

O09.81 Supervision of pregnancy resulting from assisted reproductive technology
Supervision of pregnancy resulting from in-vitro fertilization

  Excludes2 gestational carrier status (Z33.3) ◀

O09.811 Supervision of pregnancy resulting from assisted reproductive technology, first trimester ♀   M

O09.812 Supervision of pregnancy resulting from assisted reproductive technology, second trimester ♀   M

O09.813 Supervision of pregnancy resulting from assisted reproductive technology, third trimester ♀   M

O09.819 Supervision of pregnancy resulting from assisted reproductive technology, unspecified trimester ♀   M

◀ New   ◀▬ Revised   ~~deleted~~ Deleted   Excludes 1   Excludes 2   Includes   Use additional   Code first   Code also   Unspecified

OGCR Official Guidelines   X Assign placeholder X   ● Use Additional Character(s)   ▶ Manifestation Code   **Coding Clinic**

● **O09.82**   **Supervision of pregnancy with history of in utero procedure during previous pregnancy**

     O09.821   **Supervision of pregnancy with history of in utero procedure during previous pregnancy, first trimester** ♀   M

     O09.822   **Supervision of pregnancy with history of in utero procedure during previous pregnancy, second trimester** ♀   M

     O09.823   **Supervision of pregnancy with history of in utero procedure during previous pregnancy, third trimester** ♀   M

     O09.829   **Supervision of pregnancy with history of in utero procedure during previous pregnancy, unspecified trimester** ♀   M

         Excludes1   supervision of pregnancy affected by in utero procedure during current pregnancy (O35.7)

● **O09.89**   **Supervision of other high risk pregnancies**

     O09.891   **Supervision of other high risk pregnancies, first trimester** ♀   M

     O09.892   **Supervision of other high risk pregnancies, second trimester** ♀   M

     O09.893   **Supervision of other high risk pregnancies, third trimester** ♀   M

     O09.899   **Supervision of other high risk pregnancies, unspecified trimester** ♀   M

● **O09.9**   **Supervision of high risk pregnancy, unspecified**

     O09.90   **Supervision of high risk pregnancy, unspecified, unspecified trimester** ♀   M

     O09.91   **Supervision of high risk pregnancy, unspecified, first trimester** ♀   M

     O09.92   **Supervision of high risk pregnancy, unspecified, second trimester** ♀   M

     O09.93   **Supervision of high risk pregnancy, unspecified, third trimester** ♀   M

EDEMA, PROTEINURIA AND HYPERTENSIVE DISORDERS IN PREGNANCY, CHILDBIRTH AND THE PUERPERIUM (O10-O16)

● **O10**   **Pre-existing hypertension complicating pregnancy, childbirth and the puerperium**

     Includes   pre-existing hypertension with pre-existing proteinuria complicating pregnancy, childbirth and the puerperium

     Excludes2   pre-existing hypertension with superimposed pre-eclampsia complicating pregnancy, childbirth and the puerperium (O11.-)

● **O10.0**   **Pre-existing essential hypertension complicating pregnancy, childbirth and the puerperium**

     Any condition in I10 specified as a reason for obstetric care during pregnancy, childbirth or the puerperium

   ● **O10.01**   **Pre-existing essential hypertension complicating pregnancy**

     O10.011   **Pre-existing essential hypertension complicating pregnancy, first trimester** ♀   M

     O10.012   **Pre-existing essential hypertension complicating pregnancy, second trimester** ♀

     O10.013   **Pre-existing essential hypertension complicating pregnancy, third trimester** ♀   M

     O10.019   **Pre-existing essential hypertension complicating pregnancy, unspecified trimester** ♀   M

   O10.02   **Pre-existing essential hypertension complicating childbirth** ♀   M

   O10.03   **Pre-existing essential hypertension complicating the puerperium** ♀   M

● **O10.1**   **Pre-existing hypertensive heart disease complicating pregnancy, childbirth and the puerperium**

     Any condition in I11 specified as a reason for obstetric care during pregnancy, childbirth or the puerperium

     Use additional code from I11 to identify the type of hypertensive heart disease

   ● **O10.11**   **Pre-existing hypertensive heart disease complicating pregnancy**

     O10.111   **Pre-existing hypertensive heart disease complicating pregnancy, first trimester** ♀   M

     O10.112   **Pre-existing hypertensive heart disease complicating pregnancy, second trimester** ♀   M

     O10.113   **Pre-existing hypertensive heart disease complicating pregnancy, third trimester** ♀   M

     O10.119   **Pre-existing hypertensive heart disease complicating pregnancy, unspecified trimester** ♀   M

   O10.12   **Pre-existing hypertensive heart disease complicating childbirth** ♀   M

   O10.13   **Pre-existing hypertensive heart disease complicating the puerperium** ♀   M

● **O10.2**   **Pre-existing hypertensive chronic kidney disease complicating pregnancy, childbirth and the puerperium**

     Any condition in I12 specified as a reason for obstetric care during pregnancy, childbirth or the puerperium

     Use additional code from I12 to identify the type of hypertensive chronic kidney disease

   ● **O10.21**   **Pre-existing hypertensive chronic kidney disease complicating pregnancy**

     O10.211   **Pre-existing hypertensive chronic kidney disease complicating pregnancy, first trimester** ♀   M

     O10.212   **Pre-existing hypertensive chronic kidney disease complicating pregnancy, second trimester** ♀   M

     O10.213   **Pre-existing hypertensive chronic kidney disease complicating pregnancy, third trimester** ♀   M

     O10.219   **Pre-existing hypertensive chronic kidney disease complicating pregnancy, unspecified trimester** ♀   M

   O10.22   **Pre-existing hypertensive chronic kidney disease complicating childbirth** ♀   M

   O10.23   **Pre-existing hypertensive chronic kidney disease complicating the puerperium** ♀   M

● **O10.3　Pre-existing hypertensive heart and chronic kidney disease complicating pregnancy, childbirth and the puerperium**
　　Any condition in I13 specified as a reason for obstetric care during pregnancy, childbirth or the puerperium
　　Use additional code from I13 to identify the type of hypertensive heart and chronic kidney disease

　● **O10.31　Pre-existing hypertensive heart and chronic kidney disease complicating pregnancy**

　　　O10.311　Pre-existing hypertensive heart and chronic kidney disease complicating pregnancy, first trimester ♀　　M

　　　O10.312　Pre-existing hypertensive heart and chronic kidney disease complicating pregnancy, second trimester ♀　　M

　　　O10.313　Pre-existing hypertensive heart and chronic kidney disease complicating pregnancy, third trimester ♀　　M

　　　O10.319　Pre-existing hypertensive heart and chronic kidney disease complicating pregnancy, unspecified trimester ♀　M

　　O10.32　Pre-existing hypertensive heart and chronic kidney disease complicating childbirth ♀　　M

　　O10.33　Pre-existing hypertensive heart and chronic kidney disease complicating the puerperium ♀　　M

● **O10.4　Pre-existing secondary hypertension complicating pregnancy, childbirth and the puerperium**
　　Any condition in I15 specified as a reason for obstetric care during pregnancy, childbirth or the puerperium
　　Use additional code from I15 to identify the type of secondary hypertension

　● **O10.41　Pre-existing secondary hypertension complicating pregnancy**

　　　O10.411　Pre-existing secondary hypertension complicating pregnancy, first trimester ♀　　M

　　　O10.412　Pre-existing secondary hypertension complicating pregnancy, second trimester ♀　　M

　　　O10.413　Pre-existing secondary hypertension complicating pregnancy, third trimester ♀　　M

　　　O10.419　Pre-existing secondary hypertension complicating pregnancy, unspecified trimester ♀　　M

　　O10.42　Pre-existing secondary hypertension complicating childbirth ♀　　M

　　O10.43　Pre-existing secondary hypertension complicating the puerperium ♀　　M

● **O10.9　Unspecified pre-existing hypertension complicating pregnancy, childbirth and the puerperium**

　● **O10.91　Unspecified pre-existing hypertension complicating pregnancy**

　　　O10.911　Unspecified pre-existing hypertension complicating pregnancy, first trimester ♀　　M

　　　O10.912　Unspecified pre-existing hypertension complicating pregnancy, second trimester ♀　　M

　　　O10.913　Unspecified pre-existing hypertension complicating pregnancy, third trimester ♀　　M

　　　O10.919　Unspecified pre-existing hypertension complicating pregnancy, unspecified trimester ♀　　M

　　O10.92　Unspecified pre-existing hypertension complicating childbirth ♀　　M

　　O10.93　Unspecified pre-existing hypertension complicating the puerperium ♀

● **O11　Pre-existing hypertension with pre-eclampsia**
　　Includes　conditions in O10 complicated by pre-eclampsia
　　　pre-eclampsia superimposed pre-existing hypertension
　　Use additional code from O10 to identify the type of hypertension

　　O11.1　Pre-existing hypertension with pre-eclampsia, first trimester ♀　　M

　　O11.2　Pre-existing hypertension with pre-eclampsia, second trimester ♀　　M

　　O11.3　Pre-existing hypertension with pre-eclampsia, third trimester ♀　　M

　　O11.4　Pre-existing hypertension with pre-eclampsia, complicating childbirth ♀ ◀　　M

　　O11.5　Pre-existing hypertension with pre-eclampsia, complicating the puerperium ♀ ◀　　M

　　O11.9　Pre-existing hypertension with pre-eclampsia, unspecified trimester ♀　　M

● **O12　Gestational [pregnancy-induced] edema and proteinuria without hypertension**

　● **O12.0　Gestational edema**

　　　O12.00　Gestational edema, unspecified trimester ♀　　M

　　　O12.01　Gestational edema, first trimester ♀　　M

　　　O12.02　Gestational edema, second trimester ♀　　M

　　　O12.03　Gestational edema, third trimester ♀　　M

　　　O12.04　Gestational edema, complicating childbirth ♀ ◀　　M

　　　O12.05　Gestational edema, complicating the puerperium ♀ ◀　　M

　● **O12.1　Gestational proteinuria**

　　　O12.10　Gestational proteinuria, unspecified trimester ♀　　M

　　　O12.11　Gestational proteinuria, first trimester ♀　　M

　　　O12.12　Gestational proteinuria, second trimester ♀　　M

　　　O12.13　Gestational proteinuria, third trimester ♀　　M

　　　O12.14　Gestational proteinuria, complicating childbirth ♀ ◀　　M

　　　O12.15　Gestational proteinuria, complicating the puerperium ♀ ◀　　M

　● **O12.2　Gestational edema with proteinuria**

　　　O12.20　Gestational edema with proteinuria, unspecified trimester ♀　　M

　　　O12.21　Gestational edema with proteinuria, first trimester ♀　　M

　　　O12.22　Gestational edema with proteinuria, second trimester ♀　　M

　　　O12.23　Gestational edema with proteinuria, third trimester ♀　　M

　　　O12.24　Gestational edema with proteinuria, complicating childbirth ♀ ◀　　M

　　　O12.25　Gestational edema with proteinuria, complicating the puerperium ♀ ◀　　M

● **O13　Gestational [pregnancy-induced] hypertension without significant proteinuria**
　　Includes　gestational hypertension NOS
　　　transient hypertension of pregnancy ◀

　　O13.1　Gestational [pregnancy-induced] hypertension without significant proteinuria, first trimester ♀　　M

　　O13.2　Gestational [pregnancy-induced] hypertension without significant proteinuria, second trimester ♀　　M

　　O13.3　Gestational [pregnancy-induced] hypertension without significant proteinuria, third trimester ♀　　M

　　O13.4　Gestational [pregnancy-induced] hypertension without significant proteinuria, complicating childbirth ♀ ◀　　M

　　O13.5　Gestational [pregnancy-induced] hypertension without significant proteinuria, complicating the puerperium ♀ ◀　　M

　　O13.9　Gestational [pregnancy-induced] hypertension without significant proteinuria, unspecified trimester ♀　　M

◀ New　⬅ Revised　~~deleted~~ Deleted　Excludes 1　Excludes 2　Includes　Use additional　Code first　Code also　Unspecified
OGCR Official Guidelines　X Assign placeholder X　● Use Additional Character(s)　▶ Manifestation Code　Coding Clinic

● **O14   Pre-eclampsia**
    Excludes1   pre-existing hypertension with pre-eclampsia (O11)
   ● **O14.0   Mild to moderate pre-eclampsia**
      O14.00   Mild to moderate pre-eclampsia, unspecified trimester ♀   M
      O14.02   Mild to moderate pre-eclampsia, second trimester ♀   M
      O14.03   Mild to moderate pre-eclampsia, third trimester ♀   M
      O14.04   Mild to moderate pre-eclampsia, complicating childbirth ♀ ◄   M
      O14.05   Mild to moderate pre-eclampsia, complicating the puerperium ♀ ◄   M
   ● **O14.1   Severe pre-eclampsia**
      Excludes1   HELLP syndrome (O14.2-)
      H=hemolysis, EL=elevated liver enzymes, LP=low platelet count
      O14.10   Severe pre-eclampsia, unspecified trimester ♀   M
      O14.12   Severe pre-eclampsia, second trimester ♀   M
      O14.13   Severe pre-eclampsia, third trimester ♀   M
      O14.14   Severe pre-eclampsia complicating childbirth ♀ ◄   M
      O14.15   Severe pre-eclampsia, complicating the puerperium ♀ ◄   M
   ● **O14.2   HELLP syndrome**
      Severe pre-eclampsia with hemolysis, elevated liver enzymes and low platelet count (HELLP)
      O14.20   HELLP syndrome (HELLP), unspecified trimester ♀   M
      O14.22   HELLP syndrome (HELLP), second trimester ♀   M
      O14.23   HELLP syndrome (HELLP), third trimester ♀   M
      O14.24   HELLP syndrome, complicating childbirth ♀ ◄   M
      O14.25   HELLP syndrome, complicating the puerperium ♀ ◄   M
   ● **O14.9   Unspecified pre-eclampsia**
      O14.90   Unspecified pre-eclampsia, unspecified trimester ♀   M
      O14.92   Unspecified pre-eclampsia, second trimester ♀   M
      O14.93   Unspecified pre-eclampsia, third trimester ♀   M
      O14.94   Unspecified pre-eclampsia, complicating childbirth ♀ ◄   M
      O14.95   Unspecified pre-eclampsia, complicating the puerperium ♀ ◄   M

● **O15   Eclampsia**
    Includes   convulsions following conditions in O10-O14 and O16
   ● **O15.0   Eclampsia complicating pregnancy** ◄▥
      O15.00   Eclampsia complicating pregnancy, unspecified trimester ♀ ◄▥   M
      O15.02   Eclampsia complicating pregnancy, second trimester ♀ ◄▥   M
      O15.03   Eclampsia complicating pregnancy, third trimester ♀ ◄▥   M
    O15.1   Eclampsia complicating labor ♀ ◄▥   M
    O15.2   Eclampsia complicating the puerperium ♀ ◄▥   M
    O15.9   Eclampsia, unspecified as to time period ♀   M
      Eclampsia NOS

● **O16   Unspecified maternal hypertension**
    O16.1   Unspecified maternal hypertension, first trimester ♀   M
    O16.2   Unspecified maternal hypertension, second trimester ♀   M

    O16.3   Unspecified maternal hypertension, third trimester ♀   M
    O16.4   Unspecified maternal hypertension, complicating childbirth ♀ ◄   M
    O16.5   Unspecified maternal hypertension, complicating the puerperium ♀ ◄   M
    O16.9   Unspecified maternal hypertension, unspecified trimester ♀   M

OTHER MATERNAL DISORDERS PREDOMINANTLY RELATED TO PREGNANCY (O20-O29)

    Excludes2   maternal care related to the fetus and amniotic cavity and possible delivery problems (O30-O48)
           maternal diseases classifiable elsewhere but complicating pregnancy, labor and delivery, and the puerperium (O98-O99)

● **O20   Hemorrhage in early pregnancy**
    Includes   hemorrhage before completion of 20 weeks gestation
    Excludes1   pregnancy with abortive outcome (O00-O08)
    O20.0   Threatened abortion ♀   M
      Hemorrhage specified as due to threatened abortion
    O20.8   Other hemorrhage in early pregnancy ♀   M
    O20.9   Hemorrhage in early pregnancy, unspecified ♀   M

● **O21   Excessive vomiting in pregnancy**
    O21.0   Mild hyperemesis gravidarum ♀   M
      Hyperemesis gravidarum, mild or unspecified, starting before the end of the 20th week of gestation
    O21.1   Hyperemesis gravidarum with metabolic disturbance   M
      Hyperemesis gravidarum, starting before the end of the 20th week of gestation, with metabolic disturbance such as carbohydrate depletion
      Hyperemesis gravidarum, starting before the end of the 20th week of gestation, with metabolic disturbance such as dehydration
      Hyperemesis gravidarum, starting before the end of the 20th week of gestation, with metabolic disturbance such as electrolyte imbalance
    O21.2   Late vomiting of pregnancy ♀   M
      Excessive vomiting starting after 20 completed weeks of gestation
    O21.8   Other vomiting complicating pregnancy ♀   M
      Vomiting due to diseases classified elsewhere, complicating pregnancy
      Use additional code, to identify cause
    O21.9   Vomiting of pregnancy, unspecified ♀   M

● **O22   Venous complications and hemorrhoids in pregnancy**
    Excludes1   venous complications of:
         abortion NOS (O03.9)
         ectopic or molar pregnancy (O08.7)
         failed attempted abortion (O07.35)
         induced abortion (O04.85)
         spontaneous abortion (O03.89)
    Excludes2   obstetric pulmonary embolism (O88.-)
         venous complications and hemorrhoids of childbirth and the puerperium (O87.-)
   ● **O22.0   Varicose veins of lower extremity in pregnancy**
      Varicose veins NOS in pregnancy
      O22.00   Varicose veins of lower extremity in pregnancy, unspecified trimester ♀   M
      O22.01   Varicose veins of lower extremity in pregnancy, first trimester ♀   M
      O22.02   Varicose veins of lower extremity in pregnancy, second trimester ♀   M
      O22.03   Varicose veins of lower extremity in pregnancy, third trimester ♀   M

● **O22.1 Genital varices in pregnancy**
    Perineal varices in pregnancy
    Vaginal varices in pregnancy
    Vulval varices in pregnancy

    O22.10 Genital varices in pregnancy, `unspecified` trimester ♀   M

    O22.11 Genital varices in pregnancy, first trimester ♀   M

    O22.12 Genital varices in pregnancy, second trimester ♀   M

    O22.13 Genital varices in pregnancy, third trimester ♀ M

● **O22.2 Superficial thrombophlebitis in pregnancy**
    Phlebitis in pregnancy NOS
    Thrombophlebitis of legs in pregnancy
    Thrombosis in pregnancy NOS

    Use additional code to identify the superficial thrombophlebitis (I80.0-)

    O22.20 Superficial thrombophlebitis in pregnancy, `unspecified` trimester ♀   M

    O22.21 Superficial thrombophlebitis in pregnancy, first trimester ♀   M

    O22.22 Superficial thrombophlebitis in pregnancy, second trimester ♀   M

    O22.23 Superficial thrombophlebitis in pregnancy, third trimester ♀   M

● **O22.3 Deep phlebothrombosis in pregnancy**
    Deep vein thrombosis, antepartum

    Use additional code to identify the deep vein thrombosis (I82.4-, I82.5-, I82.62-. I82.72-)

    Use additional code, if applicable, for associated long-term (current) use of anticoagulants (Z79.01)

    O22.30 Deep phlebothrombosis in pregnancy, `unspecified` trimester ♀   M

    O22.31 Deep phlebothrombosis in pregnancy, first trimester ♀   M

    O22.32 Deep phlebothrombosis in pregnancy, second trimester ♀   M

    O22.33 Deep phlebothrombosis in pregnancy, third trimester ♀   M

● **O22.4 Hemorrhoids in pregnancy**

    O22.40 Hemorrhoids in pregnancy, `unspecified` trimester ♀   M

    O22.41 Hemorrhoids in pregnancy, first trimester ♀   M

    O22.42 Hemorrhoids in pregnancy, second trimester ♀   M

    O22.43 Hemorrhoids in pregnancy, third trimester ♀   M

● **O22.5 Cerebral venous thrombosis in pregnancy**
    Cerebrovenous sinus thrombosis in pregnancy

    O22.50 Cerebral venous thrombosis in pregnancy, `unspecified` trimester ♀   M

    O22.51 Cerebral venous thrombosis in pregnancy, first trimester ♀   M

    O22.52 Cerebral venous thrombosis in pregnancy, second trimester ♀   M

    O22.53 Cerebral venous thrombosis in pregnancy, third trimester ♀   M

● **O22.8 Other venous complications in pregnancy**

    ● **O22.8X** Other venous complications in pregnancy

        O22.8X1 Other venous complications in pregnancy, first trimester ♀   M

        O22.8X2 Other venous complications in pregnancy, second trimester ♀   M

        O22.8X3 Other venous complications in pregnancy, third trimester ♀   M

        O22.8X9 Other venous complications in pregnancy, `unspecified` trimester ♀   M

● **O22.9 Venous complication in pregnancy, unspecified**

Gestational phlebitis NOS
Gestational phlebopathy NOS
Gestational thrombosis NOS

    O22.90 Venous complication in pregnancy, `unspecified`, unspecified trimester ♀   M

    O22.91 Venous complication in pregnancy, `unspecified`, first trimester ♀   M

    O22.92 Venous complication in pregnancy, `unspecified`, second trimester ♀   M

    O22.93 Venous complication in pregnancy, `unspecified`, third trimester ♀   M

● **O23 Infections of genitourinary tract in pregnancy**

    Use additional code to identify organism (B95.-, B96.-)

    `Excludes2` gonococcal infections complicating pregnancy, childbirth and the puerperium (O98.2)
        infections with a predominantly sexual mode of transmission NOS complicating pregnancy, childbirth and the puerperium (O98.3)
        syphilis complicating pregnancy, childbirth and the puerperium (O98.1)
        tuberculosis of genitourinary system complicating pregnancy, childbirth and the puerperium (O98.0)
        venereal disease NOS complicating pregnancy, childbirth and the puerperium (O98.3)

● **O23.0 Infections of kidney in pregnancy**
    Pyelonephritis in pregnancy

    O23.00 Infections of kidney in pregnancy, `unspecified` trimester ♀   M

    O23.01 Infections of kidney in pregnancy, first trimester ♀   M

    O23.02 Infections of kidney in pregnancy, second trimester ♀   M

    O23.03 Infections of kidney in pregnancy, third trimester ♀   M

● **O23.1 Infections of bladder in pregnancy**

    O23.10 Infections of bladder in pregnancy, `unspecified` trimester ♀   M

    O23.11 Infections of bladder in pregnancy, first trimester ♀   M

    O23.12 Infections of bladder in pregnancy, second trimester ♀   M

    O23.13 Infections of bladder in pregnancy, third trimester ♀   M

● **O23.2 Infections of urethra in pregnancy**

    O23.20 Infections of urethra in pregnancy, `unspecified` trimester ♀   M

    O23.21 Infections of urethra in pregnancy, first trimester ♀   M

    O23.22 Infections of urethra in pregnancy, second trimester ♀   M

    O23.23 Infections of urethra in pregnancy, third trimester ♀   M

● **O23.3 Infections of other parts of urinary tract in pregnancy**

    O23.30 Infections of other parts of urinary tract in pregnancy, `unspecified` trimester ♀   M

    O23.31 Infections of other parts of urinary tract in pregnancy, first trimester ♀   M

    O23.32 Infections of other parts of urinary tract in pregnancy, second trimester ♀   M

    O23.33 Infections of other parts of urinary tract in pregnancy, third trimester ♀   M

● **O23.4 Unspecified infection of urinary tract in pregnancy**

    O23.40 `Unspecified` infection of urinary tract in pregnancy, unspecified trimester ♀   M

    O23.41 `Unspecified` infection of urinary tract in pregnancy, first trimester ♀   M

    O23.42 `Unspecified` infection of urinary tract in pregnancy, second trimester ♀   M

    O23.43 `Unspecified` infection of urinary tract in pregnancy, third trimester ♀   M

CHAPTER 15 (O00-O9A)

◀ New   ◀▬ Revised   ~~deleted~~ Deleted   Excludes 1   Excludes 2   Includes   Use additional   Code first   Code also   Unspecified

1098   **OGCR** Official Guidelines   X Assign placeholder X   ● Use Additional Character(s)   ▷ Manifestation Code   **Coding Clinic**

● **O23.5   Infections of the genital tract in pregnancy**
   ● **O23.51   Infection of cervix in pregnancy**
      O23.511   Infections of cervix in pregnancy, first trimester ♀   M
      O23.512   Infections of cervix in pregnancy, second trimester ♀   M
      O23.513   Infections of cervix in pregnancy, third trimester ♀   M
      O23.519   Infections of cervix in pregnancy, unspecified trimester ♀   M
   ● **O23.52   Salpingo-oophoritis in pregnancy**
      Oophoritis = inflammation of ovary
      Salpingitis = inflammation of fallopian tube
      Oophoritis in pregnancy
      Salpingitis in pregnancy
      O23.521   Salpingo-oophoritis in pregnancy, first trimester ♀   M
      O23.522   Salpingo-oophoritis in pregnancy, second trimester ♀   M
      O23.523   Salpingo-oophoritis in pregnancy, third trimester ♀   M
      O23.529   Salpingo-oophoritis in pregnancy, unspecified trimester ♀   M
   ● **O23.59   Infection of other part of genital tract in pregnancy**
      O23.591   Infection of other part of genital tract in pregnancy, first trimester ♀   M
      O23.592   Infection of other part of genital tract in pregnancy, second trimester ♀   M
      O23.593   Infection of other part of genital tract in pregnancy, third trimester ♀   M
      O23.599   Infection of other part of genital tract in pregnancy, unspecified trimester ♀   M
   ● **O23.9   Unspecified genitourinary tract infection in pregnancy**
      Genitourinary tract infection in pregnancy NOS
      O23.90   Unspecified genitourinary tract infection in pregnancy, unspecified trimester ♀   M
      O23.91   Unspecified genitourinary tract infection in pregnancy, first trimester ♀   M
      O23.92   Unspecified genitourinary tract infection in pregnancy, second trimester ♀   M
      O23.93   Unspecified genitourinary tract infection in pregnancy, third trimester ♀   M

OGCR Section I.C.15.g.

Diabetes mellitus in pregnancy
Diabetes mellitus is a significant complicating factor in pregnancy. Pregnant women who are diabetic should be assigned a code from category O24, Diabetes mellitus in pregnancy, childbirth, and the puerperium, first, followed by the appropriate diabetes code(s) (E08-E13) from Chapter 4.

● **O24   Diabetes mellitus in pregnancy, childbirth, and the puerperium**
   ● **O24.0   Pre-existing type 1 diabetes mellitus, in pregnancy, childbirth and the puerperium** ◀▥
      Juvenile onset diabetes mellitus, in pregnancy, childbirth and the puerperium
      Ketosis-prone diabetes mellitus in pregnancy, childbirth and the puerperium
      Use additional code from category E10 to further identify any manifestations
   ● **O24.01   Pre-existing type 1 diabetes mellitus, in pregnancy** ◀▥
      O24.011   Pre-existing type 1 diabetes mellitus, in pregnancy, first trimester ♀ ◀▥   M
      O24.012   Pre-existing type 1 diabetes mellitus, in pregnancy, second trimester ♀ ◀▥ M
      O24.013   Pre-existing type 1 diabetes mellitus, in pregnancy, third trimester ♀ ◀▥   M
      O24.019   Pre-existing type 1 diabetes mellitus, in pregnancy, unspecified trimester ♀ ◀▥   M

      O24.02   Pre-existing type 1 diabetes mellitus, in childbirth ♀ ◀▥   M
      O24.03   Pre-existing type 1 diabetes mellitus, in the puerperium ♀ ◀▥   M
   ● **O24.1   Pre-existing type 2 diabetes mellitus, in pregnancy, childbirth and the puerperium** ◀▥
      Insulin-resistant diabetes mellitus in pregnancy, childbirth and the puerperium
      Use additional code (for):
      from category E11 to further identify any manifestations
      long-term (current) use of insulin (Z79.4)
   ● **O24.11   Pre-existing type 2 diabetes mellitus, in pregnancy** ◀▥
      O24.111   Pre-existing type 2 diabetes mellitus, in pregnancy, first trimester ♀ ◀▥   M
      O24.112   Pre-existing type 2 diabetes mellitus, in pregnancy, second trimester ♀ ◀▥ M
      O24.113   Pre-existing type 2 diabetes mellitus, in pregnancy, third trimester ♀ ◀▥   M
      O24.119   Pre-existing type 2 diabetes mellitus, in pregnancy, unspecified trimester ♀ ◀▥   M
      O24.12   Pre-existing type 2 diabetes mellitus, in childbirth ♀ ◀▥   M
      O24.13   Pre-existing type 2 diabetes mellitus, in the puerperium ♀ ◀▥   M
   ● **O24.3   Unspecified pre-existing diabetes mellitus in pregnancy, childbirth and the puerperium**
      Use additional code (for):
      from category E11 to further identify any manifestation
      long-term (current) use of insulin (Z79.4)
   ● **O24.31   Unspecified pre-existing diabetes mellitus in pregnancy**
      O24.311   Unspecified pre-existing diabetes mellitus in pregnancy, first trimester ♀   M
      O24.312   Unspecified pre-existing diabetes mellitus in pregnancy, second trimester ♀   M
      O24.313   Unspecified pre-existing diabetes mellitus in pregnancy, third trimester ♀   M
      O24.319   Unspecified pre-existing diabetes mellitus in pregnancy, unspecified trimester ♀   M
      O24.32   Unspecified pre-existing diabetes mellitus in childbirth ♀   M
      O24.33   Unspecified pre-existing diabetes mellitus in the puerperium ♀   M
   ● **O24.4   Gestational diabetes mellitus**
      Diabetes mellitus arising in pregnancy
      Gestational diabetes mellitus NOS
   ● **O24.41   Gestational diabetes mellitus in pregnancy**
      O24.410   Gestational diabetes mellitus in pregnancy, diet controlled ♀   M
      O24.414   Gestational diabetes mellitus in pregnancy, insulin controlled ♀   M
      O24.415   Gestational diabetes mellitus in pregnancy, controlled by oral hypoglycemic drugs ♀ ◀   M
        Gestational diabetes mellitus in pregnancy, controlled by oral antidiabetic drugs ◀
      O24.419   Gestational diabetes mellitus in pregnancy, unspecified control ♀   M
        Coding Clinic: 2015, Q4, P34

● **O24.42 Gestational diabetes mellitus in childbirth**

    O24.420 **Gestational diabetes mellitus in childbirth, diet controlled** ♀   M

    O24.424 **Gestational diabetes mellitus in childbirth, insulin controlled** ♀   M

    O24.425 **Gestational diabetes mellitus in childbirth, controlled by oral hypoglycemic drugs** ♀ ◄   M
        Gestational diabetes mellitus in childbirth, controlled by oral antidiabetic drugs ◄

    O24.429 **Gestational diabetes mellitus in childbirth, unspecified control** ♀   M

OGCR **Section I.C.15.i.**

> Gestational (pregnancy induced) diabetes
>
> Gestational (pregnancy induced) diabetes can occur during the second and third trimester of pregnancy in women who were not diabetic prior to pregnancy. Gestational diabetes can cause complications in the pregnancy similar to those of pre-existing diabetes mellitus. It also puts the woman at greater risk of developing diabetes after the pregnancy. Codes for gestational diabetes are in subcategory O24.4, Gestational diabetes mellitus. No other code from category O24, Diabetes mellitus in pregnancy, childbirth, and the puerperium, should be used with a code from O24.4
>
> The codes under subcategory O24.4 include diet controlled, insulin controlled, **and controlled by oral hypoglycemic drugs.** If a patient with gestational diabetes is treated with both diet and insulin, only the code for insulin-controlled is required. **If a patient with gestational diabetes is treated with both diet and oral hypoglycemic medications, only the code for "controlled by oral hypoglycemic drugs" is required.** Code Z79.4, Long-term (current) use of insulin **or code Z79.84, Long-term (current) use of oral hypoglycemic drugs,** should not be assigned with codes from subcategory O24.4.
>
> An abnormal glucose tolerance in pregnancy is assigned a code from subcategory O99.81, Abnormal glucose complicating pregnancy, childbirth, and the puerperium.

● **O24.43 Gestational diabetes mellitus in the puerperium**

    O24.430 **Gestational diabetes mellitus in the puerperium, diet controlled** ♀   M

    O24.434 **Gestational diabetes mellitus in the puerperium, insulin controlled** ♀   M

    O24.435 **Gestational diabetes mellitus in puerperium, controlled by oral hypoglycemic drugs** ♀ ◄   M
        Gestational diabetes mellitus in puerperium, controlled by oral antidiabetic drugs ◄

    O24.439 **Gestational diabetes mellitus in the puerperium, unspecified control** ♀   M

● **O24.8 Other pre-existing diabetes mellitus in pregnancy, childbirth, and the puerperium**

    Use additional code (for):
      from categories E08, E09 and E13 to further identify any manifestation
      long-term (current) use of insulin (Z79.4)

● **O24.81 Other pre-existing diabetes mellitus in pregnancy**

    O24.811 **Other pre-existing diabetes mellitus in pregnancy, first trimester** ♀   M

    O24.812 **Other pre-existing diabetes mellitus in pregnancy, second trimester** ♀   M

    O24.813 **Other pre-existing diabetes mellitus in pregnancy, third trimester** ♀   M

    O24.819 **Other pre-existing diabetes mellitus in pregnancy, unspecified trimester** ♀   M

   O24.82 **Other pre-existing diabetes mellitus in childbirth** ♀   M

   O24.83 **Other pre-existing diabetes mellitus in the puerperium** ♀   M

● **O24.9 Unspecified diabetes mellitus in pregnancy, childbirth and the puerperium**

    Use additional code for long-term (current) use of insulin (Z79.4)
    Unknown whether patient was diabetic before pregnancy occurred

● **O24.91 Unspecified diabetes mellitus in pregnancy**

    O24.911 **Unspecified diabetes mellitus in pregnancy, first trimester** ♀   M

    O24.912 **Unspecified diabetes mellitus in pregnancy, second trimester** ♀   M

    O24.913 **Unspecified diabetes mellitus in pregnancy, third trimester** ♀   M

    O24.919 **Unspecified diabetes mellitus in pregnancy, unspecified trimester** ♀   M

   O24.92 **Unspecified diabetes mellitus in childbirth** ♀   M

   O24.93 **Unspecified diabetes mellitus in the puerperium** ♀   M

● **O25 Malnutrition in pregnancy, childbirth and the puerperium**

● **O25.1 Malnutrition in pregnancy**

   O25.10 **Malnutrition in pregnancy, unspecified trimester** ♀   M

   O25.11 **Malnutrition in pregnancy, first trimester** ♀   M

   O25.12 **Malnutrition in pregnancy, second trimester** ♀ M

   O25.13 **Malnutrition in pregnancy, third trimester** ♀   M

  O25.2 **Malnutrition in childbirth** ♀   M

  O25.3 **Malnutrition in the puerperium** ♀   M

● **O26 Maternal care for other conditions predominantly related to pregnancy**

● **O26.0 Excessive weight gain in pregnancy**

    Excludes2   gestational edema (O12.0, O12.2)

   O26.00 **Excessive weight gain in pregnancy, unspecified trimester** ♀   M

   O26.01 **Excessive weight gain in pregnancy, first trimester** ♀   M

   O26.02 **Excessive weight gain in pregnancy, second trimester** ♀   M

   O26.03 **Excessive weight gain in pregnancy, third trimester** ♀   M

● **O26.1 Low weight gain in pregnancy**

   O26.10 **Low weight gain in pregnancy, unspecified trimester** ♀   M

   O26.11 **Low weight gain in pregnancy, first trimester** ♀   M

   O26.12 **Low weight gain in pregnancy, second trimester** ♀   M

   O26.13 **Low weight gain in pregnancy, third trimester** ♀   M

● **O26.2 Pregnancy care for patient with recurrent pregnancy loss**

   O26.20 **Pregnancy care for patient with recurrent pregnancy loss, unspecified trimester** ♀   M

   O26.21 **Pregnancy care for patient with recurrent pregnancy loss, first trimester** ♀   M

   O26.22 **Pregnancy care for patient with recurrent pregnancy loss, second trimester** ♀   M

   O26.23 **Pregnancy care for patient with recurrent pregnancy loss, third trimester** ♀   M

◄ New   ◄ Revised   ~~deleted~~ Deleted   Excludes 1   Excludes 2   Includes   Use additional   Code first   Code also   Unspecified

OGCR Official Guidelines   X Assign placeholder X   ● Use Additional Character(s)   ▷ Manifestation Code   **Coding Clinic**

● **O26.3** **Retained intrauterine contraceptive device in pregnancy**
    O26.30   **Retained intrauterine contraceptive device in pregnancy, unspecified trimester** ♀   M
    O26.31   **Retained intrauterine contraceptive device in pregnancy, first trimester** ♀   M
    O26.32   **Retained intrauterine contraceptive device in pregnancy, second trimester** ♀   M
    O26.33   **Retained intrauterine contraceptive device in pregnancy, third trimester** ♀   M

● **O26.4** **Herpes gestationis**
    O26.40   **Herpes gestationis, unspecified trimester** ♀   M
    O26.41   **Herpes gestationis, first trimester** ♀   M
    O26.42   **Herpes gestationis, second trimester** ♀   M
    O26.43   **Herpes gestationis, third trimester** ♀   M

● **O26.5** **Maternal hypotension syndrome**
    Supine hypotensive syndrome
    O26.50   **Maternal hypotension syndrome, unspecified trimester** ♀   M
    O26.51   **Maternal hypotension syndrome, first trimester** ♀   M
    O26.52   **Maternal hypotension syndrome, second trimester** ♀   M
    O26.53   **Maternal hypotension syndrome, third trimester** ♀   M

● **O26.6** **Liver and biliary tract disorders in pregnancy, childbirth and the puerperium**
    Use additional code to identify the specific disorder
    Excludes2   hepatorenal syndrome following labor and delivery (O90.4)
   ● O26.61   **Liver and biliary tract disorders in pregnancy**
      O26.611   **Liver and biliary tract disorders in pregnancy, first trimester** ♀   M
      O26.612   **Liver and biliary tract disorders in pregnancy, second trimester** ♀   M
      O26.613   **Liver and biliary tract disorders in pregnancy, third trimester** ♀   M
      O26.619   **Liver and biliary tract disorders in pregnancy, unspecified trimester** ♀   M
    O26.62   **Liver and biliary tract disorders in childbirth** ♀   M
    O26.63   **Liver and biliary tract disorders in the puerperium** ♀   M

● **O26.7** **Subluxation of symphysis (pubis) in pregnancy, childbirth and the puerperium**
    Excludes1   traumatic separation of symphysis (pubis) during childbirth (O71.6)
   ● O26.71   **Subluxation of symphysis (pubis) in pregnancy**
      O26.711   **Subluxation of symphysis (pubis) in pregnancy, first trimester** ♀   M
      O26.712   **Subluxation of symphysis (pubis) in pregnancy, second trimester** ♀   M
      O26.713   **Subluxation of symphysis (pubis) in pregnancy, third trimester** ♀   M
      O26.719   **Subluxation of symphysis (pubis) in pregnancy, unspecified trimester** ♀   M
    O26.72   **Subluxation of symphysis (pubis) in childbirth** ♀   M
    O26.73   **Subluxation of symphysis (pubis) in the puerperium** ♀   M

● **O26.8** **Other specified pregnancy related conditions**
   ● O26.81   **Pregnancy related exhaustion and fatigue**
      O26.811   **Pregnancy related exhaustion and fatigue, first trimester** ♀   M
      O26.812   **Pregnancy related exhaustion and fatigue, second trimester** ♀   M
      O26.813   **Pregnancy related exhaustion and fatigue, third trimester** ♀   M
      O26.819   **Pregnancy related exhaustion and fatigue, unspecified trimester** ♀   M

● **O26.82** **Pregnancy related peripheral neuritis**
    O26.821   **Pregnancy related peripheral neuritis, first trimester** ♀   M
    O26.822   **Pregnancy related peripheral neuritis, second trimester** ♀   M
    O26.823   **Pregnancy related peripheral neuritis, third trimester** ♀   M
    O26.829   **Pregnancy related peripheral neuritis, unspecified trimester** ♀   M

● **O26.83** **Pregnancy related renal disease**
    Use additional code to identify the specific disorder
    O26.831   **Pregnancy related renal disease, first trimester** ♀   M
    O26.832   **Pregnancy related renal disease, second trimester** ♀   M
    O26.833   **Pregnancy related renal disease, third trimester** ♀   M
    O26.839   **Pregnancy related renal disease, unspecified trimester** ♀   M

● **O26.84** **Uterine size-date discrepancy complicating pregnancy**
    Excludes1   encounter for suspected problem with fetal growth ruled out (Z03.74)
    O26.841   **Uterine size-date discrepancy, first trimester** ♀   M
    O26.842   **Uterine size-date discrepancy, second trimester** ♀   M
    O26.843   **Uterine size-date discrepancy, third trimester** ♀   M
    O26.849   **Uterine size-date discrepancy, unspecified trimester** ♀   M

● **O26.85** **Spotting complicating pregnancy**
    O26.851   **Spotting complicating pregnancy, first trimester** ♀   M
    O26.852   **Spotting complicating pregnancy, second trimester** ♀   M
    O26.853   **Spotting complicating pregnancy, third trimester** ♀   M
    O26.859   **Spotting complicating pregnancy, unspecified trimester** ♀   M

● **O26.86** **Pruritic urticarial papules and plaques of pregnancy (PUPPP)** ♀   M
    Polymorphic eruption of pregnancy

● **O26.87** **Cervical shortening**
    Excludes1   encounter for suspected cervical shortening ruled out (Z03.75)
    O26.872   **Cervical shortening, second trimester** ♀   M
    O26.873   **Cervical shortening, third trimester** ♀   M
    O26.879   **Cervical shortening, unspecified trimester**   M

● **O26.89** **Other specified pregnancy related conditions**
    O26.891   **Other specified pregnancy related conditions, first trimester** ♀   M
    O26.892   **Other specified pregnancy related conditions, second trimester** ♀   M
    O26.893   **Other specified pregnancy related conditions, third trimester** ♀   M
      Coding Clinic: 2015, Q3, P40
    O26.899   **Other specified pregnancy related conditions, unspecified trimester** ♀   M

CHAPTER 15 (O00-O9A)

CHAPTER 15 (O00-O9A)

● O26.9   **Pregnancy related conditions, unspecified**
     O26.90   Pregnancy related conditions, unspecified, unspecified trimester ♀   M
     O26.91   Pregnancy related conditions, unspecified, first trimester ♀   M
     O26.92   Pregnancy related conditions, unspecified, second trimester ♀   M
     O26.93   Pregnancy related conditions, unspecified, third trimester ♀   M

● O28   **Abnormal findings on antenatal screening of mother**
     Excludes1   diagnostic findings classified elsewhere - see Alphabetical Index
   O28.0   Abnormal hematological finding on antenatal screening of mother ♀   M
   O28.1   Abnormal biochemical finding on antenatal screening of mother ♀   M
   O28.2   Abnormal cytological finding on antenatal screening of mother ♀   M
   O28.3   Abnormal ultrasonic finding on antenatal screening of mother ♀   M
   O28.4   Abnormal radiological finding on antenatal screening of mother ♀   M
   O28.5   Abnormal chromosomal and genetic finding on antenatal screening of mother ♀   M
   O28.8   Other abnormal findings on antenatal screening of mother ♀   M
   O28.9   Unspecified abnormal findings on antenatal screening of mother ♀   M

● O29   **Complications of anesthesia during pregnancy**
     Includes   maternal complications arising from the administration of a general, regional or local anesthetic, analgesic or other sedation during pregnancy
     Use additional code, if necessary, to identify the complication
     Excludes2   complications of anesthesia during labor and delivery (O74.-)
               complications of anesthesia during the puerperium (O89.-)
   ● O29.0   Pulmonary complications of anesthesia during pregnancy
     ● O29.01   Aspiration pneumonitis due to anesthesia during pregnancy
          Inhalation of stomach contents or secretions NOS due to anesthesia during pregnancy
          Mendelson's syndrome due to anesthesia during pregnancy
       O29.011   Aspiration pneumonitis due to anesthesia during pregnancy, first trimester ♀   M
       O29.012   Aspiration pneumonitis due to anesthesia during pregnancy, second trimester ♀   M
       O29.013   Aspiration pneumonitis due to anesthesia during pregnancy, third trimester ♀   M
       O29.019   Aspiration pneumonitis due to anesthesia during pregnancy, unspecified trimester ♀   M
     ● O29.02   Pressure collapse of lung due to anesthesia during pregnancy
       O29.021   Pressure collapse of lung due to anesthesia during pregnancy, first trimester ♀   M
       O29.022   Pressure collapse of lung due to anesthesia during pregnancy, second trimester ♀   M
       O29.023   Pressure collapse of lung due to anesthesia during pregnancy, third trimester ♀   M
       O29.029   Pressure collapse of lung due to anesthesia during pregnancy, unspecified trimester ♀   M

   ● O29.09   Other pulmonary complications of anesthesia during pregnancy
       O29.091   Other pulmonary complications of anesthesia during pregnancy, first trimester ♀
       O29.092   Other pulmonary complications of anesthesia during pregnancy, second trimester ♀   M
       O29.093   Other pulmonary complications of anesthesia during pregnancy, third trimester ♀   M
       O29.099   Other pulmonary complications of anesthesia during pregnancy, unspecified trimester ♀   M
   ● O29.1   Cardiac complications of anesthesia during pregnancy
     ● O29.11   Cardiac arrest due to anesthesia during pregnancy
       O29.111   Cardiac arrest due to anesthesia during pregnancy, first trimester ♀   M
       O29.112   Cardiac arrest due to anesthesia during pregnancy, second trimester ♀   M
       O29.113   Cardiac arrest due to anesthesia during pregnancy, third trimester ♀   M
       O29.119   Cardiac arrest due to anesthesia during pregnancy, unspecified trimester ♀   M
     ● O29.12   Cardiac failure due to anesthesia during pregnancy
       O29.121   Cardiac failure due to anesthesia during pregnancy, first trimester ♀   M
       O29.122   Cardiac failure due to anesthesia during pregnancy, second trimester ♀   M
       O29.123   Cardiac failure due to anesthesia during pregnancy, third trimester ♀   M
       O29.129   Cardiac failure due to anesthesia during pregnancy, unspecified trimester ♀   M
     ● O29.19   Other cardiac complications of anesthesia during pregnancy
       O29.191   Other cardiac complications of anesthesia during pregnancy, first trimester ♀   M
       O29.192   Other cardiac complications of anesthesia during pregnancy, second trimester ♀   M
       O29.193   Other cardiac complications of anesthesia during pregnancy, third trimester ♀   M
       O29.199   Other cardiac complications of anesthesia during pregnancy, unspecified trimester ♀   M
   ● O29.2   Central nervous system complications of anesthesia during pregnancy
     ● O29.21   Cerebral anoxia due to anesthesia during pregnancy
       O29.211   Cerebral anoxia due to anesthesia during pregnancy, first trimester ♀   M
       O29.212   Cerebral anoxia due to anesthesia during pregnancy, second trimester ♀   M
       O29.213   Cerebral anoxia due to anesthesia during pregnancy, third trimester ♀   M
       O29.219   Cerebral anoxia due to anesthesia during pregnancy, unspecified trimester ♀   M

◀ New   ◀■ Revised   ~~deleted~~ Deleted   Excludes 1   Excludes 2   Includes   Use additional   Code first   Code also   Unspecified

OGCR Official Guidelines   X Assign placeholder X   ● Use Additional Character(s)   ❱ Manifestation Code   **Coding Clinic**

1160

● **O29.29 Other central nervous system complications of anesthesia during pregnancy**
  O29.291 Other central nervous system complications of anesthesia during pregnancy, first trimester ♀ M
  O29.292 Other central nervous system complications of anesthesia during pregnancy, second trimester ♀ M
  O29.293 Other central nervous system complications of anesthesia during pregnancy, third trimester ♀ M
  O29.299 Other central nervous system complications of anesthesia during pregnancy, unspecified trimester ♀ M

● **O29.3 Toxic reaction to local anesthesia during pregnancy**
  ● **O29.3X Toxic reaction to local anesthesia during pregnancy**
    O29.3X1 Toxic reaction to local anesthesia during pregnancy, first trimester ♀ M
    O29.3X2 Toxic reaction to local anesthesia during pregnancy, second trimester ♀ M
    O29.3X3 Toxic reaction to local anesthesia during pregnancy, third trimester ♀ M
    O29.3X9 Toxic reaction to local anesthesia during pregnancy, unspecified trimester ♀ M

● **O29.4 Spinal and epidural anesthesia induced headache during pregnancy**
  O29.40 Spinal and epidural anesthesia induced headache during pregnancy, unspecified trimester ♀ M
  O29.41 Spinal and epidural anesthesia induced headache during pregnancy, first trimester ♀ M
  O29.42 Spinal and epidural anesthesia induced headache during pregnancy, second trimester ♀ M
  O29.43 Spinal and epidural anesthesia induced headache during pregnancy, third trimester ♀ M

● **O29.5 Other complications of spinal and epidural anesthesia during pregnancy**
  ● **O29.5X Other complications of spinal and epidural anesthesia during pregnancy**
    O29.5X1 Other complications of spinal and epidural anesthesia during pregnancy, first trimester ♀ M
    O29.5X2 Other complications of spinal and epidural anesthesia during pregnancy, second trimester ♀ M
    O29.5X3 Other complications of spinal and epidural anesthesia during pregnancy, third trimester ♀ M
    O29.5X9 Other complications of spinal and epidural anesthesia during pregnancy, unspecified trimester ♀ M

● **O29.6 Failed or difficult intubation for anesthesia during pregnancy**
  O29.60 Failed or difficult intubation for anesthesia during pregnancy, unspecified trimester ♀ M
  O29.61 Failed or difficult intubation for anesthesia during pregnancy, first trimester ♀ M
  O29.62 Failed or difficult intubation for anesthesia during pregnancy, second trimester ♀ M
  O29.63 Failed or difficult intubation for anesthesia during pregnancy, third trimester ♀ M

● **O29.8 Other complications of anesthesia during pregnancy**
  ● **O29.8X Other complications of anesthesia during pregnancy**
    O29.8X1 Other complications of anesthesia during pregnancy, first trimester ♀ M
    O29.8X2 Other complications of anesthesia during pregnancy, second trimester ♀ M
    O29.8X3 Other complications of anesthesia during pregnancy, third trimester ♀ M
    O29.8X9 Other complications of anesthesia during pregnancy, unspecified trimester ♀ M

● **O29.9 Unspecified complication of anesthesia during pregnancy**
  O29.90 Unspecified complication of anesthesia during pregnancy, unspecified trimester ♀ M
  O29.91 Unspecified complication of anesthesia during pregnancy, first trimester ♀ M
  O29.92 Unspecified complication of anesthesia during pregnancy, second trimester ♀ M
  O29.93 Unspecified complication of anesthesia during pregnancy, third trimester ♀ M

MATERNAL CARE RELATED TO THE FETUS AND AMNIOTIC CAVITY AND POSSIBLE DELIVERY PROBLEMS (O30-O48)

● **O30 Multiple gestation**
  Code also any complications specific to multiple gestation
  ● **O30.0 Twin pregnancy**
    ● **O30.00 Twin pregnancy, unspecified number of placenta and unspecified number of amniotic sacs**
      O30.001 Twin pregnancy, unspecified number of placenta and unspecified number of amniotic sacs, first trimester ♀ M
      O30.002 Twin pregnancy, unspecified number of placenta and unspecified number of amniotic sacs, second trimester ♀ M
      O30.003 Twin pregnancy, unspecified number of placenta and unspecified number of amniotic sacs, third trimester ♀ M
      O30.009 Twin pregnancy, unspecified number of placenta and unspecified number of amniotic sacs, unspecified trimester ♀ M
    ● **O30.01 Twin pregnancy, monochorionic/monoamniotic**
      Twin pregnancy, one placenta, one amniotic sac
      Excludes1 conjoined twins (O30.02-)
      O30.011 Twin pregnancy, monochorionic/monoamniotic, first trimester ♀ M
      O30.012 Twin pregnancy, monochorionic/monoamniotic, second trimester ♀ M
      O30.013 Twin pregnancy, monochorionic/monoamniotic, third trimester ♀ M
      O30.019 Twin pregnancy, monochorionic/monoamniotic, unspecified trimester ♀ M
    ● **O30.02 Conjoined twin pregnancy**
      O30.021 Conjoined twin pregnancy, first trimester ♀ M
      O30.022 Conjoined twin pregnancy, second trimester ♀ M
      O30.023 Conjoined twin pregnancy, third trimester ♀ M
      O30.029 Conjoined twin pregnancy, unspecified trimester ♀ M

CHAPTER 15 (O00-O9A)

● **O30.03**   **Twin pregnancy, monochorionic/diamniotic**
Twin pregnancy, one placenta, two amniotic sacs

    O30.031   Twin pregnancy, monochorionic/diamniotic, first trimester ♀   M

    O30.032   Twin pregnancy, monochorionic/diamniotic, second trimester ♀   M

    O30.033   Twin pregnancy, monochorionic/diamniotic, third trimester ♀   M

    O30.039   Twin pregnancy, monochorionic/diamniotic, unspecified trimester ♀   M

● **O30.04**   **Twin pregnancy, dichorionic/diamniotic**
Twin pregnancy, two placentae, two amniotic sacs

    O30.041   Twin pregnancy, dichorionic/diamniotic, first trimester ♀   M

    O30.042   Twin pregnancy, dichorionic/diamniotic, second trimester ♀   M

    O30.043   Twin pregnancy, dichorionic/diamniotic, third trimester ♀   M

    O30.049   Twin pregnancy, dichorionic/diamniotic, unspecified trimester ♀   M

● **O30.09**   **Twin pregnancy, unable to determine number of placenta and number of amniotic sacs**

    O30.091   Twin pregnancy, unable to determine number of placenta and number of amniotic sacs, first trimester ♀   M

    O30.092   Twin pregnancy, unable to determine number of placenta and number of amniotic sacs, second trimester ♀   M

    O30.093   Twin pregnancy, unable to determine number of placenta and number of amniotic sacs, third trimester ♀   M

    O30.099   Twin pregnancy, unable to determine number of placenta and number of amniotic sacs, unspecified trimester ♀   M

● **O30.1**   **Triplet pregnancy**

● **O30.10**   **Triplet pregnancy, unspecified number of placenta and unspecified number of amniotic sacs**

    O30.101   Triplet pregnancy, unspecified number of placenta and unspecified number of amniotic sacs, first trimester ♀   M

    O30.102   Triplet pregnancy, unspecified number of placenta and unspecified number of amniotic sacs, second trimester ♀   M

    O30.103   Triplet pregnancy, unspecified number of placenta and unspecified number of amniotic sacs, third trimester ♀   M
        Coding Clinic: 2016, Q2, P8

    O30.109   Triplet pregnancy, unspecified number of placenta and unspecified number of amniotic sacs, unspecified trimester ♀   M

● **O30.11**   **Triplet pregnancy with two or more monochorionic fetuses**

    O30.111   Triplet pregnancy with two or more monochorionic fetuses, first trimester ♀   M

    O30.112   Triplet pregnancy with two or more monochorionic fetuses, second trimester ♀   M

    O30.113   Triplet pregnancy with two or more monochorionic fetuses, third trimester ♀   M

    O30.119   Triplet pregnancy with two or more monochorionic fetuses, unspecified trimester ♀   M

● **O30.12**   **Triplet pregnancy with two or more monoamniotic fetuses**

    O30.121   Triplet pregnancy with two or more monoamniotic fetuses, first trimester ♀   M

    O30.122   Triplet pregnancy with two or more monoamniotic fetuses, second trimester ♀   M

    O30.123   Triplet pregnancy with two or more monoamniotic fetuses, third trimester ♀   M

    O30.129   Triplet pregnancy with two or more monoamniotic fetuses, unspecified trimester ♀   M

● **O30.19**   **Triplet pregnancy, unable to determine number of placenta and number of amniotic sacs**

    O30.191   Triplet pregnancy, unable to determine number of placenta and number of amniotic sacs, first trimester ♀   M

    O30.192   Triplet pregnancy, unable to determine number of placenta and number of amniotic sacs, second trimester ♀   M

    O30.193   Triplet pregnancy, unable to determine number of placenta and number of amniotic sacs, third trimester ♀   M

    O30.199   Triplet pregnancy, unable to determine number of placenta and number of amniotic sacs, unspecified trimester ♀   M

● **O30.2**   **Quadruplet pregnancy**

● **O30.20**   **Quadruplet pregnancy, unspecified number of placenta and unspecified number of amniotic sacs**

    O30.201   Quadruplet pregnancy, unspecified number of placenta and unspecified number of amniotic sacs, first trimester ♀   M

    O30.202   Quadruplet pregnancy, unspecified number of placenta and unspecified number of amniotic sacs, second trimester ♀   M

    O30.203   Quadruplet pregnancy, unspecified number of placenta and unspecified number of amniotic sacs, third trimester ♀   M

    O30.209   Quadruplet pregnancy, unspecified number of placenta and unspecified number of amniotic sacs, unspecified trimester ♀   M

◀ New   ◀◀ Revised   ~~deleted~~ Deleted   Excludes 1   Excludes 2   Includes   Use additional   Code first   Code also   Unspecified
OGCR Official Guidelines   X Assign placeholder X   ● Use Additional Character(s)   ▶ Manifestation Code   **Coding Clinic**

● **O30.21 Quadruplet pregnancy with two or more monochorionic fetuses**
- O30.211 Quadruplet pregnancy with two or more monochorionic fetuses, first trimester ♀   M
- O30.212 Quadruplet pregnancy with two or more monochorionic fetuses, second trimester ♀   M
- O30.213 Quadruplet pregnancy with two or more monochorionic fetuses, third trimester ♀   M
- O30.219 Quadruplet pregnancy with two or more monochorionic fetuses, unspecified trimester ♀   M

● **O30.22 Quadruplet pregnancy with two or more monoamniotic fetuses**
- O30.221 Quadruplet pregnancy with two or more monoamniotic fetuses, first trimester ♀   M
- O30.222 Quadruplet pregnancy with two or more monoamniotic fetuses, second trimester ♀   M
- O30.223 Quadruplet pregnancy with two or more monoamniotic fetuses, third trimester ♀   M
- O30.229 Quadruplet pregnancy with two or more monoamniotic fetuses, unspecified trimester ♀   M

● **O30.29 Quadruplet pregnancy, unable to determine number of placenta and number of amniotic sacs**
- O30.291 Quadruplet pregnancy, unable to determine number of placenta and number of amniotic sacs, first trimester ♀   M
- O30.292 Quadruplet pregnancy, unable to determine number of placenta and number of amniotic sacs, second trimester ♀   M
- O30.293 Quadruplet pregnancy, unable to determine number of placenta and number of amniotic sacs, third trimester ♀   M
- O30.299 Quadruplet pregnancy, unable to determine number of placenta and number of amniotic sacs, unspecified trimester ♀   M

● **O30.8 Other specified multiple gestation**
Multiple gestation pregnancy greater then quadruplets

● **O30.80 Other specified multiple gestation, unspecified number of placenta and unspecified number of amniotic sacs**
- O30.801 Other specified multiple gestation, unspecified number of placenta and unspecified number of amniotic sacs, first trimester ♀   M
- O30.802 Other specified multiple gestation, unspecified number of placenta and unspecified number of amniotic sacs, second trimester ♀   M
- O30.803 Other specified multiple gestation, unspecified number of placenta and unspecified number of amniotic sacs, third trimester ♀   M
- O30.809 Other specified multiple gestation, unspecified number of placenta and unspecified number of amniotic sacs, unspecified trimester ♀   M

● **O30.81 Other specified multiple gestation with two or more monochorionic fetuses**
- O30.811 Other specified multiple gestation with two or more monochorionic fetuses, first trimester ♀   M
- O30.812 Other specified multiple gestation with two or more monochorionic fetuses, second trimester ♀   M
- O30.813 Other specified multiple gestation with two or more monochorionic fetuses, third trimester ♀   M
- O30.819 Other specified multiple gestation with two or more monochorionic fetuses, unspecified trimester ♀   M

● **O30.82 Other specified multiple gestation with two or more monoamniotic fetuses**
- O30.821 Other specified multiple gestation with two or more monoamniotic fetuses, first trimester ♀   M
- O30.822 Other specified multiple gestation with two or more monoamniotic fetuses, second trimester ♀   M
- O30.823 Other specified multiple gestation with two or more monoamniotic fetuses, third trimester ♀   M
- O30.829 Other specified multiple gestation with two or more monoamniotic fetuses, unspecified trimester ♀   M

● **O30.89 Other specified multiple gestation, unable to determine number of placenta and number of amniotic sacs**
- O30.891 Other specified multiple gestation, unable to determine number of placenta and number of amniotic sacs, first trimester ♀   M
- O30.892 Other specified multiple gestation, unable to determine number of placenta and number of amniotic sacs, second trimester ♀   M
- O30.893 Other specified multiple gestation, unable to determine number of placenta and number of amniotic sacs, third trimester ♀   M
- O30.899 Other specified multiple gestation, unable to determine number of placenta and number of amniotic sacs, unspecified trimester ♀   M

● **O30.9 Multiple gestation, unspecified**
Multiple pregnancy NOS
- O30.90 Multiple gestation, unspecified, unspecified trimester ♀   M
- O30.91 Multiple gestation, unspecified, first trimester ♀   M
- O30.92 Multiple gestation, unspecified, second trimester ♀   M
- O30.93 Multiple gestation, unspecified, third trimester ♀   M

CHAPTER 15 (O00–O9A)

CHAPTER 15 (O00-O9A)

● **O31 Complications specific to multiple gestation**

    Excludes2   delayed delivery of second twin, triplet, etc. (O63.2)
                 malpresentation of one fetus or more (O32.9)
                 placental transfusion syndromes (O43.0-)

    Coding Clinic: 2012, Q4, P107

    One of the following 7th characters is to be assigned to each code under category O31. 7th character Ø is for single gestations and multiple gestations where the fetus is unspecified. 7th characters 1 through 9 are for cases of multiple gestations to identify the fetus for which the code applies. The appropriate code from category O30, Multiple gestation, must also be assigned when assigning a code from category O31 that has a 7th character of 1 through 9.

Ø	not applicable or unspecified
1	fetus 1
2	fetus 2
3	fetus 3
4	fetus 4
5	fetus 5
9	other fetus

● **O31.0 Papyraceous fetus**
    Fetus compressus

  X ● **O31.00 Papyraceous fetus, unspecified trimester** ♀   M
  X ● **O31.01 Papyraceous fetus, first trimester** ♀   M
  X ● **O31.02 Papyraceous fetus, second trimester** ♀   M
  X ● **O31.03 Papyraceous fetus, third trimester** ♀   M

● **O31.1 Continuing pregnancy after spontaneous abortion of one fetus or more**

  X ● **O31.10 Continuing pregnancy after spontaneous abortion of one fetus or more, unspecified trimester** ♀   M
  X ● **O31.11 Continuing pregnancy after spontaneous abortion of one fetus or more, first trimester** ♀   M
  X ● **O31.12 Continuing pregnancy after spontaneous abortion of one fetus or more, second trimester** ♀   M
  X ● **O31.13 Continuing pregnancy after spontaneous abortion of one fetus or more, third trimester** ♀   M

● **O31.2 Continuing pregnancy after intrauterine death of one fetus or more**

  X ● **O31.20 Continuing pregnancy after intrauterine death of one fetus or more, unspecified trimester** ♀   M
  X ● **O31.21 Continuing pregnancy after intrauterine death of one fetus or more, first trimester** ♀   M
  X ● **O31.22 Continuing pregnancy after intrauterine death of one fetus or more, second trimester** ♀   M
  X ● **O31.23 Continuing pregnancy after intrauterine death of one fetus or more, third trimester** ♀   M

● **O31.3 Continuing pregnancy after elective fetal reduction of one fetus or more**
    Continuing pregnancy after selective termination of one fetus or more

  X ● **O31.30 Continuing pregnancy after elective fetal reduction of one fetus or more, unspecified trimester** ♀   M
  X ● **O31.31 Continuing pregnancy after elective fetal reduction of one fetus or more, first trimester** ♀   M
  X ● **O31.32 Continuing pregnancy after elective fetal reduction of one fetus or more, second trimester** ♀   M
  X ● **O31.33 Continuing pregnancy after elective fetal reduction of one fetus or more, third trimester** ♀   M

● **O31.8 Other complications specific to multiple gestation**

  ● **O31.8X Other complications specific to multiple gestation**

    ● **O31.8X1 Other complications specific to multiple gestation, first trimester** ♀   M
    ● **O31.8X2 Other complications specific to multiple gestation, second trimester** ♀   M
    ● **O31.8X3 Other complications specific to multiple gestation, third trimester** ♀ M
    ● **O31.8X9 Other complications specific to multiple gestation, unspecified trimester** ♀   M

● **O32 Maternal care for malpresentation of fetus**

    Includes   the listed conditions as a reason for observation, hospitalization or other obstetric care of the mother, or for cesarean delivery before onset of labor

    Excludes1   malpresentation of fetus with obstructed labor (O64.-)

    Coding Clinic: 2012, Q4, P107

    One of the following 7th characters is to be assigned to each code under category O32. 7th character Ø is for single gestations and multiple gestations where the fetus is unspecified. 7th characters 1 through 9 are for cases of multiple gestations to identify the fetus for which the code applies. The appropriate code from category O30, Multiple gestation, must also be assigned when assigning a code from category O32 that has a 7th character of 1 through 9.

Ø	not applicable or unspecified
1	fetus 1
2	fetus 2
3	fetus 3
4	fetus 4
5	fetus 5
9	other fetus

X ● **O32.0 Maternal care for unstable lie** ♀   M
X ● **O32.1 Maternal care for breech presentation** ♀   M
    Maternal care for buttocks presentation
    Maternal care for complete breech
    Maternal care for frank breech

    Excludes1   footling presentation (O32.8)
                incomplete breech (O32.8)

X ● **O32.2 Maternal care for transverse and oblique lie** ♀   M
    Maternal care for oblique presentation
    Maternal care for transverse presentation

X ● **O32.3 Maternal care for face, brow and chin presentation** ♀   M
X ● **O32.4 Maternal care for high head at term** ♀   M
    Maternal care for failure of head to enter pelvic brim

X ● **O32.6 Maternal care for compound presentation** ♀   M
X ● **O32.8 Maternal care for other malpresentation of fetus** ♀   M
    Maternal care for footling presentation
    Maternal care for incomplete breech

X ● **O32.9 Maternal care for malpresentation of fetus, unspecified** ♀   M

● **O33 Maternal care for disproportion**

    Includes   the listed conditions as a reason for observation, hospitalization or other obstetric care of the mother, or for cesarean delivery before onset of labor

    Excludes1   disproportion with obstructed labor (O65-O66)

    O33.0 Maternal care for disproportion due to deformity of maternal pelvic bones ♀   M
    Maternal care for disproportion due to pelvic deformity causing disproportion NOS

◀ New   ◀▬ Revised   ~~deleted~~ Deleted   Excludes 1   Excludes 2   Includes   Use additional   Code first   Code also   Unspecified

OGCR Official Guidelines   X Assign placeholder X   ● Use Additional Character(s)   ▶ Manifestation Code   **Coding Clinic**

O33.1   **Maternal care for disproportion due to generally contracted pelvis** ♀   M

    Maternal care for disproportion due to contracted pelvis NOS causing disproportion

O33.2   **Maternal care for disproportion due to inlet contraction of pelvis** ♀   M

    Maternal care for disproportion due to inlet contraction (pelvis) causing disproportion

X● **O33.3**   **Maternal care for disproportion due to outlet contraction of pelvis** ♀   M

    Maternal care for disproportion due to mid-cavity contraction (pelvis)

    Maternal care for disproportion due to outlet contraction (pelvis)

    One of the following 7th characters is to be assigned to code O33.3. 7th character Ø is for single gestations and multiple gestations where the fetus is unspecified. 7th characters 1 through 9 are for cases of multiple gestations to identify the fetus for which the code applies. The appropriate code from category O3Ø, Multiple gestation, must also be assigned when assigning code O33.3 with a 7th character of 1 through 9.

Ø	not applicable or unspecified
1	fetus 1
2	fetus 2
3	fetus 3
4	fetus 4
5	fetus 5
9	other fetus

X● **O33.4**   **Maternal care for disproportion of mixed maternal and fetal origin** ♀   M

    One of the following 7th characters is to be assigned to code O33.4. 7th character Ø is for single gestations and multiple gestations where the fetus is unspecified. 7th characters 1 through 9 are for cases of multiple gestations to identify the fetus for which the code applies. The appropriate code from category O3Ø, Multiple gestation, must also be assigned when assigning code O33.4 with a 7th character of 1 through 9.

Ø	not applicable or unspecified
1	fetus 1
2	fetus 2
3	fetus 3
4	fetus 4
5	fetus 5
9	other fetus

X● **O33.5**   **Maternal care for disproportion due to unusually large fetus** ♀   M

    Maternal care for disproportion due to disproportion of fetal origin with normally formed fetus

    Maternal care for disproportion due to fetal disproportion NOS

    One of the following 7th characters is to be assigned to code O33.5. 7th character Ø is for single gestations and multiple gestations where the fetus is unspecified. 7th characters 1 through 9 are for cases of multiple gestations to identify the fetus for which the code applies. The appropriate code from category O3Ø, Multiple gestation, must also be assigned when assigning code O33.5 with a 7th character of 1 through 9.

Ø	not applicable or unspecified
1	fetus 1
2	fetus 2
3	fetus 3
4	fetus 4
5	fetus 5
9	other fetus

X● **O33.6**   **Maternal care for disproportion due to hydrocephalic fetus** ♀   M

    One of the following 7th characters is to be assigned to code O33.6. 7th character Ø is for single gestations and multiple gestations where the fetus is unspecified. 7th characters 1 through 9 are for cases of multiple gestations to identify the fetus for which the code applies. The appropriate code from category O3Ø, Multiple gestation, must also be assigned when assigning code O33.6 with a 7th character of 1 through 9.

Ø	not applicable or unspecified
1	fetus 1
2	fetus 2
3	fetus 3
4	fetus 4
5	fetus 5
9	other fetus

X● **O33.7**   **Maternal care for disproportion due to other fetal deformities** ♀   M

    Maternal care for disproportion due to fetal ascites

    Maternal care for disproportion due to fetal hydrops

    Maternal care for disproportion due to fetal meningomyelocele

    Maternal care for disproportion due to fetal sacral teratoma

    Maternal care for disproportion due to fetal tumor

    Excludes1   obstructed labor due to other fetal deformities (O66.3)

    One of the following 7th characters is to be assigned to code O33.7. 7th character Ø is for single gestations and multiple gestations where the fetus is unspecified. 7th characters 1 through 9 are for cases of multiple gestations to identify the fetus for which the code applies. The appropriate code from category O3Ø, Multiple gestation, must also be assigned when assigning code O33.7 with a 7th character of 1 through 9. ◄

Ø	not applicable or unspecified ◄
1	fetus 1 ◄
2	fetus 2 ◄
3	fetus 3 ◄
4	fetus 4 ◄
5	fetus 5 ◄
9	other fetus ◄

O33.8   **Maternal care for disproportion of other origin** ♀   M

O33.9   **Maternal care for disproportion, unspecified** ♀   M

    Maternal care for disproportion due to cephalopelvic disproportion NOS

    Maternal care for disproportion due to fetopelvic disproportion NOS

● **O34**   **Maternal care for abnormality of pelvic organs**

    Includes   the listed conditions as a reason for hospitalization or other obstetric care of the mother, or for cesarean delivery before onset of labor

    Code first any associated obstructed labor (O65.5)

    Use additional code for specific condition

● **O34.Ø**   **Maternal care for congenital malformation of uterus**

    Maternal care for double uterus ◄

    Maternal care for uterus bicornis ◄

    O34.ØØ   **Maternal care for unspecified congenital malformation of uterus, unspecified trimester** ♀   M

    O34.Ø1   **Maternal care for unspecified congenital malformation of uterus, first trimester** ♀   M

    O34.Ø2   **Maternal care for unspecified congenital malformation of uterus, second trimester** ♀   M

    O34.Ø3   **Maternal care for unspecified congenital malformation of uterus, third trimester** ♀   M

CHAPTER 15 (OØØ-O9A)

CHAPTER 15 (O00-O9A)

● **O34.1**   **Maternal care for benign tumor of corpus uteri**
> **Excludes2**   maternal care for benign tumor of cervix (O34.4-)
> maternal care for malignant neoplasm of uterus (O9A.1-)

     O34.10   **Maternal care for benign tumor of corpus uteri, unspecified trimester** ♀   M

     O34.11   **Maternal care for benign tumor of corpus uteri, first trimester** ♀   M

     O34.12   **Maternal care for benign tumor of corpus uteri, second trimester** ♀   M

     O34.13   **Maternal care for benign tumor of corpus uteri, third trimester** ♀   M

● **O34.2**   **Maternal care due to uterine scar from previous surgery**

  ● **O34.21**   **Maternal care for scar from previous cesarean delivery**

     O34.211   **Maternal care for low transverse scar from previous cesarean delivery** ♀ ◀   M

     O34.212   **Maternal care for vertical scar from previous cesarean delivery** ♀ ◀   M
> Maternal care for classical scar from previous cesarean delivery ◀

     O34.219   **Maternal care for unspecified type scar from previous cesarean delivery** ♀ ◀   M

     O34.29   **Maternal care due to uterine scar from other previous surgery** ♀   M
> Maternal care due to uterine scar from other transmural uterine incision ◀

● **O34.3**   **Maternal care for cervical incompetence**
> Maternal care for cerclage with or without cervical incompetence
> Maternal care for Shirodkar suture with or without cervical incompetence

     O34.30   **Maternal care for cervical incompetence, unspecified trimester** ♀   M

     O34.31   **Maternal care for cervical incompetence, first trimester** ♀   M

     O34.32   **Maternal care for cervical incompetence, second trimester** ♀   M

     O34.33   **Maternal care for cervical incompetence, third trimester** ♀   M

● **O34.4**   **Maternal care for other abnormalities of cervix**

     O34.40   **Maternal care for other abnormalities of cervix, unspecified trimester** ♀   M

     O34.41   **Maternal care for other abnormalities of cervix, first trimester** ♀   M

     O34.42   **Maternal care for other abnormalities of cervix, second trimester** ♀   M

     O34.43   **Maternal care for other abnormalities of cervix, third trimester** ♀   M

● **O34.5**   **Maternal care for other abnormalities of gravid uterus**

  ● **O34.51**   **Maternal care for incarceration of gravid uterus**

     O34.511   **Maternal care for incarceration of gravid uterus, first trimester** ♀   M

     O34.512   **Maternal care for incarceration of gravid uterus, second trimester** ♀   M

     O34.513   **Maternal care for incarceration of gravid uterus, third trimester** ♀   M

     O34.519   **Maternal care for incarceration of gravid uterus, unspecified trimester** ♀   M

  ● **O34.52**   **Maternal care for prolapse of gravid uterus**

     O34.521   **Maternal care for prolapse of gravid uterus, first trimester** ♀   M

     O34.522   **Maternal care for prolapse of gravid uterus, second trimester** ♀   M

     O34.523   **Maternal care for prolapse of gravid uterus, third trimester** ♀   M

     O34.529   **Maternal care for prolapse of gravid uterus, unspecified trimester** ♀   M

  ● **O34.53**   **Maternal care for retroversion of gravid uterus**

     O34.531   **Maternal care for retroversion of gravid uterus, first trimester** ♀   M

     O34.532   **Maternal care for retroversion of gravid uterus, second trimester** ♀   M

     O34.533   **Maternal care for retroversion of gravid uterus, third trimester** ♀   M

     O34.539   **Maternal care for retroversion of gravid uterus, unspecified trimester** ♀   M

  ● **O34.59**   **Maternal care for other abnormalities of gravid uterus**

     O34.591   **Maternal care for other abnormalities of gravid uterus, first trimester** ♀   M

     O34.592   **Maternal care for other abnormalities of gravid uterus, second trimester** ♀   M

     O34.593   **Maternal care for other abnormalities of gravid uterus, third trimester** ♀   M

     O34.599   **Maternal care for other abnormalities of gravid uterus, unspecified trimester** ♀   M

● **O34.6**   **Maternal care for abnormality of vagina**
> **Excludes2**   maternal care for vaginal varices in pregnancy (O22.1-)

     O34.60   **Maternal care for abnormality of vagina, unspecified trimester** ♀   M

     O34.61   **Maternal care for abnormality of vagina, first trimester** ♀   M

     O34.62   **Maternal care for abnormality of vagina, second trimester** ♀   M

     O34.63   **Maternal care for abnormality of vagina, third trimester** ♀   M

● **O34.7**   **Maternal care for abnormality of vulva and perineum**
> **Excludes2**   maternal care for perineal and vulval varices in pregnancy (O22.1-)

     O34.70   **Maternal care for abnormality of vulva and perineum, unspecified trimester** ♀   M

     O34.71   **Maternal care for abnormality of vulva and perineum, first trimester** ♀   M

     O34.72   **Maternal care for abnormality of vulva and perineum, second trimester** ♀   M

     O34.73   **Maternal care for abnormality of vulva and perineum, third trimester** ♀   M

● **O34.8**   **Maternal care for other abnormalities of pelvic organs**

     O34.80   **Maternal care for other abnormalities of pelvic organs, unspecified trimester** ♀   M

     O34.81   **Maternal care for other abnormalities of pelvic organs, first trimester** ♀   M

     O34.82   **Maternal care for other abnormalities of pelvic organs, second trimester** ♀   M

     O34.83   **Maternal care for other abnormalities of pelvic organs, third trimester** ♀   M

● **O34.9**   **Maternal care for abnormality of pelvic organ, unspecified**

     O34.90   **Maternal care for abnormality of pelvic organ, unspecified, unspecified trimester** ♀   M

     O34.91   **Maternal care for abnormality of pelvic organ, unspecified, first trimester** ♀   M

     O34.92   **Maternal care for abnormality of pelvic organ, unspecified, second trimester** ♀   M

     O34.93   **Maternal care for abnormality of pelvic organ, unspecified, third trimester** ♀   M

◀ New   ◀▦ Revised   ~~deleted~~ Deleted   Excludes 1   Excludes 2   Includes   Use additional   Code first   Code also   Unspecified

OGCR Official Guidelines   X Assign placeholder X   ● Use Additional Character(s)   ▶ Manifestation Code   **Coding Clinic**

● **O35**   **Maternal care for known or suspected fetal abnormality and damage**

> **Includes**   the listed conditions in the fetus as a reason for hospitalization or other obstetric care to the mother, or for termination of pregnancy

Code also any associated maternal condition

> **Excludes1**   encounter for suspected maternal and fetal conditions ruled out (Z03.7-)

One of the following 7th characters is to be assigned to each code under category O35. 7th character Ø is for single gestations and multiple gestations where the fetus is unspecified. 7th characters 1 through 9 are for cases of multiple gestations to identify the fetus for which the code applies. The appropriate code from category O30, Multiple gestation, must also be assigned when assigning a code from category O35 that has a 7th character of 1 through 9.

Ø	not applicable or unspecified
1	fetus 1
2	fetus 2
3	fetus 3
4	fetus 4
5	fetus 5
9	other fetus

X ● **O35.0**   **Maternal care for (suspected) central nervous system malformation in fetus** ♀   M
> Maternal care for fetal anencephaly
> Maternal care for fetal hydrocephalus
> Maternal care for fetal spina bifida
>> **Excludes2**   chromosomal abnormality in fetus (O35.1)

X ● **O35.1**   **Maternal care for (suspected) chromosomal abnormality in fetus** ♀   M

X ● **O35.2**   **Maternal care for (suspected) hereditary disease in fetus** ♀   M
>> **Excludes2**   chromosomal abnormality in fetus (O35.1)

OGCR Section I.C.15.e.l.

> Fetal Conditions Affecting the Management of the Mother
>
> 1) Code from categories O35 and O36
>
> Codes from categories O35, Maternal care for known or suspected fetal abnormality and damage, and O36, Maternal care for other fetal problems, are assigned only when the fetal condition is actually responsible for modifying the management of the mother, i.e., by requiring diagnostic studies, additional observation, special care, or termination of pregnancy. The fact that the fetal condition exists does not justify assigning a code from this series to the mother's record.
>
> 2) In utero surgery
>
> In cases when surgery is performed on the fetus, a diagnosis code from category O35, Maternal care for known or suspected fetal abnormality and damage, should be assigned identifying the fetal condition. Assign the appropriate procedure code for the procedure performed.
>
> No code from Chapter 16, the perinatal codes, should be used on the mother's record to identify fetal conditions. Surgery performed in utero on a fetus is still to be coded as an obstetric encounter.

X ● **O35.3**   **Maternal care for (suspected) damage to fetus from viral disease in mother** ♀   M
> Maternal care for damage to fetus from maternal cytomegalovirus infection
> Maternal care for damage to fetus from maternal rubella

X ● **O35.4**   **Maternal care for (suspected) damage to fetus from alcohol** ♀   M

X ● **O35.5**   **Maternal care for (suspected) damage to fetus by drugs** ♀   M
> Maternal care for damage to fetus from drug addiction

X ● **O35.6**   **Maternal care for (suspected) damage to fetus by radiation** ♀   M

X ● **O35.7**   **Maternal care for (suspected) damage to fetus by other medical procedures** ♀   M
> Maternal care for damage to fetus by amniocentesis
> Maternal care for damage to fetus by biopsy procedures
> Maternal care for damage to fetus by hematological investigation
> Maternal care for damage to fetus by intrauterine contraceptive device
> Maternal care for damage to fetus by intrauterine surgery

X ● **O35.8**   **Maternal care for other (suspected) fetal abnormality and damage** ♀   M
> Maternal care for damage to fetus from maternal listeriosis
> Maternal care for damage to fetus from maternal toxoplasmosis

X ● **O35.9**   **Maternal care for (suspected) fetal abnormality and damage, unspecified** ♀   M

● **O36**   **Maternal care for other fetal problems**

> **Includes**   the listed conditions in the fetus as a reason for hospitalization or other obstetric care of the mother, or for termination of pregnancy

> **Excludes1**   encounter for suspected maternal and fetal conditions ruled out (Z03.7-)
> placental transfusion syndromes (O43.0-)

> **Excludes2**   labor and delivery complicated by fetal stress (O77.-)

One of the following 7th characters is to be assigned to each code under category O36. 7th character Ø is for single gestations and multiple gestations where the fetus is unspecified. 7th characters 1 through 9 are for cases of multiple gestations to identify the fetus for which the code applies. The appropriate code from category O30, Multiple gestation, must also be assigned when assigning a code from category O36 that has a 7th character of 1 through 9.

Ø	not applicable or unspecified
1	fetus 1
2	fetus 2
3	fetus 3
4	fetus 4
5	fetus 5
9	other fetus

Coding Clinic: 2015, Q3, P40

● **O36.0**   **Maternal care for rhesus isoimmunization**
> Maternal care for Rh incompatibility (with hydrops fetalis)

> ● **O36.01**   **Maternal care for anti-D [Rh] antibodies**
>> ● **O36.011**   **Maternal care for anti-D [Rh] antibodies, first trimester** ♀   M
>> ● **O36.012**   **Maternal care for anti-D [Rh] antibodies, second trimester** ♀   M
>> ● **O36.013**   **Maternal care for anti-D [Rh] antibodies, third trimester** ♀   M
>> ● **O36.019**   **Maternal care for anti-D [Rh] antibodies, unspecified trimester** ♀   M

> ● **O36.09**   **Maternal care for other rhesus isoimmunization**
>> ● **O36.091**   **Maternal care for other rhesus isoimmunization, first trimester** ♀   M
>> ● **O36.092**   **Maternal care for other rhesus isoimmunization, second trimester** ♀   M
>> ● **O36.093**   **Maternal care for other rhesus isoimmunization, third trimester** ♀   M
>> Coding Clinic: 2015, Q3, P40
>> ● **O36.099**   **Maternal care for other rhesus isoimmunization, unspecified trimester** ♀   M

CHAPTER 15 (O00-O9A)

CHAPTER 15 (O00-O9A)

- ● O36.1   **Maternal care for other isoimmunization**
  Maternal care for ABO isoimmunization
  - ● O36.11   **Maternal care for Anti-A sensitization**
    Maternal care for isoimmunization NOS (with hydrops fetalis)
    - ● O36.111   **Maternal care for Anti-A sensitization, first trimester** ♀   M
    - ● O36.112   **Maternal care for Anti-A sensitization, second trimester** ♀   M
    - ● O36.113   **Maternal care for Anti-A sensitization, third trimester** ♀   M
    - ● O36.119   **Maternal care for Anti-A sensitization, unspecified trimester** ♀   M
  - ● O36.19   **Maternal care for other isoimmunization**
    Maternal care for Anti-B sensitization
    - ● O36.191   **Maternal care for other isoimmunization, first trimester** ♀   M
    - ● O36.192   **Maternal care for other isoimmunization, second trimester** ♀   M
    - ● O36.193   **Maternal care for other isoimmunization, third trimester** ♀   M
    - ● O36.199   **Maternal care for other isoimmunization, unspecified trimester** ♀   M
- ● O36.2   **Maternal care for hydrops fetalis**
  Maternal care for hydrops fetalis NOS
  Maternal care for hydrops fetalis not associated with isoimmunization
  - **Excludes1**   hydrops fetalis associated with ABO isoimmunization (O36.1-)
    hydrops fetalis associated with rhesus isoimmunization (O36.0-)
  - ● O36.20   **Maternal care for hydrops fetalis, unspecified trimester** ♀   M
  - ● O36.21   **Maternal care for hydrops fetalis, first trimester** ♀   M
  - ● O36.22   **Maternal care for hydrops fetalis, second trimester** ♀   M
  - ● O36.23   **Maternal care for hydrops fetalis, third trimester** ♀   M
- ● O36.4   **Maternal care for intrauterine death** ♀   M
  Maternal care for intrauterine fetal death NOS
  Maternal care for intrauterine fetal death after completion of 20 weeks of gestation
  Maternal care for late fetal death
  Maternal care for missed delivery
  - **Excludes1**   missed abortion (O02.1)
    stillbirth (P95)
- ● O36.5   **Maternal care for known or suspected poor fetal growth**
  - ● O36.51   **Maternal care for known or suspected placental insufficiency**
    - ● O36.511   **Maternal care for known or suspected placental insufficiency, first trimester** ♀   M
    - ● O36.512   **Maternal care for known or suspected placental insufficiency, second trimester** ♀   M
    - ● O36.513   **Maternal care for known or suspected placental insufficiency, third trimester** ♀   M
    - ● O36.519   **Maternal care for known or suspected placental insufficiency, unspecified trimester** ♀   M

- ● O36.59   **Maternal care for other known or suspected poor fetal growth**
  Maternal care for known or suspected light-for-dates NOS
  Maternal care for known or suspected small-for-dates NOS
  - ● O36.591   **Maternal care for other known or suspected poor fetal growth, first trimester** ♀   M
  - ● O36.592   **Maternal care for other known or suspected poor fetal growth, second trimester** ♀   M
  - ● O36.593   **Maternal care for other known or suspected poor fetal growth, third trimester** ♀   M
  - ● O36.599   **Maternal care for other known or suspected poor fetal growth, unspecified trimester** ♀   M
- ● O36.6   **Maternal care for excessive fetal growth**
  Maternal care for known or suspected large-for-dates
  - X ● O36.60   **Maternal care for excessive fetal growth, unspecified trimester** ♀   M
  - X ● O36.61   **Maternal care for excessive fetal growth, first trimester** ♀   M
  - X ● O36.62   **Maternal care for excessive fetal growth, second trimester** ♀   M
  - X ● O36.63   **Maternal care for excessive fetal growth, third trimester** ♀   M
- ● O36.7   **Maternal care for viable fetus in abdominal pregnancy**
  - X ● O36.70   **Maternal care for viable fetus in abdominal pregnancy, unspecified trimester** ♀   M
  - X ● O36.71   **Maternal care for viable fetus in abdominal pregnancy, first trimester** ♀   M
  - X ● O36.72   **Maternal care for viable fetus in abdominal pregnancy, second trimester** ♀   M
  - X ● O36.73   **Maternal care for viable fetus in abdominal pregnancy, third trimester** ♀   M
- ● O36.8   **Maternal care for other specified fetal problems**
  - X ● O36.80   **Pregnancy with inconclusive fetal viability** ♀   M
    Encounter to determine fetal viability of pregnancy
  - ● O36.81   **Decreased fetal movements**
    - ● O36.812   **Decreased fetal movements, second trimester** ♀   M
    - ● O36.813   **Decreased fetal movements, third trimester** ♀   M
    - ● O36.819   **Decreased fetal movements, unspecified trimester** ♀   M
  - ● O36.82   **Fetal anemia and thrombocytopenia**
    - ● O36.821   **Fetal anemia and thrombocytopenia, first trimester** ♀   M
    - ● O36.822   **Fetal anemia and thrombocytopenia, second trimester** ♀   M
    - ● O36.823   **Fetal anemia and thrombocytopenia, third trimester** ♀   M
    - ● O36.829   **Fetal anemia and thrombocytopenia, unspecified trimester** ♀   M
  - ● O36.89   **Maternal care for other specified fetal problems**
    - ● O36.891   **Maternal care for other specified fetal problems, first trimester** ♀   M
    - ● O36.892   **Maternal care for other specified fetal problems, second trimester** ♀   M
    - ● O36.893   **Maternal care for other specified fetal problems, third trimester** ♀   M
    - ● O36.899   **Maternal care for other specified fetal problems, unspecified trimester** ♀   M

◀ New   ◀■■ Revised   ~~deleted~~ Deleted   Excludes 1   Excludes 2   Includes   Use additional   Code first   Code also   Unspecified

OGCR Official Guidelines   X Assign placeholder X   ● Use Additional Character(s)   ▷ Manifestation Code   **Coding Clinic**

1110

● **O36.9**   **Maternal care for fetal problem, unspecified**
   X● **O36.90**   **Maternal care for fetal problem, unspecified, unspecified trimester** ♀   M
   X● **O36.91**   **Maternal care for fetal problem, unspecified, first trimester** ♀   M
   X● **O36.92**   **Maternal care for fetal problem, unspecified, second trimester** ♀   M
   X● **O36.93**   **Maternal care for fetal problem, unspecified, third trimester** ♀   M

● **O40**   **Polyhydramnios**
   Overabundance of amniotic fluid
   Includes   hydramnios
   Excludes1   encounter for suspected maternal and fetal conditions ruled out (Z03.7-)

One of the following 7th characters is to be assigned to each code under category O40. 7th character 0 is for single gestations and multiple gestations where the fetus is unspecified. 7th characters 1 through 9 are for cases of multiple gestations to identify the fetus for which the code applies. The appropriate code from category O30, Multiple gestation, must also be assigned when assigning a code from category O40 that has a 7th character of 1 through 9.

0	not applicable or unspecified
1	fetus 1
2	fetus 2
3	fetus 3
4	fetus 4
5	fetus 5
9	other fetus

   X● **O40.1**   **Polyhydramnios, first trimester** ♀   M
   X● **O40.2**   **Polyhydramnios, second trimester** ♀   M
   X● **O40.3**   **Polyhydramnios, third trimester** ♀   M
   X● **O40.9**   **Polyhydramnios, unspecified trimester** ♀   M

● **O41**   **Other disorders of amniotic fluid and membranes**
   Excludes1   encounter for suspected maternal and fetal conditions ruled out (Z03.7-)

One of the following 7th characters is to be assigned to each code under category O41. 7th character 0 is for single gestations and multiple gestations where the fetus is unspecified. 7th characters 1 through 9 are for cases of multiple gestations to identify the fetus for which the code applies. The appropriate code from category O30, Multiple gestation, must also be assigned when assigning a code from category O41 that has a 7th character of 1 through 9.

0	not applicable or unspecified
1	fetus 1
2	fetus 2
3	fetus 3
4	fetus 4
5	fetus 5
9	other fetus

● **O41.0**   **Oligohydramnios**
   Scant volume of amniotic fluid
   Oligohydramnios without rupture of membranes
   X● **O41.00**   **Oligohydramnios, unspecified trimester** ♀   M
   X● **O41.01**   **Oligohydramnios, first trimester** ♀   M
   X● **O41.02**   **Oligohydramnios, second trimester** ♀   M
   X● **O41.03**   **Oligohydramnios, third trimester** ♀   M

● **O41.1**   **Infection of amniotic sac and membranes**
   ● **O41.10**   **Infection of amniotic sac and membranes, unspecified**
     ● **O41.101**   **Infection of amniotic sac and membranes, unspecified, first trimester** ♀   M
     ● **O41.102**   **Infection of amniotic sac and membranes, unspecified, second trimester** ♀   M
     ● **O41.103**   **Infection of amniotic sac and membranes, unspecified, third trimester** ♀   M
     ● **O41.109**   **Infection of amniotic sac and membranes, unspecified, unspecified trimester** ♀   M
   ● **O41.12**   **Chorioamnionitis**
     ● **O41.121**   **Chorioamnionitis, first trimester** ♀   M
     ● **O41.122**   **Chorioamnionitis, second trimester** ♀   M
     ● **O41.123**   **Chorioamnionitis, third trimester** ♀   M
     ● **O41.129**   **Chorioamnionitis, unspecified trimester** ♀   M
   ● **O41.14**   **Placentitis**
     ● **O41.141**   **Placentitis, first trimester** ♀   M
     ● **O41.142**   **Placentitis, second trimester** ♀   M
     ● **O41.143**   **Placentitis, third trimester** ♀   M
     ● **O41.149**   **Placentitis, unspecified trimester** ♀   M

● **O41.8**   **Other specified disorders of amniotic fluid and membranes**
   ● **O41.8X**   **Other specified disorders of amniotic fluid and membranes**
     ● **O41.8X1**   **Other specified disorders of amniotic fluid and membranes, first trimester** ♀   M
     ● **O41.8X2**   **Other specified disorders of amniotic fluid and membranes, second trimester** ♀   M
     ● **O41.8X3**   **Other specified disorders of amniotic fluid and membranes, third trimester** ♀   M
     ● **O41.8X9**   **Other specified disorders of amniotic fluid and membranes, unspecified trimester** ♀   M

● **O41.9**   **Disorder of amniotic fluid and membranes, unspecified**
   X● **O41.90**   **Disorder of amniotic fluid and membranes, unspecified, unspecified trimester** ♀   M
   X● **O41.91**   **Disorder of amniotic fluid and membranes, unspecified, first trimester** ♀   M
   X● **O41.92**   **Disorder of amniotic fluid and membranes, unspecified, second trimester** ♀   M
   X● **O41.93**   **Disorder of amniotic fluid and membranes, unspecified, third trimester** ♀   M

● **O42**   **Premature rupture of membranes**
   ● **O42.0**   **Premature rupture of membranes, onset of labor within 24 hours of rupture**
     O42.00   **Premature rupture of membranes, onset of labor within 24 hours of rupture, unspecified weeks of gestation** ♀   M
     ● **O42.01**   **Preterm premature rupture of membranes, onset of labor within 24 hours of rupture**
      Premature rupture of membranes before 37 completed weeks of gestation
       O42.011   **Preterm premature rupture of membranes, onset of labor within 24 hours of rupture, first trimester** ♀   M
       O42.012   **Preterm premature rupture of membranes, onset of labor within 24 hours of rupture, second trimester** ♀ M
       O42.013   **Preterm premature rupture of membranes, onset of labor within 24 hours of rupture, third trimester** ♀   M
       O42.019   **Preterm premature rupture of membranes, onset of labor within 24 hours of rupture, unspecified trimester** ♀   M
     O42.02   **Full-term premature rupture of membranes, onset of labor within 24 hours of rupture** ♀   M
      Premature rupture of membranes at or after 37 completed weeks of gestation, onset of labor within 24 hours of rupture ◀▥

CHAPTER 15 (O00-O9A)

- O42.1 **Premature rupture of membranes, onset of labor more than 24 hours following rupture**
  - O42.10 **Premature rupture of membranes, onset of labor more than 24 hours following rupture, unspecified weeks of gestation** ♀   M
  - O42.11 **Preterm premature rupture of membranes, onset of labor more than 24 hours following rupture**
    Premature rupture of membranes before 37 completed weeks of gestation
    - O42.111 **Preterm premature rupture of membranes, onset of labor more than 24 hours following rupture, first trimester** ♀   M
    - O42.112 **Preterm premature rupture of membranes, onset of labor more than 24 hours following rupture, second trimester** ♀   M
    - O42.113 **Preterm premature rupture of membranes, onset of labor more than 24 hours following rupture, third trimester** ♀   M
    - O42.119 **Preterm premature rupture of membranes, onset of labor more than 24 hours following rupture, unspecified trimester** ♀   M
  - O42.12 **Full-term premature rupture of membranes, onset of labor more than 24 hours following rupture** ♀   M
    Premature rupture of membranes at or after 37 completed weeks of gestation, onset of labor more than 24 hours following rupture ◄▥
- O42.9 **Premature rupture of membranes, unspecified as to length of time between rupture and onset of labor**
  - O42.90 **Premature rupture of membranes, unspecified as to length of time between rupture and onset of labor, unspecified weeks of gestation** ♀   M
  - O42.91 **Preterm premature rupture of membranes, unspecified as to length of time between rupture and onset of labor**
    Premature rupture of membranes before 37 completed weeks of gestation
    - O42.911 **Preterm premature rupture of membranes, unspecified as to length of time between rupture and onset of labor, first trimester** ♀   M
    - O42.912 **Preterm premature rupture of membranes, unspecified as to length of time between rupture and onset of labor, second trimester** ♀   M
    - O42.913 **Preterm premature rupture of membranes, unspecified as to length of time between rupture and onset of labor, third trimester** ♀   M
    - O42.919 **Preterm premature rupture of membranes, unspecified as to length of time between rupture and onset of labor, unspecified trimester** ♀   M
  - O42.92 **Full-term premature rupture of membranes, unspecified as to length of time between rupture and onset of labor** ♀   M
    Premature rupture of membranes at or after 37 completed weeks of gestation, unspecified as to length of time between rupture and onset of labor ◄▥

- O43 **Placental disorders**
  - **Excludes2**   maternal care for poor fetal growth due to placental insufficiency (O36.5-)
    placenta previa (O44.-)
    placental polyp (O90.89)
    placentitis (O41.14-)
    premature separation of placenta [abruptio placentae] (O45.-)
  - O43.0 **Placental transfusion syndromes**
    - O43.01 **Fetomaternal placental transfusion syndrome**
      Maternofetal placental transfusion syndrome
      - O43.011 **Fetomaternal placental transfusion syndrome, first trimester** ♀   M
      - O43.012 **Fetomaternal placental transfusion syndrome, second trimester** ♀   M
      - O43.013 **Fetomaternal placental transfusion syndrome, third trimester** ♀   M
      - O43.019 **Fetomaternal placental transfusion syndrome, unspecified trimester** ♀   M
    - O43.02 **Fetus-to-fetus placental transfusion syndrome**
      - O43.021 **Fetus-to-fetus placental transfusion syndrome, first trimester** ♀   M
      - O43.022 **Fetus-to-fetus placental transfusion syndrome, second trimester** ♀   M
      - O43.023 **Fetus-to-fetus placental transfusion syndrome, third trimester** ♀   M
      - O43.029 **Fetus-to-fetus placental transfusion syndrome, unspecified trimester** ♀   M
  - O43.1 **Malformation of placenta**
    - O43.10 **Malformation of placenta, unspecified**
      Abnormal placenta NOS
      - O43.101 **Malformation of placenta, unspecified, first trimester** ♀   M
      - O43.102 **Malformation of placenta, unspecified, second trimester** ♀   M
      - O43.103 **Malformation of placenta, unspecified, third trimester** ♀   M
      - O43.109 **Malformation of placenta, unspecified, unspecified trimester** ♀ M
    - O43.11 **Circumvallate placenta**
      - O43.111 **Circumvallate placenta, first trimester** ♀   M
      - O43.112 **Circumvallate placenta, second trimester** ♀   M
      - O43.113 **Circumvallate placenta, third trimester** ♀   M
      - O43.119 **Circumvallate placenta, unspecified trimester** ♀   M
    - O43.12 **Velamentous insertion of umbilical cord**
      - O43.121 **Velamentous insertion of umbilical cord, first trimester** ♀   M
      - O43.122 **Velamentous insertion of umbilical cord, second trimester** ♀   M
      - O43.123 **Velamentous insertion of umbilical cord, third trimester** ♀   M
      - O43.129 **Velamentous insertion of umbilical cord, unspecified trimester** ♀   M
    - O43.19 **Other malformation of placenta**
      - O43.191 **Other malformation of placenta, first trimester** ♀   M
      - O43.192 **Other malformation of placenta, second trimester** ♀   M
      - O43.193 **Other malformation of placenta, third trimester** ♀   M
      - O43.199 **Other malformation of placenta, unspecified trimester** ♀   M

- **O43.2 Morbidly adherent placenta**
  Code also associated third stage postpartum hemorrhage, if applicable (O72.Ø)
  Excludes1 retained placenta (O73.-)
  - **O43.21 Placenta accreta**
    - O43.211 Placenta accreta, first trimester ♀ M
    - O43.212 Placenta accreta, second trimester ♀ M
    - O43.213 Placenta accreta, third trimester ♀ M
    - O43.219 Placenta accreta, unspecified trimester ♀ M
  - **O43.22 Placenta increta**
    - O43.221 Placenta increta, first trimester ♀ M
    - O43.222 Placenta increta, second trimester ♀ M
    - O43.223 Placenta increta, third trimester ♀ M
    - O43.229 Placenta increta, unspecified trimester ♀ M
  - **O43.23 Placenta percreta**
    - O43.231 Placenta percreta, first trimester ♀ M
    - O43.232 Placenta percreta, second trimester ♀ M
    - O43.233 Placenta percreta, third trimester ♀ M
    - O43.239 Placenta percreta, unspecified trimester ♀ M
- **O43.8 Other placental disorders**
  - **O43.81 Placental infarction**
    - O43.811 Placental infarction, first trimester ♀ M
    - O43.812 Placental infarction, second trimester ♀ M
    - O43.813 Placental infarction, third trimester ♀ M
    - O43.819 Placental infarction, unspecified trimester ♀ M
  - **O43.89 Other placental disorders**
    Placental dysfunction
    - O43.891 Other placental disorders, first trimester ♀ M
    - O43.892 Other placental disorders, second trimester ♀ M
    - O43.893 Other placental disorders, third trimester ♀ M
    - O43.899 Other placental disorders, unspecified trimester ♀ M
- **O43.9 Unspecified placental disorder**
  - O43.90 Unspecified placental disorder, unspecified trimester ♀ M
  - O43.91 Unspecified placental disorder, first trimester ♀ M
  - O43.92 Unspecified placental disorder, second trimester ♀ M
  - O43.93 Unspecified placental disorder, third trimester ♀ M
- **O44 Placenta previa**
  - **O44.Ø Complete placenta previa NOS or without hemorrhage** ◀▥
    Placenta previa NOS ◀
    - O44.00 Complete placenta previa NOS or without hemorrhage, unspecified trimester ♀ ◀▥ M
    - O44.Ø1 Complete placenta previa NOS or without hemorrhage, first trimester ♀ ◀▥ M
    - O44.Ø2 Complete placenta previa NOS or without hemorrhage, second trimester ♀ ◀▥ M
    - O44.Ø3 Complete placenta previa NOS or without hemorrhage, third trimester ♀ ◀▥ M

Figure 15-2 A. Marginal placento previa. **B.** Partial placenta previa. **C.** Total placento previa.

Item 15–3 Placenta previa is a condition in which the opening of the cervix is obstructed by the displaced placenta. The three types, marginal, partial, and total, are varying degrees of placenta displacement. Placenta abruption is the premature breaking away of the placenta from the site of the uterine implant before the delivery of the fetus.

- **O44.1 Complete placenta previa with hemorrhage** ◀▥
  Excludes1 labor and delivery complicated by hemorrhage from vasa previa (O69.4)
  - O44.10 Complete placenta previa with hemorrhage, unspecified trimester ♀ ◀▥ M
  - O44.11 Complete placenta previa with hemorrhage, first trimester ♀ ◀▥ M
  - O44.12 Complete placenta previa with hemorrhage, second trimester ♀ ◀▥ M
  - O44.13 Complete placenta previa with hemorrhage, third trimester ♀ ◀▥ M
- **O44.2 Partial placenta previa without hemorrhage** ◀
  Marginal placenta previa, NOS or without hemorrhage ◀
  - O44.20 Partial placenta previa NOS or without hemorrhage, unspecified trimester ♀ ◀ M
  - O44.21 Partial placenta previa NOS or without hemorrhage, first trimester ♀ ◀ M
  - O44.22 Partial placenta previa NOS or without hemorrhage, second trimester ♀ ◀ M
  - O44.23 Partial placenta previa NOS or without hemorrhage, third trimester ♀ ◀ M
- **O44.3 Partial placenta previa with hemorrhage** ◀
  Marginal placenta previa with hemorrhage ◀
  - O44.3Ø Partial placenta previa with hemorrhage, unspecified trimester ♀ ◀ M
  - O44.31 Partial placenta previa with hemorrhage, first trimester ♀ ◀ M
  - O44.32 Partial placenta previa with hemorrhage, second trimester ♀ ◀ M
  - O44.33 Partial placenta previa with hemorrhage, third trimester ♀ ◀ M
- **O44.4 Low lying placenta NOS or without hemorrhage** ◀
  Low implantation of placenta NOS or without hemorrhage ◀
  - O44.40 Low lying placenta NOS or without hemorrhage, unspecified trimester ♀ ◀ M
  - O44.41 Low lying placenta NOS or without hemorrhage, first trimester ♀ ◀ M
  - O44.42 Low lying placenta NOS or without hemorrhage, second trimester ♀ ◀ M
  - O44.43 Low lying placenta NOS or without hemorrhage, third trimester ♀ ◀ M
- **O44.5 Low lying placenta with hemorrhage** ◀
  Low implantation of placenta with hemorrhage ◀
  - O44.5Ø Low lying placenta with hemorrhage, unspecified trimester ♀ ◀ M
  - O44.51 Low lying placenta with hemorrhage, first trimester ♀ ◀ M
  - O44.52 Low lying placenta with hemorrhage, second trimester ♀ ◀ M
  - O44.53 Low lying placenta with hemorrhage, third trimester ♀ ◀ M

CHAPTER 15 (OØØ-O9A)

Figure 15-3 Abruptio placentae is classified according to the grade of separation of the placenta from the uterine wall. **A.** Mild separation in which hemorrhage is internal. **B.** Moderate separation in which there is external hemorrhage. **C.** Severe separation in which there is external hemorrhage and extreme separation.

● **O45**   **Premature separation of placenta [abruptio placentae]**

  ● **O45.0**   **Premature separation of placenta with coagulation defect**

    ● **O45.00**   Premature separation of placenta with coagulation defect, unspecified

        O45.001   Premature separation of placenta with coagulation defect, unspecified, first trimester ♀   M

        O45.002   Premature separation of placenta with coagulation defect, unspecified, second trimester ♀   M

        O45.003   Premature separation of placenta with coagulation defect, unspecified, third trimester ♀   M

        O45.009   Premature separation of placenta with coagulation defect, unspecified, unspecified trimester ♀   M

    ● **O45.01**   Premature separation of placenta with afibrinogenemia

         Premature separation of placenta with hypofibrinogenemia

        O45.011   Premature separation of placenta with afibrinogenemia, first trimester ♀   M

        O45.012   Premature separation of placenta with afibrinogenemia, second trimester ♀ M

        O45.013   Premature separation of placenta with afibrinogenemia, third trimester ♀ M

        O45.019   Premature separation of placenta with afibrinogenemia, unspecified trimester ♀   M

    ● **O45.02**   Premature separation of placenta with disseminated intravascular coagulation

        O45.021   Premature separation of placenta with disseminated intravascular coagulation, first trimester ♀   M

        O45.022   Premature separation of placenta with disseminated intravascular coagulation, second trimester ♀   M

        O45.023   Premature separation of placenta with disseminated intravascular coagulation, third trimester ♀   M

        O45.029   Premature separation of placenta with disseminated intravascular coagulation, unspecified trimester ♀ M

    ● **O45.09**   Premature separation of placenta with other coagulation defect

        O45.091   Premature separation of placenta with other coagulation defect, first trimester ♀   M

        O45.092   Premature separation of placenta with other coagulation defect, second trimester ♀   M

        O45.093   Premature separation of placenta with other coagulation defect, third trimester ♀   M

        O45.099   Premature separation of placenta with other coagulation defect, unspecified trimester ♀   M

  ● **O45.8**   **Other premature separation of placenta**

    ● **O45.8X**   Other premature separation of placenta

        O45.8X1   Other premature separation of placenta, first trimester ♀   M

        O45.8X2   Other premature separation of placenta, second trimester ♀   M

        O45.8X3   Other premature separation of placenta, third trimester ♀   M

        O45.8X9   Other premature separation of placenta, unspecified trimester ♀   M

  ● **O45.9**   **Premature separation of placenta, unspecified**

       Abruptio placentae NOS

        O45.90   Premature separation of placenta, unspecified, unspecified trimester ♀   M

        O45.91   Premature separation of placenta, unspecified, first trimester ♀   M

        O45.92   Premature separation of placenta, unspecified, second trimester ♀   M

        O45.93   Premature separation of placenta, unspecified, third trimester ♀   M

● **O46**   **Antepartum hemorrhage, not elsewhere classified**

    Excludes1   hemorrhage in early pregnancy (O20.-)
                intrapartum hemorrhage NEC (O67.-)
                placenta previa (O44.-)
                premature separation of placenta [abruptio placentae] (O45.-)

  ● **O46.0**   **Antepartum hemorrhage with coagulation defect**

    ● **O46.00**   Antepartum hemorrhage with coagulation defect, unspecified

        O46.001   Antepartum hemorrhage with coagulation defect, unspecified, first trimester ♀   M

        O46.002   Antepartum hemorrhage with coagulation defect, unspecified, second trimester ♀   M

        O46.003   Antepartum hemorrhage with coagulation defect, unspecified, third trimester ♀   M

        O46.009   Antepartum hemorrhage with coagulation defect, unspecified, unspecified trimester ♀   M

    ● **O46.01**   Antepartum hemorrhage with afibrinogenemia

         Antepartum hemorrhage with hypofibrinogenemia

        O46.011   Antepartum hemorrhage with afibrinogenemia, first trimester ♀   M

        O46.012   Antepartum hemorrhage with afibrinogenemia, second trimester ♀ M

        O46.013   Antepartum hemorrhage with afibrinogenemia, third trimester ♀   M

        O46.019   Antepartum hemorrhage with afibrinogenemia, unspecified trimester ♀   M

    ● **O46.02**   Antepartum hemorrhage with disseminated intravascular coagulation

        O46.021   Antepartum hemorrhage with disseminated intravascular coagulation, first trimester ♀   M

        O46.022   Antepartum hemorrhage with disseminated intravascular coagulation, second trimester ♀   M

        O46.023   Antepartum hemorrhage with disseminated intravascular coagulation, third trimester ♀   M

        O46.029   Antepartum hemorrhage with disseminated intravascular coagulation, unspecified trimester ♀ M

◄ New   ◄•• Revised   ~~deleted~~ Deleted   Excludes 1   Excludes 2   Includes   Use additional   Code first   Code also   Unspecified

OGCR Official Guidelines   X Assign placeholder X   ● Use Additional Character(s)   ▷ Manifestation Code   **Coding Clinic**

● **O46.09**   **Antepartum hemorrhage with other coagulation defect**

    O46.091   **Antepartum hemorrhage with other coagulation defect, first trimester** ♀ **M**

    O46.092   **Antepartum hemorrhage with other coagulation defect, second trimester** ♀   **M**

    O46.093   **Antepartum hemorrhage with other coagulation defect, third trimester** ♀ **M**

    O46.099   **Antepartum hemorrhage with other coagulation defect, unspecified trimester** ♀   **M**

● **O46.8**   **Other antepartum hemorrhage**

   ● **O46.8x**   **Other antepartum hemorrhage**

    O46.8x1   **Other antepartum hemorrhage, first trimester** ♀   **M**

    O46.8x2   **Other antepartum hemorrhage, second trimester** ♀   **M**

    O46.8x3   **Other antepartum hemorrhage, third trimester** ♀   **M**

    O46.8x9   **Other antepartum hemorrhage, unspecified trimester** ♀   **M**

● **O46.9**   **Antepartum hemorrhage, unspecified**

    O46.90   **Antepartum hemorrhage, unspecified, unspecified trimester** ♀   **M**

    O46.91   **Antepartum hemorrhage, unspecified, first trimester** ♀   **M**

    O46.92   **Antepartum hemorrhage, unspecified, second trimester** ♀   **M**

    O46.93   **Antepartum hemorrhage, unspecified, third trimester** ♀   **M**

● **O47**   **False labor**

Includes	Braxton Hicks contractions threatened labor
Excludes1	preterm labor (O60.-)

● **O47.0**   **False labor before 37 completed weeks of gestation**

    O47.00   **False labor before 37 completed weeks of gestation, unspecified trimester** ♀   **M**

    O47.02   **False labor before 37 completed weeks of gestation, second trimester** ♀   **M**

    O47.03   **False labor before 37 completed weeks of gestation, third trimester** ♀   **M**

   O47.1   **False labor at or after 37 completed weeks of gestation** ♀   **M**

   O47.9   **False labor, unspecified** ♀   **M**

● **O48**   **Late pregnancy**

   O48.0   **Post-term pregnancy** ♀   **M**
     Pregnancy over 40 completed weeks to 42 completed weeks gestation

   O48.1   **Prolonged pregnancy** ♀   **M**
     Pregnancy which has advanced beyond 42 completed weeks gestation

---

COMPLICATIONS OF LABOR AND DELIVERY (O60-O77)

● **O60**   **Preterm labor**

Includes	onset (spontaneous) of labor before 37 completed weeks of gestation
Excludes1	false labor (O47.0-) threatened labor NOS (O47.0-)

● **O60.0**   **Preterm labor without delivery**

    O60.00   **Preterm labor without delivery, unspecified trimester** ♀   **M**

    O60.02   **Preterm labor without delivery, second trimester** ♀   **M**

    O60.03   **Preterm labor without delivery, third trimester** ♀   **M**

● **O60.1**   **Preterm labor with preterm delivery**

One of the following 7th characters is to be assigned to each code under subcategory O60.1. 7th character 0 is for single gestations and multiple gestations where the fetus is unspecified. 7th characters 1 through 9 are for cases of multiple gestations to identify the fetus for which the code applies. The appropriate code from category O30, Multiple gestation, must also be assigned when assigning a code from subcategory O60.1 that has a 7th character of 1 through 9.

0	not applicable or unspecified
1	fetus 1
2	fetus 2
3	fetus 3
4	fetus 4
5	fetus 5
9	other fetus

Coding Clinic: 2016, Q2, P11

X ● **O60.10**   **Preterm labor with preterm delivery, unspecified trimester** ♀   **M**
     Preterm labor with delivery NOS

X ● **O60.12**   **Preterm labor second trimester with preterm delivery second trimester** ♀   **M**

X ● **O60.13**   **Preterm labor second trimester with preterm delivery third trimester** ♀   **M**

X ● **O60.14**   **Preterm labor third trimester with preterm delivery third trimester** ♀   **M**
     Coding Clinic: 2016, Q2, P10

● **O60.2**   **Term delivery with preterm labor**

One of the following 7th characters is to be assigned to each code under subcategory O60.2. 7th character 0 is for single gestations and multiple gestations where the fetus is unspecified. 7th characters 1 through 9 are for cases of multiple gestations to identify the fetus for which the code applies. The appropriate code from category O30, Multiple gestation, must also be assigned when assigning a code from subcategory O60.2 that has a 7th character of 1 through 9.

0	not applicable or unspecified
1	fetus 1
2	fetus 2
3	fetus 3
4	fetus 4
5	fetus 5
9	other fetus

X ● **O60.20**   **Term delivery with preterm labor, unspecified trimester** ♀   **M**

X ● **O60.22**   **Term delivery with preterm labor, second trimester** ♀   **M**

X ● **O60.23**   **Term delivery with preterm labor, third trimester** ♀   **M**

● **O61**   **Failed induction of labor**

   O61.0   **Failed medical induction of labor** ♀   **M**
     Failed induction (of labor) by oxytocin
     Failed induction (of labor) by prostaglandins

   O61.1   **Failed instrumental induction of labor** ♀   **M**
     Failed mechanical induction (of labor)
     Failed surgical induction (of labor)

   O61.8   **Other failed induction of labor** ♀   **M**

   O61.9   **Failed induction of labor, unspecified** ♀   **M**

● **O62**   **Abnormalities of forces of labor**

    O62.0   **Primary inadequate contractions** ♀   M
         Failure of cervical dilatation
         Primary hypotonic uterine dysfunction
         Uterine inertia during latent phase of labor

    O62.1   **Secondary uterine inertia** ♀   M
         Arrested active phase of labor
         Secondary hypotonic uterine dysfunction

    O62.2   **Other uterine inertia** ♀   M
         Atony of uterus without hemorrhage
         Atony of uterus NOS
         Desultory labor
         Hypotonic uterine dysfunction NOS
         Irregular labor
         Poor contractions
         Slow slope active phase of labor
         Uterine inertia NOS

         Excludes1   atony of uterus with hemorrhage
                         (postpartum) (O72.1)
                   postpartum atony of uterus without
                         hemorrhage (O75.89)

    O62.3   **Precipitate labor** ♀   M

    O62.4   **Hypertonic, incoordinate, and prolonged uterine**
             contractions ♀   M
         Cervical spasm
         Contraction ring dystocia
         Dyscoordinate labor
         Hour-glass contraction of uterus
         Hypertonic uterine dysfunction
         Incoordinate uterine action
         Tetanic contractions
         Uterine dystocia NOS
         Uterine spasm

         Excludes1   dystocia (fetal) (maternal) NOS (O66.9)

    O62.8   **Other abnormalities of forces of labor** ♀   M
    O62.9   **Abnormality of forces of labor, unspecified** ♀   M

● **O63**   **Long labor**
    O63.0   **Prolonged first stage (of labor)** ♀   M
    O63.1   **Prolonged second stage (of labor)** ♀   M
    O63.2   **Delayed delivery of second twin, triplet, etc.** ♀   M
    O63.9   **Long labor, unspecified** ♀   M
         Prolonged labor NOS

● **O64**   **Obstructed labor due to malposition and malpresentation of**
      fetus

         One of the following 7th characters is to be assigned to each
         code under category O64. 7th character Ø is for single
         gestations and multiple gestations where the fetus is
         unspecified. 7th characters 1 through 9 are for cases of
         multiple gestations to identify the fetus for which the code
         applies. The appropriate code from category O30, Multiple
         gestation, must also be assigned when assigning a code
         from category O64 that has a 7th character of 1 through 9.

Ø	not applicable or unspecified
1	fetus 1
2	fetus 2
3	fetus 3
4	fetus 4
5	fetus 5
9	other fetus

X ● **O64.0**   **Obstructed labor due to incomplete rotation of fetal**
             head ♀   M
         Deep transverse arrest
         Obstructed labor due to persistent occipitoiliac
            (position)
         Obstructed labor due to persistent occipitoposterior
            (position)
         Obstructed labor due to persistent occipitosacral
            (position)
         Obstructed labor due to persistent occipitotransverse
            (position)

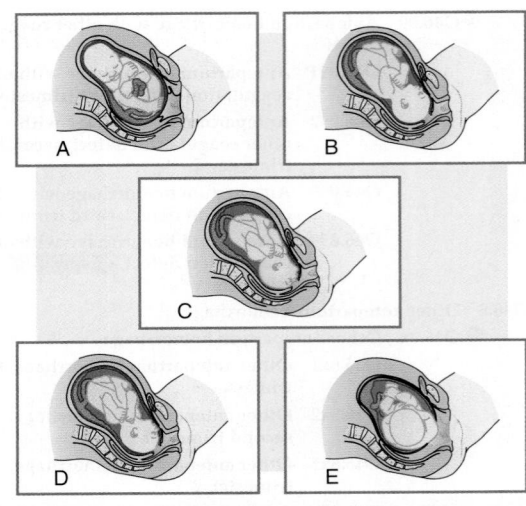

Figure 15-4   Five types of malposition and malpresentation of the fetus:
A. Breech. **B.** Vertex. **C.** Face. **D.** Brow. **E.** Shoulder.

X ● **O64.1**   **Obstructed labor due to breech presentation** ♀   M
         Obstructed labor due to buttocks presentation
         Obstructed labor due to complete breech presentation
         Obstructed labor due to frank breech presentation

X ● **O64.2**   **Obstructed labor due to face presentation** ♀   M
         Obstructed labor due to chin presentation

X ● **O64.3**   **Obstructed labor due to brow presentation** ♀   M
X ● **O64.4**   **Obstructed labor due to shoulder presentation** ♀   M
         Prolapsed arm

         Excludes1   impacted shoulders (O66.0)
                    shoulder dystocia (O66.0)

X ● **O64.5**   **Obstructed labor due to compound presentation** ♀   M
X ● **O64.8**   **Obstructed labor due to other malposition and**
             malpresentation ♀   M
         Obstructed labor due to footling presentation
         Obstructed labor due to incomplete breech presentation

X ● **O64.9**   **Obstructed labor due to malposition and**
             malpresentation, unspecified ♀   M

● **O65**   **Obstructed labor due to maternal pelvic abnormality**
    O65.0   **Obstructed labor due to deformed pelvis** ♀   M
    O65.1   **Obstructed labor due to generally contracted pelvis** ♀   M
    O65.2   **Obstructed labor due to pelvic inlet contraction** ♀   M
    O65.3   **Obstructed labor due to pelvic outlet and mid-cavity**
             contraction ♀   M
    O65.4   **Obstructed labor due to fetopelvic disproportion,**
             unspecified ♀   M

         Excludes1   dystocia due to abnormality of fetus
                    (O66.2-O66.3)

    O65.5   **Obstructed labor due to abnormality of maternal pelvic**
             organs ♀   M
         Obstructed labor due to conditions listed in O34.-

         Use additional code to identify abnormality of pelvic
            organs O34.-

    O65.8   **Obstructed labor due to other maternal pelvic**
             abnormalities ♀   M
    O65.9   **Obstructed labor due to maternal pelvic abnormality,**
             unspecified ♀   M

◀ New   ⬅ Revised   ~~deleted~~ Deleted   Excludes 1   Excludes 2   Includes   Use additional   Code first   Code also   Unspecified

1116   **OGCR** Official Guidelines   X Assign placeholder X   ● Use Additional Character(s)   ▶ Manifestation Code   **Coding Clinic**

Figure 15-5   Hydrocephalic fetus causing disproportion.

● **O66**   **Other obstructed labor**

   O66.0   **Obstructed labor due to shoulder dystocia** ♀   M
        Impacted shoulders

   O66.1   **Obstructed labor due to locked twins** ♀   M

   O66.2   **Obstructed labor due to unusually large fetus** ♀   M

   O66.3   **Obstructed labor due to other abnormalities of fetus** ♀ M
        Dystocia due to fetal ascites
        Dystocia due to fetal hydrops
        Dystocia due to fetal meningomyelocele
        Dystocia due to fetal sacral teratoma
        Dystocia due to fetal tumor
        Dystocia due to hydrocephalic fetus
        Use additional code to identify cause of obstruction

● **O66.4**   **Failed trial of labor**

   O66.40   **Failed trial of labor, unspecified** ♀   M

   O66.41   **Failed attempted vaginal birth after previous cesarean delivery** ♀   M
        Code first rupture of uterus, if applicable (O71.0-, O71.1)

   O66.5   **Attempted application of vacuum extractor and forceps** ♀   M
        Attempted application of vacuum or forceps, with subsequent delivery by forceps or cesarean delivery

   O66.6   **Obstructed labor due to other multiple fetuses** ♀   M

   O66.8   **Other specified obstructed labor** ♀   M
        Use additional code to identify cause of obstruction

   O66.9   **Obstructed labor, unspecified** ♀   M
        Dystocia NOS
        Fetal dystocia NOS
        Maternal dystocia NOS

● **O67**   **Labor and delivery complicated by intrapartum hemorrhage, not elsewhere classified**

   Excludes1   antepartum hemorrhage NEC (O46.-)
          placenta previa (O44.-)
          premature separation of placenta [abruptio placentae] (O45.-)

   Excludes2   postpartum hemorrhage (O72.-)

   O67.0   **Intrapartum hemorrhage with coagulation defect** ♀   M
        Intrapartum hemorrhage (excessive) associated with afibrinogenemia
        Intrapartum hemorrhage (excessive) associated with disseminated intravascular coagulation
        Intrapartum hemorrhage (excessive) associated with hyperfibrinolysis
        Intrapartum hemorrhage (excessive) associated with hypofibrinogenemia

   O67.8   **Other intrapartum hemorrhage** ♀   M
        Excessive intrapartum hemorrhage

   O67.9   **Intrapartum hemorrhage, unspecified** ♀   M

O68   **Labor and delivery complicated by abnormality of fetal acid-base balance** ♀   M
        Fetal acidemia complicating labor and delivery
        Fetal acidosis complicating labor and delivery
        Fetal alkalosis complicating labor and delivery
        Fetal metabolic acidemia complicating labor and delivery

   Excludes1   fetal stress NOS (O77.9)
          labor and delivery complicated by electrocardiographic evidence of fetal stress (O77.8)
          labor and delivery complicated by ultrasonic evidence of fetal stress (O77.8)

   Excludes2   abnormality in fetal heart rate or rhythm (O76)
          labor and delivery complicated by meconium in amniotic fluid (O77.0)

● **O69**   **Labor and delivery complicated by umbilical cord complications**

   One of the following 7th characters is to be assigned to each code under category O69. 7th character Ø is for single gestations and multiple gestations where the fetus is unspecified. 7th characters 1 through 9 are for cases of multiple gestations to identify the fetus for which the code applies. The appropriate code from category O3Ø, Multiple gestation, must also be assigned when assigning a code from category O69 that has a 7th character of 1 through 9.

Ø	not applicable or unspecified
1	fetus 1
2	fetus 2
3	fetus 3
4	fetus 4
5	fetus 5
9	other fetus

X ● **O69.0**   **Labor and delivery complicated by prolapse of cord** ♀   M

X ● **O69.1**   **Labor and delivery complicated by cord around neck, with compression** ♀   M
     Excludes1   labor and delivery complicated by cord around neck, without compression (O69.81)

X ● **O69.2**   **Labor and delivery complicated by other cord entanglement, with compression** ♀   M
        Labor and delivery complicated by compression of cord NOS
        Labor and delivery complicated by entanglement of cords of twins in monoamniotic sac
        Labor and delivery complicated by knot in cord
     Excludes1   labor and delivery complicated by other cord entanglement, without compression (O69.82)

X ● **O69.3**   **Labor and delivery complicated by short cord** ♀   M

X ● **O69.4**   **Labor and delivery complicated by vasa previa** ♀   M
        Labor and delivery complicated by hemorrhage from vasa previa

X ● **O69.5**   **Labor and delivery complicated by vascular lesion of cord** ♀   M
        Labor and delivery complicated by cord bruising
        Labor and delivery complicated by cord hematoma
        Labor and delivery complicated by thrombosis of umbilical vessels

● **O69.8**   **Labor and delivery complicated by other cord complications**

   X ● **O69.81**   **Labor and delivery complicated by cord around neck, without compression** ♀   M

   X ● **O69.82**   **Labor and delivery complicated by other cord entanglement, without compression** ♀   M

   X ● **O69.89**   **Labor and delivery complicated by other cord complications** ♀   M

X ● **O69.9**   **Labor and delivery complicated by cord complication, unspecified** ♀   M

● **O70**   **Perineal laceration during delivery**

   Includes   episiotomy extended by laceration
   Excludes1   obstetric high vaginal laceration alone (O71.4)

   O70.0   **First degree perineal laceration during delivery** ♀   M
        Perineal laceration, rupture or tear involving fourchette during delivery
        Perineal laceration, rupture or tear involving labia during delivery
        Perineal laceration, rupture or tear involving skin during delivery
        Perineal laceration, rupture or tear involving vagina during delivery
        Perineal laceration, rupture or tear involving vulva during delivery
        Slight perineal laceration, rupture or tear during delivery

CHAPTER 15 (O00-O9A)

Vaginal   Urethral
opening   opening

A
B
C
D

Anus

Figure 15-6 Perineal lacerations: **A.** First-degree is laceration of superficial tissues. **B.** Second-degree is limited to the pelvic floor and may involve the perineal or vaginal muscles. **C.** Third-degree involves the anal sphincter. **D.** Fourth-degree involves anal or rectal mucosa.

O70.1   **Second degree perineal laceration during delivery** ♀   M
Perineal laceration, rupture or tear during delivery as in O70.0, also involving pelvic floor
Perineal laceration, rupture or tear during delivery as in O70.0, also involving perineal muscles
Perineal laceration, rupture or tear during delivery as in O70.0, also involving vaginal muscles
Excludes1   perineal laceration involving anal sphincter (O70.2)
Coding Clinic: 2016, Q2, P34

● O70.2   **Third degree perineal laceration during delivery**
Perineal laceration, rupture or tear during delivery as in O70.1, also involving anal sphincter
Perineal laceration, rupture or tear during delivery as in O70.1, also involving rectovaginal septum
Perineal laceration, rupture or tear during delivery as in O70.1, also involving sphincter NOS
Excludes1   anal sphincter tear during delivery without third degree perineal laceration (O70.4)
perineal laceration involving anal or rectal mucosa (O70.3)

O70.20   **Third degree perineal laceration during delivery, unspecified** ♀ ◀   M
O70.21   **Third degree perineal laceration during delivery, IIIa** ♀ ◀   M
Third degree perineal laceration during delivery with less than 50% of external anal sphincter (EAS) thickness torn ◀
O70.22   **Third degree perineal laceration during delivery, IIIb** ♀ ◀   M
Third degree perineal laceration during delivery with more than 50% external anal sphincter (EAS) thickness torn ◀
O70.23   **Third degree perineal laceration during delivery, IIIc** ♀ ◀   M
Third degree perineal laceration during delivery with both external anal sphincter (EAS) and internal anal sphincter (IAS) torn ◀

O70.3   **Fourth degree perineal laceration during delivery** ♀   M
Perineal laceration, rupture or tear during delivery as in O70.2, also involving anal mucosa
Perineal laceration, rupture or tear during delivery as in O70.2, also involving rectal mucosa

O70.4   **Anal sphincter tear complicating delivery, not associated with third degree laceration** ♀   M
Excludes1   anal sphincter tear with third degree perineal laceration (O70.2)

O70.9   **Perineal laceration during delivery, unspecified** ♀   M

● O71   **Other obstetric trauma**
Includes   obstetric damage from instruments
● O71.0   **Rupture of uterus (spontaneous) before onset of labor**
Excludes1   disruption of (current) cesarean delivery wound (O90.0)
laceration of uterus, NEC (O71.81)
O71.00   **Rupture of uterus before onset of labor, unspecified trimester** ♀   M
O71.02   **Rupture of uterus before onset of labor, second trimester** ♀   M
O71.03   **Rupture of uterus before onset of labor, third trimester** ♀   M
O71.1   **Rupture of uterus during labor** ♀   M
Rupture of uterus not stated as occurring before onset of labor
Excludes1   disruption of cesarean delivery wound (O90.0)
laceration of uterus, NEC (O71.81)
O71.2   **Postpartum inversion of uterus** ♀   M
O71.3   **Obstetric laceration of cervix** ♀   M
Annular detachment of cervix
O71.4   **Obstetric high vaginal laceration alone** ♀   M
Laceration of vaginal wall without perineal laceration
Excludes1   obstetric high vaginal laceration with perineal laceration (O70.-)
O71.5   **Other obstetric injury to pelvic organs** ♀   M
Obstetric injury to bladder
Obstetric injury to urethra
Excludes2   obstetric periurethral trauma (O71.82)
O71.6   **Obstetric damage to pelvic joints and ligaments** ♀   M
Obstetric avulsion of inner symphyseal cartilage
Obstetric damage to coccyx
Obstetric traumatic separation of symphysis (pubis)
O71.7   **Obstetric hematoma of pelvis** ♀   M
Obstetric hematoma of perineum
Obstetric hematoma of vagina
Obstetric hematoma of vulva
● O71.8   **Other specified obstetric trauma**
O71.81   **Laceration of uterus, not elsewhere classified** ♀   M
O71.82   **Other specified trauma to perineum and vulva** ♀   M
Obstetric periurethral trauma
O71.89   **Other specified obstetric trauma** ♀   M
O71.9   **Obstetric trauma, unspecified** ♀   M

● O72   **Postpartum hemorrhage**
Includes   hemorrhage after delivery of fetus or infant
O72.0   **Third-stage hemorrhage** ♀   M
Hemorrhage associated with retained, trapped or adherent placenta
Retained placenta NOS
Code also type of adherent placenta (O43.2-)
O72.1   **Other immediate postpartum hemorrhage** ♀   M
Hemorrhage following delivery of placenta
Postpartum hemorrhage (atonic) NOS
Uterine atony with hemorrhage
Excludes1   uterine atony NOS (O62.2)
uterine atony without hemorrhage (O62.2)
postpartum atony of uterus without hemorrhage (O75.89)
O72.2   **Delayed and secondary postpartum hemorrhage** ♀   M
Hemorrhage associated with retained portions of placenta or membranes after the first 24 hours following delivery of placenta
Retained products of conception NOS, following delivery
O72.3   **Postpartum coagulation defects** ♀   M
Postpartum afibrinogenemia
Postpartum fibrinolysis

◀ New   ◀━ Revised   d̶e̶l̶e̶t̶e̶d̶ Deleted   Excludes 1   Excludes 2   Includes   Use additional   Code first   Code also   Unspecified
OGCR Official Guidelines   X Assign placeholder X   ▶ Use Additional Character(s)   ▶ Manifestation Code   Coding Clinic
1118

CHAPTER 15 (O00-O9A)

● **O73** **Retained placenta and membranes, without hemorrhage**
   Excludes1   placenta accreta (O43.21-)
                placenta increta (O43.22-)
                placenta percreta (O43.23-)
  O73.0 **Retained placenta without hemorrhage** ♀   M
       Adherent placenta, without hemorrhage
       Trapped placenta without hemorrhage
  O73.1 **Retained portions of placenta and membranes, without hemorrhage** ♀   M
       Retained products of conception following delivery, without hemorrhage

● **O74** **Complications of anesthesia during labor and delivery**
   Includes   maternal complications arising from the administration of a general, regional or local anesthetic, analgesic or other sedation during labor and delivery
  Use additional code, if applicable, to identify specific complication
  O74.0 **Aspiration pneumonitis due to anesthesia during labor and delivery** ♀   M
       Inhalation of stomach contents or secretions NOS due to anesthesia during labor and delivery
       Mendelson's syndrome due to anesthesia during labor and delivery
  O74.1 **Other pulmonary complications of anesthesia during labor and delivery** ♀   M
  O74.2 **Cardiac complications of anesthesia during labor and delivery** ♀   M
  O74.3 **Central nervous system complications of anesthesia during labor and delivery** ♀   M
  O74.4 **Toxic reaction to local anesthesia during labor and delivery** ♀   M
  O74.5 **Spinal and epidural anesthesia-induced headache during labor and delivery** ♀   M
  O74.6 **Other complications of spinal and epidural anesthesia during labor and delivery** ♀   M
  O74.7 **Failed or difficult intubation for anesthesia during labor and delivery** ♀   M
  O74.8 **Other complications of anesthesia during labor and delivery** ♀   M
  O74.9 **Complication of anesthesia during labor and delivery, unspecified** ♀   M

● **O75** **Other complications of labor and delivery, not elsewhere classified**
   Excludes2   puerperal (postpartum) infection (O86.-)
                puerperal (postpartum) sepsis (O85)
  O75.0 **Maternal distress during labor and delivery** ♀   M
  O75.1 **Shock during or following labor and delivery** ♀   M
       Obstetric shock following labor and delivery
  O75.2 **Pyrexia during labor, not elsewhere classified** ♀   M
  O75.3 **Other infection during labor** ♀   M
       Sepsis during labor
       Use additional code (B95-B97), to identify infectious agent
  O75.4 **Other complications of obstetric surgery and procedures** ♀   M
       Cardiac arrest following obstetric surgery or procedures
       Cardiac failure following obstetric surgery or procedures
       Cerebral anoxia following obstetric surgery or procedures
       Pulmonary edema following obstetric surgery or procedures
       Use additional code to identify specific complication
   Excludes2   complications of anesthesia during labor and delivery (O74.-)
                disruption of obstetrical (surgical) wound (O90.0-O90.1)
                hematoma of obstetrical (surgical) wound (O90.2)
                infection of obstetrical (surgical) wound (O86.0)

  O75.5 **Delayed delivery after artificial rupture of membranes** ♀   M
● **O75.8** **Other specified complications of labor and delivery**
  O75.81 **Maternal exhaustion complicating labor and delivery** ♀   M
  O75.82 **Onset (spontaneous) of labor after 37 completed weeks of gestation but before 39 completed weeks gestation, with delivery by (planned) cesarean section** ♀   M
       Delivery by (planned) cesarean section occurring after 37 completed weeks of gestation but before 39 completed weeks gestation due to (spontaneous) onset of labor
       Code first to specify reason for planned cesarean section such as:
       cephalopelvic disproportion (normally formed fetus) (O33.9)
       previous cesarean delivery (O34.21)
  O75.89 **Other specified complications of labor and delivery** ♀   M
  O75.9 **Complication of labor and delivery, unspecified** ♀   M

O76 **Abnormality in fetal heart rate and rhythm complicating labor and delivery** ♀   M
       Depressed fetal heart rate tones complicating labor and delivery
       Fetal bradycardia complicating labor and delivery
       Fetal heart rate decelerations complicating labor and delivery
       Fetal heart rate irregularity complicating labor and delivery
       Fetal heart rate abnormal variability complicating labor and delivery
       Fetal tachycardia complicating labor and delivery
       Non-reassuring fetal heart rate or rhythm complicating labor and delivery
   Excludes1   fetal stress NOS (O77.9)
                labor and delivery complicated by electrocardiographic evidence of fetal stress (O77.8)
                labor and delivery complicated by ultrasonic evidence of fetal stress (O77.8)
   Excludes2   fetal metabolic acidemia (O68)
                other fetal stress (O77.0-O77.1)

● **O77** **Other fetal stress complicating labor and delivery**
  O77.0 **Labor and delivery complicated by meconium in amniotic fluid** ♀   M
  O77.1 **Fetal stress in labor or delivery due to drug administration** ♀   M
  O77.8 **Labor and delivery complicated by other evidence of fetal stress** ♀   M
       Labor and delivery complicated by electrocardiographic evidence of fetal stress
       Labor and delivery complicated by ultrasonic evidence of fetal stress
   Excludes1   abnormality of fetal acid-base balance (O68)
                abnormality in fetal heart rate or rhythm (O76)
                fetal metabolic acidemia (O68)
  O77.9 **Labor and delivery complicated by fetal stress, unspecified** ♀   M
   Excludes1   abnormality of fetal acid-base balance (O68)
                abnormality in fetal heart rate or rhythm (O76)
                fetal metabolic acidemia (O68)

CHAPTER 15 (O00-O9A)

CHAPTER 15 (O00–O9A)

Figure 15-7 The four stages of normal delivery: **I.** Lightening, which occurs 2 to 4 weeks before birth, at which time the fetus turns with head toward the vagina. **II.** Regular contractions begin, the amniotic sac ruptures, and dilation is complete. **III.** Delivery of the head and rotation. **IV.** Expulsion of placenta.

OGCR Section I.C., Chapter 15.n.

Normal Delivery, Code O80

1) Encounter for full term uncomplicated delivery

Code O80 should be assigned when a woman is admitted for a full-term normal delivery and delivers a single, healthy infant without any complications antepartum, during the delivery, or postpartum during the delivery episode. Code O80 is always a principal diagnosis. It is not to be used if any other code from chapter 15 is needed to describe a current complication of the antenatal, delivery, or perinatal period. Additional codes from other chapters may be used with code O80 if they are not related to or are in any way complicating the pregnancy.

2) Uncomplicated delivery with resolved antepartum complication

Code O80 may be used if the patient had a complication at some point during the pregnancy, but the complication is not present at the time of the admission for delivery.

3) Outcome of delivery for O80

Z37.0, Single live brith, is the only outcome of delivery code appropriate for use with O80.

ENCOUNTER FOR DELIVERY (O80–O82)

O80 Encounter for full-term uncomplicated delivery ♀   M
Delivery requiring minimal or no assistance, with or without episiotomy, without fetal manipulation [e.g., rotation version] or instrumentation [forceps] of a spontaneous, cephalic, vaginal, full-term, single, live-born infant. This code is for use as a single diagnosis code and is not to be used with any other code from chapter 15.
Use additional code to indicate outcome of delivery (Z37.0)

O82 Encounter for cesarean delivery without indication ♀   M
Use additional code to indicate outcome of delivery (Z37.0)

COMPLICATIONS PREDOMINANTLY RELATED TO THE PUERPERIUM (O85–O92)

Excludes2   mental and behavioral disorders associated with the puerperium (F53)
obstetrical tetanus (A34)
puerperal osteomalacia (M83.0)

O85 Puerperal sepsis ♀   M
Postpartum sepsis
Puerperal peritonitis
Puerperal pyemia
Use additional code (B95–B97), to identify infectious agent
Use additional code (R65.2-) to identify severe sepsis, if applicable
Excludes1   fever of unknown origin following delivery (O86.4)
genital tract infection following delivery (O86.1-)
obstetric pyemic and septic embolism (O88.3-)
puerperal septic thrombophlebitis (O86.81)
urinary tract infection following delivery (O86.2-)
Excludes2   sepsis during labor (O75.3)

● **O86 Other puerperal infections**
Use additional code (B95–B97), to identify infectious agent
Excludes2   infection during labor (O75.3)
obstetrical tetanus (A34)

O86.0 Infection of obstetric surgical wound ♀   M
Infected cesarean delivery wound following delivery
Infected perineal repair following delivery

● **O86.1 Other infection of genital tract following delivery**
O86.11 Cervicitis following delivery ♀   M
O86.12 Endometritis following delivery ♀   M
O86.13 Vaginitis following delivery ♀   M
O86.19 Other infection of genital tract following delivery ♀   M

● **O86.2 Urinary tract infection following delivery**
O86.20 Urinary tract infection following delivery, unspecified ♀   M
Puerperal urinary tract infection NOS
O86.21 Infection of kidney following delivery ♀   M
O86.22 Infection of bladder following delivery ♀   M
Infection of urethra following delivery
O86.29 Other urinary tract infection following delivery ♀   M

O86.4 Pyrexia of unknown origin following delivery ♀   M
Puerperal infection NOS following delivery
Puerperal pyrexia NOS following delivery
Excludes2   pyrexia during labor (O75.2)

● **O86.8 Other specified puerperal infections**
O86.81 Puerperal septic thrombophlebitis ♀   M
O86.89 Other specified puerperal infections ♀   M

● **O87 Venous complications and hemorrhoids in the puerperium**
Includes   venous complications in labor, delivery and the puerperium
Excludes2   obstetric embolism (O88.-)
puerperal septic thrombophlebitis (O86.81)
venous complications in pregnancy (O22.-)

O87.0 Superficial thrombophlebitis in the puerperium ♀   M
Puerperal phlebitis NOS
Puerperal thrombosis NOS

O87.1 Deep phlebothrombosis in the puerperium ♀   M
Deep vein thrombosis, postpartum
Pelvic thrombophlebitis, postpartum
Use additional code to identify the deep vein thrombosis (I82.4-, I82.5-, I82.62-. I82.72-)
Use additional code, if applicable, for associated long-term (current) use of anticoagulants (Z79.01)

◀ New   ◀▥ Revised   ~~deleted~~ Deleted   Excludes 1   Excludes 2   Includes   Use additional   Code first   Code also   Unspecified

1120   OGCR Official Guidelines   X Assign placeholder X   ● Use Additional Character(s)   ▶ Manifestation Code   **Coding Clinic**

O87.2   **Hemorrhoids in the puerperium** ♀   M
O87.3   **Cerebral venous thrombosis in the puerperium** ♀   M
     Cerebrovenous sinus thrombosis in the puerperium
O87.4   **Varicose veins of lower extremity in the puerperium** ♀   M
O87.8   **Other venous complications in the puerperium** ♀   M
     Genital varices in the puerperium
O87.9   **Venous complication in the puerperium, unspecified** ♀   M
     Puerperal phlebopathy NOS

O88   **Obstetric embolism**
   Excludes1   embolism complicating abortion NOS (O03.2)
     embolism complicating ectopic or molar pregnancy (O08.2)
     embolism complicating failed attempted abortion (O07.2)
     embolism complicating induced abortion (O04.7)
     embolism complicating spontaneous abortion (O03.2, O03.7)

 ● **O88.0   Obstetric air embolism**
   ● **O88.01   Obstetric air embolism in pregnancy**
      O88.011   **Air embolism in pregnancy, first trimester** ♀   M
      O88.012   **Air embolism in pregnancy, second trimester** ♀   M
      O88.013   **Air embolism in pregnancy, third trimester** ♀   M
      O88.019   **Air embolism in pregnancy, unspecified trimester** ♀   M
    O88.02   **Air embolism in childbirth** ♀   M
    O88.03   **Air embolism in the puerperium** ♀   M
 ● **O88.1   Amniotic fluid embolism**
     Anaphylactoid syndrome in pregnancy
   ● **O88.11   Amniotic fluid embolism in pregnancy**
      O88.111   **Amniotic fluid embolism in pregnancy, first trimester** ♀   M
      O88.112   **Amniotic fluid embolism in pregnancy, second trimester** ♀   M
      O88.113   **Amniotic fluid embolism in pregnancy, third trimester** ♀   M
      O88.119   **Amniotic fluid embolism in pregnancy, unspecified trimester** ♀   M
    O88.12   **Amniotic fluid embolism in childbirth** ♀   M
    O88.13   **Amniotic fluid embolism in the puerperium** ♀   M
 ● **O88.2   Obstetric thromboembolism**
   ● **O88.21   Thromboembolism in pregnancy**
     Obstetric (pulmonary) embolism NOS
      O88.211   **Thromboembolism in pregnancy, first trimester** ♀   M
      O88.212   **Thromboembolism in pregnancy, second trimester** ♀   M
      O88.213   **Thromboembolism in pregnancy, third trimester** ♀   M
      O88.219   **Thromboembolism in pregnancy, unspecified trimester** ♀   M
    O88.22   **Thromboembolism in childbirth** ♀   M
    O88.23   **Thromboembolism in the puerperium** ♀   M
     Puerperal (pulmonary) embolism NOS

 ● **O88.3   Obstetric pyemic and septic embolism**
   ● **O88.31   Pyemic and septic embolism in pregnancy**
      O88.311   **Pyemic and septic embolism in pregnancy, first trimester** ♀   M
      O88.312   **Pyemic and septic embolism in pregnancy, second trimester** ♀   M
      O88.313   **Pyemic and septic embolism in pregnancy, third trimester** ♀   M
      O88.319   **Pyemic and septic embolism in pregnancy, unspecified trimester** ♀   M
    O88.32   **Pyemic and septic embolism in childbirth** ♀   M
    O88.33   **Pyemic and septic embolism in the puerperium** ♀   M
 ● **O88.8   Other obstetric embolism**
     Obstetric fat embolism
   ● **O88.81   Other embolism in pregnancy**
      O88.811   **Other embolism in pregnancy, first trimester** ♀   M
      O88.812   **Other embolism in pregnancy, second trimester** ♀   M
      O88.813   **Other embolism in pregnancy, third trimester** ♀   M
      O88.819   **Other embolism in pregnancy, unspecified trimester** ♀   M
    O88.82   **Other embolism in childbirth** ♀   M
    O88.83   **Other embolism in the puerperium** ♀   M

● O89   **Complications of anesthesia during the puerperium**
   Includes   maternal complications arising from the administration of a general, regional or local anesthetic, analgesic or other sedation during the puerperium
   Use additional code, if applicable, to identify specific complication
 ● **O89.0   Pulmonary complications of anesthesia during the puerperium**
    O89.01   **Aspiration pneumonitis due to anesthesia during the puerperium** ♀   M
     Inhalation of stomach contents or secretions NOS due to anesthesia during the puerperium
     Mendelson's syndrome due to anesthesia during the puerperium
    O89.09   **Other pulmonary complications of anesthesia during the puerperium** ♀   M
  O89.1   **Cardiac complications of anesthesia during the puerperium** ♀   M
  O89.2   **Central nervous system complications of anesthesia during the puerperium** ♀   M
  O89.3   **Toxic reaction to local anesthesia during the puerperium** ♀   M
  O89.4   **Spinal and epidural anesthesia-induced headache during the puerperium** ♀   M
  O89.5   **Other complications of spinal and epidural anesthesia during the puerperium** ♀   M
  O89.6   **Failed or difficult intubation for anesthesia during the puerperium** ♀   M
  O89.8   **Other complications of anesthesia during the puerperium** ♀   M
  O89.9   **Complication of anesthesia during the puerperium, unspecified** ♀   M

CHAPTER 15 (O00-O9A)

● O90   Complications of the puerperium, not elsewhere classified

O90.0   Disruption of cesarean delivery wound ♀   M
: Dehiscence of cesarean delivery wound

     Excludes1   rupture of uterus (spontaneous) before onset of labor (O71.0-)
                   rupture of uterus during labor (O71.1)

O90.1   Disruption of perineal obstetric wound ♀   M
: Disruption of wound of episiotomy
Disruption of wound of perineal laceration
Secondary perineal tear

O90.2   Hematoma of obstetric wound ♀   M

O90.3   Peripartum cardiomyopathy ♀   M
: Conditions in I42.- arising during pregnancy and the puerperium

     Excludes1   pre-existing heart disease complicating pregnancy and the puerperium (O99.4-)

O90.4   Postpartum acute kidney failure ♀   M
: Hepatorenal syndrome following labor and delivery

O90.5   Postpartum thyroiditis ♀   M

O90.6   Postpartum mood disturbance ♀   M
: Postpartum blues   Postpartum sadness
Postpartum dysphoria

     Excludes1   postpartum depression (F53)
                   puerperal psychosis (F53)

● O90.8   Other complications of the puerperium, not elsewhere classified

O90.81   Anemia of the puerperium ♀   M
: Postpartum anemia NOS

     Excludes1   pre-existing anemia complicating the puerperium (O99.03)

O90.89   Other complications of the puerperium, not elsewhere classified ♀   M
: Placental polyp

O90.9   Complication of the puerperium, unspecified ♀   M

● O91   Infections of breast associated with pregnancy, the puerperium and lactation

     Use additional code to identify infection

● O91.0   Infection of nipple associated with pregnancy, the puerperium and lactation

● O91.01   Infection of nipple associated with pregnancy
: Gestational abscess of nipple

O91.011   Infection of nipple associated with pregnancy, first trimester ♀   M

O91.012   Infection of nipple associated with pregnancy, second trimester ♀   M

O91.013   Infection of nipple associated with pregnancy, third trimester ♀   M

O91.019   Infection of nipple associated with pregnancy, unspecified trimester ♀   M

O91.02   Infection of nipple associated with the puerperium ♀   M
: Puerperal abscess of nipple

O91.03   Infection of nipple associated with lactation ♀ M
: Abscess of nipple associated with lactation

● O91.1   Abscess of breast associated with pregnancy, the puerperium and lactation

● O91.11   Abscess of breast associated with pregnancy
: Gestational mammary abscess
Gestational purulent mastitis
Gestational subareolar abscess

O91.111   Abscess of breast associated with pregnancy, first trimester ♀   M

O91.112   Abscess of breast associated with pregnancy, second trimester ♀   M

O91.113   Abscess of breast associated with pregnancy, third trimester ♀   M

O91.119   Abscess of breast associated with pregnancy, unspecified trimester ♀   M

O91.12   Abscess of breast associated with the puerperium ♀   M
: Puerperal mammary abscess
Puerperal purulent mastitis
Puerperal subareolar abscess

O91.13   Abscess of breast associated with lactation ♀   M
: Mammary abscess associated with lactation
Purulent mastitis associated with lactation
Subareolar abscess associated with lactation

● O91.2   Nonpurulent mastitis associated with pregnancy, the puerperium and lactation

● O91.21   Nonpurulent mastitis associated with pregnancy
: Gestational interstitial mastitis
Gestational lymphangitis of breast
Gestational mastitis NOS
Gestational parenchymatous mastitis

O91.211   Nonpurulent mastitis associated with pregnancy, first trimester ♀   M

O91.212   Nonpurulent mastitis associated with pregnancy, second trimester ♀   M

O91.213   Nonpurulent mastitis associated with pregnancy, third trimester ♀   M

O91.219   Nonpurulent mastitis associated with pregnancy, unspecified trimester ♀   M

O91.22   Nonpurulent mastitis associated with the puerperium ♀   M
: Puerperal interstitial mastitis
Puerperal lymphangitis of breast
Puerperal mastitis NOS
Puerperal parenchymatous mastitis

O91.23   Nonpurulent mastitis associated with lactation ♀   M
: Interstitial mastitis associated with lactation
Lymphangitis of breast associated with lactation
Mastitis NOS associated with lactation
Parenchymatous mastitis associated with lactation

● O92   Other disorders of breast and disorders of lactation associated with pregnancy and the puerperium

● O92.0   Retracted nipple associated with pregnancy, the puerperium, and lactation

● O92.01   Retracted nipple associated with pregnancy

O92.011   Retracted nipple associated with pregnancy, first trimester ♀   M

O92.012   Retracted nipple associated with pregnancy, second trimester ♀   M

O92.013   Retracted nipple associated with pregnancy, third trimester ♀   M

O92.019   Retracted nipple associated with pregnancy, unspecified trimester ♀   M

O92.02   Retracted nipple associated with the puerperium ♀   M

O92.03   Retracted nipple associated with lactation ♀   M

● O92.1   Cracked nipple associated with pregnancy, the puerperium, and lactation
: Fissure of nipple, gestational or puerperal

● O92.11   Cracked nipple associated with pregnancy

O92.111   Cracked nipple associated with pregnancy, first trimester ♀   M

O92.112   Cracked nipple associated with pregnancy, second trimester ♀   M

O92.113   Cracked nipple associated with pregnancy, third trimester ♀   M

O92.119   Cracked nipple associated with pregnancy, unspecified trimester ♀   M

O92.12   Cracked nipple associated with the puerperium ♀   M

O92.13   Cracked nipple associated with lactation ♀   M

◀ New   ◀▥ Revised   ~~deleted~~ Deleted   Excludes 1   Excludes 2   Includes   Use additional   Code first   Code also   Unspecified

OGCR Official Guidelines   X Assign placeholder X   ● Use Additional Character(s)   ▶ Manifestation Code   **Coding Clinic**

● **O92.2** **Other and unspecified disorders of breast associated with pregnancy and the puerperium**
     O92.20 Unspecified disorder of breast associated with pregnancy and the puerperium ♀   M
     O92.29 Other disorders of breast associated with pregnancy and the puerperium ♀   M

O92.3 **Agalactia** ♀   M
     Primary agalactia
     Excludes1 elective agalactia (O92.5)
                secondary agalactia (O92.5)
                therapeutic agalactia (O92.5)

O92.4 **Hypogalactia** ♀   M

O92.5 **Suppressed lactation** ♀   M
     Elective agalactia   Therapeutic agalactia
     Secondary agalactia
     Excludes1 primary agalactia (O92.3)

O92.6 **Galactorrhea** ♀   M

● **O92.7** **Other and unspecified disorders of lactation**
     O92.70 Unspecified disorders of lactation ♀   M
     O92.79 Other disorders of lactation ♀   M
           Puerperal galactocele

OTHER OBSTETRIC CONDITIONS, NOT ELSEWHERE CLASSIFIED (O94-O9A)

O94 **Sequelae of complication of pregnancy, childbirth, and the puerperium** ♀   M
     Note: This category is to be used to indicate conditions in O00-O77.-, O85-O94 and O98-O9A.- as the cause of late effects. The 'sequelae' include conditions specified as such, or as late effects, which may occur at any time after the puerperium.
     Code first condition resulting from (sequela) of complication of pregnancy, childbirth, and the puerperium

O98 **Maternal infectious and parasitic diseases classifiable elsewhere but complicating pregnancy, childbirth and the puerperium**
     Includes the listed conditions when complicating the pregnant state, when aggravated by the pregnancy, or as a reason for obstetric care
     Use additional code (Chapter 1), to identify specific infectious or parasitic disease
     Excludes2 herpes gestationis (O26.4-)
                infectious carrier state (O99.82-, O99.83-)
                obstetrical tetanus (A34)
                puerperal infection (O86.-)
                puerperal sepsis (O85)
                when the reason for maternal care is that the disease is known or suspected to have affected the fetus (O35-O36)

● **O98.0** **Tuberculosis complicating pregnancy, childbirth and the puerperium**
     Conditions in A15-A19
     ● **O98.01** Tuberculosis complicating pregnancy
         O98.011 Tuberculosis complicating pregnancy, first trimester ♀   M
         O98.012 Tuberculosis complicating pregnancy, second trimester ♀   M
         O98.013 Tuberculosis complicating pregnancy, third trimester ♀   M
         O98.019 Tuberculosis complicating pregnancy, unspecified trimester ♀   M
     O98.02 Tuberculosis complicating childbirth ♀   M
     O98.03 Tuberculosis complicating the puerperium ♀   M

● **O98.1** **Syphilis complicating pregnancy, childbirth and the puerperium**
     Conditions in A50-A53
     ● **O98.11** Syphilis complicating pregnancy
         O98.111 Syphilis complicating pregnancy, first trimester ♀   M
         O98.112 Syphilis complicating pregnancy, second trimester ♀   M
         O98.113 Syphilis complicating pregnancy, third trimester ♀   M
         O98.119 Syphilis complicating pregnancy, unspecified trimester ♀   M
     O98.12 Syphilis complicating childbirth ♀   M
     O98.13 Syphilis complicating the puerperium ♀   M

● **O98.2** **Gonorrhea complicating pregnancy, childbirth and the puerperium**
     Conditions in A54.-
     ● **O98.21** Gonorrhea complicating pregnancy
         O98.211 Gonorrhea complicating pregnancy, first trimester ♀   M
         O98.212 Gonorrhea complicating pregnancy, second trimester ♀   M
         O98.213 Gonorrhea complicating pregnancy, third trimester ♀   M
         O98.219 Gonorrhea complicating pregnancy, unspecified trimester ♀   M
     O98.22 Gonorrhea complicating childbirth ♀   M
     O98.23 Gonorrhea complicating the puerperium ♀   M

● **O98.3** **Other infections with a predominantly sexual mode of transmission complicating pregnancy, childbirth and the puerperium**
     Conditions in A55-A64
     ● **O98.31** Other infections with a predominantly sexual mode of transmission complicating pregnancy
         O98.311 Other infections with a predominantly sexual mode of transmission complicating pregnancy, first trimester ♀   M
         O98.312 Other infections with a predominantly sexual mode of transmission complicating pregnancy, second trimester ♀   M
         O98.313 Other infections with a predominantly sexual mode of transmission complicating pregnancy, third trimester ♀   M
         O98.319 Other infections with a predominantly sexual mode of transmission complicating pregnancy, unspecified trimester ♀   M
     O98.32 Other infections with a predominantly sexual mode of transmission complicating childbirth ♀   M
     O98.33 Other infections with a predominantly sexual mode of transmission complicating the puerperium ♀   M

● **O98.4** **Viral hepatitis complicating pregnancy, childbirth and the puerperium**
     Conditions in B15-B19
     ● **O98.41** Viral hepatitis complicating pregnancy
         O98.411 Viral hepatitis complicating pregnancy, first trimester ♀   M
         O98.412 Viral hepatitis complicating pregnancy, second trimester ♀   M
         O98.413 Viral hepatitis complicating pregnancy, third trimester ♀   M
         O98.419 Viral hepatitis complicating pregnancy, unspecified trimester ♀   M
     O98.42 Viral hepatitis complicating childbirth ♀   M
     O98.43 Viral hepatitis complicating the puerperium ♀   M

CHAPTER 15 (O00-O9A)

● **O98.5 Other viral diseases complicating pregnancy, childbirth and the puerperium**
Conditions in A80-B09, B25-B34, R87.81-, R87.82-

> **Excludes:1** human immunodeficiency virus [HIV] disease complicating pregnancy, childbirth and the puerperium (O98.7-)

  ● **O98.51 Other viral diseases complicating pregnancy**

    O98.511 Other viral diseases complicating pregnancy, first trimester ♀   M

    O98.512 Other viral diseases complicating pregnancy, second trimester ♀   M

    O98.513 Other viral diseases complicating pregnancy, third trimester ♀   M

    O98.519 Other viral diseases complicating pregnancy, unspecified trimester ♀   M

  O98.52 Other viral diseases complicating childbirth ♀   M

  O98.53 Other viral diseases complicating the puerperium ♀   M

● **O98.6 Protozoal diseases complicating pregnancy, childbirth and the puerperium**
Conditions in B50-B64

  ● **O98.61 Protozoal diseases complicating pregnancy**

    O98.611 Protozoal diseases complicating pregnancy, first trimester ♀   M

    O98.612 Protozoal diseases complicating pregnancy, second trimester ♀   M

    O98.613 Protozoal diseases complicating pregnancy, third trimester ♀   M

    O98.619 Protozoal diseases complicating pregnancy, unspecified trimester ♀   M

  O98.62 Protozoal diseases complicating childbirth ♀   M

  O98.63 Protozoal diseases complicating the puerperium ♀   M

● **O98.7 Human immunodeficiency virus [HIV] disease complicating pregnancy, childbirth and the puerperium**

> Use additional code to identify the type of HIV disease:
> Acquired immune deficiency syndrome (AIDS) (B20)
> Asymptomatic HIV status (Z21)
> HIV positive NOS (Z21)
> Symptomatic HIV disease (B20)

> **OGCR Section I.C.15.f.**

> HIV Infection in Pregnancy, Childbirth and the Puerperium
>
> During pregnancy, childbirth or the puerperium, a patient admitted because of an HIV-related illness should receive a principal diagnosis from subcategory O98.7-. Human immunodeficiency [HIV] disease complicating pregnancy, childbirth and the puerperium, followed by the code(s) for the HIV-related illness(es).
>
> Patients with asymptomatic HIV infection status admitted during pregnancy, childbirth, or the puerperium should receive codes of O98.7- and Z21, Asymptomatic human immunodeficiency virus [HIV] infection status.

  ● **O98.71 Human immunodeficiency virus [HIV] disease complicating pregnancy**

    O98.711 Human immunodeficiency virus [HIV] disease complicating pregnancy, first trimester ♀   M

    O98.712 Human immunodeficiency virus [HIV] disease complicating pregnancy, second trimester ♀   M

    O98.713 Human immunodeficiency virus [HIV] disease complicating pregnancy, third trimester ♀   M

    O98.719 Human immunodeficiency virus [HIV] disease complicating pregnancy, unspecified trimester ♀   M

  O98.72 Human immunodeficiency virus [HIV] disease complicating childbirth ♀   M

  O98.73 Human immunodeficiency virus [HIV] disease complicating the puerperium ♀   M

● **O98.8 Other maternal infectious and parasitic diseases complicating pregnancy, childbirth and the puerperium**

  ● **O98.81 Other maternal infectious and parasitic diseases complicating pregnancy**

    O98.811 Other maternal infectious and parasitic diseases complicating pregnancy, first trimester ♀   M

    O98.812 Other maternal infectious and parasitic diseases complicating pregnancy, second trimester ♀   M

    O98.813 Other maternal infectious and parasitic diseases complicating pregnancy, third trimester ♀   M

    O98.819 Other maternal infectious and parasitic diseases complicating pregnancy, unspecified trimester ♀   M

  O98.82 Other maternal infectious and parasitic diseases complicating childbirth ♀   M

  O98.83 Other maternal infectious and parasitic diseases complicating the puerperium ♀   M

● **O98.9 Unspecified maternal infectious and parasitic disease complicating pregnancy, childbirth and the puerperium**

  ● **O98.91 Unspecified maternal infectious and parasitic disease complicating pregnancy**

    O98.911 Unspecified maternal infectious and parasitic disease complicating pregnancy, first trimester ♀   M

    O98.912 Unspecified maternal infectious and parasitic disease complicating pregnancy, second trimester ♀   M

    O98.913 Unspecified maternal infectious and parasitic disease complicating pregnancy, third trimester ♀   M

    O98.919 Unspecified maternal infectious and parasitic disease complicating pregnancy, unspecified trimester ♀   M

  O98.92 Unspecified maternal infectious and parasitic disease complicating childbirth ♀   M

  O98.93 Unspecified maternal infectious and parasitic disease complicating the puerperium ♀   M

● **O99 Other maternal diseases classifiable elsewhere but complicating pregnancy, childbirth and the puerperium**

> **Includes:** conditions which complicate the pregnant state, are aggravated by the pregnancy or are a main reason for obstetric care

> Use additional code to identify specific condition

> **Excludes2** when the reason for maternal care is that the condition is known or suspected to have affected the fetus (O35-O36)

● **O99.0 Anemia complicating pregnancy, childbirth and the puerperium**
Conditions in D50-D64

> **Excludes1** anemia arising in the puerperium (O90.81)
> postpartum anemia NOS (O90.81)

  ● **O99.01 Anemia complicating pregnancy**

    O99.011 Anemia complicating pregnancy, first trimester ♀   M

    O99.012 Anemia complicating pregnancy, second trimester ♀   M

    O99.013 Anemia complicating pregnancy, third trimester ♀   M

    O99.019 Anemia complicating pregnancy, unspecified trimester ♀   M

  O99.02 Anemia complicating childbirth ♀   M

  O99.03 Anemia complicating the puerperium ♀   M

> **Excludes1** postpartum anemia not pre-existing prior to delivery (O90.81)

● **O99.1** **Other diseases of the blood and blood-forming organs and certain disorders involving the immune mechanism complicating pregnancy, childbirth and the puerperium**
Conditions in D65-D89

> **Excludes2** hemorrhage with coagulation defects (O45.-, O46.0-, O67.0, O72.3)

● **O99.11** **Other diseases of the blood and blood-forming organs and certain disorders involving the immune mechanism complicating pregnancy**

　　O99.111 Other diseases of the blood and blood-forming organs and certain disorders involving the immune mechanism complicating pregnancy, first trimester ♀　　M

　　O99.112 Other diseases of the blood and blood-forming organs and certain disorders involving the immune mechanism complicating pregnancy, second trimester ♀　　M

　　O99.113 Other diseases of the blood and blood-forming organs and certain disorders involving the immune mechanism complicating pregnancy, third trimester ♀　　M

　　O99.119 Other diseases of the blood and blood-forming organs and certain disorders involving the immune mechanism complicating pregnancy, unspecified trimester ♀　　M

　O99.12 Other diseases of the blood and blood-forming organs and certain disorders involving the immune mechanism complicating childbirth ♀　　M

　O99.13 Other diseases of the blood and blood-forming organs and certain disorders involving the immune mechanism complicating the puerperium ♀　　M

● **O99.2** **Endocrine, nutritional and metabolic diseases complicating pregnancy, childbirth and the puerperium**
Conditions in E00-E88

> **Excludes2** diabetes mellitus (O24.-)
> malnutrition (O25.-)
> postpartum thyroiditis (O90.5)

● **O99.21** **Obesity complicating pregnancy, childbirth, and the puerperium**
Use additional code to identify the type of obesity (E66.-)

　　O99.210 Obesity complicating pregnancy, unspecified trimester ♀　　M

　　O99.211 Obesity complicating pregnancy, first trimester ♀　　M

　　O99.212 Obesity complicating pregnancy, second trimester ♀　　M

　　O99.213 Obesity complicating pregnancy, third trimester ♀　　M

　　O99.214 Obesity complicating childbirth ♀　　M

　　O99.215 Obesity complicating the puerperium ♀　　M

● **O99.28** **Other endocrine, nutritional and metabolic diseases complicating pregnancy, childbirth and the puerperium**

　　O99.280 Endocrine, nutritional and metabolic diseases complicating pregnancy, unspecified trimester ♀　　M

　　O99.281 Endocrine, nutritional and metabolic diseases complicating pregnancy, first trimester ♀　　M

　　O99.282 Endocrine, nutritional and metabolic diseases complicating pregnancy, second trimester ♀　　M

　　O99.283 Endocrine, nutritional and metabolic diseases complicating pregnancy, third trimester ♀　　M

　　O99.284 Endocrine, nutritional and metabolic diseases complicating childbirth ♀　M

　　O99.285 Endocrine, nutritional and metabolic diseases complicating the puerperium ♀　　M

● **O99.3** **Mental disorders and diseases of the nervous system complicating pregnancy, childbirth and the puerperium**

● **O99.31** **Alcohol use complicating pregnancy, childbirth, and the puerperium**
Use additional code(s) from F10 to identify manifestations of the alcohol use

　　O99.310 Alcohol use complicating pregnancy, unspecified trimester ♀　　M

　　O99.311 Alcohol use complicating pregnancy, first trimester ♀　　M

　　O99.312 Alcohol use complicating pregnancy, second trimester ♀　　M

　　O99.313 Alcohol use complicating pregnancy, third trimester ♀　　M

　　O99.314 Alcohol use complicating childbirth ♀　　M

　　O99.315 Alcohol use complicating the puerperium ♀　　M

● **O99.32** **Drug use complicating pregnancy, childbirth, and the puerperium**
Use additional code(s) from F11-F16 and F18-F19 to identify manifestations of the drug use

　　O99.320 Drug use complicating pregnancy, unspecified trimester ♀　　M

　　O99.321 Drug use complicating pregnancy, first trimester ♀　　M

　　O99.322 Drug use complicating pregnancy, second trimester ♀　　M

　　O99.323 Drug use complicating pregnancy, third trimester ♀　　M

　　O99.324 Drug use complicating childbirth ♀　M

　　O99.325 Drug use complicating the puerperium ♀　　M

● **O99.33** **Tobacco use disorder complicating pregnancy, childbirth, and the puerperium** ◄▥
Smoking complicating pregnancy, childbirth, and the puerperium ◄
Use additional code from category F17 to identify type of tobacco nicotine dependence ◄

　　O99.330 Smoking (tobacco) complicating pregnancy, unspecified trimester ♀　M

　　O99.331 Smoking (tobacco) complicating pregnancy, first trimester ♀　　M

　　O99.332 Smoking (tobacco) complicating pregnancy, second trimester ♀　　M

　　O99.333 Smoking (tobacco) complicating pregnancy, third trimester ♀　　M

　　O99.334 Smoking (tobacco) complicating childbirth ♀　　M

　　O99.335 Smoking (tobacco) complicating the puerperium ♀　　M

CHAPTER 15 (O00-O9A)

● **O99.34** **Other mental disorders complicating pregnancy, childbirth, and the puerperium**
Conditions in F01-F09 and F20-F99

> **Excludes2**   postpartum mood disturbance (O90.6)
> postnatal psychosis (F53)
> puerperal psychosis (F53)

     O99.340 **Other mental disorders complicating pregnancy, unspecified trimester** ♀   M

     O99.341 **Other mental disorders complicating pregnancy, first trimester** ♀   M

     O99.342 **Other mental disorders complicating pregnancy, second trimester** ♀   M

     O99.343 **Other mental disorders complicating pregnancy, third trimester** ♀   M

     O99.344 **Other mental disorders complicating childbirth** ♀   M

     O99.345 **Other mental disorders complicating the puerperium** ♀   M

● **O99.35** **Diseases of the nervous system complicating pregnancy, childbirth, and the puerperium**
Conditions in G00-G99

> **Excludes2**   pregnancy related peripheral neuritis (O26.8-)

     O99.350 **Diseases of the nervous system complicating pregnancy, unspecified trimester** ♀   M

     O99.351 **Diseases of the nervous system complicating pregnancy, first trimester** ♀   M

     O99.352 **Diseases of the nervous system complicating pregnancy, second trimester** ♀   M

     O99.353 **Diseases of the nervous system complicating pregnancy, third trimester** ♀   M

     O99.354 **Diseases of the nervous system complicating childbirth** ♀   M

     O99.355 **Diseases of the nervous system complicating the puerperium** ♀   M

● **O99.4** **Diseases of the circulatory system complicating pregnancy, childbirth and the puerperium**
Conditions in I00-I99

> **Excludes1**   peripartum cardiomyopathy (O90.3)
> **Excludes2**   hypertensive disorders (O10-O16)
> obstetric embolism (O88.-)
> venous complications and cerebrovenous sinus thrombosis in labor, childbirth and the puerperium (O87.-)
> venous complications and cerebrovenous sinus thrombosis in pregnancy (O22.-)

● **O99.41** **Diseases of the circulatory system complicating pregnancy**
Coding Clinic: 2016, Q2, P8

     O99.411 **Diseases of the circulatory system complicating pregnancy, first trimester** ♀   M

     O99.412 **Diseases of the circulatory system complicating pregnancy, second trimester** ♀   M

     O99.413 **Diseases of the circulatory system complicating pregnancy, third trimester** ♀   M

     O99.419 **Diseases of the circulatory system complicating pregnancy, unspecified trimester** ♀   M

     O99.42 **Diseases of the circulatory system complicating childbirth** ♀   M

     O99.43 **Diseases of the circulatory system complicating the puerperium** ♀   M

● **O99.5** **Diseases of the respiratory system complicating pregnancy, childbirth and the puerperium**
Conditions in J00-J99

● **O99.51** **Diseases of the respiratory system complicating pregnancy**

     O99.511 **Diseases of the respiratory system complicating pregnancy, first trimester** ♀   M

     O99.512 **Diseases of the respiratory system complicating pregnancy, second trimester** ♀   M

     O99.513 **Diseases of the respiratory system complicating pregnancy, third trimester** ♀   M

     O99.519 **Diseases of the respiratory system complicating pregnancy, unspecified trimester** ♀   M

     O99.52 **Diseases of the respiratory system complicating childbirth** ♀   M

     O99.53 **Diseases of the respiratory system complicating the puerperium** ♀   M

● **O99.6** **Diseases of the digestive system complicating pregnancy, childbirth and the puerperium**
Conditions in K00-K93

> **Excludes2**   hemorrhoids in pregnancy (O22.4-) ◀
> liver and biliary tract disorders in pregnancy, childbirth and the puerperium (O26.6-)

● **O99.61** **Diseases of the digestive system complicating pregnancy**

     O99.611 **Diseases of the digestive system complicating pregnancy, first trimester** ♀   M

     O99.612 **Diseases of the digestive system complicating pregnancy, second trimester** ♀   M

     O99.613 **Diseases of the digestive system complicating pregnancy, third trimester** ♀   M

     O99.619 **Diseases of the digestive system complicating pregnancy, unspecified trimester** ♀   M

     O99.62 **Diseases of the digestive system complicating childbirth** ♀   M

     O99.63 **Diseases of the digestive system complicating the puerperium** ♀   M

● **O99.7** **Diseases of the skin and subcutaneous tissue complicating pregnancy, childbirth and the puerperium**
Conditions in L00-L99

> **Excludes2**   herpes gestationis (O26.4)
> pruritic urticarial papules and plaques of pregnancy (PUPPP) (O26.86)

● **O99.71** **Diseases of the skin and subcutaneous tissue complicating pregnancy**

     O99.711 **Diseases of the skin and subcutaneous tissue complicating pregnancy, first trimester** ♀   M

     O99.712 **Diseases of the skin and subcutaneous tissue complicating pregnancy, second trimester** ♀   M

     O99.713 **Diseases of the skin and subcutaneous tissue complicating pregnancy, third trimester** ♀   M

     O99.719 **Diseases of the skin and subcutaneous tissue complicating pregnancy, unspecified trimester** ♀   M

     O99.72 **Diseases of the skin and subcutaneous tissue complicating childbirth** ♀   M

     O99.73 **Diseases of the skin and subcutaneous tissue complicating the puerperium** ♀   M

◀ New   ◀▥ Revised   ~~deleted~~ Deleted   Excludes 1   Excludes 2   Includes   Use additional   Code first   Code also   Unspecified

OGCR Official Guidelines   X Assign placeholder X   ● Use Additional Character(s)   ▶ Manifestation Code   **Coding Clinic**

● **O99.8 Other specified diseases and conditions complicating pregnancy, childbirth and the puerperium**
   Conditions in D00-D48, H00-H95, M00-N99, and Q00-Q99

   Use additional code to identify condition

   Excludes2 genitourinary infections in pregnancy (O23.-)
        infection of genitourinary tract following delivery (O86.1-O86.3)
        malignant neoplasm complicating pregnancy, childbirth and the puerperium (O9A.1-)
        maternal care for known or suspected abnormality of maternal pelvic organs (O34.-)
        postpartum acute kidney failure (O90.4)
        traumatic injuries in pregnancy (O9A.2-)

● **O99.81 Abnormal glucose complicating pregnancy, childbirth and the puerperium**
    Excludes1 gestational diabetes (O24.4-)

   O99.810 Abnormal glucose complicating pregnancy ♀   M

   O99.814 Abnormal glucose complicating childbirth ♀   M

   O99.815 Abnormal glucose complicating the puerperium ♀   M

● **O99.82 Streptococcus B carrier state complicating pregnancy, childbirth and the puerperium**
    Excludes1 Carrier of streptococcus group B (GBS) in a nonpregnant woman (Z22.330) ◀

   O99.820 Streptococcus B carrier state complicating pregnancy ♀ M

   O99.824 Streptococcus B carrier state complicating childbirth ♀ M

   O99.825 Streptococcus B carrier state complicating the puerperium ♀ M

● **O99.83 Other infection carrier state complicating pregnancy, childbirth and the puerperium**
   Use additional code to identify the carrier state (Z22.-)

   O99.830 Other infection carrier state complicating pregnancy ♀ M

   O99.834 Other infection carrier state complicating childbirth ♀ M

   O99.835 Other infection carrier state complicating the puerperium ♀ M

● **O99.84 Bariatric surgery status complicating pregnancy, childbirth and the puerperium**
   Gastric banding status complicating pregnancy, childbirth and the puerperium
   Gastric bypass status for obesity complicating pregnancy, childbirth and the puerperium
   Obesity surgery status complicating pregnancy, childbirth and the puerperium

   O99.840 Bariatric surgery status complicating pregnancy, unspecified trimester ♀ M

   O99.841 Bariatric surgery status complicating pregnancy, first trimester ♀ M

   O99.842 Bariatric surgery status complicating pregnancy, second trimester ♀ M

   O99.843 Bariatric surgery status complicating pregnancy, third trimester ♀ M

   O99.844 Bariatric surgery status complicating childbirth ♀ M

   O99.845 Bariatric surgery status complicating the puerperium ♀ M

● **O99.89 Other specified diseases and conditions complicating pregnancy, childbirth and the puerperium** ♀ M

OGCR Section I.C.2.I.3.

Malignant neoplasm in a pregnant patient
When a pregnant woman has a malignant neoplasm, a code from subcategory O9A.1-, Malignant neoplasm complicating pregnancy, childbirth, and the puerperium, should be sequenced first, followed by the appropriate code from Chapter 2 to indicate the type of neoplasm.

● **O9A Maternal malignant neoplasms, traumatic injuries and abuse classifiable elsewhere but complicating pregnancy, childbirth and the puerperium**

 ● **O9A.1 Malignant neoplasm complicating pregnancy, childbirth and the puerperium**
   Conditions in C00-C96

   Use additional code to identify neoplasm

   Excludes2 maternal care for benign tumor of corpus uteri (O34.1-)
        maternal care for benign tumor of cervix (O34.4-)

  ● **O9A.11 Malignant neoplasm complicating pregnancy**

    O9A.111 Malignant neoplasm complicating pregnancy, first trimester ♀ M

    O9A.112 Malignant neoplasm complicating pregnancy, second trimester ♀ M

    O9A.113 Malignant neoplasm complicating pregnancy, third trimester ♀ M

    O9A.119 Malignant neoplasm complicating pregnancy, unspecified trimester ♀ M

   O9A.12 Malignant neoplasm complicating childbirth ♀ M

   O9A.13 Malignant neoplasm complicating the puerperium ♀ M
     Coding Clinic: 2015, Q3, P19

 ● **O9A.2 Injury, poisoning and certain other consequences of external causes complicating pregnancy, childbirth and the puerperium**
   Conditions in S00-T88, except T74 and T76

   Use additional code(s) to identify the injury or poisoning

   Excludes2 physical, sexual and psychological abuse complicating pregnancy, childbirth and the puerperium (O9A.3-, O9A.4-, O9A.5-)

  ● **O9A.21 Injury, poisoning and certain other consequences of external causes complicating pregnancy**

    O9A.211 Injury, poisoning and certain other consequences of external causes complicating pregnancy, first trimester ♀ M

    O9A.212 Injury, poisoning and certain other consequences of external causes complicating pregnancy, second trimester ♀ M

    O9A.213 Injury, poisoning and certain other consequences of external causes complicating pregnancy, third trimester ♀ M

    O9A.219 Injury, poisoning and certain other consequences of external causes complicating pregnancy, unspecified trimester ♀ M

   O9A.22 Injury, poisoning and certain other consequences of external causes complicating childbirth ♀ M

   O9A.23 Injury, poisoning and certain other consequences of external causes complicating the puerperium ♀ M

CHAPTER 15 (O00-O9A)

● **O9A.3 Physical abuse complicating pregnancy, childbirth and the puerperium**
    Conditions in T74.11 or T76.11

    Use additional code (if applicable):
      to identify any associated current injury due to physical abuse
      to identify the perpetrator of abuse (Y07.-)

    Excludes2 sexual abuse complicating pregnancy, childbirth and the puerperium (O9A.4)

  ● **O9A.31 Physical abuse complicating pregnancy**
      O9A.311 Physical abuse complicating pregnancy, first trimester ♀   M
      O9A.312 Physical abuse complicating pregnancy, second trimester ♀   M
      O9A.313 Physical abuse complicating pregnancy, third trimester ♀   M
      O9A.319 Physical abuse complicating pregnancy, unspecified trimester ♀ M

    O9A.32 Physical abuse complicating childbirth ♀   M
    O9A.33 Physical abuse complicating the puerperium ♀   M

● **O9A.4 Sexual abuse complicating pregnancy, childbirth and the puerperium**
    Conditions in T74.21 or T76.21

    Use additional code (if applicable):
      to identify any associated current injury due to sexual abuse
      to identify the perpetrator of abuse (Y07.-)

  ● **O9A.41 Sexual abuse complicating pregnancy**
      O9A.411 Sexual abuse complicating pregnancy, first trimester ♀   M
      O9A.412 Sexual abuse complicating pregnancy, second trimester ♀   M
      O9A.413 Sexual abuse complicating pregnancy, third trimester ♀   M
      O9A.419 Sexual abuse complicating pregnancy, unspecified trimester ♀   M

    O9A.42 Sexual abuse complicating childbirth ♀   M
    O9A.43 Sexual abuse complicating the puerperium ♀   M

● **O9A.5 Psychological abuse complicating pregnancy, childbirth and the puerperium**
    Conditions in T74.31 or T76.31

    Use additional code to identify the perpetrator of abuse (Y07.-)

  ● **O9A.51 Psychological abuse complicating pregnancy**
      O9A.511 Psychological abuse complicating pregnancy, first trimester ♀   M
      O9A.512 Psychological abuse complicating pregnancy, second trimester ♀   M
      O9A.513 Psychological abuse complicating pregnancy, third trimester ♀   M
      O9A.519 Psychological abuse complicating pregnancy, unspecified trimester ♀   M

    O9A.52 Psychological abuse complicating childbirth ♀ M
    O9A.53 Psychological abuse complicating the puerperium ♀   M

◀ New   ◀▥ Revised   ~~deleted~~ Deleted   Excludes 1   Excludes 2   Includes   Use additional   Code first   Code also   Unspecified

OGCR Official Guidelines   X Assign placeholder X   ● Use Additional Character(s)   ▶ Manifestation Code   **Coding Clinic**

CHAPTER 16

CERTAIN CONDITIONS ORIGINATING IN THE PERINATAL PERIOD (P00-P96)

OGCR Chapter-Specific Coding Guidelines

16. **Chapter 16: Certain Conditions Originating in the Perinatal Period (P00-P96)**
For coding and reporting purposes the perinatal period is defined as before birth through the 28th day following birth. The following guidelines are provided for reporting purposes

a. **General Perinatal Rules**

1) **Use of Chapter 16 Codes**
Codes in this chapter are <u>never</u> for use on the maternal record. Codes from Chapter 15, the obstetric chapter, are never permitted on the newborn record. Chapter 16 codes may be used throughout the life of the patient if the condition is still present.

2) **Principal Diagnosis for Birth Record**
When coding the birth episode in a newborn record, assign a code from category Z38, Liveborn infants according to place of birth and type of delivery, as the principal diagnosis. A code from category Z38 is assigned only once, to a newborn at the time of birth. If a newborn is transferred to another institution, a code from category Z38 should not be used at the receiving hospital.

A code from category Z38 is used only on the newborn record, not on the mother's record.

3) **Use of Codes from other Chapters with Codes from Chapter 16**
Codes from other chapters may be used with codes from chapter 16 if the codes from the other chapters provide more specific detail. Codes for signs and symptoms may be assigned when a definitive diagnosis has not been established. If the reason for the encounter is a perinatal condition, the code from chapter 16 should be sequenced first.

4) **Use of Chapter 16 Codes after the Perinatal Period**
Should a condition originate in the perinatal period, and continue throughout the life of the patient, the perinatal code should continue to be used regardless of the patient's age.

5) **Birth process or community acquired conditions**
If a newborn has a condition that may be either due to the birth process or community acquired and the documentation does not indicate which it is, the default is due to the birth process and the code from Chapter 16 should be used. If the condition is community-acquired, a code from Chapter 16 should not be assigned.

6) **Code all clinically significant conditions**
All clinically significant conditions noted on routine newborn examination should be coded. A condition is clinically significant if it requires:
- clinical evaluation; or
- therapeutic treatment; or
- diagnostic procedures; or
- extended length of hospital stay; or
- increased nursing care and/or monitoring; or
- has implications for future health care needs

Note: The perinatal guidelines listed above are the same as the general coding guidelines for "additional diagnoses", except for the final point regarding implications for future health care needs. Codes should be assigned for conditions that have been specified by the provider as having implications for future health care needs.

b. **Observation and Evaluation of Newborns for Suspected Conditions not Found**

1) **Assign a code from category Z05, Observation and evaluation of newborns and infants for suspected** conditions ruled out, to identify those instances when a healthy newborn is evaluated for a suspected condition that is determined after study not to be present. Do not use a code from category Z05 when the patient has identified signs or symptoms of a suspected problem; in such cases code the sign or symptom.

2) A code from category Z05 may also be assigned as a principal or first-listed code for readmissions or encounters when the code from category Z38 code no longer applies. Codes from category Z05 are for use only for healthy newborns and infants for which no condition after study is found to be present.

3) **Z05 on a birth record**
A code from category Z05 is to be used as a secondary code after the code from category Z38, Liveborn infants according to place of birth and type of delivery.

c. **Coding Additional Perinatal Diagnoses**

1) **Assigning codes for conditions that require treatment**
Assign codes for conditions that require treatment or further investigation, prolong the length of stay, or require resource utilization.

2) **Codes for conditions specified as having implications for future health care needs**
Assign codes for conditions that have been specified by the provider as having implications for future health care needs.
Note: This guideline should not be used for adult patients.

d. **Prematurity and Fetal Growth Retardation**
Providers utilize different criteria in determining prematurity. A code for prematurity should not be assigned unless it is documented. Assignment of codes in categories P05, Disorders of newborn related to slow fetal growth and fetal malnutrition, and P07, Disorders of newborn related to short gestation and low birth weight, not elsewhere classified, should be based on the recorded birth weight and estimated gestational age. Codes from category P05 should not be assigned with codes from category P07.

When both birth weight and gestational age are available, two codes from category P07 should be assigned, with the code for birth weight sequenced before the code for gestational age.

e. **Low birth weight and immaturity status**
Codes from category P07, Disorders of newborn related to short gestation and low birth weight, not elsewhere classified, are for use for a child or adult who was premature or had a low birth weight as a newborn and this is affecting the patient's current health status.
See Section I.C.21. Factors influencing health status and contact with health services, Status.

f. **Bacterial Sepsis of Newborn**
Category P36, Bacterial sepsis of newborn, includes congenital sepsis. If a perinate is documented as having sepsis without documentation of congenital or community acquired, the default is congenital and a code from category P36 should be assigned. If the P36 code includes the causal organism, an additional code from category B95, Streptococcus, Staphylococcus, and Enterococcus as the cause of diseases classified elsewhere, or B96, Other bacterial agents as the cause of diseases classified elsewhere, should not be assigned. If the P36 code does not include the causal organism, assign an additional code from category B96. If applicable, use additional codes to identify severe sepsis (R65.2-) and any associated acute organ dysfunction.

g. **Stillbirth**
Code P95, Stillbirth, is only for use in institutions that maintain separate records for stillbirths. No other code should be used with P95. Code P95 should not be used on the mother's record.

CHAPTER 16

CERTAIN CONDITIONS ORIGINATING IN THE PERINATAL PERIOD (P00-P96)

Note: Codes from this chapter are for use on newborn records only, never on maternal records.

Includes   conditions that have their origin in the fetal or perinatal period (before birth through the first 28 days after birth) even if morbidity occurs later

Excludes2   congenital malformations, deformations and chromosomal abnormalities (Q00-Q99)
endocrine, nutritional and metabolic diseases (E00-E88)
injury, poisoning and certain other consequences of external causes (S00-T88)
neoplasms (C00-D49)
tetanus neonatorum (A33)

This chapter contains the following blocks:

P00-P04	Newborn affected by maternal factors and by complications of pregnancy, labor, and delivery
P05-P08	Disorders of newborns related to length of gestation and fetal growth
P09	Abnormal findings on neonatal screening
P10-P15	Birth trauma
P19-P29	Respiratory and cardiovascular disorders specific to the perinatal period
P35-P39	Infections specific to the perinatal period
P50-P61	Hemorrhagic and hematological disorders of newborn
P70-P74	Transitory endocrine and metabolic disorders specific to newborn
P76-P78	Digestive system disorders of newborn
P80-P83	Conditions involving the integument and temperature regulation of newborn
P84	Other problems with newborn
P90-P96	Other disorders originating in the perinatal period

NEWBORN AFFECTED BY MATERNAL FACTORS AND BY COMPLICATIONS OF PREGNANCY, LABOR, AND DELIVERY (P00–P04)

Note: These codes are for use when the listed maternal conditions are specified as the cause of confirmed morbidity or potential morbidity which have their origin in the perinatal period (before birth through the first 28 days after birth). ◀▥

● **P00**   **Newborn affected by maternal conditions that may be unrelated to present pregnancy** ◀▥

Code first any current condition in newborn

Excludes2   encounter for observation of newborn for suspected diseases and conditions ruled out (Z05.-) ◀
newborn affected by maternal complications of pregnancy (P01.-) ◀
newborn affected by maternal endocrine and metabolic disorders (P70–P74)
newborn affected by noxious substances transmitted via placenta or breast milk (P04.-)

P00.0   **Newborn affected by maternal hypertensive disorders** ◀▥
Newborn affected by maternal conditions classifiable to O10-O11, O13-O16 ◀▥

P00.1   **Newborn affected by maternal renal and urinary tract diseases** ◀▥
Newborn affected by maternal conditions classifiable to N00-N39 ◀▥

P00.2   **Newborn affected by maternal infectious and parasitic diseases** ◀▥
Newborn affected by maternal infectious disease classifiable to A00-B99, J09 and J10 ◀▥

Excludes1   infections specific to the perinatal period (P35-P39)
maternal genital tract or other localized infections (P00.8)

Coding Clinic: 2015, Q3, P21

P00.3   **Newborn affected by other maternal circulatory and respiratory diseases** ◀▥
Newborn affected by maternal conditions classifiable to I00-I99, J00-J99, Q20-Q34 and not included in P00.0, P00.2 ◀▥

P00.4   **Newborn affected by maternal nutritional disorders** ◀▥
Newborn affected by maternal disorders classifiable to E40-E64 ◀▥
Maternal malnutrition NOS

P00.5   **Newborn affected by maternal injury** ◀▥
Newborn affected by maternal conditions classifiable to O9A.2- ◀▥

P00.6   **Newborn affected by surgical procedure on mother** ◀▥
Newborn affected by amniocentesis ◀▥

Excludes1   Cesarean delivery for present delivery (P03.4)
damage to placenta from amniocentesis, cesarean delivery or surgical induction (P02.1)
previous surgery to uterus or pelvic organs (P03.89)

Excludes2   newborn affected by complication of (fetal) intrauterine procedure (P96.5)

P00.7   **Newborn affected by other medical procedures on mother, not elsewhere classified** ◀▥
Newborn affected by radiation to mother ◀▥

Excludes1   damage to placenta from amniocentesis, cesarean delivery or surgical induction (P02.1)
newborn affected by other complications of labor and delivery (P03.-)

● **P00.8**   **Newborn affected by other maternal conditions** ◀▥

P00.81   **Newborn affected by periodontal disease in mother** ◀▥

P00.89   **Newborn affected by other maternal conditions** ◀▥
Newborn affected by conditions classifiable to T80-T88 ◀▥
Newborn affected by maternal genital tract or other localized infections ◀▥
Newborn affected by maternal systemic lupus erythematosus ◀▥

P00.9   **Newborn affected by unspecified maternal condition** ◀▥

● **P01**   **Newborn affected by maternal complications of pregnancy** ◀▥
Code first any current condition in newborn

Excludes2   encounter for observation of newborn for suspected diseases and conditions ruled out (Z05.-) ◀

P01.0   **Newborn affected by incompetent cervix** ◀▥

P01.1   **Newborn affected by premature rupture of membranes** ◀▥

P01.2   **Newborn affected by oligohydramnios** ◀▥

Excludes1   oligohydramnios due to premature rupture of membranes (P01.1)

P01.3   **Newborn affected by polyhydramnios** ◀▥
Excess of amniotic fluid, usually > 2000 mL
Newborn affected by hydramnios ◀▥

P01.4   **Newborn affected by ectopic pregnancy** ◀▥
Newborn affected by abdominal pregnancy ◀▥

P01.5   **Newborn affected by multiple pregnancy** ◀▥
Newborn affected by triplet (pregnancy) ◀▥
Newborn affected by twin (pregnancy) ◀▥

P01.6   **Newborn affected by maternal death** ◀▥

P01.7   **Newborn affected by malpresentation before labor** ◀▥
Newborn affected by breech presentation before labor ◀▥
Newborn affected by external version before labor ◀▥
Newborn affected by face presentation before labor ◀▥
Newborn affected by transverse lie before labor ◀▥
Newborn affected by unstable lie before labor ◀▥

P01.8   **Newborn affected by other maternal complications of pregnancy** ◀▥

P01.9   **Newborn affected by maternal complication of pregnancy, unspecified** ◀▥

◀ New   ◀▥ Revised   ~~deleted~~ Deleted   Excludes 1   Excludes 2   Includes   Use additional   Code first   Code also   Unspecified
OGCR Official Guidelines   X Assign placeholder X   ● Use Additional Character(s)   ▶ Manifestation Code   **Coding Clinic**

● **P02   Newborn affected by complications of placenta, cord and membranes** ◄▥

    Code first any current condition in newborn

    Excludes2   encounter for observation of newborn for suspected diseases and conditions ruled out (Z05.-) ◄

P02.0   Newborn affected by placenta previa ◄▥

P02.1   Newborn affected by other forms of placental separation and hemorrhage ◄▥

    Newborn affected by abruptio placenta ◄▥

    Newborn affected by accidental hemorrhage ◄▥

    Newborn affected by antepartum hemorrhage ◄▥

    Newborn affected by damage to placenta from amniocentesis, cesarean delivery or surgical induction ◄▥

    Newborn affected by maternal blood loss ◄▥

    Newborn affected by premature separation of placenta ◄▥

● **P02.2   Newborn affected by other and unspecified morphological and functional abnormalities of placenta** ◄▥

    P02.20   Newborn affected by unspecified **morphological and functional abnormalities of placenta** ◄▥

    P02.29   Newborn affected by other morphological and functional abnormalities of placenta ◄▥

        Newborn affected by placental dysfunction ◄▥

        Newborn affected by placental infarction ◄▥

        Newborn affected by placental insufficiency ◄▥

P02.3   Newborn affected by placental transfusion syndromes ◄▥

    Newborn affected by placental and cord abnormalities resulting in twin-to-twin or other transplacental transfusion ◄▥

P02.4   Newborn affected by prolapsed cord ◄▥

P02.5   Newborn affected by other compression of umbilical cord ◄▥

    Newborn affected by umbilical cord (tightly) around neck ◄▥

    Newborn affected by entanglement of umbilical cord ◄▥

    Newborn affected by knot in umbilical cord ◄▥

● **P02.6   Newborn affected by other and unspecified conditions of umbilical cord** ◄▥

    P02.60   Newborn affected by unspecified **conditions of umbilical cord** ◄▥

    P02.69   Newborn affected by other conditions of umbilical cord ◄▥

        Newborn affected by short umbilical cord ◄▥

        Newborn affected by vasa previa ◄▥

        Excludes1   newborn affected by single umbilical artery (Q27.0)

P02.7   Newborn affected by chorioamnionitis ◄▥

    Inflammation of chorion and amnion

    Newborn affected by amnionitis ◄▥

    Newborn affected by membranitis ◄▥

    Newborn affected by placentitis ◄▥

P02.8   Newborn affected by other abnormalities of membranes ◄▥

P02.9   Newborn affected by abnormality of membranes, unspecified ◄▥

● **P03   Newborn affected by other complications of labor and delivery** ◄▥

    Code first any current condition in newborn

    Excludes2   encounter for observation of newborn for suspected diseases and conditions ruled out (Z05.-) ◄

P03.0   Newborn affected by breech delivery and extraction ◄▥

P03.1   Newborn affected by other malpresentation, malposition and disproportion during labor and delivery ◄▥

    Newborn affected by contracted pelvis ◄▥

    Newborn affected by conditions classifiable to O64-O66 ◄▥

    Newborn affected by persistent occipitoposterior ◄▥

    Newborn affected by transverse lie ◄▥

P03.2   Newborn affected by forceps delivery ◄▥

P03.3   Newborn affected by delivery by vacuum extractor [ventouse] ◄▥

P03.4   Newborn affected by Cesarean delivery ◄▥

P03.5   Newborn affected by precipitate delivery ◄▥

    Newborn affected by rapid second stage ◄▥

P03.6   Newborn affected by abnormal uterine contractions ◄▥

    Newborn affected by conditions classifiable to O62.-, except O62.3 ◄▥

    Newborn affected by hypertonic labor ◄▥

    Newborn affected by uterine inertia ◄▥

● **P03.8   Newborn affected by other specified complications of labor and delivery** ◄▥

    ● **P03.81   Newborn affected by abnormality in fetal (intrauterine) heart rate or rhythm** ◄▥

        Excludes1   neonatal cardiac dysrhythmia (P29.1-)

        P03.810   Newborn affected by abnormality in fetal (intrauterine) heart rate or rhythm before the onset of labor ◄▥

        P03.811   Newborn affected by abnormality in fetal (intrauterine) heart rate or rhythm during labor ◄▥

        P03.819   Newborn affected by abnormality in fetal (intrauterine) heart rate or rhythm, unspecified **as to time of onset** ◄▥

    P03.82   Meconium passage during delivery

        Excludes1   meconium aspiration (P24.00, P24.01)

                meconium staining (P96.83)

    P03.89   Newborn affected by other specified complications of labor and delivery ◄▥

        Newborn affected by abnormality of maternal soft tissues ◄▥

        Newborn affected by conditions classifiable to O60-O75 and by procedures used in labor and delivery not included in P02.- and P03.0-P03.6 ◄▥

        Newborn affected by induction of labor ◄▥

P03.9   Newborn affected by complication of labor and delivery, unspecified ◄▥

● **P04   Newborn affected by noxious substances transmitted via placenta or breast milk** ◄▥

    Includes   nonteratogenic effects of substances transmitted via placenta

    Excludes2   congenital malformations (Q00-Q99)

        encounter for observation of newborn for suspected diseases and conditions ruled out (Z05.-) ◄

        neonatal jaundice from excessive hemolysis due to drugs or toxins transmitted from mother (P58.4)

        newborn in contact with and (suspected) exposures hazardous to health not transmitted via placenta or breast milk (Z77.-)

P04.0   Newborn affected by maternal anesthesia and analgesia in pregnancy, labor and delivery ◄▥

    Newborn affected by reactions and intoxications from maternal opiates and tranquilizers administered during labor and delivery ◄▥

P04.1   Newborn affected by other maternal medication ◄▥

    Newborn affected by cancer chemotherapy ◄▥

    Newborn affected by cytotoxic drugs ◄▥

    Excludes1   dysmorphism due to warfarin (Q86.2)

                fetal hydantoin syndrome (Q86.1)

                maternal use of drugs of addiction (P04.4-)

CHAPTER 16 (P00-P96)

CHAPTER 16 (P00-P96)

P04.2 **Newborn affected by maternal use of tobacco** ◀▥
Newborn affected by exposure in utero to tobacco smoke ◀▥
> **Excludes2** newborn exposure to environmental tobacco smoke (P96.81)

P04.3 **Newborn affected by maternal use of alcohol** ◀▥
> **Excludes1** fetal alcohol syndrome (Q86.0)

● **P04.4** **Newborn affected by maternal use of drugs of addiction** ◀▥

P04.41 **Newborn affected by maternal use of cocaine** ◀▥
'Crack baby'

P04.49 **Newborn affected by maternal use of other drugs of addiction** ◀▥
> **Excludes2** newborn affected by maternal anesthesia and analgesia (P04.0) ◀▥
> withdrawal symptoms from maternal use of drugs of addiction (P96.1)

P04.5 **Newborn affected by maternal use of nutritional chemical substances** ◀▥

P04.6 **Newborn affected by maternal exposure to environmental chemical substances** ◀▥

P04.8 **Newborn affected by other maternal noxious substances** ◀▥

P04.9 **Newborn affected by maternal noxious substance, unspecified** ◀▥

OGCR Section I.C.16.d.

Prematurity and Fetal Growth Retardation
Providers utilize different criteria in determining prematurity. A code for prematurity should not be assigned unless it is documented. Assignment of codes in categories P05, Disorders of newborn related to slow fetal growth and fetal malnutrition, and P07, Disorders of newborn related to short gestation and low birth weight, not elsewhere classified, should be based on the recorded birth weight and estimated gestational age. Codes from category P05 should not be assigned with codes from category P07.

When both birth weight and gestational age are available, two codes from category P07 should be assigned, with the code for birth weight sequenced before the code for gestational age.

A code from P05 and codes from P07.2 and P07.3 may be used to specify weeks of gestation as documented by the provider in the record.

DISORDERS OF NEWBORN RELATED TO LENGTH OF GESTATION AND FETAL GROWTH (P05-P08)

● **P05** **Disorders of newborn related to slow fetal growth and fetal malnutrition**

● **P05.0** **Newborn light for gestational age**
Newborn light-for-dates
Weight below but length above 10th percentile for gestational age ◀

P05.00 **Newborn light for gestational age, unspecified weight**

P05.01 **Newborn light for gestational age, less than 500 grams**

P05.02 **Newborn light for gestational age, 500-749 grams**

P05.03 **Newborn light for gestational age, 750-999 grams**

P05.04 **Newborn light for gestational age, 1000-1249 grams**

P05.05 **Newborn light for gestational age, 1250-1499 grams**

P05.06 **Newborn light for gestational age, 1500-1749 grams**

P05.07 **Newborn light for gestational age, 1750-1999 grams**

P05.08 **Newborn light for gestational age, 2000-2499 grams**

P05.09 **Newborn light for gestational age, 2500 grams and over** ◀
Newborn light for gestational age, other ◀

● **P05.1** **Newborn small for gestational age**
Newborn small-and-light-for-dates
Newborn small-for-dates
Weight and length below 10th percentile for gestational age ◀

P05.10 **Newborn small for gestational age, unspecified weight**

P05.11 **Newborn small for gestational age, less than 500 grams**

P05.12 **Newborn small for gestational age, 500-749 grams**

P05.13 **Newborn small for gestational age, 750-999 grams**

P05.14 **Newborn small for gestational age, 1000-1249 grams**

P05.15 **Newborn small for gestational age, 1250-1499 grams**

P05.16 **Newborn small for gestational age, 1500-1749 grams**

P05.17 **Newborn small for gestational age, 1750-1999 grams**

P05.18 **Newborn small for gestational age, 2000-2499 grams**

P05.19 **Newborn small for gestational age, other** ◀
Newborn small for gestational age, 2500 grams and over ◀

P05.2 **Newborn affected by fetal (intrauterine) malnutrition not light or small for gestational age**
Infant, not light or small for gestational age, showing signs of fetal malnutrition, such as dry, peeling skin and loss of subcutaneous tissue
> **Excludes1** newborn affected by fetal malnutrition with light for gestational age (P05.0-)
> newborn affected by fetal malnutrition with small for gestational age (P05.1-)

P05.9 **Newborn affected by slow intrauterine growth, unspecified**
Newborn affected by fetal growth retardation NOS

● **P07** **Disorders of newborn related to short gestation and low birth weight, not elsewhere classified**
Note: When both birth weight and gestational age of the newborn are available, both should be coded with birth weight sequenced before gestational age.
> **Includes** the listed conditions, without further specification, as the cause of morbidity or additional care, in newborn

● **P07.0** **Extremely low birth weight newborn**
Newborn birth weight 999 g. or less
> **Excludes1** low birth weight due to slow fetal growth and fetal malnutrition (P05.-) ◀

P07.00 **Extremely low birth weight newborn, unspecified weight**

P07.01 **Extremely low birth weight newborn, less than 500 grams**

P07.02 **Extremely low birth weight newborn, 500-749 grams**

P07.03 **Extremely low birth weight newborn, 750-999 grams**

◀ New   ◀▥ Revised   ~~deleted~~ Deleted   Excludes 1   Excludes 2   Includes   Use additional   Code first   Code also   Unspecified

OGCR Official Guidelines   X Assign placeholder X   ● Use Additional Character(s)   ▶ Manifestation Code   **Coding Clinic**

● **P07.1**   **Other low birth weight newborn**
Newborn birth weight 1000-2499 g.
> **Excludes1**   low birth weight due to slow fetal growth and fetal malnutrition (P05.-) ◄

P07.10   **Other low birth weight newborn, unspecified weight**

P07.14   **Other low birth weight newborn, 1000-1249 grams**

P07.15   **Other low birth weight newborn, 1250-1499 grams**

P07.16   **Other low birth weight newborn, 1500-1749 grams**

P07.17   **Other low birth weight newborn, 1750-1999 grams**

P07.18   **Other low birth weight newborn, 2000-2499 grams**

● **P07.2**   **Extreme immaturity of newborn**
Less than 28 completed weeks (less than 196 completed days) of gestation

P07.20   **Extreme immaturity of newborn, unspecified weeks of gestation**
Gestational age less than 28 completed weeks NOS

P07.21   **Extreme immaturity of newborn, gestational age less than 23 completed weeks**
Extreme immaturity of newborn, gestational age less than 23 weeks, 0 days

P07.22   **Extreme immaturity of newborn, gestational age 23 completed weeks**
Extreme immaturity of newborn, gestational age 23 weeks, 0 days through 23 weeks, 6 days

P07.23   **Extreme immaturity of newborn, gestational age 24 completed weeks**
Extreme immaturity of newborn, gestational age 24 weeks, 0 days through 24 weeks, 6 days

P07.24   **Extreme immaturity of newborn, gestational age 25 completed weeks**
Extreme immaturity of newborn, gestational age 25 weeks, 0 days through 25 weeks, 6 days

P07.25   **Extreme immaturity of newborn, gestational age 26 completed weeks**
Extreme immaturity of newborn, gestational age 26 weeks, 0 days through 26 weeks, 6 days

P07.26   **Extreme immaturity of newborn, gestational age 27 completed weeks**
Extreme immaturity of newborn, gestational age 27 weeks, 0 days through 27 weeks, 6 days

● **P07.3**   **Preterm [premature] newborn [other]**
28 completed weeks or more but less than 37 completed weeks (196 completed days but less than 259 completed days) of gestation
Prematurity NOS

P07.30   **Preterm newborn, unspecified weeks of gestation**

P07.31   **Preterm newborn, gestational age 28 completed weeks**
Preterm newborn, gestational age 28 weeks, 0 days through 28 weeks, 6 days

P07.32   **Preterm newborn, gestational age 29 completed weeks**
Preterm newborn, gestational age 29 weeks, 0 days through 29 weeks, 6 days

P07.33   **Preterm newborn, gestational age 30 completed weeks**
Preterm newborn, gestational age 30 weeks, 0 days through 30 weeks, 6 days

P07.34   **Preterm newborn, gestational age 31 completed weeks**
Preterm newborn, gestational age 31 weeks, 0 days through 31 weeks, 6 days

P07.35   **Preterm newborn, gestational age 32 completed weeks**
Preterm newborn, gestational age 32 weeks, 0 days through 32 weeks, 6 days

P07.36   **Preterm newborn, gestational age 33 completed weeks**
Preterm newborn, gestational age 33 weeks, 0 days through 33 weeks, 6 days

P07.37   **Preterm newborn, gestational age 34 completed weeks**
Preterm newborn, gestational age 34 weeks, 0 days through 34 weeks, 6 days

P07.38   **Preterm newborn, gestational age 35 completed weeks**
Preterm newborn, gestational age 35 weeks, 0 days through 35 weeks, 6 days

P07.39   **Preterm newborn, gestational age 36 completed weeks**
Preterm newborn, gestational age 36 weeks, 0 days through 36 weeks, 6 days

● **P08**   **Disorders of newborn related to long gestation and high birth weight**
Note: When both birth weight and gestational age of the newborn are available, priority of assignment should be given to birth weight.
> **Includes**   the listed conditions, without further specification, as causes of morbidity or additional care, in newborn

P08.0   **Exceptionally large newborn baby**
Usually implies a birth weight of 4500 g. or more
> **Excludes1**   syndrome of infant of diabetic mother (P70.1)
> syndrome of infant of mother with gestational diabetes (P70.0)

P08.1   **Other heavy for gestational age newborn**
Other newborn heavy- or large-for-dates regardless of period of gestation
Usually implies a birth weight of 4000 g. to 4499 g.
> **Excludes1**   newborn with a birth weight of 4500 or more (P08.0)
> syndrome of infant of diabetic mother (P70.1)
> syndrome of infant of mother with gestational diabetes (P70.0)

● **P08.2**   **Late newborn, not heavy for gestational age**

P08.21   **Post-term newborn**
Newborn with gestation period over 40 completed weeks to 42 completed weeks

P08.22   **Prolonged gestation of newborn**
Newborn with gestation period over 42 completed weeks (294 days or more), not heavy- or large-for-dates
Postmaturity NOS

ABNORMAL FINDINGS ON NEONATAL SCREENING (P09)

P09   **Abnormal findings on neonatal screening**
Use additional code to identify signs, symptoms and conditions associated with the screening
> **Excludes2**   nonspecific serologic evidence of human immunodeficiency virus [HIV] (R75)

CHAPTER 16 (P00-P96)

BIRTH TRAUMA (P10-P15)

● **P10**   **Intracranial laceration and hemorrhage due to birth injury**
> **Excludes1**   intracranial hemorrhage of newborn NOS (P52.9)
> intracranial hemorrhage of newborn due to anoxia or hypoxia (P52.-)
> nontraumatic intracranial hemorrhage of newborn (P52.-)

P10.0   **Subdural hemorrhage due to birth injury**
> Subdural hematoma (localized) due to birth injury
> **Excludes1**   subdural hemorrhage accompanying tentorial tear (P10.4)

P10.1   **Cerebral hemorrhage due to birth injury**

P10.2   **Intraventricular hemorrhage due to birth injury**

P10.3   **Subarachnoid hemorrhage due to birth injury**

P10.4   **Tentorial tear due to birth injury**
> *Pertaining to tentorium of cerebellum (extension of dura mater that separates cerebellum from inferior portion of occipital lobes)*

P10.8   **Other intracranial lacerations and hemorrhages due to birth injury**

P10.9   **Unspecified intracranial laceration and hemorrhage due to birth injury**

Item 16–1   The **peripheral nervous system** consists of 31 pairs of spinal nerves, 12 pairs of cranial nerves, and the autonomic nerves, which are divided into the parasympathetic and sympathetic nerves. The cranial nerves are: olfactory (I), optic (II), oculomotor (III), trochlear (IV), trigeminal (V), abducens (VI), facial (VII), vestibulocochlear (VIII), glossopharyngeal (IX), vagus (X), accessory (XI), and hypoglossal (XII).

Central Nervous System
- Brain
- Spinal cord

Peripheral Nervous System
- Cranial nerves (12)
- Spinal nerves
  cervical (8)
  thoracic (12)
  lumbar (5)
  sacral (5)
  coccyx (1)

Figure 16-1   The central nervous system consists of the brain and spinal cord. The peripheral nervous system consists of nerves that lie outside the skull and spinal cord. (From Stoy: Mosby's EMT-Basic Textbook, ed 2, St. Louis, Mosby, 2007)

● **P11**   **Other birth injuries to central nervous system**
P11.0   **Cerebral edema due to birth injury**
P11.1   **Other specified brain damage due to birth injury**
P11.2   **Unspecified brain damage due to birth injury**
P11.3   **Birth injury to facial nerve**
> Facial palsy due to birth injury
P11.4   **Birth injury to other cranial nerves**
P11.5   **Birth injury to spine and spinal cord**
> Fracture of spine due to birth injury
P11.9   **Birth injury to central nervous system, unspecified**

● **P12**   **Birth injury to scalp**
P12.0   **Cephalhematoma due to birth injury**
P12.1   **Chignon (from vacuum extraction) due to birth injury**
P12.2   **Epicranial subaponeurotic hemorrhage due to birth injury**
> Subgaleal hemorrhage
P12.3   **Bruising of scalp due to birth injury**
P12.4   **Injury of scalp of newborn due to monitoring equipment**
> Sampling incision of scalp of newborn
> Scalp clip (electrode) injury of newborn
● **P12.8**   **Other birth injuries to scalp**
    P12.81   **Caput succedaneum**
    P12.89   **Other birth injuries to scalp**
P12.9   **Birth injury to scalp, unspecified**

● **P13**   **Birth injury to skeleton**
> **Excludes2**   birth injury to spine (P11.5)
P13.0   **Fracture of skull due to birth injury**
P13.1   **Other birth injuries to skull**
> **Excludes1**   cephalhematoma (P12.0)
P13.2   **Birth injury to femur**
P13.3   **Birth injury to other long bones**
P13.4   **Fracture of clavicle due to birth injury**
P13.8   **Birth injuries to other parts of skeleton**
P13.9   **Birth injury to skeleton, unspecified**

● **P14**   **Birth injury to peripheral nervous system**
P14.0   **Erb's paralysis due to birth injury**
P14.1   **Klumpke's paralysis due to birth injury**
P14.2   **Phrenic nerve paralysis due to birth injury**
P14.3   **Other brachial plexus birth injuries**
P14.8   **Birth injuries to other parts of peripheral nervous system**
P14.9   **Birth injury to peripheral nervous system, unspecified**

● **P15**   **Other birth injuries**
P15.0   **Birth injury to liver**
> Rupture of liver due to birth injury
P15.1   **Birth injury to spleen**
> Rupture of spleen due to birth injury
P15.2   **Sternomastoid injury due to birth injury**
P15.3   **Birth injury to eye**
> Subconjunctival hemorrhage due to birth injury
> Traumatic glaucoma due to birth injury
P15.4   **Birth injury to face**
> Facial congestion due to birth injury
P15.5   **Birth injury to external genitalia**
P15.6   **Subcutaneous fat necrosis due to birth injury**
P15.8   **Other specified birth injuries**
P15.9   **Birth injury, unspecified**

◀ New   ◀▥ Revised   ~~deleted~~ Deleted   Excludes 1   Excludes 2   Includes   Use additional   Code first   Code also   Unspecified
OGCR Official Guidelines   X Assign placeholder X   ● Use Additional Character(s)   ▷ Manifestation Code   **Coding Clinic**

RESPIRATORY AND CARDIOVASCULAR DISORDERS SPECIFIC TO THE PERINATAL PERIOD (P19-P29)

● **P19**   **Metabolic acidemia in newborn**

> | Includes | metabolic acidemia in newborn |

   P19.0   **Metabolic acidemia in newborn first noted before onset of labor**

   P19.1   **Metabolic acidemia in newborn first noted during labor**

   P19.2   **Metabolic acidemia noted at birth**

   P19.9   **Metabolic acidemia, unspecified**

● **P22**   **Respiratory distress of newborn**

> | Excludes1 | respiratory arrest of newborn (P28.81)
respiratory failure of newborn NOS (P28.5) |

   P22.0   **Respiratory distress syndrome of newborn**
Cardiorespiratory distress syndrome of newborn
Hyaline membrane disease
Idiopathic respiratory distress syndrome [IRDS or RDS] of newborn
Pulmonary hypoperfusion syndrome
Respiratory distress syndrome, type I

   P22.1   **Transient tachypnea of newborn**
Idiopathic tachypnea of newborn
Respiratory distress syndrome, type II
Wet lung syndrome

   P22.8   **Other respiratory distress of newborn**

   P22.9   **Respiratory distress of newborn, unspecified**

● **P23**   Congenital pneumonia

> | Includes | infective pneumonia acquired in utero or during birth |

> | Excludes1 | neonatal pneumonia resulting from aspiration (P24.-) |

   P23.0   **Congenital pneumonia due to viral agent**
Use additional code (B97) to identify organism

> | Excludes1 | congenital rubella pneumonitis (P35.0) |

   P23.1   **Congenital pneumonia due to Chlamydia**

   P23.2   **Congenital pneumonia due to staphylococcus**

   P23.3   **Congenital pneumonia due to streptococcus, group B**

   P23.4   **Congenital pneumonia due to Escherichia coli**

   P23.5   **Congenital pneumonia due to Pseudomonas**

   P23.6   **Congenital pneumonia due to other bacterial agents**
Congenital pneumonia due to Hemophilus influenzae
Congenital pneumonia due to Klebsiella pneumoniae
Congenital pneumonia due to Mycoplasma
Congenital pneumonia due to Streptococcus, except group B
Use additional code (B95-B96) to identify organism

   P23.8   **Congenital pneumonia due to other organisms**

   P23.9   **Congenital pneumonia, unspecified**

● **P24**   **Neonatal aspiration**

> | Includes | aspiration in utero and during delivery |

●   **P24.0**   **Meconium aspiration**

> | Excludes1 | meconium passage (without aspiration) during delivery (P03.82)
meconium staining (P96.83) |

     P24.00   **Meconium aspiration without respiratory symptoms**
Meconium aspiration NOS

     P24.01   **Meconium aspiration with respiratory symptoms**
Meconium aspiration pneumonia
Meconium aspiration pneumonitis
Meconium aspiration syndrome NOS
Use additional code to identify any secondary pulmonary hypertension, if applicable (I27.2)

● **P24.1**   **Neonatal aspiration of (clear) amniotic fluid and mucus**
Neonatal aspiration of liquor (amnii)

   P24.10   **Neonatal aspiration of (clear) amniotic fluid and mucus without respiratory symptoms**
Neonatal aspiration of amniotic fluid and mucus NOS

   P24.11   **Neonatal aspiration of (clear) amniotic fluid and mucus with respiratory symptoms**
Neonatal aspiration of amniotic fluid and mucus with pneumonia
Neonatal aspiration of amniotic fluid and mucus with pneumonitis
Use additional code to identify any secondary pulmonary hypertension, if applicable (I27.2)

● **P24.2**   **Neonatal aspiration of blood**

   P24.20   **Neonatal aspiration of blood without respiratory symptoms**
Neonatal aspiration of blood NOS

   P24.21   **Neonatal aspiration of blood with respiratory symptoms**
Neonatal aspiration of blood with pneumonia
Neonatal aspiration of blood with pneumonitis
Use additional code to identify any secondary pulmonary hypertension, if applicable (I27.2)

● **P24.3**   **Neonatal aspiration of milk and regurgitated food**
Neonatal aspiration of stomach contents

   P24.30   **Neonatal aspiration of milk and regurgitated food without respiratory symptoms**
Neonatal aspiration of milk and regurgitated food NOS

   P24.31   **Neonatal aspiration of milk and regurgitated food with respiratory symptoms**
Neonatal aspiration of milk and regurgitated food with pneumonia
Neonatal aspiration of milk and regurgitated food with pneumonitis
Use additional code to identify any secondary pulmonary hypertension, if applicable (I27.2)

● **P24.8**   **Other neonatal aspiration**

   P24.80   **Other neonatal aspiration without respiratory symptoms**
Neonatal aspiration NEC

   P24.81   **Other neonatal aspiration with respiratory symptoms**
Neonatal aspiration pneumonia NEC
Neonatal aspiration with pneumonitis NEC
Neonatal aspiration with pneumonia NOS
Neonatal aspiration with pneumonitis NOS
Use additional code to identify any secondary pulmonary hypertension, if applicable (I27.2)

   P24.9   **Neonatal aspiration, unspecified**

● **P25**   **Interstitial emphysema and related conditions originating in the perinatal period**

   P25.0   **Interstitial emphysema originating in the perinatal period**

   P25.1   **Pneumothorax originating in the perinatal period**

   P25.2   **Pneumomediastinum originating in the perinatal period**

   P25.3   **Pneumopericardium originating in the perinatal period**

   P25.8   **Other conditions related to interstitial emphysema originating in the perinatal period**

CHAPTER 16 (P00-P96)

● **P26**   **Pulmonary hemorrhage originating in the perinatal period**
    Excludes1   acute idiopathic hemorrhage in infants over 28 days old (R04.81)

    P26.0   **Tracheobronchial hemorrhage originating in the perinatal period**

    P26.1   **Massive pulmonary hemorrhage originating in the perinatal period**

    P26.8   **Other pulmonary hemorrhages originating in the perinatal period**

    P26.9   **Unspecified pulmonary hemorrhage originating in the perinatal period**

● **P27**   **Chronic respiratory disease originating in the perinatal period**
    Excludes1   respiratory distress of newborn (P22.0-P22.9)

    P27.0   **Wilson-Mikity syndrome**
       Pulmonary dysmaturity

    P27.1   **Bronchopulmonary dysplasia originating in the perinatal period**

    P27.8   **Other chronic respiratory diseases originating in the perinatal period**
       Congenital pulmonary fibrosis
       Ventilator lung in newborn

    P27.9   **Unspecified chronic respiratory disease originating in the perinatal period**

● **P28**   **Other respiratory conditions originating in the perinatal period**
    Excludes1   congenital malformations of the respiratory system (Q30-Q34)

    P28.0   **Primary atelectasis of newborn**
       Failure of lungs to expand properly at birth
       Primary failure to expand terminal respiratory units
       Pulmonary hypoplasia associated with short gestation
       Pulmonary immaturity NOS

    ● **P28.1**   **Other and unspecified atelectasis of newborn**

      P28.10   **Unspecified atelectasis of newborn**
         Atelectasis of newborn NOS

      P28.11   **Resorption atelectasis without respiratory distress syndrome**
         Excludes1   resorption atelectasis with respiratory distress syndrome (P22.0)

      P28.19   **Other atelectasis of newborn**
         Partial atelectasis of newborn
         Secondary atelectasis of newborn

    P28.2   **Cyanotic attacks of newborn**
       Excludes1   apnea of newborn (P28.3-P28.4)

    P28.3   **Primary sleep apnea of newborn**
       Central sleep apnea of newborn
       Obstructive sleep apnea of newborn
       Sleep apnea of newborn NOS

    P28.4   **Other apnea of newborn**
       Apnea of prematurity
       Obstructive apnea of newborn
       Excludes1   obstructive sleep apnea of newborn (P28.3)

    P28.5   **Respiratory failure of newborn**
       Excludes1   respiratory arrest of newborn (P28.81)
                 respiratory distress of newborn (P22.0-)

    ● **P28.8**   **Other specified respiratory conditions of newborn**

      P28.81   **Respiratory arrest of newborn**

      P28.89   **Other specified respiratory conditions of newborn**
         Congenital laryngeal stridor
         Sniffles in newborn
         Snuffles in newborn
         Excludes1   early congenital syphilitic rhinitis (A50.05)

    P28.9   **Respiratory condition of newborn, unspecified**
       Respiratory depression in newborn

● **P29**   **Cardiovascular disorders originating in the perinatal period**
    Excludes1   congenital malformations of the circulatory system (Q20-Q28)

    P29.0   **Neonatal cardiac failure**

    ● **P29.1**   **Neonatal cardiac dysrhythmia**

      P29.11   **Neonatal tachycardia**

      P29.12   **Neonatal bradycardia**

    P29.2   **Neonatal hypertension**

    P29.3   **Persistent fetal circulation**
       Delayed closure of ductus arteriosus
       (Persistent) pulmonary hypertension of newborn

    P29.4   **Transient myocardial ischemia in newborn**

    ● **P29.8**   **Other cardiovascular disorders originating in the perinatal period**

      P29.81   **Cardiac arrest of newborn**

      P29.89   **Other cardiovascular disorders originating in the perinatal period**

    P29.9   **Cardiovascular disorder originating in the perinatal period, unspecified**

INFECTIONS SPECIFIC TO THE PERINATAL PERIOD (P35-P39)

Infections acquired in utero, during birth via the umbilicus, or during the first 28 days after birth

    Excludes2   asymptomatic human immunodeficiency virus [HIV] infection status (Z21)
                congenital gonococcal infection (A54.-)
                congenital pneumonia (P23.-)
                congenital syphilis (A50.-)
                human immunodeficiency virus [HIV] disease (B20)
                infant botulism (A48.51)
                infectious diseases not specific to the perinatal period (A00-B99, J09, J10.-)
                intestinal infectious disease (A00-A09)
                laboratory evidence of human immunodeficiency virus [HIV] (R75)
                tetanus neonatorum (A33)

● **P35**   **Congenital viral diseases**
    Includes   infections acquired in utero or during birth

    P35.0   **Congenital rubella syndrome**
       Congenital rubella pneumonitis

    P35.1   **Congenital cytomegalovirus infection**
       Viruses transmitted by multiple routes that cause mild/subclinical infection

    P35.2   **Congenital herpesviral [herpes simplex] infection**

    P35.3   **Congenital viral hepatitis**

    P35.8   **Other congenital viral diseases**
       Congenital varicella [chickenpox]

    P35.9   **Congenital viral disease, unspecified**

● **P36**   **Bacterial sepsis of newborn**
    Includes   congenital sepsis
    Use additional code(s), if applicable, to identify severe sepsis (R65.2-) and associated acute organ dysfunction(s)

    P36.0   **Sepsis of newborn due to streptococcus, group B**

    ● **P36.1**   **Sepsis of newborn due to other and unspecified streptococci**

      P36.10   **Sepsis of newborn due to unspecified streptococci**

      P36.19   **Sepsis of newborn due to other streptococci**

    P36.2   **Sepsis of newborn due to Staphylococcus aureus**

    ● **P36.3**   **Sepsis of newborn due to other and unspecified staphylococci**

      P36.30   **Sepsis of newborn due to unspecified staphylococci**

      P36.39   **Sepsis of newborn due to other staphylococci**

    P36.4   **Sepsis of newborn due to Escherichia coli**

    P36.5   **Sepsis of newborn due to anaerobes**

◀ New   ◀▦ Revised   ~~deleted~~ Deleted   Excludes 1   Excludes 2   Includes   Use additional   Code first   Code also   Unspecified

OGCR Official Guidelines   **X** Assign placeholder X   ● Use Additional Character(s)   ▶ Manifestation Code   **Coding Clinic**

1136

P36.8 **Other bacterial sepsis of newborn**
> Use additional code from category B96 to identify organism

P36.9 **Bacterial sepsis of newborn, unspecified**

● **P37** **Other congenital infectious and parasitic diseases**
> **Excludes2**   congenital syphilis (A50.-)
> infectious neonatal diarrhea (A00-A09)
> necrotizing enterocolitis in newborn (P77.-)
> noninfectious neonatal diarrhea (P78.3)
> ophthalmia neonatorum due to gonococcus (A54.31)
> tetanus neonatorum (A33)

P37.0 **Congenital tuberculosis**

P37.1 **Congenital toxoplasmosis**
> *Parasitic infection, often causing mild flu-like illness*
> Hydrocephalus due to congenital toxoplasmosis

P37.2 **Neonatal (disseminated) listeriosis**
> *Acquired transplacentally or during/after parturition in which symptoms are those of sepsis*

P37.3 **Congenital falciparum malaria**

P37.4 **Other congenital malaria**

P37.5 **Neonatal candidiasis**

P37.8 **Other specified congenital infectious and parasitic diseases**

P37.9 **Congenital infectious or parasitic disease, unspecified**

● **P38** **Omphalitis of newborn**
> *Inflammation of umbilicus*
> **Excludes1**   omphalitis not of newborn (L08.82)
> tetanus omphalitis (A33)
> umbilical hemorrhage of newborn (P51.-)

P38.1 **Omphalitis with mild hemorrhage**

P38.9 **Omphalitis without hemorrhage**
> Omphalitis of newborn NOS

● **P39** **Other infections specific to the perinatal period**
> Use additional code to identify organism or specific infection

P39.0 **Neonatal infective mastitis**
> **Excludes1**   breast engorgement of newborn (P83.4)
> noninfective mastitis of newborn (P83.4)

P39.1 **Neonatal conjunctivitis and dacryocystitis**
> Neonatal chlamydial conjunctivitis
> Ophthalmia neonatorum NOS
> *Neonate = newborn*
> **Excludes1**   gonococcal conjunctivitis (A54.31)

P39.2 **Intra-amniotic infection affecting newborn, not elsewhere classified**

P39.3 **Neonatal urinary tract infection**

P39.4 **Neonatal skin infection**
> Neonatal pyoderma
> **Excludes1**   pemphigus neonatorum (L00)
> staphylococcal scalded skin syndrome (L00)

P39.8 **Other specified infections specific to the perinatal period**

P39.9 **Infection specific to the perinatal period, unspecified**

HEMORRHAGIC AND HEMATOLOGICAL DISORDERS OF NEWBORN (P50-P61)

> **Excludes1**   congenital stenosis and stricture of bile ducts (Q44.3)
> Crigler-Najjar syndrome (E80.5)
> Dubin-Johnson syndrome (E80.6)
> Gilbert syndrome (E80.4)
> hereditary hemolytic anemias (D55-D58)

● **P50** **Newborn affected by intrauterine (fetal) blood loss**
> **Excludes1**   congenital anemia from intrauterine (fetal) blood loss (P61.3)

P50.0 **Newborn affected by intrauterine (fetal) blood loss from vasa previa**

P50.1 **Newborn affected by intrauterine (fetal) blood loss from ruptured cord**

P50.2 **Newborn affected by intrauterine (fetal) blood loss from placenta**

P50.3 **Newborn affected by hemorrhage into co-twin**

P50.4 **Newborn affected by hemorrhage into maternal circulation**

P50.5 **Newborn affected by intrauterine (fetal) blood loss from cut end of co-twin's cord**

P50.8 **Newborn affected by other intrauterine (fetal) blood loss**

P50.9 **Newborn affected by intrauterine (fetal) blood loss, unspecified**
> Newborn affected by fetal hemorrhage NOS

● **P51** **Umbilical hemorrhage of newborn**
> **Excludes1**   omphalitis with mild hemorrhage (P38.1)
> umbilical hemorrhage from cut end of co-twins cord (P50.5)

P51.0 **Massive umbilical hemorrhage of newborn**

P51.8 **Other umbilical hemorrhages of newborn**
> Slipped umbilical ligature NOS

P51.9 **Umbilical hemorrhage of newborn, unspecified**

● **P52** **Intracranial nontraumatic hemorrhage of newborn**
> **Includes**   intracranial hemorrhage due to anoxia or hypoxia
> **Excludes1**   intracranial hemorrhage due to birth injury (P10.-)
> intracranial hemorrhage due to other injury (S06.-)

P52.0 **Intraventricular (nontraumatic) hemorrhage, grade 1, of newborn**
> Subependymal hemorrhage (without intraventricular extension)
> Bleeding into germinal matrix

P52.1 **Intraventricular (nontraumatic) hemorrhage, grade 2, of newborn**
> Subependymal hemorrhage with intraventricular extension
> Bleeding into ventricle

● **P52.2** **Intraventricular (nontraumatic) hemorrhage, grade 3 and grade 4, of newborn**

    P52.21 **Intraventricular (nontraumatic) hemorrhage, grade 3, of newborn**
> Subependymal hemorrhage with intraventricular extension with enlargement of ventricle

    P52.22 **Intraventricular (nontraumatic) hemorrhage, grade 4, of newborn**
> Bleeding into cerebral cortex
> Subependymal hemorrhage with intracerebral extension

P52.3 **Unspecified intraventricular (nontraumatic) hemorrhage of newborn**

P52.4 **Intracerebral (nontraumatic) hemorrhage of newborn**

P52.5 **Subarachnoid (nontraumatic) hemorrhage of newborn**

P52.6 **Cerebellar (nontraumatic) and posterior fossa hemorrhage of newborn**

P52.8 **Other intracranial (nontraumatic) hemorrhages of newborn**

P52.9 **Intracranial (nontraumatic) hemorrhage of newborn, unspecified**

P53 **Hemorrhagic disease of newborn**
> Vitamin K deficiency of newborn

CHAPTER 16 (P00-P96)

● **P54 Other neonatal hemorrhages**

> **Excludes1**   newborn affected by (intrauterine) blood loss (P50.-)
> pulmonary hemorrhage originating in the perinatal period (P26.-)

P54.0 Neonatal hematemesis
Vomiting of blood

> **Excludes1**   neonatal hematemesis due to swallowed maternal blood (P78.2)

P54.1 Neonatal melena
Dark-colored feces stained with blood pigments

> **Excludes1**   neonatal melena due to swallowed maternal blood (P78.2)

P54.2 Neonatal rectal hemorrhage

P54.3 Other neonatal gastrointestinal hemorrhage

P54.4 Neonatal adrenal hemorrhage

P54.5 Neonatal cutaneous hemorrhage
Neonatal bruising
Neonatal ecchymoses
Neonatal petechiae
Neonatal superficial hematomata

> **Excludes2**   bruising of scalp due to birth injury (P12.3)
> cephalhematoma due to birth injury (P12.0)

P54.6 Neonatal vaginal hemorrhage ♀
Neonatal pseudomenses

P54.8 Other specified neonatal hemorrhages

P54.9 Neonatal hemorrhage, unspecified

● **P55 Hemolytic disease of newborn**
AKA erythroblastosis fetalis and is due to Rh isoimmunization, result of Rh blood factor incompatibilities between mother (Rh negative) and fetus (Rh positive)

P55.0 Rh isoimmunization of newborn

P55.1 ABO isoimmunization of newborn
Coding Clinic: 2015, Q3, P20

P55.8 Other hemolytic diseases of newborn

P55.9 Hemolytic disease of newborn, unspecified

● **P56 Hydrops fetalis due to hemolytic disease**
Caused by maternal sensitization to fetal blood group antigen

> **Excludes1**   hydrops fetalis NOS (P83.2)

P56.0 Hydrops fetalis due to isoimmunization

● **P56.9 Hydrops fetalis due to other and unspecified hemolytic disease**

P56.90 Hydrops fetalis due to unspecified hemolytic disease

P56.99 Hydrops fetalis due to other hemolytic disease

● **P57 Kernicterus**
High levels of bilirubin in blood, with severe neural symptoms

P57.0 Kernicterus due to isoimmunization

P57.8 Other specified kernicterus

> **Excludes1**   Crigler-Najjar syndrome (E80.5)

P57.9 Kernicterus, unspecified

● **P58 Neonatal jaundice due to other excessive hemolysis**

> **Excludes1**   jaundice due to isoimmunization (P55-P57)

P58.0 Neonatal jaundice due to bruising

P58.1 Neonatal jaundice due to bleeding

P58.2 Neonatal jaundice due to infection

P58.3 Neonatal jaundice due to polycythemia

P58.4 Neonatal jaundice due to drugs or toxins transmitted from mother or given to newborn

> *Code first poisoning due to drug or toxin, if applicable (T36-T65 with fifth or sixth character 1-4 or 6)*
> Use additional code for adverse effect, if applicable, to identify drug (T36-T50 with fifth or sixth character 5)

P58.41 Neonatal jaundice due to drugs or toxins transmitted from mother

P58.42 Neonatal jaundice due to drugs or toxins given to newborn

P58.5 Neonatal jaundice due to swallowed maternal blood

P58.8 Neonatal jaundice due to other specified excessive hemolysis

P58.9 Neonatal jaundice due to excessive hemolysis, unspecified

● **P59 Neonatal jaundice from other and unspecified causes**

> **Excludes1**   jaundice due to inborn errors of metabolism (E70-E88)
> kernicterus (P57.-)

P59.0 Neonatal jaundice associated with preterm delivery
Hyperbilirubinemia of prematurity
Jaundice due to delayed conjugation associated with preterm delivery

P59.1 Inspissated bile syndrome

● **P59.2 Neonatal jaundice from other and unspecified hepatocellular damage**

> **Excludes1**   congenital viral hepatitis (P35.3)

P59.20 Neonatal jaundice from unspecified hepatocellular damage

P59.29 Neonatal jaundice from other hepatocellular damage
Neonatal giant cell hepatitis
Neonatal (idiopathic) hepatitis

P59.3 Neonatal jaundice from breast milk inhibitor

P59.8 Neonatal jaundice from other specified causes

P59.9 Neonatal jaundice, unspecified
Neonatal physiological jaundice (intense)(prolonged) NOS
Coding Clinic: 2015, Q3, P20

P60 Disseminated intravascular coagulation of newborn
Defibrination syndrome of newborn

● **P61 Other perinatal hematological disorders**

> **Excludes1**   transient hypogammaglobulinemia of infancy (D80.7)

P61.0 Transient neonatal thrombocytopenia
Lack of sufficient numbers of circulating thrombocytes (platelets)
Neonatal thrombocytopenia due to exchange transfusion
Neonatal thrombocytopenia due to idiopathic maternal thrombocytopenia
Neonatal thrombocytopenia due to isoimmunization

P61.1 Polycythemia neonatorum
Neonate = newborn

P61.2 Anemia of prematurity

P61.3 Congenital anemia from fetal blood loss

P61.4 Other congenital anemias, not elsewhere classified
Congenital anemia NOS

P61.5 Transient neonatal neutropenia
Low levels of granulocytic neutrophilic white blood cells

> **Excludes1**   congenital neutropenia (nontransient) (D70.0)

P61.6 Other transient neonatal disorders of coagulation

P61.8 Other specified perinatal hematological disorders

P61.9 Perinatal hematological disorder, unspecified

◄ New   ◄▦ Revised   ~~deleted~~ Deleted   Excludes 1   Excludes 2   Includes   Use additional   Code first   Code also   Unspecified
OGCR Official Guidelines   X Assign placeholder X   ● Use Additional Character(s)   ▌ Manifestation Code   Coding Clinic
1138

TRANSITORY ENDOCRINE AND METABOLIC DISORDERS SPECIFIC TO NEWBORN (P70-P74)

> | Includes | transitory endocrine and metabolic disturbances caused by the infant's response to maternal endocrine and metabolic factors, or its adjustment to extrauterine environment |
> |---|---|

● **P70**   **Transitory disorders of carbohydrate metabolism specific to newborn**

    P70.0   **Syndrome of infant of mother with gestational diabetes**
Newborn (with hypoglycemia) affected by maternal gestational diabetes

> | Excludes1 | newborn (with hypoglycemia) affected by maternal (pre-existing) diabetes mellitus (P70.1) |
> |---|---|
> | | syndrome of infant of a diabetic mother (P70.1) |

    P70.1   **Syndrome of infant of a diabetic mother**
Newborn (with hypoglycemia) affected by maternal (pre-existing) diabetes mellitus

> | Excludes1 | newborn (with hypoglycemia) affected by maternal gestational diabetes (P70.0) |
> |---|---|
> | | syndrome of infant of mother with gestational diabetes (P70.0) |

    P70.2   **Neonatal diabetes mellitus**

    P70.3   **Iatrogenic neonatal hypoglycemia**

    P70.4   **Other neonatal hypoglycemia**
Transitory neonatal hypoglycemia

    P70.8   **Other transitory disorders of carbohydrate metabolism of newborn**

    P70.9   **Transitory disorder of carbohydrate metabolism of newborn, unspecified**

● **P71**   **Transitory neonatal disorders of calcium and magnesium metabolism**

    P71.0   **Cow's milk hypocalcemia in newborn**

    P71.1   **Other neonatal hypocalcemia**

> | Excludes1 | neonatal hypoparathyroidism (P71.4) |
> |---|---|

    P71.2   **Neonatal hypomagnesemia**

    P71.3   **Neonatal tetany without calcium or magnesium deficiency**
Neonatal tetany NOS

    P71.4   **Transitory neonatal hypoparathyroidism**

    P71.8   **Other transitory neonatal disorders of calcium and magnesium metabolism**

    P71.9   **Transitory neonatal disorder of calcium and magnesium metabolism, unspecified**

● **P72**   **Other transitory neonatal endocrine disorders**

> | Excludes1 | congenital hypothyroidism with or without goiter (E03.0-E03.1) |
> |---|---|
> | | dyshormogenetic goiter (E07.1) |
> | | Pendred's syndrome (E07.1) |

    P72.0   **Neonatal goiter, not elsewhere classified**
Transitory congenital goiter with normal functioning

    P72.1   **Transitory neonatal hyperthyroidism**
Neonatal thyrotoxicosis

    P72.2   **Other transitory neonatal disorders of thyroid function, not elsewhere classified**
Transitory neonatal hypothyroidism

    P72.8   **Other specified transitory neonatal endocrine disorders**

    P72.9   **Transitory neonatal endocrine disorder, unspecified**

● **P74**   **Other transitory neonatal electrolyte and metabolic disturbances**

    P74.0   **Late metabolic acidosis of newborn**

> | Excludes1 | (fetal) metabolic acidosis of newborn (P19) |
> |---|---|

    P74.1   **Dehydration of newborn**

    P74.2   **Disturbances of sodium balance of newborn**

    P74.3   **Disturbances of potassium balance of newborn**

    P74.4   **Other transitory electrolyte disturbances of newborn**

    P74.5   **Transitory tyrosinemia of newborn**

    P74.6   **Transitory hyperammonemia of newborn**

    P74.8   **Other transitory metabolic disturbances of newborn**
Amino-acid metabolic disorders described as transitory

    P74.9   **Transitory metabolic disturbance of newborn, unspecified**

DIGESTIVE SYSTEM DISORDERS OF NEWBORN (P76-P78)

● **P76**   **Other intestinal obstruction of newborn**

    P76.0   **Meconium plug syndrome**
Fetal stool obstruction in large intestine, present at birth; may be symptom of organic disease.
Meconium ileus NOS

> | Excludes1 | meconium ileus in cystic fibrosis (E84.11) |
> |---|---|

    P76.1   **Transitory ileus of newborn**
Temporary obstruction of ileus (small intestine)

> | Excludes1 | Hirschsprung's disease (Q43.1) |
> |---|---|

    P76.2   **Intestinal obstruction due to inspissated milk**
Being thickened, dried, or made less fluid

    P76.8   **Other specified intestinal obstruction of newborn**

> | Excludes1 | intestinal obstruction classifiable to K56.- |
> |---|---|

    P76.9   **Intestinal obstruction of newborn, unspecified**

● **P77**   **Necrotizing enterocolitis of newborn**

    P77.1   **Stage 1 necrotizing enterocolitis in newborn**
Necrotizing enterocolitis without pneumatosis, without perforation

    P77.2   **Stage 2 necrotizing enterocolitis in newborn**
Necrotizing enterocolitis with pneumatosis, without perforation

    P77.3   **Stage 3 necrotizing enterocolitis in newborn**
Necrotizing enterocolitis with perforation
Necrotizing enterocolitis with pneumatosis and perforation

    P77.9   **Necrotizing enterocolitis in newborn, unspecified**
Necrotizing enterocolitis in newborn, NOS

● **P78**   **Other perinatal digestive system disorders**

> | Excludes1 | cystic fibrosis (E84.0-E84.9) |
> |---|---|
> | | neonatal gastrointestinal hemorrhages (P54.0-P54.3) |

    P78.0   **Perinatal intestinal perforation**
Meconium peritonitis

    P78.1   **Other neonatal peritonitis**
Neonatal peritonitis NOS

    P78.2   **Neonatal hematemesis and melena due to swallowed maternal blood**

    P78.3   **Noninfective neonatal diarrhea**
Neonatal diarrhea NOS

 ● **P78.8**   **Other specified perinatal digestive system disorders**

      P78.81   **Congenital cirrhosis (of liver)**

      P78.82   **Peptic ulcer of newborn**

      P78.83   **Newborn esophageal reflux**
Neonatal esophageal reflux

      P78.89   **Other specified perinatal digestive system disorders**

    P78.9   **Perinatal digestive system disorder, unspecified**

CONDITIONS INVOLVING THE INTEGUMENT AND TEMPERATURE REGULATION OF NEWBORN (P80-P83)

● **P80**   **Hypothermia of newborn**

    P80.0   **Cold injury syndrome**
Severe and usually chronic hypothermia associated with a pink flushed appearance, edema and neurological and biochemical abnormalities.

> | Excludes1 | mild hypothermia of newborn (P80.8) |
> |---|---|

    P80.8   **Other hypothermia of newborn**
Mild hypothermia of newborn

    P80.9   **Hypothermia of newborn, unspecified**

CHAPTER 16 (P00-P96)

● **P81   Other disturbances of temperature regulation of newborn**
    P81.0   Environmental hyperthermia of newborn
    P81.8   Other specified disturbances of temperature regulation of newborn
    P81.9   Disturbance of temperature regulation of newborn, unspecified
            Fever of newborn NOS

● **P83   Other conditions of integument specific to newborn**
    Excludes1   congenital malformations of skin and integument (Q80-Q84)
                 hydrops fetalis due to hemolytic disease (P56.-)
                 neonatal skin infection (P39.4)
                 staphylococcal scalded skin syndrome (L00)
    Excludes2   cradle cap (L21.0)
                 diaper [napkin] dermatitis (L22)
    P83.0   Sclerema neonatorum
            Neonate = newborn
    P83.1   Neonatal erythema toxicum
            Benign, generalized, transient pustules that become firm vesicles
    P83.2   Hydrops fetalis not due to hemolytic disease
            Severe, life-threatening problem of severe edema (swelling) as result of too much fluid leaving blood and entering tissue
            Hydrops fetalis NOS
    ● **P83.3   Other and unspecified edema specific to newborn**
        P83.30   Unspecified edema specific to newborn
        P83.39   Other edema specific to newborn
    P83.4   Breast engorgement of newborn
            Noninfective mastitis of newborn
    P83.5   Congenital hydrocele ♂
    P83.6   Umbilical polyp of newborn
    P83.8   Other specified conditions of integument specific to newborn
            Bronze baby syndrome
            Neonatal scleroderma
            Urticaria neonatorum
    P83.9   Condition of the integument specific to newborn, unspecified

OTHER PROBLEMS WITH NEWBORN (P84)

P84   Other problems with newborn
            Acidemia of newborn
            Acidosis of newborn
            Anoxia of newborn NOS
            Asphyxia of newborn NOS
            Hypercapnia of newborn
            Hypoxemia of newborn
            Hypoxia of newborn NOS
            Mixed metabolic and respiratory acidosis of newborn
    Excludes1   intracranial hemorrhage due to anoxia or hypoxia (P52.-)
                 hypoxic ischemic encephalopathy [HIE] (P91.6-)
                 late metabolic acidosis of newborn (P74.0)

OTHER DISORDERS ORIGINATING IN THE PERINATAL PERIOD (P90-P96)

P90   Convulsions of newborn
    Excludes1   benign myoclonic epilepsy in infancy (G40.3-)
                 benign neonatal convulsions (familial) (G40.3-)

● **P91   Other disturbances of cerebral status of newborn**
    P91.0   Neonatal cerebral ischemia
    P91.1   Acquired periventricular cysts of newborn
    P91.2   Neonatal cerebral leukomalacia
            Degeneration of white matter adjacent to cerebral ventricles following cerebral hypoxia or brain ischemia in neonates
            Periventricular leukomalacia
    P91.3   Neonatal cerebral irritability
    P91.4   Neonatal cerebral depression
    P91.5   Neonatal coma

● **P91.6   Hypoxic ischemic encephalopathy [HIE]**
    P91.60   Hypoxic ischemic encephalopathy [HIE], unspecified
    P91.61   Mild hypoxic ischemic encephalopathy [HIE]
    P91.62   Moderate hypoxic ischemic encephalopathy [HIE]
    P91.63   Severe hypoxic ischemic encephalopathy [HIE]
    P91.8   Other specified disturbances of cerebral status of newborn
    P91.9   Disturbance of cerebral status of newborn, unspecified

● **P92   Feeding problems of newborn**
    Excludes1   feeding problems in child over 28 days old (R63.3)
    ● **P92.0   Vomiting of newborn**
            Excludes1   vomiting of child over 28 days old (R11.-)
        P92.01   Bilious vomiting of newborn
                Excludes1   bilious vomiting in child over 28 days old (R11.14)
        P92.09   Other vomiting of newborn
                Excludes1   regurgitation of food in newborn (P92.1)
    P92.1   Regurgitation and rumination of newborn
    P92.2   Slow feeding of newborn
    P92.3   Underfeeding of newborn
    P92.4   Overfeeding of newborn
    P92.5   Neonatal difficulty in feeding at breast
    P92.6   Failure to thrive in newborn
            Excludes1   failure to thrive in child over 28 days old (R62.51)
    P92.8   Other feeding problems of newborn
    P92.9   Feeding problem of newborn, unspecified

● **P93   Reactions and intoxications due to drugs administered to newborn**
    Includes   reactions and intoxications due to drugs administered to fetus affecting newborn
    Excludes1   jaundice due to drugs or toxins transmitted from mother or given to newborn (P58.4-)
                 reactions and intoxications from maternal opiates, tranquilizers and other medication (P04.0-P04.1, P04.4)
                 withdrawal symptoms from maternal use of drugs of addiction (P96.1)
                 withdrawal symptoms from therapeutic use of drugs in newborn (P96.2)
    P93.0   Grey baby syndrome
            Grey syndrome from chloramphenicol administration in newborn
    P93.8   Other reactions and intoxications due to drugs administered to newborn
            Use additional code for adverse effect, if applicable, to identify drug (T36-T50 with fifth or sixth character 5)

● **P94   Disorders of muscle tone of newborn**
    P94.0   Transient neonatal myasthenia gravis
            Excludes1   myasthenia gravis (G70.0)
    P94.1   Congenital hypertonia
    P94.2   Congenital hypotonia
            Floppy baby syndrome, unspecified
    P94.8   Other disorders of muscle tone of newborn
    P94.9   Disorder of muscle tone of newborn, unspecified

P95　Stillbirth
Deadborn fetus NOS
Fetal death of unspecified cause
Stillbirth NOS

> **Excludes1**　maternal care for intrauterine death (O36.4)
> missed abortion (O02.1)
> outcome of delivery, stillbirth (Z37.1, Z37.3,
> Z37.4, Z37.7)

OGCR Section I.C.16.g.

Stillbirth
Code P95, Stillbirth, is only for use for institutions that
maintain separate records for stillbirths. No other code
should be used with P95. Code P95 should not be used on the
mother's record.

● **P96　Other conditions originating in the perinatal period**

P96.0　Congenital renal failure
Uremia of newborn

**P96.1　Neonatal withdrawal symptoms from maternal use of
drugs of addiction**
Drug withdrawal syndrome in infant of dependent
mother
Neonatal abstinence syndrome

> **Excludes1**　reactions and intoxications from
> maternal opiates and tranquilizers
> administered during labor and
> delivery (P04.0)

**P96.2　Withdrawal symptoms from therapeutic use of drugs in
newborn**

P96.3　Wide cranial sutures of newborn
Neonatal craniotabes

**P96.5　Complication to newborn due to (fetal) intrauterine
procedure**

> **Excludes2**　newborn affected by amniocentesis
> (P00.6) ◄▭

● **P96.8　Other specified conditions originating in the perinatal
period**

**P96.81　Exposure to (parental) (environmental) tobacco
smoke in the perinatal period**

> **Excludes2**　newborn affected by in utero
> exposure to tobacco (P04.2)
> exposure to environmental
> tobacco smoke after the
> perinatal period (Z77.22)

P96.82　Delayed separation of umbilical cord

P96.83　Meconium staining

> **Excludes1**　meconium aspiration (P24.00,
> P24.01)
> meconium passage during
> delivery (P03.82)

**P96.89　Other specified conditions originating in the
perinatal period**
Use additional code to specify condition

**P96.9　Condition originating in the perinatal period,
unspecified**
Congenital debility NOS

CHAPTER 17

CONGENITAL MALFORMATIONS, DEFORMATIONS AND CHROMOSOMAL ABNORMALITIES (Q00-Q99)

CHAPTER 17 (Q00-Q99)

OGCR Chapter-Specific Coding Guidelines

17. Chapter 17: Congenital malformations, deformations, and chromosomal abnormalities (Q00-Q99)
Assign an appropriate code(s) from categories Q00-Q99, Congenital malformations, deformations, and chromosomal abnormalities when a malformation/deformation or chromosomal abnormality is documented. A malformation/deformation/or chromosomal abnormality may be the principal/first-listed diagnosis on a record or a secondary diagnosis.

When a malformation/deformation/or chromosomal abnormality does not have a unique code assignment, assign additional code(s) for any manifestations that may be present.

When the code assignment specifically identifies the malformation/deformation/or chromosomal abnormality, manifestations that are an inherent component of the anomaly should not be coded separately. Additional codes should be assigned for manifestations that are not an inherent component.

Codes from Chapter 17 may be used throughout the life of the patient. If a congenital malformation or deformity has been corrected, a personal history code should be used to identify the history of the malformation or deformity. Although present at birth, malformation/deformation/or chromosomal abnormality may not be identified until later in life. Whenever the condition is diagnosed by the physician, it is appropriate to assign a code from codes Q00-Q99.

For the birth admission, the appropriate code from category Z38, Liveborn infants, according to place of birth and type of delivery, should be sequenced as the principal diagnosis, followed by any congenital anomaly codes, Q00-Q99.

CHAPTER 17

CONGENITAL MALFORMATIONS, DEFORMATIONS AND CHROMOSOMAL ABNORMALITIES (Q00-Q99)

Note: Codes from this chapter are not for use on maternal or fetal records

Excludes2 inborn errors of metabolism (E70-E88)

This chapter contains the following blocks:

Q00-Q07	Congenital malformations of the nervous system
Q10-Q18	Congenital malformations of eye, ear, face and neck
Q20-Q28	Congenital malformations of the circulatory system
Q30-Q34	Congenital malformations of the respiratory system
Q35-Q37	Cleft lip and cleft palate
Q38-Q45	Other congenital malformations of the digestive system
Q50-Q56	Congenital malformations of genital organs
Q60-Q64	Congenital malformations of the urinary system
Q65-Q79	Congenital malformations and deformations of the musculoskeletal system
Q80-Q89	Other congenital malformations
Q90-Q99	Chromosomal abnormalities, not elsewhere classified

Figure 17-1 An infant with a large occipital encephalocele. The large skin-covered encephalocele is visible. (From Townsend: Sabiston Textbook of Surgery, ed 19, Saunders, An Imprint of Elsevier, 2012)

CONGENITAL MALFORMATIONS OF THE NERVOUS SYSTEM (Q00–Q07)

● **Q00   Anencephaly and similar malformations**

Q00.0   Anencephaly
Absence of skull with cerebral hemispheres missing or reduced to small masses attached to base of cranium
Acephaly
Acrania
Amyelencephaly
Hemianencephaly
Hemicephaly

Q00.1   Craniorachischisis
Developmental anomaly consisting of fissure of cranium and vertebral column

Q00.2   Iniencephaly
Developmental anomaly characterized by enlargement of foramen magnum and absence of laminae and spinous processes of cervical, dorsal

● **Q01   Encephalocele**
Sac-like protrusions of brain and membranes visible through an opening in skull

Includes   Arnold-Chiari syndrome, type III
encephalocystocele
encephalomyelocele
hydroencephalocele
hydromeningocele, cranial
meningocele, cerebral
meningoencephalocele

Excludes1   Meckel-Gruber syndrome (Q61.9)

Q01.0   Frontal encephalocele
Q01.1   Nasofrontal encephalocele
Q01.2   Occipital encephalocele
Q01.8   Encephalocele of other sites
Q01.9   Encephalocele, unspecified

● **Q02   Microcephaly**
Head size measures significantly below normal based on standardized charts

Includes   hydromicrocephaly
micrencephalon

Excludes1   Meckel-Gruber syndrome (Q61.9)

● **Q03   Congenital hydrocephalus**
Accumulation of cerebrospinal fluid in ventricles resulting in swelling and enlargement

Includes   hydrocephalus in newborn

Excludes1   Arnold-Chiari syndrome, type II (Q07.0-)
acquired hydrocephalus (G91.-)
hydrocephalus due to congenital toxoplasmosis (P37.1)
hydrocephalus with spina bifida (Q05.0-Q05.4)

Q03.0   Malformations of aqueduct of Sylvius
Anomaly of aqueduct of Sylvius
Obstruction of aqueduct of Sylvius, congenital
Stenosis of aqueduct of Sylvius

Q03.1   Atresia of foramina of Magendie and Luschka
Dandy-Walker syndrome

Q03.8   Other congenital hydrocephalus

Q03.9   Congenital hydrocephalus, unspecified

◀ New   ◀▥ Revised   ~~deleted~~ Deleted   Excludes 1   Excludes 2   Includes   Use additional   Code first   Code also   Unspecified
OGCR Official Guidelines   X Assign placeholder X   ● Use Additional Character(s)   ▸ Manifestation Code   **Coding Clinic**

● **Q04**   **Other congenital malformations of brain**

     Excludes1   cyclopia (Q87.0)
                      macrocephaly (Q75.3)

    Q04.0   **Congenital malformations of corpus callosum**
          Agenesis of corpus callosum

    Q04.1   **Arhinencephaly**
          Congenital absence of olfactory bulbs, tract, or nerves

    Q04.2   **Holoprosencephaly**
          Failure of cleavage of forebrain (prosencephalon) resulting in incomplete or absent cortical separation and deficits in midline facial development

    Q04.3   **Other reduction deformities of brain**
          Absence of part of brain   Agyria
          Agenesis of part of brain
             Cerebral cortex are not fully formed, brain surface is smooth
          Aplasia of part of brain
          Hydranencephaly
          Hypoplasia of part of brain
          Lissencephaly
             Congenital malformation or absence of convolutions of cerebral cortex
          Microgyria
             Malformation of brain characterized by excessive number of small convolutions (gyri) on surface
          Pachygyria
             Reduction in number of sulci of cerebrum
      Excludes1   congenital malformations of corpus callosum (Q04.0)

    Q04.4   **Septo-optic dysplasia of brain**

    Q04.5   **Megalencephaly**
          Abnormally large brain

    Q04.6   **Congenital cerebral cysts**
          Porencephaly   Schizencephaly
      Excludes1   acquired porencephalic cyst (G93.0)

    Q04.8   **Other specified congenital malformations of brain**
          Arnold-Chiari syndrome, type IV
          Macrogyria

    Q04.9   **Congenital malformation of brain, unspecified**
          Congenital anomaly NOS of brain
          Congenital deformity NOS of brain
          Congenital disease or lesion NOS of brain
          Multiple anomalies NOS of brain, congenital

● **Q05**   **Spina bifida**
     Developmental anomaly characterized by defective closure of vertebral arch, through which spinal cord and meninges may protrude

     Includes   hydromeningocele (spinal)
                  meningocele (spinal)
                  meningomyelocele
                  myelocele
                  myelomeningocele
                  rachischisis
                  spina bifida (aperta)(cystica)
                  syringomyelocele

     Use additional code for any associated paraplegia (paraparesis) (G82.2-)

     Excludes1   Arnold-Chiari syndrome, type II (Q07.0-)
                  spina bifida occulta (Q76.0)

    Q05.0   **Cervical spina bifida with hydrocephalus**

    Q05.1   **Thoracic spina bifida with hydrocephalus**
          Dorsal spina bifida with hydrocephalus
          Thoracolumbar spina bifida with hydrocephalus

    Q05.2   **Lumbar spina bifida with hydrocephalus**
          Lumbosacral spina bifida with hydrocephalus

    Q05.3   **Sacral spina bifida with hydrocephalus**

    Q05.4   **Unspecified spina bifida with hydrocephalus**

    Q05.5   **Cervical spina bifida without hydrocephalus**

    Q05.6   **Thoracic spina bifida without hydrocephalus**
          Dorsal spina bifida NOS
          Thoracolumbar spina bifida NOS

    Q05.7   **Lumbar spina bifida without hydrocephalus**
          Lumbosacral spina bifida NOS

    Q05.8   **Sacral spina bifida without hydrocephalus**

    Q05.9   **Spina bifida, unspecified**

● **Q06**   **Other congenital malformations of spinal cord**

    Q06.0   **Amyelia**
          Congenital absence of spinal cord

    Q06.1   **Hypoplasia and dysplasia of spinal cord**
          Underdevelopment of spinal cord
          Atelomyelia
             Congenitally incomplete development of spinal cord
          Myelatelia
          Myelodysplasia of spinal cord
             Defective development of spinal cord, especially lower segments

    Q06.2   **Diastematomyelia**
          Congenital anomaly, associated with spina bifida, in which spinal cord is split into halves and surrounded by dural sac

    Q06.3   **Other congenital cauda equina malformations**

    Q06.4   **Hydromyelia**
          Dilation of central canal of spinal cord with increased fluid accumulation
          Hydrorachis

    Q06.8   **Other specified congenital malformations of spinal cord**

    Q06.9   **Congenital malformation of spinal cord, unspecified**
          Congenital anomaly NOS of spinal cord
          Congenital deformity NOS of spinal cord
          Congenital disease or lesion NOS of spinal cord

● **Q07**   **Other congenital malformations of nervous system**
     Excludes2   congenital central alveolar hypoventilation syndrome (G47.35)
                  familial dysautonomia [Riley-Day] (G90.1)
                  neurofibromatosis (nonmalignant) (Q85.0-)

● **Q07.0**   **Arnold-Chiari syndrome**
     Herniation of cerebellar tonsils and vermis through foramen magnum into spinal canal
     Arnold-Chiari syndrome, type II
     Excludes1   Arnold-Chiari syndrome, type III (Q01.-)
                  Arnold-Chiari syndrome, type IV (Q04.8)

    Q07.00   **Arnold-Chiari syndrome without spina bifida or hydrocephalus**

    Q07.01   **Arnold-Chiari syndrome with spina bifida**

    Q07.02   **Arnold-Chiari syndrome with hydrocephalus**

    Q07.03   **Arnold-Chiari syndrome with spina bifida and hydrocephalus**

    Q07.8   **Other specified congenital malformations of nervous system**
          Agenesis of nerve
          Displacement of brachial plexus
          Jaw-winking syndrome
          Marcus Gunn's syndrome

    Q07.9   **Congenital malformation of nervous system, unspecified**
          Congenital anomaly NOS of nervous system
          Congenital deformity NOS of nervous system
          Congenital disease or lesion NOS of nervous system

CHAPTER 17 (Q00-Q99)

CONGENITAL MALFORMATIONS OF EYE, EAR, FACE AND NECK (Q10-Q18)

Excludes2   cleft lip and cleft palate (Q35-Q37)
congenital malformation of cervical spine (Q05.0,
Q05.5, Q67.5, Q76.0-Q76.4)
congenital malformation of larynx (Q31.-)
congenital malformation of lip NEC (Q38.0)
congenital malformation of nose (Q30.-)
congenital malformation of parathyroid gland
(Q89.2)
congenital malformation of thyroid gland (Q89.2)

● **Q10** **Congenital malformations of eyelid, lacrimal apparatus and orbit**

Excludes1   cryptophthalmos NOS (Q11.2)
cryptophthalmos syndrome (Q87.0)

Q10.0 **Congenital ptosis**
Prolapse or drooping of upper eyelid from paralysis of third nerve or from sympathetic innervations

Q10.1 **Congenital ectropion**
Outward turning of eyelid

Q10.2 **Congenital entropion**
Inward turning of eyelid

Q10.3 **Other congenital malformations of eyelid**
Ablepharon
Blepharophimosis, congenital
Coloboma of eyelid
Congenital absence or agenesis of cilia
Congenital absence or agenesis of eyelid
Congenital accessory eyelid
Congenital accessory eye muscle
Congenital malformation of eyelid NOS

Q10.4 **Absence and agenesis of lacrimal apparatus**
Congenital absence of punctum lacrimale

Q10.5 **Congenital stenosis and stricture of lacrimal duct**

Q10.6 **Other congenital malformations of lacrimal apparatus**
Congenital malformation of lacrimal apparatus NOS

Q10.7 **Congenital malformation of orbit**

● **Q11** **Anophthalmos, microphthalmos and macrophthalmos**
Absence of eye and optic pit

Q11.0 **Cystic eyeball**

Q11.1 **Other anophthalmos**
Anophthalmos NOS
Agenesis of eye
Absence of eye
Aplasia of eye

Q11.2 **Microphthalmos**
Partial absence of eye and optic pit
Cryptophthalmos NOS
Dysplasia of eye
Hypoplasia of eye
Rudimentary eye
Excludes1   cryptophthalmos syndrome (Q87.0)

Q11.3 **Macrophthalmos**
Congenital enlargement of eyes
Excludes1   macrophthalmos in congenital glaucoma (Q15.0)

● **Q12** **Congenital lens malformations**

Q12.0 **Congenital cataract**

Q12.1 **Congenital displaced lens**

Q12.2 **Coloboma of lens**

Q12.3 **Congenital aphakia**

Q12.4 **Spherophakia**
Smaller, more spherical optic lens than normal

Q12.8 **Other congenital lens malformations**
Microphakia

Q12.9 **Congenital lens malformation, unspecified**

Figure 17-2 Bilateral congenital **hydrophthalmia,** in which the eyes are very large in comparison to the other facial features due to glaucoma.

● **Q13** **Congenital malformations of anterior segment of eye**

Q13.0 **Coloboma of iris**
Coloboma NOS

Q13.1 **Absence of iris**
Aniridia
Use additional code for associated glaucoma (H42)

Q13.2 **Other congenital malformations of iris**
Anisocoria, congenital
Atresia of pupil
Congenital malformation of iris NOS
Corectopia

Q13.3 **Congenital corneal opacity**

Q13.4 **Other congenital corneal malformations**
Congenital malformation of cornea NOS
Microcornea
Peter's anomaly

Q13.5 **Blue sclera**
Condition of unusual blueness of sclera; not harmful

● **Q13.8** **Other congenital malformations of anterior segment of eye**

Q13.81 **Rieger's anomaly**
Use additional code for associated glaucoma (H42)

Q13.89 **Other congenital malformations of anterior segment of eye**

Q13.9 **Congenital malformation of anterior segment of eye, unspecified**

● **Q14** **Congenital malformations of posterior segment of eye**
Excludes2   optic nerve hypoplasia (H47.03-)

Q14.0 **Congenital malformation of vitreous humor**
Congenital vitreous opacity

Q14.1 **Congenital malformation of retina**
Congenital retinal aneurysm

Q14.2 **Congenital malformation of optic disc**
Coloboma of optic disc

Q14.3 **Congenital malformation of choroid**

Q14.8 **Other congenital malformations of posterior segment of eye**
Coloboma of the fundus

Q14.9 **Congenital malformation of posterior segment of eye, unspecified**

◀ New   ◀ Revised   ~~deleted~~ Deleted   Excludes 1   Excludes 2   Includes   Use additional   Code first   Code also   Unspecified
OGCR Official Guidelines   X Assign placeholder X   ● Use Additional Character(s)   ▶ Manifestation Code   **Coding Clinic**

● **Q15**   **Other congenital malformations of eye**
     Excludes 1   congenital nystagmus (H55.01)
              ocular albinism (E70.31-)
              optic nerve hypoplasia (H47.03-)
              retinitis pigmentosa (H35.52)

     Q15.0   **Congenital glaucoma**
          Axenfeld's anomaly
          Buphthalmos
          Congenital syndrome characterized by port-wine nevus covering portions of face and cranium
          Glaucoma of childhood
          Glaucoma of newborn
          Hydrophthalmos
          Keratoglobus, congenital, with glaucoma
          Macrocornea with glaucoma
          Macrophthalmos in congenital glaucoma
          Megalocornea with glaucoma

     Q15.8   **Other specified congenital malformations of eye**

     Q15.9   **Congenital malformation of eye, unspecified**
          Congenital anomaly of eye
          Congenital deformity of eye

● **Q16**   **Congenital malformations of ear causing impairment of hearing**
     Excludes 1   congenital deafness (H90.-)

     Q16.0   **Congenital absence of (ear) auricle**

     Q16.1   **Congenital absence, atresia and stricture of auditory canal (external)**
          Congenital atresia or stricture of osseous meatus

     Q16.2   **Absence of eustachian tube**

     Q16.3   **Congenital malformation of ear ossicles**
          Congenital fusion of ear ossicles

     Q16.4   **Other congenital malformations of middle ear**
          Congenital malformation of middle ear NOS

     Q16.5   **Congenital malformation of inner ear**
          Congenital anomaly of membranous labyrinth
          Congenital anomaly of organ of Corti

     Q16.9   **Congenital malformation of ear causing impairment of hearing, unspecified**
          Congenital absence of ear NOS

● **Q17**   **Other congenital malformations of ear**
     Excludes 1   congenital malformations of ear with impairment of hearing (Q16.0-Q16.9)
              preauricular sinus (Q18.1)

     Q17.0   **Accessory auricle**
          Accessory tragus
          Polyotia
          Preauricular appendage or tag
          Supernumerary ear
          Supernumerary lobule

     Q17.1   **Macrotia**
          Enlarged ears

     Q17.2   **Microtia**
          An abnormally small or underdeveloped external ear

     Q17.3   **Other misshapen ear**
          Pointed ear

     Q17.4   **Misplaced ear**
          Low-set ears
          Excludes 1   cervical auricle (Q18.2)

     Q17.5   **Prominent ear**
          Bat ear

     Q17.8   **Other specified congenital malformations of ear**
          Congenital absence of lobe of ear

     Q17.9   **Congenital malformation of ear, unspecified**
          Congenital anomaly of ear NOS

● **Q18**   **Other congenital malformations of face and neck**
     Excludes 1   cleft lip and cleft palate (Q35-Q37)
              conditions classified to Q67.0-Q67.4
              congenital malformations of skull and face bones (Q75.-)
              cyclopia (Q87.0)
              dentofacial anomalies [including malocclusion] (M26.-)
              malformation syndromes affecting facial appearance (Q87.0)
              persistent thyroglossal duct (Q89.2)

     Q18.0   **Sinus, fistula and cyst of branchial cleft**
          Branchial vestige
          Brachial remnants (cysts, fistula, skin tags) that are developmental anomalies

     Q18.1   **Preauricular sinus and cyst**
          Fistula of auricle, congenital
          Cervicoaural fistula
          Abnormal passage in neck originating from first branchial cleft

     Q18.2   **Other branchial cleft malformations**
          Branchial cleft malformation NOS
          Cervical auricle
          Otocephaly

     Q18.3   **Webbing of neck**
          Pterygium colli
          Thick fold of skin on side of neck

     Q18.4   **Macrostomia**
          Results from failure of union of maxillary and mandibular processes, results in abnormally large mouth

     Q18.5   **Microstomia**

     Q18.6   **Macrocheilia**
          Excessive size of lips
          Hypertrophy of lip, congenital

     Q18.7   **Microcheilia**
          Abnormal smallness of lips

     Q18.8   **Other specified congenital malformations of face and neck**
          Medial cyst of face and neck
          Medial fistula of face and neck
          Medial sinus of face and neck

     Q18.9   **Congenital malformation of face and neck, unspecified**
          Congenital anomaly NOS of face and neck

CONGENITAL MALFORMATIONS OF THE CIRCULATORY SYSTEM (Q20-Q28)

● **Q20**   **Congenital malformations of cardiac chambers and connections**
     Excludes 1   dextrocardia with situs inversus (Q89.3)
              mirror-image atrial arrangement with situs inversus (Q89.3)

     Q20.0   **Common arterial trunk**
          Persistent truncus arteriosus
          Excludes 1   aortic septal defect (Q21.4)

     Q20.1   **Double outlet right ventricle**
          Taussig-Bing syndrome

     Q20.2   **Double outlet left ventricle**

     Q20.3   **Discordant ventriculoarterial connection**
          Dextrotransposition of aorta
          Transposition of great vessels (complete)

     Q20.4   **Double inlet ventricle**
          Common ventricle
          Cor triloculare biatriatum
          Single ventricle

     Q20.5   **Discordant atrioventricular connection**
          Corrected transposition
          Levotransposition
          Ventricular inversion

     Q20.6   **Isomerism of atrial appendages**
          Isomerism of atrial appendages with asplenia or polysplenia

     Q20.8   **Other congenital malformations of cardiac chambers and connections**
          Cor binoculare

     Q20.9   **Congenital malformation of cardiac chambers and connections, unspecified**

CHAPTER 17 (Q00-Q99)

● **Q21   Congenital malformations of cardiac septa**

> **Excludes1**   acquired cardiac septal defect (I51.0)

Q21.0   Ventricular septal defect
Roger's disease

Q21.1   Atrial septal defect
Coronary sinus defect
Patent or persistent foramen ovale
Patent or persistent ostium secundum defect (type II)
Patent or persistent sinus venosus defect

Q21.2   Atrioventricular septal defect
Common atrioventricular canal
Endocardial cushion defect
Ostium primum atrial septal defect (type I)

Q21.3   Tetralogy of Fallot
Ventricular septal defect with pulmonary stenosis or atresia, dextroposition of aorta and hypertrophy of right ventricle.

Q21.4   Aortopulmonary septal defect
Aortic septal defect
Aortopulmonary window

Q21.8   Other congenital malformations of cardiac septa
Eisenmenger's defect
Pentalogy of Fallot

> **Excludes1**   Eisenmenger's complex (I27.8)
> Eisenmenger's syndrome (I27.8)

Q21.9   Congenital malformation of cardiac septum, unspecified
Septal (heart) defect NOS

● **Q22   Congenital malformations of pulmonary and tricuspid valves**

Q22.0   Pulmonary valve atresia

Q22.1   Congenital pulmonary valve stenosis

Q22.2   Congenital pulmonary valve insufficiency
Congenital pulmonary valve regurgitation

Q22.3   Other congenital malformations of pulmonary valve
Congenital malformation of pulmonary valve NOS
Supernumerary cusps of pulmonary valve

Q22.4   Congenital tricuspid stenosis
Congenital tricuspid atresia

Q22.5   Ebstein's anomaly
Malformation of tricuspid valve

Q22.6   Hypoplastic right heart syndrome

Q22.8   Other congenital malformations of tricuspid valve

Q22.9   Congenital malformation of tricuspid valve, unspecified

● **Q23   Congenital malformations of aortic and mitral valves**

Q23.0   Congenital stenosis of aortic valve
Congenital aortic atresia
Congenital aortic stenosis NOS

> **Excludes1**   congenital stenosis of aortic valve in hypoplastic left heart syndrome (Q23.4)
> congenital subaortic stenosis (Q24.4)
> supravalvular aortic stenosis (congenital) (Q25.3)

Q23.1   Congenital insufficiency of aortic valve
Bicuspid aortic valve
Congenital aortic insufficiency

Q23.2   Congenital mitral stenosis
Congenital mitral atresia

Q23.3   Congenital mitral insufficiency

Q23.4   Hypoplastic left heart syndrome

Q23.8   Other congenital malformations of aortic and mitral valves

Q23.9   Congenital malformation of aortic and mitral valves, unspecified

● **Q24   Other congenital malformations of heart**

> **Excludes1**   endocardial fibroelastosis (I42.4)

Q24.0   Dextrocardia
Heart is located in right hemithorax

> **Excludes1**   dextrocardia with situs inversus (Q89.3)
> isomerism of atrial appendages (with asplenia or polysplenia) (Q20.6)
> mirror-image atrial arrangement with situs inversus (Q89.3)

Q24.1   Levocardia
Normal position of heart but related structures on wrong side

Q24.2   Cor triatriatum
Congenital heart defect; left atrium is subdivided

Q24.3   Pulmonary infundibular stenosis
Subvalvular pulmonic stenosis

Q24.4   Congenital subaortic stenosis

Q24.5   Malformation of coronary vessels
Congenital coronary (artery) aneurysm

Q24.6   Congenital heart block

Q24.8   Other specified congenital malformations of heart
Congenital diverticulum of left ventricle
Congenital malformation of myocardium
Congenital malformation of pericardium
Malposition of heart
Uhl's disease

Q24.9   Congenital malformation of heart, unspecified
Congenital anomaly of heart
Congenital disease of heart

● **Q25   Congenital malformations of great arteries**

Q25.0   Patent ductus arteriosus
Fetal blood vessel connecting left pulmonary artery directly to descending aorta
Patent ductus Botallo
Persistent ductus arteriosus

Q25.1   Coarctation of aorta
Coarctation of aorta (preductal) (postductal)
Stenosis of aorta ◀

● **Q25.2   Atresia of aorta**

Q25.21   Interruption of aortic arch ◀
Atresia of aortic arch ◀

Q25.29   Other atresia of aorta ◀
Atresia of aorta ◀

Q25.3   Supravalvular aortic stenosis

> **Excludes1**   congenital aortic stenosis NOS (Q23.0)
> congenital stenosis of aortic valve (Q23.0)

● **Q25.4   Other congenital malformations of aorta**

> **Excludes1**   hypoplasia of aorta in hypoplastic left heart syndrome (Q23.4)

Q25.40   Congenital malformation of aorta unspecified ◀

Q25.41   Absence and aplasia of aorta ◀

Q25.42   Hypoplasia of aorta ◀

Q25.43   Congenital aneurysm of aorta ◀
Congenital aneurysm of aortic root ◀
Congenital aneurysm of aortic sinus ◀

Q25.44   Congenital dilation of aorta ◀

Q25.45   Double aortic arch ◀
Vascular ring of aorta ◀

Q25.46   Tortuous aortic arch ◀
Persistent convolutions of aortic arch ◀

Q25.47   Right aortic arch ◀
Persistent right aortic arch ◀

Q25.48   Anomalous origin of subclavian artery ◀

Q25.49   Other congenital malformations of aorta ◀

Q25.5   Atresia of pulmonary artery

Q25.6   Stenosis of pulmonary artery
Supravalvular pulmonary stenosis

◀ New   ◀▥ Revised   ~~deleted~~ Deleted   Excludes 1   Excludes 2   Includes   Use additional   Code first   Code also   Unspecified

1146   OGCR Official Guidelines   X Assign placeholder X   ● Use Additional Character(s)   ▶ Manifestation Code   **Coding Clinic**

- **Q25.7   Other congenital malformations of pulmonary artery**

  Q25.71   Coarctation of pulmonary artery

  Q25.72   Congenital pulmonary arteriovenous malformation
  > Congenital pulmonary arteriovenous aneurysm

  Q25.79   Other congenital malformations of pulmonary artery
  > Aberrant pulmonary artery
  > Agenesis of pulmonary artery
  > Congenital aneurysm of pulmonary artery
  > Congenital anomaly of pulmonary artery
  > Hypoplasia of pulmonary artery

  Q25.8   Other congenital malformations of other great arteries

  Q25.9   Congenital malformation of great arteries, unspecified

- **Q26   Congenital malformations of great veins**

  Q26.0   Congenital stenosis of vena cava
  > Congenital stenosis of vena cava (inferior)(superior)

  Q26.1   Persistent left superior vena cava

  Q26.2   Total anomalous pulmonary venous connection
  > Total anomalous pulmonary venous return [TAPVR], subdiaphragmatic
  > Total anomalous pulmonary venous return [TAPVR], supradiaphragmatic

  Q26.3   Partial anomalous pulmonary venous connection
  > Partial anomalous pulmonary venous return

  Q26.4   Anomalous pulmonary venous connection, unspecified

  Q26.5   Anomalous portal venous connection

  Q26.6   Portal vein-hepatic artery fistula

  Q26.8   Other congenital malformations of great veins
  > Absence of vena cava (inferior) (superior)
  > Azygos continuation of inferior vena cava
  > Persistent left posterior cardinal vein
  > Scimitar syndrome

  Q26.9   Congenital malformation of great vein, unspecified
  > Congenital anomaly of vena cava (inferior) (superior) NOS

- **Q27   Other congenital malformations of peripheral vascular system**

  Excludes2   anomalies of cerebral and precerebral vessels (Q28.0-Q28.3)
  > anomalies of coronary vessels (Q24.5)
  > anomalies of pulmonary artery (Q25.5-Q25.7)
  > congenital retinal aneurysm (Q14.1)
  > hemangioma and lymphangioma (D18.-)

  Q27.0   Congenital absence and hypoplasia of umbilical artery
  > Single umbilical artery

  Q27.1   Congenital renal artery stenosis

  Q27.2   Other congenital malformations of renal artery
  > Congenital malformation of renal artery NOS
  > Multiple renal arteries

- **Q27.3   Arteriovenous malformation (peripheral)**
  > Arteriovenous aneurysm

  Excludes1   acquired arteriovenous aneurysm (I77.0)

  Excludes2   arteriovenous malformation of cerebral vessels (Q28.2)
  > arteriovenous malformation of precerebral vessels (Q28.0)

  Q27.30   Arteriovenous malformation, site unspecified

  Q27.31   Arteriovenous malformation of vessel of upper limb

  Q27.32   Arteriovenous malformation of vessel of lower limb

  Q27.33   Arteriovenous malformation of digestive system vessel

  Q27.34   Arteriovenous malformation of renal vessel

  Q27.39   Arteriovenous malformation, other site

Q27.4   Congenital phlebectasia

Q27.8   Other specified congenital malformations of peripheral vascular system
> Absence of peripheral vascular system
> Atresia of peripheral vascular system
> Congenital aneurysm (peripheral)
> Congenital stricture, artery
> Congenital varix

> **Excludes1**   arteriovenous malformation (Q27.3-)

Q27.9   Congenital malformation of peripheral vascular system, unspecified
> Anomaly of artery or vein NOS

- **Q28   Other congenital malformations of circulatory system**

  Excludes1   congenital aneurysm NOS (Q27.8)
  > congenital coronary aneurysm (Q24.5)
  > ruptured cerebral arteriovenous malformation (I60.8)
  > ruptured malformation of precerebral vessels (I72.0)

  Excludes2   congenital peripheral aneurysm (Q27.8)
  > congenital pulmonary aneurysm (Q25.79)
  > congenital retinal aneurysm (Q14.1)

  Q28.0   Arteriovenous malformation of precerebral vessels
  > Congenital arteriovenous precerebral aneurysm (nonruptured)

  Q28.1   Other malformations of precerebral vessels
  > Congenital malformation of precerebral vessels NOS
  > Congenital precerebral aneurysm (nonruptured)

  Q28.2   Arteriovenous malformation of cerebral vessels
  > Arteriovenous malformation of brain NOS
  > Congenital arteriovenous cerebral aneurysm (nonruptured)

  Q28.3   Other malformations of cerebral vessels
  > Congenital cerebral aneurysm (nonruptured)
  > Congenital malformation of cerebral vessels NOS
  > Developmental venous anomaly

  Q28.8   Other specified congenital malformations of circulatory system
  > Congenital aneurysm, specified site NEC
  > Spinal vessel anomaly

  Q28.9   Congenital malformation of circulatory system, unspecified

CONGENITAL MALFORMATIONS OF THE RESPIRATORY SYSTEM (Q30-Q34)

- **Q30   Congenital malformations of nose**

  Excludes1   congenital deviation of nasal septum (Q67.4)

  Q30.0   Choanal atresia
  > Atresia of nares (anterior) (posterior)
  > Congenital stenosis of nares (anterior) (posterior)

  Q30.1   Agenesis and underdevelopment of nose
  > Congenital absent of nose

  Q30.2   Fissured, notched and cleft nose

  Q30.3   Congenital perforated nasal septum

  Q30.8   Other congenital malformations of nose
  > Accessory nose
  > Congenital anomaly of nasal sinus wall

  Q30.9   Congenital malformation of nose, unspecified

- **Q31   Congenital malformations of larynx**

  Excludes1   congenital laryngeal stridor NOS (P28.89)

  Q31.0   Web of larynx
  > Glottic web of larynx
  > Subglottic web of larynx
  > Web of larynx NOS

  Q31.1   Congenital subglottic stenosis

  Q31.2   Laryngeal hypoplasia

  Q31.3   Laryngocele

  Q31.5   Congenital laryngomalacia

CHAPTER 17 (Q00-Q99)

Q31.8   **Other congenital malformations of larynx**
        Absence of larynx
        Agenesis of larynx
        Atresia of larynx
        Congenital cleft thyroid cartilage
        Congenital fissure of epiglottis
        Congenital stenosis of larynx NEC
        Posterior cleft of cricoid cartilage

Q31.9   **Congenital malformation of larynx, unspecified**

● Q32   **Congenital malformations of trachea and bronchus**
        Excludes1   congenital bronchiectasis (Q33.4)

Q32.0   **Congenital tracheomalacia**

Q32.1   **Other congenital malformations of trachea**
        Atresia of trachea
        Congenital anomaly of tracheal cartilage
        Congenital dilatation of trachea
        Congenital malformation of trachea
        Congenital stenosis of trachea
        Congenital tracheocele

Q32.2   **Congenital bronchomalacia**

Q32.3   **Congenital stenosis of bronchus**

Q32.4   **Other congenital malformations of bronchus**
        Absence of bronchus
        Agenesis of bronchus
        Atresia of bronchus
        Congenital diverticulum of bronchus
        Congenital malformation of bronchus NOS

● Q33   **Congenital malformations of lung**

Q33.0   **Congenital cystic lung**
        Congenital cystic lung disease
        Congenital honeycomb lung
        Congenital polycystic lung disease
        Excludes1   cystic fibrosis (E84.0)
                        cystic lung disease, acquired or
                        unspecified (J98.4)

Q33.1   **Accessory lobe of lung**
        Azygos lobe (fissured), lung

Q33.2   **Sequestration of lung**

Q33.3   **Agenesis of lung**
        Congenital absence of lung (lobe)

Q33.4   **Congenital bronchiectasis**

Q33.5   **Ectopic tissue in lung**

Q33.6   **Congenital hypoplasia and dysplasia of lung**
        Excludes1   pulmonary hypoplasia associated with
                        short gestation (P28.0)

Q33.8   **Other congenital malformations of lung**

Q33.9   **Congenital malformation of lung, unspecified**

● Q34   **Other congenital malformations of respiratory system**
        Excludes2   congenital central alveolar hypoventilation
                        syndrome (G47.35)

Q34.0   **Anomaly of pleura**

Q34.1   **Congenital cyst of mediastinum**

Q34.8   **Other specified congenital malformations of respiratory
        system**
        Atresia of nasopharynx

Q34.9   **Congenital malformation of respiratory system,
        unspecified**
        Congenital absence of respiratory system
        Congenital anomaly of respiratory system NOS

Figure 17-3   Cleft palate.

CLEFT LIP AND CLEFT PALATE (Q35-Q37)

Use additional code to identify associated malformation of the
nose (Q30.2)
        Excludes1   Robin's syndrome (Q87.0)

● Q35   **Cleft palate**
        Includes   fissure of palate
                       palatoschisis
        Excludes1   cleft palate with cleft lip (Q37.-)

Q35.1   **Cleft hard palate**

Q35.3   **Cleft soft palate**

Q35.5   **Cleft hard palate with cleft soft palate**

Q35.7   **Cleft uvula**

Q35.9   **Cleft palate, unspecified**
        Cleft palate NOS

● Q36   **Cleft lip**
        Includes   cheiloschisis
                       congenital fissure of lip
                       harelip
                       labium leporinum
        Excludes1   cleft lip with cleft palate (Q37.-)

Q36.0   **Cleft lip, bilateral**

Q36.1   **Cleft lip, median**

Q36.9   **Cleft lip, unilateral**
        Cleft lip NOS

● Q37   **Cleft palate with cleft lip**
        Includes   cheilopalatoschisis

Q37.0   **Cleft hard palate with bilateral cleft lip**

Q37.1   **Cleft hard palate with unilateral cleft lip**
        Cleft hard palate with cleft lip NOS

Q37.2   **Cleft soft palate with bilateral cleft lip**

Q37.3   **Cleft soft palate with unilateral cleft lip**
        Cleft soft palate with cleft lip NOS

Q37.4   **Cleft hard and soft palate with bilateral cleft lip**

Q37.5   **Cleft hard and soft palate with unilateral cleft lip**
        Cleft hard and soft palate with cleft lip NOS

Q37.8   **Unspecified cleft palate with bilateral cleft lip**

Q37.9   **Unspecified cleft palate with unilateral cleft lip**
        Cleft palate with cleft lip NOS

◀ New   ⇚ Revised   ~~deleted~~ Deleted   Excludes 1   Excludes 2   Includes   Use additional   Code first   Code also   Unspecified

OGCR Official Guidelines   X Assign placeholder X   ● Use Additional Character(s)   ▷ Manifestation Code   **Coding Clinic**

OTHER CONGENITAL MALFORMATIONS OF THE DIGESTIVE SYSTEM (Q38-Q45)

● **Q38   Other congenital malformations of tongue, mouth and pharynx**

     Excludes1   dentofacial anomalies (M26.-)
                    macrostomia (Q18.4)
                    microstomia (Q18.5)

    Q38.0   Congenital malformations of lips, not elsewhere classified
         Congenital fistula of lip
         Congenital malformation of lip NOS
         Van der Woude's syndrome

         Excludes1   cleft lip (Q36.-)
                        cleft lip with cleft palate (Q37.-)
                        macrocheilia (Q18.6)
                        microcheilia (Q18.7)

    Q38.1   Ankyloglossia
         Restricted movement of tongue resulting in speech difficulty
         Tongue tie

    Q38.2   Macroglossia
         Excessive size of tongue
         Congenital hypertrophy of tongue

    Q38.3   Other congenital malformations of tongue
         Aglossia
         Bifid tongue
         Congenital adhesion of tongue
         Congenital fissure of tongue
         Congenital malformation of tongue NOS
         Double tongue
         Hypoglossia
         Hypoplasia of tongue
         Microglossia

    Q38.4   Congenital malformations of salivary glands and ducts
         Atresia of salivary glands and ducts
         Congenital absence of salivary glands and ducts
         Congenital accessory salivary glands and ducts
         Congenital fistula of salivary gland

    Q38.5   Congenital malformations of palate, not elsewhere classified
         Congenital absence of uvula
         Congenital malformation of palate NOS
         Congenital high arched palate

         Excludes1   cleft palate (Q35.-)
                        cleft palate with cleft lip (Q37.-)

    Q38.6   Other congenital malformations of mouth
         Congenital malformation of mouth NOS

    Q38.7   Congenital pharyngeal pouch
         Congenital diverticulum of pharynx

         Excludes1   pharyngeal pouch syndrome (D82.1)

    Q38.8   Other congenital malformations of pharynx
         Congenital malformation of pharynx NOS
         Imperforate pharynx

● **Q39   Congenital malformations of esophagus**

    Q39.0   Atresia of esophagus without fistula
         Atresia of esophagus NOS

    Q39.1   Atresia of esophagus with tracheo-esophageal fistula
         Atresia of esophagus with broncho-esophageal fistula

    Q39.2   Congenital tracheo-esophageal fistula without atresia
         Congenital tracheo-esophageal fistula NOS

    Q39.3   Congenital stenosis and stricture of esophagus

    Q39.4   Esophageal web

    Q39.5   Congenital dilatation of esophagus
         Congenital cardiospasm

    Q39.6   Congenital diverticulum of esophagus
         Congenital esophageal pouch

    Q39.8   Other congenital malformations of esophagus
         Congenital absence of esophagus
         Congenital displacement of esophagus
         Congenital duplication of esophagus

    Q39.9   Congenital malformation of esophagus, unspecified

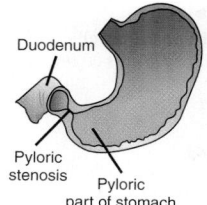

Figure 17-4   Pyloric stenosis.

Duodenum — Pyloric stenosis — Pyloric part of stomach

● **Q40   Other congenital malformations of upper alimentary tract**

    Q40.0   Congenital hypertrophic pyloric stenosis
         Congenital or infantile constriction
         Congenital or infantile hypertrophy
         Congenital or infantile spasm
         Congenital or infantile stenosis
         Congenital or infantile stricture

    Q40.1   Congenital hiatus hernia
         Congenital displacement of cardia through esophageal hiatus

         Excludes1   congenital diaphragmatic hernia (Q79.0)

    Q40.2   Other specified congenital malformations of stomach
         Congenital displacement of stomach
         Congenital diverticulum of stomach
         Congenital hourglass stomach
         Congenital duplication of stomach
         Megalogastria
         Microgastria

    Q40.3   Congenital malformation of stomach, unspecified

    Q40.8   Other specified congenital malformations of upper alimentary tract

    Q40.9   Congenital malformation of upper alimentary tract, unspecified
         Congenital anomaly of upper alimentary tract
         Congenital deformity of upper alimentary tract

● **Q41   Congenital absence, atresia and stenosis of small intestine**

     Includes   congenital obstruction, occlusion or stricture of small intestine or intestine NOS

     Excludes1   cystic fibrosis with intestinal manifestation (E84.11)
                        meconium ileus NOS (without cystic fibrosis) (P76.0)

    Q41.0   Congenital absence, atresia and stenosis of duodenum

    Q41.1   Congenital absence, atresia and stenosis of jejunum
         Apple peel syndrome
         Imperforate jejunum

    Q41.2   Congenital absence, atresia and stenosis of ileum

    Q41.8   Congenital absence, atresia and stenosis of other specified parts of small intestine

    Q41.9   Congenital absence, atresia and stenosis of small intestine, part unspecified
         Congenital absence, atresia and stenosis of intestine NOS

● **Q42   Congenital absence, atresia and stenosis of large intestine**

     Includes   congenital obstruction, occlusion and stricture of large intestine

    Q42.0   Congenital absence, atresia and stenosis of rectum with fistula

    Q42.1   Congenital absence, atresia and stenosis of rectum without fistula
         Imperforate rectum

    Q42.2   Congenital absence, atresia and stenosis of anus with fistula

    Q42.3   Congenital absence, atresia and stenosis of anus without fistula
         Imperforate anus

    Q42.8   Congenital absence, atresia and stenosis of other parts of large intestine

    Q42.9   Congenital absence, atresia and stenosis of large intestine, part unspecified

CHAPTER 17 (Q00-Q99)

CHAPTER 17 (Q00–Q99)

● **Q43   Other congenital malformations of intestine**

Q43.0   Meckel's diverticulum (displaced) (hypertrophic)
Congenital abnormality in which a pouch remains on the lower end of the small intestine
Persistent omphalomesenteric duct
Persistent vitelline duct

Q43.1   Hirschsprung's disease
Developmental disorder of enteric nervous system characterized by absence of ganglion cells in distal colon resulting in functional obstruction
Aganglionosis
Congenital (aganglionic) megacolon

Q43.2   Other congenital functional disorders of colon
Congenital dilatation of colon

Q43.3   Congenital malformations of intestinal fixation
Congenital omental, anomalous adhesions [bands]
Congenital peritoneal adhesions [bands]
Incomplete rotation of cecum and colon
Insufficient rotation of cecum and colon
Jackson's membrane
Malrotation of colon
Rotation failure of cecum and colon
Universal mesentery

Q43.4   Duplication of intestine

Q43.5   Ectopic anus
Anal opening in abnormal location

Q43.6   Congenital fistula of rectum and anus
Excludes1   congenital fistula of anus with absence, atresia and stenosis (Q42.2)
congenital fistula of rectum with absence, atresia and stenosis (Q42.0)
congenital rectovaginal fistula (Q52.2)
congenital urethrorectal fistula (Q64.73)
pilonidal fistula or sinus (L05.-)

Q43.7   Persistent cloaca
Malformation in which rectum, vagina, and urinary tract form one channel AKA congenital cloaca
Cloaca NOS

Q43.8   Other specified congenital malformations of intestine
Congenital blind loop syndrome
Congenital diverticulitis, colon
Congenital diverticulum, intestine
Dolichocolon
Megaloappendix
Megaloduodenum
Microcolon
Transposition of appendix
Transposition of colon
Transposition of intestine

Q43.9   Congenital malformation of intestine, unspecified

● **Q44   Congenital malformations of gallbladder, bile ducts and liver**

Q44.0   Agenesis, aplasia and hypoplasia of gallbladder
Congenital absence of gallbladder

Q44.1   Other congenital malformations of gallbladder
Congenital malformation of gallbladder NOS
Intrahepatic gallbladder

Q44.2   Atresia of bile ducts

Q44.3   Congenital stenosis and stricture of bile ducts

Q44.4   Choledochal cyst

Q44.5   Other congenital malformations of bile ducts
Accessory hepatic duct
Biliary duct duplication
Congenital malformation of bile duct NOS
Cystic duct duplication

Q44.6   Cystic disease of liver
Fibrocystic disease of liver

Q44.7   Other congenital malformations of liver
Accessory liver
Alagille's syndrome
Congenital absence of liver
Congenital hepatomegaly
Congenital malformation of liver NOS

● **Q45   Other congenital malformations of digestive system**
Excludes2   congenital diaphragmatic hernia (Q79.0)
congenital hiatus hernia (Q40.1)

Q45.0   Agenesis, aplasia and hypoplasia of pancreas
Congenital absence of pancreas

Q45.1   Annular pancreas

Q45.2   Congenital pancreatic cyst

Q45.3   Other congenital malformations of pancreas and pancreatic duct
Accessory pancreas
Congenital malformation of pancreas or pancreatic duct NOS
Excludes1   congenital diabetes mellitus (E10.-)
cystic fibrosis (E84.0-E84.9)
fibrocystic disease of pancreas (E84.-)
neonatal diabetes mellitus (P70.2)

Q45.8   Other specified congenital malformations of digestive system
Absence (complete) (partial) of alimentary tract NOS
Duplication of digestive system
Malposition, congenital of digestive system

Q45.9   Congenital malformation of digestive system, unspecified
Congenital anomaly of digestive system
Congenital deformity of digestive system

CONGENITAL MALFORMATIONS OF GENITAL ORGANS (Q50-Q56)

Excludes1   androgen insensitivity syndrome (E34.5-)
syndromes associated with anomalies in the number and form of chromosomes (Q90-Q99)

● **Q50   Congenital malformations of ovaries, fallopian tubes and broad ligaments**

● **Q50.0   Congenital absence of ovary**
Excludes1   Turner's syndrome (Q96.-)

Q50.01   Congenital absence of ovary, unilateral ♀

Q50.02   Congenital absence of ovary, bilateral ♀

Q50.1   Developmental ovarian cyst ♀

Q50.2   Congenital torsion of ovary ♀

● **Q50.3   Other congenital malformations of ovary**

Q50.31   Accessory ovary ♀

Q50.32   Ovarian streak ♀
Inadequate ovaries with absent follicular and hormonal function
46, XX with streak gonads

Q50.39   Other congenital malformation of ovary ♀
Congenital malformation of ovary NOS

Q50.4   Embryonic cyst of fallopian tube ♀
Fimbrial cyst

Q50.5   Embryonic cyst of broad ligament ♀
Epoophoron cyst
Parovarian cyst

Q50.6   Other congenital malformations of fallopian tube and broad ligament ♀
Absence of fallopian tube and broad ligament
Accessory fallopian tube and broad ligament
Atresia of fallopian tube and broad ligament
Congenital malformation of fallopian tube or broad ligament NOS

● **Q51**   **Congenital malformations of uterus and cervix**
    Q51.0   **Agenesis and aplasia of uterus** ♀
             Congenital absence of uterus
  ● **Q51.1**   **Doubling of uterus with doubling of cervix and vagina**
        Q51.10   **Doubling of uterus with doubling of cervix and vagina without obstruction** ♀
                Doubling of uterus with doubling of cervix and vagina NOS
        Q51.11   **Doubling of uterus with doubling of cervix and vagina with obstruction** ♀
    Q51.2   **Other doubling of uterus** ♀
             Doubling of uterus NOS
             Septate uterus, complete or partial
    Q51.3   **Bicornate uterus** ♀
             Bicornate uterus, complete or partial
             Birth defect in which uterus has two separate 'horns' that form top of uterus
    Q51.4   **Unicornate uterus** ♀
             Unicornate uterus with or without a separate uterine horn
             Uterus with only one functioning horn
             Uterus with half being undeveloped
    Q51.5   **Agenesis and aplasia of cervix** ♀
             Congenital absence of cervix
    Q51.6   **Embryonic cyst of cervix** ♀
    Q51.7   **Congenital fistulae between uterus and digestive and urinary tracts**
  ● **Q51.8**   **Other congenital malformations of uterus and cervix**
    ● **Q51.81**   **Other congenital malformations of uterus**
        Q51.810   **Arcuate uterus** ♀
                Arcuatus uterus
        Q51.811   **Hypoplasia of uterus** ♀
        Q51.818   **Other congenital malformations of uterus** ♀
                Müllerian anomaly of uterus NEC
    ● **Q51.82**   **Other congenital malformations of cervix**
        Q51.820   **Cervical duplication** ♀
        Q51.821   **Hypoplasia of cervix** ♀
        Q51.828   **Other congenital malformations of cervix** ♀
    Q51.9   **Congenital malformation of uterus and cervix, unspecified** ♀

● **Q52**   **Other congenital malformations of female genitalia**
    Q52.0   **Congenital absence of vagina** ♀
             Vaginal agenesis, total or partial
  ● **Q52.1**   **Doubling of vagina**
        Excludes1   doubling of vagina with doubling of uterus and cervix (Q51.1-)
        Q52.10   **Doubling of vagina, unspecified** ♀
                Septate vagina NOS
        Q52.11   **Transverse vaginal septum** ♀
    ● **Q52.12**   **Longitudinal vaginal septum**
          ~~Longitudinal vaginal septum with or without obstruction~~
        Q52.120   **Longitudinal vaginal septum, nonobstructing** ♀ ◄
        Q52.121   **Longitudinal vaginal septum, obstructing, right side** ♀ ◄
        Q52.122   **Longitudinal vaginal septum, obstructing, left side** ♀ ◄
        Q52.123   **Longitudinal vaginal septum, microperforate, right side** ♀ ◄
        Q52.124   **Longitudinal vaginal septum, microperforate, left side** ♀ ◄
        Q52.129   **Other and unspecified longitudinal vaginal septum** ♀ ◄
    Q52.2   **Congenital rectovaginal fistula** ♀
        Excludes1   cloaca (Q43.7)

    Q52.3   **Imperforate hymen** ♀
             Membrane (hymen) completely closes vaginal orifice
    Q52.4   **Other congenital malformations of vagina** ♀
             Canal of Nuck cyst, congenital
             Congenital malformation of vagina NOS
             Embryonic vaginal cyst
             Gartner's duct cyst
    Q52.5   **Fusion of labia** ♀
    Q52.6   **Congenital malformation of clitoris** ♀
  ● **Q52.7**   **Other and unspecified congenital malformations of vulva**
        Q52.70   **Unspecified congenital malformations of vulva** ♀
                Congenital malformation of vulva NOS
        Q52.71   **Congenital absence of vulva** ♀
        Q52.79   **Other congenital malformations of vulva** ♀
                Congenital cyst of vulva
    Q52.8   **Other specified congenital malformations of female genitalia** ♀
    Q52.9   **Congenital malformation of female genitalia, unspecified** ♀

● **Q53**   **Undescended and ectopic testicle**
  ● **Q53.0**   **Ectopic testis**
        Q53.00   **Ectopic testis, unspecified** ♂
        Q53.01   **Ectopic testis, unilateral** ♂
        Q53.02   **Ectopic testes, bilateral** ♂
  ● **Q53.1**   **Undescended testicle, unilateral**
        Q53.10   **Unspecified undescended testicle, unilateral** ♂
        Q53.11   **Abdominal testis, unilateral** ♂
        Q53.12   **Ectopic perineal testis, unilateral** ♂
  ● **Q53.2**   **Undescended testicle, bilateral**
        Q53.20   **Undescended testicle, unspecified, bilateral** ♂
        Q53.21   **Abdominal testis, bilateral** ♂
        Q53.22   **Ectopic perineal testis, bilateral** ♂
    Q53.9   **Undescended testicle, unspecified** ♂
             Cryptorchism NOS

● **Q54**   **Hypospadias**
        Birth defect of male; urethra opens in abnormal location on shaft
        Excludes1   epispadias (Q64.0)
    Q54.0   **Hypospadias, balanic** ♂
             Hypospadias, coronal
             Hypospadias, glandular
    Q54.1   **Hypospadias, penile** ♂
    Q54.2   **Hypospadias, penoscrotal** ♂
    Q54.3   **Hypospadias, perineal** ♂
    Q54.4   **Congenital chordee** ♂
             Chordee without hypospadias
    Q54.8   **Other hypospadias** ♂
             Hypospadias with intersex state
    Q54.9   **Hypospadias, unspecified** ♂

Item 17–1   Testes form in the abdomen of the male and only descend into the scrotum during normal embryonic development. "Ectopic" testes are out of their normal place or "retained" (left behind) in the abdomen. Crypto (hidden) orchism (testicle) is a major risk factor for testicular cancer.

ECTOPIC TESTES   **CRYPTORCHID TESTES**
Penile   Abdominal
Superficial inguinal   Inguinal
(most common)   Prepubic
Femoral   (most common)

Penile — Abdominal
Internal inguinal ring — Inguinal
Superficial inguinal (most common) — External inguinal ring
Femoral — Prepubic (most common)

Figure 17-5   Undescended testes and the positions of the testes in various types of cryptorchidism or abnormal paths of descent.

CHAPTER 17 (Q00-Q99)

- Q55 **Other congenital malformations of male genital organs**
  - **Excludes1** congenital hydrocele (P83.5)
    hypospadias (Q54.-)
  - Q55.0 **Absence and aplasia of testis** ♂
    Monorchism
  - Q55.1 **Hypoplasia of testis and scrotum** ♂
    Fusion of testes
  - Q55.2 **Other and unspecified congenital malformations of testis and scrotum**
    - Q55.20 **Unspecified congenital malformations of testis and scrotum** ♂
      Congenital malformation of testis or scrotum NOS
    - Q55.21 **Polyorchism** ♂
      Developmental anomaly characterized by presence of more than two testes
    - Q55.22 **Retractile testis** ♂
    - Q55.23 **Scrotal transposition** ♂
    - Q55.29 **Other congenital malformations of testis and scrotum** ♂
  - Q55.3 **Atresia of vas deferens** ♂
    Code first any associated cystic fibrosis (E84.-)
  - Q55.4 **Other congenital malformations of vas deferens, epididymis, seminal vesicles and prostate** ♂
    Absence or aplasia of prostate
    Absence or aplasia of spermatic cord
    Congenital malformation of vas deferens, epididymis, seminal vesicles or prostate NOS
  - Q55.5 **Congenital absence and aplasia of penis** ♂
  - Q55.6 **Other congenital malformations of penis**
    - Q55.61 **Curvature of penis (lateral)** ♂
    - Q55.62 **Hypoplasia of penis** ♂
      Underdevelopment penis
      Micropenis
    - Q55.63 **Congenital torsion of penis** ♂
      - **Excludes1** acquired torsion of penis (N48.82)
    - Q55.64 **Hidden penis** ♂
      Buried penis
      Concealed penis
      - **Excludes1** acquired buried penis (N48.83)
    - Q55.69 **Other congenital malformation of penis** ♂
      Congenital malformation of penis NOS
  - Q55.7 **Congenital vasocutaneous fistula** ♂
    Abnormal opening between vas deferens and skin
  - Q55.8 **Other specified congenital malformations of male genital organs** ♂
  - Q55.9 **Congenital malformation of male genital organ, unspecified** ♂
    Congenital anomaly of male genital organ
    Congenital deformity of male genital organ

- Q56 **Indeterminate sex and pseudohermaphroditism**
  Internal reproductive organs are opposite external physical characteristics.
  - **Excludes1** 46,XX true hermaphrodite (Q99.1)
    androgen insensitivity syndrome (E34.5-)
    chimera 46,XX/46,XY true hermaphrodite (Q99.0)
    female pseudohermaphroditism with adrenocortical disorder (E25.-)
    pseudohermaphroditism with specified chromosomal anomaly (Q96-Q99)
    pure gonadal dysgenesis (Q99.1)
  - Q56.0 **Hermaphroditism, not elsewhere classified**
    Ovotestis
  - Q56.1 **Male pseudohermaphroditism, not elsewhere classified** ♂
    46, XY with streak gonads
    Male pseudohermaphroditism NOS
  - Q56.2 **Female pseudohermaphroditism, not elsewhere classified** ♀
    Female pseudohermaphroditism NOS

  - Q56.3 **Pseudohermaphroditism, unspecified**
  - Q56.4 **Indeterminate sex, unspecified**
    Ambiguous genitalia

CONGENITAL MALFORMATIONS OF THE URINARY SYSTEM (Q60-Q64)

- Q60 **Renal agenesis and other reduction defects of kidney**
  - **Includes** congenital absence of kidney
    congenital atrophy of kidney
    infantile atrophy of kidney
  - Q60.0 **Renal agenesis, unilateral**
  - Q60.1 **Renal agenesis, bilateral**
  - Q60.2 **Renal agenesis, unspecified**
  - Q60.3 **Renal hypoplasia, unilateral**
  - Q60.4 **Renal hypoplasia, bilateral**
  - Q60.5 **Renal hypoplasia, unspecified**
  - Q60.6 **Potter's syndrome**

- Q61 **Cystic kidney disease**
  Cysts that develop in failing kidney due to end-stage renal disease
  - **Excludes1** acquired cyst of kidney (N28.1)
    Potter's syndrome (Q60.6)
  - Q61.0 **Congenital renal cyst**
    - Q61.00 **Congenital renal cyst, unspecified**
      Cyst of kidney NOS (congenital)
    - Q61.01 **Congenital single renal cyst**
    - Q61.02 **Congenital multiple renal cysts**
  - Q61.1 **Polycystic kidney, infantile type**
    Polycystic kidney, autosomal recessive
    - Q61.11 **Cystic dilatation of collecting ducts**
    - Q61.19 **Other polycystic kidney, infantile type**
  - Q61.2 **Polycystic kidney, adult type**
    Polycystic kidney, autosomal dominant
  - Q61.3 **Polycystic kidney, unspecified**
  - Q61.4 **Renal dysplasia**
    Multicystic dysplastic kidney
    Multicystic kidney (development)
    Multicystic kidney disease
    Multicystic renal dysplasia
    - **Excludes1** polycystic kidney disease (Q61.11-Q61.3)
  - Q61.5 **Medullary cystic kidney**
    Nephronopthisis
    Sponge kidney NOS
  - Q61.8 **Other cystic kidney diseases**
    Fibrocystic kidney
    Fibrocystic renal degeneration or disease
  - Q61.9 **Cystic kidney disease, unspecified**
    Meckel-Gruber syndrome

- Q62 **Congenital obstructive defects of renal pelvis and congenital malformations of ureter**
  - Q62.0 **Congenital hydronephrosis**
  - Q62.1 **Congenital occlusion of ureter**
    Atresia and stenosis of ureter
    - Q62.10 **Congenital occlusion of ureter, unspecified**
    - Q62.11 **Congenital occlusion of ureteropelvic junction**
    - Q62.12 **Congenital occlusion of ureterovesical orifice**
  - Q62.2 **Congenital megaureter**
    Congenital dilatation of ureter
  - Q62.3 **Other obstructive defects of renal pelvis and ureter**
    - Q62.31 **Congenital ureterocele, orthotopic**
    - Q62.32 **Cecoureterocele**
      Ectopic ureterocele
    - Q62.39 **Other obstructive defects of renal pelvis and ureter**
      Ureteropelvic junction obstruction NOS
  - Q62.4 **Agenesis of ureter**
    Congenital absence ureter

◀ New　◀▬ Revised　~~deleted~~ Deleted　Excludes 1　Excludes 2　Includes　Use additional　Code first　Code also　Unspecified
OGCR Official Guidelines　X Assign placeholder X　● Use Additional Character(s)　▌ Manifestation Code　**Coding Clinic**

Q62.5   **Duplication of ureter**
    Accessory ureter
    Double ureter

● Q62.6   **Malposition of ureter**
    Q62.60   **Malposition of ureter, unspecified**
    Q62.61   **Deviation of ureter**
    Q62.62   **Displacement of ureter**
    Q62.63   **Anomalous implantation of ureter**
       Ectopia of ureter
       Ectopic ureter
    Q62.69   **Other malposition of ureter**

Q62.7   **Congenital vesico-uretero-renal reflux**

Q62.8   **Other congenital malformations of ureter**
    Anomaly of ureter NOS

● Q63   **Other congenital malformations of kidney**
    Excludes1   congenital nephrotic syndrome (N04.-)

Q63.0   **Accessory kidney**

Q63.1   **Lobulated, fused and horseshoe kidney**

Q63.2   **Ectopic kidney**
    Congenital displaced kidney
    Malrotation of kidney

Q63.3   **Hyperplastic and giant kidney**
    Compensatory hypertrophy of kidney

Q63.8   **Other specified congenital malformations of kidney**
    Congenital renal calculi

Q63.9   **Congenital malformation of kidney, unspecified**

● Q64   **Other congenital malformations of urinary system**

Q64.0   **Epispadias** ♂
    Urethral opening somewhere on dorsum of penis
    Excludes1   hypospadias (Q54.-)

● Q64.1   **Exstrophy of urinary bladder**
    Bladder is exposed, inside out, and protrudes through abdominal wall
    Q64.10   **Exstrophy of urinary bladder, unspecified**
       Ectopia vesicae
    Q64.11   **Supravesical fissure of urinary bladder**
    Q64.12   **Cloacal extrophy of urinary bladder**
    Q64.19   **Other exstrophy of urinary bladder**
       Extroversion of bladder

Q64.2   **Congenital posterior urethral valves**

● Q64.3   **Other atresia and stenosis of urethra and bladder neck**
    Q64.31   **Congenital bladder neck obstruction**
       Congenital obstruction of vesicourethral orifice
    Q64.32   **Congenital stricture of urethra**
    Q64.33   **Congenital stricture of urinary meatus**
    Q64.39   **Other atresia and stenosis of urethra and bladder neck**
       Atresia and stenosis of urethra and bladder neck NOS

Q64.4   **Malformation of urachus**
    Cyst of urachus
    Patent urachus
    Prolapse of urachus

Q64.5   **Congenital absence of bladder and urethra**

Q64.6   **Congenital diverticulum of bladder**

● Q64.7   **Other and unspecified congenital malformations of bladder and urethra**
    Excludes1   congenital prolapse of bladder (mucosa) (Q79.4)
    Q64.70   **Unspecified congenital malformation of bladder and urethra**
       Malformation of bladder or urethra NOS
    Q64.71   **Congenital prolapse of urethra**
    Q64.72   **Congenital prolapse of urinary meatus**
    Q64.73   **Congenital urethrorectal fistula**
    Q64.74   **Double urethra**
    Q64.75   **Double urinary meatus**
    Q64.79   **Other congenital malformations of bladder and urethra**

Q64.8   **Other specified congenital malformations of urinary system**

Q64.9   **Congenital malformation of urinary system, unspecified**
    Congenital anomaly NOS of urinary system
    Congenital deformity NOS of urinary system

CONGENITAL MALFORMATIONS AND DEFORMATIONS OF THE MUSCULOSKELETAL SYSTEM (Q65-Q79)

● Q65   **Congenital deformities of hip**
    Excludes1   clicking hip (R29.4)

● Q65.0   **Congenital dislocation of hip, unilateral**
    Q65.00   **Congenital dislocation of unspecified hip, unilateral**
    Q65.01   **Congenital dislocation of right hip, unilateral**
    Q65.02   **Congenital dislocation of left hip, unilateral**

Q65.1   **Congenital dislocation of hip, bilateral**

Q65.2   **Congenital dislocation of hip, unspecified**

● Q65.3   **Congenital partial dislocation of hip, unilateral**
    Q65.30   **Congenital partial dislocation of unspecified hip, unilateral**
    Q65.31   **Congenital partial dislocation of right hip, unilateral**
    Q65.32   **Congenital partial dislocation of left hip, unilateral**

Q65.4   **Congenital partial dislocation of hip, bilateral**

Q65.5   **Congenital partial dislocation of hip, unspecified**

Q65.6   **Congenital unstable hip**
    Congenital dislocatable hip

● Q65.8   **Other congenital deformities of hip**
    Q65.81   **Congenital coxa valga**
    Q65.82   **Congenital coxa vara**
    Q65.89   **Other specified congenital deformities of hip**
       Anteversion of femoral neck
       Congenital acetabular dysplasia

Q65.9   **Congenital deformity of hip, unspecified**

● Q66   **Congenital deformities of feet**
    Excludes1   reduction defects of feet (Q72.-)
       valgus deformities (acquired) (M21.0-)
       varus deformities (acquired) (M21.1-)

Q66.0   **Congenital talipes equinovarus**
    Heel is turned inward from midline and foot is plantar flexed; AKA clubfoot

Q66.1   **Congenital talipes calcaneovarus**
    Deformity of foot in which heel is turned toward midline of body and anterior of foot is elevated

● Q66.2   **Congenital metatarsus (primus) varus**
    Angulation of first metatarsal bone toward midline of body
    Q66.21   **Congenital metatarsus primus varus** ◀
    Q66.22   **Congenital metatarsus adductus** ◀
       Congenital metatarsus varus ◀

Q66.3   **Other congenital varus deformities of feet**
    Hallux varus, congenital

Q66.4   **Congenital talipes calcaneovalgus**

● Q66.5   **Congenital pes planus**
    Congenital flat foot
    Congenital rigid flat foot
    Congenital spastic (everted) flat foot
    Excludes1   pes planus, acquired (M21.4)
    Q66.50   **Congenital pes planus, unspecified foot**
    Q66.51   **Congenital pes planus, right foot**
    Q66.52   **Congenital pes planus, left foot**

Q66.6   **Other congenital valgus deformities of feet**
    Inward angulation
    Congenital metatarsus valgus

Q66.7   **Congenital pes cavus**

Item 17–2 Equinus foot is a term referring to the hoof of a horse. The deformity is usually congenital or spastic. Talipes equinovarus is referred to as clubfoot. The foot tends to be smaller than normal, with the heel pointing downward and the forefoot turning inward. The heel cord (Achilles tendon) is tight, causing the heel to be drawn up toward the leg.

Figure 17-6 Supination and cavus deformity of forefoot. *(Courtesy Jay Cummings, MD.) (From Canale: Campbell's Operative Orthopaedics, ed 11, Mosby, Inc., 2007)*

Figure 17-7 Talipes. (From Dorland: Dorland's Illustrated Medical Dictionary, ed 31, Saunders, 2007, p 1893)

● **Q66.8 Other congenital deformities of feet**
  Q66.80 Congenital vertical talus deformity, unspecified foot
  Q66.81 Congenital vertical talus deformity, right foot
  Q66.82 Congenital vertical talus deformity, left foot
  Q66.89 Other specified congenital deformities of feet
    Congenital asymmetric talipes
    Congenital clubfoot NOS
    Congenital talipes NOS
    Congenital tarsal coalition
    Hammer toe, congenital
  Q66.9 Congenital deformity of feet, unspecified

● **Q67 Congenital musculoskeletal deformities of head, face, spine and chest**
  Excludes1 congenital malformation syndromes classified to Q87.-
    Potter's syndrome (Q60.6)
  Q67.0 Congenital facial asymmetry
  Q67.1 Congenital compression facies
  Q67.2 Dolichocephaly
    Long head dimension
  Q67.3 Plagiocephaly
    Asymmetric shape of head resulting from irregular closure of cranial sutures
  Q67.4 Other congenital deformities of skull, face and jaw
    Congenital depressions in skull
    Congenital hemifacial atrophy or hypertrophy
    Deviation of nasal septum, congenital
    Squashed or bent nose, congenital
    Excludes1 dentofacial anomalies [including malocclusion] (M26.-)
      syphilitic saddle nose (A50.5)

Figure 17-8 Mild to moderate inbowing of the lower leg. (From Jones KL: Smith's Recognizable Patterns of Human Malformation, ed 6, Philadelphia, Saunders, 2005)

  Q67.5 Congenital deformity of spine
    Congenital postural scoliosis
    Congenital scoliosis NOS
    Excludes1 infantile idiopathic scoliosis (M41.0)
      scoliosis due to congenital bony malformation (Q76.3)
  Q67.6 Pectus excavatum
    Congenital funnel chest
    Funnel-shaped chest depression
  Q67.7 Pectus carinatum
    Congenital pigeon chest
  Q67.8 Other congenital deformities of chest
    Congenital deformity of chest wall NOS

● **Q68 Other congenital musculoskeletal deformities**
  Excludes1 reduction defects of limb(s) (Q71-Q73)
  Excludes2 congenital myotonic chondrodystrophy (G71.13)
  Q68.0 Congenital deformity of sternocleidomastoid muscle
    Congenital contracture of sternocleidomastoid (muscle)
    Congenital (sternomastoid) torticollis
    Sternomastoid tumor (congenital)
  Q68.1 Congenital deformity of finger(s) and hand
    Congenital clubfinger
    Spade-like hand (congenital)
  Q68.2 Congenital deformity of knee
    Congenital dislocation of knee
    Congenital genu recurvatum
    Hyperextension of knee resulting from hypermobility
  Q68.3 Congenital bowing of femur
    Excludes1 anteversion of femur (neck) (Q65.89)
  Q68.4 Congenital bowing of tibia and fibula
  Q68.5 Congenital bowing of long bones of leg, unspecified
  Q68.6 Discoid meniscus
  Q68.8 Other specified congenital musculoskeletal deformities
    Congenital deformity of clavicle
    Congenital deformity of elbow
    Congenital deformity of forearm
    Congenital deformity of scapula
    Congenital deformity of wrist
    Congenital dislocation of elbow
    Congenital dislocation of shoulder
    Congenital dislocation of wrist

● **Q69 Polydactyly**
  AKA hyperdactyly, consists of supernumerary fingers or toes
  Q69.0 Accessory finger(s)
  Q69.1 Accessory thumb(s)
  Q69.2 Accessory toe(s)
    Accessory hallux
  Q69.9 Polydactyly, unspecified
    Supernumerary digit(s) NOS

● **Q70 Syndactyly**
  Webbing between distal phalanges of adjacent digits
  ● **Q70.0 Fused fingers**
    Complex syndactyly of fingers with synostosis
    Q70.00 Fused fingers, unspecified hand
    Q70.01 Fused fingers, right hand
    Q70.02 Fused fingers, left hand
    Q70.03 Fused fingers, bilateral

◀ New   ◀▥ Revised   ~~deleted~~ Deleted   Excludes 1   Excludes 2   Includes   Use additional   Code first   Code also   Unspecified

1154   OGCR Official Guidelines   X Assign placeholder X   ● Use Additional Character(s)   ▶ Manifestation Code   **Coding Clinic**

Figure 17-9 Polydactyly, congenital duplicated thumb. (From DeLee: DeLee and Drez's Orthopaedic Sports Medicine, ed 3, Saunders, An Imprint of Elsevier, 2009)

- Q70.1 **Webbed fingers**
  Simple syndactyly of fingers without synostosis
  - Q70.10   Webbed fingers, unspecified hand
  - Q70.11   Webbed fingers, right hand
  - Q70.12   Webbed fingers, left hand
  - Q70.13   Webbed fingers, bilateral
- Q70.2 **Fused toes**
  Complex syndactyly of toes with synostosis
  - Q70.20   Fused toes, unspecified foot
  - Q70.21   Fused toes, right foot
  - Q70.22   Fused toes, left foot
  - Q70.23   Fused toes, bilateral
- Q70.3 **Webbed toes**
  Simple syndactyly of toes without synostosis
  - Q70.30   Webbed toes, unspecified foot
  - Q70.31   Webbed toes, right foot
  - Q70.32   Webbed toes, left foot
  - Q70.33   Webbed toes, bilateral
- Q70.4 **Polysyndactyly, unspecified**
  > **Excludes 1**   specified syndactyly of hand and feet - code to specified conditions (Q70.0- -Q70.3-)
  Extra and webbed digits
- Q70.9 **Syndactyly, unspecified**
  Symphalangy NOS
- ● Q71   **Reduction defects of upper limb**
  - Q71.0   **Congenital complete absence of upper limb**
    - Q71.00   Congenital complete absence of unspecified upper limb
    - Q71.01   Congenital complete absence of right upper limb
    - Q71.02   Congenital complete absence of left upper limb
    - Q71.03   Congenital complete absence of upper limb, bilateral
  - Q71.1   **Congenital absence of upper arm and forearm with hand present**
    - Q71.10   Congenital absence of unspecified upper arm and forearm with hand present
    - Q71.11   Congenital absence of right upper arm and forearm with hand present
    - Q71.12   Congenital absence of left upper arm and forearm with hand present
    - Q71.13   Congenital absence of upper arm and forearm with hand present, bilateral
  - Q71.2   **Congenital absence of both forearm and hand**
    - Q71.20   Congenital absence of both forearm and hand, unspecified upper limb
    - Q71.21   Congenital absence of both forearm and hand, right upper limb
    - Q71.22   Congenital absence of both forearm and hand, left upper limb
    - Q71.23   Congenital absence of both forearm and hand, bilateral
  - Q71.3   **Congenital absence of hand and finger**
    - Q71.30   Congenital absence of unspecified hand and finger
    - Q71.31   Congenital absence of right hand and finger
    - Q71.32   Congenital absence of left hand and finger
    - Q71.33   Congenital absence of hand and finger, bilateral

- Q71.4   **Longitudinal reduction defect of radius**
  Clubhand (congenital)
  Radial clubhand
  - Q71.40   Longitudinal reduction defect of unspecified radius
  - Q71.41   Longitudinal reduction defect of right radius
  - Q71.42   Longitudinal reduction defect of left radius
  - Q71.43   Longitudinal reduction defect of radius, bilateral
- Q71.5   **Longitudinal reduction defect of ulna**
  - Q71.50   Longitudinal reduction defect of unspecified ulna
  - Q71.51   Longitudinal reduction defect of right ulna
  - Q71.52   Longitudinal reduction defect of left ulna
  - Q71.53   Longitudinal reduction defect of ulna, bilateral
- Q71.6   **Lobster-claw hand**
  - Q71.60   Lobster-claw hand, unspecified hand
  - Q71.61   Lobster-claw right hand
  - Q71.62   Lobster-claw left hand
  - Q71.63   Lobster-claw hand, bilateral
- Q71.8   **Other reduction defects of upper limb**
  - Q71.81   Congenital shortening of upper limb
    - Q71.811   Congenital shortening of right upper limb
    - Q71.812   Congenital shortening of left upper limb
    - Q71.813   Congenital shortening of upper limb, bilateral
    - Q71.819   Congenital shortening of unspecified upper limb
  - Q71.89   Other reduction defects of upper limb
    - Q71.891   Other reduction defects of right upper limb
    - Q71.892   Other reduction defects of left upper limb
    - Q71.893   Other reduction defects of upper limb, bilateral
    - Q71.899   Other reduction defects of unspecified upper limb
- Q71.9   **Unspecified reduction defect of upper limb**
  - Q71.90   Unspecified reduction defect of unspecified upper limb
  - Q71.91   Unspecified reduction defect of right upper limb
  - Q71.92   Unspecified reduction defect of left upper limb
  - Q71.93   Unspecified reduction defect of upper limb, bilateral
- ● Q72   **Reduction defects of lower limb**
  - Q72.0   **Congenital complete absence of lower limb**
    - Q72.00   Congenital complete absence of unspecified lower limb
    - Q72.01   Congenital complete absence of right lower limb
    - Q72.02   Congenital complete absence of left lower limb
    - Q72.03   Congenital complete absence of lower limb, bilateral
  - Q72.1   **Congenital absence of thigh and lower leg with foot present**
    - Q72.10   Congenital absence of unspecified thigh and lower leg with foot present
    - Q72.11   Congenital absence of right thigh and lower leg with foot present
    - Q72.12   Congenital absence of left thigh and lower leg with foot present
    - Q72.13   Congenital absence of thigh and lower leg with foot present, bilateral

CHAPTER 17 (Q00-Q99)

● **Q72.2** Congenital absence of both lower leg and foot

    Q72.20 Congenital absence of both lower leg and foot, unspecified lower limb

    Q72.21 Congenital absence of both lower leg and foot, right lower limb

    Q72.22 Congenital absence of both left lower leg and foot, left lower limb

    Q72.23 Congenital absence of both lower leg and foot, bilateral

● **Q72.3** Congenital absence of foot and toe(s)

    Q72.30 Congenital absence of unspecified foot and toe(s)

    Q72.31 Congenital absence of right foot and toe(s)

    Q72.32 Congenital absence of left foot and toe(s)

    Q72.33 Congenital absence of foot and toe(s), bilateral

● **Q72.4** Longitudinal reduction defect of femur

    Proximal femoral focal deficiency

    Q72.40 Longitudinal reduction defect of unspecified femur

    Q72.41 Longitudinal reduction defect of right femur

    Q72.42 Longitudinal reduction defect of left femur

    Q72.43 Longitudinal reduction defect of femur, bilateral

● **Q72.5** Longitudinal reduction defect of tibia

    Q72.50 Longitudinal reduction defect of unspecified tibia

    Q72.51 Longitudinal reduction defect of right tibia

    Q72.52 Longitudinal reduction defect of left tibia

    Q72.53 Longitudinal reduction defect of tibia, bilateral

● **Q72.6** Longitudinal reduction defect of fibula

    Q72.60 Longitudinal reduction defect of unspecified fibula

    Q72.61 Longitudinal reduction defect of right fibula

    Q72.62 Longitudinal reduction defect of left fibula

    Q72.63 Longitudinal reduction defect of fibula, bilateral

● **Q72.7** Split foot

    Q72.70 Split foot, unspecified lower limb

    Q72.71 Split foot, right lower limb

    Q72.72 Split foot, left lower limb

    Q72.73 Split foot, bilateral

● **Q72.8** Other reduction defects of lower limb

    ● **Q72.81** Congenital shortening of lower limb

        Q72.811 Congenital shortening of right lower limb

        Q72.812 Congenital shortening of left lower limb

        Q72.813 Congenital shortening of lower limb, bilateral

        Q72.819 Congenital shortening of unspecified lower limb

    ● **Q72.89** Other reduction defects of lower limb

        Q72.891 Other reduction defects of right lower limb

        Q72.892 Other reduction defects of left lower limb

        Q72.893 Other reduction defects of lower limb, bilateral

        Q72.899 Other reduction defects of unspecified lower limb

● **Q72.9** Unspecified reduction defect of lower limb

    Q72.90 Unspecified reduction defect of unspecified lower limb

    Q72.91 Unspecified reduction defect of right lower limb

    Q72.92 Unspecified reduction defect of left lower limb

    Q72.93 Unspecified reduction defect of lower limb, bilateral

● **Q73** Reduction defects of unspecified limb

    Q73.0 Congenital absence of unspecified limb(s)

        Amelia NOS

    Q73.1 Phocomelia, unspecified limb(s)

        Phocomelia NOS

        Absence/shortening of long bones primarily as a result of thalidomide

    Q73.8 Other reduction defects of unspecified limb(s)

        Longitudinal reduction deformity of unspecified limb(s)

        Ectromelia of limb NOS

        Gross hypoplasia or aplasia of one or more long bones of limb(s)

        Hemimelia of limb NOS

        Absence of one-half of long bone

        Reduction defect of limb NOS

● **Q74** Other congenital malformations of limb(s)

    Excludes1 polydactyly (Q69.-)

        reduction defect of limb (Q71-Q73)

        syndactyly (Q70.-)

    Q74.0 Other congenital malformations of upper limb(s), including shoulder girdle

        Accessory carpal bones

        Cleidocranial dysostosis

        Congenital pseudarthrosis of clavicle

        Macrodactylia (fingers)

        Madelung's deformity

        Radioulnar synostosis

        Sprengel's deformity

        Triphalangeal thumb

    Q74.1 Congenital malformation of knee

        Congenital absence of patella

        Congenital dislocation of patella

        Congenital genu valgum

        Congenital genu varum

        Rudimentary patella

        Excludes1 congenital dislocation of knee (Q68.2)

            congenital genu recurvatum (Q68.2)

            nail patella syndrome (Q87.2)

    Q74.2 Other congenital malformations of lower limb(s), including pelvic girdle

        Congenital fusion of sacroiliac joint

        Congenital malformation of ankle joint

        Congenital malformation of sacroiliac joint

        Excludes1 anteversion of femur (neck) (Q65.89)

    Q74.3 Arthrogryposis multiplex congenita

    Q74.8 Other specified congenital malformations of limb(s)

    Q74.9 Unspecified congenital malformation of limb(s)

        Congenital anomaly of limb(s) NOS

● **Q75** Other congenital malformations of skull and face bones

    Excludes1 congenital malformation of face NOS (Q18.-)

        congenital malformation syndromes classified to Q87.-

        dentofacial anomalies [including malocclusion] (M26.-)

        musculoskeletal deformities of head and face (Q67.0-Q67.4)

        skull defects associated with congenital anomalies of brain such as:

            anencephaly (Q00.0)

            encephalocele (Q01.-)

            hydrocephalus (Q03.-)

            microcephaly (Q02)

    Q75.0 Craniosynostosis

        Premature closure of sutures of skull

        Acrocephaly

        Imperfect fusion of skull

        Oxycephaly

        Trigonocephaly

    Q75.1 Craniofacial dysostosis

        Congenital deformity of head

        Crouzon's disease

◀ New   ◀▦ Revised   ~~deleted~~ Deleted   Excludes 1   Excludes 2   Includes   Use additional   Code first   Code also   Unspecified

OGCR Official Guidelines   **X** Assign placeholder X   ● Use Additional Character(s)   ▶ Manifestation Code   **Coding Clinic**

1156

Item 17–3 **Anencephalus** is a congenital deformity of the cranial vault. **Craniosynostosis,** also known as craniostenosis and stenocephaly, signifies any form of congenital deformity of the skull that results from the premature closing of the sutures of the skull. **Iniencephaly** is a deformity in which the head and neck are flexed backward to a great extent and the head is very large in comparison to the shortened body.

Figure 17-11   **A.** Spina bifida occulta. **B.** Meningocele. **C.** Myelomeningocele. **D.** Myelocystocele (syringomyelocele) or hydromyelia.

Figure 17-10 Generalized craniosynostosis in a 4-year-old girl without symptoms or signs of increased intracranial pressure. (From Bell WE, McCormick WF: Increased Intracranial Pressure in Children, ed 2, Philadelphia, WB Saunders, 1978, p 116)

Item 17–4 **Spina bifida** is a midline spinal defect in which one or more vertebrae fail to fuse, leaving an opening in the vertebral canal. When the defect is not visible, it is called spina bifida occulta, and when it is visible, it is called spina bifida cystica.

Q75.2   **Hypertelorism**

Q75.3   **Macrocephaly**
    Unusually large size of head; AKA megalocephaly

Q75.4   **Mandibulofacial dysostosis**
    Franceschetti syndrome
    Treacher Collins syndrome

Q75.5   **Oculomandibular dysostosis**
    Ossification of occular and mandibular bones

Q75.8   **Other specified congenital malformations of skull and face bones**
    Absence of skull bone, congenital
    Congenital deformity of forehead
    Platybasia

Q75.9   **Congenital malformation of skull and face bones, unspecified**
    Congenital anomaly of face bones NOS
    Congenital anomaly of skull NOS

● **Q76**   **Congenital malformations of spine and bony thorax**
    Excludes1   congenital musculoskeletal deformities of spine and chest (Q67.5-Q67.8)

Q76.0   **Spina bifida occulta**
    Excludes1   meningocele (spinal) (Q05.-)
             spina bifida (aperta) (cystica) (Q05.-)

Q76.1   **Klippel-Feil syndrome**
    Cervical fusion syndrome

Q76.2   **Congenital spondylolisthesis**
    Congenital spondylolysis
    Excludes1   spondylolisthesis (acquired) (M43.1-)
             spondylolysis (acquired) (M43.0-)

Q76.3   **Congenital scoliosis due to congenital bony malformation**
    Hemivertebra fusion or failure of segmentation with scoliosis

● Q76.4   **Other congenital malformations of spine, not associated with scoliosis**
    ● Q76.41   **Congenital kyphosis**
         Abnormal increase in convexity curvature of thoracic spinal column; AKA humpback
         Q76.411   **Congenital kyphosis, occipito-atlanto-axial region**
         Q76.412   **Congenital kyphosis, cervical region**
         Q76.413   **Congenital kyphosis, cervicothoracic region**
         Q76.414   **Congenital kyphosis, thoracic region**
         Q76.415   **Congenital kyphosis, thoracolumbar region**
         Q76.419   **Congenital kyphosis, unspecified region**

● Q76.42   **Congenital lordosis**
         An abnormal increase in curvature of lumbar spine (sway back)
         Q76.425   **Congenital lordosis, thoracolumbar region**
         Q76.426   **Congenital lordosis, lumbar region**
         Q76.427   **Congenital lordosis, lumbosacral region**
         Q76.428   **Congenital lordosis, sacral and sacrococcygeal region**
         Q76.429   **Congenital lordosis, unspecified region**

    Q76.49   **Other congenital malformations of spine, not associated with scoliosis**
         Congenital absence of vertebra NOS
         Congenital fusion of spine NOS
         Congenital malformation of lumbosacral (joint) (region) NOS
         Congenital malformation of spine NOS
         Hemivertebra NOS
         Malformation of spine NOS
         Platyspondylisis NOS
         Supernumerary vertebra NOS

Q76.5   **Cervical rib**
    Supernumerary rib in cervical region

Q76.6   **Other congenital malformations of ribs**
    Accessory rib
    Congenital absence of rib
    Congenital fusion of ribs
    Congenital malformation of ribs NOS
    Excludes1   short rib syndrome (Q77.2)

Q76.7   **Congenital malformation of sternum**
    Congenital absence of sternum
    Sternum bifidum

Q76.8   **Other congenital malformations of bony thorax**

Q76.9   **Congenital malformation of bony thorax, unspecified**

CHAPTER 17 (Q00-Q99)

● **Q77   Osteochondrodysplasia with defects of growth of tubular bones and spine**

> **Excludes1**   mucopolysaccharidosis (E76.0-E76.3)
>
> **Excludes2**   congenital myotonic chondrodystrophy (G71.13)

Q77.0   Achondrogenesis
    Hypochondrogenesis

Q77.1   Thanatophoric short stature

Q77.2   Short rib syndrome
    Asphyxiating thoracic dysplasia [Jeune]

Q77.3   Chondrodysplasia punctata
    Benign cartilaginous neoplasms

> **Excludes1**   rhizomelic chondrodysplasia punctata (E71.43)

Q77.4   Achondroplasia
    Disturbance of epiphyseal chondroblastic growth and maturation, results in dwarfism
    Hypochondroplasia
    Osteosclerosis congenita

Q77.5   Diastrophic dysplasia

Q77.6   Chondroectodermal dysplasia
    Defective development of skin, hair, teeth, with polydactyly and defect of cardiac septum
    Ellis-van Creveld syndrome

Q77.7   Spondyloepiphyseal dysplasia

Q77.8   Other osteochondrodysplasia with defects of growth of tubular bones and spine

Q77.9   Osteochondrodysplasia with defects of growth of tubular bones and spine, unspecified

● **Q78   Other osteochondrodysplasias**
    Disorder of development of bone and cartilage; common cause of dwarfism

> **Excludes2**   congenital myotonic chondrodystrophy (G71.13)

Q78.0   Osteogenesis imperfecta
    Fragilitas ossium
    Osteopsathyrosis

Q78.1   Polyostotic fibrous dysplasia
    Albright(-McCune)(-Sternberg) syndrome

Q78.2   Osteopetrosis
    Abnormally dense bone; AKA marble bones disease, ivory bones
    Albers-Schönberg syndrome
    Osteosclerosis NOS

Q78.3   Progressive diaphyseal dysplasia
    Camurati-Engelmann syndrome

Q78.4   Enchondromatosis
    Thinning of overlying cortex of bone and distorted length
    Maffucci's syndrome
    Ollier's disease

Q78.5   Metaphyseal dysplasia
    Disturbance in enchondral bone growth, causing ends of shafts to remain larger than normal in circumference
    Pyle's syndrome

Q78.6   Multiple congenital exostoses
    Diaphyseal aclasis

Q78.8   Other specified osteochondrodysplasias
    Osteopoikilosis

Q78.9   Osteochondrodysplasia, unspecified
    Chondrodystrophy NOS
    AKA skeletal dysplasia (dwarfism) caused by genetic mutations affecting hyaline cartilage capping long bones and vertebrae
    Osteodystrophy NOS

● **Q79   Congenital malformations of musculoskeletal system, not elsewhere classified**

> **Excludes2**   congenital (sternomastoid) torticollis (Q68.0)

Q79.0   Congenital diaphragmatic hernia

> **Excludes1**   congenital hiatus hernia (Q40.1)

Q79.1   Other congenital malformations of diaphragm
    Absence of diaphragm
    Congenital malformation of diaphragm NOS
    Eventration of diaphragm

Q79.2   Exomphalos
    Abdominal hernia in which part of intestine protrudes at umbilicus; AKA exomphalos and exumbilication
    Omphalocele

> **Excludes1**   umbilical hernia (K42.-)

Q79.3   Gastroschisis
    Congenital fissure of anterior abdominal wall often with protrusion of small/large intestine

Q79.4   Prune belly syndrome
    Congenital prolapse of bladder mucosa
    Eagle-Barrett syndrome

● **Q79.5   Other congenital malformations of abdominal wall**

> **Excludes1**   umbilical hernia (K42.-)

    Q79.51   Congenital hernia of bladder

    Q79.59   Other congenital malformations of abdominal wall

Q79.6   Ehlers-Danlos syndrome
    Group of inherited disorders of connective tissue; AKA cutis hyperelastica

Q79.8   Other congenital malformations of musculoskeletal system
    Absence of muscle
    Absence of tendon
    Accessory muscle
    Amyotrophia congenita
    Congenital constricting bands
    Congenital shortening of tendon
    Poland syndrome

Q79.9   Congenital malformation of musculoskeletal system, unspecified
    Congenital anomaly of musculoskeletal system NOS
    Congenital deformity of musculoskeletal system NOS

OTHER CONGENITAL MALFORMATIONS (Q80-Q89)

● **Q80   Congenital ichthyosis**
    Characterized by increased keratinization, resulting in noninflammatory scaling of skin

> **Excludes1**   Refsum's disease (G60.1)

Q80.0   Ichthyosis vulgaris

Q80.1   X-linked ichthyosis

Q80.2   Lamellar ichthyosis
    Collodion baby

Q80.3   Congenital bullous ichthyosiform erythroderma

Q80.4   Harlequin fetus

Q80.8   Other congenital ichthyosis

Q80.9   Congenital ichthyosis, unspecified

● **Q81   Epidermolysis bullosa**
    Loosening of epidermis

Q81.0   Epidermolysis bullosa simplex

> **Excludes1**   Cockayne's syndrome (Q87.1)

Q81.1   Epidermolysis bullosa letalis
    Herlitz' syndrome

Q81.2   Epidermolysis bullosa dystrophica

Q81.8   Other epidermolysis bullosa

Q81.9   Epidermolysis bullosa, unspecified

● **Q82 Other congenital malformations of skin**

     Excludes1   acrodermatitis enteropathica (E83.2)
               congenital erythropoietic porphyria (E80.0)
               pilonidal cyst or sinus (L05.-)
               Sturge-Weber (-Dimitri) syndrome (Q85.8)

Q82.0 Hereditary lymphedema
     Characterized by swelling of subcutaneous tissue caused by obstruction of lymphatic vessels and resulting edema of lymph fluid

Q82.1 Xeroderma pigmentosum
     Dry, rough, discolored state of skin, and formation of scaly desquamation

Q82.2 Mastocytosis
     Characterized by infiltrates of mast cells in tissues/organs
     Urticaria pigmentosa
     Excludes1   malignant mastocytosis (C96.2)

Q82.3 Incontinentia pigmenti
     Characterized by hyperpigmented cutaneous

Q82.4 Ectodermal dysplasia (anhidrotic)
     Absence/deficiency of tissues/structures, including teeth, hair, nails, and certain glands
     Excludes1   Ellis-van Creveld syndrome (Q77.6)

Q82.5 Congenital non-neoplastic nevus
     Birthmark NOS
     Flammeus Nevus
     Portwine Nevus
     Sanguineous Nevus
     Strawberry Nevus
     Vascular Nevus NOS
     Verrucous Nevus
     Excludes2   Café au lait spots (L81.3)
               lentigo (L81.4)
               nevus NOS (D22.-)
               araneus nevus (I78.1)
               melanocytic nevus (D22.-)
               pigmented nevus (D22.-)
               spider nevus (I78.1)
               stellar nevus (I78.1)

Q82.6 Congenital sacral dimple ◄
     Parasacral dimple ◄
     Excludes2   pilonidal cyst with abscess (L05.01) ◄
               pilonidal cyst without abscess (L05.91) ◄

Q82.8 Other specified congenital malformations of skin
     Abnormal palmar creases
     Accessory skin tags
     Benign familial pemphigus [Hailey-Hailey]
     Congenital poikiloderma
     Cutis laxa (hyperelastica)
     Dermatoglyphic anomalies
     Inherited keratosis palmaris et plantaris
     Keratosis follicularis [Darier-White]
     Excludes1   Ehlers-Danlos syndrome (Q79.6)
     Coding Clinic: 2016, Q1, P17

Q82.9 Congenital malformation of skin, unspecified

● **Q83 Congenital malformations of breast**
     Excludes2   absence of pectoral muscle (Q79.8)
               hypoplasia of breast (N64.82)
               micromastia (N64.82)

Q83.0 Congenital absence of breast with absent nipple

Q83.1 Accessory breast
     Supernumerary breast

Q83.2 Absent nipple

Q83.3 Accessory nipple
     Supernumerary nipple

Q83.8 Other congenital malformations of breast

Q83.9 Congenital malformation of breast, unspecified

● **Q84 Other congenital malformations of integument**

Q84.0 Congenital alopecia
     Congenital atrichosis

Q84.1 Congenital morphological disturbances of hair, not elsewhere classified
     Beaded hair
     Monilethrix
     Pili annulati
     Excludes1   Menkes' kinky hair syndrome (E83.0)

Q84.2 Other congenital malformations of hair
     Congenital hypertrichosis
     Congenital malformation of hair NOS
     Persistent lanugo

Q84.3 Anonychia
     Absence of nail
     Excludes1   nail patella syndrome (Q87.2)

Q84.4 Congenital leukonychia
     Opaque, whitish discoloration of nails; AKA leukopathia unguium

Q84.5 Enlarged and hypertrophic nails
     Congenital onychauxis
     Pachyonychia

Q84.6 Other congenital malformations of nails
     Congenital clubnail
     Congenital koilonychia
     Congenital malformation of nail NOS

Q84.8 Other specified congenital malformations of integument
     Aplasia cutis congenita

Q84.9 Congenital malformation of integument, unspecified
     Congenital anomaly of integument NOS
     Congenital deformity of integument NOS

● **Q85 Phakomatoses, not elsewhere classified**
     Excludes1   ataxia telangiectasia [Louis-Bar] (G11.3)
               familial dysautonomia [Riley-Day] (G90.1)

● **Q85.0 Neurofibromatosis (nonmalignant)**
     Developmental changes in nervous system and other structures, with formation of neurofibromas

     Q85.00 Neurofibromatosis, unspecified

     Q85.01 Neurofibromatosis, type 1
         Von Recklinghausen disease

     Q85.02 Neurofibromatosis, type 2
         Acoustic neurofibromatosis

     Q85.03 Schwannomatosis

     Q85.09 Other neurofibromatosis

Q85.1 Tuberous sclerosis
     Bourneville's disease
     Epiloia

Q85.8 Other phakomatoses, not elsewhere classified
     Peutz-Jeghers Syndrome
     Sturge-Weber(-Dimitri) syndrome
     von Hippel-Lindau syndrome
     Excludes1   Meckel-Gruber syndrome (Q61.9)

Q85.9 Phakomatosis, unspecified
     Hamartosis NOS

● **Q86 Congenital malformation syndromes due to known exogenous causes, not elsewhere classified**
     Excludes2   iodine-deficiency-related hypothyroidism (E00-E02)
               nonteratogenic effects of substances transmitted via placenta or breast milk (P04.-)

Q86.0 Fetal alcohol syndrome (dysmorphic)

Q86.1 Fetal hydantoin syndrome
     Meadow's syndrome

Q86.2 Dysmorphism due to warfarin

Q86.8 Other congenital malformation syndromes due to known exogenous causes

CHAPTER 17 (Q00-Q99)

● **Q87   Other specified congenital malformation syndromes affecting multiple systems**

> Use additional code(s) to identify all associated manifestations

Q87.0   **Congenital malformation syndromes predominantly affecting facial appearance**
>> Acrocephalopolysyndactyly
>> Acrocephalosyndactyly [Apert]
>> Cryptophthalmos syndrome
>> Cyclopia
>> Goldenhar syndrome
>> Moebius syndrome
>> Oro-facial-digital syndrome
>> Robin syndrome
>> Whistling face

Q87.1   **Congenital malformation syndromes predominantly associated with short stature**
>> Aarskog syndrome
>> Cockayne syndrome
>> De Lange syndrome
>> Dubowitz syndrome
>> Noonan syndrome
>> Prader-Willi syndrome
>> Robinow-Silverman-Smith syndrome
>> Russell-Silver syndrome
>> Seckel syndrome

> **Excludes1**   Ellis-van Creveld syndrome (Q77.6)
>>> Smith-Lemli-Opitz syndrome (E78.72)

Q87.2   **Congenital malformation syndromes predominantly involving limbs**
>> Holt-Oram syndrome
>> Klippel-Trenaunay-Weber syndrome
>> Nail patella syndrome
>> Rubinstein-Taybi syndrome
>> Sirenomelia syndrome
>> Thrombocytopenia with absent radius [TAR] syndrome
>> VATER syndrome

Q87.3   **Congenital malformation syndromes involving early overgrowth**
>> Beckwith-Wiedemann syndrome
>> Sotos' syndrome
>> Weaver syndrome

● Q87.4   **Marfan's syndrome**

Q87.40   **Marfan's syndrome, unspecified**

● Q87.41   **Marfan's syndrome with cardiovascular manifestations**

Q87.410   **Marfan's syndrome with aortic dilation**

Q87.418   **Marfan's syndrome with other cardiovascular manifestations**

Q87.42   **Marfan's syndrome with ocular manifestations**

Q87.43   **Marfan's syndrome with skeletal manifestation**

Q87.5   **Other congenital malformation syndromes with other skeletal changes**

● Q87.8   **Other specified congenital malformation syndromes, not elsewhere classified**

> **Excludes1**   Zellweger syndrome (E71.510)

Q87.81   **Alport syndrome**
>> *Progressive sensorineural hearing loss, progressive pyelonephritis or glomerulonephritis, and ocular defects*

>> Use additional code to identify stage of chronic kidney disease (N18.1-N18.6)

Q87.82   **Arterial tortuosity syndrome** ◀

Q87.89   **Other specified congenital malformation syndromes, not elsewhere classified**
>> Laurence-Moon (-Bardet)-Biedl syndrome

● **Q89   Other congenital malformations, not elsewhere classified**

● Q89.0   **Congenital absence and malformations of spleen**

> **Excludes1**   isomerism of atrial appendages (with asplenia or polysplenia) (Q20.6)

Q89.01   **Asplenia (congenital)**

Q89.09   **Congenital malformations of spleen**
>> Congenital splenomegaly

Q89.1   **Congenital malformations of adrenal gland**

> **Excludes1**   adrenogenital disorders (E25.-)
>>> congenital adrenal hyperplasia (E25.0)

Q89.2   **Congenital malformations of other endocrine glands**
>> Congenital malformation of parathyroid or thyroid gland
>> Persistent thyroglossal duct
>> Thyroglossal cyst

> **Excludes1**   congenital goiter (E03.0)
>>> congenital hypothyroidism (E03.1)

Q89.3   **Situs inversus**
>> *Lateral transposition of viscera of thorax and abdomen*
>> Dextrocardia with situs inversus
>> Mirror-image atrial arrangement with situs inversus
>> Situs inversus or transversus abdominalis
>> Situs inversus or transversus thoracis
>> Transposition of abdominal viscera
>> Transposition of thoracic viscera

> **Excludes1**   dextrocardia NOS (Q24.0)

Q89.4   **Conjoined twins**
>> Craniopagus
>> Dicephaly
>> Pygopagus
>> Thoracopagus

Q89.7   **Multiple congenital malformations, not elsewhere classified**
>> Multiple congenital anomalies NOS
>> Multiple congenital deformities NOS

> **Excludes1**   congenital malformation syndromes affecting multiple systems (Q87.-)

Q89.8   **Other specified congenital malformations**
>> Use additional code(s) to identify all associated manifestations

Q89.9   **Congenital malformation, unspecified**
>> Congenital anomaly NOS
>> Congenital deformity NOS

CHROMOSOMAL ABNORMALITIES, NOT ELSEWHERE CLASSIFIED (Q90-Q99)

> **Excludes2**   mitochondrial metabolic disorders (E88.4-)

● **Q90   Down syndrome**

> Use additional code(s) to identify any associated physical conditions and degree of intellectual disabilities (F70-F79)

Q90.0   **Trisomy 21, nonmosaicism (meiotic nondisjunction)**
>> *Trisomy 21, nondisjunction, accounts for 95% of Downs syndrome cases*

Q90.1   **Trisomy 21, mosaicism (mitotic nondisjunction)**

Q90.2   **Trisomy 21, translocation**

Q90.9   **Down syndrome, unspecified**
>> Trisomy 21 NOS

● **Q91   Trisomy 18 and Trisomy 13**

Q91.0   **Trisomy 18, nonmosaicism (meiotic nondisjunction)**

Q91.1   **Trisomy 18, mosaicism (mitotic nondisjunction)**

Q91.2   **Trisomy 18, translocation**

Q91.3   **Trisomy 18, unspecified**

Q91.4   **Trisomy 13, nonmosaicism (meiotic nondisjunction)**

Q91.5   **Trisomy 13, mosaicism (mitotic nondisjunction)**

Q91.6   **Trisomy 13, translocation**

Q91.7   **Trisomy 13, unspecified**

◀ New   ◀▦ Revised   ~~deleted~~ Deleted   Excludes 1   Excludes 2   Includes   Use additional   Code first   Code also   Unspecified

OGCR Official Guidelines   X Assign placeholder X   ● Use Additional Character(s)   ▶ Manifestation Code   **Coding Clinic**

● **Q92	Other trisomies and partial trisomies of the autosomes, not elsewhere classified**

> **Includes**	unbalanced translocations and insertions
> **Excludes1**	trisomies of chromosomes 13, 18, 21 (Q90-Q91)

Q92.0	**Whole chromosome trisomy, nonmosaicism (meiotic nondisjunction)**

Q92.1	**Whole chromosome trisomy, mosaicism (mitotic nondisjunction)**

Q92.2	**Partial trisomy**
	Less than whole arm duplicated
	Whole arm or more duplicated

> **Excludes1**	partial trisomy due to unbalanced translocation (Q92.5)

Q92.5	**Duplications with other complex rearrangements**
	Partial trisomy due to unbalanced translocations

> Code also any associated deletions due to unbalanced translocations, inversions and insertions (Q93.7)

● Q92.6	**Marker chromosomes**
	Trisomies due to dicentrics
	Trisomies due to extra rings
	Trisomies due to isochromosomes
	Individual with marker heterochromatin

	Q92.61	**Marker chromosomes in normal individual**
	Q92.62	**Marker chromosomes in abnormal individual**

Q92.7	**Triploidy and polyploidy**

Q92.8	**Other specified trisomies and partial trisomies of autosomes**
	Duplications identified by fluorescence in situ hybridization (FISH)
	Duplications identified by in situ hybridization (ISH)
	Duplications seen only at prometaphase

Q92.9	**Trisomy and partial trisomy of autosomes, unspecified**

● **Q93	Monosomies and deletions from the autosomes, not elsewhere classified**

Q93.0	**Whole chromosome monosomy, nonmosaicism (meiotic nondisjunction)**

Q93.1	**Whole chromosome monosomy, mosaicism (mitotic nondisjunction)**

Q93.2	**Chromosome replaced with ring, dicentric or isochromosome**

Q93.3	**Deletion of short arm of chromosome 4**
	Wolff-Hirschorn syndrome

Q93.4	**Deletion of short arm of chromosome 5**
	Cri-du-chat syndrome

Q93.5	**Other deletions of part of a chromosome**
	Angelman syndrome

Q93.7	**Deletions with other complex rearrangements**
	Deletions due to unbalanced translocations, inversions and insertions

> Code also any associated duplications due to unbalanced translocations, inversions and insertions (Q92.5)

● Q93.8	**Other deletions from the autosomes**

	Q93.81	**Velo-cardio-facial syndrome**
		Deletion 22q11.2

	Q93.88	**Other microdeletions Miller-Dieker syndrome**
		Smith-Magenis syndrome

	Q93.89	**Other deletions from the autosomes**
		Deletions identified by fluorescence in situ hybridization (FISH)
		Deletions identified by in situ hybridization (ISH)
		Deletions seen only at prometaphase

Q93.9	**Deletion from autosomes, unspecified**

● **Q95	Balanced rearrangements and structural markers, not elsewhere classified**

> **Includes**	Robertsonian and balanced reciprocal translocations and insertions

Q95.0	**Balanced translocation and insertion in normal individual**

Q95.1	**Chromosome inversion in normal individual**

Q95.2	**Balanced autosomal rearrangement in abnormal individual**

Q95.3	**Balanced sex/autosomal rearrangement in abnormal individual**

Q95.5	**Individual with autosomal fragile site**

Q95.8	**Other balanced rearrangements and structural markers**

Q95.9	**Balanced rearrangement and structural marker, unspecified**

● **Q96	Turner's syndrome**

Caused by missing or incomplete X chromosome affecting growth and sexual development

> **Excludes1**	Noonan syndrome (Q87.1)

Q96.0	**Karyotype 45, X ♀**

Q96.1	**Karyotype 46, X iso (Xq) ♀**
	Karyotype 46, isochromosome Xq

Q96.2	**Karyotype 46, X with abnormal sex chromosome, except iso (Xq) ♀**
	Karyotype 46, X with abnormal sex chromosome, except isochromosome Xq

Q96.3	**Mosaicism, 45, X/46, XX or XY ♀**

Q96.4	**Mosaicism, 45, X/other cell line(s) with abnormal sex chromosome ♀**

Q96.8	**Other variants of Turner's syndrome ♀**

Q96.9	**Turner's syndrome, unspecified ♀**

● **Q97	Other sex chromosome abnormalities, female phenotype, not elsewhere classified**

> **Excludes1**	Turner's syndrome (Q96.-)

Q97.0	**Karyotype 47, XXX ♀**

Q97.1	**Female with more than three X chromosomes ♀**

Q97.2	**Mosaicism, lines with various numbers of X chromosomes ♀**

Q97.3	**Female with 46, XY karyotype ♀**

Q97.8	**Other specified sex chromosome abnormalities, female phenotype ♀**

Q97.9	**Sex chromosome abnormality, female phenotype, unspecified ♀**

● **Q98	Other sex chromosome abnormalities, male phenotype, not elsewhere classified**

Q98.0	**Klinefelter syndrome karyotype 47, XXY ♂**

Q98.1	**Klinefelter syndrome, male with more than two X chromosomes ♂**

Q98.3	**Other male with 46, XX karyotype ♂**

Q98.4	**Klinefelter syndrome, unspecified ♂**

Q98.5	**Karyotype 47, XYY**

Q98.6	**Male with structurally abnormal sex chromosome ♂**

Q98.7	**Male with sex chromosome mosaicism ♂**

Q98.8	**Other specified sex chromosome abnormalities, male phenotype ♂**

Q98.9	**Sex chromosome abnormality, male phenotype, unspecified ♂**

● **Q99	Other chromosome abnormalities, not elsewhere classified**

Q99.0	**Chimera 46, XX/46, XY**
	Chimera 46, XX/46, XY true hermaphrodite

Q99.1	**46, XX true hermaphrodite**
	46, XX with streak gonads
	46, XY with streak gonads
	Pure gonadal dysgenesis

Q99.2	**Fragile X chromosome**
	Fragile X syndrome

Q99.8	**Other specified chromosome abnormalities**

Q99.9	**Chromosomal abnormality, unspecified**

CHAPTER 17 (Q00-Q99)

CHAPTER 18

SYMPTOMS, SIGNS AND ABNORMAL CLINICAL AND LABORATORY FINDINGS, NOT ELSEWHERE CLASSIFIED (R00-R99)

OGCR Chapter-Specific Coding Guidelines

18. **Chapter 18: Symptoms, signs, and abnormal clinical and laboratory findings, not elsewhere classified (R00-R99)**
Chapter 18 includes symptoms, signs, abnormal results of clinical or other investigative procedures, and ill-defined conditions regarding which no diagnosis classifiable elsewhere is recorded. Signs and symptoms that point to a specific diagnosis have been assigned to a category in other chapters of the classification.

a. Use of symptom codes
Codes that describe symptoms and signs are acceptable for reporting purposes when a related definitive diagnosis has not been established (confirmed) by the provider.

b. Use of a symptom code with a definitive diagnosis code
Codes for signs and symptoms may be reported in addition to a related definitive diagnosis when the sign or symptom is not routinely associated with that diagnosis, such as the various signs and symptoms associated with complex syndromes. The definitive diagnosis code should be sequenced before the symptom code.

Signs or symptoms that are associated routinely with a disease process should not be assigned as additional codes, unless otherwise instructed by the classification.

c. Combination codes that include symptoms
ICD-10-CM contains a number of combination codes that identify both the definitive diagnosis and common symptoms of that diagnosis. When using one of these combination codes, an additional code should not be assigned for the symptom.

d. Repeated falls
Code R29.6, Repeated falls, is for use for encounters when a patient has recently fallen and the reason for the fall is being investigated.

Code Z91.81, History of falling, is for use when a patient has fallen in the past and is at risk for future falls. When appropriate, both codes R29.6 and Z91.81 may be assigned together.

e. Coma scale
The coma scale codes (R40.2-) can be used in conjunction with traumatic brain injury codes, acute cerebrovascular disease or sequelae of cerebrovascular disease codes. These codes are primarily for use by trauma registries, but they may be used in any setting where this information is collected. **The coma scale may also be used to assess the status of the central nervous system for other non-trauma conditions, such as monitoring patients in the intensive care unit regardless of medical condition.** The coma scale codes should be sequenced after the diagnosis code(s).

These codes, one from each subcategory, are needed to complete the scale. The 7th character indicates when the scale was recorded. The 7th character should match for all three codes.

At a minimum, report the initial score documented on presentation at your facility. This may be a score from the emergency medicine technician (EMT) or in the emergency department. If desired, a facility may choose to capture multiple coma scale scores.

Assign code R40.24, Glasgow coma scale, total score, when only the total score is documented in the medical record and not the individual score(s).

f. Functional quadriplegia
Functional quadriplegia (code R53.2) is the lack of ability to use one's limbs or to ambulate due to extreme debility. It is not associated with neurologic deficit or injury, and code R53.2 should not be used for cases of neurologic quadriplegia. It should only be assigned if functional quadriplegia is specifically documented in the medical record.

g. SIRS due to Non-Infectious Process
The systemic inflammatory response syndrome (SIRS) can develop as a result of certain non-infectious disease processes, such as trauma, malignant neoplasm, or pancreatitis. When SIRS is documented with a noninfectious condition, and no subsequent infection is documented, the code for the underlying condition, such as an injury, should be assigned, followed by code R65.10, Systemic inflammatory response syndrome (SIRS) of non-infectious origin without acute organ dysfunction, or code R65.11, Systemic inflammatory response syndrome (SIRS) of non-infectious origin with acute organ dysfunction. If an associated acute organ dysfunction is documented, the appropriate code(s) for the specific type of organ dysfunction(s) should be assigned in addition to code R65.11. If acute organ dysfunction is documented, but it cannot be determined if the acute organ dysfunction is associated with SIRS or due to another condition (e.g., directly due to the trauma), the provider should be queried.

h. Death NOS
Code R99, Ill-defined and unknown cause of mortality, is only for use in the very limited circumstance when a patient who has already died is brought into an emergency department or other healthcare facility and is pronounced dead upon arrival. It does not represent the discharge disposition of death.

i. NIHSS Stroke Scale
The NIH stroke scale (NIHSS) codes (R29.7- -) can be used in conjunction with acute stroke codes (I63) to identify the patient's neurological status and the severity of the stroke. The stroke scale codes should be sequenced after the acute stroke diagnosis code(s).

At a minimum, report the initial score documented. If desired, a facility may choose to capture multiple stroke scale scores.

See Section I.B.14. for information concerning the medical record documentation that may be used for assignment of the NIHSS codes.

◀ New   ◀ Revised   ~~deleted~~ Deleted   Excludes 1   Excludes 2   Includes   Use additional   Code first   Code also   Unspecified

OGCR Official Guidelines   X Assign placeholder X   ● Use Additional Character(s)   ▷ Manifestation Code   **Coding Clinic**

CHAPTER 18

SYMPTOMS, SIGNS AND ABNORMAL CLINICAL AND LABORATORY FINDINGS, NOT ELSEWHERE CLASSIFIED (R00-R99)

Note: This chapter includes symptoms, signs, abnormal results of clinical or other investigative procedures, and ill-defined conditions regarding which no diagnosis classifiable elsewhere is recorded.

Signs and symptoms that point rather definitely to a given diagnosis have been assigned to a category in other chapters of the classification. In general, categories in this chapter include the less well-defined conditions and symptoms that, without the necessary study of the case to establish a final diagnosis, point perhaps equally to two or more diseases or to two or more systems of the body. Practically all categories in the chapter could be designated 'not otherwise specified', 'unknown etiology' or 'transient'. The Alphabetical Index should be consulted to determine which symptoms and signs are to be allocated here and which to other chapters. The residual subcategories, numbered .8, are generally provided for other relevant symptoms that cannot be allocated elsewhere in the classification.

The conditions and signs or symptoms included in categories R00-R94 consist of:

(a) cases for which no more specific diagnosis can be made even after all the facts bearing on the case have been investigated;

(b) signs or symptoms existing at the time of initial encounter that proved to be transient and whose causes could not be determined;

(c) provisional diagnosis in a patient who failed to return for further investigation or care;

(d) cases referred elsewhere for investigation or treatment before the diagnosis was made;

(e) cases in which a more precise diagnosis was not available for any other reason;

(f) certain symptoms, for which supplementary information is provided, that represent important problems in medical care in their own right.

Excludes2   abnormal findings on antenatal screening of mother (O28.-)

certain conditions originating in the perinatal period (P04-P96)

signs and symptoms classified in the body system chapters

signs and symptoms of breast (N63, N64.5)

This chapter contains the following blocks:

R00-R09	Symptoms and signs involving the circulatory and respiratory systems
R10-R19	Symptoms and signs involving the digestive system and abdomen
R20-R23	Symptoms and signs involving the skin and subcutaneous tissue
R25-R29	Symptoms and signs involving the nervous and musculoskeletal systems
R30-R39	Symptoms and signs involving the genitourinary system
R40-R46	Symptoms and signs involving cognition, perception, emotional state and behavior
R47-R49	Symptoms and signs involving speech and voice
R50-R69	General symptoms and signs
R70-R79	Abnormal findings on examination of blood, without diagnosis
R80-R82	Abnormal findings on examination of urine, without diagnosis
R83-R89	Abnormal findings on examination of other body fluids, substances and tissues, without diagnosis
R90-R94	Abnormal findings on diagnostic imaging and in function studies, without diagnosis
R97	Abnormal tumor markers
R99	Ill-defined and unknown cause of mortality

SYMPTOMS AND SIGNS INVOLVING THE CIRCULATORY AND RESPIRATORY SYSTEMS (R00-R09)

● **R00**   **Abnormalities of heart beat**

    Excludes1   abnormalities originating in the perinatal period (P29.1-)

    Excludes2   specified arrhythmias (I47-I49) ◄

   R00.0   **Tachycardia, unspecified**

      Rapid heart rate >100 beats

      Rapid heart beat

      Sinoauricular tachycardia NOS

      Sinus [sinusal] tachycardia NOS

      Excludes1   neonatal tachycardia (P29.11)

                     paroxysmal tachycardia (I47.-)

   R00.1   **Bradycardia, unspecified**

      Slow heart rate, <60

      Sinoatrial bradycardia

      Sinus bradycardia

      Slow heart beat

      Vagal bradycardia

      Use additional code for adverse effect, if applicable, to identify drug (T36-T50 with fifth or sixth character 5)

      Excludes1   neonatal bradycardia (P29.12)

   R00.2   **Palpitations**

      Awareness of heart beat

   R00.8   **Other abnormalities of heart beat**

   R00.9   **Unspecified abnormalities of heart beat**

- **R01   Cardiac murmurs and other cardiac sounds**
  - **Excludes1**   cardiac murmurs and sounds originating in the perinatal period (P29.8)
  - **R01.0   Benign and innocent cardiac murmurs**
    Functional cardiac murmur
  - **R01.1   Cardiac murmur, unspecified**
    Cardiac bruit NOS
    Heart murmur NOS
    Systolic murmur NOS ◀
  - **R01.2   Other cardiac sounds**
    Cardiac dullness, increased or decreased
    Precordial friction

  OGCR Section I.C.9.a.7.

  > Hypertension, Transient
  > Assign code R03.0, Elevated blood pressure reading without diagnosis of hypertension, unless patient has an established diagnosis of hypertension. Assign code O13.-, Gestational [pregnancy-induced] hypertension with significant proteinuria, or O14.-, Pre-eclampsia, for transient hypertension of pregnancy.

- **R03   Abnormal blood-pressure reading, without diagnosis**
  - **R03.0   Elevated blood-pressure reading, without diagnosis of hypertension**
    Note: This category is to be used to record an episode of elevated blood pressure in a patient in whom no formal diagnosis of hypertension has been made, or as an isolated incidental finding.
  - **R03.1   Nonspecific low blood-pressure reading**
    - **Excludes1**   hypotension (I95.-)
      maternal hypotension syndrome (O26.5-)
      neurogenic orthostatic hypotension (G90.3)

- **R04   Hemorrhage from respiratory passages**
  - **R04.0   Epistaxis**
    Hemorrhage from nose
    Nosebleed
  - **R04.1   Hemorrhage from throat**
    - **Excludes2**   hemoptysis (R04.2)
  - **R04.2   Hemoptysis**
    Blood-stained sputum
    Cough with hemorrhage
  - **R04.8   Hemorrhage from other sites in respiratory passages**
    - **R04.81   Acute idiopathic pulmonary hemorrhage in infants**   P
      AIPHI
      Acute idiopathic hemorrhage in infants over 28 days old
      - **Excludes1**   perinatal pulmonary hemorrhage (P26.-)
        von Willebrand's disease (D68.0)
    - **R04.89   Hemorrhage from other sites in respiratory passages**
      Pulmonary hemorrhage NOS
  - **R04.9   Hemorrhage from respiratory passages, unspecified**

- **R05   Cough**
  - **Excludes1**   cough with hemorrhage (R04.2)
    smoker's cough (J41.0)

- **R06   Abnormalities of breathing**
  - **Excludes1**   acute respiratory distress syndrome (J80)
    respiratory arrest (R09.2)
    respiratory arrest of newborn (P28.81)
    respiratory distress syndrome of newborn (P22.-)
    respiratory failure (J96.-)
    respiratory failure of newborn (P28.5)
  - **R06.0   Dyspnea**
    - **Excludes1**   tachypnea NOS (R06.82)
      transient tachypnea of newborn (P22.1)
    - **R06.00   Dyspnea, unspecified**
    - **R06.01   Orthopnea**
    - **R06.02   Shortness of breath**
    - **R06.09   Other forms of dyspnea**
  - **R06.1   Stridor**
    Harsh, high-pitched breath sound
    - **Excludes1**   congenital laryngeal stridor (P28.89)
      laryngismus (stridulus) (J38.5)
  - **R06.2   Wheezing**
    - **Excludes1**   Asthma (J45.-)
      Coding Clinic: 2016, Q2, P34
  - **R06.3   Periodic breathing**
    Cheyne-Stokes breathing
    An abnormal pattern of breathing with gradually increasing and decreasing tidal volume with some periods of apnea
  - **R06.4   Hyperventilation**
    - **Excludes1**   psychogenic hyperventilation (F45.8)
  - **R06.5   Mouth breathing**
    - **Excludes2**   dry mouth NOS (R68.2)
  - **R06.6   Hiccough**
    - **Excludes1**   psychogenic hiccough (F45.8)
  - **R06.7   Sneezing**
  - **R06.8   Other abnormalities of breathing**
    - **R06.81   Apnea, not elsewhere classified**
      Apnea NOS
      - **Excludes1**   apnea (of) newborn (P28.4)
        sleep apnea (G47.3-)
        sleep apnea of newborn (primary) (P28.3)
    - **R06.82   Tachypnea, not elsewhere classified**
      Tachypnea NOS
      - **Excludes1**   transitory tachypnea of newborn (P22.1)
    - **R06.83   Snoring**
    - **R06.89   Other abnormalities of breathing**
      Breath-holding (spells)
      Sighing
  - **R06.9   Unspecified abnormalities of breathing**

- **R07   Pain in throat and chest**
  - **Excludes1**   epidemic myalgia (B33.0)
  - **Excludes2**   jaw pain R68.84
    pain in breast (N64.4)
  - **R07.0   Pain in throat**
    - **Excludes1**   chronic sore throat (J31.2)
      sore throat (acute) NOS (J02.9)
    - **Excludes2**   dysphagia (R13.1-)
      pain in neck (M54.2)
  - **R07.1   Chest pain on breathing**
    Painful respiration
  - **R07.2   Precordial pain**

● **R07.8**   **Other chest pain**
     R07.81   **Pleurodynia**
         Pleurodynia NOS
         Excludes1   epidemic pleurodynia (B33.0)
     R07.82   **Intercostal pain**
     R07.89   **Other chest pain**
         Anterior chest-wall pain NOS
   R07.9   **Chest pain, unspecified**

● **R09**   **Other symptoms and signs involving the circulatory and respiratory system**
     Excludes1   acute respiratory distress syndrome (J80)
         respiratory arrest of newborn (P28.81)
         respiratory distress syndrome of newborn (P22.0)
         respiratory failure (J96.-)
         respiratory failure of newborn (P28.5)

● **R09.0**   **Asphyxia and hypoxemia**
     Excludes1   asphyxia due to carbon monoxide (T58.-)
         asphyxia due to foreign body in respiratory tract (T17.-)
         birth (intrauterine) asphyxia (P84)
         hypercapnia (R06.4)
         hyperventilation (R06.4)
         traumatic asphyxia (T71.-)
     R09.01   **Asphyxia**
     R09.02   **Hypoxemia**
   R09.1   **Pleurisy**
     Occurs when double membrane (pleura) lining chest cavity and lung surface becomes inflamed causing sharp pain on inspiration/expiration
     Excludes1   pleurisy with effusion (J90)
   R09.2   **Respiratory arrest**
     Cardiorespiratory failure
     Excludes1   cardiac arrest (I46.-)
         respiratory arrest of newborn (P28.81)
         respiratory distress of newborn (P22.0)
         respiratory failure (J96.-)
         respiratory failure of newborn (P28.5)
         respiratory insufficiency (R06.89)
         respiratory insufficiency of newborn (P28.5)
   R09.3   **Abnormal sputum**
     Abnormal amount of sputum
     Abnormal color of sputum
     Abnormal odor of sputum
     Excessive sputum
     Excludes1   blood-stained sputum (R04.2)

● **R09.8**   **Other specified symptoms and signs involving the circulatory and respiratory systems**
     R09.81   **Nasal congestion**
     R09.82   **Postnasal drip**
     R09.89   **Other specified symptoms and signs involving the circulatory and respiratory systems**
         Bruit (arterial)
         Abnormal chest percussion
         Feeling of foreign body in throat
         Friction sounds in chest
         Chest tympany
         Choking sensation
         Rales
         Wet rattling, clicking, crackling sounds on auscultation
         Weak pulse
         Excludes2   foreign body in throat (T17.2-)
         wheezing (R06.2)

SYMPTOMS AND SIGNS INVOLVING THE DIGESTIVE SYSTEM AND ABDOMEN (R10-R19)

     Excludes2   congenital or infantile pylorospasm (Q40.0) ◄
         gastrointestinal hemorrhage (K92.0-K92.2) ◄
         intestinal obstruction (K56.-) ◄
         newborn gastrointestinal hemorrhage (P54.0-P54.3) ◄
         newborn intestinal obstruction (P76.-) ◄
         pylorospasm (K31.3) ◄
         signs and symptoms involving the urinary system (R30-R39) ◄
         symptoms referable to female genital organs (N94.-) ◄
         symptoms referable to male genital organs (N48-N50) ◄

● **R10**   **Abdominal and pelvic pain**
     Excludes1   renal colic (N23)
     Excludes2   dorsalgia (M54.-)
         flatulence and related conditions (R14.-)
   R10.0   **Acute abdomen**
     Severe abdominal pain (generalized) (with abdominal rigidity)
     Excludes1   abdominal rigidity NOS (R19.3)
         generalized abdominal pain NOS (R10.84)
         localized abdominal pain (R10.1-R10.3-)

● **R10.1**   **Pain localized to upper abdomen**
     R10.10   **Upper abdominal pain, unspecified**
     R10.11   **Right upper quadrant pain**
     R10.12   **Left upper quadrant pain**
     R10.13   **Epigastric pain**
         Dyspepsia
         Excludes1   functional dyspepsia (K30)
   R10.2   **Pelvic and perineal pain**
     Excludes1   vulvodynia (N94.81)

● **R10.3**   **Pain localized to other parts of lower abdomen**
     R10.30   **Lower abdominal pain, unspecified**
     R10.31   **Right lower quadrant pain**
     R10.32   **Left lower quadrant pain**
     R10.33   **Periumbilical pain**

● **R10.8**   **Other abdominal pain**
     ● **R10.81**   **Abdominal tenderness**
         Abdominal tenderness NOS
         R10.811   **Right upper quadrant abdominal tenderness**
         R10.812   **Left upper quadrant abdominal tenderness**
         R10.813   **Right lower quadrant abdominal tenderness**
         R10.814   **Left lower quadrant abdominal tenderness**
         R10.815   **Periumbilic abdominal tenderness**
         R10.816   **Epigastric abdominal tenderness**
         R10.817   **Generalized abdominal tenderness**
         R10.819   **Abdominal tenderness, unspecified site**

CHAPTER 18 (R00-R99)

● R10.82   Rebound abdominal tenderness
   R10.821   Right upper quadrant rebound abdominal tenderness
   R10.822   Left upper quadrant rebound abdominal tenderness
   R10.823   Right lower quadrant rebound abdominal tenderness
   R10.824   Left lower quadrant rebound abdominal tenderness
   R10.825   Periumbilic rebound abdominal tenderness
   R10.826   Epigastric rebound abdominal tenderness
   R10.827   Generalized rebound abdominal tenderness
   R10.829   Rebound abdominal tenderness, unspecified site

R10.83   Colic   P
   Colic NOS
   Infantile colic
   Excludes1   colic in adult and child over 12 months old (R10.84)

R10.84   Generalized abdominal pain
   Excludes1   generalized abdominal pain associated with acute abdomen (R10.0)

R10.9   Unspecified abdominal pain

● R11   Nausea and vomiting
   Excludes1   cyclical vomiting associated with migraine (G43.A-)
                excessive vomiting in pregnancy (O21.-)
                hematemesis (K92.0)
                neonatal hematemesis (P54.0)
                newborn vomiting (P92.0-)
                psychogenic vomiting (F50.89) ◄▥▥
                vomiting associated with bulimia nervosa (F50.2)
                vomiting following gastrointestinal surgery (K91.0)

● R11.0   Nausea
   Nausea NOS
   Nausea without vomiting

● R11.1   Vomiting
   R11.10   Vomiting, unspecified
      Vomiting NOS
   R11.11   Vomiting without nausea
   R11.12   Projectile vomiting
   R11.13   Vomiting of fecal matter
   R11.14   Bilious vomiting
      Bilious emesis

● R11.2   Nausea with vomiting, unspecified
   Persistent nausea with vomiting NOS

R12   Heartburn
   Excludes1   dyspepsia NOS (R10.13)
                functional dyspepsia (K30)

● R13   Aphagia and dysphagia
   R13.0   Aphagia
      Inability to swallow
      Excludes1   psychogenic aphagia (F50.9)
● R13.1   Dysphagia
   Difficulty swallowing
   Code first, if applicable, dysphagia following cerebrovascular disease (I69. with final characters -91)
   Excludes1   psychogenic dysphagia (F45.8)
   R13.10   Dysphagia, unspecified
      Difficulty in swallowing NOS
   R13.11   Dysphagia, oral phase
   R13.12   Dysphagia, oropharyngeal phase
   R13.13   Dysphagia, pharyngeal phase
   R13.14   Dysphagia, pharyngoesophageal phase
   R13.19   Other dysphagia
      Cervical dysphagia
      Neurogenic dysphagia

● R14   Flatulence and related conditions
   Excludes1   psychogenic aerophagy (F45.8)
   R14.0   Abdominal distension (gaseous)
      Bloating
      Tympanites (abdominal) (intestinal)
   R14.1   Gas pain
   R14.2   Eructation
      Belching air from stomach through mouth
   R14.3   Flatulence

● R15   Fecal incontinence
   Includes   encopresis NOS
   Excludes1   fecal incontinence of nonorganic origin (F98.1)
   R15.0   Incomplete defecation
      Excludes1   constipation (K59.0-)
                   fecal impaction (K56.41)
   R15.1   Fecal smearing
      Fecal soiling
   R15.2   Fecal urgency
   R15.9   Full incontinence of feces
      Fecal incontinence NOS

● R16   Hepatomegaly and splenomegaly, not elsewhere classified
   Enlargement of liver or spleen
   R16.0   Hepatomegaly, not elsewhere classified
      Hepatomegaly NOS
   R16.1   Splenomegaly, not elsewhere classified
      Splenomegaly NOS
   R16.2   Hepatomegaly with splenomegaly, not elsewhere classified
      Hepatosplenomegaly NOS

R17   Unspecified jaundice
   Excludes1   neonatal jaundice (P55, P57-P59)

● R18   Ascites
   Includes   fluid in peritoneal cavity
   Excludes1   ascites in alcoholic cirrhosis (K70.31)
                ascites in alcoholic hepatitis (K70.11)
                ascites in toxic liver disease with chronic active hepatitis (K71.51)
   R18.0   Malignant ascites
      Code first malignancy, such as:
         malignant neoplasm of ovary (C56.-)
         secondary malignant neoplasm of retroperitoneum and peritoneum (C78.6)
   R18.8   Other ascites
      Ascites NOS
      Peritoneal effusion (chronic)

◄ New   ◄▥▥ Revised   d̶e̶l̶e̶t̶e̶d̶ Deleted   Excludes 1   Excludes 2   Includes   Use additional   Code first   Code also   Unspecified
OGCR Official Guidelines   X Assign placeholder X   ● Use Additional Character(s)   ▶ Manifestation Code   Coding Clinic

● **R19   Other symptoms and signs involving the digestive system and abdomen**
- **Excludes1**   acute abdomen (R10.0)

● **R19.0   Intra-abdominal and pelvic swelling, mass and lump**
- **Excludes1**   abdominal distension (gaseous) (R14.-)
  - ascites (R18.-)
- **R19.00   Intra-abdominal and pelvic swelling, mass and lump, unspecified site**
- **R19.01   Right upper quadrant abdominal swelling, mass and lump**
- **R19.02   Left upper quadrant abdominal swelling, mass and lump**
- **R19.03   Right lower quadrant abdominal swelling, mass and lump**
- **R19.04   Left lower quadrant abdominal swelling, mass and lump**
- **R19.05   Periumbilic swelling, mass or lump**
  - Diffuse or generalized umbilical swelling or mass
- **R19.06   Epigastric swelling, mass or lump**
- **R19.07   Generalized intra-abdominal and pelvic swelling, mass and lump**
  - Diffuse or generalized intra-abdominal swelling or mass NOS
  - Diffuse or generalized pelvic swelling or mass NOS
- **R19.09   Other intra-abdominal and pelvic swelling, mass and lump**

● **R19.1   Abnormal bowel sounds**
- **R19.11   Absent bowel sounds**
- **R19.12   Hyperactive bowel sounds**
- **R19.15   Other abnormal bowel sounds**
  - Abnormal bowel sounds NOS

R19.2   Visible peristalsis
- Hyperperistalsis

● **R19.3   Abdominal rigidity**
- **Excludes1**   abdominal rigidity with severe abdominal pain (R10.0)
- **R19.30   Abdominal rigidity, unspecified site**
- **R19.31   Right upper quadrant abdominal rigidity**
- **R19.32   Left upper quadrant abdominal rigidity**
- **R19.33   Right lower quadrant abdominal rigidity**
- **R19.34   Left lower quadrant abdominal rigidity**
- **R19.35   Periumbilic abdominal rigidity**
- **R19.36   Epigastric abdominal rigidity**
- **R19.37   Generalized abdominal rigidity**

R19.4   Change in bowel habit
- **Excludes1**   constipation (K59.0-)
  - functional diarrhea (K59.1)

R19.5   Other fecal abnormalities
- Abnormal stool color
- Bulky stools
- Mucus in stools
- Occult blood in feces
- Occult blood in stools
- **Excludes1**   melena (K92.1)
  - neonatal melena (P54.1)

R19.6   Halitosis

R19.7   Diarrhea, unspecified
- Diarrhea NOS
- **Excludes1**   functional diarrhea (K59.1)
  - neonatal diarrhea (P78.3)
  - psychogenic diarrhea (F45.8)

R19.8   Other specified symptoms and signs involving the digestive system and abdomen

SYMPTOMS AND SIGNS INVOLVING THE SKIN AND SUBCUTANEOUS TISSUE (R20-R23)

- **Excludes2**   symptoms relating to breast (N64.4-N64.5)

● **R20   Disturbances of skin sensation**
- **Excludes1**   dissociative anesthesia and sensory loss (F44.6)
  - psychogenic disturbances (F45.8)

R20.0   Anesthesia of skin
- *Loss of sensation*

R20.1   Hypoesthesia of skin
- *Unpleasant abnormal sensation*

R20.2   Paresthesia of skin
- *Abnormal touch sensation, including burning, prickling, often in absence of external stimulus*
- Formication   Tingling skin
- Pins and needles
- **Excludes1**   acroparesthesia (I73.8)

R20.3   Hyperesthesia

R20.8   Other disturbances of skin sensation

R20.9   Unspecified disturbances of skin sensation

R21   Rash and other nonspecific skin eruption
- **Includes**   rash NOS
- **Excludes1**   specified type of rash- code to condition
  - vesicular eruption (R23.8)

● **R22   Localized swelling, mass and lump of skin and subcutaneous tissue**
- **Includes**   subcutaneous nodules (localized) (superficial)
- **Excludes1**   abnormal findings on diagnostic imaging (R90-R93)
  - edema (R60.-)
  - enlarged lymph nodes (R59.-)
  - localized adiposity (E65)
  - swelling of joint (M25.4-)

R22.0   Localized swelling, mass and lump, head

R22.1   Localized swelling, mass and lump, neck

R22.2   Localized swelling, mass and lump, trunk
- **Excludes1**   intra-abdominal or pelvic mass and lump (R19.0-)
  - intra-abdominal or pelvic swelling (R19.0-)
- **Excludes2**   breast mass and lump (N63)

● **R22.3   Localized swelling, mass and lump, upper limb**
- **R22.30   Localized swelling, mass and lump, unspecified upper limb**
- **R22.31   Localized swelling, mass and lump, right upper limb**
- **R22.32   Localized swelling, mass and lump, left upper limb**
- **R22.33   Localized swelling, mass and lump, upper limb, bilateral**

● **R22.4   Localized swelling, mass and lump, lower limb**
- **R22.40   Localized swelling, mass and lump, unspecified lower limb**
- **R22.41   Localized swelling, mass and lump, right lower limb**
- **R22.42   Localized swelling, mass and lump, left lower limb**
- **R22.43   Localized swelling, mass and lump, lower limb, bilateral**

R22.9   Localized swelling, mass and lump, unspecified

CHAPTER 18 (R00-R99)

● **R23**   **Other skin changes**

    R23.0   **Cyanosis**

        Excludes1   acrocyanosis (I73.8)

                        cyanotic attacks of newborn (P28.2)

    R23.1   **Pallor**

           Clammy skin

    R23.2   **Flushing**

           Excessive blushing

           Code first, if applicable, menopausal and female climacteric states (N95.1)

    R23.3   **Spontaneous ecchymoses**

           Small hemorrhagic spot of skin; AKA black and blue spot

           Petechiae

        Excludes1   ecchymoses of newborn (P54.5)

                        purpura (D69.-)

    R23.4   **Changes in skin texture**

           Desquamation of skin   Scaling of skin

           Induration of skin

        Excludes1   epidermal thickening NOS (L85.9)

    R23.8   **Other skin changes**

    R23.9   **Unspecified skin changes**

SYMPTOMS AND SIGNS INVOLVING THE NERVOUS AND MUSCULOSKELETAL SYSTEMS (R25-R29)

● **R25**   **Abnormal involuntary movements**

        Excludes1   specific movement disorders (G20-G26)

                        stereotyped movement disorders (F98.4)

                        tic disorders (F95.-)

    R25.0   **Abnormal head movements**

    R25.1   **Tremor, unspecified**

        Excludes1   chorea NOS (G25.5)

                        essential tremor (G25.0)

                        hysterical tremor (F44.4)

                        intention tremor (G25.2)

    R25.2   **Cramp and spasm**

        Excludes2   carpopedal spasm (R29.0)

                        charley-horse (M62.831)

                        infantile spasms (G40.4-)

                        muscle spasm of back (M62.830)

                        muscle spasm of calf (M62.831)

    R25.3   **Fasciculation**

           Twitching NOS

    R25.8   **Other abnormal involuntary movements**

    R25.9   **Unspecified abnormal involuntary movements**

● **R26**   **Abnormalities of gait and mobility**

        Excludes1   ataxia NOS (R27.0)

                        hereditary ataxia (G11.-)

                        locomotor (syphilitic) ataxia (A52.11)

                        immobility syndrome (paraplegic) (M62.3)

    R26.0   **Ataxic gait**

           Staggering gait

    R26.1   **Paralytic gait**

           Spastic gait

    R26.2   **Difficulty in walking, not elsewhere classified**

        Excludes1   falling (R29.6)

                        unsteadiness on feet (R26.81)

        Coding Clinic: 2016, Q2, P7

● **R26.8**   **Other abnormalities of gait and mobility**

        R26.81   **Unsteadiness on feet**

        R26.89   **Other abnormalities of gait and mobility**

    R26.9   **Unspecified abnormalities of gait and mobility**

● **R27**   **Other lack of coordination**

        Excludes1   ataxic gait (R26.0)

                        hereditary ataxia (G11.-)

                        vertigo NOS (R42)

    R27.0   **Ataxia, unspecified**

        Excludes1   ataxia following cerebrovascular disease (I69. with final characters -93)

    R27.8   **Other lack of coordination**

    R27.9   **Unspecified lack of coordination**

● **R29**   **Other symptoms and signs involving the nervous and musculoskeletal systems**

    R29.0   **Tetany**

           Hyperexcitability of nerves and muscles characterized by spasm, twitching, and cramps

           Carpopedal spasm

        Excludes1   hysterical tetany (F44.5)

                        neonatal tetany (P71.3)

                        parathyroid tetany (E20.9)

                        post-thyroidectomy tetany (E89.2)

    R29.1   **Meningismus**

    R29.2   **Abnormal reflex**

        Excludes2   abnormal pupillary reflex (H57.0)

                        hyperactive gag reflex (J39.2)

                        vasovagal reaction or syncope (R55)

    R29.3   **Abnormal posture**

    R29.4   **Clicking hip**

        Excludes1   congenital deformities of hip (Q65.-)

    R29.5   **Transient paralysis**

           Code first any associated spinal cord injury (S14.0, S14.1-, S24.0, S24.1-, S34.0-, S34.1-)

        Excludes1   transient ischemic attack (G45.9)

    R29.6   **Repeated falls**

           Falling

           Tendency to fall

        Excludes2   at risk for falling (Z91.81)

                        history of falling (Z91.81)

        OGCR   Section I.C.18.d.

        Repeated falls

        Code R29.6, Repeated falls, is for use for encounters when a patient has recently fallen and the reason for the fall is being investigated.

        Code Z91.81, History of falling, is for use when a patient has fallen in the past and is at risk for future falls. When appropriate, both codes R29.6 and Z91.81 may be assigned together.

        Coding Clinic: 2016, Q2, P7

● **R29.7**   **National Institutes of Health Stroke Scale (NIHSS) score** ◀

        Code first the type of cerebral infarction (I63-) ◀

    ● **R29.70**   **NIHSS score 0-9** ◀

        R29.700   **NIHSS score 0** ◀

        R29.701   **NIHSS score 1** ◀

        R29.702   **NIHSS score 2** ◀

        R29.703   **NIHSS score 3** ◀

        R29.704   **NIHSS score 4** ◀

        R29.705   **NIHSS score 5** ◀

        R29.706   **NIHSS score 6** ◀

        R29.707   **NIHSS score 7** ◀

        R29.708   **NIHSS score 8** ◀

        R29.709   **NIHSS score 9** ◀

◀ New   ◀|||| Revised   ~~deleted~~ Deleted   Excludes 1   Excludes 2   Includes   Use additional   Code first   Code also   Unspecified

OGCR Official Guidelines   X Assign placeholder X   ● Use Additional Character(s)   ▶ Manifestation Code   **Coding Clinic**

OGCR Section I.C.18.i.

NIHSS Stroke Scale
The NIH stroke scale (NIHSS) codes (R29.7- -) can be used in conjunction with acute stroke codes (I63) to identify the patient's neurological status and the severity of the stroke. The stroke scale codes should be sequenced after the acute stroke diagnosis code(s).
At a minimum, report the initial score documented. If desired, a facility may choose to capture multiple stroke scale scores.

- **R29.71   NIHSS score 10-19** ◄
  - R29.710   NIHSS score 10 ◄
  - R29.711   NIHSS score 11 ◄
  - R29.712   NIHSS score 12 ◄
  - R29.713   NIHSS score 13 ◄
  - R29.714   NIHSS score 14 ◄
  - R29.715   NIHSS score 15 ◄
  - R29.716   NIHSS score 16 ◄
  - R29.717   NIHSS score 17 ◄
  - R29.718   NIHSS score 18 ◄
  - R29.719   NIHSS score 19 ◄
- **R29.72   NIHSS score 20-29** ◄
  - R29.720   NIHSS score 20 ◄
  - R29.721   NIHSS score 21 ◄
  - R29.722   NIHSS score 22 ◄
  - R29.723   NIHSS score 23 ◄
  - R29.724   NIHSS score 24 ◄
  - R29.725   NIHSS score 25 ◄
  - R29.726   NIHSS score 26 ◄
  - R29.727   NIHSS score 27 ◄
  - R29.728   NIHSS score 28 ◄
  - R29.729   NIHSS score 29 ◄
- **R29.73   NIHSS score 30-39** ◄
  - R29.730   NIHSS score 30 ◄
  - R29.731   NIHSS score 31 ◄
  - R29.732   NIHSS score 32 ◄
  - R29.733   NIHSS score 33 ◄
  - R29.734   NIHSS score 34 ◄
  - R29.735   NIHSS score 35 ◄
  - R29.736   NIHSS score 36 ◄
  - R29.737   NIHSS score 37 ◄
  - R29.738   NIHSS score 38 ◄
  - R29.739   NIHSS score 39 ◄
- **R29.74   NIHSS score 40-42** ◄
  - R29.740   NIHSS score 40 ◄
  - R29.741   NIHSS score 41 ◄
  - R29.742   NIHSS score 42 ◄
- **R29.8   Other symptoms and signs involving the nervous and musculoskeletal systems**
  - **R29.81   Other symptoms and signs involving the nervous system**
    - **R29.810   Facial weakness**
      Facial droop
      Excludes1   Bell's palsy (G51.0)
      facial weakness following cerebrovascular disease (I69. with final characters -92)
    - **R29.818   Other symptoms and signs involving the nervous system**

- **R29.89   Other symptoms and signs involving the musculoskeletal system**
  Excludes2   pain in limb (M79.6-)
  - **R29.890   Loss of height**
    Excludes1   osteoporosis (M80-M81)
  - **R29.891   Ocular torticollis**
    Excludes1   congenital (sterno-mastoid) torticollis Q68.0
    psychogenic torticollis (F45.8)
    spasmodic torticollis (G24.3)
    torticollis due to birth injury (P15.8)
    torticollis NOS M43.6
  - **R29.898   Other symptoms and signs involving the musculoskeletal system**
- **R29.9   Unspecified symptoms and signs involving the nervous and musculoskeletal systems**
  - **R29.90   Unspecified symptoms and signs involving the nervous system**
  - **R29.91   Unspecified symptoms and signs involving the musculoskeletal system**

SYMPTOMS AND SIGNS INVOLVING THE GENITOURINARY SYSTEM (R30-R39)

- **R30   Pain associated with micturition**
  Excludes1   psychogenic pain associated with micturition (F45.8)
  - **R30.0   Dysuria**
    Painful urination
    Strangury
  - **R30.1   Vesical tenesmus**
    Straining to urinate
  - **R30.9   Painful micturition, unspecified**
    Painful urination NOS
- **R31   Hematuria**
  Excludes1   hematuria included with underlying conditions, such as:
  acute cystitis with hematuria (N30.01)
  recurrent and persistent hematuria in glomerular diseases (N02.-)
  - **R31.0   Gross hematuria**
  - **R31.1   Benign essential microscopic hematuria**
  - **R31.2   Other microscopic hematuria**
    - **R31.21   Asymptomatic microscopic hematuria** ◄
      AMH ◄
    - **R31.29   Other microscopic hematuria** ◄
  - **R31.9   Hematuria, unspecified**
- **R32   Unspecified urinary incontinence**
  Enuresis NOS
  Excludes1   functional urinary incontinence (R39.81)
  nonorganic enuresis (F98.0)
  stress incontinence and other specified urinary incontinence (N39.3-N39.4-)
  urinary incontinence associated with cognitive impairment (R39.81)
- **R33   Retention of urine**
  Excludes1   psychogenic retention of urine (F45.8)
  - **R33.0   Drug induced retention of urine**
    Use additional code for adverse effect, if applicable, to identify drug (T36-T50 with fifth or sixth character 5)
  - **R33.8   Other retention of urine**
    Code first, if applicable, any causal condition, such as:
    enlarged prostate (N40.1)
  - **R33.9   Retention of urine, unspecified**

CHAPTER 18 (R00-R99)

R34 Anuria and oliguria

> **Excludes1**   anuria and oliguria complicating abortion or ectopic or molar pregnancy (O00-O07, O08.4)
> anuria and oliguria complicating pregnancy (O26.83-)
> anuria and oliguria complicating the puerperium (O90.4)

● **R35 Polyuria**

Passage of excessive volume of urine

Code first, if applicable, any causal condition, such as:
enlarged prostate (N40.1)

> **Excludes1**   psychogenic polyuria (F45.8)

    R35.0 Frequency of micturition
Discharge or passage of urine; AKA uresis

    R35.1 Nocturia
Urinary frequency at night

    R35.8 Other polyuria
Polyuria NOS

● **R36 Urethral discharge**

    R36.0 Urethral discharge without blood

    R36.1 Hematospermia ♂
Presence of blood in semen

    R36.9 Urethral discharge, unspecified
Penile discharge NOS
Urethrorrhea

R37 Sexual dysfunction, unspecified

● **R39 Other and unspecified symptoms and signs involving the genitourinary system**

    R39.0 Extravasation of urine
Leakage, discharge

  ● **R39.1 Other difficulties with micturition**

Code first, if applicable, any causal condition, such as:
enlarged prostate (N40.1)

       R39.11 Hesitancy of micturition

       R39.12 Poor urinary stream
Weak urinary steam

       R39.13 Splitting of urinary stream

       R39.14 Feeling of incomplete bladder emptying

       R39.15 Urgency of urination

> **Excludes1**   urge incontinence (N39.41, N39.46)

       R39.16 Straining to void

     ● **R39.19 Other difficulties with micturition**

          R39.191 Need to immediately re-void ◀

          R39.192 Position dependent micturition ◀

          R39.198 Other difficulties with micturition ◀

    R39.2 Extrarenal uremia
Prenal uremia

> **Excludes1**   uremia NOS (N19)

  ● **R39.8 Other symptoms and signs involving the genitourinary system**

       R39.81 Functional urinary incontinence
Urinary incontinence due to cognitive impairment, or severe physical disability or immobility

> **Excludes1**   stress incontinence and other specified urinary incontinence (N39.3-N39.4-)
> urinary incontinence NOS (R32)

       R39.82 Chronic bladder pain ◀

       R39.89 Other symptoms and signs involving the genitourinary system

    R39.9 Unspecified symptoms and signs involving the genitourinary system

---

SYMPTOMS AND SIGNS INVOLVING COGNITION, PERCEPTION, EMOTIONAL STATE AND BEHAVIOR (R40-R46)

> **Excludes2**   symptoms and signs constituting part of a pattern of mental disorder (F01-F99) ◀
> **Coding Clinic: 2015, Q4, P40**

● **R40 Somnolence, stupor and coma**

> **Excludes1**   neonatal coma (P91.5)
> somnolence, stupor and coma in diabetes (E08-E13)
> somnolence, stupor and coma in hepatic failure (K72.-)
> somnolence, stupor and coma in hypoglycemia (nondiabetic) (E15)

    R40.0 Somnolence
Drowsiness

> **Excludes1**   coma (R40.2-)

    R40.1 Stupor
Lowered level of consciousness
Catatonic stupor
Semicoma

> **Excludes1**   catatonic schizophrenia (F20.2)
> coma (R40.2-)
> depressive stupor (F31-F33)
> dissociative stupor (F44.2)
> manic stupor (F30.2)

OGCR Section I.C.18.e.

Coma scale

The coma scale codes (R40.2-) can be used in conjunction with traumatic brain injury codes, acute cerebrovascular disease or sequelae of cerebrovascular disease codes. These codes are primarily for use by trauma registries, but they may be used in any setting where this information is collected. **The coma scale may also be used to assess the status of the central nervous system for other non-trauma conditions, such as monitoring patients in the intensive care unit regardless of medical condition.** The coma scale codes should be sequenced after the diagnosis code(s).

These codes, one from each subcategory, are needed to complete the scale. The 7th character indicates when the scale was recorded. The 7th character should match for all three codes.

At a minimum, report the initial score documented on presentation at your facility. This may be a score from the emergency medicine technician (EMT) or in the emergency department. If desired, a facility may choose to capture multiple coma scale scores.

Assign code R40.24, Glasgow coma scale, total score, when only the total score is documented in the medical record and not the individual score(s).

● **R40.2 Coma**

Code first any associated:
fracture of skull (S02.-)
intracranial injury (S06.-)

Note: One code from each subcategory R40.21-R40-23 is required to complete the coma scale ◀▥

    R40.20 Unspecified coma
Coma NOS
Unconsciousness NOS

● **R40.21 Coma scale, eyes open**

The following appropriate 7th character is to be added to subcategory R40.21-:

0	unspecified time
1	in the field [EMT or ambulance]
2	at arrival to emergency department
3	at hospital admission
4	24 hours or more after hospital admission

Coding Clinic: 2015, Q2, P18

● **R40.211 Coma scale, eyes open, never**

● **R40.212 Coma scale, eyes open, to pain**

● **R40.213 Coma scale, eyes open, to sound**

● **R40.214 Coma scale, eyes open, spontaneous**

◀ New   ◀▥ Revised   ~~deleted~~ Deleted   Excludes 1   Excludes 2   Includes   Use additional   Code first   Code also   Unspecified

OGCR Official Guidelines   X Assign placeholder X   ● Use Additional Character(s)   ▷ Manifestation Code   **Coding Clinic**

● R40.22   **Coma scale, best verbal response**

> The following appropriate 7th character is to be added to subcategory R40.22-:

0	unspecified time
1	in the field [EMT or ambulance]
2	at arrival to emergency department
3	at hospital admission
4	24 hours or more after hospital admission

Coding Clinic: 2015, Q2, P18

● R40.221   **Coma scale, best verbal response, none**
● R40.222   **Coma scale, best verbal response, incomprehensible words**
● R40.223   **Coma scale, best verbal response, inappropriate words**
● R40.224   **Coma scale, best verbal response, confused conversation**
● R40.225   **Coma scale, best verbal response, oriented**

● R40.23   **Coma scale, best motor response**

> The following appropriate 7th character is to be added to subcategory R40.23-:

0	unspecified time
1	in the field [EMT or ambulance]
2	at arrival to emergency department
3	at hospital admission
4	24 hours or more after hospital admission

Coding Clinic: 2015, Q2, P18

● R40.231   **Coma scale, best motor response, none**
● R40.232   **Coma scale, best motor response, extension**

Glasgow Coma Scale

Eye Opening Response	
• Spontaneous--open with blinking at baseline	4 points
• To verbal stimuli, command, speech	3 points
• To pain only (not applied to face)	2 points
• No response	1 point
Verbal Response	
• Oriented	5 points
• Confused conversation, but able to answer questions	4 points
• Inappropriate words	3 points
• Incomprehensible speech	2 points
• No response	1 point
Motor Response	
• Obeys commands for movement	6 points
• Purposeful movement to painful stimulus	5 points
• Withdraws in response to pain	4 points
• Flexion in response to pain (decorticate posturing)	3 points
• Extension response in response to pain (decerebrate posturing)	2 points
• No response	1 point
Categorization:	
Coma: No eye opening, no ability to follow commands, no word verbalizations (3-8)	
Head Injury Classification:	
Severe Head Injury--GCS score of 8 or less	
Moderate Head Injury--GCS score of 9 to 12	
Mild head injury--GCS score of 13 to 15	
(Adapted from: Advanced Trauma Life Support: Course for Physicians, American College of Surgeons, 1993). http://www.bt.cdc.gov/masscasualtires/gscale.asp	

Figure 18-1

● R40.233   **Coma scale, best motor response, abnormal**
● R40.234   **Coma scale, best motor response, flexion withdrawal**
● R40.235   **Coma scale, best motor response, localizes pain**
● R40.236   **Coma scale, best motor response, obeys commands**

● R40.24   **Glasgow coma scale, total score**

> Note: Assign a code from subcategory R40.24, when only the total coma score is documented ◄
> The following appropriate 7th character is to be added to subcategory R40.24-: ◄

0	unspecified time ◄
1	in the field [EMT or ambulance] ◄
2	at arrival to emergency department ◄
3	at hospital admission ◄
4	24 hours or more after hospital admission ◄

Coding Clinic: 2015, Q2, P18

● R40.241   **Glasgow coma scale score 13-15**
● R40.242   **Glasgow coma scale score 9-12**
● R40.243   **Glasgow coma scale score 3-8**
● R40.244   **Other coma, without documented Glasgow coma scale score, or with partial score reported**

R40.3   **Persistent vegetative state**

R40.4   **Transient alteration of awareness**

● R41   **Other symptoms and signs involving cognitive functions and awareness**

> **Excludes1**   dissociative [conversion] disorders (F44.-)
> mild cognitive impairment, so stated (G31.84)

R41.0   **Disorientation, unspecified**
> Confusion NOS   Delirium NOS

R41.1   **Anterograde amnesia**

R41.2   **Retrograde amnesia**

R41.3   **Other amnesia**
> Amnesia NOS
> Memory loss NOS
>
> **Excludes1**   amnestic disorder due to known physiologic condition (F04)
> amnestic syndrome due to psychoactive substance use (F10-F19 with 5th character .6)
> mild memory disturbance due to known physiological condition (F06.8)
> transient global amnesia (G45.4)

R41.4   **Neurologic neglect syndrome**
> Asomatognosia   Left-sided neglect
> Hemi-akinesia   Sensory neglect
> Hemi-inattention   Visuospatial neglect
> Hemispatial neglect
>
> **Excludes1**   visuospatial deficit (R41.842)

● R41.8   **Other symptoms and signs involving cognitive functions and awareness**

R41.81   **Age-related cognitive decline**   A
> Senility NOS

R41.82   **Altered mental status, unspecified**
> Change in mental status NOS
>
> **Excludes1**   altered level of consciousness (R40.-)
> altered mental status due to known condition - code to condition
> delirium NOS (R41.0)

Coding Clinic: 2012, Q4, P98

CHAPTER 18 (R00-R99)

CHAPTER 18 (R00-R99)

R41.83   **Borderline intellectual functioning**
IQ level 71 to 84
> **Excludes1**   intellectual disabilities (F70-F79)

● R41.84   **Other specified cognitive deficit**
> **Excludes1**   cognitive deficits as sequelae of cerebrovascular disease (I69.01-, I69.11-, I69.21-, I69.31-, I69.81-, I69.91-) ◀

R41.840   **Attention and concentration deficit**
> **Excludes1**   attention-deficit hyperactivity disorders (F90.-)

R41.841   **Cognitive communication deficit**
R41.842   **Visuospatial deficit**
R41.843   **Psychomotor deficit**
R41.844   **Frontal lobe and executive function deficit**

R41.89   **Other symptoms and signs involving cognitive functions and awareness**
Anosognosia

R41.9   **Unspecified symptoms and signs involving cognitive functions and awareness**

R42   **Dizziness and giddiness**
Light-headedness
Vertigo NOS
> **Excludes1**   vertiginous syndromes (H81.-)
> vertigo from infrasound (T75.23)

Coding Clinic: 2015, Q4, P40

● R43   **Disturbances of smell and taste**
R43.0   **Anosmia**
Absence of sense of smell; AKA anosphresia and olfactory anesthesia

R43.1   **Parosmia**
R43.2   **Parageusia**
Perversion of sense of taste or bad taste in mouth; AKA dysgeusia

R43.8   **Other disturbances of smell and taste**
Mixed disturbance of smell and taste

R43.9   **Unspecified disturbances of smell and taste**

● R44   **Other symptoms and signs involving general sensations and perceptions**
> **Excludes1**   alcoholic hallucinations (F1.5)
> hallucinations in drug psychosis (F11-F19 with .5)
> hallucinations in mood disorders with psychotic symptoms (F30.2, F31.5, F32.3, F33.3)
> hallucinations in schizophrenia, schizotypal and delusional disorders (F20-F29)
> **Excludes2**   disturbances of skin sensation (R20.-)

R44.0   **Auditory hallucinations**
R44.1   **Visual hallucinations**
R44.2   **Other hallucinations**
R44.3   **Hallucinations, unspecified**
R44.8   **Other symptoms and signs involving general sensations and perceptions**
R44.9   **Unspecified symptoms and signs involving general sensations and perceptions**

● R45   **Symptoms and signs involving emotional state**
R45.0   **Nervousness**
Nervous tension
R45.1   **Restlessness and agitation**
R45.2   **Unhappiness**
R45.3   **Demoralization and apathy**
> **Excludes1**   anhedonia (R45.84)
R45.4   **Irritability and anger**
R45.5   **Hostility**
R45.6   **Violent behavior**
R45.7   **State of emotional shock and stress, unspecified**

R45.8   **Other symptoms and signs involving emotional state**
R45.81   **Low self-esteem**
R45.82   **Worries**
R45.83   **Excessive crying of child, adolescent or adult**
> **Excludes1**   excessive crying of infant (baby) R68.11
R45.84   **Anhedonia**
Total loss of feeling of pleasure in pleasurable acts
● R45.85   **Homicidal and suicidal ideations**
> **Excludes1**   suicide attempt (T14.91)
R45.850   **Homicidal ideations**
R45.851   **Suicidal ideations**
R45.86   **Emotional lability**
R45.87   **Impulsiveness**
R45.89   **Other symptoms and signs involving emotional state**

● R46   **Symptoms and signs involving appearance and behavior**
> **Excludes1**   appearance and behavior in schizophrenia, schizotypal and delusional disorders (F20-F29)
> mental and behavioral disorders (F01-F99)

R46.0   **Very low level of personal hygiene**
R46.1   **Bizarre personal appearance**
R46.2   **Strange and inexplicable behavior**
R46.3   **Overactivity**
R46.4   **Slowness and poor responsiveness**
> **Excludes1**   stupor (R40.1)
R46.5   **Suspiciousness and marked evasiveness**
R46.6   **Undue concern and preoccupation with stressful events**
R46.7   **Verbosity and circumstantial detail obscuring reason for contact**
● R46.8   **Other symptoms and signs involving appearance and behavior**
R46.81   **Obsessive-compulsive behavior**
> **Excludes1**   obsessive-compulsive disorder (F42-) ◀▥
R46.89   **Other symptoms and signs involving appearance and behavior**

SYMPTOMS AND SIGNS INVOLVING SPEECH AND VOICE (R47-R49)

● R47   **Speech disturbances, not elsewhere classified**
> **Excludes1**   autism (F84.0)
> cluttering (F80.81)
> specific developmental disorders of speech and language (F80.-)
> stuttering (F80.81)
● R47.0   **Dysphasia and aphasia**
R47.01   **Aphasia**
> **Excludes1**   aphasia following cerebrovascular disease (I69. with final characters -20)
> progressive isolated aphasia (G31.01)

R47.02   **Dysphasia**
Impairment in comprehension of speech, caused by left-sided brain damage
> **Excludes1**   dysphasia following cerebrovascular disease (I69. with final characters -21)

◀ New   ◀▥ Revised   ~~deleted~~ Deleted   **Excludes 1**   **Excludes 2**   **Includes**   **Use additional**   **Code first**   **Code also**   **Unspecified**

OGCR Official Guidelines   X Assign placeholder X   ● Use Additional Character(s)   ▸ Manifestation Code   **Coding Clinic**

R47.1   **Dysarthria and anarthria**
Motor speech disorder

> **Excludes 1**   dysarthria following cerebrovascular disease (I69. with final characters -22)

● R47.8   **Other speech disturbances**

> **Excludes 1**   dysarthria following cerebrovascular disease (I69. with final characters -28)

    R47.81   **Slurred speech**

▌ R47.82   *Fluency disorder in conditions classified elsewhere*
       Stuttering in conditions classified elsewhere

> *Code first underlying disease or condition, such as:*
> Parkinson's disease (G20)

> **Excludes 1**   adult onset fluency disorder (F98.5)
> childhood onset fluency disorder (F80.81)
> fluency disorder (stuttering) following cerebrovascular disease (I69. with final characters -23)

    R47.89   **Other speech disturbances**

R47.9   **Unspecified speech disturbances**

● R48   **Dyslexia and other symbolic dysfunctions, not elsewhere classified**

> **Excludes 1**   specific developmental disorders of scholastic skills (F81.-)

R48.0   **Dyslexia and alexia**

R48.1   **Agnosia**
Loss of ability to recognize objects, persons, sounds, shapes, or smells
Astereognosia (astereognosis)
Autotopagnosia

> **Excludes 1**   visual object agnosia (R48.3)

R48.2   **Apraxia**
Loss of ability to execute or carry out learned purposeful movements

> **Excludes 1**   apraxia following cerebrovascular disease (I69. with final characters -90)

R48.3   **Visual agnosia**
Prosopagnosia
Simultanagnosia (asimultagnosia)

R48.8   **Other symbolic dysfunctions**
Acalculia
Difficulty performing simple mathematical tasks resulting from neurological injury
Agraphia

R48.9   **Unspecified symbolic dysfunctions**

● R49   **Voice and resonance disorders**

> **Excludes 1**   psychogenic voice and resonance disorders (F44.4)

R49.0   **Dysphonia**
Hoarseness

R49.1   **Aphonia**
Loss of voice

● R49.2   **Hypernasality and hyponasality**

    R49.21   **Hypernasality**

    R49.22   **Hyponasality**

R49.8   **Other voice and resonance disorders**

R49.9   **Unspecified voice and resonance disorder**
Change in voice NOS
Resonance disorder NOS

GENERAL SYMPTOMS AND SIGNS (R50-R69)

● R50   **Fever of other and unknown origin**

> **Excludes 1**   chills without fever (R68.83)
> febrile convulsions (R56.0-)
> fever of unknown origin during labor (O75.2)
> fever of unknown origin in newborn (P81.9)
> hypothermia due to illness (R68.0)
> malignant hyperthermia due to anesthesia (T88.3)
> puerperal pyrexia NOS (O86.4)

R50.2   **Drug induced fever**
Use additional code for adverse effect, if applicable, to identify drug (T36-T50 with fifth or sixth character 5)

> **Excludes 1**   postvaccination (postimmunization) fever (R50.83)

● R50.8   **Other specified fever**

▌ R50.81   *Fever presenting with conditions classified elsewhere*

> *Code first underlying condition when associated fever is present, such as with:*
> leukemia (C91-C95)
> neutropenia (D70.-)
> sickle-cell disease (D57.-)

    R50.82   **Postprocedural fever**

> **Excludes 1**   postprocedural infection (T81.4-) ◀▦
> posttransfusion fever (R50.84)
> postvaccination (postimmunization) fever (R50.83)

    R50.83   **Postvaccination fever**
Postimmunization fever

    R50.84   **Febrile nonhemolytic transfusion reaction**
FNHTR
Posttransfusion fever

R50.9   **Fever, unspecified**
Fever NOS
Fever of unknown origin [FUO]
Fever with chills
Fever with rigors
Hyperpyrexia NOS
Persistent fever
Pyrexia NOS

R51   **Headache**
Facial pain NOS

> **Excludes 1**   atypical face pain (G50.1)
> migraine and other headache syndromes (G43-G44)
> trigeminal neuralgia (G50.0)

R52   **Pain, unspecified**
Acute pain NOS   Pain NOS
Generalized pain NOS

> **Excludes 1**   acute and chronic pain, not elsewhere classified (G89.-)
> localized pain, unspecified type - code to pain by site, such as:
> abdomen pain (R10.-)
> back pain (M54.9)
> breast pain (N64.4)
> chest pain (R07.1-R07.9)
> ear pain (H92.0-)
> eye pain (H57.1)
> headache (R51)
> joint pain (M25.5-)
> limb pain (M79.6-)
> lumbar region pain (M54.5)
> pelvic and perineal pain (R10.2)
> shoulder pain (M25.51-)
> spine pain (M54.-)
> throat pain (R07.0)
> tongue pain (K14.6)
> tooth pain (K08.8)
> renal colic (N23)
> pain disorders exclusively related to psychological factors (F45.41)

CHAPTER 18 (R00-R99)

● **R53   Malaise and fatigue**

    R53.0   Neoplastic (malignant) related fatigue
            Code first associated neoplasm

    R53.1   Weakness
            Asthenia NOS

            Excludes1   age-related weakness (R54)
                       muscle weakness (M62.8-)
                       sarcopenia (M62.84) ◀
                       senile asthenia (R54)

    R53.2   Functional quadriplegia
            Complete immobility due to severe physical disability
                or frailty

            Excludes1   frailty NOS (R54)
                       hysterical paralysis (F44.4)
                       immobility syndrome (M62.3)
                       neurologic quadriplegia (G82.5-)
                       quadriplegia (G82.50)

        Coding Clinic: 2016, Q2, P6

●   **R53.8   Other malaise and fatigue**

            Excludes1   combat exhaustion and fatigue (F43.0)
                       congenital debility (P96.9)
                       exhaustion and fatigue due to depressive
                           episode (F32.-)
                       exhaustion and fatigue due to excessive
                           exertion (T73.3)
                       exhaustion and fatigue due to exposure
                           (T73.2)
                       exhaustion and fatigue due to heat (T67.-)
                       exhaustion and fatigue due to pregnancy
                         (O26.8-)
                       exhaustion and fatigue due to recurrent
                         depressive episode (F33)
                       exhaustion and fatigue due to senile
                         debility (R54)

        R53.81   Other malaise
            Chronic debility
            Debility NOS
            General physical deterioration
            Malaise NOS
            Nervous debility

            Excludes1   age-related physical debility
                         (R54)

        R53.82   Chronic fatigue, unspecified
            Chronic fatigue syndrome NOS

            Excludes1   postviral fatigue syndrome
                       (G93.3)

        R53.83   Other fatigue
            Fatigue NOS   Lethargy
            Lack of energy   Tiredness

R54   Age-related physical debility
    Frailty   Senile asthenia
    Old age   Senile debility
    Senescence

    Excludes1   age-related cognitive decline (R41.81)
                 sarcopenia (M62.84) ◀
                 senile psychosis (F03)
                 senility NOS (R41.81)

R55   Syncope and collapse
    Blackout
    Fainting
    Vasovagal attack

    Excludes1   cardiogenic shock (R57.0)
                 carotid sinus syncope (G90.01)
                 heat syncope (T67.1)
                 neurocirculatory asthenia (F45.8)
                 neurogenic orthostatic hypotension (G90.3)
                 orthostatic hypotension (I95.1)
                 postprocedural shock (T81.1-)
                 psychogenic syncope (F48.8)
                 shock NOS (R57.9)
                 shock complicating or following abortion or
                     ectopic or molar pregnancy (O00-O07, O08.3)
                 shock complicating or following labor and
                     delivery (O75.1)
                 Stokes-Adams attack (I45.9)
                 unconsciousness NOS (R40.2-)

● **R56   Convulsions, not elsewhere classified**

    Excludes1   dissociative convulsions and seizures (F44.5)
                 epileptic convulsions and seizures (G40.-)
                 newborn convulsions and seizures (P90)

●   **R56.0   Febrile convulsions**

        R56.00   Simple febrile convulsions
            Febrile convulsion NOS
            Febrile seizure NOS

        R56.01   Complex febrile convulsions
            Atypical febrile seizure
            Complex febrile seizure
            Complicated febrile seizure

            Excludes1   status epilepticus (G40.901)

    R56.1   Post traumatic seizures

        Excludes1   post traumatic epilepsy (G40.-)

    R56.9   Unspecified convulsions
        Convulsion disorder   Recurrent convulsions
        Fit NOS   Seizure(s) (convulsive) NOS

● **R57   Shock, not elsewhere classified**

    Excludes1   anaphylactic shock NOS (T78.2)
                 anaphylactic reaction or shock due to adverse
                     food reaction (T78.0-)
                 anaphylactic shock due to adverse effect of
                     correct drug or medicament properly
                     administered (T88.6)
                 anaphylactic shock due to serum (T80.5-)
                 anesthetic shock (T88.3)
                 electric shock (T75.4)
                 obstetric shock (O75.1)
                 postprocedural shock (T81.1-)
                 psychic shock (F43.0)
                 septic shock (R65.21)
                 shock complicating or following ectopic or molar
                     pregnancy (O00-O07, O08.3)
                 shock due to lightning (T75.01)
                 traumatic shock (T79.4)
                 toxic shock syndrome (A48.3)

    R57.0   Cardiogenic shock

    R57.1   Hypovolemic shock
            Decreased blood volume (loss)

    R57.8   Other shock

    R57.9   Shock, unspecified
        Failure of peripheral circulation NOS
        Resulting in significant blood pressure drop

A

◀ New   ◀▪▪ Revised   ~~deleted~~ Deleted   **Excludes 1**   **Excludes 2**   **Includes**   **Use additional**   **Code first**   **Code also**   **Unspecified**

OGCR Official Guidelines   X Assign placeholder X   ● Use Additional Character(s)   ▸ Manifestation Code   **Coding Clinic**

R58   Hemorrhage, not elsewhere classified
Hemorrhage NOS

> **Excludes1**   hemorrhage included with underlying
> conditions, such as:
> acute duodenal ulcer with hemorrhage (K26.0)
> acute gastritis with bleeding (K29.01)
> ulcerative enterocolitis with rectal bleeding
> (K51.01)

● **R59   Enlarged lymph nodes**

> **Includes**   swollen glands
>
> **Excludes1**   lymphadenitis NOS (I88.9)
> acute lymphadenitis (L04.-)
> chronic lymphadenitis (I88.1)
> mesenteric (acute) (chronic) lymphadenitis (I88.0)

R59.0   Localized enlarged lymph nodes

R59.1   Generalized enlarged lymph nodes
Lymphadenopathy NOS

R59.9   Enlarged lymph nodes, unspecified

● **R60   Edema, not elsewhere classified**

> **Excludes1**   angioneurotic edema (T78.3)
> ascites (R18.-)
> cerebral edema (G93.6)
> cerebral edema due to birth injury (P11.0)
> edema of larynx (J38.4)
> edema of nasopharynx (J39.2)
> edema of pharynx (J39.2)
> gestational edema (O12.0-)
> hereditary edema (Q82.0)
> hydrops fetalis NOS (P83.2)
> hydrothorax (J94.8)
> nutritional edema (E40-E46)
> hydrops fetalis NOS (P83.2)
> newborn edema (P83.3)
> pulmonary edema (J81.-)

R60.0   Localized edema

R60.1   Generalized edema

R60.9   Edema, unspecified
Fluid retention NOS

R61   Generalized hyperhidrosis
Excessive sweating
Night sweats
Secondary hyperhidrosis

> *Code first, if applicable, menopausal and female climacteric states
> (N95.1)*
>
> **Excludes1**   focal (primary) (secondary) hyperhidrosis (L74.5-)
> Frey's syndrome (L74.52)
> localized (primary) (secondary) hyperhidrosis
> (L74.5-)

● **R62   Lack of expected normal physiological development in
childhood and adults**

> **Excludes1**   delayed puberty (E30.0)
> gonadal dysgenesis (Q99.1)
> hypopituitarism (E23.0)

R62.0   Delayed milestone in childhood   P
Delayed attainment of expected physiological
developmental stage
Late talker
Late walker

● **R62.5   Other and unspecified lack of expected normal
physiological development in childhood**

> **Excludes1**   HIV disease resulting in failure to thrive
> (B20)
> physical retardation due to malnutrition
> (E45)

**R62.50   Unspecified lack of expected normal
physiological development in childhood**
Infantilism NOS

R62.51   Failure to thrive (child)   P
Failure to gain weight

> **Excludes1**   failure to thrive in child under 28
> days old (P92.6)

R62.52   Short stature (child)
Lack of growth   Short stature NOS
Physical retardation

> **Excludes1**   short stature due to endocrine
> disorder (E34.3)

**R62.59   Other lack of expected normal physiological
development in childhood**

R62.7   Adult failure to thrive   A

● **R63   Symptoms and signs concerning food and fluid intake**

> **Excludes1**   bulimia NOS (F50.2)
> eating disorders of nonorganic origin (F50.-)
> malnutrition (E40-E46)

R63.0   Anorexia
Loss of appetite

> **Excludes1**   anorexia nervosa (F50.0-)
> loss of appetite of nonorganic origin
> (F50.89) ◀

R63.1   Polydipsia
Excessive thirst

R63.2   Polyphagia
Excessive eating   Hyperalimentation NOS

R63.3   Feeding difficulties
Feeding problem (elderly) (infant) NOS

> **Excludes1**   feeding problems of newborn (P92.-)
> infant feeding disorder of nonorganic
> origin (F98.2-)

R63.4   Abnormal weight loss

R63.5   Abnormal weight gain

> **Excludes1**   excessive weight gain in pregnancy
> (O26.0-)
> obesity (E66.-)

R63.6   Underweight

> Use additional code to identify body mass index (BMI),
> if known (Z68.-)
>
> **Excludes1**   abnormal weight loss (R63.4)
> anorexia nervosa (F50.0-)
> malnutrition (E40-E46)

**R63.8   Other symptoms and signs concerning food and fluid
intake**

R64   Cachexia
Wasting syndrome

> *Code first underlying condition, if known*
>
> **Excludes1**   abnormal weight loss (R63.4)
> nutritional marasmus (E41)

CHAPTER 18 (R00-R99)

OGCR Section I.C.18.g.

SIRS due to Non-Infectious Process

The systemic inflammatory response syndrome (SIRS) can develop as a result of certain non-infectious disease processes, such as trauma, malignant neoplasm, or pancreatitis. When SIRS is documented with a noninfectious condition, and no subsequent infection is documented, the code for the underlying condition, such as an injury, should be assigned, followed by code R65.10. Systemic inflammatory response syndrome (SIRS) of non-infectious origin without acute organ dysfunction, or code R65.11, Systemic inflammatory response syndrome (SIRS) of non-infectious origin with acute organ dysfunction. If an associated acute organ dysfunction is documented, the appropriate code(s) for the specific type of organ dysfunction(s) should be assigned in addition to code R65.11. If acute organ dysfunction is documented, but it cannot be determined if the acute organ dysfunction is associated with SIRS or due to another condition (e.g., directly due to the trauma), the provider should be queried.

● R65   **Symptoms and signs specifically associated with systemic inflammation and infection**

   ● R65.1   **Systemic inflammatory response syndrome (SIRS) of non-infectious origin**

     Code first underlying condition, such as:
     heatstroke (T67.0)
     injury and trauma (S00-T88)

     Excludes1   sepsis - code to infection
         severe sepsis (R65.2)

     R65.10   **Systemic inflammatory response syndrome (SIRS) of non-infectious origin without acute organ dysfunction**
       Systemic inflammatory response syndrome (SIRS) NOS

     R65.11   **Systemic inflammatory response syndrome (SIRS) of non-infectious origin with acute organ dysfunction**
       Use additional code to identify specific acute organ dysfunction, such as:
       acute kidney failure (N17.-)
       acute respiratory failure (J96.0-)
       critical illness myopathy (G72.81)
       critical illness polyneuropathy (G62.81)
       disseminated intravascular coagulopathy [DIC] (D65)
       encephalopathy (metabolic) (septic) (G93.41)
       hepatic failure (K72.0-)

   ● R65.2   **Severe sepsis**
     Infection with associated acute organ dysfunction
     Sepsis with acute organ dysfunction
     Sepsis with multiple organ dysfunction
     Systemic inflammatory response syndrome due to infectious process with acute organ dysfunction

     Code first underlying infection, such as:
     infection following a procedure (T81.4-)
     infections following infusion, transfusion and therapeutic injection (T80.2-)
     puerperal sepsis (O85)
     sepsis following complete or unspecified spontaneous abortion (O03.87)
     sepsis following ectopic and molar pregnancy (O08.82)
     sepsis following incomplete spontaneous abortion (O03.37)
     sepsis following (induced) termination of pregnancy (O04.87)
     sepsis NOS (A41.9)
     Use additional code to identify specific acute organ dysfunction, such as:
     acute kidney failure (N17.-)
     acute respiratory failure (J96.0-)
     critical illness myopathy (G72.81)
     critical illness polyneuropathy (G62.81)
     disseminated intravascular coagulopathy [DIC] (D65)
     encephalopathy (metabolic) (septic) (G93.41)
     hepatic failure (K72.0-)

     R65.20   **Severe sepsis without septic shock**
       Severe sepsis NOS

     R65.21   **Severe sepsis with septic shock**

● R68   **Other general symptoms and signs**

   R68.0   **Hypothermia, not associated with low environmental temperature**
     Excludes1   hypothermia NOS (accidental) (T68)
       hypothermia due to anesthesia (T88.51)
       hypothermia due to low environmental temperature (T68)
       newborn hypothermia (P80.-)

   ● R68.1   **Nonspecific symptoms peculiar to infancy**
     Excludes1   colic, infantile (R10.83)
       neonatal cerebral irritability (P91.3)
       teething syndrome (K00.7)

     R68.11   **Excessive crying of infant (baby)**   P
       Excludes1   excessive crying of child, adolescent, or adult (R45.83)

     R68.12   **Fussy infant (baby)**   P
       Irritable infant

     R68.13   **Apparent life threatening event in infant (ALTE)**   P
       Apparent life threatening event in newborn
       Code first confirmed diagnosis, if known
       Use additional code(s) for associated signs and symptoms if no confirmed diagnosis established, or if signs and symptoms are not associated routinely with confirmed diagnosis, or provide additional information for cause of ALTE

     R68.19   **Other nonspecific symptoms peculiar to infancy**   P

   R68.2   **Dry mouth, unspecified**
     Excludes1   dry mouth due to dehydration (E86.0)
       dry mouth due to sicca syndrome [Sjögren] (M35.0-)
       salivary gland hyposecretion (K11.7)

   R68.3   **Clubbing of fingers**
     Clubbing of nails
     Excludes1   congenital clubfinger (Q68.1)

   ● R68.8   **Other general symptoms and signs**
     R68.81   **Early satiety**
     R68.82   **Decreased libido**   A
       Decreased sexual desire
     R68.83   **Chills (without fever)**
       Chills NOS
       Excludes1   chills with fever (R50.9)
     R68.84   **Jaw pain**
       Mandibular pain
       Maxilla pain
       Excludes1   temporomandibular joint arthralgia (M26.62-)
     R68.89   **Other general symptoms and signs**

R69   **Illness, unspecified**
   Unknown and unspecified cases of morbidity

ABNORMAL FINDINGS ON EXAMINATION OF BLOOD, WITHOUT DIAGNOSIS (R70-R79)

   Excludes2   abnormal findings on antenatal screening of mother (O28.-)
     abnormalities of lipids (E78.-)
     abnormalities of platelets and thrombocytes (D69.-)
     abnormalities of white blood cells classified elsewhere (D70-D72)
     coagulation hemorrhagic disorders (D65-D68)
     diagnostic abnormal findings classified elsewhere —*see* Alphabetical Index
     hemorrhagic and hematological disorders of newborn (P50-P61)

● R70   **Elevated erythrocyte sedimentation rate and abnormality of plasma viscosity**
   R70.0   **Elevated erythrocyte sedimentation rate**
   R70.1   **Abnormal plasma viscosity**

● **R71**   **Abnormality of red blood cells**
> **Excludes1**   anemias (D50-D64)
> anemia of premature infant (P61.2)
> benign (familial) polycythemia (D75.0)
> congenital anemias (P61.2-P61.4)
> newborn anemia due to isoimmunization (P55.-)
> polycythemia neonatorum (P61.1)
> polycythemia NOS (D75.1)
> polycythemia vera (D45)
> secondary polycythemia (D75.1)

    R71.0   **Precipitous drop in hematocrit**
        Drop (precipitous) in hemoglobin
        Drop in hematocrit
          Blood volume that is red blood cells

    R71.8   **Other abnormality of red blood cells**
        Abnormal red-cell morphology NOS
        Abnormal red-cell volume NOS
        Anisocytosis
          Red blood cells of unequal size
        Poikilocytosis
          Red blood cells of abnormal shape

● **R73**   **Elevated blood glucose level**
> **Excludes1**   diabetes mellitus (E08-E13)
> diabetes mellitus in pregnancy, childbirth and the puerperium (O24.-)
> neonatal disorders (P70.0-P70.2)
> postsurgical hypoinsulinemia (E89.1)

  ● **R73.0**   **Abnormal glucose**
> **Excludes1**   abnormal glucose in pregnancy (O99.81-)
> diabetes mellitus (E08-E13)
> dysmetabolic syndrome X (E88.81)
> gestational diabetes (O24.4-)
> glycosuria (R81)
> hypoglycemia (E16.2)

    R73.01   **Impaired fasting glucose**
         Elevated fasting glucose

    R73.02   **Impaired glucose tolerance (oral)**
         Elevated glucose tolerance

    R73.03   **Prediabetes** ◀
         Latent diabetes ◀

    R73.09   **Other abnormal glucose**
         Abnormal glucose NOS
         Abnormal non-fasting glucose tolerance
         ~~Prediabetes~~

    R73.9   **Hyperglycemia, unspecified**

● **R74**   **Abnormal serum enzyme levels**
    R74.0   **Nonspecific elevation of levels of transaminase and lactic acid dehydrogenase [LDH]**

    R74.8   **Abnormal levels of other serum enzymes**
        Abnormal level of acid phosphatase
        Abnormal level of alkaline phosphatase
        Abnormal level of amylase
        Abnormal level of lipase [triacylglycerol lipase]

    R74.9   **Abnormal serum enzyme level, unspecified**

> **OGCR**   Section I.C.1.2.e and f.
>
> Patients with inconclusive HIV serology
> e. Patients with inconclusive HIV serology, but no definitive diagnosis or manifestations of the illness, may be assigned code R75, Inconclusive laboratory evidence of human immunodeficiency virus [HIV].
> f. Previously diagnosed HIV-related illness
> Patients with any known prior diagnosis of an HIV-related illness should be coded to B20. Once a patient has developed an HIV-related illness, the patient should always be assigned code B20 on every subsequent admission/encounter. Patients previously diagnosed with any HIV illness (B20) should never be assigned to R75 or Z21, Asymptomatic human immunodeficiency virus [HIV] infection status.

  R75   **Inconclusive laboratory evidence of human immunodeficiency virus [HIV]**
        Nonconclusive HIV-test finding in infants
> **Excludes1**   asymptomatic human immunodeficiency virus [HIV] infection status (Z21)
> human immunodeficiency virus [HIV] disease (B20)

● **R76**   **Other abnormal immunological findings in serum**
    R76.0   **Raised antibody titer**
> **Excludes1**   isoimmunization in pregnancy (O36.0-O36.1)
> isoimmunization affecting newborn (P55.-)

  ● **R76.1**   **Nonspecific reaction to test for tuberculosis**
    R76.11   **Nonspecific reaction to tuberculin skin test without active tuberculosis**
        Abnormal result of Mantoux test
        PPD positive
        Tuberculin (skin test) positive
        Tuberculin (skin test) reactor
>   **Excludes1**   nonspecific reaction to cell mediated immunity measurement of gamma interferon antigen response without active tuberculosis (R76.12)

    R76.12   **Nonspecific reaction to cell mediated immunity measurement of gamma interferon antigen response without active tuberculosis**
        Nonspecific reaction to QuantiFERON-TB test (QFT) without active tuberculosis
>   **Excludes1**   nonspecific reaction to tuberculin skin test without active tuberculosis (R76.11)
> positive tuberculin skin test (R76.11)

    R76.8   **Other specified abnormal immunological findings in serum**
        Raised level of immunoglobulins NOS

    R76.9   **Abnormal immunological finding in serum, unspecified**

● **R77**   **Other abnormalities of plasma proteins**
> **Excludes1**   disorders of plasma-protein metabolism (E88.0)

    R77.0   **Abnormality of albumin**

    R77.1   **Abnormality of globulin**
        Hyperglobulinemia NOS

    R77.2   **Abnormality of alphafetoprotein**

    R77.8   **Other specified abnormalities of plasma proteins**

    R77.9   **Abnormality of plasma protein, unspecified**

CHAPTER 18 (R00-R99)

● **R78**   **Findings of drugs and other substances, not normally found in blood**

Use additional code to identify any retained foreign body, if applicable (Z18.-)

Excludes1   mental or behavioral disorders due to psychoactive substance use (F10-F19)

R78.0   **Finding of alcohol in blood**

Use additional external cause code (Y90.-), for detail regarding alcohol level.

R78.1   **Finding of opiate drug in blood**

R78.2   **Finding of cocaine in blood**

R78.3   **Finding of hallucinogen in blood**

R78.4   **Finding of other drugs of addictive potential in blood**

R78.5   **Finding of other psychotropic drug in blood**

R78.6   **Finding of steroid agent in blood**

● **R78.7**   **Finding of abnormal level of heavy metals in blood**

   R78.71   **Abnormal lead level in blood**

     Excludes1   lead poisoning (T56.0-)

   R78.79   **Finding of abnormal level of heavy metals in blood**

● **R78.8**   **Finding of other specified substances, not normally found in blood**

   R78.81   **Bacteremia**

     Blood poisoning/bacteremia

     Excludes1   sepsis-code to specified infection ◀▥

   R78.89   **Finding of other specified substances, not normally found in blood**

     Finding of abnormal level of lithium in blood

R78.9   **Finding of unspecified substance, not normally found in blood**

● **R79**   **Other abnormal findings of blood chemistry**

Use additional code to identify any retained foreign body, if applicable (Z18.-)

Excludes1   abnormality of fluid, electrolyte or acid-base balance (E86-E87)
asymptomatic hyperuricemia (E79.0)
hyperglycemia NOS (R73.9)
hypoglycemia NOS (E16.2)
neonatal hypoglycemia (P70.3-P70.4)
specific findings indicating disorder of amino-acid metabolism (E70-E72)
specific findings indicating disorder of carbohydrate metabolism (E73-E74)
specific findings indicating disorder of lipid metabolism (E75.-)

R79.0   **Abnormal level of blood mineral**

Abnormal blood level of cobalt
Abnormal blood level of copper
Abnormal blood level of iron
Abnormal blood level of magnesium
Abnormal blood level of mineral NEC
Abnormal blood level of zinc

   Excludes1   abnormal level of lithium (R78.89)
disorders of mineral metabolism (E83.-)
neonatal hypomagnesemia (P71.2)
nutritional mineral deficiency (E58-E61)

R79.1   **Abnormal coagulation profile**

Abnormal or prolonged bleeding time
Abnormal or prolonged coagulation time
Abnormal or prolonged partial thromboplastin time [PTT]
Abnormal or prolonged prothrombin time [PT]

   Excludes1   coagulation defects (D68.-)

● **R79.8**   **Other specified abnormal findings of blood chemistry**

   R79.81   **Abnormal blood-gas level**

   R79.82   **Elevated C-reactive protein (CRP)**

   R79.89   **Other specified abnormal findings of blood chemistry**

R79.9   **Abnormal finding of blood chemistry, unspecified**

ABNORMAL FINDINGS ON EXAMINATION OF URINE, WITHOUT DIAGNOSIS (R80-R82)

Excludes1   abnormal findings on antenatal screening of mother (O28.-)
diagnostic abnormal findings classified elsewhere - see Alphabetical Index
specific findings indicating disorder of amino-acid metabolism (E70-E72)
specific findings indicating disorder of carbohydrate metabolism (E73-E74)

● **R80**   **Proteinuria**

Excludes1   gestational proteinuria (O12.1-)

R80.0   **Isolated proteinuria**

Idiopathic proteinuria

   Excludes1   isolated proteinuria with specific morphological lesion (N06.-)

R80.1   **Persistent proteinuria, unspecified**

R80.2   **Orthostatic proteinuria, unspecified**

Postural proteinuria

R80.3   **Bence Jones proteinuria**

R80.8   **Other proteinuria**

R80.9   **Proteinuria, unspecified**

Albuminuria NOS

R81   **Glycosuria**

Excludes1   renal glycosuria (E74.8)

● **R82**   **Other and unspecified abnormal findings in urine**

Includes   chromoabnormalities in urine

Use additional code to identify any retained foreign body, if applicable (Z18.-)

Excludes2   hematuria (R31.-)

R82.0   **Chyluria**

White milky urine

   Excludes1   filarial chyluria (B74.-)

R82.1   **Myoglobinuria**

Presence of myoglobin (iron containing protein) in urine

R82.2   **Biliuria**

Presence of bile pigments/salts in urine

R82.3   **Hemoglobinuria**

Presence of hemoglobin in urine

   Excludes1   hemoglobinuria due to hemolysis from external causes NEC (D59.6)
hemoglobinuria due to paroxysmal nocturnal [Marchiafava-Micheli] (D59.5)

R82.4   **Acetonuria**

Ketonuria

R82.5   **Elevated urine levels of drugs, medicaments and biological substances**

Elevated urine levels of catecholamines
Elevated urine levels of indoleacetic acid
Elevated urine levels of 17-ketosteroids
Elevated urine levels of steroids

R82.6   **Abnormal urine levels of substances chiefly nonmedicinal as to source**

Abnormal urine level of heavy metals

● **R82.7**   **Abnormal findings on microbiological examination of urine**

   Excludes1   colonization status (Z22.-)

   R82.71   **Bacteriuria** ◀

   R82.79   **Other abnormal findings on microbiological examination of urine** ◀

     Positive culture findings of urine ◀

R82.8   **Abnormal findings on cytological and histological examination of urine**

◀ New   ◀▥ Revised   ~~deleted~~ Deleted   Excludes 1   Excludes 2   Includes   Use additional   Code first   Code also   Unspecified

OGCR Official Guidelines   X Assign placeholder X   ● Use Additional Character(s)   ▶ Manifestation Code   **Coding Clinic**

● R82.9   **Other and unspecified abnormal findings in urine**

    R82.90   Unspecified **abnormal findings in urine**

    R82.91   **Other chromoabnormalities of urine**
          Chromoconversion (dipstick)
          Idiopathic dipstick converts positive for blood
            with no cellular forms in sediment

       Excludes1   hemoglobinuria (R82.3)
                  myoglobinuria (R82.1)

    R82.99   **Other abnormal findings in urine**
          Cells and casts in urine
          Crystalluria
          Melanuria

ABNORMAL FINDINGS ON EXAMINATION OF OTHER BODY FLUIDS, SUBSTANCES AND TISSUES, WITHOUT DIAGNOSIS (R83-R89)

   Excludes1   abnormal findings on antenatal screening of
            mother (O28.-)
           diagnostic abnormal findings classified elsewhere
            - see Alphabetical Index

   Excludes2   abnormal findings on examination of blood,
            without diagnosis (R70-R79)
           abnormal findings on examination of urine,
            without diagnosis (R80-R82)
           abnormal tumor markers (R97.-)

● R83   **Abnormal findings in cerebrospinal fluid**

    R83.0   **Abnormal level of enzymes in cerebrospinal fluid**

    R83.1   **Abnormal level of hormones in cerebrospinal fluid**

    R83.2   **Abnormal level of other drugs, medicaments and biological substances in cerebrospinal fluid**

    R83.3   **Abnormal level of substances chiefly nonmedicinal as to source in cerebrospinal fluid**

    R83.4   **Abnormal immunological findings in cerebrospinal fluid**

    R83.5   **Abnormal microbiological findings in cerebrospinal fluid**
          Positive culture findings in cerebrospinal fluid

       Excludes1   colonization status (Z22.-)

    R83.6   **Abnormal cytological findings in cerebrospinal fluid**

    R83.8   **Other abnormal findings in cerebrospinal fluid**
          Abnormal chromosomal findings in cerebrospinal fluid

    R83.9   Unspecified **abnormal finding in cerebrospinal fluid**

● R84   **Abnormal findings in specimens from respiratory organs and thorax**

    Includes   abnormal findings in bronchial washings
          abnormal findings in nasal secretions
          abnormal findings in pleural fluid
          abnormal findings in sputum
          abnormal findings in throat scrapings

    Excludes1   blood-stained sputum (R04.2)

    R84.0   **Abnormal level of enzymes in specimens from respiratory organs and thorax**

    R84.1   **Abnormal level of hormones in specimens from respiratory organs and thorax**

    R84.2   **Abnormal level of other drugs, medicaments and biological substances in specimens from respiratory organs and thorax**

    R84.3   **Abnormal level of substances chiefly nonmedicinal as to source in specimens from respiratory organs and thorax**

    R84.4   **Abnormal immunological findings in specimens from respiratory organs and thorax**

    R84.5   **Abnormal microbiological findings in specimens from respiratory organs and thorax**
          Positive culture findings in specimens from respiratory organs and thorax

       Excludes1   colonization status (Z22.-)

    R84.6   **Abnormal cytological findings in specimens from respiratory organs and thorax**

    R84.7   **Abnormal histological findings in specimens from respiratory organs and thorax**

    R84.8   **Other abnormal findings in specimens from respiratory organs and thorax**
          Abnormal chromosomal findings in specimens from respiratory organs and thorax

    R84.9   Unspecified **abnormal finding in specimens from respiratory organs and thorax**

● R85   **Abnormal findings in specimens from digestive organs and abdominal cavity**

    Includes   abnormal findings in peritoneal fluid
          abnormal findings in saliva

    Excludes1   cloudy peritoneal dialysis effluent (R88.0)
          fecal abnormalities (R19.5)

    R85.0   **Abnormal level of enzymes in specimens from digestive organs and abdominal cavity**

    R85.1   **Abnormal level of hormones in specimens from digestive organs and abdominal cavity**

    R85.2   **Abnormal level of other drugs, medicaments and biological substances in specimens from digestive organs and abdominal cavity**

    R85.3   **Abnormal level of substances chiefly nonmedicinal as to source in specimens from digestive organs and abdominal cavity**

    R85.4   **Abnormal immunological findings in specimens from digestive organs and abdominal cavity**

    R85.5   **Abnormal microbiological findings in specimens from digestive organs and abdominal cavity**
          Positive culture findings in specimens from digestive organs and abdominal cavity

       Excludes1   colonization status (Z22.-)

● R85.6   **Abnormal cytological findings in specimens from digestive organs and abdominal cavity**

   ● R85.61   **Abnormal cytologic smear of anus**

       Excludes1   abnormal cytological findings
                in specimens from other
                digestive organs and
                abdominal cavity (R85.69)
             carcinoma in situ of anus
                (histologically confirmed)
                (D01.3)
             anal intraepithelial neoplasia I
                [AIN I] (K62.82)
             anal intraepithelial neoplasia II
                [AIN II] (K62.82)
             anal intraepithelial neoplasia III
                [AIN III] (D01.3)
             dysplasia (mild) (moderate)
                of anus (histologically
                confirmed) (K62.82)
             severe dysplasia of anus
                (histologically confirmed)
                (D01.3)

       Excludes2   anal high risk human
                papillomavirus (HPV) DNA
                test positive (R85.81)
             anal low risk human
                papillomavirus (HPV) DNA
                test positive (R85.82)

      R85.610   **Atypical squamous cells of undetermined significance on cytologic smear of anus (ASC-US)**

      R85.611   **Atypical squamous cells cannot exclude high grade squamous intraepithelial lesion on cytologic smear of anus (ASC-H)**

      R85.612   **Low grade squamous intraepithelial lesion on cytologic smear of anus (LGSIL)**

      R85.613   **High grade squamous intraepithelial lesion on cytologic smear of anus (HGSIL)**

      R85.614   **Cytologic evidence of malignancy on smear of anus**

R85.615 Unsatisfactory cytologic smear of anus
> Inadequate sample of cytologic smear of anus

R85.616 Satisfactory anal smear but lacking transformation zone

R85.618 Other abnormal cytological findings on specimens from anus

R85.619 Unspecified abnormal cytological findings in specimens from anus
> Abnormal anal cytology NOS
> Atypical glandular cells of anus NOS

R85.69 Abnormal cytological findings in specimens from other digestive organs and abdominal cavity

R85.7 Abnormal histological findings in specimens from digestive organs and abdominal cavity

● **R85.8 Other abnormal findings in specimens from digestive organs and abdominal cavity**

R85.81 Anal high risk human papillomavirus (HPV) DNA test positive
> **Excludes1** anogenital warts due to human papillomavirus (HPV) (A63.0)
> condyloma acuminatum (A63.0)

R85.82 Anal low risk human papillomavirus (HPV) DNA test positive
> Use additional code for associated human papillomavirus (B97.7)

R85.89 Other abnormal findings in specimens from digestive organs and abdominal cavity
> Abnormal chromosomal findings in specimens from digestive organs and abdominal cavity

R85.9 Unspecified abnormal finding in specimens from digestive organs and abdominal cavity

● **R86 Abnormal findings in specimens from male genital organs**
> **Includes** abnormal findings in prostatic secretions
> abnormal findings in semen, seminal fluid
> abnormal spermatozoa
> **Excludes1** azoospermia (N46.0-)
> oligospermia (N46.1-)

R86.0 Abnormal level of enzymes in specimens from male genital organs ♂

R86.1 Abnormal level of hormones in specimens from male genital organs ♂

R86.2 Abnormal level of other drugs, medicaments and biological substances in specimens from male genital organs ♂

R86.3 Abnormal level of substances chiefly nonmedicinal as to source in specimens from male genital organs ♂

R86.4 Abnormal immunological findings in specimens from male genital organs ♂

R86.5 Abnormal microbiological findings in specimens from male genital organs ♂
> Positive culture findings in specimens from male genital organs
> **Excludes1** colonization status (Z22.-)

R86.6 Abnormal cytological findings in specimens from male genital organs ♂

R86.7 Abnormal histological findings in specimens from male genital organs ♂

R86.8 Other abnormal findings in specimens from male genital organs ♂
> Abnormal chromosomal findings in specimens from male genital organs

R86.9 Unspecified abnormal finding in specimens from male genital organs ♂

● **R87 Abnormal findings in specimens from female genital organs**
> **Includes** abnormal findings in secretion and smears from cervix uteri
> abnormal findings in secretion and smears from vagina
> abnormal findings in secretion and smears from vulva

R87.0 Abnormal level of enzymes in specimens from female genital organs ♀

R87.1 Abnormal level of hormones in specimens from female genital organs ♀

R87.2 Abnormal level of other drugs, medicaments and biological substances in specimens from female genital organs ♀

R87.3 Abnormal level of substances chiefly nonmedicinal as to source in specimens from female genital organs ♀

R87.4 Abnormal immunological findings in specimens from female genital organs ♀

R87.5 Abnormal microbiological findings in specimens from female genital organs ♀
> Positive culture findings in specimens from female genital organs
> **Excludes1** colonization status (Z22.-)

● **R87.6 Abnormal cytological findings in specimens from female genital organs**

● **R87.61 Abnormal cytological findings in specimens from cervix uteri**
> **Excludes1** abnormal cytological findings in specimens from other female genital organs (R87.69)
> abnormal cytological findings in specimens from vagina (R87.62-)
> carcinoma in situ of cervix uteri (histologically confirmed) (D06.-)
> cervical intraepithelial neoplasia I [CIN I] (N87.0)
> cervical intraepithelial neoplasia II [CIN II] (N87.1)
> cervical intraepithelial neoplasia III [CIN III] (D06.-)
> dysplasia (mild) (moderate) of cervix uteri (histologically confirmed) (N87.-)
> severe dysplasia of cervix uteri (histologically confirmed) (D06.-)
>
> **Excludes2** cervical high risk human papillomavirus (HPV) DNA test positive (R87.810)
> cervical low risk human papillomavirus (HPV) DNA test positive (R87.820)

R87.610 Atypical squamous cells of undetermined significance on cytologic smear of cervix (ASC-US) ♀

R87.611 Atypical squamous cells cannot exclude high grade squamous intraepithelial lesion on cytologic smear of cervix (ASC-H) ♀

R87.612 Low grade squamous intraepithelial lesion on cytologic smear of cervix (LGSIL) ♀

R87.613 High grade squamous intraepithelial lesion on cytologic smear of cervix (HGSIL) ♀

R87.614 Cytologic evidence of malignancy on smear of cervix ♀

R87.615 Unsatisfactory cytologic smear of cervix ♀
> Inadequate sample of cytologic smear of cervix

◀ New   ◀▬ Revised   ~~deleted~~ Deleted   Excludes 1   Excludes 2   Includes   Use additional   Code first   Code also   Unspecified

OGCR Official Guidelines   X Assign placeholder X   ● Use Additional Character(s)   ▶ Manifestation Code   **Coding Clinic**

R87.616 **Satisfactory cervical smear but lacking transformation zone** ♀

R87.618 **Other abnormal cytological findings on specimens from cervix uteri** ♀

R87.619 Unspecified **abnormal cytological findings in specimens from cervix uteri** ♀

> Abnormal cervical cytology NOS
> Abnormal Papanicolaou smear of cervix NOS
> Abnormal thin preparation smear of cervix NOS
> Atypical endocervical cells of cervix NOS
> Atypical endometrial cells of cervix NOS
> Atypical glandular cells of cervix NOS

● R87.62 **Abnormal cytological findings in specimens from vagina**

> Use additional code to identify acquired absence of uterus and cervix, if applicable (Z90.71-)

> **Excludes1** abnormal cytological findings in specimens from cervix uteri (R87.61-)
> abnormal cytological findings in specimens from other female genital organs (R87.69)
> carcinoma in situ of vagina (histologically confirmed) (D07.2)
> vaginal intraepithelial neoplasia I [VAIN I] (N89.0)
> vaginal intraepithelial neoplasia II [VAIN II] (N89.1)
> vaginal intraepithelial neoplasia III [VAIN III] (D07.2)
> dysplasia (mild) (moderate) of vagina (histologically confirmed) (N89.-)
> severe dysplasia of vagina (histologically confirmed) (D07.2)

> **Excludes2** vaginal high risk human papillomavirus (HPV) DNA test positive (R87.811)
> vaginal low risk human papillomavirus (HPV) DNA test positive (R87.821)

R87.620 **Atypical squamous cells of undetermined significance on cytologic smear of vagina (ASC-US)** ♀

R87.621 **Atypical squamous cells cannot exclude high grade squamous intraepithelial lesion on cytologic smear of vagina (ASC-H)** ♀

R87.622 **Low grade squamous intraepithelial lesion on cytologic smear of vagina (LGSIL)** ♀

R87.623 **High grade squamous intraepithelial lesion on cytologic smear of vagina (HGSIL)** ♀

R87.624 **Cytologic evidence of malignancy on smear of vagina** ♀

R87.625 **Unsatisfactory cytologic smear of vagina** ♀
> Inadequate sample of cytologic smear of vagina

R87.628 **Other abnormal cytological findings on specimens from vagina** ♀

R87.629 Unspecified **abnormal cytological findings in specimens from vagina** ♀

> Abnormal Papanicolaou smear of vagina NOS
> Abnormal thin preparation smear of vagina NOS
> Abnormal vaginal cytology NOS
> Atypical endocervical cells of vagina NOS
> Atypical endometrial cells of vagina NOS
> Atypical glandular cells of vagina NOS

R87.69 **Abnormal cytological findings in specimens from other female genital organs** ♀
> Abnormal cytological findings in specimens from female genital organs NOS

> **Excludes1** dysplasia of vulva (histologically confirmed) (N90.0-N90.3)

R87.7 **Abnormal histological findings in specimens from female genital organs** ♀

> **Excludes1** carcinoma in situ (histologically confirmed) of female genital organs (D06-D07.3)
> cervical intraepithelial neoplasia I [CIN I] (N87.0)
> cervical intraepithelial neoplasia II [CIN II] (N87.1)
> cervical intraepithelial neoplasia III [CIN III] (D06.-)
> dysplasia (mild) (moderate) of cervix uteri (histologically confirmed) (N87.-)
> dysplasia (mild) (moderate) of vagina (histologically confirmed) (N89.-)
> vaginal intraepithelial neoplasia I [VAIN I] (N89.0)
> vaginal intraepithelial neoplasia II [VAIN II] (N89.1)
> vaginal intraepithelial neoplasia III [VAIN III] (D07.2)
> severe dysplasia of cervix uteri (histologically confirmed) (D06.-)
> severe dysplasia of vagina (histologically confirmed) (D07.2)

● R87.8 **Other abnormal findings in specimens from female genital organs**

● R87.81 **High risk human papillomavirus (HPV) DNA test positive from female genital organs**

> **Excludes1** anogenital warts due to human papillomavirus (HPV) (A63.0)
> condyloma acuminatum (A63.0)

R87.810 **Cervical high risk human papillomavirus (HPV) DNA test positive** ♀

R87.811 **Vaginal high risk human papillomavirus (HPV) DNA test positive** ♀

● R87.82 **Low risk human papillomavirus (HPV) DNA test positive from female genital organs**

> Use additional code for associated human papillomavirus (B97.7)

R87.820 **Cervical low risk human papillomavirus (HPV) DNA test positive** ♀

R87.821 **Vaginal low risk human papillomavirus (HPV) DNA test positive** ♀

R87.89 **Other abnormal findings in specimens from female genital organs** ♀
> Abnormal chromosomal findings in specimens from female genital organs

R87.9 Unspecified **abnormal finding in specimens from female genital organs** ♀

CHAPTER 18 (R00-R99)

● R88   **Abnormal findings in other body fluids and substances**
     R88.0   **Cloudy (hemodialysis) (peritoneal) dialysis effluent**
     R88.8   **Abnormal findings in other body fluids and substances**

● R89   **Abnormal findings in specimens from other organs, systems and tissues**

     Includes   abnormal findings in nipple discharge
                    abnormal findings in synovial fluid
                    abnormal findings in wound secretions

     R89.0   **Abnormal level of enzymes in specimens from other organs, systems and tissues**
     R89.1   **Abnormal level of hormones in specimens from other organs, systems and tissues**
     R89.2   **Abnormal level of other drugs, medicaments and biological substances in specimens from other organs, systems and tissues**
     R89.3   **Abnormal level of substances chiefly nonmedicinal as to source in specimens from other organs, systems and tissues**
     R89.4   **Abnormal immunological findings in specimens from other organs, systems and tissues**
     R89.5   **Abnormal microbiological findings in specimens from other organs, systems and tissues**
           Positive culture findings in specimens from other organs, systems and tissues

           Excludes1   colonization status (Z22.-)

     R89.6   **Abnormal cytological findings in specimens from other organs, systems and tissues**
     R89.7   **Abnormal histological findings in specimens from other organs, systems and tissues**
     R89.8   **Other abnormal findings in specimens from other organs, systems and tissues**
           Abnormal chromosomal findings in specimens from other organs, systems and tissues
     R89.9   **Unspecified abnormal finding in specimens from other organs, systems and tissues**

ABNORMAL FINDINGS ON DIAGNOSTIC IMAGING AND IN FUNCTION STUDIES, WITHOUT DIAGNOSIS (R90-R94)

     Includes   nonspecific abnormal findings on diagnostic imaging by computerized axial tomography [CAT scan]
                    nonspecific abnormal findings on diagnostic imaging by magnetic resonance imaging [MRI][NMR]
                    nonspecific abnormal findings on diagnostic imaging by positron emission tomography [PET scan]
                    nonspecific abnormal findings on diagnostic imaging by thermography
                    nonspecific abnormal findings on diagnostic imaging by ultrasound [echogram]
                    nonspecific abnormal findings on diagnostic imaging by X-ray examination

           Excludes1   abnormal findings on antenatal screening of mother (O28.-)
                    diagnostic abnormal findings classified elsewhere - see Alphabetical Index

● R90   **Abnormal findings on diagnostic imaging of central nervous system**
     R90.0   **Intracranial space-occupying lesion found on diagnostic imaging of central nervous system**
  ● R90.8   **Other abnormal findings on diagnostic imaging of central nervous system**
         R90.81   **Abnormal echoencephalogram**
         R90.82   **White matter disease, unspecified**
         R90.89   **Other abnormal findings on diagnostic imaging of central nervous system**
              Other cerebrovascular abnormality found on diagnostic imaging of central nervous system

● R91   **Abnormal findings on diagnostic imaging of lung**
     R91.1   **Solitary pulmonary nodule**
           Coin lesion lung
           Solitary pulmonary nodule, subsegmental branch of the bronchial tree
     R91.8   **Other nonspecific abnormal finding of lung field**
           Lung mass NOS found on diagnostic imaging of lung
           Pulmonary infiltrate NOS
           Shadow, lung

● R92   **Abnormal and inconclusive findings on diagnostic imaging of breast**
     R92.0   **Mammographic microcalcification found on diagnostic imaging of breast**
           Excludes2   mammographic calcification (calculus) found on diagnostic imaging of breast (R92.1)
     R92.1   **Mammographic calcification found on diagnostic imaging of breast**
           Mammographic calculus found on diagnostic imaging of breast
     R92.2   **Inconclusive mammogram**
           Dense breasts NOS
           Inconclusive mammogram NEC
           Inconclusive mammography due to dense breasts
           Inconclusive mammography NEC
           Coding Clinic: 2015, Q1, P24
     R92.8   **Other abnormal and inconclusive findings on diagnostic imaging of breast**

● R93   **Abnormal findings on diagnostic imaging of other body structures**
     R93.0   **Abnormal findings on diagnostic imaging of skull and head, not elsewhere classified**
           Excludes1   intracranial space-occupying lesion found on diagnostic imaging (R90.0)
     R93.1   **Abnormal findings on diagnostic imaging of heart and coronary circulation**
           Abnormal echocardiogram NOS
           Abnormal heart shadow
     R93.2   **Abnormal findings on diagnostic imaging of liver and biliary tract**
           Nonvisualization of gallbladder
     R93.3   **Abnormal findings on diagnostic imaging of other parts of digestive tract**
  ● R93.4   **Abnormal findings on diagnostic imaging of urinary organs**
           Excludes2   hypertrophy of kidney (N28.81) ◄
         R93.41   **Abnormal radiologic findings on diagnostic imaging of renal pelvis, ureter, or bladder ◄**
              Filling defect of bladder found on diagnostic imaging ◄
              Filling defect of renal pelvis found on diagnostic imaging ◄
              Filling defect of ureter found on diagnostic imaging ◄
      ● R93.42   **Abnormal radiologic findings on diagnostic imaging of kidney ◄**
              R93.421   **Abnormal radiologic findings on diagnostic imaging of right kidney ◄**
              R93.422   **Abnormal radiologic findings on diagnostic imaging of left kidney ◄**
              R93.429   **Abnormal radiologic findings on diagnostic imaging of unspecified kidney ◄**
         R93.49   **Abnormal radiologic findings on diagnostic imaging of other urinary organs ◄**

◄ New   ◄ⅲ Revised   ~~deleted~~ Deleted   Excludes 1   Excludes 2   Includes   Use additional   Code first   Code also   Unspecified
OGCR Official Guidelines   X Assign placeholder X   ● Use Additional Character(s)   ▶ Manifestation Code   **Coding Clinic**

Figure 18-2   Cranial nerves. (From Patton and Thibodeau: Anatomy and physiology, ed 7, St. Louis, Mosby, 2009)

Trochlear nerve (IV)
Optic nerve (II)
Olfactory nerve (I)
Abducens nerve (VI)
Oculomotor nerve (III)
Trigeminal nerve (V)
Facial nerve (VII)
Vestibulocochlear nerve (VIII)
Glossopharyngeal nerve (IX)
Vagus nerve (X)
Accessory nerve (XI)
Hypoglossal nerve (XII)

R93.5   **Abnormal findings on diagnostic imaging of other abdominal regions, including retroperitoneum**

R93.6   **Abnormal findings on diagnostic imaging of limbs**

> **Excludes2**   abnormal finding in skin and subcutaneous tissue (R93.8)

R93.7   **Abnormal findings on diagnostic imaging of other parts of musculoskeletal system**

> **Excludes2**   abnormal findings on diagnostic imaging of skull (R93.0)

R93.8   **Abnormal findings on diagnostic imaging of other specified body structures**
> Abnormal finding by radioisotope localization of placenta
> Abnormal radiological finding in skin and subcutaneous tissue
> Mediastinal shift

R93.9   **Diagnostic imaging inconclusive due to excess body fat of patient**

● **R94**   **Abnormal results of function studies**

> **Includes**   abnormal results of radionuclide [radioisotope] uptake studies
> abnormal results of scintigraphy

● **R94.0**   **Abnormal results of function studies of central nervous system**

     R94.01   **Abnormal electroencephalogram [EEG]**

     R94.02   **Abnormal brain scan**

     R94.09   **Abnormal results of other function studies of central nervous system**

● **R94.1**   **Abnormal results of function studies of peripheral nervous system and special senses**

● **R94.11**   **Abnormal results of function studies of eye**

     R94.110   **Abnormal electro-oculogram [EOG]**

     R94.111   **Abnormal electroretinogram [ERG]**
         Abnormal retinal function study

     R94.112   **Abnormal visually evoked potential [VEP]**

     R94.113   **Abnormal oculomotor study**

     R94.118   **Abnormal results of other function studies of eye**

● **R94.12**   **Abnormal results of function studies of ear and other special senses**

     R94.120   **Abnormal auditory function study**

     R94.121   **Abnormal vestibular function study**

     R94.128   **Abnormal results of other function studies of ear and other special senses**

● **R94.13**   **Abnormal results of function studies of peripheral nervous system**

     R94.130   **Abnormal response to nerve stimulation, unspecified**

     R94.131   **Abnormal electromyogram [EMG]**

> **Excludes1**   electromyogram of eye (R94.113)

     R94.138   **Abnormal results of other function studies of peripheral nervous system**

R94.2   **Abnormal results of pulmonary function studies**
> Reduced ventilatory capacity
> Reduced vital capacity

Item 18-1   The **peripheral nervous system** consists of 31 pairs of spinal nerves, 12 pairs of cranial nerves, and the autonomic nerves, which are divided into the parasympathetic and sympathetic nerves. The cranial nerves are: olfactory (I), optic (II), oculomotor (III), trochlear (IV), trigeminal (V), abducens (VI), facial (VII), vestibulocochlear (VIII), glossopharyngeal (IX), vagus (X), accessory (XI), and hypoglossal (XII).

● R94.3 **Abnormal results of cardiovascular function studies**

  R94.30 **Abnormal result of cardiovascular function study, unspecified**

  R94.31 **Abnormal electrocardiogram [ECG] [EKG]**

  Excludes1   long QT syndrome (I45.81)

  R94.39 **Abnormal result of other cardiovascular function study**

  Abnormal electrophysiological intracardiac studies

  Abnormal phonocardiogram

  Abnormal vectorcardiogram

R94.4 **Abnormal results of kidney function studies**

  Abnormal renal function test

R94.5 **Abnormal results of liver function studies**

R94.6 **Abnormal results of thyroid function studies**

R94.7 **Abnormal results of other endocrine function studies**

  Excludes2   abnormal glucose (R73.0-)

R94.8 **Abnormal results of function studies of other organs and systems**

  Abnormal basal metabolic rate [BMR]

  Abnormal bladder function test

  Abnormal splenic function test

ABNORMAL TUMOR MARKERS (R97)

● R97 **Abnormal tumor markers**

  Elevated tumor associated antigens [TAA]

  Elevated tumor specific antigens [TSA]

  R97.0 **Elevated carcinoembryonic antigen [CEA]**

  R97.1 **Elevated cancer antigen 125 [CA 125] ♀**

● R97.2 **Elevated prostate specific antigen [PSA]**

  R97.20 **Elevated prostate specific antigen [PSA] ♂** ◄   A

  R97.21 **Rising PSA following treatment for malignant neoplasm of prostate ♂** ◄   A

  R97.8 **Other abnormal tumor markers**

ILL-DEFINED AND UNKNOWN CAUSE OF MORTALITY (R99)

R99 **Ill-defined and unknown cause of mortality**

  Death (unexplained) NOS

  Unspecified cause of mortality

  OGCR Section I.C.18.h.

  Death NOS

  Code R99, Ill-defined and unknown cause of mortality, is only for use in the very limited circumstance when a patient who has already died is brought into the emergency department or other healthcare facility and is pronounced dead upon arrival. It does not represent the discharge disposition of death.

CHAPTER 19

INJURY, POISONING AND CERTAIN OTHER CONSEQUENCES OF EXTERNAL CAUSES (S00-T88)

OGCR Chapter-Specific Coding Guidelines

19. **Chapter 19: Injury, poisoning, and certain other consequences of external causes (S00-T88)**

a. **Application of 7th Characters in Chapter 19**

Most categories in chapter 19 have a 7th character requirement for each applicable code. Most categories in this chapter have three 7th character values (with the exception of fractures): A, initial encounter, D, subsequent encounter and S, sequela. Categories for traumatic fractures have additional 7th character values. **While the patient may be seen by a new or different provider over the course of treatment for an injury, assignment of the 7th character is based on whether the patient is undergoing active treatment and not whether the provider is seeing the patient for the first time.**

For complication codes, active treatment refers to treatment for the condition described by the code, even though it may be related to an earlier precipitating problem. For example, code T84.50XA, Infection and inflammatory reaction due to unspecified internal joint prosthesis, initial encounter, is used when active treatment is provided for the infection, even though the condition relates to the prosthetic device, implant or graft that was placed at a previous encounter.

7th character "A", initial encounter is used **for each encounter where** the patient is receiving active treatment for the condition.

7th character "D" subsequent encounter is used for encounters after the patient has **completed** active treatment of the condition and is receiving routine care for the condition during the healing or recovery phase.

The aftercare Z codes should not be used for aftercare for conditions such as injuries or poisonings, where 7th characters are provided to identify subsequent care. For example, for aftercare of an injury, assign the acute injury code with the 7th character "D" (subsequent encounter).

7th character "S", sequela, is for use for complications or conditions that arise as a direct result of a condition, such as scar formation after a burn. The scars are sequelae of the burn. When using 7th character "S", it is necessary to use both the injury code that precipitated the sequela and the code for the sequela itself. The "S" is added only to the injury code, not the sequela code. The 7th character "S" identifies the injury responsible for the sequela. The specific type of sequela (e.g. scar) is sequenced first, followed by the injury code.

See Section I.B.10. Sequelae, (Late Effects)

b. **Coding of Injuries**

When coding injuries, assign separate codes for each injury unless a combination code is provided, in which case the combination code is assigned. Code T07, Unspecified multiple injuries should not be assigned in the inpatient setting unless information for a more specific code is not available. Traumatic injury codes (S00-T14.9) are not to be used for normal, healing surgical wounds or to identify complications of surgical wounds.

The code for the most serious injury, as determined by the provider and the focus of treatment, is sequenced first.

1) **Superficial injuries**

Superficial injuries such as abrasions or contusions are not coded when associated with more severe injuries of the same site.

2) **Primary injury with damage to nerves/blood vessels**

When a primary injury results in minor damage to peripheral nerves or blood vessels, the primary injury is sequenced first with additional code(s) for injuries to nerves and spinal cord (such as category S04), and/or injury to blood vessels (such as category S15). When the primary injury is to the blood vessels or nerves, that injury should be sequenced first.

c. **Coding of Traumatic Fractures**

The principles of multiple coding of injuries should be followed in coding fractures. Fractures of specified sites are coded

individually by site in accordance with both the provisions within categories S02, S12, S22, S32, S42, S49, S52, S59, S62, S72, S79, S82, S89, S92 and the level of detail furnished by medical record content.

A fracture not indicated as open or closed should be coded to closed. A fracture not indicated whether displaced or not displaced should be coded to displaced.

More specific guidelines are as follows:

1) **Initial vs. Subsequent Encounter for Fractures**

Traumatic fractures are coded using the appropriate 7th character for initial encounter (A, B, C) **for each encounter where** the patient is receiving active treatment for the fracture. The appropriate 7th character for initial encounter should also be assigned for a patient who delayed seeking treatment for the fracture or nonunion.

Fractures are coded using the appropriate 7th character for subsequent care for encounters after the patient has completed active treatment of the fracture and is receiving routine care for the fracture during the healing or recovery phase.

Care for complications of surgical treatment for fracture repairs during the healing or recovery phase should be coded with the appropriate complication codes.

Care of complications of fractures, such as malunion and nonunion, should be reported with the appropriate 7th character for subsequent care with nonunion (K, M, N,) or subsequent care with malunion (P, Q, R).

Malunion/nonunion: The appropriate 7th character for initial encounter should also be assigned for a patient who delayed seeking treatment for the fracture or nonunion.

The open fracture designations in the assignment of the 7th character for fractures of the forearm, femur and lower leg, including ankle are based on the Gustilo open fracture classification. When the Gustilo classification type is not specified for an open fracture, the 7th character for open fracture type I or II should be assigned (B, E, H, M, Q).

A code from category M80, not a traumatic fracture code, should be used for any patient with known osteoporosis who suffers a fracture, even if the patient had a minor fall or trauma, if that fall or trauma would not usually break a normal, healthy bone.

See Section I.C.13. Osteoporosis.

The aftercare Z codes should not be used for aftercare for traumatic fractures. For aftercare of a traumatic fracture, assign the acute fracture code with the appropriate 7th character.

2) **Multiple fractures sequencing**

Multiple fractures are sequenced in accordance with the severity of the fracture.

d. **Coding of Burns and Corrosions**

The ICD-10-CM makes a distinction between burns and corrosions. The burn codes are for thermal burns, except sunburns, that come from a heat source, such as a fire or hot appliance. The burn codes are also for burns resulting from electricity and radiation. Corrosions are burns due to chemicals. The guidelines are the same for burns and corrosions.

Current burns (T20-T25) are classified by depth, extent and by agent (X code). Burns are classified by depth as first degree (erythema), second degree (blistering), and third degree (full-thickness involvement). Burns of the eye and internal organs (T26-T28) are classified by site, but not by degree.

1) **Sequencing of burn and related condition codes**

Sequence first the code that reflects the highest degree of burn when more than one burn is present.

a. When the reason for the admission or encounter is for treatment of external multiple burns, sequence first the code that reflects the burn of the highest degree.

b. When a patient has both internal and external burns, the circumstances of admission govern the selection of the principal diagnosis or first-listed diagnosis.

c. When a patient is admitted for burn injuries and other related conditions such as smoke inhalation and/or respiratory failure, the circumstances of admission govern the selection of the principal or first-listed diagnosis.

2) Burns of the same local site

Classify burns of the same local site (three-character category level, T20-T28) but of different degrees to the subcategory identifying the highest degree recorded in the diagnosis.

3) Non-healing burns

Non-healing burns are coded as acute burns.

Necrosis of burned skin should be coded as a non-healed burn.

4) Infected Burn

For any documented infected burn site, use an additional code for the infection.

5) Assign separate codes for each burn site

When coding burns, assign separate codes for each burn site. Category T30, Burn and corrosion, body region unspecified is extremely vague and should rarely be used.

6) Burns and Corrosions Classified According to Extent of Body Surface Involved

Assign codes from category T31, Burns classified according to extent of body surface involved, or T32, Corrosions classified according to extent of body surface involved, when the site of the burn is not specified or when there is a need for additional data. It is advisable to use category T31 as additional coding when needed to provide data for evaluating burn mortality, such as that needed by burn units. It is also advisable to use category T31 as an additional code for reporting purposes when there is mention of a third-degree burn involving 20 percent or more of the body surface.

Categories T31 and T32 are based on the classic "rule of nines" in estimating body surface involved: head and neck are assigned nine percent, each arm nine percent, each leg 18 percent, the anterior trunk 18 percent, posterior trunk 18 percent, and genitalia one percent. Providers may change these percentage assignments where necessary to accommodate infants and children who have proportionately larger heads than adults, and patients who have large buttocks, thighs, or abdomen that involve burns.

7) Encounters for treatment of sequela of burns

Encounters for the treatment of the late effects of burns or corrosions (i.e., scars or joint contractures) should be coded with a burn or corrosion code with the 7th character "S" for sequela.

8) Sequelae with a late effect code and current burn

When appropriate, both a code for a current burn or corrosion with 7th character "A" or "D" and a burn or corrosion code with 7th character "S" may be assigned on the same record (when both a current burn and sequelae of an old burn exist). Burns and corrosions do not heal at the same rate and a current healing wound may still exist with sequela of a healed burn or corrosion.

See Section I.B.10. Sequela, (Late Effects)

9) Use of an external cause code with burns and corrosions

An external cause code should be used with burns and corrosions to identify the source and intent of the burn, as well as the place where it occurred.

e. Adverse Effects, Poisoning , Underdosing and Toxic Effects

Codes in categories T36-T65 are combination codes that include the substance that was taken as well as the intent. No additional external cause code is required for poisonings, toxic effects, adverse effects and underdosing codes.

1) Do not code directly from the Table of Drugs

Do not code directly from the Table of Drugs and Chemicals. Always refer back to the Tabular List.

2) Use as many codes as necessary to describe

Use as many codes as necessary to describe completely all drugs, medicinal or biological substances.

3) If the same code would describe the causative agent

If the same code would describe the causative agent for more than one adverse reaction, poisoning, toxic effect or underdosing, assign the code only once.

4) If two or more drugs, medicinal or biological substances

If two or more drugs, medicinal or biological substances are reported, code each individually unless a combination code is listed in the Table of Drugs and Chemicals.

5) The occurrence of drug toxicity is classified in ICD-10-CM as follows:

(a) Adverse Effect

When coding an adverse effect of a drug that has been correctly prescribed and properly administered, assign the appropriate code for the nature of the adverse effect followed by the appropriate code for the adverse effect of the drug (T36-T50). The code for the drug should have a 5th or 6th character "5" (for example T36.0X5-) Examples of the nature of an adverse effect are tachycardia, delirium, gastrointestinal hemorrhaging, vomiting, hypokalemia, hepatitis, renal failure, or respiratory failure.

(b) Poisoning

When coding a poisoning or reaction to the improper use of a medication (e.g., overdose, wrong substance given or taken in error, wrong route of administration), first assign the appropriate code from categories T36-T50. The poisoning codes have an associated intent as their 5th or 6th character (accidental, intentional self-harm, assault and undetermined). **If the intent of the poisoning is unknown or unspecified, code the intent as accidental intent. The undetermined intent is only for use if the documentation in the record specifies that the intent cannot be determined.** Use additional code(s) for all manifestations of poisonings.

If there is also a diagnosis of abuse or dependence of the substance, the abuse or dependence is assigned as an additional code.

Examples of poisoning include:

(i) Error was made in drug prescription

Errors made in drug prescription or in the administration of the drug by provider, nurse, patient, or other person.

(ii) Overdose of a drug intentionally taken If an overdose of a drug was intentionally taken or administered and resulted in drug toxicity, it would be coded as a poisoning.

(iii) Nonprescribed drug taken with correctly prescribed and properly administered drug. If a nonprescribed drug or medicinal agent was taken in combination with a correctly prescribed and properly administered drug, any drug toxicity or other reaction resulting from the interaction of the two drugs would be classified as a poisoning.

(iv) Interaction of drug(s) and alcohol. When a reaction results from the interaction of a drug(s) and alcohol, this would be classified as poisoning.

See Section I.C.4. if poisoning is the result of insulin pump malfunctions.

(c) Underdosing

Underdosing refers to taking less of a medication than is prescribed by a provider or a manufacturer's instruction. For underdosing, assign the code from categories T36-T50 (fifth or sixth character "6").

Codes for underdosing should never be assigned as principal or first-listed codes. If a patient has a relapse or exacerbation of the medical condition for which the drug is prescribed because of the reduction in dose, then the medical condition itself should be coded.

Noncompliance (Z91.12-, Z91.13-) or complication of care (Y63.6-Y63.9) codes are to be used with an underdosing code to indicate intent, if known.

(d) Toxic Effects

When a harmful substance is ingested or comes in contact with a person, this is classified as a toxic effect. The toxic effect codes are in categories T51-T65.

Toxic effect codes have an associated intent: accidental, intentional self-harm, assault and undetermined.

f. Adult and child abuse, neglect and other maltreatment

Sequence first the appropriate code from categories T74.- (Adult and child abuse, neglect and other maltreatment, confirmed) or T76.- (Adult and child abuse, neglect and other maltreatment, suspected) for abuse, neglect and other maltreatment, followed by any accompanying mental health or injury code(s).

If the documentation in the medical record states abuse or neglect it is coded as confirmed (T74.-). It is coded as suspected if it is documented as suspected (T76.-).

For cases of confirmed abuse or neglect an external cause code from the assault section (X92-**Y09**) should be added to identify the cause of any physical injuries. A perpetrator code (Y07) should be added when the perpetrator of the abuse is known. For suspected cases of abuse or neglect, do not report external cause or perpetrator code.

If a suspected case of abuse, neglect or mistreatment is ruled out during an encounter code Z04.71, Encounter for examination and observation following alleged physical adult abuse, ruled out, or code Z04.72, Encounter for examination and observation following alleged child physical abuse, ruled out, should be used, not a code from T76.

If a suspected case of alleged rape or sexual abuse is ruled out during an encounter code Z04.41, Encounter for examination and observation following alleged **adult rape** or code Z04.42, Encounter for examination and observation following alleged **child rape**, should be used, not a code from T76.

See Section I.C.15. Abuse in a pregnant patient.

g. Complications of care

1) General guidelines for complications of care

(a) Documentation of complications of care

See Section I.B.16. for information on documentation of complications of care.

2) Pain due to medical devices

Pain associated with devices, implants or grafts left in a surgical site (for example painful hip prosthesis) is assigned to the appropriate code(s) found in Chapter 19, Injury, poisoning, and certain other consequences of external causes. Specific codes for pain due to medical devices are found in the T code section of the ICD-10-CM. Use additional code(s) from category G89 to identify acute or chronic pain due to presence of the device, implant or graft (G89.18 or G89.28).

3) Transplant complications

(a) Transplant complications other than kidney

Codes under category T86, Complications of transplanted organs and tissues, are for use for both complications and rejection of transplanted organs. A transplant complication code is only assigned if the complication affects the function of the transplanted organ. Two codes are required to fully describe a transplant complication: the appropriate code from category T86 and a secondary code that identifies the complication.

Pre-existing conditions or conditions that develop after the transplant are not coded as complications unless they affect the function of the transplanted organs.

See I.C.21. for transplant organ removal status
See I.C.2. for malignant neoplasm associated with transplanted organ.

(b) Kidney transplant complications

Patients who have undergone kidney transplant may still have some form of chronic kidney disease (CKD) because the kidney transplant may not fully restore kidney function. Code T86.1- should be assigned for documented complications of a kidney transplant, such as transplant failure or rejection or other transplant complication. Code T86.1- should not be assigned for post kidney transplant patients who have chronic kidney (CKD) unless a transplant complication such as transplant failure or rejection is documented. If the documentation is unclear as to whether the patient has a complication of the transplant, query the provider.

Conditions that affect the function of the transplanted kidney, other than CKD, should be assigned a code from subcategory T86.1, Complications of transplanted organ, Kidney, and a secondary code that identifies the complication.

For patients with CKD following a kidney transplant, but who do not have a complication such as failure or rejection, *see section I.C.14. Chronic kidney disease and kidney transplant status.*

4) Complication codes that include the external cause

As with certain other T codes, some of the complications of care codes have the external cause included in the code. The code includes the nature of the complication as well as the type of procedure that caused the complication. No external cause code indicating the type of procedure is necessary for these codes.

5) Complications of care codes within the body system chapters

Intraoperative and postprocedural complication codes are found within the body system chapters with codes specific to the organs and structures of that body system. These codes should be sequenced first, followed by a code(s) for the specific complication, if applicable.

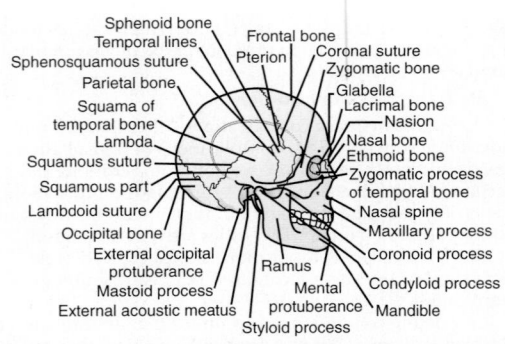

Figure 19-1 Lateral view of skull.

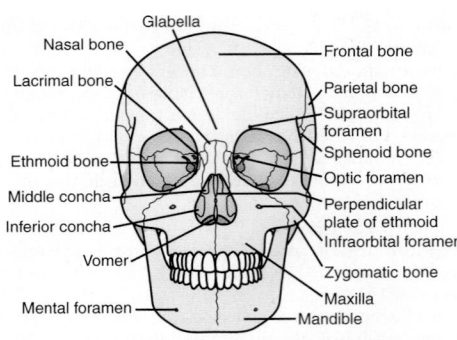

Figure 19-2 Frontal view of skull.

Figure 19-3 Anterior view of vertebral column.

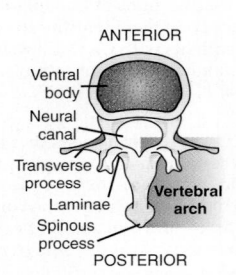

Figure 19-4 Vertebra viewed from above.

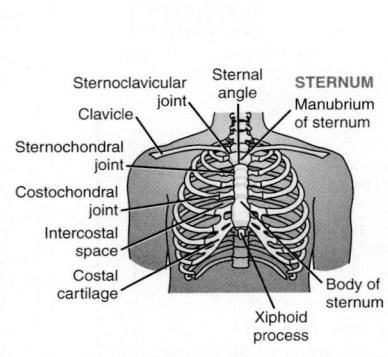

Figure 19-5 Anterior view of rib cage.

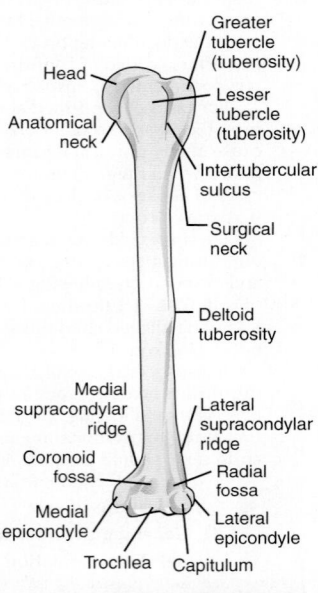

Figure 19-6 Anterior aspect of left humerus.

Figure 19-7 Anterior aspect of left radius and ulna.

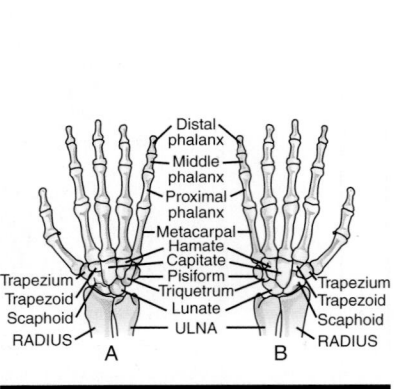

Figure 19-8 Right hand and wrist: **A.** Dorsal surface. **B.** Palmar surface.

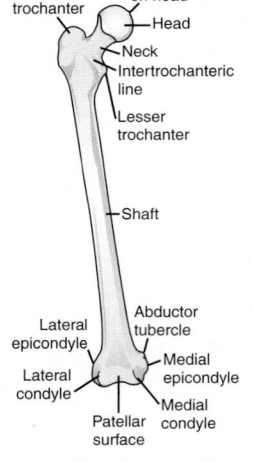

Figure 19-9 Anterior aspect of right femur.

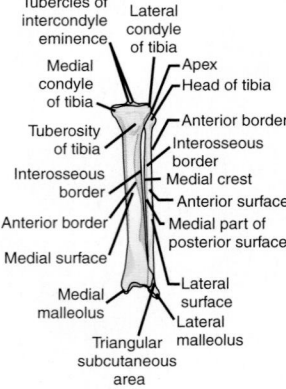

Figure 19-10 Anterior aspect of left tibia and fibula.

◀ New ◀ Revised ~~deleted~~ Deleted Excludes 1 Excludes 2 Includes Use additional Code first Code also Unspecified
OGCR Official Guidelines X Assign placeholder X ● Use Additional Character(s) ▶ Manifestation Code **Coding Clinic**

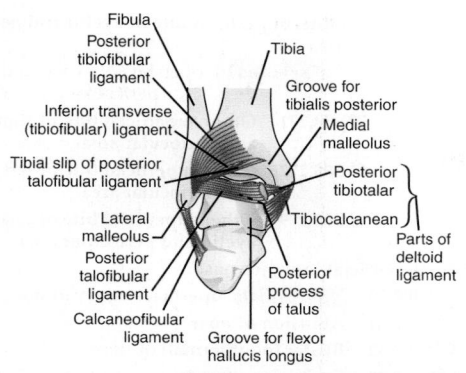

Figure 19-11 Posterior aspect of the left ankle joint.

Figure 19-12 Right foot viewed from above.

CHAPTER 19

INJURY, POISONING AND CERTAIN OTHER CONSEQUENCES OF EXTERNAL CAUSES (S00-T88)

Note: Use secondary code(s) from Chapter 20, External causes of morbidity, to indicate cause of injury. Codes within the T section that include the external cause do not require an additional external cause code.

Use additional code to identify any retained foreign body, if applicable (Z18.-)

Excludes1 birth trauma (P10-P15)
             obstetric trauma (O70-O71)

Note: The chapter uses the S-section for coding different types of injuries related to single body regions and the T-section to cover injuries to unspecified body regions as well as poisoning and certain other consequences of external causes.

This chapter contains the following blocks:

S00-S09	Injuries to the head
S10-S19	Injuries to the neck
S20-S29	Injuries to the thorax
S30-S39	Injuries to the abdomen, lower back, lumbar spine, pelvis and external genitals
S40-S49	Injuries to the shoulder and upper arm
S50-S59	Injuries to the elbow and forearm
S60-S69	Injuries to the wrist, hand, and fingers
S70-S79	Injuries to the hip and thigh
S80-S89	Injuries to the knee and lower leg
S90-S99	Injuries to the ankle and foot

T07	Injuries involving multiple body regions
T14	Injury of unspecified body region
T15-T19	Effects of foreign body entering through natural orifice
T20-T32	Burns and corrosions
T20-T25	Burns and corrosions of external body surface, specified by site
T26-T28	Burns and corrosions confined to eye and internal organs
T30-T32	Burns and corrosions of multiple and unspecified body regions
T33-T34	Frostbite
T36-T50	Poisoning by, adverse effect of and underdosing of drugs, medicaments and biological substances
T51-T65	Toxic effects of substances chiefly nonmedicinal as to source
T66-T78	Other and unspecified effects of external causes
T79	Certain early complications of trauma
T80-T88	Complications of surgical and medical care, not elsewhere classified

INJURIES TO THE HEAD (S00-S09)

Includes   injuries of ear
            injuries of eye
            injuries of face [any part]
            injuries of gum
            injuries of jaw
            injuries of oral cavity
            injuries of palate
            injuries of periocular area
            injuries of scalp
            injuries of temporomandibular joint area
            injuries of tongue
            injuries of tooth

Code also for any associated infection

Excludes2   burns and corrosions (T20-T32)
             effects of foreign body in ear (T16)
             effects of foreign body in larynx (T17.3)
             effects of foreign body in mouth NOS (T18.0)
             effects of foreign body in nose (T17.0-T17.1)
             effects of foreign body in pharynx (T17.2)
             effects of foreign body on external eye (T15.-)
             frostbite (T33-T34)
             insect bite or sting, venomous (T63.4)

● **S00** **Superficial injury of head**

Excludes1   diffuse cerebral contusion (S06.2-)
             focal cerebral contusion (S06.3-)
             injury of eye and orbit (S05.-)
             open wound of head (S01.-)

The appropriate 7th character is to be added to each code from category S00

A	initial encounter
	All encounters involving diagnosis and treatment
D	subsequent encounter
	Encounters during the healing phase
S	sequela

● **S00.0** **Superficial injury of scalp**

X● **S00.00** **Unspecified** superficial injury of scalp

X● **S00.01** **Abrasion of scalp**

X● **S00.02** **Blister (nonthermal) of scalp**

X● **S00.03** **Contusion of scalp**
                    Bruise of scalp
                    Hematoma of scalp

X● **S00.04** **External constriction of part of scalp**

X● **S00.05** **Superficial foreign body of scalp**
                    Splinter in the scalp

X● **S00.06** **Insect bite (nonvenomous) of scalp**

X● **S00.07** **Other superficial bite of scalp**

              Excludes1   open bite of scalp (S01.05)

- **S00.1 Contusion of eyelid and periocular area**
  - Black eye
  - **Excludes2** contusion of eyeball and orbital tissues (S05.1)
  - X ● **S00.10 Contusion of unspecified eyelid and periocular area**
  - X ● **S00.11 Contusion of right eyelid and periocular area**
  - X ● **S00.12 Contusion of left eyelid and periocular area**
- **S00.2 Other and unspecified superficial injuries of eyelid and periocular area**
  - **Excludes2** superficial injury of conjunctiva and cornea (S05.0-)
  - ● **S00.20 Unspecified superficial injury of eyelid and periocular area**
    - ● **S00.201 Unspecified superficial injury of right eyelid and periocular area**
    - ● **S00.202 Unspecified superficial injury of left eyelid and periocular area**
    - ● **S00.209 Unspecified superficial injury of unspecified eyelid and periocular area**
  - ● **S00.21 Abrasion of eyelid and periocular area**
    - ● **S00.211 Abrasion of right eyelid and periocular area**
    - ● **S00.212 Abrasion of left eyelid and periocular area**
    - ● **S00.219 Abrasion of unspecified eyelid and periocular area**
  - ● **S00.22 Blister (nonthermal) of eyelid and periocular area**
    - ● **S00.221 Blister (nonthermal) of right eyelid and periocular area**
    - ● **S00.222 Blister (nonthermal) of left eyelid and periocular area**
    - ● **S00.229 Blister (nonthermal) of unspecified eyelid and periocular area**
  - ● **S00.24 External constriction of eyelid and periocular area**
    - ● **S00.241 External constriction of right eyelid and periocular area**
    - ● **S00.242 External constriction of left eyelid and periocular area**
    - ● **S00.249 External constriction of unspecified eyelid and periocular area**
  - ● **S00.25 Superficial foreign body of eyelid and periocular area**
    - Splinter of eyelid and periocular area
    - **Excludes2** retained foreign body in eyelid (H02.81-)
    - ● **S00.251 Superficial foreign body of right eyelid and periocular area**
    - ● **S00.252 Superficial foreign body of left eyelid and periocular area**
    - ● **S00.259 Superficial foreign body of unspecified eyelid and periocular area**
  - ● **S00.26 Insect bite (nonvenomous) of eyelid and periocular area**
    - ● **S00.261 Insect bite (nonvenomous) of right eyelid and periocular area**
    - ● **S00.262 Insect bite (nonvenomous) of left eyelid and periocular area**
    - ● **S00.269 Insect bite (nonvenomous) of unspecified eyelid and periocular area**

- ● **S00.27 Other superficial bite of eyelid and periocular area**
  - **Excludes1** open bite of eyelid and periocular area (S01.15)
  - ● **S00.271 Other superficial bite of right eyelid and periocular area**
  - ● **S00.272 Other superficial bite of left eyelid and periocular area**
  - ● **S00.279 Other superficial bite of unspecified eyelid and periocular area**
- **S00.3 Superficial injury of nose**
  - X ● **S00.30 Unspecified superficial injury of nose**
  - X ● **S00.31 Abrasion of nose**
  - X ● **S00.32 Blister (nonthermal) of nose**
  - X ● **S00.33 Contusion of nose**
    - Bruise of nose
    - Hematoma of nose
  - X ● **S00.34 External constriction of nose**
  - X ● **S00.35 Superficial foreign body of nose**
    - Splinter in the nose
  - X ● **S00.36 Insect bite (nonvenomous) of nose**
  - X ● **S00.37 Other superficial bite of nose**
    - **Excludes1** open bite of nose (S01.25)
- **S00.4 Superficial injury of ear**
  - ● **S00.40 Unspecified superficial injury of ear**
    - ● **S00.401 Unspecified superficial injury of right ear**
    - ● **S00.402 Unspecified superficial injury of left ear**
    - ● **S00.409 Unspecified superficial injury of unspecified ear**
  - ● **S00.41 Abrasion of ear**
    - ● **S00.411 Abrasion of right ear**
    - ● **S00.412 Abrasion of left ear**
    - ● **S00.419 Abrasion of unspecified ear**
  - ● **S00.42 Blister (nonthermal) of ear**
    - ● **S00.421 Blister (nonthermal) of right ear**
    - ● **S00.422 Blister (nonthermal) of left ear**
    - ● **S00.429 Blister (nonthermal) of unspecified ear**
  - ● **S00.43 Contusion of ear**
    - Bruise of ear
    - Hematoma of ear
    - ● **S00.431 Contusion of right ear**
    - ● **S00.432 Contusion of left ear**
    - ● **S00.439 Contusion of unspecified ear**
  - ● **S00.44 External constriction of ear**
    - ● **S00.441 External constriction of right ear**
    - ● **S00.442 External constriction of left ear**
    - ● **S00.449 External constriction of unspecified ear**
  - ● **S00.45 Superficial foreign body of ear**
    - Splinter in the ear
    - ● **S00.451 Superficial foreign body of right ear**
    - ● **S00.452 Superficial foreign body of left ear**
    - ● **S00.459 Superficial foreign body of unspecified ear**
  - ● **S00.46 Insect bite (nonvenomous) of ear**
    - ● **S00.461 Insect bite (nonvenomous) of right ear**
    - ● **S00.462 Insect bite (nonvenomous) of left ear**
    - ● **S00.469 Insect bite (nonvenomous) of unspecified ear**

CHAPTER 19 (S00-T88)

● S00.47   Other superficial bite of ear
            Excludes1   open bite of ear (S01.35)
    ● S00.471   Other superficial bite of right ear
    ● S00.472   Other superficial bite of left ear
    ● S00.479   Other superficial bite of unspecified
                 ear
● S00.5   Superficial injury of lip and oral cavity
    ● S00.50   Unspecified superficial injury of lip and oral
                cavity
        ● S00.501   Unspecified superficial injury of lip
        ● S00.502   Unspecified superficial injury of oral
                     cavity
    ● S00.51   Abrasion of lip and oral cavity
        ● S00.511   Abrasion of lip
        ● S00.512   Abrasion of oral cavity
    ● S00.52   Blister (nonthermal) of lip and oral cavity
        ● S00.521   Blister (nonthermal) of lip
        ● S00.522   Blister (nonthermal) of oral cavity
    ● S00.53   Contusion of lip and oral cavity
        ● S00.531   Contusion of lip
                     Bruise of lip
                     Hematoma of oral cavity
        ● S00.532   Contusion of oral cavity
                     Bruise of lip
                     Hematoma of oral cavity
    ● S00.54   External constriction of lip and oral cavity
        ● S00.541   External constriction of lip
        ● S00.542   External constriction of oral cavity
    ● S00.55   Superficial foreign body of lip and oral cavity
        ● S00.551   Superficial foreign body of lip
                     Splinter of lip and oral cavity
        ● S00.552   Superficial foreign body of oral cavity
                     Splinter of lip and oral cavity
    ● S00.56   Insect bite (nonvenomous) of lip and oral cavity
        ● S00.561   Insect bite (nonvenomous) of lip
        ● S00.562   Insect bite (nonvenomous) of oral
                     cavity
    ● S00.57   Other superficial bite of lip and oral cavity
        ● S00.571   Other superficial bite of lip
                     Excludes1   open bite of lip
                                      (S01.551)
        ● S00.572   Other superficial bite of oral cavity
                     Excludes1   open bite of oral cavity
                                      (S01.552)
● S00.8   Superficial injury of other parts of head
           Superficial injuries of face [any part] ◄
    X ● S00.80   Unspecified superficial injury of other part of
                  head
    X ● S00.81   Abrasion of other part of head
    X ● S00.82   Blister (nonthermal) of other part of head
    X ● S00.83   Contusion of other part of head
                  Bruise of other part of head
                  Hematoma of other part of head
    X ● S00.84   External constriction of other part of head
    X ● S00.85   Superficial foreign body of other part of head
                  Splinter in other part of head
    X ● S00.86   Insect bite (nonvenomous) of other part of head
    X ● S00.87   Other superficial bite of other part of head
                  Excludes1   open bite of other part of head
                                   (S01.85)
● S00.9   Superficial injury of unspecified part of head
    X ● S00.90   Unspecified superficial injury of unspecified
                  part of head
    X ● S00.91   Abrasion of unspecified part of head
    X ● S00.92   Blister (nonthermal) of unspecified part of head
    X ● S00.93   Contusion of unspecified part of head
                  Bruise of head
                  Hematoma of head

X ● S00.94   External constriction of unspecified part of head
X ● S00.95   Superficial foreign body of unspecified part of
              head
              Splinter of head
X ● S00.96   Insect bite (nonvenomous) of unspecified part
              of head
X ● S00.97   Other superficial bite of unspecified part of
              head
              Excludes1   open bite of head (S01.95)

● S01   Open wound of head
         Code also any associated:
            injury of cranial nerve (S04.-)
            injury of muscle and tendon of head (S09.1-)
            intracranial injury (S06.-)
            wound infection
         Excludes1   open skull fracture (S02.- with 7th character B)
         Excludes2   injury of eye and orbit (S05.-)
                          traumatic amputation of part of head (S08.-)
         The appropriate 7th character is to be added to each code from
         category S01

         ┌─────────────────────────────────────┐
         │ A   initial encounter   │
         │ D   subsequent encounter   │
         │ S   sequela   │
         └─────────────────────────────────────┘

    ● S01.0   Open wound of scalp
               Excludes1   avulsion of scalp (S08.0)
        X ● S01.00   Unspecified open wound of scalp
        X ● S01.01   Laceration without foreign body of scalp
        X ● S01.02   Laceration with foreign body of scalp
                      Coding Clinic: 2015, Q1, P5-7
        X ● S01.03   Puncture wound without foreign body of scalp
        X ● S01.04   Puncture wound with foreign body of scalp
        X ● S01.05   Open bite of scalp
                      Bite of scalp NOS
                      Excludes1   superficial bite of scalp (S00.06,
                                       S00.07-)
    ● S01.1   Open wound of eyelid and periocular area
               Open wound of eyelid and periocular area with or
               without involvement of lacrimal passages
        ● S01.10   Unspecified open wound of eyelid and
                    periocular area
            ● S01.101   Unspecified open wound of right
                         eyelid and periocular area
            ● S01.102   Unspecified open wound of left
                         eyelid and periocular area
            ● S01.109   Unspecified open wound of
                         unspecified eyelid and periocular area
        ● S01.11   Laceration without foreign body of eyelid and
                    periocular area
            ● S01.111   Laceration without foreign body of
                         right eyelid and periocular area
            ● S01.112   Laceration without foreign body of
                         left eyelid and periocular area
            ● S01.119   Laceration without foreign body of
                         unspecified eyelid and periocular area
        ● S01.12   Laceration with foreign body of eyelid and
                    periocular area
            ● S01.121   Laceration with foreign body of right
                         eyelid and periocular area
            ● S01.122   Laceration with foreign body of left
                         eyelid and periocular area
            ● S01.129   Laceration with foreign body of
                         unspecified eyelid and periocular area

CHAPTER 19 (S00-T88)

CHAPTER 19 (S00-T88)

● S01.13   Puncture wound without foreign body of eyelid and periocular area
   ● S01.131   Puncture wound without foreign body of right eyelid and periocular area
   ● S01.132   Puncture wound without foreign body of left eyelid and periocular area
   ● S01.139   Puncture wound without foreign body of unspecified eyelid and periocular area

● S01.14   Puncture wound with foreign body of eyelid and periocular area
   ● S01.141   Puncture wound with foreign body of right eyelid and periocular area
   ● S01.142   Puncture wound with foreign body of left eyelid and periocular area
   ● S01.149   Puncture wound with foreign body of unspecified eyelid and periocular area

● S01.15   Open bite of eyelid and periocular area
    Bite of eyelid and periocular area NOS
    Excludes1   superficial bite of eyelid and periocular area (S00.26, S00.27)
   ● S01.151   Open bite of right eyelid and periocular area
   ● S01.152   Open bite of left eyelid and periocular area
   ● S01.159   Open bite of unspecified eyelid and periocular area

● S01.2   Open wound of nose
  X ● S01.20   Unspecified open wound of nose
  X ● S01.21   Laceration without foreign body of nose
    Coding Clinic: 2015, Q1, P5-6
  X ● S01.22   Laceration with foreign body of nose
  X ● S01.23   Puncture wound without foreign body of nose
  X ● S01.24   Puncture wound with foreign body of nose
  X ● S01.25   Open bite of nose
    Bite of nose NOS
    Excludes1   superficial bite of nose (S00.36, S00.37)

● S01.3   Open wound of ear
  ● S01.30   Unspecified open wound of ear
   ● S01.301   Unspecified open wound of right ear
   ● S01.302   Unspecified open wound of left ear
   ● S01.309   Unspecified open wound of unspecified ear
  ● S01.31   Laceration without foreign body of ear
   ● S01.311   Laceration without foreign body of right ear
   ● S01.312   Laceration without foreign body of left ear
   ● S01.319   Laceration without foreign body of unspecified ear
  ● S01.32   Laceration with foreign body of ear
   ● S01.321   Laceration with foreign body of right ear
   ● S01.322   Laceration with foreign body of left ear
   ● S01.329   Laceration with foreign body of unspecified ear
  ● S01.33   Puncture wound without foreign body of ear
   ● S01.331   Puncture wound without foreign body of right ear
   ● S01.332   Puncture wound without foreign body of left ear
   ● S01.339   Puncture wound without foreign body of unspecified ear

● S01.34   Puncture wound with foreign body of ear
   ● S01.341   Puncture wound with foreign body of right ear
   ● S01.342   Puncture wound with foreign body of left ear
   ● S01.349   Puncture wound with foreign body of unspecified ear

● S01.35   Open bite of ear
    Bite of ear NOS
    Excludes1   superficial bite of ear (S00.46, S00.47)
   ● S01.351   Open bite of right ear
   ● S01.352   Open bite of left ear
   ● S01.359   Open bite of unspecified ear

● S01.4   Open wound of cheek and temporomandibular area
  ● S01.40   Unspecified open wound of cheek and temporomandibular area
   ● S01.401   Unspecified open wound of right cheek and temporomandibular area
   ● S01.402   Unspecified open wound of left cheek and temporomandibular area
   ● S01.409   Unspecified open wound of unspecified cheek and temporomandibular area
  ● S01.41   Laceration without foreign body of cheek and temporomandibular area
   ● S01.411   Laceration without foreign body of right cheek and temporomandibular area
    Coding Clinic: 2015, Q1, P5-7
   ● S01.412   Laceration without foreign body of left cheek and temporomandibular area
   ● S01.419   Laceration without foreign body of unspecified cheek and temporomandibular area
  ● S01.42   Laceration with foreign body of cheek and temporomandibular area
   ● S01.421   Laceration with foreign body of right cheek and temporomandibular area
   ● S01.422   Laceration with foreign body of left cheek and temporomandibular area
   ● S01.429   Laceration with foreign body of unspecified cheek and temporomandibular area
  ● S01.43   Puncture wound without foreign body of cheek and temporomandibular area
   ● S01.431   Puncture wound without foreign body of right cheek and temporomandibular area
   ● S01.432   Puncture wound without foreign body of left cheek and temporomandibular area
   ● S01.439   Puncture wound without foreign body of unspecified cheek and temporomandibular area
  ● S01.44   Puncture wound with foreign body of cheek and temporomandibular area
   ● S01.441   Puncture wound with foreign body of right cheek and temporomandibular area
   ● S01.442   Puncture wound with foreign body of left cheek and temporomandibular area
   ● S01.449   Puncture wound with foreign body of unspecified cheek and temporomandibular area

◀ New   ◀|||| Revised   ~~deleted~~ Deleted   Excludes 1   Excludes 2   Includes   Use additional   Code first   Code also   Unspecified

OGCR Official Guidelines   X Assign placeholder X   ● Use Additional Character(s)   ▶ Manifestation Code   **Coding Clinic**

- **S01.45** **Open bite of cheek and temporomandibular area**
  Bite of cheek and temporomandibular area NOS
  > **Excludes2**   superficial bite of cheek and temporomandibular area (S00.86, S00.87)
  - **S01.451** **Open bite of right cheek and temporomandibular area**
  - **S01.452** **Open bite of left cheek and temporomandibular area**
  - **S01.459** **Open bite of unspecified cheek and temporomandibular area**
- **S01.5** **Open wound of lip and oral cavity**
  > **Excludes2**   tooth dislocation (S03.2)
  > tooth fracture (S02.5)
  - **S01.50** **Unspecified open wound of lip and oral cavity**
    - **S01.501** **Unspecified open wound of lip**
    - **S01.502** **Unspecified open wound of oral cavity**
  - **S01.51** **Laceration of lip and oral cavity without foreign body**
    - **S01.511** **Laceration without foreign body of lip**
    - **S01.512** **Laceration without foreign body of oral cavity**
  - **S01.52** **Laceration of lip and oral cavity with foreign body**
    - **S01.521** **Laceration with foreign body of lip**
    - **S01.522** **Laceration with foreign body of oral cavity**
  - **S01.53** **Puncture wound of lip and oral cavity without foreign body**
    - **S01.531** **Puncture wound without foreign body of lip**
    - **S01.532** **Puncture wound without foreign body of oral cavity**
  - **S01.54** **Puncture wound of lip and oral cavity with foreign body**
    - **S01.541** **Puncture wound with foreign body of lip**
    - **S01.542** **Puncture wound with foreign body of oral cavity**
  - **S01.55** **Open bite of lip and oral cavity**
    - **S01.551** **Open bite of lip**
      Bite of lip NOS
      > **Excludes1**   superficial bite of lip (S00.571)
    - **S01.552** **Open bite of oral cavity**
      Bite of oral cavity NOS
      > **Excludes1**   superficial bite of oral cavity (S00.572)
- **S01.8** **Open wound of other parts of head**
  - X **S01.80** **Unspecified open wound of other part of head**
  - X **S01.81** **Laceration without foreign body of other part of head**
  - X **S01.82** **Laceration with foreign body of other part of head**
  - X **S01.83** **Puncture wound without foreign body of other part of head**
  - X **S01.84** **Puncture wound with foreign body of other part of head**
  - X **S01.85** **Open bite of other part of head**
    Bite of other part of head NOS
    > **Excludes1**   superficial bite of other part of head (S00.85)

- **S01.9** **Open wound of unspecified part of head**
  - X **S01.90** **Unspecified open wound of unspecified part of head**
  - X **S01.91** **Laceration without foreign body of unspecified part of head**
  - X **S01.92** **Laceration with foreign body of unspecified part of head**
  - X **S01.93** **Puncture wound without foreign body of unspecified part of head**
  - X **S01.94** **Puncture wound with foreign body of unspecified part of head**
  - X **S01.95** **Open bite of unspecified part of head**
    Bite of head NOS
    > **Excludes1**   superficial bite of head NOS (S00.97)
- **S02** **Fracture of skull and facial bones**
  Note: A fracture not indicated as open or closed should be coded to closed
  The appropriate 7th character is to be added to each code from category S02

A	initial encounter for closed fracture
B	initial encounter for open fracture
D	subsequent encounter for fracture with routine healing
G	subsequent encounter for fracture with delayed healing
K	subsequent encounter for fracture with nonunion
S	sequela

  Code also any associated intracranial injury (S06.-)
  - X **S02.0** **Fracture of vault of skull**
    Fracture of frontal bone
    Fracture of parietal bone
  - **S02.1** **Fracture of base of skull**
    > **Excludes1**   orbit NOS (S02.8)
    > **Excludes2**   orbital floor (S02.3-)
    - **S02.10** **Unspecified fracture of base of skull**
      - **S02.101** **Fracture of base of skull, right side** ◀
      - **S02.102** **Fracture of base of skull, left side** ◀
      - **S02.109** **Fracture of base of skull, unspecified side** ◀
    - **S02.11** **Fracture of occiput**
      - **S02.110** **Type I occipital condyle fracture, unspecified side**
      - **S02.111** **Type II occipital condyle fracture, unspecified side**
      - **S02.112** **Type III occipital condyle fracture, unspecified side**
      - **S02.113** **Unspecified occipital condyle fracture**
      - **S02.118** **Other fracture of occiput, unspecified side**
      - **S02.119** **Unspecified fracture of occiput**
      - **S02.11A** **Type I occipital condyle fracture, right side**
      - **S02.11B** **Type I occipital condyle fracture, left side**
      - **S02.11C** **Type II occipital condyle fracture, right side**
      - **S02.11D** **Type II occipital condyle fracture, left side**
      - **S02.11E** **Type III occipital condyle fracture, right side**
      - **S02.11F** **Type III occipital condyle fracture, left side**
      - **S02.11G** **Other fracture of occiput, right side**
      - **S02.11H** **Other fracture of occiput, left side**

CHAPTER 19 (S00-T88)

X ● **S02.19** **Other fracture of base of skull**
Fracture of anterior fossa of base of skull
Fracture of ethmoid sinus
Fracture of frontal sinus
Fracture of middle fossa of base of skull
Fracture of orbital roof
Fracture of posterior fossa of base of skull
Fracture of sphenoid
Fracture of temporal bone

X ● **S02.2** **Fracture of nasal bones**

● **S02.3** **Fracture of orbital floor**
Excludes1 orbit NOS (S02.8)
Excludes2 orbital roof (S02.1-)

X ● **S02.30** **Fracture of orbital floor, unspecified side**
X ● **S02.31** **Fracture of orbital floor, right side**
X ● **S02.32** **Fracture of orbital floor, left side**

● **S02.4** **Fracture of malar, maxillary and zygoma bones**
Fracture of superior maxilla
Fracture of upper jaw (bone)
Fracture of zygomatic process of temporal bone

● **S02.40** **Fracture of malar, maxillary and zygoma bones, unspecified**
● **S02.400** Malar fracture unspecified side
● **S02.401** Maxillary fracture, unspecified side
● **S02.402** Zygomatic fracture, unspecified side
● **S02.40A** Malar fracture, right side
● **S02.40B** Malar fracture, left side
● **S02.40C** Maxillary fracture, right side
● **S02.40D** Maxillary fracture, left side
● **S02.40E** Zygomatic fracture, right side
● **S02.40F** Zygomatic fracture, left side

● **S02.41** **LeFort fracture**
● **S02.411** LeFort I fracture
● **S02.412** LeFort II fracture
● **S02.413** LeFort III fracture

X ● **S02.42** **Fracture of alveolus of maxilla**

X ● **S02.5** **Fracture of tooth (traumatic) Broken tooth**
Excludes1 cracked tooth (nontraumatic) (K03.81)

● **S02.6** **Fracture of mandible**
Fracture of lower jaw (bone)

● **S02.60** **Fracture of mandible of unspecified site**
● **S02.600** Fracture of unspecified part of body of mandible, unspecified side
● **S02.601** Fracture of unspecified part of body of right mandible
● **S02.602** Fracture of unspecified part of body of left mandible
● **S02.609** Fracture of mandible, unspecified

● **S02.61** **Fracture of condylar process of mandible**
● **S02.610** Fracture of condylar process of mandible, unspecified side
● **S02.611** Fracture of condylar process of right mandible
● **S02.612** Fracture of condylar process of left mandible

● **S02.62** **Fracture of subcondylar process of mandible**
● **S02.620** Fracture of subcondylar process of mandible, unspecified side
● **S02.621** Fracture of subcondylar process of right mandible
● **S02.622** Fracture of subcondylar process of left mandible

● **S02.63** **Fracture of coronoid process of mandible**
● **S02.630** Fracture of coronoid process of mandible, unspecified side
● **S02.631** Fracture of coronoid process of right mandible
● **S02.632** Fracture of coronoid process of left mandible

● **S02.64** **Fracture of ramus of mandible**
● **S02.640** Fracture of ramus of mandible, unspecified side
● **S02.641** Fracture of ramus of right mandible
● **S02.642** Fracture of ramus of left mandible

● **S02.65** **Fracture of angle of mandible**
● **S02.650** Fracture of angle of mandible, unspecified side
● **S02.651** Fracture of angle of right mandible
● **S02.652** Fracture of angle of left mandible

X ● **S02.66** **Fracture of symphysis of mandible**

● **S02.67** **Fracture of alveolus of mandible**
● **S02.670** Fracture of alveolus of mandible, unspecified side
● **S02.671** Fracture of alveolus of right mandible
● **S02.672** Fracture of alveolus of left mandible

X ● **S02.69** **Fracture of mandible of other specified site**

● **S02.8** **Fractures of other specified skull and facial bones**
Fracture of orbit NOS
Fracture of palate
Excludes1 fracture of orbital floor (S02.3-)
fracture of orbital roof (S02.1-)

X ● **S02.80** **Fracture of other specified skull and facial bones, unspecified side**
X ● **S02.81** **Fracture of other specified skull and facial bones, right side**
X ● **S02.82** **Fracture of other specified skull and facial bones, left side**

● **S02.9** **Fracture of unspecified skull and facial bones**
X ● **S02.91** Unspecified fracture of skull
X ● **S02.92** Unspecified fracture of facial bones

● **S03** **Dislocation and sprain of joints and ligaments of head**
Includes avulsion of joint (capsule) or ligament of head
laceration of cartilage, joint (capsule) or ligament of head
sprain of cartilage, joint (capsule) or ligament of head
traumatic hemarthrosis of joint or ligament of head
traumatic rupture of joint or ligament of head
traumatic subluxation of joint or ligament of head
traumatic tear of joint or ligament of head

Code also any associated open wound
Excludes2 Strain of muscle or tendon of head (S09.1)
The appropriate 7th character is to be added to each code from category S03

A	initial encounter
D	subsequent encounter
S	sequela

● **S03.0** **Dislocation of jaw**
Dislocation of jaw (cartilage) (meniscus)
Dislocation of mandible
Dislocation of temporomandibular (joint)
X ● **S03.00** Dislocation of jaw, unspecified side
X ● **S03.01** Dislocation of jaw, right side
X ● **S03.02** Dislocation of jaw, left side
X ● **S03.03** Dislocation of jaw, bilateral side

X ● **S03.1** **Dislocation of septal cartilage of nose**
X ● **S03.2** **Dislocation of tooth**

● **S03.4** **Sprain of jaw**
Sprain of temporomandibular (joint) (ligament)
X ● **S03.40** Sprain of jaw, unspecified side
X ● **S03.41** Sprain of jaw, right side
X ● **S03.42** Sprain of jaw, left side
X ● **S03.43** Sprain of jaw, bilateral side

X ● **S03.8** **Sprain of joints and ligaments of other parts of head**
X ● **S03.9** **Sprain of joints and ligaments of unspecified parts of head**

CHAPTER 19 (S00-T88)

◀ New   ◀▬▬ Revised   ~~deleted~~ Deleted   Excludes 1   Excludes 2   Includes   Use additional   Code first   Code also   Unspecified
OGCR Official Guidelines   X Assign placeholder X   ● Use Additional Character(s)   ▶ Manifestation Code   **Coding Clinic**

● **S04** **Injury of cranial nerve**
  The selection of side should be based on the side of the body
   being affected
  Code first any associated intracranial injury (S06.-)
  Code also any associated:
   open wound of head (S01.-)
   skull fracture (S02.-)
  The appropriate 7th character is to be added to each code from
   category S04

> A initial encounter
> D subsequent encounter
> S sequela

● **S04.0** **Injury of optic nerve and pathways**
   Use additional code to identify any visual field defect
   or blindness (H53.4-, H54)
  ● **S04.01** **Injury of optic nerve**
    Injury of 2nd cranial nerve
   ● **S04.011** **Injury of optic nerve, right eye**
   ● **S04.012** **Injury of optic nerve, left eye**
   ● **S04.019** **Injury of optic nerve, unspecified eye**
     Injury of optic nerve NOS
  X ● **S04.02** **Injury of optic chiasm**
  ● **S04.03** **Injury of optic tract and pathways**
    Injury of optic radiation
   ● **S04.031** **Injury of optic tract and pathways,
     right eye**
   ● **S04.032** **Injury of optic tract and pathways,
     left eye**
   ● **S04.039** **Injury of optic tract and pathways,
     unspecified eye**
     Injury of optic tract and pathways
     NOS
  ● **S04.04** **Injury of visual cortex**
   ● **S04.041** **Injury of visual cortex, right eye**
   ● **S04.042** **Injury of visual cortex, left eye**
   ● **S04.049** **Injury of visual cortex, unspecified eye**
     Injury of visual cortex NOS

● **S04.1** **Injury of oculomotor nerve**
   Injury of 3rd cranial nerve
  X ● **S04.10** **Injury of oculomotor nerve, unspecified side**
  X ● **S04.11** **Injury of oculomotor nerve, right side**
  X ● **S04.12** **Injury of oculomotor nerve, left side**
● **S04.2** **Injury of trochlear nerve**
   Injury of 4th cranial nerve
  X ● **S04.20** **Injury of trochlear nerve, unspecified side**
  X ● **S04.21** **Injury of trochlear nerve, right side**
  X ● **S04.22** **Injury of trochlear nerve, left side**
● **S04.3** **Injury of trigeminal nerve**
   Injury of 5th cranial nerve
  X ● **S04.30** **Injury of trigeminal nerve, unspecified side**
  X ● **S04.31** **Injury of trigeminal nerve, right side**
  X ● **S04.32** **Injury of trigeminal nerve, left side**
● **S04.4** **Injury of abducent nerve**
   Injury of 6th cranial nerve
  X ● **S04.40** **Injury of abducent nerve, unspecified side**
  X ● **S04.41** **Injury of abducent nerve, right side**
  X ● **S04.42** **Injury of abducent nerve, left side**
● **S04.5** **Injury of facial nerve**
   Injury of 7th cranial nerve
  X ● **S04.50** **Injury of facial nerve, unspecified side**
  X ● **S04.51** **Injury of facial nerve, right side**
  X ● **S04.52** **Injury of facial nerve, left side**
● **S04.6** **Injury of acoustic nerve**
   Injury of auditory nerve
   Injury of 8th cranial nerve
  X ● **S04.60** **Injury of acoustic nerve, unspecified side**
  X ● **S04.61** **Injury of acoustic nerve, right side**
  X ● **S04.62** **Injury of acoustic nerve, left side**
● **S04.7** **Injury of accessory nerve**
   Injury of 11th cranial nerve
  X ● **S04.70** **Injury of accessory nerve, unspecified side**
  X ● **S04.71** **Injury of accessory nerve, right side**
  X ● **S04.72** **Injury of accessory nerve, left side**

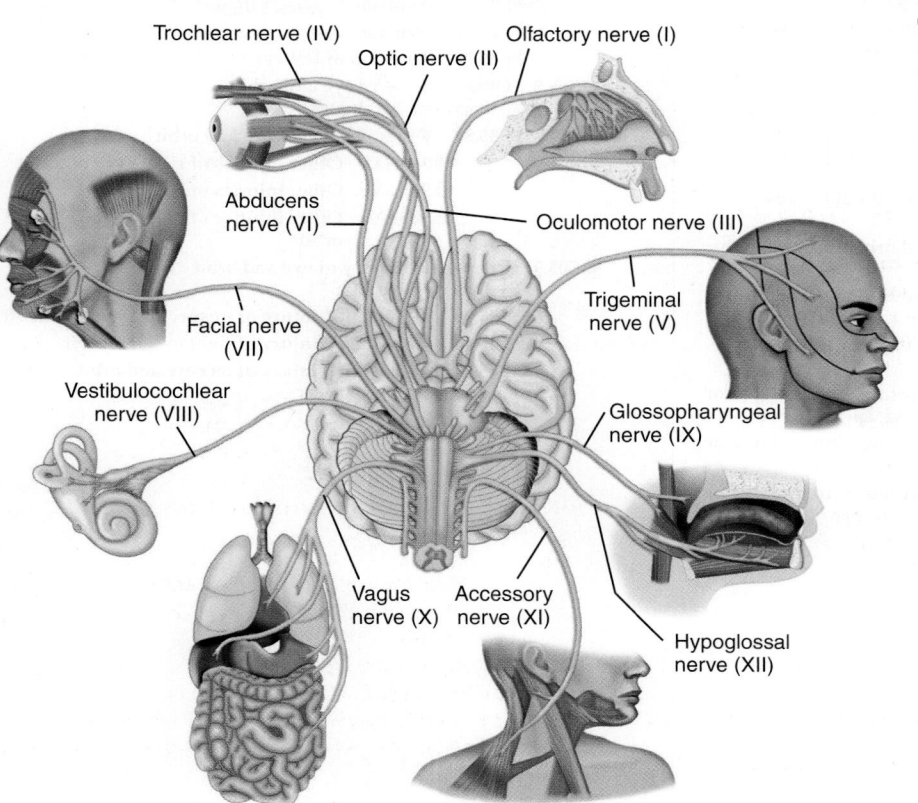

Figure 19-13 Cranial nerves. (From Patton and Thibodeau: Anatomy and physiology, ed 7, St. Louis, Mosby, 2009)

CHAPTER 19 (S00-T88)

● **S04.8   Injury of other cranial nerves**
   ● **S04.81   Injury of olfactory [1st] nerve**
     ● **S04.811   Injury of olfactory [1st] nerve, right side**
     ● **S04.812   Injury of olfactory [1st] nerve, left side**
     ● **S04.819   Injury of olfactory [1st] nerve, unspecified side**
   ● **S04.89   Injury of other cranial nerves**
     Injury of vagus [10th] nerve
     ● **S04.891   Injury of other cranial nerves, right side**
     ● **S04.892   Injury of other cranial nerves, left side**
     ● **S04.899   Injury of other cranial nerves, unspecified side**
X ● **S04.9   Injury of unspecified cranial nerve**

● **S05   Injury of eye and orbit**
   Includes   open wound of eye and orbit
   Excludes2   2nd cranial [optic] nerve injury (S04.0-)
     3rd cranial [oculomotor] nerve injury (S04.1-)
     open wound of eyelid and periocular area (S01.1-)
     orbital bone fracture (S02.1-, S02.3-, S02.8-)
     superficial injury of eyelid (S00.1-S00.2)

The appropriate 7th character is to be added to each code from category S05

   A   initial encounter
   D   subsequent encounter
   S   sequela

● **S05.0   Injury of conjunctiva and corneal abrasion without foreign body**
   Excludes1   foreign body in conjunctival sac (T15.1)
     foreign body in cornea (T15.0)
X ● **S05.00   Injury of conjunctiva and corneal abrasion without foreign body, unspecified eye**
X ● **S05.01   Injury of conjunctiva and corneal abrasion without foreign body, right eye**
X ● **S05.02   Injury of conjunctiva and corneal abrasion without foreign body, left eye**

● **S05.1   Contusion of eyeball and orbital tissues**
   Traumatic hyphema
   Excludes2   black eye NOS (S00.1)
     contusion of eyelid and periocular area (S00.1)
X ● **S05.10   Contusion of eyeball and orbital tissues, unspecified eye**
X ● **S05.11   Contusion of eyeball and orbital tissues, right eye**
X ● **S05.12   Contusion of eyeball and orbital tissues, left eye**

● **S05.2   Ocular laceration and rupture with prolapse or loss of intraocular tissue**
X ● **S05.20   Ocular laceration and rupture with prolapse or loss of intraocular tissue, unspecified eye**
X ● **S05.21   Ocular laceration and rupture with prolapse or loss of intraocular tissue, right eye**
X ● **S05.22   Ocular laceration and rupture with prolapse or loss of intraocular tissue, left eye**

● **S05.3   Ocular laceration without prolapse or loss of intraocular tissue**
   Laceration of eye NOS
X ● **S05.30   Ocular laceration without prolapse or loss of intraocular tissue, unspecified eye**
X ● **S05.31   Ocular laceration without prolapse or loss of intraocular tissue, right eye**
X ● **S05.32   Ocular laceration without prolapse or loss of intraocular tissue, left eye**

● **S05.4   Penetrating wound of orbit with or without foreign body**
   Excludes2   retained (old) foreign body following penetrating wound in orbit (H05.5-)
X ● **S05.40   Penetrating wound of orbit with or without foreign body, unspecified eye**
X ● **S05.41   Penetrating wound of orbit with or without foreign body, right eye**
X ● **S05.42   Penetrating wound of orbit with or without foreign body, left eye**

● **S05.5   Penetrating wound with foreign body of eyeball**
   Excludes2   retained (old) intraocular foreign body (H44.6-, H44.7)
X ● **S05.50   Penetrating wound with foreign body of unspecified eyeball**
X ● **S05.51   Penetrating wound with foreign body of right eyeball**
X ● **S05.52   Penetrating wound with foreign body of left eyeball**

● **S05.6   Penetrating wound without foreign body of eyeball**
   Ocular penetration NOS
X ● **S05.60   Penetrating wound without foreign body of unspecified eyeball**
X ● **S05.61   Penetrating wound without foreign body of right eyeball**
X ● **S05.62   Penetrating wound without foreign body of left eyeball**

● **S05.7   Avulsion of eye**
   Traumatic enucleation
X ● **S05.70   Avulsion of unspecified eye**
X ● **S05.71   Avulsion of right eye**
X ● **S05.72   Avulsion of left eye**

● **S05.8   Other injuries of eye and orbit**
   Lacrimal duct injury
   ● **S05.8X   Other injuries of eye and orbit**
     ● **S05.8X1   Other injuries of right eye and orbit**
     ● **S05.8X2   Other injuries of left eye and orbit**
     ● **S05.8X9   Other injuries of unspecified eye and orbit**

● **S05.9   Unspecified injury of eye and orbit**
   Injury of eye NOS
X ● **S05.90   Unspecified injury of unspecified eye and orbit**
X ● **S05.91   Unspecified injury of right eye and orbit**
X ● **S05.92   Unspecified injury of left eye and orbit**

◀ New   ◀═ Revised   deleted Deleted   Excludes 1   Excludes 2   Includes   Use additional   Code first   Code also   Unspecified

1196   OGCR Official Guidelines   X Assign placeholder X   ● Use Additional Character(s)   ▶ Manifestation Code   **Coding Clinic**

● **S06   Intracranial injury**

| **Includes** | traumatic brain injury |

Code also any associated:
    open wound of head (S01.-)
    skull fracture (S02.-)

| **Excludes1** | head injury NOS (S09.90) |

The appropriate 7th character is to be added to each code from category S06

> A   initial encounter
> D   subsequent encounter
> S   sequela

Coding Clinic: 2015, Q4, P40

● **S06.0   Concussion**
    Commotio cerebri

| **Excludes1** | concussion with other intracranial injuries classified in subcategories S06.1- to S06.6- , S06.81- and S06.82- code to specified intracranial injury ◄▒ |

● **S06.0X   Concussion**
  ● **S06.0X0   Concussion without loss of consciousness**
  ● **S06.0X1   Concussion with loss of consciousness of 30 minutes or less**
    ~~S06.0X2   Concussion with loss of consciousness of 31 minutes to 59 minutes~~
    ~~S06.0X3   Concussion with loss of consciousness of 1 hour to 5 hours 59 minutes~~
    ~~S06.0X4   Concussion with loss of consciousness of 6 hours to 24 hours~~
    ~~S06.0X5   Concussion with loss of consciousness greater than 24 hours with return to pre-existing conscious level~~
    ~~S06.0X6   Concussion with loss of consciousness greater than 24 hours without return to pre-existing conscious level with patient surviving~~
    ~~S06.0X7   Concussion with loss of consciousness of any duration with death due to brain injury prior to regaining consciousness~~
    ~~S06.0X8   Concussion with loss of consciousness of any duration with death due to other cause prior to regaining consciousness~~
  ● **S06.0X9   Concussion with loss of consciousness of** unspecified **duration**
    Concussion NOS

● **S06.1   Traumatic cerebral edema**
    Diffuse traumatic cerebral edema
    Focal traumatic cerebral edema
● **S06.1X   Traumatic cerebral edema**
  ● **S06.1X0   Traumatic cerebral edema without loss of consciousness**
    Coding Clinic: 2015, Q1, P12
  ● **S06.1X1   Traumatic cerebral edema with loss of consciousness of 30 minutes or less**
  ● **S06.1X2   Traumatic cerebral edema with loss of consciousness of 31 minutes to 59 minutes**
  ● **S06.1X3   Traumatic cerebral edema with loss of consciousness of 1 hour to 5 hours 59 minutes**
  ● **S06.1X4   Traumatic cerebral edema with loss of consciousness of 6 hours to 24 hours**
  ● **S06.1X5   Traumatic cerebral edema with loss of consciousness greater than 24 hours with return to pre-existing conscious level**
  ● **S06.1X6   Traumatic cerebral edema with loss of consciousness greater than 24 hours without return to pre-existing conscious level with patient surviving**
  ● **S06.1X7   Traumatic cerebral edema with loss of consciousness of any duration with death due to brain injury prior to regaining consciousness**
  ● **S06.1X8   Traumatic cerebral edema with loss of consciousness of any duration with death due to other cause prior to regaining consciousness**
  ● **S06.1X9   Traumatic cerebral edema with loss of consciousness of** unspecified **duration**
    Traumatic cerebral edema NOS

● **S06.2   Diffuse traumatic brain injury**
    Diffuse axonal brain injury

| **Excludes1** | traumatic diffuse cerebral edema (S06.1X-) |

● **S06.2X   Diffuse traumatic brain injury**
  ● **S06.2X0   Diffuse traumatic brain injury without loss of consciousness**
  ● **S06.2X1   Diffuse traumatic brain injury with loss of consciousness of 30 minutes or less**
  ● **S06.2X2   Diffuse traumatic brain injury with loss of consciousness of 31 minutes to 59 minutes**
  ● **S06.2X3   Diffuse traumatic brain injury with loss of consciousness of 1 hour to 5 hours 59 minutes**
  ● **S06.2X4   Diffuse traumatic brain injury with loss of consciousness of 6 hours to 24 hours**
  ● **S06.2X5   Diffuse traumatic brain injury with loss of consciousness greater than 24 hours with return to pre-existing conscious levels**
  ● **S06.2X6   Diffuse traumatic brain injury with loss of consciousness greater than 24 hours without return to pre-existing conscious level with patient surviving**
  ● **S06.2X7   Diffuse traumatic brain injury with loss of consciousness of any duration with death due to brain injury prior to regaining consciousness**
  ● **S06.2X8   Diffuse traumatic brain injury with loss of consciousness of any duration with death due to other cause prior to regaining consciousness**
  ● **S06.2X9   Diffuse traumatic brain injury with loss of consciousness of** unspecified **duration**
    Diffuse traumatic brain injury NOS

CHAPTER 19 (S00-T88)

● **S06.3**   **Focal traumatic brain injury**
     Excludes1   any condition classifiable to S06.4–S06.6
                  focal cerebral edema (S06.1)
   ● **S06.30**   **Unspecified focal traumatic brain injury**
     ● **S06.300**   Unspecified focal traumatic brain injury without loss of consciousness
     ● **S06.301**   Unspecified focal traumatic brain injury with loss of consciousness of 30 minutes or less
     ● **S06.302**   Unspecified focal traumatic brain injury with loss of consciousness of 31 minutes to 59 minutes
     ● **S06.303**   Unspecified focal traumatic brain injury with loss of consciousness of 1 hour to 5 hours 59 minutes
     ● **S06.304**   Unspecified focal traumatic brain injury with loss of consciousness of 6 hours to 24 hours
     ● **S06.305**   Unspecified focal traumatic brain injury with loss of consciousness greater than 24 hours with return to pre-existing conscious level
     ● **S06.306**   Unspecified focal traumatic brain injury with loss of consciousness greater than 24 hours without return to pre-existing conscious level with patient surviving
     ● **S06.307**   Unspecified focal traumatic brain injury with loss of consciousness of any duration with death due to brain injury prior to regaining consciousness
     ● **S06.308**   Unspecified focal traumatic brain injury with loss of consciousness of any duration with death due to other cause prior to regaining consciousness
     ● **S06.309**   Unspecified focal traumatic brain injury with loss of consciousness of unspecified duration
            Unspecified focal traumatic brain injury NOS
   ● **S06.31**   **Contusion and laceration of right cerebrum**
     ● **S06.310**   Contusion and laceration of right cerebrum without loss of consciousness
     ● **S06.311**   Contusion and laceration of right cerebrum with loss of consciousness of 30 minutes or less
     ● **S06.312**   Contusion and laceration of right cerebrum with loss of consciousness of 31 minutes to 59 minutes
     ● **S06.313**   Contusion and laceration of right cerebrum with loss of consciousness of 1 hour to 5 hours 59 minutes
     ● **S06.314**   Contusion and laceration of right cerebrum with loss of consciousness of 6 hours to 24 hours
     ● **S06.315**   Contusion and laceration of right cerebrum with loss of consciousness greater than 24 hours with return to pre-existing conscious level
     ● **S06.316**   Contusion and laceration of right cerebrum with loss of consciousness greater than 24 hours without return to pre-existing conscious level with patient surviving
     ● **S06.317**   Contusion and laceration of right cerebrum with loss of consciousness of any duration with death due to brain injury prior to regaining consciousness

     ● **S06.318**   Contusion and laceration of right cerebrum with loss of consciousness of any duration with death due to other cause prior to regaining consciousness
     ● **S06.319**   Contusion and laceration of right cerebrum with loss of consciousness of unspecified duration
            Contusion and laceration of right cerebrum NOS
   ● **S06.32**   **Contusion and laceration of left cerebrum**
     ● **S06.320**   Contusion and laceration of left cerebrum without loss of consciousness
     ● **S06.321**   Contusion and laceration of left cerebrum with loss of consciousness of 30 minutes or less
     ● **S06.322**   Contusion and laceration of left cerebrum with loss of consciousness of 31 minutes to 59 minutes
     ● **S06.323**   Contusion and laceration of left cerebrum with loss of consciousness of 1 hour to 5 hours 59 minutes
     ● **S06.324**   Contusion and laceration of left cerebrum with loss of consciousness of 6 hours to 24 hours
     ● **S06.325**   Contusion and laceration of left cerebrum with loss of consciousness greater than 24 hours with return to pre-existing conscious level
     ● **S06.326**   Contusion and laceration of left cerebrum with loss of consciousness greater than 24 hours without return to pre-existing conscious level with patient surviving
     ● **S06.327**   Contusion and laceration of left cerebrum with loss of consciousness of any duration with death due to brain injury prior to regaining consciousness
     ● **S06.328**   Contusion and laceration of left cerebrum with loss of consciousness of any duration with death due to other cause prior to regaining consciousness
     ● **S06.329**   Contusion and laceration of left cerebrum with loss of consciousness of unspecified duration
            Contusion and laceration of left cerebrum NOS
   ● **S06.33**   **Contusion and laceration of cerebrum, unspecified**
     ● **S06.330**   Contusion and laceration of cerebrum, unspecified, without loss of consciousness
     ● **S06.331**   Contusion and laceration of cerebrum, unspecified, with loss of consciousness of 30 minutes or less
     ● **S06.332**   Contusion and laceration of cerebrum, unspecified, with loss of consciousness of 31 minutes to 59 minutes
     ● **S06.333**   Contusion and laceration of cerebrum, unspecified, with loss of consciousness of 1 hour to 5 hours 59 minutes
     ● **S06.334**   Contusion and laceration of cerebrum, unspecified, with loss of consciousness of 6 hours to 24 hours
     ● **S06.335**   Contusion and laceration of cerebrum, unspecified, with loss of consciousness greater than 24 hours with return to pre-existing conscious level

◀ New   ◀▭ Revised   ~~deleted~~ Deleted   Excludes 1   Excludes 2   Includes   Use additional   Code first   Code also   Unspecified
OGCR Official Guidelines   X Assign placeholder X   ● Use Additional Character(s)   ▷ Manifestation Code   **Coding Clinic**

● **S06.336**   Contusion and laceration of cerebrum, unspecified, with loss of consciousness greater than 24 hours without return to pre-existing conscious level with patient surviving

● **S06.337**   Contusion and laceration of cerebrum, unspecified, with loss of consciousness of any duration with death due to brain injury prior to regaining consciousness

● **S06.338**   Contusion and laceration of cerebrum, unspecified, with loss of consciousness of any duration with death due to other cause prior to regaining consciousness

● **S06.339**   Contusion and laceration of cerebrum, unspecified, with loss of consciousness of unspecified duration
     Contusion and laceration of cerebrum NOS

● **S06.34**   Traumatic hemorrhage of right cerebrum
     Traumatic intracerebral hemorrhage and hematoma of right cerebrum

● **S06.340**   Traumatic hemorrhage of right cerebrum without loss of consciousness
     Coding Clinic: 2015, Q1, P12

● **S06.341**   Traumatic hemorrhage of right cerebrum with loss of consciousness of 30 minutes or less

● **S06.342**   Traumatic hemorrhage of right cerebrum with loss of consciousness of 31 minutes to 59 minutes

● **S06.343**   Traumatic hemorrhage of right cerebrum with loss of consciousness of 1 hours to 5 hours 59 minutes

● **S06.344**   Traumatic hemorrhage of right cerebrum with loss of consciousness of 6 hours to 24 hours

● **S06.345**   Traumatic hemorrhage of right cerebrum with loss of consciousness greater than 24 hours with return to pre-existing conscious level

● **S06.346**   Traumatic hemorrhage of right cerebrum with loss of consciousness greater than 24 hours without return to pre-existing conscious level with patient surviving

● **S06.347**   Traumatic hemorrhage of right cerebrum with loss of consciousness of any duration with death due to brain injury prior to regaining consciousness

● **S06.348**   Traumatic hemorrhage of right cerebrum with loss of consciousness of any duration with death due to other cause prior to regaining consciousness

● **S06.349**   Traumatic hemorrhage of right cerebrum with loss of consciousness of unspecified duration
     Traumatic hemorrhage of right cerebrum NOS

● **S06.35**   Traumatic hemorrhage of left cerebrum
     Traumatic intracerebral hemorrhage and hematoma of left cerebrum

● **S06.350**   Traumatic hemorrhage of left cerebrum without loss of consciousness

● **S06.351**   Traumatic hemorrhage of left cerebrum with loss of consciousness of 30 minutes or less

● **S06.352**   Traumatic hemorrhage of left cerebrum with loss of consciousness of 31 minutes to 59 minutes

● **S06.353**   Traumatic hemorrhage of left cerebrum with loss of consciousness of 1 hours to 5 hours 59 minutes

● **S06.354**   Traumatic hemorrhage of left cerebrum with loss of consciousness of 6 hours to 24 hours

● **S06.355**   Traumatic hemorrhage of left cerebrum with loss of consciousness greater than 24 hours with return to pre-existing conscious level

● **S06.356**   Traumatic hemorrhage of left cerebrum with loss of consciousness greater than 24 hours without return to pre-existing conscious level with patient surviving

● **S06.357**   Traumatic hemorrhage of left cerebrum with loss of consciousness of any duration with death due to brain injury prior to regaining consciousness

● **S06.358**   Traumatic hemorrhage of left cerebrum with loss of consciousness of any duration with death due to other cause prior to regaining consciousness

● **S06.359**   Traumatic hemorrhage of left cerebrum with loss of consciousness of unspecified duration
     Traumatic hemorrhage of left cerebrum NOS

● **S06.36**   Traumatic hemorrhage of cerebrum, unspecified
     Traumatic intracerebral hemorrhage and hematoma, unspecified

● **S06.360**   Traumatic hemorrhage of cerebrum, unspecified, without loss of consciousness

● **S06.361**   Traumatic hemorrhage of cerebrum, unspecified, with loss of consciousness of 30 minutes or less

● **S06.362**   Traumatic hemorrhage of cerebrum, unspecified, with loss of consciousness of 31 minutes to 59 minutes

● **S06.363**   Traumatic hemorrhage of cerebrum, unspecified, with loss of consciousness of 1 hours to 5 hours 59 minutes

● **S06.364**   Traumatic hemorrhage of cerebrum, unspecified, with loss of consciousness of 6 hours to 24 hours

● **S06.365**   Traumatic hemorrhage of cerebrum, unspecified, with loss of consciousness greater than 24 hours with return to pre-existing conscious level

● **S06.366**   Traumatic hemorrhage of cerebrum, unspecified, with loss of consciousness greater than 24 hours without return to pre-existing conscious level with patient surviving

● **S06.367**   Traumatic hemorrhage of cerebrum, unspecified, with loss of consciousness of any duration with death due to brain injury prior to regaining consciousness

● **S06.368**   Traumatic hemorrhage of cerebrum, unspecified, with loss of consciousness of any duration with death due to other cause prior to regaining consciousness

● **S06.369**   Traumatic hemorrhage of cerebrum, unspecified, with loss of consciousness of unspecified duration
     Traumatic hemorrhage of cerebrum NOS

CHAPTER 19 (S00-T88)

● S06.37   Contusion, laceration, and hemorrhage of cerebellum

● S06.370   Contusion, laceration, and hemorrhage of cerebellum without loss of consciousness

● S06.371   Contusion, laceration, and hemorrhage of cerebellum with loss of consciousness of 30 minutes or less

● S06.372   Contusion, laceration, and hemorrhage of cerebellum with loss of consciousness of 31 minutes to 59 minutes

● S06.373   Contusion, laceration, and hemorrhage of cerebellum with loss of consciousness of 1 hour to 5 hours 59 minutes

● S06.374   Contusion, laceration, and hemorrhage of cerebellum with loss of consciousness of 6 hours to 24 hours

● S06.375   Contusion, laceration, and hemorrhage of cerebellum with loss of consciousness greater than 24 hours with return to pre-existing conscious level

● S06.376   Contusion, laceration, and hemorrhage of cerebellum with loss of consciousness greater than 24 hours without return to pre-existing conscious level with patient surviving

● S06.377   Contusion, laceration, and hemorrhage of cerebellum with loss of consciousness of any duration with death due to brain injury prior to regaining consciousness

● S06.378   Contusion, laceration, and hemorrhage of cerebellum with loss of consciousness of any duration with death due to other cause prior to regaining consciousness

● S06.379   Contusion, laceration, and hemorrhage of cerebellum with loss of consciousness of unspecified duration

     Contusion, laceration, and hemorrhage of cerebellum NOS

● S06.38   Contusion, laceration, and hemorrhage of brainstem

● S06.380   Contusion, laceration, and hemorrhage of brainstem without loss of consciousness

● S06.381   Contusion, laceration, and hemorrhage of brainstem with loss of consciousness of 30 minutes or less

● S06.382   Contusion, laceration, and hemorrhage of brainstem with loss of consciousness of 31 minutes to 59 minutes

● S06.383   Contusion, laceration, and hemorrhage of brainstem with loss of consciousness of 1 hour to 5 hours 59 minutes

● S06.384   Contusion, laceration, and hemorrhage of brainstem with loss of consciousness of 6 hours to 24 hours

● S06.385   Contusion, laceration, and hemorrhage of brainstem with loss of consciousness greater than 24 hours with return to pre-existing conscious level

● S06.386   Contusion, laceration, and hemorrhage of brainstem with loss of consciousness greater than 24 hours without return to pre-existing conscious level with patient surviving

● S06.387   Contusion, laceration, and hemorrhage of brainstem with loss of consciousness of any duration with death due to brain injury prior to regaining consciousness

● S06.388   Contusion, laceration, and hemorrhage of brainstem with loss of consciousness of any duration with death due to other cause prior to regaining consciousness

● S06.389   Contusion, laceration, and hemorrhage of brainstem with loss of consciousness of unspecified duration

     Contusion, laceration, and hemorrhage of brainstem NOS

● S06.4   Epidural hemorrhage

     Situated outside dura mater
     Extradural hemorrhage NOS
     Intracranial hemorrhage due to trauma
     Extradural hemorrhage (traumatic)

● S06.4X   Epidural hemorrhage

● S06.4X0   Epidural hemorrhage without loss of consciousness

● S06.4X1   Epidural hemorrhage with loss of consciousness of 30 minutes or less

● S06.4X2   Epidural hemorrhage with loss of consciousness of 31 minutes to 59 minutes

● S06.4X3   Epidural hemorrhage with loss of consciousness of 1 hour to 5 hours 59 minutes

● S06.4X4   Epidural hemorrhage with loss of consciousness of 6 hours to 24 hours

● S06.4X5   Epidural hemorrhage with loss of consciousness greater than 24 hours with return to pre-existing conscious level

● S06.4X6   Epidural hemorrhage with loss of consciousness greater than 24 hours without return to pre-existing conscious level with patient surviving

● S06.4X7   Epidural hemorrhage with loss of consciousness of any duration with death due to brain injury prior to regaining consciousness

● S06.4X8   Epidural hemorrhage with loss of consciousness of any duration with death due to other causes prior to regaining consciousness

● S06.4X9   Epidural hemorrhage with loss of consciousness of unspecified duration

     Epidural hemorrhage NOS

● **S06.5**   **Traumatic subdural hemorrhage**
  ● **S06.5X**   **Traumatic subdural hemorrhage**
    ● **S06.5X0**   Traumatic subdural hemorrhage without loss of consciousness
      Coding Clinic: 2015, Q3, P37
    ● **S06.5X1**   Traumatic subdural hemorrhage with loss of consciousness of 30 minutes or less
    ● **S06.5X2**   Traumatic subdural hemorrhage with loss of consciousness of 31 minutes to 59 minutes
    ● **S06.5X3**   Traumatic subdural hemorrhage with loss of consciousness of 1 hour to 5 hours 59 minutes
    ● **S06.5X4**   Traumatic subdural hemorrhage with loss of consciousness of 6 hours to 24 hours
    ● **S06.5X5**   Traumatic subdural hemorrhage with loss of consciousness greater than 24 hours with return to pre-existing conscious level
    ● **S06.5X6**   Traumatic subdural hemorrhage with loss of consciousness greater than 24 hours without return to pre-existing conscious level with patient surviving
    ● **S06.5X7**   Traumatic subdural hemorrhage with loss of consciousness of any duration with death due to brain injury before regaining consciousness
    ● **S06.5X8**   Traumatic subdural hemorrhage with loss of consciousness of any duration with death due to other cause before regaining consciousness
    ● **S06.5X9**   Traumatic subdural hemorrhage with loss of consciousness of unspecified duration
      Traumatic subdural hemorrhage NOS

● **S06.6**   **Traumatic subarachnoid hemorrhage**
    Between arachnoid and pia mater
  ● **S06.6X**   **Traumatic subarachnoid hemorrhage**
    ● **S06.6X0**   Traumatic subarachnoid hemorrhage without loss of consciousness
      Coding Clinic: 2015, Q3, P37
    ● **S06.6X1**   Traumatic subarachnoid hemorrhage with loss of consciousness of 30 minutes or less
    ● **S06.6X2**   Traumatic subarachnoid hemorrhage with loss of consciousness of 31 minutes to 59 minutes
    ● **S06.6X3**   Traumatic subarachnoid hemorrhage with loss of consciousness of 1 hour to 5 hours 59 minutes
    ● **S06.6X4**   Traumatic subarachnoid hemorrhage with loss of consciousness of 6 hours to 24 hours
    ● **S06.6X5**   Traumatic subarachnoid hemorrhage with loss of consciousness greater than 24 hours with return to pre-existing conscious level
    ● **S06.6X6**   Traumatic subarachnoid hemorrhage with loss of consciousness greater than 24 hours without return to pre-existing conscious level with patient surviving
    ● **S06.6X7**   Traumatic subarachnoid hemorrhage with loss of consciousness of any duration with death due to brain injury prior to regaining consciousness
    ● **S06.6X8**   Traumatic subarachnoid hemorrhage with loss of consciousness of any duration with death due to other cause prior to regaining consciousness
    ● **S06.6X9**   Traumatic subarachnoid hemorrhage with loss of consciousness of unspecified duration
      Traumatic subarachnoid hemorrhage NOS

● **S06.8**   **Other specified intracranial injuries**
  ● **S06.81**   **Injury of right internal carotid artery, intracranial portion, not elsewhere classified**
    ● **S06.810**   Injury of right internal carotid artery, intracranial portion, not elsewhere classified without loss of consciousness
    ● **S06.811**   Injury of right internal carotid artery, intracranial portion, not elsewhere classified with loss of consciousness of 30 minutes or less
    ● **S06.812**   Injury of right internal carotid artery, intracranial portion, not elsewhere classified with loss of consciousness of 31 minutes to 59 minutes
    ● **S06.813**   Injury of right internal carotid artery, intracranial portion, not elsewhere classified with loss of consciousness of 1 hour to 5 hours 59 minutes
    ● **S06.814**   Injury of right internal carotid artery, intracranial portion, not elsewhere classified with loss of consciousness of 6 hours to 24 hours
    ● **S06.815**   Injury of right internal carotid artery, intracranial portion, not elsewhere classified with loss of consciousness greater than 24 hours with return to pre-existing conscious level
    ● **S06.816**   Injury of right internal carotid artery, intracranial portion, not elsewhere classified with loss of consciousness greater than 24 hours without return to pre-existing conscious level with patient surviving
    ● **S06.817**   Injury of right internal carotid artery, intracranial portion, not elsewhere classified with loss of consciousness of any duration with death due to brain injury prior to regaining consciousness
    ● **S06.818**   Injury of right internal carotid artery, intracranial portion, not elsewhere classified with loss of consciousness of any duration with death due to other cause prior to regaining consciousness
    ● **S06.819**   Injury of right internal carotid artery, intracranial portion, not elsewhere classified with loss of consciousness of unspecified duration
      Injury of right internal carotid artery, intracranial portion, not elsewhere classified NOS

CHAPTER 19 (S00-T88)

● S06.82   Injury of left internal carotid artery, intracranial portion, not elsewhere classified

    ● S06.820   Injury of left internal carotid artery, intracranial portion, not elsewhere classified without loss of consciousness

    ● S06.821   Injury of left internal carotid artery, intracranial portion, not elsewhere classified with loss of consciousness of 30 minutes or less

    ● S06.822   Injury of left internal carotid artery, intracranial portion, not elsewhere classified with loss of consciousness of 31 minutes to 59 minutes

    ● S06.823   Injury of left internal carotid artery, intracranial portion, not elsewhere classified with loss of consciousness of 1 hour to 5 hours 59 minutes

    ● S06.824   Injury of left internal carotid artery, intracranial portion, not elsewhere classified with loss of consciousness of 6 hours to 24 hours

    ● S06.825   Injury of left internal carotid artery, intracranial portion, not elsewhere classified with loss of consciousness greater than 24 hours with return to pre-existing conscious level

    ● S06.826   Injury of left internal carotid artery, intracranial portion, not elsewhere classified with loss of consciousness greater than 24 hours without return to pre-existing conscious level with patient surviving

    ● S06.827   Injury of left internal carotid artery, intracranial portion, not elsewhere classified with loss of consciousness of any duration with death due to brain injury prior to regaining consciousness

    ● S06.828   Injury of left internal carotid artery, intracranial portion, not elsewhere classified with loss of consciousness of any duration with death due to other cause prior to regaining consciousness

    ● S06.829   Injury of left internal carotid artery, intracranial portion, not elsewhere classified with loss of consciousness of **unspecified** duration
        Injury of left internal carotid artery, intracranial portion, not elsewhere classified NOS

● S06.89   Other specified intracranial injury
    Excludes1   concussion (S06.0X-) ◄

    ● S06.890   Other specified intracranial injury without loss of consciousness

    ● S06.891   Other specified intracranial injury with loss of consciousness of 30 minutes or less

    ● S06.892   Other specified intracranial injury with loss of consciousness of 31 minutes to 59 minutes

    ● S06.893   Other specified intracranial injury with loss of consciousness of 1 hour to 5 hours 59 minutes

    ● S06.894   Other specified intracranial injury with loss of consciousness of 6 hours to 24 hours

    ● S06.895   Other specified intracranial injury with loss of consciousness greater than 24 hours with return to pre-existing conscious level

    ● S06.896   Other specified intracranial injury with loss of consciousness greater than 24 hours without return to pre-existing conscious level with patient surviving

    ● S06.897   Other specified intracranial injury with loss of consciousness of any duration with death due to brain injury prior to regaining consciousness

    ● S06.898   Other specified intracranial injury with loss of consciousness of any duration with death due to other cause prior to regaining consciousness

    ● S06.899   Other specified intracranial injury with loss of consciousness of **unspecified** duration

● S06.9   Unspecified intracranial injury
    Brain injury NOS
    Head injury NOS with loss of consciousness
    Traumatic brain injury NOS ◄
    Excludes1   conditions classifiable to S06.0- to S06.8-code to specified intracranial injury ◄
        head injury NOS (S09.90)

  ● S06.9X   Unspecified intracranial injury

    ● S06.9X0   **Unspecified** intracranial injury without loss of consciousness

    ● S06.9X1   **Unspecified** intracranial injury with loss of consciousness of 30 minutes or less

    ● S06.9X2   **Unspecified** intracranial injury with loss of consciousness of 31 minutes to 59 minutes

    ● S06.9X3   **Unspecified** intracranial injury with loss of consciousness of 1 hour to 5 hours 59 minutes

    ● S06.9X4   **Unspecified** intracranial injury with loss of consciousness of 6 hours to 24 hours

    ● S06.9X5   **Unspecified** intracranial injury with loss of consciousness greater than 24 hours with return to pre-existing conscious level

    ● S06.9X6   **Unspecified** intracranial injury with loss of consciousness greater than 24 hours without return to pre-existing conscious level with patient surviving

    ● S06.9X7   **Unspecified** intracranial injury with loss of consciousness of any duration with death due to brain injury prior to regaining consciousness

    ● S06.9X8   **Unspecified** intracranial injury with loss of consciousness of any duration with death due to other cause prior to regaining consciousness

    ● S06.9X9   **Unspecified** intracranial injury with loss of consciousness of unspecified duration

● **S07** **Crushing injury of head**
Use additional code for all associated injuries, such as:
intracranial injuries (S06.-)
skull fractures (S02.-)

The appropriate 7th character is to be added to each code from category S07

> A　initial encounter
> D　subsequent encounter
> S　sequela

X● **S07.0** **Crushing injury of face**
X● **S07.1** **Crushing injury of skull**
X● **S07.8** **Crushing injury of other parts of head**
X● **S07.9** **Crushing injury of head, part unspecified**

● **S08** **Avulsion and traumatic amputation of part of head**
An amputation not identified as partial or complete should be coded to complete

The appropriate 7th character is to be added to each code from category S08

> A　initial encounter
> D　subsequent encounter
> S　sequela

X● **S08.0** **Avulsion of scalp**
● **S08.1** **Traumatic amputation of ear**
　● **S08.11** **Complete traumatic amputation of ear**
　　● **S08.111** **Complete traumatic amputation of right ear**
　　● **S08.112** **Complete traumatic amputation of left ear**
　　● **S08.119** **Complete traumatic amputation of unspecified ear**
　● **S08.12** **Partial traumatic amputation of ear**
　　● **S08.121** **Partial traumatic amputation of right ear**
　　● **S08.122** **Partial traumatic amputation of left ear**
　　● **S08.129** **Partial traumatic amputation of unspecified ear**
● **S08.8** **Traumatic amputation of other parts of head**
　● **S08.81** **Traumatic amputation of nose**
　　● **S08.811** **Complete traumatic amputation of nose**
　　● **S08.812** **Partial traumatic amputation of nose**
　● **S08.89** **Traumatic amputation of other parts of head**

● **S09** **Other and unspecified injuries of head**
The appropriate 7th character is to be added to each code from category S09

> A　initial encounter
> D　subsequent encounter
> S　sequela

X● **S09.0** **Injury of blood vessels of head, not elsewhere classified**
　　Excludes1　injury of cerebral blood vessels (S06.-)
　　　　　　　　injury of precerebral blood vessels (S15.-)
● **S09.1** **Injury of muscle and tendon of head**
Code also any associated open wound (S01.-)
　　Excludes2　sprain to joints and ligament of head (S03.9)
X● **S09.10** **Unspecified injury of muscle and tendon of head**
Injury of muscle and tendon of head NOS
X● **S09.11** **Strain of muscle and tendon of head**
X● **S09.12** **Laceration of muscle and tendon of head**
X● **S09.19** **Other specified injury of muscle and tendon of head**

● **S09.2** **Traumatic rupture of ear drum**
　　Excludes1　traumatic rupture of ear drum due to blast injury (S09.31-)
X● **S09.20** **Traumatic rupture of unspecified ear drum**
X● **S09.21** **Traumatic rupture of right ear drum**
X● **S09.22** **Traumatic rupture of left ear drum**
● **S09.3** **Other specified and unspecified injury of middle and inner ear**
　　Excludes1　injury to ear NOS (S09.91-)
　　Excludes2　injury to external ear (S00.4-, S01.3-, S08.1-)
　● **S09.30** **Unspecified injury of middle and inner ear**
　　● **S09.301** **Unspecified injury of right middle and inner ear**
　　● **S09.302** **Unspecified injury of left middle and inner ear**
　　● **S09.309** **Unspecified injury of unspecified middle and inner ear**
　● **S09.31** **Primary blast injury of ear**
Blast injury of ear NOS
　　● **S09.311** **Primary blast injury of right ear**
　　● **S09.312** **Primary blast injury of left ear**
　　● **S09.313** **Primary blast injury of ear, bilateral**
　　● **S09.319** **Primary blast injury of unspecified ear**
　● **S09.39** **Other specified injury of middle and inner ear**
Secondary blast injury to ear
　　● **S09.391** **Other specified injury of right middle and inner ear**
　　● **S09.392** **Other specified injury of left middle and inner ear**
　　● **S09.399** **Other specified injury of unspecified middle and inner ear**
X● **S09.8** **Other specified injuries of head**
● **S09.9** **Unspecified injury of face and head**
X● **S09.90** **Unspecified injury of head**
Head injury NOS
　　Excludes1　brain injury NOS (S06.9-)
　　　　　　　　head injury NOS with loss of consciousness (S06.9-)
　　　　　　　　intracranial injury NOS (S06.9-)
X● **S09.91** **Unspecified injury of ear**
Injury of ear NOS
X● **S09.92** **Unspecified injury of nose**
Injury of nose NOS
X● **S09.93** **Unspecified injury of face**
Injury of face NOS

INJURIES TO THE NECK (S10-S19)

Includes　injuries of nape
injuries of supraclavicular region
injuries of throat

Excludes2　burns and corrosions (T20-T32)
effects of foreign body in esophagus (T18.1)
effects of foreign body in larynx (T17.3)
effects of foreign body in pharynx (T17.2)
effects of foreign body in trachea (T17.4)
frostbite (T33-T34)
insect bite or sting, venomous (T63.4)

● **S10** **Superficial injury of neck**
The appropriate 7th character is to be added to each code from category S10

> A　initial encounter
> D　subsequent encounter
> S　sequela

X● **S10.0** **Contusion of throat**
Contusion of cervical esophagus
Contusion of larynx
Contusion of pharynx
Contusion of trachea

CHAPTER 19 (S00-T88)

● **S10.1**   **Other and unspecified superficial injuries of throat**
- X ● **S10.10**   Unspecified superficial injuries of throat
- X ● **S10.11**   Abrasion of throat
- X ● **S10.12**   Blister (nonthermal) of throat
- X ● **S10.14**   External constriction of part of throat
- X ● **S10.15**   Superficial foreign body of throat
  - Splinter in the throat
- X ● **S10.16**   Insect bite (nonvenomous) of throat
- X ● **S10.17**   Other superficial bite of throat

    Excludes1   open bite of throat (S11.85)

● **S10.8**   **Superficial injury of other specified parts of neck**
- X ● **S10.80**   Unspecified superficial injury of other specified part of neck
- X ● **S10.81**   Abrasion of other specified part of neck
- X ● **S10.82**   Blister (nonthermal) of other specified part of neck
- X ● **S10.83**   Contusion of other specified part of neck
- X ● **S10.84**   External constriction of other specified part of neck
- X ● **S10.85**   Superficial foreign body of other specified part of neck
  - Splinter in other part of neck
- X ● **S10.86**   Insect bite of other specified part of neck
- X ● **S10.87**   Other superficial bite of other specified part of neck

    Excludes1   open bite of other specified parts of neck (S11.85)

● **S10.9**   **Superficial injury of unspecified part of neck**
- X ● **S10.90**   Unspecified superficial injury of unspecified part of neck
- X ● **S10.91**   Abrasion of unspecified part of neck
- X ● **S10.92**   Blister (nonthermal) of unspecified part of neck
- X ● **S10.93**   Contusion of unspecified part of neck
- X ● **S10.94**   External constriction of unspecified part of neck
- X ● **S10.95**   Superficial foreign body of unspecified part of neck
- X ● **S10.96**   Insect bite of unspecified part of neck
- X ● **S10.97**   Other superficial bite of unspecified part of neck

● **S11**   **Open wound of neck**

    Code also any associated:
      spinal cord injury (S14.0, S14.1-)
      wound infection

    Excludes2   open fracture of vertebra (S12.- with 7th character B)

    The appropriate 7th character is to be added to each code from category S11

A	initial encounter
D	subsequent encounter
S	sequela

● **S11.0**   **Open wound of larynx and trachea**
- ● **S11.01**   Open wound of larynx

      Excludes2   open wound of vocal cord (S11.03)

- ● **S11.011**   Laceration without foreign body of larynx
- ● **S11.012**   Laceration with foreign body of larynx
- ● **S11.013**   Puncture wound without foreign body of larynx
- ● **S11.014**   Puncture wound with foreign body of larynx
- ● **S11.015**   Open bite of larynx
  - Bite of larynx NOS
- ● **S11.019**   Unspecified open wound of larynx

● **S11.02**   **Open wound of trachea**
    Open wound of cervical trachea
    Open wound of trachea NOS

    Excludes2   open wound of thoracic trachea (S27.5-)

- ● **S11.021**   Laceration without foreign body of trachea
- ● **S11.022**   Laceration with foreign body of trachea
- ● **S11.023**   Puncture wound without foreign body of trachea
- ● **S11.024**   Puncture wound with foreign body of trachea
- ● **S11.025**   Open bite of trachea
  - Bite of trachea NOS
- ● **S11.029**   Unspecified open wound of trachea

● **S11.03**   **Open wound of vocal cord**
- ● **S11.031**   Laceration without foreign body of vocal cord
- ● **S11.032**   Laceration with foreign body of vocal cord
- ● **S11.033**   Puncture wound without foreign body of vocal cord
- ● **S11.034**   Puncture wound with foreign body of vocal cord
- ● **S11.035**   Open bite of vocal cord
  - Bite of vocal cord NOS
- ● **S11.039**   Unspecified open wound of vocal cord

● **S11.1**   **Open wound of thyroid gland**
- X ● **S11.10**   Unspecified open wound of thyroid gland
- X ● **S11.11**   Laceration without foreign body of thyroid gland
- X ● **S11.12**   Laceration with foreign body of thyroid gland
- X ● **S11.13**   Puncture wound without foreign body of thyroid gland
- X ● **S11.14**   Puncture wound with foreign body of thyroid gland
- X ● **S11.15**   Open bite of thyroid gland
  - Bite of thyroid gland NOS

● **S11.2**   **Open wound of pharynx and cervical esophagus**

    Excludes1   open wound of esophagus NOS (S27.8-)

- X ● **S11.20**   Unspecified open wound of pharynx and cervical esophagus
- X ● **S11.21**   Laceration without foreign body of pharynx and cervical esophagus
- X ● **S11.22**   Laceration with foreign body of pharynx and cervical esophagus
- X ● **S11.23**   Puncture wound without foreign body of pharynx and cervical esophagus
- X ● **S11.24**   Puncture wound with foreign body of pharynx and cervical esophagus
- X ● **S11.25**   Open bite of pharynx and cervical esophagus
  - Bite of pharynx and cervical esophagus NOS

● **S11.8**   **Open wound of other specified parts of neck**
- X ● **S11.80**   Unspecified open specified wound of other part of neck
- X ● **S11.81**   Laceration without foreign body of other specified part of neck
- X ● **S11.82**   Laceration with foreign body of other specified part of neck
- X ● **S11.83**   Puncture wound without foreign body of other specified part of neck
- X ● **S11.84**   Puncture wound with foreign body of other specified part of neck
- X ● **S11.85**   Open bite of other specified part of neck
  - Bite of other part of neck NOS

    Excludes1   superficial bite of other specified part of neck (S10.87)

- X ● **S11.89**   Other open wound of other part of neck

● S11.9   Open wound of unspecified part of neck

   X ● S11.90   Unspecified open wound of unspecified part of neck

   X ● S11.91   Laceration without foreign body of unspecified part of neck

   X ● S11.92   Laceration with foreign body of unspecified part of neck

   X ● S11.93   Puncture wound without foreign body of unspecified part of neck

   X ● S11.94   Puncture wound with foreign body of unspecified part of neck

   X ● S11.95   Open bite of unspecified part of neck
          Bite of neck NOS

          Excludes1   superficial bite of neck (S10.97)

● S12   Fracture of cervical vertebra and other parts of neck

   Note: A fracture not indicated as displaced or nondisplaced should be coded to displaced

   A fracture not indicated as open or closed should be coded to closed

   Includes   fracture of cervical neural arch
             fracture of cervical spine
             fracture of cervical spinous process
             fracture of cervical transverse process
             fracture of cervical vertebral arch
             fracture of neck

   Code first any associated cervical spinal cord injury (S14.0, S14.1-)

   The appropriate 7th character is to be added to all codes from subcategories S12.0-S12.6

A	initial encounter for closed fracture
B	initial encounter for open fracture
D	subsequent encounter for fracture with routine healing
G	subsequent encounter for fracture with delayed healing
K	subsequent encounter for fracture with nonunion
S	sequela

● S12.0   Fracture of first cervical vertebra
      Atlas

   ● S12.00   Unspecified fracture of first cervical vertebra

      ● S12.000   Unspecified displaced fracture of first cervical vertebra

      ● S12.001   Unspecified nondisplaced fracture of first cervical vertebra

   X ● S12.01   Stable burst fracture of first cervical vertebra

   X ● S12.02   Unstable burst fracture of first cervical vertebra

   ● S12.03   Posterior arch fracture of first cervical vertebra

      ● S12.030   Displaced posterior arch fracture of first cervical vertebra

      ● S12.031   Nondisplaced posterior arch fracture of first cervical vertebra

   ● S12.04   Lateral mass fracture of first cervical vertebra

      ● S12.040   Displaced lateral mass fracture of first cervical vertebra

      ● S12.041   Nondisplaced lateral mass fracture of first cervical vertebra

   ● S12.09   Other fracture of first cervical vertebra

      ● S12.090   Other displaced fracture of first cervical vertebra

      ● S12.091   Other nondisplaced fracture of first cervical vertebra

● S12.1   Fracture of second cervical vertebra
      Axis

   ● S12.10   Unspecified fracture of second cervical vertebra

      ● S12.100   Unspecified displaced fracture of second cervical vertebra

      ● S12.101   Unspecified nondisplaced fracture of second cervical vertebra

● S12.11   Type II dens fracture

   ● S12.110   Anterior displaced Type II dens fracture

   ● S12.111   Posterior displaced Type II dens fracture

   ● S12.112   Nondisplaced Type II dens fracture

● S12.12   Other dens fracture

   ● S12.120   Other displaced dens fracture

   ● S12.121   Other nondisplaced dens fracture

● S12.13   Unspecified traumatic spondylolisthesis of second cervical vertebra

   ● S12.130   Unspecified traumatic displaced spondylolisthesis of second cervical vertebra

   ● S12.131   Unspecified traumatic nondisplaced spondylolisthesis of second cervical vertebra

X ● S12.14   Type III traumatic spondylolisthesis of second cervical vertebra

● S12.15   Other traumatic spondylolisthesis of second cervical vertebra

   ● S12.150   Other traumatic displaced spondylolisthesis of second cervical vertebra

   ● S12.151   Other traumatic nondisplaced spondylolisthesis of second cervical vertebra

● S12.19   Other fracture of second cervical vertebra

   ● S12.190   Other displaced fracture of second cervical vertebra

   ● S12.191   Other nondisplaced fracture of second cervical vertebra

● S12.2   Fracture of third cervical vertebra

   ● S12.20   Unspecified fracture of third cervical vertebra

      ● S12.200   Unspecified displaced fracture of third cervical vertebra

      ● S12.201   Unspecified nondisplaced fracture of third cervical vertebra

   ● S12.23   Unspecified traumatic spondylolisthesis of third cervical vertebra

      ● S12.230   Unspecified traumatic displaced spondylolisthesis of third cervical vertebra

      ● S12.231   Unspecified traumatic nondisplaced spondylolisthesis of third cervical vertebra

   X ● S12.24   Type III traumatic spondylolisthesis of third cervical vertebra

   ● S12.25   Other traumatic spondylolisthesis of third cervical vertebra

      ● S12.250   Other traumatic displaced spondylolisthesis of third cervical vertebra

      ● S12.251   Other traumatic nondisplaced spondylolisthesis of third cervical vertebra

   ● S12.29   Other fracture of third cervical vertebra

      ● S12.290   Other displaced fracture of third cervical vertebra

      ● S12.291   Other nondisplaced fracture of third cervical vertebra

● S12.3   Fracture of fourth cervical vertebra

   ● S12.30   Unspecified fracture of fourth cervical vertebra

      ● S12.300   Unspecified displaced fracture of fourth cervical vertebra

      ● S12.301   Unspecified nondisplaced fracture of fourth cervical vertebra

CHAPTER 19 (S00-T88)

- **S12.33** Unspecified traumatic spondylolisthesis of fourth cervical vertebra
  - **S12.330** Unspecified traumatic displaced spondylolisthesis of fourth cervical vertebra
  - **S12.331** Unspecified traumatic nondisplaced spondylolisthesis of fourth cervical vertebra
- X **S12.34** Type III traumatic spondylolisthesis of fourth cervical vertebra
- **S12.35** Other traumatic spondylolisthesis of fourth cervical vertebra
  - **S12.350** Other traumatic displaced spondylolisthesis of fourth cervical vertebra
  - **S12.351** Other traumatic nondisplaced spondylolisthesis of fourth cervical vertebra
- **S12.39** Other fracture of fourth cervical vertebra
  - **S12.390** Other displaced fracture of fourth cervical vertebra
  - **S12.391** Other nondisplaced fracture of fourth cervical vertebra
- **S12.4** Fracture of fifth cervical vertebra
  - **S12.40** Unspecified fracture of fifth cervical vertebra
    - **S12.400** Unspecified displaced fracture of fifth cervical vertebra
    - **S12.401** Unspecified nondisplaced fracture of fifth cervical vertebra
  - **S12.43** Unspecified traumatic spondylolisthesis of fifth cervical vertebra
    - **S12.430** Unspecified traumatic displaced spondylolisthesis of fifth cervical vertebra
    - **S12.431** Unspecified traumatic nondisplaced spondylolisthesis of fifth cervical vertebra
  - X **S12.44** Type III traumatic spondylolisthesis of fifth cervical vertebra
  - **S12.45** Other traumatic spondylolisthesis of fifth cervical vertebra
    - **S12.450** Other traumatic displaced spondylolisthesis of fifth cervical vertebra
    - **S12.451** Other traumatic nondisplaced spondylolisthesis of fifth cervical vertebra
  - **S12.49** Other fracture of fifth cervical vertebra
    - **S12.490** Other displaced fracture of fifth cervical vertebra
    - **S12.491** Other nondisplaced fracture of fifth cervical vertebra
- **S12.5** Fracture of sixth cervical vertebra
  - **S12.50** Unspecified fracture of sixth cervical vertebra
    - **S12.500** Unspecified displaced fracture of sixth cervical vertebra
    - **S12.501** Unspecified nondisplaced fracture of sixth cervical vertebra
  - **S12.53** Unspecified traumatic spondylolisthesis of sixth cervical vertebra
    - **S12.530** Unspecified traumatic displaced spondylolisthesis of sixth cervical vertebra
    - **S12.531** Unspecified traumatic nondisplaced spondylolisthesis of sixth cervical vertebra

- X **S12.54** Type III traumatic spondylolisthesis of sixth cervical vertebra
- **S12.55** Other traumatic spondylolisthesis of sixth cervical vertebra
  - **S12.550** Other traumatic displaced spondylolisthesis of sixth cervical vertebra
  - **S12.551** Other traumatic nondisplaced spondylolisthesis of sixth cervical vertebra
- **S12.59** Other fracture of sixth cervical vertebra
  - **S12.590** Other displaced fracture of sixth cervical vertebra
  - **S12.591** Other nondisplaced fracture of sixth cervical vertebra
- **S12.6** Fracture of seventh cervical vertebra
  - **S12.60** Unspecified fracture of seventh cervical vertebra
    - **S12.600** Unspecified displaced fracture of seventh cervical vertebra
    - **S12.601** Unspecified nondisplaced fracture of seventh cervical vertebra
  - **S12.63** Unspecified traumatic spondylolisthesis of seventh cervical vertebra
    - **S12.630** Unspecified traumatic displaced spondylolisthesis of seventh cervical vertebra
    - **S12.631** Unspecified traumatic nondisplaced spondylolisthesis of seventh cervical vertebra
  - X **S12.64** Type III traumatic spondylolisthesis of seventh cervical vertebra
  - **S12.65** Other traumatic spondylolisthesis of seventh cervical vertebra
    - **S12.650** Other traumatic displaced spondylolisthesis of seventh cervical vertebra
    - **S12.651** Other traumatic nondisplaced spondylolisthesis of seventh cervical vertebra
  - **S12.69** Other fracture of seventh cervical vertebra
    - **S12.690** Other displaced fracture of seventh cervical vertebra
    - **S12.691** Other nondisplaced fracture of seventh cervical vertebra
- X **S12.8** Fracture of other parts of neck

  Hyoid bone   Thyroid cartilage
  Larynx   Trachea

  The appropriate 7th character is to be added to code S12.8

A	initial encounter
D	subsequent encounter
S	sequela

- X **S12.9** Fracture of neck, unspecified

  Fracture of neck NOS
  Fracture of cervical spine NOS
  Fracture of cervical vertebra NOS

  The appropriate 7th character is to be added to code S12.9

A	initial encounter
D	subsequent encounter
S	sequela

◀ New   ◀▥ Revised   ~~deleted~~ Deleted   Excludes 1   Excludes 2   Includes   Use additional   Code first   Code also   Unspecified

OGCR Official Guidelines   X Assign placeholder X   ● Use Additional Character(s)   ▶ Manifestation Code   **Coding Clinic**

● **S13**   **Dislocation and sprain of joints and ligaments at neck level**

> **Includes**   avulsion of joint or ligament at neck level
> laceration of cartilage, joint or ligament at neck level
> sprain of cartilage, joint or ligament at neck level
> traumatic hemarthrosis of joint or ligament at neck level
> traumatic rupture of joint or ligament at neck level
> traumatic subluxation of joint or ligament at neck level
> traumatic tear of joint or ligament at neck level

Code also any associated open wound

> **Excludes2**   strain of muscle or tendon at neck level (S16.1)

The appropriate 7th character is to be added to each code from category S13

> A   initial encounter
> D   subsequent encounter
> S   sequela

X ● **S13.0**   **Traumatic rupture of cervical intervertebral disc**

> **Excludes1**   rupture or displacement (nontraumatic) of cervical intervertebral disc NOS (M50.-)

● **S13.1**   **Subluxation and dislocation of cervical vertebrae**

> Code also any associated:
>   open wound of neck (S11.-)
>   spinal cord injury (S14.1)

> **Excludes2**   fracture of cervical vertebrae (S12.0-S12.3-)

> ● **S13.10**   **Subluxation and dislocation of unspecified cervical vertebrae**
>
> > ● **S13.100**   **Subluxation of unspecified cervical vertebrae**
> >
> > ● **S13.101**   **Dislocation of unspecified cervical vertebrae**
>
> ● **S13.11**   **Subluxation and dislocation of C_0/C_1 cervical vertebrae**
> > Subluxation and dislocation of atlantooccipital joint
> > Subluxation and dislocation of atloidooccipital joint
> > Subluxation and dislocation of occipitoatloid joint
> >
> > ● **S13.110**   **Subluxation of C_0/C_1 cervical vertebrae**
> >
> > ● **S13.111**   **Dislocation of C_0/C_1 cervical vertebrae**
>
> ● **S13.12**   **Subluxation and dislocation of C_1/C_2 cervical vertebrae**
> > Subluxation and dislocation of atlantoaxial joint
> >
> > ● **S13.120**   **Subluxation of C_1/C_2 cervical vertebrae**
> >
> > ● **S13.121**   **Dislocation of C_1/C_2 cervical vertebrae**
>
> ● **S13.13**   **Subluxation and dislocation of C_2/C_3 cervical vertebrae**
> >
> > ● **S13.130**   **Subluxation of C_2/C_3 cervical vertebrae**
> >
> > ● **S13.131**   **Dislocation of C_2/C_3 cervical vertebrae**
>
> ● **S13.14**   **Subluxation and dislocation of C_3/C_4 cervical vertebrae**
> >
> > ● **S13.140**   **Subluxation of C_3/C_4 cervical vertebrae**
> >
> > ● **S13.141**   **Dislocation of C_3/C_4 cervical vertebrae**
>
> ● **S13.15**   **Subluxation and dislocation of C_4/C_5 cervical vertebrae**
> >
> > ● **S13.150**   **Subluxation of C_4/C_5 cervical vertebrae**
> >
> > ● **S13.151**   **Dislocation of C_4/C_5 cervical vertebrae**

> ● **S13.16**   **Subluxation and dislocation of C_5/C_6 cervical vertebrae**
> >
> > ● **S13.160**   **Subluxation of C_5/C_6 cervical vertebrae**
> >
> > ● **S13.161**   **Dislocation of C_5/C_6 cervical vertebrae**
>
> ● **S13.17**   **Subluxation and dislocation of C_6/C_7 cervical vertebrae**
> >
> > ● **S13.170**   **Subluxation of C_6/C_7 cervical vertebrae**
> >
> > ● **S13.171**   **Dislocation of C_6/C_7 cervical vertebrae**
>
> ● **S13.18**   **Subluxation and dislocation of C_7/T_1 cervical vertebrae**
> >
> > ● **S13.180**   **Subluxation of C_7/T_1 cervical vertebrae**
> >
> > ● **S13.181**   **Dislocation of C_7/T_1 cervical vertebrae**

● **S13.2**   **Dislocation of other and unspecified parts of neck**

> X ● **S13.20**   **Dislocation of unspecified parts of neck**
>
> X ● **S13.29**   **Dislocation of other parts of neck**

X ● **S13.4**   **Sprain of ligaments of cervical spine**

> Sprain of anterior longitudinal (ligament), cervical
> Sprain of atlanto-axial (joints)
> Sprain of atlanto-occipital (joints)
> Whiplash injury of cervical spine

X ● **S13.5**   **Sprain of thyroid region**

> Sprain of cricoarytenoid (joint) (ligament)
> Sprain of cricothyroid (joint) (ligament)
> Sprain of thyroid cartilage

X ● **S13.8**   **Sprain of joints and ligaments of other parts of neck**

X ● **S13.9**   **Sprain of joints and ligaments of unspecified parts of neck**

● **S14**   **Injury of nerves and spinal cord at neck level**

> **Note:** Code to highest level of cervical cord injury
>
> Code also any associated:
>   fracture of cervical vertebra (S12.0--S12.6.-)
>   open wound of neck (S11.-)
>   transient paralysis (R29.5)
>
> The appropriate 7th character is to be added to each code from category S14
>
> > A   initial encounter
> > D   subsequent encounter
> > S   sequela

X ● **S14.0**   **Concussion and edema of cervical spinal cord**

● **S14.1**   **Other and unspecified injuries of cervical spinal cord**

> ● **S14.10**   **Unspecified injury of cervical spinal cord**
> >
> > ● **S14.101**   **Unspecified injury at C_1 level of cervical spinal cord**
> >
> > ● **S14.102**   **Unspecified injury at C_2 level of cervical spinal cord**
> >
> > ● **S14.103**   **Unspecified injury at C_3 level of cervical spinal cord**
> >
> > ● **S14.104**   **Unspecified injury at C_4 level of cervical spinal cord**
> >
> > ● **S14.105**   **Unspecified injury at C_5 level of cervical spinal cord**
> >
> > ● **S14.106**   **Unspecified injury at C_6 level of cervical spinal cord**
> >
> > ● **S14.107**   **Unspecified injury at C_7 level of cervical spinal cord**
> >
> > ● **S14.108**   **Unspecified injury at C_8 level of cervical spinal cord**
> >
> > ● **S14.109**   **Unspecified injury at unspecified level of cervical spinal cord**
> > > Injury of cervical spinal cord NOS

- **S14.11**   Complete lesion of cervical spinal cord
  - **S14.111**   Complete lesion at C_1 level of cervical spinal cord
  - **S14.112**   Complete lesion at C_2 level of cervical spinal cord
  - **S14.113**   Complete lesion at C_3 level of cervical spinal cord
  - **S14.114**   Complete lesion at C_4 level of cervical spinal cord
  - **S14.115**   Complete lesion at C_5 level of cervical spinal cord
  - **S14.116**   Complete lesion at C_6 level of cervical spinal cord
  - **S14.117**   Complete lesion at C_7 level of cervical spinal cord
  - **S14.118**   Complete lesion at C_8 level of cervical spinal cord
  - **S14.119**   Complete lesion at unspecified level of cervical spinal cord
- **S14.12**   Central cord syndrome of cervical spinal cord
  - **S14.121**   Central cord syndrome at C_1 level of cervical spinal cord
  - **S14.122**   Central cord syndrome at C_2 level of cervical spinal cord
  - **S14.123**   Central cord syndrome at C_3 level of cervical spinal cord
  - **S14.124**   Central cord syndrome at C_4 level of cervical spinal cord
  - **S14.125**   Central cord syndrome at C_5 level of cervical spinal cord
  - **S14.126**   Central cord syndrome at C_6 level of cervical spinal cord
  - **S14.127**   Central cord syndrome at C_7 level of cervical spinal cord
  - **S14.128**   Central cord syndrome at C_8 level of cervical spinal cord
  - **S14.129**   Central cord syndrome at unspecified level of cervical spinal cord
- **S14.13**   Anterior cord syndrome of cervical spinal cord
  - **S14.131**   Anterior cord syndrome at C_1 level of cervical spinal cord
  - **S14.132**   Anterior cord syndrome at C_2 level of cervical spinal cord
  - **S14.133**   Anterior cord syndrome at C_3 level of cervical spinal cord
  - **S14.134**   Anterior cord syndrome at C_4 level of cervical spinal cord
  - **S14.135**   Anterior cord syndrome at C_5 level of cervical spinal cord
  - **S14.136**   Anterior cord syndrome at C_6 level of cervical spinal cord
  - **S14.137**   Anterior cord syndrome at C_7 level of cervical spinal cord
  - **S14.138**   Anterior cord syndrome at C_8 level of cervical spinal cord
  - **S14.139**   Anterior cord syndrome at unspecified level of cervical spinal cord
- **S14.14**   Brown-Séquard syndrome of cervical spinal cord
  - **S14.141**   Brown-Séquard syndrome at C_1 level of cervical spinal cord
  - **S14.142**   Brown-Séquard syndrome at C_2 level of cervical spinal cord
  - **S14.143**   Brown-Séquard syndrome at C_3 level of cervical spinal cord
  - **S14.144**   Brown-Séquard syndrome at C_4 level of cervical spinal cord
  - **S14.145**   Brown-Séquard syndrome at C_5 level of cervical spinal cord
  - **S14.146**   Brown-Séquard syndrome at C_6 level of cervical spinal cord
  - **S14.147**   Brown-Séquard syndrome at C_7 level of cervical spinal cord
  - **S14.148**   Brown-Séquard syndrome at C_8 level of cervical spinal cord
  - **S14.149**   Brown-Séquard syndrome at unspecified level of cervical spinal cord
- **S14.15**   Other incomplete lesions of cervical spinal cord

  Incomplete lesion of cervical spinal cord NOS
  Posterior cord syndrome of cervical spinal cord
  - **S14.151**   Other incomplete lesion at C_1 level of cervical spinal cord
  - **S14.152**   Other incomplete lesion at C_2 level of cervical spinal cord
  - **S14.153**   Other incomplete lesion at C_3 level of cervical spinal cord
  - **S14.154**   Other incomplete lesion at C_4 level of cervical spinal cord
  - **S14.155**   Other incomplete lesion at C_5 level of cervical spinal cord
  - **S14.156**   Other incomplete lesion at C_6 level of cervical spinal cord
  - **S14.157**   Other incomplete lesion at C_7 level of cervical spinal cord
  - **S14.158**   Other incomplete lesion at C_8 level of cervical spinal cord
  - **S14.159**   Other incomplete lesion at unspecified level of cervical spinal cord
- X● **S14.2**   Injury of nerve root of cervical spine
- X● **S14.3**   Injury of brachial plexus
- X● **S14.4**   Injury of peripheral nerves of neck
- X● **S14.5**   Injury of cervical sympathetic nerves
- X● **S14.8**   Injury of other specified nerves of neck
- X● **S14.9**   Injury of unspecified nerves of neck

- ● **S15**   Injury of blood vessels at neck level

  Code also any associated open wound (S11.-)

  The appropriate 7th character is to be added to each code from category S15

A	initial encounter
D	subsequent encounter
S	sequela

  - ● **S15.0**   Injury of carotid artery of neck

    Injury of carotid artery (common) (external) (internal, extracranial portion)
    Injury of carotid artery NOS

    Excludes1   injury of internal carotid artery, intracranial portion (S06.8)
    - ● **S15.00**   Unspecified injury of carotid artery
      - ● **S15.001**   Unspecified injury of right carotid artery
      - ● **S15.002**   Unspecified injury of left carotid artery
      - ● **S15.009**   Unspecified injury of unspecified carotid artery
    - ● **S15.01**   Minor laceration of carotid artery

      Incomplete transection of carotid artery
      Laceration of carotid artery NOS
      Superficial laceration of carotid artery
      - ● **S15.011**   Minor laceration of right carotid artery
      - ● **S15.012**   Minor laceration of left carotid artery
      - ● **S15.019**   Minor laceration of unspecified carotid artery

- S15.02   **Major laceration of carotid artery**
  Complete transection of carotid artery
  Traumatic rupture of carotid artery
  - S15.021   **Major laceration of right carotid artery**
  - S15.022   **Major laceration of left carotid artery**
  - S15.029   **Major laceration of unspecified carotid artery**
- S15.09   **Other specified injury of carotid artery**
  - S15.091   **Other specified injury of right carotid artery**
  - S15.092   **Other specified injury of left carotid artery**
  - S15.099   **Other specified injury of unspecified carotid artery**
- S15.1   **Injury of vertebral artery**
  - S15.10   **Unspecified injury of vertebral artery**
    - S15.101   **Unspecified injury of right vertebral artery**
    - S15.102   **Unspecified injury of left vertebral artery**
    - S15.109   **Unspecified injury of unspecified vertebral artery**
  - S15.11   **Minor laceration of vertebral artery**
    Incomplete transection of vertebral artery
    Laceration of vertebral artery NOS
    Superficial laceration of vertebral artery
    - S15.111   **Minor laceration of right vertebral artery**
    - S15.112   **Minor laceration of left vertebral artery**
    - S15.119   **Minor laceration of unspecified vertebral artery**
  - S15.12   **Major laceration of vertebral artery**
    Complete transection of vertebral artery
    Traumatic rupture of vertebral artery
    - S15.121   **Major laceration of right vertebral artery**
    - S15.122   **Major laceration of left vertebral artery**
    - S15.129   **Major laceration of unspecified vertebral artery**
  - S15.19   **Other specified injury of vertebral artery**
    - S15.191   **Other specified injury of right vertebral artery**
    - S15.192   **Other specified injury of left vertebral artery**
    - S15.199   **Other specified injury of unspecified vertebral artery**
- S15.2   **Injury of external jugular vein**
  - S15.20   **Unspecified injury of external jugular vein**
    - S15.201   **Unspecified injury of right external jugular vein**
    - S15.202   **Unspecified injury of left external jugular vein**
    - S15.209   **Unspecified injury of unspecified external jugular vein**
  - S15.21   **Minor laceration of external jugular vein**
    Incomplete transection of external jugular vein
    Laceration of external jugular vein NOS
    Superficial laceration of external jugular vein
    - S15.211   **Minor laceration of right external jugular vein**
    - S15.212   **Minor laceration of left external jugular vein**
    - S15.219   **Minor laceration of unspecified external jugular vein**

- S15.22   **Major laceration of external jugular vein**
  Complete transection of external jugular vein
  Traumatic rupture of external jugular vein
  - S15.221   **Major laceration of right external jugular vein**
  - S15.222   **Major laceration of left external jugular vein**
  - S15.229   **Major laceration of unspecified external jugular vein**
- S15.29   **Other specified injury of external jugular vein**
  - S15.291   **Other specified injury of right external jugular vein**
  - S15.292   **Other specified injury of left external jugular vein**
  - S15.299   **Other specified injury of unspecified external jugular vein**
- S15.3   **Injury of internal jugular vein**
  - S15.30   **Unspecified injury of internal jugular vein**
    - S15.301   **Unspecified injury of right internal jugular vein**
    - S15.302   **Unspecified injury of left internal jugular vein**
    - S15.309   **Unspecified injury of unspecified internal jugular vein**
  - S15.31   **Minor laceration of internal jugular vein**
    Incomplete transection of internal jugular vein
    Laceration of internal jugular vein NOS
    Superficial laceration of internal jugular vein
    - S15.311   **Minor laceration of right internal jugular vein**
    - S15.312   **Minor laceration of left internal jugular vein**
    - S15.319   **Minor laceration of unspecified internal jugular vein**
  - S15.32   **Major laceration of internal jugular vein**
    Complete transection of internal jugular vein
    Traumatic rupture of internal jugular vein
    - S15.321   **Major laceration of right internal jugular vein**
    - S15.322   **Major laceration of left internal jugular vein**
    - S15.329   **Major laceration of unspecified internal jugular vein**
  - S15.39   **Other specified injury of internal jugular vein**
    - S15.391   **Other specified injury of right internal jugular vein**
    - S15.392   **Other specified injury of left internal jugular vein**
    - S15.399   **Other specified injury of unspecified internal jugular vein**
- X S15.8   **Injury of other specified blood vessels at neck level**
- X S15.9   **Injury of unspecified blood vessel at neck level**

- S16   **Injury of muscle, fascia and tendon at neck level**
  Code also any associated open wound (S11.-)
  Excludes2   sprain of joint or ligament at neck level (S13.9)
  The appropriate 7th character is to be added to each code from category S16

A	initial encounter
D	subsequent encounter
S	sequela

- X S16.1   **Strain of muscle, fascia and tendon at neck level**
- X S16.2   **Laceration of muscle, fascia and tendon at neck level**
- X S16.8   **Other specified injury of muscle, fascia and tendon at neck level**
- X S16.9   **Unspecified injury of muscle, fascia and tendon at neck level**

CHAPTER 19 (S00-T88)

● **S17**   **Crushing injury of neck**
> Use additional code for all associated injuries, such as:
>> injury of blood vessels (S15.-)
>> open wound of neck (S11.-)
>> spinal cord injury (S14.0, S14.1-)
>> vertebral fracture (S12.0--S12.3-)
>
> The appropriate 7th character is to be added to each code from category S17

> | | |
> |---|---|
> | A | initial encounter |
> | D | subsequent encounter |
> | S | sequela |

X ● **S17.0**   Crushing injury of larynx and trachea
X ● **S17.8**   Crushing injury of other specified parts of neck
X ● **S17.9**   Crushing injury of neck, part unspecified

● **S19**   **Other and unspecified injuries of neck**
> The appropriate 7th character is to be added to each code from category S19

> | | |
> |---|---|
> | A | initial encounter |
> | D | subsequent encounter |
> | S | sequela |

  ● **S19.8**   **Other specified injuries of neck**
    X ● **S19.80**   Other specified injuries of unspecified part of neck
    X ● **S19.81**   Other specified injuries of larynx
    X ● **S19.82**   Other specified injuries of cervical trachea
>> **Excludes2**   other specified injury of thoracic trachea (S27.5-)

    X ● **S19.83**   Other specified injuries of vocal cord
    X ● **S19.84**   Other specified injuries of thyroid gland
    X ● **S19.85**   Other specified injuries of pharynx and cervical esophagus
    X ● **S19.89**   Other specified injuries of other specified part of neck
  X ● **S19.9**   Unspecified injury of neck

INJURIES TO THE THORAX (S20-S29)

> | | |
> |---|---|
> | **Includes** | injuries of breast |
> | | injuries of chest (wall) |
> | | injuries of interscapular area |

> | | |
> |---|---|
> | **Excludes2** | burns and corrosions (T20-T32) |
> | | effects of foreign body in bronchus (T17.5) |
> | | effects of foreign body in esophagus (T18.1) |
> | | effects of foreign body in lung (T17.8) |
> | | effects of foreign body in trachea (T17.4) |
> | | frostbite (T33-T34) |
> | | injuries of axilla |
> | | injuries of clavicle |
> | | injuries of scapular region |
> | | injuries of shoulder |
> | | insect bite or sting, venomous (T63.4) |

● **S20**   **Superficial injury of thorax**
> The appropriate 7th character is to be added to each code from category S20

> | | |
> |---|---|
> | A | initial encounter |
> | D | subsequent encounter |
> | S | sequela |

  ● **S20.0**   **Contusion of breast**
    X ● **S20.00**   Contusion of breast, unspecified breast
    X ● **S20.01**   Contusion of right breast
    X ● **S20.02**   Contusion of left breast

  ● **S20.1**   **Other and unspecified superficial injuries of breast**
    ● **S20.10**   **Unspecified superficial injuries of breast**
      ● **S20.101**   Unspecified superficial injuries of breast, right breast
      ● **S20.102**   Unspecified superficial injuries of breast, left breast
      ● **S20.109**   Unspecified superficial injuries of breast, unspecified breast
    ● **S20.11**   **Abrasion of breast**
      ● **S20.111**   Abrasion of breast, right breast
      ● **S20.112**   Abrasion of breast, left breast
      ● **S20.119**   Abrasion of breast, unspecified breast
    ● **S20.12**   **Blister (nonthermal) of breast**
      ● **S20.121**   Blister (nonthermal) of breast, right breast
      ● **S20.122**   Blister (nonthermal) of breast, left breast
      ● **S20.129**   Blister (nonthermal) of breast, unspecified breast
    ● **S20.14**   **External constriction of part of breast**
      ● **S20.141**   External constriction of part of breast, right breast
      ● **S20.142**   External constriction of part of breast, left breast
      ● **S20.149**   External constriction of part of breast, unspecified breast
    ● **S20.15**   **Superficial foreign body of breast**
>> Splinter in the breast

      ● **S20.151**   Superficial foreign body of breast, right breast
      ● **S20.152**   Superficial foreign body of breast, left breast
      ● **S20.159**   Superficial foreign body of breast, unspecified breast
    ● **S20.16**   **Insect bite (nonvenomous) of breast**
      ● **S20.161**   Insect bite (nonvenomous) of breast, right breast
      ● **S20.162**   Insect bite (nonvenomous) of breast, left breast
      ● **S20.169**   Insect bite (nonvenomous) of breast, unspecified breast
    ● **S20.17**   **Other superficial bite of breast**
>> **Excludes1**   open bite of breast (S21.05-)

      ● **S20.171**   Other superficial bite of breast, right breast
      ● **S20.172**   Other superficial bite of breast, left breast
      ● **S20.179**   Other superficial bite of breast, unspecified breast

  ● **S20.2**   **Contusion of thorax**
    X ● **S20.20**   Contusion of thorax, unspecified
    ● **S20.21**   **Contusion of front wall of thorax**
      ● **S20.211**   Contusion of right front wall of thorax
      ● **S20.212**   Contusion of left front wall of thorax
      ● **S20.219**   Contusion of unspecified front wall of thorax
    ● **S20.22**   **Contusion of back wall of thorax**
      ● **S20.221**   Contusion of right back wall of thorax
      ● **S20.222**   Contusion of left back wall of thorax
      ● **S20.229**   Contusion of unspecified back wall of thorax

◀ New   ◀ Revised   ~~deleted~~ Deleted   Excludes 1   Excludes 2   Includes   Use additional   Code first   Code also   Unspecified
OGCR Official Guidelines   X Assign placeholder X   ● Use Additional Character(s)   ▷ Manifestation Code   **Coding Clinic**

● **S20.3** **Other and unspecified superficial injuries of front wall of thorax**
- ● **S20.30** Unspecified superficial injuries of front wall of thorax
  - ● **S20.301** Unspecified superficial injuries of right front wall of thorax
  - ● **S20.302** Unspecified superficial injuries of left front wall of thorax
  - ● **S20.309** Unspecified superficial injuries of unspecified front wall of thorax
- ● **S20.31** Abrasion of front wall of thorax
  - ● **S20.311** Abrasion of right front wall of thorax
  - ● **S20.312** Abrasion of left front wall of thorax
  - ● **S20.319** Abrasion of unspecified front wall of thorax
- ● **S20.32** Blister (nonthermal) of front wall of thorax
  - ● **S20.321** Blister (nonthermal) of right front wall of thorax
  - ● **S20.322** Blister (nonthermal) of left front wall of thorax
  - ● **S20.329** Blister (nonthermal) of unspecified front wall of thorax
- ● **S20.34** External constriction of front wall of thorax
  - ● **S20.341** External constriction of right front wall of thorax
  - ● **S20.342** External constriction of left front wall of thorax
  - ● **S20.349** External constriction of unspecified front wall of thorax
- ● **S20.35** Superficial foreign body of front wall of thorax
  Splinter in front wall of thorax
  - ● **S20.351** Superficial foreign body of right front wall of thorax
  - ● **S20.352** Superficial foreign body of left front wall of thorax
  - ● **S20.359** Superficial foreign body of unspecified front wall of thorax
- ● **S20.36** Insect bite (nonvenomous) of front wall of thorax
  - ● **S20.361** Insect bite (nonvenomous) of right front wall of thorax
  - ● **S20.362** Insect bite (nonvenomous) of left front wall of thorax
  - ● **S20.369** Insect bite (nonvenomous) of unspecified front wall of thorax
- ● **S20.37** Other superficial bite of front wall of thorax
  - **Excludes1** open bite of front wall of thorax (S21.14)
  - ● **S20.371** Other superficial bite of right front wall of thorax
  - ● **S20.372** Other superficial bite of left front wall of thorax
  - ● **S20.379** Other superficial bite of unspecified front wall of thorax

● **S20.4** **Other and unspecified superficial injuries of back wall of thorax**
- ● **S20.40** Unspecified superficial injuries of back wall of thorax
  - ● **S20.401** Unspecified superficial injuries of right back wall of thorax
  - ● **S20.402** Unspecified superficial injuries of left back wall of thorax
  - ● **S20.409** Unspecified superficial injuries of unspecified back wall of thorax

● **S20.41** **Abrasion of back wall of thorax**
- ● **S20.411** Abrasion of right back wall of thorax
- ● **S20.412** Abrasion of left back wall of thorax
- ● **S20.419** Abrasion of unspecified back wall of thorax
- ● **S20.42** Blister (nonthermal) of back wall of thorax
  - ● **S20.421** Blister (nonthermal) of right back wall of thorax
  - ● **S20.422** Blister (nonthermal) of left back wall of thorax
  - ● **S20.429** Blister (nonthermal) of unspecified back wall of thorax
- ● **S20.44** External constriction of back wall of thorax
  - ● **S20.441** External constriction of right back wall of thorax
  - ● **S20.442** External constriction of left back wall of thorax
  - ● **S20.449** External constriction of unspecified back wall of thorax
- ● **S20.45** Superficial foreign body of back wall of thorax
  Splinter of back wall of thorax
  - ● **S20.451** Superficial foreign body of right back wall of thorax
  - ● **S20.452** Superficial foreign body of left back wall of thorax
  - ● **S20.459** Superficial foreign body of unspecified back wall of thorax
- ● **S20.46** Insect bite (nonvenomous) of back wall of thorax
  - ● **S20.461** Insect bite (nonvenomous) of right back wall of thorax
  - ● **S20.462** Insect bite (nonvenomous) of left back wall of thorax
  - ● **S20.469** Insect bite (nonvenomous) of unspecified back wall of thorax
- ● **S20.47** Other superficial bite of back wall of thorax
  - **Excludes1** open bite of back wall of thorax (S21.24)
  - ● **S20.471** Other superficial bite of right back wall of thorax
  - ● **S20.472** Other superficial bite of left back wall of thorax
  - ● **S20.479** Other superficial bite of unspecified back wall of thorax

● **S20.9** **Superficial injury of unspecified parts of thorax**
- **Excludes1** contusion of thorax NOS (S20.20)
- X ● **S20.90** Unspecified superficial injury of unspecified parts of thorax
  Superficial injury of thoracic wall NOS
- X ● **S20.91** Abrasion of unspecified parts of thorax
- X ● **S20.92** Blister (nonthermal) of unspecified parts of thorax
- X ● **S20.94** External constriction of unspecified parts of thorax
- X ● **S20.95** Superficial foreign body of unspecified parts of thorax
  Splinter in thorax NOS
- X ● **S20.96** Insect bite (nonvenomous) of unspecified parts of thorax
- X ● **S20.97** Other superficial bite of unspecified parts of thorax
  - **Excludes1** open bite of thorax NOS (S21.95)

CHAPTER 19 (S00-T88)

CHAPTER 19 (S00-T88)

Item 19-1 **Pneumothorax** is a collection of gas (positive air pressure) in the pleural space resulting in the lung collapsing. A tension pneumothorax is life-threatening and is a result of air in the pleural space causing a displacement in the mediastinal structures and cardiopulmonary function compromise. A traumatic pneumothorax results from blunt or penetrating injury that disrupts the parietal/visceral pleura. **Hemothorax** is blood or bloody fluid in the pleural cavity as a result of traumatic blood vessel rupture or inflammation of the lungs from pneumonia.

● **S21   Open wound of thorax**

Code also any associated injury such as:
injury of heart (S26.-)
injury of intrathoracic organs (S27.-)
rib fracture (S22.3-, S22.4-)
spinal cord injury (S24.0-, S24.1-)
traumatic hemothorax (S27.1)
traumatic hemopneumothorax (S27.3)
traumatic pneumothorax (S27.0)
wound infection

Excludes1   traumatic amputation (partial) of thorax (S28.1)

The appropriate 7th character is to be added to each code from category S21

A	initial encounter
D	subsequent encounter
S	sequela

● **S21.0   Open wound of breast**

● **S21.00   Unspecified open wound of breast**

● **S21.001   Unspecified open wound of right breast**

● **S21.002   Unspecified open wound of left breast**

● **S21.009   Unspecified open wound of unspecified breast**

● **S21.01   Laceration without foreign body of breast**

● **S21.011   Laceration without foreign body of right breast**

● **S21.012   Laceration without foreign body of left breast**

● **S21.019   Laceration without foreign body of unspecified breast**

● **S21.02   Laceration with foreign body of breast**

● **S21.021   Laceration with foreign body of right breast**

● **S21.022   Laceration with foreign body of left breast**

● **S21.029   Laceration with foreign body of unspecified breast**

● **S21.03   Puncture wound without foreign body of breast**

● **S21.031   Puncture wound without foreign body of right breast**

● **S21.032   Puncture wound without foreign body of left breast**

● **S21.039   Puncture wound without foreign body of unspecified breast**

● **S21.04   Puncture wound with foreign body of breast**

● **S21.041   Puncture wound with foreign body of right breast**

● **S21.042   Puncture wound with foreign body of left breast**

● **S21.049   Puncture wound with foreign body of unspecified breast**

● **S21.05   Open bite of breast**
Bite of breast NOS

Excludes1   superficial bite of breast (S20.17)

● **S21.051   Open bite of right breast**

● **S21.052   Open bite of left breast**

● **S21.059   Open bite of unspecified breast**

● **S21.1   Open wound of front wall of thorax without penetration into thoracic cavity**
Open wound of chest without penetration into thoracic cavity

● **S21.10   Unspecified open wound of front wall of thorax without penetration into thoracic cavity**

● **S21.101   Unspecified open wound of right front wall of thorax without penetration into thoracic cavity**

● **S21.102   Unspecified open wound of left front wall of thorax without penetration into thoracic cavity**

● **S21.109   Unspecified open wound of unspecified front wall of thorax without penetration into thoracic cavity**

● **S21.11   Laceration without foreign body of front wall of thorax without penetration into thoracic cavity**

● **S21.111   Laceration without foreign body of right front wall of thorax without penetration into thoracic cavity**

● **S21.112   Laceration without foreign body of left front wall of thorax without penetration into thoracic cavity**

● **S21.119   Laceration without foreign body of unspecified front wall of thorax without penetration into thoracic cavity**

● **S21.12   Laceration with foreign body of front wall of thorax without penetration into thoracic cavity**

● **S21.121   Laceration with foreign body of right front wall of thorax without penetration into thoracic cavity**

● **S21.122   Laceration with foreign body of left front wall of thorax without penetration into thoracic cavity**

● **S21.129   Laceration with foreign body of unspecified front wall of thorax without penetration into thoracic cavity**

● **S21.13   Puncture wound without foreign body of front wall of thorax without penetration into thoracic cavity**

● **S21.131   Puncture wound without foreign body of right front wall of thorax without penetration into thoracic cavity**

● **S21.132   Puncture wound without foreign body of left front wall of thorax without penetration into thoracic cavity**

● **S21.139   Puncture wound without foreign body of unspecified front wall of thorax without penetration into thoracic cavity**

● **S21.14   Puncture wound with foreign body of front wall of thorax without penetration into thoracic cavity**

● **S21.141   Puncture wound with foreign body of right front wall of thorax without penetration into thoracic cavity**

● **S21.142   Puncture wound with foreign body of left front wall of thorax without penetration into thoracic cavity**

● **S21.149   Puncture wound with foreign body of unspecified front wall of thorax without penetration into thoracic cavity**

◄ New   ◄▦ Revised   ~~deleted~~ Deleted   Excludes 1   Excludes 2   Includes   Use additional   Code first   Code also   Unspecified

1212   OGCR Official Guidelines   X Assign placeholder X   ● Use Additional Character(s)   ▶ Manifestation Code   **Coding Clinic**

● S21.15 **Open bite of front wall of thorax without penetration into thoracic cavity**
Bite of front wall of thorax NOS
> **Excludes1** superficial bite of front wall of thorax (S20.37)

● S21.151 **Open bite of right front wall of thorax without penetration into thoracic cavity**

● S21.152 **Open bite of left front wall of thorax without penetration into thoracic cavity**

● S21.159 **Open bite of unspecified front wall of thorax without penetration into thoracic cavity**

● S21.2 **Open wound of back wall of thorax without penetration into thoracic cavity**

● S21.20 **Unspecified open wound of back wall of thorax without penetration into thoracic cavity**

● S21.201 **Unspecified open wound of right back wall of thorax without penetration into thoracic cavity**

● S21.202 **Unspecified open wound of left back wall of thorax without penetration into thoracic cavity**

● S21.209 **Unspecified open wound of unspecified back wall of thorax without penetration into thoracic cavity**

● S21.21 **Laceration without foreign body of back wall of thorax without penetration into thoracic cavity**

● S21.211 **Laceration without foreign body of right back wall of thorax without penetration into thoracic cavity**

● S21.212 **Laceration without foreign body of left back wall of thorax without penetration into thoracic cavity**

● S21.219 **Laceration without foreign body of unspecified back wall of thorax without penetration into thoracic cavity**

● S21.22 **Laceration with foreign body of back wall of thorax without penetration into thoracic cavity**

● S21.221 **Laceration with foreign body of right back wall of thorax without penetration into thoracic cavity**

● S21.222 **Laceration with foreign body of left back wall of thorax without penetration into thoracic cavity**

● S21.229 **Laceration with foreign body of unspecified back wall of thorax without penetration into thoracic cavity**

● S21.23 **Puncture wound without foreign body of back wall of thorax without penetration into thoracic cavity**

● S21.231 **Puncture wound without foreign body of right back wall of thorax without penetration into thoracic cavity**

● S21.232 **Puncture wound without foreign body of left back wall of thorax without penetration into thoracic cavity**

● S21.239 **Puncture wound without foreign body of unspecified back wall of thorax without penetration into thoracic cavity**

● S21.24 **Puncture wound with foreign body of back wall of thorax without penetration into thoracic cavity**

● S21.241 **Puncture wound with foreign body of right back wall of thorax without penetration into thoracic cavity**

● S21.242 **Puncture wound with foreign body of left back wall of thorax without penetration into thoracic cavity**

● S21.249 **Puncture wound with foreign body of unspecified back wall of thorax without penetration into thoracic cavity**

● S21.25 **Open bite of back wall of thorax without penetration into thoracic cavity**
Bite of back wall of thorax NOS
> **Excludes1** superficial bite of back wall of thorax (S20.47)

● S21.251 **Open bite of right back wall of thorax without penetration into thoracic cavity**

● S21.252 **Open bite of left back wall of thorax without penetration into thoracic cavity**

● S21.259 **Open bite of unspecified back wall of thorax without penetration into thoracic cavity**

● S21.3 **Open wound of front wall of thorax with penetration into thoracic cavity**
Open wound of chest with penetration into thoracic cavity

● S21.30 **Unspecified open wound of front wall of thorax with penetration into thoracic cavity**

● S21.301 **Unspecified open wound of right front wall of thorax with penetration into thoracic cavity**

● S21.302 **Unspecified open wound of left front wall of thorax with penetration into thoracic cavity**

● S21.309 **Unspecified open wound of unspecified front wall of thorax with penetration into thoracic cavity**

● S21.31 **Laceration without foreign body of front wall of thorax with penetration into thoracic cavity**

● S21.311 **Laceration without foreign body of right front wall of thorax with penetration into thoracic cavity**

● S21.312 **Laceration without foreign body of left front wall of thorax with penetration into thoracic cavity**

● S21.319 **Laceration without foreign body of unspecified front wall of thorax with penetration into thoracic cavity**

● S21.32 **Laceration with foreign body of front wall of thorax with penetration into thoracic cavity**

● S21.321 **Laceration with foreign body of right front wall of thorax with penetration into thoracic cavity**

● S21.322 **Laceration with foreign body of left front wall of thorax with penetration into thoracic cavity**

● S21.329 **Laceration with foreign body of unspecified front wall of thorax with penetration into thoracic cavity**

CHAPTER 19 (S00–T88)

● **S21.33** Puncture wound without foreign body of front wall of thorax with penetration into thoracic cavity
- ● **S21.331** Puncture wound without foreign body of right front wall of thorax with penetration into thoracic cavity
- ● **S21.332** Puncture wound without foreign body of left front wall of thorax with penetration into thoracic cavity
- ● **S21.339** Puncture wound without foreign body of unspecified front wall of thorax with penetration into thoracic cavity

● **S21.34** Puncture wound with foreign body of front wall of thorax with penetration into thoracic cavity
- ● **S21.341** Puncture wound with foreign body of right front wall of thorax with penetration into thoracic cavity
- ● **S21.342** Puncture wound with foreign body of left front wall of thorax with penetration into thoracic cavity
- ● **S21.349** Puncture wound with foreign body of unspecified front wall of thorax with penetration into thoracic cavity

● **S21.35** Open bite of front wall of thorax with penetration into thoracic cavity
  Excludes1 superficial bite of front wall of thorax (S20.37)
- ● **S21.351** Open bite of right front wall of thorax with penetration into thoracic cavity
- ● **S21.352** Open bite of left front wall of thorax with penetration into thoracic cavity
- ● **S21.359** Open bite of unspecified front wall of thorax with penetration into thoracic cavity

● **S21.4** Open wound of back wall of thorax with penetration into thoracic cavity
- ● **S21.40** Unspecified open wound of back wall of thorax with penetration into thoracic cavity
  - ● **S21.401** Unspecified open wound of right back wall of thorax with penetration into thoracic cavity
  - ● **S21.402** Unspecified open wound of left back wall of thorax with penetration into thoracic cavity
  - ● **S21.409** Unspecified open wound of unspecified back wall of thorax with penetration into thoracic cavity
- ● **S21.41** Laceration without foreign body of back wall of thorax with penetration into thoracic cavity
  - ● **S21.411** Laceration without foreign body of right back wall of thorax with penetration into thoracic cavity
  - ● **S21.412** Laceration without foreign body of left back wall of thorax with penetration into thoracic cavity
  - ● **S21.419** Laceration without foreign body of unspecified back wall of thorax with penetration into thoracic cavity

● **S21.42** Laceration with foreign body of back wall of thorax with penetration into thoracic cavity
- ● **S21.421** Laceration with foreign body of right back wall of thorax with penetration into thoracic cavity
- ● **S21.422** Laceration with foreign body of left back wall of thorax with penetration into thoracic cavity
- ● **S21.429** Laceration with foreign body of unspecified back wall of thorax with penetration into thoracic cavity

● **S21.43** Puncture wound without foreign body of back wall of thorax with penetration into thoracic cavity
- ● **S21.431** Puncture wound without foreign body of right back wall of thorax with penetration into thoracic cavity
- ● **S21.432** Puncture wound without foreign body of left back wall of thorax with penetration into thoracic cavity
- ● **S21.439** Puncture wound without foreign body of unspecified back wall of thorax with penetration into thoracic cavity

● **S21.44** Puncture wound with foreign body of back wall of thorax with penetration into thoracic cavity
- ● **S21.441** Puncture wound with foreign body of right back wall of thorax with penetration into thoracic cavity
- ● **S21.442** Puncture wound with foreign body of left back wall of thorax with penetration into thoracic cavity
- ● **S21.449** Puncture wound with foreign body of unspecified back wall of thorax with penetration into thoracic cavity

● **S21.45** Open bite of back wall of thorax with penetration into thoracic cavity
  Bite of back wall of thorax NOS
  Excludes1 superficial bite of back wall of thorax (S20.47)
- ● **S21.451** Open bite of right back wall of thorax with penetration into thoracic cavity
- ● **S21.452** Open bite of left back wall of thorax with penetration into thoracic cavity
- ● **S21.459** Open bite of unspecified back wall of thorax with penetration into thoracic cavity

● **S21.9** Open wound of unspecified part of thorax
  Open wound of thoracic wall NOS
- X ● **S21.90** Unspecified open wound of unspecified part of thorax
- X ● **S21.91** Laceration without foreign body of unspecified part of thorax
- X ● **S21.92** Laceration with foreign body of unspecified part of thorax
- X ● **S21.93** Puncture wound without foreign body of unspecified part of thorax
- X ● **S21.94** Puncture wound with foreign body of unspecified part of thorax
- X ● **S21.95** Open bite of unspecified part of thorax
  Excludes1 superficial bite of thorax (S20.97)

◀ New   ◀▦ Revised   ~~deleted~~ Deleted   Excludes 1   Excludes 2   Includes   Use additional   Code first   Code also   Unspecified

1214   OGCR Official Guidelines   X Assign placeholder X   ● Use Additional Character(s)   ▶ Manifestation Code   **Coding Clinic**

● **S22**   **Fracture of rib(s), sternum and thoracic spine**

Note: A fracture not indicated as displaced or nondisplaced should be coded to displaced

A fracture not indicated as open or closed should be coded to closed

Includes   fracture of thoracic neural arch
fracture of thoracic spinous process
fracture of thoracic transverse process
fracture of thoracic vertebra
fracture of thoracic vertebral arch

Code first any associated:
injury of intrathoracic organ (S27.-)
spinal cord injury (S24.0-, S24.1-)

Excludes1   transection of thorax (S28.1)

Excludes2   fracture of clavicle (S42.0-)
fracture of scapula (S42.1-)

The appropriate 7th character is to be added to each code from category S22

A	initial encounter for closed fracture
B	initial encounter for open fracture
D	subsequent encounter for fracture with routine healing
G	subsequent encounter for fracture with delayed healing
K	subsequent encounter for fracture with nonunion
S	sequela

● **S22.0**   **Fracture of thoracic vertebra**

   ● **S22.00**   **Fracture of unspecified thoracic vertebra**

     ● **S22.000**   Wedge compression fracture of unspecified thoracic vertebra

     ● **S22.001**   Stable burst fracture of unspecified thoracic vertebra

     ● **S22.002**   Unstable burst fracture of unspecified thoracic vertebra

     ● **S22.008**   Other fracture of unspecified thoracic vertebra

     ● **S22.009**   Unspecified fracture of unspecified thoracic vertebra

   ● **S22.01**   **Fracture of first thoracic vertebra**

     ● **S22.010**   Wedge compression fracture of first thoracic vertebra

     ● **S22.011**   Stable burst fracture of first thoracic vertebra

     ● **S22.012**   Unstable burst fracture of first thoracic vertebra

     ● **S22.018**   Other fracture of first thoracic vertebra

     ● **S22.019**   Unspecified fracture of first thoracic vertebra

   ● **S22.02**   **Fracture of second thoracic vertebra**

     ● **S22.020**   Wedge compression fracture of second thoracic vertebra

     ● **S22.021**   Stable burst fracture of second thoracic vertebra

     ● **S22.022**   Unstable burst fracture of second thoracic vertebra

     ● **S22.028**   Other fracture of second thoracic vertebra

     ● **S22.029**   Unspecified fracture of second thoracic vertebra

   ● **S22.03**   **Fracture of third thoracic vertebra**

     ● **S22.030**   Wedge compression fracture of third thoracic vertebra

     ● **S22.031**   Stable burst fracture of third thoracic vertebra

     ● **S22.032**   Unstable burst fracture of third thoracic vertebra

     ● **S22.038**   Other fracture of third thoracic vertebra

     ● **S22.039**   Unspecified fracture of third thoracic vertebra

● **S22.04**   **Fracture of fourth thoracic vertebra**

   ● **S22.040**   Wedge compression fracture of fourth thoracic vertebra

   ● **S22.041**   Stable burst fracture of fourth thoracic vertebra

   ● **S22.042**   Unstable burst fracture of fourth thoracic vertebra

   ● **S22.048**   Other fracture of fourth thoracic vertebra

   ● **S22.049**   Unspecified fracture of fourth thoracic vertebra

● **S22.05**   **Fracture of T_5-T_6 vertebra**

   ● **S22.050**   Wedge compression fracture of T_5-T_6 vertebra

   ● **S22.051**   Stable burst fracture of T_5-T_6 vertebra

   ● **S22.052**   Unstable burst fracture of T_5-T_6 vertebra

   ● **S22.058**   Other fracture of T_5-T_6 vertebra

   ● **S22.059**   Unspecified fracture of T_5-T_6 vertebra

● **S22.06**   **Fracture of T_7-T_8 vertebra**

   ● **S22.060**   Wedge compression fracture of T_7-T_8 vertebra

   ● **S22.061**   Stable burst fracture of T_7-T_8 vertebra

   ● **S22.062**   Unstable burst fracture of T_7-T_8 vertebra

   ● **S22.068**   Other fracture of T_7-T_8 thoracic vertebra

   ● **S22.069**   Unspecified fracture of T_7-T_8 vertebra

● **S22.07**   **Fracture of T_9-T_{10} vertebra**

   ● **S22.070**   Wedge compression fracture of T_9-T_{10} vertebra

   ● **S22.071**   Stable burst fracture of T_9-T_{10} vertebra

   ● **S22.072**   Unstable burst fracture of T_9-T_{10} vertebra

   ● **S22.078**   Other fracture of T_9-T_{10} vertebra

   ● **S22.079**   Unspecified fracture of T_9-T_{10} vertebra

● **S22.08**   **Fracture of T_{11}-T_{12} vertebra**

   ● **S22.080**   Wedge compression fracture of T_{11}-T_{12} vertebra

   ● **S22.081**   Stable burst fracture of T_{11}-T_{12} vertebra

   ● **S22.082**   Unstable burst fracture of T_{11}-T_{12} vertebra

   ● **S22.088**   Other fracture of T_{11}-T_{12} vertebra

   ● **S22.089**   Unspecified fracture of T_{11}-T_{12} vertebra

● **S22.2**   **Fracture of sternum**

   X● **S22.20**   Unspecified fracture of sternum

   X● **S22.21**   Fracture of manubrium

   X● **S22.22**   Fracture of body of sternum

   X● **S22.23**   Sternal manubrial dissociation

   X● **S22.24**   Fracture of xiphoid process

● **S22.3**   **Fracture of one rib**

   X● **S22.31**   Fracture of one rib, right side

   X● **S22.32**   Fracture of one rib, left side

   X● **S22.39**   Fracture of one rib, unspecified side

● **S22.4**   **Multiple fractures of ribs**

   Fractures of two or more ribs

   Excludes1   flail chest (S22.5-)

   X● **S22.41**   Multiple fractures of ribs, right side

   X● **S22.42**   Multiple fractures of ribs, left side

   X● **S22.43**   Multiple fractures of ribs, bilateral

   X● **S22.49**   Multiple fractures of ribs, unspecified side

● X● **S22.5**   **Flail chest**

   Unstable chest due to sternum and/or rib fracture

X● **S22.9**   **Fracture of bony thorax, part unspecified**

CHAPTER 19 (S00-T88)

● **S23   Dislocation and sprain of joints and ligaments of thorax**

     Includes   avulsion of joint or ligament of thorax
           laceration of cartilage, joint or ligament of thorax
           sprain of cartilage, joint or ligament of thorax
           traumatic hemarthrosis of joint or ligament of
             thorax
           traumatic rupture of joint or ligament of thorax
           traumatic subluxation of joint or ligament of
             thorax
           traumatic tear of joint or ligament of thorax

Code also any associated open wound

     Excludes2   dislocation, sprain of sternoclavicular joint (S43.2,
             S43.6)
           strain of muscle or tendon of thorax (S29.01-)

The appropriate 7th character is to be added to each code from
category S23

> A   initial encounter
> D   subsequent encounter
> S   sequela

X ● **S23.0   Traumatic rupture of thoracic intervertebral disc**

     Excludes1   rupture or displacement (nontraumatic)
             of thoracic intervertebral disc NOS
             (M51.- with fifth character 4)

● **S23.1   Subluxation and dislocation of thoracic vertebra**

     Code also any associated
       open wound of thorax (S21.-)
       spinal cord injury (S24.0-, S24.1-)

     Excludes2   fracture of thoracic vertebrae (S22.0-)

   ● **S23.10   Subluxation and dislocation of unspecified
            thoracic vertebra**

     ● **S23.100   Subluxation of unspecified thoracic
             vertebra**

     ● **S23.101   Dislocation of unspecified thoracic
             vertebra**

   ● **S23.11   Subluxation and dislocation of T_1/T_2 thoracic
            vertebra**

     ● **S23.110   Subluxation of T_1/T_2 thoracic vertebra**
     ● **S23.111   Dislocation of T_1/T_2 thoracic vertebra**

   ● **S23.12   Subluxation and dislocation of T_2/T_3-T_3/T_4
            thoracic vertebra**

     ● **S23.120   Subluxation of T_2/T_3 thoracic vertebra**
     ● **S23.121   Dislocation of T_2/T_3 thoracic vertebra**
     ● **S23.122   Subluxation of T_3/T_4 thoracic vertebra**
     ● **S23.123   Dislocation of T_3/T_4 thoracic vertebra**

   ● **S23.13   Subluxation and dislocation of T_4/T_5-T_5/T_6
            thoracic vertebra**

     ● **S23.130   Subluxation of T_4/T_5 thoracic vertebra**
     ● **S23.131   Dislocation of T_4/T_5 thoracic vertebra**
     ● **S23.132   Subluxation of T_5/T_6 thoracic vertebra**
     ● **S23.133   Dislocation of T_5/T_6 thoracic vertebra**

   ● **S23.14   Subluxation and dislocation of T_6/T_7-T_7/T_8
            thoracic vertebra**

     ● **S23.140   Subluxation of T_6/T_7 thoracic vertebra**
     ● **S23.141   Dislocation of T_6/T_7 thoracic vertebra**
     ● **S23.142   Subluxation of T_7/T_8 thoracic vertebra**
     ● **S23.143   Dislocation of T_7/T_8 thoracic vertebra**

   ● **S23.15   Subluxation and dislocation of T_8/T_9-T_9/T_{10}
            thoracic vertebra**

     ● **S23.150   Subluxation of T_8/T_9 thoracic vertebra**
     ● **S23.151   Dislocation of T_8/T_9 thoracic vertebra**
     ● **S23.152   Subluxation of T_9/T_{10} thoracic
             vertebra**
     ● **S23.153   Dislocation of T_9/T_{10} thoracic vertebra**

● **S23.16   Subluxation and dislocation of T_{10}/T_{11}-T_{11}/T_{12}
            thoracic vertebra**

   ● **S23.160   Subluxation of T_{10}/T_{11} thoracic
            vertebra**
   ● **S23.161   Dislocation of T_{10}/T_{11} thoracic vertebra**
   ● **S23.162   Subluxation of T_{11}/T_{12} thoracic
            vertebra**
   ● **S23.163   Dislocation of T_{11}/T_{12} thoracic vertebra**

● **S23.17   Subluxation and dislocation of T_{12}/L_1 thoracic
            vertebra**

   ● **S23.170   Subluxation of T_{12}/L_1 thoracic vertebra**
   ● **S23.171   Dislocation of T_{12}/L_1 thoracic vertebra**

● **S23.2   Dislocation of other and unspecified parts of thorax**

X ● **S23.20   Dislocation of unspecified part of thorax**
X ● **S23.29   Dislocation of other parts of thorax**

X ● **S23.3   Sprain of ligaments of thoracic spine**

● **S23.4   Sprain of ribs and sternum**

X ● **S23.41   Sprain of ribs**

   ● **S23.42   Sprain of sternum**

     ● **S23.420   Sprain of sternoclavicular (joint)
            (ligament)**
     ● **S23.421   Sprain of chondrosternal joint**
     ● **S23.428   Other sprain of sternum**
     ● **S23.429   Unspecified sprain of sternum**

X ● **S23.8   Sprain of other specified parts of thorax**
X ● **S23.9   Sprain of unspecified parts of thorax**

● **S24   Injury of nerves and spinal cord at thorax level**

     Note: Code to highest level of thoracic spinal cord injury.

         Injuries to the spinal cord (S24.0 and S24.1) refer to the cord
         level and not bone level injury, and can affect nerve roots at
         and below the level given.

     Code also any associated:
       fracture of thoracic vertebra (S22.0-)
       open wound of thorax (S21.-)
       transient paralysis (R29.5)

     Excludes2   injury of brachial plexus (S14.3)

The appropriate 7th character is to be added to each code from
category S24

> A   initial encounter
> D   subsequent encounter
> S   sequela

X ● **S24.0   Concussion and edema of thoracic spinal cord**

● **S24.1   Other and unspecified injuries of thoracic spinal cord**

   ● **S24.10   Unspecified injury of thoracic spinal cord**

     ● **S24.101   Unspecified injury at T_1 level of
            thoracic spinal cord**
     ● **S24.102   Unspecified injury at T_2-T_6 level of
            thoracic spinal cord**
     ● **S24.103   Unspecified injury at T_7-T_{10} level of
            thoracic spinal cord**
     ● **S24.104   Unspecified injury at T_{11}-T_{12} level of
            thoracic spinal cord**
     ● **S24.109   Unspecified injury at unspecified level
            of thoracic spinal cord**
            Injury of thoracic spinal cord NOS

   ● **S24.11   Complete lesion of thoracic spinal cord**

     ● **S24.111   Complete lesion at T_1 level of thoracic
            spinal cord**
     ● **S24.112   Complete lesion at T_2-T_6 level of
            thoracic spinal cord**
     ● **S24.113   Complete lesion at T_7-T_{10} level of
            thoracic spinal cord**
     ● **S24.114   Complete lesion at T_{11}-T_{12} level of
            thoracic spinal cord**
     ● **S24.119   Complete lesion at unspecified level
            of thoracic spinal cord**

◀ New   ◀▥ Revised   ~~deleted~~ Deleted   Excludes 1   Excludes 2   Includes   Use additional   Code first   Code also   Unspecified

OGCR Official Guidelines   X Assign placeholder X   ● Use Additional Character(s)   ▌ Manifestation Code   **Coding Clinic**

● S24.13   Anterior cord syndrome of thoracic spinal cord
    ● S24.131   Anterior cord syndrome at T_1 level of thoracic spinal cord
    ● S24.132   Anterior cord syndrome at T_2-T_6 level of thoracic spinal cord
    ● S24.133   Anterior cord syndrome at T_7-T_{10} level of thoracic spinal cord
    ● S24.134   Anterior cord syndrome at T_{11}-T_{12} level of thoracic spinal cord
    ● S24.139   Anterior cord syndrome at unspecified level of thoracic spinal cord

● S24.14   Brown-Séquard syndrome of thoracic spinal cord
    ● S24.141   Brown-Séquard syndrome at T_1 level of thoracic spinal cord
    ● S24.142   Brown-Séquard syndrome at T_2-T_6 level of thoracic spinal cord
    ● S24.143   Brown-Séquard syndrome at T_7-T_{10} level of thoracic spinal cord
    ● S24.144   Brown-Séquard syndrome at T_{11}-T_{12} level of thoracic spinal cord
    ● S24.149   Brown-Séquard syndrome at unspecified level of thoracic spinal cord

● S24.15   Other incomplete lesions of thoracic spinal cord
     Incomplete lesion of thoracic spinal cord NOS
     Posterior cord syndrome of thoracic spinal cord
    ● S24.151   Other incomplete lesion at T_1 level of thoracic spinal cord
    ● S24.152   Other incomplete lesion at T_2-T_6 level of thoracic spinal cord
    ● S24.153   Other incomplete lesion at T_7-T_{10} level of thoracic spinal cord
    ● S24.154   Other incomplete lesion at T_{11}-T_{12} level of thoracic spinal cord
    ● S24.159   Other incomplete lesion at unspecified level of thoracic spinal cord

X● S24.2   Injury of nerve root of thoracic spine
X● S24.3   Injury of peripheral nerves of thorax
X● S24.4   Injury of thoracic sympathetic nervous system
     Injury of cardiac plexus
     Injury of esophageal plexus
     Injury of pulmonary plexus
     Injury of stellate ganglion
     Injury of thoracic sympathetic ganglion
X● S24.8   Injury of other specified nerves of thorax
X● S24.9   Injury of unspecified nerve of thorax

● S25   Injury of blood vessels of thorax
     The appropriate 7th character is to be added to each code from category S25

A	initial encounter
D	subsequent encounter
S	sequela

     Code also any associated open wound (S21.-)

● S25.0   Injury of thoracic aorta
     Injury of aorta NOS
  X● S25.00   Unspecified injury of thoracic aorta
  X● S25.01   Minor laceration of thoracic aorta
     Incomplete transection of thoracic aorta
     Laceration of thoracic aorta NOS
     Superficial laceration of thoracic aorta
  X● S25.02   Major laceration of thoracic aorta
     Complete transection of thoracic aorta
     Traumatic rupture of thoracic aorta
  X● S25.09   Other specified injury of thoracic aorta

● S25.1   Injury of innominate or subclavian artery
    ● S25.10   Unspecified injury of innominate or subclavian artery
     ● S25.101   Unspecified injury of right innominate or subclavian artery
     ● S25.102   Unspecified injury of left innominate or subclavian artery
     ● S25.109   Unspecified injury of unspecified innominate or subclavian artery
    ● S25.11   Minor laceration of innominate or subclavian artery
     Incomplete transection of innominate or subclavian artery
     Laceration of innominate or subclavian artery NOS
     Superficial laceration of innominate or subclavian artery
     ● S25.111   Minor laceration of right innominate or subclavian artery
     ● S25.112   Minor laceration of left innominate or subclavian artery
     ● S25.119   Minor laceration of unspecified innominate or subclavian artery
    ● S25.12   Major laceration of innominate or subclavian artery
     Complete transection of innominate or subclavian artery
     Traumatic rupture of innominate or subclavian artery
     ● S25.121   Major laceration of right innominate or subclavian artery
     ● S25.122   Major laceration of left innominate or subclavian artery
     ● S25.129   Major laceration of unspecified innominate or subclavian artery
    ● S25.19   Other specified injury of innominate or subclavian artery
     ● S25.191   Other specified injury of right innominate or subclavian artery
     ● S25.192   Other specified injury of left innominate or subclavian artery
     ● S25.199   Other specified injury of unspecified innominate or subclavian artery

● S25.2   Injury of superior vena cava
     Injury of vena cava NOS
  X● S25.20   Unspecified injury of superior vena cava
  X● S25.21   Minor laceration of superior vena cava
     Incomplete transection of superior vena cava
     Laceration of superior vena cava NOS
     Superficial laceration of superior vena cava
  X● S25.22   Major laceration of superior vena cava
     Complete transection of superior vena cava
     Traumatic rupture of superior vena cava
  X● S25.29   Other specified injury of superior vena cava

● S25.3   Injury of innominate or subclavian vein
    ● S25.30   Unspecified injury of innominate or subclavian vein
     ● S25.301   Unspecified injury of right innominate or subclavian vein
     ● S25.302   Unspecified injury of left innominate or subclavian vein
     ● S25.309   Unspecified injury of unspecified innominate or subclavian vein

CHAPTER 19 (S00-T88)

●S25.31   Minor laceration of innominate or subclavian vein
     Incomplete transection of innominate or subclavian vein
     Laceration of innominate or subclavian vein NOS
     Superficial laceration of innominate or subclavian vein
   ●S25.311   Minor laceration of right innominate or subclavian vein
   ●S25.312   Minor laceration of left innominate or subclavian vein
   ●S25.319   Minor laceration of unspecified innominate or subclavian vein

●S25.32   Major laceration of innominate or subclavian vein
     Complete transection of innominate or subclavian vein
     Traumatic rupture of innominate or subclavian vein
   ●S25.321   Major laceration of right innominate or subclavian vein
   ●S25.322   Major laceration of left innominate or subclavian vein
   ●S25.329   Major laceration of unspecified innominate or subclavian vein

●S25.39   Other specified injury of innominate or subclavian vein
   ●S25.391   Other specified injury of right innominate or subclavian vein
   ●S25.392   Other specified injury of left innominate or subclavian vein
   ●S25.399   Other specified injury of unspecified innominate or subclavian vein

●S25.4   Injury of pulmonary blood vessels
   ●S25.40   Unspecified injury of pulmonary blood vessels
     ●S25.401   Unspecified injury of right pulmonary blood vessels
     ●S25.402   Unspecified injury of left pulmonary blood vessels
     ●S25.409   Unspecified injury of unspecified pulmonary blood vessels

   ●S25.41   Minor laceration of pulmonary blood vessels
     Incomplete transection of pulmonary blood vessels
     Laceration of pulmonary blood vessels NOS
     Superficial laceration of pulmonary blood vessels
     ●S25.411   Minor laceration of right pulmonary blood vessels
     ●S25.412   Minor laceration of left pulmonary blood vessels
     ●S25.419   Minor laceration of unspecified pulmonary blood vessels

   ●S25.42   Major laceration of pulmonary blood vessels
     Complete transection of pulmonary blood vessels
     Traumatic rupture of pulmonary blood vessels
     ●S25.421   Major laceration of right pulmonary blood vessels
     ●S25.422   Major laceration of left pulmonary blood vessels
     ●S25.429   Major laceration of unspecified pulmonary blood vessels

●S25.49   Other specified injury of pulmonary blood vessels
   ●S25.491   Other specified injury of right pulmonary blood vessels
   ●S25.492   Other specified injury of left pulmonary blood vessels
   ●S25.499   Other specified injury of unspecified pulmonary blood vessels

●S25.5   Injury of intercostal blood vessels
   ●S25.50   Unspecified injury of intercostal blood vessels
     ●S25.501   Unspecified injury of intercostal blood vessels, right side
     ●S25.502   Unspecified injury of intercostal blood vessels, left side
     ●S25.509   Unspecified injury of intercostal blood vessels, unspecified side

   ●S25.51   Laceration of intercostal blood vessels
     ●S25.511   Laceration of intercostal blood vessels, right side
     ●S25.512   Laceration of intercostal blood vessels, left side
     ●S25.519   Laceration of intercostal blood vessels, unspecified side

   ●S25.59   Other specified injury of intercostal blood vessels
     ●S25.591   Other specified injury of intercostal blood vessels, right side
     ●S25.592   Other specified injury of intercostal blood vessels, left side
     ●S25.599   Other specified injury of intercostal blood vessels, unspecified side

●S25.8   Injury of other blood vessels of thorax
     Injury of azygos vein
     Injury of mammary artery or vein
   ●S25.80   Unspecified injury of other blood vessels of thorax
     ●S25.801   Unspecified injury of other blood vessels of thorax, right side
     ●S25.802   Unspecified injury of other blood vessels of thorax, left side
     ●S25.809   Unspecified injury of other blood vessels of thorax, unspecified side

   ●S25.81   Laceration of other blood vessels of thorax
     ●S25.811   Laceration of other blood vessels of thorax, right side
     ●S25.812   Laceration of other blood vessels of thorax, left side
     ●S25.819   Laceration of other blood vessels of thorax, unspecified side

   ●S25.89   Other specified injury of other blood vessels of thorax
     ●S25.891   Other specified injury of other blood vessels of thorax, right side
     ●S25.892   Other specified injury of other blood vessels of thorax, left side
     ●S25.899   Other specified injury of other blood vessels of thorax, unspecified side

●S25.9   Injury of unspecified blood vessel of thorax
   X●S25.90   Unspecified injury of unspecified blood vessel of thorax
   X●S25.91   Laceration of unspecified blood vessel of thorax
   X●S25.99   Other specified injury of unspecified blood vessel of thorax

◀ New   ◀▥▥ Revised   ~~deleted~~ Deleted   Excludes 1   Excludes 2   Includes   Use additional   Code first   Code also   Unspecified
OGCR Official Guidelines   X Assign placeholder X   ● Use Additional Character(s)   ▷ Manifestation Code   **Coding Clinic**

Item 19–2   **Pneumothorax** is a collection of gas (positive air pressure) in the pleural space resulting in the lung collapsing. A tension pneumothorax is life-threatening and is a result of air in the pleural space causing a displacement in the mediastinal structures and cardiopulmonary function compromise. A traumatic pneumothorax results from blunt or penetrating injury that disrupts the parietal/visceral pleura. **Hemothorax** is blood or bloody fluid in the pleural cavity as a result of traumatic blood vessel rupture or inflammation of the lungs from pneumonia.

● **S26**   **Injury of heart**

The appropriate 7th character is to be added to each code from category S26

> A   initial encounter
> D   subsequent encounter
> S   sequela

Code also any associated:
> open wound of thorax (S21.-)
> traumatic hemopneumothorax (S27.2)
> traumatic hemothorax (S27.1)
> traumatic pneumothorax (S27.0)

● **S26.0**   **Injury of heart with hemopericardium**
> *Hemopericardium: effusion of blood within pericardium*

X● **S26.00**   Unspecified injury of heart with hemopericardium

X● **S26.01**   Contusion of heart with hemopericardium

● **S26.02**   Laceration of heart with hemopericardium

> ● **S26.020**   Mild laceration of heart with hemopericardium
> > Laceration of heart without penetration of heart chamber

> ● **S26.021**   Moderate laceration of heart with hemopericardium
> > Laceration of heart with penetration of heart chamber

> ● **S26.022**   Major laceration of heart with hemopericardium
> > Laceration of heart with penetration of multiple heart chambers

X● **S26.09**   Other injury of heart with hemopericardium

● **S26.1**   **Injury of heart without hemopericardium**
> *Hemopericardium: effusion of blood within pericardium*

X● **S26.10**   Unspecified injury of heart without hemopericardium

X● **S26.11**   Contusion of heart without hemopericardium

X● **S26.12**   Laceration of heart without hemopericardium

X● **S26.19**   Other injury of heart without hemopericardium

● **S26.9**   **Injury of heart, unspecified with or without hemopericardium**
> *Hemopericardium: effusion of blood within pericardium*

X● **S26.90**   Unspecified injury of heart, unspecified with or without hemopericardium

X● **S26.91**   Contusion of heart, unspecified with or without hemopericardium

X● **S26.92**   Laceration of heart, unspecified with or without hemopericardium
> Laceration of heart NOS

X● **S26.99**   Other injury of heart, unspecified with or without hemopericardium

● **S27**   **Injury of other and unspecified intrathoracic organs**
> Code also any associated open wound of thorax (S21.-)
>
> **Excludes2**   injury of cervical esophagus (S10-S19)
> > injury of trachea (cervical) (S10-S19)

The appropriate 7th character is to be added to each code from category S27

> A   initial encounter
> D   subsequent encounter
> S   sequela

X● **S27.0**   Traumatic pneumothorax
> **Excludes1**   spontaneous pneumothorax (J93.-)

X● **S27.1**   Traumatic hemothorax

X● **S27.2**   Traumatic hemopneumothorax

● **S27.3**   Other and unspecified injuries of lung

> ● **S27.30**   Unspecified injury of lung
> > ● **S27.301**   Unspecified injury of lung, unilateral
> > ● **S27.302**   Unspecified injury of lung, bilateral
> > ● **S27.309**   Unspecified injury of lung, unspecified

> ● **S27.31**   Primary blast injury of lung
> > Blast injury of lung NOS
> > ● **S27.311**   Primary blast injury of lung, unilateral
> > ● **S27.312**   Primary blast injury of lung, bilateral
> > ● **S27.319**   Primary blast injury of lung, unspecified

> ● **S27.32**   Contusion of lung
> > ● **S27.321**   Contusion of lung, unilateral
> > ● **S27.322**   Contusion of lung, bilateral
> > ● **S27.329**   Contusion of lung, unspecified

> ● **S27.33**   Laceration of lung
> > ● **S27.331**   Laceration of lung, unilateral
> > ● **S27.332**   Laceration of lung, bilateral
> > ● **S27.339**   Laceration of lung, unspecified

> ● **S27.39**   Other injuries of lung
> > Secondary blast injury of lung
> > ● **S27.391**   Other injuries of lung, unilateral
> > ● **S27.392**   Other injuries of lung, bilateral
> > ● **S27.399**   Other injuries of lung, unspecified

● **S27.4**   **Injury of bronchus**

> ● **S27.40**   Unspecified injury of bronchus
> > ● **S27.401**   Unspecified injury of bronchus, unilateral
> > ● **S27.402**   Unspecified injury of bronchus, bilateral
> > ● **S27.409**   Unspecified injury of bronchus, unspecified

> ● **S27.41**   Primary blast injury of bronchus
> > Blast injury of bronchus NOS
> > ● **S27.411**   Primary blast injury of bronchus, unilateral
> > ● **S27.412**   Primary blast injury of bronchus, bilateral
> > ● **S27.419**   Primary blast injury of bronchus, unspecified

CHAPTER 19 (S00-T88)

CHAPTER 19 (S00-T88)

- ● S27.42   Contusion of bronchus
  - ● S27.421   Contusion of bronchus, unilateral
  - ● S27.422   Contusion of bronchus, bilateral
  - ● S27.429   Contusion of bronchus, unspecified
- ● S27.43   Laceration of bronchus
  - ● S27.431   Laceration of bronchus, unilateral
  - ● S27.432   Laceration of bronchus, bilateral
  - ● S27.439   Laceration of bronchus, unspecified
- ● S27.49   Other injury of bronchus
  Secondary blast injury of bronchus
  - ● S27.491   Other injury of bronchus, unilateral
  - ● S27.492   Other injury of bronchus, bilateral
  - ● S27.499   Other injury of bronchus, unspecified
- ● S27.5   Injury of thoracic trachea
  - X ● S27.50   Unspecified injury of thoracic trachea
  - X ● S27.51   Primary blast injury of thoracic trachea

    Blast injury of thoracic trachea NOS
  - X ● S27.52   Contusion of thoracic trachea
  - X ● S27.53   Laceration of thoracic trachea
  - X ● S27.59   Other injury of thoracic trachea
    Secondary blast injury of thoracic trachea
- ● S27.6   Injury of pleura
  - X ● S27.60   Unspecified injury of pleura
  - X ● S27.63   Laceration of pleura
  - X ● S27.69   Other injury of pleura
- ● S27.8   Injury of other specified intrathoracic organs
  - ● S27.80   Injury of diaphragm
    - ● S27.802   Contusion of diaphragm
    - ● S27.803   Laceration of diaphragm
    - ● S27.808   Other injury of diaphragm
    - ● S27.809   Unspecified injury of diaphragm
  - ● S27.81   Injury of esophagus (thoracic part)
    - ● S27.812   Contusion of esophagus (thoracic part)
    - ● S27.813   Laceration of esophagus (thoracic part)
    - ● S27.818   Other injury of esophagus (thoracic part)
    - ● S27.819   Unspecified injury of esophagus (thoracic part)
  - ● S27.89   Injury of other specified intrathoracic organs
    Injury of lymphatic thoracic duct
    Injury of thymus gland
    - ● S27.892   Contusion of other specified intrathoracic organs
    - ● S27.893   Laceration of other specified intrathoracic organs
    - ● S27.898   Other injury of other specified intrathoracic organs
    - ● S27.899   Unspecified injury of other specified intrathoracic organs
  - X ● S27.9   Injury of unspecified intrathoracic organ
- ● S28   Crushing injury of thorax, and traumatic amputation of part of thorax

  The appropriate 7th character is to be added to each code from category S28

A	initial encounter
D	subsequent encounter
S	sequela

  - X ● S28.0   Crushed chest

    Use additional code for all associated injuries

    Excludes1   flail chest (S22.5)
  - X ● S28.1   Traumatic amputation (partial) of part of thorax, except breast

- ● S28.2   Traumatic amputation of breast
  - ● S28.21   Complete traumatic amputation of breast
    Traumatic amputation of breast NOS
    - ● S28.211   Complete traumatic amputation of right breast
    - ● S28.212   Complete traumatic amputation of left breast
    - ● S28.219   Complete traumatic amputation of unspecified breast
  - ● S28.22   Partial traumatic amputation of breast
    - ● S28.221   Partial traumatic amputation of right breast
    - ● S28.222   Partial traumatic amputation of left breast
    - ● S28.229   Partial traumatic amputation of unspecified breast
- ● S29   Other and unspecified injuries of thorax

  Code also any associated open wound (S21.-)

  The appropriate 7th character is to be added to each code from category S29

A	initial encounter
D	subsequent encounter
S	sequela

  - ● S29.0   Injury of muscle and tendon at thorax level
    - ● S29.00   Unspecified injury of muscle and tendon of thorax
      - ● S29.001   Unspecified injury of muscle and tendon of front wall of thorax
      - ● S29.002   Unspecified injury of muscle and tendon of back wall of thorax
      - ● S29.009   Unspecified injury of muscle and tendon of unspecified wall of thorax
    - ● S29.01   Strain of muscle and tendon of thorax
      - ● S29.011   Strain of muscle and tendon of front wall of thorax
      - ● S29.012   Strain of muscle and tendon of back wall of thorax
      - ● S29.019   Strain of muscle and tendon of unspecified wall of thorax
    - ● S29.02   Laceration of muscle and tendon of thorax
      - ● S29.021   Laceration of muscle and tendon of front wall of thorax
      - ● S29.022   Laceration of muscle and tendon of back wall of thorax
      - ● S29.029   Laceration of muscle and tendon of unspecified wall of thorax
    - ● S29.09   Other injury of muscle and tendon of thorax
      - ● S29.091   Other injury of muscle and tendon of front wall of thorax
      - ● S29.092   Other injury of muscle and tendon of back wall of thorax
      - ● S29.099   Other injury of muscle and tendon of unspecified wall of thorax
  - X ● S29.8   Other specified injuries of thorax
  - X ● S29.9   Unspecified injury of thorax

◀ New   ◀▥▥ Revised   ~~deleted~~ Deleted   Excludes 1   Excludes 2   Includes   Use additional   Code first   Code also   Unspecified

OGCR Official Guidelines   X Assign placeholder X   ● Use Additional Character(s)   ▶ Manifestation Code   **Coding Clinic**

1220

INJURIES TO THE ABDOMEN, LOWER BACK, LUMBAR SPINE PELVIS AND EXTERNAL GENITALS (S30-S39)

Includes injuries to the abdominal wall
injuries to the anus
injuries to the buttock
injuries to the external genitalia
injuries to the flank
injuries to the groin

Excludes2 burns and corrosions (T20-T32)
effects of foreign body in anus and rectum (T18.5)
effects of foreign body in genitourinary tract (T19.-)
effects of foreign body in stomach, small intestine and colon (T18.2-T18.4)
frostbite (T33-T34)
insect bite or sting, venomous (T63.4)

● **S30** **Superficial injury of abdomen, lower back, pelvis and external genitals**

Excludes2 superficial injury of hip (S70.-)

The appropriate 7th character is to be added to each code from category S30

> A   initial encounter
> D   subsequent encounter
> S   sequela

X● **S30.0** **Contusion of lower back and pelvis**
Contusion of buttock

X● **S30.1** **Contusion of abdominal wall**
Contusion of flank
Contusion of groin

● **S30.2** **Contusion of external genital organs**

  ● **S30.20** **Contusion of unspecified external genital organ**

    ● **S30.201** **Contusion of unspecified external genital organ, male ♂**

    ● **S30.202** **Contusion of unspecified external genital organ, female ♀**

  X● **S30.21** **Contusion of penis ♂**

  X● **S30.22** **Contusion of scrotum and testes ♂**

  X● **S30.23** **Contusion of vagina and vulva ♀**

X● **S30.3** **Contusion of anus**

● **S30.8** **Other superficial injuries of abdomen, lower back, pelvis and external genitals**

  ● **S30.81** **Abrasion of abdomen, lower back, pelvis and external genitals**

    ● **S30.810** **Abrasion of lower back and pelvis**

    ● **S30.811** **Abrasion of abdominal wall**

    ● **S30.812** **Abrasion of penis ♂**

    ● **S30.813** **Abrasion of scrotum and testes ♂**

    ● **S30.814** **Abrasion of vagina and vulva ♀**

    ● **S30.815** **Abrasion of unspecified external genital organs, male ♂**

    ● **S30.816** **Abrasion of unspecified external genital organs, female ♀**

    ● **S30.817** **Abrasion of anus**

  ● **S30.82** **Blister (nonthermal) of abdomen, lower back, pelvis and external genitals**

    ● **S30.820** **Blister (nonthermal) of lower back and pelvis**

    ● **S30.821** **Blister (nonthermal) of abdominal wall**

    ● **S30.822** **Blister (nonthermal) of penis ♂**

    ● **S30.823** **Blister (nonthermal) of scrotum and testes ♂**

    ● **S30.824** **Blister (nonthermal) of vagina and vulva ♀**

    ● **S30.825** **Blister (nonthermal) of unspecified external genital organs, male ♂**

    ● **S30.826** **Blister (nonthermal) of unspecified external genital organs, female ♀**

    ● **S30.827** **Blister (nonthermal) of anus**

● **S30.84** **External constriction of abdomen, lower back, pelvis and external genitals**

  ● **S30.840** **External constriction of lower back and pelvis**

  ● **S30.841** **External constriction of abdominal wall**

  ● **S30.842** **External constriction of penis ♂**
Hair tourniquet syndrome of penis
Use additional cause code to identify the constricting item (W49.0-)

  ● **S30.843** **External constriction of scrotum and testes ♂**

  ● **S30.844** **External constriction of vagina and vulva ♀**

  ● **S30.845** **External constriction of unspecified external genital organs, male ♂**

  ● **S30.846** **External constriction of unspecified external genital organs, female ♀**

● **S30.85** **Superficial foreign body of abdomen, lower back, pelvis and external genitals**
Splinter in the abdomen, lower back, pelvis and external genitals

  ● **S30.850** **Superficial foreign body of lower back and pelvis**

  ● **S30.851** **Superficial foreign body of abdominal wall**

  ● **S30.852** **Superficial foreign body of penis ♂**

  ● **S30.853** **Superficial foreign body of scrotum and testes ♂**

  ● **S30.854** **Superficial foreign body of vagina and vulva ♀**

  ● **S30.855** **Superficial foreign body of unspecified external genital organs, male ♂**

  ● **S30.856** **Superficial foreign body of unspecified external genital organs, female ♀**

  ● **S30.857** **Superficial foreign body of anus**

● **S30.86** **Insect bite (nonvenomous) of abdomen, lower back, pelvis and external genitals**

  ● **S30.860** **Insect bite (nonvenomous) of lower back and pelvis**

  ● **S30.861** **Insect bite (nonvenomous) of abdominal wall**

  ● **S30.862** **Insect bite (nonvenomous) of penis ♂**

  ● **S30.863** **Insect bite (nonvenomous) of scrotum and testes ♂**

  ● **S30.864** **Insect bite (nonvenomous) of vagina and vulva ♀**

  ● **S30.865** **Insect bite (nonvenomous) of unspecified external genital organs, male ♂**

  ● **S30.866** **Insect bite (nonvenomous) of unspecified external genital organs, female ♀**

  ● **S30.867** **Insect bite (nonvenomous) of anus**

CHAPTER 19 (S00-T88)

● **S30.87** **Other superficial bite of abdomen, lower back, pelvis and external genitals**

> **Excludes1** open bite of abdomen, lower back, pelvis and external genitals (S31.05, S31.15, S31.25, S31.35, S31.45, S31.55)

  ● **S30.870** **Other superficial bite of lower back and pelvis**

  ● **S30.871** **Other superficial bite of abdominal wall**

  ● **S30.872** **Other superficial bite of penis** ♂

  ● **S30.873** **Other superficial bite of scrotum and testes** ♂

  ● **S30.874** **Other superficial bite of vagina and vulva** ♀

  ● **S30.875** **Other superficial bite of unspecified external genital organs, male** ♂

  ● **S30.876** **Other superficial bite of unspecified external genital organs, female** ♀

  ● **S30.877** **Other superficial bite of anus**

● **S30.9** **Unspecified superficial injury of abdomen, lower back, pelvis and external genitals**

  X● **S30.91** **Unspecified superficial injury of lower back and pelvis**

  X● **S30.92** **Unspecified superficial injury of abdominal wall**

  X● **S30.93** **Unspecified superficial injury of penis** ♂

  X● **S30.94** **Unspecified superficial injury of scrotum and testes** ♂

  X● **S30.95** **Unspecified superficial injury of vagina and vulva** ♀

  X● **S30.96** **Unspecified superficial injury of unspecified external genital organs, male** ♂

  X● **S30.97** **Unspecified superficial injury of unspecified external genital organs, female** ♀

  X● **S30.98** **Unspecified superficial injury of anus**

● **S31** **Open wound of abdomen, lower back, pelvis and external genitals**

> Code also any associated:
> spinal cord injury (S24.0, S24.1-, S34.0-, S34.1-)
> wound infection

> **Excludes1** traumatic amputation of part of abdomen, lower back and pelvis (S38.2-, S38.3)

> **Excludes2** open wound of hip (S71.00-S71.02)
> open fracture of pelvis (S32.1--S32.9 with 7th character B)

> The appropriate 7th character is to be added to each code from category S31

> | A | initial encounter |
> |---|---|
> | D | subsequent encounter |
> | S | sequela |

● **S31.0** **Open wound of lower back and pelvis**

  ● **S31.00** **Unspecified open wound of lower back and pelvis**

    ● **S31.000** **Unspecified open wound of lower back and pelvis without penetration into retroperitoneum**
> Unspecified open wound of lower back and pelvis NOS

    ● **S31.001** **Unspecified open wound of lower back and pelvis with penetration into retroperitoneum**

● **S31.01** **Laceration without foreign body of lower back and pelvis**

  ● **S31.010** **Laceration without foreign body of lower back and pelvis without penetration into retroperitoneum**
> Laceration without foreign body of lower back and pelvis NOS

  ● **S31.011** **Laceration without foreign body of lower back and pelvis with penetration into retroperitoneum**

● **S31.02** **Laceration with foreign body of lower back and pelvis**

  ● **S31.020** **Laceration with foreign body of lower back and pelvis without penetration into retroperitoneum**
> Laceration with foreign body of lower back and pelvis NOS

  ● **S31.021** **Laceration with foreign body of lower back and pelvis with penetration into retroperitoneum**

● **S31.03** **Puncture wound without foreign body of lower back and pelvis**

  ● **S31.030** **Puncture wound without foreign body of lower back and pelvis without penetration into retroperitoneum**
> Puncture wound without foreign body of lower back and pelvis NOS

  ● **S31.031** **Puncture wound without foreign body of lower back and pelvis with penetration into retroperitoneum**

● **S31.04** **Puncture wound with foreign body of lower back and pelvis**

  ● **S31.040** **Puncture wound with foreign body of lower back and pelvis without penetration into retroperitoneum**
> Puncture wound with foreign body of lower back and pelvis NOS

  ● **S31.041** **Puncture wound with foreign body of lower back and pelvis with penetration into retroperitoneum**

● **S31.05** **Open bite of lower back and pelvis**
> Bite of lower back and pelvis NOS

> **Excludes1** superficial bite of lower back and pelvis (S30.860, S30.870)

  ● **S31.050** **Open bite of lower back and pelvis without penetration into retroperitoneum**
> Open bite of lower back and pelvis NOS

  ● **S31.051** **Open bite of lower back and pelvis with penetration into retroperitoneum**

● **S31.1** **Open wound of abdominal wall without penetration into peritoneal cavity**
> Open wound of abdominal wall NOS

> **Excludes2** open wound of abdominal wall with penetration into peritoneal cavity (S31.6-)

  ● **S31.10** **Unspecified open wound of abdominal wall without penetration into peritoneal cavity**

  ● **S31.100** **Unspecified open wound of abdominal wall, right upper quadrant without penetration into peritoneal cavity**

  ● **S31.101** **Unspecified open wound of abdominal wall, left upper quadrant without penetration into peritoneal cavity**

● S31.102   Unspecified open wound of abdominal wall, epigastric region without penetration into peritoneal cavity

● S31.103   Unspecified open wound of abdominal wall, right lower quadrant without penetration into peritoneal cavity

● S31.104   Unspecified open wound of abdominal wall, left lower quadrant without penetration into peritoneal cavity

● S31.105   Unspecified open wound of abdominal wall, periumbilic region without penetration into peritoneal cavity

● S31.109   Unspecified open wound of abdominal wall, unspecified quadrant without penetration into peritoneal cavity

       Unspecified open wound of abdominal wall NOS

● S31.11   Laceration without foreign body of abdominal wall without penetration into peritoneal cavity

  ● S31.110   Laceration without foreign body of abdominal wall, right upper quadrant without penetration into peritoneal cavity

  ● S31.111   Laceration without foreign body of abdominal wall, left upper quadrant without penetration into peritoneal cavity

  ● S31.112   Laceration without foreign body of abdominal wall, epigastric region without penetration into peritoneal cavity

  ● S31.113   Laceration without foreign body of abdominal wall, right lower quadrant without penetration into peritoneal cavity

  ● S31.114   Laceration without foreign body of abdominal wall, left lower quadrant without penetration into peritoneal cavity

  ● S31.115   Laceration without foreign body of abdominal wall, periumbilic region without penetration into peritoneal cavity

  ● S31.119   Laceration without foreign body of abdominal wall, unspecified quadrant without penetration into peritoneal cavity

● S31.12   Laceration with foreign body of abdominal wall without penetration into peritoneal cavity

  ● S31.120   Laceration of abdominal wall with foreign body, right upper quadrant without penetration into peritoneal cavity

  ● S31.121   Laceration of abdominal wall with foreign body, left upper quadrant without penetration into peritoneal cavity

  ● S31.122   Laceration of abdominal wall with foreign body, epigastric region without penetration into peritoneal cavity

  ● S31.123   Laceration of abdominal wall with foreign body, right lower quadrant without penetration into peritoneal cavity

  ● S31.124   Laceration of abdominal wall with foreign body, left lower quadrant without penetration into peritoneal cavity

● S31.125   Laceration of abdominal wall with foreign body, periumbilic region without penetration into peritoneal cavity

● S31.129   Laceration of abdominal wall with foreign body, unspecified quadrant without penetration into peritoneal cavity

● S31.13   Puncture wound of abdominal wall without foreign body without penetration into peritoneal cavity

  ● S31.130   Puncture wound of abdominal wall without foreign body, right upper quadrant without penetration into peritoneal cavity

  ● S31.131   Puncture wound of abdominal wall without foreign body, left upper quadrant without penetration into peritoneal cavity

  ● S31.132   Puncture wound of abdominal wall without foreign body, epigastric region without penetration into peritoneal cavity

  ● S31.133   Puncture wound of abdominal wall without foreign body, right lower quadrant without penetration into peritoneal cavity

  ● S31.134   Puncture wound of abdominal wall without foreign body, left lower quadrant without penetration into peritoneal cavity

  ● S31.135   Puncture wound of abdominal wall without foreign body, periumbilic region without penetration into peritoneal cavity

  ● S31.139   Puncture wound of abdominal wall without foreign body, unspecified quadrant without penetration into peritoneal cavity

● S31.14   Puncture wound of abdominal wall with foreign body without penetration into peritoneal cavity

  ● S31.140   Puncture wound of abdominal wall with foreign body, right upper quadrant without penetration into peritoneal cavity

  ● S31.141   Puncture wound of abdominal wall with foreign body, left upper quadrant without penetration into peritoneal cavity

  ● S31.142   Puncture wound of abdominal wall with foreign body, epigastric region without penetration into peritoneal cavity

  ● S31.143   Puncture wound of abdominal wall with foreign body, right lower quadrant without penetration into peritoneal cavity

  ● S31.144   Puncture wound of abdominal wall with foreign body, left lower quadrant without penetration into peritoneal cavity

  ● S31.145   Puncture wound of abdominal wall with foreign body, periumbilic region without penetration into peritoneal cavity

  ● S31.149   Puncture wound of abdominal wall with foreign body, unspecified quadrant without penetration into peritoneal cavity

● **S31.15**   **Open bite of abdominal wall without penetration into peritoneal cavity**
Bite of abdominal wall NOS

> **Excludes1**   superficial bite of abdominal wall (S30.871)

  ● **S31.150**   Open bite of abdominal wall, right upper quadrant without penetration into peritoneal cavity

  ● **S31.151**   Open bite of abdominal wall, left upper quadrant without penetration into peritoneal cavity

  ● **S31.152**   Open bite of abdominal wall, epigastric region without penetration into peritoneal cavity

  ● **S31.153**   Open bite of abdominal wall, right lower quadrant without penetration into peritoneal cavity

  ● **S31.154**   Open bite of abdominal wall, left lower quadrant without penetration into peritoneal cavity

  ● **S31.155**   Open bite of abdominal wall, periumbilic region without penetration into peritoneal cavity

  ● **S31.159**   Open bite of abdominal wall, unspecified quadrant without penetration into peritoneal cavity

● **S31.2**   **Open wound of penis**

  X ● **S31.20**   Unspecified open wound of penis ♂

  X ● **S31.21**   Laceration without foreign body of penis ♂

  X ● **S31.22**   Laceration with foreign body of penis ♂

  X ● **S31.23**   Puncture wound without foreign body of penis ♂

  X ● **S31.24**   Puncture wound with foreign body of penis ♂

  X ● **S31.25**   Open bite of penis ♂
Bite of penis NOS

> **Excludes1**   superficial bite of penis (S30.862, S30.872)

● **S31.3**   **Open wound of scrotum and testes**

  X ● **S31.30**   Unspecified open wound of scrotum and testes ♂

  X ● **S31.31**   Laceration without foreign body of scrotum and testes ♂

  X ● **S31.32**   Laceration with foreign body of scrotum and testes ♂

  X ● **S31.33**   Puncture wound without foreign body of scrotum and testes ♂

  X ● **S31.34**   Puncture wound with foreign body of scrotum and testes ♂

  X ● **S31.35**   Open bite of scrotum and testes ♂
Bite of scrotum and testes NOS

> **Excludes1**   superficial bite of scrotum and testes (S30.863, S30.873)

● **S31.4**   **Open wound of vagina and vulva**

> **Excludes1**   injury to vagina and vulva during delivery (O70.-, O71.4)

  X ● **S31.40**   Unspecified open wound of vagina and vulva ♀

  X ● **S31.41**   Laceration without foreign body of vagina and vulva ♀

  X ● **S31.42**   Laceration with foreign body of vagina and vulva ♀

  X ● **S31.43**   Puncture wound without foreign body of vagina and vulva ♀

  X ● **S31.44**   Puncture wound with foreign body of vagina and vulva ♀

  X ● **S31.45**   Open bite of vagina and vulva ♀
Bite of vagina and vulva NOS

> **Excludes1**   superficial bite of vagina and vulva (S30.864, S30.874)

● **S31.5**   **Open wound of unspecified external genital organs**

> **Excludes1**   traumatic amputation of external genital organs (S38.21, S38.22)

  ● **S31.50**   Unspecified open wound of unspecified external genital organs

    ● **S31.501**   Unspecified open wound of unspecified external genital organs, male ♂

    ● **S31.502**   Unspecified open wound of unspecified external genital organs, female ♀

  ● **S31.51**   Laceration without foreign body of unspecified external genital organs

    ● **S31.511**   Laceration without foreign body of unspecified external genital organs, male ♂

    ● **S31.512**   Laceration without foreign body of unspecified external genital organs, female ♀

  ● **S31.52**   Laceration with foreign body of unspecified external genital organs

    ● **S31.521**   Laceration with foreign body of unspecified external genital organs, male ♂

    ● **S31.522**   Laceration with foreign body of unspecified external genital organs, female ♀

  ● **S31.53**   Puncture wound without foreign body of unspecified external genital organs

    ● **S31.531**   Puncture wound without foreign body of unspecified external genital organs, male ♂

    ● **S31.532**   Puncture wound without foreign body of unspecified external genital organs, female ♀

  ● **S31.54**   Puncture wound with foreign body of unspecified external genital organs

    ● **S31.541**   Puncture wound with foreign body of unspecified external genital organs, male ♂

    ● **S31.542**   Puncture wound with foreign body of unspecified external genital organs, female ♀

  ● **S31.55**   Open bite of unspecified external genital organs
Bite of unspecified external genital organs NOS

> **Excludes1**   superficial bite of unspecified external genital organs (S30.865, S30.866, S30.875, S30.876)

    ● **S31.551**   Open bite of unspecified external genital organs, male ♂

    ● **S31.552**   Open bite of unspecified external genital organs, female ♀

● **S31.6**   **Open wound of abdominal wall with penetration into peritoneal cavity**

  ● **S31.60**   Unspecified open wound of abdominal wall with penetration into peritoneal cavity

    ● **S31.600**   Unspecified open wound of abdominal wall, right upper quadrant with penetration into peritoneal cavity

    ● **S31.601**   Unspecified open wound of abdominal wall, left upper quadrant with penetration into peritoneal cavity

    ● **S31.602**   Unspecified open wound of abdominal wall, epigastric region with penetration into peritoneal cavity

● S31.603   Unspecified open wound of abdominal wall, right lower quadrant with penetration into peritoneal cavity

● S31.604   Unspecified open wound of abdominal wall, left lower quadrant with penetration into peritoneal cavity

● S31.605   Unspecified open wound of abdominal wall, periumbilic region with penetration into peritoneal cavity

● S31.609   Unspecified open wound of abdominal wall, unspecified quadrant with penetration into peritoneal cavity

● S31.61   Laceration without foreign body of abdominal wall with penetration into peritoneal cavity

● S31.610   Laceration without foreign body of abdominal wall, right upper quadrant with penetration into peritoneal cavity

● S31.611   Laceration without foreign body of abdominal wall, left upper quadrant with penetration into peritoneal cavity

● S31.612   Laceration without foreign body of abdominal wall, epigastric region with penetration into peritoneal cavity

● S31.613   Laceration without foreign body of abdominal wall, right lower quadrant with penetration into peritoneal cavity
    Coding Clinic: 2015, Q4, P37

● S31.614   Laceration without foreign body of abdominal wall, left lower quadrant with penetration into peritoneal cavity

● S31.615   Laceration without foreign body of abdominal wall, periumbilic region with penetration into peritoneal cavity

● S31.619   Laceration without foreign body of abdominal wall, unspecified quadrant with penetration into peritoneal cavity

● S31.62   Laceration with foreign body of abdominal wall with penetration into peritoneal cavity

● S31.620   Laceration with foreign body of abdominal wall, right upper quadrant with penetration into peritoneal cavity

● S31.621   Laceration with foreign body of abdominal wall, left upper quadrant with penetration into peritoneal cavity

● S31.622   Laceration with foreign body of abdominal wall, epigastric region with penetration into peritoneal cavity

● S31.623   Laceration with foreign body of abdominal wall, right lower quadrant with penetration into peritoneal cavity

● S31.624   Laceration with foreign body of abdominal wall, left lower quadrant with penetration into peritoneal cavity

● S31.625   Laceration with foreign body of abdominal wall, periumbilic region with penetration into peritoneal cavity

● S31.629   Laceration with foreign body of abdominal wall, unspecified quadrant with penetration into peritoneal cavity

● S31.63   Puncture wound without foreign body of abdominal wall with penetration into peritoneal cavity

● S31.630   Puncture wound without foreign body of abdominal wall, right upper quadrant with penetration into peritoneal cavity

● S31.631   Puncture wound without foreign body of abdominal wall, left upper quadrant with penetration into peritoneal cavity

● S31.632   Puncture wound without foreign body of abdominal wall, epigastric region with penetration into peritoneal cavity

● S31.633   Puncture wound without foreign body of abdominal wall, right lower quadrant with penetration into peritoneal cavity

● S31.634   Puncture wound without foreign body of abdominal wall, left lower quadrant with penetration into peritoneal cavity

● S31.635   Puncture wound without foreign body of abdominal wall, periumbilic region with penetration into peritoneal cavity

● S31.639   Puncture wound without foreign body of abdominal wall, unspecified quadrant with penetration into peritoneal cavity

● S31.64   Puncture wound with foreign body of abdominal wall with penetration into peritoneal cavity

● S31.640   Puncture wound with foreign body of abdominal wall, right upper quadrant with penetration into peritoneal cavity

● S31.641   Puncture wound with foreign body of abdominal wall, left upper quadrant with penetration into peritoneal cavity

● S31.642   Puncture wound with foreign body of abdominal wall, epigastric region with penetration into peritoneal cavity

● S31.643   Puncture wound with foreign body of abdominal wall, right lower quadrant with penetration into peritoneal cavity

● S31.644   Puncture wound with foreign body of abdominal wall, left lower quadrant with penetration into peritoneal cavity

● S31.645   Puncture wound with foreign body of abdominal wall, periumbilic region with penetration into peritoneal cavity

● S31.649   Puncture wound with foreign body of abdominal wall, unspecified quadrant with penetration into peritoneal cavity

- ● **S31.65**   **Open bite of abdominal wall with penetration into peritoneal cavity**
  - **Excludes1**   superficial bite of abdominal wall (S30.861, S30.871)
  - ● **S31.650**   Open bite of abdominal wall, right upper quadrant with penetration into peritoneal cavity
  - ● **S31.651**   Open bite of abdominal wall, left upper quadrant with penetration into peritoneal cavity
  - ● **S31.652**   Open bite of abdominal wall, epigastric region with penetration into peritoneal cavity
  - ● **S31.653**   Open bite of abdominal wall, right lower quadrant with penetration into peritoneal cavity
  - ● **S31.654**   Open bite of abdominal wall, left lower quadrant with penetration into peritoneal cavity
  - ● **S31.655**   Open bite of abdominal wall, periumbilic region with penetration into peritoneal cavity
  - ● **S31.659**   Open bite of abdominal wall, unspecified quadrant with penetration into peritoneal cavity
- ● **S31.8**   **Open wound of other parts of abdomen, lower back and pelvis**
  - ● **S31.80**   **Open wound of unspecified buttock**
    - ● **S31.801**   Laceration without foreign body of unspecified buttock
    - ● **S31.802**   Laceration with foreign body of unspecified buttock
    - ● **S31.803**   Puncture wound without foreign body of unspecified buttock
    - ● **S31.804**   Puncture wound with foreign body of unspecified buttock
    - ● **S31.805**   Open bite of unspecified buttock
      - Bite of buttock NOS
      - **Excludes1**   superficial bite of buttock (S30.870)
    - ● **S31.809**   Unspecified open wound of unspecified buttock
  - ● **S31.81**   **Open wound of right buttock**
    - ● **S31.811**   Laceration without foreign body of right buttock
    - ● **S31.812**   Laceration with foreign body of right buttock
    - ● **S31.813**   Puncture wound without foreign body of right buttock
    - ● **S31.814**   Puncture wound with foreign body of right buttock
    - ● **S31.815**   Open bite of right buttock
      - Bite of right buttock NOS
      - **Excludes1**   superficial bite of buttock (S30.870)
    - ● **S31.819**   Unspecified open wound of right buttock
  - ● **S31.82**   **Open wound of left buttock**
    - ● **S31.821**   Laceration without foreign body of left buttock
    - ● **S31.822**   Laceration with foreign body of left buttock
    - ● **S31.823**   Puncture wound without foreign body of left buttock
    - ● **S31.824**   Puncture wound with foreign body of left buttock
    - ● **S31.825**   Open bite of left buttock
      - Bite of left buttock NOS
      - **Excludes1**   superficial bite of buttock (S30.870)
    - ● **S31.829**   Unspecified open wound of left buttock

- ● **S31.83**   **Open wound of anus**
  - ● **S31.831**   Laceration without foreign body of anus
  - ● **S31.832**   Laceration with foreign body of anus
  - ● **S31.833**   Puncture wound without foreign body of anus
  - ● **S31.834**   Puncture wound with foreign body of anus
  - ● **S31.835**   Open bite of anus
    - Bite of anus NOS
    - **Excludes1**   superficial bite of anus (S30.877)
  - ● **S31.839**   Unspecified open wound of anus
- ● **S32**   **Fracture of lumbar spine and pelvis**
  - **Note:** A fracture not indicated as displaced or nondisplaced should be coded to displaced
  - A fracture not indicated as opened or closed should be coded to closed
  - **Includes**   fracture of lumbosacral neural arch
    - fracture of lumbosacral spinous process
    - fracture of lumbosacral transverse process
    - fracture of lumbosacral vertebra
    - fracture of lumbosacral vertebral arch
  - *Code first any associated spinal cord and spinal nerve injury (S34.-)*
  - **Excludes1**   transection of abdomen (S38.3)
  - **Excludes2**   fracture of hip NOS (S72.0-)
  - The appropriate 7th character is to be added to each code from category S32

A	initial encounter for closed fracture
B	initial encounter for open fracture
D	subsequent encounter for fracture with routine healing
G	subsequent encounter for fracture with delayed healing
K	subsequent encounter for fracture with nonunion
S	sequela

  - ● **S32.0**   **Fracture of lumbar vertebra**
    - Fracture of lumbar spine NOS
    - ● **S32.00**   **Fracture of unspecified lumbar vertebra**
      - ● **S32.000**   Wedge compression fracture of unspecified lumbar vertebra
      - ● **S32.001**   Stable burst fracture of unspecified lumbar vertebra
      - ● **S32.002**   Unstable burst fracture of unspecified lumbar vertebra
      - ● **S32.008**   Other fracture of unspecified lumbar vertebra
      - ● **S32.009**   Unspecified fracture of unspecified lumbar vertebra
    - ● **S32.01**   **Fracture of first lumbar vertebra**
      - ● **S32.010**   Wedge compression fracture of first lumbar vertebra
      - ● **S32.011**   Stable burst fracture of first lumbar vertebra
      - ● **S32.012**   Unstable burst fracture of first lumbar vertebra
      - ● **S32.018**   Other fracture of first lumbar vertebra
      - ● **S32.019**   Unspecified fracture of first lumbar vertebra

◀ New   ◀◀ Revised   ~~deleted~~ Deleted   Excludes 1   Excludes 2   Includes   Use additional   Code first   Code also   Unspecified

OGCR Official Guidelines   X Assign placeholder X   ● Use Additional Character(s)   ▶ Manifestation Code   **Coding Clinic**

● **S32.02**   Fracture of second lumbar vertebra
    ● **S32.020**   Wedge compression fracture of second lumbar vertebra
    ● **S32.021**   Stable burst fracture of second lumbar vertebra
    ● **S32.022**   Unstable burst fracture of second lumbar vertebra
    ● **S32.028**   Other fracture of second lumbar vertebra
    ● **S32.029**   Unspecified fracture of second lumbar vertebra

● **S32.03**   Fracture of third lumbar vertebra
    ● **S32.030**   Wedge compression fracture of third lumbar vertebra
    ● **S32.031**   Stable burst fracture of third lumbar vertebra
    ● **S32.032**   Unstable burst fracture of third lumbar vertebra
    ● **S32.038**   Other fracture of third lumbar vertebra
    ● **S32.039**   Unspecified fracture of third lumbar vertebra

● **S32.04**   Fracture of fourth lumbar vertebra
    ● **S32.040**   Wedge compression fracture of fourth lumbar vertebra
    ● **S32.041**   Stable burst fracture of fourth lumbar vertebra
    ● **S32.042**   Unstable burst fracture of fourth lumbar vertebra
    ● **S32.048**   Other fracture of fourth lumbar vertebra
    ● **S32.049**   Unspecified fracture of fourth lumbar vertebra

● **S32.05**   Fracture of fifth lumbar vertebra
    ● **S32.050**   Wedge compression fracture of fifth lumbar vertebra
    ● **S32.051**   Stable burst fracture of fifth lumbar vertebra
    ● **S32.052**   Unstable burst fracture of fifth lumbar vertebra
    ● **S32.058**   Other fracture of fifth lumbar vertebra
    ● **S32.059**   Unspecified fracture of fifth lumbar vertebra

● **S32.1**   Fracture of sacrum
    For vertical fractures, code to most medial fracture extension
    Use two codes if both a vertical and transverse fracture are present
    Code also any associated fracture of pelvic ring (S32.8-)

X ● **S32.10**   Unspecified fracture of sacrum
● **S32.11**   Zone I fracture of sacrum
    Vertical sacral ala fracture of sacrum
    ● **S32.110**   Nondisplaced Zone I fracture of sacrum
    ● **S32.111**   Minimally displaced Zone I fracture of sacrum

    ● **S32.112**   Severely displaced Zone I fracture of sacrum
    ● **S32.119**   Unspecified Zone I fracture of sacrum
● **S32.12**   Zone II fracture of sacrum
    Vertical foraminal region fracture of sacrum
    ● **S32.120**   Nondisplaced Zone II fracture of sacrum
    ● **S32.121**   Minimally displaced Zone II fracture of sacrum
    ● **S32.122**   Severely displaced Zone II fracture of sacrum
    ● **S32.129**   Unspecified Zone II fracture of sacrum
● **S32.13**   Zone III fracture of sacrum
    Vertical fracture into spinal canal region of sacrum
    ● **S32.130**   Nondisplaced Zone III fracture of sacrum
    ● **S32.131**   Minimally displaced Zone III fracture of sacrum
    ● **S32.132**   Severely displaced Zone III fracture of sacrum
    ● **S32.139**   Unspecified Zone III fracture of sacrum
X ● **S32.14**   Type 1 fracture of sacrum
    Transverse flexion fracture of sacrum without displacement
X ● **S32.15**   Type 2 fracture of sacrum
    Transverse flexion fracture of sacrum with posterior displacement
X ● **S32.16**   Type 3 fracture of sacrum
    Transverse extension fracture of sacrum with anterior displacement
X ● **S32.17**   Type 4 fracture of sacrum
    Transverse segmental comminution of upper sacrum
X ● **S32.19**   Other fracture of sacrum
X ● **S32.2**   Fracture of coccyx
● **S32.3**   Fracture of ilium
    Excludes1   fracture of ilium with associated disruption of pelvic ring (S32.8-)
    ● **S32.30**   Unspecified fracture of ilium
      ● **S32.301**   Unspecified fracture of right ilium
      ● **S32.302**   Unspecified fracture of left ilium
      ● **S32.309**   Unspecified fracture of unspecified ilium
    ● **S32.31**   Avulsion fracture of ilium
      ● **S32.311**   Displaced avulsion fracture of right ilium
      ● **S32.312**   Displaced avulsion fracture of left ilium
      ● **S32.313**   Displaced avulsion fracture of unspecified ilium
      ● **S32.314**   Nondisplaced avulsion fracture of right ilium
      ● **S32.315**   Nondisplaced avulsion fracture of left ilium
      ● **S32.316**   Nondisplaced avulsion fracture of unspecified ilium
    ● **S32.39**   Other fracture of ilium
      ● **S32.391**   Other fracture of right ilium
      ● **S32.392**   Other fracture of left ilium
      ● **S32.399**   Other fracture of unspecified ilium

CHAPTER 19 (S00–T88)

CHAPTER 19 (S00-T88)

● **S32.4**   **Fracture of acetabulum**

    Code also any associated fracture of pelvic ring (S32.8-)

   ● **S32.40**   Unspecified fracture of acetabulum

     ● S32.401   Unspecified fracture of right acetabulum

     ● S32.402   Unspecified fracture of left acetabulum

     ● S32.409   Unspecified fracture of unspecified acetabulum

   ● **S32.41**   Fracture of anterior wall of acetabulum

     ● S32.411   Displaced fracture of anterior wall of right acetabulum

     ● S32.412   Displaced fracture of anterior wall of left acetabulum

     ● S32.413   Displaced fracture of anterior wall of unspecified acetabulum

     ● S32.414   Nondisplaced fracture of anterior wall of right acetabulum

     ● S32.415   Nondisplaced fracture of anterior wall of left acetabulum

     ● S32.416   Nondisplaced fracture of anterior wall of unspecified acetabulum

   ● **S32.42**   Fracture of posterior wall of acetabulum

     ● S32.421   Displaced fracture of posterior wall of right acetabulum

     ● S32.422   Displaced fracture of posterior wall of left acetabulum

     ● S32.423   Displaced fracture of posterior wall of unspecified acetabulum

     ● S32.424   Nondisplaced fracture of posterior wall of right acetabulum

     ● S32.425   Nondisplaced fracture of posterior wall of left acetabulum

     ● S32.426   Nondisplaced fracture of posterior wall of unspecified acetabulum

   ● **S32.43**   Fracture of anterior column [iliopubic] of acetabulum

     ● S32.431   Displaced fracture of anterior column [iliopubic] of right acetabulum

     ● S32.432   Displaced fracture of anterior column [iliopubic] of left acetabulum

     ● S32.433   Displaced fracture of anterior column [iliopubic] of unspecified acetabulum

     ● S32.434   Nondisplaced fracture of anterior column [iliopubic] of right acetabulum

     ● S32.435   Nondisplaced fracture of anterior column [iliopubic] of left acetabulum

     ● S32.436   Nondisplaced fracture of anterior column [iliopubic] of unspecified acetabulum

   ● **S32.44**   Fracture of posterior column [ilioischial] of acetabulum

     ● S32.441   Displaced fracture of posterior column [ilioischial] of right acetabulum

     ● S32.442   Displaced fracture of posterior column [ilioischial] of left acetabulum

     ● S32.443   Displaced fracture of posterior column [ilioischial] of unspecified acetabulum

     ● S32.444   Nondisplaced fracture of posterior column [ilioischial] of right acetabulum

     ● S32.445   Nondisplaced fracture of posterior column [ilioischial] of left acetabulum

     ● S32.446   Nondisplaced fracture of posterior column [ilioischial] of unspecified acetabulum

   ● **S32.45**   Transverse fracture of acetabulum

     ● S32.451   Displaced transverse fracture of right acetabulum

     ● S32.452   Displaced transverse fracture of left acetabulum

     ● S32.453   Displaced transverse fracture of unspecified acetabulum

     ● S32.454   Nondisplaced transverse fracture of right acetabulum

     ● S32.455   Nondisplaced transverse fracture of left acetabulum

     ● S32.456   Nondisplaced transverse fracture of unspecified acetabulum

   ● **S32.46**   Associated transverse-posterior fracture of acetabulum

     ● S32.461   Displaced associated transverse-posterior fracture of right acetabulum

     ● S32.462   Displaced associated transverse-posterior fracture of left acetabulum

     ● S32.463   Displaced associated transverse-posterior fracture of unspecified acetabulum

     ● S32.464   Nondisplaced associated transverse-posterior fracture of right acetabulum

     ● S32.465   Nondisplaced associated transverse-posterior fracture of left acetabulum

     ● S32.466   Nondisplaced associated transverse-posterior fracture of unspecified acetabulum

   ● **S32.47**   Fracture of medial wall of acetabulum

     ● S32.471   Displaced fracture of medial wall of right acetabulum

     ● S32.472   Displaced fracture of medial wall of left acetabulum

     ● S32.473   Displaced fracture of medial wall of unspecified acetabulum

     ● S32.474   Nondisplaced fracture of medial wall of right acetabulum

     ● S32.475   Nondisplaced fracture of medial wall of left acetabulum

     ● S32.476   Nondisplaced fracture of medial wall of unspecified acetabulum

   ● **S32.48**   Dome fracture of acetabulum

     ● S32.481   Displaced dome fracture of right acetabulum

     ● S32.482   Displaced dome fracture of left acetabulum

     ● S32.483   Displaced dome fracture of unspecified acetabulum

     ● S32.484   Nondisplaced dome fracture of right acetabulum

     ● S32.485   Nondisplaced dome fracture of left acetabulum

     ● S32.486   Nondisplaced dome fracture of unspecified acetabulum

   ● **S32.49**   Other fracture of acetabulum

     ● S32.491   Other fracture of right acetabulum

     ● S32.492   Other fracture of left acetabulum

     ● S32.499   Other fracture of unspecified acetabulum

◀ New   ◀▥ Revised   ~~deleted~~ Deleted   Excludes 1   Excludes 2   Includes   Use additional   Code first   Code also   Unspecified

OGCR Official Guidelines   X Assign placeholder X   ● Use Additional Character(s)   ▶ Manifestation Code   **Coding Clinic**

● **S32.5 Fracture of pubis**
> **Excludes1**   fracture of pubis with associated disruption of pelvic ring (S32.8-)

  ● **S32.50 Unspecified fracture of pubis**
    ● **S32.501** Unspecified fracture of right pubis
    ● **S32.502** Unspecified fracture of left pubis
    ● **S32.509** Unspecified fracture of unspecified pubis

  ● **S32.51 Fracture of superior rim of pubis**
    ● **S32.511** Fracture of superior rim of right pubis
    ● **S32.512** Fracture of superior rim of left pubis
    ● **S32.519** Fracture of superior rim of unspecified pubis

  ● **S32.59 Other specified fracture of pubis**
    ● **S32.591** Other specified fracture of right pubis
    ● **S32.592** Other specified fracture of left pubis
    ● **S32.599** Other specified fracture of unspecified pubis

● **S32.6 Fracture of ischium**
> **Excludes1**   fracture of ischium with associated disruption of pelvic ring (S32.8-)

  ● **S32.60 Unspecified fracture of ischium**
    ● **S32.601** Unspecified fracture of right ischium
    ● **S32.602** Unspecified fracture of left ischium
    ● **S32.609** Unspecified fracture of unspecified ischium

  ● **S32.61 Avulsion fracture of ischium**
    ● **S32.611** Displaced avulsion fracture of right ischium
    ● **S32.612** Displaced avulsion fracture of left ischium
    ● **S32.613** Displaced avulsion fracture of unspecified ischium
    ● **S32.614** Nondisplaced avulsion fracture of right ischium
    ● **S32.615** Nondisplaced avulsion fracture of left ischium
    ● **S32.616** Nondisplaced avulsion fracture of unspecified ischium

  ● **S32.69 Other specified fracture of ischium**
    ● **S32.691** Other specified fracture of right ischium
    ● **S32.692** Other specified fracture of left ischium
    ● **S32.699** Other specified fracture of unspecified ischium

● **S32.8 Fracture of other parts of pelvis**
> Code also any associated:
> fracture of acetabulum (S32.4-)
> sacral fracture (S32.1-)

  ● **S32.81 Multiple fractures of pelvis with disruption of pelvic ring**
    Multiple pelvic fractures with disruption of pelvic circle
    ● **S32.810** Multiple fractures of pelvis with stable disruption of pelvic ring
    ● **S32.811** Multiple fractures of pelvis with unstable disruption of pelvic ring

  X● **S32.82 Multiple fractures of pelvis without disruption of pelvic ring**
    Multiple pelvic fractures without disruption of pelvic circle

  X● **S32.89 Fracture of other parts of pelvis**

X● **S32.9 Fracture of unspecified parts of lumbosacral spine and pelvis**
> Fracture of lumbosacral spine NOS
> Fracture of pelvis NOS
> **Coding Clinic: 2012, Q4, P93**

● **S33 Dislocation and sprain of joints and ligaments of lumbar spine and pelvis**
> **Includes**   avulsion of joint or ligament of lumbar spine and pelvis
> laceration of cartilage, joint or ligament of lumbar spine and pelvis
> sprain of cartilage, joint or ligament of lumbar spine and pelvis
> traumatic hemarthrosis of joint or ligament of lumbar spine and pelvis
> traumatic rupture of joint or ligament of lumbar spine and pelvis
> traumatic subluxation of joint or ligament of lumbar spine and pelvis
> traumatic tear of joint or ligament of lumbar spine and pelvis

> Code also any associated open wound

> **Excludes1**   nontraumatic rupture or displacement of lumbar intervertebral disc NOS (M51.-)
> obstetric damage to pelvic joints and ligaments (O71.6)

> **Excludes2**   dislocation and sprain of joints and ligaments of hip (S73.-)
> strain of muscle of lower back and pelvis (S39.01-)

> The appropriate 7th character is to be added to each code from category S33

> | A | initial encounter |
> |---|---|
> | D | subsequent encounter |
> | S | sequela |

X● **S33.0 Traumatic rupture of lumbar intervertebral disc**
> **Excludes1**   rupture or displacement (nontraumatic) of lumbar intervertebral disc NOS (M51.- with fifth character 6)

● **S33.1 Subluxation and dislocation of lumbar vertebra**
> Code also any associated:
> open wound of abdomen, lower back and pelvis (S31)
> spinal cord injury (S24.0, S24.1-, S34.0-, S34.1-)
> **Excludes2**   fracture of lumbar vertebrae (S32.0-)

  ● **S33.10 Subluxation and dislocation of unspecified lumbar vertebra**
    ● **S33.100** Subluxation of unspecified lumbar vertebra
    ● **S33.101** Dislocation of unspecified lumbar vertebra

  ● **S33.11 Subluxation and dislocation of L_1/L_2 lumbar vertebra**
    ● **S33.110** Subluxation of L_1/L_2 lumbar vertebra
    ● **S33.111** Dislocation of L_1/L_2 lumbar vertebra

  ● **S33.12 Subluxation and dislocation of L_2/L_3 lumbar vertebra**
    ● **S33.120** Subluxation of L_2/L_3 lumbar vertebra
    ● **S33.121** Dislocation of L_2/L_3 lumbar vertebra

  ● **S33.13 Subluxation and dislocation of L_3/L_4 lumbar vertebra**
    ● **S33.130** Subluxation of L_3/L_4 lumbar vertebra
    ● **S33.131** Dislocation of L_3/L_4 lumbar vertebra

  ● **S33.14 Subluxation and dislocation of L_4/L_5 lumbar vertebra**
    ● **S33.140** Subluxation of L_4/L_5 lumbar vertebra
    ● **S33.141** Dislocation of L_4/L_5 lumbar vertebra

X● **S33.2 Dislocation of sacroiliac and sacrococcygeal joint**

● **S33.3 Dislocation of other and unspecified parts of lumbar spine and pelvis**
  X● **S33.30 Dislocation of unspecified parts of lumbar spine and pelvis**
  X● **S33.39 Dislocation of other parts of lumbar spine and pelvis**

X● **S33.4 Traumatic rupture of symphysis pubis**

X● **S33.5 Sprain of ligaments of lumbar spine**

X● **S33.6**   **Sprain of sacroiliac joint**

X● **S33.8**   **Sprain of other parts of lumbar spine and pelvis**

X● **S33.9**   **Sprain of** unspecified **parts of lumbar spine and pelvis**

● **S34**   **Injury of lumbar and sacral spinal cord and nerves at abdomen, lower back and pelvis level**

Note: Code to highest level of lumbar cord injury

Injuries to the spinal cord (S34.0 and S34.1) refer to the cord level and not bone level injury, and can affect nerve roots at and below the level given.

The appropriate 7th character is to be added to each code from category S34

A	initial encounter
D	subsequent encounter
S	sequela

Code also any associated:
    fracture of vertebra (S22.0-, S32.0-)
    open wound of abdomen, lower back and pelvis (S31.-)
    transient paralysis (R29.5)

● **S34.0**   **Concussion and edema of lumbar and sacral spinal cord**

X● **S34.01**   **Concussion and edema of lumbar spinal cord**

X● **S34.02**   **Concussion and edema of sacral spinal cord**
     Concussion and edema of conus medullaris

● **S34.1**   **Other and unspecified injury of lumbar and sacral spinal cord**

● **S34.10**   **Unspecified injury to lumbar spinal cord**

● **S34.101**   **Unspecified injury to L_1 level of lumbar spinal cord**
     Unspecified injury to lumbar spinal cord level 1 ◄

● **S34.102**   **Unspecified injury to L_2 level of lumbar spinal cord**
     Unspecified injury to lumbar spinal cord level 2 ◄

● **S34.103**   **Unspecified injury to L_3 level of lumbar spinal cord**
     Unspecified injury to lumbar spinal cord level 3 ◄

● **S34.104**   **Unspecified injury to L_4 level of lumbar spinal cord**
     Unspecified injury to lumbar spinal cord level 4 ◄

● **S34.105**   **Unspecified injury to L_5 level of lumbar spinal cord**
     Unspecified injury to lumbar spinal cord level 5 ◄

● **S34.109**   **Unspecified injury to unspecified level of lumbar spinal cord**

● **S34.11**   **Complete lesion of lumbar spinal cord**

● **S34.111**   **Complete lesion of L_1 level of lumbar spinal cord**
     Complete lesion of lumbar spinal cord level 1 ◄

● **S34.112**   **Complete lesion of L_2 level of lumbar spinal cord**
     Complete lesion of lumbar spinal cord level 2 ◄

● **S34.113**   **Complete lesion of L_3 level of lumbar spinal cord**
     Complete lesion of lumbar spinal cord level 3 ◄

● **S34.114**   **Complete lesion of L_4 level of lumbar spinal cord**
     Complete lesion of lumbar spinal cord level 4 ◄

● **S34.115**   **Complete lesion of L_5 level of lumbar spinal cord**
     Complete lesion of lumbar spinal cord level 5 ◄

● **S34.119**   **Complete lesion of** unspecified **level of lumbar spinal cord**

● **S34.12**   **Incomplete lesion of lumbar spinal cord**

● **S34.121**   **Incomplete lesion of L_1 level of lumbar spinal cord**
     Incomplete lesion of lumbar spinal cord level 1 ◄

● **S34.122**   **Incomplete lesion of L_2 level of lumbar spinal cord**
     Incomplete lesion of lumbar spinal cord level 2 ◄

● **S34.123**   **Incomplete lesion of L_3 level of lumbar spinal cord**
     Incomplete lesion of lumbar spinal cord level 3 ◄

● **S34.124**   **Incomplete lesion of L_4 level of lumbar spinal cord**
     Incomplete lesion of lumbar spinal cord level 4 ◄

● **S34.125**   **Incomplete lesion of L_5 level of lumbar spinal cord**
     Incomplete lesion of lumbar spinal cord level 5 ◄

● **S34.129**   **Incomplete lesion of** unspecified **level of lumbar spinal cord**

● **S34.13**   **Other and unspecified injury to sacral spinal cord**
     Other injury to conus medullaris

● **S34.131**   **Complete lesion of sacral spinal cord**
     Complete lesion of conus medullaris

● **S34.132**   **Incomplete lesion of sacral spinal cord**
     Incomplete lesion of conus medullaris

● **S34.139**   **Unspecified injury to sacral spinal cord**
     Unspecified injury of conus medullaris

● **S34.2**   **Injury of nerve root of lumbar and sacral spine**

X● **S34.21**   **Injury of nerve root of lumbar spine**

X● **S34.22**   **Injury of nerve root of sacral spine**

X● **S34.3**   **Injury of cauda equina**

X● **S34.4**   **Injury of lumbosacral plexus**

X● **S34.5**   **Injury of lumbar, sacral and pelvic sympathetic nerves**
     Injury of celiac ganglion or plexus
     Injury of hypogastric plexus
     Injury of mesenteric plexus (inferior) (superior)
     Injury of splanchnic nerve

X● **S34.6**   **Injury of peripheral nerve(s) at abdomen, lower back and pelvis level**

X● **S34.8**   **Injury of other nerves at abdomen, lower back and pelvis level**

X● **S34.9**   **Injury of** unspecified **nerves at abdomen, lower back and pelvis level**

● **S35**   **Injury of blood vessels at abdomen, lower back and pelvis level**

The appropriate 7th character is to be added to each code from category S35

A	initial encounter
D	subsequent encounter
S	sequela

Code also any associated open wound (S31.-)

● **S35.0**   **Injury of abdominal aorta**

    Excludes1   injury of aorta NOS (S25.0)

X● **S35.00**   **Unspecified injury of abdominal aorta**

X● **S35.01**   **Minor laceration of abdominal aorta**
     Incomplete transection of abdominal aorta
     Laceration of abdominal aorta NOS
     Superficial laceration of abdominal aorta

X● **S35.02**   **Major laceration of abdominal aorta**
     Complete transection of abdominal aorta
     Traumatic rupture of abdominal aorta

X● **S35.09**   **Other injury of abdominal aorta**

◄ New   ◄ Revised   ~~deleted~~ Deleted   Excludes 1   Excludes 2   Includes   Use additional   Code first   Code also   Unspecified

OGCR Official Guidelines   X Assign placeholder X   ● Use Additional Character(s)   ▶ Manifestation Code   **Coding Clinic**

● **S35.1**   **Injury of inferior vena cava**
     Injury of hepatic vein
     Excludes1   injury of vena cava NOS (S25.2)

   X ● **S35.10**   Unspecified injury of inferior vena cava

   X ● **S35.11**   **Minor laceration of inferior vena cava**
         Incomplete transection of inferior vena cava
         Laceration of inferior vena cava NOS
         Superficial laceration of inferior vena cava

   X ● **S35.12**   **Major laceration of inferior vena cava**
         Complete transection of inferior vena cava
         Traumatic rupture of inferior vena cava

   X ● **S35.19**   **Other injury of inferior vena cava**

● **S35.2**   **Injury of celiac or mesenteric artery and branches**

   ● **S35.21**   **Injury of celiac artery**

     ● **S35.211**   **Minor laceration of celiac artery**
           Incomplete transection of celiac artery
           Laceration of celiac artery NOS
           Superficial laceration of celiac artery

     ● **S35.212**   **Major laceration of celiac artery**
           Complete transection of celiac artery
           Traumatic rupture of celiac artery

     ● **S35.218**   **Other injury of celiac artery**

     ● **S35.219**   Unspecified injury of celiac artery

   ● **S35.22**   **Injury of superior mesenteric artery**

     ● **S35.221**   **Minor laceration of superior mesenteric artery**
           Incomplete transection of superior mesenteric artery
           Laceration of superior mesenteric artery NOS
           Superficial laceration of superior mesenteric artery

     ● **S35.222**   **Major laceration of superior mesenteric artery**
           Complete transection of superior mesenteric artery
           Traumatic rupture of superior mesenteric artery

     ● **S35.228**   **Other injury of superior mesenteric artery**

     ● **S35.229**   Unspecified injury of superior mesenteric artery

   ● **S35.23**   **Injury of inferior mesenteric artery**

     ● **S35.231**   **Minor laceration of inferior mesenteric artery**
           Incomplete transection of inferior mesenteric artery
           Laceration of inferior mesenteric artery NOS
           Superficial laceration of inferior mesenteric artery

     ● **S35.232**   **Major laceration of inferior mesenteric artery**
           Complete transection of inferior mesenteric artery
           Traumatic rupture of inferior mesenteric artery

     ● **S35.238**   **Other injury of inferior mesenteric artery**

     ● **S35.239**   Unspecified injury of inferior mesenteric artery

● **S35.29**   **Injury of branches of celiac and mesenteric artery**
     Injury of gastric artery
     Injury of gastroduodenal artery
     Injury of hepatic artery
     Injury of splenic artery

   ● **S35.291**   **Minor laceration of branches of celiac and mesenteric artery**
         Incomplete transection of branches of celiac and mesenteric artery
         Laceration of branches of celiac and mesenteric artery NOS
         Superficial laceration of branches of celiac and mesenteric artery

   ● **S35.292**   **Major laceration of branches of celiac and mesenteric artery**
         Complete transection of branches of celiac and mesenteric artery
         Traumatic rupture of branches of celiac and mesenteric artery

   ● **S35.298**   **Other injury of branches of celiac and mesenteric artery**

   ● **S35.299**   Unspecified injury of branches of celiac and mesenteric artery

● **S35.3**   **Injury of portal or splenic vein and branches**

   ● **S35.31**   **Injury of portal vein**

     ● **S35.311**   **Laceration of portal vein**

     ● **S35.318**   **Other specified injury of portal vein**

     ● **S35.319**   Unspecified injury of portal vein

   ● **S35.32**   **Injury of splenic vein**

     ● **S35.321**   **Laceration of splenic vein**

     ● **S35.328**   **Other specified injury of splenic vein**

     ● **S35.329**   Unspecified injury of splenic vein

   ● **S35.33**   **Injury of superior mesenteric vein**

     ● **S35.331**   **Laceration of superior mesenteric vein**

     ● **S35.338**   **Other specified injury of superior mesenteric vein**

     ● **S35.339**   Unspecified injury of superior mesenteric vein

   ● **S35.34**   **Injury of inferior mesenteric vein**

     ● **S35.341**   **Laceration of inferior mesenteric vein**

     ● **S35.348**   **Other specified injury of inferior mesenteric vein**

     ● **S35.349**   Unspecified injury of inferior mesenteric vein

● **S35.4**   **Injury of renal blood vessels**

   ● **S35.40**   **Unspecified injury of renal blood vessel**

     ● **S35.401**   Unspecified injury of right renal artery

     ● **S35.402**   Unspecified injury of left renal artery

     ● **S35.403**   Unspecified injury of unspecified renal artery

     ● **S35.404**   Unspecified injury of right renal vein

     ● **S35.405**   Unspecified injury of left renal vein

     ● **S35.406**   Unspecified injury of unspecified renal vein

CHAPTER 19 (S00-T88)

CHAPTER 19 (S00-T88)

● S35.41　Laceration of renal blood vessel
   ● S35.411　Laceration of right renal artery
   ● S35.412　Laceration of left renal artery
   ● S35.413　Laceration of unspecified renal artery
   ● S35.414　Laceration of right renal vein
   ● S35.415　Laceration of left renal vein
   ● S35.416　Laceration of unspecified renal vein
● S35.49　Other specified injury of renal blood vessel
   ● S35.491　Other specified injury of right renal artery
   ● S35.492　Other specified injury of left renal artery
   ● S35.493　Other specified injury of unspecified renal artery
   ● S35.494　Other specified injury of right renal vein
   ● S35.495　Other specified injury of left renal vein
   ● S35.496　Other specified injury of unspecified renal vein
● S35.5　Injury of iliac blood vessels
  X ● S35.50　Injury of unspecified iliac blood vessel(s)
  ● S35.51　Injury of iliac artery or vein
    Injury of hypogastric artery or vein
   ● S35.511　Injury of right iliac artery
   ● S35.512　Injury of left iliac artery
   ● S35.513　Injury of unspecified iliac artery
   ● S35.514　Injury of right iliac vein
   ● S35.515　Injury of left iliac vein
   ● S35.516　Injury of unspecified iliac vein
  ● S35.53　Injury of uterine artery or vein
   ● S35.531　Injury of right uterine artery ♀
   ● S35.532　Injury of left uterine artery ♀
   ● S35.533　Injury of unspecified uterine artery ♀
   ● S35.534　Injury of right uterine vein ♀
   ● S35.535　Injury of left uterine vein ♀
   ● S35.536　Injury of unspecified uterine vein ♀
  X ● S35.59　Injury of other iliac blood vessels
● S35.8　Injury of other blood vessels at abdomen, lower back and pelvis level
    Injury of ovarian artery or vein
  ● S35.8X　Injury of other blood vessels at abdomen, lower back and pelvis level
   ● S35.8X1　Laceration of other blood vessels at abdomen, lower back and pelvis level
   ● S35.8X8　Other specified injury of other blood vessels at abdomen, lower back and pelvis level
   ● S35.8X9　Unspecified injury of other blood vessels at abdomen, lower back and pelvis level
● S35.9　Injury of unspecified blood vessel at abdomen, lower back and pelvis level
  X ● S35.90　Unspecified injury of unspecified blood vessel at abdomen, lower back and pelvis level
  X ● S35.91　Laceration of unspecified blood vessel at abdomen, lower back and pelvis level
  X ● S35.99　Other specified injury of unspecified blood vessel at abdomen, lower back and pelvis level

● S36　Injury of intra-abdominal organs
  The appropriate 7th character is to be added to each code from category S36

A	initial encounter
D	subsequent encounter
S	sequela

  Code also any associated open wound (S31.-)
● S36.0　Injury of spleen
  X ● S36.00　Unspecified injury of spleen
  ● S36.02　Contusion of spleen
   ● S36.020　Minor contusion of spleen
     Contusion of spleen less than 2 cm
   ● S36.021　Major contusion of spleen
     Contusion of spleen greater than 2 cm
   ● S36.029　Unspecified contusion of spleen
     Coding Clinic: 2015, Q2, P36, Q1, P11
  ● S36.03　Laceration of spleen
   ● S36.030　Superficial (capsular) laceration of spleen
     Laceration of spleen less than 1 cm
     Minor laceration of spleen
   ● S36.031　Moderate laceration of spleen
     Laceration of spleen 1 to 3 cm
     Coding Clinic: 2015, Q2, P36, Q1, P11
   ● S36.032　Major laceration of spleen
     Avulsion of spleen
     Laceration of spleen greater than 3 cm
     Massive laceration of spleen
     Multiple moderate lacerations of spleen
     Stellate laceration of spleen
   ● S36.039　Unspecified laceration of spleen
  X ● S36.09　Other injury of spleen
● S36.1　Injury of liver and gallbladder and bile duct
  ● S36.11　Injury of liver
   ● S36.112　Contusion of liver
   ● S36.113　Laceration of liver, unspecified degree
   ● S36.114　Minor laceration of liver
     Laceration involving capsule only, or, without significant involvement of hepatic parenchyma [i.e., less than 1 cm deep]
   ● S36.115　Moderate laceration of liver
     Laceration involving parenchyma but without major disruption of parenchyma [i.e., less than 10 cm long and less than 3 cm deep]
   ● S36.116　Major laceration of liver
     Laceration with significant disruption of hepatic parenchyma [i.e., greater than 10 cm long and 3 cm deep]
     Multiple moderate lacerations, with or without hematoma
     Stellate laceration of liver
   ● S36.118　Other injury of liver
   ● S36.119　Unspecified injury of liver
     Coding Clinic: 2015, Q2, P17
  ● S36.12　Injury of gallbladder
   ● S36.122　Contusion of gallbladder
   ● S36.123　Laceration of gallbladder
   ● S36.128　Other injury of gallbladder
   ● S36.129　Unspecified injury of gallbladder
  X ● S36.13　Injury of bile duct

◀ New　◀▥▥ Revised　~~deleted~~ Deleted　Excludes 1　Excludes 2　Includes　Use additional　Code first　Code also　Unspecified

OGCR Official Guidelines　X Assign placeholder X　● Use Additional Character(s)　▶ Manifestation Code　**Coding Clinic**

S36.2   Injury of pancreas
  S36.20   Unspecified injury of pancreas
    S36.200   Unspecified injury of head of pancreas
    S36.201   Unspecified injury of body of pancreas
    S36.202   Unspecified injury of tail of pancreas
    S36.209   Unspecified injury of unspecified part of pancreas
  S36.22   Contusion of pancreas
    S36.220   Contusion of head of pancreas
    S36.221   Contusion of body of pancreas
    S36.222   Contusion of tail of pancreas
    S36.229   Contusion of unspecified part of pancreas
  S36.23   Laceration of pancreas, unspecified degree
    S36.230   Laceration of head of pancreas, unspecified degree
    S36.231   Laceration of body of pancreas, unspecified degree
    S36.232   Laceration of tail of pancreas, unspecified degree
    S36.239   Laceration of unspecified part of pancreas, unspecified degree
  S36.24   Minor laceration of pancreas
    S36.240   Minor laceration of head of pancreas
    S36.241   Minor laceration of body of pancreas
    S36.242   Minor laceration of tail of pancreas
    S36.249   Minor laceration of unspecified part of pancreas
  S36.25   Moderate laceration of pancreas
    S36.250   Moderate laceration of head of pancreas
    S36.251   Moderate laceration of body of pancreas
    S36.252   Moderate laceration of tail of pancreas
    S36.259   Moderate laceration of unspecified part of pancreas
  S36.26   Major laceration of pancreas
    S36.260   Major laceration of head of pancreas
    S36.261   Major laceration of body of pancreas
    S36.262   Major laceration of tail of pancreas
    S36.269   Major laceration of unspecified part of pancreas
  S36.29   Other injury of pancreas
    S36.290   Other injury of head of pancreas
    S36.291   Other injury of body of pancreas
    S36.292   Other injury of tail of pancreas
    S36.299   Other injury of unspecified part of pancreas
S36.3   Injury of stomach
  X S36.30   Unspecified injury of stomach
  X S36.32   Contusion of stomach
  X S36.33   Laceration of stomach
  X S36.39   Other injury of stomach
S36.4   Injury of small intestine
  S36.40   Unspecified injury of small intestine
    S36.400   Unspecified injury of duodenum
    S36.408   Unspecified injury of other part of small intestine
    S36.409   Unspecified injury of unspecified part of small intestine

S36.41   Primary blast injury of small intestine
             Blast injury of small intestine NOS
    S36.410   Primary blast injury of duodenum
    S36.418   Primary blast injury of other part of small intestine
    S36.419   Primary blast injury of unspecified part of small intestine
  S36.42   Contusion of small intestine
    S36.420   Contusion of duodenum
    S36.428   Contusion of other part of small intestine
    S36.429   Contusion of unspecified part of small intestine
  S36.43   Laceration of small intestine
    S36.430   Laceration of duodenum
    S36.438   Laceration of other part of small intestine
    S36.439   Laceration of unspecified part of small intestine
  S36.49   Other injury of small intestine
    S36.490   Other injury of duodenum
    S36.498   Other injury of other part of small intestine
    S36.499   Other injury of unspecified part of small intestine
S36.5   Injury of colon
         Excludes2   injury of rectum (S36.6-)
  S36.50   Unspecified injury of colon
    S36.500   Unspecified injury of ascending [right] colon
    S36.501   Unspecified injury of transverse colon
    S36.502   Unspecified injury of descending [left] colon
    S36.503   Unspecified injury of sigmoid colon
    S36.508   Unspecified injury of other part of colon
    S36.509   Unspecified injury of unspecified part of colon
  S36.51   Primary blast injury of colon
             Blast injury of colon NOS
    S36.510   Primary blast injury of ascending [right] colon
    S36.511   Primary blast injury of transverse colon
    S36.512   Primary blast injury of descending [left] colon
    S36.513   Primary blast injury of sigmoid colon
    S36.518   Primary blast injury of other part of colon
    S36.519   Primary blast injury of unspecified part of colon
  S36.52   Contusion of colon
    S36.520   Contusion of ascending [right] colon
    S36.521   Contusion of transverse colon
    S36.522   Contusion of descending [left] colon
    S36.523   Contusion of sigmoid colon
    S36.528   Contusion of other part of colon
    S36.529   Contusion of unspecified part of colon
  S36.53   Laceration of colon
    S36.530   Laceration of ascending [right] colon
    S36.531   Laceration of transverse colon
    S36.532   Laceration of descending [left] colon
    S36.533   Laceration of sigmoid colon
    S36.538   Laceration of other part of colon
    S36.539   Laceration of unspecified part of colon

CHAPTER 19 (S00-T88)

CHAPTER 19 (S00-T88)

● S36.59   Other injury of colon
      Secondary blast injury of colon
    ● S36.590   Other injury of ascending [right] colon
    ● S36.591   Other injury of transverse colon
    ● S36.592   Other injury of descending [left] colon
    ● S36.593   Other injury of sigmoid colon
    ● S36.598   Other injury of other part of colon
    ● S36.599   Other injury of unspecified part of colon

● S36.6   Injury of rectum
  X ● S36.60   Unspecified injury of rectum
  X ● S36.61   Primary blast injury of rectum
      Blast injury of rectum NOS
  X ● S36.62   Contusion of rectum
  X ● S36.63   Laceration of rectum
  X ● S36.69   Other injury of rectum
      Secondary blast injury of rectum

● S36.8   Injury of other intra-abdominal organs
  X ● S36.81   Injury of peritoneum
  ● S36.89   Injury of other intra-abdominal organs
      Injury of retroperitoneum
    ● S36.892   Contusion of other intra-abdominal organs
    ● S36.893   Laceration of other intra-abdominal organs
    ● S36.898   Other injury of other intra-abdominal organs
      S36.899   Unspecified injury of other intra-abdominal organs

● S36.9   Injury of unspecified intra-abdominal organ
  X ● S36.90   Unspecified injury of unspecified intra-abdominal organ
  X ● S36.92   Contusion of unspecified intra-abdominal organ
  X ● S36.93   Laceration of unspecified intra-abdominal organ
  X ● S36.99   Other injury of unspecified intra-abdominal organ

● S37   Injury of urinary and pelvic organs
      Code also any associated open wound (S31.-)
      Excludes1   obstetric trauma to pelvic organs (O71.-)
      Excludes2   injury of peritoneum (S36.81)
                     injury of retroperitoneum (S36.89-)
      The appropriate 7th character is to be added to each code from category S37

A	initial encounter
D	subsequent encounter
S	sequela

● S37.0   Injury of kidney
      Excludes2   acute kidney injury (nontraumatic) (N17.9)
  ● S37.00   Unspecified injury of kidney
    ● S37.001   Unspecified injury of right kidney
    ● S37.002   Unspecified injury of left kidney
    ● S37.009   Unspecified injury of unspecified kidney
  ● S37.01   Minor contusion of kidney
      Contusion of kidney less than 2 cm
      Contusion of kidney NOS
    ● S37.011   Minor contusion of right kidney
    ● S37.012   Minor contusion of left kidney
    ● S37.019   Minor contusion of unspecified kidney

● S37.02   Major contusion of kidney
      Contusion of kidney greater than 2 cm
    ● S37.021   Major contusion of right kidney
    ● S37.022   Major contusion of left kidney
    ● S37.029   Major contusion of unspecified kidney

● S37.03   Laceration of kidney, unspecified degree
    ● S37.031   Laceration of right kidney, unspecified degree
    ● S37.032   Laceration of left kidney, unspecified degree
    ● S37.039   Laceration of unspecified kidney, unspecified degree

● S37.04   Minor laceration of kidney
      Laceration of kidney less than 1 cm
    ● S37.041   Minor laceration of right kidney
    ● S37.042   Minor laceration of left kidney
    ● S37.049   Minor laceration of unspecified kidney

● S37.05   Moderate laceration of kidney
      Laceration of kidney 1 to 3 cm
    ● S37.051   Moderate laceration of right kidney
    ● S37.052   Moderate laceration of left kidney
    ● S37.059   Moderate laceration of unspecified kidney

● S37.06   Major laceration of kidney
      Avulsion of kidney
      Laceration of kidney greater than 3 cm
      Massive laceration of kidney
      Multiple moderate lacerations of kidney
      Stellate laceration of kidney
    ● S37.061   Major laceration of right kidney
    ● S37.062   Major laceration of left kidney
    ● S37.069   Major laceration of unspecified kidney

● S37.09   Other injury of kidney
    ● S37.091   Other injury of right kidney
    ● S37.092   Other injury of left kidney
    ● S37.099   Other injury of unspecified kidney

● S37.1   Injury of ureter
  X ● S37.10   Unspecified injury of ureter
  X ● S37.12   Contusion of ureter
  X ● S37.13   Laceration of ureter
  X ● S37.19   Other injury of ureter

● S37.2   Injury of bladder
  X ● S37.20   Unspecified injury of bladder
  X ● S37.22   Contusion of bladder
  X ● S37.23   Laceration of bladder
  X ● S37.29   Other injury of bladder

● S37.3   Injury of urethra
  X ● S37.30   Unspecified injury of urethra
  X ● S37.32   Contusion of urethra
  X ● S37.33   Laceration of urethra
  X ● S37.39   Other injury of urethra

● S37.4   Injury of ovary
  ● S37.40   Unspecified injury of ovary
    ● S37.401   Unspecified injury of ovary, unilateral ♀
    ● S37.402   Unspecified injury of ovary, bilateral ♀
    ● S37.409   Unspecified injury of ovary, unspecified ♀
  ● S37.42   Contusion of ovary
    ● S37.421   Contusion of ovary, unilateral ♀
    ● S37.422   Contusion of ovary, bilateral ♀
    ● S37.429   Contusion of ovary, unspecified ♀

◀ New   ◀||| Revised   ~~deleted~~ Deleted   Excludes 1   Excludes 2   Includes   Use additional   Code first   Code also   Unspecified

OGCR Official Guidelines   X Assign placeholder X   ● Use Additional Character(s)   ▶ Manifestation Code   **Coding Clinic**

- S37.43   Laceration of ovary
  - S37.431   Laceration of ovary, unilateral ♀
  - S37.432   Laceration of ovary, bilateral ♀
  - S37.439   Laceration of ovary, unspecified ♀
- S37.49   Other injury of ovary
  - S37.491   Other injury of ovary, unilateral ♀
  - S37.492   Other injury of ovary, bilateral ♀
  - S37.499   Other injury of ovary, unspecified ♀
- S37.5   Injury of fallopian tube
  - S37.50   Unspecified injury of fallopian tube
    - S37.501   Unspecified injury of fallopian tube, unilateral ♀
    - S37.502   Unspecified injury of fallopian tube, bilateral ♀
    - S37.509   Unspecified injury of fallopian tube, unspecified ♀
  - S37.51   Primary blast injury of fallopian tube
    Blast injury of fallopian tube NOS
    - S37.511   Primary blast injury of fallopian tube, unilateral ♀
    - S37.512   Primary blast injury of fallopian tube, bilateral ♀
    - S37.519   Primary blast injury of fallopian tube, unspecified ♀
  - S37.52   Contusion of fallopian tube
    - S37.521   Contusion of fallopian tube, unilateral ♀
    - S37.522   Contusion of fallopian tube, bilateral ♀
    - S37.529   Contusion of fallopian tube, unspecified ♀
  - S37.53   Laceration of fallopian tube
    - S37.531   Laceration of fallopian tube, unilateral ♀
    - S37.532   Laceration of fallopian tube, bilateral ♀
    - S37.539   Laceration of fallopian tube, unspecified ♀
  - S37.59   Other injury of fallopian tube
    Secondary blast injury of fallopian tube
    - S37.591   Other injury of fallopian tube, unilateral ♀
    - S37.592   Other injury of fallopian tube, bilateral ♀
    - S37.599   Other injury of fallopian tube, unspecified ♀
- S37.6   Injury of uterus
  Excludes1   injury to gravid uterus (O9A.2-)
  injury to uterus during delivery (O71.-)
  - X S37.60   Unspecified injury of uterus ♀
  - X S37.62   Contusion of uterus ♀
  - X S37.63   Laceration of uterus ♀
  - X S37.69   Other injury of uterus ♀
- S37.8   Injury of other urinary and pelvic organs
  - S37.81   Injury of adrenal gland
    - S37.812   Contusion of adrenal gland
    - S37.813   Laceration of adrenal gland
    - S37.818   Other injury of adrenal gland
    - S37.819   Unspecified injury of adrenal gland
  - S37.82   Injury of prostate
    - S37.822   Contusion of prostate ♂
    - S37.823   Laceration of prostate ♂
    - S37.828   Other injury of prostate ♂
    - S37.829   Unspecified injury of prostate ♂
  - S37.89   Injury of other urinary and pelvic organ
    - S37.892   Contusion of other urinary and pelvic organ
    - S37.893   Laceration of other urinary and pelvic organ

- S37.898   Other injury of other urinary and pelvic organ
- S37.899   Unspecified injury of other urinary and pelvic organ
- S37.9   Injury of unspecified urinary and pelvic organ
  - X S37.90   Unspecified injury of unspecified urinary and pelvic organ
  - X S37.92   Contusion of unspecified urinary and pelvic organ
  - X S37.93   Laceration of unspecified urinary and pelvic organ
  - X S37.99   Other injury of unspecified urinary and pelvic organ
- S38   **Crushing injury and traumatic amputation of abdomen, lower back, pelvis and external genitals**
  An amputation not identified as partial or complete should be coded to complete

  The appropriate 7th character is to be added to each code from category S38

A	initial encounter
D	subsequent encounter
S	sequela

  - S38.0   Crushing injury of external genital organs
    Use additional code for any associated injuries
    - S38.00   Crushing injury of unspecified external genital organs
      - S38.001   Crushing injury of unspecified external genital organs, male ♂
      - S38.002   Crushing injury of unspecified external genital organs, female ♀
    - X S38.01   Crushing injury of penis ♂
    - X S38.02   Crushing injury of scrotum and testis ♂
    - X S38.03   Crushing injury of vulva ♀
  - X S38.1   Crushing injury of abdomen, lower back, and pelvis
    Use additional code for all associated injuries, such as:
    fracture of thoracic or lumbar spine and pelvis (S22.0-, S32.-)
    injury to intra-abdominal organs (S36.-)
    injury to urinary and pelvic organs (S37.-)
    open wound of abdominal wall (S31.-)
    spinal cord injury (S34.0, S34.1-)
    Excludes2   crushing injury of external genital organs (S38.0-)
  - S38.2   Traumatic amputation of external genital organs
    - S38.21   Traumatic amputation of female external genital organs
      Traumatic amputation of clitoris
      Traumatic amputation of labium (majus) (minus)
      Traumatic amputation of vulva
      - S38.211   Complete traumatic amputation of female external genital organs ♀
      - S38.212   Partial traumatic amputation of female external genital organs ♀
    - S38.22   Traumatic amputation of penis
      - S38.221   Complete traumatic amputation of penis ♂
      - S38.222   Partial traumatic amputation of penis ♂
    - S38.23   Traumatic amputation of scrotum and testis
      - S38.231   Complete traumatic amputation of scrotum and testis ♂
      - S38.232   Partial traumatic amputation of scrotum and testis ♂
  - X S38.3   Transection (partial) of abdomen

CHAPTER 19 (S00-T88)

● **S39**   **Other and unspecified injuries of abdomen, lower back, pelvis and external genitals**
Code also any associated open wound (S31.-)
Excludes2   sprain of joints and ligaments of lumbar spine and pelvis (S33.-)

The appropriate 7th character is to be added to each code from category S39

> A   initial encounter
> D   subsequent encounter
> S   sequela

● **S39.0**   **Injury of muscle, fascia and tendon of abdomen, lower back and pelvis**
  ● **S39.00**   Unspecified injury of muscle, fascia and tendon of abdomen, lower back and pelvis
    ● **S39.001** Unspecified injury of muscle, fascia and tendon of abdomen
    ● **S39.002** Unspecified injury of muscle, fascia and tendon of lower back
    ● **S39.003** Unspecified injury of muscle, fascia and tendon of pelvis
  ● **S39.01**   Strain of muscle, fascia and tendon of abdomen, lower back and pelvis
    ● **S39.011** Strain of muscle, fascia and tendon of abdomen
    ● **S39.012** Strain of muscle, fascia and tendon of lower back
    ● **S39.013** Strain of muscle, fascia and tendon of pelvis
  ● **S39.02**   Laceration of muscle, fascia and tendon of abdomen, lower back and pelvis
    ● **S39.021** Laceration of muscle, fascia and tendon of abdomen
    ● **S39.022** Laceration of muscle, fascia and tendon of lower back
    ● **S39.023** Laceration of muscle, fascia and tendon of pelvis
  ● **S39.09**   Other injury of muscle, fascia and tendon of abdomen, lower back and pelvis
    ● **S39.091** Other injury of muscle, fascia and tendon of abdomen
    ● **S39.092** Other injury of muscle, fascia and tendon of lower back
    ● **S39.093** Other injury of muscle, fascia and tendon of pelvis

● **S39.8**   **Other specified injuries of abdomen, lower back, pelvis and external genitals**
  X ● **S39.81**   Other specified injuries of abdomen
  X ● **S39.82**   Other specified injuries of lower back
  X ● **S39.83**   Other specified injuries of pelvis
  ● **S39.84**   Other specified injuries of external genitals
    ● **S39.840** Fracture of corpus cavernosum penis ♂
    ● **S39.848** Other specified injuries of external genitals

● **S39.9**   **Unspecified injury of abdomen, lower back, pelvis and external genitals**
  X ● **S39.91**   Unspecified injury of abdomen
  X ● **S39.92**   Unspecified injury of lower back
  X ● **S39.93**   Unspecified injury of pelvis
  X ● **S39.94**   Unspecified injury of external genitals

INJURIES TO THE SHOULDER AND UPPER ARM (S40-S49)

Includes   injuries of axilla injuries of scapular region
Excludes2   burns and corrosions (T20-T32)
    frostbite (T33-T34)
    injuries of elbow (S50-S59)
    insect bite or sting, venomous (T63.4)

● **S40**   **Superficial injury of shoulder and upper arm**
The appropriate 7th character is to be added to each code from category S40

> A   initial encounter
> D   subsequent encounter
> S   sequela

● **S40.0**   **Contusion of shoulder and upper arm**
  ● **S40.01**   Contusion of shoulder
    ● **S40.011** Contusion of right shoulder
    ● **S40.012** Contusion of left shoulder
    ● **S40.019** Contusion of unspecified shoulder
  ● **S40.02**   Contusion of upper arm
    ● **S40.021** Contusion of right upper arm
    ● **S40.022** Contusion of left upper arm
    ● **S40.029** Contusion of unspecified upper arm

● **S40.2**   **Other superficial injuries of shoulder**
  ● **S40.21**   Abrasion of shoulder
    ● **S40.211** Abrasion of right shoulder
    ● **S40.212** Abrasion of left shoulder
    ● **S40.219** Abrasion of unspecified shoulder
  ● **S40.22**   Blister (nonthermal) of shoulder
    ● **S40.221** Blister (nonthermal) of right shoulder
    ● **S40.222** Blister (nonthermal) of left shoulder
    ● **S40.229** Blister (nonthermal) of unspecified shoulder
  ● **S40.24**   External constriction of shoulder
    ● **S40.241** External constriction of right shoulder
    ● **S40.242** External constriction of left shoulder
    ● **S40.249** External constriction of unspecified shoulder
  ● **S40.25**   Superficial foreign body of shoulder
    Splinter in the shoulder
    ● **S40.251** Superficial foreign body of right shoulder
    ● **S40.252** Superficial foreign body of left shoulder
    ● **S40.259** Superficial foreign body of unspecified shoulder
  ● **S40.26**   Insect bite (nonvenomous) of shoulder
    ● **S40.261** Insect bite (nonvenomous) of right shoulder
    ● **S40.262** Insect bite (nonvenomous) of left shoulder
    ● **S40.269** Insect bite (nonvenomous) of unspecified shoulder
  ● **S40.27**   Other superficial bite of shoulder
    Excludes1   open bite of shoulder (S41.05)
    ● **S40.271** Other superficial bite of right shoulder
    ● **S40.272** Other superficial bite of left shoulder
    ● **S40.279** Other superficial bite of unspecified shoulder

CHAPTER 19 (S00-T88)

● **S40.8   Other superficial injuries of upper arm**
　● **S40.81   Abrasion of upper arm**
　　● S40.811   Abrasion of right upper arm
　　● S40.812   Abrasion of left upper arm
　　● S40.819   Abrasion of unspecified upper arm
　● **S40.82   Blister (nonthermal) of upper arm**
　　● S40.821   Blister (nonthermal) of right upper arm
　　● S40.822   Blister (nonthermal) of left upper arm
　　● S40.829   Blister (nonthermal) of unspecified upper arm
　● **S40.84   External constriction of upper arm**
　　● S40.841   External constriction of right upper arm
　　● S40.842   External constriction of left upper arm
　　● S40.849   External constriction of unspecified upper arm
　● **S40.85   Superficial foreign body of upper arm**
　　Splinter in the upper arm
　　● S40.851   Superficial foreign body of right upper arm
　　● S40.852   Superficial foreign body of left upper arm
　　● S40.859   Superficial foreign body of unspecified upper arm
　● **S40.86   Insect bite (nonvenomous) of upper arm**
　　● S40.861   Insect bite (nonvenomous) of right upper arm
　　● S40.862   Insect bite (nonvenomous) of left upper arm
　　● S40.869   Insect bite (nonvenomous) of unspecified upper arm
　● **S40.87   Other superficial bite of upper arm**
　　Excludes1   open bite of upper arm (S41.14)
　　Excludes2   other superficial bite of shoulder (S40.27-)
　　● S40.871   Other superficial bite of right upper arm
　　● S40.872   Other superficial bite of left upper arm
　　● S40.879   Other superficial bite of unspecified upper arm
● **S40.9   Unspecified superficial injury of shoulder and upper arm**
　● **S40.91   Unspecified superficial injury of shoulder**
　　● S40.911   Unspecified superficial injury of right shoulder
　　● S40.912   Unspecified superficial injury of left shoulder
　　● S40.919   Unspecified superficial injury of unspecified shoulder
　● **S40.92   Unspecified superficial injury of upper arm**
　　● S40.921   Unspecified superficial injury of right upper arm
　　● S40.922   Unspecified superficial injury of left upper arm
　　● S40.929   Unspecified superficial injury of unspecified upper arm

● **S41   Open wound of shoulder and upper arm**
　Code also any associated wound infection
　Excludes1   traumatic amputation of shoulder and upper arm (S48.-)
　Excludes2   open fracture of shoulder and upper arm (S42.- with 7th character B or C)
　The appropriate 7th character is to be added to each code from category S41

　┌─────────────────────────────────────┐
　│ A   initial encounter   │
　│ D   subsequent encounter   │
　│ S   sequela   │
　└─────────────────────────────────────┘

　● **S41.0   Open wound of shoulder**
　　● **S41.00   Unspecified open wound of shoulder**
　　　● S41.001   Unspecified open wound of right shoulder
　　　● S41.002   Unspecified open wound of left shoulder
　　　● S41.009   Unspecified open wound of unspecified shoulder
　　● **S41.01   Laceration without foreign body of shoulder**
　　　● S41.011   Laceration without foreign body of right shoulder
　　　● S41.012   Laceration without foreign body of left shoulder
　　　● S41.019   Laceration without foreign body of unspecified shoulder
　　● **S41.02   Laceration with foreign body of shoulder**
　　　● S41.021   Laceration with foreign body of right shoulder
　　　● S41.022   Laceration with foreign body of left shoulder
　　　● S41.029   Laceration with foreign body of unspecified shoulder
　　● **S41.03   Puncture wound without foreign body of shoulder**
　　　● S41.031   Puncture wound without foreign body of right shoulder
　　　● S41.032   Puncture wound without foreign body of left shoulder
　　　● S41.039   Puncture wound without foreign body of unspecified shoulder
　　● **S41.04   Puncture wound with foreign body of shoulder**
　　　● S41.041   Puncture wound with foreign body of right shoulder
　　　● S41.042   Puncture wound with foreign body of left shoulder
　　　● S41.049   Puncture wound with foreign body of unspecified shoulder
　　● **S41.05   Open bite of shoulder**
　　　Bite of shoulder NOS
　　　Excludes1   superficial bite of shoulder (S40.27)
　　　● S41.051   Open bite of right shoulder
　　　● S41.052   Open bite of left shoulder
　　　● S41.059   Open bite of unspecified shoulder
　● **S41.1   Open wound of upper arm**
　　● **S41.10   Unspecified open wound of upper arm**
　　　● S41.101   Unspecified open wound of right upper arm
　　　● S41.102   Unspecified open wound of left upper arm
　　　● S41.109   Unspecified open wound of unspecified upper arm

CHAPTER 19 (S00-T88)

● S41.11 Laceration without foreign body of upper arm
   ● S41.111 Laceration without foreign body of right upper arm
   ● S41.112 Laceration without foreign body of left upper arm
   ● S41.119 Laceration without foreign body of unspecified upper arm
● S41.12 Laceration with foreign body of upper arm
   ● S41.121 Laceration with foreign body of right upper arm
   ● S41.122 Laceration with foreign body of left upper arm
   ● S41.129 Laceration with foreign body of unspecified upper arm
● S41.13 Puncture wound without foreign body of upper arm
   ● S41.131 Puncture wound without foreign body of right upper arm
   ● S41.132 Puncture wound without foreign body of left upper arm
   ● S41.139 Puncture wound without foreign body of unspecified upper arm
● S41.14 Puncture wound with foreign body of upper arm
   ● S41.141 Puncture wound with foreign body of right upper arm
   ● S41.142 Puncture wound with foreign body of left upper arm
   ● S41.149 Puncture wound with foreign body of unspecified upper arm
● S41.15 Open bite of upper arm
        Bite of upper arm NOS
        Excludes1 superficial bite of upper arm (S40.87)
   ● S41.151 Open bite of right upper arm
   ● S41.152 Open bite of left upper arm
   ● S41.159 Open bite of unspecified upper arm

● S42 Fracture of shoulder and upper arm
   Note: A fracture not indicated as displaced or nondisplaced should be coded to displaced

   A fracture not indicated as open or closed should be coded to closed

   Excludes1 traumatic amputation of shoulder and upper arm (S48.-)

   The appropriate 7th character is to be added to all codes from category S42

A	initial encounter for closed fracture
B	initial encounter for open fracture
D	subsequent encounter for fracture with routine healing
G	subsequent encounter for fracture with delayed healing
K	subsequent encounter for fracture with nonunion
P	subsequent encounter for fracture with malunion
S	sequela

● S42.0 Fracture of clavicle
   ● S42.00 Fracture of unspecified part of clavicle
      ● S42.001 Fracture of unspecified part of right clavicle
      ● S42.002 Fracture of unspecified part of left clavicle
      ● S42.009 Fracture of unspecified part of unspecified clavicle
             Coding Clinic: 2012, Q4, P3

● S42.01 Fracture of sternal end of clavicle
   ● S42.011 Anterior displaced fracture of sternal end of right clavicle
   ● S42.012 Anterior displaced fracture of sternal end of left clavicle
   ● S42.013 Anterior displaced fracture of sternal end of unspecified clavicle
          Displaced fracture of sternal end of clavicle NOS
   ● S42.014 Posterior displaced fracture of sternal end of right clavicle
   ● S42.015 Posterior displaced fracture of sternal end of left clavicle
   ● S42.016 Posterior displaced fracture of sternal end of unspecified clavicle
   ● S42.017 Nondisplaced fracture of sternal end of right clavicle
   ● S42.018 Nondisplaced fracture of sternal end of left clavicle
   ● S42.019 Nondisplaced fracture of sternal end of unspecified clavicle
● S42.02 Fracture of shaft of clavicle
   ● S42.021 Displaced fracture of shaft of right clavicle
   ● S42.022 Displaced fracture of shaft of left clavicle
   ● S42.023 Displaced fracture of shaft of unspecified clavicle
   ● S42.024 Nondisplaced fracture of shaft of right clavicle
   ● S42.025 Nondisplaced fracture of shaft of left clavicle
   ● S42.026 Nondisplaced fracture of shaft of unspecified clavicle
● S42.03 Fracture of lateral end of clavicle
          Fracture of acromial end of clavicle
   ● S42.031 Displaced fracture of lateral end of right clavicle
   ● S42.032 Displaced fracture of lateral end of left clavicle
   ● S42.033 Displaced fracture of lateral end of unspecified clavicle
   ● S42.034 Nondisplaced fracture of lateral end of right clavicle
   ● S42.035 Nondisplaced fracture of lateral end of left clavicle
   ● S42.036 Nondisplaced fracture of lateral end of unspecified clavicle
● S42.1 Fracture of scapula
   ● S42.10 Fracture of unspecified part of scapula
      ● S42.101 Fracture of unspecified part of scapula, right shoulder
      ● S42.102 Fracture of unspecified part of scapula, left shoulder
      ● S42.109 Fracture of unspecified part of scapula, unspecified shoulder
   ● S42.11 Fracture of body of scapula
      ● S42.111 Displaced fracture of body of scapula, right shoulder
      ● S42.112 Displaced fracture of body of scapula, left shoulder
      ● S42.113 Displaced fracture of body of scapula, unspecified shoulder
      ● S42.114 Nondisplaced fracture of body of scapula, right shoulder
      ● S42.115 Nondisplaced fracture of body of scapula, left shoulder
      ● S42.116 Nondisplaced fracture of body of scapula, unspecified shoulder

- S42.12   Fracture of acromial process
  - S42.121   Displaced fracture of acromial process, right shoulder
  - S42.122   Displaced fracture of acromial process, left shoulder
  - S42.123   Displaced fracture of acromial process, unspecified shoulder
  - S42.124   Nondisplaced fracture of acromial process, right shoulder
  - S42.125   Nondisplaced fracture of acromial process, left shoulder
  - S42.126   Nondisplaced fracture, of acromial process, unspecified shoulder
- S42.13   Fracture of coracoid process
  - S42.131   Displaced fracture of coracoid process, right shoulder
  - S42.132   Displaced fracture of coracoid process, left shoulder
  - S42.133   Displaced fracture of coracoid process, unspecified shoulder
  - S42.134   Nondisplaced fracture of coracoid process, right shoulder
  - S42.135   Nondisplaced fracture of coracoid process, left shoulder
  - S42.136   Nondisplaced fracture of coracoid process, unspecified shoulder
- S42.14   Fracture of glenoid cavity of scapula
  - S42.141   Displaced fracture of glenoid cavity of scapula, right shoulder
  - S42.142   Displaced fracture of glenoid cavity of scapula, left shoulder
  - S42.143   Displaced fracture of glenoid cavity of scapula, unspecified shoulder
  - S42.144   Nondisplaced fracture of glenoid cavity of scapula, right shoulder
  - S42.145   Nondisplaced fracture of glenoid cavity of scapula, left shoulder
  - S42.146   Nondisplaced fracture of glenoid cavity of scapula, unspecified shoulder
- S42.15   Fracture of neck of scapula
  - S42.151   Displaced fracture of neck of scapula, right shoulder
  - S42.152   Displaced fracture of neck of scapula, left shoulder
  - S42.153   Displaced fracture of neck of scapula, unspecified shoulder
  - S42.154   Nondisplaced fracture of neck of scapula, right shoulder
  - S42.155   Nondisplaced fracture of neck of scapula, left shoulder
  - S42.156   Nondisplaced fracture of neck of scapula, unspecified shoulder
- S42.19   Fracture of other part of scapula
  - S42.191   Fracture of other part of scapula, right shoulder
  - S42.192   Fracture of other part of scapula, left shoulder
  - S42.199   Fracture of other part of scapula, unspecified shoulder

- S42.2   Fracture of upper end of humerus
  Fracture of proximal end of humerus
  Excludes2   fracture of shaft of humerus (S42.3-)
  physeal fracture of upper end of humerus (S49.0-)
  - S42.20   Unspecified fracture of upper end of humerus
    - S42.201   Unspecified fracture of upper end of right humerus
    - S42.202   Unspecified fracture of upper end of left humerus
    - S42.209   Unspecified fracture of upper end of unspecified humerus
  - S42.21   Unspecified fracture of surgical neck of humerus
    Fracture of neck of humerus NOS
    - S42.211   Unspecified displaced fracture of surgical neck of right humerus
    - S42.212   Unspecified displaced fracture of surgical neck of left humerus
    - S42.213   Unspecified displaced fracture of surgical neck of unspecified humerus
    - S42.214   Unspecified nondisplaced fracture of surgical neck of right humerus
    - S42.215   Unspecified nondisplaced fracture of surgical neck of left humerus
    - S42.216   Unspecified nondisplaced fracture of surgical neck of unspecified humerus
  - S42.22   2-part fracture of surgical neck of humerus
    - S42.221   2-part displaced fracture of surgical neck of right humerus
    - S42.222   2-part displaced fracture of surgical neck of left humerus
    - S42.223   2-part displaced fracture of surgical neck of unspecified humerus
    - S42.224   2-part nondisplaced fracture of surgical neck of right humerus
    - S42.225   2-part nondisplaced fracture of surgical neck of left humerus
    - S42.226   2-part nondisplaced fracture of surgical neck of unspecified humerus
  - S42.23   3-part fracture of surgical neck of humerus
    - S42.231   3-part fracture of surgical neck of right humerus
    - S42.232   3-part fracture of surgical neck of left humerus
    - S42.239   3-part fracture of surgical neck of unspecified humerus
  - S42.24   4-part fracture of surgical neck of humerus
    - S42.241   4-part fracture of surgical neck of right humerus
    - S42.242   4-part fracture of surgical neck of left humerus
    - S42.249   4-part fracture of surgical neck of unspecified humerus
  - S42.25   Fracture of greater tuberosity of humerus
    - S42.251   Displaced fracture of greater tuberosity of right humerus
    - S42.252   Displaced fracture of greater tuberosity of left humerus
    - S42.253   Displaced fracture of greater tuberosity of unspecified humerus
    - S42.254   Nondisplaced fracture of greater tuberosity of right humerus
    - S42.255   Nondisplaced fracture of greater tuberosity of left humerus
    - S42.256   Nondisplaced fracture of greater tuberosity of unspecified humerus

● **S42.26**   Fracture of lesser tuberosity of humerus

   ● **S42.261**   Displaced fracture of lesser tuberosity of right humerus

   ● **S42.262**   Displaced fracture of lesser tuberosity of left humerus

   ● **S42.263**   Displaced fracture of lesser tuberosity of unspecified humerus

   ● **S42.264**   Nondisplaced fracture of lesser tuberosity of right humerus

   ● **S42.265**   Nondisplaced fracture of lesser tuberosity of left humerus

   ● **S42.266**   Nondisplaced fracture of lesser tuberosity of unspecified humerus

● **S42.27**   Torus fracture of upper end of humerus

The appropriate 7th character is to be added to all codes in subcategory S42.27

A	initial encounter for closed fracture
D	subsequent encounter for fracture with routine healing
G	subsequent encounter for fracture with delayed healing
K	subsequent encounter for fracture with nonunion
P	subsequent encounter for fracture with malunion
S	sequela

   ● **S42.271**   Torus fracture of upper end of right humerus

   ● **S42.272**   Torus fracture of upper end of left humerus

   ● **S42.279**   Torus fracture of upper end of unspecified humerus

● **S42.29**   Other fracture of upper end of humerus

Fracture of anatomical neck of humerus
Fracture of articular head of humerus

   ● **S42.291**   Other displaced fracture of upper end of right humerus

   ● **S42.292**   Other displaced fracture of upper end of left humerus

   ● **S42.293**   Other displaced fracture of upper end of unspecified humerus

   ● **S42.294**   Other nondisplaced fracture of upper end of right humerus

   ● **S42.295**   Other nondisplaced fracture of upper end of left humerus

   ● **S42.296**   Other nondisplaced fracture of upper end of unspecified humerus

● **S42.3**   Fracture of shaft of humerus

Fracture of humerus NOS
Fracture of upper arm NOS

Excludes2   physeal fractures of upper end of humerus (S49.0-)
physeal fractures of lower end of humerus (S49.1-)

● **S42.30**   Unspecified fracture of shaft of humerus

   ● **S42.301**   Unspecified fracture of shaft of humerus, right arm

   ● **S42.302**   Unspecified fracture of shaft of humerus, left arm

   ● **S42.309**   Unspecified fracture of shaft of humerus, unspecified arm

● **S42.31**   Greenstick fracture of shaft of humerus

The appropriate 7th character is to be added to all codes in subcategory S42.31

A	initial encounter for closed fracture
D	subsequent encounter for fracture with routine healing
G	subsequent encounter for fracture with delayed healing
K	subsequent encounter for fracture with nonunion
P	subsequent encounter for fracture with malunion
S	sequela

   ● **S42.311**   Greenstick fracture of shaft of humerus, right arm

   ● **S42.312**   Greenstick fracture of shaft of humerus, left arm

   ● **S42.319**   Greenstick fracture of shaft of humerus, unspecified arm

● **S42.32**   Transverse fracture of shaft of humerus

   ● **S42.321**   Displaced transverse fracture of shaft of humerus, right arm

   ● **S42.322**   Displaced transverse fracture of shaft of humerus, left arm

   ● **S42.323**   Displaced transverse fracture of shaft of humerus, unspecified arm

   ● **S42.324**   Nondisplaced transverse fracture of shaft of humerus, right arm

   ● **S42.325**   Nondisplaced transverse fracture of shaft of humerus, left arm

   ● **S42.326**   Nondisplaced transverse fracture of shaft of humerus, unspecified arm

● **S42.33**   Oblique fracture of shaft of humerus

   ● **S42.331**   Displaced oblique fracture of shaft of humerus, right arm

   ● **S42.332**   Displaced oblique fracture of shaft of humerus, left arm

   ● **S42.333**   Displaced oblique fracture of shaft of humerus, unspecified arm

   ● **S42.334**   Nondisplaced oblique fracture of shaft of humerus, right arm

   ● **S42.335**   Nondisplaced oblique fracture of shaft of humerus, left arm

   ● **S42.336**   Nondisplaced oblique fracture of shaft of humerus, unspecified arm

● **S42.34**   Spiral fracture of shaft of humerus

   ● **S42.341**   Displaced spiral fracture of shaft of humerus, right arm

   ● **S42.342**   Displaced spiral fracture of shaft of humerus, left arm

   ● **S42.343**   Displaced spiral fracture of shaft of humerus, unspecified arm

   ● **S42.344**   Nondisplaced spiral fracture of shaft of humerus, right arm

   ● **S42.345**   Nondisplaced spiral fracture of shaft of humerus, left arm

   ● **S42.346**   Nondisplaced spiral fracture of shaft of humerus, unspecified arm

● **S42.35**   Comminuted fracture of shaft of humerus

   ● **S42.351**   Displaced comminuted fracture of shaft of humerus, right arm

   ● **S42.352**   Displaced comminuted fracture of shaft of humerus, left arm

   ● **S42.353**   Displaced comminuted fracture of shaft of humerus, unspecified arm

◀ New   ◀ Revised   ~~deleted~~ Deleted   Excludes 1   Excludes 2   Includes   Use additional   Code first   Code also   Unspecified

1240   OGCR Official Guidelines   X Assign placeholder X   ● Use Additional Character(s)   ▶ Manifestation Code   **Coding Clinic**

● S42.354   Nondisplaced comminuted fracture of shaft of humerus, right arm

● S42.355   Nondisplaced comminuted fracture of shaft of humerus, left arm

● S42.356   Nondisplaced comminuted fracture of shaft of humerus, unspecified arm

● S42.36   Segmental fracture of shaft of humerus

  ● S42.361   Displaced segmental fracture of shaft of humerus, right arm

  ● S42.362   Displaced segmental fracture of shaft of humerus, left arm

  ● S42.363   Displaced segmental fracture of shaft of humerus, unspecified arm

  ● S42.364   Nondisplaced segmental fracture of shaft of humerus, right arm

  ● S42.365   Nondisplaced segmental fracture of shaft of humerus, left arm

  ● S42.366   Nondisplaced segmental fracture of shaft of humerus, unspecified arm

● S42.39   Other fracture of shaft of humerus

  ● S42.391   Other fracture of shaft of right humerus

  ● S42.392   Other fracture of shaft of left humerus

  ● S42.399   Other fracture of shaft of unspecified humerus

● S42.4   Fracture of lower end of humerus
Fracture of distal end of humerus

> **Excludes2**   fracture of shaft of humerus (S42.3-)
> physeal fracture of lower end of humerus (S49.1-)

● S42.40   Unspecified fracture of lower end of humerus
Fracture of elbow NOS

  ● S42.401   Unspecified fracture of lower end of right humerus

  ● S42.402   Unspecified fracture of lower end of left humerus

  ● S42.409   Unspecified fracture of lower end of unspecified humerus

● S42.41   Simple supracondylar fracture without intercondylar fracture of humerus

  ● S42.411   Displaced simple supracondylar fracture without intercondylar fracture of right humerus

  ● S42.412   Displaced simple supracondylar fracture without intercondylar fracture of left humerus

  ● S42.413   Displaced simple supracondylar fracture without intercondylar fracture of unspecified humerus

  ● S42.414   Nondisplaced simple supracondylar fracture without intercondylar fracture of right humerus

  ● S42.415   Nondisplaced simple supracondylar fracture without intercondylar fracture of left humerus

  ● S42.416   Nondisplaced simple supracondylar fracture without intercondylar fracture of unspecified humerus

● S42.42   Comminuted supracondylar fracture without intercondylar fracture of humerus

  ● S42.421   Displaced comminuted supracondylar fracture without intercondylar fracture of right humerus

  ● S42.422   Displaced comminuted supracondylar fracture without intercondylar fracture of left humerus

  ● S42.423   Displaced comminuted supracondylar fracture without intercondylar fracture of unspecified humerus

  ● S42.424   Nondisplaced comminuted supracondylar fracture without intercondylar fracture of right humerus

  ● S42.425   Nondisplaced comminuted supracondylar fracture without intercondylar fracture of left humerus

  ● S42.426   Nondisplaced comminuted supracondylar fracture without intercondylar fracture of unspecified humerus

● S42.43   Fracture (avulsion) of lateral epicondyle of humerus

  ● S42.431   Displaced fracture (avulsion) of lateral epicondyle of right humerus

  ● S42.432   Displaced fracture (avulsion) of lateral epicondyle of left humerus

  ● S42.433   Displaced fracture (avulsion) of lateral epicondyle of unspecified humerus

  ● S42.434   Nondisplaced fracture (avulsion) of lateral epicondyle of right humerus

  ● S42.435   Nondisplaced fracture (avulsion) of lateral epicondyle of left humerus

  ● S42.436   Nondisplaced fracture (avulsion) of lateral epicondyle of unspecified humerus

● S42.44   Fracture (avulsion) of medial epicondyle of humerus

  ● S42.441   Displaced fracture (avulsion) of medial epicondyle of right humerus

  ● S42.442   Displaced fracture (avulsion) of medial epicondyle of left humerus

  ● S42.443   Displaced fracture (avulsion) of medial epicondyle of unspecified humerus

  ● S42.444   Nondisplaced fracture (avulsion) of medial epicondyle of right humerus

  ● S42.445   Nondisplaced fracture (avulsion) of medial epicondyle of left humerus

  ● S42.446   Nondisplaced fracture (avulsion) of medial epicondyle of unspecified humerus

  ● S42.447   Incarcerated fracture (avulsion) of medial epicondyle of right humerus

  ● S42.448   Incarcerated fracture (avulsion) of medial epicondyle of left humerus

  ● S42.449   Incarcerated fracture (avulsion) of medial epicondyle of unspecified humerus

● S42.45   Fracture of lateral condyle of humerus
Fracture of capitellum of humerus

  ● S42.451   Displaced fracture of lateral condyle of right humerus

  ● S42.452   Displaced fracture of lateral condyle of left humerus

  ● S42.453   Displaced fracture of lateral condyle of unspecified humerus

  ● S42.454   Nondisplaced fracture of lateral condyle of right humerus

  ● S42.455   Nondisplaced fracture of lateral condyle of left humerus

  ● S42.456   Nondisplaced fracture of lateral condyle of unspecified humerus

CHAPTER 19 (S00-T88)

● **S42.46**   **Fracture of medial condyle of humerus**
Trochlea fracture of humerus

     ● **S42.461**   **Displaced fracture of medial condyle of right humerus**

     ● **S42.462**   **Displaced fracture of medial condyle of left humerus**

     ● **S42.463**   **Displaced fracture of medial condyle of unspecified humerus**

     ● **S42.464**   **Nondisplaced fracture of medial condyle of right humerus**

     ● **S42.465**   **Nondisplaced fracture of medial condyle of left humerus**

     ● **S42.466**   **Nondisplaced fracture of medial condyle of unspecified humerus**

● **S42.47**   **Transcondylar fracture of humerus**

     ● **S42.471**   **Displaced transcondylar fracture of right humerus**

     ● **S42.472**   **Displaced transcondylar fracture of left humerus**

     ● **S42.473**   **Displaced transcondylar fracture of unspecified humerus**

     ● **S42.474**   **Nondisplaced transcondylar fracture of right humerus**

     ● **S42.475**   **Nondisplaced transcondylar fracture of left humerus**

     ● **S42.476**   **Nondisplaced transcondylar fracture of unspecified humerus**

● **S42.48**   **Torus fracture of lower end of humerus**

The appropriate 7th character is to be added to all codes in subcategory S42.48

> A   initial encounter for closed fracture
> D   subsequent encounter for fracture with routine healing
> G   subsequent encounter for fracture with delayed healing
> K   subsequent encounter for fracture with nonunion
> P   subsequent encounter for fracture with malunion
> S   sequela

     ● **S42.481**   **Torus fracture of lower end of right humerus**

     ● **S42.482**   **Torus fracture of lower end of left humerus**

     ● **S42.489**   **Torus fracture of lower end of unspecified humerus**

● **S42.49**   **Other fracture of lower end of humerus**

     ● **S42.491**   **Other displaced fracture of lower end of right humerus**

     ● **S42.492**   **Other displaced fracture of lower end of left humerus**

     ● **S42.493**   **Other displaced fracture of lower end of unspecified humerus**

     ● **S42.494**   **Other nondisplaced fracture of lower end of right humerus**

     ● **S42.495**   **Other nondisplaced fracture of lower end of left humerus**

     ● **S42.496**   **Other nondisplaced fracture of lower end of unspecified humerus**

● **S42.9**   **Fracture of shoulder girdle, part unspecified**
Fracture of shoulder NOS

X ● **S42.90**   **Fracture of unspecified shoulder girdle, part unspecified**

X ● **S42.91**   **Fracture of right shoulder girdle, part unspecified**

X ● **S42.92**   **Fracture of left shoulder girdle, part unspecified**

● **S43**   **Dislocation and sprain of joints and ligaments of shoulder girdle**

     Includes   avulsion of joint or ligament of shoulder girdle
laceration of cartilage, joint or ligament of shoulder girdle
sprain of cartilage, joint or ligament of shoulder girdle
traumatic hemarthrosis of joint or ligament of shoulder girdle
traumatic rupture of joint or ligament of shoulder girdle
traumatic subluxation of joint or ligament of shoulder girdle
traumatic tear of joint or ligament of shoulder girdle

Code also any associated open wound

     Excludes2   strain of muscle, fascia and tendon of shoulder and upper arm (S46.-)

The appropriate 7th character is to be added to each code from category S43

> A   initial encounter
> D   subsequent encounter
> S   sequela

● **S43.0**   **Subluxation and dislocation of shoulder joint**
Dislocation of glenohumeral joint
Subluxation of glenohumeral joint

     ● **S43.00**   **Unspecified subluxation and dislocation of shoulder joint**
Dislocation of humerus NOS
Subluxation of humerus NOS

         ● **S43.001**   **Unspecified subluxation of right shoulder joint**

         ● **S43.002**   **Unspecified subluxation of left shoulder joint**

         ● **S43.003**   **Unspecified subluxation of unspecified shoulder joint**

         ● **S43.004**   **Unspecified dislocation of right shoulder joint**

         ● **S43.005**   **Unspecified dislocation of left shoulder joint**

         ● **S43.006**   **Unspecified dislocation of unspecified shoulder joint**

     ● **S43.01**   **Anterior subluxation and dislocation of humerus**

         ● **S43.011**   **Anterior subluxation of right humerus**

         ● **S43.012**   **Anterior subluxation of left humerus**

         ● **S43.013**   **Anterior subluxation of unspecified humerus**

         ● **S43.014**   **Anterior dislocation of right humerus**

         ● **S43.015**   **Anterior dislocation of left humerus**

         ● **S43.016**   **Anterior dislocation of unspecified humerus**

     ● **S43.02**   **Posterior subluxation and dislocation of humerus**

         ● **S43.021**   **Posterior subluxation of right humerus**

         ● **S43.022**   **Posterior subluxation of left humerus**

         ● **S43.023**   **Posterior subluxation of unspecified humerus**

         ● **S43.024**   **Posterior dislocation of right humerus**

         ● **S43.025**   **Posterior dislocation of left humerus**

         ● **S43.026**   **Posterior dislocation of unspecified humerus**

◄ New   ◄◄ Revised   ~~deleted~~ Deleted   Excludes 1   Excludes 2   Includes   Use additional   Code first   Code also   Unspecified

OGCR Official Guidelines   X Assign placeholder X   ● Use Additional Character(s)   ▶ Manifestation Code   **Coding Clinic**

1242

● S43.03   Inferior subluxation and dislocation of humerus
  ● S43.031   Inferior subluxation of right humerus
  ● S43.032   Inferior subluxation of left humerus
  ● S43.033   Inferior subluxation of unspecified humerus
  ● S43.034   Inferior dislocation of right humerus
  ● S43.035   Inferior dislocation of left humerus
  ● S43.036   Inferior dislocation of unspecified humerus
● S43.08   Other subluxation and dislocation of shoulder joint
  ● S43.081   Other subluxation of right shoulder joint
  ● S43.082   Other subluxation of left shoulder joint
  ● S43.083   Other subluxation of unspecified shoulder joint
  ● S43.084   Other dislocation of right shoulder joint
  ● S43.085   Other dislocation of left shoulder joint
  ● S43.086   Other dislocation of unspecified shoulder joint
● S43.1   Subluxation and dislocation of acromioclavicular joint
  ● S43.10   Unspecified dislocation of acromioclavicular joint
    ● S43.101   Unspecified dislocation of right acromioclavicular joint
    ● S43.102   Unspecified dislocation of left acromioclavicular joint
    ● S43.109   Unspecified dislocation of unspecified acromioclavicular joint
  ● S43.11   Subluxation of acromioclavicular joint
    ● S43.111   Subluxation of right acromioclavicular joint
    ● S43.112   Subluxation of left acromioclavicular joint
    ● S43.119   Subluxation of unspecified acromioclavicular joint
  ● S43.12   Dislocation of acromioclavicular joint, 100%-200% displacement
    ● S43.121   Dislocation of right acromioclavicular joint, 100%-200% displacement
    ● S43.122   Dislocation of left acromioclavicular joint, 100%-200% displacement
    ● S43.129   Dislocation of unspecified acromioclavicular joint, 100%-200% displacement
  ● S43.13   Dislocation of acromioclavicular joint, greater than 200% displacement
    ● S43.131   Dislocation of right acromioclavicular joint, greater than 200% displacement
    ● S43.132   Dislocation of left acromioclavicular joint, greater than 200% displacement
    ● S43.139   Dislocation of unspecified acromioclavicular joint, greater than 200% displacement
  ● S43.14   Inferior dislocation of acromioclavicular joint
    ● S43.141   Inferior dislocation of right acromioclavicular joint
    ● S43.142   Inferior dislocation of left acromioclavicular joint
    ● S43.149   Inferior dislocation of unspecified acromioclavicular joint

● S43.15   Posterior dislocation of acromioclavicular joint
  ● S43.151   Posterior dislocation of right acromioclavicular joint
  ● S43.152   Posterior dislocation of left acromioclavicular joint
  ● S43.159   Posterior dislocation of unspecified acromioclavicular joint
● S43.2   Subluxation and dislocation of sternoclavicular joint
  ● S43.20   Unspecified subluxation and dislocation of sternoclavicular joint
    ● S43.201   Unspecified subluxation of right sternoclavicular joint
    ● S43.202   Unspecified subluxation of left sternoclavicular joint
    ● S43.203   Unspecified subluxation of unspecified sternoclavicular joint
    ● S43.204   Unspecified dislocation of right sternoclavicular joint
    ● S43.205   Unspecified dislocation of left sternoclavicular joint
    ● S43.206   Unspecified dislocation of unspecified sternoclavicular joint
  ● S43.21   Anterior subluxation and dislocation of sternoclavicular joint
    ● S43.211   Anterior subluxation of right sternoclavicular joint
    ♀ S43.212   Anterior subluxation of left sternoclavicular joint
    ● S43.213   Anterior subluxation of unspecified sternoclavicular joint
    ● S43.214   Anterior dislocation of right sternoclavicular joint
    ● S43.215   Anterior dislocation of left sternoclavicular joint
    ● S43.216   Anterior dislocation of unspecified sternoclavicular joint
  ● S43.22   Posterior subluxation and dislocation of sternoclavicular joint
    ● S43.221   Posterior subluxation of right sternoclavicular joint
    ● S43.222   Posterior subluxation of left sternoclavicular joint
    ● S43.223   Posterior subluxation of unspecified sternoclavicular joint
    ● S43.224   Posterior dislocation of right sternoclavicular joint
    ● S43.225   Posterior dislocation of left sternoclavicular joint
    ● S43.226   Posterior dislocation of unspecified sternoclavicular joint
● S43.3   Subluxation and dislocation of other and unspecified parts of shoulder girdle
  ● S43.30   Subluxation and dislocation of unspecified parts of shoulder girdle
    Dislocation of shoulder girdle NOS
    Subluxation of shoulder girdle NOS
    ● S43.301   Subluxation of unspecified parts of right shoulder girdle
    ● S43.302   Subluxation of unspecified parts of left shoulder girdle
    ● S43.303   Subluxation of unspecified parts of unspecified shoulder girdle
    ● S43.304   Dislocation of unspecified parts of right shoulder girdle
    ● S43.305   Dislocation of unspecified parts of left shoulder girdle
    ● S43.306   Dislocation of unspecified parts of unspecified shoulder girdle

CHAPTER 19 (S00-T88)

CHAPTER 19 (S00-T88)

● **S43.31**   **Subluxation and dislocation of scapula**
    ● **S43.311**   Subluxation of right scapula
    ● **S43.312**   Subluxation of left scapula
    ● **S43.313**   Subluxation of ==unspecified== scapula
    ● **S43.314**   Dislocation of right scapula
    ● **S43.315**   Dislocation of left scapula
    ● **S43.316**   Dislocation of ==unspecified== scapula

● **S43.39**   **Subluxation and dislocation of other parts of shoulder girdle**
    ● **S43.391**   Subluxation of other parts of right shoulder girdle
    ● **S43.392**   Subluxation of other parts of left shoulder girdle
    ● **S43.393**   Subluxation of other parts of ==unspecified== shoulder girdle
    ● **S43.394**   Dislocation of other parts of right shoulder girdle
    ● **S43.395**   Dislocation of other parts of left shoulder girdle
    ● **S43.396**   Dislocation of other parts of ==unspecified== shoulder girdle

● **S43.4**   **Sprain of shoulder joint**
   ● **S43.40**   Unspecified sprain of shoulder joint
    ● **S43.401**   ==Unspecified== sprain of right shoulder joint
    ● **S43.402**   ==Unspecified== sprain of left shoulder joint
    ● **S43.409**   ==Unspecified== sprain of unspecified shoulder joint
   ● **S43.41**   Sprain of coracohumeral (ligament)
    ● **S43.411**   Sprain of right coracohumeral (ligament)
    ● **S43.412**   Sprain of left coracohumeral (ligament)
    ● **S43.419**   Sprain of ==unspecified== coracohumeral (ligament)
   ● **S43.42**   Sprain of rotator cuff capsule
     Encounters during the healing phase
     Excludes1   rotator cuff syndrome (complete) (incomplete), not specified as traumatic (M75.1-)
     Excludes2   injury of tendon of rotator cuff (S46.0-)
    ● **S43.421**   Sprain of right rotator cuff capsule
    ● **S43.422**   Sprain of left rotator cuff capsule
    ● **S43.429**   Sprain of ==unspecified== rotator cuff capsule
   ● **S43.43**   Superior glenoid labrum lesion
     SLAP lesion
    ● **S43.431**   Superior glenoid labrum lesion of right shoulder
    ● **S43.432**   Superior glenoid labrum lesion of left shoulder
    ● **S43.439**   Superior glenoid labrum lesion of ==unspecified== shoulder
   ● **S43.49**   Other sprain of shoulder joint
    ● **S43.491**   Other sprain of right shoulder joint
    ● **S43.492**   Other sprain of left shoulder joint
    ● **S43.499**   Other sprain of ==unspecified== shoulder joint

● **S43.5**   **Sprain of acromioclavicular joint**
    Sprain of acromioclavicular ligament
   X ● **S43.50**   Sprain of ==unspecified== acromioclavicular joint
   X ● **S43.51**   Sprain of right acromioclavicular joint
   X ● **S43.52**   Sprain of left acromioclavicular joint

● **S43.6**   **Sprain of sternoclavicular joint**
   X ● **S43.60**   Sprain of ==unspecified== sternoclavicular joint
   X ● **S43.61**   Sprain of right sternoclavicular joint
   X ● **S43.62**   Sprain of left sternoclavicular joint

● **S43.8**   **Sprain of other specified parts of shoulder girdle**
   X ● **S43.80**   Sprain of other specified parts of ==unspecified== shoulder girdle
   X ● **S43.81**   Sprain of other specified parts of right shoulder girdle
   X ● **S43.82**   Sprain of other specified parts of left shoulder girdle

● **S43.9**   **Sprain of unspecified parts of shoulder girdle**
   X ● **S43.90**   Sprain of ==unspecified== parts of unspecified shoulder girdle
     Sprain of shoulder girdle NOS
   X ● **S43.91**   Sprain of ==unspecified== parts of right shoulder girdle
   X ● **S43.92**   Sprain of ==unspecified== parts of left shoulder girdle

● **S44**   **Injury of nerves at shoulder and upper arm level**
   Code also any associated open wound (S41.-)
   Excludes2   injury of brachial plexus (S14.3-)
   The appropriate 7th character is to be added to each code from category S44
     A   initial encounter
     D   subsequent encounter
     S   sequela

● **S44.0**   **Injury of ulnar nerve at upper arm level**
    Excludes1   ulnar nerve NOS (S54.0)
   X ● **S44.00**   Injury of ulnar nerve at upper arm level, ==unspecified== arm
   X ● **S44.01**   Injury of ulnar nerve at upper arm level, right arm
   X ● **S44.02**   Injury of ulnar nerve at upper arm level, left arm

● **S44.1**   **Injury of median nerve at upper arm level**
    Excludes1   median nerve NOS (S54.1)
   X ● **S44.10**   Injury of median nerve at upper arm level, ==unspecified== arm
   X ● **S44.11**   Injury of median nerve at upper arm level, right arm
   X ● **S44.12**   Injury of median nerve at upper arm level, left arm

● **S44.2**   **Injury of radial nerve at upper arm level**
    Excludes1   radial nerve NOS (S54.2)
   X ● **S44.20**   Injury of radial nerve at upper arm level, ==unspecified== arm
   X ● **S44.21**   Injury of radial nerve at upper arm level, right arm
   X ● **S44.22**   Injury of radial nerve at upper arm level, left arm

● **S44.3**   **Injury of axillary nerve**
   X ● **S44.30**   Injury of axillary nerve, ==unspecified== arm
   X ● **S44.31**   Injury of axillary nerve, right arm
   X ● **S44.32**   Injury of axillary nerve, left arm

● **S44.4**   **Injury of musculocutaneous nerve**
   X ● **S44.40**   Injury of musculocutaneous nerve, ==unspecified== arm
   X ● **S44.41**   Injury of musculocutaneous nerve, right arm
   X ● **S44.42**   Injury of musculocutaneous nerve, left arm

◀ New   ◀ Revised   ~~deleted~~ Deleted   Excludes 1   Excludes 2   Includes   Use additional   Code first   Code also   Unspecified
OGCR Official Guidelines   X Assign placeholder X   ● Use Additional Character(s)   ▶ Manifestation Code   **Coding Clinic**

● **S44.5**   **Injury of cutaneous sensory nerve at shoulder and upper arm level**
   X● S44.50   Injury of cutaneous sensory nerve at shoulder and upper arm level, unspecified arm
   X● S44.51   Injury of cutaneous sensory nerve at shoulder and upper arm level, right arm
   X● S44.52   Injury of cutaneous sensory nerve at shoulder and upper arm level, left arm

● **S44.8**   **Injury of other nerves at shoulder and upper arm level**
   ● S44.8X   Injury of other nerves at shoulder and upper arm level
     ● S44.8X1   Injury of other nerves at shoulder and upper arm level, right arm
     ● S44.8X2   Injury of other nerves at shoulder and upper arm level, left arm
     ● S44.8X9   Injury of other nerves at shoulder and upper arm level, unspecified arm

● **S44.9**   **Injury of unspecified nerve at shoulder and upper arm level**
   X● S44.90   Injury of unspecified nerve at shoulder and upper arm level, unspecified arm
   X● S44.91   Injury of unspecified nerve at shoulder and upper arm level, right arm
   X● S44.92   Injury of unspecified nerve at shoulder and upper arm level, left arm

● **S45**   **Injury of blood vessels at shoulder and upper arm level**
   Code also any associated open wound (S41.-)
   Excludes2   injury of subclavian artery (S25.1)
             injury of subclavian vein (S25.3)

   The appropriate 7th character is to be added to each code from category S45

A	initial encounter
D	subsequent encounter
S	sequela

● **S45.0**   **Injury of axillary artery**
   ● S45.00   Unspecified injury of axillary artery
     ● S45.001   Unspecified injury of axillary artery, right side
     ● S45.002   Unspecified injury of axillary artery, left side
     ● S45.009   Unspecified injury of axillary artery, unspecified side
   ● S45.01   Laceration of axillary artery
     ● S45.011   Laceration of axillary artery, right side
     ● S45.012   Laceration of axillary artery, left side
     ● S45.019   Laceration of axillary artery, unspecified side
   ● S45.09   Other specified injury of axillary artery
     ● S45.091   Other specified injury of axillary artery, right side
     ● S45.092   Other specified injury of axillary artery, left side
     ● S45.099   Other specified injury of axillary artery, unspecified side

● **S45.1**   **Injury of brachial artery**
   ● S45.10   Unspecified injury of brachial artery
     ● S45.101   Unspecified injury of brachial artery, right side
     ● S45.102   Unspecified injury of brachial artery, left side
     ● S45.109   Unspecified injury of brachial artery, unspecified side

   ● S45.11   Laceration of brachial artery
     ● S45.111   Laceration of brachial artery, right side
     ● S45.112   Laceration of brachial artery, left side
     ● S45.119   Laceration of brachial artery, unspecified side
   ● S45.19   Other specified injury of brachial artery
     ● S45.191   Other specified injury of brachial artery, right side
     ● S45.192   Other specified injury of brachial artery, left side
     ● S45.199   Other specified injury of brachial artery, unspecified side

● **S45.2**   **Injury of axillary or brachial vein**
   ● S45.20   Unspecified injury of axillary or brachial vein
     ● S45.201   Unspecified injury of axillary or brachial vein, right side
     ● S45.202   Unspecified injury of axillary or brachial vein, left side
     ● S45.209   Unspecified injury of axillary or brachial vein, unspecified side
   ● S45.21   Laceration of axillary or brachial vein
     ● S45.211   Laceration of axillary or brachial vein, right side
     ● S45.212   Laceration of axillary or brachial vein, left side
     ● S45.219   Laceration of axillary or brachial vein, unspecified side
   ● S45.29   Other specified injury of axillary or brachial vein
     ● S45.291   Other specified injury of axillary or brachial vein, right side
     ● S45.292   Other specified injury of axillary or brachial vein, left side
     ● S45.299   Other specified injury of axillary or brachial vein, unspecified side

● **S45.3**   **Injury of superficial vein at shoulder and upper arm level**
   ● S45.30   Unspecified injury of superficial vein at shoulder and upper arm level
     ● S45.301   Unspecified injury of superficial vein at shoulder and upper arm level, right arm
     ● S45.302   Unspecified injury of superficial vein at shoulder and upper arm level, left arm
     ● S45.309   Unspecified injury of superficial vein at shoulder and upper arm level, unspecified arm
   ● S45.31   Laceration of superficial vein at shoulder and upper arm level
     ● S45.311   Laceration of superficial vein at shoulder and upper arm level, right arm
     ● S45.312   Laceration of superficial vein at shoulder and upper arm level, left arm
     ● S45.319   Laceration of superficial vein at shoulder and upper arm level, unspecified arm
   ● S45.39   Other specified injury of superficial vein at shoulder and upper arm level
     ● S45.391   Other specified injury of superficial vein at shoulder and upper arm level, right arm
     ● S45.392   Other specified injury of superficial vein at shoulder and upper arm level, left arm
     ● S45.399   Other specified injury of superficial vein at shoulder and upper arm level, unspecified arm

CHAPTER 19 (S00-T88)

CHAPTER 19 (S00–T88)

● S45.8   Injury of other specified blood vessels at shoulder and upper arm level

  ● S45.80   Unspecified injury of other specified blood vessels at shoulder and upper arm level

    ● S45.801   Unspecified injury of other specified blood vessels at shoulder and upper arm level, right arm

    ● S45.802   Unspecified injury of other specified blood vessels at shoulder and upper arm level, left arm

    ● S45.809   Unspecified injury of other specified blood vessels at shoulder and upper arm level, unspecified arm

  ● S45.81   Laceration of other specified blood vessels at shoulder and upper arm level

    ● S45.811   Laceration of other specified blood vessels at shoulder and upper arm level, right arm

    ● S45.812   Laceration of other specified blood vessels at shoulder and upper arm level, left arm

    ● S45.819   Laceration of other specified blood vessels at shoulder and upper arm level, unspecified arm

  ● S45.89   Other specified injury of other specified blood vessels at shoulder and upper arm level

    ● S45.891   Other specified injury of other specified blood vessels at shoulder and upper arm level, right arm

    ● S45.892   Other specified injury of other specified blood vessels at shoulder and upper arm level, left arm

    ● S45.899   Other specified injury of other specified blood vessels at shoulder and upper arm level, unspecified arm

● S45.9   Injury of unspecified blood vessel at shoulder and upper arm level

  ● S45.90   Unspecified injury of unspecified blood vessel at shoulder and upper arm level

    ● S45.901   Unspecified injury of unspecified blood vessel at shoulder and upper arm level, right arm

    ● S45.902   Unspecified injury of unspecified blood vessel at shoulder and upper arm level, left arm

    ● S45.909   Unspecified injury of unspecified blood vessel at shoulder and upper arm level, unspecified arm

  ● S45.91   Laceration of unspecified blood vessel at shoulder and upper arm level

    ● S45.911   Laceration of unspecified blood vessel at shoulder and upper arm level, right arm

    ● S45.912   Laceration of unspecified blood vessel at shoulder and upper arm level, left arm

    ● S45.919   Laceration of unspecified blood vessel at shoulder and upper arm level, unspecified arm

  ● S45.99   Other specified injury of unspecified blood vessel at shoulder and upper arm level

    ● S45.991   Other specified injury of unspecified blood vessel at shoulder and upper arm level, right arm

    ● S45.992   Other specified injury of unspecified blood vessel at shoulder and upper arm level, left arm

    ● S45.999   Other specified injury of unspecified blood vessel at shoulder and upper arm level, unspecified arm

● S46   Injury of muscle, fascia and tendon at shoulder and upper arm level

  Code also any associated open wound (S41.-)

  Excludes2   injury of muscle, fascia and tendon at elbow (S56.-)
               sprain of joints and ligaments of shoulder girdle (S43.9)

  The appropriate 7th character is to be added to each code from category S46

A	initial encounter
D	subsequent encounter
S	sequela

● S46.0   Injury of muscle(s) and tendon(s) of the rotator cuff of shoulder

  ● S46.00   Unspecified injury of muscle(s) and tendon(s) of the rotator cuff of shoulder

    ● S46.001   Unspecified injury of muscle(s) and tendon(s) of the rotator cuff of right shoulder

    ● S46.002   Unspecified injury of muscle(s) and tendon(s) of the rotator cuff of left shoulder

    ● S46.009   Unspecified injury of muscle(s) and tendon(s) of the rotator cuff of unspecified shoulder

  ● S46.01   Strain of muscle(s) and tendon(s) of the rotator cuff of shoulder

    Acute onset due to trauma to rotator cuff muscle/tendon

    ● S46.011   Strain of muscle(s) and tendon(s) of the rotator cuff of right shoulder

    ● S46.012   Strain of muscle(s) and tendon(s) of the rotator cuff of left shoulder

    ● S46.019   Strain of muscle(s) and tendon(s) of the rotator cuff of unspecified shoulder

  ● S46.02   Laceration of muscle(s) and tendon(s) of the rotator cuff of shoulder

    ● S46.021   Laceration of muscle(s) and tendon(s) of the rotator cuff of right shoulder

    ● S46.022   Laceration of muscle(s) and tendon(s) of the rotator cuff of left shoulder

    ● S46.029   Laceration of muscle(s) and tendon(s) of the rotator cuff of unspecified shoulder

  ● S46.09   Other injury of muscle(s) and tendon(s) of the rotator cuff of shoulder

    ● S46.091   Other injury of muscle(s) and tendon(s) of the rotator cuff of right shoulder

    ● S46.092   Other injury of muscle(s) and tendon(s) of the rotator cuff of left shoulder

    ● S46.099   Other injury of muscle(s) and tendon(s) of the rotator cuff of unspecified shoulder

● S46.1   Injury of muscle, fascia and tendon of long head of biceps

  ● S46.10   Unspecified injury of muscle, fascia and tendon of long head of biceps

    ● S46.101   Unspecified injury of muscle, fascia and tendon of long head of biceps, right arm

    ● S46.102   Unspecified injury of muscle, fascia and tendon of long head of biceps, left arm

    ● S46.109   Unspecified injury of muscle, fascia and tendon of long head of biceps, unspecified arm

- S46.11   Strain of muscle, fascia and tendon of long head of biceps
  - S46.111   Strain of muscle, fascia and tendon of long head of biceps, right arm
  - S46.112   Strain of muscle, fascia and tendon of long head of biceps, left arm
  - S46.119   Strain of muscle, fascia and tendon of long head of biceps, unspecified arm
- S46.12   Laceration of muscle, fascia and tendon of long head of biceps
  - S46.121   Laceration of muscle, fascia and tendon of long head of biceps, right arm
  - S46.122   Laceration of muscle, fascia and tendon of long head of biceps, left arm
  - S46.129   Laceration of muscle, fascia and tendon of long head of biceps, unspecified arm
- S46.19   Other injury of muscle, fascia and tendon of long head of biceps
  - S46.191   Other injury of muscle, fascia and tendon of long head of biceps, right arm
  - S46.192   Other injury of muscle, fascia and tendon of long head of biceps, left arm
  - S46.199   Other injury of muscle, fascia and tendon of long head of biceps, unspecified arm
- S46.2   Injury of muscle, fascia and tendon of other parts of biceps
  - S46.20   Unspecified injury of muscle, fascia and tendon of other parts of biceps
    - S46.201   Unspecified injury of muscle, fascia and tendon of other parts of biceps, right arm
    - S46.202   Unspecified injury of muscle, fascia and tendon of other parts of biceps, left arm
    - S46.209   Unspecified injury of muscle, fascia and tendon of other parts of biceps, unspecified arm
  - S46.21   Strain of muscle, fascia and tendon of other parts of biceps
    - S46.211   Strain of muscle, fascia and tendon of other parts of biceps, right arm
    - S46.212   Strain of muscle, fascia and tendon of other parts of biceps, left arm
    - S46.219   Strain of muscle, fascia and tendon of other parts of biceps, unspecified arm
  - S46.22   Laceration of muscle, fascia and tendon of other parts of biceps
    - S46.221   Laceration of muscle, fascia and tendon of other parts of biceps, right arm
    - S46.222   Laceration of muscle, fascia and tendon of other parts of biceps, left arm
    - S46.229   Laceration of muscle, fascia and tendon of other parts of biceps, unspecified arm

- S46.29   Other injury of muscle, fascia and tendon of other parts of biceps
  - S46.291   Other injury of muscle, fascia and tendon of other parts of biceps, right arm
  - S46.292   Other injury of muscle, fascia and tendon of other parts of biceps, left arm
  - S46.299   Other injury of muscle, fascia and tendon of other parts of biceps, unspecified arm
- S46.3   Injury of muscle, fascia and tendon of triceps
  - S46.30   Unspecified injury of muscle, fascia and tendon of triceps
    - S46.301   Unspecified injury of muscle, fascia and tendon of triceps, right arm
    - S46.302   Unspecified injury of muscle, fascia and tendon of triceps, left arm
    - S46.309   Unspecified injury of muscle, fascia and tendon of triceps, unspecified arm
  - S46.31   Strain of muscle, fascia and tendon of triceps
    - S46.311   Strain of muscle, fascia and tendon of triceps, right arm
    - S46.312   Strain of muscle, fascia and tendon of triceps, left arm
    - S46.319   Strain of muscle, fascia and tendon of triceps, unspecified arm
  - S46.32   Laceration of muscle, fascia and tendon of triceps
    - S46.321   Laceration of muscle, fascia and tendon of triceps, right arm
    - S46.322   Laceration of muscle, fascia and tendon of triceps, left arm
    - S46.329   Laceration of muscle, fascia and tendon of triceps, unspecified arm
  - S46.39   Other injury of muscle, fascia and tendon of triceps
    - S46.391   Other injury of muscle, fascia and tendon of triceps, right arm
    - S46.392   Other injury of muscle, fascia and tendon of triceps, left arm
    - S46.399   Other injury of muscle, fascia and tendon of triceps, unspecified arm
- S46.8   Injury of other muscles, fascia and tendons at shoulder and upper arm level
  - S46.80   Unspecified injury of other muscles, fascia and tendons at shoulder and upper arm level
    - S46.801   Unspecified injury of other muscles, fascia and tendons at shoulder and upper arm level, right arm
    - S46.802   Unspecified injury of other muscles, fascia and tendons at shoulder and upper arm level, left arm
    - S46.809   Unspecified injury of other muscles, fascia and tendons at shoulder and upper arm level, unspecified arm
  - S46.81   Strain of other muscles, fascia and tendons at shoulder and upper arm level
    - S46.811   Strain of other muscles, fascia and tendons at shoulder and upper arm level, right arm
    - S46.812   Strain of other muscles, fascia and tendons at shoulder and upper arm level, left arm
    - S46.819   Strain of other muscles, fascia and tendons at shoulder and upper arm level, unspecified arm

CHAPTER 19 (S00-T88)

CHAPTER 19 (S00-T88)

● **S46.82**   Laceration of other muscles, fascia and tendons at shoulder and upper arm level

  ● **S46.821**   Laceration of other muscles, fascia and tendons at shoulder and upper arm level, right arm

  ● **S46.822**   Laceration of other muscles, fascia and tendons at shoulder and upper arm level, left arm

  ● **S46.829**   Laceration of other muscles, fascia and tendons at shoulder and upper arm level, unspecified arm

● **S46.89**   Other injury of other muscles, fascia and tendons at shoulder and upper arm level

  ● **S46.891**   Other injury of other muscles, fascia and tendons at shoulder and upper arm level, right arm

  ● **S46.892**   Other injury of other muscles, fascia and tendons at shoulder and upper arm level, left arm

  ● **S46.899**   Other injury of other muscles, fascia and tendons at shoulder and upper arm level, unspecified arm

● **S46.9**   Injury of unspecified muscle, fascia and tendon at shoulder and upper arm level

  ● **S46.90**   Unspecified injury of unspecified muscle, fascia and tendon at shoulder and upper arm level

    ● **S46.901**   Unspecified injury of unspecified muscle, fascia and tendon at shoulder and upper arm level, right arm

    ● **S46.902**   Unspecified injury of unspecified muscle, fascia and tendon at shoulder and upper arm level, left arm

    ● **S46.909**   Unspecified injury of unspecified muscle, fascia and tendon at shoulder and upper arm level, unspecified arm

  ● **S46.91**   Strain of unspecified muscle, fascia and tendon at shoulder and upper arm level

    ● **S46.911**   Strain of unspecified muscle, fascia and tendon at shoulder and upper arm level, right arm

    ● **S46.912**   Strain of unspecified muscle, fascia and tendon at shoulder and upper arm level, left arm

    ● **S46.919**   Strain of unspecified muscle, fascia and tendon at shoulder and upper arm level, unspecified arm

  ● **S46.92**   Laceration of unspecified muscle, fascia and tendon at shoulder and upper arm level

    ● **S46.921**   Laceration of unspecified muscle, fascia and tendon at shoulder and upper arm level, right arm

    ● **S46.922**   Laceration of unspecified muscle, fascia and tendon at shoulder and upper arm level, left arm

    ● **S46.929**   Laceration of unspecified muscle, fascia and tendon at shoulder and upper arm level, unspecified arm

  ● **S46.99**   Other injury of unspecified muscle, fascia and tendon at shoulder and upper arm level

    ● **S46.991**   Other injury of unspecified muscle, fascia and tendon at shoulder and upper arm level, right arm

    ● **S46.992**   Other injury of unspecified muscle, fascia and tendon at shoulder and upper arm level, left arm

    ● **S46.999**   Other injury of unspecified muscle, fascia and tendon at shoulder and upper arm level, unspecified arm

● **S47**   Crushing injury of shoulder and upper arm

   Use additional code for all associated injuries

   Excludes2   crushing injury of elbow (S57.0-)

   The appropriate 7th character is to be added to each code from category S47

A	initial encounter
D	subsequent encounter
S	sequela

X ● **S47.1**   Crushing injury of right shoulder and upper arm

X ● **S47.2**   Crushing injury of left shoulder and upper arm

X ● **S47.9**   Crushing injury of shoulder and upper arm, unspecified arm

● **S48**   Traumatic amputation of shoulder and upper arm

   An amputation not identified as partial or complete should be coded to complete

   Excludes1   traumatic amputation at elbow level (S58.0)

   The appropriate 7th character is to be added to each code from category S48

A	initial encounter
D	subsequent encounter
S	sequela

● **S48.0**   Traumatic amputation at shoulder joint

  ● **S48.01**   Complete traumatic amputation at shoulder joint

    ● **S48.011**   Complete traumatic amputation at right shoulder joint

    ● **S48.012**   Complete traumatic amputation at left shoulder joint

    ● **S48.019**   Complete traumatic amputation at unspecified shoulder joint

  ● **S48.02**   Partial traumatic amputation at shoulder joint

    ● **S48.021**   Partial traumatic amputation at right shoulder joint

    ● **S48.022**   Partial traumatic amputation at left shoulder joint

    ● **S48.029**   Partial traumatic amputation at unspecified shoulder joint

● **S48.1**   Traumatic amputation at level between shoulder and elbow

  ● **S48.11**   Complete traumatic amputation at level between shoulder and elbow

    ● **S48.111**   Complete traumatic amputation at level between right shoulder and elbow

    ● **S48.112**   Complete traumatic amputation at level between left shoulder and elbow

    ● **S48.119**   Complete traumatic amputation at level between unspecified shoulder and elbow

  ● **S48.12**   Partial traumatic amputation at level between shoulder and elbow

    ● **S48.121**   Partial traumatic amputation at level between right shoulder and elbow

    ● **S48.122**   Partial traumatic amputation at level between left shoulder and elbow

    ● **S48.129**   Partial traumatic amputation at level between unspecified shoulder and elbow

● S48.9   Traumatic amputation of shoulder and upper arm, level unspecified
    ● S48.91   Complete traumatic amputation of shoulder and upper arm, level unspecified
       ● S48.911   Complete traumatic amputation of right shoulder and upper arm, level unspecified
       ● S48.912   Complete traumatic amputation of left shoulder and upper arm, level unspecified
       ● S48.919   Complete traumatic amputation of unspecified shoulder and upper arm, level unspecified
    ● S48.92   Partial traumatic amputation of shoulder and upper arm, level unspecified
       ● S48.921   Partial traumatic amputation of right shoulder and upper arm, level unspecified
       ● S48.922   Partial traumatic amputation of left shoulder and upper arm, level unspecified
       ● S48.929   Partial traumatic amputation of unspecified shoulder and upper arm, level unspecified

● S49   Other and unspecified injuries of shoulder and upper arm
    The appropriate 7th character is to be added to each code from subcategories S49.0 and S49.1

A	initial encounter for closed fracture
D	subsequent encounter for fracture with routine healing
G	subsequent encounter for fracture with delayed healing
K	subsequent encounter for fracture with nonunion
P	subsequent encounter for fracture with malunion
S	sequela

   ● S49.0   Physeal fracture of upper end of humerus
    ● S49.00   Unspecified physeal fracture of upper end of humerus
       ● S49.001   Unspecified physeal fracture of upper end of humerus, right arm
       ● S49.002   Unspecified physeal fracture of upper end of humerus, left arm
       ● S49.009   Unspecified physeal fracture of upper end of humerus, unspecified arm
    ● S49.01   Salter-Harris Type I physeal fracture of upper end of humerus
       ● S49.011   Salter-Harris Type I physeal fracture of upper end of humerus, right arm
       ● S49.012   Salter-Harris Type I physeal fracture of upper end of humerus, left arm
       ● S49.019   Salter-Harris Type I physeal fracture of upper end of humerus, unspecified arm
    ● S49.02   Salter-Harris Type II physeal fracture of upper end of humerus
       ● S49.021   Salter-Harris Type II physeal fracture of upper end of humerus, right arm
       ● S49.022   Salter-Harris Type II physeal fracture of upper end of humerus, left arm
       ● S49.029   Salter-Harris Type II physeal fracture of upper end of humerus, unspecified arm
    ● S49.03   Salter-Harris Type III physeal fracture of upper end of humerus
       ● S49.031   Salter-Harris Type III physeal fracture of upper end of humerus, right arm
       ● S49.032   Salter-Harris Type III physeal fracture of upper end of humerus, left arm
       ● S49.039   Salter-Harris Type III physeal fracture of upper end of humerus, unspecified arm

Item 19-3 SALTER-HARRIS TYPE 1: epiphysis is completely separated from end of bone, or metaphysic growth plate remains attached to epiphysis
   SALTER-HARRIS TYPE 2: epiphysis and growth plate are partially separated from metaphysis, which is cracked—most common type
   SALTER-HARRIS TYPE 3: fracture occurring through epiphysis and separates part of epiphysis and growth plate from metaphysis fracture, usually at distal end of tibia
   SALTER-HARRIS TYPE 4: fracture runs through epiphysis, across growth plate, into metaphysic, surgery is required to restore joint surface to normal and align growth plate

    ● S49.04   Salter-Harris Type IV physeal fracture of upper end of humerus
       ● S49.041   Salter-Harris Type IV physeal fracture of upper end of humerus, right arm
       ● S49.042   Salter-Harris Type IV physeal fracture of upper end of humerus, left arm
       ● S49.049   Salter-Harris Type IV physeal fracture of upper end of humerus, unspecified arm
    ● S49.09   Other physeal fracture of upper end of humerus
       ● S49.091   Other physeal fracture of upper end of humerus, right arm
       ● S49.092   Other physeal fracture of upper end of humerus, left arm
       ● S49.099   Other physeal fracture of upper end of humerus, unspecified arm
   ● S49.1   Physeal fracture of lower end of humerus
    ● S49.10   Unspecified physeal fracture of lower end of humerus
       ● S49.101   Unspecified physeal fracture of lower end of humerus, right arm
       ● S49.102   Unspecified physeal fracture of lower end of humerus, left arm
       ● S49.109   Unspecified physeal fracture of lower end of humerus, unspecified arm
    ● S49.11   Salter-Harris Type I physeal fracture of lower end of humerus
       ● S49.111   Salter-Harris Type I physeal fracture of lower end of humerus, right arm
       ● S49.112   Salter-Harris Type I physeal fracture of lower end of humerus, left arm
       ● S49.119   Salter-Harris Type I physeal fracture of lower end of humerus, unspecified arm
    ● S49.12   Salter-Harris Type II physeal fracture of lower end of humerus
       ● S49.121   Salter-Harris Type II physeal fracture of lower end of humerus, right arm
       ● S49.122   Salter-Harris Type II physeal fracture of lower end of humerus, left arm
       ● S49.129   Salter-Harris Type II physeal fracture of lower end of humerus, unspecified arm
    ● S49.13   Salter-Harris Type III physeal fracture of lower end of humerus ◀
       ● S49.131   Salter-Harris Type III physeal fracture of lower end of humerus, right arm
       ● S49.132   Salter-Harris Type III physeal fracture of lower end of humerus, left arm
       ● S49.139   Salter-Harris Type III physeal fracture of lower end of humerus, unspecified arm

CHAPTER 19 (S00-T88)

● **S49.14**   **Salter-Harris Type IV physeal fracture of lower end of humerus**
    ● S49.141   Salter-Harris Type IV physeal fracture of lower end of humerus, right arm
    ● S49.142   Salter-Harris Type IV physeal fracture of lower end of humerus, left arm
    ● S49.149   Salter-Harris Type IV physeal fracture of lower end of humerus, unspecified arm

● **S49.19**   **Other physeal fracture of lower end of humerus**
    ● S49.191   Other physeal fracture of lower end of humerus, right arm
    ● S49.192   Other physeal fracture of lower end of humerus, left arm
    ● S49.199   Other physeal fracture of lower end of humerus, unspecified arm

● **S49.8**   **Other specified injuries of shoulder and upper arm**

The appropriate 7th character is to be added to each code in subcategory S49.8

A	initial encounter
D	subsequent encounter
S	sequela

X ● **S49.80**   Other specified injuries of shoulder and upper arm, unspecified arm
X ● **S49.81**   Other specified injuries of right shoulder and upper arm
X ● **S49.82**   Other specified injuries of left shoulder and upper arm

● **S49.9**   **Unspecified injury of shoulder and upper arm**

The appropriate 7th character is to be added to each code in subcategory S49.9

A	initial encounter
D	subsequent encounter
S	sequela

X ● **S49.90**   Unspecified injury of shoulder and upper arm, unspecified arm
X ● **S49.91**   Unspecified injury of right shoulder and upper arm
X ● **S49.92**   Unspecified injury of left shoulder and upper arm

INJURIES TO THE ELBOW AND FOREARM (S50-S59)

Excludes2   burns and corrosions (T20-T32)
       frostbite (T33-T34)
       injuries of wrist and hand (S60-S69)
       insect bite or sting, venomous (T63.4)

● **S50**   **Superficial injury of elbow and forearm**

Excludes2   superficial injury of wrist and hand (S60.-)

The appropriate 7th character is to be added to each code from category S50

A	initial encounter
D	subsequent encounter
S	sequela

● **S50.0**   **Contusion of elbow**
X ● **S50.00**   Contusion of unspecified elbow
X ● **S50.01**   Contusion of right elbow
X ● **S50.02**   Contusion of left elbow

● **S50.1**   **Contusion of forearm**
X ● **S50.10**   Contusion of unspecified forearm
X ● **S50.11**   Contusion of right forearm
X ● **S50.12**   Contusion of left forearm

● **S50.3**   **Other superficial injuries of elbow**
   ● **S50.31**   **Abrasion of elbow**
      ● S50.311   Abrasion of right elbow
      ● S50.312   Abrasion of left elbow
      ● S50.319   Abrasion of unspecified elbow
   ● **S50.32**   **Blister (nonthermal) of elbow**
      ● S50.321   Blister (nonthermal) of right elbow
      ● S50.322   Blister (nonthermal) of left elbow
      ● S50.329   Blister (nonthermal) of unspecified elbow
   ● **S50.34**   **External constriction of elbow**
      ● S50.341   External constriction of right elbow
      ● S50.342   External constriction of left elbow
      ● S50.349   External constriction of unspecified elbow
   ● **S50.35**   **Superficial foreign body of elbow**
      Splinter in the elbow
      ● S50.351   Superficial foreign body of right elbow
      ● S50.352   Superficial foreign body of left elbow
      ● S50.359   Superficial foreign body of unspecified elbow
   ● **S50.36**   **Insect bite (nonvenomous) of elbow**
      ● S50.361   Insect bite (nonvenomous) of right elbow
      ● S50.362   Insect bite (nonvenomous) of left elbow
      ● S50.369   Insect bite (nonvenomous) of unspecified elbow
   ● **S50.37**   **Other superficial bite of elbow**
      Excludes1   open bite of elbow (S51.04)
      ● S50.371   Other superficial bite of right elbow
      ● S50.372   Other superficial bite of left elbow
      ● S50.379   Other superficial bite of unspecified elbow

● **S50.8**   **Other superficial injuries of forearm**
   ● **S50.81**   **Abrasion of forearm**
      ● S50.811   Abrasion of right forearm
      ● S50.812   Abrasion of left forearm
      ● S50.819   Abrasion of unspecified forearm
   ● **S50.82**   **Blister (nonthermal) of forearm**
      ● S50.821   Blister (nonthermal) of right forearm
      ● S50.822   Blister (nonthermal) of left forearm
      ● S50.829   Blister (nonthermal) of unspecified forearm
   ● **S50.84**   **External constriction of forearm**
      ● S50.841   External constriction of right forearm
      ● S50.842   External constriction of left forearm
      ● S50.849   External constriction of unspecified forearm
   ● **S50.85**   **Superficial foreign body of forearm**
      Splinter in the forearm
      ● S50.851   Superficial foreign body of right forearm
      ● S50.852   Superficial foreign body of left forearm
      ● S50.859   Superficial foreign body of unspecified forearm
   ● **S50.86**   **Insect bite (nonvenomous) of forearm**
      ● S50.861   Insect bite (nonvenomous) of right forearm
      ● S50.862   Insect bite (nonvenomous) of left forearm
      ● S50.869   Insect bite (nonvenomous) of unspecified forearm

◀ New   ◀◖ Revised   ~~deleted~~ Deleted   Excludes 1   Excludes 2   Includes   Use additional   Code first   Code also   Unspecified

OGCR Official Guidelines   X Assign placeholder X   ● Use Additional Character(s)   ▶ Manifestation Code   **Coding Clinic**

1250

- S50.87   Other superficial bite of forearm
  - **Excludes1**   open bite of forearm (S51.84)
  - S50.871   Other superficial bite of right forearm
  - S50.872   Other superficial bite of left forearm
  - S50.879   Other superficial bite of unspecified forearm
- S50.9   Unspecified superficial injury of elbow and forearm
  - S50.90   Unspecified superficial injury of elbow
    - S50.901   Unspecified superficial injury of right elbow
    - S50.902   Unspecified superficial injury of left elbow
    - S50.909   Unspecified superficial injury of unspecified elbow
  - S50.91   Unspecified superficial injury of forearm
    - S50.911   Unspecified superficial injury of right forearm
    - S50.912   Unspecified superficial injury of left forearm
    - S50.919   Unspecified superficial injury of unspecified forearm
- S51   Open wound of elbow and forearm
  - Code also any associated wound infection
  - **Excludes1**   open fracture of elbow and forearm (S52.- with open fracture 7th character)
    - traumatic amputation of elbow and forearm (S58.-)
  - **Excludes2**   open wound of wrist and hand (S61.-)
  - The appropriate 7th character is to be added to each code from category S51

    | A | initial encounter |
    | D | subsequent encounter |
    | S | sequela |

  - S51.0   Open wound of elbow
    - S51.00   Unspecified open wound of elbow
      - S51.001   Unspecified open wound of right elbow
        - **Coding Clinic: 2012, Q4, P108**
      - S51.002   Unspecified open wound of left elbow
      - S51.009   Unspecified open wound of unspecified elbow
        - Open wound of elbow NOS
    - S51.01   Laceration without foreign body of elbow
      - S51.011   Laceration without foreign body of right elbow
      - S51.012   Laceration without foreign body of left elbow
      - S51.019   Laceration without foreign body of unspecified elbow
    - S51.02   Laceration with foreign body of elbow
      - S51.021   Laceration with foreign body of right elbow
      - S51.022   Laceration with foreign body of left elbow
      - S51.029   Laceration with foreign body of unspecified elbow
    - S51.03   Puncture wound without foreign body of elbow
      - S51.031   Puncture wound without foreign body of right elbow
      - S51.032   Puncture wound without foreign body of left elbow
      - S51.039   Puncture wound without foreign body of unspecified elbow

- S51.04   Puncture wound with foreign body of elbow
  - S51.041   Puncture wound with foreign body of right elbow
  - S51.042   Puncture wound with foreign body of left elbow
  - S51.049   Puncture wound with foreign body of unspecified elbow
- S51.05   Open bite of elbow
  - Bite of elbow NOS
  - **Excludes1**   superficial bite of elbow (S50.36, S50.37)
  - S51.051   Open bite, right elbow
  - S51.052   Open bite, left elbow
  - S51.059   Open bite, unspecified elbow
- S51.8   Open wound of forearm
  - **Excludes2**   open wound of elbow (S51.0-)
  - S51.80   Unspecified open wound of forearm
    - S51.801   Unspecified open wound of right forearm
    - S51.802   Unspecified open wound of left forearm
    - S51.809   Unspecified open wound of unspecified forearm
      - Open wound of forearm NOS
  - S51.81   Laceration without foreign body of forearm
    - S51.811   Laceration without foreign body of right forearm
    - S51.812   Laceration without foreign body of left forearm
    - S51.819   Laceration without foreign body of unspecified forearm
  - S51.82   Laceration with foreign body of forearm
    - S51.821   Laceration with foreign body of right forearm
    - S51.822   Laceration with foreign body of left forearm
    - S51.829   Laceration with foreign body of unspecified forearm
  - S51.83   Puncture wound without foreign body of forearm
    - S51.831   Puncture wound without foreign body of right forearm
    - S51.832   Puncture wound without foreign body of left forearm
    - S51.839   Puncture wound without foreign body of unspecified forearm
  - S51.84   Puncture wound with foreign body of forearm
    - S51.841   Puncture wound with foreign body of right forearm
    - S51.842   Puncture wound with foreign body of left forearm
    - S51.849   Puncture wound with foreign body of unspecified forearm
  - S51.85   Open bite of forearm
    - Bite of forearm NOS
    - **Excludes1**   superficial bite of forearm (S50.86, S50.87)
    - S51.851   Open bite of right forearm
    - S51.852   Open bite of left forearm
    - S51.859   Open bite of unspecified forearm

● **S52   Fracture of forearm**

Note: A fracture not identified as displaced or nondisplaced should be coded to displaced

A fracture not designated as open or closed should be coded to closed

The open fracture designations are based on the Gustilo open fracture classification

Excludes1   traumatic amputation of forearm (S58.-)

Excludes2   fracture at wrist and hand level (S62.-)

The appropriate 7th character is to be added to all codes from category S52

A	initial encounter for closed fracture
B	initial encounter for open fracture type I or II
	initial encounter for open fracture NOS
C	initial encounter for open fracture type IIIA, IIIB, or IIIC
D	subsequent encounter for closed fracture with routine healing
E	subsequent encounter for open fracture type I or II with routine healing
F	subsequent encounter for open fracture type IIIA, IIIB, or IIIC with routine healing
G	subsequent encounter for closed fracture with delayed healing
H	subsequent encounter for open fracture type I or II with delayed healing
J	subsequent encounter for open fracture type IIIA, IIIB, or IIIC with delayed healing
K	subsequent encounter for closed fracture with nonunion
M	subsequent encounter for open fracture type I or II with nonunion
N	subsequent encounter for open fracture type IIIA, IIIB, or IIIC with nonunion
P	subsequent encounter for closed fracture with malunion
Q	subsequent encounter for open fracture type I or II with malunion
R	subsequent encounter for open fracture type IIIA, IIIB, or IIIC with malunion
S	sequela

Coding Clinic: 2016, Q1, P33

● **S52.0   Fracture of upper end of ulna**
Fracture of proximal end of ulna

Excludes2   fracture of elbow NOS (S42.40-)
fractures of shaft of ulna (S52.2-)

● **S52.00   Unspecified fracture of upper end of ulna**

● S52.001   **Unspecified** fracture of upper end of right ulna

● S52.002   **Unspecified** fracture of upper end of left ulna

● S52.009   **Unspecified** fracture of upper end of unspecified ulna

● **S52.01   Torus fracture of upper end of ulna**

The appropriate 7th character is to be added to all codes in subcategory S52.01

A	initial encounter for closed fracture
D	subsequent encounter for fracture with routine healing
G	subsequent encounter for fracture with delayed healing
K	subsequent encounter for fracture with nonunion
P	subsequent encounter for fracture with malunion
S	sequela

● S52.011   Torus fracture of upper end of right ulna

● S52.012   Torus fracture of upper end of left ulna

● S52.019   Torus fracture of upper end of **unspecified** ulna

● **S52.02   Fracture of olecranon process without intraarticular extension of ulna**

● S52.021   Displaced fracture of olecranon process without intraarticular extension of right ulna

● S52.022   Displaced fracture of olecranon process without intraarticular extension of left ulna

● S52.023   Displaced fracture of olecranon process without intraarticular extension of **unspecified** ulna

● S52.024   Nondisplaced fracture of olecranon process without intraarticular extension of right ulna

● S52.025   Nondisplaced fracture of olecranon process without intraarticular extension of left ulna

● S52.026   Nondisplaced fracture of olecranon process without intraarticular extension of **unspecified** ulna

● **S52.03   Fracture of olecranon process with intraarticular extension of ulna**

● S52.031   Displaced fracture of olecranon process with intraarticular extension of right ulna

● S52.032   Displaced fracture of olecranon process with intraarticular extension of left ulna

● S52.033   Displaced fracture of olecranon process with intraarticular extension of **unspecified** ulna

● S52.034   Nondisplaced fracture of olecranon process with intraarticular extension of right ulna

● S52.035   Nondisplaced fracture of olecranon process with intraarticular extension of left ulna

● S52.036   Nondisplaced fracture of olecranon process with intraarticular extension of **unspecified** ulna

● **S52.04   Fracture of coronoid process of ulna**

● S52.041   Displaced fracture of coronoid process of right ulna

● S52.042   Displaced fracture of coronoid process of left ulna

● S52.043   Displaced fracture of coronoid process of **unspecified** ulna

● S52.044   Nondisplaced fracture of coronoid process of right ulna

● S52.045   Nondisplaced fracture of coronoid process of left ulna

● S52.046   Nondisplaced fracture of coronoid process of **unspecified** ulna

● **S52.09   Other fracture of upper end of ulna**

● S52.091   Other fracture of upper end of right ulna

● S52.092   Other fracture of upper end of left ulna

● S52.099   Other fracture of upper end of **unspecified** ulna

● **S52.1   Fracture of upper end of radius**
Fracture of proximal end of radius

Excludes2   physeal fractures of upper end of radius (S59.2-)
fracture of shaft of radius (S52.3-)

● **S52.10   Unspecified fracture of upper end of radius**

● S52.101   **Unspecified** fracture of upper end of right radius

● S52.102   **Unspecified** fracture of upper end of left radius

● S52.109   **Unspecified** fracture of upper end of unspecified radius

● **S52.11 Torus fracture of upper end of radius**

The appropriate 7th character is to be added to all codes in subcategory S52.11

A	initial encounter for closed fracture
D	subsequent encounter for fracture with routine healing
G	subsequent encounter for fracture with delayed healing
K	subsequent encounter for fracture with nonunion
P	subsequent encounter for fracture with malunion
S	sequela

  ● **S52.111 Torus fracture of upper end of right radius**

  ● **S52.112 Torus fracture of upper end of left radius**

  ● **S52.119 Torus fracture of upper end of unspecified radius**

● **S52.12 Fracture of head of radius**

  ● **S52.121 Displaced fracture of head of right radius**

  ● **S52.122 Displaced fracture of head of left radius**

  ● **S52.123 Displaced fracture of head of unspecified radius**

  ● **S52.124 Nondisplaced fracture of head of right radius**

  ● **S52.125 Nondisplaced fracture of head of left radius**

  ● **S52.126 Nondisplaced fracture of head of unspecified radius**

● **S52.13 Fracture of neck of radius**

  ● **S52.131 Displaced fracture of neck of right radius**

  ● **S52.132 Displaced fracture of neck of left radius**

  ● **S52.133 Displaced fracture of neck of unspecified radius**

  ● **S52.134 Nondisplaced fracture of neck of right radius**

  ● **S52.135 Nondisplaced fracture of neck of left radius**

  ● **S52.136 Nondisplaced fracture of neck of unspecified radius**

● **S52.18 Other fracture of upper end of radius**

  ● **S52.181 Other fracture of upper end of right radius**

  ● **S52.182 Other fracture of upper end of left radius**

  ● **S52.189 Other fracture of upper end of unspecified radius**

● **S52.2 Fracture of shaft of ulna**

  ● **S52.20 Unspecified fracture of shaft of ulna**
      Fracture of ulna NOS

    ● **S52.201 Unspecified fracture of shaft of right ulna**

    ● **S52.202 Unspecified fracture of shaft of left ulna**

    ● **S52.209 Unspecified fracture of shaft of unspecified ulna**

● **S52.21 Greenstick fracture of shaft of ulna**

The appropriate 7th character is to be added to all codes in subcategory S52.21

A	initial encounter for closed fracture
D	subsequent encounter for fracture with routine healing
G	subsequent encounter for fracture with delayed healing
K	subsequent encounter for fracture with nonunion
P	subsequent encounter for fracture with malunion
S	sequela

  ● **S52.211 Greenstick fracture of shaft of right ulna**

  ● **S52.212 Greenstick fracture of shaft of left ulna**

  ● **S52.219 Greenstick fracture of shaft of unspecified ulna**

● **S52.22 Transverse fracture of shaft of ulna**

  ● **S52.221 Displaced transverse fracture of shaft of right ulna**

  ● **S52.222 Displaced transverse fracture of shaft of left ulna**

  ● **S52.223 Displaced transverse fracture of shaft of unspecified ulna**

  ● **S52.224 Nondisplaced transverse fracture of shaft of right ulna**

  ● **S52.225 Nondisplaced transverse fracture of shaft of left ulna**

  ● **S52.226 Nondisplaced transverse fracture of shaft of unspecified ulna**

● **S52.23 Oblique fracture of shaft of ulna**

  ● **S52.231 Displaced oblique fracture of shaft of right ulna**

  ● **S52.232 Displaced oblique fracture of shaft of left ulna**

  ● **S52.233 Displaced oblique fracture of shaft of unspecified ulna**

  ● **S52.234 Nondisplaced oblique fracture of shaft of right ulna**

  ● **S52.235 Nondisplaced oblique fracture of shaft of left ulna**

  ● **S52.236 Nondisplaced oblique fracture of shaft of unspecified ulna**

● **S52.24 Spiral fracture of shaft of ulna**

  ● **S52.241 Displaced spiral fracture of shaft of ulna, right arm**

  ● **S52.242 Displaced spiral fracture of shaft of ulna, left arm**

  ● **S52.243 Displaced spiral fracture of shaft of ulna, unspecified arm**

  ● **S52.244 Nondisplaced spiral fracture of shaft of ulna, right arm**

  ● **S52.245 Nondisplaced spiral fracture of shaft of ulna, left arm**

  ● **S52.246 Nondisplaced spiral fracture of shaft of ulna, unspecified arm**

● **S52.25 Comminuted fracture of shaft of ulna**

  ● **S52.251 Displaced comminuted fracture of shaft of ulna, right arm**

  ● **S52.252 Displaced comminuted fracture of shaft of ulna, left arm**

  ● **S52.253 Displaced comminuted fracture of shaft of ulna, unspecified arm**

CHAPTER 19 (SØØ-T88)

● S52.254   Nondisplaced comminuted fracture of shaft of ulna, right arm

● S52.255   Nondisplaced comminuted fracture of shaft of ulna, left arm

● S52.256   Nondisplaced comminuted fracture of shaft of ulna, unspecified arm

● S52.26   Segmental fracture of shaft of ulna

  ● S52.261   Displaced segmental fracture of shaft of ulna, right arm

  ● S52.262   Displaced segmental fracture of shaft of ulna, left arm

  ● S52.263   Displaced segmental fracture of shaft of ulna, unspecified arm

  ● S52.264   Nondisplaced segmental fracture of shaft of ulna, right arm

  ● S52.265   Nondisplaced segmental fracture of shaft of ulna, left arm

  ● S52.266   Nondisplaced segmental fracture of shaft of ulna, unspecified arm

● S52.27   Monteggia's fracture of ulna
     Fracture of upper shaft of ulna with dislocation of radial head

  ● S52.271   Monteggia's fracture of right ulna

  ● S52.272   Monteggia's fracture of left ulna

  ● S52.279   Monteggia's fracture of unspecified ulna

● S52.28   Bent bone of ulna

  ● S52.281   Bent bone of right ulna

  ● S52.282   Bent bone of left ulna

  ● S52.283   Bent bone of unspecified ulna

● S52.29   Other fracture of shaft of ulna

  ● S52.291   Other fracture of shaft of right ulna

  ● S52.292   Other fracture of shaft of left ulna

  ● S52.299   Other fracture of shaft of unspecified ulna

● S52.3   Fracture of shaft of radius

 ● S52.30   Unspecified fracture of shaft of radius

  ● S52.301   Unspecified fracture of shaft of right radius

  ● S52.302   Unspecified fracture of shaft of left radius

  ● S52.309   Unspecified fracture of shaft of unspecified radius

 ● S52.31   Greenstick fracture of shaft of radius
     The appropriate 7th character is to be added to all codes in subcategory S52.31

> | | |
> |---|---|
> | A | initial encounter for closed fracture |
> | D | subsequent encounter for fracture with routine healing |
> | G | subsequent encounter for fracture with delayed healing |
> | K | subsequent encounter for fracture with nonunion |
> | P | subsequent encounter for fracture with malunion |
> | S | sequela |

  ● S52.311   Greenstick fracture of shaft of radius, right arm

  ● S52.312   Greenstick fracture of shaft of radius, left arm

  ● S52.319   Greenstick fracture of shaft of radius, unspecified arm

● S52.32   Transverse fracture of shaft of radius

  ● S52.321   Displaced transverse fracture of shaft of right radius

  ● S52.322   Displaced transverse fracture of shaft of left radius

  ● S52.323   Displaced transverse fracture of shaft of unspecified radius

  ● S52.324   Nondisplaced transverse fracture of shaft of right radius

  ● S52.325   Nondisplaced transverse fracture of shaft of left radius

  ● S52.326   Nondisplaced transverse fracture of shaft of unspecified radius

● S52.33   Oblique fracture of shaft of radius

  ● S52.331   Displaced oblique fracture of shaft of right radius

  ● S52.332   Displaced oblique fracture of shaft of left radius

  ● S52.333   Displaced oblique fracture of shaft of unspecified radius

  ● S52.334   Nondisplaced oblique fracture of shaft of right radius

  ● S52.335   Nondisplaced oblique fracture of shaft of left radius

  ● S52.336   Nondisplaced oblique fracture of shaft of unspecified radius

● S52.34   Spiral fracture of shaft of radius

  ● S52.341   Displaced spiral fracture of shaft of radius, right arm

  ● S52.342   Displaced spiral fracture of shaft of radius, left arm

  ● S52.343   Displaced spiral fracture of shaft of radius, unspecified arm

  ● S52.344   Nondisplaced spiral fracture of shaft of radius, right arm

  ● S52.345   Nondisplaced spiral fracture of shaft of radius, left arm

  ● S52.346   Nondisplaced spiral fracture of shaft of radius, unspecified arm

● S52.35   Comminuted fracture of shaft of radius

  ● S52.351   Displaced comminuted fracture of shaft of radius, right arm

  ● S52.352   Displaced comminuted fracture of shaft of radius, left arm

  ● S52.353   Displaced comminuted fracture of shaft of radius, unspecified arm

  ● S52.354   Nondisplaced comminuted fracture of shaft of radius, right arm

  ● S52.355   Nondisplaced comminuted fracture of shaft of radius, left arm

  ● S52.356   Nondisplaced comminuted fracture of shaft of radius, unspecified arm

● S52.36   Segmental fracture of shaft of radius

  ● S52.361   Displaced segmental fracture of shaft of radius, right arm

  ● S52.362   Displaced segmental fracture of shaft of radius, left arm

  ● S52.363   Displaced segmental fracture of shaft of radius, unspecified arm

  ● S52.364   Nondisplaced segmental fracture of shaft of radius, right arm

  ● S52.365   Nondisplaced segmental fracture of shaft of radius, left arm

  ● S52.366   Nondisplaced segmental fracture of shaft of radius, unspecified arm

- ● S52.37   Galeazzi's fracture
  - Fracture of lower shaft of radius with radioulnar joint dislocation
  - ● S52.371   Galeazzi's fracture of right radius
  - ● S52.372   Galeazzi's fracture of left radius
  - ● S52.379   Galeazzi's fracture of unspecified radius
- ● S52.38   Bent bone of radius
  - ● S52.381   Bent bone of right radius
  - ● S52.382   Bent bone of left radius
  - ● S52.389   Bent bone of unspecified radius
- ● S52.39   Other fracture of shaft of radius
  - ● S52.391   Other fracture of shaft of radius, right arm
  - ● S52.392   Other fracture of shaft of radius, left arm
  - ● S52.399   Other fracture of shaft of radius, unspecified arm
- ● S52.5   Fracture of lower end of radius
  - Fracture of distal end of radius
  - **Excludes2**   physeal fractures of lower end of radius (S59.2-)
  - ● S52.50   Unspecified fracture of the lower end of radius
    - ● S52.501   Unspecified fracture of the lower end of right radius
    - ● S52.502   Unspecified fracture of the lower end of left radius
    - ● S52.509   Unspecified fracture of the lower end of unspecified radius
  - ● S52.51   Fracture of radial styloid process
    - ● S52.511   Displaced fracture of right radial styloid process
    - ● S52.512   Displaced fracture of left radial styloid process
    - ● S52.513   Displaced fracture of unspecified radial styloid process
    - ● S52.514   Nondisplaced fracture of right radial styloid process
    - ● S52.515   Nondisplaced fracture of left radial styloid process
    - ● S52.516   Nondisplaced fracture of unspecified radial styloid process
  - ● S52.52   Torus fracture of lower end of radius
    - The appropriate 7th character is to be added to all codes in subcategory S52.52

A	initial encounter for closed fracture
D	subsequent encounter for fracture with routine healing
G	subsequent encounter for fracture with delayed healing
K	subsequent encounter for fracture with nonunion
P	subsequent encounter for fracture with malunion
S	sequela

  - ● S52.521   Torus fracture of lower end of right radius
  - ● S52.522   Torus fracture of lower end of left radius
  - ● S52.529   Torus fracture of lower end of unspecified radius

- ● S52.53   Colles' fracture
  - ● S52.531   Colles' fracture of right radius
  - ● S52.532   Colles' fracture of left radius
    - **Coding Clinic: 2016, Q2, P5**
  - ● S52.539   Colles' fracture of unspecified radius
- ● S52.54   Smith's fracture
  - ● S52.541   Smith's fracture of right radius
  - ● S52.542   Smith's fracture of left radius
  - ● S52.549   Smith's fracture of unspecified radius
- ● S52.55   Other extraarticular fracture of lower end of radius
  - ● S52.551   Other extraarticular fracture of lower end of right radius
  - ● S52.552   Other extraarticular fracture of lower end of left radius
  - ● S52.559   Other extraarticular fracture of lower end of unspecified radius
- ● S52.56   Barton's fracture
  - ● S52.561   Barton's fracture of right radius
  - ● S52.562   Barton's fracture of left radius
  - ● S52.569   Barton's fracture of unspecified radius
- ● S52.57   Other intraarticular fracture of lower end of radius
  - ● S52.571   Other intraarticular fracture of lower end of right radius
  - ● S52.572   Other intraarticular fracture of lower end of left radius
  - ● S52.579   Other intraarticular fracture of lower end of unspecified radius
- ● S52.59   Other fractures of lower end of radius
  - ● S52.591   Other fractures of lower end of right radius
  - ● S52.592   Other fractures of lower end of left radius
  - ● S52.599   Other fractures of lower end of unspecified radius
- ● S52.6   Fracture of lower end of ulna
  - ● S52.60   Unspecified fracture of lower end of ulna
    - ● S52.601   Unspecified fracture of lower end of right ulna
    - ● S52.602   Unspecified fracture of lower end of left ulna
    - ● S52.609   Unspecified fracture of lower end of unspecified ulna
  - ● S52.61   Fracture of ulna styloid process
    - ● S52.611   Displaced fracture of right ulna styloid process
    - ● S52.612   Displaced fracture of left ulna styloid process
    - ● S52.613   Displaced fracture of unspecified ulna styloid process
    - ● S52.614   Nondisplaced fracture of right ulna styloid process
    - ● S52.615   Nondisplaced fracture of left ulna styloid process
    - ● S52.616   Nondisplaced fracture of unspecified ulna styloid process

CHAPTER 19 (S00-T88)

CHAPTER 19 (S00–T88)

● **S52.62**   **Torus fracture of lower end of ulna**

> The appropriate 7th character is to be added to all codes in subcategory S52.62

> | | |
> |---|---|
> | A | initial encounter for closed fracture |
> | D | subsequent encounter for fracture with routine healing |
> | G | subsequent encounter for fracture with delayed healing |
> | K | subsequent encounter for fracture with nonunion |
> | P | subsequent encounter for fracture with malunion |
> | S | sequela |

> ● S52.621   **Torus fracture of lower end of right ulna**
>
> ● S52.622   **Torus fracture of lower end of left ulna**
>
> ● S52.629   **Torus fracture of lower end of unspecified ulna**

● **S52.69**   **Other fracture of lower end of ulna**

> ● S52.691   **Other fracture of lower end of right ulna**
>
> ● S52.692   **Other fracture of lower end of left ulna**
>
> ● S52.699   **Other fracture of lower end of unspecified ulna**

● **S52.9**   **Unspecified fracture of forearm**

> X ● S52.90   **Unspecified fracture of unspecified forearm**
>
> X ● S52.91   **Unspecified fracture of right forearm**
>
> X ● S52.92   **Unspecified fracture of left forearm**

● **S53**   **Dislocation and sprain of joints and ligaments of elbow**

> **Includes**   avulsion of joint or ligament of elbow
> laceration of cartilage, joint or ligament of elbow
> sprain of cartilage, joint or ligament of elbow
> traumatic hemarthrosis of joint or ligament of elbow
> traumatic rupture of joint or ligament of elbow
> traumatic subluxation of joint or ligament of elbow
> traumatic tear of joint or ligament of elbow

> Code also any associated open wound

> **Excludes2**   strain of muscle, fascia and tendon at forearm level (S56.-)

> The appropriate 7th character is to be added to each code from category S53

> | | |
> |---|---|
> | A | initial encounter |
> | D | subsequent encounter |
> | S | sequela |

● **S53.0**   **Subluxation and dislocation of radial head**

> Dislocation of radiohumeral joint
> Subluxation of radiohumeral joint

> **Excludes1**   Monteggia's fracture-dislocation (S52.27-)

> ● S53.00   **Unspecified subluxation and dislocation of radial head**
>
> > ● S53.001   **Unspecified subluxation of right radial head**
> >
> > ● S53.002   **Unspecified subluxation of left radial head**
> >
> > ● S53.003   **Unspecified subluxation of unspecified radial head**
> >
> > ● S53.004   **Unspecified dislocation of right radial head**
> >
> > ● S53.005   **Unspecified dislocation of left radial head**
> >
> > ● S53.006   **Unspecified dislocation of unspecified radial head**

● **S53.01**   **Anterior subluxation and dislocation of radial head**

> Anteriomedial subluxation and dislocation of radial head

> ● S53.011   **Anterior subluxation of right radial head**
>
> ● S53.012   **Anterior subluxation of left radial head**
>
> ● S53.013   **Anterior subluxation of unspecified radial head**
>
> ● S53.014   **Anterior dislocation of right radial head**
>
> ● S53.015   **Anterior dislocation of left radial head**
>
> ● S53.016   **Anterior dislocation of unspecified radial head**

● **S53.02**   **Posterior subluxation and dislocation of radial head**

> Posteriolateral subluxation and dislocation of radial head

> ● S53.021   **Posterior subluxation of right radial head**
>
> ● S53.022   **Posterior subluxation of left radial head**
>
> ● S53.023   **Posterior subluxation of unspecified radial head**
>
> ● S53.024   **Posterior dislocation of right radial head**
>
> ● S53.025   **Posterior dislocation of left radial head**
>
> ● S53.026   **Posterior dislocation of unspecified radial head**

● **S53.03**   **Nursemaid's elbow**

> ● S53.031   **Nursemaid's elbow, right elbow**
> > **Coding Clinic: 2015, Q1, P7-8**
>
> ● S53.032   **Nursemaid's elbow, left elbow**
>
> ● S53.033   **Nursemaid's elbow, unspecified elbow**

● **S53.09**   **Other subluxation and dislocation of radial head**

> ● S53.091   **Other subluxation of right radial head**
>
> ● S53.092   **Other subluxation of left radial head**
>
> ● S53.093   **Other subluxation of unspecified radial head**
>
> ● S53.094   **Other dislocation of right radial head**
>
> ● S53.095   **Other dislocation of left radial head**
>
> ● S53.096   **Other dislocation of unspecified radial head**

● **S53.1**   **Subluxation and dislocation of ulnohumeral joint**

> Subluxation and dislocation of elbow NOS

> **Excludes1**   dislocation of radial head alone (S53.0-)

> ● S53.10   **Unspecified subluxation and dislocation of ulnohumeral joint**
>
> > ● S53.101   **Unspecified subluxation of right ulnohumeral joint**
> >
> > ● S53.102   **Unspecified subluxation of left ulnohumeral joint**
> >
> > ● S53.103   **Unspecified subluxation of unspecified ulnohumeral joint**
> >
> > ● S53.104   **Unspecified dislocation of right ulnohumeral joint**
> >
> > ● S53.105   **Unspecified dislocation of left ulnohumeral joint**
> >
> > ● S53.106   **Unspecified dislocation of unspecified ulnohumeral joint**

● S53.11   Anterior subluxation and dislocation of ulnohumeral joint

  ● S53.111   Anterior subluxation of right ulnohumeral joint

  ● S53.112   Anterior subluxation of left ulnohumeral joint

  ● S53.113   Anterior subluxation of `unspecified` ulnohumeral joint

  ● S53.114   Anterior dislocation of right ulnohumeral joint
            Coding Clinic: 2012, Q4, P108

  ● S53.115   Anterior dislocation of left ulnohumeral joint

  ● S53.116   Anterior dislocation of `unspecified` ulnohumeral joint

● S53.12   Posterior subluxation and dislocation of ulnohumeral joint

  ● S53.121   Posterior subluxation of right ulnohumeral joint

  ● S53.122   Posterior subluxation of left ulnohumeral joint

  ● S53.123   Posterior subluxation of `unspecified` ulnohumeral joint

  ● S53.124   Posterior dislocation of right ulnohumeral joint

  ● S53.125   Posterior dislocation of left ulnohumeral joint

  ● S53.126   Posterior dislocation of `unspecified` ulnohumeral joint

● S53.13   Medial subluxation and dislocation of ulnohumeral joint

  ● S53.131   Medial subluxation of right ulnohumeral joint

  ● S53.132   Medial subluxation of left ulnohumeral joint

  ● S53.133   Medial subluxation of `unspecified` ulnohumeral joint

  ● S53.134   Medial dislocation of right ulnohumeral joint

  ● S53.135   Medial dislocation of left ulnohumeral joint

  ● S53.136   Medial dislocation of `unspecified` ulnohumeral joint

● S53.14   Lateral subluxation and dislocation of ulnohumeral joint

  ● S53.141   Lateral subluxation of right ulnohumeral joint

  ● S53.142   Lateral subluxation of left ulnohumeral joint

  ● S53.143   Lateral subluxation of `unspecified` ulnohumeral joint

  ● S53.144   Lateral dislocation of right ulnohumeral joint

  ● S53.145   Lateral dislocation of left ulnohumeral joint

  ● S53.146   Lateral dislocation of `unspecified` ulnohumeral joint

● S53.19   Other subluxation and dislocation of ulnohumeral joint

  ● S53.191   Other subluxation of right ulnohumeral joint

  ● S53.192   Other subluxation of left ulnohumeral joint

  ● S53.193   Other subluxation of `unspecified` ulnohumeral joint

  ● S53.194   Other dislocation of right ulnohumeral joint

  ● S53.195   Other dislocation of left ulnohumeral joint

  ● S53.196   Other dislocation of `unspecified` ulnohumeral joint

● S53.2   Traumatic rupture of radial collateral ligament
     Excludes1   sprain of radial collateral ligament NOS (S53.43-)

X ● S53.20   Traumatic rupture of `unspecified` radial collateral ligament

X ● S53.21   Traumatic rupture of right radial collateral ligament

X ● S53.22   Traumatic rupture of left radial collateral ligament

● S53.3   Traumatic rupture of ulnar collateral ligament
     Excludes1   sprain of ulnar collateral ligament (S53.44-)

X ● S53.30   Traumatic rupture of `unspecified` ulnar collateral ligament

X ● S53.31   Traumatic rupture of right ulnar collateral ligament

X ● S53.32   Traumatic rupture of left ulnar collateral ligament

● S53.4   Sprain of elbow
     Excludes2   traumatic rupture of radial collateral ligament (S53.2-)
                  traumatic rupture of ulnar collateral ligament (S53.3-)

  ● S53.40   Unspecified sprain of elbow

    ● S53.401   `Unspecified` sprain of right elbow

    ● S53.402   `Unspecified` sprain of left elbow

    ● S53.409   `Unspecified` sprain of unspecified elbow
                Sprain of elbow NOS

  ● S53.41   Radiohumeral (joint) sprain

    ● S53.411   Radiohumeral (joint) sprain of right elbow

    ● S53.412   Radiohumeral (joint) sprain of left elbow

    ● S53.419   Radiohumeral (joint) sprain of `unspecified` elbow

  ● S53.42   Ulnohumeral (joint) sprain

    ● S53.421   Ulnohumeral (joint) sprain of right elbow

    ● S53.422   Ulnohumeral (joint) sprain of left elbow

    ● S53.429   Ulnohumeral (joint) sprain of `unspecified` elbow

CHAPTER 19 (S00-T88)

● S53.43 Radial collateral ligament sprain
  ● S53.431 Radial collateral ligament sprain of right elbow
  ● S53.432 Radial collateral ligament sprain of left elbow
  ● S53.439 Radial collateral ligament sprain of unspecified elbow
● S53.44 Ulnar collateral ligament sprain
  ● S53.441 Ulnar collateral ligament sprain of right elbow
  ● S53.442 Ulnar collateral ligament sprain of left elbow
  ● S53.449 Ulnar collateral ligament sprain of unspecified elbow
● S53.49 Other sprain of elbow
  ● S53.491 Other sprain of right elbow
  ● S53.492 Other sprain of left elbow
  ● S53.499 Other sprain of unspecified elbow

● S54 Injury of nerves at forearm level
  Code also any associated open wound (S51.-)
  Excludes2 injury of nerves at wrist and hand level (S64.-)
  The appropriate 7th character is to be added to each code from category S54

  A initial encounter
  D subsequent encounter
  S sequela

● S54.0 Injury of ulnar nerve at forearm level
  Injury of ulnar nerve NOS
  X● S54.00 Injury of ulnar nerve at forearm level, unspecified arm
  X● S54.01 Injury of ulnar nerve at forearm level, right arm
  X● S54.02 Injury of ulnar nerve at forearm level, left arm
● S54.1 Injury of median nerve at forearm level
  Injury of median nerve NOS
  X● S54.10 Injury of median nerve at forearm level, unspecified arm
  X● S54.11 Injury of median nerve at forearm level, right arm
  X● S54.12 Injury of median nerve at forearm level, left arm
● S54.2 Injury of radial nerve at forearm level
  Injury of radial nerve NOS
  X● S54.20 Injury of radial nerve at forearm level, unspecified arm
  X● S54.21 Injury of radial nerve at forearm level, right arm
  X● S54.22 Injury of radial nerve at forearm level, left arm
● S54.3 Injury of cutaneous sensory nerve at forearm level
  X● S54.30 Injury of cutaneous sensory nerve at forearm level, unspecified arm
  X● S54.31 Injury of cutaneous sensory nerve at forearm level, right arm
  X● S54.32 Injury of cutaneous sensory nerve at forearm level, left arm
● S54.8 Injury of other nerves at forearm level
  ● S54.8X Injury of other nerves at forearm level ◀
    ● S54.8X1 Injury of other nerves at forearm level, right arm ◀
    ● S54.8X2 Injury of other nerves at forearm level, left arm ◀
    ● S54.8X9 Injury of other nerves at forearm level, unspecified arm ◀

● S54.9 Injury of unspecified nerve at forearm level
  X● S54.90 Injury of unspecified nerve at forearm level, unspecified arm
  X● S54.91 Injury of unspecified nerve at forearm level, right arm
  X● S54.92 Injury of unspecified nerve at forearm level, left arm

● S55 Injury of blood vessels at forearm level
  Code also any associated open wound (S51.-)
  Excludes2 injury of blood vessels at wrist and hand level (S65.-)
           injury of brachial vessels (S45.1-S45.2)
  The appropriate 7th character is to be added to each code from category S55

  A initial encounter
  D subsequent encounter
  S sequela

● S55.0 Injury of ulnar artery at forearm level
  ● S55.00 Unspecified injury of ulnar artery at forearm level
    ● S55.001 Unspecified injury of ulnar artery at forearm level, right arm
    ● S55.002 Unspecified injury of ulnar artery at forearm level, left arm
    ● S55.009 Unspecified injury of ulnar artery at forearm level, unspecified arm
  ● S55.01 Laceration of ulnar artery at forearm level
    ● S55.011 Laceration of ulnar artery at forearm level, right arm
    ● S55.012 Laceration of ulnar artery at forearm level, left arm
    ● S55.019 Laceration of ulnar artery at forearm level, unspecified arm
  ● S55.09 Other specified injury of ulnar artery at forearm level
    ● S55.091 Other specified injury of ulnar artery at forearm level, right arm
    ● S55.092 Other specified injury of ulnar artery at forearm level, left arm
    ● S55.099 Other specified injury of ulnar artery at forearm level, unspecified arm
● S55.1 Injury of radial artery at forearm level
  ● S55.10 Unspecified injury of radial artery at forearm level
    ● S55.101 Unspecified injury of radial artery at forearm level, right arm
    ● S55.102 Unspecified injury of radial artery at forearm level, left arm
    ● S55.109 Unspecified injury of radial artery at forearm level, unspecified arm
  ● S55.11 Laceration of radial artery at forearm level
    ● S55.111 Laceration of radial artery at forearm level, right arm
    ● S55.112 Laceration of radial artery at forearm level, left arm
    ● S55.119 Laceration of radial artery at forearm level, unspecified arm
  ● S55.19 Other specified injury of radial artery at forearm level
    ● S55.191 Other specified injury of radial artery at forearm level, right arm
    ● S55.192 Other specified injury of radial artery at forearm level, left arm
    ● S55.199 Other specified injury of radial artery at forearm level, unspecified arm

- S55.2   Injury of vein at forearm level
  - S55.20   Unspecified injury of vein at forearm level
    - S55.201   Unspecified injury of vein at forearm level, right arm
    - S55.202   Unspecified injury of vein at forearm level, left arm
    - S55.209   Unspecified injury of vein at forearm level, unspecified arm
  - S55.21   Laceration of vein at forearm level
    - S55.211   Laceration of vein at forearm level, right arm
    - S55.212   Laceration of vein at forearm level, left arm
    - S55.219   Laceration of vein at forearm level, unspecified arm
  - S55.29   Other specified injury of vein at forearm level
    - S55.291   Other specified injury of vein at forearm level, right arm
    - S55.292   Other specified injury of vein at forearm level, left arm
    - S55.299   Other specified injury of vein at forearm level, unspecified arm
- S55.8   Injury of other blood vessels at forearm level
  - S55.80   Unspecified injury of other blood vessels at forearm level
    - S55.801   Unspecified injury of other blood vessels at forearm level, right arm
    - S55.802   Unspecified injury of other blood vessels at forearm level, left arm
    - S55.809   Unspecified injury of other blood vessels at forearm level, unspecified arm
  - S55.81   Laceration of other blood vessels at forearm level
    - S55.811   Laceration of other blood vessels at forearm level, right arm
    - S55.812   Laceration of other blood vessels at forearm level, left arm
    - S55.819   Laceration of other blood vessels at forearm level, unspecified arm
  - S55.89   Other specified injury of other blood vessels at forearm level
    - S55.891   Other specified injury of other blood vessels at forearm level, right arm
    - S55.892   Other specified injury of other blood vessels at forearm level, left arm
    - S55.899   Other specified injury of other blood vessels at forearm level, unspecified arm
- S55.9   Injury of unspecified blood vessel at forearm level
  - S55.90   Unspecified injury of unspecified blood vessel at forearm level
    - S55.901   Unspecified injury of unspecified blood vessel at forearm level, right arm
    - S55.902   Unspecified injury of unspecified blood vessel at forearm level, left arm
    - S55.909   Unspecified injury of unspecified blood vessel at forearm level, unspecified arm
  - S55.91   Laceration of unspecified blood vessel at forearm level
    - S55.911   Laceration of unspecified blood vessel at forearm level, right arm
    - S55.912   Laceration of unspecified blood vessel at forearm level, left arm
    - S55.919   Laceration of unspecified blood vessel at forearm level, unspecified arm
  - S55.99   Other specified injury of unspecified blood vessel at forearm level
    - S55.991   Other specified injury of unspecified blood vessel at forearm level, right arm
    - S55.992   Other specified injury of unspecified blood vessel at forearm level, left arm
    - S55.999   Other specified injury of unspecified blood vessel at forearm level, unspecified arm
- S56   Injury of muscle, fascia and tendon at forearm level

  Code also any associated open wound (S51.-)

  Excludes2   injury of muscle, fascia and tendon at or below wrist (S66.-)

  sprain of joints and ligaments of elbow (S53.4-)

  The appropriate 7th character is to be added to each code from category S56

A	initial encounter
D	subsequent encounter
S	sequela

  - S56.0   Injury of flexor muscle, fascia and tendon of thumb at forearm level
    - S56.00   Unspecified injury of flexor muscle, fascia and tendon of thumb at forearm level
      - S56.001   Unspecified injury of flexor muscle, fascia and tendon of right thumb at forearm level
      - S56.002   Unspecified injury of flexor muscle, fascia and tendon of left thumb at forearm level
      - S56.009   Unspecified injury of flexor muscle, fascia and tendon of unspecified thumb at forearm level
    - S56.01   Strain of flexor muscle, fascia and tendon of thumb at forearm level
      - S56.011   Strain of flexor muscle, fascia and tendon of right thumb at forearm level
      - S56.012   Strain of flexor muscle, fascia and tendon of left thumb at forearm level
      - S56.019   Strain of flexor muscle, fascia and tendon of unspecified thumb at forearm level
    - S56.02   Laceration of flexor muscle, fascia and tendon of thumb at forearm level
      - S56.021   Laceration of flexor muscle, fascia and tendon of right thumb at forearm level
      - S56.022   Laceration of flexor muscle, fascia and tendon of left thumb at forearm level
      - S56.029   Laceration of flexor muscle, fascia and tendon of unspecified thumb at forearm level
    - S56.09   Other injury of flexor muscle, fascia and tendon of thumb at forearm level
      - S56.091   Other injury of flexor muscle, fascia and tendon of right thumb at forearm level
      - S56.092   Other injury of flexor muscle, fascia and tendon of left thumb at forearm level
      - S56.099   Other injury of flexor muscle, fascia and tendon of unspecified thumb at forearm level

CHAPTER 19 (S00-T88)

● S56.1　Injury of flexor muscle, fascia and tendon of other and unspecified finger at forearm level

　● S56.10　Unspecified injury of flexor muscle, fascia and tendon of other and unspecified finger at forearm level

　　● S56.101　Unspecified injury of flexor muscle, fascia and tendon of right index finger at forearm level

　　● S56.102　Unspecified injury of flexor muscle, fascia and tendon of left index finger at forearm level

　　● S56.103　Unspecified injury of flexor muscle, fascia and tendon of right middle finger at forearm level

　　● S56.104　Unspecified injury of flexor muscle, fascia and tendon of left middle finger at forearm level

　　● S56.105　Unspecified injury of flexor muscle, fascia and tendon of right ring finger at forearm level

　　● S56.106　Unspecified injury of flexor muscle, fascia and tendon of left ring finger at forearm level

　　● S56.107　Unspecified injury of flexor muscle, fascia and tendon of right little finger at forearm level

　　● S56.108　Unspecified injury of flexor muscle, fascia and tendon of left little finger at forearm level

　　● S56.109　Unspecified injury of flexor muscle, fascia and tendon of unspecified finger at forearm level

　● S56.11　Strain of flexor muscle, fascia and tendon of other and unspecified finger at forearm level

　　● S56.111　Strain of flexor muscle, fascia and tendon of right index finger at forearm level

　　● S56.112　Strain of flexor muscle, fascia and tendon of left index finger at forearm level

　　● S56.113　Strain of flexor muscle, fascia and tendon of right middle finger at forearm level

　　● S56.114　Strain of flexor muscle, fascia and tendon of left middle finger at forearm level

　　● S56.115　Strain of flexor muscle, fascia and tendon of right ring finger at forearm level

　　● S56.116　Strain of flexor muscle, fascia and tendon of left ring finger at forearm level

　　● S56.117　Strain of flexor muscle, fascia and tendon of right little finger at forearm level

　　● S56.118　Strain of flexor muscle, fascia and tendon of left little finger at forearm level

　　● S56.119　Strain of flexor muscle, fascia and tendon of finger of unspecified finger at forearm level

　● S56.12　Laceration of flexor muscle, fascia and tendon of other and unspecified finger at forearm level

　　● S56.121　Laceration of flexor muscle, fascia and tendon of right index finger at forearm level

　　● S56.122　Laceration of flexor muscle, fascia and tendon of left index finger at forearm level

　　● S56.123　Laceration of flexor muscle, fascia and tendon of right middle finger at forearm level

　　● S56.124　Laceration of flexor muscle, fascia and tendon of left middle finger at forearm level

　　● S56.125　Laceration of flexor muscle, fascia and tendon of right ring finger at forearm level

　　● S56.126　Laceration of flexor muscle, fascia and tendon of left ring finger at forearm level

　　● S56.127　Laceration of flexor muscle, fascia and tendon of right little finger at forearm level

　　● S56.128　Laceration of flexor muscle, fascia and tendon of left little finger at forearm level

　　● S56.129　Laceration of flexor muscle, fascia and tendon of unspecified finger at forearm level

　● S56.19　Other injury of flexor muscle, fascia and tendon of other and unspecified finger at forearm level

　　● S56.191　Other injury of flexor muscle, fascia and tendon of right index finger at forearm level

　　● S56.192　Other injury of flexor muscle, fascia and tendon of left index finger at forearm level

　　● S56.193　Other injury of flexor muscle, fascia and tendon of right middle finger at forearm level

　　● S56.194　Other injury of flexor muscle, fascia and tendon of left middle finger at forearm level

　　● S56.195　Other injury of flexor muscle, fascia and tendon of right ring finger at forearm level

　　● S56.196　Other injury of flexor muscle, fascia and tendon of left ring finger at forearm level

　　● S56.197　Other injury of flexor muscle, fascia and tendon of right little finger at forearm level

　　● S56.198　Other injury of flexor muscle, fascia and tendon of left little finger at forearm level

　　● S56.199　Other injury of flexor muscle, fascia and tendon of unspecified finger at forearm level

● S56.2　Injury of other flexor muscle, fascia and tendon at forearm level

　● S56.20　Unspecified injury of other flexor muscle, fascia and tendon at forearm level

　　● S56.201　Unspecified injury of other flexor muscle, fascia and tendon at forearm level, right arm

　　● S56.202　Unspecified injury of other flexor muscle, fascia and tendon at forearm level, left arm

　　● S56.209　Unspecified injury of other flexor muscle, fascia and tendon at forearm level, unspecified arm

　● S56.21　Strain of other flexor muscle, fascia and tendon at forearm level

　　● S56.211　Strain of other flexor muscle, fascia and tendon at forearm level, right arm

　　● S56.212　Strain of other flexor muscle, fascia and tendon at forearm level, left arm

　　● S56.219　Strain of other flexor muscle, fascia and tendon at forearm level, unspecified arm

◀ New　◀▥ Revised　d̶e̶l̶e̶t̶e̶d̶ Deleted　Excludes 1　Excludes 2　Includes　Use additional　Code first　Code also　Unspecified
OGCR Official Guidelines　X Assign placeholder X　● Use Additional Character(s)　▌ Manifestation Code　**Coding Clinic**

- ● S56.22   Laceration of other flexor muscle, fascia and tendon at forearm level
  - ● S56.221   Laceration of other flexor muscle, fascia and tendon at forearm level, right arm
  - ● S56.222   Laceration of other flexor muscle, fascia and tendon at forearm level, left arm
  - ● S56.229   Laceration of other flexor muscle, fascia and tendon at forearm level, unspecified arm
- ● S56.29   Other injury of other flexor muscle, fascia and tendon at forearm level
  - ● S56.291   Other injury of other flexor muscle, fascia and tendon at forearm level, right arm
  - ● S56.292   Other injury of other flexor muscle, fascia and tendon at forearm level, left arm
  - ● S56.299   Other injury of other flexor muscle, fascia and tendon at forearm level, unspecified arm
- ● S56.3   Injury of extensor or abductor muscles, fascia and tendons of thumb at forearm level
  - ● S56.30   Unspecified injury of extensor or abductor muscles, fascia and tendons of thumb at forearm level
    - ● S56.301   Unspecified injury of extensor or abductor muscles, fascia and tendons of right thumb at forearm level
    - ● S56.302   Unspecified injury of extensor or abductor muscles, fascia and tendons of left thumb at forearm level
    - ● S56.309   Unspecified injury of extensor or abductor muscles, fascia and tendons of unspecified thumb at forearm level
  - ● S56.31   Strain of extensor or abductor muscles, fascia and tendons of thumb at forearm level
    - ● S56.311   Strain of extensor or abductor muscles, fascia and tendons of right thumb at forearm level
    - ● S56.312   Strain of extensor or abductor muscles, fascia and tendons of left thumb at forearm level
    - ● S56.319   Strain of extensor or abductor muscles, fascia and tendons of unspecified thumb at forearm level
  - ● S56.32   Laceration of extensor or abductor muscles, fascia and tendons of thumb at forearm level
    - ● S56.321   Laceration of extensor or abductor muscles, fascia and tendons of right thumb at forearm level
    - ● S56.322   Laceration of extensor or abductor muscles, fascia and tendons of left thumb at forearm level
    - ● S56.329   Laceration of extensor or abductor muscles, fascia and tendons of unspecified thumb at forearm level
  - ● S56.39   Other injury of extensor or abductor muscles, fascia and tendons of thumb at forearm level
    - ● S56.391   Other injury of extensor or abductor muscles, fascia and tendons of right thumb at forearm level
    - ● S56.392   Other injury of extensor or abductor muscles, fascia and tendons of left thumb at forearm level
    - ● S56.399   Other injury of extensor or abductor muscles, fascia and tendons of unspecified thumb at forearm level
- ● S56.4   Injury of extensor muscle, fascia and tendon of other and unspecified finger at forearm level
  - ● S56.40   Unspecified injury of extensor muscle, fascia and tendon of other and unspecified finger at forearm level
    - ● S56.401   Unspecified injury of extensor muscle, fascia and tendon of right index finger at forearm level
    - ● S56.402   Unspecified injury of extensor muscle, fascia and tendon of left index finger at forearm level
    - ● S56.403   Unspecified injury of extensor muscle, fascia and tendon of right middle finger at forearm level
    - ● S56.404   Unspecified injury of extensor muscle, fascia and tendon of left middle finger at forearm level
    - ● S56.405   Unspecified injury of extensor muscle, fascia and tendon of right ring finger at forearm level
    - ● S56.406   Unspecified injury of extensor muscle, fascia and tendon of left ring finger at forearm level
    - ● S56.407   Unspecified injury of extensor muscle, fascia and tendon of right little finger at forearm level
    - ● S56.408   Unspecified injury of extensor muscle, fascia and tendon of left little finger at forearm level
    - ● S56.409   Unspecified injury of extensor muscle, fascia and tendon of unspecified finger at forearm level
  - ● S56.41   Strain of extensor muscle, fascia and tendon of other and unspecified finger at forearm level
    - ● S56.411   Strain of extensor muscle, fascia and tendon of right index finger at forearm level
    - ● S56.412   Strain of extensor muscle, fascia and tendon of left index finger at forearm level
    - ● S56.413   Strain of extensor muscle, fascia and tendon of right middle finger at forearm level
    - ● S56.414   Strain of extensor muscle, fascia and tendon of left middle finger at forearm level
    - ● S56.415   Strain of extensor muscle, fascia and tendon of right ring finger at forearm level
    - ● S56.416   Strain of extensor muscle, fascia and tendon of left ring finger at forearm level
    - ● S56.417   Strain of extensor muscle, fascia and tendon of right little finger at forearm level
    - ● S56.418   Strain of extensor muscle, fascia and tendon of left little finger at forearm level
    - ● S56.419   Strain of extensor muscle, fascia and tendon of finger, unspecified finger at forearm level

CHAPTER 19 (S00–T88)

● **S56.42**   Laceration of extensor muscle, fascia and tendon of other and unspecified finger at forearm level

     ● **S56.421**   Laceration of extensor muscle, fascia and tendon of right index finger at forearm level

     ● **S56.422**   Laceration of extensor muscle, fascia and tendon of left index finger at forearm level

     ● **S56.423**   Laceration of extensor muscle, fascia and tendon of right middle finger at forearm level

     ● **S56.424**   Laceration of extensor muscle, fascia and tendon of left middle finger at forearm level

     ● **S56.425**   Laceration of extensor muscle, fascia and tendon of right ring finger at forearm level

     ● **S56.426**   Laceration of extensor muscle, fascia and tendon of left ring finger at forearm level

     ● **S56.427**   Laceration of extensor muscle, fascia and tendon of right little finger at forearm level

     ● **S56.428**   Laceration of extensor muscle, fascia and tendon of left little finger at forearm level

     ● **S56.429**   Laceration of extensor muscle, fascia and tendon of unspecified finger at forearm level

● **S56.49**   Other injury of extensor muscle, fascia and tendon of other and unspecified finger at forearm level

     ● **S56.491**   Other injury of extensor muscle, fascia and tendon of right index finger at forearm level

     ● **S56.492**   Other injury of extensor muscle, fascia and tendon of left index finger at forearm level

     ● **S56.493**   Other injury of extensor muscle, fascia and tendon of right middle finger at forearm level

     ● **S56.494**   Other injury of extensor muscle, fascia and tendon of left middle finger at forearm level

     ● **S56.495**   Other injury of extensor muscle, fascia and tendon of right ring finger at forearm level

     ● **S56.496**   Other injury of extensor muscle, fascia and tendon of left ring finger at forearm level

     ● **S56.497**   Other injury of extensor muscle, fascia and tendon of right little finger at forearm level

     ● **S56.498**   Other injury of extensor muscle, fascia and tendon of left little finger at forearm level

     ● **S56.499**   Other injury of extensor muscle, fascia and tendon of unspecified finger at forearm level

● **S56.5**   Injury of other extensor muscle, fascia and tendon at forearm level

     ● **S56.50**   Unspecified injury of other extensor muscle, fascia and tendon at forearm level

        ● **S56.501**   Unspecified injury of other extensor muscle, fascia and tendon at forearm level, right arm

        ● **S56.502**   Unspecified injury of other extensor muscle, fascia and tendon at forearm level, left arm

        ● **S56.509**   Unspecified injury of other extensor muscle, fascia and tendon at forearm level, unspecified arm

● **S56.51**   Strain of other extensor muscle, fascia and tendon at forearm level

     ● **S56.511**   Strain of other extensor muscle, fascia and tendon at forearm level, right arm

     ● **S56.512**   Strain of other extensor muscle, fascia and tendon at forearm level, left arm

     ● **S56.519**   Strain of other extensor muscle, fascia and tendon at forearm level, unspecified arm

● **S56.52**   Laceration of other extensor muscle, fascia and tendon at forearm level

     ● **S56.521**   Laceration of other extensor muscle, fascia and tendon at forearm level, right arm

     ● **S56.522**   Laceration of other extensor muscle, fascia and tendon at forearm level, left arm

     ● **S56.529**   Laceration of other extensor muscle, fascia and tendon at forearm level, unspecified arm

● **S56.59**   Other injury of other extensor muscle, fascia and tendon at forearm level

     ● **S56.591**   Other injury of other extensor muscle, fascia and tendon at forearm level, right arm

     ● **S56.592**   Other injury of other extensor muscle, fascia and tendon at forearm level, left arm

     ● **S56.599**   Other injury of other extensor muscle, fascia and tendon at forearm level, unspecified arm

● **S56.8**   Injury of other muscles, fascia and tendons at forearm level

     ● **S56.80**   Unspecified injury of other muscles, fascia and tendons at forearm level

        ● **S56.801**   Unspecified injury of other muscles, fascia and tendons at forearm level, right arm

        ● **S56.802**   Unspecified injury of other muscles, fascia and tendons at forearm level, left arm

        ● **S56.809**   Unspecified injury of other muscles, fascia and tendons at forearm level, unspecified arm

     ● **S56.81**   Strain of other muscles, fascia and tendons at forearm level

        ● **S56.811**   Strain of other muscles, fascia and tendons at forearm level, right arm

        ● **S56.812**   Strain of other muscles, fascia and tendons at forearm level, left arm

        ● **S56.819**   Strain of other muscles, fascia and tendons at forearm level, unspecified arm

     ● **S56.82**   Laceration of other muscles, fascia and tendons at forearm level

        ● **S56.821**   Laceration of other muscles, fascia and tendons at forearm level, right arm

        ● **S56.822**   Laceration of other muscles, fascia and tendons at forearm level, left arm

        ● **S56.829**   Laceration of other muscles, fascia and tendons at forearm level, unspecified arm

◀ New   ◀━ Revised   ~~deleted~~ Deleted   Excludes 1   Excludes 2   Includes   Use additional   Code first   Code also   Unspecified

1262   **OGCR** Official Guidelines   **X** Assign placeholder X   ● Use Additional Character(s)   ▶ Manifestation Code   **Coding Clinic**

● S56.89   Other injury of other muscles, fascia and tendons at forearm level
     ● S56.891   Other injury of other muscles, fascia and tendons at forearm level, right arm
     ● S56.892   Other injury of other muscles, fascia and tendons at forearm level, left arm
     ● S56.899   Other injury of other muscles, fascia and tendons at forearm level, unspecified arm

● S56.9   Injury of unspecified muscles, fascia and tendons at forearm level
   ● S56.90   Unspecified injury of unspecified muscles, fascia and tendons at forearm level
     ● S56.901   Unspecified injury of unspecified muscles, fascia and tendons at forearm level, right arm
     ● S56.902   Unspecified injury of unspecified muscles, fascia and tendons at forearm level, left arm
     ● S56.909   Unspecified injury of unspecified muscles, fascia and tendons at forearm level, unspecified arm
   ● S56.91   Strain of unspecified muscles, fascia and tendons at forearm level
     ● S56.911   Strain of unspecified muscles, fascia and tendons at forearm level, right arm
     ● S56.912   Strain of unspecified muscles, fascia and tendons at forearm level, left arm
     ● S56.919   Strain of unspecified muscles, fascia and tendons at forearm level, unspecified arm
   ● S56.92   Laceration of unspecified muscles, fascia and tendons at forearm level
     ● S56.921   Laceration of unspecified muscles, fascia and tendons at forearm level, right arm
     ● S56.922   Laceration of unspecified muscles, fascia and tendons at forearm level, left arm
     ● S56.929   Laceration of unspecified muscles, fascia and tendons at forearm level, unspecified arm
   ● S56.99   Other injury of unspecified muscles, fascia and tendons at forearm level
     ● S56.991   Other injury of unspecified muscles, fascia and tendons at forearm level, right arm
     ● S56.992   Other injury of unspecified muscles, fascia and tendons at forearm level, left arm
     ● S56.999   Other injury of unspecified muscles, fascia and tendons at forearm level, unspecified arm

● S57   Crushing injury of elbow and forearm
     Use additional code(s) for all associated injuries
     Excludes2   crushing injury of wrist and hand (S67.-)
     The appropriate 7th character is to be added to each code from category S57

A	initial encounter
D	subsequent encounter
S	sequela

   ● S57.0   Crushing injury of elbow
     X ● S57.00   Crushing injury of unspecified elbow
     X ● S57.01   Crushing injury of right elbow
     X ● S57.02   Crushing injury of left elbow

● S57.8   Crushing injury of forearm
     X ● S57.80   Crushing injury of unspecified forearm
     X ● S57.81   Crushing injury of right forearm
     X ● S57.82   Crushing injury of left forearm

● S58   Traumatic amputation of elbow and forearm
     An amputation not identified as partial or complete should be coded to complete
     Excludes1   traumatic amputation of wrist and hand (S68.-)
     The appropriate 7th character is to be added to each code from category S58

A	initial encounter
D	subsequent encounter
S	sequela

   ● S58.0   Traumatic amputation at elbow level
     ● S58.01   Complete traumatic amputation at elbow level
       ● S58.011   Complete traumatic amputation at elbow level, right arm
       ● S58.012   Complete traumatic amputation at elbow level, left arm
       ● S58.019   Complete traumatic amputation at elbow level, unspecified arm
     ● S58.02   Partial traumatic amputation at elbow level
       ● S58.021   Partial traumatic amputation at elbow level, right arm
       ● S58.022   Partial traumatic amputation at elbow level, left arm
       ● S58.029   Partial traumatic amputation at elbow level, unspecified arm

   ● S58.1   Traumatic amputation at level between elbow and wrist
     ● S58.11   Complete traumatic amputation at level between elbow and wrist
       ● S58.111   Complete traumatic amputation at level between elbow and wrist, right arm
       ● S58.112   Complete traumatic amputation at level between elbow and wrist, left arm
       ● S58.119   Complete traumatic amputation at level between elbow and wrist, unspecified arm
     ● S58.12   Partial traumatic amputation at level between elbow and wrist
       ● S58.121   Partial traumatic amputation at level between elbow and wrist, right arm
       ● S58.122   Partial traumatic amputation at level between elbow and wrist, left arm
       ● S58.129   Partial traumatic amputation at level between elbow and wrist, unspecified arm

   ● S58.9   Traumatic amputation of forearm, level unspecified
     Excludes1   traumatic amputation of wrist (S68.-)
     ● S58.91   Complete traumatic amputation of forearm, level unspecified
       ● S58.911   Complete traumatic amputation of right forearm, level unspecified
       ● S58.912   Complete traumatic amputation of left forearm, level unspecified
       ● S58.919   Complete traumatic amputation of unspecified forearm, level unspecified
     ● S58.92   Partial traumatic amputation of forearm, level unspecified
       ● S58.921   Partial traumatic amputation of right forearm, level unspecified
       ● S58.922   Partial traumatic amputation of left forearm, level unspecified
       ● S58.929   Partial traumatic amputation of unspecified forearm, level unspecified

CHAPTER 19 (S00-T88)

Item 19-4 SALTER-HARRIS TYPE 1: epiphysis is completely separated from end of bone, or metaphysic growth plate remains attached to epiphysis

SALTER-HARRIS TYPE 2: epiphysis and growth plate are partially separated from metaphysis, which is cracked—most common type

SALTER-HARRIS TYPE 3: fracture occurring through epiphysis and separates part of epiphysis and growth plate from metaphysis fracture, usually at distal end of tibia

SALTER-HARRIS TYPE 4: fracture runs through epiphysis, across growth plate, into metaphysic, surgery is required to restore joint surface to normal and align growth plate

- **S59 Other and unspecified injuries of elbow and forearm**

  Excludes2 other and unspecified injuries of wrist and hand (S69.-)

  The appropriate 7th character is to be added to each code from subcategories S59.0, S59.1, and S59.2

A	initial encounter for closed fracture
D	subsequent encounter for fracture with routine healing
G	subsequent encounter for fracture with delayed healing
K	subsequent encounter for fracture with nonunion
P	subsequent encounter for fracture with malunion
S	sequela

  - **S59.0 Physeal fracture of lower end of ulna**
    - **S59.00 Unspecified physeal fracture of lower end of ulna**
      - S59.001 Unspecified physeal fracture of lower end of ulna, right arm
      - S59.002 Unspecified physeal fracture of lower end of ulna, left arm
      - S59.009 Unspecified physeal fracture of lower end of ulna, unspecified arm
    - **S59.01 Salter-Harris Type I physeal fracture of lower end of ulna**
      - S59.011 Salter-Harris Type I physeal fracture of lower end of ulna, right arm
      - S59.012 Salter-Harris Type I physeal fracture of lower end of ulna, left arm
      - S59.019 Salter-Harris Type I physeal fracture of lower end of ulna, unspecified arm
    - **S59.02 Salter-Harris Type II physeal fracture of lower end of ulna**
      - S59.021 Salter-Harris Type II physeal fracture of lower end of ulna, right arm
      - S59.022 Salter-Harris Type II physeal fracture of lower end of ulna, left arm
      - S59.029 Salter-Harris Type II physeal fracture of lower end of ulna, unspecified arm
    - **S59.03 Salter-Harris Type III physeal fracture of lower end of ulna**
      - S59.031 Salter-Harris Type III physeal fracture of lower end of ulna, right arm
      - S59.032 Salter-Harris Type III physeal fracture of lower end of ulna, left arm
      - S59.039 Salter-Harris Type III physeal fracture of lower end of ulna, unspecified arm
    - **S59.04 Salter-Harris Type IV physeal fracture of lower end of ulna**
      - S59.041 Salter-Harris Type IV physeal fracture of lower end of ulna, right arm
      - S59.042 Salter-Harris Type IV physeal fracture of lower end of ulna, left arm
      - S59.049 Salter-Harris Type IV physeal fracture of lower end of ulna, unspecified arm

  - **S59.09 Other physeal fracture of lower end of ulna**
    - S59.091 Other physeal fracture of lower end of ulna, right arm
    - S59.092 Other physeal fracture of lower end of ulna, left arm
    - S59.099 Other physeal fracture of lower end of ulna, unspecified arm
  - **S59.1 Physeal fracture of upper end of radius**
    - **S59.10 Unspecified physeal fracture of upper end of radius**
      - S59.101 Unspecified physeal fracture of upper end of radius, right arm
      - S59.102 Unspecified physeal fracture of upper end of radius, left arm
      - S59.109 Unspecified physeal fracture of upper end of radius, unspecified arm
    - **S59.11 Salter-Harris Type I physeal fracture of upper end of radius**
      - S59.111 Salter-Harris Type I physeal fracture of upper end of radius, right arm
      - S59.112 Salter-Harris Type I physeal fracture of upper end of radius, left arm
      - S59.119 Salter-Harris Type I physeal fracture of upper end of radius, unspecified arm
    - **S59.12 Salter-Harris Type II physeal fracture of upper end of radius**
      - S59.121 Salter-Harris Type II physeal fracture of upper end of radius, right arm
      - S59.122 Salter-Harris Type II physeal fracture of upper end of radius, left arm
      - S59.129 Salter-Harris Type II physeal fracture of upper end of radius, unspecified arm
    - **S59.13 Salter-Harris Type III physeal fracture of upper end of radius**
      - S59.131 Salter-Harris Type III physeal fracture of upper end of radius, right arm
      - S59.132 Salter-Harris Type III physeal fracture of upper end of radius, left arm
      - S59.139 Salter-Harris Type III physeal fracture of upper end of radius, unspecified arm
    - **S59.14 Salter-Harris Type IV physeal fracture of upper end of radius**
      - S59.141 Salter-Harris Type IV physeal fracture of upper end of radius, right arm
      - S59.142 Salter-Harris Type IV physeal fracture of upper end of radius, left arm
      - S59.149 Salter-Harris Type IV physeal fracture of upper end of radius, unspecified arm
    - **S59.19 Other physeal fracture of upper end of radius**
      - S59.191 Other physeal fracture of upper end of radius, right arm
      - S59.192 Other physeal fracture of upper end of radius, left arm
      - S59.199 Other physeal fracture of upper end of radius, unspecified arm
  - **S59.2 Physeal fracture of lower end of radius**
    - **S59.20 Unspecified physeal fracture of lower end of radius**
      - S59.201 Unspecified physeal fracture of lower end of radius, right arm
      - S59.202 Unspecified physeal fracture of lower end of radius, left arm
      - S59.209 Unspecified physeal fracture of lower end of radius, unspecified arm

CHAPTER 19 (S00-T88)

◀ New ◀ Revised ~~deleted~~ Deleted | Excludes 1 | Excludes 2 | Includes | Use additional | Code first | Code also | Unspecified

OGCR Official Guidelines X Assign placeholder X ● Use Additional Character(s) ▷ Manifestation Code **Coding Clinic**

● **S59.21**   **Salter-Harris Type I physeal fracture of lower end of radius**
- ● S59.211   Salter-Harris Type I physeal fracture of lower end of radius, right arm
- ● S59.212   Salter-Harris Type I physeal fracture of lower end of radius, left arm
- ● S59.219   Salter-Harris Type I physeal fracture of lower end of radius, <mark>unspecified</mark> arm

● **S59.22**   **Salter-Harris Type II physeal fracture of lower end of radius**
- ● S59.221   Salter-Harris Type II physeal fracture of lower end of radius, right arm
- ● S59.222   Salter-Harris Type II physeal fracture of lower end of radius, left arm
- ● S59.229   Salter-Harris Type II physeal fracture of lower end of radius, <mark>unspecified</mark> arm

● **S59.23**   **Salter-Harris Type III physeal fracture of lower end of radius**
- ● S59.231   Salter-Harris Type III physeal fracture of lower end of radius, right arm
- ● S59.232   Salter-Harris Type III physeal fracture of lower end of radius, left arm
- ● S59.239   Salter-Harris Type III physeal fracture of lower end of radius, <mark>unspecified</mark> arm

● **S59.24**   **Salter-Harris Type IV physeal fracture of lower end of radius**
- ● S59.241   Salter-Harris Type IV physeal fracture of lower end of radius, right arm
- ● S59.242   Salter-Harris Type IV physeal fracture of lower end of radius, left arm
- ● S59.249   Salter-Harris Type IV physeal fracture of lower end of radius, <mark>unspecified</mark> arm

● **S59.29**   **Other physeal fracture of lower end of radius**
- ● S59.291   Other physeal fracture of lower end of radius, right arm
- ● S59.292   Other physeal fracture of lower end of radius, left arm
- ● S59.299   Other physeal fracture of lower end of radius, <mark>unspecified</mark> arm

● **S59.8**   **Other specified injuries of elbow and forearm**

The appropriate 7th character is to be added to each code in subcategory S59.8

A	initial encounter
D	subsequent encounter
S	sequela

● **S59.80**   **Other specified injuries of elbow**
- ● S59.801   Other specified injuries of right elbow
- ● S59.802   Other specified injuries of left elbow
- ● S59.809   Other specified injuries of <mark>unspecified</mark> elbow

● **S59.81**   **Other specified injuries of forearm**
- ● S59.811   Other specified injuries right forearm
- ● S59.812   Other specified injuries left forearm
- ● S59.819   Other specified injuries <mark>unspecified</mark> forearm

● **S59.9**   **Unspecified injury of elbow and forearm**

The appropriate 7th character is to be added to each code in subcategory S59.9

A	initial encounter
D	subsequent encounter
S	sequela

● **S59.90**   **Unspecified injury of elbow**
- ● S59.901   <mark>Unspecified</mark> injury of right elbow
- ● S59.902   <mark>Unspecified</mark> injury of left elbow
- ● S59.909   <mark>Unspecified</mark> injury of unspecified elbow

● **S59.91**   **Unspecified injury of forearm**
- ● S59.911   <mark>Unspecified</mark> injury of right forearm
- ● S59.912   <mark>Unspecified</mark> injury of left forearm
- ● S59.919   <mark>Unspecified</mark> injury of unspecified forearm

---

INJURIES TO THE WRIST, HAND AND FINGERS (S60-S69)

Excludes2   burns and corrosions (T20-T32)
           frostbite (T33-T34)
           insect bite or sting, venomous (T63.4)

● **S60**   **Superficial injury of wrist, hand and fingers**

The appropriate 7th character is to be added to each code from category S60

A	initial encounter
D	subsequent encounter
S	sequela

● **S60.0**   **Contusion of finger without damage to nail**

     Excludes1   contusion involving nail (matrix) (S60.1)

X ● **S60.00**   **Contusion of unspecified finger without damage to nail**
          Contusion of finger(s) NOS

● **S60.01**   **Contusion of thumb without damage to nail**
- ● S60.011   Contusion of right thumb without damage to nail
- ● S60.012   Contusion of left thumb without damage to nail
- ● S60.019   Contusion of <mark>unspecified</mark> thumb without damage to nail
- ● S60.02   Contusion of index finger without damage to nail
- ● S60.021   Contusion of right index finger without damage to nail
- ● S60.022   Contusion of left index finger without damage to nail
- ● S60.029   Contusion of <mark>unspecified</mark> index finger without damage to nail

● **S60.03**   **Contusion of middle finger without damage to nail**
- ● S60.031   Contusion of right middle finger without damage to nail
- ● S60.032   Contusion of left middle finger without damage to nail
- ● S60.039   Contusion of <mark>unspecified</mark> middle finger without damage to nail

● **S60.04**   **Contusion of ring finger without damage to nail**
- ● S60.041   Contusion of right ring finger without damage to nail
- ● S60.042   Contusion of left ring finger without damage to nail
- ● S60.049   Contusion of <mark>unspecified</mark> ring finger without damage to nail

- S60.05   Contusion of little finger without damage to nail
  - S60.051   Contusion of right little finger without damage to nail
  - S60.052   Contusion of left little finger without damage to nail
  - S60.059   Contusion of unspecified little finger without damage to nail
- S60.1   Contusion of finger with damage to nail
  - X S60.10   Contusion of unspecified finger with damage to nail
  - S60.11   Contusion of thumb with damage to nail
    - S60.111   Contusion of right thumb with damage to nail
    - S60.112   Contusion of left thumb with damage to nail
    - S60.119   Contusion of unspecified thumb with damage to nail
  - S60.12   Contusion of index finger with damage to nail
    - S60.121   Contusion of right index finger with damage to nail
    - S60.122   Contusion of left index finger with damage to nail
    - S60.129   Contusion of unspecified index finger with damage to nail
  - S60.13   Contusion of middle finger with damage to nail
    - S60.131   Contusion of right middle finger with damage to nail
    - S60.132   Contusion of left middle finger with damage to nail
    - S60.139   Contusion of unspecified middle finger with damage to nail
  - S60.14   Contusion of ring finger with damage to nail
    - S60.141   Contusion of right ring finger with damage to nail
    - S60.142   Contusion of left ring finger with damage to nail
    - S60.149   Contusion of unspecified ring finger with damage to nail
  - S60.15   Contusion of little finger with damage to nail
    - S60.151   Contusion of right little finger with damage to nail
    - S60.152   Contusion of left little finger with damage to nail
    - S60.159   Contusion of unspecified little finger with damage to nail
- S60.2   Contusion of wrist and hand
  - **Excludes2**   contusion of fingers (S60.0-, S60.1-)
  - S60.21   Contusion of wrist
    - S60.211   Contusion of right wrist
    - S60.212   Contusion of left wrist
    - S60.219   Contusion of unspecified wrist
  - S60.22   Contusion of hand
    - S60.221   Contusion of right hand
    - S60.222   Contusion of left hand
    - S60.229   Contusion of unspecified hand
- S60.3   Other superficial injuries of thumb
  - S60.31   Abrasion of thumb
    - S60.311   Abrasion of right thumb
    - S60.312   Abrasion of left thumb
    - S60.319   Abrasion of unspecified thumb
  - S60.32   Blister (nonthermal) of thumb
    - S60.321   Blister (nonthermal) of right thumb
    - S60.322   Blister (nonthermal) of left thumb
    - S60.329   Blister (nonthermal) of unspecified thumb

- S60.34   External constriction of thumb
  - Hair tourniquet syndrome of thumb
  - Use additional cause code to identify the constricting item (W49.0-)
    - S60.341   External constriction of right thumb
    - S60.342   External constriction of left thumb
    - S60.349   External constriction of unspecified thumb
- S60.35   Superficial foreign body of thumb
  - Splinter in the thumb
    - S60.351   Superficial foreign body of right thumb
    - S60.352   Superficial foreign body of left thumb
    - S60.359   Superficial foreign body of unspecified thumb
- S60.36   Insect bite (nonvenomous) of thumb
  - S60.361   Insect bite (nonvenomous) of right thumb
  - S60.362   Insect bite (nonvenomous) of left thumb
  - S60.369   Insect bite (nonvenomous) of unspecified thumb
- S60.37   Other superficial bite of thumb
  - **Excludes1**   open bite of thumb (S61.05-, S61.15-)
    - S60.371   Other superficial bite of right thumb
    - S60.372   Other superficial bite of left thumb
    - S60.379   Other superficial bite of unspecified thumb
- S60.39   Other superficial injuries of thumb
  - S60.391   Other superficial injuries of right thumb
  - S60.392   Other superficial injuries of left thumb
  - S60.399   Other superficial injuries of unspecified thumb
- S60.4   Other superficial injuries of other fingers
  - S60.41   Abrasion of fingers
    - S60.410   Abrasion of right index finger
    - S60.411   Abrasion of left index finger
    - S60.412   Abrasion of right middle finger
    - S60.413   Abrasion of left middle finger
    - S60.414   Abrasion of right ring finger
    - S60.415   Abrasion of left ring finger
    - S60.416   Abrasion of right little finger
    - S60.417   Abrasion of left little finger
    - S60.418   Abrasion of other finger
      - Abrasion of specified finger with unspecified laterality
    - S60.419   Abrasion of unspecified finger
  - S60.42   Blister (nonthermal) of fingers
    - S60.420   Blister (nonthermal) of right index finger
    - S60.421   Blister (nonthermal) of left index finger
    - S60.422   Blister (nonthermal) of right middle finger
    - S60.423   Blister (nonthermal) of left middle finger
    - S60.424   Blister (nonthermal) of right ring finger
    - S60.425   Blister (nonthermal) of left ring finger
    - S60.426   Blister (nonthermal) of right little finger
    - S60.427   Blister (nonthermal) of left little finger

◀ New   ◀▥ Revised   ~~deleted~~ Deleted   Excludes 1   Excludes 2   Includes   Use additional   Code first   Code also   Unspecified

OGCR Official Guidelines   X Assign placeholder X   ● Use Additional Character(s)   ▶ Manifestation Code   **Coding Clinic**

● S60.428   **Blister (nonthermal) of other finger**
             Blister (nonthermal) of specified
                finger with unspecified
                laterality
● S60.429   **Blister (nonthermal) of unspecified
             finger**

●S60.44   **External constriction of fingers**
          Hair tourniquet syndrome of finger
          Use additional cause code to identify the
             constricting item (W49.0-)
● S60.440   **External constriction of right index
             finger**
● S60.441   **External constriction of left index
             finger**
● S60.442   **External constriction of right middle
             finger**
● S60.443   **External constriction of left middle
             finger**
● S60.444   **External constriction of right ring
             finger**
● S60.445   **External constriction of left ring
             finger**
● S60.446   **External constriction of right little
             finger**
● S60.447   **External constriction of left little
             finger**
● S60.448   **External constriction of other finger**
             External constriction of specified
                finger with unspecified
                laterality
● S60.449   **External constriction of unspecified
             finger**

●S60.45   **Superficial foreign body of fingers**
          Splinter in the finger(s)
● S60.450   **Superficial foreign body of right
             index finger**
● S60.451   **Superficial foreign body of left index
             finger**
● S60.452   **Superficial foreign body of right
             middle finger**
● S60.453   **Superficial foreign body of left
             middle finger**
● S60.454   **Superficial foreign body of right ring
             finger**
● S60.455   **Superficial foreign body of left ring
             finger**
● S60.456   **Superficial foreign body of right little
             finger**
● S60.457   **Superficial foreign body of left little
             finger**
● S60.458   **Superficial foreign body of other
             finger**
             Superficial foreign body of specified
                finger with unspecified laterality
● S60.459   **Superficial foreign body of
             unspecified finger**

●S60.46   **Insect bite (nonvenomous) of fingers**
● S60.460   **Insect bite (nonvenomous) of right
             index finger**
● S60.461   **Insect bite (nonvenomous) of left
             index finger**
● S60.462   **Insect bite (nonvenomous) of right
             middle finger**
● S60.463   **Insect bite (nonvenomous) of left
             middle finger**
● S60.464   **Insect bite (nonvenomous) of right
             ring finger**
● S60.465   **Insect bite (nonvenomous) of left ring
             finger**

● S60.466   **Insect bite (nonvenomous) of right
             little finger**
● S60.467   **Insect bite (nonvenomous) of left
             little finger**
● S60.468   **Insect bite (nonvenomous) of other
             finger**
             Insect bite (nonvenomous)
                of specified finger with
                unspecified laterality
● S60.469   **Insect bite (nonvenomous) of
             unspecified finger**

●S60.47   **Other superficial bite of fingers**
          Excludes1   open bite of fingers (S61.25-,
                          S61.35-)
● S60.470   **Other superficial bite of right index
             finger**
● S60.471   **Other superficial bite of left index
             finger**
● S60.472   **Other superficial bite of right middle
             finger**
● S60.473   **Other superficial bite of left middle
             finger**
● S60.474   **Other superficial bite of right ring
             finger**
● S60.475   **Other superficial bite of left ring
             finger**
● S60.476   **Other superficial bite of right little
             finger**
● S60.477   **Other superficial bite of left little
             finger**
● S60.478   **Other superficial bite of other finger**
             Other superficial bite of specified
                finger with unspecified
                laterality
● S60.479   **Other superficial bite of unspecified
             finger**

●S60.5   **Other superficial injuries of hand**
          Excludes2   superficial injuries of fingers (S60.3-,
                          S60.4-)
●S60.51   **Abrasion of hand**
● S60.511   **Abrasion of right hand**
● S60.512   **Abrasion of left hand**
● S60.519   **Abrasion of unspecified hand**
●S60.52   **Blister (nonthermal) of hand**
● S60.521   **Blister (nonthermal) of right hand**
● S60.522   **Blister (nonthermal) of left hand**
● S60.529   **Blister (nonthermal) of unspecified
             hand**
●S60.54   **External constriction of hand**
● S60.541   **External constriction of right hand**
● S60.542   **External constriction of left hand**
● S60.549   **External constriction of unspecified
             hand**
●S60.55   **Superficial foreign body of hand**
          Splinter in the hand
● S60.551   **Superficial foreign body of right hand**
● S60.552   **Superficial foreign body of left hand**
● S60.559   **Superficial foreign body of
             unspecified hand**
●S60.56   **Insect bite (nonvenomous) of hand**
● S60.561   **Insect bite (nonvenomous) of right
             hand**
● S60.562   **Insect bite (nonvenomous) of left
             hand**
● S60.569   **Insect bite (nonvenomous) of
             unspecified hand**

CHAPTER 19 (S00-T88)

● **S60.57** Other superficial bite of hand
        Excludes1   open bite of hand (S61.45-)
  ● S60.571   Other superficial bite of hand of right hand
  ● S60.572   Other superficial bite of hand of left hand
  ● S60.579   Other superficial bite of hand of unspecified hand

● **S60.8** Other superficial injuries of wrist
 ● **S60.81** Abrasion of wrist
  ● S60.811   Abrasion of right wrist
  ● S60.812   Abrasion of left wrist
  ● S60.819   Abrasion of unspecified wrist
 ● **S60.82** Blister (nonthermal) of wrist
  ● S60.821   Blister (nonthermal) of right wrist
  ● S60.822   Blister (nonthermal) of left wrist
  ● S60.829   Blister (nonthermal) of unspecified wrist
 ● **S60.84** External constriction of wrist
  ● S60.841   External constriction of right wrist
  ● S60.842   External constriction of left wrist
  ● S60.849   External constriction of unspecified wrist
 ● **S60.85** Superficial foreign body of wrist
    Splinter in the wrist
  ● S60.851   Superficial foreign body of right wrist
  ● S60.852   Superficial foreign body of left wrist
  ● S60.859   Superficial foreign body of unspecified wrist
 ● **S60.86** Insect bite (nonvenomous) of wrist
  ● S60.861   Insect bite (nonvenomous) of right wrist
  ● S60.862   Insect bite (nonvenomous) of left wrist
  ● S60.869   Insect bite (nonvenomous) of unspecified wrist
 ● **S60.87** Other superficial bite of wrist
       Excludes1   open bite of wrist (S61.55)
  ● S60.871   Other superficial bite of right wrist
  ● S60.872   Other superficial bite of left wrist
  ● S60.879   Other superficial bite of unspecified wrist

● **S60.9** Unspecified superficial injury of wrist, hand and fingers
 ● **S60.91** Unspecified superficial injury of wrist
  ● S60.911   Unspecified superficial injury of right wrist
  ● S60.912   Unspecified superficial injury of left wrist
  ● S60.919   Unspecified superficial injury of unspecified wrist
 ● **S60.92** Unspecified superficial injury of hand
  ● S60.921   Unspecified superficial injury of right hand
  ● S60.922   Unspecified superficial injury of left hand
  ● S60.929   Unspecified superficial injury of unspecified hand
 ● **S60.93** Unspecified superficial injury of thumb
  ● S60.931   Unspecified superficial injury of right thumb
  ● S60.932   Unspecified superficial injury of left thumb
  ● S60.939   Unspecified superficial injury of unspecified thumb

 ● **S60.94** Unspecified superficial injury of other fingers
  ● S60.940   Unspecified superficial injury of right index finger
  ● S60.941   Unspecified superficial injury of left index finger
  ● S60.942   Unspecified superficial injury of right middle finger
  ● S60.943   Unspecified superficial injury of left middle finger
  ● S60.944   Unspecified superficial injury of right ring finger
  ● S60.945   Unspecified superficial injury of left ring finger
  ● S60.946   Unspecified superficial injury of right little finger
  ● S60.947   Unspecified superficial injury of left little finger
  ● S60.948   Unspecified superficial injury of other finger
      Unspecified superficial injury of specified finger with unspecified laterality
  ● S60.949   Unspecified superficial injury of unspecified finger

● **S61** **Open wound of wrist, hand and fingers**
    Code also any associated wound infection
    Excludes1   open fracture of wrist, hand and finger (S62.- with 7th character B)
             traumatic amputation of wrist and hand (S68.-)
    The appropriate 7th character is to be added to each code from category S61

> A   initial encounter
> D   subsequent encounter
> S   sequela

● **S61.0** **Open wound of thumb without damage to nail**
       Excludes1   open wound of thumb with damage to nail (S61.1-)
 ● **S61.00** Unspecified open wound of thumb without damage to nail
  ● S61.001   Unspecified open wound of right thumb without damage to nail
  ● S61.002   Unspecified open wound of left thumb without damage to nail
  ● S61.009   Unspecified open wound of unspecified thumb without damage to nail
 ● **S61.01** Laceration without foreign body of thumb without damage to nail
  ● S61.011   Laceration without foreign body of right thumb without damage to nail
  ● S61.012   Laceration without foreign body of left thumb without damage to nail
  ● S61.019   Laceration without foreign body of unspecified thumb without damage to nail
 ● **S61.02** Laceration with foreign body of thumb without damage to nail
  ● S61.021   Laceration with foreign body of right thumb without damage to nail
  ● S61.022   Laceration with foreign body of left thumb without damage to nail
  ● S61.029   Laceration with foreign body of unspecified thumb without damage to nail

- ● S61.03   Puncture wound without foreign body of thumb without damage to nail
  - ● S61.031   Puncture wound without foreign body of right thumb without damage to nail
  - ● S61.032   Puncture wound without foreign body of left thumb without damage to nail
  - ● S61.039   Puncture wound without foreign body of unspecified thumb without damage to nail
- ● S61.04   Puncture wound with foreign body of thumb without damage to nail
  - ● S61.041   Puncture wound with foreign body of right thumb without damage to nail
  - ● S61.042   Puncture wound with foreign body of left thumb without damage to nail
  - ● S61.049   Puncture wound with foreign body of unspecified thumb without damage to nail
- ● S61.05   Open bite of thumb without damage to nail

  Bite of thumb NOS

  Excludes1   superficial bite of thumb (S60.36-, S60.37-)

  - ● S61.051   Open bite of right thumb without damage to nail
  - ● S61.052   Open bite of left thumb without damage to nail
  - ● S61.059   Open bite of unspecified thumb without damage to nail
- ● S61.1   Open wound of thumb with damage to nail
  - ● S61.10   Unspecified open wound of thumb with damage to nail
    - ● S61.101   Unspecified open wound of right thumb with damage to nail
    - ● S61.102   Unspecified open wound of left thumb with damage to nail
    - ● S61.109   Unspecified open wound of unspecified thumb with damage to nail
  - ● S61.11   Laceration without foreign body of thumb with damage to nail
    - ● S61.111   Laceration without foreign body of right thumb with damage to nail
    - ● S61.112   Laceration without foreign body of left thumb with damage to nail
    - ● S61.119   Laceration without foreign body of unspecified thumb with damage to nail
  - ● S61.12   Laceration with foreign body of thumb with damage to nail
    - ● S61.121   Laceration with foreign body of right thumb with damage to nail
    - ● S61.122   Laceration with foreign body of left thumb with damage to nail
    - ● S61.129   Laceration with foreign body of unspecified thumb with damage to nail
  - ● S61.13   Puncture wound without foreign body of thumb with damage to nail
    - ● S61.131   Puncture wound without foreign body of right thumb with damage to nail
    - ● S61.132   Puncture wound without foreign body of left thumb with damage to nail
    - ● S61.139   Puncture wound without foreign body of unspecified thumb with damage to nail

- ● S61.14   Puncture wound with foreign body of thumb with damage to nail
  - ● S61.141   Puncture wound with foreign body of right thumb with damage to nail
  - ● S61.142   Puncture wound with foreign body of left thumb with damage to nail
  - ● S61.149   Puncture wound with foreign body of unspecified thumb with damage to nail
- ● S61.15   Open bite of thumb with damage to nail

  Bite of thumb with damage to nail NOS

  Excludes1   superficial bite of thumb (S60.36-, S60.37-)

  - ● S61.151   Open bite of right thumb with damage to nail
  - ● S61.152   Open bite of left thumb with damage to nail
  - ● S61.159   Open bite of unspecified thumb with damage to nail
- ● S61.2   Open wound of other finger without damage to nail

  Excludes1   open wound of finger involving nail (matrix) (S61.3-)

  Excludes2   open wound of thumb without damage to nail (S61.0-)

  - ● S61.20   Unspecified open wound of other finger without damage to nail
    - ● S61.200   Unspecified open wound of right index finger without damage to nail
    - ● S61.201   Unspecified open wound of left index finger without damage to nail
    - ● S61.202   Unspecified open wound of right middle finger without damage to nail
    - ● S61.203   Unspecified open wound of left middle finger without damage to nail
    - ● S61.204   Unspecified open wound of right ring finger without damage to nail
    - ● S61.205   Unspecified open wound of left ring finger without damage to nail
    - ● S61.206   Unspecified open wound of right little finger without damage to nail
    - ● S61.207   Unspecified open wound of left little finger without damage to nail
    - ● S61.208   Unspecified open wound of other finger without damage to nail

      Unspecified open wound of specified finger with unspecified laterality without damage to nail
    - ● S61.209   Unspecified open wound of unspecified finger without damage to nail
  - ● S61.21   Laceration without foreign body of finger without damage to nail
    - ● S61.210   Laceration without foreign body of right index finger without damage to nail
    - ● S61.211   Laceration without foreign body of left index finger without damage to nail
    - ● S61.212   Laceration without foreign body of right middle finger without damage to nail
    - ● S61.213   Laceration without foreign body of left middle finger without damage to nail

● S61.214   Laceration without foreign body of right ring finger without damage to nail

● S61.215   Laceration without foreign body of left ring finger without damage to nail

● S61.216   Laceration without foreign body of right little finger without damage to nail

● S61.217   Laceration without foreign body of left little finger without damage to nail

● S61.218   Laceration without foreign body of other finger without damage to nail
Laceration without foreign body of specified finger with unspecified laterality without damage to nail

● S61.219   Laceration without foreign body of unspecified finger without damage to nail

●S61.22   Laceration with foreign body of finger without damage to nail

● S61.220   Laceration with foreign body of right index finger without damage to nail

● S61.221   Laceration with foreign body of left index finger without damage to nail

● S61.222   Laceration with foreign body of right middle finger without damage to nail

● S61.223   Laceration with foreign body of left middle finger without damage to nail

● S61.224   Laceration with foreign body of right ring finger without damage to nail

● S61.225   Laceration with foreign body of left ring finger without damage to nail

● S61.226   Laceration with foreign body of right little finger without damage to nail

● S61.227   Laceration with foreign body of left little finger without damage to nail

● S61.228   Laceration with foreign body of other finger without damage to nail
Laceration with foreign body of specified finger with unspecified laterality without damage to nail

● S61.229   Laceration with foreign body of unspecified finger without damage to nail

●S61.23   Puncture wound without foreign body of finger without damage to nail

● S61.230   Puncture wound without foreign body of right index finger without damage to nail

● S61.231   Puncture wound without foreign body of left index finger without damage to nail

● S61.232   Puncture wound without foreign body of right middle finger without damage to nail

● S61.233   Puncture wound without foreign body of left middle finger without damage to nail

● S61.234   Puncture wound without foreign body of right ring finger without damage to nail

● S61.235   Puncture wound without foreign body of left ring finger without damage to nail

● S61.236   Puncture wound without foreign body of right little finger without damage to nail

● S61.237   Puncture wound without foreign body of left little finger without damage to nail

● S61.238   Puncture wound without foreign body of other finger without damage to nail
Puncture wound without foreign body of specified finger with unspecified laterality without damage to nail

● S61.239   Puncture wound without foreign body of unspecified finger without damage to nail

●S61.24   Puncture wound with foreign body of finger without damage to nail

● S61.240   Puncture wound with foreign body of right index finger without damage to nail

● S61.241   Puncture wound with foreign body of left index finger without damage to nail

● S61.242   Puncture wound with foreign body of right middle finger without damage to nail

● S61.243   Puncture wound with foreign body of left middle finger without damage to nail

● S61.244   Puncture wound with foreign body of right ring finger without damage to nail

● S61.245   Puncture wound with foreign body of left ring finger without damage to nail

● S61.246   Puncture wound with foreign body of right little finger without damage to nail

● S61.247   Puncture wound with foreign body of left little finger without damage to nail

● S61.248   Puncture wound with foreign body of other finger without damage to nail
Puncture wound with foreign body of specified finger with unspecified laterality without damage to nail

● S61.249   Puncture wound with foreign body of unspecified finger without damage to nail

●S61.25   Open bite of finger without damage to nail
Bite of finger without damage to nail NOS

Excludes 1   superficial bite of finger (S60.46-, S60.47-)

● S61.250   Open bite of right index finger without damage to nail

● S61.251   Open bite of left index finger without damage to nail

● S61.252   Open bite of right middle finger without damage to nail

● S61.253   Open bite of left middle finger without damage to nail

● S61.254   Open bite of right ring finger without damage to nail

● S61.255   Open bite of left ring finger without damage to nail

● S61.256   Open bite of right little finger without damage to nail

● S61.257   Open bite of left little finger without damage to nail

● S61.258   Open bite of other finger without damage to nail
Open bite of specified finger with unspecified laterality without damage to nail

● S61.259   Open bite of unspecified finger without damage to nail

● **S61.3**   Open wound of other finger with damage to nail
   ● **S61.30**   Unspecified open wound of finger with damage to nail
      ● **S61.300**   Unspecified open wound of right index finger with damage to nail
      ● **S61.301**   Unspecified open wound of left index finger with damage to nail
      ● **S61.302**   Unspecified open wound of right middle finger with damage to nail
      ● **S61.303**   Unspecified open wound of left middle finger with damage to nail
      ● **S61.304**   Unspecified open wound of right ring finger with damage to nail
      ● **S61.305**   Unspecified open wound of left ring finger with damage to nail
      ● **S61.306**   Unspecified open wound of right little finger with damage to nail
      ● **S61.307**   Unspecified open wound of left little finger with damage to nail
      ● **S61.308**   Unspecified open wound of other finger with damage to nail
             Unspecified open wound of specified finger with unspecified laterality with damage to nail
      ● **S61.309**   Unspecified open wound of unspecified finger with damage to nail
   ● **S61.31**   Laceration without foreign body of finger with damage to nail
      ● **S61.310**   Laceration without foreign body of right index finger with damage to nail
      ● **S61.311**   Laceration without foreign body of left index finger with damage to nail
      ● **S61.312**   Laceration without foreign body of right middle finger with damage to nail
      ● **S61.313**   Laceration without foreign body of left middle finger with damage to nail
      ● **S61.314**   Laceration without foreign body of right ring finger with damage to nail
      ● **S61.315**   Laceration without foreign body of left ring finger with damage to nail
      ● **S61.316**   Laceration without foreign body of right little finger with damage to nail
      ● **S61.317**   Laceration without foreign body of left little finger with damage to nail
      ● **S61.318**   Laceration without foreign body of other finger with damage to nail
             Laceration without foreign body of specified finger with unspecified laterality with damage to nail
      ● **S61.319**   Laceration without foreign body of unspecified finger with damage to nail
   ● **S61.32**   Laceration with foreign body of finger with damage to nail
      ● **S61.320**   Laceration with foreign body of right index finger with damage to nail
      ● **S61.321**   Laceration with foreign body of left index finger with damage to nail
      ● **S61.322**   Laceration with foreign body of right middle finger with damage to nail
      ● **S61.323**   Laceration with foreign body of left middle finger with damage to nail
      ● **S61.324**   Laceration with foreign body of right ring finger with damage to nail
      ● **S61.325**   Laceration with foreign body of left ring finger with damage to nail
      ● **S61.326**   Laceration with foreign body of right little finger with damage to nail

● **S61.327**   Laceration with foreign body of left little finger with damage to nail
● **S61.328**   Laceration with foreign body of other finger with damage to nail
             Laceration with foreign body of specified finger with unspecified laterality with damage to nail
● **S61.329**   Laceration with foreign body of unspecified finger with damage to nail
● **S61.33**   Puncture wound without foreign body of finger with damage to nail
   ● **S61.330**   Puncture wound without foreign body of right index finger with damage to nail
   ● **S61.331**   Puncture wound without foreign body of left index finger with damage to nail
   ● **S61.332**   Puncture wound without foreign body of right middle finger with damage to nail
   ● **S61.333**   Puncture wound without foreign body of left middle finger with damage to nail
   ● **S61.334**   Puncture wound without foreign body of right ring finger with damage to nail
   ● **S61.335**   Puncture wound without foreign body of left ring finger with damage to nail
   ● **S61.336**   Puncture wound without foreign body of right little finger with damage to nail
   ● **S61.337**   Puncture wound without foreign body of left little finger with damage to nail
   ● **S61.338**   Puncture wound without foreign body of other finger with damage to nail
             Puncture wound without foreign body of specified finger with unspecified laterality with damage to nail
   ● **S61.339**   Puncture wound without foreign body of unspecified finger with damage to nail
● **S61.34**   Puncture wound with foreign body of finger with damage to nail
   ● **S61.340**   Puncture wound with foreign body of right index finger with damage to nail
   ● **S61.341**   Puncture wound with foreign body of left index finger with damage to nail
   ● **S61.342**   Puncture wound with foreign body of right middle finger with damage to nail
   ● **S61.343**   Puncture wound with foreign body of left middle finger with damage to nail
   ● **S61.344**   Puncture wound with foreign body of right ring finger with damage to nail
   ● **S61.345**   Puncture wound with foreign body of left ring finger with damage to nail
   ● **S61.346**   Puncture wound with foreign body of right little finger with damage to nail
   ● **S61.347**   Puncture wound with foreign body of left little finger with damage to nail
   ● **S61.348**   Puncture wound with foreign body of other finger with damage to nail
             Puncture wound with foreign body of specified finger with unspecified laterality with damage to nail
   ● **S61.349**   Puncture wound with foreign body of unspecified finger with damage to nail

CHAPTER 19 (S00–T88)

● **S61.35**   **Open bite of finger with damage to nail**
Bite of finger with damage to nail NOS

> **Excludes1**   superficial bite of finger (S60.46-, S60.47-)

    ● **S61.350**   **Open bite of right index finger with damage to nail**

    ● **S61.351**   **Open bite of left index finger with damage to nail**

    ● **S61.352**   **Open bite of right middle finger with damage to nail**

    ● **S61.353**   **Open bite of left middle finger with damage to nail**

    ● **S61.354**   **Open bite of right ring finger with damage to nail**

    ● **S61.355**   **Open bite of left ring finger with damage to nail**

    ● **S61.356**   **Open bite of right little finger with damage to nail**

    ● **S61.357**   **Open bite of left little finger with damage to nail**

    ● **S61.358**   **Open bite of other finger with damage to nail**
Open bite of specified finger with unspecified laterality with damage to nail

    ● **S61.359**   **Open bite of unspecified finger with damage to nail**

● **S61.4**   **Open wound of hand**

   ● **S61.40**   **Unspecified open wound of hand**

     ● **S61.401**   **Unspecified open wound of right hand**

     ● **S61.402**   **Unspecified open wound of left hand**

     ● **S61.409**   **Unspecified open wound of unspecified hand**

   ● **S61.41**   **Laceration without foreign body of hand**

     ● **S61.411**   **Laceration without foreign body of right hand**

     ● **S61.412**   **Laceration without foreign body of left hand**

     ● **S61.419**   **Laceration without foreign body of unspecified hand**

   ● **S61.42**   **Laceration with foreign body of hand**

     ● **S61.421**   **Laceration with foreign body of right hand**

     ● **S61.422**   **Laceration with foreign body of left hand**

     ● **S61.429**   **Laceration with foreign body of unspecified hand**

   ● **S61.43**   **Puncture wound without foreign body of hand**

     ● **S61.431**   **Puncture wound without foreign body of right hand**

     ● **S61.432**   **Puncture wound without foreign body of left hand**

     ● **S61.439**   **Puncture wound without foreign body of unspecified hand**

   ● **S61.44**   **Puncture wound with foreign body of hand**

     ● **S61.441**   **Puncture wound with foreign body of right hand**

     ● **S61.442**   **Puncture wound with foreign body of left hand**

     ● **S61.449**   **Puncture wound with foreign body of unspecified hand**

   ● **S61.45**   **Open bite of hand**
Bite of hand NOS

> **Excludes1**   superficial bite of hand (S60.56-, S60.57-)

     ● **S61.451**   **Open bite of right hand**

     ● **S61.452**   **Open bite of left hand**

     ● **S61.459**   **Open bite of unspecified hand**

● **S61.5**   **Open wound of wrist**

   ● **S61.50**   **Unspecified open wound of wrist**

     ● **S61.501**   **Unspecified open wound of right wrist**

     ● **S61.502**   **Unspecified open wound of left wrist**

     ● **S61.509**   **Unspecified open wound of unspecified wrist**

   ● **S61.51**   **Laceration without foreign body of wrist**

     ● **S61.511**   **Laceration without foreign body of right wrist**

     ● **S61.512**   **Laceration without foreign body of left wrist**

     ● **S61.519**   **Laceration without foreign body of unspecified wrist**

   ● **S61.52**   **Laceration with foreign body of wrist**

     ● **S61.521**   **Laceration with foreign body of right wrist**

     ● **S61.522**   **Laceration with foreign body of left wrist**

     ● **S61.529**   **Laceration with foreign body of unspecified wrist**

   ● **S61.53**   **Puncture wound without foreign body of wrist**

     ● **S61.531**   **Puncture wound without foreign body of right wrist**

     ● **S61.532**   **Puncture wound without foreign body of left wrist**

     ● **S61.539**   **Puncture wound without foreign body of unspecified wrist**

   ● **S61.54**   **Puncture wound with foreign body of wrist**

     ● **S61.541**   **Puncture wound with foreign body of right wrist**

     ● **S61.542**   **Puncture wound with foreign body of left wrist**

     ● **S61.549**   **Puncture wound with foreign body of unspecified wrist**

   ● **S61.55**   **Open bite of wrist**
Bite of wrist NOS

> **Excludes1**   superficial bite of wrist (S60.86-, S60.87-)

     ● **S61.551**   **Open bite of right wrist**

     ● **S61.552**   **Open bite of left wrist**

     ● **S61.559**   **Open bite of unspecified wrist**

● **S62**   **Fracture at wrist and hand level**

> **Note:** A fracture not indicated as displaced or nondisplaced should be coded to displaced
>
> A fracture not indicated as open or closed should be coded to closed

> **Excludes1**   traumatic amputation of wrist and hand (S68.-)
> **Excludes2**   fracture of distal parts of ulna and radius (S52.-)

The appropriate 7th character is to be added to each code from category S62

A	initial encounter for closed fracture
B	initial encounter for open fracture
D	subsequent encounter for fracture with routine healing
G	subsequent encounter for fracture with delayed healing
K	subsequent encounter for fracture with nonunion
P	subsequent encounter for fracture with malunion
S	sequela

● **S62.0**   **Fracture of navicular [scaphoid] bone of wrist**

   ● **S62.00**   **Unspecified fracture of navicular [scaphoid] bone of wrist**

     ● **S62.001**   **Unspecified fracture of navicular [scaphoid] bone of right wrist**

     ● **S62.002**   **Unspecified fracture of navicular [scaphoid] bone of left wrist**
Coding Clinic: 2012, Q4, P106

     ● **S62.009**   **Unspecified fracture of navicular [scaphoid] bone of unspecified wrist**

◀ New   ◀◀ Revised   ~~deleted~~ Deleted   Excludes 1   Excludes 2   Includes   Use additional   Code first   Code also   Unspecified

1272   **OGCR** Official Guidelines   X Assign placeholder X   ● Use Additional Character(s)   ▶ Manifestation Code   **Coding Clinic**

- ● S62.01   **Fracture of distal pole of navicular [scaphoid] bone of wrist**
  Fracture of volar tuberosity of navicular [scaphoid] bone of wrist
  - ● S62.011   Displaced fracture of distal pole of navicular [scaphoid] bone of right wrist
  - ● S62.012   Displaced fracture of distal pole of navicular [scaphoid] bone of left wrist
  - ● S62.013   Displaced fracture of distal pole of navicular [scaphoid] bone of unspecified wrist
  - ● S62.014   Nondisplaced fracture of distal pole of navicular [scaphoid] bone of right wrist
  - ● S62.015   Nondisplaced fracture of distal pole of navicular [scaphoid] bone of left wrist
  - ● S62.016   Nondisplaced fracture of distal pole of navicular [scaphoid] bone of unspecified wrist
- ● S62.02   **Fracture of middle third of navicular [scaphoid] bone of wrist**
  - ● S62.021   Displaced fracture of middle third of navicular [scaphoid] bone of right wrist
  - ● S62.022   Displaced fracture of middle third of navicular [scaphoid] bone of left wrist
  - ● S62.023   Displaced fracture of middle third of navicular [scaphoid] bone of unspecified wrist
  - ● S62.024   Nondisplaced fracture of middle third of navicular [scaphoid] bone of right wrist
  - ● S62.025   Nondisplaced fracture of middle third of navicular [scaphoid] bone of left wrist
  - ● S62.026   Nondisplaced fracture of middle third of navicular [scaphoid] bone of unspecified wrist
- ● S62.03   **Fracture of proximal third of navicular [scaphoid] bone of wrist**
  - ● S62.031   Displaced fracture of proximal third of navicular [scaphoid] bone of right wrist
  - ● S62.032   Displaced fracture of proximal third of navicular [scaphoid] bone of left wrist
  - ● S62.033   Displaced fracture of proximal third of navicular [scaphoid] bone of unspecified wrist
  - ● S62.034   Nondisplaced fracture of proximal third of navicular [scaphoid] bone of right wrist
  - ● S62.035   Nondisplaced fracture of proximal third of navicular [scaphoid] bone of left wrist
  - ● S62.036   Nondisplaced fracture of proximal third of navicular [scaphoid] bone of unspecified wrist
- ● S62.1   **Fracture of other and unspecified carpal bone(s)**
  - **Excludes2**   fracture of scaphoid of wrist (S62.0-)
  - ● S62.10   **Fracture of unspecified carpal bone**
    Fracture of wrist NOS
    - ● S62.101   Fracture of unspecified carpal bone, right wrist
    - ● S62.102   Fracture of unspecified carpal bone, left wrist
      Coding Clinic: 2012, Q4, P95
    - ● S62.109   Fracture of unspecified carpal bone, unspecified wrist

- ● S62.11   **Fracture of triquetrum [cuneiform] bone of wrist**
  - ● S62.111   Displaced fracture of triquetrum [cuneiform] bone, right wrist
  - ● S62.112   Displaced fracture of triquetrum [cuneiform] bone, left wrist
  - ● S62.113   Displaced fracture of triquetrum [cuneiform] bone, unspecified wrist
  - ● S62.114   Nondisplaced fracture of triquetrum [cuneiform] bone, right wrist
  - ● S62.115   Nondisplaced fracture of triquetrum [cuneiform] bone, left wrist
  - ● S62.116   Nondisplaced fracture of triquetrum [cuneiform] bone, unspecified wrist
- ● S62.12   **Fracture of lunate [semilunar]**
  - ● S62.121   Displaced fracture of lunate [semilunar], right wrist
  - ● S62.122   Displaced fracture of lunate [semilunar], left wrist
  - ● S62.123   Displaced fracture of lunate [semilunar], unspecified wrist
  - ● S62.124   Nondisplaced fracture of lunate [semilunar], right wrist
  - ● S62.125   Nondisplaced fracture of lunate [semilunar], left wrist
  - ● S62.126   Nondisplaced fracture of lunate [semilunar], unspecified wrist
- ● S62.13   **Fracture of capitate [os magnum] bone**
  - ● S62.131   Displaced fracture of capitate [os magnum] bone, right wrist
  - ● S62.132   Displaced fracture of capitate [os magnum] bone, left wrist
  - ● S62.133   Displaced fracture of capitate [os magnum] bone, unspecified wrist
  - ● S62.134   Nondisplaced fracture of capitate [os magnum] bone, right wrist
  - ● S62.135   Nondisplaced fracture of capitate [os magnum] bone, left wrist
  - ● S62.136   Nondisplaced fracture of capitate [os magnum] bone, unspecified wrist
- ● S62.14   **Fracture of body of hamate [unciform] bone**
  Fracture of hamate [unciform] bone NOS
  - ● S62.141   Displaced fracture of body of hamate [unciform] bone, right wrist
  - ● S62.142   Displaced fracture of body of hamate [unciform] bone, left wrist
  - ● S62.143   Displaced fracture of body of hamate [unciform] bone, unspecified wrist
  - ● S62.144   Nondisplaced fracture of body of hamate [unciform] bone, right wrist
  - ● S62.145   Nondisplaced fracture of body of hamate [unciform] bone, left wrist
  - ● S62.146   Nondisplaced fracture of body of hamate [unciform] bone, unspecified wrist
- ● S62.15   **Fracture of hook process of hamate [unciform] bone**
  Fracture of unciform process of hamate [unciform] bone
  - ● S62.151   Displaced fracture of hook process of hamate [unciform] bone, right wrist
  - ● S62.152   Displaced fracture of hook process of hamate [unciform] bone, left wrist
  - ● S62.153   Displaced fracture of hook process of hamate [unciform] bone, unspecified wrist
  - ● S62.154   Nondisplaced fracture of hook process of hamate [unciform] bone, right wrist
  - ● S62.155   Nondisplaced fracture of hook process of hamate [unciform] bone, left wrist
  - ● S62.156   Nondisplaced fracture of hook process of hamate [unciform] bone, unspecified wrist

● S62.16   Fracture of pisiform
   ● S62.161   Displaced fracture of pisiform, right wrist
   ● S62.162   Displaced fracture of pisiform, left wrist
   ● S62.163   Displaced fracture of pisiform, unspecified wrist
   ● S62.164   Nondisplaced fracture of pisiform, right wrist
   ● S62.165   Nondisplaced fracture of pisiform, left wrist
   ● S62.166   Nondisplaced fracture of pisiform, unspecified wrist

● S62.17   Fracture of trapezium [larger multangular]
   ● S62.171   Displaced fracture of trapezium [larger multangular], right wrist
   ● S62.172   Displaced fracture of trapezium [larger multangular], left wrist
   ● S62.173   Displaced fracture of trapezium [larger multangular], unspecified wrist
   ● S62.174   Nondisplaced fracture of trapezium [larger multangular], right wrist
   ● S62.175   Nondisplaced fracture of trapezium [larger multangular], left wrist
   ● S62.176   Nondisplaced fracture of trapezium [larger multangular], unspecified wrist

● S62.18   Fracture of trapezoid [smaller multangular]
   ● S62.181   Displaced fracture of trapezoid [smaller multangular], right wrist
   ● S62.182   Displaced fracture of trapezoid [smaller multangular], left wrist
   ● S62.183   Displaced fracture of trapezoid [smaller multangular], unspecified wrist
   ● S62.184   Nondisplaced fracture of trapezoid [smaller multangular], right wrist
   ● S62.185   Nondisplaced fracture of trapezoid [smaller multangular], left wrist
   ● S62.186   Nondisplaced fracture of trapezoid [smaller multangular], unspecified wrist

● S62.2   Fracture of first metacarpal bone
  ● S62.20   Unspecified fracture of first metacarpal bone
   ● S62.201   Unspecified fracture of first metacarpal bone, right hand
   ● S62.202   Unspecified fracture of first metacarpal bone, left hand
   ● S62.209   Unspecified fracture of first metacarpal bone, unspecified hand

  ● S62.21   Bennett's fracture
   ● S62.211   Bennett's fracture, right hand
   ● S62.212   Bennett's fracture, left hand
   ● S62.213   Bennett's fracture, unspecified hand

  ● S62.22   Rolando's fracture
   ● S62.221   Displaced Rolando's fracture, right hand
   ● S62.222   Displaced Rolando's fracture, left hand
   ● S62.223   Displaced Rolando's fracture, unspecified hand
   ● S62.224   Nondisplaced Rolando's fracture, right hand
   ● S62.225   Nondisplaced Rolando's fracture, left hand
   ● S62.226   Nondisplaced Rolando's fracture, unspecified hand

● S62.23   Other fracture of base of first metacarpal bone
   ● S62.231   Other displaced fracture of base of first metacarpal bone, right hand
   ● S62.232   Other displaced fracture of base of first metacarpal bone, left hand
   ● S62.233   Other displaced fracture of base of first metacarpal bone, unspecified hand
   ● S62.234   Other nondisplaced fracture of base of first metacarpal bone, right hand
   ● S62.235   Other nondisplaced fracture of base of first metacarpal bone, left hand
   ● S62.236   Other nondisplaced fracture of base of first metacarpal bone, unspecified hand

● S62.24   Fracture of shaft of first metacarpal bone
   ● S62.241   Displaced fracture of shaft of first metacarpal bone, right hand
   ● S62.242   Displaced fracture of shaft of first metacarpal bone, left hand
   ● S62.243   Displaced fracture of shaft of first metacarpal bone, unspecified hand
   ● S62.244   Nondisplaced fracture of shaft of first metacarpal bone, right hand
   ● S62.245   Nondisplaced fracture of shaft of first metacarpal bone, left hand
   ● S62.246   Nondisplaced fracture of shaft of first metacarpal bone, unspecified hand

● S62.25   Fracture of neck of first metacarpal bone
   ● S62.251   Displaced fracture of neck of first metacarpal bone, right hand
   ● S62.252   Displaced fracture of neck of first metacarpal bone, left hand
   ● S62.253   Displaced fracture of neck of first metacarpal bone, unspecified hand
   ● S62.254   Nondisplaced fracture of neck of first metacarpal bone, right hand
   ● S62.255   Nondisplaced fracture of neck of first metacarpal bone, left hand
   ● S62.256   Nondisplaced fracture of neck of first metacarpal bone, unspecified hand

● S62.29   Other fracture of first metacarpal bone
   ● S62.291   Other fracture of first metacarpal bone, right hand
   ● S62.292   Other fracture of first metacarpal bone, left hand
   ● S62.299   Other fracture of first metacarpal bone, unspecified hand

● S62.3   Fracture of other and unspecified metacarpal bone
   Excludes2   fracture of first metacarpal bone (S62.2-)

  ● S62.30   Unspecified fracture of other metacarpal bone
   ● S62.300   Unspecified fracture of second metacarpal bone, right hand
   ● S62.301   Unspecified fracture of second metacarpal bone, left hand
   ● S62.302   Unspecified fracture of third metacarpal bone, right hand
   ● S62.303   Unspecified fracture of third metacarpal bone, left hand
   ● S62.304   Unspecified fracture of fourth metacarpal bone, right hand
   ● S62.305   Unspecified fracture of fourth metacarpal bone, left hand
   ● S62.306   Unspecified fracture of fifth metacarpal bone, right hand
   ● S62.307   Unspecified fracture of fifth metacarpal bone, left hand

◀ New   ◀▪▪▪ Revised   d̶e̶l̶e̶t̶e̶d̶ Deleted   Excludes 1   Excludes 2   Includes   Use additional   Code first   Code also   Unspecified
OGCR Official Guidelines   X Assign placeholder X   ● Use Additional Character(s)   ▶ Manifestation Code   **Coding Clinic**

● S62.308   Unspecified fracture of other metacarpal bone
> Unspecified fracture of specified metacarpal bone with unspecified laterality

● S62.309   Unspecified fracture of unspecified metacarpal bone

● S62.31   Displaced fracture of base of other metacarpal bone

● S62.310   Displaced fracture of base of second metacarpal bone, right hand

● S62.311   Displaced fracture of base of second metacarpal bone, left hand

● S62.312   Displaced fracture of base of third metacarpal bone, right hand

● S62.313   Displaced fracture of base of third metacarpal bone, left hand

● S62.314   Displaced fracture of base of fourth metacarpal bone, right hand

● S62.315   Displaced fracture of base of fourth metacarpal bone, left hand

● S62.316   Displaced fracture of base of fifth metacarpal bone, right hand

● S62.317   Displaced fracture of base of fifth metacarpal bone, left hand

● S62.318   Displaced fracture of base of other metacarpal bone
> Displaced fracture of base of specified metacarpal bone with unspecified laterality

● S62.319   Displaced fracture of base of unspecified metacarpal bone

● S62.32   Displaced fracture of shaft of other metacarpal bone

● S62.320   Displaced fracture of shaft of second metacarpal bone, right hand

● S62.321   Displaced fracture of shaft of second metacarpal bone, left hand

● S62.322   Displaced fracture of shaft of third metacarpal bone, right hand

● S62.323   Displaced fracture of shaft of third metacarpal bone, left hand

● S62.324   Displaced fracture of shaft of fourth metacarpal bone, right hand

● S62.325   Displaced fracture of shaft of fourth metacarpal bone, left hand

● S62.326   Displaced fracture of shaft of fifth metacarpal bone, right hand

● S62.327   Displaced fracture of shaft of fifth metacarpal bone, left hand

● S62.328   Displaced fracture of shaft of other metacarpal bone
> Displaced fracture of shaft of specified metacarpal bone with unspecified laterality

● S62.329   Displaced fracture of shaft of unspecified metacarpal bone

● S62.33   Displaced fracture of neck of other metacarpal bone

● S62.330   Displaced fracture of neck of second metacarpal bone, right hand

● S62.331   Displaced fracture of neck of second metacarpal bone, left hand

● S62.332   Displaced fracture of neck of third metacarpal bone, right hand

● S62.333   Displaced fracture of neck of third metacarpal bone, left hand

● S62.334   Displaced fracture of neck of fourth metacarpal bone, right hand

● S62.335   Displaced fracture of neck of fourth metacarpal bone, left hand

● S62.336   Displaced fracture of neck of fifth metacarpal bone, right hand

● S62.337   Displaced fracture of neck of fifth metacarpal bone, left hand

● S62.338   Displaced fracture of neck of other metacarpal bone
> Displaced fracture of neck of specified metacarpal bone with unspecified laterality

● S62.339   Displaced fracture of neck of unspecified metacarpal bone

● S62.34   Nondisplaced fracture of base of other metacarpal bone

● S62.340   Nondisplaced fracture of base of second metacarpal bone, right hand

● S62.341   Nondisplaced fracture of base of second metacarpal bone, left hand

● S62.342   Nondisplaced fracture of base of third metacarpal bone, right hand

● S62.343   Nondisplaced fracture of base of third metacarpal bone, left hand

● S62.344   Nondisplaced fracture of base of fourth metacarpal bone, right hand

● S62.345   Nondisplaced fracture of base of fourth metacarpal bone, left hand

● S62.346   Nondisplaced fracture of base of fifth metacarpal bone, right hand

● S62.347   Nondisplaced fracture of base of fifth metacarpal bone, left hand

● S62.348   Nondisplaced fracture of base of other metacarpal bone
> Nondisplaced fracture of base of specified metacarpal bone with unspecified laterality

● S62.349   Nondisplaced fracture of base of unspecified metacarpal bone

● S62.35   Nondisplaced fracture of shaft of other metacarpal bone

● S62.350   Nondisplaced fracture of shaft of second metacarpal bone, right hand

● S62.351   Nondisplaced fracture of shaft of second metacarpal bone, left hand

● S62.352   Nondisplaced fracture of shaft of third metacarpal bone, right hand

● S62.353   Nondisplaced fracture of shaft of third metacarpal bone, left hand

● S62.354   Nondisplaced fracture of shaft of fourth metacarpal bone, right hand

● S62.355   Nondisplaced fracture of shaft of fourth metacarpal bone, left hand

● S62.356   Nondisplaced fracture of shaft of fifth metacarpal bone, right hand

● S62.357   Nondisplaced fracture of shaft of fifth metacarpal bone, left hand

● S62.358   Nondisplaced fracture of shaft of other metacarpal bone
> Nondisplaced fracture of shaft of specified metacarpal bone with unspecified laterality

● S62.359   Nondisplaced fracture of shaft of unspecified metacarpal bone

CHAPTER 19 (S00–T88)

● **S62.36**   **Nondisplaced fracture of neck of other metacarpal bone**
- ● **S62.360**   Nondisplaced fracture of neck of second metacarpal bone, right hand
- ● **S62.361**   Nondisplaced fracture of neck of second metacarpal bone, left hand
- ● **S62.362**   Nondisplaced fracture of neck of third metacarpal bone, right hand
- ● **S62.363**   Nondisplaced fracture of neck of third metacarpal bone, left hand
- ● **S62.364**   Nondisplaced fracture of neck of fourth metacarpal bone, right hand
- ● **S62.365**   Nondisplaced fracture of neck of fourth metacarpal bone, left hand
- ● **S62.366**   Nondisplaced fracture of neck of fifth metacarpal bone, right hand
- ● **S62.367**   Nondisplaced fracture of neck of fifth metacarpal bone, left hand
- ● **S62.368**   Nondisplaced fracture of neck of other metacarpal bone
  - Nondisplaced fracture of neck of specified metacarpal bone with unspecified laterality
- ● **S62.369**   Nondisplaced fracture of neck of unspecified metacarpal bone

● **S62.39**   **Other fracture of other metacarpal bone**
- ● **S62.390**   Other fracture of second metacarpal bone, right hand
- ● **S62.391**   Other fracture of second metacarpal bone, left hand
- ● **S62.392**   Other fracture of third metacarpal bone, right hand
- ● **S62.393**   Other fracture of third metacarpal bone, left hand
- ● **S62.394**   Other fracture of fourth metacarpal bone, right hand
- ● **S62.395**   Other fracture of fourth metacarpal bone, left hand
- ● **S62.396**   Other fracture of fifth metacarpal bone, right hand
- ● **S62.397**   Other fracture of fifth metacarpal bone, left hand
- ● **S62.398**   Other fracture of other metacarpal bone
  - Other fracture of specified metacarpal bone with unspecified laterality
- ● **S62.399**   Other fracture of unspecified metacarpal bone

● **S62.5**   **Fracture of thumb**
- ● **S62.50**   **Fracture of unspecified phalanx of thumb**
  - ● **S62.501**   Fracture of unspecified phalanx of right thumb
  - ● **S62.502**   Fracture of unspecified phalanx of left thumb
  - ● **S62.509**   Fracture of unspecified phalanx of unspecified thumb
- ● **S62.51**   **Fracture of proximal phalanx of thumb**
  - ● **S62.511**   Displaced fracture of proximal phalanx of right thumb
  - ● **S62.512**   Displaced fracture of proximal phalanx of left thumb
  - ● **S62.513**   Displaced fracture of proximal phalanx of unspecified thumb
  - ● **S62.514**   Nondisplaced fracture of proximal phalanx of right thumb
  - ● **S62.515**   Nondisplaced fracture of proximal phalanx of left thumb
  - ● **S62.516**   Nondisplaced fracture of proximal phalanx of unspecified thumb

● **S62.52**   **Fracture of distal phalanx of thumb**
- ● **S62.521**   Displaced fracture of distal phalanx of right thumb
- ● **S62.522**   Displaced fracture of distal phalanx of left thumb
- ● **S62.523**   Displaced fracture of distal phalanx of unspecified thumb
- ● **S62.524**   Nondisplaced fracture of distal phalanx of right thumb
- ● **S62.525**   Nondisplaced fracture of distal phalanx of left thumb
- ● **S62.526**   Nondisplaced fracture of distal phalanx of unspecified thumb

● **S62.6**   **Fracture of other and unspecified finger(s)**
    Excludes2   fracture of thumb (S62.5-)
- ● **S62.60**   **Fracture of unspecified phalanx of finger**
  - ● **S62.600**   Fracture of unspecified phalanx of right index finger
  - ● **S62.601**   Fracture of unspecified phalanx of left index finger
  - ● **S62.602**   Fracture of unspecified phalanx of right middle finger
  - ● **S62.603**   Fracture of unspecified phalanx of left middle finger
  - ● **S62.604**   Fracture of unspecified phalanx of right ring finger
  - ● **S62.605**   Fracture of unspecified phalanx of left ring finger
  - ● **S62.606**   Fracture of unspecified phalanx of right little finger
  - ● **S62.607**   Fracture of unspecified phalanx of left little finger
  - ● **S62.608**   Fracture of unspecified phalanx of other finger
    - Fracture of unspecified phalanx of specified finger with unspecified laterality
  - ● **S62.609**   Fracture of unspecified phalanx of unspecified finger
- ● **S62.61**   **Displaced fracture of proximal phalanx of finger**
  - ● **S62.610**   Displaced fracture of proximal phalanx of right index finger
  - ● **S62.611**   Displaced fracture of proximal phalanx of left index finger
  - ● **S62.612**   Displaced fracture of proximal phalanx of right middle finger
  - ● **S62.613**   Displaced fracture of proximal phalanx of left middle finger
  - ● **S62.614**   Displaced fracture of proximal phalanx of right ring finger
  - ● **S62.615**   Displaced fracture of proximal phalanx of left ring finger
  - ● **S62.616**   Displaced fracture of proximal phalanx of right little finger
  - ● **S62.617**   Displaced fracture of proximal phalanx of left little finger
  - ● **S62.618**   Displaced fracture of proximal phalanx of other finger
    - Displaced fracture of proximal phalanx of specified finger with unspecified laterality
  - ● **S62.619**   Displaced fracture of proximal phalanx of unspecified finger

● S62.62   Displaced fracture of medial phalanx of finger
> ● S62.620   Displaced fracture of medial phalanx of right index finger
> ● S62.621   Displaced fracture of medial phalanx of left index finger
> ● S62.622   Displaced fracture of medial phalanx of right middle finger
> ● S62.623   Displaced fracture of medial phalanx of left middle finger
> ● S62.624   Displaced fracture of medial phalanx of right ring finger
> ● S62.625   Displaced fracture of medial phalanx of left ring finger
> ● S62.626   Displaced fracture of medial phalanx of right little finger
> ● S62.627   Displaced fracture of medial phalanx of left little finger
> ● S62.628   Displaced fracture of medial phalanx of other finger
> > Displaced fracture of medial phalanx of specified finger with unspecified laterality
> ● S62.629   Displaced fracture of medial phalanx of unspecified finger

● S62.63   Displaced fracture of distal phalanx of finger
> ● S62.630   Displaced fracture of distal phalanx of right index finger
> ● S62.631   Displaced fracture of distal phalanx of left index finger
> ● S62.632   Displaced fracture of distal phalanx of right middle finger
> ● S62.633   Displaced fracture of distal phalanx of left middle finger
> ● S62.634   Displaced fracture of distal phalanx of right ring finger
> ● S62.635   Displaced fracture of distal phalanx of left ring finger
> ● S62.636   Displaced fracture of distal phalanx of right little finger
> ● S62.637   Displaced fracture of distal phalanx of left little finger
> ● S62.638   Displaced fracture of distal phalanx of other finger
> > Displaced fracture of distal phalanx of specified finger with unspecified laterality
> ● S62.639   Displaced fracture of distal phalanx of unspecified finger

● S62.64   Nondisplaced fracture of proximal phalanx of finger
> ● S62.640   Nondisplaced fracture of proximal phalanx of right index finger
> ● S62.641   Nondisplaced fracture of proximal phalanx of left index finger
> ● S62.642   Nondisplaced fracture of proximal phalanx of right middle finger
> ● S62.643   Nondisplaced fracture of proximal phalanx of left middle finger
> ● S62.644   Nondisplaced fracture of proximal phalanx of right ring finger
> ● S62.645   Nondisplaced fracture of proximal phalanx of left ring finger
> ● S62.646   Nondisplaced fracture of proximal phalanx of right little finger

> ● S62.647   Nondisplaced fracture of proximal phalanx of left little finger
> ● S62.648   Nondisplaced fracture of proximal phalanx of other finger
> > Nondisplaced fracture of proximal phalanx of specified finger with unspecified laterality
> ● S62.649   Nondisplaced fracture of proximal phalanx of unspecified finger

● S62.65   Nondisplaced fracture of medial phalanx of finger
> ● S62.650   Nondisplaced fracture of medial phalanx of right index finger
> ● S62.651   Nondisplaced fracture of medial phalanx of left index finger
> ● S62.652   Nondisplaced fracture of medial phalanx of right middle finger
> ● S62.653   Nondisplaced fracture of medial phalanx of left middle finger
> ● S62.654   Nondisplaced fracture of medial phalanx of right ring finger
> ● S62.655   Nondisplaced fracture of medial phalanx of left ring finger
> ● S62.656   Nondisplaced fracture of medial phalanx of right little finger
> ● S62.657   Nondisplaced fracture of medial phalanx of left little finger
> ● S62.658   Nondisplaced fracture of medial phalanx of other finger
> > Nondisplaced fracture of medial phalanx of specified finger with unspecified laterality
> ● S62.659   Nondisplaced fracture of medial phalanx of unspecified finger

● S62.66   Nondisplaced fracture of distal phalanx of finger
> ● S62.660   Nondisplaced fracture of distal phalanx of right index finger
> ● S62.661   Nondisplaced fracture of distal phalanx of left index finger
> ● S62.662   Nondisplaced fracture of distal phalanx of right middle finger
> ● S62.663   Nondisplaced fracture of distal phalanx of left middle finger
> ● S62.664   Nondisplaced fracture of distal phalanx of right ring finger
> ● S62.665   Nondisplaced fracture of distal phalanx of left ring finger
> ● S62.666   Nondisplaced fracture of distal phalanx of right little finger
> ● S62.667   Nondisplaced fracture of distal phalanx of left little finger
> ● S62.668   Nondisplaced fracture of distal phalanx of other finger
> > Nondisplaced fracture of distal phalanx of specified finger with unspecified laterality
> ● S62.669   Nondisplaced fracture of distal phalanx of unspecified finger

● S62.9   Unspecified fracture of wrist and hand
> X ● S62.90   Unspecified fracture of unspecified wrist and hand
> X ● S62.91   Unspecified fracture of right wrist and hand
> X ● S62.92   Unspecified fracture of left wrist and hand

CHAPTER 19 (S00–T88)

A   B

Figure 19-14 Dislocation including displacement and subluxation. (From Grainger & Allison's Diagnostic Radiology: A Textbook of Medical Imaging, ed 4, Churchill Livingstone, 2001)

● S63   **Dislocation and sprain of joints and ligaments at wrist and hand level**

Includes   avulsion of joint or ligament at wrist and hand level

laceration of cartilage, joint or ligament at wrist and hand level

sprain of cartilage, joint or ligament at wrist and hand level

traumatic hemarthrosis of joint or ligament at wrist and hand level

traumatic rupture of joint or ligament at wrist and hand level

traumatic subluxation of joint or ligament at wrist and hand level

traumatic tear of joint or ligament at wrist and hand level

Code also any associated open wound

Excludes2   strain of muscle, fascia and tendon of wrist and hand (S66.-)

The appropriate 7th character is to be added to each code from category S63

A	initial encounter
D	subsequent encounter
S	sequela

● S63.0   **Subluxation and dislocation of wrist and hand joints**

● S63.00   **Unspecified subluxation and dislocation of wrist and hand**

Dislocation of carpal bone NOS

Dislocation of distal end of radius NOS

Subluxation of carpal bone NOS

Subluxation of distal end of radius NOS

● S63.001   **Unspecified** subluxation of right wrist and hand

● S63.002   **Unspecified** subluxation of left wrist and hand

● S63.003   **Unspecified** subluxation of unspecified wrist and hand

● S63.004   **Unspecified** dislocation of right wrist and hand

● S63.005   **Unspecified** dislocation of left wrist and hand

● S63.006   **Unspecified** dislocation of unspecified wrist and hand

● S63.01   **Subluxation and dislocation of distal radioulnar joint**

● S63.011   Subluxation of distal radioulnar joint of right wrist

● S63.012   Subluxation of distal radioulnar joint of left wrist

● S63.013   Subluxation of distal radioulnar joint of **unspecified** wrist

● S63.014   Dislocation of distal radioulnar joint of right wrist

● S63.015   Dislocation of distal radioulnar joint of left wrist

● S63.016   Dislocation of distal radioulnar joint of **unspecified** wrist

● S63.02   **Subluxation and dislocation of radiocarpal joint**

● S63.021   Subluxation of radiocarpal joint of right wrist

● S63.022   Subluxation of radiocarpal joint of left wrist

● S63.023   Subluxation of radiocarpal joint of **unspecified** wrist

● S63.024   Dislocation of radiocarpal joint of right wrist

● S63.025   Dislocation of radiocarpal joint of left wrist

● S63.026   Dislocation of radiocarpal joint of **unspecified** wrist

● S63.03   **Subluxation and dislocation of midcarpal joint**

● S63.031   Subluxation of midcarpal joint of right wrist

● S63.032   Subluxation of midcarpal joint of left wrist

● S63.033   Subluxation of midcarpal joint of **unspecified** wrist

● S63.034   Dislocation of midcarpal joint of right wrist

● S63.035   Dislocation of midcarpal joint of left wrist

● S63.036   Dislocation of midcarpal joint of **unspecified** wrist

● S63.04   **Subluxation and dislocation of carpometacarpal joint of thumb**

Excludes2   interphalangeal subluxation and dislocation of thumb (S63.1-)

● S63.041   Subluxation of carpometacarpal joint of right thumb

● S63.042   Subluxation of carpometacarpal joint of left thumb

● S63.043   Subluxation of carpometacarpal joint of **unspecified** thumb

● S63.044   Dislocation of carpometacarpal joint of right thumb

● S63.045   Dislocation of carpometacarpal joint of left thumb

● S63.046   Dislocation of carpometacarpal joint of **unspecified** thumb

● S63.05   **Subluxation and dislocation of other carpometacarpal joint**

Excludes2   subluxation and dislocation of carpometacarpal joint of thumb (S63.04-)

● S63.051   Subluxation of other carpometacarpal joint of right hand

● S63.052   Subluxation of other carpometacarpal joint of left hand

● S63.053   Subluxation of other carpometacarpal joint of **unspecified** hand

● S63.054   Dislocation of other carpometacarpal joint of right hand

● S63.055   Dislocation of other carpometacarpal joint of left hand

● S63.056   Dislocation of other carpometacarpal joint of **unspecified** hand

- S63.06   Subluxation and dislocation of metacarpal (bone), proximal end
  - S63.061   Subluxation of metacarpal (bone), proximal end of right hand
  - S63.062   Subluxation of metacarpal (bone), proximal end of left hand
  - S63.063   Subluxation of metacarpal (bone), proximal end of unspecified hand
  - S63.064   Dislocation of metacarpal (bone), proximal end of right hand
  - S63.065   Dislocation of metacarpal (bone), proximal end of left hand
  - S63.066   Dislocation of metacarpal (bone), proximal end of unspecified hand
- S63.07   Subluxation and dislocation of distal end of ulna
  - S63.071   Subluxation of distal end of right ulna
  - S63.072   Subluxation of distal end of left ulna
  - S63.073   Subluxation of distal end of unspecified ulna
  - S63.074   Dislocation of distal end of right ulna
  - S63.075   Dislocation of distal end of left ulna
  - S63.076   Dislocation of distal end of unspecified ulna
- S63.09   Other subluxation and dislocation of wrist and hand
  - S63.091   Other subluxation of right wrist and hand
  - S63.092   Other subluxation of left wrist and hand
  - S63.093   Other subluxation of unspecified wrist and hand
  - S63.094   Other dislocation of right wrist and hand
  - S63.095   Other dislocation of left wrist and hand
  - S63.096   Other dislocation of unspecified wrist and hand
- S63.1   Subluxation and dislocation of thumb
  - S63.10   Unspecified subluxation and dislocation of thumb
    - S63.101   Unspecified subluxation of right thumb
    - S63.102   Unspecified subluxation of left thumb
    - S63.103   Unspecified subluxation of unspecified thumb
    - S63.104   Unspecified dislocation of right thumb
    - S63.105   Unspecified dislocation of left thumb
    - S63.106   Unspecified dislocation of unspecified thumb
  - S63.11   Subluxation and dislocation of metacarpophalangeal joint of thumb
    - S63.111   Subluxation of metacarpophalangeal joint of right thumb
    - S63.112   Subluxation of metacarpophalangeal joint of left thumb
    - S63.113   Subluxation of metacarpophalangeal joint of unspecified thumb
    - S63.114   Dislocation of metacarpophalangeal joint of right thumb
    - S63.115   Dislocation of metacarpophalangeal joint of left thumb
    - S63.116   Dislocation of metacarpophalangeal joint of unspecified thumb
  - S63.12   Subluxation and dislocation of unspecified interphalangeal joint of thumb
    - S63.121   Subluxation of unspecified interphalangeal joint of right thumb
    - S63.122   Subluxation of unspecified interphalangeal joint of left thumb

- S63.123   Subluxation of unspecified interphalangeal joint of unspecified thumb
- S63.124   Dislocation of unspecified interphalangeal joint of right thumb
- S63.125   Dislocation of unspecified interphalangeal joint of left thumb
- S63.126   Dislocation of unspecified interphalangeal joint of unspecified thumb
- S63.13   Subluxation and dislocation of proximal interphalangeal joint of thumb
  - S63.131   Subluxation of proximal interphalangeal joint of right thumb
  - S63.132   Subluxation of proximal interphalangeal joint of left thumb
  - S63.133   Subluxation of proximal interphalangeal joint of unspecified thumb
  - S63.134   Dislocation of proximal interphalangeal joint of right thumb
  - S63.135   Dislocation of proximal interphalangeal joint of left thumb
  - S63.136   Dislocation of proximal interphalangeal joint of unspecified thumb
- S63.14   Subluxation and dislocation of distal interphalangeal joint of thumb
  - S63.141   Subluxation of distal interphalangeal joint of right thumb
  - S63.142   Subluxation of distal interphalangeal joint of left thumb
  - S63.143   Subluxation of distal interphalangeal joint of unspecified thumb
  - S63.144   Dislocation of distal interphalangeal joint of right thumb
  - S63.145   Dislocation of distal interphalangeal joint of left thumb
  - S63.146   Dislocation of distal interphalangeal joint of unspecified thumb
- S63.2   Subluxation and dislocation of other finger(s)
  - **Excludes2**   subluxation and dislocation of thumb (S63.1-)
  - S63.20   Unspecified subluxation of other finger
    - S63.200   Unspecified subluxation of right index finger
    - S63.201   Unspecified subluxation of left index finger
    - S63.202   Unspecified subluxation of right middle finger
    - S63.203   Unspecified subluxation of left middle finger
    - S63.204   Unspecified subluxation of right ring finger
    - S63.205   Unspecified subluxation of left ring finger
    - S63.206   Unspecified subluxation of right little finger
    - S63.207   Unspecified subluxation of left little finger
    - S63.208   Unspecified subluxation of other finger
      Unspecified subluxation of specified finger with unspecified laterality
    - S63.209   Unspecified subluxation of unspecified finger

● **S63.21** Subluxation of metacarpophalangeal joint of finger

  ● **S63.210** Subluxation of metacarpophalangeal joint of right index finger

  ● **S63.211** Subluxation of metacarpophalangeal joint of left index finger

  ● **S63.212** Subluxation of metacarpophalangeal joint of right middle finger

  ● **S63.213** Subluxation of metacarpophalangeal joint of left middle finger

  ● **S63.214** Subluxation of metacarpophalangeal joint of right ring finger

  ● **S63.215** Subluxation of metacarpophalangeal joint of left ring finger

  ● **S63.216** Subluxation of metacarpophalangeal joint of right little finger

  ● **S63.217** Subluxation of metacarpophalangeal joint of left little finger

  ● **S63.218** Subluxation of metacarpophalangeal joint of other finger
    Subluxation of metacarpophalangeal joint of specified finger with unspecified laterality

  ● **S63.219** Subluxation of metacarpophalangeal joint of unspecified finger

● **S63.22** Subluxation of unspecified interphalangeal joint of finger

  ● **S63.220** Subluxation of unspecified interphalangeal joint of right index finger

  ● **S63.221** Subluxation of unspecified interphalangeal joint of left index finger

  ● **S63.222** Subluxation of unspecified interphalangeal joint of right middle finger

  ● **S63.223** Subluxation of unspecified interphalangeal joint of left middle finger

  ● **S63.224** Subluxation of unspecified interphalangeal joint of right ring finger

  ● **S63.225** Subluxation of unspecified interphalangeal joint of left ring finger

  ● **S63.226** Subluxation of unspecified interphalangeal joint of right little finger

  ● **S63.227** Subluxation of unspecified interphalangeal joint of left little finger

  ● **S63.228** Subluxation of unspecified interphalangeal joint of other finger
    Subluxation of unspecified interphalangeal joint of specified finger with unspecified laterality

  ● **S63.229** Subluxation of unspecified interphalangeal joint of unspecified finger

● **S63.23** Subluxation of proximal interphalangeal joint of finger

  ● **S63.230** Subluxation of proximal interphalangeal joint of right index finger

  ● **S63.231** Subluxation of proximal interphalangeal joint of left index finger

  ● **S63.232** Subluxation of proximal interphalangeal joint of right middle finger

  ● **S63.233** Subluxation of proximal interphalangeal joint of left middle finger

  ● **S63.234** Subluxation of proximal interphalangeal joint of right ring finger

  ● **S63.235** Subluxation of proximal interphalangeal joint of left ring finger

  ● **S63.236** Subluxation of proximal interphalangeal joint of right little finger

  ● **S63.237** Subluxation of proximal interphalangeal joint of left little finger

  ● **S63.238** Subluxation of proximal interphalangeal joint of other finger
    Subluxation of proximal interphalangeal joint of specified finger with unspecified laterality

  ● **S63.239** Subluxation of proximal interphalangeal joint of unspecified finger

● **S63.24** Subluxation of distal interphalangeal joint of finger

  ● **S63.240** Subluxation of distal interphalangeal joint of right index finger

  ● **S63.241** Subluxation of distal interphalangeal joint of left index finger

  ● **S63.242** Subluxation of distal interphalangeal joint of right middle finger

  ● **S63.243** Subluxation of distal interphalangeal joint of left middle finger

  ● **S63.244** Subluxation of distal interphalangeal joint of right ring finger

  ● **S63.245** Subluxation of distal interphalangeal joint of left ring finger

  ● **S63.246** Subluxation of distal interphalangeal joint of right little finger

  ● **S63.247** Subluxation of distal interphalangeal joint of left little finger

  ● **S63.248** Subluxation of distal interphalangeal joint of other finger
    Subluxation of distal interphalangeal joint of specified finger with unspecified laterality

  ● **S63.249** Subluxation of distal interphalangeal joint of unspecified finger

● **S63.25** Unspecified dislocation of other finger

  ● **S63.250** Unspecified dislocation of right index finger

  ● **S63.251** Unspecified dislocation of left index finger

  ● **S63.252** Unspecified dislocation of right middle finger

  ● **S63.253** Unspecified dislocation of left middle finger

  ● **S63.254** Unspecified dislocation of right ring finger

  ● **S63.255** Unspecified dislocation of left ring finger

  ● **S63.256** Unspecified dislocation of right little finger

  ● **S63.257** Unspecified dislocation of left little finger

● S63.258   Unspecified dislocation of other finger
> Unspecified dislocation of specified finger with unspecified laterality

● S63.259   Unspecified dislocation of unspecified finger
> Unspecified dislocation of specified finger with unspecified laterality

● S63.26   Dislocation of metacarpophalangeal joint of finger

● S63.260   Dislocation of metacarpophalangeal joint of right index finger

● S63.261   Dislocation of metacarpophalangeal joint of left index finger

● S63.262   Dislocation of metacarpophalangeal joint of right middle finger

● S63.263   Dislocation of metacarpophalangeal joint of left middle finger

● S63.264   Dislocation of metacarpophalangeal joint of right ring finger

● S63.265   Dislocation of metacarpophalangeal joint of left ring finger

● S63.266   Dislocation of metacarpophalangeal joint of right little finger

● S63.267   Dislocation of metacarpophalangeal joint of left little finger

● S63.268   Dislocation of metacarpophalangeal joint of other finger
> Dislocation of metacarpophalangeal joint of specified finger with unspecified laterality

● S63.269   Dislocation of metacarpophalangeal joint of unspecified finger

● S63.27   Dislocation of unspecified interphalangeal joint of finger

● S63.270   Dislocation of unspecified interphalangeal joint of right index finger

● S63.271   Dislocation of unspecified interphalangeal joint of left index finger

● S63.272   Dislocation of unspecified interphalangeal joint of right middle finger

● S63.273   Dislocation of unspecified interphalangeal joint of left middle finger

● S63.274   Dislocation of unspecified interphalangeal joint of right ring finger

● S63.275   Dislocation of unspecified interphalangeal joint of left ring finger

● S63.276   Dislocation of unspecified interphalangeal joint of right little finger

● S63.277   Dislocation of unspecified interphalangeal joint of left little finger

● S63.278   Dislocation of unspecified interphalangeal joint of other finger
> Dislocation of unspecified interphalangeal joint of specified finger with unspecified laterality

● S63.279   Dislocation of unspecified interphalangeal joint of unspecified finger
> Dislocation of unspecified interphalangeal joint of specified finger without specified laterality

● S63.28   Dislocation of proximal interphalangeal joint of finger

● S63.280   Dislocation of proximal interphalangeal joint of right index finger

● S63.281   Dislocation of proximal interphalangeal joint of left index finger

● S63.282   Dislocation of proximal interphalangeal joint of right middle finger

● S63.283   Dislocation of proximal interphalangeal joint of left middle finger

● S63.284   Dislocation of proximal interphalangeal joint of right ring finger

● S63.285   Dislocation of proximal interphalangeal joint of left ring finger

● S63.286   Dislocation of proximal interphalangeal joint of right little finger

● S63.287   Dislocation of proximal interphalangeal joint of left little finger

● S63.288   Dislocation of proximal interphalangeal joint of other finger
> Dislocation of proximal interphalangeal joint of specified finger with unspecified laterality

● S63.289   Dislocation of proximal interphalangeal joint of unspecified finger

● S63.29   Dislocation of distal interphalangeal joint of finger

● S63.290   Dislocation of distal interphalangeal joint of right index finger

● S63.291   Dislocation of distal interphalangeal joint of left index finger

● S63.292   Dislocation of distal interphalangeal joint of right middle finger

● S63.293   Dislocation of distal interphalangeal joint of left middle finger

● S63.294   Dislocation of distal interphalangeal joint of right ring finger

● S63.295   Dislocation of distal interphalangeal joint of left ring finger

● S63.296   Dislocation of distal interphalangeal joint of right little finger

● S63.297   Dislocation of distal interphalangeal joint of left little finger

● S63.298   Dislocation of distal interphalangeal joint of other finger
> Dislocation of distal interphalangeal joint of specified finger with unspecified laterality

● S63.299   Dislocation of distal interphalangeal joint of unspecified finger

● S63.3   Traumatic rupture of ligament of wrist

● S63.30   Traumatic rupture of unspecified ligament of wrist

● S63.301   Traumatic rupture of unspecified ligament of right wrist

● S63.302   Traumatic rupture of unspecified ligament of left wrist

● S63.309   Traumatic rupture of unspecified ligament of unspecified wrist

● S63.31   Traumatic rupture of collateral ligament of wrist
  - ● S63.311   Traumatic rupture of collateral ligament of right wrist
  - ● S63.312   Traumatic rupture of collateral ligament of left wrist
  - ● S63.319   Traumatic rupture of collateral ligament of unspecified wrist

● S63.32   Traumatic rupture of radiocarpal ligament
  - ● S63.321   Traumatic rupture of right radiocarpal ligament
  - ● S63.322   Traumatic rupture of left radiocarpal ligament
  - ● S63.329   Traumatic rupture of unspecified radiocarpal ligament

● S63.33   Traumatic rupture of ulnocarpal (palmar) ligament
  - ● S63.331   Traumatic rupture of right ulnocarpal (palmar) ligament
  - ● S63.332   Traumatic rupture of left ulnocarpal (palmar) ligament
  - ● S63.339   Traumatic rupture of unspecified ulnocarpal (palmar) ligament

● S63.39   Traumatic rupture of other ligament of wrist
  - ● S63.391   Traumatic rupture of other ligament of right wrist
  - ● S63.392   Traumatic rupture of other ligament of left wrist
  - ● S63.399   Traumatic rupture of other ligament of unspecified wrist

● S63.4   Traumatic rupture of ligament of finger at metacarpophalangeal and interphalangeal joint(s)

● S63.40   Traumatic rupture of unspecified ligament of finger at metacarpophalangeal and interphalangeal joint
  - ● S63.400   Traumatic rupture of unspecified ligament of right index finger at metacarpophalangeal and interphalangeal joint
  - ● S63.401   Traumatic rupture of unspecified ligament of left index finger at metacarpophalangeal and interphalangeal joint
  - ● S63.402   Traumatic rupture of unspecified ligament of right middle finger at metacarpophalangeal and interphalangeal joint
  - ● S63.403   Traumatic rupture of unspecified ligament of left middle finger at metacarpophalangeal and interphalangeal joint
  - ● S63.404   Traumatic rupture of unspecified ligament of right ring finger at metacarpophalangeal and interphalangeal joint
  - ● S63.405   Traumatic rupture of unspecified ligament of left ring finger at metacarpophalangeal and interphalangeal joint
  - ● S63.406   Traumatic rupture of unspecified ligament of right little finger at metacarpophalangeal and interphalangeal joint
  - ● S63.407   Traumatic rupture of unspecified ligament of left little finger at metacarpophalangeal and interphalangeal joint

  - ● S63.408   Traumatic rupture of unspecified ligament of other finger at metacarpophalangeal and interphalangeal joint
      Traumatic rupture of unspecified ligament of specified finger with unspecified laterality at metacarpophalangeal and interphalangeal joint
  - ● S63.409   Traumatic rupture of unspecified ligament of unspecified finger at metacarpophalangeal and interphalangeal joint

● S63.41   Traumatic rupture of collateral ligament of finger at metacarpophalangeal and interphalangeal joint
  - ● S63.410   Traumatic rupture of collateral ligament of right index finger at metacarpophalangeal and interphalangeal joint
  - ● S63.411   Traumatic rupture of collateral ligament of left index finger at metacarpophalangeal and interphalangeal joint
  - ● S63.412   Traumatic rupture of collateral ligament of right middle finger at metacarpophalangeal and interphalangeal joint
  - ● S63.413   Traumatic rupture of collateral ligament of left middle finger at metacarpophalangeal and interphalangeal joint
  - ● S63.414   Traumatic rupture of collateral ligament of right ring finger at metacarpophalangeal and interphalangeal joint
  - ● S63.415   Traumatic rupture of collateral ligament of left ring finger at metacarpophalangeal and interphalangeal joint
  - ● S63.416   Traumatic rupture of collateral ligament of right little finger at metacarpophalangeal and interphalangeal joint
  - ● S63.417   Traumatic rupture of collateral ligament of left little finger at metacarpophalangeal and interphalangeal joint
  - ● S63.418   Traumatic rupture of collateral ligament of other finger at metacarpophalangeal and interphalangeal joint
      Traumatic rupture of collateral ligament of specified finger with unspecified laterality at metacarpophalangeal and interphalangeal joint
  - ● S63.419   Traumatic rupture of collateral ligament of unspecified finger at metacarpophalangeal and interphalangeal joint

● S63.42   Traumatic rupture of palmar ligament of finger at metacarpophalangeal and interphalangeal joint
  - ● S63.420   Traumatic rupture of palmar ligament of right index finger at metacarpophalangeal and interphalangeal joint
  - ● S63.421   Traumatic rupture of palmar ligament of left index finger at metacarpophalangeal and interphalangeal joint

◄ New   ◄ Revised   deleted Deleted   Excludes 1   Excludes 2   Includes   Use additional   Code first   Code also   Unspecified

OGCR Official Guidelines   X Assign placeholder X   ● Use Additional Character(s)   ▶ Manifestation Code   Coding Clinic

● S63.422   Traumatic rupture of palmar
             ligament of right middle finger
             at metacarpophalangeal and
             interphalangeal joint

● S63.423   Traumatic rupture of palmar
             ligament of left middle finger
             at metacarpophalangeal and
             interphalangeal joint

● S63.424   Traumatic rupture of palmar
             ligament of right ring finger
             at metacarpophalangeal and
             interphalangeal joint

● S63.425   Traumatic rupture of palmar
             ligament of left ring finger
             at metacarpophalangeal and
             interphalangeal joint

● S63.426   Traumatic rupture of palmar
             ligament of right little finger
             at metacarpophalangeal and
             interphalangeal joint

● S63.427   Traumatic rupture of palmar
             ligament of left little finger
             at metacarpophalangeal and
             interphalangeal joint

● S63.428   Traumatic rupture of palmar
             ligament of other finger at
             metacarpophalangeal and
             interphalangeal joint
             Traumatic rupture of palmar
                ligament of specified finger
                with unspecified laterality
                at metacarpophalangeal and
                interphalangeal joint

● S63.429   Traumatic rupture of palmar
             ligament of unspecified finger
             at metacarpophalangeal and
             interphalangeal joint

● S63.43   Traumatic rupture of volar plate of finger at
            metacarpophalangeal and interphalangeal joint

● S63.430   Traumatic rupture of volar
             plate of right index finger at
             metacarpophalangeal and
             interphalangeal joint

● S63.431   Traumatic rupture of volar
             plate of left index finger at
             metacarpophalangeal and
             interphalangeal joint

● S63.432   Traumatic rupture of volar
             plate of right middle finger
             at metacarpophalangeal and
             interphalangeal joint

● S63.433   Traumatic rupture of volar
             plate of left middle finger at
             metacarpophalangeal and
             interphalangeal joint

● S63.434   Traumatic rupture of volar
             plate of right ring finger at
             metacarpophalangeal and
             interphalangeal joint

● S63.435   Traumatic rupture of volar
             plate of left ring finger at
             metacarpophalangeal and
             interphalangeal joint

● S63.436   Traumatic rupture of volar
             plate of right little finger at
             metacarpophalangeal and
             interphalangeal joint

● S63.437   Traumatic rupture of volar
             plate of left little finger at
             metacarpophalangeal and
             interphalangeal joint

● S63.438   Traumatic rupture of volar plate of
             other finger at metacarpophalangeal
             and interphalangeal joint
             Traumatic rupture of volar plate
                of specified finger with
                unspecified laterality at
                metacarpophalangeal and
                interphalangeal joint

● S63.439   Traumatic rupture of volar
             plate of unspecified finger
             at metacarpophalangeal and
             interphalangeal joint

● S63.49   Traumatic rupture of other ligament of finger at
            metacarpophalangeal and interphalangeal joint

● S63.490   Traumatic rupture of other
             ligament of right index finger
             at metacarpophalangeal and
             interphalangeal joint

● S63.491   Traumatic rupture of other
             ligament of left index finger
             at metacarpophalangeal and
             interphalangeal joint

● S63.492   Traumatic rupture of other
             ligament of right middle finger
             at metacarpophalangeal and
             interphalangeal joint

● S63.493   Traumatic rupture of other
             ligament of left middle finger
             at metacarpophalangeal and
             interphalangeal joint

● S63.494   Traumatic rupture of other
             ligament of right ring finger
             at metacarpophalangeal and
             interphalangeal joint

● S63.495   Traumatic rupture of other
             ligament of left ring finger
             at metacarpophalangeal and
             interphalangeal joint

● S63.496   Traumatic rupture of other
             ligament of right little finger
             at metacarpophalangeal and
             interphalangeal joint

● S63.497   Traumatic rupture of other
             ligament of left little finger
             at metacarpophalangeal and
             interphalangeal joint

● S63.498   Traumatic rupture of other
             ligament of other finger at
             metacarpophalangeal and
             interphalangeal joint
             Traumatic rupture of ligament
                of specified finger with
                unspecified laterality at
                metacarpophalangeal and
                interphalangeal joint

● S63.499   Traumatic rupture of other
             ligament of unspecified finger
             at metacarpophalangeal and
             interphalangeal joint

● S63.5   Other and unspecified sprain of wrist

● S63.50   Unspecified sprain of wrist

● S63.501   Unspecified sprain of right wrist
● S63.502   Unspecified sprain of left wrist
● S63.509   Unspecified sprain of unspecified
             wrist

● S63.51   Sprain of carpal (joint)

● S63.511   Sprain of carpal joint of right wrist
● S63.512   Sprain of carpal joint of left wrist
● S63.519   Sprain of carpal joint of unspecified
             wrist

- **S63.52**   Sprain of radiocarpal joint
  - **Excludes1**   traumatic rupture of radiocarpal ligament (S63.32-)
  - S63.521   Sprain of radiocarpal joint of right wrist
  - S63.522   Sprain of radiocarpal joint of left wrist
  - S63.529   Sprain of radiocarpal joint of unspecified wrist
- **S63.59**   Other specified sprain of wrist
  - S63.591   Other specified sprain of right wrist
  - S63.592   Other specified sprain of left wrist
  - S63.599   Other specified sprain of unspecified wrist
- **S63.6**   Other and unspecified sprain of finger(s)
  - **Excludes1**   traumatic rupture of ligament of finger at metacarpophalangeal and interphalangeal joint(s) (S63.4-)
  - **S63.60**   Unspecified sprain of thumb
    - S63.601   Unspecified sprain of right thumb
    - S63.602   Unspecified sprain of left thumb
    - S63.609   Unspecified sprain of unspecified thumb
  - **S63.61**   Unspecified sprain of other and unspecified finger(s)
    - S63.610   Unspecified sprain of right index finger
    - S63.611   Unspecified sprain of left index finger
    - S63.612   Unspecified sprain of right middle finger
    - S63.613   Unspecified sprain of left middle finger
    - S63.614   Unspecified sprain of right ring finger
    - S63.615   Unspecified sprain of left ring finger
    - S63.616   Unspecified sprain of right little finger
    - S63.617   Unspecified sprain of left little finger
    - S63.618   Unspecified sprain of other finger
      - Unspecified sprain of specified finger with unspecified laterality
    - S63.619   Unspecified sprain of unspecified finger
  - **S63.62**   Sprain of interphalangeal joint of thumb
    - S63.621   Sprain of interphalangeal joint of right thumb
    - S63.622   Sprain of interphalangeal joint of left thumb
    - S63.629   Sprain of interphalangeal joint of unspecified thumb
  - **S63.63**   Sprain of interphalangeal joint of other and unspecified finger(s)
    - S63.630   Sprain of interphalangeal joint of right index finger
    - S63.631   Sprain of interphalangeal joint of left index finger
    - S63.632   Sprain of interphalangeal joint of right middle finger
    - S63.633   Sprain of interphalangeal joint of left middle finger
    - S63.634   Sprain of interphalangeal joint of right ring finger
    - S63.635   Sprain of interphalangeal joint of left ring finger
    - S63.636   Sprain of interphalangeal joint of right little finger
    - S63.637   Sprain of interphalangeal joint of left little finger
    - S63.638   Sprain of interphalangeal joint of other finger
    - S63.639   Sprain of interphalangeal joint of unspecified finger
- **S63.64**   Sprain of metacarpophalangeal joint of thumb
  - S63.641   Sprain of metacarpophalangeal joint of right thumb
  - S63.642   Sprain of metacarpophalangeal joint of left thumb
  - S63.649   Sprain of metacarpophalangeal joint of unspecified thumb
- **S63.65**   Sprain of metacarpophalangeal joint of other and unspecified finger(s)
  - S63.650   Sprain of metacarpophalangeal joint of right index finger
  - S63.651   Sprain of metacarpophalangeal joint of left index finger
  - S63.652   Sprain of metacarpophalangeal joint of right middle finger
  - S63.653   Sprain of metacarpophalangeal joint of left middle finger
  - S63.654   Sprain of metacarpophalangeal joint of right ring finger
  - S63.655   Sprain of metacarpophalangeal joint of left ring finger
  - S63.656   Sprain of metacarpophalangeal joint of right little finger
  - S63.657   Sprain of metacarpophalangeal joint of left little finger
  - S63.658   Sprain of metacarpophalangeal joint of other finger
    - Sprain of metacarpophalangeal joint of specified finger with unspecified laterality
  - S63.659   Sprain of metacarpophalangeal joint of unspecified finger
- **S63.68**   Other sprain of thumb
  - S63.681   Other sprain of right thumb
  - S63.682   Other sprain of left thumb
  - S63.689   Other sprain of unspecified thumb
- **S63.69**   Other sprain of other and unspecified finger(s)
  - S63.690   Other sprain of right index finger
  - S63.691   Other sprain of left index finger
  - S63.692   Other sprain of right middle finger
  - S63.693   Other sprain of left middle finger
  - S63.694   Other sprain of right ring finger
  - S63.695   Other sprain of left ring finger
  - S63.696   Other sprain of right little finger
  - S63.697   Other sprain of left little finger
  - S63.698   Other sprain of other finger
    - Other sprain of specified finger with unspecified laterality
  - S63.699   Other sprain of unspecified finger
- **S63.8**   Sprain of other part of wrist and hand
  - **S63.8X**   Sprain of other part of wrist and hand
    - S63.8X1   Sprain of other part of right wrist and hand
    - S63.8X2   Sprain of other part of left wrist and hand
    - S63.8X9   Sprain of other part of unspecified wrist and hand
- **S63.9**   Sprain of unspecified part of wrist and hand
  - X ● **S63.90**   Sprain of unspecified part of unspecified wrist and hand
  - X ● **S63.91**   Sprain of unspecified part of right wrist and hand
  - X ● **S63.92**   Sprain of unspecified part of left wrist and hand

◀ New   ◀ Revised   deleted Deleted   Excludes 1   Excludes 2   Includes   Use additional   Code first   Code also   Unspecified

1284   OGCR Official Guidelines   X Assign placeholder X   ● Use Additional Character(s)   ▶ Manifestation Code   **Coding Clinic**

● **S64 Injury of nerves at wrist and hand level**

The appropriate 7th character is to be added to each code from category S64

> A   initial encounter
> D   subsequent encounter
> S   sequela

Code also any associated open wound (S61.-)

● **S64.0 Injury of ulnar nerve at wrist and hand level**

  X● **S64.00** Injury of ulnar nerve at wrist and hand level of unspecified arm

  X● **S64.01** Injury of ulnar nerve at wrist and hand level of right arm

  X● **S64.02** Injury of ulnar nerve at wrist and hand level of left arm

● **S64.1 Injury of median nerve at wrist and hand level**

  X● **S64.10** Injury of median nerve at wrist and hand level of unspecified arm

  X● **S64.11** Injury of median nerve at wrist and hand level of right arm

  X● **S64.12** Injury of median nerve at wrist and hand level of left arm

● **S64.2 Injury of radial nerve at wrist and hand level**

  X● **S64.20** Injury of radial nerve at wrist and hand level of unspecified arm

  X● **S64.21** Injury of radial nerve at wrist and hand level of right arm

  X● **S64.22** Injury of radial nerve at wrist and hand level of left arm

● **S64.3 Injury of digital nerve of thumb**

  X● **S64.30** Injury of digital nerve of unspecified thumb

  X● **S64.31** Injury of digital nerve of right thumb

  X● **S64.32** Injury of digital nerve of left thumb

● **S64.4 Injury of digital nerve of other and unspecified finger**

  X● **S64.40** Injury of digital nerve of unspecified finger

  ● **S64.49** Injury of digital nerve of other finger

    ● **S64.490** Injury of digital nerve of right index finger

    ● **S64.491** Injury of digital nerve of left index finger

    ● **S64.492** Injury of digital nerve of right middle finger

    ● **S64.493** Injury of digital nerve of left middle finger

    ● **S64.494** Injury of digital nerve of right ring finger

    ● **S64.495** Injury of digital nerve of left ring finger

    ● **S64.496** Injury of digital nerve of right little finger

    ● **S64.497** Injury of digital nerve of left little finger

    ● **S64.498** Injury of digital nerve of other finger
             Injury of digital nerve of specified finger with unspecified laterality

● **S64.8 Injury of other nerves at wrist and hand level**

  ● **S64.8X** Injury of other nerves at wrist and hand level

    ● **S64.8X1** Injury of other nerves at wrist and hand level of right arm

    ● **S64.8X2** Injury of other nerves at wrist and hand level of left arm

    ● **S64.8X9** Injury of other nerves at wrist and hand level of unspecified arm

● **S64.9 Injury of unspecified nerve at wrist and hand level**

  X● **S64.90** Injury of unspecified nerve at wrist and hand level of unspecified arm

  X● **S64.91** Injury of unspecified nerve at wrist and hand level of right arm

  X● **S64.92** Injury of unspecified nerve at wrist and hand level of left arm

● **S65 Injury of blood vessels at wrist and hand level**

The appropriate 7th character is to be added to each code from category S65

> A   initial encounter
> D   subsequent encounter
> S   sequela

Code also any associated open wound (S61.-)

● **S65.0 Injury of ulnar artery at wrist and hand level**

  ● **S65.00** Unspecified injury of ulnar artery at wrist and hand level

    ● **S65.001** Unspecified injury of ulnar artery at wrist and hand level of right arm

    ● **S65.002** Unspecified injury of ulnar artery at wrist and hand level of left arm

    ● **S65.009** Unspecified injury of ulnar artery at wrist and hand level of unspecified arm

  ● **S65.01** Laceration of ulnar artery at wrist and hand level

    ● **S65.011** Laceration of ulnar artery at wrist and hand level of right arm

    ● **S65.012** Laceration of ulnar artery at wrist and hand level of left arm

    ● **S65.019** Laceration of ulnar artery at wrist and hand level of unspecified arm

  ● **S65.09** Other specified injury of ulnar artery at wrist and hand level

    ● **S65.091** Other specified injury of ulnar artery at wrist and hand level of right arm

    ● **S65.092** Other specified injury of ulnar artery at wrist and hand level of left arm

    ● **S65.099** Other specified injury of ulnar artery at wrist and hand level of unspecified arm

● **S65.1 Injury of radial artery at wrist and hand level**

  ● **S65.10** Unspecified injury of radial artery at wrist and hand level

    ● **S65.101** Unspecified injury of radial artery at wrist and hand level of right arm

    ● **S65.102** Unspecified injury of radial artery at wrist and hand level of left arm

    ● **S65.109** Unspecified injury of radial artery at wrist and hand level of unspecified arm

  ● **S65.11** Laceration of radial artery at wrist and hand level

    ● **S65.111** Laceration of radial artery at wrist and hand level of right arm

    ● **S65.112** Laceration of radial artery at wrist and hand level of left arm

    ● **S65.119** Laceration of radial artery at wrist and hand level of unspecified arm

  ● **S65.19** Other specified injury of radial artery at wrist and hand level

    ● **S65.191** Other specified injury of radial artery at wrist and hand level of right arm

    ● **S65.192** Other specified injury of radial artery at wrist and hand level of left arm

    ● **S65.199** Other specified injury of radial artery at wrist and hand level of unspecified arm

CHAPTER 19 (S00-T88)

CHAPTER 19 (S00-T88)

● S65.2   Injury of superficial palmar arch
  ● S65.20   Unspecified injury of superficial palmar arch
    ● S65.201   Unspecified injury of superficial palmar arch of right hand
    ● S65.202   Unspecified injury of superficial palmar arch of left hand
    ● S65.209   Unspecified injury of superficial palmar arch of unspecified hand
  ● S65.21   Laceration of superficial palmar arch
    ● S65.211   Laceration of superficial palmar arch of right hand
    ● S65.212   Laceration of superficial palmar arch of left hand
    ● S65.219   Laceration of superficial palmar arch of unspecified hand
  ● S65.29   Other specified injury of superficial palmar arch
    ● S65.291   Other specified injury of superficial palmar arch of right hand
    ● S65.292   Other specified injury of superficial palmar arch of left hand
    ● S65.299   Other specified injury of superficial palmar arch of unspecified hand
● S65.3   Injury of deep palmar arch
  ● S65.30   Unspecified injury of deep palmar arch
    ● S65.301   Unspecified injury of deep palmar arch of right hand
    ● S65.302   Unspecified injury of deep palmar arch of left hand
    ● S65.309   Unspecified injury of deep palmar arch of unspecified hand
  ● S65.31   Laceration of deep palmar arch
    ● S65.311   Laceration of deep palmar arch of right hand
    ● S65.312   Laceration of deep palmar arch of left hand
    ● S65.319   Laceration of deep palmar arch of unspecified hand
  ● S65.39   Other specified injury of deep palmar arch
    ● S65.391   Other specified injury of deep palmar arch of right hand
    ● S65.392   Other specified injury of deep palmar arch of left hand
    ● S65.399   Other specified injury of deep palmar arch of unspecified hand
● S65.4   Injury of blood vessel of thumb
  ● S65.40   Unspecified injury of blood vessel of thumb
    ● S65.401   Unspecified injury of blood vessel of right thumb
    ● S65.402   Unspecified injury of blood vessel of left thumb
    ● S65.409   Unspecified injury of blood vessel of unspecified thumb
  ● S65.41   Laceration of blood vessel of thumb
    ● S65.411   Laceration of blood vessel of right thumb
    ● S65.412   Laceration of blood vessel of left thumb
    ● S65.419   Laceration of blood vessel of unspecified thumb
  ● S65.49   Other specified injury of blood vessel of thumb
    ● S65.491   Other specified injury of blood vessel of right thumb
    ● S65.492   Other specified injury of blood vessel of left thumb
    ● S65.499   Other specified injury of blood vessel of unspecified thumb

● S65.5   Injury of blood vessel of other and unspecified finger
  ● S65.50   Unspecified injury of blood vessel of other and unspecified finger
    ● S65.500   Unspecified injury of blood vessel of right index finger
    ● S65.501   Unspecified injury of blood vessel of left index finger
    ● S65.502   Unspecified injury of blood vessel of right middle finger
    ● S65.503   Unspecified injury of blood vessel of left middle finger
    ● S65.504   Unspecified injury of blood vessel of right ring finger
    ● S65.505   Unspecified injury of blood vessel of left ring finger
    ● S65.506   Unspecified injury of blood vessel of right little finger
    ● S65.507   Unspecified injury of blood vessel of left little finger
    ● S65.508   Unspecified injury of blood vessel of other finger
      Unspecified injury of blood vessel of specified finger with unspecified laterality
    ● S65.509   Unspecified injury of blood vessel of unspecified finger
  ● S65.51   Laceration of blood vessel of other and unspecified finger
    ● S65.510   Laceration of blood vessel of right index finger
    ● S65.511   Laceration of blood vessel of left index finger
    ● S65.512   Laceration of blood vessel of right middle finger
    ● S65.513   Laceration of blood vessel of left middle finger
    ● S65.514   Laceration of blood vessel of right ring finger
    ● S65.515   Laceration of blood vessel of left ring finger
    ● S65.516   Laceration of blood vessel of right little finger
    ● S65.517   Laceration of blood vessel of left little finger
    ● S65.518   Laceration of blood vessel of other finger
      Laceration of blood vessel of specified finger with unspecified laterality
    ● S65.519   Laceration of blood vessel of unspecified finger
  ● S65.59   Other specified injury of blood vessel of other and unspecified finger
    ● S65.590   Other specified injury of blood vessel of right index finger
    ● S65.591   Other specified injury of blood vessel of left index finger
    ● S65.592   Other specified injury of blood vessel of right middle finger
    ● S65.593   Other specified injury of blood vessel of left middle finger
    ● S65.594   Other specified injury of blood vessel of right ring finger
    ● S65.595   Other specified injury of blood vessel of left ring finger

◀ New   ◀▥ Revised   deleted Deleted   Excludes 1   Excludes 2   Includes   Use additional   Code first   Code also   Unspecified
OGCR Official Guidelines   X Assign placeholder X   ● Use Additional Character(s)   ▶ Manifestation Code   **Coding Clinic**

S65.596   Other specified injury of blood vessel of right little finger

S65.597   Other specified injury of blood vessel of left little finger

S65.598   Other specified injury of blood vessel of other finger
Other specified injury of blood vessel of specified finger with unspecified laterality

S65.599   Other specified injury of blood vessel of unspecified finger

● S65.8   Injury of other blood vessels at wrist and hand level

● S65.80   Unspecified injury of other blood vessels at wrist and hand level

S65.801   Unspecified injury of other blood vessels at wrist and hand level of right arm

S65.802   Unspecified injury of other blood vessels at wrist and hand level of left arm

S65.809   Unspecified injury of other blood vessels at wrist and hand level of unspecified arm

● S65.81   Laceration of other blood vessels at wrist and hand level

S65.811   Laceration of other blood vessels at wrist and hand level of right arm

S65.812   Laceration of other blood vessels at wrist and hand level of left arm

S65.819   Laceration of other blood vessels at wrist and hand level of unspecified arm

● S65.89   Other specified injury of other blood vessels at wrist and hand level

S65.891   Other specified injury of other blood vessels at wrist and hand level of right arm

S65.892   Other specified injury of other blood vessels at wrist and hand level of left arm

S65.899   Other specified injury of other blood vessels at wrist and hand level of unspecified arm

● S65.9   Injury of unspecified blood vessel at wrist and hand level

● S65.90   Unspecified injury of unspecified blood vessel at wrist and hand level

S65.901   Unspecified injury of unspecified blood vessel at wrist and hand level of right arm

S65.902   Unspecified injury of unspecified blood vessel at wrist and hand level of left arm

S65.909   Unspecified injury of unspecified blood vessel at wrist and hand level of unspecified arm

● S65.91   Laceration of unspecified blood vessel at wrist and hand level

S65.911   Laceration of unspecified blood vessel at wrist and hand level of right arm

S65.912   Laceration of unspecified blood vessel at wrist and hand level of left arm

S65.919   Laceration of unspecified blood vessel at wrist and hand level of unspecified arm

● S65.99   Other specified injury of unspecified blood vessel at wrist and hand level

S65.991   Other specified injury of unspecified blood vessel at wrist and hand of right arm

S65.992   Other specified injury of unspecified blood vessel at wrist and hand of left arm

S65.999   Other specified injury of unspecified blood vessel at wrist and hand of unspecified arm

● S66   Injury of muscle, fascia and tendon at wrist and hand level
Code also any associated open wound (S61.-)
Excludes2   sprain of joints and ligaments of wrist and hand (S63.-)
The appropriate 7th character is to be added to each code from category S66

A	initial encounter
D	subsequent encounter
S	sequela

● S66.0   Injury of long flexor muscle, fascia and tendon of thumb at wrist and hand level

● S66.00   Unspecified injury of long flexor muscle, fascia and tendon of thumb at wrist and hand level

S66.001   Unspecified injury of long flexor muscle, fascia and tendon of right thumb at wrist and hand level

S66.002   Unspecified injury of long flexor muscle, fascia and tendon of left thumb at wrist and hand level

S66.009   Unspecified injury of long flexor muscle, fascia and tendon of unspecified thumb at wrist and hand level

● S66.01   Strain of long flexor muscle, fascia and tendon of thumb at wrist and hand level

S66.011   Strain of long flexor muscle, fascia and tendon of right thumb at wrist and hand level

S66.012   Strain of long flexor muscle, fascia and tendon of left thumb at wrist and hand level

S66.019   Strain of long flexor muscle, fascia and tendon of unspecified thumb at wrist and hand level

● S66.02   Laceration of long flexor muscle, fascia and tendon of thumb at wrist and hand level

S66.021   Laceration of long flexor muscle, fascia and tendon of right thumb at wrist and hand level

S66.022   Laceration of long flexor muscle, fascia and tendon of left thumb at wrist and hand level

S66.029   Laceration of long flexor muscle, fascia and tendon of unspecified thumb at wrist and hand level

● S66.09   Other specified injury of long flexor muscle, fascia and tendon of thumb at wrist and hand level

S66.091   Other specified injury of long flexor muscle, fascia and tendon of right thumb at wrist and hand level

S66.092   Other specified injury of long flexor muscle, fascia and tendon of left thumb at wrist and hand level

S66.099   Other specified injury of long flexor muscle, fascia and tendon of unspecified thumb at wrist and hand level

● **S66.1** **Injury of flexor muscle, fascia and tendon of other and unspecified finger at wrist and hand level**

Excludes2 injury of long flexor muscle, fascia and tendon of thumb at wrist and hand level (S66.0-)

● **S66.10** Unspecified injury of flexor muscle, fascia and tendon of other and unspecified finger at wrist and hand level

● **S66.100** Unspecified injury of flexor muscle, fascia and tendon of right index finger at wrist and hand level

● **S66.101** Unspecified injury of flexor muscle, fascia and tendon of left index finger at wrist and hand level

● **S66.102** Unspecified injury of flexor muscle, fascia and tendon of right middle finger at wrist and hand level

● **S66.103** Unspecified injury of flexor muscle, fascia and tendon of left middle finger at wrist and hand level

● **S66.104** Unspecified injury of flexor muscle, fascia and tendon of right ring finger at wrist and hand level

● **S66.105** Unspecified injury of flexor muscle, fascia and tendon of left ring finger at wrist and hand level

● **S66.106** Unspecified injury of flexor muscle, fascia and tendon of right little finger at wrist and hand level

● **S66.107** Unspecified injury of flexor muscle, fascia and tendon of left little finger at wrist and hand level

● **S66.108** Unspecified injury of flexor muscle, fascia and tendon of other finger at wrist and hand level

Unspecified injury of flexor muscle, fascia and tendon of specified finger with unspecified laterality at wrist and hand level

● **S66.109** Unspecified injury of flexor muscle, fascia and tendon of unspecified finger at wrist and hand level

● **S66.11** Strain of flexor muscle, fascia and tendon of other and unspecified finger at wrist and hand level

● **S66.110** Strain of flexor muscle, fascia and tendon of right index finger at wrist and hand level

● **S66.111** Strain of flexor muscle, fascia and tendon of left index finger at wrist and hand level

● **S66.112** Strain of flexor muscle, fascia and tendon of right middle finger at wrist and hand level

● **S66.113** Strain of flexor muscle, fascia and tendon of left middle finger at wrist and hand level

● **S66.114** Strain of flexor muscle, fascia and tendon of right ring finger at wrist and hand level

● **S66.115** Strain of flexor muscle, fascia and tendon of left ring finger at wrist and hand level

● **S66.116** Strain of flexor muscle, fascia and tendon of right little finger at wrist and hand level

● **S66.117** Strain of flexor muscle, fascia and tendon of left little finger at wrist and hand level

● **S66.118** Strain of flexor muscle, fascia and tendon of other finger at wrist and hand level

Strain of flexor muscle, fascia and tendon of specified finger with unspecified laterality at wrist and hand level

● **S66.119** Strain of flexor muscle, fascia and tendon of unspecified finger at wrist and hand level

● **S66.12** Laceration of flexor muscle, fascia and tendon of other and unspecified finger at wrist and hand level

● **S66.120** Laceration of flexor muscle, fascia and tendon of right index finger at wrist and hand level

● **S66.121** Laceration of flexor muscle, fascia and tendon of left index finger at wrist and hand level

● **S66.122** Laceration of flexor muscle, fascia and tendon of right middle finger at wrist and hand level

● **S66.123** Laceration of flexor muscle, fascia and tendon of left middle finger at wrist and hand level

● **S66.124** Laceration of flexor muscle, fascia and tendon of right ring finger at wrist and hand level

● **S66.125** Laceration of flexor muscle, fascia and tendon of left ring finger at wrist and hand level

● **S66.126** Laceration of flexor muscle, fascia and tendon of right little finger at wrist and hand level

● **S66.127** Laceration of flexor muscle, fascia and tendon of left little finger at wrist and hand level

● **S66.128** Laceration of flexor muscle, fascia and tendon of other finger at wrist and hand level

Laceration of flexor muscle, fascia and tendon of specified finger with unspecified laterality at wrist and hand level

● **S66.129** Laceration of flexor muscle, fascia and tendon of unspecified finger at wrist and hand level

● **S66.19** Other injury of flexor muscle, fascia and tendon of other and unspecified finger at wrist and hand level

● **S66.190** Other injury of flexor muscle, fascia and tendon of right index finger at wrist and hand level

● **S66.191** Other injury of flexor muscle, fascia and tendon of left index finger at wrist and hand level

● **S66.192** Other injury of flexor muscle, fascia and tendon of right middle finger at wrist and hand level

● **S66.193** Other injury of flexor muscle, fascia and tendon of left middle finger at wrist and hand level

● **S66.194** Other injury of flexor muscle, fascia and tendon of right ring finger at wrist and hand level

● **S66.195** Other injury of flexor muscle, fascia and tendon of left ring finger at wrist and hand level

● **S66.196** Other injury of flexor muscle, fascia and tendon of right little finger at wrist and hand level

● **S66.197** Other injury of flexor muscle, fascia and tendon of left little finger at wrist and hand level

◄ New   ◄══ Revised   ~~deleted~~ Deleted   Excludes 1   Excludes 2   Includes   Use additional   Code first   Code also   Unspecified

1288   OGCR Official Guidelines   X Assign placeholder X   ● Use Additional Character(s)   ▶ Manifestation Code   **Coding Clinic**

● S66.198   Other injury of flexor muscle, fascia and tendon of other finger at wrist and hand level
> Other injury of flexor muscle, fascia and tendon of specified finger with unspecified laterality at wrist and hand level

● S66.199   Other injury of flexor muscle, fascia and tendon of unspecified finger at wrist and hand level

● S66.2   Injury of extensor muscle, fascia and tendon of thumb at wrist and hand level

● S66.20   Unspecified injury of extensor muscle, fascia and tendon of thumb at wrist and hand level

● S66.201   Unspecified injury of extensor muscle, fascia and tendon of right thumb at wrist and hand level

● S66.202   Unspecified injury of extensor muscle, fascia and tendon of left thumb at wrist and hand level

● S66.209   Unspecified injury of extensor muscle, fascia and tendon of unspecified thumb at wrist and hand level

● S66.21   Strain of extensor muscle, fascia and tendon of thumb at wrist and hand level

● S66.211   Strain of extensor muscle, fascia and tendon of right thumb at wrist and hand level

● S66.212   Strain of extensor muscle, fascia and tendon of left thumb at wrist and hand level

● S66.219   Strain of extensor muscle, fascia and tendon of unspecified thumb at wrist and hand level

● S66.22   Laceration of extensor muscle, fascia and tendon of thumb at wrist and hand level

● S66.221   Laceration of extensor muscle, fascia and tendon of right thumb at wrist and hand level

● S66.222   Laceration of extensor muscle, fascia and tendon of left thumb at wrist and hand level

● S66.229   Laceration of extensor muscle, fascia and tendon of unspecified thumb at wrist and hand level

● S66.29   Other specified injury of extensor muscle, fascia and tendon of thumb at wrist and hand level

● S66.291   Other specified injury of extensor muscle, fascia and tendon of right thumb at wrist and hand level

● S66.292   Other specified injury of extensor muscle, fascia and tendon of left thumb at wrist and hand level

● S66.299   Other specified injury of extensor muscle, fascia and tendon of unspecified thumb at wrist and hand level

● S66.3   Injury of extensor muscle, fascia and tendon of other and unspecified finger at wrist and hand level

Excludes2   injury of extensor muscle, fascia and tendon of thumb at wrist and hand level (S66.2-)

● S66.30   Unspecified injury of extensor muscle, fascia and tendon of other and unspecified finger at wrist and hand level

● S66.300   Unspecified injury of extensor muscle, fascia and tendon of right index finger at wrist and hand level

● S66.301   Unspecified injury of extensor muscle, fascia and tendon of left index finger at wrist and hand level

● S66.302   Unspecified injury of extensor muscle, fascia and tendon of right middle finger at wrist and hand level

● S66.303   Unspecified injury of extensor muscle, fascia and tendon of left middle finger at wrist and hand level

● S66.304   Unspecified injury of extensor muscle, fascia and tendon of right ring finger at wrist and hand level

● S66.305   Unspecified injury of extensor muscle, fascia and tendon of left ring finger at wrist and hand level

● S66.306   Unspecified injury of extensor muscle, fascia and tendon of right little finger at wrist and hand level

● S66.307   Unspecified injury of extensor muscle, fascia and tendon of left little finger at wrist and hand level

● S66.308   Unspecified injury of extensor muscle, fascia and tendon of other finger at wrist and hand level
> Unspecified injury of extensor muscle, fascia and tendon of specified finger with unspecified laterality at wrist and hand level

● S66.309   Unspecified injury of extensor muscle, fascia and tendon of unspecified finger at wrist and hand level

● S66.31   Strain of extensor muscle, fascia and tendon of other and unspecified finger at wrist and hand level

● S66.310   Strain of extensor muscle, fascia and tendon of right index finger at wrist and hand level

● S66.311   Strain of extensor muscle, fascia and tendon of left index finger at wrist and hand level

● S66.312   Strain of extensor muscle, fascia and tendon of right middle finger at wrist and hand level

● S66.313   Strain of extensor muscle, fascia and tendon of left middle finger at wrist and hand level

● S66.314   Strain of extensor muscle, fascia and tendon of right ring finger at wrist and hand level

● S66.315   Strain of extensor muscle, fascia and tendon of left ring finger at wrist and hand level

● S66.316   Strain of extensor muscle, fascia and tendon of right little finger at wrist and hand level

● S66.317   Strain of extensor muscle, fascia and tendon of left little finger at wrist and hand level

● S66.318   Strain of extensor muscle, fascia and tendon of other finger at wrist and hand level
> Strain of extensor muscle, fascia and tendon of specified finger with unspecified laterality at wrist and hand level

● S66.319   Strain of extensor muscle, fascia and tendon of unspecified finger at wrist and hand level

CHAPTER 19 (S00-T88)

S66.32 Laceration of extensor muscle, fascia and tendon of other and unspecified finger at wrist and hand level

S66.320 Laceration of extensor muscle, fascia and tendon of right index finger at wrist and hand level

S66.321 Laceration of extensor muscle, fascia and tendon of left index finger at wrist and hand level

S66.322 Laceration of extensor muscle, fascia and tendon of right middle finger at wrist and hand level

S66.323 Laceration of extensor muscle, fascia and tendon of left middle finger at wrist and hand level

S66.324 Laceration of extensor muscle, fascia and tendon of right ring finger at wrist and hand level

S66.325 Laceration of extensor muscle, fascia and tendon of left ring finger at wrist and hand level

S66.326 Laceration of extensor muscle, fascia and tendon of right little finger at wrist and hand level

S66.327 Laceration of extensor muscle, fascia and tendon of left little finger at wrist and hand level

S66.328 Laceration of extensor muscle, fascia and tendon of other finger at wrist and hand level
Laceration of extensor muscle, fascia and tendon of specified finger with unspecified laterality at wrist and hand level

S66.329 Laceration of extensor muscle, fascia and tendon of unspecified finger at wrist and hand level

S66.39 Other injury of extensor muscle, fascia and tendon of other and unspecified finger at wrist and hand level

S66.390 Other injury of extensor muscle, fascia and tendon of right index finger at wrist and hand level

S66.391 Other injury of extensor muscle, fascia and tendon of left index finger at wrist and hand level

S66.392 Other injury of extensor muscle, fascia and tendon of right middle finger at wrist and hand level

S66.393 Other injury of extensor muscle, fascia and tendon of left middle finger at wrist and hand level

S66.394 Other injury of extensor muscle, fascia and tendon of right ring finger at wrist and hand level

S66.395 Other injury of extensor muscle, fascia and tendon of left ring finger at wrist and hand level

S66.396 Other injury of extensor muscle, fascia and tendon of right little finger at wrist and hand level

S66.397 Other injury of extensor muscle, fascia and tendon of left little finger at wrist and hand level

S66.398 Other injury of extensor muscle, fascia and tendon of other finger at wrist and hand level
Other injury of extensor muscle, fascia and tendon of specified finger with unspecified laterality at wrist and hand level

S66.399 Other injury of extensor muscle, fascia and tendon of unspecified finger at wrist and hand level

S66.4 Injury of intrinsic muscle, fascia and tendon of thumb at wrist and hand level

S66.40 Unspecified injury of intrinsic muscle, fascia and tendon of thumb at wrist and hand level

S66.401 Unspecified injury of intrinsic muscle, fascia and tendon of right thumb at wrist and hand level

S66.402 Unspecified injury of intrinsic muscle, fascia and tendon of left thumb at wrist and hand level

S66.409 Unspecified injury of intrinsic muscle, fascia and tendon of unspecified thumb at wrist and hand level

S66.41 Strain of intrinsic muscle, fascia and tendon of thumb at wrist and hand level

S66.411 Strain of intrinsic muscle, fascia and tendon of right thumb at wrist and hand level

S66.412 Strain of intrinsic muscle, fascia and tendon of left thumb at wrist and hand level

S66.419 Strain of intrinsic muscle, fascia and tendon of unspecified thumb at wrist and hand level

S66.42 Laceration of intrinsic muscle, fascia and tendon of thumb at wrist and hand level

S66.421 Laceration of intrinsic muscle, fascia and tendon of right thumb at wrist and hand level

S66.422 Laceration of intrinsic muscle, fascia and tendon of left thumb at wrist and hand level

S66.429 Laceration of intrinsic muscle, fascia and tendon of unspecified thumb at wrist and hand level

S66.49 Other specified injury of intrinsic muscle, fascia and tendon of thumb at wrist and hand level

S66.491 Other specified injury of intrinsic muscle, fascia and tendon of right thumb at wrist and hand level

S66.492 Other specified injury of intrinsic muscle, fascia and tendon of left thumb at wrist and hand level

S66.499 Other specified injury of intrinsic muscle, fascia and tendon of unspecified thumb at wrist and hand level

S66.5 Injury of intrinsic muscle, fascia and tendon of other and unspecified finger at wrist and hand level

Excludes2 injury of intrinsic muscle, fascia and tendon of thumb at wrist and hand level (S66.4-)

S66.50 Unspecified injury of intrinsic muscle, fascia and tendon of other and unspecified finger at wrist and hand level

S66.500 Unspecified injury of intrinsic muscle, fascia and tendon of right index finger at wrist and hand level

S66.501 Unspecified injury of intrinsic muscle, fascia and tendon of left index finger at wrist and hand level

S66.502 Unspecified injury of intrinsic muscle, fascia and tendon of right middle finger at wrist and hand level

S66.503 Unspecified injury of intrinsic muscle, fascia and tendon of left middle finger at wrist and hand level

S66.504 Unspecified injury of intrinsic muscle, fascia and tendon of right ring finger at wrist and hand level

◀ New   ◀▦ Revised   ~~deleted~~ Deleted   Excludes 1   Excludes 2   Includes   Use additional   Code first   Code also   Unspecified

OGCR Official Guidelines   X Assign placeholder X   ● Use Additional Character(s)   ▶ Manifestation Code   Coding Clinic

● **S66.505**   Unspecified injury of intrinsic muscle, fascia and tendon of left ring finger at wrist and hand level

● **S66.506**   Unspecified injury of intrinsic muscle, fascia and tendon of right little finger at wrist and hand level

● **S66.507**   Unspecified injury of intrinsic muscle, fascia and tendon of left little finger at wrist and hand level

● **S66.508**   Unspecified injury of intrinsic muscle, fascia and tendon of other finger at wrist and hand level

     Unspecified injury of intrinsic muscle, fascia and tendon of specified finger with unspecified laterality at wrist and hand level

● **S66.509**   Unspecified injury of intrinsic muscle, fascia and tendon of unspecified finger at wrist and hand level

● **S66.51**   Strain of intrinsic muscle, fascia and tendon of other and unspecified finger at wrist and hand level

● **S66.510**   Strain of intrinsic muscle, fascia and tendon of right index finger at wrist and hand level

● **S66.511**   Strain of intrinsic muscle, fascia and tendon of left index finger at wrist and hand level

● **S66.512**   Strain of intrinsic muscle, fascia and tendon of right middle finger at wrist and hand level

● **S66.513**   Strain of intrinsic muscle, fascia and tendon of left middle finger at wrist and hand level

● **S66.514**   Strain of intrinsic muscle, fascia and tendon of right ring finger at wrist and hand level

● **S66.515**   Strain of intrinsic muscle, fascia and tendon of left ring finger at wrist and hand level

● **S66.516**   Strain of intrinsic muscle, fascia and tendon of right little finger at wrist and hand level

● **S66.517**   Strain of intrinsic muscle, fascia and tendon of left little finger at wrist and hand level

● **S66.518**   Strain of intrinsic muscle, fascia and tendon of other finger at wrist and hand level

     Strain of intrinsic muscle, fascia and tendon of specified finger with unspecified laterality at wrist and hand level

● **S66.519**   Strain of intrinsic muscle, fascia and tendon of unspecified finger at wrist and hand level

● **S66.52**   Laceration of intrinsic muscle, fascia and tendon of other and unspecified finger at wrist and hand level

● **S66.520**   Laceration of intrinsic muscle, fascia and tendon of right index finger at wrist and hand level

● **S66.521**   Laceration of intrinsic muscle, fascia and tendon of left index finger at wrist and hand level

● **S66.522**   Laceration of intrinsic muscle, fascia and tendon of right middle finger at wrist and hand level

● **S66.523**   Laceration of intrinsic muscle, fascia and tendon of left middle finger at wrist and hand level

● **S66.524**   Laceration of intrinsic muscle, fascia and tendon of right ring finger at wrist and hand level

● **S66.525**   Laceration of intrinsic muscle, fascia and tendon of left ring finger at wrist and hand level

● **S66.526**   Laceration of intrinsic muscle, fascia and tendon of right little finger at wrist and hand level

● **S66.527**   Laceration of intrinsic muscle, fascia and tendon of left little finger at wrist and hand level

● **S66.528**   Laceration of intrinsic muscle, fascia and tendon of other finger at wrist and hand level

     Laceration of intrinsic muscle, fascia and tendon of specified finger with unspecified laterality at wrist and hand level

● **S66.529**   Laceration of intrinsic muscle, fascia and tendon of unspecified finger at wrist and hand level

● **S66.59**   Other injury of intrinsic muscle, fascia and tendon of other and unspecified finger at wrist and hand level

● **S66.590**   Other injury of intrinsic muscle, fascia and tendon of right index finger at wrist and hand level

● **S66.591**   Other injury of intrinsic muscle, fascia and tendon of left index finger at wrist and hand level

● **S66.592**   Other injury of intrinsic muscle, fascia and tendon of right middle finger at wrist and hand level

● **S66.593**   Other injury of intrinsic muscle, fascia and tendon of left middle finger at wrist and hand level

● **S66.594**   Other injury of intrinsic muscle, fascia and tendon of right ring finger at wrist and hand level

● **S66.595**   Other injury of intrinsic muscle, fascia and tendon of left ring finger at wrist and hand level

● **S66.596**   Other injury of intrinsic muscle, fascia and tendon of right little finger at wrist and hand level

● **S66.597**   Other injury of intrinsic muscle, fascia and tendon of left little finger at wrist and hand level

● **S66.598**   Other injury of intrinsic muscle, fascia and tendon of other finger at wrist and hand level

     Other injury of intrinsic muscle, fascia and tendon of specified finger with unspecified laterality at wrist and hand level

● **S66.599**   Other injury of intrinsic muscle, fascia and tendon of unspecified finger at wrist and hand level

CHAPTER 19 (S00-T88)

● **S66.8**   **Injury of other specified muscles, fascia and tendons at wrist and hand level**

   ● **S66.80**   Unspecified injury of other specified muscles, fascia and tendons at wrist and hand level

     ● **S66.801**   Unspecified injury of other specified muscles, fascia and tendons at wrist and hand level, right hand

     ● **S66.802**   Unspecified injury of other specified muscles, fascia and tendons at wrist and hand level, left hand

     ● **S66.809**   Unspecified injury of other specified muscles, fascia and tendons at wrist and hand level, unspecified hand

   ● **S66.81**   Strain of other specified muscles, fascia and tendons at wrist and hand level

     ● **S66.811**   Strain of other specified muscles, fascia and tendons at wrist and hand level, right hand

     ● **S66.812**   Strain of other specified muscles, fascia and tendons at wrist and hand level, left hand

     ● **S66.819**   Strain of other specified muscles, fascia and tendons at wrist and hand level, unspecified hand

   ● **S66.82**   Laceration of other specified muscles, fascia and tendons at wrist and hand level

     ● **S66.821**   Laceration of other specified muscles, fascia and tendons at wrist and hand level, right hand

     ● **S66.822**   Laceration of other specified muscles, fascia and tendons at wrist and hand level, left hand

     ● **S66.829**   Laceration of other specified muscles, fascia and tendons at wrist and hand level, unspecified hand

   ● **S66.89**   Other injury of other specified muscles, fascia and tendons at wrist and hand level

     ● **S66.891**   Other injury of other specified muscles, fascia and tendons at wrist and hand level, right hand

     ● **S66.892**   Other injury of other specified muscles, fascia and tendons at wrist and hand level, left hand

     ● **S66.899**   Other injury of other specified muscles, fascia and tendons at wrist and hand level, unspecified hand

● **S66.9**   **Injury of unspecified muscle, fascia and tendon at wrist and hand level**

   ● **S66.90**   Unspecified injury of unspecified muscle, fascia and tendon at wrist and hand level

     ● **S66.901**   Unspecified injury of unspecified muscle, fascia and tendon at wrist and hand level, right hand

     ● **S66.902**   Unspecified injury of unspecified muscle, fascia and tendon at wrist and hand level, left hand

     ● **S66.909**   Unspecified injury of unspecified muscle, fascia and tendon at wrist and hand level, unspecified hand

   ● **S66.91**   Strain of unspecified muscle, fascia and tendon at wrist and hand level

     ● **S66.911**   Strain of unspecified muscle, fascia and tendon at wrist and hand level, right hand

     ● **S66.912**   Strain of unspecified muscle, fascia and tendon at wrist and hand level, left hand

     ● **S66.919**   Strain of unspecified muscle, fascia and tendon at wrist and hand level, unspecified hand

● **S66.92**   **Laceration of unspecified muscle, fascia and tendon at wrist and hand level**

     ● **S66.921**   Laceration of unspecified muscle, fascia and tendon at wrist and hand level, right hand

     ● **S66.922**   Laceration of unspecified muscle, fascia and tendon at wrist and hand level, left hand

     ● **S66.929**   Laceration of unspecified muscle, fascia and tendon at wrist and hand level, unspecified hand

   ● **S66.99**   Other injury of unspecified muscle, fascia and tendon at wrist and hand level

     ● **S66.991**   Other injury of unspecified muscle, fascia and tendon at wrist and hand level, right hand

     ● **S66.992**   Other injury of unspecified muscle, fascia and tendon at wrist and hand level, left hand

     ● **S66.999**   Other injury of unspecified muscle, fascia and tendon at wrist and hand level, unspecified hand

● **S67**   **Crushing injury of wrist, hand and fingers**

   Use additional code for all associated injuries, such as:
     fracture of wrist and hand (S62.-)
     open wound of wrist and hand (S61.-)

   The appropriate 7th character is to be added to each code from category S67

A	initial encounter
D	subsequent encounter
S	sequela

● **S67.0**   **Crushing injury of thumb**

   X ● **S67.00**   Crushing injury of unspecified thumb

   X ● **S67.01**   Crushing injury of right thumb

   X ● **S67.02**   Crushing injury of left thumb

● **S67.1**   **Crushing injury of other and unspecified finger(s)**

   Excludes2   crushing injury of thumb (S67.0-)

   X ● **S67.10**   Crushing injury of unspecified finger(s)

   ● **S67.19**   Crushing injury of other finger(s)

     ● **S67.190**   Crushing injury of right index finger

     ● **S67.191**   Crushing injury of left index finger

     ● **S67.192**   Crushing injury of right middle finger

     ● **S67.193**   Crushing injury of left middle finger

     ● **S67.194**   Crushing injury of right ring finger

     ● **S67.195**   Crushing injury of left ring finger

     ● **S67.196**   Crushing injury of right little finger

     ● **S67.197**   Crushing injury of left little finger

     ● **S67.198**   Crushing injury of other finger
       Crushing injury of specified finger with unspecified laterality

● **S67.2**   **Crushing injury of hand**

   Excludes2   crushing injury of fingers (S67.1-)
           crushing injury of thumb (S67.0-)

   X ● **S67.20**   Crushing injury of unspecified hand

   X ● **S67.21**   Crushing injury of right hand

   X ● **S67.22**   Crushing injury of left hand

● **S67.3**   **Crushing injury of wrist**

   X ● **S67.30**   Crushing injury of unspecified wrist

   X ● **S67.31**   Crushing injury of right wrist

   X ● **S67.32**   Crushing injury of left wrist

◀ New   ◀▦ Revised   ~~deleted~~ Deleted   Excludes 1   Excludes 2   Includes   Use additional   Code first   Code also   Unspecified

1292   OGCR Official Guidelines   X Assign placeholder X   ● Use Additional Character(s)   ▶ Manifestation Code   **Coding Clinic**

● **S67.4**   **Crushing injury of wrist and hand**
      Excludes1   crushing injury of hand alone (S67.2-)
                        crushing injury of wrist alone (S67.3-)
      Excludes2   crushing injury of fingers (S67.1-)
                        crushing injury of thumb (S67.0-)
   X ● **S67.40**   Crushing injury of unspecified wrist and hand
   X ● **S67.41**   Crushing injury of right wrist and hand
   X ● **S67.42**   Crushing injury of left wrist and hand
● **S67.9**   **Crushing injury of unspecified part(s) of wrist, hand and fingers**
   X ● **S67.90**   Crushing injury of unspecified part(s) of unspecified wrist, hand and fingers
   X ● **S67.91**   Crushing injury of unspecified part(s) of right wrist, hand and fingers
   X ● **S67.92**   Crushing injury of unspecified part(s) of left wrist, hand and fingers

● **S68**   **Traumatic amputation of wrist, hand and fingers**
     An amputation not identified as partial or complete should be coded to complete
     The appropriate 7th character is to be added to each code from category S68

A	initial encounter
D	subsequent encounter
S	sequela

● **S68.0**   **Traumatic metacarpophalangeal amputation of thumb**
     Traumatic amputation of thumb NOS
   ● **S68.01**   Complete traumatic metacarpophalangeal amputation of thumb
     ● **S68.011**   Complete traumatic metacarpophalangeal amputation of right thumb
     ● **S68.012**   Complete traumatic metacarpophalangeal amputation of left thumb
     ● **S68.019**   Complete traumatic metacarpophalangeal amputation of unspecified thumb
   ● **S68.02**   Partial traumatic metacarpophalangeal amputation of thumb
     ● **S68.021**   Partial traumatic metacarpophalangeal amputation of right thumb
     ● **S68.022**   Partial traumatic metacarpophalangeal amputation of left thumb
     ● **S68.029**   Partial traumatic metacarpophalangeal amputation of unspecified thumb
● **S68.1**   **Traumatic metacarpophalangeal amputation of other and unspecified finger**
     Traumatic amputation of finger NOS
     Excludes2   traumatic metacarpophalangeal amputation of thumb (S68.0-)
   ● **S68.11**   Complete traumatic metacarpophalangeal amputation of other and unspecified finger
     ● **S68.110**   Complete traumatic metacarpophalangeal amputation of right index finger
     ● **S68.111**   Complete traumatic metacarpophalangeal amputation of left index finger
     ● **S68.112**   Complete traumatic metacarpophalangeal amputation of right middle finger
     ● **S68.113**   Complete traumatic metacarpophalangeal amputation of left middle finger

     ● **S68.114**   Complete traumatic metacarpophalangeal amputation of right ring finger
     ● **S68.115**   Complete traumatic metacarpophalangeal amputation of left ring finger
     ● **S68.116**   Complete traumatic metacarpophalangeal amputation of right little finger
     ● **S68.117**   Complete traumatic metacarpophalangeal amputation of left little finger
     ● **S68.118**   Complete traumatic metacarpophalangeal amputation of other finger
         Complete traumatic metacarpophalangeal amputation of specified finger with unspecified laterality
     ● **S68.119**   Complete traumatic metacarpophalangeal amputation of unspecified finger
   ● **S68.12**   Partial traumatic metacarpophalangeal amputation of other and unspecified finger
     ● **S68.120**   Partial traumatic metacarpophalangeal amputation of right index finger
     ● **S68.121**   Partial traumatic metacarpophalangeal amputation of left index finger
     ● **S68.122**   Partial traumatic metacarpophalangeal amputation of right middle finger
     ● **S68.123**   Partial traumatic metacarpophalangeal amputation of left middle finger
     ● **S68.124**   Partial traumatic metacarpophalangeal amputation of right ring finger
     ● **S68.125**   Partial traumatic metacarpophalangeal amputation of left ring finger
     ● **S68.126**   Partial traumatic metacarpophalangeal amputation of right little finger
     ● **S68.127**   Partial traumatic metacarpophalangeal amputation of left little finger
     ● **S68.128**   Partial traumatic metacarpophalangeal amputation of other finger
         Partial traumatic metacarpophalangeal amputation of specified finger with unspecified laterality
     ● **S68.129**   Partial traumatic metacarpophalangeal amputation of unspecified finger
● **S68.4**   **Traumatic amputation of hand at wrist level**
     Traumatic amputation of hand NOS
     Traumatic amputation of wrist
   ● **S68.41**   Complete traumatic amputation of hand at wrist level
     ● **S68.411**   Complete traumatic amputation of right hand at wrist level
     ● **S68.412**   Complete traumatic amputation of left hand at wrist level
     ● **S68.419**   Complete traumatic amputation of unspecified hand at wrist level

● S68.42   Partial traumatic amputation of hand at wrist level
- ● S68.421   Partial traumatic amputation of right hand at wrist level
- ● S68.422   Partial traumatic amputation of left hand at wrist level
- ● S68.429   Partial traumatic amputation of unspecified hand at wrist level

● S68.5   Traumatic transphalangeal amputation of thumb
  Traumatic interphalangeal joint amputation of thumb
- ● S68.51   Complete traumatic transphalangeal amputation of thumb
  - ● S68.511   Complete traumatic transphalangeal amputation of right thumb
  - ● S68.512   Complete traumatic transphalangeal amputation of left thumb
  - ● S68.519   Complete traumatic transphalangeal amputation of unspecified thumb
- ● S68.52   Partial traumatic transphalangeal amputation of thumb
  - ● S68.521   Partial traumatic transphalangeal amputation of right thumb
  - ● S68.522   Partial traumatic transphalangeal amputation of left thumb
  - ● S68.529   Partial traumatic transphalangeal amputation of unspecified thumb

● S68.6   Traumatic transphalangeal amputation of other and unspecified finger
- ● S68.61   Complete traumatic transphalangeal amputation of other and unspecified finger(s)
  - ● S68.610   Complete traumatic transphalangeal amputation of right index finger
  - ● S68.611   Complete traumatic transphalangeal amputation of left index finger
  - ● S68.612   Complete traumatic transphalangeal amputation of right middle finger
  - ● S68.613   Complete traumatic transphalangeal amputation of left middle finger
  - ● S68.614   Complete traumatic transphalangeal amputation of right ring finger
  - ● S68.615   Complete traumatic transphalangeal amputation of left ring finger
  - ● S68.616   Complete traumatic transphalangeal amputation of right little finger
  - ● S68.617   Complete traumatic transphalangeal amputation of left little finger
  - ● S68.618   Complete traumatic transphalangeal amputation of other finger
    Complete traumatic transphalangeal amputation of specified finger with unspecified laterality
  - ● S68.619   Complete traumatic transphalangeal amputation of unspecified finger
- ● S68.62   Partial traumatic transphalangeal amputation of other and unspecified finger
  - ● S68.620   Partial traumatic transphalangeal amputation of right index finger
  - ● S68.621   Partial traumatic transphalangeal amputation of left index finger
  - ● S68.622   Partial traumatic transphalangeal amputation of right middle finger

- ● S68.623   Partial traumatic transphalangeal amputation of left middle finger
- ● S68.624   Partial traumatic transphalangeal amputation of right ring finger
- ● S68.625   Partial traumatic transphalangeal amputation of left ring finger
- ● S68.626   Partial traumatic transphalangeal amputation of right little finger
- ● S68.627   Partial traumatic transphalangeal amputation of left little finger
- ● S68.628   Partial traumatic transphalangeal amputation of other finger
  Partial traumatic transphalangeal amputation of specified finger with unspecified laterality
- ● S68.629   Partial traumatic transphalangeal amputation of unspecified finger

● S68.7   Traumatic transmetacarpal amputation of hand
- ● S68.71   Complete traumatic transmetacarpal amputation of hand
  - ● S68.711   Complete traumatic transmetacarpal amputation of right hand
  - ● S68.712   Complete traumatic transmetacarpal amputation of left hand
  - ● S68.719   Complete traumatic transmetacarpal amputation of unspecified hand
- ● S68.72   Partial traumatic transmetacarpal amputation of hand
  - ● S68.721   Partial traumatic transmetacarpal amputation of right hand
  - ● S68.722   Partial traumatic transmetacarpal amputation of left hand
  - ● S68.729   Partial traumatic transmetacarpal amputation of unspecified hand

● S69   Other and unspecified injuries of wrist, hand and finger(s)
  The appropriate 7th character is to be added to each code from category S69

A	initial encounter
D	subsequent encounter
S	sequela

- ● S69.8   Other specified injuries of wrist, hand and finger(s)
  - X ● S69.80   Other specified injuries of unspecified wrist, hand and finger(s)
  - X ● S69.81   Other specified injuries of right wrist, hand and finger(s)
  - X ● S69.82   Other specified injuries of left wrist, hand and finger(s)
- ● S69.9   Unspecified injury of wrist, hand and finger(s)
  - X ● S69.90   Unspecified injury of unspecified wrist, hand and finger(s)
  - X ● S69.91   Unspecified injury of right wrist, hand and finger(s)
  - X ● S69.92   Unspecified injury of left wrist, hand and finger(s)

INJURIES TO THE HIP AND THIGH (S70-S79)

Excludes2   burns and corrosions (T20-T32)
frostbite (T33-T34)
snake bite (T63.0-)
venomous insect bite or sting (T63.4-)

● **S70** **Superficial injury of hip and thigh**
The appropriate 7th character is to be added to each code from category S70

> A   initial encounter
> D   subsequent encounter
> S   sequela

● **S70.0** **Contusion of hip**
  X● **S70.00** Contusion of unspecified hip
  X● **S70.01** Contusion of right hip
  X● **S70.02** Contusion of left hip

● **S70.1** **Contusion of thigh**
  X● **S70.10** Contusion of unspecified thigh
  X● **S70.11** Contusion of right thigh
  X● **S70.12** Contusion of left thigh

● **S70.2** **Other superficial injuries of hip**
  ● **S70.21** **Abrasion of hip**
    ● **S70.211** Abrasion, right hip
    ● **S70.212** Abrasion, left hip
    ● **S70.219** Abrasion, unspecified hip
  ● **S70.22** **Blister (nonthermal) of hip**
    ● **S70.221** Blister (nonthermal), right hip
    ● **S70.222** Blister (nonthermal), left hip
    ● **S70.229** Blister (nonthermal), unspecified hip
  ● **S70.24** **External constriction of hip**
    ● **S70.241** External constriction, right hip
    ● **S70.242** External constriction, left hip
    ● **S70.249** External constriction, unspecified hip
  ● **S70.25** **Superficial foreign body of hip**
    Splinter in the hip
    ● **S70.251** Superficial foreign body, right hip
    ● **S70.252** Superficial foreign body, left hip
    ● **S70.259** Superficial foreign body, unspecified hip
  ● **S70.26** **Insect bite (nonvenomous) of hip**
    ● **S70.261** Insect bite (nonvenomous), right hip
    ● **S70.262** Insect bite (nonvenomous), left hip
    ● **S70.269** Insect bite (nonvenomous), unspecified hip
  ● **S70.27** **Other superficial bite of hip**
    Excludes1   open bite of hip (S71.05-)
    ● **S70.271** Other superficial bite of hip, right hip
    ● **S70.272** Other superficial bite of hip, left hip
    ● **S70.279** Other superficial bite of hip, unspecified hip

● **S70.3** **Other superficial injuries of thigh**
  ● **S70.31** **Abrasion of thigh**
    ● **S70.311** Abrasion, right thigh
    ● **S70.312** Abrasion, left thigh
    ● **S70.319** Abrasion, unspecified thigh
  ● **S70.32** **Blister (nonthermal) of thigh**
    ● **S70.321** Blister (nonthermal), right thigh
    ● **S70.322** Blister (nonthermal), left thigh
    ● **S70.329** Blister (nonthermal), unspecified thigh

● **S70.34** **External constriction of thigh**
  ● **S70.341** External constriction, right thigh
  ● **S70.342** External constriction, left thigh
  ● **S70.349** External constriction, unspecified thigh
● **S70.35** **Superficial foreign body of thigh**
  Splinter in the thigh
  ● **S70.351** Superficial foreign body, right thigh
  ● **S70.352** Superficial foreign body, left thigh
  ● **S70.359** Superficial foreign body, unspecified thigh
● **S70.36** **Insect bite (nonvenomous) of thigh**
  ● **S70.361** Insect bite (nonvenomous), right thigh
  ● **S70.362** Insect bite (nonvenomous), left thigh
  ● **S70.369** Insect bite (nonvenomous), unspecified thigh
● **S70.37** **Other superficial bite of thigh**
  Excludes1   open bite of thigh (S71.15)
  ● **S70.371** Other superficial bite of right thigh
  ● **S70.372** Other superficial bite of left thigh
  ● **S70.379** Other superficial bite of unspecified thigh

● **S70.9** **Unspecified superficial injury of hip and thigh**
  ● **S70.91** **Unspecified superficial injury of hip**
    ● **S70.911** Unspecified superficial injury of right hip
    ● **S70.912** Unspecified superficial injury of left hip
    ● **S70.919** Unspecified superficial injury of unspecified hip
  ● **S70.92** **Unspecified superficial injury of thigh**
    ● **S70.921** Unspecified superficial injury of right thigh
    ● **S70.922** Unspecified superficial injury of left thigh
    ● **S70.929** Unspecified superficial injury of unspecified thigh

● **S71** **Open wound of hip and thigh**
Code also any associated wound infection
Excludes1   open fracture of hip and thigh (S72.-)
             traumatic amputation of hip and thigh (S78.-)
Excludes2   bite of venomous animal (T63.-)
             open wound of ankle, foot and toes (S91.-)
             open wound of knee and lower leg (S81.-)
The appropriate 7th character is to be added to each code from category S71

> A   initial encounter
> D   subsequent encounter
> S   sequela

● **S71.0** **Open wound of hip**
  ● **S71.00** **Unspecified open wound of hip**
    ● **S71.001** Unspecified open wound, right hip
    ● **S71.002** Unspecified open wound, left hip
    ● **S71.009** Unspecified open wound, unspecified hip
  ● **S71.01** **Laceration without foreign body of hip**
    ● **S71.011** Laceration without foreign body, right hip
    ● **S71.012** Laceration without foreign body, left hip
    ● **S71.019** Laceration without foreign body, unspecified hip

- **S71.02   Laceration with foreign body of hip**
  - **S71.021   Laceration with foreign body, right hip**
  - **S71.022   Laceration with foreign body, left hip**
  - **S71.029   Laceration with foreign body, unspecified hip**
- **S71.03   Puncture wound without foreign body of hip**
  - **S71.031   Puncture wound without foreign body, right hip**
  - **S71.032   Puncture wound without foreign body, left hip**
  - **S71.039   Puncture wound without foreign body, unspecified hip**
- **S71.04   Puncture wound with foreign body of hip**
  - **S71.041   Puncture wound with foreign body, right hip**
  - **S71.042   Puncture wound with foreign body, left hip**
  - **S71.049   Puncture wound with foreign body, unspecified hip**
- **S71.05   Open bite of hip**
    Bite of hip NOS
    > **Excludes1**   superficial bite of hip (S70.26, S70.27)
  - **S71.051   Open bite, right hip**
  - **S71.052   Open bite, left hip**
  - **S71.059   Open bite, unspecified hip**
- **S71.1   Open wound of thigh**
  - **S71.10   Unspecified open wound of thigh**
    - **S71.101   Unspecified open wound, right thigh**
    - **S71.102   Unspecified open wound, left thigh**
    - **S71.109   Unspecified open wound, unspecified thigh**
  - **S71.11   Laceration without foreign body of thigh**
    - **S71.111   Laceration without foreign body, right thigh**
    - **S71.112   Laceration without foreign body, left thigh**
    - **S71.119   Laceration without foreign body, unspecified thigh**
  - **S71.12   Laceration with foreign body of thigh**
    - **S71.121   Laceration with foreign body, right thigh**
    - **S71.122   Laceration with foreign body, left thigh**
    - **S71.129   Laceration with foreign body, unspecified thigh**
  - **S71.13   Puncture wound without foreign body of thigh**
    - **S71.131   Puncture wound without foreign body, right thigh**
    - **S71.132   Puncture wound without foreign body, left thigh**
    - **S71.139   Puncture wound without foreign body, unspecified thigh**
  - **S71.14   Puncture wound with foreign body of thigh**
    - **S71.141   Puncture wound with foreign body, right thigh**
    - **S71.142   Puncture wound with foreign body, left thigh**
    - **S71.149   Puncture wound with foreign body, unspecified thigh**
  - **S71.15   Open bite of thigh**
      Bite of thigh NOS
      > **Excludes1**   superficial bite of thigh (S70.37-)
    - **S71.151   Open bite, right thigh**
    - **S71.152   Open bite, left thigh**
    - **S71.159   Open bite, unspecified thigh**

- **S72   Fracture of femur**
    Note: A fracture not indicated as displaced or nondisplaced should be coded to displaced

    A fracture not indicated as open or closed should be coded to closed

    The open fracture designations are based on the Gustilo open fracture classification
    > **Excludes1**   traumatic amputation of hip and thigh (S78.-)
    > **Excludes2**   fracture of lower leg and ankle (S82.-)
    > fracture of foot (S92.-)
    > periprosthetic fracture of prosthetic implant of hip (T84.040, T84.041)

    The appropriate 7th character is to be added to all codes from category S72

A	initial encounter for closed fracture
B	initial encounter for open fracture type I or II initial encounter for open fracture NOS
C	initial encounter for open fracture type IIIA, IIIB, or IIIC
D	subsequent encounter for closed fracture with routine healing
E	subsequent encounter for open fracture type I or II with routine healing
F	subsequent encounter for open fracture type IIIA, IIIB, or IIIC with routine healing
G	subsequent encounter for closed fracture with delayed healing
H	subsequent encounter for open fracture type I or II with delayed healing
J	subsequent encounter for open fracture type IIIA, IIIB, or IIIC with delayed healing
K	subsequent encounter for closed fracture with nonunion
M	subsequent encounter for open fracture type I or II with nonunion
N	subsequent encounter for open fracture type IIIA, IIIB, or IIIC with nonunion
P	subsequent encounter for closed fracture with malunion
Q	subsequent encounter for open fracture type I or II with malunion
R	subsequent encounter for open fracture type IIIA, IIIB, or IIIC with malunion
S	sequela

  - **S72.0   Fracture of head and neck of femur**
    > **Excludes2**   physeal fracture of upper end of femur (S79.0-)
    - **S72.00   Fracture of unspecified part of neck of femur**
        Fracture of hip NOS
        Fracture of neck of femur NOS
      - **S72.001   Fracture of unspecified part of neck of right femur**
      - **S72.002   Fracture of unspecified part of neck of left femur**
          Coding Clinic: 2015, Q4, P37, Q1, P17
      - **S72.009   Fracture of unspecified part of neck of unspecified femur**
    - **S72.01   Unspecified intracapsular fracture of femur**
        Subcapital fracture of femur
      - **S72.011   Unspecified intracapsular fracture of right femur**
      - **S72.012   Unspecified intracapsular fracture of left femur**
      - **S72.019   Unspecified intracapsular fracture of unspecified femur**

- **S72.02** **Fracture of epiphysis (separation) (upper) of femur**
  Transepiphyseal fracture of femur
  Fracture and separation across growth plate

  Excludes1   capital femoral epiphyseal fracture (pediatric) of femur (S79.01-)
  Salter-Harris Type I physeal fracture of upper end of femur (S79.01-)

  - **S72.021** Displaced fracture of epiphysis (separation) (upper) of right femur
  - **S72.022** Displaced fracture of epiphysis (separation) (upper) of left femur
  - **S72.023** Displaced fracture of epiphysis (separation) (upper) of unspecified femur
  - **S72.024** Nondisplaced fracture of epiphysis (separation) (upper) of right femur
  - **S72.025** Nondisplaced fracture of epiphysis (separation) (upper) of left femur
  - **S72.026** Nondisplaced fracture of epiphysis (separation) (upper) of unspecified femur

- **S72.03** **Midcervical fracture of femur**
  Transcervical fracture of femur NOS
  - **S72.031** Displaced midcervical fracture of right femur
  - **S72.032** Displaced midcervical fracture of left femur
  - **S72.033** Displaced midcervical fracture of unspecified femur
  - **S72.034** Nondisplaced midcervical fracture of right femur
  - **S72.035** Nondisplaced midcervical fracture of left femur
  - **S72.036** Nondisplaced midcervical fracture of unspecified femur

- **S72.04** **Fracture of base of neck of femur**
  Cervicotrochanteric fracture of femur
  - **S72.041** Displaced fracture of base of neck of right femur
  - **S72.042** Displaced fracture of base of neck of left femur
  - **S72.043** Displaced fracture of base of neck of unspecified femur
  - **S72.044** Nondisplaced fracture of base of neck of right femur
  - **S72.045** Nondisplaced fracture of base of neck of left femur
  - **S72.046** Nondisplaced fracture of base of neck of unspecified femur

- **S72.05** **Unspecified fracture of head of femur**
  Fracture of head of femur NOS
  - **S72.051** Unspecified fracture of head of right femur
  - **S72.052** Unspecified fracture of head of left femur
  - **S72.059** Unspecified fracture of head of unspecified femur

- **S72.06** **Articular fracture of head of femur**
  - **S72.061** Displaced articular fracture of head of right femur
  - **S72.062** Displaced articular fracture of head of left femur
  - **S72.063** Displaced articular fracture of head of unspecified femur
  - **S72.064** Nondisplaced articular fracture of head of right femur
  - **S72.065** Nondisplaced articular fracture of head of left femur
  - **S72.066** Nondisplaced articular fracture of head of unspecified femur

- **S72.09** **Other fracture of head and neck of femur**
  - **S72.091** Other fracture of head and neck of right femur
  - **S72.092** Other fracture of head and neck of left femur
  - **S72.099** Other fracture of head and neck of unspecified femur

- **S72.1** **Pertrochanteric fracture**
  Fracture extending close to, but not into, joint
  - **S72.10** **Unspecified trochanteric fracture of femur**
    Fracture of trochanter NOS
    - **S72.101** Unspecified trochanteric fracture of right femur
    - **S72.102** Unspecified trochanteric fracture of left femur
    - **S72.109** Unspecified trochanteric fracture of unspecified femur
  - **S72.11** **Fracture of greater trochanter of femur**
    - **S72.111** Displaced fracture of greater trochanter of right femur
    - **S72.112** Displaced fracture of greater trochanter of left femur
    - **S72.113** Displaced fracture of greater trochanter of unspecified femur
    - **S72.114** Nondisplaced fracture of greater trochanter of right femur
    - **S72.115** Nondisplaced fracture of greater trochanter of left femur
    - **S72.116** Nondisplaced fracture of greater trochanter of unspecified femur
  - **S72.12** **Fracture of lesser trochanter of femur**
    - **S72.121** Displaced fracture of lesser trochanter of right femur
    - **S72.122** Displaced fracture of lesser trochanter of left femur
    - **S72.123** Displaced fracture of lesser trochanter of unspecified femur
    - **S72.124** Nondisplaced fracture of lesser trochanter of right femur
    - **S72.125** Nondisplaced fracture of lesser trochanter of left femur
    - **S72.126** Nondisplaced fracture of lesser trochanter of unspecified femur
  - **S72.13** **Apophyseal fracture of femur**
    Pertaining to articulations between articular facets of adjacent vertebrae

    Excludes1   chronic (nontraumatic) slipped upper femoral epiphysis (M93.0-)

    - **S72.131** Displaced apophyseal fracture of right femur
    - **S72.132** Displaced apophyseal fracture of left femur
    - **S72.133** Displaced apophyseal fracture of unspecified femur
    - **S72.134** Nondisplaced apophyseal fracture of right femur
    - **S72.135** Nondisplaced apophyseal fracture of left femur
    - **S72.136** Nondisplaced apophyseal fracture of unspecified femur

CHAPTER 19 (S00-T88)

- S72.14   Intertrochanteric fracture of femur
  - S72.141   Displaced intertrochanteric fracture of right femur
  - S72.142   Displaced intertrochanteric fracture of left femur
  - S72.143   Displaced intertrochanteric fracture of unspecified femur
  - S72.144   Nondisplaced intertrochanteric fracture of right femur
  - S72.145   Nondisplaced intertrochanteric fracture of left femur
  - S72.146   Nondisplaced intertrochanteric fracture of unspecified femur
- S72.2   Subtrochanteric fracture of femur
  Subtrochanteric: inferior to trochanter
  - X S72.21   Displaced subtrochanteric fracture of right femur
  - X S72.22   Displaced subtrochanteric fracture of left femur
  - X S72.23   Displaced subtrochanteric fracture of unspecified femur
  - X S72.24   Nondisplaced subtrochanteric fracture of right femur
  - X S72.25   Nondisplaced subtrochanteric fracture of left femur
  - X S72.26   Nondisplaced subtrochanteric fracture of unspecified femur
- S72.3   Fracture of shaft of femur
  - S72.30   Unspecified fracture of shaft of femur
    - S72.301   Unspecified fracture of shaft of right femur
    - S72.302   Unspecified fracture of shaft of left femur
    - S72.309   Unspecified fracture of shaft of unspecified femur
  - S72.32   Transverse fracture of shaft of femur
    - S72.321   Displaced transverse fracture of shaft of right femur
    - S72.322   Displaced transverse fracture of shaft of left femur
    - S72.323   Displaced transverse fracture of shaft of unspecified femur
    - S72.324   Nondisplaced transverse fracture of shaft of right femur
    - S72.325   Nondisplaced transverse fracture of shaft of left femur
    - S72.326   Nondisplaced transverse fracture of shaft of unspecified femur
  - S72.33   Oblique fracture of shaft of femur
    - S72.331   Displaced oblique fracture of shaft of right femur
    - S72.332   Displaced oblique fracture of shaft of left femur
    - S72.333   Displaced oblique fracture of shaft of unspecified femur
    - S72.334   Nondisplaced oblique fracture of shaft of right femur
    - S72.335   Nondisplaced oblique fracture of shaft of left femur
    - S72.336   Nondisplaced oblique fracture of shaft of unspecified femur
  - S72.34   Spiral fracture of shaft of femur
    - S72.341   Displaced spiral fracture of shaft of right femur
    - S72.342   Displaced spiral fracture of shaft of left femur
    - S72.343   Displaced spiral fracture of shaft of unspecified femur
    - S72.344   Nondisplaced spiral fracture of shaft of right femur
    - S72.345   Nondisplaced spiral fracture of shaft of left femur
    - S72.346   Nondisplaced spiral fracture of shaft of unspecified femur
  - S72.35   Comminuted fracture of shaft of femur
    - S72.351   Displaced comminuted fracture of shaft of right femur
    - S72.352   Displaced comminuted fracture of shaft of left femur
    - S72.353   Displaced comminuted fracture of shaft of unspecified femur
    - S72.354   Nondisplaced comminuted fracture of shaft of right femur
    - S72.355   Nondisplaced comminuted fracture of shaft of left femur
    - S72.356   Nondisplaced comminuted fracture of shaft of unspecified femur
  - S72.36   Segmental fracture of shaft of femur
    - S72.361   Displaced segmental fracture of shaft of right femur
    - S72.362   Displaced segmental fracture of shaft of left femur
    - S72.363   Displaced segmental fracture of shaft of unspecified femur
    - S72.364   Nondisplaced segmental fracture of shaft of right femur
    - S72.365   Nondisplaced segmental fracture of shaft of left femur
    - S72.366   Nondisplaced segmental fracture of shaft of unspecified femur
  - S72.39   Other fracture of shaft of femur
    - S72.391   Other fracture of shaft of right femur
    - S72.392   Other fracture of shaft of left femur
    - S72.399   Other fracture of shaft of unspecified femur
- S72.4   Fracture of lower end of femur
  Fracture of distal end of femur
  Excludes2   fracture of shaft of femur (S72.3-)
                physeal fracture of lower end of femur (S79.1-)
  - S72.40   Unspecified fracture of lower end of femur
    - S72.401   Unspecified fracture of lower end of right femur
    - S72.402   Unspecified fracture of lower end of left femur
    - S72.409   Unspecified fracture of lower end of unspecified femur
  - S72.41   Unspecified condyle fracture of lower end of femur
    Condyle fracture of femur NOS
    - S72.411   Displaced unspecified condyle fracture of lower end of right femur
    - S72.412   Displaced unspecified condyle fracture of lower end of left femur
    - S72.413   Displaced unspecified condyle fracture of lower end of unspecified femur
    - S72.414   Nondisplaced unspecified condyle fracture of lower end of right femur
    - S72.415   Nondisplaced unspecified condyle fracture of lower end of left femur
    - S72.416   Nondisplaced unspecified condyle fracture of lower end of unspecified femur

- S72.42   Fracture of lateral condyle of femur
  - S72.421   Displaced fracture of lateral condyle of right femur
  - S72.422   Displaced fracture of lateral condyle of left femur
  - S72.423   Displaced fracture of lateral condyle of unspecified femur
  - S72.424   Nondisplaced fracture of lateral condyle of right femur
  - S72.425   Nondisplaced fracture of lateral condyle of left femur
  - S72.426   Nondisplaced fracture of lateral condyle of unspecified femur
- S72.43   Fracture of medial condyle of femur
  - S72.431   Displaced fracture of medial condyle of right femur
  - S72.432   Displaced fracture of medial condyle of left femur
  - S72.433   Displaced fracture of medial condyle of unspecified femur
  - S72.434   Nondisplaced fracture of medial condyle of right femur
  - S72.435   Nondisplaced fracture of medial condyle of left femur
  - S72.436   Nondisplaced fracture of medial condyle of unspecified femur
- S72.44   Fracture of lower epiphysis (separation) of femur

  Excludes1   Salter-Harris Type I physeal fracture of lower end of femur (S79.11-)

  - S72.441   Displaced fracture of lower epiphysis (separation) of right femur
  - S72.442   Displaced fracture of lower epiphysis (separation) of left femur
  - S72.443   Displaced fracture of lower epiphysis (separation) of unspecified femur
  - S72.444   Nondisplaced fracture of lower epiphysis (separation) of right femur
  - S72.445   Nondisplaced fracture of lower epiphysis (separation) of left femur
  - S72.446   Nondisplaced fracture of lower epiphysis (separation) of unspecified femur
- S72.45   Supracondylar fracture without intracondylar extension of lower end of femur

  Supracondylar fracture of lower end of femur NOS

  Excludes1   supracondylar fracture with intracondylar extension of lower end of femur (S72.46-)

  - S72.451   Displaced supracondylar fracture without intracondylar extension of lower end of right femur
  - S72.452   Displaced supracondylar fracture without intracondylar extension of lower end of left femur
  - S72.453   Displaced supracondylar fracture without intracondylar extension of lower end of unspecified femur
  - S72.454   Nondisplaced supracondylar fracture without intracondylar extension of lower end of right femur
  - S72.455   Nondisplaced supracondylar fracture without intracondylar extension of lower end of left femur
  - S72.456   Nondisplaced supracondylar fracture without intracondylar extension of lower end of unspecified femur

- S72.46   Supracondylar fracture with intracondylar extension of lower end of femur

  Excludes1   supracondylar fracture without intracondylar extension of lower end of femur (S72.45-)

  - S72.461   Displaced supracondylar fracture with intracondylar extension of lower end of right femur
  - S72.462   Displaced supracondylar fracture with intracondylar extension of lower end of left femur
  - S72.463   Displaced supracondylar fracture with intracondylar extension of lower end of unspecified femur
  - S72.464   Nondisplaced supracondylar fracture with intracondylar extension of lower end of right femur
  - S72.465   Nondisplaced supracondylar fracture with intracondylar extension of lower end of left femur
  - S72.466   Nondisplaced supracondylar fracture with intracondylar extension of lower end of unspecified femur
- S72.47   Torus fracture of lower end of femur

  The appropriate 7th character is to be added to all codes in subcategory S72.47

A	initial encounter for closed fracture
D	subsequent encounter for fracture with routine healing
G	subsequent encounter for fracture with delayed healing
K	subsequent encounter for fracture with nonunion
P	subsequent encounter for fracture with malunion
S	sequela

  - S72.471   Torus fracture of lower end of right femur
  - S72.472   Torus fracture of lower end of left femur
  - S72.479   Torus fracture of lower end of unspecified femur
- S72.49   Other fracture of lower end of femur
  - S72.491   Other fracture of lower end of right femur
  - S72.492   Other fracture of lower end of left femur
  - S72.499   Other fracture of lower end of unspecified femur
- S72.8   Other fracture of femur
  - S72.8X   Other fracture of femur
    - S72.8X1   Other fracture of right femur
    - S72.8X2   Other fracture of left femur
    - S72.8X9   Other fracture of unspecified femur
- S72.9   Unspecified fracture of femur

  Fracture of thigh NOS
  Fracture of upper leg NOS

  Excludes1   fracture of hip NOS (S72.00-, S72.01-)

  - X S72.90   **Unspecified** fracture of unspecified femur
    Coding Clinic: 2012, Q4, P94
  - X S72.91   **Unspecified** fracture of right femur
  - X S72.92   **Unspecified** fracture of left femur

● S73   Dislocation and sprain of joint and ligaments of hip

Includes   avulsion of joint or ligament of hip
laceration of cartilage, joint or ligament of hip
sprain of cartilage, joint or ligament of hip
traumatic hemarthrosis of joint or ligament of hip
traumatic rupture of joint or ligament of hip
traumatic subluxation of joint or ligament of hip
traumatic tear of joint or ligament of hip

Code also any associated open wound

Excludes2   strain of muscle, fascia and tendon of hip and thigh (S76.-)

The appropriate 7th character is to be added to each code from category S73

A	initial encounter
D	subsequent encounter
S	sequela

● S73.0   Subluxation and dislocation of hip
Out of position

Excludes2   dislocation and subluxation of hip prosthesis (T84.020, T84.021)

● S73.00   Unspecified subluxation and dislocation of hip
Dislocation of hip NOS
Subluxation of hip NOS

● S73.001   Unspecified subluxation of right hip
● S73.002   Unspecified subluxation of left hip
● S73.003   Unspecified subluxation of unspecified hip
● S73.004   Unspecified dislocation of right hip
● S73.005   Unspecified dislocation of left hip
● S73.006   Unspecified dislocation of unspecified hip

● S73.01   Posterior subluxation and dislocation of hip
● S73.011   Posterior subluxation of right hip
● S73.012   Posterior subluxation of left hip
● S73.013   Posterior subluxation of unspecified hip
● S73.014   Posterior dislocation of right hip
● S73.015   Posterior dislocation of left hip
● S73.016   Posterior dislocation of unspecified hip

● S73.02   Obturator subluxation and dislocation of hip
● S73.021   Obturator subluxation of right hip
● S73.022   Obturator subluxation of left hip
● S73.023   Obturator subluxation of unspecified hip
● S73.024   Obturator dislocation of right hip
● S73.025   Obturator dislocation of left hip
● S73.026   Obturator dislocation of unspecified hip

● S73.03   Other anterior dislocation of hip
● S73.031   Other anterior subluxation of right hip
● S73.032   Other anterior subluxation of left hip
● S73.033   Other anterior subluxation of unspecified hip
● S73.034   Other anterior dislocation of right hip
● S73.035   Other anterior dislocation of left hip
● S73.036   Other anterior dislocation of unspecified hip

● S73.04   Central dislocation of hip
● S73.041   Central subluxation of right hip
● S73.042   Central subluxation of left hip
● S73.043   Central subluxation of unspecified hip
● S73.044   Central dislocation of right hip
● S73.045   Central dislocation of left hip
● S73.046   Central dislocation of unspecified hip

● S73.1   Sprain of hip
● S73.10   Unspecified sprain of hip
● S73.101   Unspecified sprain of right hip
● S73.102   Unspecified sprain of left hip
● S73.109   Unspecified sprain of unspecified hip

● S73.11   Iliofemoral ligament sprain of hip
● S73.111   Iliofemoral ligament sprain of right hip
● S73.112   Iliofemoral ligament sprain of left hip
● S73.119   Iliofemoral ligament sprain of unspecified hip

● S73.12   Ischiocapsular (ligament) sprain of hip
● S73.121   Ischiocapsular ligament sprain of right hip
● S73.122   Ischiocapsular ligament sprain of left hip
● S73.129   Ischiocapsular ligament sprain of unspecified hip

● S73.19   Other sprain of hip
● S73.191   Other sprain of right hip
● S73.192   Other sprain of left hip
● S73.199   Other sprain of unspecified hip

● S74   Injury of nerves at hip and thigh level

Code also any associated open wound (S71.-)

Excludes2   injury of nerves at ankle and foot level (S94.-)
injury of nerves at lower leg level (S84.-)

The appropriate 7th character is to be added to each code from category S74

A	initial encounter
D	subsequent encounter
S	sequela

● S74.0   Injury of sciatic nerve at hip and thigh level
X ● S74.00   Injury of sciatic nerve at hip and thigh level, unspecified leg
X ● S74.01   Injury of sciatic nerve at hip and thigh level, right leg
X ● S74.02   Injury of sciatic nerve at hip and thigh level, left leg

● S74.1   Injury of femoral nerve at hip and thigh level
X ● S74.10   Injury of femoral nerve at hip and thigh level, unspecified leg
X ● S74.11   Injury of femoral nerve at hip and thigh level, right leg
X ● S74.12   Injury of femoral nerve at hip and thigh level, left leg

● S74.2   Injury of cutaneous sensory nerve at hip and thigh level
X ● S74.20   Injury of cutaneous sensory nerve at hip and thigh level, unspecified leg
X ● S74.21   Injury of cutaneous sensory nerve at hip and high level, right leg
X ● S74.22   Injury of cutaneous sensory nerve at hip and thigh level, left leg

● S74.8   Injury of other nerves at hip and thigh level
● S74.8X   Injury of other nerves at hip and thigh level
● S74.8X1   Injury of other nerves at hip and thigh level, right leg
● S74.8X2   Injury of other nerves at hip and thigh level, left leg
● S74.8X9   Injury of other nerves at hip and thigh level, unspecified leg

● S74.9   Injury of unspecified nerve at hip and thigh level
X ● S74.90   Injury of unspecified nerve at hip and thigh level, unspecified leg
X ● S74.91   Injury of unspecified nerve at hip and thigh level, right leg
X ● S74.92   Injury of unspecified nerve at hip and thigh level, left leg

◀ New   ◀▦ Revised   ~~deleted~~ Deleted   Excludes 1   Excludes 2   Includes   Use additional   Code first   Code also   Unspecified

OGCR Official Guidelines   X Assign placeholder X   ● Use Additional Character(s)   ▶ Manifestation Code   **Coding Clinic**

● **S75 Injury of blood vessels at hip and thigh level**

    Code also any associated open wound (S71.-)

    Excludes2 injury of blood vessels at lower leg level (S85.-)

             injury of popliteal artery (S85.0)

    The appropriate 7th character is to be added to each code from category S75

A	initial encounter
D	subsequent encounter
S	sequela

● **S75.0 Injury of femoral artery**

  ● **S75.00 Unspecified injury of femoral artery**

    ● **S75.001 Unspecified injury of femoral artery, right leg**

    ● **S75.002 Unspecified injury of femoral artery, left leg**

    ● **S75.009 Unspecified injury of femoral artery, unspecified leg**

  ● **S75.01 Minor laceration of femoral artery**

    Incomplete transection of femoral artery

    Laceration of femoral artery NOS

    Superficial laceration of femoral artery

    ● **S75.011 Minor laceration of femoral artery, right leg**

    ● **S75.012 Minor laceration of femoral artery, left leg**

    ● **S75.019 Minor laceration of femoral artery, unspecified leg**

  ● **S75.02 Major laceration of femoral artery**

    Complete transection of femoral artery

    Traumatic rupture of femoral artery

    ● **S75.021 Major laceration of femoral artery, right leg**

    ● **S75.022 Major laceration of femoral artery, left leg**

    ● **S75.029 Major laceration of femoral artery, unspecified leg**

  ● **S75.09 Other specified injury of femoral artery**

    ● **S75.091 Other specified injury of femoral artery, right leg**

    ● **S75.092 Other specified injury of femoral artery, left leg**

    ● **S75.099 Other specified injury of femoral artery, unspecified leg**

● **S75.1 Injury of femoral vein at hip and thigh level**

  ● **S75.10 Unspecified injury of femoral vein at hip and thigh level**

    ● **S75.101 Unspecified injury of femoral vein at hip and thigh level, right leg**

    ● **S75.102 Unspecified injury of femoral vein at hip and thigh level, left leg**

    ● **S75.109 Unspecified injury of femoral vein at hip and thigh level, unspecified leg**

  ● **S75.11 Minor laceration of femoral vein at hip and thigh level**

    Incomplete transection of femoral vein at hip and thigh level

    Laceration of femoral vein at hip and thigh level NOS

    Superficial laceration of femoral vein at hip and thigh level

    ● **S75.111 Minor laceration of femoral vein at hip and thigh level, right leg**

    ● **S75.112 Minor laceration of femoral vein at hip and thigh level, left leg**

    ● **S75.119 Minor laceration of femoral vein at hip and thigh level, unspecified leg**

● **S75.12 Major laceration of femoral vein at hip and thigh level**

    Complete transection of femoral vein at hip and thigh level

    Traumatic rupture of femoral vein at hip and thigh level

  ● **S75.121 Major laceration of femoral vein at hip and thigh level, right leg**

  ● **S75.122 Major laceration of femoral vein at hip and thigh level, left leg**

  ● **S75.129 Major laceration of femoral vein at hip and thigh level, unspecified leg**

  ● **S75.19 Other specified injury of femoral vein at hip and thigh level**

    ● **S75.191 Other specified injury of femoral vein at hip and thigh level, right leg**

    ● **S75.192 Other specified injury of femoral vein at hip and thigh level, left leg**

    ● **S75.199 Other specified injury of femoral vein at hip and thigh level, unspecified leg**

● **S75.2 Injury of greater saphenous vein at hip and thigh level**

    Excludes1 greater saphenous vein NOS (S85.3)

  ● **S75.20 Unspecified injury of greater saphenous vein at hip and thigh level**

    ● **S75.201 Unspecified injury of greater saphenous vein at hip and thigh level, right leg**

    ● **S75.202 Unspecified injury of greater saphenous vein at hip and thigh level, left leg**

    ● **S75.209 Unspecified injury of greater saphenous vein at hip and thigh level, unspecified leg**

  ● **S75.21 Minor laceration of greater saphenous vein at hip and thigh level**

    Incomplete transection of greater saphenous vein at hip and thigh level

    Laceration of greater saphenous vein at hip and thigh level NOS

    Superficial laceration of greater saphenous vein at hip and thigh level

    ● **S75.211 Minor laceration of greater saphenous vein at hip and thigh level, right leg**

    ● **S75.212 Minor laceration of greater saphenous vein at hip and thigh level, left leg**

    ● **S75.219 Minor laceration of greater saphenous vein at hip and thigh level, unspecified leg**

  ● **S75.22 Major laceration of greater saphenous vein at hip and thigh level**

    Complete transection of greater saphenous vein at hip and thigh level

    Traumatic rupture of greater saphenous vein at hip and thigh level

    ● **S75.221 Major laceration of greater saphenous vein at hip and thigh level, right leg**

    ● **S75.222 Major laceration of greater saphenous vein at hip and thigh level, left leg**

    ● **S75.229 Major laceration of greater saphenous vein at hip and thigh level, unspecified leg**

CHAPTER 19 (S00-T88)

● S75.29 Other specified injury of greater saphenous vein at hip and thigh level
  ● S75.291 Other specified injury of greater saphenous vein at hip and thigh level, right leg
  ● S75.292 Other specified injury of greater saphenous vein at hip and thigh level, left leg
  ● S75.299 Other specified injury of greater saphenous vein at hip and thigh level, unspecified leg

● S75.8 Injury of other blood vessels at hip and thigh level
  ● S75.80 Unspecified injury of other blood vessels at hip and thigh level
    ● S75.801 Unspecified injury of other blood vessels at hip and thigh level, right leg
    ● S75.802 Unspecified injury of other blood vessels at hip and thigh level, left leg
    ● S75.809 Unspecified injury of other blood vessels at hip and thigh level, unspecified leg
  ● S75.81 Laceration of other blood vessels at hip and thigh level
    ● S75.811 Laceration of other blood vessels at hip and thigh level, right leg
    ● S75.812 Laceration of other blood vessels at hip and thigh level, left leg
    ● S75.819 Laceration of other blood vessels at hip and thigh level, unspecified leg
  ● S75.89 Other specified injury of other blood vessels at hip and thigh level
    ● S75.891 Other specified injury of other blood vessels at hip and thigh level, right leg
    ● S75.892 Other specified injury of other blood vessels at hip and thigh level, left leg
    ● S75.899 Other specified injury of other blood vessels at hip and thigh level, unspecified leg

● S75.9 Injury of unspecified blood vessel at hip and thigh level
  ● S75.90 Unspecified injury of unspecified blood vessel at hip and thigh level
    ● S75.901 Unspecified injury of unspecified blood vessel at hip and thigh level, right leg
    ● S75.902 Unspecified injury of unspecified blood vessel at hip and thigh level, left leg
    ● S75.909 Unspecified injury of unspecified blood vessel at hip and thigh level, unspecified leg
  ● S75.91 Laceration of unspecified blood vessel at hip and thigh level
    ● S75.911 Laceration of unspecified blood vessel at hip and thigh level, right leg
    ● S75.912 Laceration of unspecified blood vessel at hip and thigh level, left leg
    ● S75.919 Laceration of unspecified blood vessel at hip and thigh level, unspecified leg
  ● S75.99 Other specified injury of unspecified blood vessel at hip and thigh level
    ● S75.991 Other specified injury of unspecified blood vessel at hip and thigh level, right leg
    ● S75.992 Other specified injury of unspecified blood vessel at hip and thigh level, left leg
    ● S75.999 Other specified injury of unspecified blood vessel at hip and thigh level, unspecified leg

● S76 Injury of muscle, fascia and tendon at hip and thigh level
  Code also any associated open wound (S71.-)
  Excludes2 injury of muscle, fascia and tendon at lower leg level (S86)
            sprain of joint and ligament of hip (S73.1)
  The appropriate 7th character is to be added to each code from category S76

A	initial encounter
D	subsequent encounter
S	sequela

  ● S76.0 Injury of muscle, fascia and tendon of hip
    ● S76.00 Unspecified injury of muscle, fascia and tendon of hip
      ● S76.001 Unspecified injury of muscle, fascia and tendon of right hip
      ● S76.002 Unspecified injury of muscle, fascia and tendon of left hip
      ● S76.009 Unspecified injury of muscle, fascia and tendon of unspecified hip
    ● S76.01 Strain of muscle, fascia and tendon of hip
      ● S76.011 Strain of muscle, fascia and tendon of right hip
      ● S76.012 Strain of muscle, fascia and tendon of left hip
      ● S76.019 Strain of muscle, fascia and tendon of unspecified hip
    ● S76.02 Laceration of muscle, fascia and tendon of hip
      ● S76.021 Laceration of muscle, fascia and tendon of right hip
      ● S76.022 Laceration of muscle, fascia and tendon of left hip
      ● S76.029 Laceration of muscle, fascia and tendon of unspecified hip
    ● S76.09 Other specified injury of muscle, fascia and tendon of hip
      ● S76.091 Other specified injury of muscle, fascia and tendon of right hip
      ● S76.092 Other specified injury of muscle, fascia and tendon of left hip
      ● S76.099 Other specified injury of muscle, fascia and tendon of unspecified hip

  ● S76.1 Injury of quadriceps muscle, fascia and tendon
    Injury of patellar ligament (tendon)
    ● S76.10 Unspecified injury of quadriceps muscle, fascia and tendon
      ● S76.101 Unspecified injury of right quadriceps muscle, fascia and tendon
      ● S76.102 Unspecified injury of left quadriceps muscle, fascia and tendon
      ● S76.109 Unspecified injury of unspecified quadriceps muscle, fascia and tendon
    ● S76.11 Strain of quadriceps muscle, fascia and tendon
      ● S76.111 Strain of right quadriceps muscle, fascia and tendon
      ● S76.112 Strain of left quadriceps muscle, fascia and tendon
      ● S76.119 Strain of unspecified quadriceps muscle, fascia and tendon
    ● S76.12 Laceration of quadriceps muscle, fascia and tendon
      ● S76.121 Laceration of right quadriceps muscle, fascia and tendon
      ● S76.122 Laceration of left quadriceps muscle, fascia and tendon
      ● S76.129 Laceration of unspecified quadriceps muscle, fascia and tendon

● S76.19   Other specified injury of quadriceps muscle, fascia and tendon
   ● S76.191   Other specified injury of right quadriceps muscle, fascia and tendon
   ● S76.192   Other specified injury of left quadriceps muscle, fascia and tendon
   ● S76.199   Other specified injury of unspecified quadriceps muscle, fascia and tendon

● S76.2   Injury of adductor muscle, fascia and tendon of thigh
  ● S76.20   Unspecified injury of adductor muscle, fascia and tendon of thigh
   ● S76.201   Unspecified injury of adductor muscle, fascia and tendon of right thigh
   ● S76.202   Unspecified injury of adductor muscle, fascia and tendon of left thigh
   ● S76.209   Unspecified injury of adductor muscle, fascia and tendon of unspecified thigh
  ● S76.21   Strain of adductor muscle, fascia and tendon of thigh
   ● S76.211   Strain of adductor muscle, fascia and tendon of right thigh
   ● S76.212   Strain of adductor muscle, fascia and tendon of left thigh
   ● S76.219   Strain of adductor muscle, fascia and tendon of unspecified thigh
  ● S76.22   Laceration of adductor muscle, fascia and tendon of thigh
   ● S76.221   Laceration of adductor muscle, fascia and tendon of right thigh
   ● S76.222   Laceration of adductor muscle, fascia and tendon of left thigh
   ● S76.229   Laceration of adductor muscle, fascia and tendon of unspecified thigh
  ● S76.29   Other injury of adductor muscle, fascia and tendon of thigh
   ● S76.291   Other injury of adductor muscle, fascia and tendon of right thigh
   ● S76.292   Other injury of adductor muscle, fascia and tendon of left thigh
   ● S76.299   Other injury of adductor muscle, fascia and tendon of unspecified thigh

● S76.3   Injury of muscle, fascia and tendon of the posterior muscle group at thigh level
  ● S76.30   Unspecified injury of muscle, fascia and tendon of the posterior muscle group at thigh level
   ● S76.301   Unspecified injury of muscle, fascia and tendon of the posterior muscle group at thigh level, right thigh
   ● S76.302   Unspecified injury of muscle, fascia and tendon of the posterior muscle group at thigh level, left thigh
   ● S76.309   Unspecified injury of muscle, fascia and tendon of the posterior muscle group at thigh level, unspecified thigh
  ● S76.31   Strain of muscle, fascia and tendon of the posterior muscle group at thigh level
   ● S76.311   Strain of muscle, fascia and tendon of the posterior muscle group at thigh level, right thigh
   ● S76.312   Strain of muscle, fascia and tendon of the posterior muscle group at thigh level, left thigh
   ● S76.319   Strain of muscle, fascia and tendon of the posterior muscle group at thigh level, unspecified thigh

● S76.32   Laceration of muscle, fascia and tendon of the posterior muscle group at thigh level
   ● S76.321   Laceration of muscle, fascia and tendon of the posterior muscle group at thigh level, right thigh
   ● S76.322   Laceration of muscle, fascia and tendon of the posterior muscle group at thigh level, left thigh
   ● S76.329   Laceration of muscle, fascia and tendon of the posterior muscle group at thigh level, unspecified thigh
  ● S76.39   Other specified injury of muscle, fascia and tendon of the posterior muscle group at thigh level
   ● S76.391   Other specified injury of muscle, fascia and tendon of the posterior muscle group at thigh level, right thigh
   ● S76.392   Other specified injury of muscle, fascia and tendon of the posterior muscle group at thigh level, left thigh
   ● S76.399   Other specified injury of muscle, fascia and tendon of the posterior muscle group at thigh level, unspecified thigh

● S76.8   Injury of other specified muscles, fascia and tendons at thigh level
  ● S76.80   Unspecified injury of other specified muscles, fascia and tendons at thigh level
   ● S76.801   Unspecified injury of other specified muscles, fascia and tendons at thigh level, right thigh
   ● S76.802   Unspecified injury of other specified muscles, fascia and tendons at thigh level, left thigh
   ● S76.809   Unspecified injury of other specified muscles, fascia and tendons at thigh level, unspecified thigh
  ● S76.81   Strain of other specified specified muscles, fascia and tendons at thigh level
   ● S76.811   Strain of other specified muscles, fascia and tendons at thigh level, right thigh
   ● S76.812   Strain of other specified muscles, fascia and tendons at thigh level, left thigh
   ● S76.819   Strain of other specified muscles, fascia and tendons at thigh level, unspecified thigh
  ● S76.82   Laceration of other specified muscles, fascia and tendons at thigh level
   ● S76.821   Laceration of other specified muscles, fascia and tendons at thigh level, right thigh
   ● S76.822   Laceration of other specified muscles, fascia and tendons at thigh level, left thigh
   ● S76.829   Laceration of other specified muscles, fascia and tendons at thigh level, unspecified thigh
  ● S76.89   Other injury of other specified muscles, fascia and tendons at thigh level
   ● S76.891   Other injury of other specified muscles, fascia and tendons at thigh level, right thigh
   ● S76.892   Other injury of other specified muscles, fascia and tendons at thigh level, left thigh
   ● S76.899   Other injury of other specified muscles, fascia and tendons at thigh level, unspecified thigh

- S76.9   Injury of unspecified muscles, fascia and tendons at thigh level
  - S76.90   Unspecified injury of unspecified muscles, fascia and tendons at thigh level
    - S76.901   Unspecified injury of unspecified muscles, fascia and tendons at thigh level, right thigh
    - S76.902   Unspecified injury of unspecified muscles, fascia and tendons at thigh level, left thigh
    - S76.909   Unspecified injury of unspecified muscles, fascia and tendons at thigh level, unspecified thigh
  - S76.91   Strain of unspecified muscles, fascia and tendons at thigh level
    - S76.911   Strain of unspecified muscles, fascia and tendons at thigh level, right thigh
    - S76.912   Strain of unspecified muscles, fascia and tendons at thigh level, left thigh
    - S76.919   Strain of unspecified muscles fascia and tendons at thigh level, unspecified thigh
  - S76.92   Laceration of unspecified muscles, fascia and tendons at thigh level
    - S76.921   Laceration of unspecified muscles, fascia and tendons at thigh level, right thigh
    - S76.922   Laceration of unspecified muscles, fascia and tendons at thigh level, left thigh
    - S76.929   Laceration of unspecified muscles, fascia and tendons at thigh level, unspecified thigh
  - S76.99   Other specified injury of unspecified muscles, fascia and tendons at thigh level
    - S76.991   Other specified injury of unspecified muscles, fascia and tendons at thigh level, right thigh
    - S76.992   Other specified injury of unspecified muscles, fascia and tendons at thigh level, left thigh
    - S76.999   Other specified injury of unspecified muscles, fascia and tendons at thigh level, unspecified thigh

- S77   Crushing injury of hip and thigh

  Use additional code(s) for all associated injuries

  Excludes2   crushing injury of ankle and foot (S97.-)
  crushing injury of lower leg (S87.-)

  The appropriate 7th character is to be added to each code from category S77

A	initial encounter
D	subsequent encounter
S	sequela

  - S77.0   Crushing injury of hip
    - X S77.00   Crushing injury of unspecified hip
    - X S77.01   Crushing injury of right hip
    - X S77.02   Crushing injury of left hip
  - S77.1   Crushing injury of thigh
    - X S77.10   Crushing injury of unspecified thigh
    - X S77.11   Crushing injury of right thigh
    - X S77.12   Crushing injury of left thigh
  - S77.2   Crushing injury of hip with thigh
    - X S77.20   Crushing injury of unspecified hip with thigh
    - X S77.21   Crushing injury of right hip with thigh
    - X S77.22   Crushing injury of left hip with thigh

- S78   Traumatic amputation of hip and thigh

  An amputation not identified as partial or complete should be coded to complete

  Excludes1   traumatic amputation of knee (S88.0-)

  The appropriate 7th character is to be added to each code from category S78

A	initial encounter
D	subsequent encounter
S	sequela

  - S78.0   Traumatic amputation at hip joint
    - S78.01   Complete traumatic amputation at hip joint
      - S78.011   Complete traumatic amputation at right hip joint
      - S78.012   Complete traumatic amputation at left hip joint
      - S78.019   Complete traumatic amputation at unspecified hip joint
    - S78.02   Partial traumatic amputation at hip joint
      - S78.021   Partial traumatic amputation at right hip joint
      - S78.022   Partial traumatic amputation at left hip joint
      - S78.029   Partial traumatic amputation at unspecified hip joint
  - S78.1   Traumatic amputation at level between hip and knee

    Excludes1   traumatic amputation of knee (S88.0-)

    - S78.11   Complete traumatic amputation at level between hip and knee
      - S78.111   Complete traumatic amputation at level between right hip and knee
      - S78.112   Complete traumatic amputation at level between left hip and knee
      - S78.119   Complete traumatic amputation at level between unspecified hip and knee
    - S78.12   Partial traumatic amputation at level between hip and knee
      - S78.121   Partial traumatic amputation at level between right hip and knee
      - S78.122   Partial traumatic amputation at level between left hip and knee
      - S78.129   Partial traumatic amputation at level between unspecified hip and knee
  - S78.9   Traumatic amputation of hip and thigh, level unspecified
    - S78.91   Complete traumatic amputation of hip and thigh, level unspecified
      - S78.911   Complete traumatic amputation of right hip and thigh, level unspecified
      - S78.912   Complete traumatic amputation of left hip and thigh, level unspecified
      - S78.919   Complete traumatic amputation of unspecified hip and thigh, level unspecified
    - S78.92   Partial traumatic amputation of hip and thigh, level unspecified
      - S78.921   Partial traumatic amputation of right hip and thigh, level unspecified
      - S78.922   Partial traumatic amputation of left hip and thigh, level unspecified
      - S78.929   Partial traumatic amputation of unspecified hip and thigh, level unspecified

Item 19–5   SALTER-HARRIS TYPE 1: epiphysis is completely separated from end of bone, or metaphysic growth plate remains attached to epiphysis
SALTER-HARRIS TYPE 2: epiphysis and growth plate are partially separated from metaphysis, which is cracked—most common type
SALTER-HARRIS TYPE 3: fracture occurring through epiphysis and separates part of epiphysis and growth plate from metaphysis fracture, usually at distal end of tibia
SALTER-HARRIS TYPE 4: fracture runs through epiphysis, across growth plate, into metaphysic, surgery is required to restore joint surface to normal and align growth plate

● **S79   Other and unspecified injuries of hip and thigh**

Note: A fracture not indicated as open or closed should be coded to closed

The appropriate 7th character is to be added to each code from subcategories S79.0 and S79.1

A	initial encounter for closed fracture
D	subsequent encounter for fracture with routine healing
G	subsequent encounter for fracture with delayed healing
K	subsequent encounter for fracture with nonunion
P	subsequent encounter for fracture with malunion
S	sequela

● **S79.0   Physeal fracture of upper end of femur**

Excludes1   apophyseal fracture of upper end of femur (S72.13-)
nontraumatic slipped upper femoral epiphysis (M93.0-)

● **S79.00   Unspecified physeal fracture of upper end of femur**

● **S79.001   Unspecified physeal fracture of upper end of right femur**

● **S79.002   Unspecified physeal fracture of upper end of left femur**

● **S79.009   Unspecified physeal fracture of upper end of unspecified femur**

● **S79.01   Salter-Harris Type I physeal fracture of upper end of femur**

Acute on chronic slipped capital femoral epiphysis (traumatic)
Acute slipped capital femoral epiphysis (traumatic)
Capital femoral epiphyseal fracture

Excludes1   chronic slipped upper femoral epiphysis (nontraumatic) (M93.02-)

● **S79.011   Salter-Harris Type I physeal fracture of upper end of right femur**

● **S79.012   Salter-Harris Type I physeal fracture of upper end of left femur**

● **S79.019   Salter-Harris Type I physeal fracture of upper end of unspecified femur**

● **S79.09   Other physeal fracture of upper end of femur**

● **S79.091   Other physeal fracture of upper end of right femur**

● **S79.092   Other physeal fracture of upper end of left femur**

● **S79.099   Other physeal fracture of upper end of unspecified femur**

● **S79.1   Physeal fracture of lower end of femur**

● **S79.10   Unspecified physeal fracture of lower end of femur**

● **S79.101   Unspecified physeal fracture of lower end of right femur**

● **S79.102   Unspecified physeal fracture of lower end of left femur**

● **S79.109   Unspecified physeal fracture of lower end of unspecified femur**

● **S79.11   Salter-Harris Type I physeal fracture of lower end of femur**

● **S79.111   Salter-Harris Type I physeal fracture of lower end of right femur**

● **S79.112   Salter-Harris Type I physeal fracture of lower end of left femur**

● **S79.119   Salter-Harris Type I physeal fracture of lower end of unspecified femur**

● **S79.12   Salter-Harris Type II physeal fracture of lower end of femur**

● **S79.121   Salter-Harris Type II physeal fracture of lower end of right femur**

● **S79.122   Salter-Harris Type II physeal fracture of lower end of left femur**

● **S79.129   Salter-Harris Type II physeal fracture of lower end of unspecified femur**

● **S79.13   Salter-Harris Type III physeal fracture of lower end of femur**

● **S79.131   Salter-Harris Type III physeal fracture of lower end of right femur**

● **S79.132   Salter-Harris Type III physeal fracture of lower end of left femur**

● **S79.139   Salter-Harris Type III physeal fracture of lower end of unspecified femur**

● **S79.14   Salter-Harris Type IV physeal fracture of lower end of femur**

● **S79.141   Salter-Harris Type IV physeal fracture of lower end of right femur**

● **S79.142   Salter-Harris Type IV physeal fracture of lower end of left femur**

● **S79.149   Salter-Harris Type IV physeal fracture of lower end of unspecified femur**

● **S79.19   Other physeal fracture of lower end of femur**

● **S79.191   Other physeal fracture of lower end of right femur**

● **S79.192   Other physeal fracture of lower end of left femur**

● **S79.199   Other physeal fracture of lower end of unspecified femur**

● **S79.8 Other specified injuries of hip and thigh**

The appropriate 7th character is to be added to each code in subcategory S79.8

A	initial encounter
D	subsequent encounter
S	sequela

● **S79.81   Other specified injuries of hip**

● **S79.811   Other specified injuries of right hip**

● **S79.812   Other specified injuries of left hip**

● **S79.819   Other specified injuries of unspecified hip**

● **S79.82   Other specified injuries of thigh**

● **S79.821   Other specified injuries of right thigh**

● **S79.822   Other specified injuries of left thigh**

● **S79.829   Other specified injuries of unspecified thigh**

● **S79.9   Unspecified injury of hip and thigh**

The appropriate 7th character is to be added to each code in subcategory S79.9

A	initial encounter
D	subsequent encounter
S	sequela

● **S79.91   Unspecified injury of hip**

● **S79.911   Unspecified injury of right hip**

● **S79.912   Unspecified injury of left hip**

● **S79.919   Unspecified injury of unspecified hip**

CHAPTER 19 (S00-T88)

- ● S79.92   Unspecified injury of thigh
  - ● S79.921   Unspecified injury of right thigh
  - ● S79.922   Unspecified injury of left thigh
  - ● S79.929   Unspecified injury of unspecified thigh

INJURIES TO THE KNEE AND LOWER LEG (S80-S89)

Excludes2   burns and corrosions (T20-T32)
              frostbite (T33-T34)
              injuries of ankle and foot, except fracture of ankle
                and malleolus (S90-S99)
              insect bite or sting, venomous (T63.4)

- ● S80   **Superficial injury of knee and lower leg**
  - **Excludes2**   superficial injury of ankle and foot (S90.-)
  - The appropriate 7th character is to be added to each code from category S80

A	initial encounter
D	subsequent encounter
S	sequela

  - ● S80.0   Contusion of knee
    - X ● S80.00   Contusion of unspecified knee
    - X ● S80.01   Contusion of right knee
    - X ● S80.02   Contusion of left knee
  - ● S80.1   Contusion of lower leg
    - X ● S80.10   Contusion of unspecified lower leg
    - X ● S80.11   Contusion of right lower leg
    - X ● S80.12   Contusion of left lower leg
  - ● S80.2   Other superficial injuries of knee
    - ● S80.21   Abrasion of knee
      - ● S80.211   Abrasion, right knee
      - ● S80.212   Abrasion, left knee
      - ● S80.219   Abrasion, unspecified knee
    - ● S80.22   Blister (nonthermal) of knee
      - ● S80.221   Blister (nonthermal), right knee
      - ● S80.222   Blister (nonthermal), left knee
      - ● S80.229   Blister (nonthermal), unspecified knee
    - ● S80.24   External constriction of knee
      - ● S80.241   External constriction, right knee
      - ● S80.242   External constriction, left knee
      - ● S80.249   External constriction, unspecified knee
    - ● S80.25   Superficial foreign body of knee
      - Splinter in the knee
      - ● S80.251   Superficial foreign body, right knee
      - ● S80.252   Superficial foreign body, left knee
      - ● S80.259   Superficial foreign body, unspecified knee
    - ● S80.26   Insect bite (nonvenomous) of knee
      - ● S80.261   Insect bite (nonvenomous), right knee
      - ● S80.262   Insect bite (nonvenomous), left knee
      - ● S80.269   Insect bite (nonvenomous), unspecified knee
    - ● S80.27   Other superficial bite of knee
      - **Excludes1**   open bite of knee (S81.05-)
      - ● S80.271   Other superficial bite of right knee
      - ● S80.272   Other superficial bite of left knee
      - ● S80.279   Other superficial bite of unspecified knee
  - ● S80.8   Other superficial injuries of lower leg
    - ● S80.81   Abrasion of lower leg
      - ● S80.811   Abrasion, right lower leg
      - ● S80.812   Abrasion, left lower leg
      - ● S80.819   Abrasion, unspecified lower leg

-      ● S80.82   Blister (nonthermal) of lower leg
  - ● S80.821   Blister (nonthermal), right lower leg
  - ● S80.822   Blister (nonthermal), left lower leg
  - ● S80.829   Blister (nonthermal), unspecified lower leg
- ● S80.84   External constriction of lower leg
  - ● S80.841   External constriction, right lower leg
  - ● S80.842   External constriction, left lower leg
  - ● S80.849   External constriction, unspecified lower leg
- ● S80.85   Superficial foreign body of lower leg
  - Splinter in the lower leg
  - ● S80.851   Superficial foreign body, right lower leg
  - ● S80.852   Superficial foreign body, left lower leg
  - ● S80.859   Superficial foreign body, unspecified lower leg
- ● S80.86   Insect bite (nonvenomous) of lower leg
  - ● S80.861   Insect bite (nonvenomous), right lower leg
  - ● S80.862   Insect bite (nonvenomous), left lower leg
  - ● S80.869   Insect bite (nonvenomous), unspecified lower leg
- ● S80.87   Other superficial bite of lower leg
  - **Excludes1**   open bite of lower leg (S81.85-)
  - ● S80.871   Other superficial bite, right lower leg
  - ● S80.872   Other superficial bite, left lower leg
  - ● S80.879   Other superficial bite, unspecified lower leg
- ● S80.9   Unspecified superficial injury of knee and lower leg
  - ● S80.91   Unspecified superficial injury of knee
    - ● S80.911   Unspecified superficial injury of right knee
    - ● S80.912   Unspecified superficial injury of left knee
    - ● S80.919   Unspecified superficial injury of unspecified knee
  - ● S80.92   Unspecified superficial injury of lower leg
    - ● S80.921   Unspecified superficial injury of right lower leg
    - ● S80.922   Unspecified superficial injury of left lower leg
    - ● S80.929   Unspecified superficial injury of unspecified lower leg

- ● S81   **Open wound of knee and lower leg**
  - Code also any associated wound infection
  - **Excludes1**   open fracture of knee and lower leg (S82.-)
  -               traumatic amputation of lower leg (S88.-)
  - **Excludes2**   open wound of ankle and foot (S91.-)
  - The appropriate 7th character is to be added to each code from category S81

A	initial encounter
D	subsequent encounter
S	sequela

  - ● S81.0   Open wound of knee
    - ● S81.00   Unspecified open wound of knee
      - ● S81.001   Unspecified open wound, right knee
      - ● S81.002   Unspecified open wound, left knee
      - ● S81.009   Unspecified open wound, unspecified knee

◄ New   ◄ Revised   ~~deleted~~ Deleted   Excludes 1   Excludes 2   Includes   Use additional   Code first   Code also   Unspecified

1306   **OGCR** Official Guidelines   X Assign placeholder X   ● Use Additional Character(s)   ▶ Manifestation Code   **Coding Clinic**

● **S81.01**   Laceration without foreign body of knee
- ● **S81.011**   Laceration without foreign body, right knee
- ● **S81.012**   Laceration without foreign body, left knee
- ● **S81.019**   Laceration without foreign body, unspecified knee

● **S81.02**   Laceration with foreign body of knee
- ● **S81.021**   Laceration with foreign body, right knee
- ● **S81.022**   Laceration with foreign body, left knee
- ● **S81.029**   Laceration with foreign body, unspecified knee

● **S81.03**   Puncture wound without foreign body of knee
- ● **S81.031**   Puncture wound without foreign body, right knee
- ● **S81.032**   Puncture wound without foreign body, left knee
- ● **S81.039**   Puncture wound without foreign body, unspecified knee

● **S81.04**   Puncture wound with foreign body of knee
- ● **S81.041**   Puncture wound with foreign body, right knee
- ● **S81.042**   Puncture wound with foreign body, left knee
- ● **S81.049**   Puncture wound with foreign body, unspecified knee

● **S81.05**   Open bite of knee
    Bite of knee NOS
> **Excludes1**   superficial bite of knee (S80.27-)
- ● **S81.051**   Open bite, right knee
- ● **S81.052**   Open bite, left knee
- ● **S81.059**   Open bite, unspecified knee

● **S81.8**   Open wound of lower leg
- ● **S81.80**   Unspecified open wound of lower leg
  - ● **S81.801**   Unspecified open wound, right lower leg
  - ● **S81.802**   Unspecified open wound, left lower leg
  - ● **S81.809**   Unspecified open wound, unspecified lower leg
- ● **S81.81**   Laceration without foreign body of lower leg
  - ● **S81.811**   Laceration without foreign body, right lower leg
  - ● **S81.812**   Laceration without foreign body, left lower leg
  - ● **S81.819**   Laceration without foreign body, unspecified lower leg
- ● **S81.82**   Laceration with foreign body of lower leg
  - ● **S81.821**   Laceration with foreign body, right lower leg
  - ● **S81.822**   Laceration with foreign body, left lower leg
  - ● **S81.829**   Laceration with foreign body, unspecified lower leg
- ● **S81.83**   Puncture wound without foreign body of lower leg
  - ● **S81.831**   Puncture wound without foreign body, right lower leg
  - ● **S81.832**   Puncture wound without foreign body, left lower leg
  - ● **S81.839**   Puncture wound without foreign body, unspecified lower leg

● **S81.84**   Puncture wound with foreign body of lower leg
- ● **S81.841**   Puncture wound with foreign body, right lower leg
- ● **S81.842**   Puncture wound with foreign body, left lower leg
- ● **S81.849**   Puncture wound with foreign body, unspecified lower leg

● **S81.85**   Open bite of lower leg
    Bite of lower leg NOS
> **Excludes1**   superficial bite of lower leg (S80.86-, S80.87-)
- ● **S81.851**   Open bite, right lower leg
- ● **S81.852**   Open bite, left lower leg
- ● **S81.859**   Open bite, unspecified lower leg

● **S82**   **Fracture of lower leg, including ankle**
> **Note:** A fracture not indicated as displaced or nondisplaced should be coded to displaced
>
> A fracture not indicated as open or closed should be coded to closed
>
> The open fracture designations are based on the Gustilo open fracture classification

> **Includes**   fracture of malleolus
> **Excludes1**   traumatic amputation of lower leg (S88.-)
> **Excludes2**   fracture of foot, except ankle (S92.-)
>   periprosthetic fracture of prosthetic implant of knee (T84.042, T84.043)

The appropriate 7th character is to be added to all codes from category S82

A	initial encounter for closed fracture
B	initial encounter for open fracture type I or II initial encounter for open fracture NOS
C	initial encounter for open fracture type IIIA, IIIB, or IIIC
D	subsequent encounter for closed fracture with routine healing
E	subsequent encounter for open fracture type I or II with routine healing
F	subsequent encounter for open fracture type IIIA, IIIB, or IIIC with routine healing
G	subsequent encounter for closed fracture with delayed healing
H	subsequent encounter for open fracture type I or II with delayed healing
J	subsequent encounter for open fracture type IIIA, IIIB, or IIIC with delayed healing
K	subsequent encounter for closed fracture with nonunion
M	subsequent encounter for open fracture type I or II with nonunion
N	subsequent encounter for open fracture type IIIA, IIIB, or IIIC with nonunion
P	subsequent encounter for closed fracture with malunion
Q	subsequent encounter for open fracture type I or II with malunion
R	subsequent encounter for open fracture type IIIA, IIIB, or IIIC with malunion
S	sequela

● **S82.0**   **Fracture of patella**
    Knee cap
- ● **S82.00**   Unspecified fracture of patella
  - ● **S82.001**   Unspecified fracture of right patella
  - ● **S82.002**   Unspecified fracture of left patella
  - ● **S82.009**   Unspecified fracture of unspecified patella

CHAPTER 19 (S00-T88)

- ● S82.01   Osteochondral fracture of patella
  - ● S82.011   Displaced osteochondral fracture of right patella
  - ● S82.012   Displaced osteochondral fracture of left patella
  - ● S82.013   Displaced osteochondral fracture of unspecified patella
  - ● S82.014   Nondisplaced osteochondral fracture of right patella
  - ● S82.015   Nondisplaced osteochondral fracture of left patella
  - ● S82.016   Nondisplaced osteochondral fracture of unspecified patella
- ● S82.02   Longitudinal fracture of patella
  - ● S82.021   Displaced longitudinal fracture of right patella
  - ● S82.022   Displaced longitudinal fracture of left patella
  - ● S82.023   Displaced longitudinal fracture of unspecified patella
  - ● S82.024   Nondisplaced longitudinal fracture of right patella
  - ● S82.025   Nondisplaced longitudinal fracture of left patella
  - ● S82.026   Nondisplaced longitudinal fracture of unspecified patella
- ● S82.03   Transverse fracture of patella
  - ● S82.031   Displaced transverse fracture of right patella
  - ● S82.032   Displaced transverse fracture of left patella
  - ● S82.033   Displaced transverse fracture of unspecified patella
  - ● S82.034   Nondisplaced transverse fracture of right patella
  - ● S82.035   Nondisplaced transverse fracture of left patella
  - ● S82.036   Nondisplaced transverse fracture of unspecified patella
- ● S82.04   Comminuted fracture of patella
  - ● S82.041   Displaced comminuted fracture of right patella
  - ● S82.042   Displaced comminuted fracture of left patella
  - ● S82.043   Displaced comminuted fracture of unspecified patella
  - ● S82.044   Nondisplaced comminuted fracture of right patella
  - ● S82.045   Nondisplaced comminuted fracture of left patella
  - ● S82.046   Nondisplaced comminuted fracture of unspecified patella
- ● S82.09   Other fracture of patella
  - ● S82.091   Other fracture of right patella
  - ● S82.092   Other fracture of left patella
  - ● S82.099   Other fracture of unspecified patella
- ● S82.1   Fracture of upper end of tibia
  - Fracture of proximal end of tibia
  - **Excludes2**   fracture of shaft of tibia (S82.2-)
    - physeal fracture of upper end of tibia (S89.0-)
  - ● S82.10   Unspecified fracture of upper end of tibia
    - ● S82.101   Unspecified fracture of upper end of right tibia
    - ● S82.102   Unspecified fracture of upper end of left tibia
    - ● S82.109   Unspecified fracture of upper end of unspecified tibia

- ● S82.11   Fracture of tibial spine
  - ● S82.111   Displaced fracture of right tibial spine
  - ● S82.112   Displaced fracture of left tibial spine
  - ● S82.113   Displaced fracture of unspecified tibial spine
  - ● S82.114   Nondisplaced fracture of right tibial spine
  - ● S82.115   Nondisplaced fracture of left tibial spine
  - ● S82.116   Nondisplaced fracture of unspecified tibial spine
- ● S82.12   Fracture of lateral condyle of tibia
  - ● S82.121   Displaced fracture of lateral condyle of right tibia
  - ● S82.122   Displaced fracture of lateral condyle of left tibia
  - ● S82.123   Displaced fracture of lateral condyle of unspecified tibia
  - ● S82.124   Nondisplaced fracture of lateral condyle of right tibia
  - ● S82.125   Nondisplaced fracture of lateral condyle of left tibia
  - ● S82.126   Nondisplaced fracture of lateral condyle of unspecified tibia
- ● S82.13   Fracture of medial condyle of tibia
  - ● S82.131   Displaced fracture of medial condyle of right tibia
  - ● S82.132   Displaced fracture of medial condyle of left tibia
  - ● S82.133   Displaced fracture of medial condyle of unspecified tibia
  - ● S82.134   Nondisplaced fracture of medial condyle of right tibia
  - ● S82.135   Nondisplaced fracture of medial condyle of left tibia
  - ● S82.136   Nondisplaced fracture of medial condyle of unspecified tibia
- ● S82.14   Bicondylar fracture of tibia
  - Fracture of tibial plateau NOS
  - ● S82.141   Displaced bicondylar fracture of right tibia
  - ● S82.142   Displaced bicondylar fracture of left tibia
  - ● S82.143   Displaced bicondylar fracture of unspecified tibia
  - ● S82.144   Nondisplaced bicondylar fracture of right tibia
  - ● S82.145   Nondisplaced bicondylar fracture of left tibia
  - ● S82.146   Nondisplaced bicondylar fracture of unspecified tibia
- ● S82.15   Fracture of tibial tuberosity
  - ● S82.151   Displaced fracture of right tibial tuberosity
  - ● S82.152   Displaced fracture of left tibial tuberosity
  - ● S82.153   Displaced fracture of unspecified tibial tuberosity
  - ● S82.154   Nondisplaced fracture of right tibial tuberosity
  - ● S82.155   Nondisplaced fracture of left tibial tuberosity
  - ● S82.156   Nondisplaced fracture of unspecified tibial tuberosity

◀ New   ◀⃝ Revised   ~~deleted~~ Deleted   Excludes 1   Excludes 2   Includes   Use additional   Code first   Code also   Unspecified

1308   **OGCR** Official Guidelines   X Assign placeholder X   ● Use Additional Character(s)   ▶ Manifestation Code   **Coding Clinic**

● **S82.16**   **Torus fracture of upper end of tibia**
The appropriate 7th character is to be added to all codes in subcategory S82.16

A	initial encounter for closed fracture
D	subsequent encounter for fracture with routine healing
G	subsequent encounter for fracture with delayed healing
K	subsequent encounter for fracture with nonunion
P	subsequent encounter for fracture with malunion
S	sequela

   ● **S82.161**   Torus fracture of upper end of right tibia
   ● **S82.162**   Torus fracture of upper end of left tibia
   ● **S82.169**   Torus fracture of upper end of unspecified tibia

● **S82.19**   **Other fracture of upper end of tibia**
   ● **S82.191**   Other fracture of upper end of right tibia
   ● **S82.192**   Other fracture of upper end of left tibia
   ● **S82.199**   Other fracture of upper end of unspecified tibia

● **S82.2**   **Fracture of shaft of tibia**
   ● **S82.20**   **Unspecified fracture of shaft of tibia**
     Fracture of tibia NOS
     ● **S82.201**   Unspecified fracture of shaft of right tibia
     ● **S82.202**   Unspecified fracture of shaft of left tibia
     ● **S82.209**   Unspecified fracture of shaft of unspecified tibia

   ● **S82.22**   **Transverse fracture of shaft of tibia**
     ● **S82.221**   Displaced transverse fracture of shaft of right tibia
     ● **S82.222**   Displaced transverse fracture of shaft of left tibia
     ● **S82.223**   Displaced transverse fracture of shaft of unspecified tibia
     ● **S82.224**   Nondisplaced transverse fracture of shaft of right tibia
     ● **S82.225**   Nondisplaced transverse fracture of shaft of left tibia
     ● **S82.226**   Nondisplaced transverse fracture of shaft of unspecified tibia

   ● **S82.23**   **Oblique fracture of shaft of tibia**
     ● **S82.231**   Displaced oblique fracture of shaft of right tibia
     ● **S82.232**   Displaced oblique fracture of shaft of left tibia
     ● **S82.233**   Displaced oblique fracture of shaft of unspecified tibia
     ● **S82.234**   Nondisplaced oblique fracture of shaft of right tibia
         Coding Clinic: 2015, Q1, P9-10
     ● **S82.235**   Nondisplaced oblique fracture of shaft of left tibia
     ● **S82.236**   Nondisplaced oblique fracture of shaft of unspecified tibia

● **S82.24**   **Spiral fracture of shaft of tibia**
     Toddler fracture
   ● **S82.241**   Displaced spiral fracture of shaft of right tibia
   ● **S82.242**   Displaced spiral fracture of shaft of left tibia
   ● **S82.243**   Displaced spiral fracture of shaft of unspecified tibia
   ● **S82.244**   Nondisplaced spiral fracture of shaft of right tibia
   ● **S82.245**   Nondisplaced spiral fracture of shaft of left tibia
   ● **S82.246**   Nondisplaced spiral fracture of shaft of unspecified tibia

● **S82.25**   **Comminuted fracture of shaft of tibia**
   ● **S82.251**   Displaced comminuted fracture of shaft of right tibia
       Coding Clinic: 2015, Q2, P6
   ● **S82.252**   Displaced comminuted fracture of shaft of left tibia
   ● **S82.253**   Displaced comminuted fracture of shaft of unspecified tibia
   ● **S82.254**   Nondisplaced comminuted fracture of shaft of right tibia
   ● **S82.255**   Nondisplaced comminuted fracture of shaft of left tibia
   ● **S82.256**   Nondisplaced comminuted fracture of shaft of unspecified tibia

● **S82.26**   **Segmental fracture of shaft of tibia**
   ● **S82.261**   Displaced segmental fracture of shaft of right tibia
   ● **S82.262**   Displaced segmental fracture of shaft of left tibia
   ● **S82.263**   Displaced segmental fracture of shaft of unspecified tibia
   ● **S82.264**   Nondisplaced segmental fracture of shaft of right tibia
   ● **S82.265**   Nondisplaced segmental fracture of shaft of left tibia
   ● **S82.266**   Nondisplaced segmental fracture of shaft of unspecified tibia

● **S82.29**   **Other fracture of shaft of tibia**
   ● **S82.291**   Other fracture of shaft of right tibia
   ● **S82.292**   Other fracture of shaft of left tibia
   ● **S82.299**   Other fracture of shaft of unspecified tibia

● **S82.3**   **Fracture of lower end of tibia**
   Excludes1   bimalleolar fracture of lower leg (S82.84-)
               fracture of medial malleolus alone (S82.5-)
               Maisonneuve's fracture (S82.86-)
               pilon fracture of distal tibia (S82.87-)
               trimalleolar fractures of lower leg (S82.85-)

● **S82.30**   **Unspecified fracture of lower end of tibia**
   ● **S82.301**   Unspecified fracture of lower end of right tibia
   ● **S82.302**   Unspecified fracture of lower end of left tibia
   ● **S82.309**   Unspecified fracture of lower end of unspecified tibia

CHAPTER 19 (S00-T88)

● S82.31 Torus fracture of lower end of tibia

The appropriate 7th character is to be added to all codes in subcategory S82.31

> A   initial encounter for closed fracture
> D   subsequent encounter for fracture with routine healing
> G   subsequent encounter for fracture with delayed healing
> K   subsequent encounter for fracture with nonunion
> P   subsequent encounter for fracture with malunion
> S   sequela

　　● S82.311 Torus fracture of lower end of right tibia
　　● S82.312 Torus fracture of lower end of left tibia
　　● S82.319 Torus fracture of lower end of unspecified tibia

● S82.39 Other fracture of lower end of tibia
　　● S82.391 Other fracture of lower end of right tibia
　　● S82.392 Other fracture of lower end of left tibia
　　　　Coding Clinic: 2015, Q1, P25
　　● S82.399 Other fracture of lower end of unspecified tibia

● S82.4 Fracture of shaft of fibula
　　Excludes2   fracture of lateral malleolus alone (S82.6-)

● S82.40 Unspecified fracture of shaft of fibula
　　● S82.401 Unspecified fracture of shaft of right fibula
　　● S82.402 Unspecified fracture of shaft of left fibula
　　● S82.409 Unspecified fracture of shaft of unspecified fibula

● S82.42 Transverse fracture of shaft of fibula
　　● S82.421 Displaced transverse fracture of shaft of right fibula
　　● S82.422 Displaced transverse fracture of shaft of left fibula
　　● S82.423 Displaced transverse fracture of shaft of unspecified fibula
　　● S82.424 Nondisplaced transverse fracture of shaft of right fibula
　　● S82.425 Nondisplaced transverse fracture of shaft of left fibula
　　● S82.426 Nondisplaced transverse fracture of shaft of unspecified fibula

● S82.43 Oblique fracture of shaft of fibula
　　● S82.431 Displaced oblique fracture of shaft of right fibula
　　● S82.432 Displaced oblique fracture of shaft of left fibula
　　● S82.433 Displaced oblique fracture of shaft of unspecified fibula
　　● S82.434 Nondisplaced oblique fracture of shaft of right fibula
　　● S82.435 Nondisplaced oblique fracture of shaft of left fibula
　　● S82.436 Nondisplaced oblique fracture of shaft of unspecified fibula

● S82.44 Spiral fracture of shaft of fibula
　　● S82.441 Displaced spiral fracture of shaft of right fibula
　　● S82.442 Displaced spiral fracture of shaft of left fibula
　　● S82.443 Displaced spiral fracture of shaft of unspecified fibula
　　● S82.444 Nondisplaced spiral fracture of shaft of right fibula
　　● S82.445 Nondisplaced spiral fracture of shaft of left fibula
　　● S82.446 Nondisplaced spiral fracture of shaft of unspecified fibula

● S82.45 Comminuted fracture of shaft of fibula
　　● S82.451 Displaced comminuted fracture of shaft of right fibula
　　● S82.452 Displaced comminuted fracture of shaft of left fibula
　　● S82.453 Displaced comminuted fracture of shaft of unspecified fibula
　　● S82.454 Nondisplaced comminuted fracture of shaft of right fibula
　　● S82.455 Nondisplaced comminuted fracture of shaft of left fibula
　　● S82.456 Nondisplaced comminuted fracture of shaft of unspecified fibula

● S82.46 Segmental fracture of shaft of fibula
　　● S82.461 Displaced segmental fracture of shaft of right fibula
　　● S82.462 Displaced segmental fracture of shaft of left fibula
　　● S82.463 Displaced segmental fracture of shaft of unspecified fibula
　　● S82.464 Nondisplaced segmental fracture of shaft of right fibula
　　● S82.465 Nondisplaced segmental fracture of shaft of left fibula
　　● S82.466 Nondisplaced segmental fracture of shaft of unspecified fibula

● S82.49 Other fracture of shaft of fibula
　　● S82.491 Other fracture of shaft of right fibula
　　● S82.492 Other fracture of shaft of left fibula
　　● S82.499 Other fracture of shaft of unspecified fibula

● S82.5 Fracture of medial malleolus
　　Excludes1   pilon fracture of distal tibia (S82.87-)
　　　　Salter-Harris type III of lower end of tibia (S89.13-)
　　　　Salter-Harris type IV of lower end of tibia (S89.14-)

X ● S82.51 Displaced fracture of medial malleolus of right tibia
X ● S82.52 Displaced fracture of medial malleolus of left tibia
X ● S82.53 Displaced fracture of medial malleolus of unspecified tibia
X ● S82.54 Nondisplaced fracture of medial malleolus of right tibia
X ● S82.55 Nondisplaced fracture of medial malleolus of left tibia
X ● S82.56 Nondisplaced fracture of medial malleolus of unspecified tibia

● **S82.6**   **Fracture of lateral malleolus**
> **Excludes1**   pilon fracture of distal tibia (S82.87-)

X● **S82.61**   Displaced fracture of lateral malleolus of right fibula

X● **S82.62**   Displaced fracture of lateral malleolus of left fibula

X● **S82.63**   Displaced fracture of lateral malleolus of unspecified fibula

X● **S82.64**   Nondisplaced fracture of lateral malleolus of right fibula

X● **S82.65**   Nondisplaced fracture of lateral malleolus of left fibula

X● **S82.66**   Nondisplaced fracture of lateral malleolus of unspecified fibula

● **S82.8**   **Other fractures of lower leg**

● **S82.81**   **Torus fracture of upper end of fibula**
> The appropriate 7th character is to be added to all codes in subcategory S82.81

> A   initial encounter for closed fracture
> D   subsequent encounter for fracture with routine healing
> G   subsequent encounter for fracture with delayed healing
> K   subsequent encounter for fracture with nonunion
> P   subsequent encounter for fracture with malunion
> S   sequela

● **S82.811**   Torus fracture of upper end of right fibula

● **S82.812**   Torus fracture of upper end of left fibula

● **S82.819**   Torus fracture of upper end of unspecified fibula

● **S82.82**   **Torus fracture of lower end of fibula**
> The appropriate 7th character is to be added to all codes in subcategory S82.82

> A   initial encounter for closed fracture
> D   subsequent encounter for fracture with routine healing
> G   subsequent encounter for fracture with delayed healing
> K   subsequent encounter for fracture with nonunion
> P   subsequent encounter for fracture with malunion
> S   sequela

● **S82.821**   Torus fracture of lower end of right fibula

● **S82.822**   Torus fracture of lower end of left fibula

● **S82.829**   Torus fracture of lower end of unspecified fibula

● **S82.83**   **Other fracture of upper and lower end of fibula**

● **S82.831**   Other fracture of upper and lower end of right fibula

● **S82.832**   Other fracture of upper and lower end of left fibula
> **Coding Clinic: 2015, Q1, P9-10**

● **S82.839**   Other fracture of upper and lower end of unspecified fibula

● **S82.84**   **Bimalleolar fracture of lower leg**

● **S82.841**   Displaced bimalleolar fracture of right lower leg

● **S82.842**   Displaced bimalleolar fracture of left lower leg

● **S82.843**   Displaced bimalleolar fracture of unspecified lower leg

● **S82.844**   Nondisplaced bimalleolar fracture of right lower leg

● **S82.845**   Nondisplaced bimalleolar fracture of left lower leg

● **S82.846**   Nondisplaced bimalleolar fracture of unspecified lower leg

● **S82.85**   **Trimalleolar fracture of lower leg**

● **S82.851**   Displaced trimalleolar fracture of right lower leg

● **S82.852**   Displaced trimalleolar fracture of left lower leg

● **S82.853**   Displaced trimalleolar fracture of unspecified lower leg

● **S82.854**   Nondisplaced trimalleolar fracture of right lower leg

● **S82.855**   Nondisplaced trimalleolar fracture of left lower leg

● **S82.856**   Nondisplaced trimalleolar fracture of unspecified lower leg

● **S82.86**   **Maisonneuve's fracture**

● **S82.861**   Displaced Maisonneuve's fracture of right leg

● **S82.862**   Displaced Maisonneuve's fracture of left leg

● **S82.863**   Displaced Maisonneuve's fracture of unspecified leg

● **S82.864**   Nondisplaced Maisonneuve's fracture of right leg

● **S82.865**   Nondisplaced Maisonneuve's fracture of left leg

● **S82.866**   Nondisplaced Maisonneuve's fracture of unspecified leg

● **S82.87**   **Pilon fracture of tibia**

● **S82.871**   Displaced pilon fracture of right tibia

● **S82.872**   Displaced pilon fracture of left tibia

● **S82.873**   Displaced pilon fracture of unspecified tibia

● **S82.874**   Nondisplaced pilon fracture of right tibia

● **S82.875**   Nondisplaced pilon fracture of left tibia

● **S82.876**   Nondisplaced pilon fracture of unspecified tibia

● **S82.89**   **Other fractures of lower leg**
> Fracture of ankle NOS

● **S82.891**   Other fracture of right lower leg

● **S82.892**   Other fracture of left lower leg

● **S82.899**   Other fracture of unspecified lower leg

● **S82.9**   **Unspecified fracture of lower leg**

X● **S82.90**   Unspecified fracture of unspecified lower leg

X● **S82.91**   Unspecified fracture of right lower leg

X● **S82.92**   Unspecified fracture of left lower leg

CHAPTER 19 (S00-T88)

● **S83**   **Dislocation and sprain of joints and ligaments of knee**

Includes   avulsion of joint or ligament of knee
laceration of cartilage, joint or ligament of knee
sprain of cartilage, joint or ligament of knee
traumatic hemarthrosis of joint or ligament of knee
traumatic rupture of joint or ligament of knee
traumatic subluxation of joint or ligament of knee
traumatic tear of joint or ligament of knee

Code also any associated open wound

Excludes1   derangement of patella (M22.0-M22.3)
injury of patellar ligament (tendon) (S76.1-)
internal derangement of knee (M23.-)
old dislocation of knee (M24.36)
pathological dislocation of knee (M24.36)
recurrent dislocation of knee (M22.0)

Excludes2   strain of muscle, fascia and tendon of lower leg (S86.-)

The appropriate 7th character is to be added to each code from category S83

> A   initial encounter
> D   subsequent encounter
> S   sequela

● **S83.0**   **Subluxation and dislocation of patella**

   ● **S83.00**   Unspecified subluxation and dislocation of patella

     ● **S83.001**   Unspecified subluxation of right patella

     ● **S83.002**   Unspecified subluxation of left patella

     ● **S83.003**   Unspecified subluxation of unspecified patella

     ● **S83.004**   Unspecified dislocation of right patella

     ● **S83.005**   Unspecified dislocation of left patella

     ● **S83.006**   Unspecified dislocation of unspecified patella

   ● **S83.01**   Lateral subluxation and dislocation of patella

     ● **S83.011**   Lateral subluxation of right patella

     ● **S83.012**   Lateral subluxation of left patella

     ● **S83.013**   Lateral subluxation of unspecified patella

     ● **S83.014**   Lateral dislocation of right patella

     ● **S83.015**   Lateral dislocation of left patella

     ● **S83.016**   Lateral dislocation of unspecified patella

   ● **S83.09**   Other subluxation and dislocation of patella

     ● **S83.091**   Other subluxation of right patella

     ● **S83.092**   Other subluxation of left patella

     ● **S83.093**   Other subluxation of unspecified patella

     ● **S83.094**   Other dislocation of right patella

     ● **S83.095**   Other dislocation of left patella

     ● **S83.096**   Other dislocation of unspecified patella

● **S83.1**   **Subluxation and dislocation of knee**

Excludes2   instability of knee prosthesis (T84.022, T84.023)

   ● **S83.10**   Unspecified subluxation and dislocation of knee

     ● **S83.101**   Unspecified subluxation of right knee

     ● **S83.102**   Unspecified subluxation of left knee

     ● **S83.103**   Unspecified subluxation of unspecified knee

     ● **S83.104**   Unspecified dislocation of right knee

     ● **S83.105**   Unspecified dislocation of left knee

     ● **S83.106**   Unspecified dislocation of unspecified knee

   ● **S83.11**   **Anterior subluxation and dislocation of proximal end of tibia**
Posterior subluxation and dislocation of distal end of femur

     ● **S83.111**   Anterior subluxation of proximal end of tibia, right knee

     ● **S83.112**   Anterior subluxation of proximal end of tibia, left knee

     ● **S83.113**   Anterior subluxation of proximal end of tibia, unspecified knee

     ● **S83.114**   Anterior dislocation of proximal end of tibia, right knee

     ● **S83.115**   Anterior dislocation of proximal end of tibia, left knee

     ● **S83.116**   Anterior dislocation of proximal end of tibia, unspecified knee

   ● **S83.12**   **Posterior subluxation and dislocation of proximal end of tibia**
Anterior dislocation of distal end of femur

     ● **S83.121**   Posterior subluxation of proximal end of tibia, right knee

     ● **S83.122**   Posterior subluxation of proximal end of tibia, left knee

     ● **S83.123**   Posterior subluxation of proximal end of tibia, unspecified knee

     ● **S83.124**   Posterior dislocation of proximal end of tibia, right knee

     ● **S83.125**   Posterior dislocation of proximal end of tibia, left knee

     ● **S83.126**   Posterior dislocation of proximal end of tibia, unspecified knee

   ● **S83.13**   Medial subluxation and dislocation of proximal end of tibia

     ● **S83.131**   Medial subluxation of proximal end of tibia, right knee

     ● **S83.132**   Medial subluxation of proximal end of tibia, left knee

     ● **S83.133**   Medial subluxation of proximal end of tibia, unspecified knee

     ● **S83.134**   Medial dislocation of proximal end of tibia, right knee

     ● **S83.135**   Medial dislocation of proximal end of tibia, left knee

     ● **S83.136**   Medial dislocation of proximal end of tibia, unspecified knee

   ● **S83.14**   Lateral subluxation and dislocation of proximal end of tibia

     ● **S83.141**   Lateral subluxation of proximal end of tibia, right knee

     ● **S83.142**   Lateral subluxation of proximal end of tibia, left knee

     ● **S83.143**   Lateral subluxation of proximal end of tibia, unspecified knee

     ● **S83.144**   Lateral dislocation of proximal end of tibia, right knee

     ● **S83.145**   Lateral dislocation of proximal end of tibia, left knee

     ● **S83.146**   Lateral dislocation of proximal end of tibia, unspecified knee

   ● **S83.19**   Other subluxation and dislocation of knee

     ● **S83.191**   Other subluxation of right knee

     ● **S83.192**   Other subluxation of left knee

     ● **S83.193**   Other subluxation of unspecified knee

     ● **S83.194**   Other dislocation of right knee

     ● **S83.195**   Other dislocation of left knee

     ● **S83.196**   Other dislocation of unspecified knee

◀ New   ◀▥ Revised   ~~deleted~~ Deleted   Excludes 1   Excludes 2   Includes   Use additional   Code first   Code also   Unspecified

1312   **OGCR** Official Guidelines   X Assign placeholder X   ● Use Additional Character(s)   ▶ Manifestation Code   **Coding Clinic**

● S83.2   Tear of meniscus, current injury

     Excludes1   old bucket-handle tear (M23.2)

● S83.20   Tear of unspecified meniscus, current injury
                    Tear of meniscus of knee NOS

    ● S83.200   Bucket-handle tear of unspecified meniscus, current injury, right knee

    ● S83.201   Bucket-handle tear of unspecified meniscus, current injury, left knee

    ● S83.202   Bucket-handle tear of unspecified meniscus, current injury, unspecified knee

    ● S83.203   Other tear of unspecified meniscus, current injury, right knee

    ● S83.204   Other tear of unspecified meniscus, current injury, left knee

    ● S83.205   Other tear of unspecified meniscus, current injury, unspecified knee

    ● S83.206   Unspecified tear of unspecified meniscus, current injury, right knee

    ● S83.207   Unspecified tear of unspecified meniscus, current injury, left knee

    ● S83.209   Unspecified tear of unspecified meniscus, current injury, unspecified knee

● S83.21   Bucket-handle tear of medial meniscus, current injury

    ● S83.211   Bucket-handle tear of medial meniscus, current injury, right knee

    ● S83.212   Bucket-handle tear of medial meniscus, current injury, left knee

    ● S83.219   Bucket-handle tear of medial meniscus, current injury, unspecified knee

● S83.22   Peripheral tear of medial meniscus, current injury

    ● S83.221   Peripheral tear of medial meniscus, current injury, right knee

    ● S83.222   Peripheral tear of medial meniscus, current injury, left knee

    ● S83.229   Peripheral tear of medial meniscus, current injury, unspecified knee

● S83.23   Complex tear of medial meniscus, current injury

    ● S83.231   Complex tear of medial meniscus, current injury, right knee

    ● S83.232   Complex tear of medial meniscus, current injury, left knee

    ● S83.239   Complex tear of medial meniscus, current injury, unspecified knee

● S83.24   Other tear of medial meniscus, current injury

    ● S83.241   Other tear of medial meniscus, current injury, right knee

    ● S83.242   Other tear of medial meniscus, current injury, left knee

    ● S83.249   Other tear of medial meniscus, current injury, unspecified knee

● S83.25   Bucket-handle tear of lateral meniscus, current injury

    ● S83.251   Bucket-handle tear of lateral meniscus, current injury, right knee

    ● S83.252   Bucket-handle tear of lateral meniscus, current injury, left knee

    ● S83.259   Bucket-handle tear of lateral meniscus, current injury, unspecified knee

● S83.26   Peripheral tear of lateral meniscus, current injury

    ● S83.261   Peripheral tear of lateral meniscus, current injury, right knee

    ● S83.262   Peripheral tear of lateral meniscus, current injury, left knee

    ● S83.269   Peripheral tear of lateral meniscus, current injury, unspecified knee

● S83.27   Complex tear of lateral meniscus, current injury

    ● S83.271   Complex tear of lateral meniscus, current injury, right knee

    ● S83.272   Complex tear of lateral meniscus, current injury, left knee

    ● S83.279   Complex tear of lateral meniscus, current injury, unspecified knee

● S83.28   Other tear of lateral meniscus, current injury

    ● S83.281   Other tear of lateral meniscus, current injury, right knee

    ● S83.282   Other tear of lateral meniscus, current injury, left knee

    ● S83.289   Other tear of lateral meniscus, current injury, unspecified knee

● S83.3   Tear of articular cartilage of knee, current

  X ● S83.30   Tear of articular cartilage of unspecified knee, current

  X ● S83.31   Tear of articular cartilage of right knee, current

  X ● S83.32   Tear of articular cartilage of left knee, current

● S83.4   Sprain of collateral ligament of knee

  ● S83.40   Sprain of unspecified collateral ligament of knee

    ● S83.401   Sprain of unspecified collateral ligament of right knee

    ● S83.402   Sprain of unspecified collateral ligament of left knee

    ● S83.409   Sprain of unspecified collateral ligament of unspecified knee

  ● S83.41   Sprain of medial collateral ligament of knee
              Sprain of tibial collateral ligament

     S83.411   Sprain of medial collateral ligament of right knee

     S83.412   Sprain of medial collateral ligament of left knee

     S83.419   Sprain of medial collateral ligament of unspecified knee

  ● S83.42   Sprain of lateral collateral ligament of knee
              Sprain of fibular collateral ligament

    ● S83.421   Sprain of lateral collateral ligament of right knee

    ● S83.422   Sprain of lateral collateral ligament of left knee

    ● S83.429   Sprain of lateral collateral ligament of unspecified knee

● S83.5   Sprain of cruciate ligament of knee

  ● S83.50   Sprain of unspecified cruciate ligament of knee

    ● S83.501   Sprain of unspecified cruciate ligament of right knee

    ● S83.502   Sprain of unspecified cruciate ligament of left knee

    ● S83.509   Sprain of unspecified cruciate ligament of unspecified knee

  ● S83.51   Sprain of anterior cruciate ligament of knee

    ● S83.511   Sprain of anterior cruciate ligament of right knee
                Coding Clinic: 2016, Q2, P4

    ● S83.512   Sprain of anterior cruciate ligament of left knee

    ● S83.519   Sprain of anterior cruciate ligament of unspecified knee

CHAPTER 19 (S00-T88)

● S83.52　Sprain of posterior cruciate ligament of knee
　　● S83.521　Sprain of posterior cruciate ligament of right knee
　　● S83.522　Sprain of posterior cruciate ligament of left knee
　　● S83.529　Sprain of posterior cruciate ligament of unspecified knee
● S83.6　Sprain of the superior tibiofibular joint and ligament
　X● S83.60　Sprain of the superior tibiofibular joint and ligament, unspecified knee
　X● S83.61　Sprain of the superior tibiofibular joint and ligament, right knee
　X● S83.62　Sprain of the superior tibiofibular joint and ligament, left knee
● S83.8　Sprain of other specified parts of knee
　● S83.8X　Sprain of other specified parts of knee
　　● S83.8X1　Sprain of other specified parts of right knee
　　● S83.8X2　Sprain of other specified parts of left knee
　　● S83.8X9　Sprain of other specified parts of unspecified knee
● S83.9　Sprain of unspecified site of knee
　X● S83.90　Sprain of unspecified site of unspecified knee
　X● S83.91　Sprain of unspecified site of right knee
　X● S83.92　Sprain of unspecified site of left knee

● S84　Injury of nerves at lower leg level
　　Code also any associated open wound (S81.-)
　　Excludes2　injury of nerves at ankle and foot level (S94.-)
　　The appropriate 7th character is to be added to each code from category S84

> A　initial encounter
> D　subsequent encounter
> S　sequela

● S84.0　Injury of tibial nerve at lower leg level
　X● S84.00　Injury of tibial nerve at lower leg level, unspecified leg
　X● S84.01　Injury of tibial nerve at lower leg level, right leg
　X● S84.02　Injury of tibial nerve at lower leg level, left leg
● S84.1　Injury of peroneal nerve at lower leg level
　X● S84.10　Injury of peroneal nerve at lower leg level, unspecified leg
　X● S84.11　Injury of peroneal nerve at lower leg level, right leg
　X● S84.12　Injury of peroneal nerve at lower leg level, left leg
● S84.2　Injury of cutaneous sensory nerve at lower leg level
　X● S84.20　Injury of cutaneous sensory nerve at lower leg level, unspecified leg
　X● S84.21　Injury of cutaneous sensory nerve at lower leg level, right leg
　X● S84.22　Injury of cutaneous sensory nerve at lower leg level, left leg
● S84.8　Injury of other nerves at lower leg level
　● S84.80　Injury of other nerves at lower leg level
　　● S84.801　Injury of other nerves at lower leg level, right leg
　　● S84.802　Injury of other nerves at lower leg level, left leg
　　● S84.809　Injury of other nerves at lower leg level, unspecified leg
● S84.9　Injury of unspecified nerve at lower leg level
　X● S84.90　Injury of unspecified nerve at lower leg level, unspecified leg
　X● S84.91　Injury of unspecified nerve at lower leg level, right leg
　X● S84.92　Injury of unspecified nerve at lower leg level, left leg

● S85　Injury of blood vessels at lower leg level
　　Code also any associated open wound (S81.-)
　　Excludes2　injury of blood vessels at ankle and foot level (S95.-)
　　The appropriate 7th character is to be added to each code from category S85

> A　initial encounter
> D　subsequent encounter
> S　sequela

● S85.0　Injury of popliteal artery
　● S85.00　Unspecified injury of popliteal artery
　　● S85.001　Unspecified injury of popliteal artery, right leg
　　● S85.002　Unspecified injury of popliteal artery, left leg
　　● S85.009　Unspecified injury of popliteal artery, unspecified leg
　● S85.01　Laceration of popliteal artery
　　● S85.011　Laceration of popliteal artery, right leg
　　● S85.012　Laceration of popliteal artery, left leg
　　● S85.019　Laceration of popliteal artery, unspecified leg
　● S85.09　Other specified injury of popliteal artery
　　● S85.091　Other specified injury of popliteal artery, right leg
　　● S85.092　Other specified injury of popliteal artery, left leg
　　● S85.099　Other specified injury of popliteal artery, unspecified leg
● S85.1　Injury of tibial artery
　● S85.10　Unspecified injury of unspecified tibial artery
　　　Injury of tibial artery NOS
　　● S85.101　Unspecified injury of unspecified tibial artery, right leg
　　● S85.102　Unspecified injury of unspecified tibial artery, left leg
　　● S85.109　Unspecified injury of unspecified tibial artery, unspecified leg
　● S85.11　Laceration of unspecified tibial artery
　　● S85.111　Laceration of unspecified tibial artery, right leg
　　● S85.112　Laceration of unspecified tibial artery, left leg
　　● S85.119　Laceration of unspecified tibial artery, unspecified leg
　● S85.12　Other specified injury of unspecified tibial artery
　　● S85.121　Other specified injury of unspecified tibial artery, right leg
　　● S85.122　Other specified injury of unspecified tibial artery, left leg
　　● S85.129　Other specified injury of unspecified tibial artery, unspecified leg
　● S85.13　Unspecified injury of anterior tibial artery
　　● S85.131　Unspecified injury of anterior tibial artery, right leg
　　● S85.132　Unspecified injury of anterior tibial artery, left leg
　　● S85.139　Unspecified injury of anterior tibial artery, unspecified leg
　● S85.14　Laceration of anterior tibial artery
　　● S85.141　Laceration of anterior tibial artery, right leg
　　● S85.142　Laceration of anterior tibial artery, left leg
　　● S85.149　Laceration of anterior tibial artery, unspecified leg

◀ New　◀▥ Revised　~~deleted~~ Deleted　Excludes 1　Excludes 2　Includes　Use additional　Code first　Code also　Unspecified
OGCR Official Guidelines　X Assign placeholder X　● Use Additional Character(s)　▶ Manifestation Code　Coding Clinic
1314

● **S85.15**   Other specified injury of anterior tibial artery
- ● **S85.151**   Other specified injury of anterior tibial artery, right leg
- ● **S85.152**   Other specified injury of anterior tibial artery, left leg
- ● **S85.159**   Other specified injury of anterior tibial artery, unspecified leg

● **S85.16**   Unspecified injury of posterior tibial artery
- ● **S85.161**   Unspecified injury of posterior tibial artery, right leg
- ● **S85.162**   Unspecified injury of posterior tibial artery, left leg
- ● **S85.169**   Unspecified injury of posterior tibial artery, unspecified leg

● **S85.17**   Laceration of posterior tibial artery
- ● **S85.171**   Laceration of posterior tibial artery, right leg
- ● **S85.172**   Laceration of posterior tibial artery, left leg
- ● **S85.179**   Laceration of posterior tibial artery, unspecified leg

● **S85.18**   Other specified injury of posterior tibial artery
- ● **S85.181**   Other specified injury of posterior tibial artery, right leg
- ● **S85.182**   Other specified injury of posterior tibial artery, left leg
- ● **S85.189**   Other specified injury of posterior tibial artery, unspecified leg

● **S85.2**   Injury of peroneal artery
- ● **S85.20**   Unspecified injury of peroneal artery
  - ● **S85.201**   Unspecified injury of peroneal artery, right leg
  - ● **S85.202**   Unspecified injury of peroneal artery, left leg
  - ● **S85.209**   Unspecified injury of peroneal artery, unspecified leg
- ● **S85.21**   Laceration of peroneal artery
  - ● **S85.211**   Laceration of peroneal artery, right leg
  - ● **S85.212**   Laceration of peroneal artery, left leg
  - ● **S85.219**   Laceration of peroneal artery, unspecified leg
- ● **S85.29**   Other specified injury of peroneal artery
  - ● **S85.291**   Other specified injury of peroneal artery, right leg
  - ● **S85.292**   Other specified injury of peroneal artery, left leg
  - ● **S85.299**   Other specified injury of peroneal artery, unspecified leg

● **S85.3**   Injury of greater saphenous vein at lower leg level
    Injury of greater saphenous vein NOS
    Injury of saphenous vein NOS
- ● **S85.30**   Unspecified injury of greater saphenous vein at lower leg level
  - ● **S85.301**   Unspecified injury of greater saphenous vein at lower leg level, right leg
  - ● **S85.302**   Unspecified injury of greater saphenous vein at lower leg level, left leg
  - ● **S85.309**   Unspecified injury of greater saphenous vein at lower leg level, unspecified leg

● **S85.31**   Laceration of greater saphenous vein at lower leg level
- ● **S85.311**   Laceration of greater saphenous vein at lower leg level, right leg
- ● **S85.312**   Laceration of greater saphenous vein at lower leg level, left leg
- ● **S85.319**   Laceration of greater saphenous vein at lower leg level, unspecified leg

● **S85.39**   Other specified injury of greater saphenous vein at lower leg level
- ● **S85.391**   Other specified injury of greater saphenous vein at lower leg level, right leg
- ● **S85.392**   Other specified injury of greater saphenous vein at lower leg level, left leg
- ● **S85.399**   Other specified injury of greater saphenous vein at lower leg level, unspecified leg

● **S85.4**   Injury of lesser saphenous vein at lower leg level
- ● **S85.40**   Unspecified injury of lesser saphenous vein at lower leg level
  - ● **S85.401**   Unspecified injury of lesser saphenous vein at lower leg level, right leg
  - ● **S85.402**   Unspecified injury of lesser saphenous vein at lower leg level, left leg
  - ● **S85.409**   Unspecified injury of lesser saphenous vein at lower leg level, unspecified leg
- ● **S85.41**   Laceration of lesser saphenous vein at lower leg level
  - ● **S85.411**   Laceration of lesser saphenous vein at lower leg level, right leg
  - ● **S85.412**   Laceration of lesser saphenous vein at lower leg level, left leg
  - ● **S85.419**   Laceration of lesser saphenous vein at lower leg level, unspecified leg
- ● **S85.49**   Other specified injury of lesser saphenous vein at lower leg level
  - ● **S85.491**   Other specified injury of lesser saphenous vein at lower leg level, right leg
  - ● **S85.492**   Other specified injury of lesser saphenous vein at lower leg level, left leg
  - ● **S85.499**   Other specified injury of lesser saphenous vein at lower leg level, unspecified leg

● **S85.5**   Injury of popliteal vein
- ● **S85.50**   Unspecified injury of popliteal vein
  - ● **S85.501**   Unspecified injury of popliteal vein, right leg
  - ● **S85.502**   Unspecified injury of popliteal vein, left leg
  - ● **S85.509**   Unspecified injury of popliteal vein, unspecified leg
- ● **S85.51**   Laceration of popliteal vein
  - ● **S85.511**   Laceration of popliteal vein, right leg
  - ● **S85.512**   Laceration of popliteal vein, left leg
  - ● **S85.519**   Laceration of popliteal vein, unspecified leg

- S85.59   Other specified injury of popliteal vein
  - S85.591   Other specified injury of popliteal vein, right leg
  - S85.592   Other specified injury of popliteal vein, left leg
  - S85.599   Other specified injury of popliteal vein, unspecified leg
- S85.8   Injury of other blood vessels at lower leg level
  - S85.80   Unspecified injury of other blood vessels at lower leg level
    - S85.801   Unspecified injury of other blood vessels at lower leg level, right leg
    - S85.802   Unspecified injury of other blood vessels at lower leg level, left leg
    - S85.809   Unspecified injury of other blood vessels at lower leg level, unspecified leg
  - S85.81   Laceration of other blood vessels at lower leg level
    - S85.811   Laceration of other blood vessels at lower leg level, right leg
    - S85.812   Laceration of other blood vessels at lower leg level, left leg
    - S85.819   Laceration of other blood vessels at lower leg level, unspecified leg
  - S85.89   Other specified injury of other blood vessels at lower leg level
    - S85.891   Other specified injury of other blood vessels at lower leg level, right leg
    - S85.892   Other specified injury of other blood vessels at lower leg level, left leg
    - S85.899   Other specified injury of other blood vessels at lower leg level, unspecified leg
- S85.9   Injury of unspecified blood vessel at lower leg level
  - S85.90   Unspecified injury of unspecified blood vessel at lower leg level
    - S85.901   Unspecified injury of unspecified blood vessel at lower leg level, right leg
    - S85.902   Unspecified injury of unspecified blood vessel at lower leg level, left leg
    - S85.909   Unspecified injury of unspecified blood vessel at lower leg level, unspecified leg
  - S85.91   Laceration of unspecified blood vessel at lower leg level
    - S85.911   Laceration of unspecified blood vessel at lower leg level, right leg
    - S85.912   Laceration of unspecified blood vessel at lower leg level, left leg
    - S85.919   Laceration of unspecified blood vessel at lower leg level, unspecified leg
  - S85.99   Other specified injury of unspecified blood vessel at lower leg level
    - S85.991   Other specified injury of unspecified blood vessel at lower leg level, right leg
    - S85.992   Other specified injury of unspecified blood vessel at lower leg level, left leg
    - S85.999   Other specified injury of unspecified blood vessel at lower leg level, unspecified leg

- S86   **Injury of muscle, fascia and tendon at lower leg level**

  Code also any associated open wound (S81.-)

  Excludes2   injury of muscle, fascia and tendon at ankle (S96.-)
  injury of patellar ligament (tendon) (S76.1-)
  sprain of joints and ligaments of knee (S83.-)

  The appropriate 7th character is to be added to each code from category S86

A	initial encounter
D	subsequent encounter
S	sequela

  - S86.0   Injury of Achilles tendon
    - S86.00   Unspecified injury of Achilles tendon
      - S86.001   Unspecified injury of right Achilles tendon
      - S86.002   Unspecified injury of left Achilles tendon
      - S86.009   Unspecified injury of unspecified Achilles tendon
    - S86.01   Strain of Achilles tendon
      - S86.011   Strain of right Achilles tendon
      - S86.012   Strain of left Achilles tendon
      - S86.019   Strain of unspecified Achilles tendon
    - S86.02   Laceration of Achilles tendon
      - S86.021   Laceration of right Achilles tendon
      - S86.022   Laceration of left Achilles tendon
      - S86.029   Laceration of unspecified Achilles tendon
    - S86.09   Other specified injury of Achilles tendon
      - S86.091   Other specified injury of right Achilles tendon
      - S86.092   Other specified injury of left Achilles tendon
      - S86.099   Other specified injury of unspecified Achilles tendon
  - S86.1   Injury of other muscle(s) and tendon(s) of posterior muscle group at lower leg level
    - S86.10   Unspecified injury of other muscle(s) and tendon(s) of posterior muscle group at lower leg level
      - S86.101   Unspecified injury of other muscle(s) and tendon(s) of posterior muscle group at lower leg level, right leg
      - S86.102   Unspecified injury of other muscle(s) and tendon(s) of posterior muscle group at lower leg level, left leg
      - S86.109   Unspecified injury of other muscle(s) and tendon(s) of posterior muscle group at lower leg level, unspecified leg
    - S86.11   Strain of other muscle(s) and tendon(s) of posterior muscle group at lower leg level
      - S86.111   Strain of other muscle(s) and tendon(s) of posterior muscle group at lower leg level, right leg
      - S86.112   Strain of other muscle(s) and tendon(s) of posterior muscle group at lower leg level, left leg
      - S86.119   Strain of other muscle(s) and tendon(s) of posterior muscle group at lower leg level, unspecified leg

● S86.12   Laceration of other muscle(s) and tendon(s) of posterior muscle group at lower leg level

   ● S86.121   Laceration of other muscle(s) and tendon(s) of posterior muscle group at lower leg level, right leg

   ● S86.122   Laceration of other muscle(s) and tendon(s) of posterior muscle group at lower leg level, left leg

   ● S86.129   Laceration of other muscle(s) and tendon(s) of posterior muscle group at lower leg level, unspecified leg

● S86.19   Other injury of other muscle(s) and tendon(s) of posterior muscle group at lower leg level

   ● S86.191   Other injury of other muscle(s) and tendon(s) of posterior muscle group at lower leg level, right leg

   ● S86.192   Other injury of other muscle(s) and tendon(s) of posterior muscle group at lower leg level, left leg

   ● S86.199   Other injury of other muscle(s) and tendon(s) of posterior muscle group at lower leg level, unspecified leg

● S86.2   Injury of muscle(s) and tendon(s) of anterior muscle group at lower leg level

   ● S86.20   Unspecified injury of muscle(s) and tendon(s) of anterior muscle group at lower leg level

     ● S86.201   Unspecified injury of muscle(s) and tendon(s) of anterior muscle group at lower leg level, right leg

     ● S86.202   Unspecified injury of muscle(s) and tendon(s) of anterior muscle group at lower leg level, left leg

     ● S86.209   Unspecified injury of muscle(s) and tendon(s) of anterior muscle group at lower leg level, unspecified leg

   ● S86.21   Strain of muscle(s) and tendon(s) of anterior muscle group at lower leg level

     ● S86.211   Strain of muscle(s) and tendon(s) of anterior muscle group at lower leg level, right leg

     ● S86.212   Strain of muscle(s) and tendon(s) of anterior muscle group at lower leg level, left leg

     ● S86.219   Strain of muscle(s) and tendon(s) of anterior muscle group at lower leg level, unspecified leg

   ● S86.22   Laceration of muscle(s) and tendon(s) of anterior muscle group at lower leg level

     ● S86.221   Laceration of muscle(s) and tendon(s) of anterior muscle group at lower leg level, right leg

     ● S86.222   Laceration of muscle(s) and tendon(s) of anterior muscle group at lower leg level, left leg

     ● S86.229   Laceration of muscle(s) and tendon(s) of anterior muscle group at lower leg level, unspecified leg

   ● S86.29   Other injury of muscle(s) and tendon(s) of anterior muscle group at lower leg level

     ● S86.291   Other injury of muscle(s) and tendon(s) of anterior muscle group at lower leg level, right leg

     ● S86.292   Other injury of muscle(s) and tendon(s) of anterior muscle group at lower leg level, left leg

     ● S86.299   Other injury of muscle(s) and tendon(s) of anterior muscle group at lower leg level, unspecified leg

● S86.3   Injury of muscle(s) and tendon(s) of peroneal muscle group at lower leg level

   ● S86.30   Unspecified injury of muscle(s) and tendon(s) of peroneal muscle group at lower leg level

     ● S86.301   Unspecified injury of muscle(s) and tendon(s) of peroneal muscle group at lower leg level, right leg

     ● S86.302   Unspecified injury of muscle(s) and tendon(s) of peroneal muscle group at lower leg level, left leg

     ● S86.309   Unspecified injury of muscle(s) and tendon(s) of peroneal muscle group at lower leg level, unspecified leg

   ● S86.31   Strain of muscle(s) and tendon(s) of peroneal muscle group at lower leg level

     ● S86.311   Strain of muscle(s) and tendon(s) of peroneal muscle group at lower leg level, right leg

     ● S86.312   Strain of muscle(s) and tendon(s) of peroneal muscle group at lower leg level, left leg

     ● S86.319   Strain of muscle(s) and tendon(s) of peroneal muscle group at lower leg level, unspecified leg

   ● S86.32   Laceration of muscle(s) and tendon(s) of peroneal muscle group at lower leg level

     ● S86.321   Laceration of muscle(s) and tendon(s) of peroneal muscle group at lower leg level, right leg

     ● S86.322   Laceration of muscle(s) and tendon(s) of peroneal muscle group at lower leg level, left leg

     ● S86.329   Laceration of muscle(s) and tendon(s) of peroneal muscle group at lower leg level, unspecified leg

   ● S86.39   Other injury of muscle(s) and tendon(s) of peroneal muscle group at lower leg level

     ● S86.391   Other injury of muscle(s) and tendon(s) of peroneal muscle group at lower leg level, right leg

     ● S86.392   Other injury of muscle(s) and tendon(s) of peroneal muscle group at lower leg level, left leg

     ● S86.399   Other injury of muscle(s) and tendon(s) of peroneal muscle group at lower leg level, unspecified leg

● S86.8   Injury of other muscles and tendons at lower leg level

   ● S86.80   Unspecified injury of other muscles and tendons at lower leg level

     ● S86.801   Unspecified injury of other muscle(s) and tendon(s) at lower leg level, right leg

     ● S86.802   Unspecified injury of other muscle(s) and tendon(s) at lower leg level, left leg

     ● S86.809   Unspecified injury of other muscle(s) and tendon(s) at lower leg level, unspecified leg

   ● S86.81   Strain of other muscles and tendons at lower leg level

     ● S86.811   Strain of other muscle(s) and tendon(s) at lower leg level, right leg

     ● S86.812   Strain of other muscle(s) and tendon(s) at lower leg level, left leg

     ● S86.819   Strain of other muscle(s) and tendon(s) at lower leg level, unspecified leg

CHAPTER 19 (S00-T88)

N Newborn Age: 0   **P** Pediatric Age: 0–17   **M** Maternity DX: 12–55   **A** Adult Age: 15–124   ♀ Females Only   ♂ Males Only   **1317**

● **S86.82**   **Laceration of other muscles and tendons at lower leg level**
  ● S86.821   Laceration of other muscle(s) and tendon(s) at lower leg level, right leg
  ● S86.822   Laceration of other muscle(s) and tendon(s) at lower leg level, left leg
  ● S86.829   Laceration of other muscle(s) and tendon(s) at lower leg level, unspecified leg
● **S86.89**   **Other injury of other muscles and tendons at lower leg level**
  ● S86.891   Other injury of other muscle(s) and tendon(s) at lower leg level, right leg
  ● S86.892   Other injury of other muscle(s) and tendon(s) at lower leg level, left leg
  ● S86.899   Other injury of other muscle(s) and tendon(s) at lower leg level, unspecified leg
● **S86.9**   **Injury of unspecified muscle and tendon at lower leg level**
  ● **S86.90**   **Unspecified injury of unspecified muscle and tendon at lower leg level**
    ● S86.901   Unspecified injury of unspecified muscle(s) and tendon(s) at lower leg level, right leg
    ● S86.902   Unspecified injury of unspecified muscle(s) and tendon(s) at lower leg level, left leg
    ● S86.909   Unspecified injury of unspecified muscle(s) and tendon(s) at lower leg level, unspecified leg
  ● **S86.91**   **Strain of unspecified muscle and tendon at lower leg level**
    ● S86.911   Strain of unspecified muscle(s) and tendon(s) at lower leg level, right leg
    ● S86.912   Strain of unspecified muscle(s) and tendon(s) at lower leg level, left leg
    ● S86.919   Strain of unspecified muscle(s) and tendon(s) at lower leg level, unspecified leg
  ● **S86.92**   **Laceration of unspecified muscle and tendon at lower leg level**
    ● S86.921   Laceration of unspecified muscle(s) and tendon(s) at lower leg level, right leg
    ● S86.922   Laceration of unspecified muscle(s) and tendon(s) at lower leg level, left leg
    ● S86.929   Laceration of unspecified muscle(s) and tendon(s) at lower leg level, unspecified leg
  ● **S86.99**   **Other injury of unspecified muscle and tendon at lower leg level**
    ● S86.991   Other injury of unspecified muscle(s) and tendon(s) at lower leg level, right leg
    ● S86.992   Other injury of unspecified muscle(s) and tendon(s) at lower leg level, left leg
    ● S86.999   Other injury of unspecified muscle(s) and tendon(s) at lower leg level, unspecified leg

● **S87**   **Crushing injury of lower leg**
  Use additional code(s) for all associated injuries
  Excludes2   crushing injury of ankle and foot (S97.-)
  The appropriate 7th character is to be added to each code from category S87

A	initial encounter
D	subsequent encounter
S	sequela

  ● **S87.0**   **Crushing injury of knee**
    X ● S87.00   Crushing injury of unspecified knee
    X ● S87.01   Crushing injury of right knee
    X ● S87.02   Crushing injury of left knee
  ● **S87.8**   **Crushing injury of lower leg**
    X ● S87.80   Crushing injury of unspecified lower leg
    X ● S87.81   Crushing injury of right lower leg
    X ● S87.82   Crushing injury of left lower leg

● **S88**   **Traumatic amputation of lower leg**
  An amputation not identified as partial or complete should be coded to complete
  Excludes1   traumatic amputation of ankle and foot (S98.-)
  The appropriate 7th character is to be added to each code from category S88

A	initial encounter
D	subsequent encounter
S	sequela

  ● **S88.0**   **Traumatic amputation at knee level**
    ● **S88.01**   **Complete traumatic amputation at knee level**
      ● S88.011   Complete traumatic amputation at knee level, right lower leg
      ● S88.012   Complete traumatic amputation at knee level, left lower leg
      ● S88.019   Complete traumatic amputation at knee level, unspecified lower leg
    ● **S88.02**   **Partial traumatic amputation at knee level**
      ● S88.021   Partial traumatic amputation at knee level, right lower leg
      ● S88.022   Partial traumatic amputation at knee level, left lower leg
      ● S88.029   Partial traumatic amputation at knee level, unspecified lower leg
  ● **S88.1**   **Traumatic amputation at level between knee and ankle**
    ● **S88.11**   **Complete traumatic amputation at level between knee and ankle**
      ● S88.111   Complete traumatic amputation at level between knee and ankle, right lower leg
      ● S88.112   Complete traumatic amputation at level between knee and ankle, left lower leg
      ● S88.119   Complete traumatic amputation at level between knee and ankle, unspecified lower leg
    ● **S88.12**   **Partial traumatic amputation at level between knee and ankle**
      ● S88.121   Partial traumatic amputation at level between knee and ankle, right lower leg
      ● S88.122   Partial traumatic amputation at level between knee and ankle, left lower leg
      ● S88.129   Partial traumatic amputation at level between knee and ankle, unspecified lower leg

◄ New   ◄▪▪ Revised   ~~deleted~~ Deleted   Excludes 1   Excludes 2   Includes   Use additional   Code first   Code also   Unspecified
OGCR Official Guidelines   X Assign placeholder X   ● Use Additional Character(s)   ▶ Manifestation Code   **Coding Clinic**

● S88.9   Traumatic amputation of lower leg, level unspecified
   ● S88.91   Complete traumatic amputation of lower leg, level unspecified
     ● S88.911   Complete traumatic amputation of right lower leg, level unspecified
     ● S88.912   Complete traumatic amputation of left lower leg, level unspecified
     ● S88.919   Complete traumatic amputation of unspecified lower leg, level unspecified
   ● S88.92   Partial traumatic amputation of lower leg, level unspecified
     ● S88.921   Partial traumatic amputation of right lower leg, level unspecified
     ● S88.922   Partial traumatic amputation of left lower leg, level unspecified
     ● S88.929   Partial traumatic amputation of unspecified lower leg, level unspecified

● S89   Other and unspecified injuries of lower leg

   Note: A fracture not indicated as open or closed should be coded to closed

   Excludes2   other and unspecified injuries of ankle and foot (S99.-)

   The appropriate 7th character is to be added to each code from subcategories S89.0, S89.1, S89.2, and S89.3

A	initial encounter for closed fracture
D	subsequent encounter for fracture with routine healing
G	subsequent encounter for fracture with delayed healing
K	subsequent encounter for fracture with nonunion
P	subsequent encounter for fracture with malunion
S	sequela

● S89.0   Physeal fracture of upper end of tibia
   ● S89.00   Unspecified physeal fracture of upper end of tibia
     ● S89.001   Unspecified physeal fracture of upper end of right tibia
     ● S89.002   Unspecified physeal fracture of upper end of left tibia
     ● S89.009   Unspecified physeal fracture of upper end of unspecified tibia
   ● S89.01   Salter-Harris Type I physeal fracture of upper end of tibia
     ● S89.011   Salter-Harris Type I physeal fracture of upper end of right tibia
     ● S89.012   Salter-Harris Type I physeal fracture of upper end of left tibia
     ● S89.019   Salter-Harris Type I physeal fracture of upper end of unspecified tibia
   ● S89.02   Salter-Harris Type II physeal fracture of upper end of tibia
     ● S89.021   Salter-Harris Type II physeal fracture of upper end of right tibia
     ● S89.022   Salter-Harris Type II physeal fracture of upper end of left tibia
     ● S89.029   Salter-Harris Type II physeal fracture of upper end of unspecified tibia
   ● S89.03   Salter-Harris Type III physeal fracture of upper end of tibia
     ● S89.031   Salter-Harris Type III physeal fracture of upper end of right tibia
     ● S89.032   Salter-Harris Type III physeal fracture of upper end of left tibia
     ● S89.039   Salter-Harris Type III physeal fracture of upper end of unspecified tibia

● S89.04   Salter-Harris Type IV physeal fracture of upper end of tibia
     ● S89.041   Salter-Harris Type IV physeal fracture of upper end of right tibia
     ● S89.042   Salter-Harris Type IV physeal fracture of upper end of left tibia
     ● S89.049   Salter-Harris Type IV physeal fracture of upper end of unspecified tibia
   ● S89.09   Other physeal fracture of upper end of tibia
     ● S89.091   Other physeal fracture of upper end of right tibia
     ● S89.092   Other physeal fracture of upper end of left tibia
     ● S89.099   Other physeal fracture of upper end of unspecified tibia

● S89.1   Physeal fracture of lower end of tibia
   ● S89.10   Unspecified physeal fracture of lower end of tibia
     ● S89.101   Unspecified physeal fracture of lower end of right tibia
     ● S89.102   Unspecified physeal fracture of lower end of left tibia
     ● S89.109   Unspecified physeal fracture of lower end of unspecified tibia
   ● S89.11   Salter-Harris Type I physeal fracture of lower end of tibia
     ● S89.111   Salter-Harris Type I physeal fracture of lower end of right tibia
     ● S89.112   Salter-Harris Type I physeal fracture of lower end of left tibia
     ● S89.119   Salter-Harris Type I physeal fracture of lower end of unspecified tibia
   ● S89.12   Salter-Harris Type II physeal fracture of lower end of tibia
     ● S89.121   Salter-Harris Type II physeal fracture of lower end of right tibia
     ● S89.122   Salter-Harris Type II physeal fracture of lower end of left tibia
     ● S89.129   Salter-Harris Type II physeal fracture of lower end of unspecified tibia
   ● S89.13   Salter-Harris Type III physeal fracture of lower end of tibia
     Excludes1   fracture of medial malleolus (adult) (S82.5-)
     ● S89.131   Salter-Harris Type III physeal fracture of lower end of right tibia
     ● S89.132   Salter-Harris Type III physeal fracture of lower end of left tibia
     ● S89.139   Salter-Harris Type III physeal fracture of lower end of unspecified tibia
   ● S89.14   Salter-Harris Type IV physeal fracture of lower end of tibia
     Excludes1   fracture of medial malleolus (adult) (S82.5-)
     ● S89.141   Salter-Harris Type IV physeal fracture of lower end of right tibia
     ● S89.142   Salter-Harris Type IV physeal fracture of lower end of left tibia
     ● S89.149   Salter-Harris Type IV physeal fracture of lower end of unspecified tibia
   ● S89.19   Other physeal fracture of lower end of tibia
     ● S89.191   Other physeal fracture of lower end of right tibia
     ● S89.192   Other physeal fracture of lower end of left tibia
     ● S89.199   Other physeal fracture of lower end of unspecified tibia

CHAPTER 19 (S00-T88)

● **S89.2   Physeal fracture of upper end of fibula**
  ● **S89.20   Unspecified physeal fracture of upper end of fibula**
    ● S89.201   Unspecified physeal fracture of upper end of right fibula
    ● S89.202   Unspecified physeal fracture of upper end of left fibula
    ● S89.209   Unspecified physeal fracture of upper end of unspecified fibula
  ● **S89.21   Salter-Harris Type I physeal fracture of upper end of fibula**
    ● S89.211   Salter-Harris Type I physeal fracture of upper end of right fibula
    ● S89.212   Salter-Harris Type I physeal fracture of upper end of left fibula
    ● S89.219   Salter-Harris Type I physeal fracture of upper end of unspecified fibula
  ● **S89.22   Salter-Harris Type II physeal fracture of upper end of fibula**
    ● S89.221   Salter-Harris Type II physeal fracture of upper end of right fibula
    ● S89.222   Salter-Harris Type II physeal fracture of upper end of left fibula
    ● S89.229   Salter-Harris Type II physeal fracture of upper end of unspecified fibula
  ● **S89.29   Other physeal fracture of upper end of fibula**
    ● S89.291   Other physeal fracture of upper end of right fibula
    ● S89.292   Other physeal fracture of upper end of left fibula
    ● S89.299   Other physeal fracture of upper end of unspecified fibula
● **S89.3   Physeal fracture of lower end of fibula**
  ● **S89.30   Unspecified physeal fracture of lower end of fibula**
    ● S89.301   Unspecified physeal fracture of lower end of right fibula
    ● S89.302   Unspecified physeal fracture of lower end of left fibula
    ● S89.309   Unspecified physeal fracture of lower end of unspecified fibula
  ● **S89.31   Salter-Harris Type I physeal fracture of lower end of fibula**
    ● S89.311   Salter-Harris Type I physeal fracture of lower end of right fibula
    ● S89.312   Salter-Harris Type I physeal fracture of lower end of left fibula
    ● S89.319   Salter-Harris Type I physeal fracture of lower end of unspecified fibula
  ● **S89.32   Salter-Harris Type II physeal fracture of lower end of fibula**
    ● S89.321   Salter-Harris Type II physeal fracture of lower end of right fibula
    ● S89.322   Salter-Harris Type II physeal fracture of lower end of left fibula
    ● S89.329   Salter-Harris Type II physeal fracture of lower end of unspecified fibula
  ● **S89.39   Other physeal fracture of lower end of fibula**
    ● S89.391   Other physeal fracture of lower end of right fibula
    ● S89.392   Other physeal fracture of lower end of left fibula
    ● S89.399   Other physeal fracture of lower end of unspecified fibula

● **S89.8   Other specified injuries of lower leg**
  The appropriate 7th character is to be added to each code in subcategory S89.8

A	initial encounter
D	subsequent encounter
S	sequela

  X ● **S89.80   Other specified injuries of unspecified lower leg**
  X ● **S89.81   Other specified injuries of right lower leg**
  X ● **S89.82   Other specified injuries of left lower leg**
● **S89.9   Unspecified injury of lower leg**
  The appropriate 7th character is to be added to each code in subcategory S89.9

A	initial encounter
D	subsequent encounter
S	sequela

  X ● **S89.90   Unspecified injury of unspecified lower leg**
  X ● **S89.91   Unspecified injury of right lower leg**
  X ● **S89.92   Unspecified injury of left lower leg**

INJURIES TO THE ANKLE AND FOOT (S90-S99)

Excludes2   burns and corrosions (T20-T32)
                 fracture of ankle and malleolus (S82.-)
                 frostbite (T33-T34)
                 insect bite or sting, venomous (T63.4)

● **S90   Superficial injury of ankle, foot and toes**
  The appropriate 7th character is to be added to each code from category S90

A	initial encounter
D	subsequent encounter
S	sequela

  ● **S90.0   Contusion of ankle**
    X ● **S90.00   Contusion of unspecified ankle**
    X ● **S90.01   Contusion of right ankle**
    X ● **S90.02   Contusion of left ankle**
  ● **S90.1   Contusion of toe without damage to nail**
    ● **S90.11   Contusion of great toe without damage to nail**
      ● S90.111   Contusion of right great toe without damage to nail
      ● S90.112   Contusion of left great toe without damage to nail
      ● S90.119   Contusion of unspecified great toe without damage to nail
    ● **S90.12   Contusion of lesser toe without damage to nail**
      ● S90.121   Contusion of right lesser toe(s) without damage to nail
      ● S90.122   Contusion of left lesser toe(s) without damage to nail
      ● S90.129   Contusion of unspecified lesser toe(s) without damage to nail
                   Contusion of toe NOS
  ● **S90.2   Contusion of toe with damage to nail**
    ● **S90.21   Contusion of great toe with damage to nail**
      ● S90.211   Contusion of right great toe with damage to nail
      ● S90.212   Contusion of left great toe with damage to nail
      ● S90.219   Contusion of unspecified great toe with damage to nail

● **S90.22**   Contusion of lesser toe with damage to nail
     ● **S90.221**   Contusion of right lesser toe(s) with damage to nail
     ● **S90.222**   Contusion of left lesser toe(s) with damage to nail
     ● **S90.229**   Contusion of unspecified lesser toe(s) with damage to nail

● **S90.3**   Contusion of foot
     Excludes2   contusion of toes (S90.1-, S90.2-)
X ● **S90.30**   Contusion of unspecified foot
       Contusion of foot NOS
X ● **S90.31**   Contusion of right foot
X ● **S90.32**   Contusion of left foot

● **S90.4**   Other superficial injuries of toe
   ● **S90.41**   Abrasion of toe
     ● **S90.411**   Abrasion, right great toe
     ● **S90.412**   Abrasion, left great toe
     ● **S90.413**   Abrasion, unspecified great toe
     ● **S90.414**   Abrasion, right lesser toe(s)
     ● **S90.415**   Abrasion, left lesser toe(s)
     ● **S90.416**   Abrasion, unspecified lesser toe(s)
   ● **S90.42**   Blister (nonthermal) of toe
     ● **S90.421**   Blister (nonthermal), right great toe
     ● **S90.422**   Blister (nonthermal), left great toe
     ● **S90.423**   Blister (nonthermal), unspecified great toe
     ● **S90.424**   Blister (nonthermal), right lesser toe(s)
     ● **S90.425**   Blister (nonthermal), left lesser toe(s)
     ● **S90.426**   Blister (nonthermal), unspecified lesser toe(s)
   ● **S90.44**   External constriction of toe
       Hair tourniquet syndrome of toe
     ● **S90.441**   External constriction, right great toe
     ● **S90.442**   External constriction, left great toe
     ● **S90.443**   External constriction, unspecified great toe
     ● **S90.444**   External constriction, right lesser toe(s)
     ● **S90.445**   External constriction, left lesser toe(s)
     ● **S90.446**   External constriction, unspecified lesser toe(s)
   ● **S90.45**   Superficial foreign body of toe
       Splinter in the toe
     ● **S90.451**   Superficial foreign body, right great toe
     ● **S90.452**   Superficial foreign body, left great toe
     ● **S90.453**   Superficial foreign body, unspecified great toe
     ● **S90.454**   Superficial foreign body, right lesser toe(s)
     ● **S90.455**   Superficial foreign body, left lesser toe(s)
     ● **S90.456**   Superficial foreign body, unspecified lesser toe(s)
   ● **S90.46**   Insect bite (nonvenomous) of toe
     ● **S90.461**   Insect bite (nonvenomous), right great toe
     ● **S90.462**   Insect bite (nonvenomous), left great toe
     ● **S90.463**   Insect bite (nonvenomous), unspecified great toe
     ● **S90.464**   Insect bite (nonvenomous), right lesser toe(s)
     ● **S90.465**   Insect bite (nonvenomous), left lesser toe(s)
     ● **S90.466**   Insect bite (nonvenomous), unspecified lesser toe(s)

● **S90.47**   Other superficial bite of toe
     Excludes1   open bite of toe (S91.15-, S91.25-)
     ● **S90.471**   Other superficial bite of right great toe
     ● **S90.472**   Other superficial bite of left great toe
     ● **S90.473**   Other superficial bite of unspecified great toe
     ● **S90.474**   Other superficial bite of right lesser toe(s)
     ● **S90.475**   Other superficial bite of left lesser toe(s)
     ● **S90.476**   Other superficial bite of unspecified lesser toe(s)

● **S90.5**   Other superficial injuries of ankle
   ● **S90.51**   Abrasion of ankle
     ● **S90.511**   Abrasion, right ankle
     ● **S90.512**   Abrasion, left ankle
     ● **S90.519**   Abrasion, unspecified ankle
   ● **S90.52**   Blister (nonthermal) of ankle
     ● **S90.521**   Blister (nonthermal), right ankle
     ● **S90.522**   Blister (nonthermal), left ankle
     ● **S90.529**   Blister (nonthermal), unspecified ankle
   ● **S90.54**   External constriction of ankle
     ● **S90.541**   External constriction, right ankle
     ● **S90.542**   External constriction, left ankle
     ● **S90.549**   External constriction, unspecified ankle
   ● **S90.55**   Superficial foreign body of ankle
       Splinter in the ankle
     ● **S90.551**   Superficial foreign body, right ankle
     ● **S90.552**   Superficial foreign body, left ankle
     ● **S90.559**   Superficial foreign body, unspecified ankle
   ● **S90.56**   Insect bite (nonvenomous) of ankle
     ● **S90.561**   Insect bite (nonvenomous), right ankle
     ● **S90.562**   Insect bite (nonvenomous), left ankle
     ● **S90.569**   Insect bite (nonvenomous), unspecified ankle
   ● **S90.57**   Other superficial bite of ankle
     Excludes1   open bite of ankle (S91.05-)
     ● **S90.571**   Other superficial bite of ankle, right ankle
     ● **S90.572**   Other superficial bite of ankle, left ankle
     ● **S90.579**   Other superficial bite of ankle, unspecified ankle

● **S90.8**   Other superficial injuries of foot
   ● **S90.81**   Abrasion of foot
     ● **S90.811**   Abrasion, right foot
     ● **S90.812**   Abrasion, left foot
     ● **S90.819**   Abrasion, unspecified foot
   ● **S90.82**   Blister (nonthermal) of foot
     ● **S90.821**   Blister (nonthermal), right foot
     ● **S90.822**   Blister (nonthermal), left foot
     ● **S90.829**   Blister (nonthermal), unspecified foot
   ● **S90.84**   External constriction of foot
     ● **S90.841**   External constriction, right foot
     ● **S90.842**   External constriction, left foot
     ● **S90.849**   External constriction, unspecified foot
   ● **S90.85**   Superficial foreign body of foot
       Splinter in the foot
     ● **S90.851**   Superficial foreign body, right foot
     ● **S90.852**   Superficial foreign body, left foot
     ● **S90.859**   Superficial foreign body, unspecified foot

CHAPTER 19 (S00-T88)

- S90.86   Insect bite (nonvenomous) of foot
  - S90.861   Insect bite (nonvenomous), right foot
  - S90.862   Insect bite (nonvenomous), left foot
  - S90.869   Insect bite (nonvenomous), unspecified foot
- S90.87   Other superficial bite of foot
  - **Excludes1**   open bite of foot (S91.35-)
  - S90.871   Other superficial bite of right foot
  - S90.872   Other superficial bite of left foot
  - S90.879   Other superficial bite of unspecified foot
- S90.9   Unspecified superficial injury of ankle, foot and toe
  - S90.91   Unspecified superficial injury of ankle
    - S90.911   Unspecified superficial injury of right ankle
    - S90.912   Unspecified superficial injury of left ankle
    - S90.919   Unspecified superficial injury of unspecified ankle
  - S90.92   Unspecified superficial injury of foot
    - S90.921   Unspecified superficial injury of right foot
    - S90.922   Unspecified superficial injury of left foot
    - S90.929   Unspecified superficial injury of unspecified foot
  - S90.93   Unspecified superficial injury of toes
    - S90.931   Unspecified superficial injury of right great toe
    - S90.932   Unspecified superficial injury of left great toe
    - S90.933   Unspecified superficial injury of unspecified great toe
    - S90.934   Unspecified superficial injury of right lesser toe(s)
    - S90.935   Unspecified superficial injury of left lesser toe(s)
    - S90.936   Unspecified superficial injury of unspecified lesser toe(s)

- S91   Open wound of ankle, foot and toes
  - Code also any associated wound infection
  - **Excludes1**   open fracture of ankle, foot and toes (S92.-with 7th character B)
  - traumatic amputation of ankle and foot (S98.-)
  - The appropriate 7th character is to be added to each code from category S91

A	initial encounter
D	subsequent encounter
S	sequela

  - S91.0   Open wound of ankle
    - S91.00   Unspecified open wound of ankle
      - S91.001   Unspecified open wound, right ankle
      - S91.002   Unspecified open wound, left ankle
      - S91.009   Unspecified open wound, unspecified ankle
    - S91.01   Laceration without foreign body of ankle
      - S91.011   Laceration without foreign body, right ankle
      - S91.012   Laceration without foreign body, left ankle
      - S91.019   Laceration without foreign body, unspecified ankle

- S91.02   Laceration with foreign body of ankle
  - S91.021   Laceration with foreign body, right ankle
  - S91.022   Laceration with foreign body, left ankle
  - S91.029   Laceration with foreign body, unspecified ankle
- S91.03   Puncture wound without foreign body of ankle
  - S91.031   Puncture wound without foreign body, right ankle
  - S91.032   Puncture wound without foreign body, left ankle
  - S91.039   Puncture wound without foreign body, unspecified ankle
- S91.04   Puncture wound with foreign body of ankle
  - S91.041   Puncture wound with foreign body, right ankle
  - S91.042   Puncture wound with foreign body, left ankle
  - S91.049   Puncture wound with foreign body, unspecified ankle
- S91.05   Open bite of ankle
  - **Excludes1**   superficial bite of ankle (S90.56-, S90.57-)
  - S91.051   Open bite, right ankle
  - S91.052   Open bite, left ankle
  - S91.059   Open bite, unspecified ankle
- S91.1   Open wound of toe without damage to nail
  - S91.10   Unspecified open wound of toe without damage to nail
    - S91.101   Unspecified open wound of right great toe without damage to nail
    - S91.102   Unspecified open wound of left great toe without damage to nail
    - S91.103   Unspecified open wound of unspecified great toe without damage to nail
    - S91.104   Unspecified open wound of right lesser toe(s) without damage to nail
    - S91.105   Unspecified open wound of left lesser toe(s) without damage to nail
    - S91.106   Unspecified open wound of unspecified lesser toe(s) without damage to nail
    - S91.109   Unspecified open wound of unspecified toe(s) without damage to nail
  - S91.11   Laceration without foreign body of toe without damage to nail
    - S91.111   Laceration without foreign body of right great toe without damage to nail
    - S91.112   Laceration without foreign body of left great toe without damage to nail
    - S91.113   Laceration without foreign body of unspecified great toe without damage to nail
    - S91.114   Laceration without foreign body of right lesser toe(s) without damage to nail
    - S91.115   Laceration without foreign body of left lesser toe(s) without damage to nail
    - S91.116   Laceration without foreign body of unspecified lesser toe(s) without damage to nail
    - S91.119   Laceration without foreign body of unspecified toe without damage to nail

◀ New   ◀▬ Revised   ~~deleted~~ Deleted   Excludes 1   Excludes 2   Includes   Use additional   Code first   Code also   Unspecified

OGCR Official Guidelines   X Assign placeholder X   ● Use Additional Character(s)   ▶ Manifestation Code   **Coding Clinic**

1322

● **S91.12** Laceration with foreign body of toe without damage to nail
- ● **S91.121** Laceration with foreign body of right great toe without damage to nail
- ● **S91.122** Laceration with foreign body of left great toe without damage to nail
- ● **S91.123** Laceration with foreign body of unspecified great toe without damage to nail
- ● **S91.124** Laceration with foreign body of right lesser toe(s) without damage to nail
- ● **S91.125** Laceration with foreign body of left lesser toe(s) without damage to nail
- ● **S91.126** Laceration with foreign body of unspecified lesser toe(s) without damage to nail
- ● **S91.129** Laceration with foreign body of unspecified toe(s) without damage to nail

● **S91.13** Puncture wound without foreign body of toe without damage to nail
- ● **S91.131** Puncture wound without foreign body of right great toe without damage to nail
- ● **S91.132** Puncture wound without foreign body of left great toe without damage to nail
- ● **S91.133** Puncture wound without foreign body of unspecified great toe without damage to nail
- ● **S91.134** Puncture wound without foreign body of right lesser toe(s) without damage to nail
- ● **S91.135** Puncture wound without foreign body of left lesser toe(s) without damage to nail
- ● **S91.136** Puncture wound without foreign body of unspecified lesser toe(s) without damage to nail
- ● **S91.139** Puncture wound without foreign body of unspecified toe(s) without damage to nail

● **S91.14** Puncture wound with foreign body of toe without damage to nail
- ● **S91.141** Puncture wound with foreign body of right great toe without damage to nail
- ● **S91.142** Puncture wound with foreign body of left great toe without damage to nail
- ● **S91.143** Puncture wound with foreign body of unspecified great toe without damage to nail
- ● **S91.144** Puncture wound with foreign body of right lesser toe(s) without damage to nail
- ● **S91.145** Puncture wound with foreign body of left lesser toe(s) without damage to nail
- ● **S91.146** Puncture wound with foreign body of unspecified lesser toe(s) without damage to nail
- ● **S91.149** Puncture wound with foreign body of unspecified toe(s) without damage to nail

● **S91.15** Open bite of toe without damage to nail
  Bite of toe NOS
  Excludes1 superficial bite of toe (S90.46-, S90.47-)
- ● **S91.151** Open bite of right great toe without damage to nail
- ● **S91.152** Open bite of left great toe without damage to nail

- ● **S91.153** Open bite of unspecified great toe without damage to nail
- ● **S91.154** Open bite of right lesser toe(s) without damage to nail
- ● **S91.155** Open bite of left lesser toe(s) without damage to nail
- ● **S91.156** Open bite of unspecified lesser toe(s) without damage to nail
- ● **S91.159** Open bite of unspecified toe(s) without damage to nail

● **S91.2** Open wound of toe with damage to nail
● **S91.20** Unspecified open wound of toe with damage to nail
- ● **S91.201** Unspecified open wound of right great toe with damage to nail
- ● **S91.202** Unspecified open wound of left great toe with damage to nail
- ● **S91.203** Unspecified open wound of unspecified great toe with damage to nail
- ● **S91.204** Unspecified open wound of right lesser toe(s) with damage to nail
- ● **S91.205** Unspecified open wound of left lesser toe(s) with damage to nail
- ● **S91.206** Unspecified open wound of unspecified lesser toe(s) with damage to nail
- ● **S91.209** Unspecified open wound of unspecified toe(s) with damage to nail

● **S91.21** Laceration without foreign body of toe with damage to nail
- ● **S91.211** Laceration without foreign body of right great toe with damage to nail
- ● **S91.212** Laceration without foreign body of left great toe with damage to nail
- ● **S91.213** Laceration without foreign body of unspecified great toe with damage to nail
- ● **S91.214** Laceration without foreign body of right lesser toe(s) with damage to nail
- ● **S91.215** Laceration without foreign body of left lesser toe(s) with damage to nail
- ● **S91.216** Laceration without foreign body of unspecified lesser toe(s) with damage to nail
- ● **S91.219** Laceration without foreign body of unspecified toe(s) with damage to nail

● **S91.22** Laceration with foreign body of toe with damage to nail
- ● **S91.221** Laceration with foreign body of right great toe with damage to nail
- ● **S91.222** Laceration with foreign body of left great toe with damage to nail
- ● **S91.223** Laceration with foreign body of unspecified great toe with damage to nail
- ● **S91.224** Laceration with foreign body of right lesser toe(s) with damage to nail
- ● **S91.225** Laceration with foreign body of left lesser toe(s) with damage to nail
- ● **S91.226** Laceration with foreign body of unspecified lesser toe(s) with damage to nail
- ● **S91.229** Laceration with foreign body of unspecified toe(s) with damage to nail

● **S91.23** Puncture wound without foreign body of toe with damage to nail
  - ● **S91.231** Puncture wound without foreign body of right great toe with damage to nail
  - ● **S91.232** Puncture wound without foreign body of left great toe with damage to nail
  - ● **S91.233** Puncture wound without foreign body of unspecified great toe with damage to nail
  - ● **S91.234** Puncture wound without foreign body of right lesser toe(s) with damage to nail
  - ● **S91.235** Puncture wound without foreign body of left lesser toe(s) with damage to nail
  - ● **S91.236** Puncture wound without foreign body of unspecified lesser toe(s) with damage to nail
  - ● **S91.239** Puncture wound without foreign body of unspecified toe(s) with damage to nail

● **S91.24** Puncture wound with foreign body of toe with damage to nail
  - ● **S91.241** Puncture wound with foreign body of right great toe with damage to nail
  - ● **S91.242** Puncture wound with foreign body of left great toe with damage to nail
  - ● **S91.243** Puncture wound with foreign body of unspecified great toe with damage to nail
  - ● **S91.244** Puncture wound with foreign body of right lesser toe(s) with damage to nail
  - ● **S91.245** Puncture wound with foreign body of left lesser toe(s) with damage to nail
  - ● **S91.246** Puncture wound with foreign body of unspecified lesser toe(s) with damage to nail
  - ● **S91.249** Puncture wound with foreign body of unspecified toe(s) with damage to nail

● **S91.25** Open bite of toe with damage to nail
  Bite of toe with damage to nail NOS
  Excludes1 superficial bite of toe (S90.46-, S90.47-)
  - ● **S91.251** Open bite of right great toe with damage to nail
  - ● **S91.252** Open bite of left great toe with damage to nail
  - ● **S91.253** Open bite of unspecified great toe with damage to nail
  - ● **S91.254** Open bite of right lesser toe(s) with damage to nail
  - ● **S91.255** Open bite of left lesser toe(s) with damage to nail
  - ● **S91.256** Open bite of unspecified lesser toe(s) with damage to nail
  - ● **S91.259** Open bite of unspecified toe(s) with damage to nail

● **S91.3** Open wound of foot
  - ● **S91.30** Unspecified open wound of foot
    - ● **S91.301** Unspecified open wound, right foot
    - ● **S91.302** Unspecified open wound, left foot
    - ● **S91.309** Unspecified open wound, unspecified foot

● **S91.31** Laceration without foreign body of foot
  - ● **S91.311** Laceration without foreign body, right foot
  - ● **S91.312** Laceration without foreign body, left foot
  - ● **S91.319** Laceration without foreign body, unspecified foot

● **S91.32** Laceration with foreign body of foot
  - ● **S91.321** Laceration with foreign body, right foot
  - ● **S91.322** Laceration with foreign body, left foot
  - ● **S91.329** Laceration with foreign body, unspecified foot

● **S91.33** Puncture wound without foreign body of foot
  - ● **S91.331** Puncture wound without foreign body, right foot
  - ● **S91.332** Puncture wound without foreign body, left foot
  - ● **S91.339** Puncture wound without foreign body, unspecified foot

● **S91.34** Puncture wound with foreign body of foot
  - ● **S91.341** Puncture wound with foreign body, right foot
  - ● **S91.342** Puncture wound with foreign body, left foot
  - ● **S91.349** Puncture wound with foreign body, unspecified foot

● **S91.35** Open bite of foot
  Excludes1 superficial bite of foot (S90.86-, S90.87-)
  - ● **S91.351** Open bite, right foot
  - ● **S91.352** Open bite, left foot
  - ● **S91.359** Open bite, unspecified foot

● **S92** **Fracture of foot and toe, except ankle**
  Note: A fracture not indicated as displaced or nondisplaced should be coded to displaced
  A fracture not indicated as open or closed should be coded to closed
  Excludes1 traumatic amputation of ankle and foot (S98.-)
  Excludes2 fracture of ankle (S82.-)
  fracture of malleolus (S82.-)
  The appropriate 7th character is to be added to each code from category S92

A	initial encounter for closed fracture
B	initial encounter for open fracture
D	subsequent encounter for fracture with routine healing
G	subsequent encounter for fracture with delayed healing
K	subsequent encounter for fracture with nonunion
P	subsequent encounter for fracture with malunion
S	sequela

● **S92.0** Fracture of calcaneus
  Heel bone   Os calcis
  Excludes2 Physeal fracture of calcaneus (S99.0-) ◀
  - ● **S92.00** Unspecified fracture of calcaneus
    - ● **S92.001** Unspecified fracture of right calcaneus
    - ● **S92.002** Unspecified fracture of left calcaneus
    - ● **S92.009** Unspecified fracture of unspecified calcaneus
  - ● **S92.01** Fracture of body of calcaneus
    - ● **S92.011** Displaced fracture of body of right calcaneus
    - ● **S92.012** Displaced fracture of body of left calcaneus

● S92.013 Displaced fracture of body of unspecified calcaneus

● S92.014 Nondisplaced fracture of body of right calcaneus

● S92.015 Nondisplaced fracture of body of left calcaneus

● S92.016 Nondisplaced fracture of body of unspecified calcaneus

● S92.02 Fracture of anterior process of calcaneus

● S92.021 Displaced fracture of anterior process of right calcaneus

● S92.022 Displaced fracture of anterior process of left calcaneus

● S92.023 Displaced fracture of anterior process of unspecified calcaneus

● S92.024 Nondisplaced fracture of anterior process of right calcaneus

● S92.025 Nondisplaced fracture of anterior process of left calcaneus

● S92.026 Nondisplaced fracture of anterior process of unspecified calcaneus

● S92.03 Avulsion fracture of tuberosity of calcaneus

● S92.031 Displaced avulsion fracture of tuberosity of right calcaneus

● S92.032 Displaced avulsion fracture of tuberosity of left calcaneus

● S92.033 Displaced avulsion fracture of tuberosity of unspecified calcaneus

● S92.034 Nondisplaced avulsion fracture of tuberosity of right calcaneus

● S92.035 Nondisplaced avulsion fracture of tuberosity of left calcaneus

● S92.036 Nondisplaced avulsion fracture of tuberosity of unspecified calcaneus

● S92.04 Other fracture of tuberosity of calcaneus

● S92.041 Displaced other fracture of tuberosity of right calcaneus

● S92.042 Displaced other fracture of tuberosity of left calcaneus

● S92.043 Displaced other fracture of tuberosity of unspecified calcaneus

● S92.044 Nondisplaced other fracture of tuberosity of right calcaneus

● S92.045 Nondisplaced other fracture of tuberosity of left calcaneus

● S92.046 Nondisplaced other fracture of tuberosity of unspecified calcaneus

● S92.05 Other extraarticular fracture of calcaneus

● S92.051 Displaced other extraarticular fracture of right calcaneus

● S92.052 Displaced other extraarticular fracture of left calcaneus

● S92.053 Displaced other extraarticular fracture of unspecified calcaneus

● S92.054 Nondisplaced other extraarticular fracture of right calcaneus

● S92.055 Nondisplaced other extraarticular fracture of left calcaneus

● S92.056 Nondisplaced other extraarticular fracture of unspecified calcaneus

● S92.06 Intraarticular fracture of calcaneus

● S92.061 Displaced intraarticular fracture of right calcaneus

● S92.062 Displaced intraarticular fracture of left calcaneus

● S92.063 Displaced intraarticular fracture of unspecified calcaneus

● S92.064 Nondisplaced intraarticular fracture of right calcaneus

● S92.065 Nondisplaced intraarticular fracture of left calcaneus

● S92.066 Nondisplaced intraarticular fracture of unspecified calcaneus

● S92.1 Fracture of talus
       Astragalus

● S92.10 Unspecified fracture of talus

● S92.101 Unspecified fracture of right talus

● S92.102 Unspecified fracture of left talus

● S92.109 Unspecified fracture of unspecified talus

● S92.11 Fracture of neck of talus

● S92.111 Displaced fracture of neck of right talus

● S92.112 Displaced fracture of neck of left talus

● S92.113 Displaced fracture of neck of unspecified talus

● S92.114 Nondisplaced fracture of neck of right talus

● S92.115 Nondisplaced fracture of neck of left talus

● S92.116 Nondisplaced fracture of neck of unspecified talus

● S92.12 Fracture of body of talus

● S92.121 Displaced fracture of body of right talus

● S92.122 Displaced fracture of body of left talus

● S92.123 Displaced fracture of body of unspecified talus

● S92.124 Nondisplaced fracture of body of right talus

● S92.125 Nondisplaced fracture of body of left talus

● S92.126 Nondisplaced fracture of body of unspecified talus

● S92.13 Fracture of posterior process of talus

● S92.131 Displaced fracture of posterior process of right talus

● S92.132 Displaced fracture of posterior process of left talus

● S92.133 Displaced fracture of posterior process of unspecified talus

● S92.134 Nondisplaced fracture of posterior process of right talus

● S92.135 Nondisplaced fracture of posterior process of left talus

● S92.136 Nondisplaced fracture of posterior process of unspecified talus

● S92.14 Dome fracture of talus

       Excludes1 osteochondritis dissecans (M93.2)

● S92.141 Displaced dome fracture of right talus

● S92.142 Displaced dome fracture of left talus

● S92.143 Displaced dome fracture of unspecified talus

● S92.144 Nondisplaced dome fracture of right talus

● S92.145 Nondisplaced dome fracture of left talus

● S92.146 Nondisplaced dome fracture of unspecified talus

- S92.15   Avulsion fracture (chip fracture) of talus
  - S92.151   Displaced avulsion fracture (chip fracture) of right talus
  - S92.152   Displaced avulsion fracture (chip fracture) of left talus
  - S92.153   Displaced avulsion fracture (chip fracture) of unspecified talus
  - S92.154   Nondisplaced avulsion fracture (chip fracture) of right talus
  - S92.155   Nondisplaced avulsion fracture (chip fracture) of left talus
  - S92.156   Nondisplaced avulsion fracture (chip fracture) of unspecified talus
- S92.19   Other fracture of talus
  - S92.191   Other fracture of right talus
  - S92.192   Other fracture of left talus
  - S92.199   Other fracture of unspecified talus
- S92.2   Fracture of other and unspecified tarsal bone(s)
  - S92.20   Fracture of unspecified tarsal bone(s)
    - S92.201   Fracture of unspecified tarsal bone(s) of right foot
    - S92.202   Fracture of unspecified tarsal bone(s) of left foot
    - S92.209   Fracture of unspecified tarsal bone(s) of unspecified foot
  - S92.21   Fracture of cuboid bone
    - S92.211   Displaced fracture of cuboid bone of right foot
    - S92.212   Displaced fracture of cuboid bone of left foot
    - S92.213   Displaced fracture of cuboid bone of unspecified foot
    - S92.214   Nondisplaced fracture of cuboid bone of right foot
    - S92.215   Nondisplaced fracture of cuboid bone of left foot
    - S92.216   Nondisplaced fracture of cuboid bone of unspecified foot
  - S92.22   Fracture of lateral cuneiform
    - S92.221   Displaced fracture of lateral cuneiform of right foot
    - S92.222   Displaced fracture of lateral cuneiform of left foot
    - S92.223   Displaced fracture of lateral cuneiform of unspecified foot
    - S92.224   Nondisplaced fracture of lateral cuneiform of right foot
    - S92.225   Nondisplaced fracture of lateral cuneiform of left foot
    - S92.226   Nondisplaced fracture of lateral cuneiform of unspecified foot
  - S92.23   Fracture of intermediate cuneiform
    - S92.231   Displaced fracture of intermediate cuneiform of right foot
    - S92.232   Displaced fracture of intermediate cuneiform of left foot
    - S92.233   Displaced fracture of intermediate cuneiform of unspecified foot
    - S92.234   Nondisplaced fracture of intermediate cuneiform of right foot
    - S92.235   Nondisplaced fracture of intermediate cuneiform of left foot
    - S92.236   Nondisplaced fracture of intermediate cuneiform of unspecified foot

- S92.24   Fracture of medial cuneiform
  - S92.241   Displaced fracture of medial cuneiform of right foot
  - S92.242   Displaced fracture of medial cuneiform of left foot
  - S92.243   Displaced fracture of medial cuneiform of unspecified foot
  - S92.244   Nondisplaced fracture of medial cuneiform of right foot
  - S92.245   Nondisplaced fracture of medial cuneiform of left foot
  - S92.246   Nondisplaced fracture of medial cuneiform of unspecified foot
- S92.25   Fracture of navicular [scaphoid] of foot
  - S92.251   Displaced fracture of navicular [scaphoid] of right foot
  - S92.252   Displaced fracture of navicular [scaphoid] of left foot
  - S92.253   Displaced fracture of navicular [scaphoid] of unspecified foot
  - S92.254   Nondisplaced fracture of navicular [scaphoid] of right foot
  - S92.255   Nondisplaced fracture of navicular [scaphoid] of left foot
  - S92.256   Nondisplaced fracture of navicular [scaphoid] of unspecified foot
- S92.3   Fracture of metatarsal bone(s)
  - **Excludes2**   Physeal fracture of metatarsal (S99.1-) ◄
  - S92.30   Fracture of unspecified metatarsal bone(s)
    - S92.301   Fracture of unspecified metatarsal bone(s), right foot
    - S92.302   Fracture of unspecified metatarsal bone(s), left foot
    - S92.309   Fracture of unspecified metatarsal bone(s), unspecified foot
  - S92.31   Fracture of first metatarsal bone
    - S92.311   Displaced fracture of first metatarsal bone, right foot
    - S92.312   Displaced fracture of first metatarsal bone, left foot
    - S92.313   Displaced fracture of first metatarsal bone, unspecified foot
    - S92.314   Nondisplaced fracture of first metatarsal bone, right foot
    - S92.315   Nondisplaced fracture of first metatarsal bone, left foot
    - S92.316   Nondisplaced fracture of first metatarsal bone, unspecified foot
  - S92.32   Fracture of second metatarsal bone
    - S92.321   Displaced fracture of second metatarsal bone, right foot
    - S92.322   Displaced fracture of second metatarsal bone, left foot
    - S92.323   Displaced fracture of second metatarsal bone, unspecified foot
    - S92.324   Nondisplaced fracture of second metatarsal bone, right foot
    - S92.325   Nondisplaced fracture of second metatarsal bone, left foot
    - S92.326   Nondisplaced fracture of second metatarsal bone, unspecified foot
  - S92.33   Fracture of third metatarsal bone
    - S92.331   Displaced fracture of third metatarsal bone, right foot
    - S92.332   Displaced fracture of third metatarsal bone, left foot
    - S92.333   Displaced fracture of third metatarsal bone, unspecified foot

● **S92.334**   Nondisplaced fracture of third metatarsal bone, right foot

● **S92.335**   Nondisplaced fracture of third metatarsal bone, left foot

● **S92.336**   Nondisplaced fracture of third metatarsal bone, unspecified foot

● **S92.34**   Fracture of fourth metatarsal bone

● **S92.341**   Displaced fracture of fourth metatarsal bone, right foot

● **S92.342**   Displaced fracture of fourth metatarsal bone, left foot

● **S92.343**   Displaced fracture of fourth metatarsal bone, unspecified foot

● **S92.344**   Nondisplaced fracture of fourth metatarsal bone, right foot

● **S92.345**   Nondisplaced fracture of fourth metatarsal bone, left foot

● **S92.346**   Nondisplaced fracture of fourth metatarsal bone, unspecified foot

● **S92.35**   Fracture of fifth metatarsal bone

● **S92.351**   Displaced fracture of fifth metatarsal bone, right foot

● **S92.352**   Displaced fracture of fifth metatarsal bone, left foot

● **S92.353**   Displaced fracture of fifth metatarsal bone, unspecified foot

● **S92.354**   Nondisplaced fracture of fifth metatarsal bone, right foot

● **S92.355**   Nondisplaced fracture of fifth metatarsal bone, left foot

● **S92.356**   Nondisplaced fracture of fifth metatarsal bone, unspecified foot

● **S92.4**   Fracture of great toe

    Excludes2   Physeal fracture of phalanx of toe (S99.2-) ◄

● **S92.40**   Unspecified fracture of great toe

● **S92.401**   Displaced unspecified fracture of right great toe

● **S92.402**   Displaced unspecified fracture of left great toe

● **S92.403**   Displaced unspecified fracture of unspecified great toe

● **S92.404**   Nondisplaced unspecified fracture of right great toe

● **S92.405**   Nondisplaced unspecified fracture of left great toe

● **S92.406**   Nondisplaced unspecified fracture of unspecified great toe

● **S92.41**   Fracture of proximal phalanx of great toe

● **S92.411**   Displaced fracture of proximal phalanx of right great toe

● **S92.412**   Displaced fracture of proximal phalanx of left great toe

● **S92.413**   Displaced fracture of proximal phalanx of unspecified great toe

● **S92.414**   Nondisplaced fracture of proximal phalanx of right great toe

● **S92.415**   Nondisplaced fracture of proximal phalanx of left great toe

● **S92.416**   Nondisplaced fracture of proximal phalanx of unspecified great toe

● **S92.42**   Fracture of distal phalanx of great toe

● **S92.421**   Displaced fracture of distal phalanx of right great toe

● **S92.422**   Displaced fracture of distal phalanx of left great toe

● **S92.423**   Displaced fracture of distal phalanx of unspecified great toe

● **S92.424**   Nondisplaced fracture of distal phalanx of right great toe

● **S92.425**   Nondisplaced fracture of distal phalanx of left great toe

● **S92.426**   Nondisplaced fracture of distal phalanx of unspecified great toe

● **S92.49**   Other fracture of great toe

● **S92.491**   Other fracture of right great toe

● **S92.492**   Other fracture of left great toe

● **S92.499**   Other fracture of unspecified great toe

● **S92.5**   Fracture of lesser toe(s)

    Excludes2   Physeal fracture of phalanx of toe (S99.2-) ◄

● **S92.50**   Unspecified fracture of lesser toe(s)

● **S92.501**   Displaced unspecified fracture of right lesser toe(s)

● **S92.502**   Displaced unspecified fracture of left lesser toe(s)

● **S92.503**   Displaced unspecified fracture of unspecified lesser toe(s)

● **S92.504**   Nondisplaced unspecified fracture of right lesser toe(s)

● **S92.505**   Nondisplaced unspecified fracture of left lesser toe(s)

● **S92.506**   Nondisplaced unspecified fracture of unspecified lesser toe(s)

● **S92.51**   Fracture of proximal phalanx of lesser toe(s)

● **S92.511**   Displaced fracture of proximal phalanx of right lesser toe(s)

● **S92.512**   Displaced fracture of proximal phalanx of left lesser toe(s)

● **S92.513**   Displaced fracture of proximal phalanx of unspecified lesser toe(s)

● **S92.514**   Nondisplaced fracture of proximal phalanx of right lesser toe(s)

● **S92.515**   Nondisplaced fracture of proximal phalanx of left lesser toe(s)

● **S92.516**   Nondisplaced fracture of proximal phalanx of unspecified lesser toe(s)

● **S92.52**   Fracture of medial phalanx of lesser toe(s)

● **S92.521**   Displaced fracture of medial phalanx of right lesser toe(s)

● **S92.522**   Displaced fracture of medial phalanx of left lesser toe(s)

● **S92.523**   Displaced fracture of medial phalanx of unspecified lesser toe(s)

● **S92.524**   Nondisplaced fracture of medial phalanx of right lesser toe(s)

● **S92.525**   Nondisplaced fracture of medial phalanx of left lesser toe(s)

● **S92.526**   Nondisplaced fracture of medial phalanx of unspecified lesser toe(s)

● **S92.53**   Fracture of distal phalanx of lesser toe(s)

● **S92.531**   Displaced fracture of distal phalanx of right lesser toe(s)

● **S92.532**   Displaced fracture of distal phalanx of left lesser toe(s)

● **S92.533**   Displaced fracture of distal phalanx of unspecified lesser toe(s)

● **S92.534**   Nondisplaced fracture of distal phalanx of right lesser toe(s)

● **S92.535**   Nondisplaced fracture of distal phalanx of left lesser toe(s)

● **S92.536**   Nondisplaced fracture of distal phalanx of unspecified lesser toe(s)

CHAPTER 19 (S00-T88)

- S92.59 Other fracture of lesser toe(s)
  - S92.591 Other fracture of right lesser toe(s)
  - S92.592 Other fracture of left lesser toe(s)
  - S92.599 Other fracture of unspecified lesser toe(s)
- S92.8 Other fracture of foot, except ankle ◄
  - S92.81 Other fracture of foot ◄
    - Sesamoid fracture of foot
    - S92.811 Other fracture of right foot
    - S92.812 Other fracture of left foot
    - S92.819 Other fracture of unspecified foot
- S92.9 Unspecified fracture of foot and toe
  - S92.90 Unspecified fracture of foot
    - S92.901 Unspecified fracture of right foot
    - S92.902 Unspecified fracture of left foot
    - S92.909 Unspecified fracture of unspecified foot
  - S92.91 Unspecified fracture of toe
    - S92.911 Unspecified fracture of right toe(s)
    - S92.912 Unspecified fracture of left toe(s)
    - S92.919 Unspecified fracture of unspecified toe(s)

- S93 Dislocation and sprain of joints and ligaments at ankle, foot and toe level

  Includes avulsion of joint or ligament of ankle, foot and toe
  laceration of cartilage, joint or ligament of ankle, foot and toe
  sprain of cartilage, joint or ligament of ankle, foot and toe
  traumatic hemarthrosis of joint or ligament of ankle, foot and toe
  traumatic rupture of joint or ligament of ankle, foot and toe
  traumatic subluxation of joint or ligament of ankle, foot and toe
  traumatic tear of joint or ligament of ankle, foot and toe

  Code also any associated open wound
  Excludes2 strain of muscle and tendon of ankle and foot (S96.-)

  The appropriate 7th character is to be added to each code from category S93

A	initial encounter
D	subsequent encounter
S	sequela

- S93.0 Subluxation and dislocation of ankle joint
  - Subluxation and dislocation of astragalus
  - Subluxation and dislocation of fibula, lower end
  - Subluxation and dislocation of talus
  - Subluxation and dislocation of tibia, lower end
  - X S93.01 Subluxation of right ankle joint
  - X S93.02 Subluxation of left ankle joint
  - X S93.03 Subluxation of unspecified ankle joint
  - X S93.04 Dislocation of right ankle joint
  - X S93.05 Dislocation of left ankle joint
  - X S93.06 Dislocation of unspecified ankle joint
- S93.1 Subluxation and dislocation of toe
  - S93.10 Unspecified subluxation and dislocation of toe
    - Dislocation of toe NOS
    - Subluxation of toe NOS
    - S93.101 Unspecified subluxation of right toe(s)
    - S93.102 Unspecified subluxation of left toe(s)
    - S93.103 Unspecified subluxation of unspecified toe(s)
    - S93.104 Unspecified dislocation of right toe(s)
    - S93.105 Unspecified dislocation of left toe(s)
    - S93.106 Unspecified dislocation of unspecified toe(s)
  - S93.11 Dislocation of interphalangeal joint
    - S93.111 Dislocation of interphalangeal joint of right great toe
    - S93.112 Dislocation of interphalangeal joint of left great toe
    - S93.113 Dislocation of interphalangeal joint of unspecified great toe
    - S93.114 Dislocation of interphalangeal joint of right lesser toe(s)
    - S93.115 Dislocation of interphalangeal joint of left lesser toe(s)
    - S93.116 Dislocation of interphalangeal joint of unspecified lesser toe(s)
    - S93.119 Dislocation of interphalangeal joint of unspecified toe(s)
  - S93.12 Dislocation of metatarsophalangeal joint
    - S93.121 Dislocation of metatarsophalangeal joint of right great toe
    - S93.122 Dislocation of metatarsophalangeal joint of left great toe
    - S93.123 Dislocation of metatarsophalangeal joint of unspecified great toe
    - S93.124 Dislocation of metatarsophalangeal joint of right lesser toe(s)
    - S93.125 Dislocation of metatarsophalangeal joint of left lesser toe(s)
    - S93.126 Dislocation of metatarsophalangeal joint of unspecified lesser toe(s)
    - S93.129 Dislocation of metatarsophalangeal joint of unspecified toe(s)
  - S93.13 Subluxation of interphalangeal joint
    - S93.131 Subluxation of interphalangeal joint of right great toe
    - S93.132 Subluxation of interphalangeal joint of left great toe
    - S93.133 Subluxation of interphalangeal joint of unspecified great toe
    - S93.134 Subluxation of interphalangeal joint of right lesser toe(s)
    - S93.135 Subluxation of interphalangeal joint of left lesser toe(s)
    - S93.136 Subluxation of interphalangeal joint of unspecified lesser toe(s)
    - S93.139 Subluxation of interphalangeal joint of unspecified toe(s)
  - S93.14 Subluxation of metatarsophalangeal joint
    - S93.141 Subluxation of metatarsophalangeal joint of right great toe
    - S93.142 Subluxation of metatarsophalangeal joint of left great toe
    - S93.143 Subluxation of metatarsophalangeal joint of unspecified great toe
    - S93.144 Subluxation of metatarsophalangeal joint of right lesser toe(s)
    - S93.145 Subluxation of metatarsophalangeal joint of left lesser toe(s)
    - S93.146 Subluxation of metatarsophalangeal joint of unspecified lesser toe(s)
    - S93.149 Subluxation of metatarsophalangeal joint of unspecified toe(s)

1328

◄ New ⬅ Revised deleted Deleted | Excludes 1 | Excludes 2 | Includes | Use additional | Code first | Code also | Unspecified

OGCR Official Guidelines X Assign placeholder X ● Use Additional Character(s) ▷ Manifestation Code Coding Clinic

● S93.3   **Subluxation and dislocation of foot**
  Excludes2   dislocation of toe (S93.1-)
  ● S93.30   **Unspecified subluxation and dislocation of foot**
      Dislocation of foot NOS
      Subluxation of foot NOS
      ● S93.301   Unspecified subluxation of right foot
      ● S93.302   Unspecified subluxation of left foot
      ● S93.303   Unspecified subluxation of unspecified foot
      ● S93.304   Unspecified dislocation of right foot
      ● S93.305   Unspecified dislocation of left foot
      ● S93.306   Unspecified dislocation of unspecified foot
  ● S93.31   **Subluxation and dislocation of tarsal joint**
      ● S93.311   Subluxation of tarsal joint of right foot
      ● S93.312   Subluxation of tarsal joint of left foot
      ● S93.313   Subluxation of tarsal joint of unspecified foot
      ● S93.314   Dislocation of tarsal joint of right foot
      ● S93.315   Dislocation of tarsal joint of left foot
      ● S93.316   Dislocation of tarsal joint of unspecified foot
  ● S93.32   **Subluxation and dislocation of tarsometatarsal joint**
      ● S93.321   Subluxation of tarsometatarsal joint of right foot
      ● S93.322   Subluxation of tarsometatarsal joint of left foot
      ● S93.323   Subluxation of tarsometatarsal joint of unspecified foot
      ● S93.324   Dislocation of tarsometatarsal joint of right foot
      ● S93.325   Dislocation of tarsometatarsal joint of left foot
      ● S93.326   Dislocation of tarsometatarsal joint of unspecified foot
  ● S93.33   **Other subluxation and dislocation of foot**
      ● S93.331   Other subluxation of right foot
      ● S93.332   Other subluxation of left foot
      ● S93.333   Other subluxation of unspecified foot
      ● S93.334   Other dislocation of right foot
      ● S93.335   Other dislocation of left foot
      ● S93.336   Other dislocation of unspecified foot
● S93.4   **Sprain of ankle**
    Injury to ligaments when one or more is stretched/torn
    Excludes2   injury of Achilles tendon (S86.0-)
  ● S93.40   **Sprain of unspecified ligament of ankle**
      Sprain of ankle NOS
      Sprained ankle NOS
      ● S93.401   Sprain of unspecified ligament of right ankle
      ● S93.402   Sprain of unspecified ligament of left ankle
      ● S93.409   Sprain of unspecified ligament of unspecified ankle
  ● S93.41   **Sprain of calcaneofibular ligament**
      ● S93.411   Sprain of calcaneofibular ligament of right ankle
      ● S93.412   Sprain of calcaneofibular ligament of left ankle
      ● S93.419   Sprain of calcaneofibular ligament of unspecified ankle

● S93.42   **Sprain of deltoid ligament**
      ● S93.421   Sprain of deltoid ligament of right ankle
      ● S93.422   Sprain of deltoid ligament of left ankle
      ● S93.429   Sprain of deltoid ligament of unspecified ankle
  ● S93.43   **Sprain of tibiofibular ligament**
      ● S93.431   Sprain of tibiofibular ligament of right ankle
      ● S93.432   Sprain of tibiofibular ligament of left ankle
      ● S93.439   Sprain of tibiofibular ligament of unspecified ankle
  ● S93.49   **Sprain of other ligament of ankle**
      Sprain of internal collateral ligament
      Sprain of talofibular ligament
      ● S93.491   Sprain of other ligament of right ankle
      ● S93.492   Sprain of other ligament of left ankle
      ● S93.499   Sprain of other ligament of unspecified ankle
● S93.5   **Sprain of toe**
  ● S93.50   **Unspecified sprain of toe**
      ● S93.501   Unspecified sprain of right great toe
      ● S93.502   Unspecified sprain of left great toe
      ● S93.503   Unspecified sprain of unspecified great toe
      ● S93.504   Unspecified sprain of right lesser toe(s)
      ● S93.505   Unspecified sprain of left lesser toe(s)
      ● S93.506   Unspecified sprain of unspecified lesser toe(s)
      ● S93.509   Unspecified sprain of unspecified toe(s)
  ● S93.51   **Sprain of interphalangeal joint of toe**
      ● S93.511   Sprain of interphalangeal joint of right great toe
      ● S93.512   Sprain of interphalangeal joint of left great toe
      ● S93.513   Sprain of interphalangeal joint of unspecified great toe
      ● S93.514   Sprain of interphalangeal joint of right lesser toe(s)
      ● S93.515   Sprain of interphalangeal joint of left lesser toe(s)
      ● S93.516   Sprain of interphalangeal joint of unspecified lesser toe(s)
      ● S93.519   Sprain of interphalangeal joint of unspecified toe(s)
  ● S93.52   **Sprain of metatarsophalangeal joint of toe**
      ● S93.521   Sprain of metatarsophalangeal joint of right great toe
      ● S93.522   Sprain of metatarsophalangeal joint of left great toe
      ● S93.523   Sprain of metatarsophalangeal joint of unspecified great toe
      ● S93.524   Sprain of metatarsophalangeal joint of right lesser toe(s)
      ● S93.525   Sprain of metatarsophalangeal joint of left lesser toe(s)
      ● S93.526   Sprain of metatarsophalangeal joint of unspecified lesser toe(s)
      ● S93.529   Sprain of metatarsophalangeal joint of unspecified toe(s)

CHAPTER 19 (S00-T88)

● S93.6   Sprain of foot
    Excludes2   sprain of metatarsophalangeal joint of toe
                 (S93.52-)
                 sprain of toe (S93.5-)
    ● S93.60   Unspecified sprain of foot
        ● S93.601   Unspecified sprain of right foot
        ● S93.602   Unspecified sprain of left foot
        ● S93.609   Unspecified sprain of unspecified foot
    ● S93.61   Sprain of tarsal ligament of foot
        ● S93.611   Sprain of tarsal ligament of right foot
        ● S93.612   Sprain of tarsal ligament of left foot
        ● S93.619   Sprain of tarsal ligament of
                     unspecified foot
    ● S93.62   Sprain of tarsometatarsal ligament of foot
        ● S93.621   Sprain of tarsometatarsal ligament of
                     right foot
        ● S93.622   Sprain of tarsometatarsal ligament of
                     left foot
        ● S93.629   Sprain of tarsometatarsal ligament of
                     unspecified foot
    ● S93.69   Other sprain of foot
        ● S93.691   Other sprain of right foot
        ● S93.692   Other sprain of left foot
        ● S93.699   Other sprain of unspecified foot
● S94   Injury of nerves at ankle and foot level
    The appropriate 7th character is to be added to each code from
        category S94

A	initial encounter
D	subsequent encounter
S	sequela

    Code also any associated open wound (S91.-)
    ● S94.0   Injury of lateral plantar nerve
        X ● S94.00   Injury of lateral plantar nerve, unspecified leg
        X ● S94.01   Injury of lateral plantar nerve, right leg
        X ● S94.02   Injury of lateral plantar nerve, left leg
    ● S94.1   Injury of medial plantar nerve
        X ● S94.10   Injury of medial plantar nerve, unspecified leg
        X ● S94.11   Injury of medial plantar nerve, right leg
        X ● S94.12   Injury of medial plantar nerve, left leg
    ● S94.2   Injury of deep peroneal nerve at ankle and foot level
            Injury of terminal, lateral branch of deep peroneal nerve
        X ● S94.20   Injury of deep peroneal nerve at ankle and foot
                     level, unspecified leg
        X ● S94.21   Injury of deep peroneal nerve at ankle and foot
                     level, right leg
        X ● S94.22   Injury of deep peroneal nerve at ankle and foot
                     level, left leg
    ● S94.3   Injury of cutaneous sensory nerve at ankle and foot level
        X ● S94.30   Injury of cutaneous sensory nerve at ankle and
                     foot level, unspecified leg
        X ● S94.31   Injury of cutaneous sensory nerve at ankle and
                     foot level, right leg
        X ● S94.32   Injury of cutaneous sensory nerve at ankle and
                     foot level, left leg
    ● S94.8   Injury of other nerves at ankle and foot level
        ● S94.8X   Injury of other nerves at ankle and foot level
            ● S94.8X1   Injury of other nerves at ankle and
                         foot level, right leg
            ● S94.8X2   Injury of other nerves at ankle and
                         foot level, left leg
            ● S94.8X9   Injury of other nerves at ankle and
                         foot level, unspecified leg

● S94.9   Injury of unspecified nerve at ankle and foot level
    X ● S94.90   Injury of unspecified nerve at ankle and foot
                 level, unspecified leg
    X ● S94.91   Injury of unspecified nerve at ankle and foot
                 level, right leg
    X ● S94.92   Injury of unspecified nerve at ankle and foot
                 level, left leg
● S95   Injury of blood vessels at ankle and foot level
    Code also any associated open wound (S91.-)
        Excludes2   injury of posterior tibial artery and vein (S85.1-,
                     S85.8-)
    The appropriate 7th character is to be added to each code from
        category S95

A	initial encounter
D	subsequent encounter
S	sequela

    ● S95.0   Injury of dorsal artery of foot
        ● S95.00   Unspecified injury of dorsal artery of foot
            ● S95.001   Unspecified injury of dorsal artery of
                         right foot
            ● S95.002   Unspecified injury of dorsal artery of
                         left foot
            ● S95.009   Unspecified injury of dorsal artery of
                         unspecified foot
        ● S95.01   Laceration of dorsal artery of foot
            ● S95.011   Laceration of dorsal artery of right
                         foot
            ● S95.012   Laceration of dorsal artery of left foot
            ● S95.019   Laceration of dorsal artery of
                         unspecified foot
        ● S95.09   Other specified injury of dorsal artery of foot
            ● S95.091   Other specified injury of dorsal artery
                         of right foot
            ● S95.092   Other specified injury of dorsal artery
                         of left foot
            ● S95.099   Other specified injury of dorsal artery
                         of unspecified foot
    ● S95.1   Injury of plantar artery of foot
        ● S95.10   Unspecified injury of plantar artery of foot
            ● S95.101   Unspecified injury of plantar artery of
                         right foot
            ● S95.102   Unspecified injury of plantar artery of
                         left foot
            ● S95.109   Unspecified injury of plantar artery of
                         unspecified foot
        ● S95.11   Laceration of plantar artery of foot
            ● S95.111   Laceration of plantar artery of right
                         foot
            ● S95.112   Laceration of plantar artery of left
                         foot
            ● S95.119   Laceration of plantar artery of
                         unspecified foot
        ● S95.19   Other specified injury of plantar artery of foot
            ● S95.191   Other specified injury of plantar
                         artery of right foot
            ● S95.192   Other specified injury of plantar
                         artery of left foot
            ● S95.199   Other specified injury of plantar
                         artery of unspecified foot

◀ New   ◀▥ Revised   ~~deleted~~ Deleted   Excludes 1   Excludes 2   Includes   Use additional   Code first   Code also   Unspecified
OGCR Official Guidelines   X Assign placeholder X   ● Use Additional Character(s)   ▶ Manifestation Code   **Coding Clinic**

● **S95.2**   **Injury of dorsal vein of foot**
   ● **S95.20**   Unspecified injury of dorsal vein of foot
     ● **S95.201**   Unspecified injury of dorsal vein of right foot
     ● **S95.202**   Unspecified injury of dorsal vein of left foot
     ● **S95.209**   Unspecified injury of dorsal vein of unspecified foot
   ● **S95.21**   Laceration of dorsal vein of foot
     ● **S95.211**   Laceration of dorsal vein of right foot
     ● **S95.212**   Laceration of dorsal vein of left foot
     ● **S95.219**   Laceration of dorsal vein of unspecified foot
   ● **S95.29**   Other specified injury of dorsal vein of foot
     ● **S95.291**   Other specified injury of dorsal vein of right foot
     ● **S95.292**   Other specified injury of dorsal vein of left foot
     ● **S95.299**   Other specified injury of dorsal vein of unspecified foot

● **S95.8**   **Injury of other blood vessels at ankle and foot level**
   ● **S95.80**   Unspecified injury of other blood vessels at ankle and foot level
     ● **S95.801**   Unspecified injury of other blood vessels at ankle and foot level, right leg
     ● **S95.802**   Unspecified injury of other blood vessels at ankle and foot level, left leg
     ● **S95.809**   Unspecified injury of other blood vessels at ankle and foot level, unspecified leg
   ● **S95.81**   Laceration of other blood vessels at ankle and foot level
     ● **S95.811**   Laceration of other blood vessels at ankle and foot level, right leg
     ● **S95.812**   Laceration of other blood vessels at ankle and foot level, left leg
     ● **S95.819**   Laceration of other blood vessels at ankle and foot level, unspecified leg
   ● **S95.89**   Other specified injury of other blood vessels at ankle and foot level
     ● **S95.891**   Other specified injury of other blood vessels at ankle and foot level, right leg
     ● **S95.892**   Other specified injury of other blood vessels at ankle and foot level, left leg
     ● **S95.899**   Other specified injury of other blood vessels at ankle and foot level, unspecified leg

● **S95.9**   **Injury of unspecified blood vessel at ankle and foot level**
   ● **S95.90**   Unspecified injury of unspecified blood vessel at ankle and foot level
     ● **S95.901**   Unspecified injury of unspecified blood vessel at ankle and foot level, right leg
     ● **S95.902**   Unspecified injury of unspecified blood vessel at ankle and foot level, left leg
     ● **S95.909**   Unspecified injury of unspecified blood vessel at ankle and foot level, unspecified leg
   ● **S95.91**   Laceration of unspecified blood vessel at ankle and foot level
     ● **S95.911**   Laceration of unspecified blood vessel at ankle and foot level, right leg
     ● **S95.912**   Laceration of unspecified blood vessel at ankle and foot level, left leg
     ● **S95.919**   Laceration of unspecified blood vessel at ankle and foot level, unspecified leg

   ● **S95.99**   Other specified injury of unspecified blood vessel at ankle and foot level
     ● **S95.991**   Other specified injury of unspecified blood vessel at ankle and foot level, right leg
     ● **S95.992**   Other specified injury of unspecified blood vessel at ankle and foot level, left leg
     ● **S95.999**   Other specified injury of unspecified blood vessel at ankle and foot level, unspecified leg

● **S96**   **Injury of muscle and tendon at ankle and foot level**
    Code also any associated open wound (S91.-)
    Excludes2   injury of Achilles tendon (S86.0-)
                 sprain of joints and ligaments of ankle and foot (S93.-)
    The appropriate 7th character is to be added to each code from category S96

A	initial encounter
D	subsequent encounter
S	sequela

   ● **S96.0**   **Injury of muscle and tendon of long flexor muscle of toe at ankle and foot level**
     ● **S96.00**   Unspecified injury of muscle and tendon of long flexor muscle of toe at ankle and foot level
       ● **S96.001**   Unspecified injury of muscle and tendon of long flexor muscle of toe at ankle and foot level, right foot
       ● **S96.002**   Unspecified injury of muscle and tendon of long flexor muscle of toe at ankle and foot level, left foot
       ● **S96.009**   Unspecified injury of muscle and tendon of long flexor muscle of toe at ankle and foot level, unspecified foot
     ● **S96.01**   Strain of muscle and tendon of long flexor muscle of toe at ankle and foot level
       ● **S96.011**   Strain of muscle and tendon of long flexor muscle of toe at ankle and foot level, right foot
       ● **S96.012**   Strain of muscle and tendon of long flexor muscle of toe at ankle and foot level, left foot
       ● **S96.019**   Strain of muscle and tendon of long flexor muscle of toe at ankle and foot level, unspecified foot
     ● **S96.02**   Laceration of muscle and tendon of long flexor muscle of toe at ankle and foot level
       ● **S96.021**   Laceration of muscle and tendon of long flexor muscle of toe at ankle and foot level, right foot
       ● **S96.022**   Laceration of muscle and tendon of long flexor muscle of toe at ankle and foot level, left foot
       ● **S96.029**   Laceration of muscle and tendon of long flexor muscle of toe at ankle and foot level, unspecified foot
     ● **S96.09**   Other injury of muscle and tendon of long flexor muscle of toe at ankle and foot level
       ● **S96.091**   Other injury of muscle and tendon of long flexor muscle of toe at ankle and foot level, right foot
       ● **S96.092**   Other injury of muscle and tendon of long flexor muscle of toe at ankle and foot level, left foot
       ● **S96.099**   Other injury of muscle and tendon of long flexor muscle of toe at ankle and foot level, unspecified foot

● S96.1 Injury of muscle and tendon of long extensor muscle of toe at ankle and foot level
- ● S96.10 Unspecified injury of muscle and tendon of long extensor muscle of toe at ankle and foot level
  - ● S96.101 Unspecified injury of muscle and tendon of long extensor muscle of toe at ankle and foot level, right foot
  - ● S96.102 Unspecified injury of muscle and tendon of long extensor muscle of toe at ankle and foot level, left foot
  - ● S96.109 Unspecified injury of muscle and tendon of long extensor muscle of toe at ankle and foot level, unspecified foot
- ● S96.11 Strain of muscle and tendon of long extensor muscle of toe at ankle and foot level
  - ● S96.111 Strain of muscle and tendon of long extensor muscle of toe at ankle and foot level, right foot
  - ● S96.112 Strain of muscle and tendon of long extensor muscle of toe at ankle and foot level, left foot
  - ● S96.119 Strain of muscle and tendon of long extensor muscle of toe at ankle and foot level, unspecified foot
- ● S96.12 Laceration of muscle and tendon of long extensor muscle of toe at ankle and foot level
  - ● S96.121 Laceration of muscle and tendon of long extensor muscle of toe at ankle and foot level, right foot
  - ● S96.122 Laceration of muscle and tendon of long extensor muscle of toe at ankle and foot level, left foot
  - ● S96.129 Laceration of muscle and tendon of long extensor muscle of toe at ankle and foot level, unspecified foot
- ● S96.19 Other specified injury of muscle and tendon of long extensor muscle of toe at ankle and foot level
  - ● S96.191 Other specified injury of muscle and tendon of long extensor muscle of toe at ankle and foot level, right foot
  - ● S96.192 Other specified injury of muscle and tendon of long extensor muscle of toe at ankle and foot level, left foot
  - ● S96.199 Other specified injury of muscle and tendon of long extensor muscle of toe at ankle and foot level, unspecified foot

● S96.2 Injury of intrinsic muscle and tendon at ankle and foot level
- ● S96.20 Unspecified injury of intrinsic muscle and tendon at ankle and foot level
  - ● S96.201 Unspecified injury of intrinsic muscle and tendon at ankle and foot level, right foot
  - ● S96.202 Unspecified injury of intrinsic muscle and tendon at ankle and foot level, left foot
  - ● S96.209 Unspecified injury of intrinsic muscle and tendon at ankle and foot level, unspecified foot
- ● S96.21 Strain of intrinsic muscle and tendon at ankle and foot level
  - ● S96.211 Strain of intrinsic muscle and tendon at ankle and foot level, right foot
  - ● S96.212 Strain of intrinsic muscle and tendon at ankle and foot level, left foot
  - ● S96.219 Strain of intrinsic muscle and tendon at ankle and foot level, unspecified foot

- ● S96.22 Laceration of intrinsic muscle and tendon at ankle and foot level
  - ● S96.221 Laceration of intrinsic muscle and tendon at ankle and foot level, right foot
  - ● S96.222 Laceration of intrinsic muscle and tendon at left ankle and foot level, left foot
  - ● S96.229 Laceration of intrinsic muscle and tendon at ankle and foot level, unspecified foot
- ● S96.29 Other specified injury of intrinsic muscle and tendon at ankle and foot level
  - ● S96.291 Other specified injury of intrinsic muscle and tendon at ankle and foot level, right foot
  - ● S96.292 Other specified injury of intrinsic muscle and tendon at ankle and foot level, left foot
  - ● S96.299 Other specified injury of intrinsic muscle and tendon at ankle and foot level, unspecified foot

● S96.8 Injury of other specified muscles and tendons at ankle and foot level
- ● S96.80 Unspecified injury of other specified muscles and tendons at ankle and foot level
  - ● S96.801 Unspecified injury of other specified muscles and tendons at ankle and foot level, right foot
  - ● S96.802 Unspecified injury of other specified muscles and tendons at ankle and foot level, left foot
  - ● S96.809 Unspecified injury of other specified muscles and tendons at ankle and foot level, unspecified foot
- ● S96.81 Strain of other specified muscles and tendons at ankle and foot level
  - ● S96.811 Strain of other specified muscles and tendons at ankle and foot level, right foot
  - ● S96.812 Strain of other specified muscles and tendons at ankle and foot level, left foot
  - ● S96.819 Strain of other specified muscles and tendons at ankle and foot level, unspecified foot
- ● S96.82 Laceration of other specified muscles and tendons at ankle and foot level
  - ● S96.821 Laceration of other specified muscles and tendons at ankle and foot level, right foot
  - ● S96.822 Laceration of other specified muscles and tendons at ankle and foot level, left foot
  - ● S96.829 Laceration of other specified muscles and tendons at ankle and foot level, unspecified foot
- ● S96.89 Other specified injury of other specified muscles and tendons at ankle and foot level
  - ● S96.891 Other specified injury of other specified muscles and tendons at ankle and foot level, right foot
  - ● S96.892 Other specified injury of other specified muscles and tendons at ankle and foot level, left foot
  - ● S96.899 Other specified injury of other specified muscles and tendons at ankle and foot level, unspecified foot

◀ New ◀▪▪▪ Revised ~~deleted~~ Deleted | Excludes 1 | Excludes 2 | Includes | Use additional | Code first | Code also | Unspecified
OGCR Official Guidelines X Assign placeholder X ● Use Additional Character(s) ▶ Manifestation Code **Coding Clinic**

● **S96.9**   **Injury of unspecified muscle and tendon at ankle and foot level**
    ● **S96.90**   Unspecified injury of unspecified muscle and tendon at ankle and foot level
       ● **S96.901**   Unspecified injury of unspecified muscle and tendon at ankle and foot level, right foot
       ● **S96.902**   Unspecified injury of unspecified muscle and tendon at ankle and foot level, left foot
       ● **S96.909**   Unspecified injury of unspecified muscle and tendon at ankle and foot level, unspecified foot
    ● **S96.91**   Strain of unspecified muscle and tendon at ankle and foot level
       ● **S96.911**   Strain of unspecified muscle and tendon at ankle and foot level, right foot
       ● **S96.912**   Strain of unspecified muscle and tendon at ankle and foot level, left foot
       ● **S96.919**   Strain of unspecified muscle and tendon at ankle and foot level, unspecified foot
    ● **S96.92**   Laceration of unspecified muscle and tendon at ankle and foot level
       ● **S96.921**   Laceration of unspecified muscle and tendon at ankle and foot level, right foot
       ● **S96.922**   Laceration of unspecified muscle and tendon at ankle and foot level, left foot
       ● **S96.929**   Laceration of unspecified muscle and tendon at ankle and foot level, unspecified foot
    ● **S96.99**   Other specified injury of unspecified muscle and tendon at ankle and foot level
       ● **S96.991**   Other specified injury of unspecified muscle and tendon at ankle and foot level, right foot
       ● **S96.992**   Other specified injury of unspecified muscle and tendon at ankle and foot level, left foot
       ● **S96.999**   Other specified injury of unspecified muscle and tendon at ankle and foot level, unspecified foot

● **S97**   **Crushing injury of ankle and foot**
    Use additional code(s) for all associated injuries
    The appropriate 7th character is to be added to each code from category S97

A	initial encounter
D	subsequent encounter
S	sequela

    ● **S97.0**   Crushing injury of ankle
      X ● **S97.00**   Crushing injury of unspecified ankle
      X ● **S97.01**   Crushing injury of right ankle
      X ● **S97.02**   Crushing injury of left ankle
    ● **S97.1**   Crushing injury of toe
       ● **S97.10**   Crushing injury of unspecified toe(s)
          ● **S97.101**   Crushing injury of unspecified right toe(s)
          ● **S97.102**   Crushing injury of unspecified left toe(s)
          ● **S97.109**   Crushing injury of unspecified toe(s)
            Crushing injury of toe NOS

● **S97.11**   Crushing injury of great toe
      ● **S97.111**   Crushing injury of right great toe
      ● **S97.112**   Crushing injury of left great toe
      ● **S97.119**   Crushing injury of unspecified great toe
    ● **S97.12**   Crushing injury of lesser toe(s)
      ● **S97.121**   Crushing injury of right lesser toe(s)
      ● **S97.122**   Crushing injury of left lesser toe(s)
      ● **S97.129**   Crushing injury of lesser toe(s), unspecified toe(s)
    ● **S97.8**   Crushing injury of foot
      X ● **S97.80**   Crushing injury of foot, unspecified side
         Crushing injury of foot NOS
      X ● **S97.81**   Crushing injury of right foot
      X ● **S97.82**   Crushing injury of left foot

● **S98**   **Traumatic amputation of ankle and foot**
    An amputation not identified as partial or complete should be coded to complete
    The appropriate 7th character is to be added to each code from category S98

A	initial encounter
D	subsequent encounter
S	sequela

    ● **S98.0**   Traumatic amputation of foot at ankle level
       ● **S98.01**   Complete traumatic amputation of foot at ankle level
          ● **S98.011**   Complete traumatic amputation of right foot at ankle level
          ● **S98.012**   Complete traumatic amputation of left foot at ankle level
          ● **S98.019**   Complete traumatic amputation of unspecified foot at ankle level
       ● **S98.02**   Partial traumatic amputation of foot at ankle level
          ● **S98.021**   Partial traumatic amputation of right foot at ankle level
          ● **S98.022**   Partial traumatic amputation of left foot at ankle level
          ● **S98.029**   Partial traumatic amputation of unspecified foot at ankle level
    ● **S98.1**   Traumatic amputation of one toe
       ● **S98.11**   Complete traumatic amputation of great toe
          ● **S98.111**   Complete traumatic amputation of right great toe
          ● **S98.112**   Complete traumatic amputation of left great toe
          ● **S98.119**   Complete traumatic amputation of unspecified great toe
       ● **S98.12**   Partial traumatic amputation of great toe
          ● **S98.121**   Partial traumatic amputation of right great toe
          ● **S98.122**   Partial traumatic amputation of left great toe
          ● **S98.129**   Partial traumatic amputation of unspecified great toe
       ● **S98.13**   Complete traumatic amputation of one lesser toe
          Traumatic amputation of toe NOS
          ● **S98.131**   Complete traumatic amputation of one right lesser toe
          ● **S98.132**   Complete traumatic amputation of one left lesser toe
          ● **S98.139**   Complete traumatic amputation of one unspecified lesser toe

● S98.14   Partial traumatic amputation of one lesser toe
   ● S98.141   Partial traumatic amputation of one right lesser toe
   ● S98.142   Partial traumatic amputation of one left lesser toe
   ● S98.149   Partial traumatic amputation of one unspecified lesser toe
● S98.2   Traumatic amputation of two or more lesser toes
   ● S98.21   Complete traumatic amputation of two or more lesser toes
      ● S98.211   Complete traumatic amputation of two or more right lesser toes
      ● S98.212   Complete traumatic amputation of two or more left lesser toes
      ● S98.219   Complete traumatic amputation of two or more unspecified lesser toes
   ● S98.22   Partial traumatic amputation of two or more lesser toes
      ● S98.221   Partial traumatic amputation of two or more right lesser toes
      ● S98.222   Partial traumatic amputation of two or more left lesser toes
      ● S98.229   Partial traumatic amputation of two or more unspecified lesser toes
● S98.3   Traumatic amputation of midfoot
   ● S98.31   Complete traumatic amputation of midfoot
      ● S98.311   Complete traumatic amputation of right midfoot
      ● S98.312   Complete traumatic amputation of left midfoot
      ● S98.319   Complete traumatic amputation of unspecified midfoot
   ● S98.32   Partial traumatic amputation of midfoot
      ● S98.321   Partial traumatic amputation of right midfoot
      ● S98.322   Partial traumatic amputation of left midfoot
      ● S98.329   Partial traumatic amputation of unspecified midfoot
● S98.9   Traumatic amputation of foot, level unspecified
   ● S98.91   Complete traumatic amputation of foot, level unspecified
      ● S98.911   Complete traumatic amputation of right foot, level unspecified
      ● S98.912   Complete traumatic amputation of left foot, level unspecified
      ● S98.919   Complete traumatic amputation of unspecified foot, level unspecified
   ● S98.92   Partial traumatic amputation of foot, level unspecified
      ● S98.921   Partial traumatic amputation of right foot, level unspecified
      ● S98.922   Partial traumatic amputation of left foot, level unspecified
      ● S98.929   Partial traumatic amputation of unspecified foot, level unspecified

● S99   Other and unspecified injuries of ankle and foot
   ● S99.0   Physeal fracture of calcaneus ◄
      The appropriate 7th character is to be added to each code from subcategories S99.0 ◄

      | A | initial encounter for closed fracture ◄ |
      | B | initial encounter for open fracture ◄ |
      | D | subsequent encounter for fracture with routine healing ◄ |
      | G | subsequent encounter for fracture with delayed healing ◄ |
      | K | subsequent encounter for fracture with nonunion ◄ |
      | P | subsequent encounter for fracture with malunion ◄ |
      | S | sequela ◄ |

      ● S99.00   Unspecified physeal fracture of calcaneus ◄
         ● S99.001   Unspecified physeal fracture of right calcaneus ◄
         ● S99.002   Unspecified physeal fracture of left calcaneus ◄
         ● S99.009   Unspecified physeal fracture of unspecified calcaneus ◄
      ● S99.01   Salter-Harris Type I physeal fracture of calcaneus ◄
         ● S99.011   Salter-Harris Type I physeal fracture of right calcaneus ◄
         ● S99.012   Salter-Harris Type I physeal fracture of left calcaneus ◄
         ● S99.019   Salter-Harris Type I physeal fracture of unspecified calcaneus ◄
      ● S99.02   Salter-Harris Type II physeal fracture of calcaneus ◄
         ● S99.021   Salter-Harris Type II physeal fracture of right calcaneus ◄
         ● S99.022   Salter-Harris Type II physeal fracture of left calcaneus ◄
         ● S99.029   Salter-Harris Type II physeal fracture of unspecified calcaneus ◄
      ● S99.03   Salter-Harris Type III physeal fracture of calcaneus ◄
         ● S99.031   Salter-Harris Type III physeal fracture of right calcaneus ◄
         ● S99.032   Salter-Harris Type III physeal fracture of left calcaneus ◄
         ● S99.039   Salter-Harris Type III physeal fracture of unspecified calcaneus ◄
      ● S99.04   Salter-Harris Type IV physeal fracture of calcaneus ◄
         ● S99.041   Salter-Harris Type IV physeal fracture of right calcaneus ◄
         ● S99.042   Salter-Harris Type IV physeal fracture of left calcaneus ◄
         ● S99.049   Salter-Harris Type IV physeal fracture of unspecified calcaneus ◄
      ● S99.09   Other physeal fracture of calcaneus ◄
         ● S99.091   Other physeal fracture of right calcaneus ◄
         ● S99.092   Other physeal fracture of left calcaneus ◄
         ● S99.099   Other physeal fracture of unspecified calcaneus ◄

◄ New   ◄▥ Revised   deleted Deleted   Excludes 1   Excludes 2   Includes   Use additional   Code first   Code also   Unspecified
OGCR Official Guidelines   X Assign placeholder X   ● Use Additional Character(s)   ▶ Manifestation Code   Coding Clinic

● **S99.1**   **Physeal fracture of metatarsal** ◄

The appropriate 7th character is to be added to each
code from subcategories S99.1 ◄

A	initial encounter for closed fracture ◄
B	initial encounter for open fracture ◄
D	subsequent encounter for fracture with routine healing ◄
G	subsequent encounter for fracture with delayed healing ◄
K	subsequent encounter for fracture with nonunion ◄
P	subsequent encounter for fracture with malunion ◄
S	sequela ◄

● **S99.10**   Unspecified physeal fracture of metatarsal ◄

● S99.101   Unspecified physeal fracture of right metatarsal ◄

● S99.102   Unspecified physeal fracture of left metatarsal ◄

● S99.109   Unspecified physeal fracture of unspecified metatarsal ◄

● **S99.11**   Salter-Harris Type I physeal fracture of metatarsal ◄

● S99.111   Salter-Harris Type I physeal fracture of right metatarsal ◄

● S99.112   Salter-Harris Type I physeal fracture of left metatarsal ◄

● S99.119   Salter-Harris Type I physeal fracture of unspecified metatarsal ◄

● **S99.12**   Salter-Harris Type II physeal fracture of metatarsal ◄

● S99.121   Salter-Harris Type II physeal fracture of right metatarsal ◄

● S99.122   Salter-Harris Type II physeal fracture of left metatarsal ◄

● S99.129   Salter-Harris Type II physeal fracture of unspecified metatarsal ◄

● **S99.13**   Salter-Harris Type III physeal fracture of metatarsal ◄

● S99.131   Salter-Harris Type III physeal fracture of right metatarsal ◄

● S99.132   Salter-Harris Type III physeal fracture of left metatarsal ◄

● S99.139   Salter-Harris Type III physeal fracture of unspecified metatarsal ◄

● **S99.14**   Salter-Harris Type IV physeal fracture of metatarsal ◄

● S99.141   Salter-Harris Type IV physeal fracture of right metatarsal ◄

● S99.142   Salter-Harris Type IV physeal fracture of left metatarsal ◄

● S99.149   Salter-Harris Type IV physeal fracture of unspecified metatarsal ◄

● **S99.19**   Other physeal fracture of metatarsal ◄

● S99.191   Other physeal fracture of right metatarsal ◄

● S99.192   Other physeal fracture of left metatarsal ◄

● S99.199   Other physeal fracture of unspecified metatarsal ◄

● **S99.2**   **Physeal fracture of phalanx of toe** ◄

The appropriate 7th character is to be added to each
code from subcategories S99.2 ◄

A	initial encounter for closed fracture ◄
B	initial encounter for open fracture ◄
D	subsequent encounter for fracture with routine healing ◄
G	subsequent encounter for fracture with delayed healing ◄
K	subsequent encounter for fracture with nonunion ◄
P	subsequent encounter for fracture with malunion ◄
S	sequela ◄

● **S99.20**   Unspecified physeal fracture of phalanx of toe ◄

● S99.201   Unspecified physeal fracture of phalanx of right toe ◄

● S99.202   Unspecified physeal fracture of phalanx of right toe ◄

● S99.209   Unspecified physeal fracture of phalanx of unspecified toe ◄

● **S99.21**   Salter-Harris Type I physeal fracture of phalanx of toe ◄

● S99.211   Salter-Harris Type I physeal fracture of phalanx of right toe ◄

● S99.212   Salter-Harris Type I physeal fracture of phalanx of left toe ◄

● S99.219   Salter-Harris Type I physeal fracture of phalanx of unspecified toe ◄

● **S99.22**   Salter-Harris Type II physeal fracture of phalanx of toe ◄

● S99.221   Salter-Harris Type II physeal fracture of phalanx of right toe ◄

● S99.222   Salter-Harris Type II physeal fracture of phalanx of left toe ◄

● S99.229   Salter-Harris Type II physeal fracture of phalanx of unspecified toe ◄

● **S99.23**   Salter-Harris Type III physeal fracture of phalanx of toe ◄

● S99.231   Salter-Harris Type III physeal fracture of phalanx of right toe ◄

● S99.232   Salter-Harris Type III physeal fracture of phalanx of left toe ◄

● S99.239   Salter-Harris Type III physeal fracture of phalanx of unspecified toe ◄

● **S99.24**   Salter-Harris Type IV physeal fracture of phalanx of toe ◄

● S99.241   Salter-Harris Type IV physeal fracture of phalanx of right toe ◄

● S99.242   Salter-Harris Type IV physeal fracture of phalanx of left toe ◄

● S99.249   Salter-Harris Type IV physeal fracture of phalanx of unspecified toe ◄

● **S99.29**   Other physeal fracture of phalanx of toe ◄

● S99.291   Other physeal fracture of phalanx of right toe ◄

● S99.292   Other physeal fracture of phalanx of left toe ◄

● S99.299   Other physeal fracture of phalanx of unspecified toe ◄

CHAPTER 19 (S00-T88)

N Newborn Age: Ø   **P** Pediatric Age: Ø–17   **M** Maternity DX: 12–55   **A** Adult Age: 15–124   ♀ Females Only   ♂ Males Only

1335

● **S99.8**   **Other specified injuries of ankle and foot**
The appropriate 7th character is to be added to each code from subcategory S99.8 ◀

A	initial encounter ◀
D	subsequent encounter ◀
S	sequela ◀

● **S99.81**   **Other specified injuries of ankle**
● **S99.811**   **Other specified injuries of right ankle**
● **S99.812**   **Other specified injuries of left ankle**
● **S99.819**   **Other specified injuries of unspecified ankle**
● **S99.82**   **Other specified injuries of foot**
● **S99.821**   **Other specified injuries of right foot**
● **S99.822**   **Other specified injuries of left foot**
● **S99.829**   **Other specified injuries of unspecified foot**

● **S99.9**   **Unspecified injury of ankle and foot**
The appropriate 7th character is to be added to each code from subcategory S99.9 ◀

A	initial encounter ◀
D	subsequent encounter ◀
S	sequela ◀

● **S99.91**   **Unspecified injury of ankle**
● **S99.911**   **Unspecified injury of right ankle**
● **S99.912**   **Unspecified injury of left ankle**
● **S99.919**   **Unspecified injury of unspecified ankle**
● **S99.92**   **Unspecified injury of foot**
● **S99.921**   **Unspecified injury of right foot**
● **S99.922**   **Unspecified injury of left foot**
● **S99.929**   **Unspecified injury of unspecified foot**

INJURY, POISONING AND CERTAIN OTHER CONSEQUENCES OF EXTERNAL CAUSES (T07-T88)

INJURIES INVOLVING MULTIPLE BODY REGIONS (T07)

Excludes1   burns and corrosions (T20-T32)
frostbite (T33-T34)
insect bite or sting, venomous (T63.4)
sunburn (L55.-)

T07   **Unspecified multiple injuries**
Excludes1   injury NOS (T14)

INJURY OF UNSPECIFIED BODY REGION (T14)

● **T14**   **Injury of unspecified body region**
Excludes1   multiple unspecified injuries (T07)
T14.8   **Other injury of unspecified body region**

Abrasion NOS	Fracture NOS
Contusion NOS	Skin injury NOS
Crush injury NOS	Vascular injury NOS

● **T14.9**   **Unspecified injury**
T14.90   **Injury, unspecified**
Injury NOS
T14.91   **Suicide attempt**
Attempted suicide NOS

EFFECTS OF FOREIGN BODY ENTERING THROUGH NATURAL ORIFICE (T15-T19)

Excludes2   foreign body accidentally left in operation wound (T81.5-)
foreign body in penetrating wound - see open wound by body region
residual foreign body in soft tissue (M79.5)
splinter, without open wound - see superficial injury by body region

● **T15**   **Foreign body on external eye**
Excludes2   foreign body in penetrating wound of orbit and eye ball (S05.4-, S05.5-)
open wound of eyelid and periocular area (S01.1-)
retained foreign body in eyelid (H02.8-)
retained (old) foreign body in penetrating wound of orbit and eye ball (H05.5-, H44.6-, H44.7-)
superficial foreign body of eyelid and periocular area (S00.25-)

The appropriate 7th character is to be added to each code from category T15

A	initial encounter
D	subsequent encounter
S	sequela

● **T15.0**   **Foreign body in cornea**
X ● **T15.00**   **Foreign body in cornea, unspecified eye**
X ● **T15.01**   **Foreign body in cornea, right eye**
X ● **T15.02**   **Foreign body in cornea, left eye**
● **T15.1**   **Foreign body in conjunctival sac**
X ● **T15.10**   **Foreign body in conjunctival sac, unspecified eye**
X ● **T15.11**   **Foreign body in conjunctival sac, right eye**
X ● **T15.12**   **Foreign body in conjunctival sac, left eye**
● **T15.8**   **Foreign body in other and multiple parts of external eye**
Foreign body in lacrimal punctum
X ● **T15.80**   **Foreign body in other and multiple parts of external eye, unspecified eye**
X ● **T15.81**   **Foreign body in other and multiple parts of external eye, right eye**
X ● **T15.82**   **Foreign body in other and multiple parts of external eye, left eye**
● **T15.9**   **Foreign body on external eye, part unspecified**
X ● **T15.90**   **Foreign body on external eye, part unspecified, unspecified eye**
X ● **T15.91**   **Foreign body on external eye, part unspecified, right eye**
X ● **T15.92**   **Foreign body on external eye, part unspecified, left eye**

● **T16**   **Foreign body in ear**
Includes   foreign body in auditory canal
The appropriate 7th character is to be added to each code from category T16

A	initial encounter
D	subsequent encounter
S	sequela

X ● **T16.1**   **Foreign body in right ear**
X ● **T16.2**   **Foreign body in left ear**
X ● **T16.9**   **Foreign body in ear, unspecified ear**

● **T17**   **Foreign body in respiratory tract**
The appropriate 7th character is to be added to each code from category T17

A	initial encounter
D	subsequent encounter
S	sequela

X ● **T17.0**   **Foreign body in nasal sinus**
X ● **T17.1**   **Foreign body in nostril**
Foreign body in nose NOS

◀ New   ◀▥ Revised   ~~deleted~~ Deleted   Excludes 1   Excludes 2   Includes   Use additional   Code first   Code also   Unspecified
OGCR Official Guidelines   X Assign placeholder X   ● Use Additional Character(s)   ▶ Manifestation Code   Coding Clinic

● **T17.2**   **Foreign body in pharynx**
     Foreign body in nasopharynx
     Foreign body in throat NOS
   ● **T17.20**   Unspecified foreign body in pharynx
     ● **T17.200**   Unspecified foreign body in pharynx causing asphyxiation
     ● **T17.208**   Unspecified foreign body in pharynx causing other injury
   ● **T17.21**   Gastric contents in pharynx
     Aspiration of gastric contents into pharynx
     Vomitus in pharynx
     ● **T17.210**   Gastric contents in pharynx causing asphyxiation
     ● **T17.218**   Gastric contents in pharynx causing other injury
   ● **T17.22**   Food in pharynx
     Bones in pharynx
     Seeds in pharynx
     ● **T17.220**   Food in pharynx causing asphyxiation
     ● **T17.228**   Food in pharynx causing other injury
   ● **T17.29**   Other foreign object in pharynx
     ● **T17.290**   Other foreign object in pharynx causing asphyxiation
     ● **T17.298**   Other foreign object in pharynx causing other injury

● **T17.3**   **Foreign body in larynx**
   ● **T17.30**   Unspecified foreign body in larynx
     ● **T17.300**   Unspecified foreign body in larynx causing asphyxiation
     ● **T17.308**   Unspecified foreign body in larynx causing other injury
   ● **T17.31**   Gastric contents in larynx
     Aspiration of gastric contents into larynx
     Vomitus in larynx
     ● **T17.310**   Gastric contents in larynx causing asphyxiation
     ● **T17.318**   Gastric contents in larynx causing other injury
   ● **T17.32**   Food in larynx
     Bones in larynx ◀▥
     Seeds in larynx
     ● **T17.320**   Food in larynx causing asphyxiation
     ● **T17.328**   Food in larynx causing other injury
   ● **T17.39**   Other foreign object in larynx
     ● **T17.390**   Other foreign object in larynx causing asphyxiation
     ● **T17.398**   Other foreign object in larynx causing other injury

● **T17.4**   **Foreign body in trachea**
   ● **T17.40**   Unspecified foreign body in trachea
     ● **T17.400**   Unspecified foreign body in trachea causing asphyxiation
     ● **T17.408**   Unspecified foreign body in trachea causing other injury
   ● **T17.41**   Gastric contents in trachea
     Aspiration of gastric contents into trachea
     Vomitus in trachea
     ● **T17.410**   Gastric contents in trachea causing asphyxiation
     ● **T17.418**   Gastric contents in trachea causing other injury
   ● **T17.42**   Food in trachea
     Bones in trachea
     Seeds in trachea
     ● **T17.420**   Food in trachea causing asphyxiation
     ● **T17.428**   Food in trachea causing other injury

   ● **T17.49**   Other foreign object in trachea
     ● **T17.490**   Other foreign object in trachea causing asphyxiation
     ● **T17.498**   Other foreign object in trachea causing other injury

● **T17.5**   **Foreign body in bronchus**
   ● **T17.50**   Unspecified foreign body in bronchus
     ● **T17.500**   Unspecified foreign body in bronchus causing asphyxiation
     ● **T17.508**   Unspecified foreign body in bronchus causing other injury
   ● **T17.51**   Gastric contents in bronchus
     Aspiration of gastric contents into bronchus
     Vomitus in bronchus
     ● **T17.510**   Gastric contents in bronchus causing asphyxiation
     ● **T17.518**   Gastric contents in bronchus causing other injury
   ● **T17.52**   Food in bronchus
     Bones in bronchus
     Seeds in bronchus
     ● **T17.520**   Food in bronchus causing asphyxiation
     ● **T17.528**   Food in bronchus causing other injury
   ● **T17.59**   Other foreign object in bronchus
     ● **T17.590**   Other foreign object in bronchus causing asphyxiation
     ● **T17.598**   Other foreign object in bronchus causing other injury

● **T17.8**   **Foreign body in other parts of respiratory tract**
     Foreign body in bronchioles
     Foreign body in lung
   ● **T17.80**   Unspecified foreign body in other parts of respiratory tract
     ● **T17.800**   Unspecified foreign body in other parts of respiratory tract causing asphyxiation
     ● **T17.808**   Unspecified foreign body in other parts of respiratory tract causing other injury
   ● **T17.81**   Gastric contents in other parts of respiratory tract
     Aspiration of gastric contents into other parts of respiratory tract
     Vomitus in other parts of respiratory tract
     ● **T17.810**   Gastric contents in other parts of respiratory tract causing asphyxiation
     ● **T17.818**   Gastric contents in other parts of respiratory tract causing other injury
   ● **T17.82**   Food in other parts of respiratory tract
     Bones in other parts of respiratory tract
     Seeds in other parts of respiratory tract
     ● **T17.820**   Food in other parts of respiratory tract causing asphyxiation
     ● **T17.828**   Food in other parts of respiratory tract causing other injury
   ● **T17.89**   Other foreign object in other parts of respiratory tract
     ● **T17.890**   Other foreign object in other parts of respiratory tract causing asphyxiation
     ● **T17.898**   Other foreign object in other parts of respiratory tract causing other injury

● **T17.9**   **Foreign body in respiratory tract, part unspecified**
   ● **T17.90**   Unspecified foreign body in respiratory tract, part unspecified
     ● **T17.900**   Unspecified foreign body in respiratory tract, part unspecified causing asphyxiation
     ● **T17.908**   Unspecified foreign body in respiratory tract, part unspecified causing other injury

● **T17.91**   **Gastric contents in respiratory tract, part unspecified**
> Aspiration of gastric contents into respiratory tract, part unspecified
> Vomitus in trachea respiratory tract, part unspecified

  ● **T17.910**   **Gastric contents in respiratory tract, part unspecified causing asphyxiation**

  ● **T17.918**   **Gastric contents in respiratory tract, part unspecified causing other injury**

● **T17.92**   **Food in respiratory tract, part unspecified**
> Bones in respiratory tract, part unspecified
> Seeds in respiratory tract, part unspecified

  ● **T17.920**   **Food in respiratory tract, part unspecified causing asphyxiation**

  ● **T17.928**   **Food in respiratory tract, part unspecified causing other injury**

● **T17.99**   **Other foreign object in respiratory tract, part unspecified**

  ● **T17.990**   **Other foreign object in respiratory tract, part unspecified in causing asphyxiation**

  ● **T17.998**   **Other foreign object in respiratory tract, part unspecified causing other injury**

● **T18**   **Foreign body in alimentary tract**
> **Excludes2**   foreign body in pharynx (T17.2-)

> The appropriate 7th character is to be added to each code from category T18

A	initial encounter
D	subsequent encounter
S	sequela

X ● **T18.0**   **Foreign body in mouth**

X ● **T18.1**   **Foreign body in esophagus**
> **Excludes2**   foreign body in respiratory tract (T17.-)

  ● **T18.10**   **Unspecified foreign body in esophagus**

    ● **T18.100**   **Unspecified foreign body in esophagus causing compression of trachea**
> Unspecified foreign body in esophagus causing obstruction of respiration

    ● **T18.108**   **Unspecified foreign body in esophagus causing other injury**

  ● **T18.11**   **Gastric contents in esophagus**
> Vomitus in esophagus

    ● **T18.110**   **Gastric contents in esophagus causing compression of trachea**
> Gastric contents in esophagus causing obstruction of respiration

    ● **T18.118**   **Gastric contents in esophagus causing other injury**

  ● **T18.12**   **Food in esophagus**
> Bones in esophagus
> Seeds in esophagus

    ● **T18.120**   **Food in esophagus causing compression of trachea**
> Food in esophagus causing obstruction of respiration

    ● **T18.128**   **Food in esophagus causing other injury**

  ● **T18.19**   **Other foreign object in esophagus**

    ● **T18.190**   **Other foreign body in esophagus causing compression of trachea**
> Other foreign body in esophagus causing obstruction of respiration
> **Coding Clinic: 2015, Q1, P24**

    ● **T18.198**   **Other foreign object in esophagus causing other injury**
> **Coding Clinic: 2015, Q1, P24**

X ● **T18.2**   **Foreign body in stomach**

X ● **T18.3**   **Foreign body in small intestine**

X ● **T18.4**   **Foreign body in colon**

X ● **T18.5**   **Foreign body in anus and rectum**
> Foreign body in rectosigmoid (junction)

X ● **T18.8**   **Foreign body in other parts of alimentary tract**

X ● **T18.9**   **Foreign body of alimentary tract, part unspecified**
> Foreign body in digestive system NOS
> Swallowed foreign body NOS

● **T19**   **Foreign body in genitourinary tract**
> **Excludes2**   complications due to implanted mesh (T83.7-)
> mechanical complications of contraceptive device (intrauterine) (vaginal) (T83.3-)
> presence of contraceptive device (intrauterine) (vaginal) (Z97.5)

> The appropriate 7th character is to be added to each code from category T19

A	initial encounter
D	subsequent encounter
S	sequela

X ● **T19.0**   **Foreign body in urethra**

X ● **T19.1**   **Foreign body in bladder**

X ● **T19.2**   **Foreign body in vulva and vagina** ♀

X ● **T19.3**   **Foreign body in uterus** ♀

X ● **T19.4**   **Foreign body in penis** ♂

X ● **T19.8**   **Foreign body in other parts of genitourinary tract**

X ● **T19.9**   **Foreign body in genitourinary tract, part unspecified**

BURNS AND CORROSIONS (T20-T32)

> **Includes**   burns (thermal) from electrical heating appliances
> burns (thermal) from electricity
> burns (thermal) from flame
> burns (thermal) from friction
> burns (thermal) from hot air and hot gases
> burns (thermal) from hot objects
> burns (thermal) from lightning
> burns (thermal) from radiation chemical burn [corrosion] (external) (internal) scalds

> **Excludes2**   erythema [dermatitis] ab igne (L59.0)
> radiation-related disorders of the skin and subcutaneous tissue (L55-L59)
> sunburn (L55.-)

OGCR   Section I.C.19.d.

> Burns and Corrosions
>
> The ICD-10-CM makes a distinction between burn and corrosions. The burn codes are for thermal burns, except sunburns, that come from a heat source, such as a fire or hot appliance. The burn codes are also for burns resulting from electricity and radiation. Corrosions are burns due to chemicals. The guidelines for burns and corrosions are the same.
>
> Current burns (T20-T25) are classified by depth, extent and by agent (X code). Burns are classified by depth as first degree (erythema), second degree (blistering), and third degree (full-thickness involvement). Burns of the eye and internal organs (T26-T28) are classified by site, but not by degree.
>
> 1) Sequencing of burn and related condition codes
>
> Sequence first the code that reflects the highest degree of burn when more than one burn is present.
>
> a. When the reason for the admission or encounter is for treatment of external multiple burns, sequence first the code that reflects the burn of the highest degree.
>
> b. When a patient has both internal and external burns, the circumstances of admission govern the selection of the principal diagnosis or first-listed diagnosis.
>
> c. When a patient is admitted for burn injuries and other related conditions such as smoke inhalation and/or respiratory failure, the circumstances of admission govern the selection of the principal or first-listed diagnosis.
>
> 2) Burns of the same local site
>
> Classify burns of the same local site (three-character category level, T20-T28) but of different degrees to the subcategory identifying the highest degree recorded in the diagnosis.

◄ New   ◄|||| Revised   ~~deleted~~ Deleted   Excludes 1   Excludes 2   Includes   Use additional   Code first   Code also   Unspecified

1338   **OGCR** Official Guidelines   X Assign placeholder X   ● Use Additional Character(s)   ▶ Manifestation Code   **Coding Clinic**

Figure 19-15 A. Second-degree burn. **B.** Third-degree burn. (From Cummings: Otolaryngology: Head & Neck Surgery, ed 4, Mosby, 2005)

BURNS AND CORROSIONS OF EXTERNAL BODY SURFACE, SPECIFIED BY SITE (T20-T25)

Includes   burns and corrosions of first degree [erythema]
burns and corrosions of second degree [blisters] [epidermal loss]
burns and corrosions of third degree [deep necrosis of underlying tissue] [full-thickness skin loss]

Use additional code from category T31 or T32 to identify extent of body surface involved

● **T20   Burn and corrosion of head, face, and neck**

Excludes2   burn and corrosion of ear drum (T28.41, T28.91)
burn and corrosion of eye and adnexa (T26.-)
burn and corrosion of mouth and pharynx (T28.0)

The appropriate 7th character is to be added to each code from category T20

A	initial encounter
D	subsequent encounter
S	sequela

● **T20.0   Burn of unspecified degree of head, face, and neck**

Use additional external cause code to identify the source, place and intent of the burn (X00-X19, X75-X77, X96-X98, Y92)

X● **T20.00   Burn of unspecified degree of head, face, and neck, unspecified site**

● **T20.01   Burn of unspecified degree of ear [any part, except ear drum]**

Excludes2   burn of ear drum (T28.41-)

● **T20.011   Burn of unspecified degree of right ear [any part, except ear drum]**

● **T20.012   Burn of unspecified degree of left ear [any part, except ear drum]**

● **T20.019   Burn of unspecified degree of unspecified ear [any part, except ear drum]**

X● **T20.02   Burn of unspecified degree of lip(s)**

X● **T20.03   Burn of unspecified degree of chin**

X● **T20.04   Burn of unspecified degree of nose (septum)**

X● **T20.05   Burn of unspecified degree of scalp [any part]**

X● **T20.06   Burn of unspecified degree of forehead and cheek**

X● **T20.07   Burn of unspecified degree of neck**

X● **T20.09   Burn of unspecified degree of multiple sites of head, face, and neck**

● **T20.1   Burn of first degree of head, face, and neck**

Use additional external cause code to identify the source, place and intent of the burn (X00-X19, X75-X77, X96-X98, Y92)

X● **T20.10   Burn of first degree of head, face, and neck, unspecified site**

● **T20.11   Burn of first degree of ear [any part, except ear drum]**

Excludes2   burn of ear drum (T28.41-)

● **T20.111   Burn of first degree of right ear [any part, except ear drum]**

● **T20.112   Burn of first degree of left ear [any part, except ear drum]**

● **T20.119   Burn of first degree of unspecified ear [any part, except ear drum]**

X● **T20.12   Burn of first degree of lip(s)**

X● **T20.13   Burn of first degree of chin**

X● **T20.14   Burn of first degree of nose (septum)**

X● **T20.15   Burn of first degree of scalp [any part]**

X● **T20.16   Burn of first degree of forehead and cheek**

X● **T20.17   Burn of first degree of neck**

X● **T20.19   Burn of first degree of multiple sites of head, face, and neck**

● **T20.2   Burn of second degree of head, face, and neck**

Use additional external cause code to identify the source, place and intent of the burn (X00-X19, X75-X77, X96-X98, Y92)

X● **T20.20   Burn of second degree of head, face, and neck, unspecified site**

● **T20.21   Burn of second degree of ear [any part, except ear drum]**

Excludes2   burn of ear drum (T28.41-)

● **T20.211   Burn of second degree of right ear [any part, except ear drum]**

● **T20.212   Burn of second degree of left ear [any part, except ear drum]**

● **T20.219   Burn of second degree of unspecified ear [any part, except ear drum]**

X● **T20.22   Burn of second degree of lip(s)**

X● **T20.23   Burn of second degree of chin**

X● **T20.24   Burn of second degree of nose (septum)**

X● **T20.25   Burn of second degree of scalp [any part]**
Coding Clinic: 2015, Q1, P19

X● **T20.26   Burn of second degree of forehead and cheek**

X● **T20.27   Burn of second degree of neck**

X● **T20.29   Burn of second degree of multiple sites of head, face, and neck**

● **T20.3   Burn of third degree of head, face, and neck**

Use additional external cause code to identify the source, place and intent of the burn (X00-X19, X75-X77, X96-X98, Y92)

X● **T20.30   Burn of third degree of head, face, and neck, unspecified site**

● **T20.31   Burn of third degree of ear [any part, except ear drum]**

Excludes2   burn of ear drum (T28.41-)

● **T20.311   Burn of third degree of right ear [any part, except ear drum]**

● **T20.312   Burn of third degree of left ear [any part, except ear drum]**
Coding Clinic: 2015, Q1, P18

● **T20.319   Burn of third degree of unspecified ear [any part, except ear drum]**

CHAPTER 19 (S00-T88)

X ● T20.32   Burn of third degree of lip(s)

X ● T20.33   Burn of third degree of chin

X ● T20.34   Burn of third degree of nose (septum)

X ● T20.35   Burn of third degree of scalp [any part]

X ● T20.36   Burn of third degree of forehead and cheek

X ● T20.37   Burn of third degree of neck

X ● T20.39   Burn of third degree of multiple sites of head, face, and neck

● T20.4   Corrosion of unspecified degree of head, face, and neck

Code first (T51-T65) to identify chemical and intent

Use additional external cause code to identify place (Y92)

X ● T20.40   Corrosion of unspecified degree of head, face, and neck, unspecified site

● T20.41   Corrosion of unspecified degree of ear [any part, except ear drum]

Excludes2   corrosion of ear drum (T28.91-)

● T20.411   Corrosion of unspecified degree of right ear [any part, except ear drum]

● T20.412   Corrosion of unspecified degree of left ear [any part, except ear drum]

● T20.419   Corrosion of unspecified degree of unspecified ear [any part, except ear drum]

X ● T20.42   Corrosion of unspecified degree of lip(s)

X ● T20.43   Corrosion of unspecified degree of chin

X ● T20.44   Corrosion of unspecified degree of nose (septum)

X ● T20.45   Corrosion of unspecified degree of scalp [any part]

X ● T20.46   Corrosion of unspecified degree of forehead and cheek

X ● T20.47   Corrosion of unspecified degree of neck

X ● T20.49   Corrosion of unspecified degree of multiple sites of head, face, and neck

● T20.5   Corrosion of first degree of head, face, and neck

Code first (T51-T65) to identify chemical and intent

Use additional external cause code to identify place (Y92)

X ● T20.50   Corrosion of first degree of head, face, and neck, unspecified site

● T20.51   Corrosion of first degree of ear [any part, except ear drum]

Excludes2   corrosion of ear drum (T28.91-)

● T20.511   Corrosion of first degree of right ear [any part, except ear drum]

● T20.512   Corrosion of first degree of left ear [any part, except ear drum]

● T20.519   Corrosion of first degree of unspecified ear [any part, except ear drum]

X ● T20.52   Corrosion of first degree of lip(s)

X ● T20.53   Corrosion of first degree of chin

X ● T20.54   Corrosion of first degree of nose (septum)

X ● T20.55   Corrosion of first degree of scalp [any part]

X ● T20.56   Corrosion of first degree of forehead and cheek

X ● T20.57   Corrosion of first degree of neck

X ● T20.59   Corrosion of first degree of multiple sites of head, face, and neck

● T20.6   Corrosion of second degree of head, face, and neck

Code first (T51-T65) to identify chemical and intent

Use additional external cause code to identify place (Y92)

X ● T20.60   Corrosion of second degree of head, face, and neck, unspecified site

● T20.61   Corrosion of second degree of ear [any part, except ear drum]

Excludes2   corrosion of ear drum (T28.91-)

● T20.611   Corrosion of second degree of right ear [any part, except ear drum]

● T20.612   Corrosion of second degree of left ear [any part, except ear drum]

● T20.619   Corrosion of second degree of unspecified ear [any part, except ear drum]

X ● T20.62   Corrosion of second degree of lip(s)

X ● T20.63   Corrosion of second degree of chin

X ● T20.64   Corrosion of second degree of nose (septum)

X ● T20.65   Corrosion of second degree of scalp [any part]

X ● T20.66   Corrosion of second degree of forehead and cheek

X ● T20.67   Corrosion of second degree of neck

X ● T20.69   Corrosion of second degree of multiple sites of head, face, and neck

● T20.7   Corrosion of third degree of head, face, and neck

Code first (T51-T65) to identify chemical and intent

Use additional external cause code to identify place (Y92)

X ● T20.70   Corrosion of third degree of head, face, and neck, unspecified site

● T20.71   Corrosion of third degree of ear [any part, except ear drum]

Excludes2   corrosion of ear drum (T28.91-)

● T20.711   Corrosion of third degree of right ear [any part, except ear drum]

● T20.712   Corrosion of third degree of left ear [any part, except ear drum]

● T20.719   Corrosion of third degree of unspecified ear [any part, except ear drum]

X ● T20.72   Corrosion of third degree of lip(s)

X ● T20.73   Corrosion of third degree of chin

X ● T20.74   Corrosion of third degree of nose (septum)

X ● T20.75   Corrosion of third degree of scalp [any part]

X ● T20.76   Corrosion of third degree of forehead and cheek

X ● T20.77   Corrosion of third degree of neck

X ● T20.79   Corrosion of third degree of multiple sites of head, face, and neck

● **T21   Burn and corrosion of trunk**

Includes   burns and corrosion of hip region

Excludes2   burns and corrosion of axilla (T22.- with fifth character 4)

burns and corrosion of scapular region (T22.- with fifth character 6)

burns and corrosion of shoulder (T22.- with fifth character 5)

The appropriate 7th character is to be added to each code from category T21

A	initial encounter
D	subsequent encounter
S	sequela

● **T21.0   Burn of unspecified degree of trunk**

Use additional external cause code to identify the source, place and intent of the burn (X00-X19, X75-X77, X96-X98, Y92)

X ● **T21.00   Burn of unspecified degree of trunk, unspecified site**

X ● **T21.01   Burn of unspecified degree of chest wall**
Burn of of unspecified degree of breast

X ● **T21.02   Burn of unspecified degree of abdominal wall**
Burn of unspecified degree of flank
Burn of unspecified degree of groin

X ● **T21.03   Burn of unspecified degree of upper back**
Burn of unspecified degree of interscapular region

X ● **T21.04   Burn of unspecified degree of lower back**

X ● **T21.05   Burn of unspecified degree of buttock**
Burn of unspecified degree of anus

X ● **T21.06   Burn of unspecified degree of male genital region ♂**
Burn of unspecified degree of penis
Burn of unspecified degree of scrotum
Burn of unspecified degree of testis

X ● **T21.07   Burn of unspecified degree of female genital region ♀**
Burn of unspecified degree of labium (majus) (minus)
Burn of unspecified degree of perineum
Burn of unspecified degree of vulva
Excludes2   burn of vagina (T28.3)

X ● **T21.09   Burn of unspecified degree of other site of trunk**

● **T21.1   Burn of first degree of trunk**

Use additional external cause code to identify the source, place and intent of the burn (X00-X19, X75-X77, X96-X98, Y92)

X ● **T21.10   Burn of first degree of trunk, unspecified site**

X ● **T21.11   Burn of first degree of chest wall**
Burn of first degree of breast

X ● **T21.12   Burn of first degree of abdominal wall**
Burn of first degree of flank
Burn of first degree of groin

X ● **T21.13   Burn of first degree of upper back**
Burn of first degree of interscapular region

X ● **T21.14   Burn of first degree of lower back**

X ● **T21.15   Burn of first degree of buttock**
Burn of first degree of anus

X ● **T21.16   Burn of first degree of male genital region ♂**
Burn of first degree of penis
Burn of first degree of scrotum
Burn of first degree of testis

X ● **T21.17   Burn of first degree of female genital region ♀**
Burn of first degree of labium (majus) (minus)
Burn of first degree of perineum
Burn of first degree of vulva
Excludes2   burn of vagina (T28.3)

X ● **T21.19   Burn of first degree of other site of trunk**

● **T21.2   Burn of second degree of trunk**

Use additional external cause code to identify the source, place and intent of the burn (X00-X19, X75-X77, X96-X98, Y92)

X ● **T21.20   Burn of second degree of trunk, unspecified site**

X ● **T21.21   Burn of second degree of chest wall**
Burn of second degree of breast

X ● **T21.22   Burn of second degree of abdominal wall**
Burn of second degree of flank
Burn of second degree of groin

X ● **T21.23   Burn of second degree of upper back**
Burn of second degree of interscapular region

X ● **T21.24   Burn of second degree of lower back**

X ● **T21.25   Burn of second degree of buttock**
Burn of second degree of anus

X ● **T21.26   Burn of second degree of male genital region ♂**
Burn of second degree of penis
Burn of second degree of scrotum
Burn of second degree of testis

X ● **T21.27   Burn of second degree of female genital region ♀**
Burn of second degree of labium (majus) (minus)
Burn of second degree of perineum
Burn of second degree of vulva
Excludes2   burn of vagina (T28.3)

X ● **T21.29   Burn of second degree of other site of trunk**

● **T21.3   Burn of third degree of trunk**

Use additional external cause code to identify the source, place and intent of the burn (X00-X19, X75-X77, X96-X98, Y92)

X ● **T21.30   Burn of third degree of trunk, unspecified site**

X ● **T21.31   Burn of third degree of chest wall**
Burn of third degree of breast
Coding Clinic: 2016, Q2, P6

X ● **T21.32   Burn of third degree of abdominal wall**
Burn of third degree of flank
Burn of third degree of groin

X ● **T21.33   Burn of third degree of upper back**
Burn of third degree of interscapular region

X ● **T21.34   Burn of third degree of lower back**

X ● **T21.35   Burn of third degree of buttock**
Burn of third degree of anus

X ● **T21.36   Burn of third degree of male genital region ♂**
Burn of third degree of penis
Burn of third degree of scrotum
Burn of third degree of testis

X ● **T21.37   Burn of third degree of female genital region ♀**
Burn of third degree of labium (majus) (minus)
Burn of third degree of perineum
Burn of third degree of vulva
Excludes2   burn of vagina (T28.3)

X ● **T21.39   Burn of third degree of other site of trunk**

● **T21.4 Corrosion of unspecified degree of trunk**
Code first (T51-T65) to identify chemical and intent
Use additional external cause code to identify place (Y92)

X ● **T21.40 Corrosion of unspecified degree of trunk, unspecified site**

X ● **T21.41 Corrosion of unspecified degree of chest wall**
Corrosion of unspecified degree of breast

X ● **T21.42 Corrosion of unspecified degree of abdominal wall**
Corrosion of unspecified degree of flank
Corrosion of unspecified degree of groin

X ● **T21.43 Corrosion of unspecified degree of upper back**
Corrosion of unspecified degree of interscapular region

X ● **T21.44 Corrosion of unspecified degree of lower back**

X ● **T21.45 Corrosion of unspecified degree of buttock**
Corrosion of unspecified degree of anus

X ● **T21.46 Corrosion of unspecified degree of male genital region ♂**
Corrosion of unspecified degree of penis
Corrosion of unspecified degree of scrotum
Corrosion of unspecified degree of testis

X ● **T21.47 Corrosion of unspecified degree of female genital region ♀**
Corrosion of unspecified degree of labium (majus) (minus)
Corrosion of unspecified degree of perineum
Corrosion of unspecified degree of vulva
Excludes2 corrosion of vagina (T28.8)

X ● **T21.49 Corrosion of unspecified degree of other site of trunk**

● **T21.5 Corrosion of first degree of trunk**
Code first (T51-T65) to identify chemical and intent
Use additional external cause code to identify place (Y92)

X ● **T21.50 Corrosion of first degree of trunk, unspecified site**

X ● **T21.51 Corrosion of first degree of chest wall**
Corrosion of first degree of breast

X ● **T21.52 Corrosion of first degree of abdominal wall**
Corrosion of first degree of flank
Corrosion of first degree of groin

X ● **T21.53 Corrosion of first degree of upper back**
Corrosion of first degree of interscapular region

X ● **T21.54 Corrosion of first degree of lower back**

X ● **T21.55 Corrosion of first degree of buttock**
Corrosion of first degree of anus

X ● **T21.56 Corrosion of first degree of male genital region ♂**
Corrosion of first degree of penis
Corrosion of first degree of scrotum
Corrosion of first degree of testis

X ● **T21.57 Corrosion of first degree of female genital region ♀**
Corrosion of first degree of labium (majus) (minus)
Corrosion of first degree of perineum
Corrosion of first degree of vulva
Excludes2 corrosion of vagina (T28.8)

X ● **T21.59 Corrosion of first degree of other site of trunk**

● **T21.6 Corrosion of second degree of trunk**
Code first (T51-T65) to identify chemical and intent
Use additional external cause code to identify place (Y92)

X ● **T21.60 Corrosion of second degree of trunk, unspecified site**

X ● **T21.61 Corrosion of second degree of chest wall**
Corrosion of second degree of breast

X ● **T21.62 Corrosion of second degree of abdominal wall**
Corrosion of second degree of flank
Corrosion of second degree of groin

X ● **T21.63 Corrosion of second degree of upper back**
Corrosion of second degree of interscapular region

X ● **T21.64 Corrosion of second degree of lower back**

X ● **T21.65 Corrosion of second degree of buttock**
Corrosion of second degree of anus

X ● **T21.66 Corrosion of second degree of male genital region ♂**
Corrosion of second degree of penis
Corrosion of second degree of scrotum
Corrosion of second degree of testis

X ● **T21.67 Corrosion of second degree of female genital region ♀**
Corrosion of second degree of labium (majus) (minus)
Corrosion of second degree of perineum
Corrosion of second degree of vulva
Excludes2 corrosion of vagina (T28.8)

X ● **T21.69 Corrosion of second degree of other site of trunk**

● **T21.7 Corrosion of third degree of trunk**
Code first (T51-T65) to identify chemical and intent
Use additional external cause code to identify place (Y92)

X ● **T21.70 Corrosion of third degree of trunk, unspecified site**

X ● **T21.71 Corrosion of third degree of chest wall**
Corrosion of third degree of breast

X ● **T21.72 Corrosion of third degree of abdominal wall**
Corrosion of third degree of flank
Corrosion of third degree of groin

X ● **T21.73 Corrosion of third degree of upper back**
Corrosion of third degree of interscapular region

X ● **T21.74 Corrosion of third degree of lower back**

X ● **T21.75 Corrosion of third degree of buttock**
Corrosion of third degree of anus

X ● **T21.76 Corrosion of third degree of male genital region ♂**
Corrosion of third degree of penis
Corrosion of third degree of scrotum
Corrosion of third degree of testis

X ● **T21.77 Corrosion of third degree of female genital region ♀**
Corrosion of third degree of labium (majus) (minus)
Corrosion of third degree of perineum
Corrosion of third degree of vulva
Excludes2 corrosion of vagina (T28.8)

X ● **T21.79 Corrosion of third degree of other site of trunk**

◀ New   ◀▥ Revised   ~~deleted~~ Deleted   Excludes 1   Excludes 2   Includes   Use additional   Code first   Code also   Unspecified

OGCR Official Guidelines   X Assign placeholder X   ● Use Additional Character(s)   ▶ Manifestation Code   **Coding Clinic**

CHAPTER 19 (S00-T88)

● **T22** Burn and corrosion of shoulder and upper limb, except wrist and hand

> **Excludes2** burn and corrosion of interscapular region (T21.-)
> burn and corrosion of wrist and hand (T23.-)
>
> The appropriate 7th character is to be added to each code from category T22

> A   initial encounter
> D   subsequent encounter
> S   sequela

● **T22.0** Burn of unspecified degree of shoulder and upper limb, except wrist and hand

> Use additional external cause code to identify the source, place and intent of the burn (X00-X19, X75-X77, X96-X98, Y92)

X ● **T22.00** Burn of unspecified degree of shoulder and upper limb, except wrist and hand, unspecified site

● **T22.01** Burn of unspecified degree of forearm
- ● **T22.011** Burn of unspecified degree of right forearm
- ● **T22.012** Burn of unspecified degree of left forearm
- ● **T22.019** Burn of unspecified degree of unspecified forearm

● **T22.02** Burn of unspecified degree of elbow
- ● **T22.021** Burn of unspecified degree of right elbow
- ● **T22.022** Burn of unspecified degree of left elbow
- ● **T22.029** Burn of unspecified degree of unspecified elbow

● **T22.03** Burn of unspecified degree of upper arm
- ● **T22.031** Burn of unspecified degree of right upper arm
- ● **T22.032** Burn of unspecified degree of left upper arm
- ● **T22.039** Burn of unspecified degree of unspecified upper arm

● **T22.04** Burn of unspecified degree of axilla
- ● **T22.041** Burn of unspecified degree of right axilla
- ● **T22.042** Burn of unspecified degree of left axilla
- ● **T22.049** Burn of unspecified degree of unspecified axilla

● **T22.05** Burn of unspecified degree of shoulder
- ● **T22.051** Burn of unspecified degree of right shoulder
- ● **T22.052** Burn of unspecified degree of left shoulder
- ● **T22.059** Burn of unspecified degree of unspecified shoulder

● **T22.06** Burn of unspecified degree of scapular region
- ● **T22.061** Burn of unspecified degree of right scapular region
- ● **T22.062** Burn of unspecified degree of left scapular region
- ● **T22.069** Burn of unspecified degree of unspecified scapular region

● **T22.09** Burn of unspecified degree of multiple sites of shoulder and upper limb, except wrist and hand
- ● **T22.091** Burn of unspecified degree of multiple sites of right shoulder and upper limb, except wrist and hand
- ● **T22.092** Burn of unspecified degree of multiple sites of left shoulder and upper limb, except wrist and hand
- ● **T22.099** Burn of unspecified degree of multiple sites of unspecified shoulder and upper limb, except wrist and hand

● **T22.1** Burn of first degree of shoulder and upper limb, except wrist and hand

> Use additional external cause code to identify the source, place and intent of the burn (X00-X19, X75-X77, X96-X98, Y92)

X ● **T22.10** Burn of first degree of shoulder and upper limb, except wrist and hand, unspecified site

● **T22.11** Burn of first degree of forearm
- ● **T22.111** Burn of first degree of right forearm
- ● **T22.112** Burn of first degree of left forearm
- ● **T22.119** Burn of first degree of unspecified forearm

● **T22.12** Burn of first degree of elbow
- ● **T22.121** Burn of first degree of right elbow
- ● **T22.122** Burn of first degree of left elbow
- ● **T22.129** Burn of first degree of unspecified elbow

● **T22.13** Burn of first degree of upper arm
- ● **T22.131** Burn of first degree of right upper arm
- ● **T22.132** Burn of first degree of left upper arm
- ● **T22.139** Burn of first degree of unspecified upper arm

● **T22.14** Burn of first degree of axilla
- ● **T22.141** Burn of first degree of right axilla
- ● **T22.142** Burn of first degree of left axilla
- ● **T22.149** Burn of first degree of unspecified axilla

● **T22.15** Burn of first degree of shoulder
- ● **T22.151** Burn of first degree of right shoulder
- ● **T22.152** Burn of first degree of left shoulder
- ● **T22.159** Burn of first degree of unspecified shoulder

● **T22.16** Burn of first degree of scapular region
- ● **T22.161** Burn of first degree of right scapular region
- ● **T22.162** Burn of first degree of left scapular region
- ● **T22.169** Burn of first degree of unspecified scapular region

● **T22.19** Burn of first degree of multiple sites of shoulder and upper limb, except wrist and hand
- ● **T22.191** Burn of first degree of multiple sites of right shoulder and upper limb, except wrist and hand
- ● **T22.192** Burn of first degree of multiple sites of left shoulder and upper limb, except wrist and hand
- ● **T22.199** Burn of first degree of multiple sites of unspecified shoulder and upper limb, except wrist and hand

N Newborn Age: 0   **P** Pediatric Age: 0–17   **M** Maternity DX: 12–55   **A** Adult Age: 15–124   ♀ Females Only   ♂ Males Only

CHAPTER 19 (S00-T88)

1343

● **T22.2 Burn of second degree of shoulder and upper limb, except wrist and hand**

Use additional external cause code to identify the source, place and intent of the burn (X00-X19, X75-X77, X96-X98, Y92)

X● **T22.20** Burn of second degree of shoulder and upper limb, except wrist and hand, **unspecified** site

● **T22.21** Burn of second degree of forearm

  ● **T22.211** Burn of second degree of right forearm

  ● **T22.212** Burn of second degree of left forearm

  ● **T22.219** Burn of second degree of **unspecified** forearm

● **T22.22** Burn of second degree of elbow

  ● **T22.221** Burn of second degree of right elbow

  ● **T22.222** Burn of second degree of left elbow

  ● **T22.229** Burn of second degree of **unspecified** elbow

● **T22.23** Burn of second degree of upper arm

  ● **T22.231** Burn of second degree of right upper arm

  ● **T22.232** Burn of second degree of left upper arm

  ● **T22.239** Burn of second degree of **unspecified** upper arm

● **T22.24** Burn of second degree of axilla

  ● **T22.241** Burn of second degree of right axilla

  ● **T22.242** Burn of second degree of left axilla

  ● **T22.249** Burn of second degree of **unspecified** axilla

● **T22.25** Burn of second degree of shoulder

  ● **T22.251** Burn of second degree of right shoulder

  ● **T22.252** Burn of second degree of left shoulder

  ● **T22.259** Burn of second degree of **unspecified** shoulder

● **T22.26** Burn of second degree of scapular region

  ● **T22.261** Burn of second degree of right scapular region

  ● **T22.262** Burn of second degree of left scapular region

  ● **T22.269** Burn of second degree of **unspecified** scapular region

● **T22.29** Burn of second degree of multiple sites of shoulder and upper limb, except wrist and hand

  ● **T22.291** Burn of second degree of multiple sites of right shoulder and upper limb, except wrist and hand

  ● **T22.292** Burn of second degree of multiple sites of left shoulder and upper limb, except wrist and hand

  ● **T22.299** Burn of second degree of multiple sites of **unspecified** shoulder and upper limb, except wrist and hand

● **T22.3 Burn of third degree of shoulder and upper limb, except wrist and hand**

Use additional external cause code to identify the source, place and intent of the burn (X00-X19, X75-X77, X96-X98, Y92)

X● **T22.30** Burn of third degree of shoulder and upper limb, except wrist and hand, **unspecified** site

● **T22.31** Burn of third degree of forearm

  ● **T22.311** Burn of third degree of right forearm

  ● **T22.312** Burn of third degree of left forearm

  ● **T22.319** Burn of third degree of **unspecified** forearm

● **T22.32** Burn of third degree of elbow

  ● **T22.321** Burn of third degree of right elbow

  ● **T22.322** Burn of third degree of left elbow

  ● **T22.329** Burn of third degree of **unspecified** elbow

● **T22.33** Burn of third degree of upper arm

  ● **T22.331** Burn of third degree of right upper arm

  ● **T22.332** Burn of third degree of left upper arm

  ● **T22.339** Burn of third degree of **unspecified** upper arm

● **T22.34** Burn of third degree of axilla

  ● **T22.341** Burn of third degree of right axilla

  ● **T22.342** Burn of third degree of left axilla

  ● **T22.349** Burn of third degree of **unspecified** axilla

● **T22.35** Burn of third degree of shoulder

  ● **T22.351** Burn of third degree of right shoulder

  ● **T22.352** Burn of third degree of left shoulder

  ● **T22.359** Burn of third degree of **unspecified** shoulder

● **T22.36** Burn of third degree of scapular region

  ● **T22.361** Burn of third degree of right scapular region

  ● **T22.362** Burn of third degree of left scapular region

  ● **T22.369** Burn of third degree of **unspecified** scapular region

● **T22.39** Burn of third degree of multiple sites of shoulder and upper limb, except wrist and hand

  ● **T22.391** Burn of third degree of multiple sites of right shoulder and upper limb, except wrist and hand

  ● **T22.392** Burn of third degree of multiple sites of left shoulder and upper limb, except wrist and hand

  ● **T22.399** Burn of third degree of multiple sites of **unspecified** shoulder and upper limb, except wrist and hand

● **T22.4 Corrosion of unspecified degree of shoulder and upper limb, except wrist and hand**

Code first (T51-T65) to identify chemical and intent

Use additional external cause code to identify place (Y92)

X● **T22.40** Corrosion of **unspecified** degree of shoulder and upper limb, except wrist and hand, unspecified site

● **T22.41** Corrosion of unspecified degree of forearm

  ● **T22.411** Corrosion of **unspecified** degree of right forearm

  ● **T22.412** Corrosion of **unspecified** degree of left forearm

  ● **T22.419** Corrosion of **unspecified** degree of unspecified forearm

● **T22.42** Corrosion of unspecified degree of elbow

  ● **T22.421** Corrosion of **unspecified** degree of right elbow

  ● **T22.422** Corrosion of **unspecified** degree of left elbow

  ● **T22.429** Corrosion of **unspecified** degree of unspecified elbow

● **T22.43** Corrosion of unspecified degree of upper arm

  ● **T22.431** Corrosion of **unspecified** degree of right upper arm

  ● **T22.432** Corrosion of **unspecified** degree of left upper arm

  ● **T22.439** Corrosion of **unspecified** degree of unspecified upper arm

◀ New   ◀ Revised   deleted Deleted   Excludes 1   Excludes 2   Includes   Use additional   Code first   Code also   Unspecified

OGCR Official Guidelines   X Assign placeholder X   ● Use Additional Character(s)   ▶ Manifestation Code   **Coding Clinic**

● **T22.44** Corrosion of unspecified degree of axilla
  ● **T22.441** Corrosion of unspecified degree of right axilla
  ● **T22.442** Corrosion of unspecified degree of left axilla
  ● **T22.449** Corrosion of unspecified degree of unspecified axilla
● **T22.45** Corrosion of unspecified degree of shoulder
  ● **T22.451** Corrosion of unspecified degree of right shoulder
  ● **T22.452** Corrosion of unspecified degree of left shoulder
  ● **T22.459** Corrosion of unspecified degree of unspecified shoulder
● **T22.46** Corrosion of unspecified degree of scapular region
  ● **T22.461** Corrosion of unspecified degree of right scapular region
  ● **T22.462** Corrosion of unspecified degree of left scapular region
  ● **T22.469** Corrosion of unspecified degree of unspecified scapular region
● **T22.49** Corrosion of unspecified degree of multiple sites of shoulder and upper limb, except wrist and hand
  ● **T22.491** Corrosion of unspecified degree of multiple sites of right shoulder and upper limb, except wrist and hand
  ● **T22.492** Corrosion of unspecified degree of multiple sites of left shoulder and upper limb, except wrist and hand
  ● **T22.499** Corrosion of unspecified degree of multiple sites of unspecified shoulder and upper limb, except wrist and hand
● **T22.5** Corrosion of first degree of shoulder and upper limb, except wrist and hand

  Code first (T51-T65) *to identify chemical and intent*
  Use additional external cause code to identify place (Y92)

  X ● **T22.50** Corrosion of first degree of shoulder and upper limb, except wrist and hand unspecified site
  ● **T22.51** Corrosion of first degree of forearm
    ● **T22.511** Corrosion of first degree of right forearm
    ● **T22.512** Corrosion of first degree of left forearm
    ● **T22.519** Corrosion of first degree of unspecified forearm
  ● **T22.52** Corrosion of first degree of elbow
    ● **T22.521** Corrosion of first degree of right elbow
    ● **T22.522** Corrosion of first degree of left elbow
    ● **T22.529** Corrosion of first degree of unspecified elbow
  ● **T22.53** Corrosion of first degree of upper arm
    ● **T22.531** Corrosion of first degree of right upper arm
    ● **T22.532** Corrosion of first degree of left upper arm
    ● **T22.539** Corrosion of first degree of unspecified upper arm
  ● **T22.54** Corrosion of first degree of axilla
    ● **T22.541** Corrosion of first degree of right axilla
    ● **T22.542** Corrosion of first degree of left axilla
    ● **T22.549** Corrosion of first degree of unspecified axilla

● **T22.55** Corrosion of first degree of shoulder
  ● **T22.551** Corrosion of first degree of right shoulder
  ● **T22.552** Corrosion of first degree of left shoulder
  ● **T22.559** Corrosion of first degree of unspecified shoulder
● **T22.56** Corrosion of first degree of scapular region
  ● **T22.561** Corrosion of first degree of right scapular region
  ● **T22.562** Corrosion of first degree of left scapular region
  ● **T22.569** Corrosion of first degree of unspecified scapular region
● **T22.59** Corrosion of first degree of multiple sites of shoulder and upper limb, except wrist and hand
  ● **T22.591** Corrosion of first degree of multiple sites of right shoulder and upper limb, except wrist and hand
  ● **T22.592** Corrosion of first degree of multiple sites of left shoulder and upper limb, except wrist and hand
  ● **T22.599** Corrosion of first degree of multiple sites of unspecified shoulder and upper limb, except wrist and hand
● **T22.6** Corrosion of second degree of shoulder and upper limb, except wrist and hand

  Code first (T51-T65) *to identify chemical and intent*
  Use additional external cause code to identify place (Y92)

  X ● **T22.60** Corrosion of second degree of shoulder and upper limb, except wrist and hand, unspecified site
  ● **T22.61** Corrosion of second degree of forearm
    ● **T22.611** Corrosion of second degree of right forearm
    ● **T22.612** Corrosion of second degree of left forearm
    ● **T22.619** Corrosion of second degree of unspecified forearm
  ● **T22.62** Corrosion of second degree of elbow
    ● **T22.621** Corrosion of second degree of right elbow
    ● **T22.622** Corrosion of second degree of left elbow
    ● **T22.629** Corrosion of second degree of unspecified elbow
  ● **T22.63** Corrosion of second degree of upper arm
    ● **T22.631** Corrosion of second degree of right upper arm
    ● **T22.632** Corrosion of second degree of left upper arm
    ● **T22.639** Corrosion of second degree of unspecified upper arm
  ● **T22.64** Corrosion of second degree of axilla
    ● **T22.641** Corrosion of second degree of right axilla
    ● **T22.642** Corrosion of second degree of left axilla
    ● **T22.649** Corrosion of second degree of unspecified axilla
  ● **T22.65** Corrosion of second degree of shoulder
    ● **T22.651** Corrosion of second degree of right shoulder
    ● **T22.652** Corrosion of second degree of left shoulder
    ● **T22.659** Corrosion of second degree of unspecified shoulder

● T22.66 Corrosion of second degree of scapular region
 ● T22.661 Corrosion of second degree of right scapular region
 ● T22.662 Corrosion of second degree of left scapular region
 ● T22.669 Corrosion of second degree of unspecified scapular region
● T22.69 Corrosion of second degree of multiple sites of shoulder and upper limb, except wrist and hand
 ● T22.691 Corrosion of second degree of multiple sites of right shoulder and upper limb, except wrist and hand
 ● T22.692 Corrosion of second degree of multiple sites of left shoulder and upper limb, except wrist and hand
 ● T22.699 Corrosion of second degree of multiple sites of unspecified shoulder and upper limb, except wrist and hand
● T22.7 Corrosion of third degree of shoulder and upper limb, except wrist and hand
   Code first (T51-T65) *to identify chemical and intent*
   Use additional external cause code to identify place (Y92)
 X ● T22.70 Corrosion of third degree of shoulder and upper limb, except wrist and hand, unspecified site
 ● T22.71 Corrosion of third degree of forearm
  ● T22.711 Corrosion of third degree of right forearm
  ● T22.712 Corrosion of third degree of left forearm
  ● T22.719 Corrosion of third degree of unspecified forearm
 ● T22.72 Corrosion of third degree of elbow
  ● T22.721 Corrosion of third degree of right elbow
  ● T22.722 Corrosion of third degree of left elbow
  ● T22.729 Corrosion of third degree of unspecified elbow
 ● T22.73 Corrosion of third degree of upper arm
  ● T22.731 Corrosion of third degree of right upper arm
  ● T22.732 Corrosion of third degree of left upper arm
  ● T22.739 Corrosion of third degree of unspecified upper arm
 ● T22.74 Corrosion of third degree of axilla
  ● T22.741 Corrosion of third degree of right axilla
  ● T22.742 Corrosion of third degree of left axilla
  ● T22.749 Corrosion of third degree of unspecified axilla
 ● T22.75 Corrosion of third degree of shoulder
  ● T22.751 Corrosion of third degree of right shoulder
  ● T22.752 Corrosion of third degree of left shoulder
  ● T22.759 Corrosion of third degree of unspecified shoulder
 ● T22.76 Corrosion of third degree of scapular region
  ● T22.761 Corrosion of third degree of right scapular region
  ● T22.762 Corrosion of third degree of left scapular region
  ● T22.769 Corrosion of third degree of unspecified scapular region

● T22.79 Corrosion of third degree of multiple sites of shoulder and upper limb, except wrist and hand
 ● T22.791 Corrosion of third degree of multiple sites of right shoulder and upper limb, except wrist and hand
 ● T22.792 Corrosion of third degree of multiple sites of left shoulder and upper limb, except wrist and hand
 ● T22.799 Corrosion of third degree of multiple sites of unspecified shoulder and upper limb, except wrist and hand

● T23 Burn and corrosion of wrist and hand
   The appropriate 7th character is to be added to each code from category T23

A	initial encounter
D	subsequent encounter
S	sequela

 ● T23.0 Burn of unspecified degree of wrist and hand
   Use additional external cause code to identify the source, place and intent of the burn (X00-X19, X75-X77, X96-X98, Y92)
  ● T23.00 Burn of unspecified degree of hand, unspecified site
   ● T23.001 Burn of unspecified degree of right hand, unspecified site
   ● T23.002 Burn of unspecified degree of left hand, unspecified site
   ● T23.009 Burn of unspecified degree of unspecified hand, unspecified site
  ● T23.01 Burn of unspecified degree of thumb (nail)
   ● T23.011 Burn of unspecified degree of right thumb (nail)
   ● T23.012 Burn of unspecified degree of left thumb (nail)
   ● T23.019 Burn of unspecified degree of unspecified thumb (nail)
  ● T23.02 Burn of unspecified degree of single finger (nail) except thumb
   ● T23.021 Burn of unspecified degree of single right finger (nail) except thumb
   ● T23.022 Burn of unspecified degree of single left finger (nail) except thumb
   ● T23.029 Burn of unspecified degree of unspecified single finger (nail) except thumb
  ● T23.03 Burn of unspecified degree of multiple fingers (nail), not including thumb
   ● T23.031 Burn of unspecified degree of multiple right fingers (nail), not including thumb
   ● T23.032 Burn of unspecified degree of multiple left fingers (nail), not including thumb
   ● T23.039 Burn of unspecified degree of unspecified multiple fingers (nail), not including thumb
  ● T23.04 Burn of unspecified degree of multiple fingers (nail), including thumb
   ● T23.041 Burn of unspecified degree of multiple right fingers (nail), including thumb
   ● T23.042 Burn of unspecified degree of multiple left fingers (nail), including thumb
   ● T23.049 Burn of unspecified degree of unspecified multiple fingers (nail), including thumb

◀ New ⬅ Revised ~~deleted~~ Deleted Excludes 1 Excludes 2 Includes Use additional Code first Code also Unspecified
OGCR Official Guidelines X Assign placeholder X ● Use Additional Character(s) ▶ Manifestation Code **Coding Clinic**

- T23.05 Burn of unspecified degree of palm
  - T23.051 Burn of unspecified degree of right palm
  - T23.052 Burn of unspecified degree of left palm
  - T23.059 Burn of unspecified degree of unspecified palm
- T23.06 Burn of unspecified degree of back of hand
  - T23.061 Burn of unspecified degree of back of right hand
  - T23.062 Burn of unspecified degree of back of left hand
  - T23.069 Burn of unspecified degree of back of unspecified hand
- T23.07 Burn of unspecified degree of wrist
  - T23.071 Burn of unspecified degree of right wrist
  - T23.072 Burn of unspecified degree of left wrist
  - T23.079 Burn of unspecified degree of unspecified wrist
- T23.09 Burn of unspecified degree of multiple sites of wrist and hand
  - T23.091 Burn of unspecified degree of multiple sites of right wrist and hand
  - T23.092 Burn of unspecified degree of multiple sites of left wrist and hand
  - T23.099 Burn of unspecified degree of multiple sites of unspecified wrist and hand
- T23.1 Burn of first degree of wrist and hand

  Use additional external cause code to identify the source, place and intent of the burn (X00-X19, X75-X77, X96-X98, Y92)
  - T23.10 Burn of first degree of hand, unspecified site
    - T23.101 Burn of first degree of right hand, unspecified site
    - T23.102 Burn of first degree of left hand, unspecified site
    - T23.109 Burn of first degree of unspecified hand, unspecified site
  - T23.11 Burn of first degree of thumb (nail)
    - T23.111 Burn of first degree of right thumb (nail)
    - T23.112 Burn of first degree of left thumb (nail)
    - T23.119 Burn of first degree of unspecified thumb (nail)
  - T23.12 Burn of first degree of single finger (nail) except thumb
    - T23.121 Burn of first degree of single right finger (nail) except thumb
    - T23.122 Burn of first degree of single left finger (nail) except thumb
    - T23.129 Burn of first degree of unspecified single finger (nail) except thumb
  - T23.13 Burn of first degree of multiple fingers (nail), not including thumb
    - T23.131 Burn of first degree of multiple right fingers (nail), not including thumb
    - T23.132 Burn of first degree of multiple left fingers (nail), not including thumb
    - T23.139 Burn of first degree of unspecified multiple fingers (nail), not including thumb

- T23.14 Burn of first degree of multiple fingers (nail), including thumb
  - T23.141 Burn of first degree of multiple right fingers (nail), including thumb
  - T23.142 Burn of first degree of multiple left fingers (nail), including thumb
  - T23.149 Burn of first degree of unspecified multiple fingers (nail), including thumb
- T23.15 Burn of first degree of palm
  - T23.151 Burn of first degree of right palm
  - T23.152 Burn of first degree of left palm
  - T23.159 Burn of first degree of unspecified palm
- T23.16 Burn of first degree of back of hand
  - T23.161 Burn of first degree of back of right hand
  - T23.162 Burn of first degree of back of left hand
  - T23.169 Burn of first degree of back of unspecified hand
- T23.17 Burn of first degree of wrist
  - T23.171 Burn of first degree of right wrist
  - T23.172 Burn of first degree of left wrist
  - T23.179 Burn of first degree of unspecified wrist
- T23.19 Burn of first degree of multiple sites of wrist and hand
  - T23.191 Burn of first degree of multiple sites of right wrist and hand
  - T23.192 Burn of first degree of multiple sites of left wrist and hand
  - T23.199 Burn of first degree of multiple sites of unspecified wrist and hand
- T23.2 Burn of second degree of wrist and hand

  Use additional external cause code to identify the source, place and intent of the burn (X00-X19, X75-X77, X96-X98, Y92)
  - T23.20 Burn of second degree of hand, unspecified site
    - T23.201 Burn of second degree of right hand, unspecified site
    - T23.202 Burn of second degree of left hand, unspecified site
    - T23.209 Burn of second degree of unspecified hand, unspecified site
  - T23.21 Burn of second degree of thumb (nail)
    - T23.211 Burn of second degree of right thumb (nail)
    - T23.212 Burn of second degree of left thumb (nail)
    - T23.219 Burn of second degree of unspecified thumb (nail)
  - T23.22 Burn of second degree of single finger (nail) except thumb
    - T23.221 Burn of second degree of single right finger (nail) except thumb
    - T23.222 Burn of second degree of single left finger (nail) except thumb
    - T23.229 Burn of second degree of unspecified single finger (nail) except thumb
  - T23.23 Burn of second degree of multiple fingers (nail), not including thumb
    - T23.231 Burn of second degree of multiple right fingers (nail), not including thumb
    - T23.232 Burn of second degree of multiple left fingers (nail), not including thumb
    - T23.239 Burn of second degree of unspecified multiple fingers (nail), not including thumb

CHAPTER 19 (S00-T88)

● T23.24   Burn of second degree of multiple fingers (nail), including thumb
- ● T23.241   Burn of second degree of multiple right fingers (nail), including thumb
- ● T23.242   Burn of second degree of multiple left fingers (nail), including thumb
- ● T23.249   Burn of second degree of unspecified multiple fingers (nail), including thumb

● T23.25   Burn of second degree of palm
- ● T23.251   Burn of second degree of right palm
- ● T23.252   Burn of second degree of left palm
- ● T23.259   Burn of second degree of unspecified palm

● T23.26   Burn of second degree of back of hand
- ● T23.261   Burn of second degree of back of right hand
- ● T23.262   Burn of second degree of back of left hand
- ● T23.269   Burn of second degree of back of unspecified hand

● T23.27   Burn of second degree of wrist
- ● T23.271   Burn of second degree of right wrist
- ● T23.272   Burn of second degree of left wrist
- ● T23.279   Burn of second degree of unspecified wrist

● T23.29   Burn of second degree of multiple sites of wrist and hand
- ● T23.291   Burn of second degree of multiple sites of right wrist and hand
- ● T23.292   Burn of second degree of multiple sites of left wrist and hand
- ● T23.299   Burn of second degree of multiple sites of unspecified wrist and hand

● T23.3   Burn of third degree of wrist and hand
> Use additional external cause code to identify the source, place and intent of the burn (X00-X19, X75-X77, X96-X98, Y92)

● T23.30   Burn of third degree of hand, unspecified site
- ● T23.301   Burn of third degree of right hand, unspecified site
  Coding Clinic: 2015, Q1, P19
- ● T23.302   Burn of third degree of left hand, unspecified site
  Coding Clinic: 2016, Q2, P5
- ● T23.309   Burn of third degree of unspecified hand, unspecified site

● T23.31   Burn of third degree of thumb (nail)
- ● T23.311   Burn of third degree of right thumb (nail)
- ● T23.312   Burn of third degree of left thumb (nail)
- ● T23.319   Burn of third degree of unspecified thumb (nail)

● T23.32   Burn of third degree of single finger (nail) except thumb
- ● T23.321   Burn of third degree of single right finger (nail) except thumb
- ● T23.322   Burn of third degree of single left finger (nail) except thumb
- ● T23.329   Burn of third degree of unspecified single finger (nail) except thumb

● T23.33   Burn of third degree of multiple fingers (nail), not including thumb
- ● T23.331   Burn of third degree of multiple right fingers (nail), not including thumb
- ● T23.332   Burn of third degree of multiple left fingers (nail), not including thumb
- ● T23.339   Burn of third degree of unspecified multiple fingers (nail), not including thumb

● T23.34   Burn of third degree of multiple fingers (nail), including thumb
- ● T23.341   Burn of third degree of multiple right fingers (nail), including thumb
- ● T23.342   Burn of third degree of multiple left fingers (nail), including thumb
- ● T23.349   Burn of third degree of unspecified multiple fingers (nail), including thumb

● T23.35   Burn of third degree of palm
- ● T23.351   Burn of third degree of right palm
- ● T23.352   Burn of third degree of left palm
- ● T23.359   Burn of third degree of unspecified palm

● T23.36   Burn of third degree of back of hand
- ● T23.361   Burn of third degree of back of right hand
- ● T23.362   Burn of third degree of back of left hand
- ● T23.369   Burn of third degree of back of unspecified hand

● T23.37   Burn of third degree of wrist
- ● T23.371   Burn of third degree of right wrist
- ● T23.372   Burn of third degree of left wrist
- ● T23.379   Burn of third degree of unspecified wrist

● T23.39   Burn of third degree of multiple sites of wrist and hand
- ● T23.391   Burn of third degree of multiple sites of right wrist and hand
- ● T23.392   Burn of third degree of multiple sites of left wrist and hand
- ● T23.399   Burn of third degree of multiple sites of unspecified wrist and hand

● T23.4   Corrosion of unspecified degree of wrist and hand
> *Code first (T51-T65) to identify chemical and intent*
> Use additional external cause code to identify place (Y92)

● T23.40   Corrosion of unspecified degree of hand, unspecified site
- ● T23.401   Corrosion of unspecified degree of right hand, unspecified site
- ● T23.402   Corrosion of unspecified degree of left hand, unspecified site
- ● T23.409   Corrosion of unspecified degree of unspecified hand, unspecified site

● T23.41   Corrosion of unspecified degree of thumb (nail)
- ● T23.411   Corrosion of unspecified degree of right thumb (nail)
- ● T23.412   Corrosion of unspecified degree of left thumb (nail)
- ● T23.419   Corrosion of unspecified degree of unspecified thumb (nail)

◀ New   ◀▥ Revised   ~~deleted~~ Deleted   Excludes 1   Excludes 2   Includes   Use additional   Code first   Code also   Unspecified

OGCR Official Guidelines   X Assign placeholder X   ● Use Additional Character(s)   ▶ Manifestation Code   **Coding Clinic**

● **T23.42**   Corrosion of unspecified degree of single finger (nail) except thumb

   ● **T23.421**   Corrosion of unspecified degree of single right finger (nail) except thumb

   ● **T23.422**   Corrosion of unspecified degree of single left finger (nail) except thumb

   ● **T23.429**   Corrosion of unspecified degree of unspecified single finger (nail) except thumb

● **T23.43**   Corrosion of unspecified degree of multiple fingers (nail), not including thumb

   ● **T23.431**   Corrosion of unspecified degree of multiple right fingers (nail), not including thumb

   ● **T23.432**   Corrosion of unspecified degree of multiple left fingers (nail), not including thumb

   ● **T23.439**   Corrosion of unspecified degree of unspecified multiple fingers (nail), not including thumb

● **T23.44**   Corrosion of unspecified degree of multiple fingers (nail), including thumb

   ● **T23.441**   Corrosion of unspecified degree of multiple right fingers (nail), including thumb

   ● **T23.442**   Corrosion of unspecified degree of multiple left fingers (nail), including thumb

   ● **T23.449**   Corrosion of unspecified degree of unspecified multiple fingers (nail), including thumb

● **T23.45**   Corrosion of unspecified degree of palm

   ● **T23.451**   Corrosion of unspecified degree of right palm

   ● **T23.452**   Corrosion of unspecified degree of left palm

   ● **T23.459**   Corrosion of unspecified degree of unspecified palm

● **T23.46**   Corrosion of unspecified degree of back of hand

   ● **T23.461**   Corrosion of unspecified degree of back of right hand

   ● **T23.462**   Corrosion of unspecified degree of back of left hand

   ● **T23.469**   Corrosion of unspecified degree of back of unspecified hand

● **T23.47**   Corrosion of unspecified degree of wrist

   ● **T23.471**   Corrosion of unspecified degree of right wrist

   ● **T23.472**   Corrosion of unspecified degree of left wrist

   ● **T23.479**   Corrosion of unspecified degree of unspecified wrist

● **T23.49**   Corrosion of unspecified degree of multiple sites of wrist and hand

   ● **T23.491**   Corrosion of unspecified degree of multiple sites of right wrist and hand

   ● **T23.492**   Corrosion of unspecified degree of multiple sites of left wrist and hand

   ● **T23.499**   Corrosion of unspecified degree of multiple sites of unspecified wrist and hand

● **T23.5**   Corrosion of first degree of wrist and hand

   Code first (T51-T65) to identify chemical and intent

   Use additional external cause code to identify place (Y92)

  ● **T23.50**   Corrosion of first degree of hand, unspecified site

   ● **T23.501**   Corrosion of first degree of right hand, unspecified site

   ● **T23.502**   Corrosion of first degree of left hand, unspecified site

   ● **T23.509**   Corrosion of first degree of unspecified hand, unspecified site

  ● **T23.51**   Corrosion of first degree of thumb (nail)

   ● **T23.511**   Corrosion of first degree of right thumb (nail)

   ● **T23.512**   Corrosion of first degree of left thumb (nail)

   ● **T23.519**   Corrosion of first degree of unspecified thumb (nail)

  ● **T23.52**   Corrosion of first degree of single finger (nail) except thumb

   ● **T23.521**   Corrosion of first degree of single right finger (nail) except thumb

   ● **T23.522**   Corrosion of first degree of single left finger (nail) except thumb

   ● **T23.529**   Corrosion of first degree of unspecified single finger (nail) except thumb

  ● **T23.53**   Corrosion of first degree of multiple fingers (nail), not including thumb

   ● **T23.531**   Corrosion of first degree of multiple right fingers (nail), not including thumb

   ● **T23.532**   Corrosion of first degree of multiple left fingers (nail), not including thumb

   ● **T23.539**   Corrosion of first degree of unspecified multiple fingers (nail), not including thumb

  ● **T23.54**   Corrosion of first degree of multiple fingers (nail), including thumb

   ● **T23.541**   Corrosion of first degree of multiple right fingers (nail), including thumb

   ● **T23.542**   Corrosion of first degree of multiple left fingers (nail), including thumb

   ● **T23.549**   Corrosion of first degree of unspecified multiple fingers (nail), including thumb

  ● **T23.55**   Corrosion of first degree of palm

   ● **T23.551**   Corrosion of first degree of right palm

   ● **T23.552**   Corrosion of first degree of left palm

   ● **T23.559**   Corrosion of first degree of unspecified palm

  ● **T23.56**   Corrosion of first degree of back of hand

   ● **T23.561**   Corrosion of first degree of back of right hand

   ● **T23.562**   Corrosion of first degree of back of left hand

   ● **T23.569**   Corrosion of first degree of back of unspecified hand

  ● **T23.57**   Corrosion of first degree of wrist

   ● **T23.571**   Corrosion of first degree of right wrist

   ● **T23.572**   Corrosion of first degree of left wrist

   ● **T23.579**   Corrosion of first degree of unspecified wrist

CHAPTER 19 (S00-T88)

- ● **T23.59** Corrosion of first degree of multiple sites of wrist and hand
  - ● **T23.591** Corrosion of first degree of multiple sites of right wrist and hand
  - ● **T23.592** Corrosion of first degree of multiple sites of left wrist and hand
  - ● **T23.599** Corrosion of first degree of multiple sites of unspecified wrist and hand
- ● **T23.6** Corrosion of second degree of wrist and hand

  Code first (T51-T65) *to identify chemical and intent*

  Use additional external cause code to identify place (Y92)
  - ● **T23.60** Corrosion of second degree of hand, unspecified site
    - ● **T23.601** Corrosion of second degree of right hand, unspecified site
    - ● **T23.602** Corrosion of second degree of left hand, unspecified site
    - ● **T23.609** Corrosion of second degree of unspecified hand, unspecified site
  - ● **T23.61** Corrosion of second degree of thumb (nail)
    - ● **T23.611** Corrosion of second degree of right thumb (nail)
    - ● **T23.612** Corrosion of second degree of left thumb (nail)
    - ● **T23.619** Corrosion of second degree of unspecified thumb (nail)
  - ● **T23.62** Corrosion of second degree of single finger (nail) except thumb
    - ● **T23.621** Corrosion of second degree of single right finger (nail) except thumb
    - ● **T23.622** Corrosion of second degree of single left finger (nail) except thumb
    - ● **T23.629** Corrosion of second degree of unspecified single finger (nail) except thumb
  - ● **T23.63** Corrosion of second degree of multiple fingers (nail), not including thumb
    - ● **T23.631** Corrosion of second degree of multiple right fingers (nail), not including thumb
    - ● **T23.632** Corrosion of second degree of multiple left fingers (nail), not including thumb
    - ● **T23.639** Corrosion of second degree of unspecified multiple fingers (nail), not including thumb
  - ● **T23.64** Corrosion of second degree of multiple fingers (nail), including thumb
    - ● **T23.641** Corrosion of second degree of multiple right fingers (nail), including thumb
    - ● **T23.642** Corrosion of second degree of multiple left fingers (nail), including thumb
    - ● **T23.649** Corrosion of second degree of unspecified multiple fingers (nail), including thumb
  - ● **T23.65** Corrosion of second degree of palm
    - ● **T23.651** Corrosion of second degree of right palm
    - ● **T23.652** Corrosion of second degree of left palm
    - ● **T23.659** Corrosion of second degree of unspecified palm

- ● **T23.66** Corrosion of second degree of back of hand
  - ● **T23.661** Corrosion of second degree back of right hand
  - ● **T23.662** Corrosion of second degree back of left hand
  - ● **T23.669** Corrosion of second degree back of unspecified hand
- ● **T23.67** Corrosion of second degree of wrist
  - ● **T23.671** Corrosion of second degree of right wrist
  - ● **T23.672** Corrosion of second degree of left wrist
  - ● **T23.679** Corrosion of second degree of unspecified wrist
- ● **T23.69** Corrosion of second degree of multiple sites of wrist and hand
  - ● **T23.691** Corrosion of second degree of multiple sites of right wrist and hand
  - ● **T23.692** Corrosion of second degree of multiple sites of left wrist and hand
  - ● **T23.699** Corrosion of second degree of multiple sites of unspecified wrist and hand
- ● **T23.7** Corrosion of third degree of wrist and hand

  Code first (T51-T65) *to identify chemical and intent*

  Use additional external cause code to identify place (Y92)
  - ● **T23.70** Corrosion of third degree of hand, unspecified site
    - ● **T23.701** Corrosion of third degree of right hand, unspecified site
    - ● **T23.702** Corrosion of third degree of left hand, unspecified site
    - ● **T23.709** Corrosion of third degree of unspecified hand, unspecified site
  - ● **T23.71** Corrosion of third degree of thumb (nail)
    - ● **T23.711** Corrosion of third degree of right thumb (nail)
    - ● **T23.712** Corrosion of third degree of left thumb (nail)
    - ● **T23.719** Corrosion of third degree of unspecified thumb (nail)
  - ● **T23.72** Corrosion of third degree of single finger (nail) except thumb
    - ● **T23.721** Corrosion of third degree of single right finger (nail) except thumb
    - ● **T23.722** Corrosion of third degree of single left finger (nail) except thumb
    - ● **T23.729** Corrosion of third degree of unspecified single finger (nail) except thumb
  - ● **T23.73** Corrosion of third degree of multiple fingers (nail), not including thumb
    - ● **T23.731** Corrosion of third degree of multiple right fingers (nail), not including thumb
    - ● **T23.732** Corrosion of third degree of multiple left fingers (nail), not including thumb
    - ● **T23.739** Corrosion of third degree of unspecified multiple fingers (nail), not including thumb

◀ New   ◀▦ Revised   ~~deleted~~ Deleted   Excludes 1   Excludes 2   Includes   Use additional   Code first   Code also   Unspecified

OGCR Official Guidelines   X Assign placeholder X   ● Use Additional Character(s)   ▶ Manifestation Code   **Coding Clinic**

● **T23.74** Corrosion of third degree of multiple fingers (nail), including thumb

    ● **T23.741** Corrosion of third degree of multiple right fingers (nail), including thumb

    ● **T23.742** Corrosion of third degree of multiple left fingers (nail), including thumb

    ● **T23.749** Corrosion of third degree of unspecified multiple fingers (nail), including thumb

● **T23.75** Corrosion of third degree of palm

    ● **T23.751** Corrosion of third degree of right palm

    ● **T23.752** Corrosion of third degree of left palm

    ● **T23.759** Corrosion of third degree of unspecified palm

● **T23.76** Corrosion of third degree of back of hand

    ● **T23.761** Corrosion of third degree of back of right hand

    ● **T23.762** Corrosion of third degree of back of left hand

    ● **T23.769** Corrosion of third degree of back of unspecified hand

● **T23.77** Corrosion of third degree of wrist

    ● **T23.771** Corrosion of third degree of right wrist

    ● **T23.772** Corrosion of third degree of left wrist

    ● **T23.779** Corrosion of third degree of unspecified wrist

● **T23.79** Corrosion of third degree of multiple sites of wrist and hand

    ● **T23.791** Corrosion of third degree of multiple sites of right wrist and hand

    ● **T23.792** Corrosion of third degree of multiple sites of left wrist and hand

    ● **T23.799** Corrosion of third degree of multiple sites of unspecified wrist and hand

● **T24** Burn and corrosion of lower limb, except ankle and foot

    Excludes2 burn and corrosion of ankle and foot (T25.-)
                  burn and corrosion of hip region (T21.-)

    The appropriate 7th character is to be added to each code from category T24

A	initial encounter
D	subsequent encounter
S	sequela

● **T24.0** Burn of unspecified degree of lower limb, except ankle and foot

    Use additional external cause code to identify the source, place and intent of the burn (X00-X19, X75-X77, X96-X98, Y92)

    ● **T24.00** Burn of unspecified degree of unspecified site of lower limb, except ankle and foot

        ● **T24.001** Burn of unspecified degree of unspecified site of right lower limb, except ankle and foot

        ● **T24.002** Burn of unspecified degree of unspecified site of left lower limb, except ankle and foot

        ● **T24.009** Burn of unspecified degree of unspecified site of unspecified lower limb, except ankle and foot

    ● **T24.01** Burn of unspecified degree of thigh

        ● **T24.011** Burn of unspecified degree of right thigh

        ● **T24.012** Burn of unspecified degree of left thigh

        ● **T24.019** Burn of unspecified degree of unspecified thigh

● **T24.02** Burn of unspecified degree of knee

    ● **T24.021** Burn of unspecified degree of right knee

    ● **T24.022** Burn of unspecified degree of left knee

    ● **T24.029** Burn of unspecified degree of unspecified knee

● **T24.03** Burn of unspecified degree of lower leg

    ● **T24.031** Burn of unspecified degree of right lower leg

    ● **T24.032** Burn of unspecified degree of left lower leg

    ● **T24.039** Burn of unspecified degree of unspecified lower leg

● **T24.09** Burn of unspecified degree of multiple sites of lower limb, except ankle and foot

    ● **T24.091** Burn of unspecified degree of multiple sites of right lower limb, except ankle and foot

    ● **T24.092** Burn of unspecified degree of multiple sites of left lower limb, except ankle and foot

    ● **T24.099** Burn of unspecified degree of multiple sites of unspecified lower limb, except ankle and foot

● **T24.1** Burn of first degree of lower limb, except ankle and foot

    Use additional external cause code to identify the source, place and intent of the burn (X00-X19, X75-X77, X96-X98, Y92)

    ● **T24.10** Burn of first degree of unspecified site of lower limb, except ankle and foot

        ● **T24.101** Burn of first degree of unspecified site of right lower limb, except ankle and foot

        ● **T24.102** Burn of first degree of unspecified site of left lower limb, except ankle and foot

        ● **T24.109** Burn of first degree of unspecified site of unspecified lower limb, except ankle and foot

    ● **T24.11** Burn of first degree of thigh

        ● **T24.111** Burn of first degree of right thigh

        ● **T24.112** Burn of first degree of left thigh

        ● **T24.119** Burn of first degree of unspecified thigh

    ● **T24.12** Burn of first degree of knee

        ● **T24.121** Burn of first degree of right knee

        ● **T24.122** Burn of first degree of left knee

        ● **T24.129** Burn of first degree of unspecified knee

    ● **T24.13** Burn of first degree of lower leg

        ● **T24.131** Burn of first degree of right lower leg

        ● **T24.132** Burn of first degree of left lower leg

        ● **T24.139** Burn of first degree of unspecified lower leg

    ● **T24.19** Burn of first degree of multiple sites of lower limb, except ankle and foot

        ● **T24.191** Burn of first degree of multiple sites of right lower limb, except ankle and foot

        ● **T24.192** Burn of first degree of multiple sites of left lower limb, except ankle and foot

        ● **T24.199** Burn of first degree of multiple sites of unspecified lower limb, except ankle and foot

● **T24.2** **Burn of second degree of lower limb, except ankle and foot**

> Use additional external cause code to identify the source, place and intent of the burn (X00-X19, X75-X77, X96-X98, Y92)

● **T24.20** **Burn of second degree of unspecified site of lower limb, except ankle and foot**

● **T24.201** Burn of second degree of unspecified site of right lower limb, except ankle and foot

● **T24.202** Burn of second degree of unspecified site of left lower limb, except ankle and foot

● **T24.209** Burn of second degree of unspecified site of unspecified lower limb, except ankle and foot

● **T24.21** **Burn of second degree of thigh**

● **T24.211** Burn of second degree of right thigh

● **T24.212** Burn of second degree of left thigh

● **T24.219** Burn of second degree of unspecified thigh

● **T24.22** **Burn of second degree of knee**

● **T24.221** Burn of second degree of right knee

● **T24.222** Burn of second degree of left knee

● **T24.229** Burn of second degree of unspecified knee

● **T24.23** **Burn of second degree of lower leg**

● **T24.231** Burn of second degree of right lower leg

● **T24.232** Burn of second degree of left lower leg

● **T24.239** Burn of second degree of unspecified lower leg

● **T24.29** **Burn of second degree of multiple sites of lower limb, except ankle and foot**

● **T24.291** Burn of second degree of multiple sites of right lower limb, except ankle and foot

● **T24.292** Burn of second degree of multiple sites of left lower limb, except ankle and foot

● **T24.299** Burn of second degree of multiple sites of unspecified lower limb, except ankle and foot

● **T24.3** **Burn of third degree of lower limb, except ankle and foot**

> Use additional external cause code to identify the source, place and intent of the burn (X00-X19, X75-X77, X96-X98, Y92)

● **T24.30** **Burn of third degree of unspecified site of lower limb, except ankle and foot**

● **T24.301** Burn of third degree of unspecified site of right lower limb, except ankle and foot

● **T24.302** Burn of third degree of unspecified site of left lower limb, except ankle and foot

● **T24.309** Burn of third degree of unspecified site of unspecified lower limb, except ankle and foot

● **T24.31** **Burn of third degree of thigh**

● **T24.311** Burn of third degree of right thigh

● **T24.312** Burn of third degree of left thigh

● **T24.319** Burn of third degree of unspecified thigh

● **T24.32** **Burn of third degree of knee**

● **T24.321** Burn of third degree of right knee

● **T24.322** Burn of third degree of left knee

● **T24.329** Burn of third degree of unspecified knee

● **T24.33** **Burn of third degree of lower leg**

● **T24.331** Burn of third degree of right lower leg

● **T24.332** Burn of third degree of left lower leg

● **T24.339** Burn of third degree of unspecified lower leg

● **T24.39** **Burn of third degree of multiple sites of lower limb, except ankle and foot**

● **T24.391** Burn of third degree of multiple sites of right lower limb, except ankle and foot

> **Coding Clinic: 2016, Q2, P5**

● **T24.392** Burn of third degree of multiple sites of left lower limb, except ankle and foot

● **T24.399** Burn of third degree of multiple sites of unspecified lower limb, except ankle and foot

● **T24.4** **Corrosion of unspecified degree of lower limb, except ankle and foot**

> *Code first (T51-T65) to identify chemical and intent*
>
> Use additional external cause code to identify place (Y92)

● **T24.40** **Corrosion of unspecified degree of unspecified site of lower limb, except ankle and foot**

● **T24.401** Corrosion of unspecified degree of unspecified site of right lower limb, except ankle and foot

● **T24.402** Corrosion of unspecified degree of unspecified site of left lower limb, except ankle and foot

● **T24.409** Corrosion of unspecified degree of unspecified site of unspecified lower limb, except ankle and foot

● **T24.41** **Corrosion of unspecified degree of thigh**

● **T24.411** Corrosion of unspecified degree of right thigh

● **T24.412** Corrosion of unspecified degree of left thigh

● **T24.419** Corrosion of unspecified degree of unspecified thigh

● **T24.42** **Corrosion of unspecified degree of knee**

● **T24.421** Corrosion of unspecified degree of right knee

● **T24.422** Corrosion of unspecified degree of left knee

● **T24.429** Corrosion of unspecified degree of unspecified knee

● **T24.43** **Corrosion of unspecified degree of lower leg**

● **T24.431** Corrosion of unspecified degree of right lower leg

● **T24.432** Corrosion of unspecified degree of left lower leg

● **T24.439** Corrosion of unspecified degree of unspecified lower leg

● **T24.49** **Corrosion of unspecified degree of multiple sites of lower limb, except ankle and foot**

● **T24.491** Corrosion of unspecified degree of multiple sites of right lower limb, except ankle and foot

● **T24.492** Corrosion of unspecified degree of multiple sites of left lower limb, except ankle and foot

● **T24.499** Corrosion of unspecified degree of multiple sites of unspecified lower limb, except ankle and foot

● **T24.5**   **Corrosion of first degree of lower limb, except ankle and foot**

> *Code first* (T51-T65) *to identify chemical and intent*
>
> Use additional external cause code to identify place (Y92)

  ● **T24.50**   Corrosion of first degree of unspecified site of lower limb, except ankle and foot

    ● **T24.501**   Corrosion of first degree of unspecified site of right lower limb, except ankle and foot

    ● **T24.502**   Corrosion of first degree of unspecified site of left lower limb, except ankle and foot

    ● **T24.509**   Corrosion of first degree of unspecified site of unspecified lower limb, except ankle and foot

  ● **T24.51**   Corrosion of first degree of thigh

    ● **T24.511**   Corrosion of first degree of right thigh

    ● **T24.512**   Corrosion of first degree of left thigh

    ● **T24.519**   Corrosion of first degree of unspecified thigh

  ● **T24.52**   Corrosion of first degree of knee

    ● **T24.521**   Corrosion of first degree of right knee

    ● **T24.522**   Corrosion of first degree of left knee

    ● **T24.529**   Corrosion of first degree of unspecified knee

  ● **T24.53**   Corrosion of first degree of lower leg

    ● **T24.531**   Corrosion of first degree of right lower leg

    ● **T24.532**   Corrosion of first degree of left lower leg

    ● **T24.539**   Corrosion of first degree of unspecified lower leg

  ● **T24.59**   Corrosion of first degree of multiple sites of lower limb, except ankle and foot

    ● **T24.591**   Corrosion of first degree of multiple sites of right lower limb, except ankle and foot

    ● **T24.592**   Corrosion of first degree of multiple sites of left lower limb, except ankle and foot

    ● **T24.599**   Corrosion of first degree of multiple sites of unspecified lower limb, except ankle and foot

● **T24.6**   **Corrosion of second degree of lower limb, except ankle and foot**

> *Code first* (T51-T65) *to identify chemical and intent*
>
> Use additional external cause code to identify place (Y92)

  ● **T24.60**   Corrosion of second degree of unspecified site of lower limb, except ankle and foot

    ● **T24.601**   Corrosion of second degree of unspecified site of right lower limb, except ankle and foot

    ● **T24.602**   Corrosion of second degree of unspecified site of left lower limb, except ankle and foot

    ● **T24.609**   Corrosion of second degree of unspecified site of unspecified lower limb, except ankle and foot

  ● **T24.61**   Corrosion of second degree of thigh

    ● **T24.611**   Corrosion of second degree of right thigh

    ● **T24.612**   Corrosion of second degree of left thigh

    ● **T24.619**   Corrosion of second degree of unspecified thigh

  ● **T24.62**   Corrosion of second degree of knee

    ● **T24.621**   Corrosion of second degree of right knee

    ● **T24.622**   Corrosion of second degree of left knee

    ● **T24.629**   Corrosion of second degree of unspecified knee

  ● **T24.63**   Corrosion of second degree of lower leg

    ● **T24.631**   Corrosion of second degree of right lower leg

    ● **T24.632**   Corrosion of second degree of left lower leg

    ● **T24.639**   Corrosion of second degree of unspecified lower leg

  ● **T24.69**   Corrosion of second degree of multiple sites of lower limb, except ankle and foot

    ● **T24.691**   Corrosion of second degree of multiple sites of right lower limb, except ankle and foot

    ● **T24.692**   Corrosion of second degree of multiple sites of left lower limb, except ankle and foot

    ● **T24.699**   Corrosion of second degree of multiple sites of unspecified lower limb, except ankle and foot

● **T24.7**   **Corrosion of third degree of lower limb, except ankle and foot**

> *Code first* (T51-T65) *to identify chemical and intent*
>
> Use additional external cause code to identify place (Y92)

  ● **T24.70**   Corrosion of third degree of unspecified site of lower limb, except ankle and foot

    ● **T24.701**   Corrosion of third degree of unspecified site of right lower limb, except ankle and foot

    ● **T24.702**   Corrosion of third degree of unspecified site of left lower limb, except ankle and foot

    ● **T24.709**   Corrosion of third degree of unspecified site of unspecified lower limb, except ankle and foot

  ● **T24.71**   Corrosion of third degree of thigh

    ● **T24.711**   Corrosion of third degree of right thigh

    ● **T24.712**   Corrosion of third degree of left thigh

    ● **T24.719**   Corrosion of third degree of unspecified thigh

  ● **T24.72**   Corrosion of third degree of knee

    ● **T24.721**   Corrosion of third degree of right knee

    ● **T24.722**   Corrosion of third degree of left knee

    ● **T24.729**   Corrosion of third degree of unspecified knee

  ● **T24.73**   Corrosion of third degree of lower leg

    ● **T24.731**   Corrosion of third degree of right lower leg

    ● **T24.732**   Corrosion of third degree of left lower leg

    ● **T24.739**   Corrosion of third degree of unspecified lower leg

  ● **T24.79**   Corrosion of third degree of multiple sites of lower limb, except ankle and foot

    ● **T24.791**   Corrosion of third degree of multiple sites of right lower limb, except ankle and foot

    ● **T24.792**   Corrosion of third degree of multiple sites of left lower limb, except ankle and foot

    ● **T24.799**   Corrosion of third degree of multiple sites of unspecified lower limb, except ankle and foot

CHAPTER 19 (S00-T88)

CHAPTER 19 (S00-T88)

● **T25   Burn and corrosion of ankle and foot**

The appropriate 7th character is to be added to each code from category T25

A	initial encounter
D	subsequent encounter
S	sequela

● **T25.0   Burn of unspecified degree of ankle and foot**

Use additional external cause code to identify the source, place and intent of the burn (X00-X19, X75-X77, X96-X98, Y92)

● **T25.01   Burn of unspecified degree of ankle**
   ● T25.011   Burn of unspecified degree of right ankle
   ● T25.012   Burn of unspecified degree of left ankle
   ● T25.019   Burn of unspecified degree of unspecified ankle

● **T25.02   Burn of unspecified degree of foot**
   Excludes2   burn of unspecified degree of toe(s) (nail) (T25.03-)
   ● T25.021   Burn of unspecified degree of right foot
   ● T25.022   Burn of unspecified degree of left foot
   ● T25.029   Burn of unspecified degree of unspecified foot

● **T25.03   Burn of unspecified degree of toe(s) (nail)**
   ● T25.031   Burn of unspecified degree of right toe(s) (nail)
   ● T25.032   Burn of unspecified degree of left toe(s) (nail)
   ● T25.039   Burn of unspecified degree of unspecified toe(s) (nail)

● **T25.09   Burn of unspecified degree of multiple sites of ankle and foot**
   ● T25.091   Burn of unspecified degree of multiple sites of right ankle and foot
   ● T25.092   Burn of unspecified degree of multiple sites of left ankle and foot
   ● T25.099   Burn of unspecified degree of multiple sites of unspecified ankle and foot

● **T25.1   Burn of first degree of ankle and foot**

Use additional external cause code to identify the source, place and intent of the burn (X00-X19, X75-X77, X96-X98, Y92)

● **T25.11   Burn of first degree of ankle**
   ● T25.111   Burn of first degree of right ankle
   ● T25.112   Burn of first degree of left ankle
   ● T25.119   Burn of first degree of unspecified ankle

● **T25.12   Burn of first degree of foot**
   Excludes2   burn of first degree of toe(s) (nail) (T25.13-)
   ● T25.121   Burn of first degree of right foot
   ● T25.122   Burn of first degree of left foot
   ● T25.129   Burn of first degree of unspecified foot

● **T25.13   Burn of first degree of toe(s) (nail)**
   ● T25.131   Burn of first degree of right toe(s) (nail)
   ● T25.132   Burn of first degree of left toe(s) (nail)
   ● T25.139   Burn of first degree of unspecified toe(s) (nail)

● **T25.19   Burn of first degree of multiple sites of ankle and foot**
   ● T25.191   Burn of first degree of multiple sites of right ankle and foot
   ● T25.192   Burn of first degree of multiple sites of left ankle and foot
   ● T25.199   Burn of first degree of multiple sites of unspecified ankle and foot

● **T25.2   Burn of second degree of ankle and foot**

Use additional external cause code to identify the source, place and intent of the burn (X00-X19, X75-X77, X96-X98, Y92)

● **T25.21   Burn of second degree of ankle**
   ● T25.211   Burn of second degree of right ankle
   ● T25.212   Burn of second degree of left ankle
   ● T25.219   Burn of second degree of unspecified ankle

● **T25.22   Burn of second degree of foot**
   Excludes2   burn of second degree of toe(s) (nail) (T25.23-)
   ● T25.221   Burn of second degree of right foot
   ● T25.222   Burn of second degree of left foot
   ● T25.229   Burn of second degree of unspecified foot

● **T25.23   Burn of second degree of toe(s) (nail)**
   ● T25.231   Burn of second degree of right toe(s) (nail)
   ● T25.232   Burn of second degree of left toe(s) (nail)
   ● T25.239   Burn of second degree of unspecified toe(s) (nail)

● **T25.29   Burn of second degree of multiple sites of ankle and foot**
   ● T25.291   Burn of second degree of multiple sites of right ankle and foot
   ● T25.292   Burn of second degree of multiple sites of left ankle and foot
   ● T25.299   Burn of second degree of multiple sites of unspecified ankle and foot

● **T25.3   Burn of third degree of ankle and foot**

Use additional external cause code to identify the source, place and intent of the burn (X00-X19, X75-X77, X96-X98, Y92)

● **T25.31   Burn of third degree of ankle**
   ● T25.311   Burn of third degree of right ankle
   ● T25.312   Burn of third degree of left ankle
   ● T25.319   Burn of third degree of unspecified ankle

● **T25.32   Burn of third degree of foot**
   Excludes2   burn of third degree of toe(s) (nail) (T25.33-)
   ● T25.321   Burn of third degree of right foot
   ● T25.322   Burn of third degree of left foot
   ● T25.329   Burn of third degree of unspecified foot

● **T25.33   Burn of third degree of toe(s) (nail)**
   ● T25.331   Burn of third degree of right toe(s) (nail)
   ● T25.332   Burn of third degree of left toe(s) (nail)
   ● T25.339   Burn of third degree of unspecified toe(s) (nail)

● **T25.39   Burn of third degree of multiple sites of ankle and foot**
   ● T25.391   Burn of third degree of multiple sites of right ankle and foot
   ● T25.392   Burn of third degree of multiple sites of left ankle and foot
   ● T25.399   Burn of third degree of multiple sites of unspecified ankle and foot

◀ New   ◀▬ Revised   ~~deleted~~ Deleted   Excludes 1   Excludes 2   Includes   Use additional   Code first   Code also   Unspecified

OGCR Official Guidelines   X Assign placeholder X   ● Use Additional Character(s)   ▷ Manifestation Code   **Coding Clinic**

T25.4   Corrosion of unspecified degree of ankle and foot

Code first (T51-T65) *to identify chemical and intent*

Use additional external cause code to identify place (Y92)

T25.41   Corrosion of unspecified degree of ankle

- **T25.411   Corrosion of unspecified degree of right ankle**
- **T25.412   Corrosion of unspecified degree of left ankle**
- **T25.419   Corrosion of unspecified degree of unspecified ankle**

T25.42   Corrosion of unspecified degree of foot

Excludes2   corrosion of unspecified degree of toe(s) (nail) (T25.43-)

- **T25.421   Corrosion of unspecified degree of right foot**
- **T25.422   Corrosion of unspecified degree of left foot**
- **T25.429   Corrosion of unspecified degree of unspecified foot**

T25.43   Corrosion of unspecified degree of toe(s) (nail)

- **T25.431   Corrosion of unspecified degree of right toe(s) (nail)**
- **T25.432   Corrosion of unspecified degree of left toe(s) (nail)**
- **T25.439   Corrosion of unspecified degree of unspecified toe(s) (nail)**

T25.49   Corrosion of unspecified degree of multiple sites of ankle and foot

- **T25.491   Corrosion of unspecified degree of multiple sites of right ankle and foot**
- **T25.492   Corrosion of unspecified degree of multiple sites of left ankle and foot**
- **T25.499   Corrosion of unspecified degree of multiple sites of unspecified ankle and foot**

T25.5   Corrosion of first degree of ankle and foot

Code first (T51-T65) *to identify chemical and intent*

Use additional external cause code to identify place (Y92)

T25.51   Corrosion of first degree of ankle

- **T25.511   Corrosion of first degree of right ankle**
- **T25.512   Corrosion of first degree of left ankle**
- **T25.519   Corrosion of first degree of unspecified ankle**

T25.52   Corrosion of first degree of foot

Excludes2   corrosion of first degree of toe(s) (nail) (T25.53-)

- **T25.521   Corrosion of first degree of right foot**
- **T25.522   Corrosion of first degree of left foot**
- **T25.529   Corrosion of first degree of unspecified foot**

T25.53   Corrosion of first degree of toe(s) (nail)

- **T25.531   Corrosion of first degree of right toe(s) (nail)**
- **T25.532   Corrosion of first degree of left toe(s) (nail)**
- **T25.539   Corrosion of first degree of unspecified toe(s) (nail)**

T25.59   Corrosion of first degree of multiple sites of ankle and foot

- **T25.591   Corrosion of first degree of multiple sites of right ankle and foot**
- **T25.592   Corrosion of first degree of multiple sites of left ankle and foot**
- **T25.599   Corrosion of first degree of multiple sites of unspecified ankle and foot**

T25.6   Corrosion of second degree of ankle and foot

Code first (T51-T65) *to identify chemical and intent*

Use additional external cause code to identify place (Y92)

T25.61   Corrosion of second degree of ankle

- **T25.611   Corrosion of second degree of right ankle**
- **T25.612   Corrosion of second degree of left ankle**
- **T25.619   Corrosion of second degree of unspecified ankle**

T25.62   Corrosion of second degree of foot

Excludes2   corrosion of second degree of toe(s) (nail) (T25.63-)

- **T25.621   Corrosion of second degree of right foot**
- **T25.622   Corrosion of second degree of left foot**
- **T25.629   Corrosion of second degree of unspecified foot**

T25.63   Corrosion of second degree of toe(s) (nail)

- **T25.631   Corrosion of second degree of right toe(s) (nail)**
- **T25.632   Corrosion of second degree of left toe(s) (nail)**
- **T25.639   Corrosion of second degree of unspecified toe(s) (nail)**

T25.69   Corrosion of second degree of multiple sites of ankle and foot

- **T25.691   Corrosion of second degree of right ankle and foot**
- **T25.692   Corrosion of second degree of left ankle and foot**
- **T25.699   Corrosion of second degree of unspecified ankle and foot**

T25.7   Corrosion of third degree of ankle and foot

Code first (T51-T65) *to identify chemical and intent*

Use additional external cause code to identify place (Y92)

T25.71   Corrosion of third degree of ankle

- **T25.711   Corrosion of third degree of right ankle**
- **T25.712   Corrosion of third degree of left ankle**
- **T25.719   Corrosion of third degree of unspecified ankle**

T25.72   Corrosion of third degree of foot

Excludes2   corrosion of third degree of toe(s) (nail) (T25.73-)

- **T25.721   Corrosion of third degree of right foot**
- **T25.722   Corrosion of third degree of left foot**
- **T25.729   Corrosion of third degree of unspecified foot**

T25.73   Corrosion of third degree of toe(s) (nail)

- **T25.731   Corrosion of third degree of right toe(s) (nail)**
- **T25.732   Corrosion of third degree of left toe(s) (nail)**
- **T25.739   Corrosion of third degree of unspecified toe(s) (nail)**

T25.79   Corrosion of third degree of multiple sites of ankle and foot

- **T25.791   Corrosion of third degree of multiple sites of right ankle and foot**
- **T25.792   Corrosion of third degree of multiple sites of left ankle and foot**
- **T25.799   Corrosion of third degree of multiple sites of unspecified ankle and foot**

BURNS AND CORROSIONS CONFINED TO EYE AND INTERNAL ORGANS (T26-T28)

● **T26**   **Burn and corrosion confined to eye and adnexa**

The appropriate 7th character is to be added to each code from category T26

A	initial encounter
D	subsequent encounter
S	sequela

● **T26.0**   **Burn of eyelid and periocular area**

Use additional external cause code to identify the source, place and intent of the burn (X00-X19, X75-X77, X96-X98, Y92)

X ● **T26.00**   Burn of unspecified eyelid and periocular area

X ● **T26.01**   Burn of right eyelid and periocular area

X ● **T26.02**   Burn of left eyelid and periocular area

● **T26.1**   **Burn of cornea and conjunctival sac**

Use additional external cause code to identify the source, place and intent of the burn (X00-X19, X75-X77, X96-X98, Y92)

X ● **T26.10**   Burn of cornea and conjunctival sac, unspecified eye

X ● **T26.11**   Burn of cornea and conjunctival sac, right eye

X ● **T26.12**   Burn of cornea and conjunctival sac, left eye

● **T26.2**   **Burn with resulting rupture and destruction of eyeball**

Use additional external cause code to identify the source, place and intent of the burn (X00-X19, X75-X77, X96-X98, Y92)

X ● **T26.20**   Burn with resulting rupture and destruction of unspecified eyeball

X ● **T26.21**   Burn with resulting rupture and destruction of right eyeball

X ● **T26.22**   Burn with resulting rupture and destruction of left eyeball

● **T26.3**   **Burns of other specified parts of eye and adnexa**

Use additional external cause code to identify the source, place and intent of the burn (X00-X19, X75-X77, X96-X98, Y92)

X ● **T26.30**   Burns of other specified parts of unspecified eye and adnexa

X ● **T26.31**   Burns of other specified parts of right eye and adnexa

X ● **T26.32**   Burns of other specified parts of left eye and adnexa

● **T26.4**   **Burn of eye and adnexa, part unspecified**

Use additional external cause code to identify the source, place and intent of the burn (X00-X19, X75-X77, X96-X98, Y92)

X ● **T26.40**   Burn of unspecified eye and adnexa, part unspecified

X ● **T26.41**   Burn of right eye and adnexa, part unspecified

X ● **T26.42**   Burn of left eye and adnexa, part unspecified

● **T26.5**   **Corrosion of eyelid and periocular area**

Code first (T51-T65) to identify chemical and intent

Use additional external cause code to identify place (Y92)

X ● **T26.50**   Corrosion of unspecified eyelid and periocular area

X ● **T26.51**   Corrosion of right eyelid and periocular area

X ● **T26.52**   Corrosion of left eyelid and periocular area

● **T26.6**   **Corrosion of cornea and conjunctival sac**

Code first (T51-T65) to identify chemical and intent

Use additional external cause code to identify place (Y92)

X ● **T26.60**   Corrosion of cornea and conjunctival sac, unspecified eye

X ● **T26.61**   Corrosion of cornea and conjunctival sac, right eye

X ● **T26.62**   Corrosion of cornea and conjunctival sac, left eye

● **T26.7**   **Corrosion with resulting rupture and destruction of eyeball**

Code first (T51-T65) to identify chemical and intent

Use additional external cause code to identify place (Y92)

X ● **T26.70**   Corrosion with resulting rupture and destruction of unspecified eyeball

X ● **T26.71**   Corrosion with resulting rupture and destruction of right eyeball

X ● **T26.72**   Corrosion with resulting rupture and destruction of left eyeball

● **T26.8**   **Corrosions of other specified parts of eye and adnexa**

Code first (T51-T65) to identify chemical and intent

Use additional external cause code to identify place (Y92)

X ● **T26.80**   Corrosions of other specified parts of unspecified eye and adnexa

X ● **T26.81**   Corrosions of other specified parts of right eye and adnexa

X ● **T26.82**   Corrosions of other specified parts of left eye and adnexa

● **T26.9**   **Corrosion of eye and adnexa, part unspecified**

Code first (T51-T65) to identify chemical and intent

Use additional external cause code to identify place (Y92)

X ● **T26.90**   Corrosion of unspecified eye and adnexa, part unspecified

X ● **T26.91**   Corrosion of right eye and adnexa, part unspecified

X ● **T26.92**   Corrosion of left eye and adnexa, part unspecified

● **T27**   **Burn and corrosion of respiratory tract**

Use additional external cause code to identify the source and intent of the burn (X00-X19, X75-X77, X96-X98)

Use additional external cause code to identify place (Y92)

The appropriate 7th character is to be added to each code from category T27

A	initial encounter
D	subsequent encounter
S	sequela

X ● **T27.0**   Burn of larynx and trachea

X ● **T27.1**   Burn involving larynx and trachea with lung

X ● **T27.2**   Burn of other parts of respiratory tract

Burn of thoracic cavity

X ● **T27.3**   Burn of respiratory tract, part unspecified

Code first (T51-T65) to identify chemical and intent for codes T27.4-T27.7

X ● **T27.4**   Corrosion of larynx and trachea

X ● **T27.5**   Corrosion involving larynx and trachea with lung

X ● **T27.6**   Corrosion of other parts of respiratory tract

X ● **T27.7**   Corrosion of respiratory tract, part unspecified

◀ New   ◀▥ Revised   ~~deleted~~ Deleted   Excludes 1   Excludes 2   Includes   Use additional   Code first   Code also   Unspecified

OGCR Official Guidelines   X Assign placeholder X   ● Use Additional Character(s)   ▶ Manifestation Code   **Coding Clinic**

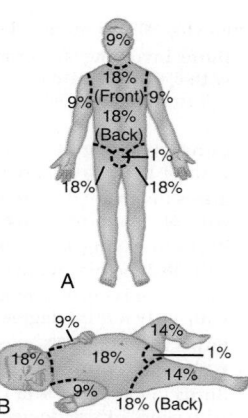

Figure 19-16   Rule of nines: percentages of total body area. (From Marx: Rosen's Emergency Medicine: Concepts and Clinical Practice, ed 6, Mosby, 2006)

●**T28**   **Burn and corrosion of other internal organs**
> Use additional external cause code to identify the source and intent of the burn (X00-X19, X75-X77, X96-X98)
> Use additional external cause code to identify place (Y92)
> The appropriate 7th character is to be added to each code from category T28
>
> | | |
> |---|---|
> | A | initial encounter |
> | D | subsequent encounter |
> | S | sequela |

X●**T28.0**   Burn of mouth and pharynx
X●**T28.1**   Burn of esophagus
X●**T28.2**   Burn of other parts of alimentary tract
X●**T28.3**   Burn of internal genitourinary organs
X●**T28.4**   Burns of other and unspecified internal organs
    X●**T28.40**   Burn of unspecified internal organ
    ●**T28.41**   Burn of ear drum
       ●**T28.411**   Burn of right ear drum
       ●**T28.412**   Burn of left ear drum
       ●**T28.419**   Burn of unspecified ear drum
    X●**T28.49**   Burn of other internal organ
>   *Code first* (T51-T65) to identify chemical and intent for T28.5-T28.9-

X●**T28.5**   Corrosion of mouth and pharynx
X●**T28.6**   Corrosion of esophagus
X●**T28.7**   Corrosion of other parts of alimentary tract
X●**T28.8**   Corrosion of internal genitourinary organs
●**T28.9**   Corrosions of other and unspecified internal organs
    X●**T28.90**   Corrosions of unspecified internal organs
    ●**T28.91**   Corrosions of ear drum
       ●**T28.911**   Corrosions of right ear drum
       ●**T28.912**   Corrosions of left ear drum
       ●**T28.919**   Corrosions of unspecified ear drum
    X●**T28.99**   Corrosions of other internal organs

OGCR Section I.C.19.d.5.

> Assign separate code for each burn site
> When coding burns, assign separate codes for each burn site. Category T30, Burn and corrosion, body region unspecified is extremely vague and should rarely be used.

BURNS AND CORROSIONS OF MULTIPLE AND UNSPECIFIED BODY REGIONS (T30-T32)

●**T30**   **Burn and corrosion, body region unspecified**
    T30.0   **Burn of unspecified body region, unspecified degree**
>   This code is not for inpatient use. Code to specified site and degree of burns
>   Burn NOS
>   Multiple burns NOS

    T30.4   **Corrosion of unspecified body region, unspecified degree**
>   This code is not for inpatient use. Code to specified site and degree of corrosion
>   Corrosion NOS
>   Multiple corrosion NOS

●**T31**   **Burns classified according to extent of body surface involved**
> **Note:** This category is to be used as the primary code only when the site of the burn is unspecified. It should be used as a supplementary code with categories T20-T25 when the site is specified.

    T31.0   **Burns involving less than 10% of body surface**
●**T31.1**   **Burns involving 10-19% of body surface**
    T31.10   **Burns involving 10-19% of body surface with 0% to 9% third degree burns**
>   Burns involving 10-19% of body surface NOS

    T31.11   **Burns involving 10-19% of body surface with 10-19% third degree burns**
●**T31.2**   **Burns involving 20-29% of body surface**
    T31.20   **Burns involving 20-29% of body surface with 0% to 9% third degree burns**
>   Burns involving 20-29% of body surface NOS

    T31.21   **Burns involving 20-29% of body surface with 10-19% third degree burns**
    T31.22   **Burns involving 20-29% of body surface with 20-29% third degree burns**
●**T31.3**   **Burns involving 30-39% of body surface**
    T31.30   **Burns involving 30-39% of body surface with 0% to 9% third degree burns**
>   Burns involving 30-39% of body surface NOS

    T31.31   **Burns involving 30-39% of body surface with 10-19% third degree burns**
    T31.32   **Burns involving 30-39% of body surface with 20-29% third degree burns**
    T31.33   **Burns involving 30-39% of body surface with 30-39% third degree burns**
●**T31.4**   **Burns involving 40-49% of body surface**
    T31.40   **Burns involving 40-49% of body surface with 0% to 9% third degree burns**
>   Burns involving 40-49% of body surface NOS

    T31.41   **Burns involving 40-49% of body surface with 10-19% third degree burns**
    T31.42   **Burns involving 40-49% of body surface with 20-29% third degree burns**
    T31.43   **Burns involving 40-49% of body surface with 30-39% third degree burns**
    T31.44   **Burns involving 40-49% of body surface with 40-49% third degree burns**

CHAPTER 19 (S00-T88)

● **T31.5   Burns involving 50-59% of body surface**

T31.50   **Burns involving 50-59% of body surface with 0% to 9% third degree burns**
Burns involving 50-59% of body surface NOS

T31.51   **Burns involving 50-59% of body surface with 10-19% third degree burns**

T31.52   **Burns involving 50-59% of body surface with 20-29% third degree burns**

T31.53   **Burns involving 50-59% of body surface with 30-39% third degree burns**

T31.54   **Burns involving 50-59% of body surface with 40-49% third degree burns**

T31.55   **Burns involving 50-59% of body surface with 50-59% third degree burns**

● **T31.6   Burns involving 60-69% of body surface**

T31.60   **Burns involving 60-69% of body surface with 0% to 9% third degree burns**
Burns involving 60-69% of body surface NOS

T31.61   **Burns involving 60-69% of body surface with 10-19% third degree burns**

T31.62   **Burns involving 60-69% of body surface with 20-29% third degree burns**

T31.63   **Burns involving 60-69% of body surface with 30-39% third degree burns**

T31.64   **Burns involving 60-69% of body surface with 40-49% third degree burns**

T31.65   **Burns involving 60-69% of body surface with 50-59% third degree burns**

T31.66   **Burns involving 60-69% of body surface with 60-69% third degree burns**

● **T31.7   Burns involving 70-79% of body surface**

T31.70   **Burns involving 70-79% of body surface with 0% to 9% third degree burns**
Burns involving 70-79% of body surface NOS

T31.71   **Burns involving 70-79% of body surface with 10-19% third degree burns**

T31.72   **Burns involving 70-79% of body surface with 20-29% third degree burns**

T31.73   **Burns involving 70-79% of body surface with 30-39% third degree burns**

T31.74   **Burns involving 70-79% of body surface with 40-49% third degree burns**

T31.75   **Burns involving 70-79% of body surface with 50-59% third degree burns**

T31.76   **Burns involving 70-79% of body surface with 60-69% third degree burns**

T31.77   **Burns involving 70-79% of body surface with 70-79% third degree burns**

● **T31.8   Burns involving 80-89% of body surface**

T31.80   **Burns involving 80-89% of body surface with 0% to 9% third degree burns**
Burns involving 80-89% of body surface NOS

T31.81   **Burns involving 80-89% of body surface with 10-19% third degree burns**

T31.82   **Burns involving 80-89% of body surface with 20-29% third degree burns**

T31.83   **Burns involving 80-89% of body surface with 30-39% third degree burns**

T31.84   **Burns involving 80-89% of body surface with 40-49% third degree burns**

T31.85   **Burns involving 80-89% of body surface with 50-59% third degree burns**

T31.86   **Burns involving 80-89% of body surface with 60-69% third degree burns**

T31.87   **Burns involving 80-89% of body surface with 70-79% third degree burns**

T31.88   **Burns involving 80-89% of body surface with 80-89% third degree burns**

● **T31.9   Burns involving 90% or more of body surface**

T31.90   **Burns involving 90% or more of body surface with 0% to 9% third degree burns**
Burns involving 90% or more of body surface NOS

T31.91   **Burns involving 90% or more of body surface with 10-19% third degree burns**

T31.92   **Burns involving 90% or more of body surface with 20-29% third degree burns**

T31.93   **Burns involving 90% or more of body surface with 30-39% third degree burns**

T31.94   **Burns involving 90% or more of body surface with 40-49% third degree burns**

T31.95   **Burns involving 90% or more of body surface with 50-59% third degree burns**

T31.96   **Burns involving 90% or more of body surface with 60-69% third degree burns**

T31.97   **Burns involving 90% or more of body surface with 70-79% third degree burns**

T31.98   **Burns involving 90% or more of body surface with 80-89% third degree burns**

T31.99   **Burns involving 90% or more of body surface with 90% or more third degree burns**

● **T32   Corrosions classified according to extent of body surface involved**

Note: This category is to be used as the primary code only when the site of the corrosion is unspecified. It may be used as a supplementary code with categories T20-T25 when the site is specified.

T32.0   Corrosions involving less than 10% of body surface

● **T32.1   Corrosions involving 10-19% of body surface**

T32.10   **Corrosions involving 10-19% of body surface with 0% to 9% third degree corrosion**
Corrosions involving 10-19% of body surface NOS

T32.11   **Corrosions involving 10-19% of body surface with 10-19% third degree corrosion**

● **T32.2   Corrosions involving 20-29% of body surface**

T32.20   **Corrosions involving 20-29% of body surface with 0% to 9% third degree corrosion**

T32.21   **Corrosions involving 20-29% of body surface with 10-19% third degree corrosion**

T32.22   **Corrosions involving 20-29% of body surface with 20-29% third degree corrosion**

● **T32.3   Corrosions involving 30-39% of body surface**

T32.30   **Corrosions involving 30-39% of body surface with 0% to 9% third degree corrosion**

T32.31   **Corrosions involving 30-39% of body surface with 10-19% third degree corrosion**

T32.32   **Corrosions involving 30-39% of body surface with 20-29% third degree corrosion**

T32.33   **Corrosions involving 30-39% of body surface with 30-39% third degree corrosion**

● **T32.4   Corrosions involving 40-49% of body surface**

T32.40   **Corrosions involving 40-49% of body surface with 0% to 9% third degree corrosion**

T32.41   **Corrosions involving 40-49% of body surface with 10-19% third degree corrosion**

T32.42   **Corrosions involving 40-49% of body surface with 20-29% third degree corrosion**

T32.43   **Corrosions involving 40-49% of body surface with 30-39% third degree corrosion**

T32.44   **Corrosions involving 40-49% of body surface with 40-49% third degree corrosion**

◀ New   ◀▥ Revised   ~~deleted~~ Deleted   Excludes 1   Excludes 2   Includes   Use additional   Code first   Code also   Unspecified
OGCR Official Guidelines   X Assign placeholder X   ● Use Additional Character(s)   ▶ Manifestation Code   **Coding Clinic**

● **T32.5**   **Corrosions involving 50-59% of body surface**

     T32.50   Corrosions involving 50-59% of body surface with 0% to 9% third degree corrosion

     T32.51   Corrosions involving 50-59% of body surface with 10-19% third degree corrosion

     T32.52   Corrosions involving 50-59% of body surface with 20-29% third degree corrosion

     T32.53   Corrosions involving 50-59% of body surface with 30-39% third degree corrosion

     T32.54   Corrosions involving 50-59% of body surface with 40-49% third degree corrosion

     T32.55   Corrosions involving 50-59% of body surface with 50-59% third degree corrosion

● **T32.6**   **Corrosions involving 60-69% of body surface**

     T32.60   Corrosions involving 60-69% of body surface with 0% to 9% third degree corrosion

     T32.61   Corrosions involving 60-69% of body surface with 10-19% third degree corrosion

     T32.62   Corrosions involving 60-69% of body surface with 20-29% third degree corrosion

     T32.63   Corrosions involving 60-69% of body surface with 30-39% third degree corrosion

     T32.64   Corrosions involving 60-69% of body surface with 40-49% third degree corrosion

     T32.65   Corrosions involving 60-69% of body surface with 50-59% third degree corrosion

     T32.66   Corrosions involving 60-69% of body surface with 60-69% third degree corrosion

● **T32.7**   **Corrosions involving 70-79% of body surface**

     T32.70   Corrosions involving 70-79% of body surface with 0% to 9% third degree corrosion

     T32.71   Corrosions involving 70-79% of body surface with 10-19% third degree corrosion

     T32.72   Corrosions involving 70-79% of body surface with 20-29% third degree corrosion

     T32.73   Corrosions involving 70-79% of body surface with 30-39% third degree corrosion

     T32.74   Corrosions involving 70-79% of body surface with 40-49% third degree corrosion

     T32.75   Corrosions involving 70-79% of body surface with 50-59% third degree corrosion

     T32.76   Corrosions involving 70-79% of body surface with 60-69% third degree corrosion

     T32.77   Corrosions involving 70-79% of body surface with 70-79% third degree corrosion

● **T32.8**   **Corrosions involving 80-89% of body surface**

     T32.80   Corrosions involving 80-89% of body surface with 0% to 9% third degree corrosion

     T32.81   Corrosions involving 80-89% of body surface with 10-19% third degree corrosion

     T32.82   Corrosions involving 80-89% of body surface with 20-29% third degree corrosion

     T32.83   Corrosions involving 80-89% of body surface with 30-39% third degree corrosion

     T32.84   Corrosions involving 80-89% of body surface with 40-49% third degree corrosion

     T32.85   Corrosions involving 80-89% of body surface with 50-59% third degree corrosion

     T32.86   Corrosions involving 80-89% of body surface with 60-69% third degree corrosion

     T32.87   Corrosions involving 80-89% of body surface with 70-79% third degree corrosion

     T32.88   Corrosions involving 80-89% of body surface with 80-89% third degree corrosion

● **T32.9**   **Corrosions involving 90% or more of body surface**

     T32.90   Corrosions involving 90% or more of body surface with 0% to 9% third degree corrosion

     T32.91   Corrosions involving 90% or more of body surface with 10-19% third degree corrosion

     T32.92   Corrosions involving 90% or more of body surface with 20-29% third degree corrosion

     T32.93   Corrosions involving 90% or more of body surface with 30-39% third degree corrosion

     T32.94   Corrosions involving 90% or more of body surface with 40-49% third degree corrosion

     T32.95   Corrosions involving 90% or more of body surface with 50-59% third degree corrosion

     T32.96   Corrosions involving 90% or more of body surface with 60-69% third degree corrosion

     T32.97   Corrosions involving 90% or more of body surface with 70-79% third degree corrosion

     T32.98   Corrosions involving 90% or more of body surface with 80-89% third degree corrosion

     T32.99   Corrosions involving 90% or more of body surface with 90% or more third degree corrosion

FROSTBITE (T33-T34)

Excludes2   hypothermia and other effects of reduced temperature (T68, T69.-)

● **T33**   **Superficial frostbite**

   Includes   frostbite with partial thickness skin loss

   The appropriate 7th character is to be added to each code from category T33

A	initial encounter
D	subsequent encounter
S	sequela

   ● **T33.0**   **Superficial frostbite of head**

     ● **T33.01**   **Superficial frostbite of ear**

       ● **T33.011**   Superficial frostbite of right ear

       ● **T33.012**   Superficial frostbite of left ear

       ● **T33.019**   Superficial frostbite of unspecified ear

   X ● **T33.02**   Superficial frostbite of nose

   X ● **T33.09**   Superficial frostbite of other part of head

X ● **T33.1**   **Superficial frostbite of neck**

X ● **T33.2**   **Superficial frostbite of thorax**

X ● **T33.3**   **Superficial frostbite of abdominal wall, lower back and pelvis**

   ● **T33.4**   **Superficial frostbite of arm**

     Excludes2   superficial frostbite of wrist and hand (T33.5-)

   X ● **T33.40**   Superficial frostbite of unspecified arm

   X ● **T33.41**   Superficial frostbite of right arm

   X ● **T33.42**   Superficial frostbite of left arm

   ● **T33.5**   **Superficial frostbite of wrist, hand, and fingers**

     ● **T33.51**   **Superficial frostbite of wrist**

       ● **T33.511**   Superficial frostbite of right wrist

       ● **T33.512**   Superficial frostbite of left wrist

       ● **T33.519**   Superficial frostbite of unspecified wrist

     ● **T33.52**   **Superficial frostbite of hand**

       Excludes2   superficial frostbite of fingers (T33.53-)

       ● **T33.521**   Superficial frostbite of right hand

       ● **T33.522**   Superficial frostbite of left hand

       ● **T33.529**   Superficial frostbite of unspecified hand

● T33.53   Superficial frostbite of finger(s)
     ● T33.531   Superficial frostbite of right finger(s)
     ● T33.532   Superficial frostbite of left finger(s)
     ● T33.539   Superficial frostbite of unspecified finger(s)

● T33.6   Superficial frostbite of hip and thigh
   X ● T33.60   Superficial frostbite of unspecified hip and thigh
   X ● T33.61   Superficial frostbite of right hip and thigh
   X ● T33.62   Superficial frostbite of left hip and thigh

● T33.7   Superficial frostbite of knee and lower leg
     Excludes2   superficial frostbite of ankle and foot (T33.8-)
   X ● T33.70   Superficial frostbite of unspecified knee and lower leg
   X ● T33.71   Superficial frostbite of right knee and lower leg
   X ● T33.72   Superficial frostbite of left knee and lower leg

● T33.8   Superficial frostbite of ankle, foot, and toe(s)
   ● T33.81   Superficial frostbite of ankle
     ● T33.811   Superficial frostbite of right ankle
     ● T33.812   Superficial frostbite of left ankle
     ● T33.819   Superficial frostbite of unspecified ankle
   ● T33.82   Superficial frostbite of foot
     ● T33.821   Superficial frostbite of right foot
     ● T33.822   Superficial frostbite of left foot
     ● T33.829   Superficial frostbite of unspecified foot
   ● T33.83   Superficial frostbite of toe(s)
     ● T33.831   Superficial frostbite of right toe(s)
     ● T33.832   Superficial frostbite of left toe(s)
     ● T33.839   Superficial frostbite of unspecified toe(s)

● T33.9   Superficial frostbite of other and unspecified sites
   X ● T33.90   Superficial frostbite of unspecified sites
     Superficial frostbite NOS
   X ● T33.99   Superficial frostbite of other sites
     Superficial frostbite of leg NOS
     Superficial frostbite of trunk NOS

● T34   Frostbite with tissue necrosis
   The appropriate 7th character is to be added to each code from category T34

> A   initial encounter
> D   subsequent encounter
> S   sequela

● T34.0   Frostbite with tissue necrosis of head
   ● T34.01   Frostbite with tissue necrosis of ear
     ● T34.011   Frostbite with tissue necrosis of right ear
     ● T34.012   Frostbite with tissue necrosis of left ear
     ● T34.019   Frostbite with tissue necrosis of unspecified ear
   X ● T34.02   Frostbite with tissue necrosis of nose
   X ● T34.09   Frostbite with tissue necrosis of other part of head

X ● T34.1   Frostbite with tissue necrosis of neck
X ● T34.2   Frostbite with tissue necrosis of thorax
X ● T34.3   Frostbite with tissue necrosis of abdominal wall, lower back and pelvis

● T34.4   Frostbite with tissue necrosis of arm
     Excludes2   frostbite with tissue necrosis of wrist and hand (T34.5-)
   X ● T34.40   Frostbite with tissue necrosis of unspecified arm
   X ● T34.41   Frostbite with tissue necrosis of right arm
   X ● T34.42   Frostbite with tissue necrosis of left arm

● T34.5   Frostbite with tissue necrosis of wrist, hand, and finger(s)
   ● T34.51   Frostbite with tissue necrosis of wrist
     ● T34.511   Frostbite with tissue necrosis of right wrist
     ● T34.512   Frostbite with tissue necrosis of left wrist
     ● T34.519   Frostbite with tissue necrosis of unspecified wrist
   ● T34.52   Frostbite with tissue necrosis of hand
     Excludes2   frostbite with tissue necrosis of finger(s) (T34.53-)
     ● T34.521   Frostbite with tissue necrosis of right hand
     ● T34.522   Frostbite with tissue necrosis of left hand
     ● T34.529   Frostbite with tissue necrosis of unspecified hand
   ● T34.53   Frostbite with tissue necrosis of finger(s)
     ● T34.531   Frostbite with tissue necrosis of right finger(s)
     ● T34.532   Frostbite with tissue necrosis of left finger(s)
     ● T34.539   Frostbite with tissue necrosis of unspecified finger(s)

● T34.6   Frostbite with tissue necrosis of hip and thigh
   X ● T34.60   Frostbite with tissue necrosis of unspecified hip and thigh
   X ● T34.61   Frostbite with tissue necrosis of right hip and thigh
   X ● T34.62   Frostbite with tissue necrosis of left hip and thigh

● T34.7   Frostbite with tissue necrosis of knee and lower leg
     Excludes2   frostbite with tissue necrosis of ankle and foot (T34.8-)
   X ● T34.70   Frostbite with tissue necrosis of unspecified knee and lower leg
   X ● T34.71   Frostbite with tissue necrosis of right knee and lower leg
   X ● T34.72   Frostbite with tissue necrosis of left knee and lower leg

● T34.8   Frostbite with tissue necrosis of ankle, foot, and toe(s)
   ● T34.81   Frostbite with tissue necrosis of ankle
     ● T34.811   Frostbite with tissue necrosis of right ankle
     ● T34.812   Frostbite with tissue necrosis of left ankle
     ● T34.819   Frostbite with tissue necrosis of unspecified ankle

- **T34.82**   Frostbite with tissue necrosis of foot
  - **T34.821**   Frostbite with tissue necrosis of right foot
  - **T34.822**   Frostbite with tissue necrosis of left foot
  - **T34.829**   Frostbite with tissue necrosis of unspecified foot
- **T34.83**   Frostbite with tissue necrosis of toe(s)
  - **T34.831**   Frostbite with tissue necrosis of right toe(s)
  - **T34.832**   Frostbite with tissue necrosis of left toe(s)
  - **T34.839**   Frostbite with tissue necrosis of unspecified toe(s)
- **T34.9**   Frostbite with tissue necrosis of other and unspecified sites
  - X **T34.90**   Frostbite with tissue necrosis of unspecified sites
    Frostbite with tissue necrosis NOS
  - X **T34.99**   Frostbite with tissue necrosis of other sites
    Frostbite with tissue necrosis of leg NOS
    Frostbite with tissue necrosis of trunk NOS

OGCR   See Section I.C.19.e.

Adverse Effects, Poisoning , Underdosing and Toxic Effects

Codes in categories T36-T65 are combination codes that include the substance that was taken as well as the intent. No additional external cause code is required for poisonings, toxic effects, adverse effects and underdosing codes.

POISONING BY, ADVERSE EFFECTS OF AND UNDERDOSING OF DRUGS MEDICAMENTS AND BIOLOGICAL SUBSTANCES (T36-T5Ø)

| **Includes** | adverse effect of correct substance properly administered
poisoning by overdose of substance
poisoning by wrong substance given or taken in error
underdosing by (inadvertently) (deliberately) taking less substance than prescribed or instructed |

Code first, for adverse effects, the nature of the adverse effect, such as:
   adverse effect NOS (T88.7)
   aspirin gastritis (K29.-)
   blood disorders (D56-D76)
   contact dermatitis (L23-L25)
   dermatitis due to substances taken internally (L27.-)
   nephropathy (N14.Ø-N14.2)

Note: The drug giving rise to the adverse effect should be identified by use of codes from categories T36-T5Ø with fifth or sixth character 5.

Use additional code(s) to specify:
   manifestations of poisoning
   underdosing or failure in dosage during medical and surgical care (Y63.6, Y63.8-Y63.9)
   underdosing of medication regimen (Z91.12-, Z91.13-)

| **Excludes1** | toxic reaction to local anesthesia in pregnancy (O29.3-) |

| **Excludes2** | abuse and dependence of psychoactive substances (F1Ø-F19)
abuse of non-dependence-producing substances (F55.-)
drug reaction and poisoning affecting newborn (PØØ-P96)
pathological drug intoxication (inebriation) (F1Ø-F19) |

- **T36**   Poisoning by, adverse effect of and underdosing of systemic antibiotics

  | **Excludes1** | antineoplastic antibiotics (T45.1-)
  locally applied antibiotic NEC (T49.Ø)
  topically used antibiotic for ear, nose and throat (T49.6)
  topically used antibiotic for eye (T49.5) |

  The appropriate 7th character is to be added to each code from category T36

A	initial encounter
D	subsequent encounter
S	sequela

  - **T36.Ø**   Poisoning by, adverse effect of and underdosing of penicillins
    - **T36.ØX**   Poisoning by, adverse effect of and underdosing of penicillins
      - **T36.ØX1**   Poisoning by penicillins, accidental (unintentional)
        Poisoning by penicillins NOS
      - **T36.ØX2**   Poisoning by penicillins, intentional self-harm
      - **T36.ØX3**   Poisoning by penicillins, assault
      - **T36.ØX4**   Poisoning by penicillins, undetermined
      - **T36.ØX5**   Adverse effect of penicillins
      - **T36.ØX6**   Underdosing of penicillins
  - **T36.1**   Poisoning by, adverse effect of and underdosing of cephalosporins and other betalactam antibiotics
    - **T36.1X**   Poisoning by, adverse effect of and underdosing of cephalosporins and other beta-lactam antibiotics
      - **T36.1X1**   Poisoning by cephalosporins and other beta-lactam antibiotics, accidental (unintentional)
        Poisoning by cephalosporins and other beta-lactam antibiotics NOS
      - **T36.1X2**   Poisoning by cephalosporins and other beta-lactam antibiotics, intentional self-harm
      - **T36.1X3**   Poisoning by cephalosporins and other beta-lactam antibiotics, assault
      - **T36.1X4**   Poisoning by cephalosporins and other beta-lactam antibiotics, undetermined
      - **T36.1X5**   Adverse effect of cephalosporins and other beta-lactam antibiotics
      - **T36.1X6**   Underdosing of cephalosporins and other beta-lactam antibiotics
  - **T36.2**   Poisoning by, adverse effect of and underdosing of chloramphenicol group
    - **T36.2X**   Poisoning by, adverse effect of and underdosing of chloramphenicol group
      - **T36.2X1**   Poisoning by chloramphenicol group, accidental (unintentional)
        Poisoning by chloramphenicol group NOS
      - **T36.2X2**   Poisoning by chloramphenicol group, intentional self-harm
      - **T36.2X3**   Poisoning by chloramphenicol group, assault
      - **T36.2X4**   Poisoning by chloramphenicol group, undetermined
      - **T36.2X5**   Adverse effect of chloramphenicol group
      - **T36.2X6**   Underdosing of chloramphenicol group

CHAPTER 19 (SØØ-T88)

● **T36.3** Poisoning by, adverse effect of and underdosing of macrolides

　● **T36.3X** Poisoning by, adverse effect of and underdosing of macrolides

　　● **T36.3X1** Poisoning by macrolides, accidental (unintentional)
　　　　　　Poisoning by macrolides NOS

　　● **T36.3X2** Poisoning by macrolides, intentional self-harm

　　● **T36.3X3** Poisoning by macrolides, assault

　　● **T36.3X4** Poisoning by macrolides, undetermined

　　● **T36.3X5** Adverse effect of macrolides

　　● **T36.3X6** Underdosing of macrolides

● **T36.4** Poisoning by, adverse effect of and underdosing of tetracyclines

　● **T36.4X** Poisoning by, adverse effect of and underdosing of tetracyclines

　　● **T36.4X1** Poisoning by tetracyclines, accidental (unintentional)
　　　　　　Poisoning by tetracyclines NOS

　　● **T36.4X2** Poisoning by tetracyclines, intentional self-harm

　　● **T36.4X3** Poisoning by tetracyclines, assault

　　● **T36.4X4** Poisoning by tetracyclines, undetermined

　　● **T36.4X5** Adverse effect of tetracyclines

　　● **T36.4X6** Underdosing of tetracyclines

● **T36.5** Poisoning by, adverse effect of and underdosing of aminoglycosides
　　　Poisoning by, adverse effect of and underdosing of streptomycin

　● **T36.5X** Poisoning by, adverse effect of and underdosing of aminoglycosides

　　● **T36.5X1** Poisoning by aminoglycosides, accidental (unintentional)
　　　　　　Poisoning by aminoglycosides NOS

　　● **T36.5X2** Poisoning by aminoglycosides, intentional self-harm

　　● **T36.5X3** Poisoning by aminoglycosides, assault

　　● **T36.5X4** Poisoning by aminoglycosides, undetermined

　　● **T36.5X5** Adverse effect of aminoglycosides

　　● **T36.5X6** Underdosing of aminoglycosides

● **T36.6** Poisoning by, adverse effect of and underdosing of rifampicins

　● **T36.6X** Poisoning by, adverse effect of and underdosing of rifampicins

　　● **T36.6X1** Poisoning by rifampicins, accidental (unintentional)
　　　　　　Poisoning by rifampicins NOS

　　● **T36.6X2** Poisoning by rifampicins, intentional self-harm

　　● **T36.6X3** Poisoning by rifampicins, assault

　　● **T36.6X4** Poisoning by rifampicins, undetermined

　　● **T36.6X5** Adverse effect of rifampicins

　　● **T36.6X6** Underdosing of rifampicins

● **T36.7** Poisoning by, adverse effect of and underdosing of antifungal antibiotics, systemically used

　● **T36.7X** Poisoning by, adverse effect of and underdosing of antifungal antibiotics, systemically used

　　● **T36.7X1** Poisoning by antifungal antibiotics, systemically used, accidental (unintentional)
　　　　　　Poisoning by antifungal antibiotics, systemically used NOS

　　● **T36.7X2** Poisoning by antifungal antibiotics, systemically used, intentional self-harm

　　● **T36.7X3** Poisoning by antifungal antibiotics, systemically used, assault

　　● **T36.7X4** Poisoning by antifungal antibiotics, systemically used, undetermined

　　● **T36.7X5** Adverse effect of antifungal antibiotics, systemically used

　　● **T36.7X6** Underdosing of antifungal antibiotics, systemically used

● **T36.8** Poisoning by, adverse effect of and underdosing of other systemic antibiotics

　● **T36.8X** Poisoning by, adverse effect of and underdosing of other systemic antibiotics

　　● **T36.8X1** Poisoning by other systemic antibiotics, accidental (unintentional)
　　　　　　Poisoning by other systemic antibiotics NOS

　　● **T36.8X2** Poisoning by other systemic antibiotics, intentional self-harm

　　● **T36.8X3** Poisoning by other systemic antibiotics, assault

　　● **T36.8X4** Poisoning by other systemic antibiotics, undetermined

　　● **T36.8X5** Adverse effect of other systemic antibiotics

　　● **T36.8X6** Underdosing of other systemic antibiotics

● **T36.9** Poisoning by, adverse effect of and underdosing of unspecified systemic antibiotic

　X ● **T36.91** Poisoning by unspecified systemic antibiotic, accidental (unintentional)
　　　　　Poisoning by systemic antibiotic NOS

　X ● **T36.92** Poisoning by unspecified systemic antibiotic, intentional self-harm

　X ● **T36.93** Poisoning by unspecified systemic antibiotic, assault

　X ● **T36.94** Poisoning by unspecified systemic antibiotic, undetermined

　X ● **T36.95** Adverse effect of unspecified systemic antibiotic

　X ● **T36.96** Underdosing of unspecified systemic antibiotic

● **T37** Poisoning by, adverse effect of and underdosing of other systemic anti-infectives and antiparasitics

　Excludes1　anti-infectives topically used for ear, nose and throat (T49.6-)
　　　anti-infectives topically used for eye (T49.5-)
　　　locally applied anti-infectives NEC (T49.0-)

　The appropriate 7th character is to be added to each code from category T37

A	initial encounter
D	subsequent encounter
S	sequela

● **T37.0** Poisoning by, adverse effect of and underdosing of sulfonamides

　● **T37.0X** Poisoning by, adverse effect of and underdosing of sulfonamides

　　● **T37.0X1** Poisoning by sulfonamides, accidental (unintentional)
　　　　　　Poisoning by sulfonamides NOS

　　● **T37.0X2** Poisoning by sulfonamides, intentional self-harm

　　● **T37.0X3** Poisoning by sulfonamides, assault

　　● **T37.0X4** Poisoning by sulfonamides, undetermined

　　● **T37.0X5** Adverse effect of sulfonamides

　　● **T37.0X6** Underdosing of sulfonamides

- **T37.1 Poisoning by, adverse effect of and underdosing of antimycobacterial drugs**
    - **Excludes1** rifampicins (T36.6-) streptomycin (T36.5-)
  - **T37.1X Poisoning by, adverse effect of and underdosing of antimycobacterial drugs**
    - **T37.1X1 Poisoning by antimycobacterial drugs, accidental (unintentional)**
      - Poisoning by antimycobacterial drugs NOS
    - **T37.1X2 Poisoning by antimycobacterial drugs, intentional self-harm**
    - **T37.1X3 Poisoning by antimycobacterial drugs, assault**
    - **T37.1X4 Poisoning by antimycobacterial drugs, undetermined**
    - **T37.1X5 Adverse effect of antimycobacterial drugs**
    - **T37.1X6 Underdosing of antimycobacterial drugs**
- **T37.2 Poisoning by, adverse effect of and underdosing of antimalarials and drugs acting on other blood protozoa**
    - **Excludes1** hydroxyquinoline derivatives (T37.8-)
  - **T37.2X Poisoning by, adverse effect of and underdosing of antimalarials and drugs acting on other blood protozoa**
    - **T37.2X1 Poisoning by antimalarials and drugs acting on other blood protozoa, accidental (unintentional)**
      - Poisoning by antimalarials and drugs acting on other blood protozoa NOS
    - **T37.2X2 Poisoning by antimalarials and drugs acting on other blood protozoa, intentional self-harm**
    - **T37.2X3 Poisoning by antimalarials and drugs acting on other blood protozoa, assault**
    - **T37.2X4 Poisoning by antimalarials and drugs acting on other blood protozoa, undetermined**
    - **T37.2X5 Adverse effect of antimalarials and drugs acting on other blood protozoa**
    - **T37.2X6 Underdosing of antimalarials and drugs acting on other blood protozoa**
- **T37.3 Poisoning by, adverse effect of and underdosing of other antiprotozoal drugs**
  - **T37.3X Poisoning by, adverse effect of and underdosing of other antiprotozoal drugs**
    - **T37.3X1 Poisoning by other antiprotozoal drugs, accidental (unintentional)**
      - Poisoning by other antiprotozoal drugs NOS
    - **T37.3X2 Poisoning by other antiprotozoal drugs, intentional self-harm**
    - **T37.3X3 Poisoning by other antiprotozoal drugs, assault**
    - **T37.3X4 Poisoning by other antiprotozoal drugs, undetermined**
    - **T37.3X5 Adverse effect of other antiprotozoal drugs**
    - **T37.3X6 Underdosing of other antiprotozoal drugs**
- **T37.4 Poisoning by, adverse effect of and underdosing of anthelminthics**
  - **T37.4X Poisoning by, adverse effect of and underdosing of anthelminthics**
    - **T37.4X1 Poisoning by anthelminthics, accidental (unintentional)**
      - Poisoning by anthelminthics NOS
    - **T37.4X2 Poisoning by anthelminthics, intentional self-harm**

- **T37.4X3 Poisoning by anthelminthics, assault**
- **T37.4X4 Poisoning by anthelminthics, undetermined**
- **T37.4X5 Adverse effect of anthelminthics**
- **T37.4X6 Underdosing of anthelminthics**
- **T37.5 Poisoning by, adverse effect of and underdosing of antiviral drugs**
    - **Excludes1** amantadine (T42.8-) cytarabine (T45.1-)
  - **T37.5X Poisoning by, adverse effect of and underdosing of antiviral drugs**
    - **T37.5X1 Poisoning by antiviral drugs, accidental (unintentional)**
      - Poisoning by antiviral drugs NOS
    - **T37.5X2 Poisoning by antiviral drugs, intentional self-harm**
    - **T37.5X3 Poisoning by antiviral drugs, assault**
    - **T37.5X4 Poisoning by antiviral drugs, undetermined**
    - **T37.5X5 Adverse effect of antiviral drugs**
    - **T37.5X6 Underdosing of antiviral drugs**
- **T37.8 Poisoning by, adverse effect of and underdosing of other specified systemic anti-infectives and antiparasitics**
    - Poisoning by, adverse effect of and underdosing of hydroxyquinoline derivatives
    - **Excludes1** antimalarial drugs (T37.2-)
  - **T37.8X Poisoning by, adverse effect of and underdosing of other specified systemic anti-infectives and antiparasitics**
    - **T37.8X1 Poisoning by other specified systemic anti-infectives and antiparasitics, accidental (unintentional)**
      - Poisoning by other specified systemic anti-infectives and antiparasitics NOS
    - **T37.8X2 Poisoning by other specified systemic anti-infectives and antiparasitics, intentional self-harm**
    - **T37.8X3 Poisoning by other specified systemic anti-infectives and antiparasitics, assault**
    - **T37.8X4 Poisoning by other specified systemic anti-infectives and antiparasitics, undetermined**
    - **T37.8X5 Adverse effect of other specified systemic anti-infectives and antiparasitics**
    - **T37.8X6 Underdosing of other specified systemic anti-infectives and antiparasitics**
- **T37.9 Poisoning by, adverse effect of and underdosing of unspecified systemic anti-infective and antiparasitics**
  - X **T37.91 Poisoning by unspecified systemic anti-infective and antiparasitics, accidental (unintentional)**
    - Poisoning by, adverse effect of and underdosing of systemic anti-infective and antiparasitics NOS
  - X **T37.92 Poisoning by unspecified systemic anti-infective and antiparasitics, intentional self-harm**
  - X **T37.93 Poisoning by unspecified systemic anti-infective and antiparasitics, assault**
  - X **T37.94 Poisoning by unspecified systemic anti-infective and antiparasitics, undetermined**
  - X **T37.95 Adverse effect of unspecified systemic anti-infective and antiparasitic**
  - X **T37.96 Underdosing of unspecified systemic anti-infectives and antiparasitics**

● **T38** **Poisoning by, adverse effect of and underdosing of hormones and their synthetic substitutes and antagonists, not elsewhere classified**

Excludes1 mineralocorticoids and their antagonists (T50.0-)
oxytocic hormones (T48.0-)
parathyroid hormones and derivatives (T50.9-)

The appropriate 7th character is to be added to each code from category T38

A	initial encounter
D	subsequent encounter
S	sequela

● **T38.0** **Poisoning by, adverse effect of and underdosing of glucocorticoids and synthetic analogues**

Excludes1 glucocorticoids, topically used (T49.-)

● **T38.0X** **Poisoning by, adverse effect of and underdosing of glucocorticoids and synthetic analogues**

● **T38.0X1** Poisoning by glucocorticoids and synthetic analogues, accidental (unintentional)
Poisoning by glucocorticoids and synthetic analogues NOS

● **T38.0X2** Poisoning by glucocorticoids and synthetic analogues, intentional self-harm

● **T38.0X3** Poisoning by glucocorticoids and synthetic analogues, assault

● **T38.0X4** Poisoning by glucocorticoids and synthetic analogues, undetermined

● **T38.0X5** Adverse effect of glucocorticoids and synthetic analogues

● **T38.0X6** Underdosing of glucocorticoids and synthetic analogues

● **T38.1** **Poisoning by, adverse effect of and underdosing of thyroid hormones and substitutes**

● **T38.1X** **Poisoning by, adverse effect of and underdosing of thyroid hormones and substitutes**

● **T38.1X1** Poisoning by thyroid hormones and substitutes, accidental (unintentional)
Poisoning by thyroid hormones and substitutes NOS

● **T38.1X2** Poisoning by thyroid hormones and substitutes, intentional self-harm

● **T38.1X3** Poisoning by thyroid hormones and substitutes, assault

● **T38.1X4** Poisoning by thyroid hormones and substitutes, undetermined

● **T38.1X5** Adverse effect of thyroid hormones and substitutes

● **T38.1X6** Underdosing of thyroid hormones and substitutes

● **T38.2** **Poisoning by, adverse effect of and underdosing of antithyroid drugs**

● **T38.2X** **Poisoning by, adverse effect of and underdosing of antithyroid drugs**

● **T38.2X1** Poisoning by antithyroid drugs, accidental (unintentional)
Poisoning by antithyroid drugs NOS

● **T38.2X2** Poisoning by antithyroid drugs, intentional self-harm

● **T38.2X3** Poisoning by antithyroid drugs, assault

● **T38.2X4** Poisoning by antithyroid drugs, undetermined

● **T38.2X5** Adverse effect of antithyroid drugs

● **T38.2X6** Underdosing of antithyroid drugs

● **T38.3** **Poisoning by, adverse effect of and underdosing of insulin and oral hypoglycemic [antidiabetic] drugs**

● **T38.3X** **Poisoning by, adverse effect of and underdosing of insulin and oral hypoglycemic [antidiabetic] drugs**

● **T38.3X1** Poisoning by insulin and oral hypoglycemic [antidiabetic] drugs, accidental (unintentional)
Poisoning by insulin and oral hypoglycemic [antidiabetic] drugs NOS

● **T38.3X2** Poisoning by insulin and oral hypoglycemic [antidiabetic] drugs, intentional self-harm

● **T38.3X3** Poisoning by insulin and oral hypoglycemic [antidiabetic] drugs, assault

● **T38.3X4** Poisoning by insulin and oral hypoglycemic [antidiabetic] drugs, undetermined

● **T38.3X5** Adverse effect of insulin and oral hypoglycemic [antidiabetic] drugs

● **T38.3X6** Underdosing of insulin and oral hypoglycemic [antidiabetic] drugs

● **T38.4** **Poisoning by, adverse effect of and underdosing of oral contraceptives**
Poisoning by, adverse effect of and underdosing of multiple- and single-ingredient oral contraceptive preparations

● **T38.4X** **Poisoning by, adverse effect of and underdosing of oral contraceptives**

● **T38.4X1** Poisoning by oral contraceptives, accidental (unintentional)
Poisoning by oral contraceptives NOS

● **T38.4X2** Poisoning by oral contraceptives, intentional self-harm

● **T38.4X3** Poisoning by oral contraceptives, assault

● **T38.4X4** Poisoning by oral contraceptives, undetermined

● **T38.4X5** Adverse effect of oral contraceptives

● **T38.4X6** Underdosing of oral contraceptives

● **T38.5** **Poisoning by, adverse effect of and underdosing of other estrogens and progestogens**
Poisoning by, adverse effect of and underdosing of estrogens and progestogens mixtures and substitutes

● **T38.5X** **Poisoning by, adverse effect of and underdosing of other estrogens and progestogens**

● **T38.5X1** Poisoning by other estrogens and progestogens, accidental (unintentional)
Poisoning by other estrogens and progestogens NOS

● **T38.5X2** Poisoning by other estrogens and progestogens, intentional self-harm

● **T38.5X3** Poisoning by other estrogens and progestogens, assault

● **T38.5X4** Poisoning by other estrogens and progestogens, undetermined

● **T38.5X5** Adverse effect of other estrogens and progestogens

● **T38.5X6** Underdosing of other estrogens and progestogens

◀ New ⬛ Revised ~~deleted~~ Deleted | Excludes 1 | Excludes 2 | Includes | Use additional | Code first | Code also | Unspecified
OGCR Official Guidelines X Assign placeholder X ● Use Additional Character(s) ▶ Manifestation Code **Coding Clinic**

- **T38.6** Poisoning by, adverse effect of and underdosing of antigonadotrophins, antiestrogens, antiandrogens, not elsewhere classified

  Poisoning by, adverse effect of and underdosing of tamoxifen

  - **T38.6X** Poisoning by, adverse effect of and underdosing of antigonadotrophins, antiestrogens, antiandrogens, not elsewhere classified

    - **T38.6X1** Poisoning by antigonadotrophins, antiestrogens, antiandrogens, not elsewhere classified, accidental (unintentional)

      Poisoning by antigonadotrophins, antiestrogens, antiandrogens, not elsewhere classified NOS

    - **T38.6X2** Poisoning by antigonadotrophins, antiestrogens, antiandrogens, not elsewhere classified, intentional self-harm

    - **T38.6X3** Poisoning by antigonadotrophins, antiestrogens, antiandrogens, not elsewhere classified, assault

    - **T38.6X4** Poisoning by antigonadotrophins, antiestrogens, antiandrogens, not elsewhere classified, undetermined

    - **T38.6X5** Adverse effect of antigonadotrophins, antiestrogens, antiandrogens, not elsewhere classified

    - **T38.6X6** Underdosing of antigonadotrophins, antiestrogens, antiandrogens, not elsewhere classified

- **T38.7** Poisoning by, adverse effect of and underdosing of androgens and anabolic congeners

  - **T38.7X** Poisoning by, adverse effect of and underdosing of androgens and anabolic congeners

    - **T38.7X1** Poisoning by androgens and anabolic congeners, accidental (unintentional)

      Poisoning by androgens and anabolic congeners NOS

    - **T38.7X2** Poisoning by androgens and anabolic congeners, intentional self-harm

    - **T38.7X3** Poisoning by androgens and anabolic congeners, assault

    - **T38.7X4** Poisoning by androgens and anabolic congeners, undetermined

    - **T38.7X5** Adverse effect of androgens and anabolic congeners

    - **T38.7X6** Underdosing of androgens and anabolic congeners

- **T38.8** Poisoning by, adverse effect of and underdosing of other and unspecified hormones and synthetic substitutes

  - **T38.80** Poisoning by, adverse effect of and underdosing of unspecified hormones and synthetic substitutes

    - **T38.801** Poisoning by unspecified hormones and synthetic substitutes, accidental (unintentional)

      Poisoning by unspecified hormones and synthetic substitutes NOS

    - **T38.802** Poisoning by unspecified hormones and synthetic substitutes, intentional self-harm

    - **T38.803** Poisoning by unspecified hormones and synthetic substitutes, assault

    - **T38.804** Poisoning by unspecified hormones and synthetic substitutes, undetermined

    - **T38.805** Adverse effect of unspecified hormones and synthetic substitutes

    - **T38.806** Underdosing of unspecified hormones and synthetic substitutes

  - **T38.81** Poisoning by, adverse effect of and underdosing of anterior pituitary [adenohypophyseal] hormones

    - **T38.811** Poisoning by anterior pituitary [adenohypophyseal] hormones, accidental (unintentional)

      Poisoning by anterior pituitary [adenohypophyseal] hormones NOS

    - **T38.812** Poisoning by anterior pituitary [adenohypophyseal] hormones, intentional self-harm

    - **T38.813** Poisoning by anterior pituitary [adenohypophyseal] hormones, assault

    - **T38.814** Poisoning by anterior pituitary [adenohypophyseal] hormones, undetermined

    - **T38.815** Adverse effect of anterior pituitary [adenohypophyseal] hormones

    - **T38.816** Underdosing of anterior pituitary [adenohypophyseal] hormones

  - **T38.89** Poisoning by, adverse effect of and underdosing of other hormones and synthetic substitutes

    - **T38.891** Poisoning by other hormones and synthetic substitutes, accidental (unintentional)

      Poisoning by other hormones and synthetic substitutes NOS

    - **T38.892** Poisoning by other hormones and synthetic substitutes, intentional self-harm

    - **T38.893** Poisoning by other hormones and synthetic substitutes, assault

    - **T38.894** Poisoning by other hormones and synthetic substitutes, undetermined

    - **T38.895** Adverse effect of other hormones and synthetic substitutes

    - **T38.896** Underdosing of other hormones and synthetic substitutes

- **T38.9** Poisoning by, adverse effect of and underdosing of other and unspecified hormone antagonists

  - **T38.90** Poisoning by, adverse effect of and underdosing of unspecified hormone antagonists

    - **T38.901** Poisoning by unspecified hormone antagonists, accidental (unintentional)

      Poisoning by unspecified hormone antagonists NOS

    - **T38.902** Poisoning by unspecified hormone antagonists, intentional self-harm

    - **T38.903** Poisoning by unspecified hormone antagonists, assault

    - **T38.904** Poisoning by unspecified hormone antagonists, undetermined

    - **T38.905** Adverse effect of unspecified hormone antagonists

    - **T38.906** Underdosing of unspecified hormone antagonists

CHAPTER 19 (S00-T88)

● T38.99   Poisoning by, adverse effect of and underdosing of other hormone antagonists

    ● T38.991   Poisoning by other hormone antagonists, accidental (unintentional)
       Poisoning by other hormone antagonists NOS

    ● T38.992   Poisoning by other hormone antagonists, intentional self-harm

    ● T38.993   Poisoning by other hormone antagonists, assault

    ● T38.994   Poisoning by other hormone antagonists, undetermined

    ● T38.995   Adverse effect of other hormone antagonists

    ● T38.996   Underdosing of other hormone antagonists

● T39   Poisoning by, adverse effect of and underdosing of nonopioid analgesics, antipyretics and antirheumatics

    The appropriate 7th character is to be added to each code from category T39

> A   initial encounter
> D   subsequent encounter
> S   sequela

   ● T39.0   Poisoning by, adverse effect of and underdosing of salicylates

    ● T39.01   Poisoning by, adverse effect of and underdosing of aspirin
       Poisoning by, adverse effect of and underdosing of acetylsalicylic acid

      ● T39.011   Poisoning by aspirin, accidental (unintentional)

      ● T39.012   Poisoning by aspirin, intentional self-harm

      ● T39.013   Poisoning by aspirin, assault

      ● T39.014   Poisoning by aspirin, undetermined

      ● T39.015   Adverse effect of aspirin
        Coding Clinic: 2016, Q1, P15

      ● T39.016   Underdosing of aspirin

    ● T39.09   Poisoning by, adverse effect of and underdosing of other salicylates

      ● T39.091   Poisoning by salicylates, accidental (unintentional)
        Poisoning by salicylates NOS

      ● T39.092   Poisoning by salicylates, intentional self-harm

      ● T39.093   Poisoning by salicylates, assault

      ● T39.094   Poisoning by salicylates, undetermined

      ● T39.095   Adverse effect of salicylates

      ● T39.096   Underdosing of salicylates

   ● T39.1   Poisoning by, adverse effect of and underdosing of 4-Aminophenol derivatives

    ● T39.1X   Poisoning by, adverse effect of and underdosing of 4-Aminophenol derivatives

      ● T39.1X1   Poisoning by 4-Aminophenol derivatives, accidental (unintentional)
        Poisoning by 4-Aminophenol derivatives NOS

      ● T39.1X2   Poisoning by 4-Aminophenol derivatives, intentional self-harm

      ● T39.1X3   Poisoning by 4-Aminophenol derivatives, assault

      ● T39.1X4   Poisoning by 4-Aminophenol derivatives, undetermined

      ● T39.1X5   Adverse effect of 4-Aminophenol derivatives

      ● T39.1X6   Underdosing of 4-Aminophenol derivatives

● T39.2   Poisoning by, adverse effect of and underdosing of pyrazolone derivatives

   ● T39.2X   Poisoning by, adverse effect of and underdosing of pyrazolone derivatives

     ● T39.2X1   Poisoning by pyrazolone derivatives, accidental (unintentional)
       Poisoning by pyrazolone derivatives NOS

     ● T39.2X2   Poisoning by pyrazolone derivatives, intentional self-harm

     ● T39.2X3   Poisoning by pyrazolone derivatives, assault

     ● T39.2X4   Poisoning by pyrazolone derivatives, undetermined

     ● T39.2X5   Adverse effect of pyrazolone derivatives

     ● T39.2X6   Underdosing of pyrazolone derivatives

● T39.3   Poisoning by, adverse effect of and underdosing of other nonsteroidal anti-inflammatory drugs [NSAID]

   ● T39.31   Poisoning by, adverse effect of and underdosing of propionic acid derivatives
     Poisoning by, adverse effect of and underdosing of fenoprofen
     Poisoning by, adverse effect of and underdosing of flurbiprofen
     Poisoning by, adverse effect of and underdosing of ibuprofen
     Poisoning by, adverse effect of and underdosing of ketoprofen
     Poisoning by, adverse effect of and underdosing of naproxen
     Poisoning by, adverse effect of and underdosing of oxaprozin

     ● T39.311   Poisoning by propionic acid derivatives, accidental (unintentional)

     ● T39.312   Poisoning by propionic acid derivatives, intentional self-harm

     ● T39.313   Poisoning by propionic acid derivatives, assault

     ● T39.314   Poisoning by propionic acid derivatives, undetermined

     ● T39.315   Adverse effect of propionic acid derivatives

     ● T39.316   Underdosing of propionic acid derivatives

   ● T39.39   Poisoning by, adverse effect of and underdosing of other nonsteroidal anti-inflammatory drugs [NSAID]

     ● T39.391   Poisoning by other nonsteroidal anti-inflammatory drugs [NSAID], accidental (unintentional)
       Poisoning by other nonsteroidal anti-inflammatory drugs NOS

     ● T39.392   Poisoning by other nonsteroidal anti-inflammatory drugs [NSAID], intentional self-harm

     ● T39.393   Poisoning by other nonsteroidal anti-inflammatory drugs [NSAID], assault

     ● T39.394   Poisoning by other nonsteroidal anti-inflammatory drugs [NSAID], undetermined

     ● T39.395   Adverse effect of other nonsteroidal anti-inflammatory drugs [NSAID]

     ● T39.396   Underdosing of other nonsteroidal anti-inflammatory drugs [NSAID]

◄ New   ◄═ Revised   ~~deleted~~ Deleted   Excludes 1   Excludes 2   Includes   Use additional   Code first   Code also   Unspecified

1366   **OGCR** Official Guidelines   **X** Assign placeholder X   ● Use Additional Character(s)   ▶ Manifestation Code   **Coding Clinic**

● T39.4 Poisoning by, adverse effect of and underdosing of antirheumatics, not elsewhere classified

> Excludes1   poisoning by, adverse effect of and underdosing of glucocorticoids (T38.0-)
> poisoning by, adverse effect of and underdosing of salicylates (T39.0-)

● T39.4X Poisoning by, adverse effect of and underdosing of antirheumatics, not elsewhere classified

● T39.4X1 Poisoning by antirheumatics, not elsewhere classified, accidental (unintentional)
> Poisoning by antirheumatics, not elsewhere classified NOS

● T39.4X2 Poisoning by antirheumatics, not elsewhere classified, intentional self-harm

● T39.4X3 Poisoning by antirheumatics, not elsewhere classified, assault

● T39.4X4 Poisoning by antirheumatics, not elsewhere classified, undetermined

● T39.4X5 Adverse effect of antirheumatics, not elsewhere classified

● T39.4X6 Underdosing of antirheumatics, not elsewhere classified

● T39.8 Poisoning by, adverse effect of and underdosing of other nonopioid analgesics and antipyretics, not elsewhere classified

● T39.8X Poisoning by, adverse effect of and underdosing of other nonopioid analgesics and antipyretics, not elsewhere classified

● T39.8X1 Poisoning by other nonopioid analgesics and antipyretics, not elsewhere classified, accidental (unintentional)
> Poisoning by other nonopioid analgesics and antipyretics, not elsewhere classified NOS

● T39.8X2 Poisoning by other nonopioid analgesics and antipyretics, not elsewhere classified, intentional self-harm

● T39.8X3 Poisoning by other nonopioid analgesics and antipyretics, not elsewhere classified, assault

● T39.8X4 Poisoning by other nonopioid analgesics and antipyretics, not elsewhere classified, undetermined

● T39.8X5 Adverse effect of other nonopioid analgesics and antipyretics, not elsewhere classified

● T39.8X6 Underdosing of other nonopioid analgesics and antipyretics, not elsewhere classified

● T39.9 Poisoning by, adverse effect of and underdosing of unspecified nonopioid analgesic, antipyretic and antirheumatic

X ● T39.91 Poisoning by unspecified nonopioid analgesic, antipyretic and antirheumatic, accidental (unintentional)
> Poisoning by nonopioid analgesic, antipyretic and antirheumatic NOS

X ● T39.92 Poisoning by unspecified nonopioid analgesic, antipyretic and antirheumatic, intentional self-harm

X ● T39.93 Poisoning by unspecified nonopioid analgesic, antipyretic and antirheumatic, assault

X ● T39.94 Poisoning by unspecified nonopioid analgesic, antipyretic and antirheumatic, undetermined

X ● T39.95 Adverse effect of unspecified nonopioid analgesic, antipyretic and antirheumatic

X ● T39.96 Underdosing of unspecified nonopioid analgesic, antipyretic and antirheumatic

● T40 Poisoning by, adverse effect of and underdosing of narcotics and psychodysleptics [hallucinogens]

> Excludes2   drug dependence and related mental and behavioral disorders due to psychoactive substance use (F10.-F19.-)

The appropriate 7th character is to be added to each code from category T40

A	initial encounter
D	subsequent encounter
S	sequela

● T40.0 Poisoning by, adverse effect of and underdosing of opium

● T40.0X Poisoning by, adverse effect of and underdosing of opium

● T40.0X1 Poisoning by opium, accidental (unintentional)
> Poisoning by opium NOS

● T40.0X2 Poisoning by opium, intentional self-harm

● T40.0X3 Poisoning by opium, assault

● T40.0X4 Poisoning by opium, undetermined

● T40.0X5 Adverse effect of opium

● T40.0X6 Underdosing of opium

● T40.1 Poisoning by and adverse effect of heroin

● T40.1X Poisoning by and adverse effect of heroin

● T40.1X1 Poisoning by heroin, accidental (unintentional)
> Poisoning by heroin NOS

● T40.1X2 Poisoning by heroin, intentional self-harm

● T40.1X3 Poisoning by heroin, assault

● T40.1X4 Poisoning by heroin, undetermined

● T40.2 Poisoning by, adverse effect of and underdosing of other opioids

● T40.2X Poisoning by, adverse effect of and underdosing of other opioids

● T40.2X1 Poisoning by other opioids, accidental (unintentional)
> Poisoning by other opioids NOS

● T40.2X2 Poisoning by other opioids, intentional self-harm

● T40.2X3 Poisoning by other opioids, assault

● T40.2X4 Poisoning by other opioids, undetermined

● T40.2X5 Adverse effect of other opioids

● T40.2X6 Underdosing of other opioids

● T40.3 Poisoning by, adverse effect of and underdosing of methadone

● T40.3X Poisoning by, adverse effect of and underdosing of methadone

● T40.3X1 Poisoning by methadone, accidental (unintentional)
> Poisoning by methadone NOS

● T40.3X2 Poisoning by methadone, intentional self-harm

● T40.3X3 Poisoning by methadone, assault

● T40.3X4 Poisoning by methadone, undetermined

● T40.3X5 Adverse effect of methadone

● T40.3X6 Underdosing of methadone

CHAPTER 19 (S00-T88)

● T40.4   Poisoning by, adverse effect of and underdosing of other synthetic narcotics

  ● T40.4X   Poisoning by, adverse effect of and underdosing of other synthetic narcotics

    ● T40.4X1   Poisoning by other synthetic narcotics, accidental (unintentional)
         Poisoning by other synthetic narcotics NOS

    ● T40.4X2   Poisoning by other synthetic narcotics, intentional self-harm

    ● T40.4X3   Poisoning by other synthetic narcotics, assault

    ● T40.4X4   Poisoning by other synthetic narcotics, undetermined

    ● T40.4X5   Adverse effect of other synthetic narcotics

    ● T40.4X6   Underdosing of other synthetic narcotics

● T40.5   Poisoning by, adverse effect of and underdosing of cocaine

  ● T40.5X   Poisoning by, adverse effect of and underdosing of cocaine

    ● T40.5X1   Poisoning by cocaine, accidental (unintentional)
         Poisoning by cocaine NOS
         Coding Clinic: 2016, Q2, P9

    ● T40.5X2   Poisoning by cocaine, intentional self-harm

    ● T40.5X3   Poisoning by cocaine, assault

    ● T40.5X4   Poisoning by cocaine, undetermined

    ● T40.5X5   Adverse effect of cocaine

    ● T40.5X6   Underdosing of cocaine

● T40.6   Poisoning by, adverse effect of and underdosing of other and unspecified narcotics

  ● T40.60   Poisoning by, adverse effect of and underdosing of unspecified narcotics

    ● T40.601   Poisoning by unspecified narcotics, accidental (unintentional)
         Poisoning by narcotics NOS

    ● T40.602   Poisoning by unspecified narcotics, intentional self-harm

    ● T40.603   Poisoning by unspecified narcotics, assault

    ● T40.604   Poisoning by unspecified narcotics, undetermined

    ● T40.605   Adverse effect of unspecified narcotics

    ● T40.606   Underdosing of unspecified narcotics

  ● T40.69   Poisoning by, adverse effect of and underdosing of other narcotics

    ● T40.691   Poisoning by other narcotics, accidental (unintentional)
         Poisoning by other narcotics NOS

    ● T40.692   Poisoning by other narcotics, intentional self-harm

    ● T40.693   Poisoning by other narcotics, assault

    ● T40.694   Poisoning by other narcotics, undetermined

    ● T40.695   Adverse effect of other narcotics

    ● T40.696   Underdosing of other narcotics

● T40.7   Poisoning by, adverse effect of and underdosing of cannabis (derivatives)

  ● T40.7X   Poisoning by, adverse effect of and underdosing of cannabis (derivatives)

    ● T40.7X1   Poisoning by cannabis (derivatives), accidental (unintentional)
         Poisoning by cannabis NOS

    ● T40.7X2   Poisoning by cannabis (derivatives), intentional self-harm

    ● T40.7X3   Poisoning by cannabis (derivatives), assault

    ● T40.7X4   Poisoning by cannabis (derivatives), undetermined

    ● T40.7X5   Adverse effect of cannabis (derivatives)

    ● T40.7X6   Underdosing of cannabis (derivatives)

● T40.8   Poisoning by and adverse effect of lysergide [LSD]

  ● T40.8X   Poisoning by and adverse effect of lysergide [LSD]

    ● T40.8X1   Poisoning by lysergide [LSD], accidental (unintentional)
         Poisoning by lysergide [LSD] NOS

    ● T40.8X2   Poisoning by lysergide [LSD], intentional self-harm

    ● T40.8X3   Poisoning by lysergide [LSD], assault

    ● T40.8X4   Poisoning by lysergide [LSD], undetermined

● T40.9   Poisoning by, adverse effect of and underdosing of other and unspecified psychodysleptics [hallucinogens]

  ● T40.90   Poisoning by, adverse effect of and underdosing of unspecified psychodysleptics [hallucinogens]

    ● T40.901   Poisoning by unspecified psychodysleptics [hallucinogens], accidental (unintentional)

    ● T40.902   Poisoning by unspecified psychodysleptics [hallucinogens], intentional self-harm

    ● T40.903   Poisoning by unspecified psychodysleptics [hallucinogens], assault

    ● T40.904   Poisoning by unspecified psychodysleptics [hallucinogens], undetermined

    ● T40.905   Adverse effect of unspecified psychodysleptics [hallucinogens]

    ● T40.906   Underdosing of unspecified psychodysleptics

  ● T40.99   Poisoning by, adverse effect of and underdosing of other psychodysleptics [hallucinogens]

    ● T40.991   Poisoning by other psychodysleptics [hallucinogens], accidental (unintentional)
         Poisoning by other psychodysleptics [hallucinogens] NOS

    ● T40.992   Poisoning by other psychodysleptics [hallucinogens], intentional self-harm

    ● T40.993   Poisoning by other psychodysleptics [hallucinogens], assault

    ● T40.994   Poisoning by other psychodysleptics [hallucinogens], undetermined

    ● T40.995   Adverse effect of other psychodysleptics [hallucinogens]

    ● T40.996   Underdosing of other psychodysleptics

◄ New   ◄ Revised   ~~deleted~~ Deleted   Excludes 1   Excludes 2   Includes   Use additional   Code first   Code also   Unspecified
OGCR Official Guidelines   X Assign placeholder X   ● Use Additional Character(s)   ▶ Manifestation Code   **Coding Clinic**

● **T41**   **Poisoning by, adverse effect of and underdosing of anesthetics and therapeutic gases**

   Excludes1   benzodiazepines (T42.4-)
            cocaine (T40.5-)
            complications of anesthesia during pregnancy
              (O29.-)
            complications of anesthesia during labor and
              delivery (O74.-)
            complications of anesthesia during the
              puerperium (O89.-) opioids (T40.0-T40.2-)

   The appropriate 7th character is to be added to each code from
     category T41

> A   initial encounter
> D   subsequent encounter
> S   sequela

● **T41.0**   **Poisoning by, adverse effect of and underdosing of inhaled anesthetics**

   Excludes1   oxygen (T41.5-)

   ● **T41.0X**   **Poisoning by, adverse effect of and underdosing of inhaled anesthetics**

     ● **T41.0X1**   **Poisoning by inhaled anesthetics, accidental (unintentional)**
                 Poisoning by inhaled anesthetics NOS

     ● **T41.0X2**   **Poisoning by inhaled anesthetics, intentional self-harm**

     ● **T41.0X3**   **Poisoning by inhaled anesthetics, assault**

     ● **T41.0X4**   **Poisoning by inhaled anesthetics, undetermined**

     ● **T41.0X5**   **Adverse effect of inhaled anesthetics**

     ● **T41.0X6**   **Underdosing of inhaled anesthetics**

● **T41.1**   **Poisoning by, adverse effect of and underdosing of intravenous anesthetics**

   Poisoning by, adverse effect of and underdosing of
     thiobarbiturates

   ● **T41.1X**   **Poisoning by, adverse effect of and underdosing of intravenous anesthetics**

     ● **T41.1X1**   **Poisoning by intravenous anesthetics, accidental (unintentional)**
                 Poisoning by intravenous anesthetics NOS

     ● **T41.1X2**   **Poisoning by intravenous anesthetics, intentional self-harm**

     ● **T41.1X3**   **Poisoning by intravenous anesthetics, assault**

     ● **T41.1X4**   **Poisoning by intravenous anesthetics, undetermined**

     ● **T41.1X5**   **Adverse effect of intravenous anesthetics**

     ● **T41.1X6**   **Underdosing of intravenous anesthetics**

● **T41.2**   **Poisoning by, adverse effect of and underdosing of other and unspecified general anesthetics**

   ● **T41.20**   **Poisoning by, adverse effect of and underdosing of unspecified general anesthetics**

     ● **T41.201**   **Poisoning by unspecified general anesthetics, accidental (unintentional)**
                 Poisoning by general anesthetics NOS

     ● **T41.202**   **Poisoning by unspecified general anesthetics, intentional self-harm**

     ● **T41.203**   **Poisoning by unspecified general anesthetics, assault**

     ● **T41.204**   **Poisoning by unspecified general anesthetics, undetermined**

     ● **T41.205**   **Adverse effect of unspecified general anesthetics**

     ● **T41.206**   **Underdosing of unspecified general anesthetics**

   ● **T41.29**   **Poisoning by, adverse effect of and underdosing of other general anesthetics**

     ● **T41.291**   **Poisoning by other general anesthetics, accidental (unintentional)**
                 Poisoning by other general anesthetics NOS

     ● **T41.292**   **Poisoning by other general anesthetics, intentional self-harm**

     ● **T41.293**   **Poisoning by other general anesthetics, assault**

     ● **T41.294**   **Poisoning by other general anesthetics, undetermined**

     ● **T41.295**   **Adverse effect of other general anesthetics**

     ● **T41.296**   **Underdosing of other general anesthetics**

● **T41.3**   **Poisoning by, adverse effect of and underdosing of local anesthetics**

   Cocaine (topical)

   Excludes2   poisoning by cocaine used as a central
                nervous system stimulant (T40.5X1-
                T40.5X4)

   ● **T41.3X**   **Poisoning by, adverse effect of and underdosing of local anesthetics**

     ● **T41.3X1**   **Poisoning by local anesthetics, accidental (unintentional)**
                 Poisoning by local anesthetics NOS

     ● **T41.3X2**   **Poisoning by local anesthetics, intentional self-harm**

     ● **T41.3X3**   **Poisoning by local anesthetics, assault**

     ● **T41.3X4**   **Poisoning by local anesthetics, undetermined**

     ● **T41.3X5**   **Adverse effect of local anesthetics**

     ● **T41.3X6**   **Underdosing of local anesthetics**

● **T41.4**   **Poisoning by, adverse effect of and underdosing of unspecified anesthetic**

   X ● **T41.41**   **Poisoning by unspecified anesthetic, accidental (unintentional)**
                 Poisoning by anesthetic NOS

   X ● **T41.42**   **Poisoning by unspecified anesthetic, intentional self-harm**

   X ● **T41.43**   **Poisoning by unspecified anesthetic, assault**

   X ● **T41.44**   **Poisoning by unspecified anesthetic, undetermined**

   X ● **T41.45**   **Adverse effect of unspecified anesthetic**

   X ● **T41.46**   **Underdosing of unspecified anesthetics**

● **T41.5**   **Poisoning by, adverse effect of and underdosing of therapeutic gases**

   ● **T41.5X**   **Poisoning by, adverse effect of and underdosing of therapeutic gases**

     ● **T41.5X1**   **Poisoning by therapeutic gases, accidental (unintentional)**
                 Poisoning by therapeutic gases NOS

     ● **T41.5X2**   **Poisoning by therapeutic gases, intentional self-harm**

     ● **T41.5X3**   **Poisoning by therapeutic gases, assault**

     ● **T41.5X4**   **Poisoning by therapeutic gases, undetermined**

     ● **T41.5X5**   **Adverse effect of therapeutic gases**

     ● **T41.5X6**   **Underdosing of therapeutic gases**

CHAPTER 19 (S00-T88)

- T42 **Poisoning by, adverse effect of and underdosing of antiepileptic, sedative-hypnotic and antiparkinsonism drugs**

  Excludes2   drug dependence and related mental and behavioral disorders due to psychoactive substance use (F1Ø.--F19.-)

  The appropriate 7th character is to be added to each code from category T42

A	initial encounter
D	subsequent encounter
S	sequela

  - T42.Ø **Poisoning by, adverse effect of and underdosing of hydantoin derivatives**
    - T42.ØX **Poisoning by, adverse effect of and underdosing of hydantoin derivatives**
      - T42.ØX1 **Poisoning by hydantoin derivatives, accidental (unintentional)**
        Poisoning by hydantoin derivatives NOS
      - T42.ØX2 **Poisoning by hydantoin derivatives, intentional self-harm**
      - T42.ØX3 **Poisoning by hydantoin derivatives, assault**
      - T42.ØX4 **Poisoning by hydantoin derivatives, undetermined**
      - T42.ØX5 **Adverse effect of hydantoin derivatives**
      - T42.ØX6 **Underdosing of hydantoin derivatives**
  - T42.1 **Poisoning by, adverse effect of and underdosing of iminostilbenes**
    Poisoning by, adverse effect of and underdosing of carbamazepine
    - T42.1X **Poisoning by, adverse effect of and underdosing of iminostilbenes**
      - T42.1X1 **Poisoning by iminostilbenes, accidental (unintentional)**
        Poisoning by iminostilbenes NOS
      - T42.1X2 **Poisoning by iminostilbenes, intentional self-harm**
      - T42.1X3 **Poisoning by iminostilbenes, assault**
      - T42.1X4 **Poisoning by iminostilbenes, undetermined**
      - T42.1X5 **Adverse effect of iminostilbenes**
      - T42.1X6 **Underdosing of iminostilbenes**
  - T42.2 **Poisoning by, adverse effect of and underdosing of succinimides and oxazolidinediones**
    - T42.2X **Poisoning by, adverse effect of and underdosing of succinimides and oxazolidinediones**
      - T42.2X1 **Poisoning by succinimides and oxazolidinediones, accidental (unintentional)**
        Poisoning by succinimides and oxazolidinediones NOS
      - T42.2X2 **Poisoning by succinimides and oxazolidinediones, intentional self-harm**
      - T42.2X3 **Poisoning by succinimides and oxazolidinediones, assault**
      - T42.2X4 **Poisoning by succinimides and oxazolidinediones, undetermined**
      - T42.2X5 **Adverse effect of succinimides and oxazolidinediones**
      - T42.2X6 **Underdosing of succinimides and oxazolidinediones**

- T42.3 **Poisoning by, adverse effect of and underdosing of barbiturates**

  Excludes1   poisoning by, adverse effect of and underdosing of thiobarbiturates (T41.1-)

  - T42.3X **Poisoning by, adverse effect of and underdosing of barbiturates**
    - T42.3X1 **Poisoning by barbiturates, accidental (unintentional)**
      Poisoning by barbiturates NOS
    - T42.3X2 **Poisoning by barbiturates, intentional self-harm**
    - T42.3X3 **Poisoning by barbiturates, assault**
    - T42.3X4 **Poisoning by barbiturates, undetermined**
    - T42.3X5 **Adverse effect of barbiturates**
    - T42.3X6 **Underdosing of barbiturates**
- T42.4 **Poisoning by, adverse effect of and underdosing of benzodiazepines**
  - T42.4X **Poisoning by, adverse effect of and underdosing of benzodiazepines**
    - T42.4X1 **Poisoning by benzodiazepines, accidental (unintentional)**
      Poisoning by benzodiazepines NOS
    - T42.4X2 **Poisoning by benzodiazepines, intentional self-harm**
    - T42.4X3 **Poisoning by benzodiazepines, assault**
    - T42.4X4 **Poisoning by benzodiazepines, undetermined**
    - T42.4X5 **Adverse effect of benzodiazepines**
    - T42.4X6 **Underdosing of benzodiazepines**
- T42.5 **Poisoning by, adverse effect of and underdosing of mixed antiepileptics**
  - T42.5X **Poisoning by, adverse effect of and underdosing of antiepileptics**
    - T42.5X1 **Poisoning by mixed antiepileptics, accidental (unintentional)**
      Poisoning by mixed antiepileptics NOS
    - T42.5X2 **Poisoning by mixed antiepileptics, intentional self-harm**
    - T42.5X3 **Poisoning by mixed antiepileptics, assault**
    - T42.5X4 **Poisoning by mixed antiepileptics, undetermined**
    - T42.5X5 **Adverse effect of mixed antiepileptics**
    - T42.5X6 **Underdosing of mixed antiepileptics**
- T42.6 **Poisoning by, adverse effect of and underdosing of other antiepileptic and sedative-hypnotic drugs**
  Poisoning by, adverse effect of and underdosing of methaqualone
  Poisoning by, adverse effect of and underdosing of valproic acid

  Excludes1   poisoning by, adverse effect of and underdosing of carbamazepine (T42.1-)

  - T42.6X **Poisoning by, adverse effect of and underdosing of other antiepileptic and sedative-hypnotic drugs**
    - T42.6X1 **Poisoning by other antiepileptic and sedative-hypnotic drugs, accidental (unintentional)**
      Poisoning by other antiepileptic and sedative-hypnotic drugs NOS
    - T42.6X2 **Poisoning by other antiepileptic and sedative-hypnotic drugs, intentional self-harm**

● T42.6X3   Poisoning by other antiepileptic and sedative-hypnotic drugs, assault

● T42.6X4   Poisoning by other antiepileptic and sedative-hypnotic drugs, undetermined

● T42.6X5   Adverse effect of other antiepileptic and sedative-hypnotic drugs

● T42.6X6   Underdosing of other antiepileptic and sedative-hypnotic drugs

● T42.7   Poisoning by, adverse effect of and underdosing of unspecified antiepileptic and sedative-hypnotic drugs

X ● T42.71   Poisoning by unspecified antiepileptic and sedative-hypnotic drugs, accidental (unintentional)

Poisoning by antiepileptic and sedative-hypnotic drugs NOS

X ● T42.72   Poisoning by unspecified antiepileptic and sedative-hypnotic drugs, intentional self-harm

X ● T42.73   Poisoning by unspecified antiepileptic and sedative-hypnotic drugs, assault

X ● T42.74   Poisoning by unspecified antiepileptic and sedative-hypnotic drugs, undetermined

X ● T42.75   Adverse effect of unspecified antiepileptic and sedative-hypnotic drugs

X ● T42.76   Underdosing of unspecified antiepileptic and sedative-hypnotic drugs

● T42.8   Poisoning by, adverse effect of and underdosing of antiparkinsonism drugs and other central muscle-tone depressants

Poisoning by, adverse effect of and underdosing of amantadine

● T42.8X   Poisoning by, adverse effect of and underdosing of antiparkinsonism drugs and other central muscle-tone depressants

● T42.8X1   Poisoning by antiparkinsonism drugs and other central muscle-tone depressants, accidental (unintentional)

Poisoning by antiparkinsonism drugs and other central muscle-tone depressants NOS

● T42.8X2   Poisoning by antiparkinsonism drugs and other central muscle-tone depressants, intentional self-harm

● T42.8X3   Poisoning by antiparkinsonism drugs and other central muscle-tone depressants, assault

● T42.8X4   Poisoning by antiparkinsonism drugs and other central muscle-tone depressants, undetermined

● T42.8X5   Adverse effect of antiparkinsonism drugs and other central muscle-tone depressants

● T42.8X6   Underdosing of antiparkinsonism drugs and other central muscle-tone depressants

● T43   Poisoning by, adverse effect of and underdosing of psychotropic drugs, not elsewhere classified

Excludes1   appetite depressants (T5Ø.5-)
barbiturates (T42.3-)
benzodiazepines (T42.4-)
methaqualone (T42.6-)
psychodysleptics [hallucinogens] (T4Ø.7-T4Ø.9-)

Excludes2   drug dependence and related mental and behavioral disorders due to psychoactive substance use (F1Ø.--F19.-)

The appropriate 7th character is to be added to each code from category T43

A	initial encounter
D	subsequent encounter
S	sequela

● T43.Ø   Poisoning by, adverse effect of and underdosing of tricyclic and tetracyclic antidepressants

● T43.Ø1   Poisoning by, adverse effect of and underdosing of tricyclic antidepressants

● T43.Ø11   Poisoning by tricyclic antidepressants, accidental (unintentional)

Poisoning by tricyclic antidepressants NOS

● T43.Ø12   Poisoning by tricyclic antidepressants, intentional self-harm

● T43.Ø13   Poisoning by tricyclic antidepressants, assault

● T43.Ø14   Poisoning by tricyclic antidepressants, undetermined

● T43.Ø15   Adverse effect of tricyclic antidepressants

● T43.Ø16   Underdosing of tricyclic antidepressants

● T43.Ø2   Poisoning by, adverse effect of and underdosing of tetracyclic antidepressants

● T43.Ø21   Poisoning by tetracyclic antidepressants, accidental (unintentional)

Poisoning by tetracyclic antidepressants NOS

● T43.Ø22   Poisoning by tetracyclic antidepressants, intentional self-harm

● T43.Ø23   Poisoning by tetracyclic antidepressants, assault

● T43.Ø24   Poisoning by tetracyclic antidepressants, undetermined

● T43.Ø25   Adverse effect of tetracyclic antidepressants

● T43.Ø26   Underdosing of tetracyclic antidepressants

CHAPTER 19 (SØØ-T88)

- **T43.1** Poisoning by, adverse effect of and underdosing of monoamine-oxidase-inhibitor antidepressants
  - **T43.1X** Poisoning by, adverse effect of and underdosing of monoamine-oxidase-inhibitor antidepressants
    - **T43.1X1** Poisoning by monoamine-oxidase-inhibitor antidepressants, accidental (unintentional)
      Poisoning by monoamine-oxidase-inhibitor antidepressants NOS
    - **T43.1X2** Poisoning by monoamine-oxidase-inhibitor antidepressants, intentional self-harm
    - **T43.1X3** Poisoning by monoamine-oxidase-inhibitor antidepressants, assault
    - **T43.1X4** Poisoning by monoamine-oxidase-inhibitor antidepressants, undetermined
    - **T43.1X5** Adverse effect of monoamine-oxidase-inhibitor antidepressants
    - **T43.1X6** Underdosing of monoamine-oxidase-inhibitor antidepressants
- **T43.2** Poisoning by, adverse effect of and underdosing of other and unspecified antidepressants
  - **T43.20** Poisoning by, adverse effect of and underdosing of unspecified antidepressants
    - **T43.201** Poisoning by unspecified antidepressants, accidental (unintentional)
      Poisoning by antidepressants NOS
    - **T43.202** Poisoning by unspecified antidepressants, intentional self-harm
    - **T43.203** Poisoning by unspecified antidepressants, assault
    - **T43.204** Poisoning by unspecified antidepressants, undetermined
    - **T43.205** Adverse effect of unspecified antidepressants
    - **T43.206** Underdosing of unspecified antidepressants
  - **T43.21** Poisoning by, adverse effect of and underdosing of selective serotonin and norepinephrine reuptake inhibitors
    Poisoning by, adverse effect of and underdosing of SSNRI antidepressants
    - **T43.211** Poisoning by selective serotonin and norepinephrine reuptake inhibitors, accidental (unintentional)
    - **T43.212** Poisoning by selective serotonin and norepinephrine reuptake inhibitors, intentional self-harm
    - **T43.213** Poisoning by selective serotonin and norepinephrine reuptake inhibitors, assault
    - **T43.214** Poisoning by selective serotonin and norepinephrine reuptake inhibitors, undetermined
    - **T43.215** Adverse effect of selective serotonin and norepinephrine reuptake inhibitors
    - **T43.216** Underdosing of selective serotonin and norepinephrine reuptake inhibitors
  - **T43.22** Poisoning by, adverse effect of and underdosing of selective serotonin reuptake inhibitors
    Poisoning by, adverse effect of and underdosing of SSRI antidepressants
    - **T43.221** Poisoning by selective serotonin reuptake inhibitors, accidental (unintentional)
    - **T43.222** Poisoning by selective serotonin reuptake inhibitors, intentional self-harm

- **T43.223** Poisoning by selective serotonin reuptake inhibitors, assault
- **T43.224** Poisoning by selective serotonin reuptake inhibitors, undetermined
- **T43.225** Adverse effect of selective serotonin reuptake inhibitors
- **T43.226** Underdosing of selective serotonin reuptake inhibitors
  - **T43.29** Poisoning by, adverse effect of and underdosing of other antidepressants
    - **T43.291** Poisoning by other antidepressants, accidental (unintentional)
      Poisoning by other antidepressants NOS
    - **T43.292** Poisoning by other antidepressants, intentional self-harm
    - **T43.293** Poisoning by other antidepressants, assault
    - **T43.294** Poisoning by other antidepressants, undetermined
    - **T43.295** Adverse effect of other antidepressants
    - **T43.296** Underdosing of other antidepressants
- **T43.3** Poisoning by, adverse effect of and underdosing of phenothiazine antipsychotics and neuroleptics
  - **T43.3X** Poisoning by, adverse effect of and underdosing of phenothiazine antipsychotics and neuroleptics
    - **T43.3X1** Poisoning by phenothiazine antipsychotics and neuroleptics, accidental (unintentional)
      Poisoning by phenothiazine antipsychotics and neuroleptics NOS
    - **T43.3X2** Poisoning by phenothiazine antipsychotics and neuroleptics, intentional self-harm
    - **T43.3X3** Poisoning by phenothiazine antipsychotics and neuroleptics, assault
    - **T43.3X4** Poisoning by phenothiazine antipsychotics and neuroleptics, undetermined
    - **T43.3X5** Adverse effect of phenothiazine antipsychotics and neuroleptics
    - **T43.3X6** Underdosing of phenothiazine antipsychotics and neuroleptics
- **T43.4** Poisoning by, adverse effect of and underdosing of butyrophenone and thiothixene neuroleptics
  - **T43.4X** Poisoning by, adverse effect of and underdosing of butyrophenone and thiothixene neuroleptics
    - **T43.4X1** Poisoning by butyrophenone and thiothixene neuroleptics, accidental (unintentional)
      Poisoning by butyrophenone and thiothixene neuroleptics NOS
    - **T43.4X2** Poisoning by butyrophenone and thiothixene neuroleptics, intentional self-harm
    - **T43.4X3** Poisoning by butyrophenone and thiothixene neuroleptics, assault
    - **T43.4X4** Poisoning by butyrophenone and thiothixene neuroleptics, undetermined
    - **T43.4X5** Adverse effect of butyrophenone and thiothixene neuroleptics
    - **T43.4X6** Underdosing of butyrophenone and thiothixene neuroleptics

◀ New   ◀═ Revised   ~~deleted~~ Deleted   Excludes 1   Excludes 2   Includes   Use additional   Code first   Code also   Unspecified
OGCR Official Guidelines   X Assign placeholder X   ● Use Additional Character(s)   ▶ Manifestation Code   **Coding Clinic**

● T43.5   **Poisoning by, adverse effect of and underdosing of other and unspecified antipsychotics and neuroleptics**

> **Excludes1**   poisoning by, adverse effect of and underdosing of rauwolfia (T46.5-)

   ● T43.50   **Poisoning by, adverse effect of and underdosing of unspecified antipsychotics and neuroleptics**

     ● T43.501   **Poisoning by unspecified antipsychotics and neuroleptics, accidental (unintentional)**
> Poisoning by antipsychotics and neuroleptics NOS

     ● T43.502   **Poisoning by unspecified antipsychotics and neuroleptics, intentional self-harm**

     ● T43.503   **Poisoning by unspecified antipsychotics and neuroleptics, assault**

     ● T43.504   **Poisoning by unspecified antipsychotics and neuroleptics, undetermined**

     ● T43.505   **Adverse effect of unspecified antipsychotics and neuroleptics**

     ● T43.506   **Underdosing of unspecified antipsychotics and neuroleptics**

   ● T43.59   **Poisoning by, adverse effect of and underdosing of other antipsychotics and neuroleptics**

     ● T43.591   **Poisoning by other antipsychotics and neuroleptics, accidental (unintentional)**
> Poisoning by other antipsychotics and neuroleptics NOS

     ● T43.592   **Poisoning by other antipsychotics and neuroleptics, intentional self-harm**

     ● T43.593   **Poisoning by other antipsychotics and neuroleptics, assault**

     ● T43.594   **Poisoning by other antipsychotics and neuroleptics, undetermined**

     ● T43.595   **Adverse effect of other antipsychotics and neuroleptics**

     ● T43.596   **Underdosing of other antipsychotics and neuroleptics**

● T43.6   **Poisoning by, adverse effect of and underdosing of psychostimulants**

> **Excludes1**   poisoning by, adverse effect of and underdosing of cocaine (T40.5-)

   ● T43.60   **Poisoning by, adverse effect of and underdosing of unspecified psychostimulant**

     ● T43.601   **Poisoning by unspecified psychostimulants, accidental (unintentional)**
> Poisoning by psychostimulants NOS

     ● T43.602   **Poisoning by unspecified psychostimulants, intentional self-harm**

     ● T43.603   **Poisoning by unspecified psychostimulants, assault**

     ● T43.604   **Poisoning by unspecified psychostimulants, undetermined**

     ● T43.605   **Adverse effect of unspecified psychostimulants**

     ● T43.606   **Underdosing of unspecified psychostimulants**

   ● T43.61   **Poisoning by, adverse effect of and underdosing of caffeine**

     ● T43.611   **Poisoning by caffeine, accidental (unintentional)**
> Poisoning by caffeine NOS

     ● T43.612   **Poisoning by caffeine, intentional self-harm**

     ● T43.613   **Poisoning by caffeine, assault**

     ● T43.614   **Poisoning by caffeine, undetermined**

     ● T43.615   **Adverse effect of caffeine**

     ● T43.616   **Underdosing of caffeine**

   ● T43.62   **Poisoning by, adverse effect of and underdosing of amphetamines**
> Poisoning by, adverse effect of and underdosing of methamphetamines

     ● T43.621   **Poisoning by amphetamines, accidental (unintentional)**
> Poisoning by amphetamines NOS

     ● T43.622   **Poisoning by amphetamines, intentional self-harm**

     ● T43.623   **Poisoning by amphetamines, assault**

     ● T43.624   **Poisoning by amphetamines, undetermined**

     ● T43.625   **Adverse effect of amphetamines**

     ● T43.626   **Underdosing of amphetamines**

   ● T43.63   **Poisoning by, adverse effect of and underdosing of methylphenidate**

     ● T43.631   **Poisoning by methylphenidate, accidental (unintentional)**
> Poisoning by methylphenidate NOS

     ● T43.632   **Poisoning by methylphenidate, intentional self-harm**

     ● T43.633   **Poisoning by methylphenidate, assault**

     ● T43.634   **Poisoning by methylphenidate, undetermined**

     ● T43.635   **Adverse effect of methylphenidate**

     ● T43.636   **Underdosing of methylphenidate**

   ● T43.69   **Poisoning by, adverse effect of and underdosing of other psychostimulants**

     ● T43.691   **Poisoning by other psychostimulants, accidental (unintentional)**
> Poisoning by other psychostimulants NOS

     ● T43.692   **Poisoning by other psychostimulants, intentional self-harm**

     ● T43.693   **Poisoning by other psychostimulants, assault**

     ● T43.694   **Poisoning by other psychostimulants, undetermined**

     ● T43.695   **Adverse effect of other psychostimulants**

     ● T43.696   **Underdosing of other psychostimulants**

● T43.8   **Poisoning by, adverse effect of and underdosing of other psychotropic drugs**

   ● T43.8X   **Poisoning by, adverse effect of and underdosing of other psychotropic drugs**

     ● T43.8X1   **Poisoning by other psychotropic drugs, accidental (unintentional)**
> Poisoning by other psychotropic drugs NOS

     ● T43.8X2   **Poisoning by other psychotropic drugs, intentional self-harm**

     ● T43.8X3   **Poisoning by other psychotropic drugs, assault**

     ● T43.8X4   **Poisoning by other psychotropic drugs, undetermined**

     ● T43.8X5   **Adverse effect of other psychotropic drugs**

     ● T43.8X6   **Underdosing of other psychotropic drugs**

CHAPTER 19 (S00-T88)

● T43.9   Poisoning by, adverse effect of and underdosing of unspecified psychotropic drug

   X ● T43.91   Poisoning by unspecified psychotropic drug, accidental (unintentional)
       Poisoning by psychotropic drug NOS

   X ● T43.92   Poisoning by unspecified psychotropic drug, intentional self-harm

   X ● T43.93   Poisoning by unspecified psychotropic drug, assault

   X ● T43.94   Poisoning by unspecified psychotropic drug, undetermined

   X ● T43.95   Adverse effect of unspecified psychotropic drug

   X ● T43.96   Underdosing of unspecified psychotropic drug

● T44   Poisoning by, adverse effect of and underdosing of drugs primarily affecting the autonomic nervous system

   The appropriate 7th character is to be added to each code from category T44

> A   initial encounter
> D   subsequent encounter
> S   sequela

● T44.0   Poisoning by, adverse effect of and underdosing of anticholinesterase agents

   ● T44.0X   Poisoning by, adverse effect of and underdosing of anticholinesterase agents

     ● T44.0X1   Poisoning by anticholinesterase agents, accidental (unintentional)
       Poisoning by anticholinesterase agents NOS

     ● T44.0X2   Poisoning by anticholinesterase agents, intentional self-harm

     ● T44.0X3   Poisoning by anticholinesterase agents, assault

     ● T44.0X4   Poisoning by anticholinesterase agents, undetermined

     ● T44.0X5   Adverse effect of anticholinesterase agents

     ● T44.0X6   Underdosing of anticholinesterase agents

● T44.1   Poisoning by, adverse effect of and underdosing of other parasympathomimetics [cholinergics]

   ● T44.1X   Poisoning by, adverse effect of and underdosing of other parasympathomimetics [cholinergics]

     ● T44.1X1   Poisoning by other parasympathomimetics [cholinergics], accidental (unintentional)
       Poisoning by other parasympathomimetics [cholinergics] NOS

     ● T44.1X2   Poisoning by other parasympathomimetics [cholinergics], intentional self-harm

     ● T44.1X3   Poisoning by other parasympathomimetics [cholinergics], assault

     ● T44.1X4   Poisoning by other parasympathomimetics [cholinergics], undetermined

     ● T44.1X5   Adverse effect of other parasympathomimetics [cholinergics]

     ● T44.1X6   Underdosing of other parasympathomimetics

● T44.2   Poisoning by, adverse effect of and underdosing of ganglionic blocking drugs

   ● T44.2X   Poisoning by, adverse effect of and underdosing of ganglionic blocking drugs

     ● T44.2X1   Poisoning by ganglionic blocking drugs, accidental (unintentional)
       Poisoning by ganglionic blocking drugs NOS

     ● T44.2X2   Poisoning by ganglionic blocking drugs, intentional self-harm

     ● T44.2X3   Poisoning by ganglionic blocking drugs, assault

     ● T44.2X4   Poisoning by ganglionic blocking drugs, undetermined

     ● T44.2X5   Adverse effect of ganglionic blocking drugs

     ● T44.2X6   Underdosing of ganglionic blocking drugs

● T44.3   Poisoning by, adverse effect of and underdosing of other parasympatholytics [anticholinergics and antimuscarinics] and spasmolytics
   Poisoning by, adverse effect of and underdosing of papaverine

   ● T44.3X   Poisoning by, adverse effect of and underdosing of other parasympatholytics [anticholinergics and antimuscarinics] and spasmolytics

     ● T44.3X1   Poisoning by other parasympatholytics [anticholinergics and antimuscarinics] and spasmolytics, accidental (unintentional)
       Poisoning by other parasympatholytics [anticholinergics and antimuscarinics] and spasmolytics NOS

     ● T44.3X2   Poisoning by other parasympatholytics [anticholinergics and antimuscarinics] and spasmolytics, intentional self-harm

     ● T44.3X3   Poisoning by other parasympatholytics [anticholinergics and antimuscarinics] and spasmolytics, assault

     ● T44.3X4   Poisoning by other parasympatholytics [anticholinergics and antimuscarinics] and spasmolytics, undetermined

     ● T44.3X5   Adverse effect of other parasympatholytics [anticholinergics and antimuscarinics] and spasmolytics

     ● T44.3X6   Underdosing of other parasympatholytics [anticholinergics and antimuscarinics] and spasmolytics

● T44.4   Poisoning by, adverse effect of and underdosing of predominantly alpha-adrenoreceptor agonists
   Poisoning by, adverse effect of and underdosing of metaraminol

   ● T44.4X   Poisoning by, adverse effect of and underdosing of predominantly alpha-adrenoreceptor agonists

     ● T44.4X1   Poisoning by predominantly alpha-adrenoreceptor agonists, accidental (unintentional)
       Poisoning by predominantly alpha-adrenoreceptor agonists NOS

     ● T44.4X2   Poisoning by predominantly alpha-adrenoreceptor agonists, intentional self-harm

     ● T44.4X3   Poisoning by predominantly alpha-adrenoreceptor agonists, assault

     ● T44.4X4   Poisoning by predominantly alpha-adrenoreceptor agonists, undetermined

     ● T44.4X5   Adverse effect of predominantly alpha-adrenoreceptor agonists

     ● T44.4X6   Underdosing of predominantly alpha-adrenoreceptor agonists

● T44.5 **Poisoning by, adverse effect of and underdosing of predominantly beta-adrenoreceptor agonists**

Excludes1 poisoning by, adverse effect of and underdosing of beta-adrenoreceptor agonists used in asthma therapy (T48.6-)

● T44.5X **Poisoning by, adverse effect of and underdosing of predominantly beta-adrenoreceptor agonists**

● T44.5X1 **Poisoning by predominantly beta-adrenoreceptor agonists, accidental (unintentional)**
Poisoning by predominantly beta-adrenoreceptor agonists NOS

● T44.5X2 **Poisoning by predominantly beta-adrenoreceptor agonists, intentional self-harm**

● T44.5X3 **Poisoning by predominantly beta-adrenoreceptor agonists, assault**

● T44.5X4 **Poisoning by predominantly beta-adrenoreceptor agonists, undetermined**

● T44.5X5 **Adverse effect of predominantly beta-adrenoreceptor agonists**

● T44.5X6 **Underdosing of predominantly beta-adrenoreceptor agonists**

● T44.6 **Poisoning by, adverse effect of and underdosing of alpha-adrenoreceptor antagonists**

Excludes1 poisoning by, adverse effect of and underdosing of ergot alkaloids (T48.0)

● T44.6X **Poisoning by, adverse effect of and underdosing of alpha-adrenoreceptor antagonists**

● T44.6X1 **Poisoning by alpha-adrenoreceptor antagonists, accidental (unintentional)**
Poisoning by alpha-adrenoreceptor antagonists NOS

● T44.6X2 **Poisoning by alpha-adrenoreceptor antagonists, intentional self-harm**

● T44.6X3 **Poisoning by alpha-adrenoreceptor antagonists, assault**

● T44.6X4 **Poisoning by alpha-adrenoreceptor antagonists, undetermined**

● T44.6X5 **Adverse effect of alpha-adrenoreceptor antagonists**

● T44.6X6 **Underdosing of alpha-adrenoreceptor antagonists**

● T44.7 **Poisoning by, adverse effect of and underdosing of beta-adrenoreceptor antagonists**

● T44.7X **Poisoning by, adverse effect of and underdosing of beta-adrenoreceptor antagonists**

● T44.7X1 **Poisoning by beta-adrenoreceptor antagonists, accidental (unintentional)**
Poisoning by beta-adrenoreceptor antagonists NOS

● T44.7X2 **Poisoning by beta-adrenoreceptor antagonists, intentional self-harm**

● T44.7X3 **Poisoning by beta-adrenoreceptor antagonists, assault**

● T44.7X4 **Poisoning by beta-adrenoreceptor antagonists, undetermined**

● T44.7X5 **Adverse effect of beta-adrenoreceptor antagonists**

● T44.7X6 **Underdosing of beta-adrenoreceptor antagonists**

● T44.8 **Poisoning by, adverse effect of and underdosing of centrally-acting and adrenergic-neuron-blocking agents**

Excludes1 poisoning by, adverse effect of and underdosing of clonidine (T46.5)
poisoning by, adverse effect of and underdosing of guanethidine (T46.5)

● T44.8X **Poisoning by, adverse effect of and underdosing of centrally-acting and adrenergic-neuron-blocking agents**

● T44.8X1 **Poisoning by centrally-acting and adrenergic-neuron-blocking agents, accidental (unintentional)**
Poisoning by centrally-acting and adrenergic-neuron-blocking agents NOS

● T44.8X2 **Poisoning by centrally-acting and adrenergic-neuron-blocking agents, intentional self-harm**

● T44.8X3 **Poisoning by centrally-acting and adrenergic-neuron-blocking agents, assault**

● T44.8X4 **Poisoning by centrally-acting and adrenergic-neuron-blocking agents, undetermined**

● T44.8X5 **Adverse effect of centrally-acting and adrenergic-neuron-blocking agents**

● T44.8X6 **Underdosing of centrally-acting and adrenergic-neuron-blocking agents**

● T44.9 **Poisoning by, adverse effect of and underdosing of other and unspecified drugs primarily affecting the autonomic nervous system**
Poisoning by, adverse effect of and underdosing of drug stimulating both alpha and beta-adrenoreceptors

● T44.90 **Poisoning by, adverse effect of and underdosing of unspecified drugs primarily affecting the autonomic nervous system**

● T44.901 **Poisoning by unspecified drugs primarily affecting the autonomic nervous system, accidental (unintentional)**
Poisoning by unspecified drugs primarily affecting the autonomic nervous system NOS

● T44.902 **Poisoning by unspecified drugs primarily affecting the autonomic nervous system, intentional self-harm**

● T44.903 **Poisoning by unspecified drugs primarily affecting the autonomic nervous system, assault**

● T44.904 **Poisoning by unspecified drugs primarily affecting the autonomic nervous system, undetermined**

● T44.905 **Adverse effect of unspecified drugs primarily affecting the autonomic nervous system**

● T44.906 **Underdosing of unspecified drugs primarily affecting the autonomic nervous system**

CHAPTER 19 (S00-T88)

● T44.99 Poisoning by, adverse effect of and underdosing of other drugs primarily affecting the autonomic nervous system

  ● T44.991 Poisoning by other drug primarily affecting the autonomic nervous system, accidental (unintentional)
    Poisoning by other drugs primarily affecting the autonomic nervous system NOS

  ● T44.992 Poisoning by other drug primarily affecting the autonomic nervous system, intentional self-harm

  ● T44.993 Poisoning by other drug primarily affecting the autonomic nervous system, assault

  ● T44.994 Poisoning by other drug primarily affecting the autonomic nervous system, undetermined

  ● T44.995 Adverse effect of other drug primarily affecting the autonomic nervous system

  ● T44.996 Underdosing of other drug primarily affecting the autonomic nervous system

● T45 Poisoning by, adverse effect of and underdosing of primarily systemic and hematological agents, not elsewhere classified

The appropriate 7th character is to be added to each code from category T45

> A initial encounter
> D subsequent encounter
> S sequela

● T45.0 Poisoning by, adverse effect of and underdosing of antiallergic and antiemetic drugs

  Excludes1 poisoning by, adverse effect of and underdosing of phenothiazine-based neuroleptics (T43.3)

  ● T45.0X Poisoning by, adverse effect of and underdosing of antiallergic and antiemetic drugs

    ● T45.0X1 Poisoning by antiallergic and antiemetic drugs, accidental (unintentional)
      Poisoning by antiallergic and antiemetic drugs NOS

    ● T45.0X2 Poisoning by antiallergic and antiemetic drugs, intentional self-harm

    ● T45.0X3 Poisoning by antiallergic and antiemetic drugs, assault

    ● T45.0X4 Poisoning by antiallergic and antiemetic drugs, undetermined

    ● T45.0X5 Adverse effect of antiallergic and antiemetic drugs

    ● T45.0X6 Underdosing of antiallergic and antiemetic drugs

● T45.1 Poisoning by, adverse effect of and underdosing of antineoplastic and immunosuppressive drugs

  Excludes1 poisoning by, adverse effect of and underdosing of tamoxifen (T38.6)

  ● T45.1X Poisoning by, adverse effect of and underdosing of antineoplastic and immunosuppressive drugs

    ● T45.1X1 Poisoning by antineoplastic and immunosuppressive drugs, accidental (unintentional)
      Poisoning by antineoplastic and immunosuppressive drugs NOS

    ● T45.1X2 Poisoning by antineoplastic and immunosuppressive drugs, intentional self-harm

    ● T45.1X3 Poisoning by antineoplastic and immunosuppressive drugs, assault

    ● T45.1X4 Poisoning by antineoplastic and immunosuppressive drugs, undetermined

    ● T45.1X5 Adverse effect of antineoplastic and immunosuppressive drugs

    ● T45.1X6 Underdosing of antineoplastic and immunosuppressive drugs

● T45.2 Poisoning by, adverse effect of and underdosing of vitamins

  Excludes2 poisoning by, adverse effect of and underdosing of nicotinic acid (derivatives) (T46.7)
    poisoning by, adverse effect of and underdosing of iron (T45.4)
    poisoning by, adverse effect of and underdosing of vitamin K (T45.7)

  ● T45.2X Poisoning by, adverse effect of and underdosing of vitamins

    ● T45.2X1 Poisoning by vitamins, accidental (unintentional)
      Poisoning by vitamins NOS

    ● T45.2X2 Poisoning by vitamins, intentional self-harm

    ● T45.2X3 Poisoning by vitamins, assault

    ● T45.2X4 Poisoning by vitamins, undetermined

    ● T45.2X5 Adverse effect of vitamins

    ● T45.2X6 Underdosing of vitamins

      Excludes1 vitamin deficiencies (E50-E56)

● T45.3 Poisoning by, adverse effect of and underdosing of enzymes

  ● T45.3X Poisoning by, adverse effect of and underdosing of enzymes

    ● T45.3X1 Poisoning by enzymes, accidental (unintentional)
      Poisoning by enzymes NOS

    ● T45.3X2 Poisoning by enzymes, intentional self-harm

    ● T45.3X3 Poisoning by enzymes, assault

    ● T45.3X4 Poisoning by enzymes, undetermined

    ● T45.3X5 Adverse effect of enzymes

    ● T45.3X6 Underdosing of enzymes

● T45.4 Poisoning by, adverse effect of and underdosing of iron and its compounds

  ● T45.4X Poisoning by, adverse effect of and underdosing of iron and its compounds

    ● T45.4X1 Poisoning by iron and its compounds, accidental (unintentional)
      Poisoning by iron and its compounds NOS

    ● T45.4X2 Poisoning by iron and its compounds, intentional self-harm

    ● T45.4X3 Poisoning by iron and its compounds, assault

    ● T45.4X4 Poisoning by iron and its compounds, undetermined

    ● T45.4X5 Adverse effect of iron and its compounds

    ● T45.4X6 Underdosing of iron and its compounds

      Excludes1 iron deficiency (E61.1)

●T45.5   Poisoning by, adverse effect of and underdosing of anticoagulants and antithrombotic drugs

     ●T45.51   Poisoning by, adverse effect of and underdosing of anticoagulants

         ●T45.511   Poisoning by anticoagulants, accidental (unintentional)
             Poisoning by anticoagulants NOS

         ●T45.512   Poisoning by anticoagulants, intentional self-harm

         ●T45.513   Poisoning by anticoagulants, assault

         ●T45.514   Poisoning by anticoagulants, undetermined

         ●T45.515   Adverse effect of anticoagulants
             Coding Clinic: 2016, Q1, P14; 2013, Q2, P35

         ●T45.516   Underdosing of anticoagulants

     ●T45.52   Poisoning by, adverse effect of and underdosing of antithrombotic drugs
         Poisoning by, adverse effect of and underdosing of antiplatelet drugs

         Excludes2   poisoning by, adverse effect of and underdosing of aspirin (T39.01-)
             poisoning by, adverse effect of and underdosing of acetylsalicylic acid (T39.01-)

         ●T45.521   Poisoning by antithrombotic drugs, accidental (unintentional)
             Poisoning by antithrombotic drug NOS

         ●T45.522   Poisoning by antithrombotic drugs, intentional self-harm

         ●T45.523   Poisoning by antithrombotic drugs, assault

         ●T45.524   Poisoning by antithrombotic drugs, undetermined

         ●T45.525   Adverse effect of antithrombotic drugs
             Coding Clinic: 2016, Q1, P15

         ●T45.526   Underdosing of antithrombotic drugs

●T45.6   Poisoning by, adverse effect of and underdosing of fibrinolysis-affecting drugs

     ●T45.60   Poisoning by, adverse effect of and underdosing of unspecified fibrinolysis-affecting drugs

         ●T45.601   Poisoning by unspecified fibrinolysis-affecting drugs, accidental (unintentional)
             Poisoning by fibrinolysis-affecting drug NOS

         ●T45.602   Poisoning by unspecified fibrinolysis-affecting drugs, intentional self-harm

         ●T45.603   Poisoning by unspecified fibrinolysis-affecting drugs, assault

         ●T45.604   Poisoning by unspecified fibrinolysis-affecting drugs, undetermined

         ●T45.605   Adverse effect of unspecified fibrinolysis-affecting drugs

         ●T45.606   Underdosing of unspecified fibrinolysis-affecting drugs

     ●T45.61   Poisoning by, adverse effect of and underdosing of thrombolytic drugs

         ●T45.611   Poisoning by thrombolytic drug, accidental (unintentional)
             Poisoning by thrombolytic drug NOS

         ●T45.612   Poisoning by thrombolytic drug, intentional self-harm

         ●T45.613   Poisoning by thrombolytic drug, assault

         ●T45.614   Poisoning by thrombolytic drug, undetermined

         ●T45.615   Adverse effect of thrombolytic drugs

         ●T45.616   Underdosing of thrombolytic drugs

     ●T45.62   Poisoning by, adverse effect of and underdosing of hemostatic drugs

         ●T45.621   Poisoning by hemostatic drug, accidental (unintentional)
             Poisoning by hemostatic drug NOS

         ●T45.622   Poisoning by hemostatic drug, intentional self-harm

         ●T45.623   Poisoning by hemostatic drug, assault

         ●T45.624   Poisoning by hemostatic drug, undetermined

         ●T45.625   Adverse effect of hemostatic drug

         ●T45.626   Underdosing of hemostatic drugs

     ●T45.69   Poisoning by, adverse effect of and underdosing of other fibrinolysis-affecting drugs

         ●T45.691   Poisoning by other fibrinolysis-affecting drugs, accidental (unintentional)
             Poisoning by other fibrinolysis-affecting drug NOS

         ●T45.692   Poisoning by other fibrinolysis-affecting drugs, intentional self-harm

         ●T45.693   Poisoning by other fibrinolysis-affecting drugs, assault

         ●T45.694   Poisoning by other fibrinolysis-affecting drugs, undetermined

         ●T45.695   Adverse effect of other fibrinolysis-affecting drugs

         ●T45.696   Underdosing of other fibrinolysis-affecting drugs

●T45.7   Poisoning by, adverse effect of and underdosing of anticoagulant antagonists, vitamin K and other coagulants

     ●T45.7X   Poisoning by, adverse effect of and underdosing of anticoagulant antagonists, vitamin K and other coagulants

         ●T45.7X1   Poisoning by anticoagulant antagonists, vitamin K and other coagulants, accidental (unintentional)
             Poisoning by anticoagulant antagonists, vitamin K and other coagulants NOS

         ●T45.7X2   Poisoning by anticoagulant antagonists, vitamin K and other coagulants, intentional self-harm

         ●T45.7X3   Poisoning by anticoagulant antagonists, vitamin K and other coagulants, assault

         ●T45.7X4   Poisoning by anticoagulant antagonists, vitamin K and other coagulants, undetermined

         ●T45.7X5   Adverse effect of anticoagulant antagonists, vitamin K and other coagulants

         ●T45.7X6   Underdosing of anticoagulant antagonist, vitamin K and other coagulants

             Excludes1   vitamin K deficiency (E56.1)

● **T45.8** **Poisoning by, adverse effect of and underdosing of other primarily systemic and hematological agents**
Poisoning by, adverse effect of and underdosing of liver preparations and other antianemic agents
Poisoning by, adverse effect of and underdosing of natural blood and blood products
Poisoning by, adverse effect of and underdosing of plasma substitute

> **Excludes2**   poisoning by, adverse effect of and underdosing of immunoglobulin (T50.Z1)
> poisoning by, adverse effect of and underdosing of iron (T45.4)
> transfusion reactions (T80.-)

● **T45.8X** **Poisoning by, adverse effect of and underdosing of other primarily systemic and hematological agents**

● **T45.8X1** **Poisoning by other primarily systemic and hematological agents, accidental (unintentional)**
Poisoning by other primarily systemic and hematological agents NOS

● **T45.8X2** **Poisoning by other primarily systemic and hematological agents, intentional self-harm**

● **T45.8X3** **Poisoning by other primarily systemic and hematological agents, assault**

● **T45.8X4** **Poisoning by other primarily systemic and hematological agents, undetermined**

● **T45.8X5** **Adverse effect of other primarily systemic and hematological agents**

● **T45.8X6** **Underdosing of other primarily systemic and hematological agents**

● **T45.9** **Poisoning by, adverse effect of and underdosing of unspecified primarily systemic and hematological agent**

X ● **T45.91** **Poisoning by unspecified primarily systemic and hematological agent, accidental (unintentional)**
Poisoning by primarily systemic and hematological agent NOS

X ● **T45.92** **Poisoning by unspecified primarily systemic and hematological agent, intentional self-harm**

X ● **T45.93** **Poisoning by unspecified primarily systemic and hematological agent, assault**

X ● **T45.94** **Poisoning by unspecified primarily systemic and hematological agent, undetermined**

X ● **T45.95** **Adverse effect of unspecified primarily systemic and hematological agent**

X ● **T45.96** **Underdosing of unspecified primarily systemic and hematological agent**

● **T46** **Poisoning by, adverse effect of and underdosing of agents primarily affecting the cardiovascular system**

> **Excludes1**   poisoning by, adverse effect of and underdosing of metaraminol (T44.4)

The appropriate 7th character is to be added to each code from category T46

A	initial encounter
D	subsequent encounter
S	sequela

● **T46.0** **Poisoning by, adverse effect of and underdosing of cardiac-stimulant glycosides and drugs of similar action**

● **T46.0X** **Poisoning by, adverse effect of and underdosing of cardiac-stimulant glycosides and drugs of similar action**

● **T46.0X1** **Poisoning by cardiac-stimulant glycosides and drugs of similar action, accidental (unintentional)**
Poisoning by cardiac-stimulant glycosides and drugs of similar action NOS

● **T46.0X2** **Poisoning by cardiac-stimulant glycosides and drugs of similar action, intentional self-harm**

● **T46.0X3** **Poisoning by cardiac-stimulant glycosides and drugs of similar action, assault**

● **T46.0X4** **Poisoning by cardiac-stimulant glycosides and drugs of similar action, undetermined**

● **T46.0X5** **Adverse effect of cardiac-stimulant glycosides and drugs of similar action**

● **T46.0X6** **Underdosing of cardiac-stimulant glycosides and drugs of similar action**

● **T46.1** **Poisoning by, adverse effect of and underdosing of calcium-channel blockers**

● **T46.1X** **Poisoning by, adverse effect of and underdosing of calcium-channel blockers**

● **T46.1X1** **Poisoning by calcium-channel blockers, accidental (unintentional)**
Poisoning by calcium-channel blockers NOS

● **T46.1X2** **Poisoning by calcium-channel blockers, intentional self-harm**

● **T46.1X3** **Poisoning by calcium-channel blockers, assault**

● **T46.1X4** **Poisoning by calcium-channel blockers, undetermined**

● **T46.1X5** **Adverse effect of calcium-channel blockers**

● **T46.1X6** **Underdosing of calcium-channel blockers**

● **T46.2** **Poisoning by, adverse effect of and underdosing of other antidysrhythmic drugs, not elsewhere classified**

> **Excludes1**   poisoning by, adverse effect of and underdosing of beta-adrenoreceptor antagonists (T44.7-)

● **T46.2X** **Poisoning by, adverse effect of and underdosing of other antidysrhythmic drugs**

● **T46.2X1** **Poisoning by other antidysrhythmic drugs, accidental (unintentional)**
Poisoning by other antidysrhythmic drugs NOS

● **T46.2X2** **Poisoning by other antidysrhythmic drugs, intentional self-harm**

● **T46.2X3** **Poisoning by other antidysrhythmic drugs, assault**

● **T46.2X4** **Poisoning by other antidysrhythmic drugs, undetermined**

● **T46.2X5** **Adverse effect of other antidysrhythmic drugs**

● **T46.2X6** **Underdosing of other antidysrhythmic drugs**

● **T46.3** **Poisoning by, adverse effect of and underdosing of coronary vasodilators**
Poisoning by, adverse effect of and underdosing of dipyridamole

> **Excludes1**   poisoning by, adverse effect of and underdosing of calcium-channel blockers (T46.1)

● **T46.3X** **Poisoning by, adverse effect of and underdosing of coronary vasodilators**

● **T46.3X1** **Poisoning by coronary vasodilators, accidental (unintentional)**
Poisoning by coronary vasodilators NOS

● **T46.3X2** **Poisoning by coronary vasodilators, intentional self-harm**

● **T46.3X3** **Poisoning by coronary vasodilators, assault**

● T46.3X4   Poisoning by coronary vasodilators, undetermined

● T46.3X5   Adverse effect of coronary vasodilators

● T46.3X6   Underdosing of coronary vasodilators

● T46.4   Poisoning by, adverse effect of and underdosing of angiotensin-converting-enzyme inhibitors

   ● T46.4X   Poisoning by, adverse effect of and underdosing of angiotensin-converting-enzyme inhibitors

      ● T46.4X1   Poisoning by angiotensin-converting-enzyme inhibitors, accidental (unintentional)
         Poisoning by angiotensin-converting-enzyme inhibitors NOS

      ● T46.4X2   Poisoning by angiotensin-converting-enzyme inhibitors, intentional self-harm

      ● T46.4X3   Poisoning by angiotensin-converting-enzyme inhibitors, assault

      ● T46.4X4   Poisoning by angiotensin-converting-enzyme inhibitors, undetermined

      ● T46.4X5   Adverse effect of angiotensin-converting-enzyme inhibitors

      ● T46.4X6   Underdosing of angiotensin-converting-enzyme inhibitors

● T46.5   Poisoning by, adverse effect of and underdosing of other antihypertensive drugs

   Excludes2   poisoning by, adverse effect of and underdosing of beta-adrenoreceptor antagonists (T44.7)
      poisoning by, adverse effect of and underdosing of calcium-channel blockers (T46.1)
      poisoning by, adverse effect of and underdosing of diuretics (T50.0-T50.2)

   ● T46.5X   Poisoning by, adverse effect of and underdosing of other antihypertensive drugs

      ● T46.5X1   Poisoning by other antihypertensive drugs, accidental (unintentional)
         Poisoning by other antihypertensive drugs NOS

      ● T46.5X2   Poisoning by other antihypertensive drugs, intentional self-harm

      ● T46.5X3   Poisoning by other antihypertensive drugs, assault

      ● T46.5X4   Poisoning by other antihypertensive drugs, undetermined

      ● T46.5X5   Adverse effect of other antihypertensive drugs

      ● T46.5X6   Underdosing of other antihypertensive drugs

● T46.6   Poisoning by, adverse effect of and underdosing of antihyperlipidemic and antiarteriosclerotic drugs

   ● T46.6X   Poisoning by, adverse effect of and underdosing of antihyperlipidemic and antiarteriosclerotic drugs

      ● T46.6X1   Poisoning by antihyperlipidemic and antiarteriosclerotic drugs, accidental (unintentional)
         Poisoning by antihyperlipidemic and antiarteriosclerotic drugs NOS

      ● T46.6X2   Poisoning by antihyperlipidemic and antiarteriosclerotic drugs, intentional self-harm

      ● T46.6X3   Poisoning by antihyperlipidemic and antiarteriosclerotic drugs, assault

      ● T46.6X4   Poisoning by antihyperlipidemic and antiarteriosclerotic drugs, undetermined

● T46.6X5   Adverse effect of antihyperlipidemic and antiarteriosclerotic drugs

● T46.6X6   Underdosing of antihyperlipidemic and antiarteriosclerotic drugs

● T46.7   Poisoning by, adverse effect of and underdosing of peripheral vasodilators
   Poisoning by, adverse effect of and underdosing of nicotinic acid (derivatives)
   Excludes1   poisoning by, adverse effect of and underdosing of papaverine (T44.3)

   ● T46.7X   Poisoning by, adverse effect of and underdosing of peripheral vasodilators

      ● T46.7X1   Poisoning by peripheral vasodilators, accidental (unintentional)
         Poisoning by peripheral vasodilators NOS

      ● T46.7X2   Poisoning by peripheral vasodilators, intentional self-harm

      ● T46.7X3   Poisoning by peripheral vasodilators, assault

      ● T46.7X4   Poisoning by peripheral vasodilators, undetermined

      ● T46.7X5   Adverse effect of peripheral vasodilators

      ● T46.7X6   Underdosing of peripheral vasodilators

● T46.8   Poisoning by, adverse effect of and underdosing of antivaricose drugs, including sclerosing agents

   ● T46.8X   Poisoning by, adverse effect of and underdosing of antivaricose drugs, including sclerosing agents

      ● T46.8X1   Poisoning by antivaricose drugs, including sclerosing agents, accidental (unintentional)
         Poisoning by antivaricose drugs, including sclerosing agents NOS

      ● T46.8X2   Poisoning by antivaricose drugs, including sclerosing agents, intentional self-harm

      ● T46.8X3   Poisoning by antivaricose drugs, including sclerosing agents, assault

      ● T46.8X4   Poisoning by antivaricose drugs, including sclerosing agents, undetermined

      ● T46.8X5   Adverse effect of antivaricose drugs, including sclerosing agents

      ● T46.8X6   Underdosing of antivaricose drugs, including sclerosing agents

● T46.9   Poisoning by, adverse effect of and underdosing of other and unspecified agents primarily affecting the cardiovascular system

   ● T46.90   Poisoning by, adverse effect of and underdosing of unspecified agents primarily affecting the cardiovascular system

      ● T46.901   Poisoning by unspecified agents primarily affecting the cardiovascular system, accidental (unintentional)

      ● T46.902   Poisoning by unspecified agents primarily affecting the cardiovascular system, intentional self-harm

      ● T46.903   Poisoning by unspecified agents primarily affecting the cardiovascular system, assault

      ● T46.904   Poisoning by unspecified agents primarily affecting the cardiovascular system, undetermined

      ● T46.905   Adverse effect of unspecified agents primarily affecting the cardiovascular system

      ● T46.906   Underdosing of unspecified agents primarily affecting the cardiovascular system

CHAPTER 19 (S00-T88)

● **T46.99** Poisoning by, adverse effect of and underdosing of other agents primarily affecting the cardiovascular system

   ● **T46.991** Poisoning by other agents primarily affecting the cardiovascular system, accidental (unintentional)

   ● **T46.992** Poisoning by other agents primarily affecting the cardiovascular system, intentional self-harm

   ● **T46.993** Poisoning by other agents primarily affecting the cardiovascular system, assault

   ● **T46.994** Poisoning by other agents primarily affecting the cardiovascular system, undetermined

   ● **T46.995** Adverse effect of other agents primarily affecting the cardiovascular system

   ● **T46.996** Underdosing of other agents primarily affecting the cardiovascular system

● **T47** Poisoning by, adverse effect of and underdosing of agents primarily affecting the gastrointestinal system

The appropriate 7th character is to be added to each code from category T47

> A   initial encounter
> D   subsequent encounter
> S   sequela

● **T47.0** Poisoning by, adverse effect of and underdosing of histamine H2-receptor blockers

  ● **T47.0X** Poisoning by, adverse effect of and underdosing of histamine H2-receptor blockers

   ● **T47.0X1** Poisoning by histamine H2-receptor blockers, accidental (unintentional)
       Poisoning by histamine H2-receptor blockers NOS

   ● **T47.0X2** Poisoning by histamine H2-receptor blockers, intentional self-harm

   ● **T47.0X3** Poisoning by histamine H2-receptor blockers, assault

   ● **T47.0X4** Poisoning by histamine H2-receptor blockers, undetermined

   ● **T47.0X5** Adverse effect of histamine H2-receptor blockers

   ● **T47.0X6** Underdosing of histamine H2-receptor blockers

● **T47.1** Poisoning by, adverse effect of and underdosing of other antacids and anti-gastric-secretion drugs

  ● **T47.1X** Poisoning by, adverse effect of and underdosing of other antacids and anti-gastric-secretion drugs

   ● **T47.1X1** Poisoning by other antacids and anti-gastric-secretion drugs, accidental (unintentional)
       Poisoning by other antacids and anti-gastric-secretion drugs NOS

   ● **T47.1X2** Poisoning by other antacids and anti-gastric-secretion drugs, intentional self-harm

   ● **T47.1X3** Poisoning by other antacids and anti-gastric-secretion drugs, assault

   ● **T47.1X4** Poisoning by other antacids and anti-gastric-secretion drugs, undetermined

   ● **T47.1X5** Adverse effect of other antacids and anti-gastric-secretion drugs

   ● **T47.1X6** Underdosing of other antacids and anti-gastric-secretion drugs

● **T47.2** Poisoning by, adverse effect of and underdosing of stimulant laxatives

  ● **T47.2X** Poisoning by, adverse effect of and underdosing of stimulant laxatives

   ● **T47.2X1** Poisoning by stimulant laxatives, accidental (unintentional)
       Poisoning by stimulant laxatives NOS

   ● **T47.2X2** Poisoning by stimulant laxatives, intentional self-harm

   ● **T47.2X3** Poisoning by stimulant laxatives, assault

   ● **T47.2X4** Poisoning by stimulant laxatives, undetermined

   ● **T47.2X5** Adverse effect of stimulant laxatives

   ● **T47.2X6** Underdosing of stimulant laxatives

● **T47.3** Poisoning by, adverse effect of and underdosing of saline and osmotic laxatives

  ● **T47.3X** Poisoning by and adverse effect of saline and osmotic laxatives

   ● **T47.3X1** Poisoning by saline and osmotic laxatives, accidental (unintentional)
       Poisoning by saline and osmotic laxatives NOS

   ● **T47.3X2** Poisoning by saline and osmotic laxatives, intentional self-harm

   ● **T47.3X3** Poisoning by saline and osmotic laxatives, assault

   ● **T47.3X4** Poisoning by saline and osmotic laxatives, undetermined

   ● **T47.3X5** Adverse effect of saline and osmotic laxatives

   ● **T47.3X6** Underdosing of saline and osmotic laxatives

● **T47.4** Poisoning by, adverse effect of and underdosing of other laxatives

  ● **T47.4X** Poisoning by, adverse effect of and underdosing of other laxatives

   ● **T47.4X1** Poisoning by other laxatives, accidental (unintentional)
       Poisoning by other laxatives NOS

   ● **T47.4X2** Poisoning by other laxatives, intentional self-harm

   ● **T47.4X3** Poisoning by other laxatives, assault

   ● **T47.4X4** Poisoning by other laxatives, undetermined

   ● **T47.4X5** Adverse effect of other laxatives

   ● **T47.4X6** Underdosing of other laxatives

● **T47.5** Poisoning by, adverse effect of and underdosing of digestants

  ● **T47.5X** Poisoning by, adverse effect of and underdosing of digestants

   ● **T47.5X1** Poisoning by digestants, accidental (unintentional)
       Poisoning by digestants NOS

   ● **T47.5X2** Poisoning by digestants, intentional self-harm

   ● **T47.5X3** Poisoning by digestants, assault

   ● **T47.5X4** Poisoning by digestants, undetermined

   ● **T47.5X5** Adverse effect of digestants

   ● **T47.5X6** Underdosing of digestants

◄ New   ◄|||| Revised   ~~deleted~~ Deleted   Excludes 1   Excludes 2   Includes   Use additional   Code first   Code also   Unspecified

OGCR Official Guidelines   X Assign placeholder X   ● Use Additional Character(s)   ▌ Manifestation Code   **Coding Clinic**

● T47.6   Poisoning by, adverse effect of and underdosing of antidiarrheal drugs

> **Excludes2**   poisoning by, adverse effect of and underdosing of systemic antibiotics and other anti-infectives (T36-T37)

  ● T47.6X   Poisoning by, adverse effect of and underdosing of antidiarrheal drugs

    ● T47.6X1   Poisoning by antidiarrheal drugs, accidental (unintentional)
> Poisoning by antidiarrheal drugs NOS

    ● T47.6X2   Poisoning by antidiarrheal drugs, intentional self-harm

    ● T47.6X3   Poisoning by antidiarrheal drugs, assault

    ● T47.6X4   Poisoning by antidiarrheal drugs, undetermined

    ● T47.6X5   Adverse effect of antidiarrheal drugs

    ● T47.6X6   Underdosing of antidiarrheal drugs

● T47.7   Poisoning by, adverse effect of and underdosing of emetics

  ● T47.7X   Poisoning by, adverse effect of and underdosing of emetics

    ● T47.7X1   Poisoning by emetics, accidental (unintentional)
> Poisoning by emetics NOS

    ● T47.7X2   Poisoning by emetics, intentional self-harm

    ● T47.7X3   Poisoning by emetics, assault

    ● T47.7X4   Poisoning by emetics, undetermined

    ● T47.7X5   Adverse effect of emetics

    ● T47.7X6   Underdosing of emetics

● T47.8   Poisoning by, adverse effect of and underdosing of other agents primarily affecting gastrointestinal system

  ● T47.8X   Poisoning by, adverse effect of and underdosing of other agents primarily affecting gastrointestinal system

    ● T47.8X1   Poisoning by other agents primarily affecting gastrointestinal system, accidental (unintentional)
> Poisoning by other agents primarily affecting gastrointestinal system NOS

    ● T47.8X2   Poisoning by other agents primarily affecting gastrointestinal system, intentional self-harm

    ● T47.8X3   Poisoning by other agents primarily affecting gastrointestinal system, assault

    ● T47.8X4   Poisoning by other agents primarily affecting gastrointestinal system, undetermined

    ● T47.8X5   Adverse effect of other agents primarily affecting gastrointestinal system

    ● T47.8X6   Underdosing of other agents primarily affecting gastrointestinal system

● T47.9   Poisoning by, adverse effect of and underdosing of unspecified agents primarily affecting the gastrointestinal system

  X ● T47.91   Poisoning by unspecified agents primarily affecting the gastrointestinal system, accidental (unintentional)
> Poisoning by agents primarily affecting the gastrointestinal system NOS

  X ● T47.92   Poisoning by unspecified agents primarily affecting the gastrointestinal system, intentional self-harm

  X ● T47.93   Poisoning by unspecified agents primarily affecting the gastrointestinal system, assault

  X ● T47.94   Poisoning by unspecified agents primarily affecting the gastrointestinal system, undetermined

  X ● T47.95   Adverse effect of unspecified agents primarily affecting the gastrointestinal system

  X ● T47.96   Underdosing of unspecified agents primarily affecting the gastrointestinal system

● T48   Poisoning by, adverse effect of and underdosing of agents primarily acting on smooth and skeletal muscles and the respiratory system

> The appropriate 7th character is to be added to each code from category T48

> | A | initial encounter |
> |---|---|
> | D | subsequent encounter |
> | S | sequela |

● T48.0   Poisoning by, adverse effect of and underdosing of oxytocic drugs

> **Excludes1**   poisoning by, adverse effect of and underdosing of estrogens, progestogens and antagonists (T38.4-T38.6)

  ● T48.0X   Poisoning by, adverse effect of and underdosing of oxytocic drugs

    ● T48.0X1   Poisoning by oxytocic drugs, accidental (unintentional)
> Poisoning by oxytocic drugs NOS

    ● T48.0X2   Poisoning by oxytocic drugs, intentional self-harm

    ● T48.0X3   Poisoning by oxytocic drugs, assault

    ● T48.0X4   Poisoning by oxytocic drugs, undetermined

    ● T48.0X5   Adverse effect of oxytocic drugs

    ● T48.0X6   Underdosing of oxytocic drugs

● T48.1   Poisoning by, adverse effect of and underdosing of skeletal muscle relaxants [neuromuscular blocking agents]

  ● T48.1X   Poisoning by, adverse effect of and underdosing of skeletal muscle relaxants [neuromuscular blocking agents]

    ● T48.1X1   Poisoning by skeletal muscle relaxants [neuromuscular blocking agents], accidental (unintentional)
> Poisoning by skeletal muscle relaxants [neuromuscular blocking agents] NOS

    ● T48.1X2   Poisoning by skeletal muscle relaxants [neuromuscular blocking agents], intentional self-harm

    ● T48.1X3   Poisoning by skeletal muscle relaxants [neuromuscular blocking agents], assault

    ● T48.1X4   Poisoning by skeletal muscle relaxants [neuromuscular blocking agents], undetermined

    ● T48.1X5   Adverse effect of skeletal muscle relaxants [neuromuscular blocking agents]

    ● T48.1X6   Underdosing of skeletal muscle relaxants [neuromuscular blocking agents]

CHAPTER 19 (S00-T88)

- **T48.2 Poisoning by, adverse effect of and underdosing of other and unspecified drugs acting on muscles**
  - **T48.20 Poisoning by, adverse effect of and underdosing of unspecified drugs acting on muscles**
    - **T48.201 Poisoning by unspecified drugs acting on muscles, accidental (unintentional)**
      Poisoning by unspecified drugs acting on muscles NOS
    - **T48.202 Poisoning by unspecified drugs acting on muscles, intentional self-harm**
    - **T48.203 Poisoning by unspecified drugs acting on muscles, assault**
    - **T48.204 Poisoning by unspecified drugs acting on muscles, undetermined**
    - **T48.205 Adverse effect of unspecified drugs acting on muscles**
    - **T48.206 Underdosing of unspecified drugs acting on muscles**
  - **T48.29 Poisoning by, adverse effect of and underdosing of other drugs acting on muscles**
    - **T48.291 Poisoning by other drugs acting on muscles, accidental (unintentional)**
      Poisoning by other drugs acting on muscles NOS
    - **T48.292 Poisoning by other drugs acting on muscles, intentional self-harm**
    - **T48.293 Poisoning by other drugs acting on muscles, assault**
    - **T48.294 Poisoning by other drugs acting on muscles, undetermined**
    - **T48.295 Adverse effect of other drugs acting on muscles**
    - **T48.296 Underdosing of other drugs acting on muscles**
- **T48.3 Poisoning by, adverse effect of and underdosing of antitussives**
  - **T48.3X Poisoning by, adverse effect of and underdosing of antitussives**
    - **T48.3X1 Poisoning by antitussives, accidental (unintentional)**
      Poisoning by antitussives NOS
    - **T48.3X2 Poisoning by antitussives, intentional self-harm**
    - **T48.3X3 Poisoning by antitussives, assault**
    - **T48.3X4 Poisoning by antitussives, undetermined**
    - **T48.3X5 Adverse effect of antitussives**
    - **T48.3X6 Underdosing of antitussives**
- **T48.4 Poisoning by, adverse effect of and underdosing of expectorants**
  - **T48.4X Poisoning by, adverse effect of and underdosing of expectorants**
    - **T48.4X1 Poisoning by expectorants, accidental (unintentional)**
      Poisoning by expectorants NOS
    - **T48.4X2 Poisoning by expectorants, intentional self-harm**
    - **T48.4X3 Poisoning by expectorants, assault**
    - **T48.4X4 Poisoning by expectorants, undetermined**
    - **T48.4X5 Adverse effect of expectorants**
    - **T48.4X6 Underdosing of expectorants**

- **T48.5 Poisoning by, adverse effect of and underdosing of other anti-common-cold drugs**
  Poisoning by, adverse effect of and underdosing of decongestants
  - **Excludes2** poisoning by, adverse effect of and underdosing of antipyretics, NEC (T39.9-)
    poisoning by, adverse effect of and underdosing of non-steroidal antiinflammatory drugs (T39.3-)
    poisoning by, adverse effect of and underdosing of salicylates (T39.0-)
  - **T48.5X Poisoning by, adverse effect of and underdosing of other anti-common-cold drugs**
    - **T48.5X1 Poisoning by other anti-common-cold drugs, accidental (unintentional)**
      Poisoning by other anti-common-cold drugs NOS
    - **T48.5X2 Poisoning by other anti-common-cold drugs, intentional self-harm**
    - **T48.5X3 Poisoning by other anti-common-cold drugs, assault**
    - **T48.5X4 Poisoning by other anti-common-cold drugs, undetermined**
    - **T48.5X5 Adverse effect of other anti-common-cold drugs**
    - **T48.5X6 Underdosing of other anti-common-cold drugs**
- **T48.6 Poisoning by, adverse effect of and underdosing of antiasthmatics, not elsewhere classified**
  Poisoning by, adverse effect of and underdosing of beta-adrenoreceptor agonists used in asthma therapy
  - **Excludes1** poisoning by, adverse effect of and underdosing of beta-adrenoreceptor agonists not used in asthma therapy (T44.5)
    poisoning by, adverse effect of and underdosing of anterior pituitary [adenohypophyseal] hormones (T38.8)
  - **T48.6X Poisoning by, adverse effect of and underdosing of antiasthmatics**
    - **T48.6X1 Poisoning by antiasthmatics, accidental (unintentional)**
      Poisoning by antiasthmatics NOS
    - **T48.6X2 Poisoning by antiasthmatics, intentional self-harm**
    - **T48.6X3 Poisoning by antiasthmatics, assault**
    - **T48.6X4 Poisoning by antiasthmatics, undetermined**
    - **T48.6X5 Adverse effect of antiasthmatics**
    - **T48.6X6 Underdosing of antiasthmatics**
- **T48.9 Poisoning by, adverse effect of and underdosing of other and unspecified agents primarily acting on the respiratory system**
  - **T48.90 Poisoning by, adverse effect of and underdosing of unspecified agents primarily acting on the respiratory system**
    - **T48.901 Poisoning by unspecified agents primarily acting on the respiratory system, accidental (unintentional)**
    - **T48.902 Poisoning by unspecified agents primarily acting on the respiratory system, intentional self-harm**
    - **T48.903 Poisoning by unspecified agents primarily acting on the respiratory system, assault**
    - **T48.904 Poisoning by unspecified agents primarily acting on the respiratory system, undetermined**

New ◀ | Revised ◀ | ~~deleted~~ Deleted | Excludes 1 | Excludes 2 | Includes | Use additional | Code first | Code also | Unspecified

OGCR Official Guidelines   X Assign placeholder X   ● Use Additional Character(s)   ▶ Manifestation Code   **Coding Clinic**

● T48.905　Adverse effect of unspecified agents primarily acting on the respiratory system
● T48.906　Underdosing of unspecified agents primarily acting on the respiratory system
● T48.99　Poisoning by, adverse effect of and underdosing of other agents primarily acting on the respiratory system
　● T48.991　Poisoning by other agents primarily acting on the respiratory system, accidental (unintentional)
　● T48.992　Poisoning by other agents primarily acting on the respiratory system, intentional self-harm
　● T48.993　Poisoning by other agents primarily acting on the respiratory system, assault
　● T48.994　Poisoning by other agents primarily acting on the respiratory system, undetermined
　● T48.995　Adverse effect of other agents primarily acting on the respiratory system
　● T48.996　Underdosing of other agents primarily acting on the respiratory system

● T49　Poisoning by, adverse effect of and underdosing of topical agents primarily affecting skin and mucous membrane and by ophthalmological, otorhinorlaryngological and dental drugs

Includes　poisoning by, adverse effect of and underdosing of glucocorticoids, topically used

The appropriate 7th character is to be added to each code from category T49

A　initial encounter
D　subsequent encounter
S　sequela

● T49.0　Poisoning by, adverse effect of and underdosing of local antifungal, anti-infective and anti-inflammatory drugs
　● T49.0X　Poisoning by, adverse effect of and underdosing of local antifungal, anti-infective and anti-inflammatory drugs
　　● T49.0X1　Poisoning by local antifungal, anti-infective and anti-inflammatory drugs, accidental (unintentional)
　　　Poisoning by local antifungal, anti-infective and anti-inflammatory drugs NOS
　　● T49.0X2　Poisoning by local antifungal, anti-infective and anti-inflammatory drugs, intentional self-harm
　　● T49.0X3　Poisoning by local antifungal, anti-infective and anti-inflammatory drugs, assault
　　● T49.0X4　Poisoning by local antifungal, anti-infective and anti-inflammatory drugs, undetermined
　　● T49.0X5　Adverse effect of local antifungal, anti-infective and anti-inflammatory drugs
　　● T49.0X6　Underdosing of local antifungal, anti-infective and anti-inflammatory drugs

● T49.1　Poisoning by, adverse effect of and underdosing of antipruritics
　● T49.1X　Poisoning by, adverse effect of and underdosing of antipruritics
　　● T49.1X1　Poisoning by antipruritics, accidental (unintentional)
　　　Poisoning by antipruritics NOS
　　● T49.1X2　Poisoning by antipruritics, intentional self-harm
　　● T49.1X3　Poisoning by antipruritics, assault
　　● T49.1X4　Poisoning by antipruritics, undetermined
　　● T49.1X5　Adverse effect of antipruritics
　　● T49.1X6　Underdosing of antipruritics

● T49.2　Poisoning by, adverse effect of and underdosing of local astringents and local detergents
　● T49.2X　Poisoning by, adverse effect of and underdosing of local astringents and local detergents
　　● T49.2X1　Poisoning by local astringents and local detergents, accidental (unintentional)
　　　Poisoning by local astringents and local detergents NOS
　　● T49.2X2　Poisoning by local astringents and local detergents, intentional self-harm
　　● T49.2X3　Poisoning by local astringents and local detergents, assault
　　● T49.2X4　Poisoning by local astringents and local detergents, undetermined
　　● T49.2X5　Adverse effect of local astringents and local detergents
　　● T49.2X6　Underdosing of local astringents and local detergents

● T49.3　Poisoning by, adverse effect of and underdosing of emollients, demulcents and protectants
　● T49.3X　Poisoning by, adverse effect of and underdosing of emollients, demulcents and protectants
　　● T49.3X1　Poisoning by emollients, demulcents and protectants, accidental (unintentional)
　　　Poisoning by emollients, demulcents and protectants NOS
　　● T49.3X2　Poisoning by emollients, demulcents and protectants, intentional self-harm
　　● T49.3X3　Poisoning by emollients, demulcents and protectants, assault
　　● T49.3X4　Poisoning by emollients, demulcents and protectants, undetermined
　　● T49.3X5　Adverse effect of emollients, demulcents and protectants
　　● T49.3X6　Underdosing of emollients, demulcents and protectants

● T49.4　Poisoning by, adverse effect of and underdosing of keratolytics, keratoplastics, and other hair treatment drugs and preparations
　● T49.4X　Poisoning by, adverse effect of and underdosing of keratolytics, keratoplastics, and other hair treatment drugs and preparations
　　● T49.4X1　Poisoning by keratolytics, keratoplastics, and other hair treatment drugs and preparations, accidental (unintentional)
　　　Poisoning by keratolytics, keratoplastics, and other hair treatment drugs and preparations NOS
　　● T49.4X2　Poisoning by keratolytics, keratoplastics, and other hair treatment drugs and preparations, intentional self-harm
　　● T49.4X3　Poisoning by keratolytics, keratoplastics, and other hair treatment drugs and preparations, assault
　　● T49.4X4　Poisoning by keratolytics, keratoplastics, and other hair treatment drugs and preparations, undetermined
　　● T49.4X5　Adverse effect of keratolytics, keratoplastics, and other hair treatment drugs and preparations
　　● T49.4X6　Underdosing of keratolytics, keratoplastics, and other hair treatment drugs and preparations

CHAPTER 19 (S00-T88)

● **T49.5** **Poisoning by, adverse effect of and underdosing of ophthalmological drugs and preparations**
  ● **T49.5X** **Poisoning by, adverse effect of and underdosing of ophthalmological drugs and preparations**
    ● **T49.5X1** **Poisoning by ophthalmological drugs and preparations, accidental (unintentional)**
      Poisoning by ophthalmological drugs and preparations NOS
    ● **T49.5X2** **Poisoning by ophthalmological drugs and preparations, intentional self-harm**
    ● **T49.5X3** **Poisoning by ophthalmological drugs and preparations, assault**
    ● **T49.5X4** **Poisoning by ophthalmological drugs and preparations, undetermined**
    ● **T49.5X5** **Adverse effect of ophthalmological drugs and preparations**
    ● **T49.5X6** **Underdosing of ophthalmological drugs and preparations**

● **T49.6** **Poisoning by, adverse effect of and underdosing of otorhinolaryngological drugs and preparations**
  ● **T49.6X** **Poisoning by, adverse effect of and underdosing of otorhinolaryngological drugs and preparations**
    ● **T49.6X1** **Poisoning by otorhinolaryngological drugs and preparations, accidental (unintentional)**
      Poisoning by otorhinolaryngological drugs and preparations NOS
    ● **T49.6X2** **Poisoning by otorhinolaryngological drugs and preparations, intentional self-harm**
    ● **T49.6X3** **Poisoning by otorhinolaryngological drugs and preparations, assault**
    ● **T49.6X4** **Poisoning by otorhinolaryngological drugs and preparations, undetermined**
    ● **T49.6X5** **Adverse effect of otorhinolaryngological drugs and preparations**
    ● **T49.6X6** **Underdosing of otorhinolaryngological drugs and preparations**

● **T49.7** **Poisoning by, adverse effect of and underdosing of dental drugs, topically applied**
  ● **T49.7X** **Poisoning by, adverse effect of and underdosing of dental drugs, topically applied**
    ● **T49.7X1** **Poisoning by dental drugs, topically applied, accidental (unintentional)**
      Poisoning by dental drugs, topically applied NOS
    ● **T49.7X2** **Poisoning by dental drugs, topically applied, intentional self-harm**
    ● **T49.7X3** **Poisoning by dental drugs, topically applied, assault**
    ● **T49.7X4** **Poisoning by dental drugs, topically applied, undetermined**
    ● **T49.7X5** **Adverse effect of dental drugs, topically applied**
    ● **T49.7X6** **Underdosing of dental drugs, topically applied**

● **T49.8** **Poisoning by, adverse effect of and underdosing of other topical agents**
  Poisoning by, adverse effect of and underdosing of spermicides
  ● **T49.8X** **Poisoning by, adverse effect of and underdosing of other topical agents**
    ● **T49.8X1** **Poisoning by other topical agents, accidental (unintentional)**
      Poisoning by other topical agents NOS
    ● **T49.8X2** **Poisoning by other topical agents, intentional self-harm**
    ● **T49.8X3** **Poisoning by other topical agents, assault**
    ● **T49.8X4** **Poisoning by other topical agents, undetermined**
    ● **T49.8X5** **Adverse effect of other topical agents**
    ● **T49.8X6** **Underdosing of other topical agents**

● **T49.9** **Poisoning by, adverse effect of and underdosing of unspecified topical agent**
  X ● **T49.91** **Poisoning by unspecified topical agent, accidental (unintentional)**
  X ● **T49.92** **Poisoning by unspecified topical agent, intentional self-harm**
  X ● **T49.93** **Poisoning by unspecified topical agent, assault**
  X ● **T49.94** **Poisoning by unspecified topical agent, undetermined**
  X ● **T49.95** **Adverse effect of unspecified topical agent**
  X ● **T49.96** **Underdosing of unspecified topical agent**

● **T50** **Poisoning by, adverse effect of and underdosing of diuretics and other and unspecified drugs, medicaments and biological substances**
  The appropriate 7th character is to be added to each code from category T50

> | | |
> |---|---|
> | A | initial encounter |
> | D | subsequent encounter |
> | S | sequela |

● **T50.0** **Poisoning by, adverse effect of and underdosing of mineralocorticoids and their antagonists**
  ● **T50.0X** **Poisoning by, adverse effect of and underdosing of mineralocorticoids and their antagonists**
    ● **T50.0X1** **Poisoning by mineralocorticoids and their antagonists, accidental (unintentional)**
      Poisoning by mineralocorticoids and their antagonists NOS
    ● **T50.0X2** **Poisoning by mineralocorticoids and their antagonists, intentional self-harm**
    ● **T50.0X3** **Poisoning by mineralocorticoids and their antagonists, assault**
    ● **T50.0X4** **Poisoning by mineralocorticoids and their antagonists, undetermined**
    ● **T50.0X5** **Adverse effect of mineralocorticoids and their antagonists**
    ● **T50.0X6** **Underdosing of mineralocorticoids and their antagonists**

● **T50.1** **Poisoning by, adverse effect of and underdosing of loop [high-ceiling] diuretics**
  ● **T50.1X** **Poisoning by, adverse effect of and underdosing of loop [high-ceiling] diuretics**
    ● **T50.1X1** **Poisoning by loop [high-ceiling] diuretics, accidental (unintentional)**
      Poisoning by loop [high-ceiling] diuretics NOS
    ● **T50.1X2** **Poisoning by loop [high-ceiling] diuretics, intentional self-harm**
    ● **T50.1X3** **Poisoning by loop [high-ceiling] diuretics, assault**

◄ New   ⬅ Revised   ~~deleted~~ Deleted   Excludes 1   Excludes 2   Includes   Use additional   Code first   Code also   Unspecified
OGCR Official Guidelines   X Assign placeholder X   ● Use Additional Character(s)   ▶ Manifestation Code   **Coding Clinic**

● T50.1X4   Poisoning by loop [high-ceiling] diuretics, undetermined

● T50.1X5   Adverse effect of loop [high-ceiling] diuretics

● T50.1X6   Underdosing of loop [high-ceiling] diuretics

● T50.2   Poisoning by, adverse effect of and underdosing of carbonic-anhydrase inhibitors, benzothiadiazides and other diuretics
     Poisoning by, adverse effect of and underdosing of acetazolamide

   ● T50.2X   Poisoning by, adverse effect of and underdosing of carbonic-anhydrase inhibitors, benzothiadiazides and other diuretics

     ● T50.2X1   Poisoning by carbonic-anhydrase inhibitors, benzothiadiazides and other diuretics, accidental (unintentional)
       Poisoning by carbonic-anhydrase inhibitors, benzothiadiazides and other diuretics NOS

     ● T50.2X2   Poisoning by carbonic-anhydrase inhibitors, benzothiadiazides and other diuretics, intentional self-harm

     ● T50.2X3   Poisoning by carbonic-anhydrase inhibitors, benzothiadiazides and other diuretics, assault

     ● T50.2X4   Poisoning by carbonic-anhydrase inhibitors, benzothiadiazides and other diuretics, undetermined

     ● T50.2X5   Adverse effect of carbonic-anhydrase inhibitors, benzothiadiazides and other diuretics

     ● T50.2X6   Underdosing of carbonic-anhydrase inhibitors, benzothiadiazides and other diuretics

● T50.3   Poisoning by, adverse effect of and underdosing of electrolytic, caloric and water-balance agents
     Poisoning by, adverse effect of and underdosing of oral rehydration salts

   ● T50.3X   Poisoning by, adverse effect of and underdosing of electrolytic, caloric and water-balance agents

     ● T50.3X1   Poisoning by electrolytic, caloric and water-balance agents, accidental (unintentional)
       Poisoning by electrolytic, caloric and water-balance agents NOS

     ● T50.3X2   Poisoning by electrolytic, caloric and water-balance agents, intentional self-harm

     ● T50.3X3   Poisoning by electrolytic, caloric and water-balance agents, assault

     ● T50.3X4   Poisoning by electrolytic, caloric and water-balance agents, undetermined

     ● T50.3X5   Adverse effect of electrolytic, caloric and water-balance agents

     ● T50.3X6   Underdosing of electrolytic, caloric and water-balance agents

● T50.4   Poisoning by, adverse effect of and underdosing of drugs affecting uric acid metabolism

   ● T50.4X   Poisoning by, adverse effect of and underdosing of drugs affecting uric acid metabolism

     ● T50.4X1   Poisoning by drugs affecting uric acid metabolism, accidental (unintentional)
       Poisoning by drugs affecting uric acid metabolism NOS

     ● T50.4X2   Poisoning by drugs affecting uric acid metabolism, intentional self-harm

     ● T50.4X3   Poisoning by drugs affecting uric acid metabolism, assault

     ● T50.4X4   Poisoning by drugs affecting uric acid metabolism, undetermined

     ● T50.4X5   Adverse effect of drugs affecting uric acid metabolism

     ● T50.4X6   Underdosing of drugs affecting uric acid metabolism

● T50.5   Poisoning by, adverse effect of and underdosing of appetite depressants

   ● T50.5X   Poisoning by, adverse effect of and underdosing of appetite depressants

     ● T50.5X1   Poisoning by appetite depressants, accidental (unintentional)
       Poisoning by appetite depressants NOS

     ● T50.5X2   Poisoning by appetite depressants, intentional self-harm

     ● T50.5X3   Poisoning by appetite depressants, assault

     ● T50.5X4   Poisoning by appetite depressants, undetermined

     ● T50.5X5   Adverse effect of appetite depressants

     ● T50.5X6   Underdosing of appetite depressants

● T50.6   Poisoning by, adverse effect of and underdosing of antidotes and chelating agents
     Poisoning by, adverse effect of and underdosing of alcohol deterrents

   ● T50.6X   Poisoning by, adverse effect of and underdosing of antidotes and chelating agents

     ● T50.6X1   Poisoning by antidotes and chelating agents, accidental (unintentional)
       Poisoning by antidotes and chelating agents NOS

     ● T50.6X2   Poisoning by antidotes and chelating agents, intentional self-harm

     ● T50.6X3   Poisoning by antidotes and chelating agents, assault

     ● T50.6X4   Poisoning by antidotes and chelating agents, undetermined

     ● T50.6X5   Adverse effect of antidotes and chelating agents

     ● T50.6X6   Underdosing of antidotes and chelating agents

● T50.7   Poisoning by, adverse effect of and underdosing of analeptics and opioid receptor antagonists

   ● T50.7X   Poisoning by, adverse effect of and underdosing of analeptics and opioid receptor antagonists

     ● T50.7X1   Poisoning by analeptics and opioid receptor antagonists, accidental (unintentional)
       Poisoning by analeptics and opioid receptor antagonists NOS

     ● T50.7X2   Poisoning by analeptics and opioid receptor antagonists, intentional self-harm

     ● T50.7X3   Poisoning by analeptics and opioid receptor antagonists, assault

     ● T50.7X4   Poisoning by analeptics and opioid receptor antagonists, undetermined

     ● T50.7X5   Adverse effect of analeptics and opioid receptor antagonists

     ● T50.7X6   Underdosing of analeptics and opioid receptor antagonists

CHAPTER 19 (S00–T88)

● **T50.8** Poisoning by, adverse effect of and underdosing of diagnostic agents

  ● **T50.8X** Poisoning by, adverse effect of and underdosing of diagnostic agents

    ● **T50.8X1** Poisoning by diagnostic agents, accidental (unintentional)
         Poisoning by diagnostic agents NOS

    ● **T50.8X2** Poisoning by diagnostic agents, intentional self-harm

    ● **T50.8X3** Poisoning by diagnostic agents, assault

    ● **T50.8X4** Poisoning by diagnostic agents, undetermined

    ● **T50.8X5** Adverse effect of diagnostic agents

    ● **T50.8X6** Underdosing of diagnostic agents

● **T50.A** Poisoning by, adverse effect of and underdosing of bacterial vaccines

  ● **T50.A1** Poisoning by, adverse effect of and underdosing of pertussis vaccine, including combinations with a pertussis component

    ● **T50.A11** Poisoning by pertussis vaccine, including combinations with a pertussis component, accidental (unintentional)

    ● **T50.A12** Poisoning by pertussis vaccine, including combinations with a pertussis component, intentional self-harm

    ● **T50.A13** Poisoning by pertussis vaccine, including combinations with a pertussis component, assault

    ● **T50.A14** Poisoning by pertussis vaccine, including combinations with a pertussis component, undetermined

    ● **T50.A15** Adverse effect of pertussis vaccine, including combinations with a pertussis component

    ● **T50.A16** Underdosing of pertussis vaccine, including combinations with a pertussis component

  ● **T50.A2** Poisoning by, adverse effect of and underdosing of mixed bacterial vaccines without a pertussis component

    ● **T50.A21** Poisoning by mixed bacterial vaccines without a pertussis component, accidental (unintentional)

    ● **T50.A22** Poisoning by mixed bacterial vaccines without a pertussis component, intentional self-harm

    ● **T50.A23** Poisoning by mixed bacterial vaccines without a pertussis component, assault

    ● **T50.A24** Poisoning by mixed bacterial vaccines without a pertussis component, undetermined

    ● **T50.A25** Adverse effect of mixed bacterial vaccines without a pertussis component

    ● **T50.A26** Underdosing of mixed bacterial vaccines without a pertussis component

● **T50.A9** Poisoning by, adverse effect of and underdosing of other bacterial vaccines

    ● **T50.A91** Poisoning by other bacterial vaccines, accidental (unintentional)

    ● **T50.A92** Poisoning by other bacterial vaccines, intentional self-harm

    ● **T50.A93** Poisoning by other bacterial vaccines, assault

    ● **T50.A94** Poisoning by other bacterial vaccines, undetermined

    ● **T50.A95** Adverse effect of other bacterial vaccines

    ● **T50.A96** Underdosing of other bacterial vaccines

● **T50.B** Poisoning by, adverse effect of and underdosing of viral vaccines

  ● **T50.B1** Poisoning by, adverse effect of and underdosing of smallpox vaccines

    ● **T50.B11** Poisoning by smallpox vaccines, accidental (unintentional)

    ● **T50.B12** Poisoning by smallpox vaccines, intentional self-harm

    ● **T50.B13** Poisoning by smallpox vaccines, assault

    ● **T50.B14** Poisoning by smallpox vaccines, undetermined

    ● **T50.B15** Adverse effect of smallpox vaccines

    ● **T50.B16** Underdosing of smallpox vaccines

  ● **T50.B9** Poisoning by, adverse effect of and underdosing of other viral vaccines

    ● **T50.B91** Poisoning by other viral vaccines, accidental (unintentional)

    ● **T50.B92** Poisoning by other viral vaccines, intentional self-harm

    ● **T50.B93** Poisoning by other viral vaccines, assault

    ● **T50.B94** Poisoning by other viral vaccines, undetermined

    ● **T50.B95** Adverse effect of other viral vaccines

    ● **T50.B96** Underdosing of other viral vaccines

● **T50.Z** Poisoning by, adverse effect of and underdosing of other vaccines and biological substances

  ● **T50.Z1** Poisoning by, adverse effect of and underdosing of immunoglobulin

    ● **T50.Z11** Poisoning by immunoglobulin, accidental (unintentional)

    ● **T50.Z12** Poisoning by immunoglobulin, intentional self-harm

    ● **T50.Z13** Poisoning by immunoglobulin, assault

    ● **T50.Z14** Poisoning by immunoglobulin, undetermined

    ● **T50.Z15** Adverse effect of immunoglobulin

    ● **T50.Z16** Underdosing of immunoglobulin

◀ New   ⬅ Revised   ~~deleted~~ Deleted   Excludes 1   Excludes 2   Includes   Use additional   Code first   Code also   Unspecified

OGCR Official Guidelines   X Assign placeholder X   ● Use Additional Character(s)   ▶ Manifestation Code   **Coding Clinic**

● **T50.Z9**   Poisoning by, adverse effect of and underdosing of other vaccines and biological substances

     ● **T50.Z91**   Poisoning by other vaccines and biological substances, accidental (unintentional)

     ● **T50.Z92**   Poisoning by other vaccines and biological substances, intentional self-harm

     ● **T50.Z93**   Poisoning by other vaccines and biological substances, assault

     ● **T50.Z94**   Poisoning by other vaccines and biological substances, undetermined

     ● **T50.Z95**   Adverse effect of other vaccines and biological substances

     ● **T50.Z96**   Underdosing of other vaccines and biological substances

● **T50.9**   Poisoning by, adverse effect of and underdosing of other and unspecified drugs, medicaments and biological substances

     ● **T50.90**   Poisoning by, adverse effect of and underdosing of unspecified drugs, medicaments and biological substances

         ● **T50.901**   Poisoning by unspecified drugs, medicaments and biological substances, accidental (unintentional)
                 Coding Clinic: 2015, Q1, P21

         ● **T50.902**   Poisoning by unspecified drugs, medicaments and biological substances, intentional self-harm

         ● **T50.903**   Poisoning by unspecified drugs, medicaments and biological substances, assault

         ● **T50.904**   Poisoning by unspecified drugs, medicaments and biological substances, undetermined

         ● **T50.905**   Adverse effect of unspecified drugs, medicaments and biological substances

         ● **T50.906**   Underdosing of unspecified drugs, medicaments and biological substances

     ● **T50.99**   Poisoning by, adverse effect of and underdosing of other drugs, medicaments and biological substances

         ● **T50.991**   Poisoning by other drugs, medicaments and biological substances, accidental (unintentional)

         ● **T50.992**   Poisoning by other drugs, medicaments and biological substances, intentional self-harm

         ● **T50.993**   Poisoning by other drugs, medicaments and biological substances, assault

         ● **T50.994**   Poisoning by other drugs, medicaments and biological substances, undetermined

         ● **T50.995**   Adverse effect of other drugs, medicaments and biological substances

         ● **T50.996**   Underdosing of other drugs, medicaments and biological substances

---

TOXIC EFFECTS OF SUBSTANCES CHIEFLY NONMEDICINAL AS TO SOURCE (T51-T65)

Note: When no intent is indicated code to accidental. Undetermined intent is only for use when there is specific documentation in the record that the intent of the toxic effect cannot be determined.

Use additional code(s): for all associated manifestations of toxic effect, such as:
respiratory conditions due to external agents (J60-J70)
personal history of foreign body fully removed (Z87.821)
to identify any retained foreign body, if applicable (Z18.-)

Excludes1   contact with and (suspected) exposure to toxic substances (Z77.-)

● **T51**   **Toxic effect of alcohol**

The appropriate 7th character is to be added to each code from category T51

A	initial encounter
D	subsequent encounter
S	sequela

● **T51.0**   **Toxic effect of ethanol**
Toxic effect of ethyl alcohol

     Excludes2   acute alcohol intoxication or 'hangover' effects (F10.129, F10.229, F10.929)
                 drunkenness (F10.129, F10.229, F10.929)
                 pathological alcohol intoxication (F10.129, F10.229, F10.929)

     ● **T51.0X**   Toxic effect of ethanol

         ● **T51.0X1**   Toxic effect of ethanol, accidental (unintentional)
                 Toxic effect of ethanol NOS

         ● **T51.0X2**   Toxic effect of ethanol, intentional self-harm

         ● **T51.0X3**   Toxic effect of ethanol, assault

         ● **T51.0X4**   Toxic effect of ethanol, undetermined

● **T51.1**   **Toxic effect of methanol**
Toxic effect of methyl alcohol

     ● **T51.1X**   Toxic effect of methanol

         ● **T51.1X1**   Toxic effect of methanol, accidental (unintentional)
                 Toxic effect of methanol NOS

         ● **T51.1X2**   Toxic effect of methanol, intentional self-harm

         ● **T51.1X3**   Toxic effect of methanol, assault

         ● **T51.1X4**   Toxic effect of methanol, undetermined

● **T51.2**   **Toxic effect of 2-Propanol**
Toxic effect of isopropyl alcohol

     ● **T51.2X**   Toxic effect of 2-Propanol

         ● **T51.2X1**   Toxic effect of 2-Propanol, accidental (unintentional)
                 Toxic effect of 2-Propanol NOS

         ● **T51.2X2**   Toxic effect of 2-Propanol, intentional self-harm

         ● **T51.2X3**   Toxic effect of 2-Propanol, assault

         ● **T51.2X4**   Toxic effect of 2-Propanol, undetermined

● **T51.3**   **Toxic effect of fusel oil**
Toxic effect of amyl alcohol
Toxic effect of butyl [1-butanol] alcohol
Toxic effect of propyl [1-propanol] alcohol

     ● **T51.3X**   Toxic effect of fusel oil

         ● **T51.3X1**   Toxic effect of fusel oil, accidental (unintentional)
                 Toxic effect of fusel oil NOS

         ● **T51.3X2**   Toxic effect of fusel oil, intentional self-harm

         ● **T51.3X3**   Toxic effect of fusel oil, assault

         ● **T51.3X4**   Toxic effect of fusel oil, undetermined

- ● T51.8   **Toxic effect of other alcohols**
  - ● T51.8X   **Toxic effect of other alcohols**
    - ● T51.8X1   **Toxic effect of other alcohols, accidental (unintentional)**
      Toxic effect of other alcohols NOS
    - ● T51.8X2   **Toxic effect of other alcohols, intentional self-harm**
    - ● T51.8X3   **Toxic effect of other alcohols, assault**
    - ● T51.8X4   **Toxic effect of other alcohols, undetermined**
- ● T51.9   **Toxic effect of unspecified alcohol**
  - X ● T51.91   **Toxic effect of unspecified alcohol, accidental (unintentional)**
  - X ● T51.92   **Toxic effect of unspecified alcohol, intentional self-harm**
  - X ● T51.93   **Toxic effect of unspecified alcohol, assault**
  - X ● T51.94   **Toxic effect of unspecified alcohol, undetermined**
- ● T52   **Toxic effect of organic solvents**

  Excludes1   halogen derivatives of aliphatic and aromatic hydrocarbons (T53.-)

  The appropriate 7th character is to be added to each code from category T52

A	initial encounter
D	subsequent encounter
S	sequela

  - ● T52.0   **Toxic effects of petroleum products**
    Toxic effects of gasoline [petrol]
    Toxic effects of kerosene [paraffin oil]
    Toxic effects of paraffin wax
    Toxic effects of ether petroleum
    Toxic effects of naphtha petroleum
    Toxic effects of spirit petroleum
    - ● T52.0X   **Toxic effects of petroleum products**
      - ● T52.0X1   **Toxic effect of petroleum products, accidental (unintentional)**
        Toxic effects of petroleum products NOS
      - ● T52.0X2   **Toxic effect of petroleum products, intentional self-harm**
      - ● T52.0X3   **Toxic effect of petroleum products, assault**
      - ● T52.0X4   **Toxic effect of petroleum products, undetermined**
  - ● T52.1   **Toxic effects of benzene**

    Excludes1   homologues of benzene (T52.2)
    nitroderivatives and aminoderivatives of benzene and its homologues (T65.3)
    - ● T52.1X   **Toxic effects of benzene**
      - ● T52.1X1   **Toxic effect of benzene, accidental (unintentional)**
        Toxic effects of benzene NOS
      - ● T52.1X2   **Toxic effect of benzene, intentional self-harm**
      - ● T52.1X3   **Toxic effect of benzene, assault**
      - ● T52.1X4   **Toxic effect of benzene, undetermined**
  - ● T52.2   **Toxic effects of homologues of benzene**
    Toxic effects of toluene [methylbenzene]
    Toxic effects of xylene [dimethylbenzene]
    - ● T52.2X   **Toxic effects of homologues of benzene**
      - ● T52.2X1   **Toxic effect of homologues of benzene, accidental (unintentional)**
        Toxic effects of homologues of benzene NOS
      - ● T52.2X2   **Toxic effect of homologues of benzene, intentional self-harm**
      - ● T52.2X3   **Toxic effect of homologues of benzene, assault**
      - ● T52.2X4   **Toxic effect of homologues of benzene, undetermined**

- ● T52.3   **Toxic effects of glycols**
  - ● T52.3X   **Toxic effects of glycols**
    - ● T52.3X1   **Toxic effect of glycols, accidental (unintentional)**
      Toxic effects of glycols NOS
    - ● T52.3X2   **Toxic effect of glycols, intentional self-harm**
    - ● T52.3X3   **Toxic effect of glycols, assault**
    - ● T52.3X4   **Toxic effect of glycols, undetermined**
- ● T52.4   **Toxic effects of ketones**
  - ● T52.4X   **Toxic effects of ketones**
    - ● T52.4X1   **Toxic effect of ketones, accidental (unintentional)**
      Toxic effects of ketones NOS
    - ● T52.4X2   **Toxic effect of ketones, intentional self-harm**
    - ● T52.4X3   **Toxic effect of ketones, assault**
    - ● T52.4X4   **Toxic effect of ketones, undetermined**
- ● T52.8   **Toxic effects of other organic solvents**
  - ● T52.8X   **Toxic effects of other organic solvents**
    - ● T52.8X1   **Toxic effect of other organic solvents, accidental (unintentional)**
      Toxic effects of other organic solvents NOS
    - ● T52.8X2   **Toxic effect of other organic solvents, intentional self-harm**
    - ● T52.8X3   **Toxic effect of other organic solvents, assault**
    - ● T52.8X4   **Toxic effect of other organic solvents, undetermined**
- ● T52.9   **Toxic effects of unspecified organic solvent**
  - X ● T52.91   **Toxic effect of unspecified organic solvent, accidental (unintentional)**
  - X ● T52.92   **Toxic effect of unspecified organic solvent, intentional self-harm**
  - X ● T52.93   **Toxic effect of unspecified organic solvent, assault**
  - X ● T52.94   **Toxic effect of unspecified organic solvent, undetermined**
- ● T53   **Toxic effect of halogen derivatives of aliphatic and aromatic hydrocarbons**

  The appropriate 7th character is to be added to each code from category T53

A	initial encounter
D	subsequent encounter
S	sequela

  - ● T53.0   **Toxic effects of carbon tetrachloride**
    Toxic effects of tetrachloromethane
    - ● T53.0X   **Toxic effects of carbon tetrachloride**
      - ● T53.0X1   **Toxic effect of carbon tetrachloride, accidental (unintentional)**
        Toxic effects of carbon tetrachloride NOS
      - ● T53.0X2   **Toxic effect of carbon tetrachloride, intentional self-harm**
      - ● T53.0X3   **Toxic effect of carbon tetrachloride, assault**
      - ● T53.0X4   **Toxic effect of carbon tetrachloride, undetermined**

◀ New   ◀▦ Revised   ~~deleted~~ Deleted   **Excludes 1**   **Excludes 2**   **Includes**   **Use additional**   **Code first**   **Code also**   **Unspecified**

OGCR Official Guidelines   X Assign placeholder X   ● Use Additional Character(s)   ▌ Manifestation Code   **Coding Clinic**

1388

● **T53.1**   **Toxic effects of chloroform**
     Toxic effects of trichloromethane
   ● **T53.1X**   **Toxic effects of chloroform**
     ● **T53.1X1**   **Toxic effect of chloroform, accidental (unintentional)**
         Toxic effects of chloroform NOS
     ● **T53.1X2**   **Toxic effect of chloroform, intentional self-harm**
     ● **T53.1X3**   **Toxic effect of chloroform, assault**
     ● **T53.1X4**   **Toxic effect of chloroform, undetermined**
● **T53.2**   **Toxic effects of trichloroethylene**
     Toxic effects of trichloroethene
   ● **T53.2X**   **Toxic effects of trichloroethylene**
     ● **T53.2X1**   **Toxic effect of trichloroethylene, accidental (unintentional)**
         Toxic effects of trichloroethylene NOS
     ● **T53.2X2**   **Toxic effect of trichloroethylene, intentional self-harm**
     ● **T53.2X3**   **Toxic effect of trichloroethylene, assault**
     ● **T53.2X4**   **Toxic effect of trichloroethylene, undetermined**
● **T53.3**   **Toxic effects of tetrachloroethylene**
     Toxic effects of perchloroethylene
     Toxic effect of tetrachloroethene
   ● **T53.3X**   **Toxic effects of tetrachloroethylene**
     ● **T53.3X1**   **Toxic effect of tetrachloroethylene, accidental (unintentional)**
         Toxic effects of tetrachloroethylene NOS
     ● **T53.3X2**   **Toxic effect of tetrachloroethylene, intentional self-harm**
     ● **T53.3X3**   **Toxic effect of tetrachloroethylene, assault**
     ● **T53.3X4**   **Toxic effect of tetrachloroethylene, undetermined**
● **T53.4**   **Toxic effects of dichloromethane**
     Toxic effects of methylene chloride
   ● **T53.4X**   **Toxic effects of dichloromethane**
     ● **T53.4X1**   **Toxic effect of dichloromethane, accidental (unintentional)**
         Toxic effects of dichloromethane NOS
     ● **T53.4X2**   **Toxic effect of dichloromethane, intentional self-harm**
     ● **T53.4X3**   **Toxic effect of dichloromethane, assault**
     ● **T53.4X4**   **Toxic effect of dichloromethane, undetermined**
● **T53.5**   **Toxic effects of chlorofluorocarbons**
   ● **T53.5X**   **Toxic effects of chlorofluorocarbons**
     ● **T53.5X1**   **Toxic effect of chlorofluorocarbons, accidental (unintentional)**
         Toxic effects of chlorofluorocarbons NOS
     ● **T53.5X2**   **Toxic effect of chlorofluorocarbons, intentional self-harm**
     ● **T53.5X3**   **Toxic effect of chlorofluorocarbons, assault**
     ● **T53.5X4**   **Toxic effect of chlorofluorocarbons, undetermined**

● **T53.6**   **Toxic effects of other halogen derivatives of aliphatic hydrocarbons**
   ● **T53.6X**   **Toxic effects of other halogen derivatives of aliphatic hydrocarbons**
     ● **T53.6X1**   **Toxic effect of other halogen derivatives of aliphatic hydrocarbons, accidental (unintentional)**
         Toxic effects of other halogen derivatives of aliphatic hydrocarbons NOS
     ● **T53.6X2**   **Toxic effect of other halogen derivatives of aliphatic hydrocarbons, intentional self-harm**
     ● **T53.6X3**   **Toxic effect of other halogen derivatives of aliphatic hydrocarbons, assault**
     ● **T53.6X4**   **Toxic effect of other halogen derivatives of aliphatic hydrocarbons, undetermined**
● **T53.7**   **Toxic effects of other halogen derivatives of aromatic hydrocarbons**
   ● **T53.7X**   **Toxic effects of other halogen derivatives of aromatic hydrocarbons**
     ● **T53.7X1**   **Toxic effect of other halogen derivatives of aromatic hydrocarbons, accidental (unintentional)**
         Toxic effects of other halogen derivatives of aromatic hydrocarbons NOS
     ● **T53.7X2**   **Toxic effect of other halogen derivatives of aromatic hydrocarbons, intentional self-harm**
     ● **T53.7X3**   **Toxic effect of other halogen derivatives of aromatic hydrocarbons, assault**
     ● **T53.7X4**   **Toxic effect of other halogen derivatives of aromatic hydrocarbons, undetermined**
● **T53.9**   **Toxic effects of unspecified halogen derivatives of aliphatic and aromatic hydrocarbons**
   X ● **T53.91**   **Toxic effect of unspecified halogen derivatives of aliphatic and aromatic hydrocarbons, accidental (unintentional)**
   X ● **T53.92**   **Toxic effect of unspecified halogen derivatives of aliphatic and aromatic hydrocarbons, intentional self-harm**
   X ● **T53.93**   **Toxic effect of unspecified halogen derivatives of aliphatic and aromatic hydrocarbons, assault**
   X ● **T53.94**   **Toxic effect of unspecified halogen derivatives of aliphatic and aromatic hydrocarbons, undetermined**

● **T54**   **Toxic effect of corrosive substances**
     The appropriate 7th character is to be added to each code from category T54

A	initial encounter
D	subsequent encounter
S	sequela

● **T54.0**   **Toxic effects of phenol and phenol homologues**
   ● **T54.0X**   **Toxic effects of phenol and phenol homologues**
     ● **T54.0X1**   **Toxic effect of phenol and phenol homologues, accidental (unintentional)**
         Toxic effects of phenol and phenol homologues NOS
     ● **T54.0X2**   **Toxic effect of phenol and phenol homologues, intentional self-harm**
     ● **T54.0X3**   **Toxic effect of phenol and phenol homologues, assault**
     ● **T54.0X4**   **Toxic effect of phenol and phenol homologues, undetermined**

CHAPTER 19 (S00-T88)

CHAPTER 19 (S00-T88)

● T54.1   Toxic effects of other corrosive organic compounds
- ● T54.1X   Toxic effects of other corrosive organic compounds
  - ● T54.1X1   Toxic effect of other corrosive organic compounds, accidental (unintentional)
    - Toxic effects of other corrosive organic compounds NOS
  - ● T54.1X2   Toxic effect of other corrosive organic compounds, intentional self-harm
  - ● T54.1X3   Toxic effect of other corrosive organic compounds, assault
  - ● T54.1X4   Toxic effect of other corrosive organic compounds, undetermined

● T54.2   Toxic effects of corrosive acids and acid-like substances
- Toxic effects of hydrochloric acid
- Toxic effects of sulfuric acid
- ● T54.2X   Toxic effects of corrosive acids and acid-like substances
  - ● T54.2X1   Toxic effect of corrosive acids and acid-like substances, accidental (unintentional)
    - Toxic effects of corrosive acids and acid-like substances NOS
  - ● T54.2X2   Toxic effect of corrosive acids and acid-like substances, intentional self-harm
  - ● T54.2X3   Toxic effect of corrosive acids and acid-like substances, assault
  - ● T54.2X4   Toxic effect of corrosive acids and acid-like substances, undetermined

● T54.3   Toxic effects of corrosive alkalis and alkali-like substances
- Toxic effects of potassium hydroxide
- Toxic effects of sodium hydroxide
- ● T54.3X   Toxic effects of corrosive alkalis and alkali-like substances
  - ● T54.3X1   Toxic effect of corrosive alkalis and alkali-like substances, accidental (unintentional)
    - Toxic effects of corrosive alkalis and alkali-like substances NOS
  - ● T54.3X2   Toxic effect of corrosive alkalis and alkali-like substances, intentional self-harm
  - ● T54.3X3   Toxic effect of corrosive alkalis and alkali-like substances, assault
  - ● T54.3X4   Toxic effect of corrosive alkalis and alkali-like substances, undetermined

● T54.9   Toxic effects of unspecified corrosive substance
- X ● T54.91   Toxic effect of unspecified corrosive substance, accidental (unintentional)
- X ● T54.92   Toxic effect of unspecified corrosive substance, intentional self-harm
- X ● T54.93   Toxic effect of unspecified corrosive substance, assault
- X ● T54.94   Toxic effect of unspecified corrosive substance, undetermined

● T55   Toxic effect of soaps and detergents
- The appropriate 7th character is to be added to each code from category T55

A	initial encounter
D	subsequent encounter
S	sequela

- ● T55.0   Toxic effect of soaps
  - ● T55.0X   Toxic effect of soaps
    - ● T55.0X1   Toxic effect of soaps, accidental (unintentional)
      - Toxic effect of soaps NOS
    - ● T55.0X2   Toxic effect of soaps, intentional self-harm
    - ● T55.0X3   Toxic effect of soaps, assault
    - ● T55.0X4   Toxic effect of soaps, undetermined
- ● T55.1   Toxic effect of detergents
  - ● T55.1X   Toxic effect of detergents
    - ● T55.1X1   Toxic effect of detergents, accidental (unintentional)
      - Toxic effect of detergents NOS
    - ● T55.1X2   Toxic effect of detergents, intentional self-harm
    - ● T55.1X3   Toxic effect of detergents, assault
    - ● T55.1X4   Toxic effect of detergents, undetermined

● T56   Toxic effect of metals
- **Includes**   toxic effects of fumes and vapors of metals
  - toxic effects of metals from all sources, except medicinal substances
- Use additional code to identify any retained metal foreign body, if applicable (Z18.0-, T18.1-)
- **Excludes1**   arsenic and its compounds (T57.0)
  - manganese and its compounds (T57.2)
- The appropriate 7th character is to be added to each code from category T56

A	initial encounter
D	subsequent encounter
S	sequela

- ● T56.0   Toxic effects of lead and its compounds
  - ● T56.0X   Toxic effects of lead and its compounds
    - ● T56.0X1   Toxic effect of lead and its compounds, accidental (unintentional)
      - Toxic effects of lead and its compounds NOS
    - ● T56.0X2   Toxic effect of lead and its compounds, intentional self-harm
    - ● T56.0X3   Toxic effect of lead and its compounds, assault
    - ● T56.0X4   Toxic effect of lead and its compounds, undetermined
- ● T56.1   Toxic effects of mercury and its compounds
  - ● T56.1X   Toxic effects of mercury and its compounds
    - ● T56.1X1   Toxic effect of mercury and its compounds, accidental (unintentional)
      - Toxic effects of mercury and its compounds NOS
    - ● T56.1X2   Toxic effect of mercury and its compounds, intentional self-harm
    - ● T56.1X3   Toxic effect of mercury and its compounds, assault
    - ● T56.1X4   Toxic effect of mercury and its compounds, undetermined

◀ New   ◀▓ Revised   ~~deleted~~ Deleted   Excludes 1   Excludes 2   Includes   Use additional   Code first   Code also   Unspecified

1390   OGCR Official Guidelines   X Assign placeholder X   ● Use Additional Character(s)   ▶ Manifestation Code   **Coding Clinic**

● **T56.2**   Toxic effects of chromium and its compounds
   ● **T56.2X**   Toxic effects of chromium and its compounds
     ● **T56.2X1**   Toxic effect of chromium and its compounds, accidental (unintentional)
       Toxic effects of chromium and its compounds NOS
     ● **T56.2X2**   Toxic effect of chromium and its compounds, intentional self-harm
     ● **T56.2X3**   Toxic effect of chromium and its compounds, assault
     ● **T56.2X4**   Toxic effect of chromium and its compounds, undetermined

● **T56.3**   Toxic effects of cadmium and its compounds
   ● **T56.3X**   Toxic effects of cadmium and its compounds
     ● **T56.3X1**   Toxic effect of cadmium and its compounds, accidental (unintentional)
       Toxic effects of cadmium and its compounds NOS
     ● **T56.3X2**   Toxic effect of cadmium and its compounds, intentional self-harm
     ● **T56.3X3**   Toxic effect of cadmium and its compounds, assault
     ● **T56.3X4**   Toxic effect of cadmium and its compounds, undetermined

● **T56.4**   Toxic effects of copper and its compounds
   ● **T56.4X**   Toxic effects of copper and its compounds
     ● **T56.4X1**   Toxic effect of copper and its compounds, accidental (unintentional)
       Toxic effects of copper and its compounds NOS
     ● **T56.4X2**   Toxic effect of copper and its compounds, intentional self-harm
     ● **T56.4X3**   Toxic effect of copper and its compounds, assault
     ● **T56.4X4**   Toxic effect of copper and its compounds, undetermined

● **T56.5**   Toxic effects of zinc and its compounds
   ● **T56.5X**   Toxic effects of zinc and its compounds
     ● **T56.5X1**   Toxic effect of zinc and its compounds, accidental (unintentional)
       Toxic effects of zinc and its compounds NOS
     ● **T56.5X2**   Toxic effect of zinc and its compounds, intentional self-harm
     ● **T56.5X3**   Toxic effect of zinc and its compounds, assault
     ● **T56.5X4**   Toxic effect of zinc and its compounds, undetermined

● **T56.6**   Toxic effects of tin and its compounds
   ● **T56.6X**   Toxic effects of tin and its compounds
     ● **T56.6X1**   Toxic effect of tin and its compounds, accidental (unintentional)
       Toxic effects of tin and its compounds NOS
     ● **T56.6X2**   Toxic effect of tin and its compounds, intentional self-harm
     ● **T56.6X3**   Toxic effect of tin and its compounds, assault
     ● **T56.6X4**   Toxic effect of tin and its compounds, undetermined

● **T56.7**   Toxic effects of beryllium and its compounds
   ● **T56.7X**   Toxic effects of beryllium and its compounds
     ● **T56.7X1**   Toxic effect of beryllium and its compounds, accidental (unintentional)
       Toxic effects of beryllium and its compounds NOS
     ● **T56.7X2**   Toxic effect of beryllium and its compounds, intentional self-harm
     ● **T56.7X3**   Toxic effect of beryllium and its compounds, assault
     ● **T56.7X4**   Toxic effect of beryllium and its compounds, undetermined

● **T56.8**   Toxic effects of other metals
   ● **T56.81**   Toxic effect of thallium
     ● **T56.811**   Toxic effect of thallium, accidental (unintentional)
       Toxic effect of thallium NOS
     ● **T56.812**   Toxic effect of thallium, intentional self-harm
     ● **T56.813**   Toxic effect of thallium, assault
     ● **T56.814**   Toxic effect of thallium, undetermined
   ● **T56.89**   Toxic effects of other metals
     ● **T56.891**   Toxic effect of other metals, accidental (unintentional)
       Toxic effects of other metals NOS
     ● **T56.892**   Toxic effect of other metals, intentional self-harm
     ● **T56.893**   Toxic effect of other metals, assault
     ● **T56.894**   Toxic effect of other metals, undetermined

● **T56.9**   Toxic effects of unspecified metal
   X ● **T56.91**   Toxic effect of unspecified metal, accidental (unintentional)
   X ● **T56.92**   Toxic effect of unspecified metal, intentional self-harm
   X ● **T56.93**   Toxic effect of unspecified metal, assault
   X ● **T56.94**   Toxic effect of unspecified metal, undetermined

● **T57**   Toxic effect of other inorganic substances
   The appropriate 7th character is to be added to each code from category T57

> | A | initial encounter |
> | D | subsequent encounter |
> | S | sequela |

● **T57.0**   Toxic effect of arsenic and its compounds
   ● **T57.0X**   Toxic effect of arsenic and its compounds
     ● **T57.0X1**   Toxic effect of arsenic and its compounds, accidental (unintentional)
       Toxic effect of arsenic and its compounds NOS
     ● **T57.0X2**   Toxic effect of arsenic and its compounds, intentional self-harm
     ● **T57.0X3**   Toxic effect of arsenic and its compounds, assault
     ● **T57.0X4**   Toxic effect of arsenic and its compounds, undetermined

CHAPTER 19 (S00-T88)

● **T57.1**   **Toxic effect of phosphorus and its compounds**
    Excludes1   organophosphate insecticides (T60.0)
   ● **T57.1X**   **Toxic effect of phosphorus and its compounds**
     ● **T57.1X1**   **Toxic effect of phosphorus and its compounds, accidental (unintentional)**
        Toxic effect of phosphorus and its compounds NOS
     ● **T57.1X2**   **Toxic effect of phosphorus and its compounds, intentional self-harm**
     ● **T57.1X3**   **Toxic effect of phosphorus and its compounds, assault**
     ● **T57.1X4**   **Toxic effect of phosphorus and its compounds, undetermined**

● **T57.2**   **Toxic effect of manganese and its compounds**
   ● **T57.2X**   **Toxic effect of manganese and its compounds**
     ● **T57.2X1**   **Toxic effect of manganese and its compounds, accidental (unintentional)**
        Toxic effect of manganese and its compounds NOS
     ● **T57.2X2**   **Toxic effect of manganese and its compounds, intentional self-harm**
     ● **T57.2X3**   **Toxic effect of manganese and its compounds, assault**
     ● **T57.2X4**   **Toxic effect of manganese and its compounds, undetermined**

● **T57.3**   **Toxic effect of hydrogen cyanide**
   ● **T57.3X**   **Toxic effect of hydrogen cyanide**
     ● **T57.3X1**   **Toxic effect of hydrogen cyanide, accidental (unintentional)**
        Toxic effect of hydrogen cyanide NOS
     ● **T57.3X2**   **Toxic effect of hydrogen cyanide, intentional self-harm**
     ● **T57.3X3**   **Toxic effect of hydrogen cyanide, assault**
     ● **T57.3X4**   **Toxic effect of hydrogen cyanide, undetermined**

● **T57.8**   **Toxic effect of other specified inorganic substances**
   ● **T57.8X**   **Toxic effect of other specified inorganic substances**
     ● **T57.8X1**   **Toxic effect of other specified inorganic substances, accidental (unintentional)**
        Toxic effect of other specified inorganic substances NOS
     ● **T57.8X2**   **Toxic effect of other specified inorganic substances, intentional self-harm**
     ● **T57.8X3**   **Toxic effect of other specified inorganic substances, assault**
     ● **T57.8X4**   **Toxic effect of other specified inorganic substances, undetermined**

● **T57.9**   **Toxic effect of unspecified inorganic substance**
   X ● **T57.91**   **Toxic effect of unspecified inorganic substance, accidental (unintentional)**
   X ● **T57.92**   **Toxic effect of unspecified inorganic substance, intentional self-harm**
   X ● **T57.93**   **Toxic effect of unspecified inorganic substance, assault**
   X ● **T57.94**   **Toxic effect of unspecified inorganic substance, undetermined**

● **T58**   **Toxic effect of carbon monoxide**
    Includes   asphyxiation from carbon monoxide
       toxic effect of carbon monoxide from all sources
   The appropriate 7th character is to be added to each code from category T58

A	initial encounter
D	subsequent encounter
S	sequela

● **T58.0**   **Toxic effect of carbon monoxide from motor vehicle exhaust**
     Toxic effect of exhaust gas from gas engine
     Toxic effect of exhaust gas from motor pump
   X ● **T58.01**   **Toxic effect of carbon monoxide from motor vehicle exhaust, accidental (unintentional)**
   X ● **T58.02**   **Toxic effect of carbon monoxide from motor vehicle exhaust, intentional self-harm**
   X ● **T58.03**   **Toxic effect of carbon monoxide from motor vehicle exhaust, assault**
   X ● **T58.04**   **Toxic effect of carbon monoxide from motor vehicle exhaust, undetermined**

● **T58.1**   **Toxic effect of carbon monoxide from utility gas**
     Toxic effect of acetylene
     Toxic effect of gas NOS used for lighting, heating, cooking
     Toxic effect of water gas
   X ● **T58.11**   **Toxic effect of carbon monoxide from utility gas, accidental (unintentional)**
   X ● **T58.12**   **Toxic effect of carbon monoxide from utility gas, intentional self-harm**
   X ● **T58.13**   **Toxic effect of carbon monoxide from utility gas, assault**
   X ● **T58.14**   **Toxic effect of carbon monoxide from utility gas, undetermined**

● **T58.2**   **Toxic effect of carbon monoxide from incomplete combustion of other domestic fuels**
     Toxic effect of carbon monoxide from incomplete combustion of coal, coke, kerosene, wood
   ● **T58.2X**   **Toxic effect of carbon monoxide from incomplete combustion of other domestic fuels**
     ● **T58.2X1**   **Toxic effect of carbon monoxide from incomplete combustion of other domestic fuels, accidental (unintentional)**
     ● **T58.2X2**   **Toxic effect of carbon monoxide from incomplete combustion of other domestic fuels, intentional self-harm**
     ● **T58.2X3**   **Toxic effect of carbon monoxide from incomplete combustion of other domestic fuels, assault**
     ● **T58.2X4**   **Toxic effect of carbon monoxide from incomplete combustion of other domestic fuels, undetermined**

● **T58.8**   **Toxic effect of carbon monoxide from other source**
     Toxic effect of carbon monoxide from blast furnace gas
     Toxic effect of carbon monoxide from fuels in industrial use
     Toxic effect of carbon monoxide from kiln vapor
   ● **T58.8X**   **Toxic effect of carbon monoxide from other source**
     ● **T58.8X1**   **Toxic effect of carbon monoxide from other source, accidental (unintentional)**
     ● **T58.8X2**   **Toxic effect of carbon monoxide from other source, intentional self-harm**
     ● **T58.8X3**   **Toxic effect of carbon monoxide from other source, assault**
     ● **T58.8X4**   **Toxic effect of carbon monoxide from other source, undetermined**

◄ New   ◀◀ Revised   ~~deleted~~ Deleted   Excludes 1   Excludes 2   Includes   Use additional   Code first   Code also   Unspecified

1392   OGCR Official Guidelines   X Assign placeholder X   ● Use Additional Character(s)   ▶ Manifestation Code   **Coding Clinic**

● T58.9   Toxic effect of carbon monoxide from unspecified source

   X ● T58.91   Toxic effect of carbon monoxide from unspecified source, accidental (unintentional)

   X ● T58.92   Toxic effect of carbon monoxide from unspecified source, intentional self-harm

   X ● T58.93   Toxic effect of carbon monoxide from unspecified source, assault

   X ● T58.94   Toxic effect of carbon monoxide from unspecified source, undetermined

● T59   Toxic effect of other gases, fumes and vapors

   Includes   aerosol propellants

   Excludes1   chlorofluorocarbons (T53.5)

   The appropriate 7th character is to be added to each code from category T59

     A   initial encounter
     D   subsequent encounter
     S   sequela

● T59.0   Toxic effect of nitrogen oxides

   ● T59.0X   Toxic effect of nitrogen oxides

     ● T59.0X1   Toxic effect of nitrogen oxides, accidental (unintentional)
       Toxic effect of nitrogen oxides NOS

     ● T59.0X2   Toxic effect of nitrogen oxides, intentional self-harm

     ● T59.0X3   Toxic effect of nitrogen oxides, assault

     ● T59.0X4   Toxic effect of nitrogen oxides, undetermined

● T59.1   Toxic effect of sulfur dioxide

   ● T59.1X   Toxic effect of sulfur dioxide

     ● T59.1X1   Toxic effect of sulfur dioxide, accidental (unintentional)
       Toxic effect of sulfur dioxide NOS

     ● T59.1X2   Toxic effect of sulfur dioxide, intentional self-harm

     ● T59.1X3   Toxic effect of sulfur dioxide, assault

     ● T59.1X4   Toxic effect of sulfur dioxide, undetermined

● T59.2   Toxic effect of formaldehyde

   ● T59.2X   Toxic effect of formaldehyde

     ● T59.2X1   Toxic effect of formaldehyde, accidental (unintentional)
       Toxic effect of formaldehyde NOS

     ● T59.2X2   Toxic effect of formaldehyde, intentional self-harm

     ● T59.2X3   Toxic effect of formaldehyde, assault

     ● T59.2X4   Toxic effect of formaldehyde, undetermined

● T59.3   Toxic effect of lacrimogenic gas
   Toxic effect of tear gas

   ● T59.3X   Toxic effect of lacrimogenic gas

     ● T59.3X1   Toxic effect of lacrimogenic gas, accidental (unintentional)
       Toxic effect of lacrimogenic gas NOS

     ● T59.3X2   Toxic effect of lacrimogenic gas, intentional self-harm

     ● T59.3X3   Toxic effect of lacrimogenic gas, assault

     ● T59.3X4   Toxic effect of lacrimogenic gas, undetermined

● T59.4   Toxic effect of chlorine gas

   ● T59.4X   Toxic effect of chlorine gas

     ● T59.4X1   Toxic effect of chlorine gas, accidental (unintentional)
       Toxic effect of chlorine gas NOS

     ● T59.4X2   Toxic effect of chlorine gas, intentional self-harm

     ● T59.4X3   Toxic effect of chlorine gas, assault

     ● T59.4X4   Toxic effect of chlorine gas, undetermined

● T59.5   Toxic effect of fluorine gas and hydrogen fluoride

   ● T59.5X   Toxic effect of fluorine gas and hydrogen fluoride

     ● T59.5X1   Toxic effect of fluorine gas and hydrogen fluoride, accidental (unintentional)
       Toxic effect of fluorine gas and hydrogen fluoride NOS

     ● T59.5X2   Toxic effect of fluorine gas and hydrogen fluoride, intentional self-harm

     ● T59.5X3   Toxic effect of fluorine gas and hydrogen fluoride, assault

     ● T59.5X4   Toxic effect of fluorine gas and hydrogen fluoride, undetermined

● T59.6   Toxic effect of hydrogen sulfide

   ● T59.6X   Toxic effect of hydrogen sulfide

     ● T59.6X1   Toxic effect of hydrogen sulfide, accidental (unintentional)
       Toxic effect of hydrogen sulfide NOS

     ● T59.6X2   Toxic effect of hydrogen sulfide, intentional self-harm

     ● T59.6X3   Toxic effect of hydrogen sulfide, assault

     ● T59.6X4   Toxic effect of hydrogen sulfide, undetermined

● T59.7   Toxic effect of carbon dioxide

   ● T59.7X   Toxic effect of carbon dioxide

     ● T59.7X1   Toxic effect of carbon dioxide, accidental (unintentional)
       Toxic effect of carbon dioxide NOS

     ● T59.7X2   Toxic effect of carbon dioxide, intentional self-harm

     ● T59.7X3   Toxic effect of carbon dioxide, assault

     ● T59.7X4   Toxic effect of carbon dioxide, undetermined

● T59.8   Toxic effect of other specified gases, fumes and vapors

   ● T59.81   Toxic effect of smoke
     Smoke inhalation

     Excludes2   toxic effect of cigarette (tobacco) smoke (T65.22-)

     ● T59.811   Toxic effect of smoke, accidental (unintentional)
       Toxic effect of smoke NOS

     ● T59.812   Toxic effect of smoke, intentional self-harm

     ● T59.813   Toxic effect of smoke, assault

     ● T59.814   Toxic effect of smoke, undetermined

   ● T59.89   Toxic effect of other specified gases, fumes and vapors

     ● T59.891   Toxic effect of other specified gases, fumes and vapors, accidental (unintentional)

     ● T59.892   Toxic effect of other specified gases, fumes and vapors, intentional self-harm

     ● T59.893   Toxic effect of other specified gases, fumes and vapors, assault

     ● T59.894   Toxic effect of other specified gases, fumes and vapors, undetermined

CHAPTER 19 (S00-T88)

● **T59.9**   **Toxic effect of unspecified gases, fumes and vapors**
   X ● **T59.91**   Toxic effect of unspecified gases, fumes and vapors, accidental (unintentional)
   X ● **T59.92**   Toxic effect of unspecified gases, fumes and vapors, intentional self-harm
   X ● **T59.93**   Toxic effect of unspecified gases, fumes and vapors, assault
   X ● **T59.94**   Toxic effect of unspecified gases, fumes and vapors, undetermined

● **T60**   **Toxic effect of pesticides**
    Includes   toxic effect of wood preservatives
    The appropriate 7th character is to be added to each code from category T60

> A   initial encounter
> D   subsequent encounter
> S   sequela

● **T60.0**   **Toxic effect of organophosphate and carbamate insecticides**
   ● **T60.0X**   Toxic effect of organophosphate and carbamate insecticides
     ● **T60.0X1**   Toxic effect of organophosphate and carbamate insecticides, accidental (unintentional)
         Toxic effect of organophosphate and carbamate insecticides NOS
     ● **T60.0X2**   Toxic effect of organophosphate and carbamate insecticides, intentional self-harm
     ● **T60.0X3**   Toxic effect of organophosphate and carbamate insecticides, assault
     ● **T60.0X4**   Toxic effect of organophosphate and carbamate insecticides, undetermined

● **T60.1**   **Toxic effect of halogenated insecticides**
    Excludes1   chlorinated hydrocarbon (T53.-)
   ● **T60.1X**   Toxic effect of halogenated insecticides
     ● **T60.1X1**   Toxic effect of halogenated insecticides, accidental (unintentional)
         Toxic effect of halogenated insecticides NOS
     ● **T60.1X2**   Toxic effect of halogenated insecticides, intentional self-harm
     ● **T60.1X3**   Toxic effect of halogenated insecticides, assault
     ● **T60.1X4**   Toxic effect of halogenated insecticides, undetermined

● **T60.2**   **Toxic effect of other insecticides**
   ● **T60.2X**   Toxic effect of other insecticides
     ● **T60.2X1**   Toxic effect of other insecticides, accidental (unintentional)
         Toxic effect of other insecticides NOS
     ● **T60.2X2**   Toxic effect of other insecticides, intentional self-harm
     ● **T60.2X3**   Toxic effect of other insecticides, assault
     ● **T60.2X4**   Toxic effect of other insecticides, undetermined

● **T60.3**   **Toxic effect of herbicides and fungicides**
   ● **T60.3X**   Toxic effect of herbicides and fungicides
     ● **T60.3X1**   Toxic effect of herbicides and fungicides, accidental (unintentional)
         Toxic effect of herbicides and fungicides NOS
     ● **T60.3X2**   Toxic effect of herbicides and fungicides, intentional self-harm
     ● **T60.3X3**   Toxic effect of herbicides and fungicides, assault
     ● **T60.3X4**   Toxic effect of herbicides and fungicides, undetermined

● **T60.4**   **Toxic effect of rodenticides**
    Excludes1   strychnine and its salts (T65.1)
            thallium (T56.81-)
   ● **T60.4X**   Toxic effect of rodenticides
     ● **T60.4X1**   Toxic effect of rodenticides, accidental (unintentional)
         Toxic effect of rodenticides NOS
     ● **T60.4X2**   Toxic effect of rodenticides, intentional self-harm
     ● **T60.4X3**   Toxic effect of rodenticides, assault
     ● **T60.4X4**   Toxic effect of rodenticides, undetermined

● **T60.8**   **Toxic effect of other pesticides**
   ● **T60.8X**   Toxic effect of other pesticides
     ● **T60.8X1**   Toxic effect of other pesticides, accidental (unintentional)
         Toxic effect of other pesticides NOS
     ● **T60.8X2**   Toxic effect of other pesticides, intentional self-harm
     ● **T60.8X3**   Toxic effect of other pesticides, assault
     ● **T60.8X4**   Toxic effect of other pesticides, undetermined

● **T60.9**   **Toxic effect of unspecified pesticide**
   X ● **T60.91**   Toxic effect of unspecified pesticide, accidental (unintentional)
   X ● **T60.92**   Toxic effect of unspecified pesticide, intentional self-harm
   X ● **T60.93**   Toxic effect of unspecified pesticide, assault
   X ● **T60.94**   Toxic effect of unspecified pesticide, undetermined

● **T61**   **Toxic effect of noxious substances eaten as seafood**
    Excludes1   allergic reaction to food, such as:
         anaphylactic reaction or shock due to adverse food reaction (T78.0-)
         bacterial foodborne intoxications (A05.-)
         dermatitis (L23.6, L25.4, L27.2)
         food protein-induced enterocolitis syndrome (K52.21) ◄
         food protein-induced enteropathy (K52.22) ◄
         gastroenteritis (noninfective) (K52.29) ◄
         toxic effect of aflatoxin and other mycotoxins (T64)
         toxic effect of cyanides (T65.0-)
         toxic effect of harmful algae bloom (T65.82-)
         toxic effect of hydrogen cyanide (T57.3-)
         toxic effect of mercury (T56.1-)
         toxic effect of red tide (T65.82-)
    The appropriate 7th character is to be added to each code from category T61

> A   initial encounter
> D   subsequent encounter
> S   sequela

● **T61.0**   **Ciguatera fish poisoning**
   X ● **T61.01**   Ciguatera fish poisoning, accidental (unintentional)
   X ● **T61.02**   Ciguatera fish poisoning, intentional self-harm
   X ● **T61.03**   Ciguatera fish poisoning, assault
   X ● **T61.04**   Ciguatera fish poisoning, undetermined

● **T61.1**   **Scombroid fish poisoning**
    Histamine-like syndrome
   X ● **T61.11**   Scombroid fish poisoning, accidental (unintentional)
   X ● **T61.12**   Scombroid fish poisoning, intentional self-harm
   X ● **T61.13**   Scombroid fish poisoning, assault
   X ● **T61.14**   Scombroid fish poisoning, undetermined

● **T61.7　Other fish and shellfish poisoning**
　● **T61.77　Other fish poisoning**
　　● **T61.771　Other fish poisoning, accidental (unintentional)**
　　● **T61.772　Other fish poisoning, intentional self-harm**
　　● **T61.773　Other fish poisoning, assault**
　　● **T61.774　Other fish poisoning, undetermined**
　● **T61.78　Other shellfish poisoning**
　　● **T61.781　Other shellfish poisoning, accidental (unintentional)**
　　● **T61.782　Other shellfish poisoning, intentional self-harm**
　　● **T61.783　Other shellfish poisoning, assault**
　　● **T61.784　Other shellfish poisoning, undetermined**
● **T61.8　Toxic effect of other seafood**
　● **T61.8X　Toxic effect of other seafood**
　　● **T61.8X1　Toxic effect of other seafood, accidental (unintentional)**
　　● **T61.8X2　Toxic effect of other seafood, intentional self-harm**
　　● **T61.8X3　Toxic effect of other seafood, assault**
　　● **T61.8X4　Toxic effect of other seafood, undetermined**
● **T61.9　Toxic effect of unspecified seafood**
　X ● **T61.91　Toxic effect of unspecified seafood, accidental (unintentional)**
　X ● **T61.92　Toxic effect of unspecified seafood, intentional self-harm**
　X ● **T61.93　Toxic effect of unspecified seafood, assault**
　X ● **T61.94　Toxic effect of unspecified seafood, undetermined**

● **T62　Toxic effect of other noxious substances eaten as food**

　Excludes1　allergic reaction to food, such as:
　　　　　anaphylactic shock (reaction) due to adverse food reaction (T78.0-)
　　　　　dermatitis (L23.6, L25.4, L27.2)
　　　　　food protein-induced enterocolitis syndrome (K52.21) ◀
　　　　　food protein-induced enteropathy (K52.22) ◀
　　　　　gastroenteritis (noninfective) (K52.29) ◀
　　　　bacterial food borne intoxications (A05.-)
　　　toxic effect of aflatoxin and other mycotoxins (T64)
　　　toxic effect of cyanides (T65.0-)
　　　toxic effect of hydrogen cyanide (T57.3-)
　　　toxic effect of mercury (T56.1-)

　The appropriate 7th character is to be added to each code from category T62

A	initial encounter
D	subsequent encounter
S	sequela

● **T62.0　Toxic effect of ingested mushrooms**
　● **T62.0X　Toxic effect of ingested mushrooms**
　　● **T62.0X1　Toxic effect of ingested mushrooms, accidental (unintentional)**
　　　　Toxic effect of ingested mushrooms NOS
　　● **T62.0X2　Toxic effect of ingested mushrooms, intentional self-harm**
　　● **T62.0X3　Toxic effect of ingested mushrooms, assault**
　　● **T62.0X4　Toxic effect of ingested mushrooms, undetermined**

● **T62.1　Toxic effect of ingested berries**
　● **T62.1X　Toxic effect of ingested berries**
　　● **T62.1X1　Toxic effect of ingested berries, accidental (unintentional)**
　　　　Toxic effect of ingested berries NOS
　　● **T62.1X2　Toxic effect of ingested berries, intentional self-harm**
　　● **T62.1X3　Toxic effect of ingested berries, assault**
　　● **T62.1X4　Toxic effect of ingested berries, undetermined**
● **T62.2　Toxic effect of other ingested (parts of) plant(s)**
　● **T62.2X　Toxic effect of other ingested (parts of) plant(s)**
　　● **T62.2X1　Toxic effect of other ingested (parts of) plant(s), accidental (unintentional)**
　　　　Toxic effect of other ingested (parts of) plant(s) NOS
　　● **T62.2X2　Toxic effect of other ingested (parts of) plant(s), intentional self-harm**
　　● **T62.2X3　Toxic effect of other ingested (parts of) plant(s), assault**
　　● **T62.2X4　Toxic effect of other ingested (parts of) plant(s), undetermined**
● **T62.8　Toxic effect of other specified noxious substances eaten as food**
　● **T62.8X　Toxic effect of other specified noxious substances eaten as food**
　　● **T62.8X1　Toxic effect of other specified noxious substances eaten as food, accidental (unintentional)**
　　　　Toxic effect of other specified noxious substances eaten as food NOS
　　● **T62.8X2　Toxic effect of other specified noxious substances eaten as food, intentional self-harm**
　　● **T62.8X3　Toxic effect of other specified noxious substances eaten as food, assault**
　　● **T62.8X4　Toxic effect of other specified noxious substances eaten as food, undetermined**
● **T62.9　Toxic effect of unspecified noxious substance eaten as food**
　X ● **T62.91　Toxic effect of unspecified noxious substance eaten as food, accidental (unintentional)**
　　　　Toxic effect of unspecified noxious substance eaten as food NOS
　X ● **T62.92　Toxic effect of unspecified noxious substance eaten as food, intentional self-harm**
　X ● **T62.93　Toxic effect of unspecified noxious substance eaten as food, assault**
　X ● **T62.94　Toxic effect of unspecified noxious substance eaten as food, undetermined**

● **T63　Toxic effect of contact with venomous animals and plants**

　Includes　bite or touch of venomous animal
　　　　　pricked or stuck by thorn or leaf

　Excludes2　ingestion of toxic animal or plant (T61.-, T62.-)

　The appropriate 7th character is to be added to each code from category T63

A	initial encounter
D	subsequent encounter
S	sequela

● **T63.0　Toxic effect of snake venom**
　● **T63.00　Toxic effect of unspecified snake venom**
　　● **T63.001　Toxic effect of unspecified snake venom, accidental (unintentional)**
　　　　Toxic effect of unspecified snake venom NOS
　　● **T63.002　Toxic effect of unspecified snake venom, intentional self-harm**
　　● **T63.003　Toxic effect of unspecified snake venom, assault**
　　● **T63.004　Toxic effect of unspecified snake venom, undetermined**

- ● **T63.Ø1**   Toxic effect of rattlesnake venom
  - ● **T63.Ø11**   Toxic effect of rattlesnake venom, accidental (unintentional)
    - Toxic effect of rattlesnake venom NOS
  - ● **T63.Ø12**   Toxic effect of rattlesnake venom, intentional self-harm
  - ● **T63.Ø13**   Toxic effect of rattlesnake venom, assault
  - ● **T63.Ø14**   Toxic effect of rattlesnake venom, undetermined
- ● **T63.Ø2**   Toxic effect of coral snake venom
  - ● **T63.Ø21**   Toxic effect of coral snake venom, accidental (unintentional)
    - Toxic effect of coral snake venom NOS
  - ● **T63.Ø22**   Toxic effect of coral snake venom, intentional self-harm
  - ● **T63.Ø23**   Toxic effect of coral snake venom, assault
  - ● **T63.Ø24**   Toxic effect of coral snake venom, undetermined
- ● **T63.Ø3**   Toxic effect of taipan venom
  - ● **T63.Ø31**   Toxic effect of taipan venom, accidental (unintentional)
    - Toxic effect of taipan venom NOS
  - ● **T63.Ø32**   Toxic effect of taipan venom, intentional self-harm
  - ● **T63.Ø33**   Toxic effect of taipan venom, assault
  - ● **T63.Ø34**   Toxic effect of taipan venom, undetermined
- ● **T63.Ø4**   Toxic effect of cobra venom
  - ● **T63.Ø41**   Toxic effect of cobra venom, accidental (unintentional)
    - Toxic effect of cobra venom NOS
  - ● **T63.Ø42**   Toxic effect of cobra venom, intentional self-harm
  - ● **T63.Ø43**   Toxic effect of cobra venom, assault
  - ● **T63.Ø44**   Toxic effect of cobra venom, undetermined
- ● **T63.Ø6**   Toxic effect of venom of other North and South American snake
  - ● **T63.Ø61**   Toxic effect of venom of other North and South American snake, accidental (unintentional)
    - Toxic effect of venom of other North and South American snake NOS
  - ● **T63.Ø62**   Toxic effect of venom of other North and South American snake, intentional self-harm
  - ● **T63.Ø63**   Toxic effect of venom of other North and South American snake, assault
  - ● **T63.Ø64**   Toxic effect of venom of other North and South American snake, undetermined
- ● **T63.Ø7**   Toxic effect of venom of other Australian snake
  - ● **T63.Ø71**   Toxic effect of venom of other Australian snake, accidental (unintentional)
    - Toxic effect of venom of other Australian snake NOS
  - ● **T63.Ø72**   Toxic effect of venom of other Australian snake, intentional self-harm
  - ● **T63.Ø73**   Toxic effect of venom of other Australian snake, assault
  - ● **T63.Ø74**   Toxic effect of venom of other Australian snake, undetermined

- ● **T63.Ø8**   Toxic effect of venom of other African and Asian snake
  - ● **T63.Ø81**   Toxic effect of venom of other African and Asian snake, accidental (unintentional)
    - Toxic effect of venom of other African and Asian snake NOS
  - ● **T63.Ø82**   Toxic effect of venom of other African and Asian snake, intentional self-harm
  - ● **T63.Ø83**   Toxic effect of venom of other African and Asian snake, assault
  - ● **T63.Ø84**   Toxic effect of venom of other African and Asian snake, undetermined
- ● **T63.Ø9**   Toxic effect of venom of other snake
  - ● **T63.Ø91**   Toxic effect of venom of other snake, accidental (unintentional)
    - Toxic effect of venom of other snake NOS
  - ● **T63.Ø92**   Toxic effect of venom of other snake, intentional self-harm
  - ● **T63.Ø93**   Toxic effect of venom of other snake, assault
  - ● **T63.Ø94**   Toxic effect of venom of other snake, undetermined
- ● **T63.1**   Toxic effect of venom of other reptiles
  - ● **T63.11**   Toxic effect of venom of gila monster
    - ● **T63.111**   Toxic effect of venom of gila monster, accidental (unintentional)
      - Toxic effect of venom of gila monster NOS
    - ● **T63.112**   Toxic effect of venom of gila monster, intentional self-harm
    - ● **T63.113**   Toxic effect of venom of gila monster, assault
    - ● **T63.114**   Toxic effect of venom of gila monster, undetermined
  - ● **T63.12**   Toxic effect of venom of other venomous lizard
    - ● **T63.121**   Toxic effect of venom of other venomous lizard, accidental (unintentional)
      - Toxic effect of venom of other venomous lizard NOS
    - ● **T63.122**   Toxic effect of venom of other venomous lizard, intentional self-harm
    - ● **T63.123**   Toxic effect of venom of other venomous lizard, assault
    - ● **T63.124**   Toxic effect of venom of other venomous lizard, undetermined
  - ● **T63.19**   Toxic effect of venom of other reptiles
    - ● **T63.191**   Toxic effect of venom of other reptiles, accidental (unintentional)
      - Toxic effect of venom of other reptiles NOS
    - ● **T63.192**   Toxic effect of venom of other reptiles, intentional self-harm
    - ● **T63.193**   Toxic effect of venom of other reptiles, assault
    - ● **T63.194**   Toxic effect of venom of other reptiles, undetermined
- ● **T63.2**   Toxic effect of venom of scorpion
  - ● **T63.2X**   Toxic effect of venom of scorpion
    - ● **T63.2X1**   Toxic effect of venom of scorpion, accidental (unintentional)
      - Toxic effect of venom of scorpion NOS
    - ● **T63.2X2**   Toxic effect of venom of scorpion, intentional self-harm

◀ New   ◀▪▪ Revised   ~~deleted~~ Deleted   Excludes 1   Excludes 2   Includes   Use additional   Code first   Code also   Unspecified

OGCR Official Guidelines   X Assign placeholder X   ▶ Use Additional Character(s)   ▶ Manifestation Code   **Coding Clinic**

● T63.2X3   Toxic effect of venom of scorpion, assault
● T63.2X4   Toxic effect of venom of scorpion, undetermined

● T63.3   Toxic effect of venom of spider
   ● T63.30   Toxic effect of unspecified spider venom
     ● T63.301   Toxic effect of unspecified spider venom, accidental (unintentional)
     ● T63.302   Toxic effect of unspecified spider venom, intentional self-harm
     ● T63.303   Toxic effect of unspecified spider venom, assault
     ● T63.304   Toxic effect of unspecified spider venom, undetermined
   ● T63.31   Toxic effect of venom of black widow spider
     ● T63.311   Toxic effect of venom of black widow spider, accidental (unintentional)
     ● T63.312   Toxic effect of venom of black widow spider, intentional self-harm
     ● T63.313   Toxic effect of venom of black widow spider, assault
     ● T63.314   Toxic effect of venom of black widow spider, undetermined
   ● T63.32   Toxic effect of venom of tarantula
     ● T63.321   Toxic effect of venom of tarantula, accidental (unintentional)
     ● T63.322   Toxic effect of venom of tarantula, intentional self-harm
     ● T63.323   Toxic effect of venom of tarantula, assault
     ● T63.324   Toxic effect of venom of tarantula, undetermined
   ● T63.33   Toxic effect of venom of brown recluse spider
     ● T63.331   Toxic effect of venom of brown recluse spider, accidental (unintentional)
     ● T63.332   Toxic effect of venom of brown recluse spider, intentional self-harm
     ● T63.333   Toxic effect of venom of brown recluse spider, assault
     ● T63.334   Toxic effect of venom of brown recluse spider, undetermined
   ● T63.39   Toxic effect of venom of other spider
     ● T63.391   Toxic effect of venom of other spider, accidental (unintentional)
     ● T63.392   Toxic effect of venom of other spider, intentional self-harm
     ● T63.393   Toxic effect of venom of other spider, assault
     ● T63.394   Toxic effect of venom of other spider, undetermined

● T63.4   Toxic effect of venom of other arthropods
   ● T63.41   Toxic effect of venom of centipedes and venomous millipedes
     ● T63.411   Toxic effect of venom of centipedes and venomous millipedes, accidental (unintentional)
     ● T63.412   Toxic effect of venom of centipedes and venomous millipedes, intentional self-harm
     ● T63.413   Toxic effect of venom of centipedes and venomous millipedes, assault
     ● T63.414   Toxic effect of venom of centipedes and venomous millipedes, undetermined

   ● T63.42   Toxic effect of venom of ants
     ● T63.421   Toxic effect of venom of ants, accidental (unintentional)
     ● T63.422   Toxic effect of venom of ants, intentional self-harm
     ● T63.423   Toxic effect of venom of ants, assault
     ● T63.424   Toxic effect of venom of ants, undetermined
   ● T63.43   Toxic effect of venom of caterpillars
     ● T63.431   Toxic effect of venom of caterpillars, accidental (unintentional)
     ● T63.432   Toxic effect of venom of caterpillars, intentional self-harm
     ● T63.433   Toxic effect of venom of caterpillars, assault
     ● T63.434   Toxic effect of venom of caterpillars, undetermined
   ● T63.44   Toxic effect of venom of bees
     ● T63.441   Toxic effect of venom of bees, accidental (unintentional)
     ● T63.442   Toxic effect of venom of bees, intentional self-harm
     ● T63.443   Toxic effect of venom of bees, assault
     ● T63.444   Toxic effect of venom of bees, undetermined
   ● T63.45   Toxic effect of venom of hornets
     ● T63.451   Toxic effect of venom of hornets, accidental (unintentional)
     ● T63.452   Toxic effect of venom of hornets, intentional self-harm
     ● T63.453   Toxic effect of venom of hornets, assault
     ● T63.454   Toxic effect of venom of hornets, undetermined
   ● T63.46   Toxic effect of venom of wasps
       Toxic effect of yellow jacket
     ● T63.461   Toxic effect of venom of wasps, accidental (unintentional)
     ● T63.462   Toxic effect of venom of wasps, intentional self-harm
     ● T63.463   Toxic effect of venom of wasps, assault
     ● T63.464   Toxic effect of venom of wasps, undetermined
   ● T63.48   Toxic effect of venom of other arthropod
     ● T63.481   Toxic effect of venom of other arthropod, accidental (unintentional)
     ● T63.482   Toxic effect of venom of other arthropod, intentional self-harm
     ● T63.483   Toxic effect of venom of other arthropod, assault
     ● T63.484   Toxic effect of venom of other arthropod, undetermined

● T63.5   Toxic effect of contact with venomous fish
     Excludes2   poisoning by ingestion of fish (T61.-)
   ● T63.51   Toxic effect of contact with stingray
     ● T63.511   Toxic effect of contact with stingray, accidental (unintentional)
     ● T63.512   Toxic effect of contact with stingray, intentional self-harm
     ● T63.513   Toxic effect of contact with stingray, assault
     ● T63.514   Toxic effect of contact with stingray, undetermined

● T63.59   Toxic effect of contact with other venomous fish
- ● T63.591   Toxic effect of contact with other venomous fish, accidental (unintentional)
- ● T63.592   Toxic effect of contact with other venomous fish, intentional self-harm
- ● T63.593   Toxic effect of contact with other venomous fish, assault
- ● T63.594   Toxic effect of contact with other venomous fish, undetermined

● T63.6   Toxic effect of contact with other venomous marine animals

> **Excludes1**   sea-snake venom (T63.Ø9)
>
> **Excludes2**   poisoning by ingestion of shellfish (T61.78-)

- ● T63.61   Toxic effect of contact with Portugese Man-o-war
  Toxic effect of contact with bluebottle
  - ● T63.611   Toxic effect of contact with Portugese Man-o-war, accidental (unintentional)
  - ● T63.612   Toxic effect of contact with Portugese Man-o-war, intentional self-harm
  - ● T63.613   Toxic effect of contact with Portugese Man-o-war, assault
  - ● T63.614   Toxic effect of contact with Portugese Man-o-war, undetermined
- ● T63.62   Toxic effect of contact with other jellyfish
  - ● T63.621   Toxic effect of contact with other jellyfish, accidental (unintentional)
  - ● T63.622   Toxic effect of contact with other jellyfish, intentional self-harm
  - ● T63.623   Toxic effect of contact with other jellyfish, assault
  - ● T63.624   Toxic effect of contact with other jellyfish, undetermined
- ● T63.63   Toxic effect of contact with sea anemone
  - ● T63.631   Toxic effect of contact with sea anemone, accidental (unintentional)
  - ● T63.632   Toxic effect of contact with sea anemone, intentional self-harm
  - ● T63.633   Toxic effect of contact with sea anemone, assault
  - ● T63.634   Toxic effect of contact with sea anemone, undetermined
- ● T63.69   Toxic effect of contact with other venomous marine animals
  - ● T63.691   Toxic effect of contact with other venomous marine animals, accidental (unintentional)
  - ● T63.692   Toxic effect of contact with other venomous marine animals, intentional self-harm
  - ● T63.693   Toxic effect of contact with other venomous marine animals, assault
  - ● T63.694   Toxic effect of contact with other venomous marine animals, undetermined

● T63.7   Toxic effect of contact with venomous plant
- ● T63.71   Toxic effect of contact with venomous marine plant
  - ● T63.711   Toxic effect of contact with venomous marine plant, accidental (unintentional)
  - ● T63.712   Toxic effect of contact with venomous marine plant, intentional self-harm
  - ● T63.713   Toxic effect of contact with venomous marine plant, assault
  - ● T63.714   Toxic effect of contact with venomous marine plant, undetermined

● T63.79   Toxic effect of contact with other venomous plant
- ● T63.791   Toxic effect of contact with other venomous plant, accidental (unintentional)
- ● T63.792   Toxic effect of contact with other venomous plant, intentional self-harm
- ● T63.793   Toxic effect of contact with other venomous plant, assault
- ● T63.794   Toxic effect of contact with other venomous plant, undetermined

● T63.8   Toxic effect of contact with other venomous animals
- ● T63.81   Toxic effect of contact with venomous frog

  > **Excludes1**   contact with nonvenomous frog (W62.Ø)

  - ● T63.811   Toxic effect of contact with venomous frog, accidental (unintentional)
  - ● T63.812   Toxic effect of contact with venomous frog, intentional self-harm
  - ● T63.813   Toxic effect of contact with venomous frog, assault
  - ● T63.814   Toxic effect of contact with venomous frog, undetermined
- ● T63.82   Toxic effect of contact with venomous toad

  > **Excludes1**   contact with nonvenomous toad (W62.1)

  - ● T63.821   Toxic effect of contact with venomous toad, accidental (unintentional)
  - ● T63.822   Toxic effect of contact with venomous toad, intentional self-harm
  - ● T63.823   Toxic effect of contact with venomous toad, assault
  - ● T63.824   Toxic effect of contact with venomous toad, undetermined
- ● T63.83   Toxic effect of contact with other venomous amphibian

  > **Excludes1**   contact with nonvenomous amphibian (W62.9)

  - ● T63.831   Toxic effect of contact with other venomous amphibian, accidental (unintentional)
  - ● T63.832   Toxic effect of contact with other venomous amphibian, intentional self-harm
  - ● T63.833   Toxic effect of contact with other venomous amphibian, assault
  - ● T63.834   Toxic effect of contact with other venomous amphibian, undetermined
- ● T63.89   Toxic effect of contact with other venomous animals
  - ● T63.891   Toxic effect of contact with other venomous animals, accidental (unintentional)
  - ● T63.892   Toxic effect of contact with other venomous animals, intentional self-harm
  - ● T63.893   Toxic effect of contact with other venomous animals, assault
  - ● T63.894   Toxic effect of contact with other venomous animals, undetermined

● T63.9   Toxic effect of contact with unspecified venomous animal
- X ● T63.91   Toxic effect of contact with unspecified venomous animal, accidental (unintentional)
- X ● T63.92   Toxic effect of contact with unspecified venomous animal, intentional self-harm
- X ● T63.93   Toxic effect of contact with unspecified venomous animal, assault
- X ● T63.94   Toxic effect of contact with unspecified venomous animal, undetermined

CHAPTER 19 (SØØ-T88)

● **T64   Toxic effect of aflatoxin and other mycotoxin food contaminants**
     The appropriate 7th character is to be added to each code from
     category T64

A	initial encounter
D	subsequent encounter
S	sequela

● **T64.0   Toxic effect of aflatoxin**
     X● **T64.01   Toxic effect of aflatoxin, accidental
                     (unintentional)**
     X● **T64.02   Toxic effect of aflatoxin, intentional self-harm**
     X● **T64.03   Toxic effect of aflatoxin, assault**
     X● **T64.04   Toxic effect of aflatoxin, undetermined**
● **T64.8   Toxic effect of other mycotoxin food contaminants**
     X● **T64.81   Toxic effect of other mycotoxin food
                     contaminants, accidental (unintentional)**
     X● **T64.82   Toxic effect of other mycotoxin food
                     contaminants, intentional self-harm**
     X● **T64.83   Toxic effect of other mycotoxin food
                     contaminants, assault**
     X● **T64.84   Toxic effect of other mycotoxin food
                     contaminants, undetermined**

● **T65   Toxic effect of other and unspecified substances**
     The appropriate 7th character is to be added to each code from
     category T65

A	initial encounter
D	subsequent encounter
S	sequela

● **T65.0   Toxic effect of cyanides**
     Excludes1   hydrogen cyanide (T57.3-)
     ● **T65.0X   Toxic effect of cyanides**
          ● **T65.0X1   Toxic effect of cyanides, accidental
                          (unintentional)**
                          Toxic effect of cyanides NOS
          ● **T65.0X2   Toxic effect of cyanides, intentional
                          self-harm**
          ● **T65.0X3   Toxic effect of cyanides, assault**
          ● **T65.0X4   Toxic effect of cyanides,
                          undetermined**
● **T65.1   Toxic effect of strychnine and its salts**
     ● **T65.1X   Toxic effect of strychnine and its salts**
          ● **T65.1X1   Toxic effect of strychnine and its salts,
                          accidental (unintentional)**
                          Toxic effect of strychnine and its
                          salts NOS
          ● **T65.1X2   Toxic effect of strychnine and its salts,
                          intentional self-harm**
          ● **T65.1X3   Toxic effect of strychnine and its salts,
                          assault**
          ● **T65.1X4   Toxic effect of strychnine and its salts,
                          undetermined**
● **T65.2   Toxic effect of tobacco and nicotine**
     Excludes2   nicotine dependence (F17.-)
     ● **T65.21   Toxic effect of chewing tobacco**
          ● **T65.211   Toxic effect of chewing tobacco,
                          accidental (unintentional)**
                          Toxic effect of chewing tobacco NOS
          ● **T65.212   Toxic effect of chewing tobacco,
                          intentional self-harm**
          ● **T65.213   Toxic effect of chewing tobacco,
                          assault**
          ● **T65.214   Toxic effect of chewing tobacco,
                          undetermined**

● **T65.22   Toxic effect of tobacco cigarettes**
          Toxic effect of tobacco smoke
          Use additional code for exposure to second
             hand tobacco smoke (Z57.31, Z77.22)
     ● **T65.221   Toxic effect of tobacco cigarettes,
                     accidental (unintentional)**
                     Toxic effect of tobacco cigarettes
                     NOS
     ● **T65.222   Toxic effect of tobacco cigarettes,
                     intentional self-harm**
     ● **T65.223   Toxic effect of tobacco cigarettes,
                     assault**
     ● **T65.224   Toxic effect of tobacco cigarettes,
                     undetermined**
● **T65.29   Toxic effect of other tobacco and nicotine**
     ● **T65.291   Toxic effect of other tobacco and
                     nicotine, accidental (unintentional)**
                     Toxic effect of other tobacco and
                     nicotine NOS
     ● **T65.292   Toxic effect of other tobacco and
                     nicotine, intentional self-harm**
     ● **T65.293   Toxic effect of other tobacco and
                     nicotine, assault**
     ● **T65.294   Toxic effect of other tobacco and
                     nicotine, undetermined**
● **T65.3   Toxic effect of nitroderivatives and aminoderivatives of
             benzene and its homologues**
          Toxic effect of anilin [benzenamine]
          Toxic effect of nitrobenzene
          Toxic effect of trinitrotoluene
     ● **T65.3X   Toxic effect of nitroderivatives and
                    aminoderivatives of benzene and its
                    homologues**
          ● **T65.3X1   Toxic effect of nitroderivatives
                          and aminoderivatives of benzene
                          and its homologues, accidental
                          (unintentional)**
                          Toxic effect of nitroderivatives and
                          aminoderivatives of benzene
                          and its homologues NOS
          ● **T65.3X2   Toxic effect of nitroderivatives and
                          aminoderivatives of benzene and its
                          homologues, intentional self-harm**
          ● **T65.3X3   Toxic effect of nitroderivatives and
                          aminoderivatives of benzene and its
                          homologues, assault**
          ● **T65.3X4   Toxic effect of nitroderivatives and
                          aminoderivatives of benzene and its
                          homologues, undetermined**
● **T65.4   Toxic effect of carbon disulfide**
     ● **T65.4X   Toxic effect of carbon disulfide**
          ● **T65.4X1   Toxic effect of carbon disulfide,
                          accidental (unintentional)**
                          Toxic effect of carbon disulfide NOS
          ● **T65.4X2   Toxic effect of carbon disulfide,
                          intentional self-harm**
          ● **T65.4X3   Toxic effect of carbon disulfide,
                          assault**
          ● **T65.4X4   Toxic effect of carbon disulfide,
                          undetermined**

CHAPTER 19 (S00-T88)

● **T65.5** **Toxic effect of nitroglycerin and other nitric acids and esters**
     Toxic effect of 1,2,3-Propanetriol trinitrate

   ● **T65.5X** **Toxic effect of nitroglycerin and other nitric acids and esters**

     ● **T65.5X1** **Toxic effect of nitroglycerin and other nitric acids and esters, accidental (unintentional)**
         Toxic effect of nitroglycerin and other nitric acids and esters NOS

     ● **T65.5X2** **Toxic effect of nitroglycerin and other nitric acids and esters, intentional self-harm**

     ● **T65.5X3** **Toxic effect of nitroglycerin and other nitric acids and esters, assault**

     ● **T65.5X4** **Toxic effect of nitroglycerin and other nitric acids and esters, undetermined**

● **T65.6** **Toxic effect of paints and dyes, not elsewhere classified**

   ● **T65.6X** **Toxic effect of paints and dyes, not elsewhere classified**

     ● **T65.6X1** **Toxic effect of paints and dyes, not elsewhere classified, accidental (unintentional)**
         Toxic effect of paints and dyes NOS

     ● **T65.6X2** **Toxic effect of paints and dyes, not elsewhere classified, intentional self-harm**

     ● **T65.6X3** **Toxic effect of paints and dyes, not elsewhere classified, assault**

     ● **T65.6X4** **Toxic effect of paints and dyes, not elsewhere classified, undetermined**

● **T65.8** **Toxic effect of other specified substances**

   ● **T65.81** **Toxic effect of latex**

     ● **T65.811** **Toxic effect of latex, accidental (unintentional)**
         Toxic effect of latex NOS

     ● **T65.812** **Toxic effect of latex, intentional self-harm**

     ● **T65.813** **Toxic effect of latex, assault**

     ● **T65.814** **Toxic effect of latex, undetermined**

   ● **T65.82** **Toxic effect of harmful algae and algae toxins**
     Toxic effect of (harmful) algae bloom NOS
     Toxic effect of blue-green algae bloom
     Toxic effect of brown tide
     Toxic effect of cyanobacteria bloom
     Toxic effect of Florida red tide
     Toxic effect of pfiesteria piscicida
     Toxic effect of red tide

     ● **T65.821** **Toxic effect of harmful algae and algae toxins, accidental (unintentional)**
         Toxic effect of harmful algae and algae toxins NOS

     ● **T65.822** **Toxic effect of harmful algae and algae toxins, intentional self-harm**

     ● **T65.823** **Toxic effect of harmful algae and algae toxins, assault**

     ● **T65.824** **Toxic effect of harmful algae and algae toxins, undetermined**

   ● **T65.83** **Toxic effect of fiberglass**

     ● **T65.831** **Toxic effect of fiberglass, accidental (unintentional)**
         Toxic effect of fiberglass NOS

     ● **T65.832** **Toxic effect of fiberglass, intentional self-harm**

     ● **T65.833** **Toxic effect of fiberglass, assault**

     ● **T65.834** **Toxic effect of fiberglass, undetermined**

   ● **T65.89** **Toxic effect of other specified substances**

     ● **T65.891** **Toxic effect of other specified substances, accidental (unintentional)**
         Toxic effect of other specified substances NOS

     ● **T65.892** **Toxic effect of other specified substances, intentional self-harm**

     ● **T65.893** **Toxic effect of other specified substances, assault**

     ● **T65.894** **Toxic effect of other specified substances, undetermined**

● **T65.9** **Toxic effect of unspecified substance**

   X ● **T65.91** **Toxic effect of `unspecified` substance, accidental (unintentional)**
     Poisoning NOS

   X ● **T65.92** **Toxic effect of `unspecified` substance, intentional self-harm**

   X ● **T65.93** **Toxic effect of `unspecified` substance, assault**

   X ● **T65.94** **Toxic effect of `unspecified` substance, undetermined**

OTHER AND UNSPECIFIED EFFECTS OF EXTERNAL CAUSES (T66-T78)

● **T66** **Radiation sickness, `unspecified`**

   Excludes1   specified adverse effects of radiation, such as:
     burns (T20-T31)
     leukemia (C91-C95)
     radiation gastroenteritis and colitis (K52.0)
     radiation pneumonitis (J70.0)
     radiation related disorders of the skin and subcutaneous tissue (L55-L59)
     sunburn (L55.-)

   The appropriate 7th character is to be added to code T66

A	initial encounter
D	subsequent encounter
S	sequela

● **T67** **Effects of heat and light**

   Excludes1   erythema [dermatitis] ab igne (L59.0)
     malignant hyperpyrexia due to anesthesia (T88.3)
     radiation-related disorders of the skin and subcutaneous tissue (L55-L59)

   Excludes2   burns (T20-T31)
     sunburn (L55.-)
     sweat disorder due to heat (L74-L75)

   The appropriate 7th character is to be added to each code from category T67

A	initial encounter
D	subsequent encounter
S	sequela

   X ● **T67.0** **Heatstroke and sunstroke**
     Heat apoplexy
     Heat pyrexia
     Siriasis
     Thermoplegia
     Use additional code(s) to identify any associated complications of heatstroke, such as:
     coma and stupor (R40.-)
     systemic inflammatory response syndrome (R65.1-)

   X ● **T67.1** **Heat syncope**
     Heat collapse

   X ● **T67.2** **Heat cramp**

   X ● **T67.3** **Heat exhaustion, anhydrotic**
     Heat prostration due to water depletion

     Excludes1   heat exhaustion due to salt depletion (T67.4)

◀ New   ⇐ Revised   ~~deleted~~ Deleted   Excludes 1   Excludes 2   Includes   Use additional   Code first   Code also   Unspecified

OGCR Official Guidelines   X Assign placeholder X   ● Use Additional Character(s)   ▶ Manifestation Code   **Coding Clinic**

1400

X● **T67.4** **Heat exhaustion due to salt depletion**
     Heat prostration due to salt (and water) depletion

X● **T67.5** **Heat exhaustion, unspecified**
     Heat prostration NOS

X● **T67.6** **Heat fatigue, transient**

X● **T67.7** **Heat edema**

X● **T67.8** **Other effects of heat and light**

X● **T67.9** **Effect of heat and light, unspecified**

X●**T68** **Hypothermia**
     Accidental hypothermia
     Hypothermia NOS
     Use additional code to identify source of exposure:
        Exposure to excessive cold of man-made origin (W93)
        Exposure to excessive cold of natural origin (X31)

     Excludes1   hypothermia following anesthesia (T88.51)
                hypothermia not associated with low
                   environmental temperature (R68.0)
                hypothermia of newborn (P80.-)

     Excludes2   frostbite (T33-T34)

     The appropriate 7th character is to be added to code T68

A	initial encounter
D	subsequent encounter
S	sequela

● **T69** **Other effects of reduced temperature**
     Use additional code to identify source of exposure:
        Exposure to excessive cold of man-made origin (W93)
        Exposure to excessive cold of natural origin (X31)

     Excludes2   frostbite (T33-T34)

     The appropriate 7th character is to be added to each code from
     category T69

A	initial encounter
D	subsequent encounter
S	sequela

  ● **T69.0** **Immersion hand and foot**
    ● **T69.01** **Immersion hand**
      ● **T69.011** **Immersion hand, right hand**
      ● **T69.012** **Immersion hand, left hand**
      ● **T69.019** **Immersion hand, unspecified hand**
    ● **T69.02** **Immersion foot**
         Trench foot
      ● **T69.021** **Immersion foot, right foot**
      ● **T69.022** **Immersion foot, left foot**
      ● **T69.029** **Immersion foot, unspecified foot**

X● **T69.1** **Chilblains**

X● **T69.8** **Other specified effects of reduced temperature**

X● **T69.9** **Effect of reduced temperature, unspecified**

● **T70** **Effects of air pressure and water pressure**
     The appropriate 7th character is to be added to each code from
     category T70

A	initial encounter
D	subsequent encounter
S	sequela

X● **T70.0** **Otitic barotrauma**
     Aero-otitis media
     Effects of change in ambient atmospheric pressure or
       water pressure on ears

X● **T70.1** **Sinus barotrauma**
     Aerosinusitis
     Effects of change in ambient atmospheric pressure on
       sinuses

● **T70.2** **Other and unspecified effects of high altitude**
     Excludes2   polycythemia due to high altitude (D75.1)

X● **T70.20** **Unspecified effects of high altitude**

X● **T70.29** **Other effects of high altitude**
     Alpine sickness
     Anoxia due to high altitude
     Barotrauma NOS
     Hypobaropathy
     Mountain sickness

X● **T70.3** **Caisson disease [decompression sickness]**
     Compressed-air disease
     Diver's palsy or paralysis

X● **T70.4** **Effects of high-pressure fluids**
     Hydraulic jet injection (industrial)
     Pneumatic jet injection (industrial)
     Traumatic jet injection (industrial)

X● **T70.8** **Other effects of air pressure and water pressure**

X● **T70.9** **Effect of air pressure and water pressure, unspecified**

● **T71** **Asphyxiation**
     Mechanical suffocation
     Traumatic suffocation

     Excludes1   acute respiratory distress (syndrome) (J80)
                anoxia due to high altitude (T70.2)
                asphyxia NOS (R09.01)
                asphyxia from carbon monoxide (T58.-)
                asphyxia from inhalation of food or foreign body
                   (T17.-)
                asphyxia from other gases, fumes and vapors
                   (T59.-)
                respiratory distress (syndrome) in newborn
                   (P22.-)

     The appropriate 7th character is to be added to each code from
     category T71

A	initial encounter
D	subsequent encounter
S	sequela

● **T71.1** **Asphyxiation due to mechanical threat to breathing**
     Suffocation due to mechanical threat to breathing

  ● **T71.11** **Asphyxiation due to smothering under pillow**

    ● **T71.111** **Asphyxiation due to smothering under pillow, accidental**
         Asphyxiation due to smothering under pillow NOS

    ● **T71.112** **Asphyxiation due to smothering under pillow, intentional self-harm**

    ● **T71.113** **Asphyxiation due to smothering under pillow, assault**

    ● **T71.114** **Asphyxiation due to smothering under pillow, undetermined**

  ● **T71.12** **Asphyxiation due to plastic bag**

    ● **T71.121** **Asphyxiation due to plastic bag, accidental**
         Asphyxiation due to plastic bag NOS

    ● **T71.122** **Asphyxiation due to plastic bag, intentional self-harm**

    ● **T71.123** **Asphyxiation due to plastic bag, assault**

    ● **T71.124** **Asphyxiation due to plastic bag, undetermined**

CHAPTER 19 (S00-T88)

● **T71.13**   **Asphyxiation due to being trapped in bed linens**

   ● **T71.131**   Asphyxiation due to being trapped in bed linens, accidental

         Asphyxiation due to being trapped in bed linens NOS

   ● **T71.132**   Asphyxiation due to being trapped in bed linens, intentional self-harm

   ● **T71.133**   Asphyxiation due to being trapped in bed linens, assault

   ● **T71.134**   Asphyxiation due to being trapped in bed linens, undetermined

● **T71.14**   **Asphyxiation due to smothering under another person's body (in bed)**

   ● **T71.141**   Asphyxiation due to smothering under another person's body (in bed), accidental

         Asphyxiation due to smothering under another person's body (in bed) NOS

   ● **T71.143**   Asphyxiation due to smothering under another person's body (in bed), assault

   ● **T71.144**   Asphyxiation due to smothering under another person's body (in bed), undetermined

● **T71.15**   **Asphyxiation due to smothering in furniture**

   ● **T71.151**   Asphyxiation due to smothering in furniture, accidental

         Asphyxiation due to smothering in furniture NOS

   ● **T71.152**   Asphyxiation due to smothering in furniture, intentional self-harm

   ● **T71.153**   Asphyxiation due to smothering in furniture, assault

   ● **T71.154**   Asphyxiation due to smothering in furniture, undetermined

● **T71.16**   **Asphyxiation due to hanging**

         Hanging by window shade cord

         Use additional code for any associated injuries, such as:

           crushing injury of neck (S17.-)

           fracture of cervical vertebrae (S12.0-S12.2-)

           open wound of neck (S11.-)

   ● **T71.161**   Asphyxiation due to hanging, accidental

         Asphyxiation due to hanging NOS

         Hanging NOS

   ● **T71.162**   Asphyxiation due to hanging, intentional self-harm

   ● **T71.163**   Asphyxiation due to hanging, assault

   ● **T71.164**   Asphyxiation due to hanging, undetermined

● **T71.19**   **Asphyxiation due to mechanical**

         Threat to breathing due to other causes

   ● **T71.191**   Asphyxiation due to mechanical threat to breathing due to other causes, accidental

         Asphyxiation due to other causes NOS

   ● **T71.192**   Asphyxiation due to mechanical threat to breathing due to other causes, intentional self-harm

   ● **T71.193**   Asphyxiation due to mechanical threat to breathing due to other causes, assault

   ● **T71.194**   Asphyxiation due to mechanical threat to breathing due to other causes, undetermined

● **T71.2**   **Asphyxiation due to systemic oxygen deficiency due to low oxygen content in ambient air**

         Suffocation due to systemic oxygen deficiency due to low oxygen content in ambient air

 X ● **T71.20**   Asphyxiation due to systemic oxygen deficiency due to low oxygen content in ambient air due to unspecified cause

 X ● **T71.21**   Asphyxiation due to cave-in or falling earth

         Use additional code for any associated cataclysm (X34-X38)

  ● **T71.22**   Asphyxiation due to being trapped in a car trunk

   ● **T71.221**   Asphyxiation due to being trapped in a car trunk, accidental

   ● **T71.222**   Asphyxiation due to being trapped in a car trunk, intentional self-harm

   ● **T71.223**   Asphyxiation due to being trapped in a car trunk, assault

   ● **T71.224**   Asphyxiation due to being trapped in a car trunk, undetermined

  ● **T71.23**   Asphyxiation due to being trapped in a (discarded) refrigerator

   ● **T71.231**   Asphyxiation due to being trapped in a (discarded) refrigerator, accidental

   ● **T71.232**   Asphyxiation due to being trapped in a (discarded) refrigerator, intentional self-harm

   ● **T71.233**   Asphyxiation due to being trapped in a (discarded) refrigerator, assault

   ● **T71.234**   Asphyxiation due to being trapped in a (discarded) refrigerator, undetermined

 X ● **T71.29**   Asphyxiation due to being trapped in other low oxygen environment

 X ● **T71.9**   **Asphyxiation due to unspecified cause**

         Suffocation (by strangulation) due to unspecified cause

         Suffocation NOS

         Systemic oxygen deficiency due to low oxygen content in ambient air due to unspecified cause

         Systemic oxygen deficiency due to mechanical threat to breathing due to unspecified cause

         Traumatic asphyxia NOS

● **T73**   **Effects of other deprivation**

         The appropriate 7th character is to be added to each code from category T73

A	initial encounter
D	subsequent encounter
S	sequela

 X ● **T73.0**   **Starvation**

         Deprivation of food

 X ● **T73.1**   **Deprivation of water**

 X ● **T73.2**   **Exhaustion due to exposure**

 X ● **T73.3**   **Exhaustion due to excessive exertion**

         Exhaustion due to overexertion

 X ● **T73.8**   **Other effects of deprivation**

 X ● **T73.9**   **Effect of deprivation, unspecified**

●T74   **Adult and child abuse, neglect and other maltreatment, confirmed**

> Use additional code, if applicable, to identify any associated current injury
>
> Use additional external cause code to identify perpetrator, if known (Y07.-)
>
> **Excludes1**   abuse and maltreatment in pregnancy (O9A.3-, O9A.4-, O9A.5-)
>   adult and child maltreatment, suspected (T76.-)
>
> The appropriate 7th character is to be added to each code from category T74

> | | |
> |---|---|
> | A | initial encounter |
> | D | subsequent encounter |
> | S | sequela |

●**T74.0**   **Neglect or abandonment, confirmed**

   X● **T74.01**   **Adult neglect or abandonment, confirmed**   A

   X● **T74.02**   **Child neglect or abandonment, confirmed**   P

●**T74.1**   **Physical abuse, confirmed**

>   **Excludes2**   sexual abuse (T74.2-)

   X● **T74.11**   **Adult physical abuse, confirmed**   A

   X● **T74.12**   **Child physical abuse, confirmed**   P

>   **Excludes2**   shaken infant syndrome (T74.4)

●**T74.2**   **Sexual abuse, confirmed**
> Rape, confirmed
> Sexual assault, confirmed

   X● **T74.21**   **Adult sexual abuse, confirmed**   A

   X● **T74.22**   **Child sexual abuse, confirmed**   P

●**T74.3**   **Psychological abuse, confirmed**

   X● **T74.31**   **Adult psychological abuse, confirmed**   A

   X● **T74.32**   **Child psychological abuse, confirmed**   P

X● **T74.4**   **Shaken infant syndrome**   P

●**T74.9**   **Unspecified maltreatment, confirmed**

   X● **T74.91**   **Unspecified adult maltreatment, confirmed**   A

   X● **T74.92**   **Unspecified child maltreatment, confirmed**   P

●T75   **Other and unspecified effects of other external causes**

> **Excludes1**   adverse effects NEC (T78.-)
>
> **Excludes2**   burns (electric) (T20-T31)
>
> The appropriate 7th character is to be added to each code from category T75

> | | |
> |---|---|
> | A | initial encounter |
> | D | subsequent encounter |
> | S | sequela |

●**T75.0**   **Effects of lightning**
> Struck by lightning

   X● **T75.00**   **Unspecified effects of lightning**
> Struck by lightning NOS

   X● **T75.01**   **Shock due to being struck by lightning**

   X● **T75.09**   **Other effects of lightning**

>   Use additional code for other effects of lightning

X● **T75.1**   **Unspecified effects of drowning and nonfatal submersion**
> Immersion

>   **Excludes1**   specified effects of drowning code to effects

●**T75.2**   **Effects of vibration**

   X● **T75.20**   **Unspecified effects of vibration**

   X● **T75.21**   **Pneumatic hammer syndrome**

   X● **T75.22**   **Traumatic vasospastic syndrome**

   X● **T75.23**   **Vertigo from infrasound**

>   **Excludes1**   vertigo NOS (R42)

   X● **T75.29**   **Other effects of vibration**

X● **T75.3**   **Motion sickness**
> Airsickness   Travel sickness
> Seasickness
>
> Use additional external cause code to identify vehicle or type of motion (Y92.81-, Y93.5-)

X● **T75.4**   **Electrocution**
> Shock from electric current
> Shock from electroshock gun (taser)

●**T75.8**   **Other specified effects of external causes**

   X● **T75.81**   **Effects of abnormal gravitation [G] forces**

   X● **T75.82**   **Effects of weightlessness**

   X● **T75.89**   **Other specified effects of external causes**

●T76   **Adult and child abuse, neglect and other maltreatment, suspected**

> Use additional code, if applicable, to identify any associated current injury
>
> **Excludes1**   adult and child maltreatment, confirmed (T74.-)
>   suspected abuse and maltreatment in pregnancy (O9A.3-, O9A.4-, O9A.5-)
>   suspected adult physical abuse, ruled out (Z04.71)
>   suspected adult sexual abuse, ruled out (Z04.41)
>   suspected child physical abuse, ruled out (Z04.72)
>   suspected child sexual abuse, ruled out (Z04.42)
>
> The appropriate 7th character is to be added to each code from category T76

> | | |
> |---|---|
> | A | initial encounter |
> | D | subsequent encounter |
> | S | sequela |

●**T76.0**   **Neglect or abandonment, suspected**

   X● **T76.01**   **Adult neglect or abandonment, suspected**   A

   X● **T76.02**   **Child neglect or abandonment, suspected**   P

●**T76.1**   **Physical abuse, suspected**

   X● **T76.11**   **Adult physical abuse, suspected**   A

   X● **T76.12**   **Child physical abuse, suspected**   P

●**T76.2**   **Sexual abuse, suspected**
> Rape, suspected
> Sexual abuse, suspected

>   **Excludes1**   alleged abuse, ruled out (Z04.7)

   X● **T76.21**   **Adult sexual abuse, suspected**   A

   X● **T76.22**   **Child sexual abuse, suspected**   P

●**T76.3**   **Psychological abuse, suspected**

   X● **T76.31**   **Adult psychological abuse, suspected**   A

   X● **T76.32**   **Child psychological abuse, suspected**   P

●**T76.9**   **Unspecified maltreatment, suspected**

   X● **T76.91**   **Unspecified adult maltreatment, suspected**   A

   X● **T76.92**   **Unspecified child maltreatment, suspected**   P

● T78   Adverse effects, not elsewhere classified

> **Excludes2**   complications of surgical and medical care NEC (T80-T88)

> The appropriate 7th character is to be added to each code from category T78

> | A | initial encounter |
> |---|---|
> | D | subsequent encounter |
> | S | sequela |

● T78.0   Anaphylactic reaction due to food
> Anaphylactic reaction due to adverse food reaction
> Anaphylactic shock or reaction due to nonpoisonous foods
> Anaphylactoid reaction due to food

X ● **T78.00   Anaphylactic reaction due to unspecified food**

X ● **T78.01   Anaphylactic reaction due to peanuts**

X ● **T78.02   Anaphylactic reaction due to shellfish (crustaceans)**

X ● **T78.03   Anaphylactic reaction due to other fish**

X ● **T78.04   Anaphylactic reaction due to fruits and vegetables**

X ● **T78.05   Anaphylactic reaction due to tree nuts and seeds**

> > **Excludes2**   anaphylactic reaction due to peanuts (T78.01) ◀

X ● **T78.06   Anaphylactic reaction due to food additives**

X ● **T78.07   Anaphylactic reaction due to milk and dairy products**

X ● **T78.08   Anaphylactic reaction due to eggs**

X ● **T78.09   Anaphylactic reaction due to other food products**

X ● **T78.1   Other adverse food reactions, not elsewhere classified**
> Use additional code to identify the type of reaction, if applicable ◀▥

> > **Excludes1**   anaphylactic reaction or shock due to adverse food reaction (T78.0-)
> > anaphylactic reaction due to food (T78.0-)
> > bacterial food borne intoxications (A05.-)

> > **Excludes2**   allergic and dietetic gastroenteritis and colitis (K52.29) ◀▥
> > allergic rhinitis due to food (J30.5)
> > dermatitis due to food in contact with skin (L23.6, L24.6, L25.4)
> > dermatitis due to ingested food (L27.2)
> > food protein-induced enterocolitis syndrome (K52.21) ◀
> > food protein-induced enteropathy (K52.22) ◀

X ● **T78.2   Anaphylactic shock, unspecified**
> *Occurs when allergic response triggers large quantities of histamines, prostaglandins, leukotrienes resulting in systemic vasodilation*
> Allergic shock
> Anaphylactic reaction
> Anaphylaxis

> > **Excludes1**   anaphylactic reaction or shock due to adverse effect of correct medicinal substance properly administered (T88.6)
> > anaphylactic reaction or shock due to adverse food reaction (T78.0-)
> > anaphylactic reaction or shock due to serum (T80.5-)

X ● **T78.3   Angioneurotic edema**
> Allergic angioedema
> Giant urticaria
> *Vascular disorder resulting from abnormalities of autonomic nervous system fibers supplying blood vessels*
> Quincke's edema

> > **Excludes1**   serum urticaria (T80.6-)
> > urticaria (L50.-)

● T78.4   Other and unspecified allergy

> **Excludes1**   specified types of allergic reaction such as:
> > allergic diarrhea (K52.29) ◀▥
> > allergic gastroenteritis and colitis (K52.29) ◀▥
> > dermatitis (L23-L25, L27.-)
> > food protein-induced enterocolitis syndrome (K52.21) ◀
> > food protein-induced enteropathy (K52.22) ◀
> > hay fever (J30.1)

X ● **T78.40   Allergy, unspecified**
> Allergic reaction NOS
> Hypersensitivity NOS

X ● **T78.41   Arthus phenomenon**
> Arthus reaction

X ● **T78.49   Other allergy**

X ● **T78.8   Other adverse effects, not elsewhere classified**

CERTAIN EARLY COMPLICATIONS OF TRAUMA (T79)

● T79   Certain early complications of trauma, not elsewhere classified

> **Excludes2**   acute respiratory distress syndrome (J80)
> complications occurring during or following medical procedures (T80-T88)
> complications of surgical and medical care NEC (T80-T88)
> newborn respiratory distress syndrome (P22.0)

> The appropriate 7th character is to be added to each code from category T79

> | A | initial encounter |
> |---|---|
> | D | subsequent encounter |
> | S | sequela |

X ● **T79.0   Air embolism (traumatic)**
> > **Excludes1**   air embolism complicating abortion or ectopic or molar pregnancy (O00-O07, O08.2)
> > air embolism complicating pregnancy, childbirth and the puerperium (O88.0)
> > air embolism following infusion, transfusion, and therapeutic injection (T80.0)
> > air embolism following procedure NEC (T81.7-)

X ● **T79.1   Fat embolism (traumatic)**
> > **Excludes1**   fat embolism complicating:
> > abortion or ectopic or molar pregnancy (O00-O07, O08.2)
> > pregnancy, childbirth and the puerperium (O88.8)

X ● **T79.2   Traumatic secondary and recurrent hemorrhage and seroma**

◀ New   ◀▥ Revised   ~~deleted~~ Deleted   Excludes 1   Excludes 2   Includes   Use additional   Code first   Code also   Unspecified
OGCR Official Guidelines   X Assign placeholder X   ● Use Additional Character(s)   ▷ Manifestation Code   **Coding Clinic**

X● T79.4   Traumatic shock
Shock (immediate) (delayed) following injury

> **Excludes1**   anaphylactic shock due to adverse food
> reaction (T78.0-)
> anaphylactic shock due to correct
> medicinal substance properly
> administered (T88.6)
> anaphylactic shock due to serum (T80.5-)
> anaphylactic shock NOS (T78.2)
> anesthetic shock (T88.2)
> electric shock (T75.4)
> nontraumatic shock NEC (R57.-)
> obstetric shock (O75.1)
> postprocedural shock (T81.1-)
> septic shock (R65.21)
> shock complicating abortion or ectopic or
> molar pregnancy (O00-O07, O08.3)
> shock due to lightning (T75.01)
> shock NOS (R57.9)

X● T79.5   Traumatic anuria
Crush syndrome
Renal failure following crushing

X● T79.6   Traumatic ischemia of muscle
Traumatic rhabdomyolysis
Volkmann's ischemic contracture

> **Excludes2**   anterior tibial syndrome (M76.8)
> compartment syndrome (traumatic)
> (T79.A-)
> nontraumatic ischemia of muscle (M62.2-)

X● T79.7   Traumatic subcutaneous emphysema

> **Excludes1**   emphysema NOS (J43)
> emphysema (subcutaneous) resulting
> from a procedure (T81.82)

● T79.A   Traumatic compartment syndrome

> **Excludes1**   fibromyalgia (M79.7)
> nontraumatic compartment syndrome
> (M79.A-)
> traumatic ischemic infarction of muscle
> (T79.6)

X● T79.A0   Compartment syndrome, unspecified
Compartment syndrome NOS

**● T79.A1   Traumatic compartment syndrome of upper
extremity**
Traumatic compartment syndrome of shoulder,
arm, forearm, wrist, hand, and fingers

    **● T79.A11   Traumatic compartment syndrome of
right upper extremity**

    **● T79.A12   Traumatic compartment syndrome of
left upper extremity**

    **● T79.A19   Traumatic compartment syndrome of
unspecified upper extremity**

**● T79.A2   Traumatic compartment syndrome of lower
extremity**
Traumatic compartment syndrome of hip,
buttock, thigh, leg, foot, and toes

    **● T79.A21   Traumatic compartment syndrome of
right lower extremity**

    **● T79.A22   Traumatic compartment syndrome of
left lower extremity**

    **● T79.A29   Traumatic compartment syndrome of
unspecified lower extremity**

X● T79.A3   Traumatic compartment syndrome of abdomen

X● T79.A9   Traumatic compartment syndrome of other sites

X● T79.8   Other early complications of trauma

X● T79.9   Unspecified early complication of trauma

COMPLICATIONS OF SURGICAL AND MEDICAL CARE NOT ELSEWHERE CLASSIFIED (T80-T88)

> Use additional code for adverse effect, if applicable, to identify
> drug (T36-T50 with fifth or sixth character 5)

> Use additional code(s) to identify the specified condition
> resulting from the complication.

> Use additional code to identify devices involved and details of
> circumstances (Y62-Y82)

> **Excludes2**   any encounters with medical care for
> postprocedural conditions in which no
> complications are present, such as:
> artificial opening status (Z93.-)
> closure of external stoma (Z43.-)
> fitting and adjustment of external prosthetic
> device (Z44.-)
> burns and corrosions from local applications and
> irradiation (T20-T32)
> complications of surgical procedures during
> pregnancy, childbirth and the puerperium
> (O00-O9A)
> mechanical complication of respirator [ventilator]
> (J95.850)
> poisoning and toxic effects of drugs and
> chemicals (T36-T65 with fifth or sixth
> character 1-4 or 6)
> postprocedural fever (R50.82)
> specified complications classified elsewhere,
> such as:
> cerebrospinal fluid leak from spinal puncture
> (G97.0)
> colostomy malfunction (K94.0-)
> disorders of fluid and electrolyte imbalance
> (E86-E87)
> functional disturbances following cardiac
> surgery (I97.0-I97.1)
> intraoperative and postprocedural
> complications of specified body systems
> (D78.-, E36.-, E89.-, G97.3-, G97.4, H59.3-,
> H59.-, H95.2-, H95.3, I97.4-, I97.5, J95.6-,
> J95.7, K91.6-, L76.-, M96.-, N99.-)
> ostomy complications (J95.0-, K94.-, N99.5-)
> postgastric surgery syndromes (K91.1)
> postlaminectomy syndrome NEC (M96.1)
> postmastectomy lymphedema syndrome
> (I97.2)
> postsurgical blind-loop syndrome (K91.2)
> ventilator associated pneumonia (J95.851)

**● T80   Complications following infusion, transfusion and therapeutic
injection**

> **Includes**   complications following perfusion
> **Excludes2**   bone marrow transplant rejection (T86.01)
> febrile nonhemolytic transfusion reaction (R50.84)
> fluid overload due to transfusion (E87.71)
> posttransfusion purpura (D69.51)
> transfusion associated circulatory overload
> (TACO) (E87.71)
> transfusion (red blood cell) associated
> hemochromatosis (E83.111)
> transfusion related acute lung injury (TRALI)
> (J95.84)

> The appropriate 7th character is to be added to each code from
> category T80

> | A | initial encounter |
> |---|---|
> | D | subsequent encounter |
> | S | sequela |

**X● T80.0   Air embolism following infusion, transfusion and
therapeutic injection**

X● **T80.1 Vascular complications following infusion, transfusion and therapeutic injection**
Use additional code to identify the vascular complication

Excludes2 extravasation of vesicant agent (T80.81-)
infiltration of vesicant agent (T80.81-)
vascular complications specified as due to prosthetic devices, implants and grafts (T82.8- T83.8-, T84.8-, T85.8-) ◀
postprocedural vascular complications (T81.7-)

● **T80.2 Infections following infusion, transfusion and therapeutic injection**
Use additional code to identify the specific infection, such as:
sepsis (A41.9)
Use additional code (R65.2-) to identify severe sepsis, if applicable

Excludes2 infections specified as due to prosthetic devices, implants and grafts (T82.6-T82.7, T83.5-T83.6, T84.5-T84.7, T85.7)
postprocedural infections (T81.4-) ◀

● **T80.21 Infection due to central venous catheter**
Infection due to pulmonary artery catheter (Swan-Ganz catheter) ◀

● **T80.211 Bloodstream infection due to central venous catheter**
Catheter-related bloodstream infection (CRBSI) NOS
Central line-associated bloodstream infection (CLABSI)
Bloodstream infection due to Hickman catheter
Bloodstream infection due to peripherally inserted central catheter (PICC)
Bloodstream infection due to portacath (port-a-cath)
Bloodstream infection due to pulmonary artery catheter ◀
Bloodstream infection due to triple lumen catheter
Bloodstream infection due to umbilical venous catheter

● **T80.212 Local infection due to central venous catheter**
Exit or insertion site infection
Local infection due to Hickman catheter
Local infection due to peripherally inserted central catheter (PICC)
Local infection due to portacath (port-a-cath)
Local infection due to pulmonary artery catheter ◀
Local infection due to triple lumen catheter
Local infection due to umbilical venous catheter
Port or reservoir infection
Tunnel infection

● **T80.218 Other infection due to central venous catheter**
Other central line-associated infection
Other infection due to Hickman catheter
Other infection due to peripherally inserted central catheter (PICC)
Other infection due to portacath (port-a-cath)
Other infection due to pulmonary artery catheter ◀
Other infection due to triple lumen catheter
Other infection due to umbilical venous catheter

● **T80.219 Unspecified infection due to central venous catheter**
Central line-associated infection NOS
Unspecified infection due to Hickman catheter
Unspecified infection due to peripherally inserted central catheter (PICC)
Unspecified infection due to portacath (port-a-cath)
Unspecified infection due to pulmonary artery catheter ◀
Unspecified infection due to triple lumen catheter
Unspecified infection due to umbilical venous catheter

X● **T80.22 Acute infection following transfusion, infusion, or injection of blood and blood products**

X● **T80.29 Infection following other infusion, transfusion and therapeutic injection**

● **T80.3 ABO incompatibility reaction due to transfusion of blood or blood products**
Excludes1 minor blood group antigens reactions (Duffy) (E) (K(ell)) (Kidd) (Lewis) (M) (N) (P) (S) (T80.A)

X● **T80.30 ABO incompatibility reaction due to transfusion of blood or blood products, unspecified**
ABO incompatibility blood transfusion NOS
Reaction to ABO incompatibility from transfusion NOS

● **T80.31 ABO incompatibility with hemolytic transfusion reaction**

● **T80.310 ABO incompatibility with acute hemolytic transfusion reaction**
ABO incompatibility with hemolytic transfusion reaction less than 24 hours after transfusion
Acute hemolytic transfusion reaction (AHTR) due to ABO incompatibility

● **T80.311 ABO incompatibility with delayed hemolytic transfusion reaction**
ABO incompatibility with hemolytic transfusion reaction 24 hours or more after transfusion
Delayed hemolytic transfusion reaction (DHTR) due to ABO incompatibility

CHAPTER 19 (S00-T88)

◀ New ◀ Revised ~~deleted~~ Deleted Excludes 1 Excludes 2 Includes Use additional Code first Code also Unspecified
OGCR Official Guidelines X Assign placeholder X ● Use Additional Character(s) ▶ Manifestation Code Coding Clinic

● T80.319   **ABO incompatibility with hemolytic transfusion reaction, unspecified**
ABO incompatibility with hemolytic transfusion reaction at unspecified time after transfusion
Hemolytic transfusion reaction (HTR) due to ABO incompatibility NOS

X ● T80.39   **Other ABO incompatibility reaction due to transfusion of blood or blood products**
Delayed serologic transfusion reaction (DSTR) from ABO incompatibility
Other ABO incompatible blood transfusion
Other reaction to ABO incompatible blood transfusion

● T80.4   **Rh incompatibility reaction due to transfusion of blood or blood products**
Reaction due to incompatibility of Rh antigens (C) (c) (D) (E) (e)

X ● T80.40   **Rh incompatibility reaction due to transfusion of blood or blood products, unspecified**
Reaction due to Rh factor in transfusion NOS
Rh incompatible blood transfusion NOS

● T80.41   **Rh incompatibility with hemolytic transfusion reaction**

● T80.410   **Rh incompatibility with acute hemolytic transfusion reaction**
Acute hemolytic transfusion reaction (AHTR) due to Rh incompatibility
Rh incompatibility with hemolytic transfusion reaction less than 24 hours after transfusion

● T80.411   **Rh incompatibility with delayed hemolytic transfusion reaction**
Delayed hemolytic transfusion reaction (DHTR) due to Rh incompatibility
Rh incompatibility with hemolytic transfusion reaction 24 hours or more after transfusion

● T80.419   **Rh incompatibility with hemolytic transfusion reaction, unspecified**
Rh incompatibility with hemolytic transfusion reaction at unspecified time after transfusion
Hemolytic transfusion reaction (HTR) due to Rh incompatibility NOS

X ● T80.49   **Other Rh incompatibility reaction due to transfusion of blood or blood products**
Delayed serologic transfusion reaction (DSTR) from Rh incompatibility
Other reaction to Rh incompatible blood transfusion

● T80.A   **Non-ABO incompatibility reaction due to transfusion of blood or blood products**
Reaction due to incompatibility of minor antigens (Duffy) (Kell) (Kidd) (Lewis) (M) (N) (P) (S)

X ● T80.A0   **Non-ABO incompatibility reaction due to transfusion of blood or blood products, unspecified**
Non-ABO antigen incompatibility reaction from transfusion NOS

● T80.A1   **Non-ABO incompatibility with hemolytic transfusion reaction**

● T80.A10   **Non-ABO incompatibility with acute hemolytic transfusion reaction**
Acute hemolytic transfusion reaction (AHTR) due to non-ABO incompatibility
Non-ABO incompatibility with hemolytic transfusion reaction less than 24 hours after transfusion

● T80.A11   **Non-ABO incompatibility with delayed hemolytic transfusion reaction**
Delayed hemolytic transfusion reaction (DHTR) due to non-ABO incompatibility
Non-ABO incompatibility with hemolytic transfusion reaction 24 or more hours after transfusion

● T80.A19   **Non-ABO incompatibility with hemolytic transfusion reaction, unspecified**
Hemolytic transfusion reaction (HTR) due to non-ABO incompatibility NOS
Non-ABO incompatibility with hemolytic transfusion reaction at unspecified time after transfusion

X ● T80.A9   **Other non-ABO incompatibility reaction due to transfusion of blood or blood products**
Delayed serologic transfusion reaction (DSTR) from non-ABO incompatibility
Other reaction to non-ABO incompatible blood transfusion

● T80.5   **Anaphylactic reaction due to serum**
Allergic reaction due to serum
Anaphylactic shock due to serum
Anaphylactoid reaction due to serum
Anaphylaxis due to serum

Excludes1   ABO incompatibility reaction due to transfusion of blood or blood products (T80.3-)
allergic reaction or shock NOS (T78.2)
anaphylactic reaction or shock NOS (T78.2)
anaphylactic reaction or shock due to adverse effect of correct medicinal substance properly administered (T88.6)
other serum reaction (T80.6-)

X ● T80.51   **Anaphylactic reaction due to administration of blood and blood products**

X ● T80.52   **Anaphylactic reaction due to vaccination**

X ● T80.59   **Anaphylactic reaction due to other serum**

CHAPTER 19 (S00-T88)

● **T80.6**   **Other serum reactions**
      Intoxication by serum   Serum sickness
      Protein sickness   Serum urticaria
      Serum rash

      Excludes2   serum hepatitis (B16-B19) ◀▥

   X ● **T80.61**   **Other serum reaction due to administration of blood and blood products**

   X ● **T80.62**   **Other serum reaction due to vaccination**

   X ● **T80.69**   **Other serum reaction due to other serum**

● **T80.8**   **Other complications following infusion, transfusion and therapeutic injection**

   ● **T80.81**   **Extravasation of vesicant agent**
          Infiltration of vesicant agent

     ● **T80.810**   **Extravasation of vesicant antineoplastic chemotherapy**
            Infiltration of vesicant antineoplastic chemotherapy

     ● **T80.818**   **Extravasation of other vesicant agent**
            Infiltration of other vesicant agent

   X ● **T80.89**   **Other complications following infusion, transfusion and therapeutic injection**
          Delayed serologic transfusion reaction (DSTR), unspecified incompatibility

          Use additional code to identify graft-versus-host reaction, if applicable, (D89.81-)

● **T80.9**   **Unspecified complication following infusion, transfusion and therapeutic injection**

   X ● **T80.90**   **Unspecified complication following infusion and therapeutic injection**

   ● **T80.91**   **Hemolytic transfusion reaction, unspecified incompatibility**

      Excludes1   ABO incompatibility with hemolytic transfusion reaction (T80.31-)
            Non-ABO incompatibility with hemolytic transfusion reaction (T80.A1-)
            Rh incompatibility with hemolytic transfusion reaction (T80.41-)

     ● **T80.910**   **Acute hemolytic transfusion reaction, unspecified incompatibility**

     ● **T80.911**   **Delayed hemolytic transfusion reaction, unspecified incompatibility**

     ● **T80.919**   **Hemolytic transfusion reaction, unspecified incompatibility, unspecified as acute or delayed**
            Hemolytic transfusion reaction NOS

   X ● **T80.92**   **Unspecified transfusion reaction**
          Transfusion reaction NOS

● **T81**   **Complications of procedures, not elsewhere classified**
      Use additional code for adverse effect, if applicable, to identify drug (T36-T50 with fifth or sixth character 5)

      Excludes2   complications following immunization (T88.0-T88.1)
            complications following infusion, transfusion and therapeutic injection (T80.-)
            complications of transplanted organs and tissue (T86.-)
            poisoning and toxic effects of drugs and chemicals (T36-T65 with fifth or sixth character 1-4 or 6)
            specified complications classified elsewhere, such as:
                complication of prosthetic devices, implants and grafts (T82-T85)
                dermatitis due to drugs and medicaments (L23.3, L24.4, L25.1, L27.0-L27.1)
                endosseous dental implant failure (M27.6-)
                floppy iris syndrome (IFIS) (intraoperative) H21.81
                intraoperative and postprocedural complications of specific body system (D78.-, E36.-, E89.-, G97.3-, G97.4, H59.3-, H59.-, H95.2-, H95.3, I97.4-, I97.5, J95, K91.-, L76.-, M96.-, N99.-)
                ostomy complications (J95.0-, K94.-, N99.5-)
                plateau iris syndrome (post-iridectomy) (postprocedural) H21.82

      The appropriate 7th character is to be added to each code from category T81

A	initial encounter
D	subsequent encounter
S	sequela

● **T81.1**   **Postprocedural shock**
      Shock during or resulting from a procedure, not elsewhere classified

      Excludes1   anaphylactic shock NOS (T78.2)
            anaphylactic shock due to correct substance properly administered (T88.6)
            anaphylactic shock due to serum (T80.5-)
            anesthetic shock (T88.2)
            electric shock (T75.4)
            obstetric shock (O75.1)
            septic shock (R65.21)
            shock following abortion or ectopic or molar pregnancy (O00-O07, O08.3)
            traumatic shock (T79.4)

   X ● **T81.10**   **Postprocedural shock unspecified**
          Collapse NOS during or resulting from a procedure, not elsewhere classified
          Postprocedural failure of peripheral circulation
          Postprocedural shock NOS

   X ● **T81.11**   **Postprocedural cardiogenic shock**

   X ● **T81.12**   **Postprocedural septic shock**
          Postprocedural endotoxic shock resulting from a procedure, not elsewhere classified ◀▥
          Postprocedural gram-negative shock resulting from a procedure, not elsewhere classified ◀▥

          Code first underlying infection
          Use additional code, to identify any associated acute organ dysfunction, if applicable

   X ● **T81.19**   **Other postprocedural shock**
          Postprocedural hypovolemic shock

◀ New   ◀▥ Revised   ~~deleted~~ Deleted   Excludes 1   Excludes 2   Includes   Use additional   Code first   Code also   Unspecified

1408   **OGCR** Official Guidelines   X Assign placeholder X   ● Use Additional Character(s)   ▶ Manifestation Code   **Coding Clinic**

● **T81.3**   **Disruption of wound, not elsewhere classified**
Disruption of any suture materials or other closure methods

     Excludes1   breakdown (mechanical) of permanent sutures (T85.612)
                   displacement of permanent sutures (T85.622)
                   disruption of cesarean delivery wound (O90.0)
                   disruption of perineal obstetric wound (O90.1)
                   mechanical complication of permanent sutures NEC (T85.692)

X ● **T81.30**   **Disruption of wound, unspecified**
            Disruption of wound NOS

X ● **T81.31**   **Disruption of external operation (surgical) wound, not elsewhere classified**

     Excludes1   dehiscence of amputation stump (T87.81)
           Dehiscence of operation wound NOS
           Disruption of operation wound NOS
           Disruption or dehiscence of closure of cornea
           Disruption or dehiscence of closure of mucosa
           Disruption or dehiscence of closure of skin and subcutaneous tissue
           Full-thickness skin disruption or dehiscence
           Superficial disruption or dehiscence of operation wound
           Coding Clinic: 2015, Q1, P20

X ● **T81.32**   **Disruption of internal operation (surgical) wound, not elsewhere classified**
           Deep disruption or dehiscence of operation wound NOS
           Disruption or dehiscence of closure of internal organ or other internal tissue
           Disruption or dehiscence of closure of muscle or muscle flap
           Disruption or dehiscence of closure of ribs or rib cage
           Disruption or dehiscence of closure of skull or craniotomy
           Disruption or dehiscence of closure of sternum or sternotomy
           Disruption or dehiscence of closure of tendon or ligament
           Disruption or dehiscence of closure of superficial or muscular fascia

X ● **T81.33**   **Disruption of traumatic injury wound repair**
           Disruption or dehiscence of closure of traumatic laceration (external) (internal)

X ● **T81.4**   **Infection following a procedure**
           Intra-abdominal abscess following a procedure
           Postprocedural infection, not elsewhere classified
           Sepsis following a procedure
           Stitch abscess following a procedure
           Subphrenic abscess following a procedure
           Wound abscess following a procedure

           Use additional code to identify infection

           Use additional code (R65.2-) to identify severe sepsis, if applicable

     Excludes1   obstetric surgical wound infection (O86.0)
                   postprocedural fever NOS (R50.82)
                   postprocedural retroperitoneal abscess (K68.11)

     Excludes2   bleb associated endophthalmitis (H59.4-)
                   infection due to infusion, transfusion and therapeutic injection (T80.2-)
                   infection due to prosthetic devices, implants and grafts (T82.6-T82.7, T83.5-T83.6, T84.5-T84.7, T85.7)
         Coding Clinic: 2015, Q4, P37

● **T81.5**   **Complications of foreign body accidentally left in body following procedure**

● **T81.50**   **Unspecified complication of foreign body accidentally left in body following procedure**

   ● **T81.500**   Unspecified complication of foreign body accidentally left in body following surgical operation

   ● **T81.501**   Unspecified complication of foreign body accidentally left in body following infusion or transfusion

   ● **T81.502**   Unspecified complication of foreign body accidentally left in body following kidney dialysis

   ● **T81.503**   Unspecified complication of foreign body accidentally left in body following injection or immunization

   ● **T81.504**   Unspecified complication of foreign body accidentally left in body following endoscopic examination

   ● **T81.505**   Unspecified complication of foreign body accidentally left in body following heart catheterization

   ● **T81.506**   Unspecified complication of foreign body accidentally left in body following aspiration, puncture or other catheterization

   ● **T81.507**   Unspecified complication of foreign body accidentally left in body following removal of catheter or packing

   ● **T81.508**   Unspecified complication of foreign body accidentally left in body following other procedure

   ● **T81.509**   Unspecified complication of foreign body accidentally left in body following unspecified procedure

● **T81.51**   **Adhesions due to foreign body accidentally left in body following procedure**

   ● **T81.510**   **Adhesions due to foreign body accidentally left in body following surgical operation**

   ● **T81.511**   **Adhesions due to foreign body accidentally left in body following infusion or transfusion**

   ● **T81.512**   **Adhesions due to foreign body accidentally left in body following kidney dialysis**

   ● **T81.513**   **Adhesions due to foreign body accidentally left in body following injection or immunization**

   ● **T81.514**   **Adhesions due to foreign body accidentally left in body following endoscopic examination**

   ● **T81.515**   **Adhesions due to foreign body accidentally left in body following heart catheterization**

   ● **T81.516**   **Adhesions due to foreign body accidentally left in body following aspiration, puncture or other catheterization**

   ● **T81.517**   **Adhesions due to foreign body accidentally left in body following removal of catheter or packing**

   ● **T81.518**   **Adhesions due to foreign body accidentally left in body following other procedure**

   ● **T81.519**   **Adhesions due to foreign body accidentally left in body following unspecified procedure**

● **T81.52**   **Obstruction due to foreign body accidentally left in body following procedure**

  ● **T81.520**   Obstruction due to foreign body accidentally left in body following surgical operation

  ● **T81.521**   Obstruction due to foreign body accidentally left in body following infusion or transfusion

  ● **T81.522**   Obstruction due to foreign body accidentally left in body following kidney dialysis

  ● **T81.523**   Obstruction due to foreign body accidentally left in body following injection or immunization

  ● **T81.524**   Obstruction due to foreign body accidentally left in body following endoscopic examination

  ● **T81.525**   Obstruction due to foreign body accidentally left in body following heart catheterization

  ● **T81.526**   Obstruction due to foreign body accidentally left in body following aspiration, puncture or other catheterization

  ● **T81.527**   Obstruction due to foreign body accidentally left in body following removal of catheter or packing

  ● **T81.528**   Obstruction due to foreign body accidentally left in body following other procedure

  ● **T81.529**   Obstruction due to foreign body accidentally left in body following unspecified procedure

● **T81.53**   **Perforation due to foreign body accidentally left in body following procedure**

  ● **T81.530**   Perforation due to foreign body accidentally left in body following surgical operation

  ● **T81.531**   Perforation due to foreign body accidentally left in body following infusion or transfusion

  ● **T81.532**   Perforation due to foreign body accidentally left in body following kidney dialysis

  ● **T81.533**   Perforation due to foreign body accidentally left in body following injection or immunization

  ● **T81.534**   Perforation due to foreign body accidentally left in body following endoscopic examination

  ● **T81.535**   Perforation due to foreign body accidentally left in body following heart catheterization

  ● **T81.536**   Perforation due to foreign body accidentally left in body following aspiration, puncture or other catheterization

  ● **T81.537**   Perforation due to foreign body accidentally left in body following removal of catheter or packing

  ● **T81.538**   Perforation due to foreign body accidentally left in body following other procedure

  ● **T81.539**   Perforation due to foreign body accidentally left in body following unspecified procedure

● **T81.59**   **Other complications of foreign body accidentally left in body following procedure**

  Excludes2   obstruction or perforation due to prosthetic devices and implants intentionally left in body (T82.0-T82.5, T83.0-T83.4, T83.7, T84.0-T84.4, T85.0-T85.6)

  ● **T81.590**   Other complications of foreign body accidentally left in body following surgical operation

  ● **T81.591**   Other complications of foreign body accidentally left in body following infusion or transfusion

  ● **T81.592**   Other complications of foreign body accidentally left in body following kidney dialysis

  ● **T81.593**   Other complications of foreign body accidentally left in body following injection or immunization

  ● **T81.594**   Other complications of foreign body accidentally left in body following endoscopic examination

  ● **T81.595**   Other complications of foreign body accidentally left in body following heart catheterization

  ● **T81.596**   Other complications of foreign body accidentally left in body following aspiration, puncture or other catheterization

  ● **T81.597**   Other complications of foreign body accidentally left in body following removal of catheter or packing

  ● **T81.598**   Other complications of foreign body accidentally left in body following other procedure

  ● **T81.599**   Other complications of foreign body accidentally left in body following unspecified procedure

● **T81.6**   **Acute reaction to foreign substance accidentally left during a procedure**

  Excludes2   complications of foreign body accidentally left in body cavity or operation wound following procedure (T81.5-)

X ● **T81.60**   Unspecified acute reaction to foreign substance accidentally left during a procedure

X ● **T81.61**   Aseptic peritonitis due to foreign substance accidentally left during a procedure
       Chemical peritonitis

X ● **T81.69**   Other acute reaction to foreign substance accidentally left during a procedure

---

◀ New   ◀═ Revised   ~~deleted~~ Deleted   Excludes 1   Excludes 2   Includes   Use additional   Code first   Code also   Unspecified

OGCR Official Guidelines   X Assign placeholder X   ● Use Additional Character(s)   ▷ Manifestation Code   **Coding Clinic**

● **T81.7**   **Vascular complications following a procedure, not elsewhere classified**
Air embolism following procedure NEC
Phlebitis or thrombophlebitis resulting from a procedure

> **Excludes1**   embolism complicating abortion or ectopic or molar pregnancy (O00-O07, O08.2)
embolism complicating pregnancy, childbirth and the puerperium (O88.-)
traumatic embolism (T79.0)

> **Excludes2**   embolism due to prosthetic devices, implants and grafts (T82.8, T83.81, T84.8-, T85.1-) ◀━
embolism following infusion, transfusion and therapeutic injection (T80.0)

● **T81.71**   Complication of artery following a procedure, not elsewhere classified

     ● **T81.710**   Complication of mesenteric artery following a procedure, not elsewhere classified

     ● **T81.711**   Complication of renal artery following a procedure, not elsewhere classified

     ● **T81.718**   Complication of other artery following a procedure, not elsewhere classified

     ● **T81.719**   Complication of unspecified artery following a procedure, not elsewhere classified

X ● **T81.72**   Complication of vein following a procedure, not elsewhere classified

● **T81.8**   **Other complications of procedures, not elsewhere classified**

> **Excludes2**   hypothermia following anesthesia (T88.51)
malignant hyperpyrexia due to anesthesia (T88.3)

X ● **T81.81**   Complication of inhalation therapy

X ● **T81.82**   Emphysema (subcutaneous) resulting from a procedure

X ● **T81.83**   Persistent postprocedural fistula

X ● **T81.89**   Other complications of procedures, not elsewhere classified
> Use additional code to specify complication, such as:
> postprocedural delirium (F05)

X ● **T81.9**   Unspecified complication of procedure

● **T82**   **Complications of cardiac and vascular prosthetic devices, implants and grafts**

> **Excludes2**   failure and rejection of transplanted organs and tissue (T86.-)

The appropriate 7th character is to be added to each code from category T82

A	initial encounter
D	subsequent encounter
S	sequela

● **T82.0**   **Mechanical complication of heart valve prosthesis**
Mechanical complication of artificial heart valve

> **Excludes1**   mechanical complication of biological heart valve graft (T82.22-)

X ● **T82.01**   Breakdown (mechanical) of heart valve prosthesis

X ● **T82.02**   Displacement of heart valve prosthesis
Malposition of heart valve prosthesis

X ● **T82.03**   Leakage of heart valve prosthesis

X ● **T82.09**   Other mechanical complication of heart valve prosthesis
Obstruction (mechanical) of heart valve prosthesis
Perforation of heart valve prosthesis
Protrusion of heart valve prosthesis

● **T82.1**   **Mechanical complication of cardiac electronic device**

● **T82.11**   Breakdown (mechanical) of cardiac electronic device

     ● **T82.110**   Breakdown (mechanical) of cardiac electrode

     ● **T82.111**   Breakdown (mechanical) of cardiac pulse generator (battery)

     ● **T82.118**   Breakdown (mechanical) of other cardiac electronic device

     ● **T82.119**   Breakdown (mechanical) of unspecified cardiac electronic device

● **T82.12**   Displacement of cardiac electronic device
Malposition of cardiac electronic device

     ● **T82.120**   Displacement of cardiac electrode

     ● **T82.121**   Displacement of cardiac pulse generator (battery)

     ● **T82.128**   Displacement of other cardiac electronic device

     ● **T82.129**   Displacement of unspecified cardiac electronic device

● **T82.19**   Other mechanical complication of cardiac electronic device
Leakage of cardiac electronic device
Obstruction of cardiac electronic device
Perforation of cardiac electronic device
Protrusion of cardiac electronic device

     ● **T82.190**   Other mechanical complication of cardiac electrode

     ● **T82.191**   Other mechanical complication of cardiac pulse generator (battery)

     ● **T82.198**   Other mechanical complication of other cardiac electronic device

     ● **T82.199**   Other mechanical complication of unspecified cardiac device

● **T82.2**   **Mechanical complication of coronary artery bypass graft and biological heart valve graft**

> **Excludes1**   mechanical complication of artificial heart valve prosthesis (T82.0-)

● **T82.21**   Mechanical complication of coronary artery bypass graft

     ● **T82.211**   Breakdown (mechanical) of coronary artery bypass graft

     ● **T82.212**   Displacement of coronary artery bypass graft
Malposition of coronary artery bypass graft

     ● **T82.213**   Leakage of coronary artery bypass graft

     ● **T82.218**   Other mechanical complication of coronary artery bypass graft
Obstruction, mechanical of coronary artery bypass graft
Perforation of coronary artery bypass graft
Protrusion of coronary artery bypass graft

● **T82.22** **Mechanical complication of biological heart valve graft**
  ● **T82.221** **Breakdown (mechanical) of biological heart valve graft**
  ● **T82.222** **Displacement of biological heart valve graft**
     Malposition of biological heart valve graft
  ● **T82.223** **Leakage of biological heart valve graft**
  ● **T82.228** **Other mechanical complication of biological heart valve graft**
     Obstruction of biological heart valve graft
     Perforation of biological heart valve graft
     Protrusion of biological heart valve graft

● **T82.3** **Mechanical complication of other vascular grafts**
  ● **T82.31** **Breakdown (mechanical) of other vascular grafts**
    ● **T82.310** **Breakdown (mechanical) of aortic (bifurcation) graft (replacement)**
    ● **T82.311** **Breakdown (mechanical) of carotid arterial graft (bypass)**
    ● **T82.312** **Breakdown (mechanical) of femoral arterial graft (bypass)**
    ● **T82.318** **Breakdown (mechanical) of other vascular grafts**
    ● **T82.319** **Breakdown (mechanical) of** unspecified **vascular grafts**
  ● **T82.32** **Displacement of other vascular grafts**
     Malposition of other vascular grafts
    ● **T82.320** **Displacement of aortic (bifurcation) graft (replacement)**
    ● **T82.321** **Displacement of carotid arterial graft (bypass)**
    ● **T82.322** **Displacement of femoral arterial graft (bypass)**
    ● **T82.328** **Displacement of other vascular grafts**
    ● **T82.329** **Displacement of** unspecified **vascular grafts**
  ● **T82.33** **Leakage of other vascular grafts**
    ● **T82.330** **Leakage of aortic (bifurcation) graft (replacement)**
    ● **T82.331** **Leakage of carotid arterial graft (bypass)**
    ● **T82.332** **Leakage of femoral arterial graft (bypass)**
    ● **T82.338** **Leakage of other vascular grafts**
    ● **T82.339** **Leakage of** unspecified **vascular graft**
  ● **T82.39** **Other mechanical complication of other vascular grafts**
     Obstruction (mechanical) of other vascular grafts
     Perforation of other vascular grafts
     Protrusion of other vascular grafts
    ● **T82.390** **Other mechanical complication of aortic (bifurcation) graft (replacement)**
    ● **T82.391** **Other mechanical complication of carotid arterial graft (bypass)**
    ● **T82.392** **Other mechanical complication of femoral arterial graft (bypass)**
    ● **T82.398** **Other mechanical complication of other vascular grafts**
    ● **T82.399** **Other mechanical complication of** unspecified **vascular grafts**

● **T82.4** **Mechanical complication of vascular dialysis catheter**
   Mechanical complication of hemodialysis catheter
   | Excludes1 | mechanical complication of intraperitoneal dialysis catheter (T85.62) |
   X ● **T82.41** **Breakdown (mechanical) of vascular dialysis catheter**
   X ● **T82.42** **Displacement of vascular dialysis catheter**
     Malposition of vascular dialysis catheter
   X ● **T82.43** **Leakage of vascular dialysis catheter**
   X ● **T82.49** **Other complication of vascular dialysis catheter**
     Obstruction (mechanical) of vascular dialysis catheter
     Perforation of vascular dialysis catheter
     Protrusion of vascular dialysis catheter

● **T82.5** **Mechanical complication of other cardiac and vascular devices and implants**
   | Excludes2 | mechanical complication of epidural and subdural infusion catheter (T85.61) |
  ● **T82.51** **Breakdown (mechanical) of other cardiac and vascular devices and implants**
    ● **T82.510** **Breakdown (mechanical) of surgically created arteriovenous fistula**
    ● **T82.511** **Breakdown (mechanical) of surgically created arteriovenous shunt**
    ● **T82.512** **Breakdown (mechanical) of artificial heart**
    ● **T82.513** **Breakdown (mechanical) of balloon (counterpulsation) device**
    ● **T82.514** **Breakdown (mechanical) of infusion catheter**
    ● **T82.515** **Breakdown (mechanical) of umbrella device**
    ● **T82.518** **Breakdown (mechanical) of other cardiac and vascular devices and implants**
    ● **T82.519** **Breakdown (mechanical) of** unspecified **cardiac and vascular devices and implants**
  ● **T82.52** **Displacement of other cardiac and vascular devices and implants**
     Malposition of other cardiac and vascular devices and implants
    ● **T82.520** **Displacement of surgically created arteriovenous fistula**
    ● **T82.521** **Displacement of surgically created arteriovenous shunt**
    ● **T82.522** **Displacement of artificial heart**
    ● **T82.523** **Displacement of balloon (counterpulsation) device**
    ● **T82.524** **Displacement of infusion catheter**
    ● **T82.525** **Displacement of umbrella device**
    ● **T82.528** **Displacement of other cardiac and vascular devices and implants**
    ● **T82.529** **Displacement of** unspecified **cardiac and vascular devices and implants**
  ● **T82.53** **Leakage of other cardiac and vascular devices and implants**
    ● **T82.530** **Leakage of surgically created arteriovenous fistula**
    ● **T82.531** **Leakage of surgically created arteriovenous shunt**
    ● **T82.532** **Leakage of artificial heart**
    ● **T82.533** **Leakage of balloon (counterpulsation) device**
    ● **T82.534** **Leakage of infusion catheter**
    ● **T82.535** **Leakage of umbrella device**
    ● **T82.538** **Leakage of other cardiac and vascular devices and implants**
    ● **T82.539** **Leakage of** unspecified **cardiac and vascular devices and implants**

● **T82.59**   **Other mechanical complication of other cardiac and vascular devices and implants**
     Obstruction (mechanical) of other cardiac and vascular devices and implants
     Perforation of other cardiac and vascular devices and implants
     Protrusion of other cardiac and vascular devices and implants

   ● **T82.590**   **Other mechanical complication of surgically created arteriovenous fistula**

   ● **T82.591**   **Other mechanical complication of surgically created arteriovenous shunt**

   ● **T82.592**   **Other mechanical complication of artificial heart**

   ● **T82.593**   **Other mechanical complication of balloon (counterpulsation) device**

   ● **T82.594**   **Other mechanical complication of infusion catheter**

   ● **T82.595**   **Other mechanical complication of umbrella device**

   ● **T82.598**   **Other mechanical complication of other cardiac and vascular devices and implants**

   ● **T82.599**   **Other mechanical complication of unspecified cardiac and vascular devices and implants**

X ● **T82.6**   **Infection and inflammatory reaction due to cardiac valve prosthesis**
     Use additional code to identify infection

X ● **T82.7**   **Infection and inflammatory reaction due to other cardiac and vascular devices, implants and grafts**
     Use additional code to identify infection

● **T82.8**   **Other specified complications of cardiac and vascular prosthetic devices, implants and grafts**

   ● **T82.81**   **Embolism due to cardiac and vascular prosthetic devices, implants and grafts** ◀▥

     ● **T82.817**   **Embolism due to cardiac prosthetic devices, implants and grafts**
        Coding Clinic: 2015, Q1, P20

     ● **T82.818**   **Embolism due to vascular prosthetic devices, implants and grafts**

   ● **T82.82**   **Fibrosis due to cardiac and vascular prosthetic devices, implants and grafts** ◀▥

     ● **T82.827**   **Fibrosis due to cardiac prosthetic devices, implants and grafts**

     ● **T82.828**   **Fibrosis due to vascular prosthetic devices, implants and grafts**

   ● **T82.83**   **Hemorrhage due to cardiac and vascular prosthetic devices, implants and grafts** ◀▥

     ● **T82.837**   **Hemorrhage due to cardiac prosthetic devices, implants and grafts**

     ● **T82.838**   **Hemorrhage due to vascular prosthetic devices, implants and grafts**

   ● **T82.84**   **Pain due to cardiac and vascular prosthetic devices, implants and grafts** ◀▥

     ● **T82.847**   **Pain due to cardiac prosthetic devices, implants and grafts**

     ● **T82.848**   **Pain due to vascular prosthetic devices, implants and grafts**

   ● **T82.85**   **Stenosis due to cardiac and vascular prosthetic devices, implants and grafts** ◀▥

     ● **T82.855**   **Stenosis of coronary artery stent** ◀
        In-stent stenosis (restenosis) of coronary artery stent ◀
        Restenosis of coronary artery stent ◀

     ● **T82.856**   **Stenosis of peripheral vascular stent** ◀
        In-stent stenosis (restenosis) of peripheral vascular stent ◀
        Restenosis of peripheral vascular stent ◀

     ● **T82.857**   **Stenosis of other cardiac prosthetic devices, implants and grafts**

     ● **T82.858**   **Stenosis of other vascular prosthetic devices, implants and grafts**

   ● **T82.86**   **Thrombosis of cardiac and vascular prosthetic devices, implants and grafts**

     ● **T82.867**   **Thrombosis due to cardiac prosthetic devices, implants and grafts**

     ● **T82.868**   **Thrombosis due to vascular prosthetic devices, implants and grafts**

   ● **T82.89**   **Other specified complication of cardiac and vascular prosthetic devices, implants and grafts**

     ● **T82.897**   **Other specified complication of cardiac prosthetic devices, implants and grafts**

     ● **T82.898**   **Other specified complication of vascular prosthetic devices, implants and grafts**

X ● **T82.9**   **Unspecified complication of cardiac and vascular prosthetic device, implant and graft**

● **T83**   **Complications of genitourinary prosthetic devices, implants and grafts**

   Excludes2   failure and rejection of transplanted organs and tissue (T86.-)

   The appropriate 7th character is to be added to each code from category T83

A	initial encounter
D	subsequent encounter
S	sequela

   ● **T83.0**   **Mechanical complication of urinary catheter** ◀▥

     Excludes2   complications of stoma of urinary tract (N99.5-)

     ● **T83.01**   **Breakdown (mechanical) of urinary catheter** ◀▥

       ● **T83.010**   **Breakdown (mechanical) of cystostomy catheter**

       ● **T83.011**   **Breakdown (mechanical) of indwelling urethral catheter**

       ● **T83.012**   **Breakdown (mechanical) of nephrostomy catheter**

       ● **T83.018**   **Breakdown (mechanical) of other urinary catheter** ◀▥
          Breakdown (mechanical) of Hopkins catheter
          Breakdown (mechanical) of ileostomy catheter
          Breakdown (mechanical) urostomy catheter

● **T83.02**   **Displacement of urinary catheter** ◀▥
     Malposition of urinary catheter ◀▥

   ● **T83.020**   **Displacement of cystostomy catheter**

   ● **T83.021**   **Displacement of indwelling urethral catheter**

   ● **T83.022**   **Displacement of nephrostomy catheter**

   ● **T83.028**   **Displacement of other urinary catheter** ◀▥
       Displacement of Hopkins catheter ◀
       Displacement of ileostomy catheter ◀
       Displacement of urostomy catheter ◀

● **T83.03**   **Leakage of urinary catheter** ◀▥

   ● **T83.030**   **Leakage of cystostomy catheter**

   ● **T83.031**   **Leakage of indwelling urethral catheter**

   ● **T83.032**   **Leakage of nephrostomy catheter**

   ● **T83.038**   **Leakage of other urinary catheter** ◀▥
       Leakage of Hopkins catheter ◀
       Leakage of ileostomy catheter ◀
       Leakage of urostomy catheter ◀

● **T83.09**   **Other mechanical complication of urinary catheter** ◀▥
     Obstruction (mechanical) of urinary catheter ◀▥
     Perforation of urinary catheter ◀▥
     Protrusion of urinary catheter ◀▥

   ● **T83.090**   **Other mechanical complication of cystostomy catheter**

   ● **T83.091**   **Other mechanical complication of indwelling urethral catheter**

   ● **T83.092**   **Other mechanical complication of nephrostomy catheter**

   ● **T83.098**   **Other mechanical complication of other urinary catheter** ◀▥
       Other mechanical complication of Hopkins catheter ◀
       Other mechanical complication of ileostomy catheter ◀
       Other mechanical complication of urostomy catheter ◀

● **T83.1**   **Mechanical complication of other urinary devices and implants**

   ● **T83.11**   **Breakdown (mechanical) of other urinary devices and implants**

     ● **T83.110**   **Breakdown (mechanical) of urinary electronic stimulator device**

> **Excludes2**   Breakdown (mechanical) of electrode (lead) for sacral nerve neurostimulator (T85.111) ◀
> Breakdown (mechanical) of implanted electronic sacral neurostimulator, pulse generator or receiver (T85.113) ◀

     ● **T83.111**   **Breakdown (mechanical) of implanted urinary sphincter**

     ● **T83.112**   **Breakdown (mechanical) of indwelling ureteral stent**

     ● **T83.113**   **Breakdown (mechanical) of other urinary stents**
       Breakdown (mechanical) of ileal conduit stent ◀
       Breakdown (mechanical) of nephroureteral stent ◀

     ● **T83.118**   **Breakdown (mechanical) of other urinary devices and implants**

● **T83.12**   **Displacement of other urinary devices and implants**
     Malposition of other urinary devices and implants

   ● **T83.120**   **Displacement of urinary electronic stimulator device**

> **Excludes2**   Displacement of electrode (lead) for sacral nerve neurostimulator (T85.121) ◀
> Displacement of implanted electronic sacral neurostimulator, pulse generator or receiver (T85.123) ◀

   ● **T83.121**   **Displacement of implanted urinary sphincter**

   ● **T83.122**   **Displacement of indwelling ureteral stent**

   ● **T83.123**   **Displacement of other urinary stents**
       Displacement of ileal conduit stent ◀
       Displacement of nephroureteral stent ◀

   ● **T83.128**   **Displacement of other urinary devices and implants**

● **T83.19**   **Other mechanical complication of other urinary devices and implants**
     Leakage of other urinary devices and implants
     Obstruction (mechanical) of other urinary devices and implants
     Perforation of other urinary devices and implants
     Protrusion of other urinary devices and implants

   ● **T83.190**   **Other mechanical complication of urinary electronic stimulator device**

> **Excludes2**   Other mechanical complication of electrode (lead) for sacral nerve neurostimulator (T85.191) ◀
> Other mechanical complication of implanted electronic sacral neurostimulator, pulse generator or receiver (T85.193) ◀

   ● **T83.191**   **Other mechanical complication of implanted urinary sphincter**

   ● **T83.192**   **Other mechanical complication of indwelling ureteral stent**

   ● **T83.193**   **Other mechanical complication of other urinary stent**
       Other mechanical complication of ileal conduit stent ◀
       Other mechanical complication of nephroureteral stent ◀

   ● **T83.198**   **Other mechanical complication of other urinary devices and implants**

● **T83.2**   **Mechanical complication of graft of urinary organ**

   X ● **T83.21**   **Breakdown (mechanical) of graft of urinary organ**

   X ● **T83.22**   **Displacement of graft of urinary organ**
     Malposition of graft of urinary organ

   X ● **T83.23**   **Leakage of graft of urinary organ**

   X ● **T83.24**   **Erosion of graft of urinary organ**

◀ New   ◀▥ Revised   ~~deleted~~ Deleted   Excludes 1   Excludes 2   Includes   Use additional   Code first   Code also   Unspecified

1414   OGCR Official Guidelines   X Assign placeholder X   ● Use Additional Character(s)   ▶ Manifestation Code   **Coding Clinic**

X ● **T83.25**   **Exposure of graft of urinary organ**

X ● **T83.29**   **Other mechanical complication of graft of urinary organ**

Obstruction (mechanical) of graft of urinary organ

Perforation of graft of urinary organ

Protrusion of graft of urinary organ

● **T83.3**   **Mechanical complication of intrauterine contraceptive device**

X ● **T83.31**   **Breakdown (mechanical) of intrauterine contraceptive device ♀**

X ● **T83.32**   **Displacement of intrauterine contraceptive device ♀**

Malposition of intrauterine contraceptive device

Missing string of intrauterine contraceptive device ◄

X ● **T83.39**   **Other mechanical complication of intrauterine contraceptive device ♀**

Leakage of intrauterine contraceptive device

Obstruction (mechanical) of intrauterine contraceptive device

Perforation of intrauterine contraceptive device

Protrusion of intrauterine contraceptive device

● **T83.4**   **Mechanical complication of other prosthetic devices, implants and grafts of genital tract**

● **T83.41**   **Breakdown (mechanical) of other prosthetic devices, implants and grafts of genital tract**

● **T83.410**   **Breakdown (mechanical) of implanted penile prosthesis ♂**

Breakdown (mechanical) of penile prosthesis cylinder ◄

Breakdown (mechanical) of penile prosthesis pump ◄

Breakdown (mechanical) of penile prosthesis reservoir ◄

● **T83.411**   **Breakdown (mechanical) of implanted testicular prosthesis** ◄

● **T83.418**   **Breakdown (mechanical) of other prosthetic devices, implants and grafts of genital tract**

● **T83.42**   **Displacement of other prosthetic devices, implants and grafts of genital tract**

Malposition of other prosthetic devices, implants and grafts of genital tract

● **T83.420**   **Displacement of implanted penile prosthesis ♂**

Displacement of penile prosthesis cylinder ◄

Displacement of penile prosthesis pump ◄

Displacement of penile prosthesis reservoir ◄

● **T83.421**   **Displacement of implanted testicular prosthesis** ◄

● **T83.428**   **Displacement of other prosthetic devices, implants and grafts of genital tract**

● **T83.49**   **Other mechanical complication of other prosthetic devices, implants and grafts of genital tract**

Leakage of other prosthetic devices, implants and grafts of genital tract

Obstruction, mechanical of other prosthetic devices, implants and grafts of genital tract

Perforation of other prosthetic devices, implants and grafts of genital tract

Protrusion of other prosthetic devices, implants and grafts of genital tract

● **T83.490**   **Other mechanical complication of implanted penile prosthesis ♂**

Other mechanical complication of penile prosthesis cylinder ◄

Other mechanical complication of penile prosthesis pump ◄

Other mechanical complication of penile prosthesis reservoir ◄

● **T83.491**   **Other mechanical complication of implanted testicular prosthesis**

● **T83.498**   **Other mechanical complication of other prosthetic devices, implants and grafts of genital tract**

● **T83.5**   **Infection and inflammatory reaction due to prosthetic device, implant and graft in urinary system**

Use additional code to identify infection

● **T83.51**   **Infection and inflammatory reaction due to urinary catheter**

> **Excludes2**   complications of stoma of urinary tract (N99.5-)

● **T83.510**   **Infection and inflammatory reaction due to cystostomy catheter**

● **T83.511**   **Infection and inflammatory reaction due to indwelling urethral catheter**

● **T83.512**   **Infection and inflammatory reaction due to nephrostomy catheter**

● **T83.518**   **Infection and inflammatory reaction due to other urinary catheter**

Infection and inflammatory reaction due to Hopkins catheter ◄

Infection and inflammatory reaction due to ileostomy catheter ◄

Infection and inflammatory reaction due to urostomy catheter ◄

● **T83.59**   **Infection and inflammatory reaction due to prosthetic device, implant and graft in urinary system**

● **T83.590**   **Infection and inflammatory reaction due to implanted urinary neurostimulation device**

> **Excludes2**   Infection and inflammatory reaction due to electrode lead of sacral nerve neurostimulator (T85.732) ◄
>
> Infection and inflammatory reaction due to pulse generator or receiver of sacral nerve neurostimulator (T85.734) ◄

● **T83.591**   **Infection and inflammatory reaction due to implanted urinary sphincter**

● **T83.592**   **Infection and inflammatory reaction due to indwelling ureteral stent**

● **T83.593**   **Infection and inflammatory reaction due to other urinary stents**

Infection and inflammatory reaction due to ileal conduit stents ◄

Infection and inflammatory reaction due to nephroureteral stent ◄

● **T83.598**   **Infection and inflammatory reaction due to other prosthetic device, implant and graft in urinary system**

CHAPTER 19 (S00–T88)

● **T83.6** **Infection and inflammatory reaction due to prosthetic device, implant and graft in genital tract**
> Use additional code to identify infection

● **T83.61** **Infection and inflammatory reaction due to implanted penile prosthesis**
>> Infection and inflammatory reaction due to penile prosthesis cylinder ◀
>> Infection and inflammatory reaction due to penile prosthesis pump ◀
>> Infection and inflammatory reaction due to penile prosthesis reservoir ◀

● **T83.62** **Infection and inflammatory reaction due to implanted testicular prosthesis**

● **T83.69** **Infection and inflammatory reaction due to other prosthetic device, implant and graft in genital tract**

● **T83.7** **Complications due to implanted mesh and other prosthetic materials**

● **T83.71** **Erosion of implanted mesh and other prosthetic materials to surrounding organ or tissue**

● **T83.711** **Erosion of implanted vaginal mesh to surrounding organ or tissue ♀ ◀⃜**
>> Erosion of implanted vaginal mesh into pelvic floor muscles ◀⃜

● **T83.712** **Erosion of implanted urethral mesh to surrounding organ or tissue**
>> Erosion of implanted female urethral sling ◀
>> Erosion of implanted male urethral sling ◀
>> Erosion of implanted urethral mesh into pelvic floor muscles ◀

● **T83.713** **Erosion of implanted urethral bulking agent to surrounding organ or tissue**

● **T83.714** **Erosion of implanted ureteral bulking agent to surrounding organ or tissue**

● **T83.718** **Erosion of other implanted mesh to organ or tissue**

● **T83.719** **Erosion of other prosthetic materials to surrounding organ or tissue**

● **T83.72** **Exposure of implanted mesh and other prosthetic materials into surrounding organ or tissue**
> Extrusion of implanted mesh ◀

● **T83.721** **Exposure of implanted vaginal mesh into vagina ♀ ◀⃜**
>> Exposure of implanted vaginal mesh through vaginal wall ◀⃜

● **T83.722** **Exposure of implanted urethral mesh into urethra**
>> Exposure of implanted female urethral sling ◀
>> Exposure of implanted male urethral sling ◀
>> Exposure of implanted urethral mesh through urethral wall ◀

● **T83.723** **Exposure of implanted urethral bulking agent into urethra**

● **T83.724** **Exposure of implanted ureteral bulking agent into ureter**

● **T83.728** **Exposure of other implanted mesh into organ or tissue**

● **T83.729** **Exposure of other prosthetic materials into organ or tissue**

X ● **T83.79** **Other specified complications due to other genitourinary prosthetic materials**

● **T83.8** **Other specified complications of genitourinary prosthetic devices, implants and grafts**

X ● **T83.81** **Embolism due to genitourinary prosthetic devices, implants and grafts**

X ● **T83.82** **Fibrosis due to genitourinary prosthetic devices, implants and grafts**

X ● **T83.83** **Hemorrhage due to genitourinary prosthetic devices, implants and grafts**

X ● **T83.84** **Pain due to genitourinary prosthetic devices, implants and grafts**

X ● **T83.85** **Stenosis due to genitourinary prosthetic devices, implants and grafts**

X ● **T83.86** **Thrombosis due to genitourinary prosthetic devices, implants and grafts**

X ● **T83.89** **Other specified complication of genitourinary prosthetic devices, implants and grafts**

X ● **T83.9** **Unspecified complication of genitourinary prosthetic device, implant and graft**

● **T84** **Complications of internal orthopedic prosthetic devices, implants and grafts**

> **Excludes2** failure and rejection of transplanted organs and tissues (T86.-)
> fracture of bone following insertion of orthopedic implant, joint prosthesis or bone plate (M96.6)

> The appropriate 7th character is to be added to each code from category T84

A	initial encounter
D	subsequent encounter
S	sequela

● **T84.0** **Mechanical complication of internal joint prosthesis**

● **T84.01** **Broken internal joint prosthesis**
>> Breakage (fracture) of prosthetic joint
>> Broken prosthetic joint implant

> **Excludes1** periprosthetic joint implant fracture (T84.04)

● **T84.010** **Broken internal right hip prosthesis**

● **T84.011** **Broken internal left hip prosthesis**

● **T84.012** **Broken internal right knee prosthesis**

● **T84.013** **Broken internal left knee prosthesis**

● **T84.018** **Broken internal joint prosthesis, other site**
>> Use additional code to identify the joint (Z96.6-)

● **T84.019** **Broken internal joint prosthesis, unspecified site**

● **T84.02** **Dislocation of internal joint prosthesis**
>> Instability of internal joint prosthesis
>> Subluxation of internal joint prosthesis

● **T84.020** **Dislocation of internal right hip prosthesis**

● **T84.021** **Dislocation of internal left hip prosthesis**

● **T84.022** **Instability of internal right knee prosthesis**

● **T84.023** **Instability of internal left knee prosthesis**

● **T84.028** **Dislocation of other internal joint prosthesis**
>> Use additional code to identify the joint (Z96.6-)

● **T84.029** **Dislocation of unspecified internal joint prosthesis**

◀ New   ◀⃜ Revised   ~~deleted~~ Deleted   Excludes 1   Excludes 2   Includes   Use additional   Code first   Code also   Unspecified

1416   OGCR Official Guidelines   X Assign placeholder X   ● Use Additional Character(s)   ▶ Manifestation Code   **Coding Clinic**

● **T84.03 Mechanical loosening of internal prosthetic joint**
    Aseptic loosening of prosthetic joint
- ● **T84.030 Mechanical loosening of internal right hip prosthetic joint**
- ● **T84.031 Mechanical loosening of internal left hip prosthetic joint**
- ● **T84.032 Mechanical loosening of internal right knee prosthetic joint**
- ● **T84.033 Mechanical loosening of internal left knee prosthetic joint**
- ● **T84.038 Mechanical loosening of other internal prosthetic joint**
    Use additional code to identify the joint (Z96.6-)
- ● **T84.039 Mechanical loosening of unspecified internal prosthetic joint**

~~T84.04 Periprosthetic fracture around internal prosthetic joint~~
- ~~T84.040 Periprosthetic fracture around internal prosthetic right hip joint~~
- ~~T84.041 Periprosthetic fracture around internal prosthetic left hip joint~~
- ~~T84.042 Periprosthetic fracture around internal prosthetic right knee joint~~
- ~~T84.043 Periprosthetic fracture around internal prosthetic left knee joint~~
- ~~T84.048 Periprosthetic fracture around other internal prosthetic joint~~
- ~~T84.049 Periprosthetic fracture around unspecified internal prosthetic joint~~

● **T84.05 Periprosthetic osteolysis of internal prosthetic joint**
    Use additional code to identify major osseous defect, if applicable (M89.7-)
- ● **T84.050 Periprosthetic osteolysis of internal prosthetic right hip joint**
- ● **T84.051 Periprosthetic osteolysis of internal prosthetic left hip joint**
- ● **T84.052 Periprosthetic osteolysis of internal prosthetic right knee joint**
- ● **T84.053 Periprosthetic osteolysis of internal prosthetic left knee joint**
- ● **T84.058 Periprosthetic osteolysis of other internal prosthetic joint**
    Use additional code to identify the joint (Z96.6-)
- ● **T84.059 Periprosthetic osteolysis of unspecified internal prosthetic joint**

● **T84.06 Wear of articular bearing surface of internal prosthetic joint**
- ● **T84.060 Wear of articular bearing surface of internal prosthetic right hip joint**
- ● **T84.061 Wear of articular bearing surface of internal prosthetic left hip joint**
- ● **T84.062 Wear of articular bearing surface of internal prosthetic right knee joint**
- ● **T84.063 Wear of articular bearing surface of internal prosthetic left knee joint**
- ● **T84.068 Wear of articular bearing surface of other internal prosthetic joint**
    Use additional code to identify the joint (Z96.6-)
- ● **T84.069 Wear of articular bearing surface of unspecified internal prosthetic joint**

● **T84.09 Other mechanical complication of internal joint prosthesis**
    Prosthetic joint implant failure NOS
- ● **T84.090 Other mechanical complication of internal right hip prosthesis**
- ● **T84.091 Other mechanical complication of internal left hip prosthesis**
- ● **T84.092 Other mechanical complication of internal right knee prosthesis**
- ● **T84.093 Other mechanical complication of internal left knee prosthesis**
- ● **T84.098 Other mechanical complication of other internal joint prosthesis**
    Use additional code to identify the joint (Z96.6-)
- ● **T84.099 Other mechanical complication of unspecified internal joint prosthesis**

● **T84.1 Mechanical complication of internal fixation device of bones of limb**
    Excludes2 mechanical complication of internal fixation device of bones of feet (T84.2-)
    mechanical complication of internal fixation device of bones of fingers (T84.2-)
    mechanical complication of internal fixation device of bones of hands (T84.2-)
    mechanical complication of internal fixation device of bones of toes (T84.2-)
- ● **T84.11 Breakdown (mechanical) of internal fixation device of bones of limb**
  - ● **T84.110 Breakdown (mechanical) of internal fixation device of right humerus**
  - ● **T84.111 Breakdown (mechanical) of internal fixation device of left humerus**
  - ● **T84.112 Breakdown (mechanical) of internal fixation device of bone of right forearm**
  - ● **T84.113 Breakdown (mechanical) of internal fixation device of bone of left forearm**
  - ● **T84.114 Breakdown (mechanical) of internal fixation device of right femur**
  - ● **T84.115 Breakdown (mechanical) of internal fixation device of left femur**
  - ● **T84.116 Breakdown (mechanical) of internal fixation device of bone of right lower leg**
  - ● **T84.117 Breakdown (mechanical) of internal fixation device of bone of left lower leg**
  - ● **T84.119 Breakdown (mechanical) of internal fixation device of unspecified bone of limb**
- ● **T84.12 Displacement of internal fixation device of bones of limb**
    Malposition of internal fixation device of bones of limb
  - ● **T84.120 Displacement of internal fixation device of right humerus**
  - ● **T84.121 Displacement of internal fixation device of left humerus**
  - ● **T84.122 Displacement of internal fixation device of bone of right forearm**
  - ● **T84.123 Displacement of internal fixation device of bone of left forearm**
  - ● **T84.124 Displacement of internal fixation device of right femur**
  - ● **T84.125 Displacement of internal fixation device of left femur**
  - ● **T84.126 Displacement of internal fixation device of bone of right lower leg**
  - ● **T84.127 Displacement of internal fixation device of bone of left lower leg**
  - ● **T84.129 Displacement of internal fixation device of unspecified bone of limb**

CHAPTER 19 (S00-T88)

- T84.19 **Other mechanical complication of internal fixation device of bones of limb**
  Obstruction (mechanical) of internal fixation device of bones of limb
  Perforation of internal fixation device of bones of limb
  Protrusion of internal fixation device of bones of limb
  - T84.190 **Other mechanical complication of internal fixation device of right humerus**
  - T84.191 **Other mechanical complication of internal fixation device of left humerus**
  - T84.192 **Other mechanical complication of internal fixation device of bone of right forearm**
  - T84.193 **Other mechanical complication of internal fixation device of bone of left forearm**
  - T84.194 **Other mechanical complication of internal fixation device of right femur**
  - T84.195 **Other mechanical complication of internal fixation device of left femur**
  - T84.196 **Other mechanical complication of internal fixation device of bone of right lower leg**
  - T84.197 **Other mechanical complication of internal fixation device of bone of left lower leg**
  - T84.199 **Other mechanical complication of internal fixation device of** unspecified **bone of limb**
- T84.2 **Mechanical complication of internal fixation device of other bones**
  - T84.21 **Breakdown (mechanical) of internal fixation device of other bones**
    - T84.210 **Breakdown (mechanical) of internal fixation device of bones of hand and fingers**
    - T84.213 **Breakdown (mechanical) of internal fixation device of bones of foot and toes**
    - T84.216 **Breakdown (mechanical) of internal fixation device of vertebrae**
    - T84.218 **Breakdown (mechanical) of internal fixation device of other bones**
  - T84.22 **Displacement of internal fixation device of other bones**
    Malposition of internal fixation device of other bones
    - T84.220 **Displacement of internal fixation device of bones of hand and fingers**
    - T84.223 **Displacement of internal fixation device of bones of foot and toes**
    - T84.226 **Displacement of internal fixation device of vertebrae**
    - T84.228 **Displacement of internal fixation device of other bones**

- T84.29 **Other mechanical complication of internal fixation device of other bones**
  Obstruction (mechanical) of internal fixation device of other bones
  Perforation of internal fixation device of other bones
  Protrusion of internal fixation device of other bones
  - T84.290 **Other mechanical complication of internal fixation device of bones of hand and fingers**
  - T84.293 **Other mechanical complication of internal fixation device of bones of foot and toes**
  - T84.296 **Other mechanical complication of internal fixation device of vertebrae**
  - T84.298 **Other mechanical complication of internal fixation device of other bones**
- T84.3 **Mechanical complication of other bone devices, implants and grafts**
  Excludes2   other complications of bone graft (T86.83-)
  - T84.31 **Breakdown (mechanical) of other bone devices, implants and grafts**
    - T84.310 **Breakdown (mechanical) of electronic bone stimulator**
    - T84.318 **Breakdown (mechanical) of other bone devices, implants and grafts**
  - T84.32 **Displacement of other bone devices, implants and grafts**
    Malposition of other bone devices, implants and grafts
    - T84.320 **Displacement of electronic bone stimulator**
    - T84.328 **Displacement of other bone devices, implants and grafts**
  - T84.39 **Other mechanical complication of other bone devices, implants and grafts**
    Obstruction (mechanical) of other bone devices, implants and grafts
    Perforation of other bone devices, implants and grafts
    Protrusion of other bone devices, implants and grafts
    - T84.390 **Other mechanical complication of electronic bone stimulator**
    - T84.398 **Other mechanical complication of other bone devices, implants and grafts**
- T84.4 **Mechanical complication of other internal orthopedic devices, implants and grafts**
  - T84.41 **Breakdown (mechanical) of other internal orthopedic devices, implants and grafts**
    - T84.410 **Breakdown (mechanical) of muscle and tendon graft**
    - T84.418 **Breakdown (mechanical) of other internal orthopedic devices, implants and grafts**
  - T84.42 **Displacement of other internal orthopedic devices, implants and grafts**
    Malposition of other internal orthopedic devices, implants and grafts
    - T84.420 **Displacement of muscle and tendon graft**
    - T84.428 **Displacement of other internal orthopedic devices, implants and grafts**

◀ New   ◀▥ Revised   ~~deleted~~ Deleted   Excludes 1   Excludes 2   Includes   Use additional   Code first   Code also   Unspecified
OGCR Official Guidelines   X Assign placeholder X   ● Use Additional Character(s)   ▶ Manifestation Code   **Coding Clinic**

● **T84.49** **Other mechanical complication of other internal orthopedic devices, implants and grafts**
Mechanical complication of other internal orthopedic devices, implants and grafts NOS
Obstruction (mechanical) of other internal orthopedic devices, implants and grafts
Perforation of other internal orthopedic devices, implants and grafts
Protrusion of other internal orthopedic devices, implants and grafts

● **T84.490** **Other mechanical complication of muscle and tendon graft**

● **T84.498** **Other mechanical complication of other internal orthopedic devices, implants and grafts**

● **T84.5** **Infection and inflammatory reaction due to internal joint prosthesis**
Use additional code to identify infection
Coding Clinic: 2015, Q1, P16

X ● **T84.50** **Infection and inflammatory reaction due to unspecified internal joint prosthesis**
Coding Clinic: 2015, Q1, P3

X ● **T84.51** **Infection and inflammatory reaction due to internal right hip prosthesis**
Coding Clinic: 2015, Q4, P36

X ● **T84.52** **Infection and inflammatory reaction due to internal left hip prosthesis**
Coding Clinic: 2015, Q1, P16-17

X ● **T84.53** **Infection and inflammatory reaction due to internal right knee prosthesis**

X ● **T84.54** **Infection and inflammatory reaction due to internal left knee prosthesis**

X ● **T84.59** **Infection and inflammatory reaction due to other internal joint prosthesis**

● **T84.6** **Infection and inflammatory reaction due to internal fixation device**
Use additional code to identify infection

X ● **T84.60** **Infection and inflammatory reaction due to internal fixation device of unspecified site**

● **T84.61** **Infection and inflammatory reaction due to internal fixation device of arm**

● **T84.610** **Infection and inflammatory reaction due to internal fixation device of right humerus**

● **T84.611** **Infection and inflammatory reaction due to internal fixation device of left humerus**

● **T84.612** **Infection and inflammatory reaction due to internal fixation device of right radius**

● **T84.613** **Infection and inflammatory reaction due to internal fixation device of left radius**

● **T84.614** **Infection and inflammatory reaction due to internal fixation device of right ulna**

● **T84.615** **Infection and inflammatory reaction due to internal fixation device of left ulna**

● **T84.619** **Infection and inflammatory reaction due to internal fixation device of unspecified bone of arm**

● **T84.62** **Infection and inflammatory reaction due to internal fixation device of leg**

● **T84.620** **Infection and inflammatory reaction due to internal fixation device of right femur**

● **T84.621** **Infection and inflammatory reaction due to internal fixation device of left femur**

● **T84.622** **Infection and inflammatory reaction due to internal fixation device of right tibia**

● **T84.623** **Infection and inflammatory reaction due to internal fixation device of left tibia**

● **T84.624** **Infection and inflammatory reaction due to internal fixation device of right fibula**

● **T84.625** **Infection and inflammatory reaction due to internal fixation device of left fibula**

● **T84.629** **Infection and inflammatory reaction due to internal fixation device of unspecified bone of leg**

X ● **T84.63** **Infection and inflammatory reaction due to internal fixation device of spine**

X ● **T84.69** **Infection and inflammatory reaction due to internal fixation device of other site**

● **T84.7** **Infection and inflammatory reaction due to other internal orthopedic prosthetic devices, implants and grafts**
Use additional code to identify infection

● **T84.8** **Other specified complications of internal orthopedic prosthetic devices, implants and grafts**

X ● **T84.81** **Embolism due to internal orthopedic prosthetic devices, implants and grafts**

X ● **T84.82** **Fibrosis due to internal orthopedic prosthetic devices, implants and grafts**

X ● **T84.83** **Hemorrhage due to internal orthopedic prosthetic devices, implants and grafts**

X ● **T84.84** **Pain due to internal orthopedic prosthetic devices, implants and grafts**

X ● **T84.85** **Stenosis due to internal orthopedic prosthetic devices, implants and grafts**

X ● **T84.86** **Thrombosis due to internal orthopedic prosthetic devices, implants and grafts**

X ● **T84.89** **Other specified complication of internal orthopedic prosthetic devices, implants and grafts**

X ● **T84.9** **Unspecified complication of internal orthopedic prosthetic device, implant and graft**

● **T85** **Complications of other internal prosthetic devices, implants and grafts**
Excludes2   failure and rejection of transplanted organs and tissue (T86.-)
The appropriate 7th character is to be added to each code from category T85

A	initial encounter
D	subsequent encounter
S	sequela

● **T85.0** **Mechanical complication of ventricular intracranial (communicating) shunt**

X ● **T85.01** **Breakdown (mechanical) of ventricular intracranial (communicating) shunt**

X ● **T85.02** **Displacement of ventricular intracranial (communicating) shunt**
Malposition of ventricular intracranial (communicating) shunt

X ● **T85.03** **Leakage of ventricular intracranial (communicating) shunt**

X ● **T85.09** **Other mechanical complication of ventricular intracranial (communicating) shunt**
Obstruction (mechanical) of ventricular intracranial (communicating) shunt
Perforation of ventricular intracranial (communicating) shunt
Protrusion of ventricular intracranial (communicating) shunt

CHAPTER 19 (S00-T88)

● **T85.1**   **Mechanical complication of implanted electronic stimulator of nervous system**

  ● **T85.11**   **Breakdown (mechanical) of implanted electronic stimulator of nervous system**

    ● **T85.110**   **Breakdown (mechanical) of implanted electronic neurostimulator of brain electrode (lead)**

    ● **T85.111**   **Breakdown (mechanical) of implanted electronic neurostimulator of peripheral nerve electrode (lead)**

       Breakdown of electrode (lead) for cranial nerve neurostimulators ◀

       Breakdown of electrode (lead) for gastric neurostimulator ◀

       Breakdown of electrode (lead) for sacral nerve neurostimulator ◀

       Breakdown of electrode (lead) for vagal nerve neurostimulators ◀

    ● **T85.112**   **Breakdown (mechanical) of implanted electronic neurostimulator of spinal cord electrode (lead)**

    ● **T85.113**   **Breakdown (mechanical) of implanted electronic neurostimulator, generator**

       Breakdown (mechanical) of implanted electronic neurostimuator generator, brain, peripheral, gastric, spinal ◀

       Breakdown (mechanical) of implanted electronic sacral neurostimulator, pulse generator or receiver ◀

    ● **T85.118**   **Breakdown (mechanical) of other implanted electronic stimulator of nervous system**

  ● **T85.12**   **Displacement of implanted electronic stimulator of nervous system**

    Malposition of implanted electronic stimulator of nervous system

    ● **T85.120**   **Displacement of implanted electronic neurostimulator of brain electrode (lead)**

    ● **T85.121**   **Displacement of implanted electronic neurostimulator of peripheral nerve electrode (lead)**

       Displacement of electrode (lead) for cranial nerve neurostimulators ◀

       Displacement of electrode (lead) for gastric neurostimulator ◀

       Displacement of electrode (lead) for sacral nerve neurostimulator ◀

       Displacement of electrode (lead) for vagal nerve neurostimulators ◀

    ● **T85.122**   **Displacement of implanted electronic neurostimulator of spinal cord electrode (lead)**

    ● **T85.123**   **Displacement of implanted electronic neurostimulator, generator**

       Displacement of implanted electronic neurostimulator generator, brain, peripheral, gastric, spinal ◀

       Displacement of implanted electronic sacral neurostimulator, pulse generator or receiver ◀

    ● **T85.128**   **Displacement of other implanted electronic stimulator of nervous system**

● **T85.19**   **Other mechanical complication of implanted electronic stimulator of nervous system**

    Leakage of implanted electronic stimulator of nervous system

    Obstruction (mechanical) of implanted electronic stimulator of nervous system

    Perforation of implanted electronic stimulator of nervous system

    Protrusion of implanted electronic stimulator of nervous system

  ● **T85.190**   **Other mechanical complication of implanted electronic neurostimulator of brain electrode (lead)**

  ● **T85.191**   **Other mechanical complication of implanted electronic neurostimulator of peripheral nerve electrode (lead)**

    Other mechanical complication of electrode (lead) for cranial nerve neurostimulators ◀

    Other mechanical complication of electrode (lead) for gastric neurostimulator ◀

    Other mechanical complication of electrode (lead) for sacral nerve neurostimulator ◀

    Other mechanical complication of electrode (lead) for vagal nerve neurostimulators ◀

  ● **T85.192**   **Other mechanical complication of implanted electronic neurostimulator of spinal cord electrode (lead)**

  ● **T85.193**   **Other mechanical complication of implanted electronic neurostimulator, generator**

    Other mechanical complication of implanted electronic neurostimulator generator, brain, peripheral, gastric, spinal ◀

    Other mechanical complication of implanted electronic sacral neurostimulator, pulse generator or receiver ◀

  ● **T85.199**   **Other mechanical complication of other implanted electronic stimulator of nervous system**

● **T85.2**   **Mechanical complication of intraocular lens**

  X ● **T85.21**   **Breakdown (mechanical) of intraocular lens**

  X ● **T85.22**   **Displacement of intraocular lens**

    Malposition of intraocular lens

  X ● **T85.29**   **Other mechanical complication of intraocular lens**

    Obstruction (mechanical) of intraocular lens

    Perforation of intraocular lens

    Protrusion of intraocular lens

● **T85.3**   **Mechanical complication of other ocular prosthetic devices, implants and grafts**

  Excludes2   other complications of corneal graft (T86.84-)

  ● **T85.31**   **Breakdown (mechanical) of other ocular prosthetic devices, implants and grafts**

    ● **T85.310**   **Breakdown (mechanical) of prosthetic orbit of right eye**

    ● **T85.311**   **Breakdown (mechanical) of prosthetic orbit of left eye**

    ● **T85.318**   **Breakdown (mechanical) of other ocular prosthetic devices, implants and grafts**

◀ New   ◀═ Revised   ~~deleted~~ Deleted   Excludes 1   Excludes 2   Includes   Use additional   Code first   Code also   Unspecified

OGCR Official Guidelines   X Assign placeholder X   ● Use Additional Character(s)   ▌ Manifestation Code   **Coding Clinic**

1420

● **T85.32**   **Displacement of other ocular prosthetic devices, implants and grafts**
Malposition of other ocular prosthetic devices, implants and grafts

   ● **T85.320**   **Displacement of prosthetic orbit of right eye**

   ● **T85.321**   **Displacement of prosthetic orbit of left eye**

   ● **T85.328**   **Displacement of other ocular prosthetic devices, implants and grafts**

● **T85.39**   **Other mechanical complication of other ocular prosthetic devices, implants and grafts**
Obstruction (mechanical) of other ocular prosthetic devices, implants and grafts
Perforation of other ocular prosthetic devices, implants and grafts
Protrusion of other ocular prosthetic devices, implants and grafts

   ● **T85.390**   **Other mechanical complication of prosthetic orbit of right eye**

   ● **T85.391**   **Other mechanical complication of prosthetic orbit of left eye**

   ● **T85.398**   **Other mechanical complication of other ocular prosthetic devices, implants and grafts**

● **T85.4**   **Mechanical complication of breast prosthesis and implant**

   X ● **T85.41**   **Breakdown (mechanical) of breast prosthesis and implant**

   X ● **T85.42**   **Displacement of breast prosthesis and implant**
Malposition of breast prosthesis and implant

   X ● **T85.43**   **Leakage of breast prosthesis and implant**

   X ● **T85.44**   **Capsular contracture of breast implant**

   X ● **T85.49**   **Other mechanical complication of breast prosthesis and implant**
Obstruction (mechanical) of breast prosthesis and implant
Perforation of breast prosthesis and implant
Protrusion of breast prosthesis and implant

● **T85.5**   **Mechanical complication of gastrointestinal prosthetic devices, implants and grafts**

   ● **T85.51**   **Breakdown (mechanical) of gastrointestinal prosthetic devices, implants and grafts**

     ● **T85.510**   **Breakdown (mechanical) of bile duct prosthesis**

     ● **T85.511**   **Breakdown (mechanical) of esophageal anti-reflux device**

     ● **T85.518**   **Breakdown (mechanical) of other gastrointestinal prosthetic devices, implants and grafts**

   ● **T85.52**   **Displacement of gastrointestinal prosthetic devices, implants and grafts**
Malposition of gastrointestinal prosthetic devices, implants and grafts

     ● **T85.520**   **Displacement of bile duct prosthesis**

     ● **T85.521**   **Displacement of esophageal anti-reflux device**

     ● **T85.528**   **Displacement of other gastrointestinal prosthetic devices, implants and grafts**

● **T85.59**   **Other mechanical complication of gastrointestinal prosthetic devices, implants and**
Obstruction, mechanical of gastrointestinal prosthetic devices, implants and grafts
Perforation of gastrointestinal prosthetic devices, implants and grafts
Protrusion of gastrointestinal prosthetic devices, implants and grafts

   ● **T85.590**   **Other mechanical complication of bile duct prosthesis**

   ● **T85.591**   **Other mechanical complication of esophageal anti-reflux device**

   ● **T85.598**   **Other mechanical complication of other gastrointestinal prosthetic devices, implants and grafts**

● **T85.6**   **Mechanical complication of other specified internal and external prosthetic devices, implants and grafts**

   ● **T85.61**   **Breakdown (mechanical) of other specified internal prosthetic devices, implants and grafts**

     ● **T85.610**   **Breakdown (mechanical) of cranial or spinal infusion catheter**
Breakdown (mechanical) of epidural infusion catheter ◄
Breakdown (mechanical) of intrathecal infusion catheter ◄
Breakdown (mechanical) of subarachnoid infusion catheter ◄
Breakdown (mechanical) of subdural infusion catheter ◄

     ● **T85.611**   **Breakdown (mechanical) of intraperitoneal dialysis catheter**

       Excludes1   mechanical complication of vascular dialysis catheter (T82.4-)

     ● **T85.612**   **Breakdown (mechanical) of permanent sutures**

       Excludes1   mechanical complication of permanent (wire) suture used in bone repair (T84.1-T84.2)

     ● **T85.613**   **Breakdown (mechanical) of artificial skin graft and decellularized allodermis**
Failure of artificial skin graft and decellularized allodermis
Non-adherence of artificial skin graft and decellularized allodermis
Poor incorporation of artificial skin graft and decellularized allodermis
Shearing of artificial skin graft and decellularized allodermis

     ● **T85.614**   **Breakdown (mechanical) of insulin pump**

     ● **T85.615**   **Breakdown (mechanical) of other nervous system device, implant or graft**
Breakdown (mechanical) of intrathecal infusion pump ◄

     ● **T85.618**   **Breakdown (mechanical) of other specified internal prosthetic devices, implants and grafts**

● T85.62   **Displacement of other specified internal prosthetic devices, implants and grafts**
    Malposition of other specified internal prosthetic devices, implants and grafts

   ● T85.620   **Displacement of cranial or spinal infusion catheter**
      Displacement of epidural infusion catheter ◀
      Displacement of intrathecal infusion catheter ◀
      Displacement of subarachnoid infusion catheter ◀
      Displacement of subdural infusion catheter ◀

   ● T85.621   **Displacement of intraperitoneal dialysis catheter**
      Excludes1   mechanical complication of vascular dialysis catheter (T82.4-)

   ● T85.622   **Displacement of permanent sutures**
      Excludes1   mechanical complication of permanent (wire) suture used in bone repair (T84.1-T84.2)

   ● T85.623   **Displacement of artificial skin graft and decellularized allodermis**
      Dislodgement of artificial skin graft and decellularized allodermis
      Displacement of artificial skin graft and decellularized allodermis

   ● T85.624   **Displacement of insulin pump**

   ● T85.625   **Displacement of other nervous system device, implant or graft**
      Displacement of intrathecal infusion pump ◀

   ● T85.628   **Displacement of other specified internal prosthetic devices, implants and grafts**
      Coding Clinic: 2015, Q1, P15

● T85.63   **Leakage of other specified internal prosthetic devices, implants and grafts**

   ● T85.630   **Leakage of cranial or spinal infusion catheter**
      Leakage of epidural infusion catheter ◀
      Leakage of intrathecal infusion catheter ◀
      Leakage of subdural infusion catheter ◀
      Leakage of subarachnoid infusion catheter ◀

   ● T85.631   **Leakage of intraperitoneal dialysis catheter**
      Excludes1   mechanical complication of vascular dialysis catheter (T82.4)

   ● T85.633   **Leakage of insulin pump**

   ● T85.635   **Leakage of other nervous system device, implant or graft**
      Leakage of intrathecal infusion pump ◀

   ● T85.638   **Leakage of other specified internal prosthetic devices, implants and grafts**

● T85.69   **Other mechanical complication of other specified internal prosthetic devices, implants and grafts**
    Obstruction, mechanical of other specified internal prosthetic devices, implants and grafts
    Perforation of other specified internal prosthetic devices, implants and grafts
    Protrusion of other specified internal prosthetic devices, implants and grafts

   ● T85.690   **Other mechanical complication of cranial or spinal infusion catheter**
      Other mechanical complication of epidural infusion catheter ◀
      Other mechanical complication of intrathecal infusion catheter ◀
      Other mechanical complication of subarachnoid infusion catheter ◀
      Other mechanical complication of subdural infusion catheter ◀

   ● T85.691   **Other mechanical complication of intraperitoneal dialysis catheter**
      Excludes1   mechanical complication of vascular dialysis catheter (T82.4)

   ● T85.692   **Other mechanical complication of permanent sutures**
      Excludes1   mechanical complication of permanent (wire) suture used in bone repair (T84.1-T84.2)

   ● T85.693   **Other mechanical complication of artificial skin graft and decellularized allodermis**

   ● T85.694   **Other mechanical complication of insulin pump**

   ● T85.695   **Other mechanical complication of other nervous system device, implant or graft**
      Other mechanical complication of intrathecal infusion pump ◀

   ● T85.698   **Other mechanical complication of other specified internal prosthetic devices, implants and grafts**
      Mechanical complication of nonabsorbable surgical material NOS

● T85.7   **Infection and inflammatory reaction due to other internal prosthetic devices, implants and grafts**
    Use additional code to identify infection

X ● T85.71   **Infection and inflammatory reaction due to peritoneal dialysis catheter**

X ● T85.72   **Infection and inflammatory reaction due to insulin pump**

● T85.73   **Infection and inflammatory reaction due to nervous system devices, implants and graft**

   ● T85.730   **Infection and inflammatory reaction due to ventricular intracranial (communicating) shunt**

   ● T85.731   **Infection and inflammatory reaction due to implanted electronic neurostimulator of brain, electrode (lead)**

CHAPTER 19 (S00-T88)

● **T85.732** **Infection and inflammatory reaction due to implanted electronic neurostimulator of peripheral nerve, electrode (lead)**
Infection and inflammatory reaction due to electrode (lead) for cranial nerve neurostimulators
Infection and inflammatory reaction due to electrode (lead) for gastric neurostimulator ◀
Infection and inflammatory reaction due to electrode (lead) for sacral nerve neurostimulator ◀
Infection and inflammatory reaction due to electrode (lead) for vagal nerve neurostimulators ◀

● **T85.733** **Infection and inflammatory reaction due to implanted electronic neurostimulator of spinal cord, electrode (lead)** ◀

● **T85.734** **Infection and inflammatory reaction due to implanted electronic neurostimulator, generator** ◀
Generator pocket infection ◀

● **T85.735** **Infection and inflammatory reaction due to cranial or spinal infusion catheter** ◀
Infection and inflammatory reaction due to epidural catheter ◀
Infection and inflammatory reaction due to intrathecal infusion catheter ◀
Infection and inflammatory reaction due to subarachnoid catheter ◀
Infection and inflammatory reaction due to subdural catheter ◀

● **T85.738** **Infection and inflammatory reaction due to other nervous system device, implant or graft** ◀
Infection and inflammatory reaction due to intrathecal infusion pump ◀

X ● **T85.79** **Infection and inflammatory reaction due to other internal prosthetic devices, implants and grafts**

● **T85.8** **Other specified complications of internal prosthetic devices, implants and grafts, not elsewhere classified**

● **T85.81** **Embolism due to internal prosthetic devices, implants and grafts, not elsewhere classified**
   ● **T85.810** **Embolism due to nervous system prosthetic devices, implants and grafts**
   ● **T85.818** **Embolism due to other internal prosthetic devices, implants and grafts**

● **T85.82** **Fibrosis due to internal prosthetic devices, implants and grafts, not elsewhere classified**
   ● **T85.820** **Fibrosis due to nervous system prosthetic devices, implants and grafts**
   ● **T85.828** **Fibrosis due to other internal prosthetic devices, implants and grafts**

● **T85.83** **Hemorrhage due to internal prosthetic devices, implants and grafts, not elsewhere classified**
   ● **T85.830** **Hemorrhage due to nervous system prosthetic devices, implants and grafts**
   ● **T85.838** **Hemorrhage due to other internal prosthetic devices, implants and grafts**

● **T85.84** **Pain due to internal prosthetic devices, implants and grafts, not elsewhere classified**
   ● **T85.840** **Pain due to nervous system prosthetic devices, implants and grafts**
   ● **T85.848** **Pain due to other internal prosthetic devices, implants and grafts**

● **T85.85** **Stenosis due to internal prosthetic devices, implants and grafts, not elsewhere classified**
   ● **T85.850** **Stenosis due to nervous system prosthetic devices, implants and grafts**
   ● **T85.858** **Stenosis due to other internal prosthetic devices, implants and grafts**

● **T85.86** **Thrombosis due to internal prosthetic devices, implants and grafts, not elsewhere classified**
   ● **T85.860** **Thrombosis due to nervous system prosthetic devices, implants and grafts**
   ● **T85.868** **Thrombosis due to other internal prosthetic devices, implants and grafts**

● **T85.89** **Other specified complication of internal prosthetic devices, implants and grafts, not elsewhere classified**
   ● **T85.890** **Other specified complication of nervous system prosthetic devices, implants and grafts**
   ● **T85.898** **Other specified complication of other internal prosthetic devices, implants and grafts**

X ● **T85.9** **Unspecified complication of internal prosthetic device, implant and graft**
Complication of internal prosthetic device, implant and graft NOS

● **T86** **Complications of transplanted organs and tissue**
Use additional code to identify other transplant complications, such as:
graft-versus-host disease (D89.81-)
malignancy associated with organ transplant (C80.2)
post-transplant lymphoproliferative disorders (PTLD) (D47.Z1)

● **T86.0** **Complications of bone marrow transplant**
T86.00 **Unspecified complication of bone marrow transplant**
T86.01 **Bone marrow transplant rejection**
T86.02 **Bone marrow transplant failure**
T86.03 **Bone marrow transplant infection**
T86.09 **Other complications of bone marrow transplant**

● **T86.1** **Complications of kidney transplant**
T86.10 **Unspecified complication of kidney transplant**
T86.11 **Kidney transplant rejection**
T86.12 **Kidney transplant failure**
   Coding Clinic: 2013, Q1, P24
T86.13 **Kidney transplant infection**
   Use additional code to specify infection
T86.19 **Other complication of kidney transplant**

CHAPTER 19 (S00-T88)

OGCR Section I.C.19.g.3.

Organ Transplant Complications

Transplant Complications

(a) Transplant complications other than kidney

Codes under category T86, Complications of transplanted organs and tissues, are for use for both complications and rejection of transplanted organs. A transplant complication code is only assigned if the complication affects the function of the transplanted organ. Two codes are required to fully describe a transplant complication: the appropriate code from category T86 and a secondary code that identifies the complication.

Pre-existing conditions or conditions that develop after the transplant are not coded as complications unless they affect the function of the transplanted organs.

See I.C.21 for transplant organ removal status

See I.C.2 for malignant neoplasm associated with transplanted organ.

● **T86.2** **Complications of heart transplant**
     Excludes1 complication of:
                 artificial heart device (T82.5)
                 heart-lung transplant (T86.3)
     T86.20 **Unspecified** complication of heart transplant
     T86.21 **Heart transplant rejection**
     T86.22 **Heart transplant failure**
     T86.23 **Heart transplant infection**
         Use additional code to specify infection
   ● T86.29 **Other complications of heart transplant**
     T86.290 **Cardiac allograft vasculopathy**
         Excludes1 atherosclerosis of coronary arteries (I25.75-, I25.76-, I25.81-)
     T86.298 **Other complications of heart transplant**
● **T86.3** **Complications of heart-lung transplant**
     T86.30 **Unspecified** complication of heart-lung transplant
     T86.31 **Heart-lung transplant rejection**
     T86.32 **Heart-lung transplant failure**
     T86.33 **Heart-lung transplant infection**
         Use additional code to specify infection
     T86.39 **Other complications of heart-lung transplant**
● **T86.4** **Complications of liver transplant**
     T86.40 **Unspecified** complication of liver transplant
     T86.41 **Liver transplant rejection**
     T86.42 **Liver transplant failure**
     T86.43 **Liver transplant infection**
         Use additional code to identify infection, such as:
             Cytomegalovirus (CMV) infection (B25.-)
     T86.49 **Other complications of liver transplant**
● **T86.5** **Complications of stem cell transplant**
     Complications from stem cells from peripheral blood
     Complications from stem cells from umbilical cord

● **T86.8** **Complications of other transplanted organs and tissues**
   ● T86.81 **Complications of lung transplant**
     Excludes1 complication of heart-lung transplant (T86.3-)
     T86.810 **Lung transplant rejection**
     T86.811 **Lung transplant failure**
     T86.812 **Lung transplant infection**
         Use additional code to specify infection
     T86.818 **Other complications of lung transplant**
     T86.819 **Unspecified** complication of lung transplant
   ● T86.82 **Complications of skin graft (allograft) (autograft)**
     Excludes2 complication of artificial skin graft (T85.693)
     T86.820 **Skin graft (allograft) rejection**
     T86.821 **Skin graft (allograft) (autograft) failure**
     T86.822 **Skin graft (allograft) (autograft) infection**
         Use additional code to specify infection
     T86.828 **Other complications of skin graft (allograft) (autograft)**
     T86.829 **Unspecified** complication of skin graft (allograft) (autograft)
   ● T86.83 **Complications of bone graft**
     Excludes2 mechanical complications of bone graft (T84.3-)
     T86.830 **Bone graft rejection**
     T86.831 **Bone graft failure**
     T86.832 **Bone graft infection**
         Use additional code to specify infection
     T86.838 **Other complications of bone graft**
     T86.839 **Unspecified** complication of bone graft
   ● T86.84 **Complications of corneal transplant**
     Excludes2 mechanical complications of corneal graft (T85.3-)
     T86.840 **Corneal transplant rejection**
     T86.841 **Corneal transplant failure**
     T86.842 **Corneal transplant infection**
         Use additional code to specify infection
     T86.848 **Other complications of corneal transplant**
     T86.849 **Unspecified** complication of corneal transplant
   ● T86.85 **Complication of intestine transplant**
     T86.850 **Intestine transplant rejection**
     T86.851 **Intestine transplant failure**
     T86.852 **Intestine transplant infection**
         Use additional code to specify infection
     T86.858 **Other complications of intestine transplant**
     T86.859 **Unspecified** complication of intestine transplant

◀ New   ◀▥ Revised   ~~deleted~~ Deleted   Excludes 1   Excludes 2   Includes   Use additional   Code first   Code also   Unspecified

OGCR Official Guidelines   X Assign placeholder X   ● Use Additional Character(s)   ▶ Manifestation Code   **Coding Clinic**

● **T86.89** **Complications of other transplanted tissue**
Transplant failure or rejection of pancreas

  T86.890 **Other transplanted tissue rejection**

  T86.891 **Other transplanted tissue failure**

  T86.892 **Other transplanted tissue infection**
Use additional code to specify infection

  T86.898 **Other complications of other transplanted tissue**

  T86.899 **Unspecified complication of other transplanted tissue**

● **T86.9** **Complication of unspecified transplanted organ and tissue**

  T86.90 **Unspecified complication of unspecified transplanted organ and tissue**

  T86.91 **Unspecified transplanted organ and tissue rejection**

  T86.92 **Unspecified transplanted organ and tissue failure**

  T86.93 **Unspecified transplanted organ and tissue infection**
Use additional code to specify infection

  T86.99 **Other complications of unspecified transplanted organ and tissue**

● **T87** **Complications peculiar to reattachment and amputation**

● **T87.0** **Complications of reattached (part of) upper extremity**

  ● **T87.0X** **Complications of reattached (part of) upper extremity**

    T87.0X1 **Complications of reattached (part of) right upper extremity**

    T87.0X2 **Complications of reattached (part of) left upper extremity**

    T87.0X9 **Complications of reattached (part of) unspecified upper extremity**

● **T87.1** **Complications of reattached (part of) lower extremity**

  ● **T87.1X** **Complications of reattached (part of) lower extremity**

    T87.1X1 **Complications of reattached (part of) right lower extremity**

    T87.1X2 **Complications of reattached (part of) left lower extremity**

    T87.1X9 **Complications of reattached (part of) unspecified lower extremity**

  T87.2 **Complications of other reattached body part**

● **T87.3** **Neuroma of amputation stump**

  T87.30 **Neuroma of amputation stump, unspecified extremity**

  T87.31 **Neuroma of amputation stump, right upper extremity**

  T87.32 **Neuroma of amputation stump, left upper extremity**

  T87.33 **Neuroma of amputation stump, right lower extremity**

  T87.34 **Neuroma of amputation stump, left lower extremity**

● **T87.4** **Infection of amputation stump**

  T87.40 **Infection of amputation stump, unspecified extremity**

  T87.41 **Infection of amputation stump, right upper extremity**

  T87.42 **Infection of amputation stump, left upper extremity**

  T87.43 **Infection of amputation stump, right lower extremity**

  T87.44 **Infection of amputation stump, left lower extremity**

● **T87.5** **Necrosis of amputation stump**

  T87.50 **Necrosis of amputation stump, unspecified extremity**

  T87.51 **Necrosis of amputation stump, right upper extremity**

  T87.52 **Necrosis of amputation stump, left upper extremity**

  T87.53 **Necrosis of amputation stump, right lower extremity**

  T87.54 **Necrosis of amputation stump, left lower extremity**

● **T87.8** **Other complications of amputation stump**

  T87.81 **Dehiscence of amputation stump**

  T87.89 **Other complications of amputation stump**
Amputation stump contracture
Amputation stump contracture of next proximal joint
Amputation stump flexion
Amputation stump edema
Amputation stump hematoma

    Excludes2 phantom limb syndrome (G54.6-G54.7)

● **T87.9** **Unspecified complications of amputation stump**

● **T88** **Other complications of surgical and medical care, not elsewhere classified**

  Excludes2 complication following infusion, transfusion and therapeutic injection (T80.-)
complication following procedure NEC (T81.-)
complications of anesthesia in labor and delivery (O74.-)
complications of anesthesia in pregnancy (O29.-)
complications of anesthesia in puerperium (O89.-)
complications of devices, implants and grafts (T82-T85)
complications of obstetric surgery and procedure (O75.4)
dermatitis due to drugs and medicaments (L23.3, L24.4, L25.1, L27.0-L27.1)
poisoning and toxic effects of drugs and chemicals (T36-T65 with fifth or sixth character 1-4 or 6)
specified complications classified elsewhere

The appropriate 7th character is to be added to each code from category T88

A	initial encounter
D	subsequent encounter
S	sequela

X ● **T88.0** **Infection following immunization**
Sepsis following immunization

X ● **T88.1** **Other complications following immunization, not elsewhere classified**
Generalized vaccinia
Rash following immunization

  Excludes1 vaccinia not from vaccine (B08.011)

  Excludes2 anaphylactic shock due to serum (T80.5-)
other serum reactions (T80.6-)
postimmunization arthropathy (M02.2)
postimmunization encephalitis (G04.02)
postimmunization fever (R50.83)

X ● **T88.2** **Shock due to anesthesia**
Use additional code for adverse effect, if applicable, to identify drug (T41.- with fifth or sixth character 5)

  Excludes1 complications of anesthesia (in):
labor and delivery (O74.-)
pregnancy (O29.-)
puerperium (O89.-)
postprocedural shock NOS (T81.1-)

CHAPTER 19 (S00-T88)

X● **T88.3** **Malignant hyperthermia due to anesthesia**

> Use additional code for adverse effect, if applicable, to identify drug (T41.- with fifth or sixth character 5)

X● **T88.4** **Failed or difficult intubation**

X● **T88.5** **Other complications of anesthesia**

> Use additional code for adverse effect, if applicable, to identify drug (T41.- with fifth or sixth character 5)

X● **T88.51** **Hypothermia following anesthesia**

X● **T88.52** **Failed moderate sedation during procedure**

> Failed conscious sedation during procedure

> **Excludes2**　personal history of failed moderate sedation (Z92.83)

X● **T88.53** **Unintended awareness under general anesthesia during procedure** ◀

> **Excludes2**　personal history of unintended awareness under general anesthesia (Z92.84) ◀

X● **T88.59** **Other complications of anesthesia**

X● **T88.6** **Anaphylactic reaction due to adverse effect of correct drug or medicament properly administered**

> Anaphylactic shock due to adverse effect of correct drug or medicament properly administered
> Anaphylactoid reaction NOS

> Use additional code for adverse effect, if applicable, to identify drug (T36-T50 with fifth or sixth character 5)

> **Excludes1**　anaphylactic reaction due to serum (T80.5-)
> anaphylactic shock or reaction due to adverse food reaction (T78.0-)

X● **T88.7** **Unspecified adverse effect of drug or medicament**

> Drug hypersensitivity NOS
> Drug reaction NOS

> Use additional code for adverse effect, if applicable, to identify drug (T36-T50 with fifth or sixth character 5)

> **Excludes1**　specified adverse effects of drugs and medicaments (A00-R94 and T80-T88.6, T88.8)

X● **T88.8** **Other specified complications of surgical and medical care, not elsewhere classified**

> Use additional code to identify the complication

X● **T88.9** **Complication of surgical and medical care, unspecified**

CHAPTER 19 (S00-T88)

CHAPTER 20

EXTERNAL CAUSES OF MORBIDITY
(V00-Y99)

OGCR Chapter-Specific Coding Guidelines

20. Chapter 20: External Causes of Morbidity (V00-Y99)
The external causes of morbidity codes should never be sequenced as the first-listed or principal diagnosis.

External cause codes are intended to provide data for injury research and evaluation of injury prevention strategies. These codes capture how the injury or health condition happened (cause), the intent (unintentional or accidental; or intentional, such as suicide or assault), the place where the event occurred the activity of the patient at the time of the event, and the person's status (e.g., civilian, military).

There is no national requirement for mandatory ICD-10-CM external cause code reporting. Unless a provider is subject to a state-based external cause code reporting mandate or these codes are required by a particular payer, reporting of ICD-10-CM codes in Chapter 20, External Causes of Morbidity, is not required. In the absence of a mandatory reporting requirement, providers are encouraged to voluntarily report external cause codes, as they provide valuable data for injury research and evaluation of injury prevention strategies.

a. General External Cause Coding Guidelines

1) Used with any code in the range of A00.0-T88.9, Z00-Z99
An external cause code may be used with any code in the range of A00.0-T88.9, Z00-Z99, classification that is a health condition due to an external cause. Though they are most applicable to injuries, they are also valid for use with such things as infections or diseases due to an external source, and other health conditions, such as a heart attack that occurs during strenuous physical activity.

2) External cause used for length of treatment
Assign the external cause code, with the appropriate 7th character (initial encounter, subsequent encounter or sequela) for each encounter for which the injury or condition is being treated.

Most categories in chapter 20 have a 7th character requirement for each applicable code. Most categories in this chapter have three 7th character values: A, initial encounter, D, subsequent encounter and S, sequela. While the patient may be seen by a new or different provider over the course of treatment for an injury or condition, assignment of the 7th character for external cause should match the 7th character of the code assigned for the associated injury or condition for the encounter.

3) Use the full range of external cause codes
Use the full range of external cause codes to completely describe the cause, the intent, the place of occurrence and if applicable, the activity of the patient at the time of the event, and the patient's status, for all injuries, and other health conditions due to an external cause.

4) Assign as many external cause codes as necessary
Assign as many external cause codes as necessary to fully explain each cause. If only one external code can be recorded, assign the code most related to the principal diagnosis.

5) The selection of the appropriate external cause code
The selection of the appropriate external cause code is guided by the Alphabetic Index of External Causes and by Inclusion and Exclusion notes in the Tabular List.

6) External cause code can never be a principal diagnosis
An external cause code can never be a principal (first-listed) diagnosis.

7) Combination external cause codes
Certain of the external cause codes are combination codes that identify sequential events that result in an injury, such as a fall which results in striking against an object. The injury may be due to either event or both. The combination external cause code used should correspond to the sequence of events regardless of which caused the most serious injury.

8) No external cause code needed in certain circumstances
No external cause code from Chapter 20 is needed if the external cause and intent are included in a code from another chapter (e.g. T36.0X1- Poisoning by penicillins, accidental (unintentional)).

b. Place of Occurrence Guideline
Codes from category Y92, Place of occurrence of the external cause, are secondary codes for use after other external cause codes to identify the location of the patient at the time of injury or other condition.

Generally, a place of occurrence code is **assigned** only once, at the initial encounter for treatment. **However, in the rare instance that a new injury occurs during hospitalization, an additional place of occurrence code may be assigned.** No 7th characters are used for Y92. Only one code from Y92 should be recorded on a medical record.

Do not use place of occurrence code Y92.9 if the place is not stated or is not applicable.

c. Activity Code
Assign a code from category Y93, Activity code, to describe the activity of the patient at the time the injury or other health condition occurred.

An activity code is used only once, at the initial encounter for treatment. Only one code from Y93 should be recorded on a medical record.

The activity codes are not applicable to poisonings, adverse effects, misadventures or sequela.

Do not assign Y93.9, Unspecified activity, if the activity is not stated.

A code from category Y93 is appropriate for use with external cause and intent codes if identifying the activity provides additional information about the event.

d. Place of Occurrence, Activity, and Status Codes Used with other External Cause Code
When applicable, place of occurrence, activity, and external cause status codes are sequenced after the main external cause code(s). Regardless of the number of external cause codes assigned, there should be only one place of occurrence code, one activity code, and one external cause status code assigned to an encounter.

e. If the Reporting Format Limits the Number of External Cause Codes

If the reporting format limits the number of external cause codes that can be used in reporting clinical data, report the code for the cause/intent most related to the principal diagnosis. If the format permits capture of additional external cause codes, the cause/intent, including medical misadventures, of the additional events should be reported rather than the codes for place, activity, or external status.

f. Multiple External Cause Coding Guidelines

More than one external cause code is required to fully describe the external cause of an illness or injury. The assignment of external cause codes should be sequenced in the following priority:

If two or more events cause separate injuries, an external cause code should be assigned for each cause. The first-listed external cause code will be selected in the following order:

External codes for child and adult abuse take priority over all other external cause codes.

See Section I.C.19., Child and Adult abuse guidelines.

External codes for terrorism events take priority over all other external cause codes except child and adult abuse.

External cause codes for cataclysmic events take priority over all other external cause codes except child and adult abuse and terrorism.

External cause codes for transport accidents take priority over all other external cause codes except cataclysmic events, child and adult abuse and terrorism.

Activity and external cause status codes are assigned following all causal (intent) external cause codes.

The first-listed external cause code should correspond to the cause of the most serious diagnosis due to an assault, accident, or self-harm, following the order of hierarchy listed above.

g. Child and Adult Abuse Guideline

Adult and child abuse, neglect and maltreatment are classified as assault. Any of the assault codes may be used to indicate the external cause of any injury resulting from the confirmed abuse.

For confirmed cases of abuse, neglect and maltreatment, when the perpetrator is known, a code from Y07, Perpetrator of maltreatment and neglect, should accompany any other assault codes.

See Section I.C.19. Adult and child abuse, neglect and other maltreatment

h. Unknown or Undetermined Intent Guideline

If the intent (accident, self-harm, assault) of the cause of an injury or other condition is unknown or unspecified, code the intent as accidental intent. All transport accident categories assume accidental intent.

1) Use of undetermined intent

External cause codes for events of undetermined intent are only for use if the documentation in the record specifies that the intent cannot be determined.

i. Sequelae (Late Effects) of External Cause Guidelines

1) Sequelae external cause codes

Sequela are reported using the external cause code with the 7th character "S" for sequela. These codes should be used with any report of a late effect or sequela resulting from a previous injury.

See Section I.B.10. Sequela, (Late Effects)

2) Sequela external cause code with a related current injury

A sequela external cause code should never be used with a related current nature of injury code.

3) Use of sequela external cause codes for subsequent visits

Use a late effect external cause code for subsequent visits when a late effect of the initial injury is being treated. Do not use a late effect external cause code for subsequent visits for follow-up care (e.g., to assess healing, to receive rehabilitative therapy) of the injury when no late effect of the injury has been documented.

j. Terrorism Guidelines

1) Cause of injury identified by the Federal Government (FBI) as terrorism

When the cause of an injury is identified by the Federal Government (FBI) as terrorism, the first-listed external cause code should be a code from category Y38, Terrorism. The definition of terrorism employed by the FBI is found at the inclusion note at the beginning of category Y38. Use additional code for place of occurrence (Y92.-). More than one Y38 code may be assigned if the injury is the result of more than one mechanism of terrorism.

2) Cause of an injury is suspected to be the result of terrorism

When the cause of an injury is suspected to be the result of terrorism a code from category Y38 should not be assigned. Suspected cases should be classified as assault.

3) Code Y38.9, Terrorism, secondary effects

Assign code Y38.9, Terrorism, secondary effects, for conditions occurring subsequent to the terrorist event. This code should not be assigned for conditions that are due to the initial terrorist act.

It is acceptable to assign code Y38.9 with another code from Y38 if there is an injury due to the initial terrorist event and an injury that is a subsequent result of the terrorist event.

k. External cause status

A code from category Y99, External cause status, should be assigned whenever any other external cause code is assigned for an encounter, including an Activity code, except for the events noted below. Assign a code from category Y99, External cause status, to indicate the work status of the person at the time the event occurred. The status code indicates whether the event occurred during military activity, whether a non-military person was at work, whether an individual including a student or volunteer was involved in a non-work activity at the time of the causal event.

A code from Y99, External cause status, should be assigned, when applicable, with other external cause codes, such as transport accidents and falls. The external cause status codes are not applicable to poisonings, adverse effects, misadventures or late effects.

Do not assign a code from category Y99 if no other external cause codes (cause, activity) are applicable for the encounter.

An external cause status code is used only once, at the initial encounter for treatment. Only one code from Y99 should be recorded on a medical record.

Do not assign code Y99.9, Unspecified external cause status, if the status is not stated.

CHAPTER 20

EXTERNAL CAUSES OF MORBIDITY (V00-Y99)

Note: This chapter permits the classification of environmental events and circumstances as the cause of injury, and other adverse effects. Where a code from this section is applicable, it is intended that it shall be used secondary to a code from another chapter of the Classification indicating the nature of the condition. Most often, the condition will be classifiable to Chapter 19, Injury, poisoning and certain other consequences of external causes (S00-T88). Other conditions that may be stated to be due to external causes are classified in Chapters I to XVIII. For these conditions, codes from Chapter 20 should be used to provide additional information as to the cause of the condition.

This chapter contains the following blocks:

V00-X58	Accidents
V00-V99	Transport accidents
V00-V09	Pedestrian injured in transport accident
V10-V19	Pedal cycle rider injured in transport accident
V20-V29	Motorcycle rider injured in transport accident
V30-V39	Occupant of three-wheeled motor vehicle injured in transport accident
V40-V49	Car occupant injured in transport accident
V50-V59	Occupant of pick-up truck or van injured in transport accident
V60-V69	Occupant of heavy transport vehicle injured in transport accident
V70-V79	Bus occupant injured in transport accident
V80-V89	Other land transport accidents
V90-V94	Water transport accidents
V95-V97	Air and space transport accidents
V98-V99	Other and unspecified transport accidents
W00-X58	Other external causes of accidental injury
W00-W19	Slipping, tripping, stumbling and falls
W20-W49	Exposure to inanimate mechanical forces
W50-W64	Exposure to animate mechanical forces
W65-W74	Accidental non-transport drowning and submersion
W85-W99	Exposure to electric current, radiation and extreme ambient air temperature and pressure
X00-X08	Exposure to smoke, fire and flames
X10-X19	Contact with heat and hot substances
X30-X39	Exposure to forces of nature
X50	Overexertion and strenuous or repetitive movements ◀
X52, X58	Accidental exposure to other specified factors
X71-X83	Intentional self-harm
X92-Y09 ◀	Assault
Y21-Y33	Event of undetermined intent
Y35-Y38	Legal intervention, operations of war, military operations, and terrorism
Y62-Y84	Complications of medical and surgical care
Y62-Y69	Misadventures to patients during surgical and medical care
Y70-Y82	Medical devices associated with adverse incidents in diagnostic and therapeutic use
Y83-Y84	Surgical and other medical procedures as the cause of abnormal reaction of the patient, or of later complication, without mention of misadventure at the time of the procedure
Y90-Y99	Supplementary factors related to causes of morbidity classified elsewhere

ACCIDENTS (V00-X58)

TRANSPORT ACCIDENTS (V00-V99)

Note: This section is structured in 12 groups. Those relating to land transport accidents (V00-V89) reflect the victim's mode of transport and are subdivided to identify the victim's 'counterpart' or the type of event. The vehicle of which the injured person is an occupant is identified in the first two characters since it is seen as the most important factor to identify for prevention purposes. A transport accident is one in which the vehicle involved must be moving or running or in use for transport purposes at the time of the accident. ◀

Use additional code to identify:
Airbag injury (W22.1)
Type of street or road (Y92.4-)
Use of cellular telephone and other electronic equipment at the time of the transport accident (Y93.C-)

Excludes1 agricultural vehicles in stationary use or maintenance (W31.-)
assault by crashing of motor vehicle (Y03.-)
automobile or motor cycle in stationary use or maintenance - code to type of accident
crashing of motor vehicle, undetermined intent (Y32)
intentional self-harm by crashing of motor vehicle (X82)

Excludes2 transport accidents due to cataclysm (X34-X38)

Note: Definitions related to transport accidents: ◀

(a) A transport accident (V00-V99) is any accident involving a device designed primarily for, or used at the time primarily for, conveying persons or good from one place to another. ◀

(b) A public highway [trafficway] or street is the entire width between property lines (or other boundary lines) of land open to the public as a matter of right or custom for purposes of moving persons or property from one place to another. A roadway is that part of the public highway designed, improved and customarily used for vehicular traffic.

(c) A traffic accident is any vehicle accident occurring on the public highway [i.e., originating on, terminating on, or involving a vehicle partially on the highway]. A vehicle accident is assumed to have occurred on the public highway unless another place is specified, except in the case of accidents involving only off-road motor vehicles, which are classified as nontraffic accidents unless the contrary is stated.

(d) A nontraffic accident is any vehicle accident that occurs entirely in any place other than a public highway.

(e) A pedestrian is any person involved in an accident who was not at the time of the accident riding in or on a motor vehicle, railway train, streetcar or animal-drawn or other vehicle, or on a pedal cycle or animal. This includes, a person changing a tire, working on a parked car, or a person on foot. It also includes the user of a pedestrian conveyance such as a baby-stroller, ice-skates, skis, sled, roller skates, a skateboard, nonmotorized or motorized wheelchair, motorized mobility scooter, or nonmotorized scooter. ◀

(f) A driver is an occupant of a transport vehicle who is operating or intending to operate it.

(g) A passenger is any occupant of a transport vehicle other than the driver, except a person traveling on the outside of the vehicle.

(h) A person on the outside of a vehicle is any person being transported by a vehicle but not occupying the space normally reserved for the driver or passengers, or the space intended for the transport of property. This includes a person travelling on the bodywork, bumper, fender, roof, running board or step of a vehicle, as well as, hanging on the outside of the vehicle. ◀

(i) A pedal cycle is any land transport vehicle operated solely by nonmotorized pedals including a bicycle or tricycle.

(j) A pedal cyclist is any person riding a pedal cycle or in a sidecar or trailer attached to a pedal cycle.

CHAPTER 20 (V01-Y99)

(k) A motorcycle is a two-wheeled motor vehicle with one or two riding saddles and sometimes with a third wheel for the support of a sidecar. The sidecar is considered part of the motorcycle. This includes a moped, motor scooter, or motorized bicycle. ◄▥

(l) A motorcycle rider is any person riding a motorcycle or in a sidecar or trailer attached to the motorcycle.

(m) A three-wheeled motor vehicle is a motorized tricycle designed primarily for on-road use. This includes a motor-driven tricycle, a motorized rickshaw, or a three-wheeled motor car.

(n) A car [automobile] is a four-wheeled motor vehicle designed primarily for carrying up to 7 persons. A trailer being towed by the car is considered part of the car. It does not include a van or minivan—see definition (o) ◄▥

(o) A pick-up truck or van is a four or six-wheeled motor vehicle designed for carrying passengers as well as property or cargo weighing less than the local limit for classification as a heavy goods vehicle, and not requiring a special driver's license. This includes a minivan and a sport-utility vehicle (SUV).

(p) A heavy transport vehicle is a motor vehicle designed primarily for carrying property, meeting local criteria for classification as a heavy goods vehicle in terms of weight and requiring a special driver's license.

(q) A bus (coach) is a motor vehicle designed or adapted primarily for carrying more than 10 passengers, and requiring a special driver's license.

(r) A railway train or railway vehicle is any device, with or without freight or passenger cars coupled to it, designed for traffic on a railway track. This includes subterranean (subways) or elevated trains.

(s) A streetcar is a device designed and used primarily for transporting passengers within a municipality, running on rails, usually subject to normal traffic control signals, and operated principally on a right-of-way that forms part of the roadway. This includes a tram or trolley that runs on rails. A trailer being towed by a streetcar is considered part of the streetcar.

(t) A special vehicle mainly used on industrial premises is a motor vehicle designed primarily for use within the buildings and premises of industrial or commercial establishments. This includes battery-powered airport passenger vehicles or baggage/mail trucks, forklifts, coal-cars in a coal mine, logging cars and trucks used in mines or quarries. ◄▥

(u) A special vehicle mainly used in agriculture is a motor vehicle designed specifically for use in farming and agriculture (horticulture), to work the land, tend and harvest crops and transport materials on the farm. This includes harvesters, farm machinery and tractor and trailers.

(v) A special construction vehicle is a motor vehicle designed specifically for use on construction and demolition sites. This includes bulldozers, diggers, earth levellers, dump trucks, backhoes, front-end loaders, pavers, and mechanical shovels.

(w) A special all-terrain vehicle is a motor vehicle of special design to enable it to negotiate over rough or soft terrain, snow or sand. Examples of special design are high construction, special wheels and tires, tracks, and support on a cushion of air. This includes snow mobiles, all-terrain vehicles (ATV), and dune buggies. It does not include passenger vehicle designated as sport utility vehicles (SUV). ◄▥

(x) A watercraft is any device designed for transporting passengers or goods on water. This includes motor or sail boats, ships, and hovercraft.

(y) An aircraft is any device for transporting passengers or goods in the air. This includes hot-air balloons, gliders, helicopters and airplanes.

(z) A military vehicle is any motorized vehicle operating on a public roadway owned by the military and being operated by a member of the military.

PEDESTRIAN INJURED IN TRANSPORT ACCIDENT (V00-V09)

Includes   person changing tire on transport vehicle
person examining engine of vehicle broken down in (on side of) road

Excludes1   fall due to non-transport collision with other person (W03)
pedestrian on foot falling (slipping) on ice and snow (W00.-)
struck or bumped by another person (W51)

● **V00   Pedestrian conveyance accident**

Use additional place of occurrence and activity external cause codes, if known (Y92.-, Y93.-)

Excludes1   collision with another person without fall (W51)
fall due to person on foot colliding with another person on foot (W03)
fall from non-moving wheelchair, nonmotorized scooter and motorized mobility scooter without collision (W05.-)
pedestrian (conveyance) collision with other land transport vehicle (V01-V09)
pedestrian on foot falling (slipping) on ice and snow (W00.-)

The appropriate 7th character is to be added to each code from category V00

A	initial encounter
D	subsequent encounter
S	sequela

● **V00.0   Pedestrian on foot injured in collision with pedestrian conveyance**

X ● **V00.01   Pedestrian on foot injured in collision with roller-skater**

X ● **V00.02   Pedestrian on foot injured in collision with skateboarder**

X ● **V00.09   Pedestrian on foot injured in collision with other pedestrian conveyance**

● **V00.1   Rolling-type pedestrian conveyance accident**

Excludes1   accident with babystroller (V00.82-)
accident with wheelchair (powered) (V00.81-)
accident with motorized mobility scooter (V00.83-)

● **V00.11   In-line roller-skate accident**

● **V00.111   Fall from in-line roller-skates**

● **V00.112   In-line roller-skater colliding with stationary object**

● **V00.118   Other in-line roller-skate accident**

Excludes1   roller-skater collision with other land transport vehicle (V01-V09 with 5th character 1)

● **V00.12   Non-in-line roller-skate accident**

● **V00.121   Fall from non-in-line roller-skates**

● **V00.122   Non-in-line roller-skater colliding with stationary object**

● **V00.128   Other non-in-line roller-skating accident**

Excludes1   roller-skater collision with other land transport vehicle (V01-V09 with 5th character 1)

◄ New   ◄▥ Revised   ~~deleted~~ Deleted   Excludes 1   Excludes 2   Includes   Use additional   Code first   Code also   Unspecified

OGCR Official Guidelines   X Assign placeholder X   ● Use Additional Character(s)   ▌ Manifestation Code   **Coding Clinic**

●**V00.13**   **Skateboard accident**
- ●**V00.131**   **Fall from skateboard**
- ●**V00.132**   **Skateboarder colliding with stationary object**
- ●**V00.138**   **Other skateboard accident**
  - **Excludes1**   skateboarder collision with other land transport vehicle (V01-V09 with 5th character 2)

●**V00.14**   **Scooter (nonmotorized) accident**
- **Excludes1**   motorscooter accident (V20-V29)
- ●**V00.141**   **Fall from scooter (nonmotorized)**
- ●**V00.142**   **Scooter (nonmotorized) colliding with stationary object**
- ●**V00.148**   **Other scooter (nonmotorized) accident**
  - **Excludes1**   scooter (non-motorized) collision with other land transport vehicle (V01-V09 with fifth character 9)

●**V00.15**   **Heelies accident**
Rolling shoe
Wheeled shoe
Wheelies accident
- ●**V00.151**   **Fall from heelies**
- ●**V00.152**   **Heelies colliding with stationary object**
- ●**V00.158**   **Other heelies accident**

●**V00.18**   **Accident on other rolling-type pedestrian conveyance**
- ●**V00.181**   **Fall from other rolling-type pedestrian conveyance**
- ●**V00.182**   **Pedestrian on other rolling-type pedestrian conveyance colliding with stationary object**
- ●**V00.188**   **Other accident on other rolling-type pedestrian conveyance**

●**V00.2**   **Gliding-type pedestrian conveyance accident**
- ●**V00.21**   **Ice-skates accident**
  - ●**V00.211**   **Fall from ice-skates**
  - ●**V00.212**   **Ice-skater colliding with stationary object**
  - ●**V00.218**   **Other ice-skates accident**
    - **Excludes1**   ice-skater collision with other land transport vehicle (V01-V09 with 5th digit 9)
- ●**V00.22**   **Sled accident**
  - ●**V00.221**   **Fall from sled**
  - ●**V00.222**   **Sledder colliding with stationary object**
  - ●**V00.228**   **Other sled accident**
    - **Excludes1**   sled collision with other land transport vehicle (V01-V09 with 5th digit 9)

●**V00.28**   **Other gliding-type pedestrian conveyance accident**
- ●**V00.281**   **Fall from other gliding-type pedestrian conveyance**
- ●**V00.282**   **Pedestrian on other gliding-type pedestrian conveyance colliding with stationary object**
- ●**V00.288**   **Other accident on other gliding-type pedestrian conveyance**
  - **Excludes1**   gliding-type pedestrian conveyance collision with other land transport vehicle (V01-V09 with 5th digit 9)

●**V00.3**   **Flat-bottomed pedestrian conveyance accident**
- ●**V00.31**   **Snowboard accident**
  - ●**V00.311**   **Fall from snowboard**
  - ●**V00.312**   **Snowboarder colliding with stationary object**
  - ●**V00.318**   **Other snowboard accident**
    - **Excludes1**   snowboarder collision with other land transport vehicle (V01-V09 with 5th digit 9)
- ●**V00.32**   **Snow-ski accident**
  - ●**V00.321**   **Fall from snow-skis**
    - Coding Clinic: 2015, Q1, P12
  - ●**V00.322**   **Snow-skier colliding with stationary object**
  - ●**V00.328**   **Other snow-ski accident**
    - **Excludes1**   snow-skier collision with other land transport vehicle (V01-V09 with 5th digit 9)
- ●**V00.38**   **Other flat-bottomed pedestrian conveyance accident**
  - ●**V00.381**   **Fall from other flat-bottomed pedestrian conveyance**
  - ●**V00.382**   **Pedestrian on other flat-bottomed pedestrian conveyance colliding with stationary object**
  - ●**V00.388**   **Other accident on other flat-bottomed pedestrian conveyance**

●**V00.8**   **Accident on other pedestrian conveyance**
- ●**V00.81**   **Accident with wheelchair (powered)**
  - ●**V00.811**   **Fall from moving wheelchair (powered)**
    - **Excludes1**   fall from non-moving wheelchair (W05.0)
  - ●**V00.812**   **Wheelchair (powered) colliding with stationary object**
  - ●**V00.818**   **Other accident with wheelchair (powered)**
- ●**V00.82**   **Accident with babystroller**
  - ●**V00.821**   **Fall from babystroller**
  - ●**V00.822**   **Babystroller colliding with stationary object**
  - ●**V00.828**   **Other accident with babystroller**

● V00.83 **Accident with motorized mobility scooter**

   ● V00.831 **Fall from motorized mobility scooter**

      Excludes1   fall from non-moving motorized mobility scooter (W05.2)

   ● V00.832 **Motorized mobility scooter colliding with stationary object**

   ● V00.838 **Other accident with motorized mobility scooter**

● V00.89 **Accident on other pedestrian conveyance**

   ● V00.891 **Fall from other pedestrian conveyance**

   ● V00.892 **Pedestrian on other pedestrian conveyance colliding with stationary object**

   ● V00.898 **Other accident on other pedestrian conveyance**

      Excludes1   other pedestrian (conveyance) collision with other land transport vehicle (V01-V09 with 5th digit 9)

● V01 **Pedestrian injured in collision with pedal cycle**

The appropriate 7th character is to be added to each code from category V01

A	initial encounter
D	subsequent encounter
S	sequela

● V01.0 **Pedestrian injured in collision with pedal cycle in nontraffic accident**

X ● V01.00 **Pedestrian on foot injured in collision with pedal cycle in nontraffic accident**
Pedestrian NOS injured in collision with pedal cycle in nontraffic accident

X ● V01.01 **Pedestrian on roller-skates injured in collision with pedal cycle in nontraffic accident**

X ● V01.02 **Pedestrian on skateboard injured in collision with pedal cycle in nontraffic accident**

X ● V01.09 **Pedestrian with other conveyance injured in collision with pedal cycle in nontraffic accident**
Pedestrian with babystroller injured in collision with pedal cycle in nontraffic accident
Pedestrian in wheelchair (powered) injured in collision with pedal cycle in nontraffic accident
Pedestrian in motorized mobility scooter injured in collision with pedal cycle in nontraffic accident
Pedestrian on ice-skates injured in collision with pedal cycle in nontraffic accident
Pedestrian on nonmotorized scooter injured in collision with pedal cycle in nontraffic accident
Pedestrian on sled injured in collision with pedal cycle in nontraffic accident
Pedestrian on snowboard injured in collision with pedal cycle in nontraffic accident
Pedestrian on snow-skis injured in collision with pedal cycle in nontraffic accident

● V01.1 **Pedestrian injured in collision with pedal cycle in traffic accident**

X ● V01.10 **Pedestrian on foot injured in collision with pedal cycle in traffic accident**
Pedestrian NOS injured in collision with pedal cycle in traffic accident

X ● V01.11 **Pedestrian on roller-skates injured in collision with pedal cycle in traffic accident**

X ● V01.12 **Pedestrian on skateboard injured in collision with pedal cycle in traffic accident**

X ● V01.19 **Pedestrian with other conveyance injured in collision with pedal cycle in traffic accident**
Pedestrian with babystroller injured in collision with pedal cycle in traffic accident
Pedestrian in wheelchair (powered) injured in collision with pedal cycle in traffic accident
Pedestrian in motorized mobility scooter injured in collision with pedal cycle in traffic accident
Pedestrian on ice-skates injured in collision with pedal cycle in traffic accident
Pedestrian on nonmotorized scooter injured in collision with pedal cycle in traffic accident
Pedestrian on sled injured in collision with pedal cycle in traffic accident
Pedestrian on snowboard injured in collision with pedal cycle in traffic accident
Pedestrian on snow-skis injured in collision with pedal cycle in traffic accident

● V01.9 **Pedestrian injured in collision with pedal cycle, unspecified whether traffic or nontraffic accident**

X ● V01.90 **Pedestrian on foot injured in collision with pedal cycle, unspecified whether traffic or nontraffic accident**
Pedestrian NOS injured in collision with pedal cycle, unspecified whether traffic or nontraffic accident

X ● V01.91 **Pedestrian on roller-skates injured in collision with pedal cycle, unspecified whether traffic or nontraffic accident**

X ● V01.92 **Pedestrian on skateboard injured in collision with pedal cycle, unspecified whether traffic or nontraffic accident**

X ● V01.99 **Pedestrian with other conveyance injured in collision with pedal cycle, unspecified whether traffic or nontraffic accident**
Pedestrian with babystroller injured in collision with pedal cycle, unspecified whether traffic or nontraffic accident
Pedestrian in wheelchair (powered) injured in collision with pedal cycle, unspecified whether traffic or nontraffic accident
Pedestrian in motorized mobility scooter injured in collision with pedal cycle, unspecified whether traffic or nontraffic accident
Pedestrian on ice-skates injured in collision with pedal cycle unspecified, whether traffic or nontraffic accident
Pedestrian on nonmotorized scooter injured in collision with pedal cycle, unspecified whether traffic or nontraffic accident
Pedestrian on sled injured in collision with pedal cycle unspecified, whether traffic or nontraffic accident
Pedestrian on snowboard injured in collision with pedal cycle, unspecified whether traffic or nontraffic accident
Pedestrian on snow-skis injured in collision with pedal cycle, unspecified whether traffic or nontraffic accident

◀ New   ◀▦ Revised   ~~deleted~~ Deleted   Excludes 1   Excludes 2   Includes   Use additional   Code first   Code also   Unspecified

OGCR Official Guidelines   X Assign placeholder X   ● Use Additional Character(s)   ▶ Manifestation Code   **Coding Clinic**

● **V02**   **Pedestrian injured in collision with two- or three-wheeled motor vehicle**

The appropriate 7th character is to be added to each code from category V02

A	initial encounter
D	subsequent encounter
S	sequela

● **V02.0**   **Pedestrian injured in collision with two- or three-wheeled motor vehicle in nontraffic accident**

X ● **V02.00**   **Pedestrian on foot injured in collision with two- or three-wheeled motor vehicle in nontraffic accident**

Pedestrian NOS injured in collision with two- or three-wheeled motor vehicle in nontraffic accident

X ● **V02.01**   **Pedestrian on roller-skates injured in collision with two- or three-wheeled motor vehicle in nontraffic accident**

X ● **V02.02**   **Pedestrian on skateboard injured in collision with two- or three-wheeled motor vehicle in nontraffic accident**

X ● **V02.09**   **Pedestrian with other conveyance injured in collision with two- or three-wheeled motor vehicle in nontraffic accident**

Pedestrian with babystroller injured in collision with two- or three-wheeled motor vehicle in nontraffic accident

Pedestrian on ice-skates injured in collision with two- or three-wheeled motor vehicle in nontraffic accident

Pedestrian in wheelchair (powered) injured in collision with two- or three-wheeled motor vehicle in nontraffic accident

Pedestrian in motorized mobility scooter injured in collision with two- or three-wheeled motor vehicle in nontraffic accident

Pedestrian on nonmotorized scooter injured in collision with two- or three-wheeled motor vehicle in nontraffic accident

Pedestrian on sled injured in collision with two- or three-wheeled motor vehicle in nontraffic accident

Pedestrian on snowboard injured in collision with two- or three-wheeled motor vehicle in nontraffic accident

Pedestrian on snow-skis injured in collision with two- or three-wheeled motor vehicle in nontraffic accident

● **V02.1**   **Pedestrian injured in collision with two- or three-wheeled motor vehicle in traffic accident**

X ● **V02.10**   **Pedestrian on foot injured in collision with two- or three-wheeled motor vehicle in traffic accident**

Pedestrian NOS injured in collision with two- or three-wheeled motor vehicle in traffic accident

X ● **V02.11**   **Pedestrian on roller-skates injured in collision with two- or three-wheeled motor vehicle in traffic accident**

X ● **V02.12**   **Pedestrian on skateboard injured in collision with two- or three-wheeled motor vehicle in traffic accident**

X ● **V02.19**   **Pedestrian with other conveyance injured in collision with two- or three-wheeled motor vehicle in traffic accident**

Pedestrian with babystroller injured in collision with two- or three-wheeled motor vehicle in traffic accident

Pedestrian in wheelchair (powered) injured in collision with two- or three-wheeled motor vehicle in traffic accident

Pedestrian in motorized mobility scooter injured in collision with two- or three-wheeled motor vehicle in traffic accident

Pedestrian on ice-skates injured in collision with two- or three-wheeled motor vehicle in traffic accident

Pedestrian on nonmotorized scooter injured in collision with two- or three-wheeled motor vehicle in traffic accident

Pedestrian on sled injured in collision with two- or three-wheeled motor vehicle in traffic accident

Pedestrian on snowboard injured in collision with two- or three-wheeled motor vehicle in traffic accident

Pedestrian on snow-skis injured in collision with two- or three-wheeled motor vehicle in traffic accident

● **V02.9**   **Pedestrian injured in collision with two- or three-wheeled motor vehicle, unspecified whether traffic or nontraffic accident**

X ● **V02.90**   **Pedestrian on foot injured in collision with two- or three-wheeled motor vehicle, unspecified whether traffic or nontraffic accident**

Pedestrian NOS injured in collision with two- or three-wheeled motor vehicle, unspecified whether traffic or nontraffic accident

X ● **V02.91**   **Pedestrian on roller-skates injured in collision with two- or three-wheeled motor vehicle, unspecified whether traffic or nontraffic accident**

X ● **V02.92**   **Pedestrian on skateboard injured in collision with two- or three-wheeled motor vehicle, unspecified whether traffic or nontraffic accident**

X ● **V02.99** **Pedestrian with other conveyance injured in collision with two- or three-wheeled motor vehicle, unspecified whether traffic or nontraffic accident**

Pedestrian with babystroller injured in collision with two- or three-wheeled motor vehicle, unspecified whether traffic or nontraffic accident

Pedestrian in wheelchair (powered) injured in collision with two- or three-wheeled motor vehicle, unspecified whether traffic or nontraffic accident

Pedestrian in motorized mobility scooter injured in collision with two- or three-wheeled motor vehicle, unspecified whether traffic or nontraffic accident

Pedestrian on ice-skates injured in collision with two- or three-wheeled motor vehicle, unspecified whether traffic or nontraffic accident

Pedestrian on nonmotorized scooter injured in collision with two- or three-wheeled motor vehicle, unspecified whether traffic or nontraffic accident

Pedestrian on sled injured in collision with two- or three-wheeled motor vehicle, unspecified whether traffic or nontraffic accident

Pedestrian on snowboard injured in collision with two- or three-wheeled motor vehicle, unspecified whether traffic or nontraffic accident

Pedestrian on snow-skis injured in collision with two- or three-wheeled motor vehicle, unspecified whether traffic or nontraffic accident

● **V03** **Pedestrian injured in collision with car, pick-up truck or van**

The appropriate 7th character is to be added to each code from category V03

A	initial encounter
D	subsequent encounter
S	sequela

● **V03.0** **Pedestrian injured in collision with car, pick-up truck or van in nontraffic accident**

X ● **V03.00** **Pedestrian on foot injured in collision with car, pick-up truck or van in nontraffic accident**

Pedestrian NOS injured in collision with car, pick-up truck or van in nontraffic accident

X ● **V03.01** **Pedestrian on roller-skates injured in collision with car, pick-up truck or van in nontraffic accident**

X ● **V03.02** **Pedestrian on skateboard injured in collision with car, pick-up truck or van in nontraffic accident**

X ● **V03.09** **Pedestrian with other conveyance injured in collision with car, pick-up truck or van in nontraffic accident**

Pedestrian with babystroller injured in collision with car, pick-up truck or van in nontraffic accident

Pedestrian in wheelchair (powered) injured in collision with car, pick-up truck or van in nontraffic accident

Pedestrian in motorized mobility scooter injured in collision with car, pick-up truck or van in nontraffic accident

Pedestrian on ice-skates injured in collision with car, pick-up truck or van in nontraffic accident

Pedestrian on nonmotorized scooter injured in collision with car, pick-up truck or van in nontraffic accident

Pedestrian on sled injured in collision with car, pick-up truck or van in nontraffic accident

Pedestrian on snowboard injured in collision with car, pick-up truck or van in nontraffic accident

Pedestrian on snow-skis injured in collision with car, pick-up truck or van in nontraffic accident

● **V03.1** **Pedestrian injured in collision with car, pick-up truck or van in traffic accident**

X ● **V03.10** **Pedestrian on foot injured in collision with car, pick-up truck or van in traffic accident**

Pedestrian NOS injured in collision with car, pick-up truck or van in traffic accident

X ● **V03.11** **Pedestrian on roller-skates injured in collision with car, pick-up truck or van in traffic accident**

X ● **V03.12** **Pedestrian on skateboard injured in collision with car, pick-up truck or van in traffic accident**

X ● **V03.19** **Pedestrian with other conveyance injured in collision with car, pick-up truck or van in traffic accident**

Pedestrian with babystroller injured in collision with car, pick-up truck or van in traffic accident

Pedestrian in wheelchair (powered) injured in collision with car, pick-up truck or van in traffic accident

Pedestrian in motorized mobility scooter injured in collision with car, pick-up truck or van in traffic accident

Pedestrian on ice-skates injured in collision with car, pick-up truck or van in traffic accident

Pedestrian on nonmotorized scooter injured in collision with car, pick-up truck or van in traffic accident

Pedestrian on sled injured in collision with car, pick-up truck or van in traffic accident

Pedestrian on snowboard injured in collision with car, pick-up truck or van in traffic accident

Pedestrian on snow-skis injured in collision with car, pick-up truck or van in traffic accident

● **V03.9**   **Pedestrian injured in collision with car, pick-up truck or van, unspecified whether traffic or nontraffic accident**

    X ● **V03.90**   **Pedestrian on foot injured in collision with car, pick-up truck or van, unspecified whether traffic or nontraffic accident**

       Pedestrian NOS injured in collision with car, pick-up truck or van, unspecified whether traffic or nontraffic accident

    X ● **V03.91**   **Pedestrian on roller-skates injured in collision with car, pick-up truck or van, unspecified whether traffic or nontraffic accident**

    X ● **V03.92**   **Pedestrian on skateboard injured in collision with car, pick-up truck or van, unspecified whether traffic or nontraffic accident**

    X ● **V03.99**   **Pedestrian with other conveyance injured in collision with car, pick-up truck or van, unspecified whether traffic or nontraffic accident**

       Pedestrian with babystroller injured in collision with car, pick-up truck or van, unspecified whether traffic or nontraffic accident

       Pedestrian in wheelchair (powered) injured in collision with car, pick-up truck or van, unspecified whether traffic or nontraffic accident

       Pedestrian in motorized mobility scooter injured in collision with car, pick-up truck or van, unspecified whether traffic or nontraffic accident

       Pedestrian on ice-skates injured in collision with car, pick-up truck or van, unspecified whether traffic or nontraffic accident

       Pedestrian on nonmotorized scooter injured in collision with car, pick-up truck or van, unspecified whether traffic or nontraffic accident

       Pedestrian on sled injured in collision with car, pick-up truck or van in nontraffic accident

       Pedestrian on snowboard injured in collision with car, pick-up truck or van, unspecified whether traffic or nontraffic accident

       Pedestrian on snow-skis injured in collision with car, pick-up truck or van, unspecified whether traffic or nontraffic accident

● **V04**   **Pedestrian injured in collision with heavy transport vehicle or bus**

    Excludes1   pedestrian injured in collision with military vehicle (V09.01, V09.21)

    The appropriate 7th character is to be added to each code from category V04

      A   initial encounter
      D   subsequent encounter
      S   sequela

● **V04.0**   **Pedestrian injured in collision with heavy transport vehicle or bus in nontraffic accident**

    X ● **V04.00**   **Pedestrian on foot injured in collision with heavy transport vehicle or bus in nontraffic accident**

       Pedestrian NOS injured in collision with heavy transport vehicle or bus in nontraffic accident

    X ● **V04.01**   **Pedestrian on roller-skates injured in collision with heavy transport vehicle or bus in nontraffic accident**

    X ● **V04.02**   **Pedestrian on skateboard injured in collision with heavy transport vehicle or bus in nontraffic accident**

    X ● **V04.09**   **Pedestrian with other conveyance injured in collision with heavy transport vehicle or bus in nontraffic accident**

       Pedestrian with babystroller injured in collision with heavy transport vehicle or bus in nontraffic accident

       Pedestrian in wheelchair (powered) injured in collision with heavy transport vehicle or bus in nontraffic accident

       Pedestrian in motorized mobility scooter injured in collision with heavy transport vehicle or bus in nontraffic accident

       Pedestrian on ice-skates injured in collision with heavy transport vehicle or bus in nontraffic accident

       Pedestrian on nonmotorized scooter injured in collision with heavy transport vehicle or bus in nontraffic accident

       Pedestrian on sled injured in collision with heavy transport vehicle or bus in nontraffic accident

       Pedestrian on snowboard injured in collision with heavy transport vehicle or bus in nontraffic accident

       Pedestrian on snow-skis injured in collision with heavy transport vehicle or bus in nontraffic accident

● **V04.1**   **Pedestrian injured in collision with heavy transport vehicle or bus in traffic accident**

    X ● **V04.10**   **Pedestrian on foot injured in collision with heavy transport vehicle or bus in traffic accident**

       Pedestrian NOS injured in collision with heavy transport vehicle or bus in traffic accident

    X ● **V04.11**   **Pedestrian on roller-skates injured in collision with heavy transport vehicle or bus in traffic accident**

    X ● **V04.12**   **Pedestrian on skateboard injured in collision with heavy transport vehicle or bus in traffic accident**

    X ● **V04.19**   **Pedestrian with other conveyance injured in collision with heavy transport vehicle or bus in traffic accident**

       Pedestrian with babystroller injured in collision with heavy transport vehicle or bus in traffic accident

       Pedestrian in wheelchair (powered) injured in collision with heavy transport vehicle or bus in traffic accident

       Pedestrian in motorized mobility scooter injured in collision with heavy transport vehicle or bus in traffic accident

       Pedestrian on ice-skates injured in collision with heavy transport vehicle or bus in traffic accident

       Pedestrian on nonmotorized scooter injured in collision with heavy transport vehicle or bus in traffic accident

       Pedestrian on sled injured in collision with heavy transport vehicle or bus in traffic accident

       Pedestrian on snowboard injured in collision with heavy transport vehicle or bus in traffic accident

       Pedestrian on snow-skis injured in collision with heavy transport vehicle or bus in traffic accident

CHAPTER 20 (V01-Y99)

● **V04.9 Pedestrian injured in collision with heavy transport vehicle or bus, unspecified whether traffic or nontraffic accident**

X ● V04.90 **Pedestrian on foot injured in collision with heavy transport vehicle or bus, unspecified whether traffic or nontraffic accident**
Pedestrian NOS injured in collision with heavy transport vehicle or bus, unspecified whether traffic or nontraffic accident

X ● V04.91 **Pedestrian on roller-skates injured in collision with heavy transport vehicle or bus, unspecified whether traffic or nontraffic accident**

X ● V04.92 **Pedestrian on skateboard injured in collision with heavy transport vehicle or bus, unspecified whether traffic or nontraffic accident**

X ● V04.99 **Pedestrian with other conveyance injured in collision with heavy transport vehicle or bus, unspecified whether traffic or nontraffic accident**
Pedestrian with babystroller injured in collision with heavy transport vehicle or bus, unspecified whether traffic or nontraffic accident
Pedestrian in wheelchair (powered) injured in collision with heavy transport vehicle or bus, unspecified whether traffic or nontraffic accident
Pedestrian in motorized mobility scooter injured in collision with heavy transport vehicle or bus, unspecified whether traffic or nontraffic accident
Pedestrian on ice-skates injured in collision with heavy transport vehicle or bus, unspecified whether traffic or nontraffic accident
Pedestrian on nonmotorized scooter injured in collision with heavy transport vehicle or bus, unspecified whether traffic or nontraffic accident
Pedestrian on sled injured in collision with heavy transport vehicle or bus, unspecified whether traffic or nontraffic accident
Pedestrian on snowboard injured in collision with heavy transport vehicle or bus, unspecified whether traffic or nontraffic accident
Pedestrian on snow-skis injured in collision with heavy transport vehicle or bus, unspecified whether traffic or nontraffic accident

● **V05 Pedestrian injured in collision with railway train or railway vehicle**

The appropriate 7th character is to be added to each code from category V05

> A   initial encounter
> D   subsequent encounter
> S   sequela

● **V05.0 Pedestrian injured in collision with railway train or railway vehicle in nontraffic accident**

X ● V05.00 **Pedestrian on foot injured in collision with railway train or railway vehicle in nontraffic accident**
Pedestrian NOS injured in collision with railway train or railway vehicle in nontraffic accident

X ● V05.01 **Pedestrian on roller-skates injured in collision with railway train or railway vehicle in nontraffic accident**

X ● V05.02 **Pedestrian on skateboard injured in collision with railway train or railway vehicle in nontraffic accident**

X ● V05.09 **Pedestrian with other conveyance injured in collision with railway train or railway vehicle in nontraffic accident**
Pedestrian with babystroller injured in collision with railway train or railway vehicle in nontraffic accident
Pedestrian in wheelchair (powered) injured in collision with railway train or railway vehicle in nontraffic accident
Pedestrian in motorized mobility scooter injured in collision with railway train or railway vehicle in nontraffic accident
Pedestrian on ice-skates injured in collision with railway train or railway vehicle in nontraffic accident
Pedestrian on nonmotorized scooter injured in collision with railway train or railway vehicle in nontraffic accident
Pedestrian on sled injured in collision with railway train or railway vehicle in nontraffic accident
Pedestrian on snowboard injured in collision with railway train or railway vehicle in nontraffic accident
Pedestrian on snow-skis injured in collision with railway train or railway vehicle in nontraffic accident

● **V05.1 Pedestrian injured in collision with railway train or railway vehicle in traffic accident**

X ● V05.10 **Pedestrian on foot injured in collision with railway train or railway vehicle in traffic accident**
Pedestrian NOS injured in collision with railway train or railway vehicle in traffic accident

X ● V05.11 **Pedestrian on roller-skates injured in collision with railway train or railway vehicle in traffic accident**

X ● V05.12 **Pedestrian on skateboard injured in collision with railway train or railway vehicle in traffic accident**

X ● V05.19 **Pedestrian with other conveyance injured in collision with railway train or railway vehicle in traffic accident**
Pedestrian with babystroller injured in collision with railway train or railway vehicle in traffic accident
Pedestrian in wheelchair (powered) injured in collision with railway train or railway vehicle in traffic accident
Pedestrian in motorized mobility scooter injured in collision with railway train or railway vehicle in traffic accident
Pedestrian on ice-skates injured in collision with railway train or railway vehicle in traffic accident
Pedestrian on nonmotorized scooter injured in collision with railway train or railway vehicle in traffic accident
Pedestrian on sled injured in collision with railway train or railway vehicle in traffic accident
Pedestrian on snowboard injured in collision with railway train or railway vehicle in traffic accident
Pedestrian on snow-skis injured in collision with railway train or railway vehicle in traffic accident

◄ New   ◄⊪ Revised   ~~deleted~~ Deleted   Excludes 1   Excludes 2   Includes   Use additional   Code first   Code also   Unspecified

1436   OGCR Official Guidelines   X Assign placeholder X   ● Use Additional Character(s)   ▶ Manifestation Code   **Coding Clinic**

● **V05.9** **Pedestrian injured in collision with railway train or railway vehicle, unspecified whether traffic or nontraffic accident**

X ● **V05.90** **Pedestrian on foot injured in collision with railway train or railway vehicle, unspecified whether traffic or nontraffic accident**
    Pedestrian NOS injured in collision with railway train or railway vehicle, unspecified whether traffic or nontraffic accident

X ● **V05.91** **Pedestrian on roller-skates injured in collision with railway train or railway vehicle, unspecified whether traffic or nontraffic accident**

X ● **V05.92** **Pedestrian on skateboard injured in collision with railway train or railway vehicle, unspecified whether traffic or nontraffic accident**

X ● **V05.99** **Pedestrian with other conveyance injured in collision with railway train or railway vehicle, unspecified whether traffic or nontraffic accident**
    Pedestrian with babystroller injured in collision with railway train or railway vehicle, unspecified whether traffic or nontraffic
    Pedestrian in wheelchair (powered) injured in collision with railway train or railway vehicle, unspecified whether traffic or nontraffic
    Pedestrian in motorized mobility scooter injured in collision with railway train or railway vehicle, unspecified whether traffic or nontraffic
    Pedestrian on ice-skates injured in collision with railway train or railway vehicle, unspecified whether traffic or nontraffic
    Pedestrian on nonmotorized scooter injured in collision with railway train or railway vehicle, unspecified whether traffic or nontraffic
    Pedestrian on sled injured in collision with railway train or railway vehicle, unspecified whether traffic or nontraffic
    Pedestrian on snowboard injured in collision with railway train or railway vehicle, unspecified whether traffic or nontraffic
    Pedestrian on snow-skis injured in collision with railway train or railway vehicle, unspecified whether traffic or nontraffic

● **V06** **Pedestrian injured in collision with other nonmotor vehicle**

    Includes   collision with animal-drawn vehicle, animal being ridden, nonpowered streetcar

    Excludes1   pedestrian injured in collision with pedestrian conveyance (V00.0-)

    The appropriate 7th character is to be added to each code from category V06

    A   initial encounter
    D   subsequent encounter
    S   sequela

● **V06.0** **Pedestrian injured in collision with other nonmotor vehicle in nontraffic accident**

X ● **V06.00** **Pedestrian on foot injured in collision with other nonmotor vehicle in nontraffic accident**
    Pedestrian NOS injured in collision with other nonmotor vehicle in nontraffic accident

X ● **V06.01** **Pedestrian on roller-skates injured in collision with other nonmotor vehicle in nontraffic accident**

X ● **V06.02** **Pedestrian on skateboard injured in collision with other nonmotor vehicle in nontraffic accident**

X ● **V06.09** **Pedestrian with other conveyance injured in collision with other nonmotor vehicle in nontraffic accident**
    Pedestrian with babystroller injured in collision with other nonmotor vehicle in nontraffic accident
    Pedestrian in wheelchair (powered) injured in collision with other nonmotor vehicle in nontraffic accident
    Pedestrian in motorized mobility scooter injured in collision with other nonmotor vehicle in nontraffic accident
    Pedestrian on ice-skates injured in collision with other nonmotor vehicle in nontraffic accident
    Pedestrian on nonmotorized scooter injured in collision with other nonmotor vehicle in nontraffic accident
    Pedestrian on sled injured in collision with other nonmotor vehicle in nontraffic accident
    Pedestrian on snowboard injured in collision with other nonmotor vehicle in nontraffic accident
    Pedestrian on snow-skis injured in collision with other nonmotor vehicle in nontraffic accident

● **V06.1** **Pedestrian injured in collision with other nonmotor vehicle in traffic accident**

X ● **V06.10** **Pedestrian on foot injured in collision with other nonmotor vehicle in traffic accident**
    Pedestrian NOS injured in collision with other nonmotor vehicle in traffic accident

X ● **V06.11** **Pedestrian on roller-skates injured in collision with other nonmotor vehicle in traffic accident**

X ● **V06.12** **Pedestrian on skateboard injured in collision with other nonmotor vehicle in traffic accident**

X ● **V06.19** **Pedestrian with other conveyance injured in collision with other nonmotor vehicle in traffic accident**
    Pedestrian with babystroller injured in collision with other nonmotor vehicle in nontraffic accident
    Pedestrian in wheelchair (powered) injured in collision with other nonmotor vehicle in traffic accident
    Pedestrian in motorized mobility scooter injured in collision with other nonmotor vehicle in traffic accident
    Pedestrian on ice-skates injured in collision with other nonmotor vehicle in traffic accident
    Pedestrian on nonmotorized scooter injured in collision with other nonmotor vehicle in traffic accident
    Pedestrian on sled injured in collision with other nonmotor vehicle in traffic accident
    Pedestrian on snowboard injured in collision with other nonmotor vehicle in traffic accident
    Pedestrian on snow-skis injured in collision with other nonmotor vehicle in traffic accident

● V06.9   Pedestrian injured in collision with other nonmotor vehicle, unspecified whether traffic or nontraffic accident

   X ● V06.90   Pedestrian on foot injured in collision with other nonmotor vehicle, unspecified whether traffic or nontraffic accident

       Pedestrian NOS injured in collision with other nonmotor vehicle, unspecified whether traffic or nontraffic accident

   X ● V06.91   Pedestrian on roller-skates injured in collision with other nonmotor vehicle, unspecified whether traffic or nontraffic accident

   X ● V06.92   Pedestrian on skateboard injured in collision with other nonmotor vehicle, unspecified whether traffic or nontraffic accident

   X ● V06.99   Pedestrian with other conveyance injured in collision with other nonmotor vehicle, unspecified whether traffic or nontraffic accident

       Pedestrian with babystroller injured in collision with other nonmotor vehicle, unspecified whether traffic or nontraffic accident

       Pedestrian in wheelchair (powered) injured in collision with other nonmotor vehicle, unspecified whether traffic or nontraffic accident

       Pedestrian in motorized mobility scooter injured in collision with other nonmotor vehicle, unspecified whether traffic or nontraffic accident

       Pedestrian on ice-skates injured in collision with other nonmotor vehicle, unspecified whether traffic or nontraffic accident

       Pedestrian on nonmotorized scooter injured in collision with other nonmotor vehicle, unspecified whether traffic or nontraffic accident

       Pedestrian on sled injured in collision with other nonmotor vehicle, unspecified whether traffic or nontraffic accident

       Pedestrian on snowboard injured in collision with other nonmotor vehicle, unspecified whether traffic or nontraffic accident

       Pedestrian on snow-skis injured in collision with other nonmotor vehicle, unspecified whether traffic or nontraffic accident

● V09   Pedestrian injured in other and unspecified transport accidents

   The appropriate 7th character is to be added to each code from category V09

A	initial encounter
D	subsequent encounter
S	sequela

   ● V09.0   Pedestrian injured in nontraffic accident involving other and unspecified motor vehicles

     X ● V09.00   Pedestrian injured in nontraffic accident involving unspecified motor vehicles

     X ● V09.01   Pedestrian injured in nontraffic accident involving military vehicle

     X ● V09.09   Pedestrian injured in nontraffic accident involving other motor vehicles

       Pedestrian injured in nontraffic accident by special vehicle

   X ● V09.1   Pedestrian injured in unspecified nontraffic accident

   ● V09.2   Pedestrian injured in traffic accident involving other and unspecified motor vehicles

     X ● V09.20   Pedestrian injured in traffic accident involving unspecified motor vehicles

     X ● V09.21   Pedestrian injured in traffic accident involving military vehicle

     X ● V09.29   Pedestrian injured in traffic accident involving other motor vehicles

   X ● V09.3   Pedestrian injured in unspecified traffic accident

   X ● V09.9   Pedestrian injured in unspecified transport accident

PEDAL CYCLE RIDER INJURED IN TRANSPORT ACCIDENT (V10-V19)

   Includes   any non-motorized vehicle, excluding an animal-drawn vehicle, or a sidecar or trailer attached to the pedal cycle

   Excludes2   rupture of pedal cycle tire (W37.0)

● V10   Pedal cycle rider injured in collision with pedestrian or animal

   Excludes1   pedal cycle rider collision with animal-drawn vehicle or animal being ridden (V16.-)

   The appropriate 7th character is to be added to each code from category V10

A	initial encounter
D	subsequent encounter
S	sequela

   X ● V10.0   Pedal cycle driver injured in collision with pedestrian or animal in nontraffic accident

   X ● V10.1   Pedal cycle passenger injured in collision with pedestrian or animal in nontraffic accident

   X ● V10.2   Unspecified pedal cyclist injured in collision with pedestrian or animal in nontraffic accident

   X ● V10.3   Person boarding or alighting a pedal cycle injured in collision with pedestrian or animal

   X ● V10.4   Pedal cycle driver injured in collision with pedestrian or animal in traffic accident

   X ● V10.5   Pedal cycle passenger injured in collision with pedestrian or animal in traffic accident

   X ● V10.9   Unspecified pedal cyclist injured in collision with pedestrian or animal in traffic accident

● V11   Pedal cycle rider injured in collision with other pedal cycle

   The appropriate 7th character is to be added to each code from category V11

A	initial encounter
D	subsequent encounter
S	sequela

   X ● V11.0   Pedal cycle driver injured in collision with other pedal cycle in nontraffic accident

   X ● V11.1   Pedal cycle passenger injured in collision with other pedal cycle in nontraffic accident

   X ● V11.2   Unspecified pedal cyclist injured in collision with other pedal cycle in nontraffic accident

   X ● V11.3   Person boarding or alighting a pedal cycle injured in collision with other pedal cycle

   X ● V11.4   Pedal cycle driver injured in collision with other pedal cycle in traffic accident

   X ● V11.5   Pedal cycle passenger injured in collision with other pedal cycle in traffic accident

   X ● V11.9   Unspecified pedal cyclist injured in collision with other pedal cycle in traffic accident

● **V12** **Pedal cycle rider injured in collision with two- or three-wheeled motor vehicle**

    The appropriate 7th character is to be added to each code from category V12

> A   initial encounter
> D   subsequent encounter
> S   sequela

X● **V12.0** Pedal cycle driver injured in collision with two- or three-wheeled motor vehicle in nontraffic accident

X● **V12.1** Pedal cycle passenger injured in collision with two- or three-wheeled motor vehicle in nontraffic accident

X● **V12.2** Unspecified pedal cyclist injured in collision with two- or three-wheeled motor vehicle in nontraffic accident

X● **V12.3** Person boarding or alighting a pedal cycle injured in collision with two- or three-wheeled motor vehicle

X● **V12.4** Pedal cycle driver injured in collision with two- or three-wheeled motor vehicle in traffic accident

X● **V12.5** Pedal cycle passenger injured in collision with two- or three-wheeled motor vehicle in traffic accident

X● **V12.9** Unspecified pedal cyclist injured in collision with two- or three-wheeled motor vehicle in traffic accident

● **V13** **Pedal cycle rider injured in collision with car, pick-up truck or van**

    The appropriate 7th character is to be added to each code from category V13

> A   initial encounter
> D   subsequent encounter
> S   sequela

X● **V13.0** Pedal cycle driver injured in collision with car, pick-up truck or van in nontraffic accident

X● **V13.1** Pedal cycle passenger injured in collision with car, pick-up truck or van in nontraffic accident

X● **V13.2** Unspecified pedal cyclist injured in collision with car, pick-up truck or van in nontraffic accident

X● **V13.3** Person boarding or alighting a pedal cycle injured in collision with car, pick-up truck or van

X● **V13.4** Pedal cycle driver injured in collision with car, pick-up truck or van in traffic accident

X● **V13.5** Pedal cycle passenger injured in collision with car, pick-up truck or van in traffic accident

X● **V13.9** Unspecified pedal cyclist injured in collision with car, pick-up truck or van in traffic accident

● **V14** **Pedal cycle rider injured in collision with heavy transport vehicle or bus**

    Excludes1   pedal cycle rider injured in collision with military vehicle (V19.81)

    The appropriate 7th character is to be added to each code from category V14

> A   initial encounter
> D   subsequent encounter
> S   sequela

X● **V14.0** Pedal cycle driver injured in collision with heavy transport vehicle or bus in nontraffic accident

X● **V14.1** Pedal cycle passenger injured in collision with heavy transport vehicle or bus in nontraffic accident

X● **V14.2** Unspecified pedal cyclist injured in collision with heavy transport vehicle or bus in nontraffic accident

X● **V14.3** Person boarding or alighting a pedal cycle injured in collision with heavy transport vehicle or bus

X● **V14.4** Pedal cycle driver injured in collision with heavy transport vehicle or bus in traffic accident

X● **V14.5** Pedal cycle passenger injured in collision with heavy transport vehicle or bus in traffic accident

X● **V14.9** Unspecified pedal cyclist injured in collision with heavy transport vehicle or bus in traffic accident

● **V15** **Pedal cycle rider injured in collision with railway train or railway vehicle**

    The appropriate 7th character is to be added to each code from category V15

> A   initial encounter
> D   subsequent encounter
> S   sequela

X● **V15.0** Pedal cycle driver injured in collision with railway train or railway vehicle in nontraffic accident

X● **V15.1** Pedal cycle passenger injured in collision with railway train or railway vehicle in nontraffic accident

X● **V15.2** Unspecified pedal cyclist injured in collision with railway train or railway vehicle in nontraffic accident

X● **V15.3** Person boarding or alighting a pedal cycle injured in collision with railway train or railway vehicle

X● **V15.4** Pedal cycle driver injured in collision with railway train or railway vehicle in traffic accident

X● **V15.5** Pedal cycle passenger injured in collision with railway train or railway vehicle in traffic accident

X● **V15.9** Unspecified pedal cyclist injured in collision with railway train or railway vehicle in traffic accident

● **V16** **Pedal cycle rider injured in collision with other nonmotor vehicle**

    Includes   collision with animal-drawn vehicle, animal being ridden, streetcar

    The appropriate 7th character is to be added to each code from category V16

> A   initial encounter
> D   subsequent encounter
> S   sequela

X● **V16.0** Pedal cycle driver injured in collision with other nonmotor vehicle in nontraffic accident

X● **V16.1** Pedal cycle passenger injured in collision with other nonmotor vehicle in nontraffic accident

X● **V16.2** Unspecified pedal cyclist injured in collision with other nonmotor vehicle in nontraffic accident

X● **V16.3** Person boarding or alighting a pedal cycle injured in collision with other nonmotor vehicle in nontraffic accident

X● **V16.4** Pedal cycle driver injured in collision with other nonmotor vehicle in traffic accident

X● **V16.5** Pedal cycle passenger injured in collision with other nonmotor vehicle in traffic accident

X● **V16.9** Unspecified pedal cyclist injured in collision with other nonmotor vehicle in traffic accident

● **V17** **Pedal cycle rider injured in collision with fixed or stationary object**

    The appropriate 7th character is to be added to each code from category V17

> A   initial encounter
> D   subsequent encounter
> S   sequela

X● **V17.0** Pedal cycle driver injured in collision with fixed or stationary object in nontraffic accident

X● **V17.1** Pedal cycle passenger injured in collision with fixed or stationary object in nontraffic accident

X● **V17.2** Unspecified pedal cyclist injured in collision with fixed or stationary object in nontraffic accident

X● **V17.3** Person boarding or alighting a pedal cycle injured in collision with fixed or stationary object

X● **V17.4** Pedal cycle driver injured in collision with fixed or stationary object in traffic accident

X● **V17.5** Pedal cycle passenger injured in collision with fixed or stationary object in traffic accident

X● **V17.9** Unspecified pedal cyclist injured in collision with fixed or stationary object in traffic accident

CHAPTER 20 (V01-Y99)

● **V18**   **Pedal cycle rider injured in noncollision transport accident**

> **Includes**   fall or thrown from pedal cycle (without antecedent collision)
> overturning pedal cycle NOS
> overturning pedal cycle without collision

> The appropriate 7th character is to be added to each code from category V18

> | | |
> |---|---|
> | A | initial encounter |
> | D | subsequent encounter |
> | S | sequela |

X ● **V18.0**   Pedal cycle driver injured in noncollision transport accident in nontraffic accident

X ● **V18.1**   Pedal cycle passenger injured in noncollision transport accident in nontraffic accident

X ● **V18.2**   Unspecified pedal cyclist injured in noncollision transport accident in nontraffic accident

X ● **V18.3**   Person boarding or alighting a pedal cycle injured in noncollision transport accident

X ● **V18.4**   Pedal cycle driver injured in noncollision transport accident in traffic accident

X ● **V18.5**   Pedal cycle passenger injured in noncollision transport accident in traffic accident

X ● **V18.9**   Unspecified pedal cyclist injured in noncollision transport accident in traffic accident

● **V19**   **Pedal cycle rider injured in other and unspecified transport accidents**

> The appropriate 7th character is to be added to each code from category V19

> | | |
> |---|---|
> | A | initial encounter |
> | D | subsequent encounter |
> | S | sequela |

● **V19.0**   Pedal cycle driver injured in collision with other and unspecified motor vehicles in nontraffic accident

   X ● **V19.00**   Pedal cycle driver injured in collision with unspecified motor vehicles in nontraffic accident

   X ● **V19.09**   Pedal cycle driver injured in collision with other motor vehicles in nontraffic accident

● **V19.1**   Pedal cycle passenger injured in collision with other and unspecified motor vehicles in nontraffic accident

   X ● **V19.10**   Pedal cycle passenger injured in collision with unspecified motor vehicles in nontraffic accident

   X ● **V19.19**   Pedal cycle passenger injured in collision with other motor vehicles in nontraffic accident

● **V19.2**   Unspecified pedal cyclist injured in collision with other and unspecified motor vehicles in nontraffic accident

   X ● **V19.20**   Unspecified pedal cyclist injured in collision with unspecified motor vehicles in nontraffic accident
       Pedal cycle collision NOS, nontraffic

   X ● **V19.29**   Unspecified pedal cyclist injured in collision with other motor vehicles in nontraffic accident

X ● **V19.3**   Pedal cyclist (driver) (passenger) injured in unspecified nontraffic accident
     Pedal cycle accident NOS, nontraffic
     Pedal cyclist injured in nontraffic accident NOS

● **V19.4**   Pedal cycle driver injured in collision with other and unspecified motor vehicles in traffic accident

   X ● **V19.40**   Pedal cycle driver injured in collision with unspecified motor vehicles in traffic accident

   X ● **V19.49**   Pedal cycle driver injured in collision with other motor vehicles in traffic accident

● **V19.5**   Pedal cycle passenger injured in collision with other and unspecified motor vehicles in traffic accident

   X ● **V19.50**   Pedal cycle passenger injured in collision with unspecified motor vehicles in traffic accident

   X ● **V19.59**   Pedal cycle passenger injured in collision with other motor vehicles in traffic accident

● **V19.6**   Unspecified pedal cyclist injured in collision with other and unspecified motor vehicles in traffic accident

   X ● **V19.60**   Unspecified pedal cyclist injured in collision with unspecified motor vehicles in traffic accident
       Pedal cycle collision NOS (traffic)

   X ● **V19.69**   Unspecified pedal cyclist injured in collision with other motor vehicles in traffic accident

● **V19.8**   Pedal cyclist (driver) (passenger) injured in other specified transport accidents

   X ● **V19.81**   Pedal cyclist (driver) (passenger) injured in transport accident with military vehicle

   X ● **V19.88**   Pedal cyclist (driver) (passenger) injured in other specified transport accidents

X ● **V19.9**   Pedal cyclist (driver) (passenger) injured in unspecified traffic accident
     Pedal cycle accident NOS

MOTORCYCLE RIDER INJURED IN TRANSPORT ACCIDENT (V20-V29)

> **Includes**   moped motorcycle with sidecar motorized bicycle motor scooter

> **Excludes1**   three-wheeled motor vehicle (V30-V39)

● **V20**   **Motorcycle rider injured in collision with pedestrian or animal**

> **Excludes1**   motorcycle rider collision with animal-drawn vehicle or animal being ridden (V26.-)

> The appropriate 7th character is to be added to each code from category V20

> | | |
> |---|---|
> | A | initial encounter |
> | D | subsequent encounter |
> | S | sequela |

X ● **V20.0**   Motorcycle driver injured in collision with pedestrian or animal in nontraffic accident

X ● **V20.1**   Motorcycle passenger injured in collision with pedestrian or animal in nontraffic accident

X ● **V20.2**   Unspecified motorcycle rider injured in collision with pedestrian or animal in nontraffic accident

X ● **V20.3**   Person boarding or alighting a motorcycle injured in collision with pedestrian or animal

X ● **V20.4**   Motorcycle driver injured in collision with pedestrian or animal in traffic accident

X ● **V20.5**   Motorcycle passenger injured in collision with pedestrian or animal in traffic accident

X ● **V20.9**   Unspecified motorcycle rider injured in collision with pedestrian or animal in traffic accident

● **V21**   **Motorcycle rider injured in collision with pedal cycle**

> The appropriate 7th character is to be added to each code from category V21

> | | |
> |---|---|
> | A | initial encounter |
> | D | subsequent encounter |
> | S | sequela |

X ● **V21.0**   Motorcycle driver injured in collision with pedal cycle in nontraffic accident

X ● **V21.1**   Motorcycle passenger injured in collision with pedal cycle in nontraffic accident

X ● **V21.2**   Unspecified motorcycle rider injured in collision with pedal cycle in nontraffic accident

X ● **V21.3**   Person boarding or alighting a motorcycle injured in collision with pedal cycle

X ● **V21.4**   Motorcycle driver injured in collision with pedal cycle in traffic accident

X ● **V21.5**   Motorcycle passenger injured in collision with pedal cycle in traffic accident

X ● **V21.9**   Unspecified motorcycle rider injured in collision with pedal cycle in traffic accident

◀ New   ⬅ Revised   ~~deleted~~ Deleted   Excludes 1   Excludes 2   Includes   Use additional   Code first   Code also   Unspecified

1440   **OGCR** Official Guidelines   X Assign placeholder X   ● Use Additional Character(s)   ▶ Manifestation Code   **Coding Clinic**

● **V22**   **Motorcycle rider injured in collision with two- or three-wheeled motor vehicle**

    The appropriate 7th character is to be added to each code from category V22

A	initial encounter
D	subsequent encounter
S	sequela

X● **V22.0**   Motorcycle driver injured in collision with two- or three-wheeled motor vehicle in nontraffic accident

X● **V22.1**   Motorcycle passenger injured in collision with two- or three-wheeled motor vehicle in nontraffic accident

X● **V22.2**   Unspecified motorcycle rider injured in collision with two- or three-wheeled motor vehicle in nontraffic accident

X● **V22.3**   Person boarding or alighting a motorcycle injured in collision with two- or three-wheeled motor vehicle

X● **V22.4**   Motorcycle driver injured in collision with two- or three-wheeled motor vehicle in traffic accident

X● **V22.5**   Motorcycle passenger injured in collision with two- or three-wheeled motor vehicle in traffic accident

X● **V22.9**   Unspecified motorcycle rider injured in collision with two- or three-wheeled motor vehicle in traffic accident

● **V23**   **Motorcycle rider injured in collision with car, pick-up truck or van**

    The appropriate 7th character is to be added to each code from category V23

A	initial encounter
D	subsequent encounter
S	sequela

X● **V23.0**   Motorcycle driver injured in collision with car, pick-up truck or van in nontraffic accident

X● **V23.1**   Motorcycle passenger injured in collision with car, pick-up truck or van in nontraffic accident

X● **V23.2**   Unspecified motorcycle rider injured in collision with car, pick-up truck or van in nontraffic accident

X● **V23.3**   Person boarding or alighting a motorcycle injured in collision with car, pick-up truck or van

X● **V23.4**   Motorcycle driver injured in collision with car, pick-up truck or van in traffic accident

X● **V23.5**   Motorcycle passenger injured in collision with car, pick-up truck or van in traffic accident

X● **V23.9**   Unspecified motorcycle rider injured in collision with car, pick-up truck or van in traffic accident

● **V24**   **Motorcycle rider injured in collision with heavy transport vehicle or bus**

    Excludes1   motorcycle rider injured in collision with military vehicle (V29.81)

    The appropriate 7th character is to be added to each code from category V24

A	initial encounter
D	subsequent encounter
S	sequela

X● **V24.0**   Motorcycle driver injured in collision with heavy transport vehicle or bus in nontraffic accident

X● **V24.1**   Motorcycle passenger injured in collision with heavy transport vehicle or bus in nontraffic accident

X● **V24.2**   Unspecified motorcycle rider injured in collision with heavy transport vehicle or bus in nontraffic accident

X● **V24.3**   Person boarding or alighting a motorcycle injured in collision with heavy transport vehicle or bus

X● **V24.4**   Motorcycle driver injured in collision with heavy transport vehicle or bus in traffic accident

X● **V24.5**   Motorcycle passenger injured in collision with heavy transport vehicle or bus in traffic accident

X● **V24.9**   Unspecified motorcycle rider injured in collision with heavy transport vehicle or bus in traffic accident

● **V25**   **Motorcycle rider injured in collision with railway train or railway vehicle**

    The appropriate 7th character is to be added to each code from category V25

A	initial encounter
D	subsequent encounter
S	sequela

X● **V25.0**   Motorcycle driver injured in collision with railway train or railway vehicle in nontraffic accident

X● **V25.1**   Motorcycle passenger injured in collision with railway train or railway vehicle in nontraffic accident

X● **V25.2**   Unspecified motorcycle rider injured in collision with railway train or railway vehicle in nontraffic accident

X● **V25.3**   Person boarding or alighting a motorcycle injured in collision with railway train or railway vehicle

X● **V25.4**   Motorcycle driver injured in collision with railway train or railway vehicle in traffic accident

X● **V25.5**   Motorcycle passenger injured in collision with railway train or railway vehicle in traffic accident

X● **V25.9**   Unspecified motorcycle rider injured in collision with railway train or railway vehicle in traffic accident

● **V26**   **Motorcycle rider injured in collision with other nonmotor vehicle**

    Includes   collision with animal-drawn vehicle, animal being ridden, streetcar

    The appropriate 7th character is to be added to each code from category V26

A	initial encounter
D	subsequent encounter
S	sequela

X● **V26.0**   Motorcycle driver injured in collision with other nonmotor vehicle in nontraffic accident

X● **V26.1**   Motorcycle passenger injured in collision with other nonmotor vehicle in nontraffic accident

X● **V26.2**   Unspecified motorcycle rider injured in collision with other nonmotor vehicle in nontraffic accident

X● **V26.3**   Person boarding or alighting a motorcycle injured in collision with other nonmotor vehicle

X● **V26.4**   Motorcycle driver injured in collision with other nonmotor vehicle in traffic accident

X● **V26.5**   Motorcycle passenger injured in collision with other nonmotor vehicle in traffic accident

X● **V26.9**   Unspecified motorcycle rider injured in collision with other nonmotor vehicle in traffic accident

● **V27**   **Motorcycle rider injured in collision with fixed or stationary object**

    The appropriate 7th character is to be added to each code from category V27

A	initial encounter
D	subsequent encounter
S	sequela

X● **V27.0**   Motorcycle driver injured in collision with fixed or stationary object in nontraffic accident

X● **V27.1**   Motorcycle passenger injured in collision with fixed or stationary object in nontraffic accident

X● **V27.2**   Unspecified motorcycle rider injured in collision with fixed or stationary object in nontraffic accident

X● **V27.3**   Person boarding or alighting a motorcycle injured in collision with fixed or stationary object

X● **V27.4**   Motorcycle driver injured in collision with fixed or stationary object in traffic accident

X● **V27.5**   Motorcycle passenger injured in collision with fixed or stationary object in traffic accident

X● **V27.9**   Unspecified motorcycle rider injured in collision with fixed or stationary object in traffic accident

CHAPTER 20 (V01-Y99)

● **V28   Motorcycle rider injured in noncollision transport accident**

Includes	fall or thrown from motorcycle (without antecedent collision)
	overturning motorcycle NOS
	overturning motorcycle without collision

The appropriate 7th character is to be added to each code from category V28

A	initial encounter
D	subsequent encounter
S	sequela

X ● **V28.0   Motorcycle driver injured in noncollision transport accident in nontraffic accident**

X ● **V28.1   Motorcycle passenger injured in noncollision transport accident in nontraffic accident**

X ● **V28.2   Unspecified motorcycle rider injured in noncollision transport accident in nontraffic accident**

X ● **V28.3   Person boarding or alighting a motorcycle injured in noncollision transport accident**

X ● **V28.4   Motorcycle driver injured in noncollision transport accident in traffic accident**

X ● **V28.5   Motorcycle passenger injured in noncollision transport accident in traffic accident**

X ● **V28.9   Unspecified motorcycle rider injured in noncollision transport accident in traffic accident**

● **V29   Motorcycle rider injured in other and unspecified transport accidents**

The appropriate 7th character is to be added to each code from category V29

A	initial encounter
D	subsequent encounter
S	sequela

Coding Clinic: 2015, Q3, P20

● **V29.0   Motorcycle driver injured in collision with other and unspecified motor vehicles in nontraffic accident**

X ● **V29.00   Motorcycle driver injured in collision with unspecified motor vehicles in nontraffic accident**

X ● **V29.09   Motorcycle driver injured in collision with other motor vehicles in nontraffic accident**

● **V29.1   Motorcycle passenger injured in collision with other and unspecified motor vehicles in nontraffic accident**

X ● **V29.10   Motorcycle passenger injured in collision with unspecified motor vehicles in nontraffic accident**

X ● **V29.19   Motorcycle passenger injured in collision with other motor vehicles in nontraffic accident**

● **V29.2   Unspecified motorcycle rider injured in collision with other and unspecified motor vehicles in nontraffic accident**

X ● **V29.20   Unspecified motorcycle rider injured in collision with unspecified motor vehicles in nontraffic accident**
Motorcycle collision NOS, nontraffic

X ● **V29.29   Unspecified motorcycle rider injured in collision with other motor vehicles in nontraffic accident**

X ● **V29.3   Motorcycle rider (driver) (passenger) injured in unspecified nontraffic accident**
Motorcycle accident NOS, nontraffic
Motorcycle rider injured in nontraffic accident NOS

● **V29.4   Motorcycle driver injured in collision with other and unspecified motor vehicles in traffic accident**

X ● **V29.40   Motorcycle driver injured in collision with unspecified motor vehicles in traffic accident**

X ● **V29.49   Motorcycle driver injured in collision with other motor vehicles in traffic accident**

● **V29.5   Motorcycle passenger injured in collision with other and unspecified motor vehicles in traffic accident**

X ● **V29.50   Motorcycle passenger injured in collision with unspecified motor vehicles in traffic accident**

X ● **V29.59   Motorcycle passenger injured in collision with other motor vehicles in traffic accident**

● **V29.6   Unspecified motorcycle rider injured in collision with other and unspecified motor vehicles in traffic accident**

X ● **V29.60   Unspecified motorcycle rider injured in collision with unspecified motor vehicles in traffic accident**
Motorcycle collision NOS (traffic)

X ● **V29.69   Unspecified motorcycle rider injured in collision with other motor vehicles in traffic accident**

● **V29.8   Motorcycle rider (driver) (passenger) injured in other specified transport accidents**

X ● **V29.81   Motorcycle rider (driver) (passenger) injured in transport accident with military vehicle**

X ● **V29.88   Motorcycle rider (driver) (passenger) injured in other specified transport accidents**

X ● **V29.9   Motorcycle rider (driver) (passenger) injured in unspecified traffic accident**
Motorcycle accident NOS

OCCUPANT OF THREE-WHEELED MOTOR VEHICLE INJURED IN TRANSPORT ACCIDENT (V30-V39)

Includes	motorized tricycle
	motorized rickshaw
	three-wheeled motor car
Excludes1	all-terrain vehicles (V86.-)
	motorcycle with sidecar (V20-V29)
	vehicle designed primarily for off-road use (V86.-)

● **V30   Occupant of three-wheeled motor vehicle injured in collision with pedestrian or animal**

Excludes1	three-wheeled motor vehicle collision with animal-drawn vehicle or animal being ridden (V36.-)

The appropriate 7th character is to be added to each code from category V30

A	initial encounter
D	subsequent encounter
S	sequela

X ● **V30.0   Driver of three-wheeled motor vehicle injured in collision with pedestrian or animal in nontraffic accident**

X ● **V30.1   Passenger in three-wheeled motor vehicle injured in collision with pedestrian or animal in nontraffic accident**

X ● **V30.2   Person on outside of three-wheeled motor vehicle injured in collision with pedestrian or animal in nontraffic accident**

X ● **V30.3   Unspecified occupant of three-wheeled motor vehicle injured in collision with pedestrian or animal in nontraffic accident**

X ● **V30.4   Person boarding or alighting a three-wheeled motor vehicle injured in collision with pedestrian or animal**

X ● **V30.5   Driver of three-wheeled motor vehicle injured in collision with pedestrian or animal in traffic accident**

X ● **V30.6   Passenger in three-wheeled motor vehicle injured in collision with pedestrian or animal in traffic accident**

X ● **V30.7   Person on outside of three-wheeled motor vehicle injured in collision with pedestrian or animal in traffic accident**

X ● **V30.9   Unspecified occupant of three-wheeled motor vehicle injured in collision with pedestrian or animal in traffic accident**

◀ New   ◀◀ Revised   ~~deleted~~ Deleted   Excludes 1   Excludes 2   Includes   Use additional   Code first   Code also   Unspecified

OGCR Official Guidelines   X Assign placeholder X   ● Use Additional Character(s)   ▶ Manifestation Code   **Coding Clinic**

● **V31   Occupant of three-wheeled motor vehicle injured in collision with pedal cycle**

> The appropriate 7th character is to be added to each code from category V31

A	initial encounter
D	subsequent encounter
S	sequela

X● **V31.0** Driver of three-wheeled motor vehicle injured in collision with pedal cycle in nontraffic accident

X● **V31.1** Passenger in three-wheeled motor vehicle injured in collision with pedal cycle in nontraffic accident

X● **V31.2** Person on outside of three-wheeled motor vehicle injured in collision with pedal cycle in nontraffic accident

X● **V31.3** Unspecified occupant of three-wheeled motor vehicle injured in collision with pedal cycle in nontraffic accident

X● **V31.4** Person boarding or alighting a three-wheeled motor vehicle injured in collision with pedal cycle

X● **V31.5** Driver of three-wheeled motor vehicle injured in collision with pedal cycle in traffic accident

X● **V31.6** Passenger in three-wheeled motor vehicle injured in collision with pedal cycle in traffic accident

X● **V31.7** Person on outside of three-wheeled motor vehicle injured in collision with pedal cycle in traffic accident

X● **V31.9** Unspecified occupant of three-wheeled motor vehicle injured in collision with pedal cycle in traffic accident

● **V32   Occupant of three-wheeled motor vehicle injured in collision with two- or three-wheeled motor vehicle**

> The appropriate 7th character is to be added to each code from category V32

A	initial encounter
D	subsequent encounter
S	sequela

X● **V32.0** Driver of three-wheeled motor vehicle injured in collision with two- or three-wheeled motor vehicle in nontraffic accident

X● **V32.1** Passenger in three-wheeled motor vehicle injured in collision with two- or three-wheeled motor vehicle in nontraffic accident

X● **V32.2** Person on outside of three-wheeled motor vehicle injured in collision with two- or three-wheeled motor vehicle in nontraffic accident

X● **V32.3** Unspecified occupant of three-wheeled motor vehicle injured in collision with two- or three-wheeled motor vehicle in nontraffic accident

X● **V32.4** Person boarding or alighting a three-wheeled motor vehicle injured in collision with two- or three-wheeled motor vehicle

X● **V32.5** Driver of three-wheeled motor vehicle injured in collision with two- or three-wheeled motor vehicle in traffic accident

X● **V32.6** Passenger in three-wheeled motor vehicle injured in collision with two- or three-wheeled motor vehicle in traffic accident

X● **V32.7** Person on outside of three-wheeled motor vehicle injured in collision with two- or three-wheeled motor vehicle in traffic accident

X● **V32.9** Unspecified occupant of three-wheeled motor vehicle injured in collision with two- or three-wheeled motor vehicle in traffic accident

● **V33   Occupant of three-wheeled motor vehicle injured in collision with car, pick-up truck or van**

> The appropriate 7th character is to be added to each code from category V33

A	initial encounter
D	subsequent encounter
S	sequela

X● **V33.0** Driver of three-wheeled motor vehicle injured in collision with car, pick-up truck or van in nontraffic accident

X● **V33.1** Passenger in three-wheeled motor vehicle injured in collision with car, pick-up truck or van in nontraffic accident

X● **V33.2** Person on outside of three-wheeled motor vehicle injured in collision with car, pick-up truck or van in nontraffic accident

X● **V33.3** Unspecified occupant of three-wheeled motor vehicle injured in collision with car, pick-up truck or van in nontraffic accident

X● **V33.4** Person boarding or alighting a three-wheeled motor vehicle injured in collision with car, pick-up truck or van

X● **V33.5** Driver of three-wheeled motor vehicle injured in collision with car, pick-up truck or van in traffic accident

X● **V33.6** Passenger in three-wheeled motor vehicle injured in collision with car, pick-up truck or van in traffic accident

X● **V33.7** Person on outside of three-wheeled motor vehicle injured in collision with car, pick-up truck or van in traffic accident

X● **V33.9** Unspecified occupant of three-wheeled motor vehicle injured in collision with car, pick-up truck or van in traffic accident

● **V34   Occupant of three-wheeled motor vehicle injured in collision with heavy transport vehicle or bus**

> **Excludes1**   occupant of three-wheeled motor vehicle injured in collision with military vehicle (V39.81)

> The appropriate 7th character is to be added to each code from category V34

A	initial encounter
D	subsequent encounter
S	sequela

X● **V34.0** Driver of three-wheeled motor vehicle injured in collision with heavy transport vehicle or bus in nontraffic accident

X● **V34.1** Passenger in three-wheeled motor vehicle injured in collision with heavy transport vehicle or bus in nontraffic accident

X● **V34.2** Person on outside of three-wheeled motor vehicle injured in collision with heavy transport vehicle or bus in nontraffic accident

X● **V34.3** Unspecified occupant of three-wheeled motor vehicle injured in collision with heavy transport vehicle or bus in nontraffic accident

X● **V34.4** Person boarding or alighting a three-wheeled motor vehicle injured in collision with heavy transport vehicle or bus

X● **V34.5** Driver of three-wheeled motor vehicle injured in collision with heavy transport vehicle or bus in traffic accident

X● **V34.6** Passenger in three-wheeled motor vehicle injured in collision with heavy transport vehicle or bus in traffic accident

X● **V34.7** Person on outside of three-wheeled motor vehicle injured in collision with heavy transport vehicle or bus in traffic accident

X● **V34.9** Unspecified occupant of three-wheeled motor vehicle injured in collision with heavy transport vehicle or bus in traffic accident

CHAPTER 20 (V01-Y99)

● V35 Occupant of three-wheeled motor vehicle injured in collision with railway train or railway vehicle

The appropriate 7th character is to be added to each code from category V35

A	initial encounter
D	subsequent encounter
S	sequela

X ● **V35.0** Driver of three-wheeled motor vehicle injured in collision with railway train or railway vehicle in nontraffic accident

X ● **V35.1** Passenger in three-wheeled motor vehicle injured in collision with railway train or railway vehicle in nontraffic accident

X ● **V35.2** Person on outside of three-wheeled motor vehicle injured in collision with railway train or railway vehicle in nontraffic accident

X ● **V35.3** Unspecified occupant of three-wheeled motor vehicle injured in collision with railway train or railway vehicle in nontraffic accident

X ● **V35.4** Person boarding or alighting a three-wheeled motor vehicle injured in collision with railway train or railway vehicle

X ● **V35.5** Driver of three-wheeled motor vehicle injured in collision with railway train or railway vehicle in traffic accident

X ● **V35.6** Passenger in three-wheeled motor vehicle injured in collision with railway train or railway vehicle in traffic accident

X ● **V35.7** Person on outside of three-wheeled motor vehicle injured in collision with railway train or railway vehicle in traffic accident

X ● **V35.9** Unspecified occupant of three-wheeled motor vehicle injured in collision with railway train or railway vehicle in traffic accident

● V36 Occupant of three-wheeled motor vehicle injured in collision with other nonmotor vehicle

Includes collision with animal-drawn vehicle, animal being ridden, streetcar

The appropriate 7th character is to be added to each code from category V36

A	initial encounter
D	subsequent encounter
S	sequela

X ● **V36.0** Driver of three-wheeled motor vehicle injured in collision with other nonmotor vehicle in nontraffic accident

X ● **V36.1** Passenger in three-wheeled motor vehicle injured in collision with other nonmotor vehicle in nontraffic accident

X ● **V36.2** Person on outside of three-wheeled motor vehicle injured in collision with other nonmotor vehicle in nontraffic accident

X ● **V36.3** Unspecified occupant of three-wheeled motor vehicle injured in collision with other nonmotor vehicle in nontraffic accident

X ● **V36.4** Person boarding or alighting a three-wheeled motor vehicle injured in collision with other nonmotor vehicle

X ● **V36.5** Driver of three-wheeled motor vehicle injured in collision with other nonmotor vehicle in traffic accident

X ● **V36.6** Passenger in three-wheeled motor vehicle injured in collision with other nonmotor vehicle in traffic accident

X ● **V36.7** Person on outside of three-wheeled motor vehicle injured in collision with other nonmotor vehicle in traffic accident

X ● **V36.9** Unspecified occupant of three-wheeled motor vehicle injured in collision with other nonmotor vehicle in traffic accident

● V37 Occupant of three-wheeled motor vehicle injured in collision with fixed or stationary object

The appropriate 7th character is to be added to each code from category V37

A	initial encounter
D	subsequent encounter
S	sequela

X ● **V37.0** Driver of three-wheeled motor vehicle injured in collision with fixed or stationary object in nontraffic accident

X ● **V37.1** Passenger in three-wheeled motor vehicle injured in collision with fixed or stationary object in nontraffic accident

X ● **V37.2** Person on outside of three-wheeled motor vehicle injured in collision with fixed or stationary object in nontraffic accident

X ● **V37.3** Unspecified occupant of three-wheeled motor vehicle injured in collision with fixed or stationary object in nontraffic accident

X ● **V37.4** Person boarding or alighting a three-wheeled motor vehicle injured in collision with fixed or stationary object

X ● **V37.5** Driver of three-wheeled motor vehicle injured in collision with fixed or stationary object in traffic accident

X ● **V37.6** Passenger in three-wheeled motor vehicle injured in collision with fixed or stationary object in traffic accident

X ● **V37.7** Person on outside of three-wheeled motor vehicle injured in collision with fixed or stationary object in traffic accident

X ● **V37.9** Unspecified occupant of three-wheeled motor vehicle injured in collision with fixed or stationary object in traffic accident

● V38 Occupant of three-wheeled motor vehicle injured in noncollision transport accident

Includes fall or thrown from three-wheeled motor vehicle overturning of three-wheeled motor vehicle NOS overturning of three-wheeled motor vehicle without collision

The appropriate 7th character is to be added to each code from category V38

A	initial encounter
D	subsequent encounter
S	sequela

X ● **V38.0** Driver of three-wheeled motor vehicle injured in noncollision transport accident in nontraffic accident

X ● **V38.1** Passenger in three-wheeled motor vehicle injured in noncollision transport accident in nontraffic accident

X ● **V38.2** Person on outside of three-wheeled motor vehicle injured in noncollision transport accident in nontraffic accident

X ● **V38.3** Unspecified occupant of three-wheeled motor vehicle injured in noncollision transport accident in nontraffic accident

X ● **V38.4** Person boarding or alighting a three-wheeled motor vehicle injured in noncollision transport accident

X ● **V38.5** Driver of three-wheeled motor vehicle injured in noncollision transport accident in traffic accident

X ● **V38.6** Passenger in three-wheeled motor vehicle injured in noncollision transport accident in traffic accident

X ● **V38.7** Person on outside of three-wheeled motor vehicle injured in noncollision transport accident in traffic accident

X ● **V38.9** Unspecified occupant of three-wheeled motor vehicle injured in noncollision transport accident in traffic accident

CHAPTER 20 (V01-Y99)

◀ New   ◀▥ Revised   ~~deleted~~ Deleted   Excludes 1   Excludes 2   Includes   Use additional   Code first   Code also   Unspecified

OGCR Official Guidelines   X Assign placeholder X   ● Use Additional Character(s)   ▶ Manifestation Code   **Coding Clinic**

● **V39   Occupant of three-wheeled motor vehicle injured in other and unspecified transport accidents**

The appropriate 7th character is to be added to each code from category V39

> A   initial encounter
> D   subsequent encounter
> S   sequela

● **V39.0   Driver of three-wheeled motor vehicle injured in collision with other and unspecified motor vehicles in nontraffic accident**

  X ● **V39.00   Driver of three-wheeled motor vehicle injured in collision with unspecified motor vehicles in nontraffic accident**

  X ● **V39.09   Driver of three-wheeled motor vehicle injured in collision with other motor vehicles in nontraffic accident**

● **V39.1   Passenger in three-wheeled motor vehicle injured in collision with other and unspecified motor vehicles in nontraffic accident**

  X ● **V39.10   Passenger in three-wheeled motor vehicle injured in collision with unspecified motor vehicles in nontraffic accident**

  X ● **V39.19   Passenger in three-wheeled motor vehicle injured in collision with other motor vehicles in nontraffic accident**

● **V39.2   Unspecified occupant of three-wheeled motor vehicle injured in collision with other and unspecified motor vehicles in nontraffic accident**

  X ● **V39.20   Unspecified occupant of three-wheeled motor vehicle injured in collision with unspecified motor vehicles in nontraffic accident**
> Collision NOS involving three-wheeled motor vehicle, nontraffic

  X ● **V39.29   Unspecified occupant of three-wheeled motor vehicle injured in collision with other motor vehicles in nontraffic accident**

  X ● **V39.3   Occupant (driver) (passenger) of three-wheeled motor vehicle injured in unspecified nontraffic accident**
> Accident NOS involving three-wheeled motor vehicle, nontraffic
> Occupant of three-wheeled motor vehicle injured in nontraffic accident NOS

● **V39.4   Driver of three-wheeled motor vehicle injured in collision with other and unspecified motor vehicles in traffic accident**

  X ● **V39.40   Driver of three-wheeled motor vehicle injured in collision with unspecified motor vehicles in traffic accident**

  X ● **V39.49   Driver of three-wheeled motor vehicle injured in collision with other motor vehicles in traffic accident**

● **V39.5   Passenger in three-wheeled motor vehicle injured in collision with other and unspecified motor vehicles in traffic accident**

  X ● **V39.50   Passenger in three-wheeled motor vehicle injured in collision with unspecified motor vehicles in traffic accident**

  X ● **V39.59   Passenger in three-wheeled motor vehicle injured in collision with other motor vehicles in traffic accident**

● **V39.6   Unspecified occupant of three-wheeled motor vehicle injured in collision with other and unspecified motor vehicles in traffic accident**

  X ● **V39.60   Unspecified occupant of three-wheeled motor vehicle injured in collision with unspecified motor vehicles in traffic accident**
> Collision NOS involving three-wheeled motor vehicle (traffic)

  X ● **V39.69   Unspecified occupant of three-wheeled motor vehicle injured in collision with other motor vehicles in traffic accident**

● **V39.8   Occupant (driver) (passenger) of three-wheeled motor vehicle injured in other specified transport accidents**

  X ● **V39.81   Occupant (driver) (passenger) of three-wheeled motor vehicle injured in transport accident with military vehicle**

  X ● **V39.89   Occupant (driver) (passenger) of three-wheeled motor vehicle injured in other specified transport accidents**

  X ● **V39.9   Occupant (driver) (passenger) of three-wheeled motor vehicle injured in unspecified traffic accident**
> Accident NOS involving three-wheeled motor vehicle

CAR OCCUPANT INJURED IN TRANSPORT ACCIDENT (V40-V49)

> **Includes**   a four-wheeled motor vehicle designed primarily for carrying passengers
> automobile (pulling a trailer or camper)

> **Excludes1**   bus (V50-V59)
> minibus (V50-V59)
> minivan (V50-V59)
> motorcoach (V70-V79)
> pick-up truck (V50-V59)
> sport utility vehicle (SUV) (V50-V59)

● **V40   Car occupant injured in collision with pedestrian or animal**

> **Excludes1**   car collision with animal-drawn vehicle or animal being ridden (V46.-)

The appropriate 7th character is to be added to each code from category V40

> A   initial encounter
> D   subsequent encounter
> S   sequela

  X ● **V40.0   Car driver injured in collision with pedestrian or animal in nontraffic accident**

  X ● **V40.1   Car passenger injured in collision with pedestrian or animal in nontraffic accident**

  X ● **V40.2   Person on outside of car injured in collision with pedestrian or animal in nontraffic accident**

  X ● **V40.3   Unspecified car occupant injured in collision with pedestrian or animal in nontraffic accident**

  X ● **V40.4   Person boarding or alighting a car injured in collision with pedestrian or animal**

  X ● **V40.5   Car driver injured in collision with pedestrian or animal in traffic accident**

  X ● **V40.6   Car passenger injured in collision with pedestrian or animal in traffic accident**

  X ● **V40.7   Person on outside of car injured in collision with pedestrian or animal in traffic accident**

  X ● **V40.9   Unspecified car occupant injured in collision with pedestrian or animal in traffic accident**

● **V41   Car occupant injured in collision with pedal cycle**

The appropriate 7th character is to be added to each code from category V41

> A   initial encounter
> D   subsequent encounter
> S   sequela

  X ● **V41.0   Car driver injured in collision with pedal cycle in nontraffic accident**

  X ● **V41.1   Car passenger injured in collision with pedal cycle in nontraffic accident**

  X ● **V41.2   Person on outside of car injured in collision with pedal cycle in nontraffic accident**

  X ● **V41.3   Unspecified car occupant injured in collision with pedal cycle in nontraffic accident**

  X ● **V41.4   Person boarding or alighting a car injured in collision with pedal cycle**

  X ● **V41.5   Car driver injured in collision with pedal cycle in traffic accident**

  X ● **V41.6   Car passenger injured in collision with pedal cycle in traffic accident**

CHAPTER 20 (V01-Y99)

X● **V41.7** Person on outside of car injured in collision with pedal cycle in traffic accident

X● **V41.9** Unspecified car occupant injured in collision with pedal cycle in traffic accident

● **V42** Car occupant injured in collision with two- or three-wheeled motor vehicle

> The appropriate 7th character is to be added to each code from category V42

> | A | initial encounter |
> |---|---|
> | D | subsequent encounter |
> | S | sequela |

X● **V42.0** Car driver injured in collision with two- or three-wheeled motor vehicle in nontraffic accident

X● **V42.1** Car passenger injured in collision with two- or three-wheeled motor vehicle in nontraffic accident

X● **V42.2** Person on outside of car injured in collision with two- or three-wheeled motor vehicle in nontraffic accident

X● **V42.3** Unspecified car occupant injured in collision with two- or three-wheeled motor vehicle in nontraffic accident

X● **V42.4** Person boarding or alighting a car injured in collision with two- or three-wheeled motor vehicle

X● **V42.5** Car driver injured in collision with two- or three-wheeled motor vehicle in traffic accident

X● **V42.6** Car passenger injured in collision with two- or three-wheeled motor vehicle in traffic accident

X● **V42.7** Person on outside of car injured in collision with two- or three-wheeled motor vehicle in traffic accident

X● **V42.9** Unspecified car occupant injured in collision with two- or three-wheeled motor vehicle in traffic accident

● **V43** Car occupant injured in collision with car, pick-up truck or van

> The appropriate 7th character is to be added to each code from category V43

> | A | initial encounter |
> |---|---|
> | D | subsequent encounter |
> | S | sequela |

● **V43.0** Car driver injured in collision with car, pick-up truck or van in nontraffic accident

X● **V43.01** Car driver injured in collision with sport utility vehicle in nontraffic accident

X● **V43.02** Car driver injured in collision with other type car in nontraffic accident

X● **V43.03** Car driver injured in collision with pick-up truck in nontraffic accident

X● **V43.04** Car driver injured in collision with van in nontraffic accident

● **V43.1** Car passenger injured in collision with car, pick-up truck or van in nontraffic accident

X● **V43.11** Car passenger injured in collision with sport utility vehicle in nontraffic accident

X● **V43.12** Car passenger injured in collision with other type car in nontraffic accident

X● **V43.13** Car passenger injured in collision with pick-up in nontraffic accident

X● **V43.14** Car passenger injured in collision with van in nontraffic accident

● **V43.2** Person on outside of car injured in collision with car, pick-up truck or van in nontraffic accident

X● **V43.21** Person on outside of car injured in collision with sport utility vehicle in nontraffic accident

X● **V43.22** Person on outside of car injured in collision with other type car in nontraffic accident

X● **V43.23** Person on outside of car injured in collision with pick-up truck in nontraffic accident

X● **V43.24** Person on outside of car injured in collision with van in nontraffic accident

● **V43.3** Unspecified car occupant injured in collision with car, pick-up truck or van in nontraffic accident

X● **V43.31** Unspecified car occupant injured in collision with sport utility vehicle in nontraffic accident

X● **V43.32** Unspecified car occupant injured in collision with other type car in nontraffic accident

X● **V43.33** Unspecified car occupant injured in collision with pick-up truck in nontraffic accident

X● **V43.34** Unspecified car occupant injured in collision with van in nontraffic accident

● **V43.4** Person boarding or alighting a car injured in collision with car, pick-up truck or van

X● **V43.41** Person boarding or alighting a car injured in collision with sport utility vehicle

X● **V43.42** Person boarding or alighting a car injured in collision with other type car

X● **V43.43** Person boarding or alighting a car injured in collision with pick-up truck

X● **V43.44** Person boarding or alighting a car injured in collision with van

● **V43.5** Car driver injured in collision with car, pick-up truck or van in traffic accident

X● **V43.51** Car driver injured in collision with sport utility vehicle in traffic accident

X● **V43.52** Car driver injured in collision with other type car in traffic accident

X● **V43.53** Car driver injured in collision with pick-up truck in traffic accident

X● **V43.54** Car driver injured in collision with van in traffic accident

● **V43.6** Car passenger injured in collision with car, pick-up truck or van in traffic accident

X● **V43.61** Car passenger injured in collision with sport utility vehicle in traffic accident
    Coding Clinic: 2015, Q1, P5-7

X● **V43.62** Car passenger injured in collision with other type car in traffic accident

X● **V43.63** Car passenger injured in collision with pick-up truck in traffic accident

X● **V43.64** Car passenger injured in collision with van in traffic accident

● **V43.7** Person on outside of car injured in collision with car, pick-up truck or van in traffic accident

X● **V43.71** Person on outside of car injured in collision with sport utility vehicle in traffic accident

X● **V43.72** Person on outside of car injured in collision with other type car in traffic accident

X● **V43.73** Person on outside of car injured in collision with pick-up truck in traffic accident

X● **V43.74** Person on outside of car injured in collision with van in traffic accident

● **V43.9** Unspecified car occupant injured in collision with car, pick-up truck or van in traffic accident

X● **V43.91** Unspecified car occupant injured in collision with sport utility vehicle in traffic accident

X● **V43.92** Unspecified car occupant injured in collision with other type car in traffic accident

X● **V43.93** Unspecified car occupant injured in collision with pick-up truck in traffic accident

X● **V43.94** Unspecified car occupant injured in collision with van in traffic accident

● **V44**   **Car occupant injured in collision with heavy transport vehicle or bus**

> **Excludes1**   car occupant injured in collision with military vehicle (V49.81)
>
> The appropriate 7th character is to be added to each code from category V44
>
> | | |
> |---|---|
> | A | initial encounter |
> | D | subsequent encounter |
> | S | sequela |

X ● **V44.0**   Car driver injured in collision with heavy transport vehicle or bus in nontraffic accident

X ● **V44.1**   Car passenger injured in collision with heavy transport vehicle or bus in nontraffic accident

X ● **V44.2**   Person on outside of car injured in collision with heavy transport vehicle or bus in nontraffic accident

X ● **V44.3**   Unspecified car occupant injured in collision with heavy transport vehicle or bus in nontraffic accident

X ● **V44.4**   Person boarding or alighting a car injured in collision with heavy transport vehicle or bus

X ● **V44.5**   Car driver injured in collision with heavy transport vehicle or bus in traffic accident

X ● **V44.6**   Car passenger injured in collision with heavy transport vehicle or bus in traffic accident

X ● **V44.7**   Person on outside of car injured in collision with heavy transport vehicle or bus in traffic accident

X ● **V44.9**   Unspecified car occupant injured in collision with heavy transport vehicle or bus in traffic accident

● **V45**   **Car occupant injured in collision with railway train or railway vehicle**

> The appropriate 7th character is to be added to each code from category V45
>
> | | |
> |---|---|
> | A | initial encounter |
> | D | subsequent encounter |
> | S | sequela |

X ● **V45.0**   Car driver injured in collision with railway train or railway vehicle in nontraffic accident

X ● **V45.1**   Car passenger injured in collision with railway train or railway vehicle in nontraffic accident

X ● **V45.2**   Person on outside of car injured in collision with railway train or railway vehicle in nontraffic accident

X ● **V45.3**   Unspecified car occupant injured in collision with railway train or railway vehicle in nontraffic accident

X ● **V45.4**   Person boarding or alighting a car injured in collision with railway train or railway vehicle

X ● **V45.5**   Car driver injured in collision with railway train or railway vehicle in traffic accident

X ● **V45.6**   Car passenger injured in collision with railway train or railway vehicle in traffic accident

X ● **V45.7**   Person on outside of car injured in collision with railway train or railway vehicle in traffic accident

X ● **V45.9**   Unspecified car occupant injured in collision with railway train or railway vehicle in traffic accident

● **V46**   **Car occupant injured in collision with other nonmotor vehicle**

> **Includes**   collision with animal-drawn vehicle, animal being ridden, streetcar
>
> The appropriate 7th character is to be added to each code from category V46
>
> | | |
> |---|---|
> | A | initial encounter |
> | D | subsequent encounter |
> | S | sequela |

X ● **V46.0**   Car driver injured in collision with other nonmotor vehicle in nontraffic accident

X ● **V46.1**   Car passenger injured in collision with other nonmotor vehicle in nontraffic accident

X ● **V46.2**   Person on outside of car injured in collision with other nonmotor vehicle in nontraffic accident

X ● **V46.3**   Unspecified car occupant injured in collision with other nonmotor vehicle in nontraffic accident

X ● **V46.4**   Person boarding or alighting a car injured in collision with other nonmotor vehicle

X ● **V46.5**   Car driver injured in collision with other nonmotor vehicle in traffic accident

X ● **V46.6**   Car passenger injured in collision with other nonmotor vehicle in traffic accident

X ● **V46.7**   Person on outside of car injured in collision with other nonmotor vehicle in traffic accident

X ● **V46.9**   Unspecified car occupant injured in collision with other nonmotor vehicle in traffic accident

● **V47**   **Car occupant injured in collision with fixed or stationary object**

> The appropriate 7th character is to be added to each code from category V47
>
> | | |
> |---|---|
> | A | initial encounter |
> | D | subsequent encounter |
> | S | sequela |

X ● **V47.0**   Car driver injured in collision with fixed or stationary object in nontraffic accident

> ~~V47.01   Driver of sport utility vehicle injured in collision with fixed or stationary object in nontraffic accident~~
>
> ~~V47.02   Driver of other type car injured in collision with fixed or stationary object in nontraffic accident~~

X ● **V47.1**   Car passenger injured in collision with fixed or stationary object in nontraffic accident

> ~~V47.11   Passenger of sport utility vehicle injured in collision with fixed or stationary object in nontraffic accident~~
>
> ~~V47.12   Passenger of other type car injured in collision with fixed or stationary object in nontraffic accident~~

X ● **V47.2**   Person on outside of car injured in collision with fixed or stationary object in nontraffic accident

X ● **V47.3**   Unspecified car occupant injured in collision with fixed or stationary object in nontraffic accident

> ~~V47.31   Unspecified occupant of sport utility vehicle injured in collision with fixed or stationary object in nontraffic accident~~
>
> ~~V47.32   Unspecified occupant of other type car injured in collision with fixed or stationary object in nontraffic accident~~

X ● **V47.4**   Person boarding or alighting a car injured in collision with fixed or stationary object

X ● **V47.5**   Car driver injured in collision with fixed or stationary object in traffic accident

> ~~V47.51   Driver of sport utility vehicle injured in collision with fixed or stationary object in traffic accident~~
>
> ~~V47.52   Driver of other type car injured in collision with fixed or stationary object in traffic accident~~

X ● **V47.6**   Car passenger injured in collision with fixed or stationary object in traffic accident

> ~~V47.61   Passenger of sport utility vehicle injured in collision with fixed or stationary object in traffic accident~~
>
> ~~V47.62   Passenger of other type car injured in collision with fixed or stationary object in traffic accident~~

X ● **V47.7**   Person on outside of car injured in collision with fixed or stationary object in traffic accident

X ● **V47.9**   Unspecified car occupant injured in collision with fixed or stationary object in traffic accident

> ~~V47.91   Unspecified occupant of sport utility vehicle injured in collision with fixed or stationary object in traffic accident~~
>
> ~~V47.92   Unspecified occupant of other type car injured in collision with fixed or stationary object in traffic accident~~

● V48   Car occupant injured in noncollision transport accident

> **Includes**   overturning car NOS
> overturning car without collision

The appropriate 7th character is to be added to each code from category V48

> A   initial encounter
> D   subsequent encounter
> S   sequela

X● V48.0   Car driver injured in noncollision transport accident in nontraffic accident

X● V48.1   Car passenger injured in noncollision transport accident in nontraffic accident

X● V48.2   Person on outside of car injured in noncollision transport accident in nontraffic accident

X● V48.3   Unspecified car occupant injured in noncollision transport accident in nontraffic accident

X● V48.4   Person boarding or alighting a car injured in noncollision transport accident

X● V48.5   Car driver injured in noncollision transport accident in traffic accident

X● V48.6   Car passenger injured in noncollision transport accident in traffic accident

X● V48.7   Person on outside of car injured in noncollision transport accident in traffic accident

X● V48.9   Unspecified car occupant injured in noncollision transport accident in traffic accident

● V49   Car occupant injured in other and unspecified transport accidents

The appropriate 7th character is to be added to each code from category V49

> A   initial encounter
> D   subsequent encounter
> S   sequela

● V49.0   Driver injured in collision with other and unspecified motor vehicles in nontraffic accident

X● V49.00   Driver injured in collision with unspecified motor vehicles in nontraffic accident

X● V49.09   Driver injured in collision with other motor vehicles in nontraffic accident

● V49.1   Passenger injured in collision with other and unspecified motor vehicles in nontraffic accident

X● V49.10   Passenger injured in collision with unspecified motor vehicles in nontraffic accident

X● V49.19   Passenger injured in collision with other motor vehicles in nontraffic accident

● V49.2   Unspecified car occupant injured in collision with other and unspecified motor vehicles in nontraffic accident

X● V49.20   Unspecified car occupant injured in collision with unspecified motor vehicles in nontraffic accident
> Car collision NOS, nontraffic

X● V49.29   Unspecified car occupant injured in collision with other motor vehicles in nontraffic accident

X● V49.3   Car occupant (driver) (passenger) injured in unspecified nontraffic accident
> Car accident NOS, nontraffic
> Car occupant injured in nontraffic accident NOS

● V49.4   Driver injured in collision with other and unspecified motor vehicles in traffic accident

X● V49.40   Driver injured in collision with unspecified motor vehicles in traffic accident

X● V49.49   Driver injured in collision with other motor vehicles in traffic accident

● V49.5   Passenger injured in collision with other and unspecified motor vehicles in traffic accident

X● V49.50   Passenger injured in collision with unspecified motor vehicles in traffic accident

X● V49.59   Passenger injured in collision with other motor vehicles in traffic accident

● V49.6   Unspecified car occupant injured in collision with other and unspecified motor vehicles in traffic accident

X● V49.60   Unspecified car occupant injured in collision with unspecified motor vehicles in traffic accident
> Car collision NOS (traffic)

X● V49.69   Unspecified car occupant injured in collision with other motor vehicles in traffic accident

● V49.8   Car occupant (driver) (passenger) injured in other specified transport accidents

X● V49.81   Car occupant (driver) (passenger) injured in transport accident with military vehicle

X● V49.88   Car occupant (driver) (passenger) injured in other specified transport accidents

X● V49.9   Car occupant (driver) (passenger) injured in unspecified traffic accident
> Car accident NOS
> **Coding Clinic: 2015, Q1, P11**

OCCUPANT OF PICK-UP TRUCK OR VAN INJURED IN TRANSPORT ACCIDENT (V50-V59)

> **Includes**   a four- or six-wheel motor vehicle designed primarily for carrying passengers and property but weighing less than the local limit for classification as a heavy goods vehicle
> minibus
> minivan
> sport utility vehicle (SUV)
> truck
> van

> **Excludes1**   heavy transport vehicle (V60-V69)

● V50   Occupant of pick-up truck or van injured in collision with pedestrian or animal

> **Excludes1**   pick-up truck or van collision with animal-drawn vehicle or animal being ridden (V56.-)

The appropriate 7th character is to be added to each code from category V50

> A   initial encounter
> D   subsequent encounter
> S   sequela

X● V50.0   Driver of pick-up truck or van injured in collision with pedestrian or animal in nontraffic accident

X● V50.1   Passenger in pick-up truck or van injured in collision with pedestrian or animal in nontraffic accident

X● V50.2   Person on outside of pick-up truck or van injured in collision with pedestrian or animal in nontraffic accident

X● V50.3   Unspecified occupant of pick-up truck or van injured in collision with pedestrian or animal in nontraffic accident

X● V50.4   Person boarding or alighting a pick-up truck or van injured in collision with pedestrian or animal

X● V50.5   Driver of pick-up truck or van injured in collision with pedestrian or animal in traffic accident

X● V50.6   Passenger in pick-up truck or van injured in collision with pedestrian or animal in traffic accident

X● V50.7   Person on outside of pick-up truck or van injured in collision with pedestrian or animal in traffic accident

X● V50.9   Unspecified occupant of pick-up truck or van injured in collision with pedestrian or animal in traffic accident

◀ New   ◀▥ Revised   ~~deleted~~ Deleted   Excludes 1   Excludes 2   Includes   Use additional   Code first   Code also   Unspecified
OGCR Official Guidelines   X Assign placeholder X   ● Use Additional Character(s)   ▸ Manifestation Code   **Coding Clinic**

● **V51** **Occupant of pick-up truck or van injured in collision with pedal cycle**

   The appropriate 7th character is to be added to each code from category V51

A	initial encounter
D	subsequent encounter
S	sequela

X● **V51.0** Driver of pick-up truck or van injured in collision with pedal cycle in nontraffic accident

X● **V51.1** Passenger in pick-up truck or van injured in collision with pedal cycle in nontraffic accident

X● **V51.2** Person on outside of pick-up truck or van injured in collision with pedal cycle in nontraffic accident

X● **V51.3** Unspecified occupant of pick-up truck or van injured in collision with pedal cycle in nontraffic accident

X● **V51.4** Person boarding or alighting a pick-up truck or van injured in collision with pedal cycle

X● **V51.5** Driver of pick-up truck or van injured in collision with pedal cycle in traffic accident

X● **V51.6** Passenger in pick-up truck or van injured in collision with pedal cycle in traffic accident

X● **V51.7** Person on outside of pick-up truck or van injured in collision with pedal cycle in traffic accident

X● **V51.9** Unspecified occupant of pick-up truck or van injured in collision with pedal cycle in traffic accident

● **V52** **Occupant of pick-up truck or van injured in collision with two- or three-wheeled motor vehicle**

   The appropriate 7th character is to be added to each code from category V52

A	initial encounter
D	subsequent encounter
S	sequela

X● **V52.0** Driver of pick-up truck or van injured in collision with two- or three-wheeled motor vehicle in nontraffic accident

X● **V52.1** Passenger in pick-up truck or van injured in collision with two- or three-wheeled motor vehicle in nontraffic accident

X● **V52.2** Person on outside of pick-up truck or van injured in collision with two- or three-wheeled motor vehicle in nontraffic accident

X● **V52.3** Unspecified occupant of pick-up truck or van injured in collision with two- or three-wheeled motor vehicle in nontraffic accident

X● **V52.4** Person boarding or alighting a pick-up truck or van injured in collision with two- or three-wheeled motor vehicle

X● **V52.5** Driver of pick-up truck or van injured in collision with two- or three-wheeled motor vehicle in traffic accident

X● **V52.6** Passenger in pick-up truck or van injured in collision with two- or three-wheeled motor vehicle in traffic accident

X● **V52.7** Person on outside of pick-up truck or van injured in collision with two- or three-wheeled motor vehicle in traffic accident

X● **V52.9** Unspecified occupant of pick-up truck or van injured in collision with two- or three-wheeled motor vehicle in traffic accident

● **V53** **Occupant of pick-up truck or van injured in collision with car, pick-up truck or van**

   The appropriate 7th character is to be added to each code from category V53

A	initial encounter
D	subsequent encounter
S	sequela

X● **V53.0** Driver of pick-up truck or van injured in collision with car, pick-up truck or van in nontraffic accident

X● **V53.1** Passenger in pick-up truck or van injured in collision with car, pick-up truck or van in nontraffic accident

X● **V53.2** Person on outside of pick-up truck or van injured in collision with car, pick-up truck or van in nontraffic accident

X● **V53.3** Unspecified occupant of pick-up truck or van injured in collision with car, pick-up truck or van in nontraffic accident

X● **V53.4** Person boarding or alighting a pick-up truck or van injured in collision with car, pick-up truck or van

X● **V53.5** Driver of pick-up truck or van injured in collision with car, pick-up truck or van in traffic accident

X● **V53.6** Passenger in pick-up truck or van injured in collision with car, pick-up truck or van in traffic accident

X● **V53.7** Person on outside of pick-up truck or van injured in collision with car, pick-up truck or van in traffic accident

X● **V53.9** Unspecified occupant of pick-up truck or van injured in collision with car, pick-up truck or van in traffic accident

● **V54** **Occupant of pick-up truck or van injured in collision with heavy transport vehicle or bus**

   Excludes1   occupant of pick-up truck or van injured in collision with military vehicle (V59.81)

   The appropriate 7th character is to be added to each code from category V54

A	initial encounter
D	subsequent encounter
S	sequela

X● **V54.0** Driver of pick-up truck or van injured in collision with heavy transport vehicle or bus in nontraffic accident

X● **V54.1** Passenger in pick-up truck or van injured in collision with heavy transport vehicle or bus in nontraffic accident

X● **V54.2** Person on outside of pick-up truck or van injured in collision with heavy transport vehicle or bus in nontraffic accident

X● **V54.3** Unspecified occupant of pick-up truck or van injured in collision with heavy transport vehicle or bus in nontraffic accident

X● **V54.4** Person boarding or alighting a pick-up truck or van injured in collision with heavy transport vehicle or bus

X● **V54.5** Driver of pick-up truck or van injured in collision with heavy transport vehicle or bus in traffic accident

X● **V54.6** Passenger in pick-up truck or van injured in collision with heavy transport vehicle or bus in traffic accident

X● **V54.7** Person on outside of pick-up truck or van injured in collision with heavy transport vehicle or bus in traffic accident

X● **V54.9** Unspecified occupant of pick-up truck or van injured in collision with heavy transport vehicle or bus in traffic accident

CHAPTER 20 (V01-Y99)

● **V55**   **Occupant of pick-up truck or van injured in collision with railway train or railway vehicle**

> The appropriate 7th character is to be added to each code from category V55

> A   initial encounter
> D   subsequent encounter
> S   sequela

X ● **V55.0**   Driver of pick-up truck or van injured in collision with railway train or railway vehicle in nontraffic accident

X ● **V55.1**   Passenger in pick-up truck or van injured in collision with railway train or railway vehicle in nontraffic accident

X ● **V55.2**   Person on outside of pick-up truck or van injured in collision with railway train or railway vehicle in nontraffic accident

X ● **V55.3**   Unspecified occupant of pick-up truck or van injured in collision with railway train or railway vehicle in nontraffic accident

X ● **V55.4**   Person boarding or alighting a pick-up truck or van injured in collision with railway train or railway vehicle

X ● **V55.5**   Driver of pick-up truck or van injured in collision with railway train or railway vehicle in traffic accident

X ● **V55.6**   Passenger in pick-up truck or van injured in collision with railway train or railway vehicle in traffic accident

X ● **V55.7**   Person on outside of pick-up truck or van injured in collision with railway train or railway vehicle in traffic accident

X ● **V55.9**   Unspecified occupant of pick-up truck or van injured in collision with railway train or railway vehicle in traffic accident

● **V56**   **Occupant of pick-up truck or van injured in collision with other nonmotor vehicle**

> **Includes**   collision with animal-drawn vehicle, animal being ridden, streetcar

> The appropriate 7th character is to be added to each code from category V56

> A   initial encounter
> D   subsequent encounter
> S   sequela

X ● **V56.0**   Driver of pick-up truck or van injured in collision with other nonmotor vehicle in nontraffic accident

X ● **V56.1**   Passenger in pick-up truck or van injured in collision with other nonmotor vehicle in nontraffic accident

X ● **V56.2**   Person on outside of pick-up truck or van injured in collision with other nonmotor vehicle in nontraffic accident

X ● **V56.3**   Unspecified occupant of pick-up truck or van injured in collision with other nonmotor vehicle in nontraffic accident

X ● **V56.4**   Person boarding or alighting a pick-up truck or van injured in collision with other nonmotor vehicle

X ● **V56.5**   Driver of pick-up truck or van injured in collision with other nonmotor vehicle in traffic accident

X ● **V56.6**   Passenger in pick-up truck or van injured in collision with other nonmotor vehicle in traffic accident

X ● **V56.7**   Person on outside of pick-up truck or van injured in collision with other nonmotor vehicle in traffic accident

X ● **V56.9**   Unspecified occupant of pick-up truck or van injured in collision with other nonmotor vehicle in traffic accident

● **V57**   **Occupant of pick-up truck or van injured in collision with fixed or stationary object**

> The appropriate 7th character is to be added to each code from category V57

> A   initial encounter
> D   subsequent encounter
> S   sequela

X ● **V57.0**   Driver of pick-up truck or van injured in collision with fixed or stationary object in nontraffic accident

X ● **V57.1**   Passenger in pick-up truck or van injured in collision with fixed or stationary object in nontraffic accident

X ● **V57.2**   Person on outside of pick-up truck or van injured in collision with fixed or stationary object in nontraffic accident

X ● **V57.3**   Unspecified occupant of pick-up truck or van injured in collision with fixed or stationary object in nontraffic accident

X ● **V57.4**   Person boarding or alighting a pick-up truck or van injured in collision with fixed or stationary object

X ● **V57.5**   Driver of pick-up truck or van injured in collision with fixed or stationary object in traffic accident

X ● **V57.6**   Passenger in pick-up truck or van injured in collision with fixed or stationary object in traffic accident

X ● **V57.7**   Person on outside of pick-up truck or van injured in collision with fixed or stationary object in traffic accident

X ● **V57.9**   Unspecified occupant of pick-up truck or van injured in collision with fixed or stationary object in traffic accident

● **V58**   **Occupant of pick-up truck or van injured in noncollision transport accident**

> **Includes**   overturning pick-up truck or van NOS
> overturning pick-up truck or van without collision

> The appropriate 7th character is to be added to each code from category V58

> A   initial encounter
> D   subsequent encounter
> S   sequela

X ● **V58.0**   Driver of pick-up truck or van injured in noncollision transport accident in nontraffic accident

X ● **V58.1**   Passenger in pick-up truck or van injured in noncollision transport accident in nontraffic accident

X ● **V58.2**   Person on outside of pick-up truck or van injured in noncollision transport accident in nontraffic accident

X ● **V58.3**   Unspecified occupant of pick-up truck or van injured in noncollision transport accident in nontraffic accident

X ● **V58.4**   Person boarding or alighting a pick-up truck or van injured in noncollision transport accident

X ● **V58.5**   Driver of pick-up truck or van injured in noncollision transport accident in traffic accident

X ● **V58.6**   Passenger in pick-up truck or van injured in noncollision transport accident in traffic accident

X ● **V58.7**   Person on outside of pick-up truck or van injured in noncollision transport accident in traffic accident

X ● **V58.9**   Unspecified occupant of pick-up truck or van injured in noncollision transport accident in traffic accident

◀ New   ◀▥ Revised   ~~deleted~~ Deleted   Excludes 1   Excludes 2   Includes   Use additional   Code first   Code also   Unspecified

1450   **OGCR** Official Guidelines   X Assign placeholder X   ● Use Additional Character(s)   ▶ Manifestation Code   **Coding Clinic**

● **V59**   **Occupant of pick-up truck or van injured in other and unspecified transport accidents**

> The appropriate 7th character is to be added to each code from category V59

> | | |
> |---|---|
> | A | initial encounter |
> | D | subsequent encounter |
> | S | sequela |

● **V59.0**   **Driver of pick-up truck or van injured in collision with other and unspecified motor vehicles in nontraffic accident**

   X● **V59.00**   Driver of pick-up truck or van injured in collision with unspecified motor vehicles in nontraffic accident

   X● **V59.09**   Driver of pick-up truck or van injured in collision with other motor vehicles in nontraffic accident

● **V59.1**   **Passenger in pick-up truck or van injured in collision with other and unspecified motor vehicles in nontraffic accident**

   X● **V59.10**   Passenger in pick-up truck or van injured in collision with unspecified motor vehicles in nontraffic accident

   X● **V59.19**   Passenger in pick-up truck or van injured in collision with other motor vehicles in nontraffic accident

● **V59.2**   **Unspecified occupant of pick-up truck or van injured in collision with other and unspecified motor vehicles in nontraffic accident**

   X● **V59.20**   Unspecified occupant of pick-up truck or van injured in collision with unspecified motor vehicles in nontraffic accident
      Collision NOS involving pick-up truck or van, nontraffic

   X● **V59.29**   Unspecified occupant of pick-up truck or van injured in collision with other motor vehicles in nontraffic accident

X● **V59.3**   **Occupant (driver) (passenger) of pick-up truck or van injured in unspecified nontraffic accident**
      Accident NOS involving pick-up truck or van, nontraffic
      Occupant of pick-up truck or van injured in nontraffic accident NOS

● **V59.4**   **Driver of pick-up truck or van injured in collision with other and unspecified motor vehicles in traffic accident**

   X● **V59.40**   Driver of pick-up truck or van injured in collision with unspecified motor vehicles in traffic accident

   X● **V59.49**   Driver of pick-up truck or van injured in collision with other motor vehicles in traffic accident

● **V59.5**   **Passenger in pick-up truck or van injured in collision with other and unspecified motor vehicles in traffic accident**

   X● **V59.50**   Passenger in pick-up truck or van injured in collision with unspecified motor vehicles in traffic accident

   X● **V59.59**   Passenger in pick-up truck or van injured in collision with other motor vehicles in traffic accident

● **V59.6**   **Unspecified occupant of pick-up truck or van injured in collision with other and unspecified motor vehicles in traffic accident**

   X● **V59.60**   Unspecified occupant of pick-up truck or van injured in collision with unspecified motor vehicles in traffic accident
      Collision NOS involving pick-up truck or van (traffic)

   X● **V59.69**   Unspecified occupant of pick-up truck or van injured in collision with other motor vehicles in traffic accident

X● **V59.8**   **Occupant (driver) (passenger) of pick-up truck or van injured in other specified transport accidents**

   X● **V59.81**   Occupant (driver) (passenger) of pick-up truck or van injured in transport accident with military vehicle

   X● **V59.88**   Occupant (driver) (passenger) of pick-up truck or van injured in other specified transport accidents

X● **V59.9**   **Occupant (driver) (passenger) of pick-up truck or van injured in unspecified traffic accident**
      Accident NOS involving pick-up truck or van

OCCUPANT OF HEAVY TRANSPORT VEHICLE INJURED IN TRANSPORT ACCIDENT (V60-V69)

> **Includes**   18 wheeler
>   armored car
>   panel truck
>
> **Excludes1**   bus
>   motorcoach

● **V60**   **Occupant of heavy transport vehicle injured in collision with pedestrian or animal**

> **Excludes1**   heavy transport vehicle collision with animal-drawn vehicle or animal being ridden (V66.-)

> The appropriate 7th character is to be added to each code from category V60

> | | |
> |---|---|
> | A | initial encounter |
> | D | subsequent encounter |
> | S | sequela |

   X● **V60.0**   Driver of heavy transport vehicle injured in collision with pedestrian or animal in nontraffic accident

   X● **V60.1**   Passenger in heavy transport vehicle injured in collision with pedestrian or animal in nontraffic accident

   X● **V60.2**   Person on outside of heavy transport vehicle injured in collision with pedestrian or animal in nontraffic accident

   X● **V60.3**   Unspecified occupant of heavy transport vehicle injured in collision with pedestrian or animal in nontraffic accident

   X● **V60.4**   Person boarding or alighting a heavy transport vehicle injured in collision with pedestrian or animal

   X● **V60.5**   Driver of heavy transport vehicle injured in collision with pedestrian or animal in traffic accident

   X● **V60.6**   Passenger in heavy transport vehicle injured in collision with pedestrian or animal in traffic accident

   X● **V60.7**   Person on outside of heavy transport vehicle injured in collision with pedestrian or animal in traffic accident

   X● **V60.9**   Unspecified occupant of heavy transport vehicle injured in collision with pedestrian or animal in traffic accident

● **V61**   **Occupant of heavy transport vehicle injured in collision with pedal cycle**

> The appropriate 7th character is to be added to each code from category V61

> | | |
> |---|---|
> | A | initial encounter |
> | D | subsequent encounter |
> | S | sequela |

   X● **V61.0**   Driver of heavy transport vehicle injured in collision with pedal cycle in nontraffic accident

   X● **V61.1**   Passenger in heavy transport vehicle injured in collision with pedal cycle in nontraffic accident

   X● **V61.2**   Person on outside of heavy transport vehicle injured in collision with pedal cycle in nontraffic accident

   X● **V61.3**   Unspecified occupant of heavy transport vehicle injured in collision with pedal cycle in nontraffic accident

   X● **V61.4**   Person boarding or alighting a heavy transport vehicle injured in collision with pedal cycle while boarding or alighting

   X● **V61.5**   Driver of heavy transport vehicle injured in collision with pedal cycle in traffic accident

X● **V61.6** Passenger in heavy transport vehicle injured in collision with pedal cycle in traffic accident

X● **V61.7** Person on outside of heavy transport vehicle injured in collision with pedal cycle in traffic accident

X● **V61.9** Unspecified occupant of heavy transport vehicle injured in collision with pedal cycle in traffic accident

●**V62** Occupant of heavy transport vehicle injured in collision with two- or three-wheeled motor vehicle

The appropriate 7th character is to be added to each code from category V62

A	initial encounter
D	subsequent encounter
S	sequela

X● **V62.0** Driver of heavy transport vehicle injured in collision with two- or three-wheeled motor vehicle in nontraffic accident

X● **V62.1** Passenger in heavy transport vehicle injured in collision with two- or three-wheeled motor vehicle in nontraffic accident

X● **V62.2** Person on outside of heavy transport vehicle injured in collision with two- or three-wheeled motor vehicle in nontraffic accident

X● **V62.3** Unspecified occupant of heavy transport vehicle injured in collision with two- or three-wheeled motor vehicle in nontraffic accident

X● **V62.4** Person boarding or alighting a heavy transport vehicle injured in collision with two- or three-wheeled motor vehicle

X● **V62.5** Driver of heavy transport vehicle injured in collision with two- or three-wheeled motor vehicle in traffic accident

X● **V62.6** Passenger in heavy transport vehicle injured in collision with two- or three-wheeled motor vehicle in traffic accident

X● **V62.7** Person on outside of heavy transport vehicle injured in collision with two- or three-wheeled motor vehicle in traffic accident

X● **V62.9** Unspecified occupant of heavy transport vehicle injured in collision with two- or three-wheeled motor vehicle in traffic accident

●**V63** Occupant of heavy transport vehicle injured in collision with car, pick-up truck or van

The appropriate 7th character is to be added to each code from category V63

A	initial encounter
D	subsequent encounter
S	sequela

X● **V63.0** Driver of heavy transport vehicle injured in collision with car, pick-up truck or van in nontraffic accident

X● **V63.1** Passenger in heavy transport vehicle injured in collision with car, pick-up truck or van in nontraffic accident

X● **V63.2** Person on outside of heavy transport vehicle injured in collision with car, pick-up truck or van in nontraffic accident

X● **V63.3** Unspecified occupant of heavy transport vehicle injured in collision with car, pick-up truck or van in nontraffic accident

X● **V63.4** Person boarding or alighting a heavy transport vehicle injured in collision with car, pick-up truck or van

X● **V63.5** Driver of heavy transport vehicle injured in collision with car, pick-up truck or van in traffic accident

X● **V63.6** Passenger in heavy transport vehicle injured in collision with car, pick-up truck or van in traffic accident

X● **V63.7** Person on outside of heavy transport vehicle injured in collision with car, pick-up truck or van in traffic accident

X● **V63.9** Unspecified occupant of heavy transport vehicle injured in collision with car, pick-up truck or van in traffic accident

●**V64** Occupant of heavy transport vehicle injured in collision with heavy transport vehicle or bus

Excludes1 occupant of heavy transport vehicle injured in collision with military vehicle (V69.81)

The appropriate 7th character is to be added to each code from category V64

A	initial encounter
D	subsequent encounter
S	sequela

X● **V64.0** Driver of heavy transport vehicle injured in collision with heavy transport vehicle or bus in nontraffic accident

X● **V64.1** Passenger in heavy transport vehicle injured in collision with heavy transport vehicle or bus in nontraffic accident

X● **V64.2** Person on outside of heavy transport vehicle injured in collision with heavy transport vehicle or bus in nontraffic accident

X● **V64.3** Unspecified occupant of heavy transport vehicle injured in collision with heavy transport vehicle or bus in nontraffic accident

X● **V64.4** Person boarding or alighting a heavy transport vehicle injured in collision with heavy transport vehicle or bus while boarding or alighting

X● **V64.5** Driver of heavy transport vehicle injured in collision with heavy transport vehicle or bus in traffic accident

X● **V64.6** Passenger in heavy transport vehicle injured in collision with heavy transport vehicle or bus in traffic accident

X● **V64.7** Person on outside of heavy transport vehicle injured in collision with heavy transport vehicle or bus in traffic accident

X● **V64.9** Unspecified occupant of heavy transport vehicle injured in collision with heavy transport vehicle or bus in traffic accident

●**V65** Occupant of heavy transport vehicle injured in collision with railway train or railway vehicle

The appropriate 7th character is to be added to each code from category V65

A	initial encounter
D	subsequent encounter
S	sequela

X● **V65.0** Driver of heavy transport vehicle injured in collision with railway train or railway vehicle in nontraffic accident

X● **V65.1** Passenger in heavy transport vehicle injured in collision with railway train or railway vehicle in nontraffic accident

X● **V65.2** Person on outside of heavy transport vehicle injured in collision with railway train or railway vehicle in nontraffic accident

X● **V65.3** Unspecified occupant of heavy transport vehicle injured in collision with railway train or railway vehicle in nontraffic accident

X● **V65.4** Person boarding or alighting a heavy transport vehicle injured in collision with railway train or railway vehicle

X● **V65.5** Driver of heavy transport vehicle injured in collision with railway train or railway vehicle in traffic accident

X● **V65.6** Passenger in heavy transport vehicle injured in collision with railway train or railway vehicle in traffic accident

X● **V65.7** Person on outside of heavy transport vehicle injured in collision with railway train or railway vehicle in traffic accident

X● **V65.9** Unspecified occupant of heavy transport vehicle injured in collision with railway train or railway vehicle in traffic accident

◀ New　◀▦ Revised　deleted Deleted　Excludes 1　Excludes 2　Includes　Use additional　Code first　Code also　Unspecified
OGCR Official Guidelines　X Assign placeholder X　● Use Additional Character(s)　▶ Manifestation Code　**Coding Clinic**

● **V66 Occupant of heavy transport vehicle injured in collision with other nonmotor vehicle**

> | **Includes** | collision with animal-drawn vehicle, animal being ridden, streetcar |
> |---|---|

> The appropriate 7th character is to be added to each code from category V66

> | A | initial encounter |
> |---|---|
> | D | subsequent encounter |
> | S | sequela |

X ● **V66.0 Driver of heavy transport vehicle injured in collision with other nonmotor vehicle in nontraffic accident**

X ● **V66.1 Passenger in heavy transport vehicle injured in collision with other nonmotor vehicle in nontraffic accident**

X ● **V66.2 Person on outside of heavy transport vehicle injured in collision with other nonmotor vehicle in nontraffic accident**

X ● **V66.3 Unspecified occupant of heavy transport vehicle injured in collision with other nonmotor vehicle in nontraffic accident**

X ● **V66.4 Person boarding or alighting a heavy transport vehicle injured in collision with other nonmotor vehicle**

X ● **V66.5 Driver of heavy transport vehicle injured in collision with other nonmotor vehicle in traffic accident**

X ● **V66.6 Passenger in heavy transport vehicle injured in collision with other nonmotor vehicle in traffic accident**

X ● **V66.7 Person on outside of heavy transport vehicle injured in collision with other nonmotor vehicle in traffic accident**

X ● **V66.9 Unspecified occupant of heavy transport vehicle injured in collision with other nonmotor vehicle in traffic accident**

● **V67 Occupant of heavy transport vehicle injured in collision with fixed or stationary object**

> The appropriate 7th character is to be added to each code from category V67

> | A | initial encounter |
> |---|---|
> | D | subsequent encounter |
> | S | sequela |

X ● **V67.0 Driver of heavy transport vehicle injured in collision with fixed or stationary object in nontraffic accident**

X ● **V67.1 Passenger in heavy transport vehicle injured in collision with fixed or stationary object in nontraffic accident**

X ● **V67.2 Person on outside of heavy transport vehicle injured in collision with fixed or stationary object in nontraffic accident**

X ● **V67.3 Unspecified occupant of heavy transport vehicle injured in collision with fixed or stationary object in nontraffic accident**

X ● **V67.4 Person boarding or alighting a heavy transport vehicle injured in collision with fixed or stationary object**

X ● **V67.5 Driver of heavy transport vehicle injured in collision with fixed or stationary object in traffic accident**

X ● **V67.6 Passenger in heavy transport vehicle injured in collision with fixed or stationary object in traffic accident**

X ● **V67.7 Person on outside of heavy transport vehicle injured in collision with fixed or stationary object in traffic accident**

X ● **V67.9 Unspecified occupant of heavy transport vehicle injured in collision with fixed or stationary object in traffic accident**

● **V68 Occupant of heavy transport vehicle injured in noncollision transport accident**

> | **Includes** | overturning heavy transport vehicle NOS overturning heavy transport vehicle without collision |
> |---|---|

> The appropriate 7th character is to be added to each code from category V68

> | A | initial encounter |
> |---|---|
> | D | subsequent encounter |
> | S | sequela |

X ● **V68.0 Driver of heavy transport vehicle injured in noncollision transport accident in nontraffic accident**

X ● **V68.1 Passenger in heavy transport vehicle injured in noncollision transport accident in nontraffic accident**

X ● **V68.2 Person on outside of heavy transport vehicle injured in noncollision transport accident in nontraffic accident**

X ● **V68.3 Unspecified occupant of heavy transport vehicle injured in noncollision transport accident in nontraffic accident**

X ● **V68.4 Person boarding or alighting a heavy transport vehicle injured in noncollision transport accident**

X ● **V68.5 Driver of heavy transport vehicle injured in noncollision transport accident in traffic accident**

X ● **V68.6 Passenger in heavy transport vehicle injured in noncollision transport accident in traffic accident**

X ● **V68.7 Person on outside of heavy transport vehicle injured in noncollision transport accident in traffic accident**

X ● **V68.9 Unspecified occupant of heavy transport vehicle injured in noncollision transport accident in traffic accident**

● **V69 Occupant of heavy transport vehicle injured in other and unspecified transport accidents**

> The appropriate 7th character is to be added to each code from category V69

> | A | initial encounter |
> |---|---|
> | D | subsequent encounter |
> | S | sequela |

● **V69.0 Driver of heavy transport vehicle injured in collision with other and unspecified motor vehicles in nontraffic accident**

    X ● **V69.00 Driver of heavy transport vehicle injured in collision with unspecified motor vehicles in nontraffic accident**

    X ● **V69.09 Driver of heavy transport vehicle injured in collision with other motor vehicles in nontraffic accident**

● **V69.1 Passenger in heavy transport vehicle injured in collision with other and unspecified motor vehicles in nontraffic accident**

    X ● **V69.10 Passenger in heavy transport vehicle injured in collision with unspecified motor vehicles in nontraffic accident**

    X ● **V69.19 Passenger in heavy transport vehicle injured in collision with other motor vehicles in nontraffic accident**

● **V69.2 Unspecified occupant of heavy transport vehicle injured in collision with other and unspecified motor vehicles in nontraffic accident**

    X ● **V69.20 Unspecified occupant of heavy transport vehicle injured in collision with unspecified motor vehicles in nontraffic accident**

        Collision NOS involving heavy transport vehicle, nontraffic

    X ● **V69.29 Unspecified occupant of heavy transport vehicle injured in collision with other motor vehicles in nontraffic accident**

X● **V69.3** Occupant (driver) (passenger) of heavy transport vehicle injured in unspecified nontraffic accident
  Accident NOS involving heavy transport vehicle, nontraffic
  Occupant of heavy transport vehicle injured in nontraffic accident NOS

● **V69.4** Driver of heavy transport vehicle injured in collision with other and unspecified motor vehicles in traffic accident

  X● **V69.40** Driver of heavy transport vehicle injured in collision with unspecified motor vehicles in traffic accident

  X● **V69.49** Driver of heavy transport vehicle injured in collision with other motor vehicles in traffic accident

● **V69.5** Passenger in heavy transport vehicle injured in collision with other and unspecified motor vehicles in traffic accident

  X● **V69.50** Passenger in heavy transport vehicle injured in collision with unspecified motor vehicles in traffic accident

  X● **V69.59** Passenger in heavy transport vehicle injured in collision with other motor vehicles in traffic accident

● **V69.6** Unspecified occupant of heavy transport vehicle injured in collision with other and unspecified motor vehicles in traffic accident

  X● **V69.60** Unspecified occupant of heavy transport vehicle injured in collision with unspecified motor vehicles in traffic accident
    Collision NOS involving heavy transport vehicle (traffic)

  X● **V69.69** Unspecified occupant of heavy transport vehicle injured in collision with other motor vehicles in traffic accident

● **V69.8** Occupant (driver) (passenger) of heavy transport vehicle injured in other specified transport accidents

  X● **V69.81** Occupant (driver) (passenger) of heavy transport vehicle injured in transport accidents with military vehicle

  X● **V69.88** Occupant (driver) (passenger) of heavy transport vehicle injured in other specified transport accidents

X● **V69.9** Occupant (driver) (passenger) of heavy transport vehicle injured in unspecified traffic accident
  Accident NOS involving heavy transport vehicle

BUS OCCUPANT INJURED IN TRANSPORT ACCIDENT (V70-V79)

Includes motorcoach
Excludes1 minibus (V50-V59)

● **V70** Bus occupant injured in collision with pedestrian or animal
  Excludes1 bus collision with animal-drawn vehicle or animal being ridden (V76.-)

  The appropriate 7th character is to be added to each code from category V70

A	initial encounter
D	subsequent encounter
S	sequela

  X● **V70.0** Driver of bus injured in collision with pedestrian or animal in nontraffic accident

  X● **V70.1** Passenger on bus injured in collision with pedestrian or animal in nontraffic accident

  X● **V70.2** Person on outside of bus injured in collision with pedestrian or animal in nontraffic accident

  X● **V70.3** Unspecified occupant of bus injured in collision with pedestrian or animal in nontraffic accident

  X● **V70.4** Person boarding or alighting from bus injured in collision with pedestrian or animal

  X● **V70.5** Driver of bus injured in collision with pedestrian or animal in traffic accident

  X● **V70.6** Passenger on bus injured in collision with pedestrian or animal in traffic accident

  X● **V70.7** Person on outside of bus injured in collision with pedestrian or animal in traffic accident

  X● **V70.9** Unspecified occupant of bus injured in collision with pedestrian or animal in traffic accident

● **V71** Bus occupant injured in collision with pedal cycle
  The appropriate 7th character is to be added to each code from category V71

A	initial encounter
D	subsequent encounter
S	sequela

  X● **V71.0** Driver of bus injured in collision with pedal cycle in nontraffic accident

  X● **V71.1** Passenger on bus injured in collision with pedal cycle in nontraffic accident

  X● **V71.2** Person on outside of bus injured in collision with pedal cycle in nontraffic accident

  X● **V71.3** Unspecified occupant of bus injured in collision with pedal cycle in nontraffic accident

  X● **V71.4** Person boarding or alighting from bus injured in collision with pedal cycle

  X● **V71.5** Driver of bus injured in collision with pedal cycle in traffic accident

  X● **V71.6** Passenger on bus injured in collision with pedal cycle in traffic accident

  X● **V71.7** Person on outside of bus injured in collision with pedal cycle in traffic accident

  X● **V71.9** Unspecified occupant of bus injured in collision with pedal cycle in traffic accident

● **V72** Bus occupant injured in collision with two- or three-wheeled motor vehicle
  The appropriate 7th character is to be added to each code from category V72

A	initial encounter
D	subsequent encounter
S	sequela

  X● **V72.0** Driver of bus injured in collision with two- or three-wheeled motor vehicle in nontraffic accident

  X● **V72.1** Passenger on bus injured in collision with two- or three-wheeled motor vehicle in nontraffic accident

  X● **V72.2** Person on outside of bus injured in collision with two- or three-wheeled motor vehicle in nontraffic accident

  X● **V72.3** Unspecified occupant of bus injured in collision with two- or three-wheeled motor vehicle in nontraffic accident

  X● **V72.4** Person boarding or alighting from bus injured in collision with two- or three-wheeled motor vehicle

  X● **V72.5** Driver of bus injured in collision with two- or three-wheeled motor vehicle in traffic accident

  X● **V72.6** Passenger on bus injured in collision with two- or three-wheeled motor vehicle in traffic accident

  X● **V72.7** Person on outside of bus injured in collision with two- or three-wheeled motor vehicle in traffic accident

  X● **V72.9** Unspecified occupant of bus injured in collision with two- or three-wheeled motor vehicle in traffic accident

● **V73** **Bus occupant injured in collision with car, pick-up truck or van**

The appropriate 7th character is to be added to each code from category V73

> A   initial encounter
> D   subsequent encounter
> S   sequela

X● **V73.0** Driver of bus injured in collision with car, pick-up truck or van in nontraffic accident

X● **V73.1** Passenger on bus injured in collision with car, pick-up truck or van in nontraffic accident

X● **V73.2** Person on outside of bus injured in collision with car, pick-up truck or van in nontraffic accident

X● **V73.3** Unspecified occupant of bus injured in collision with car, pick-up truck or van in nontraffic accident

X● **V73.4** Person boarding or alighting from bus injured in collision with car, pick-up truck or van

X● **V73.5** Driver of bus injured in collision with car, pick-up truck or van in traffic accident

X● **V73.6** Passenger on bus injured in collision with car, pick-up truck or van in traffic accident

X● **V73.7** Person on outside of bus injured in collision with car, pick-up truck or van in traffic accident

X● **V73.9** Unspecified occupant of bus injured in collision with car, pick-up truck or van in traffic accident

● **V74** **Bus occupant injured in collision with heavy transport vehicle or bus**

Excludes1 bus occupant injured in collision with military vehicle (V79.81)

The appropriate 7th character is to be added to each code from category V74

> A   initial encounter
> D   subsequent encounter
> S   sequela

X● **V74.0** Driver of bus injured in collision with heavy transport vehicle or bus in nontraffic accident

X● **V74.1** Passenger on bus injured in collision with heavy transport vehicle or bus in nontraffic accident

X● **V74.2** Person on outside of bus injured in collision with heavy transport vehicle or bus in nontraffic accident

X● **V74.3** Unspecified occupant of bus injured in collision with heavy transport vehicle or bus in nontraffic accident

X● **V74.4** Person boarding or alighting from bus injured in collision with heavy transport vehicle or bus

X● **V74.5** Driver of bus injured in collision with heavy transport vehicle or bus in traffic accident

X● **V74.6** Passenger on bus injured in collision with heavy transport vehicle or bus in traffic accident

X● **V74.7** Person on outside of bus injured in collision with heavy transport vehicle or bus in traffic accident

X● **V74.9** Unspecified occupant of bus injured in collision with heavy transport vehicle or bus in traffic accident

● **V75** **Bus occupant injured in collision with railway train or railway vehicle**

The appropriate 7th character is to be added to each code from category V75

> A   initial encounter
> D   subsequent encounter
> S   sequela

X● **V75.0** Driver of bus injured in collision with railway train or railway vehicle in nontraffic accident

X● **V75.1** Passenger on bus injured in collision with railway train or railway vehicle in nontraffic accident

X● **V75.2** Person on outside of bus injured in collision with railway train or railway vehicle in nontraffic accident

X● **V75.3** Unspecified occupant of bus injured in collision with railway train or railway vehicle in nontraffic accident

X● **V75.4** Person boarding or alighting from bus injured in collision with railway train or railway vehicle

X● **V75.5** Driver of bus injured in collision with railway train or railway vehicle in traffic accident

X● **V75.6** Passenger on bus injured in collision with railway train or railway vehicle in traffic accident

X● **V75.7** Person on outside of bus injured in collision with railway train or railway vehicle in traffic accident

X● **V75.9** Unspecified occupant of bus injured in collision with railway train or railway vehicle in traffic accident

● **V76** **Bus occupant injured in collision with other nonmotor vehicle**

Includes collision with animal-drawn vehicle, animal being ridden, streetcar

The appropriate 7th character is to be added to each code from category V76

> A   initial encounter
> D   subsequent encounter
> S   sequela

X● **V76.0** Driver of bus injured in collision with other nonmotor vehicle in nontraffic accident

X● **V76.1** Passenger on bus injured in collision with other nonmotor vehicle in nontraffic accident

X● **V76.2** Person on outside of bus injured in collision with other nonmotor vehicle in nontraffic accident

X● **V76.3** Unspecified occupant of bus injured in collision with other nonmotor vehicle in nontraffic accident

X● **V76.4** Person boarding or alighting from bus injured in collision with other nonmotor vehicle

X● **V76.5** Driver of bus injured in collision with other nonmotor vehicle in traffic accident

X● **V76.6** Passenger on bus injured in collision with other nonmotor vehicle in traffic accident

X● **V76.7** Person on outside of bus injured in collision with other nonmotor vehicle in traffic accident

X● **V76.9** Unspecified occupant of bus injured in collision with other nonmotor vehicle in traffic accident

● **V77** **Bus occupant injured in collision with fixed or stationary object**

The appropriate 7th character is to be added to each code from category V77

> A   initial encounter
> D   subsequent encounter
> S   sequela

X● **V77.0** Driver of bus injured in collision with fixed or stationary object in nontraffic accident

X● **V77.1** Passenger on bus injured in collision with fixed or stationary object in nontraffic accident

X● **V77.2** Person on outside of bus injured in collision with fixed or stationary object in nontraffic accident

X● **V77.3** Unspecified occupant of bus injured in collision with fixed or stationary object in nontraffic accident

X● **V77.4** Person boarding or alighting from bus injured in collision with fixed or stationary object

X● **V77.5** Driver of bus injured in collision with fixed or stationary object in traffic accident

X● **V77.6** Passenger on bus injured in collision with fixed or stationary object in traffic accident

X● **V77.7** Person on outside of bus injured in collision with fixed or stationary object in traffic accident

X● **V77.9** Unspecified occupant of bus injured in collision with fixed or stationary object in traffic accident

CHAPTER 20 (V01-Y99)

● **V78 Bus occupant injured in noncollision transport accident**

> **Includes**   overturning bus NOS
>   overturning bus without collision
>
> The appropriate 7th character is to be added to each code from category V78
>
> | A | initial encounter |
> |---|---|
> | D | subsequent encounter |
> | S | sequela |

X ● **V78.0 Driver of bus injured in noncollision transport accident in nontraffic accident**

X ● **V78.1 Passenger on bus injured in noncollision transport accident in nontraffic accident**

X ● **V78.2 Person on outside of bus injured in noncollision transport accident in nontraffic accident**

X ● **V78.3 Unspecified occupant of bus injured in noncollision transport accident in nontraffic accident**

X ● **V78.4 Person boarding or alighting from bus injured in noncollision transport accident**

X ● **V78.5 Driver of bus injured in noncollision transport accident in traffic accident**

X ● **V78.6 Passenger on bus injured in noncollision transport accident in traffic accident**

X ● **V78.7 Person on outside of bus injured in noncollision transport accident in traffic accident**

X ● **V78.9 Unspecified occupant of bus injured in noncollision transport accident in traffic accident**

● **V79 Bus occupant injured in other and unspecified transport accidents**

> The appropriate 7th character is to be added to each code from category V79
>
> | A | initial encounter |
> |---|---|
> | D | subsequent encounter |
> | S | sequela |

● **V79.0 Driver of bus injured in collision with other and unspecified motor vehicles in nontraffic accident**

X ● **V79.00 Driver of bus injured in collision with unspecified motor vehicles in nontraffic accident**

X ● **V79.09 Driver of bus injured in collision with other motor vehicles in nontraffic accident**

● **V79.1 Passenger on bus injured in collision with other and unspecified motor vehicles in nontraffic accident**

X ● **V79.10 Passenger on bus injured in collision with unspecified motor vehicles in nontraffic accident**

X ● **V79.19 Passenger on bus injured in collision with other motor vehicles in nontraffic accident**

● **V79.2 Unspecified bus occupant injured in collision with other and unspecified motor vehicles in nontraffic accident**

X ● **V79.20 Unspecified bus occupant injured in collision with unspecified motor vehicles in nontraffic accident**
> Bus collision NOS, nontraffic

X ● **V79.29 Unspecified bus occupant injured in collision with other motor vehicles in nontraffic accident**

X ● **V79.3 Bus occupant (driver) (passenger) injured in unspecified nontraffic accident**
> Bus accident NOS, nontraffic
> Bus occupant injured in nontraffic accident NOS

● **V79.4 Driver of bus injured in collision with other and unspecified motor vehicles in traffic accident**

X ● **V79.40 Driver of bus injured in collision with unspecified motor vehicles in traffic accident**

X ● **V79.49 Driver of bus injured in collision with other motor vehicles in traffic accident**

● **V79.5 Passenger on bus injured in collision with other and unspecified motor vehicles in traffic accident**

X ● **V79.50 Passenger on bus injured in collision with unspecified motor vehicles in traffic accident**

X ● **V79.59 Passenger on bus injured in collision with other motor vehicles in traffic accident**

● **V79.6 Unspecified bus occupant injured in collision with other and unspecified motor vehicles in traffic accident**

X ● **V79.60 Unspecified bus occupant injured in collision with unspecified motor vehicles in traffic accident**
> Bus collision NOS (traffic)

X ● **V79.69 Unspecified bus occupant injured in collision with other motor vehicles in traffic accident**

● **V79.8 Bus occupant (driver) (passenger) injured in other specified transport accidents**

X ● **V79.81 Bus occupant (driver) (passenger) injured in transport accidents with military vehicle**

X ● **V79.88 Bus occupant (driver) (passenger) injured in other specified transport accidents**

X ● **V79.9 Bus occupant (driver) (passenger) injured in unspecified traffic accident**
> Bus accident NOS

OTHER LAND TRANSPORT ACCIDENTS (V80-V89)

● **V80 Animal-rider or occupant of animal-drawn vehicle injured in transport accident**

> The appropriate 7th character is to be added to each code from category V80
>
> | A | initial encounter |
> |---|---|
> | D | subsequent encounter |
> | S | sequela |

● **V80.0 Animal-rider or occupant of animal drawn vehicle injured by fall from or being thrown from animal or animal-drawn vehicle in noncollision accident**

● **V80.01 Animal-rider injured by fall from or being thrown from animal in noncollision accident**

● **V80.010 Animal-rider injured by fall from or being thrown from horse in noncollision accident**

● **V80.018 Animal-rider injured by fall from or being thrown from other animal in noncollision accident**

X ● **V80.02 Occupant of animal-drawn vehicle injured by fall from or being thrown from animal-drawn vehicle in noncollision accident**
> Overturning animal-drawn vehicle NOS
> Overturning animal-drawn vehicle without collision

● **V80.1 Animal-rider or occupant of animal-drawn vehicle injured in collision with pedestrian or animal**

> **Excludes1**   animal-rider or animal-drawn vehicle collision with animal-drawn vehicle or animal being ridden (V80.7)

X ● **V80.11 Animal-rider injured in collision with pedestrian or animal**

X ● **V80.12 Occupant of animal-drawn vehicle injured in collision with pedestrian or animal**

● **V80.2 Animal-rider or occupant of animal-drawn vehicle injured in collision with pedal cycle**

X ● **V80.21 Animal-rider injured in collision with pedal cycle**

X ● **V80.22 Occupant of animal-drawn vehicle injured in collision with pedal cycle**

◀ New   ◀◀ Revised   ~~deleted~~ Deleted   Excludes 1   Excludes 2   Includes   Use additional   Code first   Code also   Unspecified

OGCR Official Guidelines   X Assign placeholder X   ● Use Additional Character(s)   ▶ Manifestation Code   **Coding Clinic**

● V80.3 Animal-rider or occupant of animal-drawn vehicle injured in collision with two- or three-wheeled motor vehicle

X ● V80.31 Animal-rider injured in collision with two- or three-wheeled motor vehicle

X ● V80.32 Occupant of animal-drawn vehicle injured in collision with two- or three-wheeled motor vehicle

● V80.4 Animal-rider or occupant of animal-drawn vehicle injured in collision with car, pick-up truck, van, heavy transport vehicle or bus

Excludes1   animal-rider injured in collision with military vehicle (V80.910)
             occupant of animal-drawn vehicle injured in collision with military vehicle (V80.920)

X ● V80.41 Animal-rider injured in collision with car, pick-up truck, van, heavy transport vehicle or bus

X ● V80.42 Occupant of animal-drawn vehicle injured in collision with car, pick-up truck, van, heavy transport vehicle or bus

● V80.5 Animal-rider or occupant of animal-drawn vehicle injured in collision with other specified motor vehicle

X ● V80.51 Animal-rider injured in collision with other specified motor vehicle

X ● V80.52 Occupant of animal-drawn vehicle injured in collision with other specified motor vehicle

● V80.6 Animal-rider or occupant of animal-drawn vehicle injured in collision with railway train or railway vehicle

X ● V80.61 Animal-rider injured in collision with railway train or railway vehicle

X ● V80.62 Occupant of animal-drawn vehicle injured in collision with railway train or railway vehicle

● V80.7 Animal-rider or occupant of animal-drawn vehicle injured in collision with other nonmotor vehicles

● V80.71 Animal-rider or occupant of animal-drawn vehicle injured in collision with animal being ridden

● V80.710 Animal-rider injured in collision with other animal being ridden

● V80.711 Occupant of animal-drawn vehicle injured in collision with animal being ridden

● V80.72 Animal-rider or occupant of animal-drawn vehicle injured in collision with other animal-drawn vehicle

● V80.720 Animal-rider injured in collision with animal-drawn vehicle

● V80.721 Occupant of animal-drawn vehicle injured in collision with other animal-drawn vehicle

● V80.73 Animal-rider or occupant of animal-drawn vehicle injured in collision with streetcar

● V80.730 Animal-rider injured in collision with streetcar

● V80.731 Occupant of animal-drawn vehicle injured in collision with streetcar

● V80.79 Animal-rider or occupant of animal-drawn vehicle injured in collision with other nonmotor vehicles

● V80.790 Animal-rider injured in collision with other nonmotor vehicles

● V80.791 Occupant of animal-drawn vehicle injured in collision with other nonmotor vehicles

● V80.8 Animal-rider or occupant of animal-drawn vehicle injured in collision with fixed or stationary object

X ● V80.81 Animal-rider injured in collision with fixed or stationary object

X ● V80.82 Occupant of animal-drawn vehicle injured in collision with fixed or stationary object

● V80.9 Animal-rider or occupant of animal-drawn vehicle injured in other and unspecified transport accidents

● V80.91 Animal-rider injured in other and unspecified transport accidents

● V80.910 Animal-rider injured in transport accident with military vehicle

● V80.918 Animal-rider injured in other transport accident

● V80.919 Animal-rider injured in unspecified transport accident
        Animal rider accident NOS

● V80.92 Occupant of animal-drawn vehicle injured in other and unspecified transport accidents

● V80.920 Occupant of animal-drawn vehicle injured in transport accident with military vehicle

● V80.928 Occupant of animal-drawn vehicle injured in other transport accident

● V80.929 Occupant of animal-drawn vehicle injured in unspecified transport accident
        Animal-drawn vehicle accident NOS

● V81 Occupant of railway train or railway vehicle injured in transport accident

Includes   derailment of railway train or railway vehicle
             person on outside of train

Excludes1   streetcar (V82.-)

The appropriate 7th character is to be added to each code from category V81

A	initial encounter
D	subsequent encounter
S	sequela

X ● V81.0 Occupant of railway train or railway vehicle injured in collision with motor vehicle in nontraffic accident

Excludes1   occupant of railway train or railway vehicle injured due to collision with military vehicle (V81.83)

X ● V81.1 Occupant of railway train or railway vehicle injured in collision with motor vehicle in traffic accident

Excludes1   occupant of railway train or railway vehicle injured due to collision with military vehicle (V81.83)

X ● V81.2 Occupant of railway train or railway vehicle injured in collision with or hit by rolling stock

X ● V81.3 Occupant of railway train or railway vehicle injured in collision with other object
        Railway collision NOS

X ● V81.4 Person injured while boarding or alighting from railway train or railway vehicle

X ● V81.5 Occupant of railway train or railway vehicle injured by fall in railway train or railway vehicle

X ● V81.6 Occupant of railway train or railway vehicle injured by fall from railway train or railway vehicle

X ● V81.7 Occupant of railway train or railway vehicle injured in derailment without antecedent collision

CHAPTER 20 (V01-Y99)

● **V81.8 Occupant of railway train or railway vehicle injured in other specified railway accidents**

  X ● **V81.81 Occupant of railway train or railway vehicle injured due to explosion or fire on train**

  X ● **V81.82 Occupant of railway train or railway vehicle injured due to object falling onto train**
       Occupant of railway train or railway vehicle injured due to falling earth onto train
       Occupant of railway train or railway vehicle injured due to falling rocks onto train
       Occupant of railway train or railway vehicle injured due to falling snow onto train
       Occupant of railway train or railway vehicle injured due to falling trees onto train

  X ● **V81.83 Occupant of railway train or railway vehicle injured due to collision with military vehicle**

  X ● **V81.89 Occupant of railway train or railway vehicle injured due to other specified railway accident**

X ● **V81.9 Occupant of railway train or railway vehicle injured in** `unspecified` **railway accident**
     Railway accident NOS

● **V82 Occupant of powered streetcar injured in transport accident**

    `Includes`   interurban electric car
                person on outside of streetcar
                tram (car)
                trolley (car)

    `Excludes1`   bus (V70-V79)
                motorcoach (V70-V79)
                nonpowered streetcar (V76.-)
                train (V81.-)

The appropriate 7th character is to be added to each code from category V82

A	initial encounter
D	subsequent encounter
S	sequela

X ● **V82.0 Occupant of streetcar injured in collision with motor vehicle in nontraffic accident**

X ● **V82.1 Occupant of streetcar injured in collision with motor vehicle in traffic accident**

X ● **V82.2 Occupant of streetcar injured in collision with or hit by rolling stock**

X ● **V82.3 Occupant of streetcar injured in collision with other object**
    `Excludes1`   collision with animal-drawn vehicle or animal being ridden (V82.8)

X ● **V82.4 Person injured while boarding or alighting from streetcar**

X ● **V82.5 Occupant of streetcar injured by fall in streetcar**
    `Excludes1`   fall in streetcar:
                 while boarding or alighting (V82.4)
                 with antecedent collision (V82.0-V82.3)

X ● **V82.6 Occupant of streetcar injured by fall from streetcar**
    `Excludes1`   fall from streetcar:
                 while boarding or alighting (V82.4)
                 with antecedent collision (V82.0-V82.3)

X ● **V82.7 Occupant of streetcar injured in derailment without antecedent collision**
    `Excludes1`   occupant of streetcar injured in derailment with antecedent collision (V82.0-V82.3)

X ● **V82.8 Occupant of streetcar injured in other specified transport accidents**
     Streetcar collision with military vehicle
     Streetcar collision with train or nonmotor vehicles

X ● **V82.9 Occupant of streetcar injured in** `unspecified` **traffic accident**
     Streetcar accident NOS

● **V83 Occupant of special vehicle mainly used on industrial premises injured in transport accident**

    `Includes`   battery-powered airport passenger vehicle
                battery-powered truck (baggage) (mail)
                coal-car in mine
                forklift (truck)
                logging car
                self-propelled industrial truck
                station baggage truck (powered)
                tram, truck, or tub (powered) in mine or quarry

    `Excludes1`   special construction vehicles (V85.-)
                special industrial vehicle in stationary use or maintenance (W31.-)

The appropriate 7th character is to be added to each code from category V83

A	initial encounter
D	subsequent encounter
S	sequela

X ● **V83.0 Driver of special industrial vehicle injured in traffic accident**

X ● **V83.1 Passenger of special industrial vehicle injured in traffic accident**

X ● **V83.2 Person on outside of special industrial vehicle injured in traffic accident**

X ● **V83.3** `Unspecified` **occupant of special industrial vehicle injured in traffic accident**

X ● **V83.4 Person injured while boarding or alighting from special industrial vehicle**

X ● **V83.5 Driver of special industrial vehicle injured in nontraffic accident**

X ● **V83.6 Passenger of special industrial vehicle injured in nontraffic accident**

X ● **V83.7 Person on outside of special industrial vehicle injured in nontraffic accident**

X ● **V83.9** `Unspecified` **occupant of special industrial vehicle injured in nontraffic accident**
     Special-industrial-vehicle accident NOS

● **V84 Occupant of special vehicle mainly used in agriculture injured in transport accident**

    `Includes`   self-propelled farm machinery
                tractor (and trailer)

    `Excludes1`   animal-powered farm machinery accident (W30.8-)
                contact with combine harvester (W30.0)
                special agricultural vehicle in stationary use or maintenance (W30.-)

The appropriate 7th character is to be added to each code from category V84

A	initial encounter
D	subsequent encounter
S	sequela

X ● **V84.0 Driver of special agricultural vehicle injured in traffic accident**

X ● **V84.1 Passenger of special agricultural vehicle injured in traffic accident**

X ● **V84.2 Person on outside of special agricultural vehicle injured in traffic accident**

X ● **V84.3** `Unspecified` **occupant of special agricultural vehicle injured in traffic accident**

X ● **V84.4 Person injured while boarding or alighting from special agricultural vehicle**

X ● **V84.5 Driver of special agricultural vehicle injured in nontraffic accident**

X ● **V84.6 Passenger of special agricultural vehicle injured in nontraffic accident**

X ● **V84.7 Person on outside of special agricultural vehicle injured in nontraffic accident**

X ● **V84.9** `Unspecified` **occupant of special agricultural vehicle injured in nontraffic accident**
     Special-agricultural vehicle accident NOS

◀ New   ◀◀ Revised   ~~deleted~~ Deleted   `Excludes 1`   `Excludes 2`   `Includes`   `Use additional`   `Code first`   `Code also`   `Unspecified`

1458   **OGCR** Official Guidelines   X Assign placeholder X   ● Use Additional Character(s)   ▶ Manifestation Code   **Coding Clinic**

● **V85**   **Occupant of special construction vehicle injured in transport accident**

Includes	bulldozer
	digger
	dump truck
	earth-leveller
	mechanical shovel
	road-roller

Excludes1	special industrial vehicle (V83.-)
	special construction vehicle in stationary use or maintenance (W31.-)

The appropriate 7th character is to be added to each code from category V85

A	initial encounter
D	subsequent encounter
S	sequela

X● **V85.0**   **Driver of special construction vehicle injured in traffic accident**

X● **V85.1**   **Passenger of special construction vehicle injured in traffic accident**

X● **V85.2**   **Person on outside of special construction vehicle injured in traffic accident**

X● **V85.3**   **Unspecified occupant of special construction vehicle injured in traffic accident**

X● **V85.4**   **Person injured while boarding or alighting from special construction vehicle**

X● **V85.5**   **Driver of special construction vehicle injured in nontraffic accident**

X● **V85.6**   **Passenger of special construction vehicle injured in nontraffic accident**

X● **V85.7**   **Person on outside of special construction vehicle injured in nontraffic accident**

X● **V85.9**   **Unspecified occupant of special construction vehicle injured in nontraffic accident**
     Special-construction-vehicle accident NOS

● **V86**   **Occupant of special all-terrain or other off-road motor vehicle, injured in transport accident**

Excludes1	special all-terrain vehicle in stationary use or maintenance (W31.-)
	sport-utility vehicle (V50-V59)
	three-wheeled motor vehicle designed for on-road use (V30-V39)

The appropriate 7th character is to be added to each code from category V86

A	initial encounter
D	subsequent encounter
S	sequela

● **V86.0**   **Driver of special all-terrain or other off-road motor vehicle injured in traffic accident**

X● **V86.01**   **Driver of ambulance or fire engine injured in traffic accident**

X● **V86.02**   **Driver of snowmobile injured in traffic accident**

X● **V86.03**   **Driver of dune buggy injured in traffic accident**

X● **V86.04**   **Driver of military vehicle injured in traffic accident**

X● **V86.09**   **Driver of other off-road special all-terrain or other off-road vehicle injured in traffic accident**
     Driver of dirt bike injured in traffic accident
     Driver of go cart injured in traffic accident
     Driver of golf cart injured in traffic accident

● **V86.1**   **Passenger of special all-terrain or other off-road motor vehicle injured in traffic accident**

X● **V86.11**   **Passenger of ambulance or fire engine injured in traffic accident**

X● **V86.12**   **Passenger of snowmobile injured in traffic accident**

X● **V86.13**   **Passenger of dune buggy injured in traffic accident**

X● **V86.14**   **Passenger of military vehicle injured in traffic accident**

X● **V86.19**   **Passenger of other off-road special all-terrain or other off-road off-road motor vehicle injured in traffic accident**
     Passenger of dirt bike injured in traffic accident
     Passenger of go cart injured in traffic accident
     Passenger of golf cart injured in traffic accident

● **V86.2**   **Person on outside of special all-terrain or other off-road motor vehicle injured in traffic accident**

X● **V86.21**   **Person on outside of ambulance or fire engine injured in traffic accident**

X● **V86.22**   **Person on outside of snowmobile injured in traffic accident**

X● **V86.23**   **Person on outside of dune buggy injured in traffic accident**

X● **V86.24**   **Person on outside of military vehicle injured in traffic accident**

X● **V86.29**   **Person on outside of other special all-terrain or off-road motor vehicle injured in traffic accident**
     Person on outside of dirt bike injured in traffic accident
     Person on outside of go cart in traffic accident
     Person on outside of golf cart injured in traffic accident

● **V86.3**   **Unspecified occupant of special all-terrain or other off-road motor vehicle injured in traffic accident**

X● **V86.31**   **Unspecified occupant of ambulance or fire engine injured in traffic accident**

X● **V86.32**   **Unspecified occupant of snowmobile injured in traffic accident**

X● **V86.33**   **Unspecified occupant of dune buggy injured in traffic accident**

X● **V86.34**   **Unspecified occupant of military vehicle injured in traffic accident**

X● **V86.39**   **Unspecified occupant of other special all-terrain or other off-road motor vehicle injured in traffic accident**
     Unspecified occupant of dirt bike injured in traffic accident
     Unspecified occupant of go cart injured in traffic accident
     Unspecified occupant of golf cart injured in traffic accident

● **V86.4**   **Person injured while boarding or alighting from special all-terrain or other off-road motor vehicle**

X● **V86.41**   **Person injured while boarding or alighting from ambulance or fire engine**

X● **V86.42**   **Person injured while boarding or alighting from snowmobile**

X● **V86.43**   **Person injured while boarding or alighting from dune buggy**

X● **V86.44**   **Person injured while boarding or alighting from military vehicle**

X● **V86.49**   **Person injured while boarding or alighting from other special all-terrain or other off-road motor vehicle**
     Person injured while boarding or alighting from dirt bike
     Person injured while boarding or alighting from go cart
     Person injured while boarding or alighting from golf cart

CHAPTER 20 (V01-Y99)

● V86.5   Driver of special all-terrain or other off-road motor vehicle injured in nontraffic accident

X● V86.51   Driver of ambulance or fire engine injured in nontraffic accident

X● V86.52   Driver of snowmobile injured in nontraffic accident

X● V86.53   Driver of dune buggy injured in nontraffic accident

X● V86.54   Driver of military vehicle injured in nontraffic accident

X● V86.59   Driver of other off-road special all-terrain or other off-road motor vehicle injured in nontraffic accident
   Driver of dirt bike injured in nontraffic accident
   Driver of go cart injured in nontraffic accident
   Driver of golf cart injured in nontraffic accident

● V86.6   Passenger of special all-terrain or other off-road motor vehicle injured in nontraffic accident

X● V86.61   Passenger of ambulance or fire engine injured in nontraffic accident

X● V86.62   Passenger of snowmobile injured in nontraffic accident

X● V86.63   Passenger of dune buggy injured in nontraffic accident

X● V86.64   Passenger of military vehicle injured in nontraffic accident

X● V86.69   Passenger of other special all-terrain or other off-road vehicle injured in nontraffic accident
   Passenger of dirt bike injured in nontraffic accident
   Passenger of go cart injured in nontraffic accident
   Passenger of golf cart injured in nontraffic accident

● V86.7   Person on outside of special all-terrain or other off-road motor vehicle injured in nontraffic accident

X● V86.71   Person on outside of ambulance or fire engine injured in nontraffic accident

X● V86.72   Person on outside of snowmobile injured in nontraffic accident

X● V86.73   Person on outside of dune buggy injured in nontraffic accident

X● V86.74   Person on outside of military vehicle injured in nontraffic accident

X● V86.79   Person on outside of other special all-terrain or other off-road motor vehicles injured in nontraffic accident
   Person on outside of dirt bike injured in nontraffic accident
   Person on outside of go cart injured in nontraffic accident
   Person on outside of golf cart injured in nontraffic accident

● V86.9   Unspecified occupant of special all-terrain or other off-road motor vehicle injured in nontraffic accident

X● V86.91   Unspecified occupant of ambulance or fire engine injured in nontraffic accident

X● V86.92   Unspecified occupant of snowmobile injured in nontraffic accident

X● V86.93   Unspecified occupant of dune buggy injured in nontraffic accident

X● V86.94   Unspecified occupant of military vehicle injured in nontraffic accident

X● V86.99   Unspecified occupant of other off-road special all-terrain or other off-road motor vehicle injured in nontraffic accident
   All-terrain motor-vehicle accident NOS
   Off-road motor-vehicle accident NOS
   Other motor-vehicle accident NOS
   Unspecified occupant of dirt bike injured in nontraffic accident
   Unspecified occupant of go cart injured in nontraffic accident
   Unspecified occupant of golf cart injured in nontraffic accident
   Unspecified occupant of race car injured in nontraffic accident

● V87   Traffic accident of specified type but victim's mode of transport unknown

   Excludes1   collision involving:
      pedal cycle (V10-V19)
      pedestrian (V01-V09)

   The appropriate 7th character is to be added to each code from category V87

A	initial encounter
D	subsequent encounter
S	sequela

X● V87.0   Person injured in collision between car and two- or three-wheeled powered vehicle (traffic)

X● V87.1   Person injured in collision between other motor vehicle and two- or three-wheeled motor vehicle (traffic)

X● V87.2   Person injured in collision between car and pick-up truck or van (traffic)

X● V87.3   Person injured in collision between car and bus (traffic)

X● V87.4   Person injured in collision between car and heavy transport vehicle (traffic)

X● V87.5   Person injured in collision between heavy transport vehicle and bus (traffic)

X● V87.6   Person injured in collision between railway train or railway vehicle and car (traffic)

X● V87.7   Person injured in collision between other specified motor vehicles (traffic)

X● V87.8   Person injured in other specified noncollision transport accidents involving motor vehicle (traffic)

X● V87.9   Person injured in other specified (collision) (noncollision) transport accidents involving nonmotor vehicle (traffic)

● V88   Nontraffic accident of specified type but victim's mode of transport unknown

   Excludes1   collision involving:
      pedal cycle (V10-V19)
      pedestrian (V01-V09)

   The appropriate 7th character is to be added to each code from category V88

A	initial encounter
D	subsequent encounter
S	sequela

X● V88.0   Person injured in collision between car and two- or three-wheeled motor vehicle, nontraffic

X● V88.1   Person injured in collision between other motor vehicle and two- or three-wheeled motor vehicle, nontraffic

X● V88.2   Person injured in collision between car and pick-up truck or van, nontraffic

X● **V88.3** **Person injured in collision between car and bus, nontraffic**

X● **V88.4** **Person injured in collision between car and heavy transport vehicle, nontraffic**

X● **V88.5** **Person injured in collision between heavy transport vehicle and bus, nontraffic**

X● **V88.6** **Person injured in collision between railway train or railway vehicle and car, nontraffic**

X● **V88.7** **Person injured in collision between other specified motor vehicle, nontraffic**

X● **V88.8** **Person injured in other specified noncollision transport accidents involving motor vehicle, nontraffic**

X● **V88.9** **Person injured in other specified (collision) (noncollision) transport accidents involving nonmotor vehicle, nontraffic**

● **V89** **Motor- or nonmotor-vehicle accident, type of vehicle unspecified**

The appropriate 7th character is to be added to each code from category V89

> A   initial encounter
> D   subsequent encounter
> S   sequela

X● **V89.0** **Person injured in unspecified motor-vehicle accident, nontraffic**
Motor-vehicle accident NOS, nontraffic

X● **V89.1** **Person injured in unspecified nonmotor-vehicle accident, nontraffic**
Nonmotor-vehicle accident NOS (nontraffic)

X● **V89.2** **Person injured in unspecified motor-vehicle accident, traffic**
Motor-vehicle accident [MVA] NOS
Road (traffic) accident [RTA] NOS

X● **V89.3** **Person injured in unspecified nonmotor-vehicle accident, traffic**
Nonmotor-vehicle traffic accident NOS

X● **V89.9** **Person injured in unspecified vehicle accident**
Collision NOS

WATER TRANSPORT ACCIDENTS (V90-V94)

● **V90** **Drowning and submersion due to accident to watercraft**
Excludes1 civilian water transport accident involving military watercraft (V94.81-)
fall into water not from watercraft (W16.-)
military watercraft accident in military or war operations (Y36.0-, Y37.0-)
water-transport–related drowning or submersion without accident to watercraft (V92.-)

The appropriate 7th character is to be added to each code from category V90

> A   initial encounter
> D   subsequent encounter
> S   sequela

● **V90.0** **Drowning and submersion due to watercraft overturning**

X● **V90.00** **Drowning and submersion due to merchant ship overturning**

X● **V90.01** **Drowning and submersion due to passenger ship overturning**
Drowning and submersion due to ferry-boat overturning
Drowning and submersion due to liner overturning

X● **V90.02** **Drowning and submersion due to fishing boat overturning**

X● **V90.03** **Drowning and submersion due to other powered watercraft overturning**
Drowning and submersion due to hovercraft (on open water) overturning
Drowning and submersion due to jet ski overturning

X● **V90.04** **Drowning and submersion due to sailboat overturning**

X● **V90.05** **Drowning and submersion due to canoe or kayak overturning**

X● **V90.06** **Drowning and submersion due to (nonpowered) inflatable craft overturning**

X● **V90.08** **Drowning and submersion due to other unpowered watercraft overturning**
Drowning and submersion due to windsurfer overturning

X● **V90.09** **Drowning and submersion due to unspecified watercraft overturning**
Drowning and submersion due to boat NOS overturning
Drowning and submersion due to ship NOS overturning
Drowning and submersion due to watercraft NOS overturning

● **V90.1** **Drowning and submersion due to watercraft sinking**

X● **V90.10** **Drowning and submersion due to merchant ship sinking**

X● **V90.11** **Drowning and submersion due to passenger ship sinking**
Drowning and submersion due to ferry-boat sinking
Drowning and submersion due to liner sinking

X● **V90.12** **Drowning and submersion due to fishing boat sinking**

X● **V90.13** **Drowning and submersion due to other powered watercraft sinking**
Drowning and submersion due to hovercraft (on open water) sinking
Drowning and submersion due to jet ski sinking

X● **V90.14** **Drowning and submersion due to sailboat sinking**

X● **V90.15** **Drowning and submersion due to canoe or kayak sinking**

X● **V90.16** **Drowning and submersion due to (nonpowered) inflatable craft sinking**

X● **V90.18** **Drowning and submersion due to other unpowered watercraft sinking**

X● **V90.19** **Drowning and submersion due to unspecified watercraft sinking**
Drowning and submersion due to boat NOS sinking
Drowning and submersion due to ship NOS sinking
Drowning and submersion due to watercraft NOS sinking

● **V90.2** **Drowning and submersion due to falling or jumping from burning watercraft**

X● **V90.20** **Drowning and submersion due to falling or jumping from burning merchant ship**

X● **V90.21** **Drowning and submersion due to falling or jumping from burning passenger ship**
Drowning and submersion due to falling or jumping from burning ferry-boat
Drowning and submersion due to falling or jumping from burning liner

X● **V90.22** **Drowning and submersion due to falling or jumping from burning fishing boat**

X● **V90.23** **Drowning and submersion due to falling or jumping from other burning powered watercraft**
Drowning and submersion due to falling and jumping from burning hovercraft (on open water)
Drowning and submersion due to falling and jumping from burning jet ski

X● **V90.24** **Drowning and submersion due to falling or jumping from burning sailboat**

X● **V90.25** **Drowning and submersion due to falling or jumping from burning canoe or kayak**

X● **V90.26** **Drowning and submersion due to falling or jumping from burning (nonpowered) inflatable craft**

X● **V90.27** **Drowning and submersion due to falling or jumping from burning water-skis**

X● **V90.28** **Drowning and submersion due to falling or jumping from other burning unpowered watercraft**
Drowning and submersion due to falling and jumping from burning surf-board
Drowning and submersion due to falling and jumping from burning windsurfer

X● **V90.29** **Drowning and submersion due to falling or jumping from unspecified burning watercraft**
Drowning and submersion due to falling or jumping from burning boat NOS
Drowning and submersion due to falling or jumping from burning ship NOS
Drowning and submersion due to falling or jumping from burning watercraft NOS

● **V90.3** **Drowning and submersion due to falling or jumping from crushed watercraft**

X● **V90.30** **Drowning and submersion due to falling or jumping from crushed merchant ship**

X● **V90.31** **Drowning and submersion due to falling or jumping from crushed passenger ship**
Drowning and submersion due to falling and jumping from crushed ferry-boat
Drowning and submersion due to falling and jumping from crushed liner

X● **V90.32** **Drowning and submersion due to falling or jumping from crushed fishing boat**

X● **V90.33** **Drowning and submersion due to falling or jumping from other crushed powered watercraft**
Drowning and submersion due to falling and jumping from crushed hovercraft
Drowning and submersion due to falling and jumping from crushed jet ski

X● **V90.34** **Drowning and submersion due to falling or jumping from crushed sailboat**

X● **V90.35** **Drowning and submersion due to falling or jumping from crushed canoe or kayak**

X● **V90.36** **Drowning and submersion due to falling or jumping from crushed (nonpowered) inflatable craft**

X● **V90.37** **Drowning and submersion due to falling or jumping from crushed water-skis**

X● **V90.38** **Drowning and submersion due to falling or jumping from other crushed unpowered watercraft**
Drowning and submersion due to falling and jumping from crushed surf-board
Drowning and submersion due to falling and jumping from crushed windsurfer

X● **V90.39** **Drowning and submersion due to falling or jumping from crushed unspecified watercraft**
Drowning and submersion due to falling and jumping from crushed boat NOS
Drowning and submersion due to falling and jumping from crushed ship NOS
Drowning and submersion due to falling and jumping from crushed watercraft NOS

● **V90.8** **Drowning and submersion due to other accident to watercraft**

X● **V90.80** **Drowning and submersion due to other accident to merchant ship**

X● **V90.81** **Drowning and submersion due to other accident to passenger ship**
Drowning and submersion due to other accident to ferry-boat
Drowning and submersion due to other accident to liner

X● **V90.82** **Drowning and submersion due to other accident to fishing boat**

X● **V90.83** **Drowning and submersion due to other accident to other powered watercraft**
Drowning and submersion due to other accident to hovercraft (on open water)
Drowning and submersion due to other accident to jet ski

X● **V90.84** **Drowning and submersion due to other accident to sailboat**

X● **V90.85** **Drowning and submersion due to other accident to canoe or kayak**

X● **V90.86** **Drowning and submersion due to other accident to (nonpowered) inflatable craft**

X● **V90.87** **Drowning and submersion due to other accident to water-skis**

X● **V90.88** **Drowning and submersion due to other accident to other unpowered watercraft**
Drowning and submersion due to other accident to surf-board
Drowning and submersion due to other accident to windsurfer

X● **V90.89** **Drowning and submersion due to other accident to unspecified watercraft**
Drowning and submersion due to other accident to boat NOS
Drowning and submersion due to other accident to ship NOS
Drowning and submersion due to other accident to watercraft NOS

● **V91** **Other injury due to accident to watercraft**

Includes any injury except drowning and submersion as a result of an accident to watercraft

Excludes1 civilian water transport accident involving military watercraft (V94.81-)
military watercraft accident in military or war operations (Y36, Y37.-)

Excludes2 drowning and submersion due to accident to watercraft (V90.-)

The appropriate 7th character is to be added to each code from category V91

A	initial encounter
D	subsequent encounter
S	sequela

● **V91.0** **Burn due to watercraft on fire**

Excludes1 burn from localized fire or explosion on board ship without accident to watercraft (V93.-)

X● **V91.00** **Burn due to merchant ship on fire**

X● **V91.01** **Burn due to passenger ship on fire**
Burn due to ferry-boat on fire
Burn due to liner on fire

X● **V91.02** **Burn due to fishing boat on fire**

X● **V91.03** **Burn due to other powered watercraft on fire**
Burn due to hovercraft (on open water) on fire
Burn due to jet ski on fire

X● **V91.04** **Burn due to sailboat on fire**

X● **V91.05** **Burn due to canoe or kayak on fire**

X● **V91.06** **Burn due to (nonpowered) inflatable craft on fire**

X● **V91.07** **Burn due to water-skis on fire**

X● **V91.08** **Burn due to other unpowered watercraft on fire**

X● **V91.09** **Burn due to unspecified watercraft on fire**
Burn due to boat NOS on fire
Burn due to ship NOS on fire
Burn due to watercraft NOS on fire

● **V91.1**   **Crushed between watercraft and other watercraft or other object due to collision**
> Crushed by lifeboat after abandoning ship in a collision
>
> **Note:** Select the specified type of watercraft that the victim was on at the time of the collision.

X● **V91.10**   **Crushed between merchant ship and other watercraft or other object due to collision**

X● **V91.11**   **Crushed between passenger ship and other watercraft or other object due to collision**
> Crushed between ferry-boat and other watercraft or other object due to collision
> Crushed between liner and other watercraft or other object due to collision

X● **V91.12**   **Crushed between fishing boat and other watercraft or other object due to collision**

X● **V91.13**   **Crushed between other powered watercraft and other watercraft or other object due to collision**
> Crushed between hovercraft (on open water) and other watercraft or other object due to collision
> Crushed between jet ski and other watercraft or other object due to collision

X● **V91.14**   **Crushed between sailboat and other watercraft or other object due to collision**

X● **V91.15**   **Crushed between canoe or kayak and other watercraft or other object due to collision**

X● **V91.16**   **Crushed between (nonpowered) inflatable craft and other watercraft or other object due to collision**

X● **V91.18**   **Crushed between other unpowered watercraft and other watercraft or other object due to collision**
> Crushed between surfboard and other watercraft or other object due to collision
> Crushed between windsurfer and other watercraft or other object due to collision

X● **V91.19**   **Crushed between** unspecified **watercraft and other watercraft or other object due to collision**
> Crushed between boat NOS and other watercraft or other object due to collision
> Crushed between ship NOS and other watercraft or other object due to collision
> Crushed between watercraft NOS and other watercraft or other object due to collision

● **V91.2**   **Fall due to collision between watercraft and other watercraft or other object**
> Fall while remaining on watercraft after collision
>
> **Note:** Select the specified type of watercraft that the victim was on at the time of the collision.
>
> **Excludes1**   crushed between watercraft and other watercraft and other object due to collision (V91.1-)
> drowning and submersion due to falling from crushed watercraft (V90.3-)

X● **V91.20**   **Fall due to collision between merchant ship and other watercraft or other object**

X● **V91.21**   **Fall due to collision between passenger ship and other watercraft or other object**
> Fall due to collision between ferry-boat and other watercraft or other object
> Fall due to collision between liner and other watercraft or other object

X● **V91.22**   **Fall due to collision between fishing boat and other watercraft or other object**

X● **V91.23**   **Fall due to collision between other powered watercraft and other watercraft or other object**
> Fall due to collision between hovercraft (on open water) and other watercraft or other object
> Fall due to collision between jet ski and other watercraft or other object

X● **V91.24**   **Fall due to collision between sailboat and other watercraft or other object**

X● **V91.25**   **Fall due to collision between canoe or kayak and other watercraft or other object**

X● **V91.26**   **Fall due to collision between (nonpowered) inflatable craft and other watercraft or other object**

X● **V91.29**   **Fall due to collision between** unspecified **watercraft and other watercraft or other object**
> Fall due to collision between boat NOS and other watercraft or other object
> Fall due to collision between ship NOS and other watercraft or other object
> Fall due to collision between watercraft NOS and other watercraft or other object

● **V91.3**   **Hit or struck by falling object due to accident to watercraft**
> Hit or struck by falling object (part of damaged watercraft or other object) after falling or jumping from damaged watercraft
>
> **Excludes2**   drowning or submersion due to fall or jumping from damaged watercraft (V90.2-, V90.3-)

X● **V91.30**   **Hit or struck by falling object due to accident to merchant ship**

X● **V91.31**   **Hit or struck by falling object due to accident to passenger ship**
> Hit or struck by falling object due to accident to ferry-boat
> Hit or struck by falling object due to accident to liner

X● **V91.32**   **Hit or struck by falling object due to accident to fishing boat**

X● **V91.33**   **Hit or struck by falling object due to accident to other powered watercraft**
> Hit or struck by falling object due to accident to hovercraft (on open water)
> Hit or struck by falling object due to accident to jet ski

X● **V91.34**   **Hit or struck by falling object due to accident to sailboat**

X● **V91.35**   **Hit or struck by falling object due to accident to canoe or kayak**

X● **V91.36**   **Hit or struck by falling object due to accident to (nonpowered) inflatable craft**

X● **V91.37**   **Hit or struck by falling object due to accident to water-skis**
> Hit by water-skis after jumping off of waterskis

X● **V91.38**   **Hit or struck by falling object due to accident to other unpowered watercraft**
> Hit or struck by surf-board after falling off damaged surf-board
> Hit or struck by object after falling off damaged windsurfer

X● **V91.39**   **Hit or struck by falling object due to accident to** unspecified **watercraft**
> Hit or struck by falling object due to accident to boat NOS
> Hit or struck by falling object due to accident to ship NOS
> Hit or struck by falling object due to accident to watercraft NOS

- ● V91.8   Other injury due to other accident to watercraft
  - X ● V91.80   **Other injury due to other accident to merchant ship**
  - X ● V91.81   **Other injury due to other accident to passenger ship**
    - Other injury due to other accident to ferry-boat
    - Other injury due to other accident to liner
  - X ● V91.82   **Other injury due to other accident to fishing boat**
  - X ● V91.83   **Other injury due to other accident to other powered watercraft**
    - Other injury due to other accident to hovercraft (on open water)
    - Other injury due to other accident to jet ski
  - X ● V91.84   **Other injury due to other accident to sailboat**
  - X ● V91.85   **Other injury due to other accident to canoe or kayak**
  - X ● V91.86   **Other injury due to other accident to (nonpowered) inflatable craft**
  - X ● V91.87   **Other injury due to other accident to water-skis**
  - X ● V91.88   **Other injury due to other accident to other unpowered watercraft**
    - Other injury due to other accident to surf-board
    - Other injury due to other accident to windsurfer
  - X ● V91.89   **Other injury due to other accident to** `unspecified` **watercraft**
    - Other injury due to other accident to boat NOS
    - Other injury due to other accident to ship NOS
    - Other injury due to other accident to watercraft NOS

- ● V92   **Drowning and submersion due to accident on board watercraft, without accident to watercraft**
  - `Excludes1`   civilian water transport accident involving military watercraft (V94.81-)
    - drowning or submersion due to accident to watercraft (V90-V91)
    - drowning or submersion of diver who voluntarily jumps from boat not involved in an accident (W16.711, W16.721)
    - fall into water without watercraft (W16.-)
    - military watercraft accident in military or war operations (Y36, Y37)

  The appropriate 7th character is to be added to each code from category V92

A	initial encounter
D	subsequent encounter
S	sequela

- ● V92.0   **Drowning and submersion due to fall off watercraft**
  - Drowning and submersion due to fall from gangplank of watercraft
  - Drowning and submersion due to fall overboard watercraft
  - `Excludes2`   hitting head on object or bottom of body of water due to fall from watercraft (V94.0-)
  - X ● V92.00   **Drowning and submersion due to fall off merchant ship**
  - X ● V92.01   **Drowning and submersion due to fall off passenger ship**
    - Drowning and submersion due to fall off ferry-boat
    - Drowning and submersion due to fall off liner
  - X ● V92.02   **Drowning and submersion due to fall off fishing boat**

- X ● V92.03   **Drowning and submersion due to fall off other powered watercraft**
  - Drowning and submersion due to fall off hovercraft (on open water)
  - Drowning and submersion due to fall off jet ski
- X ● V92.04   **Drowning and submersion due to fall off sailboat**
- X ● V92.05   **Drowning and submersion due to fall off canoe or kayak**
- X ● V92.06   **Drowning and submersion due to fall off (nonpowered) inflatable craft**
- X ● V92.07   **Drowning and submersion due to fall off water-skis**
  - `Excludes1`   drowning and submersion due to falling off burning water-skis (V90.27)
    - drowning and submersion due to falling off crushed water-skis (V90.37)
    - hit by boat while water-skiing NOS (V94.X)
- X ● V92.08   **Drowning and submersion due to fall off other unpowered watercraft**
  - Drowning and submersion due to fall off surf-board
  - Drowning and submersion due to fall off windsurfer
  - `Excludes1`   drowning and submersion due to fall off burning unpowered watercraft (V90.28)
    - drowning and submersion due to fall off crushed unpowered watercraft (V90.38)
    - drowning and submersion due to fall off damaged unpowered watercraft (V90.88)
    - drowning and submersion due to rider of nonpowered watercraft being hit by other watercraft (V94.-)
    - other injury due to rider of nonpowered watercraft being hit by other watercraft (V94.-)
- X ● V92.09   **Drowning and submersion due to fall off** `unspecified` **watercraft**
  - Drowning and submersion due to fall off boat NOS
  - Drowning and submersion due to fall off ship NOS
  - Drowning and submersion due to fall off watercraft NOS

- ● V92.1   **Drowning and submersion due to being thrown overboard by motion of watercraft**
  - `Excludes1`   drowning and submersion due to fall off surf-board (V92.08)
    - drowning and submersion due to fall off water-skis (V92.07)
    - drowning and submersion due to fall off windsurfer (V92.08)
  - X ● V92.10   **Drowning and submersion due to being thrown overboard by motion of merchant ship**
  - X ● V92.11   **Drowning and submersion due to being thrown overboard by motion of passenger ship**
    - Drowning and submersion due to being thrown overboard by motion of ferry-boat
    - Drowning and submersion due to being thrown overboard by motion of liner

X● **V92.12** **Drowning and submersion due to being thrown overboard by motion of fishing boat**

X● **V92.13** **Drowning and submersion due to being thrown overboard by motion of other powered watercraft**
     Drowning and submersion due to being thrown overboard by motion of hovercraft

X● **V92.14** **Drowning and submersion due to being thrown overboard by motion of sailboat**

X● **V92.15** **Drowning and submersion due to being thrown overboard by motion of canoe or kayak**

X● **V92.16** **Drowning and submersion due to being thrown overboard by motion of (nonpowered) inflatable craft**

X● **V92.19** **Drowning and submersion due to being thrown overboard by motion of unspecified watercraft**
     Drowning and submersion due to being thrown overboard by motion of boat NOS
     Drowning and submersion due to being thrown overboard by motion of ship NOS
     Drowning and submersion due to being thrown overboard by motion of watercraft NOS

●**V92.2** **Drowning and submersion due to being washed overboard from watercraft**
     Code first any associated cataclysm (X37.0-)

X● **V92.20** **Drowning and submersion due to being washed overboard from merchant ship**

X● **V92.21** **Drowning and submersion due to being washed overboard from passenger ship**
     Drowning and submersion due to being washed overboard from ferry-boat
     Drowning and submersion due to being washed overboard from liner

X● **V92.22** **Drowning and submersion due to being washed overboard from fishing boat**

X● **V92.23** **Drowning and submersion due to being washed overboard from other powered watercraft**
     Drowning and submersion due to being washed overboard from hovercraft (on open water)
     Drowning and submersion due to being washed overboard from jet ski

X● **V92.24** **Drowning and submersion due to being washed overboard from sailboat**

X● **V92.25** **Drowning and submersion due to being washed overboard from canoe or kayak**

X● **V92.26** **Drowning and submersion due to being washed overboard from (nonpowered) inflatable craft**

X● **V92.27** **Drowning and submersion due to being washed overboard from water-skis**
     Excludes1   drowning and submersion due to fall off water-skis (V92.07)

X● **V92.28** **Drowning and submersion due to being washed overboard from other unpowered watercraft**
     Drowning and submersion due to being washed overboard from surf-board
     Drowning and submersion due to being washed overboard from windsurfer

X● **V92.29** **Drowning and submersion due to being washed overboard from unspecified watercraft**
     Drowning and submersion due to being washed overboard from boat NOS
     Drowning and submersion due to being washed overboard from ship NOS
     Drowning and submersion due to being washed overboard from watercraft NOS

●**V93** **Other injury due to accident on board watercraft, without accident to watercraft**
     Excludes1   civilian water transport accident involving military watercraft (V94.81-)
     other injury due to accident to watercraft (V91.-)
     military watercraft accident in military or war operations (Y36, Y37.-)
     Excludes2   drowning and submersion due to accident on board watercraft, without accident to watercraft (V92.-)

The appropriate 7th character is to be added to each code from category V93

> A   initial encounter
> D   subsequent encounter
> S   sequela

●**V93.0** **Burn due to localized fire on board watercraft**
     Excludes1   burn due to watercraft on fire (V91.0-)

X● **V93.00** **Burn due to localized fire on board merchant vessel**

X● **V93.01** **Burn due to localized fire on board passenger vessel**
     Burn due to localized fire on board ferry-boat
     Burn due to localized fire on board liner

X● **V93.02** **Burn due to localized fire on board fishing boat**

X● **V93.03** **Burn due to localized fire on board other powered watercraft**
     Burn due to localized fire on board hovercraft
     Burn due to localized fire on board jet ski

X● **V93.04** **Burn due to localized fire on board sailboat**

X● **V93.09** **Burn due to localized fire on board unspecified watercraft**
     Burn due to localized fire on board boat NOS
     Burn due to localized fire on board ship NOS
     Burn due to localized fire on board watercraft NOS

●**V93.1** **Other burn on board watercraft**
     Burn due to source other than fire on board watercraft
     Excludes1   burn due to watercraft on fire (V91.0-)

X● **V93.10** **Other burn on board merchant vessel**

X● **V93.11** **Other burn on board passenger vessel**
     Other burn on board ferry-boat
     Other burn on board liner

X● **V93.12** **Other burn on board fishing boat**

X● **V93.13** **Other burn on board other powered watercraft**
     Other burn on board hovercraft
     Other burn on board jet ski

X● **V93.14** **Other burn on board sailboat**

X● **V93.19** **Other burn on board unspecified watercraft**
     Other burn on board boat NOS
     Other burn on board ship NOS
     Other burn on board watercraft NOS

●**V93.2** **Heat exposure on board watercraft**
     Excludes1   exposure to man-made heat not aboard watercraft (W92)
     exposure to natural heat while on board watercraft (X30)
     exposure to sunlight while on board watercraft (X32)
     Excludes2   burn due to fire on board watercraft (V93.0-)

X● **V93.20** **Heat exposure on board merchant ship**

X● **V93.21** **Heat exposure on board passenger ship**
     Heat exposure on board ferry-boat
     Heat exposure on board liner

X● **V93.22** **Heat exposure on board fishing boat**

X● **V93.23** **Heat exposure on board other powered watercraft**
     Heat exposure on board hovercraft

CHAPTER 20 (V01-Y99)

X● **V93.24** **Heat exposure on board sailboat**

X● **V93.29** **Heat exposure on board unspecified watercraft**
Heat exposure on board boat NOS
Heat exposure on board ship NOS
Heat exposure on board watercraft NOS

● **V93.3** **Fall on board watercraft**
  Excludes1   fall due to collision of watercraft (V91.2-)

X● **V93.30** **Fall on board merchant ship**

X● **V93.31** **Fall on board passenger ship**
Fall on board ferry-boat
Fall on board liner

X● **V93.32** **Fall on board fishing boat**

X● **V93.33** **Fall on board other powered watercraft**
Fall on board hovercraft (on open water)
Fall on board jet ski

X● **V93.34** **Fall on board sailboat**

X● **V93.35** **Fall on board canoe or kayak**

X● **V93.36** **Fall on board (nonpowered) inflatable craft**

X● **V93.38** **Fall on board other unpowered watercraft**

X● **V93.39** **Fall on board unspecified watercraft**
Fall on board boat NOS
Fall on board ship NOS
Fall on board watercraft NOS

● **V93.4** **Struck by falling object on board watercraft**
Hit by falling object on board watercraft
  Excludes1   struck by falling object due to accident to watercraft (V91.3)

X● **V93.40** **Struck by falling object on merchant ship**

X● **V93.41** **Struck by falling object on passenger ship**
Struck by falling object on ferry-boat
Struck by falling object on liner

X● **V93.42** **Struck by falling object on fishing boat**

X● **V93.43** **Struck by falling object on other powered watercraft**
Struck by falling object on hovercraft

X● **V93.44** **Struck by falling object on sailboat**

X● **V93.48** **Struck by falling object on other unpowered watercraft**

X● **V93.49** **Struck by falling object on unspecified watercraft**

● **V93.5** **Explosion on board watercraft**
Boiler explosion on steamship
  Excludes2   fire on board watercraft (V93.0-)

X● **V93.50** **Explosion on board merchant ship**

X● **V93.51** **Explosion on board passenger ship**
Explosion on board ferry-boat
Explosion on board liner

X● **V93.52** **Explosion on board fishing boat**

X● **V93.53** **Explosion on board other powered watercraft**
Explosion on board hovercraft
Explosion on board jet ski

X● **V93.54** **Explosion on board sailboat**

X● **V93.59** **Explosion on board unspecified watercraft**
Explosion on board boat NOS
Explosion on board ship NOS
Explosion on board watercraft NOS

● **V93.6** **Machinery accident on board watercraft**
  Excludes1   machinery explosion on board watercraft (V93.4-)
machinery fire on board watercraft (V93.0-)

X● **V93.60** **Machinery accident on board merchant ship**

X● **V93.61** **Machinery accident on board passenger ship**
Machinery accident on board ferry-boat
Machinery accident on board liner

X● **V93.62** **Machinery accident on board fishing boat**

X● **V93.63** **Machinery accident on board other powered watercraft**
Machinery accident on board hovercraft

X● **V93.64** **Machinery accident on board sailboat**

X● **V93.69** **Machinery accident on board unspecified watercraft**
Machinery accident on board boat NOS
Machinery accident on board ship NOS
Machinery accident on board watercraft NOS

● **V93.8** **Other injury due to other accident on board watercraft**
Accidental poisoning by gases or fumes on watercraft

X● **V93.80** **Other injury due to other accident on board merchant ship**

X● **V93.81** **Other injury due to other accident on board passenger ship**
Other injury due to other accident on board ferry-boat
Other injury due to other accident on board liner

X● **V93.82** **Other injury due to other accident on board fishing boat**

X● **V93.83** **Other injury due to other accident on board other powered watercraft**
Other injury due to other accident on board hovercraft
Other injury due to other accident on board jet ski

X● **V93.84** **Other injury due to other accident on board sailboat**

X● **V93.85** **Other injury due to other accident on board canoe or kayak**

X● **V93.86** **Other injury due to other accident on board (nonpowered) inflatable craft**

X● **V93.87** **Other injury due to other accident on board water-skis**
Hit or struck by object while waterskiing

X● **V93.88** **Other injury due to other accident on board other unpowered watercraft**
Hit or struck by object while surfing
Hit or struck by object while on board windsurfer

X● **V93.89** **Other injury due to other accident on board unspecified watercraft**
Other injury due to other accident on board boat NOS
Other injury due to other accident on board ship NOS
Other injury due to other accident on board watercraft NOS

● **V94** **Other and unspecified water transport accidents**
  Excludes1   military watercraft accidents in military or war operations (Y36, Y37)

The appropriate 7th character is to be added to each code from category V94

> A   initial encounter
> D   subsequent encounter
> S   sequela

X● **V94.0** **Hitting object or bottom of body of water due to fall from watercraft**
  Excludes2   drowning and submersion due to fall from watercraft (V92.0-)

● **V94.1** **Bather struck by watercraft**
Swimmer hit by watercraft

X● **V94.11** **Bather struck by powered watercraft**

X● **V94.12** **Bather struck by nonpowered watercraft**

◀ New   ◀|||| Revised   deleted Deleted   Excludes 1   Excludes 2   Includes   Use additional   Code first   Code also   Unspecified
OGCR Official Guidelines   X Assign placeholder X   ● Use Additional Character(s)   ▷ Manifestation Code   **Coding Clinic**

● **V94.2**   **Rider of nonpowered watercraft struck by other watercraft**

   X ● **V94.21**   **Rider of nonpowered watercraft struck by other nonpowered watercraft**
      Canoer hit by other nonpowered watercraft
      Surfer hit by other nonpowered watercraft
      Windsurfer hit by other nonpowered watercraft

   X ● **V94.22**   **Rider of nonpowered watercraft struck by powered watercraft**
      Canoer hit by motorboat
      Surfer hit by motorboat
      Windsurfer hit by motorboat

● **V94.3**   **Injury to rider of (inflatable) watercraft being pulled behind other watercraft**

   X ● **V94.31**   **Injury to rider of (inflatable) recreational watercraft being pulled behind other watercraft**
      Injury to rider of inner-tube pulled behind motor boat

   X ● **V94.32**   **Injury to rider of non-recreational watercraft being pulled behind other watercraft**
      Injury to occupant of dingy being pulled behind boat or ship
      Injury to occupant of life-raft being pulled behind boat or ship

X ● **V94.4**   **Injury to barefoot water-skier**
      Injury to person being pulled behind boat or ship

● **V94.8**   **Other water transport accident**

   ● **V94.81**   **Water transport accident involving military watercraft**

     ● **V94.810**   **Civilian watercraft involved in water transport accident with military watercraft**
       Passenger on civilian watercraft injured due to accident with military watercraft

     ● **V94.811**   **Civilian in water injured by military watercraft**

     ● **V94.818**   **Other water transport accident involving military watercraft**

   X ● **V94.89**   **Other water transport accident**

X ● **V94.9**   **Unspecified water transport accident**
      Water transport accident NOS

AIR AND SPACE TRANSPORT ACCIDENTS (V95-V97)

Excludes1   military aircraft accidents in military or war operations (Y36, Y37)

● **V95**   **Accident to powered aircraft causing injury to occupant**
   The appropriate 7th character is to be added to each code from category V95

> A   initial encounter
> D   subsequent encounter
> S   sequela

● **V95.0**   **Helicopter accident injuring occupant**

   X ● **V95.00**   **Unspecified helicopter accident injuring occupant**

   X ● **V95.01**   **Helicopter crash injuring occupant**

   X ● **V95.02**   **Forced landing of helicopter injuring occupant**

   X ● **V95.03**   **Helicopter collision injuring occupant**
      Helicopter collision with any object, fixed, movable or moving

   X ● **V95.04**   **Helicopter fire injuring occupant**

   X ● **V95.05**   **Helicopter explosion injuring occupant**

   X ● **V95.09**   **Other helicopter accident injuring occupant**

● **V95.1**   **Ultralight, microlight or powered-glider accident injuring occupant**

   X ● **V95.10**   **Unspecified ultralight, microlight or powered-glider accident injuring occupant**

   X ● **V95.11**   **Ultralight, microlight or powered-glider crash injuring occupant**

   X ● **V95.12**   **Forced landing of ultralight, microlight or powered-glider injuring occupant**

   X ● **V95.13**   **Ultralight, microlight or powered-glider collision injuring occupant**
      Ultralight, microlight or powered-glider collision with any object, fixed, movable or moving

   X ● **V95.14**   **Ultralight, microlight or powered-glider fire injuring occupant**

   X ● **V95.15**   **Ultralight, microlight or powered-glider explosion injuring occupant**

   X ● **V95.19**   **Other ultralight, microlight or powered-glider accident injuring occupant**

● **V95.2**   **Other private fixed-wing aircraft accident injuring occupant**

   X ● **V95.20**   **Unspecified accident to other private fixed-wing aircraft, injuring occupant**

   X ● **V95.21**   **Other private fixed-wing aircraft crash injuring occupant**

   X ● **V95.22**   **Forced landing of other private fixed-wing aircraft injuring occupant**

   X ● **V95.23**   **Other private fixed-wing aircraft collision injuring occupant**
      Other private fixed-wing aircraft collision with any object, fixed, movable or moving

   X ● **V95.24**   **Other private fixed-wing aircraft fire injuring occupant**

   X ● **V95.25**   **Other private fixed-wing aircraft explosion injuring occupant**

   X ● **V95.29**   **Other accident to other private fixed-wing aircraft injuring occupant**

● **V95.3**   **Commercial fixed-wing aircraft accident injuring occupant**

   X ● **V95.30**   **Unspecified accident to commercial fixed-wing aircraft injuring occupant**

   X ● **V95.31**   **Commercial fixed-wing aircraft crash injuring occupant**

   X ● **V95.32**   **Forced landing of commercial fixed-wing aircraft injuring occupant**

   X ● **V95.33**   **Commercial fixed-wing aircraft collision injuring occupant**
      Commercial fixed-wing aircraft collision with any object, fixed, movable or moving

   X ● **V95.34**   **Commercial fixed-wing aircraft fire injuring occupant**

   X ● **V95.35**   **Commercial fixed-wing aircraft explosion injuring occupant**

   X ● **V95.39**   **Other accident to commercial fixed-wing aircraft injuring occupant**

● **V95.4**   **Spacecraft accident injuring occupant**

   X ● **V95.40**   **Unspecified spacecraft accident injuring occupant**

   X ● **V95.41**   **Spacecraft crash injuring occupant**

   X ● **V95.42**   **Forced landing of spacecraft injuring occupant**

   X ● **V95.43**   **Spacecraft collision injuring occupant**
      Spacecraft collision with any object, fixed, moveable or moving

   X ● **V95.44**   **Spacecraft fire injuring occupant**

   X ● **V95.45**   **Spacecraft explosion injuring occupant**

   X ● **V95.49**   **Other spacecraft accident injuring occupant**

X ● **V95.8**   **Other powered aircraft accidents injuring occupant**

X ● **V95.9**   **Unspecified aircraft accident injuring occupant**
      Aircraft accident NOS
      Air transport accident NOS

● **V96　Accident to nonpowered aircraft causing injury to occupant**

The appropriate 7th character is to be added to each code from category V96

> A　initial encounter
> D　subsequent encounter
> S　sequela

● **V96.0　Balloon accident injuring occupant**
- X ● **V96.00** Unspecified balloon accident injuring occupant
- X ● **V96.01** Balloon crash injuring occupant
- X ● **V96.02** Forced landing of balloon injuring occupant
- X ● **V96.03** Balloon collision injuring occupant
  - Balloon collision with any object, fixed, moveable or moving
- X ● **V96.04** Balloon fire injuring occupant
- X ● **V96.05** Balloon explosion injuring occupant
- X ● **V96.09** Other balloon accident injuring occupant

● **V96.1　Hang-glider accident injuring occupant**
- X ● **V96.10** Unspecified hang-glider accident injuring occupant
- X ● **V96.11** Hang-glider crash injuring occupant
- X ● **V96.12** Forced landing of hang-glider injuring occupant
- X ● **V96.13** Hang-glider collision injuring occupant
  - Hang-glider collision with any object, fixed, moveable or moving
- X ● **V96.14** Hang-glider fire injuring occupant
- X ● **V96.15** Hang-glider explosion injuring occupant
- X ● **V96.19** Other hang-glider accident injuring occupant

● **V96.2　Glider (nonpowered) accident injuring occupant**
- X ● **V96.20** Unspecified glider (nonpowered) accident injuring occupant
- X ● **V96.21** Glider (nonpowered) crash injuring occupant
- X ● **V96.22** Forced landing of glider (nonpowered) injuring occupant
- X ● **V96.23** Glider (nonpowered) collision injuring occupant
  - Glider (nonpowered) collision with any object, fixed, moveable or moving
- X ● **V96.24** Glider (nonpowered) fire injuring occupant
- X ● **V96.25** Glider (nonpowered) explosion injuring occupant
- X ● **V96.29** Other glider (nonpowered) accident injuring occupant

- X ● **V96.8** Other nonpowered-aircraft accidents injuring occupant
  - Kite carrying a person accident injuring occupant
- X ● **V96.9** Unspecified nonpowered-aircraft accident injuring occupant
  - Nonpowered-aircraft accident NOS

● **V97　Other specified air transport accidents**

The appropriate 7th character is to be added to each code from category V97

> A　initial encounter
> D　subsequent encounter
> S　sequela

- X ● **V97.0** Occupant of aircraft injured in other specified air transport accidents
  - Fall in, on or from aircraft in air transport accident
  - **Excludes1**　accident while boarding or alighting aircraft (V97.1)
- X ● **V97.1** Person injured while boarding or alighting from aircraft

● **V97.2　Parachutist accident**
- X ● **V97.21** Parachutist entangled in object
  - Parachutist landing in tree
- X ● **V97.22** Parachutist injured on landing
- X ● **V97.29** Other parachutist accident

● **V97.3　Person on ground injured in air transport accident**
- X ● **V97.31** Hit by object falling from aircraft
  - Hit by crashing aircraft
  - Injured by aircraft hitting house
  - Injured by aircraft hitting car
- X ● **V97.32** Injured by rotating propeller
- X ● **V97.33** Sucked into jet engine
- X ● **V97.39** Other injury to person on ground due to air transport accident

● **V97.8　Other air transport accidents, not elsewhere classified**

> **Excludes1**　aircraft accident NOS (V95.9)
> exposure to changes in air pressure during ascent or descent (W94.-)

- ● **V97.81** Air transport accident involving military aircraft
  - ● **V97.810** Civilian aircraft involved in air transport accident with military aircraft
    - Passenger in civilian aircraft injured due to accident with military aircraft
  - ● **V97.811** Civilian injured by military aircraft
  - ● **V97.818** Other air transport accident involving military aircraft
- X ● **V97.89** Other air transport accidents, not elsewhere classified
  - Injury from machinery on aircraft

OTHER AND UNSPECIFIED TRANSPORT ACCIDENTS (V98-V99)

> **Excludes1**　vehicle accident, type of vehicle unspecified (V89.-)

● **V98　Other specified transport accidents**

The appropriate 7th character is to be added to each code from category V98

> A　initial encounter
> D　subsequent encounter
> S　sequela

- X ● **V98.0** Accident to, on or involving cable-car, not on rails
  - Caught or dragged by cable-car, not on rails
  - Fall or jump from cable-car, not on rails
  - Object thrown from or in cable-car, not on rails
- X ● **V98.1** Accident to, on or involving land-yacht
- X ● **V98.2** Accident to, on or involving ice yacht
- X ● **V98.3** Accident to, on or involving ski lift
  - Accident to, on or involving ski chair-lift
  - Accident to, on or involving ski-lift with gondola
- X ● **V98.8** Other specified transport accidents

X ● **V99　Unspecified transport accident**

The appropriate 7th character is to be added to code V99

> A　initial encounter
> D　subsequent encounter
> S　sequela

OTHER EXTERNAL CAUSES OF ACCIDENTAL INJURY (W00-X58)

SLIPPING, TRIPPING, STUMBLING AND FALLS (W00-W19)

Excludes1   assault involving a fall (Y01-Y02)
fall from animal (V80.-)
fall (in) (from) machinery (in operation) (W28-W31)
fall (in) (from) transport vehicle (V01-V99)
intentional self-harm involving a fall (X80-X81)

Excludes2   at risk for fall (history of fall) Z91.81
fall (in) (from) burning building (X00.-)
fall into fire (X00-X04, X08-X09)

● **W00**   **Fall due to ice and snow**

    Includes   pedestrian on foot falling (slipping) on ice and snow

    Excludes1   fall on (from) ice and snow involving pedestrian conveyance (V00.-)
fall from stairs and steps not due to ice and snow (W10.-)

The appropriate 7th character is to be added to each code from category W00

> A   initial encounter
> D   subsequent encounter
> S   sequela

X● **W00.0**   **Fall on same level due to ice and snow**
      Coding Clinic: 2016, Q2, P5

X● **W00.1**   **Fall from stairs and steps due to ice and snow**

X● **W00.2**   **Other fall from one level to another due to ice and snow**

X● **W00.9**   **Unspecified fall due to ice and snow**

● **W01**   **Fall on same level from slipping, tripping and stumbling**

    Includes   fall on moving sidewalk

    Excludes1   fall due to bumping (striking) against object (W18.0-)
fall in shower or bathtub (W18.2-)
fall on same level NOS (W18.30)
fall on same level from slipping, tripping and stumbling due to ice or snow (W00.0)
fall off or from toilet (W18.1-)
slipping, tripping and stumbling NOS (W18.40)
slipping, tripping and stumbling without falling (W18.4-)

The appropriate 7th character is to be added to each code from category W01

> A   initial encounter
> D   subsequent encounter
> S   sequela

X● **W01.0**   **Fall on same level from slipping, tripping and stumbling without subsequent striking against object**
      Falling over animal

● **W01.1**   **Fall on same level from slipping, tripping and stumbling with subsequent striking against object**

   X● **W01.10**   **Fall on same level from slipping, tripping and stumbling with subsequent striking against unspecified object**

   ● **W01.11**   **Fall on same level from slipping, tripping and stumbling with subsequent striking against sharp object**

     ● **W01.110**   **Fall on same level from slipping, tripping and stumbling with subsequent striking against sharp glass**

     ● **W01.111**   **Fall on same level from slipping, tripping and stumbling with subsequent striking against power tool or machine**

     ● **W01.118**   **Fall on same level from slipping, tripping and stumbling with subsequent striking against other sharp object**

     ● **W01.119**   **Fall on same level from slipping, tripping and stumbling with subsequent striking against unspecified sharp object**

   ● **W01.19**   **Fall on same level from slipping, tripping and stumbling with subsequent striking against other object**

     ● **W01.190**   **Fall on same level from slipping, tripping and stumbling with subsequent striking against furniture**

     ● **W01.198**   **Fall on same level from slipping, tripping and stumbling with subsequent striking against other object**

X● **W03**   **Other fall on same level due to collision with another person**
      Fall due to non-transport collision with other person

    Excludes1   collision with another person without fall (W51)
crushed or pushed by a crowd or human stampede (W52)
fall involving pedestrian conveyance (V00-V09)
fall due to ice or snow (W00)
fall on same level NOS (W18.30)

The appropriate 7th character is to be added to code W03

> A   initial encounter
> D   subsequent encounter
> S   sequela

Coding Clinic: 2015, Q1, P9-10; 2012, Q4, P108

X● **W04**   **Fall while being carried or supported by other persons**
      Accidentally dropped while being carried

The appropriate 7th character is to be added to code W04

> A   initial encounter
> D   subsequent encounter
> S   sequel

● **W05**   **Fall from non-moving wheelchair, nonmotorized scooter and motorized mobility scooter**

    Excludes1   fall from moving wheelchair (powered) (V00.811)
fall from moving motorized mobility scooter (V00.831)
fall from nonmotorized scooter (V00.141)

The appropriate 7th character is to be added to each code from category W05

> A   initial encounter
> D   subsequent encounter
> S   sequela

X● **W05.0**   **Fall from non-moving wheelchair**

X● **W05.1**   **Fall from non-moving nonmotorized scooter**

X● **W05.2**   **Fall from non-moving motorized mobility scooter**

CHAPTER 20 (V01-Y99)

X ● **W06 Fall from bed**
> The appropriate 7th character is to be added to code W06

A	initial encounter
D	subsequent encounter
S	sequela

X ● **W07 Fall from chair**
> The appropriate 7th character is to be added to code W07

A	initial encounter
D	subsequent encounter
S	sequela

X ● **W08 Fall from other furniture**
> The appropriate 7th character is to be added to code W08

A	initial encounter
D	subsequent encounter
S	sequela

● **W09 Fall on and from playground equipment**
> **Excludes1**   fall involving recreational machinery (W31)
>
> The appropriate 7th character is to be added to each code from category W09

A	initial encounter
D	subsequent encounter
S	sequela

X ● **W09.0 Fall on or from playground slide**
X ● **W09.1 Fall from playground swing**
X ● **W09.2 Fall on or from jungle gym**
X ● **W09.8 Fall on or from other playground equipment**

● **W10 Fall on and from stairs and steps**
> **Excludes1**   fall from stairs and steps due to ice and snow (W00.1)
>
> The appropriate 7th character is to be added to each code from category W10

A	initial encounter
D	subsequent encounter
S	sequela

X ● **W10.0 Fall (on) (from) escalator**
X ● **W10.1 Fall (on) (from) sidewalk curb**
X ● **W10.2 Fall (on) (from) incline**
> Fall (on) (from) ramp
X ● **W10.8 Fall (on) (from) other stairs and steps**
X ● **W10.9 Fall (on) (from) unspecified stairs and steps**

X ● **W11 Fall on and from ladder**
> The appropriate 7th character is to be added to code W11

A	initial encounter
D	subsequent encounter
S	sequela

X ● **W12 Fall on and from scaffolding**
> The appropriate 7th character is to be added to code W12

A	initial encounter
D	subsequent encounter
S	sequela

● **W13 Fall from, out of or through building or structure**
> The appropriate 7th character is to be added to each code from category W13

A	initial encounter
D	subsequent encounter
S	sequela

X ● **W13.0 Fall from, out of or through balcony**
> Fall from, out of or through railing
X ● **W13.1 Fall from, out of or through bridge**
X ● **W13.2 Fall from, out of or through roof**
X ● **W13.3 Fall through floor**
X ● **W13.4 Fall from, out of or through window**
> **Excludes2**   fall with subsequent striking against sharp glass (W01.110)
X ● **W13.8 Fall from, out of or through other building or structure**
> Fall from, out of or through viaduct
> Fall from, out of or through wall
> Fall from, out of or through flag-pole
X ● **W13.9 Fall from, out of or through building, not otherwise specified**
> **Excludes1**   collapse of a building or structure (W20.-)
> fall or jump from burning building or structure (X00.-)

X ● **W14 Fall from tree**
> The appropriate 7th character is to be added to code W14

A	initial encounter
D	subsequent encounter
S	sequela

X ● **W15 Fall from cliff**
> The appropriate 7th character is to be added to code W15

A	initial encounter
D	subsequent encounter
S	sequela

● **W16 Fall, jump or diving into water**
> **Excludes1**   accidental non-watercraft drowning and submersion not involving fall (W65-W74)
> effects of air pressure from diving (W94.-)
> fall into water from watercraft (V90-V94)
> hitting an object or against bottom when falling from watercraft (V94.0)
>
> **Excludes2**   striking or hitting diving board (W21.4)
>
> The appropriate 7th character is to be added to each code from category W16

A	initial encounter
D	subsequent encounter
S	sequela

● **W16.0 Fall into swimming pool**
> Fall into swimming pool NOS
> **Excludes1**   fall into empty swimming pool (W17.3)
● **W16.01 Fall into swimming pool striking water surface**
● **W16.011 Fall into swimming pool striking water surface causing drowning and submersion**
> **Excludes1**   drowning and submersion while in swimming pool without fall (W67)
● **W16.012 Fall into swimming pool striking water surface causing other injury**

◄ New   ◄┅ Revised   ~~deleted~~ Deleted   Excludes 1   Excludes 2   Includes   Use additional   Code first   Code also   Unspecified

OGCR Official Guidelines   X Assign placeholder X   ● Use Additional Character(s)   ▶ Manifestation Code   **Coding Clinic**

● **W16.02 Fall into swimming pool striking bottom**
   ● **W16.021 Fall into swimming pool striking bottom causing drowning and submersion**
       Excludes1   drowning and submersion while in swimming pool without fall (W67)
   ● **W16.022 Fall into swimming pool striking bottom causing other injury**

● **W16.03 Fall into swimming pool striking wall**
   ● **W16.031 Fall into swimming pool striking wall causing drowning and submersion**
       Excludes1   drowning and submersion while in swimming pool without fall (W67)
   ● **W16.032 Fall into swimming pool striking wall causing other injury**

● **W16.1 Fall into natural body of water**
    Fall into lake
    Fall into open sea
    Fall into river
    Fall into stream
   ● **W16.11 Fall into natural body of water striking water surface**
      ● **W16.111 Fall into natural body of water striking water surface causing drowning and submersion**
          Excludes1   drowning and submersion while in natural body of water without fall (W69)
      ● **W16.112 Fall into natural body of water striking water surface causing other injury**
   ● **W16.12 Fall into natural body of water striking bottom**
      ● **W16.121 Fall into natural body of water striking bottom causing drowning and submersion**
          Excludes1   drowning and submersion while in natural body of water without fall (W69)
      ● **W16.122 Fall into natural body of water striking bottom causing other injury**
   ● **W16.13 Fall into natural body of water striking side**
      ● **W16.131 Fall into natural body of water striking side causing drowning and submersion**
          Excludes1   drowning and submersion while in natural body of water without fall (W69)
      ● **W16.132 Fall into natural body of water striking side causing other injury**

● **W16.2 Fall in (into) filled bathtub or bucket of water**
   ● **W16.21 Fall in (into) filled bathtub**
       Excludes1   fall into empty bathtub (W18.2)
      ● **W16.211 Fall in (into) filled bathtub causing drowning and submersion**
          Excludes1   drowning and submersion while in filled bathtub without fall (W65)
      ● **W16.212 Fall in (into) filled bathtub causing other injury**

● **W16.22 Fall in (into) bucket of water**
   ● **W16.221 Fall in (into) bucket of water causing drowning and submersion**
   ● **W16.222 Fall in (into) bucket of water causing other injury**

● **W16.3 Fall into other water**
    Fall into fountain
    Fall into reservoir
   ● **W16.31 Fall into other water striking water surface**
      ● **W16.311 Fall into other water striking water surface causing drowning and submersion**
          Excludes1   drowning and submersion while in other water without fall (W73)
      ● **W16.312 Fall into other water striking water surface causing other injury**
   ● **W16.32 Fall into other water striking bottom**
      ● **W16.321 Fall into other water striking bottom causing drowning and submersion**
          Excludes1   drowning and submersion while in other water without fall (W73)
      ● **W16.322 Fall into other water striking bottom causing other injury**
   ● **W16.33 Fall into other water striking wall**
      ● **W16.331 Fall into other water striking wall causing drowning and submersion**
          Excludes1   drowning and submersion while in other water without fall (W73)
      ● **W16.332 Fall into other water striking wall causing other injury**

● **W16.4 Fall into unspecified water**
   X ● **W16.41 Fall into unspecified water causing drowning and submersion**
   X ● **W16.42 Fall into unspecified water causing other injury**

● **W16.5 Jumping or diving into swimming pool**
   ● **W16.51 Jumping or diving into swimming pool striking water surface**
      ● **W16.511 Jumping or diving into swimming pool striking water surface causing drowning and submersion**
          Excludes1   drowning and submersion while in swimming pool without jumping or diving (W67)
      ● **W16.512 Jumping or diving into swimming pool striking water surface causing other injury**
   ● **W16.52 Jumping or diving into swimming pool striking bottom**
      ● **W16.521 Jumping or diving into swimming pool striking bottom causing drowning and submersion**
          Excludes1   drowning and submersion while in swimming pool without jumping or diving (W67)
      ● **W16.522 Jumping or diving into swimming pool striking bottom causing other injury**

CHAPTER 20 (V01-Y99)

● **W16.53** **Jumping or diving into swimming pool striking wall**

    ● **W16.531** **Jumping or diving into swimming pool striking wall causing drowning and submersion**

         Excludes1   drowning and submersion while in swimming pool without jumping or diving (W67)

    ● **W16.532** **Jumping or diving into swimming pool striking wall causing other injury**

● **W16.6** **Jumping or diving into natural body of water**

     Jumping or diving into lake
     Jumping or diving into open sea
     Jumping or diving into river
     Jumping or diving into stream

  ● **W16.61** **Jumping or diving into natural body of water striking water surface**

    ● **W16.611** **Jumping or diving into natural body of water striking water surface causing drowning and submersion**

         Excludes1   drowning and submersion while in natural body of water without jumping or diving (W69)

    ● **W16.612** **Jumping or diving into natural body of water striking water surface causing other injury**

  ● **W16.62** **Jumping or diving into natural body of water striking bottom**

    ● **W16.621** **Jumping or diving into natural body of water striking bottom causing drowning and submersion**

         Excludes1   drowning and submersion while in natural body of water without jumping or diving (W69)

    ● **W16.622** **Jumping or diving into natural body of water striking bottom causing other injury**

● **W16.7** **Jumping or diving from boat**

     Excludes1   fall from boat into water - see watercraft accident (V90-V94)

  ● **W16.71** **Jumping or diving from boat striking water surface**

    ● **W16.711** **Jumping or diving from boat striking water surface causing drowning and submersion**

    ● **W16.712** **Jumping or diving from boat striking water surface causing other injury**

  ● **W16.72** **Jumping or diving from boat striking bottom**

    ● **W16.721** **Jumping or diving from boat striking bottom causing drowning and submersion**

    ● **W16.722** **Jumping or diving from boat striking bottom causing other injury**

● **W16.8** **Jumping or diving into other water**

     Jumping or diving into fountain
     Jumping or diving into reservoir

  ● **W16.81** **Jumping or diving into other water striking water surface**

    ● **W16.811** **Jumping or diving into other water striking water surface causing drowning and submersion**

         Excludes1   drowning and submersion while in other water without jumping or diving (W73)

    ● **W16.812** **Jumping or diving into other water striking water surface causing other injury**

  ● **W16.82** **Jumping or diving into other water striking bottom**

    ● **W16.821** **Jumping or diving into other water striking bottom causing drowning and submersion**

         Excludes1   drowning and submersion while in other water without jumping or diving (W73)

    ● **W16.822** **Jumping or diving into other water striking bottom causing other injury**

  ● **W16.83** **Jumping or diving into other water striking wall**

    ● **W16.831** **Jumping or diving into other water striking wall causing drowning and submersion**

         Excludes1   drowning and submersion while in other water without jumping or diving (W73)

    ● **W16.832** **Jumping or diving into other water striking wall causing other injury**

● **W16.9** **Jumping or diving into unspecified water**

   X ● **W16.91** **Jumping or diving into unspecified water causing drowning and submersion**

   X ● **W16.92** **Jumping or diving into unspecified water causing other injury**

● **W17** **Other fall from one level to another**

     The appropriate 7th character is to be added to each code from category W17

A	initial encounter
D	subsequent encounter
S	sequela

X ● **W17.0** **Fall into well**

X ● **W17.1** **Fall into storm drain or manhole**

X ● **W17.2** **Fall into hole**

     Fall into pit

X ● **W17.3** **Fall into empty swimming pool**

     Excludes1   fall into filled swimming pool (W16.0-)

X ● **W17.4** **Fall from dock**

● **W17.8** **Other fall from one level to another**

   X ● **W17.81** **Fall down embankment (hill)**

   X ● **W17.82** **Fall from (out of) grocery cart**

     Fall due to grocery cart tipping over

   X ● **W17.89** **Other fall from one level to another**

     Fall from cherry picker
     Fall from lifting device
     Fall from mobile elevated work platform [MEWP]
     Fall from sky lift
     Coding Clinic: 2015, Q2, P6

◀ New   ⬅ Revised   ~~deleted~~ Deleted   Excludes 1   Excludes 2   Includes   Use additional   Code first   Code also   Unspecified

OGCR Official Guidelines   X Assign placeholder X   Use Additional Character(s)   ▶ Manifestation Code   **Coding Clinic**

● **W18   Other slipping, tripping and stumbling and falls**

The appropriate 7th character is to be added to each code from category W18

A	initial encounter
D	subsequent encounter
S	sequela

● **W18.0   Fall due to bumping against object**

Striking against object with subsequent fall

> **Excludes1**   fall on same level due to slipping, tripping, or stumbling with subsequent striking against object (W01.1-)

X ● **W18.00   Striking against unspecified object with subsequent fall**

X ● **W18.01   Striking against sports equipment with subsequent fall**

X ● **W18.02   Striking against glass with subsequent fall**

X ● **W18.09   Striking against other object with subsequent fall**

● **W18.1   Fall from or off toilet**

X ● **W18.11   Fall from or off toilet without subsequent striking against object**

Fall from (off) toilet NOS

X ● **W18.12   Fall from or off toilet with subsequent striking against object**

X ● **W18.2   Fall in (into) shower or empty bathtub**

> **Excludes1**   fall in full bathtub causing drowning or submersion (W16.21-)

● **W18.3   Other and unspecified fall on same level**

X ● **W18.30   Fall on same level, unspecified**

X ● **W18.31   Fall on same level due to stepping on an object**

Fall on same level due to stepping on an animal

> **Excludes1**   slipping, tripping and stumbling without fall due to stepping on animal (W18.41)

X ● **W18.39   Other fall on same level**

● **W18.4   Slipping, tripping and stumbling without falling**

> **Excludes1**   collision with another person without fall (W51)

X ● **W18.40   Slipping, tripping and stumbling without falling, unspecified**

X ● **W18.41   Slipping, tripping and stumbling without falling due to stepping on object**

Slipping, tripping and stumbling without falling due to stepping on animal

> **Excludes1**   slipping, tripping and stumbling with fall due to stepping on animal (W18.31)

X ● **W18.42   Slipping, tripping and stumbling without falling due to stepping into hole or opening**

X ● **W18.43   Slipping, tripping and stumbling without falling due to stepping from one level to another**

X ● **W18.49   Other slipping, tripping and stumbling without falling**

X ● **W19   Unspecified fall**

Accidental fall NOS

The appropriate 7th character is to be added to code W19

A	initial encounter
D	subsequent encounter
S	sequela

Coding Clinic: 2012, Q4, P95

EXPOSURE TO INANIMATE MECHANICAL FORCES (W20-W49)

> **Excludes1**   assault (X92-Y09) ◀▥
> contact or collision with animals or persons (W50-W64)
> exposure to inanimate mechanical forces involving military or war operations (Y36.-, Y37.-)
> intentional self-harm (X71-X83)

● **W20   Struck by thrown, projected or falling object**

Code first any associated:
cataclysm (X34-X39)
lightning strike (T75.00)

> **Excludes1**   falling object in machinery accident (W24, W28-W31)
> falling object in transport accident (V01-V99)
> object set in motion by explosion (W35-W40)
> object set in motion by firearm (W32-W34)
> struck by thrown sports equipment (W21.-)

The appropriate 7th character is to be added to each code from category W20

A	initial encounter
D	subsequent encounter
S	sequela

X ● **W20.0   Struck by falling object in cave-in**

> **Excludes2**   asphyxiation due to cave-in (T71.21)

X ● **W20.1   Struck by object due to collapse of building**

> **Excludes1**   struck by object due to collapse of burning building (X00.2, X02.2)

X ● **W20.8   Other cause of strike by thrown, projected or falling object**

> **Excludes1**   struck by thrown sports equipment (W21.-)

● **W21   Striking against or struck by sports equipment**

> **Excludes1**   assault with sports equipment (Y08.0-)
> striking against or struck by sports equipment with subsequent fall (W18.01)

The appropriate 7th character is to be added to each code from category W21

A	initial encounter
D	subsequent encounter
S	sequela

● **W21.0   Struck by hit or thrown ball**

X ● **W21.00   Struck by hit or thrown ball, unspecified type**

X ● **W21.01   Struck by football**

X ● **W21.02   Struck by soccer ball**

X ● **W21.03   Struck by baseball**

X ● **W21.04   Struck by golf ball**

X ● **W21.05   Struck by basketball**

X ● **W21.06   Struck by volleyball**

X ● **W21.07   Struck by softball**

X ● **W21.09   Struck by other hit or thrown ball**

● **W21.1   Struck by bat, racquet or club**

X ● **W21.11   Struck by baseball bat**

X ● **W21.12   Struck by tennis racquet**

X ● **W21.13   Struck by golf club**

X ● **W21.19   Struck by other bat, racquet or club**

● **W21.2 Struck by hockey stick or puck**
   ● **W21.21 Struck by hockey stick**
      ● **W21.210 Struck by ice hockey stick**
      ● **W21.211 Struck by field hockey stick**
   ● **W21.22 Struck by hockey puck**
      ● **W21.220 Struck by ice hockey puck**
      ● **W21.221 Struck by field hockey puck**
● **W21.3 Struck by sports foot wear**
   X ● **W21.31 Struck by shoe cleats**
      Stepped on by shoe cleats
   X ● **W21.32 Struck by skate blades**
      Skated over by skate blades
   X ● **W21.39 Struck by other sports foot wear**
X ● **W21.4 Striking against diving board**
   Use additional code for subsequent falling into water, if applicable (W16.-)
● **W21.8 Striking against or struck by other sports equipment**
   X ● **W21.81 Striking against or struck by football helmet**
   X ● **W21.89 Striking against or struck by other sports equipment**
X ● **W21.9 Striking against or struck by** `unspecified` **sports equipment**

● **W22 Striking against or struck by other objects**
   `Excludes1`   striking against or struck by object with subsequent fall (W18.09)

   The appropriate 7th character is to be added to each code from category W22

> A   initial encounter
> D   subsequent encounter
> S   sequela

   ● **W22.0 Striking against stationary object**
      `Excludes1`   striking against stationary sports equipment (W21.8)
   X ● **W22.01 Walked into wall**
   X ● **W22.02 Walked into lamppost**
   X ● **W22.03 Walked into furniture**
   ● **W22.04 Striking against wall of swimming pool**
      ● **W22.041 Striking against wall of swimming pool causing drowning and submersion**
         `Excludes1`   drowning and submersion while swimming without striking against wall (W67)
      ● **W22.042 Striking against wall of swimming pool causing other injury**
   X ● **W22.09 Striking against other stationary object**
   ● **W22.1 Striking against or struck by automobile airbag**
   X ● **W22.10 Striking against or struck by** `unspecified` **automobile airbag**
   X ● **W22.11 Striking against or struck by driver side automobile airbag**
   X ● **W22.12 Striking against or struck by front passenger side automobile airbag**
   X ● **W22.19 Striking against or struck by other automobile airbag**
X ● **W22.8 Striking against or struck by other objects**
   Striking against or struck by object NOS
   `Excludes1`   struck by thrown, projected or falling object (W20.-)

● **W23 Caught, crushed, jammed or pinched in or between objects**
   `Excludes1`   injury caused by cutting or piercing instruments (W25-W27)
      injury caused by firearms malfunction (W32.1, W33.1-, W34.1-)
      injury caused by lifting and transmission devices (W24.-)
      injury caused by machinery (W28-W31)
      injury caused by nonpowered hand tools (W27.-)
      injury caused by transport vehicle being used as a means of transportation (V01-V99)
      injury caused by struck by thrown, projected or falling object (W20.-)

   The appropriate 7th character is to be added to each code from category W23

> A   initial encounter
> D   subsequent encounter
> S   sequela

   X ● **W23.0 Caught, crushed, jammed, or pinched between moving objects**
   X ● **W23.1 Caught, crushed, jammed, or pinched between stationary objects**

● **W24 Contact with lifting and transmission devices, not elsewhere classified**
   `Excludes1`   transport accidents (V01-V99)
   The appropriate 7th character is to be added to each code from category W24

> A   initial encounter
> D   subsequent encounter
> S   sequela

   X ● **W24.0 Contact with lifting devices, not elsewhere classified**
      Contact with chain hoist
      Contact with drive belt
      Contact with pulley (block)
   X ● **W24.1 Contact with transmission devices, not elsewhere classified**
      Contact with transmission belt or cable

X ● **W25 Contact with sharp glass**
   Code first any associated:
      injury due to flying glass from explosion or firearm discharge (W32-W40)
      transport accident (V00-V99)
   `Excludes1`   fall on same level due to slipping, tripping and stumbling with subsequent striking against sharp glass (W01.10)
      striking against sharp glass with subsequent fall (W18.02)
   `Excludes2`   glass embedded in skin (W45) ◄
   The appropriate 7th character is to be added to code W25

> A   initial encounter
> D   subsequent encounter
> S   sequela

● **W26 Contact with other sharp objects** ◄▬
   `Excludes2`   sharp object(s) embedded in skin (W45) ◄
   The appropriate 7th character is to be added to each code from category W26

> A   initial encounter
> D   subsequent encounter
> S   sequela

   X ● **W26.0 Contact with knife**
      `Excludes1`   contact with electric knife (W29.1)
   X ● **W26.1 Contact with sword or dagger**
   X ● **W26.2 Contact with edge of stiff paper** ◄
      Paper cut ◄
   X ● **W26.8 Contact with other sharp object(s), not elsewhere classified** ◄
      Contact with tin can lid ◄
   X ● **W26.9 Contact with** `unspecified` **sharp object(s)** ◄

◄ New   ◄▬ Revised   ~~deleted~~ Deleted   `Excludes 1`   `Excludes 2`   `Includes`   `Use additional`   `Code first`   `Code also`   `Unspecified`

OGCR Official Guidelines   X Assign placeholder X   ● Use Additional Character(s)   ▶ Manifestation Code   **Coding Clinic**

● **W27 Contact with nonpowered hand tool**

The appropriate 7th character is to be added to each code from category W27

A	initial encounter
D	subsequent encounter
S	sequela

X● **W27.0 Contact with workbench tool**
Contact with auger
Contact with axe
Contact with chisel
Contact with handsaw
Contact with screwdriver

X● **W27.1 Contact with garden tool**
Contact with hoe
Contact with nonpowered lawn mower
Contact with pitchfork
Contact with rake

X● **W27.2 Contact with scissors**

X● **W27.3 Contact with needle (sewing)**
   Excludes1   contact with hypodermic needle (W46.-)

X● **W27.4 Contact with kitchen utensil**
Contact with fork
Contact with ice-pick
Contact with can-opener NOS

X● **W27.5 Contact with paper-cutter**

X● **W27.8 Contact with other nonpowered hand tool**
Contact with nonpowered sewing machine
Contact with shovel

X● **W28 Contact with powered lawn mower**
Powered lawn mower (commercial) (residential)
   Excludes1   contact with nonpowered lawn mower (W27.1)
   Excludes2   exposure to electric current (W86.-)
The appropriate 7th character is to be added to code W28

A	initial encounter
D	subsequent encounter
S	sequela

● **W29 Contact with other powered hand tools and household machinery**
   Excludes1   contact with commercial machinery (W31.82)
     contact with hot household appliance (X15)
     contact with nonpowered hand tool (W27.-)
     exposure to electric current (W86)
The appropriate 7th character is to be added to each code from category W29

A	initial encounter
D	subsequent encounter
S	sequela

X● **W29.0 Contact with powered kitchen appliance**
Contact with blender
Contact with can-opener
Contact with garbage disposal
Contact with mixer

X● **W29.1 Contact with electric knife**

X● **W29.2 Contact with other powered household machinery**
Contact with electric fan
Contact with powered dryer (clothes) (powered) (spin)
Contact with washing-machine
Contact with sewing machine

X● **W29.3 Contact with powered garden and outdoor hand tools and machinery**
Contact with chainsaw
Contact with edger
Contact with garden cultivator (tiller)
Contact with hedge trimmer
Contact with other powered garden tool
   Excludes1   contact with powered lawn mower (W28)

X● **W29.4 Contact with nail gun**

X● **W29.8 Contact with other powered powered hand tools and household machinery**
Contact with do-it-yourself tool NOS

● **W30 Contact with agricultural machinery**
   Includes   animal-powered farm machine
   Excludes1   agricultural transport vehicle accident (V01-V99)
     explosion of grain store (W40.8)
     exposure to electric current (W86.-)
The appropriate 7th character is to be added to each code from category W30

A	initial encounter
D	subsequent encounter
S	sequela

X● **W30.0 Contact with combine harvester**
Contact with reaper
Contact with thresher

X● **W30.1 Contact with power take-off devices (PTO)**

X● **W30.2 Contact with hay derrick**

X● **W30.3 Contact with grain storage elevator**
   Excludes1   explosion of grain store (W40.8)

● **W30.8 Contact with other specified agricultural machinery**

X● **W30.81 Contact with agricultural transport vehicle in stationary use**
Contact with agricultural transport vehicle under repair, not on public roadway
   Excludes1   agricultural transport vehicle accident (V01-V99)

X● **W30.89 Contact with other specified agricultural machinery**

X● **W30.9 Contact with unspecified agricultural machinery**
Contact with farm machinery NOS

● **W31 Contact with other and unspecified machinery**
   Excludes1   contact with agricultural machinery (W30.-)
     contact with machinery in transport under own power or being towed by a vehicle (V01-V99)
     exposure to electric current (W86)
The appropriate 7th character is to be added to each code from category W31

A	initial encounter
D	subsequent encounter
S	sequela

X● **W31.0 Contact with mining and earth-drilling machinery**
Contact with bore or drill (land) (seabed)
Contact with shaft hoist
Contact with shaft lift
Contact with undercutter

X● **W31.1 Contact with metalworking machines**
Contact with abrasive wheel
Contact with forging machine
Contact with lathe
Contact with mechanical shears
Contact with metal drilling machine
Contact with milling machine
Contact with power press
Contact with rolling-mill
Contact with metal sawing machine

X● **W31.2 Contact with powered woodworking and forming machines**
Contact with band saw
Contact with bench saw
Contact with circular saw
Contact with molding machine
Contact with overhead plane
Contact with powered saw
Contact with radial saw
Contact with sander
   Excludes1   nonpowered woodworking tools (W27.0)

CHAPTER 20 (V01-Y99)

X● **W31.3** **Contact with prime movers**
Contact with gas turbine
Contact with internal combustion engine
Contact with steam engine
Contact with water driven turbine

● **W31.8** **Contact with other specified machinery**

X● **W31.81** **Contact with recreational machinery**
Contact with roller-coaster

X● **W31.82** **Contact with other commercial machinery**
Contact with commercial electric fan
Contact with commercial kitchen appliances
Contact with commercial powered dryer
(clothes) (powered) (spin)
Contact with commercial washing-machine
Contact with commercial sewing machine

Excludes1   contact with household
machinery (W29.-)
contact with powered lawn
mower (W28)

X● **W31.83** **Contact with special construction vehicle in
stationary use**
Contact with special construction vehicle
under repair, not on public roadway

Excludes1   special construction vehicle
accident (V01-V99)

X● **W31.89** **Contact with other specified machinery**

X● **W31.9** **Contact with unspecified machinery**
Contact with machinery NOS

● **W32** **Accidental handgun discharge and malfunction**

Includes   accidental discharge and malfunction of gun for
single hand use
accidental discharge and malfunction of pistol
accidental discharge and malfunction of revolver
handgun discharge and malfunction NOS

Excludes1   accidental airgun discharge and malfunction
(W34.010, W34.110)
accidental BB gun discharge and malfunction
(W34.010, W34.110)
accidental pellet gun discharge and malfunction
(W34.010, W34.110)
accidental shotgun discharge and malfunction
(W33.01, W33.11)
assault by handgun discharge (X93)
handgun discharge involving legal intervention
(Y35.0-)
handgun discharge involving military or war
operations (Y36.4-)
intentional self-harm by handgun discharge (X72)
Very pistol discharge and malfunction (W34.09,
W34.19)

The appropriate 7th character is to be added to each code from
category W32

A   initial encounter
D   subsequent encounter
S   sequela

X● **W32.0** **Accidental handgun discharge**
X● **W32.1** **Accidental handgun malfunction**
Injury due to explosion of handgun (parts)
Injury due to malfunction of mechanism or component
of handgun
Injury due to recoil of handgun
Powder burn from handgun

● **W33** **Accidental rifle, shotgun and larger firearm discharge and
malfunction**

Includes   rifle, shotgun and larger firearm discharge and
malfunction NOS

Excludes1   accidental airgun discharge and malfunction
(W34.010, W34.110)
accidental BB gun discharge and malfunction
(W34.010, W34.110)
accidental handgun discharge and malfunction
(W32.-)
accidental pellet gun discharge and malfunction
(W34.010, W34.110)
assault by rifle, shotgun and larger firearm
discharge (X94)
firearm discharge involving legal intervention
(Y35.0-)
firearm discharge involving military or war
operations (Y36.4-)
intentional self-harm by rifle, shotgun and larger
firearm discharge (X73)

The appropriate 7th character is to be added to each code from
category W33

A   initial encounter
D   subsequent encounter
S   sequela

● **W33.0** **Accidental rifle, shotgun and larger firearm discharge**

X● **W33.00** **Accidental discharge of unspecified larger
firearm**
Discharge of unspecified larger firearm NOS

X● **W33.01** **Accidental discharge of shotgun**
Discharge of shotgun NOS

X● **W33.02** **Accidental discharge of hunting rifle**
Discharge of hunting rifle NOS

X● **W33.03** **Accidental discharge of machine gun**
Discharge of machine gun NOS

X● **W33.09** **Accidental discharge of other larger firearm**
Discharge of other larger firearm NOS

● **W33.1** **Accidental rifle, shotgun and larger firearm malfunction**
Injury due to explosion of rifle, shotgun and larger
firearm (parts)
Injury due to malfunction of mechanism or component
of rifle, shotgun and larger firearm
Injury due to piercing, cutting, crushing or pinching
due to (by) slide trigger mechanism, scope or other
gun part
Injury due to recoil of rifle, shotgun and larger firearm
Powder burn from rifle, shotgun and larger firearm

X● **W33.10** **Accidental malfunction of unspecified larger
firearm**
Malfunction of unspecified larger firearm NOS

X● **W33.11** **Accidental malfunction of shotgun**
Malfunction of shotgun NOS

X● **W33.12** **Accidental malfunction of hunting rifle**
Malfunction of hunting rifle NOS

X● **W33.13** **Accidental malfunction of machine gun**
Malfunction of machine gun NOS

X● **W33.19** **Accidental malfunction of other larger firearm**
Malfunction of other larger firearm NOS

CHAPTER 20 (V01-Y99)

◄ New   ◄▥ Revised   ~~deleted~~ Deleted   Excludes 1   Excludes 2   Includes   Use additional   Code first   Code also   Unspecified
OGCR Official Guidelines   X Assign placeholder X   ● Use Additional Character(s)   ▷ Manifestation Code   **Coding Clinic**

● **W34   Accidental discharge and malfunction from other and unspecified firearms and guns**

> The appropriate 7th character is to be added to each code from category W34

> | | |
> |---|---|
> | A | initial encounter |
> | D | subsequent encounter |
> | S | sequela |

● **W34.0   Accidental discharge from other and unspecified firearms and guns**

   X● **W34.00   Accidental discharge from unspecified firearms or gun**

> Discharge from firearm NOS
> Gunshot wound NOS
> Shot NOS
> **Coding Clinic: 2015, Q1, P17**

   ● **W34.01   Accidental discharge of gas, air or spring-operated guns**

     ● **W34.010   Accidental discharge of airgun**

> Accidental discharge of BB gun
> Accidental discharge of pellet gun

     ● **W34.011   Accidental discharge of paintball gun**

> Accidental injury due to paintball discharge

     ● **W34.018   Accidental discharge of other gas, air or spring-operated gun**

   X● **W34.09   Accidental discharge from other specified firearms**

> Accidental discharge from Very pistol [flare]

● **W34.1   Accidental malfunction from other and unspecified firearms and guns**

   X● **W34.10   Accidental malfunction from unspecified firearms or gun**

> Firearm malfunction NOS

   ● **W34.11   Accidental malfunction of gas, air or spring-operated guns**

     ● **W34.110   Accidental malfunction of airgun**

> Accidental malfunction of BB gun
> Accidental malfunction of pellet gun

     ● **W34.111   Accidental malfunction of paintball gun**

> Accidental injury due to paintball gun malfunction

     ● **W34.118   Accidental malfunction of other gas, air or spring-operated gun**

   X● **W34.19   Accidental malfunction from other specified firearms**

> Accidental malfunction from Very pistol [flare]

X● **W35   Explosion and rupture of boiler**

> **Excludes1**   explosion and rupture of boiler on watercraft (V93.4)

> The appropriate 7th character is to be added to code W35

> | | |
> |---|---|
> | A | initial encounter |
> | D | subsequent encounter |
> | S | sequela |

● **W36   Explosion and rupture of gas cylinder**

> The appropriate 7th character is to be added to each code from category W36

> | | |
> |---|---|
> | A | initial encounter |
> | D | subsequent encounter |
> | S | sequela |

X● **W36.1   Explosion and rupture of aerosol can**

X● **W36.2   Explosion and rupture of air tank**

X● **W36.3   Explosion and rupture of pressurized-gas tank**

X● **W36.8   Explosion and rupture of other gas cylinder**

X● **W36.9   Explosion and rupture of unspecified gas cylinder**

● **W37   Explosion and rupture of pressurized tire, pipe or hose**

> The appropriate 7th character is to be added to each code from category W37

> | | |
> |---|---|
> | A | initial encounter |
> | D | subsequent encounter |
> | S | sequela |

X● **W37.0   Explosion of bicycle tire**

X● **W37.8   Explosion and rupture of other pressurized tire, pipe or hose**

X● **W38   Explosion and rupture of other specified pressurized devices**

> The appropriate 7th character is to be added to code W38

> | | |
> |---|---|
> | A | initial encounter |
> | D | subsequent encounter |
> | S | sequela |

X● **W39   Discharge of firework**

> The appropriate 7th character is to be added to code W39

> | | |
> |---|---|
> | A | initial encounter |
> | D | subsequent encounter |
> | S | sequela |

● **W40   Explosion of other materials**

> **Excludes1**   assault by explosive material (X96)
>   explosion involving legal intervention (Y35.1-)
>   explosion involving military or war operations (Y36.0-, Y36.2-)
>   intentional self-harm by explosive material (X75)

> The appropriate 7th character is to be added to each code from category W40

> | | |
> |---|---|
> | A | initial encounter |
> | D | subsequent encounter |
> | S | sequela |

X● **W40.0   Explosion of blasting material**

> Explosion of blasting cap
> Explosion of detonator
> Explosion of dynamite
> Explosion of explosive (any) used in blasting operations

X● **W40.1   Explosion of explosive gases**

> Explosion of acetylene
> Explosion of butane
> Explosion of coal gas
> Explosion in mine NOS
> Explosion of explosive gas
> Explosion of fire damp
> Explosion of gasoline fumes
> Explosion of methane
> Explosion of propane

X● **W40.8   Explosion of other specified explosive materials**

> Explosion in dump NOS
> Explosion in factory NOS
> Explosion in grain store
> Explosion in munitions

> **Excludes1**   explosion involving legal intervention (Y35.1-)
>   explosion involving military or war operations (Y36.0-, Y36.2-)

X● **W40.9   Explosion of unspecified explosive materials**

> Explosion NOS

● **W42   Exposure to noise**

> The appropriate 7th character is to be added to each code from category W42

> | | |
> |---|---|
> | A | initial encounter |
> | D | subsequent encounter |
> | S | sequela |

X● **W42.0   Exposure to supersonic waves**

X● **W42.9   Exposure to other noise**

> Exposure to sound waves NOS

CHAPTER 20 (V01-Y99)

CHAPTER 20 (V01-Y99)

● **W45 Foreign body or object entering through skin**

Includes foreign body or object embedded in skin ◀
nail embedded in skin ◀

Excludes2 contact with hand tools (nonpowered) (powered) (W27-W29)
contact with other sharp object(s) (W26.-) ◀▥
contact with sharp glass (W25.-)
struck by objects (W20-W22)

The appropriate 7th character is to be added to each code from category W45

A	initial encounter
D	subsequent encounter
S	sequela

X ● **W45.0 Nail entering through skin**

~~W45.1 Paper entering through skin~~
~~Paper cut~~

~~W45.2 Lid of can entering through skin~~

X ● **W45.8 Other foreign body or object entering through skin**
Splinter in skin NOS

● **W46 Contact with hypodermic needle**

The appropriate 7th character is to be added to each code from category W46

A	initial encounter
D	subsequent encounter
S	sequela

X ● **W46.0 Contact with hypodermic needle**
Hypodermic needle stick NOS

X ● **W46.1 Contact with contaminated hypodermic needle**

● **W49 Exposure to other inanimate mechanical forces**

Includes exposure to abnormal gravitational [G] forces
exposure to inanimate mechanical forces NEC

Excludes1 exposure to inanimate mechanical forces involving military or war operations (Y36.-, Y37.-)

The appropriate 7th character is to be added to each code from category W49

A	initial encounter
D	subsequent encounter
S	sequela

● **W49.0 Item causing external constriction**

X ● **W49.01 Hair causing external constriction**

X ● **W49.02 String or thread causing external constriction**

X ● **W49.03 Rubber band causing external constriction**

X ● **W49.04 Ring or other jewelry causing external constriction**

X ● **W49.09 Other item causing external constriction**

X ● **W49.9 Exposure to other inanimate mechanical forces**

EXPOSURE TO ANIMATE MECHANICAL FORCES (W50-W64)

Excludes1 toxic effect of contact with venomous animals and plants (T63.-)

● **W50 Accidental hit, strike, kick, twist, bite or scratch by another person**

Includes hit, strike, kick, twist, bite, or scratch by another person NOS

Excludes1 assault by bodily force (Y04)
struck by objects (W20-W22)

The appropriate 7th character is to be added to each code from category W50

A	initial encounter
D	subsequent encounter
S	sequela

X ● **W50.0 Accidental hit or strike by another person**
Hit or strike by another person NOS

X ● **W50.1 Accidental kick by another person**
Kick by another person NOS

X ● **W50.2 Accidental twist by another person**
Twist by another person NOS
Coding Clinic: 2015, Q1, P8

X ● **W50.3 Accidental bite by another person**
Human bite
Bite by another person NOS

X ● **W50.4 Accidental scratch by another person**
Scratch by another person NOS

X ● **W51 Accidental striking against or bumped into by another person**

Excludes1 assault by striking against or bumping into by another person (Y04.2)
fall due to collision with another person (W03)

The appropriate 7th character is to be added to code W51

A	initial encounter
D	subsequent encounter
S	sequela

X ● **W52 Crushed, pushed or stepped on by crowd or human stampede**
Crushed, pushed or stepped on by crowd or human stampede with or without fall

The appropriate 7th character is to be added to code W52

A	initial encounter
D	subsequent encounter
S	sequela

● **W53 Contact with rodent**

Includes contact with saliva, feces or urine of rodent

The appropriate 7th character is to be added to each code from category W53

A	initial encounter
D	subsequent encounter
S	sequela

● **W53.0 Contact with mouse**

X ● **W53.01 Bitten by mouse**

X ● **W53.09 Other contact with mouse**

● **W53.1 Contact with rat**

X ● **W53.11 Bitten by rat**

X ● **W53.19 Other contact with rat**

● **W53.2 Contact with squirrel**

X ● **W53.21 Bitten by squirrel**

X ● **W53.29 Other contact with squirrel**

● **W53.8 Contact with other rodent**

X ● **W53.81 Bitten by other rodent**

X ● **W53.89 Other contact with other rodent**

● **W54 Contact with dog**

Includes contact with saliva, feces or urine of dog

The appropriate 7th character is to be added to each code from category W54

A	initial encounter
D	subsequent encounter
S	sequela

X ● **W54.0 Bitten by dog**

X ● **W54.1 Struck by dog**
Knocked over by dog

X ● **W54.8 Other contact with dog**

◀ New   ◀▥ Revised   ~~deleted~~ Deleted   Excludes 1   Excludes 2   Includes   Use additional   Code first   Code also   Unspecified

OGCR Official Guidelines   X Assign placeholder X   ● Use Additional Character(s)   ▶ Manifestation Code   **Coding Clinic**

● **W55 Contact with other mammals**

     Includes   contact with saliva, feces or urine of mammal

     Excludes1   animal being ridden - see transport accidents

                   bitten or struck by dog (W54)

                   bitten or struck by rodent (W53.-)

                   contact with marine mammals (W56.X-)

     The appropriate 7th character is to be added to each code from category W55

        A   initial encounter
        D   subsequent encounter
        S   sequela

● **W55.0 Contact with cat**

   X● **W55.01 Bitten by cat**

   X● **W55.03 Scratched by cat**

   X● **W55.09 Other contact with cat**

● **W55.1 Contact with horse**

   X● **W55.11 Bitten by horse**

   X● **W55.12 Struck by horse**

   X● **W55.19 Other contact with horse**

● **W55.2 Contact with cow**

       Contact with bull

   X● **W55.21 Bitten by cow**

   X● **W55.22 Struck by cow**

          Gored by bull

   X● **W55.29 Other contact with cow**

● **W55.3 Contact with other hoof stock**

       Contact with goats

       Contact with sheep

   X● **W55.31 Bitten by other hoof stock**

   X● **W55.32 Struck by other hoof stock**

          Gored by goat

          Gored by ram

   X● **W55.39 Other contact with other hoof stock**

● **W55.4 Contact with pig**

   X● **W55.41 Bitten by pig**

   X● **W55.42 Struck by pig**

   X● **W55.49 Other contact with pig**

● **W55.5 Contact with raccoon**

   X● **W55.51 Bitten by raccoon**

   X● **W55.52 Struck by raccoon**

   X● **W55.59 Other contact with raccoon**

● **W55.8 Contact with other mammals**

   X● **W55.81 Bitten by other mammals**

   X● **W55.82 Struck by other mammals**

   X● **W55.89 Other contact with other mammals**

● **W56 Contact with nonvenomous marine animal**

     Excludes1   contact with venomous marine animal (T63.-)

     The appropriate 7th character is to be added to each code from category W56

        A   initial encounter
        D   subsequent encounter
        S   sequela

● **W56.0 Contact with dolphin**

   X● **W56.01 Bitten by dolphin**

   X● **W56.02 Struck by dolphin**

   X● **W56.09 Other contact with dolphin**

● **W56.1 Contact with sea lion**

   X● **W56.11 Bitten by sea lion**

   X● **W56.12 Struck by sea lion**

   X● **W56.19 Other contact with sea lion**

● **W56.2 Contact with orca**

       Contact with killer whale

   X● **W56.21 Bitten by orca**

   X● **W56.22 Struck by orca**

   X● **W56.29 Other contact with orca**

● **W56.3 Contact with other marine mammals**

   X● **W56.31 Bitten by other marine mammals**

   X● **W56.32 Struck by other marine mammals**

   X● **W56.39 Other contact with other marine mammals**

● **W56.4 Contact with shark**

   X● **W56.41 Bitten by shark**

   X● **W56.42 Struck by shark**

   X● **W56.49 Other contact with shark**

● **W56.5 Contact with other fish**

   X● **W56.51 Bitten by other fish**

   X● **W56.52 Struck by other fish**

   X● **W56.59 Other contact with other fish**

● **W56.8 Contact with other nonvenomous marine animals**

   X● **W56.81 Bitten by other nonvenomous marine animals**

   X● **W56.82 Struck by other nonvenomous marine animals**

   X● **W56.89 Other contact with other nonvenomous marine animals**

X● **W57 Bitten or stung by nonvenomous insect and other nonvenomous arthropods**

     Excludes1   contact with venomous insects and arthropods (T63.2-, T63.3-, T63.4-)

     The appropriate 7th character is to be added to code W57

        A   initial encounter
        D   subsequent encounter
        S   sequela

● **W58 Contact with crocodile or alligator**

     The appropriate 7th character is to be added to each code from category W58

        A   initial encounter
        D   subsequent encounter
        S   sequela

● **W58.0 Contact with alligator**

   X● **W58.01 Bitten by alligator**

   X● **W58.02 Struck by alligator**

   X● **W58.03 Crushed by alligator**

   X● **W58.09 Other contact with alligator**

● **W58.1 Contact with crocodile**

   X● **W58.11 Bitten by crocodile**

   X● **W58.12 Struck by crocodile**

   X● **W58.13 Crushed by crocodile**

   X● **W58.19 Other contact with crocodile**

● **W59 Contact with other nonvenomous reptiles**

     Excludes1   contact with venomous reptile (T63.0-, T63.1-)

     The appropriate 7th character is to be added to each code from category W59

        A   initial encounter
        D   subsequent encounter
        S   sequela

● **W59.0 Contact with nonvenomous lizards**

   X● **W59.01 Bitten by nonvenomous lizards**

   X● **W59.02 Struck by nonvenomous lizards**

   X● **W59.09 Other contact with nonvenomous lizards**

          Exposure to nonvenomous lizards

CHAPTER 20 (V01-Y99)

● **W59.1   Contact with nonvenomous snakes**
   X● **W59.11   Bitten by nonvenomous snake**
   X● **W59.12   Struck by nonvenomous snake**
   X● **W59.13   Crushed by nonvenomous snake**
   X● **W59.19   Other contact with nonvenomous snake**

● **W59.2   Contact with turtles**
   Excludes1   contact with tortoises (W59.8-)
   X● **W59.21   Bitten by turtle**
   X● **W59.22   Struck by turtle**
   X● **W59.29   Other contact with turtle**
       Exposure to turtles

● **W59.8   Contact with other nonvenomous reptiles**
   X● **W59.81   Bitten by other nonvenomous reptiles**
   X● **W59.82   Struck by other nonvenomous reptiles**
   X● **W59.83   Crushed by other nonvenomous reptiles**
   X● **W59.89   Other contact with other nonvenomous reptiles**

X● **W60   Contact with nonvenomous plant thorns and spines and sharp leaves**
   Excludes1   contact with venomous plants (T63.X7-)
   The appropriate 7th character is to be added to code W60

A	initial encounter
D	subsequent encounter
S	sequela

● **W61   Contact with birds (domestic) (wild)**
   Includes   contact with excreta of birds
   The appropriate 7th character is to be added to each code from category W61

A	initial encounter
D	subsequent encounter
S	sequela

● **W61.0   Contact with parrot**
   X● **W61.01   Bitten by parrot**
   X● **W61.02   Struck by parrot**
   X● **W61.09   Other contact with parrot**
       Exposure to parrots

● **W61.1   Contact with macaw**
   X● **W61.11   Bitten by macaw**
   X● **W61.12   Struck by macaw**
   X● **W61.19   Other contact with macaw**
       Exposure to macaws

● **W61.2   Contact with other psittacines**
   X● **W61.21   Bitten by other psittacines**
   X● **W61.22   Struck by other psittacines**
   X● **W61.29   Other contact with other psittacines**
       Exposure to other psittacines

● **W61.3   Contact with chicken**
   X● **W61.32   Struck by chicken**
   X● **W61.33   Pecked by chicken**
   X● **W61.39   Other contact with chicken**
       Exposure to chickens

● **W61.4   Contact with turkey**
   X● **W61.42   Struck by turkey**
   X● **W61.43   Pecked by turkey**
   X● **W61.49   Other contact with turkey**

● **W61.5   Contact with goose**
   X● **W61.51   Bitten by goose**
   X● **W61.52   Struck by goose**
   X● **W61.59   Other contact with goose**

● **W61.6   Contact with duck**
   X● **W61.61   Bitten by duck**
   X● **W61.62   Struck by duck**
   X● **W61.69   Other contact with duck**

● **W61.9   Contact with other birds**
   X● **W61.91   Bitten by other birds**
   X● **W61.92   Struck by other birds**
   X● **W61.99   Other contact with other birds**
       Contact with bird NOS

● **W62   Contact with nonvenomous amphibians**
   Excludes1   contact with venomous amphibians (T63.81-R63.83)
   The appropriate 7th character is to be added to each code from category W62

A	initial encounter
D	subsequent encounter
S	sequela

   X● **W62.0   Contact with nonvenomous frogs**
   X● **W62.1   Contact with nonvenomous toads**
   X● **W62.9   Contact with other nonvenomous amphibians**

X● **W64   Exposure to other animate mechanical forces**
   Includes   exposure to nonvenomous animal NOS
   Excludes1   contact with venomous animal (T63.-)
   The appropriate 7th character is to be added to code W64

A	initial encounter
D	subsequent encounter
S	sequela

ACCIDENTAL NON-TRANSPORT DROWNING AND SUBMERSION (W65-W74)

   Excludes1   accidental drowning and submersion due to fall into water (W16.-)
       accidental drowning and submersion due to water transport accident (V90.-, V92.-)
   Excludes2   accidental drowning and submersion due to cataclysm (X34-X39)

X● **W65   Accidental drowning and submersion while in bathtub**
   Excludes1   accidental drowning and submersion due to fall in (into) bathtub (W16.211)
   The appropriate 7th character is to be added to code W65

A	initial encounter
D	subsequent encounter
S	sequela

X● **W67   Accidental drowning and submersion while in swimming pool**
   Excludes1   accidental drowning and submersion due to fall into swimming pool (W16.011, W16.021, W16.031)
       accidental drowning and submersion due to striking into wall of swimming pool (W22.041)
   The appropriate 7th character is to be added to code W67

A	initial encounter
D	subsequent encounter
S	sequela

X● **W69   Accidental drowning and submersion while in natural water**
   Accidental drowning and submersion while in lake
   Accidental drowning and submersion while in open sea
   Accidental drowning and submersion while in river
   Accidental drowning and submersion while in stream
   Excludes1   accidental drowning and submersion due to fall into natural body of water (W16.111, W16.121, W16.131)
   The appropriate 7th character is to be added to code W69

A	initial encounter
D	subsequent encounter
S	sequela

◀ New   ◀▦ Revised   ~~deleted~~ Deleted   Excludes 1   Excludes 2   Includes   Use additional   Code first   Code also   Unspecified

1480   OGCR Official Guidelines   X Assign placeholder X   ● Use Additional Character(s)   ▸ Manifestation Code   **Coding Clinic**

X⬤**W73**   **Other specified cause of accidental non-transport drowning and submersion**
>Accidental drowning and submersion while in quenching tank
>Accidental drowning and submersion while in reservoir
>
>**Excludes1**   accidental drowning and submersion due to fall into other water (W16.311, W16.321, W16.331)
>
>The appropriate 7th character is to be added to code W73

> | | |
> |---|---|
> | A | initial encounter |
> | D | subsequent encounter |
> | S | sequela |

X⬤**W74**   **Unspecified cause of accidental drowning and submersion**
>Drowning NOS
>
>The appropriate 7th character is to be added to code W74

> | | |
> |---|---|
> | A | initial encounter |
> | D | subsequent encounter |
> | S | sequela |

EXPOSURE TO ELECTRIC CURRENT, RADIATION AND EXTREME AMBIENT AIR TEMPERATURE AND PRESSURE (W85-W99)

Excludes1   exposure to:
>failure in dosage of radiation or temperature during surgical and medical care (Y63.2-Y63.5)
>lightning (T75.0-)
>natural cold (X31)
>natural heat (X30)
>natural radiation NOS (X39)
>radiological procedure and radiotherapy (Y84.2)
>sunlight (X32)

X⬤**W85**   **Exposure to electric transmission lines**
>Broken power line
>
>The appropriate 7th character is to be added to code W85

> | | |
> |---|---|
> | A | initial encounter |
> | D | subsequent encounter |
> | S | sequela |

⬤**W86**   **Exposure to other specified electric current**
>The appropriate 7th character is to be added to each code from category W86

> | | |
> |---|---|
> | A | initial encounter |
> | D | subsequent encounter |
> | S | sequela |

X⬤ **W86.0**   **Exposure to domestic wiring and appliances**

X⬤ **W86.1**   **Exposure to industrial wiring, appliances and electrical machinery**
>Exposure to conductors
>Exposure to control apparatus
>Exposure to electrical equipment and machinery
>Exposure to transformers

X⬤ **W86.8**   **Exposure to other electric current**
>Exposure to wiring and appliances in or on farm (not farmhouse)
>Exposure to wiring and appliances outdoors
>Exposure to wiring and appliances in or on public building
>Exposure to wiring and appliances in or on residential institutions
>Exposure to wiring and appliances in or on schools

⬤**W88**   **Exposure to ionizing radiation**
>**Excludes1**   exposure to sunlight (X32)
>
>The appropriate 7th character is to be added to each code from category W88

> | | |
> |---|---|
> | A | initial encounter |
> | D | subsequent encounter |
> | S | sequela |

X⬤ **W88.0**   **Exposure to X-rays**

X⬤ **W88.1**   **Exposure to radioactive isotopes**

X⬤ **W88.8**   **Exposure to other ionizing radiation**

⬤**W89**   **Exposure to man-made visible and ultraviolet light**
>**Includes**   exposure to welding light (arc)
>**Excludes1**   exposure to sunlight (X32) ◄
>
>The appropriate 7th character is to be added to each code from category W89

> | | |
> |---|---|
> | A | initial encounter |
> | D | subsequent encounter |
> | S | sequela |

X⬤ **W89.0**   **Exposure to welding light (arc)**

X⬤ **W89.1**   **Exposure to tanning bed**

X⬤ **W89.8**   **Exposure to other man-made visible and ultraviolet light**

X⬤ **W89.9**   **Exposure to unspecified man-made visible and ultraviolet light**

⬤**W90**   **Exposure to other nonionizing radiation**
>**Excludes1**   exposure to sunlight (X32)
>
>The appropriate 7th character is to be added to each code from category W90

> | | |
> |---|---|
> | A | initial encounter |
> | D | subsequent encounter |
> | S | sequela |

X⬤ **W90.0**   **Exposure to radiofrequency**

X⬤ **W90.1**   **Exposure to infrared radiation**

X⬤ **W90.2**   **Exposure to laser radiation**

X⬤ **W90.8**   **Exposure to other nonionizing radiation**

X⬤**W92**   **Exposure to excessive heat of man-made origin**
>The appropriate 7th character is to be added to code W92

> | | |
> |---|---|
> | A | initial encounter |
> | D | subsequent encounter |
> | S | sequela |

⬤**W93**   **Exposure to excessive cold of man-made origin**
>The appropriate 7th character is to be added to each code from category W93

> | | |
> |---|---|
> | A | initial encounter |
> | D | subsequent encounter |
> | S | sequela |

⬤ **W93.0**   **Contact with or inhalation of dry ice**

     X⬤ **W93.01**   **Contact with dry ice**

     X⬤ **W93.02**   **Inhalation of dry ice**

⬤ **W93.1**   **Contact with or inhalation of liquid air**

     X⬤ **W93.11**   **Contact with liquid air**
>Contact with liquid hydrogen
>Contact with liquid nitrogen

     X⬤ **W93.12**   **Inhalation of liquid air**
>Inhalation of liquid hydrogen
>Inhalation of liquid nitrogen

X⬤ **W93.2**   **Prolonged exposure in deep freeze unit or refrigerator**

X⬤ **W93.8**   **Exposure to other excessive cold of man-made origin**

● W94   **Exposure to high and low air pressure and changes in air pressure**

     The appropriate 7th character is to be added to each code from category W94

> A   initial encounter
> D   subsequent encounter
> S   sequela

X ● W94.0   Exposure to prolonged high air pressure

● W94.1   **Exposure to prolonged low air pressure**

     X ● W94.11   Exposure to residence or prolonged visit at high altitude

     X ● W94.12   Exposure to other prolonged low air pressure

● W94.2   **Exposure to rapid changes in air pressure during ascent**

     X ● W94.21   Exposure to reduction in atmospheric pressure while surfacing from deep-water diving

     X ● W94.22   Exposure to reduction in atmospheric pressure while surfacing from underground

     X ● W94.23   Exposure to sudden change in air pressure in aircraft during ascent

     X ● W94.29   Exposure to other rapid changes in air pressure during ascent

● W94.3   **Exposure to rapid changes in air pressure during descent**

     X ● W94.31   Exposure to sudden change in air pressure in aircraft during descent

     X ● W94.32   Exposure to high air pressure from rapid descent in water

     X ● W94.39   Exposure to other rapid changes in air pressure during descent

X ● W99   **Exposure to other man-made environmental factors**

     The appropriate 7th character is to be added to code W99

> A   initial encounter
> D   subsequent encounter
> S   sequela

EXPOSURE TO SMOKE, FIRE AND FLAMES (X00-X08)

Excludes1   arson (X97)

Excludes2   explosions (W35-W40)
           lightning (T75.0-)
           transport accident (V01-V99)

● X00   **Exposure to uncontrolled fire in building or structure**

     Includes   conflagration in building or structure

     Code first any associated cataclysm

     Excludes2   exposure to ignition or melting of nightwear (X05)
                 exposure to ignition or melting of other clothing and apparel (X06.-)
                 exposure to other specified smoke, fire and flames (X08.-)

     The appropriate 7th character is to be added to each code from category X00

> A   initial encounter
> D   subsequent encounter
> S   sequela

X ● X00.0   Exposure to flames in uncontrolled fire in building or structure
         Coding Clinic: 2016, Q2, P5-6; 2015, Q1, P19

X ● X00.1   Exposure to smoke in uncontrolled fire in building or structure

X ● X00.2   Injury due to collapse of burning building or structure in uncontrolled fire

         Excludes1   injury due to collapse of building not on fire (W20.1)

X ● X00.3   Fall from burning building or structure in uncontrolled fire

X ● X00.4   Hit by object from burning building or structure in uncontrolled fire

X ● X00.5   Jump from burning building or structure in uncontrolled fire

X ● X00.8   Other exposure to uncontrolled fire in building or structure

● X01   **Exposure to uncontrolled fire, not in building or structure**

     Includes   exposure to forest fire

     The appropriate 7th character is to be added to each code from category X01

> A   initial encounter
> D   subsequent encounter
> S   sequela

X ● X01.0   Exposure to flames in uncontrolled fire, not in building or structure

X ● X01.1   Exposure to smoke in uncontrolled fire, not in building or structure

X ● X01.3   Fall due to uncontrolled fire, not in building or structure

X ● X01.4   Hit by object due to uncontrolled fire, not in building or structure

X ● X01.8   Other exposure to uncontrolled fire, not in building or structure

● X02   **Exposure to controlled fire in building or structure**

     Includes   exposure to fire in fireplace exposure to fire in stove

     The appropriate 7th character is to be added to each code from category X02

> A   initial encounter
> D   subsequent encounter
> S   sequela

X ● X02.0   Exposure to flames in controlled fire in building or structure

X ● X02.1   Exposure to smoke in controlled fire in building or structure

X ● X02.2   Injury due to collapse of burning building or structure in controlled fire

         Excludes1   injury due to collapse of building not on fire (W20.1)

X ● X02.3   Fall from burning building or structure in controlled fire

X ● X02.4   Hit by object from burning building or structure in controlled fire

X ● X02.5   Jump from burning building or structure in controlled fire

X ● X02.8   Other exposure to controlled fire in building or structure

● X03   **Exposure to controlled fire, not in building or structure**

     Includes   exposure to bon fire exposure to camp fire exposure to trash fire

     The appropriate 7th character is to be added to each code from category X03

> A   initial encounter
> D   subsequent encounter
> S   sequela

X ● X03.0   Exposure to flames in controlled fire, not in building or structure
         Coding Clinic: 2015, Q1, P19

X ● X03.1   Exposure to smoke in controlled fire, not in building or structure

X ● X03.3   Fall due to controlled fire, not in building or structure

X ● X03.4   Hit by object due to controlled fire, not in building or structure

X ● X03.8   Other exposure to controlled fire, not in building or structure

◀ New   ◀▦ Revised   ~~deleted~~ Deleted   Excludes 1   Excludes 2   Includes   Use additional   Code first   Code also   Unspecified

OGCR Official Guidelines   X Assign placeholder X   ● Use Additional Character(s)   ▶ Manifestation Code   **Coding Clinic**

1482

X ● **X04**   **Exposure to ignition of highly flammable material**
Exposure to ignition of gasoline
Exposure to ignition of kerosene
Exposure to ignition of petrol

    Excludes2   exposure to ignition or melting of nightwear (X05)
             exposure to ignition or melting of other clothing and apparel (X06)

The appropriate 7th character is to be added to code X04

A	initial encounter
D	subsequent encounter
S	sequela

Coding Clinic: 2016, Q2, P4

X ● **X05**   **Exposure to ignition or melting of nightwear**

    Excludes2   exposure to uncontrolled fire in building or structure (X00.-)
             exposure to uncontrolled fire, not in building or structure (X01.-)
             exposure to controlled fire in building or structure (X02.-)
             exposure to controlled fire, not in building or structure (X03.-)
             exposure to ignition of highly flammable materials (X04.-)

The appropriate 7th character is to be added to code X05

A	initial encounter
D	subsequent encounter
S	sequela

● **X06**   **Exposure to ignition or melting of other clothing and apparel**

    Excludes2   exposure to uncontrolled fire in building or structure (X00.-)
             exposure to uncontrolled fire, not in building or structure (X01.-)
             exposure to controlled fire in building or structure (X02.-)
             exposure to controlled fire, not in building or structure (X03.-)
             exposure to ignition of highly flammable materials (X04.-)

The appropriate 7th character is to be added to each code from category X06

A	initial encounter
D	subsequent encounter
S	sequela

X ● **X06.0**   **Exposure to ignition of plastic jewelry**
X ● **X06.1**   **Exposure to melting of plastic jewelry**
X ● **X06.2**   **Exposure to ignition of other clothing and apparel**
X ● **X06.3**   **Exposure to melting of other clothing and apparel**

● **X08**   **Exposure to other specified smoke, fire and flames**
The appropriate 7th character is to be added to each code from category X08

A	initial encounter
D	subsequent encounter
S	sequela

● **X08.0**   **Exposure to bed fire**
Exposure to mattress fire

X ● **X08.00**   **Exposure to bed fire due to** unspecified **burning material**
X ● **X08.01**   **Exposure to bed fire due to burning cigarette**
        Coding Clinic: 2015, Q1, P19
X ● **X08.09**   **Exposure to bed fire due to other burning material**

● **X08.1**   **Exposure to sofa fire**
X ● **X08.10**   **Exposure to sofa fire due to** unspecified **burning material**
X ● **X08.11**   **Exposure to sofa fire due to burning cigarette**
X ● **X08.19**   **Exposure to sofa fire due to other burning material**

● **X08.2**   **Exposure to other furniture fire**
X ● **X08.20**   **Exposure to other furniture fire due to** unspecified **burning material**
X ● **X08.21**   **Exposure to other furniture fire due to burning cigarette**
X ● **X08.29**   **Exposure to other furniture fire due to other burning material**

X ● **X08.8**   **Exposure to other specified smoke, fire and flames**

CONTACT WITH HEAT AND HOT SUBSTANCES (X10-X19)

    Excludes1   exposure to excessive natural heat (X30)
             exposure to fire and flames (X00-X09)

● **X10**   **Contact with hot drinks, food, fats and cooking oils**
The appropriate 7th character is to be added to each code from category X10

A	initial encounter
D	subsequent encounter
S	sequela

X ● **X10.0**   **Contact with hot drinks**
X ● **X10.1**   **Contact with hot food**
X ● **X10.2**   **Contact with fats and cooking oils**

● **X11**   **Contact with hot tap-water**

    Includes   contact with boiling tap-water
               contact with boiling water NOS

    Excludes1   contact with water heated on stove (X12)

The appropriate 7th character is to be added to each code from category X11

A	initial encounter
D	subsequent encounter
S	sequela

X ● **X11.0**   **Contact with hot water in bath or tub**
    Excludes1   contact with running hot water in bath or tub (X11.1)
X ● **X11.1**   **Contact with running hot water**
Contact with hot water running out of hose
Contact with hot water running out of tap
X ● **X11.8**   **Contact with other hot tap-water**
Contact with hot water in bucket
Contact with hot tap-water NOS

X ● **X12**   **Contact with other hot fluids**
Contact with water heated on stove
    Excludes1   hot (liquid) metals (X18)
The appropriate 7th character is to be added to code X12

A	initial encounter
D	subsequent encounter
S	sequela

● **X13**   **Contact with steam and other hot vapors**
The appropriate 7th character is to be added to each code from category X13

A	initial encounter
D	subsequent encounter
S	sequela

X ● **X13.0**   **Inhalation of steam and other hot vapors**
X ● **X13.1**   **Other contact with steam and other hot vapors**

CHAPTER 20 (V01-Y99)

● **X14**   **Contact with hot air and other hot gases**

The appropriate 7th character is to be added to each code from category X14

A	initial encounter
D	subsequent encounter
S	sequela

X ● **X14.0**   **Inhalation of hot air and gases**

X ● **X14.1**   **Other contact with hot air and other hot gases**

● **X15**   **Contact with hot household appliances**

Excludes1   contact with heating appliances (X16)
contact with powered household appliances (W29.-)
exposure to controlled fire in building or structure due to household appliance (X02.8)
exposure to household appliances electrical current (W86.0)

The appropriate 7th character is to be added to each code from category X15

A	initial encounter
D	subsequent encounter
S	sequela

X ● **X15.0**   **Contact with hot stove (kitchen)**

X ● **X15.1**   **Contact with hot toaster**

X ● **X15.2**   **Contact with hotplate**

X ● **X15.3**   **Contact with hot saucepan or skillet**

X ● **X15.8**   **Contact with other hot household appliances**
Contact with cooker
Contact with kettle
Contact with light bulbs

X ● **X16**   **Contact with hot heating appliances, radiators and pipes**

Excludes1   contact with powered appliances (W29.-)
exposure to controlled fire in building or structure due to appliance (X02.8)
exposure to industrial appliances electrical current (W86.1)

The appropriate 7th character is to be added to code X16

A	initial encounter
D	subsequent encounter
S	sequela

X ● **X17**   **Contact with hot engines, machinery and tools**

Excludes1   contact with hot heating appliances, radiators and pipes (X16)
contact with hot household appliances (X15)

The appropriate 7th character is to be added to code X17

A	initial encounter
D	subsequent encounter
S	sequela

X ● **X18**   **Contact with other hot metals**
Contact with liquid metal

The appropriate 7th character is to be added to code X18

A	initial encounter
D	subsequent encounter
S	sequela

X ● **X19**   **Contact with other heat and hot substances**

Excludes1   objects that are not normally hot, e.g., an object made hot by a house fire (X00-X09)

The appropriate 7th character is to be added to code X19

A	initial encounter
D	subsequent encounter
S	sequela

EXPOSURE TO FORCES OF NATURE (X30-X39)

X ● **X30**   **Exposure to excessive natural heat**
Exposure to excessive heat as the cause of sunstroke
Exposure to heat NOS

Excludes1   excessive heat of man-made origin (W92)
exposure to man-made radiation (W89)
exposure to sunlight (X32)
exposure to tanning bed (W89)

The appropriate 7th character is to be added to code X30

A	initial encounter
D	subsequent encounter
S	sequela

X ● **X31**   **Exposure to excessive natural cold**
Excessive cold as the cause of chilblains NOS
Excessive cold as the cause of immersion foot or hand
Exposure to cold NOS
Exposure to weather conditions

Excludes1   cold of man-made origin (W93.-)
contact with or inhalation of dry ice (W93.-)
contact with or inhalation of liquefied gas (W93.-)

The appropriate 7th character is to be added to code X31

A	initial encounter
D	subsequent encounter
S	sequela

X ● **X32**   **Exposure to sunlight**

Excludes1   ~~radiation-related disorders of the skin and subcutaneous tissue (L55-L59)~~
man-made radiation (tanning bed) (W89)

The appropriate 7th character is to be added to code X32

A	initial encounter
D	subsequent encounter
S	sequela

X ● **X34**   **Earthquake**

Excludes2   tidal wave (tsunami) due to earthquake (X37.41)

The appropriate 7th character is to be added to code X34

A	initial encounter
D	subsequent encounter
S	sequela

X ● **X35**   **Volcanic eruption**

Excludes2   tidal wave (tsunami) due to volcanic eruption (X37.41)

The appropriate 7th character is to be added to code X35

A	initial encounter
D	subsequent encounter
S	sequela

● **X36**   **Avalanche, landslide and other earth movements**

Includes   victim of mudslide of cataclysmic nature

Excludes1   earthquake (X34)

Excludes2   transport accident involving collision with avalanche or landslide not in motion (V01-V99)

The appropriate 7th character is to be added to each code from category X36

A	initial encounter
D	subsequent encounter
S	sequela

X ● **X36.0**   **Collapse of dam or man-made structure causing earth movement**

X ● **X36.1**   **Avalanche, landslide, or mudslide**

◄ New   ◄ Revised   ~~deleted~~ Deleted   Excludes 1   Excludes 2   Includes   Use additional   Code first   Code also   Unspecified

OGCR Official Guidelines   X Assign placeholder X   ● Use Additional Character(s)   ▶ Manifestation Code   **Coding Clinic**

● **X37**   **Cataclysmic storm**

> The appropriate 7th character is to be added to each code from category X37

> | | |
> |---|---|
> | A | initial encounter |
> | D | subsequent encounter |
> | S | sequela |

X● **X37.0**   **Hurricane**
> Storm surge   Typhoon

X● **X37.1**   **Tornado**
> Cyclone   Twister

X● **X37.2**   **Blizzard (snow) (ice)**

X● **X37.3**   **Dust storm**

● **X37.4**   **Tidalwave**

     X● **X37.41**   **Tidal wave due to earthquake or volcanic eruption**
> Tidal wave NOS
> Tsunami

     X● **X37.42**   **Tidal wave due to storm**

     X● **X37.43**   **Tidal wave due to landslide**

X● **X37.8**   **Other cataclysmic storms**
> Cloudburst
> Torrential rain
>
> **Excludes2**   flood (X38)

X● **X37.9**   **Unspecified cataclysmic storm**
> Storm NOS
>
> **Excludes1**   collapse of dam or man-made structure causing earth movement (X39.0)

X● **X38**   **Flood**
> Flood arising from remote storm
> Flood of cataclysmic nature arising from melting snow
> Flood resulting directly from storm
>
> **Excludes1**   collapse of dam or man-made structure causing earth movement (X39.0)
>   tidal wave NOS (X37.41)
>   tidal wave caused by storm (X37.2)

> The appropriate 7th character is to be added to code X38

> | | |
> |---|---|
> | A | initial encounter |
> | D | subsequent encounter |
> | S | sequela |

● **X39**   **Exposure to other forces of nature**

> The appropriate 7th character is to be added to each code from category X39

> | | |
> |---|---|
> | A | initial encounter |
> | D | subsequent encounter |
> | S | sequela |

● **X39.0**   **Exposure to natural radiation**
> **Excludes1**   contact with and (suspected) exposure to radon and other naturally occuring radiation (Z77.123)◄⫻
>   exposure to man-made radiation (W88-W90)
>   exposure to sunlight (X32)

     X● **X39.01**   **Exposure to radon**

     X● **X39.08**   **Exposure to other natural radiation**

X● **X39.8**   **Other exposure to forces of nature**

●**X50**   **Overexertion and strenuous or repetitive movements** ◄

> The appropriate 7th character is to be added to each code from category X50◄

> | | |
> |---|---|
> | A | initial encounter ◄ |
> | D | subsequent encounter ◄ |
> | S | sequela ◄ |

X● **X50.0**   **Overexertion from strenuous movement or load** ◄
> Lifting heavy objects ◄
> Lifting weights ◄

X● **X50.1**   **Overexertion from prolonged static or awkward postures** ◄
> Prolonged bending ◄
> Prolonged kneeling ◄
> Prolonged reaching ◄
> Prolonged sitting ◄
> Prolonged standing ◄
> Prolonged twisting ◄
> Static bending ◄
> Static kneeling ◄
> Static reaching ◄
> Static sitting ◄
> Static standing ◄
> Static twisting ◄

X● **X50.3**   **Overexertion from repetitive movements** ◄
> Use of hand as hammer ◄
>
> **Excludes2**   Overuse from prolonged static or awkward postures (X50.1) ◄

X● **X50.9**   **Other and unspecified overexertion or strenuous movements or postures** ◄
> Contact pressure ◄
> Contact stress ◄

X● **X52**   **Prolonged stay in weightless environment**
> Weightlessness in spacecraft (simulator)

> The appropriate 7th character is to be added to code X52

> | | |
> |---|---|
> | A | initial encounter |
> | D | subsequent encounter |
> | S | sequela |

X● **X58**   **Exposure to other specified factors**
> Accident NOS
> Exposure NOS

> The appropriate 7th character is to be added to code X58

> | | |
> |---|---|
> | A | initial encounter |
> | D | subsequent encounter |
> | S | sequela |

Purposely self-inflicted injury
Suicide (attempted)

● **X71**   **Intentional self-harm by drowning and submersion**

> The appropriate 7th character is to be added to each code from category X71

> | | |
> |---|---|
> | A | initial encounter |
> | D | subsequent encounter |
> | S | sequela |

X● **X71.0**   **Intentional self-harm by drowning and submersion while in bathtub**

X● **X71.1**   **Intentional self-harm by drowning and submersion while in swimming pool**

X● **X71.2**   **Intentional self-harm by drowning and submersion after jump into swimming pool**

CHAPTER 20 (V01-Y99)

CHAPTER 20 (VØ1-Y99)

X● **X71.3**   **Intentional self-harm by drowning and submersion in natural water**

X● **X71.8**   **Other intentional self-harm by drowning and submersion**

X● **X71.9**   **Intentional self-harm by drowning and submersion, unspecified**

X●**X72**   **Intentional self-harm by handgun discharge**
Intentional self-harm by gun for single hand use
Intentional self-harm by pistol
Intentional self-harm by revolver

> **Excludes1**   Very pistol (X74.8)

The appropriate 7th character is to be added to code X72

A	initial encounter
D	subsequent encounter
S	sequela

●**X73**   **Intentional self-harm by rifle, shotgun and larger firearm discharge**

> **Excludes1**   airgun (X74.Ø1)

The appropriate 7th character is to be added to each code from category X73

A	initial encounter
D	subsequent encounter
S	sequela

X● **X73.Ø**   **Intentional self-harm by shotgun discharge**

X● **X73.1**   **Intentional self-harm by hunting rifle discharge**

X● **X73.2**   **Intentional self-harm by machine gun discharge**

X● **X73.8**   **Intentional self-harm by other larger firearm discharge**

X● **X73.9**   **Intentional self-harm by unspecified larger firearm discharge**

●**X74**   **Intentional self-harm by other and unspecified firearm and gun discharge**

The appropriate 7th character is to be added to each code from category X74

A	initial encounter
D	subsequent encounter
S	sequela

●**X74.Ø**   **Intentional self-harm by gas, air or spring-operated guns**

X● **X74.Ø1**   **Intentional self-harm by airgun**
Intentional self-harm by BB gun discharge
Intentional self-harm by pellet gun discharge

X● **X74.Ø2**   **Intentional self-harm by paintball gun**

X● **X74.Ø9**   **Intentional self-harm by other gas, air or spring-operated gun**

X● **X74.8**   **Intentional self-harm by other firearm discharge**
Intentional self-harm by Very pistol [flare] discharge

X● **X74.9**   **Intentional self-harm by unspecified firearm discharge**

X●**X75**   **Intentional self-harm by explosive material**

The appropriate 7th character is to be added to code X75

A	initial encounter
D	subsequent encounter
S	sequela

X●**X76**   **Intentional self-harm by smoke, fire and flames**

The appropriate 7th character is to be added to code X76

A	initial encounter
D	subsequent encounter
S	sequela

●**X77**   **Intentional self-harm by steam, hot vapors and hot objects**

The appropriate 7th character is to be added to each code from category X77

A	initial encounter
D	subsequent encounter
S	sequela

X● **X77.Ø**   **Intentional self-harm by steam or hot vapors**

X● **X77.1**   **Intentional self-harm by hot tap water**

X● **X77.2**   **Intentional self-harm by other hot fluids**

X● **X77.3**   **Intentional self-harm by hot household appliances**

X● **X77.8**   **Intentional self-harm by other hot objects**

X● **X77.9**   **Intentional self-harm by unspecified hot objects**

●**X78**   **Intentional self-harm by sharp object**

The appropriate 7th character is to be added to each code from category X78

A	initial encounter
D	subsequent encounter
S	sequela

X● **X78.Ø**   **Intentional self-harm by sharp glass**

X● **X78.1**   **Intentional self-harm by knife**

X● **X78.2**   **Intentional self-harm by sword or dagger**

X● **X78.8**   **Intentional self-harm by other sharp object**

X● **X78.9**   **Intentional self-harm by unspecified sharp object**

X●**X79**   **Intentional self-harm by blunt object**

The appropriate 7th character is to be added to code X79

A	initial encounter
D	subsequent encounter
S	sequela

X●**X80**   **Intentional self-harm by jumping from a high place**
Intentional fall from one level to another

The appropriate 7th character is to be added to code X8Ø

A	initial encounter
D	subsequent encounter
S	sequela

●**X81**   **Intentional self-harm by jumping or lying in front of moving object**

The appropriate 7th character is to be added to each code from category X81

A	initial encounter
D	subsequent encounter
S	sequela

X● **X81.Ø**   **Intentional self-harm by jumping or lying in front of motor vehicle**

X● **X81.1**   **Intentional self-harm by jumping or lying in front of (subway) train**

X● **X81.8**   **Intentional self-harm by jumping or lying in front of other moving object**

●**X82**   **Intentional self-harm by crashing of motor vehicle**

The appropriate 7th character is to be added to each code from category X82

A	initial encounter
D	subsequent encounter
S	sequela

X● **X82.Ø**   **Intentional collision of motor vehicle with other motor vehicle**

X● **X82.1**   **Intentional collision of motor vehicle with train**

X● **X82.2**   **Intentional collision of motor vehicle with tree**

X● **X82.8**   **Other intentional self-harm by crashing of motor vehicle**

◀ New   ⬅ Revised   ~~deleted~~ Deleted   Excludes 1   Excludes 2   Includes   Use additional   Code first   Code also   Unspecified

OGCR Official Guidelines   X Assign placeholder X   ● Use Additional Character(s)   ▶ Manifestation Code   **Coding Clinic**

1486

● **X83   Intentional self-harm by other specified means**

> **Excludes1**   intentional self-harm by poisoning or contact
> with toxic substance - see Table of Drugs and
> Chemicals

> The appropriate 7th character is to be added to each code from
> category X83

A	initial encounter
D	subsequent encounter
S	sequela

X● **X83.0   Intentional self-harm by crashing of aircraft**
X● **X83.1   Intentional self-harm by electrocution**
X● **X83.2   Intentional self-harm by exposure to extremes of cold**
X● **X83.8   Intentional self-harm by other specified means**

ASSAULT (X92-Y09) ◀

> **Includes**   homicide injuries inflicted by another person
> with intent to injure or kill, by any means

> **Excludes1**   injuries due to legal intervention (Y35.-)
> injuries due to operations of war (Y36.-)
> injuries due to terrorism (Y38.-)

● **X92   Assault by drowning and submersion**

> The appropriate 7th character is to be added to each code from
> category X92

A	initial encounter
D	subsequent encounter
S	sequela

X● **X92.0   Assault by drowning and submersion while in bathtub**
X● **X92.1   Assault by drowning and submersion while in
swimming pool**
X● **X92.2   Assault by drowning and submersion after push into
swimming pool**
X● **X92.3   Assault by drowning and submersion in natural water**
X● **X92.8   Other assault by drowning and submersion**
X● **X92.9   Assault by drowning and submersion, unspecified**

X● **X93   Assault by handgun discharge**

> Assault by discharge of gun for single hand use
> Assault by discharge of pistol
> Assault by discharge of revolver

> **Excludes1**   Very pistol (X95.8)

> The appropriate 7th character is to be added to code X93

A	initial encounter
D	subsequent encounter
S	sequela

● **X94   Assault by rifle, shotgun and larger firearm discharge**

> **Excludes1**   airgun (X95.01)

> The appropriate 7th character is to be added to each code from
> category X94

A	initial encounter
D	subsequent encounter
S	sequela

X● **X94.0   Assault by shotgun**
X● **X94.1   Assault by hunting rifle**
X● **X94.2   Assault by machine gun**
X● **X94.8   Assault by other larger firearm discharge**
X● **X94.9   Assault by unspecified larger firearm discharge**

● **X95   Assault by other and unspecified firearm and gun discharge**

> The appropriate 7th character is to be added to each code from
> category X95

A	initial encounter
D	subsequent encounter
S	sequela

● **X95.0   Assault by gas, air or spring-operated guns**
X● **X95.01   Assault by airgun discharge**
> Assault by BB gun discharge
> Assault by pellet gun discharge
X● **X95.02   Assault by paintball gun discharge**
X● **X95.09   Assault by other gas, air or spring-operated gun**
X● **X95.8   Assault by other firearm discharge**
> Assault by very pistol [flare] discharge
X● **X95.9   Assault by unspecified firearm discharge**

● **X96   Assault by explosive material**

> **Excludes1**   incendiary device (X97)
> terrorism involving explosive material (Y38.2-)

> The appropriate 7th character is to be added to each code from
> category X96

A	initial encounter
D	subsequent encounter
S	sequela

X● **X96.0   Assault by antipersonnel bomb**

> **Excludes1**   antipersonnel bomb use in military or
> war (Y36.2-)

X● **X96.1   Assault by gasoline bomb**
X● **X96.2   Assault by letter bomb**
X● **X96.3   Assault by fertilizer bomb**
X● **X96.4   Assault by pipe bomb**
X● **X96.8   Assault by other specified explosive**
X● **X96.9   Assault by unspecified explosive**

X● **X97   Assault by smoke, fire and flames**

> Assault by arson
> Assault by cigarettes
> Assault by incendiary device

> The appropriate 7th character is to be added to code X97

A	initial encounter
D	subsequent encounter
S	sequela

● **X98   Assault by steam, hot vapors and hot objects**

> The appropriate 7th character is to be added to each code from
> category X98

A	initial encounter
D	subsequent encounter
S	sequela

X● **X98.0   Assault by steam or hot vapors**
X● **X98.1   Assault by hot tap water**
X● **X98.2   Assault by hot fluids**
X● **X98.3   Assault by hot household appliances**
X● **X98.8   Assault by other hot objects**
X● **X98.9   Assault by unspecified hot objects**

CHAPTER 20 (V01-Y99)

● **X99**   **Assault by sharp object**
     Excludes1   assault by strike by sports equipment (Y08.0-)
     The appropriate 7th character is to be added to each code from category X99

     | A | initial encounter |
     | D | subsequent encounter |
     | S | sequela |

X ● **X99.0**   **Assault by sharp glass**
X ● **X99.1**   **Assault by knife**
X ● **X99.2**   **Assault by sword or dagger**
X ● **X99.8**   **Assault by other sharp object**
X ● **X99.9**   **Assault by unspecified sharp object**
       Assault by stabbing NOS

X ● **Y00**   **Assault by blunt object**
     Excludes1   assault by strike by sports equipment (Y08.0)
     The appropriate 7th character is to be added to code Y00

     | A | initial encounter |
     | D | subsequent encounter |
     | S | sequela |

X ● **Y01**   **Assault by pushing from high place**
     The appropriate 7th character is to be added to code Y01

     | A | initial encounter |
     | D | subsequent encounter |
     | S | sequela |

● **Y02**   **Assault by pushing or placing victim in front of moving object**
     The appropriate 7th character is to be added to each code from category Y02

     | A | initial encounter |
     | D | subsequent encounter |
     | S | sequela |

X ● **Y02.0**   **Assault by pushing or placing victim in front of motor vehicle**
X ● **Y02.1**   **Assault by pushing or placing victim in front of (subway) train**
X ● **Y02.8**   **Assault by pushing or placing victim in front of other moving object**

● **Y03**   **Assault by crashing of motor vehicle**
     The appropriate 7th character is to be added to each code from category Y03

     | A | initial encounter |
     | D | subsequent encounter |
     | S | sequela |

X ● **Y03.0**   **Assault by being hit or run over by motor vehicle**
X ● **Y03.8**   **Other assault by crashing of motor vehicle**

● **Y04**   **Assault by bodily force**
     Excludes1   assault by:
         submersion (X92.-)
         use of weapon (X93-X95, X99, Y00)
     The appropriate 7th character is to be added to each code from category Y04

     | A | initial encounter |
     | D | subsequent encounter |
     | S | sequela |

X ● **Y04.0**   **Assault by unarmed brawl or fight**
X ● **Y04.1**   **Assault by human bite**
X ● **Y04.2**   **Assault by strike against or bumped into by another person**
X ● **Y04.8**   **Assault by other bodily force**
       Assault by bodily force NOS

OGCR Section I.C.19.f.

Adult and child abuse, neglect and other maltreatment
Sequence first the appropriate code from categories T74.- or T76.- for abuse, neglect and other maltreatment, followed by any accompanying mental health or injury code(s).

If the documentation in the medical record states abuse or neglect it is coded as confirmed. It is coded as suspected if it is documented as suspected.

For cases of confirmed abuse or neglect an external cause code from the assault section (X92-Y08) should be added to identify the cause of any physical injuries. A perpetrator code (Y07) should be added when the perpetrator of the abuse is known. For suspected cases of abuse or neglect, do not report external cause or perpetrator code.

If a suspected case of abuse, neglect or mistreatment is ruled out during an encounter code Z04.71, Encounter for examination and observation following alleged physical adult abuse, ruled out, or code Z04.72, Encounter for examination and observation following alleged child physical abuse, ruled out, should be used, not a code from T76.

If a suspected case of alleged rape or sexual abuse is ruled out during an encounter code Z04.41, Encounter for examination and observation following alleged physical adult abuse, ruled out, or code Z04.42, Encounter for examination and observation following alleged rape or sexual abuse, ruled out, should be used, not a code from T76.

● **Y07**   **Perpetrator of assault, maltreatment and neglect**
     Note: Codes from this category are for use only in cases of confirmed abuse (T74.-)
       Selection of the correct perpetrator code is based on the relationship between the perpetrator and the victim
     Includes   perpetrator of abandonment
         perpetrator of emotional neglect
         perpetrator of mental cruelty
         perpetrator of physical abuse
         perpetrator of physical neglect
         perpetrator of sexual abuse
         perpetrator of torture

● **Y07.0**   **Spouse or partner, perpetrator of maltreatment and neglect**
       Spouse or partner, perpetrator of maltreatment and neglect against spouse or partner
     Y07.01   **Husband, perpetrator of maltreatment and neglect**
     Y07.02   **Wife, perpetrator of maltreatment and neglect**
     Y07.03   **Male partner, perpetrator of maltreatment and neglect**
     Y07.04   **Female partner, perpetrator of maltreatment and neglect**

● **Y07.1**   **Parent (adoptive) (biological), perpetrator of maltreatment and neglect**
     Y07.11   **Biological father, perpetrator of maltreatment and neglect**
     Y07.12   **Biological mother, perpetrator of maltreatment and neglect**
     Y07.13   **Adoptive father, perpetrator of maltreatment and neglect**
     Y07.14   **Adoptive mother, perpetrator of maltreatment and neglect**

● **Y07.4**   **Other family member, perpetrator of maltreatment and neglect**
     ● **Y07.41**   **Sibling, perpetrator of maltreatment and neglect**
       Excludes1   stepsibling, perpetrator of maltreatment and neglect (Y07.435, Y07.436)
       Y07.410   **Brother, perpetrator of maltreatment and neglect**
       Y07.411   **Sister, perpetrator of maltreatment and neglect**

◀ New   ◀══ Revised   ~~deleted~~ Deleted   Excludes 1   Excludes 2   Includes   Use additional   Code first   Code also   Unspecified
OGCR Official Guidelines   X Assign placeholder X   ● Use Additional Character(s)   ▶ Manifestation Code   **Coding Clinic**
1488

● **Y07.42**   Foster parent, perpetrator of maltreatment and neglect

    Y07.420   Foster father, perpetrator of maltreatment and neglect

    Y07.421   Foster mother, perpetrator of maltreatment and neglect

● **Y07.43**   Stepparent or stepsibling, perpetrator of maltreatment and neglect

    Y07.430   Stepfather, perpetrator of maltreatment and neglect

    Y07.432   Male friend of parent (co-residing in household), perpetrator of maltreatment and neglect

    Y07.433   Stepmother, perpetrator of maltreatment and neglect

    Y07.434   Female friend of parent (co-residing in household), perpetrator of maltreatment and neglect

    Y07.435   Stepbrother, perpetrator or maltreatment and neglect

    Y07.436   Stepsister, perpetrator of maltreatment and neglect

● **Y07.49**   Other family member, perpetrator of maltreatment and neglect

    Y07.490   Male cousin, perpetrator of maltreatment and neglect

    Y07.491   Female cousin, perpetrator of maltreatment and neglect

    Y07.499   Other family member, perpetrator of maltreatment and neglect

● **Y07.5**   Non-family member, perpetrator of maltreatment and neglect

    Y07.50   Unspecified non-family member, perpetrator of maltreatment and neglect

● **Y07.51**   Daycare provider, perpetrator of maltreatment and neglect

    Y07.510   At-home childcare provider, perpetrator of maltreatment and neglect

    Y07.511   Daycare center childcare provider, perpetrator of maltreatment and neglect

    Y07.512   At-home adultcare provider, perpetrator of maltreatment and neglect

    Y07.513   Adultcare center provider, perpetrator of maltreatment and neglect

    Y07.519   Unspecified daycare provider, perpetrator of maltreatment and neglect

● **Y07.52**   Healthcare provider, perpetrator of maltreatment and neglect

    Y07.521   Mental health provider, perpetrator of maltreatment and neglect

    Y07.528   Other therapist or healthcare provider, perpetrator of maltreatment and neglect

        Nurse perpetrator of maltreatment and neglect

        Occupational therapist perpetrator of maltreatment and neglect

        Physical therapist perpetrator of maltreatment and neglect

        Speech therapist perpetrator of maltreatment and neglect

    Y07.529   Unspecified healthcare provider, perpetrator of maltreatment and neglect

    Y07.53   Teacher or instructor, perpetrator of maltreatment and neglect

        Coach, perpetrator of maltreatment and neglect

    Y07.59   Other non-family member, perpetrator of maltreatment and neglect

    Y07.9   Unspecified perpetrator of maltreatment and neglect

● **Y08**   Assault by other specified means

The appropriate 7th character is to be added to each code from category Y08

A	initial encounter
D	subsequent encounter
S	sequela

● **Y08.0**   Assault by strike by sport equipment

X ● **Y08.01**   Assault by strike by hockey stick

X ● **Y08.02**   Assault by strike by baseball bat

X ● **Y08.09**   Assault by strike by other specified type of sport equipment

● **Y08.8**   Assault by other specified means

X ● **Y08.81**   Assault by crashing of aircraft

X ● **Y08.89**   Assault by other specified means

● **Y09**   Assault by unspecified means

Assassination (attempted) NOS
Homicide (attempted) NOS
Manslaughter (attempted) NOS
Murder (attempted) NOS

EVENT OF UNDETERMINED INTENT (Y21-Y33)

Undetermined intent is only for use when there is specific documentation in the record that the intent of the injury cannot be determined. If no such documentation is present, code to accidental (unintentional)

● **Y21**   Drowning and submersion, undetermined intent

The appropriate 7th character is to be added to each code from category Y21

A	initial encounter
D	subsequent encounter
S	sequela

X ● **Y21.0**   Drowning and submersion while in bathtub, undetermined intent

X ● **Y21.1**   Drowning and submersion after fall into bathtub, undetermined intent

X ● **Y21.2**   Drowning and submersion while in swimming pool, undetermined intent

X ● **Y21.3**   Drowning and submersion after fall into swimming pool, undetermined intent

X ● **Y21.4**   Drowning and submersion in natural water, undetermined intent

X ● **Y21.8**   Other drowning and submersion, undetermined intent

X ● **Y21.9**   Unspecified drowning and submersion, undetermined intent

X ● **Y22**   Handgun discharge, undetermined intent

Discharge of gun for single hand use, undetermined intent
Discharge of pistol, undetermined intent
Discharge of revolver, undetermined intent

Excludes2   very pistol (Y24.8)

The appropriate 7th character is to be added to code Y22

A	initial encounter
D	subsequent encounter
S	sequela

CHAPTER 20 (V01-Y99)

● **Y23**   **Rifle, shotgun and larger firearm discharge, undetermined intent**

     Excludes2   airgun (Y24.Ø)

     The appropriate 7th character is to be added to each code from category Y23

A	initial encounter
D	subsequent encounter
S	sequela

X ● **Y23.Ø**   Shotgun discharge, undetermined intent
X ● **Y23.1**   Hunting rifle discharge, undetermined intent
X ● **Y23.2**   Military firearm discharge, undetermined intent
X ● **Y23.3**   Machine gun discharge, undetermined intent
X ● **Y23.8**   Other larger firearm discharge, undetermined intent
X ● **Y23.9**   Unspecified larger firearm discharge, undetermined intent

● **Y24**   **Other and unspecified firearm discharge, undetermined intent**

     The appropriate 7th character is to be added to each code from category Y24

A	initial encounter
D	subsequent encounter
S	sequela

X ● **Y24.Ø**   Airgun discharge, undetermined intent
       BB gun discharge, undetermined intent
       Pellet gun discharge, undetermined intent
X ● **Y24.8**   Other firearm discharge, undetermined intent
       Paintball gun discharge, undetermined intent
       Very pistol [flare] discharge, undetermined intent
X ● **Y24.9**   Unspecified firearm discharge, undetermined intent

X ● **Y25**   **Contact with explosive material, undetermined intent**

     The appropriate 7th character is to be added to code Y25

A	initial encounter
D	subsequent encounter
S	sequela

X ● **Y26**   **Exposure to smoke, fire and flames, undetermined intent**

     The appropriate 7th character is to be added to code Y26

A	initial encounter
D	subsequent encounter
S	sequela

● **Y27**   **Contact with steam, hot vapors and hot objects, undetermined intent**

     The appropriate 7th character is to be added to each code from category Y27

A	initial encounter
D	subsequent encounter
S	sequela

X ● **Y27.Ø**   Contact with steam and hot vapors, undetermined intent
X ● **Y27.1**   Contact with hot tap water, undetermined intent
X ● **Y27.2**   Contact with hot fluids, undetermined intent
X ● **Y27.3**   Contact with hot household appliance, undetermined intent
X ● **Y27.8**   Contact with other hot objects, undetermined intent
X ● **Y27.9**   Contact with unspecified hot objects, undetermined intent

● **Y28**   **Contact with sharp object, undetermined intent**

     The appropriate 7th character is to be added to each code from category Y28

A	initial encounter
D	subsequent encounter
S	sequela

X ● **Y28.Ø**   Contact with sharp glass, undetermined intent
X ● **Y28.1**   Contact with knife, undetermined intent
X ● **Y28.2**   Contact with sword or dagger, undetermined intent
X ● **Y28.8**   Contact with other sharp object, undetermined intent
X ● **Y28.9**   Contact with unspecified sharp object, undetermined intent

X ● **Y29**   **Contact with blunt object, undetermined intent**

     The appropriate 7th character is to be added to code Y29

A	initial encounter
D	subsequent encounter
S	sequela

X ● **Y30**   **Falling, jumping or pushed from a high place, undetermined intent**

     Victim falling from one level to another, undetermined intent

     The appropriate 7th character is to be added to code Y30

A	initial encounter
D	subsequent encounter
S	sequela

X ● **Y31**   **Falling, lying or running before or into moving object, undetermined intent**

     The appropriate 7th character is to be added to code Y31

A	initial encounter
D	subsequent encounter
S	sequela

X ● **Y32**   **Crashing of motor vehicle, undetermined intent**

     The appropriate 7th character is to be added to code Y32

A	initial encounter
D	subsequent encounter
S	sequela

X ● **Y33**   **Other specified events, undetermined intent**

     The appropriate 7th character is to be added to code Y33

A	initial encounter
D	subsequent encounter
S	sequela

◄ New   ◄⊪ Revised   ~~deleted~~ Deleted   Excludes 1   Excludes 2   Includes   Use additional   Code first   Code also   Unspecified

OGCR Official Guidelines   X Assign placeholder X   ● Use Additional Character(s)   ▶ Manifestation Code   **Coding Clinic**

149Ø

LEGAL INTERVENTION, OPERATIONS OF WAR, MILITARY OPERATIONS, AND TERRORISM (Y35-Y38)

● Y35   **Legal intervention**

Includes	any injury sustained as a result of an encounter with any law enforcement official, serving in any capacity at the time of the encounter, whether on-duty or off-duty. Includes: injury to law enforcement official, suspect and bystander

The appropriate 7th character is to be added to each code from category Y35

A	initial encounter
D	subsequent encounter
S	sequela

● Y35.0   **Legal intervention involving firearm discharge**

  ● Y35.00   **Legal intervention involving unspecified firearm discharge**
      Legal intervention involving gunshot wound
      Legal intervention involving shot NOS

    ● Y35.001   Legal intervention involving unspecified firearm discharge, law enforcement official injured

    ● Y35.002   Legal intervention involving unspecified firearm discharge, bystander injured

    ● Y35.003   Legal intervention involving unspecified firearm discharge, suspect injured

  ● Y35.01   **Legal intervention involving injury by machine gun**

    ● Y35.011   Legal intervention involving injury by machine gun, law enforcement official injured

    ● Y35.012   Legal intervention involving injury by machine gun, bystander injured

    ● Y35.013   Legal intervention involving injury by machine gun, suspect injured

  ● Y35.02   **Legal intervention involving injury by handgun**

    ● Y35.021   Legal intervention involving injury by handgun, law enforcement official injured

    ● Y35.022   Legal intervention involving injury by handgun, bystander injured

    ● Y35.023   Legal intervention involving injury by handgun, suspect injured

  ● Y35.03   **Legal intervention involving injury by rifle pellet**

    ● Y35.031   Legal intervention involving injury by rifle pellet, law enforcement official injured

    ● Y35.032   Legal intervention involving injury by rifle pellet, bystander injured

    ● Y35.033   Legal intervention involving injury by rifle pellet, suspect injured

  ● Y35.04   **Legal intervention involving injury by rubber bullet**

    ● Y35.041   Legal intervention involving injury by rubber bullet, law enforcement official injured

    ● Y35.042   Legal intervention involving injury by rubber bullet, bystander injured

    ● Y35.043   Legal intervention involving injury by rubber bullet, suspect injured

● Y35.09   **Legal intervention involving other firearm discharge**

    ● Y35.091   Legal intervention involving other firearm discharge, law enforcement official injured

    ● Y35.092   Legal intervention involving other firearm discharge, bystander injured

    ● Y35.093   Legal intervention involving other firearm discharge, suspect injured

● Y35.1   **Legal intervention involving explosives**

  ● Y35.10   **Legal intervention involving unspecified explosives**

    ● Y35.101   Legal intervention involving unspecified explosives, law enforcement official injured

    ● Y35.102   Legal intervention involving unspecified explosives, bystander injured

    ● Y35.103   Legal intervention involving unspecified explosives, suspect injured

  ● Y35.11   **Legal intervention involving injury by dynamite**

    ● Y35.111   Legal intervention involving injury by dynamite, law enforcement official injured

    ● Y35.112   Legal intervention involving injury by dynamite, bystander injured

    ● Y35.113   Legal intervention involving injury by dynamite, suspect injured

  ● Y35.12   **Legal intervention involving injury by explosive shell**

    ● Y35.121   Legal intervention involving injury by explosive shell, law enforcement official injured

    ● Y35.122   Legal intervention involving injury by explosive shell, bystander injured

    ● Y35.123   Legal intervention involving injury by explosive shell, suspect injured

  ● Y35.19   **Legal intervention involving other explosives**
      Legal intervention involving injury by grenade
      Legal intervention involving injury by mortar bomb

    ● Y35.191   Legal intervention involving other explosives, law enforcement official injured

    ● Y35.192   Legal intervention involving other explosives, bystander injured

    ● Y35.193   Legal intervention involving other explosives, suspect injured

● Y35.2   **Legal intervention involving gas**
    Legal intervention involving asphyxiation by gas
    Legal intervention involving poisoning by gas

  ● Y35.20   **Legal intervention involving unspecified gas**

    ● Y35.201   Legal intervention involving unspecified gas, law enforcement official injured

    ● Y35.202   Legal intervention involving unspecified gas, bystander injured

    ● Y35.203   Legal intervention involving unspecified gas, suspect injured

● Y35.21   Legal intervention involving injury by tear gas
    ● Y35.211   Legal intervention involving injury by tear gas, law enforcement official injured
    ● Y35.212   Legal intervention involving injury by tear gas, bystander injured
    ● Y35.213   Legal intervention involving injury by tear gas, suspect injured
● Y35.29   Legal intervention involving other gas
    ● Y35.291   Legal intervention involving other gas, law enforcement official injured
    ● Y35.292   Legal intervention involving other gas, bystander injured
    ● Y35.293   Legal intervention involving other gas, suspect injured
● Y35.3   Legal intervention involving blunt objects
        Legal intervention involving being hit or struck by blunt object
    ● Y35.30   Legal intervention involving unspecified blunt objects
        ● Y35.301   Legal intervention involving unspecified blunt objects, law enforcement official injured
        ● Y35.302   Legal intervention involving unspecified blunt objects, bystander injured
        ● Y35.303   Legal intervention involving unspecified blunt objects, suspect injured
    ● Y35.31   Legal intervention involving baton
        ● Y35.311   Legal intervention involving baton, law enforcement official injured
        ● Y35.312   Legal intervention involving baton, bystander injured
        ● Y35.313   Legal intervention involving baton, suspect injured
    ● Y35.39   Legal intervention involving other blunt objects
        ● Y35.391   Legal intervention involving other blunt objects, law enforcement official injured
        ● Y35.392   Legal intervention involving other blunt objects, bystander injured
        ● Y35.393   Legal intervention involving other blunt objects, suspect injured
● Y35.4   Legal intervention involving sharp objects
        Legal intervention involving being cut by sharp objects
        Legal intervention involving being stabbed by sharp objects
    ● Y35.40   Legal intervention involving unspecified sharp objects
        ● Y35.401   Legal intervention involving unspecified sharp objects, law enforcement official injured
        ● Y35.402   Legal intervention involving unspecified sharp objects, bystander injured
        ● Y35.403   Legal intervention involving unspecified sharp objects, suspect injured
    ● Y35.41   Legal intervention involving bayonet
        ● Y35.411   Legal intervention involving bayonet, law enforcement official injured
        ● Y35.412   Legal intervention involving bayonet, bystander injured
        ● Y35.413   Legal intervention involving bayonet, suspect injured

● Y35.49   Legal intervention involving other sharp objects
    ● Y35.491   Legal intervention involving other sharp objects, law enforcement official injured
    ● Y35.492   Legal intervention involving other sharp objects, bystander injured
    ● Y35.493   Legal intervention involving other sharp objects, suspect injured
● Y35.8   Legal intervention involving other specified means
    ● Y35.81   Legal intervention involving manhandling
        ● Y35.811   Legal intervention involving manhandling, law enforcement official injured
        ● Y35.812   Legal intervention involving manhandling, bystander injured
        ● Y35.813   Legal intervention involving manhandling, suspect injured
    ● Y35.89   Legal intervention involving other specified means
        ● Y35.891   Legal intervention involving other specified means, law enforcement official injured
        ● Y35.892   Legal intervention involving other specified means, bystander injured
        ● Y35.893   Legal intervention involving other specified means, suspect injured
● Y35.9   Legal intervention, means unspecified
    X ● Y35.91   Legal intervention, means unspecified, law enforcement official injured
    X ● Y35.92   Legal intervention, means unspecified, bystander injured
    X ● Y35.93   Legal intervention, means unspecified, suspect injured

● Y36   Operations of war
    Includes   injuries to military personnel and civilians caused by war, civil insurrection, and peacekeeping missions
    Excludes1   injury to military personnel occurring during peacetime military operations (Y37.-)
                military vehicles involved in transport accidents with non-military vehicle during peacetime (V09.01, V09.21, V19.81, V29.81, V39.81, V49.81, V59.81, V69.81, V79.81)
    The appropriate 7th character is to be added to each code from category Y36

A	initial encounter
D	subsequent encounter
S	sequela

    ● Y36.0   War operations involving explosion of marine weapons
            Weapons and military watercraft
        ● Y36.00   War operations involving explosion of unspecified marine weapon
                War operations involving underwater blast NOS
            ● Y36.000   War operations involving explosion of unspecified marine weapon, military personnel
            ● Y36.001   War operations involving explosion of unspecified marine weapon, civilian
        ● Y36.01   War operations involving explosion of depth-charge
            ● Y36.010   War operations involving explosion of depth-charge, military personnel
            ● Y36.011   War operations involving explosion of depth-charge, civilian

- Y36.02 **War operations involving explosion of marine mine**
  War operations involving explosion of marine mine, at sea or in harbor
  - Y36.020 **War operations involving explosion of marine mine, military personnel**
  - Y36.021 **War operations involving explosion of marine mine, civilian**
- Y36.03 **War operations involving explosion of sea-based artillery shell**
  - Y36.030 **War operations involving explosion of sea-based artillery shell, military personnel**
  - Y36.031 **War operations involving explosion of sea-based artillery shell, civilian**
- Y36.04 **War operations involving explosion of torpedo**
  - Y36.040 **War operations involving explosion of torpedo, military personnel**
  - Y36.041 **War operations involving explosion of torpedo, civilian**
- Y36.05 **War operations involving accidental detonation of onboard marine weapons**
  - Y36.050 **War operations involving accidental detonation of onboard marine weapons, military personnel**
  - Y36.051 **War operations involving accidental detonation of onboard marine weapons, civilian**
- Y36.09 **War operations involving explosion of other marine weapons**
  - Y36.090 **War operations involving explosion of other marine weapons, military personnel**
  - Y36.091 **War operations involving explosion of other marine weapons, civilian**
- Y36.1 **War operations involving destruction of aircraft**
  - Y36.10 **War operations involving unspecified destruction of aircraft**
    - Y36.100 **War operations involving unspecified destruction of aircraft, military personnel**
    - Y36.101 **War operations involving unspecified destruction of aircraft, civilian**
  - Y36.11 **War operations involving destruction of aircraft due to enemy fire or explosives**
    War operations involving destruction of aircraft due to air to air missile
    War operations involving destruction of aircraft due to explosive placed on aircraft
    War operations involving destruction of aircraft due to rocket propelled grenade [RPG]
    War operations involving destruction of aircraft due to small arms fire
    War operations involving destruction of aircraft due to surface to air missile
    - Y36.110 **War operations involving destruction of aircraft due to enemy fire or explosives, military personnel**
    - Y36.111 **War operations involving destruction of aircraft due to enemy fire or explosives, civilian**
  - Y36.12 **War operations involving destruction of aircraft due to collision with other aircraft**
    - Y36.120 **War operations involving destruction of aircraft due to collision with other aircraft, military personnel**
    - Y36.121 **War operations involving destruction of aircraft due to collision with other aircraft, civilian**

- Y36.13 **War operations involving destruction of aircraft due to onboard fire**
  - Y36.130 **War operations involving destruction of aircraft due to onboard fire, military personnel**
  - Y36.131 **War operations involving destruction of aircraft due to onboard fire, civilian**
- Y36.14 **War operations involving destruction of aircraft due to accidental detonation of onboard munitions and explosives**
  - Y36.140 **War operations involving destruction of aircraft due to accidental detonation of onboard munitions and explosives, military personnel**
  - Y36.141 **War operations involving destruction of aircraft due to accidental detonation of onboard munitions and explosives, civilian**
- Y36.19 **War operations involving other destruction of aircraft**
  - Y36.190 **War operations involving other destruction of aircraft, military personnel**
  - Y36.191 **War operations involving other destruction of aircraft, civilian**
- Y36.2 **War operations involving other explosions and fragments**

  Excludes1   war operations involving explosion of aircraft (Y36.1-)
  war operations involving explosion of marine weapons (Y36.0-)
  war operations involving explosion of nuclear weapons (Y36.5-)
  war operations involving explosion occurring after cessation of hostilities (Y36.8-)

  - Y36.20 **War operations involving unspecified explosion and fragments**
    War operations involving air blast NOS
    War operations involving blast NOS
    War operations involving blast fragments NOS
    War operations involving blast wave NOS
    War operations involving blast wind NOS
    War operations involving explosion NOS
    War operations involving explosion of bomb NOS
    - Y36.200 **War operations involving unspecified explosion and fragments, military personnel**
    - Y36.201 **War operations involving unspecified explosion and fragments, civilian**
  - Y36.21 **War operations involving explosion of aerial bomb**
    - Y36.210 **War operations involving explosion of aerial bomb, military personnel**
    - Y36.211 **War operations involving explosion of aerial bomb, civilian**
  - Y36.22 **War operations involving explosion of guided missile**
    - Y36.220 **War operations involving explosion of guided missile, military personnel**
    - Y36.221 **War operations involving explosion of guided missile, civilian**

● **Y36.23** **War operations involving explosion of improvised explosive device [IED]**
    War operations involving explosion of person-borne improvised explosive device [IED]
    War operations involving explosion of vehicle-borne improvised explosive device [IED]
    War operations involving explosion of roadside improvised explosive device [IED]

  ● **Y36.230** **War operations involving explosion of improvised explosive device [IED], military personnel**

  ● **Y36.231** **War operations involving explosion of improvised explosive device [IED], civilian**

● **Y36.24** **War operations involving explosion due to accidental detonation and discharge of own munitions or munitions launch device**

  ● **Y36.240** **War operations involving explosion due to accidental detonation and discharge of own munitions or munitions launch device, military personnel**

  ● **Y36.241** **War operations involving explosion due to accidental detonation and discharge of own munitions or munitions launch device, civilian**

● **Y36.25** **War operations involving fragments from munitions**

  ● **Y36.250** **War operations involving fragments from munitions, military personnel**

  ● **Y36.251** **War operations involving fragments from munitions, civilian**

● **Y36.26** **War operations involving fragments of improvised explosive device [IED]**
    War operations involving fragments of person-borne improvised explosive device [IED]
    War operations involving fragments of vehicle-borne improvised explosive device [IED]
    War operations involving fragments of roadside improvised explosive device [IED]

  ● **Y36.260** **War operations involving fragments of improvised explosive device [IED], military personnel**

  ● **Y36.261** **War operations involving fragments of improvised explosive device [IED], civilian**

● **Y36.27** **War operations involving fragments from weapons**

  ● **Y36.270** **War operations involving fragments from weapons, military personnel**

  ● **Y36.271** **War operations involving fragments from weapons, civilian**

● **Y36.29** **War operations involving other explosions and fragments**
    War operations involving explosion of grenade
    War operations involving explosions of land mine
    War operations involving shrapnel NOS

  ● **Y36.290** **War operations involving other explosions and fragments, military personnel**

  ● **Y36.291** **War operations involving other explosions and fragments, civilian**

● **Y36.3** **War operations involving fires, conflagrations and hot substances**
    War operations involving smoke, fumes, and heat from fires, conflagrations and hot substances

  Excludes1 war operations involving fires and conflagrations aboard military aircraft (Y36.1-)
      war operations involving fires and conflagrations aboard military watercraft (Y36.0-)
      war operations involving fires and conflagrations caused indirectly by conventional weapons (Y36.2-)
      war operations involving fires and thermal effects of nuclear weapons (Y36.53-)

  ● **Y36.30** **War operations involving unspecified fire, conflagration and hot substance**

    ● **Y36.300** **War operations involving unspecified fire, conflagration and hot substance, military personnel**

    ● **Y36.301** **War operations involving unspecified fire, conflagration and hot substance, civilian**

  ● **Y36.31** **War operations involving gasoline bomb**
    War operations involving incendiary bomb
    War operations involving petrol bomb

    ● **Y36.310** **War operations involving gasoline bomb, military personnel**

    ● **Y36.311** **War operations involving gasoline bomb, civilian**

  ● **Y36.32** **War operations involving incendiary bullet**

    ● **Y36.320** **War operations involving incendiary bullet, military personnel**

    ● **Y36.321** **War operations involving incendiary bullet, civilian**

  ● **Y36.33** **War operations involving flamethrower**

    ● **Y36.330** **War operations involving flamethrower, military personnel**

    ● **Y36.331** **War operations involving flamethrower, civilian**

  ● **Y36.39** **War operations involving other fires, conflagrations and hot substances**

    ● **Y36.390** **War operations involving other fires, conflagrations and hot substances, military personnel**

    ● **Y36.391** **War operations involving other fires, conflagrations and hot substances, civilian**

● **Y36.4** **War operations involving firearm discharge and other forms of conventional warfare**

  ● **Y36.41** **War operations involving rubber bullets**

    ● **Y36.410** **War operations involving rubber bullets, military personnel**

    ● **Y36.411** **War operations involving rubber bullets, civilian**

  ● **Y36.42** **War operations involving firearms pellets**

    ● **Y36.420** **War operations involving firearms pellets, military personnel**

    ● **Y36.421** **War operations involving firearms pellets, civilian**

● **Y36.43**   **War operations involving other firearms discharge**
    War operations involving bullets NOS

    Excludes1   war operations involving munitions fragments (Y36.25-)
              war operations involving incendiary bullets (Y36.32-)

   ● **Y36.430**   **War operations involving other firearms discharge, military personnel**

   ● **Y36.431**   **War operations involving other firearms discharge, civilian**

● **Y36.44**   **War operations involving unarmed hand to hand combat**

    Excludes1   war operations involving combat using blunt or piercing object (Y36.45-)
              war operations involving intentional restriction of air and airway (Y36.46-)
              war operations involving unintentional restriction of air and airway (Y36.47-)

   ● **Y36.440**   **War operations involving unarmed hand to hand combat, military personnel**

   ● **Y36.441**   **War operations involving unarmed hand to hand combat, civilian**

● **Y36.45**   **War operations involving combat using blunt or piercing object**

   ● **Y36.450**   **War operations involving combat using blunt or piercing object, military personnel**

   ● **Y36.451**   **War operations involving combat using blunt or piercing object, civilian**

● **Y36.46**   **War operations involving intentional restriction of air and airway**

   ● **Y36.460**   **War operations involving intentional restriction of air and airway, military personnel**

   ● **Y36.461**   **War operations involving intentional restriction of air and airway, civilian**

● **Y36.47**   **War operations involving unintentional restriction of air and airway**

   ● **Y36.470**   **War operations involving unintentional restriction of air and airway, military personnel**

   ● **Y36.471**   **War operations involving unintentional restriction of air and airway, civilian**

● **Y36.49**   **War operations involving other forms of conventional warfare**

   ● **Y36.490**   **War operations involving other forms of conventional warfare, military personnel**

   ● **Y36.491**   **War operations involving other forms of conventional warfare, civilian**

● **Y36.5**   **War operations involving nuclear weapons**
    War operations involving dirty bomb NOS

   ● **Y36.50**   **War operations involving unspecified effect of nuclear weapon**

     ● **Y36.500**   **War operations involving unspecified effect of nuclear weapon, military personnel**

     ● **Y36.501**   **War operations involving unspecified effect of nuclear weapon, civilian**

● **Y36.51**   **War operations involving direct blast effect of nuclear weapon**
    War operations involving blast pressure of nuclear weapon

   ● **Y36.510**   **War operations involving direct blast effect of nuclear weapon, military personnel**

   ● **Y36.511**   **War operations involving direct blast effect of nuclear weapon, civilian**

● **Y36.52**   **War operations involving indirect blast effect of nuclear weapon**
    War operations involving being thrown by blast of nuclear weapon
    War operations involving being struck or crushed by blast debris of nuclear weapon

   ● **Y36.520**   **War operations involving indirect blast effect of nuclear weapon, military personnel**

   ● **Y36.521**   **War operations involving indirect blast effect of nuclear weapon, civilian**

● **Y36.53**   **War operations involving thermal radiation effect of nuclear weapon**
    War operations involving direct heat from nuclear weapon
    War operation involving fireball effects from nuclear weapon

   ● **Y36.530**   **War operations involving thermal radiation effect of nuclear weapon, military personnel**

   ● **Y36.531**   **War operations involving thermal radiation effect of nuclear weapon, civilian**

● **Y36.54**   **War operation involving nuclear radiation effects of nuclear weapon**
    War operation involving acute radiation exposure from nuclear weapon
    War operation involving exposure to immediate ionizing radiation from nuclear weapon
    War operation involving fallout exposure from nuclear weapon
    War operation involving secondary effects of nuclear weapons

   ● **Y36.540**   **War operation involving nuclear radiation effects of nuclear weapon, military personnel**

   ● **Y36.541**   **War operation involving nuclear radiation effects of nuclear weapon, civilian**

● **Y36.59**   **War operation involving other effects of nuclear weapons**

   ● **Y36.590**   **War operation involving other effects of nuclear weapons, military personnel**

   ● **Y36.591**   **War operation involving other effects of nuclear weapons, civilian**

● **Y36.6**   **War operations involving biological weapons**

   ● **Y36.6X**   **War operations involving biological weapons**

     ● **Y36.6X0**   **War operations involving biological weapons, military personnel**

     ● **Y36.6X1**   **War operations involving biological weapons, civilian**

● **Y36.7   War operations involving chemical weapons and other forms of unconventional warfare**

    Excludes1   war operations involving incendiary devices (Y36.3-, Y36.5-)

  ● **Y36.7X   War operations involving chemical weapons and other forms of unconventional warfare**

    ● **Y36.7XØ   War operations involving chemical weapons and other forms of unconventional warfare, military personnel**

    ● **Y36.7X1   War operations involving chemical weapons and other forms of unconventional warfare, civilian**

● **Y36.8   War operations occurring after cessation of hostilities**

    War operations classifiable to categories Y36.Ø-Y36.8 but occurring after cessation of hostilities

  ● **Y36.81   Explosion of mine placed during war operations but exploding after cessation of hostilities**

    ● **Y36.81Ø   Explosion of mine placed during war operations but exploding after cessation of hostilities, military personnel**

    ● **Y36.811   Explosion of mine placed during war operations but exploding after cessation of hostilities, civilian**

  ● **Y36.82   Explosion of bomb placed during war operations but exploding after cessation of hostilities**

    ● **Y36.82Ø   Explosion of bomb placed during war operations but exploding after cessation of hostilities, military personnel**

    ● **Y36.821   Explosion of bomb placed during war operations but exploding after cessation of hostilities, civilian**

  ● **Y36.88   Other war operations occurring after cessation of hostilities**

    ● **Y36.88Ø   Other war operations occurring after cessation of hostilities, military personnel**

    ● **Y36.881   Other war operations occurring after cessation of hostilities, civilian**

  ● **Y36.89   Unspecified war operations occurring after cessation of hostilities**

    ● **Y36.89Ø   Unspecified war operations occurring after cessation of hostilities, military personnel**

    ● **Y36.891   Unspecified war operations occurring after cessation of hostilities, civilian**

● **Y36.9   Other and unspecified war operations**

  X ● **Y36.9Ø   War operations, unspecified**

  X ● **Y36.91   War operations involving unspecified weapon of mass destruction [WMD]**

  X ● **Y36.92   War operations involving friendly fire**

● **Y37   Military operations**

    Includes   Injuries to military personnel and civilians occurring during peacetime on military property and during routine military exercises and operations

    Excludes1   military aircraft involved in aircraft accident with civilian aircraft (V97.81-)

        military vehicles involved in transport accident with civilian vehicle (VØ9.Ø1, VØ9.21, V19.81, V29.81, V39.81, V49.81, V59.81, V69.81, V79.81)

        military watercraft involved in water transport accident with civilian watercraft (V94.81-)

        war operations (Y36.-)

The appropriate 7th character is to be added to each code from category Y37

A	initial encounter
D	subsequent encounter
S	sequela

● **Y37.Ø   Military operations involving explosion of marine weapons**

  ● **Y37.ØØ   Military operations involving explosion of unspecified marine weapon**

    Military operations involving underwater blast NOS

    ● **Y37.ØØØ   Military operations involving explosion of unspecified marine weapon, military personnel**

    ● **Y37.ØØ1   Military operations involving explosion of unspecified marine weapon, civilian**

  ● **Y37.Ø1   Military operations involving explosion of depth-charge**

    ● **Y37.Ø1Ø   Military operations involving explosion of depth-charge, military personnel**

    ● **Y37.Ø11   Military operations involving explosion of depth-charge, civilian**

  ● **Y37.Ø2   Military operations involving explosion of marine mine**

    Military operations involving explosion of marine mine, at sea or in harbor

    ● **Y37.Ø2Ø   Military operations involving explosion of marine mine, military personnel**

    ● **Y37.Ø21   Military operations involving explosion of marine mine, civilian**

  ● **Y37.Ø3   Military operations involving explosion of sea-based artillery shell**

    ● **Y37.Ø3Ø   Military operations involving explosion of sea-based artillery shell, military personnel**

    ● **Y37.Ø31   Military operations involving explosion of sea-based artillery shell, civilian**

  ● **Y37.Ø4   Military operations involving explosion of torpedo**

    ● **Y37.Ø4Ø   Military operations involving explosion of torpedo, military personnel**

    ● **Y37.Ø41   Military operations involving explosion of torpedo, civilian**

  ● **Y37.Ø5   Military operations involving accidental detonation of onboard marine weapons**

    ● **Y37.Ø5Ø   Military operations involving accidental detonation of onboard marine weapons, military personnel**

    ● **Y37.Ø51   Military operations involving accidental detonation of onboard marine weapons, civilian**

◀ New   ⬅ Revised   ~~deleted~~ Deleted   Excludes 1   Excludes 2   Includes   Use additional   Code first   Code also   Unspecified

OGCR Official Guidelines   X Assign placeholder X   ● Use Additional Character(s)   ▶ Manifestation Code   **Coding Clinic**

● Y37.09 Military operations involving explosion of other marine weapons
- ● Y37.090 Military operations involving explosion of other marine weapons, military personnel
- ● Y37.091 Military operations involving explosion of other marine weapons, civilian

● Y37.1 Military operations involving destruction of aircraft
- ● Y37.10 Military operations involving unspecified destruction of aircraft
  - ● Y37.100 Military operations involving unspecified destruction of aircraft, military personnel
  - ● Y37.101 Military operations involving unspecified destruction of aircraft, civilian
- ● Y37.11 Military operations involving destruction of aircraft due to enemy fire or explosives
  Military operations involving destruction of aircraft due to air to air missile
  Military operations involving destruction of aircraft due to explosive placed on aircraft
  Military operations involving destruction of aircraft due to rocket propelled grenade [RPG]
  Military operations involving destruction of aircraft due to small arms fire
  Military operations involving destruction of aircraft due to surface to air missile
  - ● Y37.110 Military operations involving destruction of aircraft due to enemy fire or explosives, military personnel
  - ● Y37.111 Military operations involving destruction of aircraft due to enemy fire or explosives, civilian
- ● Y37.12 Military operations involving destruction of aircraft due to collision with other aircraft
  - ● Y37.120 Military operations involving destruction of aircraft due to collision with other aircraft, military personnel
  - ● Y37.121 Military operations involving destruction of aircraft due to collision with other aircraft, civilian
- ● Y37.13 Military operations involving destruction of aircraft due to onboard fire
  - ● Y37.130 Military operations involving destruction of aircraft due to onboard fire, military personnel
  - ● Y37.131 Military operations involving destruction of aircraft due to onboard fire, civilian
- ● Y37.14 Military operations involving destruction of aircraft due to accidental detonation of onboard munitions and explosives
  - ● Y37.140 Military operations involving destruction of aircraft due to accidental detonation of onboard munitions and explosives, military personnel
  - ● Y37.141 Military operations involving destruction of aircraft due to accidental detonation of onboard munitions and explosives, civilian
- ● Y37.19 Military operations involving other destruction of aircraft
  - ● Y37.190 Military operations involving other destruction of aircraft, military personnel
  - ● Y37.191 Military operations involving other destruction of aircraft, civilian

● Y37.2 Military operations involving other explosions and fragments
    Excludes1 military operations involving explosion of aircraft (Y37.1-)
                military operations involving explosion of marine weapons (Y37.0-)
                military operations involving explosion of nuclear weapons (Y37.5-)
- ● Y37.20 Military operations involving unspecified explosion and fragments
  Military operations involving air blast NOS
  Military operations involving blast NOS
  Military operations involving blast fragments NOS
  Military operations involving blast wave NOS
  Military operations involving blast wind NOS
  Military operations involving explosion NOS
  Military operations involving explosion of bomb NOS
  - ● Y37.200 Military operations involving unspecified explosion and fragments, military personnel
  - ● Y37.201 Military operations involving unspecified explosion and fragments, civilian
- ● Y37.21 Military operations involving explosion of aerial bomb
  - ● Y37.210 Military operations involving explosion of aerial bomb, military personnel
  - ● Y37.211 Military operations involving explosion of aerial bomb, civilian
- ● Y37.22 Military operations involving explosion of guided missile
  - ● Y37.220 Military operations involving explosion of guided missile, military personnel
  - ● Y37.221 Military operations involving explosion of guided missile, civilian
- ● Y37.23 Military operations involving explosion of improvised explosive device [IED]
  Military operations involving explosion of person-borne improvised explosive device [IED]
  Military operations involving explosion of vehicle-borne improvised explosive device [IED]
  Military operations involving explosion of roadside improvised explosive device [IED]
  - ● Y37.230 Military operations involving explosion of improvised explosive device [IED], military personnel
  - ● Y37.231 Military operations involving explosion of improvised explosive device [IED], civilian
- ● Y37.24 Military operations involving explosion due to accidental detonation and discharge of own munitions or munitions launch device
  - ● Y37.240 Military operations involving explosion due to accidental detonation and discharge of own munitions or munitions launch device, military personnel
  - ● Y37.241 Military operations involving explosion due to accidental detonation and discharge of own munitions or munitions launch device, civilian

● Y37.25   Military operations involving fragments from munitions
   ● Y37.250   Military operations involving fragments from munitions, military personnel
   ● Y37.251   Military operations involving fragments from munitions, civilian

● Y37.26   Military operations involving fragments of improvised explosive device [IED]
   Military operations involving fragments of person-borne improvised explosive device [IED]
   Military operations involving fragments of vehicle-borne improvised explosive device [IED]
   Military operations involving fragments of roadside improvised explosive device [IED]
   ● Y37.260   Military operations involving fragments of improvised explosive device [IED], military personnel
   ● Y37.261   Military operations involving fragments of improvised explosive device [IED], civilian

● Y37.27   Military operations involving fragments from weapons
   ● Y37.270   Military operations involving fragments from weapons, military personnel
   ● Y37.271   Military operations involving fragments from weapons, civilian

● Y37.29   Military operations involving other explosions and fragments
   Military operations involving explosion of grenade
   Military operations involving explosions of land mine
   Military operations involving shrapnel NOS
   ● Y37.290   Military operations involving other explosions and fragments, military personnel
   ● Y37.291   Military operations involving other explosions and fragments, civilian

● Y37.3   Military operations involving fires, conflagrations and hot substances
   Military operations involving smoke, fumes, and heat from fires, conflagrations and hot substances
   Excludes1   military operations involving fires and conflagrations aboard military aircraft (Y37.1-)
   military operations involving fires and conflagrations aboard military watercraft (Y37.0-)
   military operations involving fires and conflagrations caused indirectly by conventional weapons (Y37.2-)
   military operations involving fires and thermal effects of nuclear weapons (Y36.53-)

   ● Y37.30   Military operations involving unspecified fire, conflagration and hot substance
      ● Y37.300   Military operations involving unspecified fire, conflagration and hot substance, military personnel
      ● Y37.301   Military operations involving unspecified fire, conflagration and hot substance, civilian

   ● Y37.31   Military operations involving gasoline bomb
      Military operations involving incendiary bomb
      Military operations involving petrol bomb
      ● Y37.310   Military operations involving gasoline bomb, military personnel
      ● Y37.311   Military operations involving gasoline bomb, civilian

● Y37.32   Military operations involving incendiary bullet
   ● Y37.320   Military operations involving incendiary bullet, military personnel
   ● Y37.321   Military operations involving incendiary bullet, civilian

● Y37.33   Military operations involving flamethrower
   ● Y37.330   Military operations involving flamethrower, military personnel
   ● Y37.331   Military operations involving flamethrower, civilian

● Y37.39   Military operations involving other fires, conflagrations and hot substances
   ● Y37.390   Military operations involving other fires, conflagrations and hot substances, military personnel
   ● Y37.391   Military operations involving other fires, conflagrations and hot substances, civilian

● Y37.4   Military operations involving firearm discharge and other forms of conventional warfare
   ● Y37.41   Military operations involving rubber bullets
      ● Y37.410   Military operations involving rubber bullets, military personnel
      ● Y37.411   Military operations involving rubber bullets, civilian

   ● Y37.42   Military operations involving firearms pellets
      ● Y37.420   Military operations involving firearms pellets, military personnel
      ● Y37.421   Military operations involving firearms pellets, civilian

   ● Y37.43   Military operations involving other firearms discharge
      Military operations involving bullets NOS
      Excludes1   military operations involving munitions fragments (Y37.25-)
      military operations involving incendiary bullets (Y37.32-)
      ● Y37.430   Military operations involving other firearms discharge, military personnel
      ● Y37.431   Military operations involving other firearms discharge, civilian

   ● Y37.44   Military operations involving unarmed hand to hand combat
      Excludes1   military operations involving combat using blunt or piercing object (Y37.45-)
      military operations involving intentional restriction of air and airway (Y37.46-)
      military operations involving unintentional restriction of air and airway (Y37.47-)
      ● Y37.440   Military operations involving unarmed hand to hand combat, military personnel
      ● Y37.441   Military operations involving unarmed hand to hand combat, civilian

   ● Y37.45   Military operations involving combat using blunt or piercing object
      ● Y37.450   Military operations involving combat using blunt or piercing object, military personnel
      ● Y37.451   Military operations involving combat using blunt or piercing object, civilian

◄ New   ◄|||| Revised   ~~deleted~~ Deleted   Excludes 1   Excludes 2   Includes   Use additional   Code first   Code also   Unspecified
OGCR Official Guidelines   X Assign placeholder X   ● Use Additional Character(s)   ❱ Manifestation Code   **Coding Clinic**

● Y37.46 **Military operations involving intentional restriction of air and airway**
  ● Y37.460 **Military operations involving intentional restriction of air and airway, military personnel**
  ● Y37.461 **Military operations involving intentional restriction of air and airway, civilian**
● Y37.47 **Military operations involving unintentional restriction of air and airway**
  ● Y37.470 **Military operations involving unintentional restriction of air and airway, military personnel**
  ● Y37.471 **Military operations involving unintentional restriction of air and airway, civilian**
● Y37.49 **Military operations involving other forms of conventional warfare**
  ● Y37.490 **Military operations involving other forms of conventional warfare, military personnel**
  ● Y37.491 **Military operations involving other forms of conventional warfare, civilian**
● Y37.5 **Military operations involving nuclear weapons**
    Military operation involving dirty bomb NOS
  ● Y37.50 **Military operations involving unspecified effect of nuclear weapon**
    ● Y37.500 **Military operations involving unspecified effect of nuclear weapon, military personnel**
    ● Y37.501 **Military operations involving unspecified effect of nuclear weapon, civilian**
  ● Y37.51 **Military operations involving direct blast effect of nuclear weapon**
      Military operations involving blast pressure of nuclear weapon
    ● Y37.510 **Military operations involving direct blast effect of nuclear weapon, military personnel**
    ● Y37.511 **Military operations involving direct blast effect of nuclear weapon, civilian**
  ● Y37.52 **Military operations involving indirect blast effect of nuclear weapon**
      Military operations involving being thrown by blast of nuclear weapon
      Military operations involving being struck or crushed by blast debris of nuclear weapon
    ● Y37.520 **Military operations involving indirect blast effect of nuclear weapon, military personnel**
    ● Y37.521 **Military operations involving indirect blast effect of nuclear weapon, civilian**
  ● Y37.53 **Military operations involving thermal radiation effect of nuclear weapon**
      Military operations involving direct heat from nuclear weapon
      Military operation involving fireball effects from nuclear weapon
    ● Y37.530 **Military operations involving thermal radiation effect of nuclear weapon, military personnel**
    ● Y37.531 **Military operations involving thermal radiation effect of nuclear weapon, civilian**

● Y37.54 **Military operation involving nuclear radiation effects of nuclear weapon**
    Military operation involving acute radiation exposure from nuclear weapon
    Military operation involving exposure to immediate ionizing radiation from nuclear weapon
    Military operation involving fallout exposure from nuclear weapon
    Military operation involving secondary effects of nuclear weapons
  ● Y37.540 **Military operation involving nuclear radiation effects of nuclear weapon, military personnel**
  ● Y37.541 **Military operation involving nuclear radiation effects of nuclear weapon, civilian**
● Y37.59 **Military operation involving other effects of nuclear weapons**
  ● Y37.590 **Military operation involving other effects of nuclear weapons, military personnel**
  ● Y37.591 **Military operation involving other effects of nuclear weapons, civilian**
● Y37.6 **Military operations involving biological weapons**
  ● Y37.6X **Military operations involving biological weapons**
    ● Y37.6X0 **Military operations involving biological weapons, military personnel**
    ● Y37.6X1 **Military operations involving biological weapons, civilian**
● Y37.7 **Military operations involving chemical weapons and other forms of unconventional warfare**
    Excludes1 military operations involving incendiary devices (Y36.3-, Y36.5-)
  ● Y37.7X **Military operations involving chemical weapons and other forms of unconventional warfare**
    ● Y37.7X0 **Military operations involving chemical weapons and other forms of unconventional warfare, military personnel**
    ● Y37.7X1 **Military operations involving chemical weapons and other forms of unconventional warfare, civilian**
● Y37.9 **Other and unspecified military operations**
  X ● Y37.90 **Military operations, unspecified**
  X ● Y37.91 **Military operations involving unspecified weapon of mass destruction [WMD]**
  X ● Y37.92 **Military operations involving friendly fire**

CHAPTER 20 (VØ1-Y99)

● **Y38   Terrorism**

These codes are for use to identify injuries resulting from the unlawful use of force or violence against persons or property to intimidate or coerce a government, the civilian population, or any segment thereof, in furtherance of political or social objective

Use additional code for place of occurrence (Y92.-)

The appropriate 7th character is to be added to each code from category Y38

> A   initial encounter
> D   subsequent encounter
> S   sequela

● **Y38.0   Terrorism involving explosion of marine weapons**

Terrorism involving depth-charge
Terrorism involving marine mine
Terrorism involving mine NOS, at sea or in harbor
Terrorism involving sea-based artillery shell
Terrorism involving torpedo
Terrorism involving underwater blast

● **Y38.0X   Terrorism involving explosion of marine weapons**

● **Y38.0X1   Terrorism involving explosion of marine weapons, public safety official injured**

● **Y38.0X2   Terrorism involving explosion of marine weapons, civilian injured**

● **Y38.0X3   Terrorism involving explosion of marine weapons, terrorist injured**

● **Y38.1   Terrorism involving destruction of aircraft**

Terrorism involving aircraft burned
Terrorism involving aircraft exploded
Terrorism involving aircraft being shot down
Terrorism involving aircraft used as a weapon

● **Y38.1X   Terrorism involving destruction of aircraft**

● **Y38.1X1   Terrorism involving destruction of aircraft, public safety official injured**

● **Y38.1X2   Terrorism involving destruction of aircraft, civilian injured**

● **Y38.1X3   Terrorism involving destruction of aircraft, terrorist injured**

● **Y38.2   Terrorism involving other explosions and fragments**

Terrorism involving antipersonnel (fragments) bomb
Terrorism involving blast NOS
Terrorism involving explosion NOS
Terrorism involving explosion of breech block
Terrorism involving explosion of cannon block
Terrorism involving explosion (fragments) of artillery shell
Terrorism involving explosion (fragments) of bomb
Terrorism involving explosion (fragments) of grenade
Terrorism involving explosion (fragments) of guided missile
Terrorism involving explosion (fragments) of land mine
Terrorism involving explosion of mortar bomb
Terrorism involving explosion of munitions
Terrorism involving explosion (fragments) of rocket
Terrorism involving explosion (fragments) of shell
Terrorism involving shrapnel
Terrorism involving mine NOS, on land

Excludes1   terrorism involving explosion of nuclear weapon (Y38.5)
terrorism involving suicide bomber (Y38.81)

● **Y38.2X   Terrorism involving other explosions and fragments**

● **Y38.2X1   Terrorism involving other explosions and fragments, public safety official injured**

● **Y38.2X2   Terrorism involving other explosions and fragments, civilian injured**

● **Y38.2X3   Terrorism involving other explosions and fragments, terrorist injured**

● **Y38.3   Terrorism involving fires, conflagration and hot substances**

Terrorism involving conflagration NOS
Terrorism involving fire NOS
Terrorism involving petrol bomb

Excludes1   terrorism involving fire or heat of nuclear weapon (Y38.5)

● **Y38.3X   Terrorism involving fires, conflagration and hot substances**

● **Y38.3X1   Terrorism involving fires, conflagration and hot substances, public safety official injured**

● **Y38.3X2   Terrorism involving fires, conflagration and hot substances, civilian injured**

● **Y38.3X3   Terrorism involving fires, conflagration and hot substances, terrorist injured**

● **Y38.4   Terrorism involving firearms**

Terrorism involving carbine bullet
Terrorism involving machine gun bullet
Terrorism involving pellets (shotgun)
Terrorism involving pistol bullet
Terrorism involving rifle bullet
Terrorism involving rubber (rifle) bullet

● **Y38.4X   Terrorism involving firearms**

● **Y38.4X1   Terrorism involving firearms, public safety official injured**

● **Y38.4X2   Terrorism involving firearms, civilian injured**

● **Y38.4X3   Terrorism involving firearms, terrorist injured**

● **Y38.5   Terrorism involving nuclear weapons**

Terrorism involving blast effects of nuclear weapon
Terrorism involving exposure to ionizing radiation from nuclear weapon
Terrorism involving fireball effect of nuclear weapon
Terrorism involving heat from nuclear weapon

● **Y38.5X   Terrorism involving nuclear weapons**

● **Y38.5X1   Terrorism involving nuclear weapons, public safety official injured**

● **Y38.5X2   Terrorism involving nuclear weapons, civilian injured**

● **Y38.5X3   Terrorism involving nuclear weapons, terrorist injured**

● **Y38.6   Terrorism involving biological weapons**

Terrorism involving anthrax
Terrorism involving cholera
A serious, often deadly, infectious disease of small intestine
Terrorism involving smallpox

● **Y38.6X   Terrorism involving biological weapons**

● **Y38.6X1   Terrorism involving biological weapons, public safety official injured**

● **Y38.6X2   Terrorism involving biological weapons, civilian injured**

● **Y38.6X3   Terrorism involving biological weapons, terrorist injured**

● **Y38.7   Terrorism involving chemical weapons**

Terrorism involving gases, fumes, chemicals
Terrorism involving hydrogen cyanide
Terrorism involving phosgene
Terrorism involving sarin

● **Y38.7X   Terrorism involving chemical weapons**

● **Y38.7X1   Terrorism involving chemical weapons, public safety official injured**

● **Y38.7X2   Terrorism involving chemical weapons, civilian injured**

● **Y38.7X3   Terrorism involving chemical weapons, terrorist injured**

◀ New   ◀▬ Revised   ~~deleted~~ Deleted   Excludes 1   Excludes 2   Includes   Use additional   Code first   Code also   Unspecified
OGCR Official Guidelines   X Assign placeholder X   ● Use Additional Character(s)   ▶ Manifestation Code   **Coding Clinic**

- Y38.8   **Terrorism involving other and unspecified means**
  - Y38.80   **Terrorism involving unspecified means**
    Terrorism NOS
  - Y38.81   **Terrorism involving suicide bomber**
    - Y38.811   **Terrorism involving suicide bomber, public safety official injured**
    - Y38.812   **Terrorism involving suicide bomber, civilian injured**
  - Y38.89   **Terrorism involving other means**
    Terrorism involving drowning and submersion
    Terrorism involving lasers
    Terrorism involving piercing or stabbing instruments
    - Y38.891   **Terrorism involving other means, public safety official injured**
    - Y38.892   **Terrorism involving other means, civilian injured**
    - Y38.893   **Terrorism involving other means, terrorist injured**
- Y38.9   **Terrorism, secondary effects**
  > **Note:** This code is for use to identify conditions occurring subsequent to a terrorist attack not those that are due to the initial terrorist attack.
  - Y38.9X   **Terrorism, secondary effects**
    - Y38.9X1   **Terrorism, secondary effects, public safety official injured**
    - Y38.9X2   **Terrorism, secondary effects, civilian injured categories**

COMPLICATIONS OF MEDICAL AND SURGICAL CARE (Y62-Y84)

Includes	complications of medical devices surgical and medical procedures as the cause of abnormal reaction of the patient, or of later complication, without mention of misadventure at the time of the procedure

MISADVENTURES TO PATIENTS DURING SURGICAL AND MEDICAL CARE (Y62-Y69)

Excludes1	surgical and medical procedures as the cause of abnormal reaction of the patient, without mention of misadventure at the time of the procedure (Y83-Y84) ◄
Excludes2	breakdown or malfunctioning of medical device (during procedure) (after implantation) (ongoing use) (Y70-Y82)

- Y62   **Failure of sterile precautions during surgical and medical care**
  - Y62.0   **Failure of sterile precautions during surgical operation**
  - Y62.1   **Failure of sterile precautions during infusion or transfusion**
  - Y62.2   **Failure of sterile precautions during kidney dialysis and other perfusion**
  - Y62.3   **Failure of sterile precautions during injection or immunization**
  - Y62.4   **Failure of sterile precautions during endoscopic examination**
  - Y62.5   **Failure of sterile precautions during heart catheterization**
  - Y62.6   **Failure of sterile precautions during aspiration, puncture and other catheterization**
  - Y62.8   **Failure of sterile precautions during other surgical and medical care**
  - Y62.9   **Failure of sterile precautions during unspecified surgical and medical care**

- Y63   **Failure in dosage during surgical and medical care**

Excludes2	accidental overdose of drug or wrong drug given in error (T36-T50)

  - Y63.0   **Excessive amount of blood or other fluid given during transfusion or infusion**
  - Y63.1   **Incorrect dilution of fluid used during infusion**
  - Y63.2   **Overdose of radiation given during therapy**
  - Y63.3   **Inadvertent exposure of patient to radiation during medical care**
  - Y63.4   **Failure in dosage in electroshock or insulin-shock therapy**
  - Y63.5   **Inappropriate temperature in local application and packing**
  - Y63.6   **Underdosing and nonadministration of necessary drug, medicament or biological substance**
  - Y63.8   **Failure in dosage during other surgical and medical care**
  - Y63.9   **Failure in dosage during unspecified surgical and medical care**

- Y64   **Contaminated medical or biological substances**
  - Y64.0   **Contaminated medical or biological substance, transfused or infused**
  - Y64.1   **Contaminated medical or biological substance, injected or used for immunization**
  - Y64.8   **Contaminated medical or biological substance administered by other means**
  - Y64.9   **Contaminated medical or biological substance administered by unspecified means**
    Administered contaminated medical or biological substance NOS

- Y65   **Other misadventures during surgical and medical care**
  - Y65.0   **Mismatched blood in transfusion**
  - Y65.1   **Wrong fluid used in infusion**
  - Y65.2   **Failure in suture or ligature during surgical operation**
  - Y65.3   **Endotracheal tube wrongly placed during anesthetic procedure**
  - Y65.4   **Failure to introduce or to remove other tube or instrument**
  - Y65.5   **Performance of wrong procedure (operation)**
    - Y65.51   **Performance of wrong procedure (operation) on correct patient**
      Wrong device implanted into correct surgical site

Excludes1	performance of correct procedure (operation) on wrong side or body part (Y65.53)

    - Y65.52   **Performance of procedure (operation) on patient not scheduled for surgery**
      Performance of procedure (operation) intended for another patient
      Performance of procedure (operation) on wrong patient
    - Y65.53   **Performance of correct procedure (operation) on wrong side or body part**
      Performance of correct procedure (operation) on wrong side
      Performance of correct procedure (operation) on wrong site
  - Y65.8   **Other specified misadventures during surgical and medical care**

- Y66   **Nonadministration of surgical and medical care**
  Premature cessation of surgical and medical care

Excludes1	DNR status (Z66) palliative care (Z51.5)

- Y69   **Unspecified misadventure during surgical and medical care**

MEDICAL DEVICES ASSOCIATED WITH ADVERSE INCIDENTS IN DIAGNOSTIC AND THERAPEUTIC USE (Y70-Y82)

Includes breakdown or malfunction of medical devices (during use) (after implantation) (ongoing use)

Excludes2 breakdown or malfunctioning of medical device (after implantation) (during procedure) (ongoing use) (Y70-Y82) ◄
later complications following use of medical devices without breakdown or malfunctioning of device (Y83-Y84) ◄
misadventure to patients during surgical and medical care, classifiable to (Y62-Y69) ◄
surgical and other medical procedures as the cause of abnormal reaction of the patient, or of later complication, without mention of misadventure at the time of the procedure (Y83-Y84) ◄

● Y70 **Anesthesiology devices associated with adverse incidents**
- Y70.0 Diagnostic and monitoring anesthesiology devices associated with adverse incidents
- Y70.1 Therapeutic (nonsurgical) and rehabilitative anesthesiology devices associated with adverse incidents
- Y70.2 Prosthetic and other implants, materials and accessory anesthesiology devices associated with adverse incidents
- Y70.3 Surgical instruments, materials and anesthesiology devices (including sutures) associated with adverse incidents
- Y70.8 Miscellaneous anesthesiology devices associated with adverse incidents, not elsewhere classified

● Y71 **Cardiovascular devices associated with adverse incidents**
- Y71.0 Diagnostic and monitoring cardiovascular devices associated with adverse incidents
- Y71.1 Therapeutic (nonsurgical) and rehabilitative cardiovascular devices associated with adverse incidents
- Y71.2 Prosthetic and other implants, materials and accessory cardiovascular devices associated with adverse incidents
- Y71.3 Surgical instruments, materials and cardiovascular devices (including sutures) associated with adverse incidents
- Y71.8 Miscellaneous cardiovascular devices associated with adverse incidents, not elsewhere classified

● Y72 **Otorhinolaryngological devices associated with adverse incidents**
- Y72.0 Diagnostic and monitoring otorhinolaryngological devices associated with adverse incidents
- Y72.1 Therapeutic (nonsurgical) and rehabilitative otorhinolaryngological devices associated with adverse incidents
- Y72.2 Prosthetic and other implants, materials and accessory otorhinolaryngological devices associated with adverse incidents
- Y72.3 Surgical instruments, materials and otorhinolaryngological devices (including sutures) associated with adverse incidents
- Y72.8 Miscellaneous otorhinolaryngological devices associated with adverse incidents, not elsewhere classified

● Y73 **Gastroenterology and urology devices associated with adverse incidents**
- Y73.0 Diagnostic and monitoring gastroenterology and urology devices associated with adverse incidents
- Y73.1 Therapeutic (nonsurgical) and rehabilitative gastroenterology and urology devices associated with adverse incidents
- Y73.2 Prosthetic and other implants, materials and accessory gastroenterology and urology devices associated with adverse incidents
- Y73.3 Surgical instruments, materials and gastroenterology and urology devices (including sutures) associated with adverse incidents
- Y73.8 Miscellaneous gastroenterology and urology devices associated with adverse incidents, not elsewhere classified

● Y74 **General hospital and personal-use devices associated with adverse incidents**
- Y74.0 Diagnostic and monitoring general hospital and personal-use devices associated with adverse incidents
- Y74.1 Therapeutic (nonsurgical) and rehabilitative general hospital and personal-use devices associated with adverse incidents
- Y74.2 Prosthetic and other implants, materials and accessory general hospital and personal-use devices associated with adverse incidents
- Y74.3 Surgical instruments, materials and general hospital and personal-use devices (including sutures) associated with adverse incidents
- Y74.8 Miscellaneous general hospital and personal-use devices associated with adverse incidents, not elsewhere classified

● Y75 **Neurological devices associated with adverse incidents**
- Y75.0 Diagnostic and monitoring neurological devices associated with adverse incidents
- Y75.1 Therapeutic (nonsurgical) and rehabilitative neurological devices associated with adverse incidents
- Y75.2 Prosthetic and other implants, materials and neurological devices associated with adverse incidents
- Y75.3 Surgical instruments, materials and neurological devices (including sutures) associated with adverse incidents
- Y75.8 Miscellaneous neurological devices associated with adverse incidents, not elsewhere classified

● Y76 **Obstetric and gynecological devices associated with adverse incidents**
- Y76.0 Diagnostic and monitoring obstetric and gynecological devices associated with adverse incidents ♀
- Y76.1 Therapeutic (nonsurgical) and rehabilitative obstetric and gynecological devices associated with adverse incidents ♀
- Y76.2 Prosthetic and other implants, materials and accessory obstetric and gynecological devices associated with adverse incidents ♀
- Y76.3 Surgical instruments, materials and obstetric and gynecological devices (including sutures) associated with adverse incidents ♀
- Y76.8 Miscellaneous obstetric and gynecological devices associated with adverse incidents, not elsewhere classified ♀

◄ New   ◄▥ Revised   deleted Deleted   Excludes 1   Excludes 2   Includes   Use additional   Code first   Code also   Unspecified
1502
OGCR Official Guidelines   X Assign placeholder X   ● Use Additional Character(s)   ▷ Manifestation Code   Coding Clinic

● **Y77**   Ophthalmic devices associated with adverse incidents

    Y77.0   Diagnostic and monitoring ophthalmic devices associated with adverse incidents

    Y77.1   Therapeutic (nonsurgical) and rehabilitative ophthalmic devices associated with adverse incidents

    Y77.2   Prosthetic and other implants, materials and accessory ophthalmic devices associated with adverse incidents

    Y77.3   Surgical instruments, materials and ophthalmic devices (including sutures) associated with adverse incidents

    Y77.8   Miscellaneous ophthalmic devices associated with adverse incidents, not elsewhere classified

● **Y78**   Radiological devices associated with adverse incidents

    Y78.0   Diagnostic and monitoring radiological devices associated with adverse incidents

    Y78.1   Therapeutic (nonsurgical) and rehabilitative radiological devices associated with adverse incidents

    Y78.2   Prosthetic and other implants, materials and accessory radiological devices associated with adverse incidents

    Y78.3   Surgical instruments, materials and radiological devices (including sutures) associated with adverse incidents

    Y78.8   Miscellaneous radiological devices associated with adverse incidents, not elsewhere classified

● **Y79**   Orthopedic devices associated with adverse incidents

    Y79.0   Diagnostic and monitoring orthopedic devices associated with adverse incidents

    Y79.1   Therapeutic (nonsurgical) and rehabilitative orthopedic devices associated with adverse incidents

    Y79.2   Prosthetic and other implants, materials and accessory orthopedic devices associated with adverse incidents

    Y79.3   Surgical instruments, materials and orthopedic devices (including sutures) associated with adverse incidents

    Y79.8   Miscellaneous orthopedic devices associated with adverse incidents, not elsewhere classified

● **Y80**   Physical medicine devices associated with adverse incidents

    Y80.0   Diagnostic and monitoring physical medicine devices associated with adverse incidents

    Y80.1   Therapeutic (nonsurgical) and rehabilitative physical medicine devices associated with adverse incidents

    Y80.2   Prosthetic and other implants, materials and accessory physical medicine devices associated with adverse incidents

    Y80.3   Surgical instruments, materials and physical medicine devices (including sutures) associated with adverse incidents

    Y80.8   Miscellaneous physical medicine devices associated with adverse incidents, not elsewhere classified

● **Y81**   General- and plastic-surgery devices associated with adverse incidents

    Y81.0   Diagnostic and monitoring general- and plastic-surgery devices associated with adverse incidents

    Y81.1   Therapeutic (nonsurgical) and rehabilitative general- and plastic-surgery devices associated with adverse incidents

    Y81.2   Prosthetic and other implants, materials and accessory general- and plastic-surgery devices associated with adverse incidents

    Y81.3   Surgical instruments, materials and general- and plastic-surgery devices (including sutures) associated with adverse incidents

    Y81.8   Miscellaneous general- and plastic-surgery devices associated with adverse incidents, not elsewhere classified

● **Y82**   Other and unspecified medical devices associated with adverse incidents

    Y82.8   Other medical devices associated with adverse incidents

    Y82.9   Unspecified medical devices associated with adverse incidents

---

SURGICAL AND OTHER MEDICAL PROCEDURES AS THE CAUSE OF ABNORMAL REACTION OF THE PATIENT, OR OF LATER COMPLICATION, WITHOUT MENTION OF MISADVENTURE AT THE TIME OF THE PROCEDURE (Y83-Y84)

Excludes1   misadventures to patients during surgical and medical care, classifiable to (Y62-Y69)

Excludes2   breakdown or malfunctioning of medical device (after implantation) (during procedure) (ongoing use) (Y70-Y82) ◄

● **Y83**   Surgical operation and other surgical procedures as the cause of abnormal reaction of the patient, or of later complication, without mention of misadventure at the time of the procedure

    Y83.0   Surgical operation with transplant of whole organ as the cause of abnormal reaction of the patient, or of later complication, without mention of misadventure at the time of the procedure

    Y83.1   Surgical operation with implant of artificial internal device as the cause of abnormal reaction of the patient, or of later complication, without mention of misadventure at the time of the procedure

    Y83.2   Surgical operation with anastomosis, bypass or graft as the cause of abnormal reaction of the patient, or of later complication, without mention of misadventure at the time of the procedure

    Y83.3   Surgical operation with formation of external stoma as the cause of abnormal reaction of the patient, or of later complication, without mention of misadventure at the time of the procedure

    Y83.4   Other reconstructive surgery as the cause of abnormal reaction of the patient, or of later complication, without mention of misadventure at the time of the procedure

    Y83.5   Amputation of limb(s) as the cause of abnormal reaction of the patient, or of later complication, without mention of misadventure at the time of the procedure

    Y83.6   Removal of other organ (partial) (total) as the cause of abnormal reaction of the patient, or of later complication, without mention of misadventure at the time of the procedure

    Y83.8   Other surgical procedures as the cause of abnormal reaction of the patient, or of later complication, without mention of misadventure at the time of the procedure

    Y83.9   Surgical procedure, unspecified as the cause of abnormal reaction of the patient, or of later complication, without mention of misadventure at the time of the procedure

● **Y84**   Other medical procedures as the cause of abnormal reaction of the patient, or of later complication, without mention of misadventure at the time of the procedure

    Y84.0   Cardiac catheterization as the cause of abnormal reaction of the patient, or of later complication, without mention of misadventure at the time of the procedure

    Y84.1   Kidney dialysis as the cause of abnormal reaction of the patient, or of later complication, without mention of misadventure at the time of the procedure

    Y84.2   Radiological procedure and radiotherapy as the cause of abnormal reaction of the patient, or of later complication, without mention of misadventure at the time of the procedure

    Y84.3   Shock therapy as the cause of abnormal reaction of the patient, or of later complication, without mention of misadventure at the time of the procedure

    Y84.4   Aspiration of fluid as the cause of abnormal reaction of the patient, or of later complication, without mention of misadventure at the time of the procedure

    Y84.5   Insertion of gastric or duodenal sound as the cause of abnormal reaction of the patient, or of later complication, without mention of misadventure at the time of the procedure

    Y84.6   Urinary catheterization as the cause of abnormal reaction of the patient, or of later complication, without mention of misadventure at the time of the procedure

    Y84.7   Blood-sampling as the cause of abnormal reaction of the patient, or of later complication, without mention of misadventure at the time of the procedure

CHAPTER 20 (V01-Y99)

Y84.8 Other medical procedures as the cause of abnormal reaction of the patient, or of later complication, without mention of misadventure at the time of the procedure

Y84.9 Medical procedure, unspecified as the cause of abnormal reaction of the patient, or of later complication, without mention of misadventure at the time of the procedure

---

SUPPLEMENTARY FACTORS RELATED TO CAUSES OF MORBIDITY CLASSIFIED ELSEWHERE (Y90-Y99)

Note: These categories may be used to provide supplementary information concerning causes of morbidity. They are not to be used for single-condition coding.

● **Y90** Evidence of alcohol involvement determined by blood alcohol level

Code first any associated alcohol related disorders (F10)

Y90.0 Blood alcohol level of less than 20 mg/100 ml
Y90.1 Blood alcohol level of 20-39 mg/100 ml
Y90.2 Blood alcohol level of 40-59 mg/100 ml
Y90.3 Blood alcohol level of 60-79 mg/100 ml
Y90.4 Blood alcohol level of 80-99 mg/100 ml
Y90.5 Blood alcohol level of 100-119 mg/100 ml
Y90.6 Blood alcohol level of 120-199 mg/100 ml
Y90.7 Blood alcohol level of 200-239 mg/100 ml
Y90.8 Blood alcohol level of 240 mg/100 ml or more
Y90.9 Presence of alcohol in blood, level not specified

OGCR Section I.C.20.b.

Place of Occurrence Guideline

Codes from category Y92, Place of occurrence of the external cause, are secondary codes for use after other external cause codes to identify the location of the patient at the time of injury or other condition.

Generally, a place of occurrence code is assigned only once, at the initial encounter for treatment. However, in the rare instance that a new injury occurs during hospitalization, an additional place of occurrence code may be assigned. No 7th characters are used for Y92. Only one code from Y92 should be recorded on a medical record. A place of occurrence code should be used in conjunction with an activity code, Y93.

Do not use place of occurrence code Y92.9 if the place is not stated or is not applicable.

● **Y92** Place of occurrence of the external cause

The following category is for use, when relevant, to identify the place of occurrence of the external cause. Use in conjunction with an activity code.

Place of occurrence should be recorded only at the initial encounter for treatment

● **Y92.0** Non-institutional (private) residence as the place of occurrence of the external cause

> **Excludes1** abandoned or derelict house (Y92.89)
> home under construction but not yet occupied (Y92.6-)
> institutional place of residence (Y92.1-)

● **Y92.00** Unspecified non-institutional (private) residence as the place of occurrence of the external cause

Y92.000 Kitchen of unspecified non-institutional (private) residence as the place of occurrence of the external cause

Y92.001 Dining room of unspecified non-institutional (private) residence as the place of occurrence of the external cause

Y92.002 Bathroom of unspecified non-institutional (private) residence single-family (private) house as the place of occurrence of the external cause

Y92.003 Bedroom of unspecified non-institutional (private) residence as the place of occurrence of the external cause

Y92.007 Garden or yard of unspecified non-institutional (private) residence as the place of occurrence of the external cause

Y92.008 Other place in unspecified non-institutional (private) residence as the place of occurrence of the external cause

Y92.009 Unspecified place in unspecified non-institutional (private) residence as the place of occurrence of the external cause

Home (NOS) as the place of occurrence of the external cause

● **Y92.01** Single-family non-institutional (private) house as the place of occurrence of the external cause

Farmhouse as the place of occurrence of the external cause

> **Excludes1** barn (Y92.71)
> chicken coop or hen house (Y92.72)
> farm field (Y92.73)
> orchard (Y92.74)
> single family mobile home or trailer (Y92.02-)
> slaughter house (Y92.86)

Y92.010 Kitchen of single-family (private) house as the place of occurrence of the external cause

Y92.011 Dining room of single-family (private) house as the place of occurrence of the external cause

Y92.012 Bathroom of single-family (private) house as the place of occurrence of the external cause

Y92.013 Bedroom of single-family (private) house as the place of occurrence of the external cause

Y92.014 Private driveway to single-family (private) house as the place of occurrence of the external cause

Y92.015 Private garage of single-family (private) house as the place of occurrence of the external cause

Y92.016 Swimming pool in single-family (private) house or garden as the place of occurrence of the external cause

Y92.017 Garden or yard in single-family (private) house as the place of occurrence of the external cause

Y92.018 Other place in single-family (private) house as the place of occurrence of the external cause

Y92.019 Unspecified place in single-family (private) house as the place of occurrence of the external cause

● Y92.02   Mobile home as the place of occurrence of the external cause

     Y92.020   Kitchen in mobile home as the place of occurrence of the external cause

     Y92.021   Dining room in mobile home as the place of occurrence of the external cause

     Y92.022   Bathroom in mobile home as the place of occurrence of the external cause

     Y92.023   Bedroom in mobile home as the place of occurrence of the external cause

     Y92.024   Driveway of mobile home as the place of occurrence of the external cause

     Y92.025   Garage of mobile home as the place of occurrence of the external cause

     Y92.026   Swimming pool of mobile home as the place of occurrence of the external cause

     Y92.027   Garden or yard of mobile home as the place of occurrence of the external cause

     Y92.028   Other place in mobile home as the place of occurrence of the external cause

     Y92.029   Unspecified place in mobile home as the place of occurrence of the external cause

● Y92.03   Apartment as the place of occurrence of the external cause

     Condominium as the place of occurrence of the external cause

     Co-op apartment as the place of occurrence of the external cause

     Y92.030   Kitchen in apartment as the place of occurrence of the external cause

     Y92.031   Bathroom in apartment as the place of occurrence of the external cause

     Y92.032   Bedroom in apartment as the place of occurrence of the external cause

     Y92.038   Other place in apartment as the place of occurrence of the external cause

     Y92.039   Unspecified place in apartment as the place of occurrence of the external cause

● Y92.04   Boarding-house as the place of occurrence of the external cause

     Y92.040   Kitchen in boarding-house as the place of occurrence of the external cause

     Y92.041   Bathroom in boarding-house as the place of occurrence of the external cause

     Y92.042   Bedroom in boarding-house as the place of occurrence of the external cause

     Y92.043   Driveway of boarding-house as the place of occurrence of the external cause

     Y92.044   Garage of boarding-house as the place of occurrence of the external cause

     Y92.045   Swimming pool of boarding-house as the place of occurrence of the external cause

     Y92.046   Garden or yard of boarding-house as the place of occurrence of the external cause

     Y92.048   Other place in boarding-house as the place of occurrence of the external cause

     Y92.049   Unspecified place in boarding-house as the place of occurrence of the external cause

● Y92.09   Other non-institutional residence as the place of occurrence of the external cause

     Y92.090   Kitchen in other non-institutional residence as the place of occurrence of the external cause

     Y92.091   Bathroom in other non-institutional residence as the place of occurrence of the external cause

     Y92.092   Bedroom in other non-institutional residence as the place of occurrence of the external cause

     Y92.093   Driveway of other non-institutional residence as the place of occurrence of the external cause

     Y92.094   Garage of other non-institutional residence as the place of occurrence of the external cause

     Y92.095   Swimming pool of other non-institutional residence as the place of occurrence of the external cause

     Y92.096   Garden or yard of other non-institutional residence as the place of occurrence of the external cause

     Y92.098   Other place in other non-institutional residence as the place of occurrence of the external cause

     Y92.099   Unspecified place in other non-institutional residence as the place of occurrence of the external cause

● Y92.1   Institutional (nonprivate) residence as the place of occurrence of the external cause

     Y92.10   Unspecified residential institution as the place of occurrence of the external cause

● Y92.11   Children's home and orphanage as the place of occurrence of the external cause

     Y92.110   Kitchen in children's home and orphanage as the place of occurrence of the external cause

     Y92.111   Bathroom in children's home and orphanage as the place of occurrence of the external cause

     Y92.112   Bedroom in children's home and orphanage as the place of occurrence of the external cause

     Y92.113   Driveway of children's home and orphanage as the place of occurrence of the external cause

     Y92.114   Garage of children's home and orphanage as the place of occurrence of the external cause

     Y92.115   Swimming pool of children's home and orphanage as the place of occurrence of the external cause

     Y92.116   Garden or yard of children's home and orphanage as the place of occurrence of the external cause

     Y92.118   Other place in children's home and orphanage as the place of occurrence of the external cause

     Y92.119   Unspecified place in children's home and orphanage as the place of occurrence of the external cause

CHAPTER 20 (V01-Y99)

● **Y92.12** Nursing home as the place of occurrence of the external cause
> Home for the sick as the place of occurrence of the external cause
> Hospice as the place of occurrence of the external cause

Y92.120 Kitchen in nursing home as the place of occurrence of the external cause

Y92.121 Bathroom in nursing home as the place of occurrence of the external cause

Y92.122 Bedroom in nursing home as the place of occurrence of the external cause

Y92.123 Driveway of nursing home as the place of occurrence of the external cause

Y92.124 Garage of nursing home as the place of occurrence of the external cause

Y92.125 Swimming pool of nursing home as the place of occurrence of the external cause

Y92.126 Garden or yard of nursing home as the place of occurrence of the external cause

Y92.128 Other place in nursing home as the place of occurrence of the external cause

Y92.129 Unspecified place in nursing home as the place of occurrence of the external cause

● **Y92.13** Military base as the place of occurrence of the external cause
> **Excludes 1**   military training grounds (Y92.83)

Y92.130 Kitchen on military base as the place of occurrence of the external cause

Y92.131 Mess hall on military base as the place of occurrence of the external cause

Y92.133 Barracks on military base as the place of occurrence of the external cause

Y92.135 Garage on military base as the place of occurrence of the external cause

Y92.136 Swimming pool on military base as the place of occurrence of the external cause

Y92.137 Garden or yard on military base as the place of occurrence of the external cause

Y92.138 Other place on military base as the place of occurrence of the external cause

Y92.139 Unspecified place military base as the place of occurrence of the external cause

● **Y92.14** Prison as the place of occurrence of the external cause

Y92.140 Kitchen in prison as the place of occurrence of the external cause

Y92.141 Dining room in prison as the place of occurrence of the external cause

Y92.142 Bathroom in prison as the place of occurrence of the external cause

Y92.143 Cell of prison as the place of occurrence of the external cause

Y92.146 Swimming pool of prison as the place of occurrence of the external cause

Y92.147 Courtyard of prison as the place of occurrence of the external cause

Y92.148 Other place in prison as the place of occurrence of the external cause

Y92.149 Unspecified place in prison as the place of occurrence of the external cause

● **Y92.15** Reform school as the place of occurrence of the external cause

Y92.150 Kitchen in reform school as the place of occurrence of the external cause

Y92.151 Dining room in reform school as the place of occurrence of the external cause

Y92.152 Bathroom in reform school as the place of occurrence of the external cause

Y92.153 Bedroom in reform school as the place of occurrence of the external cause

Y92.154 Driveway of reform school as the place of occurrence of the external cause

Y92.155 Garage of reform school as the place of occurrence of the external cause

Y92.156 Swimming pool of reform school as the place of occurrence of the external cause

Y92.157 Garden or yard of reform school as the place of occurrence of the external cause

Y92.158 Other place in reform school as the place of occurrence of the external cause

Y92.159 Unspecified place in reform school as the place of occurrence of the external cause

● **Y92.16** School dormitory as the place of occurrence of the external cause
> **Excludes 1**   reform school as the place of occurrence of the external cause (Y92.15-)
> school buildings and grounds as the place of occurrence of the external cause (Y92.2-)
> school sports and athletic areas as the place of occurrence of the external cause (Y92.3-)

Y92.160 Kitchen in school dormitory as the place of occurrence of the external cause

Y92.161 Dining room in school dormitory as the place of occurrence of the external cause

Y92.162 Bathroom in school dormitory as the place of occurrence of the external cause

Y92.163 Bedroom in school dormitory as the place of occurrence of the external cause

Y92.168 Other place in school dormitory as the place of occurrence of the external cause

Y92.169 Unspecified place in school dormitory as the place of occurrence of the external cause

● **Y92.19**   **Other specified residential institution as the place of occurrence of the external cause**

     Y92.190   **Kitchen in other specified residential institution as the place of occurrence of the external cause**

     Y92.191   **Dining room in other specified residential institution as the place of occurrence of the external cause**

     Y92.192   **Bathroom in other specified residential institution as the place of occurrence of the external cause**

     Y92.193   **Bedroom in other specified residential institution as the place of occurrence of the external cause**

     Y92.194   **Driveway of other specified residential institution as the place of occurrence of the external cause**

     Y92.195   **Garage of other specified residential institution as the place of occurrence of the external cause**

     Y92.196   **Pool of other specified residential institution as the place of occurrence of the external cause**

     Y92.197   **Garden or yard of other specified residential institution as the place of occurrence of the external cause**

     Y92.198   **Other place in other specified residential institution as the place of occurrence of the external cause**

     Y92.199   **Unspecified place in other specified residential institution as the place of occurrence of the external cause**

● **Y92.2**   **School, other institution and public administrative area as the place of occurrence of the external cause**

     Building and adjacent grounds used by the general public or by a particular group of the public

     Excludes1   building under construction as the place of occurrence of the external cause (Y92.6)

            residential institution as the place of occurrence of the external cause (Y92.1)

            school dormitory as the place of occurrence of the external cause (Y92.16-)

            sports and athletics area of schools as the place of occurrence of the external cause (Y92.3-)

● **Y92.21**   **School (private) (public) (state) as the place of occurrence of the external cause**

     Y92.210   **Daycare center as the place of occurrence of the external cause**

     Y92.211   **Elementary school as the place of occurrence of the external cause**

            Kindergarten as the place of occurrence of the external cause

     Y92.212   **Middle school as the place of occurrence of the external cause**

     Y92.213   **High school as the place of occurrence of the external cause**

            Coding Clinic: 2012, Q4, P108

     Y92.214   **College as the place of occurrence of the external cause**

            University as the place of occurrence of the external cause

     Y92.215   **Trade school as the place of occurrence of the external cause**

     Y92.218   **Other school as the place of occurrence of the external cause**

     Y92.219   **Unspecified school as the place of occurrence of the external cause**

Y92.22   **Religious institution as the place of occurrence of the external cause**

     Church as the place of occurrence of the external cause

     Mosque as the place of occurrence of the external cause

     Synagogue as the place of occurrence of the external cause

● **Y92.23**   **Hospital as the place of occurrence of the external cause**

     Excludes1   ambulatory (outpatient) health services establishments (Y92.53-)

            home for the sick as the place of occurrence of the external cause (Y92.12-)

            hospice as the place of occurrence of the external cause (Y92.12-)

            nursing home as the place of occurrence of the external cause (Y92.12-)

     Y92.230   **Patient room in hospital as the place of occurrence of the external cause**

     Y92.231   **Patient bathroom in hospital as the place of occurrence of the external cause**

     Y92.232   **Corridor of hospital as the place of occurrence of the external cause**

     Y92.233   **Cafeteria of hospital as the place of occurrence of the external cause**

     Y92.234   **Operating room of hospital as the place of occurrence of the external cause**

     Y92.238   **Other place in hospital as the place of occurrence of the external cause**

     Y92.239   **Unspecified place in hospital as the place of occurrence of the external cause**

● **Y92.24**   **Public administrative building as the place of occurrence of the external cause**

     Y92.240   **Courthouse as the place of occurrence of the external cause**

     Y92.241   **Library as the place of occurrence of the external cause**

     Y92.242   **Post office as the place of occurrence of the external cause**

     Y92.243   **City hall as the place of occurrence of the external cause**

     Y92.248   **Other public administrative building as the place of occurrence of the external cause**

● **Y92.25**   **Cultural building as the place of occurrence of the external cause**

     Y92.250   **Art gallery as the place of occurrence of the external cause**

     Y92.251   **Museum as the place of occurrence of the external cause**

     Y92.252   **Music hall as the place of occurrence of the external cause**

     Y92.253   **Opera house as the place of occurrence of the external cause**

     Y92.254   **Theater (live) as the place of occurrence of the external cause**

     Y92.258   **Other cultural public building as the place of occurrence of the external cause**

Y92.26   **Movie house or cinema as the place of occurrence of the external cause**

Y92.29   **Other specified public building as the place of occurrence of the external cause**

     Assembly hall as the place of occurrence of the external cause

     Clubhouse as the place of occurrence of the external cause

CHAPTER 20 (V01-Y99)

● Y92.3   **Sports and athletics area as the place of occurrence of the external cause**

    ● Y92.31   **Athletic court as the place of occurrence of the external cause**

       Excludes1   tennis court in private home or garden (Y92.09)

       Y92.310   **Basketball court as the place of occurrence of the external cause**

       Y92.311   **Squash court as the place of occurrence of the external cause**

       Y92.312   **Tennis court as the place of occurrence of the external cause**

       Y92.318   **Other athletic court as the place of occurrence of the external cause**

    ● Y92.32   **Athletic field as the place of occurrence of the external cause**

       Y92.320   **Baseball field as the place of occurrence of the external cause**

       Y92.321   **Football field as the place of occurrence of the external cause**

       Y92.322   **Soccer field as the place of occurrence of the external cause**

       Y92.328   **Other athletic field as the place of occurrence of the external cause**
          Cricket field as the place of occurrence of the external cause
          Hockey field as the place of occurrence of the external cause

    ● Y92.33   **Skating rink as the place of occurrence of the external cause**

       Y92.330   **Ice skating rink (indoor) (outdoor) as the place of occurrence of the external cause**

       Y92.331   **Roller skating rink as the place of occurrence of the external cause**

    Y92.34   **Swimming pool (public) as the place of occurrence of the external cause**

       Excludes1   swimming pool in private home or garden (Y92.016)

    Y92.39   **Other specified sports and athletic area as the place of occurrence of the external cause**
       Golf-course as the place of occurrence of the external cause
       Gymnasium as the place of occurrence of the external cause
       Riding-school as the place of occurrence of the external cause
       Stadium as the place of occurrence of the external cause

● Y92.4   **Street, highway and other paved roadways as the place of occurrence of the external cause** ◀▬

       Excludes1   private driveway of residence (Y92.014, Y92.024, Y92.043, Y92.093, Y92.113, Y92.123, Y92.154, Y92.194)

    ● Y92.41   **Street and highway as the place of occurrence of the external cause**

       Y92.410   **Unspecified street and highway as the place of occurrence of the external cause**
          Road NOS as the place of occurrence of the external cause

       Y92.411   **Interstate highway as the place of occurrence of the external cause**
          Freeway as the place of occurrence of the external cause
          Motorway as the place of occurrence of the external cause

       Y92.412   **Parkway as the place of occurrence of the external cause**

       Y92.413   **State road as the place of occurrence of the external cause**

       Y92.414   **Local residential or business street as the place of occurrence of the external cause**

       Y92.415   **Exit ramp or entrance ramp of street or highway as the place of occurrence of the external cause**

    ● Y92.48   **Other paved roadways as the place of occurrence of the external cause**

       Y92.480   **Sidewalk as the place of occurrence of the external cause**

       Y92.481   **Parking lot as the place of occurrence of the external cause**

       Y92.482   **Bike path as the place of occurrence of the external cause**

       Y92.488   **Other paved roadways as the place of occurrence of the external cause**

● Y92.5   **Trade and service area as the place of occurrence of the external cause**

       Excludes1   garage in private home (Y92.015)
          schools and other public administration buildings (Y92.2-)

    ● Y92.51   **Private commercial establishments as the place of occurrence of the external cause**

       Y92.510   **Bank as the place of occurrence of the external cause**

       Y92.511   **Restaurant or café as the place of occurrence of the external cause**

       Y92.512   **Supermarket, store or market as the place of occurrence of the external cause**

       Y92.513   **Shop (commercial) as the place of occurrence of the external cause**

    ● Y92.52   **Service areas as the place of occurrence of the external cause**

       Y92.520   **Airport as the place of occurrence of the external cause**

       Y92.521   **Bus station as the place of occurrence of the external cause**

       Y92.522   **Railway station as the place of occurrence of the external cause**

       Y92.523   **Highway rest stop as the place of occurrence of the external cause**

       Y92.524   **Gas station as the place of occurrence of the external cause**
          Petroleum station as the place of occurrence of the external cause
          Service station as the place of occurrence of the external cause

    ● Y92.53   **Ambulatory health services establishments as the place of occurrence of the external cause**

       Y92.530   **Ambulatory surgery center as the place of occurrence of the external cause**
          Outpatient surgery center, including that connected with a hospital as the place of occurrence of the external cause
          Same day surgery center, including that connected with a hospital as the place of occurrence of the external cause

       Y92.531   **Health care provider office as the place of occurrence of the external cause**
          Physician office as the place of occurrence of the external cause

       Y92.532   **Urgent care center as the place of occurrence of the external cause**

       Y92.538   **Other ambulatory health services establishments as the place of occurrence of the external cause**

Y92.59   **Other trade areas as the place of occurrence of the external cause**
  Office building as the place of occurrence of the external cause
  Casino as the place of occurrence of the external cause
  Garage (commercial) as the place of occurrence of the external cause
  Hotel as the place of occurrence of the external cause
  Radio or television station as the place of occurrence of the external cause
  Shopping mall as the place of occurrence of the external cause
  Warehouse as the place of occurrence of the external cause

● Y92.6   **Industrial and construction area as the place of occurrence of the external cause**

Y92.61   **Building [any] under construction as the place of occurrence of the external cause**

Y92.62   **Dock or shipyard as the place of occurrence of the external cause**
  Dockyard as the place of occurrence of the external cause
  Dry dock as the place of occurrence of the external cause
  Shipyard as the place of occurrence of the external cause

Y92.63   **Factory as the place of occurrence of the external cause**
  Factory building as the place of occurrence of the external cause
  Factory premises as the place of occurrence of the external cause
  Industrial yard as the place of occurrence of the external cause

Y92.64   **Mine or pit as the place of occurrence of the external cause**
  Mine as the place of occurrence of the external cause

Y92.65   **Oil rig as the place of occurrence of the external cause**
  Pit (coal) (gravel) (sand) as the place of occurrence of the external cause

Y92.69   **Other specified industrial and construction area as the place of occurrence of the external cause**
  Gasworks as the place of occurrence of the external cause
  Power-station (coal) (nuclear) (oil) as the place of occurrence of the external cause
  Tunnel under construction as the place of occurrence of the external cause
  Workshop as the place of occurrence of the external cause

● Y92.7   **Farm as the place of occurrence of the external cause**
  Ranch as the place of occurrence of the external cause
  Excludes1   farmhouse and home premises of farm (Y92.01-)

Y92.71   **Barn as the place of occurrence of the external cause**

Y92.72   **Chicken coop as the place of occurrence of the external cause**
  Hen house as the place of occurrence of the external cause

Y92.73   **Farm field as the place of occurrence of the external cause**

Y92.74   **Orchard as the place of occurrence of the external cause**

Y92.79   **Other farm location as the place of occurrence of the external cause**

● Y92.8   **Other places as the place of occurrence of the external cause**

● Y92.81   **Transport vehicle as the place of occurrence of the external cause**
  Excludes1   transport accidents (V00-V99)

Y92.810   **Car as the place of occurrence of the external cause**

Y92.811   **Bus as the place of occurrence of the external cause**

Y92.812   **Truck as the place of occurrence of the external cause**

Y92.813   **Airplane as the place of occurrence of the external cause**

Y92.814   **Boat as the place of occurrence of the external cause**

Y92.815   **Train as the place of occurrence of the external cause**

Y92.816   **Subway car as the place of occurrence of the external cause**

Y92.818   **Other transport vehicle as the place of occurrence of the external cause**

● Y92.82   **Wilderness area**

Y92.820   **Desert as the place of occurrence of the external cause**

Y92.821   **Forest as the place of occurrence of the external cause**

Y92.828   **Other wilderness area as the place of occurrence of the external cause**
  Swamp as the place of occurrence of the external cause
  Mountain as the place of occurrence of the external cause
  Marsh as the place of occurrence of the external cause
  Prairie as the place of occurrence of the external cause

● Y92.83   **Recreation area as the place of occurrence of the external cause**

Y92.830   **Public park as the place of occurrence of the external cause**

Y92.831   **Amusement park as the place of occurrence of the external cause**

Y92.832   **Beach as the place of occurrence of the external cause**
  Seashore as the place of occurrence of the external cause

Y92.833   **Campsite as the place of occurrence of the external cause**

Y92.834   **Zoological garden (zoo) as the place of occurrence of the external cause**

Y92.838   **Other recreation area as the place of occurrence of the external cause**

Y92.84   **Military training ground as the place of occurrence of the external cause**

Y92.85   **Railroad track as the place of occurrence of the external cause**

Y92.86   **Slaughter house as the place of occurrence of the external cause**

Y92.89   **Other specified places as the place of occurrence of the external cause**
  Derelict house as the place of occurrence of the external cause

OGCR Section I.C.20.b.

Do not use place of occurrence code Y92.9 if the place is not stated or is not applicable.

Y92.9   **Unspecified** place or not applicable

OGCR See Section I.C.20.c.

Activity Code

Assign a code from category Y93, Activity code, to describe the activity of the patient at the time the injury or other health condition occurred.

An activity code is used only once, at the initial encounter for treatment. Only one code from Y93 should be recorded on a medical record.

The activity codes are not applicable to poisonings, adverse effects, misadventures or sequela.

Do not assign Y93.9, Unspecified activity, if the activity is not stated.

A code from category Y93 is appropriate for use with external cause and intent codes if identifying the activity provides additional information about the event.

● **Y93 Activity codes**

Note: Category Y93 is provided for use to indicate the activity of the person seeking healthcare for an injury or health condition, such as a heart attack while shoveling snow, which resulted from, or was contributed to, by the activity. These codes are appropriate for use for both acute injuries, such as those from chapter 19, and conditions that are due to the long-term, cumulative effects of an activity, such as those from chapter 13. They are also appropriate for use with external cause codes for cause and intent if identifying the activity provides additional information on the event. These codes should be used in conjunction with codes for external cause status (Y99) and place of occurrence (Y92).

This section contains the following broad activity categories:

Y93.0	Activities involving walking and running
Y93.1	Activities involving water and water craft
Y93.2	Activities involving ice and snow
Y93.3	Activities involving climbing, rappelling, and jumping off
Y93.4	Activities involving dancing and other rhythmic movement
Y93.5	Activities involving other sports and athletics played individually
Y93.6	Activities involving other sports and athletics played as a team or group
Y93.7	Activities involving other specified sports and athletics
Y93.A	Activities involving other cardiorespiratory exercise
Y93.B	Activities involving other muscle strengthening exercises
Y93.C	Activities involving computer technology and electronic devices
Y93.D	Activities involving arts and handcrafts
Y93.E	Activities involving personal hygiene and interior property and clothing maintenance
Y93.F	Activities involving caregiving
Y93.G	Activities involving food preparation, cooking and grilling
Y93.H	Activities involving exterior property and land maintenance, building and construction
Y93.I	Activities involving roller coasters and other types of external motion
Y93.J	Activities involving playing musical instrument
Y93.K	Activities involving animal care
Y93.8	Activities, other specified
Y93.9	Activity, unspecified

● **Y93.0 Activities involving walking and running**

> **Excludes1** Activity, walking an animal (Y93.K1)
> Activity, walking or running on a treadmill (Y93.A1)

Y93.01 Activity, walking, marching and hiking
Activity, walking, marching and hiking on level or elevated terrain

> **Excludes1** activity, mountain climbing (Y93.31)

Y93.02 Activity, running

● **Y93.1 Activities involving water and water craft**

> **Excludes1** activities involving ice (Y93.2-)

Y93.11 Activity, swimming

Y93.12 Activity, springboard and platform diving

Y93.13 Activity, water polo

Y93.14 Activity, water aerobics and water exercise

Y93.15 Activity, underwater diving and snorkeling
Activity, SCUBA diving

Y93.16 Activity, rowing, canoeing, kayaking, rafting and tubing
Activity, canoeing, kayaking, rafting and tubing in calm and turbulent water

Y93.17 Activity, water skiing and wake boarding

Y93.18 Activity, surfing, windsurfing and boogie boarding
Activity, water sliding

Y93.19 Activity, other involving water and watercraft
Activity involving water NOS
Activity, parasailing
Activity, water survival training and testing

● **Y93.2 Activities involving ice and snow**

> **Excludes1** activity, shoveling ice and snow (Y93.H1)

Y93.21 Activity, ice skating
Activity, figure skating (singles) (pairs)
Activity, ice dancing

> **Excludes1** activity, ice hockey (Y93.22)

Y93.22 Activity, ice hockey

Y93.23 Activity, snow (alpine) (downhill) skiing, snow boarding, sledding, tobogganing and snow tubing

> **Excludes1** activity, cross country skiing (Y93.24)

Y93.24 Activity, cross country skiing
Activity, nordic skiing

Y93.29 Activity, other activity involving ice and snow
Activity, activity involving ice and snow NOS

● **Y93.3 Activities involving climbing, rappelling and jumping off**

> **Excludes1** activity, hiking on level or elevated terrain (Y93.01)
> activity, jumping rope (Y93.56)
> activity, trampoline jumping (Y93.44)

Y93.31 Activity, mountain climbing, rock climbing and wall climbing

Y93.32 Activity, rappelling

Y93.33 Activity, BASE jumping
Activity, building, Antenna, Span, Earth jumping

Y93.34 Activity, bungee jumping

Y93.35 Activity, hang gliding

Y93.39 Activity, other activity involving climbing, rappelling and jumping off

● **Y93.4 Activities involving dancing and other rhythmic movement**

> **Excludes1** activity, martial arts (Y93.75)

Y93.41 Activity, dancing
Coding Clinic: 2012, Q4, P108

Y93.42 Activity, yoga

Y93.43 Activity, gymnastics
Activity, rhythmic gymnastics

> **Excludes1** activity, trampolining (Y93.44)

Y93.44 Activity, trampolining

Y93.45 Activity, cheerleading

Y93.49 Activity, other involving dancing and other rhythmic movements

◀ New   ◀▥ Revised   ~~deleted~~ Deleted   Excludes 1   Excludes 2   Includes   Use additional   Code first   Code also   Unspecified

1510   OGCR Official Guidelines   X Assign placeholder X   ● Use Additional Character(s)   ▶ Manifestation Code   **Coding Clinic**

● **Y93.5   Activities involving other sports and athletics played individually**

     Excludes1   activity, dancing (Y93.41)
                      activity, gymnastic (Y93.43)
                      activity, trampolining (Y93.44)
                      activity, yoga (Y93.42)

     Y93.51   Activity, roller skating (inline) and skateboarding

     Y93.52   Activity, horseback riding

     Y93.53   Activity, golf

     Y93.54   Activity, bowling

     Y93.55   Activity, bike riding

     Y93.56   Activity, jumping rope

     Y93.57   Activity, non-running track and field events

         Excludes1   activity, running (any form) (Y93.02)

     Y93.59   Activity, other involving other sports and athletics played individually

         Excludes1   activities involving climbing, rappelling, and jumping (Y93.3-)
                      activities involving ice and snow (Y93.2-)
                      activities involving walking and running (Y93.0-)
                      activities involving water and watercraft (Y93.1-)

● **Y93.6   Activities involving other sports and athletics played as a team or group**

     Excludes1   activity, ice hockey (Y93.22)
                      activity, water polo (Y93.13)

     Y93.61   Activity, American tackle football
          Activity, football NOS

     Y93.62   Activity, American flag or touch football

     Y93.63   Activity, rugby

     Y93.64   Activity, baseball
          Activity, softball

     Y93.65   Activity, lacrosse and field hockey
          Coding Clinic: 2015, Q1, P9

     Y93.66   Activity, soccer

     Y93.67   Activity, basketball

     Y93.68   Activity, volleyball (beach) (court)

     Y93.6A   Activity, physical games generally associated with school recess, summer camp and children
          Activity, capture the flag
          Activity, dodge ball
          Activity, four square
          Activity, kickball

     Y93.69   Activity, other involving other sports and athletics played as a team or group
          Cricket

● **Y93.7   Activities involving other specified sports and athletics**

     Y93.71   Activity, boxing

     Y93.72   Activity, wrestling

     Y93.73   Activity, racquet and hand sports
          Activity, handball
          Activity, racquetball
          Activity, squash
          Activity, tennis

     Y93.74   Activity, frisbee
          Activity, ultimate frisbee

     Y93.75   Activity, martial arts
          Activity, combatives

     Y93.79   Activity, other specified sports and athletics

         Excludes1   sports and athletics activities specified in categories Y93.0-Y93.6

● **Y93.A   Activities involving other cardiorespiratory exercise**
      Activities involving physical training

     Y93.A1   Activity, exercise machines primarily for cardiorespiratory conditioning
          Activity, elliptical and stepper machines
          Activity, stationary bike
          Activity, treadmill

     Y93.A2   Activity, calisthenics
          Activity, jumping jacks
          Activity, warm up and cool down

     Y93.A3   Activity, aerobic and step exercise

     Y93.A4   Activity, circuit training

     Y93.A5   Activity, obstacle course
          Activity, challenge course
          Activity, confidence course

     Y93.A6   Activity, grass drills
          Activity, guerilla drills

     Y93.A9   Activity, other involving other cardiorespiratory exercise

         Excludes1   activities involving cardiorespiratory exercise specified in categories Y93.0-Y93.7

● **Y93.B   Activity involving other muscle strengthening exercises**

     Y93.B1   Activity, exercise machines primarily for muscle strengthening

     Y93.B2   Activity, push-ups, pull-ups, sit-ups

     Y93.B3   Activity, free weights
          Activity, barbells
          Activity, dumbbells

     Y93.B4   Activity, pilates

     Y93.B9   Activity, other involving other muscle strengthening exercises

         Excludes1   activities involving muscle strengthening specified in categories Y93.0-Y93.A

● **Y93.C   Activities involving computer technology and electronic devices**

     Excludes1   activity, electronic musical keyboard or instruments (Y93.J-)

     Y93.C1   Activity, computer keyboarding
          Activity, electronic game playing using keyboard or other stationary device

     Y93.C2   Activity, hand held interactive electronic device
          Activity, cellular telephone and communication device
          Activity, electronic game playing using interactive device

         Excludes1   activity, electronic game playing using keyboard or other stationary device (Y93.C1)

     Y93.C9   Activity, other involving computer technology and electronic devices

● **Y93.D   Activities involving arts and handcrafts**

     Excludes1   activities involving playing musical instrument (Y93.J-)

     Y93.D1   Knitting and crocheting

     Y93.D2   Sewing

     Y93.D3   Furniture building and finishing
          Furniture repair

     Y93.D9   Activity, other involving arts and handcrafts

CHAPTER 20 (V01-Y99)

● **Y93.E**   **Activities involving personal hygiene and interior property and clothing maintenance**

     Excludes1   activities involving cooking and grilling (Y93.G-)

          activities involving exterior property and land maintenance, building and construction (Y93.H-)

          activity involving caregiving (Y93.F-)

          activity, dishwashing (Y93.G1)

          activity, food preparation (Y93.G1)

          activity, gardening (Y93.H2)

   Y93.E1 **Activity, personal bathing and showering**

   Y93.E2 **Activity, laundry**

   Y93.E3 **Activity, vacuuming**

   Y93.E4 **Activity, ironing**

   Y93.E5 **Activity, floor mopping and cleaning**

   Y93.E6 **Activity, residential relocation**

       Activity, packing up and unpacking involved in moving to a new residence

   Y93.E8 **Activity, other personal hygiene activity**

   Y93.E9 **Activity, other household maintenance**

● **Y93.F**   **Activities involving person providing caregiving**

     Activity involving the provider of caregiving

   Y93.F1 **Activity, caregiving involving bathing**

   Y93.F2 **Activity, caregiving involving lifting**

   Y93.F9 **Activity, other caregiving**

● **Y93.G**   **Activities involving food preparation, cooking and grilling**

   Y93.G1 **Activity, food preparation and clean up**

       Activity, dishwashing

   Y93.G2 **Activity, grilling and smoking food**

   Y93.G3 **Activity, cooking and baking**

       Activity, use of stove, oven and microwave oven

   Y93.G9 **Activity, other activity involving cooking and grilling**

● **Y93.H**   **Activities involving property and land maintenance, building and construction**

   Y93.H1 **Activity, digging, shoveling and raking**

       Activity, dirt digging

       Activity, raking leaves

       Activity, snow shoveling

   Y93.H2 **Activity, gardening and landscaping**

       Activity, pruning, trimming shrubs, weeding

   Y93.H3 **Activity, building and construction**

   Y93.H9 **Activity, other activity involving property and land maintenance, building and construction**

● **Y93.I**   **Activities involving roller coasters and other types of external motion**

   Y93.I1 **Activity, rollercoaster riding**

   Y93.I9 **Activity, other involving external motion**

● **Y93.J**   **Activities involving playing musical instrument**

     Activity involving playing electric musical instrument

   Y93.J1 **Activity, piano playing**

       Activity, musical keyboard (electronic) playing

   Y93.J2 **Activity, drum and other percussion instrument playing**

   Y93.J3 **Activity, string instrument playing**

   Y93.J4 **Activity, winds and brass instrument playing**

● **Y93.K**   **Activities involving animal care**

     Excludes1   activity, horseback riding (Y93.52)

   Y93.K1 **Activity, walking an animal**

   Y93.K2 **Activity, milking an animal**

   Y93.K3 **Activity, grooming and shearing an animal**

   Y93.K9 **Activity, other activity involving animal care**

● **Y93.8**   **Other activity**

   Y93.81 **Activity, refereeing a sports activity**

   Y93.82 **Activity, spectator at an event**

   Y93.83 **Activity, rough housing and horseplay**

       Coding Clinic: 2015, Q1, P8

   Y93.84 **Activity, sleeping**

   Y93.85 **Activity, choking game** ◄

       Activity, blackout game ◄

       Activity, fainting game ◄

       Activity, pass out game ◄

   Y93.89 **Activity, other specified**

OGCR See Section I.C.20.c.

   Do not assign Y93.9, Unspecified activity, if the activity is not stated.

● **Y93.9**   **Activity, unspecified**

Y95   **Nosocomial condition**

● **Y99**   **External cause status**

   Note: A single code from category Y99 should be used in conjunction with the external cause code(s) assigned to a record to indicate the status of the person at the time the event occurred.

   Y99.0   **Civilian activity done for income or pay**

     Civilian activity done for financial or other compensation

     Excludes1   military activity (Y99.1)

          volunteer activity (Y99.2)

   Y99.1   **Military activity**

     Excludes1   activity of off duty military personnel (Y99.8)

   Y99.2   **Volunteer activity**

     Excludes1   activity of child or other family member assisting in compensated work of other family member (Y99.8)

   Y99.8   **Other external cause status**

     Activity NEC

     Activity of child or other family member assisting in compensated work of other family member

     Hobby not done for income

     Leisure activity

     Off-duty activity of military personnel

     Recreation or sport not for income or while a student

     Student activity

     Excludes1   civilian activity done for income or compensation (Y99.0)

          military activity (Y99.1)

     Coding Clinic: 2012, Q4, P108

   Y99.9   **Unspecified external cause status**

◄ New   ◄▬ Revised   ~~deleted~~ Deleted   Excludes 1   Excludes 2   Includes   Use additional   Code first   Code also   Unspecified

OGCR Official Guidelines   X Assign placeholder X   ● Use Additional Character(s)   ▶ Manifestation Code   Coding Clinic

CHAPTER 21

FACTORS INFLUENCING HEALTH STATUS AND CONTACT WITH HEALTH SERVICES (Z00-Z99)

OGCR Chapter-Specific Coding Guidelines

21. **Chapter 21: Factors influencing health status and contact with health services (Z00-Z99)**
Note: The chapter specific guidelines provide additional information about the use of Z codes for specified encounters.

a. **Use of Z codes in any healthcare setting**
Z codes are for use in any healthcare setting. Z codes may be used as either a first-listed (principal diagnosis code in the inpatient setting) or secondary code, depending on the circumstances of the encounter. Certain Z codes may only be used as first-listed or principal diagnosis.

b. **Z Codes indicate a reason for an encounter**
Z codes are not procedure codes. A corresponding procedure code must accompany a Z code to describe any procedure performed.

c. **Categories of Z Codes**

1) **Contact/Exposure**
Category Z20 indicates contact with, and suspected exposure to, communicable diseases. These codes are for patients who do not show any sign or symptom of a disease but are suspected to have been exposed to it by close personal contact with an infected individual or are in an area where a disease is epidemic.

Category Z77, **Other contact with and (suspected) exposures hazardous to health,** indicates contact with and suspected exposures hazardous to health.

Contact/exposure codes may be used as a first-listed code to explain an encounter for testing, or, more commonly, as a secondary code to identify a potential risk.

2) **Inoculations and vaccinations**
Code Z23 is for encounters for inoculations and vaccinations. It indicates that a patient is being seen to receive a prophylactic inoculation against a disease. Procedure codes are required to identify the actual administration of the injection and the type(s) of immunizations given. Code Z23 may be used as a secondary code if the inoculation is given as a routine part of preventive health care, such as a well-baby visit.

3) **Status**
Status codes indicate that a patient is either a carrier of a disease or has the sequelae or residual of a past disease or condition. This includes such things as the presence of prosthetic or mechanical devices resulting from past treatment. A status code is informative, because the status may affect the course of treatment and its outcome. A status code is distinct from a history code. The history code indicates that the patient no longer has the condition.

A status code should not be used with a diagnosis code from one of the body system chapters, if the diagnosis code includes the information provided by the status code. For example, code Z94.1, Heart transplant status, should not be used with a code from subcategory T86.2, Complications of heart transplant. The status code does not provide additional information. The complication code indicates that the patient is a heart transplant patient.

For encounters for weaning from a mechanical ventilator, assign a code from subcategory J96.1, Chronic respiratory failure, followed by code Z99.11, Dependence on respirator [ventilator] status.

The status Z codes/categories are:

Z14   Genetic carrier
Genetic carrier status indicates that a person carries a gene, associated with a particular disease, which may be passed to offspring who may develop that disease. The person does not have the disease and is not at risk of developing the disease.

Z15   Genetic susceptibility to disease Genetic susceptibility indicates that a person has a gene that increases the risk of that person developing the disease.

Codes from category Z15 should not be used as principal or first-listed codes. If the patient has the condition to which he/she is susceptible, and that condition is the reason for the encounter, the code for the current condition should be sequenced first. If the patient is being seen for follow-up after completed treatment for this condition, and the condition no longer exists, a follow-up

code should be sequenced first, followed by the appropriate personal history and genetic susceptibility codes. If the purpose of the encounter is genetic counseling associated with procreative management, code Z31.5, Encounter for genetic counseling, should be assigned as the first-listed code, followed by a code from category Z15. Additional codes should be assigned for any applicable family or personal history.

Z16   Resistance to antimicrobial drugs
This code indicates that a patient has a condition that is resistant to antimicrobial drug treatment. Sequence the infection code first.

Z17   Estrogen receptor status

Z18   Retained foreign body fragments

Z19   **Hormone sensitivity malignancy status**

Z21   Asymptomatic HIV infection status This code indicates that a patient has tested positive for HIV but has manifested no signs or symptoms of the disease.

Z22   Carrier of infectious disease Carrier status indicates that a person harbors the specific organisms of a disease without manifest symptoms and is capable of transmitting the infection.

Z28.3   Underimmunization status

Z33.1   Pregnant state, incidental This code is a secondary code only for use when the pregnancy is in no way complicating the reason for visit. Otherwise, a code from the obstetric chapter is required.

Z66   Do not resuscitate
This code may be used when it is documented by the provider that a patient is on do not resuscitate status at any time during the stay.

Z67   Blood type

Z68   Body mass index (BMI)
As with all other secondary diagnosis codes, the BMI codes should only be assigned when they meet the definition of a reportable diagnosis (see Section III, Reporting Additional Diagnoses).

Z74.01   Bed confinement status

Z76.82   Awaiting organ transplant status

Z78   Other specified health status
Code Z78.1, Physical restraint status, may be used when it is documented by the provider that a patient has been put in restraints during the current encounter. Please note that this code should not be reported when it is documented by the provider that a patient is temporarily restrained during a procedure.

Z79   Long-term (current) drug therapy
Codes from this category indicate a patient's continuous use of a prescribed drug (including such things as aspirin therapy) for the long-term treatment of a condition or for prophylactic use. It is not for use for patients who have addictions to drugs. This subcategory is not for use of medications for detoxification or maintenance programs to prevent withdrawal symptoms in patients with drug dependence (e.g., methadone maintenance for opiate dependence). Assign the appropriate code for the drug dependence instead.

Assign a code from Z79 if the patient is receiving a medication for an extended period as a prophylactic measure (such as for the prevention of deep vein thrombosis) or as treatment of a chronic condition (such as arthritis) or a disease requiring a lengthy course of treatment (such as cancer). Do not assign a code from category Z79 for medication being administered for a brief period of time to treat an acute illness or injury (such as a course of antibiotics to treat acute bronchitis).

Z88   Allergy status to drugs, medicaments and biological substances Except: Z88.9, Allergy status to unspecified drugs, medicaments and biological substances status

Z89   Acquired absence of limb

Z90   Acquired absence of organs, not elsewhere classified

Z91.0-   Allergy status, other than to drugs and biological substances

Z92.82   Status post administration of tPA (rtPA) in a different facility within the last 24 hours prior to admission to a current facility Assign code Z92.82, Status post administration of tPA (rtPA) in a different facility within the last 24 hours prior to admission to current facility, as a secondary diagnosis when a patient is received by transfer into a facility and documentation indicates they were administered tissue plasminogen activator (tPA) within the last 24 hours prior to admission to the current facility. This guideline applies even if the patient is still receiving the tPA at the time they are received into the current facility. The appropriate code for the condition for which the tPA was administered (such as cerebrovascular disease or myocardial infarction) should be assigned first. Code Z92.82 is only applicable to the receiving facility record and not to the transferring facility record.

Z93	Artificial opening status
Z94	Transplanted organ and tissue status
Z95	Presence of cardiac and vascular implants and grafts
Z96	Presence of other functional implants
Z97	Presence of other devices
Z98	Other postprocedural states

Assign code Z98.85, Transplanted organ removal status, to indicate that a transplanted organ has been previously removed. This code should not be assigned for the encounter in which the transplanted organ is removed. The complication necessitating removal of the transplant organ should be assigned for that encounter.

See section I.C.19. for information on the coding of organ transplant complications.

| Z99 | Dependence on enabling machines and devices, not elsewhere classified |

Note: Categories Z89-Z90 and Z93-Z99 are for use only if there are no complications or malfunctions of the organ or tissue replaced, the amputation site or the equipment on which the patient is dependent.

4) History (of)

There are two types of history Z codes, personal and family. Personal history codes explain a patient's past medical condition that no longer exists and is not receiving any treatment, but that has the potential for recurrence, and therefore may require continued monitoring.

Family history codes are for use when a patient has a family member(s) who has had a particular disease that causes the patient to be at higher risk of also contracting the disease.

Personal history codes may be used in conjunction with follow-up codes and family history codes may be used in conjunction with screening codes to explain the need for a test or procedure. History codes are also acceptable on any medical record regardless of the reason for visit. A history of an illness, even if no longer present, is important information that may alter the type of treatment ordered.

The history Z code categories are:

Z80	Family history of primary malignant neoplasm
Z81	Family history of mental and behavioral disorders
Z82	Family history of certain disabilities and chronic diseases (leading to disablement)
Z83	Family history of other specific disorders
Z84	Family history of other conditions
Z85	Personal history of malignant neoplasm
Z86	Personal history of certain other diseases
Z87	Personal history of other diseases and conditions
Z91.4-	Personal history of psychological trauma, not elsewhere classified
Z91.5	Personal history of self-harm
Z91.8-	Other specified personal risk factors, not elsewhere classified Exception: Z91.83, Wandering in diseases classified elsewhere
Z92	Personal history of medical treatment Except: Z92.0, Personal history of contraception Except: Z92.82, Status post administration of tPA (rtPA) in a different facility within the last 24 hours prior to admission to a current facility

5) Screening

Screening is the testing for disease or disease precursors in seemingly well individuals so that early detection and treatment can be provided for those who test positive for the disease (e.g., screening mammogram).

The testing of a person to rule out or confirm a suspected diagnosis because the patient has some sign or symptom is a diagnostic examination, not a screening. In these cases, the sign or symptom is used to explain the reason for the test.

A screening code may be a first-listed code if the reason for the visit is specifically the screening exam. It may also be used as an additional code if the screening is done during

an office visit for other health problems. A screening code is not necessary if the screening is inherent to a routine examination, such as a pap smear done during a routine pelvic examination.

Should a condition be discovered during the screening then the code for the condition may be assigned as an additional diagnosis.

The Z code indicates that a screening exam is planned. A procedure code is required to confirm that the screening was performed.

The screening Z codes/categories:

Z11	Encounter for screening for infectious and parasitic diseases
Z12	Encounter for screening for malignant neoplasms
Z13	Encounter for screening for other diseases and disorders Except: Z13.9, Encounter for screening, unspecified
Z36	Encounter for antenatal screening for mother

6) Observation

There are **three** observation Z code categories. They are for use in very limited circumstances when a person is being observed for a suspected condition that is ruled out. The observation codes are not for use if an injury or illness or any signs or symptoms related to the suspected condition are present. In such cases the diagnosis/symptom code is used with the corresponding external cause code.

The observation codes are to be used as principal diagnosis only. **The only exception to this is when the principal diagnosis is required to be a code from category Z38, Liveborn infants according to place of birth and type of delivery. Then a code from category Z05, Encounter for observation and evaluation of newborn for suspected diseases and conditions ruled out, is sequenced after the Z38 code.** Additional codes may be used in addition to the observation code but only if they are unrelated to the suspected condition being observed.

Codes from subcategory Z03.7 Encounter for suspected maternal and fetal conditions ruled out, may either be used as a first-listed or as an additional code assignment depending on the case. They are for use in very limited circumstances on a maternal record when an encounter is for a suspected maternal or fetal condition that is ruled out during that encounter (for example, a maternal or fetal condition may be suspected due to an abnormal test result). These codes should not be used when the condition is confirmed. In those cases, the confirmed condition should be coded. In addition, these codes are not for use if an illness or any signs or symptoms related to the suspected condition or problem are present. In such cases the diagnosis/symptom code is used.

Additional codes may be used in addition to the code from subcategory Z03.7, but only if they are unrelated to the suspected condition being evaluated.

Codes from subcategory Z03.7 may not be used for encounters for antenatal screening of mother. *See Section I.C.21. Screening.*

For encounters for suspected fetal condition that are inconclusive following testing and evaluation, assign the appropriate code from category O35, O36, O40 or O41.

The observation Z code categories:

Z03	Encounter for medical observation for suspected diseases and conditions ruled out
Z04	Encounter for examination and observation for other reasons Except: Z04.9, Encounter for examination and observation for unspecified reason
Z05	**Encounter for observation and evaluation of newborn for suspected diseases and conditions ruled out**

7) Aftercare

Aftercare visit codes cover situations when the initial treatment of a disease has been performed and the patient requires continued care during the healing or recovery phase, or for the long-term consequences of the disease. The aftercare Z code should not be used if treatment is directed at a current, acute disease. The diagnosis code is to be used in these cases.

Exceptions to this rule are codes Z51.0, Encounter for antineoplastic radiation therapy, and codes from subcategory Z51.1, Encounter for antineoplastic chemotherapy and immunotherapy. These codes are to be first-listed, followed by the diagnosis code when a patient's encounter is solely

◀ New ◀▪▪ Revised ~~deleted~~ Deleted | Excludes 1 | Excludes 2 | Includes | Use additional | Code first | Code also | Unspecified

OGCR Official Guidelines X Assign placeholder X ● Use Additional Character(s) ▶ Manifestation Code **Coding Clinic**

to receive radiation therapy, chemotherapy, or immunotherapy for the treatment of a neoplasm. If the reason for the encounter is more than one type of antineoplastic therapy, code Z51.0 and a code from subcategory Z51.1 may be assigned together, in which case one of these codes would be reported as a secondary diagnosis.

The aftercare Z codes should also not be used for aftercare for injuries. For aftercare of an injury, assign the acute injury code with the appropriate 7th character (for subsequent encounter).

The aftercare codes are generally first-listed to explain the specific reason for the encounter. An aftercare code may be used as an additional code when some type of aftercare is provided in addition to the reason for admission and no diagnosis code is applicable. An example of this would be the closure of a colostomy during an encounter for treatment of another condition.

Aftercare codes should be used in conjunction with other aftercare codes or diagnosis codes to provide better detail on the specifics of an aftercare encounter visit, unless otherwise directed by the classification. Should a patient receive multiple types of antineoplastic therapy during the same encounter, code Z51.0, Encounter for antineoplastic radiation therapy, and codes from subcategory Z51.1, Encounter for antineoplastic chemotherapy and immunotherapy, may be used together on a record. The sequencing of multiple aftercare codes depends on the circumstances of the encounter.

Certain aftercare Z code categories need a secondary diagnosis code to describe the resolving condition or sequelae. For others, the condition is included in the code title.

Additional Z code aftercare category terms include fitting and adjustment, and attention to artificial openings.

Status Z codes may be used with aftercare Z codes to indicate the nature of the aftercare. For example code Z95.1, Presence of aortocoronary bypass graft, may be used with code Z48.812, Encounter for surgical aftercare following surgery on the circulatory system, to indicate the surgery for which the aftercare is being performed. A status code should not be used when the aftercare code indicates the type of status, such as using Z43.0, Encounter for attention to tracheostomy, with Z93.0, Tracheostomy status.

The aftercare Z category/codes:

Z42	Encounter for plastic and reconstructive surgery following medical procedure or healed injury
Z43	Encounter for attention to artificial openings
Z44	Encounter for fitting and adjustment of external prosthetic device
Z45	Encounter for adjustment and management of implanted device
Z46	Encounter for fitting and adjustment of other devices
Z47	Orthopedic aftercare
Z48	Encounter for other postprocedural aftercare
Z49	Encounter for care involving renal dialysis
Z51	Encounter for other aftercare **and medical care**

8) Follow-up

The follow-up codes are used to explain continuing surveillance following completed treatment of a disease, condition, or injury. They imply that the condition has been fully treated and no longer exists. They should not be confused with aftercare codes, or injury codes with a 7th character for subsequent encounter, that explain ongoing care of a healing condition or its sequelae. Follow-up codes may be used in conjunction with history codes to provide the full picture of the healed condition and its treatment. The follow-up code is sequenced first, followed by the history code.

A follow-up code may be used to explain multiple visits. Should a condition be found to have recurred on the follow-up visit, then the diagnosis code for the condition should be assigned in place of the follow-up code.

The follow-up Z code categories:

Z08	Encounter for follow-up examination after completed treatment for malignant neoplasm
Z09	Encounter for follow-up examination after completed treatment for conditions other than malignant neoplasm
Z39	Encounter for maternal postpartum care and examination

9) Donor

Codes in category Z52, Donors of organs and tissues, are used for living individuals who are donating blood or other body tissue.

These codes are only for individuals donating for others, not for self-donations. They are not used to identify cadaveric donations.

10) Counseling

Counseling Z codes are used when a patient or family member receives assistance in the aftermath of an illness or injury, or when support is required in coping with family or social problems. They are not used in conjunction with a diagnosis code when the counseling component of care is considered integral to standard treatment.

The counseling Z codes/categories:

Z30.0-	Encounter for general counseling and advice on contraception
Z31.5	Encounter for genetic counseling
Z31.6-	Encounter for general counseling and advice on procreation
Z32.2	Encounter for childbirth instruction
Z32.3	Encounter for childcare instruction
Z69	Encounter for mental health services for victim and perpetrator of abuse
Z70	Counseling related to sexual attitude, behavior and orientation
Z71	Persons encountering health services for other counseling and medical advice, not elsewhere classified
Z76.81	Expectant mother prebirth pediatrician visit

11) Encounters for Obstetrical and Reproductive Services

See Section I.C.15. Pregnancy, Childbirth, and the Puerperium, for further instruction on the use of these codes.

Z codes for pregnancy are for use in those circumstances when none of the problems or complications included in the codes from the Obstetrics chapter exist (a routine prenatal visit or postpartum care). Codes in category Z34, Encounter for supervision of normal pregnancy, are always first listed and are not to be used with any other code from the OB chapter.

Codes in category Z3A, Weeks of gestation, may be assigned to provide additional information about the pregnancy. **Category Z3A codes should not be assigned for pregnancies with abortive outcomes (categories O00-O08), elective termination of pregnancy (code Z33.32), nor for postpartum conditions, as category Z3A is not applicable to these conditions.** The date of the admission should be used to determine weeks of gestation for inpatient admissions that encompass more than one gestational week.

The outcome of delivery, category Z37, should be included on all maternal delivery records. It is always a secondary code. Codes in category Z37 should not be used on the newborn record.

Z codes for family planning (contraceptive) or procreative management and counseling should be included on an obstetric record either during the pregnancy or the postpartum stage, if applicable.

Z codes/categories for obstetrical and reproductive services:

Z30	Encounter for contraceptive management
Z31	Encounter for procreative management
Z32.2	Encounter for childbirth instruction
Z32.3	Encounter for childcare instruction
Z33	Pregnant state
Z34	Encounter for supervision of normal pregnancy
Z36	Encounter for antenatal screening of mother
Z3A	Weeks of gestation
Z37	Outcome of delivery
Z39	Encounter for maternal postpartum care and examination
Z76.81	Expectant mother prebirth pediatrician visit

12) Newborns and Infants

See Section I.C.16. Newborn (Perinatal) Guidelines, for further instruction on the use of these codes.

Newborn Z codes/categories:

Z76.1	Encounter for health supervision and care of foundling
Z00.1-	Encounter for routine child health examination
Z38	Liveborn infants according to place of birth and type of delivery

13) Routine and administrative examinations

The Z codes allow for the description of encounters for routine examinations, such as, a general check-up, or, examinations for administrative purposes, such as, a pre-employment physical. The codes are not to be used if the examination is for diagnosis of a suspected condition or for treatment purposes. In such cases the diagnosis code is used. During a routine exam, should a diagnosis or condition be discovered, it should be coded as an additional code. Pre-existing and chronic conditions and history codes may also be included as additional codes as long as the examination is for administrative purposes and not focused on any particular condition.

Some of the codes for routine health examinations distinguish between "with" and "without" abnormal findings. Code assignment depends on the information that is known at the time the encounter is being coded. For example, if no abnormal findings were found during the examination, but the encounter is being coded before test results are back, it is acceptable to assign the code for "without abnormal findings." When assigning a code for "with abnormal findings," additional code(s) should be assigned to identify the specific abnormal finding(s).

Pre-operative examination and pre-procedural laboratory examination Z codes are for use only in those situations when a patient is being cleared for a procedure or surgery and no treatment is given.

The Z codes/categories for routine and administrative examinations:

Z00	Encounter for general examination without complaint, suspected or reported diagnosis
Z01	Encounter for other special examination without complaint, suspected or reported diagnosis
Z02	Encounter for administrative examination Except: Z02.9, Encounter for administrative examinations, unspecified
Z32.0-	Encounter for pregnancy test

14) Miscellaneous Z codes

The miscellaneous Z codes capture a number of other health care encounters that do not fall into one of the other categories. Certain of these codes identify the reason for the encounter; others are for use as additional codes that provide useful information on circumstances that may affect a patient's care and treatment.

Prophylactic Organ Removal

For encounters specifically for prophylactic removal of an organ (such as prophylactic removal of breasts due to a genetic susceptibility to cancer or a family history of cancer), the principal or first-listed code should be a code from category Z40, Encounter for prophylactic surgery, followed by the appropriate codes to identify the associated risk factor (such as genetic susceptibility or family history).

If the patient has a malignancy of one site and is having prophylactic removal at another site to prevent either a new primary malignancy or metastatic disease, a code for the malignancy should also be assigned in addition to a code from subcategory Z40.0, Encounter for prophylactic surgery for risk factors related to malignant neoplasms. A Z40.0 code should not be assigned if the patient is having organ removal for treatment of a malignancy, such as the removal of the testes for the treatment of prostate cancer.

Miscellaneous Z codes/categories:

Z28	Immunization not carried out Except: Z28.3, Underimmunization status
Z29	**Encounter for other prophylactic measures**
Z40	Encounter for prophylactic surgery
Z41	Encounter for procedures for purposes other than remedying health state Except: Z41.9, Encounter for procedure for purposes other than remedying health state, unspecified
Z53	Persons encountering health services for specific procedures and treatment, not carried out
Z55	Problems related to education and literacy
Z56	Problems related to employment and unemployment
Z57	Occupational exposure to risk factors
Z58	Problems related to physical environment
Z59	Problems related to housing and economic circumstances
Z60	Problems related to social environment
Z62	Problems related to upbringing
Z63	Other problems related to primary support group, including family circumstances
Z64	Problems related to certain psychosocial circumstances
Z65	Problems related to other psychosocial circumstances

Z72	Problems related to lifestyle Note: These codes should be assigned only when the documentation specifies that the patient has an associated problem
Z73	Problems related to life management difficulty
Z74	Problems related to care provider dependency Except: Z74.01, Bed confinement status
Z75	Problems related to medical facilities and other health care
Z76.0	Encounter for issue of repeat prescription
Z76.3	Healthy person accompanying sick person
Z76.4	Other boarder to healthcare facility
Z76.5	Malingerer [conscious simulation]
Z91.1-	Patient's noncompliance with medical treatment and regimen
Z91.83	Wandering in diseases classified elsewhere
Z91.89	Other specified personal risk factors, not elsewhere classified

15) Nonspecific Z codes

Certain Z codes are so non-specific, or potentially redundant with other codes in the classification, that there can be little justification for their use in the inpatient setting. Their use in the outpatient setting should be limited to those instances when there is no further documentation to permit more precise coding. Otherwise, any sign or symptom or any other reason for visit that is captured in another code should be used.

Nonspecific Z codes/categories:

Z02.9	Encounter for administrative examinations, unspecified
Z04.9	Encounter for examination and observation for unspecified reason
Z13.9	Encounter for screening, unspecified
Z41.9	Encounter for procedure for purposes other than remedying health state, unspecified
Z52.9	Donor of unspecified organ or tissue
Z86.59	Personal history of other mental and behavioral disorders
Z88.9	Allergy status to unspecified drugs, medicaments and biological substances status
Z92.0	Personal history of contraception

16) Z Codes That May Only be Principal/First-Listed Diagnosis

The following Z codes/categories may only be reported as the principal/first-listed diagnosis, except when there are multiple encounters on the same day and the medical records for the encounters are combined:

Z00	Encounter for general examination without complaint, suspected or reported diagnosis Except: Z00.6
Z01	Encounter for other special examination without complaint, suspected or reported diagnosis
Z02	Encounter for administrative examination
Z03	Encounter for medical observation for suspected diseases and conditions ruled out
Z04	Encounter for examination and observation for other reasons
Z33.2	Encounter for elective termination of pregnancy
Z31.81	Encounter for male factor infertility in female patient
Z31.83	Encounter for assisted reproductive fertility procedure cycle
Z31.84	Encounter for fertility preservation procedure
Z34	Encounter for supervision of normal pregnancy
Z39	Encounter for maternal postpartum care and examination
Z38	Liveborn infants according to place of birth and type of delivery
Z42	Encounter for plastic and reconstructive surgery following medical procedure or healed injury
Z51.0	Encounter for antineoplastic radiation therapy
Z51.1-	Encounter for antineoplastic chemotherapy and immunotherapy
Z52	Donors of organs and tissues Except: Z52.9, Donor of unspecified organ or tissue
Z76.1	Encounter for health supervision and care of foundling
Z76.2	Encounter for health supervision and care of other healthy infant and child
Z99.12	Encounter for respirator [ventilator] dependence during power failure

◀ New   ◀▭▭ Revised   ~~deleted~~ Deleted   Excludes 1   Excludes 2   Includes   Use additional   Code first   Code also   Unspecified

OGCR Official Guidelines   X Assign placeholder X   ● Use Additional Character(s)   ▶ Manifestation Code   **Coding Clinic**

CHAPTER 21

FACTORS INFLUENCING HEALTH STATUS AND CONTACT WITH HEALTH SERVICES (Z00-Z99)

Note: Z codes represent reasons for encounters. A corresponding procedure code must accompany a Z code if a procedure is performed. Categories Z00-Z99 are provided for occasions when circumstances other than a disease, injury or external cause classifiable to categories A00-Y89 are recorded as 'diagnoses' or 'problems.' This can arise in two main ways:

(a) When a person who may or may not be sick encounters the health services for some specific purpose, such as to receive limited care or service for a current condition, to donate an organ or tissue, to receive prophylactic vaccination (immunization), or to discuss a problem which is in itself not a disease or injury.

(b) When some circumstance or problem is present which influences the person's health status but is not in itself a current illness or injury.

This chapter contains the following blocks:

Z00-Z13	Persons encountering health services for examination
Z14-Z15	Genetic carrier and genetic susceptibility to disease
Z16	Resistance to antimicrobial drugs
Z17	Estrogen receptor status
Z18	Retained foreign body fragments
Z19	Hormone sensitivity malignancy status ◀
Z20-Z29	Persons with potential health hazards related to communicable diseases ◀
Z30-Z39	Persons encountering health services in circumstances related to reproduction
Z40-Z53	Encounters for other specific health care
Z55-Z65	Persons with potential health hazards related to socioeconomic and psychosocial circumstances
Z66	Do not resuscitate status
Z67	Blood type
Z68	Body mass index (BMI)
Z69-Z76	Persons encountering health services in other circumstances
Z77-Z99	Persons with potential health hazards related to family and personal history and certain conditions influencing health status

PERSONS ENCOUNTERING HEALTH SERVICES FOR EXAMINATIONS (Z00-Z13)

Note: Nonspecific abnormal findings disclosed at the time of these examinations are classified to categories R70-R94.

Excludes1   examinations related to pregnancy and reproduction (Z30-Z36, Z39.-)

● **Z00**   **Encounter for general examination without complaint, suspected or reported diagnosis**

Excludes1   encounter for examination for administrative purposes (Z02.-)

Excludes2   encounter for pre-procedural examinations (Z01.81-)
special screening examinations (Z11-Z13)

● **Z00.0**   **Encounter for general adult medical examination**
Encounter for adult periodic examination (annual) (physical) and any associated laboratory and radiologic examinations

Excludes1   encounter for examination of sign or symptom - code to sign or symptom general health check-up of infant or child (Z00.12.-)

Z00.00   **Encounter for general adult medical examination without abnormal findings**   A
Encounter for adult health check-up NOS
Coding Clinic: 2016, Q1, P37

Z00.01   **Encounter for general adult medical examination with abnormal findings**   A
Use additional code to identify abnormal findings
Coding Clinic: 2016, Q1, P36

● **Z00.1**   **Encounter for newborn, infant and child health examinations**

● **Z00.11**   **Newborn health examination**
Health check for child under 29 days old
Use additional code to identify any abnormal findings

Excludes1   health check for child over 28 days old (Z00.12-)

Z00.110   **Health examination for newborn under 8 days old**   N
Health check for newborn under 8 days old

Z00.111   **Health examination for newborn 8 to 28 days old**   N
Health check for newborn 8 to 28 days old
Newborn weight check

● **Z00.12**   **Encounter for routine child health examination**
Encounter for development testing of infant or child
Health check (routine) for child over 28 days old

Excludes1   health check for child under 29 days old (Z00.11-)
health supervision of foundling or other healthy infant or child (Z76.1-Z76.2)
newborn health examination (Z00.11-)

Z00.121   **Encounter for routine child health examination with abnormal findings**   P
Use additional code to identify abnormal findings
Coding Clinic: 2016, Q1, P34-35

Z00.129   **Encounter for routine child health examination without abnormal findings**   P
Encounter for routine child health examination NOS
Coding Clinic: 2016, Q1, P34

Z00.2   **Encounter for examination for period of rapid growth in childhood**   P

Z00.3   **Encounter for examination for adolescent development state**   P
Encounter for puberty development state

Z00.5   **Encounter for examination of potential donor of organ and tissue**

Z00.6   **Encounter for examination for normal comparison and control in clinical research program**
Examination of participant or control in clinical research program

● **Z00.7**   **Encounter for examination for period of delayed growth in childhood**

Z00.70   **Encounter for examination for period of delayed growth in childhood without abnormal findings**   P

Z00.71   **Encounter for examination for period of delayed growth in childhood with abnormal findings**   P
Use additional code to identify abnormal findings

Z00.8   **Encounter for other general examination**
Encounter for health examination in population surveys

● **ZØ1 Encounter for other special examination without complaint, suspected or reported diagnosis**

   Includes   routine examination of specific system

   Note: Codes from category ZØ1 represent the reason for the encounter. A separate procedure code is required to identify any examinations or procedures performed.

   Excludes1   encounter for examination for administrative purposes (ZØ2.-)
      encounter for examination for suspected conditions, proven not to exist (ZØ3.-)
      encounter for laboratory and radiologic examinations as a component of general medical examinations (ZØØ.Ø-)
      encounter for laboratory, radiologic and imaging examinations for sign(s) and symptom(s) - code to the sign(s) or symptom(s)

   Excludes2   screening examinations (Z11-Z13)

● **ZØ1.Ø Encounter for examination of eyes and vision**

   Excludes1   examination for driving license (ZØ2.4)

   ZØ1.ØØ Encounter for examination of eyes and vision without abnormal findings
      Encounter for examination of eyes and vision NOS

   ZØ1.Ø1 Encounter for examination of eyes and vision with abnormal findings
      Use additional code to identify abnormal findings

● **ZØ1.1 Encounter for examination of ears and hearing**

   ZØ1.1Ø Encounter for examination of ears and hearing without abnormal findings
      Encounter for examination of ears and hearing NOS

   ● **ZØ1.11 Encounter for examination of ears and hearing with abnormal findings**

      ZØ1.11Ø Encounter for hearing examination following failed hearing screening

      ZØ1.118 Encounter for examination of ears and hearing with other abnormal findings
        Use additional code to identify abnormal findings

   ZØ1.12 Encounter for hearing conservation and treatment

● **ZØ1.2 Encounter for dental examination and cleaning**

   ZØ1.2Ø Encounter for dental examination and cleaning without abnormal findings
      Encounter for dental examination and cleaning NOS

   ZØ1.21 Encounter for dental examination and cleaning with abnormal findings
      Use additional code to identify abnormal findings

● **ZØ1.3 Encounter for examination of blood pressure**

   ZØ1.3Ø Encounter for examination of blood pressure without abnormal findings
      Encounter for examination of blood pressure NOS

   ZØ1.31 Encounter for examination of blood pressure with abnormal findings
      Use additional code to identify abnormal findings

● **ZØ1.4 Encounter for gynecological examination**

   Excludes2   pregnancy examination or test (Z32.Ø-)
      routine examination for contraceptive maintenance (Z3Ø.4-)

   ● **ZØ1.41 Encounter for routine gynecological examination**
      Encounter for general gynecological examination with or without cervical smear
      Encounter for gynecological examination (general) (routine) NOS
      Encounter for pelvic examination (annual) (periodic)
      Use additional code:
        for screening for human papillomavirus, if applicable (Z11.51)
        for screening vaginal pap smear, if applicable (Z12.72)
        to identify acquired absence of uterus, if applicable (Z9Ø.71-)

      Excludes1   gynecologic examination status-post hysterectomy for malignant condition (ZØ8)
        screening cervical pap smear not a part of a routine gynecological examination (Z12.4)

      ZØ1.411 Encounter for gynecological examination (general) (routine) with abnormal findings ♀
        Use additional code to identify any abnormal findings ◀

      ZØ1.419 Encounter for gynecological examination (general) (routine) without abnormal findings ♀

   ZØ1.42 Encounter for cervical smear to confirm findings of recent normal smear following initial abnormal smear ♀

● **ZØ1.8 Encounter for other specified special examinations**

   ● **ZØ1.81 Encounter for preprocedural examinations**
      Encounter for preoperative examinations
      Encounter for radiological and imaging examinations as part of preprocedural examination

      ZØ1.81Ø Encounter for preprocedural cardiovascular examination

      ZØ1.811 Encounter for preprocedural respiratory examination

      ZØ1.812 Encounter for preprocedural laboratory examination
        Blood and urine tests prior to treatment or procedure

      ZØ1.818 Encounter for other preprocedural examination
        Encounter for preprocedural examination NOS
        Encounter for examinations prior to antineoplastic chemotherapy

   ZØ1.82 Encounter for allergy testing
      Excludes1   encounter for antibody response examination (ZØ1.84)

   ZØ1.83 Encounter for blood typing
      Encounter for Rh typing

   ZØ1.84 Encounter for antibody response examination
      Encounter for immunity status testing
      Excludes1   encounter for allergy testing (ZØ1.82)

   ZØ1.89 Encounter for other specified special examinations

● **Z02**   **Encounter for administrative examination**

    Z02.0   **Encounter for examination for admission to educational institution**
        Encounter for examination for admission to preschool (education)
        Encounter for examination for re-admission to school following illness or medical treatment

    Z02.1   **Encounter for pre-employment examination**

    Z02.2   **Encounter for examination for admission to residential institution**
        Excludes1   examination for admission to prison (Z02.89)

    Z02.3   **Encounter for examination for recruitment to armed forces**

    Z02.4   **Encounter for examination for driving license**

    Z02.5   **Encounter for examination for participation in sport**
        Excludes1   blood-alcohol and blood-drug test (Z02.83)

    Z02.6   **Encounter for examination for insurance purposes**

●   **Z02.7**   **Encounter for issue of medical certificate**
        Excludes1   encounter for general medical examination (Z00-Z01, Z02.0-Z02.6, Z02.8-Z02.9)

        Z02.71   **Encounter for disability determination**
            Encounter for issue of medical certificate of incapacity
            Encounter for issue of medical certificate of invalidity

        Z02.79   **Encounter for issue of other medical certificate**

●   **Z02.8**   **Encounter for other administrative examinations**

        Z02.81   **Encounter for paternity testing**

        Z02.82   **Encounter for adoption services**

        Z02.83   **Encounter for blood-alcohol and blood-drug test**
            Use additional code for findings of alcohol or drugs in blood (R78.-)

        Z02.89   **Encounter for other administrative examinations**
            Encounter for examination for admission to prison
            Encounter for examination for admission to summer camp
            Encounter for immigration examination
            Encounter for naturalization examination
            Encounter for premarital examination
            Excludes1   health supervision of foundling or other healthy infant or child (Z76.1-Z76.2)

    Z02.9   **Encounter for administrative examinations, unspecified**

OGCR Section II.C.21.c.6.

Observation

There are **three** observation Z code categories. They are for use in very limited circumstances when a person is being observed for a suspected condition that is ruled out. The observation codes are not for use if an injury or illnesses or any signs or symptoms related to the suspected condition are present. In such cases the diagnosis/symptom code is used with the corresponding external cause code.

The observation codes are to be used as principal diagnosis only. **The only exception to this is when the principal diagnosis is required to be a code from category Z38, Liveborn infants according to place of birth and type of delivery. Then a code from category Z05, Encounter for observation and evaluation of newborn for suspected diseases and conditions ruled out, is sequenced after the Z38 code.** Additional codes may be used in addition to the observation code but only if they are unrelated to the suspected condition being observed.

Codes from subcategory Z03.7 Encounter for suspected maternal and fetal conditions ruled out, may either be used as a first listed or as an additional code assignment depending on the case. They are for use in very limited circumstances on a maternal record when an encounter is for a suspected maternal or fetal condition that is ruled out during that encounter (for example, a maternal or fetal condition may be suspected due to an abnormal test result). These codes should not be used when the condition is confirmed. In those cases, the confirmed condition should be coded. In addition, these codes are not for use if an illness or any signs or symptoms related to the suspected condition or problem are present. In such cases the diagnosis/symptom code is used.

Additional codes may be used in addition to the code from subcategory Z03.7, but only if they are unrelated to the suspected condition being evaluated.

Codes from subcategory Z03.7 may not be used for encounters for antenatal screening of mother. *See Section I.C.21. Screening.*

For encounters for suspected fetal condition that are inconclusive following testing and evaluation, assign the appropriate code from category O35, O36, O40 or O41.

The observation Z code categories:

Z03   Encounter for medical observation for suspected diseases and conditions ruled out

Z04   Encounter for examination and observation for other reasons
      Except: Z04.9, Encounter for examination and observation for unspecified reason

Z05   **Encounter for observation and evaluation of newborn for suspected diseases and conditions ruled out**

● **Z03**   **Encounter for medical observation for suspected diseases and conditions ruled out**
        This category is to be used when a person without a diagnosis is suspected of having an abnormal condition, without signs or symptoms, which requires study, but after examination and observation, is ruled out. This category is also for use for administrative and legal observation status.

        Excludes1   contact with and (suspected) exposures hazardous to health (Z77.-)
                newborn observation for suspected condition, ruled out (P00-P04)
                person with feared complaint in whom no diagnosis is made (Z71.1)
                signs or symptoms under study - code to signs or symptoms

    Z03.6   **Encounter for observation for suspected toxic effect from ingested substance ruled out**
        Encounter for observation for suspected adverse effect from drug
        Encounter for observation for suspected poisoning

● **Z03.7** **Encounter for suspected maternal and fetal conditions ruled out**

Encounter for suspected maternal and fetal conditions not found

Excludes1 known or suspected fetal anomalies affecting management of mother, not ruled out (O26.-, O35.-, O36.-, O40.-, O41.-)

Z03.71 **Encounter for suspected problem with amniotic cavity and membrane ruled out ♀** M

Encounter for suspected oligohydramnios ruled out

Encounter for suspected polyhydramnios ruled out

Z03.72 **Encounter for suspected placental problem ruled out ♀** M

Z03.73 **Encounter for suspected fetal anomaly ruled out ♀** M

Z03.74 **Encounter for suspected problem with fetal growth ruled out ♀** M

Z03.75 **Encounter for suspected cervical shortening ruled out ♀** M

Z03.79 **Encounter for other suspected maternal and fetal conditions ruled out ♀** M

● **Z03.8** **Encounter for observation for other suspected diseases and conditions ruled out**

● **Z03.81** **Encounter for observation for suspected exposure to biological agents ruled out**

Z03.810 **Encounter for observation for suspected exposure to anthrax ruled out**

Z03.818 **Encounter for observation for suspected exposure to other biological agents ruled out**

Z03.89 **Encounter for observation for other suspected diseases and conditions ruled out**

● **Z04** **Encounter for examination and observation for other reasons**

Includes encounter for examination for medicolegal reasons

This category is to be used when a person without a diagnosis is suspected of having an abnormal condition, without signs or symptoms, which requires study, but after examination and observation, is ruled-out. This category is also for use for administrative and legal observation status.

Z04.1 **Encounter for examination and observation following transport accident**

Excludes1 encounter for examination and observation following work accident (Z04.2)

Z04.2 **Encounter for examination and observation following work accident**

Z04.3 **Encounter for examination and observation following other accident**

● **Z04.4** **Encounter for examination and observation following alleged rape**

Encounter for examination and observation of victim following alleged rape

Encounter for examination and observation of victim following alleged sexual abuse

Z04.41 **Encounter for examination and observation following alleged adult rape** A

Suspected adult rape, ruled out

Suspected adult sexual abuse, ruled out

Z04.42 **Encounter for examination and observation following alleged child rape** P

Suspected child rape, ruled out

Suspected child sexual abuse, ruled out

Z04.6 **Encounter for general psychiatric examination, requested by authority**

● **Z04.7** **Encounter for examination and observation following alleged physical abuse**

Z04.71 **Encounter for examination and observation following alleged adult physical abuse** A

Suspected adult physical abuse, ruled out

Excludes1 confirmed case of adult physical abuse (T74.-)

encounter for examination and observation following alleged adult sexual abuse (Z04.41)

suspected case of adult physical abuse, not ruled out (T76.-)

Z04.72 **Encounter for examination and observation following alleged child physical abuse** P

Suspected child physical abuse, ruled out

Excludes1 confirmed case of child physical abuse (T74.-)

encounter for examination and observation following alleged child sexual abuse (Z04.42)

suspected case of child physical abuse, not ruled out (T76.-)

Z04.8 **Encounter for examination and observation for other specified reasons**

Encounter for examination and observation for request for expert evidence

Z04.9 **Encounter for examination and observation for unspecified reason**

Encounter for observation NOS

● **Z05** **Encounter for observation and evaluation of newborn for suspected diseases and conditions ruled out** ◄

This category is to be used for newborns, within the neonatal period (the first 28 days of life), who are suspected of having an abnormal condition unrelated to exposure from the mother or the birth process, but without signs or symptoms, and which, after examination and observation, is ruled out. ◄

Excludes2 newborn observation for suspected condition, related to exposure from the mother or birth process (P00-P04) ◄

Z05.0 **Observation and evaluation of newborn for suspected cardiac condition ruled out** ◄

Z05.1 **Observation and evaluation of newborn for suspected infectious condition ruled out** ◄

Z05.2 **Observation and evaluation of newborn for suspected neurological condition ruled out** ◄

Z05.3 **Observation and evaluation of newborn for suspected respiratory condition ruled out** ◄

● **Z05.4** **Observation and evaluation of newborn for suspected genetic, metabolic or immunologic condition ruled out** ◄

Z05.41 **Observation and evaluation of newborn for suspected genetic condition ruled out** ◄

Z05.42 **Observation and evaluation of newborn for suspected metabolic condition ruled out** ◄

Z05.43 **Observation and evaluation of newborn for suspected immunologic condition ruled out** ◄

Z05.5 **Observation and evaluation of newborn for suspected gastrointestinal condition ruled out** ◄

Z05.6 **Observation and evaluation of newborn for suspected genitourinary condition ruled out** ◄

● **Z05.7** **Observation and evaluation of newborn for suspected skin, subcutaneous, musculoskeletal and connective tissue condition ruled out** ◄

Z05.71 **Observation and evaluation of newborn for suspected skin and subcutaneous tissue condition ruled out** ◄

Z05.72 **Observation and evaluation of newborn for suspected musculoskeletal condition ruled out** ◄

Z05.73 **Observation and evaluation of newborn for suspected connective tissue condition ruled out** ◄

◄ New   ◄◄ Revised   ~~deleted~~ Deleted   Excludes 1   Excludes 2   Includes   Use additional   Code first   Code also   Unspecified

OGCR Official Guidelines   X Assign placeholder X   ● Use Additional Character(s)   ▶ Manifestation Code   **Coding Clinic**

Z05.8   **Observation and evaluation of newborn for other specified suspected condition ruled out** ◄

Z05.9   **Observation and evaluation of newborn for unspecified suspected condition ruled out** ◄

OGCR   See Section II.C.21.c.8.

> The follow-up codes are used to explain continuing surveillance following completed treatment of a disease, condition, or injury. They imply that the condition has been fully treated and no longer exists. They should not be confused with aftercare codes, or injury codes with 7th character "D," that explain ongoing care of a healing condition or its sequelae. Follow-up codes may be used in conjunction with history codes to provide the full picture of the healed condition and its treatment. The follow-up code is sequenced first, followed by the history code.
>
> A follow-up code may be used to explain multiple visits. Should a condition be found to have recurred on the follow-up visit, then the diagnosis code for the condition should be assigned in place of the follow-up code.
>
> The follow-up Z code categories:
>
> Z08   Encounter for follow-up examination after completed treatment for malignant neoplasm
>
> Z09   Encounter for follow-up examination after completed treatment for conditions other than malignant neoplasm
>
> Z39   Encounter for maternal postpartum care and examination

Z08   **Encounter for follow-up examination after completed treatment for malignant neoplasm**
Medical surveillance following completed treatment
Use additional code to identify any acquired absence of organs (Z90.-)
Use additional code to identify the personal history of malignant neoplasm (Z85.-)
Excludes1   aftercare following medical care (Z43-Z49, Z51)

Z09   **Encounter for follow-up examination after completed treatment for conditions other than malignant neoplasm**
Medical surveillance following completed treatment
Use additional code to identify any applicable history of disease code (Z86.-. Z87.-)
Excludes1   aftercare following medical care (Z43-Z49, Z51)
surveillance of contraception (Z30.4-)
surveillance of prosthetic and other medical devices (Z44-Z46)
Coding Clinic: 2015, Q1, P8

OGCR   Section II.C.21.c.5.

> Screening
>
> Screening is the testing for disease or disease precursors in seemingly well individuals so that early detection and treatment can be provided for those who test positive for the disease (e.g., screening mammogram).
>
> The testing of a person to rule out or confirm a suspected diagnosis because the patient has some sign or symptom is a diagnostic examination, not a screening. In these cases, the sign or symptom is used to explain the reason for the test.
>
> A screening code may be a first listed code if the reason for the visit is specifically the screening exam. It may also be used as an additional code if the screening is done during an office visit for other health problems. A screening code is not necessary if the screening is inherent to a routine examination, such as a pap smear done during a routine pelvic examination.
>
> Should a condition be discovered during the screening then the code for the condition may be assigned as an additional diagnosis.
>
> The Z code indicates that a screening exam is planned. A procedure code is required to confirm that the screening was performed.
>
> The screening Z codes /categories:
>
> Z11   Encounter for screening for infectious and parasitic diseases
>
> Z12   Encounter for screening for malignant neoplasms
>
> Z13   Encounter for screening for other diseases and disorders
> Except: Z13.9, Encounter for screening, unspecified
>
> Z36   Encounter for antenatal screening for mother

● **Z11**   **Encounter for screening for infectious and parasitic diseases**
Screening is the testing for disease or disease precursors in asymptomatic individuals so that early detection and treatment can be provided for those who test positive for the disease.
Excludes1   encounter for diagnostic examination - code to sign or symptom

Z11.0   **Encounter for screening for intestinal infectious diseases**

Z11.1   **Encounter for screening for respiratory tuberculosis**

Z11.2   **Encounter for screening for other bacterial diseases**

Z11.3   **Encounter for screening for infections with a predominantly sexual mode of transmission**
Excludes2   encounter for screening for human immunodeficiency virus [HIV] (Z11.4)
encounter for screening for human papillomavirus (Z11.51)

Z11.4   **Encounter for screening for human immunodeficiency virus [HIV]**

● **Z11.5**   **Encounter for screening for other viral diseases**
Excludes2   encounter for screening for viral intestinal disease (Z11.0)

Z11.51   **Encounter for screening for human papillomavirus (HPV)**

Z11.59   **Encounter for screening for other viral diseases**

Z11.6   **Encounter for screening for other protozoal diseases and helminthiases**
Diseases or infestations caused by parasitic worms
Excludes2   encounter for screening for protozoal intestinal disease (Z11.0)

Z11.8   **Encounter for screening for other infectious and parasitic diseases**
Encounter for screening for chlamydia
Encounter for screening for rickettsial
Encounter for screening for spirochetal
Encounter for screening for mycoses

Z11.9   **Encounter for screening for infectious and parasitic diseases, unspecified**

● **Z12**   **Encounter for screening for malignant neoplasms**
Screening is the testing for disease or disease precursors in asymptomatic individuals so that early detection and treatment can be provided for those who test positive for the disease.
Use additional code to identify any family history of malignant neoplasm (Z80.-)
Excludes1   encounter for diagnostic examination - code to sign or symptom

Z12.0   **Encounter for screening for malignant neoplasm of stomach**

● **Z12.1**   **Encounter for screening for malignant neoplasm of intestinal tract**

Z12.10   **Encounter for screening for malignant neoplasm of intestinal tract, unspecified**

Z12.11   **Encounter for screening for malignant neoplasm of colon**
Encounter for screening colonoscopy NOS

Z12.12   **Encounter for screening for malignant neoplasm of rectum**

Z12.13   **Encounter for screening for malignant neoplasm of small intestine**

Z12.2   **Encounter for screening for malignant neoplasm of respiratory organs**

● **Z12.3**   **Encounter for screening for malignant neoplasm of breast**

Z12.31   **Encounter for screening mammogram for malignant neoplasm of breast**
Excludes1   inconclusive mammogram (R92.2)
Coding Clinic: 2015, Q1, P24

Z12.39   **Encounter for other screening for malignant neoplasm of breast**

CHAPTER 21 (Z00-Z99)

Z12.4 Encounter for screening for malignant neoplasm of cervix ♀
> Encounter for screening pap smear for malignant neoplasm of cervix
>> **Excludes1** when screening is part of general gynecological examination (Z01.4-)
>> **Excludes2** encounter for screening for human papillomavirus (Z11.51) ◄

Z12.5 Encounter for screening for malignant neoplasm of prostate ♂

Z12.6 Encounter for screening for malignant neoplasm of bladder

● **Z12.7** Encounter for screening for malignant neoplasm of other genitourinary organs

Z12.71 Encounter for screening for malignant neoplasm of testis ♂

Z12.72 Encounter for screening for malignant neoplasm of vagina ♀
> Vaginal pap smear status - post hysterectomy for non-malignant condition
> Use additional code to identify acquired absence of uterus (Z90.71-)
>> **Excludes1** vaginal pap smear status - post hysterectomy for malignant conditions (Z08)

Z12.73 Encounter for screening for malignant neoplasm of ovary ♀

Z12.79 Encounter for screening for malignant neoplasm of other genitourinary organs

● **Z12.8** Encounter for screening for malignant neoplasm of other sites

Z12.81 Encounter for screening for malignant neoplasm of oral cavity

Z12.82 Encounter for screening for malignant neoplasm of nervous system

Z12.83 Encounter for screening for malignant neoplasm of skin

Z12.89 Encounter for screening for malignant neoplasm of other sites

Z12.9 Encounter for screening for malignant neoplasm, site unspecified

● **Z13** Encounter for screening for other diseases and disorders
> Screening is the testing for disease or disease precursors in asymptomatic individuals so that early detection and treatment can be provided for those who test positive for the disease.
>> **Excludes1** encounter for diagnostic examination - code to sign or symptom

Z13.0 Encounter for screening for diseases of the blood and blood-forming organs and certain disorders involving the immune mechanism

Z13.1 Encounter for screening for diabetes mellitus

● **Z13.2** Encounter for screening for nutritional, metabolic and other endocrine disorders

Z13.21 Encounter for screening for nutritional disorder

● **Z13.22** Encounter for screening for metabolic disorder

Z13.220 Encounter for screening for lipoid disorders
> Encounter for screening for cholesterol level
> Encounter for screening for hypercholesterolemia
> Encounter for screening for hyperlipidemia

Z13.228 Encounter for screening for other metabolic disorders

Z13.29 Encounter for screening for other suspected endocrine disorder
>> **Excludes1** encounter for screening for diabetes mellitus (Z13.1)

Z13.4 Encounter for screening for certain developmental disorders in childhood   P
> Encounter for screening for developmental handicaps in early childhood
>> **Excludes1** routine development testing of infant or child (Z00.1-)

Z13.5 Encounter for screening for eye and ear disorders
>> **Excludes2** encounter for general hearing examination (Z01.1-)
>> encounter for general vision examination (Z01.0-)

Z13.6 Encounter for screening for cardiovascular disorders

● **Z13.7** Encounter for screening for genetic and chromosomal anomalies
>> **Excludes1** genetic testing for procreative management (Z31.4-)

Z13.71 Encounter for nonprocreative screening for genetic disease carrier status

Z13.79 Encounter for other screening for genetic and chromosomal anomalies

● **Z13.8** Encounter for screening for other specified diseases and disorders
>> **Excludes2** screening for malignant neoplasms (Z12.-)

● **Z13.81** Encounter for screening for digestive system disorders

Z13.810 Encounter for screening for upper gastrointestinal disorder

Z13.811 Encounter for screening for lower gastrointestinal disorder
>> **Excludes1** encounter for screening for intestinal infectious disease (Z11.0)

Z13.818 Encounter for screening for other digestive system disorders

● **Z13.82** Encounter for screening for musculoskeletal disorder

Z13.820 Encounter for screening for osteoporosis

Z13.828 Encounter for screening for other musculoskeletal disorder

Z13.83 Encounter for screening for respiratory disorder NEC
>> **Excludes1** encounter for screening for respiratory tuberculosis (Z11.1)

Z13.84 Encounter for screening for dental disorders

● **Z13.85** Encounter for screening for nervous system disorders

Z13.850 Encounter for screening for traumatic brain injury

Z13.858 Encounter for screening for other nervous system disorders

Z13.88 Encounter for screening for disorder due to exposure to contaminants
>> **Excludes1** those exposed to contaminants without suspected disorders (Z57-Z77.-)

Z13.89 Encounter for screening for other disorder
> Encounter for screening for genitourinary disorders

Z13.9 Encounter for screening, unspecified

◄ New   ◄▥ Revised   ~~deleted~~ Deleted   Excludes 1   Excludes 2   Includes   Use additional   Code first   Code also   Unspecified
OGCR Official Guidelines   X Assign placeholder X   ● Use Additional Character(s)   ▶ Manifestation Code   **Coding Clinic**

CHAPTER 21 (Z00-Z99)

GENETIC CARRIER AND GENETIC SUSCEPTIBILITY TO DISEASE (Z14-Z15)

- **Z14**   **Genetic carrier**
  - **Z14.0**   **Hemophilia A carrier**
    - **Z14.01**   **Asymptomatic hemophilia A carrier**
    - **Z14.02**   **Symptomatic hemophilia A carrier**
  - **Z14.1**   **Cystic fibrosis carrier**
  - **Z14.8**   **Genetic carrier of other disease**

- **Z15**   **Genetic susceptibility to disease**
  - **Excludes1**   chromosomal anomalies (Q90-Q99)
  - **Includes**   confirmed abnormal gene
  - Use additional code, if applicable, for any associated family history of the disease (Z80-Z84)
  - **Z15.0**   **Genetic susceptibility to malignant neoplasm**
    - *Code first if applicable, any current malignant neoplasm (C00-C75, C81-C96)*
    - Use additional code, if applicable, for any personal history of malignant neoplasm (Z85.-)
    - **Z15.01**   **Genetic susceptibility to malignant neoplasm of breast**
    - **Z15.02**   **Genetic susceptibility to malignant neoplasm of ovary ♀**
    - **Z15.03**   **Genetic susceptibility to malignant neoplasm of prostate ♂**
    - **Z15.04**   **Genetic susceptibility to malignant neoplasm of endometrium ♀**
    - **Z15.09**   **Genetic susceptibility to other malignant neoplasm**
  - **Z15.8**   **Genetic susceptibility to other disease**
    - **Z15.81**   **Genetic susceptibility to multiple endocrine neoplasia [MEN]**
      - **Excludes1**   multiple endocrine neoplasia [MEN] syndromes (E31.2-)
    - **Z15.89**   **Genetic susceptibility to other disease**

RESISTANCE TO ANTIMICROBIAL DRUGS (Z16)

- **Z16**   **Resistance to antimicrobial drugs**
  - **Note:** The codes in this category are provided for use as additional codes to identify the resistance and non-responsiveness of a condition to antimicrobial drugs.
  - *Code first the infection*
  - **Excludes1**   Methicillin resistant Staphylococcus aureus infection (A49.02)
    - Methicillin resistant Staphylococcus aureus infection in diseases classified elsewhere (B95.62)
    - Methicillin resistant Staphylococcus aureus pneumonia (J15.212)
    - Sepsis due to Methicillin resistant Staphylococcus aureus (A41.02)
  - **Z16.1**   **Resistance to beta lactam antibiotics**
    - **Z16.10**   **Resistance to unspecified beta lactam antibiotics**
    - **Z16.11**   **Resistance to penicillins**
      - Resistance to amoxicillin
      - Resistance to ampicillin
    - **Z16.12**   **Extended spectrum beta lactamase (ESBL) resistance**
    - **Z16.19**   **Resistance to other specified beta lactam antibiotics**
      - Resistance to cephalosporins
  - **Z16.2**   **Resistance to other antibiotics**
    - **Z16.20**   **Resistance to unspecified antibiotic**
      - Resistance to antibiotics NOS
    - **Z16.21**   **Resistance to vancomycin**
    - **Z16.22**   **Resistance to vancomycin related antibiotics**
    - **Z16.23**   **Resistance to quinolones and fluoroquinolones**
    - **Z16.24**   **Resistance to multiple antibiotics**

- **Z16.29**   **Resistance to other single specified antibiotic**
  - Resistance to aminoglycosides
  - Resistance to macrolides
  - Resistance to sulfonamides
  - Resistance to tetracyclines
- **Z16.3**   **Resistance to other antimicrobial drugs**
  - **Excludes1**   resistance to antibiotics (Z16.1-, Z16.2-)
  - **Z16.30**   **Resistance to unspecified antimicrobial drugs**
    - Drug resistance NOS
  - **Z16.31**   **Resistance to antiparasitic drug(s)**
    - Resistance to quinine and related compounds
  - **Z16.32**   **Resistance to antifungal drug(s)**
  - **Z16.33**   **Resistance to antiviral drug(s)**
  - **Z16.34**   **Resistance to antimycobacterial drug(s)**
    - Resistance to tuberculostatics
    - **Z16.341**   **Resistance to single antimycobacterial drug**
      - Resistance to antimycobacterial drug NOS
    - **Z16.342**   **Resistance to multiple antimycobacterial drugs**
  - **Z16.35**   **Resistance to multiple antimicrobial drugs**
    - **Excludes1**   Resistance to multiple antibiotics only (Z16.24)
  - **Z16.39**   **Resistance to other specified antimicrobial drug**

ESTROGEN RECEPTOR STATUS (Z17)

- **Z17**   **Estrogen receptor status**
  - *Code first malignant neoplasm of breast (C50.-)*
  - **Z17.0**   **Estrogen receptor positive status [ER+]**
  - **Z17.1**   **Estrogen receptor negative status [ER-]**

RETAINED FOREIGN BODY FRAGMENTS (Z18)

- **Z18**   **Retained foreign body fragments**
  - **Includes**   embedded fragment (status)
    - embedded splinter (status)
    - retained foreign body status
  - **Excludes1**   artificial joint prosthesis status (Z96.6-)
    - foreign body accidentally left during a procedure (T81.5-)
    - foreign body entering through orifice (T15-T19)
    - in situ cardiac device (Z95.-)
    - organ or tissue replaced by means other than transplant (Z96.-, Z97.-)
    - organ or tissue replaced by transplant (Z94.-)
    - personal history of retained foreign body fully removed Z87.821
    - superficial foreign body (non-embedded splinter) - code to superficial foreign body, by site
  - **Z18.0**   **Retained radioactive fragments**
    - **Z18.01**   **Retained depleted uranium fragments**
    - **Z18.09**   **Other retained radioactive fragments**
      - Other retained depleted isotope fragments
      - Retained nontherapeutic radioactive fragments
  - **Z18.1**   **Retained metal fragments**
    - **Excludes1**   retained radioactive metal fragments (Z18.01-Z18.09)
    - **Z18.10**   **Retained metal fragments, unspecified**
      - Retained metal fragment NOS
    - **Z18.11**   **Retained magnetic metal fragments**
    - **Z18.12**   **Retained nonmagnetic metal fragments**
  - **Z18.2**   **Retained plastic fragments**
    - Acrylics fragments
    - Diethylhexylphthalates fragments
    - Isocyanate fragments
  - **Z18.3**   **Retained organic fragments**
    - **Z18.31**   **Retained animal quills or spines**
    - **Z18.32**   **Retained tooth**
    - **Z18.33**   **Retained wood fragments**
    - **Z18.39**   **Other retained organic fragments**

CHAPTER 21 (Z00-Z99)

● **Z18.8**   **Other specified retained foreign body**

    Z18.81   Retained glass fragments

    Z18.83   Retained stone or crystalline fragments
              Retained concrete or cement fragments

    Z18.89   Other specified retained foreign body fragments

Z18.9   Retained foreign body fragments, unspecified material

HORMONE SENSITIVITY MALIGNANCY STATUS (Z19) ◀

● **Z19**   **Hormone sensitivity malignancy status** ◀

    Code first malignant neoplasm —*see* Table of Neoplasms, by site, malignant ◀

    Z19.1   Hormone sensitive malignancy status ◀

    Z19.2   Hormone resistant malignancy status ◀
              Castrate resistant prostate malignancy status ◀

PERSONS WITH POTENTIAL HEALTH HAZARDS RELATED TO COMMUNICABLE DISEASES (Z20-Z29) ◀▥

● **Z20**   **Contact with and (suspected) exposure to communicable diseases**

    Excludes1   carrier of infectious disease (Z22.-)
              diagnosed current infectious or parasitic disease - see Alphabetic Index

    Excludes2   personal history of infectious and parasitic diseases (Z86.1-)

● **Z20.0**   **Contact with and (suspected) exposure to intestinal infectious diseases**

    Z20.01   Contact with and (suspected) exposure to intestinal infectious diseases due to Escherichia coli (E. coli)

    Z20.09   Contact with and (suspected) exposure to other intestinal infectious diseases

Z20.1   Contact with and (suspected) exposure to tuberculosis

Z20.2   Contact with and (suspected) exposure to infections with a predominantly sexual mode of transmission

Z20.3   Contact with and (suspected) exposure to rabies

Z20.4   Contact with and (suspected) exposure to rubella

Z20.5   Contact with and (suspected) exposure to viral hepatitis

Z20.6   Contact with and (suspected) exposure to human immunodeficiency virus [HIV]

    Excludes1   asymptomatic human immunodeficiency virus [HIV]
              HIV infection status (Z21)

Z20.7   Contact with and (suspected) exposure to pediculosis, acariasis and other infestations

● **Z20.8**   **Contact with and (suspected) exposure to other communicable diseases**

    ● **Z20.81**   Contact with and (suspected) exposure to other bacterial communicable diseases

        Z20.810   Contact with and (suspected) exposure to anthrax

        Z20.811   Contact with and (suspected) exposure to meningococcus

        Z20.818   Contact with and (suspected) exposure to other bacterial communicable diseases

    ● **Z20.82**   Contact with and (suspected) exposure to other viral communicable diseases

        Z20.820   Contact with and (suspected) exposure to varicella

        Z20.828   Contact with and (suspected) exposure to other viral communicable diseases

    Z20.89   Contact with and (suspected) exposure to other communicable diseases

Z20.9   Contact with and (suspected) exposure to unspecified communicable disease

● **Z21**   **Asymptomatic human immunodeficiency virus [HIV] infection status**
    HIV positive NOS

    Code first Human immunodeficiency virus [HIV] disease complicating pregnancy, childbirth and the puerperium, if applicable (O98.7-)

    Excludes1   acquired immunodeficiency syndrome (B20)
              contact with human immunodeficiency virus [HIV] (Z20.6)
              exposure to human immunodeficiency virus [HIV] (Z20.6)
              human immunodeficiency virus [HIV] disease (B20)
              inconclusive laboratory evidence of human immunodeficiency virus [HIV] (R75)

● **Z22**   **Carrier of infectious disease**

    Includes   colonization status
              suspected carrier

    Excludes2   carrier of viral hepatitis (B18.-) ◀

    Z22.0   Carrier of typhoid

    Z22.1   Carrier of other intestinal infectious diseases

    Z22.2   Carrier of diphtheria

  ● **Z22.3**   **Carrier of other specified bacterial diseases**

    Z22.31   Carrier of bacterial disease due to meningococci

    ● **Z22.32**   Carrier of bacterial disease due to staphylococci

        Z22.321   Carrier or suspected carrier of Methicillin susceptible Staphylococcus aureus
              MSSA colonization

        Z22.322   Carrier or suspected carrier of Methicillin resistant Staphylococcus aureus
              MRSA colonization

    ● **Z22.33**   Carrier of bacterial disease due to streptococci

        Z22.330   Carrier of Group B streptococcus

            Excludes1   Carrier of streptococcus group B (GBS) complicating pregnancy, childbirth and the puerperium (O99.82-) ◀

        Z22.338   Carrier of other streptococcus

    Z22.39   Carrier of other specified bacterial diseases

    Z22.4   Carrier of infections with a predominantly sexual mode of transmission

    ~~Z22.5~~   ~~Carrier of viral hepatitis~~

        ~~Z22.50~~   ~~Carrier of unspecified viral hepatitis~~

        ~~Z22.51~~   ~~Carrier of viral hepatitis B~~
           ~~Hepatitis B surface antigen [HBsAg] carrier~~

        ~~Z22.52~~   ~~Carrier of viral hepatitis C~~

        ~~Z22.59~~   ~~Carrier of other viral hepatitis~~

    Z22.6   Carrier of human T-lymphotropic virus type-1 [HTLV-1] infection

    Z22.8   Carrier of other infectious diseases

    Z22.9   Carrier of infectious disease, unspecified

Z23   **Encounter for immunization**

    Code first any routine childhood examination

    Note: Procedure codes are required to identify the types of immunizations given.

◀ New   ◀▥ Revised   ~~deleted~~ Deleted   Excludes 1   Excludes 2   Includes   Use additional   Code first   Code also   Unspecified

OGCR Official Guidelines   X Assign placeholder X   ● Use Additional Character(s)   ▶ Manifestation Code   **Coding Clinic**

● **Z28   Immunization not carried out and underimmunization status**

     Includes   vaccination not carried out

● **Z28.0   Immunization not carried out because of contraindication**

     Z28.01   Immunization not carried out because of acute illness of patient

     Z28.02   Immunization not carried out because of chronic illness or condition of patient

     Z28.03   Immunization not carried out because of immune compromised state of patient

     Z28.04   Immunization not carried out because of patient allergy to vaccine or component

     Z28.09   Immunization not carried out because of other contraindication

● **Z28.1   Immunization not carried out because of patient decision for reasons of belief or group pressure**

     Immunization not carried out because of religious belief

● **Z28.2   Immunization not carried out because of patient decision for other and unspecified reason**

     Z28.20   Immunization not carried out because of patient decision for unspecified reason

     Z28.21   Immunization not carried out because of patient refusal

     Z28.29   Immunization not carried out because of patient decision for other reason

   Z28.3   Underimmunization status

     Delinquent immunization status

     Lapsed immunization schedule status

● **Z28.8   Immunization not carried out for other reason**

     Z28.81   Immunization not carried out due to patient having had the disease

     Z28.82   Immunization not carried out because of caregiver refusal

       Immunization not carried out because of guardian refusal

       Immunization not carried out because of parent refusal

       Excludes1   immunization not carried out because of caregiver refusal because of religious belief (Z28.1)

     Z28.89   Immunization not carried out for other reason

   Z28.9   Immunization not carried out for unspecified reason

● **Z29   Encounter for other prophylactic measures** ◄

     Excludes1   desensitization to allergens (Z51.6) ◄

                     prophylactic surgery (Z40.-) ◄

● **Z29.1   Encounter for prophylactic immunotherapy** ◄

     Encounter for administration of immunoglobulin ◄

     Z29.11   Encounter for prophylactic immunotherapy for respiratory syncytial virus (RSV) ◄

     Z29.12   Encounter for prophylactic antivenin ◄

     Z29.13   Encounter for prophylactic Rho(D) immune globulin ◄

     Z29.14   Encounter for prophylactic rabies immune globin ◄

   Z29.3   Encounter for prophylactic fluoride administration ◄

   Z29.8   Encounter for other specified prophylactic measures ◄

   Z29.9   Encounter for prophylactic measures, unspecified ◄

PERSONS ENCOUNTERING HEALTH SERVICES IN CIRCUMSTANCES RELATED TO REPRODUCTION (Z30-Z39)

● **Z30   Encounter for contraceptive management**

● **Z30.0   Encounter for general counseling and advice on contraception**

● **Z30.01   Encounter for initial prescription of contraceptives**

     Excludes1   encounter for surveillance of contraceptives (Z30.4-)

     Z30.011   Encounter for initial prescription of contraceptive pills ♀

     Z30.012   Encounter for prescription of emergency contraception ♀

       Encounter for postcoital contraception

     Z30.013   Encounter for initial prescription of injectable contraceptive ♀

     Z30.014   Encounter for initial prescription of intrauterine contraceptive device ♀

       Excludes1   encounter for insertion of intrauterine contraceptive device (Z30.430, Z30.432)

     Z30.015   Encounter for initial prescription of vaginal ring hormonal contraceptive ♀ ◄

     Z30.016   Encounter for initial prescription of transdermal patch hormonal contraceptive device ◄

     Z30.017   Encounter for initial prescription of implantable subdermal contraceptive ◄

     Z30.018   Encounter for initial prescription of other contraceptives ♀

       Encounter for initial prescription of barrier contraception ◄

       Encounter for initial prescription of diaphragm ◄

     Z30.019   Encounter for initial prescription of contraceptives, unspecified ♀

   Z30.02   Counseling and instruction in natural family planning to avoid pregnancy

   Z30.09   Encounter for other general counseling and advice on contraception

     Encounter for family planning advice NOS

   Z30.2   Encounter for sterilization

● **Z30.4   Encounter for surveillance of contraceptives**

     Z30.40   Encounter for surveillance of contraceptives, unspecified

     Z30.41   Encounter for surveillance of contraceptive pills ♀

       Encounter for repeat prescription for contraceptive pill

     Z30.42   Encounter for surveillance of injectable contraceptive ♀

● **Z30.43   Encounter for surveillance of intrauterine contraceptive device**

     Z30.430   Encounter for insertion of intrauterine contraceptive device ♀

     Z30.431   Encounter for routine checking of intrauterine contraceptive device ♀

     Z30.432   Encounter for removal of intrauterine contraceptive device ♀

     Z30.433   Encounter for removal and reinsertion of intrauterine contraceptive device ♀

       Encounter for replacement of intrauterine contraceptive device

CHAPTER 21 (Z00-Z99)

Z30.44 Encounter for surveillance of vaginal ring hormonal contraceptive device ♀ ◄

Z30.45 Encounter for surveillance of transdermal patch hormonal contraceptive device ♀ ◄

Z30.46 Encounter for surveillance of implantable subdermal contraceptive ♀ ◄
Encounter for checking, reinsertion or removal of implantable subdermal contraceptive ◄

Z30.49 Encounter for surveillance of other contraceptives ♀
Encounter for surveillance of barrier contraception ◄
Encounter for surveillance of diaphragm ◄

Z30.8 Encounter for other contraceptive management
Encounter for postvasectomy sperm count
Encounter for routine examination for contraceptive maintenance
> **Excludes1** sperm count following sterilization reversal (Z31.42)
> sperm count for fertility testing (Z31.41)

Z30.9 Encounter for contraceptive management, unspecified

● **Z31** Encounter for procreative management
> **Excludes1** complications associated with artificial fertilization (N98.-)
> female infertility (N97.-)
> male infertility (N46.-)

Z31.0 Encounter for reversal of previous sterilization

● **Z31.4** Encounter for procreative investigation and testing
> **Excludes1** postvasectomy sperm count (Z30.8)

Z31.41 Encounter for fertility testing
Encounter for fallopian tube patency testing
Encounter for sperm count for fertility testing

Z31.42 Aftercare following sterilization reversal
Sperm count following sterilization reversal

● **Z31.43** Encounter for genetic testing of female for procreative management
Use additional code for recurrent pregnancy loss, if applicable (N96, O26.2-)
> **Excludes1** nonprocreative genetic testing (Z13.7-)

Z31.430 Encounter of female for testing for genetic disease carrier status for procreative management ♀

Z31.438 Encounter for other genetic testing of female for procreative management ♀

● **Z31.44** Encounter for genetic testing of male for procreative management
> **Excludes1** nonprocreative genetic testing (Z13.7-)

Z31.440 Encounter of male for testing for genetic disease carrier status for procreative management ♂

Z31.441 Encounter for testing of male partner of patient with recurrent pregnancy loss ♂   A

Z31.448 Encounter for other genetic testing of male for procreative management ♂ A

Z31.49 Encounter for other procreative investigation and testing

Z31.5 Encounter for genetic counseling

● **Z31.6** Encounter for general counseling and advice on procreation

Z31.61 Procreative counseling and advice using natural family planning

Z31.62 Encounter for fertility preservation counseling
Encounter for fertility preservation counseling prior to cancer therapy
Encounter for fertility preservation counseling prior to surgical removal of gonads

Z31.69 Encounter for other general counseling and advice on procreation

Z31.7 Encounter for procreative management and counseling for gestational carrier ◄
> **Excludes1** pregnant state, gestational carrier (Z33.3) ◄

● **Z31.8** Encounter for other procreative management

Z31.81 Encounter for male factor infertility in female patient ♀

Z31.82 Encounter for Rh incompatibility status ♀
Coding Clinic: 2015, Q3, P40

Z31.83 Encounter for assisted reproductive fertility procedure cycle ♀
Patient undergoing in vitro fertilization cycle
Use additional code to identify the type of infertility
> **Excludes1** pre-cycle diagnosis and testing - code to reason for encounter

Z31.84 Encounter for fertility preservation procedure
Encounter for fertility preservation procedure prior to cancer therapy
Encounter for fertility preservation procedure prior to surgical removal of gonads

Z31.89 Encounter for other procreative management

Z31.9 Encounter for procreative management, unspecified

● **Z32** Encounter for pregnancy test and childbirth and childcare instruction

● **Z32.0** Encounter for pregnancy test

Z32.00 Encounter for pregnancy test, result unknown ♀
Encounter for pregnancy test NOS

Z32.01 Encounter for pregnancy test, result positive ♀   M

Z32.02 Encounter for pregnancy test, result negative ♀

Z32.2 Encounter for childbirth instruction

Z32.3 Encounter for childcare instruction
Encounter for prenatal or postpartum childcare instruction

● **Z33** Pregnant state

Z33.1 Pregnant state, incidental ♀   M
Pregnant state NOS
> **Excludes1** complications of pregnancy (O00-O9A)
> pregnant state, gestational carrier (Z33.3) ◄

Z33.2 Encounter for elective termination of pregnancy ♀   M
> **Excludes1** early fetal death with retention of dead fetus (O02.1)
> late fetal death (O36.4)
> spontaneous abortion (O03)

Z33.3 Pregnant state, gestational carrier ♀ ◄
> **Excludes1** encounter for procreative management and counseling for gestational carrier (Z31.7) ◄

● **Z34** Encounter for supervision of normal pregnancy
> **Excludes1** any complication of pregnancy (O00-O9A)
> encounter for pregnancy test (Z32.0-)
> encounter for supervision of high risk pregnancy (O09.-)

● **Z34.0** Encounter for supervision of normal first pregnancy

Z34.00 Encounter for supervision of normal first pregnancy, unspecified trimester ♀   M

Z34.01 Encounter for supervision of normal first pregnancy, first trimester ♀   M

Z34.02 Encounter for supervision of normal first pregnancy, second trimester ♀   M

Z34.03 Encounter for supervision of normal first pregnancy, third trimester ♀   M

| First trimester (0 to 14 weeks) | Second trimester (14 to 28 weeks) | Third trimester (28 weeks to delivery) |

Figure 21-1 Trimesters. (From Shiland, Betsy J. Medical Terminology & Anatomy for ICD-10 Coding, ed 2, Mosby, 2015)

- ● **Z34.8** **Encounter for supervision of other normal pregnancy**
  - **Z34.80** Encounter for supervision of other normal pregnancy, unspecified trimester ♀　　M
  - **Z34.81** Encounter for supervision of other normal pregnancy, first trimester ♀　　M
  - **Z34.82** Encounter for supervision of other normal pregnancy, second trimester ♀　　M
  - **Z34.83** Encounter for supervision of other normal pregnancy, third trimester ♀　　M
- ● **Z34.9** **Encounter for supervision of normal pregnancy, unspecified**
  - **Z34.90** Encounter for supervision of normal pregnancy, unspecified, unspecified trimester ♀　　M
  - **Z34.91** Encounter for supervision of normal pregnancy, unspecified, first trimester ♀　　M
  - **Z34.92** Encounter for supervision of normal pregnancy, unspecified, second trimester ♀　　M
  - **Z34.93** Encounter for supervision of normal pregnancy, unspecified, third trimester ♀　　M
- **Z36** **Encounter for antenatal screening of mother** ♀　　M
  - **Excludes1** abnormal findings on antenatal screening of mother (O28.-)
    diagnostic examination - code to sign or symptom
    encounter for suspected maternal and fetal conditions ruled out (Z03.7-)
    suspected fetal condition affecting management of pregnancy - code to condition in Chapter 15
  - **Excludes2** genetic counseling and testing (Z31.43-, Z31.5)
    routine prenatal care (Z34)
- ● **Z3A** **Weeks of gestation**
  - **Note:** Codes from category Z3A are for use, only on the maternal record, to indicate the weeks of gestation of the pregnancy, if known. ◀
  - *Code first complications of pregnancy, childbirth and the puerperium (O00-O9A)*
  - Coding Clinic: 2013, Q2, P33
  - ● **Z3A.0** **Weeks of gestation of pregnancy, unspecified or less than 10 weeks**
    - **Z3A.00** Weeks of gestation of pregnancy not specified ♀　　M
    - **Z3A.01** Less than 8 weeks gestation of pregnancy ♀　　M
    - **Z3A.08** 8 weeks gestation of pregnancy ♀　　M
    - **Z3A.09** 9 weeks gestation of pregnancy ♀　　M

- ● **Z3A.1** **Weeks of gestation of pregnancy, weeks 10-19**
  - **Z3A.10** 10 weeks gestation of pregnancy ♀　　M
  - **Z3A.11** 11 weeks gestation of pregnancy ♀　　M
  - **Z3A.12** 12 weeks gestation of pregnancy ♀　　M
  - **Z3A.13** 13 weeks gestation of pregnancy ♀　　M
  - **Z3A.14** 14 weeks gestation of pregnancy ♀　　M
  - **Z3A.15** 15 weeks gestation of pregnancy ♀　　M
  - **Z3A.16** 16 weeks gestation of pregnancy ♀　　M
  - **Z3A.17** 17 weeks gestation of pregnancy ♀　　M
  - **Z3A.18** 18 weeks gestation of pregnancy ♀　　M
  - **Z3A.19** 19 weeks gestation of pregnancy ♀　　M
- ● **Z3A.2** **Weeks of gestation of pregnancy, weeks 20-29**
  - **Z3A.20** 20 weeks gestation of pregnancy ♀　　M
  - **Z3A.21** 21 weeks gestation of pregnancy ♀　　M
  - **Z3A.22** 22 weeks gestation of pregnancy ♀　　M
  - **Z3A.23** 23 weeks gestation of pregnancy ♀　　M
  - **Z3A.24** 24 weeks gestation of pregnancy ♀　　M
  - **Z3A.25** 25 weeks gestation of pregnancy ♀　　M
  - **Z3A.26** 26 weeks gestation of pregnancy ♀　　M
  - **Z3A.27** 27 weeks gestation of pregnancy ♀　　M
  - **Z3A.28** 28 weeks gestation of pregnancy ♀　　M
  - **Z3A.29** 29 weeks gestation of pregnancy ♀　　M
- ● **Z3A.3** **Weeks of gestation of pregnancy, weeks 30-39**
  - **Z3A.30** 30 weeks gestation of pregnancy ♀　　M
  - **Z3A.31** 31 weeks gestation of pregnancy ♀　　M
  - **Z3A.32** 32 weeks gestation of pregnancy ♀　　M
  - **Z3A.33** 33 weeks gestation of pregnancy ♀　　M
  - **Z3A.34** 34 weeks gestation of pregnancy ♀　　M
  - **Z3A.35** 35 weeks gestation of pregnancy ♀　　M
  - **Z3A.36** 36 weeks gestation of pregnancy ♀　　M
  - **Z3A.37** 37 weeks gestation of pregnancy ♀　　M
  - **Z3A.38** 38 weeks gestation of pregnancy ♀　　M
    Coding Clinic: 2016, Q2, P34
  - **Z3A.39** 39 weeks gestation of pregnancy ♀　　M
- ● **Z3A.4** **Weeks of gestation of pregnancy, weeks 40 or greater**
  - **Z3A.40** 40 weeks gestation of pregnancy ♀　　M
  - **Z3A.41** 41 weeks gestation of pregnancy ♀　　M
  - **Z3A.42** 42 weeks gestation of pregnancy ♀　　M
  - **Z3A.49** Greater than 42 weeks gestation of pregnancy ♀　　M
- ● **Z37** **Outcome of delivery**
  - This category is intended for use as an additional code to identify the outcome of delivery on the mother's record. It is not for use on the newborn record.
  - **Excludes1** stillbirth (P95)
  - **Z37.0** Single live birth ♀　　M
    Coding Clinic: 2016, Q2, P34
  - **Z37.1** Single stillbirth ♀　　M
  - **Z37.2** Twins, both liveborn ♀　　M
  - **Z37.3** Twins, one liveborn and one stillborn ♀　　M
  - **Z37.4** Twins, both stillborn ♀　　M
  - ● **Z37.5** **Other multiple births, all liveborn**
    - **Z37.50** Multiple births, unspecified, all liveborn ♀　　M
    - **Z37.51** Triplets, all liveborn ♀　　M
    - **Z37.52** Quadruplets, all liveborn ♀　　M
    - **Z37.53** Quintuplets, all liveborn ♀　　M
    - **Z37.54** Sextuplets, all liveborn ♀　　M
    - **Z37.59** Other multiple births, all liveborn ♀　　M

CHAPTER 21 (Z00-Z99)

● **Z37.6 Other multiple births, some liveborn**
    Z37.60 Multiple births, unspecified, some liveborn ♀ M
    Z37.61 Triplets, some liveborn ♀   M
    Z37.62 Quadruplets, some liveborn ♀   M
    Z37.63 Quintuplets, some liveborn ♀   M
    Z37.64 Sextuplets, some liveborn ♀   M
    Z37.69 Other multiple births, some liveborn ♀   M
  Z37.7 Other multiple births, all stillborn ♀   M
  Z37.9 Outcome of delivery, unspecified ♀   M
    Multiple birth NOS
    Single birth NOS

● **Z38 Liveborn infants according to place of birth and type of delivery**
  This category is for use as the principal code on the initial record of a newborn baby. It is to be used for the initial birth record only. It is not to be used on the mother's record.
  Coding Clinic: 2015, Q2, P15

● **Z38.0 Single liveborn infant, born in hospital**
  Single liveborn infant, born in birthing center or other health care facility
    Z38.00 Single liveborn infant, delivered vaginally N
    Z38.01 Single liveborn infant, delivered by cesarean N
  Z38.1 Single liveborn infant, born outside hospital N
  Z38.2 Single liveborn infant, unspecified as to place of birth N
    Single liveborn infant NOS
● **Z38.3 Twin liveborn infant, born in hospital**
    Z38.30 Twin liveborn infant, delivered vaginally N
    Z38.31 Twin liveborn infant, delivered by cesarean N
  Z38.4 Twin liveborn infant, born outside hospital N
  Z38.5 Twin liveborn infant, unspecified as to place of birth N
● **Z38.6 Other multiple liveborn infant, born in hospital**
    Z38.61 Triplet liveborn infant, delivered vaginally N
    Z38.62 Triplet liveborn infant, delivered by cesarean N
    Z38.63 Quadruplet liveborn infant, delivered vaginally N
    Z38.64 Quadruplet liveborn infant, delivered by cesarean N
    Z38.65 Quintuplet liveborn infant, delivered vaginally N
    Z38.66 Quintuplet liveborn infant, delivered by cesarean N
    Z38.68 Other multiple liveborn infant, delivered vaginally N
    Z38.69 Other multiple liveborn infant, delivered by cesarean N
  Z38.7 Other multiple liveborn infant, born outside hospital N
  Z38.8 Other multiple liveborn infant, unspecified as to place of birth N

● **Z39 Encounter for maternal postpartum care and examination**
  Z39.0 Encounter for care and examination of mother immediately after delivery ♀   M
    Care and observation in uncomplicated cases when the delivery occurs outside a healthcare facility
    Excludes1 care for postpartum complication - see Alphabetic index
  Z39.1 Encounter for care and examination of lactating mother ♀   M
    Encounter for supervision of lactation
    Excludes1 disorders of lactation (O92.-)
  Z39.2 Encounter for routine postpartum follow-up ♀   M

ENCOUNTERS FOR OTHER SPECIFIC HEALTH CARE (Z40-Z53)

Categories Z40-Z53 are intended for use to indicate a reason for care. They may be used for patients who have already been treated for a disease or injury, but who are receiving aftercare or prophylactic care, or care to consolidate the treatment, or to deal with a residual state

Excludes2 follow-up examination for medical surveillance after treatment (Z08-Z09)

● **Z40 Encounter for prophylactic surgery**
  Excludes1 organ donations (Z52.-)
    therapeutic organ removal - code to condition
● **Z40.0 Encounter for prophylactic surgery for risk factors related to malignant neoplasms**
  Admission for prophylactic organ removal
  Use additional code to identify risk factor
    Z40.00 Encounter for prophylactic removal of unspecified organ
    Z40.01 Encounter for prophylactic removal of breast
    Z40.02 Encounter for prophylactic removal of ovary ♀
    Z40.09 Encounter for prophylactic removal of other organ
  Z40.8 Encounter for other prophylactic surgery
  Z40.9 Encounter for prophylactic surgery, unspecified

● **Z41 Encounter for procedures for purposes other than remedying health state**
  Z41.1 Encounter for cosmetic surgery
    Encounter for cosmetic breast implant
    Encounter for cosmetic procedure
    Excludes1 encounter for plastic and reconstructive surgery following medical procedure or healed injury (Z42.-)
    encounter for post-mastectomy breast implantation (Z42.1)
  Z41.2 Encounter for routine and ritual male circumcision ♂
  Z41.3 Encounter for ear piercing
  Z41.8 Encounter for other procedures for purposes other than remedying health state
  Z41.9 Encounter for procedure for purposes other than remedying health state, unspecified

● **Z42 Encounter for plastic and reconstructive surgery following medical procedure or healed injury**
  Excludes1 encounter for cosmetic plastic surgery (Z41.1)
    encounter for plastic surgery for treatment of current injury - code to relevent injury
  Z42.1 Encounter for breast reconstruction following mastectomy   A
    Excludes1 deformity and disproportion of reconstructed breast (N65.1-)
  Z42.8 Encounter for other plastic and reconstructive surgery following medical procedure or healed injury

◄ New ◄▬ Revised ~~deleted~~ Deleted | Excludes 1 | Excludes 2 | Includes | Use additional | Code first | Code also | Unspecified
OGCR Official Guidelines   X Assign placeholder X   ● Use Additional Character(s)   ▶ Manifestation Code   **Coding Clinic**

● **Z43**   **Encounter for attention to artificial openings**

    Includes   closure of artificial openings
                      passage of sounds or bougies through artificial
                          openings
                      reforming artificial openings
                      removal of catheter from artificial openings
                      toilet or cleansing of artificial openings

    Excludes1   artificial opening status only, without need for
                        care (Z93.-)
                      complications of external stoma (J95.0-, K94.-,
                        N99.5-)

    Excludes2   fitting and adjustment of prosthetic and other
                        devices (Z44-Z46)

    Z43.0   Encounter for attention to tracheostomy

    Z43.1   Encounter for attention to gastrostomy

    Z43.2   Encounter for attention to ileostomy

    Z43.3   Encounter for attention to colostomy

    Z43.4   Encounter for attention to other artificial openings of digestive tract

    Z43.5   Encounter for attention to cystostomy

    Z43.6   Encounter for attention to other artificial openings of urinary tract
                Encounter for attention to nephrostomy
                Encounter for attention to ureterostomy
                Encounter for attention to urethrostomy

    Z43.7   Encounter for attention to artificial vagina

    Z43.8   Encounter for attention to other artificial openings

    Z43.9   Encounter for attention to unspecified artificial opening

● **Z44**   **Encounter for fitting and adjustment of external prosthetic device**

    Includes   removal or replacement of external prosthetic
                      device

    Excludes1   malfunction or other complications of device - see
                        Alphabetical Index presence of prosthetic
                        device (Z97.-)

● **Z44.0**   **Encounter for fitting and adjustment of artificial arm**

    ● **Z44.00**   Encounter for fitting and adjustment of unspecified artificial arm

        Z44.001   Encounter for fitting and adjustment of unspecified right artificial arm

        Z44.002   Encounter for fitting and adjustment of unspecified left artificial arm

        Z44.009   Encounter for fitting and adjustment of unspecified artificial arm, unspecified arm

    ● **Z44.01**   Encounter for fitting and adjustment of complete artificial arm

        Z44.011   Encounter for fitting and adjustment of complete right artificial arm

        Z44.012   Encounter for fitting and adjustment of complete left artificial arm

        Z44.019   Encounter for fitting and adjustment of complete artificial arm, unspecified arm

    ● **Z44.02**   Encounter for fitting and adjustment of partial artificial arm

        Z44.021   Encounter for fitting and adjustment of partial artificial right arm

        Z44.022   Encounter for fitting and adjustment of partial artificial left arm

        Z44.029   Encounter for fitting and adjustment of partial artificial arm, unspecified arm

● **Z44.1**   **Encounter for fitting and adjustment of artificial leg**

    ● **Z44.10**   Encounter for fitting and adjustment of unspecified artificial leg

        Z44.101   Encounter for fitting and adjustment of unspecified right artificial leg

        Z44.102   Encounter for fitting and adjustment of unspecified left artificial leg

        Z44.109   Encounter for fitting and adjustment of unspecified artificial leg, unspecified leg

    ● **Z44.11**   Encounter for fitting and adjustment of complete artificial leg

        Z44.111   Encounter for fitting and adjustment of complete right artificial leg

        Z44.112   Encounter for fitting and adjustment of complete left artificial leg

        Z44.119   Encounter for fitting and adjustment of complete artificial leg, unspecified leg

    ● **Z44.12**   Encounter for fitting and adjustment of partial artificial leg

        Z44.121   Encounter for fitting and adjustment of partial artificial right leg

        Z44.122   Encounter for fitting and adjustment of partial artificial left leg

        Z44.129   Encounter for fitting and adjustment of partial artificial leg, unspecified leg

● **Z44.2**   **Encounter for fitting and adjustment of artificial eye**

    Excludes1   mechanical complication of ocular prosthesis (T85.3)

    Z44.20   Encounter for fitting and adjustment of artificial eye, unspecified

    Z44.21   Encounter for fitting and adjustment of artificial right eye

    Z44.22   Encounter for fitting and adjustment of artificial left eye

● **Z44.3**   **Encounter for fitting and adjustment of external breast prosthesis**

    Excludes1   complications of breast implant (T85.4-)
                        encounter for adjustment or removal of
                        breast implant (Z45.81-)
                      encounter for initial breast implant
                        insertion for cosmetic breast
                        augmentation (Z41.1)
                      encounter for breast reconstruction
                        following mastectomy (Z42.1)

    Z44.30   Encounter for fitting and adjustment of external breast prosthesis, unspecified breast

    Z44.31   Encounter for fitting and adjustment of external right breast prosthesis

    Z44.32   Encounter for fitting and adjustment of external left breast prosthesis

    Z44.8   Encounter for fitting and adjustment of other external prosthetic devices

    Z44.9   Encounter for fitting and adjustment of unspecified external prosthetic device

CHAPTER 21 (Z00-Z99)

● **Z45 Encounter for adjustment and management of implanted device**

   Includes   removal or replacement of implanted device

   Excludes 1   malfunction or other complications of device - see Alphabetical Index

                  presence of prosthetic and other devices (Z95-Z97)

   Excludes 2   encounter for fitting and adjustment of non-implanted device (Z46.-)

  ● **Z45.0 Encounter for adjustment and management of cardiac device**

    ● **Z45.01 Encounter for adjustment and management of cardiac pacemaker**

        Encounter for adjustment and management of cardiac resynchronization therapy pacemaker (CRT-P) ◄

        Excludes 1   encounter for adjustment and management of automatic implantable cardiac defibrillator with synchronous cardiac pacemaker (Z45.02)

        Z45.010 Encounter for checking and testing of cardiac pacemaker pulse generator [battery]

            Encounter for replacing cardiac pacemaker pulse generator [battery]

        Z45.018 Encounter for adjustment and management of other part of cardiac pacemaker

    Z45.02 Encounter for adjustment and management of automatic implantable cardiac defibrillator

        Encounter for adjustment and management of automatic implantable cardiac defibrillator with synchronous cardiac pacemaker

        Encounter for adjustment and management of cardiac resynchronization therapy defibrillator (CRT-D) ◄

    Z45.09 Encounter for adjustment and management of other cardiac device

  Z45.1 Encounter for adjustment and management of infusion pump

  Z45.2 Encounter for adjustment and management of vascular access device

    Encounter for adjustment and management of vascular catheters

    Excludes 1   encounter for adjustment and management of renal dialysis catheter (Z49.01)

  ● **Z45.3 Encounter for adjustment and management of implanted devices of the special senses**

    Z45.31 Encounter for adjustment and management of implanted visual substitution device

    ● **Z45.32 Encounter for adjustment and management of implanted hearing device**

        Excludes 1   encounter for fitting and adjustment of hearing aide (Z46.1)

        Z45.320 Encounter for adjustment and management of bone conduction device

        Z45.321 Encounter for adjustment and management of cochlear device

        Z45.328 Encounter for adjustment and management of other implanted hearing device

● **Z45.4 Encounter for adjustment and management of implanted nervous system device**

    Z45.41 Encounter for adjustment and management of cerebrospinal fluid drainage device

        Encounter for adjustment and management of cerebral ventricular (communicating) shunt

    Z45.42 Encounter for adjustment and management of neuropacemaker (brain) (peripheral nerve) (spinal cord)

    Z45.49 Encounter for adjustment and management of other implanted nervous system device

● **Z45.8 Encounter for adjustment and management of other implanted devices**

  ● **Z45.81 Encounter for adjustment or removal of breast implant**

    Encounter for elective implant exchange (different material) (different size)

    Encounter removal of tissue expander without synchronous insertion of permanent implant

    Excludes 1   complications of breast implant (T85.4-)

            encounter for initial breast implant insertion for cosmetic breast augmentation (Z41.1)

            encounter for breast reconstruction following mastectomy (Z42.1)

    Z45.811 Encounter for adjustment or removal of right breast implant

    Z45.812 Encounter for adjustment or removal of left breast implant

    Z45.819 Encounter for adjustment or removal of unspecified breast implant

  Z45.82 Encounter for adjustment or removal of myringotomy device (stent) (tube)

  Z45.89 Encounter for adjustment and management of other implanted devices

  Z45.9 Encounter for adjustment and management of unspecified implanted device

● **Z46 Encounter for fitting and adjustment of other devices**

   Includes   removal or replacement of other device

   Excludes 1   malfunction or other complications of device - see Alphabetical Index

   Excludes 2   encounter for fitting and management of implanted devices (Z45.-)

            issue of repeat prescription only (Z76.0)

            presence of prosthetic and other devices (Z95-Z97)

  Z46.0 Encounter for fitting and adjustment of spectacles and contact lenses

  Z46.1 Encounter for fitting and adjustment of hearing aid

    Excludes 1   encounter for adjustment and management of implanted hearing device (Z45.32-)

  Z46.2 Encounter for fitting and adjustment of other devices related to nervous system and special senses

    Excludes 2   encounter for adjustment and management of implanted nervous system device (Z45.4-)

            encounter for adjustment and management of implanted visual substitution device (Z45.31)

  Z46.3 Encounter for fitting and adjustment of dental prosthetic device

    Encounter for fitting and adjustment of dentures

  Z46.4 Encounter for fitting and adjustment of orthodontic device

◄ New   ⬛ Revised   ~~deleted~~ Deleted   Excludes 1   Excludes 2   Includes   Use additional   Code first   Code also   Unspecified

OGCR Official Guidelines   X Assign placeholder X   ● Use Additional Character(s)   ▸ Manifestation Code   **Coding Clinic**

● **Z46.5** **Encounter for fitting and adjustment of other gastrointestinal appliance and device**
> **Excludes1** encounter for attention to artificial openings of digestive tract (Z43.1-Z43.4)

    Z46.51 **Encounter for fitting and adjustment of gastric lap band**

    Z46.59 **Encounter for fitting and adjustment of other gastrointestinal appliance and device**

Z46.6 **Encounter for fitting and adjustment of urinary device**
> **Excludes2** attention to artificial openings of urinary tract (Z43.5, Z43.6)

● **Z46.8** **Encounter for fitting and adjustment of other specified devices**

    Z46.81 **Encounter for fitting and adjustment of insulin pump**
> Encounter for insulin pump instruction and training
> Encounter for insulin pump titration

    Z46.82 **Encounter for fitting and adjustment of non-vascular catheter**

    Z46.89 **Encounter for fitting and adjustment of other specified devices**
> Encounter for fitting and adjustment of wheelchair

Z46.9 **Encounter for fitting and adjustment of unspecified device**

● **Z47** **Orthopedic aftercare**
> **Excludes1** aftercare for healing fracture - code to fracture with 7th character D

Z47.1 **Aftercare following joint replacement surgery**
> Use additional code to identify the joint (Z96.6-)

Z47.2 **Encounter for removal of internal fixation device**
> **Excludes1** encounter for adjustment of internal fixation device for fracture treatment - code to fracture with appropriate 7th character
> encounter for removal of external fixation device - code to fracture with 7th character D
> infection or inflammatory reaction to internal fixation device (T84.6-)
> mechanical complication of internal fixation device (T84.1-)

● **Z47.3** **Aftercare following explantation of joint prosthesis**
> Aftercare following explantation of joint prosthesis, staged procedure
> Encounter for joint prosthesis insertion following prior explantation of joint prosthesis
> Coding Clinic: 2015, Q1, P17

    Z47.31 **Aftercare following explantation of shoulder joint prosthesis**
> **Excludes1** acquired absence of shoulder joint following prior explantation of shoulder joint prosthesis (Z89.23-)
> shoulder joint prosthesis explantation status (Z89.23-)

    Z47.32 **Aftercare following explantation of hip joint prosthesis**
> **Excludes1** acquired absence of hip joint following prior explantation of hip joint prosthesis (Z89.62-)
> hip joint prosthesis explantation status (Z89.62-)
> Coding Clinic: 2015, Q1, P17

    Z47.33 **Aftercare following explantation of knee joint prosthesis**
> **Excludes1** acquired absence of knee joint following prior explantation of knee prosthesis (Z89.52-)
> knee joint prosthesis explantation status (Z89.52-)

Z47.8 **Encounter for other orthopedic aftercare**

    Z47.81 **Encounter for orthopedic aftercare following surgical amputation**
> Use additional code to identify the limb amputated (Z89.-)

    Z47.82 **Encounter for orthopedic aftercare following scoliosis surgery**

    Z47.89 **Encounter for other orthopedic aftercare**
> Coding Clinic: 2015, Q1, P8

● **Z48** **Encounter for other postprocedural aftercare**
> **Excludes1** encounter for follow-up examination after completed treatment (Z08-Z09)
> **Excludes2** encounter for attention to artificial openings (Z43.-)
> encounter for fitting and adjustment of prosthetic and other devices (Z44-Z46)

● **Z48.0** **Encounter for attention to dressings, sutures and drains**
> **Excludes1** encounter for planned postprocedural wound closure (Z48.1)

    Z48.00 **Encounter for change or removal of nonsurgical wound dressing**
> Encounter for change or removal of wound dressing NOS

    Z48.01 **Encounter for change or removal of surgical wound dressing**
> Coding Clinic: 2015, Q4, P38

    Z48.02 **Encounter for removal of sutures**
> Encounter for removal of staples
> Coding Clinic: 2015, Q1, P6

    Z48.03 **Encounter for change or removal of drains**

Z48.1 **Encounter for planned postprocedural wound closure**
> **Excludes1** encounter for attention to dressings and sutures (Z48.0-)

● **Z48.2** **Encounter for aftercare following organ transplant**

    Z48.21 **Encounter for aftercare following heart transplant**

    Z48.22 **Encounter for aftercare following kidney transplant**

    Z48.23 **Encounter for aftercare following liver transplant**

    Z48.24 **Encounter for aftercare following lung transplant**

● **Z48.28** **Encounter for aftercare following multiple organ transplant**

      Z48.280 **Encounter for aftercare following heart-lung transplant**

      Z48.288 **Encounter for aftercare following multiple organ transplant**

● **Z48.29** **Encounter for aftercare following other organ transplant**

      Z48.290 **Encounter for aftercare following bone marrow transplant**

      Z48.298 **Encounter for aftercare following other organ transplant**

Z48.3 **Aftercare following surgery for neoplasm**
> Use additional code to identify the neoplasm

CHAPTER 21 (Z00-Z99)

● **Z48.8　Encounter for other specified postprocedural aftercare**
　　● **Z48.81　Encounter for surgical aftercare following surgery on specified body systems**
　　　　These codes identify the body system requiring aftercare. They are for use in conjunction with other aftercare codes to fully explain the aftercare encounter. The condition treated should also be coded if still present.

　　　　Excludes1　aftercare for injury - code the injury with 7th character D
　　　　　　aftercare following surgery for neoplasm (Z48.3)

　　　　Excludes2　aftercare following organ transplant (Z48.2-)
　　　　　　orthopedic aftercare (Z47.-)

　　　　Z48.810　Encounter for surgical aftercare following surgery on the sense organs

　　　　Z48.811　Encounter for surgical aftercare following surgery on the nervous system
　　　　　　Excludes2　encounter for surgical aftercare following surgery on the sense organs (Z48.810)

　　　　Z48.812　Encounter for surgical aftercare following surgery on the circulatory system
　　　　　　Coding Clinic: 2012, Q4, P96

　　　　Z48.813　Encounter for surgical aftercare following surgery on the respiratory system

　　　　Z48.814　Encounter for surgical aftercare following surgery on the teeth or oral cavity

　　　　Z48.815　Encounter for surgical aftercare following surgery on the digestive system
　　　　　　Coding Clinic: 2015, Q4, P38

　　　　Z48.816　Encounter for surgical aftercare following surgery on the genitourinary system
　　　　　　Excludes1　encounter for aftercare following sterilization reversal (Z31.42)

　　　　Z48.817　Encounter for surgical aftercare following surgery on the skin and subcutaneous tissue
　　　　　　Coding Clinic: 2015, Q1, P6

　　Z48.89　Encounter for other specified surgical aftercare

● **Z49　Encounter for care involving renal dialysis**
　　Code also associated end stage renal disease (N18.6)
　　● **Z49.0　Preparatory care for renal dialysis**
　　　　Encounter for dialysis instruction and training
　　　Z49.01　Encounter for fitting and adjustment of extracorporeal dialysis catheter
　　　　　Removal or replacement of renal dialysis catheter
　　　　　Toilet or cleansing of renal dialysis catheter
　　　Z49.02　Encounter for fitting and adjustment of peritoneal dialysis catheter
　　● **Z49.3　Encounter for adequacy testing for dialysis**
　　　Z49.31　Encounter for adequacy testing for hemodialysis
　　　Z49.32　Encounter for adequacy testing for peritoneal dialysis
　　　　　Encounter for peritoneal equilibration test

● **Z51　Encounter for other aftercare and medical care** ◀▥
　　Code also condition requiring care
　　Excludes1　follow-up examination after treatment (Z08-Z09)
　　Z51.0　Encounter for antineoplastic radiation therapy
　　● **Z51.1　Encounter for antineoplastic chemotherapy and immunotherapy**
　　　　Excludes2　encounter for chemotherapy and immunotherapy for nonneoplastic condition-code to condition
　　　Z51.11　Encounter for antineoplastic chemotherapy
　　　　　Coding Clinic: 2015, Q3, P19
　　　Z51.12　Encounter for antineoplastic immunotherapy
　　Z51.5　Encounter for palliative care
　　Z51.6　Encounter for desensitization to allergens ◀
　　● **Z51.8　Encounter for other specified aftercare**
　　　　Excludes1　holiday relief care (Z75.5)
　　　Z51.81　Encounter for therapeutic drug level monitoring
　　　　　Code also any long-term (current) drug therapy (Z79.-)
　　　　　Excludes1　encounter for blood-drug test for administrative or medicolegal reasons (Z02.83)
　　　Z51.89　Encounter for other specified aftercare
　　　　　Coding Clinic: 2012, Q4, P96-97

● **Z52　Donors of organs and tissues**
　　Includes　autologous and other living donors
　　Excludes1　cadaveric donor - omit code examination of potential donor (Z00.5)
　　Coding Clinic: 2012, Q4, P100
　　● **Z52.0　Blood donor**
　　　● **Z52.00　Unspecified blood donor**
　　　　Z52.000　Unspecified donor, whole blood
　　　　Z52.001　Unspecified donor, stem cells
　　　　Z52.008　Unspecified donor, other blood
　　　● **Z52.01　Autologous blood donor**
　　　　Z52.010　Autologous donor, whole blood
　　　　Z52.011　Autologous donor, stem cells
　　　　Z52.018　Autologous donor, other blood
　　　● **Z52.09　Other blood donor**
　　　　　Volunteer donor
　　　　Z52.090　Other blood donor, whole blood
　　　　Z52.091　Other blood donor, stem cells
　　　　Z52.098　Other blood donor, other blood
　　● **Z52.1　Skin donor**
　　　Z52.10　Skin donor, unspecified
　　　Z52.11　Skin donor, autologous
　　　Z52.19　Skin donor, other
　　● **Z52.2　Bone donor**
　　　Z52.20　Bone donor, unspecified
　　　Z52.21　Bone donor, autologous
　　　Z52.29　Bone donor, other
　　Z52.3　Bone marrow donor
　　Z52.4　Kidney donor
　　Z52.5　Cornea donor
　　Z52.6　Liver donor
　　　　Coding Clinic: 2012, Q4, P100

● **Z52.8**   **Donor of other specified organs or tissues**
     ● **Z52.81**   **Egg (Oocyte) donor**
         Z52.810   **Egg (Oocyte) donor under age 35, anonymous recipient** ♀
             Egg donor under age 35 NOS
         Z52.811   **Egg (Oocyte) donor under age 35, designated recipient** ♀
         Z52.812   **Egg (Oocyte) donor age 35 and over, anonymous recipient** ♀
             Egg donor age 35 and over NOS
         Z52.813   **Egg (Oocyte) donor age 35 and over, designated recipient** ♀
         Z52.819   **Egg (Oocyte) donor, unspecified** ♀
     Z52.89   **Donor of other specified organs or tissues**
● **Z52.9**   **Donor of unspecified organ or tissue**
         Donor NOS

● **Z53**   **Persons encountering health services for specific procedures and treatment, not carried out**
     ● **Z53.0**   **Procedure and treatment not carried out because of contraindication**
         Z53.01   **Procedure and treatment not carried out due to patient smoking**
         Z53.09   **Procedure and treatment not carried out because of other contraindication**
     Z53.1   **Procedure and treatment not carried out because of patient's decision for reasons of belief and group pressure**
     ● **Z53.2**   **Procedure and treatment not carried out because of patient's decision for other and unspecified reasons**
         Z53.20   **Procedure and treatment not carried out because of patient's decision for unspecified reasons**
         Z53.21   **Procedure and treatment not carried out due to patient leaving prior to being seen by health care provider**
         Z53.29   **Procedure and treatment not carried out because of patient's decision for other reasons**
     ● **Z53.3**   **Procedure converted to open procedure** ◄
         Z53.31   **Laparoscopic surgical procedure converted to open procedure** ◄
         Z53.32   **Thoracoscopic surgical procedure converted to open procedure** ◄
         Z53.33   **Arthroscopic surgical procedure converted to open procedure** ◄
         Z53.39   **Other specified procedure converted to open procedure** ◄
     Z53.8   **Procedure and treatment not carried out for other reasons**
     Z53.9   **Procedure and treatment not carried out, unspecified reason**

PERSONS WITH POTENTIAL HEALTH HAZARDS RELATED TO SOCIOECONOMIC AND PSYCHOSOCIAL CIRCUMSTANCES (Z55-Z65)

● **Z55**   **Problems related to education and literacy**
     Excludes1   disorders of psychological development (F80-F89)
     Z55.0   **Illiteracy and low-level literacy**
     Z55.1   **Schooling unavailable and unattainable**
     Z55.2   **Failed school examinations**
     Z55.3   **Underachievement in school**
     Z55.4   **Educational maladjustment and discord with teachers and classmates**
     Z55.8   **Other problems related to education and literacy**
         Problems related to inadequate teaching
     Z55.9   **Problems related to education and literacy, unspecified**
         Academic problems NOS

● **Z56**   **Problems related to employment and unemployment**
     Excludes2   occupational exposure to risk factors (Z57.-)
             problems related to housing and economic circumstances (Z59.-)
     Z56.0   **Unemployment, unspecified**
     Z56.1   **Change of job**   **A**
     Z56.2   **Threat of job loss**
     Z56.3   **Stressful work schedule**
     Z56.4   **Discord with boss and workmates**
     Z56.5   **Uncongenial work environment**
         Difficult conditions at work
     Z56.6   **Other physical and mental strain related to work**
     ● **Z56.8**   **Other problems related to employment**
         Z56.81   **Sexual harassment on the job**
         Z56.82   **Military deployment status**
             Individual (civilian or military) currently deployed in theater or in support of military war, peacekeeping and humanitarian operations
         Z56.89   **Other problems related to employment**
     Z56.9   **Unspecified problems related to employment**
         Occupational problems NOS

● **Z57**   **Occupational exposure to risk factors**
     Z57.0   **Occupational exposure to noise**
     Z57.1   **Occupational exposure to radiation**
     Z57.2   **Occupational exposure to dust**
     ● **Z57.3**   **Occupational exposure to other air contaminants**
         Z57.31   **Occupational exposure to environmental tobacco smoke**
             Excludes2   exposure to environmental tobacco smoke (Z77.22)
         Z57.39   **Occupational exposure to other air contaminants**
     Z57.4   **Occupational exposure to toxic agents in agriculture**
         Occupational exposure to solids, liquids, gases or vapors in agriculture
     Z57.5   **Occupational exposure to toxic agents in other industries**
         Occupational exposure to solids, liquids, gases or vapors in other industries
     Z57.6   **Occupational exposure to extreme temperature**
     Z57.7   **Occupational exposure to vibration**
     Z57.8   **Occupational exposure to other risk factors**
     Z57.9   **Occupational exposure to unspecified risk factor**

● **Z59**   **Problems related to housing and economic circumstances**
     Excludes2   problems related to upbringing (Z62.-)
     Z59.0   **Homelessness**
     Z59.1   **Inadequate housing**
         Lack of heating
         Restriction of space
         Technical defects in home preventing adequate care
         Unsatisfactory surroundings
         Excludes1   problems related to the natural and physical environment (Z77.1-)
     Z59.2   **Discord with neighbors, lodgers and landlord**
     Z59.3   **Problems related to living in residential institution**
         Boarding-school resident
         Excludes1   institutional upbringing (Z62.2)
     Z59.4   **Lack of adequate food and safe drinking water**
         Inadequate drinking water supply
         Excludes1   effects of hunger (T73.0)
             inappropriate diet or eating habits (Z72.4)
             malnutrition (E40-E46)
     Z59.5   **Extreme poverty**
     Z59.6   **Low income**
     Z59.7   **Insufficient social insurance and welfare support**

CHAPTER 21 (Z00-Z99)

CHAPTER 21 (Z00-Z99)

Z59.8   **Other problems related to housing and economic circumstances**
Foreclosure on loan
Isolated dwelling
Problems with creditors

Z59.9   **Problem related to housing and economic circumstances, unspecified**

● **Z60**   **Problems related to social environment**

Z60.0   **Problems of adjustment to life-cycle transitions**
Empty nest syndrome
Phase of life problem
Problem with adjustment to retirement [pension]

Z60.2   **Problems related to living alone**

Z60.3   **Acculturation difficulty**
Problem with migration
Problem with social transplantation

Z60.4   **Social exclusion and rejection**
Exclusion and rejection on the basis of personal characteristics, such as unusual physical appearance, illness or behavior.

> **Excludes1**   target of adverse discrimination such as for racial or religious reasons (Z60.5)

Z60.5   **Target of (perceived) adverse discrimination and persecution**

> **Excludes1**   social exclusion and rejection (Z60.4)

Z60.8   **Other problems related to social environment**

Z60.9   **Problem related to social environment, unspecified**

● **Z62**   **Problems related to upbringing**

> **Includes**   current and past negative life events in childhood
> current and past problems of a child related to upbringing

> **Excludes2**   maltreatment syndrome (T74.-)
> problems related to housing and economic circumstances (Z59.-)

Z62.0   **Inadequate parental supervision and control**

Z62.1   **Parental overprotection**

● **Z62.2**   **Upbringing away from parents**

> **Excludes1**   problems with boarding school (Z59.3)

Z62.21   **Child in welfare custody**   P
Child in care of non-parental family member
Child in foster care

> **Excludes2**   problem for parent due to child in welfare custody (Z63.5)

Z62.22   **Institutional upbringing**
Child living in orphanage or group home

Z62.29   **Other upbringing away from parents**

Z62.3   **Hostility towards and scapegoating of child**   P

Z62.6   **Inappropriate (excessive) parental pressure**

● **Z62.8**   **Other specified problems related to upbringing**

● **Z62.81**   **Personal history of abuse in childhood**

Z62.810   **Personal history of physical and sexual abuse in childhood**

> **Excludes1**   current child physical abuse (T74.12, T76.12)
> current child sexual abuse (T74.22, T76.22)

Z62.811   **Personal history of psychological abuse in childhood**

> **Excludes1**   current child psychological abuse (T74.32, T76.32)

Z62.812   **Personal history of neglect in childhood**

> **Excludes1**   current child neglect (T74.02, T76.02)

Z62.819   **Personal history of unspecified abuse in childhood**

> **Excludes1**   current child abuse NOS (T74.92, T76.92)

● **Z62.82**   **Parent-child conflict**

Z62.820   **Parent-biological child conflict**
Parent-child problem NOS

Z62.821   **Parent-adopted child conflict**

Z62.822   **Parent-foster child conflict**

● **Z62.89**   **Other specified problems related to upbringing**

Z62.890   **Parent-child estrangement NEC**

Z62.891   **Sibling rivalry**

Z62.898   **Other specified problems related to upbringing**

Z62.9   **Problem related to upbringing, unspecified**

● **Z63**   **Other problems related to primary support group, including family circumstances**

> **Excludes2**   maltreatment syndrome (T74.-, T76)
> parent-child problems (Z62.-)
> problems related to negative life events in childhood (Z62.-)
> problems related to upbringing (Z62.-)

Z63.0   **Problems in relationship with spouse or partner**

> **Excludes1**   counseling for spousal or partner abuse problems (Z69.1)
> counseling related to sexual attitude, behavior, and orientation (Z70.-)

Z63.1   **Problems in relationship with in-laws**

● **Z63.3**   **Absence of family member**

> **Excludes1**   absence of family member due to disappearance and death (Z63.4)
> absence of family member due to separation and divorce (Z63.5)

Z63.31   **Absence of family member due to military deployment**
Individual or family affected by other family member being on military deployment

> **Excludes1**   family disruption due to return of family member from military deployment (Z63.71)

Z63.32   **Other absence of family member**

Z63.4   **Disappearance and death of family member**
Assumed death of family member
Bereavement

Z63.5   **Disruption of family by separation and divorce**
Marital estrangement

Z63.6   **Dependent relative needing care at home**

● **Z63.7**   **Other stressful life events affecting family and household**

Z63.71   **Stress on family due to return of family member from military deployment**
Individual or family affected by family member having returned from military deployment (current or past conflict)

Z63.72   **Alcoholism and drug addiction in family**

Z63.79   **Other stressful life events affecting family and household**
Anxiety (normal) about sick person in family
Health problems within family
Ill or disturbed family member
Isolated family

◀ New   ◀≣ Revised   ~~deleted~~ Deleted   Excludes 1   Excludes 2   Includes   Use additional   Code first   Code also   Unspecified
OGCR Official Guidelines   X Assign placeholder X   ● Use Additional Character(s)   ▶ Manifestation Code   **Coding Clinic**

Z63.8   Other specified problems related to primary support group
> Family discord NOS
> Family estrangement NOS
> High expressed emotional level within family
> Inadequate family support NOS
> Inadequate or distorted communication within family

Z63.9   Problem related to primary support group, unspecified
> Relationship disorder NOS

● **Z64   Problems related to certain psychosocial circumstances**

    Z64.0   Problems related to unwanted pregnancy ♀

    Z64.1   Problems related to multiparity ♀

    Z64.4   Discord with counselors
> Discord with probation officer
> Discord with social worker

● **Z65   Problems related to other psychosocial circumstances**

    Z65.0   Conviction in civil and criminal proceedings without imprisonment

    Z65.1   Imprisonment and other incarceration

    Z65.2   Problems related to release from prison

    Z65.3   Problems related to other legal circumstances
> Arrest
> Child custody or support proceedings
> Litigation
> Prosecution

    Z65.4   Victim of crime and terrorism
> Victim of torture

    Z65.5   Exposure to disaster, war and other hostilities
> **Excludes1**   target of perceived discrimination or persecution (Z60.5)

    Z65.8   Other specified problems related to psychosocial circumstances

    Z65.9   Problem related to unspecified psychosocial circumstances

DO NOT RESUSCITATE STATUS (Z66)

Z66   Do not resuscitate
> DNR status

BLOOD TYPE (Z67)

● **Z67   Blood type**
> Coding Clinic: 2015, Q3, P40

  ● **Z67.1   Type A blood**

    Z67.10   Type A blood, Rh positive

    Z67.11   Type A blood, Rh negative

  ● **Z67.2   Type B blood**

    Z67.20   Type B blood, Rh positive

    Z67.21   Type B blood, Rh negative

  ● **Z67.3   Type AB blood**

    Z67.30   Type AB blood, Rh positive

    Z67.31   Type AB blood, Rh negative

  ● **Z67.4   Type O blood**

    Z67.40   Type O blood, Rh positive

    Z67.41   Type O blood, Rh negative

  ● **Z67.9   Unspecified blood type**

    Z67.90   Unspecified blood type, Rh positive

    Z67.91   Unspecified blood type, Rh negative
> Coding Clinic: 2015, Q3, P40

BODY MASS INDEX [BMI] (Z68)

OGCR Section I.B.14.

General Coding Guidelines

14. Documentation for BMI, *Depth of* Non-pressure ulcers, Pressure Ulcer Stages, **Coma Scale,** *and NIH Stroke Scale*

For the Body Mass Index (BMI), depth of non-pressure chronic ulcers, pressure ulcer stage, **coma scale, and NIH stroke scale (NIHSS) codes,** code assignment may be based on medical record documentation from clinicians who are not the patient's provider (i.e., physician or other qualified healthcare practitioner legally accountable for establishing the patient's diagnosis), since this information is typically documented by other clinicians involved in the care of the patient (e.g., a dietitian often documents the BMI, a nurse often documents the pressure ulcer stages, **and an emergency medical technician often documents the coma scale).** However, the associated diagnosis (such as overweight, obesity, **acute stroke,** or pressure ulcer) must be documented by the patient's provider. If there is conflicting medical record documentation, either from the same clinician or different clinicians, the patient's attending provider should be queried for clarification.

The BMI, **coma scale, and NIHSS** codes should only be reported as secondary diagnoses.

● **Z68   Body mass index [BMI]**
> Kilograms per meters squared

> **Note:** BMI adult codes are for use for persons 21 years of age or older.

> BMI pediatric codes are for use for persons 2-20 years of age. These percentiles are based on the growth charts published by the Centers for Disease Control and Prevention (CDC)

    Z68.1   Body mass index (BMI) 19 or less, adult   A

  ● **Z68.2   Body mass index (BMI) 20-29, adult**

    Z68.20   Body mass index (BMI) 20.0-20.9, adult   A

    Z68.21   Body mass index (BMI) 21.0-21.9, adult   A

    Z68.22   Body mass index (BMI) 22.0-22.9, adult   A

    Z68.23   Body mass index (BMI) 23.0-23.9, adult   A

    Z68.24   Body mass index (BMI) 24.0-24.9, adult   A

    Z68.25   Body mass index (BMI) 25.0-25.9, adult   A

    Z68.26   Body mass index (BMI) 26.0-26.9, adult   A

    Z68.27   Body mass index (BMI) 27.0-27.9, adult   A

    Z68.28   Body mass index (BMI) 28.0-28.9, adult   A

    Z68.29   Body mass index (BMI) 29.0-29.9, adult   A

  ● **Z68.3   Body mass index (BMI) 30-39, adult**

    Z68.30   Body mass index (BMI) 30.0-30.9, adult   A

    Z68.31   Body mass index (BMI) 31.0-31.9, adult   A

    Z68.32   Body mass index (BMI) 32.0-32.9, adult   A

    Z68.33   Body mass index (BMI) 33.0-33.9, adult   A

    Z68.34   Body mass index (BMI) 34.0-34.9, adult   A

    Z68.35   Body mass index (BMI) 35.0-35.9, adult   A

    Z68.36   Body mass index (BMI) 36.0-36.9, adult   A

    Z68.37   Body mass index (BMI) 37.0-37.9, adult   A

    Z68.38   Body mass index (BMI) 38.0-38.9, adult   A

    Z68.39   Body mass index (BMI) 39.0-39.9, adult   A

  ● **Z68.4   Body mass index (BMI) 40 or greater, adult**

    Z68.41   Body mass index (BMI) 40.0-44.9, adult   A

    Z68.42   Body mass index (BMI) 45.0-49.9, adult   A

    Z68.43   Body mass index (BMI) 50-59.9, adult   A

    Z68.44   Body mass index (BMI) 60.0-69.9, adult   A

    Z68.45   Body mass index (BMI) 70 or greater, adult   A

● **Z68.5** **Body mass index (BMI) pediatric**

    Z68.51 Body mass index (BMI) pediatric, less than 5th percentile for age

    Z68.52 Body mass index (BMI) pediatric, 5th percentile to less than 85th percentile for age

    Z68.53 Body mass index (BMI) pediatric, 85th percentile to less than 95th percentile for age

    Z68.54 Body mass index (BMI) pediatric, greater than or equal to 95th percentile for age

PERSONS ENCOUNTERING HEALTH SERVICES IN OTHER CIRCUMSTANCES (Z69-Z76)

● **Z69** **Encounter for mental health services for victim and perpetrator of abuse**

    Includes counseling for victims and perpetrators of abuse

● **Z69.0** **Encounter for mental health services for child abuse problems**

  ● **Z69.01** **Encounter for mental health services for parental child abuse**

    Z69.010 Encounter for mental health services for victim of parental child abuse   P

    Z69.011 Encounter for mental health services for perpetrator of parental child abuse

      Excludes1 encounter for mental health services for non-parental child abuse (Z69.02-)

  ● **Z69.02** **Encounter for mental health services for non-parental child abuse**

    Z69.020 Encounter for mental health services for victim of non-parental child abuse   P

    Z69.021 Encounter for mental health services for perpetrator of non- parental child abuse

● **Z69.1** **Encounter for mental health services for spousal or partner abuse problems**

    Z69.11 Encounter for mental health services for victim of spousal or partner abuse

    Z69.12 Encounter for mental health services for perpetrator of spousal or partner abuse

● **Z69.8** **Encounter for mental health services for victim or perpetrator of other abuse**

    Z69.81 Encounter for mental health services for victim of other abuse
      Encounter for rape victim counseling

    Z69.82 Encounter for mental health services for perpetrator of other abuse

● **Z70** **Counseling related to sexual attitude, behavior and orientation**

    Includes encounter for mental health services for sexual attitude, behavior and orientation

    Excludes2 contraceptive or procreative counseling (Z30-Z31)

Z70.0 **Counseling related to sexual attitude**

Z70.1 **Counseling related to patient's sexual behavior and orientation**
    Patient concerned regarding impotence
    Patient concerned regarding non-responsiveness
    Patient concerned regarding promiscuity
    Patient concerned regarding sexual orientation

Z70.2 **Counseling related to sexual behavior and orientation of third party**
    Advice sought regarding sexual behavior and orientation of child
    Advice sought regarding sexual behavior and orientation of partner
    Advice sought regarding sexual behavior and orientation of spouse

Z70.3 **Counseling related to combined concerns regarding sexual attitude, behavior and orientation**

Z70.8 **Other sex counseling**
    Encounter for sex education

Z70.9 **Sex counseling, unspecified**

● **Z71** **Persons encountering health services for other counseling and medical advice, not elsewhere classified**

    Excludes2 contraceptive or procreation counseling (Z30-Z31)
      sex counseling (Z70.-)

Z71.0 **Person encountering health services to consult on behalf of another person**
    Person encountering health services to seek advice or treatment for non-attending third party

    Excludes2 anxiety (normal) about sick person in family (Z63.7)
      expectant (adoptive) parent(s) pre-birth pediatrician visit (Z76.81)

Z71.1 **Person with feared health complaint in whom no diagnosis is made**
    Person encountering health services with feared condition which was not demonstrated
    Person encountering health services in which problem was normal state
    'Worried well'

    Excludes1 medical observation for suspected diseases and conditions proven not to exist (Z03.-)

Z71.2 **Person consulting for explanation of examination or test findings**

Z71.3 **Dietary counseling and surveillance**
    Use additional code for any associated underlying medical condition
    Use additional code to identify body mass index (BMI), if known (Z68.-)

● **Z71.4** **Alcohol abuse counseling and surveillance**
    Use additional code for alcohol abuse or dependence (F10.-)

    Z71.41 Alcohol abuse counseling and surveillance of alcoholic

    Z71.42 Counseling for family member of alcoholic
      Counseling for significant other, partner, or friend of alcoholic

● **Z71.5** **Drug abuse counseling and surveillance**
    Use additional code for drug abuse or dependence (F11-F16, F18-F19)

    Z71.51 Drug abuse counseling and surveillance of drug abuser

    Z71.52 Counseling for family member of drug abuser
      Counseling for significant other, partner, or friend of drug abuser

Z71.6 **Tobacco abuse counseling**
    Use additional code for nicotine dependence (F17.-)

Z71.7 **Human immunodeficiency virus [HIV] counseling**

● **Z71.8** **Other specified counseling**

    Excludes2 counseling for contraception (Z30.0-)
      counseling for genetics (Z31.5)
      counseling for procreative management (Z31.6-)

    Z71.81 Spiritual or religious counseling

    Z71.89 Other specified counseling

Z71.9 **Counseling, unspecified**
    Encounter for medical advice NOS

CHAPTER 21 (Z00-Z99)

● **Z72**   **Problems related to lifestyle**
    Excludes2   problems related to life-management difficulty (Z73.-)
              problems related to socioeconomic and psychosocial circumstances (Z55-Z65)

    Z72.0   **Tobacco use**
        Tobacco use NOS
        Excludes1   history of tobacco dependence (Z87.891)
                nicotine dependence (F17.2-)
                tobacco dependence (F17.2-)
                tobacco use during pregnancy (O99.33-)

    Z72.3   **Lack of physical exercise**

    Z72.4   **Inappropriate diet and eating habits**
        Excludes1   behavioral eating disorders of infancy or childhood (F98.2.-F98.3)
                eating disorders (F50.-)
                lack of adequate food (Z59.4)
                malnutrition and other nutritional deficiencies (E40-E64)

● **Z72.5**   **High risk sexual behavior**
        Promiscuity
        Excludes1   paraphilias (F65)

    Z72.51   **High risk heterosexual behavior**

    Z72.52   **High risk homosexual behavior**

    Z72.53   **High risk bisexual behavior**

    Z72.6   **Gambling and betting**
        Excludes1   compulsive or pathological gambling (F63.0)

● **Z72.8**   **Other problems related to lifestyle**
    ● **Z72.81**   **Antisocial behavior**
        Excludes1   conduct disorders (F91.-)
        Z72.810   **Child and adolescent antisocial behavior**   P
                Antisocial behavior (child) (adolescent) without manifest psychiatric disorder
                Delinquency NOS
                Group delinquency
                Offenses in the context of gang membership
                Stealing in company with others
                Truancy from school
        Z72.811   **Adult antisocial behavior**   A
                Adult antisocial behavior without manifest psychiatric disorder

    ● **Z72.82**   **Problems related to sleep**
        Z72.820   **Sleep deprivation**
                Lack of adequate sleep
            Excludes1   insomnia (G47.0-)
        Z72.821   **Inadequate sleep hygiene**
                Bad sleep habits
                Irregular sleep habits
                Unhealthy sleep wake schedule
            Excludes1   insomnia (F51.0-, G47.0-)

    Z72.89   **Other problems related to lifestyle**
        Self-damaging behavior

    Z72.9   **Problem related to lifestyle, unspecified**

● **Z73**   **Problems related to life management difficulty**
    Excludes2   problems related to socioeconomic and psychosocial circumstances (Z55-Z65)

    Z73.0   **Burn-out**

    Z73.1   **Type A behavior pattern**

    Z73.2   **Lack of relaxation and leisure**

    Z73.3   **Stress, not elsewhere classified**
        Physical and mental strain NOS
        Excludes1   stress related to employment or unemployment (Z56.-)

    Z73.4   **Inadequate social skills, not elsewhere classified**

    Z73.5   **Social role conflict, not elsewhere classified**

    Z73.6   **Limitation of activities due to disability**
        Excludes1   care-provider dependency (Z74.-)

● **Z73.8**   **Other problems related to life management difficulty**
    ● **Z73.81**   **Behavioral insomnia of childhood**
        Z73.810   **Behavioral insomnia of childhood, sleep-onset association type**   P
        Z73.811   **Behavioral insomnia of childhood, limit setting type**   P
        Z73.812   **Behavioral insomnia of childhood, combined type**   P
        Z73.819   **Behavioral insomnia of childhood, unspecified type**   P

    Z73.82   **Dual sensory impairment**

    Z73.89   **Other problems related to life management difficulty**

    Z73.9   **Problem related to life management difficulty, unspecified**

● **Z74**   **Problems related to care provider dependency**
    Excludes2   dependence on enabling machines or devices NEC (Z99.-)

● **Z74.0**   **Reduced mobility**
    Z74.01   **Bed confinement status**
        Bedridden
    Z74.09   **Other reduced mobility**
        Chairridden
        Reduced mobility NOS
        Excludes2   wheelchair dependence (Z99.3)

    Z74.1   **Need for assistance with personal care**

    Z74.2   **Need for assistance at home and no other household member able to render care**

    Z74.3   **Need for continuous supervision**

    Z74.8   **Other problems related to care provider dependency**

    Z74.9   **Problem related to care provider dependency, unspecified**

● **Z75**   **Problems related to medical facilities and other health care**

    Z75.0   **Medical services not available in home**
        Excludes1   no other household member able to render care (Z74.2)

    Z75.1   **Person awaiting admission to adequate facility elsewhere**

    Z75.2   **Other waiting period for investigation and treatment**

    Z75.3   **Unavailability and inaccessibility of health care facilities**
        Excludes1   bed unavailable (Z75.1)

    Z75.4   **Unavailability and inaccessibility of other helping agencies**

    Z75.5   **Holiday relief care**

    Z75.8   **Other problems related to medical facilities and other health care**

    Z75.9   **Unspecified problem related to medical facilities and other health care**

CHAPTER 21 (Z00-Z99)

CHAPTER 21 (Z00-Z99)

● **Z76**   **Persons encountering health services in other circumstances**

Z76.0   **Encounter for issue of repeat prescription**

Encounter for issue of repeat prescription for appliance

Encounter for issue of repeat prescription for medicaments

Encounter for issue of repeat prescription for spectacles

> **Excludes2**   issue of medical certificate (Z02.7)
> repeat prescription for contraceptive (Z30.4-)

Z76.1   **Encounter for health supervision and care of foundling**

Z76.2   **Encounter for health supervision and care of other healthy infant and child**   P

Encounter for medical or nursing care or supervision of healthy infant under circumstances such as adverse socioeconomic conditions at home

Encounter for medical or nursing care or supervision of healthy infant under circumstances such as awaiting foster or adoptive placement

Encounter for medical or nursing care or supervision of healthy infant under circumstances such as maternal illness

Encounter for medical or nursing care or supervision of healthy infant under circumstances such as number of children at home preventing or interfering with normal care

Z76.3   **Healthy person accompanying sick person**

Z76.4   **Other boarder to healthcare facility**

> **Excludes1**   homelessness (Z59.0)

Z76.5   **Malingerer [conscious simulation]**

Person feigning illness (with obvious motivation)

> **Excludes1**   factitious disorder (F68.1-)
> peregrinating patient (F68.1-)

● **Z76.8**   **Persons encountering health services in other specified circumstances**

Z76.81   **Expectant parent(s) prebirth pediatrician visit**

Pre-adoption pediatrician visit for adoptive parent(s)

Z76.82   **Awaiting organ transplant status**

Patient waiting for organ availability

Z76.89   **Persons encountering health services in other specified circumstances**

Persons encountering health services NOS

PERSONS WITH POTENTIAL HEALTH HAZARDS RELATED TO FAMILY AND PERSONAL HISTORY AND CERTAIN CONDITIONS INFLUENCING HEALTH STATUS (Z77-Z99)

Code also any follow-up examination (Z08-Z09)

● **Z77**   **Other contact with and (suspected) exposures hazardous to health**

> **Includes**   contact with and (suspected) exposures to potential hazards to health

> **Excludes2**   contact with and (suspected) exposure to communicable diseases (Z20.-)
> exposure to (parental) (environmental) tobacco smoke in the perinatal period (P96.81)
> newborn affected by noxious substances transmitted via placenta or breast milk (P04.-) ◄▥
> occupational exposure to risk factors (Z57.-)
> retained foreign body (Z18.-)
> retained foreign body fully removed (Z87.821)
> toxic effects of substances chiefly nonmedicinal as to source (T51-T65)

● **Z77.0**   **Contact with and (suspected) exposure to hazardous, chiefly nonmedicinal, chemicals**

● **Z77.01**   **Contact with and (suspected) exposure to hazardous metals**

Z77.010   **Contact with and (suspected) exposure to arsenic**

Z77.011   **Contact with and (suspected) exposure to lead**

Z77.012   **Contact with and (suspected) exposure to uranium**

> **Excludes1**   retained depleted uranium fragments (Z18.01)

Z77.018   **Contact with and (suspected) exposure to other hazardous metals**

Contact with and (suspected) exposure to chromium compounds

Contact with and (suspected) exposure to nickel dust

● **Z77.02**   **Contact with and (suspected) exposure to hazardous aromatic compounds**

Z77.020   **Contact with and (suspected) exposure to aromatic amines**

Z77.021   **Contact with and (suspected) exposure to benzene**

Z77.028   **Contact with and (suspected) exposure to other hazardous aromatic compounds**

Aromatic dyes NOS

Polycyclic aromatic hydrocarbons

● **Z77.09**   **Contact with and (suspected) exposure to other hazardous, chiefly nonmedicinal, chemicals**

Z77.090   **Contact with and (suspected) exposure to asbestos**

Z77.098   **Contact with and (suspected) exposure to other hazardous, chiefly nonmedicinal, chemicals**

Dyes NOS

● **Z77.1**   **Contact with and (suspected) exposure to environmental pollution and hazards in the physical environment**

● **Z77.11**   **Contact with and (suspected) exposure to environmental pollution**

Z77.110   **Contact with and (suspected) exposure to air pollution**

Z77.111   **Contact with and (suspected) exposure to water pollution**

Z77.112   **Contact with and (suspected) exposure to soil pollution**

Z77.118   **Contact with and (suspected) exposure to other environmental pollution**

● **Z77.12**   **Contact with and (suspected) exposure to hazards in the physical environment**

Z77.120   **Contact with and (suspected) exposure to mold (toxic)**

Z77.121   **Contact with and (suspected) exposure to harmful algae and algae toxins**

Contact with and (suspected) exposure to (harmful) algae bloom NOS

Contact with and (suspected) exposure to blue-green algae bloom

Contact with and (suspected) exposure to brown tide

Contact with and (suspected) exposure to cyanobacteria bloom

Contact with and (suspected) exposure to Florida red tide

Contact with and (suspected) exposure to pfiesteria piscicida

Contact with and (suspected) exposure to red tide

Z77.122   **Contact with and (suspected) exposure to noise**

◄ New   ◄▥ Revised   ~~deleted~~ Deleted   Excludes 1   Excludes 2   Includes   Use additional   Code first   Code also   Unspecified

OGCR Official Guidelines   X Assign placeholder X   ● Use Additional Character(s)   ▶ Manifestation Code   **Coding Clinic**

Z77.123 **Contact with and (suspected) exposure to radon and other naturally occuring radiation**

    Excludes2 radiation exposure as the cause of a confirmed condition (W88-W90, X39.0-)
       radiation sickness NOS (T66)

Z77.128 **Contact with and (suspected) exposure to other hazards in the physical environment**

● Z77.2 **Contact with and (suspected) exposure to other hazardous substances**

Z77.21 **Contact with and (suspected) exposure to potentially hazardous body fluids**

Z77.22 **Contact with and (suspected) exposure to environmental tobacco smoke (acute) (chronic)**
    Exposure to second hand tobacco smoke (acute) (chronic)
    Passive smoking (acute) (chronic)
    Excludes1 nicotine dependence (F17.-) tobacco use (Z72.0)
    Excludes2 occupational exposure to environmental tobacco smoke (Z57.31)

Z77.29 **Contact with and (suspected) exposure to other hazardous substances**
    Coding Clinic: 2016, Q2, P34

Z77.9 **Other contact with and (suspected) exposures hazardous to health**

● Z78 **Other specified health status**
    Excludes2 asymptomatic human immunodeficiency virus [HIV] infection status (Z21)
       postprocedural status (Z93-Z99)
       sex reassignment status (Z87.890)

Z78.0 **Asymptomatic menopausal state** ♀   A
    Menopausal state NOS
    Postmenopausal status NOS
    Excludes2 symptomatic menopausal state (N95.1)

Z78.1 **Physical restraint status**
    Excludes1 physical restraint due to a procedure - omit code

Z78.9 **Other specified health status**

● Z79 **Long term (current) drug therapy**
    Includes long term (current) drug use for prophylactic purposes
    Code also any therapeutic drug level monitoring (Z51.81)
    Excludes2 drug abuse and dependence (F11-F19)
       drug use complicating pregnancy, childbirth, and the puerperium (O99.32-)
       long term (current) use of oral antidiabetic drugs (Z79.84) ◄
       long term (current) use of oral hypoglycemic drugs (Z79.84) ◄

● Z79.0 **Long term (current) use of anticoagulants and antithrombotics/antiplatelets**
    Excludes2 long term (current) use of aspirin (Z79.82)

Z79.01 **Long term (current) use of anticoagulants**

Z79.02 **Long term (current) use of antithrombotics/antiplatelets**

Z79.1 **Long term (current) use of non-steroidal anti-inflammatories (NSAID)**
    Excludes2 long term (current) use of aspirin (Z79.82)

Z79.2 **Long term (current) use of antibiotics**

Z79.3 **Long term (current) use of hormonal contraceptives**
    Long term (current) use of birth control pill or patch

Z79.4 **Long term (current) use of insulin**

● Z79.5 **Long term (current) use of steroids**

Z79.51 **Long term (current) use of inhaled steroids**

Z79.52 **Long term (current) use of systemic steroids**

● Z79.8 **Other long term (current) drug therapy**

● Z79.81 **Long term (current) use of agents affecting estrogen receptors and estrogen levels**
    Code first, if applicable:
    malignant neoplasm of breast (C50.-)
    malignant neoplasm of prostate (C61)
    Use additional code, if applicable, to identify:
    estrogen receptor positive status (Z17.0)
    family history of breast cancer (Z80.3)
    genetic susceptibility to malignant neoplasm (cancer) (Z15.0-)
    personal history of breast cancer (Z85.3)
    personal history of prostate cancer (Z85.46)
    postmenopausal status (Z78.0)
    Excludes1 hormone replacement therapy (postmenopausal) (Z79.890)

Z79.810 **Long term (current) use of selective estrogen receptor modulators (SERMs)**
    Long term (current) use of raloxifene (Evista)
    Long term (current) use of tamoxifen (Nolvadex)
    Long term (current) use of toremifene (Fareston)

Z79.811 **Long term (current) use of aromatase inhibitors**
    Long term (current) use of anastrozole (Arimidex)
    Long term (current) use of exemestane (Aromasin)
    Long term (current) use of letrozole (Femara)

Z79.818 **Long term (current) use of other agents affecting estrogen receptors and estrogen levels**
    Long term (current) use of estrogen receptor downregulators
    Long term (current) use of fulvestrant (Faslodex)
    Long term (current) use of gonadotropin-releasing hormone (GnRH) agonist
    Long term (current) use of goserelin acetate (Zoladex)
    Long term (current) use of leuprolide acetate (leuprorelin) (Lupron)
    Long term (current) use of megestrol acetate (Megace)

Z79.82 **Long term (current) use of aspirin**

Z79.83 **Long term (current) use of bisphosphonates**

Z79.84 **Long term (current) use of oral hypoglycemic drugs** ◄
    Long term (current) use of oral antidiabetic drugs ◄
    Excludes2 long term (current) use of insulin (Z79.4) ◄

● Z79.89 **Other long term (current) drug therapy**

Z79.890 **Hormone replacement therapy (postmenopausal)**

Z79.891 **Long term (current) use of opiate analgesic**
    Long term (current) use of methadone for pain management
    Excludes1 methadone use NOS (F11.9-) ◄
       use of methadone for treatment of heroin addiction (F11.2-)

Z79.899 **Other long term (current) drug therapy**
    Coding Clinic: 2015, Q4, P34, Q3, P21

CHAPTER 21 (Z00-Z99)

CHAPTER 21 (Z00-Z99)

● **Z80   Family history of primary malignant neoplasm**

Z80.0   Family history of malignant neoplasm of digestive organs
Conditions classifiable to C15-C26

Z80.1   Family history of malignant neoplasm of trachea, bronchus and lung
Conditions classifiable to C33-C34

Z80.2   Family history of malignant neoplasm of other respiratory and intrathoracic organs
Conditions classifiable to C30-C32, C37-C39

Z80.3   Family history of malignant neoplasm of breast
Conditions classifiable to C50.-

● **Z80.4   Family history of malignant neoplasm of genital organs**
Conditions classifiable to C51-C63

   Z80.41   Family history of malignant neoplasm of ovary

   Z80.42   Family history of malignant neoplasm of prostate

   Z80.43   Family history of malignant neoplasm of testis

   Z80.49   Family history of malignant neoplasm of other genital organs

● **Z80.5   Family history of malignant neoplasm of urinary tract**
Conditions classifiable to C64-C68

   Z80.51   Family history of malignant neoplasm of kidney

   Z80.52   Family history of malignant neoplasm of bladder

   Z80.59   Family history of malignant neoplasm of other urinary tract organ

Z80.6   Family history of leukemia
Conditions classifiable to C91-C95

Z80.7   Family history of other malignant neoplasms of lymphoid, hematopoietic and related tissues
Conditions classifiable to C81-C90, C96.-

Z80.8   Family history of malignant neoplasm of other organs or systems
Conditions classifiable to C00-C14, C40-C49, C69-C79

Z80.9   Family history of malignant neoplasm, unspecified
Conditions classifiable to C80.1

● **Z81   Family history of mental and behavioral disorders**

Z81.0   Family history of intellectual disabilities
Conditions classifiable to F70-F79

Z81.1   Family history of alcohol abuse and dependence
Conditions classifiable to F10.-

Z81.2   Family history of tobacco abuse and dependence
Conditions classifiable to F17.-

Z81.3   Family history of other psychoactive substance abuse and dependence
Conditions classifiable to F11-F16, F18-F19

Z81.4   Family history of other substance abuse and dependence
Conditions classifiable to F55

Z81.8   Family history of other mental and behavioral disorders
Conditions classifiable elsewhere in F01-F99

● **Z82   Family history of certain disabilities and chronic diseases (leading to disablement)**

Z82.0   Family history of epilepsy and other diseases of the nervous system
Conditions classifiable to G00-G99

Z82.1   Family history of blindness and visual loss
Conditions classifiable to H54.-

Z82.2   Family history of deafness and hearing loss
Conditions classifiable to H90-H91

Z82.3   Family history of stroke
Conditions classifiable to I60-I64

● **Z82.4   Family history of ischemic heart disease and other diseases of the circulatory system**
Conditions classifiable to I00-I52, I65-I99

   Z82.41   Family history of sudden cardiac death

   Z82.49   Family history of ischemic heart disease and other diseases of the circulatory system

Z82.5   Family history of asthma and other chronic lower respiratory diseases
Conditions classifiable to J40-J47

   Excludes2   family history of other diseases of the respiratory system (Z83.6)

● **Z82.6   Family history of arthritis and other diseases of the musculoskeletal system and connective tissue**
Conditions classifiable to M00-M99

   Z82.61   Family history of arthritis

   Z82.62   Family history of osteoporosis

   Z82.69   Family history of other diseases of the musculoskeletal system and connective tissue

● **Z82.7   Family history of congenital malformations, deformations and chromosomal abnormalities**
Conditions classifiable to Q00-Q99

   Z82.71   Family history of polycystic kidney

   Z82.79   Family history of other congenital malformations, deformations and chromosomal abnormalities

Z82.8   Family history of other disabilities and chronic diseases leading to disablement, not elsewhere classified

● **Z83   Family history of other specific disorders**

   Excludes2   contact with and (suspected) exposure to communicable disease in the family (Z20.-)

Z83.0   Family history of human immunodeficiency virus [HIV] disease
Conditions classifiable to B20

Z83.1   Family history of other infectious and parasitic diseases
Conditions classifiable to A00-B19, B25-B94, B99

Z83.2   Family history of diseases of the blood and blood-forming organs and certain disorders involving the immune mechanism
Conditions classifiable to D50-D89

Z83.3   Family history of diabetes mellitus
Conditions classifiable to E08-E13

● **Z83.4   Family history of other endocrine, nutritional and metabolic diseases**
Conditions classifiable to E00-E07, E15-E88

   Z83.41   Family history of multiple endocrine neoplasia [MEN] syndrome

   Z83.42   Family history of familial hypercholesterolemia ◀

   Z83.49   Family history of other endocrine, nutritional and metabolic diseases

● **Z83.5   Family history of eye and ear disorders**

   ● **Z83.51   Family history of eye disorders**
   Conditions classifiable to H00-H53, H55-H59

      Excludes2   family history of blindness and visual loss (Z82.1)

      Z83.511   Family history of glaucoma

      Z83.518   Family history of other specified eye disorder

   Z83.52   Family history of ear disorders
   Conditions classifiable to H60-H83, H92-H95

      Excludes2   family history of deafness and hearing loss (Z82.2)

Z83.6   Family history of other diseases of the respiratory system
Conditions classifiable to J00-J39, J60-J99

   Excludes2   family history of asthma and other chronic lower respiratory diseases (Z82.5)

● **Z83.7**   **Family history of diseases of the digestive system**
Conditions classifiable to K00-K93

     Z83.71   **Family history of colonic polyps**
         Excludes1   family history of malignant neoplasm of digestive organs (Z80.0)

     Z83.79   **Family history of other diseases of the digestive system**

● **Z84**   **Family history of other conditions**

     Z84.0   **Family history of diseases of the skin and subcutaneous tissue**
Conditions classifiable to L00-L99

     Z84.1   **Family history of disorders of kidney and ureter**
Conditions classifiable to N00-N29

     Z84.2   **Family history of other diseases of the genitourinary system**
Conditions classifiable to N30-N99

     Z84.3   **Family history of consanguinity**

● **Z84.8**   **Family history of other specified conditions**

     Z84.81   **Family history of carrier of genetic disease**

     Z84.82   **Family history of sudden infant death syndrome ◄**
         Family history of SIDS ◄

     Z84.89   **Family history of other specified conditions**

● **Z85**   **Personal history of malignant neoplasm**
Code first any follow-up examination after treatment of malignant neoplasm (Z08)
Use additional code to identify:
   alcohol use and dependence (F10.-)
   exposure to environmental tobacco smoke (Z77.22)
   history of tobacco dependence (Z87.891) ◄▥
   occupational exposure to environmental tobacco smoke (Z57.31)
   tobacco dependence (F17.-)
   tobacco use (Z72.0)
     Excludes2   personal history of benign neoplasm (Z86.01-)
             personal history of carcinoma-in-situ (Z86.00-)

● **Z85.0**   **Personal history of malignant neoplasm of digestive organs**

     Z85.00   **Personal history of malignant neoplasm of** unspecified **digestive organ**

     Z85.01   **Personal history of malignant neoplasm of esophagus**
Conditions classifiable to C15

     ● **Z85.02**   **Personal history of malignant neoplasm of stomach**

         Z85.020   **Personal history of malignant carcinoid tumor of stomach**
Conditions classifiable to C7A.092

         Z85.028   **Personal history of other malignant neoplasm of stomach**
Conditions classifiable to C16

     ● **Z85.03**   **Personal history of malignant neoplasm of large intestine**

         Z85.030   **Personal history of malignant carcinoid tumor of large intestine**
Conditions classifiable to C7A.022-C7A.025, C7A.029

         Z85.038   **Personal history of other malignant neoplasm of large intestine**
Conditions classifiable to C18

     ● **Z85.04**   **Personal history of malignant neoplasm of rectum, rectosigmoid junction, and anus**

         Z85.040   **Personal history of malignant carcinoid tumor of rectum**
Conditions classifiable to C7A.026

         Z85.048   **Personal history of other malignant neoplasm of rectum, rectosigmoid junction, and anus**
Conditions classifiable to C19-C21

     Z85.05   **Personal history of malignant neoplasm of liver**
Conditions classifiable to C22

● **Z85.06**   **Personal history of malignant neoplasm of small intestine**

     Z85.060   **Personal history of malignant carcinoid tumor of small intestine**
Conditions classifiable to C7A.01-

     Z85.068   **Personal history of other malignant neoplasm of small intestine**
Conditions classifiable to C17

     Z85.07   **Personal history of malignant neoplasm of pancreas**
Conditions classifiable to C25

     Z85.09   **Personal history of malignant neoplasm of other digestive organs**

● **Z85.1**   **Personal history of malignant neoplasm of trachea, bronchus and lung**

     ● **Z85.11**   **Personal history of malignant neoplasm of bronchus and lung**

         Z85.110   **Personal history of malignant carcinoid tumor of bronchus and lung**
Conditions classifiable to C7A.090

         Z85.118   **Personal history of other malignant neoplasm of bronchus and lung**
Conditions classifiable to C34

     Z85.12   **Personal history of malignant neoplasm of trachea**
Conditions classifiable to C33

● **Z85.2**   **Personal history of malignant neoplasm of other respiratory and intrathoracic organs**

     Z85.20   **Personal history of malignant neoplasm of** unspecified **respiratory organ**

     Z85.21   **Personal history of malignant neoplasm of larynx**
Conditions classifiable to C32

     Z85.22   **Personal history of malignant neoplasm of nasal cavities, middle ear, and accessory sinuses**
Conditions classifiable to C30-C31

     ● **Z85.23**   **Personal history of malignant neoplasm of thymus**

         Z85.230   **Personal history of malignant carcinoid tumor of thymus**
Conditions classifiable to C7A.091

         Z85.238   **Personal history of other malignant neoplasm of thymus**
Conditions classifiable to C37

     Z85.29   **Personal history of malignant neoplasm of other respiratory and intrathoracic organs**

     Z85.3   **Personal history of malignant neoplasm of breast**
Conditions classifiable to C50.-

● **Z85.4**   **Personal history of malignant neoplasm of genital organs**
Conditions classifiable to C51-C63

     Z85.40   **Personal history of malignant neoplasm of** unspecified **female genital organ ♀**

     Z85.41   **Personal history of malignant neoplasm of cervix uteri ♀**

     Z85.42   **Personal history of malignant neoplasm of other parts of uterus ♀**

     Z85.43   **Personal history of malignant neoplasm of ovary ♀**

     Z85.44   **Personal history of malignant neoplasm of other female genital organs ♀**

     Z85.45   **Personal history of malignant neoplasm of** unspecified **male genital organ ♂**

     Z85.46   **Personal history of malignant neoplasm of prostate ♂**

     Z85.47   **Personal history of malignant neoplasm of testis ♂**

CHAPTER 21 (Z00-Z99)

CHAPTER 21 (Z00-Z99)

Z85.48   Personal history of malignant neoplasm of epididymis ♂

Z85.49   Personal history of malignant neoplasm of other male genital organs ♂

● Z85.5   Personal history of malignant neoplasm of urinary tract
Conditions classifiable to C64-C68

Z85.50   Personal history of malignant neoplasm of unspecified urinary tract organ

Z85.51   Personal history of malignant neoplasm of bladder

● Z85.52   Personal history of malignant neoplasm of kidney

    Excludes1   personal history of malignant neoplasm of renal pelvis (Z85.53)

    Z85.520   Personal history of malignant carcinoid tumor of kidney
Conditions classifiable to C7A.093

    Z85.528   Personal history of other malignant neoplasm of kidney
Conditions classifiable to C64

Z85.53   Personal history of malignant neoplasm of renal pelvis

Z85.54   Personal history of malignant neoplasm of ureter

Z85.59   Personal history of malignant neoplasm of other urinary tract organ

Z85.6   Personal history of leukemia
Conditions classifiable to C91-C95

    Excludes1   leukemia in remission C91.0-C95.9 with 5th character 1

● Z85.7   Personal history of other malignant neoplasms of lymphoid, hematopoietic and related tissues

Z85.71   Personal history of Hodgkin lymphoma
Conditions classifiable to C81

Z85.72   Personal history of non-Hodgkin lymphomas
Conditions classifiable to C82-C85

Z85.79   Personal history of other malignant neoplasms of lymphoid, hematopoietic and related tissues
Conditions classifiable to C88-C90, C96

    Excludes1   multiple myeloma in remission (C90.01)
plasma cell leukemia in remission (C90.11)
plasmacytoma in remission (C90.21)

● Z85.8   Personal history of malignant neoplasms of other organs and systems
Conditions classifiable to C00-C14, C40-C49, C69-C75, C7A.098, C76-C79 ◄▦

● Z85.81   Personal history of malignant neoplasm of lip, oral cavity, and pharynx

    Z85.810   Personal history of malignant neoplasm of tongue

    Z85.818   Personal history of malignant neoplasm of other sites of lip, oral cavity, and pharynx

    Z85.819   Personal history of malignant neoplasm of unspecified site of lip, oral cavity, and pharynx

● Z85.82   Personal history of malignant neoplasm of skin

    Z85.820   Personal history of malignant melanoma of skin
Conditions classifiable to C43

    Z85.821   Personal history of Merkel cell carcinoma
Conditions classifiable to C4A

    Z85.828   Personal history of other malignant neoplasm of skin
Conditions classifiable to C44

● Z85.83   Personal history of malignant neoplasm of bone and soft tissue

    Z85.830   Personal history of malignant neoplasm of bone

    Z85.831   Personal history of malignant neoplasm of soft tissue

        Excludes2   personal history of malignant neoplasm of skin (Z85.82-)

● Z85.84   Personal history of malignant neoplasm of eye and nervous tissue

    Z85.840   Personal history of malignant neoplasm of eye

    Z85.841   Personal history of malignant neoplasm of brain

    Z85.848   Personal history of malignant neoplasm of other parts of nervous tissue

● Z85.85   Personal history of malignant neoplasm of endocrine glands

    Z85.850   Personal history of malignant neoplasm of thyroid

    Z85.858   Personal history of malignant neoplasm of other endocrine glands

Z85.89   Personal history of malignant neoplasm of other organs and systems

Z85.9   Personal history of malignant neoplasm, unspecified
Conditions classifiable to C7A.00, C80.1

● Z86   Personal history of certain other diseases
Code first any follow-up examination after treatment (Z09)

● Z86.0   Personal history of in-situ and benign neoplasms and neoplasms of uncertain behavior

    Excludes2   personal history of malignant neoplasms (Z85.-)

● Z86.00   Personal history of in-situ neoplasm
Conditions classifiable to D00-D09 ◄

    Z86.000   Personal history of in-situ neoplasm of breast

    Z86.001   Personal history of in-situ neoplasm of cervix uteri ♀
Personal history of cervical intraepithelial neoplasia III [CIN III] ◄

    Z86.008   Personal history of in-situ neoplasm of other site
Personal history of vaginal intraepithelial neoplasia III [VAIN III] ◄
Personal history of vulvar intraepithelial neoplasia III [VIN III] ◄

● Z86.01   Personal history of benign neoplasm

    Z86.010   Personal history of colonic polyps

    Z86.011   Personal history of benign neoplasm of the brain

    Z86.012   Personal history of benign carcinoid tumor

    Z86.018   Personal history of other benign neoplasm

Z86.03   Personal history of neoplasm of uncertain behavior

◄ New   ◄▦ Revised   ~~deleted~~ Deleted   Excludes 1   Excludes 2   Includes   Use additional   Code first   Code also   Unspecified

OGCR Official Guidelines   X Assign placeholder X   ● Use Additional Character(s)   ▶ Manifestation Code   **Coding Clinic**

● **Z86.1 Personal history of infectious and parasitic diseases**
Conditions classifiable to A00-B89, B99

> **Excludes1**   personal history of infectious diseases specific to a body system sequelae of infectious and parasitic diseases (B90-B94)

Z86.11 Personal history of tuberculosis

Z86.12 Personal history of poliomyelitis

Z86.13 Personal history of malaria

Z86.14 Personal history of Methicillin resistant Staphylococcus aureus infection
Personal history of MRSA infection

Z86.19 Personal history of other infectious and parasitic diseases

Z86.2 Personal history of diseases of the blood and blood-forming organs and certain disorders involving the immune mechanism
Conditions classifiable to D50-D89

● **Z86.3 Personal history of endocrine, nutritional and metabolic diseases**
Conditions classifiable to E00-E88

Z86.31 Personal history of diabetic foot ulcer

> **Excludes2**   current diabetic foot ulcer (E08.621, E09.621, E10.621, E11.621, E13.621)

Z86.32 Personal history of gestational diabetes ♀
Personal history of conditions classifiable to O24.4-

> **Excludes1**   gestational diabetes mellitus in current pregnancy (O24.4-)

Z86.39 Personal history of other endocrine, nutritional and metabolic disease

● **Z86.5 Personal history of mental and behavioral disorders**
Conditions classifiable to F40-F59

Z86.51 Personal history of combat and operational stress reaction   A

Z86.59 Personal history of other mental and behavioral disorders

● **Z86.6 Personal history of diseases of the nervous system and sense organs**
Conditions classifiable to G00-G99, H00-H95

Z86.61 Personal history of infections of the central nervous system
Personal history of encephalitis
Personal history of meningitis

Z86.69 Personal history of other diseases of the nervous system and sense organs

● **Z86.7 Personal history of diseases of the circulatory system**
Conditions classifiable to I00-I99

> **Excludes2**   old myocardial infarction (I25.2)
> personal history of anaphylactic shock (Z87.892)
> postmyocardial infarction syndrome (I24.1)

● **Z86.71 Personal history of venous thrombosis and embolism**

Z86.711 Personal history of pulmonary embolism

Z86.718 Personal history of other venous thrombosis and embolism

Z86.72 Personal history of thrombophlebitis

Z86.73 Personal history of transient ischemic attack (TIA), and cerebral infarction without residual deficits
Personal history of prolonged reversible ischemic neurological deficit (PRIND)
Personal history of stroke NOS without residual deficits

> **Excludes1**   personal history of traumatic brain injury (Z87.820)
> sequelae of cerebrovascular disease (I69.-)

Coding Clinic: 2012, Q4, P3

Z86.74 Personal history of sudden cardiac arrest
Personal history of sudden cardiac death successfully resuscitated

Z86.79 Personal history of other diseases of the circulatory system

● **Z87 Personal history of other diseases and conditions**
Code first any follow-up examination after treatment (Z09)

● **Z87.0 Personal history of diseases of the respiratory system**
Conditions classifiable to J00-J99

Z87.01 Personal history of pneumonia (recurrent)

Z87.09 Personal history of other diseases of the respiratory system

● **Z87.1 Personal history of diseases of the digestive system**
Conditions classifiable to K00-K93

Z87.11 Personal history of peptic ulcer disease

Z87.19 Personal history of other diseases of the digestive system

Z87.2 Personal history of diseases of the skin and subcutaneous tissue
Conditions classifiable to L00-L99

> **Excludes2**   personal history of diabetic foot ulcer (Z86.31)

● **Z87.3 Personal history of diseases of the musculoskeletal system and connective tissue**
Conditions classifiable to M00-M99

> **Excludes2**   personal history of (healed) traumatic fracture (Z87.81)

● **Z87.31 Personal history of (healed) nontraumatic fracture**

Z87.310 Personal history of (healed) osteoporosis fracture
Personal history of (healed) fragility fracture
Personal history of (healed) collapsed vertebra due to osteoporosis

Z87.311 Personal history of (healed) other pathological fracture
Personal history of (healed) collapsed vertebra NOS

> **Excludes2**   personal history of osteoporosis fracture (Z87.310)

Z87.312 Personal history of (healed) stress fracture
Personal history of (healed) fatigue fracture

Z87.39 Personal history of other diseases of the musculoskeletal system and connective tissue

● **Z87.4　Personal history of diseases of genitourinary system**
　　Conditions classifiable to N00-N99

　● **Z87.41　Personal history of dysplasia of the female genital tract**

　　　　Excludes1　personal history of intraepithelial neoplasia III of female genital tract (Z87.001, Z87.008) ◄
　　　　　　　　personal history of malignant neoplasm of female genital tract (Z85.40-Z85.44)

　　　Z87.410　Personal history of cervical dysplasia ♀

　　　Z87.411　Personal history of vaginal dysplasia ♀

　　　Z87.412　Personal history of vulvar dysplasia ♀

　　Z87.42　Personal history of other diseases of the female genital tract ♀

　● **Z87.43　Personal history of diseases of male genital organs**

　　　Z87.430　Personal history of prostatic dysplasia ♂

　　　　　Excludes1　personal history of malignant neoplasm of prostate (Z85.46)

　　　Z87.438　Personal history of other diseases of male genital organs ♂

　● **Z87.44　Personal history of diseases of urinary system**

　　　Excludes1　personal history of malignant neoplasm of cervix uteri (Z85.41)

　　　Z87.440　Personal history of urinary (tract) infections

　　　Z87.441　Personal history of nephrotic syndrome

　　　Z87.442　Personal history of urinary calculi
　　　　　　Personal history of kidney stones

　　　Z87.448　Personal history of other diseases of urinary system

● **Z87.5　Personal history of complications of pregnancy, childbirth and the puerperium**
　　Conditions classifiable to O00-O9A

　　Excludes2　recurrent pregnancy loss (N96)

　　Z87.51　Personal history of pre-term labor ♀

　　　　Excludes1　current pregnancy with history of pre-term labor (O09.21-)

　　Z87.59　Personal history of other complications of pregnancy, childbirth and the puerperium ♀
　　　　Personal history of trophoblastic disease

● **Z87.7　Personal history of (corrected) congenital malformations**
　　Conditions classifiable to Q00-Q89 that have been repaired or corrected

　　Excludes1　congenital malformations that have been partially corrected or repair but which still require medical treatment - code to condition

　　Excludes2　other postprocedural states (Z98.-)
　　　　personal history of medical treatment (Z92.-)
　　　　presence of cardiac and vascular implants and grafts (Z95.-)
　　　　presence of other devices (Z97.-)
　　　　presence of other functional implants (Z96.-)
　　　　transplanted organ and tissue status (Z94.-)

　● **Z87.71　Personal history of (corrected) congenital malformations of genitourinary system**

　　　Z87.710　Personal history of (corrected) hypospadias ♂

　　　Z87.718　Personal history of other specified (corrected) congenital malformations of genitourinary system

　● **Z87.72　Personal history of (corrected) congenital malformations of nervous system and sense organs**

　　　Z87.720　Personal history of (corrected) congenital malformations of eye

　　　Z87.721　Personal history of (corrected) congenital malformations of ear

　　　Z87.728　Personal history of other specified (corrected) congenital malformations of nervous system and sense organs

　● **Z87.73　Personal history of (corrected) congenital malformations of digestive system**

　　　Z87.730　Personal history of (corrected) cleft lip and palate

　　　Z87.738　Personal history of other specified (corrected) congenital malformations of digestive system

　　Z87.74　Personal history of (corrected) congenital malformations of heart and circulatory system

　　Z87.75　Personal history of (corrected) congenital malformations of respiratory system

　　Z87.76　Personal history of (corrected) congenital malformations of integument, limbs and musculoskeletal system

　● **Z87.79　Personal history of other (corrected) congenital malformations**

　　　Z87.790　Personal history of (corrected) congenital malformations of face and neck

　　　Z87.798　Personal history of other (corrected) congenital malformations

● **Z87.8　Personal history of other specified conditions**

　　Excludes2　personal history of self harm (Z91.5)

　　Z87.81　Personal history of (healed) traumatic fracture

　　　　Excludes2　personal history of (healed) nontraumatic fracture (Z87.31-)

　● **Z87.82　Personal history of other (healed) physical injury and trauma**
　　　Conditions classifiable to S00-T88, except traumatic fractures

　　　Z87.820　Personal history of traumatic brain injury

　　　　　Excludes1　personal history of transient ischemic attack (TIA), and cerebral infarction without residual deficits (Z86.73)

　　　Z87.821　Personal history of retained foreign body fully removed

　　　Z87.828　Personal history of other (healed) physical injury and trauma

　● **Z87.89　Personal history of other specified conditions**

　　　Z87.890　Personal history of sex reassignment

　　　Z87.891　Personal history of nicotine dependence

　　　　Excludes1　current nicotine dependence (F17.2-)

　　　Z87.892　Personal history of anaphylaxis
　　　　　Code also allergy status such as:
　　　　　allergy status to drugs, medicaments and biological substances (Z88.-)
　　　　　allergy status, other than to drugs and biological substances (Z91.0-)

　　　Z87.898　Personal history of other specified conditions
　　　　　Coding Clinic: 2013, Q1, P21

◄ New　◄▥ Revised　~~deleted~~ Deleted　| Excludes 1 |　| Excludes 2 |　| Includes |　| Use additional |　| Code first |　| Code also |　| Unspecified |

OGCR Official Guidelines　X Assign placeholder X　● Use Additional Character(s)　▶ Manifestation Code　**Coding Clinic**

● **Z88**   **Allergy status to drugs, medicaments and biological substances**

     Excludes2   allergy status, other than to drugs and biological substances (Z91.0-)

     Z88.0   Allergy status to penicillin

     Z88.1   Allergy status to other antibiotic agents status

     Z88.2   Allergy status to sulfonamides status
           Coding Clinic: 2015, Q3, P23

     Z88.3   Allergy status to other anti-infective agents status

     Z88.4   Allergy status to anesthetic agent status

     Z88.5   Allergy status to narcotic agent status

     Z88.6   Allergy status to analgesic agent status

     Z88.7   Allergy status to serum and vaccine status

     Z88.8   Allergy status to other drugs, medicaments and biological substances status

     Z88.9   Allergy status to unspecified drugs, medicaments and biological substances status

● **Z89**   **Acquired absence of limb**

     Includes   amputation status
           postprocedural loss of limb
           post-traumatic loss of limb

     Excludes1   acquired deformities of limbs (M20-M21)
                congenital absence of limbs (Q71-Q73)

● **Z89.0**   **Acquired absence of thumb and other finger(s)**

    ● **Z89.01**   **Acquired absence of thumb**

        Z89.011   Acquired absence of right thumb

        Z89.012   Acquired absence of left thumb

        Z89.019   Acquired absence of unspecified thumb

    ● **Z89.02**   **Acquired absence of other finger(s)**

        Excludes2   acquired absence of thumb (Z89.01-)

        Z89.021   Acquired absence of right finger(s)

        Z89.022   Acquired absence of left finger(s)

        Z89.029   Acquired absence of unspecified finger(s)

● **Z89.1**   **Acquired absence of hand and wrist**

    ● **Z89.11**   **Acquired absence of hand**

        Z89.111   Acquired absence of right hand

        Z89.112   Acquired absence of left hand

        Z89.119   Acquired absence of unspecified hand

    ● **Z89.12**   **Acquired absence of wrist**
           Disarticulation at wrist

        Z89.121   Acquired absence of right wrist

        Z89.122   Acquired absence of left wrist

        Z89.129   Acquired absence of unspecified wrist

● **Z89.2**   **Acquired absence of upper limb above wrist**

    ● **Z89.20**   **Acquired absence of upper limb, unspecified level**

        Z89.201   Acquired absence of right upper limb, unspecified level

        Z89.202   Acquired absence of left upper limb, unspecified level

        Z89.209   Acquired absence of unspecified upper limb, unspecified level
               Acquired absence of arm NOS

    ● **Z89.21**   **Acquired absence of upper limb below elbow**

        Z89.211   Acquired absence of right upper limb below elbow

        Z89.212   Acquired absence of left upper limb below elbow

        Z89.219   Acquired absence of unspecified upper limb below elbow

    ● **Z89.22**   **Acquired absence of upper limb above elbow**
           Disarticulation at elbow

        Z89.221   Acquired absence of right upper limb above elbow

        Z89.222   Acquired absence of left upper limb above elbow

        Z89.229   Acquired absence of unspecified upper limb above elbow

    ● **Z89.23**   **Acquired absence of shoulder**
           Acquired absence of shoulder joint following explantation of shoulder joint prosthesis, with or without presence of antibiotic-impregnated cement spacer

        Z89.231   Acquired absence of right shoulder

        Z89.232   Acquired absence of left shoulder

        Z89.239   Acquired absence of unspecified shoulder

● **Z89.4**   **Acquired absence of toe(s), foot, and ankle**

    ● **Z89.41**   **Acquired absence of great toe**

        Z89.411   Acquired absence of right great toe

        Z89.412   Acquired absence of left great toe

        Z89.419   Acquired absence of unspecified great toe

    ● **Z89.42**   **Acquired absence of other toe(s)**

        Excludes2   acquired absence of great toe (Z89.41-)

        Z89.421   Acquired absence of other right toe(s)

        Z89.422   Acquired absence of other left toe(s)

        Z89.429   Acquired absence of other toe(s), unspecified side

    ● **Z89.43**   **Acquired absence of foot**

        Z89.431   Acquired absence of right foot

        Z89.432   Acquired absence of left foot

        Z89.439   Acquired absence of unspecified foot

    ● **Z89.44**   **Acquired absence of ankle**
           Disarticulation of ankle

        Z89.441   Acquired absence of right ankle

        Z89.442   Acquired absence of left ankle

        Z89.449   Acquired absence of unspecified ankle

● **Z89.5**   **Acquired absence of leg below knee**

    ● **Z89.51**   **Acquired absence of leg below knee**

        Z89.511   Acquired absence of right leg below knee

        Z89.512   Acquired absence of left leg below knee

        Z89.519   Acquired absence of unspecified leg below knee

    ● **Z89.52**   **Acquired absence of knee**
           Acquired absence of knee joint following explantation of knee joint prosthesis, with or without presence of antibiotic-impregnated cement spacer

        Z89.521   Acquired absence of right knee

        Z89.522   Acquired absence of left knee

        Z89.529   Acquired absence of unspecified knee

● Z89.6   **Acquired absence of leg above knee**
   ● Z89.61   **Acquired absence of leg above knee**
      Acquired absence of leg NOS
      Disarticulation at knee
      Z89.611   **Acquired absence of right leg above knee**
      Z89.612   **Acquired absence of left leg above knee**
      Z89.619   **Acquired absence of unspecified leg above knee**
   ● Z89.62   **Acquired absence of hip**
      Acquired absence of hip joint following explantation of hip joint prosthesis, with or without presence of antibiotic-impregnated cement spacer
      Disarticulation at hip
      Z89.621   **Acquired absence of right hip joint**
      Z89.622   **Acquired absence of left hip joint**
      Z89.629   **Acquired absence of unspecified hip joint**
   Z89.9   **Acquired absence of limb, unspecified**

● Z90   **Acquired absence of organs, not elsewhere classified**
   Includes   postprocedural or post-traumatic loss of body part NEC
   Excludes1   congenital absence - see Alphabetical Index
   Excludes2   postprocedural absence of endocrine glands (E89.-)
   ● Z90.0   **Acquired absence of part of head and neck**
      Z90.01   **Acquired absence of eye**
      Z90.02   **Acquired absence of larynx**
      Z90.09   **Acquired absence of other part of head and neck**
        Acquired absence of nose
        Excludes2   teeth (K08.1)
   ● Z90.1   **Acquired absence of breast and nipple**
      Z90.10   **Acquired absence of unspecified breast and nipple**
      Z90.11   **Acquired absence of right breast and nipple**
      Z90.12   **Acquired absence of left breast and nipple**
      Z90.13   **Acquired absence of bilateral breasts and nipples**
   Z90.2   **Acquired absence of lung [part of]**
   Z90.3   **Acquired absence of stomach [part of]**
   ● Z90.4   **Acquired absence of other specified parts of digestive tract**
      ● Z90.41   **Acquired absence of pancreas**
        Code also exocrine pancreatic insufficiency (K86.81) ◄
        Use additional code to identify any associated:
        insulin use (Z79.4)
        diabetes mellitus, postpancreatectomy (E13.-)
        Z90.410   **Acquired total absence of pancreas**
          Acquired absence of pancreas NOS
        Z90.411   **Acquired partial absence of pancreas**
      Z90.49   **Acquired absence of other specified parts of digestive tract**
   Z90.5   **Acquired absence of kidney**
   Z90.6   **Acquired absence of other parts of urinary tract**
      Acquired absence of bladder

● Z90.7   **Acquired absence of genital organ(s)**
   Excludes1   personal history of sex reassignment (Z87.890)
   Excludes2   female genital mutilation status (N90.81-)
   ● Z90.71   **Acquired absence of cervix and uterus**
      Z90.710   **Acquired absence of both cervix and uterus ♀**
        Acquired absence of uterus NOS
        Status post total hysterectomy
      Z90.711   **Acquired absence of uterus with remaining cervical stump ♀**
        Status post partial hysterectomy with remaining cervical stump
      Z90.712   **Acquired absence of cervix with remaining uterus ♀**
   ● Z90.72   **Acquired absence of ovaries**
      Z90.721   **Acquired absence of ovaries, unilateral ♀**
      Z90.722   **Acquired absence of ovaries, bilateral ♀**
   Z90.79   **Acquired absence of other genital organ(s)**
   ● Z90.8   **Acquired absence of other organs**
      Z90.81   **Acquired absence of spleen**
      Z90.89   **Acquired absence of other organs**

● Z91   **Personal risk factors, not elsewhere classified**
   Excludes2   contact with and (suspected) exposures hazardous to health (Z77.-)
      exposure to pollution and other problems related to physical environment (Z77.1-)
      occupational exposure to risk factors (Z57.-)
      personal history of physical injury and trauma (Z87.81, Z87.82-)
   ● Z91.0   **Allergy status, other than to drugs and biological substances**
      Excludes2   allergy status to drugs, medicaments, and biological substances (Z88.-)
      ● Z91.01   **Food allergy status**
        Excludes2   food additives allergy status (Z91.02)
        Z91.010   **Allergy to peanuts**
        Z91.011   **Allergy to milk products**
          Excludes1   lactose intolerance (E73.-)
        Z91.012   **Allergy to eggs**
        Z91.013   **Allergy to seafood**
          Allergy to shellfish
          Allergy to octopus or squid ink
        Z91.018   **Allergy to other foods**
          Allergy to nuts other than peanuts
      Z91.02   **Food additives allergy status**
      ● Z91.03   **Insect allergy status**
        Z91.030   **Bee allergy status**
        Z91.038   **Other insect allergy status**
      ● Z91.04   **Nonmedicinal substance allergy status**
        Z91.040   **Latex allergy status**
          Latex sensitivity status
        Z91.041   **Radiographic dye allergy status**
          Allergy status to contrast media used for diagnostic X-ray procedure
        Z91.048   **Other nonmedicinal substance allergy status**
      Z91.09   **Other allergy status, other than to drugs and biological substances**

◄ New   ◄▥ Revised   ~~deleted~~ Deleted   Excludes 1   Excludes 2   Includes   Use additional   Code first   Code also   Unspecified

OGCR Official Guidelines   X Assign placeholder X   ● Use Additional Character(s)   ▶ Manifestation Code   **Coding Clinic**

● **Z91.1** **Patient's noncompliance with medical treatment and regimen**

    Z91.11 **Patient's noncompliance with dietary regimen**

    ● **Z91.12** **Patient's intentional underdosing of medication regimen**

        Code first underdosing of medication (T36-T50) with fifth or sixth character 6

        Excludes1   adverse effect of prescribed drug taken as directed - code to adverse effect
                         poisoning (overdose) - code to poisoning

        Z91.120 **Patient's intentional underdosing of medication regimen due to financial hardship**

        Z91.128 **Patient's intentional underdosing of medication regimen for other reason**

    ● **Z91.13** **Patient's unintentional underdosing of medication regimen**

        Code first underdosing of medication (T36-T50) with fifth or sixth character 6

        Excludes1   adverse effect of prescribed drug taken as directed - code to adverse effect
                         poisoning (overdose) - code to poisoning

        Z91.130 **Patient's unintentional underdosing of medication regimen due to age-related debility**

        Z91.138 **Patient's unintentional underdosing of medication regimen for other reason**

    Z91.14 **Patient's other noncompliance with medication regimen**

        Patient's underdosing of medication NOS

    Z91.15 **Patient's noncompliance with renal dialysis**

    Z91.19 **Patient's noncompliance with other medical treatment and regimen**

● **Z91.4** **Personal history of psychological trauma, not elsewhere classified**

    ● **Z91.41** **Personal history of adult abuse**

        Excludes2   personal history of abuse in childhood (Z62.81-)

        Z91.410 **Personal history of adult physical and sexual abuse**   A

            Excludes1   current adult physical abuse (T74.11, T76.11)
                           current adult sexual abuse (T74.21, T76.11)

        Z91.411 **Personal history of adult psychological abuse**   A

        Z91.412 **Personal history of adult neglect**   A

            Excludes1   current adult neglect (T74.01, T76.01)

        Z91.419 **Personal history of unspecified adult abuse**   A

    Z91.49 **Other personal history of psychological trauma, not elsewhere classified**

● **Z91.5** **Personal history of self-harm**

    Personal history of parasuicide
    Personal history of self-poisoning
    Personal history of suicide attempt

● **Z91.8** **Other specified personal risk factors, not elsewhere classified**

    Z91.81 **History of falling**

        At risk for falling

    Z91.82 **Personal history of military deployment**   A

        Individual (civilian or military) with past history of military war, peacekeeping and humanitarian deployment (current or past conflict)

        Returned from military deployment

    ▸ **Z91.83** *Wandering in diseases classified elsewhere*

        Code first underlying disorder such as:
        Alzheimer's disease (G30.-)
        autism or pervasive developmental disorder (F84.-)
        intellectual disabilities (F70-F79)
        unspecified dementia with behavioral disturbance (F03.9-)

    Z91.89 **Other specified personal risk factors, not elsewhere classified**

● **Z92** **Personal history of medical treatment**

    Excludes2   postprocedural states (Z98.-)

    Z92.0 **Personal history of contraception**

        Excludes1   counseling or management of current contraceptive practices (Z30.-)
                         long term (current) use of contraception (Z79.3)
                         presence of (intrauterine) contraceptive device (Z97.5)

    ● **Z92.2** **Personal history of drug therapy**

        Excludes2   long term (current) drug therapy (Z79.-)

        Z92.21 **Personal history of antineoplastic chemotherapy**

        Z92.22 **Personal history of monoclonal drug therapy**

        Z92.23 **Personal history of estrogen therapy**

       ● **Z92.24** **Personal history of steroid therapy**

            Z92.240 **Personal history of inhaled steroid therapy**

            Z92.241 **Personal history of systemic steroid therapy**

                Personal history of steroid therapy NOS

        Z92.25 **Personal history of immunosupression therapy**

            Excludes2   personal history of steroid therapy (Z92.24)

        Z92.29 **Personal history of other drug therapy**

    Z92.3 **Personal history of irradiation**

        Personal history of exposure to therapeutic radiation

        Excludes1   exposure to radiation in the physical environment (Z77.12)
                         occupational exposure to radiation (Z57.1)

    ● **Z92.8** **Personal history of other medical treatment**

        Z92.81 **Personal history of extracorporeal membrane oxygenation (ECMO)**

        Z92.82 **Status post administration of tPA (rtPA) in a different facility within the last 24 hours prior to admission to current facility**

            Code first condition requiring tPA administration, such as:
            acute cerebral infarction (I63.-)
            acute myocardial infarction (I21.-, I22.-)

        Z92.83 **Personal history of failed moderate sedation**

        Personal history of failed conscious sedation

        Excludes2   failed moderate sedation during procedure (T88.52)

CHAPTER 21 (Z00-Z99)

CHAPTER 21 (Z00-Z99)

Z92.84   Personal history of unintended awareness under general anesthesia ◄

> **Excludes2**   unintended awareness under general anesthesia during procedure (T88.53) ◄

Z92.89   Personal history of other medical treatment

● **Z93   Artificial opening status**

> **Excludes1**   artificial openings requiring attention or management (Z43.-)
> complications of external stoma (J95.0-, K94.-, N99.5-)

Z93.0   Tracheostomy status

Z93.1   Gastrostomy status

Z93.2   Ileostomy status

Z93.3   Colostomy status

Z93.4   Other artificial openings of gastrointestinal tract status

● **Z93.5   Cystostomy status**

Z93.50   Unspecified cystostomy status

Z93.51   Cutaneous-vesicostomy status

Z93.52   Appendico-vesicostomy status

Z93.59   Other cystostomy status

Z93.6   Other artificial openings of urinary tract status
Nephrostomy status
Ureterostomy status
Urethrostomy status

Z93.8   Other artificial opening status

Z93.9   Artificial opening status, unspecified

● **Z94   Transplanted organ and tissue status**

> **Includes**   organ or tissue replaced by heterogenous or homogenous transplant

> **Excludes1**   complications of transplanted organ or tissue - see Alphabetical Index

> **Excludes2**   presence of vascular grafts (Z95.-)

Z94.0   Kidney transplant status

Z94.1   Heart transplant status

> **Excludes1**   artificial heart status (Z95.812)
> heart-valve replacement status (Z95.2-Z95.4)

Z94.2   Lung transplant status

Z94.3   Heart and lungs transplant status

Z94.4   Liver transplant status

Z94.5   Skin transplant status
Autogenous skin transplant status

Z94.6   Bone transplant status

Z94.7   Corneal transplant status

● **Z94.8   Other transplanted organ and tissue status**

Z94.81   Bone marrow transplant status

Z94.82   Intestine transplant status

Z94.83   Pancreas transplant status

Z94.84   Stem cells transplant status

Z94.89   Other transplanted organ and tissue status

Z94.9   Transplanted organ and tissue status, unspecified

● **Z95   Presence of cardiac and vascular implants and grafts**

> **Excludes1**   complications of cardiac and vascular devices, implants and grafts (T82.-)

Z95.0   Presence of cardiac pacemaker
Presence of cardiac resynchronization therapy (CRT-P) pacemaker ◄

> **Excludes1**   adjustment or management of cardiac device (Z45.0-) ◄
> adjustment or management of cardiac pacemaker (Z45.0)
> presence of automatic (implantable) cardiac defibrillator with synchronous cardiac pacemaker (Z95.810)

Z95.1   Presence of aortocoronary bypass graft
Presence of coronary artery bypass graft ◄

Z95.2   Presence of prosthetic heart valve
Presence of heart valve NOS

Z95.3   Presence of xenogenic heart valve

Z95.4   Presence of other heart-valve replacement

Z95.5   Presence of coronary angioplasty implant and graft

> **Excludes1**   coronary angioplasty status without implant and graft (Z98.61)

● **Z95.8   Presence of other cardiac and vascular implants and grafts**

● **Z95.81   Presence of other cardiac implants and grafts**

Z95.810   Presence of automatic (implantable) cardiac defibrillator
Presence of automatic (implantable) cardiac defibrillator with synchronous cardiac pacemaker
Presence of cardiac resynchronization therapy defibrillator (CRT-D) ◄
Presence of cardioverter-defibrillator (ICD) ◄

Z95.811   Presence of heart assist device

Z95.812   Presence of fully implantable artificial heart

Z95.818   Presence of other cardiac implants and grafts

● **Z95.82   Presence of other vascular implants and grafts**

Z95.820   Peripheral vascular angioplasty status with implants and grafts

> **Excludes1**   peripheral vascular angioplasty without implant and graft (Z98.62)

Z95.828   Presence of other vascular implants and grafts
Presence of intravascular prosthesis NEC

Z95.9   Presence of cardiac and vascular implant and graft, unspecified

◄ New   ◄ Revised   ~~deleted~~ Deleted   Excludes 1   Excludes 2   Includes   Use additional   Code first   Code also   Unspecified
OGCR Official Guidelines   X Assign placeholder X   ● Use Additional Character(s)   ▷ Manifestation Code   **Coding Clinic**

● **Z96** **Presence of other functional implants**
  Excludes2 complications of internal prosthetic devices, implants and grafts (T82-T85)
  fitting and adjustment of prosthetic and other devices (Z44-Z46)
  Z96.0 **Presence of urogenital implants**
  Z96.1 **Presence of intraocular lens**
    Presence of pseudophakia
● **Z96.2** **Presence of otological and audiological implants**
    Z96.20 **Presence of otological and audiological implant, unspecified**
    Z96.21 **Cochlear implant status**
    Z96.22 **Myringotomy tube(s) status**
    Z96.29 **Presence of other otological and audiological implants**
      Presence of bone-conduction hearing device
      Presence of eustachian tube stent
      Stapes replacement
  Z96.3 **Presence of artificial larynx**
● **Z96.4** **Presence of endocrine implants**
    Z96.41 **Presence of insulin pump (external) (internal)**
    Z96.49 **Presence of other endocrine implants**
  Z96.5 **Presence of tooth-root and mandibular implants**
● **Z96.6** **Presence of orthopedic joint implants**
    Z96.60 **Presence of unspecified orthopedic joint implant**
  ● **Z96.61** **Presence of artificial shoulder joint**
      Z96.611 **Presence of right artificial shoulder joint**
      Z96.612 **Presence of left artificial shoulder joint**
      Z96.619 **Presence of unspecified artificial shoulder joint**
  ● **Z96.62** **Presence of artificial elbow joint**
      Z96.621 **Presence of right artificial elbow joint**
      Z96.622 **Presence of left artificial elbow joint**
      Z96.629 **Presence of unspecified artificial elbow joint**
  ● **Z96.63** **Presence of artificial wrist joint**
      Z96.631 **Presence of right artificial wrist joint**
      Z96.632 **Presence of left artificial wrist joint**
      Z96.639 **Presence of unspecified artificial wrist joint**
  ● **Z96.64** **Presence of artificial hip joint**
      Hip-joint replacement (partial) (total)
      Z96.641 **Presence of right artificial hip joint**
      Z96.642 **Presence of left artificial hip joint**
        Coding Clinic: 2015, Q1, P16
      Z96.643 **Presence of artificial hip joint, bilateral**
      Z96.649 **Presence of unspecified artificial hip joint**
  ● **Z96.65** **Presence of artificial knee joint**
      Z96.651 **Presence of right artificial knee joint**
      Z96.652 **Presence of left artificial knee joint**
      Z96.653 **Presence of artificial knee joint, bilateral**
      Z96.659 **Presence of unspecified artificial knee joint**
  ● **Z96.66** **Presence of artificial ankle joint**
      Z96.661 **Presence of right artificial ankle joint**
      Z96.662 **Presence of left artificial ankle joint**
      Z96.669 **Presence of unspecified artificial ankle joint**

● **Z96.69** **Presence of other orthopedic joint implants**
    Z96.691 **Finger-joint replacement of right hand**
    Z96.692 **Finger-joint replacement of left hand**
    Z96.693 **Finger-joint replacement, bilateral**
    Z96.698 **Presence of other orthopedic joint implants**
  Z96.7 **Presence of other bone and tendon implants**
    Presence of skull plate
● **Z96.8** **Presence of other specified functional implants**
    Z96.81 **Presence of artificial skin**
    Z96.89 **Presence of other specified functional implants**
  Z96.9 **Presence of functional implant, unspecified**
● **Z97** **Presence of other devices**
  Excludes1 complications of internal prosthetic devices, implants and grafts (T82-T85)
  fitting and adjustment of prosthetic and other devices (Z44-Z46)
  Excludes2 presence of cerebrospinal fluid drainage device (Z98.2)
  Z97.0 **Presence of artificial eye**
● **Z97.1** **Presence of artificial limb (complete) (partial)**
    Z97.10 **Presence of artificial limb (complete) (partial), unspecified**
    Z97.11 **Presence of artificial right arm (complete) (partial)**
    Z97.12 **Presence of artificial left arm (complete) (partial)**
    Z97.13 **Presence of artificial right leg (complete) (partial)**
    Z97.14 **Presence of artificial left leg (complete) (partial)**
    Z97.15 **Presence of artificial arms, bilateral (complete) (partial)**
    Z97.16 **Presence of artificial legs, bilateral (complete) (partial)**
  Z97.2 **Presence of dental prosthetic device (complete) (partial)**
    Presence of dentures (complete) (partial)
  Z97.3 **Presence of spectacles and contact lenses**
  Z97.4 **Presence of external hearing-aid**
  Z97.5 **Presence of (intrauterine) contraceptive device ♀**
    Excludes1 checking, reinsertion or removal of implantable subdermal contraceptive (Z30.46) ◄
      checking, reinsertion or removal of intrauterine contraceptive device (Z30.43-) ◄
  Z97.8 **Presence of other specified devices**
● **Z98** **Other postprocedural states**
  Excludes2 aftercare (Z43-Z49, Z51)
  follow-up medical care (Z08-Z09)
  postprocedural complication - see Alphabetical Index
  Z98.0 **Intestinal bypass and anastomosis status**
    Excludes2 bariatric surgery status (Z98.84)
    gastric bypass status (Z98.84)
    obesity surgery status (Z98.84)
  Z98.1 **Arthrodesis status**
  Z98.2 **Presence of cerebrospinal fluid drainage device**
    Presence of CSF shunt
  Z98.3 **Post therapeutic collapse of lung status**
    Code first underlying disease
● **Z98.4** **Cataract extraction status**
    Use additional code to identify intraocular lens implant status (Z96.1)
    Excludes1 aphakia (H27.0)
    Z98.41 **Cataract extraction status, right eye**
    Z98.42 **Cataract extraction status, left eye**
    Z98.49 **Cataract extraction status, unspecified eye**

● Z98.5   Sterilization status

     Excludes1   female infertility (N97.-)
                  male infertility (N46.-)

   Z98.51   Tubal ligation status ♀

   Z98.52   Vasectomy status ♂   A

● Z98.6   Angioplasty status

   Z98.61   Coronary angioplasty status

     Excludes1   coronary angioplasty status with
                  implant and graft (Z95.5)

   Z98.62   Peripheral vascular angioplasty status

     Excludes1   peripheral vascular angioplasty
                  status with implant and
                  graft (Z95.820)

● Z98.8   Other specified postprocedural states

 ● Z98.81   Dental procedure status

     Z98.810   Dental sealant status

     Z98.811   Dental restoration status
                Dental crown status
                Dental fillings status

     Z98.818   Other dental procedure status

   Z98.82   Breast implant status

     Excludes1   breast implant removal status
                  (Z98.86)

   Z98.83   Filtering (vitreous) bleb after glaucoma surgery status

     Excludes1   inflammation (infection) of
                  postprocedural bleb
                  (H59.4-)

   Z98.84   Bariatric surgery status
           Gastric banding status
           Gastric bypass status for obesity
           Obesity surgery status

     Excludes1   bariatric surgery status
                  complicating pregnancy,
                  childbirth, or the
                  puerperium (O99.84)

     Excludes2   intestinal bypass and
                  anastomosis status (Z98.0)

   Z98.85   Transplanted organ removal status
           Transplanted organ previously removed due to
           complication, failure, rejection or infection

     Excludes1   encounter for removal of
                  transplanted organ
                  -code to complication of
                  transplanted organ (T86.-)

   Z98.86   Personal history of breast implant removal

 ● Z98.87   Personal history of in utero procedure

     Z98.870   Personal history of in utero procedure during pregnancy ♀

     Excludes2   complications from in
                  utero procedure
                  for current
                  pregnancy
                  (O35.7)
                  supervision of current
                  pregnancy with
                  history of in
                  utero procedure
                  during previous
                  pregnancy
                  (O09.82-)

     Z98.871   Personal history of in utero procedure while a fetus

● Z98.89   Other specified postprocedural states

   Z98.890   Other specified postprocedural states ◄
          Personal history of surgery, not
           elsewhere classified ◄

   Z98.891   History of uterine scar from previous surgery ◄

     Excludes1   Maternal care due to
                  uterine scar from
                  previous surgery
                  (O34.2-) ◄

● Z99   Dependence on enabling machines and devices, not elsewhere classified

     Excludes1   cardiac pacemaker status (Z95.0)

   Z99.0   Dependence on aspirator

● Z99.1   Dependence on respirator
          Dependence on ventilator

   Z99.11   Dependence on respirator [ventilator] status
          Coding Clinic: 2015, Q1, P21

   Z99.12   Encounter for respirator [ventilator] dependence during power failure

     Excludes1   mechanical complication of
                  respirator [ventilator]
                  (J95.850)

   Z99.2   Dependence on renal dialysis
          Hemodialysis status
          Peritoneal dialysis status
          Presence of arteriovenous shunt for dialysis
          Renal dialysis status NOS

     Excludes1   encounter for fitting and adjustment of
                  dialysis catheter (Z49.0-)

     Excludes2   noncompliance with renal dialysis
                  (Z91.15) ◄

     Coding Clinic: 2016, Q1, P13

   Z99.3   Dependence on wheelchair
          Wheelchair confinement status
          Code first cause of dependence, such as:
          muscular dystrophy (G71.0)
          obesity (E66.-)

● Z99.8   Dependence on other enabling machines and devices

   Z99.81   Dependence on supplemental oxygen
          Dependence on long-term oxygen

   Z99.89   Dependence on other enabling machines and devices
          Dependence on machine or device NOS

◄ New   ◄◄ Revised   ~~deleted~~ Deleted   Excludes 1   Excludes 2   Includes   Use additional   Code first   Code also   Unspecified

OGCR Official Guidelines   X Assign placeholder X   ● Use Additional Character(s)   ▶ Manifestation Code   Coding Clinic